Primary Care Medicine

SIXTH EDITION

Primary Care Medicine
OFFICE EVALUATION AND MANAGEMENT OF THE ADULT PATIENT

Allan H. Goroll, M.D., MACP
Professor of Medicine
Harvard Medical School
Physician
Massachusetts General Hospital
Boston, Massachusetts

Albert G. Mulley, Jr., M.D., M.P.P.
Chief, General Medicine Division
Massachusetts General Hospital
Associate Professor of Medicine
Harvard Medical School
Boston, Massachusetts

Wolters Kluwer | Lippincott Williams & Wilkins
Health

Philadelphia • Baltimore • New York • London
Buenos Aires • Hong Kong • Sydney • Tokyo

Acquisitions Editor: Sonya Seigafuse
Managing Editor: Ryan Shaw
Project Manager: Nicole Walz
Senior Manufacturing Manager: Benjamin Rivera
Marketing Manager: Kimberly Schonberger
Design Coordinator: Risa Clow
Production Services: Aptara, Inc.

© 2009 by LIPPINCOTT WILLIAMS & WILKINS, a Wolters Kluwer business
© 2006 and 2000 by Lippincott Williams & Wilkins
© 1995, 1987, and 1981 by JB Lippincott
530 Walnut Street
Philadelphia, PA 19106

Printed in China.

Library of Congress Cataloging-in-Publication Data

Primary care medicine : office evaluation and management of the adult patient / [edited by] Allan H. Goroll, Albert G. Mulley Jr. — 6th ed.
    p. ; cm.
  Includes bibliographical references and index.
  ISBN 978-0-7817-7513-7
  ISBN 0-7817-7513-2
 1. Family medicine.   2. Ambulatory medical care.   I. Goroll, Allan H.   II. Mulley, Albert G.
  [DNLM: 1. Primary Health Care—methods.   2. Ambulatory Care—methods.
W 84.6 P94916 2009]
  RC46.G56 2009
  616—dc22

                                                 2008045935

                            10 9 8 7 6 5 4 3 2

Dedicated with gratitude to our parents Frances and Jacob Goroll, and Genevieve and Albert Mulley, who formed us with their encouragement, support, and unabiding love. And to all primary care health professionals, present and future, who are the backbone and heart of our health care delivery system.

Jeremy S. Abramson, MD
Instructor
Department of Medicine
Harvard Medical School
Boston, Massachusetts
Clinical Director
Center for Lymphoma
Massachusetts General Hospital Cancer Center
Boston, Massachusetts

Audrey Ahuero, MD
Massachusetts Eye and Ear Infirmary
Boston, Massachusetts

Ernie-Paul Barrette, MD
MetroHealth Medical Center
Cleveland, Ohio

Michael J. Barry, MD
Professor of Medicine
Harvard Medical School
Chief
General Medicine Unit
Massachusetts General Hospital
Boston, Massachusetts

Arthur J. Barsky, MD
Professor of Psychiatry
Harvard Medical School
Director of Psychiatric Research
Brigham & Women's Hospital
Boston, Massachusetts

Hasan Bazari, MD
Renal Unit
Massachusetts General Hospital
Boston, Massachusetts

Kristie Bennett, OD
Ophthalmic Consultants of Boston, Inc.
Boston, Massachusetts

Neil Bhattacharyya, MD
Assistant Professor of Otology & Laryngology
Harvard Medical School
Attending Surgeon
Brigham and Women's Hospital
Division of Otolaryngology
Boston, Massachusetts

J. Andrew Billings, MD
Co-Director, Center for Palliative Care
Associate Professor of Medicine
Harvard Medical School
Director
Palliative Care Service
Founders House
Massachusetts General Hospital
Boston, Massachusetts

Shanna Birnbaum, MD
Massachusetts General Hospital
Internal Medicine Associates
Wang Ambulatory Center
Boston, Massachusetts

Stephen L. Boswell, MD
Assistant Professor of Medicine
Department of Medicine
Harvard Medical School
President & CEO
Fenway Health
Boston, Massachusetts

Ilana Monica Braun, MD
Instructor
Department of Psychiatry
Harvard Medical School
Attending
Department of Psychiatry
Massachusetts General Hospital
Boston, Massachusetts

David C. Brewster, MD
Department of Surgery
Massachusetts General Hospital
Boston, Massachusetts

Jeffrey William Clark, MD
Hematology/Oncology Associates
Massachusetts General Hospital
Boston, Massachusetts

Tina Cleary, MD
Ophthalmic Consultants of Boston, Inc.
Boston, Massachusetts

Cornelia Cremens, MD
Massachusetts General Hospital
Geriatrics Unit
Boston, Massachusetts

Benjamin T. Davis, MD
Massachusetts General Hospital
Infectious Disease Unit
Boston, Massachusetts

Thomas F. Delaney, MD
Associate Radiation Oncologist
Department of Radiation Oncology
Massachusetts General Hospital
Boston, Massachusetts

Jules L. Dienstag, MD
Carl W. Walter Professor of Medicine
Dean for Medical Education
Harvard Medical School Physician
Gastrointestinal Unit (Medical Services)
Massachusetts General Hospital
Boston, Massachusetts

Leslie Fang, MD
Massachusetts General Hospital
Boston, Massachusetts

Laura C. Fine, MD
Ophthalmic Consultants of Boston, Inc.
Boston, Massachusetts

Mason W. Freeman, MD
Massachusetts General Hospital
Lipid Metabolism Unit
Boston, Massachusetts

Lawrence S. Friedman, MD
Chief of Medicine
Newton-Wellesley Hospital
Newton, Massachusetts
Professor of Medicine
Harvard Medical School
Boston, Massachusetts

Nicolletta Fynn-Thompson, MD
Ophthalmic Consultants of Boston, Inc.
50 Staniford St. Suite 600
Boston, Massachusetts

Ellie J.C. Goldstein, MD
Clinical Professor of Medicine
UCLA School of Medicine
Los Angeles, California
Director of Infection Control
Kindred Hospital-LA
Los Angeles, California

John D. Goodson, MD
Associate Professor of Medicine
Harvard Medical School
Physician
Department of Medicine
Massachusetts General Hospital
Boston, Massachusetts

Claus Hamann, MD
MGH-Senior Health
Boston, Massachusetts

Eleanor Z. Hanna, PhD
Associate Director for Special Projects and Centers
Office of Research on Women's Health
Office of the Director
National Institutes of Health
Bethesda, Maryland

Mark Hatton, MD
Ophthalmic Consultants of Boston, Inc.
Boston, Massachusetts

Gale S. Haydock, MD
Wang Ambulatory Care Center
Massachusetts General Hospital
Boston, Massachusetts

Carolyn C. Hintlian, MPH, MBA, RD, LDN
Consulting Nutritionist
Boston Nutrition Downtown
Administrative Manager
MGH Biostatistics Center
Massachusetts General Hospital
Boston, Massachusetts

James W. Hung, MD
Ophthalmic Consultants of Boston, Inc.
Boston, Massachusetts

Elaine M. Hylek, MD
Massachusetts General Hospital
General Internal Medicine Unit
Boston, Massachusetts

Michael A. Jenike, MD
Massachusetts General Hospital
Department of Psychiatry
Obsessive Compulsive Disorders Unit
Charlestown, Massachusetts

Jesse B. Jupiter, MD
Hansjorg Wyss Professor
Department of Orthopaedic Surgery
Harvard Medical School
Chief, Hand and Upper Limb
Orthopaedic Surgery
Massachusetts General Hospital
Boston, Massachusetts

John P. Kelly, MD, DMD
Associate Clinical Professor
Department of Surgery
Yale School of Medicine
Section Chief
Oral and Maxillofacial Surgery
Hospital of St. Raphael
New Haven, Connecticut

Linda A. King, MD
Assistant Professor of Medicine
Section of Palliative Care and Medical Ethics
University of Pittsburgh Medical Center
Pittsburgh, Pennsylvania

William A. Kormos, MD
Massachusetts General Hospital
Wang Ambulatory Care Center
Boston, Massachusetts

Eric L. Krakauer, MD, PhD
Attending Physician
Palliative Care Service
Massachusetts General Hospital
Instructor
Departments of Medicine and Social Medicine
Harvard Medical School
Boston, Massachusetts

Regina C. LaRocque, MD, MPH
Instructor in Medicine
Harvard Medical School
Division of Infectious Diseases
Massachusetts General Hospital
Boston, Massachusetts

Richard R. Liberthson, MD
Department of Cardiology
Massachusetts General Hospital
Boston, Massachusetts

Charles J. McCabe, MD
Associate Chief
Emergency Associates
Massachusetts General Hospital
Boston, Massachusetts

Kenneth L. Minaker, MD
MGH-Senior Health
100 Charles River Plaza, 5th floor
Boston, Massachusetts

William E. Minichiello, EdD
Psychologist
Massachusetts General Hospital
Associate Professor of Psychology
Department of Psychiatry
Harvard Medical School
Boston, Massachusetts

L. Christine Oliver, MD
Assistant Clinical Professor
Department of Medicine
Harvard Medical School
Associate Physician
Massachusetts General Hospital
Boston, Massachusetts

Amy A. Pruitt, MD
Associate Professor
Department of Neurology
University of Pennsylvania
Department of Neurology
Hospital of the University of Pennsylvania
Philadelphia, Pennsylvania

Scott L. Rauch, MD
Associate Chief of Psychiatry
Neuroscience Research
Massachusetts General Hospital
Charlestown, Massachusetts

Claudia U. Richter, MD
Clinical Instructor
Department of Ophthalmology
Harvard Medical School
Boston, Massachusetts

James M. Richter, MD
Caritas Christi Health Care System
Boston, Massachusetts

Nancy A. Rigotti, MD
Professor of Medicine
Harvard Medical School
Director
Tobacco Research and Treatment Center
Massachusetts General Hospital
Boston, Massachusetts

Lawrence Ronan, MD
Massachusetts General Hospital
Internal Medicine Associates
Ambulatory Care Center
Boston, Massachusetts

Edward T. Ryan, MD
Associate Professor of Medicine
Harvard Medical School
Associate Professor of Immunology & Infectious Diseases
Harvard School of Public Health
Director, Immunization Center
Division of Infectious Diseases
Massachusetts General Hospital
Boston, Massachusetts

Peter C. Schalock, MD
Instructor
Department of Dermatology
Harvard Medical School
Boston, Massachusetts
Assistant in Dermatology
Department of Dermatology
Massachusetts General Hospital Cancer Center
Boston, Massachusetts

Linda C. Shafer, MD
Instructor
Department of Psychiatry
Harvard Medical School
Psychiatrist
Department of Psychiatry
Massachusetts General Hospital
Boston, Massachusetts

David Slovik, MD
Chief of Medicine
Spaulding Rehabilitation Hospital
Boston, Massachusetts

Arthur Sober, MD
Massachusetts General Hospital
Dermatology Associates
Ambulatory Care Center
Boston, Massachusetts

John T. Stoeckle, MD
Massachusetts General Hospital
Boston, Massachusetts

Katherine K. Treadway, MD
Wang Ambulatory Care Center
Massachusetts General Hospital
Boston, Massachusetts

Jeff Weilburg, MD
Department of Psychiatry
Wang Ambulatory Care Center
Massachusetts General Hospital
Boston, Massachusetts

John J. Worthington, III, MD
Staff Psychiatrist
Clinical Psychopharmacology Unit
Department of Psychiatry
Massachusetts General Hospital
Boston, Massachusetts

Patrick S. Yachimski, MD, MPH
Advanced Endoscopy Fellow
Brigham & Women's Hospital
Massachusetts General Hospital
Harvard Medical School
Boston, Massachusetts

■ PREFACE

At this challenging yet very exciting time for primary care, we are pleased to offer the sixth edition of *Primary Care Medicine*. There is a nascent renaissance in primary care emerging, supported by powerful evidence that well delivered primary care improves health status, lowers health care costs, and reduces health disparities. Society's renewed demand for access to comprehensive, patient-centered primary care is spawning fundamental reforms in practice and payment, with an emphasis on value over volume and increasing engagement of the patient as a partner in care. It is in this context that *Primary Care Medicine* seeks to provide the information needed to deliver personalized, evidence-based, cost-effective care. This has been our mission from day 1 of the first edition over a quarter century ago, and it is now more important than ever before. We have written *Primary Care Medicine* to function not only as a reference text for learners but also as a decision support tool for busy practitioners, utilizing Web-based electronic delivery for point-of-care use. We continue our basic approach of presenting information in a tightly written problem-based format that focuses on key clinical decisions and combines pathophysiology, social science, and best clinical studies to construct evidence-based recommendations for evaluation, management, and patient education. We incorporate current consensus guidelines but try to go beyond them to help you customize care for individual patients. Cost-effectiveness considerations, especially as regards diagnostic imaging and prescribing are top priorities, as are indications for timely referral and hospital admission, critical responsibilities for the primary care clinician.

Like each of our previous editions, the sixth edition is thoroughly rewritten, incorporating nearly 3,000 important new references that define important advances in screening, diagnostics, and treatment relevant to achieving improved outcomes. To help you with this daunting exponential increase in knowledge, we attempt to put these new developments in context and provide perspective so the primary care physician does not feel buffeted by the latest information, typically brought to one's attention by a patient who brings in a media report. Moreover, in this age of direct-to-consumer advertising and unregulated promotion of self-care remedies, we critically examine often-unsubstantiated claims with the best available scientific evidence to help you practice rationally and inform your patients effectively.

For us, *Primary Care Medicine* has been and continues to be a labor of love, and we thank the generations of learners and practitioners who have helped make it a standard in the field.

Allan H. Goroll, MD
Albert G. Mulley, Jr. MD, MPP
Boston, Massachusetts
October 2008

■ ACKNOWLEDGMENTS

Over the preceding five editions, many individuals have generously participated in the writing of this book. Listing all of them here is not feasible; however, we would like to single out those former contributors who completed their contributions to the book with the fifth edition, given the importance of their work to the collective effort of preparing this edition. These persons and the chapters they previously authored include: Drs. John D. Stoeckle and Linda L. Emanuel for Chapter 1, Dr. John D. Stoeckle for Chapter 39, Robert A. Hughes for Chapter 83, Michael A. Jenike for the Appendix to Chapter 173, William V. Shellow and his colleagues Adam M. Rotunda, Delphine J. Lee, and Noah Craft for the Dermatology section consisting of Chapters 178-197, Eric Kortz for the Appendix Section 12, and Patrick L. Lillard for Chapter 235.

We also are much indebted to our devoted section editors for their extraordinary writing contributions, including Drs. James M. Richter for gastroenterology, Jeffrey W. Clark for oncology, David M. Slovik for Endocrinology, Amy A. Pruitt for Neurology, Peter C. Schalock for Dermatology, Claudia U. Richter for Ophthalmology, and Neil Bhattacharyya for ENT.

Finally, we want to acknowledge the professionalism and commitment to publishing quality of our collaborating editors Sonya Seigafuse and Ryan Shaw at our publisher Lippincott Williams & Wilkins. We are grateful for the opportunity to have authored now six beautifully produced editions with this distinguished publisher.

■ FOREWORD TO THE FIRST EDITION

Physicians have traditionally provided direct, initial, comprehensive care for patients as well as continuity of care. In the past two decades the growing proportion of specialist physicians has endangered this traditional role of the physician. The development of highly technologic, tertiary, inpatient medical care has preoccupied the attention of our teaching institutions. Coping with the increased armamentarium of diagnostic and therapeutic interventions has distracted some physicians from traditional roles in patient care. The primary care movement has been a national response to this situation aimed at providing more physicians skilled in dealing wisely and humanely with illness in their patients and providing the overall supervision and continuity of medical care that we expect of good generalists. It encourages these physicians to know their patients as human and social beings as well as bearers of organ pathology. Promotion of prevention as well as the practice of curing is an important part of primary care.

The concerns which have led to renewed attention of the medical profession to primary care medicine have had a very salutary effect on our teaching institutions. There has been a resurgence of training in the ambulatory setting. Medical students and residents have learned that many illnesses formerly thought to require hospitalization can be effectively managed in the ambulatory setting. As usual, this is not an original discovery; rather, it is a return to the emphasis that was very much a part of training programs in the earlier decades of this century.

Primary Care Medicine has grown out of the experiences of a group of young physicians who have pioneered in the rebirth of primary care medicine within the Harvard medical community. They have organized primary care practices which have served as training sites for other physicians and health workers. They have examined their own practices, as well as the published experience of others, in order to provide within this text a synthesis of the best available information for ambulatory management of adult medical patients. Their discussions are brief and practical rather than exhaustive, but the interested reader is provided with a key annotated bibliography which directs him to further sources of information. This book is not meant to compete with the traditional exhaustive textbook of Medicine. Rather, its brief, clear discussions and analyses of current knowledge are prepared for the busy practitioner who daily encounters many problems for which he needs to quickly know the best available answers.

To whom is the book addressed? To the primary care physician, of course. It will be his bible—a valuable source of guidance and of solace in innumerable management situations. But it is becoming increasingly evident that the medical subspecialist devotes a considerable portion of his practice time to the provision of first contact and continuous care of the medical needs of his patients. This book will, therefore, find a welcome place on the desk of both the medical subspecialist and the medical generalist and is addressed to everyone engaged in the clinical practice of adult Medicine.

Alexander Leaf, M.D.
Jackson Professor of Medicine
Harvard Medical School; and
Chief, Medical Services
Massachusetts General Hospital
Boston, Massachusetts
April 1981

■ CONTENTS

PART III ▪ CARDIOVASCULAR PROBLEMS

PART VIII ■ GYNECOLOGIC PROBLEMS

PART IX ■ GENITOURINARY PROBLEMS

PART X ■ MUSCULOSKELETAL PROBLEMS

PART XI ■ NEUROLOGIC PROBLEMS

PART XII ■ DERMATOLOGIC PROBLEMS

PART XIII ■ OPHTHALMOLOGIC PROBLEMS

PART XIV ■ EAR, NOSE, AND THROAT PROBLEMS

PART XV ■ PSYCHIATRIC PROBLEMS

PART XVI ■ ALLIED FIELDS

Primary Care Medicine

CHAPTER 1 ■ THE PRACTICE OF PRIMARY CARE

JOHN D. STOECKLE

DEFINITIONS OF PRIMARY CARE (1–3)

From the perspective of practice, primary care can be defined by its several clinical tasks: (a) medical diagnosis and treatment, (b) psychological diagnosis and treatment, (c) personal support of patients of all backgrounds in all stages of illness, (d) communication of information about prevention, diagnosis, treatment, and prognosis, and (e) prevention and care of chronic disease and disability through risk assessment, health education, early disease detection, preventive treatment, and behavioral change. These tasks are a clinical or operational definition of the work of primary care practitioners.

Besides this clinical definition of primary care, there are other definitions that derive from organizational, functional, professional, and academic perspectives. For example, in the past, some policy planners defined primary care as a *level of community-based medical services* provided in offices, clinics, neighborhood health centers, group practices, schools, and factories. These first-contact primary care community-based services were considered less technical compared with secondary care (consultant or specialty services) and with tertiary care (hospital services). Whereas such a three-tier organizational definition of health services once provided a scheme for the allocation of public resources, such distinctions in site and content of care are blurred today as diagnostic and treatment technologies have been decentralized to ambulatory practices for both primary and specialty use. If practices also engage in community interventions besides individual treatment, the resulting care has been defined as *community-oriented primary care,* which few practices do. For another definition, Alpert and Charney (1) looked at important *patient care functions* of primary care practitioners—namely, to provide access, continuity, and coordination. Although this definition is useful in describing the functions performed by primary care practitioners for patients, it does not define the tasks of their clinical work. From the standpoint of professionalism, primary care has been defined as a *specialty* concentrating on general medical skills and knowledge for illnesses treated outside of the hospital but with fewer skills in the special diagnostic and treatment technologies that characterize specialization. This definition has been useful in designing the curriculum for training in the specialties of primary care—general internal medicine, combined medicine–pediatrics, general pediatrics, and family practice. In medical schools, primary care may be implicitly defined as an *academic interdepartmental discipline* with social, behavioral, and administrative research interests in the organization of practice, the behaviors of patients and doctors, and the uses and outcomes of health services.

Although each of these definitions represents a particular perspective about primary care, the clinical tasks of care explain much of the primary care physician's day-to-day work with patients. In providing care, the rationales of these tasks are noted.

TASKS AND THEIR RATIONALES

Medical Diagnosis and Treatment (4–6)

Medical diagnosis and treatment are central tasks, but alone they do not provide the care of patients, as ancient and modern writings consistently affirm. Nonetheless, the primary clinician must certainly be knowledgeable about disease and must exercise judgment in determining the scope, site, and pace of the medical workup to provide the patient accurate diagnosis and treatment. For this task, the practitioner learns the patient's history of illness, performs the physical exam, makes appropriate use of tests and therapies from evidence-based studies, considers the needs for consultative advice and shared care with specialist colleagues, and, in this process, shares and negotiates decisions with the patient. The methods developed in clinical epidemiology and decision analysis that can help the clinician rationally choose among a sometimes bewildering array of diagnostic and therapeutic options are discussed in Chapters 2 and 5. Application of these methods has proved difficult in many primary care settings in the absence of system support. Diagnostic and therapeutic decision support systems have been developed to support physicians in these complex tasks, with varying degrees of measurable success. In many cases, the need for adoption and consistent use of these systems by clinicians is the major challenge to realizing better decision quality.

Psychological Diagnosis and Treatment and Personal Support (7,8)

Psychological diagnosis, treatment, and personal support are tasks of both medicine's art and its science. The mixed roots of these tasks derive from the biopsychosocial definition of clinical medicine; from studies that have documented the physiologic, even immune effects of emotions; from studies of outcomes of medical–surgical treatment that brings emotional distress; and from surveys that show a high frequency of psychosocial illness in patients seeking medical help. The recognition of the patient's anxiety and/or depression helps in the interpretation of bodily complaints, in using communication skills for emotional relief, and in shared decision making about treatment choices. In addition, the patient's defenses, personality style, and cultural roots also help the clinician to provide meaningful support and respond appropriately to the patient's emotional needs. Such psychotherapeutic aspects of clinical practice derive from continuing studies of doctor–patient communication by clinicians and social scientists. Modern studies of outcomes of medical and surgical treatment have included quality-of-life measures, in which emotional states, especially depression, have significant effect.

Eliciting and Addressing Patient Expectations and Requests (9–11)

Eliciting and addressing patient expectations of and requests for care are important because they often play a major part in patients' decisions to seek medical help, in their adherence to treatment plans, and in their satisfaction with care. In studies of illness behavior and patients' use of doctors, social scientists have viewed the following patient expectations as explanations of their decisions to see a doctor: to enhance status by seeing socially important professionals; to achieve catharsis of grief, anger, and despair; to obtain sanction for failure to cope; and to find understanding and control of illness through medical scientific explanations. Along with these expectations about care and treatment are often latent traditional medical ones—for example, that the doctor (or medicine) cures disease and has techniques for its control and relief, topics about which patients are better informed today. Such expectations not only explain decisions to seek care, but also are useful topics to address in the tasks of personal support and communication of information about illness. Clinical studies by Lazare and colleagues (10) separated *requests* from expectations. Requests are specific, concrete helping actions and behaviors that patients want. These studies demonstrated that prompt recognition and negotiation of requests benefited both patient and doctor. The doctor's interest in ascertaining what treatment the patient wants indicates a reciprocity that is associated with greater satisfaction and adherence to medical advice. Continuing care, referral, discharge, informed consent, and end-of-life preferences are some of the many decisions negotiated through an understanding of patient requests. Practitioners need to both elicit and respond to them.

Communication of Information about Illness (12–15)

To inform, explain, reassure, and advise patients are essential to primary care. These communication tasks often depend on knowledge of the patient's *attributions*, that is, what the patient thinks is the cause of illness. If the patient's attributions differ from the doctor's and are not uncovered, the patient's anxieties may not be relieved, nor will the doctor's explanation be accepted. In responding to the needs of the patient, what is told to the patient about the illness may be ineffective if the patient's interpretation of the illness has not been elicited.

Mechanic's (13) study, for example, suggested that patients with bodily complaints may go to the primary care doctor not only for relief of physical discomfort, but also to learn what is causing their complaints and to be reassured that the causes are less serious than feared. This is a common office experience of the practitioner. Such confirmation or correction of the patient's attributions is a kind of "attribution therapy." From a broader perspective, Kleinman (12) assigned to attributions a major function in all medical care systems—namely, the con-

trol of illness through the explanation of its cause. In effect, the doctor's clinical or scientific explanations of illness provide labels, names, and models so that the patient can feel that the illness can be understood and controlled, regardless of its technical treatment. In essence, the patient's beliefs about the illness need to be elicited so that they can be used in explanation, education, and reassurance, even more so today with the cultural diversity of the population seeking medical aid.

Care of the Chronically Ill (16,17)

Care of the chronically ill draws heavily on the continuity and coordination of primary care. Here, obtaining patient compliance with or adherence to an agreed course of management is essential because most long-term treatment now takes place without daily medical supervision, and most of that treatment requires self-administering drugs and undertaking behaviors necessary to monitor disease and slow progression or prevent exacerbations. To improve adherence to therapy, it has become increasingly important to learn about the *patient's views of treatment* and actual self-treatment. The record on adherence to treatment is not good (see later discussion). A wide discrepancy between what the patient is prescribed and what he or she does typifies the literature on "following the doctor's orders." The problem of compliance, however, is becoming as much one relating to practitioners as to patients. Patient outcomes depend on getting the patient to "take medicines," whereas practice outcomes depend on getting the doctor to prescribe appropriately to all patients needing treatment in his or her practice panel, where many gaps may appear in prescribing effective therapy. Even without office visits, information technologies can facilitate the communication of reminders about treatment to improve compliance, given that much information and advice at the visit may be soon forgotten. Knowledge about patients' levels of motivation and confidence regarding advised behavior changes can also be used to design more effective support to help them overcome barriers to compliance and self-management (see later discussion).

Prevention of Disease and Disability (18)

Preventing disease and disability depends heavily on assessing and communicating risk coupled with achieving the behavior change necessary to reduce any risks that can be altered (e.g., smoking, violence, alcohol, drugs, diet). With early interventions for risk and risky behavior through health education, behavioral change, and preventive treatment, some of the expected morbidity, disability, and mortality can be prevented. The practitioner needs to know which conditions and risk factors are worth screening for and how best to detect and effectively manage them (see Chapter 3). Primary care clinicians can also use their understanding of the epidemiology of disease and risks of the entire practice population and its community base to institute preventive programs both inside and outside of the practice.

A less commonly considered but no less important aspect of prevention involves attention to the patient's *social network* because illness is often precipitated by a disruption of interpersonal relationships. Learning about a patient's social network can reveal stresses at work and home that might be illness precipitants and make it possible to relieve them by support and counseling. If loss or separation has occurred, the task of helping the patient to reestablish a supportive network can be shared with family, social workers, nurses, and home services personnel.

USING THE DOCTOR–PATIENT PARTNERSHIP (5,19–25)

Personal Care

The ideal and need for personal care, now called patient-centered care, remain. This means that therapeutic regimens must not only be evidence based, but they also must be made acceptable to patients of diverse backgrounds, ages, levels of education, and views of illness and treatments.

The Basis for Partnership

The doctor–patient relationship is a partnership in which the physician engages the patient's participation in care in the following ways:

1. Attends all patients with unconditional regard.
2. Educates patients so that they are well informed, and elicits their preferences among possible diagnostic testing and treatment alternatives to engage them in shared decision making and compliance in treatment.
3. Negotiates patients' choices, decisions, and requests, including possible conflict in the relationship or in the practice organization.
4. Provides helping actions and communications that are patient centered by eliciting and responding to patients' feelings, concerns, and perspectives about their illness and care.
5. Promotes health education, self-help, and preventive behaviors by communicating information about risks.

Recognizing Communication Barriers

Today, the patient population is older and more multicultural, trends that are predicted to continue as the United States remains an open society and longevity increases with better control and prevention of chronic disease. Patient care requires understanding patients' varied cultural backgrounds, and, for older patients, assessing and responding to any impairments to communication. In the clinical interview, the doctor often needs the skills of a trained interpreter, not just the help of a family member. With older patients, the need is to assess visual, auditory, vocal, and cognitive functions to determine whether there are factors that might be limiting effective communication and to devise aids and tactics to cope with such barriers.

Making Use of Communication Technologies

With modern information technologies (especially through the Internet), patients often access information on disease management and obtain mutual support online from disease-specific groups. Recent data suggest that such Internet-informed patients more often than not fail to share their Internet search findings with their primary care physician, so there may be a potential information divide in the doctor–patient relationship. To prevent such a division, several steps are recommended. The physician should (a) ask patients about Internet use when reviewing their condition and its treatment; (b) review the information they obtained, helping them put it in context; (c) build on their desire for accurate medical information by providing suggestions for further reading; and (d) help them to obtain reliable information, directing them to authoritative websites.

ENHANCING ADHERENCE IN THE DOCTOR–PATIENT PARTNERSHIP (26–30)

Adherence has been defined as the extent to which patient behavior with regard to taking medications, following a diet, modifying behavior, or attending clinical appointments is consistent with medical advice. As such, it is synonymous with the terms *compliance* and *concordance*, although some see these terms as more and less judgmental, respectively, than adherence. Depending on the behavior advised, nonadherence may be reported in as many as 80% of patients. Obviously, this is troublesome. Patients' adherence to medication regimens is critical in effectively and efficiently treating medical disorders, as is their adoption and learning of appropriate behaviors (with regard to eating, exercise, smoking, drinking, relaxation, and use of drugs) for preventing disease and exacerbations of chronic conditions. Furthermore, nonadherence also reflects failures of communication and of collaboration in tasks that neither doctor nor patient can accomplish alone.

Adherence can be improved by practitioner–patient communication that includes careful explanation combined with a search for sources of motivation, which are often different for different patients. Different patients also face different barriers to behavior change. Identifying these barriers, as well as sources of support, with the patient can lead to strategies for overcoming obstacles and providing necessary confidence. The clinician's goal should be to enhance both motivation and confidence and thereby improve patient adherence and health outcomes.

Elements of a Strategy

The education and communication strategies and techniques helpful in facilitating compliance begin with the doctor–patient relationship. A positive, mutually respectful doctor–patient relationship is important in making the patient ready to receive patient education and negotiate the goals and means of treatment. Moreover, the physician's explanations and educational efforts, in turn, contribute to that relationship. Specific strategies focus on motivation, specific and tailored medical advice, ongoing dialogue, and collaboration in monitoring the condition and its treatment. The following are strategies the physician should undertake.

Motivation

1. Describe immediate and long-term treatment benefits along with health risk and cost. If possible, present treatment options and acknowledge whether the rationale for the recommendation may differ from the patient's views and preferred course of action.
2. Assist patients in identifying sources of motivation and clarifying their priorities. In chronically ill patients with multiple comorbid conditions, it is often necessary to recognize that many things compete for the time and attention that they can realistically devote to their self-care. In such cases, priority setting is critical.
3. Use his or her expertise, experience, and relationship not only to assert expectations for patient compliance, but also to offer support in identifying and overcoming perceived barriers to adherence.

Specific and Tailored Medical Advice

1. Adapt instructions to the patient's language and knowledge level, responding to any misconceptions about the condition and its treatment.
2. Make directions explicit, simple, personalized, and operational (how many, what kind, and when to take pills; organize pill taking into the routine of the patient's everyday life).
3. Use multiple modes of communication, both verbal and written instructions, and, when available, audiovisual materials that reinforce general knowledge about treatment. Enlist other members of the clinical team in providing instructions; also recruit family in the educational process.

Ongoing Dialogue

1. Have the patient paraphrase his or her understanding of the medical advice given and the rationale for it.
2. Have the patient talk through how medical advice will be carried out, naming obstacles and identifying sources of support for overcoming obstacles.
3. Jointly plan return visits, phone calls, and additional reviews with the clinical team (nurse practitioners, physician assistants) if needed.

Collaborative Monitoring and Care

1. At return visits, review the patient's compliance, again eliciting the rationale along with the problems the patient has experienced in treatment.
2. Use information to reexplain or redesign treatment, and reinforce adherence to advised behaviors with an affirming attitude.
3. Encourage and help to organize the patient's self-monitoring of treatment (e.g., blood pressure measurements).
4. Be sure that the patient knows how to respond to symptoms and signs that may signal exacerbations of the condition or treatment side effects. Agree on a written response plan.

All too often these approaches are not used to create collaborative relationships between clinicians and patients or caregivers. The missed opportunities are costly for everyone.

ASSURING PROFESSIONALISM IN PRIMARY CARE

In carrying out clinical tasks and in forging partnerships with patients, practitioners must attend to their performance not only along the dimensions of clinical competence and effectiveness, but also with due regard for the ethical obligations of a professional.

Confidentiality (31)

Trust—the *sine qua non* of the patient–doctor relationship—requires that patients' confidences be kept by the physician. This need is recognized in the law as part of the constitutional right to privacy, and was underscored in the Health Insurance Privacy and Protection Act. Physicians should be able to reassure the patient who is concerned about confidentiality of the primacy and privacy of the patient–doctor relationship. However, there are some limits to this confidentiality that should be understood by the patient.

Limits to Confidentiality

Confidentiality is limited by clinician's responsibility *to protect third parties from harm*, as may occur, for example, when a patient reveals to a psychiatrist a plan to murder someone. Balancing obligations to the patient with obligations to a third party depends on an assessment of relative harms. One such example is the reporting of a sexually transmitted disease, including AIDS, to the patient's sexual contact(s). State requirements vary. Persuading the patient to reveal the information directly to the third party often allows the discharge of all obligations to the third party with minimal damage to the patient–doctor alliance. Occasionally, confidentiality must be breached when it is *in the best interests of the patient*, although this rule should be used sparingly. The physician should reveal the minimum that is necessary in such situations.

Sometimes, the *physician's role* or *responsibility* limits the ability to keep a patient's confidence. A physician employed by a company, school, military unit, or court has split allegiances, which the patient must be made aware of at the outset. Medical information must be reported to insurance companies in many cases, but not all, and the consent of the patient is always required before this can occur. More subtle constraints on confidentiality can arise when *medical records* are readily accessed by other employees, such as those in a billing office. Policies and procedures for affording extra protection to patients who may be known to employees are indicated. Physicians may receive *court subpoenas*, in response to which they must appear in court with the appropriate information. A patient's privilege to bar the physician from testifying may be invoked, but it can be overruled by the court.

Sharing of Information within the Limits of Confidentiality

Sharing of information about a patient among members of the health care team is rarely problematic. However, the risk of breaches rises as the number of persons included in the health care team increases. Patient information used for teaching rounds or publication should be carefully safeguarded against any identifying features.

Involving family or friends in a patient's care is often in the best interests of the patient, but sharing patient information with them requires the patient's explicit permission. When family members reveal information relevant to the patient that they ask the physician to withhold from the patient, the request cannot be honored, and the family should be made aware of this obligation ahead of time if possible. The conflict may be resolved by persuading the family of the inadvisability of such secrecy.

Patient Information in Electronic Databases

The use of computer-based records and central support systems has raised important questions about how to maintain the proper confidentiality of patient records in large electronic systems. Among other concerns, protective measures must still allow the desirable use of information, for example, for systematic quality improvement or approved research activities. The issue is largely an institutional policy matter, and quality improvement and research information in many cases can be pursued without a breach of patient confidentiality by the use of only deidentified, aggregate data. However, physicians should be sure that the institution in which they work provides suitable confidentiality protection in the electronic medium and that physicians and others abide by the protective measures.

These should include the use of personal identification codes for access to computers that hold patient information.

Improperly Motivated Requests for Confidentiality

On rare occasions, requests for confidentiality may come from patients with seductive, suicidal, hostile, or criminal intentions. When this is the case, the physician should involve a colleague as consultant and document the encounter. These steps will serve to protect the physician from such charges as sexual misconduct, harboring a fugitive, or facilitating a suicide. They also help to preserve good judgment and justified levels of confidentiality, and they free the physician from the intimidating nature of the secret.

Avoiding Financial Conflicts (32,33)

Major medical ethics codes all note the need to avoid the financial exploitation of patients, many of whom are in situations such that they would spend unfair amounts of money in the hope of securing their health. Physicians should charge, or help ensure that their institutions charge, fees that are not exorbitant. Reimbursement claims should honestly describe the service rendered and should avoid claiming for subcomponents of the service for the purpose of securing a higher reimbursement rate.

Self-employed and group-practice physicians working within fee-for-service systems need to avoid arrangements such as self-referrals and kickbacks. Such arrangements include those in which physicians refer patients to facilities in which the physician has a financial interest or to other physicians who pay the referring physician a referral fee, and those in which physicians receive payment from a drug company for each prescription written for a specified drug. Primary care physicians should also be aware of financial incentives to provide procedures and injectable drugs fixed by specialist colleagues to whom they refer patients.

Physicians often face financial incentives that may influence their treatment decisions. Primary care physicians should do what they can to be sure that financial incentives are (a) a relatively small proportion of a physician's income, (b) paid relatively infrequently, (c) shared by a group of physicians rather than applied to individuals, and (d) designed in such a way that they foster good patient care. A useful rule of thumb may be to ask the following question: Would the physician be embarrassed to disclose the incentive arrangement to the patient? These standards may minimize the inappropriate influence of incentives. If incentive systems deviate from professional standards, physicians can work within the institution to effect change and if necessary can also decline to receive inappropriate incentives.

Informed Consent (34)

Informed consent is much more than a legal document. In fact, a signed document in the absence of a valid discussion with the physician is unlikely to be of legal benefit. Informed consent is a continuing part of the patient–physician relationship and involves the giving and interpretation of information, deliberation, and shared decision making. As such, informed consent represents an integral part of the continuing therapeutic alliance. Informed consent is required for most nonemergent decisions, whether routine or major.

Required Components of Information Giving and Consent

Laws and legal opinions have defined the following required components of information giving: The patient must receive a description of the *nature of the treatment*, the associated risks (both major and frequent), and their expected time of occurrence. It is neither reasonable nor appropriate for the physician to furnish an exhaustive catalogue of risks; the physician's role is to provide relevant information and judgment. The *expected benefits* and *alternative treatments* should also be reviewed relative to the recommended action.

Each component of informed consent can be pursued to varying levels of intensity. The courts initially adopted a *standard of practice* criterion in which the physician was expected to provide information according to the standards of current practice in the community. Later, the criterion shifted toward providing what a hypothetical *reasonable person* would want to know. A mixed standard is now in general use. In practice, valid consent is most likely to be given when information giving is tailored to suit the needs of the individual patient.

Consent also has required components. First, there must be an *understanding of the information* by the patient. A practical means of assessing understanding is to ask the patient about concerns and expectations; the responses can guide further information giving. Second, the decision must be *voluntary*. However, persuasion is appropriate in some circumstances, and physicians need not feel constrained from expressing their best medical judgment.

Research Consent

Research consent requires that particular attention be paid to the patient's sense of volunteerism and understanding. The design of the study protocol must be fully understood. Randomized, controlled trials require patients to take the chance of receiving the standard treatment instead of what may be the preferred treatment. In some trials, patients also take the chance of receiving placebo treatment, and in double-blind studies, the patient's physician will not know which treatment the patient is receiving. The benefit to patients in the control arm may be limited to close monitoring.

Patients must understand that the physician may have conflicting interests. For example, there may be a gain in collegiality, career advancement, or even material benefit. Many of these interests are inevitable and acceptable, but they must be fully disclosed and discussed with the patient. Reassurance of a true primary commitment of the physician to the patient should be possible. If such a primary commitment to the patient is lacking, the patient should be transferred to another physician for care or should not participate in the research protocol.

Advance Directives for Health Care (35–45)

The term *advance directives* refers to provisions made by patients to direct their health care in case of future incompetence. Advance directives are written statements and can include a living will and the designation of a proxy decision maker (sometimes referred to as *durable power of attorney for health care*). Ideally, advance directives combine both modalities. They are inactive until such time as incompetence occurs.

The Office Discussion

For the sake of clear communication, advance directives should be completed in the context of a discussion with the patient and witnessed by the person who will be the designated proxy decision maker. Ambulatory patients have been found to be very receptive to advance planning and often expect physicians to take the initiative. When structured around the completion of an advance directive document, the core discussion can be expected to take about 15 to 30 minutes. Interval follow-up discussions are appropriate and particularly relevant at times of a significant change in the patient's health or personal circumstances. Although it is common to undertake advance planning for the elderly and seriously ill, planning for the young and healthy can be quite worthwhile. Planning discussions can be regarded as a good investment of time, in that they can make subsequent difficult decisions more efficient. Moreover, they help to build a quality relationship of shared decision making around the patient's goals and the physician's expertise and efforts at health promotion.

As important as any other components of advance care planning are the education and sense of readiness provided to the patient, the proxy, and the physician. These discussions foster a sense of participation and consensus, and consign documents and legalities to their proper role as necessary but peripheral components.

Choosing a Document

Using a standardized, worksheet-type document or the outline of a document can be very helpful. A well-designed worksheet facilitates discussion. Many facilities have recommended documents available, and some generic documents have been designed to be binding in all states. Usually, there are separate documents for a written statement of preferences and for the designation of a proxy, although more-efficient documents combining the two exist. If a patient has a document already drawn up, the physician should review it with the patient. Patients should be advised that advance directives can elect for intervention as well as withdrawal or withholding of treatment, depending on the situation. Treatment decisions should be as specific as possible and linked to statements regarding the goals of intervention and general values of health care.

Legal Considerations

Federal law requires that patients be informed of hospital policy regarding living wills at the time of admission and be asked whether they have any advance directives drawn up. This information must be entered into the medical record. Advance directives must be honored under law as a statement of the patient's autonomous wishes. Rarely, there may be a conflict between a patient's wishes and local statutes. For example, some states restrict the withdrawal of nutrition and hydration to terminally ill patients, which potentially prevents withdrawal from some patients, such as those in a persistent vegetative state. The patient should be informed whether such conflict exists. Conflicts related to differences in values between the patient and the physician should be discussed fully so that they can be resolved before problematic decisions arise. An inability to resolve the conflict is cause for asking the patient to agree to transfer of care should the circumstances in question arise.

Patients who are Confused or Refuse Care (31,35,36,39)

Many treatment refusals arise from fear, perceived loss of control, distrust, or anger. Discussing patient concerns in a receptive, respectful manner that also offers the patient some choices and a sense of control often suffices to reverse the refusal. Treatment refusal may be a result of patient incompetence, but other refusals may be well reasoned and valid.

Right to Refuse Care

The right to refuse medical care is strongly endorsed by the law as part of a constitutional right to privacy. The U.S. Supreme Court has affirmed that this right exists for competent patients, incompetent patients with explicit preferences, and even incompetent patients without explicit preferences (although the right is more difficult to implement in this circumstance). Treatments that have been determined in case law to be terminable range from mechanical respiration to artificial nutrition and hydration. The Patient Self-Determination Act of 1990 requires that patients be reminded on enrollment in or admission to a health care facility of their right to accept or refuse medical treatment.

However, the right to refuse care is *not absolute*. It can be limited by opposing interests. Some states invoke their interest in preserving life to restrict withholding or withdrawing of life-sustaining treatments from incompetent patients unless they are terminally ill or, in some states, in a hopeless or persistent vegetative state. The need to protect minors may limit a competent patient's right to refuse treatment.

Declaring and Determining Incompetence

If a patient's refusal of care appears to be related to mental or psychological incompetence(s), the patient can be declared incompetent, and the refusal can be overridden. Incompetence is commonly declared by the physician, sometimes with the help of a consulting psychiatrist. Review by an institutional ethics committee or even the judiciary should be considered if (a) a question arises about who should be the surrogate decision maker for the patient, (b) legal action is current or anticipated, or (c) the case involves the termination of life-sustaining treatment in the absence of a valid advance directive to that effect.

Determining incompetence involves assessing inability to make the individual decision at hand. Competence is not an all-or-nothing state. A patient may be competent for some decisions but incompetent for others. There are four minimum standards of competence: The patient must (a) be able to *communicate a choice*, (b) have an adequate *factual understanding* of information relevant to the decision (e.g., be able to paraphrase the information), (c) *appreciate the implications* of the decision, and (d) be able to *manipulate relevant information rationally*. Rational manipulation refers to the ability to understand, for example, not only that nontreatment of a gangrenous limb may result in death, but also that death means the end of life.

If incompetence is determined, a proxy decision maker should be appointed. Generally, this person should be someone other than the physician who will be responsible for speaking with the physician on behalf of the patient.

Sexual Boundaries and the Patient–Physician Relationship (46)

The intimacy of the patient–physician encounter and the trust required for the therapeutic encounter together require that personal boundaries be clear and well maintained. One such boundary concerns sexual behavior. A unanimous standard throughout major traditions in medicine is that physicians should not engage in sexual relations with their patients. Variations in opinion tend to relate to matters of definition—what exactly constitutes a sexual touch, for instance—and to questions such as whether the prohibition applies to former patients.

In general, physicians should stay well away from sexual behavior in the professional context and avoid behavior that tests any fine distinctions. One allegation of sexual misconduct can end a medical career. If any concerns arise—for instance, if the physician's instincts suggest that such feelings exist on either side and certainly if a patient makes sexual overtures— some of the following steps may help. Involve a chaperone, especially during the physical examination of any sexual region of the anatomy. Ask a colleague on your team for additional insight; a nurse may be able to provide important feedback about patient perceptions. Consult a physician colleague; apart from receiving helpful advice, shared information is less likely to become a coercive secret.

CHANGE AND THE ENDURING PRINCIPLES OF PRIMARY CARE MEDICINE (47–50)

This text, which addresses knowledge for the clinical tasks of primary care internal medicine, appears at a time when many social, technological, economic, and political changes are transforming primary care practice, indeed health care in general. As so many commentators and practitioners have noted, medical diagnosis and treatment, doctor–patient relationships, psychosocial care, the organization of medical practice, the design of practitioners' work, the government support of health care, and a market economy are no longer as they were in the primary care movement of the 1960s, which promised more general medical care in society and, it was hoped, a personal doctor for everyone. The following areas of change are worth noting.

Diagnosis and Treatment

Scientific advances in medicine continue to bring great promise of improved clinical care and better health for individuals and populations. However, the widespread introduction of direct-to-consumer marketing of services, as well as drugs and devices, has created much hype alongside any legitimate hope. There is ample evidence to suggest that patients receive more diagnostic and therapeutic interventions than they would choose if they had more realistic expectations and more than is good for them. This tendency to believe that more is better and to assume value in new services and products needs to be tempered. The primary care clinician is well positioned to help patients avoid the negative unintended consequences of highly specialized, technologically sophisticated medicine when it is administered uncritically.

Group Practice and Corporate Organization

Medical work today is often in the context of group practices, often in corporate organizations where practitioners are employed or where practitioners are contracted under health insurance plans for services. Diagnoses, risk assessments, and treatments are more guideline driven and evidence based for assuring high standards and cost control, and treatments are now monitored not only for appropriate individual use, but also for their needed use in medical practices and community

populations where the adoption of new, effective treatments may be slow or neglected. Monitoring a doctor's prescribing compliance in his or her practice panel has become a proactive effort to improve outcomes. Compliance in treatment is now as much the doctor's job as it once was deemed only the patient's. Such monitoring of disease management from within and by practices rather than from outside is being accepted in an organizational and professional spirit of improving the care of patients.

Partnership Relationship

Doctor–patient relationships, once dominated by the professional, are now partnerships for shared decision making in which doctors transmit more information to empower patients, and patients actively seek health information for shared decision making with the doctor or for engaging in self-help. Patients seeking diagnostic and treatment advice from the doctor are also being informed from outside of the partnership by drug firms on what to take and ask the doctor for, by hospital systems on where to go and what they offer, by health plans on what care is approved, and on the Internet on their diagnosis and treatment. Whereas patients are better informed, they may still seek consultations for review, advice, and negotiation in shared decision making. Doctors must become comfortable in this partnership role with its shared decision making. Skills in this area are now an important element of teaching for medical students, residents, and practitioners.

Psychosocial Care

Medicine's art has also expanded from knowing the patient as a person and providing helping emotional relief, to demonstrating competence in communication skills for the many information needs of patients for, among others, (a) diagnosis and treatment, (b) informed consent, (c) risk assessment (alcohol, smoking, violence, sexual activity) for behavioral change, (d) end-of-life-care, and (e) cultural understandings. In the care of the patient, the communications for such informing acts are being carried out in whole or in part by primary care practitioners along with physician assistants, social workers, nurses, clinical psychologists, practice colleagues, and consultants. Patients also seek support from other patients through self-help support groups, including some based on the Internet. The doctor's psychosocial care in the office, at the bedside, and on the phone can be reinforced when shared more widely in the health professions, even though it is viewed as diminished by short face-to-face encounters in productivity-driven practices. Group visits with patients dealing with similar problems have proved to be an efficient way to combine doctor–patient communication and support with patient–patient support.

Practice Productivity

In a market economy, not only have medical practices become more organized in corporate groups, but also the work of the practitioner has become productivity driven to meet economic goals. In this process, the care of the patient is often deskilled, then divided with other health care professionals, and, with care also more technical, more is also shared with specialist colleagues. With productivity demands, patient–doctor encounters are often shorter, or seem so, with care more divided and interprofessional, now shared with part-time practice colleagues, specialist consultants, physician assistants, and nurse practitioners. Thus, continuing relationships or encounters of the primary doctor and the patient may be diminished.

For long-term care of the very disabled, care may not only be divided and exchanged with other health professionals, but it also may be transferred to distant staff of other treatment institutions (nursing homes, rehab centers, home care services). With such division, the doctor's knowledge of the patient as a person may be reduced and important long-term contacts interrupted, for example, by transferring care to hospitalists, not attending patients, or not being present through the crisis of an acute illness. Despite such division of care, interprofessional communication using electronic records is connecting providers, not only for carrying out shared care and reducing errors, but also for maintaining a spirit of professional colleagueship. Despite those communication barriers, use of telemedicine, the telephone, e-mail, and other innovations such as open scheduling and group visits may help to keep doctors and patients connected. The adoption of these patient–doctor communication technologies may be slow when the traditional office visit is the only transaction of the partnership that is paid.

Domain of Primary Care

Along with these technological, social, and economic changes have come some uncertainties about the domains or boundaries of general medicine amid increasing subspecialization. With the hospitalist movement, the practitioner loses first-hand learning of the patient's experience of acute illness and the opportunity to learn medicine on the job from consultant colleagues. The shared patient management of the primary physician with the subspecialist for chronic disease and disabilities may also be lessened when subspecialists join together in specialized disease centers (back, cancer, breast) that promise comprehensive services for a narrow range of conditions. Even as more patients are empowered by diagnostic-treatment information, they may come to the primary practitioner better informed but still uncertain, or they may bypass the primary practitioner and seek subspecialist care directly, and lose continuity. Indeed, the clinical domain of primary care may seem uncertain even with diagnostic–treatment technologies decentralized to ambulatory practices for shared care with many colleagues.

Yet there are new opportunities. With new molecular genetic risk detection and more medical therapies, the domain of general internal medicine care may shift to a medicine of health education and risk detection and reduction. With new therapies for preventing, treating, and rehabilitating chronic disease and disability, the domain of primary care medicine may be chronic disease management with medical, behavioral, and community interventions. Whereas primary care functions may now be split from the primary care doctor alone, new interprofessional teams or groups for patient needs of access, coordination, and continuity for clinical tasks may result in new directions for the organization of the work of primary care.

Policy and Politics

Despite improvements and changes, the promise of primary care goes unfulfilled when so many people are uninsured. Indeed, the improvement in primary care requires not only new knowledge for its tasks, new organizations of practice and of medical work, and new communication competencies of practitioners with new programs of public education, but also access to care for everyone. That is not likely without a program of universal insurance. Primary care medicine is political, too.

Local Reforms

Despite these many changes and policy uncertainties driving health care, the profession has the following opportunities to experiment locally in the improvement of primary care:

1. The redesign of practice work with teams.
2. The organization of collaborative care with specialists.
3. The continued improvement in communication with patients to foster more effective shared decision making and collaborative care of chronic disease.
4. The development of special services for the needs of patients from diverse cultural backgrounds.
5. The continued assessment of practice outcomes for the improvement of treatment.

A.G.M.

Annotated Bibliography

1. Alpert JJ, Charney E. The education of physicians for primary care (DHEW Publication No. 74-31B). Washington, DC: U.S. Government Printing Office, 1975. (*One of the original functional definitions of primary care.*)
2. McWhinney IR. General practice as an academic discipline. Lancet 1966;1:419. (*Defines primary care from an academic perspective.*)
3. Mullan F, Epstein L. Community oriented primary care: new reliance in a changing world. Am J Public Health 2002;92:1748. (*Reviews the benefits and opportunities.*)
4. Freeman AC, Sweeney K. Why general practitioners do not implement evidence: qualitative study. BMJ 2001;323:1. (*Practitioners' feelings about their relationships with patients have an important role in modifying how clinical evidence is applied.*)
5. Hunt DL, Haynes RB, Hanna SE, et al. Effects of computer-based clinical decision support systems on physician behaviour and patient outcomes: a systematic review. JAMA 1998;280:1339. (*A very useful overview.*)
6. Mulley AG. Applying effectiveness and outcomes research to clinical practice. In: Heitoff HA, Lohr KM, eds. Effectiveness and outcomes in health care. Washington, DC: National Academy Press, 1990. (*A very useful overview.*)
7. Balaint M. The doctor, the patient and the illness. New York: International Universities Press, 1957. (*A classic study of the British general practitioner's negotiations with patients about diagnosis and treatment.*)
8. Kahana RJ, Bibring GL. Personality types in medical management. In: Zinberg NE, ed. Psychiatry and medical practice in a general hospital. New York: International Universities Press, 1965. (*A classic discussion of the use of defense mechanisms derived from personality assessment in treatment.*)
9. Kravitz RL, Cope OW, Bhrany V, et al. Internal medicine patients' expectations for care at office visits. J Gen Intern Med 1994;9:75. (*There has been rapid evolution in requests and needs.*)
10. Lazare A, Cohen F, Mignone R, et al. The walk-in patient as a customer: a key dimension in evaluation and treatment. Am J Orthopsychiatry 1972;42:872. (*A classic article introducing the concept of the patient as "customer."*)
11. Shuval JT, Antonovsky A, Davies AM. Social function of medical practice: doctor–patient relationship in Israel. San Francisco: Jossey-Bass, 1970. (*An analysis of the rates and reasons for medical visits; provides a typology of the uses of medical visits.*)
12. Kleinman AM. Toward a comparative study of medical systems: an integrated approach to the study of the relationship of medicine and culture. Sci Med Man 1973;1:55. (*A study that examines the specific and general significance of attributions.*)
13. Mechanic D. Social psychological factors affecting the presentation of bodily complaints. N Engl J Med 1972;286:1132. (*A sociological study that examines the factors influencing a patient's decision to seek medical help.*)

14. Xuegin G, Henderson G. Rethinking ethnicity and health care. Springfield: Charles C Thomas, 1999. (*A comprehensive discussion of the increasingly important role of ethnicity in patient care.*)

15. Zaborenko RN, Zaborenko L, Hengea RA. The psychodynamics of physicianhood. Psychiatry 1970;33:102. (*An illustration of the importance of understanding patients' defenses and personalities and the uses this knowledge may have in the treatment relationship.*)

16. Bodenheimer T, Wagner EH, Grumbach K. Electronic technology. A spark to revitalize primary care? JAMA 2003;290:259. (*Details the obstacles that must be overcome to realize the benefits of e-health in primary care.*)

17. Bodenheimer T, Wagner EH, Grumbach K. Improving primary care for patients with chronic disease: the chronic care model. JAMA 2002;288:1909. (*A very useful overview.*)

18. McKinlay JB. Social networks, lay consultation and help-seeking behavior. Social Forces 1973;51:275. (*Uses networks to explain differences in help-seeking behavior.*)

19. Diaz JA, Griffith RA, Ng JJ, et al. Patients' use of the Internet for medical information. J Gen Intern Med 2002;17:180. (*A survey study of primary care practice, finding that patient use is high but that patients usually do not discuss their findings with their doctor.*)

20. Elwyn G, Edwards A, Kinnersley P. Shared decision-making in primary care: the neglected second half of the consultation. Br J Gen Pract 1999;49:477. (*Reviews the process of decision making with patients.*)

21. Kanfert JM, Dutsch RW. Communication through interpreters in health care: ethical dilemmas arising from differences in class, culture, language, and power. J Clin Ethics 1994;8:71. (*Addresses the problems that language and cultural differences bring to the patient care setting.*)

22. Quill TE, Brody H. Physician recommendations and patient autonomy: finding a balance between physician power and patient choice. Ann Intern Med 1996;125:763. (*Provides recommendations that promote collaboration.*)

23. Stoeckle JD, Ronan LJ, Emanuel L, et al. Doctoring together: a physician's guide to manners, duties and communication in the shared care of patients. Boston: Massachusetts General Hospital, 2003. (*Reflections on interpersonal behaviors and communications.*)

24. Waitzkin H, Stoeckle JD. The communication of information about illness: clinical, sociological and methodological considerations. In: Lipowski ZJ, ed. Advances in psychosomatic medicine: psychosocial aspects of physical illness, Vol. 8. Basel: Karger, 1972. (*Discusses the role of communication in the patient–doctor relationship and a review of the research on communication in medical practice.*)

25. Woloshin S, Bickell NA, Schwartz LM, et al. Language barriers in medicine in the US. JAMA 1995;273:724. (*Reviews the role of language in medical encounters.*)

26. Kaplan SH, Greenfield S, Gandek B, et al. Characteristics of physicians with participatory decision-making styles. Ann Intern Med 1996;124:497. (*Documents the qualities and benefits of participatory decision making.*)

27. McDonald HP, Garg AX, Haynes RB. Interventions to enhance patient adherence to medication prescriptions. JAMA 2002;288:2868. (*A scientific review of 33 studies evaluating efforts to improve adherence; results are found to be inconsistent; more effective means and better research are needed.*)

28. Quill TE, Brody H. Physician recommendations and patient autonomy: finding a balance between physician power and patient choice. Ann Intern Med 1996;125:763. (*Provides recommendations that promote collaboration.*)

29. Sackett DL, Snow JC. The magnitude of compliance and non-compliance. In: Haynes R, Sackett D, eds. Compliance in health care. Baltimore: Johns Hopkins University Press, 1979. (*One of many useful chapters in this book devoted to both academic and practical aspects of the compliance issue.*)

30. Schroeder K, Fahey T, Ebrahim S. How can we improve adherence to blood pressure–lowering medication in ambulatory care? Arch Intern Med 2004;164:722. (*Reducing the number of daily doses appears to increase adherence, but the effect on blood pressure is unclear; motivational strategies and complex strategies appear to be promising.*)

31. American College of Physicians. Ethics manual, 4th ed. Ann Intern Med 1997;128:576. (*A practical guide to clinical practice from a leading professional organization.*)

32. Armour BS, Pitts MM, Maclean R, et al. The effect of explicit financial incentives on physician behavior. Arch Intern Med 2001;161:1261. (*A literature review suggesting that financial incentives reduce physicians' resource utilization, but evidence is poor.*)

33. Kassirer JP. Managed care and the morality of the marketplace. N Engl J Med 1995;333:50. (*An editorial on the market-driven approach to health care reform and its moral implications.*)

34. Applebaum PS, Lidz CW, Meisel A. Informed consent: legal theory and clinical practice. New York: Oxford University Press, 1987. (*An excellent resource for theory, relevant case law, and clinical guidance regarding informed consent.*)

35. American Medical Association. Education for physicians in end-of-life care (EPEC) curriculum. Chicago: American Medical Association, 1999. (*A 16-module instructional text on end-of-life care, including a discussion of advance care planning.*)

36. Dunn PM, Levinson W. Discussing futility with patients and families. J Gen Intern Med 1996;11:689. (*A practical approach to this difficult conversation.*)

37. Emanuel LL, Barry MJ, Stoeckle JD, et al. Advance directives for medical care: a case for greater use. N Engl J Med 1991;324:889. (*Discussion of performing scenario-based advance planning in a reasonable amount of office time.*)

38. Singer PA, Martin DK, Lavery JV, et al. Reconceptualizing advance care planning from the patient's perspective. Arch Intern Med 1998;158:879. (*A slightly different perspective is provided, with an emphasis on the role of relationships in the advance planning exercise.*)

39. Emanuel EJ. A review of the ethical and legal aspects of terminating medical care. Am J Med 1988;84:291. (*Discusses issues of competence, use of advance directives, and types of care terminated.*)

40. Gramelspacher GP, Xiao-Hua Z, Hanna MP, et al. Preferences of physicians and their patients for end-of-life care. J Gen Intern Med 1997;12:346. (*Explores the differences and areas of agreement.*)

41. Lynn J, Nolan K, Kabcenell A, et al. Reforming care for persons near the end of life: the promise of quality improvement. Ann Intern Med 2002;137:117. (*Discusses the need for systems-minded thinking for improving end-of-life care.*)

42. Martin DK, Emanuel LL, et al. Planning for the end of life. BMJ 2000;356:1672. (*Addresses the goals and assessment of advance care planning.*)

43. Meisel A, Snyder L, Quill T. Seven legal barriers to end-of-life care: myths, realities, and grains of truth. JAMA 2000;284:2495. (*There is no moral distinction between withholding and withdrawing care.*)

44. Tsevat J, Cook F, Green ML, et al. Health values of the seriously ill. Ann Intern Med 1995;122:514. (*Prospective, longitudinal, multicenter study showing wider variations than surrogates believed.*)

45. Wenger NS, Rosenfeld K. Quality indicators for end-of-life care in vulnerable elders. Ann Intern Med 2001;135:677–685. (*Effective advance care plans are a quality measure.*)

46. Johnson SH. Judicial review of disciplinary action for sexual misconduct in the practice of medicine. JAMA 1993;270:1596. (*The problem from the judicial perspective.*)

47. Showstack T, Sox H, eds. The future of primary care. Ann Intern Med 2003;138:242. (*A review of changes and potential improvements, with contributions by several authors.*)

48. Bodenheimer T. Primary care—will it survive? N Engl J Med 2006;355:862. (*Describes the growing demands on primary care and the decline in interest in such careers among trainees, referencing policy approaches to reverse the trends.*)

49. Woo B. Primary care—the best job in medicine? N Engl J Med 2006;355:864. (*Describes the growing demands on primary care and the decline in interest in such careers among trainees, referencing policy approaches to reverse the trends.*)

50. Bodenheimer T. Coordinating care—a perilous journey through the health care system. N Engl J Med.2008;358:1064. (*Details importance of coordination of services through primary care.*)

CHAPTER 2 ■ SELECTION AND INTERPRETATION OF DIAGNOSTIC TESTS

Diagnostic tests are often essential to patient care. Although the history and physical examination remain the foundation of a clinical database and sometimes suffice, the limits to what we can know about a patient are continually expanding with the addition of new diagnostic tests. These tests have many uses: (a) to make a diagnosis in a patient known to be sick, (b) to provide prognostic information for a patient with known disease, (c) to identify a person with subclinical disease or at risk for subsequent development of disease, and (d) to monitor ongoing therapy. The ultimate objective is to reduce morbidity and mortality. However, physicians and patients must avoid pitfalls along the way that can result from misuse or misinterpretation of laboratory tests.

UNCERTAINTY AND DIAGNOSTIC DECISION MAKING (1–7)

Pitfalls are more likely to be avoided if the physician appreciates the inherent uncertainty and probabilistic nature of the diagnostic process and understands the relationship between the characteristics of a diagnostic test and those of the patient(s) being tested. Sometimes a diagnosis is evident when a patient presents with a pathognomonic constellation of signs and symptoms. The proportion of diagnoses that can be so recognized increases with the physician's experience and knowledge.

In many cases, however, presenting signs or symptoms are not specific. Instead, they can be explained by a number of diagnoses, each with distinctly different implications for the patient's health. In these cases, on completion of the history and physical examination, the clinician considers a list of conditions, referred to as the *differential diagnosis*, which might explain the findings. The diagnoses can then be ranked to reflect an implicit assignment of probabilities to each. Such a ranking can be thought of as the physician's index of suspicion for each condition, based on knowledge and past experience with similar patients. The purpose of subsequent laboratory testing is to refine the initial probability estimates and, in the process, to revise the differential diagnosis. The probability of any particular disease on the revised list will depend on its probability of being present before testing and the validity of the information provided by test results.

Often the physician will focus on the presence or absence of a single disease. For example, is the chest pain caused by coronary insufficiency or not? Is the sore throat due to pharyngitis caused by group A beta-hemolytic streptococci or not? Elements of the history and physical exam provide a basis for estimating the probability of the condition in question. Dull substernal pain or pressure radiating to the left arm makes coronary insufficiency more likely. Sharp pain and tenderness make it less likely. Fever, tonsillar exudates, or tender anterior lymphadenopathy make group A beta-hemolytic streptococci infection more likely. Cough makes it less likely. This process may lower the probability below a threshold for action in which the most prudent course is to move on and behave as if the condition is not present. Alternatively, the evolving diagnostic process may raise the probability high enough to simply get on with treatment. If the probability is between these two thresholds, further diagnostic testing is warranted. This threshold approach is illustrated in Fig. 2.1. Implicit in the approach are three distinguishable tasks: (a) Estimate the pretest probability of disease based on characteristics of the patient, including symptoms and signs; (b) revise the probability of disease based on new information, including results of diagnostic tests; and (c) know where the probability thresholds are—how low does the probability have to be to behave as if the condition is not present, and how high does it have to be to behave as if it is?

VOCABULARY OF DIAGNOSTIC TEST INTERPRETATION (1,3,4–8)

Terminology is important in diagnostic test interpretation. Clinical pathologists often focus on a test's accuracy and precision. *Accuracy* is the degree of closeness of the measurement made to the true value, as measured by some alternative gold standard or reference test. *Precision* is a test's ability to give nearly the same result in repeated determinations. Clinicians, on the other hand, are more concerned with the ability of a test result to discriminate between persons with and persons without a given disease or condition; this discriminating ability can be characterized by a test's sensitivity and specificity. *Sensitivity* is the probability that a test result will be positive when the test is applied to a person who actually has the disease. *Specificity* is the probability that a test result will be negative when the test is applied to a person who actually does not have the disease. A perfectly sensitive test can rule out disease if the result is negative. A perfectly specific test can rule in disease if the result is positive. Because most tests are neither perfectly sensitive nor perfectly specific, the result must be interpreted probabilistically rather than categorically.

Often there is a tradeoff that can be made between the sensitivity and the specificity of a test. More-stringent criteria for making a diagnosis, or behaving as if the condition is present, will have lower sensitivity and higher specificity than less-stringent criteria. The most graphic examples of this principle involve tests that provide quantitative results, such as the measurement of serum prostate-specific antigen (PSA) when the diagnosis of prostate cancer is being considered. The general case is illustrated in Fig. 2.2. Note that the "normal" values for the test results are all too often derived from frequency distributions of results among apparently well persons; the potential tradeoff between sensitivity and specificity is not considered.

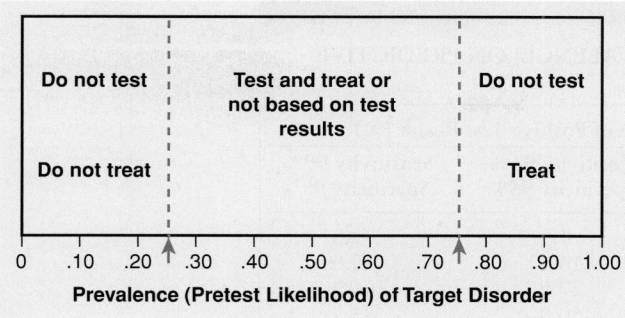

FIGURE 2.1. The threshold approach to decision making can be illustrated with a continuous probability of disease ranging from 0.0 to 1.0. Pretest probability can be estimated based on demographic variables, as well as symptoms and signs. Diagnostic test results can be thought of as new information that revises the probability of disease, leading to the decision to not treat if the revised probability is sufficiently low or to treat if the resulting probability is sufficiently high. Thresholds depend on the consequences of correct and incorrect diagnostic classifications. (From Sackett DL, Haynes RB, Guyatt GH, et al. Clinical epidemiology: a basic science for clinical medicine, 2nd ed. Boston: Little, Brown, 1991, with permission.)

Although sensitivity and specificity are important considerations in selecting a test, the probabilities they measure are not in themselves what ordinarily concern the physician and the patient after the test result has returned. Both are concerned with the following questions: If the result is positive, what is the probability that disease is present? If the result is negative, what is the probability that the patient is indeed disease-free? These probabilities are known respectively as the *predictive value positive* and the *predictive value negative*. They are determined not only by the sensitivity and the specificity of the test, but also by the probability of the disease being present before the test was ordered.

Relationships between sensitivity and specificity and positive and negative predictive values can be better understood by referring to a two-by-two table (Fig. 2.3). The two columns indicate the presence or absence of disease (note that a gold standard of diagnosis is assumed), and the two rows indicate positive or negative test results. Any given patient with a test

		Disease		
		Present	Absent	
Test	Positive	*a*	*b*	*a* + *b*
	Negative	*c*	*d*	*c* + *d*
		a + *c*	*b* + *d*	*a* + *b* + *c* + *d*

Definitions

Sensitivity:	$\dfrac{a}{a+c}$		False-negative rate:	$\dfrac{c}{a+c}$	
Specificity:	$\dfrac{d}{b+d}$		False-positive rate:	$\dfrac{b}{b+d}$	
Predictive value positive:	$\dfrac{a}{a+b}$		False-alarm rate:	$\dfrac{b}{a+b}$	
Predictive value negative:	$\dfrac{d}{c+d}$		False-reassurance rate:	$\dfrac{c}{c+d}$	

FIGURE 2.3. The two-by-two table clarifies relationships between test characteristics (sensitivity and specificity) and the predictive values of positive and negative test results. Clinicians interpreting a diagnostic test can fill in the table if they are aware of the sensitivity and the specificity of the test and a patient's (population's) pretest probability (prevalence) of disease. The pretest probability is *a* + *c*, and 1 − the pretest probability is *b* + *d*. Multiplying *a* + *c* by the sensitivity provides the value for *a*, and multiplying *b* + *d* by the specificity provides the value for *d*. Values for cell *c* and cell *b* can be determined by simple subtraction. With the cells filled in, the predictive value of a negative or positive test result can be calculated easily. It is worth noting that this calculation method is precisely equivalent to Bayes's theorem of conditional probability.

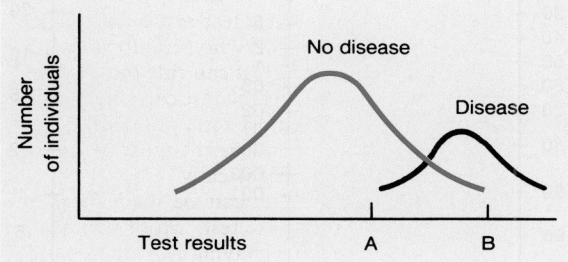

FIGURE 2.2. Hypothetical distribution of test results among patients with and without disease. Because the distributions overlap, the test is far from perfect. If all patients with values to the right of A are said to have "positive" results, the test will be 100% sensitive but will have a low specificity. If only those patients with values to the right of B are said to have "positive" results, the test will be 100% specific but will have a low sensitivity. The choice of a cutoff value between A and B should depend on the relative importance of true- and false-positive and true- and false-negative results.

result could be included in one of the four cells labeled *a, b, c,* or *d*. Definitions of sensitivity, specificity, predictive value positive, and predictive value negative can be restated by using these labels. It is important to note that each of these four ratios has a complement. The complement of sensitivity (1 − sensitivity) is referred to as the *false-negative rate,* whereas the complement of specificity (1 − specificity) is referred to as the *false-positive rate.* These terms have often been used ambiguously in the medical literature; the false-negative rate is confused with the complement of the predictive value negative, which is *best* termed the *false-reassurance rate*; the false-positive rate is confused with the complement of the predictive value positive, which is *best* termed the *false-alarm rate.*

INTERPRETING TEST RESULTS: REVISING DIAGNOSTIC PROBABILITIES (1–8)

When clinicians interpret test results, they usually process the information informally. Rarely is a pad and pencil or a calculator used to revise probability estimates explicitly. However, sometimes the revision of diagnostic probabilities is counterintuitive; for instance, it has been shown that most clinicians rely too heavily on positive test results when the pretest probability or disease prevalence is low.

Attention to the two-by-two table indicates why predictive values are crucially dependent on disease prevalence. This is particularly true when one is using a test to screen for a rare disease. If a disease is rare, even a very small false-positive rate (which is, remember, the complement of specificity) is

TABLE 2.1

EFFECT OF PRIOR PROBABILITY (PREVALENCE) ON PREDICTIVE VALUE OF POSITIVE TEST RESULTS

Prior Probability (Prevalence) (%)	Predictive Value of Positive Test Result (%)		
	Sensitivity 90%, Specificity 90%	Sensitivity 95%, Specificity 95%	Sensitivity 99%, Specificity 99%
0.1	0.9	1.9	9.0
1	8.3	16.1	50.0
2	15.5	27.9	66.9
5	32.1	50.0	83.9
50	90.0	95.0	99.0

multiplied by a very large relative number—that is, $(b + d)$ is much greater than $(a + c)$. Therefore, b will be surprisingly large relative to a, and the predictive value positive will be counterintuitively low. Examples of this effect are evident in Table 2.1.

Consider the example of a noninvasive test to detect coronary disease applied to a 50-year-old man with a history of atypical chest pain. Based on test evaluations reported in the literature, the sensitivity and the specificity of the test can be estimated at 80% and 90%, respectively. Based on symptoms and risk factors, the clinician estimates that the patient's pretest probability of coronary disease is 0.20. (This is the same as saying that the prevalence of coronary disease in a population of similar patients would be 20%.)

According to Fig. 2.3, with a pretest probability of 0.20, $a + c = 0.20$ and $b + d = 0.80$. Multiplying 0.20 by 0.8 (the sensitivity) gives a value of 0.16 for a (subtraction gives a value of 0.04 for c). Multiplying 0.80 by 0.9 (the specificity) gives a value of 0.72 for d (again, subtraction gives 0.08 for b). The predictive value positive, then, is 0.16/0.24, or 0.67. The predictive value negative is 0.72/0.76, or 0.95.

Clinicians can use another method to revise probabilities quickly to test their intuition. It requires an understanding of *odds* as well as probability. If p is the probability that a particular disease is present, the ratio of p to $(1 - p)$, or $p/(1 - p)$, is called the *odds favoring that disease*. The *odds against that disease* being present are represented by $(1 - p)/p$. Just as one can estimate the pretest probability of disease before diagnostic tests are performed, one can express that estimate as the pretest odds.

Pretest odds can be revised simply by multiplying a ratio called the *likelihood ratio*, which is the relative occurrence of the test result among persons with and without disease—that is, the probability of the result (either positive or negative or a particular range of values) given the presence of disease divided by the probability of that result given the absence of disease. Note that the positive likelihood ratio is nothing more (or less) than the ratio of sensitivity to the false-positive rate (i.e., 1 – specificity). The negative likelihood ratio is the ratio of the false-negative rate (i.e., 1 – sensitivity) to the specificity. Likelihood ratios therefore include all of the information contained in estimates of sensitivity and specificity. When the pretest odds of a disease are multiplied by the positive likelihood ratio, the result—sometimes termed the *posttest odds*—represents the odds favoring disease, given the test result.

Returning to the example, we see that the previously mentioned patient with atypical chest pain could have his chances of having coronary disease expressed as odds rather than a probability. A probability of 0.20 is equivalent to odds of 1/4

(0.20/0.80). The likelihood ratio for a test with a sensitivity of 0.8 and a specificity of 0.9 is 8 [0.8/(1 – 0.9)]. The pretest odds of disease can be converted to the posttest odds of disease following a positive test result simply by multiplying by the positive likelihood ratio: $1/4 \times 8 = 2$. Note that the posttest odds ratio of 2:1 is equivalent to the posttest probability of 0.67.

For some, it is easier to revise probabilities in the clinical setting using sensitivities and specificities. For others, it is easier to do so by using likelihood ratios. A nomogram can be helpful until one gets used to converting from probabilities to odds and back again (Fig. 2.4). Likelihood ratios also have the advantage of capturing more clinical data from the patient's particular test results. Whereas estimates of sensitivity and specificity usually rely on a dichotomous positive–negative result threshold,

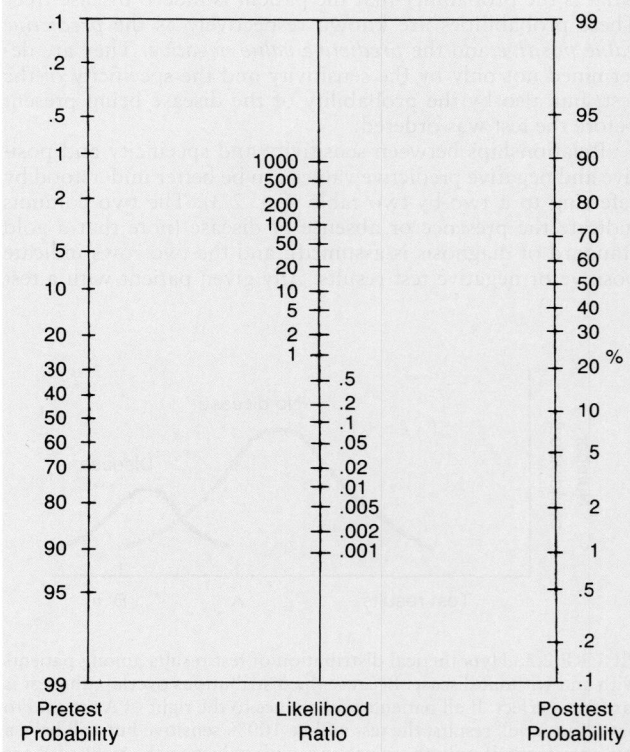

FIGURE 2.4. A nomogram for applying likelihood ratios. (Adapted from Fagan TJ. Nomogram for Bayes' theorem [Letter]. N Engl J Med 1975;293:257, with permission.)

different likelihood ratios can be determined for different ranges of test results. For example, a high serum PSA level will have a higher positive likelihood ratio than a moderate elevation. The degree of elevation will then be reflected in the revised probability of prostate cancer.

WHERE DOES THE INFORMATION COME FROM? (9–20)

One of the reasons clinicians are reluctant to take a quantitative approach to diagnostic test interpretation is that such an approach suggests a precision that belies our uncertainty about pretest probabilities and about the sensitivity and specificity of even commonly used tests. The estimation of pretest probability hinges on epidemiologic information about the incidence and the prevalence of various diseases, modified on the basis of patient characteristics and presenting symptoms. This kind of information is all too rarely presented in the medical literature. Estimates are necessarily uncertain.

There is also uncertainty about the sensitivity and the specificity of tests. Rarely are these values presented in medical texts, and test evaluations in the medical literature can sometimes be misleading. The clinician should be familiar with some of the reasons why a test rarely performs as well in general use as it does during the evaluation study that appears in a medical journal.

False-Positive Rate and Pretest Probability: Overestimating Predictive Values

Clinical heterogeneity and the resulting importance of the pretest probability of disease in an individual patient (or the prevalence of disease in a population of such patients) for determining the predictive values of a test are often not fully appreciated and may lead to disappointment in the clinical performance of the test. Consider how, during its initial evaluation, the sensitivity and the specificity of a test might be estimated. Two groups of patients are assembled. One consists of patients known to have the disease in question as defined by some gold standard or reference test (represented by $a + c$ in Fig. 2.3). The other consists of persons without disease based on the same reference test (represented by $b + d$). The test being evaluated is then applied to both populations. The proportion of those with disease who have a positive result $[a/(a + c)]$ provides an estimate of the test's sensitivity. The proportion of those without the disease who have a negative result $[d/(b + d)]$ gives an estimate of the test's specificity. Our confidence that these estimates of sensitivity and specificity are accurate increases with the number of people in each group tested. The investigator can most efficiently maximize confidence in the estimates of both sensitivity and specificity by applying the test to disease and nondisease groups of equal size. It is not surprising, therefore, that many tests have been evaluated by applying them to populations in which disease and nondisease occur with equal frequency, or nearly so.

If sensitivity, specificity, and predictive values are sufficiently high in such an evaluation study, the test is proposed for general use. What happens when the test is adopted and applied in a general population in which the disease is much less likely to be present than nondisease? The sensitivity and the specificity should remain the same, but the predictive value positive will necessarily fall, and its complement, the false-alarm rate, will

necessarily increase. This phenomenon is most important when the disease in question is rare, as is evident in Table 2.1.

Defining Disease for Diagnostic Test Evaluation: The Gold Standard Problem

To evaluate a diagnostic test, an investigator must be able to distinguish between persons with and without disease by some alternative method. Often, this gold standard reference test is more invasive or more expensive than the newer, proposed test being evaluated. (The newer test would not be worth evaluating if it did not confer some advantage for patient or clinician.) Sometimes, a reference test is not readily available. If the disease is one with a short, predictable, natural history (e.g., pancreatic cancer), an investigator may resort to follow-up, defining the absence of disease by morbidity-free survival during a specified period. If, however, the disease has a highly variable natural history (e.g., coronary disease and most rheumatologic disorders), the follow-up approach becomes impractical. Instead, the investigator must rely on more-arbitrary and often more-subjective criteria to define disease, including combinations of tests, signs, and symptoms. Herein lies a potential pitfall that can affect the accuracy of the estimates of sensitivity and specificity. If the diagnostic criteria are not assessed independently of the test being evaluated, the sensitivity, the specificity, or both will be overestimated.

The problem occurs in its most obvious form when a positive test result leads the investigator to a more extensive search for disease than was applied to those with a negative test result. A related problem occurs when the test and the diagnostic criteria are very similar biologic measures. This will result in overly optimistic estimates of sensitivity and specificity. For example, to the extent that false-negative results of a test that is being evaluated are correlated with false-negative results of a test that contributes to the diagnostic criteria used as a gold standard, the sensitivity of the new test will be overestimated. To the extent that false-positive results are correlated with false-positive results, the specificity of the new test will be overestimated.

The Narrow-Spectrum Problem: Overestimating Sensitivity When the "Disease" Group Is Too Sick

When investigators assemble a group known to have the disease in question by means of some reference test, they may choose patients with unequivocal diagnostic (gold standard) findings. In doing so, they may select a severely ill group that is not representative of the disease in the general population—that is, they will focus on too narrow a spectrum of disease.

Consider a group of investigators evaluating a noninvasive test for coronary artery disease, such as an electrocardiographically monitored exercise tolerance test. To be sure that they are dealing with true coronary disease, the investigators include only people with unequivocal prior myocardial infarction or with classic angina symptoms. By using their chosen criteria for a positive test result, they determine that the sensitivity of the test is 90%. What they (and the readers of their report) may not realize is that the test is more sensitive when coronary disease is extensive (two- or three-vessel disease rather than single-vessel disease) or severe (99% stenosis rather than 80% stenosis) and that their gold standard criteria selected for patients with extensive or severe disease. When the test is used to detect less extensive disease producing more equivocal symptoms in the general population, its sensitivity will prove disappointing. Note that the sensitivity estimate provided by the evaluation is accurate for the narrow spectrum of disease severity found in the test population. The disappointment comes when that estimate is generalized inappropriately to include those with less-severe disease.

The Comorbidity Problem: Overestimating Specificity When the "No-Disease" Group Is Too Well

In the same way that investigators can assemble a "disease" group that is sicker than the population to which the test will eventually be applied, they can assemble a "no-disease" group that is too healthy. Many tests will perform better when used to discriminate between disease A and no disease than when used to discriminate between disease A, on one hand, and diseases B through Z, on the other. Consider an investigator who chooses to estimate the sensitivity and the specificity of guaiac testing as a screening test for colonic cancer. The investigator knows about the spectrum problem and includes in the "disease" group people with early cancers. For the "no-disease" group, medical school students are selected. It should be clear that this choice of controls provides an estimate of specificity that is higher than could be expected when the test is generally applied to a population including older individuals more likely to have a nonmalignant source of occult bleeding. Obviously, the controls should not have the target disease (e.g., colon cancer). However, if all comorbid conditions that the test might confuse with the disease (e.g., peptic ulcer disease, diverticular disease) are also excluded from the control population, the investigator's estimate of specificity will be too optimistic.

Investigators can guard against such disappointments by drawing their "disease" and "no-disease" populations from the target population in which the test will eventually be used. The spectrum of disease that should be detected in the target population should be represented in the "disease" group. Comorbid conditions that might be confused with that disease should be included in the "no-disease" control group. Such an effectiveness evaluation of a diagnostic test might be preceded by a simpler study comparing very sick with completely well persons. If the test cannot discriminate between the very sick and the very well in such an efficacy study, the more difficult effectiveness trial need not be undertaken. The clinician can guard against being misled by reports of a test's efficacy by carefully considering the populations in which a test has been evaluated and not generalizing the results inappropriately to larger, more heterogeneous groups.

How Does the Test Compare with Others?

A final reason for disappointment with the application of apparently promising tests is failure to consider adequately a test's potential role in the constellation of tests that is already available. Does the new test provide new information? Does it obviate the need for more-invasive or more-expensive tests?

To answer these questions, the clinician should have a good sense of how to compare two different tests. Comparative estimates of sensitivity and specificity must account for the implicit or explicit choice of criteria or cutoff level for distinguishing "normal" from "abnormal." Estimating the range of sensitiv-

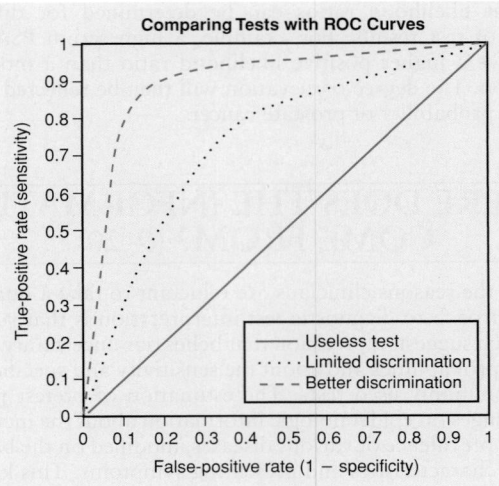

FIGURE 2.5. Receiver-operating-characteristic (ROC) curves are plots of sensitivity (true-positive rate) against 1– specificity (false-positive rate) for a diagnostic test. The ROC "curve" for a perfect test would extend from the origin to the upper left corner and then to the right. The "curve" for a useless test would be the diagonal extending from the origin. Curves close to the diagonal have limited discriminating ability; those extending to the upper left quadrant have better discriminating ability.

ities and specificities achievable with more- or less-stringent criteria or cutoffs is one approach to this problem. This range of possible sensitivity–specificity pairs can be plotted to produce a receiver-operating-characteristic (ROC) curve that allows formal comparison of the discriminating ability of multiple tests as well as informal observations regarding the relative performance of tests in the most clinically relevant ranges of sensitivity–specificity. This can be seen in Fig. 2.5.

Estimates of sensitivity and specificity may be more or less precise, and precision is often not addressed in published evaluations of diagnostic tests. Confidence in precision of a test may vary across the range of sensitivity–specificity pairs. Precision improves when the results of multiple studies evaluating the same tests can be pooled, but this pooling can be misleading if heterogeneity among study populations and methods is not adequately considered, and it always entails some statistical challenges.

WHICH TESTS SHOULD WE USE? (1,3–24)

Perfect tests are rare. Clinicians must choose among tests with imperfect sensitivity and specificity. The physician frequently has some choice about the sensitivity and specificity of a test. Obviously, alternative tests—usually those that are more costly or invasive—may be more sensitive and more specific. A new technology or an improved skill in interpretation may improve both measures, extending the ROC curve upward and to the left. Often, however, as depicted in Figs. 2.2 and 2.5, the physician can increase specificity only by accepting a decrease in sensitivity, essentially choosing a point on the ROC curve. There is ample evidence to suggest that clinicians do not make these choices systematically and with due consideration for the impact on patient outcomes. There is also evidence that system support and behavioral interventions can have a positive impact on diagnostic decision quality.

The stakes are high for clinicians and patients when the decisions about test use are poorly considered. How high should the troponin level be before a patient is told he or she has had a heart attack? What level of PSA warrants a biopsy of a man's prostate? Such questions cannot be answered responsibly without considering fully the benefits of true-positive and true-negative results, as well as the harms of false-positive and false-negative results. These judgments depend on the interplay between disease prognosis and effectiveness of therapy. It has been demonstrated that providing information about test results and their implications *before* the test is performed increases the reassurance value of subsequent test findings and can reduce symptoms. Nowhere are these issues more evident than in decisions about screening and health maintenance. Their critical consideration is addressed in the following chapters.

A.G.M.

Annotated Bibliography

1. Black ER, Barry MJ. Diagnostic strategies for common medical problems. Philadelphia: American College of Physicians, 1999. (*A superb resource. Includes information about prior probabilities and sensitivity and specificity of tests, and recommends well-reasoned strategies.*)
2. Elstein AS, Schwarz A. Evidence base of clinical diagnosis: clinical problem solving and diagnostic decision making: selective review of the cognitive literature. BMJ 2002;324:729. (*Reviews cognitive processes involved in diagnostic decision making.*)
3. Griner PF, Mayewski RJ, Mushlin AI, et al. Selection and interpretation of diagnostic tests and procedures: principles and applications. Ann Intern Med 1981;94[4 Pt 2]:557. (*A very well presented primer with many good examples.*)
4. Pauker SG, Kassirer JP. The threshold approach to clinical decision making. N Engl J Med 1980;302:1109. (*Elegant and thoughtful explication of a rational approach to diagnosis; a seminal paper.*)
5. Reid MC, Lane DA, Feinstein AR. Academic calculations versus clinical judgments: practicing physicians' use of quantitative measures of test accuracy. Am J Med 1998;104:374. (*Clinicians in this telephone survey avoided any quantitative approaches to the interpretation of diagnostic tests.*)
6. Puhan MA, Steurer J, Bachmann LM, et al. A randomized trial of ways to describe test accuracy: the effect on physicians' post-test probability estimates. Ann Intern Med 2005;143:184. (*Presentation of likelihood ratios did not affect posttest probability estimates as much as presentation of corresponding sensitivities and specificities.*)
7. Sox HC Jr. Common diagnostic tests: use and interpretation, 2nd ed. Philadelphia: American College of Physicians, 1990. (*An excellent volume with introductory chapters on diagnostic reasoning and probability theory followed by 16 chapters on specific tests.*)
8. Jaeschke R, Guyatt G, Sackett DL. Users' guide to the medical literature. III. How to use an article about a diagnostic test. A. Are the results of the study valid? B. What are the results and will they help me in caring for my patients? JAMA 1994;271:389. (*Part of an extensive series designed to provide practical applications of clinical epidemiology for the practitioner.*)
9. Vecchio TJ. Predictive value of a single diagnostic test in unselected populations. N Engl J Med 1966;274:1171. (*Early article pointing out the importance of prevalence to predictive value.*)
10. Knottnerus JA, van Weel C, Muris JW. Evaluation of diagnostic procedures. BMJ 2002;324:477. (*Provides a succinct review of vocabulary and methodologic issues as the first in a series of five articles.*)
11. Bossuyt PM, Reitsma JB, Bruns DE, et al. Towards complete and accurate reporting of studies of diagnostic accuracy: the STARD initiative. BMJ 2003;326:41. (*Presents consensus standards for the reporting of studies designed to evaluate diagnostic tests.*)
12. Deeks J. Systematic reviews of evaluations of diagnostic and screening tests. BMJ 2001;323:157. (*Reviews methodology for pooling the results of evaluations and related problems in applying results to practices.*)
13. Lijmer JG, Mol BW, Heisterkamp S, et al. Empirical evidence of design-related bias in studies of diagnostic tests. JAMA 1999; 282:1061. (*Demonstrates the extent of bias.*)
14. Mulherin SA, Miller WC. Spectrum bias or spectrum effect? Subgroup variation in diagnostic test evaluation. Ann Intern Med 2002;137:598. (*Stresses the importance of clinical heterogeneity in the design and interpretation of diagnostic test evaluations.*)
15. Ransohoff DF, Feinstein AR. Problems of spectrum and bias in evaluating the efficacy of diagnostic tests. N Engl J Med 1978;299:926. (*Classic review of problems in disease definition and population selection that may affect evaluations of diagnostic tests.*)
16. Sackett DL, Haynes RB. Evidence base of clinical diagnosis: the architecture of diagnostic research. BMJ 2002;324:539. (*Offers phase I through phase IV terminology to distinguish among evaluation studies.*)
17. Whiting P, Rutjes AWS, Reitsma JB, et al. Sources of variation and bias in studies of diagnostic accuracy. Ann Intern Med 2004;140:189. (*Systematic review detailing the sources of bias and estimating the impact of each source on sensitivity, specificity, and overall accuracy.*)
18. Tatsioni A, Zarin DA, Aronson N, et al. Challenges in systematic reviews of diagnostic technologies. Ann Intern Med 2005;142:1048. (*Reviews challenges related to finding relevant studies, assessing methodologic quality, and dealing with studies in different populations or using different outcome measures.*)
19. Lord SJ, Irwig L, Simes J. When is measuring sensitivity and specificity sufficient to evaluate a diagnostic test, and when do we need randomized trials? Ann Intern Med 2006;144:850-855. (*Points out that the answer to this question depends primarily on whether a more sensitive test detects cases that have the same spectrum of disease and/or the same responsiveness to therapy.*)
20. Harper R, Reeves B. Reporting of precision of estimates for diagnostic accuracy: a review. BMJ 1999;318:1322. (*Observes that confidence intervals are presented for sensitivity and specificity all too infrequently.*)
21. Solomon DH, Hashimoto H, Daltroy L, et al. Techniques to improve physicians' use of diagnostic tests: a new conceptual framework. JAMA 1998;280:2020. (*Papers generally claim success for behavioral interventions.*)
22. Verstappen WHJM, van der Weijden T. Effect of a practice-based strategy on test ordering performance of primary care physicians. JAMA 2003;289:2407. (*Guidelines, feedback, and social interaction had a modest effect.*)
23. Centor RM. Signal detectability: the use of ROC curves and their analyses. Med Decision Making 1999;11:102. (*Excellent review for the clinician, which also includes statistical considerations.*)
24. Petrie KJ, Muller JT, Schirmbeck F, et al. Effect of providing information about normal test results on patients' reassurance: randomized controlled trial. BMJ 2007;334:352. (*Education of patients about the implications of test results before the test is performed improves rates of reassurance and symptom relief.*)

CHAPTER 3 ■ HEALTH MAINTENANCE AND THE ROLE OF SCREENING

Public interest in health maintenance or, more positively, health enhancement has grown dramatically in recent years. Many Americans have demonstrated their interest in exercise, good dietary habits, maintenance of appropriate body weight, and stress reduction. Increased enthusiasm stems from the growing awareness of associations between elements of lifestyle and health. Despite reliable evidence and public acceptance of these associations, however, many people continue to indulge in self-destructive habits such as smoking, overeating, and alcohol abuse. For instance, in recent years we have seen a dramatic increase in the prevalence of obesity and the incidence of type 2 diabetes. Efforts to alter such behavior are often frustratingly ineffective. Patients who seek reassurance from physician visits that include routine screening procedures often persist in behavior that greatly increases their risk of morbidity.

Physicians must acknowledge their primary role in prevention as that of educators. Accurate information regarding risk factors is most likely to reinforce health-enhancing behavior and alter self-destructive behavior. Physicians must appreciate the potential for behavior modification and familiarize themselves with local resources that can help patients to identify and overcome barriers to healthy behavior. Routine screening for specific diseases—the health maintenance activity most closely identified with the physician—should be performed selectively. The limits of screening tests, as well as their potential health benefits, should be clearly understood by every primary care physician.

Specific risk factors and screening tests are discussed in subsequent chapters. This chapter focuses on the following question: What makes a disease or risk factor worth screening for? The relationship between prevalence and the predictive value of a test is particularly important in the screening situation (see Chapter 2). Because the physician should be more interested in improving health outcomes for patients than in simply providing them with diagnoses, elements of the natural history of the disease and of the effectiveness of therapy are critically important.

CRITERIA FOR SCREENING (1–6)

Whether a screening policy results in improved health outcomes depends on the characteristics of the disease(s), the test(s), and the patient population. These are summarized in Table 3.1.

NATURAL HISTORY OF THE DISEASE AND EFFECTIVENESS OF THERAPY (3)

Screening tests are performed to identify asymptomatic disease. The alternative is to wait until the patient presents with symptoms and then make a diagnosis. The question then is: What makes a disease worth diagnosing early? The practical objective of screening is prevention of morbidity and mortality, not simply early diagnosis. There is little benefit to the patient, and perhaps considerable harm, in advancing the time of diagnosis of a disease for which earlier treatment does not influence outcome.

The importance of the natural history of the disease and the effectiveness of therapy can be illustrated by considering Fig. 3.1. As it shows schematically, some variable time after the biologic onset of a disease, a diagnosis is possible with the use of a screening test. This is followed by another variable time period during which the patient has no symptoms. Usually, a short time after symptoms appear, the clinical diagnosis is made. Eventually, after the course of therapy has been selected and completed, there is an identifiable clinical outcome that can range from cure and complete health to death.

Often, outcome depends somewhat on the point during the natural history of the disease at which therapy is initiated. This is clearest in the case of localized versus metastatic cancer. Many tumors can be readily excised, and the patient cured of the disease, during early stages. The opportunity for cure is often lost when tumor spread makes excision or other local therapy impractical. The "escape from cure" may not be as dramatic as the point of tumor metastasis; a disease may simply become more refractory to therapy, which increases the likelihood of morbid complications. The practical purpose of screening is to advance the time of the diagnosis to a point in the natural history of the disease when a relative or absolute "escape from cure" is less likely to have occurred.

Although the natural history of any disease varies a great deal among persons afflicted, some generalizations are worthwhile. If an "escape from cure" generally occurs at point A in Fig. 3.1 or at any point before available screening tests can detect the disease in question, the value of screening must be questioned. The most common result will be bad news sooner for the patient but no difference in outcome. If "escape from cure" routinely occurs after symptoms appear (e.g., at point C), screening may be valuable but can likely be supplanted by patient and professional education programs aimed at ensuring early presentation and prompt diagnosis. Diseases in which "escape from cure" generally occurs after the disease is detectable but while it remains asymptomatic (e.g., at point B) are the most appropriate targets of screening efforts.

Several points about the evaluation of screening programs can also be made with reference to Fig. 3.1. Critics of indiscriminate screening point out that the benefits of a screening program can easily be overestimated if the relationship between time of diagnosis and natural history is not understood. One fallacy results from neglecting the importance of *lead time* when evaluating the effect of screening on subsequent survival.

TABLE 3.1

CRITERIA FOR SCREENING

Characteristics of the Disease
  Significant effect on quality or length of life
  Prevalence sufficiently high to justify costs
  Acceptable methods of treatment available
  Asymptomatic period during which detection and
    treatment significantly reduce morbidity and mortality
  Treatment in the asymptomatic phase yields a better
    therapeutic result than treatment delayed until
    symptoms appear
Characteristics of the Test
  Sufficiently sensitive to detect disease during the
    asymptomatic period
  Sufficiently specific to provide acceptable predictive value
    positive
  Acceptable to patients
Characteristics of the Population Screened
  Sufficiently high disease prevalence
  Accessibility
  Compliance with subsequent diagnostic tests and necessary
    therapy

Because screening has the potential to advance the time of diagnosis from one point in the natural history to another and because survival is, by necessity, measured from the time of diagnosis rather than from the time of onset, the survival of patients whose diseases are detected by screening should be expected to be longer than that of patients who present symptomatically. Extensive follow-up data on many patients allow approximation of the average length of time by which the diagnosis is advanced by screening. This illusory gain in survival—the lead time—can then be subtracted from any measured difference in survival duration to learn the true benefits of the screening program.

The second fallacy that can lead to overestimation of screening benefits depends on the variability in natural history among individual cases of the same disease. Patients who have less-aggressive disease and so spend more time in a detectable but asymptomatic stage are, other things being equal, more likely to have their disease detected by a screening test than are patients with more aggressive disease. If patients with indolent, asymptomatic disease are more likely to have an indolent

clinical course after diagnosis, patients with disease diagnosed by screening should be expected to have longer survival rates than patients who present symptomatically. Arguments about the effect of such biologic determinism versus that of advancing the time of diagnosis have most frequently been raised with regard to breast and prostate cancers, but they apply generally to all screening. This potential bias toward prolonged survival among patients with disease detected by screening tests has been called *time-linked bias sampling*. An extreme form of this phenomenon is *overdiagnosis*. Overdiagnosis occurs when disease that would not have been diagnosed during the patient's lifetime is diagnosed because a screening test was performed. This is the case for most prostate cancers detected by screening and for approximately half of all cases of ductal carcinoma *in situ* of the breast.

None of these arguments is meant to deny the value of screening for treatable disease. They simply advise caution in interpreting apparently favorable results based on unsophisticated measures of effectiveness.

VALIDITY OF AVAILABLE SCREENING TESTS AND POPULATIONS SCREENED (1–6)

Diseases worth identifying usually have a relatively low prevalence in the asymptomatic population. As a result, the specificity of the diagnostic test used is the principal determinant of the predictive value positive of the test. Tests that may be very useful in diagnosis when the prior probability of disease is 10% or 20% may produce an unacceptable number of false-positive results when used in a screening situation. Such nonspecificity has been referred to as the *cost of a screening test*. The costs, including morbidity and patient concern, of diagnostic evaluations among patients with false-positive screening results can far outweigh other costs of a screening program. The sensitivity and the specificity of the screening test, costs, and patient acceptability are critical considerations in the decision to screen for disease.

The importance of disease prevalence in determining the predictive value positive is one basis for the use of risk factors in screening policy. By limiting screening to a high-risk population, the physician in effect increases the prevalence of the disease in the population tested (and increases the prior probability of the disease in any individual patient), thereby

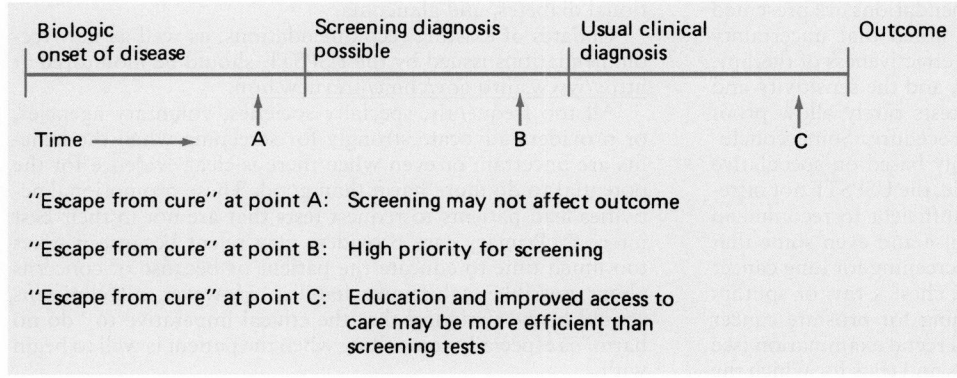

FIGURE 3.1. Relationships between screening and natural history of disease.

increasing the predictive value positive and decreasing the false-alarm rate and the number of false-positive results.

HEALTH MAINTENANCE: WHAT IS APPROPRIATE? (1–10)

Periodic health evaluation has been recommended with varying degrees of enthusiasm throughout the twentieth century and into the twenty-first. Many patients believe in its value; the majority of Americans feel that more health resources should be expended on preventive efforts. Increasingly, employers, many of whom were long enamored of the "executive physical," are advocating checkups as part of wellness programs, and "welcome to Medicare" visits have been instituted for beneficiaries who have just reached eligibility. However, the value of periodic examinations and specific preventive measures has also long been questioned. Evidence regarding the effectiveness of periodic examinations, measured in terms of decreased morbidity and mortality, is fragmentary. A systematic review of the effects of the periodic health evaluation published in 2007 found that the evidence supported only the conclusions that such scheduled visits improved the delivery of some recommended preventive services and may lessen patient worry. But these findings beg questions about which preventive services are recommended for whom and why, and about the source of the worry that may be lessened by the routine trip to the doctor.

Clearly, routine examinations should be tailored to the individual patient. Although the importance of the characteristics of the patient, the diseases, and the test in determining appropriate prevention strategies must be recognized, summary recommendations can be useful. A number of reviews, each applying the criteria discussed in this chapter, have offered recommendations for preventive health care. The recommendations have come from the American Cancer Society, the American College of Physicians, the Canadian Task Force on the Periodic Health Examination, and the U.S. Preventive Services Task Force (USPSTF), with the latter receiving the most attention of late due to its ongoing commitment to refining processes and methods and making the rationale for those refinements, as well as for specific recommendations, known to clinicians.

Relatively few conditions have received general endorsement as targets for screening among *asymptomatic* persons *without* specific *risk factors*. These are summarized in Table 3.2. The rationales for these recommendations are presented in the subsequent chapters noted in the table. Table 3.3 provides a summary of recommendations that have been made for other preventive services that are warranted in selected patients. Again, the rationales for these recommendations are presented in subsequent chapters. It should be noted that uncertainty about both the natural history and the effectiveness of therapy, the importance of specific risk factors, and the sensitivity and the specificity of potential screening tests rarely allow proof of the effectiveness of a screening procedure. Some conclusions and recommendations, necessarily based on speculative data, remain controversial. For example, the USPSTF not infrequently concludes that evidence is insufficient to recommend for or against many tests that are in use and even some that have been endorsed by other groups. Screening for lung cancer with low-dose computed tomography, chest x-ray, or sputum cytology (see Chapter 37) and screening for prostate cancer with prostate-specific antigen or digital rectal examination (see Chapter 126) are among the conditions and tests for which the

TABLE 3.2

CONDITIONS THAT WARRANT PERIODIC EVALUATION IN ALL PATIENTS OF APPROPRIATE AGE AND GENDER

Disease	Comment
Hypertension	See Chapters 14, 19, and 26
Hyperlipidemia	See Chapters 5 and 27
Smoking	See Chapter 54
Colon cancer	See Chapter 56
Breast cancer	See Chapter 106
Cervical cancer	See Chapter 107
Osteoporosis	See Chapter 144
Depression	See Chapter 227
Alcoholism	See Chapter 228
Obesity	See Chapter 233

USPSTF has found evidence to be insufficient. In some cases, a recommendation for a narrow segment of the population will inappropriately be used more broadly. An example of a recently issued recommendation with this potential is the recommendation for a one-time ultrasound screen for abdominal aortic aneurysm among men age 65 to 75 years who have ever smoked cigarettes. The USPSTF makes no recommendation for men who have never smoked and recommends against screening for women.

Some clinicians perform, and some groups advocate for, screening when available evidence suggests that the harms may outweigh the benefits. For example, the USPSTF recommends against routine screening with resting electrocardiography, exercise treadmill test, or electron-beam computed tomography scanning for coronary calcium for either the presence of severe coronary artery stenosis or the prediction of coronary heart disease events in adults at low risk for such events, and finds evidence insufficient to recommend screening in adults with higher risk. Among the conditions for which the USPSTF recommends against routine screening in all populations because there is sufficient evidence to conclude that harms are likely to outweigh benefits are the following: bladder cancer, pancreatic cancer, testicular cancer, peripheral artery disease, and genital herpes. As already noted, the USPSTF concluded that evidence is insufficient to recommend for or against routine screening for either lung cancer or prostate cancer. The list of adult conditions for which this is the case also includes oral cancer, skin cancer, hepatitis C, intimate partner violence, dementia, suicide risk, thyroid disease, bacterial vaginosis in pregnancy, gestational diabetes, and glaucoma.

Updates of existing recommendations, as well as new recommendations issued by the USPSTF, should be monitored at http://www.ahrq.gov/clinic/prevnew.htm.

All too frequently, specialty societies, voluntary agencies, or providers advocate strongly for screening when the benefits are uncertain or even when there is clear evidence for the potential to do more harm than good. These promotional activities lead patients to request tests that are not in their best interests. Primary care providers may relent because it takes too much time to educate the patient or because of concerns about possible malpractice liability. However, all clinicians should be ever mindful that the ethical imperative to "do no harm" is especially compelling when the patient is well to begin with.

TABLE 3.3

CONDITIONS THAT WARRANT PERIODIC EVALUATION IN SELECTED PATIENTS

Condition	Risk Factor	Comment
Rubella susceptibility	Anticipated pregnancy; occupation (health care worker)	See Chapter 6
Human immunodeficiency virus infection	Pregnancy; men who have had sex with men after 1975; men and women who have had unprotected sex with multiple partners; injection drug use; blood transfusions 1978–1985	See Chapter 7
Endocarditis susceptibility	Prosthetic cardiac valve; previous endocarditis; certain congenital heart defects; certain heart transplant recipients	See Chapter 16
Rheumatic fever susceptibility	Rheumatic fever history	See Chapter 17
Tuberculosis (PPD reactivity)	Occupational exposure; travel exposure	See Chapters 38 and 49
Occupational lung disease	Occupational exposure	See Chapter 39
Hepatitis B infection	Pregnancy	See Chapter 57
Anemia	Pregnancy	See Chapter 77
Sickle cell trait	African American of childbearing age	Genetic counseling must be acceptable; see Chapter 78
Thyroid cancer	Radiation of head and neck	See Chapter 94
Diabetes (type 2)	Hypertension; hyperlipidemia	See Chapter 93
Endometrial cancer	Exogenous estrogens	See Chapter 109
Syphilis	Pregnancy; MSM; men and women who engage in high-risk sexual activity; commercial sex workers; persons who exchange sex for drugs; persons in adult correctional facilities	See Chapter 124
Chlamydial genitourinary infection	Sexually active women age ≤25 yr at increased risk, marked by being unmarried, African American, having new or multiple sex partners, prior history of STD, having cervical ectopy, or using barrier contraceptives inconsistently Pregnant women age ≤25 yr	See Chapter 125
Bacteriuria	Pregnancy	See Chapter 127

MSM, men who have sex with men; PPD, purified protein derivative; STD, sexually transmitted disease.

PATIENT EDUCATION AND OTHER APPROACHES TO IMPROVE SCREENING AND HEALTH MAINTENANCE (11–15)

It has been shown that patients have highly exaggerated expectations for the benefits of screening and exhibit important variations in their attitudes and preferences. It is the clinician's responsibility to educate the patient about the limitations of screening such that expectations are reasonable and to respect their informed preferences. This can be difficult because of the complexity of the issues and the extent to which "early detection" has been promoted uncritically in some circles. Decision aids have been shown to be highly effective in informing patients about their screening options, sometimes with dramatic effects on rates at which people choose to be screened when the evidence is contradictory and benefits and harms uncertain. There is also evidence that customization of risk communication can increase the use of warranted screening for cancers and cardiovascular risk factors. The manner in which information is conveyed, and especially the way in which risks and benefits are framed by the clinician, can have a profound effect on patients' decisions. Clinicians should be aware of the subtle biases that can unintentionally persuade or dissuade patients from taking a particular course of action (see Chapter 4).

The clinician must also be mindful of the potential to help patients to avoid preventable morbidity and early death by taking the time to provide advice and counsel about behavior and lifestyle. Patients often need specific advice, not only about the use of alcohol, tobacco, and harmful substances, but also about diet, exercise, sexual practices, and injury prevention. Such discussions should be carefully crafted and personalized to each patient's level of motivation to change behavior and confidence in his or her ability to do so. These conversations have the potential to produce a far greater effect on health and longevity than do specific screening tests and procedures.

The efforts of the individual primary physician, although important, are insufficient to ensure that patients take maximal advantage of available effective preventive services such as immunization and screening that is known to be effective. Meta-analysis of controlled trials examining strategies for optimizing the use of preventive services identified systematic organizational measures as central to the effort. The most effective of these measures include establishment of separate clinics devoted to prevention, a planned prevention care visit, and assignment of nonphysicians to perform specific prevention activities. Next-best approaches involve removal of financial barriers and offering of patient reminders. Less benefit was observed from education of patients and health care professionals and from feedback to providers. The take-home message: It takes a "systems" approach.

A.G.M.

Annotated Bibliography

1. Canadian Task Force on the Periodic Health Examination. Canadian guide to clinical preventive healthcare. Ottawa: Canada Communications Group, 1994. (*A compendium of evidence-based recommendations.*)
2. Canadian Task Force on the Periodic Health Examination. Canadian guide to clinical preventive healthcare. Available at: http://www.ctfphc.org/. (*Web site with more than 125 recommendations posted since 1994, including 24 topics published since 2000.*)
3. Feinleb M, Zelen M. Some pitfalls in the evaluation of screening programs. Arch Environ Health 1969;19:412. (*Classic review of problems with predictive value positive, lead time, and time-linked bias sampling.*)
4. Frame PS, Carlson SJ. A critical review of periodic health screening using specific screening criteria, Part 1: selected diseases of respiratory, cardiovascular, and central nervous systems; Part 2: selected endocrine, metabolic, and gastrointestinal diseases; Part 3: selected diseases of the genitourinary system; Part 4: selected miscellaneous diseases. J Fam Pract 1975;2:29, 123, 189, 283. (*Cited for its historical significance; truly groundbreaking critical examination, ahead of its time.*)
5. U.S. Preventive Services Task Force. Guide to clinical preventive services (AHRQ Publication No. 06-0588, June 2006). Rockville, MD: Agency for Healthcare Research and Quality, 2006. http://www.ahrq.gov/clinic/pocketgd.htm. (*Superb summary of evidence for selected conditions in pocket guide format, also available as a download for a PDA.*)
6. U.S. Preventive Services Task Force. Guide to clinical preventive services: new releases. Rockville, MD: Agency for Healthcare Research and Quality. Available at: http://www.ahrq.gov/clinic/prevnew.htm (*Recommendations for new topics are posted on this website.*)
7. Guirguis-Blake J, Calonge N, Miller T, et al. Current processes of the U.S. Preventive Services Task Force: refining evidence-based recommendation development. Ann Intern Med 2007;147:117. (*Summarizes recent changes in the recommendation development process, including mechanism for prioritizing topics for review.*)
8. Barton M, Miller T, Wolff T, et al. How to read the new recommendation statement: methods update from the U.S. Preventive Services Task Force. Ann Intern Med 2007;147:123. (*Describes changes in format, including standardization of format.*)
9. Han PKJ. Historical changes in the objectives of the periodic health examination. Ann Intern Med 1998;127:910. (*Traces the history of the periodic health examination, detailing reasons for enthusiasm and bases for skepticism about its effect on outcomes.*)
10. Boulware LE, Marinopoulos S, Phillips KA, et al. Systematic review: the value of the periodic health evaluation. Ann Intern Med 2007;146:289. (*The periodic examination improves delivery of some recommended procedures and may decrease patient worry.*)
11. Schwarz LM, Woloshin S, Fowler FJ Jr, et al. Enthusiasm for cancer screening in the United States. JAMA 2004;291:71. (*Documents the exaggerated expectations among U.S. adults about the benefits of cancer screening; also indicates important variations in attitudes and preferences.*)
12. Edwards A, Unigwe S, Elwyn G, et al. Personalised risk communication for informed decision making about entering screening programs (Cochrane review). In: The Cochrane library, Issue 3. Oxford: Update Software, 2004. (*Personalized risk communication seems to increase the use of screening, but it is not clear that decisions are more informed.*)
13. O'Connor AM, Stacey D, Entwistle V, et al. Decision aids for people facing health treatment or screening decisions (Cochrane review). In: The Cochrane library, Issue 3. Oxford: Update Software, 2004. (*Decision aids can help patients to make better-informed choices that are more consistent with their values.*)
14. Sox HC. Straight talk about disease prevention. Ann Intern Med 2007;146:891. (*Insight about the importance of framing effects when discussing risk and risk reduction with patients.*)
15. Stone EG, Morton SC, Hulscher ME, et al. Interventions that increase use of adult immunization and cancer screening services: a meta-analysis. Ann Intern Med 2002;136:641. (*A meta-analysis showing that organizational changes and a systems-based approach to care are the best measures.*)

CHAPTER 4 ■ ESTIMATING AND COMMUNICATING RISK AND PROGNOSIS

Diagnosis is a process of classification. A constellation of symptoms, signs, and test results is given a label, and the patient who presents with those characteristics is implicitly grouped with other patients who have presented with similar findings. What makes the classification process and the resulting label so significant for both patient and clinician is what it implies about the future. Will symptoms persist, get worse, or resolve spontaneously? What other health outcomes can be expected? Will therapeutic interventions improve chances for a good outcome?

Similar questions arise when a patient is found to have a risk factor that increases the likelihood of future disease. How great is the risk? What are the chances of avoiding the anticipated bad outcome, either because of efforts to lower risk or by good fortune? To answer such questions, the primary care physician must understand the methods by which valid information about prognosis and risk is derived from the experience of previous patients. Doctor–patient dialogues about the implications of an illness or risk factor are often momentous for patients. Information about an uncertain future must be communicated with clarity, compassion, and an appreciation for the uniqueness of each patient's needs.

RISK AND PROGNOSIS: PREDICTING THE PATIENT'S FUTURE (1–6)

The source for information about the future of any particular patient is the collective experience with previous patients with the same condition. The accuracy of the information so derived depends on the manner in which that experience is collected and recorded and on the degree of similarity between the patient at hand and past patients who have been followed over time.

Theoretically, the best mechanism for studying prognosis would be to characterize patients carefully at the time of diagnosis (or when a risk factor is identified) with regard to disease stage and severity, presence or absence of any comorbid conditions, and other factors that could be expected to have an impact on outcome. Because such factors are often systematically influenced by the pattern of patient referral, the setting in which patients are seen and the manner in which they happened to be there would be described. All patients would be examined with the same level of scrutiny at the time they entered the cohort and during subsequent follow-up examinations. Relevant outcomes, and criteria by which they would be measured, would be specified in advance. Those conducting follow-up examinations would be unaware of baseline differences among patients so as not to be influenced by expected associations between these variables and outcomes. All patients would be followed, and their status with regard to outcomes would be known at the time the experience was analyzed. The impact of different baseline characteristics on relevant outcomes would be examined by reporting experience for different subgroups or developing statistical models. The predictive validity of these models would be tested in separate samples of patients.

Rarely, if ever, is it possible to meet all of these methodologic objectives. As a result, much of the research that clinicians rely on for information about risk and prognosis is potentially misleading. To avoid being misled and misleading patients, clinicians must understand the biases that can be introduced when suboptimal methods are used to gather information to help predict the future.

When the outcomes of interest are rare events, it may not be feasible to assemble a cohort large enough, and follow it long enough, to accumulate sufficient experience to provide useful estimates of prognosis or risk. Alternatively, patients who have already experienced the outcome can be identified as cases and their past histories can be examined to identify events or *exposures* that may have conferred risk and may be of prognostic value. *Control* patients without the outcome of interest can also be questioned about the same exposures. Comparison of the rates of exposure among cases and controls can produce an estimate of the degree of risk associated with the exposure. The *odds ratio* is an estimate of the *relative risk* that is very accurate when the disease or outcome in question is rare. This retrospective case–control approach places a heavy burden on the investigator and sources of information to ensure that similar degrees of scrutiny are applied to the histories of cases and controls. Selective recollection of the past, often with greater vigilance stimulated by the outcome of interest, can produce misleading estimates of risk and prognosis.

Even if patients with a particular risk factor or diagnosis are identified prospectively and followed forward in time, biases that can lead to faulty conclusions may be introduced. Perhaps the most important bias for primary care physicians to recognize has been termed *referral filter bias*. It occurs frequently as a result of the fact that patients in many published reports have been described because they have been referred to academic centers. Such patients often have complicating characteristics and exhibit a worse prognosis than do patients who are drawn from an entire population or a representative sample of a population. Similar problems arise when patients are selected for study based on particular test results. Patients with more-worrisome signs and symptoms may be more likely to be tested and more likely to fare poorly over time. Alternatively, patients who are tested may have better access to medical care and fare better than average as a result.

Differences in the ways patients are followed over time can also introduce important biases. Patients lost to follow-up may be different from those who remain in the cohort. A conservative approach to estimating prognosis when some patients are lost to follow-up before the relevant outcome has occurred is to assume that *all* lost patients experienced the outcome and then, in contrast, to assume that *no* lost patients experienced it. The first assumption produces an *upper-bound estimate,* with lost patients included in both numerator and denominator; the second produces a *lower-bound estimate,* with lost patients included only in the denominator.

Even when patients are successfully followed over time, biases can be introduced by the selective use of tests and other outcome measures or by the expectations of clinicians who are aware of patient characteristics that may or may not have real prognostic significance. Statistical models that have not been validated on independent samples may mistake random variations among characteristics and outcomes for important prognostic associations.

DESCRIBING THE RISK OF FUTURE DISEASE (7–20)

People are generally very interested in the risk of untoward events and ways to reduce risks. Despite the high level of interest, there is a great deal of confusion about the meaning of quantitative expressions of risk. This confusion often carries over to conversations between doctors and patients. An important source of confusion is the distinction between *relative* and *absolute* risk. The effect of risk factors is usually expressed as a relative risk or risk ratio—that is, the incidence of disease among people with the risk factor divided by the incidence among people without the factor (often estimated as the odds ratio from a case–control study). However, for the individual patient with the risk factor, the incidence of disease—the absolute risk of the outcome—may be more useful. For example, a patient may have a 20- or 30-fold increased risk for a rare disease but still face less than a 1% absolute risk for development of that disease in his or her lifetime. Another way of conveying the implications of a risk factor is to cite the attributable risk, which is the difference between the incidence among exposed people and the incidence among those who are not exposed.

Such distinctions are also important in weighing the harms and benefits of interventions designed to reduce risk. Treating hypertension may well reduce the risk of stroke by 40% (the relative risk reduction). However, doctor and patient should also understand that the baseline risk of stroke during the next 10 years might be as low as 1% for some patients with mild hypertension. This means that the benefit of risk reduction, or the risk difference attributable to the untreated mild hypertension, is the difference between 1.0% and 0.6%, or 0.4%. Another approach to summarizing this kind of data is to cite the number of patients one would need to treat to have the desired effect in a single patient. Returning to the hypertension example, treating 1,000 patients would reduce the number of strokes from 10 to 6, and so 250 people with mild hypertension would have to be treated to avoid 1 stroke.

There are other considerations that need attention. It has been shown that patients respond differently when the same information is presented in either a positive or a negative way. For example, people are more inclined to favor an action that is described as having a 99% survival rate than if it is described as having a 1% mortality rate. These differences in response are called framing effects. Framing effects cannot be avoided. Presenting information both positively and negatively, either verbally or using a simple graphic, can balance framing effects and thereby support unbiased decision making. Patients often find it difficult to interpret quantitative information when the events being considered produce highly emotional reactions and seem all too imminent. Under these circumstances, empathy and reassurance that all that can be done will be done are important communication tools.

DESCRIBING OUTCOMES OVER TIME DURING AN UNCERTAIN FUTURE (4,8–11,13–20)

The diagnosis of a particular condition is generally much more predictive of future outcomes than the identification of risk factors. Outcomes are more frequent and are often described as simple rates. The proportion of people with a particular condition who eventually die of that disease is the *case fatality rate.* Describing the proportion of people alive at a particular point in time after diagnosis (e.g., the 5-year survival rate) can give some indication of prognosis. Alternatively, investigators and clinicians might refer to the duration of survival that occurs on average (e.g., mean survival) or the duration in survival for one half of the population (e.g., median survival). Simple rates and durations have the advantage of being easy to remember and communicate. However, valuable information is lost when prognosis—the distribution of uncertain events over time—is summarized by a single rate or duration. The more complete picture of prognosis is captured in a *survival curve* (Fig. 4.1).

Survival curves are often used to display the proportion of a cohort surviving over time, but the same technique can be used to display the occurrence, or lack thereof, of other events, such as onset of symptoms or recurrence of disease. Survival curves are constructed by plotting sequentially calculated probabilities of survival (or freedom from events) over time. The decrease

in the height of the curve at any time period depends on the proportion of the remaining cohort who experience the event during that period, with patients lost to follow-up excluded from the denominator. Sometimes, the proportion of people who experience events, rather than the proportion who are event free, is plotted on the vertical axis. Such *cumulative incidence curves,* or *cumulative hazard curves,* convey the same information.

It is important to recognize that comparisons between survival curves (e.g., comparing results for two different treatment approaches) can be made by citing the difference in vertical distance (proportion surviving) at a particular point in time (e.g., differences in the 5-year survival) or the difference in horizontal distance for a particular proportion of the population, usually one half. This difference in median survival is often referred to as the difference in life expectancy. It is also important to recognize that two survival curves representing outcomes for two treatment approaches can cross, meaning that survival is more likely at one point in time with one treatment and more likely at another point in time with the other treatment. This is not uncommon for surgical and medical interventions that confer high early mortality risk but also confer a reduction in subsequent risk that accumulates over time.

Because survival curves display serial estimates that are based on the experience of fewer and fewer people as events and loss to follow-up deplete the denominator, the clinician can be more confident in the estimates displayed on the left part of the curve than in those on the right. The distant future is more uncertain than the near term. However, when a new diagnosis of serious disease is made, it is often the near term that is of greatest interest to the patient. A cumulative recurrence risk of 30% may be frightening to the woman with early-stage breast cancer, and this may be a case in which use of the simple rate to express prognosis is a disservice. The more complete picture presented by a survival curve, including attention to the low annual incidence of recurrence in the near term, may be more helpful to the patient. Graphical displays of outcomes over time have been developed specifically to support patients' informed decisions. Such decision aids have been shown to provide patients with more realistic expectations about the future.

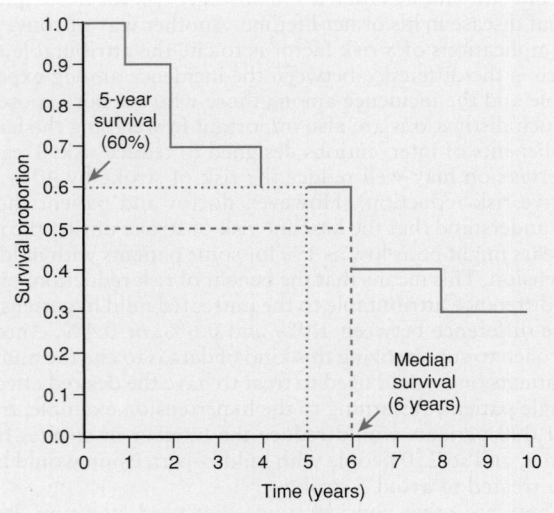

FIGURE 4.1. A survival curve is a plot of the proportion of subjects surviving (vertical axis) against the duration of observation (horizontal axis). Summary statistics may include the proportion of people surviving at a particular point in time, such as 5-year survival (in this case 60%; see dotted line), or the duration of survival for a particular proportion, such as median survival (in this case 6 years; see dashed line). With larger numbers of subjects, the curve becomes smoother as the series of downward steps become less visible.

THE UNIQUENESS OF EACH PATIENT (9,10,14,19)

Descriptions of risk and prognosis should be provided to patients with an appreciation for the uniqueness of each person and his or her predicament. Different people respond differently to the same risk. A 1% risk for stroke during a 5- or 10-year period may be threatening to some but inconsequential to others. This can be explained by the very real competing risks that different people face because of other medical conditions or the environment in which they live. Similarly, different people have different attitudes about tradeoffs between the present or near future and the distant future. Putting up with side effects or inconvenience now for some *possible* benefit in the future makes good sense to some but little sense to others. Again, competing risks explain some of these differences.

Different people also respond differently to the same health outcome. Symptoms that may be easy for one person to tolerate can be impossible for another. It is especially important that the primary care physician assist patients in understanding that the impact of a particular health state on health-related quality of life can be very personal. Helping patients accurately to imagine future health states and what they will mean for them is a difficult but critically important responsibility of the primary physician.

Another important difference among patients relates to their desire for information about the future. Many demand such information. Others would rather not know details about prognosis, even when that means that they must defer to the clinician for important decisions. As in other aspects of patient education, respect for the patient's autonomy and personal values during the communication of information about illness and its implications for the future requires a negotiated approach to patient care.

A.G.M.

Annotated Bibliography

1. Concato J, Feinstein AR, Holford TR. The risk of determining risk with multivariable models. Ann Intern Med 1993;118:201. (*Reviews principles and standards for the application of multivariable statistical methods in the general medical literature.*)
2. Laupacis A, Wells G, Richardson WS, et al. Users' guide to the medical literature. V. How to use an article about prognosis. JAMA 1994; 272:234. (*A systematic approach to practical application of the literature.*)
3. Hayden JA, Cote P, Bombardier C. Evaluation of the quality of prognosis studies in systematic reviews. Ann Intern Med 2006;144:427. (*Describes six sources of bias in systematic reviews related to prognosis and finds that few reviews assessed the impact of confounding.*)
4. Steiner JF. Talking about treatment: the language of populations and the language of individuals. Ann Intern Med 1999;130:618. (*Makes important distinctions that are helpful in communicating with patients.*)
5. Wasson JH, Sox HC, Neff RK, et al. Clinical prediction rules: applications and methodological standards. N Engl J Med 1985;313:793. (*Provides a checklist for methodologic standards for studies that purport to define prognostic variables.*)
6. Reilly BM, Evans AT. Translating clinical research into clinical practice: impact of using prediction rules to make decisions. Ann Intern Med 2006;144:201. (*Reviews standards of evidence for developing and evaluating prediction rules, including the need to measure both efficacy and effectiveness in assessing impact.*)
7. Laupacis A, Sackett DL, Roberts RS. An assessment of clinically useful measures of the consequences of treatment. N Engl J Med 1988;318:1728. (*An analysis of alternative approaches to summarizing effectiveness data, including the number needed to treat, or NNT.*)
8. Halvorsen PA, Selmer R, Kristiansen IS. Different ways to describe the benefits of risk-reducing treatments: a randomized trial. Ann Intern Med 2007;146:848. (*Treatment effects expressed in terms of NNT yielded higher consent rates than did those expressed as equivalent postponements.*)
9. Sox HC. Straight talk about disease prevention. Ann Intern Med 2007;146:891. (*Insight into the importance of framing effects when discussing risk and risk reduction with patients.*)
10. Edwards A, Elwyn G, Mulley A. Explaining risks: turning numerical data into meaningful pictures. BMJ 2002;324:827. (*Describes approaches to communicating risk more effectively.*)
11. Hembroff LA, Holmes-Rovner M, Wills CE. Treatment decision-making and the form of risk communication: results of a factorial survey. BMC Med

Inform Decision Making 2004;4:20. (*A standard strategy of presenting absolute risk information may improve patient decision making.*)
12. Kristiansen IS, Gyrd-Hansen D, Nexøe J, et al. Number needed to treat: easily understood and intuitively meaningful? Theoretical considerations and a randomized trial. J Clin Epidemiol 2002;55(9):888. (*The proportion of people consenting to the hypothetical drug was about 80%, irrespective of whether the NNT was set at 10, 25, 50, 100, 200, or 400.*)
13. Gigerenzer G, Edwards A. Simple tools for understanding risks: from innumeracy to insight. BMJ 2003;327:741. (*Argues against the use of single event probabilities, conditional probabilities, and relative risks, and suggests alternatives.*)
14. O'Connor A, Legare F, Stacey D. Risk communication in practice: the contribution of decision aids. BMJ 2003;327:736. (*Summarizes the use of risk communication for discrete decisions and to motivate behavior change for risk reduction.*)
15. Weymiller AJ, Montori VM, Jones LA, et al. Helping patients with type 2 diabetes mellitus make treatment decisions: statin choice randomized trial. Arch Intern Med 2007;167:1076. (*A decision aid enhanced decision making about statin drugs and may have favorably affected drug adherence.*)
16. Paling J. Strategies to help patients understand risks. BMJ 2003;327:745. (*Argues for absolute numbers, positive and negative framing, and the use of pictures to communicate and improve relationship with the patient.*)
17. Schwartz L, Woloshin S, Welch G. Risk communication in clinical practice: putting cancer in context. J Natl Cancer Inst Mongr 1999;25:124. (*Guidelines for communicating cancer risk and prognosis.*)
18. Edwards A, Unigwe S, Elwyn G, et al. Personalised risk communication for informed decision making about entering screening programs (Cochrane review). In: The Cochrane library, Issue 3. Oxford: Update Software, 2004. (*Personalized risk communication seems to increase the use of screening, but it is not clear that decisions are better informed.*)
19. O'Connor AM, Stacey D, Entwistle V, et al. Decision aids for people facing health treatment or screening decisions (Cochrane review). In: The Cochrane library, Issue 3. Oxford: Update Software, 2004. (*Decision aids can help patients to play an active role in screening decisions.*)
20. Brundage M, Feldman-Stewart D, Leis A, et al. Communicating quality of life information to cancer patients: a study of six presentation formats. J Clin Oncol 2005;23(28):6949. (*Patients generally prefer a simple linear representation of group mean health-related quality-of-life scores and can accurately interpret data presented in this format more than 98% of the time, irrespective of their age group and educational level.*)

CHAPTER 5 ■ CHOOSING AMONG TREATMENT OPTIONS

Although discerning diagnosis and accurate prognosis are essential to effective patient care, the process of choosing among treatment options can have the greatest effect on the relief of suffering and the prolongation of life. The right choice depends on accurate information about the effects of various treatment strategies on health outcomes. Will symptoms be relieved or at least reduced? Will serious complications of disease be averted by timely intervention, or will treatment side effects or complications decrease the quality or length of life? Treatment choices also depend on patients' preferences for different possible health outcomes and on their attitudes toward risks or their willingness to endure morbidity now for some possible future benefit. As noted in Chapter 4, different patients have different preferences and attitudes toward risks and time tradeoffs. Effective therapeutic decision making therefore requires both a strong clinical knowledge base and the communication skills necessary to gain an empathic understanding of the individual patient's wants and needs.

WHAT WE KNOW ABOUT TREATMENT EFFECTIVENESS

The cumulative knowledge base about the effectiveness of treatments of human disease is prodigious. Nonetheless, the use of many of the most common therapeutic interventions in clinical practice is not supported by evidence derived from clinical trials. Clinicians often rely on their experience with similar patients, supplemented by published case series, to estimate the likelihood of relevant health outcomes with different treatments. This less-than-rigorous approach produces different opinions about treatment effectiveness, which lead to wide variations in clinical practices for ostensibly similar patients. Because of less-stringent regulatory control, the knowledge gaps are generally greater with devices and surgical procedures than with drugs. For example, discectomy for lumbar disk disease was first described in 1934. Nevertheless, the first randomized trial was published in 1983 and included only 60 surgical patients. The collective experience of the millions of patients who have undergone discectomy worldwide contributed relatively little to our knowledge. Similarly, transurethral prostatectomy represented the standard of care for benign prostatic hyperplasia for 40 years before publication of a clinical trial.

RANDOMIZED CLINICAL TRIALS AND TREATMENT EFFECTIVENESS (1–11)

Even when randomized trials are performed, uncertainty remains about the effectiveness of treatment for a specific patient. This in part reflects the methods used in clinical trials to measure the isolated effects of the treatment being studied. Explicit inclusion and exclusion criteria are often applied to ensure that the study population is homogeneous to minimize the effect of patient-specific variables on outcomes. Patients with severe disease or important comorbid conditions are often excluded. Others may be excluded because of age or sex. Patients who meet criteria are then randomized to one of two or more carefully defined treatment strategies. Barriers are erected to discourage patients from switching from one treatment to another, and other steps are taken to preserve the integrity of the treatments.

The course of patients in well-conducted randomized trials is carefully monitored, with equal attention given to patients regardless of treatment, and their outcomes are determined by means of explicit, predefined measures. Ideally, both patients and those who measure outcomes are unaware of the treatment assignment, even if this requires the use of placebos or sham procedures. Otherwise, expectations may have a real effect on perceived treatment outcomes and be interpreted as specific effects of treatment.

All of these steps serve to protect the validity of the trial as a test of the hypothesis that the treatments compared in the trial have different effects on outcome. However, these same steps often limit the applicability or generalizability of the study

findings to patients for whom the study treatment might be considered. The clinician must be concerned both about the internal validity of the trial as a test of the hypothesis about treatment effectiveness and its external validity, that is, the extent to which results are applicable to the patients seen in practice, who may be quite different from patients in the trial.

Treatments may also vary from one setting to another. This is especially true for surgical procedures and for "complex interventions," which are defined by the British Medical Research Council as those that are built up from a number of components, which may act both independently and interdependently. Regarding surgery, many studies have suggested that the volume of particular procedures performed in a hospital and/or by particular surgeons is inversely related to mortality rate. One study indicated that these differences in risk can be quite significant clinically for complex procedures, including pancreatectomy, esophagectomy, and pneumonectomy. Other characteristics of hospitals and of particular surgeons have been studied less well.

In the case of complex interventions, the effectiveness can vary significantly with the context of the environment in which it is designed and implemented. This is often the case when the intervention involves comanagement of the disease by clinician and patient or caregiver.

Concerns are also raised when there are multiple goals, either stated or unstated, for a particular trial. All trials involve potential tradeoffs in the welfare of trial participants and those future patients who would benefit from the highest achievable scientific validity of the study. Different perspectives exist on appropriate times to stop trials early because of apparent benefit, thereby forgoing the more precise estimates of benefit and harm.

Some trials are designed to compare a new agent and an established agent and prove not a greater benefit, but rather noninferiority to the active-control agent. Such noninferiority may justify a change to the new agent when it has other advantages related to cost, convenience or safety, but in an age of direct-to-consumer promotion of new drugs through highly selective presentation of evidence, there may be reason for concern.

A similar concern about the construction of trials that may allow for misleading conclusions derives from the use of "composite endpoints," made up of one or more of several events of interest, as the primary outcome of a trial. The advantage of using a composite endpoint is an increased event rate and increased power of the trial for a given number of patients. However, some events, such as all-cause or disease-specific death, may be uniformly important to all patients, whereas other events, such as new onset of angina, might be less important, and this might be variably so among patients. Trials using composite endpoints can be misleading if the number of more important events is small and the magnitude of effect varies across elements.

SYSTEMATIC REVIEWS AND TREATMENT EFFECTIVENESS (12–16)

All too frequently, individual trials may not be large enough to provide definitive answers to clinical questions. Increasingly, data from multiple trials are being combined in meta-analyses to allow careful systematic interpretation of the evidence. With the proliferation of randomized trials in the last decade, systematic reviews, or meta-analyses, have become the gold standard for treatment effectiveness. However, systematic reviews have their own problems in design, conduct, and interpretation. For example, to combine results of trials that measure the same outcome on different scales (e.g., one of several depression scales or quality-of-life measures), the author of a systematic review must calculate the standardized mean difference for each trial. Although the statistical process is straightforward, it has been shown that errors in data abstraction capable of significantly altering results are not uncommon.

There are other challenges in combining the results of different trials. There may be evident *clinical heterogeneity* of the patient populations, the intervention, or both. Interventions designed to support patients in decision making or self-management often vary from one trial to another and from one setting to another. In other cases, the populations and interventions may seem similar, but the results of trials may not be not consistent with one another. This *statistical heterogeneity* can be seen in a "forest plot" of trial results or determined with statistical tests for heterogeneity that produce a high *P*-value when heterogeneity is low and a low *P*-value when heterogeneity is high. If heterogeneity is high, it may be explained by unappreciated clinical differences, methodologic problems, of publication bias. The meta-analysis can proceed using a random-effects model rather than a fixed-effects model. This means that because of the heterogeneity, the effects of treatment are assumed to vary around an overall average treatment effect rather than the same common fixed effect. However, in situations of high heterogeneity, the clinician interpreting the systematic review may want to step back and ask whether it made sense to combine the trials that were included.

Despite the problems that sometimes arise in combining studies, systematic reviews provide a great resource for the clinician who strives to make the most of clinical knowledge in the care of patients. A prodigious amount of work has been done under a number of different auspices; most notable are those of the Cochrane Collaboration (see later discussion, under Making the Most of Available Resources). That work is necessarily ongoing. Even the most robust of systematic reviews is always at risk of going out of date. One study found a mean duration of "survival" without the need for updating of 5.5 years for a cohort of 100 systematic reviews. However, 23% were in need of revision within 2 years and 15% within 1 year. There is also a need to make the results of systematic reviews more accessible to clinicians and policy makers. Standardized formats for different audiences have been proposed and are increasingly being used.

OTHER STUDIES OF TREATMENT EFFECTIVENESS (17–25)

Randomized trials are not always necessary. When a new treatment has unprecedented or dramatic effects, such as penicillin for pneumococcal pneumonia or pacemaker insertion for life-threatening bradycardia, a trial is neither necessary nor desirable. When results of trials would be helpful because treatment effects are more equivocal, they are often not available. Randomized trials are costly, time-consuming, and poorly accepted by many clinicians and patients. Sometimes, a trial is obsolete before it is completed because the experimental treatment has been modified or replaced by a newer approach or technology.

For all of these reasons, clinicians must rely on data from observational studies in addition to those from randomized trial results. However, great caution must be used in the application of conclusions of observational studies to patient care.

Differences in patient characteristics among different treatment groups may lead to erroneous conclusions about treatment effectiveness. Although there have been important advances in the use of statistical methods to control for such different prognostic factors in an attempt to isolate the treatment effect, the investigator can control only for those factors that are anticipated and measured. Observational studies complement randomized trials. They can be used to design efficient and targeted trials and to assess the generalizability of trial results. However, the clinician should be mindful of the quality of evidence when making treatment choices and should recognize that there is often no substitute for a well-conducted randomized trial.

THE EFFECT OF PATIENTS' EXPECTATIONS ON OUTCOMES (23,24)

There is ample evidence demonstrating that patients' expectations regarding the effectiveness of a treatment have a profound influence on the outcome of that treatment. It is not at all unusual for patients receiving inactive agents (placebos) or sham surgical procedures to report an improvement in symptoms. For example, as much as two thirds of the symptom improvement appreciated by patients taking finasteride for benign prostatic hyperplasia was reported by those assigned to placebo in double-blind, randomized trials. Furthermore, improvements in objective outcomes, such as mortality rates, have been reported following the use of placebo agents or sham surgical procedures. There are also examples of studies in which patients who have sufficiently high expectations to comply faithfully with a prescribed regimen do better than patients who do not. These compliance effects occur regardless of whether the regimen includes an active agent or actual procedure. It is likely that the effect of patients' expectation plays a substantial role in the perceived effectiveness of many interventions, including those termed "complementary" or "alternative" because they are outside the mainstream of what is taught in medical schools. An important task of primary care is to teach patients the rules of evidence that are critical to the scientific basis of health services, ideally with an open-minded approach to the patients' attributions and understandings of science.

TREATMENT CHOICE AND PATIENT VALUES (26–29)

Even if the probabilities of outcomes contingent on alternative treatment choices can be estimated precisely, there is still much work to be done to ensure a wise treatment choice for a particular patient. Consider the predicament of the 75-year-old man who is bothered by nocturia and urinary frequency resulting from benign prostatic hyperplasia. He can live with his symptoms, but this means accepting a diminished quality of life. He may choose to try a medical approach, such as finasteride or an α-blocker, with the hope of a modest relief of symptoms. Alternatively, surgical therapy offers a good chance of more dramatic symptom relief but also confers a small but real risk of a catastrophic event that could result in death. Surgery also puts the patient at risk for complications, such as incontinence or sexual dysfunction, that can diminish the quality of life as much as or more than nocturia and frequency.

The probabilities of these outcomes are critically important to the decision. Equally important, however, is how the patient feels about the outcomes. Different men feel differently about tradeoffs between urinary function and sexual function, and they have different attitudes toward the small risk of perioperative death. These personal value judgments are often as important in determining the "right" choice as the probabilities that are derived from clinical research. The right choice, therefore, requires careful communication between clinician and patient about what the possible outcomes will mean for that patient's quality of life, especially when the patient has never experienced the outcomes.

MAKING THE MOST OF AVAILABLE RESOURCES (30–34)

The tasks of accessing and using the best available evidence about treatment effectiveness, tailored to the clinical circumstances of particular patients, are extraordinarily difficult. Fortunately, new resources have been developed to support clinicians in this role and to facilitate communication between clinicians and patients. Many of these resources are available on the Internet, either free or for modest fees. The National Library of Medicine's popular search engine PubMed offers access to more than 17 million references and abstracts from more than 5,000 journals published since 1966. During its tenth-anniversary year in 2007, PubMed supported an average of three million searches per day. Efficient search strategies have been devised for articles about prognosis, diagnosis, therapy, and other elements of clinical care. Other valuable sources include compendia of evidence reviews developed by professional societies and by federally funded centers of research. Links to such resources, including the National Guideline Clearinghouse, can be found at http://www.ahrq.gov. Many believe that the evidence summaries produced by members of the Cochrane Collaboration set the standard for quality. Abstracts of these reviews can be seen at http://www.cochrane.org, where full reviews are also accessible.

Commercial firms are making evidence more efficiently accessible by aggregating material protected by copyright, including multiple journals that do not provide free Internet access, and providing full-text access for an institutional license or a single-user subscription fee (e.g., Ovid). Further accessibility is provided by meta-search engines (e.g., Skolar), which range across both public domain resources such as PubMed and the National Guideline Clearinghouse, as well as material protected by copyright, including the full-text Cochrane reviews and even collections of leading textbooks.

Many sites designed primarily for professionals also include resources for patients. The site http://www.ahrq.gov has links to consumer information, as does http://www.cochrane.org and the very useful http://www.informedhealthonline.org. In addition to these general sources of information, decision aids have been developed for patients facing specific decisions that may be difficult because of the tradeoffs among different treatment choices. Such decision aids have proven most effective when they are fully integrated in the clinical workflow and when use is facilitated by high-quality decision counseling to help patients understand the potential risks, benefits, and uncertainties of clinical practice. A Cochrane Review Group has found that decision aids increase patient knowledge, lead to more realistic expectations about the future, and can help patients to make decisions that reflect their personal preferences. Examples can be found at http://decisionaid.ohri.ca/ and http://www.collaborativecare.net.

Making the most of the vast knowledge base that should inform clinical practice can be facilitated by these kinds of resources; they are well leveraged to great effect on behalf of patients in many settings. However, there is great need for more integration of interventions and strategies for informing, educating, and engaging patients in the treatment decisions that so affect their lives. There should be no higher priority for the primary care practitioner.

A.G.M.

Annotated Bibliography

1. Guyatt G, Sackett D, Taylor DW, et al. Determining optimal therapy-randomized trials in individual patients. N Engl J Med 1986;314:889. (*A persuasive argument for blinded, placebo-controlled, crossover trials in individual patients to evaluate the specific effects of medical treatments more critically.*)
2. Localio AR, Berlin JA, TenHave TR, et al. Adjustments for center in multicenter studies: an overview. Ann Intern Med 2001;135:112. (*Highlights issues related to variations among treatment effects in different centers, as well as analytic options.*)
3. Moher D, Jones A, Lepage L, et al. Use of the CONSORT statement and quality of reports of randomized trials: a comparative before-and-after evaluation. JAMA 2001;285:1992. (*The use of the Consolidated Standards of Reporting Trials [CONSORT] statement and standards improved quality.*)
4. Van Spall HGC, Toren A, Kiss A, et al. Eligibility criteria of randomized controlled trials published in high-impact general medical journals: a systematic sampling review. JAMA 2007;297:1233. (*Among 283 trials, common medical conditions formed the basis for exclusion in 81%, and age did so in 72%; most exclusion criteria were deemed unjustified in the context of the intervention.*)
5. Birkmeyer JD, Siewers AE, Finlayson EVA, et al. Hospital volume and surgical mortality in the United States. N Engl J Med 2002;346:1128. (*A higher mortality risk exists at lower-volume hospitals, strikingly so for some procedures, including pancreatectomy, esophagectomy, and pneumonectomy.*)
6. Campbell NC, Murray E, Darbyshire J, et al. Designing and evaluating complex interventions to improve health care. BMJ 2007;334:455-459. (*Advice based on the British Medical Research Council framework, with examples to clarify elements of design and conduct of studies.*)

7. Perera R, Yudkin K. A graphical method for depicting randomized trials of complex interventions. BMJ 2007;334:127. (*The use of boxes and circles to represents different elements of complex interventions helps to clarify an analysis; a picture is worth….*)
8. Mueller PS, Montori VM, Bassler D, et al. Ethical issues in stopping randomized trials early because of apparent benefit. Ann Intern Med 2007;146:878. (*Argues that "stopping rules" should not be used because of the resulting exaggeration of efficacy estimates and the lost opportunity to assess harms.*)
9. Goodman SN. Stopping at nothing? Some dilemmas of data monitoring in clinical trials. Ann Intern Med 2007;146:882. (*A critique of the argument that "stopping rules" should not be used because of the resulting exaggeration of efficacy estimates and the lost opportunity to assess harms.*)
10. Kaul S, Diamond GA. Good enough: a primer on the analysis and interpretation of noninferiority trials. Ann Intern Med. 2006;145:62. (*Identifies the prerequisites for trials designed to establish therapeutic noninferiority between new and standard, active-control treatment and finds that eight recently published noninferiority trials are wanting.*)
11. Ferreira-Gonzalez I, Busse JW, Heels-Ansdell D, et al. Problems with use of composite end points in cardiovascular trials: systematic review of randomized controlled trials. BMJ 2007;334:786. (*Makes the important observation that the outcome elements of composite endpoints exhibit very large gradients in importance to patients and that higher event rates and/or larger treatment effects associated with less important outcomes can result in misleading conclusions about the effect of treatment.*)
12. Oxman AD, Cook DJ, Guyatt GH, et al. Users' guide to the medical literature. VI. How to use an overview. JAMA 1994;272:1367. (*Practical advice*

about how to use the literature, in this case, by interpreting increasingly prevalent systematic overviews.)

13. Gotzsche PC, Hrobjartsson A, Maric K, et al. Data extraction errors in meta-analyses that use standardized mean differences. JAMA 2007;298:430. (*Errors are the rule rather than the exception among meta-analyses that require standardization of effect size by calculating the standard mean difference.*)

14. Fletcher J. What is heterogeneity and is it important? BMJ 2007;334:94. (*A succinct review of the detection and significance of clinical heterogeneity and statistical heterogeneity when conducting and interpreting systematic reviews.*)

15. Shojania KG, Sampson M, Ansari MT, et al. How quickly do systematic reviews go out of date? A survival analysis. Ann Intern Med 2007;147:224. (*Among 100 systematic reviews, the median survival free of a signal for updating was 5.5 years; a signal occurred within 2 years for 23% and within 1 year for 15%.*)

16. Laupacis A, Straus S. Systematic reviews: time to address clinical and policy relevance as well as methodological rigor. Ann Intern Med 2007;147:273. (*Recounts the shortcomings in the presentation of systematic reviews that limit effect and offers some suggestions, including three different standardized formats for different audiences.*)

17. Glasziou P, Chalmers I, Rawlins M, et al. When are randomized trials unnecessary? Picking signal from noise. BMJ 2007;334:349. (*An analytic approach to determining when observations speak for themselves.*)

18. Glasziou P, Vandenbrouke J, Chalmers I, et al. Education and debate: assessing the quality of research. BMJ 2004;328:39. (*A thoughtful stocktaking of benefits and limitations of research hierarchies.*)

19. Benson K, Hartz AJ. A comparison of observational studies and randomized, controlled trials. N Engl J Med 2000;342:1878. (*Estimates of treatment effects from well-designed observational studies were similar to those of randomized, controlled trials.*)

20. Concato J, Shah N, Horwitz RI, et al. Randomized, controlled trials, observational studies, and the hierarchy of research designs. N Engl J Med 2000;342:1887. (*The results of well-designed observational studies do not systematically overestimate treatment effects compared with randomized, controlled trials.*)

21. Radford MJ, Foody JM. How do observational studies expand the evidence base for therapy? JAMA 2001;286:1228. (*An editorial describing the use of propensity analysis to minimize the effect of confounding in an analysis of aspirin use and all-cause mortality.*)

22. Smith GCS, Pell JP. Parachute use to prevent death and major trauma related to gravitational challenge: systematic review of randomised controlled trials. BMJ 2003;327:1459. (*A tongue-firmly-in-cheek reminder that there are other ways to learn than just the randomized, controlled trial.*)

23. Jackson JL, Kroenke K. The effect of unmet expectations among adults presenting with physical symptoms. Ann Intern Med 2001;134:889. (*Prognostic and diagnostic interactions may be highly valued but are often not provided; when provided, they may be associated with better symptom relief and functional states.*)

24. Kaptchuk TJ. The placebo effect in alternative medicine: can the performance of a healing ritual have clinical significance? Ann Intern Med 2002;136:817. (*Noteworthy for its explication of performance efficacy, with lessons for the conventional practitioner.*)

25. McAlister FA, Straus SE, Guyatt GH, et al. Users' guides to the medical literature: XX. Integrating research evidence with the care of the individual patient. JAMA 2000;283:2829. (*Reviews the approach to estimating patient-specific benefit and risk and incorporating the patient's values.*)

26. Mulley AG. Assessing patients' utilities: can the ends justify the means? Med Care 1989;27:S269. (*A somewhat technical discussion of the role of patients' preferences and their measurement in clinical decision making.*)

27. Hunt DL, Jaeschke R, McKibbon KA, et al. Users' guides to the medical literature: XXI. Using electronic health information resources in evidence-based practice. JAMA 2000;283:1875. (*Describes electronic resources for accessing evidence.*)

28. Sheridan SL, Pignone MP, Lewis CL. A randomized comparison of patients' understanding of number needed to treat and other common risk reduction formats. J Gen Intern Med 2003;18:884. (*Patients are best able to interpret the benefits of treatment when presented in a relative risk reduction format with a baseline risk of disease; absolute risk reduction also is easily interpreted, but number needed to treat is often misinterpreted.*)

29. Halvorsen PA, Selmer R, Kristiansen IS. Different ways to describe the benefits of risk-reducing treatments: a randomized trial. Ann Intern Med 2007;146:848-56. (*Treatment effects expressed in terms of number needed to treat yielded higher consent rates than did those expressed as equivalent postponements.*)

30. Weymiller AJ, Montori VM, Jones LA, et al. Helping patients with type 2 diabetes mellitus make treatment decisions: statin choice randomized trial. Arch Intern Med 2007;167:1076. (*A decision aid enhanced decision making about statin drugs and may have favorably affected drug adherence.*)

31. O'Connor AM, Stacey D, Entwistle V, et al. Decision aids for people facing health treatment or screening decisions (Cochrane review). In: The Cochrane library, Issue 3. Oxford: Update Software, 2004. (*Decision aids can help patients to make better-informed choices that are more consistent with their values.*)

32. Woolf SH, Chan ECY, Harris R, et al. Promoting informed choice: transforming health care to dispense knowledge for decision making. Ann Intern Med 2005;143:293. (*Makes a strong argument for coupling information with high-quality decision counseling to help patients understand the potential risks, benefits, and uncertainties of clinical options.*)

33. Lomas J. The in-between world of knowledge brokering. BMJ 2007;334:129. (*A fascinating argument for the need for an "intermediary" in order for research findings effectively to influence health services delivery.*)

34. Coulter A, Ellins J. Effectiveness of strategies for informing, educating and involving patients. BMJ 2007;335:24. (*A succinct and authoritative analytic summary of a much more extensive review online at* http://www.pickereurope.org.)

CHAPTER 6 ■ IMMUNIZATION

REGINA C. LAROCQUE AND EDWARD T. RYAN

Immunization is the most cost-effective means of preventing infectious diseases. Immunizations are grouped into five major categories: (a) routine vaccinations of childhood and adolescence, (b) routine vaccinations of adulthood (Tables 6.1 and 6.2), (c) postexposure prophylactic immunizations, (d) travel-related immunizations, and (e) work-related/special circumstance immunizations. Of these, administration of vaccines during childhood has been most successful; fewer than 100 children die each year of vaccine-preventable illnesses in the

United States. In comparison, 50,000 to 70,000 adults die each year in the United States of vaccine-preventable illnesses.

Compared with responses in young adults or children, responses are often lower in elderly or immunocompromised persons; however, vaccines still induce clinically meaningful protective immunity in most adult populations. Vaccine administration in adults is safe. Most adverse reactions from parenteral injections occur at the injection site and include induration, erythema, and tenderness; low-grade fever and mild constitutional

TABLE 6.1

SUMMARY OF RECOMMENDATIONS FOR ROUTINE ADULT IMMUNIZATIONS

Vaccine Name and Route	For Whom Recommended	Schedule (Any Vaccine Can Be Given with Another)	Contraindications and Precautions (Mild Illness not a Contraindication)
Influenza Inactivated influenza vaccine	■ Anyone wishing to reduce the likelihood of becoming ill with influenza	■ Given every year	**Contraindications:** ■ Previous anaphylactic reaction to this vaccine, to any of its components, or to eggs
■ Give IM	■ Adults ≥50 yr of age; Children 6 months–18 yr of age	■ In the temperate Northern Hemisphere, October–November is the optimal time to receive an annual flu shot to maximize protection, but the vaccine may be given at any time during the influenza season (typically December–March) or at other times when the risk of influenza exists	**Precautions:** ■ Moderate or severe acute illness ■ History of Guillain-Barré syndrome within 6 wk of previous administration of inactivated influenza vaccine ■ Pregnancy and breast-feeding are not contraindications to the use of this vaccine
	■ People 6 mo–50 yr of age with medical problems such as heart disease, lung disease, diabetes, renal dysfunction, hemoglobinopathies, immunosuppression; people living in long-term care facilities		
	■ Persons with any condition that compromises respiratory function or the handling of respiratory secretions, or that can increase the risk of aspiration		
	■ People >6 mo of age working or living with at-risk people		
	■ All health care workers and those who provide key community services		
	■ Women who will be pregnant during the influenza season		
	■ Household contacts and out-of-home caregivers of children ages 0–59 mo		
	■ Persons traveling to areas where influenza activity exists or among people from areas of the world where there is current influenza activity		
	■ Students or other persons in institutional settings		

Vaccine	Indications	Contraindications/Precautions
Live attenuated influenza vaccine ■ Give intranasally	■ Healthy, nonpregnant individuals aged ≤49 yr with an indication or desire for influenza vaccination	■ Same as for inactivated influenza vaccine, except that the live attenuated vaccine may be given as soon as it is available ■ If the LAIV and MMR, yellow fever or varicella vaccines are not given on the same day, then space them at least 28 days apart	**Contraindications:** ■ Previous anaphylactic reaction to this vaccine, to any of its components, or to eggs ■ Pregnancy, asthma, reactive airways disease or other chronic disorder of the cardiac or pulmonary systems; an underlying medical condition, including diabetes, renal disease, or hemoglobinopathy; a known or suspected immune deficiency disease or receipt of immunosuppressive therapy; history of Guillain-Barré syndrome. ■ Close contact with severely immunosuppressed persons
Pneumococcal polysaccharide (PPV23) ■ Give IM or SC	■ Adults >65 yr of age	■ Routinely given as one-time dose; administer if previous vaccination history is unknown	**Contraindications:** ■ Previous anaphylactic reaction to this vaccine or to any of its components. **Precautions:** ■ Moderate or severe acute illness
	■ People 2–64 yr of age who have chronic illness or other risk factors, including chronic cardiac or pulmonary diseases, chronic liver disease, alcoholism, diabetes mellitus, or CSF leaks, and persons living in special environments or social settings (including Alaska natives and certain Native American populations); those at highest risk of fatal pneumococcal infection are persons with anatomic or functional asplenia (including sickle cell disease); immunocompromised persons, including those with HIV infection, leukemia, lymphoma, Hodgkin's disease, multiple myeloma, generalized malignancy, chronic renal failure, or nephrotic syndrome; those receiving immunosuppressive chemotherapy (including corticosteroids); those who have received an organ or bone marrow transplant; and candidates for or recipients of cochlear implants	■ One-time revaccination is recommended 5 yr later for people at highest risk of fatal pneumococcal infection or rapid antibody loss (e.g., renal disease) and for people >65 yr if the first dose was given before age 65 and 5 yr or more have elapsed since previous dose	

(Continued)

TABLE 6.1

SUMMARY OF RECOMMENDATIONS FOR ROUTINE ADULT IMMUNIZATIONS (*Continued*)

Vaccine Name and Route	For Whom Recommended	Schedule (Any Vaccine Can Be Given with Another)	Contraindications and Precautions (Mild Illness not a Contraindication)
Hepatitis B (Hep B) ■ Give IM Brands may be used interchangeably	■ All persons through 18 years; any adult wishing to obtain immunity ■ High-risk adults, including household contacts and sex partners of HbsAg-positive persons; users of illicit injectable drugs; sexually active persons not in a long-term, mutually monogamous relationship; men who have sex with men; people with HIV or recently diagnosed STDs; patients in hemodialysis units and patients with renal disease that may result in dialysis; recipients of certain blood products; health care workers and public safety workers who are exposed to blood; clients and staff of institutions for the developmentally disabled; inmates of long-term correctional facilities; certain international travelers *Note:* Prior serologic testing may be recommended, depending on the specific level of risk or likelihood of previous exposure. ■ Persons with chronic liver disease. *Note:* Perform serologic screening for people who have emigrated from endemic areas. When HbsAg-positive persons are identified, offer them appropriate disease management; in addition, screen their household members and intimate contacts and give the first dose of vaccine at the same visit; if found susceptible, complete the vaccine series	■ Three doses are needed on a 0-, 1-, 6-mo schedule ■ Alternate timing options for vaccination include 0, 2, and 4 mo and 0, 1, and 4 mo ■ There must be 4 wk between doses 1 and 2, and 8 wk between doses 2 and 3; overall, there must be at least 4 mo between doses 1 and 3 ■ Schedule for those who have fallen behind: if the series is delayed between doses, do not start the series over; continue from where it was left off *Note:* Fixed combination of the A and B vaccines should be given on a 0-, 1-, 6-mo schedule or on an accelerated schedule of 0, 7, and 21–30 d and a booster dose at 12 mo	**Contraindications:** ■ Previous anaphylactic reaction to this vaccine or to any of its components
Hepatitis A (Hep A)	■ People who travel or work outside the United States, northern and western Europe, New Zealand, Australia, Canada, and Japan	■ Two doses are needed	**Contraindications:** ■ Previous anaphylactic reaction to this vaccine or to any of its components.

Indications	Schedule	Contraindications/Precautions
People with chronic liver disease, including people with hepatitis C virus infection, people with hepatitis B who have chronic liver disease, illicit drug users, men who have sex with men, people with clotting factor disorders, people who work with hepatitis A virus in experimental lab settings (this does not refer to routine medical laboratories), and food handlers when health authorities or private employers determine vaccination to be cost-effective	The minimum interval between doses 1 and 2 is 6 mo	**Precautions:** ■ Moderate or severe acute illness.
■ Give IM ■ Anyone wishing to obtain immunity to hepatitis A Brands may be used interchangeably	■ If dose 2 is delayed, do not repeat dose 1; just give dose 2	■ Safety in pregnancy has not been determined, so benefits must be weighed against potential risks
Td, Tdap (tetanus, diphtheria, pertussis) ■ All adults who lack a history of a primary series containing at least 3 doses of tetanus- and diphtheria- containing vaccine	■ For persons who are unvaccinated or behind, complete the primary series with Td (spaced 0, 1- to 2-, and 6- to 12-mo intervals); one dose of Tdap may be used for any dose if ages 19–64 yr	**Contraindications:** ■ Previous anaphylactic reaction to this vaccine or to any of its components
■ After the primary series has been completed, a booster dose is recommended every 10 yr	■ Give Td booster every 10 yr after the primary series has been completed; for adults ages 19–64 yr, a one-time dose of Tdap is recommended to replace the next Td	■ For Tdap only, history of encephalopathy within 7 days following DTP/DTaP
■ A booster dose of tetanus- and diphtheria-containing toxoid as early as 5 yr later may be needed for the purpose of wound management, so consult ACIP recommendations	■ Intervals of 2 yr or less between Td and Tdap may be used if needed	**Precautions:** ■ Moderate or severe acute illness
For Tdap only: ■ All adults age <65 years who have not received Tdap		■ Unstable neurologic condition
■ Health care workers who have direct patient contact and have not received Tdap	*Note:* The 2 Tdap products are licensed for different age groups: Adacel (sanofi pasteur) for use in persons ages 11–64 yr and Boostrix (Glaxo-SmithKline) for use in persons ages 10–18 yr	■ Guillain-Barré syndrome within 6 wk of receiving tetanus toxoid–containing vaccine ■ History of Arthus reaction after a previous dose of tetanus- and/or diphtheria toxoid–containing vaccine, including MCV4

(*Continued*)

TABLE 6.1

SUMMARY OF RECOMMENDATIONS FOR ROUTINE ADULT IMMUNIZATIONS (*Continued*)

Vaccine Name and Route	For Whom Recommended	Schedule (Any Vaccine Can Be Given with Another)	Contraindications and Precautions (Mild Illness not a Contraindication)
	■ Adults in contact with infants younger than 12 mo who have not received Tdap		*Note:* Td is preferred when tetanus and diphtheria protection is required during pregnancy; health care providers can choose to administer Tdap instead of Td to add protection against pertussis in situations with increased risk for pertussis; when Td or Tdap is administered during pregnancy, the second or third trimester is preferred
■ Polio (IPV) ■ Give IM or SC	■ Not routinely recommended for persons >18 yr of age *Note:* Adults living in the United States who never received or completed a primary series of polio vaccine need not be vaccinated unless they intend to travel to areas where exposure to wild-type virus is likely; previously vaccinated adults should receive one booster dose if traveling to polio-endemic areas.	■ Refer to ACIP recommendations regarding unique situations, schedules, and dosing information	**Contraindications:** ■ Previous anaphylactic or neurologic reaction to this vaccine or to any of its components **Precautions:** ■ Moderate or severe acute illness.
■ Varicella (chickenpox) ■ Give SC	■ All adults without evidence of immunity *Note:* Evidence of immunity is defined as a history of two doses of varicella vaccine; born in the United States before 1980 (exception: health care personnel and pregnant women); a history of varicella disease or herpes zoster based on health care provider diagnosis; laboratory evidence of immunity; and/or laboratory confirmation of disease	■ Two doses are needed ■ Dose 2 is given 4–8 wk after dose 1 ■ If the second dose is delayed, do not repeat dose 1; Just give dose 2	■ Pregnancy **Contraindications:** ■ Previous anaphylactic reaction to this vaccine or to any of its components ■ Pregnancy or possibility of pregnancy within 4 wk ■ Persons immunocompromised because of malignancies and primary or acquired cellular immunodeficiency including HIV/AIDS *Note:* For those on high-dose immunosuppressive therapy, consult ACIP recommendations regarding delay time

Precautions:
- Moderate or severe acute illness
- Manufacturer recommends that salicylates be avoided for 6 wk after administration of varicella vaccine because of a theoretical risk of Reye's syndrome

- If the varicella vaccine and either MMR, live attenuated influenza vaccine, or yellow fever vaccine are not given on the same day, then space them at least 28 d apart
- If blood, plasma, and/or immune globulin were given in past 11 mo, consult the ACIP guidelines regarding time to wait before vaccinating

Herpes zoster (shingles)

Give SC

Note: The varicella and the herpes zoster vaccine are *not* to be used interchangeably; the herpes zoster vaccine contains more than 10 times the amount of live virus as the varicella vaccine

- All persons age ≥60 yr who do not have contraindications

Contraindications:
- Previous anaphylactic reaction to this vaccine or to any of its components
- Pregnancy or possibility of pregnancy within 4 wk (Manufacturer recommends 3 mo.)
- Persons immunocompromised because of malignancies and primary or acquired cellular immunodeficiency, including HIV/AIDS

- The zoster vaccine should not be administered to individuals who have never had chickenpox or shingles; such individuals should have serologic testing; if negative, they should receive the varicella vaccine

Precautions:
- Moderate or severe acute illness

(Continued)

TABLE 6.1

SUMMARY OF RECOMMENDATIONS FOR ROUTINE ADULT IMMUNIZATIONS (*Continued*)

Vaccine Name and Route	For Whom Recommended	Schedule (Any Vaccine Can Be Given with Another)	Contraindications and Precautions (Mild Illness not a Contraindication)
Meningococcal	■ College freshmen living in dormitories ■ All persons 11–18 yr of age	■ One dose is needed	**Contraindications:** ■ Previous anaphylactic or neurologic reaction to the vaccine or to any of its components, including diphtheria toxoid (for MCV4)
Meningococcal conjugate vaccine (MCV4) ■ Give IM	■ Persons with anatomic or functional asplenia or with terminal complement component deficiencies ■ Persons who travel to or reside in countries in which meningococcal disease is hyperendemic or epidemic (e.g., the "meningitis belt" of sub-Saharan Africa)	■ If previous vaccine was MPSV, revaccinate after 5 yr if risk continues ■ Revaccination after MCV4 is not recommended	**Precautions:** ■ Moderate or severe acute illness ■ For MCV4 only, history of Guillain-Barré syndrome
Meningococcal polysaccharide vaccine (MPSV) ■ Give SC		■ MCV4 is preferred over MPSV for persons age ≤55 yr, although MPSV is an acceptable alternative	
Measles, mumps, rubella (MMR) ■ Give SC	■ Adults born in 1957 or later (especially those born outside the United States) should receive at least one dose of MMR if there is no serologic proof of immunity or documentation of a dose given on or after the first birthday ■ Persons in high-risk groups, such as health care personnel, students entering college and other post–high school educational institutions, and international travelers, should receive a total of two doses ■ Adults born before 1957 are usually considered immune, but proof of immunity (serology or vaccination) may be desirable for health care personnel ■ Women of child-bearing age who do not have acceptable evidence of rubella immunity or vaccination	■ One or two doses are needed ■ If dose 2 is recommended, give it no sooner than 4 wk after dose 1 ■ If MMR and other live viral vaccines are not given on the same day, then space them at least 28 d apart ■ If a pregnant woman is found to be rubella susceptible, administer MMR postpartum	**Contraindications:** ■ Previous anaphylactic reaction to this vaccine or to any of its components ■ Pregnancy or possibility of pregnancy within 4 wk ■ Persons immunocompromised because of cancer, leukemia, lymphoma, or immunosuppressive drug therapy, including high-dose steroids or radiation therapy *Note:* HIV positivity is *not* a contraindication to MMR except for those who are severely immunocompromised

Precautions:

- If blood, plasma, and/or immune globulin were given in past 11 mo, see ACIP recommendations regarding time to wait before vaccinating
- Moderate or severe acute illness
- History of thrombocytopenia or thrombocytopenic purpura

Note: If PPD (tuberculosis skin test) and MMR are both needed but not given on same day, delay PPD for 4–6 wk after MMR

Contraindications:

- Previous anaphylactic reaction to this vaccine or to any of its components

Precautions:

- Data on vaccination in pregnancy are limited; vaccination should be delayed until after completion of the pregnancy

Human papillomavirus (HPV)	■ All previously unvaccinated girls and women age 9–26 yr	■ Three doses are needed on a 0-, 2-, 6-mo schedule ■ The minimum interval between doses 1 and 2 is 4 wk and between doses 2 and 3 is 12 wk

Detailed Advisory Committee on Immunization Practices recommendations can be found at http://www.cdc.gov/vaccines/.
ACIP, Advisory Committee on Immunization Practices; CSF, cerebrospinal fluid; HbsAg, hepatitis B surface antigen; IM, intramuscular; MCV4, meningococcal conjugate vaccine; ; MMR, measles, mumps, rubella; MPSV, meningococcal polysaccharide vaccine; PPD, purified protein derivative; PPV23, 23-valent polysaccharide vaccine; SC, subcutaneous; STD, sexually transmitted disease.
Adapted from Immunization Action Coalition. Summary of recommendations for adult immunization, 2008, with permission. Available at: http://www.immunize.org/catg.d/p2011b.htm. Technical content of the Immunization Action Coalition table was reviewed by the Centers for Disease Control and Prevention.

TABLE 6.2

RECOMMENDED ADULT IMMUNIZATION SCHEDULE

Vaccine	Age 19–49 yr	Age 50–64 yr	Age ≥65 yr
Tetanus, diphtheria, pertussis (Td/Tdap)	1-dose Td booster every 10 yr		
	Substitute 1 dose of Tdap or Td		
Human papillomavirus (HPV)	3 doses (females up to 26 yr)		
Measles, mumps, rubella (MMR)	1 or 2 doses	1 dose	
Varicella	2 doses		
Influenza	1 dose annually	1 dose annually	
Pneumococcal polysaccharide (PPV23)	1 or 2 doses		1 dose
Hepatitis A	2 doses		
Hepatitis B	3 doses		
Meningococcal	1 or more doses		
Zoster			1 dose

Open boxes: For all persons in this category who meet the age requirements and who lack evidence of immunity. Shaded boxes: Recommended if some other risk factor is present (e.g., on the basis of medical, occupational, lifestyle, or other indications)
For detailed recommendations on all vaccines, refer to the text.
The zoster vaccine should not be administered to individuals who have never had chickenpox; such individuals should receive the varicella vaccine.
Adapted from U.S. Department of Health and Human Services, Centers for Disease Control and Prevention. Recommended adult immunization schedule by vaccine and age group, October 2007–September 2008.

symptoms may also occur. Severe complications such as anaphylactic shock occur in fewer than 1 in 1 million inoculations. Individuals with a high likelihood of having severe reactions can usually be identified before the administration of a specific agent. Although most people born in the United States receive standard immunizations during childhood, approximately 1 in 10 persons currently living in the United States was born in another country. Many of these people have been incompletely immunized.

GENERAL PRINCIPLES OF IMMUNIZATION (1–4)

Types of Immunization

Immunizations can be either *active* or *passive*.

Active Immunization

Active immunization entails the administration of a *vaccine* (live attenuated microorganisms, killed microorganisms, or purified proteins or polysaccharides of microorganisms) or a *toxoid* (a deactivated toxin). Active immunization often provides long-term (lasting for years or, less frequently, for life) protective immunity; however, meaningful immunity is often not achieved until 2 to 4 weeks after vaccination. Vaccines that are live attenuated versions of an infectious agent are usually more efficacious and provide longer-lasting immunity than do nonliving vaccines. Similarly, polysaccharide-based vaccines are in general less immunogenic than protein-based vaccines; how-

ever, the coupling of polysaccharide antigens to "carrier" proteins may markedly increase immunologic responses against polysaccharide components.

Passive Immunization

Passive immunization entails the administration of preformed antibody (such as immunoglobulin). Passive immunization results in immediate protective immunity, but such immunity is short term (usually lasting for only 3 to 6 months).

Administration

A host of strategies are available for administration.

Technique

With a few exceptions, most vaccines may be administered simultaneously. An adult can usually tolerate the administration of up to four vaccines (two vaccines administered separately in each deltoid area) in a given appointment. Adults should be vaccinated in the *deltoid area* of their upper extremities. Because of unreliable absorption, inoculations (other than certain immunoglobulin preparations) should not be administered in the gluteal region. A new syringe and needle should be used for each vaccination/immunization. If more than one live attenuated viral vaccine (e.g., measles, mumps, and rubella; varicella or herpes zoster; yellow fever) is indicated, the vaccines should be administered on the same day (at different injection sites) or at least 4 weeks apart. When live vaccines are administered on different days sooner than 4 weeks apart, immunologic responses may decrease.

Combining Passive and Active Immunization

Immunoglobulin preparations (and immunoglobulin-containing blood products) should not be administered with live viral vaccines when the immunoglobulin preparation contains antibodies directed against such viruses. If a patient requires both an immunoglobulin preparation and a live viral vaccine, the live viral vaccine should be administered at least 2 weeks before the immunoglobulin preparation (if possible). If the immunoglobulin preparation is administered first, 3 to 11 months (usually 3 to 6 months) should elapse before the live viral vaccine is administered. The duration of inhibition of a live viral vaccine is related to the dose of immunoglobulin given. (Specific recommendations can be found in Table 1.2, Health Information for International Travel 2008, "The Yellow Book.") Simultaneous administration of immunoglobulin preparations and all or any of the nonliving vaccines is not problematic. Persons with immunoglobulin A deficiency should not receive immunoglobulin preparations unless the risk of illness clearly outweighs the risk anaphylaxis.

Allergic Reactions

A person who has an anaphylactic reaction to *eggs* or *egg proteins* should not receive vaccines grown in chick-egg embryos or cell cultures. For special circumstances, vaccine desensitization protocols are available. Gastric or intestinal discomfort after eating eggs is not a contraindication to receiving these vaccines. Vaccines sometimes contain low levels of antibiotics that may trigger an allergic reaction. No vaccine that is available in the United States contains penicillin, so an allergy to penicillin does not contraindicate the use of any vaccine in the United States. However, the measles, mumps, and rubella (MMR), varicella, herpes zoster, and inactivated polio virus (IPV) vaccines do contain low levels of *neomycin;* individuals with a history of anaphylactic reactions to neomycin should not receive these vaccines. IPV should also not be administered to individuals with a history of anaphylactic reactions to *polymyxin B* or *streptomycin.*

If an individual has a history of a reaction to any vaccine, the repeated administration of that vaccine should be carefully weighed against the risk and severity of the illness in that individual and the severity of the previous reaction.

Vaccination during Pregnancy and Breast-Feeding

Generally, live attenuated viral vaccines should not be administered to pregnant women because of the theoretical risk of transmission of the vaccine virus to the fetus (Table 6.3). A woman who receives a live attenuated viral vaccine should be advised to avoid pregnancy for 1 month following MMR, varicella, herpes zoster, or yellow fever vaccination. Pregnancy in a household contact is not a contraindication to vaccine administration, except to varicella and herpes zoster vaccines if the pregnant woman is not immune to varicella (on theoretical grounds), or (also on theoretical grounds) live influenza vaccine if the pregnant woman did not receive the corresponding inactivated influenza vaccine at least 2 to 4 weeks previously. Most live vaccines have not been demonstrated to be secreted in breast milk. Only the rubella vaccine has been reported to be transmitted through breast milk, and this attenuated virus has not been known to be harmful in the nursing infant. Whether the varicella vaccine is excreted in human breast milk and, if so, whether the infant could be infected are not known. Therefore, varicella vaccine may be considered for a nursing mother. Breast-feeding is therefore not a contraindication to vaccine administration, with the exception of the smallpox vaccine.

Vaccination of Immunocompromised Persons

Severely immunocompromised persons should not receive vaccines of *live attenuated viruses* (Table 6.4). Moreover, an individual with an immunocompromised household contact should not receive the varicella, herpes zoster, or live attenuated influenza vaccine because person-to-person transmission may occur. The MMR vaccine, however, may be administered to individuals infected with the human immunodeficiency virus who are not severely immunocompromised. All vaccines of *inactivated viruses* may be safely administered to immunocompromised individuals, although immune responses may be less than optimal. Anecdotal historical reports associated administration of a tetanus toxoid–containing vaccine (the tetanus–diphtheria [Td] vaccine) with organ rejection in transplant recipients, but causality was not established, and organ transplantation is not considered a contraindication to receiving tetanus toxoid–containing vaccines.

Misconceptions about Contraindications

Mild or moderate *local reactions* to a previous vaccination (including tenderness, redness, or swelling at the injection site or a low-grade fever) are not contraindications to subsequent vaccination. Neither are mild respiratory, intestinal, or *flu-like illnesses, low-grade fever*, and a history of recent illness contraindications to vaccine administration. Current antibiotic therapy is a contraindication only to the administration of the oral typhoid vaccine (an attenuated bacterial strain that is killed by antibiotics); all other vaccines may be administered to an individual receiving antibiotics. With the exception of allergies to neomycin, streptomycin, or polymyxin B, allergies to antibiotics are not a contraindication to vaccine administration. For individuals in whom a vaccine is otherwise indicated, a history of seizures is not a contraindication to vaccine administration, nor is a history of a non–vaccine-associated chronic demyelinating condition (such as multiple sclerosis or Guillain-Barré syndrome); many such individuals are at increased risk for a number of vaccine-preventable illnesses. In light of recent reports of Guillain-Barré syndrome after receipt of the meningococcal conjugate vaccine (MCV4), persons with a history of Guillain-Barré syndrome who are not in a high-risk group for invasive meningococcal disease should not receive MCV4 until more data are available. Of note, current data are not sufficient to determine whether MCV increases the risk of Guillain-Barré syndrome in persons receiving the vaccine.

Record Keeping

The National Childhood Vaccine Injury Act of 1986 requires that all health care providers who administer MMR vaccines (in any combination), polio vaccines, or diphtheria, pertussis, and tetanus vaccines (in any combination) maintain immunization records and contact the Centers for Disease Control and Prevention (CDC) and the Food and Drug Administration (FDA) if an adverse reaction occurs (http://www.vaers.hhs.gov). This is true even if a vaccine is administered to an adult. Records should include the date,

TABLE 6.3

SUMMARY OF RECOMMENDATIONS ON IMMUNIZATION OF PREGNANT WOMEN

Vaccine	Should Be Considered If Otherwise Indicated	Contraindicated During Pregnancy	Comment
Routine			
Hepatitis A			Safety during pregnancy has not been determined; the risk associated with vaccination should be weighed against the risk for hepatitis A in pregnant women who may be at high risk for exposure
Hepatitis B	X		Pregnant women who are identified as being at risk for hepatitis B virus infection during pregnancy should be vaccinated
Human papillomavirus			Not recommended for use in pregnancy; if a woman is found to be pregnant after initiation of the vaccination series, the remainder of the three-dose regimen should be delayed until after completion of the pregnancy
Influenza (inactivated)	Recommended		
Influenza (live attenuated)*		X	
Measles*		X	
Meningococcal (MCV4)			No data are available on safety during pregnancy
Mumps*		X	
Pneumococcal (PPV23)			The safety of PPV23 during the first trimester of pregnancy has not been evaluated, although no adverse consequences have been reported among newborns whose mothers were inadvertently vaccinated during pregnancy
Polio (IPV)			Vaccination of pregnant women should be avoided on theoretical grounds
Rubella*		X	Rubella-susceptible women who are not vaccinated because they may be pregnant should be counseled about the risk for congenital rubella syndrome and the importance of being vaccinated as soon as they are no longer pregnant
Tetanus-diphtheria (Td)	X		Although no evidence exists that Td is teratogenic, waiting until the second trimester of pregnancy to administer Td is a reasonable precaution for minimizing any concern about the theoretical possibility of such reactions
Tetanus-diphtheria-pertussis (Tdap)			ACIP recommends Td when tetanus and diphtheria protection is required during pregnancy; health care providers can choose to administer Tdap instead of Td to add protection against pertussis in situations with increased risk for pertussis: pregnant adolescents, pregnant health care personnel, pregnant child care providers, or pregnant women employed in an institution or living in a community with increased pertussis activity; when Tdap is administered during pregnancy, the second or third trimester is preferred
Varicella*		X	
Zoster		X	
Travel and Other			
Herpes zoster*		X	
Japanese encephalitis (JE)			Pregnant women who must travel to an area where risk of JE is high should be vaccinated when the theoretical risks of immunization are outweighed by the risk of infection to the mother and developing fetus
Meningococcal (MPSV)	X		Studies of vaccination with MPSV during pregnancy have not documented adverse effects among either pregnant women or newborns
Rabies	X		Pregnancy is not considered a contraindication to postexposure prophylaxis; if the risk of exposure to rabies is substantial, preexposure prophylaxis might also be indicated during pregnancy
Typhoid (parenteral and oral*)			No data have been reported on the use of any of the typhoid vaccines among pregnant women
Yellow fever*		X	The safety of yellow fever vaccination during pregnancy has not been established, and the vaccine should be administered only if travel to an endemic area is unavoidable and if an increased risk for exposure exists; if international travel requirements are the only reason to vaccinate a pregnant woman rather than an increased risk of infection, efforts should be made to obtain a waiver letter

ACIP, Advisory Committee on Immunization Practices.
Asterisk indicates a live attenuated vaccine. Generally, live-virus vaccines are contraindicated for pregnant women because of the theoretical risk of transmission of the vaccine virus to the fetus. If a live-virus vaccine is inadvertently given to a pregnant woman or if a woman becomes pregnant within 4 wk after vaccination, she should be counseled about the potential effects on the fetus. Vaccination is not ordinarily an indication to terminate the pregnancy. Women should be counseled to avoid pregnancy for 4 wk after vaccination with a live-virus vaccine.
Adapted from U.S. Department of Health and Human Services, Centers for Disease Control and Prevention. Guidelines for vaccinating pregnant women, 2008.

TABLE 6.4

SUMMARY OF ADVISORY COMMITTEE ON IMMUNIZATION PRACTICES RECOMMENDATIONS ON IMMUNIZATION OF ADULTS WITH MEDICAL CONDITIONS

	Congenital Immunodeficiency, Leukemia, Lymphoma, Generalized Malignancy, Cerebrospinal Fluid Leaks; Therapy with Alkylating Agents, Antimetabolites, Radiation, or High-Dose, Long-Term Corticosteroids	Diabetes, Heart Disease, Chronic Pulmonary Disease, Chronic Alcoholism	Asplenia (Including Elective Splenectomy and Terminal Complement Component Deficiencies)	Chronic Liver Disease, Recipients of Clotting Factor Concentrates	Kidney Failure, End-Stage Renal Disease, Recipients of Hemodialysis	Human Immunodeficiencies Virus CD4 and T Lymphocyte Count < 200 cells/μl	Human Immunodeficiencies Virus CD4 and T Lymphocyte Count ≥ 200 cells/μl	Health Care Workers
Tetanus, diphtheria, pertussis (Td/Tdap)	R	R	R	R	R	R	R	R
Human papillomavirus	R	R	R	R	R	R	R	R
Measles, mumps, rubella	C	R	R	R	R	C	R	R
Varicella	C	R	R	R	R	C	R	R
Influenza (inactivated)[a]	R	R	I	R	R	C	R	R
Pneumococcal polysaccharide	R	R	R	R	R	R	R	I
Hepatitis A	I	I	I	R	I	I	I	I
Hepatitis B	I	I	I	R	R	R	R	R
Meningococcal	I	I	R	I	I	I	I	I
Zoster	C	R	R	R	R	C	R	R

C, contraindicated; I, recommended if another risk factor is present; R, recommended for all persons in this category who meet the age requirements and who lack evidence of immunity.

The zoster vaccine should not be administered to individuals who have never had chicken pox; such individuals should receive the varicella vaccine.

[a] The inactivated influenza vaccine is preferred over the live attenuated vaccine for use in individuals with chronic medical conditions or with immune compromise or in health care workers.

Adapted from U.S. Department of Health and Human Services, Centers for Disease Control and Prevention. Recommended adult immunization schedule, by vaccine and medical and other indications, October 2007–September 2008.

name of the vaccine, manufacturer, lot number, inoculation site, route of administration, and name of the person administering the vaccine. All clinically significant postvaccination reactions should be reported, not just those required by law. Federal law also requires the distribution of vaccine information statements (VIS) to persons (even adults) receiving certain vaccines (MMR, polio, diphtheria, pertussis, and tetanus vaccines in any combination). VIS can be accessed at http://www.cdc.gov/vaccines/pubs/vis/default.htm or http://www.immunize.org/vis (VIS sheets are available in approximately 30 languages).

SPECIFIC IMMUNIZATION PROGRAMS (1–4)

Tetanus

Despite the fact that almost half of all individuals older than 60 years of age lack protective levels of serum anti–tetanus toxin antibodies, fewer than 100 cases of tetanus occur each year in the United States. Almost all cases of tetanus reported in the United States occur in adults who did not complete a primary tetanus immunization series or who did not receive appropriate treatment for a tetanus-prone wound. Prevention of tetanus should, therefore, concentrate on primary vaccination and proper postexposure immunization (Table 6.5); immigrants and elderly persons are most likely not to have received a primary immunization series.

The antitetanus vaccines contain a formaldehyde-treated toxoid (detoxified toxin). Tetanus toxoid is available as a single-antigen preparation, combined with diphtheria toxoid as a pediatric vaccine (DT) or an adult vaccine (Td), and combined with both diphtheria toxoid and acellular pertussis vaccine (DTaP or Tdap for pediatric and adult vaccines, respectively). Pediatric formulations (DT and DTaP) contain a similar amount of tetanus toxoid as adult Td but contain three to four times as much diphtheria toxoid (letter capitalization denotes a higher quantity of that antigen). In adults, Td or Tdap should be administered rather than tetanus toxoid alone because of the additional coverage provided against diphtheria and per-

tussis. It is recommended that all adults receive a Td vaccine every 10 years following a primary series. Adults aged 19 to 64 years, particularly postpartum women, household or close contacts of children less than 1 year of age, and health care personnel, should receive a single dose of Tdap to replace Td for booster immunization if they have not previously received Tdap. Tdap is currently licensed for one-dose administration. The more common reactions to Td and Tdap vaccines include erythema, induration, and tenderness at the inoculation site. Appropriate postexposure antitetanus prophylaxis is required regardless of vaccination regimen (Table 6.5).

Adults who require a primary antitetanus series should receive an intramuscular dose of Tdap, to be followed by subsequent immunizations with Td at 4 weeks and then again 6 to 12 months after the second inoculation. There is no need to repeat doses if the schedule is interrupted.

Diphtheria

In the United States, diphtheria in adults is rare (fewer than 10 cases per year), especially among adults who have received a complete primary series, even if it has been more than 10 years since the administration of a diphtheria booster. More than half of American adults lack protective levels of anti–diphtheria toxin antibodies. Unfortunately, diphtheria remains endemic in many parts of the world, and in 1990 to 1995 there were large outbreaks in the states of the former Soviet Union. International travelers should receive Tdap (or Td) vaccine if it has been longer than 10 years since their last booster antidiphtheria immunization. Diphtheria antitoxin of equine origin may be used to treat diphtheria.

Pertussis

Pertussis is an acute, infectious cough illness that remains endemic in the United States despite longstanding routine childhood pertussis vaccination. Infants less than 12 months of age are more likely to suffer from pertussis-related morbidity and mortality than older age groups. Adults presenting with a severe or persistent cough should be suspected of having pertussis infection (see Chapter 52). Because the number of reported

---

TABLE 6.5

WOUND MANAGEMENT AFTER EXPOSURE: TETANUS

History of Tetanus Toxoid (Doses)	Clean, Minor Wound		All Other Wounds[a]	
	Tdap, Td, or DTaP[b]	TIG[c]	Tdap, Td, or DTaP[b]	TIG[c]
Unknown or <3	Yes	No	Yes	Yes
≥3[d]	No[e]	No	No[f]	No

DtaP, tetanus-diphtheria-pertussis, pediatric; Td, tetanus-diphtheria; Tdap, tetanus-diphtheria-pertussis, adult; TIG, tetanus immunoglobulin.
[a] Such as, but not limited to, wounds contaminated with dirt, feces, soil, and saliva; puncture wounds and avulsions; and wounds resulting from missiles, crushing, burns, or frostbite.
[b] Tdap is preferred to Td for adolescents and adults aged 11–64 yr who have never received Tdap. Td is preferred to tetanus toxoid for adults who received Tdap previously or when Tdap is not available. DTaP is indicated for children <7 yr old.
[c] Equine tetanus antitoxin should be used when TIG is not available.
[d] If only three doses of toxoid have been received, a fourth dose of toxoid, preferably an adsorbed toxoid, should be given.
[e] Yes, if >10 yr since last tetanus toxoid–containing vaccine dose.
[f] Yes, if >5 yr since last tetanus toxoid–containing vaccine dose.
Adapted from Centers for Disease Control and Prevention. Health information for international travel ["The yellow book"]. Atlanta: U.S. Department of Health and Human Services, Public Health Service, 2008.

pertussis cases has steadily increased in adolescents and adults in the United States since the 1980s, a single booster immunization with the acellular pertussis vaccine in combination with the tetanus and diphtheria toxoids (Tdap) is now recommended for adults aged 19 to 64 years of age. Postpartum women and other adults who anticipate close contact with an infant less than 12 months of age should be particularly targeted to receive Tdap. An interval of 2 years from the last dose of Td is suggested to reduce the risk for local and systemic reactions after vaccination; however, shorter intervals may be used. Two formulations of Tdap are available. Adacel (sanofi pasteur) is licensed for use in persons age 11 to 64 years; Boostrix (GlaxoSmithKline) is licensed for use in adolescents but not among persons 19 years or older.

Measles, Mumps, and Rubella

Measles and rubella (MR); measles, mumps, and rubella (MMR); and measles, mumps, rubella, and varicella (MMRV) vaccines are available (the latter is only approved for use in children 12 months to 12 years of age). Adults immune to one or more components of the combination vaccines may still receive the MMR vaccine. The MMR vaccines (in any combination) should not be administered to pregnant women or to severely immunocompromised persons; women of childbearing age should be cautioned to avoid pregnancy for 1 month after vaccination. Individuals with a history of severe allergic reaction to eggs should not receive vaccines containing measles or mumps components, nor should the vaccine be administered to individuals with anaphylactic reactions to neomycin. Individuals who have received immunoglobulin preparations or blood or blood products in the preceding 3 to 11 months may not generate adequate immune responses to vaccination.

Measles

In most circumstances, use of the MMR vaccine is preferred. Persons born before 1957 in the United States are assumed to be immune to measles because of the very high likelihood of exposure; such persons do not require serologic evaluation for antibody unless they are health care workers. In the United States, measles is no longer an indigenous disease. Almost all cases are primarily or secondarily related to travel or importation. After a single inoculation of the live attenuated measles vaccine (in any combination), protective antibody levels develop in approximately 90% to 95% of individuals. The remaining 5% to 10% remain at risk for measles. A second dose of the vaccine will result in protective immunity in almost all of these individuals. Those immunized between 1963 and 1967 may have received an inactivated measles vaccine and should receive the live viral vaccine.

Preexposure Immunization. Because of a resurgence of measles, it is recommended that persons born after 1956 who are attending *postsecondary educational institutions*, who are *health care professionals*, or who are *traveling to a foreign country* receive two doses of live attenuated MMR vaccine (or live attenuated measles monovalent vaccine), separated by at least 1 month, unless they have a physician-documented case of measles or serologic confirmation of measles antibody. Many secondary schools now require documentation of two vaccinations against measles. It is more cost-effective to administer the two doses of the vaccine to all individuals than to screen patients for a serologic response after a single vaccination.

Postexposure Prophylaxis. A susceptible individual exposed to someone with measles should receive intramuscular *immunoglobulin* (0.25 mL/kg, maximum of 15 mL) followed 6 months later by live measles vaccine. Administration of immunoglobulin may prevent or modify infection if given within 6 days of exposure. The vaccine itself may afford some protection if administered within 72 hours of exposure. Postexposure immunoglobulin should also be administered to severely immunocompromised individuals exposed to active measles (regardless of immunization history). Because measles vaccination may temporarily suppress tuberculin reactivity, any tuberculosis skin testing should be performed on the day of vaccination or at least 4 to 6 weeks later.

Mumps

In 2006, a multistate mumps outbreak began that has to date resulted in more than 6,000 reported cases in the United States. Many cases have occurred among college students who had received one or two doses of MMR vaccine. Mumps vaccination is indicated for adults born after 1956 who have not received at least one live mumps vaccine, have not had a physician-documented case of mumps, or who lack serologic evidence of immunity. A second dose of mumps vaccine is now recommended for school-age children and for adults at high risk of exposure, including health care personnel, international travelers, and students at post–high school educational institutions. The combined MMR vaccine is recommended for both doses. Administration of immunoglobulin or vaccine after exposure to mumps has not been documented to be of clinical efficacy.

Rubella

Protective immunity develops in almost all individuals after a single vaccination with a live attenuated rubella vaccine. Routine vaccination with MMR is sufficient in almost all cases. Because rubella causes considerable morbidity if acquired during pregnancy, special emphasis should be placed on identifying susceptible women of childbearing age (especially among immigrant populations). Susceptible women should receive the rubella vaccine before they become pregnant or after they have delivered. Health care workers without antibody evidence of immunity should also be immunized. The vaccine is well tolerated, although mild and transient arthralgias or arthritis may occur.

Polio

In the United States, the parenterally administered *inactivated polio vaccine* (IPV) has replaced the live *oral polio vaccine* (OPV) because the approximately 5 to 10 cases of poliomyelitis that occurred each year in the United States following eradication of wild-type polio were caused by OPV (risk in recipients or household contacts of recipients was 1 per 500,000 first doses administered). IPV does not cause poliomyelitis. Although OPV is not commercially available in the United States, it is still commonly used in many countries, and although the World Health Organization (WHO) has targeted polio for eradication, it is still active in a number of regions (especially southern Asia and sub-Saharan Africa). As such, paralytic poliomyelitis could recur in epidemic fashion in the United States if population-based immunity is allowed to wane.

Routine polio vaccination of adults in the United States is not recommended. Individuals planning to travel to Africa or areas of Asia should have completed a primary series within 10 years or completed a primary series and received at least one booster immunization as an adult. The clinical efficacy of additional boosters is unknown. *Laboratory workers* and *health care professionals* who are exposed to wild-type polio virus should also be vaccinated. A three-vaccine primary series of IPV may be administered to an adult at 0 and at 4 to 8 weeks and at least 4 weeks (preferably 6 to 12 months) after the second inoculation.

Contraindications

IPV should not be administered to individuals with a history of anaphylactic reactions to streptomycin, polymyxin B, or neomycin. A prior episode of polio (caused by one strain of polio virus) is not a contraindication to receiving IPV (protective against three strains of polio virus).

Influenza

Approximately 20,000 to 50,000 people die of influenza each year in the United States. Most of these deaths occur in persons 65 years of age or older, with those having cardiopulmonary conditions at greatest risk. Two versions of the influenza vaccine exist. A parenteral vaccine is composed of inactivated viruses formulated yearly to include two influenza virus type A strains and one type B strain. Contrary to popular belief, this vaccine does not cause influenza. In young adults, the vaccine is quite effective at reducing the severity of clinical illness and time lost from work. In older persons, there is a 30% to 40% reduction in overall clinical illness and a decrease in pneumonia, hospitalization, and deaths from influenza. Despite these benefits, vaccination rates fall short. A live attenuated influenza virus vaccine has also been approved for use in the United States (FluMist, MedImmune). It is administered intranasally and has only been approved for use in individuals 2 to 49 years of age who are not immunocompromised (i.e., the population least at risk of severe complications of influenza).

Indications and Timing

The influenza vaccine is recommended for all individuals older than the age of 50 years. Pregnant women and individuals with chronic illness, including cardiopulmonary disease, diabetes, renal dysfunction, immunosuppression, and other disorders that compromise respiratory function, should also receive annual vaccination, regardless of age. The vaccine can also be offered to anyone who wishes to avoid the flu, including close contacts of persons at high risk for complications of influenza. In the continental United States, administration should be between October and mid-November, but the vaccine may be administered at any time during the flu season. Although the influenza season is usually well defined in the temperate United States, influenza outbreaks occur at different times throughout the world. Influenza is most common from April to September in the temperate Southern Hemisphere and occurs year-round in the tropics. Protection begins 1 to 2 weeks after inoculation and continues for 6 months. The duration of protective immunity in frail, elderly, or immunocompromised individuals may be shorter. During a community outbreak of influenza, drugs effective against influenza viruses may have a useful adjunctive role (see Chapter 52).

Side Effects and Contraindications

Transient low-grade fever, myalgia, and malaise may occur after immunization with the inactivated vaccine. Individuals with a history of influenza vaccine–associated Guillain-Barré syndrome should not receive the inactivated influenza vaccine; no instances of Guillain-Barré syndrome have been reported among recipients of the live attenuated vaccine. The risk of the influenza vaccine in individuals with a history of Guillain-Barré syndrome not associated with influenza vaccination is controversial. Such persons may be at high risk for severe influenza. Neither the live attenuated nor the inactivated influenza vaccines should be administered to individuals with a history of anaphylactic reactions to eggs or egg products. The live attenuated vaccine should not be used in immunosuppressed and pregnant individuals or their household contacts or in those with asthma, reactive airways disease, or other chronic pulmonary diseases. Due to the risk of transmission, individuals who receive the live attenuated influenza virus vaccine should avoid contact with immunocompromised individuals for at least 2 weeks.

Avian Influenza

Water-birds are the natural reservoir of influenza viruses. Avian influenza viruses may cross the species barrier to infect humans, either directly or through intermediate hosts such as pigs. A global outbreak of highly pathogenic avian influenza caused by H5N1 virus is in progress. H5N1 has caused the deaths of millions of birds and has also been associated with isolated cases of human disease and death, particularly in Asia and the Middle East. Limited, inefficient, and unsustained human-to-human spread of H5N1 has occurred, but there is concern that the virus could gain the capacity to infect and spread between humans more easily. Vaccines produced annually for seasonal influenza will not protect against such newly emergent viral strains. An inactivated monovalent two-dose H5N1 influenza virus vaccine has been developed for use in persons 18 to 64 years of age. This vaccine is being purchased and stockpiled exclusively by governments and health agencies in preparation for a possible response to a global pandemic of H5N1 influenza.

Pneumococcal Pneumonia

More than 50,000 cases and more than 4,000 deaths due to invasive pneumococcal disease are estimated to occur annually in the United States. At least half of these deaths occur in adults who had an indication for pneumococcal vaccination. The current pneumococcal polysaccharide vaccine for adult administration (PPV23, Pneumovax 23, Merck) contains capsular polysaccharide components of 23 pneumococcal types; these account for approximately 80% to 90% of invasive pneumococcal infections and include the six serotypes most frequently associated with antibiotic resistance. Because antibiotic resistance is rapidly rising, immunization is of increasing importance. A pneumococcal seven-valent vaccine conjugated to diphtheria CRM 197 protein (PCV7, Prevnar, Wyeth) is also licensed for use in children in the United States. Since the introduction of PCV7 in 2000, the rate of invasive pneumococcal disease due to vaccine serotypes in children younger than 5 years of age has declined by 94%, and among adults, invasive pneumococcal disease has decreased by more than 50%, suggesting herd immunity attributable to the use of PCV7 in children.

Efficacy

PPV23 reduces the incidence of pneumococcal bacteremia and pneumonia among individuals who are able to generate a good antibody response. Overall, the vaccine is 60% to 80% effective at preventing bacteremia. It has not been shown to decrease mortality. Efficacy in immunosuppressed individuals is less well defined.

Indications

Severe disease is most likely to develop in persons older than 65 years of age and those with cardiopulmonary disease, immunocompromise, diabetes, alcoholism, or hepatic or renal failure, and such individuals should receive the vaccine. The vaccine should be administered at least 2 weeks before elective splenectomy or immunosuppression (if possible). Alaskan natives, African American adults, and certain Native American populations are also at increased risk. As of 2003, it was estimated that only 64% of the elderly have been vaccinated with PPV23. Hospitalization represents an opportunity to vaccinate high-risk persons, and coadministration (at different sites) with influenza vaccine should also be considered because the target groups for the two vaccines overlap.

Because not all persons manifest a full antibody response on first vaccination and because antibody levels may decline with time, a single booster vaccination is recommended if 5 or more years have elapsed since first vaccination and if first immunization occurred before 65 years of age, although the utility of booster vaccination has not been definitively established.

Safety

PPV23 is safe; most reactions are minor and occur at the inoculation site. Severe allergic reactions are rare but might become more frequent with subsequent immunization. Pneumococcal and influenza vaccines may be administered at separate inoculation sites during a single office visit.

Haemophilus influenzae Infection

Before the introduction of the *Haemophilus influenzae* type b conjugate vaccine (Hib), most cases of invasive *H. influenzae* disease in children were caused by *H. influenzae* capsular type b, but with the application of Hib vaccine, most cases now represent non–type b disease. A number of Hib vaccines are available, all linking a polysaccharide molecule (polyribosyl-ribotol phosphate) to a carrier protein to increase immunogenicity. The vaccine is often administered to individuals with functional or anatomic asplenia or immunoglobulin deficiencies because such persons have a higher incidence of invasive disease caused by encapsulated organisms. However, definitive benefit has not been established in these individuals, perhaps because many already have humoral immunity against *H. influenzae* type b organisms.

Meningococcal Disease

Meningococcal disease is endemic throughout the world, and large epidemics may occur globally. In the United States, meningococcal infection is usually caused by *Neisseria meningitidis* serogroup B or C and occurs as isolated cases or as small outbreaks. Two meningococcal vaccines are available for use in the United States. The meningococcal polysaccharide vaccine (MPSV, Menomune, sanofi pasteur) is quadrivalent for serogroups A, C, Y, and W-135. In 2005, a meningococcal conjugate vaccine (MCV, Menactra, sanofi pasteur) that contains *N. meningitidis* serogroups A, C, Y, and W-135 capsular polysaccharide antigens individually conjugated to diphtheria toxoid protein was licensed for use among persons aged 11 to 55 years. The conjugate vaccine is expected to provide a longer duration of protection than MPSV and to reduce asymptomatic carriage of *N. meningitidis*, and it is replacing the pure polysaccharide vaccine.

Indications and Timing

Routine immunization of young adolescents aged 11 to 12 years with MCV is recommended, with catch-up vaccination before high school entry for those who have not previously been immunized. Meningococcal vaccination is recommended for those at increased risk of meningococcal disease, including persons with anatomic or functional asplenia and those with terminal complement deficiencies. In addition, the vaccine should be recommended for travelers who visit certain areas of the world during "meningitis season" (e.g., the Sahel region of sub-Saharan Africa during the dry winter months, December through June) or who will visit an area of the world experiencing a meningococcal outbreak. Saudi Arabia requires documentation of meningococcal vaccination from individuals entering the country on religious pilgrimage. MCV is preferred for routine vaccination of adolescents and for those at increased risk of meningococcal disease. MPSV is an acceptable alternative for individuals aged 11 to 55 years when MCV is not available. Both vaccines are well tolerated; most adverse reactions are mild and local. The need for booster vaccination after MPSV is not well characterized but may be indicated for those individuals who remain at high risk for infection. Revaccination may be considered 3 to 5 years after receipt of the first dose of MPSV, and MCV should be used for revaccination of those aged 11 to 55 years. Revaccination after receipt of MCV is not recommended.

Safety

As of September 2006, 15 confirmed cases of Guillain-Barré syndrome (GBS) occurring in persons 11 to 19 years of age following receipt of the MCV vaccine had been reported to the CDC. Data are insufficient to determine whether MCV increases the risk of GBS among recipients of the vaccine, particularly because the expected background population rates of GBS are not precisely known. Postlicensure surveillance is ongoing, and the CDC recommends continuation of current vaccination strategies. However, until this issue is clarified, persons with a history of GBS who are not in a high-risk group for invasive meningococcal disease should not receive MCV. Such individuals at high risk should receive MPSV instead.

Human Papilloma Virus

Genital infection with human papilloma virus (HPV) is the most common sexually transmitted infection in the United States. The majority of infections cause no clinical symptoms and are self-limited; however, persistent infection with oncogenic types of the virus (types 16 and 18 in >70% of cases) may result in cervical cancer. HPV infection is also the cause of other anogenital cancers and genital warts. A quadrivalent vaccine (Gardasil, Merck) prepared from HPV types 6, 11, 16, and 18 was recently licensed in the United States. The vaccine is effective in preventing persistent HPV infection, cervical cancer precursor lesions, vaginal and vulvar cancer precursor lesions, and genital warts caused by the HPV types included in the vaccine among females who have not already been infected with the respective HPV type. Longer-term follow-up is in progress to ascertain whether these promising results translate into prevention of cervical cancer and related deaths.

Indications and Timing

The HPV vaccine should be given in a three-dose series, with the second and third doses administered 2 and 6 months, respectively, after the first dose. The Advisory Committee on Immunization Practices (ACIP) recommends routine vaccination of girls aged 11 to 12 years. Vaccine can be administered to those as young as age 9 years, and catch-up immunization is recommended for females aged 13 to 26 years who have not been previously vaccinated. HPV vaccination is not a substitute for routine cervical cancer screening because not all HPV types that cause cervical cancer are included in the vaccine. The HPV vaccine is not licensed for use in males; efficacy studies regarding the use of HPV vaccine in males are ongoing.

Varicella (Chickenpox)

The complication rate of primary varicella infection (*chickenpox*) is higher in adults than in children; pneumonitis, hepatitis, encephalitis, and death are more frequent. Approximately 5% of American adults are not immune; the rate is higher among those born outside the United States. Since the varicella vaccine became a routine vaccine of childhood, the incidence of varicella infection has fallen rapidly in the United States. The varicella vaccine is a live attenuated viral vaccine that is most immunogenic in children (Varivax, Merck). The vaccine is administered twice, the second inoculation 4 to 8 weeks after the first. The vaccine is not completely protective, but a 70% reduction in the expected number of cases is achieved. When the vaccine is administered to adults who have a high frequency of exposure (through a household contact), approximately 27% of adults report breakthrough chickenpox but of a mild nature. The efficacy of the vaccine for protection against the complications of chickenpox (including encephalitis, hepatitis, and pneumonitis) has not been assessed, but it may well be protective. The need for booster vaccination has not been established.

Indications

The vaccine should be administered to all adults without evidence of immunity. The majority of adults who do not report a history of chickenpox have serologic evidence of a previous episode of varicella. The serum of adults who deny a previous episode of chickenpox should be screened for antivaricella antibodies. The vaccine should not be administered to immunocompromised individuals or to pregnant women. Women who receive the vaccine should be advised to avoid pregnancy for 1 month after receiving it. Individuals who have received immunoglobulin preparations or blood or blood products within the previous 3 to 11 months may not adequately respond to the vaccine. The vaccine should not be administered to individuals with an anaphylactic reaction to neomycin. The vaccine requires storage at a temperature below −15°C.

Adverse Effects

The vaccine is well tolerated by most individuals. Common reactions are local in nature: A temperature of 37.7°C (100°F) or higher will develop in approximately 10% of individuals after the first or second vaccination; 25% to 30% will complain of local erythema, tenderness, and swelling at the inoculation site; in 3%, a *localized varicella-like rash* will develop at the injection site after the first inoculation, and such a rash will develop after the second inoculation in approximately 1%. Rashes occur 1 to 3 weeks after inoculation. A *generalized varicella-like rash* may occur in 3% to 5% after the first inoculation and in 1% after the second. The median number of lesions in such individuals is five.

Precautions

The vaccine strain of the virus has been *transmitted* to susceptible contacts. Persons receiving vaccine should avoid contact with immunocompromised individuals who lack immunity to varicella and with susceptible pregnant women. The manufacturer advises that such precautions be taken for 6 weeks after inoculation and that vaccinated individuals avoid contact with newborn infants of mothers who lack a documented history of chickenpox or laboratory evidence of prior varicella. The manufacturer also advises that *salicylate products* not be administered for 6 weeks after vaccination because of the theoretical risk of *Reye's syndrome*. In a number of individuals who have received the varicella vaccine, *herpes zoster infection* (shingles) has subsequently developed. In some of these cases, viral cultures disclosed the presence of wild-type varicella virus, demonstrating the incomplete protective efficacy of the vaccine.

Postexposure Prophylaxis

If susceptible pregnant or immunocompromised individuals are exposed to varicella, they should ideally receive intramuscular *varicella zoster immunoglobulin* (VZIG) (125 U/10 kg; maximum dose, 625 U), although there have been recent supply and availability issues with VZIG. For susceptible individuals who are neither immunocompromised nor pregnant, postexposure use of the varicella vaccine may be beneficial. The varicella vaccine appears to be effective in preventing chickenpox and in reducing the severity of the disease if used within 3 and possibly up to 5 days after exposure. The vaccine should not be administered concomitantly with varicella immunoglobulin.

Herpes Zoster (Shingles)

Reactivation of latent varicella infection results in herpes zoster (shingles). Aging and immunosuppression are associated with recurrent disease, and 10% to 20% of individuals with a history of varicella may develop shingles at some point during their life. Herpes zoster typically manifests as a unilateral vesicular eruption in the distribution of a sensory nerve, but generalized skin lesions and central nervous system, pulmonary, and hepatic involvement may also occur in immunocompromised persons. Zostavax (Merck), a preparation of the live attenuated varicella vaccine formulated for the prevention of shingles, was licensed for use in the United States in 2006. Use of the herpes zoster vaccine among individuals of age 60 years and older has been shown to reduce the incidence of herpes zoster and postherpetic neuralgia. Efficacy of the vaccine corresponds with age at immunization. In prelicensure studies, administration of the herpes zoster vaccine was associated with a 66% reduction in zoster-related illness in individuals 60 to 70 years of age and a 55% reduction in individuals older than 70 years of age over a mean of 3 years of follow-up.

Indications

Recommendations for the use of the herpes zoster vaccine are in development. The ACIP provisionally recommends a single dose of the herpes zoster vaccine for immunocompetent adults 60 years of age and older, whether or not they report a prior episode of herpes zoster. Persons with chronic medical conditions may be vaccinated unless a contraindication exists for their condition. The vaccine should not be administered to immunocompromised individuals.

Precautions

The zoster vaccine contains more than 10 times the amount of live attenuated varicella virus as does the varicella vaccine. The zoster vaccine should not be administered to individuals who have never had varicella (chickenpox); such individuals should receive the varicella vaccine.

Hepatitis B

Hepatitis B vaccines contain recombinant, noninfectious hepatitis B surface antigen. Two monovalent hepatitis B vaccines are available in the United States: Engerix-B (GlaxoSmithKline Kline) and Recombivax HB (Merck). They may be used interchangeably, even in a primary inoculation. A combination hepatitis B and hepatitis A vaccine is also available (Twinrix, Glaxo SmithKline). Three doses of hepatitis B antigen–containing vaccine induce protective antibodies in more than 90% of healthy young adults. Antibody responses decline with increasing age and are lower in immunocompromised individuals.

Indications

Because it has been difficult to carry out vaccination among many high-risk groups, immunization against hepatitis B has been introduced in the *standard childhood vaccine series*. Nonetheless, high-risk unvaccinated adults should still be offered vaccination, especially individuals likely to comply, such as those with occupational or other exposure to blood or body fluids and the household and sexual contacts of hepatitis B virus carriers. Other high-risk groups include intravenous drug users, those with multiple sexual partners, men who have sex with men, and individuals with a recent history of a sexually transmitted disease. The hepatitis B vaccine should be considered for long-term overseas travelers, especially for those who may be exposed to blood or bodily secretions through employment or sexual contact. The prevalence of hepatitis B infection is much higher, and the carrier state and chronic active hepatitis are much more frequent, in Asia, Africa, and Latin America than in the United States.

Postexposure Prophylaxis

Postexposure prophylaxis should be administered to individuals with mucous membrane or percutaneous exposure to blood or bodily secretions of individuals known or suspected of being acutely infected with hepatitis B or of being a hepatitis B carrier. Intramuscular hepatitis B immunoglobulin (0.06 mL/kg) should be administered immediately after exposure, ideally within 6 days. The vaccine series should also be started.

Administration

The vaccines may be administered to adults in three doses (usually at 0, 1, and 6 months), although other vaccination regimens may be employed. The Engerix-B vaccine may also be administered at 0, 1, 2, and 12 months; this accelerated regimen results in a more rapid increase in the serum anti–hepatitis B response. The Recombivax HB vaccine is approved as a two-dose series given 4 to 6 months apart in adolescents of age 11 to 15 years, and Twinrix is approved not only for administration at 0, 1, 6 months, but also for an accelerated schedule of 0, 7 and 21 to 30 days, followed by a booster dose at 12 months. Larger anti–hepatitis B vaccine doses (two to four times the normal adult dose) or an increased number of doses are required to induce protective antibody in many hemodialysis patients and may also be necessary in other immunocompromised persons. The hepatitis B vaccines should routinely be administered intramuscularly in adults in the deltoid muscle; injection in the buttock has been associated with a lower antibody response.

Postimmunization Serologic Testing

Postimmunization serologic testing for hepatitis B surface antibody should be performed in individuals who are immunocompromised, 30 years of age or older when they receive the vaccine, or at high risk for ongoing exposure to hepatitis B, including health care workers. Those who do not respond to the vaccine should repeat the complete three-dose inoculation series (rebooting); serum should then be rechecked for antibody. Those who remain serologically negative after administration of six hepatitis B vaccines should be considered "nonimmune." Such persons may be chronically infected with hepatitis B, and their serum should be tested for hepatitis B surface antigen. Routine rebooting or serologic evaluation of individuals who respond to the vaccine is not recommended. Hemodialysis patients should receive a primary series and should have anti–hepatitis B surface antigen antibody responses measured annually. Booster immunizations should be administered to these individuals if the anti–hepatitis B surface antigen antibody level declines to less than 10 mIU/mL.

Adverse Effects

The hepatitis B vaccines are well tolerated, with a mild local reaction at the injection site being the most common adverse event. The risk for Guillain-Barré syndrome or multiple sclerosis is not increased.

Hepatitis A

The ACIP recommends routine immunization of children with two doses of hepatitis A vaccine beginning at 1 year of age. Vaccination should also be considered for high-risk groups (e.g., men who have sex with men, users of illegal drugs, those regularly receiving clotting factor transfusions, and persons with chronic liver disease). Food handlers and day care workers should also consider vaccination. The vaccine is also frequently administered before travel to countries other than major industrialized nations.

Preparations and Administration

Two versions of the monovalent vaccine are available in the United States: Havrix (GlaxoSmithKline) and Vaqta (Merck). The vaccines are administered to adults in a two-dose primary series at 0 and 6 to 12 months (HAVRIX) or at 0 and 6 to 18 months (VAQTA). A three-dose series for children and adolescents is also available. Protective antibody levels that persist for 6 to 12 months are achieved in more than 95% of recipients after a single dose. Protective levels that last for more than 10 years can be induced with the second immunization.

Individuals who require immediate and full protection have historically received *immunoglobulin* intramuscularly (0.02 mL/kg if short-term protection of 1 to 2 months is required, and 0.06 mL/kg if long-term protection of 3 to 5 months is required). Recent data suggest that administration of hepatitis A vaccine may not be inferior to gamma globulin when given to healthy 2–40 year olds. Hepatitis A vaccine and immunoglobulin may also be administered simultaneously at distinct inoculation sites. Individuals who have been exposed to a person with hepatitis A (e.g., close household or sexual contact of an individual with active hepatitis A, restaurant outbreak) should receive *postexposure prophylaxis* with either intramuscular immunoglobulin (0.02 mL/kg), or, if otherwise healthy and are

2–40 years of age, with hepatitis A vaccine. Immunoglobulin prophylaxis given more than 2 weeks after exposure is unlikely to be of benefit and is not indicated. A combination hepatitis A and hepatitis B vaccine is available in the United States (Twinrix, GlaxoSmithKline). It is administered at 0, 1, and 6 months or on an accelerated schedule of 0, 7, and 21 to 30 days, followed by a booster dose at 12 months. This combination vaccine contains half the amount of inactivated hepatitis A virus as monovalent hepatitis A vaccine, and if the combination vaccine is being administered to travelers or other individuals who will have a defined exposure to hepatitis A, at least two doses of the combination vaccine should be administered before exposure occurs.

Rabies

Rabies is a potentially fatal viral infection transmitted in the saliva of animals, usually through a bite. More rarely, cases result from the contamination of wounds with saliva of a rabies-infected animal; aerosol transmission occurs in special circumstances (e.g., research laboratories, bat-infested caves). Although dog bites account for the majority of rabies cases throughout the world, dog bites account for a minority (38%) of human rabies cases in the United States (and in 50% of such cases, the dog bite occurred overseas). Most rabies in the United States occurs in nondomesticated animals, especially bats, skunks, foxes, coyotes, raccoons, and woodchucks. Rabies should be considered in any case of *rapidly progressive encephalitis,* even in individuals who do not have a history of an animal bite. Therapy is preventive in nature and should be administered as either preexposure or, more commonly, postexposure prophylaxis.

Indications

Persons bitten by infected animals should receive *postexposure prophylaxis.* The risk of transmission of rabies through a ferret bite approximates that associated with a dog or a cat bite. Because bat bites can be small, may not be recalled, and may be missed on physical examination, rabies postexposure prophylaxis is recommended for individuals who have a bat exposure and cannot exclude a bat bite. Such situations might include an individual who awakens in a room with a bat, someone who

is unresponsive in a room with a bat (unconscious or intoxicated), or a person in a room with a bat who cannot report an exposure (e.g., a small child).

Postexposure Prophylaxis

Postexposure prophylaxis consists of three crucial steps (Table 6.6):

- First, the wound should be immediately and thoroughly *cleaned* and extensively *irrigated* with soap and water. Cleaning the wound with iodine or alcohol is not sufficient.
- Second, 20 IU of *rabies human immunoglobulin* (HRIG) per kilogram should be administered to individuals with an exposure who have not previously received a complete preexposure or postexposure series of tissue culture–derived rabies vaccine (or another type of rabies vaccine and had serologic confirmation of immunity). The entire HRIG dose should be instilled directly into the animal bite. If the entire HRIG dose cannot be instilled into the wound, as much of the dose that can be administered should be locally instilled and the remainder inoculated intramuscularly at a site distinct from the vaccine inoculation. If there is more than one animal bite, the HRIG dose should be divided equally among sites.
- Third, all individuals should receive *rabies vaccine* (a 1-mL dose of any of the rabies vaccines administered intramuscularly in the deltoid). If an individual has received a rabies primary vaccine series approved in the United States, that individual should receive two rabies boosters (days 0 and 3). Individuals who have not previously received such rabies vaccines should receive five doses (days 0, 3, 7, 14, and 28). HRIG and rabies vaccine should never be administered at the same site or with the same syringe.

Vaccine Preparations and Administration

Three rabies vaccines are approved in the United States—the human diploid-cell rabies vaccine (HDCV; sanofi pasteur), the rabies vaccine adsorbed (RVA; GlaxoSmithKline), and the purified chick-embryo cell culture (PCEC) rabies vaccine (RabAvert and Rabipur, Novartis)—although only HDCV and PCEC are commercially available. When postexposure prophylaxis is administered, no more than the recommended dose of HRIG should be administered because HRIG may partially suppress

TABLE 6.6

POSTEXPOSURE IMMUNIZATION FOR RABIES

Immunization Status	Vaccine/Product	Dose	Number of Doses	Schedule (Days)	Route
Not previously immunized	RIG	20 IU/kg body weight	1	0	Infiltrated at bite site (if possible); remainder intramuscular
	and				
	HDCV or PCEC	1.0 mL	5	0, 3, 7, 14, 28	Intramuscular
Previously immunized[a,b]	HDCV or PCEC	1.0 mL	2	0, 3	Intramuscular

RIG; rabies immune globulin; HDCV; human diploid-cell rabies vaccine; PCEC, purified chick-embryo cell rabies vaccine.
All postexposure prophylaxis should begin with immediate, thorough cleansing of all wounds with soap and water.
[a]Preexposure immunization with HDCV or PCEC; prior postexposure prophylaxis with HDCV or PCEC; or persons previously immunized with any other type of rabies vaccine and a documented history of positive antibody response to the prior vaccination.
[b]RIG should not be administered.
Adapted from Centers for Disease Control and Prevention. Health information for international travel ["The yellow book"]. Atlanta: U.S. Department of Health and Human Services, Public Health Service, 2008.

the antibody response to rabies vaccine. Tetanus prophylaxis should be considered.

Adverse Effects

Most reactions to rabies vaccine are local and mild. Serum sickness–type reactions may occur, especially with multiple boosting doses of HDCV or RVA; the PCEC vaccine is rarely associated with such reactions. The PCEC rabies vaccine may be used for booster vaccination regardless of the identity of the primary vaccination series. HRIG available in the United States appears to be safe. The safety of antirabies immunoglobulin preparations (human and rabbit) manufactured overseas has not been formally evaluated. Because rabies is a fatal illness, pregnancy should not be considered a contraindication to postexposure prophylaxis if it is indicated.

Preexposure Prophylaxis

Individuals who may be at risk for rabies should consider receiving preexposure prophylaxis, including those who work with animals, laboratory researchers who work with rabies virus, travelers who plan on spending a prolonged period of time in enzootic areas, and possibly short-term travelers who will be in rabies-enzootic areas without access to medical care (Table 6.7). Preexposure rabies vaccination consists of three 1-mL dose immunizations administered intramuscularly in the deltoid on days 0, 7, and 21 or 28. Antibody levels should be regularly checked in persons with ongoing exposure to rabies, and booster vaccinations should be administered as needed. Further information may be obtained from the CDC or from the local department of public health, which may have an on-call rabies specialist.

Typhoid

Because most cases of typhoid reported in the United States each year are acquired abroad, typhoid vaccine use is targeted for travelers to areas endemic for *Salmonella enterica* serova Typhi infection, especially when long-term nonhotel stays are planned. Individuals at highest risk of typhoid are travelers who will be visiting friends or family in the developing world, especially individuals who will be overseas for 3 to 4 weeks or longer. Two typhoid vaccines are available in the United States.

A recombinant vaccine comprised of purified capsular polysaccharide Vi antigen (Typhim Vi, sanofi pasteur) is approved for individuals 2 years of age or older. It is administered as a single dose and provides approximately 60% to 75% protection for 2 years.

An oral typhoid vaccine, based on a live attenuated strain of *Salmonella enterica* serova Typhi (Ty21a), is also available (Vivotif Berna, Swiss Serum and Vaccine Institute). The oral

---

TABLE 6.7

PREEXPOSURE IMMUNIZATION FOR RABIES

Risk Category	Nature of Risk	Typical Populations	Preexposure Regimen
Continuous	Virus present continuously, often in high concentrations; Specific exposures likely to go unrecognized; Bite, nonbite, or aerosol exposure	Rabies research laboratory workers,[a] rabies biologics production workers	Primary course: Serologic testing every 6 mo; booster vaccination if antibody titer is below acceptable level[b]
Frequent	Exposure usually episodic with source recognized, but exposure might also be unrecognized; Bite, nonbite, or aerosol exposure possible	Rabies diagnostic laboratory workers,[a] cavers, veterinarians and staff, and animal control and wildlife workers in rabies epizootic areas	Primary course: Serologic testing every 2 yr; booster vaccination if antibody titer is below acceptable level[b]
Infrequent (greater than general population)	Exposure nearly always episodic with source recognized; Bite or nonbite exposure	Veterinarians, animal control and wildlife workers in areas with low rabies rates; veterinary students; and travelers visiting areas where rabies is enzootic and immediate access to appropriate medical care, including biologics, is limited	Primary course: no serologic testing or booster vaccination
Rare (general population)	Exposure always episodic, with source recognized	U.S. population at large, including individuals in rabies-epizootic areas	No preexposure immunization necessary

Preexposure immunization consists of three doses of human diploid cell vaccine (HDCV), purified chick-embryo cell culture vaccine (PCEC), or rabies vaccine adsorbed (RVA), 1.0 mL, intramuscular (i.e., deltoid area), one each on days 0, 7, and 21 or 28. Administration of routine booster doses of vaccine depends on exposure risk category as noted above. Patients who are immunosuppressed by disease or medications should postpone preexposure vaccinations and consider avoiding activities for which rabies preexposure prophylaxis is indicated. When this course is not possible, immunosuppressed persons who are at risk for rabies should have their antibody titers checked after vaccination.
[a]Judgment of relative risk and extra monitoring of vaccination status of laboratory workers is the responsibility of the laboratory supervisor (see U.S. Department of Health and Human Services. Biosafety in microbiological and biomedical laboratories. Washington DC: U.S. Government Printing Office, 1999. Available at: http://bmbl.od.nih.gov/).
[b]Preexposure booster immunization consists of one dose of HDCV, PCEC, or RVA, 1.0 mL/dose (deltoid area). Minimum acceptable antibody level is complete virus neutralization at a 1 : 5 serum dilution by the rapid fluorescent focus inhibition test. A booster dose should be administered if titer falls below this level.

vaccine may be used in individuals 6 years of age or older and is approved in the United States as a single pill every other day for four doses (days 0, 2, 4, and 6). It provides approximately 60% to 75% protection for 5 years and is well tolerated by most individuals. (In the United Kingdom, the same vaccine is approved as a three-dose series.) Patients should be reminded to keep their vaccine refrigerated between doses, although studies have shown that the oral vaccine remains potent even if it remains stored at room temperature for up to 24 hours. Mild intestinal upset is the most common adverse event after oral administration. The oral vaccine should be taken with cool liquid 1 hour before a meal. Immunocompromised individuals and those with chronic inflammatory bowel disease should not receive the oral vaccine, nor should persons taking antimicrobial agents (antibiotics or antimalarial agents).

Japanese Encephalitis

Japanese encephalitis (JE) is a mosquito-borne viral infection that exists throughout eastern, southeastern, and southern Asia. In most individuals who become infected, encephalitis or severe illness does not develop, but when it does, the death rate is 25%, and the rate of severe neurologic sequelae is 50%. The disease occurs in rural environments and is transmitted by a mosquito vector that normally feeds on pigs and birds. Individuals from the United States at highest risk are those staying longer than 30 days in rural areas (usually in an Asian locale with extensive rice farming and pig husbandry) during the appropriate mosquito season (May through October in many areas of Asia, but year-round in endemic tropical areas). The overall risk to a traveler is approximately 1 in 1 million; however, this risk may increase to greater than 1 in 20,000 per week for high-risk travel. Risk may be markedly decreased through the use of protective clothing and insect repellents, especially during late afternoon.

The current JE vaccine (JE-VAS, sanofi pasteur), a formalin-inactivated product derived from infected mouse brains, is administered in a three-dose primary series (days 0, 7, and 14 or 30). Booster inoculation may be administered every 2 years. New JE vaccines are being developed. The most common adverse effects to the current JE vaccine are local, but mild constitutional symptoms may develop in up to 10% of cases. In 0.6% of recipients, the vaccine may cause *urticaria, angioedema, respiratory distress, hypotension*, and *anaphylaxis*. Most allergic reactions may be treated with antihistamines and corticosteroids; epinephrine and supportive care may be required. Severe reactions usually occur within 1 day of vaccination but have occurred as long as 2 weeks after administration of any of the three inoculations. Individuals with a history of severe allergic reactions, angioedema, or urticaria are at highest risk for severe reactions. Ideally, individuals who receive the vaccine should have access to medical care for at least 10 days after completion of the vaccine series. Consequently, the vaccine series ideally needs to be started at least 24 days before departure if the accelerated vaccination course of 0, 7, and 14 days is used.

Yellow Fever

Yellow fever is a mosquito-borne hemorrhagic viral illness that is often fatal; it is endemic in sub-Saharan Africa and tropical Latin America. The live attenuated virus vaccine (YF-VAX, sanofi pasteur) is, at present, the only immunization legally required for crossing some international borders. Contraindications to immunization include allergy to eggs, immunocompromise, and pregnancy. Women who receive the vaccine should be advised not to become pregnant for 1 month after vaccination. The vaccine is administered only through WHO-approved centers. State departments of public health and the CDC keep a list of such sites (http://www.cdc.gov). Individuals who require yellow fever vaccination should be directed to a yellow fever vaccination center. Immunized individuals will receive a WHO vaccination certificate. The vaccination record becomes "acceptable" to immigration officers 10 days after the vaccine has been administered. The vaccine is effective for 10 years. Vaccination is recommended for individuals traveling to or living in endemic areas. Countries may require documentation of yellow fever vaccination, even from individuals who only pass through endemic areas. Countries reporting yellow fever are posted by the WHO and the CDC; a listing can be accessed at http://www.cdc.gov.

Most reactions to yellow fever vaccine are local in nature. However, two important systemic adverse reactions to yellow fever vaccine can occur: yellow fever vaccine–associated neurologic disease and yellow fever vaccine–associated viscerotropic disease. Yellow fever vaccine–associated neurologic disease includes encephalitis and autoimmune neurologic disease, particularly Guillain-Barré syndrome and acute disseminated encephalomyelitis. The overall reported rate of yellow fever vaccine–associated neurologic disease in the United States is estimated to be 0.5 per 100,000 doses distributed. Because of the risk for vaccine-associated encephalitis, the vaccine should never be administered to children 4 months of age or younger and rarely (if ever) to children 4 to 9 months of age. Yellow fever vaccine–associated viscerotropic disease has been increasingly recognized in the last 10 years among recipients of yellow fever vaccines in a number of countries and irrespective of vaccine manufacturer. The syndrome of fever and multiple-organ-system failure is clinically and pathologically similar to naturally acquired yellow fever and has only been reported in first-time recipients of the vaccine. Since 1996, 12 cases of yellow fever vaccine–associated viscerotropic disease have occurred in the United States, and at least an additional 24 suspected cases have been identified worldwide. The risk of viscerotropic disease appears to be higher for individuals older than 60 years of age (11 of the 12 cases in the United States were reported in individuals older than the age of 60 years). Thymic disorders may also predispose to viscerotropic disease, and individuals with a history of thymic disorders should not be vaccinated. Crude estimates of the risk of viscerotropic disease following vaccination are 1.8 cases per 100,000 doses of vaccine for individuals 60 years of age or older and 0.3 to 0.5 cases per 100,000 doses of vaccine for individuals younger than 60 years of age. Less severe systemic reactions to the yellow fever vaccine are more common and may include a flulike illness that may occur 5 to 10 days after vaccination. If an individual is proceeding to an endemic yellow fever area and the vaccine is contraindicated, a yellow fever waiver certificate may be issued from the WHO yellow fever vaccination center. Immunocompromised individuals and pregnant women who will live long term in a highly endemic yellow fever area of the world should carefully weigh the risk of vaccination versus the risk of illness. A desensitization protocol is available for individuals with a history of a severe allergy to eggs. The effectiveness of the yellow fever vaccine is not affected by the administration of immunoglobulin.

Tuberculosis

Bacille Calmette-Guérin (BCG) is a live attenuated strain of *Mycobacterium bovis* that is used in *children* throughout the world to prevent tuberculosis. Vaccine trials in *adults* have yielded conflicting results, in part due to the use of different strains of BCG. Overall, the vaccine may be approximately 30% to 50% effective. Most immigrants to the United States will have received the BCG vaccine as children. A positive tuberculin skin test result, however, should not be ascribed to BCG vaccination in any individual, regardless of the country of origin. If required, molecular immunological essays are available which may differentiate positive skin reactions due to previous BCG vaccination from previous tuberculosis. In the United States, where the prevention of tuberculosis rests on the proper identification and treatment of exposed individuals, BCG is rarely administered to protect individuals against tuberculosis (see Chapter 49), and at present the vaccine is not commercially available in the United States. The vaccine may be considered for individuals exposed to multidrug-resistant tuberculosis, including health care workers who practice in certain prison settings or in certain overseas clinics. It may also be useful for those who cannot receive preventive therapy but have close contact with an individual with active, untreated disease or with disease that is ineffectively treated or multidrug resistant. The vaccine is administered intradermally; ulceration and prolonged discharge at the site of vaccination, regional adenitis, and osteitis may occur in up to 20% of vaccine recipients. Disseminated BCG may develop in immunocompromised individuals who receive the vaccine.

Other Vaccines

A number of other vaccines exist but are not routinely commercially available in the United States. These include vaccines against smallpox (vaccinia), anthrax, cholera, plague, and typhus. Acquisition and administration of many of these vaccines require regulatory approval, and these vaccines should only be administered to individuals in targeted populations. A vaccine against tick-borne encephalitis is also available in Europe and Russia.

ACKNOWLEDGMENTS

This work was supported in part by grants U19 CI000514 from the Centers for Disease Control and Prevention and K01 TW07144 from the Fogarty International Center (R.C.L.) and by a Claflin Distinguished Scholar Award from the Massachusetts General Hospital (R.C.L.).

WEBSITES/INTERNET RESOURCES

http://www.cdc.gov
Main site for immunization-related resources and information.

http://www.cdc.gov/vaccines/
Excellent central resource page of the National Immunization Program/Centers for Disease Control and Prevention [CDC]. Includes links to vaccine information statements, recommendations of the Advisory Committee on Immunization Practices, the "Pink Book," vaccine safety information, tabular summaries of recommendations for adults, adolescents, and children, and other resources.

http://www.cdc.gov/od/science/iso/about_iso.htm
Vaccine safety website.

http://www.hhs.gov/nvpo/
National Vaccine Program Office website.

http://www.cdc.gov/travel
Review of travel-related vaccines. Includes the complete "Yellow Book" online.

http://www.cdc.gov/vaccines/pubs/ACIP-list.htm
Up-to-date Advisory Committee on Immunization Practices statements that review immunizations against infectious diseases; includes definitive recommendations for each immunization.

http://www.cdc.gov/mmwr
Morbidity and Mortality Weekly Report online (free). Publishes vaccine updates and recommendations.

http://www.nfid.org/
Website of the National Foundation for Infectious Diseases.

http://www.who.int/
World Health Organization. Lists infectious disease outbreaks and immunization recommendations.

http://www.immunize.org
Site maintained by the Immunization Action Coalition (IAC), a nonprofit organization; the site includes/accesses many immunization-related resources (patient education resources, policy statements, contact numbers for each state's immunization program office, links to other sites). The IAC also produces two newsletters that cover immunization-related updates and developments: Needle Tips and Vaccinate Adults. These publications are free. All materials are reviewed by the CDC. The IAC can be contacted at 1573 Selby Avenue, Suite 234, St. Paul, MN 55104-6328. Telephone: 651-647-9008/9; e-mail: admin@immunize.org.

http://www.cdc.gov/nip/publications/preg_guide.htm
Includes CDC guidelines for vaccinating pregnant women.

Annotated Bibliography

1. Centers for Disease Control and Prevention. Epidemiology and prevention of vaccine-preventable diseases ["The pink book"], 10th ed. Atkinson W, Hamborsky J, McIntyre L, et al., eds. Washington, DC: Public Health Foundation, 2007. Available at: http://www.cdc.gov/vaccines/pubs/pinkbook/default.htm. (*Practical vaccine information.*)

2. Pickering LK, ed. Red book: 2006 report of the Committee on Infectious Diseases, 27th ed. Elk Grove Village, IL: American Academy of Pediatrics, 2006. (*Overview of infectious diseases; considers incubation periods, clinical manifestations, and preventive measures, including immunization and postexposure prophylaxis.*)

3. Centers for Disease Control and Prevention. Health information for international travel 2008 ["The yellow book"]. Atlanta: U.S. Department of Health and Human Services, Public Health Service, 2007. Available at: http://wwwn.cdc.gov/travel/contentYellowBook.aspx. (*The standard reference from the Centers for Disease Control and Prevention on travel-related immunizations.*)

4. Plotkin SA, Orenstein WA, ed. Vaccines, 5th ed. Philadelphia: Saunders, Elsevier, 2008. (*A definitive and comprehensive vaccine text.*)

CHAPTER 7 ■ SCREENING FOR HIV-1 INFECTION

STEPHEN L. BOSWELL

INTRODUCTION

Knowledge of human immunodeficiency virus (HIV) infection status in the asymptomatic period permits infected persons to seek potentially beneficial medical treatment in a timely fashion, including antiretroviral agents and other medications that decrease the risk of developing opportunistic infections (see Chapter 13). These measures delay the onset of acquired immunodeficiency syndrome (AIDS) and prolong survival. In addition, early identification of HIV-1 infection can increase the effectiveness of tuberculin skin testing and thus improve tuberculosis screening and prophylaxis (see Chapter 49). Appropriate counseling, an essential part of screening for HIV-1 infection, may help some individuals prevent HIV-1 transmission by modifying their behavior. However, indiscriminate testing, especially among patients at very low risk for HIV-1 infection, raises the chance of a false-positive result and its attendant psychosocial morbidity. The primary care physician should know how best to advise the patient who asks about HIV-1 testing and whom to recommend for testing.

ASSESSING THE RISK FOR HIV-1 INFECTION (1–5)

In the United States, it is estimated that more than 1 million people are infected with HIV-1. A related retrovirus, HIV-2, can also cause immune dysfunction, although it is generally less pathogenic than HIV-1. HIV-2 is distributed primarily in West Africa, but cases are increasingly being identified in the United States. Those at highest risk of infection with HIV-1 are men with a history of homosexual or bisexual activity (approximately 50% of those infected); intravenous drug users and their sexual contacts (approximately 25% of those infected); the sexual contacts of homosexual or bisexual men; persons who received blood and blood products between 1978 and 1985; and children born to infected women. The risk of directly acquiring HIV-1 infection through processed blood or selected blood products (plasma and clotting factor concentrates) has dramatically decreased since 1985 as a consequence of the widespread screening of those who donate blood and plasma, the use of serologic tests for HIV, and the viral inactivation of various plasma products.

Knowledge of the epidemiology of HIV-1 infection is necessary to estimate the pretest probability of HIV-1 infection in the person for whom screening is being considered. Attention to the pretest probability estimate is important to the decision to screen. Placing too much weight on the high sensitivity and specificity of HIV-1 antibody testing and ignoring the pretest probability is a common error (see Chapters 2 and 3).

The pretest probability of HIV-1 infection in a given patient is a function of the patient's previous risk behavior and the geographic location of the behavior. The testing setting, too, may be helpful in assessing the likelihood of infection. Settings characterized by high seroprevalence include sexually transmitted disease clinics, psychiatric hospitals, homeless shelters, alcohol rehabilitation facilities, and inner-city emergency departments. These factors should be weighed when assessing the need for HIV-1 testing.

When assessing the behavioral risk factors for acquiring HIV-1 infection in an individual patient the following questions are particularly useful in clinical practice. Has the patient:

- had sex with someone known to have HIV-1 or AIDS?
- had a history of sexually transmitted diseases?
- had sex with many men or women or had sex with someone who has had sex with many men or women?
- had sex with someone who has used needles to take drugs?
- shared needles or works to take drugs?
- had a history of receiving blood transfusions or clotting factor between 1978 and 1985?

If the answer to any of these questions is yes, then the patient and physician should give serious consideration of having HIV-1 antibody testing performed.

ROUTINE HIV TESTING (1,6–7)

In 2006, in an effort to ensure that more HIV-positive people would know their HIV status, the Centers for Disease Control and Prevention (CDC) recommended routine HIV screening of adults, adolescents, and pregnant women in health care settings in the United States. These guidelines emphasized the importance of reducing barriers to HIV testing in the clinical setting.

The public health imperative supporting this approach is based on the observation that approximately 25% of the 1 million individuals infected with HIV in the United States are unaware of their infection. They are unable to take advantage of the treatments that can keep them healthy and extend their lives. They are also unaware of the need to protect their sex or drug-use partners from becoming infected. Studies have demonstrated that many infected individuals decrease behaviors that transmit infection to others once they are aware of their HIV status. In addition, medical treatment lowers HIV viral load and may reduce the risk of transmission to others.

Important aspects of these new recommendations include the following:

- HIV screening is recommended for patients in all health care settings after the patient is notified that testing will be performed unless the patient declines (opt-out screening).
- Persons at high risk of HIV infection should be screened for HIV at least annually.
- Separate written consent for HIV testing should not be required; general consent for medical care should be considered sufficient to encompass consent for HIV testing.
- Prevention counseling should not be required with HIV diagnostic testing or as part of HIV screening programs in health care settings.
- HIV screening should be part of the routine panel of prenatal screening tests for all pregnant women.
- Repeat screening in the third trimester is recommended in certain jurisdictions with elevated rates of HIV infection among pregnant women.

Full implementation of these guidelines requires changes in existing laws in many states and localities. It is essential that the practicing physician be familiar with current law in his or her locality before adopting the CDC guidelines in clinical practice. Legislation pertaining to HIV/AIDS has been enacted in every state and in the District of Columbia, and specific requirements related to informed consent and pretest counseling differ among states. In many jurisdictions, statutory and other regulatory impediments exist to opt-out screening and changes to procedures for counseling, written consent, confirmatory testing, and communication of HIV test results.

TESTING FOR HIV-1 INFECTION (1,3–13)

Viral Dynamics and the Immunologic Response to HIV-1 (1,9–11)

After transmission of HIV-1, there is usually a 2- to 8-week period before the acute retroviral syndrome develops. This flulike illness occurs in 50% to 90% of infected individuals, lasts 2 to 4 weeks, and resolves spontaneously. Coincident with the acute illness, high-grade viremia develops: Titers of 50 to 100 million particles per milliliter have been reported. Viral titers begin to fall 2 to 3 weeks after the onset of acute symptoms, usually before an HIV-1 antibody response can be detected. This observation suggests that a response other than HIV-1 antibody may be responsible for the initial control of virus replication. Recent evidence suggests a central role for HIV-1–specific cell-mediated immunity in the control of virus replication during primary HIV-1 infection. Serial measurement of proliferative responses to HIV-1 antigens using $CD4^+$ lymphocytes from acutely infected individuals demonstrated a strong inverse correlation between the generation of HIV-specific $CD4^+$ lymphocyte helper cells and plasma HIV-1 RNA levels. Similarly, among long-term nonprogressors the highest HIV-specific proliferative responses had the lowest plasma HIV-1 RNA levels.

Although the presence of symptoms is common among those who are acutely infected, the infection often goes unrecognized in the primary care setting because of the similarity of the symptoms to those of other common illnesses. Physicians should maintain a high level of suspicion for HIV infection in all patients presenting with a compatible syndrome. A careful evaluation of the patient's risk behaviors during the 3-month period prior to presentation should be obtained for all such patients. When appropriate, laboratory testing should be performed. This testing may include measurement of HIV RNA by HIV polymerase chain reaction or HIV B-DNA and HIV antibody. Although HIV RNA measurement is the preferred method of testing, a test for p24 antigen can be used when RNA testing is not readily available. A negative p24 antigen test does not rule out acute infection, however.

HIV-1 Antibody Assays (1,12,13)

Diagnosis of HIV-1 infection is most frequently accomplished by detection of specific antibodies against viral antigens in serum. Recently, diagnostic testing using saliva and urine has been developed. *Enzyme immunoassays (EIAs)* for HIV-1 detection were first developed in 1985. Although EIAs are easily automated, inexpensive, and well suited for testing large numbers of samples, they can nonspecifically bind antibodies and produce false-positive results in patients exposed to other infections or vaccines. The assays have improved from first-generation tests that used viral lysates as a source of viral antigens to the current third-generation tests using recombinant DNA proteins coated on paper strips, beads, and microplate wells. The most advanced assays have reported sensitivity and specificity of greater than 99.9% in serum from individuals with known HIV-1 infection and uninfected controls.

Rapid serologic screening tests have been developed for office use, including *HIV antigen–coated gelatin* or *latex particle agglutination assays*. These tests can be performed quickly (in some cases <10 minutes), but they still require Western blot confirmation. Data suggest that some particle agglutination assays may be slightly less sensitive and specific than EIA in moderate- or high-titer samples. Additional rapid screening assays using dipsticks and other technologies are available. Based on comparing EIA with several of these rapid assays, data suggest that the rapid assays can be significantly less sensitive when testing low-antibody-titer samples. This may be a particular problem during primary HIV-1 infection when antibodies against selected antigens may not yet be present or may be present at very low titer. In general, EIA with confirmatory *Western blot* is the preferred screening test.

An important limitation of the HIV-1 screening assays used in the United States is that they often detect a single subtype of HIV-1. HIV-1 has significant genetic variability. It can be categorized into major groups (M) and outlier groups (O). Group M can be further divided into subtypes or clades A through J. These clades have significant geographic variability. Many conventional assays for HIV-1 screening were developed using a group M, subtype B virus, the predominate clade in the United States and Europe. Consequently, their ability to detect geographically diverse subtypes has limitations. Several manufacturers are attempting to address this issue by adding non–subtype B peptides to their assays, but it should be remembered that the geography of HIV-1 acquisition can affect the accuracy of HIV-1 screening.

Body fluids other than blood may be used to determine an individual's HIV-1 status. Oral fluids and urine may contain antibodies against HIV-1. Recently, the U.S. Food and Drug Administration (FDA) approved several tests using these fluids. The *OraSure* test collects oral mucosal transudate via a cotton swab that is inserted into the mouth for 2 to 5 minutes. The swab is then packaged and sent to a reference laboratory for standard EIA and Western blot confirmation. This test has demonstrated better than 99% sensitivity and specificity when compared with standard Western blot confirmation. The

OraQuick test is a rapid fingerstick whole-blood test for HIV. It detects HIV-1 antibodies, requires only a drop of blood, and can produce a result in 20 minutes.

In an effort to widen testing options further, kits specifically designed to be used in the home have been developed. One such kit, *Home Access System* (Home Access Health Corp.), uses blood collected using a lancet. The blood is blotted onto a test card, mailed to a reference laboratory, and tested using a standard EIA and confirmatory Western blot. Within 1 week, the individual may retrieve results by calling an automated system that stores results by a specific number assigned to each kit. A counselor is available to discuss a negative result, if desired. A call for a positive result is connected immediately to a telephone counselor who will discuss the results with the individual.

A *positive EIA test* should be confirmed by *Western blot* testing. Relative to EIA, the Western blot is slower, more labor intensive, and much more expensive, but it is able to measure specific HIV-1 antibodies and thus enhance the specificity of testing. It detects antibodies directed at specific HIV-1 proteins (core, envelope, and polymerase) after their separation by gel electrophoresis.

For the licensed Western blot, interpretation of reactive and nonreactive tests is based on data from clinical studies submitted to FDA for licensure. A test is considered positive with this Western blot if antibodies to multiple virus-specific protein bands are present, that is, p24, p31, and either gp41 or gp160. If fewer bands are present, the test is considered indeterminate; it is interpreted as negative only if no bands are present on the blot. When these criteria are used for interpreting test results, the probability of either a false-positive or a false-negative result is extremely small. It should be noted, however, that as many as 15% to 20% of tests on persons at low risk for HIV-1 infection may be described as indeterminate. Sera from persons recently infected with HIV-1 also may produce an indeterminate Western blot pattern. For such persons, a repeat Western blot on a second specimen obtained after the initial specimen often yields a positive blot pattern within 6 months. Conversely, follow-up testing of uninfected persons whose serum had an indeterminate blot pattern on initial testing usually will show no change in the banding pattern. Serum from some HIV-infected persons who have advanced immunodeficiency may have an indeterminate pattern because of a loss of antibodies to nonenvelope proteins. In spite of the existence of a licensed Western blot test, many laboratories continue to use unlicensed tests because of cost and the stringent criteria required for interpreting the licensed test. The performance characteristics of the unlicensed tests have not been uniformly subjected to the same rigorous scrutiny required for licensure by the FDA. Although recommendations for standardization have been published, the extent to which these are followed is unknown. Information about production standards, interlot variability, or validation of criteria used for interpretation often is not available. The absence of standardization and appropriate quality controls may result in a lower sensitivity or specificity and, thus, a higher probability of inaccurate results.

Other Tests (1,8,12,13)

Tests for virus and viral components are readily available in the United States. These tests include *virus culture, p24 antigen assays, polymerase chain reaction assays,* and *signal amplification assays.* In general, these assays are not used for the initial diagnosis of HIV-1 infection in the adult.

Virus culture is time consuming, costly, difficult to standardize, and relatively insensitive. Assays for p24 antigen are hampered by the low prevalence of antigen during the asymptomatic phase of HIV-1 infection. Polymerase chain reaction and signal amplification assays have a high false-positive rate and are not suitable for screening in most circumstances. Surrogate markers do not test directly for virus and antibody. The most common is the CD4$^+$ lymphocyte count, which is useful for assessing prognosis and therapeutic decision making, but it should not be used as an indirect method of determining whether a patient is HIV-1 infected.

Test Interpretation—Minimizing False Positives and False Negatives (1)

When testing for the presence of HIV-1 antibodies and interpreting the results, it is necessary to consider the timing of antibody responses to HIV-1 infection (Fig. 7.1), the sensitivity and specificity of the enzyme-linked immunosorbent assay (ELISA) and Western blot tests, and the pretest probability of the person being tested. For example, a negative ELISA test in a patient with a pretest probability of 0.1% (1 in 1,000) virtually rules out the diagnosis of HIV-1 infection. However, the same test result in a person with a 50% pretest probability of HIV-1 infection does not drop the posttest probability to zero (in biologic terms, testing might be occurring before the appearance of antibody). Conversely, a positive ELISA test result in a person with a low pretest probability (0.1%) produces a posttest probability of only 40%, necessitating confirmatory testing.

A major objective is to limit the risk of a false-positive result and its potentially adverse psychological and social consequences. Pretest counseling is especially important for the low-risk person who needs to be informed of the risk of a false-positive result. It is often advisable to repeat a positive ELISA if it occurs in an individual with no identifiable risk factor or from a site that performs anonymous testing. There is always the finite possibility of laboratory error or sample mislabeling. Confirmatory testing with the Western blot test is essential and a standard procedure in most laboratories.

A negative Western blot result in the setting of a positive ELISA and a small pretest probability of HIV-1 rules out HIV-1

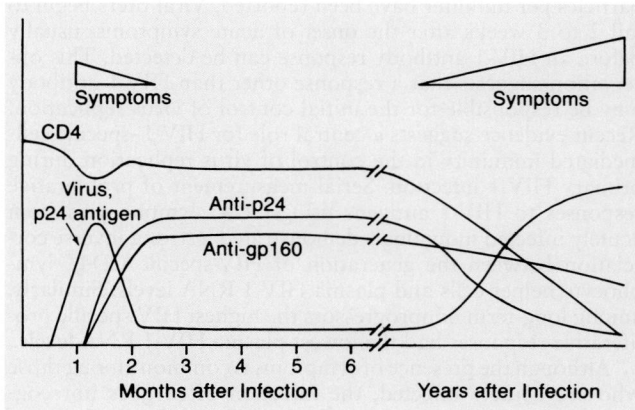

FIGURE 7.1. Natural history of HIV-1 infection. (Adapted from Clark SJ, Saag MS, Decker WD, et al. High titers of cytopathic virus in plasma of patients with symptomatic primary HIV-1 infection. N Engl J Med 324;00:951, with permission.)

infection. A positive Western blot following a positive ELISA virtually rules in the diagnosis of HIV-1 infection, even among persons with a low pretest probability, but an "indeterminate" result can be problematic.

Despite the enhanced specificity afforded by adding the Western blot to the testing sequence, a small but important proportion (15% to 20%) of individuals with a positive ELISA result will test "indeterminate." The most frequent cause of an indeterminate Western blot result is the presence of a single band of antibody, usually against p24. In high-risk individuals, this may reflect ongoing seroconversion. Low-risk persons with this result are virtually never infected. Repeat testing should take place within 2 to 6 months of the initial indeterminate result. If the individual is HIV-1 infected, a positive ELISA will usually be accompanied by two or more positive bands on the Western blot. Among low-risk persons, the single band will frequently persist. In general, low-risk individuals with indeterminate test results should be reassured that HIV-1 infection is unlikely.

False-negative test results most frequently occur when testing is performed during the window period—usually within 6 months after viral transmission. Alternative methods of identifying HIV-1 infection are available in cases in which further clarification is desirable. These include polymerase chain reaction, viral culture, and detection of p24 antigen. These tests should not be used in place of antibody testing, but occasionally they may be useful.

Repeat Screening (1)

Repeated screening at 6- to 12-month intervals is indicated for those who continue to practice high-risk behavior. An essential part of HIV-1 testing is the provision of HIV-1 counseling. Careful instruction should be given to all persons in how to minimize the risk of HIV-1 transmission.

RECOMMENDATIONS (1)

- Patients at high risk for HIV-1 disease should be screened (Table 7.1).
- High-risk patients who are negative but continue high-risk behavior should be rescreened every 6 to 12 months.
- Patients at low risk who are donors of blood, semen, or organs should also be screened.
- Test result interpretation must take into account pretest probability, sensitivity and specificity of testing methods,

TABLE 7.1

CENTERS FOR DISEASE CONTROL AND PREVENTION RECOMMENDATIONS FOR HIV SEROLOGIC TESTING

HIV screening is recommended for patients in all health care settings after the patient is notified that testing will be performed unless the patient declines (opt-out screening). It is essential that the practicing physician be familiar with current law in his or her locality before adopting this recommendation in clinical practice.

Annual screening should be performed with ongoing risk factors:
- Persons who have sexually transmitted diseases
- High-risk individuals: intravenous drug users, sexually active gay and bisexual men, hemophiliacs, regular sexual partners of persons in these categories and persons with known HIV infection; lower-incidence groups include prostitutes and persons who received transfusions during 1978–1985
- Persons who consider themselves at risk or request the test
- Recipient and source of blood and body fluid exposures; body fluids besides blood considered at risk include semen, vaginal secretions, cerebrospinal fluid, synovial fluid, pleural fluid, peritoneal fluid, pericardial fluid, amniotic fluid, and any bloody body fluid; body fluids not considered at risk are feces, nasal secretions, sputum, saliva, sweat, tears, urine, and vomitus, unless they contain visible blood
- Health care workers who perform exposure-prone invasive procedures
- Donors of blood, semen, and organs

and timing of the testing in relation to time of possible infection.
- Patient education regarding HIV-1 transmission and HIV-1 risk reduction should be part of every screening effort.
- Once a diagnosis of HIV-1 infection is established, the patient should be referred to a clinician with specialized expertise in HIV-1 medicine.
- Confidentiality should be protected of those who are tested.
- Local, state, and federal regulations and policies that govern provision of HIV testing should be followed.
- Clinicians should be alert to the possibility of the acute retroviral syndrome when evaluating patients with a compatible symptom complex.

Annotated Bibliography

1. Branson BM, Handsfield HH, Lampe MA, et al. (2006). Revised recommendations for HIV testing of adults, adolescents, and pregnant women in health-care settings. MMWR 55(RR-14):1. (*Recommends HIV testing for all health care providers in the public and private sectors, including those working in hospital emergency departments, urgent care clinics, inpatient services, substance abuse treatment clinics, public health clinics, community clinics, correctional health care facilities, and primary care settings.*)
2. Epidemiology of HIV/AIDS—United States, 1981–2005. MMWR 2006;55(21):589. (*Reviews risk factors and prevalences.*)
3. HIV counseling and testing—United States, 1993. MMWR1995;44(9):169. (*An examination of the variations in rates of use of private and public HIV counseling and testing sites by state.*)
4. Liddicoat RV, Horton NJ, Urban R, et al. Assessing missed opportunities for HIV testing in medical settings. J Gen Intern Med 2004;19:349. (*Missed opportunities for HIV testing are frequent.*)

5. Walensky RP, Weinstein MC, Kimmel AD, et al. Routine human immunodeficiency virus testing: an economic evaluation of current guidelines. Am J Med 2005;118:292. (*Routine inpatient HIV screening programs are not only cost-effective, but also would likely remain so at a prevalence of undiagnosed HIV infection 10 times lower than the ≥1% threshold recommended at the time.*)
6. Fisher AH, Hanssens C, Schulman DI. The CDC's routine HIV testing recommendation: legally, not so routine. HIV AIDS Policy Law Rev 2006;11(2-3):17. (*The authors argue that the CDC's recommendation to do away with specific written informed consent for HIV tests is based on a false assumption that informed consent constitutes a barrier to HIV testing.*)
7. Greenwald JL, Hall J, Skulnick PR. Approaching the CDC's guidelines on the HIV testing of inpatients: physician-referral versus nonreferral-based testing. AIDS Patient Care STDS 2006;20(5):311. (*Routinely offering HIV tests to inpatients yields higher testing rates than physician*

referral–based systems and increases the number of patients who know their HIV status.)

8. Greenwald JL, Burstein GR, Pincus J, et al. A rapid review of rapid HIV antibody tests. Curr Infect Dis Rep 2006;8(2):125. (*Reviews the operating and performance characteristics, quality assurance and laboratory requirements, and HIV counseling implications of the available rapid HIV tests.*)

9. Henrard DR, Daar E, Farzadegas H, et al. Virologic and immunologic characterization of symptomatic and asymptomatic primary HIV-1 infection. J Acquir Immune Defic Syndr Hum Retrovirol 1995;9:305. (*Immunologic control of viremia early after infection is important determinant of subsequent course.*)

10. Coco A, Kleinhans E. Prevalence of primary HIV infection in symptomatic ambulatory patients. Ann Fam Med 2005;3:400. (*Patients complaining of fever and other visit reasons consistent with primary HIV infection had a*

disease prevalence of 0.66% [0.57% to 1.02%], those with rash had a prevalence of 0.50% [0.31% to 0.82%], and those with pharyngitis had a prevalence of 0.16% [0.11% to 0.22%].)

11. Flanigan T, Tashima KT. Diagnosis of acute HIV infection: it's time to get moving! Ann Intern Med 2001;134:75. (*Methods of diagnosing acute infection are reviewed.*)

12. Paul SM, Grimes-Dennis J, Burr CK, et al. Rapid diagnostic testing for HIV. Clinical implications. N J Med 2003;100(9 Suppl):11. (*Succinct review of implications.*)

13. Hu DJ, Dondero TJ, Rayfield MA, et al. The emerging genetic diversity of HIV. The importance of global surveillance for diagnostics, research, and prevention. JAMA 1996;275(3):210. (*The existence of highly divergent strains of HIV that are not reliably detected by a number of commonly used diagnostic tests underscores the need for effective surveillance.*)

CHAPTER 8 ■ EVALUATION OF CHRONIC FATIGUE

Chronic fatigue is one of the most common complaints in primary care practice, with a reported frequency in excess of 20%. It can also be one of the more frustrating problems to assess because it is a sensitive but nonspecific indicator of underlying medical pathology and psychological distress. Regardless of cause, the patient typically reports having a lack of energy, being listless, and being too tired to participate in family, work, or even leisure activities. Many patients speculate that they have a vitamin or mineral deficiency and self-treat accordingly before coming for evaluation. Others fear an underlying malignancy, endocrine disorder, or serious infection (e.g., HIV infection, tuberculosis, hepatitis, "chronic mono") and request extensive testing and/or treatment.

Most patients bothered by chronic fatigue come to the primary physician looking for an organic cause, especially those with a rather abrupt onset of symptoms. Although most studies of chronic fatigue find the vast majority of cases to have a psychological basis (e.g., depression), few patients initially report psychological symptoms, and if they do, they view such symptoms as secondary to a medical illness. Attempts by the physician to address psychological issues may be misinterpreted by the patient as not being taken seriously. Thus, the primary physician has the difficult tasks of sorting through a vast number of potential etiologies and patient concerns, determining what proportion of the problem is physiologic and what part is psychological, and helping the patient to understand and deal effectively with the underlying condition and its consequences.

PATHOPHYSIOLOGY AND CLINICAL PRESENTATION (1–17)

Almost all illnesses are capable of causing fatigue; however, a few are noteworthy for the prominence of the symptom in the clinical presentation.

Psychological Etiologies

As just noted, fatigue is an important somatic symptom of depression, often coexisting with early-morning awakening, appetite and sexual disturbances, and multiple bodily complaints. Abnormalities of central nervous system neurotransmitter metabolism and function are believed to play a major role in the pathogenesis of depression (see Chapter 227). Chronic anxiety may result in generalized fatigue, in part because it interferes with obtaining adequate physical and psychological rest. Patients report trouble falling asleep and a host of associated bodily complaints. Many maintain their neck muscles in a constantly tensed state, which gives rise to occipital–nuchal headaches. Seemingly unprovoked episodes of palpitations, difficulty breathing, and chest tightness may occur, especially in those whose anxiety is accompanied by a panic disorder (see Chapter 226).

Patients in whom somatization represents an underlying personality disorder may complain of chronic fatigue, often accompanied by a host of other refractory symptoms. Such individuals have a lifelong history of bodily complaints that elude diagnosis and treatment. Their symptoms are a cross they bear in a crude attempt to achieve a modicum of self-esteem (see Chapter 230).

Medications

Many of the medications used to treat anxiety, depression, and insomnia can cause fatigue by virtue of their sedating side effects. When used in excess, they may actually worsen the patient's symptoms and sense of fatigue rather than alleviate them. Of the *antidepressants*, the *tricyclics* and *trazodone* are among the most sedating, which makes them useful when agitation or insomnia is a problem, but they can also lead to a feeling of being "knocked out" (see Chapter 227). Inappropriate use of *hypnotics* or *anxiolytics* (e.g., *antihistamines*, such as diphenhydramine and chlorpheniramine, and *benzodiazepines*) may produce excessive sedation or, paradoxically, exacerbate difficulty in falling or staying asleep (see Chapters 226 and 232). *Centrally acting antihypertensive agents* (e.g., reserpine, methyldopa, clonidine) may precipitate fatigue, and reserpine in doses greater than 0.5 mg/d can cause depression in patients with a prior history of the condition. On the other hand, beta-blockers do not significantly increase the risk of depression and result in only a small increase in the risk of fatigue—on the order of 18 cases per 1,000 patient-years—regardless of lipid solubility and central nervous system penetration.

Endocrine Disturbances

Endocrine disturbances are important, treatable precipitants. Dysfunction of the thyroid, adrenal, pituitary, parathyroid, or endocrine pancreas can be subtle in onset, starting out inconspicuously as fatigue, perhaps accompanied by more specific symptoms. For example, *hypothyroidism* may present as fatigue, perhaps in association with weight gain, dry skin, mild hoarseness, or cold intolerance (see Chapter 104). In the elderly, *hyperthyroidism* may take an atypical form (apathetic hyperthyroidism) characterized by fatigue, marked weight loss, apathy, and otherwise unexplained atrial fibrillation (see Chapter 103). Patients with *Addison's disease* manifest an insidious onset of fatigue in conjunction with weight loss, vague gastrointestinal upset, postural hypotension, and eventually hyperpigmentation. *Panhypopituitarism* from postpartum hemorrhage or a tumor of the sellar region can cause fatigue. The postpartum patient fails to lactate or resume menstruation; lassitude, decreased libido, and loss of axillary and pubic hair ensue. Later, symptoms of hypothyroidism may develop. The patient with a pituitary tumor may note galactorrhea and amenorrhea (see Chapter 100). Poorly controlled *diabetes mellitus* may present as fatigue accompanied by polyuria when glycosuria is severe enough to produce caloric wasting and volume depletion (see Chapter 102). The condition is easy to overlook when fatigue dominates the clinical presentation and obscures the more characteristic features of hyperglycemia (see Chapter 102). Similarly, fatigue may be the initial symptom of *hyperparathyroidism* and other causes of *hypercalcemia*.

Renal and Hepatic Disturbances

Chronic renal failure may present inconspicuously with fatigue and few localizing symptoms or signs aside from laboratory findings of azotemia, mild anemia, impaired renal concentrating ability, and an abnormal urinary sediment (see Chapter 142). *Hepatocellular failure* is an important source of lassitude. Jaundice, ascites, petechiae, asterixis, spider angiomata, and other signs of hepatic insufficiency usually contribute to the clinical picture. However, in anicteric hepatitis and mild forms of chronic hepatitis, jaundice may be minimal or absent while fatigue is prominent; the same holds for the prodromal phase of acute viral hepatitis (see Chapters 70 and 71).

Hematologic and Oncologic Etiologies

Iron deficiency is often blamed for fatigue, although the correlation between iron-deficiency anemia and fatigue is poor, especially when the anemia is mild (see Chapter 79). In a double-blind study of menstruating women with mild anemia resulting from iron deficiency, no significant difference was noted between the effects of iron and of placebo on fatigue. The relation between severe anemia (hematocrit <20) and fatigue is more direct. Lassitude prevails, at times in association with exertional dyspnea or with postural hypotension when blood loss is acute.

Occult malignancy is a much-feared etiology. Although fatigue and lassitude accompany most cancers, pancreatic carcinoma is the archetypal example of a tumor that may present initially as marked fatigue with few localizing symptoms. Severe weight loss, depression, and apathy may also dominate the clinical picture before other manifestations of the malignancy become evident. Malignancies causing *hypercalcemia* (e.g., breast cancer, myeloma) may present with fatigue, although usually the hypercalcemia is a late development.

Cardiopulmonary Disease

The hallmark of fatigue associated with cardiopulmonary disease is a history of exertional dyspnea. Fatigue sometimes dominates the clinical presentation of patients with chronic *congestive heart failure* or *chronic lung disease*, especially when patients with heart failure are treated aggressively for symptoms of pulmonary congestion (see Chapters 32 and 47). *Sleep apnea* is an often overlooked pulmonary cause of chronic fatigue. Daytime sleepiness, excessive snoring, irregular breathing, disturbed sleep, and hemoglobin desaturation are characteristic. If untreated, sleep apnea may progress to pulmonary hypertension (see Chapter 46).

Infectious Diseases

Profound fatigue, low-grade fever, and lymphadenopathy are the hallmarks of a number of much-feared infectious etiologies, including *mononucleosis*, viral *hepatitis*, and *HIV* infection. Other viral illnesses, such as *cytomegalovirus* infection and the possibly *postviral chronic fatigue syndrome* (as discussed later), may also present in this way. *Tuberculosis* and *subacute bacterial endocarditis* are important infectious etiologies of fatigue in which few localizing symptoms may be present. A history of cough, night sweats, HIV infection, or exposure is sometimes elicited from the patient with tuberculosis (see Chapter 49). Recent dental work, a heart murmur, and intravenous drug abuse are risk factors for subacute bacterial endocarditis. *Lyme disease* is noteworthy for fatigue accompanied by joint complaints, headache, and low-grade fever (see Chapter 160).

Connective Tissue Disease and Other Forms of Immune Dysfunction

Marked fatigue may dominate the initial clinical presentation of most rheumatoid diseases, before characteristic inflammatory connective tissue manifestations become evident (see Chapter 156).

Chronic Fatigue Syndrome

Chronic fatigue syndrome (CFS) is an idiopathic condition characterized by new onset of persistent or relapsing fatigue lasting at least 6 consecutive months in patients with no prior history of such fatigue. Associated symptoms may include migratory arthralgias, myalgias, sore throat, tender lymph nodes, new generalized headache, unrefreshing sleep, postexertional malaise, and impaired memory or concentration. The initial presentation may be flulike, but unlike the typical symptoms of postviral fatigue, these symptoms persist far beyond 1 to 2 months. CFS accounts for about 5% to 10% of all cases of chronic fatigue. Peak prevalence is among persons of age 20 to 50 years. Women outnumber men by 3 to 1; however, the condition is not restricted to white, middle-class women.

The mechanism of CFS is unknown. The most consistent finding of CFS etiologic studies has been the inconsistency of results. Early, uncontrolled studies revealed intriguing suggestions of Epstein–Barr virus (EBV) reactivation, immunologic dysfunction, and even chronic *Candida* infection. The findings encouraged early etiologic designations such as "chronic mononucleosis," "chronic fatigue and immune dysfunction syndrome," and "chronic candidiasis." Attempts at treatment with antiviral agents, immunoglobulin injections, and systemic antifungal agents proved ineffective when studied in controlled fashion. Moreover, subsequent controlled studies found many CFS patients with no evidence of EBV infection or reactivation, immunologic dysfunction, or chronic candidal infection. Still, some investigators continue to explore the relation between stress (a known risk factor for CFS), immune modulation, and reactivation of latent viruses, with an eye toward how these conditions might trigger neuroendocrine responses.

Current research focuses on neuroendocrinologic mechanisms. Interest derives from the observation that neurally mediated hypotension occurs with increased frequency in CFS patients; however, questions remain as to whether this is a cause or an effect of the deconditioning that occurs in CFS patients. Placebo-controlled, double-blinded studies of hydrocortisone, fludrocortisone, and a combination of the two fail to demonstrate significant improvement in symptoms. An association with fibromyalgia has been noted, but it is unclear whether this represents a common pathophysiology or overlapping diagnostic criteria (see Chapter 159). Similarly, there is an increased prevalence of other nonexclusionary chronic fatiguing illnesses such as irritable bowel syndrome, chronic pelvic pain, multiple chemical sensitivities, and temporomandibular joint dysfunction.

Some view CFS as predominantly a psychiatric condition, given the high prevalence of concurrent psychiatric disease, particularly somatization disorder, found in CFS patients subjected to detailed psychiatric study (range, 20% to 70%). Others argue that this association might be simply a consequence of the original diagnostic criteria for CFS, which had many features overlapping with those of somatization disorder (see later discussion). However, population-based studies reveal a significant association between increased levels of multiple types of childhood trauma and clinically confirmed CFS, as well as an association between higher emotional instability or self-reported stress in the premorbid period and risk for the condition. Studies of twins find that genetic influences may play a role in mediating both personality style and expression of the disorder.

Risk of suicidality and a high prevalence of major depression in CFS patients are no higher than what is found in patients with other chronic disabling diseases. In addition, the physical manifestations noted here are atypical for such psychiatric disorders as depression and anxiety, and the anhedonia, guilt, and low motivation that characterize depression are infrequent in CFS. In fact, many of these patients are highly motivated and work hard to deal with their illness.

DIFFERENTIAL DIAGNOSIS

Although the list of conditions that may present with fatigue is extensive, most cases have a strong overlay of anxiety, depression, or both, even when the cause is medical. Fatigue, of course, may accompany any illness, but those listed in Table 8.1 are notable for the prominence of lassitude in the clinical presentation. Depression and associated psychiatric conditions account for about two thirds of cases of persistent fatigue subjected to comprehensive medical and psychological evaluation. Another one fourth of cases remain idiopathic, having some but not enough features to qualify as CFS. About 5% meet the Centers for Disease Control and Prevention (CDC) criteria for

TABLE 8.1

SOME CONDITIONS PRESENTING AS CHRONIC FATIGUE

Psychological
  Depression
  Anxiety
  Somatization disorder
Pharmacologic
  Hypnotics
  Antihypertensives
  Antidepressants
  Tranquilizers
  Drug abuse and drug withdrawal
Endocrine—Metabolic
  Hypothyroidism
  Diabetes mellitus
  Apathetic hyperthyroidism of the elderly
  Pituitary insufficiency
  Hyperparathyroidism or hypercalcemia of any origin
  Addison's disease
  Chronic renal failure
  Hepatocellular failure
Neoplastic—Hematologic
  Occult malignancy (e.g., pancreatic cancer)
  Severe anemia
Infectious
  Endocarditis
  Tuberculosis
  Mononucleosis
  Hepatitis
  Parasitic disease
  HIV infection
  Cytomegalovirus infection
Cardiopulmonary
  Chronic congestive heart failure
  Chronic obstructive pulmonary disease
Connective Tissue Disease—Immune Hyperreactivity
  Rheumatoid disease
  Chronic fatigue syndrome
Disturbed Sleep
  Sleep apnea
  Esophageal reflux
  Allergic rhinitis
  Psychological etiologies (see earlier entries)

chronic fatigue syndrome, and 3% turn out to be previously unrecognized medical disorders.

WORKUP (9–18)

In most instances, the evaluation of fatigue can be conveniently performed in the office. Two or three visits may be needed to establish the underlying etiology; at times, the patient may insist that medical illness be ruled out before agreeing to discuss psychosocial matters.

History

The inquiry should begin with a thorough description of the fatigue to be sure that the patient is not confusing focal neuromuscular disease with generalized lassitude. Because depression underlies many cases of fatigue, it is essential to check for its somatic manifestations, such as early-morning awakening, alteration of appetite, and multisystem functional complaints. It is also important to ask about significant losses, history of childhood abuse, low self-esteem, and occurrence of crying spells and suicidal thoughts. Anxiety is suggested by unresolved conflict, persistent nervousness, recurrent bouts of excessive uneasiness, and trouble falling asleep. A lifelong history of refractory bodily complaints that defy diagnosis and treatment should raise suspicion of a personality disturbance.

Any abuse of hypnotics or tranquilizers needs to be ascertained and considered as a cause of disturbed sleep and resultant fatigue. Fatigue in the elderly patient should not be ascribed to age; an underlying psychogenic or medical illness is likely. A history of fever, sweats, weight loss, and adenopathy points toward smoldering infection and occult neoplasm. Symptoms suggesting a metabolic or endocrinologic cause include polyuria, polydipsia, changes in skin pigmentation and texture, hoarseness, cold intolerance, nausea, and abnormal menses. Symmetric joint pain and morning stiffness are clues to underlying rheumatoid disease.

Checking into factors that might disturb sleep can lead to detection of treatable causes such as sleep apnea (see Chapter 46), esophageal reflux (see Chapter 61), and allergic rhinitis (see Chapter 222).

The past medical history should be investigated for anemia, rheumatic fever, mononucleosis, heart murmur, recurrent urinary tract infection, proteinuria, liver disease, alcohol and drug abuse, and depression. Epidemiologic considerations ought to include exposure to tuberculosis, mononucleosis, and hepatitis; any risk factors for AIDS are important to note (see Chapter 13). Travel to areas where parasitic infections are endemic, work in meat-packing industries or on a farm, and a sudden common source outbreak of illness are other potentially important epidemiologic clues.

A full listing of the patient's medications should be obtained. Often overlooked are over-the-counter antihistamines that patients use for sleep, allergies, and colds. The list should be reviewed for centrally acting antihypertensive agents, hypnotics, and psychotropic agents.

Physical Examination

Vital signs including postural pulse and blood pressure, temperature, and weight should be determined. If no fever is noted on examination in the office but it is suggested by history, then a 10 P.M. reading at home is indicated. Skin is assessed for change in pigmentation, purpura, dryness, rash, jaundice, and pallor. Endocarditis may first be suggested by the finding of splinter hemorrhages or petechiae. Fundoscopic examination may reveal Roth's spots, diabetic retinopathy, or even, in rare instances, a tuberculoma. The sclerae are observed for icterus. If examination of the pharynx reveals petechiae at the junction of the hard and the soft palate, mononucleosis ought to be considered. The thyroid is checked for goiter.

Careful examination of all lymph nodes is essential; size, degree of tenderness, and distribution should be noted. Diffuse adenopathy suggests malignancy and infection, and is sometimes a sign of HIV infection (see Chapter 12). Breasts should be checked for masses because breast cancer and its attendant hypercalcemia may present as fatigue. The lungs are examined for rales, consolidation, and effusion and the heart for murmurs, rubs, gallops, and rhythm disturbances. Unexplained atrial fibrillation in the elderly may be a manifestation of apathetic hyperthyroidism.

The abdomen is palpated for organomegaly, masses, ascites, and hepatic tenderness. The rectal examination includes a look for masses, prostatic pathology, and occult blood. The genitalia should be checked for masses suggestive of malignancy and tenderness indicative of infection. The joints are assessed for signs of inflammation. A complete neurologic examination is necessary to ensure that the patient's fatigue is not a manifestation of neuromuscular disease. Any tenderness, atrophy, focal weakness, or fasciculations in the muscles are noted. Deep tendon reflexes that have a slow relaxation phase are suggestive of hypothyroidism. Even visual field testing is important because a pituitary lesion may produce a bitemporal hemianopsia. Mental status assessment is critical, including observation of affect, thinking, judgment, and memory. Formal testing for suicidality is indicated (see Chapter 227) because of the high prevalence of depression in this patient population.

Laboratory Tests

In the overtly depressed patient with an otherwise completely normal history and physical examination, there is no need to proceed with an extensive laboratory workup for occult medical illness. A *complete blood count* (CBC) and *erythrocyte sedimentation rate* (ESR) are often ordered for screening purposes. The CBC, particularly if accompanied by a look at the peripheral smear and differential, may provide important clues to underlying infection, inflammatory disease, hepatocellular failure, or malignancy. Unfortunately, the ESR has not proved to be sensitive or specific enough to help in detecting or ruling out occult illness. Consequently, many physicians no longer order the ESR, whereas others continue to use it with the intent of acting on it only if the result is markedly elevated (e.g., >75 mm/hr).

A particularly difficult situation is the patient with no evidence of depression as a primary cause and an unrevealing history and physical examination. Here, a few extra serum *chemistries* (calcium, albumin, blood urea nitrogen, creatinine, glucose, and transaminase–aminotransferase) are warranted to help rule out clinically subtle conditions that may present as fatigue, such as hypercalcemia, mild renal failure, early diabetes mellitus, and anicteric hepatitis. A *thyrotropin* (TSH) test is worth considering because thyroid disease represents a very treatable cause that can have a very subtle presentation, and the improved TSH assay is very sensitive for the detection of most forms of hyperthyroidism and hypothyroidism. The elderly fatigued patient with weight loss and unexplained atrial fibrillation is a prime candidate for a TSH determination. Other thyroid indices add little and should not be obtained unless the TSH level is abnormal (see Chapters 103 and 104).

Patients with recent onset of persisting fatigue and adenopathy should undergo a *heterophile test* for acute mononucleosis. However, viral antibody titers (with the exception of testing for viral hepatitis and HIV infection) are of no known utility in patients with undiagnosed chronic fatigue. Ordering a battery of viral antibody titers was popular when CFS was thought to be caused by chronic EBV infection or reactivation of other viruses. Without a proven etiologic role for viruses in CFS, viral titers proved to be useless and sometimes misleading, especially when results were "positive" in a patient with severe depression who refused to accept a psychiatric diagnosis. The same holds true for *Candida* and fungal testing. *Lyme titers* are also of little use in the absence of other evidence suggestive of Lyme disease, such as polyarthritis, history of tick bite, or erythema chronicum migrans (see Chapter 160). Testing for viral hepatitis is clearly indicated in those with a transaminase elevation, and *HIV testing* is appropriate when diffuse adenopathy or a history of high-risk behavior is present.

Neuroimaging studies have been used investigationally in persons with CFS to assess regional brain function. Positron emission tomography and single-photon emission computed tomography have demonstrated areas of brain hypometabolism and hypoperfusion, respectively, in CFS patients. Because the specificity and pathophysiologic significance of these findings remain to be determined, these imaging techniques are not indicated at present for the workup of chronic fatigue or diagnosis of CFS.

Diagnosis of Chronic Fatigue Syndrome

No test or set of tests is diagnostic for CFS. Diagnosis is based on clinical findings and the ruling out of other etiologies. A working case definition was developed by the CDC in 1988 to provide a more uniform basis for identifying and studying patients with CFS. Patients had to fulfill two major criteria plus either six symptom criteria and two physical criteria or eight symptom criteria (Table 8.2).

Despite the development of a case definition, studies continued to produce unacceptably inconsistent results, suggesting that the case definition was producing too much heterogeneity in CFS populations and too much overlap with somatization disorders. In 1994, the CDC sponsored a revision of the case definition (Table 8.2). Two major criteria were eliminated: (a) more than 50% reduction in activity because it is too difficult to quantify, and (b) absence of any psychiatric disease because nonpsychotic depression and anxiety are frequent in CFS. In addition, the number of minor criteria was reduced from eight to four (Table 8.2) to reduce overlap with somatization disorder.

TABLE 8.2

CENTERS FOR DISEASE CONTROL AND PREVENTION CASE DEFINITION CRITERIA FOR CHRONIC FATIGUE SYNDROME

	1988 Criteria	1994 Criteria
Major Criteria		
New onset	+	+
No previous history	+	+
Duration >6 mo	+	+
Does not improve with bed rest	+	+
All other illnesses excluded	+	+
Activity reduction >50%	+	−
All psychiatric illnesses excluded	+	+/−
Minor Criteria	Need 8 of 14	Need 4 of 8
Sore throat	+	+
Painful lymph nodes	+	+
Muscle discomfort	+	+
Prolonged fatigue after exercise	+	+
Generalized (new) headache	+	+
Migratory arthralgias	+	+
Impaired concentration or memory	+	+
Unrefreshing sleep	+	+
Low-grade fever	+	−
Generalized weakness	+	−
Acute onset	+	−
Documented low-grade fever	+	−
Documented nonexudative pharyngitis	+	−
Documented palpable or tender lymph nodes	+	−
Subclassifications		
Presence of comorbid conditions (depression)	None	Yes
Current level of fatigue	None	Yes
Duration of fatigue	None	Yes
Current level of physical function	None	Yes

From Levine PH. Chronic fatigue syndrome comes of age. Am J Med 1997;105:35, with permission.

Subgroup classifications were recommended to facilitate identification for the study of patients who might have similar prognoses and responses to therapy. Subgrouping criteria include comorbid conditions, severity of fatigue, duration, and current level of physical function. Finally, a designation of idiopathic chronic fatigue was proposed for the substantial number of persons with unexplained fatigue meeting some but not all of the criteria for chronic fatigue syndrome.

Clinicians need to keep in mind that case definitions are only consensus views intended to facilitate research. Although such definitions can be used for clinical diagnosis, they are not based on scientifically established criteria and remain somewhat arbitrary, requiring clinical judgment for proper use in patient care. Until the etiology of CFS is better understood, these shortcomings will have to be taken into consideration when the working definition is used for diagnostic purposes. (The reader is urged to watch the literature closely for further developments.)

PATIENT EDUCATION

It is often useful to determine patients' views of their illness before proceeding with patient education so that the explanation will address patient concerns and perspectives. Patients who have a medical view of their condition are more receptive to a biologic explanation for their symptoms, even if the cause is psychogenic. However, one must be careful not to evoke a misleading medical explanation, such as "viral infection" or "immune dysfunction," especially in the setting of a suspected or possible psychogenic etiology, because this might cause a patient to delay or refuse psychiatric intervention. Patients with evidence of underlying psychogenic disease need an especially thorough review of the evidence for their diagnosis and a careful explanation of their symptoms because many come to the physician thinking they have a medical problem. For example, reviewing the diagnostic criteria for depression and describing the neurochemical mechanisms by which depression leads to fatigue (see Chapter 227) can be helpful.

The attention given to CFS in the lay press often necessitates addressing the issue of its likelihood and some of its purported, although unfounded, causes (e.g., EBV infection, yeast infection, immune dysfunction). Many patients with a psychogenic etiology prefer to cling to this diagnosis as an acceptable explanation of their psychophysiologic symptoms rather than face a diagnosis of depression, anxiety, or somatization disorder. In addition to a careful workup, a respectful, sympathetic, open-minded approach is essential (see Chapter 230).

SYMPTOMATIC RELIEF

When the cause of chronic fatigue is endocrinologic, metabolic, or infectious, treatment needs to be etiologic. Similarly, chronic fatigue due to a sleep disorder related to sleep apnea, reflux, or allergic rhinitis should be treated by attending to the underlying pathophysiology (see Chapters 46, 61, and 222). Fatigue due to malignancy is multifactorial, necessitating a host of measures, including use of antidepressants when depression is prominent (see Chapter 87). In general, disabling fatigue associated with depression is an indication for antidepressant therapy. For younger persons, a minimally sedating tricyclic agent taken before bed (e.g., *nortriptyline* 25 mg every evening at bedtime) can be helpful; for older patients, a generic SSRI antidepressant (e.g., *fluoxetine* 20 mg in the morning) may be better tolerated (see Chapter 227). The sleep disorder of depression may respond well to these small starting doses, with fatigue dissipating as the patients gets a better night's sleep (see Chapter 232).

Fatigue due to an anxiety disorder may initially respond to benzodiazepine therapy, but long-term use of these anxiolytics can lead to abuse, dependency, and worsening of symptoms. The anxiolytic effect of selective serotonin reuptake inhibitor (SSRI) antidepressants can be very useful in persons with an anxiety disorder, obviating or at least reducing the need for chronic benzodiazepine use. Starting with a combined program of a generic SSRI and a long-acting benzodiazepine (e.g., *fluoxetine* 20 mg in the morning and *clonazepam* 0.5 mg twice daily) provides prompt and sustained symptomatic relief and allows discontinuation of the benzodiazepine in about 4 to 6 weeks as the SSRI takes effect (see Chapter 226).

If fatigue results from sleep disturbed by sleep apnea, reflux, or allergic rhinitis, then treatment should be directed toward the underlying pathophysiology (see Chapters 46, 61, and 222).

APPROACH TO THE PATIENT WITH CHRONIC FATIGUE SYNDROME (12,13,19–25)

For patients who meet the criteria for chronic fatigue syndrome, the physician should emphasize the legitimacy of the patient's symptoms and summarize the workup, its rationale, and its findings. Also useful is a review of the idiopathic nature of the illness, its generally self-limited course, and often favorable response to simple measures (see later discussion). Establishing a partnership with the patient is key to successful management. Certain beliefs and behaviors known to perpetuate disability and lead to a worse outcome in CFS must be addressed, particularly the view that a purely physical disease mechanism is present that is unresponsive to intervention and that exercise is harmful. Such beliefs and associated behaviors contribute to resignation, anxiety, and depression and exacerbate deconditioning and the feeling of fatigue. At times, referral for formal cognitive–behavioral therapy is worth pursuing to achieve the educational and behavioral goals so important to recovery (see further discussion). It is important that any new symptoms or signs be investigated thoroughly and not simply attributed to CFS.

Some of the best results have been achieved with *cognitive–behavioral therapy*, a nonpharmacologic treatment that focuses on identifying and reversing beliefs and coping mechanisms that perpetuate disability and block recovery. More than 75% of patients experience a return to normal daily activity by 12 months, in comparison with 25% randomized to standard medical care alone. Although this approach does not directly address the underlying etiology of CFS (which remains unknown), it does seek to deal with ideas and behaviors that encourage passivity and hinder self-help and symptomatic improvement. Treatment begins by elucidating the patient's beliefs about the illness and by exploring the behaviors that follow from these beliefs. Patients marked by helplessness and passivity are targeted for change during a series of sessions in which the therapist works in partnership with the patient. The goal is to have the patient regain a sense of control and active participation in recovery. Although most studies of cognitive–behavioral therapy in CFS involve formally trained therapists, there is no theoretical reason why the primary care physician cannot conduct the basic steps of the program (Table 8.3).

TABLE 8.3

BASIC STEPS IN COGNITIVE–BEHAVIORAL THERAPY

1. Problem assessment and formulation
2. Identification of beliefs and coping behaviors that perpetuate illness-related disability
3. Development of more adaptive beliefs and coping behaviors
4. Patient testing of new approach to the illness and adopting it if it works
5. Consolidating gains and planning further self-help

From Sharpe M. Cognitive behavior therapy for chronic fatigue syndrome: efficacy and implications. Am J Med 1998;105:104S, with permission.

A basic part of the cognitive–behavioral program is a gentle, graded exercise program. Some have even speculated that exercise is the key element, but exercise in the absence of a cognitive component leads to a high dropout rate. Those bothered by disordered sleep may benefit from low-dose antidepressant therapy (e.g., 25 mg of nortriptyline at bedtime, 10 to 20 mg of doxepin at bedtime, or 10 mg of paroxetine every morning). Higher doses do not appear to confer better results. Nonsteroidal antiinflammatory drugs provide symptomatic relief in patients bothered by myalgias, arthralgias, or headache.

A host of enthusiastic reports from uncontrolled studies have appeared claiming marked benefit from the use of liver extract, antifungal therapy, antiviral drugs, vitamins, immunoglobulin infusions, fatty acids, adrenal corticosteroids (e.g., hydrocortisone and fludrocortisone), and anticholinesterases. Almost without exception, none has proved beneficial when subjected to randomized, double-blind, placebo-controlled study. Definitive etiologic therapy will have to await a better understanding of CFS pathophysiology. Fortunately, its symptoms are often self-limited, frequently improving or even clearing within 12 to 18 months. A strong patient–doctor alliance is essential, not only for providing support, but also for protecting the patient from unnecessary testing and unproven therapies.

A.H.G.

Annotated Bibliography

1. Kroenke K, Wood DR, Mangelsdorff, et al. Chronic fatigue in primary care. JAMA 1988;260:929. (*Documents a high prevalence of persistence and functional impairment.*)
2. Jason LA, Richman JA, Rademaker AW, et al. A community-based study of chronic fatigue syndrome. Arch Intern Med 1999;159:2129 (*A point-prevalence study of >28,000 Chicago residents; highest prevalences are found among women but are spread across ethnic groups.*)
3. Manu P, Lane TJ, Mathews DA. The frequency of the chronic fatigue syndrome in patients with symptoms of persistent fatigue. Ann Intern Med 1988;109:554. (*The prevalence was only 5%, which indicates that the condition is actually quite uncommon among those presenting with fatigue.*)
4. Croog SH, Levine S, Testa A, et al. The effects of antihypertensive therapy on the quality of life. N Engl J Med 1986;314:1657. (*The incidence of fatigue was about 5% in persons taking the antihypertensive agents methyldopa and propranolol.*)
5. Ko DT, Hebert PR, Coffey CS, et al. Beta-block therapy and symptoms of depression, fatigue, and sexual dysfunction. JAMA 2002;288:351. (*A meta-analysis of 15 randomized trials; there was a small but significant annual increase in risk of fatigue.*)
6. Aurbach G, Mallette L, Patten B, et al. Hyperparathyroidism: recent studies. NIH conference. Ann Intern Med 1973;79:566. (*Fatigue headed the list of symptoms reported in 57 cases of primary hyperparathyroidism; 24% reported the problem.*)
7. Thomas F, Mazzaferri E, Skillman T. Apathetic thyrotoxicosis: a distinctive clinical and laboratory entity. Ann Intern Med 1970;72:679. (*A classic article identifying the condition; patients are typically elderly and depressed, and they exhibit marked weight loss and otherwise unexplained atrial fibrillation.*)
8. Wood M, Elwood P. Symptoms of iron deficiency anemia: a community survey. Br J Prev Soc Med 1966;20:117. (*Correlation between hemoglobin concentration and symptoms was poor; iron therapy produced no statistically significant improvement in symptoms.*)
9. Fukuda K, Straus SE, Hickie I, et al. The chronic fatigue syndrome: a comprehensive approach to its definition and study. Ann Intern Med 1994;121:953. (*The current Centers for Disease Control and Prevention consensus working definition of the syndrome and recommendations for evaluation and study.*)
10. Heim C, Wagner D, Maloney E, et al. Early adverse experience and risk for chronic fatigue syndrome: results from a population-based study. Arch Gen Psychiatry 2006;63:1258. (*An epidemiologic case–control study finding a significant correlation between childhood psychiatric trauma and the risk of developing chronic fatigue syndrome.*)
11. Holmes GP, Kaplan JE, Gantz NM, et al. Chronic fatigue syndrome: a working case definition. Ann Intern Med 1988;108:387. (*The original working case definition of chronic fatigue syndrome.*)
12. Kato K, Sullivan PF, Evengard B, et al. Premorbid predictors of chronic fatigue. Arch Gen Psychiatry 2006;63:1267. (*Prospective epidemiologic twin study; finds that the premorbid psychological state predicts chronic fatigue risk.*)
13. Dismukes WE, Wade JS, Lee JY, et al. A randomized, double-blind trial of nystatin therapy for the candidiasis hypersensitivity syndrome. N Engl J Med 1990;323:1717. (*Strong evidence against yeast infection as the cause of the chronic fatigue syndrome.*)
14. Freeman R, Komaroff AL. Does the chronic fatigue syndrome involve the autonomic nervous system? Am J Med 1997;102:357. (*Evidence supporting autonomic dysfunction but not distinguishing between deconditioning and an autonomic neuropathy.*)
15. Kendell RE. Chronic fatigue, viruses, and depression. Lancet 1991;337:160. (*An editorial summing up the evidence favors the view that most patients reporting chronic fatigue have depression, and a few might have some kind of postviral syndrome.*)
16. Gold D, Bowden R, Sixbey J, et al. Chronic fatigue: a prospective clinical and virologic study. JAMA 1990;264:48. (*Isolated Epstein–Barr virus [EBV] was no more frequent in patients with chronic fatigue than it was in healthy controls, and improvement in patients with chronic fatigue was not associated with any change in EBV levels.*)
17. Goldenberg DL, Simms RW, Geiger A, et al. High frequency of fibromyalgia in patients with chronic fatigue syndrome seen in a primary care practice. Arthritis Rheum 1990;33:381. (*An interesting association, but its significance is unclear.*)
18. Sox HC, Liang MH. The erythrocyte sedimentation rate. Ann Intern Med 1986;104:515. (*A critical review arguing the test is not a useful screening procedure in most instances.*)
19. Blockmans D, Persoons P, Van Houdenhove B, et al. Combination therapy with hydrocortisone and fludrocortisone does not improve symptoms in chronic fatigue syndrome: a randomized placebo controlled, double-blind trial. Am J Med 2003;114:736. (*A well-designed study finding no benefit.*)
20. Kaslow JE, Rucker L, Onishi R. Liver extract–folic acid–cyanocobalamin vs. placebo for chronic fatigue syndrome. Arch Intern Med 1989;149:2501. (*A double-blind, placebo-controlled, crossover study showing no benefit.*)
21. Rowe PC, Calkins H, DeBusk K, et al. Fludrocortisone acetate to treat neurally mediated hypotension in chronic fatigue syndrome. JAMA 2001;285:52. (*A randomized, double-blinded, placebo-controlled trial; treatment was no better than placebo.*)
22. Vollmer-Conna U, Hicki I, Hadzi-Pavlovic D, et al. Intravenous immunoglobulin is ineffective in the treatment of patients with chronic fatigue syndrome. Am J Med 1997;103:38. (*A randomized, double-blind study showing no benefit.*)
23. Whiting P, Bagnall WP, Sowden AJ, et al. Interventions for the treatment and management of chronic fatigue syndrome. A systematic review. JAMA 2001;286:1360. (*A systematic review of nearly 40 controlled studies of treatment; best results were found for cognitive–behavioral therapy.*)
24. Sharpe M. Cognitive behavior therapy for chronic fatigue syndrome: efficacy and implications. Am J Med 1998;105(3A):104s. (*Best summary of the approach; nearly 75% of patients achieve a return to normal daily activity by 12 months.*)
25. Blacker CV Russel, Greenwood DT, Wesnes R, et al. Effect of galantamine hydrobromide in chronic fatigue syndrome: a randomized controlled trial. JAMA 2004;292:1195. (*Placebo-controlled randomized controlled trial; no benefit found.*)

CHAPTER 9 ■ EVALUATION OF WEIGHT LOSS

Involuntary weight loss, which can be defined as an unexplained sustained weight loss of 5% or more over a 6- to 12-month period, is a sensitive, although nonspecific, complaint, which can be a harbinger of serious underlying pathology and poor prognosis, especially in the elderly. Reports of prevalence range from 3% to 10%, with frequency greatest among the elderly. Unexplained weight loss often suggests the presence of worrisome underlying pathology, yet a substantial fraction of patients turns out to be free of serious organic illness. For example, in a series of patients with involuntary weight loss followed for 1 year, 50% either died or deteriorated during the course of the study; however, another 35% were well at the time of follow-up. Involuntary weight loss in excess of 2.5 kg (about 5.5 lb) over 6 to 12 months is usually considered a reasonable threshold for evaluation because more than 95% of patients with an organic etiology will have lost at least that much weight. However, unless extreme, the amount of weight loss is not predictive of an organic etiology. In many cases of weight loss, accompanying symptoms readily suggest the cause, but when a marked fall in weight is the sole or predominant complaint, the assessment can be difficult. Underlying malignancy, chronic inflammatory disease, serious infection, and depression represent primary concerns. The primary physician needs to determine at the time of initial presentation who requires an extensive medical evaluation and who can be followed expectantly.

PATHOPHYSIOLOGY AND CLINICAL PRESENTATION

Pathophysiology (1–10)

Involuntary weight loss represents a state of malnutrition, which can be subdivided pathophysiologically into mechanisms of *starvation* and *cachexia*. Although frank clinical states of starvation or cachexia are often not evident, one of these pathophysiologic mechanisms is likely to be operational in cases of involuntary weight loss. In both, there is reduced caloric intake resulting in weight loss, but in starvation, resting energy expenditure, protein synthesis, and protein degradation are reduced, whereas in cachexia, these parameters are markedly increased. In starvation, fat is lost preferentially; in cachexia, loss of muscle mass is prominent.

Cachexia

The pathophysiology of cachexia starts with tissue injury triggering the release of proinflammatory cytokines (e.g., interleukins, tumor necrosis factor), which in turn stimulate synthesis of binding proteins, complement, apoproteins, fibrinogen, C-reactive protein, and other inflammatory mediators. Skeletal muscle is sacrificed to provide the essential amino acids needed to support the increased protein synthesis. Resting metabolism increases to supply the additional energy necessary for proteolysis and synthesis of new protein. Cytokine release also reduces appetite and contributes to the anorexia and fatigue that are prominent in conditions associated with cachexia.

Starvation

In contrast, starvation's pathophysiology entails mobilization and metabolism of stored fat in conjunction with reductions in energy expenditure, protein synthesis, and protein degradation.

Caloric Deficit and Volume Depletion

Regardless of underlying pathophysiology, caloric deficit is a common denominator in cases of weight loss, initially targeting fat stores. The principal mechanisms resulting in caloric deficits are *reduced food intake, malabsorption, excess nutrient loss,* and *increased caloric requirements.* When the number of calories available for utilization falls below daily needs, weight is lost; 1 lb of fat is consumed for every 3,500-cal deficit. Loss of fluid and dehydration will also register as a fall in weight, with about 1 kg (2.2 lb) lost for every liter removed and not replaced.

Anorexia

The mechanisms of anorexia include those associated with the pathologic conditions leading to cachexia (see earlier) as well as with polypharmacy, pain, and depression (e.g., increased corticotropin-releasing factor). In the elderly, the normal physiology of aging may contribute, producing reductions in smell and taste and increases in the appetite-suppressing hormones leptin (from decreased testosterone) and cholecystokinin. Moreover, there is less gastric distensibility (producing early satiety) and more social isolation. Unpalatable diets, especially those that are very low in sodium, may contribute.

Clinical Presentation (1–10)

Although the clinical features of the underlying etiology usually dominate the presentation, a few features may suggest the underlying pathophysiology. For example, disproportionate loss of muscle mass and increased resting heart rate suggest cachexia, whereas relative preservation of muscle mass and a slow pulse suggest starvation. *Reduced intake* is suggested clinically by anorexia or disinterest in food. *Malabsorption* can cause foul-smelling, bulky, greasy stools in advanced cases; subtle changes in stool consistency and frequency are noted earlier (see Chapter 64). *Excessive loss* may present as recurrent vomiting, profuse diarrhea, polyuria, or fistulous drainage. *Increased demand* may be manifested by signs of underlying infection, inflammation, metabolic excess, or malignancy.

Although many of the illnesses that cause weight loss produce readily evident clinical manifestations, some conditions have presentations that are notoriously subtle and may involve little more than unexplained weight loss and vague systemic or functional complaints. These deserve special elaboration.

Major Depression

Major depression is the leading cause of unexplained weight loss, especially in the elderly, in whom the condition accounts for up to 30% of cases. As frequent as it is, depression is often overlooked unless specifically considered. Somatic manifestations include appetite disturbance, early-morning awakening, multiple bodily complaints, and fatigue; anhedonia, low self-esteem, feelings of guilt, and suicidal thoughts are among the characteristic psychological features. The death of a loved one, social isolation, and poverty are important psychosocial precipitants (see Chapter 227).

Dementia

Dementia is an increasingly important etiology of weight loss in the frail elderly and often contributes to social isolation and depression. Early manifestations may be subtle and include cessation of regular shopping and failure to prepare meals or to come to dinner in social settings (see Chapter 173).

Eating Disorders

Eating disorders often involve covert behaviors. The patient suffering from *anorexia nervosa* may deny any disturbance of appetite yet persist in restricting food intake to the point of cachexia. Prevalence is highest among adolescent girls and young women. They decide to diet to an extreme degree, are preoccupied with a phobic concern about being fat, and are motivated by a relentless pursuit of thinness. Dieting persists because its psychological gratifications outweigh those derived from the intake of food. Paradoxically, the patient often reports feeling well and initially appears bright and undisturbed by the weight loss; anorexia is usually denied. At times, a few specific foods are the only ones consumed (e.g., vegetable juices). Amenorrhea is invariable and appears shortly after weight loss begins. A variant of anorexia nervosa consists of surreptitiously induced vomiting following engorgement with food; hypokalemic alkalosis results (see Chapter 234).

Carcinoma of the Pancreas

Carcinoma of the pancreas is the prototypical *occult neoplasm* associated with dramatic weight loss. Weight loss is found in 79% to 90% of patients at the time of diagnosis and averages 15 to 20 lb. The degree of weight loss does not seem to correlate with size, location, or extent of disease. Aversion to food is more typical of this malignancy than is true anorexia. In many instances, weight loss precedes all other symptoms; once jaundice and abdominal pain supervene, the tumor is usually far advanced. Many other gastrointestinal malignancies as well as *ovarian cancer* may follow a similar clinical course.

HIV Infection

HIV infection can result in profound weight loss. There may be inadequate intake resulting from dysphagia, depression, or medication. Early satiety can result from gastrointestinal invasion by lymphoma, Kaposi's sarcoma, or *Mycobacterium avium–intracellulare* infection. Weight loss in the setting of adequate caloric intake suggests disseminated infection by *M. avium–intracellulare* or cytomegalovirus as well as occult malignancy. Often, the later stages of AIDS are characterized by a *wasting syndrome*, which includes loss of more than 10% of baseline weight, recurrent fever, and persistent diarrhea. The pathophysiologic mechanisms of cachexia (see earlier discussion) may play important roles, as might hypogonadism (see Chapter 13).

Celiac Sprue

Celiac sprue and other gastrointestinal causes of malabsorption may present nonspecifically in their early phases with subtle weight loss and vague gastrointestinal or extraintestinal complaints. The textbook presentation of steatorrhea may not become evident until much later. Common manifestations include modest weight loss, unexplained iron-deficiency anemia, aphthous stomatitis, malaise, fatigue, nocturnal diarrhea, flatulence, and lactose deficiency (see Chapter 64). Stools are noted to be a bit softer and more frequent than usual, and a diagnosis of irritable bowel syndrome may be entertained mistakenly because of abdominal discomfort and bloating. Mild forms of inflammatory bowel disease may also be mistaken for irritable bowel syndrome (see Chapter 64).

Early Crohn's Disease

Early Crohn's disease in adolescents has been noted on occasion to begin inconspicuously with anorexia predominating. *Blind-loop syndrome* and *giardiasis* may also have indolent presentations with weight loss and vague abdominal discomfort; however, changes in stools are usually present also, with patients reporting mushy, foul-smelling bowel movements (see Chapter 58).

Diabetes Mellitus

Diabetes mellitus is commonly found in overweight adults, but it may be the cause of weight loss when there is substantial wasting of calories from marked glycosuria. In addition, young male insulin-dependent diabetic patients are sometimes plagued by diarrhea, which exacerbates fluid and nutrient losses; true malabsorption has been noted in a few cases (see Chapter 102).

Hyperthyroidism

Hyperthyroidism that is clinically overt is an obvious cause of weight loss due to increased caloric demand; however, *apathetic hyperthyroidism* of the elderly may be mistaken for malignancy because weight loss is profound and the patient appears listless. The typical symptoms of excess thyroid hormone are absent, and unexplained atrial fibrillation is often present (see Chapter 103).

Vasculitis

Vasculitis, like HIV infection, is an archetypical example of unexplained weight loss due to tissue injury and cachexic pathophysiology. Resting metabolism is increased due to stepped-up synthesis of cytokines and other immunomodulators. A host of nonspecific systemic symptoms may predominate, triggered by the high circulating levels of these inflammatory mediators. Low-grade fever, malaise, anorexia, night sweats, apathy, and even depression may predominate. High levels of C-reactive protein and a markedly elevated erythrocyte sedimentation rate are characteristic and important clues to the diagnosis. More-specific symptoms and signs suggesting the underlying etiology include palpable purpura, joint swelling and warmth, cranial artery tenderness, microscopic hematuria, and proteinuria (see Chapters 161 and 179).

Patients with an *underlying medical cause* for their weight loss usually present with symptoms and signs that strongly suggest organic illness. In a Veterans Administration study of 91 patients with involuntary weight loss, the cause in the overwhelming majority was readily diagnosed on the basis of the initial history and physical examination; only 1 patient had a truly occult malignancy (see later discussion).

DIFFERENTIAL DIAGNOSIS (3,4,6–8)

The extensive list of causes of involuntary weight loss can be grouped pathophysiologically. Decreased intake, impaired absorption, increased loss, and excess demand are the principal mechanisms around which the differential can be organized (Table 9.1). Almost any illness can cause involuntary weight

TABLE 9.1

SOME IMPORTANT CAUSES OF WEIGHT LOSS

Decreased Intake
  HIV infection, AIDS
  Depression, bereavement
  Anxiety
  Poor dentition, loss of taste
  Esophageal disease
  Gastrointestinal disease worsened by food (e.g., peptic ulcer)
  Drugs (e.g., digitalis excess, quinidine, amphetamines, nonsteroidal antiinflammatory drugs, antitumor agents)
  Hypercalcemia
  Alcoholism
  Prodrome of viral hepatitis
  Hypokalemia
  Uremia
  Malignancy
  Chronic congestive heart failure
  Chronic inflammatory disease
  Anorexia nervosa
  Social isolation, poverty
  Dementia
Impaired Absorption
  Cholestasis
  Pancreatic insufficiency
  Postgastrectomy
  Small-bowel disease
  Parasitic infection (e.g., giardiasis)
  Blind-loop syndrome
  Drugs (e.g., cholestyramine, cathartics)
  AIDS
Increased Nutrient Loss
  Uncontrolled diabetes mellitus
  Persistent diarrhea
  Recurrent vomiting
  Drainage from a fistulous tract
Excess Demand
  Hyperthyroidism
  Fever
  Malignancy
  Emotional states (e.g., mania)
  Amphetamine abuse

loss; Table 9.1 emphasizes those conditions seen in the ambulatory setting that may present as unexplained loss of weight. Studies from primary care practices find depression to be the leading cause of unexplained weight loss, with prevalence reported in the range of 15% to 30%. Among the elderly, psychosocial factors such as loss of a spouse, social isolation, and poverty can exacerbate inadequate food intake resulting from depression. Occult malignancy, although much feared in the elderly, is usually a distant runner-up, with half the prevalence of depression. In some series, therapeutic diets, particularly those for hyperlipidemia and diabetes, also rank high in the list of causes, followed by uncontrolled diabetes and oropharyngeal problems. In the elderly, immobility, poor dentition, dementia, side effects of medication, and a decrease in sense of taste are additional causative factors that require consideration.

In high-risk populations, it is important to keep in mind serious infectious etiologies such as HIV, hepatitis C, and tuberculosis. Autoimmune disease and depression also require consideration, especially in the context of vague gastrointestinal symptoms or a preponderance of systemic or multisystem complaints.

In the elderly, essential components of the differential besides organic disease states include polypharmacy (e.g., digoxin, nonsteroidal antiinflammatory drugs [NSAIDs], theophylline), depression, dementia, social isolation, swallowing problems, poor dentition, tremor (making it difficult to eat), unpalatable diets, and inability to shop for food.

WORKUP (3,5,6,8–14)

Overall Strategy

The overall strategy is to conduct a clinical assessment that focuses on defining the underlying mechanism of weight loss so that further investigation can proceed in a logical and parsimonious fashion. Attention to the history and physical examination—including psychosocial aspects and mental status examination—is essential to accurate diagnosis and cost-effective testing. Although occult malignancy is always a concern and deserves consideration, especially in elderly persons, its workup should not preclude careful inquiry into depression, early dementia, and social isolation, which can reduce the percentage of undiagnosed cases from about 25% to 7%.

Despite a careful history and physical examination, some cases remain unexplained and are sometimes labeled *isolated involuntary weight loss*. Because extensive testing for unexplained weight loss can be arduous, expensive, and not clearly related to improved outcomes, it is helpful to formulate a pretest estimate of risk for important underlying pathology. In older undiagnosed patients, the use of a few simple screening blood tests (to be described) has proven helpful in formulating this estimate and in deciding whether more extensive testing is warranted.

History

The first task is to document that weight loss has indeed occurred and to determine its extent. In some settings, almost half of patients do not prove to have lost weight once available records have been checked. In the absence of recorded weights, meaningful historical data include a change in clothing size, the ability to report an exact weight change, and confirmation of the history by a family member.

The history can be used to help identify the mechanism(s) responsible for the decline in weight by obtaining the details of daily food intake (including calorie count) and inquiring into the presence of any appetite disturbance, dysphagia, odynophagia, steatorrhea, diarrhea, vomiting, polyuria, or symptoms of a hypermetabolic state.

When *decreased intake* is suspected, one needs to inquire into the somatic and affective symptoms of depression (see Chapter 227). Other areas of questioning should include checking for nausea and vomiting, abdominal pain, melena, early satiety, excessive use of alcohol (see Chapter 228), exposure to and risk factors for hepatitis, poor dentition, oral candidiasis, aphthous ulcers, discomfort induced by eating, medication use, history of renal or liver disease, and anxiety. Risk factors for HIV infection should also be explored (see Chapter 13). If the patient is a young woman, anorexia nervosa should be considered, and a gentle inquiry into eating habits, self-image, and attitudes about weight is indicated (see Chapter 234). Family members should also be questioned.

In the *frail elderly*, questions about social isolation, bereavement, physical impairment, poor dentition, and poverty can be of critical importance in identifying impediments to adequate food intake. Family members should be asked about memory loss, behavioral changes, and other manifestations of dementia. A review of drug use in the elderly is also essential because of the large number of medications prescribed and their potential for inducing anorexia and gastrointestinal upset. In addition, patients should be checked for a loss of taste, which is sometimes responsible for poor intake in the elderly. Use of validated questionnaires to screen for anorexia in the elderly and predict risk of weight loss focus on overall appetite, onset of feeling full when eating, taste of food, and number of meals per day.

When *impairment of absorption* is suspected, inquiries are made into other gastrointestinal symptoms, previous gastrointestinal surgery, the character of the stools, jaundice, history of pancreatitis, travel to an area known for giardiasis or other parasites, symptoms of inflammatory bowel disease (see Chapter 73), and manifestations of vitamin malabsorption (e.g., pallor, easy bruising, paresthesias, sore tongue). Increased nutrient loss is assessed historically by ascertaining the quality and quantity of material lost in addition to the frequency and duration of the condition. Of major importance is checking for symptoms of diabetic enteropathy (diarrhea in conjunction with polyuria and polydipsia).

When *excess demand* is under consideration, the patient needs to be questioned about fever, other systemic symptoms, manifestations of malignancy, symptoms of hyperthyroidism, history of amphetamine abuse (see Chapter 235), chronic anxiety (see Chapter 226), manic states, HIV disease (see Chapter 13), and autoimmune conditions (see Chapters 145, 161, and 179).

Physical Examination

The examination should begin with an accurate weight determination, followed by the notation of any wasting, apathetic appearance, fever, tachycardia, pallor, ecchymoses, purpura (palpable and not), jaundice, stigmata of hyperthyroidism or hepatocellular failure, or signs of Kaposi's sarcoma. Next, the head and neck are examined for cranial artery tenderness, glossitis, stomatitis, poor dentition, goiter, and lymphadenopathy. The lungs and heart are examined for crackles, wheezes, consolidation, effusion, cardiomegaly, murmur, and a third heart sound. The abdomen is studied for surgical scars, organomegaly, hyperactive bowel sounds, focal tenderness, distention, ascites, and masses. The rectum is examined for masses, tenderness, discharge, blood, and the appearance of the stool. The neurologic examination includes a check for signs of vitamin B$_{12}$ deficiency suggestive of terminal ileal disease (see Chapter 79), as well as any tremor, manic or depressive affect, or signs of dementia.

Laboratory Testing

Because the number of potential investigations is enormous, laboratory testing should be selective to avoid being wasteful, burdensome, and misleading. The history and physical examination will usually identify the basic mechanism(s) of weight loss and suggest specific causes that can be confirmed or ruled out by further investigation.

Decreased Intake

When decreased intake is manifested by a markedly reduced appetite accompanied by nausea, it is worth obtaining a few selected serum chemistries, including measurement of *calcium*, *potassium*, *creatinine*, *transaminase*, and *amylase*, to check for a possible gastrointestinal or metabolic precipitant. Patients with such symptoms who are taking a digitalis preparation, quinidine, or any other drug that can cause gastrointestinal upset at toxic levels should have a *serum drug concentration* determined. If NSAIDs are being taken, they should be stopped. Those not taking an NSAID should be considered for endoscopic or radiologic evaluation of the upper gastrointestinal tract and *Helicobacter* testing (see Chapter 68). In the HIV-infected patient, endoscopy may be indicated to search for upper gastrointestinal mucosal erosion (see Chapter 13).

Impaired Absorption

Stool should be obtained for gross and microscopic examination and guaiac testing performed. A *qualitative stool fat* examination, in which fecal material is stained for neutral fat, is a basic step in the workup of suspected malabsorption. If doubt persists, a 72-hour stool collection for *quantitative stool fat* provides more precise information, with values of less than 8 g/d ruling out malabsorption. The *serum carotene* level is another useful marker of fat absorption. Its absorption is independent of pancreatic function, so a normal level in the setting of malabsorption suggests pancreatic dysfunction. Similarly, the D-*xylose* test can help to distinguish pancreatic dysfunction from small-bowel disease because D-xylose absorption also does not require pancreatic enzyme activity (see Chapter 74). An elevated *serum amylase* or the radiologic demonstration of *pancreatic calcification* indicates pancreatitis (see Chapter 72), but a *secretin stimulation test* may be necessary to assess pancreatic exocrine function better. Sprue and blind-loop syndrome are the most common forms of small-bowel pathology responsible for malabsorption. A small-bowel radiologic *contrast study* might be suggestive, but a *small-bowel biopsy* is necessary for the diagnosis of sprue; an abnormal *carbon-14 glycolate breath test* will help to document bacterial overgrowth, although usually the test is unnecessary. For the diagnosis of *giardiasis*, a *stool sample for ova and parasites* suffices in many instances. Because parasites are passed intermittently, three or more stools on alternate days should be examined. Because the cysts are hardy, a fresh stool specimen is not required. Trophozoites are more likely to be found in acute cases. Examination of a duodenal aspirate or jejunal biopsy specimen is resorted to when suspicion is high but stool findings are negative. Although these tests are more productive, they are cumbersome; some clinicians instead advocate a diagnostic trial of an antigiardial drug such as metronidazole.

Increased Nutrient Loss

Any patient suspected of having diabetes mellitus should have a *urinalysis* for glycosuria. Marked glycosuria should be present in the patient with weight loss caused by diabetes.

Excess Demand

Suspicion of hyperthyroidism necessitates a *thyrotropin* determination, especially in the elderly, apathetic patient with unexplained atrial fibrillation and weight loss (see Chapter 103). In the febrile HIV patient with adequate caloric intake, the weight loss likely represents excessive demand; *cultures* of blood and stool for *acid-fast bacilli* and of blood and urine for *cytomegalovirus* are required.

Isolated Involuntary Weight Loss

One of the most difficult diagnostic issues encountered in the workup of weight loss concerns the possibility of *occult malignancy* in a person with "isolated" disease (history and physical are unrevealing). About 25% to 40% of such cases eventually prove to have cancer. Deciding when to embark on a search for tumor requires an estimate not only of the likelihood of finding a malignancy, but also of the chances that it will be treatable. Unfortunately, by the time weight loss has occurred, most malignancies are rather far advanced, and the effect of detection on survival is minimal (median survival about 2 months; few live longer than 1 year). Nonetheless, making a diagnosis of cancer can reduce uncertainty and as such may be considered worth the effort.

Use of a panel of simple blood tests has been explored as a practical means of determining who should undergo more extensive testing. The combination of *complete blood cell count, erythrocyte sedimentation rate, aspartate aminotransferase, alanine aminotransferase, gamma-glutamyltranspeptidase, alkaline phosphatase, and serum albumin* was found in one study to have a high sensitivity (95%) but low specificity (35%) for diagnosis of cancer in older persons with unexplained weight loss. Negative results on this battery of studies greatly reduced the probability of finding malignancy (only 3 of 97 cancers missed); a positive result helped to identify patients who would benefit from further investigation (starting with abdominal ultrasound in those with abnormal liver enzymes). In a primary care study of elderly patients with undiagnosed weight loss, the yield of unselected application of computed tomography was very low in the absence of clinical evidence of underlying disease.

SYMPTOMATIC THERAPY
(1,3,6,9,11,15–19)

The best approach is to treat etiologically, but the first task is to ensure that food is available to the patient, particularly the elderly person, who may be too isolated, impoverished, infirm, or depressed to take in adequate calories. It is estimated that the intake of 10% to 15% of elderly persons is less than 1,000 kcal/d. Ensuring at least one palatable hot meal per day is essential and can usually be arranged with the help of local social service agencies.

Underlying Medical Illness

Most medical causes of weight loss must be addressed etiologically. However, there are important exceptions to this generalization. Sometimes, the severe anorexia associated with malignancy or use of antitumor agents can be overcome by pharmacologic means, such as use of *megestrol* (see later discussion and Chapter 91). *Dronabinol (tetrahydrocannabinol)* is reserved for persons with anorexia or nausea associated with chemotherapy or terminal illness but is less effective for weight loss than megestrol. The poor intake seen with *hepatitis* can be improved by providing *small, frequent feedings*, especially in the morning, when nausea is less severe (see Chapter 70).

Maldigestion resulting from *pancreatic insufficiency* can be compensated for by the use of oral *pancreatic enzyme preparations* (see Chapter 72). The bacterial overgrowth of blind-loop syndrome responds to oral *broad-spectrum antibiotic therapy* (e.g., 250 mg of *tetracycline* four times daily or 250 mg of *amoxicillin* three times daily), given for multiple 10-day courses or for 3 or 4 days each week indefinitely. Caloric supplements may be necessary (see later discussion).

Malabsorption resulting in weight loss can be countered with caloric supplements in the form of *medium-chain triglyceride/dextrose preparations*. Initially, 3 oz are given with each meal; gradually this is increased to 6 oz, including supplements between meals. If *sprue* is suspected, a *gluten-free diet* can be tried empirically. *Fat-soluble vitamin supplements* are also needed in cases of malabsorption to prevent malnutrition, even though caloric intake may be replenished. The fat-soluble vitamins A, D, and K are the most likely to be depleted. Daily requirements in such cases are 25,000 to 50,000 U for vitamin A, 30,000 U for vitamin D, and 4 to 12 g for oral vitamin K. Monthly *vitamin B_{12}* injections of 1,000 mcg are needed for terminal ileal disease presenting with megaloblastic anemia (see Chapter 82). Methods for controlling excessive vomiting and diarrhea are helpful (see Chapters 59 and 64).

Depression

Appetite disturbances associated with depression in younger patients are often amenable to *tricyclic* therapy, whereas *selective serotonin reuptake inhibitor* treatment is better tolerated in older patients; faster onset of action may occur with use of the atypical antidepressant *mirtazapine* at low dose in the elderly (e.g., 15 mg every night at bedtime; see Chapter 227).

Anorexia in the Elderly

In addition to attempting to treat etiologically and ensuring access to food, a number of supplementary measures are worth considering. Liquid *caloric supplements* (e.g., Ensure, Sustical, Boost, etc.) between meals can reduce the risk of weight loss. Socialization efforts can be important. *Flavor enhancers* have also proved helpful. *Appetite stimulants* (e.g., *megestrol*) can be considered when all else has failed; use produces weight gain but increases the risk of thromboembolism, especially in sedentary persons. As a progestational glucocorticosteroid, it also can suppress the adrenal–pituitary axis, necessitating glucocorticosteroid supplementation in acute illness or stress. A new formulation of megestrol does not require food intake for absorption, making it useful in severe anorexia.

INDICATIONS FOR REFERRAL AND ADMISSION

Referral to a dietician can be very helpful for both diagnosis and design of the treatment program, especially in the elderly with weight loss in the absence of serious underlying illness or major depression. Anyone with an unexplained weight loss in excess of 15 kg is likely to have a life-threatening condition and requires prompt hospitalization. The AIDS patient with unexplained weight loss may also benefit from some form of inpatient care while undergoing further evaluation. Any person with substantial weight loss who is suspected of having anorexia nervosa should be hospitalized and seen by a psychiatrist experienced in dealing with anorexia because this, too, can be a life-threatening condition (see Chapter 234). When malabsorption is documented by 72-hour stool fat assessment, consultation with a gastroenterologist should coincide with proceeding to further assessment. HIV patients with weight loss can certainly be evaluated by their primary care physician, provided that the physician is familiar with the evaluation of such patients. Otherwise, referral is indicated.

A.H.G.

Annotated Bibliography

1. Bach MC, Howell DA, Valenti AJ. Aphthous ulceration of the gastrointestinal tract in patients with AIDS. Ann Intern Med 1990;112:465. (*An important cause of decreased intake resulting from odynophagia and dysphagia.*)
2. Farrell RJ, Kelly CP. Celiac sprue. N Engl J Med 2002;346:180. (*Excellent review of sprue with emphasis on subtleties of presentation.*)
3. Kotler DP. Cachexia. Ann Intern Med 2000;133:622. (*Comprehensive review with emphasis on disease mechanisms; 121 references.*)
4. Morley JE. Decreased food intake with aging. J Gerontol Med Sci 2001;56A:81 (*Evidence for a physiology of anorexia in the elderly.*)
5. Marton KI, Sox HC, Krupp JR. Involuntary weight loss: diagnostic and prognostic significance. Ann Intern Med 1981;5:568. (*A classic paper describing a prospective study attempting to identify predictors of serious pathology and poor prognosis.*)
6. Roland Y, Kim, M-J, Gammack JK, et al. Office management of weight loss in older persons. Am J Med 2006;119:1019. (*Includes excellent review of mechanisms of anorexia.*)
7. Thomas FB, Mazzaferri EL, Skillman TG. Apathetic thyrotoxicosis: a distinctive clinical and laboratory entity. Ann Intern Med 1970;72:679. (*Classic article describing this syndrome, which is characterized by marked weight loss, apathy, and unexplained atrial fibrillation in the elderly.*)
8. Thompson MP, Morris LK. Unexplained weight loss in the ambulatory elderly. J Am Geriatr Soc 1991;39:497. (*A study of patients from seven primary care centers; depression was the most common cause; malignancy was next; many cases remained undiagnosed; computed tomography was low in yield.*)
9. Wallace JI, Schwartz RS. Involuntary weight loss in elderly outpatients: recognition, etiologies, and treatment. Clin Geriatr Med 1997;13:1717. (*Outpatient study finding that cancer, gastrointestinal disease, and psychiatric problems are the leading causes in this setting.*)
10. Wilson MMG, Vaswani S, Liu D, et al. Prevalence and causes of undernutrition in medical outpatients. Am J Med 1998;104:56. (*A population study from primary care practice; prevalence is 11% in patients 65 years and older and 7% in younger persons; leading causes in the elderly include depression, poorly controlled diabetes, and occult cancer; etiology is often unrecognized, although readily identifiable.*)
11. Greene JB. Clinical approach to weight loss in the patient with AIDS. Gastroenterol Clin North Am 1988;17:573. (*A very useful algorithm for guiding the potentially complex workup in the AIDS patient.*)
12. Hernandez JL, Riancho JA, Matorras P, et al. Clinical evaluation for cancer in patients with involuntary weight loss without specific symptoms. Am J Med 2003;114:631. (*A cohort study of 306 patients; examines the utility of a set of simple blood tests to help determine need for further workup for occult malignancy.*)
13. Ryan ME, Olsen WA. A diagnostic approach to malabsorption syndromes. Clin Gastroenterol 1983;12:533. (*A pathophysiologic approach.*)
14. Wilson MM, Thomas DR, Rubenstein LZ, et al. Appetite assessment: simple appetite questionnaire predicts weight loss in community-swelling adults and nursing home residents. Am J Clin Nutr 2005;82:1074. (*Validation of a screening instrument for anorexia and risk of weight loss.*)
15. Morley JE. Orexigenic and anabolic agents. Clin Geriatr Med 2002;18:853. (*Review of factors reducing appetite and causing weight loss in the elderly.*)
16. Morley JE, Silver AJ, Fiatarone M, et al. Nutrition and the elderly. J Am Geriatr Soc 1986;34:823. (*A review of critical factors often overlooked.*)
17. Milne AC, Potter J, Avenell A. Protein and energy supplementation in elderly people at risk for malnutrition. Cochrane Database Syst Rev 2002;(3):CD003288. (*Evidence of efficacy.*)
18. Mathey MF, Siebelink E, De Graaf C, et al. Flavor enhancement of foods improves intake and nutritional status of elderly nursing home patients. J Gerontol Med Sci 2001;56:M200. (*A very practical idea.*)
19. Berenstein EG, Ortiz A. Megestrol acetate for the treatment of anorexia–cachexia syndrome. Cochrane Database Syst Rev 2005(2):CD004310. (*Systematic review of efficacy.*)

CHAPTER 10 ■ EVALUATION OF OVERWEIGHT AND OBESITY

Overweight and obesity have become major health concerns in modern postindustrial societies, affecting an estimated 55% of Americans older than the age of 20 years. Community-based study finds the long-term risk of becoming overweight greater than 50% and the risk of becoming obese in excess of 25%. The personal and social costs are enormous, approaching $100 billion annually when medical complications, lost wages, and expenditures for weight reduction efforts are taken into account, not to mention the accompanying emotional pain, social stigmatization, and discrimination that may ensue.

Excessive weight, through its promotion of the metabolic syndrome, is a major risk factor for cardiovascular disease, type 2 diabetes mellitus, dyslipidemia, and hypertension, and it is also associated with increased risks of stroke, heart failure, cancer, and premature death. In addition, obese patients manifest heightened risks of impaired pulmonary function (including sleep apnea), osteoarthritis, gallbladder disease, and surgical complications.

The tasks for the primary physician in the evaluation of patients with excess weight include not only an attempt to identify etiologic factors, but also a careful assessment of weight status and fat distribution as risk factors for major disease. This chapter focuses on the diagnostic evaluation; see Chapter 233 for the approach to treatment.

PATHOPHYSIOLOGY AND CLINICAL PRESENTATION (1–17)

Definitions

The preferred definitions of overweight and obesity are based on *body mass index* (BMI) determinations, which approximate total body fat content and correlate with disease risk (Table 10.1). *Overweight* is defined as a BMI of 25 to 29.9 kg/m^2. *Obesity* is defined as a BMI greater than 30 kg/m^2, and *morbid obesity* as a BMI greater than 40 kg/m^2 (Table 10.1).

Physiology

Caloric intake and energy expenditure are linked through hypothalamic regulation of appetite and metabolism. The hypothalamus integrates a complex and redundant set of afferent signals, including *leptin,* released from adipose tissue; *norepinephrine,* from the autonomic nervous system; *epinephrine, insulin, androgens, glucocorticoids, progesterone,* and *estrogens,* from endocrine glands; *peptide YY, glucagon, cholecystokinin, bombesin peptides, neurotensin, growth hormone–releasing hormone, somatostatin,* and *glucose,* from the gastrointestinal tract; and *dopamine, gamma-aminobutyric acid, ghlanin, opioids, growth hormone–releasing factor, somatostatin,* and *serotonin,* from the central nervous system. The efferent output from the hypothalamus controls energy expenditure and appetite by the release of *alpha-melanocyte-stimulating hormone* (alpha-MSH), *norepinephrine, serotonin, neuropeptide Y, glucagon-like peptide I, thyrotropic hormone,* and *corticotropin-releasing hormone,* which act on the autonomic nervous system and the thyroid gland. Increasingly appreciated as a factor in appetite control is the role of alpha-MSH on the *melanocortin 4 receptor* (MC4R), which, when stimulated, suppresses appetite.

Pathophysiology

Obesity is often the consequence of physical inactivity, especially in persons with an underlying disturbance in metabolism, appetite control, or dietary composition. In most instances, the etiology is multifactorial, although one factor may predominate. Susceptibility is influenced by genetic determinants that were once advantageous in regard to evolution, such as those that reduce energy expenditure or encourage the intake of energy-rich foods. However, such inherited traits can be counterproductive to good health in postindustrial societies, in which physical demands are greatly reduced and high-calorie food is plentiful and inexpensive.

Physical Inactivity

Physical inactivity emerges as a leading cause of obesity in modern society, underscored by the increasing prevalence of obesity despite a decline in average daily caloric intake. When daily life makes few physical demands, caloric needs drop precipitously, which leads to an epidemic of excess weight, even among those without major genetic susceptibility to weight gain. Some genetic variability in the propensity for exercise has been described, which may contribute to inactivity in some.

Metabolic Factors

Metabolic factors are important, genetically determined contributors to excessive weight and include resting energy expenditure, thermic effect of food, and exercise-induced energy

---

TABLE 10.1

DEFINITION AND CLASSIFICATION OF EXCESS WEIGHT

Class	BMI (kg/m^2)	Waist Circumference[a]	Relative Risk[b]
Normal	18.5–24.9	Normal	Normal
		Increased	Increased
Overweight	25.0–29.9	Normal	Increased
		Increased	High
Obese	30.0–34.9	Normal	High
		Increased	Very High
	35.0–39.9	Normal	Very high
		Increased	Very high
Obese, morbid	40.0+	All are increased	Extremely high

BMI, body mass index.
[a]Increased, >102 cm (40 in.) in men, >88 cm (35 in.) in women.
[b]For diabetes type 2, hypertension, coronary artery disease.
Adapted from Expert Panel on the Identification, Evaluation, and Treatment of Overweight and Obesity in Adults. Executive summary of the clinical guidelines on the identification, evaluation, and treatment of overweight and obesity in adults. Arch Intern Med 1998;158:1855, with permission.

expenditure. Among these, a reduction in energy utilization with exercise correlates the most strongly with risk for weight gain. From 9- to 30-fold variations have been observed. Because exercise-induced energy expenditure accounts for about 30% of total energy demand, any genetic propensity for reduced energy expenditure with exertion could substantially increase the risk for obesity.

Dietary Composition

Dietary composition actually plays a much smaller role than might be expected. In most persons, changing the percentages of dietary fat, protein, and carbohydrate *without* changing the number of calories consumed has little or no influence on the development of obesity. Diets high in fat contribute to obesity mostly because they are rich in calories, not because they are rich in fat. Despite claims to the contrary by those promoting weight-loss diets, there is no evidence that dietary composition alone is a major determinant of obesity for the vast majority of persons. Almost all weight loss diets work by restricting total calories (see Chapter 233). The *timing of food intake* may contribute modestly to obesity; eating once daily, particularly before going to bed, predisposes to the accumulation of adipose tissue in some persons.

Appetite Disturbances

Appetite disturbances have long been suspected as a cause of obesity. Many obese individuals appear to eat without satiety. This has led to intensive study of appetite regulation and its disruption. In some, there appears to be resistance to normal appetite controls, such as the appetite suppressant *leptin*, serum levels of which actually increase in obese subjects. In some obese persons, the postprandial production of appetite suppressing *gut hormone fragment polypeptide YY* (PYY) is reduced compared with normal controls. In others, there is genetic alteration of the MC4R (see later discussion). In some animals, the effects of appetite suppressants can be overcome by providing easy access to palatable, energy-rich foods.

Genetic Factors

Genetic factors, as noted earlier, play a substantial role by influencing energy utilization, appetite, food preferences, and even propensity for physical activity. The importance of genetic factors is underscored by findings from studies of twins, families, and adoptees, which reveal a strong relation between weight class of adoptees and their biologic parents but none between adoptees and their adopted parents. Parental obesity doubles the risk for adult obesity in obese and nonobese children younger than the age of 10 years. Obese children younger than the age of 3 years who have an obese parent have a very high risk for adult obesity, but they experience no increase in risk if neither parent is obese. The alpha-MSH/MC4R axis appears important in some cases of morbid obesity. Patients with a mutation in the MC4R gene manifest hyperphagia, binge eating, and morbid obesity. Genetic factors are estimated to account for nearly 50% of the risk of becoming overweight and even more for becoming obese.

Developmental and Environmental Factors

Developmental and environmental factors, manifested by parental influences and childhood environment, contribute to the development of adult obesity. As the age of the child increases, the influence of environment increases. At ages greater than 10 years, heredity becomes a less-dominant determinant of adult obesity, and environment increases in importance.

Persons growing up in the current era of plentiful, inexpensive high-calorie fast food are at greater risk of obesity than are cohorts from earlier eras. Teenagers, especially, consume large amounts of such food, with potentially serious long-term consequences. Natural history studies find a strong relation between increased weight during the teenage and young adult years and risk of becoming frankly obese later in life. Those who become obese tend to remain obese their entire lives.

Psychological and Behavioral Factors

Psychological and behavioral factors have long been thought to be important; however, there is no known psychological explanation for why reactive hyperphagia develops in some persons as a response to emotional stress, whereas anorexia is the reaction of others. Considerable research has been unable to determine any particular personality organization or cluster of psychological defense mechanisms clearly linked to obesity. Nonetheless, psychological problems frequently contribute to the onset and perpetuation of obesity-inducing behavioral changes. For example, some individuals characteristically overeat in response to stress, loss, or frustration. Those with the *night-eating syndrome*, characterized by insomnia, massive late-evening "refrigerator raids," and morning anorexia, also experience particular emotional distress when they try to reform their eating behaviors. Usually, coinciding social stresses are present as well. The appetite disturbance associated with *major depression* may lead to either an increase or a decrease in weight.

Social Factors

Social factors are key determinants of the frequency and nature of feasts, timing of meals, role and meaning of food, types of foods consumed, and norms of appearance. In U.S. society, excess weight occurs far more frequently among minorities and the socioeconomically disadvantaged than among others. Young African American and Hispanic women are 2.1 and 1.5 times, respectively, more likely to become obese than are young white women. Whether this difference represents dietary preference, socially motivated behavior, or interactional factors is unclear. In certain occupations, such as wrestling, obesity is a help, not a hindrance. In former times, corpulence was a sign of prosperity and was cultivated by bankers and businessmen.

Clinical Presentation

Most cases of overweight and obesity occur independent of an underlying medical condition, although they may exacerbate or lead to illness. Onset of exogenous obesity is often evident by early adulthood and tends to persist. Those who are overweight by their early 20s are at considerable risk of developing frank obesity by their late 30s. Persons with an underlying hereditary etiology usually manifest obesity before age 10 years.

In 5% to 10% of adult cases, an underlying medical condition or medication that affects energy expenditure, fuel utilization, appetite, or physical activity may be responsible. Often, the mechanism is an effect on one of the substances involved in regulating energy intake or expenditure (see earlier discussion).

Pharmacologic Agents

Pharmacologic agents prescribed for clinical conditions other than obesity may cause weight gain. *Beta-blockers* and *central sympatholytics* (e.g., clonidine) can decrease metabolic rate and energy expenditure. *Glucocorticosteroids* cause hypertrophic obesity in a characteristic truncal pattern. *Antidepressants*, such as the *tricyclics* and *selective serotonin reuptake inhibitors*, and some *antihistamines* (e.g., cyproheptadine) act as appetite stimulants. Weight gain is also common with oral contraceptive use.

Endocrine Disturbances

Endocrine disturbances are more often the result, rather than the cause, of excess weight. However, *hypothyroidism* (see Chapter 104) has been found to account for up to 5% of cases in some series. *Cushing's syndrome* is a rare cause and is usually accompanied by characteristic features of truncal obesity and peripheral muscle wasting. *Stein–Leventhal syndrome*—polycystic ovaries, absent menses, moderate hirsutism, and hyperinsulinism (see Chapter 112)—often goes unrecognized as an endocrinologic form of obesity; the precise mechanism of the obesity is unknown. *Eunuchism* may also be associated with obesity. Of great concern is the marked increase in frequency of insulin resistance and its attendant *metabolic syndrome*, characterized by hyperinsulinism, elevated triglycerides, and low high-density-lipoprotein (HDL) cholesterol, all important risk factors for diabetes, hypertension, and cardiovascular disease. Serum insulin and triglyceride levels are elevated, and HDL cholesterol is reduced.

Neurologic Causes

Neurologic causes of obesity are usually not cryptic; they mostly result from *hypothalamic injury*, as occurs with craniopharyngiomas, encephalitis, or trauma. Visual field defects or headaches are usually present. Two rare types of neurologic disease without obvious central nervous system symptoms have been described. Kleine–Levin syndrome consists of periodic hyperphagia and hypersomnia. A second syndrome is characterized by preoccupation with food and accompanying electroencephalographic abnormalities that respond to phenytoin.

Mental Illness

Mental illness may be heralded by weight gain. The appetite disturbance of *major depression* is one of the cardinal manifestations of the condition and may be a presenting complaint (see Chapter 227).

DIFFERENTIAL DIAGNOSIS (18)

The causes of obesity can be primary or secondary, with the latter being medical conditions that result in obesity. Some forms of secondary weight gain are a consequence of salt retention and fluid overload rather than an increase in fat cell mass. Among the important causes of sodium retention are congestive heart failure, severe hepatocellular disease, and renal failure (see Chapters 32, 71, and 142). Primary forms of obesity can be classified by their underlying pathophysiology. The vast majority of cases are primary in nature. An etiologic/pathophysiologic diagnosis is essential to the design of an effective management program (Table 10.2).

WORKUP (18–21)

Particular attention should be paid to detection and early intervention in persons at greatest risk for becoming obese, namely overweight teenagers and young adults, especially women from minority groups.

TABLE 10.2

IMPORTANT CAUSES OF OBESITY

Primary
Psychological factors
  Depression
  Anxiety
  Frustration
Biologic factors
  Reduced thermogenesis
  Increased fat cell mass
  Autonomic dysfunction
  Altered hypothalamic set-point
  Single large daily meal taken before bedtime
  Decreased energy expenditure
  Drugs (e.g., tricyclic antidepressants, oral contraceptives, corticosteroids, phenothiazines)
Genetic influences
  Familial obesity
Social and occupational factors
  Lower socioeconomic class
  Social/occupational situation
Secondary
Endocrine disease
  Hypothyroidism
  Stein–Leventhal syndrome
  Cushing's syndrome
Neurologic disease
  Hypothalamic injury (e.g., trauma, encephalitis, craniopharyngioma)

A principal objective of the overweight/obesity evaluation is to determine how much risk the weight problem confers. The risk assessment begins with an estimate of the amount and distribution of fat, followed by a consideration of other risk factors and underlying conditions that add to morbidity and mortality risks; it concludes with estimates of relative and absolute risk. Additional components of the workup pertinent to management include elucidation of the underlying mechanism(s) responsible for the patient's weight problem, detection of any underlying illnesses presenting as weight excess, and assessment of the patient's motivation to lose weight.

Weight Assessment

To establish whether an individual has a weight problem that poses a health risk, an estimation of the *amount* and *distribution* of fat is required. Both are independent determinants of disease risk. Fat distribution is particularly important, even among persons who are not obese.

Measurement of Body Fat

This is best accomplished by calculating the BMI. The BMI determination assumes that weight is measured with shoes and heavy clothing removed. If weight is obtained with shoes and all clothing on, then 5 lb should be subtracted for men and 3 lb for women. The BMI is calculated by taking the weight in kilograms and dividing it by the square of the height in meters (or by multiplying by 703 the weight in pounds divided by the square of the height in inches). This ratio of weight to height actually calculates total body mass rather than fat mass, but it correlates highly with the amount of body fat and its associated health risks except in very muscular individuals, who might be falsely labeled as overweight with use of the BMI. The BMI range of 20 to 24.9 is classified as "normal" because no actuarial increase in disease mortality is noted within it. Mortality begins to increase as the BMI exceeds 25, and it is here that health professionals should be concerned. Most expert consensus panels recommend that health professionals adopt the BMI as the preferred measure for evaluating weight status because it provides the best estimate of disease risk (Fig. 10.1 and Table 10.1).

Height and Weight Tables

Height and weight tables have the advantage of simplicity. However, there are serious limitations to their use. Standard charts typically list "ideal" or desired weights based on actuarial data, yet it is not weight per se that minimizes morbidity or the incidence of disease. The person having a significant percentage of lean body mass, such as a physical laborer, may well exceed "ideal" body weight, yet not be obese. On the other hand, some individuals may be within the

TABLE 10.3

OPTIMAL WEIGHTS, IN POUNDS, FOR ADULTS AGES 25 YEARS AND OLDER (LIGHT CLOTHING)

Height (In Shoes) (ft, in.)	Small Frame	Medium Frame	Large Frame
Men			
5 2	112–120	118–129	126–141
5 3	115–123	121–133	129–144
5 4	118–126	124–136	132–148
5 5	121–129	127–139	135–152
5 6	124–133	130–143	138–156
5 7	128–137	134–147	142–161
5 8	132–141	138–152	147–166
5 9	136–145	142–156	151–170
5 10	140–150	146–160	155–174
5 11	144–154	150–165	159–179
6 0	148–158	154–170	164–184
6 1	152–162	158–175	168–189
6 2	156–167	162–180	173–194
6 3	160–171	167–185	178–199
6 4	164–175	172–190	182–204
Women			
4 10	92–98	96–107	104–119
4 11	94–101	98–110	106–122
5 0	96–104	101–113	109–125
5 1	99–107	104–116	112–128
5 2	102–110	107–119	115–131
5 3	105–113	110–122	118–134
5 4	108–116	113–126	121–138
5 5	111–119	116–130	125–142
5 6	114–123	120–135	129–146
5 7	118–127	124–139	133–150
5 8	122–131	128–143	137–154
5 9	126–135	132–147	141–158
5 10	130–140	136–151	145–163
5 11	134–144	140–155	149–168
6 0	138–148	144–159	153–173

Optimal weights are considered to be those associated with the lowest mortality rates (derived from actuarial data, Metropolitan Life Insurance Company).

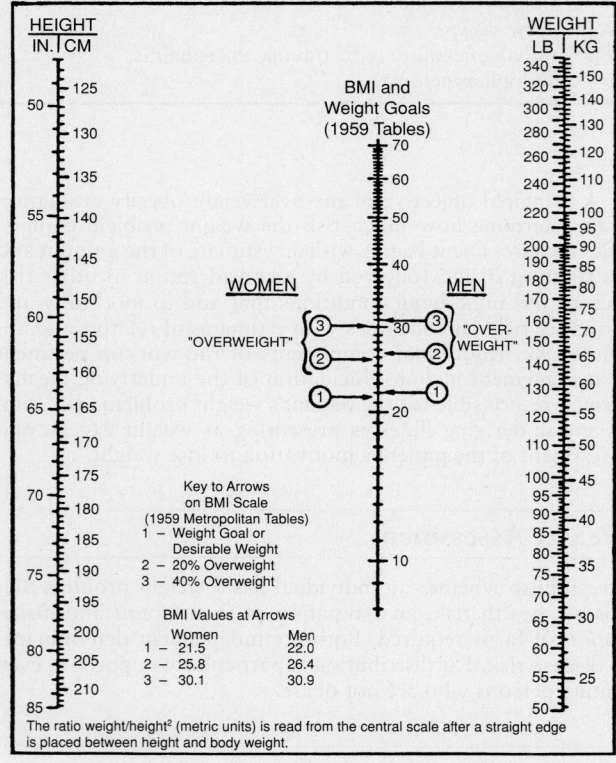

FIGURE 10.1. Nomogram for body mass index (BMI) (kg/m^2). Weights and heights are without clothing. With clothes, add 5 lb (2.3 kg) for men and 3 lb (1.4 kg) for women. Add 1 in. (2.5 cm) in height for shoes. (From New weight standards for men and women. J Am Diet Assoc 1985;85:1119, with permission. Based on data from Metropolitan Life Insurance Company. New weight standards for men and women. Stat Bull Metrop Life Insur Co 1959;40:1.)

ideal range but have non–insulin-dependent diabetes mellitus, hypertension, or other conditions that would benefit from weight reduction. The Metropolitan Life Insurance Company publishes revised reference weights in an attempt to isolate the effect of weight alone on longevity; individuals with major diseases, such as cancer, diabetes, or heart disease, are omitted from the study (Table 10.3). Life tables, based only on mortality, ignore possible nonfatal risks associated with increased weight.

Height and Weight Formulas

Height and weight formulas are sometimes used to determine ideal body weight and estimate the degree of obesity, but they provide only the crudest of estimates and should not be used to set goals for weight reduction. They are provided here only because they are sometimes referred to (appropriate weight goals for patients can be determined only by a thorough analysis of their medical history and physical findings, supplemented by appropriate laboratory evaluation):

■ Female weight: Allow 100 lb for first 5 ft of height plus 5 lb for each additional inch.

■ Male weight: Allow 106 lb for first 5 ft of height plus 6 lb for each additional inch.

Some use the measurement of *skinfold thickness* to quantify adiposity. Calipers are used to measure skinfold thickness in the triceps and subscapular regions. However, reliability can be a problem when skinfold measurements are used because body fat increases with age, grossly obese patients are difficult to measure, and results vary among providers using the calipers.

Bioelectric Impedance Analysis

Bioelectric impedance analysis is sometimes used to measure body fat. Electrodes are applied to one arm and leg, and the impedance is measured. Impedance is proportional to the aqueous composition of the body. Formulas are used to estimate the percentage of fat in the body. Although accurate, this method is expensive and not readily available.

The old-fashioned *eyeball test* remains a mainstay of assessment: If a person looks fat, he or she is likely to be fat. However, quantification and correlation with risk are crude with this commonsense method.

Measurement of Fat Distribution

The other independent determinant of health risk associated with excess weight is fat distribution, which can be quantified by measuring *waist circumference*. The circumference of the waist is obtained at the narrowest area above the umbilicus. Measurements in excess of gender-specific cutoffs (>102 cm, or 40 in., in men and >88 cm, or 35 in., in women) confer an increased relative risk of disease morbidity and mortality (see Table 10.3). The effect of fat distribution on risk is so strong that waist circumference is important even in persons who are not technically overweight. However, in morbidly obese patients, waist circumference is always exceeded, and the measurement confers no additional risk.

The *ratio* of *waist* or *abdominal circumference* to *hip* or *gluteal circumference* provides an even more precise quantitative index of regional fat distribution. The hip circumference is measured at the maximal gluteal protrusion. Individuals with excess upper body fat (android obesity) are at higher risk for diabetes, atherosclerosis, and stroke than are those who have more adipose tissue in the hips, buttocks, and thighs (gynecoid obesity). In quantitative terms, individuals with waist-to-hip ratios greater than 0.8 for women and 1.0 for men have an increased risk for coronary disease.

Estimation of Disease Risk

One begins with determinations of total body fat and fat distribution, represented respectively by BMI and waist circumference. These parameters correlate well with *relative risk*, especially among persons younger than the age of 65 years (see Table 10.3). Relative risk from obesity is greatest among younger persons and declines somewhat with advancing age. Determination of the *absolute risk* associated with obesity requires checking for underlying *coronary heart disease*

(see Chapter 20), *type 2 diabetes mellitus* (see Chapter 93), *noncoronary atherosclerotic disease* (see Chapters 23 and 171), *hypertension* (see Chapter 19), and *sleep apnea* (see Chapter 46), in addition to the end-organ injuries that may result from them (see Chapters 26, 30, 35, 46, and 102). The cardiovascular risk assessment is enhanced by screening for principal risk factors such as *hyperlipidemia* (see Chapter 15), *hypertension* (see Chapter 14), *smoking* (see Chapter 54), and premature coronary disease in first-degree relatives. Calculations of absolute risk are possible from a consideration of these factors (see Chapters 26 and 27). Searches for *osteoarthritis* (see Chapter 146), *cholelithiasis* (see Chapter 69), and *stress incontinence* also help to predict risk of weight-related consequences.

Assessment of Etiology and Consequences

As important as risk assessment is, etiologic factors and health consequences deserve attention because they are relevant to the approach to management.

History

An extensive weight history should include age of onset of obesity, weight status of parents and siblings, and any identifiable circumstances associated with the onset of obesity. Although dietary composition per se is not a risk factor for obesity, dietary composition and quantity need to be ascertained to determine total caloric intake. A high-fat diet is likely to provide excessive calories. Because physical inactivity is a major precipitant of excess weight, the patient's daily activities should be elucidated in detail to estimate daily energy requirements. Proclivity toward exercise should also be ascertained. A careful review of ongoing psychological and situational stresses is essential and should include screening for depression (see Chapter 227). Any recent attempts at smoking cessation should be reviewed for effect on weight. The social and cultural dimensions of the history should be explored for their possible contribution to weight gain.

Even in a patient without obvious medical pathology, a workup that screens for underlying endocrinologic and neurologic diseases is essential, as is a check for drug-induced causes. The history requires a thorough neuroendocrine review of symptoms: fatigue, unexplained weight gain, cold intolerance, hoarseness, change in skin and hair texture, amenorrhea, hirsutism, easy bruising, weakness, visual disturbances, and headache. Medications are reviewed for agents that may stimulate appetite or affect metabolism, such as antidepressants, oral contraceptives, corticosteroids, phenothiazines, antithyroid medications, beta-blockers, and insulin.

A review of systems for the consequences of obesity should include inquiry into chest pain, shortness of breath, polyuria, polydipsia, impotence, numbness, limb pain or coldness, transient neurologic deficits, daytime sleepiness, apneic periods at night, and pain in weight-bearing joints.

The Physical Examination

The physical examination includes a check for such etiologic clues as moon facies, hirsutism, dry and thickened skin, coarse hair, truncal obesity, pigmented striae, goiter, adnexal masses, lack of secondary sex characteristics, delayed relaxation of ankle jerks, and visual field deficits. The physical examination should include a search for the consequences of obesity, including blood pressure elevation, diabetic retinopathic changes, carotid bruits, obstruction of soft tissues in the upper airway, cor pulmonale, rales, cardiac enlargement, degenerative changes in the hips and knees, and signs of peripheral arterial insufficiency and peripheral neuropathy.

Laboratory Testing

Laboratory testing includes two components: the diagnosis of an underlying medical etiology and the detection of metabolic consequences. A strategy of routinely testing for all possible medical causes in the absence of suggestive clinical findings adds to expenses and increases the risk of generating a high percentage of false-positive results (see Chapter 2). Nonetheless, some clinicians routinely screen for hypothyroidism with a *thyrotropin* determination because the test is sensitive, the condition has a relatively high frequency, and the clinical presentation of hypothyroidism can be very subtle (see Chapter 104).

The laboratory evaluation is most productive when directed at causes suggested by the history and the physical examination. For example, the obese patient suspected of having Cushing's syndrome because of truncal obesity, peripheral wasting, and pigmented striae is a reasonable candidate for an overnight *1-mg dexamethasone suppression test*. If headaches accompanied by a visual field disturbance are present, then *computed tomography* of the sella turcica is needed to check for the possibility of a pituitary tumor (see Chapter 100). Measures of energy expenditure, thermogenesis, autonomic function, fat cell count, and metabolic set-point are relegated to the research laboratory. Similarly, genetic testing and assays for such appetite suppressant factors as leptins, alpha-MSH, MC4R, and PYY remain confined to the study setting but may be useful in the future.

Testing for *insulin resistance* and its metabolic consequences is essential to identifying those persons at increased cardiovascular risk. About half of obese persons will have evidence of insulin resistance. *Fasting glucose* and *lipid profile* (see Chapter 15) are essential determinations. *Serum insulin* levels provide a more direct measurement of hyperinsulinism, but assays are not well standardized. The *plasma triglyceride* level (>130 mg/dL) and ratio of *triglyceride to high-density-lipoprotein cholesterol* (>3.0) provide the best approximation of insulin levels and correlate with cardiovascular risk, as does the better-established ratio of *total cholesterol to HDL cholesterol* (<4.5). These results help to detect *metabolic syndrome* and identify those persons at greatest cardiovascular risk and who are likely to benefit most from weight reduction.

Patients bothered by daytime sleepiness and a history of excessive snoring and disturbed sleep resulting from irregular breathing should be considered for a formal *sleep study* (see Chapter 46).

MANAGEMENT

See Chapter 233.

INDICATIONS FOR REFERRAL

Patients who are morbidly obese and demonstrate such adverse sequelae as marked respiratory compromise, disabling arthritis, or symptomatic coronary disease require consultation for consideration of a very low calorie diet under the supervision of persons experienced in its implementation (see Chapter 233). Referral for consideration of surgical approaches to treatment may also be indicated in such persons. Obstructive sleep apnea in patients with mild-to-moderate obesity may not require such extreme measures, but pulmonary consultation in conjunction with a weight-loss program is indicated (see Chapter 46).

PATIENT EDUCATION

Most patients come for evaluation out of concern for an underlying medical condition or a genetic determinant. The vast majority has no such cause and need to know that inactivity and caloric excess are the principal reasons for their weight gain. Although they may have genetically determined risk factors, such as a proclivity for high-fat food, reduced exercise-related energy expenditure, or a defect in appetite suppression, they will benefit when the physician reemphasizes the overwhelming importance of exercise and an active lifestyle to weight control, as well as modest restriction in caloric intake (see Chapter 233). The occasional patient whose obesity is driven predominantly by heredity (both parents obese, onset before age 3 years) appreciates knowing that the weight problem is not a consequence of defective character. For the vast majority of patients, the education process begins by drawing attention away from diets, medical conditions, and "metabolism problems" and to the importance of exercise. The goals are to provide the patient with an estimate of the disease risk posed by the excessive weight and an assessment of the factors contributing to it.

RECOMMENDATIONS

- Make overweight detection and early intervention an important goal of the health maintenance/prevention agenda for teenagers and young adults. Focus efforts on those at greatest risk for becoming obese, namely overweight teenagers and young adult women from minority groups.
- Begin the weight assessment by determining the amount of body fat and fat distribution, which independently correlate with the relative risk associated with excess weight.
- Estimate body fat content by calculating the BMI (body weight in kilograms divided by the square of the height in meters).
- Determine fat distribution by measuring the waist circumference at the narrowest area above the umbilicus.
- Estimate the relative risk of cardiovascular disease, type 2 diabetes, and hypertension from these determinations.
- Search for major cardiovascular risk factors and for evidence of end-organ damage to determine the absolute risk of cardiovascular morbidity and mortality.
- Check the history and the physical examination for etiologic factors, ranging from familial propensity and early age of onset to dietary excess, physical inactivity, and underlying medical and psychological conditions.
- Restrict laboratory testing to investigating etiologic hypotheses suggested by the history and the physical examination and to assessing cardiovascular risk associated with metabolic syndrome; include measurement of fasting triglycerides and HDL cholesterol.
- Provide the patient with an assessment of the factors contributing to excessive weight and with an estimate of disease risk posed by the obesity so that a customized management plan can be formulated (see Chapter 233).

A.H.G.

Annotated Bibliography

1. Flegal KM, Carroll MD, Ogden CL, et al. Prevalence and trends in obesity among US adults, 1999–2000. JAMA 2002;288:1723. (*Documents the epidemic proportions of the problem.*)
2. Hu FB, Willett WC, Tricia L, et al. Adiposity as compared with physical activity in predicting mortality among women. N Engl J Med 2004;351:2694. (*Data from the Nurses' Health Study; both increased adiposity and decreased exercise were found to be independent predictors of death.*)
3. Peeters A, Barendregt JJ, Willendens F, et al. Obesity in adulthood and its consequences for life expectancy: a life table analysis. Ann Intern Med 2003;138:24. (*A prospective cohort study from the Framingham Study; finds large decreases in life expectancy and increases in early mortality.*)
4. Calle EE, Rodriguez C, Walker-Thurmond, et al. Overweight, obesity, and mortality from cancer in a prospectively studied cohort of U.S. adults. N Engl J Med 2003;348:1625. (*Large prospective population study; increased weight was associated with an increase in death from all cancers.*)
5. van Dam R, Willett WC, Manson JE, et al. The relationship between overweight in adolescence and premature death in women. Ann Intern Med 145:91. (*Data from the Nurses' Health Study; moderate adiposity was associated with increased premature death.*)
6. Vasan RS, Pencian MJ, Cobain M, et al. Estimated risks for developing obesity in the Framingham Heart Study. Ann Intern Med 2005;143:473. (*Data from a major epidemiologic study showing high long-term risk exceeding 50% of becoming overweight and 25% of becoming obese.*)
7. Wilson PWF, D'Agostina RB, Sullivan L, et al. Overweight and obesity as determinants of cardiovascular risk: the Framingham experience. Arch Intern Med 2002;162:1867. (*Prospective cohort study from the Framingham Study; cardiovascular risk was strongly associated with overweight status.*)
8. Kurth T, Gaziano JM, Berger K, et al. Body mass index and the risk of stroke in men. Arch Intern Med 2002;162:2557. (*Prospective cohort study from the Physicians' Health Study; there was a significant increase in stroke risk with increasing body mass index [BMI].*)
9. Kenchaiah S, Evans JC, Levy D, et al. Obesity and the risk of heart failure. N Engl J Med 2003;347:305. (*Prospective cohort study from the Framingham Heart Study; an increased BMI was associated with an increased risk of heart failure.*)
10. Rosenbaum M, Leibel RL, Hirsch J. Obesity. N Engl J Med 1997;337:396. (*Review of the physiology and pathophysiology of weight control.*)
11. Liebel RL, Hirsch J, Appel BE, et al. Energy intake required to maintain body weight is not affected by wide variation in diet composition. Am J Clin Nutr 1992;55:350. (*Best evidence that what a person eats is less important than the total number of calories.*)
12. Silva JE. The thermogenic effect of thyroid hormone and its clinical implications. Ann Intern Med 2003;139:205. (*Review of physiology of thyroid hormone and its contribution to energy homeostasis.*)
13. Weinsier RL, Hunter GR, Heini AF, et al. The etiology of obesity: relative contributions of metabolic factors, diet, and physical activity. Am J Med 1998;105:145. (*An analysis of data arguing that physical activity appears to be the most important determinant of obesity in postindustrial societies.*)
14. Korner J, Leibel RL. To eat or not to eat—how the gut talks to the brain. N Engl J Med 2003;349:926. (*Succinct discussion of appetite control mechanisms and their potential roles in obesity.*)
15. List JF, Habener JF. Defective melanocortin 4 receptors in hyperphagia and morbid obesity. N Engl J Med 2003;348:1160. (*An editorial summarizing new studies on genetic causes of obesity.*)
16. Hu FB, Li TY, Colditz GA, et al. Television watching and other sedentary behaviors in relation to risk of obesity and type 2 diabetes mellitus in women. JAMA 2003;289:1785. (*Prospective cohort study from the Nurses' Health Study; sedentary behavior was found to be a major risk factor.*)
17. McTigue KM, Garrett JM, Popkin BM. The natural history of the development of obesity in a cohort of young U.S. adults between 1981 and 1998. Ann Intern Med 2002;136:857. (*A long-term prospective cohort study finding that the risk of frank obesity was greatest in overweight young persons.*)
18. Expert Panel on the Identification, Evaluation, and Treatment of Overweight and Obesity in Adults. Executive summary of the clinical guidelines on the identification, evaluation, and treatment of overweight and obesity in adults. Arch Intern Med 1998;158:1855. (*Evidence-based consensus panel recommendations.*)
19. Janssen I, Katzmarzyk PT, Ross R. Body mass index, waist circumference, and health risk: evidence in support of current National Institutes of Health guidelines. Arch Intern Med 2002;162:2074. (*Finds waist circumference correlates well with risk.*)
20. Rexrode KM, Carey VJ, Hennekens CH, et al. Abdominal adiposity and coronary heart disease in women. JAMA 1998;280:1843. (*Data from the Nurses' Health Study showing increased waist circumference to be an independent risk factor for coronary disease, even in persons who have a normal BMI.*)
21. McLaughlin T, Abbasi F, Cheal K, et al. Use of metabolic markers to identify overweight individuals who are insulin resistant. Ann Intern Med 2003;139:802. (*A cross-sectional study identifying fasting triglyceride level and ratio of triglycerides to high-density-lipoprotein cholesterol as the best proxies for insulin determination and detection of insulin resistance.*)

CHAPTER 11 ■ EVALUATION OF FEVER

Since antiquity, fever has been recognized as a cardinal manifestation of disease. Indeed, people identify fever as a sign of illness more readily than they recognize the importance of most other symptoms. In addition to causing concern, the presence of fever usually raises high therapeutic expectations. In the popular mind today, fever is equated with infection, and infections are expected to respond to the administration of antibiotics. As a result, the physician is faced with the challenge of defining the cause of the fever, instituting appropriate therapy, and explaining the reasons for limiting antibiotic use to bacterial infections. Persistent or relapsing fevers are among the most difficult of diagnostic challenges, necessitating an appreciation for the spectrum of causes and a thoughtful strategic approach to workup.

PATHOPHYSIOLOGY AND CLINICAL PRESENTATION (1,2)

"Normal" Body Temperature and the Definition of Fever

Popular lore notwithstanding, 98.6°F (37°C) is *not* normal body temperature. In fact, there is no single normal value; like so many other biologic phenomena, body temperature displays a circadian rhythm. In healthy individuals, mean rectal temperatures vary from a low of about 97°F (36.1°C) in early morning to a high of about 99.3°F (37.4°C) in late afternoon.

In children, the normal range may be even greater. Moreover, physiologic factors such as exercise and the menstrual cycle can further alter body temperature. In practical terms, understanding the diurnal rhythm of body temperature is important for two reasons. First, many patients have been unnecessarily subjected to extensive workups and even psychologically incapacitated in the erroneous quest for a cause of deviation from the mythical "normal" temperature of 98.6°F. Second, the fever of disease states is superimposed on the normal cycle so that fevers are generally highest in the evening and lowest in the morning. As a result, frequent temperature recordings throughout the day are required to monitor fever in sick patients. The absence of fever in a single office visit does not exclude a febrile illness. A temperature in excess of 38.3°C is the standard definition of fever.

Mechanism of Fever

Fever ensues as a consequence of infection or tissue injury. The cytokines (e.g., interleukins, tumor necrosis factor) comprise the endogenous pyrogens; microbial surface components account for most of the exogenous ones. The latter evoke fever either directly or through stimulation of the endogenous pyrogens. The final common pathway is triggering of increased prostaglandin E_2 levels in thermoregulatory parts of the hypothalamus. Fever stimulates some components of the immune response and inhibits further release of pyrogenic mediators. Antipyretic drugs owe much of their efficacy to suppression of prostaglandin formation.

Clinical Manifestations of Fever

The presenting complaints of the febrile patient may be explained by the underlying disease process or by the fever itself. The signs and symptoms of fever vary tremendously. Some patients are asymptomatic; more often, they have a sensation of warmth or flushing. Malaise and fatigue are common. The hypothalamus, acting through somatic efferent nerves, increases muscle tone to generate heat and raise body temperature; many febrile patients experience *myalgias* as a result.

These same factors account for one of the most dramatic manifestations of fever: the *shaking chill* or *rigor*. It is taught that rigor is a manifestation of bacteremia, but in fact, any stimulus that raises the hypothalamic set-point rapidly may produce a rigor. Patients experiencing a rigor exhibit uncontrolled violent shaking and trembling, and they characteristically heap themselves with blankets even as their temperatures are shooting up. This phenomenon also has a physiologic basis. Despite their high central or core temperature, these patients subjectively feel cold because their surface temperature is reduced. To generate fever in response to hypothalamic stimuli, cutaneous vasoconstriction occurs, skin temperature falls, and cold receptors in the skin sense this as cold. Quite the reverse occurs during defervescence; body temperature falls in response to cutaneous vasodilation, and drenching sweats typically terminate an episode of fever.

Other manifestations of temperature elevation include central nervous system symptoms that range from a mild inability to concentrate to *confusion*, *delirium*, or even *stupor*, especially in the elderly or debilitated patient. High fevers (104°F to 106°F) may produce *convulsions* in infants and young children without any primary neurologic disorder. Increased cardiac output is an invariable consequence of fever, and *tachycardia* typically accompanies fever. Tachycardia is so usual that its absence should lead one to suspect uncommon problems such as typhoid fever, in which relative bradycardia is typical (for unknown reasons), drug fever, and factitious fever. Patients with underlying heart disease may respond to the high-output stress of fever with angina or heart failure.

Another sign of fever is the so-called fever blister—*labial herpes simplex*. The problem is probably not precipitated by fever per se, for it is much more common in some infections, such as pneumococcal pneumonia and meningococcal meningitis, than in other febrile states. Because fever accompanies infection so frequently, numerous investigators have tried to determine whether fever has any protective or beneficial role. There are a few circumstances, such as central nervous system syphilis, in which elevations of body temperature may exceed the thermal tolerance of the infectious agent. In fact, induced fever was once a form of therapy for syphilis. In several animal models, fever enhances recovery from experimental infections; however, there is no such proven clinical benefit from fever in humans.

Consequences of Fever

Is fever detrimental? Most otherwise healthy individuals can tolerate temperatures up to 105°F (40.5°C) without ill effects, although even in these individuals, symptoms often warrant therapy. In children, high fevers should be suppressed because convulsions may occur. Patients with heart disease should also receive antipyretic therapy. Each increase of 1°F in temperature increases the basal metabolic rate by 7%, which results in increased demands on the heart, so that myocardial ischemia, failure, or even shock can ensue. In addition, extreme hyperthermia beyond 108°F (42.1°C) may cause direct cellular damage. Vascular endothelium seems particularly susceptible to such damage, and disseminated intravascular coagulation frequently accompanies extreme hyperthermia. Other structures that may be directly damaged are the brain, muscle, and heart. Finally, metabolic derangements such as hypoxia, acidosis, and sometimes hyperkalemia can result from extreme pyrexia and, in turn, further contribute to coma, seizures, arrhythmias, or hypotension, which can be lethal. Nevertheless, patients have survived temperatures of up to 108°F without demonstrable organ damage, although mortality in this temperature range is appreciable. Body temperatures as high as 113°F have been demonstrated in humans, but these have been uniformly lethal.

DIFFERENTIAL DIAGNOSIS (2–9,12,14–16)

Many inflammatory, infectious, neoplastic, and hypersensitivity processes can produce fever. Most *acute fevers* encountered in the office setting are of obvious causes such as upper respiratory or urinary tract infection. Viral illnesses, drug allergy (especially to antibiotics), and connective tissue disease are other important precipitants.

Recurrent or intermittent fever is most characteristic of infectious conditions with cyclic features, such as malaria, hepatitis B, leptospirosis, brucellosis, and disseminated fungal infection. Migration of intraluminal parasites (as in schistosomiasis, amebiasis, and trypanosomiasis) can lead to intermittent fever, as can cell lysis by intracellular parasites (e.g., *Bartonella* and

Ehrlichia). A cyclic pattern of high fevers for 1 to 2 weeks alternating with afebrile periods suggests the pathognomonic *Pel–Ebstein fever* of Hodgkin's disease. Included in the list of causes for periodic fevers are the *hereditary periodic fevers*, which include *familial Mediterranean fever, hyperimmunoglobulin D (IgD) syndrome*, and *tumor necrosis factor (TNF)-receptor–associated periodic syndrome*. All produce recurrent episodes of fever and are associated with a positive family history.

Travel-related fever in a Northern Hemisphere resident returning from a stay in the tropics is a common clinical problem. Whereas respiratory infections and bacterial enteritis are common causes in returning travelers (11% and 6%, respectively), tropical diseases are also a major concern, with the differential diagnosis being destination dependent (Table 11.1). In those returning from Africa, *malaria* is the predominant cause (35%), followed by *rickettsial infection* (5%), *dengue fever* (4%), and *schistosomiasis* (3%). In those having visited tropical Asia, dengue fever accounts for 12%, malaria 9%, and enteric fever 4%. Persons presenting months after travel often have malaria as the cause. Nearly 24% of cases are of unknown etiology but are invariably associated with a favorable outcome.

Unexplained persistent fever can be a major diagnostic challenge. "Fevers of unknown origin" (FUOs) are defined as those persisting for 3 weeks, exceeding temperatures of 101°F, and eluding 1 week of intensive diagnostic study. The spectrum of illness depends on the setting. In reported series of immunocompetent FUO patients encountered in the outpatient community setting, noninfectious inflammatory conditions accounted for about one third of cases, followed by infection and ma-

TABLE 11.1

FEVER IN PERSONS RETURNING FROM TRAVEL TO THE TROPICS

Tropical Diseases	**39%**[a]
Malaria (falciparum and nonfalciparum)	28%
Rickettsial infection (typhus, African tick bite fever)	3%
Dengue fever	3%
Acute schistosomiasis	2%
Enteric fever (*Salmonella typhi* and *S. paratyphi*)	1%
Cosmopolitan Infections	**34%**
Respiratory tract infections	11%
Bacterial enteritis	6%
Infectious mononucleosis–like syndromes	4%
Soft tissue infection	4%
Genitorurinary infection	3%
Tuberculosis	2%
Unknown Causes	**24%**
No focus of infection	9%
Symptoms of enteritis	8%
Symptoms of upper respiratory tract infection	7%
Noninfectious Causes	**2%**
Cardiorespiratory compromise	
New significant cardiac murmurs	
Petechial eruption	
Marked leukocytosis or leucopenia	

[a]Highly destination dependent.
Adapted from Bottieu E, Clerinx J, Schrooten W, et al. Etiology and outcome of fever after a stay in the tropics. Arch Intern Med 2006;166:1642, with permission.

TABLE 11.2

CAUSES OF FEVER OF UNDETERMINED ORIGIN

"The Big Three"
Infections (20%–40%)
  Systemic
    Tuberculosis (miliary)
    Infective endocarditis (subacute)
    Miscellaneous infections: cytomegalovirus infection, toxoplasmosis, brucellosis, psittacosis, gonococcemia, chronic meningococcemia, disseminated mycoses
  Localized
    Hepatic infections (liver abscess, cholangitis)
    Other visceral infections (pancreatic, tuboovarian, and pericholecystic abscesses; empyema of gallbladder)
    Intraperitoneal infections (subhepatic, subphrenic, paracolic, appendiceal, pelvic, and other abscesses)
    Urinary tract infections (pyelonephritis, renal carbuncle, perinephric abscess, prostatic abscess)
Neoplasms (7%–20%), especially lymphomas, leukemias, renal cell carcinoma, atrial myomas, and cancers metastatic to bone or liver
Collagen-vascular and other multisystem disease (15%–25%), including temporal arteritis and juvenile rheumatoid arthritis as well as systemic lupus erythematosus, rheumatoid arthritis, polyarteritis nodosa, Wegener's granulomatosis, mixed connective tissue disease, sarcoidosis
Less-Common Causes (5%–15%)
  Noninfectious granulomatous diseases (e.g., granulomatous hepatitis)
  Inflammatory bowel disease
  Pulmonary embolization
  Drug fever
  Factitious fever
  Hepatic cirrhosis with active hepatocellular necrosis
  Miscellaneous uncommon diseases (familial Mediterranean fever, Whipple's disease)
  Undiagnosed

Modified from Jacoby GA, Swartz MN. Fever of unknown origin. N Engl J Med 1973;289:1407, with permission.

lignancy (Table 11.2). Up to one third of cases remain undiagnosed after comprehensive workup, but only a small percentage of these eventually prove life threatening (usually from hematologic malignancy). Most cases of FUO represent unusual presentations of common diseases rather than rare conditions. The spectrum of FUO disease has expanded in the last three decades. HIV infection raises a whole new set of diagnostic possibilities (e.g., *Pneumocystis* pneumonia or *Mycobacteria avium* infection; see Chapter 13 and Table 11.3), as does immunosuppression from cancer chemotherapy, intravenous drug abuse, and the increasing use of prosthetic devices.

WORKUP (3,5,6,9,10,12,13,17,18)

The acutely febrile patient presents a common but demanding problem in differential diagnosis. In most cases, a careful history and physical examination will reveal the diagnostic clues so that laboratory studies can be used selectively. The evaluation of persistent fever can be more demanding. The initial

TABLE 11.3

FEVER OF UNKNOWN ORIGIN IN PATIENTS WITH HIV INFECTION OR CANCER

HIV Patients
  Infectious (75% of cases)
    Mycobacterial infection (*Mycobacterium tuberculosis,*
      M. avium complex)
    Cytomegalovirus infection
    Toxoplasmosis
    Pneumocystis infection
    Cryptococcal infection
    Salmonella infection
    Aspergillosis
    Herpes zoster
    Underlying HIV infection
  Noninfectious (10%)
    Lymphoma (non-Hodgkin's)
    Drug fever
  Unexplained (15%)
Cancer Patients
  Infection (50%), usually as a consequence of neutropenia
    Gram-negative bacilli
    Fungi
Malignancy
Extension and widespread dissemination of underlying
  malignancy

Adapted from Hirschman JV. Fever of unknown origin in adults. Clin Infect Dis 1997;24:291, with permission.

TABLE 11.4

FEBRILE PATIENTS WHO REQUIRE SPECIAL ATTENTION

Vulnerable Hosts
  Age (very young or very old)
  Corticosteroid or immunosuppressive therapy
  Serious underlying diseases (neutropenia sickle cell anemia,
    diabetes, cirrhosis, advanced chronic obstructive
    pulmonary disease, renal failure, malignancies, AIDS)
  Implanted prosthetic device (hert valves, joint prostheses)
  Intravenous drug abuse
Toxic Patients
  Rigors, prostration, extreme pyrexia
  Hypotension, oliguria
  Central nervous system abnormalities
  Cardiorespiratory compromise
  New significant cardiac murmurs
  Petechial eruption
Marked leukocytosis or leukopenia

office evaluation should help to determine the proper pace of diagnostic testing and the need for therapeutic intervention. If the illness is insidious in onset and only slowly progressive or if the patient is nontoxic and clinically stable, one may proceed with the workup in a deliberate manner on an ambulatory basis, using serial clinical observations and time as key diagnostic tools. On the other hand, if the patient is a compromised host or is acutely ill and toxic, several immediate diagnostic studies are mandatory, and treatment may be required even before all the results are available; hospitalization is usually necessary in such cases. Table 11.4 lists some factors that should prompt an aggressive approach to diagnosis and therapy.

Febrile illnesses are most commonly acute processes that are either readily diagnosed and treated (common bacterial infections) or self-limited despite the lack of a specific diagnosis (viral infections, allergic reactions). However, patients will occasionally present with undiagnosed fevers, fulfilling the classic criterion for FUO. In both situations, the keys to diagnosis are a careful history and a meticulous physical examination, which almost always suggest the diagnosis and guide the rational use of imaging studies and other diagnostic modalities.

History

The infectious disease history should stress several items not routinely emphasized: (a) host factors, (b) epidemiology, (c) symptomatology, and (d) drug history.

Host Factors

One should determine whether patients are basically healthy or have an underlying disease that may render them unusually susceptible to infection. Patients taking *corticosteroids* or other *immunosuppressive agents* are especially vulnerable to infection. Patients with hematologic and other *malignancies, HIV infection, chronic liver disease, diabetes mellitus, neutropenia,* or *sickle cell anemia* may become infected with unusual opportunistic pathogens or may fail to respond normally to common infectious agents. Individuals with implanted *prosthetic devices*, such as artificial heart valves or hip prostheses, are also at increased risk for serious infection. Finally, patients with a *past history* of certain infectious processes, such as pyelonephritis, may be prone to relapses or recurrences of similar problems.

Epidemiology

Epidemiologic inquiry is often very productive. Inquiry is necessary about *high-risk sexual activity* in screening for HIV infection, *travel* in determining exposure to parasitic infections, and *intravenous drug abuse* for estimating risk of endocarditis and viral hepatitis. *Malaria* should be a consideration in patients developing fever months after travel to the tropics. Less-obvious factors, such as *animal contacts*, may be of great importance. Vectors of infection can be found even among household pets, such as cats (cat-scratch disease and *Pasteurella multocida* cellulitis from bites or scratches, toxoplasmosis from fecal contamination), parakeets (psittacosis), and turtles (salmonellosis). A history of *bites* by stray dogs, skunks, or bats may suggest the possibility of rabies. Animal contacts can also provide exposure to insect vectors such as *ticks. Homelessness* places patients at great risk for a host of infectious etiologies, including tuberculosis, HIV infection, viral hepatitis, right-sided endocarditis from intravenous drug abuse, and even louse-borne infections such as the one caused by *Bartonella quintana*, the notorious organism responsible for trench fever in World War I.

An inquiry into what is "going around" in the *community* may be helpful. A very localized outbreak of a flulike illness or atypical pneumonia may be a clue to *Legionella* infection (see Chapter 52). Being exposed to or part of a *population with a high incidence* of tuberculosis (see Chapter 49), HIV infection (see Chapter 13), or viral hepatitis (see Chapter 70) raises the risk of contracting the infection. Intravenous drug abusers are at notoriously high risk for such conditions in addition to bacterial endocarditis. The patient's *occupation* is also sometimes revealing. For example, abattoir workers may be exposed to brucellosis, leather workers to anthrax, and gardeners to sporotrichosis.

Persons with one of the hereditary periodic fever syndromes commonly report onset of an attack in the context of inflammatory system stress, which may be as inapparent as localized trauma, immunization, or minor surgical intervention.

Symptomatology

Symptomatology may serve to pinpoint the site of infection. *Localizing symptoms* should be sought. They include rash, headache, cranial tenderness, sinus discomfort, ear pain, toothache, sore throat, tender thyroid gland, breast mass or tenderness, pleuritic chest pain, cough, dyspnea, abdominal pain, flank pain, dysuria, vaginal discharge, pelvic pain, anorectal or perineal discomfort, testicular pain, bone pain, joint swelling, joint stiffness or pain, calf or vein tenderness, neck stiffness, focal neurologic deficit, and alteration in consciousness. The *pattern of fever* can be useful diagnostically. Periodicity suggests parasitic etiologies, Hodgkin's disease, and hereditary syndromes such as familial Mediterranean fever (FMF), hyper-IgD syndrome (HIDs), and TNF-receptor–associated periodic syndrome. The latter are further suggested by initial onset at a young age and a host of concurrent symptoms due of inflammatory hyperactivity, such as those of serositis (monoarthritis, pleuritis, peritonitis, and rash) in FMF and cervical lymphadenopathy and abdominal pain in HIDs.

Medications

A full review of all drug use and any substance abuse (see Chapter 235) is essential. Is the patient taking any medications that may be responsible for fever as a manifestation of hypersensitivity? Does the patient have any drug allergies? Has the patient been taking antibiotics, which can alter susceptibility to infection by favoring drug-resistant organisms or mask infection by rendering the patient culture-negative? Is there an underlying problem (e.g., renal failure) that may alter the choice of therapeutic agents and lead to the use of a less-common agent? If fever persists beyond 3 days of stopping all possible offending drugs, then the chances of the fever being drug induced are markedly reduced.

Family History

Persons with periodic fevers lasting up to 1 week and interspersed with long asymptomatic periods should be asked about a family history of such episodes. Most persons with one of the hereditary periodic fevers (FMF, HIDs, TNF-receptor–associated periodic syndrome) have a positive family history, as well as onset before adulthood.

Physical Examination

Vital signs should be determined in all cases. Fever is an important but nonspecific sign of infection; some patients with infections are afebrile, whereas others may have a fever resulting from noninfectious causes, such as hypersensitivity states, lymphoreticular malignancies, autoimmune disease, and disorders of inflammatory mediators. The shaking chill or rigor may suggest bacteremia, but other etiologies may trigger release of the same mediators that produce rigors. In the neonate or in occasional adults with overwhelming sepsis, hypothermia may be present. Respiratory distress may signal pulmonary infection, pleuritis, or septic shock, and hypotension may be the presenting finding leading to a diagnosis of sepsis.

The skin and mucous membranes may provide crucial information. To cite some examples: Petechial eruptions on the skin suggest meningococcemia or Rocky Mountain spotted fever, and those at the junction of the hard and the soft palate occur with infectious mononucleosis. Pustular lesions raise the question of gonococcemia (see Chapter 137) or staphylococcal endocarditis. Splinter hemorrhages and conjunctival petechiae herald endocarditis. Ecthyma gangrenosa is a hallmark of *Pseudomonas* septicemia. Macular or vesicular eruptions occur with viral infections, and bullae with *Vibrio vulnificus* infection. Erythema chronicum migrans is an important sign of Lyme disease. Erysipilis-like skin eruptions on the shins or feet are characteristic of FMF.

The *sinuses* should be percussed for tenderness and transilluminated for evidence of sinusitis. In the elderly, the *scalp* is palpated for the tender arteries of cranial arteritis. The optic *fundi* are examined for the retinopathy of connective tissue disease (see Chapter 146), the Roth spots of endocarditis, and the choroidal tubercles of miliary tuberculosis and *Candida* septicemia. The *tympanic membranes* should be examined for effusion and erythema and the oral cavity for tonsillar pathology, tooth abscess, and salivary gland tenderness. The *neck* is checked for thyroid gland tenderness and local adenopathy. Careful examination of all the *lymph nodes* for enlargement may provide a very important clue to etiology, as might the distribution of the adenopathy (see Chapter 12).

The *breasts* are examined for masses, tenderness, and nipple discharge. The *chest* is noted for rubs and signs of consolidation and effusion. A careful *heart* examination for murmurs and rubs is essential. The *abdomen* is checked for organomegaly, masses, tenderness, guarding, rebound, and tenderness of the costovertebral angle.

The *genitorectal area* is all too frequently overlooked, yet it is often a source of key information. A woman without an obvious source of fever must have a careful pelvic examination with a search for cervical discharge, adnexal tenderness, and mass lesions (see Chapter 114). In men, the prostate and testicles need to be checked gently for tenderness and masses and the penis for discharge and rash (see Chapter 136). The rectal examination should include evaluation for discharge, tenderness, and masses (see Chapter 66), and the stool should be tested for occult blood.

Musculoskeletal examination may suggest inflammation or infection of the bone or joints if swelling, increased warmth, or tenderness is present. The *lower extremities* are examined for evidence of phlebitis (asymmetric swelling, calf tenderness, palpable cord). The *neurologic evaluation* should include a look for signs of meningeal irritation, the presence of focal deficits, and disturbances in mentation.

Laboratory Studies

If the history and physical examination findings provide strong indications of an infectious process, laboratory studies can be used selectively to confirm or refute the clinical diagnosis. For example, in the patient with an obvious viral upper respiratory infection, no studies are necessary. In patients with bronchitis, a sputum smear and culture may be all that is required, but if pneumonia is a possibility, a chest radiograph and complete blood cell count (CBC) are minimal additional requirements (see Chapter 52). In the patient with probable lower urinary tract infection, a urinalysis and perhaps a culture may suffice, but if there is concern about upper tract infection, especially as a complication of obstruction, then renal function tests, blood cultures, renal ultrasonography, and intravenous pyelography deserve serious consideration (see Chapter 133).

In other patients, however, more extensive tests are needed to establish a diagnosis when the cause of fever remains unknown. Although such studies must be individualized, the approach to the diagnosis of an obscure fever should include the following.

Complete Blood Cell Count, Differential, and Sedimentation Rate

Leukocytosis and a "shift to the left" suggest but do not prove bacterial infection. Toxic granulations, Döhle's bodies, and vacuoles in polymorphonuclear leukocytes suggest bacterial sepsis but are not entirely specific. In most instances, the erythrocyte sedimentation rate (ESR) lacks the sensitivity and specificity needed for it to serve as an adequate means of detecting or ruling out such causes of fever as tumor, connective tissue disease, and infection. Although a very elevated ESR is an invitation to additional testing and may be a clue to a specific process such as temporal arteritis (see Chapter 161), many elevations are a consequence of trivial conditions unrelated to the cause of fever. The ESR should be ordered and interpreted cautiously and not be viewed as a screening test for "disease." The same pertains to *C-reactive protein,* another nonspecific marker of inflammation.

Urinalysis

Pyuria strongly suggests urinary tract infection. Gram's stain of the unspun urine specimen can be diagnostic (see Chapter 127). Isolated hematuria may be a clue to an underlying glomerular disease or urinary tract malignancy, such as hypernephroma, which is notoriously difficult to diagnose early and a classic FUO etiology.

Radiographic Studies

Chest radiographs may detect infiltrates, effusions, masses, or nodes even in the absence of abnormalities on physical examination, whereas *kidney–ureter–bladder* and upright abdominal films can disclose air–fluid levels in the bowel. *Ultrasonographic* or *computed tomographic* (CT) study may eventually be needed if an abscess or tumor is suspected (see later discussion). *Plain films of bone* will show diagnostic changes of osteomyelitis after 10 to 14 days; for earlier diagnosis, one should consider *radionuclide bone scanning* and *magnetic resonance imaging* (MRI).

Blood Chemistries

The blood sugar determination is helpful in a search for previously unsuspected diabetes mellitus. The test is also important in evaluating the significance of the sugar concentration in various body fluids. Liver function tests are useful in helping to define obscure sources of fever. For example, transaminase elevation suggests hepatitis, and isolated rises in alkaline phosphatase point to infiltration of the liver.

Examination of Body Fluids

If there is any possibility of meningitis, a lumbar puncture is mandatory. Aspiration and study of pleural effusions, ascitic fluid, or joint effusions may be diagnostic. Such specimens should be examined directly by cell counts and stains (see later discussion). Sugar and protein determinations help to differentiate etiologies; in general, bacterial, mycobacterial, and fungal infections produce low sugar and high protein levels in body fluid.

Cultures

If the patient has a heart murmur or a prosthetic heart valve or other implantable device or appears seriously ill, *blood cultures* should be obtained. Having three sets of two blood cultures from separate venipunctures maximizes test sensitivity. Most patients should have cultures taken of *urine* (clean-catch or catheterized specimen) and *sputum*. If other body fluids are obtainable, they should be cultured. Special mycobacterial and fungal media are required for culturing if the patient is a compromised host or has undergone prolonged antibiotic therapy. Anaerobic cultures are important when one is dealing with a possible abscess or other infection of the pulmonary, gastrointestinal, or pelvic regions.

Microscopic Evaluation

Any body fluid that can be obtained should be examined by the *Gram's stain* technique. Sputum, urine, wound exudates, cerebrospinal fluid, pleural fluid, ascitic fluid, and joint fluid often reveal the cause of infection on Gram's stain. Even Gram's stains of the stool may be helpful in certain situations, such as acute diarrhea (see Chapter 64). The presence of bacteria in a specimen of body fluid that is normally sterile is presumptive evidence of infection. This is particularly true when one is examining the spun sediment obtained from cerebrospinal fluid. Likewise, bacteria are not found in normal ascitic, joint, or pleural fluid. The presence of bacteria in unspun urine correlates well with significant urinary tract infection. However, Gram's stains must be examined and interpreted with a certain amount of caution. For example, if one sees epithelial cells in a sputum specimen, one can be certain that the specimen contains mouth organisms and is not representative of conditions in the tracheobronchial tree. In such instances, one should obtain a better sputum sample. In the presence of bacterial pneumonia, the sputum usually contains many polymorphonuclear leukocytes and a large number of bacteria. *Acid-fast stains* are required to visualize mycobacteria (see Chapter 49), and specially stained *wet mounts* of body fluids can be useful in uncovering numerous types of fungal infections.

Immunologic Studies

In selected instances, serologic testing for evidence of infection can be of great help. Examples include suspected HIV infection (*enzyme-linked immunosorbent assay* and *Western blot testing;* see Chapter 13), rheumatic fever and other streptococcal infections (*anti-DNAase B titers*), infectious mononucleosis (*heterophile test*), and *Salmonella* (*Widal titers*). Skin tests (especially the *tuberculin test*) can provide confirmatory evidence and need to be considered when clinical findings are suggestive. Testing for *antinuclear antibody (ANA)*, *rheumatoid factor (RF)*, and *antinucleoprotein cystoplasmic antibody* may help in the diagnosis of suspected connective tissue, rheumatoid, and vasculitic diseases. The presence of rheumatoid factor or immune complexes can be clues to "culture-negative" endocarditis or underlying connective tissue disease (see Chapter 146). Very high levels of *IgD* (>100 IU/mL) and *IgA* are characteristic of the hyper-IgD syndrome. In the diagnosis of obscure fevers, it is often useful to freeze and save an "acute-phase serum" for later comparison with a "convalescent serum."

Genetic Studies—Molecular Testing

Testing for specific gene mutations is an emerging technology that holds considerable promise, especially for diagnosis of the hereditary periodic fevers. Currently, FMF is a clinical diagnosis, but screening for common mutations in the MEFV gene (M694V, V726A, V680I, E148Q, V694I) holds promise as a diagnostic modality. In the hyper-IgD syndrome, there are mutations in the gene for mevalonate kinase; screening for the V3771 mutation may be diagnostically useful.

Undiagnosed Fever—Fever of Unknown Origin (3,5–10,12,14,15,17)

Overall Approach

Cases of persistent or relapsing fever that elude initial investigation pose one of internal medicine's greatest diagnostic challenges. Because the list of possible etiologies includes important infectious, inflammatory, and malignant conditions, a concerted effort at further investigation is warranted. However, it is essential to proceed in a logical, stepwise fashion guided by pretest probabilities because uncritical ordering of the ever-increasing number of available tests and procedures raises the risk of subjecting patients to unnecessary risk, expense, and false-positive results. The search for evidence-based approaches to investigation of undiagnosed fever continues, with some data emerging on the test characteristics, yield, and safety of common modalities (see later discussion).

Before embarking on an extended FUO workup, it is first necessary to reconfirm the persistence of fever and rule out a drug-induced etiology. All potentially offending medications should have been stopped early in the workup of fever and daily temperatures taken. Only if temperature elevations continue beyond 72 hours of stopping all medications should the fever be considered non-drug related. If the fever remains undiagnosed despite a week of investigation (including CBC, differential, aspartate aminotransferase, alanine aminotransferase, ANA, RF, blood cultures × 3, HIV serology, urinalysis and culture, chest x-ray, and serology for cytomegalovirus and mononucleosis), then attention should be directed at the most common causes of FUO, listed in Table 11.2. Of note, most modern series on FUO in immunocompetent persons find that the vast majority of cases are due to a rather limited number of conditions. Of the infectious etiologies, the most common are abdominal abscess, endocarditis, and tuberculosis. Leading the list of noninfectious inflammatory conditions are systemic lupus, polymyalgia rheumatica/temporal arteritis, sarcoidosis, adult juvenile rheumatoid arthritis, Crohn's disease, and deep vein thrombophlebitis. Most of the cases due to malignancy are a result of lymphoma or leukemia.

The history remains the best source of clues to the diagnosis. In a study from the community hospital setting, the history, physical examination, and basic laboratory studies supplemented by serologic testing revealed the diagnosis in more than 85% of instances. Should the diagnosis remain elusive, then consideration of a sequential approach to further workup is reasonable, using those tests proven to be both safe and of highest yield in the setting of FUO, including abdominal CT scan, technetium nuclear scan, cardiac ultrasound, Doppler ultrasound, temporal artery biopsy, and, if the patient is deteriorating, liver biopsy.

Imaging Studies

Imaging deserves consideration.

Computed Tomography of the Abdomen. This is one of the first studies that should be considered, demonstrating a high yield (19% in one retrospective series) due largely to its ability to detect two of the leading causes of FUO: abdominal abscess and lymphoma. Normal CT of the abdomen is very helpful in ruling out serious intraabdominal and retroperitoneal pathology.

Radionuclide Imaging. Radionuclide imaging can be helpful for detection of inflammation or infection; however, nuclear scanning tends to be more specific than sensitive, limiting its usefulness in ruling out such conditions. Technetium is the best radionuclide for use in FUO assessment, with excellent specificity (90% to 95%) but disappointing sensitivity (40% to 75%) for identification of a focus of inflammation or infection. Positive likelihood ratios range from 5 to 12. Radiation exposure is less than that for CT scanning. Use of other radionuclides does not improve test performance.

Doppler Ultrasound of the Lower Extremities. Doppler ultrasound of the lower extremities is excellent for detection of deep venous thrombosis (DVT). Sensitivity and specificity for clot above the knee are very high (see Chapter 35). Because DVT accounts for only about 5% of FUO cases, the use of Doppler ultrasound should be reserved for those with risk factors or clinical suspicion. Test morbidity is nil.

Echocardiography. Echocardiography, especially by the transesophageal approach, should be considered when blood cultures are negative but endocarditis is still a clinical consideration. Sensitivity and specificity are in the 95% to 100% range for detection of valvular vegetations. Transthoracic echocardiography has considerably lower sensitivity (60% to 65%) but similar specificity.

MRI. MRI may localize an abscess or malignancy that has invaded bone and detect disease earlier than radionuclide imaging or plain films of the bone. Compared to CT of the abdomen, MRI is more expensive and usually not significantly better for detection of abscess or lymphadenopathy to justify its much greater cost; however, there is no radiation exposure, and in some instances, it can add additional information and help to confirm suspicious findings. Its role in workup for FUO has not been formally studied, nor has the role of bone scan.

Biopsy

Temporal Artery Biopsy. It contributes to workup in older patients, especially if they have symptoms suggestive of polymyalgia rheumatica, which may be overlooked or dismissed as nonspecific complaints (see Chapter 161). *Color-duplex ultrasonography* helps to identify an optimal biopsy site and in some instances is used as a noninvasive alternative for diagnosis. Yield of biopsy has been reported to be in excess of 15% in cases of FUO involving elderly patients due to the high prevalence of the disease in this population. The biopsy is safe, with rare instances of facial nerve injury leading to droop.

Liver Biopsy. Liver biopsy may detect a granulomatous or neoplastic process. Yield is reported to be about 15% and not necessarily predicted by abnormalities on physical examination or liver function testing. Risk of complications is as high as 3 per 1,000, and risk of death is up to 1 per 1,000. Patients who are clinically deteriorating should be considered for liver biopsy.

Bone Marrow Aspiration and Biopsy. Bone marrow aspiration and biopsy are prime considerations when hematologic malignancy is a consideration, but they contribute little when searching for occult infection; diagnostic yield of *bone marrow culture* has been found to be too low to justify the procedure due to its cost and morbidity.

Lumbar Puncture. A *lumbar puncture* is unlikely to help unless nuchal rigidity or neurologic abnormalities are present.

Surgical Exploration. Surgical exploration played a role in the pre-CT, pre–skinny-needle-biopsy era for patients who were deteriorating. It has largely been replaced by these much less invasive approaches to diagnosis. *Laparoscopy* is a last resort, sometimes undertaken in undiagnosed patients who are deteriorating, but there are no data in the post-CT era that address its yield.

Therapeutic Trials

The only essential principal therapeutic trial is halting all potentially offending and unnecessary mediations to rule out a drug-induced fever. There are no data that justify empiric trials of antibiotics (including antituberculosis drugs) or antiinflammatory agents (including steroids) in patients who present in the office setting. Patients who appear seriously ill, immunocompromised, and at high risk of infection may qualify for consideration of empiric antibiotic therapy, but such persons should be admitted to the hospital and treated under close observation with a definite predetermined endpoint.

The Second Look

Despite the array of sophisticated technology available for the study of febrile illnesses, the history and physical examination remain the keys to diagnosis in most cases. Time can be a most valuable diagnostic tool. Unless the patient is progressively deteriorating, it may be advisable to interrupt the workup for a period of clinical observation, possibly with the aid of symptomatic therapy such as antipyretics. A second look, beginning with the history and physical examination, may then be fruitful.

Unexplained Fever in High-Risk Patients (with HIV Infection or Cancer)

The risk for infection is markedly increased in patients with HIV infection (especially when $CD4^+$ cell counts fall below $100/cm^3$) and in those with cancer complicated by neutropenia. Opportunistic organisms dominate the list of causes (Table 11.3). A careful history and physical examination remain the cornerstone of assessment. When the cause remains unclear, laboratory testing should include blood cultures for bacteria, fungi, and mycobacteria. If blood cultures are negative but the suspicion of mycobacterial and fungal infection persists, then liver and bone marrow biopsies with cultures are indicated. Serum cryptococcal antigen testing provides a sensitive means of identifying disseminated infection. In cancer patients, unexplained fever also suggests dissemination of malignancy. Chest CT with contrast can be useful when intrathoracic spread (including involvement of mediastinal lymph nodes) is a concern, and abdominal CT with contrast can help to detect spread to the liver and retroperitoneal nodes. Lymph node enlargement should trigger consideration of node biopsy.

SYMPTOMATIC THERAPY (3,9,11,13,16,19–22)

The best therapy is obviously to *treat the underlying cause*. However, antipyretic therapy may provide comfort and prevent complications. The first issue, of course, is to determine whether fever should be treated. An elevated temperature itself does not necessarily call for therapy. However, if unpleasant symptoms are present, the patient has a limited cardiac reserve, or the complications of fever are imminent, antipyretics should be administered. Antipyretic therapy depends on the use of both chemical agents and physical methods. The most effective antipyretic drugs are the *salicylates* and *acetaminophen*; both appear to act on the hypothalamus to lower the thermal set-point, presumably by inhibiting prostaglandin E_2 synthesis. Although parenteral salicylates are available, oral or rectal administration of either aspirin or acetaminophen is preferable. Doses of up to 1.2 g of either drug may be given to adults to initiate antipyretic therapy. In addition to their intrinsic toxicities (for acetaminophen, liver toxicity; for aspirin, bleeding), it must be remembered that both aspirin and acetaminophen occasionally produce an exaggerated response, with hypothermia and even dangerous hypotension. Patients with typhoid fever or Hodgkin's disease and elderly and debilitated patients seem to be at somewhat greater risk for this uncommon complication.

Physical cooling is also extremely effective. At the simplest level, undressing and exposing the patient to a cool ambient temperature will allow cooling by radiation; a bedside fan will promote cooling by convection also. Sponging with cool water or alcohol is helpful and promotes evaporation. With extreme elevations ($>106°F$), more drastic measures are necessary, and hospitalization is urgent. *Immersion in an ice water bath* is the most efficient of these methods and may be indicated in hyperthermic emergencies, such as heat stroke. All methods of physical cooling present the risk for hypothermic overresponse and should therefore be discontinued when the body temperature begins to fall below critical levels.

Hyperthermic emergencies are rare, but fever is common and most often presents as an unpleasant symptom rather than a medical crisis. It seems appropriate, therefore, to conclude with a comment about patient comfort. Although fever causes discomfort in most patients, physical cooling produces discomfort in virtually all of them; often, the treatment is remembered as far worse than the illness itself. As a result, these measures should be employed only when fever itself presents medical problems. The same is true to a lesser extent with aspirin and acetaminophen. In particular, many patients find rapid rises and falls of temperature very distressing; therefore, administering antipyretics every 4 hours for the first day or two of treatment may be preferable to waiting for the fever to spike.

Neutropenic patients with cancer undergoing chemotherapy are at great risk for life-threatening infection and require urgent empiric antibiotic therapy before a pathogen is identified. Prompt hospital admission is indicated in this setting for immediate administration of a broad-spectrum cidal antibiotic program, usually involving an *aminoglycoside* and a *beta-lactam*. *Ciprofloxacin* plus a *beta-lactam* is a reasonable alternative regimen in persons who have not had prior exposure to a fluoroquinolone for prophylaxis and in settings where fluoroquinolone resistance is uncommon. Persistence of fever in such patients should trigger consideration of adding antifungal coverage. Amphotericin B, its lipid formulations, and the triazoles (e.g., fluconazole, itraconazole) have been used but are suboptimal due to limited spectrum and associated drug toxicity. Echinocandin antifungal agents (e.g., caspofungin) offer promise of improved outcomes, being at least as effective and better tolerated in head-to-head study.

INDICATIONS FOR ADMISSION AND CONSULTATION

Patients who appear toxic, frail, or immunocompromised should be admitted promptly and infectious disease consultation obtained. Initiation of empiric board-spectrum antibiotic therapy needs prompt consideration. In cases of weight loss and debilitation, early hospitalization should also be considered. Moreover, when fever remains elevated above 101°F for weeks and ambulatory diagnostic efforts have been unsuccessful, it is often beneficial to bring the patient into the hospital for closer evaluation, documentation of fever, and infectious disease consultation.

PATIENT EDUCATION (1)

Whenever fever is suspected in the ambulatory setting, the patient should be instructed to keep a record of temperatures, preferably rectal, taken each evening, when elevations are most likely to occur. The patient needs to be reassured that there is nothing abnormal about temperatures in the range of 97.0°F to 99.3°F.

A.H.G.

Annotated Bibliography

1. Hirschman JV. Normal body temperature. JAMA 1992;267:414. (*A discussion of patients who claim that their normal temperature is <98.6°F.*)
2. Bottieu E, Clerinx J, Schrooten W, et al. Etiology and outcome of fever after a stay in the tropics. Arch Intern Med 2006;166:1642. (*In a series of 1,743 patients presenting to this European center with fever after travel in the tropics, causes depended on destination, and malaria was high on the list.*)
3. Wilder-Smith A, Schwartz E. Dengue in travelers. N Engl J Med 2005;353:924. (*Excellent general review; 73 references.*)
4. Vanderschueren S, Knockaert D, Adriaessens T, et al. From prolonged febrile illness to fever of unknown origin: the challenge continues. Arch Intern Med 2003;163:1033. (*A large prospective cohort study of immunocompetent patients with fever of unknown origin, many of whom presented in the outpatient setting; provides an updated perspective on the differential diagnosis.*)
5. Drenth JPH, van der Meer JWM. Hereditary periodic fever. N Engl J Med 2001;345:1748. (*Comprehensive review of this important class of etiologies; 78 references.*)
6. Hirschman JV. Fever of unknown origin in adults. Clin Infect Dis 1997;24:291. (*Updated review of the problem, extending the classic approach of earlier writers and incorporating newer diagnostic approaches.*)
7. Jacoby GA, Swartz MN. Fever of undetermined origin. N Engl J Med 1973;289:1407. (*A still-useful classic review of the etiologies that should be considered in the patient with fever of unknown origin.*)
8. Kazanjian PH. Fever of unknown origin: review of 86 patients treated in community hospitals. Clin Infect Dis 1992;15:968. (*Unlike most series, which derive from referral centers, this one reports on etiologies seen in community settings.*)
9. Kearney RA, Eisen HJ, Wolf JE. Nonvalvular infections of the cardiovascular system. Ann Intern Med 1994;121:219. (*Very useful discussion of the risk factors, clinical presentation, diagnosis, and treatment of these often difficult-to-detect causes of unexplained fever.*)
10. Knockaert DC, Vanneste LJ, Vanneste SB, et al. Fever of unknown origin in the 1980s. Arch Intern Med 1992;152:51. (*An update of the originally described diagnostic spectrum to include the advent of HIV-related diseases.*)
11. Kumar KL, Reuler JB. Drug fever. West J Med 1986;144:753. (*Still one of the best reviews of drug fever, especially of its clinical presentations.*)
12. Larson EB, Featherstone HJ, Petersdorf RG. Fever of undetermined origin: diagnosis and follow-up of 105 cases. Medicine (Baltimore) 1982;61:269. (*An update of the original 1961 review; cancer was the leading cause.*)
13. Lew DP, Waldvogel FA. Osteomyelitis. N Engl J Med 1997;336:999. (*Review of this important etiology of persistent fever; 62 references.*)
14. Petersdorf RG. Fever of unknown origin: an old friend revisited. Arch Intern Med 1992;154:21. (*An editorial commenting on the changing pattern of etiologies cited in the Knockaert et al. study.*)
15. Petersdorf RG, Beeson PB. Fever of unexplained origin: report on 100 cases. Medicine (Baltimore) 1961;40:1. (*The classic article on fever of unknown origin; it details a logical diagnostic approach that is still useful.*)
16. Simon HB. Current concepts: hyperthermia. N Engl J Med 1993;329:483. (*Review of noninfectious causes of fever.*)
17. Mourad O, Palda V, Detsky A. A comprehensive evidence-based approach to fever of unknown origin. Arch Intern Med 2003;163:545. (*A systematic review of the utility of available diagnostic studies.*)
18. Sox HC, Liang MH. The erythrocyte sedimentation rate. Ann Intern Med 1986;104:515. (*A critical review of the test, arguing that it is not a useful screening procedure.*)
19. Aronofff DM, Neilson EG. Antipyretics: mechanisms of action and clinical use in fever suppression. Am J Med 2001;111:304. (*Best review and thoughtful approach to the use of antipyretics; 96 references.*)
20. Bliziotis IA, Michalopoulos A, Kasia SK, et al. Ciprofloxacin vs an aminoglycoside in combination with a beta-lactam for the treatment of febrile neutropenia: a meta-analysis of randomized controlled trials. Mayo Clin Proc 2005;80:1146. (*Finds ciprofloxacin a reasonable alternative to aminoglycoside therapy for use in combination with a beta-lactam antibiotic.*)
21. DiNubile MJ. Acute fevers of unknown origin. Arch Intern Med 1993;153:2525. (*A plea for restraint in the empiric use of antibiotics when etiology is unknown.*)
22. Walsh TJ, Teppler H, Donowitz GR, et al. Caspofungin versus liposomal amphotericin B for empirical antifungal therapy in patients with persistent fever and neutropenia. N Engl J Med 2004;351:1391. (*Caspofungin was found to be superior and better tolerated in this randomized, controlled trial involving immunocompromised patients.*)

CHAPTER 12 ■ EVALUATION OF LYMPHADENOPATHY

Of the nearly 600 lymph nodes throughout the body, only a few are normally palpable, including small nodes in the submandibular, axillary, and inguinal regions. Nevertheless, lymphadenopathy is a very common presenting symptom. Most often, adenopathy indicates benign, self-limited disease; this is particularly true in children and young adults, who are more prone to reactive lymphatic hyperplasia. Despite this, patient concern is often substantial because of worry about serious infectious processes (e.g., AIDS) on one hand and neoplastic diseases on the other. A systematic evaluation of lymphadenopathy will provide both reassurance and a correct diagnosis. A critical decision for the primary physician is when to refer the patient for a lymph node biopsy.

PATHOPHYSIOLOGY AND CLINICAL PRESENTATION (1–5)

Pathophysiology

As part of the lymphoreticular system, normal lymph nodes play an essential role in host defense, often reacting to threat with a hyperplastic response that usually resolves within 1 month of resolution of the underlying stimulus. Sometimes, a degree of hyperplasia may persist leaving some residual enlargement, especially if the nodal response was marked or the stimulus was severe or prolonged. Pathologic enlargement ensues when inflammation or infiltration overtakes the node. If the underlying disease is well localized, the accompanying adenopathy tends to be focal and limited to the area of involvement. If the illness is widespread or systemic, generalized adenopathy may ensue.

Clinical Presentation

Size and Quality

Most nodes are not normally palpable in healthy individuals, except for the small lymph nodes in the neck, axilla, and groin. Palpable nodes in other regions or any node greater than 1 cm in size should be regarded as potentially abnormal, especially if they persist for more than 1 month in the absence of an obvious explanation. Size alone is not itself diagnostic of the underlying pathology, but nodes greater than 3 cm suggest neoplastic disease. The presentation of pathologic nodal enlargement can range from painless to tender, soft to hard, and mobile to fixed. Although soft, freely moveable nodes are more characteristic of nonmalignant nodal disease, early malignant involvement may present in similar fashion. Tenderness is not unique to adenopathy due to inflammation; rapidly expanding malignant nodes and those with intranodal hemorrhage may also be painful, as may the nodes of Hodgkin's disease after intake of alcohol.

Accompanying Symptoms

"B" symptoms (recurrent fevers >38.3°C, night sweats, weight loss) are characteristic of the lymphomas, especially Hodgkin's disease, and carry a worse prognosis (see Chapter 84). Such symptoms may also occur in systemic infections. Fever alone can occur across the full spectrum of etiologies of lymphadenopathy. Lymphangetic streaking is a hallmark of infection in the area of drainage. Accompanying splenomegaly is limited to infectious mononucleosis, lymphomas, and lymphocytic leukemias.

Distribution

The location of the adenopathy is directly related to etiology.

Generalized. Widespread lymph node enlargement results from systemic processes, such as infection, malignancy, hypersensitivity, and sometimes even metabolic disease with node infiltration. The adenopathy associated with infection may be caused by the disease itself (e.g., HIV infection) or to secondary infection (e.g., with cytomegalovirus). It may result from an illness that first produces localized adenopathy (e.g., cat-scratch disease). At the intersection of neoplastic and reactive lymphadenopathy is Castleman's disease, a rare, idiopathic, atypical lymphoproliferative disease that can be localized or multicentric. Its clinical presentation can mimic that of lymphoma and HIV disease. Localized disease has a benign clinical course, but multicentric disease produces disseminated lymphadenopathy, systemic symptoms, and an increased risk for infection and cancer.

Cervical. Most cervical adenopathy is a consequence of head or neck infection, but lymphomas (especially Hodgkin's disease) have a predilection for beginning in the cervical or supraclavicular nodes. Submandibular nodal enlargement, perhaps the most common type of adenopathy, typically results from pharyngitis (viral, streptococcal, gonococcal) or oral cavity infection. Preauricular adenopathy may be a component of "occuloglandular fevers" due to adenoviral conjunctivitis, sarcoidosis, tularemia, cat-scratch disease, and other processes. Posterior auricular or posterior cervical adenopathy frequently reflects infections of the scalp but may also be prominent in systemic processes, such as rubella or toxoplasmosis.

Supraclavicular. Isolated supraclavicular node enlargement is indicative of lymphoma or metastatic cancer. The right supraclavicular nodes drain the mediastinum, esophagus, and thorax, whereas the left supraclavicular system (Virchow's node) serves the thoracic duct, which conducts flow from the abdomen.

Axillary. Breast cancer is the chief concern, but nodes in the axilla also become enlarged in response to infection of the upper extremities.

Hilar. *Bilateral hilar adenopathy* in an asymptomatic patient raises the possibilities of sarcoidosis and fungal exposure. Unilateral hilar disease suggests lymphoma, cancer, and granulomatous disease, as does bilateral disease in a symptomatic patient or one with abnormal physical findings.

Abdominal. Most isolated mesenteric lymph node enlargement is due to adenocarcinoma of the gut. Isolated retroperitoneal adenopathy is a manifestation of Hodgkin's disease, other lymphomas, metastatic adenocarcinoma, tuberculosis, bladder cancer, and leukemias. A palpable periumbilical abdominal node (the Sister Joseph nodule) is a noted sign of metastatic gastric adenocarcinoma.

Inguinal. Nodes in this area are often palpable in healthy persons, especially if they walk barefoot, but these nodes can enlarge substantially in infections of the genitalia or perineum and in infections of the lower extremities. Cancers are also important causes of inguinal adenopathy, particularly lymphoma, melanoma, and squamous cell carcinomas of the genitalia.

Epitrochlear. Enlargement of these nodes traditionally suggested the generalized adenopathy of secondary syphilis—the proverbial sailor's handshake supposedly included a check for epitrochlear nodes—but topping the list of modern etiologies are lymphoma, chronic lymphocytic leukemia, infectious mononucleosis, and HIV infection, usually in the setting of more-generalized nodal involvement. Local hand infections may also trigger epitrochlear enlargement.

Other Lymphatic Abnormalities

In addition to lymphadenopathy, abnormalities of the lymphatic system may present in other ways. *Lymphangitis*, appearing as red, warm streaks along the course of superficial lymphatic networks, suggests an acute inflammatory response to pyogenic infection in the drainage area; staphylococci and streptococci are frequently responsible. *Lymphadenitis*, presenting as a tender, warm, soft, rapidly enlarging node, has a similar significance and often reflects acute pyogenic infection of the node itself. An idiopathic variant, necrotizing lymphadenitis (*Kikuchi's disease*), causes self-limited tender cervical adenopathy. *Lymphedema* results from the interruption of lymphatic drainage; surgical node dissection, radiotherapy, or fibrosis caused by chronic infections such as filariasis or lymphogranuloma venereum are causes of lymphedema.

DIFFERENTIAL DIAGNOSIS (1,6)

The causes of lymphadenopathy can be conveniently considered in terms of location of the enlarged nodes (Table 12.1). In children and young adults, most adenopathy is a result of reactive hyperplasia and is less likely to represent serious pathology than it is in adults. In persons less than the age of 30 years, the cause proves to be benign in 80% of cases; in persons greater than age 50 years, the rate of benign disease falls to 40%.

WORKUP (1,2,6–13)

History and Physical Examination

A number of basic questions arise in the evaluation of lymphadenopathy, which can be readily addressed by a careful history and physical examination:

1. Is the palpable mass indeed a lymph node? A variety of other structures, including enlarged parotid glands, cervical hygromas, thyroglossal and branchial cysts, hemangiomas, abscesses, lipomas, and other tumors, may on occasion be confused with lymphadenopathy.
2. Is the lymphadenopathy acute or chronic? Clearly, lymph node enlargement resulting from acute viral or pyogenic infection becomes less likely as the days and weeks pass, and granulomatous inflammation (sarcoidosis, tuberculosis, fungal infection) and neoplastic disease become greater worries. Even so, chronicity alone is not always a harbinger of serious disease because on occasion reactive hyperplasia can persist for many months.
3. What is the character of the enlarged node itself? Tender, mobile nodes most often reflect lymphadenitis or lymphatic hyperplasia in response to acute inflammation. Firm, rubbery, nontender nodes may be found in lymphoma. Painless, stone-hard, fixed, matted nodes suggest metastatic carcinoma.
4. Is the adenopathy localized or generalized? Numerous systemic processes that include *infections* (e.g., infectious mononucleosis and other viral infections, toxoplasmosis, secondary syphilis), *hypersensitivity reactions* (serum sickness, reactions to phenytoin [Dilantin] and other drugs, and vasculitis, including systemic lupus erythematosus and rheumatoid arthritis), *metabolic diseases* (hyperthyroidism and various lipidoses), and *neoplasia* (especially leukemia) can produce generalized lymphadenopathy. However, Hodgkin's disease is usually unicentric in origin and spreads to contiguous regional nodes, so that generalized adenopathy is rare except in very advanced disease. Although certain non-Hodgkin's lymphomas may be multicentric, generalized adenopathy is also a late finding and is usually asymmetric, unlike the earlier and more symmetric adenopathy of some leukemias, such as chronic lymphocytic leukemia.
5. Are there associated systemic or localizing symptoms or signs? Fever, rash, weight loss, sore throat, dental pain, genital inflammation, and infections of the extremities are clues that may be particularly helpful. Of these symptoms, night sweats and weight loss suggest granulomatous and neoplastic disease. Ear, nose, and throat symptoms suggest reactive lymphatic hyperplasia secondary to viral or localized bacterial infection. A careful examination of the skin for a primary inoculation site may provide the clue to a diagnosis of cat-scratch disease or tularemia. A check for scalp infections, dermatophytes, and scabies is also needed. The liver and spleen are carefully examined; organomegaly may be an important clue for mononucleosis, sarcoidosis, or malignancy. Sternal tenderness may be present in leukemia.
6. Are there unusual epidemiologic clues? To cite some examples, in patients exposed to cats, cat-scratch disease or toxoplasmosis, which can also result from eating poorly cooked meat, may develop. Travel to the southwestern United States may suggest the possibility of plague. An appropriate travel history or exposure to bird droppings may suggest fungal infection, as may lacerations sustained during gardening in

TABLE 12.1

IMPORTANT CAUSES OF LYMPHADENOPATHY

Generalized Lymphadenopathy	Localized Lymphadenopathy
Infections	**Anterior Auricular**
Mononucleosis	Viral conjunctivitis
AIDS	Trachoma, posterior auricular
AIDS-related complex	Rubella
Toxoplasmosis	Scalp infection
Secondary syphilis	**Submandibular or Cervical (Unilateral)**
Hypersensitivity Reactions	Buccal cavity infection
Serum sickness	Pharyngitis (can be bilateral)
Phenytoin and other drugs	Nasopharyngeal tumor
Vasculitis, lupus, rheumatoid arthritis	Thyroid malignancy
Metabolic Disease	**Cervical Bilateral**
Hyperthyroidism	Mononucleosis
Lipidoses	Sarcoidosis
Neoplasia	Toxoplasmosis
Leukemia	Pharyngitis
Hodgkin's disease (advanced stages)	**Supraclavicular, Right**
Non-Hodgkin's lymphoma	Pulmonary malignancy
	Mediastinal malignancy
	Esophageal malignancy
	Supraclavicular, Left
	Intraabdominal malignancy
	Renal malignancy
	Testicular or ovarian malignancy
	Axillary
	Breast malignancy or infection
	Upper extremity infection
	Epitrochlear
	Syphilis (bilateral)
	Hand infection (unilateral)
	Inguinal
	Syphilis
	Genital herpes
	Lymphogranuloma venereum
	Chancroid
	Lower extremity or local infection
	Any Region
	Cat-scratch fever
	Hodgkin's disease
	Non-Hodgkin's lymphoma
	Leukemia
	Metastatic cancer
	Sarcoidosis
	Granulomatous infections
	Hilar Adenopathy, Bilateral
	Sarcoidosis
	Fungal infection (histoplasmosis, coccidioidomycosis)
	Lymphoma
	Bronchogenic carcinoma
	Tuberculosis
	Hilar Adenopathy, Unilateral
	Lymphoma
	Bronchogenic carcinoma
	Tuberculosis
	Sarcoidosis

the case of sporotrichosis. Contact with wild rodents can result in tularemia, as can tick bites. A history of exposure to tuberculosis may be an important clue to scrofula. More commonly, community outbreaks can provide clues to the diagnosis of streptococcal pharyngitis or rubella, whereas a history of sexual exposure may raise the question of gonorrhea, syphilis, genital herpes, or lymphogranuloma.

Laboratory Studies

Laboratory studies need not be very elaborate. A *complete blood cell count* with *differential* often provides useful information and is almost always indicated. For example, atypical lymphocytosis suggests mononucleosis, other viral infections, and toxoplasmosis; granulocytosis is indicative of pyogenic infection; eosinophilia raises the question of a hypersensitivity reaction; and pancytopenia is consistent with marrow suppression by tumor and HIV infection.

Other studies are based on the clinical presentation of the lymphadenopathy. A variety of blood chemistries may help in selected cases. Elevations of *uric acid* may reflect lymphoma or other hematologic malignancies. *Serum liver chemistries* (especially the *alkaline phosphatase* level) provide objective parameters to follow. Although such abnormalities are nonspecific, they do suggest liver involvement, which can be further evaluated by biopsy.

Localized Adenopathy

If pharyngitis and cervical or submandibular adenopathy are present, a *throat culture* is mandatory. It should be remembered that although these specimens are routinely processed for streptococci, a special Thayer–Martin medium also must be used if gonococci are suspected. *Urethral* or *cervical cultures* and smears should also be obtained if gonorrhea is a potential cause of inguinal lymphadenopathy. *Blood cultures* are indicated in the rare cases of suspected plague, tularemia, or brucellosis or if the clinical picture suggests staphylococcal or streptococcal lymphadenitis. Biopsy may be necessary to rule out lymphoma and Hodgkin's disease if the adenopathy is progressive and the remainder of the workup is unrevealing (see later discussion).

On occasion, lymphomatous retroperitoneal or intraabdominal nodes may enlarge enough to present as an abdominal mass. When lymphoma is a serious possibility, or when staging is necessary in known lymphoma or Hodgkin's disease, *abdominal computed tomography* (CT) can be used to detect enlargement of the retroperitoneal nodes; *bone marrow biopsy* may provide a tissue diagnosis (see Chapter 84).

Generalized Adenopathy

Serologic tests can be of great value. The *heterophile test* and *serologic tests for syphilis* are obvious examples. In addition, a serum sample from the acute phase of the illness can be frozen to be submitted with a later, convalescent-phase serum specimen for antibody titers against viruses, fungi, and toxoplasmosis. Brucellosis can also be diagnosed serologically. Serologic tests, including those for *antinuclear antibodies* and *rheumatoid factor*, may suggest a noninfectious process, such as collagen vascular disease.

Hilar Adenopathy

Tuberculin skin testing with purified protein derivative (PPD) and the *angiotensin-converting enzyme* (ACE) determination can facilitate the assessment. If the results of both are negative and the patient is white, then bronchoscopy and mediastinoscopy may be necessary to rule out lymphoma. If the patient is ACE-positive and PPD-negative, then the probability is very high that sarcoidosis is the cause, and there is little need for further evaluation. If the patient is ACE-negative and PPD-positive, then primary tuberculosis is likely. Reliable skin tests are also available for coccidioidomycosis and tularemia. On the other hand, cutaneous anergy may suggest sarcoidosis or lymphoma, but this is a nonspecific finding. Skin testing can be very helpful in the diagnosis of cat-scratch disease, but, as with the Kveim test, the necessary antigen is available only on a research basis in selected centers.

Among radiologic studies, the *chest radiograph* is particularly valuable because hilar adenopathy may be present in patients with enlargement of peripheral nodes. Hilar adenopathy may also be detected on chest radiograph in the absence of peripheral lymphadenopathy. Sarcoidosis, lymphoma, fungal infection, tuberculosis, or metastatic carcinoma (particularly from a lung primary) should be among the diagnostic considerations. CT can provide additional definition. *Mediastinoscopy* may be required for tissue diagnosis, although not in asymptomatic patients with bilateral hilar adenopathy and clear lung fields, who most likely have sarcoidosis or a fungal exposure.

Lymph Node Biopsy

Biopsy is the most direct approach to the diagnosis of lymphadenopathy. Sometimes, careful *observation* for a period of time may be diagnostically useful before biopsy is undertaken. In many cases of benign lymphadenopathy, the nodes will regress spontaneously even if no etiologic diagnosis has been made. However, some lymphomas may regress transiently and simulate a more benign etiology.

Indications. If undiagnosed adenopathy persists during a period of weeks to months, especially if the nodes are enlarging or if neoplastic disease remains a concern, then consideration of node biopsy is indicated. In one retrospective study, weight loss, night sweats, nodes greater than 2 cm, and abnormal chest radiographic findings were the strongest predictors of important disease before biopsy. In radiologic series, nodes greater than 1 cm in the thoracic and retroperitoneal regions that persisted for more than 1 month were likely to be pathologic.

Approaches and Yield. When possible, *excisional biopsy* is preferred. It is more accurate than needle biopsy and higher yielding. *Fine-needle aspiration* has an accuracy of 75% for non-Hodgkin's lymphoma and 85% for metastatic carcinoma compared to excisional biopsy. In persons with an accessible peripheral node, excision is preferred to skinny-needle aspiration, especially when it is necessary to distinguish lymphoid hyperplasia from lymphoma. However, skinny-needle sampling can be helpful in settings in which surgical biopsy may be problematic, such as with pancreatic or thyroid disease. When possible, core-needle biopsy is preferred to skinny-needle aspiration. Suspicious nodes revealing *atypical hyperplasia* require consideration of follow-up examination; a small but substantial percentage of such cases eventually prove to be due to lymphoma. In the case of fluctuant nodes, *needle aspiration* can be used to diagnose infectious processes in some cases.

Choice of Node. The node to be sampled should be selected with care. When multiple nodes are enlarged, the largest node is the preferred target. If generalized adenopathy is present, it is best to avoid inguinal or axillary nodes if possible because reactive hyperplasia in these areas may make interpretation difficult. In general, enlarged *supraclavicular nodes* have the highest diagnostic yield.

Complications. The majority of excisional biopsies are not technically demanding and can be accomplished under local anesthesia. Nonetheless, this is an invasive procedure and should be employed only when simpler approaches have failed to give a diagnosis and suspicion of a therapeutically important cause remains (e.g., tuberculosis, lymphoma, cancer, sarcoidosis, cat-scratch disease). Complications include spinal accessory nerve injury in posterior cervical biopsy and facial nerve injury in biopsy of the parotid area.

Processing of Biopsy Specimen. Proper processing is essential to maximizing diagnostic yield. Alerting the pathologist to the diagnostic considerations is essential to assuring optimal processing. Immunohistochemical staining of frozen tissue and flow cytometry improve the detection of lymphoma, Hodgkin's disease, and other malignancies. When infection is a concern, tissue should be submitted for appropriate bacteriologic smears and cultures in addition to histologic study. Touch preparations may be useful. Special stains for bacteria, mycobacteria, and fungi may be helpful, as may specific stains for unusual processes, such as periodic acid-Schiff stains for Whipple's disease or lipidosis and Congo red stains for amyloid. The interpretation of lymph node pathology can be quite difficult and requires careful study by experienced observers. With such study, benign processes such as toxoplasmosis or cat-scratch disease can be suspected histologically, and detailed analysis of serial sections may reveal lymphomas that are not diagnosed with less intensive pathologic study.

Follow-up/Empiric Treatment

Empiric therapy with antibiotics or steroids is not recommended unless there is a diagnosis of high probability that is evident and the treatment is specific to it. If pathologic study reveals reactive hyperplasia or is nondiagnostic, patients should be followed carefully because up to 25% may eventually exhibit an illness responsible for the lymphadenopathy, most often lymphoma.

Evaluation of Lymphadenopathy in the HIV-Infected Patient

In most patients who are HIV-positive, the lymphadenopathy represents follicular hyperplasia in response to HIV infection. However, the list of possible causes includes lymphoma, mycobacterial and viral infections, Kaposi's sarcoma, and other cancers (see Chapter 13). The principles for evaluation and biopsy are similar to those for the non-HIV patient, with the proviso that the probability of serious underlying pathology is increased. Suggested criteria for lymph node biopsy in these patients include a diameter greater than 2 cm, rapidly enlarging or asymmetric adenopathy, constitutional symptoms, and intrathoracic adenopathy on chest radiograph. When these rather restrictive criteria are used and needle aspiration is the mode of biopsy, yields of less than 50% have been reported, with most patients having follicular hyperplasia.

INDICATIONS FOR REFERRAL

Any patient suspected of harboring a malignancy should have a consultation with an oncologist or oncologic surgeon to consider further the need for biopsy and to determine the best approach to obtaining a tissue diagnosis. Simply arranging for the biopsy of an accessible node may fail to achieve a diagnosis and will subject the patient to an unnecessary invasive procedure. Consultation may also be useful if one is thinking about a period of observation and wants to be sure that this represents a reasonable approach.

A.H.G.

Annotated Bibliography

1. Habermann TM, Steensma DP. Lymphadenopathy. Mayo Clin Proc 2000;75:723. (*Excellent traditional review, especially as regards differential diagnosis and workup; 154 references.*)
2. Pangalis GA, Vassilakopoulos TP, Boussiotis VA, et al. Clinical approach to lymphadenopathy. Semin Oncol 1993;20:570. (*Finds that nodes >1.5 cm in diameter deserve evaluation.*)
3. Dorfman RE, Alpern MB, Gross BH, et al. Upper abdominal lymph nodes: criteria for normal size determined with CT. Radiology 1991;180:319. (*Nodes >1.0 cm are likely to be pathologic.*)
4. Tompkins DC, Steigbigel RT. Rochalimaea's role in cat-scratch disease and bacillary angiomatosis. Ann Intern Med 1993;118:388. (*Editorial useful for its terse review of the criteria for diagnosis of cat-scratch disease, an important infectious cause of localized and diffuse lymphadenopathy.*)
5. Herrad J, Cabanillas F, Rice L, et al. The clinical behavior of localized and multicentric Castleman disease. Ann Intern Med 1998;128:657. (*Best review of this idiopathic condition, which has both reactive and neoplastic characteristics and can mimic lymphoma.*)
6. Greenfield S, Jordan MC. The clinical investigation of lymphadenopathy in primary care practice. JAMA 1978;240:1388. (*A still-useful algorithm for the workup of peripheral lymphadenopathy in the ambulatory setting.*)
7. Slap GB, Brooks JSJ, Schwartz JS. When to perform biopsies of enlarged peripheral lymph nodes in young patients. JAMA 1984;252:1321. (*A retrospective study of 123 patients up to the age of 25 years who underwent lymph node biopsy. A predictive model was developed to determine before biopsy which patients were likely to have "treatable" causes of adenopathy.*)
8. Slap GB, Connor JL, Wigton RS, et al. Validation of a model to identify young patients for lymph node biopsy. JAMA 1986;255:2768. (*Follow-up study testing the model in ref. 7 found that it performed well.*)
9. Gupta AK, Nayar M, Chandra M. Reliability and limitations of fine needle aspiration cytology of lymphadenopathies: an analysis of 1261 cases. Acta Cytol 1991;35:777. (*Finds utility, but not as high yielding as excision.*)
10. Battista AF. Complications of biopsy of the cervical lymph nodes. Surg Gynecol Obstet 1991;173:142. (*Biopsy is not without its risks, which are reviewed here.*)
11. Pinkus GS. Needle biopsy in malignant lymphoma. J Clin Oncol 1996;14:2415. (*An editorial arguing that excisional biopsy is preferred.*)
12. Knowles DM. Immunophenotypic and immunogenotypic approaches useful in distinguishing benign and malignant lymphoid proliferation. Semin Oncol 1993;20:583. (*Summary of modern methods.*)
13. Schroer KR, Fransilla KO. Atypical hyperplasia of lymph nodes: a follow-up study. Cancer 1979;44:115. (*Cohort study; 6% to 25% of participants were found within a few months to have lymphoma, cancer, connective tissue disease, or infection.*)

CHAPTER 13 ■ APPROACH TO THE PATIENT WITH HUMAN IMMUNODEFICIENCY VIRUS (HIV) INFECTION

STEPHEN L. BOSWELL

Despite the fact that a cure remains elusive, the management of the patient infected with *human immunodeficiency virus (HIV)* has improved significantly in recent years. Most care is now conducted in the outpatient setting, even for patients with *acquired immunodeficiency syndrome (AIDS)*. Earlier intervention, new therapies, and innovative strategies to prevent secondary infections have significantly decreased morbidity and increased survival. With the shift in management to the outpatient setting, primary care physicians have assumed an increasingly central role in the comprehensive care of the HIV-infected patient; they are responsible for initial diagnosis, counseling, prevention of spread, initiation of antiviral and prophylactic therapies, outpatient treatment of secondary infection, determination of need for hospitalization, and provision of supportive care in the late stages of illness. This requires that the primary care physician be knowledgeable about HIV risk behaviors, disease manifestations, laboratory techniques, current therapy, and prophylaxis strategies. It is recommended that an expert be involved in the care of all patients who are HIV infected. This can be accomplished by an expert primary care clinician or by an expert consultant.

SURVEILLANCE CASE DEFINITION AND EPIDEMIOLOGY OF HIV INFECTION AND AIDS (1–6)

Case Definitions

HIV Infection

The Centers for Disease Control and Prevention (CDC) criteria for HIV infection (HIV or HIV-2) in patients older than 18 months of age include the following:

- A positive result on a screening test for *HIV antibody* (e.g., repeatedly reactive enzyme immunoassay), followed by a positive result on a confirmatory test for HIV antibody (e.g., Western blot or immunofluorescence antibody test), *or*
- A positive result or report of a detectable quantity on any of the following HIV virologic (nonantibody) tests: HIV nucleic acid (DNA or RNA) detection (e.g., *DNA polymerase chain reaction [PCR]* or *plasma HIV RNA*); HIV *p24 antigen* test, including neutralization assay; and HIV isolation (viral culture).

AIDS

In 1993, the CDC revised the criteria for the definition of AIDS to incorporate clinical presentations in women and heterosexuals and advances in understanding the significance of counts of CD4+ lymphocytes (also known as helper T lymphocytes or CD4 cells). This CDC surveillance definition of AIDS requires the following:

- *CD4+ T-lymphocyte count less than 200 cells/mm^3* and laboratory evidence of HIV infection, *or*
- Presence of an *AIDS-indicator disease* (*candidiasis* of the esophagus, trachea, bronchi, or lungs; *invasive cervical cancer*; extrapulmonary *coccidiomycosis*; extrapulmonary *cryptococcosis*; *cryptosporidiosis* with diarrhea for more than 1 month; *cytomegalovirus infection* of any organ other than the liver, spleen, or lymph nodes; *herpes simplex* infection with mucocutaneous ulcer for more than 1 month or bronchitis, pneumonitis, or esophagitis; extrapulmonary *histoplasmosis*; *HIV-associated dementia*; *HIV-associated wasting*; *isosporiasis* with diarrhea for more than 1 month; *Kaposi's sarcoma* in a patient younger than 60 years of age; disseminated *Mycobacterium avium*; pulmonary or extrapulmonary *tuberculosis*; *Pneumocystis jiroveci* pneumonia; *recurrent bacterial pneumonia*; progressive *multifocal leukoencephalopath*y; recurrent *Salmonella septicemia* (nontyphoid); and *toxoplasmosis*) and laboratory evidence of *HIV infection.*

Epidemiology

HIV infection is a pandemic. It has become the world's leading infectious cause of death, a position previously held by tuberculosis. In 2006 alone, an estimated 2.9 million people died of AIDS-related causes worldwide. It has moved to this position from relative obscurity when 5 cases of AIDS were reported in Los Angeles in 1981. HIV has spread most rapidly in Asia and sub-Saharan Africa, with more than 8.6 million and 24.7 million cases, respectively. The epidemic continues to expand in South America but appears to have slowed significantly in North America and Europe. In developing countries, the virus is spread primarily through heterosexual contact and affects males and females on a more equal basis than in Western countries.

In the United States, more than 1 million individuals are now infected with HIV, and the numbers continue to rise. In spite of this fact, the death rate from AIDS has dropped significantly in most Western countries in the last several years. This is attributable to significant improvements in medical treatment. The African American and Hispanic communities are increasingly affected. The epidemic appears to have started to climb again in the gay population after having plateaued for several years. The incidence of HIV infection continues to rise in injection-drug users, women, and persons who have acquired HIV through heterosexual contact.

In the United States, those at highest risk of infection are *men who have sex with men (MSM)*; *intravenous drug users* and their sexual contacts; the *sexual contacts* of MSM; persons who received blood and *blood products prior to 1985*; and *children* born to infected women. The risk of directly acquiring HIV infection through processed blood or selected blood products (plasma and clotting factor concentrates) has dramatically decreased since 1985 as a consequence of the widespread screening of those who donate blood and plasma, the use of serologic tests for HIV, and the viral inactivation of various plasma products.

AIDS is only part of the much larger epidemic of HIV infection. For every person who is living with AIDS in the United States, there is another individual who is HIV infected with minimal or no symptoms. Such individuals often present to health care providers for problems related to high-risk activity (e.g., intravenous drug use), unaware that they are carrying HIV. These encounters provide a critical opportunity to teach about HIV infection.

PATHOPHYSIOLOGY, CLINICAL PRESENTATION, AND COURSE (7–15)

Pathophysiology

The *human immunodeficiency virus* is an RNA retrovirus that includes a core protein (p24), a reverse transcriptase, an HIV protease, and envelope glycoproteins. Isolates of HIV differ genetically and antigenically, particularly in regard to envelope proteins (a feature that has complicated development of an effective vaccine).

HIV is transmitted through *sexual contact, parenteral exposure* to blood and selected blood products, and *maternal transmission* (via breast milk and perinatal transmission). Once the virus enters the body, it attaches to the surface of *CD4⁺ T lymphocytes*. These helper T lymphocytes are the target of HIV by virtue of the virus's affinity for receptors on their surface. Once attached, the virus enters the lymphocyte and uncoats. Its RNA is transcribed to DNA by reverse transcriptase. The DNA may remain in the cytoplasm or become integrated into the host cell genome, where it can remain latent until some stimulus triggers replication of virus.

Billions of viral particles are produced in an untreated infected person each day. Most of these viral particles are produced by activated $CD4^+$ lymphocytes, which are killed when the virus enters the lytic stage of infection. These cells are central to the maintenance of immunocompetence. With damage to the CD4 cell population, patients are at increased risk for clinical manifestations directly associated with the disease, including HIV encephalopathy and HIV-associated wasting. As HIV infection progresses, the risks of opportunistic infections and neoplasm increase. Death occurs most frequently because of wasting, opportunistic infection, or neoplasm.

Clinical Presentations and Course

HIV infection in humans is a continuum that can be crudely broken into four phases: (a) primary HIV infection, (b) asymptomatic infection, (c) symptomatic infection excluding acquired immunodeficiency syndrome (AIDS), and (d) AIDS. The rate of disease progression varies from person to person and appears to depend on both viral and host factors. In general, the use of antiretroviral therapy and chemoprophylaxis of opportunistic infection have a profound effect on the pace of disease progression.

Primary Infection

This first phase of the illness is brief and consists of a *mononucleosis-like syndrome*. It occurs 1 to 4 weeks after transmission. In the initial years of the epidemic, the syndrome was not recognized, but after the development of serologic tests, it became possible to link HIV to this clinical syndrome. The syndrome consists of fever, sweats, lethargy, malaise, myalgias, arthralgias, headaches, photophobia, diarrhea, sore throat, lymphadenopathy, and a truncal maculopapular rash. It is of sudden onset and lasts 3 to 14 days. More than 50% of individuals infected with HIV experience one or more of these symptoms. Less frequently, neurologic signs and symptoms occur, such as those of meningoencephalitis, myelopathy, peripheral neuropathy, and Guillain–Barré syndrome. The most common neurologic symptoms in primary HIV infection are headache and photophobia. The symptoms that most markedly differentiate seroconversion subjects from control subjects are *swollen lymph nodes*, truncal or generalized *rash, depression*, irritability, anorexia, *weight loss*, and *retroorbital pain*. Unfortunately, these symptoms are not specific for primary HIV infection.

Asymptomatic Seropositivity

This second phase of HIV infection is the longest of the four phases and is also the most variable. Without treatment, this phase typically lasts *4 to 8 years* and is distinguished by the lack of overt evidence of HIV infection.

Symptomatic Seropositivity (Pre-AIDS)

The onset of the third phase of HIV infection ushers in the first physical evidence of immune system dysfunction. *Persistent generalized lymphadenopathy* is often an early sign of this phase. *Localized fungal infections* of the toes, fingernails, and mouth frequently occur. Among women, recalcitrant *vaginal yeast* and *trichomonal infections* often recur. *Oral hairy leukoplakia*, one of the most commonly missed signs of HIV infection, is very prevalent and typically found on the tongue. Cutaneous manifestations of this phase of illness include widespread *warts, molluscum contagiosum*, exacerbations of *psoriasis*, and *seborrheic dermatitis*. Multidermatomal *herpes zoster* and an increased severity or frequency of *herpes simplex* infections can occur. Constitutional symptoms including *night sweats, weight loss*, and *diarrhea* are often seen. Without treatment, the duration of this phase is typically *1 to 3 years*.

Acquired Immunodeficiency Syndrome

AIDS is characterized by significant immune suppression. This suppression leads to the development of disseminated opportunistic infections and unusual malignancies. Pulmonary, gastrointestinal, neurologic, and systemic symptoms are common.

Pneumocystis jiroveci Pneumonia. This is among the most common infections in AIDS patients, with an attack rate of almost 80% in patients not receiving primary prophylaxis (see later discussion). Fever, night sweats, malaise, and weight loss typically precede the onset of pulmonary symptoms by days to weeks. A dry cough may be the first pulmonary manifestation, followed by shortness of breath. Diffuse infiltrates on chest radiograph, widening alveolar–arteriolar oxygen gradient (>30 mm Hg), and a low oxygen pressure (<50 mm Hg) are associated with reduced survival.

Fungal Infections. Pulmonary and disseminated forms of invasive fungal infection with *Cryptococcus neoformans, Histoplasma capsulatum,* and *Coccidioides immitis* are other hallmarks of AIDS. Cryptococcal infection occurs throughout the United States and often presents subtly, with headache, fever, and malaise. Altered mentation and stiff neck are absent in most cases. At times, pulmonary complaints dominate the clinical picture of cryptococcal infection. Pulmonary and systemic complaints are prominent in patients with histoplasmosis or coccidiomycosis. Infiltrates on chest film of a patient living in an endemic area suggest the diagnosis; splenomegaly can be marked in histoplasmosis.

Mycobacterial Infections. Mycobacterial infections, both pulmonary and disseminated, are consequences of falling CD4 cell counts. HIV-seropositive patients with latent *Mycobacterium tuberculosis (TB)* infection are at increased risk of reactivation and dissemination. Meningeal involvement is the most common form of disseminated disease. Many strains isolated from AIDS patients demonstrate multiple-drug resistance (see Chapter 49). *Mycobacterium avium intracellulare* infection accompanies very advanced disease. The clinical presentation is one of wasting, fever, sweats, diarrhea, and weight loss. Blood cultures are often positive.

Recurrent Bacterial Pneumonia. Recurrent bacterial pneumonia (two or more episodes per year) is a more recently appreciated manifestation of AIDS. The presentations and organisms are typical of those for bacterial pneumonia, with positive sputum cultures and infiltrates on chest radiograph. Such pneumonias are 20 times more common in HIV patients with low CD4 cell counts (< 200 cells/mm^3) than in those with normal counts. The recurrent development of such pneumonias represents significant immunosuppression.

Cytomegalovirus (CMV) Infection. CMV infection, often due to reactivation of latent disease, is common in AIDS. *Retinitis,* presenting as unilateral visual loss or floaters and, if untreated, progressing to bilateral disease and blindness, afflicts about 5% to 10% of AIDS patients. Exudates and hemorrhages are noted on fundoscopic examination. Esophagitis, gastritis, and colitis also may develop.

Enteric Infection. Enteric infections cause much morbidity for AIDS patients and typically present as weight loss, cramping pain, and large-volume diarrhea. *Salmonella, Shigella,* and *Campylobacter* are the leading causes, with the last two more characteristically presenting with bloody diarrhea and leukocytes on Wright's stain of a fecal smear. *Cryptosporidia,* a protozoan, is an important cause of diarrhea in AIDS patients in undeveloped areas of the world.

HIV Wasting Syndrome. This syndrome is characterized by profound involuntary loss of more than 10% of body weight in conjunction with either chronic diarrhea (two or more stools per day for >1 month) or fever and persistent weakness for a similar period in the absence of another cause.

Neurologic Injury. Nerve damage from HIV infection ranges from mild *peripheral neuropathy* causing paresthesias to *encephalopathy* with debilitating dementia. The virus appears to be neurotropic, causing significant neurologic injury in up to 30% of AIDS patients. *AIDS dementia* results from direct injury to neurons from HIV invasion of the central nervous system (CNS). Early on, there may be only minor impairment of cognitive or motor function, but in later stages, frank dementia and disabling motor disturbances ensue. Neuroimaging studies may show diffuse atrophic changes.

Opportunistic CNS Infections. *Toxoplasmosis* is one of the most common of these. Most *Toxoplasma gondii* disease represents the reactivation of latent infection. About one third of patients who are immunoglobulin G (IgG) seropositive experience reactivation. CNS involvement can cause symptoms both of a mass lesion (discrete deficits, headache) and encephalitis (fever, altered mental status). The images on scanning by computed tomography or magnetic resonance imaging are characteristic: multiple (more than three) contrast-enhanced mass lesions in the basal ganglia and subcortical white matter.

Syphilis. Syphilis is of increased likelihood in HIV patients with a history of high-risk sexual behavior, and it may take an atypical or accelerated course, including CNS spread.

Malignancies. A consequence of the reduction in cellular immunity, Kaposi's sarcoma, non-Hodgkin's lymphoma, and primary CNS lymphoma occur with greatly increased frequency in the setting of HIV infection and serve to define the onset of AIDS. *Kaposi's sarcoma* is characterized by raised violaceous nonblanching plaques or nodules on the skin or mucus membranes. Visceral involvement may occur, presenting as hematemesis, melena, or hematochezia. A mass lesion on neuroimaging study may represent a *primary CNS lymphoma,* especially in a patient free of the encephalopathic findings that occur with toxoplasmosis of the CNS. Such lymphomas are rare except in the context of HIV infection. There is a 10-fold increase in the incidence of *cervical dysplasia* in HIV-seropositive women. The development of *invasive cervical cancer* is indicative of severe immune compromise.

Skin Conditions. In addition to Kaposi's sarcoma, other skin conditions are an important source of morbidity. They range from severe *seborrheic dermatitis* to *cellulitis* and *drug eruptions.* Frequency increases with worsening of immune function. Drug reactions are particularly common, with trimethoprim-sulfamethoxazole, dapsone-trimethoprim, and aminopenicillins most often implicated.

Lipodystrophy Syndrome. Fat distribution changes, including *central fat gain* and *peripheral fat loss* in association with *insulin resistance* and *dyslipidemia,* have been associated with HIV infection and highly active antiretroviral therapy. The relationship between antiretroviral therapy and these changes remains complex and poorly understood, but several antiretrovirals (e.g., the dideoxynucleosides stavudine, didanosine, and zalcitabine) are associated with peripheral and facial fat loss, and the protease inhibitors appear to be most closely linked to central (abdominal and dorsocervical spine) fat accumulation.

Prognosis

Prognosis strongly correlates with CD4 cell count and is inversely related to HIV viral load. Asymptomatic HIV-seropositive patients with CD4 cell counts greater than 500 cells/mm^3 and a low viral load may remain otherwise healthy without treatment for many years. However, as HIV infection progresses, patients are at increased risk for clinical manifestations directly associated with the disease (see prior discussion). Most frequently, death is caused by opportunistic infection or malignancy. Increasingly, comorbid conditions such as hepatitis C infection are playing an important role in HIV mortality. Earlier intervention in HIV infection postpones the onset of AIDS and improves overall survival and quality of life (see later discussion).

DIAGNOSIS (1,5)

Diagnosis of HIV Infection

The diagnosis of HIV infection is usually made serologically, by the presence of persistent HIV antibody positivity (Table 13.1). Alternative diagnostic methods include virus isolation and HIV antigen detection. The very sensitive *ELISA* method (enzyme-linked immunosorbent assay) is used for HIV antibody screening, with positive tests subjected to the more specific *Western blot analysis* for confirmation. Sensitivity and specificity of the ELISA are in the range of 99%. Most infected patients produce antibody to HIV within 6 to 8 weeks of transmission. Fifty percent have a positive result by 3 to 4 weeks, and nearly all have detectable antibody by 6 months. Occasionally, it is necessary to attempt direct detection of the virus (using such methods as viral culture, polymerase chain reaction, HIV signal amplification [branched DNA assay], or p24Ag) when clinical suspicion of acute HIV infection is high but standard screening tests are negative.

Diagnosis of AIDS

The diagnosis of AIDS has little bearing on clinical management and is useful primarily for historical and epidemiologic reasons (Table 13.1). When the HIV epidemic was first recognized, the diagnosis of AIDS was predominantly a clinical one, based on the identification of an *indicator condition*. However, the initial AIDS definition emphasized conditions seen in HIV-infected gay men and omitted attention to CD4 cell count and to presentations in other populations, such as women and heterosexuals. These shortcomings were addressed in the 1993

TABLE 13.1

LABORATORY TESTING

Test	Indication for Baseline Test	Test Frequency
HIV serology	All patients without written documentation of positive serology	Baseline only
CBC/Diff/Plt	All patients	As indicated
Chemistry	All patients	As indicated
CD4$^+$ T cell count	All patients	Every 3–4 mo
HIV RNA (viral load)	All patients	Every 1–4 mo
RPR or VDRL	All patients	Yearly
PPD	All patients without history of (+)PPD, TB treatment, or prophylaxis	Consider yearly PPD for those at high risk
Toxoplasma IgG	All patients	As indicated
Varicella IgG	All patients	Baseline
CMV IgG	All patients	Baseline
HAA	All patients	Baseline
HBsAg	All patients	Baseline and as indicated
HbsAb and/or HbcAb	All patients	Baseline
Anti-HCV	All patients	Baseline and as indicated
G-6-PD	Nonwhite patients	Baseline
Papanicolaou smear (cervical)	All women	Yearly
Papanicolaou smear (anal)	Consider in patients with anal complaints; consider in MSM on annual basis	
CXR	All patients	As indicated

CBC/Diff /Plt, complete blood count/differential/platelet count; CMV, cytomegalovirus; CXR, chest x-ray; G-6-PD, glucose-6-phosphate dehydrogenase; HAA, hepatitis-associated antigen; HbcAb, hepatitis B core antibody; HbsAb, hepatitis B surface antibody; HCV, hepatitis C virus; IgG, immunoglobulin G; PPD, purified protein derivative; RPR, rapid plasma reagin; TB, tuberculosis; VDRL, Venereal Disease Research Laboratory.

CDC surveillance definition of AIDS (see prior discussion), which expanded the list of indicator conditions to include *pulmonary TB*, invasive *cervical cancer*, and *recurrent pneumonia* in patients who are HIV seropositive. In addition, the importance of immune status is acknowledged in these diagnostic criteria, with HIV-seropositive patients having a *CD4 cell* count less than 200 included among those considered to have AIDS.

WORKUP (7,9,10,13–20)

Once a diagnosis of HIV infection has been made, the goals of the workup are to identify the stage of illness, determine prognosis, and promptly identify complications of immunoincompetence. Progression of immune system damage is a major concern. Patients with falling CD4 cell counts and high viral loads (>100,000 copies/mL) are at particularly high risk and should be treated promptly and followed closely.

History

The initial interview of the HIV-infected patient should seek information about *infections*, *malignancies*, and *exposures* that may indicate ongoing immune dysfunction or the potential for comorbid conditions. A review of sexual practices helps to define special categories of risk, such as *men who have sex with men*.

Past Medical History

Past medical history is carefully reviewed for a previous diagnosis of herpetic infections; aseptic meningitis; recurrent sinusitis; skin problems such as folliculitis, staphylococcal infections, psoriasis, molluscum contagiosum, warts, persistent tinea, or seborrhea; recurrent bacterial pneumonia due to encapsulated organisms (*Haemophilus influenzae*, pneumococci); oral and vaginal candidiasis; abnormal Papanicolaou smear results; sexually transmitted diseases (if there is a history of syphilis, the details of treatment and serologic titers should be carefully documented); hepatitis B infection or vaccination; hepatitis C infection; TB (including history of skin testing, exposures, chest radiographs, vaccination, prophylaxis, and treatment); and gastrointestinal infections with parasitic organisms or bacterial pathogens. A travel history may be useful in assessing the risk of exposure to histoplasmosis and coccidiomycosis.

Review of Systems

Because HIV infection is usually a multisystem disease, the review of systems takes on particular importance. It begins with inquiry into *systemic symptoms* (fever, chills, drenching night sweats, fatigue, weight loss), which may be manifestations of acute infection or more advanced disease. *Skin* complaints should be reviewed, particularly reports of violaceous nodules or plaques, pustules, petechiae, groin rashes, or herpetic lesions. Moving to the *head, eyes, ears, nose, and throat* review, it is important to ask about sinus pain and any purulent drainage, sore throat, coated tongue, and white patches in the pharynx. Inquiry into *lymphadenopathy* may prove informative.

The *pulmonary* review includes a check for dyspnea, persistent dry or productive cough, and hemoptysis. A nonproductive cough of recent onset in conjunction with dyspnea on exertion should raise suspicion for pneumocystis pneumonia. Patients should be asked about *gastrointestinal* symptoms, especially odynophagia (painful swallowing suggestive of fungal esophagitis), abdominal pain, nausea, vomiting, diarrhea, melena, hematochezia, hematemesis, tenesmus, and perianal pain. Diarrhea and tenesmus suggest large-bowel pathology. Cramping periumbilical pain, diarrhea, and increased flatus point to a small-bowel process. Early satiety, anorexia, and weight loss may be manifestations of gastrointestinal lymphoma. Genitourinary involvement is screened by inquiry into abnormal vaginal bleeding or discharge, dyspareunia, urinary frequency, dysuria, and hematuria.

The *neurologic* review is critical. Unilateral headache becoming more generalized in conjunction with a stiff neck suggests the spread of a parameningeal focus of infection into the CNS. New onset of lateralized weakness or numbness, especially if accompanied by a worsening unilateral headache, raises the question of a mass lesion (lymphoma, toxoplasmosis, brain abscess). Monocular visual field disturbances and floaters are characteristic complaints in patients with CMV retinitis. Diplopia and homonymous hemianopsia may indicate a CNS infection or malignancy. Numbness or tingling in the fingers or toes points to a peripheral neuropathy or myelopathy.

Neuropsychiatric difficulties raise the question of AIDS dementia. Suggestive symptoms include cognitive problems, difficulty with concentration, memory loss, insomnia, apathy, social isolation, and alterations in mood, especially depression. When accompanied by fever and delirium, they are more likely to be the consequence of an encephalopathy, but such difficulties may also occur as a consequence of a reactive depression. Distinguishing among these conditions can sometimes be difficult and may require neuropsychiatric testing and other diagnostic tests.

Physical Examination

The physical examination is directed toward signs of immunocompromise and its consequences. It includes a careful inspection of the skin, sinuses, eyes, oral cavity, lymph nodes, chest, abdomen, pelvis, and central and peripheral nervous systems. In addition, vital signs should be obtained and carefully recorded. Subtle but persistent unintended weight loss occurs frequently in HIV infection and can be one of the earliest manifestations of disease progression, secondary infection, or malignancy.

Skin

Attention to the skin examination is warranted because skin is a frequently affected organ. *Kaposi's sarcoma* (especially prevalent in gay men), *warts, molluscum contagiosum, psoriasis, seborrheic dermatitis*, and *fungal infections* of the skin and nails are especially common. A painless, persistent, raised purple lesion, especially if there is more than one such lesion, may be Kaposi's sarcoma and warrants biopsy. Severe facial seborrhea, scars from recurrent herpetic infections, and premature graying are among the subtler signs of immunocompromise.

Head, Eyes, Ears, Nose, and Throat

The sinuses are noted for tenderness, failure to transilluminate, and purulent discharge. Fundoscopic examination may reveal retinal exudates, hemorrhages, or cotton-wool spots suggestive of CMV infection. The exudate is typically pale and with associated hemorrhage; it usually begins peripherally and may be difficult to visualize during routine funduscopic examination.

Careful examination of the oral cavity is essential, looking for signs of oral hairy *leukoplakia*, *thrush*, mucosal *petechiae*, *stomatitis*, *gingivitis*, and *Kaposi's sarcoma*. Thrush is an important indicator of disease progression. The most common form is *pseudomembranous candidiasis*, removable white plaques on any oral mucosal surface. *Atrophic oral candidiasis* appears as smooth, red patches on the hard or soft palate, buccal mucosa, or dorsal surface of the tongue. These may be easily missed without careful inspection. Rarely, candidiasis can occur in a leukoplakia-like form consisting of white lesions that cannot be wiped off but regress with prolonged antifungal therapy. This form of *Candida* infection can easily be confused with oral hairy leukoplakia and is distinguished primarily by its response to therapy (biopsy is rarely warranted). *Angular cheilitis* caused by *Candida* can appear as erythema, cracks, and fissures at the corner of the mouth. This may require the addition of a topical antifungal cream for adequate treatment. Mucosal petechiae can be the sole evidence of HIV-associated thrombocytopenia. *Kaposi's sarcoma* often produces oral lesions on the hard and soft palate and gingiva. Aphthous stomatitis may be easily confused with stomatitis due to herpes simplex or CMV infections. Biopsy may be required to distinguish them. Lymphoma may appear as a mass or ulcer(s), most commonly seen in the peritonsillar region.

Lymph Nodes

Periodic examination is indicated because adenopathy may be an important sign of disease progression. If lymphadenopathy occurs in two or more noncontiguous extrainguinal sites, persists for longer than 3 months, and no cause other than HIV can be found, it is referred to as *persistent generalized lymphadenopathy (PGL)*. Occasionally, *splenomegaly* may be found in association with PGL. Asymmetric, large, firm, tender nodes may be evidence of malignancy or secondary infection and often require biopsy.

Chest, Abdomen, Rectum, and Genitalia

The lungs are examined for signs of consolidation, pleural inflammation, and effusion. The heart is checked for murmurs and rubs. The abdomen is noted for enlargement of the liver or spleen and for localized tenderness. Genital and rectal examinations are essential in all patients. Although evidence suggests that Papanicolaou test sensitivity may be reduced among HIV-infected women, it is recommended that it be performed semiannually because of the greatly increased risk of invasive cervical cancer. Lymphoma, squamous cell carcinoma, CMV infection, and acyclovir-resistant herpes simplex infections are examples of unresponsive anorectal lesions that may require biopsy for diagnosis. Anoscopy or sigmoidoscopy may be necessary to diagnose rectal or colonic lesions or diarrhea. Evidence suggests that the risk of anal cancer in MSM is approximately 80 times that of the general population. Like cervical cancer, anal cancer is strongly associated with human papilloma virus infection. Screening for anal cancer using anal brushings (*anal Pap smear*) has been advocated by some experts, but this recommendation has not yet found its way into established guidelines. Annual visual inspection and digital rectal exam are recommended. Consider an anal Pap for any anorectal complaint and annual anal Pap smears for all HIV-positive MSM. Repeat the smear in 6 to 12 months if the initial test was low grade and refer to a colorectal surgeon for anal colposcopy and biopsy for high-grade results.

Neurologic Examination

One should check regularly for meningeal irritation, focal neurologic deficits, and changes in mental status. Evidence for peripheral neuropathy, myelopathy, and myopathy should be sought because these are common and often treatable abnor-

malities. A detailed mental status examination may aid in the early detection of AIDS dementia.

Laboratory Testing

Laboratory testing plays an essential role, not only in workup and monitoring, but also in deciding on the nature and timing of therapy (Table 13.1). Testing is used to identify those patients who might benefit from special interventions (e.g., hepatitis B vaccine for those who are negative for both hepatitis B surface antibody and hepatitis B core antibody). In other instances, it may reveal hidden medical problems that can be treated (e.g., interferon-α for the treatment of chronic hepatitis C infection). Decisions regarding the initiation of antiretroviral therapy and *Pneumocystis carinii* pneumonia (PCP) prophylaxis are largely based on laboratory tests, especially the CD4 cell count (see later discussion). Increasingly, the effectiveness of antiretroviral therapy is being measured by CD4 cell count and HIV viral load.

Initial Testing of the HIV-Seropositive Patient

Complete blood count and *platelet count* are essential. Anemia of chronic disease, lymphopenia, and thrombocytopenia are common among HIV-infected patients, especially those patients with advanced disease. Idiopathic thrombocytopenia is sometimes seen in the acute phase of HIV infection. Macrocytic anemia occurs in patients receiving certain reverse transcriptase inhibitors. Marrow suppression with pancytopenia may develop in the context of invasion by lymphoma or disseminated fungal infection. Proper workup may require measurement of serum iron, ferritin, folate, and vitamin B_{12} concentrations (see Chapter 79). When assessing the cause of anemia, it should be recognized that the measurement of mean corpuscular volume may be confounded by the macrocytosis that commonly occurs when patients are taking zidovudine and stavudine.

Before initiating any drug therapies, baseline *serum chemistries* (electrolytes, blood urea nitrogen, creatinine, transaminase, alkaline phosphatase) may help to identify drug toxicities and comorbid conditions such as HIV- or drug-related renal insufficiency and liver damage due to alcohol or viral hepatitis.

Serologic testing for syphilis is essential because of its high prevalence among HIV-infected individuals. False-positive tests are not uncommon and can be excluded with a confirmatory fluorescent treponemal antibody-absorption test. The natural history of syphilis may be altered by HIV infection, and therefore careful attention to a history and prior treatment for syphilis is essential. If a history of syphilis cannot be documented or if a positive result is accompanied by neurologic signs or symptoms, further workup including a lumbar puncture is advocated by most authorities (see Chapter 124 and Chapter 141). Patients who experience therapeutic failure or who cannot receive standard therapy with benzathine penicillin should undergo lumbar puncture also. Interpretation of cerebrospinal fluid (CSF) results may be difficult, however. CSF Venereal Disease Research Laboratory testing is insensitive, and the mononuclear pelocytosis and elevated CSF protein are frequently elevated in HIV infection without neurosyphilis.

Toxoplasma gondii IgG serology may be helpful in identifying those individuals who would benefit from chemoprophylaxis to prevent reactivation. This prophylaxis is recommended in guidelines on opportunistic infection prevention released by the U.S. Public Health Service and the Infectious Disease Society of America. Estimates have placed the risk of developing toxoplasmic encephalitis in an HIV-infected, *Toxoplasma-*

seropositive patient at between 20% and 50%. Seropositive patients should receive prophylaxis against toxoplasmosis when the CD4+ lymphocyte count drops to less than 100 cells/mm³.

CMV culturing has little role in managing the HIV-seropositive asymptomatic patient. However, *CMV serology* should be obtained. Patients who are CMV seronegative should be given CMV-negative or leukocyte-reduced cellular blood products only.

All HIV-seropositive patients should have an *intermediate-strength purified protein derivative (PPD)* tuberculin skin test unless they have previously been documented to be PPD positive, have a history of TB, or have received the bacillus Calmette–Guérin vaccine. This test should be interpreted as positive if the area of induration is *greater than 5 mm* (modified Mantoux test). Routine anergy testing is no longer recommended because of its poor predictive value and because prophylaxis in anergic individuals has been relatively ineffective. *Screening for hepatitis B* (see Chapter 57) should be performed to determine the need for immunization. *Hepatitis C screening* may help to identify patients who might benefit from therapy. *Hepatitis A* vaccine can be safely given in HIV-infected patients and should be considered in patients without evidence of prior exposure.

Glucose-6-phosphate dehydrogenase (G-6-PD) deficiency is a genetic condition that predisposes individuals to hemolysis when exposed to oxidant drugs. Dapsone, primaquine, and sulfonamides are examples of oxidant drugs that are frequently used in HIV-infected patients. The most common variants of G-6-PD deficiency occur in two forms. The first, Gd^{A-}, occurs in approximately 10% of black men and 1% to 2% of black women. The second, Gd^{med}, occurs in men from the Mediterranean region, India, and Southeast Asia. The hemolysis associated with Gd^{med} can be life threatening, whereas that associated with Gd^{A-} is milder and more self-limited. Individuals at risk should be screened with a G-6-PD level either at baseline or before initiating therapy with an oxidant drug.

Formal *neuropsychiatric testing* may be needed to document AIDS dementia and is best conducted by a technician experienced in the assessment of HIV-infected patients.

Screening for pelvic inflammatory disease and *cervical cancer* is indicated. HIV-infected women have an elevated risk for pelvic inflammatory disease, *Candida* vaginitis, and cervical dysplasia. The last-named condition may progress more rapidly as immunodeficiency progresses and can lead to invasive cervical carcinoma. All HIV-infected women should have a baseline pelvic examination with *Pap smear*. The use of routine *colposcopy* is controversial, but the test should be performed in women with abnormal Pap smears or history of vaginal condylomata. They should be repeated at least annually in asymptomatic women. More frequent evaluations are recommended in women with abnormalities and with more advanced disease.

Screening for anal cancer with an *anal Pap smear* should be considered in men who have sex with men because of their increased risk.

Assessing Degree of Immunocompromise, and Prognosis

The *CD4 cell count* and *plasma HIV RNA* levels provide complementary information.

CD4 Cell Count. The CD4 cell count is the best single indicator of the risk of disease progression. Left untreated, approximately 30% of patients with a CD4 cell count lower than 200 cells/mm³ develop AIDS within 1 year. Thirty-nine percent of such patients with a count between 200 and 350 cells/mm³ develop AIDS within 3 years. Untreated individuals with CD4 cell counts greater than 350 cells/mm³ have a 14% chance of developing AIDS within 3 years. CD4 cell count is used to determine when to initiate antiretroviral therapy and PCP prophylaxis. Finally, CD4 cell count is useful in assessing the response to antiretroviral therapy. The primary care physician must be aware of factors that can affect CD4 cell count. These include diurnal variation, the use of corticosteroids, intercurrent illness, inter- and intralaboratory variation, coinfection with human T-cell lymphotropic virus type 1, and variation in the components of the white blood cell count. *The CD4 percentage* is less subject to variation than the absolute CD4 cell count and may be a more suitable measure of immune status. A CD4 cell count greater than 500 cells/mm³ is believed to be equivalent to a CD4 percentage greater than 29%; a count between 200 and 499 cells/mm³ is equivalent to a percentage of 14% to 28%, and a count lower than 200 cells/mm³ is equivalent to a percentage lower than 14%.

Quantitative Virology ("Viral Load"). Viral load assays include *HIV RNA PCR, branched-chain DNA (HIV bDNA)*, and *nucleic acid sequence–based amplification*. Plasma HIV RNA levels provide complementary prognostic information to the CD4+ count and serve an essential role in determining the response to antiretroviral therapy. Commercially available assays can detect virus levels as low as 20 to 50 copies/mL. In general, viral load measurements are highest (>100,000 copies/mL) during the acute retroviral syndrome and during advanced disease. They are often lowest (100 to 100,000 copies/mL) during the asymptomatic phase of HIV infection. Many factors can influence viral load measurement, including concomitant illness and recent vaccination. In these circumstances, viral load measurement should be deferred for several weeks or months.

Changes in HIV RNA level on the initiation of therapy correlate strongly with prognosis. For a change in viral load to be clinically significant, it must be at least 3-fold. A reduction of more than 10-fold in RNA level is associated with a significant reduction in the risk of disease progression. Failure to obtain such a reduction within 8 weeks of initiation should trigger consideration of modifying the regimen. Viremia should continue to decline and usually reaches its nadir by week 16. The speed of viral load decline is affected by the baseline CD4 cell count, the initial viral load, the potency of the regimen, medication adherence, prior exposure to antiretrovirals, and the presence of opportunistic infections. These individual differences should be considered when monitoring the effect of therapy. Optimal antiretroviral therapy will push viral load to less than 50 copies/mL by 6 months.

Measurement of plasma HIV RNA levels and CD4 cell count should be performed at the time of diagnosis and every 3 months thereafter. Less frequent evaluation may be reasonable in those with a high CD4+ T cell count, whereas more frequent evaluation may be reasonable in those with more advanced disease and in whom therapy is being changed.

Other tests have been studied for value in assessing prognosis (*infectious HIV titers, syncytium-inducing viral phenotype, ratio of CD4 to CD8 lymphocytes, β_2-microglobulin, neopterin, and HIV p24 antigen*). None has proven as useful as the CD4+ and HIV RNA determinations.

Diagnosis of Conditions Indicative of AIDS

As noted earlier, the diagnosis of AIDS depends principally on the identification of an indicator condition or on finding in an HIV-seropositive patient a CD4 cell count lower than 200 cells/mm³. Although clinical findings help in making a presumptive diagnosis of an indicator condition, definitive diagnosis depends on laboratory confirmation. Diagnostic modalities include histologic or cytologic study, culturing, serologic study, neuroimaging, and endoscopy.

Pneumocystitis Pneumonia and TB. All seropositive individuals whose PPD status is unknown should have a 5–tuberculin unit *PPD* planted. HIV individuals are judged positive if there is *5 mm or more of induration* (see Chapter 38). Workup for a HIV patient with new respiratory symptoms and a CD4 cell count lower than 200 cells/mm³ includes a *chest radiograph* and an *induced sputum.* The sputum should be sent for *Gram's stain,* routine *culture, mycobacterial stain and culture, fungal wet prep and culture,* and *immunofluorescent stain for Pneumocystis jiroveci. Oximetry* and *arterial blood gases* may provide additional information. If the radiograph reveals a bilateral interstitial infiltrate and the sputum Gram's stain is not diagnostic of a specific etiology, the patient should be treated presumptively for PCP while awaiting immunofluorescent stains.

Candidiasis. Candidiasis is diagnosed by direct observation or microscopy but not from culture because *Candida* is a common contaminant.

HIV Encephalopathy. The diagnosis of HIV encephalopathy is one of exclusion, requiring examination of cerebrospinal fluid and neuroimaging to rule out other causes.

HIV Wasting Syndrome. HIV wasting syndrome is another diagnosis of exclusion, necessitating a search for cancer, TB, cryptosporidiosis, and other specific forms of enteritis before concluding it is the cause.

PRINCIPLES OF MANAGEMENT
(7,9,13,14,19–34)

The major components of therapy are vaccination, antiretroviral agents, prophylaxis and treatment of opportunistic infec-

tions, and counseling. Each plays a major role. Although the disease remains invariably fatal pending the development of curative therapy, a comprehensive and humanely administered treatment program can do much to preserve quality of life and reduce suffering.

Vaccination

An HIV-seropositive adult (especially if the CD4 cell count is >200 cells/mm³) should be vaccinated to the degree possible (Table 13.2). However, caution should be used when considering the use of many live-virus vaccines because the patient may already be immunocompromised. All HIV-seropositive individuals should receive the *pneumococcal polysaccharide vaccine,* the *influenza vaccine* (yearly), and the *hepatitis B vaccine* (if not already antibody positive). *Hepatitis A vaccine* should be given to patients with chronic viral hepatitis who are *hepatitis A antibody* negative, MSM who are *hepatitis A antibody* negative, travelers to endemic areas for *hepatitis A,* and those with other chronic liver disease. In addition, a *tetanus–diphtheria booster* should be given if one has not been received within the last 10 years. The immunogenicity of these vaccines in HIV patients has been called into question, especially in more advanced disease (CD4⁺ T cell count <200 cells/mm³). Consequently, vaccination should be conducted as early in HIV infection as possible (Table 13.2).

Initial Antiretroviral Therapy

Candidates for Treatment

Antiretroviral therapy (Table 13.3) should be considered in (a) any patient with a history of an AIDS-defining illness or a CD4 cell count less than 350 cells/mm³, equivalent to a percentage of 14%, and (b) regardless of CD4 cell count, any HIV patient who is pregnant, has HIV-associated nephropathy, or has

TABLE 13.2

IMMUNIZATIONS

Vaccine	Indication	Frequency
Pneumovax	All patients without a history of prior vaccination	Consider repeat after 5–6 yr
Hepatitis A vaccine	All patients with negative HAA, especially those with chronic hepatitis B and hepatitis C infections	One series only
Hepatitis B vaccine	Patients with negative HBsAb or HbcAb	One series only
Human papillomavirus	Recommended for females ages 9–26. Not recommended during pregnancy	One series
Influenza vaccine	All patients as clinically appropriate	Yearly
Measles, mumps, rubella	Patients born after 1957 and never vaccinated; patients vaccinated between 1963 and 1967; avoid vaccination when CD4 count is <200 cells/mm³	Once
Meningococcal vaccine	College students, military recruits, people without a spleen	Once
Tetanus booster	Patients without tetanus booster in previous 10 yr	Every 10 yr
Varicella vaccine	People born before 1980 DO NOT need vaccine. Avoid vaccination when CD4 count is <200 cells/mm³. Not recommended during pregnancy	One series
Travel vaccines	Travel to endemic areas; generally considered safe except oral polio, yellow fever, and live oral typhoid (live vaccines); case-by-case use of these vaccines may be considered when CD4 count is >350 cells/mm³ (data are limited)	As indicated

HAA, hepatitis-associated antigen; HbcAb, hepatitis B core antibody; HbsAb, hepatitis B surface antibody.

TABLE 13.3

RECOMMENDED ANTIRETROVIRAL AGENTS FOR TREATMENT-NAIVE PATIENTS

	Nonnucleoside Reverse Transcriptase Inhibitors or Boosted/Unboosted Protease Inhibitors	Nucleoside Reverse Transcriptase Inhibitors
Preferred	Efavirenz Atazanavir + ritonavir Fosamprenavir + ritonavir, twice daily Lopinavir + ritonavir, twice daily	Tenofovir/emtricitabine Zidovudine/lamivudine
Alternative	Nevirapine Atazanavir Fosamprenavir Fosamprenavir + ritonavir, daily Lopinavir/ritonavir, daily	Abacavir/lamivudine Didanosine + lamivudine or emtricitabine

hepatitis B infection. For those HIV-infected individuals who have not had an AIDS-defining illness and have an absolute CD4 cell count greater than or equal to 350 cells/mm^3 treatment may be considered on a case-by-case basis. If treatment is deferred, the patient should be carefully followed with reevaluation of plasma HIV RNA concentration and CD4 cell counts every 3 months. Persistent and significant increases in plasma HIV RNA concentrations or drops in CD4 cell count should precipitate the initiation of antiretroviral therapy.

Once antiretroviral therapy has started, careful attention must be paid to assisting the patient in maintaining adherence. This can be a particularly difficult problem if the patient feels healthy before initiating therapy. The problem is further exacerbated by the multiple side effects of many antiretrovirals. Individuals embarking on antiretroviral therapy must understand that adherence to the regimen is essential to the ultimate success of therapy.

Choice of Initial Regimen

Choice should be based on the goal of reducing and maintaining the plasma HIV RNA concentration as low as possible. This will forestall the development of viral resistance, drug failure, and disease progression. One should bear in mind that the *higher the plasma HIV RNA* concentration prior to initiating therapy, the more potent the antiretroviral regimen must be to suppress it. In tailoring antiretroviral therapy to individual patients, several factors need consideration, including *overlapping toxicities*, *pharmacokinetic interactions*, *absence of cross-resistance*, and *drug sequencing* that preserves future antiretroviral options (see Guidelines for the Use of Antiretroviral Agents in HIV-Infected Adults and Adolescents, which is available at http://aidsinfo.nih.gov/contentfiles/AdultandAdolescentGL.pdf).

Table 13.3 lists drugs approved by the U.S. Food and Drug Administration for the treatment of HIV infection. The most-studied initial therapies are three-drug regimens that involve *two nucleoside reverse transcriptase inhibitors (NRTIs)* and either a *nonnucleoside reverse transcriptase inhibitor (NNRTI)* or a *protease inhibitor (PI)* (Table 13.3). Starting triple-drug regimens currently recommended in major consensus guidelines (e.g., those from the U.S. Department of Health and Human Services and the International AIDS Society-USA) involve *two nucleoside analogues* (one of which is either lamivudine or emtricitabine) and at least *one protease inhibitor* (usually boosted with low-dose ritonavir) or an *NNRTI*.

If a patient's disease is advanced or his or her plasma HIV RNA concentration is very elevated, a highly active regimen using at least one potent protease inhibitor or efavirenz should be used. Nevirapine, delavirdine, and efavirenz, if used as part of an initial regimen, should be used in combinations that will decrease the plasma HIV RNA concentration below detection. Resistance to these drugs develops quickly if significant viral replication occurs in their presence.

Subsequent Antiretroviral Therapy and Changes in Regimen

Changes in antiretroviral therapy may be necessary due to treatment failure or drug toxicity (Table 13.4). When considering a change in antiretrovirals, a distinction between *drug failure* and *drug toxicity* is essential. Patients sometimes request an interruption of treatment.

Treatment Failure

Treatment failure occurs when viral load significantly increases or fails to achieve the desired reduction, when CD4 cell count decreases significantly, or when clinical progression occurs. If a new regimen fails to achieve a 3- to 6-fold reduction in viral load by 4 weeks or less than a 10-fold reduction by 8 weeks, a change in therapy should be considered. If a regimen achieves the 4- and 8-week goals but fails to suppress viral load to undetectable levels by 4 to 6 months, a careful reevaluation of the patient's regimen should occur.

Failure may occur for several reasons, including viral resistance to one or more antiretroviral agents, altered absorption or metabolism of one or more agents, altered pharmacokinetics due to drug interactions, and poor patient adherence to a regimen. Before changing antiretroviral therapy, it is important to understand the reason(s) for the failure of the current regimen.

Drug Resistance. Viral genotyping and/or phenotyping are essential to making drug choices in initial therapy and in treatment failure. Table 13.5 lists several scenarios in which resistance testing may be of assistance. These assays generally assess the predominant viral quasispecies circulating in plasma. It should be remembered that resistant variants selected by drug pressure may quickly contract to a level below the threshold of detection in plasma when selective pressure is removed. These variants remain and will return to detectable levels quickly if selection pressure is reapplied. It is for these reasons that the assessment of resistance should incorporate the evaluation of all previously performed resistance testing. The interpretation of resistance assays requires expert input. In addition to using

TABLE 13.4

U.S. FOOD AND DRUG ADMINISTRATION–APPROVED ANTIRETROVIRALS BY CLASS

Nucleoside/Nucleotide Reverse Transcriptase Inhibitors
Abacavir
Didanosine
Emtricitabine
Lamivudine
Stavudine
Tenofovir
Zalcitabine
Zidovudine
Combivir (zidovudine + lamivudine)
Epzicom (abacavir + lamivudine)
Trizivir (zidovudine + lamivudine + abacavir)
Truvada (tenofovir + emtricitabine)

Nonnucleoside Reverse Transcriptase Inhibitors
Delavirdine
Efavirenz
Nevirapine

Protease Inhibitors
Amprenavir
Atazanavir
Darunavir
Fosamprenavir
Indinavir
Lopinavir/ritonavir
Nelfinavir
Ritonavir
Saquinavir
Tipranavir

Fusion Inhibitor
Enfuvirtide

Entry Inhibitor
Maraviroc

Integrase Inhibitor
Raltegravir

Cross-Class Combinations
Atripla (efavirenz/tenofovir/emtricitabine)

resistance testing to guide drug choice after treatment failure, it should be noted that genotypic resistance testing should be performed in all treatment-naive patients entering clinical care, regardless of whether antiretroviral therapy is to be initiated.

Shift in Viral Tropism. An increasingly recognized cause of treatment failure for drugs that block a specific binding molecule is a shift in viral tropism from one binding molecule to another. HIV gains entry to cells via attachment to the CD4 receptor followed by binding to either the CCR5 or CXCR4 molecules and fusion of the viral and cellular membranes. The CCR5 inhibitors prevent HIV entry into target cells by binding to the CCR5 receptor. Whereas the majority of patients harbor CCR5-utilizing virus, the majority of untreated patients eventually exhibit a shift in coreceptor tropism from CCR5 to either CXCR4 or both CCR5 and CXCR4. Tropism testing prior to the initiation of a CCR5 antagonist, such as maraviroc, should be performed. Coreceptor tropism testing might also be considered for patients exhibiting virologic failure on maraviroc (or any CCR5 inhibitor).

Changing the Regimen. In the case of drug failure due to resistance, a detailed history of current and past antiretroviral agents is essential. In this situation, agents with as little overlapping resistance as possible should be sought (see the previously cited Guidelines for the Use of Antiretroviral Agents in HIV-Infected Adults and Adolescents). At least two and preferably three new agents should be used. As the patient becomes more "drug experienced," the task of minimizing overlapping resistance becomes more difficult, and one must rely extensively on viral resistance testing, plasma viral load, and CD4+ T cell count response to inform drug choices. Consulting an HIV specialist is often quite helpful when considering changes in antiretroviral therapy.

Drug Toxicity and Hypersensitivity

When drug toxicity is the reason for considering a change in regimen, it is appropriate to substitute one or more agents from the *same antiretroviral class* with potency similar to the original agent but with a different side-effect profile (see the previously cited Guidelines for the Use of Antiretroviral Agents in HIV-Infected Adults and Adolescents). When abacavir triggers a hypersensitivity reaction, HLA testing should be considered.

TABLE 13.5

RECOMMENDATIONS FOR THE USE OF HIV DRUG-RESISTANCE ASSAYS

Clinical Situation	Rationale
Recommended	
Treatment-naive HIV infection	Transmitted resistant mutations may be more readily detected at a time point more proximal to the time of infection
Virologic failure during antiretroviral therapy	Assess the role of resistance to failure and assist in selecting subsequent regimen
Suboptimal suppression after initiation of antiretroviral therapy	Assess the role of resistance to failure and assist in selecting subsequent regimen
Not Typically Recommended	
After discontinuation of antiretroviral therapy	Once selective pressure is removed, drug-resistant mutations may not be detected with current assays
Plasma viral load <1,000 copies/mL	Available resistance assays cannot be reliably preformed when viral load is <1,000 copies/mL

Evaluation for HLA-B*5701. The *abacavir hypersensitivity reaction* is a multiorgan clinical syndrome most frequently seen within the initial 6 weeks of abacavir treatment. It is characterized by acute onset of high fever, diffuse skin rash, malaise, nausea, headache, myalgia, chills, diarrhea, vomiting, abdominal pain, dyspnea, arthralgias, and respiratory symptoms (pharyngitis, dyspnea/tachypnea). This reaction has been reported in 5% to 8% of patients taking the drug. Discontinuation usually terminates symptoms. Subsequent rechallenge can cause a rapid, severe, and even life-threatening recurrence. There is a highly significant association between abacavir hypersensitivity reaction and the presence of the MHC class I allele HLA-B*5701. It is recommended that HLA-B*5701 testing be performed prior to initiating abacavir therapy to reduce the risk of hypersensitivity reaction. HLA-B*5701–positive patients should not be prescribed abacavir, and the positive status should be recorded as an abacavir allergy in the patient's medical record. When HLA-B*5701 screening is not readily available, it remains reasonable to initiate abacavir with appropriate clinical counseling and monitoring for any signs of abacavir-associated hypersensitivity reaction.

Interruption of Treatment

Adverse effects, expense, and demands of compliance often cause patients to request an interruption of treatment, especially if they appear to be in remission. Others may simply stop treatment without making a request for permission to do so. Randomized study of the effects of interrupting treatment in persons with CD4 cell counts of less than 350 cells/mm³ and restarting only when counts fell below 250 cells/mm³ showed significant increases in the risk of death and opportunistic in-

fection and no reduction in the risk of treatment-related adverse events. Other approaches to treatment holidays might be considered, but the risks should be clearly understood and interruption not encouraged.

Special Situations

There are several situations that warrant specific comment with regard to the use of antiretroviral therapy: primary infection, postexposure prophylaxis, and perinatal transmission.

Primary HIV Infection

Primary infection may represent an opportunity significantly to alter the course of HIV disease for an infected individual. Short-term improvements in viral load and CD4⁺ T cell count have been reported when antiretroviral therapy is given during primary infection, but these data are limited. Some experts recommend antiretroviral therapy for all patients who demonstrate laboratory evidence of primary infection (detectable HIV RNA in plasma together with a negative or indeterminate HIV antibody test). If a clinical trial for acute infection is unavailable or is declined by the patient, a regimen may be selected from the options available for treating established infection (Table 13.4).

Postexposure Prophylaxis

The use of antiretroviral agents to prevent transmission resulting from high-risk exposures remains an option, both in the occupational setting and after high-risk activity (Tables 13.6 and 13.7).

TABLE 13.6

RECOMMENDATIONS FOR POSTEXPOSURE PROPHYLAXIS (PEP)

Exposure Type	HIV-Positive, Class 1[a]	HIV-Positive, Class 2[a]	Infection Status of Source		HIV-Negative
			Source of Unknown HIV Status[b]	Unknown Source[c]	
Less severe[d]	Recommend basic 2-drug PEP	Recommend expanded ≥3-drug	Generally, no PEP warranted; however, consider basic 2-drug PEP[e] for source with HIV risk factors[f]	Generally, no PEP warranted: however, consider basic 2-drug PEP[e] in settings in which exposure to HIV-infected persons is likely	No PEP warranted
More severe[g]	Recommend expended 3-drug PEP	Recommend expanded ≥3-drug PEP	Generally, no PEP warranted: however, consider basic 2-drug PEP[e] for source with HIV risk factors[f]	Generally, no PEP warranted: however, consider basic 2-drug PEP[e] in settings in which exposure to HIV-infected persons is likely	No PEP warranted

[a]HIV-positive class 1—asymptomatic HIV infection or known low viral load (e.g., <1,500 ribonucleic acid copie/mL). HIV-positive, class 2—symptomatic HIV infection, acquired immunodeficiency syndrome, acute seroconvision, or known high viral load. If drug resistance is a concern, obtain expect consultation. Initiation of PEP should not be delayed pending expert consultation, and, because expert consultation alone cannot substitute for face-to-face counseling, resources should be available to provide immediated evaluation and follow-up care for all exposures.
[b]For example, deceased source person with no samples available for HIV testing.
[c]For example, a needle from a sharps disposal container.
[d]For example, solid needle or superficial injury.
[e]The recommendation "consider PEP" indicates that PEP is optional; a decision to initiate the PEP should be based on a discussion between the exposed person and the treating clinician regarding the riske versus benefits of PEP.
[f]If PEP is offered and administered and the source is later determined to be HIV-negative, PEP should be discontinued.
[g]For example, large-bore hollow needle, deep puncture, visible blood on device, or needle used in patient's artery or vein.
Adopted from Panlilio AL, Cardo DM, Grohskopf LA, et al., Updated U.S. Public Health Service Guidelines for the Management of Occupational Exposures to HIV and Recommendations for Postexposure Propylaxis. (MMWR Morb Mortal Wkly Rep). 2005:54(RR09);1, with permission.

TABLE 13.7

RECOMMENDED HIV POSTEXPOSURE PROPHYLAXIS (PEP) FOR MUCOUS MEMBRANE EXPOSURES AND NONINTACT SKIN EXPOSURES

Exposure Type	HIV-Positive, Class 1[a]	HIV-Positive, Class 2[a]	Infection Status of Source		HIV Negative
			Source of Unknown HIV Status[b]	Unknown Source[c]	
Small volume[d]	Consider basic 2-drug PEP[e]	Recommend basic 2-drug PEP	Generally no PEP warranted[f]	Generally, no PEP warranted	No-PEP warranted
Large volume[g]	Recommend basic 2-drug PEP	Recommend expanded ≥3-drug PEP	Generally, no PEP warranted; however, consider basic 2-drug PEP[e] for source with HIV risk factors[f]	Generally, no PEP warranted; however, consider basic 2-drug PEP[e] in settings in which exposure to HIV-infected persons is likely	No-PEP warranted

For skin exposures, follow-up is indicated only if evidence exists of compromised skin integrity (e.g., dermatitis, abrasion, or open wound).
[a]HIV-positive class 1—asymptomatic HIV infection or known low viral load (e.g., <1,500 ribonucleic acid copies/mL). HIV-positive, class 2—symptomatic HIV infection, AIDS, acute seroconversion, or known high viral load. If drug resistance is a concern, obtain expert consultation. Initiation of PEP should not be delayed pending expert consultation, and because expert consultation alone cannot substitute for face-to-face counseling, resources should be available to provide immediate evaluation and follow-up care for all exposures.
[b]For example, deceased source person with no samples available for HIV testing.
[c]For example, splash from inappropriately disposed blood.
[d]For example, a few drops.
[e]The recommendation "consider PEP" indicates that PEP is optional; a decision to initiate the PEP should be based on a discussion between the exposed person and the treting clinician regarding the risks versus benefits of PEP.
[f]If PEP is offered and administered and the source is later determined to be HIV-negative, PEP should be discontinued.
[g]For example, a major blood splash.
Adopted from Panlilio AL, Cardo DM, Grohskopf LA, et al., Updated U.S. Public Health Service Guidelines for the Management of Occupational Exposures to HIV and Recommendations for Postexposure Propylaxis. (MMWR Morb Mortal Wkly Rep). 2005:54(RR09);1, with permission.

Occupational Exposure. Prophylactic antiretroviral treatment in the occupational setting has been widely accepted for several years. Guidelines should be followed (updated U.S. Public Health Service guidelines for the management of occupational exposures to HBV, HCV, and HIV and recommendations for postexposure prophylaxis available at: http://aidsinfo. nih.gov/Guidelines/Default.aspx?MenuItem=Guidelines). The risk of seroconversion for accidental exposure is very low— 0.36% of exposures of health care workers in the largest series; none had broken skin or mucus membrane exposure. About one third took zidovudine after exposure; one seroconverted despite zidovudine prophylaxis. There are no placebo-controlled, randomized trial data available. In their absence, a consensus treatment protocol has been established as part of a multicenter open study. Data are pending.

In the absence of definitive data, the decision to administer antiretroviral prophylaxis must be individualized and shared with the patient. In counseling the patient, one should take into account the severity of the exposure, the very low risk of seroconversion, the fact that such therapy does not provide absolute protection, the high incidence of drug side effects, and the need for frequent monitoring.

High-Risk Sexual and Other Nonoccupational Exposures. Antiretroviral prophylaxis for *high-risk sexual exposures, injection-drug use*, and other nonoccupational exposures (referred to as *nonoccupational postexposure prophylaxis [nPEP]*) is being studied. The Centers for Disease Control guidelines recommend against the use of nPEP where the exposure risk is negligible or when the duration of time since exposure exceeds 72 hours. In cases in which the source patient is known to be positive, the duration of time since exposure is less than 72 hours, and the exposure risk is not negligible, antiretroviral therapy is recommended. If the source patient's HIV status is unknown, the duration of time since exposure is less than 72 hours, and the exposure risk is not negligible, a case-by-case determination is recommended. If treatment is given, its duration should be 4 weeks. The regimens recommended for nPEP are similar to the regimens recommended for the treatment of HIV infection, although no evidence indicates that any specific antiretroviral medication or combination of medications is optimal for use as nPEP. Information pertaining to the effectiveness and safety of regimens used for postexposure prophylaxis is limited.

Preventing Perinatal Transmission

Zidovudine and nevirapine have been shown significantly to decrease the likelihood of HIV transmission in the perinatal setting. No other antiretrovirals have been demonstrated to reduce the likelihood of vertical HIV transmission. Therefore, whenever possible, zidovudine and/or nevirapine should be included as a component of any antiretroviral regimen used during pregnancy. It should be noted that nevirapine has been associated with an increased risk of hepatoxicity in women with pre-nevirapine CD4 cell count of greater than 250 cells/mm[3]. Therefore, in nevirapine-naive pregnant women with CD4 cell counts greater than 250 cells/mm[3], nevirapine should not be initiated as a component of a combination regimen in most circumstances. Efavirenz should be avoided in pregnancy especially during the first trimester due to its teratogenic effects. Didanosine and stavudine should not be used in combination during pregnancy because of an increased risk of lactic acidosis with hepatic steatosis and/or pancreatitis after prolonged use. Due to a recent report of a potential toxic byproduct, ethyl methanesulfonate, found in nelfinavir, it is recommended that nelfinavir not be used in pregnant women or in women anticipating conception. With these considerations in mind, regimens selected to treat HIV-infected adults and adolescents should be applied to preventing perinatal transmission.

Prevention and Treatment of Metabolic Disturbances and Fat and Muscle Disorders

The prevention and treatment of the muscle-wasting and lipodystrophy syndromes seen in the era of highly active antiretroviral therapy remain problematic due to a limited understanding of the underlying mechanisms and the inadvisability of compromising highly active antiretroviral therapy (see earlier discussion). Nonetheless, some measures show promise.

Muscle Wasting. *Anabolic steroids* (e.g., *testosterone*) in combination with *resistance training* can increase lean body mass in hypogonadal men with AIDS-related muscle wasting, but most men with the condition have normal serum testosterone levels. In such persons, testosterone administration, although also capable of increasing muscle and lean body mass, subjects them to adverse changes in lipid profile that increase cardiovascular risk. Isotonic resistance exercise has the advantage of exerting its beneficial effects independent of testosterone and lowering cardiovascular risk. Studies examining the use of *growth-hormone-releasing hormone (GHRH)* have produced promising results that include an increase in lean body mass and a decrease in truncal fat but not significant changes in insulin, glucose, or lipid profiles.

Lipodystrophy. *Metformin* and *rosiglitazone* have been studied for use in lipodystrophy, with the former improving insulin sensitivity and the latter increasing peripheral subcutaneous fat; however, metformin may aggravate peripheral fat loss, and there is concern about increased cardiovascular risk associated with glitazone therapy (see Chapter 102). Because highly active antiretroviral therapy has been associated with increased insulin resistance, one might consider substituting agents if insulin resistance becomes a problem; however, such substitution might compromise disease control. The reduction in growth hormone noted in these patients has stimulated testing *GHRH*, which shows an ability to help restore normal fat distribution; however, beneficial effects on insulin resistance and lipids have been less notable and expense would be very high. The use of *growth hormone* is complicated by impaired glucose metabolism, fluid retention, and joint pain. Cosmetic concerns and the absence of effective therapy have led some patients to consider injectable filler to compensate for the loss of facial subcutaneous fat. Management of dyslipidemia (elevated triglycerides, low high-density-lipoprotein cholesterol, elevated low-density-lipoprotein cholesterol) requires treating these abnormalities specifically (see Chapter 27).

Opportunistic Infection: Prophylaxis and Treatment

Prophylaxis and prompt treatment of opportunistic infection can significantly lessen disease morbidity and need for hospitalization. Several of the most common infections are discussed here. These include PCP, TB, toxoplasmosis, and candidiasis.

Pneumocystis jiroveci Pneumonia

This is the most common pulmonary infection in HIV-infected adults. Adults with CD4 cell counts less than 200 cells/mm^3 (or <14% of total lymphocytes) or a history of oropharyngeal candidiasis should receive PCP prophylaxis. Several prophylaxis regimens are available. *Trimethoprim–sulfamethoxazole (TMS)* is the preferred agent. One double-strength tablet per day is recommended. However, one single-strength tablet per day is also effective and may be better tolerated. TMS at a dose of one double-strength tablet per day confers cross-protection against *T. gondii* and some common respiratory bacterial pathogens. For most patients, it is well tolerated, but a substantial proportion of patients experience adverse reactions—primarily fever and rash—necessitating desensitization or consideration of an alternative means of PCP prophylaxis. Desensitization to TMS can be used successfully in up to 70% of patients who experience these reactions.

Dapsone (50 to 100 mg once daily) is an effective prophylactic agent for PCP. This is a very inexpensive drug with a long half-life. Less frequent dosing may be effective, but such dosing schemes may decrease overall adherence.

Aerosolized pentamidine (300 mg once every 4 weeks via a Respirgard II nebulizer) has also been shown to be effective in preventing PCP, although not quite to the same degree as TMS. When breakthroughs occur, they may have an upper lobe predominance. The dissemination of *Pneumocystis jiroveci* to other tissues has been reported. Individuals with active TB should not receive aerosolized pentamidine because this greatly increases the risk of TB among health care providers giving the therapy.

Atovaquone (1,500 mg each day) is comparable to aerosolized pentamidine in effectiveness but is substantially more expensive.

Effective *oral therapies* for PCP include *TMS, dapsone–trimethoprim, atovaquone,* and *clindamycin–primaquine.* If the patient appears clinically stable and is not in respiratory distress, treatment can be initiated on an outpatient basis. Careful follow-up is essential.

One of the most effective and easily tolerated of these regimens is dapsone (75 to 100 mg/d in an average-sized adult) combined with trimethoprim (15 mg/kg per day in three or four divided doses). TMS (15 mg/kg per day by trimethoprim content, in three or four divided doses) is effective but causes more adverse reactions than dapsone–trimethoprim. Clindamycin–primaquine may be used in patients who are unable to tolerate dapsone–trimethoprim or TMS. G-6-PD–deficient (Gd^{med}) patients should not receive dapsone, TMS, or primaquine. Effective intravenous therapies include TMS, trimetrexate, and *pentamidine.*

Oral corticosteroid therapy should be used when a significant alveolar–arterial oxygen gradient (>30 mm Hg) is present, provided it is started within 72 hours of the initiation of treatment. Later therapy has not been shown to improve outcome. If a patient is in respiratory distress or has a significant alveolar–arterial gradient, hospitalization should be considered.

Tuberculosis and Atypical Mycobacteria

Several regimens may be used for prophylaxis of tuberculosis in this setting. These include *isoniazid* (INH) 300 mg each day with 50 mg of pyridoxine for 9 months; 900 mg of *isoniazid* with 100 mg of pyridoxine given twice weekly for 9 months; and, if no PI or NNRTI is being given as part of the patient's antiretroviral regimen, *rifampin* 600 mg given with pyrazinamide 15 to 20 mg/kg daily for 2 months. If a concomitant PI or NNRTI is being given, rifabutin is generally substituted for rifampin. The rifabutin dose must be tailored to the particular choice of PI and/or NNRTI. Many authorities suggest that an anergic individual with a history of positive PPD also should receive a course of isoniazid.

As noted previously, the use of aerosolized pentamidine may induce coughing and thereby facilitate transmission of undiagnosed pulmonary TB from HIV-infected patients to persons sharing the same breathing space during or after treatment. The potential for transmission of TB depends on the prevalence of TB infection in the HIV-infected population being served and on such factors as room ventilation, the number of infectious droplet nuclei generated by the patient, and duration of exposure. Specially ventilated facilities are required to deliver the drug safely.

The development of *active TB* in the HIV patient is a problem made even more serious because of the associated risk of *multidrug-resistant strains.* Such patients require very careful attention to respiratory precautions (see Chapter 49).

Prophylaxis of *Mycobacterium avium* complex (MAC) infection should be instituted for those with CD4$^+$ T cell count of less than 50 cells/mm^3. *Clarithromycin* (500 mg/d) and *azithromycin* (1,200 mg given once each week) are the preferred prophylactic agents. In addition to their prophylactic activity against MAC, clarithromycin and azithromycin may provide protection against respiratory bacterial infections.

Treatment of MAC infection requires multiple drugs. One of the most effective regimens is composed of clarithromycin (500 mg given every 12 hours) and ethambutol (15 mg per kilogram of body weight given daily) with or without rifabutin (300 mg/d). Azithromycin may be substituted for clarithromycin at a dose of 500 to 600 mg/d.

Toxoplasmosis

Trimethoprim–sulfamethoxazole (one single-strength tablet daily or one double-strength tablet three times each week) or *dapsone–pyrimethamine (dapsone* 50 mg/d + *pyrimethamine* 50 mg/wk + *folinic acid* 25 mg/wk or *dapsone* 200 mg/wk + *pyrimethamine* 75 mg/wk + *folinic acid* 25 mg/wk) appears to provide effective chemoprophylaxis in patients seropositive for *T. gondii* who have CD4 cell counts lower than 100 cells/mm^3. For those individuals who are not seropositive, the thorough cooking of meat and careful hand washing after contact with raw meat should be emphasized. Furthermore, cat owners should clean litter boxes while wearing gloves and practice careful hand washing afterward or have another person perform this chore. If the individual is a gardener, he or she should be encouraged to use gloves while enjoying this pastime. Patients with encephalitis require hospitalization for initiation of sulfadiazine, pyrimethamine, and leucovorin (*pyrimethamine* 100- to 200-mg loading dose, then 50 to 100 mg/d + *folinic acid* 10 mg/d orally + *sulfadiazine* or *trisulfapyrimidine* 4 to 8 g/d for at least 6 weeks). Alternative regimens involving the use of *pyrimethamine* and *folinic acid* with *clindamycin, azithromycin, clarithromycin,* or *atovaquone* can also be used.

Candidal Infection

Candidal infection occurs frequently in HIV-infected individuals, especially as the CD4$^+$ T cell count drops to less than 200 cells/mm^3. Thrush, esophageal candidiasis, and vaginitis are the most common forms of this infection. Although prophylaxis of thrush is not routinely recommended, occasionally chronic maintenance therapy is required to stem recurrent infections. Topical agents for *oral candidiasis* are effective and well tolerated. One 10-mg *clotrimazole troche* held in the mouth for 15 to 30 minutes three times each day is effective. *Chlorhexidine gluconate* may be useful, especially among patients with significant gingivitis and periodontitis. *Nystatin* is available in either an oral suspension or a pastille. Nystatin oral pastilles (200,000 U), one pastille taken three times each day, or nystatin suspension (100,000 U/mL), 15-mL swish-and-swallow six times per day, can also be used.

Esophageal candidiasis is treated with systemic therapy. *Fluconazole* (200 mg given once daily for 2 to 3 weeks) is one of the most effective therapies. *Itraconazole* (100 to 200 mg given twice daily or 100- to 200-mg oral suspension given once daily) may also be used for this purpose. Amphotericin B with or without *flucytosine* may be required for infections unresponsive to either fluconazole or itraconazole.

Vulvovaginal candidiasis is a common problem for HIV-infected women. It tends to occur earlier in HIV infection than does oral candidiasis. Again, there are several agents available for *prophylaxis:* intravaginal *miconazole* suppository (200 mg taken for 3 days or cream [2%] taken for 7 days), *clotrimazole* (cream [1%] taken for 7 to 14 days, 100-mg tabs taken daily for 7 days or 100-mg tabs taken twice daily for 3 days or 500 mg taken once), or *fluconazole* (150-mg tab taken orally once). Maintenance therapy may be required to prevent frequent relapse (*ketoconazole* 100 mg given daily, *fluconazole* 50 to 100 mg given daily, or *fluconazole* 200 mg given weekly).

Cytomegalovirus

Ganciclovir, foscarnet, cidofovir, and *fomivirsen* are the drugs approved for treatment of CMV *retinitis. Foscarnet (60 mg/kg intravenously every 8 hours or 90 mg/kg intravenously every 12 hours for 14 to 21 days)* has been shown to be superior to *ganciclovir* in patients with normal renal function. For patients with impaired renal function, *ganciclovir* (5 mg/kg intravenously twice daily for 14 to 21 days) is preferred. However, granulocyte counts have to be monitored closely because both cause granulocytopenia. It should be noted that data suggest that alternating or combining *ganciclovir* and *foscarnet* may be less toxic and more active against CMV compared to foscarnet alone. An intraocular *ganciclovir* release device (*Vitrasert*) can also be used for local treatment. *Cidofovir* (5 mg/kg intravenously once weekly for 2 weeks followed by 5 mg/kg intravenously every 2 weeks with 2 g of probenecid given 3 hours before each dose and 1 g at 2 and 8 hours after each dose) and *fomivirsen* (330 mg by intravitreal injection on day 1 and day 15, then monthly) may also be used but should not be considered first-line therapy; these are best prescribed by specialists.

Extraocular CMV disease may be treated with *ganciclovir* and *foscarnet* at doses similar to those used for ocular disease. In general, induction therapy is generally given for a longer period (3 to 6 weeks) in extraocular disease. Maintenance therapy should be considered, especially after reinduction and relapse.

PATIENT EDUCATION AND SUPPORT

As with other chronic diseases, understanding the patient's existing *support network* and helping the patient develop additional supports can be very important. It is often helpful if the patient can link up with infected peers to share experiences and concerns; this helps to minimize isolation, loneliness, and fear. Depression is extremely common in patients diagnosed with HIV infection. Appropriate screening and intervention is essential (see Chapter 227).

In many localities, there are special *community resources* to aid HIV-infected patients with legal, social, and financial issues pertaining to the infection. It is important for every physician who cares for these individuals to identify these resources.

An open discussion of *safe-sex measures* with HIV-seropositive individuals and their sexual partners is essential.

These steps are useful in preventing transmission of not only HIV, but also other sexually transmitted diseases.

Adherence to antiretroviral therapy is essential to its ultimate success. The physician plays an important role in both assessing adherence and assisting patients to maintain the highest possible level of adherence.

INDICATIONS FOR ADMISSION AND CONSULTATION

Although outpatient care is preferred for many elements of HIV management, there are several instances in which prompt hospitalization is essential. The patient with signs or symptoms suggestive of significant pulmonary, CNS, or disseminated infection (especially that which may be due to severe *Pneumocystis* pneumonia, tuberculosis, atypical mycobacteria, syphilis, toxoplasmosis, histoplasmosis, coccidiomycosis, *Cryptococcus*, CMV, and decompensated hepatitis C infection) may require prompt hospital admission and infectious disease consultation. Outpatient treatment may be possible later, even for the administration of parenteral therapy, but treatment should be initiated in the hospital. Also requiring immediate hospitalization is the suicidal patient, particularly one who admits to having made specific plans for suicide. Urgent psychiatric consultation is essential. When appropriate, referral for *hospice care* should be considered. At this stage of illness, hospital admissions should be kept to a minimum except as needed for purposes of providing comfort.

Annotated Bibliography

1. Buehler JW, Ward JW. A new definition for AIDS surveillance. Ann Intern Med 1993;118:390. (*An editorial on the implications of the expanded surveillance definition.*)
2. Centers for Disease Control and Prevention (CDC). HIV/AIDS Surveillance Report, 2004, Vol. 16. Atlanta: U.S. Department of Health and Human Services, Centers for Disease Control and Prevention; 2005. (*Authoritative epidemiologic data.*)
3. Geberding JL. Occupational exposure to HIV in health care settings. N Engl J Med 2003;348:826. (*A very useful clinical review; 38 references.*)
4. Hader SL, Smith DK, Moore JS, et al. HIV infection in women in the United States: status at the millennium. JAMA 2001;285:1186. (*An excellent review of epidemiologic data; 91 references.*)
5. Revised classification system for HIV infection and expanded surveillance case definition for AIDS among adolescents and adults, 1993. MMWR Morb Mortal Wkly Rep 1992;41(RR-17):1. (*Centers for Disease Control and Prevention [CDC] criteria for the diagnosis and classification of HIV infection and AIDS.*)
6. Valleroy LA, MacKellar DA, Karon JM, et al. HIV prevalence and associated risks in young men who have sex with men. JAMA 2000;284:198 (*An epidemiologic study; finds disturbing evidence that the prevalence is high and increasing, especially among minorities.*)
7. Antman K, Change Y. Kaposi's sarcoma. N Engl J Med 2000;342:1027. (*A comprehensive review; 112 references.*)
8. Bodasing N, Fox R. HIV-associated lipodystrophy syndrome: description and pathogenesis. J Infect Dis 2003;187:149. (*An excellent description of this important and increasingly appreciated syndrome.*)
9. Chen XM, Keithly JS, Paya C, et al. Cryptosporidiosis. N Engl J Med 2002;346:1723. (*A useful review of this pathogen, which strikes HIV-infected patients; 50 references.*)
10. Ellerabrock TV, Chiasson MA, Bush TJ, et al. Incidence of cervical squamous intraepithelial lesion in HIV-infected women. JAMA 2000;283:1031. (*A prospective cohort study; 1 in 5 patients developed lesions within 3 years; the results underscore the importance of surveillance.*)
11. Graziosi C, Soudeyns H, Rizzardi GP, et al. Immunopathogenesis of HIV infection. AIDS Res Hum Retroviruses 1998;Suppl 2:S135. (*A useful overview of viral biology.*)
12. Ho DD, Neumann AU, Perelson AS, et al. Rapid turnover of plasma virions and CD4 lymphocytes in HIV infection. Nature 1995;373:123. (*An important contribution to the understanding of pathogenesis.*)
13. Little RF, Gurierrwez M, Jaffe ES, et al. HIV-associated non-Hodgkin's lymphoma: incidence, presentation, and prognosis. JAMA 2001;285:1880. (*A grand-rounds review of this important complication of HIV infection; 60 references.*)
14. Morse CG, Kovacs JA. Metabolic and skeletal complications of HIV infection. JAMA 2006;296:844. (*A very lucid case-based review; 95 references.*)
15. Navia BA, Jordan BD, Price RW. The AIDS dementia complex. I: Clinical features. Ann Neurol 1986;19:517. (*An important and debilitating accompaniment of advanced disease that must be distinguished from more treatable forms of central nervous system deterioration.*)
16. Hughes MD, Johnson VA, Hirsch MS, et al. Monitoring plasma HIV RNA levels in addition to CD4+ lymphocyte count improves assessment of antiretroviral therapeutic response. Ann Intern Med 1997;126:929. (*Documents the contribution of monitoring the viral load.*)
17. Levine AM. Evaluation and management of HIV-infected women. Ann Intern Med 2002;136:228. (*An extremely helpful review for the clinician; 150 references.*)
18. Mellors JW, Rinaldo CR Jr, Gupta P, et al. Prognosis in HIV infection predicted by the quantity of virus in plasma. Science 1996;272:1167. (*Documents the added value of measuring the viral load for predicting prognosis.*)
19. O'Brien WA, Hartigan PM, Martin D, et al. Changes in plasma HIV RNA and CD4+ lymphocyte counts and the risk of progression to AIDS. N Engl J Med 1996;334:426. (*Treatment-induced changes in HIV-1 RNA and CD4 cell counts are valid predictors of prognosis.*)
20. U.S. Department of Health and Human Services. A guide to primary care for people with HIV/AIDS, 2004 edition. Available at: http://www.hab.hrsa.gov/tools/primarycareguide/index.htm.
21. U.S. Department of Health and Human Services. A guide to the clinical care of women with HIV/AIDS, 2005 edition. Available at http://hab.hrsa.gov/publications/womencare05/.
22. Benson CA, Kaplan JE, Masur H, et al. Treating opportunistic infections among HIV-infected adults and adolescents: recommendations from CDC, the National Institutes of Health, and the HIV Medicine Association/Infectious Diseases Society of America. MMWR Morb Mortal Wkly Rep 2004;53(RR-15):1.
23. Grinspoon S, Corcoran C, Parlman K, et al. Effects of testosterone and progressive resistance training in eugonadal men with AIDS wasting: a randomized trial. Ann Intern Med 2000;133:348. (*A randomized, controlled trial; resistance exercise produced an independent benefit; testosterone also helped but was associated with potentially adverse effects.*)
24. Panel on Antiretroviral Guidelines for Adults and Adolescents, Department of Health and Human Services. Guidelines for the use of antiretroviral agents in HIV-1–infected adults and adolescents. January 29, 2008. Available at: http://aidsinfo.nih.gov/contentfiles/AdultandAdolescentGL.pdf. (*The most recent recommendations for the use of antiretrovirals and detailed information on available agents.*)
25. Hirsch MS, Brun-Vezinet F, D'Aquila RT, et al. Antiretroviral drug resistance testing in adult HIV-1 infection: recommendations of an International AIDS Society-USA Panel. JAMA 2000;283:2417.
26. Incorporating HIV prevention into the medical care of persons living with HIV. Recommendations of CDC, the Health Resources and Services Administration, the National Institutes of Health, and the HIV Medicine Association of the Infectious Diseases Society of America, 2003. MMWR Morb Mortal Wkly Rep 2003;52(RR-12):1.
27. Kaplan JE, Masur H, Holmes KK, et al. Guidelines for preventing opportunistic infections among HIV-infected persons—2002. Recommendations of the U.S. Public Health Service and the Infectious Diseases Society of America. MMWR Morb Mortal Wkly Rep 2002; 51(RR-8):1.
28. Kurman RJ, Henson DE, Herbst AL, et al. Interim guidelines for management of abnormal cervical cytology. JAMA 1994;271:1866. (*Increased surveillance is needed because of the increased risk of cancer.*)
29. Panlilio AL, Cardo DM, Grohskopf LA, et al. Updated U.S. Public Health Service guidelines for the management of occupational exposures to HIV and recommendations for postexposure prophylaxis. MMWR Morb Mortal Wkly Rep 2005;54(RR-09):1.
30. U.S. Public Health Service Task Force. Recommendations for use of antiretroviral drugs in pregnant HIV-infected women for maternal health and interventions to reduce perinatal HIV transmission in the United States, 2007. Available at: http://aidsinfo.nih.gov/contentfiles/PerinatalGL.pdf.
31. Smith DK, Grohskopf LA, Black RJ, et al. Antiretroviral postexposure prophylaxis after sexual, injection-drug use, or other nonoccupational exposure

to HIV in the United States: recommendations from the U.S. Department of Health and Human Services. MMWR Morb Mortal Wkly Rep 2005; 54(RR-2):1.

32. The Strategies for Management of Antiretroviral Therapy (SMART) Study Group. CD4+ count–guided interruption of antiretroviral treatment. N Engl J Med 2006;355:2283. (*A randomized, controlled trial, showing an increased risk of death and opportunistic infection in the group with interrupted therapy.*)

33. Treisman GJ, Angelino AF, Hutton HE. Psychiatric issues in the management of patients with HIV infection. JAMA 2001;286:2857. (*A grand-rounds review underscoring the importance of identifying and addressing psychiatric issues.*)

34. Updated U.S. Public Health Service guidelines for the management of occupational exposures to HBV, HCV, and HIV and recommendations for postexposure prophylaxis. Available at: http://aidsinfo.nih.gov/Guidelines/Default.aspx?MenuItem=Guidelines.

SECTION 3 ■ CARDIOVASCULAR PROBLEMS

CHAPTER 14 ■ SCREENING FOR HYPERTENSION

KATHARINE K. TREADWAY

Hypertension can be considered the most significant condition the practitioner concerned with health maintenance will meet in clinical practice, accounting for more than 35 million office visits a year in the United States. The size of the affected population is staggering—approximately 20% of adults in the United States have hypertension. Among the elderly, the prevalence is even higher. Excess morbidity and mortality caused by hypertension have been well documented. Over the last 30 years, efforts to educate both physicians and the general public about the importance of identifying and treating high blood pressure and the improved options for treatment have resulted in improved blood pressure control and a significant decrease in morbidity and mortality from cardiovascular disease and stroke. Despite this progress, the National Health and Nutrition Examination Survey (NHANES III) indicated that 31% of hypertensive individuals remain unaware of their hypertension, 17% are aware but are not being treated, and 29% are being treated but not controlled—leaving only 23% who are being treated and controlled. In an analysis of NHANES III, Hyman and Pavlik concluded that the lack of access to medical care did not explain the small number of treated and controlled hypertensive patients. Indeed, "undiagnosed hypertension and treated but uncontrolled hypertension occurred largely under the watchful eye of the health care system." The elderly, who represent the fastest-growing segment of the population, have the smallest proportion of adequately controlled blood pressure, and yet this is the group with the highest rates of cardiovascular complications. It behooves all internists to be expert in the evaluation, management, and treatment of hypertension.

The U.S. Preventive Services Task Force has recently reaffirmed its recommendation that all adults 18 years of age and older should be routinely screened for hypertension based on the clear evidence of benefit of detection and treatment in reducing the complications of this condition.

The evaluation and management of the identified hypertensive patient are presented in Chapters 19 and 26, respectively. This chapter reviews the epidemiology of high blood pressure, its importance as a risk factor, its measurement, and the evidence for the effectiveness of therapy.

EPIDEMIOLOGY AND RISK FACTORS FOR THE DEVELOPMENT OF HYPERTENSION (1–15)

Of the 50 million Americans who are hypertensive, approximately 70% fall into stage 1 (diastolic blood pressure [DBP] 90 to 99, systolic blood pressure [SBP] 140 to 159 mm Hg), as defined by the Joint National Committee on Prevention, Detection, Evaluation and Management of High Blood Pressure (JNC VII). Most estimates of the prevalence of hypertension derive from the National Health and Nutrition Examination Surveys of the early 1960s and late 1970s. Subsequent, smaller surveys have both substantiated prevalence estimates and confirmed that age, race, and gender significantly affect prevalence.

Age (6,7)

Systolic and diastolic blood pressures rise steadily with age into the fifth and sixth decades, when the rate of increase levels off. By then, the prevalence of hypertension approaches 50%. The lifetime risk for developing hypertension in individuals older than 55 years is 90%. The complication risk also rises steadily with age. For individuals older than 50 years, the systolic pressure is a greater predictor of complication risk than the diastolic pressure. In the elderly, pulse pressure (the difference between systolic and diastolic pressures) is an independent predictor of cardiovascular disease. Systolic hypertension, which in former years was considered benign, confers significant risk.

Gender (8,9)

Men in all age groups have a higher prevalence of hypertension than women. In the third and fourth decades, it is more than twice as common among men as among women. The ratio decreases with advancing age, so that by age 60 years, there is only a slight male predominance. Men have substantially higher complication rates than women until 5 to 10 years after menopause, when the rates become similar. The Framingham Study demonstrated that for the major complications of hypertension, the risk of developing cardiovascular complications in mildly hypertensive women approximately equals that of normotensive men. The postulated mechanisms for this reduced risk in women include the beneficial effects of estrogen on vasculature and the different hemodynamic profile of premenopausal hypertensive women, which includes a lower peripheral resistance and higher cardiac output. After menopause, estrogen levels fall, the hemodynamic profile shifts to one of high peripheral resistance and normal cardiac output, and by age 70 years, the incidences of stroke and coronary disease in women approach those of men.

Race (10)

There is a marked *increase* in the prevalence of hypertension among *African Americans*. Compared with whites, the overall prevalence ratio is 2:1. It is higher in young adults and lower in the elderly. Severe hypertension occurs nearly five times more often than in whites. In addition, the complication rate for any given blood pressure is significantly higher. For example, compared with white hypertensive patients, African Americans have an 80% higher mortality from stroke, a 50% higher mortality from heart disease, and a 320% higher incidence of end-stage renal failure. Whether this represents as-yet undefined differences in the underlying pathophysiology of hypertension in African Americans or inadequate access to medical care is unclear, although it is likely that both factors play a role.

Obesity (11–13)

The prevalence increases in obese patients, as does the prevalence of hyperlipidemia and type 2 diabetes mellitus. The association of these three conditions has been attributed to the presence of relative insulin resistance, which may cause hypertension in some patients (see Chapter 19). Data from the Nurses' Health Study demonstrated that women who gained more than 20 lb after age 18 years had a fivefold increase in the risk of developing hypertension compared with those who did not gain weight. Conversely, women who were at higher body mass index levels at age 18 years and lost 5 to 10 lb had about half of the risk of developing hypertension. In a recent study of short-term predictors of increases in blood pressure, a weight gain of 5% or an increase in waist circumference of 1 inch or more was associated with a significant increase in blood pressure. In addition, obesity is associated with the development of obstructive sleep apnea, another independent risk factor for the development of hypertension.

Other Risk Factors (14,15)

Hypertension is much more likely to occur in patients with a *positive family history*. It is increasingly clear that hypertension may be caused by a variety of genetic mutations. In addition, environmental factors affect the onset and severity of hypertension. *Increased salt intake* correlates with increased prevalence in large populations, although not in individuals. An individual's prior or current salt intake per se is not a predictor of blood pressure level. *Alcohol* intake in excess of 2 oz/d is linked to hypertension. This appears to be related to alcohol's ability to stimulate the release of corticotropin-releasing factor from the hypothalamus, which increases central nervous system sympathetic activity, causing a rise in blood pressure. *Caffeine* intake may cause an acute increase in blood pressure but does not appear to effect the prevalence of hypertension generally. *Sedentary lifestyle* has been associated with an increase in the risk of developing hypertension. The role of *psychological stress* and its concomitant sympathetic stimulation appears to be variable and possibly a function of underlying differences in susceptibility. *Cigarette smoking*, an important risk factor in its own right, is not positively associated with increased blood pressure, but hypertensive smokers are at significantly greater risk of developing cardiovascular complications than are hypertensive nonsmokers. Analgesic use in populations of healthy men did not correlate with an increased risk of developing hypertension. In a study of the effect of drinking green tea on the risk of developing high blood pressure, those who drank 120 mL or more a day for a year had a 46% reduction.

HYPERTENSION AS A RISK FACTOR FOR CARDIOVASCULAR MORBIDITY AND MORTALITY (16)

The complications of hypertension may be divided into *hypertensive risks*—those that result directly from the presence of high blood pressure—and *atherosclerotic risks*—those for which hypertension is one of several risk factors. The major hypertensive complications are *stroke, congestive heart failure, renal failure,* and *left ventricular hypertrophy.* The Framingham Study showed hypertension to be the dominant predictor of congestive heart failure, with a sixfold increase in incidence among hypertensive individuals.

The atherosclerotic complications are coronary artery disease, cerebrovascular disease, and peripheral vascular disease. The risk of developing any of these complications rises gradually over *all* levels of blood pressure, doubling for every 20 mm Hg rise in systolic pressure and 10 mm Hg rise in diastolic pressure over a range of blood pressure from 115/75 to 185/115 mm Hg. The risk in a given individual for developing atherosclerotic complications varies enormously, depending on what other risk factors are present.

Although hypertension remains one of the principal atherosclerotic risk factors for the development of coronary artery disease, the additive effects from smoking, hypercholesterolemia, glucose intolerance, and left ventricular hypertrophy are also extremely important (see Chapters 15, 54, and 93). For example, the chance of a 40-year-old man with moderate hypertension alone developing ischemic heart disease over a 10-year period is about 9%, but it rises to 70% if all coronary risk factors are present.

NATURAL HISTORY OF HYPERTENSION AND EFFECTIVENESS OF TREATMENT (17–24)

Natural History

With rare exceptions, hypertension is an *asymptomatic* condition. The natural history is one of *insidious* damage that is most often clinically silent for a decade or more. It typically begins between the ages of 35 and 55 years, often preceded by a period of lability. Those patients with blood pressures at the high end of normal (130 to 140/85 to 90 mm Hg) are twice as likely to develop hypertension than those with lower pressures. About 70% of hypertensive patients fall into stage 1; this group accounts for more than 58% of the excess cardiovascular mortality attributable to hypertension. About 20% of stage 1 hypertensive patients will progress to higher stages if left untreated, and about 1% will go on to develop malignant hypertension. About 15% to 30% will become spontaneously normotensive, although we have no way to identify in which patients this will occur.

Effectiveness of Treatment (18–24)

Convincing evidence for vigorous *early treatment* of hypertension began to appear 40 years ago with publication of the landmark Veterans Administration Cooperative Study, the first large-scale, placebo-controlled, randomized, prospective study. It followed patients with *moderate to severe hypertension* and found that rates of major nonfatal events and cardiovascular death fell with treatment more than 10-fold among those with severe hypertension and 3-fold among those with moderate pressure elevations. Treatment was most effective in reducing risks of stroke and congestive heart failure.

Later randomized studies expanded these initial findings, and meta-analyses of such studies confirmed the efficacy of treatment and expanded the spectrum of illness to mild to moderate hypertension. With the extensive literature now available, there is no longer any doubt that the treatment of hypertension reduces the complications of hypertension: stroke, coronary artery disease, congestive heart failure, and progression of renal disease.

Findings also indicate that benefit from blood pressure reduction increases with the severity of blood pressure elevation. African Americans and those older than 50 years of age benefit most, and young white women benefit least. This difference in benefit can be explained by the lower level of overall cardiovascular risk in young white women. Treating *systolic hypertension in the elderly* significantly lowers the risk of stroke and coronary disease.

Although the benefits of treating hypertension appear to be clear, it is interesting to note that mildly hypertensive patients whose blood pressure spontaneously reverts to normal seem to do even better than those whose pressure is lowered by medication. This finding was first noted in the landmark Australian study of mild hypertensive patients, in which almost half of the placebo group became spontaneously normotensive over the 5-year period of the study. Such patients had fewer complications than those who achieved a similar level of blood pressure with medication.

In sum, the benefit of lowering blood pressure is real, reducing all of the major complications of hypertension significantly. In most studies, the *benefit* from treatment of hypertension appears *within 2 to 3 years of initiation of therapy.*

Decision to Treat

Whereas all hypertensive patients should be instructed in methods of nonpharmacologic blood pressure control, the decision to initiate pharmacologic therapy is based on an estimate of *overall cardiovascular risk.* Such an estimate requires consideration not only of blood pressure, but also of age, race, gender, smoking habits, hypercholesterolemia, diabetes, and family history of hypertensive or cardiac complications, as well as the presence or absence of target-organ damage (see Chapter 26).

SCREENING METHODS (25)

Measurement of Blood Pressure

Blood pressure should be measured at each health encounter. Although the process of identifying patients with hypertension seems to be relatively straightforward, there are numerous pitfalls in measuring blood pressure that can be avoided by the proper screening protocol. All personnel responsible for recording blood pressures should be aware of the sources of measurement error. Effective screening technique includes having the patient *rest for 5 minutes* before measurement is made. The pressure should be taken in both arms while the patient is *seated comfortably with back and arm supported and feet on the ground. Two or more readings* are taken, separated by 2 minutes. If these readings differ by more than 5 mm Hg, then *additional readings* should be taken. Patients should refrain from smoking or drinking a caffeinated beverage at least 30 minutes before a determination. Note should be made whether the patient is cold, anxious, has a full bladder, or has recently exercised because any of these factors may transiently elevate pressure.

Reliable equipment and its proper use are important. *Mercury bulb manometers* are best; *aneroid or digital manometers,* if used, should be checked and recalibrated regularly. The cuff should be placed as high on the arm as possible and the arm supported and positioned at *heart level* while the pressure is taken. *Cuff size* must be adequate to avoid falsely elevated readings. The *width* of the cuff's inflatable bladder should be greater than *two thirds* of the arm width and its *length* greater than *two thirds* of the arm *circumference.* Using a standard-size cuff in a muscular or obese adult will result in a reading that is as much as 10 mm Hg higher than the true blood pressure. To avoid this error, a large adult-sized cuff should be used in such patients. Although most auscultate using the diaphragm of the stethoscope, the *bell* is recommended for its superior transmission of the low-pitched sounds that characterize the last of the Korotkoff sounds.

Systolic pressure is defined as the point at which sound is first heard (Korotkoff 1). *Diastolic pressure* is taken at the point at which sound *disappears* (Korotkoff 5) rather than when it changes in quality (Korotkoff 4). The *averages* of two successive measurements in each arm are recorded. Variability of blood pressure may be related to recent physical activity, emotional state, or body position. Although such factors must be kept in mind, the predictive value of the "casual" blood pressure determination has been validated. Nonetheless, the diagnosis of hypertension should not be made on the basis of a single reading.

CONCLUSIONS AND RECOMMENDATIONS

- Hypertension is an extremely common condition and the strongest predictor of subsequent cardiovascular and cerebrovascular morbidity and mortality. It is usually asymptomatic, with insidious damage to target organs occurring if left untreated.
- A large segment of the hypertensive population will benefit from treatment and show significant reductions in the rates of stroke, congestive heart failure, renal failure, and coronary disease. Absolute risk reduction from treatment is a function of pretreatment risk.
- Detection is simple, reliable, and inexpensive. All adults should be screened for hypertension. Its detection and treatment are among the foremost responsibilities of the primary care physician (see also Chapter 19 for diagnostic evaluation and Chapter 26 for treatment).

Annotated Bibliography

1. National Center for Health Statistics. Plan and operation of the Third National Health and Nutrition Examination Survey, 1988–94. Vital and health statistics, Ser. 1, No. 32. (DHHS Publication no. [PHS] 94-1308). Washington, DC: U.S. Government Printing Office, 1994. (*National hypertension statistics.*)
2. Hyman DJ, Pavlik VN. Characteristics of patients with uncontrolled hypertension in the United States. N Engl J Med 2001;345:479. (*An analysis of factors contributing to poor levels of blood pressure control, concluding that access to medical care was not a major factor.*)
3. Lloyd-Jones DM, Evans, JC, Levy, D. Hypertension in adults across the age spectrum. JAMA 2005;294:466. (*An analysis of current rates of hypertension treatment and control in the very elderly.*)
4. U.S. Preventive Services Task Force. Screening for high blood pressure: U.S. Preventive Services Task Force reaffirmation recommendation statement. Ann Intern Med 2007;147:783. (*Reaffirms value of screening.*)
5. The seventh report of the Joint National Committee on Prevention, Detection, Evaluation and Treatment of High Blood Pressure: the JNC VII report. JAMA 2003;289:2560. (*The most recent update of a major consensus report.*)
6. Vasan RS, Beiser A, Larson MG, et al. Residual lifetime risk of developing hypertension in middle-aged women and men. The Framingham Heart Study. JAMA 2002;287:1003. (*Data representing a high residual risk of developing hypertension.*)
7. Blacher J, Staessen JA, Girerd X, et al. Pulse pressure not mean pressure determines cardiovascular risk in older hypertensive patients. Arch Intern Med 2000;160:1085. (*The presence of significant risk is indicated by elevated pulse pressure in elderly hypertensive patients.*)
8. Kannel WB. Blood pressure as a cardiovascular risk factor: prevention and treatment. JAMA 1996;275:1571. (*An analysis of hypertension as a significant risk factor for cardiovascular disease based on the Framingham data.*)
9. Messerli FH, Garavaglia GE, Schmieder RE. Disparate cardiovascular findings in men and women with essential hypertension. Ann Int Med 1987;107:158. (*A comparison of hemodynamic patterns in hypertensive men and women.*)
10. The sixth report of the Joint National Committee on Prevention, Detection, Evaluation and Treatment of High Blood Pressure (JNC VI). Arch Intern Med 1997;157:2413. (*A major consensus report, supplemented by JNC VII in 2003.*)
11. Reaven GM, Lithell H, Landsberg I. Hypertension and associated metabolic abnormalities—the role of insulin resistance and the sympathoadrenal system. N Engl J Med 1996;334:374. (*One of the classic papers describing the links among obesity, diabetes, and hypertension based on insulin resistance.*)
12. Huang Z, Willett WC, Manson JE, et al. Body weight, weight change, and risk for hypertension. Ann Intern Med 1998;128:81. (*Important data from the Nurses' Study confirming the importance of weight and the development of hypertension.*)
13. Aiyer AN, Kip KE, Mulukutla SR, et al. Predictors of short term increases in blood pressure in a community-based population. Am J Med 2007;120:960 (*Data supporting the high importance of weight as a risk factor for developing hypertension.*)
14. Oparil S, Zamin MA, Calhoun DA. Pathogenesis of hypertension. Ann Intern Med 2003;139:761. (*An excellent review article on current theories on the pathogenesis of hypertension.*)
15. Randin D, Vollenweider P, Tappy L, et al. Suppression of alcohol induced hypertension by dexamethasone. N Engl J Med 1995;332:1733. (*Data supporting the role of the central nervous system in alcohol-induced hypertension.*)
16. Kannel WB, Hartland MC, McNamara PM. Framingham: lessons in cardiovascular epidemiology. Ann Intern Med 1976;85:447. (*A classic paper analyzing the effect of associated risk factors in the development of the major cardiovascular complications in hypertensive adults.*)
17. Vasan RS, Larson MG, Leip EP, et al. Assessment of frequency of progression to hypertension in non-hypertensive participants in the Framingham Heart Study. Lancet 2001;358:1682. (*Documents the risk of high-normal hypertension.*)
18. Veterans Administration Cooperative Study Group on Antihypertensive Agents. Effects of treatment on morbidity in hypertension. I. Results in patients with diastolic blood pressures averaging 115 through 129 mm Hg. JAMA 1967;202:1028. (*This and refs. 19 and 20 report the original randomized, prospective trials that established the benefit of treating hypertension.*)
19. Veterans Administration Cooperative Study Group on Antihypertensive Agents. Effects of treatment on morbidity in hypertension. II. Results in patients with diastolic blood pressure averaging 90 through 114 mm Hg. JAMA 1970;213:1143. (*This and refs. 18 and 20 report the original randomized, prospective trials that established the benefit of treating hypertension.*)
20. Veterans Administration Cooperative Study Group on Antihypertensive Agents. Effects of treatment on morbidity in hypertension. III. Influence of age, diastolic pressure, and prior cardiovascular disease. Further analysis of side effects. Circulation 1972;45:901. (*This and refs. 18 and 19 report the original randomized, prospective trials that established the benefit of treating hypertension.*)
21. Psaty BM, Smith NL, Siscovick DS, et al. Health outcomes associated with antihypertensive therapies used as first line agents: a systematic review and meta-analysis. JAMA 1997;277:739. (*A meta-analysis of randomized, controlled trials demonstrating the benefit of treating hypertension for the reduction of cardiovascular complications.*)
22. Gueyffier F, Boutitie F, Boissel J, et al. Effect of anti-hypertensive drug treatment on cardiovascular outcomes in men and women. Ann Intern Med 1997;126:761. (*A major meta-analysis of randomized, controlled trials; treatment benefit was the same for men and women and was a function of pretreatment cardiovascular risk.*)
23. Systolic Hypertension in the Elderly Program (SHEP) Cooperative Research Group. Prevention of stroke by antihypertensive drug treatment in older persons with isolated systolic hypertension. JAMA 1991;265:3255. (*The treatment of isolated systolic hypertension reduced the risk of stroke in the elderly.*)
24. Management Committee. Untreated mild hypertension. Lancet 1980;1:1195. (*A report demonstrating that outcomes were superior in mild hypertensive patients who became spontaneously normotensive compared with those requiring medication to reach similar levels of blood pressure.*)
25. Frohlich ED, Grim C, Labarthe DR, et al. Report of a special task force appointed by the Steering Committee, American Heart Association: recommendations for human blood pressure determinations by sphygmomanometers. Hypertension 1988;11:209A. (*Consensus panel recommendations on technique.*)

CHAPTER 15 ■ SCREENING FOR HYPERLIPIDEMIA

G. SHERRY HAYDOCK AND MASON W. FREEMAN

Coronary heart disease (CHD) is the leading cause of death in American men and women, making identification and treatment of its risk factors a major health care priority. Major independent risk factors include smoking, hypertension, diabetes mellitus, advanced age, family history of coronary artery disease, and the common *dyslipidemias* (elevated low-density-lipoprotein [LDL] cholesterol and low high-density-lipoprotein [HDL] cholesterol). Other dyslipidemias that may contribute to risk include hypertriglyceridemia and increased lipoprotein (a) [Lp(a)]. *C-reactive protein (CRP)*, an acute-phase reactant that increases during inflammation, is a moderate predictor for CHD risk independent of other major CHD risk factors. Elevations in plasma *homocysteine* also appear to confer some independent risk for CHD.

Proper CHD screening is the responsibility of all primary care physicians and requires attention to several questions: Which abnormalities truly increase coronary risk? To what degree will lowering them reduce such risk? How are they best measured? At what age should screening be initiated and for how long? This chapter addresses the CHD risk associated with the dyslipidemias and elevated levels of Lp(a), C-reactive protein, and homocysteine. (See Chapter 14 for a discussion of screening for hypertension, Chapter 54 for smoking, and Chapter 93 for diabetes screening.)

DYSLIPIDEMIAS (1–4)

Seventeen percent of all adults older than 20 years of age have a total serum cholesterol concentration in excess of 240 mg/dL, a level associated with an accelerating risk of CHD. Fifty percent of the adult population has total cholesterol levels exceeding 200 mg/dL, the level considered desirable. Patient and professional awareness of the importance of hypercholesterolemia has contributed to a modest reduction in mean total cholesterol over the last two decades, but the problem remains widespread. Screening for hyperlipidemia is a key element in the primary and secondary prevention of CHD.

RISK FACTORS FOR HYPERLIPIDEMIA (1–6)

Age

Cholesterol levels increase with age. Total cholesterol increases, on the average, more than 2 mg/dL per year during early adulthood and continues increasing but at a lesser rate until age 65 years, after which it declines slightly. Men 45 years or older

and women aged 55 years or older are considered to have age as a risk factor for CHD.

Gender

Men have higher total cholesterol levels than women until age 50 years and an approximately twofold higher risk of developing CHD. Women carry a higher proportion of cholesterol in the form of HDL cholesterol (primarily HDL_2). At the onset of menopause, women exhibit an increase in cholesterol and an increased risk of CHD. Hormone replacement is no longer believed to be protective for CHD. As women move into their mid-60s and beyond, their risk of developing CHD approaches that of men of the same age.

Genetic Factors

Primary lipid disorders arising from a *monogenic* (single gene) abnormality account for only a small fraction of patients with hyperlipidemia. These relatively uncommon genetic disorders are, however, frequently responsible for the most severe hyperlipidemias. These are, in turn, associated with the most aggressive forms of coronary artery disease. Because these disorders are more likely to affect the immediate relatives of an affected patient than are complex polygenic conditions, family screening should be performed in the relatives of patients suspected of harboring these genetic mutations.

Diet

A diet high in *saturated fatty acids* raises total and LDL cholesterol. Total and LDL cholesterol are also increased by dietary *cholesterol*, but the effect is smaller than that of saturated fatty acids. *Caloric excess* resulting in obesity has more of an effect on triglycerides than on cholesterol and can contribute to insulin resistance, which is associated with CHD. *Alcohol* has little effect on total cholesterol levels, but it can cause an acute rise in triglycerides among people with hypertriglyceridemia. Moderate alcohol ingestion also causes a rise in HDL levels.

Medications

Antihypertensive agents that adversely affect lipid levels can compromise the effort to reduce CHD risk. *Thiazides may* increase LDL cholesterol, at least temporarily, when taken in full doses. The effect is hypothesized to account for the shortfall in reduction in mortality found among hypertensive patients treated with thiazides (see Chapter 26). *Beta-blockers may* cause modest reductions in HDL cholesterol and increase serum triglyceride levels. *Exogenous estrogens* increase HDL_2 and can cause extreme triglyceride increases in patients with preexisting, moderate hypertriglyceridemia. *Corticosteroids* and HIV *protease inhibitors* can also dramatically elevate serum lipids.

Exercise, Weight, Smoking, and Concurrent Diseases

Activity, weight loss, and smoking cessation increase HDL cholesterol. *Diabetics* commonly have a lipid disorder characterized by high triglycerides and low HDL cholesterol levels. *Hypothyroidism*, *nephrotic syndrome*, *and obstructive liver disease* are important causes of secondary hypercholesterolemia, characterized by increases in total and LDL cholesterol levels and, not infrequently, increased triglycerides as well.

Family History

A family history of CHD is considered a risk factor when it occurs in a first-degree relative in men less than the age of 55 years and in women less than the age of 65 years.

HYPERLIPIDEMIA AS A RISK FACTOR FOR CORONARY HEART DISEASE (1–4,6–13)

Total Cholesterol

Both epidemiologic and prospective studies have demonstrated that hypercholesterolemia is an independent risk factor for the development of CHD. Coronary risk increases curvilinearly with increasing total cholesterol levels, even within the "normal" range. Over the usually encountered range of total cholesterol values (180 to 300 mg/dL), risk increases by an average of four- to fivefold. Risk begins to accelerate more sharply when the total cholesterol level exceeds 240 mg/dL. LDL is, in the majority of cases, the underlying cause of elevated levels of total cholesterol and is most closely linked with the development of CHD.

Low-Density-Lipoprotein Cholesterol

The positive relationship between total cholesterol and CHD risk derives mainly from the atherogenic LDL cholesterol component. Because the LDL cholesterol accounts for about two thirds of the total cholesterol in the typical patient, the total cholesterol concentration is generally used as a proxy for LDL cholesterol. *Current guidelines define LDL levels of less than 100 mg/dL as optimal. Treatment goals for LDL depend on the presence of coronary disease or other risk factors such as diabetes, smoking, hypertension, family history of coronary disease, peripheral vascular disease, active carotid disease, abdominal aortic aneurysm, low HDL levels or increased age.* LDL serum levels in excess of 160 mg/dL are associated with significant increases in CHD risk.

Small, dense LDL particles are considered to be more atherogenic that larger forms of LDL. Small, dense forms are associated with high triglyceride levels. From a clinical standpoint, routine screening for LDL size is not indicated.

Lp(a) is a modified form of LDL. It consists of an LDL particle attached to a protein of variable size, called "apoprotein little a." It appears in most (but not all) studies to contribute independently to CHD risk. Serum levels are genetically determined. Lp(a) is believed to be thrombogenic in nature. Lp(a) competes with the binding of plasminogen and promotes clot formation. The absence of any studies demonstrating that a reduction in Lp(a) levels results in improved clinical outcomes has kept this marker from being routinely assayed. Niacin has been shown to reduce Lp(a), and thus it may be useful to measure Lp(a) levels in patients with intermediate CHD risk if an elevated level would tip the scale in favor of using niacin to treat the patient's other lipid abnormalities.

High-Density-Lipoprotein Cholesterol

The relation of the HDL cholesterol level to CHD risk is an inverse one. HDL cholesterol exerts a protective effect that is at least as strong as the atherogenic effect of LDL. For every 10-mg/dL increment in HDL cholesterol concentration, there is a 50% decrease in coronary risk. An HDL cholesterol level lower than 40 mg/dL has come to be recognized as a major independent risk factor for CHD. A level in excess of 60 mg/dL is considered a "negative" risk factor (see Chapter 27). A low HDL cholesterol increases CHD risk across the full range of total and LDL cholesterol concentrations, with recent data indicating that HDL is a significant inverse predictor of cardiovascular events even in patients with LDL values less than 70 mg/dL. Conversely, it is possible for a person with an elevated total cholesterol to be at low risk for CHD by virtue of having a very high HDL cholesterol (60 to 100 mg/dL). The determination of a *total-to-HDL cholesterol ratio* helps to distinguish such low-risk individuals from others with elevated total cholesterol. The Framingham Study showed that the ratio was a strong predictor of risk. A ratio of 5 approximates the average or standard risk, with ratios of 10 and 20 denoting double and triple the risk. A ratio of 4.5 or less is considered desirable.

High-density lipoprotein particles are functionally heterogeneous and vary in size, density, and composition. Inflammation can reduce protective effects by modifying the major apolipoprotein within HDL, *apolipoprotein A-I*, rendering it proinflammatory and atherogenic. In addition, *apolipoprotein A-II*, another component of HDL, has been shown to be proatherogenic in animal models. Subcomponents (e.g., apolipoprotein A-1) are more difficult and expensive to measure, and their added contribution to the estimation of CHD risk does not yet appear to warrant their additional cost.

Triglycerides

The importance of *hypertriglyceridemia* to cardiovascular risk was, for a long time, controversial. In univariate analysis, it is consistently associated with increased CHD risk, but in multivariate analysis, most of this risk is lost when the contribution of HDL cholesterol is factored out. Because high serum levels of triglycerides causally contribute to lowered HDL levels, however, one cannot conclude that hypertriglyceridemia is unimportant. The latest National Cholesterol Education Program (NCEP) guidelines place increased emphasis on measuring and treating hypertriglyceridemia. This emphasis may be particularly important when the hypertriglyceridemia is accompanied by a large waist circumference (>40 inches for men and >35 inches for women). This combination, often associated with the *metabolic syndrome*, may be a better marker of insulin resistance and the risk of coronary disease than the triglyceride level alone.

Metabolic Syndrome

The metabolic syndrome increases the risk of coronary artery disease at any level of LDL. It is a metabolic disorder associated with obesity and insulin resistance. The diagnosis of metabolic syndrome is made when individuals have three or more of the following clinical characteristics: abdominal obesity (waist circumference in men of >40 inches and in women of >35 inches), triglycerides of greater than 150 mg/dL, low levels of HDL cholesterol (men <40 mg/dL, women <50 mg/dL), blood pressure of greater than 135/85 mm Hg, and a fasting glucose of greater than 110. This syndrome is associated with obesity and inactivity.

Age, Hyperlipidemia, and Risk

For young men (younger than age 35 years) and premenopausal women, elevated total and LDL cholesterol levels increase the *long-term risk* of developing CHD. However, *short-term* CHD risk among those with even moderately high LDL cholesterol levels (160 to 220 mg/dL) but no other CHD risk factors remains relatively low. On the other hand, the presence of additional CHD risk factors, particularly diabetes or family history of early CHD, appears to increase short-term risk, as does the development of a very high LDL cholesterol level (220 mg/dL).

CHD risk due to hypercholesterolemia in the *elderly* is also incompletely defined. The relative risk of CHD observed in men 60 to 79 years of age with marked hypercholesterolemia is about 1.5. This relative risk is lower than that in comparably hypercholesterolemic patients younger than 60 years of age. The difference is believed to be related to the high prevalence of already established CHD, hypertension, and diabetes in this age group. Among hyperlipidemic elderly patients with established CHD, the relative risk of a new coronary event is just as high as in younger patients. Because the elderly have the highest rates of coronary disease in the population (85% of individuals dying of CHD are 65 years or older), the aggressiveness with which to screen older individuals is a topic of debate in the prevention field.

EFFECTIVENESS OF TREATMENT (1–4,14–24)

Nonpharmacologic Measures

Decreases in the intake of cholesterol and saturated fat in controlled settings can *reduce total and LDL cholesterol* levels by 30% or more, but this magnitude of reduction is rarely achieved in clinical practice. LDL cholesterol levels are lowered by an average of 10% when reasonably intensive diets are used in the outpatient setting. Dietary measures may also produce a small (approximately 5%) reduction in HDL cholesterol concentration, although the overall total-to-HDL ratio typically still improves. Weight loss (if the patient is obese), aerobic exercise, and smoking cessation can raise the HDL cholesterol level and facilitate the dietary lowering of LDL cholesterol. These

measures also reduce CHD risk by decreasing blood pressure and glucose intolerance. Caloric and fat restrictions and control of diabetes lower triglyceride levels, an effect enhanced by the restriction or elimination of alcohol. In patients with moderate to severe hypertriglyceridemia, even modest alcohol intake can be a significant factor. The CHD risk tradeoff between alcohol's HDL- and triglyceride-raising properties has not been well studied. Reductions in CHD risk follow from cholesterol lowering and amelioration of other risk factors.

Addition of Pharmacologic Measures

Adding drug therapy to a diet and exercise program enhances the lipid-lowering effort. Reductions two to three times greater (25% to 60%) than those achieved by dietary measures alone are attainable and associated with a further lowering of CHD risk. The reduction is most evident among patients with established CHD—a *secondary prevention* effect—with CHD mortality reduced by greater than 40% and all-cause mortality by 30%. In addition, a halt to *plaque progression* and a modest amount of plaque regression have been demonstrated in patients with established CHD treated aggressively with medical therapy. Pharmacologic therapy for hypercholesterolemic individuals without clinically evident CHD (so-called *primary prevention*) also reduces CHD risk. Reductions of approximately 30% in rates of nonfatal infarction, death from CHD, and death from all forms of cardiovascular disease have been achieved in medically treated men and women with moderate increases in their LDL cholesterol levels (LDL levels of 150 to 190 mg/dL). The cardiovascular benefit of these interventions with the hydroxy-3-methylglutaryl coenzyme A reductase inhibitor class of drugs ("statins") has not been associated with any increase in noncardiac deaths (an earlier concern, not borne out in large-scale prospective clinical trials).

Measurement of Cholesterol (1–4,25)

The total blood cholesterol is the sum of the cholesterol concentrations contained in the three major circulating lipoproteins (HDL, LDL, and very-low-density lipoproteins [VLDLs]). Thus, total cholesterol is equal to LDL cholesterol plus HDL cholesterol plus VLDL cholesterol. Most laboratories measure total cholesterol and HDL cholesterol directly, calculate the VLDL concentration by dividing the triglyceride concentration by 5 (as long as triglyceride is <400 mg/dL), and then mathematically deriving the LDL cholesterol concentration.

The accuracy of determinations of total cholesterol and its fractions can vary considerably. In general, elevated levels of cholesterol obtained through the finger stick method should be confirmed with a fasting cholesterol profile that includes total cholesterol, HDL, LDL, and triglyceride level. Not all laboratories ensure the accuracy of results. Acceptable laboratories are those with instruments calibrated to the standards of the Centers for Disease Control and Prevention, with a margin of error (coefficient of variation) of 3% for a total cholesterol measurement. Given the variability among labs, it is recommended that patients have serial testing performed in the same lab.

Chronic stress or serious illness might cause the cholesterol levels to fall significantly. Thus, it is best to measure lipid levels in patients when they have recovered from any acute infections, illnesses that result in tissue necrosis, or surgical procedures.

Screening

Screening recommendations have changed considerably in recent years. The most recent NCEP Adult Treatment Panel recommends that all patients older than the age of 20 years be screened with a fasting lipid profile. This includes a total cholesterol, HDL cholesterol, LDL cholesterol, and a triglyceride level. If these values are normal, repeat screening should be performed in 5 years. For high-risk patients, such as those with a strong family history of coronary disease, screening for other risk factors should be considered. Additional testing could include high-sensitivity CRP, homocysteine, and Lp(a) levels where available. For low-risk patients who are non-fasting it is reasonable to perform a total and HDL cholesterol alone. If these values are greater than 200 mg/dL or less than 40 mg/dL, respectively, the patient should return for a complete fasting profile. NCEP treatment guidelines are based on the LDL cholesterol level, the presence of other risk factors, and the 10-year risk of developing coronary disease (see Chapter 27).

The issue of cholesterol screening in the *elderly* also remains somewhat unsettled. It is clearly indicated for those at high risk for CHD (multiple CHD risk factors, established CHD, other clinically evident atherosclerotic disease) who are otherwise well. Screening lower-risk, healthy individuals older than 70 years of age is of unknown value but likely to be beneficial, given the high prevalence of silent CHD in the population. The subgroup analyses that have been done in the population greater than 65 years enrolled in the statin trials demonstrate clear benefits to treatment. The percentage reduction in events in patients with known heart disease treated with lipid-lowering medication is the same in patients greater and less than age 65 years. At what point an elderly person is beyond the age at which primary prevention of CHD should be considered is a topic that is little informed by any data. Many clinicians feel that screening is appropriate for healthy elderly individuals who do not appear to have a lifespan limited by other medical conditions.

What to Measure When Screening

A fasting determination of total, HDL, and LDL cholesterol and serum triglyceride should be performed on patients after a 12- to 14-hour fast. Patients may drink water, black tea, or coffee and should take their medications. If the triglycerides are greater than 400 mg/dL, the LDL cannot be accurately determined by the usual laboratory method. It can be measured by ultracentrifugation or by a variety of newer direct LDL assay tests. If one routinely uses a direct LDL assay in patients, it is worth remembering that these assays were generally not used in the major outcomes trials, and so discrepant calculated and direct LDL values warrant clarification by the assay lab. Patients who fail to fast for a lipid profile will have calculated LDL cholesterol results that typically underestimate their true LDL value in proportion to the rise in serum triglycerides associated with the nonfasting state.

C-REACTIVE PROTEIN (26,27)

CRP is an acute-phase reactant that increases in the setting of inflammation. It is produced by hepatocytes and activates both complement and endothelial cells. Recent interest in atherosclerosis as an inflammatory process has drawn attention to CRP as a possible marker/risk factor for CHD events. Associations between CRP elevations and cardiovascular events in persons with CHD have been observed, leading some to suggest that screening for CRP might improve the determination of CHD risk and outcomes.

Association with Coronary Heart Disease Risk

In some case–control studies and meta-analyses of prospective studies, CRP appears to stand as an independent risk factor for CHD.

In a study of apparently healthy men, the level of high-sensitivity CRP was predictive of long-term risk of first myocardial infarction, ischemic stroke, peripheral vascular disease, and all-cause mortality. In a similar study, CRP appeared to add to the predictive value of total and HDL cholesterol in determining risk of first myocardial infarction. Data from the Women's Health Study, a large, prospective epidemiologic study, found the CRP level to be an independent predictor of CHD events that was more powerful than the level of LDL cholesterol. Women in the highest quartile for CRP concentration had a relative risk of 2.3 for a CHD event, compared to a relative risk of 1.5 for women in the highest LDL cholesterol quartile. In addition, CRP appeared to identify a separate population of high-risk persons not identified by LDL cholesterol. On the other hand, the predictive power of CRP diminishes somewhat when other CHD risk factors are taken into account, and CRP elevations are also found in persons with central adiposity and insulin resistance, known CHD risk factors that might be responsible for some of the effects associated with CRP. A recent larger-scale study of CRP levels and CHD confirmed that it is an independent risk factor but showed it to be less powerful than LDL cholesterol in predicting cardiovascular outcomes.

Measurement

Because only modest elevations in CRP are associated with substantial increases in CHD risk, it is essential to be able to measure subtle elevations in CRP. A high-sensitivity assay has been validated, providing this capability. Standard, low-sensitivity CRP assays are of no value in estimating the CHD risk. There is documented variability in CRP levels. If CRP is to be followed, it is best to obtain serial values and follow trends.

Effectiveness of Treatment

A critical determinant of the validity and utility of a risk factor for screening is evidence of a survival benefit associated with treatment of the risk factor. There are no randomized, prospective studies examining the effect of CRP lowering on CHD risk. In fact, the best means of lowering CRP levels remains unclear. Of interest is the finding that statin drugs appear to be most effective in persons with elevations in CRP, suggesting that their survival benefit might be due in part to CRP reduction. Treating other risk factors for coronary heart disease such as smoking, diabetes, inactivity, hypertension, and obesity will reduce CRP levels.

Selection of Persons to Screen

In the absence of definitive evidence that treatment of CRP elevations reduces CHD risk, there is disagreement as to whether to screen for CRP. Those who are impressed with the available epidemiologic data feel that all adults should be screened. Others want evidence from prospective studies of improved outcomes before recommending CRP screening; they suggest for now that available resources be directed at aggressively identifying and better treating the more well-established CHD risk factors. Taking a selective approach, one might reserve CRP measurement for those patients who would undergo a change in therapy based on the degree of risk suggested by the CRP measurement (e.g., the low- to intermediate-risk individual who would be started on aspirin or a statin if the CRP measurement suggested heightened risk).

HOMOCYSTEINE (28,29)

Children who are homozygous for homocysteinuria develop premature atherosclerotic disease, and early retrospective case–control studies suggested a substantially enhanced risk of CHD events in adults with abnormally high plasma levels.

Association with Coronary Heart Disease Risk

Compared to early retrospective data, meta-analyses combining data from prospective studies confirmed that elevated homocysteine levels were associated with enhanced CHD risk. Although the risk was significant and independent of other CHD risk factors, it was substantially less than initially suggested by retrospective studies.

Measurement

A relatively inexpensive measurement of plasma homocysteine is available. Levels should be drawn when patients are fasting.

Effectiveness of Treatment

Treating patients with elevated levels of homocysteine with folate and B vitamins is no longer recommended and should be avoided. In the Norwegian Vitamin Trial, treating patients with folic acid and B vitamins in the setting of an acute myocardial infarction showed a trend toward an increase in cardiovascular events.

Patient Selection

Widespread screening is not warranted, but in some situations measurement of homocysteine may deserve consideration. For example, young adults with a strongly positive family history of CHD, especially in the absence of known CHD risk factors, and those with premature vascular disease may be reasonable candidates for screening if an elevated level affects the decision to initiate drug therapy.

CONCLUSIONS AND RECOMMENDATIONS

Hyperlipidemia

- Hypercholesterolemia is a problem of substantial proportions in the United States and a major risk factor for CHD.
- Elevations in levels of total cholesterol or LDL cholesterol and reduction in HDL cholesterol are strongly positive independent risk factors for the development of CHD in persons younger than 65 years of age.
- Diet, exercise, smoking cessation, weight loss, treatment of underlying conditions such as diabetes, and drug therapy are effective measures for the treatment of lipid abnormalities associated with CHD risk.
- Reductions in CHD morbidity and mortality have been demonstrated with treatment, particularly in high-risk hyperlipidemic patients such as those with established CHD, but also in hyperlipidemic men and women without clinical evidence of CHD.
- A complete fasting lipid profile should be performed at least every 5 years in persons older than 20 years of age. Those at increased risk of CHD because of smoking, diabetes, hypertension, a family history of premature CHD, or symptomatic noncoronary atheromatous disease require more frequent screening.
- Elderly persons are reasonable candidates for cholesterol screening, provided that their overall clinical condition would warrant the treatment of hypercholesterolemia.
- The ratio of total cholesterol to HDL cholesterol should be calculated. A ratio lower than 4.5 is desirable.
- The value of measuring biologically important risk factors such as Lp(a) and certain apolipoproteins is yet to be demonstrated.
- If the finger-stick screening serum total cholesterol is greater than 200 mg/dL, then a repeat determination using venipuncture and laboratory techniques is indicated for confirmation. Further testing and treatment are based on the patient's age and risk factor profile (see Chapter 27).

C-Reactive Protein

- CRP appears to be an independent risk factor for CHD events, particularly in women.
- The association between CHD risk and CRP elevation in women is strong, but the latest data contradict earlier findings that showed CRP levels to be better than LDL cholesterol at predicting event risk.
- There are no definitive data from long-term, randomized clinical trials proving that lowering CRP reduces the risk of CHD events. The best way to reduce CRP is not clear, but statins are effective in reducing CRP levels in patients with elevated lipid values.
- Pending definitive evidence of benefit, CRP screening should be applied selectively in instances in which the results will change management. If it is measured, the high-sensitivity assay must be used.

Homocysteine

- Elevations in homocysteine are associated with a statistically significant but modest increase in the risk of CHD events.
- Folic acid supplementation does lower homocysteine levels but is no longer believed to be of benefit in patients with elevated levels of homocysteine and should be avoided.

- Smoking cessation may decrease levels of homocysteine and should be encouraged.
- Widespread screening is not warranted at this time, but selective screening may be worth consideration if drug therapy is being considered when there is a strong family history of CHD, onset of CHD is premature, or in the case of a patient with CHD but no identifiable risk factors.

Annotated Bibliography

1. Executive summary of the third report of the National Cholesterol Education Program (NCEP) Expert Panel on Detection, Evaluation, and Treatment of High Blood Cholesterol in Adults (Adult Treatment Panel III). JAMA 2001;2486. (*Updated recommendations including the addition of plant sterols and viscous fibers to a lipid-lowering diet.*)
2. Expert Panel on Detection, Evaluation, and Treatment of High Blood Cholesterol in Adults. Summary of the second report. JAMA 1993;269:3015. (*Major consensus panel recommendations, revising those of the 1988 report; there is more emphasis on total coronary heart disease [CHD] risk and the importance of high-density lipoprotein [HDL].*)
3. National Cholesterol Education Program. Report of the Expert Panel on Detection, Evaluation, and Treatment of High Blood Cholesterol in Adults. Arch Intern Med 1988;148:36. (*A consensus panel report; urges screening all adults for total cholesterol every 5 years.*)
4. National Cholesterol Education Program Adult Treatment Panel. Prevalence of high blood cholesterol among US adults. JAMA 1993;269:3009. (*The best available epidemiologic data, indicating that 20% of Americans have a cholesterol level of ≥240 mg/dL; 50% have a cholesterol level of ≥200 mg/dL.*)
5. Kraus WE, Houmard JA, Duscha BD, et al. Effects of the amount and intensity of exercise on plasma lipoproteins. N Engl J Med 2002;347:1483. (*Exercise had a beneficial effect on lipoprotein profile, most clearly with higher amounts and higher intensity of exercise.*)
6. Wilson PWF, D'Agostino R, et al. Prediction of coronary heart disease using risk factor categories. Circulation 1998;97:1837. (*Using data from the Framingham Heart Study, the authors generated prediction algorithms that permit a more quantitative assessment of coronary artery disease risk.*)
7. Criqui MH, Heiss G, Cohn R, et al. Plasma triglyceride level and mortality from coronary heart disease. N Engl J Med 1993;328:1220. (*Found no independent association with CHD risk.*)
8. Brunzell JD. Hypertriglyceridemia. N Engl J Med. 2007;357:1009. (*A review including a good discussion of the assessment of risk.*)
9. Kannel WB. High-density lipoproteins: epidemiologic profile and risks of coronary artery disease. Am J Cardiol 1983;52:9B. (*A classic epidemiologic study establishing the contribution of the individual values and ratios of total cholesterol, HDL cholesterol, and low-density-lipoprotein [LDL] cholesterol toward predicting cardiovascular risk.*)
10. Singh IM, Shishehbor MH, Ansell BJ. High-density lipoprotein as a therapeutic target. JAMA 2007;298:786-98. (*A good review of the role of HDL in metabolism and risk prediction, as well as the response of HDL levels to intervention, concluding that evidence for aggressive intervention is only modest.*)
11. Klag KJ, Ford DE, Mead LA, et al. Serum cholesterol in young men and subsequent cardiovascular disease. N Engl J Med 1993;328:313. (*A strong association was found between serum cholesterol level in early life and CHD in midlife.*)
12. Rubin SM, Sidney S, Black DM. High blood cholesterol in elderly men and the excess risk for coronary heart disease. Ann Intern Med 1990;113:916. (*The relative risk was 1.5, indicating that cholesterol is an independent risk factor for cardiovascular mortality.*)
13. Stampfer MJ, Sacks FM, Salvini S, et al. A prospective study of cholesterol, apolipoproteins, and the risk of myocardial infarction. N Engl J Med 1991;325:373. (*HDL cholesterol was important in predicting the risk for myocardial infarction; the ratio of total to HDL cholesterol was especially useful; a one-unit change in the ratio was associated with a 53% change in risk.*)
14. Brown G, Albers JJ, Fisher LD, et al. Regression of coronary artery disease as a result of intensive lipid-lowering therapy. N Engl J Med 1990;323:1289. (*Significant plaque regression was documented in coronary arteries in this angiographic study of intensive therapy.*)
15. Hunninghake DB, Stein EA, Dujovne CA, et al. The efficacy of intensive dietary therapy alone or combined with lovastatin in outpatients with hypercholesterolemia. N Engl J Med 1993;328:1213. (*Diet alone provided only a 5% LDL reduction; medication added another 27%.*)
16. Jenkins DJA, Kendall CWC, Marchie A, et al. Effects of a dietary portfolio of cholesterol-lowering foods vs lovastatin on serum lipids and C-reactive protein. JAMA 2003;290:502. (*A diet high in plant sterols, viscous fiber, and almonds is as effective in lowering LDL and C-reactive protein [CRP] as a starting dose of lovastatin.*)
17. Law MR, Wald NJ, Rudnicka AR. Quantifying effect of statins on low density lipoprotein cholesterol, ischaemic heart disease, and stroke: systematic review and meta-analysis. BMJ 2003;326:1. (*A systematic review, documenting a very low statin side-effect rate.*)
18. Lipid Research Clinics Program. The Lipid Research Clinics Coronary Primary Prevention Trial. JAMA 1984;251:351. (*A significant reduction was observed in the incidence of coronary heart disease by lowering the total cholesterol and LDL cholesterol in asymptomatic middle-aged men with primary hypercholesterolemia.*)
19. Moore THM, Bartlett C, Burke MA, et al. Statins for preventing cardiovascular disease (Cochrane review). In: The Cochrane library, Issue 1. Oxford: Update Software, 2003. (*A systematic review.*)
20. Pignone M, Phillips C, Mulrow C. Use of lipid lowering drugs for primary prevention of coronary heart disease: meta-analysis of randomized trials. BMJ 2000;321:1. (*Drug treatment reduced the odds of coronary heart disease by 30% but did not affect all-cause mortality.*)
21. Scandinavian Simvastatin Survival Study Group. Randomized trial of cholesterol lowering in 4444 patients with coronary heart disease: the Scandinavian Survival Study. Lancet 1994;344:1383. (*A major randomized study of the efficacy of secondary prevention, showing a 42% reduction in CHD mortality and no increased risk of noncardiac death.*)
22. Shepherd J, Cobbe SM, Ford I, et al. Prevention of coronary heart disease with pravastatin in men with hypercholesterolemia. N Engl J Med 1995;333:1301. (*A randomized, placebo-controlled, prospective trial of men without CHD examining the efficacy of statin therapy for primary prevention; finds approximately 30% reductions in rates of nonfatal infarction, CHD death, and cardiovascular death.*)
23. Sacks FM, Pfeffer MA, Moye LA, et al. The effect of pravastatin on coronary events after myocardial infarction in patients with average cholesterol levels. Cholesterol and Recurrent Events Trial Investigators. N Engl J Med 1996; 335:1001. (*Reports the benefit of treating older patients with statins.*)
24. Walsh JME, Pignone M. Drug treatment of hyperlipidemia in women. JAMA 2004;291:2243. (*Drug treatment reduces the risk for CHD event for those with CHD; there was insufficient power to detect a benefit for women without CHD.*)
25. Kafonek SD, Donovan L, Lovejoy KL, et al. Biologic variation of lipids and lipoproteins in fingerstick blood. Clin Chem 1996;42:2002. (*The biologic variability in serum lipids is greater than the analytic variability, but desktop analyzer accuracy still falls somewhat short of the guidelines suggested by the National Cholesterol Education Program.*)
26. Mosca L. C-reactive protein—to screen or not to screen? N Engl J Med 2002;347:1615. (*An editorial arguing for restraint in screening for CRP until its usefulness is confirmed by randomized, prospective trials.*)
27. Ridker PM, Rifai N, Rose L, et al. Comparison of C-reactive protein and low-density lipoprotein cholesterol levels in the prediction of first cardiovascular events. N Engl J Med 2002;347:1557. (*Prospective epidemiologic data from the Women's Health Study, finding a strong independent association with CHD event risk.*)
28. The Homocysteine Studies Collaborative. Homocysteine and risk of ischemic heart disease and stroke: a meta-analysis. JAMA 2002;288:2015. (*A methodologically rigorous review of prospective observational studies, finding that the association was real but less powerful than previously reported in retrospective studies, especially when adjusting for other CHD risk factors.*)
29. Bonaa JH, Njolstad I, Rasmussen N, et al. Homocysteine lowering and cardiovascular events after acute myocardial infarction. N Engl J Med 2006; 354:1578. (*Found a trend of increased risk of cardiac events when patients were treated with B vitamins.*)

CHAPTER 16 ■ INFECTIVE ENDOCARDITIS PROPHYLAXIS

Once universally fatal, infective endocarditis remains a serious disease, with a mortality rate of about 25%. The pathogenesis of endocarditis suggests that individual infections might be prevented by judicious use of prophylactic antibiotics, yet the incidence of this infection has not changed much despite the widespread availability of antibiotics and efforts to promote their use prophylactically. Recent data directly question the effectiveness of prophylaxis among patients undergoing dental procedures, and it has become clear that the frequency of bacteremia from routine daily practices is far greater than that associated with any identifiable procedure. In the absence of clear evidence for effectiveness from randomized trials, there is the real concern that widespread use of antibiotic prophylaxis could do more harm than good. As a result, recent recommendations from the American Heart Association and others advocate prophylaxis only among patients with the highest-risk cardiac conditions who undergo procedures that involve manipulation of gingival tissue or perforation of the oral mucosa. The primary care provider should understand the rationale for prophylaxis and its limitations to properly apply these recommendations. Patient education is essential to improving the likelihood of compliance when prophylaxis is indicated.

EPIDEMIOLOGY AND RISK FACTORS (1–13)

During the last several decades, there has been a shift in the incidence of endocarditis to older age groups; the current mean age is about 50 years. Men predominate in those older than 50 years; in people younger than 50 years, the gender ratio is more nearly equal.

Risk Factors

Individual risk of endocarditis is typically viewed as a function of cardiac conditions that predispose the person to endocarditis and the risk of high-grade or sustained bacteremia induced by dental or medical procedures. However, 50% or more of cases of endocarditis occur in the absence of underlying heart disease, and spontaneous transient bacteremia confers far greater cumulative risk among susceptible individuals than do dental or medical procedures. Clearly, all individuals have some finite risk of developing endocarditis. Because of the difficulty in predicting who is most susceptible and when, it has been estimated that no more than 6% of endocarditis cases can be prevented. The number of patients that would need to be treated to prevent a single case is extraordinarily high. The risk of endocarditis among persons with high- and moderate-risk predisposing cardiac conditions has been estimated at 1 in 46,000 procedures with antibiotic prophylaxis and 1 in 150,000 without antibiotic prophylaxis. Nonetheless, the historical inclination to prescribe antibiotics prior to procedures has a strong influence on physician practice and patient expectations, and the morbidity and mortality of endocarditis may well be sufficient justification to use such preventive measures discerningly for patients at the highest levels of risk.

Predisposing Cardiac Conditions

In the preantibiotic era, chronic rheumatic heart disease was the underlying lesion in up to 90% of endocarditis cases. Now prosthetic cardiac valves, previous endocarditis (recurrence rate as high as 10%), complex congenital heart disease, and surgically constructed pulmonary shunts are the high-risk cardiac lesions (Table 16.1). Moderate risk is associated with other cardiac anomalies, including rheumatic and other acquired valvular disease, idiopathic hypertrophic subaortic stenosis, and mitral valve prolapse. Until recently, many authorities, including the authors of the 1997 American Heart Association (AHA) guidelines, recommended that prophylactic antibiotics be prescribed in these patients as well. That is also true for the European recommendations published in 2004. However, the recognition that endocarditis often occurs without known predisposing cardiac disease and that cumulative risk of bacteremia due to routine daily activities is much greater than that attributed to procedures led to the revised 2007 AHA recommendation that only those with the highest-risk cardiac lesions (Table 16.1) receive antibiotic prophylaxis.

TABLE 16.1

CARDIAC CONDITIONS WITH HIGHEST RISK FOR ENDOCARDITIS

Prosthetic heart valve(s)
History of endocarditis
Congenital heart disease (CHD)
    Unrepaired cyanotic CHD, including palliative shunts and conduits
    Completely repaired defect with prosthetic material or device, placed either by surgery or catheter intervention during the first 6 mo after repair (during which endothelialization occurs)
    Repaired CHD with residual defects at the site or adjacent to the site of a prosthetic patch or prosthetic device (which inhibit endothelialization)
Cardiac transplantation recipients who develop cardiac valvulopathy

Procedures That Induce Bacteremia

Data on incidence of bacteremia with procedures are fragmentary, but it is clear that risk is greatest with *dental procedures* that involve manipulation of gingival tissue or the perforation of the oral mucosa. Tooth extraction (10% to 100%) and periodontal surgery (36% to 88%) have the highest reported incidence rates, but bacteremia has also been documented during routine activities, including tooth brushing and flossing (20% to 68%), using toothpicks or waterpicks (7% to 50%), and even chewing food (7% to 51%).

Case reports suggest increasing incidence of endocarditis after *body piercing*, especially tongue piercing, but it is unclear whether prophylaxis or prompt treatment of postpiercing local infection is most effective in lowering risk. Endocarditis risk is minimal with coronary artery bypass graft surgery or placement of pacemakers or implanted defibrillators. Some nondental procedures also have a substantial incidence of subsequent bacteremia, but others have little. Bacteremia rates are sufficiently high to warrant recommendations for prophylaxis before *procedures* on the *respiratory tract* or *infected skin*, skin structures, or *musculoskeletal tissue* for patients with the highest-risk cardiac conditions. Antibiotic administration solely to prevent endocarditis is no longer recommended before genitourinary or gastrointestinal tract procedures.

NATURAL HISTORY OF ENDOCARDITIS AND EFFECTIVENESS OF THERAPY (1,3,13–25)

Natural History

Untreated endocarditis is uniformly fatal. Current mortality rates are approximately 10% with natural valves and 25% to 65% with prosthetic valves. Mortality also varies with the infecting organism, with rates of 4% to 16% for *viridans* streptococci, 15% to 25% for enterococci, and 25% to 47% for staphylococci. Death often follows congestive heart failure, arterial emboli, myocardial infarction, myocardial abscesses, or other complications.

Effectiveness of Therapy

The best estimates of protective efficacy for antibiotic therapy derive from case–control studies and range from 48% to 91%. There are no data from prospective trials in part because of the very large number of patients needed and difficulties in identifying patients at risk and detecting transient bacteremias. Most recommendations for prophylactic antibiotic regimens are based primarily on experience with experimental animal models.

RISK OF PROPHYLACTIC THERAPY (1,3,14)

For penicillin prophylaxis, the risk of serious reaction is very small in patients without previous allergy or a history of rheumatic fever—about 1 to 4 per 100,000. The risk of death caused by serious penicillin reaction has been estimated at 1 to 2 per 100,000 patients receiving the drug. Less information is available concerning risks associated with other prophylactic antibiotics, including amoxicillin, which is now recommended because it is better absorbed from the gastrointestinal tract and provides higher and more-sustained serum levels. Surveys have identified very few serious reactions to other oral regimens, including clindamycin. Even with parenteral regimens including aminoglycosides, there is little toxicity when the drug is given for the brief period necessary for adequate prophylaxis.

IDENTIFYING PATIENTS AT RISK (1,3,20–25)

Until recently a history of any congenital or rheumatic heart disease and presence of a murmur indicative of hemodynamically significant disease was believed to indicate a predisposing cardiac condition with risk high enough to justify antibiotic prophylaxis for procedures that induced bacteremia. Echocardiographic studies were done to assess murmurs or to document hypertrophic cardiomyopathy or the presence of valve calcification, either of which was considered an indication for prophylaxis. The most difficult cases were those in which risk appeared to be intermediate, as with mitral valve prolapse or with an isolated systolic murmur without a helpful history or other cardiac findings (see Chapter 21). Physicians frequently ordered echocardiograms for the express purpose of deciding whether to advise antibiotics for prophylaxis prior to dental or other procedures. Bacterial endocarditis prophylaxis for this moderate-risk group became increasingly controversial, however, as risk–benefit analyses suggested that expected morbidity and mortality associated with penicillin therapy outweighed the benefits of prevention. Nevertheless, many clinicians continued to recommend prophylaxis, and patients who had been so advised in the past expected to receive it. The most recent revision of the AHA recommendations substantially changes clinical practice. Endocarditis prophylaxis is now recommended *only for those heart conditions that confer the highest risk of bacterial endocarditis* (Table 16.1). It is no longer recommended for those in the moderate-risk and negligible-risk categories. Prophylaxis is indicated before dental procedures that involve manipulation of gingival tissue or the periapical region of teeth or the perforation of the oral mucosa. Prophylaxis is also recommended for patients with the highest-risk heart conditions who have procedures on the respiratory tract or on infected skin or musculoskeletal tissue. Genitourinary or gastrointestinal tract procedures are no longer considered indications for antibiotic prophylaxis.

CONCLUSIONS AND RECOMMENDATIONS (20–25)

Clinical effectiveness of endocarditis prophylaxis is difficult to demonstrate definitively, and there is an absence of evidence for an association between dental procedures and subsequent endocarditis. Nonetheless, vigorous preventive efforts have been considered justified in the past for a wide range of risk-conferring heart conditions and for a wide range of procedures. Consensus recommendations for prophylactic regimens have been revised to focus on a narrower range of the highest-risk heart conditions (Table 16.1) and a narrower range of procedures, principally dental procedures that involve manipulation of gingival tissue or the perforation of the oral mucosa.

TABLE 16.2

PROPHYLACTIC REGIMENS FOR DENTAL PROCEDURES

Situation	Agent	Regimen[a]
Oral	Amoxicillin	Adults: 2.0 g; children: 50 mg/kg orally 1 hr before procedure
Unable to take oral medications	Ampicillin	Adults: 2.0 g IM or IV; children: 50 mg/kg IM or IV within 30 min before procedure
Allergic to penicillins or ampicillin—oral	Cephalexin[b] or other first- or second-generation oral cephalosporin in equivalent doses	Adults: 2.0 g; children; 50 mg/kg orally 1 hr before procedure
	or Clindamycin	Adults: 600 mg; children: 20 mg/kg orally 1 hr before procedure
	or Azithromycin or clarithromycin	Adults: 500 mg; children: 15 mg/kg orally 1 hr before procedure
Allergic to penicillin and unable to take oral medications	Cefazolin or ceftriaxone[b]	Adults: 1.0 g; children: 50 mg/kg IM or IV within 30 min before procedure
	or Clindamycin	Adults: 600 mg; children: 20 mg/kg IM or IV within 30 min before procedure

IM, intramuscularly; IV, intravenously.
[a]Total children's dose should not exceed adult dose.
[b]Cephalosporins should not be used in individuals with immediate-type hypersensitivity reaction (urticaria, angioedema, or anaphylaxis) to penicillins.

Table 16.2 lists recommended regimens. As in all preventive efforts, patient education is extremely important. Patients who have been advised to take prophylaxis in the past who do not have a highest-risk heart condition will likely need a careful explanation of the rationale for their no longer requiring it. All patients with any identifiable risk should be urged to maintain a high level of oral health to minimize the potential for recurrent bacteremia. Patients who have a highest-risk heart condition and are receiving rheumatic fever prophylaxis must understand that their continuous therapy will not protect them from endocarditis.

A.G.M.

Annotated Bibliography

1. Durack DT. Prevention of infective endocarditis. N Engl J Med 1995;332:38. (*Sound, concise review of the rationale and supporting literature.*)
2. Dhawan V. Infective endocarditis in elderly patients. Clin Infect Dis 2002;34:806. (*Reviews epidemiology, clinical presentation, and treatment in the elderly.*)
3. Mylonakis E, Calderwood SB. Infective endocarditis in adults. N Engl J Med 2001;345:1318. (*Excellent review.*)
4. Doyle EF, Spagnuolo M, Taranta A, et al. The risk of bacterial endocarditis during antirheumatic prophylaxis. JAMA 1967;201:807. (*Sixteen cases were reported during 3,615 patient-years of antirheumatic prophylaxis.*)
5. Durack DT. Antibiotics for prevention of endocarditis during dentistry: time to scale back? Ann Intern Med 1998;129:829. (*Succinct review of the evolution of recommendations in anticipation of current scaled-back list of indications.*)
6. Everett ED, Hirschman JV. Transient bacteremia and endocarditis prophylaxis. A review. Medicine (Baltimore) 1977;56:61. (*Review of incidence data for bacteremia associated with relevant clinical procedures.*)
7. Hoen B, Alla F, Selton-Suty C, et al. Changing profile of infective endocarditis. Results of a 1-year survey in France. JAMA 2002;288:75. (*Nearly half of all cases were in people with no known prior heart disease.*)
8. Millar BC, Moore JE. Antibiotic prophylaxis, body piercing and infective endocarditis. J Antimicrob Chemother 2004;53:123. (*Reviews case reports of endocarditis after body piercing.*)
9. Duval X, Alla F, Hoen B, et al. Estimated risk of endocarditis in adults with predisposing cardiac conditions undergoing dental procedures with or without antibiotic prophylaxis. Clin Infect Dis 2006;42:e102. (*Risks of endocarditis were estimated to be 1 in 46,000 for unprotected procedures [1 in 10,700 and 1 in 54,300 for subjects with prosthetic and native valve predisposing conditions, respectively] and 1 in 150,000 for protected procedures.*)
10. Strom BL, Abrutyn E, Berlin JA, et al. Dental and cardiac risk factors for infective endocarditis. Ann Intern Med 1998;129:761. (*Dental treatment is not a risk factor for endocarditis, but cardiac valvular abnormalities are strong risk factors.*)
11. Strom BL, Abrutyn E, Berlin JA, et al. Risk factors for infective endocarditis: oral hygiene and nondental exposures. Circulation 2000;102:2842. (*No association with pulmonary, gastrointestinal, cardiac, or genitourinary procedures in this case–control study.*)
12. Singh SM, Joyner CD, Alter DA. The importance of echocardiography in physicians' support of endocarditis prophylaxis. Arch Intern Med 2006;166:549. (*Physicians strongly support the use of echocardiography in endocarditis prophylaxis decision making, but its importance relative to other factors varies across specialties.*)
13. Ivert TS, Dismukes WE, Cobbs CG, et al. Prosthetic valve endocarditis. Circulation 1984;69:223. (*High risk of both early and late endocarditis with prosthetic valves, especially mechanical prostheses and prior native valve endocarditis.*)
14. Kaufman DW, Kelly JP. Risk of anaphylaxis in a hospital population in relation to the use of various drugs: an international study. Pharmacoepidemiol Drug Safety 2003;12:202. (*The incidence of anaphylaxis related to oral amoxicillin is estimated at 6 cases per 10,000; for parentally administered penicillin, it is 32 cases per 10,000.*)
15. Dajani AS, Bawdon RE, Berry MC. Oral amoxicillin as prophylaxis for endocarditis: what is the optimal dose? Clin Infect Dis 1994;18:157. (*Adequate serum levels are achieved with a single 2.0-g dose.*)
16. Imperiale TF, Horwitz RI. Does prophylaxis prevent postdental infective endocarditis? A controlled evaluation of protective efficacy. Am J Med 1990;88:131. (*A 91% protective efficacy for antibiotic prophylaxis is estimated.*)
17. Oliver R, Roberts GJ, Hooper L. Penicillins for the prophylaxis of bacterial endocarditis in dentistry (Cochrane Review). In: The Cochrane library, Issue 3. Oxford: Update Software, 2003. (*Systematic review of effectiveness that relies heavily on ref. 19.*)
18. Van der Meer JT, Van Wijk W, Thompson J, et al. Efficacy of antibiotic prophylaxis for prevention of native-valve endocarditis. Lancet 1992;339:135. (*A 49% protective efficacy is found.*)

19. Dajani AS, Taubert KA, Wilson W, et al. Prevention of bacterial endocarditis. Recommendations by the American Heart Association. JAMA 1997;277:1794. (*Latest recommendations; a simplified approach designed to increase compliance and reduce adverse effects.*)

20. Wilson W, Taubert KA, Gewitz M, et al. Prevention of infective endocarditis. Guidelines from the American Heart Association. Circulation 2007;115:1. (*New recommendations limit indications to highest-risk heart conditions and to dental procedures or those involving infected skin or musculoskeletal tissues.*)

21. Gould FK, Elliott TSJ, Foweraker J, et al. Guidelines for the prevention of endocarditis: report of the Working Party of the British Society for Antimicrobial Chemotherapy. J Antimicrob Chemother 2006;57:1035. (*In the absence of evidence, a compromise recommendation for prophylaxis only for those patients in whom the risk of developing endocarditis is high and, if infected, would carry a particularly high mortality: prophylaxis for dental treatment restricted to patients with history of previous endocarditis, cardiac valve replacement, or those with a surgically constructed systemic or pulmonary shunt or conduit.*)

22. Task FM, Horstkotte D, Follath F, et al. Guidelines on prevention, diagnosis and treatment of infective endocarditis executive summary: the Task Force on Infective Endocarditis of the European Society of Cardiology. Eur Heart J 2004;25:267. (*A tightening of indications but still recommends prophylaxis for moderate-risk cardiac conditions, as well as highest-risk conditions.*)

23. Delahaye F, Wong J, Mills PG. Infective endocarditis: a comparison of international guidelines. Heart 2007;93:524. (*Documents an international trend toward more restricted indications.*)

24. Agha Z, Lofgren RP, VanRuiswyk JV. Is antibiotic prophylaxis for bacterial endocarditis cost-effective? Med Decision Making 2005;25:308. (*Contrary to recommendations, deems ampicillin and amoxicillin not as cost-effective as clarithromycin and cephalexin.*)

25. Pocock SB, Chen KT. Obstet Gynecol 2006;108:280. Inappropriate use of antibiotic prophylaxis to prevent infective endocarditis in obstetric patients. (*Only 3% of patients who received prophylactic antibiotics had high-risk cardiac indications, and another 3% had moderate-risk indications.*)

CHAPTER 17 ■ RHEUMATIC FEVER PROPHYLAXIS

Despite a decline in incidence that began before the availability of antibiotics, rheumatic fever and rheumatic heart disease remain significant causes of preventable morbidity. Localized resurgences occurred in the United States during the early 1990s and equally affected adults and children, the well-to-do and the disadvantaged. Increased frequency of international travel to and from places where rheumatic fever remains a leading cause of heart diseases is also common. Primary prevention depends on appropriate diagnosis and effective treatment of group A streptococcal pharyngitis (see Chapter 220). Vaccination against streptococcal infection may be possible in the future, but current preventive measures depend on discriminating use of antibiotics to treat pharyngitis.

The prophylactic use of antibiotics has been shown to be effective for primary prevention during epidemics among closed populations. The major role of antibiotic prophylaxis, however, is in prevention of second attacks. The risk of recurrence after streptococcal infection is especially high in patients with evidence of carditis. Continuous streptococcal prophylaxis in patients with prior rheumatic fever is the major means of preventing the cardiac sequelae of rheumatic fever recurrences. It is the task of the primary physician to identify patients who would benefit from such prophylaxis and to provide the instruction necessary for long-term adherence.

EPIDEMIOLOGY AND RISK FACTORS (1–7)

The epidemiology of rheumatic fever parallels that of streptococcal infection. Rare in children younger than 5 years of age, it is most common in older children and adolescents. Incidence decreases after adolescence; cases after age 40 years are very rare. There is no clear predilection by gender.

Although a genetic predisposition has not been proven, an association between certain human leukocyte antigens and rheumatic diseases has been identified, at least among white patients. Heterogeneity in the immune response to a specific streptococcal cell-wall antigen, the group A carbohydrate, has been demonstrated, but predictors of the hyperimmune response associated with the clinical sequelae of rheumatic fever have not been identified.

Racial differences in the incidence of rheumatic fever exist but disappear when socioeconomic status is considered; crowded living conditions are an important variable. Crowding may also explain the high incidence in cold climates and during winter months in temperate climates.

All demographic risk factors are heavily outweighed by a previous history of rheumatic fever. The likelihood of an attack after streptococcal infection is at least five times higher among individuals with previous rheumatic fever.

NATURAL HISTORY OF RHEUMATIC FEVER AND EFFECTIVENESS OF THERAPY (8–18)

Rheumatic fever follows between 0.5% and 3.0% of ineffectively treated cases of group A streptococcal (GAS) upper respiratory infections. Diagnosis and appropriate antibiotic therapy started within 9 days of the onset of the sore throat will prevent rheumatic fever in most cases. Guidelines have been

TABLE 17.1

RISK OF RECURRENT RHEUMATIC FEVER AFTER GROUP A STREPTOCOCCAL INFECTION

	Recurrence of Streptococcal Infection (%)
Interval Since Onset of Last Rheumatic Episode (yr)	
<2	28
2–5	15
>5	10
Number of Previous Attacks of Rheumatic Fever	
≥ 2	27
1	14
Rheumatic Heart Disease	
Not present	13
Present	26

Modified from Spagnuolo M, Pasternack B, Taranta A, et al. Risk of rheumatic fever recurrences after streptococcal infections. N Engl J Med 1971;285:641, with permission.

ing rheumatic fever recurrences. Three antibiotic regimens have gained general acceptance:

1. Benzathine penicillin G, 1,200,000 units (600,000 units if body weight <30 kg) intramuscularly every 3 or 4 weeks.
2. Sulfadiazine, 1 g/d orally (500 mg if body weight <30 kg).
3. Penicillin G, 250 mg orally twice a day.

Although the effectiveness of erythromycin (250 mg orally twice a day) has not been studied as extensively, it is recommended for the patient allergic to both penicillin and sulfonamides. The classic study comparing the effectiveness of these three regimens in preventing streptococcal infection and rheumatic fever is summarized in Table 17.2. Some reports suggest that failure rates may be higher when benzathine penicillin injections are administered every 4 weeks rather than every 3 weeks, and a Cochrane Review found that injections every 2 or 3 weeks are more effective than monthly injections. Because adherence is more difficult with the greater frequency, some have suggested monthly doses of 1,800,000 units or even 2,400,000 units, depending on patient weight, but further study is needed.

There is no real basis for firm guidelines regarding the duration of continuous antibiotic prophylaxis after an episode of rheumatic fever. According to the World Health Organization, patients with any evidence of carditis should be treated for 10 years or until age 25 years, whichever is longer, and carditis with sequelae of significant valvular disease or valve replacement warrants lifelong prophylaxis. However, factors that influence the likelihood of rheumatic recurrence after infection that have already been reviewed must be kept in mind. Within limits, the physician can estimate the risk of exposure of a particular patient to streptococcal infection. For example, parents of young children, teachers and other school personnel, health care providers, and military personnel are at high risk.

developed to assist in estimating the probability of GAS infection and treating it appropriately (see Chapters 50 and 220). Such efforts cannot be expected to eliminate rheumatic disease, however, because of the high proportion of streptococcal infections that are subclinical. Approximately one third of patients with primary rheumatic fever have no history of preceding respiratory infections. Another one third have symptoms but do not seek medical care. Many in the remaining one third are ineffectively diagnosed or treated.

Among all patients with GAS infection and a history of previous rheumatic fever, the recurrence rate is 15%. More specific rates can be estimated for subgroups, depending on the number of previous rheumatic attacks, the interval since the last attack, and whether there was evidence of carditis. Specific attack rates are summarized in Table 17.1.

Because of these high secondary attack rates and the ubiquity of the streptococcus, *continuous* antibiotic prophylaxis of streptococcal infection is the only feasible method of prevent-

RISKS OF ANTIBIOTIC PROPHYLAXIS (19,20)

The risks of penicillin administration are discussed in Chapter 16 on endocarditis prophylaxis. It should be emphasized that, in a large series, reactions after parenteral administration were no more common than those after oral therapy.

TABLE 17.2

PROPHYLAXIS AND ATTACK RATES OF STREPTOCOCCAL INFECTION AND RHEUMATIC FEVER RECURRENCES

	Oral Sulfadiazine (1 G/D)	Oral Penicillin G (200,000 Units Daily)	Intramuscular Benzathine Penicillin G (1.2 Million Units Every 4 wk)
Number of patient-yr	576	545	560
Number of streptococcal infections	138	113	34
(rate/100 patient-yr)	(24.0)	(20.7)	(6.1)
Number of rheumatic fever recurrences	16	30	2
(rate/100 patient-yr)	(2.8)	(5.5)	(0.4)

Modified from Wood H, Feinstein AR, Tarant A, et al. Rheumatic fever in children and adolescents. III. Comparative effectiveness of three prophylaxis regimens in preventing streptococcal infections and rheumatic recurrences. Ann Intern Med 1964;60:31, with permission.

CONCLUSIONS AND RECOMMENDATIONS (13,15,16)

- Primary prevention of rheumatic fever depends on accurate diagnosis and treatment of symptomatic streptococcal upper respiratory infections. Prevention of rheumatic fever recurrences depends on continuous streptococcal prophylaxis of the patients at risk.
- Injections of benzathine penicillin G (1,200,000 units intramuscularly) every 2 or 3 weeks provide the most effective prophylaxis and are recommended in patients with a high risk of both streptococcal exposure and a rheumatic recurrence after infection. Acceptable oral regimens in adult patients at lower risk include sulfadiazine, 1 g/d orally; or penicillin G, 250 mg orally twice daily; or erythromycin, 250 mg orally twice daily (in patients allergic to both penicillin and sulfa drugs).
- The duration of prophylaxis should be based on the risk incurred by the particular patient.
- All patients with rheumatic fever should be treated until age 25 years or for 10 years (whichever is longer) after an episode that includes carditis. Prophylaxis in patients with rheumatic heart disease with sequelae of significant valvular disease or at high risk of streptococcal exposure should be continued indefinitely.

A.G.M.

Annotated Bibliography

1. Carapetis JR, McDonald M, Wilson NJ. Acute rheumatic fever. Lancet 2005;366:155. (*Excellent, exhaustive review; >200 references.*)
2. Cilliers AM. Rheumatic fever and its management. BMJ 2006;333:1153. (*Succinct review with discussions of pathogenesis, as well as primary and secondary prevention.*)
3. World Health Organization. Rheumatic fever and rheumatic heart disease: report of a WHO expert consultation. Geneva. 29 October–1 November 2001. WHO Tech Rep Ser 2001;923. (*Monograph addressing all aspects of rheumatic fever with recommendations for control efforts in developed as well as developing countries; available at: www.who.int/cardiovascular_diseases/resources/trs923/en/.*)
4. Rammelkamp CH, Wannamaker LW, Denny FW. The epidemiology and prevention of rheumatic fever—1952. Bull N Y Acad Med 1997;74:119. (*The classic article reprinted for its historical interest.*)
5. Spagnuolo M, Pasternack B, Taranta A. Risk of rheumatic fever recurrences after streptococcal infections. N Engl J Med 1971;285:641. (*Data are reviewed in this chapter in Table 17.1.*)
6. Stollerman GH. Variation in group A streptococci and the prevalence of rheumatic fever: a half-century vigil. Ann Intern Med 1993;118:467. (*Editorial providing historical perspective on rheumatic fever and its prevention.*)
7. Stollerman GH. Rheumatic fever. Lancet 1997;349:935. (*A master's review.*)
8. Berrios X, del Campo E, Guzman B, et al. Discontinuing rheumatic fever prophylaxis in selected adolescents and young adults. A prospective study. Ann Intern Med 1993;118:401. (*Documents the relatively low risk of recurrence—0.7 case per 100 person-years—when prophylaxis was discontinued in selected patients in Chile.*)
9. Kaplan EL. Pathogenesis of acute rheumatic fever and rheumatic heart disease: evasive after half a century of clinical, epidemiological, and laboratory investigation. Heart 2005;91:3-4. (*Argues for greater research focus on the autoreactive antibodies to elucidate pathogenesis.*)
10. Breese BB, Disney FA. Penicillin in the treatment of streptococcal infections. A comparison of effectiveness of five different oral and one parenteral form. N Engl J Med 1958;259:57. (*No difference was found in reaction rates between intramuscular and oral use.*)
11. Cooper RJ, Hoffman JR, Bartlett JG, et al. Principles of appropriate antibiotic use for acute pharyngitis in adults. Ann Intern Med 2001;134:509. (*Advises testing and treatment decisions based on the presence of zero to four Centor criteria.*)
12. Currie BJ. Are currently recommended doses of benzathine penicillin G adequate for secondary prophylaxis of rheumatic fever? Pediatrics 1996;97:989. (*Because failure rates may be higher with 1,200,000 units every 4 weeks compared with every 3 weeks, higher doses are suggested if a 4-week interval is used.*)
13. Dajni DA, Taubert K, Ferrieri P, et al. Treatment of acute streptococcal pharyngitis and prevention of rheumatic fever: a statement for health professionals. Committee on Rheumatic Fever, Endocarditis, and Kawasaki Disease of the Council on Cardiovascular Disease in the Young, the American Heart Association. Pediatrics 1995;96:758. (*Update of the recommendations issued in 1988.*)
14. Feinstein AR, Spagnuolo M, Jonas S, et al. Prophylaxis of recurrent rheumatic fever. Therapeutic-continuous oral penicillin vs monthly injections. JAMA 1968;206:565. (*One of several classic trials by this group. Monthly injections are much more effective.*)
15. Manyemba J, Mayosi BM. Intramuscular penicillin is more effective then oral penicillin in secondary prevention of rheumatic fever—a systematic review. S Afr Med J 2003;93:212. (*Succinct version of a Cochrane Review highlighting the finding that injections every 2 or 3 weeks are more effective than injections every 4 weeks.*)
16. Manyemba J, Mayosi BM. Penicillin for secondary prevention of rheumatic fever (Cochrane Review). In: The Cochrane library, Issue 3. Oxford: Update Software, 2003. (*Full report of a systematic review.*)
17. Schwartz RH, Wientzen RL, Pedreira F, et al. Penicillin V for group A pharyngeal tonsillitis. JAMA 1981;246:1790. (*A randomized, controlled trial demonstrating a treatment failure rate of 31% for patients treated for 7 days compared with a rate of 18% for those treated for 10 days.*)
18. Wood HF, Feinstein AR, Taranta A, et al. Rheumatic fever in children and adolescents. III. Comparative effectiveness of three prophylaxis regimens in preventing streptococcal infections and rheumatic recurrences. Ann Intern Med 1964;60:31. (*Data are reviewed in this chapter in Table 17.2.*)
19. International Rheumatic Fever Study Group. Allergic reactions to long-term benzathine penicillin prophylaxis for rheumatic fever. Lancet 1991;337:1308. (*The risk was found to be very low.*)
20. McFarland RB. Reactions to benzathine penicillin. N Engl J Med 1958;259:62. (*A reaction rate of 1.3% after a single injection in 12,858 naval recruits.*)

CHAPTER 18 ■ EXERCISE FOR PREVENTION OF CARDIOVASCULAR DISEASE

When performed regularly and properly, exercise has a powerful protective effect against coronary artery disease, effective for both primary prevention and secondary prevention. Exercise also provides significant benefits for many of the chronic diseases that affect U.S. society, including hypertension, stroke, type 2 diabetes, osteoporosis, and common cancers (e.g., those of the colon, breast, and female reproductive tract). Despite these benefits, only about 22% of U.S. adults exercise at recommended levels. Sedentary living imposes a relative risk of dying from coronary artery disease of 1.9. The magnitude of this excess relative risk approaches that of smoking (2.5), elevated cholesterol (2.4), and hypertension (2.1). Because sedentary living is two to three times more prevalent than any of these other risk factors, it can be argued that physical inactivity is the single largest contributor to the epidemic of coronary artery disease. About 250,000 excess deaths in the United States each year can be attributed to lack of exercise.

The primary care physician can have a powerful motivating effect on patients by educating them about the benefits and approaches to exercise. One needs to identify those patients at risk for exercise-induced complications and prescribe a personalized exercise program that is safe and effective. Also important are identification, initial treatment, and appropriate referral of exercise-related problems.

PHYSIOLOGY AND CLINICAL EFFECTS OF EXERCISE (1–16)

Physiology

Physical work may involve either *aerobic* or *anaerobic* metabolism, and it may rely on either isotonic or isometric muscular activity. Energy must be generated continuously during exercise because the total amount of stored adenosine triphosphate in muscles can sustain only 10 seconds of maximal exertion. The production of new adenosine triphosphate requires metabolism of muscle glycogen. The availability of oxygen determines whether this metabolism will be aerobic or anaerobic. When oxygen supply is adequate, metabolism is aerobic and glycogen is completely metabolized to pyruvate and then to water and CO_2 through the Krebs cycle.

With increasing exercise intensity, the ability of the lungs to take up oxygen and of the heart and blood vessels to deliver it to muscle cells is exceeded, and metabolism becomes anaerobic. The costs of anaerobic metabolism are substantial. Anaerobic metabolism is inefficient; it generates only one third as much energy from each gram of glycogen, and it increases production of lactic acid, resulting in muscle cramps, fatigue, and dyspnea. Lactic acid is buffered by bicarbonate, resulting in increased CO_2 production and hyperventilation. Clinically, an abrupt rise in respiratory rate indicates that the anaerobic threshold has been crossed. Endurance training can be expected to increase the anaerobic threshold, thus allowing more work to be performed under favorable aerobic conditions.

Aerobic and Anaerobic Exercise

The goal of training is to improve cardiovascular function and muscular efficiency. The type of exercise is critical. Although maximal exertion (used in anaerobic training) is beneficial to certain competitive athletes, the cornerstone of training for fitness is endurance or *aerobic exercise* using large muscle groups in continuous rhythmic activity for prolonged periods. *Jogging* and *brisk walking* are ideal for this. Other good training activities include *bicycling, swimming, cross-country skiing, rowing,* and *rope jumping.* These activities provide *isotonic exercise,* whereby skeletal muscle fibers shorten in length with little change in tension. Heart rate and cardiac output increase, but peripheral vascular resistance falls.

In contrast, sports that depend on very brief bursts of intense activity, such as weight lifting, provide *isometric exercise,* in which muscle tension increases with little change in fiber length. Such exercise produces a marked increase in peripheral vascular resistance and blood pressure with little increase in cardiac output. The hypertensive response can be hazardous to patients with cardiovascular disease. Because arm work has a greater tendency to produce tachycardia and hypertension than does an equivalent degree of leg work, it is particularly important to limit the resistance level in arm exercises for patients with hypertension or heart disease. However, modest resistance training in elderly men and women and persons with cardiovascular disease can improve aerobic capacity and treadmill time to exhaustion, in part through improved muscle strength. In a prospective cohort study of men older than 40 to 75 years, resistance training was associated with reduced coronary heart disease (CHD) risk, perhaps as a consequence of its beneficial effect on body fat, glycemic control, and lipids. Sports that allow prolonged periods of inactivity, such as baseball and golf, are poor for cardiopulmonary conditioning. Similarly, although activities providing sustained but gentle muscular effort, such as yoga, can be important parts of a fitness program because they are excellent for promoting flexibility and strength, they are poor tools for attaining cardiopulmonary fitness.

Effects of Exercise

The effects of regular exercise can be classified in terms of cardiovascular, musculoskeletal, metabolic, and psychological functions. Regular endurance-type exercise improves cardiovascular performance and tends to lower blood pressure, body fat, weight, and serum triglycerides while elevating serum high-density lipoproteins. Physical fitness may also assist in the psychological response to stress. The more intense and frequent the exercise, the greater is the benefit, especially in measures of conditioning and biomarkers of cardiovascular risk, but even modest amounts of physical activity, including informal daily activity, improve survival.

Cardiovascular

Exercise provides major cardiovascular benefits.

Cardiovascular Performance. Cardiovascular performance improves markedly. Aerobic exercise requires an increase in the body's oxygen consumption, which is made possible by increased oxygen uptake by pulmonary ventilation, increased oxygen delivery by the heart and the peripheral circulation, and increased oxygen extraction by muscle. Endurance training enhances the efficiency of these processes by both central and peripheral mechanisms. At rest and at submaximal work loads, the fit individual has a slower heart rate than does the untrained person. Stroke volume is increased so that cardiac output for a given work load is unchanged. Although the achievable maximum heart rate is not increased by training, the maximum cardiac output and maximum oxygen consumption are greatly enhanced, so that the well-trained individuals can both attain higher work loads and sustain them for longer periods before becoming exhausted. *Left ventricular diastolic function* also improves, and risk of sudden death from *arrhythmias* decreases.

Myocardial Oxygen Demand. Myocardial oxygen demand for a given work load decreases. This diminution is made possible by the lower heart rate and lower systolic blood pressure that accompany physical conditioning, which can be of particular benefit to the patient with angina, because this "double product" of heart rate × blood pressure determines the angina threshold (see Chapter 30).

Slowing of Atherosclerosis. Slowing of atherosclerosis is observed. Independent of beneficial effects on lipids and blood pressure (see later discussion), exercise has been shown in middle-aged men to slow progression of early atherosclerosis (as measured by changes over time in carotid intima–media thickness). It is associated with improvements in *fibrinolytic activity*, *platelet adhesiveness*, and *C-reactive protein levels*. Endothelial vasodilator function also improves.

Blood Pressure Reduction. Blood pressure reduction is a major benefit. Systolic pressure normally increases during aerobic exercise, but this rise tends to be slightly less in the fit individual. More important, total peripheral resistance decreases as a result of improved muscle blood flow and decreased circulating catecholamine levels. The net result in trained individuals is *lower blood pressure*, both during exercise and at rest. Because this effect is actually more prominent in hypertensive subjects, endurance training can be an important non-pharmacologic treatment for the control of mild-to-moderate hypertension (see Chapter 26). In the elderly, exercise programs reduce diastolic pressure, but systolic pressure appears to be more refractory to lowering, perhaps because of aortic stiffness.

Peripheral Vascular Effects. *Capillary blood flow* to muscle is increased. Muscle fibers increase in volume, and muscle strength and endurance are enhanced. Muscle mitochondria increase in size and number, and respiratory enzymes increase. As a result, muscle oxygen extraction is improved. Training

also improves neuromuscular coordination and musculoskeletal efficiency.

Metabolic

The observed metabolic benefits are especially important to lowering the risk of atherosclerotic disease.

Hyperlipidemia. Although some improvements in lipid profile, such as a marked increase in high-density-lipoprotein (HDL) cholesterol, require considerable intensity and duration of exercise, others (e.g., reductions in low-density-lipoprotein [LDL] cholesterol and triglycerides) occur with just modest increases in physical activity.

Truncal Obesity and Its Associated Syndrome X. *Truncal obesity* and its associated *syndrome X* respond very favorably to exercise. The adverse metabolic consequences of glucose intolerance, hyperinsulinism, hypertriglyceridemia, and low-HDL cholesterol all improve with physical activity. Some of the improvement appears independent of effect on weight, suggesting a direct effect on etiologic mechanisms of hyperinsulinism. Sedentary living increases the risk of developing *glucose intolerance* and *type 2 diabetes,* and good cardiorespiratory fitness reduces it. The risk associated with lack of exercise appears independent of other known risk factors.

Basal Metabolic Rate. Basal metabolic rate increases, helping to achieve sustained *weight loss* when combined with a program of modest caloric restriction. Percentage and distribution of *body fat* respond favorably, with particular reductions noted in harmful truncal obesity. *Weight control* is an important motivating factor for many runners. An average jogger can be expected to consume about 600 calories in 1 hour of running. Other endurance activities have similar effects (Table 18.1). Although exercise alone will produce only a slow reduction in total body weight, the percentage of body fat decreases more rapidly, resulting in visible increases in muscle tone. Perhaps most important, fit people often become motivated to adhere to dietary patterns that will permit sustained weight control.

Psychological State

Most individuals who engage in regular exercise develop an *improved self-image*. This can be of great importance in the rehabilitation of patients with ischemic heart disease (see Chapter 31) and can also be used to help motivate healthy individuals to modify other risk factors by following a prudent diet and discontinuing smoking. The recreational aspects of exercise tend to lessen anxiety and depression. Running is being studied as a tool for the treatment of depression, and early results in small groups of patients are encouraging. Nevertheless, the so-called runner's high proves elusive or illusionary for many joggers. Although exercise has many psychological benefits, it is hardly a panacea. Patients can be encouraged to exercise for both psychological and physical gains, but they must have realistic expectations.

Morbidity and Mortality

Epidemiologic studies find that poor cardiovascular fitness and inactivity confer about the same or even greater degree of risk for cardiovascular morbidity and mortality as does smoking, hyperlipidemia, or hypertension and that increasing physical activity and fitness exert a strong reduction in such risk. Even modest activity started later in life results in significant reductions in cardiovascular risk. Randomized, controlled trials of

TABLE 18.1

APPROXIMATE METABOLIC EXPENDITURES ASSOCIATED WITH SELECTED ACTIVITIES

Average Energy Output	Activity
1 met	Resting
1.5–2 mets	Working at a desk
2–2.5 kcal/min	Standing
	Strolling (1 mile/hr)
2–3 mets	Level walking (2 miles/hr)
2.5–4 kcal/min	Level biking (5 miles/hr)
	Playing golf (power cart)
3–4 mets	Walking (3 miles/hr)
4–5 kcal/min	Bicycling (6 miles/hr)
	Playing badminton
	Doing housework
4–5 mets	Playing golf (carrying clubs)
5–6 kcal/min	Dancing
	Playing tennis (doubles)
	Raking leaves
	Doing calisthenics
5–6 mets	Walking (4 miles/hr)
6–7 kcal/min	Bicycling (10 miles/hr)
	Skating
	Shoveling garden soil
	Engaging in average sexual activity
6–7 mets	Walking briskly (5 miles/hr)
7–8 kcal/min	Playing tennis (singles)
	Shoveling snow
	Downhill skiing
	Water skiing
7–8 mets	Jogging (5 miles/hr)
8–10 kcal/min	Bicycling (12 miles/hr)
	Playing basketball
	Canoeing
	Mountain climbing
	Ditch digging
	Playing touch football
8–9 mets	Jogging (6 miles/hr)
10–11 kcal/min	Cross-country skiing
	Playing squash or handball (recreational)
>10 mets	Playing squash or handball (competitive)
>11 kcal/min	Running 6 miles/hr: 10 mets
	Running 8 miles/hr: 13.5 mets
	Running 10 miles/hr: 17 mets

Note: Energy output is expressed in mets. One met is the energy expended at rest and equals 3.5 mL O_2/kg body weight/min. Calorie consumption values are for a 70-kg person.
Modified from Fox SM, Naughty JP, Gorman DA. Physical activity and cardiovascular health. III. The exercise prescription; frequency and type of activity. Mod Concepts Cardiovasc Dis 1972;41:6, with permission.

exercise in high-risk persons confirm these important benefits in high-risk groups. The findings pertain to both men and women, to the obese and the nonobese, and to those with and without other cardiovascular risk factors. Risks of diabetes and hypertension are also reduced, as is all-cause mortality, principally from reduction in risk of cancer. Concerns by skeptics that genetic factors and self-selection might account for some of the observed benefits were allayed by studies of twins showing marked reductions in mortality for both occasional exercisers and for conditioned exercisers compared with their genetically identical counterparts who were sedentary. College varsity sports participation (a marker of initial fitness and genetic endowment) conferred no protective effect unless exercise was continued in later years.

As noted, the degree of exercise need not be extreme. Simply maintaining a *physically active lifestyle* can be expected to reduce the cardiovascular risk by as much as 35% to 70%. Whereas exercise is most effective when commenced early in life, physical activity confers benefit even if initiated later in life. The initiation of even light-to-moderate exercise can reduce all-cause mortality by 45%, even after adjusting for potential confounders. Even gardening for more than 60 minutes a week was associated with a 68% lower risk of primary cardiac arrests and walking with a 73% risk reduction as compared with a sedentary lifestyle. Among elderly men, walking more than 2 miles a day reduces the mortality rate by nearly 50% compared with those who walk less than 1 mile a day.

Although these studies concentrate on the role of exercise in the *primary prevention* of cardiovascular disease, attention is also being directed to the role of physical training in the treatment of patients with established atherosclerotic heart disease (*secondary prevention*; see Chapter 31). Independent meta-analyses of prospective trials of exercise in the treatment of coronary artery disease demonstrated a 20% to 25% decrease in overall mortality in the exercise group; fatal reinfarction and total cardiovascular deaths were also significantly reduced in the exercise group, but nonfatal reinfarctions were no different in the exercise and control groups.

Other Benefits

Although the greatest protective effect of exercise is on the cardiovascular system, reducing the risk of heart attack, sudden cardiac death, stroke, and hypertension, there are other important benefits of habitual exercise. Women who begin exercising in early adulthood experience nearly a 50% reduction in their lifetime risk of *breast* and *reproductive cancer*. Physically active men have a significantly lower risk of *colon cancer*. Exercise increases bone density, helping to prevent *osteoporosis* (see Chapter 146). Patients with *chronic obstructive lung disease* (see Chapter 47) and *peripheral vascular disease* (see Chapter 34) achieve symptomatic and functional improvements.

MEDICAL SCREENING OF POTENTIAL EXERCISERS (17–22)

Medical screening of the prospective participant and prescription of an appropriate exercise program are essential for the person who has been inactive. In addition, all adults planning to engage in vigorous activity (including young persons who want to participate in competitive athletics) should be screened for underlying heart disease before beginning. Risk of sudden cardiac death with vigorous exertion is increased, but absolute risk is very small, even in men older than 40 years of age (on the order of 1 death per 1 to 2 million episodes of exercise) and decreases with conditioning. The goal is to reduce the risk of sudden cardiac death. Any decision to restrict a young person from engaging in competitive sports or other vigorous activity should be based on firm evidence because of the potentially devastating social and psychological effects the restriction may have. A cardiac consultation is warranted for young persons who the primary care physician deems in need of restriction.

The initial screening effort does not need to entail elaborate laboratory testing, but a careful and detailed *cardiovascular history* and *physical examination* are essential. The value of the *resting electrocardiogram* (ECG) for detection of coronary disease in asymptomatic healthy persons is nil, but the test is warranted in asymptomatic young persons who plan to engage in competitive athletics for its ability to detect conduction, rhythm, voltage, and repolarization anomalies that can be clues to important underlying myocardial disease. Even *exercise stress testing* for detection of silent coronary disease is of limited utility in healthy asymptomatic persons but should be considered in those with risk factors for coronary heart disease (see later discussion).

What to Look For

In Older Persons

Subclinical *coronary artery disease*, with its associated risks of infarction, rhythm disturbances, and pump failure, is the major concern for men older than 45 years and for postmenopausal women seeking to start an exercise program, particularly if previously inactive. In persons with a history of hypertension, *left ventricular hypertrophy* represents an important consideration; the remodeling of the left ventricle puts the patient at increased risk for ischemia and dysrhythmias. Clinically "silent" *valvular heart disease* should be kept in mind, particularly aortic stenosis and mitral stenosis; a previously unappreciated hemodynamically significant lesion could pose a risk during exercise (see Chapter 33).

In Younger Persons

When evaluating younger persons who seek to engage in competitive athletics, it is important to check not only for the *major valvular diseases* (e.g., *aortic stenosis*, *mitral stenosis*, and *mitral valve prolapse*; see Chapters 21 and 33) and rhythm disturbances (see Chapter 25), but also for *hypertrophic cardiomyopathy* and *arrhythmogenic right ventricular cardiomyopathy,* two uncommon, often-unsuspected conditions that are important causes of sudden death in competitive athletes. The presence of any one of these conditions may be relatively silent or heralded by such findings as palpitations on exertion, syncope or near-syncope, lightheadedness, exertional dyspnea chest discomfort, a family history of heart disease or of sudden cardiac death, voltage and ST- and T-wave abnormalities on ECG, and atrial or ventricular premature beats or frank dysrhythmias. A high index of suspicion is warranted.

Hypertrophic cardiomyopathy may be mistaken for the "athlete's heart" seen in persons who engage in strenuous anaerobic exercise. However, a history of effort syncope or near-syncope, a family history of cardiac sudden death, a systolic heart murmur that increases with maneuvers that decrease left ventricular volume (see Chapter 21), and marked increase in voltages, prominent Q waves, and deep negative T waves on resting ECG should make one suspicious of hypertrophic disease. Cardiac ultrasound is required. Diagnostic findings differentiating this condition from athlete's heart include asymmetric wall thickening, involvement of the right and left ventricles, total wall thickness greater than 13 mm, and outflow tract obstruction. Heavy exertion should be restricted and a cardiac consultation obtained.

Arrhythmogenic right ventricular cardiomyopathy is rare but, as noted, has been found to be an important cause of arrhythmogenic death in younger persons who engage in competitive sports. Suggestive findings include a family history of sudden cardiac death, palpitations on exertion, inverted T waves in the right precordial leads on ECG, and ventricular premature beats with a left-bundle-branch pattern.

Anomalous origin of coronary artery is another leading cause of sudden death in athletes. It is typically asymptomatic and difficult to detect premorbidly.

History

The first step is a detailed personal and family history. Each patient should be carefully questioned about symptoms that suggest cardiovascular disease, including chest pain, palpitations, dyspnea, undue fatigue, near-syncope, syncope, and claudication. It is very important to review health habits in detail, with special attention to previous exercise patterns, smoking, diet, and the use of oral contraceptive agents. Of particular importance in the family history is the presence of coronary heart disease, peripheral vascular disease, hypertension, stroke, diabetes, syncope, or sudden death.

Physical Examination

Several components of the physical examination deserve emphasis. Height and weight should be recorded and used to calculate the *body mass index* or to measure the percentage body fat (see Chapter 10). *Postural signs* (pulse and blood pressure taken supine and standing) should be obtained at rest and after modest exertion (stair climbing or sit-ups). The *chest* is examined for rales, wheezes, and rhonchi, and the *heart* for cardiomegaly, S3, S4, abnormalities of the second heart sound, murmurs, and rhythm disturbances. The *peripheral pulses* and *abdomen* should be palpated to exclude atherosclerotic disease and an aortic aneurysm. The musculoskeletal system should be evaluated both to exclude significant pathology and to determine whether specific flexibility or strengthening exercises are required as part of the training program.

Laboratory Studies

Testing should begin with a check for atherosclerotic risk factors and include serum *glucose*, *lipid profile*, *homocysteine*, and *C-reactive protein*. Serum *hemoglobin* and *creatinine* can also be helpful. For persons older than 40 years of age (especially those with cardiac risk factors or a family history of heart disease), a *resting ECG* is helpful to check for ischemia, left ventricular hypertrophy, and disturbances of rate and rhythm. Young persons who are going to engage in competitive athletics and who have a history of heart murmur, palpitations, dyspnea, undue fatigue, syncope, or lightheadedness or a family history of sudden death, premature heart disease, or dysrhythmias might also benefit from a resting ECG.

If the screening workup discloses evidence suggesting increased risk of underlying heart disease, then *cardiac ultrasound* and *exercise stress testing* are mandatory considerations before an exercise program is initiated. When there is suspicion of valvular disease or cardiomyopathy, ultrasound should precede stress testing. Even if preliminary screening reveals no evidence of heart disease, stress testing may be helpful for asymptomatic patients with multiple cardiac risk factors, especially if they have been sedentary. Some argue that stress testing may be a prudent precursor in men older than 50 years of age and in women older than 60 years of age who are considering a vigorous exercise program, even if they are asymptomatic and apparently healthy, because atherosclerotic heart disease is so prevalent in our society. However, it must be remembered that stress testing has a very low predictive value in persons with a low pretest probability of coronary artery disease (see Chapter 36). Other uses of stress testing are to evaluate the individual's exercise capacity and establish the maximal and target heart rates for use in the exercise prescription. Patients who report exercise-induced lightheadedness or palpitations need stress testing to check for exercise-induced dysrhythmias and drops in blood pressure. *Holter monitoring* might also be helpful in the assessment.

In special cases, additional studies may be desirable, such as *forced expiratory volume in 1 second*, *vital capacity*, and *arterial blood gases* in patients with subjective dyspnea or suspected pulmonary disease. Specialized *ergometric testing* can determine maximal oxygen consumption, total work capacity, and other physiologic parameters.

Classification

Medical screening and exercise testing allow the physician to assign each patient to one of three categories:

1. *No restrictions, no supervision*: Individuals with normal studies can undertake an exercise program without medical supervision. Even in these healthy people, individualized exercise prescriptions and guidance regarding training techniques and safety precautions will be of great value.
2. *Some restrictions, some supervision*: Patients with ischemic heart disease, moderate hypertension, or moderate chronic obstructive lung disease will benefit from graded exercise programs, but they should be referred to a specialized exercise rehabilitation program that can provide medical supervision and facilities for emergency treatment. However, if structured rehabilitation is not available, milder forms of exercise without medical supervision can still be recommended (e.g., walking, stationary bicycling) with appropriate precautions.
3. *Marked restrictions or exclusion, marked supervision*: Physical exertion is relatively contraindicated in the presence of poorly controlled congestive heart failure, ventricular irritability, hypertension, diabetes, or epilepsy, although patients with these conditions can sometimes be enrolled in supervised programs if their conditions respond to medical therapy. Patients with left ventricular or aortic aneurysms or hemodynamically significant aortic valve disease should be excluded from exercise programs.

EXERCISE PRESCRIPTION (23–31)

Role of the Primary Physician

Given the significant contributions of exercise to reducing cardiovascular and all-cause morbidity and mortality, it is imperative that primary physicians counsel their patients on the importance of exercise and help them to find forms and amounts of exercise that will be safe, beneficial, enjoyable, and sustainable over prolonged periods of time. Imposing an exercise program is much less effective than finding out what the patient is willing and interested in doing. Helping the patient to incorporate an exercise program into a busy lifestyle is critical. Whereas formal workouts are essential for optimal fitness and physical performance, modest levels of informal physical activity incorporated into daily living can have significant health benefits, especially in persons who are inactive. For patients who are interested and capable, the physician should be prepared to prescribe a program of fitness training.

Basic Elements of the Fitness Program

The basic elements of the fitness program include frequency, intensity, and duration of exercise.

Frequency

As few as three exercise sessions per week will develop and maintain fitness; five sessions per week provide near-maximum benefit. Hence, the exercise prescription should call for at least three periods of exercise each week. Many individuals prefer a routine of daily activity; this is an excellent choice, but it is advisable to schedule easier and harder workouts on alternate days to prevent injuries and allow the muscles to recover.

Intensity and Duration

In general, the health benefits of exercise are proportional to the intensity and duration of activity; however, as pointed out by the results of the Nurses' Health Study, maximum reductions in coronary risk do not necessarily require attainment of maximum cardiopulmonary fitness. Moderate degrees of exercise appear to provide the same degree of protection as vigorous activity, at least in middle-aged women. Even very modest exercise can produce significant reductions in cardiovascular risk compared with inactive persons, belying the "no-pain, no-gain" motto.

Intensity and duration of training are closely related. Equal degrees of fitness can be attained through less intense exercise sustained over a longer period or through more vigorous effort for shorter periods. Maximum cardiopulmonary fitness can be attained by 15 to 60 minutes of continuous aerobic exercises that are strenuous enough to raise the heart rate to 60% to 80% of maximum or the oxygen uptake to 50% to 85% of maximum.

Designing the Program

The first task is to decide the objective(s) of the exercise program. If it is to achieve conditioning, which provides the maximum benefit, then a formal program should be designed. If the modest goal of cardiovascular risk reduction without full conditioning is deemed more appropriate, then a program of informal exercise can be laid out in which aerobic activities (e.g., walking, taking the stairs, gardening) are built into the person's daily routine. The next step might be a more specific program of walking three to five times per week.

Those who seek conditioning need a more structured exercise prescription. Goals must be attained very slowly and gradually, and the physician's exercise prescription should provide a practical means of attaining them. Both the starting point and the rate of progression depend on the health, age, and fitness of the participant. As a rule of thumb, the beginner should plan to exercise aerobically for 10 to 12 minutes at a pace sufficient to increase heart rate to 60% to 80% of maximum without producing breathlessness.

The Warm-up Period

Each aerobic workout session begins with a 5- to 10-minute warm-up period. At the beginning of exercise, even the well-conditioned athlete experiences some degree of dyspnea due to anaerobic metabolism. It takes 45 to 90 seconds for cardiac output to increase enough to meet the new work load and provide the "second wind." A warm-up period will minimize this initial anaerobic period and also allow muscles to loosen and stretch out, which prevents many injuries. For the runner, the warm-up period should consist of stretching exercise, calisthenics, and a gradual progression from walking to slow jogging to running.

The Initial Training Period

As noted, the actual training period should initially consist of a total of 10 to 12 minutes of exercise, alternating periods of effort with periods of recovery. This is easily accomplished by alternating full-intensity exercise with low-intensity exercise. For example, an unfit or older individual might alternate 1 minute of full exercising with 1 minute of gentle exercise, repeating this cycle 10 to 12 times during each training day.

The Cool-down Period

The cool-down period completes the exercise prescription and consists of 5 to 10 minutes of walking and stretching exercises. This helps to maintain venous return and sustains cardiac output, preventing hypotension and hypoperfusion from vasodilation, which occurs for dissipation of heat. Very hot or very cold showers should be avoided.

Advancing the Program

Once initial goals are met—perhaps at the end of 10 to 20 sessions over 2 to 3 weeks— the program can be advanced to 2 minutes of full exercise alternating with 2 minutes of gentle exercise, with six cycles in each session. After this is mastered, the exercise ritual can be extended to 3 or 4 minutes with only 1 or 2 minutes of rest for three or four cycles and then to two 6-minute runs with 1 or 2 minutes of walking in between. By the end of 1 or 2 months, most individuals can expect to be able to exercise for 10 to 20 minutes continuously.

Advancing the Duration of Exercise

Although the young and athletic person will progress more rapidly than the older or unfit one, it is important to urge restraint. One of the most common causes of orthopedic injuries is attempting too much too quickly. Once a base of 10 to 20 minutes of exercise is well established, further progress can be encouraged. It is reasonable to increase time or distance by a rate of about 10% per week. This can be accomplished by extending one or two sessions while preserving some short-distance days or by gradually extending each session. At the end of 4 to 6 months, 3 to 4 miles of jogging or equivalent exercise 3 to 5 days per week will provide maximum conditioning. Feelings of accomplishment and well-being usually provide motivation for sustained participation, often at even higher levels. Three to 4 hours of exercise per week provides the maximum longevity benefits.

It is important to emphasize, as noted earlier, that achievement of high levels of conditioning are not necessary to realize significant reductions in cardiovascular and all-cause morbidity and mortality. As little as 20 minutes of aerobic exercise three times per week is sufficient to achieve significant risk reduction and some degree of conditioning.

Advancing the Intensity of Exercise

The most precise readily available measure of intensity is the *heart rate*. Patients should work at a pace sufficient to raise the pulse to 60% to 80% of maximum. If exercise testing has been performed, an observed maximal heart rate can be used for this calculation. In the absence of such data, the maximal heart rate can be estimated for healthy individuals by subtracting the age from 220. As a rough guide, the target of 60% to 80% of this maximum translates to 130 to 150 beats per minute for younger persons and to 110 to 125 beats per minute for older ones. Patients can be taught to count their carotid or radial pulse just before and immediately after exercise and to adjust their pace to attain and maintain the target heart rate. For persons who find it difficult or unpleasant to take their pulse, intensity of effort can be roughly gauged by the *"talking" pace*—the intensity sufficient to feel one is working hard while still able to talk to a companion without feeling dyspneic. It can be very helpful to have patients keep a daily record of these figures together with the time and approximate distance covered. As training progresses, a more rapid pace will be required to achieve the target heart rate.

PATIENT EDUCATION (21,32,33)

Motivating the Patient

Patients need to know that next to smoking, hypertension, and hypercholesterolemia, inactivity is one of the most important treatable cardiac risk factors. Many do not appreciate that exercise not only can help them to look, feel, and work better, but also can reduce overall coronary morbidity and mortality. Also helpful is emphasizing that even modest amounts of activity (including informal exercise such as gardening) can provide substantial health benefits, and that moderate exercise (e.g., walking at a moderate pace) can be as effective in reducing coronary risk as vigorous activity. This helps patients to find enjoyable activities that can be incorporated into their daily life and facilitates motivation. The goal is to have them take up and sustain a program of endurance-type activity. Most important to success is choosing a form of exercise that is enjoyable and readily incorporated into daily living.

Focusing on Safety

Exercise is not without risk, and patients need to know what to look for and how to respond. There is no question that exercise can precipitate cardiac arrhythmias and myocardial ischemia in persons with underlying *heart disease*. Sudden death is a tragic, although infrequent, complication of exercise. Careful medical screening of potential exercisers (see earlier discussion) and design of an appropriate individualized exercise prescription are essential to patient safety. In addition, detailed review of cardiac warning signs (chest pressure, dizziness, lightheadedness, dyspnea, palpitations, unusual fatigue, nausea, diaphoresis) is critical along with advice to stop exercising immediately if such symptoms develop. One must be sure that the patient will not continue exercising or rationalize the symptoms away by misattributing them to such harmless causes as "indigestion" or "gas." Meticulous supervision of high-risk individuals and use of closely controlled conditioning programs have enabled survivors of myocardial infarctions to engage safely in aerobic exercise, even marathon running.

Some exercisers encounter exercise-induced *asthma*, particularly during cold weather. Advising use of a face mask that warms inspired air often suffices; sometimes prophylactic treatment with inhaled cromolyn, albuterol, or montelukast is necessary and helpful (see Chapter 48). Extreme environmental conditions may also produce thermal stress ranging from frostbite to heat stroke. Here, too, prevention is the best therapy.

The physician should be able to advise the exerciser about appropriate fluid intake, clothing, acclimatization, and safe duration of exposure and exercise. Similar advice prevents dehydration and electrolyte depletion.

Musculoskeletal injuries are very common and result from overuse, inflexibility, and muscle imbalance (see Chapters 152 and 154). Overuse is prevented by gradual increases in exercise; inflexibility and imbalance are avoided by stretching and strengthening (see later discussion). Providing advice about equipment and technique can also help to lessen the risk of injury (see later discussion).

Practical Advice for the Beginning Exerciser

Food and Fluid Intake

It is best to avoid exercise within 2 hours of a substantial meal. Despite many claims to the contrary, no specific dietary programs are required for exercise. The obese person should restrict calories to reduce weight, whereas the lean individual may require increased caloric intake to maintain weight. Competitive athletes believe that increased carbohydrate intake during the 3 days before a competitive endurance event helps to improve performance, and there is some experimental evidence suggesting that such "carbohydrate loading" does increase muscle glycogen content. Adequate fluid intake is essential, particularly in warm weather, because the sensation of thirst lags behind volume depletion. It is best to begin drinking small amounts before thirst becomes overt. Water is excellent, although some athletes prefer balanced electrolyte solutions or even carbonated beverages.

Climate

Thermal stress presents a potentially serious threat. When confronted with an abrupt change in climate, the exerciser should sharply reduce distance and speed for several days until acclimatization is achieved. In warm, humid weather, outdoor exercise should be confined to early morning or evening hours or shady locations, distances and speed should be reduced, fluids should be taken at frequent intervals during the run, and clothing should be light colored and lightweight. Environmental temperatures between 50°F and 60°F are ideal for exercising in shorts and T shirts. Between 40°F and 50°F, a warm-up suit is generally sufficient; below 40°F, gloves or mittens and a hat are important. Multiple layers of thin, flexible clothing are better than a single bulky garment. Woolen fabrics are ideal, but a soft cotton layer should be next to the skin. An extra layer of thermal underwear is vital for temperatures below 30°F, and if winds are strong or temperatures drop below 15°F, an additional layer such as a turtleneck, extra shorts, and possibly a ski mask are required. Again, distances should be reduced in bitter cold, and it is particularly important to avoid wet conditions, which can lead to frostbite, especially of the feet.

Air Pollutants

Air pollutants may cause irritation of the upper and lower respiratory tract, and carbon monoxide can impair oxygenation and precipitate angina. One should avoid jogging or biking on heavily traveled roads, during rush hours, and on days when temperature inversions increase air pollution.

Safety

Safety is of utmost importance. The runner and walker should run facing the flow of cars. Sidewalks are preferred; although country roads are appealing, it is desirable to stay with a companion in isolated areas in case of injury. Daytime exercise is safer because one is more visible to cars and can see road hazards more easily. Bright-colored clothing should be encouraged, and, at night, reflectorized vests are mandatory. Dogs are best avoided by means of an impromptu detour, but if this is not possible, they can generally be intimidated by a firm command to "go home" or by the threat of a stick or stone.

Equipment

One of the advantages of jogging and walking is that elaborate equipment is not required; however, good athletic *shoes* are essential. Many excellent shoes are available; the choice should be dictated by fit, comfort, and support rather than by endorsements or ratings. The toe box should provide enough room for dorsiflexion during take-off, the sole should be flexible and provide adequate cushioning, and the heel should be fairly snug without exerting pressure on the Achilles tendon. Most good athletic shoes are costly but are durable and useful for reducing the risk of injury. Good shoes are important; other items ranging from stopwatches to designer sweat suits are optional to say the least.

Orthotics and other orthopedic devices are sometimes helpful for refractory problems. Patients with overuse injuries who fail to limit their activity may require a splint or cast to enforce inactivity, even if immobilization is not actually necessary for healing. The use of such devices requires referral to an orthopedist or podiatrist skilled in treating runners' musculoskeletal problems.

Stretching

Aerobic exercise programs may produce asymmetric muscular development. In runners, the calf, hamstring, and Achilles tendon can become overdeveloped and/or shortened and tight. Hill running and sprinting may produce similar effects on the quadriceps and hip flexors. A regular program of stretching exercises is essential to promote flexibility and balanced muscular development. These exercises are ideal for the warm-up and cool-down periods before and after exercise.

Stretching routines are almost as numerous and varied as runners themselves. Four exercises are of particular value: the Achilles tendon and soleus stretch (Fig. 18.1), the hamstring stretch (Fig. 18.2), the quadriceps stretch (Fig. 18.3), and the hip and side stretch (Fig. 18.4).

With increased training, more stretching will be necessary. In addition to flexibility, balanced muscular strength can be important. Bent-knee sit-ups are particularly valuable in strengthening abdominal muscles and preventing "side stitches." Upper extremity strength is surprisingly important; push-ups are the simplest upper extremity exercise. For older persons, low-resistance, high-repetition weight training is extremely helpful for maintaining muscle mass and bone density during the aging progress.

Exercise is not a panacea, but it has many cardiopulmonary, metabolic, and psychological benefits. The physician has a crucial role in motivating, screening, and preventing problems. Periodic return visits may be necessary for dealing with various running-related problems. These visits afford the opportunity for the physician to counsel patience and persistence. Joggers who get through the difficult 2 or 3 months at the beginning of training are likely to develop running habits that are both enjoyable and healthful.

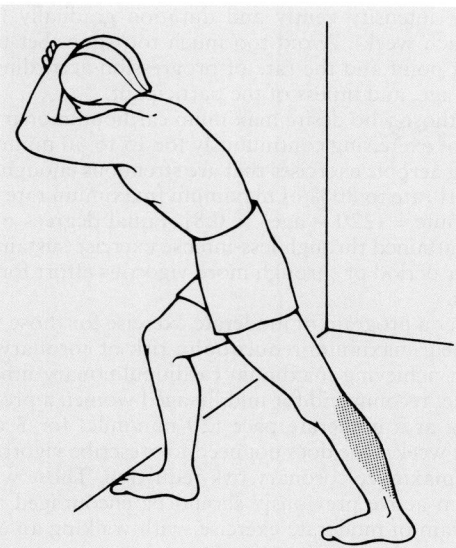

FIGURE 18.1. Calf, Achilles tendon, and soleus stretch. Stand 3 ft from a wall with one foot forward, leaning forward to support your upper body by resting your forearms against the wall. Bend the forward leg at the knee. Keep the rear leg straight with the heel on the floor, and slowly press your hips forward until you feel the calf stretch. Hold for 15 seconds. Relax and then repeat with the rear knee slightly bent so that you feel the Achilles tendon stretch. Repeat with the other leg forward.

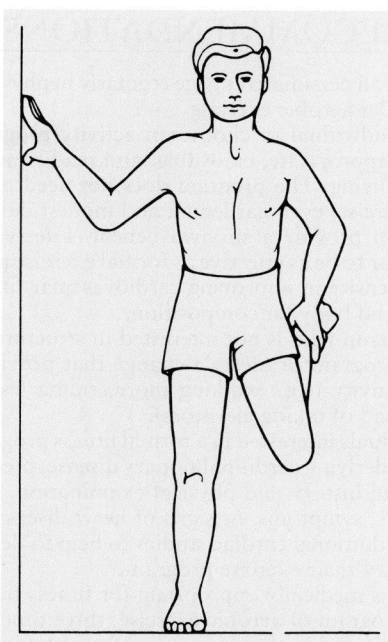

FIGURE 18.3. Quadriceps stretch. Stand at arm's length from a wall with your feet parallel to the wall. Rest your hand on the wall for support. Hold your ankle in your free hand, and pull the foot back and up until the heel touches the buttocks, while leaning slightly forward from the waist. Repeat with the other leg.

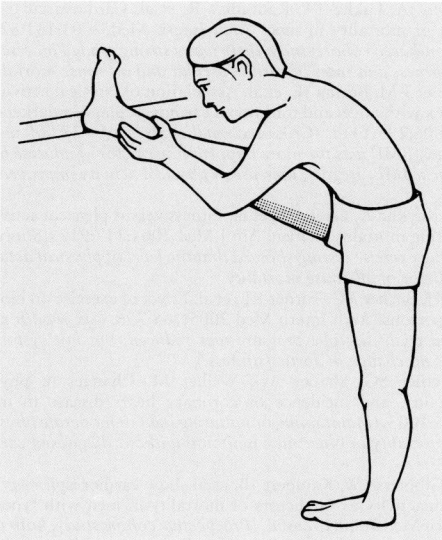

FIGURE 18.2. Hamstring stretch. Rest one leg on a sturdy table or desk. Keeping both legs straight, slowly bend forward at the waist so that you feel the hamstring stretch. Hold for 30 seconds. Repeat with the other leg up.

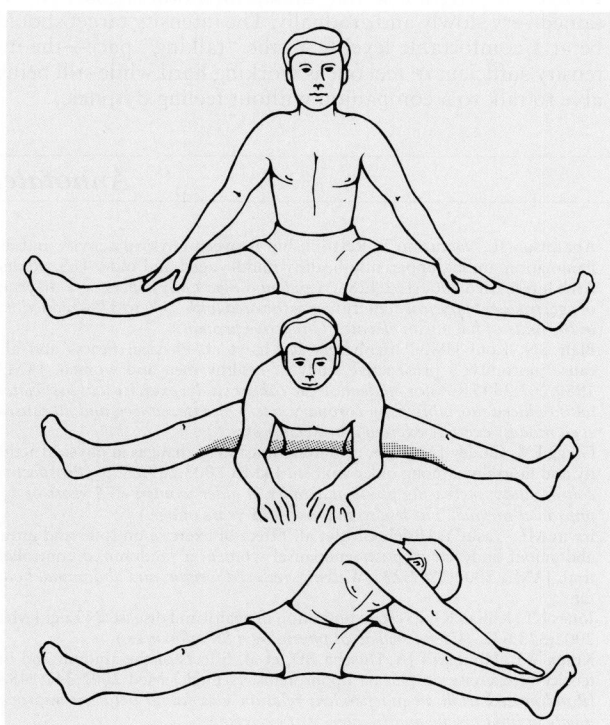

FIGURE 18.4. Hip and side stretch. Sit on the floor and spread your legs as far apart as possible. With your legs and back straight, bend forward from the waist until you feel a stretch at the inner thighs. Hold for 20 seconds. Relax, then twist at the waist, and lean to touch your right hand to your left foot. Hold for 20 seconds. Repeat on the other side.

RECOMMENDATIONS

- Encourage all persons to engage regularly in physical activity that provides aerobic exercise.
- Help the individual to choose an activity program that is medically appropriate, enjoyable, and readily incorporated into daily living. The program does not need to be one of formal exercise; even gardening and modest daily informal activity can provide a survival benefit. Lifestyle interventions appear to be as effective as formal exercise programs of similar intensity in improving cardiovascular fitness, blood pressure, and body fat composition.
- For the person who is not interested in structured training, design a program of lifestyle change that provides regular aerobic activity (e.g., walking more, riding less; climbing stairs instead of taking elevators).
- For individuals interested in a formal fitness program, screen first for underlying cardiopulmonary disease, predominantly by a careful history and physical examination. Those with risk factors, symptoms, or signs of heart disease are candidates for additional cardiac studies to help to determine the safe limits of their exercise program.
- For persons medically appropriate for fitness training, prescribe a program of aerobic exercise, three times per week. Start with 5 minutes for warm-up, 10 to 12 minutes for exercise, and 5 minutes for cooling down. As a rule of thumb, the beginner should plan to exercise aerobically for 10 to 12 minutes at a pace sufficient to increase heart rate to 60% to 80% of maximum without producing breathlessness.
- Design the program so that the optimal fitness goals are attained very slowly and gradually. The intensity target should be at a comfortable level (e.g., the "talking" pace—the intensity sufficient to feel one is working hard while still being able to talk to a companion without feeling dyspneic).
- Increase intensity gently and duration gradually (e.g., by 10% each week). Avoid too much too soon. Set both the starting point and the rate of progression according to the health, age, and fitness of the participant.
- Set for those who desire maximum cardiopulmonary fitness a goal of exercising continuously for 15 to 60 minutes, performing aerobic exercises that are strenuous enough to raise the heart rate to 80% of maximum [maximum rate in beats per minute = $(220 - \text{age}) \times 0.8$]. Equal degrees of fitness can be attained through less-intense exercise sustained over a longer period or through more-vigorous effort for shorter periods.
- Consider a program of moderate exercise for those who desire a near-maximum reduction in risk of coronary disease without achieving maximum cardiopulmonary fitness. For example, recommend for middle-aged women a program of walking at a moderate pace (20 min/mile) for 3 or more hours a week. One does not need to prescribe vigorous exercise to maximize coronary risk reduction. Those who have not been active previously should be encouraged to begin a program of moderate exercise, with walking an excellent and practical suggestion.
- For persons engaged in a program of fitness training, recommend a minimum of three sessions per week to develop and maintain fitness; recommend five sessions per week for those interested in maximum benefit.
- For those who prefer a routine of daily activity, recommend easier and harder workouts on alternate days to prevent injuries and allow the muscles to recover.
- Review cardiac warning signs (chest pressure, dizziness, lightheadedness, dyspnea, palpitations, unusual fatigue, nausea, diaphoresis). Teach all exercisers to stop activity immediately if such symptoms develop and call for assistance.

A.H.G.

Annotated Bibliography

1. Abramson JL, Vaccarino V. Relationship between physical activity and inflammation among apparently healthy middle-aged and older U.S. adults. Arch Intern Med 2002;162:1286. (*Epidemiologic study in persons >40 years of age; frequent physical activity was associated with 23% to 37% reductions in the odds of having an elevated C-reactive protein.*)
2. Blair SN, Kohl HW, Paffenbarger RS Jr, et al. Physical fitness and all-cause mortality: a prospective study of healthy men and women. JAMA 1989;262:2395. (*Major epidemiologic cohort study; exercise was associated with reduced mortality from coronary artery disease, cancer, and all causes; even modest exercise exerted a protective effect.*)
3. Gregg EW, Cauley JA, Stone, et al. Relationship of changes in physical activity and mortality among older women. JAMA 2003;289:2379. (*Prospective cohort study; increasing physical activity in older women <75 years of age improved survival, but less so in those >75 years of age.*)
4. Irwin ML, Yasui Y, Ulrich CM, et al. Effect of exercise on total and intra-abdominal body fat in postmenopausal women: a randomized controlled trial. JAMA 2003;289:323. (*Walking, reduced weight, and abdominal body fat.*)
5. Jones NL, Killian KJ. Exercise limitation in health and disease. N Engl J Med 2002;343:632. (*Useful review of physiology; 86 references.*)
6. Kraus WE, Houmard JA, Duscha BD, et al. Effects of the amount and intensity of exercise on plasma lipoproteins. N Engl J Med 2002;347:1483. (*Randomized trial; an independent relation was found between improvements in lipid profile and frequency of exercise.*)
7. Kujcla UM, Kaprio J, Sarna S. Relationship of leisure-time physical activity and mortality. JAMA 1998;275:440. (*The Finnish Twin Cohort Study; physical activity is associated with reduced mortality even after genetic and other familial factors are taken into account.*)
8. Lakka TA, Laukkanen JA, Rauramaa R, et al. Cardiorespiratory fitness and the progression of carotid atherosclerosis in middle-aged men Ann Intern Med 2001;134:12. (*Prospective cohort study; fitness was correlated with a slower progression of early atherosclerosis.*)
9. Laukkanen JA, Lakka TA, Rauramaa R, et al. Cardiovascular fitness as a predictor of mortality in men. Arch Intern Med 2001;161:825. (*Finnish population-based cohort study; there was a strong graded inverse correlation between fitness and rates of cardiovascular and all-cause mortality.*)
10. Mora S, Lee I-M, Buring JE, et al. Association of physical activity and body mass index with novel and traditional cardiovascular biomarkers in women. JAMA 2006;295:1412. (*Cross-sectional analysis of >27,000 women; body mass index [BMI] was the more important predictor of adverse findings, but within each BMI category, increase in physical activity improved biomarker profile.*)
11. Myers J, Kaykha A, George S, et al. Fitness versus physical activity patterns in predicting mortality in men. Am J Med 2004;117:912. (*Study in persons undergoing exercise testing showed that the level of physical activity was the best predictor of all-cause mortality.*)
12. Stewart KJ, Bacher AC, Turner KL, et al. Effect of exercise on blood pressure in older persons. Arch Intern Med 2005;165:756. (*Six-month randomized, controlled trial; diastolic pressure was reduced, but not systolic pressure; there was no change in aortic stiffness.*)
13. Wannamethee SG, Shaper AG, Walker M. Changes in physical activity, mortality, and incidence of coronary heart disease in men. Lancet 1998;315:1603. (*Maintaining or initiating light or moderate physical activity reduces mortality in older men with and without diagnosed cardiovascular disease.*)
14. Wei M, Gibbons LW, Kampert JB, et al. Low cardiorespiratory fitness and physical inactivity as predictors of mortality in men with type 2 diabetes. Ann Intern Med 2000;132:605. (*Prospective cohort study; both factors were found to be independent predictors of all-cause mortality.*)
15. Wei M, Gibbons LW, Mitchell TL, et al. The association between cardiorespiratory fitness and impaired fasting glucose and type 2 diabetes mellitus in men. Ann Intern Med 1999;130:89. (*A population-based prospective study in middle-aged white men showing low fitness to be an independent risk factor for type 2 diabetes after correcting for known risk factors.*)

16. Whelton SP, Chin A, Xin X, et al. Effect of aerobic exercise on blood pressure: a meta-analysis of randomized controlled trials. Ann Intern Med 2002;136:493. (*Exercise reduces pressure in both hypertensive and normotensive persons and is independent of weight loss.*)

17. Alpert CM, Mittleman MA, Chae CU, et al. Triggering of sudden death from cardiac causes by vigorous exertion. N Engl J Med 2000;343:1355. (*Prospective nested-case-crossover study of participants in the Physicians' Health Study; the relative risk of sudden death increased with vigorous exertion, but habitual vigorous exercise reduced the risk.*)

18. Burke AD, Farb A, Malcom GT. Plaque rupture and sudden death related to exertion in men with coronary disease. JAMA 1999;281:921. (*Important insight into the mechanism of sudden death during exercise.*)

19. Corrado D, Basso C, Schiavon M, et al. Screening for hypertrophic cardiomyopathy in young adults. N Engl J Med 1998;339:364. (*An epidemiologic study of a community-based screening program; findings suggest that lives can be saved, especially when there is an effort to detect hypertrophic cardiomyopathy.*)

20. Maron BJ. Cardiovascular risks to young persons on the athletic field. Ann Intern Med 1998;129:379. (*A review of sudden death in athletes with current U.S. recommendations for screening.*)

21. Siscovick DS, Ekelund LG, Johnson JL, et al. Sensitivity of exercise electrocardiography for acute cardiac events during moderate and strenuous physical activity. Arch Intern Med 1991;151:325. (*A submaximal electrocardiographic exercise stress test was not sensitive in asymptomatic hypercholesterolemic men.*)

22. Whang W, Manson JE, Hu FB, et al. Physical exertion, exercise and sudden cardiac death in women. JAMA 2006;295:1399. (*Prospective case-crossover study; sudden death is extremely rare during exercise, and regular exercise significantly reduces this risk, as well as the overall long-term risk of sudden death.*)

23. Duncan GE, Anton SD, Sydeman SJ, et al. Prescribing exercise at varied levels of intensity and frequency: a randomized trial. Arch Intern Med 2005;165:2362. (*A comparison of four regimens; the moderate-intensity/high-frequency program and high-intensity/low-frequency programs produced the best results in terms of cardiorespiratory fitness.*)

24. Dunn AL, Marcus BH, Kampert JB. Comparison of the lifestyle and structured intervention to increase physical activity and cardiorespiratory fitness: a randomized trial. JAMA 1999;281:327. (*Lifestyle interventions and structured training are both effective in promoting fitness and reducing risk factors.*)

25. Hakin AA, Petrovitch H, Burchfiel CM. Effects of walking on mortality among nonsmoking retired men. N Engl J Med 1998;338:94. (*Walking works.*)

26. Lane NA, Bloch DA, Hubert HB, et al. Running, osteoarthritis, and bone density: initial 2-year longitudinal study. Am J Med 1990;88:452. (*Running increases bone density without producing osteoarthritis.*)

27. Lee IM, Rexrode KM, Cook NR, et al. Physical activity and coronary heart disease in women: is "no pain, no gain" passé? JAMA 2001;285:1447. (*Cohort study of subjects from the Women's Health Study; found that even light-to-moderate activity was associated with reduced coronary heart disease risk, even in persons at high risk.*)

28. Manson JE, Greenland P, LaCroix AZ, et al. Walking compared with vigorous exercise for the prevention of cardiovascular events in women. N Engl J Med 2002;347:716. (*Prospective study finding that both walking and vigorous exercise were protective for postmenopausal women, even those at high risk.*)

29. Manson JE, Hu FB, Rich-Edwards JW, et al. A prospective study of walking as compared with vigorous exercise in the prevention of coronary heart disease in women. N Engl J Med 1999;341:651. (*A prospective epidemiologic study from the Nurses' Health Study database; moderately paced walking 3 hours per week reduced coronary risk to the same degree as more vigorous exercise.*)

30. Tanasescu M, Leitzmann MF, Rimm EB, et al. Exercise type and intensity in relation to coronary heart disease in men. JAMA 2002;288:1994. (*Prospective cohort study; all types of exercise, including weight training, proved beneficial; increased intensity provided independent benefit.*)

31. Vincent KR, Braith RW, Feldman RA, et al. Improving cardiorespiratory endurance following 6 months of resistance exercise in elderly men and women. Arch Intern Med 2002;162:673. (*Even some resistance exercise is helpful in improving endurance in the elderly and women.*)

32. Activity Trial Research Group. Effects of physical activity counseling in primary care: the Activity Counseling Trial. JAMA 2001;286:677. (*A randomized trial showing benefit from interactive and behavioral measures over and above simple advice and written educational materials.*)

33. Simon HB. Patient-directed nonprescription approaches to cardiovascular disease. Arch Intern Med 1994;154:2283. (*A review of lifestyle and nonprescription interventions.*)

CHAPTER 19 ■ EVALUATION OF HYPERTENSION

KATHARINE K. TREADWAY

Hypertension significantly increases the risk of developing coronary disease, heart failure, renal failure, and stroke. Risk further increases dramatically in the presence of smoking, glucose intolerance, hyperlipidemia, left ventricular hypertrophy (LVH), male gender, African American race, or increasing age. Treatment of hypertension greatly reduces its morbidity and mortality risks.

The first priority for the primary care physician when finding an elevated blood pressure is to confirm the diagnosis by checking to be sure that proper technique is used and by obtaining multiple blood pressure determinations. After confirmation, the evaluation focuses on three major tasks. The first task is to *rule out any secondary causes*. Although more than 95% of patients have primary disease (no clearly definable underlying cause), a search for a secondary etiology is important because if such a cause is present, treatment may need to be etiologic to be effective. The second task is to *assess the severity of disease* because risk and type of treatment program derive from the degree of pressure elevation and amount of target-organ (end-organ) damage. The third task is to *identify any concurrent cardiovascular risk factors* because their presence will affect the threshold for initiating therapy and the nature of the treatment program. Attempts to determine the principal underlying pathophysiology have proven elusive, although when it becomes feasible to do so, the results should facilitate diagnosis and further rationalize treatment.

DEFINITION AND CLASSIFICATION OF HYPERTENSION (1)

Definition

The definition of hypertension is somewhat arbitrary because actuarial data show that morbidity and mortality related to complications of hypertension increase almost linearly with increasing levels of either systolic blood pressure (SBP) or diastolic blood pressure (DBP). Hence, no critical level of blood pressure exists beyond which risk becomes highly magnified. In the United States, hypertension is defined as a systolic pressure of 140 mm Hg or greater and a diastolic pressure of 90 mm Hg or greater. Once diagnosed, risk must be further refined for each patient. The risk of hypertension derives not only from the absolute level of blood pressure, but also from the presence or absence of other cardiovascular risk factors. Factors besides hypertension identified by the Framingham Study as significant contributors to cardiovascular risk include cigarette smoking, elevated serum cholesterol, a low high-density-lipoprotein (HDL) cholesterol, glucose intolerance, and electrocardiographic evidence of LVH with strain. In addition, African American race, male gender, and age greater than 50 years need to be taken into account. A patient with borderline hypertension, a moderately elevated serum cholesterol level, and a history of smoking has a fivefold higher risk of incurring cardiovascular disease than a patient with borderline hypertension alone.

Classification

The Joint National Committee on Prevention, Detection, Evaluation and Treatment of High Blood Pressure (JNC), a national consensus group, has issued several reports that include recommendations of the classification of hypertension. In its most recent report, JNC VII, it continued to recommend eliminating the traditional designations of "mild," "moderate," and "severe" hypertension to avoid the misleading notion than mild hypertension is not a significant health risk. Instead, they designate three stages:

- Prehypertension: DBP 80 to 89 mm Hg, SBP 120 to 139 mm Hg
- Stage 1: DBP 90 to 99 mm Hg, SBP 140 to 159 mm Hg
- Stage 2: DBP 100 mm Hg or greater, SBP 160 mm Hg or greater

Prehypertension is designated to highlight both the increased risk of developing sustained hypertension in this group and the increased risk of cardiovascular complications. This is especially true for those with diabetes, the obese, and African Americans (Table 19.1).

PATHOPHYSIOLOGY AND CLINICAL PRESENTATION (1–21)

Pathophysiology

Control of blood pressure and the pathophysiology of hypertension are still incompletely understood. It has become increasingly clear that hypertension is a polygenic disorder with probable variable penetrance and phenotype in which environment may play a modifying role. Thus, it represents a complex interaction of multiple genetic and environmental factors playing varyingly significant roles in particular patients. Because there is a strong familial predisposition to hypertension, much of the pathophysiology is likely to be an expression of inherited defects in the regulation of blood pressure. There are probably several mechanistic subtypes of "primary" hypertension. It is also likely that several abnormal mechanisms are present in any one individual. Although several single-gene mutations have been found, the prevalence of these in the hypertensive

TABLE 19.1

CLASSIFICATION OF BLOOD PRESSURE FOR ADULTS AGED 18 YEARS AND OLDER

Category	Systolic (mm Hg)	Diastolic (mm Hg)
Normal[a]	<130	<85
High normal	130–139	85–89
Hypertension[b]		
Stage 1 (mild)	140–159	90–99
Stage 2 (moderate)	160–179	100–109
Stage 3 (severe)	>180	>110

Criteria represent individuals not taking antihypertensive drugs and not acutely ill. When systolic and diastolic pressures fall into different categories, the higher category should be selected to classify the individual's blood pressure status. For instance, 160/92 mm Hg should be classified as stage 2, and 180/120 mm Hg should be classified as stage 4. Isolated systolic hypertension is defined as a systolic blood pressure of $\geq$140 mm Hg and a diastolic blood pressure of <90 mm Hg and staged appropriately (e.g., 170/85 mm Hg is defined as stage 2 isolated systolic hypertension). In addition to classifying stages of hypertension on the basis of average blood pressure levels, the clinician should specify the presence or absence of target-organ disease and additional risk factors. For example, a patient with diabetes and a blood pressure of 142/94 mm Hg plus left ventricular hypertrophy should be classified as having "stage 1 hypertension with target-organ disease (left ventricular hypertrophy) and with another major risk factor (diabetes)." This specificity is important for risk classification and management.
[a]Optimal blood pressure with respect to cardiovascular risk is <120 mm Hg systolic and <80 mm Hg diastolic. However, unusually low readings should be evaluated for clinical significance.
[b]Based on the average of two or more readings taken at each of two or more visits after an initial screening.
From The Joint National Committee on Detection, Evaluation and Treatment of High Blood Pressure. Sixth report of the Joint National Committee on Detection, Evaluation, and Treatment of High Blood Pressure (JNC VI). Arch Intern Med 1997;157:2413, with permission.

population is rare. It is usually not possible to identify specific etiologic mechanisms in a given case. Nonetheless, several elements deserve elaboration and provide a rational basis for evaluation and therapy.

Primary Determinants and Control of Blood Pressure

Primary determinants of blood pressure are *cardiac output* and *peripheral resistance*. Each is affected in turn by a variety of factors, which have multiple control points (Fig. 19.1).

Renal Mechanisms. The kidney plays a major if not controlling role through its handling of *salt and water excretion*; other renal mechanisms play modulating roles. Many, if not all, hypertensive individuals have some degree of salt sensitivity, and many of these have an inherited defect in the ability of the kidney to excrete excess sodium. This leads to an increase in intravascular volume that is corrected by an-as-yet unidentified factor—the putative "natriuretic hormone"—that inhibits the Na^+-K^+-ATPase pump. The net result is an increase in intracellular sodium, which raises free intracellular calcium. The rise in intracellular calcium heightens vascular tone and elevates blood pressure. Natriuresis is effected at the cost of a higher resting blood pressure.

In addition, in salt-sensitive patients, a high sodium intake has been associated with higher levels of and increased responsiveness to *norepinephrine*. This helps to explain the relationship between sodium intake and blood pressure in the individual hypertensive patient. In addition, salt-sensitive

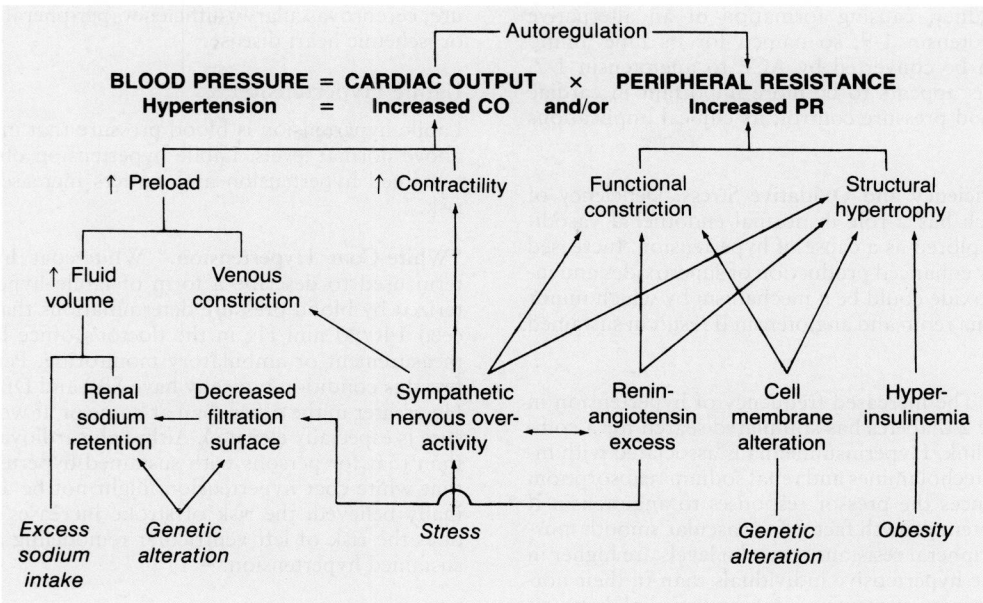

FIGURE 19.1. Factors involved in the control of blood pressure. (From Kaplan NM. Clinical hypertension, 5th ed. Baltimore: Williams & Wilkins, 1990:57, with permission.)

hypertension might also be induced by subtle renal injury caused by excess angiotensin II or excess catecholamines.

Recently, studies have indicated that a proportion of patients with hypertension have levels of aldosterone that, while still in the physiologic range, are higher than those predicted for the level of blood pressure. Offspring of patients with hypertension who have higher physiologic levels of aldosterone have been shown to have a higher risk of developing hypertension.

Reduction in *number of nephrons* has been identified as a risk factor for essential hypertension in whites. Nephron number is determined during fetal development.

Catecholamines. Catecholamines affect blood pressure regulation both centrally via the vasomotor centers in the brain and peripherally through the action of the sympathetic nervous system. They *increase peripheral resistance* and *cardiac output. Sympathetic hyperactivity* has been suggested as playing a primary role in the development of hypertension in some patients. *Pheochromocytoma* provides a model for secondary hypertension based on excessive catecholamines. In borderline hypertension, there are subgroups with a defect in autonomic control that results in excessive sympathetic and reduced parasympathetic activity. An exaggerated pressor response to external stressful stimuli has been demonstrated in some hypertensive patients and in their normotensive offspring. Also described are "hyperkinetic" hypertensive patients, who are generally young and present with tachycardia and elevated cardiac output; their hypertension may reflect the interaction of an underlying predisposition and various environmental stimuli.

Psychosocial Factors. Type A personality, depression, and anxiety have been linked to increased risk of hypertension, probably in part through their effects on catecholamines. In the most ambitious long-term study of suspected psychosocial precipitants, time urgency/impatience and hostility were found independently to correlate in dose–response fashion with the long-term risk of hypertension. Achievement striving/competitiveness, anxiety, and depression were not as strongly predictive.

Renin–Angiotensin System. *Renin* is normally secreted by the kidney's juxtaglomerular apparatus in response to decreased intravascular volume, decreased perfusion pressure, β-adrenergic stimulation, or hypokalemia. It acts on *angiotensinogen* (a decapeptide produced in the liver) to form *angiotensin I,* which is converted in the lung by *angiotensin-converting enzyme* (ACE) to *angiotensin II,* a potent vasoconstrictor. Angiotensin II also acts on the adrenal cortex to release *aldosterone,* which increases sodium and water reabsorption in the nephron's distal tubule, raising intravascular volume.

The precise pathophysiologic role of renin in hypertension appears to be far more complex than initially described and much remains to be understood. In patients with primary hypertension, about 15% have a high renin level, the remainder showing normal or low levels. Renin may be inappropriately high in some hypertensive patients, perhaps due to a defect in adrenal cortical responsiveness to angiotensin II, chronically elevating aldosterone production, sodium retention, and intravascular volume. Most patients with renovascular hypertension due to fibromuscular hyperplasia manifest elevated renin levels, but not necessarily those with renal artery stenosis due to atherosclerotic disease. There are also local renin–angiotensin systems within the brain, heart, kidney, endothelium, and placenta, which may play a significant role in the development of hypertension and in some of its consequences.

Angiotensin II may also contribute to the adverse effects of hypertension through its deleterious effects on cardiac muscle and vessel walls, where it is a potent stimulus to inflammation and fibrosis. It also interferes with nitric oxide–dependent vascular dilation and probably plays a role in the development of arteriolar dysfunction and hypertrophy, which can increase peripheral resistance. A second form of angiotensin-converting enzyme (ACE2) is expressed in the vascular endothelium of the heart and kidney, causing formation of an alternative angiotensin (angiotensin 1-9, so named for its nine amino acids), which can be converted by ACE to angiotensin 1-7, a vasodilator. This appears to be more important in cardiac function than blood pressure control; its clinical implications are unclear.

Nitric Oxide Deficiency and Oxidative Stress. Deficiency of nitric oxide (which has a role in normal endothelial vasodilation) is being explored as a cause of hypertension. Increased oxidative stress by enhanced production of superoxides and inhibition of nitric oxide could be a mechanism by which minor elevations in plasma renin and angiotensin II result in sustained hypertension.

Hyperinsulinism. The increased frequency of hypertension in patients with type 2 diabetes has stimulated search for a common mechanistic link. Hyperinsulinemia is associated with increased plasma catecholamines and renal sodium reabsorption. Insulin also enhances the pressor responses to angiotensin II and serves as a potent growth factor for vascular smooth muscle, increasing peripheral resistance. Insulin levels are higher in obese, nondiabetic hypertensive individuals than in their normotensive counterparts, suggesting a mechanistic link between obesity and hypertension. Relative insulin resistance has also been identified in nonobese, hypertensive patients and in nonhypertensive, nonobese offspring of hypertensive parents, suggesting that elevated insulin levels may also occur as a consequence of a genetic defect.

Calcium. Increased intracellular calcium appears to increase vascular tone. Alteration in calcium binding at the cellular level may lead to increased levels of free intracellular calcium with a resultant increase in vascular tone.

Alteration of Cell Membrane Function. A variety of abnormalities in cellular sodium transport has been demonstrated to occur in some hypertensive patients. These include the Na^+–Li^+ countertransport system, the Na^+–H^+ exchange, the Na^+–K^+ ATPase pump, and the Na^+–K^+–Cl^- cotransport systems, among many others. The result of these abnormal transport systems is to increase intracellular sodium.

Clinical Presentations

Primary or "Essential" Hypertension

Primary or "essential" hypertension accounts for at least 95% of cases. Onset is usually between ages 30 and 50 years, except for isolated *systolic hypertension*, which is typically a disease of the elderly. Often, a family history of hypertension can be elicited. For almost all patients, onset is gradual and at the stage 1 level at the time of diagnosis. Patients with uncomplicated disease are asymptomatic. Some patients report fatigue, headache, lightheadedness, flushing, or epistaxis, but the correlation between symptoms and blood pressure is poor, except in patients with dangerous elevations in pressure. The rare syndrome of hypertensive *encephalopathy* occurs in the setting of *malignant hypertension*, in which DBP rises rapidly above 130 mm Hg, accompanied by manifestations of increased intracranial pressure (restlessness, confusion, somnolence, blurred vision, nausea, vomiting, blurred disc margins, retinal hemorrhages) and heart failure (dyspnea, rales, third heart sound). Most patients remain asymptomatic unless end-organ damage develops and causes symptoms of congestive failure, renal failure, cerebrovascular insufficiency, peripheral vascular disease, or ischemic heart disease.

Labile Hypertension

Labile hypertension is blood pressure that intermittently rises above normal levels. Labile hypertension often progresses to sustained hypertension and confers increased cardiovascular risk.

"White-Coat Hypertension." White-coat hypertension is a term used to describe a form of labile hypertension characterized by blood pressure determinations that persistently exceed 140/90 mm Hg in the doctor's office but not on home measurement or ambulatory monitoring. Persons who manifest this condition typically have SBP and DBP at least 10 mm Hg greater in the office than at home or at work. Systolic pressure is especially elevated. Although cardiovascular risk is less than that for persons with sustained hypertension, it appears that white-coat hypertension might not be as benign as originally believed; the risk of stroke increases after 6 years, as does the risk of left ventricular remodeling and transition to sustained hypertension.

Pseudohypertension

Pseudohypertension occurs in elderly persons with very stiff brachial arteries secondary to fibrosis and atherosclerotic change. The vessel walls resist compression by the blood pressure cuff, resulting in very high sphygmomanometer readings for systolic pressure, which markedly exceed the true intraarterial pressure and simulate severe hypertension. Suggestive of the condition is the absence of target-organ changes (no retinopathy, ventricular hypertrophy, nephropathy). *Osler's maneuver* (inflating the cuff above the measured SBP and seeing whether a nonpulsatile radial artery can be palpated) is purported to be helpful in confirming the condition, but its efficacy is unproven.

Pseudorefractory Hypertension

Pseudorefractory hypertension, a form of apparently refractory disease, has been described in patients who manifest a marked vasoconstrictor response to blood pressure determinations performed with an arm cuff. Their predominant elevation is in DBP, compared with the white-coat hypertensive patient, who responds with a rise in SBP. Such patients are apt to be mistaken for truly refractory hypertensive individuals because pressures may remain elevated both in the office and at home. The tip-off to this condition is the absence of end-organ damage (e.g., normal fundi, normal cardiac ultrasound) despite the apparent persistence of hypertension.

Secondary Hypertension

These forms of hypertension have definable etiologies (Table 19.2), occur within a wide age range, and are often abrupt in onset and severe in magnitude; family history is commonly negative. Certain forms of secondary hypertension may be heralded by specific symptoms. For example, *leg claudication* may be a manifestation of *coarctation of the aorta* that causes lower-extremity ischemia. *Refractory hypertension* may be a manifestation of *renal artery stenosis*, particularly in older persons with atherosclerotic disease elsewhere or in young persons at increased risk of *fibromuscular hyperplasia*. *Hirsutism* or *easy bruising* may herald *Cushing's syndrome*. Paroxysms of excessive *perspiration*, *headaches*, or *palpitations* are experienced by almost all patients with *pheochromocytoma*; about half have

TABLE 19.2

PRIMARY VERSUS SECONDARY HYPERTENSION: SPECIFIC SCREENING PROTOCOLS

Cause (Prevalence, %)[a]	Screen	Confirmation
Coarctation (NA)	Arm and leg blood pressure, chest radiograph	Echocardiography or CT
Cushing's syndrome (0.1)	Cushingoid appearance; 1-mg dexamethasone-suppression test	
Drug-induced syndrome (0.8)	History: amphetamines, oral contraceptives, estrogens, corticosteroids, licorice, thyroid hormone	
Increased intracranial pressure (NA)	Neurologic evaluation	
Pheochromocytoma (0.2)	History of paroxysmal hypertension, headache, perspiration, palpitations or fixed diastolic blood pressure >130 mm Hg; 24-hr urinary metanephrine or VMA	Catecholamine levels, CT angiography
Primary aldosteronism (Conn's or idiopathic) (0.1)	Serum K^+, serum aldosterone: plasma renin >50:1	Inhibition and stimulation of aldosterone and renin secretion
Renal disease (2.4)	History of congenital disease, diabetes, proteinuria, pyelonephritis, obstruction; urinalysis; BUN or creatinine	Creatinine clearance, IVP, ultrasound, biopsy
Renovascular disease (1.0)	Clinical prediction rule, captopril renal scan and/or MRA (see Table 19.3)	Angiography and differential renal vein renins

BUN, blood urea nitrogen; CT, computed tomography; IVP, intravenous pyelogram; MRA, magnetic resonance angiography; NA, not available; VMA, vanillylmandelic acid.
[a]Adapted from Danielson M, Dammstrom B. The prevalence of secondary and curable hypertension. Acta Med Scand 1981;209:451.

sustained hypertension as well. *Hypokalemia* may ensue from *primary aldosteronism* and trigger *muscle cramps, weakness,* and *polyuria.* In mild *hyperaldosteronism,* overt *hypokalemia* may be absent despite the presence of refractory hypertension. *Tachycardia, systolic hypertension,* and *heat intolerance* are the hallmarks of *hyperthyroidism. Hypothyroidism* may cause an elevation of diastolic pressure.

Renal Artery Stenosis. Most renal artery stenosis occurs in the context of systemic atherosclerotic disease, manifested not only by the onset or worsening of hypertension, but also by signs and symptoms of atherosclerotic disease elsewhere (e.g., femoral or carotid bruit, angina, intermittent claudication). It may be heralded by a *renal bruit, abrupt onset* or *worsening of hypertension,* or *refractoriness to treatment* (despite a three-drug medical regimen). It may occur in association with *renal insufficiency,* with rising creatinine in the setting of good blood pressure control, or secondary to the use of ACE inhibitors (when disease is bilateral). *"Flash pulmonary edema"* in the patient with reasonably preserved left ventricular function may be another presentation. About 10% of cases are due to *fibromuscular hyperplasia,* an entity most commonly affecting the media of the renal artery and occurring typically in young women with no family history of hypertensive disease who present abruptly with difficult-to-control hypertension.

Coarctation of the Aorta. Coarctation is suggested by the presence of reduced pulses in the lower extremities in a person with elevated arm pressures. The suspicion is enhanced by finding reduced blood pressure measurements in the lower extremities and a delay in pulse transmission on simultaneous palpation of radial and femoral pulses. In severe cases, a flow murmur may be audible over the anterior chest or back.

Primary Hyperaldosteronism. Primary hyperaldosteronism is usually suggested by otherwise unexplained *hypokalemia* or excessive potassium requirements in a person taking diuretics. In about half of cases, a solitary adrenal adenoma may be demonstrated by computed tomography scan; hyperplasia accounts for the other half. Untreated hypertensive patients with primary hyperaldosteronism demonstrate an inappropriately high *ratio of plasma aldosterone to plasma renin* (>20). The associated hypertension may be refractory to standard therapy.

Cushing's Syndrome. Cushing's syndrome is often heralded by its characteristic clinical features (e.g., truncal obesity, facial plethora, violaceous abdominal striae, proximal muscle thinning and weakness, "buffalo hump"), but the presentation may be more subtle.

Pheochromocytoma. Paroxysmal sympathetic discharge (drenching sweats, headache, palpitations, tachycardia, chest and abdominal pain, nausea, tremor, blanching, and flushing) in conjunction with hypertension characterizes the condition. Sustained hypertension occurs in about half of cases and helps to differentiate the condition from other transient causes of catecholamine excess. In about 10% of cases the condition is part of a multiple endocrine neoplasia syndrome (e.g., types 2a and 2b, in which there can be medullary thyroid carcinoma or hyperparathyroidism).

DIFFERENTIAL DIAGNOSIS (1,2,4)

At least 95% of new hypertensive patients encountered in primary care practice have primary or essential disease. Secondary causes account for the remainder, with one large study showing renal failure accounting for 2.4%, renovascular disease for 1.0%, primary aldosteronism for 1.0%, drugs for 0.8%, pheochromocytoma for 0.2%, and Cushing's syndrome for 0.1%. Coarctation of the aorta is usually detected earlier in life and rarely presents as unexplained adult-onset hypertension (see Table 19.2).

WORKUP (1,2,4,7,15,22–35)

The goals of the evaluation include firmly establishing the diagnosis; ruling out secondary causes; and determining the severity of the pressure elevation, the degree of target-organ damage, and the degree of overall cardiovascular risk.

Establishing the Diagnosis

Measurement of Blood Pressure

Blood pressure is properly measured in both arms while the patient is seated comfortably, with feet on the floor, and after resting for 5 minutes. Coffee intake and smoking should be halted at least 30 minutes before taking the pressure. The cuff should be placed on the bared upper arm, which is supported by the examiner at heart level. The Korotkoff sounds are best listened for by using the *stethoscope bell* rather than the diaphragm; the bell better transmits low-pitched sounds. The average of two successive measurements in each arm is recorded. Diastolic pressure is taken at the point at which sound disappears (Korotkoff 5) rather than when it changes in quality (Korotkoff 4). Cuff size must be adequate to avoid falsely elevated readings (cuff width greater than two thirds of arm width, length of inflatable portion greater than two thirds of arm circumference). In the elderly, the pressure should also be taken with the patient standing to detect any postural changes. Any auscultatory gap (loss and reappearance of the Korotkoff sounds) should be noted because it correlates with arterial stiffness and carotid atherosclerosis, known predictors of increased cardiovascular risk.

Number of Blood Pressure Determinations and Settings

The use of proper technique for the measurement of the blood pressure is essential (see Chapter 14 and later discussion). Except in patients with severely elevated blood pressure, the diagnosis of hypertension should almost always be based on *multiple determinations* of blood pressure, preferably not only on different visits, but also by different personnel and in different settings. As noted earlier, there is a tendency for blood pressures to be higher when taken by a physician than when taken by a nurse or other medical worker. Repeating the blood pressure at the end of the visit can also be informative because pressures are likely to be less elevated at the end of a visit than at the beginning. Studies comparing the correlation of LVH with pressures obtained in the physician's office, at home, and at work show that *work-site readings* correlate best with degree of LVH.

Home and Office Determinations

Teaching the patient to check his or her pressure at home and at work can greatly facilitate diagnosis and management, but home determinations should be viewed as an adjunct, not as a replacement for office-based measurements. Home determinations are diagnostically useful when there is concern that the office reading might represent white-coat hypertension caused by patient anxiety; because they are typically lower at home, readings in excess of 138/85 mm Hg are considered elevated. If home measurement is undertaken, the patient's technique and equipment (aneroid or automated electronic manometer) should be checked and calibrated against readings obtained with a properly calibrated office sphygmomanometer. The mechanical aneroid manometers available commercially are simple, inexpensive, and accurate but need to be checked frequently. Finger monitors and wrist cuffs, although convenient and easy to use, are not accurate and not recommended. If home monitoring proves to be sufficiently accurate, one can consider using such determinations to facilitate management (see Chapter 26).

Ambulatory Blood Pressure Monitoring

Although blood pressure determinations obtained in clinical settings are powerful independent predictors of cardiovascular risk, they may over- or underestimate the true risk. Ambulatory monitoring provides the opportunity to observe blood pressure over a full diurnal cycle under conditions of normal daily living and to refine the risk determination, especially when there are discrepancies in readings between those obtained in the office and at home.

The typical monitoring device consists of a belt-worn inflation mechanism, timer, and recorder attached by plastic tubing to a blood pressure cuff. The cuff is applied and left on during the 24 hours of monitoring, inflated automatically every 15 to 30 minutes. The correlation between office and ambulatory measurements is moderate (0.5 to 0.7), with low office readings often higher on ambulatory monitoring and high readings typically lower.

When there is a marked discrepancy between home and office pressures (e.g., suspected white-coat hypertension) or a wide variation in pressures obtained throughout the day, 24-hour ambulatory monitoring may be useful. Such monitoring, with its ability to determine both *mean blood pressure* and *diurnal pattern* (loss of which increases risk and is referred to as *"nondipping"*) appears to be the most accurate way to assess blood pressure, with no regression to the mean and better correlation with left ventricular mass than casual blood pressures.

Under study conditions, patients who undergo ambulatory monitoring and adjustment of therapy based on its findings need less intensive therapy (however, costs are not reduced, due to the expense of the monitoring; see Chapter 26). Ambulatory monitoring also allows the identification of patients who lose their normal diurnal variation in blood pressure, which confers increased risk. The cost-effectiveness of ambulatory monitoring remains to be established; the procedure is approved for Medicare reimbursement only for the evaluation of suspected white-coat hypertension.

History

Key items facilitating the determination of etiology include age of onset, level at time of onset, family history, medications taken, and response to therapy. Sudden onset at a young age, very high pressure, no family history, and refractoriness to treatment suggest a secondary cause. One also checks for contributing factors (e.g., prior renal disease, salt and alcohol excess, cocaine abuse, and recent weight gain) and reviews medications for agents that may elevate blood pressure or exacerbate hypertension (e.g., amphetamines, oral contraceptives, corticosteroids, excess thyroid hormone, over-the-counter sympathomimetics, and nonsteroidal antiinflammatory drugs [including cyclooxygenase-2 inhibitors]). Taking note of additional cardiovascular risk factors (e.g., smoking, hypercholesterolemia, diabetes, obesity) and of symptoms or history of cardiovascular disease, heart failure, peripheral vascular disease, or stroke helps to determine overall risk, which is essential to guiding therapy (see Chapter 26).

Awareness of the symptoms associated with secondary etiologies is essential. Complaints such as hirsutism, easy bruising, paroxysms of palpitations and sweats, weakness, muscle cramps, and leg claudication should all suggest a secondary form of hypertension. Other clues to a secondary cause—especially renovascular disease—are onset at the extremes of age, rapid and severe course, and refractoriness to medication (see later discussion).

Physical Examination

After a careful determination of the blood pressure (see previous discussion), the remainder of the physical examination focuses on weight and pulse measurements; the skin for stigmata of Cushing's syndrome, chronic renal failure, or neurofibromatosis; fundoscopy for arteriolar narrowing, increased vascular tortuosity, arteriovenous nicking, hemorrhages, or exudates; the thyroid for enlargement or nodularity; carotid pulses for bruits or diminution of pulse; lungs for signs of heart failure; heart for left ventricular lift and S_4 and S_3 heart sounds; peripheral vasculature for pulses, bruits, and abnormalities in bilateral arm and leg pressure measurements and simultaneous radial and femoral pulse palpation; abdomen for masses and bruits; and the neurologic exam for focal deficits.

Initial Laboratory Studies

The laboratory evaluation of high blood pressure has three purposes: (a) to ascertain the degree of end-organ damage resulting from hypertension, (b) to identify patients at high risk for the development of cardiovascular complications, and (c) to screen for secondary, possibly reversible forms of the disease.

Despite the wide array of sophisticated diagnostic techniques now readily available, there is increasing evidence that the diagnosis of secondary hypertension can be made accurately and economically by the alert physician on the basis of a careful history, a physical examination, and only a few simple diagnostic tests. Extensive laboratory evaluation of patients with high blood pressure is unwarranted.

Initial studies need include little more than a *complete blood count, urinalysis, blood urea nitrogen* (BUN), *creatinine, potassium, calcium (with albumin), fasting blood sugar, total and high-density-lipoprotein cholesterol,* and *electrocardiogram* (ECG). The urinalysis, BUN, and creatinine can provide evidence of primary renal disease (e.g., azotemia, proteinuria, active sediment) and of the extent of renal compromise (rise in creatinine). Fasting blood sugar, serum cholesterol, and ECG provide data regarding cardiovascular risk and the presence of left atrial enlargement and ventricular hypertrophy. Serum potassium is a valuable screening test for primary aldosteronism and should be known before pharmacologic therapy is instituted. The total cost of these determinations is reasonable. In most patients, evaluation can and should stop here.

More-extensive routine laboratory evaluation of patients with high blood pressure has come under a great deal of criticism. The yield in the absence of clinical evidence for a secondary cause is low, and such testing is not cost-effective. It was hoped that *renin profiling* would help to identify the underlying pathophysiology in patients with primary disease, guide the workup for secondary causes, and rationalize the selection of therapy. However, the use of renin profiling has not demonstrated benefit and is not recommended, even in suspected renovascular hypertension, because most cases in older persons are not renin dependent (see later discussion).

Echocardiography for the detection of LVH has been useful in research studies, with the presence of LVH associated with an increased risk of cardiovascular complications. However, its routine use adds little to the assessment, except in the setting of refractory hypertension, in which definitive evidence of end-organ hypertrophy helps one to distinguish between true and apparent refractoriness to therapy (see Chapter 26). When the need to search for LVH is less pressing (e.g., in the patient with newly encountered blood pressure elevation), the ECG can provide a reasonable although less sensitive estimate. Of interest, however, is the finding from the Framingham data that the presence of LVH on ECG confers higher risk than that found only on ECG.

Laboratory Evaluation for Suspected Secondary Causes of Hypertension

Patients at somewhat higher risk for secondary hypertension include those with abrupt onset (especially if female and younger than 35 years of age, without a family history of hypertension, or older than age 50 years and with evidence of diffuse atherosclerosis), with severe hypertension (DBP of >110 mm Hg), or with failure to respond to maximum medical therapy despite full compliance. Fortunately, in most patients at high risk for secondary hypertension, a specific diagnosis will be suggested by history and physical examination, supplemented by a few well-chosen laboratory studies (see Table 19.2).

Cushing's Syndrome

The initial test of choice is the 24-hour urinary free cortisol. A finding of greater than 250 mcg/d is virtually diagnostic; a level greater than the upper limit of normal (65 mcg/d) in a person with characteristic clinical features strongly supports the diagnosis, but a reading of less than this rules out the condition. Persons with clinically suspected disease need an assessment of corticotropin (ACTH) dependence, which can be performed by simultaneous late-evening determinations of plasma *ACTH* and *cortisol*. An elevated cortisol and an inappropriately normal or elevated ACTH indicates an ACTH-producing source; an elevated cortisol and a suppressed ACTH level (<5 pg/mL) suggests an autonomous adrenal or ectopic source. Alternatively, an overnight 1-mg dexamethasone-suppression test can be performed (1 mg is taken at midnight, and an 8 a.m. plasma cortisol is obtained). A cortisol level greater than 5 mcg/dL is suggestive of an autonomous gland, but false positives are common (due to obesity, stress, depression, or alcohol excess).

Coarctation of the Aorta

As noted earlier, coarctation is suggested by the presence of reduced pulses in the lower extremities in a person with elevated arm pressures, especially by finding reduced blood pressure measurements in the lower extremities and a delay in pulse transmission on simultaneous palpation of radial and femoral pulses. A *chest radiograph* may show *rib notching*.

Confirmation can be obtained by *echocardiography* or *chest computed tomography* (CT).

Pheochromocytoma

Plasma and 24-hour urine collections for catecholamines and their metabolites constitute available testing options. Determination of *plasma free metanephrines* performed after the patient has been supine for 20 minutes has the best-demonstrated test characteristics (sensitivity 99%, specificity 89%). Because it measures catecholamine metabolites, it is less subject to transient catecholamine fluctuations and therefore is superior to *plasma catecholamines* (sensitivity 84%, specificity 81%). Measurement of *urinary fractionated metanephrines* has high sensitivity (97%) but low specificity (69%). The test characteristics of *urinary total metanephrines* (sensitivity 77%, specificity 93%), *urinary vanillylmandelic acid* (sensitivity 64%, specificity 95%), and *urinary catecholamines* (sensitivity 86%, specificity 88%) fall in between.

Measurement of plasma free metanephrines has emerged as the test of choice. If the test is not available, two consecutive 24-hour urine collections for determination of urine vanillylmandelic acid or total metanephrines is a reasonable substitute. By virtue of their high specificity and improved sensitivity when repeated while the patient is symptomatic, they give few false positives and can be used to rule out the diagnosis; two positive urine tests have a high predictive value for the presence of pheochromocytoma.

Combining different urinary tests does not improve test yield because the sensitivities and specificities of the tests are nearly identical. Methyldopa can falsely elevate metanephrines. If urinary screening for pheochromocytoma is positive, then one can proceed to *CT of the adrenal glands*—sensitivity is about 90% for lesions larger than 1 cm in diameter—or *magnetic resonance imaging* (MRI; sensitivity >95%). CT or MRI should be limited to patients whose urine tests positive and should never be used as a screening test for pheochromocytoma because innocent adrenal masses having nothing to do with hypertension are common.

Primary Hyperaldosteronism

Primary hyperaldosteronism is usually suggested by otherwise unexplained *hypokalemia* or excessive potassium requirements in a person taking diuretics. Untreated hypertensive patients with primary hyperaldosteronism demonstrate an inappropriately high *ratio of plasma aldosterone to plasma renin* (>20). Measuring the ratio is a reasonable screening test for suspected primary hyperaldosteronism. It is critical that serum potassium is normalized and that ACE inhibitors and angiotensin-receptor blockers be stopped for at least 2 weeks prior to testing. Confirmation requires measurements of aldosterone secretion in the setting of *sodium loading* and *sodium depletion,* which are best performed by referral to an endocrinologist. Of interest is recent evidence suggesting that hyperaldosteronism is much more common than previously thought and that hypokalemia is not necessarily present in milder forms. In one referral practice, the prevalence of excess aldosterone was reported at 24%. This suggests that testing for this should be done routinely in patients with *refractory hypertension.*

Renovascular Hypertension

The decision to proceed with workup for renovascular hypertension entails a complex set of considerations, including difficulty managing the patient's hypertension, candidacy for interventional treatment, and likelihood of response. When these are combined with an estimate of pretest probability, one can decide how best to proceed. A potentially useful prediction rule based on clinical features of renovascular hypertension has been developed to help determine pretest probability (Table 19.3). Sensitivity and specificity for this prediction rule are about 70% and 90%, respectively. Use of the pretest probability estimate can help determine who requires testing, how aggressive the workup needs to be, test selection, and test interpretation. Noninvasive approaches to diagnosis can be very helpful and often obviate the need for invasive study, but test sensitivity is often insufficient to rule out the condition in patients with a high pretest probability. Choice of test often depends on local expertise and availability.

Doppler (Duplex) Ultrasonography. Doppler ultrasonography represents a relatively low-cost, noninvasive approach to diagnosis, providing both imaging and physiologic information. Systolic velocity is increased in an area of narrowing. Because it is operator dependent, the test's operating characteristics vary with the skill of the operator. Reports from academic centers of high sensitivity and specificity (e.g., 85% and 95%, respectively) are typically much greater than results achieved in everyday practice (e.g., sensitivity and specificity 76% and 75%, respectively), where operator experience is likely to be more limited.

The test is particularly useful as a first step in evaluation of patients suspected of renal artery stenosis, especially if operator skill is high. It has the advantages of relatively low cost and no need for a dye load, which can be injurious to the ischemic kidney. In persons with moderate to low pretest probability (<20%), the high negative predictive value of the test (>90%) helps to rule out renal artery stenosis and obviate the need for more expensive, more invasive testing. However, in persons with moderate to high pretest probability (>50%), negative predictive value is insufficient to rule out the condition—one

---

TABLE 19.3

CLINICAL FEATURES SUGGESTIVE OF RENAL ARTERY STENOSIS

Highly Suggestive Features
Deteriorating control in a compliant, longstanding
   hypertensive patient (atherosclerotic disease)
Deterioration in renal function during
   angiotensin-converting-enzyme–inhibitor therapy (bilateral
   disease)
Abrupt onset of hypertension in a young woman with no
   family history (fibromuscular hyperplasia)

Additionally Predictive Features (for added diagnostic sensitivity and specificity)
Advancing age
Abdominal bruit
Increasing serum creatinine
Current or former smoking
Concurrent atherosclerotic disease
Recent onset of hypertension
Elevated serum cholesterol

Based on Krijnen P, van Jaarsveld BC, Steyerberg EW, et al. A clinical prediction rule for renal artery stenosis. Ann Intern Med 1998;129: 705.

might do better proceeding directly to more definitive imaging. Other limitations include compromise of study quality by obesity and bowel gas.

Magnetic Resonance Angiography. *Magnetic resonance angiography* (MRA) offers a more sensitive, more specific means of identifying anatomically significant renal artery stenosis; sensitivity approaches 90% and specificity 95% under optimal study conditions (less so in everyday clinical settings—78% and 88%, respectively—and even less for persons with fibromuscular hyperplasia). False positives can occur in the setting of motion artifact and tortuous vessels. Imaging of distal branches is limited, reducing test sensitivity. Cost is very high, and a dye load is required; the gadolinium contrast agent is less nephrotoxic than iodinated dyes used in CT scanning but is not risk-free in compromised kidneys. No significant physiologic information is provided.

CT Angiography. CT angiography has test characteristics similar to those of MRA and is less expensive than MRA, but its requirement for a substantial iodinated dye load makes it more problematic, especially in persons with underlying renal insufficiency who are at risk for dye-induced renal injury.

Captopril Renal Scan. The captopril renal scan is less sensitive than MR or CT angiography but provides physiologically useful information that can help to predict the likelihood of response to revascularization. In some instances, it is used to complement the anatomic information provided by noninvasive angiographic study. Radionuclide is injected 1 hour after an oral 50-mg dose of captopril. Captopril enhances the differences in glomerular filtration between normal and hypoperfused kidneys. Reports of sensitivity average 75% (range 68% to 94%) and of sensitivity 70% (range 59% to 92%). Some of the observed variation may be the result of less rigorous control of medication prior to testing (diuretics, ACE inhibitors, and angiotensin-receptor blockers must be stopped at least 5 days and ideally 1 to 2 weeks before testing to maximize test performance, but these medications may affect results even if they are stopped for a significantly longer period). The test is less useful in the setting of renal insufficiency or bilateral stenoses.

Renal Arteriography. The gold standard test remains the digital subtraction renal arteriogram. Because of the risks associated with this catheterization-dependent test, including its invasiveness, potentially nephrotoxic dye load, and cholesterol emboli, it should be reserved for patients in whom less invasive testing does not suffice (e.g., high pretest probability but negative noninvasive study negative). *Renal vein renins* can be obtained during the catheterization procedure to provide physiologic data to facilitate the interpretation of the anatomic findings.

Risk Stratification

Incorporating the findings of the workup for cardiovascular risk factors, clinically overt cardiovascular disease, and target-organ damage into a risk profile helps to guide therapy (see Chapter 26). The most important factors predicting cardiovascular risk include the presence of diabetes mellitus, clinical cardiovascular disease, and target-organ damage. Damage to target organs (manifested by hypertensive retinopathic changes, signs of LVH with remodeling, and proteinuria or renal insufficiency) indicates a significant risk of subsequent cardiovascular morbidity and mortality. Similarly, manifestations of overt cardiovascular disease (e.g., angina, claudication, congestive heart failure, stroke, carotid bruit) portend poor outcome if hypertension remains untreated. The JNC VI identifies three risk categories of increasing severity (A, B, and C) based on these determinants, which can be used to guide clinical decision making:

- Risk group A (no additional risk): no cardiovascular risk factors; no clinical cardiovascular disease or target-organ damage
- Risk group B (moderate addition risk): at least one risk factor, not including diabetes, clinical cardiovascular disease, or target-organ disease
- Risk group C (marked additional risk): clinical cardiovascular disease or target-organ disease or diabetes, with or without other risk factors

Combining these risk categories with the stage of hypertension provides a rational guide to the urgency of therapy and the intensity of the treatment program (see Chapter 26).

RECOMMENDATIONS (1,2,4,22)

- On encountering blood pressure elevation, confirm the diagnosis, but do not test for underlying pathophysiology (except in cases of suspected secondary hypertension; see later discussion) because such testing is not yet sufficiently accurate to aid in clinical decision making.
- Check for and rule out any clinically suggested secondary causes.
- Assess the severity of the blood pressure elevation.
- Identify any target-organ (end-organ) damage.
- Identify any and all concurrent cardiovascular risk factors, including clinically overt cardiovascular disease.
- Combine these risk determinations into an overall estimate of cardiovascular risk.
- Consider a workup for secondary causes and complications of hypertension when there are suggestive clinical circumstances (e.g., refractoriness to treatment, sudden worsening) or clinical findings (e.g., persistent hypokalemia, left ventricular hypertrophy).

Annotated Bibliography

1. The seventh report of the Joint National Committee on Prevention, Detection, Evaluation and Treatment of High Blood Pressure: the JNC VII Report. JAMA 2003;289:2560. (*An update of this major consensus initiative.*)
2. The Joint National Committee on Detection, Evaluation and Treatment of High Blood Pressure. Sixth report of the Joint National Committee on Detection, Evaluation, and Treatment of High Blood Pressure (JNC VI). Arch Intern Med 1997;157:2413. (*A major consensus report.*)
3. Adrogue HJ, Madias NE. Sodium and potassium in the pathogenesis of hypertension. N Engl J Med 2007;356:1966. (*A good review of pathophysiology; 98 references.*)
4. Calhoun DA, Jones D, Textor S, et al. Resistant hypertension: diagnosis, evaluation, and treatment: a scientific statement from the American Heart Association Professional Education Committee of the Council for High Blood Pressure Research. Hypertension 2008;51:1403. (*Consensus recommendations.*)

5. Chaudhry SI, Krumholz HM, Foody JM. Systolic hypertension in older persons. JAMA 2004;292:1074. (*Identifies an important risk factor.*)

6. Chobanian AV. Isolated systolic hypertension in the elderly. N Engl J Med 2007;357:789. (*A clinically focused discussion, noting the importance of detection and evaluation.*)

7. Ganguly A. Primary aldosteronism. N Engl J Med 1998;339:1828. (*An excellent review of hyperaldosteronism, including the approach to its diagnosis.*)

8. Johnson RJ, Herrera-Acosta J, Schreiner GF, et al. Subtle acquired renal injury as a mechanism of salt-sensitive hypertension. N Engl J Med 2002;346:913. (*A review of renal mechanisms contributing to the development of essential hypertension.*)

9. Keller G, Zimmer G, Mall G, et al. Nephron number in patients with primary hypertension. N Engl J Med 2003;348:101. (*Identifies another contributing factor.*)

10. Lerman CE, Brody DS, Hui T, et al. The white-coat hypertension response: prevalence and predictors. J Gen Intern Med 1987;4:226. (*Thirty-nine percent of patients were found to manifest this response, especially the elderly and those with the least hostility on psychological testing.*)

11. Nieto FJ, Young TB, Lind BK, et al., for the Sleep Heart Health Study. Association of sleep-disordered breathing, sleep apnea, and hypertension in a large community-based study. JAMA 2000;283:1829. (*Epidemiologic evidence for the importance of sleep apnea as a cause of hypertension.*)

12. Oparil S, Zamin MA, Calhoun DA. Pathogenesis of hypertension. Ann Intern Med 2003;139:761. (*An excellent review of current theories of the pathogenesis of hypertension.*)

13. Reaven GM, Lithell H, Landesberg I. Hypertension and associated metabolic abnormalities—the role of insulin resistance and the sympathoadrenal system. N Engl J Med 1996;334:374. (*A classic paper describing the links among obesity, diabetes, and hypertension based on insulin resistance.*)

14. Richard B. Devereux RB, Wachtell K, et al. Prognostic significance of left ventricular mass change during treatment of hypertension. JAMA 2004; 292: 2350. (*The condition correlated with important cardiovascular outcomes.*)

15. Safian RD, Textor. Renal-artery stenosis. N Engl J Med 2001;344:431. (*A comprehensive review; 89 references.*)

16. Thomas GD, Zhang W, Victor RG. Nitric oxide deficiency as a cause of clinical hypertension: promising new drug targets for refractory hypertension. JAMA 2001:285:2055. (*Summarizes data on oxidative stress.*)

17. Vasan RS, Evans JC, Larson MG, et al. Serum aldosterone and the incidence of hypertension in nonhypertensive persons. N Engl J Med 2004;351:33. (*Evidence of the role of "normal" aldosterone levels in the development of hypertension.*)

18. Wachtell K, Ibsen H, Olsen MH, et al. Albuminuria and cardiovascular risk in hypertensive patients with left ventricular hypertrophy: the LIFE Study. Ann Intern Med 2003;139:901. (*The finding of microalbuminuria was associated with an increased risk of cardiovascular morbidity and mortality in this high-risk population.*)

19. Weiss NS. Relation of high blood pressure to headache, epistaxis, and selected other symptoms. N Engl J Med 1972;287:631. (*A classic paper, finding no clear relation between these symptoms and the level of blood pressure; emphasizes that all but malignant hypertension is usually asymptomatic.*)

20. Windelmayer WC, Stampfer MJ, Willett WC, et al. Habitual caffeine intake and the risk of hypertension in women. JAMA 2005;294:2330. (*A major epidemiologic study, failing to find a relationship with coffee intake but finding it with caffeinated cola beverages.*)

21. Yan LL, Liu K, Matthews KA, et al. Psychosocial factors and risk of hypertension: The Coronary Artery Risk Development in Young Adults (CARDIA) Study. JAMA 2003;290:2138. (*A population-based, prospective, observational study of >3,300 persons with a 15-year-follow-up; risk was confirmed.*)

22. American College of Physicians. Automated ambulatory blood pressure and self-measured blood pressure monitoring devices: their role in the diagnosis and management of hypertension. Ann Intern Med 1993;118:889. (*A position paper suggesting that these methods have an adjunctive role in selected situations but cannot be recommended for widespread use.*)

23. Baker RH, Ende J. Confounders of auscultatory blood pressure measurement. J Gen Intern Med 1995;10:223. (*A very practical review; 65 references.*)

24. Ferguson RK. Cost and yield of the hypertensive evaluation: experience of a community-based referral clinic. Ann Intern Med 1975;82:761. (*Its conclusions are still valid; emphasizes that secondary hypertension can be detected on the basis of a careful examination and only a few simple diagnostic tests.*)

25. Frohlich ED, Grim C, Labarthe DR, et al. Report of a special task force appointed by the Steering Committee, American Heart Association. Recommendations for human blood pressure determinations by sphygmomanometers. Hypertension 1988;11:209A. (*A critical review of technique.*)

26. Krijnen P, van Jaarsveld BC, Steyerberg EW, et al. A clinical prediction rule for renal artery stenosis. Ann Intern Med 1998;129:705. (*A well-designed effort that provides a set of clinical criteria as sensitive and specific as scintigraphy.*)

27. Landers JWM, Pacak K, Walther MM, et al. Biochemical diagnosis of pheochromocytoma: which test is best? JAMA 2002;287:1427. (*A large, multicenter cohort study; the measurement of plasma free metanephrines was found to be the best test.*)

28. Mejia AD, Egan BM, Schork NJ, et al. Artifacts in measurement of blood pressure and lack of target organ involvement in patients with treatment-resistant hypertension. Ann Intern Med 1990;112:270. (*Identifies three types of artifacts in the measurement of blood pressure in patients who appear to be refractory to treatment.*)

29. Messerli FH. Osler's maneuver, pseudohypertension, and true hypertension in the elderly. Am J Med 1986;80:906. (*Addresses the problem of accurately measuring blood pressure in older persons with stiff brachial arteries.*)

30. Pickering TG, Shimbo D, Haas D. Ambulatory blood-pressure monitoring. N Engl J Med 2006;354:2368. (*An excellent review with a good discussion of indications for use; 47 references.*)

31. Staessen JA, Byttebier G, Buntinx F, et al. Antihypertensive treatment based on conventional or ambulatory blood pressure measurement: a randomized controlled trial. JAMA 1997;278:1065. (*The approach allowed less intensive treatment with no compromise of blood pressure control or inhibition of left ventricular hypertrophy, but there was no reduction in cost either.*)

32. Radermacher J, Chavan A, Bleck J, et al. Use of Doppler ultrasonography to predict the outcome of therapy for renal-artery stenosis. N Engl J Med 2001;344:410. (*The utility of Doppler ultrasonography in both the diagnosis and prediction of the response to repair of renal artery stenosis.*)

33. Vasbinder CBC, Neiemans PJ, Kessels AGH, et al. Accuracy of computed tomographic angiography and magnetic resonance angiography for diagnosing renal artery stenosis. Ann Intern Med 2004;141:674. (*Finds that sensitivity was often lacking.*)

34. Whittles RM, Kaplan EL, Roizen MF. Sensitivity of diagnostic and localization tests for pheochromocytoma in clinical practice. Arch Intern Med 2000;160:2521. (*Examines test performance characteristics under everyday conditions; magnetic resonance imaging was better than computed tomography for localization.*)

35. Wong TY, Mitchell P. Hypertensive retinopathy. N Engl J Med 2004;351:2310. (*Excellent discussion and pictures of these important findings.*)

CHAPTER 20 ■ EVALUATION OF CHEST PAIN

The patient who presents with chest pain in the outpatient setting poses a diagnostic challenge. The spectrum of diagnostic possibilities ranges from life-threatening cardiac, pulmonary, and aortic etiologies to esophageal and musculoskeletal causes. Harmless conditions may mimic more serious disease. Atypical chest pain can be especially problematic. The primary physician must be skilled in quickly and accurately differentiating the patient who requires immediate hospitalization from the person who can be safely evaluated in the outpatient setting. Initial decision making depends predominantly on a careful assessment of the history supplemented, when possible, by a check for a few key physical and electrocardiographic findings. Further testing must be selected judiciously to avoid generating false-positive results.

PATHOPHYSIOLOGY AND CLINICAL PRESENTATION (1–12)

Chest pain may arise from chest wall, intrathoracic, abdominal, or even psychophysiologic sources.

Chest Wall

Pain originating in the chest wall is usually due to musculoskeletal pathology, although occasionally nerve injury is responsible. Because it is of somatic origin, the pain can be pinpointed by the patient, who may use the "*pointing sign*" (one or two fingers locating a specific painful site on the chest wall). Although uncommon, the sign has been found to have a specificity of 98% and a positive predictive value of 88% for nonischemic disease among persons presenting to the emergency room with chest pain.

Chest wall pain is characteristically aggravated by deep inspiration, cough, direct palpation, and movement. Common sites of involvement are the costochondral and chondrosternal junctions. Duration ranges from a few seconds to several days and quality from sharp to dull or aching. Sometimes the patient complains of tightness. Vigorous and unaccustomed exertion can lead to muscular and ligamentous strain, which may account for some cases. Other cases are due to costochondritis (Tietze's syndrome), which is an inflammatory condition that causes localized swelling, erythema, warmth, and tenderness at the costochondral or chondrosternal junction. Rib fracture may produce a similar picture, although location is different, and there is a history of antecedent trauma or metastatic cancer. Of interest, there is an increased frequency of musculoskeletal pain in patients with angina, which causes a potentially confusing clinical presentation.

Nerve injury due to a recrudescence of *herpes zoster* infection can be very painful, with a dermatomal distribution being characteristic. The pain may precede the typical rash (picturesquely described as "dew drops on a rose petal"; see Chapter 193) by 3 to 5 days. Neurologic complaints range from hypoesthesia to dysesthesia and hyperesthesia. In the elderly, the pain may persist for months, long after the rash resolves.

Nerve injury from *cervical root compression* (see Chapter 148) due to cervical spine disease or a *thoracic outlet syndrome* can produce pain in the chest and upper arm, superficially resembling angina. In the outlet syndrome, a cervical rib may compress part of the brachial plexus, resulting in motor and sensory deficits in an ulnar distribution at the same time that there is discomfort in the chest and upper arm (see Chapter 167).

Lungs and Pleura

Inflammation or distention of the pleura produces true "pleuritic pain," which is worsened by deep inspiration and cough but relatively unaffected by movement or palpation. A host of causes can trigger the inflammatory process, including *pneumonia, pulmonary embolization with infarction, neoplasm, uremia,* and *connective tissue disease.* The more florid the inflammation, the greater is the pain. An infectious origin is more likely to cause pain than is a low-grade serositis associated with connective tissue disease.

Pneumococcal Pneumonia and Pulmonary Tuberculosis

Pneumococcal pneumonia and pulmonary tuberculosis are the archetypical pneumonias associated with pleural involvement. The onset of symptoms in pneumococcal pneumonia (fever, chills, cough, sputum production, pleuritic chest pain) may be acute and mimic pulmonary embolization (see Chapter 52).

Pulmonary Embolization

Pulmonary embolization can cause pleuritic pain, especially when embolization leads to parenchymal infarction and pleural reaction. Pleural rub, effusion, low-grade fever, and hemoptysis also herald pulmonary infarction with pleural involvement. However, in some instances, the pain may be less clearly pleuritic and is often absent; it is estimated that fewer than 10% of all embolic episodes are accompanied by chest pain. The classic cardiopulmonary manifestations of embolization—dyspnea, *tachypnea,* and *tachycardia*—are nearly universal but may be short lived. *Hypoxemia* and oxygen desaturation may or may not be present, depending on the degree of mismatch between ventilation and perfusion. Severe embolization can cause acute *pulmonary hypertension* manifested by systemic hypotension, jugular venous distention, an accentuated pulmonic component of the second heart sound, acute tricuspid regurgitation, chest x-ray abnormalities, and electrocardiographic manifestations of acute right heart strain (see later discussion).

Spontaneous Pneumothorax

Spontaneous pneumothorax stretches the pleura and results in acute onset of pleuritic pain and dyspnea. The condition occurs in young persons and those with emphysema, in which there can be rupture of a bleb. If the pneumothorax is large, deviation of the trachea may be observed.

Pleurodynia

Pleurodynia is a self-limited source of pleuritic pain, most commonly in children and young adults, and is associated with a respiratory viral infection, such as that due to Coxsackie virus B. A typical viral syndrome precedes the acute onset of chest pain. Chest pain in the setting of a viral upper respiratory infection may also occur from cough-initiated injury to the chest wall or from bronchospasm. Young healthy persons sometimes note a sudden sharp pleuritic episode relieved by taking a deep breath, referred to as the *precordial-catch syndrome.* Its mechanism is unclear, but a transient folding of the pleura on itself is hypothesized.

Heart and Pericardium

Angina Pectoris

Angina pectoris due to occlusive *coronary artery disease* is the most important cardiac source of chest pain. Coronary perfusion may be similarly compromised by critical *aortic stenosis* leading to angina (see Chapter 33). The classic hallmarks of angina are its sudden onset with exertion, emotional stress, or eating (usually a very large meal) and its relief within minutes by rest or nitroglycerin. Patients usually describe their chest pain as a squeezing, heaviness, or pressure, although it may be burning or sharp. The quality of the pain is not diagnostic, and many patients state the sensation is more a "discomfort" than a true pain. Radiation to the jaw, neck, shoulder, arm, back, or upper abdomen is common and may present in the absence of chest symptoms. At times, the arm is reported to feel numb or tingling. Autonomic epiphenomena such as diaphoresis and nausea may accompany the episode, as may dyspnea if there is transient pump failure or marked anxiety. Episodes last 2 to 20 minutes. Prompt response to nitroglycerin is characteristic; relief is usually obtained within 5 minutes. Often patients make gestures in describing their chest pain. Those traditionally associated with ischemia include the *Levine sign* (clenched fist brought to the chest), the *palm sign* (extended palm touching the chest), and the *arm sign* (touching the left arm with the right hand). Prevalences in prospective observational study of patients presenting to the emergency room with chest pain were 11%, 35%, and 16%, respectively; sensitivities for coronary artery disease were low (9%, 38%, and 16%, respectively) and specificities were higher (84%, 67%, and 78%, respectively), but positive predictive values were modest (50%, 65%, and 55%, respectively) and contributed little to refining the pretest probability.

Gender and racial differences in presentation have been explored. The clinical presentation of myocardial ischemia in *women*, particularly women younger than the age of 60 years, can differ from that in men. Chest pain is more likely to be absent or atypical (see later discussion) and may be overshadowed by exertional fatigue, shortness of breath, diaphoresis, arm tingling, jaw discomfort, nausea, or other epiphenomena of ischemia that are easy to dismiss as "noncardiac." Diabetes mellitus is a major risk factor for the early onset of ischemic heart disease in women. With regard to the effect of race on presentation, acute chest pain presentations appear to be similar among whites and African Americans.

Unstable Angina

Unstable angina is one of the *acute coronary syndromes*, along with *non–Q-wave myocardial infarction* and *Q-wave myocardial infarction*. All are important causes of coronary chest pain and result from acute plaque rupture, which triggers platelet activation, thrombin clot formation, and active vasoconstriction. The clinical presentations of unstable angina include onset of new chest pain within the last 2 months severe enough to inhibit activity; established angina now increasing in frequency, severity, and duration (*crescendo angina*) and occurring with progressively less provocation; and development of *rest pain* or *nocturnal angina* in a person with a previously stable anginal pattern. Immediate mortality risk is high (up to 4%) but declines after 1 to 2 weeks. Clinical features associated with greatest risk include rest pain in excess of 20 minutes, signs of pump failure (hypotension, rales, S_3), new or worsening mitral regurgitation, and 1 mm or more of ST-segment change with pain.

Women with unstable angina are less likely than men to present with acute ST-segment elevation indicative of vessel-occluding infarction. Compared with men presenting with unstable angina, they are older and more likely to have diabetes, hypertension, and prior heart failure, and they typically present hours later into the episode.

Myocardial Infarction

Myocardial infarction is typically heralded by chest pain exceeding that of unstable angina, but the presentation is often more subtle or even silent, particularly in diabetics, the elderly, and women. Bad prognostic signs include heart failure, hy-

potension, mitral regurgitation, ST-segment elevation, and a new left-bundle-branch block. Onset of *postinfarction angina* is also associated with high risk.

Variant Angina

Variant angina, as originally described by Prinzmetal, refers to anginal pain occurring exclusively at rest in conjunction with transient ST-segment elevation on electrocardiogram (ECG). Classically, this syndrome was associated with coronary artery spasm at the site of high-grade proximal fixed stenosis. However, other forms of coronary disease may produce a similar clinical picture, and coronary vasospasm may present in ways other than Prinzmetal's description. *Cocaine abuse* can trigger ischemia by precipitating coronary vasoconstriction, increasing myocardial oxygen demand, and enhancing platelet aggregation. It may present as angina in a young person with no other coronary heart disease (CHD) risk factors.

Atypical Angina (Atypical Chest Pain)

Atypical angina is a term used to denote angina-like chest pain that differs in location, quality, or other characteristics from more typical angina yet is still suggestive by virtue of similar precipitants, timing, or other features. Some define the term more precisely, indicating the presence of any two of angina's three cardinal features (substernal location, exercise precipitation, prompt relief by rest or nitroglycerin). As many as 50% of such patients who come to angiography prove to have coronary disease. Among the remainder, there appear to be increased incidences of panic disorder, major depression, esophageal disease, and coronary microcirculatory dysfunction. The mechanisms for many of these causes are not well understood, but recent interest has focused on the coronary microcirculation.

Coronary Microvascular Dysfunction (Microvascular Angina, Coronary Syndrome X)

Coronary microvascular dysfunction (microvascular angina, coronary syndrome X) has been noted among patients with typical angina who exhibit an ischemic response to exercise stress testing yet have entirely normal coronary angiograms. Proposed mechanisms include abnormal microvascular responses to autonomic and biochemical stimuli. Patients experience typical anginal chest pain and reductions in subendocardial perfusion in response to adenosine infusion. Prognosis is good and similar to that for normal persons without coronary disease. A few patients develop mild left ventricular dysfunction or conduction abnormalities. Microvascular dysfunction provides a possible explanation for the chest pain of patients with *hypertrophic cardiomyopathy*.

Mitral Valve Prolapse

Mitral valve prolapse is notorious for its association with atypical chest pain. The commonly held view of a link between the two has been challenged by recent studies controlling more stringently for selection bias. Some argue that the apparent association is due to an increased frequency of underlying psychopathology, such as panic disorder (see later discussion), which may trigger chest pain. Symptoms of autonomic dysfunction (e.g., palpitations, sweating, dizziness) may sometimes accompany the chest pain and simulate an ischemic attack.

Pericarditis

Pericarditis may present with pleuritic pain, resulting from spread of the inflammatory process from the relatively insensitive pericardium to the adjacent pain-sensitive parietal pleura. The pain is sharp, aggravated by respiratory activity, and sometimes precipitated by swallowing if the posterior aspect of the heart is involved. When the diaphragmatic surface of the pericardium is involved, pain will be referred to the tip of the shoulder. Change in position may alter the pain. Patients often note a lessening of pain on sitting up and leaning forward. Pericarditis can also produce a second type of pain that mimics angina. Its most diagnostic physical finding is a two- or three-component friction rub.

A vexing pericardial problem is the development of chest pain after coronary bypass surgery. The return of typical angina raises the specter of graft occlusion, but pleuritic pain suggests the *postpericardiotomy syndrome*.

Aorta

Aortic dissection is a must-not-miss cause of chest pain. Almost invariably (70% to 90% of cases), it begins with sudden onset of severe chest or interscapular pain, maximal from the start, and tearing or ripping in quality. If it begins in the chest, it may radiate to the interscapular region, neck, jaw, lower back, or even down into the legs. Associated symptoms include neurologic deficits from cutoff of blood supply to the brain, spinal cord, or limb. Loss or diminution of a major peripheral pulse is a key physical finding, as are new onset of aortic insufficiency and pericardial tamponade due to dissection into the aortic root.

Esophagus

Esophageal pain can be the great mimicker of anginal chest pain, producing chest discomfort that can resemble angina in quality, location, radiation, and even precipitants (e.g., exposure to cold, exertion). Unlike angina, esophageal chest pain is more likely to persist as a dull sensation for several hours after an acute attack and may occur with swallowing. The pain sometimes radiates to the interscapular region. The chest pain may occur spontaneously or in the context of meals or *acid reflux* (manifested by retrosternal burning that may be brought on by a large meal, lying down, or bending over and is relieved by antacids). Some patients report *dysphagia* as an accompanying symptom. In some instances, studies of esophageal function reveal *motor dysfunction* (e.g., nonpropulsive contractions or "spasm") and acid reflux from the stomach. Nitrates and calcium-channel blockers may provide relief in such cases, as they do for angina. Some patients with atypical chest pain and normal coronary angiograms manifest both esophageal spasm and microcirculatory dysfunction, raising the intriguing possibility of a generalized disorder of smooth muscle reactivity.

About half of patients with noncardiac (i.e., angiogram-negative) angina-like chest pain report no concurrent dysphagia or heartburn and manifest no signs of reflux or motor dysfunction on detailed esophageal testing. In the past, such chest pain was labeled as "*noncardiac chest pain of unknown etiology*"; however, controlled studies using impedance planimetry reveal esophageal *hypersensitivity, hyperreactivity*, and *stiffness* in a large proportion of previously undiagnosed patients. These findings suggest a *sensory* or "*nociceptive*" etiology to much noncardiac chest pain. It appears that, in such patients, normal degrees of esophageal distention result in exaggerated perceptions of pain and in hyperreactivity.

Other Gastrointestinal Tract Sources

An attack of acute *cholecystitis* may resemble angina by producing substernal discomfort that responds to nitrates, which reduce cystic duct spasm. On rare occasions, *pancreatitis* or *peptic ulcer disease* produces substernal chest pain. Even a patient with gaseous distention of the bowel in the area of the splenic flexure may complain of precordial discomfort.

Psychiatric Causes

Dramatic chest pain presentations are common among patients with underlying psychopathology. In addition to presentations that may be clinically indistinguishable from angina, patients with *anxiety* or *depression* often describe feelings of chest heaviness or tightness that can last for hours to days, unrelated to exertion and unrelieved by rest. In patients with anxiety disorders, this sensation may be accompanied by a feeling of inability to take in a deep breath. When there is associated hyperventilation, the resulting hypocapnia leaves the patient lightheaded and the extremities tingling.

Cardiac neurosis may lead to reports of chest pain mimicking angina. At other times, the patient misinterprets a noncardiac chest sensation. Patients with a *personality disorder* and *somatization* may describe almost any form of chest pain, including some suggestive of angina. A lifelong pattern of multiple refractory bodily complaints is characteristic (see Chapter 230). *Malingering* represents a conscious effort to feign illness for secondary gain. The hallmark is inconsistency of the story. Although other forms of psychogenic chest pain may bring secondary benefits to the patient, there is no premeditated attempt to deceive.

Depression and *panic disorder* can be sources of atypical chest pain. Patients with such conditions tend to be younger, more often female, more apt to have a higher number of accompanying autonomic symptoms, more bothered by phobias, and more likely to describe an atypical form of chest pain than those with chest pain and a positive coronary angiogram.

DIFFERENTIAL DIAGNOSIS

The differential diagnosis of chest pain can be organized along anatomic lines, as outlined in Table 20.1. Must-not-miss diagnoses include CHD, critical aortic stenosis, aortic dissection, pneumothorax, cholecystitis, pericarditis, and pleuritis from pneumonia, embolization, or cancer. Underdiagnosis and delay in diagnosis of CHD is a problem in women younger than the age of 60 years because their clinical presentations may be atypical or ignored. A high index of suspicion is warranted in such persons, especially when there is preexisting diabetes, which is a major risk factor for the early development of CHD in women. Underdiagnosis of CHD is also a problem for African Americans presenting with chest pain.

WORKUP (2,3,8,13–42)

The first priority is to determine the *need for emergent hospitalization*. This requires estimating the likelihood of myocardial ischemia, aortic dissection, and pulmonary embolization, conditions that place the patient at high risk for a potentially life-threatening complication. Timeliness of the assessment is of the utmost importance because outcome often depends on prompt intervention. In many instances, the decision to

TABLE 20.1

DIFFERENTIAL DIAGNOSIS OF CHEST PAIN

Chest Wall
- Muscular disorders
  - Muscle spasm (precordial-catch syndrome)
  - Pleurodynia
  - Muscle strain
- Skeletal disorders
  - Costochondritis (Tietze's syndrome)
  - Rib fracture
  - Metastatic disease of bone
  - Cervical or thoracic spine disease
- Neurologic disorders
  - Herpes zoster infection or postherpetic pain
  - Nerve root compression

Cardiopulmonary
- Cardiac disorders
  - Pericarditis
  - Myocardial ischemia
  - Prolapsed mitral valve
- Pleuropulmonary disorders
  - Pleurisy of any origin
  - Pneumothorax
  - Pulmonary embolization with infarction
  - Pneumonitis
  - Bronchospasm

Aortic
- Dissecting aortic aneurysm

Gastrointestinal
- Esophageal disorders
  - Reflux
  - Spasm
- Others
  - Cholecystitis
  - Peptic ulcer disease
  - Pancreatitis
  - Splenic flexure gas

Psychogenic
- Anxiety (with or without hyperventilation)
- Cardiac neurosis
- Malingering
- Depression

immediately hospitalize will need to be made by history alone, often on the basis of a telephone call by the patient. Delaying hospitalization is a major cause of poor outcome. Delays tend to be particularly prevalent among women and African Americans. Postmenopausal women presenting with ischemic chest pain are one-third less likely to be admitted to the hospital than men with the same degree of cardiac risk.

An efficient triage strategy for initial decision making is one that determines and stratifies chest pain risk on the basis of presenting history supplemented by physical examination, ECG, and on occasion chest x-ray (if available and deemed necessary). Predictions of risk based on this approach have proven to be extremely powerful and can be used to determine who will benefit most from prompt hospitalization and aggressive testing. Extensively testing low-probability patients for ischemia, dissection, and embolization is not only wasteful, it also leads to a high false-alarm rate with its attendant adverse consequences. Although there may be psychological pressure to proceed to elaborate diagnostic studies in all patients with chest

pain, only those with at least a modest pretest probability (e.g., at least 20%) of serious pathology benefit from such testing (see Chapter 2). The provision of meaningful reassurance does not usually require exhaustive testing, but it is aided by a careful clinical assessment (see the section Patient Education and Indications for Referral).

History

Estimating Probability of Coronary Disease by History

A careful chest pain description is critical. The prevalence of angiographically confirmed CHD approaches 90% in persons with a classic story for angina (see prior discussion). Prevalence declines to less than 15% in those coming to catheterization who have nonanginal chest pain. In the Framingham Study, patients presenting with new onset of definite angina had a relative risk of a coronary event over 2 years of 3.7 for men and 5.9 for women. Relative risk for those with possible angina fell to 3.0 for men and 2.9 for women, and it fell to 1.3 for men and 0.8 for women with nonanginal chest pain.

Among the features of the chest pain description with the greatest discriminant value are its *timing* in relation to *precipitating* and *alleviating factors*. Quality, location, radiation, and intensity of pain are notoriously nonspecific. Precordial pain radiating down the left arm can occur with almost any cause of chest pain. A common pitfall in taking the history is to provide classic descriptions of chest pain to the patient who cannot give a quick, crisp account of his or her chest pain. Under the duress of the physician's interrogation, the patient may agree to one of these neat descriptions, leading to a false-positive diagnosis. The initial vagueness may have been more useful. As noted earlier, gestures traditionally associated with coronary disease, such as the *Levine sign*, have only modest predictive value that are usually insufficient to change the probability of coronary disease based on more-predictive clinical features.

Past medical history is reviewed for major *cardiac risk factors* (e.g., hypertension, diabetes, smoking, hypercholesterolemia, and obesity). Inquiry into cocaine use is essential, especially in young persons presenting with ischemia-like chest pain. *Family history* is checked for *premature coronary disease*. Note is also taken of patient *age* and *gender*. Postmenopausal women with coronary artery disease have an especially poor prognosis. Awareness of the potential biasing effects of gender and race on clinical thinking is critical to avoiding them. Race and gender have been found to be independent determinants of how patients are assessed. Because there are no differences in acute chest pain presentations among whites and African Americans, the chest pain presentation can be evaluated without the need to adjust for race. However, differences in CHD presentation between sexes need to be kept in mind. Women are often underdiagnosed, in part because the story may be atypical or vague (e.g., exertional fatigue, arm tingling, nausea, shortness of breath). A high index of suspicion for CHD is required in women younger than the age of 60 years presenting with chest pain, especially if they have preexisting diabetes (which negates the beneficial effects of estrogen).

Checking for Acute Coronary Syndrome

Any person with angina-like pain and cardiac risk factors should be asked if the pain is of *greater than 20 minutes'* duration, *crescendo* in pattern, now occurring at *rest* or at *night* and with exertion, of *new onset* (especially if severe enough to limit activity), or associated with *dyspnea*. An answer of "yes" to any of these questions on telephone triage should prompt immediate hospitalization by ambulance because the risk of an acute coronary syndrome is sufficiently high and time is of the utmost importance. If evaluated in the office, the patient needs only a brief physical examination and ECG (only if immediately available; see later discussion) to complete the initial assessment.

Considering Noncardiac Etiologies in Persons with Angina-Like Pain

Some elements of the history suggestive of coronary disease are also important for the other causes they suggest. Pain brought on by exertion and relieved by rest is certainly indicative of angina, but psychogenic disease and even esophageal spasm may behave in a similar fashion, necessitating at least consideration of these alternative diagnoses. A check for anxiety, depression, panic episodes, headache, nervousness, weakness, fatigue, and lifelong history of multiple bodily complaints may help to identify a psychogenic origin. Heartburn, dysphagia, symptoms associated with meals, and an absence of CHD risk factors raise the possibility of esophageal disease. Recurrent episodes that last hours to days provide further evidence of a noncardiac origin. Prompt response to nitroglycerin is another characteristic feature of CHD, but esophageal spasm, coronary microvascular disease, cystic duct spasm, and even some psychogenic etiologies may also respond to nitrates. Chest pain brought on by eating may be due to angina, but in the absence of other risk factors for CHD, one needs to consider gastroesophageal or pancreaticobiliary pathology. As noted earlier, response to nitroglycerin is not necessarily helpful in differentiation.

Checking for Aortic Dissection

Attention to onset, radiation, and associated symptoms is critical for early identification of aortic dissection. One checks for *sudden* onset; *maximum* intensity from the start (often described as a catastrophic presentation of tearing or searing pain); radiation into the *interscapular* region, *jaw, neck*, or down into the *lower back* or *legs*; and any accompanying *new neurologic deficit or syncopal episode*. Such a presentation should strongly suggest acute dissection of the thoracic aorta and warrant consideration of immediate hospitalization. Past medical history is reviewed for atherosclerotic risk factors, existing vascular disease, blunt trauma to the chest, and connective tissue disease (e.g., Marfan's syndrome). Although many less serious conditions can cause chest pain that radiates into the back (esophageal pathology being the most common), the seriousness of aortic dissection mandates a careful review of the history and risk factors. From 70% to 90% of cases exhibit the characteristically dramatic presentation, but 10% to 30% are more subtle in their manifestations, necessitating a high index of suspicion for the condition.

Evaluating Pleuritic Pain

Pain worsened by deep inspiration or cough is a hallmark of pleural irritation, but such pain is also suggestive of pericarditis and chest wall pathology. Even aortic dissection may cause pain worsened by movement due to respiration. Focal *chest wall tenderness* worsened by movement quickly narrows the differential to a chest wall origin. In the absence of focal chest wall pain, one needs to search promptly for evidence of intrathoracic pathology. Inquiry is needed into fever, cough, sputum production, tuberculosis exposure, hemoptysis, smoking, HIV exposure or high-risk behavior, unilateral leg edema, calf tender-

ness, shortness of breath, past history of embolization, recent orthopedic surgery, and oral contraceptive use. Pneumothorax should come to mind when pleuritic pain is *sudden* in onset and accompanied by *dyspnea* in a young patient with a previous history of pneumothorax or when the patient has longstanding bullous emphysema. Precordial-catch syndrome is suggested by brief, self-limited episodes in an otherwise healthy young person. Pleuritic pain worsened by turning but relieved by *sitting up and leaning forward* is indicative of pericarditis, which can be further assessed by physical examination. Attention to *the context* of the patient's pleuritic pain often suggests the diagnosis. Onset in a person with known metastatic cancer may be due to a pathologic fracture, pleural metastasis, or pulmonary embolization. The same pain in an otherwise healthy young person with new onset of a dry cough, low-grade fever, and myalgias is consistent with viral-induced pleurodynia and muscle soreness from coughing.

Estimating the pretest probability of pulmonary embolization is a critical task in the evaluation of the chest pain patient who also presents with acute shortness of breath. Studies using multivariate analysis have identified key elements of the history that make important independent contributions to the probability of pulmonary embolization (Table 20.2). These include sudden onset or sudden worsening of dyspnea, pleuritic or noncardiac (nonretrosternal) chest pain, hemoptysis, asymmetric leg edema or pain, and the presence of risk factors for thromboembolism (history of prior thromboembolic disease; strongly positive family history of thromboembolism; recent immobilization; recent surgery, particularly orthopedic surgery; concurrent malignancy; lower-extremity paralysis). High fever, preexisting cardiopulmonary disease, and evidence for an alternative etiology reduce the pretest probability. Determination of the pretest probability helps in decisions regarding subsequent workup for thromboembolism (see later discussion).

Physical Examination

In cases of acute chest pain in which the history is very suggestive of unstable angina, pulmonary embolization, or aortic dissection, the decision immediately to hospitalize can be made on the basis of history alone. There is no reason to delay admission. In the setting of less acute chest pain or a more ambiguous story, the physical examination can provide important evidence pertinent to the differential diagnosis and the assessment of risk.

General appearance and vital signs can be telling. *Tachypnea* and *tachycardia* in a person with acute pleuritic pain are suggestive of pulmonary embolization, whereas an anxious, sighing, hyperventilating individual who complains of constant chest tightness is more likely to be suffering from an anxiety disorder. Blood pressure is noted for elevation (an important risk factor for cardiovascular disease), for *hypotension* (a bad prognostic sign in acute coronary syndromes and pulmonary embolization), and for *asymmetry* in the arms (a sign of thoracic aortic dissection).

The *skin* is checked for cyanosis, herpetic rash, pallor, jaundice, and xanthomata. Examination of the *fundi* may provide evidence of atherosclerotic, diabetic, or hypertensive disease. In the *neck*, the *carotid pulse* is palpated for diminution or loss when considering thoracic aortic dissection and for delay in upstroke when assessing for hemodynamically significant aortic stenosis. In addition, *jugular venous pressure* is determined; jugular venous distention may be noted in the setting of pump

TABLE 20.2

ESTIMATION OF THE PRETEST PROBABILITY OF PULMONARY EMBOLISM—THE WELLS SCORE

Clinical Feature	Score
Clinical signs and symptoms of DVT (objectively measured leg swelling and pain with palpation in the deep-vein system)	3.0
Heart rate >100 beats/min	1.5
Immobilization for 3 or more consecutive days (bed rest except to go to the bathroom) or surgery in previous 4 wk	1.5
Previous objectively diagnosed pulmonary embolism or DVT	1.5
Hemoptysis	1.0
Cancer (with treatment within last 6 mo or palliative treatment)	1.0
Pulmonary embolism likely or more likely than alternative diagnoses (based on history, physical examination, chest x-ray, ECG, and O_2 level)	3.0
Pretest Probability	
Low: <2.0	
Intermediate: 2.0–6.0	
High: >6.0	

Adopted from Stein PD, Fowler SE, Goodman LR, et al. Multidetector computer tomography for acute pulmonary embolism. N Engl J Med 2006;354:2317, based on data from Wells PS, Anderson DR, Rodger M, et al. Excluding pulmonary embolism at the bedside without diagnostic imaging: management of patients with suspect pulmonary embolism presenting to the emergency department by using a simple clinical model and D-dimer. Ann Intern Med 2001;135:98, with permission.

failure due to acute ischemia, acute pulmonary hypertension due to severe pulmonary embolization, and cardiac tamponade associated with pericarditis.

The *chest wall* is examined carefully in the person reporting "pleuritic" pain, beginning with inspection for signs of trauma and the *rash of herpes zoster* and palpation for swelling and focal tenderness. If pain is elicited, it is important to be sure the pain on palpation is identical to the patient's presenting complaint.

One should next listen to the *lungs for a pleural friction rub* during inspiration and expiration and note any signs of consolidation or effusion. *Hyperresonance, absent breath sounds,* and *tracheal deviation* suggest a significant pneumothorax that requires immediate attention, especially if the patient is also tachycardic, hypotensive, and cyanotic. Checking for *rales* (crackles) in the patient with angina assesses the possibility of ischemic left ventricular dysfunction (another sign of pump failure and poor prognosis).

On examination of the *heart*, the left ventricular impulse is observed and noted for signs of hypertrophy (indicative of significant aortic stenosis, longstanding hypertension, or a hypertrophic cardiomyopathy). Signs of ischemic myocardial dysfunction, such as *loss of physiologic splitting* of the second heart sound, development of an S_4, and presence of an S_3, are sought; they may be transient, occurring only during chest pain, but their presence suggests considerable myocardium at risk. Listening for the *systolic ejection murmur* of aortic stenosis should not be forgotten in the patient with angina nor should the *systolic regurgitant murmur* of mitral regurgitation due to papillary muscle ischemia. Although the relation between mitral valve prolapse and chest pain is questionable, checking for its hallmark *midsystolic click* and *late-systolic murmur* are indicated in persons with atypical chest pain. If the chest pain is pleuritic, then carefully listening for the two- to three-component *precordial friction rub* of pericarditis is indicated, as is checking for an accentuated pulmonic component of the second heart sound and a new tricuspid regurgitant murmur

indicative of acute pulmonary hypertension from severe pulmonary embolization.

The *abdomen* is checked for epigastric and *right upper quadrant tenderness* (especially when evidence suggests gastric or hepatobiliary disease) and for masses (particularly an abdominal *aneurysm* in the context of suspected dissection). The *legs* require careful examination for unilateral edema and other signs of phlebitis (see Chapter 22), a potential source of pulmonary embolization in the person presenting with pleuritic pain. All *peripheral pulses* are checked, noting any absences and evidence of acute ischemia, which might occur with an aortic dissection. The *spine* is palpated for areas of tenderness along the cervical and thoracic segments, and the *neurologic* examination needs to include a check for new focal deficits, another possible clue to dissection.

Laboratory Studies

Outpatient Testing versus Immediate Transport to the Emergency Room

Although laboratory studies can be helpful, one should not delay the decision to urgently transport the patient to the nearest emergency room (ER) when the clinical picture suggests unstable angina, acute pulmonary embolization, aortic dissection, or large pneumothorax. In fact, any delay brought about by taking time to obtain "nice-to-have" but not essential diagnostic studies in the office could be life threatening. Only those studies that are essential to immediate decision making should be considered. Even an ECG may be superfluous in the face of a good story for unstable angina because a normal study would not change the decision to get the patient quickly to the nearest ER. Obviously, an ECG is essential to ER decision making and should be obtained within minutes of the patient's arrival, but initial triage decisions made outside the hospital will be based largely on the patient's story.

Test Selection

An accurate estimation of pretest probability is essential to the workup of chest pain, especially as it pertains to effective test selection and interpretation (see Chapter 2). The number of "must-not-miss" conditions is large, and there is considerable pressure on the clinician to test extensively and exhaustively. The risks inherent in ignoring the pretest probability are poor test selection and misinterpretation of test results (see Chapter 2) leading to diagnostic errors and potentially harmful management decisions. Accurate estimation of pretest probability is afforded by focusing on the key history and physical examination findings noted earlier.

Another potential source of error in test selection is diagnostic bias associated with the patient's sociodemographic status (e.g., race, gender, social group). Physician responses to the chest pain presentation are sometimes affected by such factors and need to be kept in mind. For example, African American women are 60% less likely to be referred for cardiac catheterization than are white men with the same pretest risk of coronary disease. Women and nonwhites are less likely to be hospitalized when presenting with acute ischemia.

Testing for Suspected Coronary Artery Disease

The approach to laboratory workup for coronary disease is determined by the condition's pretest probability and an appreciation for the sensitivity, specificity, and cost of available tests (Table 20.3).

High Pretest Probability: Unstable Angina Presentation. As noted earlier, the very high probability patient (multiple CHD risk factors, history very suggestive of *unstable angina*) requires *immediate hospitalization* without delay. Additional outpatient testing is unwarranted.

Electrocardiogram. Once the patient arrives in the emergency room, a *resting ECG* is critical to initial decision making, which is used in most critical pathways for optimal emergency room triage of chest pain patients. Any ST- or T-wave changes indicative of ischemia are an indication for prompt consideration of therapy, be it thrombolytic or revascularization (see later discussion). Proceeding directly to *coronary angiography* is more cost-effective than stress testing in such very high probability patients with ECG changes.

A normal ECG is not by itself sufficient evidence for discharge of the high-probability patient, but a shortened period of observation (e.g., 6 hours) followed by *stress testing* is being applied in some centers to safely minimize the length of stay for patients with no ECG changes and normal serum levels of markers of myocardial injury (e.g., *creatine kinase* and *troponins*). Exclusionary criteria for early stress testing include ongoing chest pain, signs of heart failure, and elevations in creatine phosphokinase or troponin levels.

Creatine Kinase MB Isozyme and Cardiac Troponins T and I. Creatine kinase MB isozyme (CK-MB) and cardiac troponins T and I are macromolecular markers of myocardial injury that facilitate the emergent evaluation of chest pain, especially in patients with high or intermediate pretest probability. In cases of infarction, the CK-MB level usually begins to rise within 4 hours of myocardial injury, almost always turns positive by 12 to 24 hours, and then begins to decline unless there is reinfarction. Although sensitivity is high, specificity is not as good because other causes of myocardial injury can also cause CK-MB elevation. Cardiac troponins T and I provide enhanced sensitivity and specificity for the detection of myocardial injury and are more predictive of future coronary events. Levels rise at the same rate as CK-MB but persist for days, making the test less useful for the detection of reinfarction. Rapid assays for troponins T and I show respective sensitivities at 6 hours of 94% and 100% and specificities of 89% and 83% in persons with normal electrocardiograms. Although troponin T is excreted renally, renal insufficiency does not impair its predictive value. It is common practice to obtain CK-MB and troponin levels simultaneously and serially, although some authorities suggest reserving troponin determinations for situations in which clinical suspicion persists despite normal ECG and CK-MB levels.

Experimental Markers. The search continues for additional markers that can independently contribute to the coronary risk assessment, particularly in the ER setting, where the goal is not to discharge a patient at risk. The *C-reactive protein, erythrocyte sedimentation rate,* and *myeloperoxidase* (which derives from activated leukocytes, which are believed to be pathophysiologically important in vulnerable plaques) have shown some promise in providing additional predictive value in persons presenting with ischemic chest pain, a nondiagnostic ECG, and normal levels of CK-MB and troponins. Further confirmation of these findings is required before they can be recommended for routine use in the workup of chest pain.

TABLE 20.3

SENSITIVITY, SPECIFICITY, AND COSTS OF STRESS TESTS FOR THE DETECTION OF CORONARY DISEASE

Test Type	Sensitivity	Specificity	Sensitivity for Three-Vessel/Left-Main Disease	Relative Cost
Electrocardiographic	0.68	0.77	0.86	1.0
Echocardiographic	0.76	0.88	0.94	2.5
Thallium imaging, planar only	0.79	0.73	0.93	2.0
SPECT scanning	0.88	0.77	0.98	4.0
PET scanning	0.91	0.82	?	14.0

PET, positron emission tomography; SPECT, single-photon emission computed tomography.
From Garber AM, Solomon NA. Cost-effectiveness of alternative test strategies for the diagnosis of coronary artery disease. Ann Intern Med 1999;130:719, with permission.

High Pretest Probability: Stable Angina Presentation. The patient with CHD risk factors and a clinical presentation that is classic for *stable angina* does not need any testing to establish the diagnosis of coronary disease (the pretest probability is already >90%). Instead, the role of testing is to *estimate prognosis and stratify risk*, which inform the selection of initial treatment (i.e., revascularization vs. medical therapy; see Chapter 30). A well-recognized prognostic determinant is the *amount of myocardium at risk*, which can be assessed by electrocardiographic, radionuclide, or echocardiographic stress testing (see later discussion and Chapters 30 and 36). A less well-recognized risk factor is prior silent myocardial infarction, which may be detected by resting ECG (new Q waves or new ST- or T-wave changes since the last ECG) or *cardiac ultrasound* (segmental wall akinesis). Postinfarction angina is a sign of potentially severe coronary disease, especially in persons with prior silent infarction (16-fold increase in mortality risk).

Intermediate Pretest Probability: Story Suggestive of Unstable Angina. The initial approach to this patient is the same as for the high-probability patient, that is, immediate emergency room assessment (see prior discussion).

Intermediate Pretest Probability: Story Suggestive of Stable Angina. Patients in this category typically have a single cardiac risk factor and give a history of atypical chest pain that is noncrescendo in pattern. In such persons, a *resting ECG* may be helpful, but nonemergent *stress testing* is needed if the resting ECG is nondiagnostic. Several modalities are available for stress testing.

Stress Testing. *Electrocardiographic* stress testing (see also Chapter 36) provides excellent sensitivity and specificity for the detection of high-risk coronary disease (i.e., left-main, left-main-equivalent, or three-vessel disease) at low cost, but false positives occur in younger women, sensitivity is lower in the setting of less serious forms of coronary disease, and the test cannot be interpreted adequately unless the resting ECG is normal. *Stress echocardiography* can be performed by bicycle exercise or dobutamine stimulation; the cost is somewhat higher than with ECG, but sensitivity and specificity are better (see Chapter 36). *Radionuclide imaging with thallium* or *technetium sestamibi* uses planar scanning and, more recently, *single-photon emission computed tomography* (SPECT), which enhances sensitivity and specificity by providing three-dimensional views. It can be performed by treadmill exercising or adenosine injection, which causes a steal phenomenon and enhances differences in uptake. Increased sensitivity is achieved with radionuclide imaging but at increased cost.

Positron emission tomography (PET) is the most sensitive and specific test for coronary insufficiency, but it is also the most expensive and is still limited in availability. Overall, sensitivity for the detection of coronary disease by stress testing ranges from 0.68 for ECG to 0.91 for PET, but all stress tests are very sensitive for the detection of left-main, left-main-equivalent, and three-vessel coronary disease, with sensitivities ranging from 0.86 for ECG stress testing to 0.98 for SPECT. Electrocardiographic stress testing is by far the lowest in cost but is also slightly less sensitive and specific than other modalities. Cost-effectiveness analyses identify ECG and echocardiographic stress testing as the most cost-effective for diagnosis of coronary disease in chest pain patients with an intermediate pretest probability of coronary disease. SPECT may also be cost-effective in settings in which its cost is lower than average. The increased sensitivity and specificity associated with PET scanning are insufficient to overcome its very high cost (see Chapter 36).

Ambulatory Electrocardiographic Monitoring. Ambulatory electrocardiographic monitoring is not recommended because specificity is low and the false-positive rate is high.

Computed Tomography of the Coronary Arteries. Computed tomography (CT) of the coronary arteries has been proposed as an adjunctive means of assessing CHD risk, but its role remains to be precisely determined. The test is based on the ability of CT to detect and quantify coronary artery calcification, producing a *coronary artery calcium score* (CACS) that correlates with the degree of atherosclerosis. In studies of sensitivity and specificity in symptomatic persons undergoing coronary angiography, CT performs about the same as stress testing in predicting coronary disease. However, unlike stress testing, it does not provide physiologic information. When used in asymptomatic persons in conjunction with the *Framingham risk score* (FRS)—which uses age, gender, blood pressure, total and high-density-lipoprotein cholesterols, glucose, and smoking history to assess CHD risk—the CACS only enhances CHD risk prediction in patients judged to be at intermediate risk by the FRS (i.e., FRS between 10 and 20), providing a 3% to 9% increase in predicted 10-year CHD risk.

Unfortunately, the CT cannot rule out the presence of coronary disease; its false-negative rate is about 4% in asymptomatic persons, which is due to the presence of "soft" atherosclerotic plaque not detectable by CT. Such soft plaque is less stable than calcified plaque and more likely to rupture; it is the very lesion most likely to present as unstable angina. Thus, a "negative" CT scan could be as misleading as a "positive" test. The advent of *multidetector CT* offers the promise of improved sensitivity and specificity, and preliminary data are encouraging (sensitivity as high as 95% and specificity approaching 100%), but prospective validation study in patients presenting with chest pain is needed before the test can be recommended for routine use.

Low Pretest Probability. The patient with clearly nonanginal chest pain, no CHD risk factors, and a normal cardiac examination has such a low probability of CHD that testing is likely to generate only negative or false-positive results and excessive medical bills. Even a CHD test with high sensitivity and specificity will perform poorly and produce an excessive proportion of false-positive results if it is applied to a person with a very low pretest probability of CHD (see Chapters 2 and 36).

Occasionally, a *resting ECG* is obtained to reassure the very anxious low-risk patient. Performing this low-cost test has been found to speed the resumption of normal activity in the overly concerned patient without greatly increasing cost. This approach should not be used unless there is strong patient need for some "objective" reassurance and the patient is warned beforehand that a positive result is most likely to be a false positive. As lay knowledge of testing modalities for coronary disease increases, requests among low-risk patients for stress testing are likely to escalate but should be rebuffed because such testing will only increase cost without improving diagnostic accuracy.

Testing for Suspected Esophageal Disease

The obvious case of esophageal disease (retrosternal burning, difficulty swallowing) requires no testing unless the symptoms are refractory, in which case a search for malignancy is indicated (see Chapter 60). More problematic diagnostically is the patient with angina-like pain, a normal cardiac evaluation (including angiography), and no esophageal symptoms. As many as 20% of patients with pain suspicious enough to warrant coronary angiography have been shown to have esophageal disorders. A convincing diagnosis of esophageal disease might save the patient a cardiac catheterization.

Many provocative tests and esophageal function studies are available, including *manometry*, 24-hour *pH monitoring*, *edrophonium* provocation, and *acid perfusion* (see Chapter 60 for details). Although initial reports promoted their usefulness in the evaluation of chest pain, more carefully controlled study has failed to detect differences in esophageal function, either between periods of pain and no pain or between asymptomatic, healthy control subjects and patients. In about 25% of patients, edrophonium chloride or acid provocation will trigger pain in patients and not in control subjects, but there is no difference in motor response. Either motor dysfunction is not the etiology in most esophageal cases or the tests of motor function are not very good. In either case, there seems to be little rationale for their routine application. Recent reports suggest that measuring the response to *esophageal distention* better differentiates patients from control subjects. Distention testing is still a research tool and not available for clinical use, but the future trend in diagnosis of esophageal chest pain is likely to be toward the identification of altered nociception and a heightened sensory response.

Testing Strategy for Suspected Pulmonary Embolization

Just as for coronary disease, workup for suspected pulmonary embolization rests heavily on the assessment of pretest probability, readily determined by attention to key clinical features with or without the results a few simple preliminary tests (see later discussion). When used to determine the need for further testing and anticoagulation, this probabilistic (Bayesian) approach greatly facilitates decision making by enhancing diagnostic accuracy and readily differentiating low-risk persons, who require little additional workup, from those at intermediate or high risk, who need further consideration of pulmonary embolization. Simply subjecting all suspected persons irrespective of their pretest probability to the full battery of tests for pulmonary embolization is wasteful and often counterproductive, generating high false-positive rates and potentially subjecting persons to inappropriate anticoagulation.

Determining Pretest Probability (The Wells and Revised Geneva Scores). Rapid, accurate classification of patients into categories of low, intermediate, and high pretest probability can be achieved by attention to validated prediction rules based on key clinical findings and the results of a few simple preliminary tests that have been found to be independent predictors of risk.

The Wells Score (Table 20.2). This prediction rule is the most widely used and best validated for determining pretest probability of pulmonary embolism. It uses a combination of clinical/historical predictors, physician probability estimate of alternative explanations, and findings on chest x-ray, ECG, and pulse oximetry or arterial blood gas determination. Prospective validation testing of the rule finds 3-month rates of pulmonary embolism of approximately 1.5% to 3.5% among patients classified clinically as "low risk," compared with 16% to 28% for those categorized as "intermediate risk" and 38% to 78% for those labeled "high risk."

Of the screening laboratory determinations incorporated into the Wells score (i.e., ECG, chest x-ray, pulse oximetry/arterial blood gases), no single abnormal test result is diagnostic, nor is a normal finding sufficient to rule out embolization, but the results of these simple tests can contribute independently to the probability estimate. *Chest x-ray* findings are usually nonspecific, but fewer than 15% of patients with

proven pulmonary embolization have normal chest x-rays. The most common findings are *unilateral pleural effusion* and *atelectasis*. More specific but much less common radiologic manifestations include abrupt amputation of a hilar artery and a wedge-shaped *pleural-based infiltrate* ("*Hampton's hump*"); both are seen in blockade of a large vessel.

In the setting of pulmonary embolization, *ECG changes* are also common but usually nonspecific; *minor abnormalities in ST and T waves* are noted in upward of 70% of cases with no history of prior cardiovascular disease. Even more suggestive are findings associated with acute right heart strain, including the classic $S_1 Q_3 T_3$ pattern, *new right-bundle-branch block*, and *inverted T waves* in leads *V1 to V4*, believed due to posterior ischemia from compression of the right coronary artery in the setting of right ventricular overload.

Pulse oximetry and *arterial blood gas* determinations can be helpful, especially when *hypoxemia* is noted, but a normal oxygen level does not rule out embolization. Hypoxemia requiring *substantial oxygen supplementation* (>40% fraction of inspired oxygen) is suggestive of significant embolization. *The Revised Geneva Score* (Table 20.4) attempts to overcome perceived limitations of the Wells score by focusing entirely on risk factors, symptoms, and clinical signs and not relying on physician probability estimates, oxygen determinations, or findings from ECG or chest x-ray. Validation testing shows rates of embolism of 8% in the low-risk group, 28% in the intermediate category, and 75% in the high probability group. Compared to the Wells score, it appears to have a slightly higher false-negative rate, as might be expected because it relies exclusively on history and physical examination findings.

Low Pretest Probability—D-Dimer Testing. When pretest probability is low, a *d-dimer* determination is the test of choice (Fig. 20.1). A negative result (<500 ng/dL) reduces the probability of pulmonary embolism to less than 0.5% (negative

TABLE 20.4

REVISED GENEVA SCORE FOR THE PRETEST PROBABILITY OF PULMONARY EMBOLISM

Variable	Points
Risk factors	
Age >65 yr	1
Previous DVT or PE	3
Surgery under general anesthesia or fracture of lower limb within 1 mo	2
Active malignant condition	2
Symptoms	
Unilateral lower-limb pain	3
Hemoptysis	2
Clinical signs	
Heart rate 74–94 beats/min	3
Heart rate >94 beats/min	5
Pain on lower-limb deep venous palpation and unilateral edema	4
Clinical Probability	
Low	0–3 total
Intermediate	4–10 total
High	>10 total

DVT, deep venous thrombosis; PE, pulmonary embolism.
Adapted from Le Gal G, Righini M, Pierre-Marie R, et al. Prediction of pulmonary embolism in the emergency department: the revised Geneva Score. Ann Intern Med 2006;144:165, with permission.

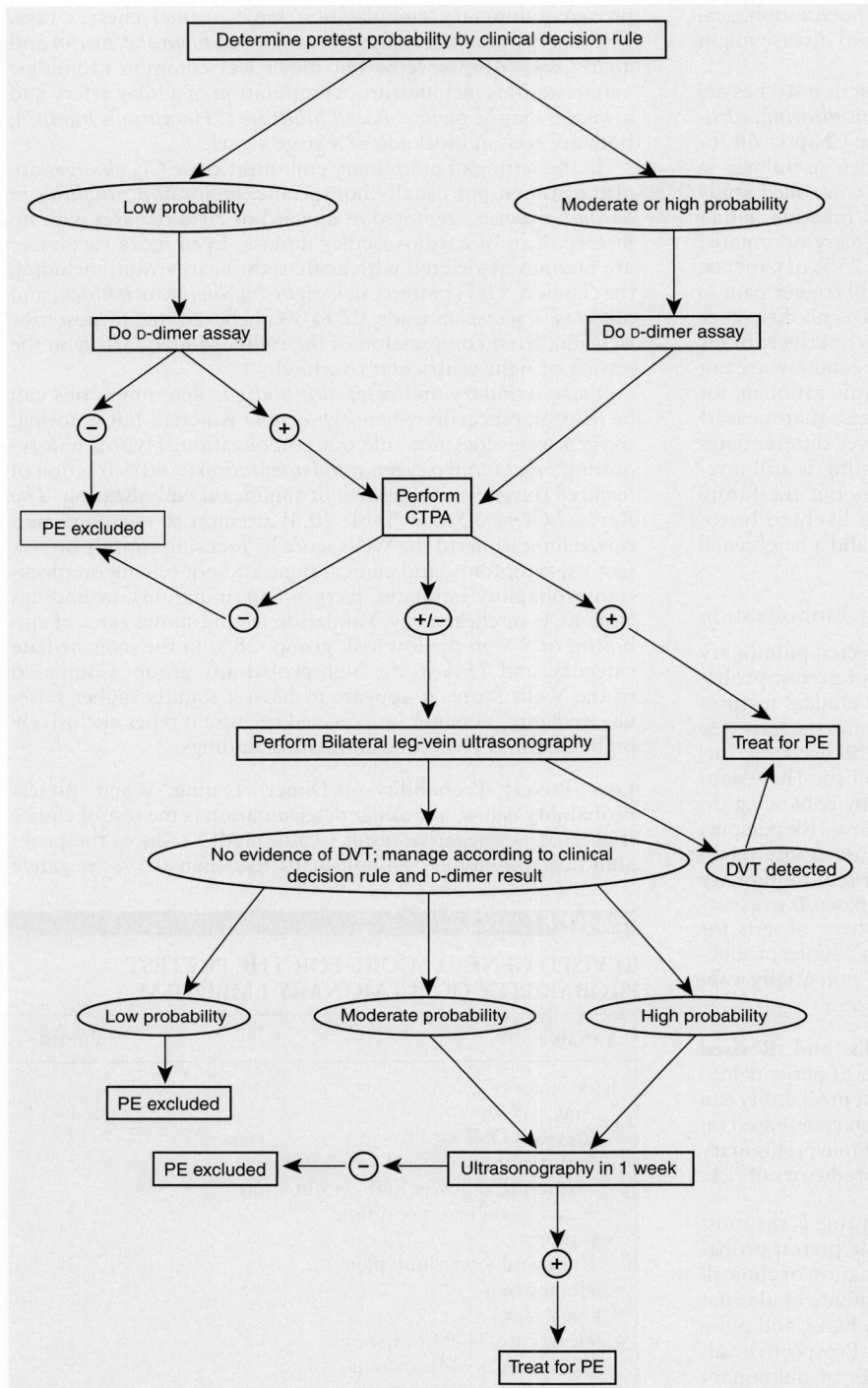

FIGURE 20.1. Diagnostic algorithm for the initial evaluation of patients with suspected pulmonary embolism. Plus and minus signs indicate positive and negative test results, respectively. CTPA, computed tomographic pulmonary angiogram; DVT, deep vein thrombosis; PE, pulmonary embolism; VQ, ventilation/perfusion lung scan. (From Wells PS, Anderson DR, Rodger M, et al. Emergency diagnosis of pulmonary embolism. Ann Intern Med 2001;135:100, with permission.)

predictive value >99.5%) and obviates the need for further testing. In a multicenter, randomized, controlled trial, none of 182 persons with low pretest probability and a negative D-dimer test without additional testing developed evidence of pulmonary embolization during follow-up; 1 of 185 who had additional testing did. Because D-dimer lacks specificity, additional testing (see later discussion) is needed when a D-dimer result is "positive" (i.e., >500 ng/dL).

D-*Dimer.* D-Dimer is a degradation product of cross-linked fibrin. Its formation occurs in the context of ongoing thrombosis and fibrinolysis, making its measurement a potentially sensitive indicator of active venous thrombosis and thromboembolization. Sensitivity in the setting of pulmonary embolism ranges from 85% to 100%, depending on the assay used. Specificity is not high (40% to 68%) and declines with advancing age because D-dimer acts as an acute-phase reactant, increasing in response to any event that induces fibrinolysis, such as inflammation, cancer, or trauma.

There are two widely available assays. The enzyme-linked immunosorbent assay is more sensitive but less specific and must be performed in the laboratory and takes about 3 to 4 hours. A rapid bedside whole-blood assay (SimpliRED) is slightly less sensitive but more specific, cutting down on the number of false positives and is more useful in settings in which the principal task is to rule out embolization. Of concern are reports of unsatisfactory performance of the whole-blood assay in cancer patients, in whom a negative result has not been found reliably to exclude deep vein thrombosis. These test characteristics make the D-dimer determination the test of choice for rapidly ruling out pulmonary embolization in patients with a low pretest probability.

Although a negative result in a low-probability patient obviates the need for further testing, a positive test needs to be interpreted in the context of the overall clinical setting and probability estimate. Patients with a low to intermediate pretest probability and a positive D-dimer test need consideration of further testing (see Intermediate Pretest Probability), whereas those with a very low pretest probability and a elevated D-dimer level might be followed expectantly without more immediate testing, especially if there is an alternative explanation for the D-dimer elevation (e.g., acute inflammation).

Intermediate Pretest Probability—Multidetector Computed Tomographic Angiography, Ventilation/Perfusion Radionuclide Scanning, and Venous imaging. The workup of this diagnostically challenging group, which often presents in the outpatient setting, has undergone a sea change in recent years as multidetector computed tomographic angiography (CTA) has rapidly replaced radionuclide ventilation/perfusion (V/Q) scanning. Unlike V/Q scanning with its often poor specificity and large percentages of "indeterminate" or "intermediate" results, CTA scanning produces clearly interpretable results in greater than 90% of cases and high levels of specificity. Its use often shortens the time to diagnosis by eliminating most of the supplementary testing commonly needed with V/Q scanning.

Multidetector CT angiography. The test is rapid, comfortable for patients (requires <10 seconds of breath holding), widely available in the community-hospital setting, and rarely inconclusive due to poor image quality. In the landmark Prospective Investigation of Pulmonary Embolism Diagnosis (PIOPED) II study, a positive CTA result in persons with intermediate pretest probability had a positive predictive value in excess of 90%. Although sensitivity was only 83% in the PIOPED study, the negative predictive value among intermediate-probability patients was greater than 90%, and only about 2% of patients with a negative CTA developed evidence of pulmonary embolism in 3 months of follow-up (suggesting that most of the emboli missed were clinically insignificant).

These performance characteristics and outcomes suggest the test can be used as a stand-alone study in this patient population. However, when the CTA result is greatly discordant with the pretest probability, other testing may be necessary. For example, when it is negative in a person with a high pretest probability, the test's negative predictive value is only 60%, and additional study is indicated (see later discussion of CT venography, as well as the subsection High Pretest Probability). Not surprisingly, the test performs poorly in persons with a low pretest probability (positive predictive value 58%); it should not be ordered in such patients because the false-positive rate is so high. CTA requires intravenous administration of iodinated contrast material, necessitating attention to hydration status,

renal function, and history of underlying kidney disease. Radiation exposure is considerable, which should be taken into account, especially when embolism is being considered in younger persons and pregnant women. Early *single-detector (helical) CTA* was too insensitive to be recommended for widespread use and has been replaced by multidetector systems.

CT Venography (CTV). Venous phase CT study of the pelvis and lower extremities provides excellent imaging of the pelvic and leg veins and a convenient means of clot detection. It can be performed following the angiographic phase of the CTA study to enhance test sensitivity. In PIOPED II, such imaging improved CTA test sensitivity by about 7 percentage points to 90%. The test may be useful when substantial clinical suspicion remains despite a negative or indeterminate CTA result, but the test is probably not cost-effective as a routine adjunct to CTA because, despite the increase in sensitivity, its contribution to the predictive value in PIOPED II was minimal over CTA in persons with intermediate pretest probability. Whether the additional expense and radiation exposure associated with routinely performing CVT with every CTA study are justified remains to be determined. Of note, adding CTV did add 22 percentage points to the negative predictive value (increasing it from 60% to 82%) of a negative test in persons with a high pretest probability.

V/Q Scan. Radionuclide imaging remains widely available and worth considering when CT angiography is unavailable, contraindicated, or equivocal. In conjunction with pretest probability determination and Doppler ultrasound scanning in PIOPED I, V/Q testing reduced the need for invasive pulmonary angiography (the previously standard diagnostic test) by nearly 40%. In selected instances, positive and negative predictive values reach into the 90% to 95% range. In the setting of an indeterminate CTA/CTV and intermediate pretest probability, a "negative" V/Q scan can rule out the diagnosis of pulmonary embolization; a positive or high-probability study confirms the diagnosis. When an indeterminate or non–high-probability V/Q test result is encountered in a patient with an intermediate pretest probability, *venous Doppler ultrasound and D-dimer* testing can help to refine the posttest probability assessment. If the ultrasound is negative and the D-dimer test is negative, then embolism is ruled out and no further testing is indicated, but if the D-dimer test is positive, then serial ultrasound testing over the next week to 10 days is a reasonable way to ensure the absence of deep vein thrombosis and a low risk of embolization.

Unfortunately, the V/Q scans of a large proportion of patients produce either equivocal results or findings that are discordant with pretest probabilities. In the PIOPED I study, the largest single group of patients included those with scans of "intermediate" probability, in whom embolization could be neither ruled in nor ruled out. High false-positive rates are especially prevalent in patients with preexisting lung disease and in the elderly. In PIOPED I, 44% of patients with a high-probability scan and a low pretest probability had no embolization by angiography. False negatives are also a problem; in PIOPED 40% of patients with a "low-probability" scan and a high pretest probability proved to have pulmonary embolization by angiography.

These high rates of false positives and false negatives among selected groups of patients and the large number of indeterminate scans reflect shortcomings in the sensitivity and the specificity of the test. Even if one assumed that any abnormality on the scan was a positive test, sensitivity would still be only about 90% and specificity just 10%. In a major randomized trial comparing V/Q to CTA, CTA proved superior in identifying emboli and at least as good in ruling out the diagnosis of embolization. Nonetheless, V/Q scanning remains widely available and particularly helpful in ruling out embolization when it is negative in a person with an intermediate pretest probability. The test appears to be safe in *pregnant women*, particularly after the first trimester.

Compression Venous Ultrasound of the Lower Extremities. Compression Doppler venous ultrasound of the lower extremities has been used to provide some of the specificity lacking in V/Q scanning and D-dimer testing. The test is very specific and sensitive for the detection of symptomatic deep vein thrombosis in the proximal veins (sensitivity 95% and specificity 96%). The application of serial ultrasound had been found to be especially useful in patients with a moderate pretest probability and indeterminate V/Q scan findings. In this setting, a normal serial ultrasound rules out the diagnosis or at least obviates the need for immediate anticoagulation or angiography; a positive study rules it in, which again avoids the need for pulmonary angiography.

Because almost all pulmonary thromboemboli originate from the deep proximal veins of the legs, venous ultrasound has been proposed as a means of improving the noninvasive diagnosis of embolization. However, the sensitivity of a single study is limited because up to 40% of patients with embolism have no detectable clot remaining in the proximal venous system after initial embolization. To overcome this limitation, serial studies are done over 1 to 2 weeks. In most instances, a clot needs to reform in the leg before reembolization. Thus, the sensitivity of the test for the risk of embolization can be greatly enhanced by performing serial ultrasound studies. Even if the diagnosis of embolism cannot be confirmed initially, the risk of reembolization can be estimated by serial study. Using serial ultrasound in conjunction with V/Q scanning and pretest probability for embolism, Canadian investigators made an accurate diagnosis in more than 96% of cases for suspected embolism; the false-negative rate was only 0.6%, with angiography needed in only 3.7% of cases.

High Pretest Probability. Such patients should be admitted and promptly heparinized pending the results of testing. Multidetector *CT angiography* has largely replaced *V/Q scanning* as the initial test of choice (Fig. 20.1). A "high-probability" CTA or V/Q scan confirms the diagnosis, demonstrating a positive predictive value of greater than 95% in the setting of a high pretest probability; no additional testing is required. A negative CTA study does not rule out embolization in high-probability patients (negative predictive value only 60%, even for multidetector CTA); additional testing is required, including consideration of CTV, V/Q scanning, and venous ultrasound (see prior discussion); pulmonary angiography remains an option if other testing is inconclusive.

Pulmonary Angiography. Pulmonary angiography remains the gold standard for the diagnosis of pulmonary embolism and should be used when definitive diagnosis is essential, urgent, and not available from noninvasive testing. Refinements in pretest probability determination and advances in noninvasive imaging have greatly reduced the need for this invasive study, which is fraught with discomfort and complications, including a large iodinated dye load, the need for right heart catheterization and prolonged breath holding, flushing, coughing, and nonsustained ventricular tachycardia. Due to difficulty with breath holding and coughing, images can be blurred and difficult to read; even under good conditions, interpreting changes beyond those in third-order vessels can be challenging. Conse-

quently, noninvasive study is preferred and angiography relegated to a backup status.

Testing for Suspected Pulmonary Infection and Other Nonembolic Causes of Pleuritic Chest Pain

The *chest x-ray* is the initial test of choice. Pneumococcal pneumonia and tuberculosis often present with acute pleuritic chest pain and may be mistaken clinically for pulmonary embolism. Consequently, any patient with pleuritic pain, sputum production, and an infiltrate of chest film should also have both *Gram's* and *acid-fast stains* made. A pleural effusion may also be detected on chest film. Any nonloculated pleural effusion of unknown etiology should be tapped, Gram's stained, cultured, examined microscopically, and sent for cell count, glucose, lactic dehydrogenase, and protein determinations (see Chapter 43). *Suspicion of pneumothorax* is also an indication for a chest film, but if radiography is not immediately available and the patient is in respiratory distress, decompression should not be delayed.

When *pericarditis* is under consideration, an ECG is essential. However, the ECG changes of early repolarization—a harmless finding seen in young men—may closely resemble those of acute pericarditis. The presence of concave ST-segment elevations in both limb and precordial leads and the presence of PR-segment depressions in the precordial leads, if they occur in the limb leads, distinguish pericarditis from early repolarization. *Cardiac ultrasonography* may reveal a pericardial effusion. An antinuclear antibody, blood urea nitrogen, and tuberculin skin test are indicated when the cause of pericarditis is not readily evident.

Suspected Aortic Dissection

A *chest x-ray*, which may demonstrate a widened mediastinum (especially in traumatic aortic rupture), is sometimes performed for screening purposes, but if dissection is truly suspected on clinical grounds, then emergency admission for aortic angiography is indicated. Delaying admission to obtain a chest film is unwise. Patients with traumatic aortic dissection may also be well served by *transesophageal ultrasonography*, which is preferred to transthoracic ultrasonography, which is less sensitive for detecting disease in the aortic arch. *CT with contrast* is useful when the aortogram is not available or is negative yet clinical suspicion remains high. Many now proceed directly to CT because it is less invasive and can be done on shorter notice than angiography. *Magnetic resonance imaging* can also detect dissection and provides another noninvasive alternative to contrast angiography.

Other Conditions

Only a few *musculoskeletal* disorders require chest radiography, including suspected rib fractures and cervical or thoracic spine disease. If a *gastrointestinal* cause is suspected, a contrast study may be in order. The ECG may show T-wave depression in cholecystitis and pancreatitis, which may mistakenly be interpreted as evidence of coronary disease.

The anxious patient with *psychogenic* pain may find a chest radiograph and/or ECG reassuring. In most instances, however, a thorough history and careful physical examination combined with a detailed explanation should suffice. Repeating tests "just to be sure" may begin to undermine the patient's confidence in the physician's explanation and even heighten anxiety, especially if there are repeat studies.

It is important to realize that as many as 10% to 15% of cases remain undiagnosed, even after careful and thorough evaluation. Nevertheless, in such instances it is still possible to rule out the presence of an acutely serious etiology. Most patients with chest pain that initially eludes diagnosis can be followed expectantly for the time being.

SYMPTOMATIC RELIEF

Relief of pain must be based on an etiologic diagnosis. Simply to suppress the pain with analgesics or sedatives before a diagnosis is made may hide important clues and endanger the patient. However, musculoskeletal forms of chest pain may benefit from analgesia, especially if the patient is splinting and not ventilating adequately. When the diagnosis of costochondritis is certain, local injection with lidocaine into the point of maximal tenderness can provide dramatic relief. An antacid regimen or histamine$_2$-blocker therapy in conjunction with other antireflux and acid-reducing measures is helpful in patients with esophagitis. Nitrates and calcium-channel blockers are sometimes of benefit to patients with esophageal spasm (see Chapter 61). Patients with depression or panic disorder require specific therapy directed at the underlying psychopathology; failure to treat etiologically may result in prolonged refractory disability from the chest pain (see Chapters 226 and 227).

PATIENT EDUCATION AND INDICATIONS FOR REFERRAL

Teaching Recognition of Acute Coronary Syndromes

The availability of effective early interventions for acute coronary syndromes and the risk of delay necessitate that patients be taught to recognize the symptoms and to call for help immediately. Those with multiple cardiac risk factors or known heart disease deserve top priority for such an educational intervention. Knowledge of key symptoms, especially duration in excess of 20 minutes, new rest pain, and epiphenomena of ischemia (e.g., diaphoresis, nausea, jaw or neck pain, lightheadedness) is weak, particularly among socioeconomically disadvantaged groups, minorities, the elderly, and younger patients. Patients should be instructed to call for an ambulance and not delay. Delay has been documented in up to 50% of cases and often compromises outcome. The importance of minimizing delay in presentation makes patient education and telephone triage important tools. Practices should be organized to handle telephone calls related to chest pain without delay.

Providing Explanation and Meaningful Reassurance

A detailed review of clinical findings and their meaning is as essential to the effective evaluation of chest pain as is a correct diagnosis. When a harmless etiology is identified, it is not enough to dismiss the chest pain as "nothing to worry about" because the symptom is associated with too many fears for such words to suffice. Meaningful reassurance requires eliciting a patient's concerns about his or her chest pain and addressing these concerns by specifically reviewing the pertinent clinical findings. Failure to do so may lead to unnecessary activity restrictions (e.g., fear of engaging in sexual relations, favorite sports, or important work activities) or trigger requests for otherwise unnecessary testing. Patients making repeated visits, asking for referrals, or requesting elaborate testing usually harbor unexplored concerns. The effort taken to provide meaningful explanation is usually well worth the time in terms of patient appreciation, cost containment, and risk management.

INDICATIONS FOR ADMISSION AND REFERRAL (43–45)

As noted earlier, immediate referral to the nearest emergency room is essential to achieving the best possible outcome for the patient with any clinical or laboratory evidence for an acute coronary syndrome, pulmonary embolization, aortic dissection, or large pneumothorax. Key features include a story of unstable angina, sudden onset of severe tearing or searing chest pain with radiation into the back, new pleuritic chest pain in a patient with risk factors for pulmonary embolization or pneumothorax, severe dyspnea, signs of respiratory or hemodynamic compromise, and ischemic ECG changes with pain. Physician errors in triage are most prevalent among patients who are female, nonwhite, present with a chief complaint of dyspnea, or have a normal or nondiagnostic ECG.

Persons who present with acute ST-segment elevation suggestive of acute myocardial infarction require consideration of immediate referral to a center capable of performing angioplasty because outcomes are often better than those achieved by thrombolysis, especially when more than 3 hours have elapsed since the onset of symptoms or time from referral to angioplasty can be less than 2 hours. Referral to the nearest emergency room for thrombolysis is reasonable when time from onset of symptoms to administration of tissue plasminogen activator will be less than 3 hours. For the chest pain patient who presents to the office with evidence of postinfarction angina or ECG findings of prior silent infarction, plans should be made for prompt hospital admission and cardiac consultation—such patients are at high risk. Acute chest pain in the context of cocaine use is also an indication for immediate hospitalization, even in a young person with no other cardiac risk factors. Referral for drug counseling should not be overlooked; it, too, is critical to a successful outcome (see Chapter 235). Patients at risk for a life-threatening chest pain etiology should be taught to recognize key symptoms and instructed to call 911 first if symptoms are acutely severe, even before calling the primary care physician.

Outpatient workup is reasonable for the patient with a low to intermediate probability of pulmonary embolization, provided there are no signs of respiratory or hemodynamic compromise and the appropriate initial testing (e.g., D-dimer determination, V/Q scan, venous ultrasound) can be completed within 2 to 3 hours. For the patient with pleuritic chest pain due to pneumonia, knowledge of the clinical features predictive of a complication is necessary to determine candidacy for admission (see Chapter 52). The utility of referral for esophageal function testing appears to be limited, but endoscopy or barium swallow should be considered if there is refractory reflux or dysphagia. The patient with panic disorder or depression severe enough to cause disabling chest pain symptoms will benefit from psychiatric referral (see Chapters 226 and 227).

RECOMMENDATIONS

- Perform a triage history focusing on evidence for acute coronary syndrome, pulmonary embolization, aortic dissection, tension pneumothorax, and acute cardiopulmonary compromise.
- Arrange immediate transport to the nearest ER by ambulance for the high-risk chest pain patient. Address common mistakes that cause delay and add to risk, such as reluctance

of the patient to call an ambulance or having the patient be driven by a friend or a family member or driving himself or herself.

- If the initial history is not strongly indicative of one of these etiologies, then proceed to evaluate the patient in the office with a more detailed history and careful physical examination, supplemented by ECG, chest x-ray, and pulse oximetry, if available.
- Select the appropriate strategy for subsequent testing based on the pretest probability for the conditions in question. Be aware of common biases based on patient age, gender, and race.
- In formulating the initial differential diagnosis from these data, include a pretest estimate of the "must-not-miss" etiologies (i.e., myocardial ischemia, pulmonary embolization, aortic dissection, tension pneumothorax) and base immediate decision making and the optimal locus and approach to further workup on these probability estimates.

For Suspected Coronary Artery Disease

- *Low pretest probability*: Explain why the chest pain is unlikely to be of cardiac origin, and consider obtaining a resting ECG if it will help to reassure the patient.
- *Intermediate pretest probability*: If the presentation is suggestive of unstable angina, proceed to immediate hospitalization and emergency room triage protocols. If the presentation is one of "stable" (i.e., noncrescendo) chest pain, proceed on a nonemergent basis to stress testing. Obtain either exercise ECG (if the resting ECG is normal) or exercise echocardiography; both are reasonably cost-effective. If other noninvasive modalities (e.g., radionuclide stress testing) are available locally at lower cost or with enhanced sensitivity and specificity, then their use may also be cost-effective and should be considered.
- *High pretest probability*: If the presentation is very suggestive of unstable angina, proceed to immediate hospitalization and emergency room triage protocols. For patients with ECG changes on arrival in the emergency room, immediate angiography without prior noninvasive testing appears to be the more cost-effective diagnostic approach. For those whose presentation is indicative of stable angina, proceed to nonemergent stress testing for determination of the amount of myocardium at risk (see Chapter 36 for test selection).
- To minimize delay in hospitalization, teach the high-risk patient and family the symptoms of acute coronary syndromes,

and instruct them to call 911 immediately if such symptoms occur.

- Reduce requests for unnecessary testing in low-risk patients by eliciting a patient's concerns about his or her chest pain, performing a detailed history and physical examination, obtaining an ECG, and addressing patient concerns by a careful review of clinical findings.
- Omit routine use of esophageal studies in the assessment of chest pain in patients who are ruled out for coronary disease.

For Suspected Pulmonary Embolization

- *Low pretest probability*: Obtain a D-dimer determination. A negative test rules out embolism. A D-dimer level greater than 500 ng/dL necessitates additional testing, with multidetector CT angiography or serial venous ultrasounds a reasonable next step.
- *Intermediate pretest probability*: Begin with CT angiography. If positive, admit for heparin anticoagulation. If negative, proceed to the venous phase of the CT study and perform CT venography of the pelvis and lower extremities. If negative, clinically significant disease is ruled out; follow expectantly. If CT angiography is not available, obtain V/Q scanning. A normal V/Q scan rules out the diagnosis; a high-probability study rules it in. A nondiagnostic V/Q result should be followed by D-dimer and serial venous ultrasound testing. If initial ultrasound is negative and D-dimer testing is positive, then serially repeat ultrasound over 1 week. If ultrasound is negative and D-dimer is negative, then embolism is excluded.
- *High pretest probability*: Admit to the hospital and begin anticoagulation, pending the results of testing. Obtain CT angiography. If it is positive, continue anticoagulation. If it is negative, proceed to CT venography. If it is negative, consider V/Q scanning and venous ultrasound. If the V/Q scan is positive, continue anticoagulation; if it is totally normal, consider cessation of anticoagulation. If it is indeterminate, follow with serial venous ultrasound and D-dimer testing. If the ultrasound is positive, the diagnosis is confirmed; if it is negative or equivocal and D-dimer testing is positive, then consider angiography. If D-dimer testing and venous ultrasound are negative, cease anticoagulation and follow with serial venous ultrasound testing over the next week.

A.H.G.

Annotated Bibliography

1. Daton W, Hall ML, Russo J. Chest pain: relationship of psychiatric illness to coronary arteriographic results. Am J Med 1988;84:1. (*There is a greatly increased incidence of major depression and panic disorder in patients with angiographically negative chest pain.*)
2. DeSanctis RW, Dorochazi RB, Austen WG, et al. Aortic dissection. N Engl J Med 1987;317:1060. (*A classic review, with emphasis on clinical features; 83 references.*)
3. Epstein SE, Gerber LH, Borer JS. Chest wall syndrome. JAMA 1979;241:226. (*The best description of the condition and the physical maneuvers that might elicit the pain associated with it.*)
4. Hochman JS, Tamis JE, Thompson TD, et al. Sex, clinical presentation, and outcome in patients with acute coronary syndromes. N Engl J Med 1999;341:2793. (*Data from the GUSTO IIb [Global Utilization of Streptokinase and t-PA for Occluded Coronary Arteries] study, showing gender-based differences in presentation and outcomes.*)
5. Kayser HL. Tietze's syndrome—a literature review. Am J Med 1956;21:982. (*A classic review; points out the often epidemic nature of the illness.*)
6. Kirshenbaum HD, Ockene IS, Alpert JS, et al. The spectrum of coronary artery spasm. JAMA 1981;246:354. (*An early paper emphasizing the variability of clinical presentation and the difficulties of diagnosis.*)
7. Kloner RA, Rexkalla SH. Cocaine and the heart. N Engl J Med 2003;348:487. (*A succinct summary of acute and chronic effects; a major cause of ischemic chest pain in young persons.*)
8. Marcus GM, Cohen J, Varosy PD, et al. The utility of gestures in patients with chest discomfort. Am J Med 2007;120:83. (*A prospective observational study; utility for the most commonly noted signs was found to be low, evidencing poor test characteristics.*)
9. Panting JR, Gatehouse PD, Yang GZ, et al. Abnormal subendocardial perfusion in cardiac syndrome X detected by cardiovascular magnetic resonance imaging. N Engl J Med 2002;346:1948. (*Evidence for microvascular dysfunction*).
10. Rao SSC, Gregersen H, Hayek B, et al. Unexplained chest pain: the hypersensitive, hyperreactive, and poorly compliant esophagus. Ann Intern Med 1996;124:950. (*Finds reductions in threshold for pain and*

compliance and enhanced reactivity to distention compared with controls.)

11. Sahn SA, Heffner JE. Spontaneous pneumothorax. N Engl J Med 2000;342:868. (*A practical review; 85 references.*)

12. Wexler L. Studies of acute coronary syndromes in women—lessons for everyone. N Engl J Med 1999;341:275. (*An editorial summing up what is known about the differences between men and women and the implications of these differences for the treatment of all patients.*)

13. Anderson DR, Kahn SR, Rodger MA, et al. Computed tomographic pulmonary angiography vs ventilation-perfusion lung scanning in patients with suspected pulmonary embolism: a randomized controlled trial. JAMA 2007;298:2743. (*Finds that multidetector computed tomography is the better of the two tests for diagnosis and at least as good for ruling out significant disease.*)

14. Bholasingh R, Cornel JH, Kamp O, et al. The prognostic value of markers of inflammation in patients with troponin-negative chest pain before discharge from the emergency room. Am J Med 2003;115:521. (*A prospective cohort study; both tests provided independent predictive value for future coronary events.*)

15. Chan WS, Ray JG, Murray S, et al. Suspected pulmonary embolism in pregnancy. Arch Intern Med 2002;162:1170. (*An observational cohort study; the prevalence of embolization was low; ventilation/perfusion [V/Q] scanning appeared to be safe for the fetus.*)

16. Eisner MD. Before diagnostic testing for pulmonary embolism: estimating the prior probability of disease. Am J Med 2003;114:232. (*An editorial emphasizing the ability and importance of making a pretest probability estimate.*)

17. Diamond GA, Forrester JS. Analysis of probability as an aid in the clinical diagnosis of coronary artery disease. N Engl J Med 1979;300:1350. (*A classic paper on the importance of pretest probability in diagnosis, particularly for coronary disease.*)

18. Feldman RL. Ambulatory electrocardiographic monitoring: the test for ischemia? Ann Intern Med 1988;109:608. (*An editorial urging caution in the use of this approach for the detection of ischemia, pointing out many problems in interpreting ST-segment depression.*)

19. Frobert O, Funch-Jensen P, Bagger JP. Diagnostic value of esophageal studies in patients with angina-like chest pain and normal coronary angiograms. Ann Intern Med 1996;124:959. (*A controlled study; no difference was found between patients and controls in 24-hour esophageal monitoring studies and/or provocation testing; the authors question the routine use of such testing in patients with noncardiac chest pain.*)

20. Garber AM, Solomon NA. Cost-effectiveness of alternative test strategies for the diagnosis of coronary artery disease. Ann Intern Med 1999;130:719. (*A meta-analysis and cost-effectiveness study; echocardiography and single-photon emission computed tomography were the most cost-effective tests when the pretest probability is intermediate; immediate angiography was best for those with a high pretest probability.*)

21. Goldhaber SZ. Multislice computer tomography for pulmonary embolism. N Engl J Med 2005;352:1812. (*An editorial comparing this new technology to previous diagnostic methods.*)

22. Kearon C, Ginsberg JS, Douketis J, et al. An evaluation of d-dimer in the diagnosis of pulmonary embolism: a randomized trial. Ann Intern Med 2006;144:812. (*Multicenter randomized, controlled trial; none of 182 persons with low pretest probability and a negative d-dimer test without additional testing developed evidence of pulmonary embolization during follow-up, compared with 1 of 185 who had additional testing.*)

23. Kearon C, Ginsberg JS, Douketis J, et al. An evaluation of D-dimer in the diagnosis of pulmonary embolism: a randomized trial. Ann Intern Med 2006;144:812. (*A large-scale, randomized, controlled trial; persons with a low pretest probability for pulmonary embolism by the Wells rule and a negative d-dimer test can forgo additional testing because their 6-month risk of embolization is zero.*)

24. Kearon C, Ginsberg JS, Hirsh J. The role of venous ultrasonography in the diagnosis of suspected deep venous thrombosis and pulmonary embolism. Ann Intern Med 1998;129:1044. (*Reviews the evidence for the efficacy of the test in the diagnosis of pulmonary embolization.*)

25. Krulp MJHA, Leclercq MGL, van der Heul C, et al. Diagnostic strategies for excluding pulmonary embolism in clinical outcome studies: a systematic review. Ann Intern Med 2003;138:138. (*Examines data on approaches that use pretest probability plus simple tests, finding substantial accuracy and efficacy.*)

26. Kuntz KM, Fleischmann KE, Hunink MGM, et al. Cost-effectiveness of diagnostic strategies for patients with chest pain. Ann Intern Med 1999;130:709. (*An excellent decision-analysis study; electrocardiogram and echo stress testing proved the most cost-effective in persons with an intermediate pretest probability of coronary disease.*)

27. Lange RA, Hillis LD. Acute pericarditis. N Engl J Med 2004;351:2195. (*A clinical review with an especially good section on diagnosis; 43 references.*)

28. Lee TH, Goldman L. Evaluation of the patient with acute chest pain. N Engl J Med 2000;342:1187. (*A practical review of initial clinical evaluation and immediate management, with emphasis on the diagnosis of ischemic disease.*)

29. Le Gal G, Righini M, Pierre-Marie R, et al. Prediction of pulmonary embolism in the emergency department: the revised Geneva Score. Ann Intern Med 2006;144:165. (*A derivation and external validation study of this probability estimate for pulmonary embolism.*)

30. Perrier A, Pierre-Marie R, Sanchez O, et al. Multidetector-row computer tomography in suspected pulmonary embolism. N Engl J Med 2005;352:1760. (*A prospective cohort study, finding a 1.5% false-negative rate when combined with a pretest probability estimate and D-dimer testing.*)

31. Perrier A, Howarth N, Didier D, et al. Performance of helical tomography in unselected outpatients with suspected pulmonary embolism. Ann Intern Med 2001;135:88. (*A prospective observational study; sensitivity was 70%, specificity was 91%, the false-negative rate was 5%, and the false-positive rate was 7% for this older computed tomographic testing modality.*)

32. Pope JH, Aufderheide TP, Ruthhazer R, et al. Missed diagnoses of acute cardiac ischemia in the emergency department. N Engl J Med 2000;342:1163. (*A prospective cohort study identifying, by multivariate analysis, the causes of missed diagnosis.*)

33. Pryor DB, Shaw L, McCants CB, et al. Value of the history and physical in identifying patients at increased risk of coronary disease. Ann Intern Med 1993;118:81. (*A clinical assessment effectively predicted the coronary heart disease risk and the need for further study.*)

34. Righini M, Goehring C, Bounameaux K, et al. Effects of age on the performance of common diagnostic tests for pulmonary embolism. Am J Med 2000;109:357. (*A cross-sectional study, finding that test yields and results were affected by age.*)

35. Robin ED. Overdiagnosis and overtreatment of pulmonary embolism. Ann Intern Med 1977;87:775. (*A classic discussion of the shortcomings of lung scans and arterial blood gases.*)

36. Schulman KA, Berline JA, Harless W, et al. The effect of race and sex on physicians' recommendations for cardiac catheterization. N Engl J Med 1999;340:618. (*A videotape study of simulated patients; race and sex were powerful independent predictors of risk assessment and management recommendations.*)

37. Stein PD, Fowler SE, Goodman LR, et al. for the PIOPED II Investigators. Multidetector computer tomography for acute pulmonary embolism. N Engl J Med 2006;354:2317. (*The PIOPED [Prospective Investigation of Pulmonary Embolism Diagnosis] II study, a major prospective, multicenter validation study of this diagnostic methodology; sensitivity was 83%, and specificity was 96%; when the approach was combined with computed tomographic venography, sensitivity increased to 90%.*)

38. Stein PD, Beemath A, Kayali F, et al. Multidetector computed tomography for the diagnosis of coronary artery disease: a systematic review. Am J Med 2006;119:203. (*A study finding that the average test sensitivity was 95% to 100% for significant coronary disease; the average specificity was 84% to 100%.*)

39. The PIOPED Investigators. Value of the ventilation/perfusion scan in acute pulmonary embolism: results of the Prospective Investigation of Pulmonary Embolism Diagnosis (PIOPED). JAMA 1990;263:2753. (*A classic study of the sensitivity and specificity of V/Q scanning.*)

40. Wells PS, Anderson DR, Rodger M, et al. Excluding pulmonary embolism at the bedside without diagnostic imaging: management of patients with suspect pulmonary embolism presenting to the emergency department by using a simple clinical model and D-dimer. Ann Intern Med 2001;135:98. (*A prospective cohort study, demonstrating the safety and the efficacy of combining pretest probability and D-dimer testing; the negative predictive value of the test was 99.5% in low-risk patients, obviating the need for further testing.*)

41. Wells PS, Ginsberg JS, Anderson DR, et al. Use of a clinical model for safe management of patients with suspected pulmonary embolism. Ann Intern Med 1998;129:997. (*A multicenter prospective cohort study demonstrating the efficacy and the safety of combining clinical assessment of pretest probability, V/Q scanning, and venous ultrasound to evaluate persons for pulmonary embolization.*)

42. Writing Group for the Christopher Study Investigators. Effectiveness of managing suspected pulmonary embolism using an algorithm combining clinical probability, D-dimer testing, and computed tomography. JAMA 2006;295:172. (*A prospective cohort study for validation of this workup algorithm in 3,300 Dutch patients presenting with suspected pulmonary embolism; the strategy was found to be effective and low in risk.*)

43. Andersen HR, Nielson TT, Rasmussen K, et al. A comparison of coronary angioplasty with fibrinolytic therapy in acute myocardial infarction. N Engl J Med 2003;249:733. (*A randomized trial in the community setting; angioplasty produced superior outcomes, despite the need to transfer patients to an invasive-therapy center.*)

44. Braunwald E, Antman EM, Beasley JW, et al. ACC/AHA guidelines for the management of patients with unstable angina and non-ST-segment elevation myocardial infarction: executive summary and recommendations: a report of the American College of Cardiology/American Heart Association Task Force on Practice Guidelines (Committee on Management of Patients with Unstable Angina). J Am Coll Cardiol 2002;40:1366. (*Consensus recommendations.*)

45. Dracup K, Alonzo AA, Atkins JM, et al. The Physician's role in minimizing prehospital delay in patients at high risk for acute myocardial infarction: recommendations from the National Heart Attack Alert Program. Ann Intern Med 1997;126:645. (*Strategies for minimizing delay in hospitalization.*)

CHAPTER 21 ■ EVALUATION OF THE ASYMPTOMATIC SYSTOLIC MURMUR

In the outpatient setting, systolic murmurs are often noted incidentally in otherwise asymptomatic patients. Although many asymptomatic murmurs are due to conditions of no prognostic significance, the absence of symptoms does not rule out the presymptomatic phase of potentially serious pathology, such as tight aortic stenosis. The primary physician should be able to conduct an effective clinical assessment in the office that differentiates the harmless murmur from one that requires additional investigation. Early detection of clinically silent but prognostically important disease is critical to optimizing outcomes and to identifying patients who require close follow-up. Routinely ordering a cardiac ultrasound examination on every patient discovered to have a systolic heart murmur is both expensive and unnecessary, but selective use can be very helpful. This chapter focuses on clinical and ultrasound assessment of the asymptomatic patient (see Chapters 20, 24, 25, 33, and 40 for detailed discussions of evaluation and management of symptomatic patients with structural heart disease).

PATHOPHYSIOLOGY AND CLINICAL PRESENTATION (1–11)

Systolic murmurs can be divided into two broad categories: ejection and regurgitant (see also Chapter 33). *Ejection murmurs* result from turbulent flow of blood across the ventricular outflow tracts during systole. They are characteristically crescendo–decrescendo, medium to low pitched, and heard best at the base of the heart, beginning after the first heart sound and ending before the second. *Regurgitation murmurs* represent backflow of blood due to incompetence of the mitral or tricuspid valve or the ventricular septum. They are typically higher in pitch, heard best at the apex or mid-sternal border, holosystolic or mid-systolic to late systolic in timing, and, like ejection murmurs, crescendo–decrescendo in pattern (unless rheumatic in origin, in which case the intensity is constant).

Ejection murmurs are common and often occur in the absence of heart disease. However, absence of symptoms does not mean absence of important underlying pathology. Regurgitant murmurs are associated with some abnormality of the mitral or tricuspid valve apparatus, valve ring, or septum, but the underlying lesion is not always of clinical significance.

Ejection Murmurs

"Physiologic" Murmurs

"Physiologic" murmurs occur when there is increased ejection velocity across a normal valve creating turbulence. Causes of increased velocity include fever, anemia, pregnancy, hyperthyroidism, exercise, and conditions associated with a large stroke volume (e.g., aortic regurgitation, bradycardia, atrial septal defect [ASD]). Dilation of the aorta, as in hypertension or aging, may also produce a flow murmur by causing turbulent flow in the dilated segment.

"Innocent" Murmurs

"Innocent" murmurs occur in normal hearts under resting conditions. The origin of such murmurs is a subject of debate, with recent evidence pointing to the aortic root. Because there is no obstruction in the outflow tract, the murmur reflects the normal ejection pattern of blood from the ventricles and is early systolic and crescendo–decrescendo. Because chamber pressures are normal, there is normal splitting of heart sounds. Valves are normal; there are no adventitious sounds or other murmurs.

Early Aortic and Pulmonic Valve Disease

Early aortic and pulmonic valve disease may produce murmurs identical to physiologic ones, except that the former are often accompanied by an early systolic *ejection click*. In *pulmonic stenosis*, the murmur increases with inspiration, and the pulmonic component of the second sound is delayed as the disease progresses, widening the splitting of the second heart sound. With increasing stenosis, ejection murmurs usually become louder and more prolonged, with peak intensity occurring later in systole. In hemodynamically significant aortic stenosis, a sustained left ventricular heave develops, the carotid upstroke becomes delayed and lower in amplitude (the *parvus et tardus* pattern), and the second heart sound becomes softer and single as the aortic closing sound decreases.

Calcific Aortic Stenosis

Calcific aortic stenosis is the most common cause of aortic stenosis in the elderly. Onset is in the fourth decade if the underlying valve is bicuspid and in the sixth to eighth decades if the valve is an otherwise normal tricuspid one. Most patients present with symptoms of advanced disease (angina, heart failure, syncope) because the condition often goes unrecognized in the asymptomatic phase. Early diagnosis is often made difficult by the speed of disease progression and the deceptively subtle and atypical physical findings in elderly persons with hemodynamically significant disease. Valve calcification can progress rapidly, leading to hemodynamically significant outflow tract obstruction in as little as 1 to 2 years. Unlike other forms of aortic stenosis, the murmur at the base may reappear at the apex as a higher-pitched sound and simulate mitral regurgitation (*Gallavardin's phenomenon*). In addition, the left ventricular lift associated with hemodynamically significant disease may be less prominent due to myocardial decompensation, and the carotid upstroke may be normal if the carotid artery is stiff due to age.

Aortic Sclerosis

Aortic sclerosis, also referred to as *aortic valve thickening*, is a precursor of calcific aortic stenosis, with 1-year risk of progression reported to be in excess of 15%. It is prevalent in the elderly (found in 40% of persons >75 years of age) and characterized by thickening of the aortic valve leaflets without causing outflow obstruction. Nonetheless, the condition is associated with an increased risk of cardiovascular morbidity and mortality, believed related to its association with atherosclerotic risk factors; however, only concurrent calcification of the mitral valve annulus has proven to be predictive of progression to hemodynamically significant aortic stenosis (perhaps reflective of a generalized process).

Hypertrophic Cardiomyopathy (Idiopathic Hypertrophic Subaortic Stenosis)

Hypertrophic cardiomyopathy produces an ejection quality murmur by dynamically obstructing the left ventricular outflow tract. Displacement of the mitral valve may also occur dynamically and cause regurgitation. The ejection murmur is affected by the size of the left ventricular cavity and contractility. Maneuvers that decrease cavity size (e.g., Valsalva) increase obstruction and intensify the murmur. When there is marked obstruction, the murmur lasts through most of systole, and its peak is delayed beyond mid-systole. Some patients are prone to tachyarrhythmias. The electrocardiogram (ECG) shows high voltage.

Atrial Septal Defects

Atrial septal defects produce physiologic murmurs due to increased right ventricular stroke volume. However, unlike other physiologic murmurs, there is often wide and fixed splitting of the second sound due to left-to-right shunting of blood and a delay in right ventricular ejection.

Patients with physiologic or innocent murmurs are generally asymptomatic from a cardiac standpoint and usually have no previous history of heart disease. Patients with mild varieties of aortic or pulmonic stenosis hypertrophic cardiomyopathy or a small ASD may be asymptomatic as well. In patients with aortic stenosis, onset of symptoms (e.g., angina, dyspnea, postural lightheadedness) is usually a late development indicating advanced disease (see Chapter 33).

Regurgitant Murmurs

Regurgitant murmurs of the arterioventricular valves may be *holosystolic* or *late systolic*, depending on the anatomy and function of the compromised valve apparatus.

Holosystolic Regurgitant Mitral Murmurs

Holosystolic regurgitant mitral murmurs usually occur with conditions that render the mitral valve incompetent throughout systole and include *rheumatic mitral valve disease*, *bacterial endocarditis*, severe cases of *dilated cardiomyopathy*, *papillary muscle rupture*, and *endocardial fibrosis* of the valve surface. The latter has been associated with prolonged, high-dose use of the diet-pill combination *phentermine/fenfluramine* (see Chapter 234). The purported mechanism of valve fibrosis is excessive serotonergic effects on valve endocardial metabolism leading to clinically significant incompetence of mitral, tricuspid, and aortic valves.

Tricuspid Regurgitation

Tricuspid regurgitation due to valve injury or right ventricular dilation produces a murmur similar in quality and timing to that of mitral regurgitation but is heard best along the left sternal border rather than the apex and characteristically increasing with inspiration.

Ventricular Septal Defect

Another mechanism of holosystolic murmur is left-to-right shunting, as occurs with ventricular septal defect (VSD). The holosystolic murmur of VSD is heard best at the left sternal border as a consequence of turbulence from the left-to-right shunting of blood. With prolonged shunting and resultant increase in right ventricular pressure, the pressure gradient and degree of shunting may decline and with it the intensity of the murmur. It is differentiated from tricuspid regurgitation by maneuvers that increase afterload (see later discussion).

Late-Systolic Regurgitant Murmur

Late-systolic regurgitant murmurs result from valve incompetence that develops as systole progresses. Mid- to late-systolic murmurs are characteristic of the mitral regurgitation due to mitral valve prolapse (MVP) and papillary muscle dysfunction associated with ischemic heart disease.

Mitral valve prolapse is the most common cause of an asymptomatic mitral regurgitant murmur in the outpatient setting. The condition is characterized by myxomatous degeneration of the valve leaflets and chordae due to abnormal glucosaminoglycan composition, making them weaker and more likely to stretch and prolapse. In the Framingham Study, the prevalence was initially reported to be as high as 17% among young women and 4% among young men. Use of more-stringent echocardiographic criteria and avoidance of selection bias has refined and reduced the estimated prevalence to 2.4%, with little difference between young men and young women. MVP, with its late-systolic murmur, is often preceded by a click as the redundant mitral valve leaflets prolapse into the atrium during late systole. Most patients with MVP have no other signs or symptoms of heart disease, although an important minority experience atypical chest pain, dysrhythmias, or dyspnea. In a few instances, particularly in older men, hemodynamically significant mitral regurgitation occurs. Asthenic builds in both men and women have been associated with MVP, as has small breast size in women. Nonspecific T-wave changes, particularly inferior lead T-wave inversion, have been described. Diagnosis is confirmed by finding definite prolapse of mitral valve leaflets in the parasternal long-axis view on two-dimensional (B-mode) ultrasound study.

DIFFERENTIAL DIAGNOSIS (12)

The differential diagnosis can be listed according to the underlying pathophysiology. Thus, systolic ejection murmurs can be classified as innocent, physiologic, aortic, and pulmonic. Regurgitant murmurs may be caused by incompetence of the mitral or tricuspid valves or by a VSD (Table 21.1). Of note, some patients have more than one cause present; in a study of patients coming to ultrasound, 28% had evidence of "combined heart disease."

WORKUP (3,6–8,12–23)

Differentiating Systolic Regurgitant Murmurs from Ejection Murmurs

In many instances, the distinction can be made early in the evaluation by physical examination. Doing so helps to narrow the

TABLE 21.1

DIFFERENTIAL DIAGNOSIS OF SYSTOLIC EJECTION MURMUR

Innocent Murmurs

Physiologic Murmurs
  Exercise or emotion
  Fever
  Anemia
  Hyperthyroidism
  Conditions with large stroke volumes: atrial septal defect,
    aortic regurgitation, bradycardia
  Pregnancy

Aortic Murmurs
  Aortic stenosis
  Hypertrophic cardiomyopathy
  Sub- and supravalvular fixed stenoses

Pulmonic Murmurs
  Pulmonic stenosis

Mitral Regurgitation Murmurs
  Rheumatic mitral insufficiency
  Mitral valve prolapse syndrome
  Congenital mitral valve disease
  Rupture of chordae tendineae
  Papillary muscle dysfunction
  Left atrial myxoma
  Dilated mitral valve ring

Tricuspid Regurgitation Murmurs
  Rheumatic tricuspid insufficiency
  Dilated tricuspid valve ring

Ventricular Septal Defect

differential diagnosis (Table 21.1) and focus the workup. The murmur's *timing*, *quality*, and *location* are among the most important differentiating features. As noted earlier, ejection-quality murmurs are typically harsh, best heard with the bell, usually loudest at the base, and radiate into the neck and down to the apex. In elderly patients with calcific aortic stenosis, the murmur may be higher pitched and maximal at the apex, mimicking mitral regurgitation. The systolic regurgitant murmurs of mitral and tricuspid regurgitation are characteristically high pitched, well localized to the apex or left sternal border (unless very loud), and pansystolic or late systolic (and sometimes preceded by a click). All ejection murmurs and most regurgitant murmurs (except for those of rheumatic origin) have a crescendo–decrescendo pattern, making this feature of little use in differentiation. Similarly, finding of electrocardiographic evidence of hypertrophy does not rule out a regurgitant etiology because some degree of eccentric hypertrophy often develops in compensated mitral regurgitation.

A few additional murmur characteristics and responses to *maneuvers* can be helpful diagnostically. Ejection murmurs change in intensity with heart *rate* and length of the cardiac cycle, becoming softer with increases in rate and louder as rate decreases. Regurgitant murmurs change little if at all with heart rate. *Handgrip* and other maneuvers that increase systolic pressure (e.g., *transient arterial occlusion* by inflation of blood pressure cuffs applied to both arms) markedly augment the intensity of the regurgitant murmurs of mitral regurgitation and VSD. Right-sided heart murmurs can be differentiated from left-sided ones by the augmentation in intensity that occurs with quiet *inspiration*.

Cardiac ultrasound examination is sometimes necessary for differentiating regurgitant disease from causes of an ejection murmur, especially in the context of concurrent left ventricular dysfunction, involvement of multiple valves, or cardiomyopathy. The test, particularly when performed in conjunction with a Doppler study, is also an important adjunct for assessment of disease severity; it should be considered when there is clinical suspicion of a hemodynamically significant lesion (see later discussion).

Assessment of Ejection Murmurs

Separating Harmless Causes from More Serious Pathology

Attention to *timing*, *quality*, *intensity*, and *location* is helpful. *Innocent* and *physiologic murmurs* are usually mid-range in frequency, less than 3/6 in intensity, peak in early to mid-systole, stop long before S2, and are heard best at the base, although they can radiate to neck and apex. Valsalva and standing decrease their intensity. The second sound is normally split and of normal intensity; there are no clicks, heaves, S3, S4, or other murmurs. The ECG and *chest radiograph* are normal. Signs of anemia, fever, hyperthyroidism, and anxiety should be sought.

The murmurs resulting from *ASD* and *hemodynamically insignificant aortic* and *pulmonic stenoses* may resemble physiologic murmurs. However, in most cases of ASD there is widened and fixed splitting of S2, and in more than 90% of cases there is a conduction defect of the *right-bundle-branch* type, producing a QRS and lead V1 with an RSR prime configuration. A normal ECG and normal splitting of S2 indicate that an ASD is unlikely. When one is in doubt, an echocardiogram can be used to look for abnormal septal motion and right ventricular enlargement; a normal study rules out the diagnosis. *Mild aortic stenosis* in the young patient may be impossible to distinguish from a physiologic murmur; the presence of an ejection click is an important clue to the former.

Clinical assessment is usually sufficient to distinguish the functional or innocent murmur from that due to underlying pathology. Sensitivity of the physical examination appears to equal that of ultrasound is this respect, making ultrasound confirmation unnecessary when clinical certainty is high.

Estimating the Severity of Aortic Stenosis

As aortic stenosis progresses and becomes more hemodynamically significant, the murmur typically gets louder and peaks later in systole, the second heart sound decreases in intensity as the aortic closure sound fades, a left ventricular lift develops, a thrill may be palpable, and the carotid upstroke becomes delayed and diminished in intensity. Evidence of left ventricular hypertrophy may appear on ECG (e.g., increased voltage, strain pattern), although the test is not a sensitive indicator.

A high index of suspicion is necessary both for the detection of *calcific aortic stenosis in the elderly* and the estimation of its severity. One needs to remember to listen at the apex and at the base and not to be lulled into a false sense of security by the softness of the murmur, the absence of a vigorous left ventricular heave, or the normality of the carotid upstroke. Its presentation as a medium- to high-pitched musical murmur, heard best at the apex, may lead to confusion with mitral regurgitation. Helping to differentiate it from mitral regurgitation is the decrease in the murmur's intensity with increase in heart rate; in mitral regurgitation, there is no change in the murmur with heart rate. Clinical detection of hemodynamically significant disease can be particularly difficult in the context of declining left ventricular function, which may blunt many of the characteristic physical findings of severe stenosis. However, such patients usually have dyspnea or other symptoms (see Chapter 33), which should help raise the index of suspicion.

Cardiac ultrasound is indicated when physical examination raises the question of important outflow-tract obstruction—the fact that the patient is asymptomatic does not rule out hemodynamically significant disease. Confirmation of suspected valvular and subvalvular obstruction to left ventricular outflow and accurate estimation of its severity can be accurately accomplished echocardiographically, especially when performed in conjunction with a continuous-wave *Doppler study*. For aortic stenosis, reasonably accurate estimates can often be obtained of valve area and pressure gradient across the valve. Severe stenosis is defined as a mean gradient in excess of 40 mm Hg with a calculated valve area less than 0.75 cm^2. A valve area in the range of 0.76 to 1.1 cm^2 and a gradient in the range of 15 to 39 mm Hg define moderate disease. Overestimates of severity can occur in the setting of low flow. The degree of valve calcification noted on echocardiography corresponds to the severity of stenosis.

Ultrasound performed in the setting of aortic stenosis can provide additional information that may be useful, including estimation of ejection fraction and detection of hemodynamically significant aortic regurgitation. Diastolic regurgitant murmurs are often missed in the setting of prominent systolic murmurs, with even experienced examiners demonstrating no more than 40% sensitivity for clinical recognition of hemodynamically significant aortic insufficiency.

Recognition of Idiopathic Hypertrophic Subaortic Stenosis

Several maneuvers help to differentiate the systolic ejection murmur associated with this type of cardiomyopathy from other ejection murmurs. Most distinctive are the murmur's responses to *squatting*, passive *leg elevation*, and *Valsalva*, maneuvers that affect left ventricular chamber size through their effects on venous return. A lessening of venous return decreases chamber size and increases obstruction to outflow by the hypertrophic heart muscle. This is why Valsalva (bearing down against a closed glottis) results in an increase in the intensity of the murmur. With passive leg elevation and with change from standing to squatting, the murmur of hypertrophic disease characteristically *decreases* as venous return rises. Although sometimes the murmur may not change substantially with increasing venous return, any clear-cut increase in the murmur under such circumstances rules out hypertrophic cardiomyopathy. The murmur peaks around mid-systole, which helps to distinguish it from those innocent murmurs that peak earlier. Other features of the murmur include maximal intensity along the left sternal border and a brisk *carotid upstroke* that is sometimes *bisferiens* (bifid) in quality. *Cardiac ultrasound* is indicated when the diagnosis is suspected on clinical grounds. Moreover, the study may reveal mitral regurgitation, which is sometimes present in the setting of this hypertrophic cardiomyopathy.

Recognition of Pulmonic Stenosis

Hemodynamically significant pulmonic stenosis is suggested by a prolonged and loud murmur (greater than 3/6) that characteristically increases with *inspiration,* wide splitting or absence of the pulmonic component of the second heart sound, an ejection click that decreases with inspiration, a right ventricular

lift, evidence of pulmonary artery dilation on chest film, and prominent R wave in V1 indicative of right ventricular hypertrophy. A normal ECG and an early systolic murmur rule out significant pulmonic stenosis. Mild hemodynamically insignificant pulmonic stenosis may be indistinguishable from an innocent murmur, but usually no therapy is indicated, and therefore misdiagnosis is of little consequence.

Summary

The key components of the initial evaluation of the systolic ejection murmur in the asymptomatic patient include attention to carotid upstroke; left and right ventricular impulses; second heart sound; clicks; the quality, timing, intensity, and location of the murmur; and the effects of provocative maneuvers that affect venous return, heart rate, and systemic resistance. ECG and chest radiograph may be helpful. Cardiac ultrasound examination in conjunction with Doppler study is indicated if there is clinical suspicion of hemodynamically significant disease or the diagnosis remains in doubt and there are adverse consequences to not identifying the lesion. Of note, aortic regurgitation is often missed clinically in the setting of aortic stenosis.

Assessment of Regurgitant Systolic Murmurs

The *timing* and *location* of the regurgitant murmur are among the most helpful features diagnostically. The response to a number of simple bedside maneuvers can also provide useful information.

Holosystolic Murmurs

A holosystolic murmur suggests rheumatic or cardiomyopathic *mitral insufficiency, tricuspid insufficiency,* or a VSD. The murmur of classic mitral insufficiency is best heard at the apex and radiates laterally into the axilla; it varies little with cycle length or with respiration but increases markedly with *handgrip* and other maneuvers that transiently increase systemic resistance (e.g., bilateral blood pressure cuff inflation). With chronic increase in volume load, there is likely to be palpable enlargement of the left ventricle. Because multivalve involvement is the rule and heart failure may occur, a careful listening for other murmurs and a check for signs of heart failure (e.g., rales, third heart sound) are in order. However, a third heart sound is quite common in mitral regurgitation and not as predictive of systolic dysfunction as it is in other forms of heart disease.

Differentiating Tricuspid from Mitral Insufficiency. One notes the effect of *respiration* on the murmur. The systolic regurgitant murmur of tricuspid insufficiency increases with quiet inspiration and sustained abdominal pressure (applied to the right upper quadrant to compress the liver). Moreover, it is usually loudest at the lower left sternal border, but when the right ventricle is very large, it may be heard at the apex. It does not radiate well to the axilla. Intensity is strongly influenced by respiration, increasing at the beginning of inspiration and fading during early expiration. The presence of *hepatojugular reflux* is very suggestive and should be checked.

Identifying Ventricular Septal Defect. The holosystolic murmur of VSD can be heard best at the sternal border and does not radiate to the axilla. Intensity does not vary with respiration, but, like mitral regurgitation, it is increased with Valsalva, handgrip, and blood pressure cuff application. The murmur often has some mid-systolic accentuation and may be confused with an ejection murmur. Like mitral regurgitation, intensity of the murmur increases markedly with handgrip and other maneuvers that increase systemic resistance.

Late-Systolic Murmurs

MVP is characterized by a mid- to late-systolic murmur preceded by a mid-systolic click. Some forms of *papillary muscle dysfunction* will also result in a mitral regurgitant murmur of similar timing, usually in the setting of anteroseptal ischemia. Suspicion of MVP is reinforced by hearing a mid-systolic click, which tends to move toward the first heart sound with standing (a maneuver that reduces left ventricular volume and softens the murmur). The MVP murmur may occur in the absence of a click. The intensity of the suspected MVP murmur should be noted. The louder the murmur, the more hemodynamically significant is the regurgitation and the greater are the risks of endocarditis and other cardiovascular complications. Handgrip or Valsalva maneuver may increase the intensity of the murmur. Increasing duration of the murmur is a sign of worsening prolapse. Development of a holosystolic murmur without a systolic click in a person with known MVP is associated with an increased risk of an adverse event.

Testing for Mitral Valve Prolapse. An *echocardiogram* can confirm MVP when uncertainty persists. Minor degrees of valve prolapse are normal. One should insist that ultrasound criteria are met before giving the patient a diagnosis of MVP. The major criterion is *systolic displacement* of one or both valve leaflets into the left atrium beyond the plane of the mitral annulus in the parasternal long-axis view on two-dimensional (B-mode) ultrasound study. *Valve thickening* and *redundancy* are other features, but a *nonclassic form of MVP* has been described in which there is no thickening, little risk for endocarditis, and little hemodynamically significant regurgitation. Ultrasound can differentiate the two and thus may help with cardiac risk stratification, although a very small risk of embolic stroke is similar in both forms. Indiscriminate use of echocardiography is to be avoided. Searching for "silent" MVP in the patient with vague chest pains and an entirely normal cardiac examination is of no value. Use of ultrasound in suspected MVP can facilitate diagnosis, but the contribution to outcome remains to be demonstrated. In most instances, the change in management engendered involves initiation of endocarditis prophylaxis (see Chapter 16). However, Doppler echocardiographic studies suggest that audible, and especially loud, systolic regurgitant murmurs are very likely to represent hemodynamically significant disease. An ultrasound examination is indicated when such a murmur is encountered.

PATIENT EDUCATION AND INDICATIONS FOR REFERRAL

Patient Education

When the murmur is determined to be innocent or hemodynamically insignificant after careful evaluation, it is essential to provide detailed explanation as part of the delivery of meaningful reassurance. Marked concern and even distrust may be precipitated by a perfunctory explanation that "it's harmless and nothing serious," especially if detailed auscultation continues to be conducted on subsequent visits. Concern about a murmur that is left incompletely explained can lead to unnecessary self-restriction of activity. Reassurance should include a discussion of the cause of the murmur, its significance, and prognosis. Informing the patient of other possible causes considered and ruled out is particularly helpful to the well-educated or medically curious patient and can obviate the demand for unnecessary testing or referral. The patient with a harmless murmur should be specifically told that there is no need to restrict activity or undergo further evaluation at the present time.

Aortic Stenosis

Asymptomatic persons found to have aortic stenosis (especially the elderly) should be informed of the importance of regular follow-up examinations and taught to watch for the symptoms of hemodynamically significant disease (i.e., postural lightheadedness, angina, exertional dyspnea), with instructions given to report them immediately should they occur (also see Chapter 33).

Mitral Valve Prolapse

Counseling is particularly important for the patient with insignificant MVP. Patients should be informed that MVP is a heterogeneous condition, and that most of them at no increased risk for cardiac complications. Those with readily audible MVP regurgitant murmurs should be advised about the need for endocarditis prophylaxis (see Chapter 16).

Indications for Referral

The person with hemodynamically significant aortic stenosis (valve area <0.9 cm^2) needs close follow-up, annual echocardiography, and consideration of cardiac consultation if stenosis continues to progress, even in the absence of symptoms. Onset of symptoms makes the referral urgent (see Chapter 33). Worsening exertional dyspnea in the patient with rheumatic, ischemic, or cardiomyopathic mitral regurgitation is also an indication for prompt cardiac consultation because it suggests that the left ventricle is decompensating (see Chapter 33). Annual echocardiography has been recommended for asymptomatic persons with hemodynamically significant mitral regurgitation, with referral indicated if there is progressive enlargement of the left ventricle or a fall in ejection fraction below 60%. Referral is also needed for the patient with tricuspid regurgitation and worsening hepatojugular reflux and other signs of right-sided failure. Patients with particularly loud murmurs of MVP suggestive of hemodynamically significant disease should be referred for cardiac consultation after undergoing ultrasound examination for confirmation. Most such patients can be reassured that they are at no increased risk and that progression to more serious disease is very rare. Prompt referral is indicated for the rare MVP patient with complex ventricular irritability, prolonged QT intervals, a family history of sudden death, or a transient ischemic event.

RECOMMENDATIONS

- Begin by determining whether the systolic murmur is regurgitant or ejection in quality by attention to the murmur's location, quality, and timing.
- Differentiate right-sided from left-sided pathology by observing response of the murmur to inspiration.
- If the murmur is ejection in quality, distinguish between innocent/physiologic murmurs and those due to structural heart disease.

- For left-sided ejection murmurs, distinguish between aortic stenosis and hypertrophic cardiomyopathy.
- If aortic stenosis is suspected, estimate clinical severity by physical examination and obtain Doppler cardiac ultrasound in those persons with physical findings suggestive of hemodynamically significant disease.
- Follow patients with calcific aortic stenosis closely, and repeat ultrasound examination periodically.
- If there is evidence of hypertrophic cardiomyopathy (idiopathic hypertrophic subaortic stenosis) by physical examination, order Doppler cardiac ultrasound to confirm.
- For holosystolic murmurs, differentiate by physical examination between arteriovenous valve regurgitation and VSD; if arteriovenous valve regurgitation is suspected, determine whether the murmur is mitral or pulmonic. Obtain Doppler ultrasound if there is clinical evidence of hemodynamically significant regurgitation.
- For late-systolic murmurs, differentiate between MVP and valve regurgitation due to papillary muscle dysfunction. If hemodynamically significant MVP is suspected, obtain Doppler ultrasound to confirm.
- Refer for cardiac consultation any patient found to have severe aortic stenosis or any other hemodynamically significant lesion with poor prognosis (e.g., hypertrophic cardiomyopathy, mitral regurgitation with falling ejection fraction).
- Provide detailed reassurance to patients with harmless lesions to minimize demand for unnecessary testing, and make clear to patients with hemodynamically significant disease the need for close follow-up.

A.H.G.

Annotated Bibliography

1. Barber JE, Kasper FK, Ratliff NB, et al. Mechanical properties of myxomatous mitral valves. J Thorac Cardiovasc Surg 2001;122:955. (*Abnormal glycosaminoglycan composition is responsible for abnormal mechanical properties.*)
2. Brenner SJ, Duffy CI, Thomas JD. Progression of aortic stenosis in 394 patients. J Am Coll Cardiol 1995;25:305. (*A serial Doppler ultrasound study with a 3-year mean duration of follow-up; documents the speed with which progression can occur in elderly patients.*)
3. Carabello BA, Crawford FA. Valvular heart disease. N Engl J Med 1997;337:32. (*Excellent review, which emphasizes pathophysiology and timely detection of a clinically important disease.*)
4. Connolly HM, Crary JL, McGoon MD, et al. Valvular heart disease associated with fenfluramine–phentermine. N Engl J Med 1997;337:581. (*Major report on valvular damage associated with the use of this once-popular diet-pill combination.*)
5. Cosmi JE, Kort S, Tunick PA, et al. The risk of development of aortic stenosis in patients with "benign" aortic valve thickening. Arch Intern Med 2002;1162:2345. (*Retrospective study; the risk of progression exceeds 15% over 1 year; examines predictors of progression.*)
6. Devereaux RB, Kramer-Fox R, Kligfield P. Mitral valve prolapse: causes, clinical manifestations, and management. Ann Intern Med 1989;111:305. (*Comprehensive review; 172 references.*)
7. Finegam RE, Gianelly RD, Harrison DC. Aortic stenosis in the elderly: relevance of age to diagnosis and treatment. N Engl J Med 1969;281:1261. (*An important classic paper; physical findings such as carotid upstroke and quality and location of the murmur may be misleading in assessing aortic stenosis in the elderly.*)
8. Freed LA, Levy D, Levine RA, et al. Prevalence and clinical outcome of mitral valve prolapse. N Engl J Med. 1999;341:1. (*A reconsideration of epidemiologic data based on echocardiographic criteria.*)
9. Lombard TJ, Selzer A. Valvular aortic stenosis. Ann Intern Med 1987;106:292. (*Clinical presentations of 397 patients, with emphasis on disease in the elderly.*)
10. Otto CM, Lind BK, Kitzman DW, et al. Association of aortic valve sclerosis with cardiovascular mortality and morbidity in the elderly. N Engl J Med. 1999;341:142. (*Evidence for increased risk of adverse cardiovascular events.*)
11. Stein PD, Sabbah H. Aortic origin of innocent murmur. Am J Cardiol 1977;39:665. (*Presents extensive data for an aortic origin.*)
12. Attenhofer-Jost CH, Turina J, Mayer K, et al. Echocardiography in the evaluation of systolic murmurs of unknown cause. Am J Med 2000;108:614. (*Cohort study comparing the diagnostic accuracy of physical examination with echocardiography; a physical exam is excellent for distinguishing functional from hemodynamically significant disease but less sensitive in a number of other situations.*)
13. Carabello BA. Aortic stenosis. N Engl J Med 2001;346:677. (*Practical review for the clinician, with emphasis on decision making; 32 references.*)
14. Etchells E, Bell C, Robb K. Does this patient have an abnormal systolic murmur? JAMA 1997;277:564. (*A comprehensive literature review of the evidence for the accuracy and precision of clinical findings in the diagnosis of systolic murmurs.*)
15. Etchells E, Glenns V, Shadowitz S, et al. A bedside clinical prediction rule for detecting moderate or severe aortic stenosis. J Gen Intern Med 1998;13:699. (*A cross-sectional study confirming the efficacy of physical examination in identifying and ruling out hemodynamically significant aortic stenosis.*)
16. Folland ED, Kriegel BJ, Henderson WG, et al. Implications of third heart sounds in patients with valvular heart disease. N Engl J Med 1992;327:458. (*Indicative of failure in aortic stenosis but not necessarily in mitral regurgitation.*)
17. Heckerling PS, Wiener SL, Moses VK, et al. Accuracy of precordial percussion in detecting cardiomegaly. Am J Med 1991;91:328. (*Not often performed but found to be surprisingly useful.*)
18. Lembo NJ, Dell'Italia LJ, Crawford MH, et al. Bedside diagnosis of systolic murmurs. N Engl J Med 1988;318:1572. (*One of the few studies providing sensitivity and specificity data on diagnostic maneuvers.*)
19. Maisel AS, Atwood JE, Goldberger AL. Hepatojugular reflux: useful in the bedside diagnosis of tricuspid regurgitation. Ann Intern Med 1984;101:781. (*Specificity 100%, sensitivity 66% in detecting tricuspid regurgitation; increase in murmur intensity with deep inspiration was as specific and more sensitive.*)
20. Maron BJ, Bonow RO, Cannon RO 3rd, et al. Hypertrophic cardiomyopathy: interrelations of clinical manifestations, pathophysiology, and therapy. Parts 1 and 2. N Engl J Med 1987;316:844. (*Best discussion of correlations between pathophysiology and clinical findings.*)
21. Nishimura RA, McGoon MD, Shub C, et al. Echocardiographically documented mitral valve prolapse: long-term follow-up of 237 patients. N Engl J Med 1985;313:1305. (*Identifies a low-risk subgroup.*)
22. Shaver JA. Cardiac auscultation: a cost-effective diagnostic skill. Curr Probl Cardiol 1995;20:447. (*Evidence for the utility of a careful clinical examination.*)
23. Tribouilloy CM, Enriquez-Sarano M, Mohty D, et al. Pathophysiologic determinants of third heart sounds: a prospective clinical and Doppler echocardiographic study. Am J Med 2001;111:96. (*Prospective cohort study; S3 is indicative of serious underlying hemodynamic and valvular dysfunction.*)

CHAPTER 22 ■ EVALUATION OF LEG EDEMA

Leg edema can be a bothersome complaint and an initial symptom of serious underlying disease. Acute onset of unilateral swelling raises the question of deep vein thrombophlebitis (DVT), which must be addressed promptly. Bilateral disease is particularly common in the elderly and often a manifestation of chronic venous insufficiency, congestive heart failure, or venodilating medications; however, pulmonary hypertension may account for as much as one fifth of cases and usually goes unrecognized. Noninvasive methods, particularly venous and cardiac ultrasound, have greatly facilitated evaluation, but the clinical estimation of pretest probability is essential to optimal test selection and interpretation. Especially important to the pretest assessment of unilateral edema is knowledge of the incidence, risk factors, symptoms, and signs of DVT. In bilateral edema, awareness of the potential contributions from often overlooked etiologies (such as pulmonary hypertension and use of nonsteroidal antiinflammatory drugs [NSAIDs]) can inform the clinical assessment and guide workup.

PATHOPHYSIOLOGY AND CLINICAL PRESENTATION (1–16)

Edema is defined as an increase in extracellular volume. It develops if hydrostatic pressure exceeds colloid oncotic pressure, capillary permeability increases, or lymphatic drainage becomes impaired. Hydrostatic pressure is a function of intravascular volume, blood pressure, and venous outflow. Colloid oncotic pressure depends on the serum albumin concentration. Inflammation and thrombosis may follow, especially in the setting of poor venous blood flow and hypercoagulability.

Decreased Oncotic Pressure

Decreased oncotic pressures are usually due to *hypoalbuminemia*, which can occur secondary to malnutrition, hepatocellular failure, or excess renal or gastrointestinal loss of albumin. The resultant fall in intravascular volume from excessive transudation of fluid stimulates salt retention. This compensatory effort to maintain adequate intravascular volume leads to further edema formation because the underlying oncotic deficit remains. Edema sets in when the serum albumin concentration falls to less than 2.5 g/100 mL. Leg swelling due to hypoalbuminemia is typically bilateral, pitting, and sometimes accompanied by edema of the face and eyelids (especially on awakening).

Increased Hydrostatic Pressure

Increased hydrostatic pressure may result from excessive *fluid retention* (as seen with congestive heart failure or drugs such as NSAIDs and corticosteroids), *impairment of venous outflow* from *venous valvular incompetence*, DVT, or *pulmonary hypertension* (which may be a consequence of sleep apnea, left heart failure, or chronic obstructive lung disease). Venodilating drugs (such as *nifedipine* and other *calcium-channel blockers*) may lead to an increase in hydrostatic pressure as blood pools in the lower extremities. A localized increase in hydrostatic pressure develops in the legs during prolonged standing, especially if the valves in the leg veins are incompetent. Increased hydrostatic pressure due to fluid retention produces bilaterally symmetric edema, whereas swelling due to venous insufficiency may be asymmetric and accompanied by varicosities and other signs of venous disease, such as stasis dermatitis, ulcers, and brawny induration. Unilateral lower leg edema can also result from venous compression by a *popliteal (Baker's) cyst*. A *stroke* that causes paresis in one leg may result in unilateral edema due to reductions in vascular tone and venous and lymphatic drainage; thrombophlebitis may ensue.

Increased Capillary Permeability

Increased capillary permeability is another mechanism of leg edema and is associated with immunologic injury, infection, inflammation, or trauma. A permeability defect is also believed to be responsible for *idiopathic edema*, a poorly understood but common problem seen almost exclusively in women. Although some patients report a periodicity to the problem that seems to parallel the menstrual cycle, careful studies have failed to find sufficient evidence to warrant the label *cyclic edema*. The condition is especially aggravated by hot weather and standing, more so than occurs with venous insufficiency. Transient abdominal distention is common, and weight may fluctuate by several pounds over the course of the day. The disorder is not progressive, but it can cause considerable discomfort. It is often accompanied by headache, fatigue, anxiety, and other functional symptoms. Some patients are bothered by nocturia.

Lymphatic Obstruction

Lymphatic obstruction hinders reabsorption of interstitial fluid. The swelling usually starts in the feet and progresses upward; often the problem is unilateral. The edema of lymphatic obstruction tends to have a brawny quality and evidences little pitting, except in its early stages. Recumbence provides only minor relief compared with edema from other causes.

Inflammation and Hypercoagulability

Inflammation secondary to changes in blood flow plays an important and increasingly appreciated role in chronic venous disease. Valvular incompetence compromises pulsatile venous flow, reducing or eliminating the normal shear stresses on endothelial cells that inhibit the release of inflammatory mediators. Such loss of normal pulsatile flow, and especially its reversal, promotes an inflammatory response that enhances the risk of thrombosis in compromised veins.

Hypercoagulability also increases the risk of thrombosis. *Acquired hypercoagulability* is seen with active *cancer*, illnesses associated with the production of *antiphospholipid antibodies*, recent plaster cast/prolonged *immobilization*, and recent major *surgery* (especially of the hip or knee). Even prolonged sitting in cramped conditions as occurs on extended *airplane flights* in coach seating increases the risk of DVT, mostly in persons with preexisting risk factors.

In a significant proportion of cases, venous thrombosis develops without a clear-cut precipitant. As noted, inflammation leading to phlebitis may ensue from loss of normal pulsatile venous flow. *Hereditary hypercoagulability* often exacerbates the situation. The most common hereditary contributor to hypercoagulability is *factor V Leiden mutation*, which is found in heterozygous form in up to 20% of some European populations. Others mutations include deficiency of *protein S, protein C*, or *antithrombin III*; *prothrombin gene mutation*; and *homocysteinemia* (see Chapter 35). Patients with factor V Leiden mutations have odds ratios for DVT of about 3 if they are heterozygous (a relatively weak risk factor) and 18 if they are homozygous, but when the mutation is present in conjunction with other hereditary and acquired risk factors, the absolute 10-year risk of DVT can be as high as 10% in heterozygotes and 50% in homozygotes.

Estrogen and *progestin* increase the risk of DVT by two- to threefold and are additive to other risk factors such as obesity, factor V Leiden mutation, and age. There is some suggestion that esterified estrogens do not increase the DVT risk compared to conjugated estrogens, but this observation requires confirmation; the addition of progestin negates this beneficial difference.

DVT may have a very subtle presentation, with acute onset of unilateral or asymmetric leg edema as the only manifestation. Such textbook findings as calf tenderness, palpable cord, and positive Homan's sign are often absent. The findings most predictive of significant DVT are swelling of the entire leg, asymmetric leg edema (>3 cm difference in calf circumferences), pitting edema of the involved leg, tenderness along deep veins, and prominent collateral superficial veins. Most clots due to thrombophlebitis form in the small veins of the calf; 20% to 30% propagate proximally into the popliteal and femoral veins of the knee and thigh. Clot below the knee poses little risk of pulmonary embolization (<3%), but extension above the knee markedly increases the chances (upward of 40%). A *ruptured Baker's cyst* may mimic DVT by causing acute pain and swelling in the calf and popliteal fossa in a person with preexisting degenerative knee arthritis.

DIFFERENTIAL DIAGNOSIS
(1,2,7,11)

The differential diagnosis of edema can be organized according to clinical presentations and pathophysiologic mechanisms (Table 22.1). The list of etiologies for bilateral edema is particularly extensive. In primary care practice, the leading causes of bilateral disease include venous insufficiency, heart failure, pulmonary hypertension, and hypoalbuminemia; pulmonary hypertension is the most commonly missed diagnosis. Certain infiltrative conditions may be mistaken for edema, such as pretibial myxedema seen with hyperthyroidism and lipedema (a familial bilateral deposition of excess fat in the lower extrem-

TABLE 22.1

IMPORTANT CAUSES OF LEG EDEMA

Unilateral or Asymmetric Swelling
  Increased hydrostatic pressure
    Deep vein thrombophlebitis
    Venous insufficiency
    Popliteal (Baker's) cyst
  Increased capillary permeability
    Cellulitis
    Trauma
  Lymphatic obstruction (local)
  Mimicking conditions
    Ruptured Baker's cyst of the knee
    Lipedema (when asymmetric)
Bilateral Swelling
  Decreased oncotic pressure
    Malnutrition
    Hepatocellular failure
    Nephrotic syndrome
    Protein-losing enteropathy
  Increased hydrostatic pressure
    Congestive heart failure
    Renal failure
    Use of salt-retaining drugs (e.g., corticosteroids, estrogens)
    Venous insufficiency
    Pulmonary hypertension and premenstrual state
    Pregnancy
  Increased capillary permeability
    Systemic vasculitis
    Idiopathic edema
    Allergic reactions
  Lymphatic obstruction (retroperitoneal or generalized)
  Mimicking conditions
    Lipedema (symmetric)

ities). A ruptured Baker's cyst of the knee may mimic DVT of the calf.

WORKUP (1,2,7,10,11,17–30)

Diagnosis of leg edema can be challenging. The initial clinical impression often undergoes revision on laboratory testing, underscoring the difficulty in making an accurate diagnosis on the basis of history and physical examination alone. In a study from primary care practice, venous insufficiency was overdiagnosed clinically and heart failure and pulmonary hypertension markedly underdiagnosed. Nonetheless, attention to clinical features is critical to making the best possible pretest probability assessment, which is essential to test selection and interpretation.

History

The distribution of the swelling should be ascertained because it helps to focus the differential diagnosis.

Unilateral or Asymmetric Leg Edema

If edema is reported to be predominantly unilateral or asymmetric, the patient should be questioned about the major risk factors for DVT, especially those found to contribute independently to risk, such as concurrent malignancy, recent paralysis or plaster-cast immobilization, 3 or more days of being bedridden, major surgery (especially of the hip or knee) within the preceding 3 months, and prior history of DVT. Also useful for risk assessment are estrogen use and family history of DVT (suggestive of an inherited hypercoagulable state). Any report of localized tenderness along deep veins, swelling of the entire leg, and marked asymmetry of the swelling should also be noted and confirmed by physical examination (see later discussion).

Bilateral Edema

If the edema is reportedly *bilateral and symmetric*, then it is important to check not only for a history of venous insufficiency, but also for dyspnea on exertion; orthopnea; paroxysmal nocturnal dyspnea; severe snoring; daytime sleepiness; interrupted sleep; chronic productive cough; a history of cardiac, pulmonary, renal, or hepatic failure; malnutrition; and use of such drugs as nifedipine, other vasodilators, NSAIDs, and corticosteroids. A report of acute facial swelling suggests an allergic reaction or hypoalbuminemia if the swelling is more chronic.

Physical Examination

The first priority is to confirm the distribution of the problem. Careful measurement of calf and thigh diameters is also very helpful.

Unilateral or Asymmetric Leg Edema

In unilateral edema, if the swelling is predominantly limited to one leg, the limb should be examined for tenderness, redness, increased warmth, varicosities, and a palpable thrombosed vein. Unfortunately, the often-cited classic signs of DVT (i.e., calf tenderness, palpable cord, positive Homan's sign) are neither very sensitive nor specific; unilateral edema may be the only clue aside from a history of risk factors. Nonetheless, a difference in calf circumferences of more than 3 cm is an independent predictor of DVT, as are tenderness along deep veins, swelling of the entire leg, pitting edema, and prominence of collateral superficial veins. Encountering three or more of these findings in a patient with risk factors for DVT is associated with a pretest probability for DVT of about 75%. If edema is prominent but pitting is only minimal, it suggests that lymphatic obstruction might be the cause.

The knee should be checked for evidence of degenerative disease and an accompanying Baker's cyst in the popliteal fossa, which may impair venous outflow. In the setting of suspected DVT, a ruptured Baker's cyst should be considered in the differential because it may cause acute calf pain, swelling, and tenderness, mimicking thrombophlebitis.

Bilateral Edema

The patient with bilateral leg edema should have the blood pressure measured for hypertension, which might be a sign of renal failure. The skin is checked for evidence of chronic cardiopulmonary disease (cyanosis, clubbing) and for signs of hepatocellular failure (jaundice, spider angiomata, ecchymoses); the jugular veins for distention; the chest for rales, wheezes, and effusion; the heart for signs of pulmonary hypertension (a right ventricular heave or right ventricular S_3, increased prominence of P_2, widened splitting of S_2) and signs of heart failure (S_3, abnormal splitting of S_2); and the abdomen for hepatojugular reflux and ascites. Any lymphadenopathy

should be noted. Lipidema should not be confused with leg edema; the deposits of adipose tissue produce no pitting or induration.

Pretest Probability Estimation for Deep Venous Thrombosis

Although no single historical or physical finding is diagnostic or exclusionary for DVT, a reasonable estimate of pretest probability can be formulated by attention to those clinical features that have been found to be independent determinants of DVT risk. Wells and colleagues developed and prospectively validated the most widely used prediction rule based on these determinants (Table 22.2). Such a probability estimate can help to guide test ordering, ensuring intensive study of patients deemed at considerable risk and limiting the need for most testing in those at low risk.

In the original validation studies done under research conditions, persons with "low-risk" Wells scores demonstrated DVT rates of only 3% on follow-up; those with "high-risk" scores had as much as a 50% prevalence of venous thrombosis. In community-based study of the Wells rule, ruling out DVT proved more difficult, with 12% of those in the low-risk group having DVT. These findings underscore the importance of supplementing the probability estimate with clinical judgment and at least a modicum of laboratory testing, particularly when the results of the prediction rule appear to conflict with clinical judgment.

Laboratory Studies

Laboratory testing is informed by the pretest probability estimate, particularly in the case of unilateral leg edema and suspected deep vein thrombosis.

TABLE 22.2

THE WELLS RULE FOR THE CLINICAL PREDICTION OF DEEP VEIN THROMBOPHLEBITIS

Clinical Feature	Score
History	
Active cancer	1
Paralysis, paresis, or recent plaster immobilization of lower extremity	1
Recently bedridden for >3 d or major surgery within 4 wk	1
Physical Examination	
Localized tenderness along deep veins	1
Swelling of entire leg	1
Calf swelling >3 cm difference in circumference compared to uninvolved leg	1
Pitting edema in the involved leg	1
Collateral superficial veins (nonvaricose)	1
Clinical Assessment	
Alternative diagnosis as or more likely than DVT	−2

Pretest probability of deep vein thrombosis: high if the score is ≥3 points, intermediate if the score is 1–2 points, and low if the score is ≤0 points.
Adapted from Wells PS, Anderson DR, Bormanis J, et al. Value of assessment of pretest probability of deep vein thrombosis in clinical management. Lancet 1997;350:1795, with permission.

Unilateral or Asymmetric Leg Edema

The principal goal of testing is the detection of DVT above the knee, which is associated with a markedly increased risk of pulmonary embolization compared to the presence of a clot below the knee, where DVT risk is less than 3%. High test sensitivity and specificity are required in this setting, not only to rule out DVT in patients who test negative, but also to justify the initiation of anticoagulation in those who test positive. Noninvasive testing modalities (e.g., D-*dimer determination, Doppler ultrasound, plethysmography*) have largely replaced invasive *venography*, the traditional gold standard. When used in conjunction with probability estimates (e.g., the Wells rule; see Table 22.2), such testing can yield high levels of predictive value and limit the need for invasive study and extensive testing.

D-Dimer Determination. D-Dimer testing now occupies a central role in the evaluation of suspected DVT, particularly for ruling out the condition in low-risk persons. It uses monoclonal antibody to detect D-dimer, which is the final degradation product of thrombosis-induced fibrinolysis. The original enzyme-linked immunosorbent assay for D-dimer had a very high sensitivity for DVT (approximately 95%), but its usefulness was limited by its lack of specificity and cumbersomeness (it took hours to perform and had to be done in batches). Its poor specificity produced a very high false-alarm rate, particularly in the setting of conditions in which DVT risk is increased (e.g., malignancy, infection, inflammation, vasculitis, trauma, hemorrhage, and surgery). The newer, quantitative D-dimer assays using automated latex-agglutination methods and the qualitative whole-blood red-cell agglutination tests provide improved convenience (they can be done on single samples in minutes) and enhanced specificity (approximately 70%) without marked sacrifice of sensitivity (85%), cutting down on but not eliminating false positives.

When used in conjunction with the Wells score for pretest-probability determination, the D-dimer demonstrates strong predictive value, especially for ruling out DVT. A negative study in a low-risk patient has a very high negative predictive value (>99.5%) and obviates the need for further testing. A positive study in a low-risk person is associated with a 15% rate of DVT and helps to identify those who require additional testing. Use of D-dimer testing in conjunction with pretest probability determination has reduced the need for additional studies by nearly 40% without any sacrifice in diagnostic accuracy; it makes for a rapid, cost-effective approach to initial laboratory workup in persons with a low pretest probability of DVT who need the condition definitively ruled out.

Doppler Venous Ultrasound. Doppler venous ultrasound provides a sensitive and specific means of detecting deep venous thrombosis above the knee. When used in conjunction with pretest probability assessment, it is the initial test of choice in patients with an intermediate or high pretest probability of DVT. A positive test rules-in the diagnosis; a negative result greatly reduces the probability of DVT but requires follow-up if the patient is other than "low risk" (see later discussion.)

Current ultrasound testing for DVT uses the combination of *two-dimensional (B-mode) ultrasonography* and *color-flow Doppler* (so-called *triplex scanning*), which has proven practical and highly sensitive and specific for the diagnosis of DVT. Failure of the vein to compress during ultrasound scanning is highly correlated with DVT. At times, direct visualization of the clot is possible. Doppler study measures blood flow, helping to identify the vein and any reduction in flow due to the clot. Computerized color enhancement of flow facilitates test performance and interpretation; without color-flow enhancement (so-called *"duplex" scanning*) the interpretation is more technician dependent. For the detection of thrombophlebitis above the knee, sensitivity and specificity of triplex scanning range from 97% to 99%. Duplex ultrasound is currently the minimum standard for ultrasound testing for DVT.

For thrombophlebitis below the knee (which accounts for about 20% of symptomatic DVT), sensitivity and specificity fall to 80% because as many as 40% of calf-vein studies are technically unsuccessful due to poor sound penetration; successful below-the-knee studies have the same sensitivity and specificity as those above the knee. Because embolic risk for DVT below the knee is very low (<3%), the clinical significance of this reduced sensitivity is relatively low. However, a below-the-knee clot can propagate above the knee, usually within the ensuing week. Consequently, a negative triplex study in a person with an intermediate or high pretest probability necessitates additional study. The standard approach has been to repeat the Doppler/ultrasound study in 1 week. Alternatively, a D-dimer study can be obtained at the time of the initial ultrasound study; if it is negative, no further testing is performed. Outcomes of the two approaches have proven comparable (negative predictive value 98% to 99%).

The disadvantages of relying on ultrasound as the initial test for DVT are cost, operator dependence, inconvenience (with the occasional need to repeat the study), and difficulty imaging pelvic veins. Ultrasound utilization can be minimized by using the complementary approach of pretest probability determination and D-dimer testing. As noted earlier, a person with a low pretest probability of DVT and a negative D-dimer test has a less than 1% chance of DVT and requires no further testing. A person with an intermediate pretest probability and a negative Doppler ultrasound study can skip repeat ultrasound if D-dimer testing is negative. Doppler ultrasound is a useful initial test for suspected DVT of the upper extremities (sensitivity 82%, specificity 82%). Patients who manifest reduced flow without incompressibility (the hallmark of DVT) require consideration for venography.

Impedance Plethysmography. Impedance plethysmography remains a widely used noninvasive approach to the diagnosis of DVT that has performance characteristics similar to those of ultrasound when performed by experienced operators. It detects changes in leg volume that follow respiration and inflation and deflation of a thigh blood pressure cuff. In DVT, the normal pattern is altered and detectable by plethysmography. In most reports, test sensitivity ranges from 83% to 93% and specificity from 83% to 97%, but some figures are in the range of 65% to 70% for tests performed in outpatients. The test is somewhat technician dependent, accounting for some of the variation reported in test performance figures. Calf-vein and nonobstructing thrombi are not well detected. Sensitivity can be enhanced by serial studies, which are obtained if there is suspicion of propagation. The test is useful for the detection of recurrent thrombophlebitis because an abnormal test usually reverts to normal 3 months after the initiation of anticoagulant therapy. When specificity in a particular laboratory is less than 90%, then the predictive value of a positive test for DVT in a patient with unilateral leg edema is in the range of 75% to 80%, which is not high enough to justify anticoagulation without further confirmatory testing. A negative test in a patient suspected on clinical grounds of having DVT should be followed either by a venogram or by serial plethysmography studies 2 and 4 days after the initial study.

Venography. Venography remains the gold standard test for the detection of acute deep vein occlusion. When performed and interpreted by an experienced radiologist, it is nearly 100% sensitive and specific. However, it is invasive, expensive, often painful, requires considerable expertise to perform and interpret, and includes a small (2% to 3%) risk of inducing thrombosis or a hypersensitivity reaction to the contrast medium. Moreover, as many as 25% of patients who are candidates for venography have unsuccessful studies. Hospitalization is usually required. These disadvantages plus the advent of sensitive noninvasive methods have relegated venography to a backup role in the evaluation for DVT, mostly for cases in which noninvasive study is technically difficult (e.g., after knee or hip replacement).

In the case of suspected *lymphedema*, venography is the test of first choice for detecting a cause of lymphatic obstruction and should be obtained before lymphangiography is attempted. Severe lymphatic obstruction may interfere with attaining a satisfactory lymphangiogram. Venography is indicated in the evaluation of *DVT of the upper extremities* when Doppler ultrasound shows isolated flow abnormalities but no venous incompressibility.

Magnetic Resonance Imaging Testing. Magnetic resonance direct thrombus imaging (MRDTI) is an investigational approach to the diagnosis of DVT. The reported sensitivity for all leg DVTs is about 96%, and specificity is 90%; for DVT restricted to the calf, its sensitivity and specificity are greater than those for other noninvasive modalities (92% and 90%, respectively). For DVT above the calf, the test characteristics are about the same as or slightly better than those for Doppler ultrasound. As impressive as these results are, MRI is a very expensive technology and its advantages over other, much less expensive modalities remain to be demonstrated. However, special circumstances, such as persons in full-length casts and pregnant women with suspected pelvic DVT, in whom the pelvic veins cannot be visualized by ultrasound, might warrant consideration of MRDTI in lieu of venography.

Computed Tomographic Venography (CTV). The venous phase of CT angiography has yielded excellent images of the pelvic and lower-extremity veins and the ready detection of clots. In the study of patients presenting with suspected pulmonary embolism, CVT has demonstrated superior sensitivity for the detection of DVT compared to ultrasound, but the clinical benefit of this enhanced sensitivity remains to be demonstrated. The test is expensive, requires a large dye load, and is usually performed only when there are indications for CT angiography (see Chapter 20).

Testing for Hypercoagulability. When DVT is confirmed and family history suggests a genetic propensity to DVT or there are no obvious risk factors to account for the episode, then testing for *hypercoagulability* deserves consideration because the results help to determine the risk of recurrence and the need for prolonged anticoagulation (see Chapter 35).

Bilateral Leg Edema

Laboratory testing is critical in bilateral leg edema because the underlying etiology may not be apparent from the history and physical examination alone. The initial laboratory evaluation might start off with a *chest film* in search of heart failure and pleural fluid, a *urinalysis* for the detection of albuminuria, a check of the *serum albumin* for hypoalbuminemia, and determinations of the serum *creatinine* and *blood urea nitrogen* for evidence of renal insufficiency. If the serum albumin is low and

there is no albuminuria, then measurements of the prothrombin time and liver function testing are indicated for further documentation of hepatocellular failure (see Chapter 71). If the serum albumin is low and protein is detected in the urine, a *24-hour urine collection* for albumin and creatinine is indicated (see Chapter 130).

When the diagnosis of bilateral leg edema remains inapparent, a *cardiac ultrasound with Doppler* should be considered, especially in persons older than the age of 45 years. The test provides an excellent noninvasive approach to the detection of heart failure, whether due to systolic or diastolic dysfunction, and to the identification of pulmonary hypertension that might otherwise escape notice. The underrecognition of heart failure and pulmonary hypertension as causes of bilateral leg edema in primary care practice necessitates attention to these possible etiologies. If pulmonary hypertension is suggested by cardiac ultrasound, then consideration of sleep apnea is indicated because of its high prevalence among adults and the subtlety of its presentation (see Chapter 46).

PATIENT EDUCATION AND SYMPTOMATIC THERAPY (4)

When edema is due to increased hydrostatic pressure or decreased oncotic pressure, a number of simple measures can provide the patient some symptomatic relief. The patient should be advised to *restrict salt intake*, avoid prolonged standing or prolonged sitting with the legs dependent, elevate the legs whenever possible, and avoid wearing garments that might restrict venous return (e.g., garters and girdles). Proper *support stockings* might provide some added benefit. Particular consideration should be given to the prevention of DVT during long airplane trips in which the patient is likely to sit in a cramped seat for many hours. The risk of asymptomatic calf DVT has been found to be as high as 12% after very long trips. Avoiding prolonged sitting should be urged, and consideration should also be given to the use of elastic compression stockings. The latter have been found to markedly reduce the risk of developing a calf DVT, although there may be a small increase in the risk of superficial thrombophlebitis.

If possible, the use of salt-retaining drugs should be discontinued or minimized. Severe edema may require *diuretic therapy* (see Chapter 35 for details on the therapy of venous insufficiency). Lymphatic obstruction and increased capillary permeability do not respond well to these measures.

Patients with idiopathic edema are sometimes helped by salt restriction, support hose, elevation, and diuretic use in the early evening. In addition to diuretics, other drugs have been reported to be useful, including propranolol and captopril. It is important to reassure the patient with this condition that the edema poses no threat to health. Furthermore, idiopathic edema often runs a self-limited course, subsiding spontaneously over a few months to several years.

Patients with chronic leg edema should be instructed to call the physician at the first sign of a unilateral increase in swelling or pain because they are at increased risk of thrombophlebitis.

RECOMMENDATIONS

For Unilateral or Markedly Asymmetric Leg Edema

- Review history for risk factors for DVT (e.g., active malignancy, recent paralysis or plaster casting, prolonged immobilization, recent major surgery [especially of the hip or knee], current estrogen/progesterone use, family history of DVT).

- Check the physical examination for key signs of DVT (e.g., difference in calf circumferences of >3 cm, tenderness along deep veins, palpable cord, pitting edema of the entire leg, prominence of collateral superficial veins).
- Estimate the pretest probability of DVT based on history and physical examination; calculate the Wells score.
- In patients with a low Wells score indicative of low pretest probability, obtain a D-dimer test to rule out DVT. If the test is negative, no further testing is necessary. If it is positive, proceed to further testing.
- For those in whom the DVT pretest probability is intermediate or high, proceed initially to Doppler venous ultrasound or plethysmography of the involved limb.
  - If positive, begin anticoagulation.
  - If negative, repeat the ultrasound in 1 week or obtain D-dimer testing at the time of the initial ultrasound testing.

- If D-dimer testing is negative, follow expectantly.
- If D-dimer testing is positive, consider additional testing such as repeat ultrasound in 1 week or proceed directly to venography.

For Bilateral Leg Edema

- Review history for symptoms of venous insufficiency, heart failure, and chronic pulmonary disease, especially sleep apnea. Also check for a history of renal or hepatic disease, malnutrition, and the use of venodilating drugs as calcium-channel blockers.
- Check serum albumin; if it is normal and no other etiology is evident, obtain cardiac ultrasound for the detection of subclinical heart failure and pulmonary hypertension.

A.H.G.

Annotated Bibliography

1. Bergan JJ, Schmid-Schoenbein GW, Coleridge-Smith PD, et al. Chronic venous disease. N Engl J Med 2006;355:488. (*An excellent review of pathophysiology; 100 references.*)
2. Blankfield RP, Finkelhor RS, Alexander JJ, et al. Etiology and diagnosis of bilateral leg edema in primary care. Am J Med 1998;105:192. (*A study from primary care practice showing marked underrecognition of heart failure and pulmonary hypertension as causes of bilateral leg edema; argues for more use of cardiac ultrasonography in the workup.*)
3. Chew HK, Wun T, Harvey D, et al. Incidence of venous thromboembolism and its effect on survival among patients with common cancers. Arch Intern Med 2006;166:458. (*Cancer registry data showing that onset during the first year was associated with an increased risk of death.*)
4. Cushman M, Kuller LH, Prentice R, et al. Estrogen plus progestin and risk of venous thrombosis. JAMA 2004;292:1573. (*Data from the Women's Health Initiative randomized, controlled trial; finds that combination therapy doubles the risk, and increases the risk associated with other risk factors.*)
5. Heit JA, Kobbervig CE, James AH, et al. Trends in incidence of venous thromboembolism during pregnancy or postpartum: a 30-year population-based study. Ann Intern Med 2005;143:697. (*A population-based cohort study; finds the highest risk to be in the postpartum period.*)
6. Juul K, Tybjaerg-Hansen A, Schnohr P, et al. Factor V Leiden and the risk of venous thromboembolism in the adult Danish population. Ann Intern Med 2004;140:330. (*A population cohort study; hazard ratios were found to be considerably lower than previously thought.*)
7. Lansfeld M, Matteson B, Johnson W, wt al. Baker's cyst mimicking the symptoms of deep vein thrombosis: diagnosis with venous duplex scanning. J Vasc Surg 1997;25:658. (*An observational cohort study, finding a 3% incidence of Baker's cysts in persons clinically suspected of having deep vein thrombosis [DVT].*)
8. Rexrode KM, Manson JE. Are some types of hormone therapy safer than others? Lessons from the estrogen and thromboembolism risk study. Circulation. 2007;115:820. (*A useful editorial summarizing the known differences in risk among hormone replacement therapy preparations.*)
9. Philbrick JT, Becker DM. Calf deep venous thrombosis. A wolf in sheep's clothing? Arch Intern Med 1988;148:2131. (*From 20% to 30% of patients with calf-vein thrombosis have proximal propagation.*)
10. Rodeghiero F, Tosetto A. Activated protein C resistance and factor V Leiden mutation are independent risk factors for venous thromboembolism. Ann Intern Med 1999;130:643. (*These hypercoagulable states account for up to 15% of cases of DVT, making attention to these states of potential importance in the evaluation of DVT, especially the recurrent form.*)
11. Rudkin GH, Miller TA. Lipidema: a clinical entity distinct from lymphedema. Plast Reconstr Surg 1994;94:841. (*A good clinical description of this common mimicking etiology.*)
12. Scurr JH, Machin SJ, Bailey-King S, et al. Frequency and prevention of symptomless deep-vein thrombosis in long-haul flights: a randomized trial. Lancet 2001;357:1485. (*Elastic compression stockings reduced the rate of DVT from 12% to 0% but increased the risk of superficial thrombophlebitis.*)
13. Schwarz T, Siegert G, Oettler W, et al. Venous thrombosis after long-haul flights. Arch Intern Med 2003;163:2759. (*A case–control study; flights of longer than 8 hours were associated with an increased risk (relative risk 2.83)*

of calf DVT; episodes occurred exclusively in persons with well-established risk factors.)
14. Smith SL, Heckbert SR, Lemaitre RN, et al. Esterified estrogens and conjugated equine estrogens and the risk of venous thrombosis. JAMA 2004;292:1581. (*A population-based case–control study; no increase in risk was found with esterified estrogens, compared to an increased risk for conjugated estrogens.*)
15. Stein PD, Beemeth A, Olson RE. Obesity as a risk factor in venous thromboembolism. Am J Med 2005;118:978. (*An observational study, finding a relative risk of 2.50 for DVT in both men and women.*)
16. White RH, Chew HK, Phou H, et al. Incidence of venous thromboembolism in the year before the diagnosis of cancer in 528693 adults. Arch Intern Med 2005;165:1782. (*Data from the California Cancer Registry; almost all cases were associated with a diagnosis of metastatic-stage disease appearing within 4 months; the results suggest little benefit from a workup for early cancer at the time of DVT presentation.*)
17. Anderson DR, Lensing AWA, Wells PS, et al. Limitations of impedance plethysmography in the diagnosis of clinically suspected deep-vein thrombosis. Ann Intern Med 1993;118:25. (*A study in outpatients, reporting a lower sensitivity than what is widely quoted.*)
18. Baarslag HJ, van Beek JR, Koopman MMW, et al. Prospective study of color duplex ultrasonography compared with contrast venography in patients suspect of having deep venous thrombosis of the upper extremities. Ann Intern Med 2001;136:865. (*A study finding that ultrasound is the initial test of choice.*)
19. Bates SM, Kearon C, Crowther M, et al. A diagnostic strategy involving a quantitative latex D-dimer assay reliably excludes deep venous thrombosis. Ann Intern Med 2003;138:787. (*A prospective cohort study; a negative test ruled out DVT.*)
20. Fraser DG, Moody AR, Morgan PS, et al. Diagnosis of lower-limb deep venous thrombosis: a prospective blinded study of magnetic resonance direct thrombus imaging. Ann Intern Med 2002;136:89. (*A study of the characteristics of this experimental diagnostic test for DVT.*)
21. Ginsberg JS, Kearon C, Kouketis J, et al. The use of D-dimer testing and impedance plethysmographic examination in patients with clinical indications of deep vein thrombosis. Arch Intern Med 1997;157:1077. (*Using the new whole-blood assay, the combination of tests had a negative predictive value of 98.5%.*)
22. Goodacre S, Sutton AJ, Simpson FC. Meta-analysis: the value of clinical assessment in the diagnosis of deep venous thrombosis. Ann Intern Med 2006;143:129. (*No single sign or symptom was found to be diagnostic, but a low Wells score plus a negative dimer test ruled out DVT.*)
23. Kearon C, Ginsberg JS, Douketis J, et al. A randomized trial of diagnostic strategies after normal proximal vein ultrasonography for suspected deep venous thrombosis: D-dimer testing compared with repeated ultrasonography. Ann Intern Med 2005;142:490. (*A randomized, controlled trial, finding that d-dimer testing was equal to repeat ultrasonography.*)
24. Langfeld M, Matteson B, Johnson W, et al. Baker's cyst mimicking the symptoms of deep venous thrombosis: diagnosis with venous duplex ultrasound. J Vasc Surg 1997;25:658. (*A cohort study, finding that 3% of patients undergoing ultrasound for DVT actually had a ruptured Baker's cyst.*)

25. Lensing AWA, Prandoni P, Brandjes D, et al. Detection of deep-vein thrombosis by real-time B-mode ultrasonography. N Engl J Med 1989;320:342. (*Sensitivity was 100% and specificity was 99% for a clot above the knee; they both fell to 80% for a clot below the knee.*)

26. Oudega R, Hoes AW, Moons KGM. The Wells rule does not adequately rule out deep venous thrombosis in primary care patients. Ann Intern Med 2005;143:100. (*A prospective cross-sectional study from everyday practice, finding a much higher false-positive rate [12%] than was previously reported [3%]; the rate fell to 2.9% when the Wells rule was used in conjunction with d-dimer testing [compared to 0.9% previously reported].*)

27. Perone N, Bounameaux H, Perrier A, et al. Comparison of four strategies for diagnosing deep vein thrombosis: a cost effectiveness analysis. Am J Med 2001;110:33. (*A decision-analysis study, finding that the combination of d-dimer and selective ultrasound testing was the most cost-effective approach.*)

28. Rathbun SW, Witsett TL, Raskob GE. Negative D-dimer result to exclude recurrent deep venous thrombosis: a management tool. Ann Intern Med 2004;141:839. (*A prospective cohort study, finding a false-negative rate of 1% in this population.*)

29. Wells PS, Anderson DR, Rodger M, et al. Evaluation of D-dimer in the diagnosis of suspected deep-vein thrombosis. N Engl J Med 2003;349:1227. (*A large-scale prospective cohort study; the combination of d-dimer testing and the pretest probability accurately ruled out DVT.*)

30. Wells PS, Anderson DR, Bormanis J, et al. Value of assessment of pretest probability of deep vein thrombosis in clinical management. Lancet 1997;350:1795. (*The best available prediction model for guiding test ordering and interpretation in patients suspected of having DVT.*)

CHAPTER 23 ■ EVALUATION OF ARTERIAL INSUFFICIENCY OF THE LOWER EXTREMITIES

DAVID C. BREWSTER

For older persons, arterial circulation to the lower extremity is a key determinant of functional status and ability to remain independent. Peripheral arterial disease of the lower extremities is an important cause of disability and usually a manifestation of systemic atherosclerosis. It is more common in men and increases in prevalence with age. The condition affects a large segment of the elderly population, many of whom are asymptomatic during the early stages of their illness. With progression, intermittent claudication ensues, experienced by about 5% of the U.S. population older than 55 years of age and by greater than 20% of those older than 75 years of age.

Proper clinical management requires the physician first to recognize the manifestations of ischemic disease and carefully evaluate its severity. Patients with mild to moderate vascular insufficiency can be managed quite effectively by conservative measures (see Chapter 34), yet in many instances, the diagnosis goes unrecognized until late stages. Those with acute ischemia or more-severe chronic ischemia that threatens to cause tissue necrosis require more intensive investigation and often surgery (see Chapter 34).

The primary physician must be able to differentiate between patients with arterial insufficiency and those with exertional limb pain due to other causes (e.g., radiculopathy, spinal stenosis). Moreover, one needs to know the indications for and the limitations of the newer noninvasive techniques for evaluating blood flow and the indications for arteriography and referral for consideration of revascularization.

PATHOPHYSIOLOGY AND CLINICAL PRESENTATION (1–5)

Risk Factors and Associated Conditions

The principal risk factors are those of atherosclerotic disease (see Chapter 27), with *cigarette smoking* and *diabetes mellitus* making the greatest contributions. Because these risk factors are the same as those for *coronary artery disease* and *cerebrovascular disease,* it is not surprising to find increased prevalences of these conditions in persons with peripheral artery disease. The probability of encountering symptomatic cardiovascular disease in patients with peripheral artery insufficiency is about 30%; more than 60% prove to have underlying cardiovascular disease when subjected to diagnostic testing. Peripheral artery disease is an independent risk factor for the development of atherosclerotic disease elsewhere.

Reduction in Flow

Occlusive disease generally becomes symptomatic by the gradual reduction of blood flow to the involved extremity or organ. Symptoms finally occur when a critical arterial stenosis is reached. Pressure and blood flow are not significantly diminished until at least 75% of the cross-sectional area of the vessel lumen is obliterated by the disease process. This is approximately equivalent to a 50% reduction in lumen diameter. More-severe stenoses or even total occlusions may remain essentially asymptomatic as long as collateral circulation maintains sufficient blood flow around a lesion to satisfy the metabolic demands of the distal limb at rest and during exercise. Development of ischemic symptoms in the leg implies either inadequate collateral circulation or additional occlusive disease distal to the particular collateral bed. Thus, lesions in the aortoiliac segment may cause little difficulty unless, as is commonly the case, there is an associated disease in the femoropopliteal arterial territory.

Distribution of Disease

Atherosclerotic plaques producing stenosis or occlusion of the arterial lumen are often segmentally distributed, with a predilection for arterial bifurcations. The infrarenal abdominal aorta and aortic bifurcation are common sites of disease, as are the iliac and femoral artery bifurcations. Diabetic patients seem prone to the onset of arteriosclerosis at an earlier age and often have a more distal distribution of occlusive arterial lesions involving the infrapopliteal, tibial, and small runoff vessels.

Early Manifestations

The first sign of impaired arterial circulation is usually *intermittent claudication* (from the Latin *claudicare*, to limp), a manifestation of reduced arterial blood flow that remains adequate at rest but inadequate during exercise. During exercise, the metabolic demands of skeletal muscle in the legs require a 5- to 10-fold increase in blood flow and oxygen delivery. In patients with occlusive disease of major conduit vessels, the requisite increase in blood flow cannot be achieved, and a supply-and-demand mismatch occurs, resulting in muscle ischemia and pain. With the cessation of activity, metabolic demand quickly returns to baseline and symptoms abate.

Patients report pain or discomfort in the lower extremity brought on by walking and relieved by stopping. Discomfort is usually described as a cramping or aching that steadily increases in severity as the distance or speed of walking increases and is frequently worse when walking up an incline. Most characteristically, it involves the calf muscles as a result of disease in the superficial femoral artery, the most common location of lower-extremity obliterative disease. However, claudication may also be noted in more-proximal muscle groups of the hip, thigh, and buttock area when there is aortoiliac involvement.

Later Manifestations

As the severity of the occlusive process worsens, blood flow becomes inadequate for tissue needs even at rest, resulting in the manifestations of more severe arterial insufficiency: *ischemic rest pain* and tissue *necrosis* (ischemic ulceration or gangrene). Rest pain typically occurs at night from leg elevation associated with lying in bed. Patients classically describe ischemic rest pain as an "ache," "pain," "numbness," or "squeezing," most often in the toes and arch of the foot. It may awaken them from sleep and ease when the leg is placed in a dependent position (e.g., dangling the leg over the bedside or standing and walking about). Simple gravitational effects improve arteriolar flow and lessen ischemia.

Ischemic ulcers are painful and appear as punched-out lesions on the dorsum or lateral aspect of the foot. A hallmark of ischemic ulceration is intense pain associated with the lesion.

Clinical Variants

Peripheral arterial insufficiency has three basic anatomic variations, although any number may be present in a given patient. Aortoiliac disease is most common in patients who smoke or have hypercholesterolemia. Claudication in the buttock or thigh is characteristic. The femoral pulses are absent or diminished, but pedal pulses may be intact. *Femoropopliteal disease* accounts for two thirds of cases and presents as calf pain with exertion. Femoral pulses may be preserved, but popliteal and pedal pulses are absent or diminished. *Tibioperoneal occlusion* is a disease of diabetics and older patients. Skin ulcers and atrophic skin changes are common.

Clinical Course and Prognosis

The natural history and associated clinical course of peripheral arterial disease are quite variable and often favorable. In the Framingham Study population, only one third of those developing claudication went on to have persistent symptoms; the remainder experienced remission or transient symptoms. However, 15% of those presenting with severe disease required amputation over the ensuing 2 years. Persistent smokers and diabetics have the worst prognoses.

Any consideration of prognosis for this atherosclerotic disease has to include the substantial risks of *cardiovascular morbidity* and *mortality*, which are increased fivefold compared with persons without peripheral arterial disease.

DIFFERENTIAL DIAGNOSIS (5)

The differential diagnosis of lower-extremity ischemia includes vascular and nonvascular etiologies (Table 23.1). Besides *atherosclerotic disease*, lower-extremity ischemia may also be caused by *arterial embolism, dissection, trauma, thrombosis of an aneurysm*, or *thromboangiitis obliterans (Buerger's disease)*. *Reflex sympathetic dystrophy* may cause transient coldness, blanching, and pain. *Venous disease* may lead to discomfort and painless superficial skin ulceration.

Musculoskeltal conditions may mimic the symptoms of arterial insufficiency. Pain in the hip, thigh, or knee region with walking is a frequent consequence of *degenerative joint disease* of the hip or knee, *lumbar disk disease* with *radiculopathy* (sciatica, cauda equina syndrome; see Chapter 147), *spinal stenosis* (pseudoclaudication; see Chapter 147), and *Paget's disease*. Muscular etiologies include *nocturnal leg cramps*, which are commonly mistaken for ischemic pain in being localized to the calf but differ, in that symptoms are exclusively a nighttime phenomenon. *Myositis* and *drug-induced muscle discomfort* (as seen with statin use) may cause pain in the quadriceps and calves, simulating ischemic pain, but associated with focal muscle tenderness to palpation and present at rest as well as with

TABLE 23.1

DIFFERENTIAL DIAGNOSIS OF LOWER-EXTREMITY CLAUDICATION

Vascular Causes
  Atherosclerotic disease
  Systemic embolization
  Buerger's disease (thromboangiitis obliterans)
  Dissection
  Trauma
  Thrombosis of an aneurysm
  Arteritis
  Reflex sympathetic dystrophy
  Venous disease

Nonvascular Causes
  Sciatica and other radiculopathies
  Hip or knee osteoarthritis
  Paget's disease
  Cauda equina syndrome
  Spinal stenosis
  Nocturnal leg cramps
  Myositis and drug-induced muscle discomfort
  Diabetic neuropathy

exertion. Overall, clues that help to differentiate these etiologies from vascular disease include pain not clearly related to a predictable amount of exercise and not promptly relieved by cessation of activity.

Diabetic neuropathy can be difficult to differentiate from ischemic rest pain, particularly in a patient with diminished or absent pulses. In both conditions, a burning, constant ache is often present in the forefoot and toes. The presence of paresthesias in addition to pain suggests a neurologic source. True ischemic rest pain is usually worse with elevation and frequently is relieved somewhat by dependency of the limb. Such features may be used in differentiation. In all such instances, noninvasive studies during exercise may be of substantial help in the differential diagnosis.

WORKUP (5–15)

The diagnosis of peripheral vascular disease and an accurate assessment of its level and severity may be made by a careful history and physical examination to an extent not usually possible in many other disease states. Although no single feature is absolutely diagnostic or exclusionary of peripheral arterial disease, combinations of readily elicited clinical findings can provide a very high level of predictive value. The availability of effective treatment for peripheral vascular disease makes it mandatory that early and accurate diagnosis be established before end-stage problems develop and threaten limb loss.

History

Intermittent claudication is the hallmark of vascular insufficiency and, by multivariate analysis, an independent predictor of the disease. A reliable story for its presence significantly increases the likelihood of the diagnosis (the likelihood ratio [LR] is 3.30; Table 23.2). The absence of claudication does not rule out the diagnosis (LR 0.89), but it does markedly lower the probability of moderate to severe ischemic disease.

A cramp or ache in the calf or thigh muscles that is reproducibly brought on by *walking a predictable distance* should be suspect, especially if the discomfort is relieved within minutes by simply stopping. The location of the pain may help to localize the occlusive process. In some instances of proximal disease, the pain may be located principally in the hip or buttock region, causing confusion with other neuroorthopedic conditions such as spinal stenosis and lumbar radiculopathy. If the walking distance required to produce the pain varies considerably from day to day or if the patient must sit or lie down for more than several minutes to obtain relief, the physician should suspect a nonvascular cause, such as spinal stenosis. Weight-bearing and other activities that extend the lumbar spine will aggravate the pain of spinal stenosis. Similarly, the pain should involve the same areas consistently and not different portions of the leg from day to day. Crampy pain occurring in the calf at rest, particularly at night, rarely signifies a vascular problem. The triad of discomfort brought on by exercise, relief achieved within 2 to 5 minutes by stopping, and ability to walk the same distance again once the discomfort ceases is strongly suggestive of vascular insufficiency.

Complaints of *pain at rest* and with exercise suggest more advanced ischemia. A history of prior claudication is almost always obtained in such patients unless the distribution of the occlusive process is quite distal or in small vessels only. Ischemic rest pain typically involves the toes or forefoot, not the calf or thigh. It is usually improved with dependency of the limb and therefore is worse at night. Pain that is not confined to the distal foot, that is better with elevation, or that occurs in a patient without intermittent claudication should alert the physician to look for other possible causes, such as diabetic neuropathy or a neuroorthopedic problem.

Symptoms of tissue necrosis will usually be quite apparent. Peripheral *gangrene* without prior symptoms should raise the possibility of embolic disease or small-vessel occlusions due to conditions other than chronic arteriosclerosis. In patients with leg ulceration, historical clues suggesting a traumatic, dermatologic, or venous origin should also be sought; many leg and foot ulcers are not ischemic in origin.

A complete history should include questioning for sexual difficulties. Erectile *impotence*, long associated with severe aortoiliac occlusive disease, has been termed the *Leriche syndrome* after the French surgeon who first reported its significance in 1923. Finally, it is of utmost importance to note the existence of known risk factors for arteriosclerosis (e.g., family history, smoking, diabetes mellitus, hypertension, lipid disorders) and related problems in the coronary and cerebrovascular systems indicative of the systemic nature of the atherosclerosis.

Physical Examination

Examination can help to confirm, localize, and establish the severity of the arterial lesion. Findings that independently

---

TABLE 23.2

DIFFERENTIATING TRUE CLAUDICATION FROM PSEUDOCLAUDICATION

Clinical Feature	Claudication	Pseudoclaudication
Character of discomfort	Cramping, tightness, tiredness, aching	Same + tingling, weakness, clumsiness
Location	Buttock, hip, thigh, calf, foot	Same
Exercise induced	Yes	Yes
Distance to pain	Same each time	Variable
Occurs with standing	No	Yes
Relief	With cessation of walking	With sitting or position change

Adapted from Krajewski LP, Olin JW. Atherosclerosis of the aorta and lower-extremity arteries. In: Young JR, Olin JW, Bartholomew JR, eds. Peripheral vascular disease, 2nd ed. St. Louis: Yearbook, 1996:208, with permission.

predict disease include abnormal pedal pulses and femoral artery bruits.

Palpation of peripheral pulses is the keystone of the examination. Palpation of the abdomen for the aortic pulsation and of both extremities for femoral, popliteal, posterior tibial, and dorsalis pedis pulses should be routine in all patients. Reduced or absent pulses in the symptomatic region substantially increases the probability of hemodynamically significant peripheral arterial disease (LR 4.70); finding normal pulses markedly reduces the likelihood (LR 0.38). Local factors such as edema or marked obesity may hinder palpation. Abnormally prominent pulsations suggest aneurysmal disease.

Auscultation of the aortic, iliac (2 cm lateral to the umbilicus), femoral, and popliteal regions should always be performed; the finding of a *bruit* markedly increases the probability of peripheral arterial disease (LR 5.60); its absence significantly lowers the probability only when absent in all arteries of the symptomatic limb (LR 0.39)—the absence of a single bruit has little diagnostic meaning, in part because marked reduction of flow in a severely stenotic or occluded vessel will not produce a bruit. Exercise may greatly intensify femoral bruits, making this a potentially useful maneuver.

Skin and *integument changes* can contribute to diagnosis. *Coolness to touch* in the symptomatic leg increases pretest probability (LR 5.90), as can *discolored skin* (LR 2.80) and *wounds* or *ulcers* (LR 5.90). Arterial ulcers appear as painful "punched-out lesions, often about the malleolus or involving the toes. Absence of such findings does little to rule out arterial disease (LR 0.84). *Rubor on dependency* is a classic manifestation of severe disease; *atrophic skin*, toe *hair loss*, and *nail changes* are less reliable indicators of chronic arterial insufficiency.

Maneuvers may help to elucidate ischemic disease. *Prolonged capillary filling time* (>5 seconds to refill after 5 seconds of plantar compression of the big toe, especially when one side is compared with the other) is suggestive of moderate to severe disease (LR 1.90). *Pallor on leg elevation (Buerger's test)* involves having the patient raise the leg to 90 degrees while supine, then passively lower the leg and noting the angle at which color returns; the test is positive if the "angle of circulatory sufficiency" is less than 0 degrees (i.e., the leg must hang below the table).

Careful spine, hip, knee, and neurologic examinations are important to rule out nonvascular causes of exertional lower-extremity pain (see Chapters 147 and 172).

Laboratory Studies

History and physical examination are usually sufficient to establish the diagnosis and provide a rough estimate of severity. In patients with mild to moderate disease free of limb-threatening ischemia or unacceptable activity limitations, no further investigation is necessary other than evaluation for potential *risk factors* such as hypertension, hyperlipidemia, smoking, and diabetes (see Chapters 14, 15, 54, and 93, respectively). Blood sugar determination may detect a previously undiagnosed diabetic, but there is still no firm evidence that tight control of the serum glucose level prevents or ameliorates macrovascular disease (see Chapter 102).

In patients with premature atherosclerotic disease but no evident precipitants, the possibility of *hyperhomocysteinemia* deserves consideration. The relation between this inborn error of metabolism and vascular disease has been established. Diagnosis is suggested by elevated serum homocysteine levels after overnight methionine loading.

Noninvasive Vascular Studies

These are indicated if the diagnosis or degree of impairment is uncertain or if the disease appears to be clinically severe enough to warrant consideration of surgical correction. A host of noninvasive testing methods is available, ranging from segmental blood pressure measurements to Doppler and two-dimensional ultrasound techniques. These methods are becoming widely available and are relatively simple to use, inexpensive compared with angiography, and without risk or discomfort to the patient. Such tests may be extremely helpful in establishing a vascular etiology for complaints of pain in the leg and in quantifying clinical impressions, which are often somewhat imprecise. Because they can be used repeatedly, such tests are also particularly helpful in evaluating improvement or deterioration of the patient's condition over time and in assessing the benefit of various forms of treatment or operation.

It should be emphasized that these methods are meant not to replace or lessen the value of a good history and physical examination, but rather to supplement them and provide such additional information as site and severity of stenosis.

Handheld Doppler. The advent of handheld Doppler devices makes it possible to incorporate Doppler testing into the initial primary care office assessment. A peripheral arterial disease score has been validated and can be calculated on the basis of the quality of the palpated posterior tibial artery pulse (normal, reduced, absent), number of auscultated Doppler pulse components (0, 1, 2, or 3), and history of myocardial infarction. The maximum possible score is 10 (for both legs); a score of less than 6 is associated with a high probability of disease (LR 7.80). The testing helps to improve the identification of patients who need a formal determination of the ankle/brachial index.

Ankle/Brachial Index. *Segmental blood pressure* measurements are taken at the arm, upper thigh, above and below the knee, and above the ankle with the patient supine. A *Doppler* device measures systolic pressure in each location. Normally, there is an increase in pressure as the pressure wave moves distally. A reduction in pressure suggests arterial occlusion. Sensitivity and specificity are maximized by determining the *ankle/brachial ratio or index* (a ratio of the systolic pressure found in the posterior tibial–dorsalis pedis arteries divided by the pressure in the brachial artery). An index of less than 0.9 has a 95% sensitivity in patients with angiographically proven disease and a 100% specificity in normal individuals. The test gives a better estimate of functional capacity than do symptoms of claudication, and the results have value as independent predictors of cardiovascular morbidity and mortality. Despite the value and simplicity of the test, it is infrequently used routinely by clinicians.

Segmental pressures can be used as a screening test for further evaluation and in gauging severity. A ratio of less than 0.8 correlates with moderate disease, 0.6 with severe or multilevel disease, and less than 0.4 with severe disease and a high risk of complications. The test is not reliable in patients with calcified vessels (e.g., diabetics).

Pulse–Volume Recordings. Pulse–volume recordings are particularly useful for the assessment of distal vascular disease, especially in patients with stiff vessels. Doppler and plethysmographic methods are used. The patient with stiff vessels and distal disease may have a normal ankle pressure, but the normally sharp pulse–volume waveform becomes blunted with obstruction. Sensitivity is improved when treadmill exercise is added to the examination. Diabetics, who tend to have stiff vessels and distal disease, are good candidates for pulse–volume recording.

Duplex Ultrasound Scanning. Duplex ultrasound scanning combines two-dimensional (B-mode) real-time ultrasound with pulsed Doppler to provide more-precise anatomic and flow data than are available from other methods. The ultrasound probe is placed over specific vessels to measure the velocity of flow. B-mode ultrasound identifies the site and nature of the stenosis. Adding *color-flow enhancement* (triplex scanning) improves test performance. Triplex scanning has a sensitivity and specificity well greater than 90%; those for duplex scanning are a bit less. Although such examinations are somewhat time consuming, require expensive equipment and experienced examiners, and lack the ability to provide detailed anatomic data on the location of stenoses or occlusions, they do provide sufficient information for most initial clinical decision making.

Magnetic Resonance Angiography. Magnetic resonance (MR) technology has been developed and studied as a means of improving the noninvasive imaging of the arteries of the lower extremity, with a goal of achieving the anatomic detail of traditional angiography. Meta-analysis of MR techniques for imaging the peripheral arterial tree found sensitivity and specificity approaching 95%, especially when three-dimensional techniques and gadolinium enhancement were used. Because standardization has not yet been developed and the procedure is expensive, MR angiography cannot yet be considered a replacement for traditional angiography; however, the procedure is promising and has important advantages (including better imaging of the distal vasculature, absence of a dye load, and no need for arterial puncture). Its principal contribution is likely to be as a noninvasive substitute for traditional angiography in the preoperative assessment.

Preoperative Studies

When surgery is being contemplated, one needs to determine the precise anatomy of the occlusive disease. Although *contrast arteriography* has little place in the initial diagnostic evaluation of arterial insufficiency, its contribution remains substantial in the assessment of the patient who is being considered for revascularization (see Chapter 34). The procedure is used for precise localization of the disease process and proper selection of the most appropriate invasive procedure. A major disadvantage and risk associated with arteriography is acute *dye-induced renal failure*. Patients with peripheral vascular disease commonly have concurrent renal vascular disease or renal dysfunction, making them especially vulnerable to acute renal failure on exposure to a large iodinated contrast load. Arteriography should also be used with caution in persons with other forms of underlying renal disease and in persons with a history of allergy to iodine or iodinated radiologic contrast agents.

Magnetic resonance angiography (MRA) provides a noninvasive alternative, free of the risk of dye-induced acute renal failure or allergic reaction. It is particularly helpful in patients with a history of severe allergic reactions to iodinated contrast, renal insufficiency, or other contraindications to conventional catheter arteriography. Further advances in MRA using noniodinated contrast hold promise for providing an even more effective diagnostic alternative to conventional contrast arteriography for the preoperative assessment.

Screening

Screening for peripheral arterial disease is indicated in asymptomatic persons with a substantially increased pretest probability of disease, including those with diabetes, age greater than 70 years, or a history of ischemic heart disease, stroke, hypercholesterolemia, smoking (current or past), or hypertension. Simple approaches to screening include asking about claudication, listening for a femoral bruit, and, palpating for a pulse abnormality. The presence of a femoral bruit increases disease probability (LR 4.80), as do claudication (LR 3.30) and a palpably abnormal pulse (LR 3.10). The absence of such findings is associated with a reduced pretest probability, especially for moderate to severe disease.

INDICATIONS FOR REFERRAL AND ADMISSION (5)

Although most patients with mild to moderate lower extremity occlusive disease can be well managed conservatively (see Chapter 34), those with pain that markedly limits daily activities and significantly impairs lifestyle may benefit from referral for consultation with an experienced vascular surgeon to review the treatment options, including revascularization. patients with evidence of more advanced disease (ischemic rest pain, nonhealing ischemic ulcerations) need prompt referral for revascularization due to the high likelihood of amputation and limb loss without revascularization. The noninvasive vascular laboratory may be very helpful in providing objective data to help define patients with critical ischemia and the need for prompt revascularization (Table 23.3). Patients with gangrenous lesions of the lower extremities or an infected ischemic ulcer require prompt hospital admission, particularly if they are diabetic.

TABLE 23.3

INDICATIONS FOR SURGICAL REFERRAL

Severe (disabling) intermittent claudication; ankle systolic pressure <50 mm Hg after exercise; cannot complete standard 5-min treadmill exercise study
Persistent ischemic rest pain; resting ankle systolic pressure <50 mm Hg
Ischemic ulceration or gangrene of foot/toes

Annotated References

1. Clarke R, Daly L, Robinson K, et al. Hyperhomocysteinemia: an independent risk factor for vascular disease. N Engl J Med 1991;324:1149. (*Documents this condition to be an independent and important risk factor for premature vascular disease.*)
2. Criqui MH, Langer RD, Fronek A, et al. Mortality over a period of 10 years in patients with peripheral arterial disease. N Engl J Med 1992;326:381. (*The ankle/brachial index values serve as independent predictors of cardiovascular morbidity and mortality.*)
3. Guralnik JM, Ferrucci L, Simonsick EM, et al. Lower extremity function in persons over the age of 70 years as a predictor of subsequent disability. N Engl J Med 1995;332:556. (*Documents the importance of lower-extremity function to the maintenance of independence.*)

4. McDermott MM, Kerwin DR, Liu K, et al. Prevalence and significance of unrecognized lower extremity peripheral arterial disease in general medicine practice. J Gen Intern Med 2001;16:384. (*A population study, finding that prevalence was high, and recognition was low.*)

5. Weitz JI, Byrne Clagett GP, et al. Diagnosis and treatment of chronic arterial insufficiency of the lower extremities: a critical review. Circulation 1996;94:3026. (*A useful and informative review relative to the incidence, natural history, and outcomes of treatment.*)

6. Cambria RP, Brewster DC, Kaufman JA, et al. Magnetic resonance angiography in the management of lower extremity arterial occlusive disease: a prospective study. J Vasc Surg 1997;25:380. (*Evaluation of the utility and accuracy of magnetic resonance angiography.*)

7. Criqui MH, Fronek A, Klauber MR, et al. The sensitivity, specificity, and predictive value of traditional clinical evaluation of peripheral arterial disease: results from noninvasive testing in a defined population. Circulation 1985;71:240. (*Lack of a posterior tibial pulse was the best clinical predictor of peripheral vascular disease.*)

8. Farkough ME, Oddone EZ, Simel DL. Improving the clinical examination for a low ankle–brachial index. Int J Angiol 2002;11:41. (*Presents a practical scoring system using physical examination and handheld Doppler testing for determining who needs further evaluation.*)

9. Khan NA, Rahim SA, Simel DL, et al. Does the clinical examination predict lower extremity peripheral artery disease? JAMA 2006;295:536. (*A superb review that is part of the very useful Rational Clinical Examination series.*)

10. Koelemay MJW, Lijmer JG, Stoker J, et al. Magnetic resonance angiography for the evaluation of lower extremity arterial disease: a meta-analysis. JAMA 2001;285:1338. (*Sensitivity and specificity are 94% for three-dimensional gadolinium-enhanced scanning.*)

11. McDermott MM, Greenland P, Liu K, et al. The ankle–brachial index is associated with leg function and physical activity: the walking and leg circulation study. Ann Intern Med 2002;136:873. (*The test correlated better with leg circulatory function than did symptoms.*)

12. McGee SR, Boyko EJ. Physical examination and chronic lower-extremity ischemia. Arch Intern Med 1998;158:1364. (*A critical literature review identifying the features of the examination that were most useful in determining the presence and the distribution of ischemia.*)

13. McLafferty RB, Dunnington GL, Mattos MA, et al. Factors affecting the diagnosis of peripheral vascular disease before surgery. J Vasc Surg 2000;31:870. (*Found very infrequent routine use of the brachial/ankle index.*)

14. Muribito JM, Evans JC, Larson MG, et al. The ankle–brachial index in the elderly and risk of stroke, coronary disease, and death. The Framingham Study. Arch Intern Med 2003;163:1939. (*A prospective cohort study; a low score was associated with a significant risk of stroke and transient ischemic attack.*)

15. Whelan JF, Barry JH, Moir JD. Color flow Doppler ultrasonography: comparison with peripheral arteriography for the investigation of peripheral vascular disease. J Clin Ultrasound 1992;20:369. (*Presents data on sensitivity and specificity.*)

CHAPTER 24 ■ EVALUATION OF SYNCOPE

Syncope denotes reversible loss of consciousness due to transiently insufficient cerebral perfusion and can be among the most difficult of conditions to evaluate because the story may be vague and findings subtle. Nonetheless, a thoughtful basic workup can uncover the cause in one half to two thirds of instances and also identify those individuals who need additional investigation. Of particular importance is identification of underlying cardiovascular disease because of its attendant increase in morbidity and mortality. Even "harmless" causes of syncope may put the patient at risk for serious injury and need to be identified and addressed.

PATHOPHYSIOLOGY AND CLINICAL PRESENTATION (1–14)

The pathophysiologic common denominator of syncope is transiently inadequate cerebral perfusion. Mechanisms compromising cerebral perfusion operate through neural, cardiac, and cerebrovascular pathways. Medication often plays a contributing role, especially in the elderly.

Neurally Mediated Syncope

The normal compensatory responses to standing up are increased sympathetic activity leading to vasoconstriction, tachycardia, increased contractility, and withdrawal of vagal tone. Catecholamines are released, as are vasoconstricting and volume-retaining hormones (e.g., renin, vasopressin). In neu-

rally mediated syncope, there is a defect in this compensatory mechanism.

Vasovagal (Neurocardiogenic) Syncope

Vasovagal syncope accounts for the largest percentage of cases. Although it is the most common cause of syncope in otherwise healthy young persons, it occurs in all age groups. Its hallmarks are inappropriate *bradycardia* and *vasodilation* due to an increase in vagal tone and interruption of normal sympathetic responses. The resultant bradycardia and vasodilation cause systemic blood pressure to plummet, compromising cerebral perfusion and leading to loss of consciousness.

Purported triggers of the heightened vagal activity include psychological distress, excess venous pooling, hypersensitivity of organ mechanoreceptors (in heart, esophagus, bladder, and respiratory tract), and the *Bezold–Jarisch reflex* (an extra strong cardiac contraction in reaction to decreased preload). The latter is a brainstem-mediated autonomic reflex that increases vagal tone, inhibits sympathetic activity, and results in reduced cardiac contractility, bradycardia, and peripheral vasodilation. Central nervous system modulators (e.g., serotonin, adenosine, opioids, and beta-endorphins) may also play a role in this reflex, perhaps mediating the vasovagal response to emotional distress and other cortical stimuli. The myocardium and conduction system are normal in such persons, accounting for the excellent prognosis. The seemingly paradoxical use of beta-blockers in treatment of this condition aims to inhibit the Bezold–Jarisch reflex by blunting the initial myocardial response. Anticholinergic agents are also used.

Clinical presentations can be quite variable, but in most instances, the episode occurs in the upright or standing position or during exercise. Although some patients (particularly the elderly) may report no premonitory symptoms, most experience *prodromal autonomic symptoms* of sweating, epigastric queasiness or nausea, lightheadedness, dizziness, blurred or dimmed vision, weakness or extreme fatigue, and occasionally a feeling of depersonalization. The patient feels restless and unable to concentrate. Yawning, sighing, or hyperventilation may be noted. The onset of premonitory symptoms may help to prevent a drop attack and resultant injury. The unconscious patient appears ashen or pale, cold, and diaphoretic with dilated pupils. At the outset, the heart rate may be rapid, but it slows markedly as the process unfolds. The presence of pallor and diaphoresis is paradoxical, but both may be prominent and reflect the high circulating levels of epinephrine found in this state of otherwise marked sympathetic inhibition. Such features make for a very distressing clinical presentation, mimicking serious cardiovascular disease. After several minutes, full consciousness is regained, although weakness, sweatiness, and nausea may persist. In the elderly, there may be some retrograde amnesia, but control of bladder and bowels is never lost, helping to differentiate the episode from a seizure. Tilt-table study can reproduce the symptoms in susceptible persons, with many reporting a prodrome of blurred vision, vertigo, tinnitus, and nausea when tested (see later discussion).

Sometimes the hypotension and hypoperfusion that occur are so profound that cerebral hypoxia and seizure activity (*convulsive syncope*) ensue. This convulsive syncope is distinct from loss of consciousness that accompanies a generalized seizure disorder and does not respond to antiseizure medication.

Situational Syncopes

Situational syncopes can be considered variants of vasovagally mediated disease, precipitated by factors that reduce venous return. The inciting event may be a coughing spell, voiding, straining at stool, pain, or emotional stress. *Posttussive syncope* is characterized by loss of consciousness following a prolonged bout of forceful coughing. Men with chronic bronchitis are most often affected. The precipitant of the vasovagal response is believed to involve decreased cardiac output due to decreased venous return. In addition, there may be increased cerebral vascular resistance secondary to hypocapnia and compression of cerebral vessels by an increase in cerebrospinal fluid pressure. Prolonged Valsalva maneuvers have a similar effect—the increase in intrathoracic pressure impedes venous return. *Postmicturition syncope* takes place in the context of emptying a distended bladder. The typical setting involves a man who has gotten up at night to urinate after consuming considerable amounts of alcohol. Consciousness is lost without much warning. Drainage of ascitic fluid or a distended bladder may produce a similar effect. Valsalva plays an important role in *postdefecation syncope*, in which straining decreases venous return and sets in motion the vasovagal reflex response. *Pain* and *acute psychological distress* can trigger a similar vasovagal response.

Psychiatric disease probably represents a class of vasovagal variants mediated by central factors. The precise pathophysiology is incompletely understood, but underlying psychopathology is becoming increasingly appreciated as an important etiologic factor, especially in investigations of syncope of unknown origin. *Generalized anxiety disorder*, *panic disorder*, and *depression* are frequently found in populations of such patients who have no evidence of heart disease. Their fainting spells often resolve with treatment of the underlying psychopathology.

Prevalence is greatest in younger persons with frequent syncopal episodes, in those who never sustain injury from their loss of consciousness, and in patients who present with multiple somatic and psychiatric symptoms, such as fear, anxiousness, nausea, lightheadedness, and numbness. Reproduction of symptoms by 2 to 3 minutes of open-mouth hyperventilation is characteristic. *Hysteria* may result in apparent loss of consciousness; the spell is a *conversion reaction* characterized by graceful fainting to the floor or couch; frequent presence of an audience; normal pulse, skin color, and blood pressure; and an emotionally detached description of the episode.

Dysautonomia

Dysautonomia represents a pathophysiologic common denominator for a spectrum of conditions that produce an inadequate autonomic response leading to *postural hypotension* (>20 mm Hg decrease in systolic pressure, >10 mm Hg decrease in diastolic pressure) and reduced cerebral perfusion pressure. Patients typically develop symptoms on standing, especially in the setting of reduced effective intravascular volume (e.g., dehydration, vasodilating drugs, acute blood loss, excessive venous pooling). The patient experiences orthostatic hypotension because reflex vasoconstriction and increase in heart rate fail to occur. Unlike the vasovagal etiologies, there is no slowing of heart rate, but heart rate typically remains inappropriately slow for the degree of blood pressure fall. Hypotension progresses over seconds to minutes until perfusion is inadequate for maintenance of consciousness. During the presyncopal period, there is no increase in heart rate or other signs of autonomic response (e.g., pallor, nausea, or sweating). The period of syncope is brief, and consciousness returns promptly. Near-syncope is common among these patients, as are impotence and bladder and bowel disturbances.

The most common cause of autonomic insufficiency is *diabetes mellitus*, but it may also occur in the context of *advancing age*, neurodegenerative disease (e.g., *Shy–Drager syndrome*) (orthostasis, parkinsonism, cerebellar ataxia), *alcohol abuse*, and *medications*. Leading the list of offending agents are the *antihypertensives* (e.g., angiotensin-converting-enzyme inhibitors, angiotensin-receptor blockers, beta-blockers, alpha-blockers, calcium-channel blockers, diuretics). *Tricyclic antidepressants* are also associated with postural hypotension and syncope in the elderly.

Postprandial hypotension is a form of postural hypotension analogous to autonomic insufficiency. It is defined as a 20-mm Hg decrease in systolic pressure within 2 hours of beginning a meal. Prevalence is greatest among elderly hypertensive patients. Postulated mechanisms range from inadequacies in sympathetic response and baroreceptor function to excessive insulin-induced and vasopeptide-induced vasodilation and splanchnic pooling. Consequences may be serious and include falls, syncope, angina, and stroke.

Neuropathic postural tachycardia syndrome is a variant of orthostatic hypotension, characterized by anxiety, lightheadedness, dimming of vision, confusion, and a dramatic rise in heart rate that occurs on standing. The limbs turn bluish red. Outright syncope occurs in about half of patients. Although symptoms are postural, there is no marked decrease in blood pressure. The underlying pathophysiology involves partial sympathetic denervation in the legs, leading to excessive pooling of blood in the lower extremities. Circulating levels of catecholamines are high. Symptoms are relieved by lying down or sitting. The condition is most commonly found among young women, and there may be concurrent mitral valve prolapse, irritable bowel syndrome, or chronic fatigue syndrome.

Carotid Sinus Hypersensitivity

Carotid sinus hypersensitivity represents a form of neurocardiogenic syncope that occurs most commonly in elderly persons with underlying atherosclerotic disease. Massage of the carotid sinus can trigger long *asystolic pauses*. Digitalis administration seems to aggravate the condition. Carotid sinus hypersensitivity may also cause a vasodepressor form of syncope in which heart rate remains unchanged but there is vasodilation and hypotension. Actions that lead to compression of the carotid sinus (wearing a tight collar, turning the head, or shaving) characteristically cause symptoms, which include lightheadedness, sweating, pallor, and nausea, followed by fainting. When the predominant mechanism is asystole, the loss of consciousness can be precipitous.

Cerebrovascular Disease

Syncope can be a consequence of *vertebrobasilar insufficiency* of the midbrain affecting the reticular activating system or, in the rare instance, of total or near-total occlusion of the carotid arteries with concurrent compromise of the circle of Willis. Lesser degrees of obstruction may contribute to minor lightheadedness on standing and can be aggravated by use of antihypertensive agents and volume depletion. Patients with substantial cerebrovascular disease often have evidence of previous strokes manifested by focal neurologic deficits. A *transient ischemic attack* involving the vertebrobasilar circulation may lead to syncope by temporarily depriving the brainstem's reticular activating system of adequate perfusion. Brainstem neurologic deficits typically accompany or precede the loss of consciousness.

Subclavian steal syndrome can compromise cerebral blood flow when occlusion of the proximal subclavian artery leads to reversal of flow in the adjacent vertebral artery. When vascular resistance in the arm falls, for example, during exercise, flow is redirected away from the brain, and ischemic symptoms may ensue.

Heart Disease

Structural Heart Disease

Aortic stenosis and *hypertrophic cardiomyopathy* can result in syncope when they cause hemodynamically significant obstruction of the left ventricular outflow tract (see Chapter 33). The characteristic clinical picture is one of *effort syncope*, with loss of consciousness in the context of vigorous exercise and sweating. The latter contributes to hemodynamic compromise by causing vasodilation and a drop in venous return. A vicious cycle of inability to raise cardiac output and falling venous return can lead to hypotension, loss of consciousness, and even sudden death. Syncope in the setting of known aortic stenosis carries a very poor prognosis (see Chapter 33). Total blockade of the mitral orifice from an *atrial myxoma* and massive *pulmonary embolization* leading to *acute pulmonary hypertension* can have similar consequences. Loss of consciousness comes with little warning. *Anomalous origin of a coronary artery* from the coronary sinus places a patient at risk for kinking or twisting of the artery, especially during vigorous exercise, and can cause syncope or even sudden death. Premonitory symptoms may be absent, but sometimes there is a history of exercise-induced chest pain or syncope.

Cardiac Dysrhythmias

Cardiac dysrhythmias may precipitate sudden loss of consciousness with none of the premonitory manifestations of neurocardiogenic syncope. At times, palpitations are reported to precede the syncopal event. Once effective systoles have ceased, less than 5 seconds of consciousness remains. Palpitations are sometimes reported, and loss of consciousness can occur while the patient is supine. Important dysrhythmias associated with syncope include *complete heart block* (Stokes–Adams attacks) and *ventricular tachycardia* (VT) (see Chapter 29). Most persons with VT have evidence of underlying heart disease (*ischemia, cardiomyopathy, QT prolongation*), but in others, the heart may appear normal (see Chapter 29). Important clinical clues of a serious arrhythmic etiology in those without overt heart disease include a history of palpitations (particularly exercise induced) and a family history of syncope or sudden death. The clinical picture of those with VT may include exercise-induced palpitations and dyspnea in addition to syncope.

Occasionally, a *supraventricular tachycardia* (e.g., paroxysmal supraventricular tachycardia or, less commonly, atrial fibrillation or flutter) with a very rapid ventricular response rate will sufficiently compromise cardiac output to result in near or complete syncope (see Chapter 28). Common precipitants of supraventricular tachyarrhythmias include ischemia, sick sinus syndrome, digitalis toxicity, and the preexcitation syndromes. Patients with chronic bifascicular and trifascicular block are more likely to have syncopal attacks, but those with syncope have not been found to have an increased risk of sudden death.

Nonsyncopal Causes of Loss of Consciousness

Seizures

Seizures differ from causes of syncope in that the loss of consciousness derives from an electrical disturbance rather than inadequate cerebral perfusion. The typical clinical presentation is unique, with aura, postictal symptoms, incontinence, and tonic–clonic movements often dominating the clinical picture. However, akinetic petit mal attacks have few of these features, although normal blood pressure and pulse help to distinguish them from seizures having cardiovascular causes (see Chapter 170). As noted previously, convulsions may occur in the setting of vagally mediated cerebral hypoperfusion in the absence of an underlying seizure disorder.

Metabolic Factors

Metabolic factors (e.g., hypoxia, hypocarbia, hypoglycemia) are more likely to alter consciousness than to cause actual syncope. Restlessness, confusion, and anxiety are prominent and precede loss of consciousness. When hyperventilation is responsible, the patient first complains of a smothering or suffocating feeling in conjunction with paresthesias in the limbs and circumorally (see Chapter 226). Syncope may take place while the patient is sitting or lying down. *Hypoglycemia* rarely causes loss of consciousness but always needs to be considered, especially in diabetics taking insulin or sulfonylureas (see Chapter 97).

Prognosis

The prognosis for syncope due to underlying cardiac disease is much worse (1-year mortality rates of 18% to 33%) than that for noncardiac or unexplained syncope (1-year mortality rates of 6% to 12%). In the elderly with unexplained syncope, the mortality rate nearly doubles. However, recurrence rates are similar for both categories (about 18% for the first year and 33% overall), and recurrence is not a risk factor for adverse outcome.

Examination of community-based populations (e.g., the Framingham Heart Study) finds that syncope due to underlying heart or neurologic disease makes an independent contribution to adverse outcome. In the Framingham Heart Study population, multivariable-adjusted hazard ratios for death from any cause, myocardial infarction, and fatal or nonfatal stroke were often significantly increased in persons experiencing syncope and having underlying heart or neurologic disease. For heart disease–related syncope, the hazard ratios (HRs) were 2.01, 2.66, and 2.01, respectively; for neurologic disease–related syncope (excluding vasovagal causes but including seizure), the HRs were 1.54, 0.79, and 2.96, respectively. There was no increase in risk for persons with vasovagal, orthostatic, or medication-induced syncope. Those with syncope of unknown etiology had an intermediate prognosis (HRs 1.32, 1.31, 0.66, respectively), probably reflecting the spectrum of underlying disease in this group. These data underscore the importance of identifying persons with a cardiac cause of syncope.

DIFFERENTIAL DIAGNOSIS
(4,5,9,10,13,14)

Important causes of syncope are listed in Table 24.1. Data from community-based epidemiologic study find vasovagal, situational, orthostatic, and medication-induced disease accounting for 45% of cases, cardiac disease for 10%, cerebrovascular disease for 4%, and seizure for another 4%, with the remaining 37% undiagnosed. In studies that added tilt-table testing and psychiatric assessment, at least half of the unexplained cases demonstrated evidence of a neurocardiogenic (vasova-

TABLE 24.1

IMPORTANT CAUSES OF SYNCOPE

Neurally Mediated
  Vasovagal
  Situational (posttussive, postprandial, postmicturition, stress)
  Psychiatric conditions (panic and generalized anxiety disorders, depression, somatization, hysteria)
  Dysautonomias (age, antihypertensive agents, diabetes, neurodegenerative disorders, neuropathic postural tachycardia syndrome
  Carotid sinus hypersensitivity

Cardiac
  Aortic outflow tract obstruction (aortic stenosis, hypertrophic cardiomyopathy)
  Dysrhythmias (Stokes–Adams attacks, ventricular tachycardia, rapid supraventricular tachycardia)
  Acute obstruction (massive pulmonary embolization, left atrial myxoma)
  Anomalous origin of coronary arteries

Neurologic/Cerebrovascular
  Cerebrovascular disease (severe diffuse; vertebrobasilar)
  Subclavian steal syndrome
  Seizures (not true syncope)
  Metabolic (not true syncope)

gal) mechanism, and many of the remainder had a psychiatric etiology (generalized anxiety, panic disorder, depression). In the elderly, the prevalence of cardiac disease among patients presenting with syncope increases to about 33%.

WORKUP (3,4,6,9,10,14–33)

Evaluation Strategy

Initial Workup

The principal task initially is to differentiate between cardiac and noncardiac etiologies because prognosis is poorest for those with underlying heart disease. A *detailed history*, *focused physical examination*, and the *resting 12-lead electrocardiogram* (ECG) are the most valuable elements of the initial evaluation. These elements alone provide a diagnosis in at about 50% of cases and suggest the diagnosis in many others. The physician and patient should appreciate that routinely ordering a battery of "syncope tests" is not only wasteful and ineffective, but also more likely to produce false-positive results than true-positive ones when ordered in the context of a low pretest probability for the condition in question.

Subsequent Testing

For the 50% of patients who remain incompletely diagnosed after the initial history, physical, and ECG, the key priority is detection of underlying heart disease, with the approach to evaluation guided by pretest probability. *Exercise stress testing* and *echocardiogram* are worth consideration in patients with clinical clues suggestive of structural heart disease (e.g., exertional symptoms such as chest pain, palpitations, heart murmur, S3 or S4, abnormal ECG). Detection of a dysrhythmia in such persons is also a priority, especially if the clinical story is suggestive (palpitations, sudden brief loss of consciousness without warning); *Holter monitoring* and *electrophysiologic study* are the tests of choice. *Continuous-loop electrocardiographic recording* is worth considering in patients who have no evidence of structural heart disease but report palpitations and have frequent syncopal episodes. Persons free of organic heart disease who have infrequent syncopal episodes and suspected neurocardiogenic (vasovagal) syncope are the best candidates for *tilt-table testing*. *Psychiatric evaluation* is indicated for patients with frequent events, no heart disease, and no injury from their spells. Such an approach results in a diagnosis in most patients. Fortunately, the prognosis for patients with a single unexplained episode of syncope is excellent. Nonetheless, a detailed search for underlying heart disease is essential and a major priority in the evaluation. The importance of a careful history and a physical examination cannot be overemphasized.

History

The differentiation of cardiac and neurologic disease from less worrisome etiologies begins with a *thorough description* of the syncopal event and its surrounding circumstances. The absence of premonitory symptoms in the presyncopal period is consistent with a sudden fall in cardiac output or the abrupt onset of generalized seizure activity. Nausea, diaphoresis, pallor, and lightheadedness are more typical of reflex and vascular causes. If recall of premonitory details is sketchy, one should be careful about interrogating the patient too vigorously with leading questions because the absence of associated or prodromal symptoms may have important diagnostic meaning. Although a seizure disorder may present with sudden loss of consciousness and no warning, more typically there are some vague premonitory symptoms and the characteristic tonic–clonic movements and sphincter incontinence.

Identification of precipitants requires asking about emotional upsets, crowded and hot surroundings, sudden standing (especially in elderly hypertensive patients after a meal), prolonged and forceful coughing, Valsalva maneuvers, micturition, vigorous exercise, hyperventilation, and symptoms of acute blood loss. Effort syncope raises the question of hemodynamically significant ventricular outflow tract obstruction. Exertional chest pain is another important clue of underlying organic heart disease. Position just before syncope is worth noting because loss of consciousness while recumbent argues against a reflex or vascular mechanism. A check of medications is always in order and especially productive in the assessment of the elderly person presenting with syncope.

Reports from witnesses should be sought whenever possible. Activity, position, complaints, and appearance before syncope and duration of the episode, associated motor activity, and behavior on regaining consciousness deserve attention. Some observers even report pulse and respirations. A seizure disorder is usually not difficult to distinguish from cardiac syncope because of the preceding aura, motor activity, incontinence, and postical symptoms of confusion, drowsiness, and paresis. However, when there are no motor manifestations, as in akinetic petit mal seizures, the differentiation may be impossible to make by history alone.

The *past medical history* should be searched for prior syncope, infarction, heart murmur, and use of cardioactive medications. A history of diabetes, stroke, use of antihypertensive agents, prolonged bedrest, impotence, and bladder and bowel incontinence should be checked for when the patient reports lightheadedness or syncope on standing. In young persons, reviewing past and recent history for prior episodes of syncope helps to identify those at increased risk of sudden death from prolonged QT syndrome (risk increases with number of distant and recent episodes).

Family history also deserves attention, with the focus on syncopal episodes and sudden death at an early age, suggesting cardiomyopathy or prolonged QT syndrome.

It is important not to mistake other conditions for true loss of consciousness. Vertigo (see Chapter 166), neuroglycopenic symptoms (see Chapter 97), and the lightheadedness associated with anxiety and other psychiatric conditions (see Chapters 226 and 227) are sometimes confused with syncope or near-syncope. On the other hand, reports of the combination of psychiatric and somatic symptoms (e.g., lightheadedness, anxiousness, numbness, nausea) in a patient with otherwise unexplained loss of consciousness should suggest an underlying psychiatric etiology. Checking for a history or current symptoms of anxiety, depression, panic, and somatization disorders can suggest an otherwise unapparent cause.

Physical Examination

The emphasis is again on the cardiovascular system. *Postural signs* provide essential information. *Blood pressure* and *pulse* are first measured in both arms with the patient lying supine for about 5 minutes and again on standing up. Most patients who demonstrate a postural fall in blood pressure will do so within 30 to 60 seconds of assuming the standing position. However, it may be necessary to wait as long as 5 minutes. Recent studies have found that 95% of cases with postural hypotension will be detected within 2 minutes of standing and most within 30 to 60 seconds. The skin is checked for pallor and ecchymoses (the latter, a sign of trauma from a seizure). Torso and head, including the tongue, require scrutiny for signs of trauma sustained during a motor seizure.

Carotid pulses are auscultated for bruits and gently palpated for volume and carotid upstroke (see Chapter 33). If there is no evidence of carotid artery disease, one can *massage* the carotid and observe for reflex bradycardia (asystole of >3 seconds) and hypotension. The maneuver is indicated when a hypersensitive carotid sinus reflex is suspected, as in elderly patients with unexplained falls. However, because it may also cut off blood supply and cause syncope when there is severe cerebral occlusive disease, it should not be attempted in such patients.

The neck veins are noted for distention and the chest for rales and rhonchi. The *heart* is palpated for heaves and thrills and is auscultated for clicks and murmurs with the patient in the supine, decubitus, and sitting positions. Systolic murmurs should be evaluated for evidence of aortic stenosis, asymmetric septal hypertrophy, and mitral valve prolapse (see Chapter 21). A variable diastolic murmur raises the question of atrial myxoma. Neurologic assessment includes a search for focal deficits indicative of prior stroke, a check for vestibular dysfunction, and a careful mental status examination that focuses on manifestations of depression and anxiety disorders.

Provocative maneuvers are particularly helpful in identifying conditions that alter consciousness but do not cause syncope. Asking the patient to voluntarily hyperventilate or undergo the Baranay maneuver (see Chapter 166) may reproduce symptoms and confirm a clinical suspicion. Exercising the arm is worthwhile if subclavian steal syndrome is suspected.

Laboratory Studies

As noted earlier, routinely ordering a battery of "syncope tests" is wasteful and ineffective. Although one does not want to miss an underlying cardiac etiology, test selection should still reflect consideration of the pretest probability of heart disease. Test yield in patients with a very low pretest probability of heart disease is extremely low, and the risk of false positives is high (see Chapters 2, 20, and 36). Neither an ECG nor other laboratory study is necessary when the history strongly suggests a harmless vasovagal episode, the physical examination is normal, and the patient has no risk factors for organic heart disease. However, when the cause is not evident, underlying heart disease needs to be ruled out, and ECG, stress testing, and echocardiogram deserve consideration, as does arrhythmia detection.

Electrocardiogram

Most patients should have an ECG performed at the time of initial evaluation because detection of underlying heart disease is a major priority of the diagnostic workup. One needs to check not only for ischemic changes, heart block, and tachyarrhythmias, but also for more subtle clues such as a short PR interval, QT-interval prolongation, axis shift, increased voltage, and delta waves. Overall, the electrocardiogram is diagnostic in less than 5% of cases but still needs to be checked in most cases because of the importance of detecting underlying heart disease. Even young persons require testing because of the possibility of prolonged-QT syndrome.

Exercise Stress Testing

Exercise stress testing may bring out arrhythmias not found during Holter monitoring, but even more useful is the test's sensitivity for the diagnosis of ischemic heart disease (see Chapter 36). Patients with atherosclerotic risk factors who report chest pain before syncope or effort syncope or have an abnormal resting ECG suggestive of ischemic disease are prime candidates for stress testing. However, patients with effort syncope should not be subjected to stress testing until after echocardiography has been performed to rule out obstruction of the left ventricular outflow tract because persons with critical aortic stenosis or hypertrophic cardiomyopathy are at risk of sudden death with vigorous physical exercise. Routine use of stress testing to rule out "silent" heart disease in the absence of clinical or electrocardiographic evidence yields little and increases cost.

Echocardiography

Echocardiography can provide key diagnostic information in patients suspected of valvular or structural heart disease because of effort syncope, chest pain, palpitations, systolic ejection murmur, systolic click, abnormal carotid upstroke with transmitted bruit, or an abnormal ECG. It is also the noninvasive test of choice if a left atrial myxoma is suspected. In the absence of clinical evidence for heart disease, routine echocardiography usually contributes little to the assessment (yield <5%). As noted previously, syncope patients who are going to have a stress test should be subjected to echocardiogram before stress testing if there is any clinical suggestion of obstruction to the left ventricular outflow tract (e.g., systolic ejection murmur).

Neurovascular Ultrasound

Yield is very low, especially in persons without evidence of focal neurologic deficit by history or physical examination; however, persons with a carotid bruit or a focal deficit have a significantly greater chance of having a clinically important lesion discovered on ultrasound testing. Nonetheless, discovery of a lesion etiologically linked to syncope is very uncommon (<2%).

Holter Monitoring

If the ECG is unrevealing but an arrhythmia, transient heart block, or other form of underlying heart disease is still suspected on clinical grounds (e.g., history of palpitations, sudden loss of consciousness without warning, effort syncope, chest pain), then a 24-hour ambulatory ECG recording (Holter monitor) deserves consideration. Holter monitoring has become an almost routine part of the syncope workup, especially in patients who remain undiagnosed after initial history, physical examination, and resting ECG, because abnormalities found on Holter can contribute to overall risk assessment. Yet the yield of the test is low, with arrhythmia-related symptoms occurring in less than 5% of patients studied and syncope or presyncope occurring without an associated arrhythmia in 15%.

Although the correlation between symptoms and Holter findings is often not strong, Holter study can provide an independent assessment of risk for underlying heart disease and sudden death. Syncopal patients with frequent premature ventricular contractions (>10 per hour), repetitive premature ventricular contractions (32 in a row), or sinus pauses (>2 seconds) on Holter monitoring have an increased risk of sudden death and overall mortality that is independent of other factors. Patients with these findings constitute a high-risk subgroup that deserves further cardiac evaluation. There may be an increase in yield of arrhythmias detected if Holter monitoring is extended to 48 hours, but many arrhythmias are asymptomatic and of unclear significance.

Continuous-Loop (Event) Recording

Continuous-loop (event) recording for detection of symptomatic arrhythmias is made feasible with *patient-activated intermittent recorders*. By virtue of their *continuous-loop* technology, these recorders can capture the previous several minutes of cardiac rhythm and detect a symptom-producing dysrhythmia shortly after it has occurred, provided the patient is capable of activating the unit. Continuous-loop recording may be useful in persons with relatively frequent syncopal episodes, but overall yield is quite low (8% to 20%); up to one fourth of patients have a normal study during symptoms. The test can be helpful for detection of bradyarrhythmias when Holter monitoring and electrophysiologic study are unrevealing (see later discussion).

Electrophysiologic Study

Electrophysiologic study (EPS) has been advocated for detecting arrhythmogenic causes of syncope, particularly *ventricular tachycardia*, in persons with suspected underlying heart disease when Holter monitoring results are nondiagnostic. The value of EPS in the assessment of patients with structural heart disease and fixed conduction defects is well documented, but its sensitivity and specificity for identifying transient rhythm disturbances, especially *bradyarrhythmias*, in patients with unexplained syncope have been disappointing.

The detection of ventricular tachycardia and hemodynamically significant bradycardia are the principal reasons for performing EPS. Consequently, prime candidates are patients with an increased risk of such an arrhythmia (e.g., persons with previous myocardial infarction, ischemic heart disease, or congestive heart failure). To improve EPS performance, criteria for better patient selection have been sought. In the largest study, patients with evidence of underlying organic heart disease and frequent premature ventricular contractions on resting ECG were at increased risk for sustained ventricular tachycardia during EPS. Those with first-degree arterioventricular block, bundle-branch block, or sinus bradycardia on resting ECG were at increased risk of a hemodynamically significant bradyarrhythmia during EPS. Overall, 87% of patients with at least one of these clinical risk factors had an important outcome on EPS, whereas the EPS was normal in 95% of patients with none of these risk factors. Holter findings may also prove predictive, but data are limited.

Although invasive and very expensive (requiring cardiac catheterization), EPS may be preferred to outpatient Holter monitoring in elderly persons with syncope and conduction disease on ECG because another episode might result in serious injury. Another reason for consideration of EPS is presence of preexcitation (short PR interval, <0.12 seconds) on ECG. Such patients are at increased risk of sustained rapid supraventricular tachycardia with hypotension. Patients with unexplained syncope but no evidence of structural heart disease and a normal ECG are not likely to benefit from EPS. The test should not be considered a routine part of a workup of syncope of unknown origin.

Upright Tilt Testing

The growing appreciation of neurocardiogenic mechanisms of syncope has stimulated interest in provocative maneuvers such as upright tilt testing. The best candidates are patients in whom heart disease has been ruled out and a vasovagal mechanism is suspected on the basis of the clinical history (e.g., premonitory nausea and flushing). The test is predicated on the hypothesis that in susceptible persons, the decrease in venous return from placement on a tilt table brought up to 60 degrees elevation will trigger the potent reflex responses that lead to neurocardiogenic syncope (see prior discussion). *Isoproterenol* infusion is added to enhance sensitivity and speed the test if tilting without isoproterenol produces no response after 15 minutes. Use of *nitrates* provides similar enhancement of sensitivity. Criteria for a positive test vary and include hypotension and bradycardia, but reproduction of the patient's syncope and associated symptoms is the sine qua non of a diagnostic study.

Sensitivity ranges from about 65% to 80%, enhanced by isoproterenol infusion. *Specificity* is 90% without isoproterenol and decreases to 75% when it is infused because of false-positive responses, particularly in young healthy persons. Most authorities recommend first performing the tilt test without isoproterenol infusion, reserving it for patients with a negative initial study who have premonitory symptoms suggestive of a vasovagal mechanism. In older patients, tilt testing with isoproterenol can be conducted safely, but prior stress testing is recommended to rule out underlying ischemia, which might be exacerbated by isoproterenol infusion.

Tilt-table testing is sometimes helpful in uncovering underlying psychopathology, such as a conversion reaction, in which the apparent loss of consciousness occurs during testing but without hypotension or bradycardia.

Other Studies

The *electroencephalogram* has repeatedly been shown to be of little use in evaluating syncope in the absence of either a history suggestive of seizure or neurologic deficits. Even when a seizure disorder is present, the routine electroencephalogram has a sensitivity of only 50%. Sleep studies and photic stimulation may improve sensitivity to 80% (see Chapter 170). Similarly, neuroimaging studies (computed tomography, magnetic resonance imaging) should generally be reserved for patients with focal seizures or defects on neurologic examination (in one study, 7 of 20 patients with and none of 17 patients without such findings had abnormalities detected on computed tomography).

Random *blood sugar* determinations are of little use in documenting hypoglycemia; a blood sugar at the time of symptoms is better (see Chapter 97). Arterial *blood gases* can detect hypocarbia when hyperventilation is suspected and hypoxia when ventilation/perfusion mismatching is of concern. However, such testing is usually unnecessary because the etiologies responsible for such blood gas abnormalities are usually self-evident.

Patients with Unexplained Syncope

When the foregoing evaluation ends without an answer other than the absence of evidence for serious underlying cardiac or neurologic pathology, then a period of watchful waiting can be considered. Patients with a fully negative evaluation are at low risk for an occult life-threatening etiology and sudden death. Those with a rare event can be reassured and followed expectantly.

Patients with Frequent Recurrences

Frequent syncopal attacks of unknown etiology are difficult to manage with a watchful-waiting approach. Recurrent episodes beg for an explanation. Patients with unexplained disease despite a full assessment benefit from close follow-up and careful reassessment for new clues by careful history and physical examination at the time of recurrences. *Hospitalization* for observation in persons with very frequent syncopal attacks may

help to guide further evaluation by providing the opportunity directly to observe an episode.

Assessment for a psychiatric etiology (e.g., generalized anxiety disorder, panic disorder, depression) should be considered in younger persons with frequent episodes, in those who never sustain injury from their loss of consciousness, and in those with multiple bodily complaints and symptoms of anxiousness (e.g., numbness, nausea, constant lightheadedness, fearfulness). Screening instruments for anxiety and depression (see Chapters 226 and 227) are useful for initial assessment, as is the *hyperventilation maneuver*, in which the patient breathes rapidly and deeply with mouth open for 2 to 3 minutes. The development of syncope or near-syncope in response to hyperventilation has a positive predictive value of greater than 50% for a psychiatric etiology. *Tilt-table testing* for persons with suspected hysteria (in which syncope represents a conversion reaction) may reveal the characteristic apparent loss of consciousness in the absence of changes in vital signs.

Elderly Patients with Unexplained Syncope

In many instances, the etiology is not one single factor, but a combination (e.g., blunted autonomic responsiveness, medications, dehydration, underlying heart disease). A review of current medications is always in order, as is that of the circumstances of each syncopal event (e.g., standing after a meal, urination, or a bowel movement). Because the prevalence of cardiovascular disease is high in this age group, reconsideration of the common etiologies (e.g., coronary disease, heart failure, conduction-system disease, other dysrhythmias) and less-common etiologies (e.g., calcific aortic stenosis, carotid sinus hypersensitivity) is in order (see prior discussion). If not already performed, carotid sinus massage should be carried out, provided there is no evidence of ongoing cardiovascular or cerebrovascular disease, such as recent myocardial infarction, carotid bruit, recent stroke, or ventricular arrhythmias. The rationale for performing carotid massage is that persons with a positive test (asystole >3 seconds in response to massage) appear to benefit from implantation of a demand pacemaker. As noted earlier, neurovascular ultrasonography is of low yield without a history of focal deficit or carotid bruit.

SYMPTOMATIC THERAPY AND PATIENT EDUCATION
(3,6,9,24,28,34)

Symptomatic Measures

The most effective therapies are those that are etiologic, particularly treatments that address serious underlying cardiac pathology (e.g., see Chapters 28 to 30, 32, and 33). A number of symptomatic measures help patients with less-threatening conditions, which are still important to treat because of their impact on the quality of daily life.

Orthostatic Hypotension

The first priority is to review all medications and reduce or eliminate those that are likely to exacerbate the problem (e.g., diuretics, vasodilators, beta-blockers, hypnotics). A number of simple measures deserve emphasis. One teaches the patient to avoid abrupt postural changes by sitting on the edge of the bed in the morning before getting up and to elevate the head of the bed at night to counter the reflex hypertension that occurs when supine. Girdles, garters, and other constricting garments should not be worn if they decrease venous return, but elastic stockings may be helpful. One can advise the patient to avoid prolonged standing and to contract the calf muscles when standing to increase venous blood flow. Liberalization of salt intake is useful; *fludrocortisone* (0.1 to 1.0 mg daily) may be necessary. Patients with severe orthostatic hypotension due to multiple-system failure or pure autonomic dysfunction may require additional treatment. Agents to be considered include *phenylpropanolamine* in low doses, *midodrine*, *indomethacin*, and *yohimbine*. Careful testing is required because responses are very idiosyncratic.

Postprandial Hypotension

Simple measures include smaller and more frequent meals, liberalized salt intake, adequate fluid intake, reduction in carbohydrate content of meals, patient education regarding the risk of falling up to 90 minutes after eating, avoidance of prolonged sitting, avoidance of standing still after a meal, encouraging a walk after eating, and avoidance of alcohol before or with meals. In addition, the aforementioned measures for management of orthostatic hypotension can be implemented. Agonists (e.g., *phenylephrine* every 6 to 12 hours) are sometimes used but of questionable safety in elderly persons. Caffeine is of little benefit. The somatostatin analogue octreotide (50 µg subcutaneously, 1/2 hour before meals) can be considered, but only for the most seriously affected persons because a painful injection is required to administer the substance.

Neurocardiogenic Syncope

Patients with confirmed neurocardiogenic disease may be candidates for a trial of a *beta-blocker* (e.g., metoprolol) or *disopyramide*. The role of *demand pacing* in such cases is unresolved; some nonrandomized studies suggest a benefit in up to one fourth of patients, but there are no randomized trials. Loosening the collar is sometimes helpful for the person with a *hypersensitive carotid sinus* reflex; demand pacing can be considered if simpler measures fail. A demand pacemaker is indicated only when heart block or severe bradycardia has been proven responsible for syncope. Empiric pacing in patients with undiagnosed recurrent episodes is to be discouraged.

Underlying Psychiatric Illness

The treatment of any underlying anxiety disorder, depression, or panic disorder results in a significant reduction in syncopal episodes and is strongly recommended (see Chapters 226 and 227).

Patient Education

The patient without evidence of underlying cardiac or neurologic disease can be reassured, even if syncopal episodes continue. Mortality does not increase with recurrent episodes, as long as there continues to be no evidence of underlying cardiac or neurologic disease. The value of a thoughtful workup in conjunction with thorough explanation should not be underestimated in helping patients with unexplained syncope to remain active. If serious heart and neurologic diseases have been ruled out, further evaluation can safely proceed on an outpatient basis even though the cause may remain undetermined. Family members and close friends should be instructed to take careful note of all events surrounding the syncopal period, including appearance, position, activity, complaints, and behavior. They might even be taught to palpate the radial or femoral pulse to provide data on heart rate and rhythm during an episode.

INDICATIONS FOR ADMISSION

It is safest to hospitalize patients with syncope who have any clinical evidence suggesting underlying heart disease, including those with a history of effort syncope, chest pain, known coronary or valvular disease, systolic ejection murmur, abnormal resting ECG, or severe postural drop in blood pressure. Similarly, persons with evidence indicating the possibility of cerebrovascular disease or a seizure disorder (e.g., carotid bruit, prior stroke, witnessed seizure activity, or suggestive symptoms) are best served by hospitalization. Although many elderly patients benefit from an inpatient evaluation because of the increased probability of underlying cardiovascular disease, not all do, especially when the circumstances are clearly situational (e.g., postprandial, postmicturition). Admission to the hospital for observation of the obscure case is a difficult decision, but, as noted earlier, it is most useful if episodes are frequent enough to provide opportunity for observing one.

RECOMMENDATIONS (4,13,14)

- Begin the evaluation with a comprehensive history and a focused physical examination that emphasize detection of underlying heart disease; obtain a resting ECG.
- In younger persons, pay particular attention to risk factors for sudden cardiac death due to the prolonged-QT syndrome, including recent and prior history of recurrent syncopal attacks and QT_c prolongation greater than 530 msec.
- Base further test selection on the pretest likelihood of underlying heart disease.

For Intermediate-to-High Pretest Probability of Serious Underlying Heart Disease

- Conduct the initial evaluation in the hospital, and include Holter monitoring or EPS (if there is high suspicion of ventricular tachycardia), supplemented by stress testing and/or echocardiography.

For Low Pretest Probability of Serious Underlying Heart Disease

- Conduct the assessment in the outpatient setting and include continuous-loop event monitoring (especially for persons with structurally normal hearts, a history of palpitations, and frequent episodes), psychiatric testing (especially for younger persons with frequent episodes in the absence of evidence for heart disease, for those with multiple somatic and psychiatric symptoms, and for those with no injury from syncopal episodes), and tilt-table testing (especially for persons with infrequent episodes who have no evidence of underlying heart disease and a story suggestive of neurocardiogenic [vasovagal] syncope or conversion reaction).
- Also consider conducting the initial evaluation on an inpatient basis for persons suspected of having a seizure disorder or stroke and for the frail elderly person who sustains a serious injury from a first syncopal episode.

A.H.G.

Annotated References

1. Abboud FM. Neurocardiogenic syncope. N Engl J Med 1993;328:1117. (*A very concise and excellent summary of pathophysiology, plus an editorial on the clinical implications.*)

2. Atkins D, Hanusa B, Sefcik T, et al. Syncope and orthostatic hypotension. Am J Med 1991;91:179. (*Orthostatic hypotension was found to be very common in patients with syncope and present in most within 2 minutes of standing; those with greater degrees of orthostasis tended to have fewer syncopal recurrences.*)

3. Fenton A, Hammill SC, Rea RF, et al. Vasovagal syncope. Ann Intern Med 2000;133:714. (*A systematic review; 90 references.*)

4. Goldschlarger N, Epstein AE, Grubb BP, et al. Etiologic considerations in the patient with syncope and an apparently normal heart. Arch Intern Med 2003;163:151. (*A review of causes in this subgroup and guidelines; 39 references.*)

5. Goldstein DS, Robertson D, Esler M, et al. Dysautonomias: clinical disorders of the autonomic nervous system. Ann Intern Med 2002:137:753. (*A National Institutes of Health conference on pathophysiology.*)

6. Hobbs JB, Peterson DR, Moss AJ, et al. Risk of aborted cardiac arrest or sudden cardiac death during adolescence in the long-QT syndrome. JAMA 2006;296:1249. (*Prospective cohort study identifying risk factors such as timing and frequency of syncope and degree of QT prolongation.*)

7. Jacob G, Costa F, Shannon J, et al. The neuropathic postural tachycardia syndrome. N Engl J Med 2000;343:1008. (*Mechanism of the syndrome; finds partial sympathetic denervation in the legs.*)

8. Jansen RWMM, Lipsitz LA. Postprandial hypotension: epidemiology, pathophysiology, and clinical management. Ann Intern Med 1995;122:286. (*A literature review finding such hypotension to be very common in the elderly and a potential cause of falls and syncope.*)

9. Kapoor WN. Syncope. N Engl J Med 2000;343:1856. (*Very useful review, especially for its critical look at yields of history, physical examination, and laboratory studies; 45 references.*)

10. Kapoor W, Snustad D, Peterson J, et al. Syncope in the elderly. Am J Med 1989;80:419. (*The elderly have an increased risk of underlying heart disease and overall mortality.*)

11. McIntosh SJ, Lawson J, Henry RA. Clinical characteristics of vasodepressor, cardioinhibitory, and mixed carotid sinus syndrome in the elderly. Am J Med 1993;95:203. (*A cause of unexplained falls in the elderly.*)

12. Soteriades ES, Evans JC, Larson MG, et al. Incidence and prognosis of syncope. N Engl J Med 2002;347:878. (*Data from the Framingham Heart Study; increased risk was associated with cardiac causes of syncope.*)

13. Linzer M, Yang EH, Estes M III, et al. Diagnosing syncope. Part 1. Value of history, physical examination, and electrocardiography. Ann Intern Med 1997;126:989. (*A literature review and position paper outlining a clinical guideline in which history, physical examination, and electrocardiogram [ECG] are recommended as the core the evaluation.*)

14. Linzer M, Yang EH, Estes M III, et al. Diagnosing syncope. Part 2. Unexplained syncope. Ann Intern Med 1997;127:76. (*A literature review and position paper on approaches to testing the 50% of patients who remain undiagnosed after history, physical examination, and ECG.*)

15. Almquist A, Goldenberg IF, Milstein S, et al. Provocation of bradycardia and hypotension by isoproterenol and upright posture in patients with unexplained syncope. N Engl J Med 1989;320:346. (*Tilt testing and isoproterenol reproduced symptoms in patients who otherwise had unexplained syncope after exhaustive evaluation.*)

16. Brignole M, Menozzi C, Gianfranchi L, et al. Carotid sinus massage, eyeball compression, and head-up tilt test in patients with syncope of uncertain origin and in healthy control subjects. Am Heart J 1991;122:1644. (*Data supporting the utility of carotid sinus massage in elderly persons with syncope.*)

17. Calkins H, Byrne M, El-Atassi R, et al. The economic burden of unrecognized vasodepressor syncope. Am J Med 1993;95:473. (*Much unnecessary testing greatly increases the cost of evaluation.*)

18. Fujimura O, Yee R, Klein GJ. The diagnostic sensitivity of electrophysiologic testing in patients with syncope caused by transient bradycardia. N Engl J Med 1989;321:1703. (*Sensitivity and specificity were disappointingly low in patients with proven bradyarrhythmic syncope.*)

19. Grubb BP. Neurocardiogenic syncope. N Engl J Med 2005;352:1004. (*Thoughtful, clinically focused review of evaluation and management; 53 references.*)

20. Joran J, Shannon JR, Biaggioni I, et al. Contrasting actions of pressor agents in severe autonomic failure. Am J Med 1998;105:116. (*A placebo-controlled trial comparing the effects of phenylpropanolamine, midodrine, caffeine, indomethacin, and yohimbine.*)

21. Kapoor WN. Back to the basics for the workup of syncope. J Gen Intern Med 1994;10:695. (*An editorial emphasizing the value of the history, physical examination, and limited testing.*)

22. Kapoor WN, Brant N. Evaluation of syncope by upright tilt testing with isoproterenol. Ann Intern Med 1992;116:358. (*A controlled study in young persons showing that the test had a low specificity, with high rates of positive responses in both syncopal patients and controls; dampens enthusiasm for the test.*)

23. Kapoor W, Cha R, Peterson JR, et al. Prolonged electrocardiographic monitoring in patients with syncope. Am J Med 1987;82:20. (*Patients with syncope and frequent or repetitive ventricular premature beats or sinus pauses had an increased risk of overall mortality and sudden death.*)

24. Kapoor WN, Peterson J, Wieand HS, et al. Diagnostic and prognostic implications of recurrences in patients with syncope. Am J Med 1987;83:700. (*Recurrences are common but not a predictor of mortality, sudden death, or etiology.*)

25. Kapoor WN, Smith M, Miller NL. Upright tilt-table testing in evaluating syncope: a comprehensive literature review. Am J Med 1994;97:78. (*Finds the test useful when it can reproduce symptoms in persons who have had cardiac causes ruled out.*)

26. Linzer M, Pritchett ELC, Pontinen M, et al. Incremental diagnostic yield of loop electrocardiographic recorders in unexplained syncope. Am J Cardiol 1990;66:214. (*Yield was modest: <20%.*)

27. Linzer M, Prystowsky EN, Divine GW, et al. Predicting outcomes of electrophysiologic studies of patients with unexplained syncope. J Gen Intern Med 1991;6:113. (*Identifies predictors of a positive electrophysiologic study and thus selection criteria for those who should be studied.*)

28. Lipsitz LA. Syncope in the elderly. Ann Intern Med 1983;99:92. (*An extensive clinical review stressing the selective use of diagnostic tests in evaluating syncope as well as attention to drug effects and treatment of symptomatic abnormalities.*)

29. Novak V, Novak P, Opfer-Gehrking TL, et al. Clinical and laboratory indices that enhance the diagnosis of postural tachycardia syndrome. Mayo Clin Proc 1998;73:1141. (*An approach to better characterization of this syndrome.*)

30. Recchia D, Barzilai B. Echocardiography in the evaluation of patients with syncope. J Gen Intern Med 1995;10:649. (*Yield was around 5% in patients with low pretest probability.*)

31. Sarasin FP, Louis-Simonet M, Carballo D, et al. Prospective evaluation of patients with syncope: a population-based study. Am J Med 2001;111:177. (*A prospective cohort study; diagnostic yield was 76%; ECG was helpful in risk stratification.*)

32. Schnipper JL, Ackerman RH, Krier JB, et al. Diagnostic yield and utility of neurovascular ultrasonography in the evaluation of patients with syncope. Mayo Clin Proc 2005;80:480. (*Retrospective cohort study of 140 patients; the yield was low except in persons with focal deficits or bruit.*)

33. Spitzer RL, Williams JB, Kroenke K, et al. Utility of a new procedure for diagnosing mental disorder in primary care. The PRIME 1000 study. JAMA 1994;272:1749. (*Presents the evidence for the usefulness of hyperventilation and screening instruments in testing for psychiatric disorders.*)

34. Benditt DG, Petersen M, Lurie KG, et al. Cardiac pacing for prevention of recurrent vasovagal syncope. Ann Intern Med 1995;122:204. (*A systematic review of the evidence, finding many gaps, but some indication of benefit in selected patients.*)

CHAPTER 25 ■ EVALUATION OF PALPITATIONS

The patient with palpitations reports a disquieting awareness of his or her heartbeat, which may be described as a "pounding," "racing," "skipping," "flopping," or "fluttering" sensation. It is disconcerting and often incites fear, although many cases seen in the office setting occur among persons with no serious underlying heart disease. The evaluation of palpitations by the primary physician focuses on differentiating the high-risk person in need of an intensive evaluation and possible cardiology referral from the low-risk individual who can be reassured after a screening assessment. The primary physician needs to be familiar with the telltale manifestations of worrisome dysrhythmias and the indications for and limitations of methodologies for their detection and evaluation.

PATHOPHYSIOLOGY AND CLINICAL PRESENTATION (1–17)

Healthy individuals are usually unaware of their resting heartbeat, but persons suffering from somatization disorders (see Chapter 230) may find the normally imperceptible heartbeat of daily life an unpleasant sensation. For most, awareness of heartbeat typically ensues when there is a sudden change in rate or rhythm, increase in stroke volume or contractility, or unusual cardiac movement within the thorax. Although acute changes in heart rate or rhythm may be noted, chronic dysrhythmias often go unnoticed. Disturbances of heartbeat may originate supraventricularly or ventricularly. Increased *automaticity* and *reentry* are among the basic mechanisms. The dysrhythmia itself may confer increased risk or represent a manifestation of underlying heart disease.

Supraventricular Dysrhythmias

As a group, arrhythmias originating in the atrium or junction tend to be less worrisome than those that originate in the ventricles, but atrial dysrhythmias may be manifestations of important underlying heart disease and sometimes can cause hemodynamic compromise or predispose to other complications (e.g., systemic embolization), making them important to identify and address.

Atrial Premature Beats

Premature atrial beats (APCs) are usually imperceptible, but awareness of a rhythm disturbance derives from the pause in rhythm, increased ventricular filling time, and the resultant forceful beat that follows the premature beat. A "turning over" or "flopping" of the heart may be reported. Premature atrial beats tend to be most noticeable when the heart rate is slow and the patient is lying in bed supine or in the left lateral decubitus position. If there is atrioventricular dissociation

and atrial contraction occurs against a closed arterioventricular valve, then a "pounding in the neck" or a sudden bulging of the neck veins (jugular *cannon venous A waves*) may also be noted.

Atrial premature beats are a common occurrence of everyday life and often increase in frequency with the use of caffeine, nicotine, or alcohol. In most instances, they are harmless, but they can trigger a rapid reentrant tachycardia in susceptible persons and may represent increased atrial automaticity due to underlying heart disease (e.g., ischemia, cardiomyopathy, advancing valvular disease). Characteristic electrocardiographic (ECG) features include a premature and abnormally configured P wave followed by a narrow QRS complex and a resetting of the sinoatrial (SA) node before the next sinus-conducted beat (resulting in a "noncompensatory" pause in heart rhythm). If the APC occurs while the ventricles are still partially refractory, there may be aberrant conduction through the ventricle resulting in a widened QRS. Such *APCs with aberrancy* can mimic ventricular premature beats but are usually differentiated from the latter by a preceding P wave and the absence of a full compensatory pause.

Sinus Tachycardia

Excess adrenergic stimulation results in increased contractility and sinus tachycardia, which may present as palpitations with a fast regular rhythm. Onset can be abrupt; resolution is usually more gradual. A constant rapid pounding at rest is felt by patients with *hyperkinetic states* (e.g., fever, severe anemia, hyperthyroidism, anxiety, agitated depression) due to the catecholamine-induced increase in contractility and stroke volume. Patients with anxiety-induced palpitations often have an underlying *panic disorder* (see Chapter 226); typically, they have difficulty telling whether the palpitations or the anxiety came first. Unappreciated is the high frequency of other supraventricular dysrhythmias in this group of patients (see later discussion). An uncommon variant of sinus tachycardia, *inappropriate sinus tachycardia*, is believed to represent a hypersensitivity to catecholamine stimulation. *Hyperthyroidism* may have a palpitation presentation similar to that of anxiety (see Chapter 103); it may also cause atrial fibrillation (see later discussion). In rare instances, the source of adrenergic outpouring is a *pheochromocytoma*. Its incidence is less than 0.1%, with about half of cases presenting as paroxysms of palpitations, hypertension, perspiration, tremor, nervousness, and other signs of adrenergic stimulation. Episodes are often spontaneous in origin but may be triggered by emotion and thus mimic an anxiety attack. An *insulin reaction* can produce a similar clinical picture (see Chapter 102), driven by an outpouring of catecholamines. A regular rhythm without tachycardia is noted in cases of valvular disease accompanied by large stroke volumes, as in *aortic regurgitation*.

Supraventricular Tachycardias

Attacks of palpitations that are regular in rhythm and rapid in rate may also be due to paroxysmal *supraventricular tachycardia* (SVT), sometimes referred to as *paroxysmal atrial tachycardia*. There are two basic mechanisms. In *atrioventricular nodal tachycardia*, which is the most common SVT, there are two functionally distinct conduction pathways in the nodal area, which enable a reentrant circuit to develop, producing ventricular response rates as high as 160 to 180 beats/min. If the atria in this rhythm disturbance are unaffected by the nodal rhythm disturbance, there can be arterioventricular nodal dissociation manifested as rapid regular pounding in the neck. The condition is considerably more common in women than men and occurs in a wide variety of patients, including those with normal hearts, sick-sinus syndrome, mitral valve prolapse and other forms of valvular disease, coronary artery disease, and cardiomyopathy. Onset may occur in the setting of emotional stress (e.g., panic attack). Some patients note that standing up after bending over may bring on an episode that can be terminated by lying down.

In the second form of SVT with a regular rhythm, *atrioventricular reciprocating tachycardia*, there is a large macrorentrant circuit, which involves the atrium, the arterioventricular node, an accessory pathway (e.g., the bundle of Kent or James), and the ventricle. The *preexcitation syndromes* (so-called because of their short electrocardiographic PR intervals), *Wolff–Parkinson–White* (WPW) and *Lown–Ganong–Levine* syndromes, operate by the reciprocating mechanism. An electrocardiographic hallmark of WPW is the delta wave at the beginning of the QRS, indicative of aberrant conduction through the accessory bundle; the QRS may be widened considerably during a run of SVT and mimic a ventricular dysrhythmia, especially when WPW is complicated by a very rapid ventricular response rate, as in atrial flutter or atrial fibrillation (see later discussion). Any SVT with a very rapid ventricular response rate may seriously compromise cardiac output in a patient with underlying heart disease and cause chest pain, dyspnea, profound weakness, or even loss of consciousness.

The onset of SVT is characteristically sudden and may be precipitated by excess *alcohol*, *emotional upset*, or strenuous *exertion*. Caffeinated beverages are less of a risk factor. SVTs may be initiated by the occurrence of premature beats that alter conduction in the normal pathway. Paroxysms cease when the conducting properties of the reentrant circuit are disturbed by changes in vagal tone, hence the report by patients of ability to terminate attacks by undertaking the Valsalva maneuver. Resolution is typically abrupt. Syncope is uncommon but may occur at the outset if the rate is very rapid and/or there is acute vasodilation.

Some of the conditions associated with SVT are responsible for other dysrhythmias as well. For example, almost half of patients with *sick-sinus syndrome* experience *heart block* or marked *bradycardia* in addition to bouts of SVT.

Paroxysmal Atrial Fibrillation

The sudden onset of palpitations with an irregularly irregular rhythm and rapid rate typifies *paroxysmal atrial fibrillation*, which occurs in a host of settings, including *acute alcohol excess* ("holiday heart"), *infection, hyperthyroidism, sick-sinus syndrome, WPW syndrome, cardiomyopathy*, and acute worsening of *ischemia* or *congestive heart failure*; the condition is also found among otherwise healthy young people ("lone" *atrial fibrillation*). High levels of circulating catecholamines may trigger atrial fibrillation, especially in someone with underlying organic heart disease. A common precipitant is exercise or the termination of exercise with its surge of vagal tone. Chronic atrial fibrillation usually does not produce palpitations. An irregularly irregular tachycardia may also be seen if there are runs of *multifocal atrial tachycardia* (MAT), which takes place in the context of severe pulmonary disease, particularly when there is an acute fall in oxygen tension or pH. Frequent atrial or ventricular premature contractions can lead to a similarly irregular rhythm and rapid rate.

Ventricular Dysrhythmias

Ventricular dysrhythmias often occur in the context of worrisome underlying heart disease and may be a harbinger of hemodynamic collapse and sudden death. However, not all ventricular rhythm disturbances are associated with increased cardiac morbidity and mortality.

Ventricular Premature Beats

Like most premature beats, those originating in the ventricles are often felt as a consequence of the forceful beat that follows the pause and increased ventricular filling after the premature beat (see prior discussion). Cannon "a" waves may also ensue and be felt as an impulse in the neck. Electrocardiographically, ventricular premature beats (VPBs) are characterized by a widened QRS, no preceding P wave, and the presence of a full *compensatory pause* (there is usually no resetting of the SA node, so the next ventricular depolarization must await the next regular discharge from the SA node). Electrocardiographic differentiation of VPBs from APCs with aberrancy can be challenging because both cause a widened QRS, but the absence of a preceding P wave, the presence of a full compensatory pause, and a QRS duration greater than 140 msec are helpful. VPBs of right ventricular origin have a left-bundle pattern to the QRS; those arising from the left have a right-bundle pattern.

In the absence of overt underlying heart disease, most VPBs (even when frequent or complex) have little prognostic significance. Even when they occur during exercise stress testing, VPBs do not appear independently to confer a significant increase in cardiac risk, although the arrhythmia may be a sign of underlying cardiovascular disease. However, frequent VPBs that occur principally during the *recovery phase* of stress testing do confer an independent and significant increase in long-term mortality risk (the hazard ratio approaches 1.5). Such recovery-phase ventricular irritability (which is believed to be related to attenuated vagal reactivation) is also associated with reduced ejection fraction.

Ventricular Tachycardia

Ventricular tachycardia is among the most worrisome of dysrhythmias related to palpitations, and is associated in some instances with the risk of sudden death. Nonetheless, not all ventricular tachycardia represents life-threatening disease. *Nonsustained ventricular tachycardia* (NSVT) may occur in otherwise normal persons (*idiopathic ventricular tachycardia*), as well as in those with underlying heart disease. In truly normal subjects, NSVT is not associated with an increased risk of sudden death; however, any NSVT that compromises cardiac output may lead to dizziness, near-syncope, or loss of consciousness. Potentially serious VT may occur in the context of clinically evident heart disease, as well as in patients with important hereditary defects but little evidence of structural pathology.

VT in the Setting of Overt Heart Disease. Most worrisome are runs of nonsustained or sustained VT occurring in the context of overt *underlying heart disease*. Such patients have an increased risk of sudden death, especially those with *ischemic heart disease*, *hypertensive heart disease* with left ventricular remodeling, *dilated and hypertrophic cardiomyopathies*, and hemodynamically significant *valvular disease*. The clinical picture is usually dominated by manifestations of the underlying heart disease but may include palpitations, near-syncope, and syncope. Such patients have a lowered threshold for VT and are especially susceptible to *hypokalemia*, *hypomagnesemia*, and *medications* that predispose to dysrhythmias (e.g., *digitalis, methylxanthines, tricyclics*).

VT in the Setting of a Normal-Appearing Heart. More difficult to recognize are patients with VT who manifest little evidence of underlying heart disease but still have an increased risk of an adverse cardiac event. Some have otherwise clinically silent heart disease (e.g., ischemia, cardiomyopathy); others harbor genetic mutations or acquire a predisposition to serious ventricular dysrhythmias by virtue of medication use or metabolic disruption. Clues to this underlying pathophysiology include the use of drugs that impair repolarization, a family history of early sudden death, recurrent syncopal episodes, and exercise-induced VT. Included in this group are persons with a prolonged QT interval, right ventricular outflow tract VT, right ventricular cardiomyopathy, and Brugada's syndrome.

Prolonged-QT Syndrome. Prolonged-QT syndrome is increasingly being recognized as an important cause of VT, particularly the potentially lethal polymorphic ventricular tachycardias referred to as *torsades de pointes*. Prolongation of the QT interval represents a disorder of myocardial repolarization, which may be acquired or hereditary. In hereditary forms, mutations in sodium- and potassium-channel genes (designated LQT1 to 6) result in a spectrum of repolarization abnormalities and susceptibility to VT and torsades (Fig. 25.1).

In acquired forms, precipitants to QT prolongation include *bradycardia*, older *age*, *left ventricular* (LV) *dysfunction*, ischemia, hypertrophy, *medications*, *hypokalemia*, *hypomagnesemia*, *hypothyroidism*, *liquid protein diets*, and *eating disorders* that cause *starvation*. The ECG criteria for QT prolongation are a corrected QT interval of greater than 450 msec in men and of greater than 460 msec in women. Other ECG features include T-wave alternans, notched T waves, and prominent U waves.

Risks of VT and cardiac death vary greatly among persons with hereditary forms of the condition; the overall risk is about 5%. The risk varies with the site of mutation, degree of QT prolongation, and gender. In patients with a history of syncope, 10-year mortality rates approach 50%. Precipitants include severe emotional stress and very vigorous exercise. In acquired forms, a number of medications have been implicated, including the antihistamines *terfenadine* and *astemizole* (especially when taken in excess or concurrently with agents that impair mitochondrial cytochrome P450 activity), as well as *class IA* and *class III antiarrhythmics*, *macrolide antibiotics*, *antipsychotics*, *antifungal agents*, and *tricyclic antidepressants*. Persons with a hereditary predisposition to QT prolongation are believed to be especially susceptible to drug-induced disease.

Right Ventricular Outflow Tract VT. Right ventricular outflow tract VT occurs in persons without evidence of structural heart disease. The VT originates from the septal portion of the right ventricular outflow tract. Patients may report exercise-induced palpitations, dyspnea, or syncope. The right ventricu-

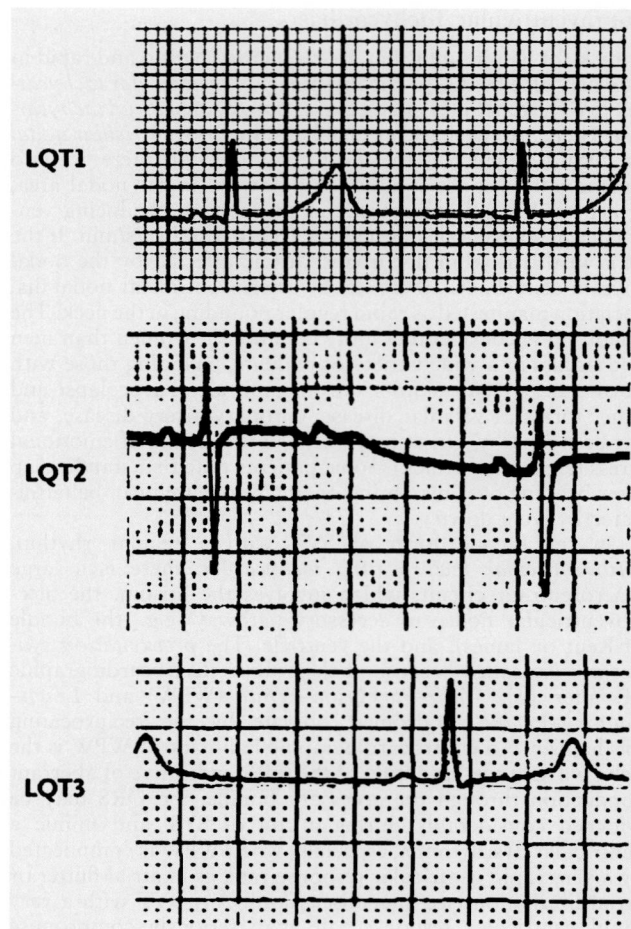

FIGURE 25.1. Electrocardiograms of commonly inherited forms of long-QT syndrome. The LQT1 form of the long-QT syndrome is associated with a broad T wave (no shortening of the QT interval during exercise). LQT2 is associated with low-amplitude, often bifid, T waves. LQT3 is associated with a long isoelectric segment and a narrow-based, tall T wave. (Adapted from Roden DM. Long-QT syndrome. N Engl J Med 2008;358:169, with permission.)

lar origin of the VT is manifested by its left-bundle pattern on ECG.

The Brugada Syndrome. The Brugada syndrome is a hereditary, autosomal-dominant syndrome due to a mutation in a gene important to the functioning of the heart's sodium channels. Male patients outnumber female patients by 9:1. Affected persons manifest no overt heart disease, but they may have a family history of sudden death, and their electrocardiograms may show characteristic features of right-bundle-branch block and ST-segment elevation in leads V1 to V3. Affected persons have a high rate of sudden death, especially during sleep. Mortality is high (up to 10%/yr).

Right Ventricular Cardiomyopathy (Arrhythmogenic Right Ventricular Cardiomyopathy). Right ventricular cardiomyopathy is a subtle cardiomyopathic cause of VT with an increased risk of sudden death. Right ventricular muscle is replaced with fibro-fatty tissue. Besides sudden death, affected persons, typically in their 20s to 30s, may experience syncope or report exercise- or non–exercise-induced palpitations due to VT. The ECG may show T-wave inversions in leads V1 to V3 and right-bundle-branch block (with or without ST-segment elevation), which is believed to be due to poor conduction through the involved fibro-fatty myocardium of the right ventricle. On stress testing, there can be ventricular ectopy with a left-bundle pattern, indicative of a right ventricular origin of the VPBs. The echocardiogram may reveal a dilated, poorly contractile right ventricle. Magnetic resonance imaging scanning reveals fatty displacement of normal myocardial tissue.

DIFFERENTIAL DIAGNOSIS (18)

The causes of palpitations can be listed in terms of their clinical presentation (Tables 25.1 and 25.2).

WORKUP (1–4,6–8,11,14,15,18–25)

Although determining the nature of the heartbeat disturbance helps to identify etiology and prognosis, the key determinants of prognosis are the presence, the type, and the severity of underlying heart disease. Consequently, a search for cardiac pathology is a high priority.

TABLE 25.1

IMPORTANT CAUSES OF PALPITATIONS

Isolated Single Palpitations
  Premature atrial or ventricular beats
  The beat after a blocked beat
  The beat after a compensatory pause
Paroxysmal Episodes with Abrupt Onset and Resolution (Rate Usually Rapid)
  Rhythm irregular
    Paroxysmal atrial fibrillation
    Paroxysmal atrial tachycardia with variable block
    Frequent atrial or ventricular premature beats
    Multifocal atrial tachycardia
  Rhythm regular
    Supraventricular tachycardias with constant block 1:1 conduction
Paroxysmal Episodes with Less-Abrupt Onset or Resolution (Rhythm Usually Regular, Rate Rapid)
  Exertion
  Emotion
    Drug side effect (e.g., sympathomimetics, theophylline compounds)
  Stimulant use (coffee, tea, tobacco)
  Insulin reaction
  Pheochromocytoma
Persistent Palpitations at Rest with Regular Rhythm (Rate Normal, Slow, or Rapid)
  Aortic or mitral regurgitation
  Large ventricular septal defect
  Bradycardia
  Severe anemia
  Hyperthyroidism (may also cause atrial fibrillation)
  Pregnancy
  Fever
  Marked volume depletion
  Anxiety neurosis

History

Eliciting a complete *description* of the patient's palpitations can be very helpful, including mode of onset, frequency, rate, rhythm, duration, termination, associated symptoms, precipitants and alleviating factors, and family history of syncope or sudden death. Unfortunately, many patients are unable to give an accurate or detailed account of their symptoms. The more hypochondriacal or somatizing the patient, the poorer is the correlation between symptoms and Holter monitoring results; however, reports of fluttering, stopping, or beating irregularly are predictive of finding an arrhythmia. The relation of the onset of symptoms to exertion can aid in separating the anxious individual, whose symptoms may occur at rest and are usually not worsened by exertion, from the patient with heart disease and impaired exercise tolerance. Palpitations brought on by exercise or stress suggests underlying heart disease. In the absence of symptoms of overt heart disease, the past medical history should be reviewed for cardiac risk factors; hereditary etiologies should be included in the differential, especially if there is a family history of syncope or early sudden death. Identification of precipitants such as emotional upset, stimulant intake, fever, pregnancy, volume depletion, and severe anemia is essential because their recognition can contribute to the design of proper therapy. Inquiry into symptoms of an insulin reaction (see Chapter 102) and hyperthyroidism (see Chapter 103) may also prove productive.

Any isolated thumping or flip-flopping in the chest suggests an atrial or ventricular premature beat. Associated *pounding in the neck* is indicative of arterioventricular (AV) dissociation, as seen with atrial or ventricular premature beats that result in AV dissociation. *Sudden onset* and *sudden cessation* of rapid regular heartbeats are characteristic of nodal and reentrant SVT and NSVT, whereas more gradual onset and cessation characterize sinus tachycardia (see Table 25.2) Onset in conjunction with a panic attack is indicative not only of sinus tachycardia, but also of nodal reentrant tachycardia, as is onset with standing up after bending over and cessation with lying down.

Inquiries into concurrent dyspnea, chest pain, lightheadedness, near-syncope, and syncope are essential both for etiology and assessment of hemodynamic severity. Syncope suggests VT or a very fast SVT with hemodynamic compromise; chest pain and dyspnea may also be signs of marked hemodynamic compromise. Also critical are a detailed review of risk factors for coronary disease, prior cardiac history (e.g., heart murmur, rheumatic fever, myocardial infarction), and family history of heart disease and early onset of syncope or sudden death. Although one should not mistake symptoms of anxiety, such as chest tightness and air hunger at rest, for evidence of organic heart disease, the presence of anxiety symptoms does not rule out a worrisome dysrhythmia. Nonetheless, assessment is not complete without specific inquiry into symptoms of panic and somatization disorders (see Chapters 226 and 230).

The use of all cardiotonic drugs should be detailed, including antiarrhythmics, digitalis preparations, theophylline compounds, sympathomimetics, and anticholinergics. Drugs associated with QT prolongation also need to be reviewed: antiarrhythmics, terfenadine, astemizole, macrolide antibiotics, ketoconazole, itraconazole, phenothiazines, and tricyclic antidepressants (Table 25.3). Many over-the-counter decongestants and diet pills contain catecholamines or theophylline derivatives; their abuse may be responsible for symptoms. The history should include inquiry into alcohol abuse (see Chapter 228), a common precipitant of paroxysmal SVT.

TABLE 25.2

DIFFERENTIATING CAUSES OF RAPID HEART BEAT

Type of Tachyarrhythmia	Typical Age at Onset of Symptoms	Underlying Condition	Usual Presentation	Finding on Baseline ECG
Paroxysmal SVT	Allages	None(normal heart)	Abrupt onset and termination of regular palpirations, diaphoresis	Preexcitation common in AVRT
Atrial fibrillation; atrial flutter, multifocal atrial tachycardia	≥60 yr	Heart diseases common (hypertension, ischemic or valvular heart disease)	Abrupt onset of paroxysmal, irregular palpitations symptoms sometimes persistent and occasionally mild or absent	Signs of left ventricular hypertrophy; nonspecific repolarization abnormalities common
Sinus tachycardia	10–30 yrs	None (normal heart)	Progressive onset and termination of palpitations	Normal
Ventricular tachycardia[b]	≥50 yrs	Ischemic heart disease	Abrupt onset and termination of regular palpitations, syncope, or sudden death from cardiac causes	Pathologic Q waves common

Atrial fibrillation and atrial flutter are not included in the category.
AVRT, atrioventricular reentrant tachycardia ; ECG, electrocardiogram; SVT, supraventricular tachycardia.
Adapted from Delacrètaz E. Supraventricular tachycardia, N Engl J med 2006;354:1039, with permission.
[a]In adults, sinus tachycardia is occasionally secondary to hyperthyroidism, anemia, infection, and heart failure. Sinus tachycardia may cause symptoms that can be difficult to differentiate from those due to tachyarrhythmia.
[b]Occasionally, ventricular tachycardia occurs in adults with no structural heart disease and is benign.

Physical Examination

Important observations include determination of the blood pressure for elevation, marked postural change, and widened pulse pressure. The apical pulse is noted for rate and rhythm disturbances; relying on the peripheral pulse may be misleading when there is a pulse deficit, as occurs in atrial fibrillation or premature beats. The temperature should be recorded. The skin is examined for pallor and signs of hyperthyroidism and anemia; the eyes for exophthalmos; the neck for goiter; the carotid pulse for upstroke; the jugular venous pulse for distention and cannon "a" waves; the chest for rales, rhonchi, wheezes, and dullness; the heart for heaves, thrills, clicks, murmurs, rubs, and third heart sound; and the extremities for edema and calf tenderness. The finding of a systolic ejection murmur along the left sternal border should be followed by examining its response to Valsalva maneuver; an increase in intensity suggests hypertrophic cardiomyopathy. Response to modest exercise should also be noted because a number of dysrhythmias may be triggered by it. Finally, the mental status examination should include checking for manifestations of anxiety, depression, panic disorder, somatization, and substance abuse (see Chapters 226 to 228, 230, and 235). In addition to possibly providing important diagnostic information, the careful, unhurried physical examination can be of considerable use in reassuring the worried patient.

Laboratory Studies

A few basic hematologic and chemistry studies contribute to the assessment of etiology and risk. Patients with signs of a hyperkinetic state require a *hemoglobin* determination to rule out a significant anemia and a *thyrotropin* (TSH) test to rule out hyperthyroidism. Patients with underlying heart disease, digitalis preparation use, or QT prolongation should have a check of the serum *potassium, calcium, magnesium,* and *TSH* (for hypothyroidism). A serum cardiac glycoside level (e.g., for *digoxin*) is equally important to rule out toxic accumulation of the drug. A finger-stick *blood glucose* can be diagnostic in the setting of a suspected insulin reaction triggering hypoglycemia (see Chapter 102). When there is sufficient clinical evidence to warrant consideration of pheochromocytoma, a 24-hour *urine for vanillylmandelic acid* can be helpful (see Chapter 26). Most of the remainder of the laboratory workup is directed toward identifying the rhythm disturbance and detecting underlying heart disease.

Resting Electrocardiogram

Most if not all patients with palpitations should have a resting 12-lead ECG. Even if physical examination is completely normal and no disturbances of rate or rhythm are noted on the ECG, one might detect a manifestation of underlying heart disease. Specifically, the ECG needs to be studied for axis shift, short PR interval (<0.12 seconds), abnormal P-wave morphology including signs of atrial enlargement, QRS widening, increase in QRS voltage, prominent septal Q waves, prolonged QT interval, delta waves, and ST- and T-wave changes. If a dysrhythmia is noted, it is worth obtaining a 2-minute rhythm strip to better characterize the rhythm disturbance. The anxiety-laden person often insists on having an ECG and finds comfort in a normal result; unfortunately, in many cases, the reassurance is only transient.

Measuring the QT Interval. When there is concern about QT prolongation as a precipitant of VT, the QT interval should

TABLE 25.3

MEDICATIONS ASSOCIATED WITH PROLONGATION OF THE QT INTERVAL

Very Probable
  Antiarrhythmics
    Amiodarone
    Disopyramide
    Sotalol
    Quinidine
    Ibutilide
  Antipsychotics
    Thioridazine
Probable
  Antipsychotics
    Pimozide
    Ziprasidone
Possible in High-Risk Patients
  Antibiotics
    Clarithromycin, erythromycin (other macrolides less likely)
    Pentamidine
    Gatifloxacin, sparfloxacin
    Sparfloxacin (other floxacins less likely)
  Antipsychotics
    Chlorpromazine
    Haloperidol
    Risperidone
    Olanzapine
  Antidepressants
    Amitriptyline
    Desipramine
    Imipramine
    Sertraline (other SSRIs less likely)
    Venlafaxine

Adapted from Al-Khatib SM, Lapointe NMA, Kramer JM, et al. What clinicians should know about the QT interval. JAMA 2003;289:2120, with permission.

be measured and the corrected QT interval (QT_c) calculated. Although there are no universally accepted standards for measurement of the QT interval or for determination of the QT_c, most authorities recommend that the interval be measured manually, taking the average of three to five QT intervals as measured in one of the limb leads from the start of the Q wave to the end of the T wave. If there is a large U wave merging with the T wave, then it should be included in the measurement. Because the QT interval varies with heart rate, a QT_c determination is also required. However, there is no consensus on the best approach to making correction. A commonly used correction formula is to divide the QT interval by the square root of the R-R interval (the Bazett formula). This correction seems to be reliable, except at high heart rates. In cases of suspected hereditary disease, the *pattern of QT prolongation* can be helpful diagnostically (Fig. 25.1).

Ambulatory Electrocardiographic Monitoring

Patients whose palpitations are accompanied by evidence of *underlying heart disease* are the best candidates for ambulatory monitoring because they are more likely to have a clinically significant arrhythmia. So long as they are not experiencing syncope, near-syncope, heart failure, or angina in association with their palpitations, they can undergo an outpatient evaluation that includes ambulatory monitoring (persons with such symptoms require consideration for admission and prompt cardiac consultation). The utility of ambulatory monitoring in otherwise healthy patients who complain solely of palpitations remains less clear, although the reassurance value of such testing can be considerable if typical symptoms occur in the presence of a normal ECG recording.

The most cost-effective approach to ambulatory monitoring is the use of an *event recorder* rather than *Holter monitoring* because most episodes of palpitations are relatively infrequent. A 2-week monitoring period using a continuous-loop event recorder yields more diagnoses at lower cost than does 48-hour Holter monitoring or 4 weeks of event recording. The only drawback to the continuous-loop event recorder is that it requires patient activation, which can be a problem if the dysrhythmia incapacitates the patient. Although monitoring may be continuous, preservation of the ECG record is usually limited to a few minutes about the time of activation. Most units use continuous-loop recording technology, although more-advanced storage technologies are under development. Some permit telephone transmission of the rhythm disturbance. Intermittent ECG recorders allow prolonged monitoring at reasonable cost in patients with relatively infrequent episodes of palpitations. Ambulatory monitoring has been disappointing as a method for detecting ischemia.

The yield from Holter monitoring is greatest in patients with daily symptoms. Patients are asked to keep a diary to ascertain the relationship between symptoms and rhythm disturbances. Because atrial and ventricular premature beats and short runs of SVT are common in normal asymptomatic patients, a positive test requires a clear-cut correlation between symptoms reported in the patient log and ECG findings. Most studies of Holter monitoring show a very high incidence of recorded "abnormalities" but a very poor correlation between ECG findings and reported symptoms. The patient who experiences typical symptoms but no concurrent rhythm disturbances during the Holter monitoring can be reassured. The patient who fails to have a symptomatic episode during Holter monitoring—a common occurrence—may be scheduled for a repeat study; however, yield is low in patients whose initial Holter study is normal and frequency of episodes is low. The cost of repeat Holter monitoring can be high.

One of the more disconcerting findings on event monitoring is a *wide-QRS tachycardia*. Although not usually encountered in the outpatient setting, it may be found on an event monitoring and needs to be addressed to determine whether it represents a rather harmless *SVT with aberrancy* or a more ominous *ventricular tachycardia*. Findings associated with a ventricular origin include a history of heart disease, evidence of an old myocardial infarction on a resting ECG, arterioventricular dissociation (which is often absent but can be diagnostic if present), a QRS duration of more than 160 msec if there is a right-bundle-branch pattern or more than 140 msec if the pattern is left bundle, a combination of left-bundle-branch block and right-axis deviation, extreme left-axis deviation (less than −90 to +180 degrees), and a different QRS pattern during tachycardia than on resting ECG in patients with preexisting bundle-branch block. The combination of these findings provides reasonable sensitivity and specificity; most single findings are relatively weak discriminants.

Exercise Stress Testing

Stress testing can help both in detecting dysrhythmias and in establishing safe limits for physical activity. The diagnostic yield for ventricular irritability is actually greater with Holter monitoring, but stress testing sometimes brings out ventricular dysrhythmias that do not appear on ambulatory monitoring, suggesting that these studies might be complementary. The best candidates for exercise stress testing are those who report palpitations occurring during or immediately after exercise. Among the arrhythmias detected by stress testing are SVTs, atrial fibrillation, and ventricular tachycardias. Although ventricular ectopy that occurs during stress testing does not independently contribute to cardiac risk, that which develops in the recovery phase does. To ensure patient safety, it is best to rule out hemodynamically significant aortic stenosis, hypertrophic cardiomyopathy, and QT prolongation before proceeding with exercise testing because these conditions are associated with an increased risk of an adverse event during or just after the stress test. Alternatively, one can ask the patient to exercise during ambulatory monitoring, but if there is a history of exercise-induced syncope, a family history of sudden death, or concern about serious underlying heart disease, it is best to order a formal exercise stress test performed under the supervision of a consulting cardiologist. Stress testing may also be indicated if palpitations occur in the context of angina-like chest pain, suggesting either an ischemic mechanism or sufficient hemodynamic compromise to result in ischemia (see Chapters 20 and 36).

Echocardiography

Patients suspected of having ischemic, valvular, or cardiomyopathic disease on the basis of history, physical examination, or ECG should undergo echocardiography for the diagnosis and determination of disease severity (see Chapters 2, 30, 32, and 33). Echocardiography should also be considered in persons with VT who have no apparent underlying heart disease because subtle wall and wall-motion abnormalities may be detected suggesting cardiomyopathy. Routine ordering of cardiac ultrasound in the absence of clinical suspicion is of little utility and only increases the cost of evaluation.

Electrophysiologic Study

Palpitations leading to syncope or near-syncope raise the question of a major rhythm disturbance (e.g., very rapid SVT, ventricular tachycardia, complete heart block). When occurring in the context of underlying organic heart disease, such arrhythmias have an especially poor prognosis (see Chapters 28 and 29). Electrophysiologic study (EPS) can help to uncover such arrhythmias and their pathologic mechanisms. The search for a focus of malignant arrhythmogenicity also helps to guide treatment. The value of EPS in syncopal patients who have significant organic heart disease is well documented, but sensitivity and specificity for identifying important arrhythmias or conduction-system disturbances in syncopal patients without signs of underlying heart disease have been disappointing. EPS remains an important diagnostic modality in the evaluation of patients with suspected ventricular tachycardia or documented heart block. Careful patient selection is essential (see Chapters 24 and 29). EPS is very expensive and not without risk because it includes the induction of potentially dangerous dysrhythmias. The study requires prior cardiac and electrophysiologic consultation, cardiac catheterization, sophisticated equipment, and a highly trained and experienced staff.

Genetic Testing

The increasing appreciation for the role of genetic mutations in the causation of cardiac dysrhythmias adds genetic testing to the list of available diagnostic tools. Identification of the LQT mutation locus is likely to play a role in treating persons with hereditary *long-QT syndrome* because it appears that risk stratification is facilitated by consideration of the responsible gene mutation (the risk with mutation in LQT2 or LQT3 is greater than that with mutation in LQT1). Such genetic testing can be especially helpful as part of the evaluation of family members of a young patient who suffered a sudden death and in whom long-QT interval is suspected. The reader is urged to watch for developments in gene mutation testing because they are likely to facilitate diagnosis and risk stratification.

PATIENT EDUCATION AND SYMPTOMATIC RELIEF
(2–6,12,13,25–27)

Patient Education

Persons with palpitations who present to physicians are usually both worried about the meaning of their symptoms and eager to have them relieved.

Providing Reassurance

When palpitations prove to be no more than a manifestation of excessive bodily concern or a harmless dysrhythmia with no adverse consequences, efforts should be made to provide meaningful reassurance. Failure to do so is likely to lead to unnecessary limitation of activity and demands for additional testing or referrals to specialists. Hasty or perfunctory words of comfort are worthless. A careful history and physical examination, combined with eliciting and responding directly to patient concerns, views, and requests (within reason), must take place before the patient can be told that the palpitations are harmless. Such reassurance may be all that is needed, especially when combined with advice to increase physical activity and cut down on alcohol, smoking, and stress. Ambulatory monitoring or exercise stress testing may have a role in helping to reassure the overly anxious patient. Directly addressing any underlying psychopathology may be required (see Chapters 226, 227, and 230).

Prevention

Patients appreciate advice regarding the avoidance of precipitants. Those with underlying heart disease or exercise-induced dysrhythmias benefit from being given parameters for safe physical exertion. Persons with underlying heart disease or a family history of syncope or early sudden death and those with hereditary QT-interval prolongation should be warned about the use of drugs that can prolong the QT interval (Table 25.3). Avoidance of "natural" ephedra-containing compounds (now banned by the U.S. Food and Drug Administration) and other nonessential sympathomimetics (e.g., over-the-counter decongestants and diet pills) should be stressed. Those who drink excessive amounts of caffeinated beverages should be advised to cut down on consumption, but absolute cessation does not appear to be necessary.

Symptomatic Management

Proper management of dysrhythmias in patients *with underlying heart disease* requires identifying and treating the underlying pathophysiology (see Chapters 28 to 30, 32, and 33). For patients with *no underlying heart disease* who find their symptoms intolerable, the following subsections give simple measures worth considering.

Atrial and Ventricular Premature Beats

All nonessential drugs capable of causing palpitations (e.g., *sympathomimetics* in decongestants) should be stopped. Stimulants should be avoided, especially those with potent adrenergic effects (e.g., *ephedra*). The role of *caffeine* in precipitating cardiac arrhythmias and the usefulness of restricting its intake in symptomatic patients has been debated for decades. Unless the patient clearly reports caffeine-induced symptoms, data show benefit only for restricting excessive intake (more than five cups a day). *Relaxation techniques* may be recommended for persons with anxiety-related palpitations and *cognitive–behavioral therapy* for those with somatization disorder (see Chapters 226 and 230). If palpitations related to premature beats persist and remain symptomatically bothersome, pharmacologic measures can be considered, such as a trial of low-dose of β-blocker therapy (e.g., atenolol or metoprolol, 25 to 50 mg/d). β-Blocker therapy can decrease the frequency of atrial or ventricular premature beats to tolerable levels.

Supraventricular Tachycardia and Sinus Tachycardia

Detailed discussion of treatment for SVT is presented in Chapter 28, but a few simple measures in addition to those mentioned for premature beats are worth noting. *Vagal maneuvers* are often effective in halting SVT. *Valsalva* and *carotid sinus massage* (in the absence of carotid disease) can be taught to the patient and suggested as the first line of therapy after the onset of an attack. Prophylaxis of SVT attacks can be accomplished by avoiding known precipitants, such as alcohol and stimulants. If a panic attack disorder is the cause of episodes of palpitations, one can consider β-blockade, a minor tranquilizer, or an antidepressant (see Chapter 226).

Symptomatic treatment of sinus tachycardia necessitates correcting the underlying precipitant (e.g., anemia [see Chapter 82], volume depletion, hyperthyroidism [see Chapter 103], fever [see Chapter 11], and congestive failure [see Chapter 32]). Patients with hypoglycemic episodes need an adjustment in their insulin regimen and/or dietary program (see Chapter 102). Treatment of MAT requires correction of the underlying pulmonary problem rather than the use of antiarrhythmic drugs. Improvement in oxygenation and pH status is essential.

Ventricular Tachycardia

Symptomatic VT episodes, especially those that cause syncope, require serious attention, even when there is no threat of sudden death. β-Blockers are often the first line of pharmacologic therapy, including use in persons with hereditary forms of the prolonged-QT syndrome (see Chapter 29).

INDICATIONS FOR ADMISSION AND REFERRAL
(2,3,7–10,14,15,25–27)

Admission

Patients with palpitations associated with syncope, near-syncope, angina-like chest pain, or true dyspnea are candidates for prompt inpatient evaluation, especially if they have evidence of underlying organic heart disease. Hospitalization is also indicated if a patient with known heart disease demonstrates runs of ventricular tachycardia, even if these are not sustained or hemodynamically compromising; mortality risk is high. Patients with SVT who manifest hemodynamic compromise (e.g., fall in blood pressure, dyspnea, angina, near-syncope) also need prompt hospital admission. Persons with VT and a family history of early sudden death should be considered for admission and electrophysiologic study.

Referral

Patients with underlying heart disease and palpitations leading to syncope, near-syncope, chest pain, or dyspnea require cardiac consultation for the consideration of electrophysiologic study, as do those with underlying heart disease and episodes of ventricular tachycardia (sustained or nonsustained), whether hemodynamically compromising or not. All such patients are at high risk and likely to benefit from EPS both diagnostically and often therapeutically (see Chapters 28 and 29).

A.H.G.

Annotated Bibliography

1. Akhtar M, Shenasa M, Jazayeri M, et al. Wide QRS complex tachycardia. Ann Intern Med 1988;109:905. (*The vast majority of cases proved to be ventricular in origin; a good discussion of criteria for distinguishing between supraventricular and ventricular sources.*)
2. Al-Khatib SM, Lapointe NMA, Kramer JM, et al. What clinicians should know about the QT interval. JAMA 2003;289:2120. (*A practical review for the clinician, focusing on medication-induced QT prolongation; 58 references.*)
3. Barnett PA, Peter CT, Swan HJC, et al. The frequency and prognostic significance of electrocardiographic abnormalities in clinically normal individuals. Prog Cardiovasc Dis 1981;23:299. (*Normal individuals have a high incidence of arrhythmias; a provocative discussion of what constitutes "normal."*)
4. Barsky AJ, Cleary PD, Coeytaux RR, et al. Psychiatric disorders in medical outpatients complaining of palpitations. J Gen Intern Med 1994;9:306. (*Panic disorder accounted for palpitations in nearly 20% of patients.*)
5. Barsky AJ, Clearly PD, Barnett MC, et al. The accuracy of symptoms reporting by patients complaining of palpitations. Am J Med 1994;97:214. (*The more hypochondriacal or somatizing the patient, the poorer was the correlation between symptoms and Holter monitoring results; however, reports of fluttering, stopping, or beating irregularly were predictive of an arrhythmia.*)
6. Cohen EJ, Klatsky AL, Armstrong MA. Alcohol use and supraventricular arrhythmia. Am J Cardiol 1988;62:971. (*Alcohol excess precipitates a host of supraventricular tachycardias [SVTs].*)
7. Elhendy A, Chandrasekaran K, Gersh BJ, et al. Functional and prognostic significance of exercise-induced ventricular arrhythmias in patients with suspected coronary artery disease. Am J Cardiol 2002;95. (*Evidence raising the question of increased risk in this population.*)
8. Frolkis JP, Pothier CE, Blackstone EH, et al. Frequent ventricular ectopy after exercise as a predictor of death. N Engl J Med 2003;348:781. (*A cohort study; frequent ectopy in the recovery phase of stress testing was associated with an increased risk of death; the adjusted hazard ratio was 1.5.*)
9. Jouven X, Sureik M, Desnos M, et al. Long-term outcome in asymptomatic men with exercise-induced premature ventricular depolarizations. N Engl J Med 2000;343:826. (*A cohort study suggesting increased long-term risk; the relative risk was 3.0.*)
10. Kennedy HL, Whitlock JA, Sprague MK, et al. Long-term follow-up of symptomatic healthy subjects with frequent and complex ventricular ectopy. N Engl J Med 1985;312:193. (*No increased risk was found of cardiac morbidity or mortality.*)

11. Lessmeier TJ, Gamperlin D, Johnson-Liddon V, et al. Unrecognized paroxysmal supraventricular tachycardia: potential for misdiagnosis as panic disorder. Arch Intern Med 1997;157:537. (*Panic disorder was very common among patients with electrophysiologic study–proven SVT.*)

12. Lowenstein SR, Gabow PA, Cramer J, et al. The role of alcohol in new onset atrial fibrillation. Arch Intern Med 1983;143:1882. (*Among 40 cases of new-onset atrial fibrillation, alcohol caused or contributed to approximately two thirds; 90% of these converted spontaneously to sinus rhythm within 24 hours.*)

13. Myers MG. Caffeine and cardiac arrhythmias. Ann Intern Med 1991;114:147. (*Reviews the evidence for and against a causative role; moderate intake appears to have little effect, even in patients with heart disease.*)

14. Naccarelli GV, Antzelevitch C. The Brugada syndrome: clinical genetic, cellular, and molecular abnormalities. Am J Med 2001;110:573. (*Excellent review of this often-fatal arrhythmic syndrome in otherwise normal hearts, which is caused by a mutation in sodium-channel proteins.*)

15. Priori SG, Schwartz PJ, Napolitano C, et al. Risk stratification in the long-QT interval syndrome. N Engl J Med 2003;348:19. (*A risk-stratification study using genetic mutation analysis of potassium- and sodium-channel genes.*)

16. Roden DM. Long-QT syndrome. N Engl J Med 2008;358:169. (*A case-based review; 59 references.*)

17. Tan HL, Hou CJ, Lauer MR, et al. Electrophysiologic mechanisms of the long QT syndromes and torsade de pointes. Ann Intern Med 1995;122:701. (*An excellent review of the condition.*)

18. Delacrétaz E. Supraventricular tachycardia. N Engl J Med 2006;354:1039. (*An excellent clinical review; 49 references.*)

19. DiMarco JP, Philbrick JT. Use of ambulatory electrocardiographic (Holter) monitoring. Ann Intern Med 1990;113:53. (*A comprehensive and critical review focusing on advantages and limitations of Holter monitoring; 139 references.*)

20. Kapoor WN, Cha R, Peterson JR, et al. Prolonged electrocardiographic monitoring in patients with syncope. Am J Med 1987;82:20. (*Patients with syncope and frequent or repetitive ventricular premature beats or sinus pauses had an increased risk of overall mortality.*)

21. Kinlay S, Leitch JW, Neil A, et al. Cardiac event recorders yield more diagnoses and are more cost-effective than 48-hour Holter monitoring in patients with palpitations: a controlled clinical trial. Ann Intern Med 1996;124:16. (*A randomized crossover study; the title says it all.*)

22. Krol RB, Morady F, Flaker S, et al. Electrophysiologic testing in patients with unexplained syncope: clinical and noninvasive predictors of outcome. J Am Coll Cardiol 1987;10:358. (*Predictors include previous myocardial infarction, low ejection fraction, and conduction abnormalities on electrocardiogram.*)

23. Shen WK, Holmes DR, Hammill SC. Transtelephonic monitoring: documentation of transient cardiac rhythm disturbances. Mayo Clin Proc 1987;62:109. (*Another method for capturing infrequent but potentially important episodes.*)

24. Simetbaum PJ, Kim KY, Josephson ME, et al. Diagnostic yield and optimal duration of continuous-loop event monitoring for the diagnosis of palpitations. Ann Intern Med 1998;128:890. (*A prospective cohort study; the yield was found to drop off markedly after 2 weeks.*)

25. Weber BE, Kapoor WN. Evaluation and outcomes of patients with palpitations. Am J Med 1996;100:138. (*Although psychiatric disorders are common, true arrhythmic etiologies need to be ruled out.*)

26. Varma N, Josephson ME. Therapy of "idiopathic" ventricular tachycardia. J Cardiovasc Electrophysiol 1997;8:104. (*Includes good descriptions of pathophysiology and clinical presentations.*)

27. Zipes DP, Camm AJ, Borggrefe M, et al. ACC/AHA/ESC 2006 guidelines for management of patients with ventricular arrhythmias and the prevention of sudden cardiac death: a report of the American College of Cardiology/American Heart Association Task Force and the European Society of Cardiology Committee for Practice Guidelines (writing committee to develop Guidelines for Management of Patients with Ventricular Arrhythmias and the Prevention of Sudden Cardiac Death): developed in collaboration with the European Heart Rhythm Association and the Heart Rhythm Society. Circulation 2006;114:e385. (*Consensus recommendations for patients with long QT interval.*)

APPENDIX 25.1: EVALUATION OF ATRIAL FIBRILLATION IN THE OUTPATIENT SETTING

Atrial fibrillation (AF) is one of several dysrhythmias that can produce an irregularly irregular heartbeat. It is often a manifestation of underlying heart disease but sometimes is discovered in a patient with no overt cardiac pathology. Many patients tolerate the arrhythmia well and can be evaluated thoroughly and safely in the outpatient setting, although the etiology does not necessarily need to be harmless. The primary care physician needs to determine whether it is safe to conduct the assessment in the office setting and how to carry out a cost-efficient evaluation.

PATHOPHYSIOLOGY AND CLINICAL PRESENTATION (1–12)

The postulated electrophysiologic mechanisms of AF include focal automaticity and a complex form of reentry. Factors that may precipitate or perpetuate AF include increased atrial size, increased atrial pressure, varying repolarization times of neighboring areas of atrial myocardium, and occurrence of atrial premature beats during the vulnerable period of an atrial cycle. Increases in circulating catecholamines may precipitate atrial premature beats and AF. Ischemia and disease of the sinoatrial nodes also predispose to atrial dysrhythmias by suppressing the SA node and allowing other atrial foci to fire. Epidemiologic data from the Framingham Study reveal that heart failure and rheumatic heart disease are the most powerful predictors of AF and hypertension the most commonly associated condition, suggesting that myocardial damage and left atrial dilation are important precursors of the condition.

The hallmarks of AF are the characteristic electrocardiographic findings of an *irregularly irregular ventricular rhythm* and *atrial fibrillatory waves*. The fibrillatory waves range in appearance from fine, irregular undulations of the baseline to very coarse waves. The QRS duration is usually normal but may widen with aberrant conduction and simulate ventricular tachyarrhythmias. The ST segments and T waves may be abnormal in appearance if there is rapid ventricular response, underlying heart disease, or use of digitalis.

AF can present as a paroxysmal or chronic dysrhythmia, both with and without evidence of underlying heart disease. Its incidence in community settings is about 2% over 20 years. The overwhelming majority of AF patients have underlying heart disease at the time of onset. AF is often a sign of advanced heart disease; onset is associated with a twofold increase in mortality.

Some patients with incidentally discovered AF are asymptomatic; however, if the AF is paroxysmal or the ventricular rate is very rapid, *palpitations* may be reported. If cardiac output falls precipitously, symptoms of *heart failure* may occur. Rapid rate may also lead to myocardial *ischemia* in patients with underlying coronary artery disease. Systemic *embolization* may be the first sign of AF and present as an acute neurologic or peripheral vascular event. An increasingly common cause of transient AF is *coronary artery bypass graft* surgery. Usually, the AF is self-limited and resolves during the recovery period.

A number of acute noncardiac conditions can precipitate AF in the absence of clinically apparent heart disease; these include acute *alcohol intoxication*, *decompensated* chronic obstructive lung disease, pneumonia, and *pulmonary embolization*. However, AF does not always occur in the context of overt heart disease or an acute event such as sudden pulmonary decompensation. The entities associated with seemingly isolated bouts of AF deserve particular attention because detection is sometimes difficult, and therapy is different from that for most other causes of AF.

Lone Atrial Fibrillation

"Lone" AF (LAF) is used to denote AF in patients without clinically evident heart disease. In about two thirds of cases, the condition presents as isolated or recurrent episodes of paroxysmal AF; in the remainder, the AF is chronic. Studies of military recruits found its prevalence to be about 1 in 10,000. LAF is a harmless condition in young people; they characteristically experience episodes precipitated by emotional stress, alcohol, use of stimulants, or smoking. Detailed investigations have failed to reveal underlying heart disease, chamber enlargement, or risk of embolization. The prognosis in young patients is excellent, with no increased risk of stroke. In those older than 60 years with LAF, there is a moderate increase in stroke risk, which is believed to be due to silent progression of atherosclerotic disease. Older LAF patients with hypertension have a high stroke risk and should probably not be designated as having LAF but rather as having AF with underlying hypertensive heart disease.

Alcoholic Cardiomyopathy

The early stages of alcoholic cardiomyopathy may present as paroxysms of AF triggered by binge drinking. The distinction between this condition and lone fibrillation triggered by alcohol (*holiday heart*) may be difficult but is suggested by the finding of cardiomegaly even in the absence of heart failure. Abstinence can halt or even reverse the condition, but continued drinking leads to progression and, in some individuals, chronic AF.

Tachycardia–Bradycardia Syndrome

Also known as *sick-sinus syndrome*, this is an important and sometimes subtle cause of AF. The exact cause of this condition is unknown but is believed to be related to diffuse degeneration of conducting-system tissue. Patients exhibit sinus node dysfunction, often in conjunction with arterioventricular nodal disease and lack of an adequate escape mechanism. Atrial tachyarrhythmias may alternate with symptomatic bradycardia and sinus arrest. Clinical presentations include palpitations, lightheadedness, and syncope. At times, the first manifestation may be a paroxysm of AF. Identification is most important because treatment directed only toward the AF may worsen the bradyarrhythmia (see Chapter 28). Paroxysmal AF due to sick-sinus syndrome is associated with an increased risk of thromboembolism.

Wolff–Parkinson–White Syndrome

WPW is a preexcitation syndrome that produces a host of supraventricular and ventricular dysrhythmias, particularly paroxysms of AF associated with a very rapid ventricular response rate. In fact, a ventricular rate greater than 200 beats/min in the absence of another cause for AF should make one suspicious of WPW. The condition is believed to be at least partially congenital in nature and characterized by rapid atrioventricular conduction over an accessory pathway (*the Kent bundle*). This anomalous conduction pathway bypasses the arterioventricular node and produces preexcitation, manifested by the characteristic baseline ECG findings of a *shortened PR interval (<0.12 seconds)* and *delta waves at the onset of the QRS*. Some WPW patients have normal baseline ECGs and show anomalous conduction only during tachyarrhythmias, making electrocardiographic identification difficult. During rapid AF, there may be a widening of the QRS, mimicking ventricular fibrillation. The reported incidence of AF among patients with WPW ranges from 11% to 39%. WPW is an important cause of AF to recognize because the AF may actually worsen with digitalis therapy (see Chapter 28) and has the potential to degenerate into ventricular tachycardia and fibrillation.

Apathetic Hyperthyroidism of the Elderly

AF that appears to occur in the absence of underlying heart disease may be due to hyperthyroidism, especially in the elderly. In the most florid form of this presentation, patients may manifest marked apathy suggesting depression or impressive weight loss that may simulate occult malignancy (see Chapter 103). Sometimes, AF is the predominant manifestation. The usual signs and symptoms of thyrotoxicosis are absent. The AF is difficult to control with standard modes of antiarrhythmic therapy but usually reverts to sinus rhythm with the correction of the hyperthyroid state (see Chapter 28).

After Cardiac Surgery

AF is common after cardiac surgery, with reported frequencies ranging from 10% to 65%. Onset is typically on the second or third postoperative day and may persist for up to 1 month. Purported mechanisms include reentry, triggered by atrial premature beats that result from surgical intervention and the associated physical and metabolic disruptions. Factors that slow atria conduction (as manifested by a prolonged P-wave duration) may facilitate the reentry and development of AF. Atria ischemia is not believed to play a major role. Postoperative AF is associated with increased 30-day and 6-month mortality, but this may reflect AF being a marker for serious underlying heart disease. Postoperative AF predisposes to an increased risk of embolic stroke, a need for a permanent pacemaker, and prolonged hospitalization. Preoperative predictors include hypertension, previous heart failure, and previous AF.

DIFFERENTIAL DIAGNOSIS

AF is only one of a number of dysrhythmias that present as an irregularly irregular pulse. Frequent atrial premature beats, MAT, SVTs with variable block, sinus arrhythmia, and frequent ventricular premature beats all may produce an irregular rhythm. The most common cause of AF in the community setting is hypertensive heart disease; however, only those hypertensive patients with evidence of left ventricular hypertrophy are likely to develop AF. The major causes of AF are listed in Table 25.4.

TABLE 25.4

IMPORTANT CAUSES OF ATRIAL FIBRILLATION

Paroxysmal Atrial Fibrillation
"Lone" fibrillation
Acute ischemia
Alcohol intoxication and early alcoholic cardiomyopathy
Sick-sinus syndrome
Wolff–Parkinson–White syndrome
Acute pulmonary embolization
Acute pericarditis
Acute pulmonary decompensation
Acute heart failure
Any cause of chronic atrial fibrillation

Sustained Atrial Fibrillation
Advanced rheumatic mitral valve disease
Chronic congestive heart failure
Advanced aortic valve disease
Advanced hypertensive heart disease
Coronary artery disease
Advanced cardiomyopathy
Congenital heart disease
Apathetic hyperthyroidism of the elderly
Sick-sinus syndrome
"Lone" fibrillation
Constrictive pericarditis
Digitalis toxicity (rarely)

WORKUP (11–13)

The diagnosis of AF is based on the characteristic *ECG findings* of an irregular ventricular response and atrial fibrillatory waves. These fibrillatory waves range from barely perceptible, irregular undulations of the ECG baseline to very coarse waves. The standard lead best suited for detection of atrial activity is lead V_1, followed by leads II, III, and AVF. Occasionally, the routine 12-lead ECG will show no atrial activity; in such instances, one can check lead V_3R for evidence of atrial activity or infer the diagnosis of AF based on the characteristic ventricular response pattern and a QRS of normal duration. MAT, paroxysmal atrial tachycardia, atrial flutter with variable block, frequent atrial premature beats, and sinus arrhythmia all produce rhythms that can resemble AF, but the presence of P waves or flutter waves on ECG separates them from AF. If the ventricular response rate is too rapid to reveal atrial activity, *vagal maneuvers* and gentle *carotid sinus massage* can be attempted (provided there is no evidence of carotid artery disease) to slow the rate and uncover any hidden fibrillatory or P waves.

History

The young patient with a paroxysm of AF should be questioned about a prior history of such episodes, excess intake of stimulants and alcohol, emotional stress, fever, heart murmur, and chest pain. Older patients should be queried about preexisting heart disease, hypertension, chest pain, dyspnea, cough, calf pain, leg edema, fever, lightheadedness, near-syncope, loss of consciousness, weight loss, depression, history of heart murmur or rheumatic fever, and any prior attacks of palpitations. A careful drug history should be taken with emphasis on al-

cohol abuse (see Chapter 228). Any use of digitalis should be noted; however, digitalis toxicity only rarely results in AF. A longstanding history of attacks dating from young adulthood suggests WPW syndrome. The presence of marked weight loss and depression in an elderly patient with unexplained AF points to apathetic hyperthyroidism. The older patient with episodes of altered consciousness may suffer from sick-sinus syndrome.

Physical Examination

In addition to noting heart rate, blood pressure, respiratory rate, jugular venous pulse, and other signs of hemodynamic status, the physician should check the patient for apathetic appearance, evidence of marked weight loss, cyanosis, goiter, wheezes, friction rub, heart murmur, calf tenderness, asymmetric leg edema, and signs of alcohol intoxication. The most common cause of "silent" mitral valve disease is failure to listen specifically for the murmurs of mitral stenosis and mitral regurgitation. Placing the patient in the left lateral decubitus position may be necessary to appreciate the murmurs. Only in rare instances are the murmurs of mitral valve disease truly inaudible (see Chapter 33).

Laboratory Studies

The *ECG* often provides useful information beyond the identification of the arrhythmia. A ventricular response rate greater than 200 beats/min suggests WPW syndrome, as does a widened QRS due to aberrant conduction; delta waves may be seen within some of the aberrantly conducted beats. The appearance of the fibrillatory waves on ECG provides some hints of etiology. Coarse fibrillatory waves are most typical of AF resulting from rheumatic heart disease and other causes of marked left atrial enlargement, whereas fine fibrillatory waves are more common in cases due to atherosclerotic and hypertensive heart diseases. The ST- and T-wave segments should be checked for evidence of ischemia, strain, digitalis effect, and pericarditis (see Chapter 20). Advanced valvular and hypertensive forms of heart disease are suggested by finding ECG evidence of left ventricular hypertrophy.

A cardiogram taken after return to sinus rhythm should be checked for a shortened PR interval and delta waves diagnostic of WPW syndrome. Occasionally, preexcitation is concealed on the resting ECG, so the ECG of some WPW patients appears normal; in such instances, the diagnosis of WPW syndrome can be difficult. Other clues to WPW syndrome include a ventricular response rate during AF of greater than 200 beats/min and delta waves distorting the QRS complex.

A rhythm strip sometimes reveals sinus node disease, but often a 24-hour *Holter monitor* will be needed to detect the episodes of bradycardia and tachycardia that characterize the sick-sinus syndrome. *Chest radiograph* is the best simple test for determining heart failure, cardiomegaly, and intrapulmonary pathology. Cardiomegaly may be the only evidence of an underlying cardiomyopathy. *Echocardiogram* provides an excellent noninvasive means of further evaluating suspected valvular, congenital, cardiomyopathic, and pericardial forms of heart disease. However, the cost-effectiveness of ordering an echocardiogram routinely in the workup of AF to search for an occult high-risk cause such as mitral stenosis remains a subject of debate. The elderly apathetic patient with unexplained AF requires measurement of *thyrotropin* level to rule out

Step 1

Age, yr	Points
55	0
56	1
57	2
58–59	3
60	4
61	5
62	6
63	7
64–65	8
66	9
67	10
68	11
69	12
70–71	13
72	14
73	15
74	16
75	17
76–77	18
78	19
79	20
80	21
81	22
82–83	23
84	24
85	25
86	26
87	27
88	28
89	29
90–91	30
92	31
93	32
94	33

Step 2

Systolic Blood Pressure, mm Hg	Points
<120	0
120–139	1
140–159	2
160–179	3
>179	5

Step 3

Diabetes	Points
No	0
Yes	4

Step 4

Smoker	Points
No	0
Yes	5

Step 5

Prior MI or CHF	Points
No	0
Yes	6

Step 6

Murmur	Points
No	0
Yes	4

Step 7

ECG LVH	Points
No	0
Yes	2

Step 8

Add Up Points From Steps 1 Through 7

Look Up Predicted 5-Year Risk of Stroke or Death in Table

Predicted 5-Year Risk of Stroke or Death

Total Points	5-Year Risk, %
0	8
1	9
2–3	10
4	11
5	12
6	13
7	15
8	16
9	17
10	19
11	20
12	22
13	24
14	26
15	28
16	30
17	32
18	35
19	37
20	40
21	43
22	46
23	49
24	52
25	55
26	58
27	61
28	65
29	68
30	71
31	75
32	78
≥33	>80

FIGURE 25.2. Risk score for stroke or death in patients with atrial fibrillation. The point-based system approximates the more precise equation-based risk function provided as an Excel spreadsheet available at http://www.nhlbi.nih.gov/about/framingham/stroke.htm. The point-based risk estimate may differ from the equation-based one, particularly for patients with uncommon combinations of characteristics. CHF, congestive heart failure; ECG LVH, electrocardiographic left ventricular hypertrophy; MI, myocardial infarction. (From Wang TJ, Massaro JM, Levy K, et al. A risk score for predicting stroke or death in individuals with new-onset atrial fibrillation in the community. JAMA 2003;290:1049, with permission.)

hyperthyroidism (see Chapter 103). Although AF is a very uncommon manifestation of digitalis toxicity, a serum *digoxin level* is probably worth checking when no other cause is apparent and the patient is known to be taking the drug.

In summary, the evaluation can be performed on an outpatient basis if the patient is tolerating the rhythm well and there is no evidence of failure, ischemia, or embolization. A careful history and physical examination, supplemented by ECG, chest radiograph, and, in selected instances, an echocardiogram complete the evaluation in most patients. Patients with AF of unknown cause should be studied further for evidence of sick-sinus syndrome, apathetic hyperthyroidism, alcoholic cardiomyopathy, and WPW syndrome.

Risk Stratification

A critical task evaluation of AF is the determination of risk for stroke and death. Such risk stratification facilitates decision making, especially with regard to the appropriate aggressiveness of therapy and the need for chronic anticoagulation (see Chapter 28). Numerous risk-stratification schemes have been developed. A potentially useful one for outpatient practice derives from community-based data from the Framingham Heart Study. Although yet to be validated on a prospective sample, the risk-scoring system uses readily available parameters that have been found on multivariate analysis to be independent predictors of outcome. They include age, systolic blood pressure, diabetes, smoking, heart murmur, heart failure or prior myocardial infarction, and evidence of left ventricular hypertrophy on ECG (Fig. 25.2).

INDICATIONS FOR ADMISSION (14)

Once the diagnosis of AF is established, one needs to determine whether workup can proceed on an outpatient basis. Prompt hospital admission is needed for the patient with evidence of acute congestive heart failure, ischemia, embolization, hypotension, or a very rapid ventricular response rate (>150 to 170 beats/min). If there is no hemodynamic compromise, an outpatient workup can commence.

A.H.G.

Annotated Bibliography

1. Brand FN, Abbott RD, Kannel WB, et al. Characteristics and prognosis of lone atrial fibrillation: 30-year follow-up in the Framingham Study. JAMA 1985;254:3449. (*A fourfold increase in stroke risk was noted, but patients were older and had more cardiovascular risk factors than patients in other studies of lone atrial fibrillation [AF].*).

2. Campbell RWF, Smith RA, Gallagher JJ, et al. Atrial fibrillation in the pre-excitation syndrome. Am J Cardiol 1977;40:514. (*AF due to preexcitation syndromes can cause very rapid and aberrantly conducted ventricular responses; ventricular dysrhythmias can sometimes result.*)

3. Engel TR, Luck JC. Effect of whiskey on atrial vulnerability and "holiday heart." J Am Coll Cardiol 1983;1:816. (*Alcohol enhanced vulnerability to AF in patients without clinical evidence of cardiomyopathy or heart failure.*)

4. Ettinger PO, Wu DF, De La Cruz C Jr, et al. Arrhythmias and the "holiday heart": alcohol-associated cardiac rhythm disorders. Am Heart J 1978;895:955. (*Paroxysmal AF may be a sign of early alcoholic cardiomyopathy and be induced by binge drinking.*)

5. Forfar JC, Miller HC, Toft AD. Occult thyrotoxicosis: a correctable cause of "idiopathic" atrial fibrillation. Am J Cardiol 1979;44:9. (*A classic paper; 10 of 75 patients presenting with AF of unknown cause were hyperthyroid.*)

6. Hanson HH, Rutledge, DI. Auricular fibrillation in normal hearts. N Engl J Med 1949;240:947. (*Another classic paper; describes the entity of "lone fibrillation."*)

7. Kannel WB, Abbott RD, Savage DD, et al. Epidemiologic features of chronic atrial fibrillation: the Framingham Study. N Engl J Med 1982;306:1018. (*A major epidemiologic study; heart failure and rheumatic heart disease were the most powerful predictive precursors of chronic AF; chronic AF was associated with a doubling of overall and cardiovascular mortality.*)

8. Kopecky SL, Gersh BJ, McGoon MD, et al. The natural history of lone atrial fibrillation: a population-based study over three decades. N Engl J Med 1987;317:669. (*A retrospective study of patients <60 years of age, showing that lone AF was associated with a very low risk of stroke.*)

9. Kopecky SL, Gersh BJ, McGoon MD, et al. Lone atrial fibrillation in elderly persons: a marker for cardiovascular risk. Arch Intern Med 1999;159:1118. (*A population-based study in Olmsted County, Minnesota; the risk of stroke increased in patients >60 years of age.*)

10. Maisel WH, Rawn JD, Stevenson WG. Atrial fibrillation after cardiac surgery. Ann Intern Med 2001;135:1061. (*A systematic review; 104 references.*)

11. Wang TJ, Massaro JM, Levy K, et al. A risk score for predicting stroke or death in individuals with new-onset atrial fibrillation in the community. JAMA 2003;290:1049. (*A major prospective, community-based epidemiologic cohort study; risk categories are developed to help guide therapy.*)

12. Culler MR, Boone JA, Gazes PC. Fibrillatory wave size as a clue to etiologic diagnosis. Am Heart J 1983;66:425. (*Coarse atrial fibrillatory waves were found most frequently in patients with mitral valve disease and left atrial enlargement; it was also noted in "lone" AF and hyperthyroidism.*)

13. Desbiens NA. Should all patients with atrial fibrillation be screened with echocardiography? J Gen Intern Med 1992;7:131. (*A decision-analysis study on the efficacy of routinely screening AF patients by echocardiography for unrecognized mitral stenosis; the benefit was small, and screening was not recommended.*)

14. Shlofmitz RA, Hirsch BE, Meyer BR. New onset atrial fibrillation. J Gen Intern Med 1986;1:139. (*A retrospective study, showing that urgent hospitalization is rarely necessary.*)

CHAPTER 26 ■ MANAGEMENT OF HYPERTENSION

KATHARINE K. TREADWAY

Hypertension is one of the few conditions in medicine that can be readily detected and effectively treated in the asymptomatic period before irreparable harm is done. It ranks as a leading risk factor for cardiovascular disease and as a major reason for office visits and the prescription of medication. Cardiovascular disease is the leading cause of death in the United States. Of these deaths, 83% are caused by myocardial infarction and 17% are from stroke. There has been a steady decline in cardiovascular death over the last three decades, at least some of which is attributable to the lowering of blood pressure in the general population. The frequency and importance of hypertension demand that the primary physician be expert in its management and capable of designing a regimen that is safe, effective, and well tolerated.

PRINCIPLES OF MANAGEMENT

Confirmation of Diagnosis, Staging, and Risk Stratification (1–7)

The first tasks are to confirm the diagnosis and estimate the overall cardiovascular risk. This guides program design, which

includes nonpharmacologic and pharmacologic interventions.

Confirming the Diagnosis

Because treatment of hypertension is likely to be lifelong, care must be taken to establish the diagnosis by correct blood pressure measurement and evaluation for possible contributing factors and secondary causes (see Chapters 14 and 19).

Staging

The assessment for treatment-program design includes staging by degree of blood pressure elevation (Table 26.1 and Chapter 19). The Joint National Committee on Prevention, Detection, Evaluation and Treatment of High Blood Pressure (JNC) has recommended eliminating the traditional designations of "*mild*," "*moderate*," and "*severe*" hypertension to avoid the misleading notion than mild hypertension is not a significant health risk. Instead, three stages are designated:

■ *Prehypertension*: systolic blood pressure (SBP) 120 to 139 mm Hg; diastolic blood pressure (DBP) 80 to 89 mm Hg
■ *Stage 1 hypertension*: SBP 140 to 159 mm Hg; DBP 90 to 99 mm Hg

TABLE 26.1

MANAGEMENT OF HYPERTENSION BY BLOOD PRESSURE STAGE AND RISK GROUP

Blood Pressure Stage	Risk Group A	Risk Group B	Risk Group C
Prehypertension (SBP 130–139 mm Hg or DBP 85–89 mm Hg)	Lifestyle modification	Lifestyle modification	Drug prescription if diabetes mellitus, congestive heart failure, or renal insufficiency; lifestyle modification
Stage 1 (SBP 140–159 mm Hg or DBP 90–99 mm Hg)	Lifestyle modification (up to 12 mo)	Lifestyle modification (up to 6 mo); initial drug prescription for patients with multiple risks	Drug prescription, lifestyle modification
Stage 2 (SBP ≥160 mm Hg or DBP ≥100 mm Hg)	Drug prescription, lifestyle modification	Drug prescription, lifestyle modification	Drug prescription, lifestyle modification

Goals of therapy:
In most patients: <140/90 mm Hg
In diabetic patients: <130/85 mm Hg
In patients with renal failure and proteinuria (>1 g in 24 hr): <125/75 mm Hg
In elderly patients with severe systolic hypertension: systolic blood pressure <160 mm Hg is reasonable if attempts to reach 140 mm Hg result in intolerable side effects

Risk group A, no major risk factors, no target-organ damage/clinical cardiovascular disease. Risk group B, at least one major risk factor, not diabetes mellitus, no target-organ damage/clinical cardiovascular disease. Risk group C, target-organ damage/clinical cardiovascular disease and/or diabetes mellitus with or without other risk factors. Major risk factors: smoking, dyslipidemia, diabetes mellitus, age >60 yr, male gender, postmenopausal women, family history.
SBP = Systolic blood pressure; DBP = Diastolic blood pressure.
Adapted from Chobanian AV, Bakris GL, Cushman WC, et al. The seventh report of the Joint National Committee on Prevention, Detection, Evaluation and Treatment of High Blood Pressure: the JNC VII report. JAMA 2003:289;2560, with permission.

■ *Stage 2 hypertension*: SBP 160 mm Hg or greater; DBP 100 mm Hg or greater

Isolated Systolic Hypertension. Isolated elevations in systolic blood pressure (>140 mm Hg) confer significant cardiovascular risk, especially in older persons, regardless of the diastolic pressure. JNC underscores that "in persons older than 50 years, systolic blood pressure of more than 140 mm Hg is a much more important cardiovascular disease risk factor than diastolic BP." In the elderly, a large pulse pressure is an independent predictor of cardiovascular risk.

Prehypertension. There is no threshold blood pressure for cardiovascular risk. The risk of cardiovascular complications begins at pressures as low as 115/75 mm Hg and doubles with every 20–mm Hg increment of SBP and every 10–mm Hg increment for DBP. Persons with blood pressures in the so-called "prehypertension" range are at increased risk for developing sustained hypertension and cardiovascular complications. Cardiovascular risk is greatest in persons with concurrent diabetes, heart failure, renal insufficiency, or preexisting coronary artery disease. Although not all patients with prehypertension will go on to develop sustained elevation of blood pressure, a large percentage do. Those at highest risk for developing sustained hypertension can be identified by attention to age, sex, systolic and diastolic blood pressure, body mass index, parental hypertension, and smoking history.

Estimating Total Cardiovascular Risk

Because the ultimate goal of antihypertensive therapy is to reduce cardiovascular morbidity and mortality, the design of the treatment program must take into account the patient's *total cardiovascular risk*, not simply the elevation in blood pressure. This assessment will determine the pace, intensity, and scope of treatment. The task requires determining the *degree of blood pressure elevation* and identifying other *cardiovascular risk factors* (e.g., smoking, diabetes, hypercholesterolemia, age, gender, and family history), as well as any manifestations of *target-organ disease* (e.g., left ventricular hypertrophy with remodeling [LVH], retinopathy, nephrosclerosis, congestive heart failure [CHF], coronary artery disease, stroke, and peripheral vascular disease [see Chapter 19]). For any level of blood pressure elevation, the presence of such features dramatically raises the coronary disease risk from hypertension (e.g., from 9% over 10 years for a 40-year-old man with stage 1 hypertension to 70% for the same 40-year-old man if he also has elevated total cholesterol, a low high-density-lipoprotein [HDL] cholesterol, diabetes, and LVH and smokes [see Appendix 26.1]). Because the risk of hypertension varies significantly depending on what other risk factors are present, the JNC has proposed an algorithm to guide treatment decisions. It should be noted that the presence of diabetes confers such a significant risk that it is treated as equivalent to the presence of overt cardiovascular disease (Table 26.1).

Even modest elevation in blood pressure greatly increases risk, a very important fact from a population perspective. Most excess cardiovascular mortality from hypertension in the United States derives from patients with stage 1 disease (formerly referred to as "mild"), accounting for almost 80% of the hypertensive population and almost 60% of the excess cardiovascular mortality attributable to hypertension. Blood pressures in this range are not benign.

Nonpharmacologic Measures (1,2,4,8–19)

All patients are candidates for nonpharmacologic measures, which represent the foundation of treatment regimens for all stages. The principal nonpharmacologic measures include *exercise* (see Chapter 18), *salt restriction, reduction of excess weight* (see Chapter 233), and the use of a *diet* rich in potassium, magnesium, and calcium (*the Dietary Approaches to Stop Hypertension [DASH] diet*). These proven measures should be the foundation of every treatment program and also serve as an excellent means of primary prevention. *Elimination of excess alcohol intake* is also important. *Behavioral therapies* demonstrate an ability modestly to reduce pressure elevations but do not appear sufficient as the sole means of therapy in most patients. All nonpharmacologic measures should continue even if drug therapy needs to be instituted because they enhance its effectiveness and allow for the use of fewer medications at lower doses.

Exercise

Of the nonpharmacologic therapies, exercise is one of the most effective and should be a cornerstone of antihypertensive management. Its use may obviate the need for pharmacologic intervention in persons with mild hypertension, as evidenced by a study of aerobic and circuit weight training three times per week for 10 weeks, which revealed blood pressure reductions comparable to those achieved with β-blocker or calcium-channel-blocker therapy obviating chronic drug treatment. Aerobic exercise provides multiple cardiovascular benefits, including weight reduction, cardiovascular conditioning, and improved lipid profile (see Chapter 18). In patients with mild uncomplicated hypertension, it should be a cornerstone. Candidates for a vigorous exercise program should undergo cardiac stress testing first (see Chapter 18).

Salt Restriction

Salt restriction is one of the mainstays of nonpharmacologic therapy for all hypertensive patients, regardless of underlying pathophysiology, although the degree of benefit is rather modest when examined by meta-analysis of randomized trials (i.e., 3 to 5 mm Hg for SBP, 2 to 3 mm Hg for DBP). Although it is clear that individuals vary in their degree of salt sensitivity, *African Americans* and the *elderly*, who tend to have low-renin, volume-expanded hypertension, appear to respond particularly well to sodium restriction. Because we lack effective ways of identifying those most likely to respond to sodium restriction, all patients should be instructed in either a *no-added-salt diet* (4 g sodium/d) or a *low-sodium diet* (2 g/d), depending on their volume status. Not only may salt restriction alone provide adequate control in some mild cases, but it also can profoundly affect the efficacy of pharmacologic therapy. Patients receiving diuretics who had an unrestricted salt intake showed a blood pressure reduction of 4%, compared with a 15% reduction for those restricting their sodium intake.

Weight Reduction and Other Dietary Measures

Weight reduction achieves significant decreases in blood pressure, even if ideal weight is not reached. This effect is independent of salt intake. All patients who are more than 15% above their ideal body weight should be urged to lose weight. In the Trial of Antihypertensive Interventions and Management study, patients receiving placebo who lost 4.5 kg or more of weight had the same reduction in pressure as those who maintained their usual diet and were treated with chlorthalidone or atenolol. The relation between obesity and blood pressure is particularly strong among young to middle-aged adults. Weight loss is especially important in patients with central adiposity (hip-to-waist ratio >0.85 in women and >0.95 in men). Such patients have a higher incidence of hypertension, diabetes, and hyperlipidemia and a higher risk of cardiovascular disease. Weight loss in this group therefore reduces multiple risk factors simultaneously.

DASH Diet and Other Dietary Measures. A dietary program rich in fruits, vegetables, and low-fat dairy products and limited in sodium (3 g/d), alcohol, and saturated fat makes an independent contribution to the treatment and prevention of hypertension even without achieving weight loss. Such a diet (sometimes referred to as the *DASH diet* for the study for which it was designed) is also rich in calcium, magnesium, and potassium. It demonstrates reductions of 11.4 mm Hg in SBP and 5.5 mm Hg in DBP. In mildly hypertensive participants, the DASH diet appears to be more effective than prescribing potassium, calcium, or magnesium supplements and demonstrates benefit across a broad spectrum of patient groups. Benefit is enhanced when the DASH diet is paired with additional salt restriction and other nonpharmacologic measures.

Observational studies find a modest reduction in blood pressure with the substitution of plant protein, specifically *soy*, for animal protein. *Coffee* consumption per se is not associated with an increased risk of hypertension, but the consumption of *caffeinated cola drinks* is, suggesting a possible benefit from limiting their intake.

Reduction in Excess Alcohol Consumption

Excessive alcohol intake is a frequent cause of "refractory" hypertension. Epidemiologic data also indicate a relationship between excess alcohol consumption and the risk of hypertension; daily intake in men of 2 oz of 100 proof whiskey, 10 oz of wine, or 24 oz of beer or more significantly increases the risk of becoming hypertensive; amounts are smaller for women.

Moderate alcohol consumption need not be curtailed. Alcohol intake of less than 1 oz/d equivalent may result in a modest decrease in blood pressure. Consumption of 2 oz or less per day has been linked to a decreased risk of myocardial infarction but not of cardiovascular death.

Behavioral Therapies

Behavioral therapies such as *relaxation techniques* and biofeedback programs have been recommended for lowering blood pressure. Small-scale studies suggested a modest benefit, especially in patients with mild pressure elevations, but a rigorous meta-analysis of available studies found little specific benefit. Although behavioral techniques were superior to no therapy, they provided no more benefit than self-monitoring or sham techniques.

Comprehensive Lifestyle Modification

Comprehensive lifestyle modification can reduce blood pressure and cardiovascular risk. A randomized trial of multiple lifestyle interventions (PREMIER) that included the DASH diet, weight loss, exercise, and restriction of sodium and alcohol produced significant reductions in blood pressure, both in persons with mild hypertension and those with prehypertension. The magnitude of reductions approached that associated with single-drug pharmacologic therapy. The study underscored that, with comprehensive lifestyle modification, the development and progression of hypertension could be countered by nonpharmacologic means.

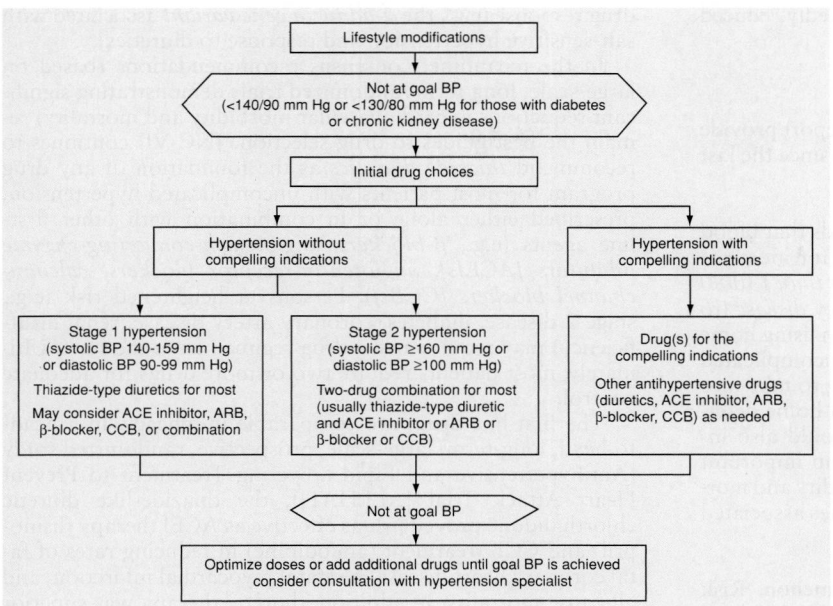

FIGURE 26.1. Algorithm for the treatment of hypertension. ACE, angiotensin-converting enzyme; ARB, angiotensin-receptor blocker; BP, blood pressure; CCB, calcium-channel blocker. (From Chobanian AV, Bakris GL, Cushman WC, et al. The seventh report of the Joint National Committee on Prevention, Detection, Evaluation and Treatment of High Blood Pressure: the JNC VII report. JAMA 2003;289:2560, with permission.)

Pharmacologic Therapy: Basic Issues
(1,20–27)

When to Initiate Drug Therapy

Pharmacologic measures require consideration when comprehensive lifestyle measures prove inadequate or when overall cardiovascular risk is high (Fig. 26.1 and Table 26.2). Persons with stage 2 hypertension, target-organ damage, diabetes, or multiple cardiovascular risk factors (especially diabetes) should begin pharmacologic therapy at the outset. For others, pharmacologic treatment can usually be deferred for weeks to months while the lifestyle modifications previously enumerated are instituted. If blood pressure does not normalize within 6 months, pharmacologic therapy should be initiated. Patients at the lowest level of risk (e.g., age <50 years, stage 1 disease, no diabetes, and no other cardiovascular risk factors or signs of target-organ involvement) can probably delay pharmacologic therapy for 6 to 12 months while nonpharmacologic measures are tried (Fig. 26.1 and Table 26.1). On the other hand, pharmacologic therapy in *elderly patients* with *isolated systolic hypertension* should not be ignored, because patients older than 50 years of age have, as noted, a significantly increased risk of

TABLE 26.2

LIFESTYLE MODIFICATIONS FOR MANAGING HYPERTENSION

Modification	Recommendation	Approximate Blood Pressure Reduction, Range (mm Hg)
Weight reduction	Maintain normal body weight (BMI, 18.5–24.9)	5–20 per 10-kg weight loss
Adopt DASH eating plan	Consume a diet rich in fruits, vegetables, and low-fat dairy products with a reduced content of saturated and total fat	8–14
Dietary sodium reduction	Reduce dietary sodium intake to ≤100 mEq/L (2.4 g sodium or 6 g sodium chloride)	2–8
Physical activity	Engage in regular aerobic physical activity such as brisk walking (at least 30 min/d most days of the week)	4–9
Moderation of alcohol consumption	Limit consumption to ≤2 drinks per day (1 oz or 30 mL of ethanol, e.g., 24 oz of beer, 10 oz of wine, or 3 oz of 80 proof whiskey) in most men and ≤1 drink per day in women and lighter-weight persons	2–4

BMI, body mass index calculated as weight in kilograms divided by the square of height in meters; DASH, Dietary Approaches to Stop Hypertension.
For overall cardiovascular risk reduction, the patient should stop smoking. The effects of implementing these modification are dose and time dependent and could be higher for some individuals.
Adapted from Chobanian AV, Bakris GL, Cushman WC, et al. The seventh report of the Joint National Committee on Prevention, Detection, Evaluation and Treatment of High Blood Pressure: the JNC VII report. JAMA 2003;289:2560, with permission.

cardiovascular complications, which can be markedly reduced with drug treatment.

Goals, Intensity, and Duration of Treatment

Consensus guidelines from the more recent JNC report provide helpful parameters, as do data that have emerged since the last report.

Treatment Goals. The JNC VII report recommends that blood pressure be lowered to *less than 140/90 mm Hg* for most patients with uncomplicated hypertension and to *less than 130/80 mm Hg* in persons with *diabetes* or *chronic kidney disease* (to slow progression to end-stage renal disease). When using home monitoring devices, the blood pressure goal for uncomplicated patients should be set at less than 135/85 mm Hg to take into account the lower readings typically recorded on home determinations (see Chapter 19). Treatment goals should also include *reduction in left ventricular hypertrophy*, an important and treatable contributor to cardiovascular morbidity and mortality; reduction in LV mass is accretive to outcomes associated with blood pressure reduction.

Intensity and Significance of the "J-Curve" Phenomenon. Risk reduction appears to parallel the degree of reduction in blood pressure along a continuum of levels. However, the significance of the so-called "J-curve" phenomenon—an apparent increase in cardiovascular morbidity and mortality associated with marked decrease in blood pressure—has been a source of debate. Of particular concern is a marked reduction in diastolic blood pressure, because most coronary perfusion takes place during diastole. In large-scale observational study of blood pressure treatment in hypertensive patients with coronary artery disease (an expectedly vulnerable population), the risk of all-cause death and myocardial infarction began to increase as diastolic pressure decreased, especially at less than 70 mm Hg; however, there was no increase in the risk of stroke. This finding and data from meta-analysis study suggest that particular attention be paid to diastolic pressure during the treatment of hypertensive patients with known coronary disease and that care be taken not to lower diastolic pressure too aggressively.

Duration. Because there is no cure for essential hypertension, drug treatment is often *lifelong*. Nonetheless, some patients with very mild hypertension may be able to stop medication, provided they continue nonpharmacologic measures and successfully control other risk factors. Even patients with substantial hypertension who require multidrug regimens may be candidates for a reduction in drug therapy. Patients with stage 1 disease whose blood pressure is well controlled with pressures in the 120/80 mm Hg range for some months may be gradually weaned off medication with the caveats that they need to continue nonpharmacologic measures and should be monitored periodically because pressures can slowly rise months after stopping therapy.

Selection of Initial Agent(s)

Pharmacologic therapy for essential hypertension remains largely empiric, guided in part by results of major prospective trials and a few generalizations about underlying mechanisms (e.g., sodium retention is common in the elderly and African Americans). Rapid advances in pharmacogenetics hold promise for a much more targeted and individualized approach to prescribing by improving the detection of underlying mechanisms and genetic polymorphisms that determine disease course and drug response (e.g., the *α-adducin gene variant* associated with salt-sensitive hypertension and response to diuretics).

In the meantime, consensus recommendations (based on large-scale, long-term randomized trials demonstrating significant reductions in cardiovascular morbidity and mortality) remain the best guides to drug selection. JNC VII continues to recommend *thiazide diuretics* as the foundation of any drug program for most patients with uncomplicated hypertension, prescribed either alone or in combination with other first-line agents (e.g., *β-blockers, angiotensin-converting-enzyme inhibitors [ACEIs], angiotensin-receptor blockers, calcium-channel blockers [CCBs]*). Persons at heightened risk (e.g., stage 2 disease, diabetes, coronary artery disease, renal insufficiency) may require a two-drug regimen from the start. Ultimately, most patients require two or more drugs for adequate control.

The first-line drugs are comparable in efficacy. In a head-to-head, long-term, large-scale, prospective, randomized study (Antihypertensive and Lipid-Lowering Treatment to Prevent Heart Attack Trial [ALLHAT]), the thiazide-like diuretic chlorthalidone proved just as effective as ACEI therapy (lisinopril) and CCB treatment (amlodipine) in reducing rates of fatal coronary heart disease, nonfatal myocardial infarction, and all-cause mortality. In addition, diuretic therapy was superior to amlodipine in lowering the risk of heart failure and better than lisinopril at reducing the risks of heart failure, stroke, and combined forms of cardiovascular disease. Results were consistent across racial groups, with no significant differences in outcomes for blacks compared to nonblacks as regards benefits from thiazide-like diuretics compared to other first-line agents. ALLHAT also uncovered an unappreciated increase in risk of heart failure in older men taking the previously recommended first-line *α-blocker agent* doxazosin.

Regardless of the medical regimen selected, all nonpharmacologic measures should be continued because they enhance the effectiveness of drug therapy and allow for the use of fewer medications at lower doses.

Selection of Subsequent Agents

As long as there is a partial response to initial therapy, the dose of the first agent should be increased as necessary and as tolerated to achieve the desired blood pressure. If there is an initial response but target blood pressure has not been achieved, the dose may be further increased or a low dose of an agent from *another first-line class* can be *added*. However, if there is *no response* to the initial dose, then *switching* to a drug from *another first-line class* is recommended rather than adding a second agent. Although monotherapy suffices in some cases, most patients will require two or more medications to reach the goal. If thiazide is not the first drug, it should almost always be the second agent used because it enhances the effectiveness of all other antihypertensive agents.

Cost Containment

Primary care physicians must consider affordability in the design of the antihypertensive regimen. Without attention to cost, the financial burden of a lifelong pharmacologic program can easily become so great that patients fill only part of a prescription or cut frequency or dose, compromising compliance and threatening blood pressure control. Fortunately, most thiazides, β-blockers, and ACEIs are now available generically at much reduced cost, as are many CCBs; only the angiotensin-receptor blockers remain largely nongeneric, but that will change soon (Table 26.3).

TABLE 26.3

ANTIHYPERTENSIVE DRUGS

Class	Drug	Initial/Maximum Dose (mg/d)	Frequency	Relative Cost
Diuretics	Thiazide type			
	Hydrochlorothiazide (generic)	12.5/50	qd/bid	1
	Esidrix			4
	Microzide			12
	Chlorothiazide (generic)	125/500	qd/bid	1.5
	Diuril			4
	Chlorthalidone (generic)	12.5/50	qd	1
	Hygroton			22
	Indapamide (generic)	1.25/5	qd	11
	Lozol			26
	Metolazone (generic)	1.25/5	qd	17
	Mykrox	0.5/1		22
	Potassium sparing			
	Triamterene (Dyrenium)	50–150	qd/bid	11
	Spironolactone	12.5–100	qd/bid	10
	Aldactazide			13
	Amiloride	5–10	qd/bid	11
	Midamor			15
	Combination			
	Hydrochlorothiazide 25 mg/triamterene 37.5 mg		qd/bid	7
	Dyazide			14
	Maxide			15
	Hydrochlorothiazide 50 mg/amiloride 5 mg		qd	2
	Moduretic			18
	Hydrochlorothiazide 25 mg/spironolactone 25 mg		qd/bid	10
	Aldactazide			14
	Loop			
	Furosemide	20/320	qd/tid	1
	Lasix			5
	Ethacrynic acid (Edecrin)	25/100	qd/tid	10
	Bumetanide	0.5/5	qd/tid	4
	Torsemide (Demadex)	5–20	qd/bid	15
β-Blockers	Atenolol	25–100	qd/bid	
	Tenormin			31
	Betaxolol (Kerlone)	5–40	qd	26
	Bisoprolol (Zebeta)	5–20	qd	32
	Metoprolol	50–200	qd/bid	2
	Lopressor			19
	Toprol XL	50–400	qd	16
	Nadolol	20–240	qd	14
	Corgard			36
	Propranolol	40–240	bid	1
	Inderal			32
	Inderal LA			28
	Timolol	10–40	bid	31
	Blocadren			28
β-Blockers with Intrinsic Sympathetic Activity	Acebutolol	200–1	qd/bid	24
	Sectral	200	qd	35
	Carteolol	2.5–10	qd	31
	Penbutolol (Levatol)	20	bid	37
	Pindolol	10–60	8	
	Visken	59		
α/β-Blockers	Carvedilol (Coreg)	12.5–50	bid	92
	Labetalol (generic)	200–1,200	bid	28
	Normodyne			33
	Trandate			33

continued

TABLE 26.3

ANTIHYPERTENSIVE DRUGS (*Continued*)

Class	Drug	Initial/Maximum Dose (mg/d)	Frequency	Relative Cost
Angiotensin-Converting-Enzyme Inhibitors (ACEIs)	Benazepril (Lotensin)	10–40	qd/bid	23
	Captopril (generic)	12.5–150	bid/tid	1
	Capoten			26
	Enalapril (Vasotec)	2.5–40	qd/bid	24
	Fosinopril (Monopril)	10–40	qd/bid	26
	Lisinopril (Prinivil)	5–40	qd	26
	(Zestril)			26
	Moexipril (Univasc)	7.5–30	qd/bid	17
	Quinapril (Accupril)	5–80	qd/bid	28
	Ramipril (Altace)	1.25–20	qd/bid	22
	Trandolapril (Mavik)	1–4	qd	20
Angiotensin-Receptor Antagonists	Candesartan cilexetil (Atacand)	8–32	qd	36
	Irbesartan (Avapro)	150–300	qd	36
	Losartan (Cozaar)	25–100	qd/bid	37
	Telmisartan (Micardis)	40–80	qd	38
	Valsartan (Diovan)	80–320	qd	36
	Side effects: same as ACEIs but do not cause cough			
Calcium-Channel Blockers	Dihydropyridines			
	Amlodipine (Norvasc)	2.5–10	qd	40
	Felodipine (Plendil)	2.5–10	qd	29
	Extended release			
	Isradipine (DynaCirc CR)	5–10	qd	37
	Nicardipine (Cardene SR)	60–120	bid	40
	Nifedipine (Adalat CL)	30–90	qd	31
	(Procardia XL)			42
	Nisoldipine (Sular)	10–60	qd	27
	Nondihydropyridines	120–360	bid	48
	Diltiazem (extended release)			
	Cardizem SR			54
	Cardizem CD	120–360	qd	35
	Dilacor XR	120–480	qd	35
	Diltia XT	120–480	qd	27
	Tiamate	120–480	qd	52
	Tiazac	120–480	qd	28
	Verapamil (extended release)	120–480	qd/bid	35
	Calan SR			32
	Isoptin SR			32
	Verelan			37
	Covera HS	180–480	qd	35
α-Blockers[a]	Prazosin (generic)	1–20	bid/tid	2
	(Minipress)			14
	Terazosin (Hytrin)	1–20	qd	51
	Doxazosin (Cardura)	1–16	qd	30
Sympatholytics (Central)	Clonidine	0.1–0.6	bid/tid	1
	Catapres			20
	Catapres TTS (transdermal)	1 patch weekly, 0.1–0.3		
	Guanabenz	4–64	bid	12
	Wytensin			24
	Guafacine (Isurelim)	1–3	qd	19
	Tenex			32
	Methyldopa	250–2,000	bid	4
	Aldomet			18
Sympatholytics (Peripheral)	Guanethidine (Ismelin)	10–50	qd	18
	Guanadrel (Hylorel)	10–75	bid	22
	Reserpine	0.05–01	qd	1

continued

TABLE 26.3

ANTIHYPERTENSIVE DRUGS (*Continued*)

Class	Drug	Initial/Maximum Dose (mg/d)	Frequency	Relative Cost
Vasodilator (Direct)	Hydralazine	40–200	qd/bid	3
	Apresoline			30
	Minoxidil	2.5–40	qd/bid	3
	Loniten			17
Combination	Benazepril 5, 10, 20 mg/HCTZ 6.25, 12.5, or 25 mg		qd	24
Preparations	Lotensin HCT			
(Selected)	Captopril 25 or 50 mg/HCTZ 15 or 25 mg		qd	22
ACEIs/Diuretics	Capozide			28
	Enalapril 5 or 10 mg/HCTZ 12.5 or 25 mg			33
	Vaseretic			
	Lisinopril 10 or 20 mg/HCTZ 12.5 or 25 mg			
	Prinzide			31
	Zestoretic			29
	Moexipril 7.5 or 15 mg/HCTZ 12.5 or 25 mg			
	Uniretic			17
Angiotensin	Losartan 50 or 100 mg/HCTZ 12.5 or 25 mg			
II–Receptor	Hyzaar			37
Antagonists and	Valsartan 80–160 mg/HCTZ 12.5 mg			
Diuretics	Diovan HCT			36

bid, twice daily; HCTZ, hydrochlorothiazide; qd, daily; tid, thrice daily.
[a]First dose at bedtime.

The reaffirmation of the effectiveness of thiazides in randomized, prospective, head-to-head study should help to control the cost of treatment. Their very low cost, ease of use, and excellent efficacy across a wide range of patients make them an essential consideration for every hypertensive treatment program. Additional approaches to minimizing cost include substituting a *sustained-release preparation* if it is less expensive than a multidose regimen, staying with a less expensive, older antihypertensive agent if it is reasonably effective and well tolerated, and using the lowest dose possible.

Pharmacologic Therapy: First-Line Agents (1,6,28–43)

Thiazide Diuretics

These agents are experiencing a renaissance of use as the first choice for pharmacologic therapy, based on findings from the landmark ALLHAT study (see prior discussion), which documented long-term outcomes equal to or better than those achieved with ACEIs, CCBs, or α-blockers (there were no direct comparisons with β-blockers). The thiazide-like agent chlorthalidone produced comparable reductions in blood pressure and LVH and similar or superior reductions in risks of cardiovascular morbidity and mortality. Such proven efficacy, combined with safety and extremely low cost, make thiazides a compelling first choice for the pharmacologic management of hypertension (Table 26.3).

Mechanism of Action. Thiazides enhance sodium excretion, resulting in a reduced intravascular volume and reduced peripheral resistance (presumably by lowering intracellular sodium in vascular smooth muscle cells). Potassium excretion is increased, and uric acid and calcium excretions are decreased.

Adverse Effects. *Potassium wasting* is a consequence of the drug's effect on the distal renal tubule and is exacerbated by high salt intake. Clinically significant *hypercalcemia* is exceedingly rare, although a decrease in calcium excretion does occur and can be beneficial in patients with osteoporosis or calcium-containing renal stones (see Chapter 135). *Hyperglycemia* is usually mild and infrequent at low doses used in hypertension. Mild *hyperuricemia* may occur but usually not to the degree that necessitates the discontinuation of therapy. A transient increase in *low-density-lipoprotein (LDL) cholesterol* has been noted. Thiazides may cause *rash*, especially a photosensitizing type, and rarely may precipitate pancreatitis. Allergy to sulfonamide antibiotics is not associated with allergy to thiazides because there is no cross-reactivity between the two classes of drugs. Most adverse metabolic effects can be minimized or eliminated by restricting the dose to the equivalent of 25 mg/d or less of hydrochlorothiazide. Higher doses generally offer little increase in efficacy while increasing the likelihood of metabolic effects.

Monitoring. Checking the serum *potassium* regularly and correcting even mild hypokalemia are essential in a person with underlying cardiac disease, particularly one bothered by dysrhythmias or taking digoxin (see Chapters 29 and 32). Hypokalemia can be prevented by concomitant salt restriction, increased dietary potassium, and, when necessary, the addition of potassium-sparing agents or supplements (see Chapter 32). Potassium levels should be maintained in the normal range.

Severe degrees of hypokalemia may cause muscle weakness. The serum *glucose* requires close monitoring when thiazides are used in a diabetic, and the *uric acid* should be watched if the patient has clinical gout. There is no need to monitor LDL cholesterol or serum calcium.

β-Blockers

These agents are highly effective in reducing cardiovascular morbidity and mortality, generally well tolerated, and relatively low in cost. They provide secondary prevention following myocardial infarction and help to reverse left ventricular remodeling but appear to be less effective in controlling blood pressure in the elderly, who should not start with a β-blocker unless there is concurrent coronary artery disease.

Mechanism of Action. Their precise mode of blood pressure reduction remains unclear, but β-blockers reduce cardiac output, renin and catecholamine release, central sympathetic activity, and peripheral resistance.

Adverse Effects. Side effects attributable to β-blockade include bradycardia, fatigue, decreased exercise tolerance, and increased airway resistance. Thus, these agents should be avoided in persons with conduction-system disease and active bronchospastic conditions, but carefully selected persons with coronary disease (see Chapter 30) and heart failure (see Chapter 32) may actually benefit from their use. β-Blockers can modestly increase insulin resistance and slightly reduce HDL cholesterol, side effects that do not seem to cancel their beneficial effects on hypertension and overall cardiovascular risk.

Anecdotal and observational data have attributed neuropsychiatric side effects (*depression*, *sexual dysfunction*, *cognitive impairment*) to β-blocker use. However, prospective, randomized trials have failed to confirm these observations or the theory that the degree of lipid solubility and central nervous system penetration might correlate with the risk of neuropsychiatric side effects. In fact, failure to control blood pressure is a risk factor for dementia in older persons. Some persons report *nightmares* with β-blocker use.

Preparations. All appear to be equally effective for the treatment of hypertension, although differences in their cardioselectivity and intrinsic sympathomimetic activity can be used to advantage. *Cardioselectivity* (greater effect on β_1-adrenergic receptors of the heart than on β_2-receptors of blood vessels and bronchi) is preferred in hypertensive patients with a history of bronchospastic disease (i.e., asthma, chronic obstructive pulmonary disease). Low-dose cardioselective β-blocker therapy is not contraindicated in such persons (see Chapter 48), but cardioselectivity is a relative quality that declines as dose increases. During exacerbations of bronchospastic disease, even cardioselective β-blockers may not be tolerated. *Atenolol* and *metoprolol* are examples of the commonly used cardioselective β-blockers. *Nebivolol*, a new β-blocker touted as being more β_1-selective and therefore more vasodilating and better tolerated than other β-blockers, is expensive and yet to be proven more advantageous over generically available drugs in this class or in other classes.

Some β-blockers have *intrinsic sympathomimetic activity* (e.g., *pindolol, acebutolol, carvedilol*), which cause less bradycardia and less disruption of lipid and carbohydrate metabolism. They help to maintain cardiac output with exercise, allowing cardiac conditioning. They are comparable with other β-blockers in ability to lower blood pressure. The β-blocker *labetalol* is unique in that it has both α- and β-blocking

actions, with about one fourth of the potency of propranolol and one sixth of the potency of phentolamine. Its rapid onset of action has made it useful for use in hypertensive emergencies—especially when given parenterally—but its chronic oral use has been limited by tendencies to cause orthostatic hypotension, sexual dysfunction, and hepatocellular injury.

Angiotensin-Converting-Enzyme Inhibitors

ACEIs are the class of choice in patients with type 1 or type 2 diabetes because of their demonstrated protective effect on the kidney. In addition, they have been shown to reduce cardiovascular mortality in patients with heart failure and in those with myocardial infarction complicated by systolic dysfunction, as well as in high-risk patients without systolic dysfunction. They reverse left ventricular remodeling and hypertrophy due to hypertension.

Mechanism of Action. These drugs block the conversion of renin-activated angiotensin I to angiotensin II (ATII), a potent vasoconstrictor that also stimulates the production of aldosterone. In addition, they inhibit the breakdown of bradykinin, itself a vasodilator, which also stimulates the production of vasodilatory prostaglandins. At least some of the effects of these drugs are related to their effect on local angiotensin systems in key organs (e.g., heart and kidney). The blockade of ATII results in suppression not only of its vasoconstricting effects and its effect on aldosterone release, but also its adverse effects on myocardium and the vasculature, which facilitate vascular inflammation and impaired vasodilation.

Adverse Effects. The most troublesome side effect is an annoying *dry cough* that occurs in about 10% to 20% of patients. It is mostly nocturnal, described as an irritation in the throat, and believed to be linked to the effect of the drug on bradykinin metabolism, causing kinin levels to build up in persons who metabolize slowly. Angioedema has also been linked to the kinin-buildup mechanism. About half of patients who experience the cough find it severe enough to warrant discontinuation of the medication. Switching to another ACEI rarely solves the problem. Uncommon side effects include *rash*, *taste disturbances*, and *agranulocytosis*, an extremely rare complication prevalent only at very high doses.

Because the ACEIs block the production of aldosterone, they can lead to *hyperkalemia* when used in conjunction with a potassium-sparing diuretic, potassium supplementation, or nonsteroidal antiinflammatory drugs. Potentially fatal hyperkalemia has been reported in diabetic patients with hyporeninemic/hypoaldosteronemic hypertension. Close monitoring of the serum potassium is indicated in such situations.

ACEIs preserve renal function in hypertensive diabetics and in any hypertensive patient with renal insufficiency by lowering intraglomerular pressure and hence slowing the progression to end-stage renal disease. Because of this beneficial effect, *creatinine may rise* following the institution of ACEIs in this setting. This is not due to a toxic effect on the kidney. Up to a 35% rise in creatinine is acceptable. If creatinine rises higher than this, the ACEI should be stopped and consideration given to the possible presence of bilateral renal artery stenosis. The originally reported *glomerular injury* is very rare, except at the extremely high doses used in early clinical trials. However, patients with *renal failure* are still at risk for glomerular injury when large doses are used, necessitating careful monitoring of renal function.

The blockade of the local renin–angiotensin system in the placenta is believed to be responsible for the adverse effects these drugs have on the developing fetus, presumably by impairing *placental blood flow*. They are absolutely contraindicated in pregnancy.

Preparations. There are many ACEIs on the market, differing predominantly in cost and duration of action. Generic formulations are widely available and the least expensive (Table 26.3).

Angiotensin II–Receptor Blockers (ARBs)

This class of drugs blocks the angiotensin II receptor, thus inhibiting the vasoconstrictive effects of angiotensin II and the associated stimulation of aldosterone production. These agents have no effect on bradykinin metabolism, which probably accounts for the absence of the cough that may accompany ACEI therapy. Aside from the lack of cough, their side effects resemble those of ACEIs. Emerging data from studies in diabetics and persons with heart failure suggest that ARBs are comparable to ACEIs in preserving renal function, reversing left ventricular remodeling, and lowering cardiovascular morbidity and mortality (see Chapters 32 and 102). They appear to be more effective than β-blockers in preventing cardiovascular morbidity and death in persons without cardiovascular disease. Because of their high cost due to lack of generic availability, they should be reserved for patients intolerant to ACEIs because of cough or angioedema.

Calcium-Channel Blockers

These agents are generally well tolerated and effective in lowering blood pressure, particularly in African American patients and the elderly. ALLHAT demonstrated the efficacy of the CCB amlodipine in reducing cardiovascular morbidity and mortality, but results were not as good as those achieved by the use of a diuretic, especially with regard to heart failure. In addition, this class of antihypertensives has been the subject of significant controversy since the publication of retrospective data suggesting an increased incidence of myocardial infarction and sudden death associated with their use. These data derived from studies of short-acting preparations (especially nifedipine and its congeners), with speculation that their rapid onset and offset of action may have resulted in wide swings in blood pressure, increasing sympathetic tone and ultimately myocardial oxygen demand. The short-acting versions of these drugs are not recommended. There has been no indication of increased coronary morbidity in studies of long-acting CCB preparations. These drugs appear to be useful in improving glomerular filtration rate in patients with renal insufficiency; however, it remains unclear whether these agents prolong the time to dialysis. Brand-name formulations are very expensive.

Mechanism of Action. CCBs impede the entry of calcium in heart and vascular smooth muscle cells, resulting in a decreased cellular calcium concentration, which reduces vascular smooth muscle contraction and lowers peripheral resistance. These agents also have a mild natriuretic effect, making them potentially useful in patients with sodium retention (e.g., the elderly and African Americans). None adversely affects lipids or insulin sensitivity, and all reduce LVH.

Adverse Effects of Individual CCBs. There is considerable variation in action and side effects among the CCBs.

Amlodipine. Amlodipine is among the most widely prescribed of the CCBs, replacing many of the earlier agents in this class because it produces *less reflex tachycardia* and *less negative* *inotropy*. *Peripheral edema* occurs (and can be substantial in persons with preexisting venous insufficiency) but usually to a lesser degree than with vasodilating CCBs. Amlodipine is comparable to thiazide diuretic therapy in achieving most major endpoints, except for being associated with a slightly higher rate of *heart failure* in high-risk hypertensive patients.

Nifedipine. Nifedipine and its *dihydropyridine* congeners (e.g., *nicardipine, isradipine, felodipine, amlodipine*) are potent vasodilators that manifest negative inotropic effects *in vitro* but clinically cause little net reduction in cardiac output. Their main drawbacks are *reflex tachycardia* and *peripheral edema* secondary to vasodilation. As noted earlier, retrospective study suggests an increased risk of *myocardial infarction* and *cardiac sudden death* associated with use of the short-acting dihydropyridine formulations, which are known to trigger reflex sympathetic activation. Occasionally, *headache* and *flushing* may be troublesome. In a small number of patients, *esophageal reflux* can become a problem secondary to relaxation of the lower esophageal sphincter.

Verapamil. Verapamil is available generically at low cost. Its main disadvantages are *negative inotropy* and *conduction-system disturbances*, leading to *arterioventricular* (AV) *nodal block* and *bradycardia*; the drug should not be used in patients with heart failure or suspected conduction-system disease. On the other hand, it is very useful for rate control in patients with hypertension in the setting of atrial fibrillation with a rapid ventricular response rate. Leg edema is usually not a problem unless heart failure worsens, but *constipation, headache,* and *dizziness* can be problematic.

Diltiazem. Diltiazem falls between nifedipine and verapamil, having mildly negative net effects on inotropy and conduction, but it is less likely than nifedipine to cause leg edema. Efficacy is enhanced by the addition of a small dose of thiazide diuretic. The drug can cause some AV nodal block and should not be used in the setting of bradycardia.

α-Blockers

These drugs act peripherally at vascular postsynaptic α-adrenergic receptors, causing arteriolar and venous dilation. Because they affect both the arterial and venous systems, they cause less reflex tachycardia than pure arterial vasodilators (see later discussion). They help to reverse left ventricular remodeling. Their use as a first-line drug in older hypertensive men with concurrent prostatism has been popular because they provide symptomatic relief of obstructive urinary symptoms (see Chapter 138), but the finding of a significant increase in risk of *heart failure* associated with α-blocker (*doxazosin*) use among such men in the ALLHAT study has removed this class from the list of first-line drugs. Risk is attenuated but not eliminated with concurrent use of an additional first-line agent to ensure the achievement of target blood pressure.

The principal side effect of α-blocker therapy is *postural hypotension*, most prominent with use of older α-blockers (e.g., *prazosin, terazosin*) in elderly patients and those taking diuretics. Such patients could experience profound postural hypotension leading to syncope 1 to 3 hours after the initial dose, necessitating starting with a low dose at bedtime and having the patient stay supine for at least 3 hours. The newer, longer-acting preparations (e.g., *doxazosin*) are less likely to cause first-dose syncope; however, even with doxazosin, postural lightheadedness is still a problem, affecting about one fifth of patients and becoming more likely as dose exceeds 1 mg/d.

α-Blockers have no adverse effects on lipids; in fact, they slightly raise HDL cholesterol and modestly reduce LDL cholesterol (both on the order of 3% to 5%). Recommendations on how these agents should be used in combination with other first-line agents await further study.

Combination Therapy

Almost all of the classes of first-line drugs mentioned earlier may be used in combination to enhance blood pressure control. Especially effective is adding a thiazide diuretic to a non-thiazide monotherapy program; even small doses (e.g., 12.5 to 25 mg/d of hydrochlorothiazide) can be very helpful. Adding an ARB to ACEI monotherapy can enhance reduction in blood pressure, but adding a thiazide provides a similar benefit and at much lower cost. Caution should be used when combining verapamil and a β-blocker in a person with underlying heart disease because of their additive suppressive effects on left ventricular function (see Chapter 32).

Pharmacologic Therapy: Second-Line Agents (1)

The second-line agents are worth considering when the list of first-line agents has been exhausted; however, most have features that make them less desirable, and in most instances, control can be achieved with combination use of first-line drugs. Consequently, they should not take precedence over a first-line drug. Second-line agents are generally reserved for patients who are refractory to combinations of first-line agents or who have special underlying conditions such as renal failure. They include the loop diuretics, distal tubular diuretics, centrally acting sympatholytics, and the older peripheral vasodilators (Table 26.3).

Loop and Potassium-Sparing Diuretics

Loop diuretics (*furosemide, ethacrynic acid, bumetanide*) are reserved for patients with evidence of renal insufficiency (creatinine clearance <30% of normal) or with allergy to thiazides. They are typically used in conjunction with *minoxidil* (see later discussion).

Distal tubular diuretics (e.g., *spironolactone, triamterene, amiloride*) are weak antihypertensive agents used predominantly in combination with thiazides to spare potassium loss. The combination preparations are widely promoted, but it is best to avoid starting with such a fixed combination until the necessary thiazide dose has been established. Hypertensive patients who must avoid hypokalemia (e.g., those taking digitalis, experiencing ventricular irritability, or suffering from organic heart disease) are the best candidates. Other indications are mineralocorticoid hypertension, thiazide hypersensitivity, and severe gout. These drugs must be used with extreme *caution* in patients with *renal insufficiency, ACEI use,* or insulin-dependent *diabetes* with renin deficiency, in which cases the risk of serious *hyperkalemia* is substantial. The tendency of spironolactone to cause *gynecomastia* limits its use in hypertension to patients with primary hyperaldosteronism. A new, selective aldosterone antagonist, *eplerenone,* has been approved for congestive heart failure; approval for use in hypertension is pending, It shows promise when combined with a thiazide in salt-sensitive hypertensive patients.

Centrally Acting Sympatholytics

Methyldopa, clonidine, and *guanabenz* are centrally acting sympatholytics that reduce blood pressure by stimulating central α-adrenergic receptors, which in turn reduce sympathetic outflow to the heart and vasculature. Because they cause secondary *sodium retention* and generally require the use of a diuretic, they should be considered as second-line agents. Although all of these agents frequently cause drowsiness, fatigue, and impotence, lower doses are often quite well tolerated, even in the elderly. Methyldopa occasionally causes fever, acute or chronic hepatitis, and a Coombs-positive hemolytic anemia. Clonidine (and sometimes methyldopa) is more likely to cause sedation, dry mouth, and *rebound hypertension* with abrupt cessation of therapy. A slow-release transdermal clonidine patch is available and convenient but very expensive and commonly irritating to the skin. Low-dose clonidine (0.1 mg) given as a once-daily dose before bed is well tolerated in the elderly. Guanabenz and guanfacine are similar to clonidine in action and side effects.

Reserpine is one of the oldest antihypertensive agents, acting as a postganglionic adrenergic antagonist. Its advantages are low cost, good efficacy, and once-daily dose. Significant side effects include *severe depression,* nightmares, drowsiness, nasal congestion, gastrointestinal disturbances, and bradycardia.

Older Arterial Vasodilators

These drugs are rarely used because of the availability of better tolerated and more effective agents. The older arterial vasodilators (e.g., *hydralazine, minoxidil*) act directly to relax arterial smooth muscle. Disadvantages include reflex tachycardia, sodium and water retention, and short duration of action, necessitating frequent dosing. *Hydralazine* is typically used as a third-line agent in combination with a β-blocker and a diuretic agent. It can cause headache, dizziness, and a lupus-like syndrome, especially in doses exceeding 200 mg/d. Reflex tachycardia may exacerbate angina. *Minoxidil* is an extremely potent vasodilator and should be used only in patients with moderately severe hypertension uncontrolled by other medications (see later discussion). Both a β-blocker and a loop diuretic must be used with it. Salt and water retention may be marked, requiring high doses of furosemide. Hypertrichosis is common and has led to the drug's topical use for hair loss. Rare adverse effects include pericardial effusion and even cardiac tamponade.

New Agents: Direct Renin Inhibitors

Aliskiren (Tekturna) is the first approved *direct renin inhibitor.* It reduces plasma renin activity, inhibiting the production of angiotensin I and II. When used alone, it can achieve reductions in blood pressure of 8 to 15 mm Hg systolic and 8 to 11 mm Hg diastolic, or about the same as ARBs. It is generally well tolerated in clinical trials, although experience is limited. Because many hypertensive patients do not experience elevations in serum renin, it remains unclear who is best served by this medication and how to best select patients who might benefit. Side effects include cough and diarrhea, which occur in less than 3% of patients. When used alone it does not cause *hyperkalemia,* but when it is combined with an ACEI, hyperkalemia rates increase to 5%. It has modest additive effects when combined with hydrochlorothiazide (HCTZ), an ACEI, or an ARB but has not been studied in combination with other antihypertensive agents. It is expensive, costing about $70 a month. Its role in the treatment of hypertension has not been defined.

Special Situations (1,3,7,44–59)

Refractory Hypertension

Patients are considered refractory if they fail to achieve target blood pressure reductions despite full doses of a three-drug regimen.

Etiologies. The most common causes are *poor compliance, alcohol excess,* and *obesity* (Table 26.4). In addition, blood pressure becomes increasingly difficult to control in the presence of *deteriorating renal function.* Additional etiologies include *renal artery stenosis, sleep apnea,* and the other *secondary causes of hypertension* (see Chapter 19). Often the cause is a *suboptimal treatment regimen,* such as one that ignores lifestyle measures or contains little or no diuretic for the degree of salt intake and sodium retention present. Nonprescription agents are a potential source of difficulty. Over-the-counter use of sympathomimetic *decongestants, nonsteroidal antiinflammatory agents,* and *exogenous estrogens* are easily overlooked pharmacologic causes. Use of ephedra-containing products and herbal supplements with adrenergic activity (e.g., ginseng) may make important contributions.

Occasionally, the cause is *pseudorefractoriness* due to the anxiety of the office visit (so-called *"white-coat" hypertension*) or to a marked vasoconstrictor response to blood pressure determination performed with an arm cuff. In the former, the act of taking the blood pressure produces a rise predominantly in the systolic blood pressure; in the latter, the rise is predominantly in the diastolic pressure (see Chapter 19).

Assessment. Medication compliance, weight gain, salt and alcohol excess, and use of other drugs should be observed. Pill counts are the best compliance check. A history of nocturia or ankle edema is suggestive of volume overload from excessive salt intake or deterioration of cardiac or renal function. Obstructive sleep apnea in the obese patient may cause refractory hypertension and should be evaluated in the appropriate patient. History and physical examination are performed to check for signs of secondary etiologies (see Chapter 19), target-organ damage, and volume overload. If white-coat hypertension is suspected, blood pressures should be taken by the patient at home and at work, after the patient's technique is checked in the office. *Continuous ambulatory monitoring* may also be of use in this situation (see Chapter 19). However, even if a pseudorefractory etiology is suspected, it should not be grounds for truncating a workup for end-organ damage. Even white-coat hypertension is associated with an increased risk of LVH and diastolic dysfunction.

TABLE 26.4

SOME IMPORTANT CAUSES OF REFRACTORY HYPERTENSION

Improper blood pressure measurement
Poor compliance with treatment regimen
Excess alcohol consumption
Volume overload and inadequate use of diuretics
Intake of competing nonprescription substances
  (decongestants, ephedra, ginseng)
Unrecognized secondary causes (renal artery stenosis, sleep
  apnea, adrenal adenoma)

If there is no clinical evidence of a secondary cause, then a check of the serum sodium, potassium, blood urea nitrogen, creatinine, and urinalysis should suffice for evidence of renal injury. The *echocardiogram,* a sensitive measure of cardiac target-organ effects, can also help to differentiate between true refractoriness leading to target-organ damage and pseudorefractoriness.

Patients with refractory hypertension believed due to white-coat response and without evidence of target-organ changes can be watched for the development of such changes and, in the meantime, be prescribed a program of diet and exercise. Those who remain refractory with no evident cause and manifest target-organ changes require additional measures.

Empiric Therapy. If the workup rules out a definite cause, then an empirical trial of both intensive nonpharmacologic and pharmacologic measures is in order. The patient should be placed on a 2-Na/d, reduced-calorie DASH diet; restricted to 1 oz of alcohol per day, and prescribed an aerobic exercise program. In addition, a multidrug regimen is indicated to ensure that each major pathophysiologic mechanism of hypertension is addressed; for example, volume overload: diuretics, aldosterone antagonists; sympathetic overactivity: β-blockers; vascular resistance: ACEI or ARBs; smooth-muscle constriction: dihydropyridine calcium-channel blockers. Using a new agent with a different mechanism of action than previously prescribed can help to overcome compensatory responses to the initial program. If the standard diuretic, ACEI/ARB, β-blocker, CCB program fails, adding an aldosterone antagonist may be helpful, especially if the patient has heart failure (monitor closely for hyperkalemia). Other measures include giving doses of drugs twice daily. Sometimes a simple dose increase will suffice, such as advancing the diuretic dose beyond the usual range (e.g., HCTZ from 25 mg/d to 50 mg/d) or adding a loop diuretic if there is renal insufficiency. In more than half of instances, the cause turns out to be inadequate diuretic therapy. The patient is instructed to monitor pressure at home and should be followed closely.

If these measures fail, then before escalating the medication program, one should consider consultation with a hypertension specialist. The review is likely to include rechecking for any secondary causes and making recommendations for additional treatment measures, such as use of a β-blocker with concurrent α-blocking activity (e.g., labetalol, carvedilol), a centrally acting agent (e.g., clonidine, reserpine, α-blocker), or a direct vasodilator (hydralazine, minoxidil). Use of a direct vasodilator necessitates the addition of a β-blocker and a loop diuretic to offset the resultant edema and tachycardia.

Treatment of Renal Artery Hypertension

Renal artery hypertension due to atherosclerotic renal artery stenosis is an important cause of difficult-to-control hypertension in the elderly. The advent of noninvasive imaging studies has facilitated identification (see Chapter 19). Although revascularization might be necessary both for the control of blood pressure and the preservation of renal function, long-term observational studies in elderly persons with moderately severe stenosis find a surprisingly good renal prognosis with conservative therapy (medication only). Nevertheless, the overall mortality risk in this group of patients is high due to the high prevalence of underlying cardiovascular disease. A randomized trial of angioplasty compared with drug therapy finds no significant difference in outcomes. Although revascularization by angioplasty is of acceptable risk when done by experienced operators, it does not appear to offer any advantages in terms of blood pressure control or renal function over initial medical therapy. Hypertensive patients with atherosclerotic renal artery stenosis should be followed closely and treated initially with antihypertensive medication. Those who fail medical therapy due to grossly inadequate blood pressure control or worsening of renal function are reasonable candidates for consideration of revascularization, especially if hypertension is complicated by flash pulmonary edema, high-serum creatinine with bilateral disease, or very tight stenosis.

Hypertension Associated with Estrogen Use

Hypertension occurs rarely in young women on oral contraceptives since the advent of low-dose estrogen pills. There is no evidence that hormone replacement therapy causes an elevation in blood pressure, and these drugs may be used in the hypertensive patient to treat disabling menopausal symptoms.

Hypertension in Pregnancy

Hypertension that develops during pregnancy may represent either *preexisting hypertension* or *preeclampsia.*

Preexisting Hypertension. Pressure elevations that appear before 20 weeks of gestation are almost always due to preexisting disease. Some preexisting hypertension improves during pregnancy because of the hemodynamic changes that occur at this time. Such patients may terminate therapy for the duration of their pregnancy, but pressures should be followed closely, as should the urinalysis for the early development of proteinuria (a powerful predictor of adverse outcomes). Other patients require the continuation of treatment. The goal of lowering blood pressure in patients with preexisting disease is the safety of the mother. There is no fetal benefit to blood pressure reduction; antihypertensive drugs do not cure or reverse preeclampsia.

The usual threshold for initiating antihypertensive medication is a DBP exceeding 100 mm Hg. For DBPs between 90 and 100 mg Hg, *modest sodium restriction* and increased *rest* often suffice. If they do not, and blood pressure continues to rise, then beginning *methyldopa,* a *β-blocker,* or *hydralazine* is safe and effective in pregnancy. *ACEIs are contraindicated* due to the dependence of placental blood flow on the intrauterine renin–angiotensin system. Diuretics are generally avoided during pregnancy. β-Blockers, calcium-channel blockers, and α-blockers may be used, although guidelines await further study.

Preeclampsia. It appears that alterations in circulating angiogenic proteins (e.g., placental growth factor) and antiangiogenic proteins (e.g., endoglin) cause endothelial dysfunction that may contribute to the development of preeclampsia. Work is ongoing to determine whether serum levels of these substances can be used as biomarkers to predict the development of preeclampsia.

Preeclampsia is heralded by blood pressure *of greater than 140/90 mm Hg, edema,* and *proteinuria* all appearing in the *third trimester.* The typical patient is a very young primigravida, but multiple births, diabetes, and hydatidiform mole contribute to risk. Change of partner is not a risk factor, but prolongation of the interval between pregnancies is. At 17 to 20 weeks of gestation, a resting blood pressure of greater than 110/75 mm Hg (sitting) or greater than 100/65 mm Hg (left lateral decubitus position) suggests an increased risk of developing preeclampsia because normally the pressure is lower at this time of pregnancy. If DBP rises above 90 mm Hg, *bedrest* is initiated and hospitalization considered.

Most antihypertensive medications safe for use in pregnancy are appropriate for the treatment of preeclampsia. Low-dose aspirin does not prevent preeclampsia. *Nitroprusside* is given in severe cases that require hospitalization. The use of volume expansion remains controversial. *Diuretics and salt restriction are to be avoided* because these patients usually are intravascularly volume constricted. Such treatment might aggravate the condition by further stimulating the renin–angiotensin–aldosterone axis. *Magnesium sulfate* is the treatment of choice for the prevention of seizures associated with eclampsia and is superior to the CCB nimodipine for the prevention of eclampsia. Use of vitamin C and E supplements does not reduce the risk of preeclampsia.

Hypertension in the Elderly

Isolated systolic hypertension (SBP >140 mm Hg), a common finding in the elderly, significantly increases the risk of cardiovascular morbidity and mortality in persons older than the age of 65 years. In fact, SBP is among the most powerful predictors; treatment lowers the risk. The goals of therapy are to reduce SBP to less than 140 mm Hg and DBP to less than 90 mm Hg.

Nonpharmacologic Therapy. The elderly tend to have low-renin, volume-overload hypertension and exhibit considerable sensitivity to salt intake. For those with very modest pressure elevations, one can begin with *salt restriction,* a gentle exercise program, and *weight reduction* if they are overweight. Many elderly patients respond well to a 2-g/d low-sodium diet. Reduction of excess *alcohol* intake to no more than 1 oz/d is also important and occasionally overlooked. Nonpharmacologic measures can lower pressure by as much as 10 mm Hg.

Pharmacologic Therapy. When drug treatment is necessary, a *thiazide* diuretic is the drug of choice for initial therapy. It is best to start with a low dose (e.g., hydrochlorothiazide 12.5 to 25.0 mg/d) and increase the dose gradually. Increments should be small to avoid rapid lowering of pressure and postural hypotension, which can lead to lightheadedness and falls. In general, the elderly do not tolerate aggressive diuretic therapy or β-blockers as well as younger patients. A review of 10 β-blocker trials in the elderly found their use often failed to achieve adequate control or reductions in cardiovascular risk.

ACEIs are a reasonable consideration as initial therapy in elderly men. In randomized trial of initial antihypertensive therapy in elderly patients, ACEI actually proved superior to thiazides. Other drugs likely to cause marked postural hypotension (e.g., α-blockers) or daytime sedation (centrally acting sympatholytic agents, e.g., methyldopa, clonidine) are also less desirable. Cardiovascular risk reduction with the use of calcium-channel blockers has been demonstrated in elderly diabetics with systolic hypertension; results in nondiabetics are less impressive.

The African American Patient

Hypertension is more prevalent in African Americans (38.2%), more commonly of the low-renin, salt-sensitive variety, and more likely to be accompanied by target-organ damage than in whites. The high prevalence of obesity, smoking, and salt excess contribute, as does decreased access to medical care. African Americans show three times the risk of developing renal insufficiency, even when treated. They respond particularly well to *sodium restriction, weight loss,* and *smoking cessation.* Thiazide diuretics are the drug class of first choice, achieving the best cardiovascular outcomes in head-to-head comparison with ACE inhibitors and calcium-channel blockers. Most patients require combination therapy for adequate control. *Calcium-channel blockers* are effective, although their use greatly increases the cost of treatment, which, in turn, might compromise long-term compliance. *ACEIs* and *β-blockers* are somewhat less effective, perhaps because of the low-renin physiology prevalent in this population. However, they should be used in situations in which their efficacy has been established (e.g., ACEIs in diabetes, β-blockers following myocardial infarction). Higher doses may be required to achieve the desired effect.

The Diabetic Patient

Control of hypertension is particularly important in diabetics because the risks of stroke, cardiovascular disease, and renal failure are particularly high. Blood pressure should be brought to levels less than 135/85 mm Hg and less than 130/80 mm Hg in persons with microalbuminuria. *ACEIs* are the drug class of choice because they decrease proteinuria and slow the progression of diabetic nephropathy as well as lower blood pressure. *ARBs* have much the same benefits and should be used in patients who cannot tolerate ACEI therapy because of cough or angioedema. *Calcium-channel blockers* also may be protective of the kidney; they are generally well tolerated and effective in lowering blood pressure and decreasing cardiovascular risk in elderly diabetics with systolic hypertension. Although *thiazide* diuretics may slightly worsen glucose intolerance and hyperlipidemia, these adverse effects can be minimized or avoided by using small doses (e.g., 12.5 to 25 mg/d of hydrochlorothiazide). *Beta-blockers* are not contraindicated in patients taking insulin, but a relatively cardioselective preparation (e.g., *atenolol* or *metoprolol*) is preferred because it is less likely to mask catecholamine-induced hypoglycemic symptoms.

The Patient with Chronic Renal Failure

Hypertension can lead to renal injury and exacerbate it. Blood pressure control is essential to the preservation of renal function in persons with chronic renal failure, particularly those with diabetic nephropathy (see Chapter 102). However, acute lowering of elevated blood pressure, especially to the recommended level of less than 125/80 mm Hg for persons with renal failure, can result in an acute nonprogressive increase in serum creatinine. This rise in serum creatinine is hemodynamic in origin (a consequence of reduction in intraglomerular pressure) and independent of type of antihypertensive agent used. It is neither a manifestation of drug-induced renal injury nor an indication to cut back on antihypertensive therapy (a common mistake in the treatment of hypertension in chronic renal failure).

Choice of Agents. Adequate control of blood pressure in persons with chronic renal failure may require a multidrug regimen. *ACEIs* and *ARBs* effectively lower blood pressure, reduce proteinuria, and help to preserve renal function. They are contraindicated when the cause of renal dysfunction is significant bilateral renal artery stenosis (>70% occlusion) and should be temporarily reduced in dose or held in the setting of acute severe volume depletion, where they may exacerbate reduction in glomerular filtration. Caution is also required when these agents are prescribed in the setting of hyperkalemia, but adding a low dose of a *thiazide* or *loop diuretic* can help to minimize the risk of hyperkalemia and helps to treat any associated volume retention. When the serum creatinine rises to greater than 2.5 mg/dL, sodium retention occurs, which can lead to

the exacerbation of blood pressure. *Furosemide* and/or *metolazone* can help to counter this sodium retention and reduce blood pressure. The use of potent diuretic therapy in conjunction with an ACEI or an ARB in renal failure requires careful attention to volume status; excessive diuresis can worsen renal function.

β-Blockers and *calcium-channel blockers* are also effective and can be added to the antihypertensive program. β-Blockers have no adverse effect on renal hemodynamics or glomerular filtration, but dihydropyridine calcium-channel blockers may blunt intrarenal vascular autoregulation. Nondihydropyridine calcium-channel blockers exert a beneficial effect on renal function that is enhanced when they are used in combination with an ACEI or an ARB; dihydropyridine use in renal failure is reasonable if it is combined with ACEI or ARB therapy. *Vasodilators* such as *minoxidil*, in combination with a loop diuretic and a β-blocker, may be necessary in refractory cases.

Other Measures. A *reduced-protein* diet (40 to 45 g/d) and *salt restriction* (2 g/d) help to preserve renal function and control blood pressure. A careful review of all other medications is essential (including over-the-counter agents); all *nonsteroidal antiinflammatory drugs* should be eliminated because their inhibition of prostaglandins can adversely affect intrarenal hemodynamics, compromise renal function, and impair potassium excretion.

The Stroke Patient

The control of hypertension is a critical goal in reducing the risk of recurrent stroke. Overtreatment is a common concern, especially in the acute poststroke phase in which reductions in pressure that are too rapid or too vigorous can lead to cerebral hypoperfusion. However, undertreatment is much more common, posing greater long-term risk. There is no evidence that treatment should vary by type of stroke or that the J-curve phenomenon applies to stroke risk. Gradual, steady blood pressure reduction over time that achieves maximum control without postural hypotension is the objective; stroke risk can be significantly reduced.

PATIENT EDUCATION (60)

Patient education is essential to ensuring *compliance*. Because it is a silent condition, hypertension does not always command the full attention of patients. The high cost of medication, high frequency of doses, and drug side effects further compromise compliance. Nonetheless, some educational and behavioral efforts can enhance patient cooperation. Educationally, one needs to review the cardiovascular consequences of untreated hypertension and the ability of treatment greatly to reduce the risk. Knowledge of the importance of nonpharmacologic measures is also critical and reassuring to many. That weight reduction, smoking cessation, and decrease in sodium intake may allow reduction or even elimination of antihypertensive medication can serve as a powerful motivating force.

One of the best approaches to improving compliance is to have the patient monitor blood pressure at home. Teaching the patient to perform *home blood pressure determinations* can foster considerable interest in blood pressure control, greatly stimulate adherence to a treatment program, and contribute to improved control. Effective home monitoring may even decrease the need for some office visits.

Medication side effects need to be addressed. Sexual dysfunction, fatigue, and depression have long bothered hypertensive patients who require drug therapy and lead many to stop their medication, often without notifying the physician. It is essential to specifically inquire about potential side effects, including symptoms of sexual dysfunction (see Chapter 229) and depression (see Chapter 227) before and after initiation of a medical regimen and to incorporate the findings into the design of the patient's program. Patients may be reluctant to raise these issues. Use of a medication that does not interfere with sexual capacity or mental function (e.g., an ACEI such as captopril) may be indicated (see prior discussion).

INDICATIONS FOR REFERRAL AND ADMISSION

Immediate hospitalization is indicated for patients with evidence of *malignant hypertension* (DBP >130 mm Hg, retinal hemorrhages, papilledema, mental status changes, heart failure). Referral may be useful for patients with refractory hypertension of unknown etiology (see prior discussion), a suspected secondary cause, or worsening renal failure in the setting of adequate control.

THERAPEUTIC RECOMMENDATIONS (1)

For All Patients (Fig. 26.1)

- Prescribe a no-added-salt diet (2 to 3 g/d) that is low in saturated fat and rich in fruits, vegetables, and low-fat dairy products; consider greater sodium restriction in patients who are likely to have volume-overload hypertension (e.g., African Americans, the elderly).
- Advise weight reduction (especially if the patient is >15% above ideal weight).
- Limit alcohol intake to 1 oz/d.
- Insist on complete smoking cessation (see Chapter 54).
- Prescribe an exercise program (see Chapter 18).

For Patients with Prehypertension (SBP 120 to 139 mm Hg, DBP 80 to 89 mm Hg)

- Recommend weight loss, exercise, salt restriction, dietary modification, and reduction of alcohol intake.
- Consider drug therapy in persons at very high risk for complications from hypertension (e.g., those with congestive heart failure, diabetes mellitus, or renal insufficiency) who do not achieve better blood pressure control with lifestyle modification alone.

For Patients with Stage 1 Hypertension (SBP 140 to 159 mm Hg, DBP 90 to 99 mm Hg), No Additional Cardiovascular Risk Factors, and No Signs of Target-Organ Disease (Fig. 26.1 and Tables 26.1 and 26.2)

- Institute full nonpharmacologic measures.
- Repeat blood pressure determinations regularly over the next 6 months.

- If improvement is noted (DBP <90 mm Hg, SBP <140 mm Hg), then continue nonpharmacologic measures and monitor blood pressure every 3 months.
- If there is no improvement after 6 to 12 months of nonpharmacologic therapy or if it fails to lower the blood pressure (DBP <90 mm Hg, SBP <140 mm Hg), then add a first-line antihypertensive agent to the nonpharmacologic program, starting with either a thiazide (e.g., HCTZ 25 mg/d) or a generic formulation of a β-blocker (e.g., atenolol 25 mg/d).

For Patients with Stage 1 Hypertension and Additional Cardiovascular Risk Factors or Signs of Target-Organ Disease (Fig. 26.1 and Table 26.1)

- Immediately institute a full nonpharmacologic program.
- Repeat blood pressure determinations regularly over 3 months.
- If blood pressure is not normalized after 3 months, then add first-line antihypertensive therapy (thiazide or a β-blocker; see prior discussion) to the nonpharmacologic program.

For Patients with Stage 2 Hypertension (DBP 100 mm Hg or Less, SBP 160 mm Hg or Greater), Especially If Accompanied by Cardiovascular Risk Factors or Target-Organ Damage

- Immediately institute a full nonpharmacologic program.
- If blood pressure is not normalized after 1 to 2 months, then add a first-line antihypertensive therapy (see prior discussion) to the nonpharmacologic program and advance the pharmacologic program as needed.
- Monitor blood pressure closely.

Initiation and Advancement of Pharmacologic Therapy

- Begin pharmacologic therapy with a first-line agent, preferably a diuretic or a β-blocker.
- Choose an agent based on a consideration of the patient's overall clinical situation (see later discussion), and start with a modest dose. In most cases, this will be a thiazide diuretic (e.g., HCTZ 12.5 to 25 mg/d).
- If pressure is not at goal within 1 month of initiating drug therapy, either increase the dose (e.g., to HCTZ 25 mg/d if 12.5 mg is used initially) or add a second first-line agent, and recheck in 4 weeks.
- If there is no response despite increasing dose, then switch to another first-line drug from a different class (e.g., a generic formulation of a β-blocker, such as atenolol, 25 mg/d).
- If there is only a partial response, then the choice is either further to increase the dose or to add a low dose of another first-line drug from a different class (e.g., add HCTZ 12.5 to 25 mg/d or a β-blocker).
- Once pressure normalizes, recheck blood pressure at 3- to 6-month intervals. When stability has been confirmed and sodium and potassium levels and renal function are stable, pressures can safely be rechecked every 6 months unless other complication factors are present.

- If a two-drug regimen using two first-line agents from different classes does not suffice, select a third drug from a new class. A particularly effective three-drug regimen is an ACEI, a thiazide diuretic, and a β-blocker.
- Consider a sustained-release formulation if it is likely to increase compliance and reduce the cost of a daily program.

First-Line Agents for Initial Use

- *Thiazides.* Consider for almost all patients; they are especially useful in those likely to have volume-overload hypertension (e.g., the elderly, African Americans, persons with nocturia or leg edema); they are an effective low-cost therapy, and enhance the antihypertensive effects of β-blockers, calcium-channel blockers, and ACEIs. Limit doses to modest amounts (e.g., HCTZ 12.5 to 25 mg/d) to minimize adverse metabolic effects, particularly in patients with marked hypercholesterolemia, poorly controlled diabetes, symptomatic gout, cardiac arrhythmias, or severe underlying coronary disease. Regularly monitor serum potassium, especially in persons with underlying heart disease.
- *β-Blockers.* Consider, often in conjunction with a thiazide diuretic, especially in those with concurrent coronary artery disease or high cardiovascular risk; they are not as effective or as well tolerated in the elderly. Choose a relatively cardioselective preparation (e.g., atenolol or metoprolol). Prescribe generic formulations (e.g., metoprolol, atenolol) to keep costs low. Avoid in patients with severe bronchospasm or nonischemic heart failure.
- *ACEIs.* Consider as the initial drug of choice, often in conjunction with low dose of thiazide diuretic for the treatment of hypertension in patients with diabetes, heart failure with systolic dysfunction, or underlying coronary heart disease. They are also useful in patients with volume overload, underlying sexual dysfunction, depression, and intolerance to the central nervous system effects of other antihypertensive agents. They may be used alone or in combination with a diuretic or a β-blocker, which enhance their effectiveness; they are contraindicated in pregnancy, bilateral renal artery stenosis, and renal failure. Monitor renal function and serum potassium, especially in patients with underlying renal dysfunction. Prescribe generic formulations (captopril, lisinopril) to minimize cost. Can substitute an *ARB* if ACEIs are not well tolerated due to cough or angioedema.
- *Calcium-Channel Blockers.* Consider as an adjunct to thiazides and ACEIs, especially in patients with volume-overload hypertension (e.g., the elderly, African Americans) and in diabetics. Short-acting preparations should not be used because of concerns about the increased risk of myocardial infarction and cardiac sudden death. Use cautiously in patients with conduction defects, especially if they are already taking a β-blocker. Avoid if possible in patients bothered by peripheral edema; short-acting agents are contraindicated in heart failure. If their use is unavoidable, consider an agent with the least adverse peripheral vascular and cardiovascular effects (e.g., amlodipine).

Annotated Bibliography

1. Chobanian AV, Bakris GL, Cushman WC, et al. The seventh report of the Joint National Committee on Prevention, Detection, Evaluation and Treatment of High Blood Pressure: the JNC VII report. JAMA 2003;289:2560. (*The most recent version of this major consensus report.*)
2. Beulens JWJ, Rimm EB, Ascherio A, et al. Alcohol consumption and risk for coronary heart disease among men with hypertension. Ann Intern Med 2007;146:10. (*A prospective cohort study; moderate consumption lowered the risk for myocardial infarction but not for death.*)
3. Blacher J, Staessen JA, Girerd X, et al. Pulse pressure not mean pressure determines cardiovascular risk in older hypertensive patients. Arch Intern Med 2000;160:1205. (*Provides evidence that high pulse pressure is a marker of significant increase in cardiovascular risk in the elderly.*)
4. Julius S, Nesbitt SD, Egan BM, et al., for the Trial of Preventing Hypertension (TROPHY) Study Investigators. N Engl J Med 2006;354:1685. (*A randomized, controlled trial [RCT]; two thirds of untreated prehypertension patients developed stage 1 hypertension; angiotensin II–receptor blocker therapy helped to prevent it.*)
5. Neaton JD, Grimm RH, Prineas RJ, et al., Treatment of Mild Hypertension Study. JAMA 1993;270:713. (*A landmark study, demonstrating benefits in relation to major outcomes.*)
6. Nissen SE, Tuzcu EM, Libby P, et al., for the CAMELOT Investigators. Effect of antihypertensive agents on cardiovascular events in patients with coronary disease and normal blood pressure: the CAMELOT Study: a randomized controlled trial. JAMA 2004;292:2217. (*Amlodipine and, to a lesser extent, enalapril reduced the risk of cardiovascular events.*)
7. Systolic Hypertension in the Elderly Program (SHEP) Cooperative Research Group. Prevention of stroke by antihypertensive drug treatment in older persons with isolated systolic hypertension. JAMA 1991;265:3255. (*The original study documenting that the treatment of isolated systolic hypertension reduces the risk of stroke in the elderly.*)
8. Appel LJ, Champagne CM, Harsha DW, et al. Writing Group of the PREMIER Collaborative Research Group. Effects of comprehensive lifestyle modification on blood pressure control: main results of the PREMIER clinical trial. JAMA 2003;289:2083. (*RCT comparing an intensive behavioral intervention—the Dietary Approaches to Stop Hypertension [DASH] diet and lifestyle changes—against advice only in persons with prehypertension; a significant reduction in blood pressure was achieved.*)
9. Appel LJ, Moore TJ, Obarzanek E, et al. A clinical trial of the effects of dietary patterns on blood pressure. N Engl J Med 1997;336:1117. (*A randomized trial of the DASH diet [rich in vegetables and fruits and low in saturated fat] in normotensive and mildly hypertensive patients; this approach significantly reduced blood pressure.*)
10. Eisenberg DM, Delbanco TL, Berkey CS, et al. Cognitive behavioral techniques for hypertension: are they effective? Ann Intern Med 1993;118:964. (*A meta-analysis incorporating data from the limited number of available well-designed studies; found no benefit over placebo.*)
11. Elmer PJ, Obarzanek E, Vollmer WM, et al. for the PREMIER Collaborative Research Group. Effects of comprehensive lifestyle modification on diet, weight, physical fitness, and blood pressure control: 18-month results of a randomized trial. Ann Intern Med 2006;144:485. (*RCT; using a multicomponent behavioral intervention that included the DASH diet, patients with prehypertension and stage 1 disease were able to sustain lifestyle modifications that reduced risk.*)
12. He J, Gu D, Wu X, et al. Effect of soybean protein on blood pressure: a randomized, controlled trial. Ann Intern Med 2005;143:1. (*RCT; there was a 4-mm Hg reduction in systolic pressure and a 2-mm Hg reduction in diastolic pressure.*)
13. Kelemen MH, Effron MB, Valenti SA, et al. Exercise training combined with antihypertensive drug therapy. JAMA 1990;263:2766. (*Exercise was just as effective as drug therapy and obviated the need for medication in mildly hypertensive patients.*)
14. MacMahon SW, Norton RN. Alcohol and hypertension. Ann Intern Med 1986;105:124. (*An editorial summarizing the evidence linking the two conditions and recommending a limit of <2 oz/d.*)
15. National High Blood Pressure Education Program Working Group. Report on primary prevention of hypertension. Arch Intern Med 1993;153:186. (*A major review of nonpharmacologic measures; 327 references.*)
16. Sacks FM, Svetkey LP, Vollmer WM, et al. Effects on blood pressure of reduced dietary sodium and the Dietary Approaches to Stop Hypertension (DASH) diet. N Engl J Med 2001;344:3. (*A major randomized, controlled trial of dietary therapy.*)
17. Vollmer WM, Sacks FM, Ard J, et al. Effects of diet and sodium intake on blood pressure: subgroup analysis of the DASH-Sodium Trial. Ann

Intern Med 2001;135:1019. (*The DASH diet was effective across diverse subgroups.*)

18. Wassertheil-Smoller S, Oberman A, Blaufox MD, et al. The Trial of Antihypertensive Interventions and Management (TAIM) study. Am J Hypertens 1992;5:37. (*A trial demonstrating the benefit of weight loss in the control of blood pressure.*)

19. Writing Group of the Premier Collaborative Research Group. Effects of comprehensive lifestyle modification on blood pressure control: main results of the PREMIER clinical trial. JAMA 2003;289:2083. (*A randomized trial; lifestyle modification works.*)

20. Boutitie F, Gueyffier F, Pocock S, et al. J-shaped relationship between blood pressure and mortality in hypertensive patients: new insights from a meta-analysis of individual-patient data. Ann Intern Med 2002;136:438. (*A meta-analysis; risk increases at low pressures due to underlying illness.*)

21. Davis BR, Cutler JA, Furberg, et al. Relationship of antihypertensive treatment regimens and change in blood pressure to risk for heart failure in hypertensive patients randomly assigned to doxazosin or chlorthalidone: further analyses from the ALLHAT trial. Ann Intern Med 2002;137:313. (*The heart failure risk with doxazosin is attenuated but not eliminated by adding other antihypertensive agents.*)

22. Devereux RB, Wachtell K, Gerdts E, et al. Prognostic significance of left ventricular mass change during treatment of hypertension. JAMA 2004;292:2350. (*A prospective cohort study; reduction in left ventricular mass was accretive to improvements in outcome.*)

23. Messerli FH, Mancia G, Conti CR, et al. Dogma disputed: can aggressively lowering blood pressure in hypertensive patients with coronary artery disease can be dangerous? Ann Intern Med 2006;144:884. (*A secondary analysis of a large international study of an angiotensin-converting-enzyme inhibitor [ACEI] vs. a calcium-channel blocker [CCB]; found that the risk was increased with a marked lowering of diastolic blood pressure—a J-curve effect.*)

24. Okin PM, Wachtell K, Devereux RB, et al. Regression of electrocardiographic left ventricular hypertrophy and decreased incidence of new-onset atrial fibrillation in patients with hypertension. JAMA 2006;296:1242. (*RCT; treatment aimed at reducing left ventricular hypertrophy reduced the atrial fibrillation risk independent of the degree of blood pressure reduction or treatment modality.*)

25. Psaty BM, Smith NL, Heckbert SR, et al. Diuretic therapy, the α-adducin gene variant, and the risk of myocardial infarction or stroke in persons with treated hypertension. JAMA 2002;287:1680. (*A case–control study examining the relation of genetic polymorphism to response to treatment.*)

26. Schmieder RE, Rockstroh JK, Messerli FZ. Antihypertensive therapy: to stop or not to stop? JAMA 1991;265:1566. (*A review of the evidence for cessation of therapy; 80 references.*)

27. Strom BJ, Schinnar R, Apter AJ, et al. Absence of cross-reactivity between sulfonamide antibiotics and sulfonamide nonantibiotics. N Engl J Med 2003;349:1628. (*A prospective cohort study; no risk of cross-allergic reaction was found.*)

28. Abernathy DR, Schwartz JB. Drug therapy: calcium antagonist drugs. N Engl J Med 1999;341:1447. (*An excellent review.*)

29. Goodfriend TL, Elliott ME, Catt KJ. Angiotensin receptors and their antagonists. N Engl J Med 1996;334:1649. (*An excellent review of the mechanism of action of this class of antihypertensive.*)

30. Lacourciere Y, Belanger A, Godin C, et al. Long term comparison of losartan and enalapril on kidney function in hypertensive type 2 diabetics with early nephropathy. Kidney Int 2000;58:762. (*Demonstration of similar renoprotective effects between ACEIs and angiotensin-receptor blockers.*)

31. Jafar TH, Schmid CH, Landa M, et al. Angiotensin converting enzyme inhibitors and progression of non-diabetic renal disease. Ann Intern Med 2001;135:73. (*The protective renal effect of ACEIs extends to hypertensive nondiabetic patients with renal dysfunction.*)

32. Lewis EJ, Hunsicker LG, Bain RP, et al. The effect of angiotensin converting enzyme inhibition on diabetic nephropathy. N Engl J Med 1993;329:1456. (*Demonstrates the protective effect of ACEIs on renal function in hypertensive diabetics.*)

33. Messerli FH, Grossman E, Goldbourt U. Are beta-blockers efficacious as first line therapy for hypertension in the elderly? JAMA 1998;279:1903. (*Evidence that the answer is that they are probably not efficacious.*)

34. Perez-Stable EJ, Halliday R, Gardiner PS, et al. The effects of propranolol on cognitive function and quality of life: a randomized trial among patients with diastolic hypertension. Am J Med 2000;108:359. (*No adverse effects were found.*)

35. Pfeffer MA, Braunwald E, Moye LA, et al. Effect of captopril on mortality and morbidity in patients with left ventricular dysfunction after myocardial infarction. N Engl J Med 1992;327:669. (*A landmark study finding reductions in morbidity and mortality.*)

36. Psaty BM, Lumly T, Furberg CD, et al. Health outcomes associated with antihypertensive therapies used as first line agents. JAMA 2003;289:2534. (*A meta-analysis of numerous trials demonstrating the benefits of low-dose diuretic therapy.*)

37. Psaty BM, Heckbert SR, Koepsell TD, et al. The risk of myocardial infarction associated with antihypertensive drug therapies. JAMA 1995;274:620.

(*A report from the Puget Sound Health Co-operative on the increase in myocardial infarction in patients treated with short-acting CCBs.*)

38. Thurman JM, Schrier RW. Comparative effects of angiotensin-converting enzyme inhibitors and angiotensin receptor blockers on blood pressure and the kidney. Am J Med 2003;114:588. (*A useful review; 85 references.*)

39. The ALLHAT Officers and Coordinators for the ALLHAT Collaborative Research Group. Major outcomes in high-risk hypertensive patients randomized to angiotensin-converting enzyme inhibitor or calcium channel blocker vs diuretic: the Antihypertensive and Lipid-Lowering Treatment to Prevent Heart Attack Trial (ALLHAT). JAMA 2002;288:2981. (*A major head-to-head RCT, finding that thiazides were superior to ACEIs and CCBs as initial agents in high-risk patients.*)

40. The ALLHAT Officers and Coordinators for the ALLHAT Collaborative Research Group. Major cardiovascular events in hypertensive patients randomized to doxazosin vs. chlorthalidone: the Anti-hypertensive and Lipid-lowering Treatment to Prevent Heart Attack Trial (ALLTHAT). JAMA 2000;283:1967. (*RCT; doxazosin failed to reduce the risk of congestive heart failure.*)

41. The Heart Outcomes Prevention/Evaluation Study Investigators. Effects of an angiotensin converting enzyme inhibitor, ramipril, on cardiovascular events in high risk patients. N Eng J Med 2000;342:1459. (*A major trial further demonstrating the benefits of ACEIs in high-risk cardiovascular patients.*)

42. Wing LM, Reid CM, Ryan P, et al. A comparison of outcomes with angiotensin converting enzyme inhibitors and diuretics for hypertension in the elderly. N Engl J Med 2003;348:583 (*A report of the Second National Australian Blood Pressure Trial; ACEIs were superior to diuretics in preventing cardiovascular disease in elderly men but not in women.*)

43. Wright JT Jr, Dunn JK, Cutler JA, et al. for the ALLHAT Collaborative Research Group. Outcomes in hypertensive black and nonblack patients treated with chlorthalidone, amlodipine, and lisinopril. JAMA 2005;293:1595. (*More findings from a landmark RCT; thiazide-like diuretics gave the best outcome results in all racial groups, including blacks.*)

44. Logan AG, Perlikowski SM, Mente A, et al. High prevalence of unrecognized sleep apnea in drug-resistant hypertension. J Hypertens 2001;19:2271. (*An important cause of "refractory" hypertension.*)

45. Calhoun DA, Jones D, Textor S, et al. Resistant hypertension: diagnosis, evaluation, and treatment: a scientific statement from the American Heart Association Professional Education Committee of the Council for High Blood Pressure Research. Hypertension 2008;51:1403. (*Consensus recommendations.*)

46. Moser M, Setaro JF. Resistant or difficult-to-control hypertension. N Engl J Med 2006;355:385. (*A useful review and practical approach; 37 references.*)

47. Balk E, Raman G, Chung M, et al. Comparative effectiveness of management strategies for renal artery stenosis: a systematic review. Ann Intern Med 2006;145:901. (*No one approach proved to be superior.*)

48. Ritz E, Mann JFE. Renal angioplasty for lowering blood pressure. N Engl J Med 2000;342:1042. (*An editorial summarizing the available data, finding little benefit over medical therapy, except in limited situations.*)

49. van Jaarsveld BC, Krijnen P, Pieterman H, et al. The effect of balloon angioplasty on hypertension in atherosclerotic renal-artery stenosis. N Engl J Med 2000;342:1007. (*A randomized trial; angioplasty was no better than medical therapy.*)

50. Staessen JA, Thijs L, Birkenhager WH, et al. Update on the Systolic Hypertension in Europe (Sys-Eur) Trial. Hypertension 1999;33:1476. (*A major European trial; the treatment of systolic hypertension reduces cardiovascular risk.*)

51. Wing LMH, Reid CM, Ryan P, et al. A comparison of outcomes with angiotensin-converting enzyme inhibitors and diuretics for hypertension in the elderly. N Engl J Med 2003;348:483. (*Starting with ACEI rather than thiazide diuretic resulted in a better outcome in men.*)

52. Palmer BF. Renal dysfunction complicating the treatment of hypertension. N Engl J Med 2002;347:1256. (*A succinct review of the relevant pathophysiology and clinical implications; 44 references.*)

53. Belfort MA, Anthony J, Saade GR, et al. A comparison of magnesium sulfate and nimodipine for the prevention of eclampsia. N Engl J Med 2003;348:304. (*A randomized trial; magnesium sulfate was better.*)

54. Cunningham FG, Lindheimer MD. Hypertension in pregnancy. N Engl J Med 1992;326:927. (*A still-useful review; 61 references.*)

55. Levine RJ, Lam C, Qian C, et al. Soluble endoglin and other circulating antiangiogenic factors in preeclampsia. N Engl J Med 2006;355:992. (*The identification of pathogenic factors.*)

56. National High Blood Pressure Education Program Working Group. Report on high blood pressure in pregnancy. Am J Obstet Gynecol 1990;163:1689. (*A comprehensive consensus report.*)

57. Rumbold AR, Crowther CA, Haaslam RR, et al. Vitamins C and E and the risks of preeclampsia and prenatal complications. N Engl J Med 2006;354:1796. (*RCT, finding no benefit.*)

58. Skjaeven R, Wilcox AJ, Lie R. The interval between pregnancies and the risk of preeclampsia. N Engl J Med 2002;346:33. (*An epidemiologic study; the interval between pregnancies increases the risk, but a change in partners does not.*)

59. Paul SL, Thrift AF. Control of hypertension 5 years after stroke in the North East Melbourne Stroke Incidence Study. Hypertension 2006;48:260. (*Documents the common phenomenon of undertreatment.*)

60. Roumie CL, Elasy TA, Greevy R, et al. Improving blood pressure control through provider education, provider alerts, and patient education. Ann Intern Med 2006;1145:165. (*RCT; patient education proved to be the most effective means of improving control.*)

APPENDIX 26.1: CORONARY HEART DISEASE RISK FACTOR PREDICTION CHART

TABLE 1

FIND POINTS FOR EACH RISK FACTOR

Women				Men				HDL-C	Pts	Total C	Pts	SBP (mm Hg)	Pts	Other	Pts
Age (yr)	Pts	Age (yr)	Pts	Age (yr)	Pts	Age (yr)	Pts								
30	−12	47–48	5	30	−2	57–59	13	25–26	7	139–151	−3	98–104	−2	Cigarettes	4
31	−11	49–50	6	31	−1	60–61	14	27–29	6	152–166	−2	105–112	−1	Diabetic male	3
32	−9	51–52	7	32–33	0	62–64	15	30–32	5	167–182	−1	113–120	0	Diabetic female	6
33	−8	53–55	8	34	1	65–67	16	33–35	4	183–199	0	121–129	1	ECG LVH	9
34	−6	56–60	9	35–36	2	68–70	17	36–38	3	200–219	1	130–139	2		
35	−5	61–67	10	37–38	3	71–73	18	39–42	2	220–239	2	140–149	3	0 Pts for each No	
36	−4	68–74	11	39	4	74	19	43–46	1	240–262	3	150–160	4		
37	−3			40–41	5			47–50	0	263–288	4	161–172	5		
38	−2			42–43	6			51–55	−1	289–315	5	173–185	6		
39	−1			44–45	7			56–60	−2	316–330	6				
40	0			46–47	8			61–66	−3						
41	1			48–49	9			67–73	−4						
42–43	2			50–51	10			74–80	−5						
44	3			52–52	11			81–87	−6						
45–46	4			55–56	12			88–96	−7						

TABLE 2

SUM POINTS FOR ALL RISK FACTORS

——— + ——— + ——— + ——— + ——— + ——— + ——— = ———
Age   HDL-C   Total C   SBP   Smoker   Diabetes   ECG LVH   Point Total

Note: Minus points/subtract from total.

3. LOOK UP RISK CORRESPONDING TO POINT TOTAL   #### 4. COMPARE WITH AVERAGE 10-YR RISK

Probability (%)			Probability (%)			Probability (%)			Probability (%)			Probability (%)		
Pts	5 Yr	10 Yr	Pts	5 Yr	10 Yr	Pts	5 Yr	10 Yr	Pts	5 Yr	10 Yr	Age	Women	Men
≤1	<1	<2	10	2	6	19	8	16	28	19	33	30–34	<1	3
2	1	2	11	3	6	20	8	18	29	20	36	35–39	1	5
3	1	2	12	3	7	21	9	19	30	22	38	40–44	2	6
4	1	2	13	3	8	22	11	21	31	24	40	45–49	5	10
5	1	3	14	4	9	23	12	23	32	25	42	50–54	8	14
6	1	3	15	5	10	24	13	25				55–59	12	16
7	1	4	16	5	12	25	14	27				60–64	13	21
8	2	4	17	6	13	26	16	29				65–69	9	30
9	2	5	18	7	14	27	17	31				70–74	12	24

C, cholesterol; ECG, electrocardiogram; HDL, high-density lipoprotein; LVH, left ventricular hypertension; Pts, points; SBP, systolic blood pressure.
Prepared with the help of William B. Kannel, M.D., professor of medicine and public health, and Ralph D'Agostino, Ph.D., head, Department of Mathematics, Boston University, Boston, Massachusetts; Keaven Anderson, Ph.D., statistician, National Heart, Lung, and Blood Institute, Framingham, Massachusetts; Daniel McGee, Ph.D., associate professor, University of Arizona, Tucson, Arizona.
From American Heart Association. Risk Factor Prediction Kit, Dallas, TX: 1990, with permission.

CHAPTER 27 ■ APPROACH TO THE PATIENT WITH A LIPID DISORDER

MASON W. FREEMAN

Over the last two decades, evidence has accumulated demonstrating that treatment of hypercholesterolemia can reduce atherosclerosis and its attendant cardiovascular complications (see Chapter 15). These findings have heightened physician and patient awareness of the importance of hypercholesterolemia. The primary care physician needs to be capable of evaluating hypercholesterolemia and of designing and implementing a treatment program that effectively uses dietary treatment, exercise, weight loss, and, when necessary, cholesterol-lowering drugs.

PATHOPHYSIOLOGY (1–17)

The production of atherogenic lipoproteins and the induction of atheromatous plaques by those lipoproteins involve distinct pathways. The presence of an elevated serum cholesterol level does not, by itself, guarantee the development of atherosclerotic lesions that will become clinically important any more than a normal cholesterol concentration ensures plaque-free coronary arteries. The formation and subsequent rupture of atherosclerotic lesions, leading to the acute coronary syndromes of unstable angina and myocardial infarction, depend on complex cellular and metabolic interactions. Serum lipids, inflammatory cells recruited to the sites of lipid deposition, the normal cellular constituents of the artery wall, and components of the blood coagulation system all contribute to the pathogenesis of atherosclerosis and its clinical consequences.

Lipoproteins

An understanding of lipoproteins and their metabolism helps guide physicians in evaluating and treating lipid disorders. To circulate in the aqueous environment of the blood, nonpolar lipids such as cholesterol and triglyceride are complexed with proteins and the more polar phospholipids into spheres called *lipoproteins*. The protein components of the lipoproteins are known as *apoproteins*, which play both structural and functional roles in the metabolism of lipid particles. Genetically inherited mutations in either the structure of apoproteins or the receptors that bind them account for many of the most severe forms of hyperlipidemia. The lipoproteins are usually divided into four major classes based on particle density, which is a reflection of their relative protein and lipid content: *chylomicrons, very-low-density lipoproteins (VLDLs); low-density lipoproteins (LDLs);* and *high-density lipoproteins (HDLs)*. There are also subdivisions and minor classes of lipoproteins (Table 27.1).

Chylomicrons

Chylomicrons derive from dietary fat and carry triglycerides throughout the body. They have the lowest density of all lipoproteins and float to the top of a plasma specimen left in the refrigerator overnight. The chylomicron itself is probably not atherogenic, but the role of the triglyceride-depleted chylomicron remnant is uncertain. Triglyceride makes up most of the chylomicron and is removed by the action of lipoprotein lipase. Patients deficient in this enzyme or its cofactors (insulin and apolipoprotein CII) have very high serum triglyceride levels and increased risk of acute pancreatitis.

Very-Low-Density Lipoproteins

VLDLs are also triglyceride rich and are acted on by lipoprotein lipase. Their function is to carry triglycerides synthesized in the liver and intestines to capillary beds in adipose tissue and muscle, where they are hydrolyzed. After removal of their triglyceride, VLDL remnants can be further metabolized to LDLs. The atherogenicity of native VLDL is controversial, but the metabolism of VLDL to atherogenic lipoproteins is not in doubt. VLDLs serve as acceptors of cholesterol transferred from HDLs, possibly accounting in part for the inverse relation between HDL cholesterol and VLDL triglyceride. The serum enzyme cholesterol ester transfer protein (CETP) mediates this transfer process, and inhibitors of CETP raise HDL cholesterol levels. It is not clear whether such inhibitors favorably alter the development of atherosclerosis, despite the substantial impact they have on raising HDL levels.

Low-Density Lipoproteins

LDLs are the major carriers of cholesterol in humans. They carry cholesterol to tissues and deliver it via receptors on the cell surface that bind and internalize the LDL particle. LDLs are the lipoproteins most clearly implicated in atherogenesis. LDL levels are increased in individuals who consume large amounts of saturated fat and/or cholesterol. There are also several Mendelian genetic disorders that result in increased LDL levels. These disorders encompass mutations that produce defective LDL receptors (familial hypercholesterolemia) or mutant proteins that interact with the LDL receptor (PCSK9 and autosomal recessive hypercholesterolemia proteins). LDL levels can also result from genetically encoded abnormalities in the structure of LDL's major protein constituent, apoprotein B (familial defective Apo B). Finally, there are non-Mendelian, polygenic disorders that cause increases in LDL.

When serum LDLs exceed a threshold concentration, they traverse the endothelial wall and can become trapped in the arterial intima. There, they may undergo oxidation, aggregation, or other modifications that enhance their uptake by

TABLE 27.1

LIPOPROTEIN COMPOSITION

Lipoprotein	Protein	Cholesterol	Cholesterol Ester %	Phospholipid	TG
VLDL	10.4	5.8	13.9	15.2	53.4
IDL	17.8	6.5	22.5	21.7	31.4
LDL	25.0	8.6	41.9	20.9	3.5
HDL$_2$	42.6	5.2	20.3	30.1	2.2
HDL$_3$	54.9	2.6	16.1	25.0	1.4
Chylomicrons	1–2	1–3	2–4	3–8	80–95

Values are percentage of composition by weight. HDL, high-density lipoprotein; IDL, intermediate-density lipoprotein; LDL, low-density lipoprotein; TG, triglycerides; VLDL, very-low-density lipoprotein.

macrophages. The accumulation of lipid in macrophages that has derived from native and modified LDL uptake appears to be an important initiating step in atherogenesis. The association of serum total cholesterol with coronary heart disease (CHD) is predominantly a reflection of the role of LDL because LDL cholesterol constitutes the bulk of serum cholesterol in most humans. Many well-designed studies demonstrate that lowering the LDL cholesterol can dramatically reduce subsequent coronary events and all-cause mortality in hypercholesterolemic patients.

High-Density Lipoproteins

HDLs appear to function in peripheral tissues as an acceptor of free cholesterol that has been transported out of the cellular membrane. The cholesterol is esterified and stored in the central core of the HDLs and may be further metabolized. This movement of cholesterol from peripheral cells back to HDLs and then ultimately to the liver for excretion is termed *reverse cholesterol transport*. The activity of this pathway may explain why patients with very high HDL levels have a reduced risk of developing CHD, even if their LDL levels are elevated. Recent investigations have also attributed direct antiinflammatory and antioxidant properties to HDLs, apparently mediated by an extremely complex mixture of proteins carried in HDLs that may vary in individuals with differing risks of coronary disease. *Apolipoprotein A1* is the major apoprotein of HDL, and its level also inversely correlates with the risk of CHD.

Women have higher levels of HDL cholesterol than men, in part because of their higher estrogen levels. Exercise increases HDL, whereas obesity, hypertriglyceridemia, and smoking lower HDL. In several epidemiologic studies, the HDL cholesterol concentration is the most powerful lipid predictor of CHD risk, but therapies that raise HDL cholesterol levels have proven difficult to develop, and the significance of such an intervention on coronary disease outcomes is uncertain. There is a growing appreciation of the complexity of the role of HDLs in atherosclerosis, which has led to the view that simply raising HDL cholesterol levels, unlike lowering LDL cholesterol values, may not reliably translate into a clinical benefit.

Dietary Influences

Dietary fat and cholesterol have a substantial influence on serum cholesterol and LDL cholesterol levels. Saturated fat intake has a greater effect on serum cholesterol than does dietary cholesterol intake. For each increase in percentage of total calo-

ries contributed by saturated fats, serum cholesterol increases by a factor of 2.16, whereas the serum cholesterol increases by only 0.068 times the percentage increase in dietary cholesterol. This relationship is summarized in the equation of Hegsted:

$$\text{Change in total cholesterol} = 2.16\Delta S - 1.65\Delta P + 0.068\Delta C$$

where ΔS, ΔP, and ΔC are the changes in the percentage of total calories contributed by saturated fats, polyunsaturated fats, and cholesterol, respectively. Fats are characterized by their constituent fatty acid composition. The fatty acids are characterized as saturated, polyunsaturated, or monounsaturated. The state of saturation refers to the number of carbon–carbon double bonds contained in the fatty acid.

Saturated Fatty Acids

These fatty acids can raise LDL cholesterol, in part by altering the LDL receptor's catabolic activity. The long-chain saturated fatty acids common to the U.S. diet—lauric (12 carbons), myristic (14 carbons), palmitic (16 carbons), and stearic (18 carbons)—have no double bonds and are not essential dietary components for human growth and development. Not all saturated fatty acids trigger rises in LDL cholesterol. For example, stearic acid and some shorter-chain fatty acids (caproic and caprylic) do not. In the typical U.S. diet, about one third of the saturated fat content of the diet derives from *meat* and meat products, whereas another third comes from *dairy products* and eggs and 10% from baked goods. Vegetable oils also may contain saturated fat (see Appendix 27.1), especially the so-called *"tropical oils"* (coconut and palm) and cocoa butter, which are commonly used in commercial food preparation. Even when unsaturated oils (see later discussion) are used in processed foods, they usually undergo *"partial hydrogenation,"* which adds back hydrogens to the carbon–carbon double bonds, eliminating some double bonds and making the fatty acids more saturated. This saturation process is performed to make these oils more solid at room temperature, but it also makes them more hypercholesterolemic.

Monounsaturated Fatty Acids

Monounsaturated fatty acids are present in all animal and vegetable fats. The most common dietary form is *oleic acid*, which is plentiful in peanuts, almonds, olives, and avocados. Oils derived from these sources neither raise nor lower LDL cholesterol by themselves, although cholesterol and CHD risk fall if they are used as substitutes for saturated fat. Mediterranean diets rich in *olive oil* and other sources of monounsaturated fatty acids appear to be relatively nonatherogenic, even though they are not low in fat.

Polyunsaturated Fatty Acids (PUFAs)

Unlike saturated and monounsaturated fatty acids, PUFAs are not synthesized by the body. They must be present in the diet and are referred to as *essential fatty acids*. The location of the first double bond from the methyl end of the molecule determines the nomenclature of the PUFAs. The major dietary fatty acids contain either an n-6 or n-3 first double bond. *Linoleic* and *arachidonic acids* are the common *omega-6 PUFAs*, found in considerable quantities in *liquid vegetable oils* (sunflower, safflower, corn, and soybean). The *omega-3 fatty acids* are represented by linoleic acid (found in canola oil and leafy vegetables) and the *omega-3 fish oils* (eicosapentanoic and docosahexanoic acids). The latter attracted considerable interest when epidemiologic studies found a link between their consumption and reduced rates of CHD mortality.

When vegetable oils rich in PUFAs are subjected to *partial hydrogenation* in commercial food processing, not only do some of their double carbon bonds get converted to single bonds, but shifts from the *cis* configuration into the *trans* configuration also occur, which increases the atherogenicity and associated CHD risk of these fats. Intake of such substances increases LDL cholesterol, lipoprotein(a), and triglycerides and reduces HDL cholesterol. Data from the Nurses' Health Study suggest that replacing *trans* unsaturated fats in the diet with polyunsaturated fats can reduce CHD risk by nearly 60%, a much greater reduction than that achieved by reducing overall fat intake. Studies in which the total fat content of the diet has been lowered have not shown consistently reproducible benefits on serum cholesterol levels and/or coronary disease outcomes. This may be because most attempts to reduce total fat lead to reductions in both saturated and unsaturated fat intake, producing no net benefit. Current evidence suggests that only reductions of saturated and *trans* fat intake would be beneficial.

Cholesterol

As the Hegsted formula indicates, dietary cholesterol has a much smaller effect than saturated fatty acids on raising total cholesterol. For every additional 100 mg of dietary cholesterol consumed per day, the serum cholesterol will rise by about 8 to 10 mg/dL. However, *organ meats* (e.g., brain, kidney, heart, sweetbreads) and *egg yolks* are concentrated sources of dietary cholesterol (see Appendix 27.2) and can have a substantial effect on serum cholesterol levels. Although *shellfish* contain moderate amounts of cholesterol, they have relatively small amounts of saturated fat and are sources of omega-3 PUFAs. Cholesterol is absent from food derived from plants. Plant stanols and sterols can actually block cholesterol absorption in the intestine, and a commercially available margarine containing the plant stanol sitostanol is available as a cholesterol-lowering agent. It reduces serum cholesterol levels by 10% to 15%. Recently released National Cholesterol Education Program (NCEP) guidelines (Adult Treatment Panel III [ATP III]) encourage the use of these plant stanols in dietary programs aimed at reducing blood cholesterol levels.

Other Dietary Factors

Low-fat, high-carbohydrate diets can reduce HDL cholesterol and increase triglycerides. Especially in obese persons, increased total caloric intake may induce overproduction of VLDL triglycerides while reducing HDL cholesterol levels. Data from the Nurses' Health Study suggest that *substituting carbohydrate for saturated fat* in the diet may reduce CHD risk by about 15%, but *substituting carbohydrate for polyunsaturated fat* may increase CHD risk by >50%. There is no evidence that either dietary carbohydrate (whether simple sugars or complex ones) or protein significantly affects LDL cholesterol.

The *fiber* content of food has generated much interest. *Insoluble fiber* (typically cellulose found in wheat bran) has no cholesterol-lowering effect, although it is beneficial for lowering the risk of diverticular disease and colon cancer (see Chapter 65). *Soluble fiber* (pectins, certain gums, psyllium) has received much attention in the lay press stimulated by claims about *oat bran*, which contains the gum β-glycan. Initial studies were encouraging, but subsequent data suggested that the cholesterol decreases observed were no greater than those found with the use of insoluble fiber and probably resulted from the replacement of dietary fat in the diet rather than from a direct effect on lipid metabolism. When studied in patients already taking a low-fat diet, high–soluble fiber intake appeared to lower serum cholesterol by a modest amount (3% to 7%).

Lifestyle Contributions

Lack of exercise and *caloric excess* are epidemic in the United States and major contributors to lipid abnormalities and CHD risk. The *obesity* that results from an unhealthy lifestyle leads to the *metabolic syndrome*, characterized by hyperinsulinism and elevations in triglycerides, reductions in HDL cholesterol, and increases in LDL cholesterol; in addition, blood pressure rises along with the risk of developing type 2 diabetes. The net result is a marked increase in CHD risk.

WORKUP (3–7,10,12–14,16–19; See Also Chapter 15)

Diagnosis

The diagnosis of hypercholesterolemia should always be based on *repeat measurements* of serum lipids because combined analytic and biologic variations in serum lipids range from 10% to 20%. A single measurement should never be viewed as sufficient for a diagnosis of hypercholesterolemia. A *venous sample* processed in a laboratory meeting Centers for Disease Control and Prevention standards for cholesterol determination (see Chapter 15) is recommended.

Whereas earlier guidelines often recommended a stepped approach to performing lipid analyses in patients, the ATP III guidelines now suggest that a fasting lipid profile be done at the initial assessment whenever possible (Table 27.2). A *fasting* venous sample for determination of *serum cholesterol*, *HDL cholesterol*, and *triglycerides* (with calculation of LDL cholesterol derived from these determinations; see later discussion) constitutes the traditional lipid profile and the basis for estimating VLDL cholesterol and calculating LDL cholesterol. The results characterize the lipid disorder and guide treatment decisions. If a fasting lipid profile cannot be readily arranged, then a practical alternative in persons at low CHD risk is to obtain nonfasting determinations of total cholesterol and HDL cholesterol and reserve for a full lipid profile only those

TABLE 27.2

INITIAL CLASSIFICATION AND RECOMMENDED FOLLOW-UP BASED ON TOTAL CHOLESTEROL

Classification, mg/dL	
<200	Desirable blood cholesterol
200–239	Borderline-high blood cholesterol
≥240	High blood cholesterol
Recommended Follow-up	
Total cholesterol, <200 mg/dL	Repeat within 5 yr
Total cholesterol, 200–239 mg/dL	
Without definite CHD or two other CHD risk factors (one of which can be male sex)	Dietary information and recheck annually
With definite CHD or two other CHD risk factors (one of which can be male sex)	Lipoprotein analysis; further action based on LDL cholesterol level
Total cholesterol ≥240 mg/dL	

CHD, coronary heart disease; LDL, low-density lipoprotein.
From Report of the National Cholesterol Education Program. Expert Panel on Detection, Evaluation, and Treatment of High Blood Cholesterol in Adults. Arch Intern Med 1988;148:36, with permission.

persons with a nonfasting total cholesterol >200 mg/dL or an HDL cholesterol <40 mg/dL (see Chapter 15).

Estimation of VLDL cholesterol and *calculation of LDL cholesterol* are derived from measurements of total and HDL cholesterol levels and the triglyceride concentration using the following formula:

$$\text{LDL cholesterol} = \text{total cholesterol} - (\text{HDL cholesterol} + \text{triglyceride}/5)$$

The triglyceride/5 factor represents a close estimate of VLDL cholesterol and derives from the observation that VLDL cholesterol is usually 20% of the serum triglyceride value. The validity of this formula for estimating LDL cholesterol has been confirmed by direct LDL cholesterol measurement and remains fairly accurate so long as the total triglyceride is <400 mg/dL. A *fasting* sample is required for accurate results because chylomicrons appearing in the blood after a meal do not contain the same ratio of triglyceride to cholesterol found in VLDL. If the triglyceride level is >400 mg/dL, the LDL cholesterol can be determined accurately only by more sophisticated and expensive methods. These methods include immunologic and nuclear magnetic resonance quantitation of LDL, gel filtration techniques, and ultracentrifugation. The added cost of these measures generally argues against their routine use, but they can be useful in patients with elevated triglycerides or unusual clinical presentations.

Excluding Secondary Causes

Before embarking on a treatment plan, one must exclude conditions that might secondarily lead to hyperlipidemia. The most important are *hypothyroidism*, *nephrotic syndrome*, and *diabetes* (Table 27.3), which are best screened for by a serum thyroid-stimulating hormone, urine dipstick for protein, and serum glucose, respectively (see Chapters 93, 104, and 130). Drugs can affect lipid levels as well, with LDL elevations occurring with *thiazide* use and triglyceride levels rising with *beta-blockers*. Postmenopausal *estrogen replacement* lowers LDL and increases HDL and triglyceride. Antiviral protease

inhibitors used in the treatment of AIDS often cause hyperlipidemia as well.

Classification

The original *Fredrickson classification* scheme is of limited utility now that a better understanding of the genetics of these diseases has emerged. However, no unified classification of comparable simplicity has replaced it. For most clinical purposes, it is probably simplest to separate patients into three broad categories: those with *elevated cholesterol*, those with *elevated cholesterol and triglyceride*, and those with *elevated triglyceride* only. Table 27.3 summarizes the likely diagnoses under these broad categories. The possibility of a genetic disorder should be considered if extremes of any lipid level are encountered or if there is a history of premature CHD in the patient or family.

Risk Stratification

Risk stratification (Tables 27.4 and 27.5) can be of considerable help to both patient and physician, helping to provide an evidence-based rationale for choice and intensity of treatment. Benefit from treatment of hypercholesterolemia is closely linked to the degree of pretreatment CHD risk, making a careful assessment of that risk essential.

Role of Established CHD Risk Factors in Risk Stratification

The CHD risk assessment should be a comprehensive one, including but also extending beyond lipid levels to consideration of all major established risk factors, including *hypertension*, *smoking*, *diabetes*, *family history of premature CHD*, *age*, *sex*, and presence of *established CHD* or *other atherosclerotic disease* (e.g., peripheral arterial insufficiency, symptomatic carotid disease). Diabetes is increasingly recognized as a major risk factor for CHD events, nearly equivalent to established CHD. The appreciation for *elevated HDL cholesterol* as a factor in

TABLE 27.3

CLASSIFICATION OF LIPOPROTEIN DISORDERS

Name	Primary Disorder	Secondary Disorder	Lipoprotein Involved	Xanthomas
Increased Triglycerides and Cholesterol				
Combined hyperlipidemia	UNKNOWN	Hypothyroidism	DL and VLDL	None
Remnant hyperlipidemia	Familial dysbetal-ipoproteinemia	Hypothyroidism SLE	IDL	Tuberous, palmar, tuboeruptive
Increased Cholesterol				
Familial hypercholesterolemia	DL receptor defects		LDL	Tendon
Combined hyperlipidemia	Unknown	Hypothyroidism Nephrotic syndrome	LDL	
Polygenic hypercholesterolemia	Unknown	Hypothyroidism	LDL	
Familial hyperalphalipoproteinemia	Unknown		HDL	
Increased Triglycerides				
Exogenous hypertriglyceridemia Apo C-II deficiency	LPL deficiency			
PL inhibition	SLE	Chylomicrons	Tuboeruptive	
Endogenous hyperTG	Familial hyperTG	Diabetes Dysglobulinemia Uremia Nephrotic syndrome Lipodystrophies Steroids Alcohol Estrogen Hypothyroidism	VLDL	Usually none
Mixed hypertriglyceridemia	Familial hyperTG LPL deficiency Apo C-II deficiency	Same as for endogenous hyperTG	VLDL and chylomicrons	Tuboeruptive

Apo, apolipoprotein; hyperTG, hypertriglycidemia; IDL, intermediate-density lipoprotein; LDL, low-density lipoprotein; LPL, lipoprotein lipase; SLE, systemic lupus erythematosus; VLDL, very-low-density lipoprotein.

reducing CHD risk has led to its designation as a "negative risk factor"; conversely, a *low HDL cholesterol* has been added to the list of positive risk factors (Table 27.5).

A gradient of CHD risk has been defined by the NCEP expert panel, taking into account the degree of LDL elevation and the presence of other CHD risk factors (Tables 27.4 and 27.5). For a given elevation in LDL cholesterol level, patients considered at highest risk are those with established CHD or other atherosclerotic disease, as well as patients with diabetes mellitus. Next come patients without CHD or diabetes mellitus who have two or more CHD risk factors, followed by those having no CHD and fewer than two CHD risk factors.

TABLE 27.4

CORONARY HEART DISEASE (CHD) RISK ASSOCIATED WITH LIPOPROTEIN CHOLESTEROL ABNORMALITIES

Lipoprotein-Cholesterol	Level (mg/dL)	Estimated CHD Risk
LDL cholesterol	<130	Low
	130–159	Moderate
	≥160	High
HDL cholesterol	>65 (and total cholesterol/HDL ratio >4.5)	Low
	<35 (and total cholesterol/HDL ratio >4.5)	Moderate-high
VLDL cholesterol	50–100 (or fasting triglycerides 250–500)	Low
	>100 (or fasting triglycerides >500)	?

The presence of additional coronary heart disease risk factors greatly increases the risk for any level of lipoprotein cholesterol. HDL, high-density lipoprotein; LDL, low-density lipoprotein; VLDL, very-low-density lipoprotein.

TABLE 27.5

CORONARY HEART DISEASE RISK FACTORS AND CORONARY HEART DISEASE RISK STATUS

Risk Factors Other Than Elevated LDL Cholesterol Level

Age >45 yr for men; age >55 yr or premature menopause for women without estrogen replacement

Family history of premature CHD (definite myocardial infarction or sudden death in first-degree male relative before age 55 yr or before age 65 yr in female first-degree relative)

Current cigarette smoking

Hypertension (systolic >140 mm Hg or diastolic >90 mm Hg)

Low HDL cholesterol (<35 mg/dL)

Diabetes mellitus

CHD Risk Status (Highest to Lowest)

Clinically evident CHD or other atherosclerotic disease (peripheral arterial insufficiency, symptomatic carotid artery disease)

No CHD but two or more CHD risk factors in addition to hypercholesterolemia

No CHD and fewer than two other CHD risk factors in addition to hypercholesterolemia

No CHD, no risk factors

CHD, coronary heart disease; HDL, high-density lipoprotein; LDL, low-density lipoprotein.
Adapted from Summary of the Second Report of the National Cholesterol Education Program Expert Panel on Detection, Evaluation, and Treatment of High Blood Cholesterol in Adults. JAMA 1993;269:3015, with permission.

Other Risk Factors

Risk stratification by use of the established risk factors accounts for up to 80% of observed CHD risk. Efforts to identify other independent risk factors for CHD are ongoing.

Triglycerides. Elevations in triglycerides have long been suspected as a CHD risk factor, but only recently has evidence been accumulating to suggest an independent contribution to risk and not just an epiphenomenon of the metabolic syndrome and low HDL cholesterol. The degree of risk that is emerging is modest, which might account for the conflicting findings in the literature, but the most recent meta-analysis found the relative risk for CHD to be 1.7 when comparing persons in the top triglyceride quartile with those in the bottom one. Risk appears greatest in young persons, women, and those with diabetes.

C-Reactive Protein. C-reactive protein (CRP) (see also Chapter 15) is an acute-phase protein that is primarily produced in the liver in response to elevations in blood cytokines, such as interleukin-6 and tumor necrosis factor-α. The inflammatory nature of the developing atherosclerotic lesion provides a plausible link between production of activating cytokines in the atheroma and the generation of hepatically produced CRP. Although there are some studies that suggest that CRP may play a direct role in exacerbating atherosclerosis, this evidence is not yet compelling. At present, the link between CRP and atherosclerosis risk should be seen as associative rather than causal. This distinction means that a therapy that lowers CRP may well reflect an improvement in a patient's CHD risk, but that improvement is not due to the lower CRP level.

A substantial body of epidemiologic evidence supports CRP as an independent predictor of CHD events in both men and women. CRP has also been used as a prognostic indicator in patients presenting with both acute coronary syndromes and more stable, chronic coronary disease. In some subgroups (such as older women with intermediate CHD risk), the CRP level appears to be as predictive as LDL cholesterol, but overall the association between CHD risk and CRP elevation appears to be less pronounced than originally proposed (relative risk on the order of 1.5 vs. previous estimates of 2.0 to 2.5) and weaker than that for several of the more established CHD risk factors (e.g., LDL cholesterol, smoking history, hypertension). Moreover, a few large studies have challenged the value of using CRP levels when CHD risk is adjusted for the other established risk factors. There are no definitive data yet from long-term randomized clinical trials proving that lowering CRP reduces the risk of CHD events, nor is it clear how best to reduce CRP. Statin therapy can lead to reduced CRP levels, and studies with these drugs in patients with coronary disease have shown that the patients with the best CRP reductions have better cardiovascular outcomes than individuals with lesser CRP responses. Those outcomes appear to be independent of LDL lowering, with patients who have the greatest reductions in both LDL and CRP having the best outcomes.

The optimum use of a CRP level to determine cardiovascular risk is a matter of considerable debate, but its determination may be helpful in selective instances in which the results will change management of established treatable CHD risk factors (e.g., motivate the patient to make substantive lifestyle changes or trigger more-aggressive pharmacologic treatment of modifiable CHD risk factors). If CRP levels are determined, at least two values, obtained several weeks apart, should be measured using a reliable, *high-sensitivity assay*.

Homocysteine. Elevations in homocysteine (see also Chapter 15) appear to be associated with statistically significant but clinically modest increases in the risk of atherosclerotic events affecting the cerebral, peripheral, and coronary vessels. Early data suggesting a more powerful association with atherosclerosis and ability to reduce homocysteine levels with vitamin supplementation (*folate*, B_{12}, and B_6) led to a period of enthusiasm for screening and treating hyperhomocysteinemia, especially in persons with established CHD. However, prospective, randomized trials of vitamin supplementation failed to achieve any reduction in risk of CHD events, either in those with established CHD or as a primary preventive therapy. In some studies, paradoxical increases in CHD risk were observed. Therefore, routine measurement and treatment of homocysteine levels is not warranted at this time, but selective testing may be worth consideration (e.g., strong family history of CHD, premature onset of CHD, or CHD with no identifiable risk factors).

Genetic Risk Factors. Genetic risk factors are an area of active research, promising to help better explain the important family-history component of CHD risk. The literature should be watched for applications of this research to clinical practice.

PRINCIPLES OF MANAGEMENT (1,2,7,9,11,13,15,17,19–53)

Overall Approach

The goals are to reduce coronary morbidity and mortality. Both *primary prevention* (reducing the risk of having a first

TREATMENT RECOMMENDATIONS

Patient Category	Initial LDL Level (mg/dL)	LDL Goal (mg/dL)
Dietary Therapy		
No CHD, <2 risk factors	>160	<160
No CHD, >2 risk factors	>130	<130
With CHD	>100	<100
Add Drug Treatment		
No CHD, <2 risk factors	>190	<160
No CHD, >2 risk factors	>160	<130
With CHD	>130	<100

CHD, coronary heart disease; LDL, low-density lipoprotein.
Adapted from Summary of the Second Report of the National Cholesterol Education Program Expert Panel on Detection, Evaluation, and Treatment of High Blood Cholesterol in Adults. JAMA 1993;269:3015, with permission.

coronary event) and *secondary prevention* (reducing the risk of a new coronary event in a person with established CHD) are sought. The most impressive reductions in risk are achieved in patients at greatest risk (see later discussion), and the greatest reductions are being increasingly realized with *intensive lipid-lowering therapy* in such persons.

The growing appreciation of the importance of lipid abnormalities and the benefits of treating them stimulated the National Institutes of Health to sponsor the third formulation of the ATP III guidelines of the NCEP. Many of the treatment recommendations generated by that expert panel are included in what follows.

As noted earlier, the approach to the treatment of hyperlipidemia is guided by an *assessment of total CHD risk*, not just the lipid abnormality. For a given degree of LDL cholesterol elevation, the threshold for initiation of therapy decreases, and the intensity of therapy increases with increasing CHD risk.

The NCEP treatment recommendations follow directly from the degree of estimated CHD risk. Dietary modification is the sole mode of therapy for patients at the lower end of the CHD risk spectrum, whereas pharmacologic measures are reserved for patients at higher risk or for those who fail dietary intervention (Table 27.6). Additional considerations include possible adverse effects of long-term pharmacologic therapy (an issue when dealing with young persons) and appropriateness of the patient for treatment (an issue in the frail elderly and seriously ill). Dietary modification, complemented by exercise and weight reduction, is the core of the lipid treatment program, with pharmacologic therapy reserved for those at higher risk and for persons failing behavioral therapies.

Dietary Modification, Exercise, and Weight Loss

Dietary modification remains the cornerstone, effective for both treatment and prevention of hypercholesterolemia. As suggested by the Hegsted equation given earlier, the greatest contributor to hypercholesterolemia is the consumption of saturated fat, with excess cholesterol contributing to a lesser extent. *Reductions in total fat, saturated fat, partially hydrogenated unsaturated fatty acids,* and dietary *cholesterol* are

recommended for all adults. Because the benefits of reducing total fat are unproven, it is more critical that lipid-lowering diet plans *substitute* foods that provide *polyunsaturated and monounsaturated fats* for those rich in saturated and *trans* unsaturated fat.

In conjunction with *exercise* and *weight loss* (which contribute to reductions in lipid levels and ameliorate other cardiac risk factors), dietary modification provides an excellent nonpharmacologic means of improving the patient's lipid profile and reducing CHD risk. The adverse effects are nil, making it the safest of treatments for hypercholesterolemia and especially well suited for persons with only a modest increase in CHD risk (e.g., hypercholesterolemic young men and premenopausal women with no other CHD risk factors). Even for high-risk patients, dietary therapies are central to the treatment program, and almost always have an additive effect to pharmacologic treatments.

Efficacy

Decreases in intake of cholesterol and saturated fat in controlled settings can reduce total and LDL cholesterol by 15% to 30%, but the reductions average about 10% when similarly intensive dietary programs are prescribed for outpatient use. Substituting polyunsaturates and monounsaturates for saturated and unsaturated fats appear to be the most important steps in reducing CHD risk by dietary intervention. Data from the Nurses' Health Study provide the best available estimates of expected changes in CHD risk from various dietary substitutions:

- Substituting polyunsaturated fat for saturated fat: 42% *decrease* in CHD risk (for every 5% of total calories)
- Substituting polyunsaturated fat for *trans* unsaturated fat: 57% *decrease* in CHD risk (for every 2% of total calories)
- Substituting carbohydrate for saturated fat: 17% *decrease* in CHD risk
- Substituting carbohydrate for polyunsaturated fat and monounsaturated fat: 20% to 60% *increase* in CHD risk

Note that not all substitutions are beneficial. Simply substituting carbohydrate for all fat might not be the best dietary strategy for reducing CHD because beneficial polyunsaturates would also be eliminated as well.

The net effects of various dietary substitutions are related in part to their effects on CHD risk factors, including HDL cholesterol, LDL cholesterol, triglycerides, lipoproteins, and platelets and clotting factors. For example, substituting total fat intake with carbohydrate may produce a small (approximately 5%) reduction in HDL cholesterol, although the overall total-to-HDL cholesterol ratio typically still improves. Caloric and fat restrictions are also effective in lowering triglyceride levels, an effect enhanced by the prohibition of alcohol. Reductions in CHD risk parallel the degree of cholesterol lowering and reduction of other risk factors.

Response to dietary modification is determined to some extent by the etiology of the hypercholesterolemia. When the phase I diet (see later discussion) is prescribed for outpatient use in patients other than those with monogenic hypercholesterolemia, the total and LDL cholesterol levels fall by 5% to 15%, respectively. Typically, the total serum cholesterol level will fall to 140 to 160 mg/dL in normal individuals consuming a very-low-fat (5% to 10% of total calories) diet. More modest but still useful reductions can be expected from less stringent diets. In the setting of a metabolic ward study, there is wide variability in the magnitude of LDL cholesterol reductions achieved by lowering saturated fat intake, ranging from <5% to >50%.

TABLE 27.7

AMERICAN HEART ASSOCIATION THREE-PHASE DIETARY PLAN

	Average U.S. Diet	Phase I	Phase II	Phase III
Total fat (as % total calories)	40–45	30	25	20
Saturated	17	10	~6	~3
Monounsaturated	18	10	~9	~7
Polyunsaturated	7	10	~10	~10
Protein (as % total calories)	15–20	15	15	15
Carbohydrate (as % total calories)	40–45	55	60	65
Dietary cholesterol, mg	500	300	200–250	100–150

Patients with severe monogenic hypercholesterolemias rarely respond to diet alone, whereas other individuals consuming a high-fat diet may demonstrate marked benefit.

Phased Approach to Dietary Modification

The phased approach, as exemplified by the American Heart Association's three-phase dietary plan, maximizes adherence. Total fat, saturated fat, and cholesterol intake are gradually reduced with partial replacement by polyunsaturated fats (which by the Hegsted equation have a modest cholesterol-lowering effect). Excess dietary saturated and *trans* unsaturated fats are supplanted by the use of polyunsaturated and monounsaturated fats and by complex carbohydrates (fruits, vegetables, cereals, pasta, grains, and legumes).

Phase I Diet. Given the high prevalence of undesirable cholesterol levels in the U.S. population, it is recommended that all Americans adopt the phase I diet (Table 27.7):

- *Total fat* as a percentage of total calories is reduced to *30%* from an average 40% to 45%.
- *Saturated fat* is reduced to 10% of total calories.
- *Polyunsaturated fat* is increased to 10% of calories.
- *Dietary cholesterol intake* is reduced from 500 to 300 mg/d.
- *Protein* is held constant.
- The *omega-6 PUFAs* found in vegetable oils should not exceed 10% of calories because they may lower HDL cholesterol.

The phase I diet usually does not require a dramatic alteration in eating habits and can be readily adopted by most persons. It is important to note that much of the polyunsaturated fat found in "low-cholesterol, low-fat" processed food products is partially hydrogenated, converting otherwise beneficial vegetable oils into the undesirable *trans* unsaturated configuration. Such processed food products should not be considered a substitute for saturated fat, but neither should saturated fat be considered a healthier alternative to such products and trigger reverting back to lard-based or tropical oil–based processed foods.

Phase II Diet. The phase II diet (Table 27.7) entails more effort because it goes beyond eliminating the obvious sources of fat and cholesterol. It is indicated for patients who do not achieve adequate results with a phase I diet and for patients at highest CHD risk (e.g., established CHD).

If just the phase I dietary interventions were widely implemented, the overall incidence of CHD in the population would likely fall significantly. The recommended percentages of fat intake in the diet must be translated into real menus and food recommendations if good compliance with these recommendations is to be realized. The counsel of a dietitian is often benefi-

cial, particularly if a phase II diet is indicated. A good working knowledge of the fat content of common foods is essential for patient, family, and health care team (see Appendix 27.3). A number of "heart-healthy" cookbooks are on the market to help patients in their food choices and preparation. The use of faddish cholesterol cookbooks should be discouraged because these often do not promote sustainable healthy eating habits. Increasingly, restaurants are offering heart-healthy menu choices, and patients should be encouraged to select them.

Low-Carbohydrate Diets

The observation that high-carbohydrate intake can stimulate weight gain and raise triglyceride levels has led to interest in low-carbohydrate diets. Unfortunately, one of the more popular low-carbohydrate diets (i.e., the *Atkins diet*) substitutes liberal amounts of saturated fat for carbohydrates. Although short-term (6- to 12-month) studies of obese persons using such diets demonstrate weight loss, reduction in triglycerides, and improved glucose tolerance, there remain concerns about the long-term durability and cardiovascular safety of the low-carbohydrate/liberal–saturated fat approach. More studies are needed, including long-term term trials and examination of modest carbohydrate restriction in conjunction with limitations on saturated fat.

Nonprescription Dietary Supplements

Nonprescription dietary supplements are no substitute for dietary reduction in saturated fat and cholesterol. Nonetheless, they are popular with patients, even though they can be expensive. These include omega-3 fish oil tablets, "antioxidant" vitamins, and garlic and yeast preparations.

Omega-3 Fish Oils. Preliminary data from prospective studies of omega-3 fish oil supplements are encouraging, but they are too limited to serve as the basis for dietary recommendations. These fats can lower serum triglycerides, but they do not improve LDL or HDL cholesterol levels. Their effect on CHD risk could be secondary to effects on cardiac ion channels affecting sudden death or inflammatory signal transduction pathways rather than serum lipid levels. They can alter clotting; impairment of clotting has been noted with the use of high doses.

Antioxidant" Vitamins. Vitamins C, E, and β-carotene (the so-called "antioxidant vitamins") do not lower cholesterol levels, but they are capable of increasing LDL resistance to oxidative change and theoretically might reduce the risk of arterial wall injury. Early small-scale human studies and several large observational epidemiologic investigations of vitamin E suggested a possible reduction in CHD risk, but prospective, large-scale, randomized trials have failed to confirm a significant benefit; the same pertains to vitamin C. The typical dose of vitamin E used in these studies was 400 to 800 IU/d. A meta-analysis of vitamin E therapy indicated that doses of >400 IU/d are associated with higher all-cause mortality. There is no evidence that β-carotene reduces CHD events, and some data suggest an association with lung neoplasms. Based on current data, the use of antioxidant vitamins C, E, and β-carotene for the prevention of CHD is not recommended.

Garlic, Fiber, and Yeast Supplements.   One half to one clove of *garlic* a day may produce a modest (5%) reduction in serum cholesterol, but powder and oil preparations have not consistently demonstrated significant benefit. Use of fiber preparations such as *psyllium* (10 g/d) also provides modest benefit, as does the *soluble fiber* in oat-containing cereals. *Red yeast extracts* contain a cholesterol synthesis inhibitor that is a member of the statin family and can lower LDL 10% to 15%. Alcohols contained in sugar cane (policanosols) were initially reported to reduce LDL cholesterol by 20% to 30%, but a randomized trial of this therapy failed to confirm this effect.

Exercise and Weight Loss

ATP III emphasizes exercise and weight reduction as complements to dietary therapy and essential components of a comprehensive nonpharmacologic program. They are helpful not only in correcting lipid abnormalities, but also in reducing other CHD risk factors and total CHD risk. For example, exercise raises the level of HDL cholesterol, decreases blood pressure, and increases the efficiency of peripheral oxygen extraction (see Chapter 18). Weight loss efforts can lower fat intake, reduce the risk of diabetes mellitus, and decrease myocardial work.

Pharmacologic Therapy: Principles

Dietary modification is not uniformly effective in achieving target reductions in LDL cholesterol or desired increases in HDL cholesterol. Addition of drug therapy to a diet and exercise program should be considered in high-risk patients whose lipid abnormalities remain inadequately controlled despite intensive dietary efforts. Use of lipid-lowering therapy in patients at lower levels of risk has become increasingly common due to the publication of large-scale trials showing impressive reductions in CHD morbidity and mortality in patients without established coronary disease (i.e., primary prevention studies) and modest levels of hypercholesterolemia. Many lipid experts are treating more aggressively than is recommended by the ATP III guidelines, using outcomes studies published after the guidelines were generated to justify this approach.

Effectiveness and Safety

The addition of drug therapy to a diet and exercise program can greatly enhance lipid-lowering results and lead to significant reductions in *nonfatal* and *fatal cardiac events* (i.e., myocardial infarction, revascularization, cardiac death). Reductions in *all-cause mortality* have also been demonstrated in lipid-lowering drug trials, particularly in higher-risk populations. With intensive drug therapy, the rate of plaque progression falls, and modest *plaque regression* can be demonstrated in major coronary vessels and systemic arteries. There is evidence that lipid-lowering medication (statins) also can reduce the *risk of stroke* in persons with atherosclerotic carotid disease.

The reductions in CHD events noted in patients with established atherosclerotic disease (*secondary prevention*) who take statins are substantial; 30% to 40% reductions in coronary morbidity and mortality are commonly reported. In addi-

tion, benefit also accrues to persons with no clinical evidence of CHD and only moderate increases in nonlipid CHD risk factors, whose reductions in rates of fatal and nonfatal coronary events with use of pharmacologic therapy (*primary prevention*) are on the order of 20% to 30%.

An early concern about an increased risk of cancer and violent deaths with use of some lipid-lowering agents has failed to materialize in major prospective, randomized, placebo-controlled studies. In four of the largest such trials conducted, using several different members of the statin class of drugs and collectively involving tens of thousands of patients (the 4S-Scandinavian, West of Scotland, AFCAPS/TexCAPS, and LIPID studies), no increase in rates of cancer or noncardiac deaths were reproducibly observed. However, each class of drug therapies has important adverse effects that need to be taken into account when considering pharmacologic intervention (see later discussion). With the trend toward more aggressive lowering of LDL cholesterol comes an increase in risk of drug side effects as larger drug doses are prescribed.

Candidacy

The risk-to-benefit ratio for pharmacologic therapy appears to be most favorable in patients at greatest CHD risk and least favorable in those at lowest risk. Because most data derive from studies involving *middle-aged men* and *postmenopausal women* with *established CHD* or *multiple CHD risk factors*, one must often extrapolate to estimate effects in other populations. In the *elderly*, high CHD risk is common, and the benefit noted in high-risk, middle-aged patients has been found also to accrue to elderly persons at similar risk (Heart Protection Study). Treatment recommendations by NCEP are based on total CHD risk that includes lipid profile and associated cardiac risk factors.

For *young men* (age <35 years) and *premenopausal women* at *marked CHD risk* (e.g., LDL cholesterol >220 mg/dL, or potent CHD risk factors such as diabetes mellitus or strong family history of premature CHD), the potential gain from use of lipid-lowering medication almost certainly outweighs any speculative long-term risks. Early concerns over very-long-term use of statins, which formerly argued against treating younger individuals, have diminished. The first statin was approved more than 20 years ago; no evidence has emerged to suggest that chronic use leads to any unexpected adverse events. In women of childbearing age, the potential teratogenicity of statin therapy must always be kept in mind when prescribing that class of lipid-lowering agent. The exercise of good clinical judgment is essential in these circumstances.

Lower-risk young persons with no CHD risk factors other than hypercholesterolemia are best considered for nonpharmacologic therapy first because their short-term risk of CHD is quite low. Whether early initiation of LDL cholesterol–lowering therapies in such young individuals would be beneficial has not been tested, but persons with lifelong very low levels of LDL cholesterol due to genetic mutations in an LDL-receptor regulatory protein manifest a strikingly low rate of CHD.

Pharmacologic Therapy—Treatment Thresholds, Goals, and Monitoring

Treatment Thresholds

Current guidelines derive from the consensus views of the NCEP panel and, for the first time, reflect the data generated by the many lipid-lowering trials done in the mid to late 1990s.

For Those with Two or More CHD Risk Factors. The NCEP recommends initiating drug therapy if the *LDL cholesterol remains above 130 mg/dL* after lifestyle modifications have been made if the 10-year risk of a new CHD event is 10% to 20%. If two or more risk factors are present, but the 10-year risk probability is <10%, an LDL cut-point of 160 mg/dL is used. The 10-year risk probabilities are determined by a formula derived from Framingham Heart Study epidemiologic data. It is available at the National Heart Lung Blood Institute web page (http://www.nhlbi.nih.gov).

For Those with Fewer Than 2 CHD Risk Factors. Drug therapy is definitively recommended for *LDL cholesterol levels above 190 mg/dL* and considered optional for those with values between 160 and 190 mg/dL. More recent clinical trials have shown improved outcomes at even lower LDL cut-points, making the NCEP recommendations a relatively conservative guide to the initiation of lipid therapy.

For Those with Isolated Low HDL Cholesterol. Although epidemiologic data show a strong inverse relation between HDL level and CHD risk, there are no data yet from large-scale, randomized, prospective clinical trials showing that raising HDL cholesterol alone significantly reduces CHD mortality. However, treatment of patients with low HDL levels with statins does seem to lower CHD morbidity. Generally healthy middle-aged and elderly persons with low HDL cholesterol and "normal" LDL cholesterol demonstrate a significant reduction in the risk of a first acute major coronary event (e.g., myocardial infarction, unstable angina) when treated with a statin drug (e.g., the AFCAPS/TexCAPS trial). Such findings suggest that even persons with modest increases in CHD risk—as manifested by advancing age and an isolated low HDL cholesterol—might benefit from pharmacologic therapy. The mechanism of the benefit may be other than the effect on HDL cholesterol because in the AFCAPS/TexCAPS study, HDL cholesterol rose only 6%.

Effect of Threshold on Cost-Effectiveness. Lowering the threshold for drug therapy below that recommended by the new NCEP guidelines could be justified on the basis of recent outcome studies, but the cost-effectiveness of such an approach remains to be established. Because results are typically reported in terms of reduction in relative risk, the magnitude of the benefit to lower-risk patients may sometimes appear inflated. Absolute risk certainly becomes an issue in younger patient populations, in which a 20% to 30% reduction in relative risk may represent only a modest clinical achievement (i.e., if the absolute risk of having a CHD event over the next 10 years is only 2%, a 20% reduction results in the absolute risk falling to 1.6%).

Treatment Goals

The ultimate treatment goal is *reduction in CHD risk*; the immediate one is *reduction of LDL cholesterol*. Target levels have been lowered, reflecting the improvement in outcomes associated with lower lipid levels.

For Primary Prevention. For primary prevention (no established CHD), the NCEP target is an *LDL cholesterol level <130 mg/dL*, although ATP III now defines an optimal LDL as one that is *<100 mg/dL*, especially for persons at higher risk (see Recommendations).

For Secondary Prevention. For *secondary prevention* (established CHD), the goal in this high-risk group is an LDL cholesterol level *<100 mg/dL*, with some researchers recommending intensive lipid-lowering therapy to achieve a level of *<70 mg/dL*, particularly for persons at highest risk. In support of aggressive lipid lowering are data from trials of persons with stable CHD and LDL cholesterol of less than 130 mg/dL who demonstrate significant reductions in the risk of major CHD events, stroke, and hospitalization for heart failure when intensive lipid-lowering therapy is used to bring the LDL cholesterol down to *70 mg/dL*; however, no reductions in overall or CHD mortality were achieved in one such study, and aminotransferase elevations increased sixfold (from 0.2% to 1.2%). Debate over the utility of intensive lipid lowering to achieve an LDL cholesterol <70 mg/dL is ongoing; more data will be forthcoming and should help to inform the debate.

Use of Non-HDL Cholesterol as Treatment Goal. The latest NCEP guidelines introduced the concept of *elevated non-HDL cholesterol* levels. Non-HDL cholesterol is determined by subtracting the HDL cholesterol value from the total cholesterol value. Patients with high triglyceride levels will have elevations in their VLDL cholesterol, which in turn contributes to a higher non-HDL cholesterol level. For patients with high triglyceride levels ATP III suggests substituting a non-HDL cholesterol goal in place of the LDL cholesterol goal and setting the cut-point 30 mg/dL higher than the LDL cut point. This 30-point differential derives from the Friedewald formula, in which VLDL cholesterol is represented by the triglyceride value divided by 5 (i.e., 150/5 = 30). Thus, as the triglyceride level rises above 150 mg/dL, the VLDL contribution to the non-HDL cholesterol rises above 30 mg/ dL.

Pharmacologic Therapy—Available Agents

Design of a pharmacologic regimen must take into account the patient's degree of *CHD risk*, the nature of the *lipoprotein abnormality*, and a drugs' *mechanisms of action* and *side effects*. The best program is one that addresses and fits well into the patient's overall clinical state. A large degree of individualization is necessary. The range of available drugs is extensive, varying greatly in cost, effect on cholesterol fractions, efficacy, and side effects (Table 27.8).

3-Hydroxy-3-methylglutaryl Coenzyme A Reductase Inhibitors (Statins)

These agents have become first-line drug therapy because of their effectiveness, patient acceptability, and increasingly favorable safety record. They block the rate-limiting enzyme for cholesterol synthesis, 3-hydroxy-3-methylglutaryl coenzyme A reductase. This inhibition decreases intracellular cholesterol and increases *clearance of LDL*. Serum LDL levels fall by 20% to 60%, depending on dose and preparation. They reduce plaque progression and in some circumstances can even induce plaque regression. HDL levels generally stay the same or increase slightly (2% to 10%). Statins also influence thrombotic and inflammatory mechanisms, effects whose importance remains to be proven. These nonlipid effects of statins may account for some of the surprising CHD prevention efficacy seen in persons with lower LDL cholesterol levels (see later discussion).

Cost and Cost-Effectiveness. Cost and cost-effectiveness are important considerations in selecting statin therapy because

TABLE 27.8

DRUGS USED TO TREAT HYPERLIPIDEMIA

Name	Indications	Effects	Dose	Side Effects	Relative Cost (Starting Dose)[a]
Bile acid sequestrants	↑LDL	↓LDL;	8–24 g/d	Constipation, heartburn, bloating	14.2
Cholestyramine		↓or no change	10–30 g/d		12.3
Colestipol		HDL	1250–3,750 mg/d		
Colesevalam					
HMG-CoA reductase inhibitors	↑LDL	↓LDL; ↑ ↓VLDL (minor)		↑Transaminases; myositis	
Atorvastatin			10–80 mg/d		7.2
Fluvastatin			20–80 mg/d		4.8
Lovastatin[b]			20–80 mg/d		9.0
Pravastatin			20–80 mg/d		8.3
Simvastatin			10–80 mg/d		14.7
Rosuvastatin			5–40 mg/dL		
Niacin (nicotinic acid)	↑LDL; ↑VLDL ↓HDL	↓LDL; ↑HDL; ↓VLDL ↓VLDL; ↑HDL;	1.5–8 g/d	Flushing, pruritus, peptic ulcer disease, hyperglycemia, rashes ? + gallstones potentiates warfarin	1.0 4.3
Gemfibrozil	↑VLDL	↑LDL (if TG high)	600–1,200 mg/d		
Fenofibrate	↑VLDL		44–45 mg/d		
Fish oils (omega-3 fatty acids)	↑VLDL	↓VLDL; ↑↓LDL	? >2–3 g of omega-3 fatty acids/d	Platelet inhibition	0.5

HDL, high-density lipoprotein; HMG-CoA, 3-hydroxy-3-methylglutaryl coenzyme A; LDL, low-density lipoprotein; TG, triglycerides; VLDL, very-low-density lipoprotein.
[a]Initial dose.
[b]Cost is for the nongeneric formulation; the generic formulation should be considerably less expensive when it becomes available.

use is likely to be measured in years. Substantial reductions in cost of statin therapy have resulted from brand-name formulations coming off patent and becoming available generically, including *lovastatin, pravastatin,* and *simvastatin.* Ability to lower LDL cholesterol is another important consideration. *Simvastatin, atorvastatin,* and *rosuvastatin* give the greatest LDL cholesterol reduction at U.S. Food and Drug Administration (FDA)–approved dosing levels. Within this group of three, the rank order of LDL cholesterol–reducing activity is simvastatin < atorvastatin < rosuvastatin. LDL reductions of 50% to 65% can be achieved with these drugs.

Cost-effectiveness studies find that the cost savings from reduced rates of cardiac events, time lost from productive work, and premature death partly offset the cost of treatment, making even the cost of brand-name statins economically viable. Formal cost-effectiveness analyses of a nongeneric statin examined the cost per year of life gained and found that statin therapy was cost-effective in men and women over a broad spectrum of ages and cholesterol ranges. The cost per year of life gained was less than half of that for other cost-effective preventive measures such as mammography. With the advent of generic statins, the cost of effective lipid-lowering therapy has plummeted, making the argument for the cost-effectiveness of their use in treating moderate- and high-risk CHD patients even stronger.

Dosing. Starting dose is typically 5 to 20 mg/d, with the most potent drugs started at 5 or 10 mg/d. The maximum dose is currently 80 mg/d for lovastatin, simvastatin, fluvastatin, ator-

vastatin, and pravastatin. The maximum dose of rosuvastatin is 40 mg/d. The shorter-acting agents (e.g. lovastatin) are best taken at night, the time of peak cholesterol synthesis, but all drugs work satisfactorily even if taken once daily in the morning.

Adverse Effects. Asymptomatic *hepatocellular dysfunction* manifested by an increase in serum levels of hepatocellular enzymes (e.g., aspartate and alanine aminotransferases) is among the most common adverse effects. Incidence ranges from about 3% for any elevation to <1% for elevations greater than three times the upper limit of normal. All such increases are reversible with cessation of therapy, which should be considered when liver enzyme levels continue to rise or reach more than three times the upper limit of normal. Transaminase monitoring is strongly recommended, with initial measurements made after 1 to 2 months of therapy and follow-up measurements made at 6 months and 1 year. The lack of new onset of liver toxicity after 1 year of therapy has led many to advocate limited monitoring after 1 year. Although there are no formal guidelines for the use of statins in patients with baseline elevations of liver transaminases, several studies indicate that they can be used in this setting.

Harmless elevations in *muscle enzymes* (e.g., creatine phosphokinase <10 times the upper limit of normal) occur in about 0.6% of cases and require no action in an asymptomatic patient. Myalgias without creatine phosphokinase elevations also occur with statin use, making routine monitoring of creatine phosphokinase of limited value. Myalgias are probably underreported in patients on statins, particularly in the elderly, because the symptom is frequently attributed to arthritis or muscle stiffness associated with the aging process. Patients should be questioned about increased muscle discomfort when placed on statins, and drug holidays may need to be instituted to clarify complaints.

Symptomatic *myositis* with demonstrable muscle breakdown is much less common, but the risk is increased with high-dose therapy and when other lipid-lowering agents are used in conjunction with statin therapy. Statin monotherapy has been reported to cause *rhabdomyolysis* and renal failure, but it is more common in the setting of concurrent *gemfibrozil* use. Dual therapy with niacin can also increase myositis. Joint use of a statin and a fibrate (either gemfibrozil or fenofibrate) should be done only with great caution and probably only by a lipid specialist. Because of an FDA warning against this combination, pharmacists will often not fill a prescription that places a patient on both drugs without first calling the physician. The voluntary withdrawal of cerivastatin from the market in 2001 was prompted by reports of rhabdomyolysis when the drug was used alone or, more commonly, in combination with a fibrate. This event will likely increase the vigilance of pharmacists in responding to combination therapy prescriptions.

As noted earlier, initial concerns about an increase in non-CHD mortality (e.g., from cancer, suicide, or violence) were raised by early meta-analyses, but large-scale prospective studies of statins show no evidence for such adverse effects.

Choice of Agent. Most lipid experts believe that all of the statins will reduce coronary events in proportion to their efficacy in lowering LDL cholesterol, but not all statins have been proven to do so. The best studies of effect on important clinical outcomes (e.g., nonfatal myocardial infarction, cardiac death) have been performed using simvastatin, pravastatin, lovastatin, and atorvastatin; rosuvastatin has been found to reduce atheroma volume in both carotid and coronary arteries, suggesting that it too would lower cardiovascular event rates. Statins not only reduce coronary events, but also lower all-cause mortality. Patients who require modest reductions in LDL cholesterol (≤25%) can be started on any of the statins with the expectation that the reduction will be achieved. Those with marked LDL elevations and high overall CHD risk require more intensive therapy (>40% reductions), which is best carried out by using one of the more potent statins discussed earlier.

In the setting of *acute coronary syndromes* (e.g., new onset of myocardial infarction or unstable angina), studies comparing high-dose atorvastatin (80 mg/d) to either moderate-dose pravastatin (40 mg/d; PROVE-IT trial) or placebo (MIRACL trial) revealed significant reductions in subsequent coronary events for the atorvastatin patients when treated shortly after hospital admission. Higher-dose simvastatin applied in a similar situation failed to demonstrate a comparable early benefit, but differences in patient populations (atorvastatin patients were much more likely to have had angioplasty prior to the statin therapy) may have accounted for some of the observed differences. Nonetheless, high-dose atorvastatin (80 mg/d) is currently favored by many in the setting of an acute coronary syndrome admission. Further study is needed to see whether benefit accrues with the use of other statins at high doses in the acute coronary syndrome setting.

Niacin

This inexpensive, first-line agent contributes to dyslipidemia therapy by virtue of its unique ability to markedly *raise HDL cholesterol* (on the order of 15% to 35%), as well as *lower LDL cholesterol* (by 5% to 25%), converting small LDL cholesterol particles to more buoyant, less atherogenic forms. Niacin also *lowers triglycerides* (by 20% to 50%). Its exact mechanism of action is unknown, although the recent discovery of the niacin receptor should help to elucidate it. Mobilization of free fatty acids from fat tissue to the liver appears to be inhibited.

In the Coronary Drug Project involving high-risk persons (e.g., prior myocardial infarction), niacin produced significant reductions in new myocardial infarction (26%), stroke (24%), and death (11%). In addition, reduction in all-cause mortality appears to result from use in patients with established CHD. In *combination* with *colestipol* or a *statin*, it can slow or reverse progression of atheromatous plaque in coronary arteries. Although effective, niacin therapy often requires high doses (1.5 to 3.0 g/d) to attain the desired results. Use in combination with a statin (which can also raise HDL cholesterol) may allow for somewhat lower doses.

Adverse Effects. The most bothersome and limiting side effect is acute prostaglandin-mediated vasodilation leading to *flushing* and sometimes *lightheadedness*. Vasodilation is a consequence of a high-capacity early route of niacin metabolism that involves conjugation with glycine to produce nicotinuric acid, which triggers the prostaglandin-mediated vasodilation. Tolerance to flushing develops over time and allows slow advancement of dose. The annoying side effect can also be lessened by starting with a low dose (e.g., 100 mg three times daily), using an extended-release preparation (see later discussion), taking once-daily pretreatment with a nonsteroidal antiinflammatory drug (e.g., aspirin 325 mg or ibuprofen 200 mg, 30 to 60 minutes before first dose), and taking niacin with meals.

Hepatotoxicity is the other major concern, related to nonconjugative metabolism of the drug to nicotinamide and pyrimidines. Risk of hepatotoxicity is greatest with the use of *sustained-release* preparations (18 to 24 hours' duration), which are metabolized predominantly by the nonconjugative route. Risk is minimized by taking an intermediate-release formulation (8 to 10 hours' duration), which optimizes metabolism through both pathways. Periodic monitoring of liver function (e.g., aspartate aminotransferase determination) is required with niacin use. Other adverse effects include exacerbation of *gout* and slight worsening of *glucose intolerance*, necessitating an occasional check of uric acid and glucose. *Rashes*, *dry skin*, and occasionally *acanthosis nigricans* may accompany niacin use. Lanolin cream helps the former, and prompt cessation clears the latter. Some patients experience gastrointestinal upset.

Preparations. As a B-complex vitamin (nicotinic acid), niacin is available without prescription in *immediate-release* and *sustained-release* forms. Although least costly, these are associated with the highest frequency of flushing and hepatotoxicity, respectively. A prescription is required for the *intermediate-release* preparation (also referred to as "*extended-release*" niacin [e.g., *Niaspan*]), which is the best tolerated but most expensive formulation. Its use should be considered in persons who cannot tolerate the immediate-release preparation or in whom there is concern about risk of hepatoxicity. If an inexpensive, well-tolerated, immediate-release brand of niacin is found, the patient should stay with it; changing brands might not be as well tolerated. A formulation that incorporates a prostaglandin inhibitor with niacin is under development; if it proves safe and effective, it could mitigate the flushing problem.

Bile Acid Sequestrants (Cholestyramine, Colestipol, Colesevelam)

These nonabsorbable agents have been first-line pharmacologic therapy for many years, with an established record of safety. They are very useful for patients who are not at great CHD risk but in whom diet alone fails to lower LDL cholesterol to target levels. They are also of benefit in individuals who are statin intolerant. Although not as cost-effective as the statins or niacin, they are very effective when used in combination with them to treat high-risk patients with severe hypercholesterolemia. The sequestrants bind bile acids in the gut and interrupt their normal enterohepatic circulation. The resultant shunting of cholesterol in the liver to bile acid production leads to a fall in total and LDL cholesterol levels. However, triglyceride levels often rise with this class of drugs, particularly if moderate hypertriglyceridemia antedates the initiation of the therapy. Cholestyramine and colestipol are prescribed as powders that are dissolved in liquid. Colesevelam, which comes as a 625-mg pill, also binds biliary lipids in the gastrointestinal tract and has comparable effects on the serum cholesterol. Ezetimibe (see later discussion) has largely supplanted the use of the bile acid resins as cholesterol absorption inhibitors. There are insufficient data to know whether the resins would contribute to additional LDL lowering if added to ezetimibe, although some small-scale studies report a benefit.

Adverse Effects. The bile sequestrants are nonabsorbable resins whose major *side effects* are gastrointestinal—*constipation, bloating, heartburn,* and *nausea.* A high-fiber diet or psyllium supplement and use of these agents just before a meal will usually ameliorate the gastrointestinal upset. The potential to *impede absorption of certain drugs* (e.g., digoxin, thyroxin, warfarin, tetracycline, phenobarbital) necessitates that bile sequestrants not be taken until at least 1 hour after or 4 hours before these other drugs. In rare instances, steatorrhea and malabsorption of the fat-soluble vitamins (A, D, E, and K) can occur. The usual starting dose is one scoop of the powdered form of the drug (4 g of cholestyramine, 5 g of colestipol) in a large glass of water twice a day. Dose can be increased to a total of three scoops twice daily. A newer formulation of cholestyramine, which is significantly less gritty (Lo-Cholest), can be tried if the texture of the generic drug formulation should prove unacceptable. Colesevelam is given as six 625-mg tablets a day, given in once- or twice-a-day dosing.

Ezetimibe (Zetia)

Like the bile acid sequestrants, ezetimibe blocks cholesterol absorption from the gut. Unlike the sequestrants, it appears to inhibit cholesterol transport by interfering with a specific transporter protein required for this activity, rather than interfering with micellar solubilization of lipid. This difference permits ezetimibe to be given in milligram rather than gram doses, and it does not interfere with the absorption of other drugs and fat-soluble vitamins. The ease of use and tolerability of ezetimibe has led to its use in many of the same circumstances in which bile acid sequestrants were formerly used. As a single agent, ezetimibe lowers LDL cholesterol 15% to 20%. When used in conjunction with a statin, it typically provides an additional 15% reduction in the LDL cholesterol level, resulting in LDL cholesterol lowering that can exceed that achieved with the highest dose of any single statin.

Preparations. Ezetimibe is available as a brand-name agent (Zetia) and in multiple fixed-dose *combinations* with *simvastatin* (Vytorin). Although the simvastatin is a generic agent, the combination with ezetimibe results in this preparation carrying a brand-name cost. An unconfirmed increase in cardiovascular risk has been observed in patients taking this combination during a research study.

Fibrates (Gemfibrozil and Fenofibrate)

Because these drugs lower LDL cholesterol much less effectively than the statins, they are not considered first-line drugs for the treatment of hypercholesterolemia. Nonetheless, they do have specific uses. They *decrease VLDL* synthesis and enhance its clearance. They also *raise HDL cholesterol,* most prominently in patients who have concomitant *triglyceride elevations.* The effect on LDL cholesterol is variable, although an 8% to 15% reduction can be seen in patients who do not have markedly elevated VLDL levels. Both fibrate agents are generally well tolerated, but they can increase bile cholesterol content, raising the risk of gallstone formation and potentiating the effect of warfarin. The FDA has issued a warning about their use in *combination with statins* because *rhabdomyolysis* has occurred when gemfibrozil and a statin are used concurrently. An earlier drug in this class, clofibrate, was taken off the market because of reports of *increased mortality* associated with its use. Although the FDA has approved both fibrates, these agents have yet to demonstrate a reduction in all-cause mortality when used to treat patients with CHD. Although an often-quoted Veteran's Administration hospital gemfibrozil study of men with low HDL cholesterol did show improvement in coronary outcomes, fibrates are used in treating lipid disorders primarily to lower triglyceride values that are high enough (>500 mg/dl) to put the patient at risk for pancreatitis.

Cholesterol Ester Transfer Protein (CEPT) Inhibitors

CEPT inhibitors are under active study as treatment for raising HDL cholesterol in persons with low levels. The first drug in this class, torcetrapib, was effective in significantly raising HDL cholesterol, but also increased blood pressure and failed to halt disease progression. More research is needed to determine whether this adverse effect is drug specific or associated with all CEPT agents.

Agents of No Proven Benefit in Lowering CHD Risk

In postmenopausal women, *estrogen replacement therapy* is effective in lowering LDL cholesterol and raising HDL cholesterol. Major retrospective epidemiologic studies suggested a lowering of CHD risk with estrogen or estrogen/progestin use; for a time, hormone replacement therapy was popular for CHD prophylaxis in postmenopausal women. However, several large-scale, prospective, randomized trials of estrogen or estrogen/progestin failed to confirm any benefit in postmenopausal women in reducing cardiovascular morbidity or mortality; in the Women's Health Initiative study, slight increases in nonfatal myocardial infarction and death were noted, particularly in older women taking combination therapy. The estrogen-only arm of the same trial was terminated in 2004, again with no benefit on CHD morbidity or mortality detected, but, unlike the dual-hormone-therapy treatment, no increase in CHD was found. Consequently, despite the beneficial impact on serum lipids, hormone replacement therapy can no longer be recommended as a standard therapy for the prevention of CHD. A possible role in the treatment of incapacitating menopausal symptoms remains (see Chapter 118).

Policosanol, a mixture of very-long-chain aliphatic alcohols purified from sugar cane wax (whose main component is octacosanol), is promoted as a "natural substance" for lowering LDL cholesterol. Well-designed, placebo-controlled trials of both standard and high doses failed to demonstrate benefit in lowering LDL cholesterol.

Monitoring

Measurement of the LDL cholesterol level, beginning about 6 to 8 weeks after initiation of therapy and then every 3 to 4 months until control is established, represents the principal approach to monitoring treatment efficacy. Afterward, every 6 to 12 months is usually sufficient. More frequent monitoring for the development of abnormalities in serum chemistries (e.g., liver enzymes) may be indicated when using certain pharmacologic agents such as statins and niacin (see earlier discussion).

Treatment in the Elderly

The prevalence of hypercholesterolemia is greatest in those >65 years of age. As in other age groups, elevations in total and LDL cholesterol predict increased cardiovascular risk. However, the statistical risk relationship is not as strong as in younger patients, due in part to the frequent occurrence of other important risk factors in the elderly (e.g., diabetes, hypertension). Despite the modestly lower relative CHD risk of an elevated LDL cholesterol in an older patient, the absolute or attributable risk of an elevated LDL level is higher because CHD prevalence is substantially greater in the elderly. Thus, the benefit of lowering LDL levels in the elderly can have an even greater effect on outcomes than it does in younger patients. Several factors favor treatment. Life expectancy continues to lengthen, and the quality of life in the elderly also has steadily improved.

Treating individuals in their late 60s and 70s with statins has been shown to reduce CHD and stroke, two of the major causes of mortality in that age group. With the advent of better-tolerated cholesterol-lowering medications, the risks of adverse effects and their negative effect on quality of life have declined. Although many elderly patients may have other advanced diseases that make CHD prevention appear to be irrelevant, those who are vigorous and have a considerable life expectancy can benefit substantially from lipid-lowering therapies for the primary and secondary prevention of CHD.

Dietary Measures

Dietary therapy of hypercholesterolemia in the elderly is similar to that for all adults and should be carried out as the first step in treatment, although dietary measures do not always suffice by themselves. *Carbohydrate* should not replace most *fat* in the diet; instead, *polyunsaturates* and *monounsaturates* should be increased moderately, keeping the *omega-6 polyunsaturated fatty acids* found in vegetable oils below 10% of calories. For the elderly, modifications of the usual low-saturated-fat diet are needed to ensure adequate calcium intake for prevention of osteoporosis. Use of skim milk and low-fat and nonfat yogurts are examples of ways to maintain *calcium* intake while cutting down on saturated fat. Maintaining adequate *protein* intake is also essential, which means that lean cuts of red meat should be allowed in addition to fish and skinless chicken to ensure palatability of the diet. *High fiber* is essential for good bowel function and cannot hurt the cholesterol-lowering effort.

Pharmacologic Therapy

Because dietary therapy alone frequently fails to achieve the goal of LDL cholesterol <130 mg/dL, drug treatment must often be considered.

Statin therapy is indicated when aggressive lowering of LDL cholesterol is needed. The statins have also proven to be useful for primary prevention in elderly persons with low HDL cholesterol and average LDL cholesterol. These drugs are well tolerated in the elderly, with minor diarrhea, myalgias, and occasional sleep disturbances being the most common problems. Minor transaminase elevations are common; they are usually asymptomatic and not a cause for discontinuation unless they exceed three times normal. However, regular transaminase monitoring is required throughout the course of therapy. As noted earlier, initial concerns about an increased risk of malignancy have been proven to be unfounded in large-scale, prospective, long-term follow-up studies. Statins are recommended as first-line drug therapy for hypercholesterolemia in the elderly.

The *bile sequestrants* are safe but can cause considerable gastrointestinal upset, especially constipation. Increasing dietary fiber helps. Because sequestrants can impair drug absorption, their use in elderly patients must include instruction to take other medications at least 1 hour before or 4 hours after sequestrant use. Among the drugs that might be affected by sequestrants are warfarin, propranolol, digitalis preparations, thyroxin, and antibiotics. Although low-dose sequestrants are a reasonable choice for pharmacologic therapy, the availability of ezetimibe has provided a better-tolerated alternative to statins.

Niacin is effective, although not always well tolerated. Its advantages over statins are its ability to also raise HDL cholesterol and its low cost. The incidence of side effects in the elderly is high, with flushing, gastrointestinal upset, dry mouth, and dry eyes being particularly annoying. The drug may exacerbate peptic ulcer disease, elevate transaminases, and trigger arrhythmias and hypotension. Multiple daily doses are usually required if the nonprescription forms are used. The once-daily formulation of niacin, Niaspan, has some distinct advantages, but is associated with a higher cost than the nonprescription formulations.

PATIENT EDUCATION

Diet and Exercise

The importance of patient education in the management of hyperlipidemia cannot be overemphasized because treatment starts with alterations in the patient's eating and exercise habits (see Chapters 18 and 233). The first step in therapy should be a careful review of the rationale for treating hypercholesterolemia, followed by a discussion of basic dietary principles for lowering cholesterol. Consultation with a dietitian can be very helpful. Many patients are surprised to learn that dietary fat is more atherogenic than dietary cholesterol (witness the patient who eats cholesterol-free potato chips with abandon). Reviewing the saturated fat and *trans* fat content of foods regularly consumed by the patient is quite worthwhile. At times, simply removing a few grossly offending foods from the diet (e.g., processed snack foods, cheese, grossly fatty meats, cold cuts, fried food) ensures a good start to a change in eating habits. More comprehensive diet planning can be aided by discussion with the nurse or dietitian, facilitated by written material such as those produced by the American Heart Association. Periodic visits to check diet, weight, and cholesterol are excellent, although often overlooked, means of facilitating compliance and providing reinforcement.

Regarding Medications

Patients need to understand the rationale for their medical program and the details of its proper use and side effects. Some mistakenly believe their drug program is curative and stop treatment after a few months of therapy. Others harbor exaggerated concerns about adverse drug effects and stop medication prematurely. Cost is another factor that often limits compliance, necessitating a strategy that takes into account the patient's insurance coverage for medication. However, careful studies find that the adequacy of insurance does not by itself explain the nearly 40% fall-off in compliance that occurs over 5 years among patients prescribed lipid-lowering medication. Choice of agent, comorbidity, and socioeconomic status also play important roles, underscoring the importance of comprehensive and ongoing patient education.

INDICATIONS FOR REFERRAL

To the Dietician

Patients prescribed a dietary program should have a consultation with a dietitian if they are unclear about the food choices they should make or if compliance with the diet is problematic. Dieticians can provide educational materials, food preparation advice, and the periodic feedback that patients often need permanently to change their eating habits.

To the Lipid Specialist

Patients with high-risk lipid profiles who do not respond to diet plus one or two first-line drugs and those with extremes of any lipoprotein level or a family history of premature coronary disease (before age 55 years) should be considered for referral to a physician expert in diagnosis and treatment of lipid disorders. Some genetic disorders are particularly refractory to standard therapies, and patients with these conditions will benefit from consideration of genetic links and more complex treatment regimens that are the province of a lipid specialist. Identification of affected family members can also be accomplished. Lipid research laboratories can often categorize specific genetic abnormalities through testing not routinely available in most clinical laboratories. Ultracentrifugation of lipoproteins, polymerase chain reaction amplification of DNA, and cell-based receptor and enzymatic assays can be used to help pinpoint the cause and screen other family members for the problem. Although these more sophisticated tests may not yet translate into different therapeutic options, they often help to clarify family questions about the risks of CHD in related individuals and are likely to influence therapeutic options in the years ahead.

THERAPEUTIC RECOMMENDATIONS (17,27)

Effective reduction of CHD risk requires identifying and aggressively treating all CHD risk factors responsive to medical intervention, including smoking, hypertension, diabetes, and obesity (see Chapters 26, 54, 102, and 233). Focusing on hyperlipidemia alone is insufficient. In treating hypercholesterolemia, one should determine total CHD risk (Tables 27.4 and 27.5) and treat accordingly (Table 27.6).

High Risk (Established CHD, Diabetes Mellitus, or Other CHD Equivalent; LDL Cholesterol 160 mg/dL plus Two CHD Risk Factors, or LDL Cholesterol Greater Than 190 mg/dL and No Other CHD Risk Factors)

- Start with dietary restriction of total fat intake to no more than 20% of calories, substituting polyunsaturated and monounsaturated fats for saturated fat, partially hydrogenated unsaturated fat, and cholesterol. Highly motivated individuals may avoid the need for lifelong medication by strict adherence to phase II or phase III dietary programs, achieving LDL reductions of 40 to 80 mg/dL. Allow 4 to 6 months for implementation of dietary lifestyle changes. Even if dietary change does not bring LDL cholesterol down to desired levels, diet will enhance the effect from lipid-lowering therapy.

- Initiate pharmacologic therapy if goals for LDL cholesterol reduction have not been met by diet alone. For most patients, a statin preparation is the drug of first choice.

- Minimize the cost of statin therapy by matching statin preparation with degree of LDL cholesterol reduction needed. For example, if an LDL cholesterol reduction of >35% is required, consider starting simvastatin 20 mg/d (see earlier discussion); if an LDL cholesterol reduction of <35% is needed, then almost all of the statins can be used, and one of the generic statins (lovastatin, pravastatin, simvastatin) is likely to be most cost-effective.

- Consider niacin (average dose, 1.5 to 3.0 g/d) as an alternative choice, if LDL cholesterol elevation is accompanied by low HDL cholesterol (<40 mg/dL).

- Consider adding a second agent in patients with high CHD risk who fail adequately to respond to diet plus maximal doses of a single agent. The bile resins (e.g., cholestyramine or colestipol, one to two scoops twice daily) or ezetimibe are well suited to combination programs. One should generally avoid the combination of a statin plus gemfibrozil because of the increased risk of rhabdomyolysis and the combination of a statin plus full doses of niacin because of increased risk of myositis.

- Consider an LDL cholesterol goal of <70 mg/dL for those with at highest risk (established CHD, diabetes mellitus, or other CHD equivalents); aim for an LDL cholesterol of <100 mg/dL for all patients in the high-risk category, with the exception of those with no other CHD risk factors besides markedly elevated LDL cholesterol, for whom the goal is an LDL cholesterol of <130 mg/dL.

Moderate Risk (LDL Cholesterol 130 to 159 mg/dL plus Two CHD Risk Factors or LDL Cholesterol 160 to 189 mg/dL and No Other CHD Risk Factors)

- Begin with dietary therapy. In patients with large intakes of saturated fat and cholesterol, the phase I diet can produce sufficient reductions in cholesterol of 20 to 40 mg/dL. More aggressive dietary fat restriction (phase II diet) may be needed in those who do not respond adequately. PUFAs should be increased moderately but to no more than 10% of total calories. The minimum goal is a reduction of LDL cholesterol to <130 mg/dL in patients with two or more

CHD risk factors and to well <160 mg/dL in those with fewer than two risk factors.

- Drug therapy to lower LDL cholesterol can be considered in patients who fail to respond to lifestyle changes and continue to have an LDL cholesterol >160 mg/dL; the benefit of such an approach has been demonstrated in statin trials, but the cost-effectiveness remains to be established.

Modest Risk (Isolated Low HDL Cholesterol [<40 mg/dL]; LDL Cholesterol Not Elevated)

- Prescribe nonpharmacologic measures that can increase HDL cholesterol, including aerobic exercise, smoking cessation, and weight loss if obese. Such actions can increase HDL by 5 to 15 mg/dL.
- Prescribe a phase I diet, in which saturated fat, cholesterol, and partially hydrogenated vegetable oils are restricted and replaced by monounsaturated and polyunsaturated fats.
- Use clinical judgment in considering pharmacologic treatment if nonpharmacologic measures prove to be insufficient.
- Although the NCEP does not yet recommend pharmacologic correction of an isolated HDL cholesterol, pay attention to total CHD risk. In patients with multiple cardiac risk factors and a low HDL cholesterol, consider statin therapy for middle-aged and elderly persons; consider niacin as an additional option, especially for younger persons who tolerate the drug better than do the elderly; and always take into account HDL cholesterol level when designing a pharmacologic program for persons with LDL cholesterol elevation.

Elevation in Triglycerides (Fasting Triglycerides >200 mg/dL)

Patients with Isolated Elevation in Triglycerides (+/− Low HDL Cholesterol)

- Because no consensus exists on the need for treatment, exercise clinical judgment.
- Begin with a program of lifestyle modification (lowering caloric intake, increasing exercise).

- Consider adding fibrate pharmacologic treatment (e.g., gemfibrozil, 600 mg twice daily, or fenofibrate, 48 to 145 mg/d) in patients with a concomitantly low HDL cholesterol (<40 mg/dL).
- Keep in mind that evidence for the efficacy of lowering CHD risk with the use of triglyceride-lowering therapy is modest; avoid using a fibrate in conjunction with a statin (increased risk of rhabdomyolysis).
- Fibrates do have an established role in reducing the risk of pancreatitis in persons with isolated very high triglyceride levels (>500 to 800 mg/dL).
- Substitute a non-HDL cholesterol level as the goal in place of the LDL cholesterol, setting the cut-point 30 mg/dL higher than the LDL cut point.

Patients with Concomitantly Low HDL-Cholesterol and Elevated LDL-Cholesterol

- Prescribe lifestyle modifications of diet and exercise.
- Begin an aggressive lipid-lowering program with a statin program, possibly in conjunction with niacin; the combination of a statin plus niacin is particularly effective in lowering CHD risk in such patients.

All Patients

- Emphasize the importance of lifestyle changes in diet and exercise.
- Fully explain the condition and the rationale for the treatment program to ensure compliance; reemphasize the importance of dietary modification, exercise, and compliance with any drug program that might be necessary. Customize the patient-education and treatment programs to the needs and capabilities of the patient.
- Address patient concerns, especially those regarding the long-term use of lipid-lowering medications or dietary modifications. Enlist the services of a dietician if there are concerns or questions regarding dietary changes.
- Consider for referral to a lipid specialist patients with high-risk lipid profiles who do not respond to diet plus one or two first-line drugs, those with extremes of any lipoprotein level, or a family history of premature coronary disease (before age 55 years).

Annotated Bibliography

1. Ashen MD. Blumenthal RS. Low HDL cholesterol levels. N Engl J Med 2005;353:1252. (*A useful clinical review including treatment options; 52 references.*)
2. Brunzell JD. Hypertriglyceridemia. N Engl J Med 2007;357:1009. (*A review of the value of, and options for, lowering elevated serum triglycerides.*)
3. Criqui MH, Heiss G, Cohn R, et al. Plasma triglyceride level and mortality from coronary heart disease. N Engl J Med 1993;328:1220. (*No independent association with risk for coronary heart disease [CHD] was found, but a relation to low high-density lipoprotein [HDL]was noted.*)
4. Criqui MH. Triglycerides and coronary heart disease revisited (again). Ann Intern Med 2007;147:425. (*An editorial reviewing the evidence for the role of triglycerides in CHD risk and the benefit of treating elevations.*)
5. Danesh J, Wheeler J, Hirschfield G, et al. C-reactive protein and other circulating markers of inflammation in the prediction of coronary heart disease. N Engl J Med 2004;350:1387. (*Data suggesting that the degree of risk is less than originally suspected.*)
6. Eikelboom JW, Lonn E, Genest J Jr, et al. Homocyst(e)ine and cardiovascular disease: a critical review of the epidemiologic evidence. Ann Intern Med 1999;131:363. (*A systematic review finding strong epidemiologic evidence for an association, but no proof that treatment lowers CHD risk.*)
7. Heart Protection Study Collaborative Group. MRC/BHF Heart Protection Study of cholesterol-lowering with simvastatin in 5963 people with diabetes:

a randomized placebo-controlled trial. Lancet 2003;361:2005. (*Establishes the benefit of lipid lowering in diabetics and underscores the contribution of diabetes to CHD risk.*)
8. Hu FB, Stampfer MJ, Manson JE, et al. Dietary fat intake and the risk of coronary heart disease in women. N Engl J Med 1997;337:1491. (*Major prospective epidemiologic study found that replacing saturated and transunsaturated fats with polyunsaturated fat produced a greater reduction in coronary disease risk than did reducing overall fat intake.*)
9. Jenkins DJA, Uolever TMS, Venketshwer R, et al. Effect on blood lipids of very high intakes of fiber in diets low in saturated fat and cholesterol. N Engl J Med 1993;329:21. (*Foods rich in soluble fiber can lower cholesterol.*)
10. Klag KJ, Ford DE, Mead LA, et al. Serum cholesterol in young men and subsequent cardiovascular disease. N Engl J Med 1993;328:313. (*Strong association found between serum cholesterol level in early life and CHD in midlife.*)
11. Mensink RP, Katan M. Effect of dietary trans fatty acids on high-density and low-density lipoprotein cholesterol levels in healthy subjects. N Engl J Med 1991;323:439. (*Partially hydrogenated unsaturated fatty acids of processed foods were found to promote undesirable lipid levels as much as or more than the saturated fatty acids they were intended to replace.*)
12. Nygard O, Nordrehaug JE, Refsum H, et al. Plasma homocysteine levels and mortality in patients with coronary artery disease. N Engl J Med

1997;337:230. (*Original epidemiologic data suggesting that homocysteine elevation is an independent predictor of CHD mortality.*)

13. Ridker PM, Cannon CP, Morrow D, et al. C-reactive protein levels and outcomes after statin therapy. N Engl J Med 2005;352:20. (*Outcomes were better in persons who experienced reductions in C-reactive protein [CRP] with statin therapy.*)

14. Ridker PM, Rifai N, Rose L, et al. Comparison of C-reactive protein and low-density lipoprotein cholesterol levels in the prediction of first cardiovascular events. N Engl J Med 2002;347:1557. (*Evidence that CRP is an independent risk factor, possibly of the same magnitude as that for LDL cholesterol; see also ref. 5.*)

15. The Lipid Research Clinics Coronary Primary Prevention Trial results. I. Reduction in incidence of coronary heart disease. JAMA1984;251:351,365. (*Two classic papers from a landmark study establishing the effect of lipid lowering on CHD risk.*)

16. Tirosh A, Rudich A, Shochat T, et al. Changes in triglyceride levels and risk for coronary heart disease in young men. Ann Intern Med 2007;147:377. (*Cohort observational study found a decrease in triglyceride levels associated with a reduction in CHD risk.*)

17. Expert Panel on Detection, Evaluation, and Treatment of High Blood Cholesterol in Adults (Adult Treatment Panel III). Executive summary of the third report of the National Cholesterol Education Program (NCEP) Expert Panel on Detection, Evaluation, and Treatment of High Blood Cholesterol in Adults. JAMA 2001;285:2486. (*Major consensus recommendations.*)

18. Ridker, PM, Rifai N, Clearfield M, et al. Measurement of C-reactive protein for the targeting of statin therapy in the primary prevention of acute coronary events. N Engl J Med 2001;344:1959. (*Case for the use of C-reactive protein to help guide treatment.*)

19. Ridker PM, Cannon CP, Morrow D, et al. for the Prove IT-TIMI 22 Investigators. C-reactive protein and outcomes after statin therapy. N Engl J Med 2005;352:20. (*Cross-sectional study providing evidence for the importance of C-reactive protein in determining clinical outcomes among patients treated with statin therapy.*)

20. Brown BG, Zhao ZQ, Chait A, et al. Simvastatin and niacin, antioxidant vitamins, or the combination for the prevention of coronary disease. N Engl J Med 2001;345:1583. (*Randomized, controlled trial [RCT] showed no added benefit from antioxidant vitamins.*)

21. Cannon CP, Braunwald E, McCabe CH, et al. Comparison of intensive and moderate lipid lowering with statins after acute coronary syndromes. N Engl J Med 2004;350:1495. (*RCT in very high risk patients showed that secondary prevention with intensive therapy was superior to moderate lipid lowering.*)

22. Denke MA, Grundy SM. Hypercholesterolemia in the elderly: resolving the treatment dilemma. Ann Intern Med 1990;112:780. (*A detailed review of the risks and benefits favors the treatment of high-risk patients; 83 references.*)

23. Downs JR, Clearfield M, Weis S, et al. Primary prevention of acute coronary events with lovastatin in men and women with average cholesterol levels: results of AFCAPS/TexCAPS. JAMA 1998;279:1615. (*Major RCT on primary prevention in healthy middle-aged and elderly patients with low HDL and normal LDL showed a 37% reduction in CHD risk demonstrated over 5 years of follow-up.*)

24. Frick MH, Elo O, Haapa K, et al. Helsinki Heart Study: primary-prevention trial with gemfibrozil in middle-aged men with dyslipidemia. Safety of treatment, changes in risk factors, and incidence of coronary heart disease. N Engl J Med 1987;317:1237. (*Original major study showing benefit for this class of drugs.*)

25. Graham DJ, Staffa JA, Shatin D, et al. Incidence of hospitalized rhabdomyolysis in patients treated with lipid-lowering drugs. JAMA 2004;292:2585. (*Cohort study showing that the risk was risk low and similar for monotherapy with statins but was increased with statin–fibrate combination therapy.*)

26. Grodstein F, Stampfer MJ, Colditz GA, et al. Postmenopausal hormone therapy and mortality. N Engl J Med 1997;336:1769. (*Original epidemiologic data suggesting a lower risk of death, later contradicted by prospective, randomized trials.*)

27. Grundy SM, Cleeman JI, Bairey CN, et al. Implications of recent clinical trials for the National Cholesterol Education Program Adult Treatment Panel III guidelines. Circulation 2004;110:227. (*Evidence-based consensus revisions of the guidelines, based on emerging data from major RCTs of intensive therapy in high-risk patients, suggesting optional lowering of LDL-cholesterol treatment thresholds and goals in such patients.*)

28. Hayward RA, Hofer TP, Vijan S. Narrative review: lack of evidence for recommended low-density lipoprotein treatment targets: a solvable problem. Ann Intern Med 2006;145:520. (*A provocative reanalysis of lipid-lowering trials for the prevention of coronary events in high-risk individuals that concludes that although the benefits of statin therapy are unequivocal in individuals with LDL levels <130 mg/dL, there is no evidence that titrating the dose to achieve a very low LDL target value is beneficial.*)

29. Heart Protection Study Collaborative Group. MRC/BHF Heart Protection Study of antioxidant vitamin supplementation in 20,536 high-risk individuals: a randomised placebo-controlled trial. Lancet 2002;360:23. (*Large RCT with 5-year follow-up; no benefit demonstrated from vitamins C and E and beta-carotene.*)

30. Heart Protection Collaborative Study Group. MRC/BHF Heart Protection Study of cholesterol lowering with simvastatin in 20,536 high-risk individuals: a randomised placebo-controlled trial. Lancet 2002;360:7. (*Major RCT showing a significant reduction in the risk in high-risk persons, including those with diabetes.*)

31. Henkin Y, Oberman A, Hurst DC, et al. Niacin revisited: clinical observations on an important but underutilized drug. Am J Med 1991;91:239. (*Makes the case for more use of this effective inexpensive drug, but notes dose-related toxicities.*)

32. Hulley S, Grady S, Bush T, et al. Randomized trial of estrogen plus progestin for secondary prevention of coronary heart disease in postmenopausal women. JAMA 1998;280:605. (*RCT; no benefit of hormone replacement therapy on survival in women with established coronary disease.*)

33. Hunninghake DB, Stein EA, Dujovne CA, et al. The efficacy of intensive dietary therapy alone or combined with lovastatin in outpatients with hypercholesterolemia. N Engl J Med 1993;328:1213. (*Diet alone provided only a 5% LDL reduction; medication added another 27%.*)

34. Isaacsohn JL, Moser M, Stein EA, et al. Garlic powder and plasma lipids and lipoproteins: a multicenter, randomized, placebo-controlled trial. Arch Intern Med 1998;158:1189. (*Garlic powder was given at a dose of 900 mg/d for 12 weeks; no significant differences were noted compared to the group prescribed placebo.*)

35. Johannesson M, Jonsson B, Kjekshus J, et al. Cost effectiveness of simvastatin treatment to lower cholesterol levels in patients with coronary heart disease. N Engl J Med 1997;336:332. (*Data from the 4S study showing simvastatin treatment is cost effective in men and women over a wide range of ages and cholesterol elevations.*)

36. Keech A, Simes, RJ, Barter P, et al. Effects of long-term fenofibrate therapy on cardiovascular events in 9795 people with type 2 diabetes mellitus (the FIELD study): randomised controlled trial. Lancet 2005;366:1849. (*A study of nearly 10,000 patients that showed no benefit on overall CHD mortality or overall mortality, despite a reduction in nonfatal myocardial infarction; the result calls into question the value of using fenofibrate to lower moderate triglyceride elevations in type 2 diabetics.*)

37. LaRosa JC, Grundy SM, Waters DD, et al. for the Treating to New Target (TNT) investigators. Intensive lipid lowering with atorvastatin in patients with stable coronary disease. N Engl J Med 2005;352:1425. (*Major RCT of intensive lipid lowering in high-risk persons with LDL cholesterol <130 mg/dL found no reductions in CHD mortality or overall mortality but significant reductions in major coronary events, stroke, and hospitalization for congestive heart failure.*)

38. LIPID Study. Prevention of cardiovascular events and death with pravastatin in patients with coronary heart disease and a broad range of initial cholesterol levels. The Long- Term Intervention with Pravastatin in Ischaemic Disease Study Group. N Engl J Med 1998;339:1349. (*RCT; treatment of modestly elevated LDL cholesterol levels improved cardiovascular mortality by 24% and overall mortality was reduced 22%; no increase in breast cancer was noted.*)

39. Neil HA, DeMicco DA, Luo D, et al. Analysis of efficacy and safety in patients aged 65-75 years at randomization: Collaborative Atorvastatin Diabetes Study (CARDS). Diabetes Care 2006;29:2378 . (*A post-hoc analysis that demonstrated that the benefits of LDL lowering in the older cohorts was similar to that seen in the younger study subjects.*)

40. Nissen SE, Tuzcu EM, Schoenhagen P, et al. Effect of intensive compared with moderate lipid-lowering therapy on progression of coronary atherosclerosis: a randomized controlled trial. JAMA 2004;291:1071. (*Found that intensive lipid lowering prevented the progression of atherosclerosis.*)

41. Pearson TA, Patel RV. The quest for a cholesterol-decreasing diet. Should we subtract, substitute, or supplement. Ann Intern Med 1993;119:627. (*An editorial arguing for reduction in fat intake as the primary therapy; good review of dietary supplements.*)

42. Pierce LR, Wysowski DK, Gross TP. Myopathy and rhabdomyolysis associated with lovastatin–gemfibrozil combination therapy. JAMA 1990;264:71. (*Documents this serious complication; the combination is generally to be avoided.*)

43. Pitt B, Waters D, Brown WV, et al., for the Atorvastatin vs. Revasculazation Treatment Investigators. Aggressive lipid-lowering therapy compared angioplasty in stable coronary artery disease. N Engl J Med 1999;341:70. (*Atorvastatin at least as effective as angioplasty for reducing the rate of coronary events.*)

44. Rossouw, JE, Anderson GL, Prentice RL, et al. Risks and benefits of estrogen plus progestin in healthy postmenopausal women: principal results from the Women's Health Initiative randomized controlled trial. JAMA 2002;288:321. (*No cardiovascular benefit was found.*)

45. Rubins HB, Robins SJ, Collins D, et al., for the Veterans Affairs High-Density Lipoprotein Cholesterol Intervention Trial Study Group. Gemfibrozil for the secondary prevention of coronary heart disease in men with low levels of high-density lipoprotein cholesterol. N Engl J Med 1999;341:410. (*RCT demonstrating reductions in the risks of infarction and death.*)

46. Sacks FM, Pfeffer MA, Moye LA, et al. The effect of pravastatin on coronary events after myocardial infarction in patients with average cholesterol levels. N Engl J Med 1996;335:1001. (*An important extension of the Scandinavian*

Simvastatin Study, in that patients with much lower LDL cholesterol values were chosen for cholesterol lowering; improved cardiovascular mortality was noted.)

47. Scandinavian Simvastatin Survival Study Group. Randomized trial of cholesterol lowering in 4444 patients with coronary heart disease: the Scandinavian Survival Study. Lancet 1994;344:1383. (*The first major RCT of statin efficacy in patients with CHD, showing a 42% reduction in CHD mortality and a 30% reduction in all-cause mortality with no increased risk of noncardiac death.*)

48. Schaefer EJ, Lamon-Fava S, Ausman LM, et al. Individual variability in lipoprotein cholesterol response to NCEP step 2 diets. Am J Clin Nutr 1997;65:823. (*A metabolic ward study of a step 2 diet showing an impressive reduction in serum cholesterol levels in the whole study group on average, but the variability between individuals was quite substantial.*)

49. Shepherd J, Cobbe SM, Ford I, et al. Prevention of coronary heart disease with pravastatin in men with hypercholesterolemia. N Engl J Med 1995;333:1301. (*RCT—the West of Scotland Study—showing approximately 30% reductions in the rates of nonfatal infarction, CHD death, and cardiovascular death in men without CHD but with multiple risk factors.*)

50. Sprecher DL, Harris BV, Goldberg AC, et al. Efficacy of psyllium in reducing serum cholesterol levels in hypercholesterolemic patients on high or low-fat diets. Ann Intern Med 1993;119:545. (*A 5% to 10% lowering was achieved in both groups.*)

51. Stern L, Iqbal N, Seshadri P, et al. The effects of low-carbohydrate versus conventional weight loss diets in severely obese adults: one-year follow-up of a randomized trial. Ann Intern Med 2004:140:778. (*Triglycerides were reduced and glucose intolerance was improved; there was no major change in LDL cholesterol.*)

52. Topol EJ. Intensive statin therapy—a sea change in cardiovascular prevention. N Engl J Med 2004;350:1562. (*An editorial summarizing the data in support of intensive therapy and lower LDL-cholesterol target levels.*)

53. Whitney EJ, Krasuski RA, Personius BE, et al. A randomized trial of a strategy for increasing high-density lipoprotein cholesterol levels: effects on progression of coronary heart disease and clinical events. Ann Intern Med 2005;142:95. (*Placebo-controlled RCT; a combination program halted angiographic disease progression and showed a trend toward preventing coronary events.*)

APPENDIX 27.1

FATTY ACID COMPOSITION OF COMMONLY CONSUMED FOODS (AS PERCENTAGE OF TOTAL FATTY ACIDS)

Food	Saturated	Monounsaturated	Polyunsaturated
Butter, cream, milk	65	30	5
Beef	46	48	6
Bacon and pork	38	50	12
Lard	42	45	13
Chicken	33	39	28
Fish	29	31	40
Coconut oil	92	6	2
Palm kernel oil	86	12	2
Cocoa butter	63	34	3
Olive oil	15	76	9
Peanut oil	20	48	32
Cottonseed oil	27	20	53
Soybean oil	16	24	60
Corn oil	13	26	61
Sunflower seed oil	11	22	67
Safflower seed oil	10	13	77

APPENDIX 27.2

CHOLESTEROL CONTENT OF COMMON FOODS

Food	Amount of Food	Cholesterol Content (mg)	Food	Amount of Food	Cholesterol Content (mg)
Brains	3.5 oz (100 g)	>2,000	Beef	3.5 oz	65
Liver, chicken	3.5 oz	555	Pork	3.5 oz	62
Kidney	3.5 oz	375	Clams	3.5 oz	50
Liver, beef	3.5 oz	300	Flounder	3.5 oz	50
Caviar	1 tbsp	>300	Oysters	3.5 oz	50
Egg yolk	1	252	Ice cream (regular)	1 cup	40
Shrimp	3.5 oz	150	Butter	1 tbsp	35
Crab	3.5 oz	100	Scallops	3.5 oz	35
Mackerel	3.5 oz	95	Milk, whole	1 cup	14
Lobster (cooked)	3.5 oz	85	Milk, 2%	1 cup	9
Cheese, cheddar	3.5 oz	84	Milk, skim	1 cup	2
Veal	3.5 oz	70	Margarine	1 tbsp	0
Chicken, breast	3.5 oz	67			

APPENDIX 27.3

FAT CONTENT OF MEATS, POULTRY, FISH, AND OTHER PROTEIN SOURCES, 3-OUNCE PORTIONS

	Total Fat (g)	Saturated Fat (g)	Calories	Cholesterol (mg)
Red Meat				
Veal top round (roasted)	2.9	1.0	127	88
Pork tenderloin (roasted)	4.1	1.4	133	67
Beef top round (broiled)	4.2	1.4	153	71
Beef eye of round (roasted)	4.2	1.5	143	59
Pork sirloin chop, boneless (broiled)	5.7	1.5	156	78
Pork loin roast, boneless (roasted)	6.4	2.4	160	66
Lamb leg (roasted)	6.6	2.3	162	78
Pork loin chop, bone in (broiled)	6.9	2.5	165	70
Beef tenderloin (broiled)	8.5	3.2	179	71
Frankfurter, beef and pork (boiled)	24.8	9.1	272	42
Pork sausage, country style (cooked)	26.5	9.2	314	71
Poultry				
Turkey breast, skinless (roasted)	2.7	0.9	133	59
Chicken breast, skinless (roasted)	3.0	0.9	140	72
Turkey thigh, skinless (roasted)	6.1	2.1	159	72
Chicken thigh, skinless (roasted)	9.3	2.6	178	81
Chicken breast, skin on (fried)	11.2	3.0	221	72
Duck, skin on (roasted)	24.1	8.2	286	71
Fish and Seafood				
Lobster meat (cooked)	0.5	<0.1	83	61
Scallops, bay or sea (raw)	0.6	<0.1	75	28
Cod (broiled)	0.7	0.1	89	47
Shrimp (moist heat cooked)	0.9	0.2	84	166
Flounder (broiled)	1.3	0.3	99	58
Crab, Alaska king (steamed)	1.3	0.1	82	45
Oysters (eastern, raw)	2.1	0.5	59	47
Tuna, white (canned in water)	2.1	0.6	116	36
Trout, rainbow (broiled)	3.7	0.7	128	62
Tuna, light (canned in oil)	7.0	1.3	168	15
Salmon, sockeye (broiled)	9.3	1.6	184	74
Other				
Tofu/bean curd	4.1	0.6	65	0
Eggs (hard boiled)	9.5	2.8	134	466
American cheese food (pasteurized process)	20.9	13.1	279	54
Cheddar cheese	28.2	17.9	343	89
Peanuts (roasted in shell)	41.4	7.3	495	0
Peanut butter	43.5	7.2	502	0

Source: Department of Agriculture, Agricultural Research Service. Composition of foods: dairy and egg products (Agriculture Handbook no. 8-1). Washington, DC: Author, 1976; Department of Agriculture, Agricultural Research Service. Composition of foods: poultry products (Agriculture Handbook no. 8-5). Washington, DC: Author, 1979; Department of Agriculture, Agricultural Research Service. Composition of foods: sausages and luncheon meats (Agriculture Handbook no. 8-7). Washington, DC: Author, 1980; Department of Agriculture, Agricultural Research Service. Composition of foods: pork products (Agriculture Handbook no. 8-10, rev.). Washington, DC: Author, 1992; Department of Agriculture, Agricultural Research Service. Composition of foods: nut and seed products (Agriculture Handbook no. 8-12). Washington, DC: Author, 1984; Department of Agriculture, Agricultural Research Service, Composition of foods: beef products (Agriculture Handbook no. 8-13, rev.). Washington, DC: Author, 1990; Department of Agriculture, Agricultural Research Service, Composition of foods: finfish and shellfish products (Agriculture Handbook no. 8-15). Washington, DC: Author, 1987; Department of Agriculture, Agricultural Research Service, Composition of foods: legumes and legume products (Agriculture Handbook no. 8-16). Washington, DC: Author, 1986; Department of Agriculture, Agricultural Research Service, Composition of foods: lamb, veal, and game products (Agriculture Handbook no. 8-17). Washington DC: Author, 1989; Highland View Hospital–Case Western Reserve University Nutrient Data Base.

CHAPTER 28 ■ OUTPATIENT MANAGEMENT OF ATRIAL FIBRILLATION

Atrial fibrillation (AF) is becoming an increasingly frequent problem, due in large part to the aging of the population. In patients older than the age of 80 years, the community prevalence approaches 9%. Many patients with new onset of AF present as outpatients, some asymptomatically and others with complaints suggestive of hemodynamic compromise. The first tasks are to ensure adequate rate control and identify and attend to underlying precipitants and etiologies. The focus then shifts to design and implementation of a risk-adjusted program of stroke prophylaxis to counter the high risk of embolic stroke.

PATHOPHYSIOLOGY, CLINICAL PRESENTATION, AND COURSE (1–18)

AF may be paroxysmal or chronic. Delayed atrial conduction and ectopic foci (including those originating from the pulmonary veins) contribute to the problem. Paroxysms typically occur in patients with lone atrial fibrillation, sick sinus syndrome, or Wolff–Parkinson–White (WPW) syndrome and during exacerbations of cardiomyopathic, valvular, and ischemic forms of organic heart disease. Advanced forms of these conditions often result in chronic AF. AF may also be triggered by hyperthyroidism. Although chronic fibrillation may be a manifestation of serious organic heart disease and represent an increase in overall risk, chronicity is not the prime determinant of embolic risk. As identified by the Framingham Study, the prime determinants of stroke and death risk in AF patients are advancing age, increasing systolic blood pressure, diabetes, smoking, and evidence of underlying heart disease (prior myocardial infarction or heart failure, heart murmur, left ventricular hypertrophy on electrocardiogram). Risk stratification can be carried out by attention to these factors (see later discussion and Chapter 25).

Lone Atrial Fibrillation

Lone AF is characterized by the occurrence of atrial fibrillation in the absence of clinically evident heart disease or cardiovascular risk factors. In about two thirds of cases, the condition presents as isolated or recurrent episodes of paroxysmal AF; in the remainder, the AF is chronic. Survival rates and stroke risks are similar regardless of whether the lone AF episodes are paroxysmal or chronic. Lone AF may be annoying and sometimes frightening, but the key question is the risk of embolization that it confers. In patients <60 years, survival and embolic risk are no different from those of a population of similar age; however, in patients >60 years, there is nearly a fourfold increase in relative risk of stroke, probably due to the increased probability of underlying cardiovascular risk fac-

tors in older patients with seemingly "lone" AF. Thus, lone AF appears to pose little risk, but only if the patient is relatively young and has no other cardiovascular risk factors. Recent study in idiopathic AF patients identified somatic mutations in the connexin 40 gene, which codes for an atrial gap-junction protein believed to be important in atrial conduction. Such findings suggest a possible genetic molecular basis for the condition.

Apathetic Hyperthyroidism of the Elderly

Clinically inapparent hyperthyroidism may be mistaken for lone AF because there may be little evidence of organic heart disease, and the typical symptoms and signs of hyperthyroidism can also be absent. Sometimes, the clinical presentation more closely resembles depression or occult malignancy, with significant weight loss, marked apathy, and unexplained AF dominating the clinical picture. Diagnosis is made by ruling out underlying organic heart disease and finding the thyrotropin to be undetectable and the free thyroxin index or total tri-iodothyronine substantially elevated (see Chapters 8 and 103). Treatment directed at the hyperthyroidism usually terminates the AF. Although uncommon, this eminently treatable form of AF should not be missed. Stroke risk is minimal if there is no accompanying organic heart disease.

Underlying Heart Disease

Patients with AF in the context of underlying heart disease have a much more serious problem. Not only is the risk of embolization significantly increased, but the AF may also lead to hemodynamic compromise. Chronic atrial fibrillation in such patients usually reflects serious cardiac pathology. In the Framingham Study, onset of atrial fibrillation and *heart failure* were closely linked. Furthermore, the development of chronic AF corresponded with a doubling of cardiovascular mortality.

Some conditions that cause AF also manifest concurrent disease of the conducting system, further increasing risk. For example, patients with the *tachycardia–bradycardia (sick-sinus) syndrome* have sinus node dysfunction, often in conjunction with atrioventricular nodal disease and lack of an adequate escape mechanism. Characteristic presentations include episodes of atrial fibrillation with a slow ventricular response rate and bouts of severe bradycardia leading to syncope or near-syncope.

Paroxysms of rapid AF and other supraventricular tachycardias are characteristic of *WPW syndrome*. In this condition, an accessory connection between the atrium and the ventricle (e.g., the Kent bundle) leads to preexcitation (short PR interval, delta waves) and a host of supraventricular dysrhythmias. The AF may be associated with a very fast ventricular response rate facilitated by rapid antegrade conduction over the accessory conduction pathway. There may be a widening of the QRS, mimicking ventricular fibrillation. In rare instances, the rapid ventricular response can degenerate into true ventricular fibrillation and sudden death. Fortunately, the risk of such serious ventricular dysrhythmias is very low in previously asymptomatic WPW patients, in part because the accessory pathways tend to lose antegrade conductivity over time.

An episode of AF in a patient with preexisting heart disease may be precipitated by such factors as *acute heart failure, ischemia, fever, infection, hypoxia,* or *hypovolemia.* Correction of the precipitant often results in at least a temporary return to sinus rhythm. If there is a *valvular, cardiomyopathic,* or *ischemic process* that continues unabated, the paroxysms of AF may become more frequent and prolonged, culminating in chronic AF. AF is particularly common in patients with mitral valve disease, due to rather early onset of increased left atrial pressure and size. AF is much less common in disease of the aortic valve; when it does occur, it signifies very severe advanced disease (see Chapter 33). Increases in *pulse pressure* indicative of aortic stiffness increase risk of AF, presumably by increasing cardiac load.

Alcohol has been implicated as a major precipitant of AF. Binge drinking may induce paroxysms of AF and ventricular dysrhythmias (so-called *holiday heart* disease). Although there may be no overt evidence of underlying heart disease, there is some debate as to how normal the hearts really are of patients who experience alcohol-induced arrhythmias. Chronic alcohol abuse can lead to *alcoholic cardiomyopathy,* which may present as paroxysmal AF during binge drinking. As drinking continues, the cardiomyopathy progresses, and the AF becomes more established. The condition is potentially reversible with total abstinence.

Systemic Embolization and Stroke

Both epidemiologic and prospective studies have documented an increased risk of systemic embolization and stroke in patients with AF. Most emboli derive from thrombus formation due to stasis in the left atrial appendage. The resulting strokes are often large and particularly devastating. It used to be thought that increased risk applied only to patients with AF caused by *rheumatic mitral valve disease* (relative risk increased nearly 15-fold), but community-based studies have identified lesser but still significant increases (e.g., 4- to 5-fold) in stroke risk for all AF patients with *underlying heart disease.* Average stroke risk from AF in the absence of valvular heart disease approaches 5%/yr. Independent predictors of high risk for stroke or systemic embolization in nonrheumatic AF patients include *clinical congestive heart failure or systolic dysfunction, previous thromboembolism, systolic hypertension* (>160 mm Hg), and *age >75 years if a woman.* Prospective transthoracic echocardiographic (ECG) study confirms that left ventricular (LV) dysfunction is an independent predictor of stroke risk, and transesophageal echocardiographic (TEE) studies find that *thrombus in the left atrium* or *left atrial appendage* also powerfully predicts embolic risk.

Atherosclerotic risk factors (e.g., *diabetes, hypertension*) markedly increase the risk of systemic embolization and stroke in persons with AF, perhaps by contributing to development of *complex atherosclerotic plaque* in the transverse portion of the thoracic *aorta,* found in TEE studies to be an independent risk factor for embolic stroke.

Data from the Framingham Study suggest that risk of stroke is greatest at the onset of AF, with >25% of AF-associated strokes occurring shortly after onset. In addition, patients with AF have twice the likelihood of having a recurrence of stroke within the first 6 months compared with patients with stroke and no AF. Patients with *paroxysmal AF* have roughly the same stroke risk as those with chronic AF. Stroke risk with *atrial flutter* is lower than with AF, but many persons with atrial flutter subsequently go on to develop AF.

Reduction in Cardiac Output and Risk of Death

The decrease in ventricular filling and loss of atrial contraction that result from AF lead to a fall in cardiac output and a rise in pulmonary capillary wedge pressure. When these are substantial, shortness of breath and reduced exercise tolerance may ensue. Rapid AF is especially likely to trigger hemodynamic compromise and heart failure. Cardiomyopathic changes are sometimes a consequence of rapid AF, further compromising cardiac output and exacerbating symptoms.

Although AF is often a proxy for underlying heart disease, it is also an independent predictor of reduced long-term survival. In the community setting, persons with AF have a risk-factor adjusted odds ratio for mortality of 1.5 for women and 1.9 for men compared with those in sinus rhythm.

PRINCIPLES OF MANAGEMENT

Before proceeding to address issues of management, it is important to confirm the diagnosis of AF. Many ECG recorders now come with software algorithms that automatically produce reports of rhythm disorders. Errors in diagnosis of AF are frequent; reported false- positive rates by such software algorithms approach 20%. Any automated reading needs confirmation by manual review of the relevant tracing.

Once AF is confirmed, the immediate tasks are determination of ventricular response rate, assessment of its hemodynamic consequences (heart rate being an important determinant of hemodynamic state and myocardial oxygen demand), and establishment of rate control. Whether to continue with rate control or attempt cardioversion requires consideration. Attention then turns to determining stroke risk and selecting an appropriate means of stroke prophylaxis.

Assessment of Ventricular Response Rate and Hemodynamic State

The assessment starts with checking quickly for symptoms and signs of hemodynamic compromise (e.g., exertional dyspnea, chest pain, lightheadedness, systolic hypotension, tachycardia, tachypnea, vasoconstricted extremities, jugular venous distention, rales, third heart sound) in conjunction with ECG and chest x-ray, if necessary. One needs to evaluate heart rate by checking the apical pulse (radial pulse may not be accurate) both at rest and after mild exertion (e.g., 5 to 10 sit-ups or standing up 5 to 10 times from a chair). Ventricular rate may appear well controlled at rest when there is little adrenergic stimulation but rise markedly with mild effort.

Patients with little evidence of hemodynamic compromise and only modest elevation in ventricular response rate can continue their evaluation and management planning on an outpatient basis (see Chapter 25, Appendix). Those with evidence of hemodynamic compromise (e.g., hypotension, acute heart failure, acute ischemia) or extremely rapid ventricular response rate (>150 beats/min) require immediate hospitalization for consideration of intravenous pharmacotherapy or, if severely compromised, *electrical cardioversion.*

Establishment of Rate Control (19–24)

The goal for ventricular response rate is a resting apical pulse of <85 beats/min and of <110 beats/min after mild exercise. Treatment is largely pharmacologic, although non-pharmacologic measures (e.g., atrioventricular node ablation with ventricular pacing) provide options in refractory situations. Pharmacologic options include beta-blockade, calcium-channel blockers, and digoxin. Choice of agent is informed by consideration of the patient's underlying pathophysiology.

Beta-Blockers

Beta-blocking agents and calcium-channel blockers have supplanted digoxin as the drugs of choice for rate control in AF largely because of their superior efficacy in settings of high adrenergic stimulation. Beta-blockers slow ventricular response by increasing the refractoriness of the atrioventricular node and blocking the β-adrenergic effect of catecholamines on heart rate. Unlike digoxin, they do not require vagal tone to slow ventricular response rate, making them particularly useful when exercise, situational stress, hyperthyroidism, fever, hypoxemia, or ischemia is responsible for the tachyarrhythmia. Although negatively inotropic, beta-blockers may even be used with benefit (albeit cautiously) for AF in the setting of congestive heart failure (see Chapter 32).

Calcium-Channel Blockers

Like beta-blockers, a number of calcium-channel blockers have proven useful for AF rate control, especially in the acute setting. *Verapamil* is the prototypical calcium-channel blocker used in AF; its ability to prolong the refractory period and the conduction time of atrioventricular nodal tissue reduces the ventricular response rate. *Diltiazem* acts similarly, although not quite as potently; its advantage is less negative inotropy. Unlike digoxin, calcium-channel blockers do not require vagal tone to be maximally effective, and consequently they control AF under circumstances that ordinarily would be refractory to digoxin (i.e., high sympathetic tone). Caution is required when using these calcium-channel blockers in the setting of underlying left ventricular failure or conduction system disease (e.g., sick sinus syndrome) because they may exacerbate failure or lead to extreme bradycardia. These agents are contraindicated in WPW syndrome due to their tendency to enhance conduction through the accessory pathway (see later discussion). Use of short-acting preparations in the setting of congestive heart failure is associated with an increased risk of cardiac death (see Chapter 32). In general, sustained-release formulations appear to be better tolerated than short-acting ones (see Chapter 26), especially for continuous use.

Digoxin

Although no longer considered the cornerstone of pharmacologic therapy for AF, digoxin can still play an important role in rate control, especially in persons whose AF is a consequence of LV dysfunction (see Chapter 32). In the setting of a failing left ventricle, digoxin's positive inotropic effects may help to lessen the stimulus for fibrillation. However, the drug's dependence on vagal tone for full effect and the high level of adrenergic stimulation common to situations that trigger paroxysms of AF or worsen rate control conspire to limit its utility.

Limitations. Digoxin tends to be ineffective in slowing heart rate when *vagal tone* is low and adrenergic stimulation is high, such as during exercise, stress, fever, hypovolemia, hyperthyroidism, ischemia, or hypoxia. Control may appear adequate at rest, but with exercise or other forms of sympathetic stimulation, the ventricular response rate rises precipitously. Moreover, in the absence of heart failure, digoxin neither restores sinus rhythm nor maintains sinus rhythm and does little to reduce the frequency and severity of paroxysmal AF episodes. Electrophysiologic studies show that the drug actually shortens the atrial refractory period and may contribute to the persistence of AF. By facilitating conduction through the bypass tract and shortening its refractory period, digoxin may exacerbate AF due to WPW syndrome. Careful case selection and close monitoring of therapy are critical to safe and effective digoxin use (see also Chapter 32).

Adverse Effects. The narrow therapeutic index for digoxin also discourages its use. Subtle dysrhythmic manifestations of digitalis toxicity in the setting of AF include *regularization* of AF, a manifestation of *junctional tachycardia*, and frequent *ventricular premature beats*. The latter should not be confused on electrocardiogram with the widened QRS complexes caused by the *Ashmann phenomenon* (prolonged relative refractory period in the beat after a long RR interval). Although ventricular response rate provides a "bioassay" of digitalis effect and makes frequent sampling of digoxin levels unnecessary, watching for changes in rhythm can be very informative. Whenever there is suspicion of digitalis toxicity, digoxin should be held and a serum level checked.

Choice of Agent

Selection of the proper agent for rate control requires an etiologic diagnosis (see Chapter 25). As noted previously, empiric therapy without regard for the underlying pathophysiology risks hemodynamic worsening. The importance of this principle is underscored by the approaches required to establish rate control in heart failure, WPW syndrome, sick sinus syndrome, and hyperthyroidism.

WPW Syndrome. WPW syndrome requires special mention because of the small but important risk of hemodynamic compromise associated with the disorder and standard approaches to rate control. WPW patients with very rapid ventricular rates and hemodynamic deterioration during an attack of AF should be hospitalized, promptly referred to a cardiologist, and treated with urgent *electrical cardioversion*. WPW patients with occasional bouts of AF that are well tolerated and self-limited require no treatment so long as the shortest RR interval during an attack is >180 msec; a shorter interval is associated with an increased risk of ventricular fibrillation. No restrictions on activity are necessary. *Digoxin and calcium-channel blockers should not be used* because they encourage conduction through the accessory pathway by blocking conduction through the atrioventricular node. Future episodes of AF are prevented by the use of antiarrhythmic agents such as *amiodarone* or *radiofrequency ablation*. Inpatient electrophysiologic testing is used to help judge which agent is most likely to provide optimal control of ventricular rate during AF. *Beta-blockers* are sometimes helpful in protecting against recurrent episodes of

AF but should also be subjected to electrophysiologic study before being used in patients with potentially serious attacks of AF. Cardiac consultation is essential.

Tachycardia–Bradycardia (Sick Sinus) Syndrome. Patients with the tachycardia–bradycardia form of *sick sinus syndrome* pose a therapeutic dilemma: Although their AF usually responds well to *beta-blockade, verapamil,* or *digoxin,* these therapies may seriously exacerbate episodes of bradycardia by further suppressing conduction through the atrioventricular node. Consequently, implantation of a *demand pacemaker* is often necessary for patients with symptomatic tachycardia–bradycardia syndrome.

Hyperthyroidism. AF caused by *hyperthyroidism* responds best to beta-blockade, although definitive treatment of the underlying thyroid disease (see Chapter 103) is essential to successful prevention of future episodes of AF. At times, elective cardioversion (see later discussion) is necessary to restore sinus rhythm after successful treatment of the hyperthyroidism.

Heart Failure. Patients with AF due to congestive failure may benefit from the judicious application of digoxin and beta-blockade. Both agents can slow ventricular response rate and enhance myocardial performance. Digoxin's directly positive inotropic effects improve cardiac output in the failing heart while slowing conduction through the junction. Although beta-blockade is negatively inotropic, its ability to slow ventricular response rate and lessen myocardial oxygen demand may have the net effect of improving ventricular performance, particularly in persons with AF due to underlying ischemic heart disease (see Chapter 32).

Refractory Rapid AF. Patients who fail to respond to or cannot tolerate pharmacologic therapy for rate control and remain symptomatic pose a problem. Options include *cardioversion* followed by measures to maintain sinus rhythm (so-called *rhythm control;* see later discussion) and *ablation of the atrioventricular node* in conjunction with placement of a permanent *ventricular pacemaker.* Ablation of the atrial reentrant circuit causing AF has been performed both surgically (the *maze procedure*) and by *radiofrequency* techniques during electrophysiologic study. With ablation, the atria continue to fibrillate (necessitating stroke prophylaxis; see later discussion), but ventricular function, exercise tolerance, and quality of life all improve, and there is no adverse effect on long-term survival. For pharmacologically refractory patients who require rate control but do not need the atrial boost to cardiac output, ablation remains an option if other measures fail.

Rhythm Control (21,25–33)

Rate Control Versus Rhythm Control

One of the longstanding debates regarding AF management has been the issue of rate control versus rhythm control (i.e., restoration of sinus rhythm). Restoration of sinus rhythm used to be considered a priority, and much effort was expended in trying to achieve it. The balance of opinion has tilted in favor of rate control, based on findings from major European and North American trials and increasing appreciation for the adverse proarrhythmic potential of available antiarrhythmic agents (see Chapter 29). The landmark studies revealed no survival advantage or reduction in cardiovascular morbidity for rhythm control compared with rate control. With rhythm

control, there were more adverse drug reactions and hospitalizations. These studies do not eliminate cardioversion or ablation therapy as treatment options—their study populations were skewed toward persons at high risk for reversion to AF—but their findings do lessen enthusiasm for routinely seeking restoration of sinus rhythm for all newly discovered AF patients. Nonetheless, rhythm control does have some potential advantages: Stroke risk can be reduced (although not eliminated due to risk of relapse), bothersome palpitations eradicated, and exercise tolerance improved.

Etiologic treatment of the underlying pathophysiology is the first step toward restoration and maintenance of sinus rhythm. Of particular importance is control of any hypertension, ischemia, heart failure, or hyperthyroidism (see Chapters 26, 30, 32, and 103). If the patient is hemodynamically stable, elective electrical or chemical cardioversion can then proceed, usually performed on an inpatient basis (see standard texts), followed by long-term maintenance of sinus rhythm.

Candidates for Rhythm Control

Persons who become unacceptably symptomatic from their AF despite efforts at rate control, either because of disturbing palpitations (e.g., young persons with anatomically normal hearts) or hemodynamic compromise, are reasonable candidates for consideration of rhythm control. The best candidates are those whose underlying pathophysiology lends itself to maintenance of sinus rhythm at low risk (blood pressure well controlled, left atrium not markedly enlarged, LV function preserved). Higher-risk patients may require consideration if they have difficulty tolerating the hemodynamic consequences of their AF despite pharmacologic measures. Desire to avoid anticoagulation is usually not an adequate rationale; anticoagulation often needs to be continued due to the substantial risk of reversion to AF, particularly in those with significant underlying heart disease (see later discussion).

Reestablishment of Sinus Rhythm: Elective Cardioversion

Both pharmacologic and electrical approaches to restoration of sinus rhythm are available. Choice of method depends on the best judgment of the consulting cardiologist and the type of local expertise available. Both *amiodarone* and *sotalol* (see later discussion) prove effective pharmacologic choices that can be used both with and without electrical cardioversion. Issues of candidacy, timing, and need for anticoagulation benefit from input by the primary physician.

Candidacy. Patients experiencing *exercise intolerance* from the hemodynamic compromise associated with loss of atrial contraction should be considered for cardioversion. Other determinants of candidacy are degree of stroke risk and likelihood of remaining in sinus rhythm. A recent cost-effectiveness analysis found that cardioversion was superior to chronic anticoagulation when there was high or moderate-to-high embolic risk. The best predictors of successful cardioversion and sustained maintenance of sinus rhythm are *duration of AF* and *age.* AF of recent onset due to an acute stress (e.g., alcohol binge, pneumonia) often reverts spontaneously. At the other end of the spectrum, AF of >1 year is difficult to cardiovert and to sustain as sinus rhythm, probably as a consequence of atrial fibrosis that occurs over time. Fibrosis is also believed to be at least part of the reason that age is a predictor of outcome. *Atrial size* is associated inversely with outcome, but often size appears to be more a reflection of AF duration than an independent predictor of success or failure. Nonetheless, a normal left atrial size is associated with a high probability of successful cardioversion and maintenance of sinus rhythm, whereas a left atrial diameter of >60 mm retains independent predictive value as a sign of poor outcome. Other factors that have been identified as predictors of poor outcome include advanced *mitral stenosis*, other forms of rheumatic heart disease, and chronic *congestive heart failure*; however, with the exception of these conditions, etiology is usually not a powerful predictor of responsiveness to cardioversion.

Timing of Elective Cardioversion: Need for Prior Anticoagulation.
Timing of elective cardioversion is affected by the risk of embolization due to dislodgement of poorly organized left atrial clot on restoration of coordinated atrial contraction. Estimates of embolization risk in the absence of prior anticoagulation range from 3% to 6%. The conventional approach to elective cardioversion is to delay the procedure for 4 weeks, during which time the patient is anticoagulated with warfarin (international normalized ratio [INR] of 2 to 3); this prevents new clot formation and allows sufficient time for any preexisting clot to organize. Under this approach, early cardioversion without oral anticoagulation is reserved for persons in hemodynamic distress and those with onset of AF of <48 hours, whose risk of thrombus formation is very low. Most patients with AF who present in the outpatient setting do so in little hemodynamic distress and with either unknown time of onset or >48 hours later. Such persons require consideration of need for prophylactic anticoagulation before the procedure.

Advances in the detection of clot in the left atrium now provide an early cardioversion option. Using TEE, one can sensitively test for presence of clot in the left atrium and left atrial appendage. If clot is absent, one can proceed directly to elective cardioversion with just brief periprocedural heparinization but no delay for oral anticoagulation. Compared with conventional elective cardioversion, the TEE approach has the same low embolic risk and similar rates of death, maintenance of sinus rhythm, and functional status; risk of hemorrhagic events is reduced, and success rate for restoration of sinus rhythm is improved. TEE is especially useful in persons who have a relative contraindication to oral anticoagulation and obviates the delay in cardioversion. Disadvantages include cost and requirements for skilled operators and specialized equipment.

Need for Postcardioversion Anticoagulation.
Both conventional and TEE approaches to elective cardioversion require at least 1 month of postcardioversion oral anticoagulation due to the risk of late embolization related to atrial instability and slow return of full atrial contractility. The indications, optimal intensity, proper duration, and cost-effectiveness of longer-term anticoagulation after cardioversion remain to be determined. Persons deemed at high risk for relapse are best maintained on anticoagulation for an extended period until it becomes clear that they are unlikely to relapse. Some physicians use aspirin for stroke prophylaxis after cardioversion in persons of low to moderate stroke risk.

Maintenance of Sinus Rhythm

Persons deemed at low risk for relapse can be cardioverted without being prescribed maintenance antiarrhythmic therapy; their chances of remaining in sinus rhythm are good. If they relapse, they can be recardioverted and started on a program of antiarrhythmic medication. Persons at *high risk* of relapse (e.g., those with previous relapse, marked left atrial enlargement, advanced underlying heart disease, and high voltage required

for cardioversion) have a high (50% to 70%) 6- to 12-month rate of relapse and are likely to need antiarrhythmic therapy right from the start and maintained indefinitely. A number of agents are available.

Amiodarone. Of available agents, amiodarone is among the most effective pharmacologic agents for maintenance of sinus rhythm, with a reported median time to recurrence of 487 days— seven times longer than that for sotalol (except in persons with ischemic heart disease, in whom times to recurrence are similar). When used in low doses ($\leq$200 mg/d), it reduces the AF recurrence rate by half to 35% (compared to 63% for other antiarrhythmics) and produces little proarrhythmic activity, increased risk of sudden death, or impairment of contractility. Consequently, it can be used in the setting of heart failure. Because it is effective for restoring sinus rhythm, it is also being used increasingly as a first-line agent for chemical cardioversion in the inpatient setting. The drug's ability to slow atrioventricular conduction makes it useful for reducing ventricular response rate during recurrences of AF.

Side effects are numerous but usually not severe enough to warrant termination of therapy. Important adverse effects include *pulmonary toxicity* (interstitial changes related to total dose), *thyroid suppression* (due to the iodine in amiodarone), *acute gastrointestinal upset*, *chronic constipation*, *corneal cysts*, and *neurologic dysfunction* (tremor, ataxia, peripheral neuropathy). The drug *potentiates* the effect of *warfarin* and may cause minor *abnormalities in liver function tests*, but frank hepatocellular injury is rare. Although amiodarone can increase the QT interval, it confers very little risk of torsades de pointes compared with other atrial antiarrhythmics (see later discussion). *Dronedarone*, an amiodarone-like agent developed to have similar efficacy without the pulmonary, thyroid, and hepatic toxicities, is undergoing study.

Sotalol. This drug belongs to the class IC antiarrhythmics but also has beta-blocking qualities. It demonstrates efficacy comparable to that of amiodarone in maintaining sinus rhythm in patients with AF due to ischemic heart disease. Sotalol's beta-blocking activity may result in marked bradycardia, fatigue, dizziness, and dyspnea, making its use in heart failure or sinus node disease problematic.

Beta-Blockers. Beta-blockers are helpful for maintenance of sinus rhythm in cases in which marked adrenergic stimulation is associated with precipitation or persistence of AF. Persons with underlying ischemic heart disease may be especially good candidates (see Chapter 30), and even persons with congestive heart failure may benefit when small doses are used and the patient is closely monitored (see Chapter 32).

Flecainide, Propafenone. These other *class IC antiarrhythmics* offered the hope of superior atrial stabilizing activity, but their negative inotropy and proarrhythmic effects have limited their use in persons with underlying heart disease. They can prolong the QT interval and increase the risk of torsades de pointes.

Quinidine and Disopyramide. Amiodarone and sotalol have relegated traditional atrial antiarrhythmics such as *quinidine* and *disopyramide* to secondary and tertiary roles for maintenance of sinus rhythm. The proarrhythmic and gastrointestinal side effects of quinidine and its suboptimal efficacy ($\geq$50% relapse rate) discourage its use. Of greatest concern is quinidine's propensity to cause *QT prolongation* and polymorphic ventricular tachycardias (e.g., *torsades de pointes*), which are associated with increased risks of *syncope* and *sudden death*.

Disopyramide has also been displaced as a first-line agent because of its disappointing efficacy, *negative inotropy*, and *anticholinergic side effects*.

Options If Pharmacologic Rhythm Control Fails

A number of options are available, ranging from focusing on rate control to using ablation techniques and implantable devices.

Focusing on Rate Control. As noted, there is no demonstrated survival advantage for rhythm control over rate control. Consequently, if the patient asymptomatically relapses back into AF despite antiarrhythmic therapy, then switching priorities from rhythm control to rate control is reasonable. If at a later time there is improvement in the patient's underlying heart disease, cardioversion can be reconsidered.

Implantable Devices. Patients who fail antiarrhythmic therapy and cannot tolerate AF are reasonable candidates for consideration of an implantable device. *Atrial pacing* can reduce the frequency of AF episodes by as much as 50% in persons with paroxysmal AF. High-frequency "burst" pacing can terminate up to 25% of episodes. Persons with sick sinus syndrome (who may already be candidates for pacemaker implantation for severe bradycardia) appear to be promising candidates for atrial pacing as a means of preventing recurrent AF. Prospective study is ongoing; randomized trials of atrial pacing versus no pacing are needed.

Termination of AF episodes can also be achieved by use of an *implantable atrial/ventricular defibrillator*. Many patients with ventricular arrhythmias requiring defibrillator implantation also have paroxysms of AF, making placement of a combined device a reasonable consideration. Such defibrillators have been approved by the U.S. Food and Drug Administration for use in persons with symptomatic, drug-refractory AF. These devices also have the capacity to provide rapid atrial burst pacing, often obviating the need for atrial defibrillation (which can be painful).

Pulmonary Vein Ablation. Many ectopic foci triggering AF are believed to arise from within the pulmonary vein. Electrophysiologists have tried identification and ablation of the responsible source(s) with some success (e.g., reports of 1-year rates of 74% for maintenance of sinus rhythm without antiarrhythmic medication). However, localization can be difficult (especially when there are multiple sources necessitating prolonged cardiac catheterization), and stricture of the pulmonary vein may ensue from the ablation procedure. Work is ongoing to better define the role of ablation in management of chronic AF; long-term randomized trials are needed. Pulmonary vein ablation should not yet be considered a first-line therapy.

Stroke Prophylaxis (1,6,9,14–18,34–46)

One of the most feared consequences of AF is systemic embolization resulting in stroke. Average risk among persons with nonvalvular AF in community settings is close to 5%/yr. Not only is risk of stroke high, but so is stroke severity, due to the many large thromboemboli originating from the left atrium and left atrial appendage. Nonetheless, stroke risk is not the same for all AF patients, and bleeding risk from anticoagulant therapy can be substantial (averaging 2%/yr under properly monitored anticoagulation but rising substantially in selected subgroups; see later discussion and Chapter 83). Risk stratifi-

cation helps to match risks and benefits and differentiate those who will benefit for anticoagulation from those who will not.

Assessment of Stroke Risk

Data from prospective, community-based epidemiologic studies (e.g., the Framingham Heart Study) and randomized trials involving hospitalized patients with new onset of AF (e.g., Stroke Prevention in Atrial Fibrillation [SPAF]) have been used to develop risk-stratification systems for classifying individual patients. The Framingham scoring system for estimating AF stroke risk (Fig. 28.1) appears to be particularly relevant for outpatient use. Both stratification systems identify similar, readily accessible clinical features that represent independent risk factors for stroke in newly diagnosed AF patients. Stratifying patients into high-, intermediate-, and low-risk categories helps to identify who must, might, and need not be anticoagulated. Although not yet fully validated by long-term prospective studies, these stratification schemes can facilitate the choice of approach to stroke prophylaxis, helping to balance risk versus benefit.

Risk Factors for Stroke in AF. The classic risk factor was rheumatic mitral valve disease, with an annual stroke risk of nearly 15%. In the Framingham Heart Study, the key determinants of stroke risk in persons without valvular disease were *age, gender, systolic blood pressure, diabetes*, and *prior stroke or transient ischemic attack*. In their study of a hospitalized cohort, the SPAF investigators arrived at a nearly identical set of risk factors, but also identified *heart failure* as an important predictor. Embolic stroke risk is not solely a function of AF; it is also related to overall atherosclerotic risk, as manifested by inclusion of atherosclerotic risk factors in both scoring systems and by the findings in other studies that complex plaque formation in the aortic arch and carotid vessels is also highly correlated with stroke risk.

Calculating and Stratifying Risk and Risk Stratification. The Framingham system places individuals along a continuum of estimated 5-year stroke risk (Fig. 28.1). The SPAF system divides AF patients into high-, moderate-, and low-risk categories based on 1-year stroke risk:

- High risk/strong candidate for anticoagulation: 1-year stroke risk is 6% to 8% (e.g., multiple high-risk features such as prior stroke, systolic blood pressure >160 mm Hg, heart failure, female gender, age >75 years).
- Moderate risk/optional candidacy for anticoagulation: 1-year stroke risk is 3% to 4% (e.g., hypertension without any high-risk features).
- Low risk/not candidate for anticoagulation: 1-year risk is 1% to 1.5% (e.g., no hypertension, no high-risk features).

Weighing risks of stroke and bleeding (see later discussion) helps to inform decisions regarding stroke prophylaxis. SPAF III confirmed in a prospective, randomized study that high-risk patients derive the most benefit from warfarin anticoagulation compared with those of intermediate or low risk. With further confirmation from long-term prospective validation studies, risk stratification should become an essential tool for individualizing stroke prevention in AF.

Warfarin Anticoagulation

Long-term warfarin anticoagulation represents one of the few well-established evidence-based approaches to stroke prophylaxis in AF. The coumarin oral anticoagulants are extremely effective for prevention of clot formation due to stasis and/or

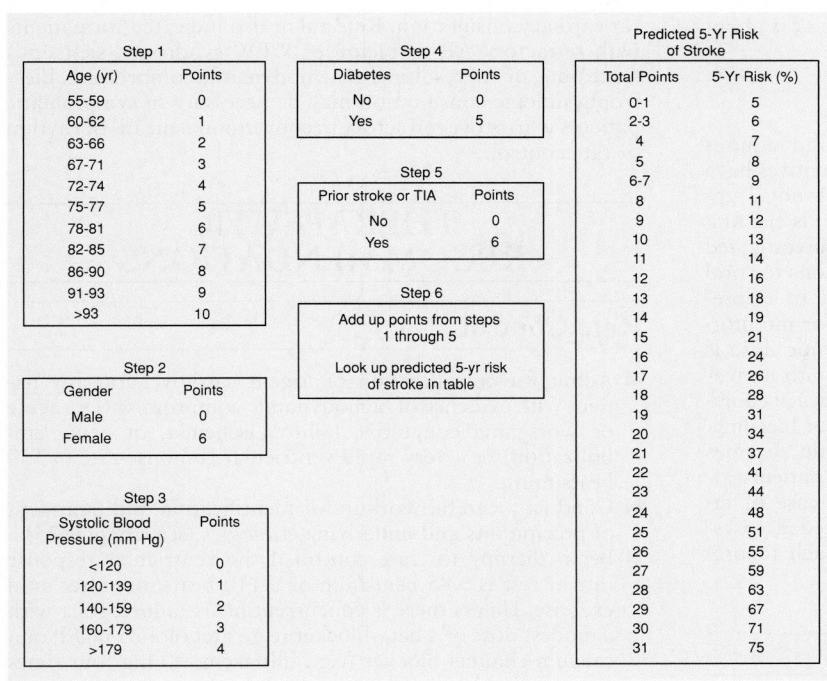

Step 1	
Age (yr)	Points
55-59	0
60-62	1
63-66	2
67-71	3
72-74	4
75-77	5
78-81	6
82-85	7
86-90	8
91-93	9
>93	10

Step 2	
Gender	Points
Male	0
Female	6

Step 3	
Systolic Blood Pressure (mm Hg)	Points
<120	0
120-139	1
140-159	2
160-179	3
>179	4

Step 4	
Diabetes	Points
No	0
Yes	5

Step 5	
Prior stroke or TIA	Points
No	0
Yes	6

Step 6
Add up points from steps 1 through 5
Look up predicted 5-yr risk of stroke in table

Predicted 5-Yr Risk of Stroke

Total Points	5-Yr Risk (%)
0-1	5
2-3	6
4	7
5	8
6-7	9
8	11
9	12
10	13
11	14
12	16
13	18
14	19
15	21
16	24
17	26
18	28
19	31
20	34
21	37
22	41
23	44
24	48
25	51
26	55
27	59
28	63
29	67
30	71
31	75

FIGURE 28.1. Calculating the risk score for stroke in atrial fibrillation. The point-based risk estimate approximates the more precise equation-based risk function provided as an Excel spreadsheet available at http://www.nhlbi.nih.gov/about/framingham/stroke.htm. The point-based risk estimate may differ from the equation-based one, particularly for patients with uncommon combinations of characteristics. TIA, transient ischemic attack. (From Wang TJ, Massaro JM, Levy K, et al. A risk score for predicting stroke or death in individuals with new-onset atrial fibrillation in the community. JAMA 2003;290:1049, with permission.)

endothelial damage (as occurs in the left atrium and left atrial appendage of AF patients with underlying heart disease). Warfarin anticoagulation significantly reduces the risk of systemic embolization and stroke, not only in persons with AF due to valvular rheumatic heart disease, but also in those with nonrheumatic heart disease. Risk is lowered by greater than two thirds. Most strokes that do occur in the context of warfarin anticoagulation are associated with noncompliance. Modern well-monitored, community-based oral anticoagulation programs help to ensure safety and minimize the risk of major hemorrhage, which averages 2%/yr in such settings. Nevertheless, the benefit must always be balanced by consideration of risk for major bleeding, which is small in population studies but needs to be individualized. Absolute increase in the risk of major extracranial hemorrhage was 0.3%/yr in meta-analytic study; the risk of intracranial hemorrhage was small with warfarin (absolute risk 0.2%/yr).

Assessment of Bleeding Risk (See Also Chapter 83). The most feared bleeding complication is *intracranial hemorrhage.* Annual incidence is 1.8% in persons older than the age of 75 years and increases by a factor of 1.5 for each 0.5 increase in INR over the goal of 2 to 3. Noncompliance and falls increase the risk of intracranial hemorrhage. History of recent intracranial hemorrhage is a contraindication to warfarin therapy. The risk of major *upper gastrointestinal hemorrhage* in a person with a recently resolved upper gastrointestinal bleed who has been tested and treated for any *Helicobacter pylori* infection is 1.2%/yr; the risk with concurrent nonsteroidal antiinflammatory therapy is 4.5%/yr (2.3%/yr with concurrent proton pump inhibitor use or cyclooxygenase-2 agent).

Patient Selection. In general, most persons at high risk for stroke due to AF will benefit from warfarin anticoagulation despite these bleeding risks, but moderate-risk persons might not and require careful weighing of stroke and bleeding risks. Low-risk patients are usually not candidates for warfarin. Other considerations include patient willingness and ability to comply with the demands of proper medication use and monitoring. Persons who poorly comply due to psychosocial factors (e.g., substance abuse, psychiatric illness) have an increased risk of adverse events (observed adjusted risk ratios in the range of 1.4 to 2.4). Similarly, elderly persons with AF prone to falls have a 10-fold increase in the risk of traumatic intracranial hemorrhage with warfarin therapy; nonetheless those with multiple stroke risk factors show a net benefit from anticoagulation.

Intensity of Warfarin Therapy. The optimal intensity of anticoagulation for maximizing reductions in stroke frequency and severity is an *INR of 2 to 3.* Lower-dose therapy (INR 1.5 to 1.9) provides significantly less prophylaxis without significantly reducing the risk of major bleeding. Higher-dose therapy (INR 3 to 4) markedly increases the risk of major bleeding without any appreciable improvement in stroke prophylaxis.

Dosing. There is wide variation among patients in dose response to warfarin, making dosing a trial and error process. Genotyping offers promise for identifying low- and high-dose haplotypes in the gene that encodes for vitamin K epoxide reductase complex 1 (VKORC1).

Initiating and Monitoring Therapy. See Chapter 83.

Aspirin

Low- to moderate-risk patients with nonvalvular AF treated with aspirin (325 mg/d) experience a very low rate of embolic events, approaching that of patients without AF. Because aspirin is less likely to cause cerebral hemorrhage than warfarin, it is preferable in this low-risk setting. However, when used in higher-risk patients, even in combination with low-dose warfarin, aspirin does not provide the same protection as does standard-dose warfarin (INR 2 to 3). Risk is reduced by about

22%, compared to 66% with warfarin. Bleeding risk is about one half of that of warfarin.

Direct Thrombin Inhibitors

Because warfarin therapy involves a bleeding risk and requires dose adjustment and coagulation monitoring, alternatives have been sought for patients with nonvalvular AF. A novel approach is direct thrombin inhibition; *ximelagatran* is the first of the direct thrombin inhibitors being extensively investigated for use in nonvalvular AF, as well as other indications for oral anticoagulation. It prolongs the prothrombin time in a dose-related predictable manner, eliminating the need for monitoring prothrombin time INR when a fixed therapeutic dose is used. In large-scale, randomized trial in patients with nonvalvular AF (SPORTIF V), the drug demonstrated efficacy equivalent to that of warfarin and slightly lower risks of bleeding, but significant transient increases in serum hepatic enzymes (alanine transaminase) occurred in about 6% of patients after 1 to 2 months of treatment, as well as one case of fatal liver failure. More data on safety will be needed to establish the role for this potentially useful approach to oral anticoagulation.

PATIENT EDUCATION

The young patient with paroxysmal AF who is free of underlying heart disease needs to be fully reassured to prevent cardiac neurosis and the unnecessary restriction of activity. Such patients should be instructed to quit smoking, avoid sleep deprivation, and limit the use of alcohol and stimulants. They often benefit from the use of relaxation techniques (see Chapter 226) at times of stress. WPW patients whose episodes of AF are brief, infrequent, and well tolerated can also be reassured and encouraged to remain fully active. Patients with AF secondary to alcohol abuse and evolving cardiomyopathy need to be informed of the risk of alcoholic cardiomyopathy and should be strongly urged to abstain from alcohol. In addition, patients at risk for AF from any other cause should be advised to use caution in their social drinking because excess intake may increase vulnerability to AF (see Chapters 25 and 228).

The cornerstone of safe, successful antiarrhythmic and anticoagulant therapies is patient education. Providing the rationale for treatment, addressing patient concerns (e.g., that drug treatment might be habit forming or injurious to the heart), and identifying potential barriers to compliance (e.g., cost of medication) are essential. Without causing undo alarm, patients and household members also need to be made aware of the symptoms and signs of hemodynamic compromise and adverse drug effects and instructed to report them promptly.

INDICATIONS FOR ADMISSION AND REFERRAL

Patients unable to tolerate their AF due to congestive heart failure or ischemia should be immediately hospitalized. The same is true if the ventricular response rate is extremely rapid (>150 to 170 beats/min). Electrical cardioversion may be urgent. Hospitalization is also indicated for patients refractory to medical therapy and those with new onset of embolization. Patients who are candidates for elective cardioversion need at least a temporary stay, even if only for the day. Patients deemed possible candidates for elective cardioversion should be referred for cardiac consultation. Referral is also indicated for patients with refractory AF, suspicion of WPW syndrome, sick sinus syndrome, or AF resulting in hemodynamic compromise. Electrophysiologic consultation may be necessary in symptomatic patients who prove refractory to conventional means of rhythm or rate control.

THERAPEUTIC RECOMMENDATIONS

Rate Control

■ Admit for consideration of urgent cardioversion any patient with evidence of hemodynamic compromise (i.e., acute or worsening congestive failure, ischemia, or acute embolization) or a very rapid ventricular response rate (>150 beats/min).

■ Conduct a careful workup for identification and treatment of precipitants and underlying etiologies (see Chapter 25).

■ Begin therapy for rate control if the ventricular response rate at rest is >85 beats/min or >110 beats/min after mild exercise. Unless there is concurrent heart failure, start with a modest dose of a beta-blocker (e.g., atenolol 25 mg/d) or a calcium-channel blocker (e.g., diltiazem, 30 mg four times a day, switching to a sustained-release formulation once an effective dose is established). In the setting of left ventricular systolic dysfunction, consider digoxin and/or very cautious low-dose use of a beta-blocker and avoid calcium-channel blockers (see Chapter 32).

■ In the setting of *WPW* and other preexcitation syndromes, refer for consideration of electrophysiologic study and ablative therapy; do not treat with digoxin or calcium-channel blockers because of their tendency to enhance conduction through accessory pathways. Young patients with brief and infrequent bouts of AF due to WPW need not be treated if episodes are well tolerated and the shortest RR interval is >180 msec.

■ In the setting of *sick sinus syndrome*, use considerable caution in the initiation of rate-control therapy because such patients are especially susceptible to symptomatic bradycardia; if marked bradycardia occurs on the initiation of such therapy, then refer for consideration of pacemaker implantation.

■ If rate control is difficult to achieve, recheck for failure, ischemia, fever, hypovolemia, hypoxia, recurrent pulmonary embolization, hyperthyroidism, and WPW syndrome. Treatment should be directed at the underlying condition. Hospitalize and refer to cardiology if the AF is not well tolerated and requires consideration of cardioversion and other interventional approaches.

Rhythm Control

■ Admit for consideration of *urgent cardioversion* any patient with evidence of *hemodynamic compromise* (i.e., acute or worsening congestive failure, ischemia, or acute embolization) or a *very rapid ventricular response rate* (>150 beats/min).

■ Conduct a careful workup for identification and treatment of precipitants and underlying etiologies (see Chapter 25).

■ Consider referring for *elective cardioversion* patients with *bothersome palpitations*, *reduced exercise tolerance*, or *failure to achieve rate control*. The best candidates are those likely to maintain sinus rhythm at low risk (blood pressure well controlled, left atrium not markedly enlarged, LV function well preserved). The worst candidates are those with a high probability of unresponsiveness or relapse (e.g., AF of >1 year duration, marked left atrial enlargement, rheumatic etiology, heart failure).

■ For candidates with AF of <48 hours' duration, proceed to *elective cardioversion with heparinization only.*

■ For candidates with AF of >48 hours' duration or with AF of *unknown duration,* prescribe *oral anticoagulation* for 1 month before *elective cardioversion.* Alternatively, obtain *TEE study* for the determination of *left atrial clot;* in the absence of clot, proceed to *cardioversion without need for oral anticoagulation.*

■ Prescribe *chronic antiarrhythmic pharmacologic therapy* (e.g., amiodarone 100 to 200 mg/d) after cardioversion for those who are at *high risk for relapse* (e.g., previous relapse, marked left atrial enlargement, advanced underlying heart disease, heart failure, high voltage required for cardioversion). For patients prescribed *amiodarone,* monitor *liver function* tests and *thyrotropin* every 6 months.

■ Prescribe *warfarin* anticoagulation for at least 4 weeks' postcardioversion and consider long-term warfarin therapy in those at *high risk for relapse and stroke.*

■ Refer those with *frequent symptomatic recurrences* of AF despite antiarrhythmic therapy for consideration of *interventional approaches* (e.g., ablation, pacing, defibrillator placement), especially if recurrences are not well tolerated hemodynamically.

Stroke Prophylaxis

■ Conduct stroke *risk stratification* by taking into account the patient's age, gender, systolic blood pressure, left ventricular function, diabetes status, and prior history of stroke (see Fig. 28.1). Assess *bleeding risk* as well.

■ Initiate chronic *warfarin* oral anticoagulation for all AF patients at *high risk* for stroke, unless there is a serious contraindication to warfarin (see Chapter 83).

■ Prescribe an adjustable-dose *warfarin* program that achieves a prothrombin time of 2.0 to 3.0 INR.

■ Weigh the risks and benefits for *moderate-risk* patients, and individualize the decision to anticoagulate. *Low-risk* patients are not candidates.

■ Prescribe enteric-coated *aspirin* (325 mg/d) for those not deemed to be candidates for warfarin therapy or who refuse it; those with concurrent atherosclerotic risk factors are likely to benefit most.

■ For those at *high risk* for systemic embolization (e.g., prior embolization or stroke, systolic dysfunction, significant left atrial mural thrombus, or female gender plus age >75 years), consider *elective cardioversion, atrial pacing, ablative therapy,* and other means of *maintaining sinus rhythm* to help reduce stroke risk, but continue oral anticoagulation even if sinus rhythm is restored.

A.H.G.

Annotated Bibliography

1. Atrial Fibrillation Investigators. Echocardiographic predictors of stroke in patients with atrial fibrillation: a prospective study of 1066 patients from 3 clinical trials. Arch Intern Med 1998;158:1316. (*Identifies left ventricular dysfunction as an independent predictor.*)

2. Bogun F, Anh D, Kalahasty F, et al. Misdiagnosis of atrial fibrillation and its clinical consequences. Am J Med 2004;117:636. (*A high false-positive rate was noted with the use of automated electrocardiogram readings.*)

3. Brand FN, Abbott RD, Kannel WB, et al. Characteristics and prognosis of lone atrial fibrillation: 30-year follow-up in the Framingham Study. JAMA 1985;254:3449. (*A fourfold increase in stroke risk was noted, but patients were older and had more cardiovascular risk factors than patients in other studies of lone atrial fibrillation [AF].*)

4. Engel TR, Luck JC. Effect of whiskey on atrial vulnerability and "holiday heart." J Am Coll Cardiol 1983;1:816. (*Alcohol enhanced vulnerability to AF in patients without clinical evidence of cardiomyopathy or heart failure.*)

5. Frost L, Vestergaard P. Alcohol and risk of atrial fibrillation or flutter. Arch Intern Med 2004;164:1933. (*Large Danish cohort study; a modest increase in risk was found, but only in men.*)

6. Go AS, Hylek EM, Phillips KA, et al. Prevalence of diagnosed atrial fibrillation in adults: national implications for rhythm management and stroke prevention: the AnTicoagulation and Risk Factors in Atrial Fibrillation (ATRIA) study. JAMA 2001;285:2370. (*Cross-sectional epidemiologic study; confirms that AF is common in the elderly.*)

7. Haissaguerre M, Jais P, Shah D, et al. Spontaneous initiation of atrial fibrillation by ectopic beats originating in the pulmonary veins. N Engl J Med 1998;339:659. (*Evidence for an extraatrial source for most triggering beats and the use of ablation as therapy.*)

8. Gollob MH, Jones DL, Krahn AD, et al. Somatic mutations in the connexin 40 gene (GJA5) in atrial fibrillation. N Engl J Med 2006;354:2677. (*A possible molecular basis for idiopathic AF.*)

9. Hart RG, Halperin JL, Pearce LA, et al. Lessons from the Stroke Prevention in Atrial Fibrillation Trials. Ann Intern Med 2003;138:831. (*A summary of these landmark studies, including risk stratification for stroke and approach to stroke prevention.*)

10. Kannel WB, Abbott RD, Savage DD, et al. Epidemiologic features of chronic atrial fibrillation: the Framingham Study. N Engl J Med 1982;306:1018. (*A major epidemiologic study; heart failure and rheumatic heart disease were the most powerful predictive precursors of chronic AF; chronic AF was associated with a doubling of cardiovascular and overall mortality.*)

11. Kopecky SL, Gersh BJ, McGoon MD, et al. The natural history of lone atrial fibrillation: a population-based study over three decades. N Engl J Med 1987;317:669. (*A retrospective study of patients younger than the age of 60 years showing that lone AF was associated with a very low risk of stroke.*)

12. Maisel WH, Rawn JD, Stevenson WG. Atrial fibrillation after cardiac surgery. Ann Intern Med 2001;135:1061. (*Systematic review; 104 references.*)

13. Mitchell GF, Vasan RS, Keyes MJ, et al. Pulse pressure and risk of new-onset atrial fibrillation. JAMA 2007;297:709. (*Increased pulse pressure was found to be associated with a significant independent increase in risk of AF.*)

14. Stollberger C, Chnupa P, Kronik G, et al. Transesophageal echocardiography to assess embolic risk in patients with atrial fibrillation. Ann Intern Med 1998;128:630. (*A multicenter observational study identifying important risk factors for embolic stroke in AF, including thrombus in the left atrium, hypertension, previous stroke, and advancing age.*)

15. The Stroke Prevention in Atrial Fibrillation Investigators. Predictors of thromboembolism in atrial fibrillation. Ann Intern Med 1992;116:1. (*A two-part study; recent congestive heart failure, hypertension, previous embolism, left ventricular dysfunction, and left atrial enlargement were independent predictors of stroke risk.*)

16. The Stroke Prevention in Atrial Fibrillation Investigators. Transesophageal echocardiographic correlates of thromboembolism in high-risk patients with nonvalvular atrial fibrillation. Ann Intern Med 1998;128:639. (*A prospective observational study finding that left atrial thrombus and complex aortic atherosclerotic plaque detected by transesophageal electrocardiography are highly correlated with the risk of subsequent thromboembolism.*)

17. Wang TJ, Massaro JM, Levy K, et al. A risk score for predicting stroke or death in individuals with new-onset atrial fibrillation in the community. JAMA 2003;290:1049. (*Major prospective, community-based epidemiologic cohort study; risk categories are developed to help guide therapy.*)

18. Wolf PA, Kannel WB, McGee DL, et al. Duration of atrial fibrillation and imminence of stroke: the Framingham Study. Stroke 1983;14:664. (*Important epidemiology data; risk of embolic stroke was found to be maximal at the onset of AF, independent of other risk factors for stroke, and substantial even in AF patients without rheumatic mitral disease; recurrence was twice as likely in patients with AF.*)

19. Cooper JM, Katcher MS, Orlov MV. Implantable devices for the treatment of atrial fibrillation. N Engl J Med 2002;346:2062. (*Useful review of this emerging approach to treatment; 68 references.*)

20. Falk RH, Leavitt JI. Digoxin for atrial fibrillation: a drug whose time has gone? Ann Intern Med 1991;114:573. (*A review critical of digoxin, which emphasizes its shortcomings in the treatment of AF; 22 references.*)

21. Fuster V, Ryden LE, Asinger RW, et al. ACC/AHA/ESC guidelines for the management of patients with atrial fibrillation. J Am Coll Cardiol 2001;38:1231. (*Consensus recommendations.*)

22. Grace AA, Camm AJ. Quinidine. N Engl J Med 1998;338:35. (*Excellent review of this long-prescribed drug; addresses its uses and limitations in AF; 105 references.*)

23. Ozcan C, Jahangir A, Friedman JP, et al. Long-term survival after ablation of the atrioventricular node and implantation of the permanent pacemaker in patients with atrial fibrillation. N Engl J Med 2001;344:1043. (*Prospective case–control study; no reduction in long-term survival was noted.*)

24. Rawles JM, Metcalfe MJ, Jennings K. Time occurrence, duration and ventricular rate of paroxysmal atrial fibrillation: the effect of digoxin. Br Heart J 1990;63:225. (*Digoxin was observed in this Holter monitoring study to have little effect on preventing recurrences, slowing the rate at the onset of a paroxysm, or terminating episodes.*)

25. Falk RH. Proarrhythmia in patients treated for atrial fibrillation or flutter. Ann Intern Med 1992;117:141. (*A review of the potential for dysrhythmias from drugs used to treat AF.*)

26. Falk RH. Management of atrial fibrillation—radical reform or modest modification? N Engl J Med 2002;347:1883. (*An editorial assessing the significance of new evidence in support of rate control over rhythm control.*)

27. Klein AL, Grimm RA, Murray, et al. Use of transesophageal echocardiography to guide cardioversion in patients with atrial fibrillation. N Engl J Med 2001;344:1411. (*Major randomized, controlled trial [RCT]; use of transesophageal electrocardiography was found to be an effective alternative to conventional management.*)

28. Oral H, Pappone C, Chugh A, et al. Circumferential pulmonary-vein ablation for chronic atrial fibrillation. N Engl J Med 2006;354:934. (*RCT demonstrating 74% efficacy in achieving sustained sinus rhythm without pharmacologic therapy.*)

29. Roy D, Talajic M, Connolly S, et al. Amiodarone to prevent recurrence of atrial fibrillation. N Engl J Med 2000;342:913. (*Multicenter RCT; amiodarone was superior to sotalol and propafenone.*)

30. The Atrial Fibrillation Follow-up Investigation of Rhythm Management (AFFIRM) Investigators. A comparison of rate control and rhythm control in patients with atrial fibrillation. N Engl J Med 2002;347:1825. (*Major RCT; rate control was superior to rhythm control.*)

31. Van Gelder IC, Hagens VE, Bosker HA, et al. A comparison of rate control and rhythm control in patients with recurrent persistent atrial fibrillation. N Engl J Med 2002;347:1834. (*Landmark European RCT; rate control was equal to rhythm control.*)

32. Weigner MJ, Caulfield TA, Danias PG, et al. Risk for clinical thromboembolism associated with conversion to sinus rhythm in patients with atrial fibrillation lasting less than 48 hours. Ann Intern Med 1997;126:615. (*A prospective observational study finding that cardioversion-related risk was nil.*)

33. Zimetbaum P. Amiodarone for atrial fibrillation. N Engl J Med 2007;356:935. (*Clinically oriented review.*)

34. Boston Area Anticoagulation Trial for Atrial Fibrillation Investigators. The effect of low-dose warfarin on the risk of stroke in patients with non-rheumatic atrial fibrillation. N Engl J Med 1990;323:1505. (*One of several major randomized trials demonstrating the benefit of an international normalized ratio [INR] of 2 to 3 in patients with chronic or paroxysmal AF.*)

35. Gage BF, Birman-Deych E, Kerzner R, et al. Incidence of intracranial hemorrhage in patients with atrial fibrillation who are prone to fall. Am J Med 2005;118:612. (*Prospective observational study with a control cohort; those with a high risk of falls had 10 times the rate of traumatic intracranial hemorrhage, but nonetheless showed a net benefit from anticoagulation if they had multiple stroke risk factors.*)

36. Gage BF, Cardinalli AB, Albers GW, et al. Cost-effectiveness of warfarin and aspirin for prophylaxis of stroke in patients with nonvalvular atrial fibrillation. JAMA 1995;274:1839. (*Data supporting the cost-effectiveness of warfarin.*)

37. Go AS, Hylek EM, Borowsky LH, et al. Warfarin use among ambulatory patients with nonvalvular atrial fibrillation: the AnTicoagulation and Risk Factor in Atrial Fibrillation (ATRIA) Study. Ann Intern Med 1999;131:927. (*A cross-sectional study of a health maintenance organization population; documented marked underutilization of warfarin in ideal candidates.*)

38. Hart RG, Pearce LA, Aguilar MI. Meta-analysis: antithrombotic therapy to prevent stroke in patients who have nonvalvular atrial fibrillation. Ann Intern Med 2007;146:857. (*Meta-analysis; warfarin was the best treatment.*)

39. Hylek EM, Go AS, Chang Y, et al. Effect of intensity of oral anticoagulation on stroke severity and mortality in atrial fibrillation. N Engl J Med 2003;349:1019. (*Large cohort study; INR >2.0 produced the best outcomes, associated with reductions in stroke severity and mortality.*)

40. Rieder MJ, Reiner AP, Gage BF, et al. Effect of VKORC1 haplotypes on transcriptional regulation of warfarin dose. N Engl J Med 2005;352:2285. (*Retrospective study found that genotyping was able to stratify patients into high-, intermediate-, and low-dose warfarin groups.*)

41. Schauer DP, Moomaw CJ, Wess M, et al. Psychosocial risk factors for adverse outcomes in patients with nonvalvular atrial fibrillation receiving warfarin. J Gen Intern Med 2005;20:1114. (*Retrospective cohort study showing increased risk of adverse events.*)

42. Singer DE. Randomized trials of warfarin for atrial fibrillation. N Engl J Med 1992;327:1451. (*A fine editorial succinctly summarizing the known and unknown.*)

43. Singh BN, Singh SN, Reda DJ, et al. Amiodarone versus sotalol for atrial fibrillation. N Engl J Med 2005;322:1861. (*Major RCT of 665 patients; both drugs were similarly efficacious in achieving rhythm control, but amiodarone was better for maintaining sinus rhythm, except in those with coronary disease, in which case sotalol was equally effective.*)

44. SPORTIF Executive Steering Committee for the SPORTIF V Investigators. Ximelagatran vs warfarin for stroke prevention in patients with nonvalvular atrial fibrillation. JAMA 2005;293:690. (*Large-scale RCT; efficacy was comparable, but there was an increased risk of hepatocellular toxicity with ximelagatran.*)

45. The Stroke Prevention in Atrial Fibrillation Investigators. Adjusted-dose warfarin versus low-intensity, fixed-dose warfarin plus aspirin for high-risk patients with atrial fibrillation: Stroke Prevention in Atrial Fibrillation III randomized clinical trial. Lancet 1996;348:633. (*A trial finding that adjusted-dose therapy was superior to low-intensity therapy plus aspirin.*)

46. The Stroke Prevention in Atrial Fibrillation Investigators. Patients with nonvalvular atrial fibrillation at low risk of stroke during treatment with aspirin: Stroke Prevention in Atrial Fibrillation III Study. JAMA 1998;279:1273. (*A prospective cohort study identifying AF patients at low risk for subsequent embolic complications.*)

CHAPTER 29 ■ MANAGEMENT OF VENTRICULAR IRRITABILITY IN THE AMBULATORY SETTING

The discovery of ventricular ectopy in the outpatient setting raises concerns about serious underlying heart disease and the possibilities of cardiac arrest and sudden death. At issue is how much danger the ventricular irritability poses, a critical determination because treatment is also fraught with risk. In some instances, pharmacologic suppression of ventricular irritability may actually increase risk of sudden death rather than reduce it. Management of ventricular ectopy is shifting from reliance on antiarrhythmic drugs to implantation of cardioverter–defibrillators, which have demonstrated promising results in preventing cardiac arrest and sudden death. Determining the optimal approach to management in this period of change requires close consultation with a cardiologist experienced in treating ventricular dysrhythmias. The primary care physician's principal tasks are to identify high-risk patients, arrange timely cardiac consultation, help patients to choose the treatment option best suited to their needs, and monitor therapy. Knowledge of the relative benefits of antiarrhythmic drugs and implantable defibrillators is essential to therapeutic decision making. Close monitoring and long-term follow-up by the primary physician help to ensure safe and effective management.

CLINICAL PRESENTATION AND COURSE (1–15)

Premature ventricular contractions (PVCs) are ubiquitous and commonly found among patients both with and without underlying heart disease. In studies of the general population, at least one PVC per routine electrocardiogram (ECG) was found in 1% of Air Force recruits, 4% of life insurance applicants, 7% of men >34 years of age, and 40% to 75% of normal persons subjected to 24 to 48 hours of continuous ambulatory (Holter) monitoring. The incidence and prevalence of PVCs increase with age and with exercise. There is no evidence that moderate intake of caffeine increases the frequency or severity of ventricular dysrhythmias in normal individuals or patients with heart disease, even those with preexisting serious ventricular ectopy.

In the ambulatory setting, ventricular irritability usually presents in one of several ways: as an incidental finding on routine examination or ECG; as an ECG finding in a patient being evaluated for palpitations, dizziness, or syncope; or as a complication of underlying heart disease noted on resting ECG, exercise stress test, or Holter monitoring. *Frequent PVCs* are defined as >60 ectopic beats/hr; *complex ventricular ectopy* is characterized by multiforms, repetitive forms, bigeminy, or R on T. *Ventricular tachycardia* (VT) refers to three or more PVCs in a row; in the *monomorphic* type, all QRS complexes are identical; in *polymorphic* VT (e.g., torsades de pointes),

the QRS complexes are all different. *Nonsustained VT* refers to brief, self-limited runs of VT; *sustained VT* persists in the absence of intervention. Prognosis is a function of the presence and severity of any underlying heart disease and the nature of the ventricular ectopic activity.

Benign Ventricular Arrhythmias

Initially, prospective studies of large populations of ambulatory men were believed to have shown a correlation between PVCs on routine ECG and subsequent sudden death; however, when these results were reexamined controlling for other cardiac risk factors, PVCs were not found to be an independent determinant of cardiac death in the general population. *Asymptomatic healthy* subjects, even those with frequent or complex PVCs, showed *no increased mortality* on long-term follow-up. Regardless of the presence and persistence of worrisome ventricular irritability, such patients have prognoses no different from those of other healthy people; there is no increased risk of cardiac death.

Other natural history surveys also emphasized that in the absence of hypertension, angina, history of myocardial infarction, heart failure, cardiomegaly on chest x-ray or ECG signs of ischemia, left ventricular (LV) hypertrophy, or bundle-branch block, people with PVCs are at no greater risk for cardiac death than the general population.

Potentially Adverse Ventricular Arrhythmias

In comparison with patients free of underlying heart disease, the situation is more worrisome for patients with a variety of cardiac problems.

In the Setting of Recent Myocardial Infarction

In the Coronary Drug Project study of >2,000 survivors of myocardial infarction, the occurrence of even a *single PVC* on a routine ECG taken 3 months or more after the infarct was associated with a *doubling* of the *mortality rate* during the 3-year follow-up period. The features most predictive of mortality are *high frequency* of PVCs (>30/hr over a 24-hour period) and presence of *complex* ventricular ectopy, especially repetitive beats (33 consecutive complexes). Prognosis is particularly poor in the setting of a *failing left ventricle* (ejection fraction <0.4). For patients with recent myocardial infarction, reduced ejection fraction, and nonsustained VT, the rate for cardiac arrest or sudden death approaches 20% at 2 years and exceeds 30% at 5 years.

237

In the Setting of Remote Myocardial Infarction

In this context, the frequency and complexity of PVCs also influence prognosis. The absence of ventricular irritability on a 1-hour ECG recording performed 3 to 9 months postinfarction is associated with a 6% risk of sudden cardiac death over 5 years, compared with 12% in patients with unifocal PVCs and 25% in those with complex ventricular ectopy. *Complex ventricular ectopy* (e.g., multifocal PVCs, nonsustained VT) has the strongest influence on risk for sudden cardiac death in this population (see later discussion).

In the Setting of Other Forms of Underlying Heart Disease

The situation is similar in other forms of heart disease that cause myocardial scarring and abnormal wall motion. Patients with hypertrophic or congestive *cardiomyopathy*, hemodynamically significant *valvular disease*, congenital heart disease with ventricular hypertrophy, hypertensive *LV hypertrophy*, and *revascularization* or *valve surgery* have been found to be at significantly increased risk of sudden death if they experience frequent or complex PVCs, especially in the context of a *reduced ejection fraction*. The ventricular ectopy is not merely a manifestation of the underlying heart disease, but is an independent predictor of prognosis. *QT interval prolongation*, be it congenital or acquired, predisposes to malignant ventricular dysrhythmias (e.g., torsades de pointes; see later discussion). Patients with *substance abuse*, particularly *cocaine* and *alcohol*, may manifest ventricular dysrhythmias due to underlying myocardial injury.

In the Recovery Phase of Exercise Stress Testing

Frequent or complex ventricular ectopy that occurs during the *recovery period of exercise* stress testing may have a worrisome prognosis. In a large-scale observational study from the Cleveland Clinic, patients who manifested frequent (≥ 7 beats/min) or complex ventricular ectopy during the recovery period of exercise stress testing had an increased risk of death (adjusted hazard ratio, 1.5) that was independent of other cardiac risk factors. Ventricular ectopy that occurred during stress testing but not in the recovery period did not confer similar independent mortality risk when corrected for confounding variables. Patients with frequent ventricular ectopy during recovery had increased risk of underlying coronary disease and left ventricular systolic dysfunction.

Malignant Ventricular Arrhythmias

The main determinants of adverse prognosis in patients with ventricular ectopy are the presence of underlying heart disease and a failing left ventricle (see prior discussion). Each of these factors is an independent predictor of survival. The complexity of the ventricular ectopy is also a determinant of prognosis, especially in patients with heart disease and LV failure, where VT portends an especially high risk of cardiac sudden death.

Nonsustained Ventricular Tachycardia

Nonsustained VT is a worrisome arrhythmia characterized by runs of VT that spontaneously revert to sinus rhythm within several beats. Unless there is hemodynamic compromise, nonsustained VT may be asymptomatic. In the context of *chronic coronary artery disease and LV dysfunction*, it represents a malignant form of electrical instability that is an independent risk factor for sudden death, increasing risk fivefold to 30% at 2 years. It has a more benign form, found in young patients with *no demonstrable heart disease* and characterized by resolution with exercise, no associated symptoms, and a regular, relatively slow rate (<150 beats/min) with uniform cycle length and QRS morphology.

Recurrent Sustained Ventricular Tachycardia

Recurrent sustained VT is a very dangerous ventricular arrhythmia, especially when it occurs in the context of *LV dysfunction*. Untreated, the 1-year mortality rate is about 40%; prognosis is poorest in symptomatic patients with compromised LV function. The arrhythmia is characterized by repeated episodes of VT, some of which may persist for up to several hours. Many patients become symptomatic due to a fall in cardiac output, which can lead to syncope, near-syncope, angina, or dyspnea. Coronary artery disease and cardiomyopathy account for almost 90% of cases. About 1% of postinfarction patients experience this arrhythmia during the first year of follow-up.

Torsades de Pointes

Torsades de pointes is a rapid, polymorphic VT that often deteriorates into ventricular fibrillation. The characteristic feature is a QRS axis that twists about the ECG baseline, going from positive to negative and back again. The arrhythmia occurs in the context of *QT-interval prolongation*, whether congenital or acquired. This is a very malignant ventricular dysrhythmia most commonly seen as an *acquired* condition in patients with electrolyte abnormalities (especially hypokalemia or hypomagnesemia) and use of drugs that prolong the QT interval (Table 29.1). Risk increases with electrolyte abnormalities, use of antiarrhythmics, or when an agent that prolongs the QT interval is used in conjunction with one that impairs its mitochondrial metabolism (Table 29.1). In the *congenital form* of QT prolongation, patients are young and have no evidence of structural heart disease but may have a family history of early (before age 30 years) sudden death in first-degree relatives, a personal history of prior syncope (especially in the setting of stress) or deafness, and ECG findings of QT prolongation, T-wave alternans, and notched T waves in at least three leads.

Probability of Occult Heart Disease in Asymptomatic Persons with Premature Ventricular Contractions

As long as the asymptomatic patient with PVCs has no evidence of underlying heart disease, the prognosis appears fine, but what is the probability of occult heart disease in an otherwise apparently healthy patient presenting with frequent or complex PVCs? The best approximation is that risk is not high. In a study of such patients subjected to coronary catheterization and angiography, only one fourth were found to have significant coronary artery disease (defined as >50% luminal narrowing). The characteristics of the ventricular ectopy did not differentiate those with coronary disease from those without it. These asymptomatic patients were treated with modest doses of beta-blocking agents and had normal survival rates after 5 years of follow-up. On the other hand, patients with syncope of unknown origin who manifest complex ventricular irritability and signs of underlying heart disease have a high risk of further syncope and cardiac death, especially if they demonstrate inducible sustained VT on electrophysiologic study.

TABLE 29.1

SOME DRUGS ASSOCIATED WITH PROLONGATION OF THE QT INTERVAL

Psychotropic agents
    Amitriptyline
    Imipramine
    Desipramine
    Haloperidol
    Thioridazine
    Pimozide
    Clozapine
Antiarrhythmics
    Procainamide
    Quinidine
    Disopyramide
Antifungal agents
    Ketoconazole
    Itraconazole
Antibiotics
    Erythromycin
    Clarithromycin
Antihistamines
    Terfenadine
    Astemizole
Prokinetic agents
    Cisapride
Antitumor agents
    Tamoxifen

Effect was enhanced by the concurrent use of drugs that inhibit cytochrome P450 enzymes (e.g., selective serotonin reuptake inhibitors, quinolone antibiotics, calcium-channel blockers, antiretroviral agents, amiodarone).
Adapted from Liu BA, Juurlink DN. Drugs and the QT interval—caveat doctor. N Engl J Med 2004;351:1053.

PRINCIPLES OF MANAGEMENT
(1,6,9,14–41)

Major progress has been made in the prevention of sudden death from malignant ventricular irritability. The approach to management has undergone fundamental change as treatment has shifted from pharmacologic therapy to the use of *implantable cardioverter–defibrillators* (ICDs). Prospective, randomized trials comparing ICDs with the best of antiarrhythmic agents find that the implantable devices are superior for primary and secondary prevention of cardiac sudden death in high-risk patients (average relative risk approximately 0.5). However, benefit over drug therapy is less pronounced in persons at lesser risk, necessitating careful patient selection. The traditional antiarrhythmics have been supplanted by amiodarone and beta-blockers, which are largely free of the proarrhythmic effects (see later discussion) that have compromised pharmacotherapy outcomes.

Candidacy for Treatment: Patient Selection

Risk stratification is essential to treatment selection because only those at highest risk benefit from ICD and/or antiarrhythmic pharmacotherapy. However, risk stratification remains rudimentary because there are no prospectively validated risk-stratification rules. Consensus recommendations regarding candidacy for an ICD and pharmacologic therapy are based on extrapolation from the findings of major randomized trials (Table 29.2).

The spectrum of patients qualifying for treatment has narrowed considerably with the appreciation that conventional antiarrhythmic agents (especially class I drugs—*quinidine, procainamide, disopyramide, mexiletine,* and *tocainide,* and even the newer class IC agents—*flecainide* and *moricizine*) increase risk of sudden death, probably as a consequence of their *proarrhythmic potential*. No longer are patients with complex ventricular irritability and underlying heart disease considered appropriate candidates for antiarrhythmic drug therapy (beyond beta-blockade) if they are asymptomatic and have preserved LV function. If their LV function declines, amiodarone may be considered; otherwise, attempts to suppress ventricular ectopy have largely ceased. The one exception is use of amiodarone and beta-blockade in very-high-risk patients who have a contraindication for ICD implantation (e.g., terminal illness, end-stage heart failure, VT or ventricular fibrillation [VF] due to correctable cause).

In sum, the realizations that rates of dysrhythmic sudden death may be (a) markedly reduced by ICD (and, to a lesser extent, by amiodarone therapy), but only in those at highest risk, and (b) worsened by conventional antiarrhythmic drugs, which have greatly increased the threshold for treatment of ventricular ectopy, have led to the recommendation that only patients at highest risk from ventricular dysrhythmic disease (e.g., prior cardiac arrest; very-high-risk hereditary condition; symptomatic or inducible sustained VT, especially in the context of recent myocardial infarction; and reduced ejection fraction) should be considered for prophylactic measures.

Identification of Candidates for Treatment

Clinical Features and Basic Testing

Patients who present in the outpatient setting with complex ventricular irritability, especially nonsustained VT, should be evaluated thoroughly for *underlying heart disease*, *LV dysfunction*, and *QT prolongation* (see Chapters 20, 24, and 25), features that are associated with increased risk of cardiac sudden death.

History should check for syncope, chest pain, dyspnea, hypertension, coronary risk factors, and family history of early sudden death and premature coronary disease. Medications should be reviewed for drugs that may prolong the QT interval or inhibit their metabolism (Table 29.1); risk is increased when several are taken concurrently. Screening for substance abuse, particularly cocaine and alcohol, should not be overlooked.

Physical examination concentrates on blood pressure, findings of LV hypertrophy (heave, S4) and LV dysfunction (jugular venous distention, crackles, S3), and other manifestations of atherosclerotic disease (arterial bruits, diminished peripheral pulses, enlarged abdominal aorta). *Laboratory testing* should include a *resting ECG* for etiologically important clues (e.g., left ventricular hypertrophy, prior infarction, prolonged QT interval, right-bundle-branch block, and ST elevation in lead V1 [Brugada syndrome]). *Chest x-ray* can confirm congestive failure. An *echocardiogram* is useful for determination of ejection fraction and detection of wall motion abnormalities when there is suspicion of cardiomyopathy, heart failure, or ischemia. A *toxic screen* for cocaine and its metabolites may be indicated when there is clinical suspicion of substance abuse.

TABLE 29.2

CANDIDACY FOR TREATMENT ACCORDING TO RISK OF CARDIAC SUDDEN DEATH

Risk	Treatment Modality
Very High Risk	
Prior cardiac arrest due to VT or VF	ICD
Sustained VT + structural heart disease	ICD
Unexplained syncope + inducible sustained VT or VF, or advanced structural heart disease and no other cause found	ICD
CHD + LV dysfunction + inducible sustained VT	ICD
Myocardial infarction + marked LV dysfunction (EF <30%)	ICD
Inherited condition with stress-induced syncope or family history of early sudden death (e.g., long-QT syndrome, Brugada syndrome, hypertrophic cardiomyopathy)	ICD
Moderate Risk	
CHD, LV dysfunction, and asymptomatic nonsustained VT (but no inducible sustained VT)	Amiodarone ± beta-blocker
Low to Moderate Risk	
CHD, LV dysfunction, VEA, but no inducible nonsustained or sustained VT	Beta-blocker

CHD, coronary heart disease; EF, ejection fraction; ICD, implantable cardioverter–defibrillator; LV, left ventricular; VF, ventricular fibrillation; VT, ventricular tachycardia; VEA, ventricular ectopic activity. Adapted from DiMarco JP. Implantable cardioverters–defibrillators. N Engl J Med 2003;349:1836, and Goldschlarger N, Epstein AE, Naccarelli G, et al. Practical guidelines for physicians who treat patients with amiodarone. Arch Intern Med 2000;160:1741, with permission.

Exercise Stress Testing

As noted earlier, development of complex ventricular ectopy in the recovery phase of exercise stress testing has been noted independently to predict increased risk of cardiac death (relative risk 1.5) and may also be helpful in detection of underlying coronary heart disease (see Chapter 36).

Electrophysiologic Study

Electrophysiologic study (EPS) is an invasive procedure, requiring formal cardiac catheterization and an experienced staff. Inducibility of sustained VT correlates well with risks of clinically sustained VT, cardiac arrest, cardiac sudden death, and benefit from cardioverter–defibrillator implantation. Consequently, the study is often performed to help identify candidates for defibrillator implantation. Those who should be referred for consideration of EPS include patients with asymptomatic nonsustained VT who have evidence of *underlying heart disease* and a *reduced ejection fraction* (<0.40). Nearly 40% of such patients demonstrate inducible sustained VT and improved survival from defibrillator implantation. Others in whom EPS facilitates decision making are those with syncope of unknown origin who manifest clinical findings suggestive of a cardiac etiology (see prior discussion). Less compelling is the need for EPS in those with documented VT accompanied by *hemodynamic compromise* (syncope, near-syncope, angina, dyspnea). EPS to determine antiarrhythmic ability to suppress induced VT has been abandoned with the finding that suppression does not correlate with outcome. Studies are undergoing to better determine the indications for this very expensive and invasive procedure and simpler alternatives to predict outcome and benefit from therapy.

Ambulatory Monitoring

The importance of detecting VT has stimulated some to consider ambulatory monitoring to screen all potentially high-risk patients (i.e., those with recent myocardial infarction, hypertrophic cardiomyopathy, or congestive heart failure). However, except for those with syncope or a family history of early sudden death, such screening has not changed outcomes and is not recommended at this time.

Selection and Initiation of Therapy

Choice of Treatment (Table 29.2)

As noted earlier, very-high-risk patients are the best candidates for prophylactic measures against dysrhythmia-induced cardiac sudden death. The approach of choice in such patients is *implantation of a cardioverter–defibrillator,* which produces a 50% reduction in relative risk of sudden cardiac death compared to *amiodarone with or without beta-blockade* (the best available pharmacologic therapy, which reduces dysrhythmic events by nearly 60% and death by about 15% to 20%). A combination of ICD and pharmacotherapy is commonly used to reduce the number of uncomfortable defibrillatory discharges (see later discussion).

Implantable Cardioverter–Defibrillators

Available technology involves implantation of a pacemaker-sized device using procedures similar to those for pacemakers (e.g., subclavian or cephalic vein insertion, subcutaneous or submuscular left pectoral generator implantation). A complex right ventricular lead is used for sensing and pacing; a coiling of this lead delivers any needed shock. The unit discharges a high-voltage shock in response to detecting ventricular fibrillation or rapid VT and begins pacing when slower monomorphic VT is detected. Maximum output is up to 30 J; the amount needed for defibrillation is between 5 and 15 J. Dual-chamber models better discriminate between ventricular and supraventricular tachyarrhythmias and allow dual-chamber pacing. Implantation is associated with a small risk of infection (2%); perioperative morality is <1%. Inappropriate shocks from mistaking supraventricular tachyarrhythmias for VT are the most common operational complication, occurring in about 20% of patients. Inappropriate firing can be terminated by placing a magnet over the device box, which should be done during any resuscitation efforts. Battery depletion is rare; battery life ranges from 5 to 9 years depending on the amount of discharging required. After implantation, there is no increased risk of endocarditis and no need for endocarditis prophylaxis.

Indications and Contraindications. Implantation is used both for primary and secondary prevention of life-threatening ventricular dysrhythmias, particularly in very-high-risk persons (Table 29.2). The indications are in a state of evolution as the full scope of benefit continues to be updated by the results of ongoing prospective, randomized trials. Contraindications include use for dysrhythmias triggered by a *self-limited event* (e.g., acute myocardial infarction), *completely correctable event* (e.g., electrolyte or metabolic disturbances), *unexplained syncope* in the absence of structural heart disease or inducible VT or VF, and *refractory disease* necessitating frequent shocks in a person with <1 year of life expectancy.

Effect on Quality of Life. Most patients adapt well, but the shock can be uncomfortable, described as similar to putting one's hand in an electrical socket. Frequent shocks can be very demoralizing and upsetting, necessitating additional measures (e.g., reprogramming, addition of pharmacologic therapy). About 15% of patients experience brief syncope due to delay in cardioversion. The risk of a recurrence decreases with time, reaching a nadir 6 months after an episode. It is at this time that most authorities allow resumption of driving if the patient is asymptomatic (Table 29.3). Of note, the accident rate attributable to an arrhythmia reported in persons with an ICD

implanted for prior symptomatic VT was 0.4% per patient-year, lower than the normal accident rate.

Precautions. Some forms of *electromagnetic exposure* are contraindicated, such as *magnetic resonance imaging*. Microwave ovens pose no hazard, nor do airport security gates or brief passes of a handheld wand to detect metal objects, but security staff should be informed on the device's presence before the person passes through. Cellular digital phones do not interfere with operation of the device, but it is recommended that they not be carried or placed within 6 in. of the unit. Concurrent use of drugs such as amiodarone and beta-blockers may require resetting of thresholds.

Cost-Effectiveness. ICDs are very expensive. Cost-effectiveness analyses confirm that mortality is reduced but costs increase. Cost-effectiveness is comparable to, but on the high end of the spectrum of, that of accepted therapies (e.g., about $70,000 per quality-adjusted life-year) and best in persons with low ejection fractions (<0.30).

Pharmacologic Therapy

As noted earlier, antiarrhythmic therapy is no longer the primary treatment modality for very-high-risk patients with ventricular irritability, having been superseded by the ICD. Nonetheless, pharmacologic treatment can still make important contributions, both as an adjunct to ICD therapy and as primary treatment for intermediate-risk persons (Table 29.2) and those at very high risk who refuse or have a contraindication to ICD use. Although all antiarrhythmic drugs can suppress ventricular ectopy, their net effect on survival has been disappointing. At best, modest reductions (10% to 20%) in overall mortality have been achieved (as with amiodarone in very-high-risk patients), but more commonly the result is no benefit over placebo or even an increase in mortality (as found in studies of class IC drugs). Consequently, drug therapy is increasingly relegated to a second-line role for prevention of cardiac arrest and sudden death. In addition, the practice of testing for and seeking to eliminate observable or inducible ventricular irritability with antiarrhythmic drugs is being abandoned because it does not correlate with outcomes. The pharmacologic agents that show the best-defined contributions to outcomes

TABLE 29.3

CONSENSUS DRIVING PROHIBITIONS WITH VENTRICULAR TACHYCARDIA

Arrhythmia Type	Private Vehicle	Commercial Vehicle
Nonsustained ventricular tachycardia	B_3,[a] A[b]	B_6,[a] A[b]
Sustained ventricular tachycardia	B_6, B_3^c	C, B_6^c
Ventricular fibrillation	B_6	C

A, no restrictions; B, restriction for a defined period of months (given by the subscript) of arrhythmia-free interval after the initiation of therapy (implantable cardioverter–defibrillator and/or amiodarone); C, total restriction with presenting arrhythmia.
[a]Symptoms of impaired consciousness with arrhythmia (before treatment).
[b]No impairment of consciousness with arrhythmia.
[c]Idiopathic ventricular tachycardia (normal coronary arteries, normal ventricular function) and no impairment of consciousness.
Adapted from Epstein AE, Miles WM, Benditt DG, et al. Personal and public safety issues related to arrhythmias that may affect consciousness: implications for regulation and physician recommendations: a medical/scientific statement from the American Heart Association and the North American Society of Pacing and Electrophysiology. Circulation 1996;94:1147, with permission.

are the beta-blockers and the class III antiarrhythmic amiodarone.

Beta-Blockers. Beta-blocking agents increase the fibrillatory threshold and reduce the risk of ventricular fibrillation and sudden death (see also Chapters 26 and 30). These agents—referred to as *class II antiarrhythmics*—are safe and especially useful when the ventricular dysrhythmia is caused by underlying ischemic heart disease. At least some of the benefit associated with class III antiarrhythmics (e.g., sotalol, amiodarone) has been attributed to their adrenergic-blocking activity.

Beta-blockers are among the few drugs proven to reduce mortality in patients with coronary artery disease (see Chapter 30). Not only do they reduce the risk of sudden death, they also reduce overall mortality. Unlike other drugs with antiarrhythmic properties, the beta-blockers have no proarrhythmic effects. They are also useful for the suppression of symptomatic ventricular irritability related to digitalis toxicity, exercise, emotional stress, prolonged QT-interval syndromes, and tricyclic antidepressants.

These features make beta-blockers ideal for the prevention of sudden death in patients with malignant ventricular irritability due to coronary artery disease and other conditions that respond to beta-blockade. By suppressing the rate of VT and episodes of sustained VT, they also help to reduce the frequency of shocks in persons with ICDs, particularly in those with underlying coronary heart disease. *Combined use* with *amiodarone* has shown synergy and is a reasonable alternative to ICD therapy in high-risk persons who have a contraindication to or reject device implantation.

Amiodarone. Amiodarone, a class III antiarrhythmic, blocks a number of cellular ionic channels and also exerts noncompetitive antiadrenergic effects, thus manifesting effects of both class I and class II antiarrhythmic agents. When used in high-risk patients, the drug demonstrates a significant reduction (29%) in risk of arrhythmic sudden death and a more modest reduction (13%) in overall mortality. Patients who present with symptomatic sustained VT or prior ventricular fibrillation arrest who cannot undergo or refuse cardioverter–defibrillator implantation are reasonable candidates for amiodarone therapy. For asymptomatic patients with preserved LV function and frequent or complex PVCs or nonsustained VT, there is no evidence of survival benefit.

Initiation and Adjustment of Dose. Loading doses are usually required because the drug is distributed in the fat. When started in the outpatient setting, the daily dose is typically 800 to 1,600 mg/d, scaling back to 400 to 600 mg/d after 2 to 3 weeks and tapering to 200 to 300 mg/d if there are adverse effects. Doses of 200 mg/d are often ineffective for adequate control of serious ventricular ectopy (unlike use of the drug for atrial fibrillation), but if reductions to this level are needed due to side effects, then adding a beta-blocker can help. Because the drug is hepatically metabolized, it does not need to be scaled back in the setting of renal insufficiency. Lower loading and maintenance doses are appropriate in the elderly and women. Serum levels are needed only in the context of suspected drug toxicity or breakthrough ventricular dysrhythmias necessitating consideration of change in dose; routine monitoring of serum levels contributes little.

Adverse Effects and Monitoring. Despite being well tolerated, amiodarone has a number of adverse effects, most of which are related to dose and duration of therapy. *Drug–drug interactions* are the most important and can be substantial: Amiodarone increases the serum levels of *digoxin*, *warfarin*, and a number of other drugs; monitoring of drug effects, serum levels, and dosing are necessary when amiodarone is used. *Pulmonary fibrosis*, usually preceded by a reversible patchy pneumonitis presenting as a dry cough, occurs in up to 20% of patients; chest x-ray can be obtained to document the problem, and discontinuation usually suffices. *Corneal deposits*, presenting as a visual halo at night, usually do not interfere with vision and disappear with drug discontinuation; *blurred vision* and *photophobia* may also occur; *optic neuritis* is rare, but visual complaints require consideration of ophthalmologic consultation. *Gastrointestinal upset* (including constipation) is common, as are minor increases in *liver enzymes*, but clinically significant *hepatitis* occurs in 4% of patients; liver enzymes should be monitored twice yearly. *Ataxia, tremor*, and *peripheral neuropathy* may also develop and resolve with dose reduction. The drug contains an iodinated segment that can interfere with thyroid metabolism and may lead to *hypothyroidism*; twice-yearly thyroid-stimulating hormone monitoring is indicated. *Skin changes* are typical after prolonged use and include *bluish discoloration* about the eyes; resultant *photosensitivity* benefits from the use of sunblock.

Amiodarone has little or no proarrhythmic activity, even though it commonly prolongs the *QT interval*. Effect on inotropy is minimal. Impairment of sinus or atrioventricular (AV) node function occurs in about 5% of users, who may experience *bradycardia* or *AV block*; care is needed when it is used in persons with nodal or conduction-system disease or in conjunction with beta-blockade. Similarly, there are important *drug–device interactions* that require attention. Amiodarone may slow the rate of VT below that detected by the ICD and may increase the defibrillatory threshold. Electrophysiologic study may be required after loading of amiodarone.

Overall, amiodarone is effective and reasonably well tolerated when used carefully and knowledgeably.

Sotalol. Sotalol has a combination of nonselective beta-blocking affects and electrophysiologic features common to class III antiarrhythmics, making it a theoretically attractive agent and, indeed, it is effective in suppressing serious ventricular ectopy. However, it prolongs the QT interval, subjecting patients to the risk of torsades de pointes, especially if accompanied by hypokalemia or hypomagnesemia. The risk of torsades accounts for the failure of the drug to reduce mortality in some controlled trials and limits its usefulness.

Class I Antiarrhythmics. The traditional antiarrhythmics in this class (*procainamide,quinidine,disopyramide*) and the more modern ones (e.g., *mexiletine, tocainide*, and the class Ic agents *flecainide* and *moricizine*) have been largely supplanted by ICD therapy and use of amiodarone and beta-blockers. Although effective in suppressing ventricular ectopy, the class I drugs manifest proarrhythmic potential that compromises their ability to reduce risk of cardiac sudden death and, in some instances, actually increases it.

Omega-3 Polyunsaturated Fatty Acid Supplements and other Dietary Measures

Omega-3 polyunsaturated fatty acids, found in oily fish and fish oil supplements, appear to stabilize myocardial cell membrane electrical activity, exerting an effect on sodium channels similar to that of class I antiarrhythmics. Reductions in rates of sudden death (but not of myocardial infarction) have been observed in placebo-controlled, randomized trials of patients with recent myocardial infarction treated with fish oil supplements. Such findings have prompted recommendations of two servings of oily fish per week for the general population and 1 g/d of omega-3 fish oil supplement in persons with coronary artery disease. However, more recent studies failed to demonstrate any major reductions in risk of VT/VF or sudden death in persons with ICDs and a history of malignant VT or VF, and in some instances there was suggestion of a proarrhythmic effect. The differences in results may be related to the populations studied: Those with recent myocardial infarction (<3 months) appear to benefit most; those without recent myocardial infarction show little or no benefit.

Caffeine restriction may cut down on the frequency of minor ventricular irritability, but there is no evidence that it has any effect on important outcomes or that moderate intake of caffeinated beverages is harmful to patients with serious ventricular irritability.

Radiofrequency Catheter Ablative Therapy

Catheter ablation is most successful in persons with VT who have no evidence of underlying structural heart disease (90% cure rate) and in those with VT involving a reentrant mechanism. Persons with VT due to coronary disease have a much lower response rate (<50%). The mapping component of the procedure can only be performed when there is hemodynamic stability during the induction of VT, a situation that is infrequent in persons with structural heart disease.

Monitoring Therapy

The primary physician plays an important role in monitoring, being in close contact with the patient and often the first to encounter a problem with control or an adverse effect of treatment.

For Patients Treated with a Cardioverter–Defibrillator

Monitoring such patients is relatively simple because the devices have built-in monitoring and storage capacity. At the time of a visit to the cardiologist, the memory can be downloaded for study. The patient should be questioned about the number of shocks experienced and the number and type of any other symptomatic events. The device is "interrogated" for assessment of battery status and lead function.

For Patients Treated Pharmacologically

In addition to monitoring for the adverse effects of amiodarone use (see prior discussion), the primary physician can do much to ensure safety and minimize iatrogenic complications. Periodic checks and maintenance of *serum potassium* and *magnesium* levels are essential to minimizing their proarrhythmic contributions, as is avoidance of drugs that markedly prolong the *QT interval* (see Chapter 25). Any concurrent use of amiodarone and digoxin necessitates close monitoring of *serum digoxin level* and careful digoxin dose adjustment. The previous standard of regularly repeated EPS or ambulatory Holter monitoring has been invalidated by the lack of correlation between suppression of ventricular irritability and outcomes. However, those experiencing syncope, near-syncope, worsening dyspnea, or crescendo angina need prompt attention (see Chapters 20, 24, and 25).

Out-of-Hospital Defibrillation by Lay Persons

Although emergency medicine is beyond the scope of this book, a few comments about out-of-hospital defibrillation by lay persons may be helpful. For example, families of high-risk patients who do not have an implantable defibrillator may ask about purchasing an automated external device. Use of automated external defibrillators by lay persons can save lives, especially when defibrillation is performed within 5 minutes of onset of symptoms. This finding has led to the installation of these units in airplanes and in many public sites. The automated units can differentiate VT/VF from rhythms not requiring defibrillation, limiting unnecessary shocks. Success is best if defibrillation is carried out within 5 minutes of onset of symptoms and the person has some prior training. If defibrillation is delayed for >5 minutes, it is recommended that cardiopulmonary resuscitation measures be instituted first before shocking (so-called "priming the pump"). The earlier the defibrillation, the more likely it is to be successful.

INDICATIONS FOR REFERRAL AND ADMISSION

Any patient found to have sustained VT complicated by symptoms of hemodynamic compromise (dyspnea, near-syncope, angina) should be emergently admitted to the hospital and referred to a cardiologist skilled in performing EPS and treating life-threatening ventricular irritability. The same pertains to a patient with acute syncope who presents with features suggestive of a serious cardiac rhythm disturbance (i.e., syncopal episode with <5 seconds of warning, other symptoms of pump dysfunction, no major residual symptoms during recovery). A bit less urgent is the case of asymptomatic nonsustained VT, but risk is still very high, and referral for consideration of EPS is indicated when there is a history of recent myocardial infarction and evidence of LV dysfunction. Asymptomatic patients with normal LV function who manifest complex ventricular ectopy other than sustained VT are not candidates for treatment and do not require admission or referral, although cardiac consultation may be done for reassurance. Increasingly frequent ICD discharges are an indication for cardiac consultation.

PATIENT EDUCATION

Patients and their families need to know the prognostic meaning of the ventricular irritability so that they can respond appropriately. Putting the problem in context avoids over- and underresponding. Those with harmless forms of ventricular irritability can be reassured that the palpitations and abnormal ECG have no implications for long-term survival, which helps to prevent cardiac neurosis and unnecessary restriction of activity. Patients with high-risk disease benefit from full disclosure of prognosis, as well as the favorable outcome afforded by treatment, helping to lessen anxiety and enhance compliance and willingness to put up with the side effects from drugs and ICDs. Those with ICDs need to be fully informed about driving, cell phone use, and other precautions regarding electromagnetic interference (see prior discussion).

Prohibition from driving is one of the most impairing quality-of-life consequences of malignant ventricular irritability. Restrictions are intended for those with high-risk ventricular dysrhythmias, unless there is a known, completely reversible cause (e.g., severe electrolyte abnormality, drug toxicity, or electrocution). Guidelines (Table 29.3) are understandably conservative and may overstate the risk because data are limited. Of note, a recent study of secondary prophylaxis (persons with a prior symptomatic VT/VF episode) found that patients who felt well enough to drive often ignored their physician's advice and demonstrated a disease/treatment-attributable accident rate below that of the general public.

CONCLUSIONS AND THERAPEUTIC RECOMMENDATIONS

- The main independent determinants of prognosis in patients with ventricular ectopy are the presence of underlying heart disease and a failing left ventricle. The complexity of the ventricular ectopy is also an independent determinant of prognosis, especially in patients with heart disease and LV failure; sustained VT portends an especially high risk of cardiac sudden death.
- Patients with underlying heart disease, LV dysfunction, and sustained VT are at very high risk of sudden death and require prompt admission and cardiac consultation, especially if they experience arrhythmia-induced symptoms of hemodynamic compromise.
- Treatment is indicated for these patients and is best initiated in the inpatient setting, in collaboration with a cardiologist skilled in treating malignant ventricular arrhythmias. Outpatient assessment and initiation of therapy may be possible in asymptomatic persons with nonsustained VT, but cardiac consultation is warranted, especially in persons with underlying heart disease.
- Patients presenting with ventricular ectopy should be evaluated for underlying heart disease, LV dysfunction, and QT prolongation (with associated review of potentially contributing medications; see Table 29.2).
- Those presenting with nonsustained VT in the setting of recent myocardial infarction and reduced ejection fraction should be considered for EPS for inducible sustained VT, an indication for prophylactic measures.
- Patients presenting with syncope and clinical evidence suggesting a cardiac etiology are also candidates for EPS to test for inducible sustained VT; checking for QT prolongation is also indicated.
- The principal goals of treatment are prevention of symptomatic sustained VT, cardiac arrest, and sudden cardiac death.

- Evidence-based recommendations limit the treatment of ventricular ectopy to those at very high or moderate to high risk of cardiac sudden death and favor ICD use over pharmacotherapy in most instances (see Table 29.1).
- Beta-blocker therapy is indicated for all patients with malignant ventricular irritability due to underlying coronary artery disease, especially for persons who have had a myocardial infarction.
- The antiarrhythmic of choice is amiodarone due to its proven ability to reduce the risk of sudden death and its low risks of proarrhythmic activity and LV impairment. High-risk patients who refuse or are not candidates for cardioverter–defibrillator implantation can be considered for amiodarone therapy.
- Because amiodarone therapy is associated with potentially adverse side effects (most of which are reversible with timely dose reduction or discontinuation) and with important drug–drug and drug–device interactions, it should be undertaken and maintained only by knowledgeable practitioners.
- Holter monitoring and EPS testing after initiation of antiarrhythmic therapy to check for ability to suppress inducible VT are no longer recommended because results do not correlate with outcomes.
- Patients with symptomatic VT without structural heart disease are potential candidates for catheter radioablation.
- Use of fish oil supplements (e.g., 1 g/d of omega-3 fatty acids) is worth consideration in persons with ventricular dysrhythmias and recent (<3 months) myocardial infarction, but efficacy of use in others remains to be established.
- Monitoring should include checking for hemodynamic compromise (near-syncope, dyspnea, angina), number of shocks (in persons with defibrillators), ECG for QT-interval prolongation and new dysrhythmias, and serum levels for potassium, magnesium, creatinine, transaminase, and drug concentrations (especially if antiarrhythmic toxicity is suspected).
- Detailed patient education is essential to maximize compliance, safety, and quality of life; guidelines for driving an automobile need to be reviewed (Table 29.3).

A.H.G.

Annotated Bibliography

1. Al-Khatib SM, LaPointe NMA, Kramer JM, et al. What clinicians should know about the QT interval. JAMA 2003;289:2120. (*Practical review; 58 references.*)
2. Bigger JT. Definition of benign versus malignant ventricular arrhythmias. Am J Cardiol 1983;52:47C. (*Excellent review of the various forms of ventricular irritability and the degree of risk associated with each.*)
3. Bikkina M, Larson MG, Levy D. Prognostic implications of asymptomatic ventricular arrhythmias: the Framingham Heart Study. Ann Intern Med 1992;117:990. (*Important epidemiologic data; there is increased risk of myocardial infarction or death from coronary disease.*)
4. Buxton AE, Lee KL, DiCarlo L, et al. Electrophysiologic testing to identify patients with coronary artery disease who are at risk for sudden death. N Engl J Med 2000;342:1937. (*The ability to induce sustained ventricular tachycardia [VT] is associated with an increased risk of sudden death.*)
5. Frolkis JP, Pothier CE, Blackstone EH, et al. Frequent ventricular ectopy after exercise as a predictor of death. N Engl J Med 2003;348:781. (*A large-scale observational study from the Cleveland Clinic; an increased risk of death was found among persons with frequent or complex ventricular ectopy during the recovery phase of exercise stress testing.*)
6. Huikuri HV, Castellanos A, Myerburg RJ. Sudden death due to cardiac arrhythmias. N Engl J Med 2001;345:1473. (*Outstanding review of etiology, epidemiology, evaluation, and prevention; 97 references.*)
7. Kennedy HL, Pescarmona J, Bouchard RJ, et al. Coronary artery status of apparently healthy subjects with frequent and complex ventricular ectopy. Ann Intern Med 1980;92:179. (*One fourth of apparently healthy patients being followed for complex and frequent ventricular ectopic activity [VEA] were found to have significant coronary stenosis; no clinical features of the ectopy differentiated them.*)
8. Kennedy HL, Whitlock JA, Sprague MK. Long-term follow-up of asymptomatic healthy subjects with frequent and complex ventricular ectopy. N Engl J Med 1985;312:1983. (*An important study; regardless of the presence of frequent and complex ventricular irritability, no increase in mortality was found among these healthy patients; the mean follow-up was 6.5 years.*)
9. Lange RA, Hillis LD. Cardiovascular complications of cocaine use. N Engl J Med 2001;345:351. (*Review of the adverse cardiovascular effects, including ventricular dysrhythmias.*)
10. Liperoti R, Gambassi F, Lapane KL, et al. Conventional and atypical antipsychotics and the risk of hospitalization for ventricular arrhythmias or cardiac arrest. Arch Intern Med 2005;165:696. (*Case–control study finding that conventional but not atypical antipsychotics were associated with increased risk.*)
11. Liu BA, Juurlink DN. Drugs and the QT interval—caveat doctor. N Engl J Med 2004;351:1053. (*Editorial reviewing drugs that prolong the QT interval and those that exacerbate the problem by inhibiting their metabolism.*)

12. McLenachan JM, Henderson E, Morris KI, et al. Ventricular arrhythmias in patients with hypertensive left ventricular hypertrophy. N Engl J Med 1987;317:787. (*Documents the increased frequency of complex ventricular irritability in such patients.*)

13. Meyers MG. Caffeine and cardiac arrhythmias. Ann Intern Med 1991;114:147. (*Critical literature review; there was no evidence of harm, even among those with preexisting serious VEA.*)

14. Ray WA, Murray KT, Meredith S, et al. Oral erythromycin and the risk of sudden death from cardiac causes. N Engl J Med 2004;351:1089. (*Cohort study; the risk was significantly increased, especially among those using oral erythromycin and a cytochrome inhibitor.*)

15. Ruskin J. Ventricular extrasystoles in healthy subjects. N Engl J Med 1985;312:238. (*An editorial summarizing current knowledge and pinpointing areas of continued uncertainty.*)

16. Akiyama T, Powell JL, Mitchell LB, et al. Resumption of driving after life-threatening ventricular tachyarrhythmia. N Engl J Med 2001;345:391. (*Retrospective cohort study; finds that the risk is low in those treated with an implantable cardioverter–defibrillator or an antiarrhythmic drug.*)

17. Amiodarone Trials Meta-Analysis Investigators. Effect of prophylactic amiodarone on mortality after acute myocardial infarction and in congestive heart failure: meta-analysis of individual data from 6500 patients in randomized trials. Lancet 1997;350:1417. (*Detects a significant reduction [29%] in the risk of arrhythmic sudden death and a more modest reduction [13%] in overall mortality.*)

18. Antiarrhythmics versus Implantable Defibrillators (AVID) Investigators. A comparison of antiarrhythmic-drug therapy with implantable defibrillators in patients resuscitated from near-fatal ventricular arrhythmias. N Engl J Med 1997;337:1576. (*In this group of very-high-risk patients, survival was enhanced by defibrillator therapy but not by antiarrhythmic drug.*)

19. Bigger JT. Prophylactic use of implanted cardiac defibrillators in patients at high risk for ventricular arrhythmias after coronary-artery bypass graft surgery. N Engl J Med 1997;337:1569. (*The CABG PATCH study, a randomized trial showing no benefit in survival for persons with a reduced ejection fraction and an abnormal resting electrocardiogram.*)

20. Boutitie F, Boissel JP, Connolly SJ, et al. Amiodarone interaction with beta-blockers: analysis of the merged EMIAT and CAMIAT databases. Circulation 1999;82:91. (*A subgroup analysis combining data from two large prospective trials suggesting a synergistic effect with improved survival in postinfarction patients.*)

21. Brouwer IA, Zock PL, Camm AJ, et al. Effect of fish oil on ventricular tachyarrhythmia and death in patients with implantable cardioverter defibrillators: the Study on Omega-3 Fatty Acids and Ventricular Arrhythmia (SOFA) randomized trial. JAMA 2006;295:2613. (*randomized, controlled trial [RCT]; no major benefit was noted in this group of patients without recent myocardial infarction.*)

22. Buxton AD, Lee KL, Fisher JD, et al. A randomized study of the prevention of sudden death in patients with coronary artery disease. N Engl J Med 1999;341:1882. (*RCT; an implantable defibrillator reduced the risk of sudden death, but antiarrhythmic pharmacotherapy did not, in these patients with nonsustained VT, heart failure, inducible VT, and recent infarction.*)

23. Buxton AE. Antiarrhythmic drugs: good for premature ventricular complexes but bad for patients? Ann Intern Med 1992;116:420. (*An editorial; reviews the disappointing results with class IC antiarrhythmics; they are more proarrhythmic than suppressive; a good discussion of the implications.*)

24. Cairns JA, Connolly SJ, Roberts RS, et al. Randomized trial of outcome after myocardial infarction in patients with frequent or repetitive premature depolarizations: CAMIAT. Lancet 1997; 349. (*The risk of sudden death was significantly reduced with amiodarone use, but only a trend toward reduction in total mortality was found in this major Canadian trial.*)

25. DiMarco JP. Implantable cardioverter–defibrillators. N Engl J Med 2003;349:1836. (*Comprehensive review for the generalist reader; 79 references.*)

26. Echt DS, Liebson PR, Mitchell B, et al. Mortality and morbidity in patients receiving encainide, flecainide, or placebo: the Cardiac Arrhythmia Suppression Trial. N Engl J Med 1991;324:781. (*Major RCT of class I antiarrhythmic therapy in mildly symptomatic patients with complex ventricular ectopy, coronary artery disease, and reduced ejection fraction; demonstrated an excessive incidence of arrhythmic deaths and proarrhythmic effects in up to 10% of patients.*)

27. Ezekowitz JA, Armstrong PW, McAlister FA. Implantable cardioverter defibrillators in primary and secondary prevention: a systematic review of randomized, controlled trials. Ann Intern Med 2003:138:445. (*The procedure was found to be effective for the prevention of sudden death, but the magnitude of the benefit was related to the underlying risk of sudden death.*)

28. Goldschlarger N, Epstein A, Friedman P, et al. Environmental and drug effects on patients with pacemakers and implantable cardioverter/defibrillators: a practical guide to patient treatment. Arch Intern Med 2001;161:649. (*Helpful information for patients and their primary physicians.*)

29. Gruppo Italiano per lo Studio della Sopravivenza nell'Infarto Miocardico. Dietary supplementation with n-3 polyunsaturated fatty acids and vitamin E after myocardial infarction: results of the GISSA-Prevenzione trial. Lancet 1999;354:447. (*The use of fish oil supplement was associated with a significant reduction in the rate of sudden death in this population with recent myocardial infarction.*)

30. Kendall MJ, Lynch KP, Hjalmarson A, et al. Beta-blockers and sudden cardiac death. Ann Intern Med 1995;123:358. (*A systematic review finding marked benefit, greater than with any other treatment modality.*)

31. Marchlinski FE, Zada ES, Deely MP, et al. Concomitant device and drug therapy: current trends, potential benefits, and adverse interactions. Am J Cardiol 1999;84(Suppl):69R. (*A review of the current state of concomitant use; some data, much interest, a number of concerns; a good paper for coming attractions.*)

32. Mason JW, et al. A comparison of electrophysiologic testing with Holter monitoring to predict arrhythmic drug efficacy for ventricular tachycardias. N Engl J Med 1993;329:445. (*Holter monitoring was more predictive of efficacy in this first large prospective, randomized trial of the two methods; however, there was a very narrow spectrum of patients, and both methods failed to predict the 50% recurrence rate of VT at 2 years.*)

33. Moss AJ, Zareba W, Hall WJ, et al. Prophylactic implantation of a defibrillator in patients with myocardial infarction and reduced ejection fraction. N Engl J Med 2002;346:877. (*RCT; there was a 31% reduction in death from all causes.*)

34. Nattel S, Singh B. Evolution, mechanisms, and classification of antiarrhythmic drugs. Am J Cardiol 1999 (Suppl)84:11R. (*Excellent review and summary.*)

35. Powell AC, Gold MR, Brooks R, et al. Electrophysiologic response to moricizine in patients with sustained ventricular arrhythmias. Ann Intern Med 1992;116:382. (*Another of the promising class IC antiarrhythmics proves to be ineffective in suppressing VT and manifests proarrhythmic activity; failure of suppressibility to predict outcome.*)

36. Raitt MH, Connor WE, Morris C, et al. Fish oil supplementation and risk of ventricular tachycardia and ventricular fibrillation in patients with implantable defibrillators: a randomized controlled trial. JAMA 2005;293:2884. (*No benefit was noted, and the question of proarrhythmic effect was raised.*)

37. Sanders GD, Hlatky MA, Every NR, et al. Potential cost-effectiveness of prophylactic use of the implantable cardioverter defibrillator or amiodarone after myocardial infarction. Ann Intern Med 2001;135:870. (*Analysis indicates effectiveness at an acceptable cost in persons with reduced ejection fraction.*)

38. The DAVID Trial Investigators. Dual-chamber pacing or ventricular backup pacing in patients with an implantable defibrillator: the Dual Chamber and VVI Implantable Defibrillator (DAVID) Trial. JAMA 2002;288:3115. (*Dual-chamber pacing was found to offer no advantages and some disadvantages.*)

39. The Public Access Defibrillation Trial Investigators. Public-access defibrillation and survival after out-of-hospital cardiac arrest. N Engl J Med 2004;351:637. (*Improved survival was found.*)

40. Wik L, Hansen TB, Fylling F, et al. Delaying defibrillation to give basic cardiopulmonary resuscitation to patients with out-of-hospital ventricular fibrillation: a randomized trial. JAMA 2003;289:1389. (*RCT; cardiopulmonary resuscitation offered no benefit if defibrillation was performed within 5 minutes of onset but was advantageous if the delay in defibrillation was >5 minutes.*)

41. Zimetbaum PJ, Josephson ME. The evolving role of ambulatory arrhythmia monitoring in general clinical practice. Ann Intern Med 1999;120:848. (*A detailed review, which includes evidence showing little benefit as a screening test for VT in asymptomatic patients with underlying heart disease.*)

CHAPTER 30 ■ MANAGEMENT OF CHRONIC STABLE ANGINA

Several million Americans suffer from coronary heart disease (CHD), and more than 600,000 die each year from the condition and its complications. Even for patients with chronic stable angina—the form of CHD most commonly encountered in the office setting—the annual risk of cardiovascular death, stroke, or myocardial infarction is high (4% to 5%); adding in hospitalizations for cardiac complications raises the rate to 15%. The array of treatment modalities is extensive, ranging from aspirin, nitrates, beta-blocking agents, calcium-channel blockers, and angiotensin-converting-enzyme (ACE) inhibitors to angioplasty, stenting, and coronary bypass surgery. These medical and surgical approaches are complemented by exercise and aggressive treatment of underlying cardiovascular risk factors such as hypercholesterolemia, hypertension, smoking, and diabetes. The goals of therapy include symptom relief, preserved quality of life, improved exercise capacity, prevention of infarction, and, ultimately, improved survival, all of which can often be accomplished by a well-designed medical regimen.

Designing the basic medical regimen of the patient with stable coronary heart disease and knowing when referral for consideration of revascularization is indicated are among the important responsibilities of the primary care physician. The popularity of minimally invasive revascularization procedures (i.e., angioplasty and stenting) and the strong economic incentives to perform them necessitate in-depth knowledge by the primary care physician of the indications and limitations of all treatment modalities, as well as a good working relationship with a consulting cardiologist.

PATHOPHYSIOLOGY (1–3)

Angina is a symptomatic manifestation of *myocardial ischemia* (MI), which occurs when oxygen demand exceeds available vascular supply. Symptoms include chest, back, arm, or neck pain, characteristically brought on by exertion, meals, or stress and relieved promptly by nitroglycerin or rest (see Chapter 20). *Anginal equivalents* include exertional dyspnea (common in women, who may not experience chest pain) and dysrhythmias, also the consequence of myocardial ischemia and resultant left ventricular (LV) dysfunction. There is also a growing appreciation for the frequency and importance of *silent myocardial ischemia*, defined as objectively documented ischemia occurring in the absence of symptoms. On the basis of results from exercise stress testing and ambulatory monitoring, it is estimated that more than half of patients with chronic stable angina experience episodes of silent ischemia. Contrary to the traditional association of silent ischemia with diabetes, controlled studies find silent ischemia to be no more frequent in diabetics than in nondiabetics. The mechanism(s) remain to be elucidated, but clinical significance is no less important than symptomatic angina.

Atherosclerotic Disease

Most cases of chronic stable angina are related to fixed atherosclerotic lesions narrowing the major coronary vessels. A series of stepwise thrombotic events is believed to account for much of the atherosclerotic occlusion that occurs in the large epicardial arteries. These lesions may develop as a consequence of episodes of acute *thrombosis*, in which activated *platelets* and other elements of the clotting system appear to play major roles, triggered by reactive endothelial injury in areas of cholesterol deposition. The association of thrombotic risk with elevation of *C-reactive protein* has called attention to the possible role of *inflammation* and *inflammatory mediators*. Many, if not most, episodes of *acute coronary insufficiency* (*unstable angina*) and *infarction* are associated with acute thrombosis, often occurring at an ulcerated, eccentrically located, or ruptured plaque, not necessarily at a site of severe stenosis.

Coronary Vasospasm

The restriction of coronary blood supply may also ensue from coronary vasospasm, which is believed to be related to a loss of normal endothelial vasoregulatory activity. The coronary endothelium appears to cease production of vasoactive peptides and prostaglandins, leaving vascular smooth muscle unopposed and susceptible to spasm. It has been documented in patients both with and without underlying atherosclerotic disease and sometimes presents as *variant angina* (rest pain, ST-segment elevation). Prevalence is about 3% in patients undergoing coronary angiography with ergonovine stimulation, but the true prevalence is estimated to be far greater. Spasm is suspected of playing a role in acute myocardial infarction and triggering anginal episodes. *Cigarette smoking* and hyperlipidemia appear to interfere with normal endothelial activity, and other precipitants include *stress, cold, α-adrenergic stimulation in the setting of beta-blockade, abrupt nitrate withdrawal, ergonovine, cocaine use*, and direct mechanical irritation from *cardiac catheterization*.

Left Ventricular Outflow Obstruction

Aortic valve disease can lead to angina when hemodynamically significant valvular *stenosis* or *calcific obstruction* of coronary ostia results in inadequate coronary perfusion (see Chapter 33). Angina may also be a manifestation of *hypertrophic cardiomyopathy*, developing as a consequence of significant LV outflow tract obstruction, increased myocardial oxygen demand by a hypertrophied myocardium, and inadequate vascular supply (see Appendix 33.1).

Microvascular Disease

Coronary microvascular dysfunction, characterized by inappropriately vasoconstrictive responses to autonomic and biochemical stimuli, can increase total resistance and reduce myocardial perfusion. The significance of these findings is unclear, but they have been found with increased frequency among patients with the combination of atypical angina, an ischemic response to exercise stress testing, and a normal coronary angiogram. The terms *microvascular angina* and *syndrome X* have been applied to such persons. More study is needed, but the findings suggest a possible explanation for the ischemic chest pain of patients with *hypertrophic cardiomyopathy*. Diabetics with hyperinsulinism may also be at increased risk for microvascular disease.

Increased Myocardial Oxygen Demand

Regardless of etiology, ischemic episodes are often triggered or aggravated by conditions that increase myocardial oxygen demand (e.g., *hyperthyroidism*, *fever*, *left ventricular hypertrophy*) or decrease oxygen supply (e.g., *severe anemia*, *respiratory insufficiency*). A circadian susceptibility to ischemic events has been identified, with the morning hours being the time of greatest risk. Mechanism(s) are unknown, but the phenomenon can be blocked by beta-blockers or aspirin.

NATURAL HISTORY, PROGNOSIS, AND RISK STRATIFICATION (4–10)

Although the clinical course of some patients may extend over 15 to 20 years, most patients with chronic stable angina are at a considerably increased risk of cardiovascular death.

Determinants of Prognosis and Risk

With so many therapeutic options available (including a number that confer considerable risk), it is becoming increasingly important to risk-stratify patients with chronic stable coronary disease. Among the best-established factors affecting prognosis are the *number* and the *location* of coronary artery *stenoses*. Combined angiographic data obtained before the widespread use of bypass surgery reveal that patients with significant disease in one vessel have a mean annual mortality rate of 2.2%. This increases to a rate of 4.5% to 7.0% if the lesion involves the *left main* coronary artery. High-grade proximal stenosis of the left anterior descending artery has a prognosis similar to that of left-main disease and is sometimes referred to as a *left-main equivalent* lesion. With stenosis of two vessels, the mean annual mortality rate is 6.8%; the rate rises to 11.4% for *three-vessel disease*.

Prognosis also closely correlates with the *severity of ischemia*, as measured by radionuclide or echocardiographic imaging and by electrocardiographic changes during exercise stress testing (see Chapter 36), regardless of whether the disease is symptomatic or silent. Other major independent determinants of increased risk are *LV dysfunction* (i.e., reduced ejection fraction; see Chapter 32), *LV diastolic dysfunction*, *LV hypertrophy*, *ventricular ectopy* (see Chapter 29), an *intercurrent ischemic event* within the last 6 months, and *cigarette smoking*. The onset of angina in a patient with *hemodynami-*

cally significant aortic stenosis reduces mean survival to about 2 to 3 years (see Chapter 33).

Many *CHD risk factors* are powerful independent determinants of prognosis. *Smoking, diabetes mellitus, hypertension, hypercholesterolemia, low high-density-lipoprotein cholesterol,* and *age* (45 years or older in men, 55 years or older in women) are well documented for their effect on prognosis in patients with stable angina due to atherosclerotic coronary artery disease. However, the fact that these risk factors do not account for all cardiovascular risk has stimulated searches for other determinants of risk and prognosis. *Hyperhomocysteinemia* emerged from preliminary epidemiologic studies as a transiently popular risk-factor candidate, but subsequent epidemiologic studies and failure of homocysteine-lowering treatment to reduce risk (see Chapters 27 and 31) have tempered enthusiasm for this purported risk factor. *Brain (B-type) natriuretic peptides* (N-terminal prohormone of BNP [NT-proBNP], which are released from cardiac myocytes in the setting of increased LV myocardial stretch due to LV dysfunction or ischemia and which may also alter vascular smooth muscle function) have been found to have independent predictive value, even in the setting of normal standard measures of LV function and inflammation.

Determining near-term risk is also of value and a source of active study. Preliminary work finds that serum elevations in biomarkers of inflammation (*C-reactive protein, amyloid A*) and thrombosis (*d-dimer*) can help predict short-term prognosis (1 to 2 years) in persons with established atherosclerotic disease. There is no significant correlation with longer-term risk (>2 years).

The natural history of *coronary artery spasm* is highly variable, reflecting the heterogeneity of patients with this condition. An important variable is the presence of underlying atherosclerotic disease. If spasm occurs in the absence of fixed stenoses, the prognosis is relatively good (e.g., no mortality, 39% remission over 6 years). Some investigators even suggest that spasm may be a temporary condition; however, myocardial infarction, heart block, and malignant arrhythmias have been documented. The prognosis of patients with spasm in the setting of underlying coronary stenosis is a function of the coronary anatomy; patients with multivessel disease are at greatest risk. Whether the risk is significantly enhanced by the presence of spasm is not yet known.

Risk Stratification

Risk stratification is essential to choosing wisely among the wide range of available treatment modalities. Most patients can be classified clinically into high-, intermediate-, and low-risk categories, supplementing the assessment when there is uncertainty with *stress testing* and *echocardiography* (see Tables 30.1 and 30.2; also see Chapters 20 and 36). Refinements using some of the newer biomarkers noted earlier (e.g., D-dimer, high-sensitivity C-reactive protein, NT-proBNP) show promise but need further validation.

Patients suspected of being at high risk need referral for the consideration of coronary bypass surgery. Persons classified as being at intermediate risk may also be candidates for revascularization (bypass vs. angioplasty/stenting) but on an elective basis and predominantly for the improved control of anginal symptoms (there is little evidence of reduced mortality). Low-risk patients (normal electrocardiogram [ECG], no evidence of heart failure, and no history of MI) with well-controlled symptoms can be followed expectantly and need not be restudied for 3 years. Urgent and full reassessment of risk is indicated

TABLE 30.1

RISK STRATIFICATION FOR PATIENTS WITH STABLE ANGINA

Low Risk
 No angina currently or minimal angina
 Normal left ventricular function (normal ejection fraction)
 Small amount of myocardium at risk (probable single-vessel disease)
Moderate Risk
 Moderate angina
 Normal left ventricular function (normal ejection fraction)
 Moderate amount of myocardium at risk (probable two-vessel or proximal left anterior descending artery disease)
High Risk
 Severe angina
 Extensive amount of myocardium at risk (probable three-vessel, left-main, or "left-main equivalent" disease)
 Impaired left ventricular function (ejection fraction <0.40)

when there a change in clinical status (e.g., change in anginal pattern, development of symptoms suggestive of heart failure).

PRINCIPLES OF MANAGEMENT

The principal goals are to improve functional capacity and quality of life and reduce the risks of adverse cardiac events and death. Measures that control *atherosclerotic risk factors*, improve *oxygen supply*, and reduce *oxygen demand* help to achieve these objectives. The institution of diet and exercise programs (see Chapters 18 and 31), beta-blockade, ACE inhibition, and platelet inhibition are central to this effort, as are aggressive treatment of hypercholesterolemia, hypertension, diabetes, and smoking; revascularization is sometimes necessary. Nitrates and calcium-channel blockers can enhance the control of symptoms and improve exercise tolerance. Also critical are attention to exacerbating factors such as *heart failure* (see Chapter 32), *aortic outflow tract obstruction* (see Chapter 33), *hyperthyroidism* (see Chapter 103), *anemia* (see Chapter 82), and hypoxemic *chronic lung diseases* (see Chapters 46 and 47).

To maximize patient safety, the aggressiveness of intervention should be proportional to the patient's degree of risk (see Table 30.1 and Chapter 20). Often the choices are stated as if they were mutually exclusive, but most of the time they are complementary. Even if revascularization is chosen, medical therapy remains the foundation of management. Surveys of CHD patients in primary care practices often find the underuse of therapies with proven survival benefit (e.g., beta-blockers, ACE inhibitors, aspirin, lipid lowering). A common error is to focus on the relief of angina and revascularization while ignoring aggressive reduction in overall cardiovascular risk.

Treatment of Atherosclerotic Risk Factors and Precipitants of Angina (4,10–16)

Atherosclerotic Risk Factors

The importance of treating atherosclerotic risk factors cannot be overemphasized. Patients with coronary disease have five times the risk of a coronary event. Secondary preventive efforts can improve quality of life, reduce the risk of coro-

TABLE 30.2

RISK ASSESSMENT FOR PATIENTS WITH STABLE CORONARY DISEASE BASED ON RESULTS OF NONINVASIVE TESTING

High Risk (>3% annual mortality rate)
 Severe resting left ventricular dysfunction (left ventricular ejection fraction <0.35)
 High-risk exercise electrocardiogram score (Duke score, ≤–10)
 Severe left ventricular dysfunction during cardiac exercise imaging (left ventricular ejection fraction <0.35)
 Large perfusion defect during stress myocardial perfusion imaging (particularly if anterior)
 Multiple perfusion defects of moderate size during stress myocardial perfusion imaging
 Large, fixed defect with left ventricular dilation or increased lung uptake using rest radionuclide angiography with thallium
 Moderate defect with left ventricular dilation or increased lung uptake during stress myocardial perfusion imaging with thallium
 Defect in more than two segments with a low heart rate (<120 beats/min) or with a low dose of dobutamine (≤10 mg/kg of body weight per minute) during stress echocardiography
 Evidence of extensive ischemia during stress echocardiography
Intermediate Risk (1%–3% annual mortality rate)
 Mild or moderate resting left ventricular dysfunction (left ventricular ejection fraction, 0.35–0.49)
 Intermediate-risk exercise electrocardiogram score (Duke treadmill score, –10 to 4)
 Moderate defects without left ventricular dilation or increased lung uptake during stress myocardial perfusion imaging
 Limited defects involving two or fewer segments only at doses of dobutamine >10 mg/kg per minute during stress echocardiography
Low Risk (<1% annual mortality rate)
 Low-risk exercise electrocardiogram score (Duke treadmill score, ≥5 or >4)
 Normal or small defect at rest or during stress with myocardial perfusion imaging
 Normal wall motion or no change in limited wall-motion abnormalities during stress echocardiography

Each test result is an independent predictor of the risk for death. There is little understanding about how to predict risk by combining test results, except that when more than one test result is present, the result predicting a higher risk should be used to guide decisions.
Adapted from Williams SV, Fihn SD, Gibbons RJ. Guidelines for the management of patients with chronic stable angina: diagnosis and risk stratification. Ann Intern Med 2001;135:530, with permission.

nary events, obviate the need for revascularization, and prolong survival. Marked reductions in cardiovascular morbidity and mortality are achievable with control of *hypertension* (see Chapter 26), lowering of *low-density-lipoprotein* (LDL) *cholesterol* (see Chapter 27), and cessation of *smoking* (see Chapter 54). *Weight reduction* (see Chapter 233) and tightening of *glycemic control* in patients with diabetes (see Chapter 102) are also critical. Central to these efforts is attention to *diet* (see Chapters 27, 31, and 233) and *exercise* (see Chapters 18, 31, and 233). *Exercise* can significantly improve functional status and outcomes by enhancing skeletal muscle efficiency, decreasing heart rate and blood pressure, enhancing morale, and fostering an improved sense of well-being (see Chapters 18 and 31).

Reducing elevations in *homocysteine, C-reactive protein,* and *triglycerides* and raising *HDL cholesterol* may also turn out to be helpful, although this is not as firmly established by prospective long-term study (see Chapters 27 and 31) as is treatment of other atherosclerotic risk factors.

The magnitude of morbidity and mortality reductions from the treatment of atherosclerotic risk factors can approach 30% to 50%, frequently equaling or exceeding that of other measures and mandating that it be a central part of all management programs in persons with coronary disease. A randomized trial of aggressive lipid-lowering therapy compared with angioplasty in patients with mild to moderate stable angina (atorvastatin vs. revascularization treatment) found that lipid lowering was equal to if not better than angioplasty with regard to reducing the frequency of future cardiac events.

Common Precipitants

Attention to precipitants is essential not only for symptomatic relief, but also for reducing morbidity and mortality.

Smoking. Smoking is not only a major CHD risk factor, but it is also a precipitant of angina. The absorbed nicotine increases blood pressure and heart rate, thus increasing myocardial oxygen demand. Nicotine may also cause vasospasm, and the rise in carboxyhemoglobin from smoke inhalation cuts down on oxygen delivery. Even passive smoking (from being in a smoke-filled room) can reduce exercise tolerance in patients with stable angina. Cessation of smoking can be psychologically stressful and physically uncomfortable, but the immediate and long-term benefits greatly outweigh the short-term discomfort. The development of symptomatic coronary disease may provide a potent stimulus to smoking cessation; the effort often succeeds when the physician takes a strong interest in achieving it (see Chapter 54).

Hypertension. Hypertension can exacerbate angina by raising myocardial oxygen demand through its effect on afterload. Its treatment can improve the symptomatic control of angina, as well as markedly reduce the risks of MI and death (see Chapter 26).

Psychological Stress. Stress is well recognized as an important precipitant, but only recently has it been appreciated how common stress-induced ischemia is in patients with coronary artery disease. Episodes of silent ischemia and symptomatic ischemia have been documented in stressful situations. Public speaking and difficult mental tasks can induce as much symptomatic and silent ischemia as exertion in patients with coronary artery disease. High levels of life stress and social isolation are independent predictors of death from coronary disease. The role of personality style, such as so-called *type A behavior*, remains a subject of debate, although the evidence from studies of mental stress suggests that coronary patients who have a low tolerance for frustrating circumstances might be expected to have an increased likelihood of ischemic stress responses.

Addressing the psychosocial stresses that the anginal patient encounters is critical. An adequate evaluation includes a thorough psychosocial history with emphasis on those factors contributing to stress and social isolation. Urging the hard-driving,

impatient person to change personality style is counterproductive, but counseling on means of coping with frustration and introducing simple *relaxation techniques* (see Appendix 226.1) may be better appreciated. If acute anxiety or situational stress is known predictably to precipitate severe chest pain or significant silent ischemia, occasional prophylactic use of a *minor tranquilizer* may be warranted. However, frequent benzodiazepine use in the absence of a true anxiety disorder is strongly discouraged because it can lead to tolerance and even addiction (see Chapter 226); furthermore, tranquilizer use is no substitute for an adequate medical regimen. *Beta-blocker* therapy can be quite effective in limiting the adverse cardiac effects of anxiety by blocking the attendant adrenergic discharge.

Depression and Anxiety. Depression and anxiety are common responses to the diagnosis of coronary disease; they can impair not only the patient's psychological sense of well-being, but also the physiologic responses to medical and interventional therapies. Moreover, anxiety is a risk factor for cardiac sudden death, and depression is a more powerful predictor of heart disease than is personality style. After 1 year of proper therapy for angina, any untreated anxiety or depression correlates more closely with exercise capacity and functional status than the severity of the underlying coronary disease. Despite receiving and complying with proper antianginal regimens, patients with these psychological states manifest more physical incapacity than patients free of active depression or anxiety. The close link between these states and functional status makes it imperative to check for and treat anxiety and depression (see Chapters 226 and 227) at the time of initial CHD workup and again during implementation of the antianginal program. Patients who fail to respond to what seems to be a properly instituted cardiac regimen should be evaluated for an underlying affective disorder.

Other Precipitants

One needs to check for and address severe *anemia* (see Chapter 82), *hyperthyroidism* (see Chapter 103), *heart failure* (see Chapter 32), and *hypoxemia* due to lung disease (see Chapters 46 and 47). All are capable of worsening both symptomatic and silent myocardial ischemia in the context of underlying coronary disease. Neither *coffee* nor *caffeine* consumption has been shown to increase the risk of coronary disease, although an oft-quoted epidemiologic study found a minor trend toward increased risk in patients consuming more than four cups of decaffeinated coffee per day.

Beta-Adrenergic Blocking Agents (17–27)

Beta-blockers reduce the *frequency* of angina (especially that induced by exercise), improve *exercise tolerance*, reduce the risk of *cardiac sudden death*, and prolong *survival* (especially in patients surviving myocardial infarction; there are 45% reductions in sudden death and 20% reductions in all-cause mortality). In patients with stable coronary disease, beta-blockers can also reduce the frequency of silent ischemia and other coronary events. The benefits of beta-blockade derive principally from the lowering of myocardial oxygen consumption through reductions in *contractility, blood pressure,* and *heart rate*. Beta-blockade also raises the *ventricular fibrillatory threshold* and, in slowing the heart rate, provides more time for *diastolic filling*, a key determinant of myocardial perfusion. Coronary *plaque regression* has been documented. Despite these proven benefits, beta-blockers continue to be underused, especially in the elderly.

Categorization and Preparations

Beta-blockers can be categorized according to their relative cardioselectivity, lipid solubility, intrinsic agonist activity, and alpha-blocking capacity. Available preparations include generic and brand versions, with the latter accounting for many of the sustained-release formulations.

Cardioselectivity refers to the degree of preferential affinity for β_1 receptors, which predominate in the heart and are the principal target of antianginal therapy. Beta-blockers that lack cardioselectivity are more likely at low doses to cause side effects associated with β_2 blockade (bronchospasm, peripheral vasoconstriction, and inhibition of glycogenolysis; see later discussion). Cardioselectivity fades as doses increase. At low to intermediate doses, cardioselectivity is demonstrated by *atenolol, metoprolol, acebutolol, betaxolol,* and *bisoprolol.* *Lipid solubility* affects absorption, metabolism, serum half-life, and the degree to which an agent crosses the blood–brain barrier. The more lipid-soluble an agent is, the more rapid is its absorption, the shorter is its half-life, and the more likely it is to enter the central nervous system (CNS). Lipid-soluble preparations are, for the most part, hepatically metabolized. The most lipid-soluble beta-blockers include propranolol, followed by metoprolol and then pindolol; the least lipid-soluble agents include atenolol and nadolol. Although it was originally believed that lipid solubility predicted the degree of CNS side effects (depression, psychomotor retardation), this has not been confirmed by randomized, controlled trials (see later discussion).

Agonist activity is an intrinsic characteristic of *pindolol, acebutolol, carvedilol, labetalol,* and *penbutolol.* At low doses, these drugs show some sympatholytic action and tend to cause less reduction in heart rate, contractility, and conduction than other beta-blockers. Consequently, they are worth considering in patients who develop symptomatic bradycardia with the use of standard beta-blockers. However, as doses increase, these agonist effects are overpowered by the underlying beta-blocking activity.

Alpha-blocking activity is a feature of *labetalol* and *carvedilol.* This characteristic makes these agents useful in situations in which potent afterload reduction is desired, as in hypertension and congestive heart failure. Labetalol combines nonselective beta-blockade with agonist activity and alpha-blocking action; it is used predominantly in hypertensive patients. Adverse effects include greater degrees of postural hypotension and sexual dysfunction than seen with most other beta-blockers. Carvedilol offers nonselective beta-blockade in conjunction with alpha-blockade; in addition, it prevents upregulation of cardiac beta receptors, reduces cardiac norepinephrine, and demonstrates antioxidant effects. The drug is approved by the U.S. Food and Drug Administration (FDA) for use in heart failure, in which it has been shown to reduce morbidity and mortality (see Chapter 32).

Preparations span the spectrum of duration of action from about 6 hours for generic propranolol to 24 hours for sustained-release metoprolol. Most beta-blockers are available generically, having come off patent years ago, which makes for considerable cost savings. Convenience and compliance can be enhanced by the use of a once-daily formulation, but the cost is increased substantially because many of these are brand-name formulations of generic agents.

Adverse Effects

Many side effects are directly attributable to the consequences of beta-blockade on organ systems that require beta stimulation for normal functioning. The risk is greatest when there is underlying organ-system dysfunction. Heart failure, heart block, and severe bronchospasm are among the most worrisome of potential adverse effects, but the risk can be minimized by careful prescribing and monitoring. In most instances, some degree of beta-blockade can be instituted, especially if cardioselective agents are used. Abrupt withdrawal of beta-blocker therapy can lead to rebound adrenergic stimulation and its attendant adverse consequences.

Heart Failure. Heart failure may develop or worsen in patients with preexisting LV dysfunction. Not all patients with a reduced ejection fraction necessarily worsen; those with heart failure due to coronary disease may actually improve (see Chapter 32), but careful monitoring is essential. Concurrent use of other negatively inotropic drugs (e.g., verapamil, disopyramide) should be eliminated or at least minimized.

Heart Block. Patients with underlying conduction-system disease may experience symptomatic *bradycardia* or *heart block* due to a slowing of the sinoatrial node and atrioventricular conduction; sinus arrest may ensue in such patients. A preparation with some intrinsic beta-agonist activity may be preferred if a beta-blocker is to be used in the setting of underlying conduction-system disease. Close monitoring is critical to safe use in persons with underlying conduction-system disease.

Coronary Vasoconstriction. Coronary vasoconstriction is a theoretical concern in patients with coronary disease, especially in those with atherosclerotic disease complicated by vasospasm and in those with purely vasospastic disease. Clinically, it is rarely a problem. In fact, beta-blockers have actually been proved to be useful in patients with variant angina, although they are usually prescribed in conjunction with coronary vasodilators such as nitrates or calcium-channel blockers. The observed benefit of beta-blockers in settings of suspected coronary vasoconstriction is believed to be related to their favorable effects on platelet aggregation, oxygen demand, and other factors contributing to vasospasm or angina.

Peripheral Vasoconstriction. Peripheral vasoconstriction can occur with beta-blocker therapy, particularly in patients who suffer from vasospastic Raynaud's disease. However, as long as a low-dose cardioselective program is used, the Raynaud's patient can usually tolerate beta-blocker treatment. Similarly, patients with peripheral atherosclerotic arterial disease rarely suffer a compromise in limb perfusion when taking a beta-blocker (see Chapter 34).

Bronchospasm. By blocking β_2 receptors, nonselective beta-blockers (and all preparations when used in full doses) may trigger bronchospasm, the most serious side effect of beta-blocker use. Bronchospasm may occur in any patient with a history of bronchospastic disease, even if the patient is asymptomatic at the time of initiating therapy. Many regard asthma as a relative contraindication to beta-blocker use, but careful use is possible in patients with inactive or well-controlled bronchospastic disease, so long as doses are kept low and a cardioselective agent is used. Nonetheless, caution and careful monitoring of flow rates are advised because even low doses of a relatively cardioselective agent can worsen bronchospasm in a patient with asthma.

Blunted Response to Hypoglycemia. Beta-blockers blunt the adrenergic response to hypoglycemia. This may impair patient recognition of a hypoglycemic episode in patients taking insulin or potent oral agents and, in theory, prolong the duration of hypoglycemia by inhibiting catecholamine-induced glycogenolysis and glucose mobilization. In practice, prolongation of hypoglycemia is rare, and diabetics have a very high risk of cardiovascular morbidity and mortality that is markedly reduced by beta-blocker therapy. Consequently, beta-blocker use is not contraindicated in diabetics, even in those taking insulin, but careful dosing and cardioselectivity are required, as are detailed patient education and careful program design (see Chapter 102).

CNS Side Effects and Depression. Early anecdotal reports described cognitive problems, depression, sexual dysfunction, altered sleep, nightmares, and fatigue associated with beta-blocker use. These problems appeared particularly frequently with the use of propranolol (the first beta-blocker to become available) and in the elderly; however, randomized, controlled trials found no increase in the risk for depression and revealed only a very small absolute risk for fatigue or sexual dysfunction (<1%). Although it was hypothesized that risk was related to use of lipid-soluble preparations such as propranolol, no such association has been confirmed. Concern about these potential side effects appears overstated and should not be used as a basis for denying a trial of carefully monitored beta-blocker therapy.

Rebound. Abrupt *withdrawal* of beta-blockade can precipitate an exacerbation of *angina, acute coronary insufficiency*, or even *infarction*. It has been hypothesized that an *"upregulation" of beta-adrenergic receptors* results from long-term blockade and makes these patients more sensitive to unopposed beta-adrenergic stimulation. Onset is characteristically within 2 to 6 days after the abrupt cessation of therapy. Concern about withdrawal often occurs in the perioperative setting, in which medications might have been held for surgery. About 10% of stable anginal patients experience a serious *rebound* in symptoms when beta-blockade is suddenly terminated. Infarction and death may occur. Those at greatest risk are patients on large doses who have achieved much benefit from beta-blockade. Withholding beta-blockers for up to 48 hours can be done without risking any increase in angina. Patients who experience an exacerbation usually do so 2 to 6 days after the abrupt discontinuation of therapy. Tapering therapy over the course of 1 to 2 weeks can minimize a withdrawal reaction.

Lipids. Although beta-blocker use (especially of nonselective agents) may cause a modest increase in serum triglycerides and a small reduction in serum high-density-lipoprotein (HDL) cholesterol, there is no evidence that these effects are clinically significant. Moreover, both animal and human studies demonstrate beta-blocker inhibition of serum factors and vessel wall stresses important to atherogenesis.

Choice of Agent

The choice of agent should be based predominantly on cost, the need for cardioselectivity, and the duration of action. Generically available formulations (e.g., propranolol, metoprolol, atenolol) are 1/10 to 1/30 the cost of brand-name beta-blockers. Cardioselectivity deserves consideration in patients with asthma, peripheral vascular disease, or neuropsychiatric problems. The duration of action becomes important for maximizing compliance, which is facilitated by the use of agents that can be administered on a once-daily or twice-daily basis. The combination of low cost, cardioselectivity, and prolonged duration of action makes generic preparations of *metoprolol* and *atenolol* the preferred beta-blockers for most patients with

coronary disease. An agent with some intrinsic beta-agonist activity (e.g., generic *pindolol*) may be worth considering in anginal patients with conduction-system disease or sinus node dysfunction bothered by symptomatic bradycardia when taking a beta-blocker without such activity. The presence of heart failure does not need to be a contraindication to beta-blocker use; both long-acting metoprolol and carvedilol have demonstrated the ability to improve survival in patients with heart failure (see Chapter 32).

Titration of Dose

Beta-blocker therapy requires the titration of dose against the *resting* and *exercise heart rates*. Lowering the resting heart rate to about 60 beats/min is usually considered evidence of sufficient beta-blockade but may not be a reliable indicator in elderly patients. A subset of patients do not achieve adequate control of their angina at this level of beta-blockade. Further increases in dose (and a slower resting heart rate) may be necessary to prevent chest pain. Such bradycardia is often well tolerated hemodynamically. Typical target heart rates are 50 to 60 beats/min at rest, with an increase to 70 to 80 beats/min with moderate exercise and to no more than 100 beats/min with vigorous exercise. The true measures of adequate therapy remain the suppression of angina and the improvement of exercise tolerance. Times of maximum diurnal adrenergic activity (early morning and early evening) are the ones most important to cover with beta-blockade because they are times when risks of cardiac events are greatest.

Angiotensin-Converting-Enzyme Inhibitors (28–31)

Angiotensin-converting-enzyme inhibitors (ACEIs) have emerged as a cornerstone of CHD management, demonstrating significant reductions in cardiovascular *morbidity* and *mortality* in persons with high CHD risk, independent of effects on heart failure and blood pressure.

Effect on CHD Morbidity and Mortality

Reductions of 20% to 30% in the risk of cardiac death, infarction, and stroke were observed in the Heart Outcomes Prevention Evaluation (HOPE) trial in high-risk persons with preserved LV function, half of whom had stable angina; similar and confirmatory findings were provided by the European Trial on the Reduction of Cardiac Events with Perindopril in Stable Coronary Artery Disease (EUROPA) in persons at lower risk for adverse CHD events. The observed benefits appear independent of blood pressure reduction, aspirin use, beta-blockers, lipid-lowering agents, and antihypertensive drugs, suggesting a unique mode of action beyond the inhibition of angiotensin-induced vasoconstriction. One explanatory hypothesis links the observed benefits to drug-stimulated increases in vascular tissue kinins and their effects on endothelial physiology, including vasodilation, tissue thromboplastin production, nitric oxide levels, prostacyclin synthesis, and oxidative stress. ACE inhibitors have shown the ability to limit vascular smooth muscle proliferation, plaque rupture, and LV hypertrophy and to improve vascular endothelial function and fibrinolysis. The accumulating evidence of survival benefit recommends ACE inhibition to all patients with CHD, irrespective of LV function. Combination with beta-blockade appears to enhance benefit and limit risk even further.

Adverse Effects

The most common adverse effect is *dry cough*, which is believed to be related to the drug-induced increase in tissue bradykinins, triggering a nagging dry cough in about 5% to 10% of patients. *Angioedema* is also seen and may have a similar mechanism. *Renal dysfunction* may occur in the context of bilateral renal artery stenosis (see Chapters 26 and 32) but is usually not a concern. The potential for an adverse *drug–drug interaction* with *aspirin* has been a concern. Post hoc analyses of studies performed for other reasons suggest a possible reduction in cardiovascular benefit when the two drugs are taken together. Speculation centers on aspirin-induced inhibition of prostaglandin synthesis blunting the beneficial kinin-triggered effects on blood vessels. Even with the blunting of the ACEI effect, the net benefit of taking the two agents together still exceeds that of not using them, leading most experts to believe that it would be premature to withhold aspirin in the context of ACE inhibitor therapy. The literature should be followed closely.

Angiotensin-Receptor Blockers as Alternatives

Angiotensin-receptor blockers (ARBs) exhibit many of the same properties as ACEIs and are often considered as an alternative by virtue of their ability to counter the action of angiotensin II without causing the potentially bothersome side effects of cough and angioedema. If these kinin-related effects are important to the observed ACEI benefit in CHD (see prior discussion), then their absence in ARB therapy may reduce their utility for management in stable angina. Prospective trials are under way to help address this question.

Preparations and Dosing

See Chapters 26 and 32.

Antiplatelet Therapy and Oral Anticoagulation (32–36)

Appreciation for the roles of platelets, clotting factors, fibrinolysis, and vascular reactivity in coronary artery disease has focused attention on the inhibition of platelet function and thrombus formation.

Antiplatelet Therapy

Of the conventional platelet inhibitors (e.g., aspirin, dipyridamole, sulfinpyrazone), only *aspirin* has proven to be consistently effective in reducing cardiac risk; dipyridamole increases the risk of exercise-induced ischemia; *clopidogrel* has shown promise.

Aspirin. Aspirin reduces the risk of myocardial infarction and death in persons with *chronic stable angina*. In the Swedish Angina Pectoris Aspirin Trial, the combined endpoint of MI and death was reduced by greater than 30%. In the Physicians' Health Study, an 87% reduction in the risk of myocardial infarction and a trend toward a reduced risk of death from infarction were observed. Aggregated data find a 22% overall reduction in the risk of ischemic events. There is a trend toward an increase in the risk of hemorrhagic stroke. Aspirin therapy does not prevent the onset of angina, and reports of *aspirin resistance* associated with an increased risk of coronary events have emerged for patients with chronic stable angina.

Clopidogrel (Plavix). This inhibitor of adenosine diphosphate–dependent activation of the platelet glycoprotein IIb/IIIa complex impairs platelet aggregation. In the only head-to-head comparison with aspirin in high-risk CHD patients, it proved to be slightly better in reducing the combined risk of MI, death, and stroke (the relative risk decreased by about 9%). Rates of bleeding complications were comparable. There have been no confirmatory studies, and the drug is far more expensive than aspirin; consequently, it is reserved for use in CHD patients who cannot take aspirin. In patients who have undergone angioplasty, clopidogrel in combination with aspirin is prescribed to prevent thrombosis, especially in patients undergoing stent implantation; chronic therapy is recommended for those receiving drug-eluting stents (see later discussion).

Oral Anticoagulation

Meta-analysis of major randomized, controlled trials of *warfarin* therapy in patients with CHD reveals significant reductions in myocardial infarction, stroke, and cardiovascular death with high-intensity (International Normalized Ratio [INR] 2.8 to 4.5) oral anticoagulation. Risks of infarction and stroke are reduced with moderate-intensity (INR 2.0 to 3.0) therapy. Low-intensity therapy (INR 1.5) reduces the risk over and above that achieved by aspirin in persons with CHD risk factors, but there are no trials in persons with stable angina. The benefits of high- and moderate-intensity anticoagulation approximate those seen with the use of aspirin, but the risk of bleeding is increased in proportion to the intensity of oral anticoagulation.

Nitrates (18,37–42)

Once a mainstay of anginal therapy, nitrates have been relegated to a supporting role with the realization that they do not improve survival. Nonetheless, they continue to be useful for the symptomatic control of angina and are moderately effective in lessening coronary vasospasm.

Mechanism of Action

Nitrates are vasodilators that act predominantly on the *venous capacitance vessels,* although they have a lesser effect on the *arterial bed.* Their mechanism of action involves the release of nitric oxide, which relaxes vascular smooth muscle. Nitrates have no direct chronotropic or inotropic effects but decrease myocardial oxygen demand by *reducing preload* through a lowering of LV filling pressure and end-diastolic volume. They also have a favorable but lesser effect on *afterload,* modestly reducing systemic blood pressure. Regional myocardial perfusion may be improved by the ability of nitrates to *dilate epicardial coronary arteries* (including stenotic segments) and collateral vessels, but there is little effect on the smaller resistance arteries, thus preventing a steal phenomenon from developing (as seen with short-acting dihydropyridine calcium-channel blockers).

Adverse Effects and Contraindications

Headache, hypotension, and tolerance are among the problems associated with nitrate use.

Headache. Headache is the most common side effect. It is typically throbbing, as a consequence of vasodilation. It is most prominent at the outset of nitrate therapy and typically abates with continued nitrate use without loss of hemodynamic benefit. It may recur on abrupt cessation of chronic nitrate use.

Headache can be particularly problematic for anginal patients who also suffer from migraine headache; adding beta-blockade to the program can help to limit the headache.

Hypotension. The risk of severe hypotension is associated with cotemporaneous use of nitrates and vasodilator agents prescribed for erectile dysfunction (e.g., sildenafil [Viagra]). The potential for hypotension persists for 24 hours after the last nitrate dose. Such use is contraindicated in persons with coronary disease due to the risk of hypotension-induced ischemic injury. The venodilation can also be harmful in persons with critical aortic stenosis, who require a high filling pressure to maintain cardiac output. Nitrates can also increase the degree of outflow tract obstruction in hypertrophic cardiomyopathy, leading to hypotension and syncope. The fall in blood pressure from vasodilation typically triggers a reflex tachycardia that can increase myocardial oxygen demand in CHD patients; concurrent use of beta-blockade helps to minimize the rise in heart rate.

Nitrate Tolerance. Tolerance is associated with chronic therapy and is believed to be related to sulfhydryl depletion in vascular endothelial cells, leading to blunted peripheral and coronary vasodilatory responses to nitrates. The problem is both dose and time dependent, occurring after as little as 7 to 10 days of continuous intermediate-dose nitrate use (e.g., 24-hour application of a 5-mg transdermal nitroglycerin patch or around-the-clock use of 30 mg of isosorbide). The common denominator is insufficient time for adequate nitrate washout. Prevention requires a daily nitrate-free period of 10 to 12 hours. Combining nitrate therapy with the use of a beta-blocker or calcium-channel blocker can help to control angina during the nitrate-free period.

Nitrate Preparations

Nitrate preparations range from the very short acting to those offering more sustained effect.

Sublingual Nitroglycerin (TNG) Tablets. This inexpensive preparation provides quick (30 seconds to 3 minutes), effective relief from anginal pain and, when taken prophylactically, improvement in exercise tolerance. The principal drawback is short duration of action (30 minutes). TNG must be taken sublingually because oral doses are inactivated hepatically on first pass through the portal circulation. The drug is volatile, necessitating storage in a tightly capped amber vial in a cool place. Once opened, the contents remain maximally effective for no more than 3 to 6 months. The absence of tongue burning with use may indicate a loss of activity and a reason for lack of response.

Aerosolized TNG Spray. The aerosol delivers 0.4 mg of rapidly absorbed TNG to the surface of the tongue from a metered-dose aerosol canister. The onset, duration, and efficacy of a single dose resemble those of a 0.4-mg sublingual TNG tablet. Each canister contains about 200 doses and retains efficacy for up to 3 years. The cost per dose is substantially greater than for TNG tablets, but the extended shelf life helps to reduce waste and total cost. The spray is a reasonable alternative for patients who wear dentures or have dry mucous membranes. Proper use requires accurately directing the spray to the tongue and not inhaling it.

Isosorbide Dinitrate. Isosorbide dinitrate provides more sustained vasodilation and better anginal prophylaxis. Single oral doses of 20 to 40 mg significantly improve hemodynamic parameters and exercise tolerance. The onset of action is 15 to 30 minutes; the clinical duration is 4 to 8 hours. The optimal *dosage schedule* is two or three times a day, timed eccentrically to provide a 12-hour nitrate-free period that minimizes the risk of nitrate tolerance. A sustained-release preparation (12-hour half-life) is available but not recommended because of uneven intestinal absorption and the risk of nitrate tolerance (unless used only once daily). Both *chewable* and *sublingual* isosorbide preparations are also available, providing more rapid onset of action (5 to 15 minutes) but shorter duration (2 hours) and increased cost.

Isosorbide Mononitrate. Isosorbide mononitrate provides longer-acting nitrate than isosorbide dinitrate. When given twice daily, it can provide up to 12 hours of antianginal activity. A large once-daily dose of the sustained-release formulation can give up to 12 hours of relief. Isosorbide mononitrate offers no significant advantage over generic isosorbide dinitrate for the control of chronic stable angina, except convenience. The mononitrate costs 10 times more per day than the generic dinitrate preparation. The heavily promoted feature of reduced risk of nitrate tolerance with mononitrate use is probably true, but less expensive means of accomplishing this objective are relatively easy to devise.

Nitroglycerin Ointment. This preparation offers an inexpensive and effective method for providing long-acting anginal prophylaxis (up to 6 hours), but the ointment can be messy and irritating to the skin if it is applied to the same area throughout the day; it is best suited for nocturnal use.

Transdermal Nitroglycerin Patch. The patch can deliver nitroglycerin for 24 hours in a convenient-to-use but relatively expensive form. Proper use to avoid nitrate tolerance requires putting the patch on in the morning and removing it in the early evening. In patients who have been using patches for months to years, termination is best conducted in a tapering fashion to avoid the precipitation of a nitrate withdrawal syndrome.

Initiation of Therapy

Long-acting nitrate therapy should be introduced gradually; starting with too large a dose produces severe vascular headaches that force many patients to stop their medication. Beginning with a low-dose program (e.g., 5 mg of isosorbide three times a day) and advancing it slowly over 1 to 2 weeks, one can achieve substantial nitrate doses without significant headache. The dose is increased until customary activity can be undertaken without angina, the heart rate at rest rises by 10 to 15 beats/min, or blood pressure falls to the point of causing postural lightheadedness. The development of headache is not a reliable therapeutic endpoint because this side effect usually disappears with the continuation of therapy. Patients with migraine headaches may be very intolerant of nitrates, but combining nitrate therapy with a beta-blocking agent can often overcome this difficulty, especially if the beta-blocker is started first. Combination with a beta-blocker can also provide anginal prophylaxis during the nitrate-free periods required for the prevention of nitrate tolerance.

Contributions to Management

Nitrates provide effective relief of anginal pain and improvement in exercise tolerance in patients with stable angina who are not adequately controlled by beta-blockade alone. Combining nitrate use with beta-blockade takes advantage of their complementary hemodynamic effects and helps to maximize the control of angina along with a reduction in mortality at low cost. Nitrates remain a first-line agent in patients with *variant angina* due to coronary vasospasm.

Calcium-Channel Blockers (18,19,25,43–47)

Calcium-channel blockers remain popular because they are well tolerated and effective for the control of symptoms, but enthusiasm for their use as first-line agents in chronic stable angina has waned with the realization that they do not improve survival and sometimes can increase the risks of MI and cardiac death.

Mechanisms of Action

These agents inhibit calcium transport via blockade of L-type and/or T-type calcium channels in cellular membranes of myocardial, vascular, and nonvascular smooth muscle tissues. In the heart, calcium-channel blockade *reduces inotropy* and *slows conduction*; in vascular tissue, the result is *vasodilation*, which may be accompanied by *reflex tachycardia*. Responses of vascular smooth muscle to angiotensin II and catecholamines are blunted. The net effects range from coronary and systemic vasodilation to decreases in myocardial contractility and conductivity. Coronary vasodilation improves perfusion in patients prone to coronary vasospasm. In most stable anginal patients, symptomatic benefit is believed to derive from a reduction in myocardial oxygen demand brought about by reductions in contractility, filling pressure (preload), and systemic blood pressure (afterload).

Classification

The different classes of calcium-channel blockers are distinguished by their binding site within the L channel and by their relative clinical effects on myocardial, conducting-system, and vascular functions. They all cause vasodilation and a lowering of blood pressure, but the degree of pressure reduction varies, as does the net effect on contractility and conduction.

Dihydropyridines (e.g., Nifedipine, Nicardipine, Amlodipine). Nifedipine is the prototypical agent of this class. Those approved for use in stable angina include nifedipine, nicardipine, and amlodipine. Only amlodipine and the long-acting formulation of nifedipine are recommended for use because of the concerns regarding the safety of short-acting calcium-channel blockers. Nifedipine is the most active vasodilator of all the calcium-channel blockers. Its main effect is arterial. Both coronary and peripheral arterial dilation result, making this agent especially useful for patients with coronary vasospasm and hypertension (see Chapter 26).

First-Generation Dihydropyridines (e.g., Nifedipine). Nifedipine is negatively inotropic, but the net negative effect on LV function is blunted by a strong beta-adrenergic reflex (leading to tachycardia and increased contractility) in response to the arterial vasodilation. In some patients, a marked *reflex tachycardia* occurs with the use of the short-acting preparation. Its potent vasodilating effects produce a higher incidence of *flushing, hypotension, dizziness, leg edema,* and *headache* than occurs with other drugs in its class. Nifedipine has no clinically significant suppressant effect on the sinoatrial or atrioventricular nodes, making it safe for use in patients with underlying conduction-system disease. It is also effective for the symptomatic treatment of chronic stable angina and variant angina.

Because of concerns about an increased risk of sudden cardiac death and marked reflex tachycardia with the use of short-acting dihydropyridines, only the sustained-release preparation of nifedipine is recommended for use in chronic stable angina.

Second-Generation Dihydropyridines (e.g., Nicardipine, Isradipine, Felodipine, Nisoldipine). Second-generation dihydropyridines are marketed predominantly as antihypertensive agents and promoted for their *vascular selectivity* because they do not affect atrioventricular or sinoatrial node activity. They are available in sustained-release formulations. Like nifedipine, these induce arterial dilation and an initial reflex tachycardia, often necessitating the concurrent use of a beta-blocker. Side effects are similar to those of nifedipine (flushing, peripheral edema, headache, lightheadedness). They are less negatively inotropic than earlier calcium-channel blockers, but they are still contraindicated in the setting of concurrent chronic heart failure.

Amlodipine. This late-generation, long-acting dihydropyridine manifests few of the adverse hemodynamic effects of earlier drugs in its class, producing little impairment of contractility, conductivity, or stimulation of neurohumoral reflexes (no reflex tachycardia). Its use in the setting of LV dysfunction does not appear to increase the rates of MI or cardiac death (see Chapter 32).

Phenylalkylamines (e.g., Verapamil). Verapamil is the prototype in this class, which has the most pronounced net effect on myocardial contractility and atrioventricular conduction. Even though they effectively reduce afterload, they can precipitate *heart failure* in patients with underlying LV dysfunction and cause *heart block* in patients with conduction-system disease, which contraindicates their use in patients with severe LV failure or marked conduction-system disease. This potent ability to slow atrioventricular conduction has made verapamil extremely useful for the acute treatment of supraventricular tachycardias (see Chapter 28). Constipation and leg edema are consequences of its dilating effect on gastrointestinal and venous smooth muscle.

Benzothiazepines (e.g., Diltiazem). Benzothiazepines are the prototypes and among the better tolerated of the calcium-channel blockers. Although diltiazem more closely resembles verapamil than nifedipine, its pharmacologic profile is unique. Compared with verapamil, it causes a greater slowing of the sinoatrial node but has less influence on the atrioventricular junction, contractility, and vascular tone. In studies of its effects on mortality and reinfarction in post–myocardial infarction patients, there was no overall improvement in either mortality or reinfarction; patients with LV dysfunction showed increased rates of adverse outcomes, suggesting that any possible benefit is limited to those with preserved LV function.

T-Type Calcium-Channel Blockers. T-type channels are found in vascular smooth muscle and conduction-system tissue but not in ventricular myocardium. The result is coronary and peripheral vascular dilation but no impairment of myocardial contractility. *Mibefradil* blocks not only the L-type calcium channel, but also the T-type (transient) calcium channel; however, it was withdrawn from the market due to a high frequency of adverse drug–drug interactions.

Adverse Effects

As noted earlier, increased risks of *myocardial infarction* and *cardiac death* have been reported in patient populations taking short-acting calcium-channel blockers. Findings from several retrospective, prospective, and meta-analytic studies have shown a significant increase in the relative risk of myocardial infarction and cardiac death (relative risk, 1.5 to 1.6). Proposed mechanisms of this mortality risk include increased myocardial oxygen demand from *reflex tachycardia* and decreased coronary perfusion from an acute *drop in filling pressure*. The extent of risk associated with longer-acting, second-generation preparations remains to be defined by prospective, randomized trials.

The use of calcium-channel blockers in *heart failure* has proven to be problematic, increasing the risks of worsening heart failure, life-threatening arrhythmias, myocardial infarction, and death when used in patients with chronic LV dysfunction. The mechanisms responsible for these cardiac complications are poorly understood. It was believed that the reflex tachycardia and negative inotropic effects of many of these agents were responsible, but even the use of sustained-release preparations and agents with little effect on the left ventricle manifest the risk (except for amlodipine, which is among the least negatively inotropic; see Chapter 32).

As noted, *heart block* and *sinoatrial node suppression* may occur or be exacerbated with use of verapamil- and diltiazem-like agents in persons with underlying conduction-system disease. Calcium-channel blockers with marked effects on noncardiac smooth muscle (e.g., dihydropyridines, verapamil) produce the highest incidence of *peripheral edema, flushing*, and *postural hypotension*, but some degree of leg edema can be seen with almost any of these drugs.

Selection of Agent

The selection of an individual agent needs to take into account cost, convenience, and the status of the patient's left ventricle, conducting system, and venous tone.

Cost and Convenience. From a cost-effectiveness perspective, calcium-channel blockers do not rank highly, but their long-acting formulations make for convenient once- or twice-daily dosing and enhanced safety of use (see prior discussion). Cost remains an issue. Even the generic sustained-release formulations are as much as 5 times the cost of generic beta-blockers; brand-name formulations are 10 to 25 times more expensive.

Use in the Setting of LV Dysfunction. Caution is advised, in view of the increased risk of adverse cardiac outcomes in patients with heart failure, especially those treated with negatively inotropic calcium-channel blockers such as verapamil, but also with most drugs in this class. Only *amlodipine* appears to be reasonably well tolerated in anginal patients with severe chronic LV dysfunction (ejection fraction <30%). However, amlodipine does not improve survival and carries a 5% risk of inducing pulmonary edema. An *ACE inhibitor* (see prior discussion and Chapter 32) is a better choice in settings of LV dysfunction.

Use in the Setting of Sinus-Node or Conduction-System Disease. Calcium-channel blockers that suppress conduction and/or sinus-node function (e.g., verapamil, diltiazem) should be avoided or used with caution in this setting, especially if beta-blockers, digoxin, or other drugs that have similar effects on nodal and conduction tissue are being taken. Late-generation dihydropyridines (e.g., amlodipine) are preferred.

Use in the Setting of Peripheral Edema. Venodilation and a worsening of leg edema can be problematic in persons with preexisting venous insufficiency. Avoiding the use of calcium-channel blockers with major venodilating effects (e.g., dihydropyridines) may help to limit the risk of worsening edema, but the problem is inherent with almost all drugs in this class.

Contributions to Management

Calcium-channel blockers can contribute to the management of chronic stable angina by providing additional symptomatic improvement (e.g., a reduced frequency of anginal episodes, a prolongation of exercise tolerance, and a decrease in nitrate requirements) in persons taking beta-blockers and nitrates. They are equivalent to nitrates in these capabilities and superior in that they do not require a 12-hour "washout period" (see prior discussion), enabling uninterrupted 24-hour control of symptoms. Although they are symptomatically beneficial, calcium-channel blockers have yet to demonstrate any reduction in rates of myocardial infarction, need for revascularization, cardiac sudden death, or overall mortality; moreover, the relative risk of adverse cardiac outcomes increases with their use in heart failure and with the use of short-acting preparations.

Consequently, these relatively expensive drugs are best reserved for patients with preserved LV function who do not achieve adequate symptomatic relief with beta-blockade and nitrates. Their addition to the medical program can enhance exercise tolerance and reduce the frequency and severity of anginal episodes. As effective long-acting coronary vasodilators, they are also very helpful in persons with *coronary vasospasm* (e.g., *variant angina*). In persons with stubborn vasospastic disease, they can be added to nitrate therapy, but with care because of the potential for hypotension and worsening angina. The combination of a *calcium-channel blocker* plus *nitrates* is occasionally worth considering in very symptomatic patients who *cannot tolerate beta-blockade* (e.g., those with severe bronchospastic disease). The calcium-channel blocker should be one that blunts reflex tachycardia (e.g., diltiazem or verapamil).

Their ability to slow conduction through the atrioventricular node makes these agents potentially useful in anginal patients with *supraventricular tachyarrhythmias* (see Chapters 25 and 28), but caution is warranted if they are used in the context of preexisting beta-blockade due to the risks of severe bradycardia and impaired contractility. In sum, their high cost and inability to improve survival relegate calcium-channel blockers to a secondary role in management of stable angina.

Revascularization (48–76)

Revascularization provides opportunities to improve coronary blood flow, symptomatic control of angina, and exercise tolerance. In high-risk patients, revascularization also achieves reductions in rates of infarction and cardiac death that are superior to those seen with medical therapy. The principal revascularization modalities are *coronary artery bypass graft (CABG)* surgery and *percutaneous coronary intervention (PCI), which includes percutaneous transluminal coronary angioplasty (PTCA)* and *stenting*. Coronary revascularization has become one of the most commonly performed invasive therapies in the United States. Although final decisions regarding revascularization are the province of the consulting cardiologist and cardiac surgeon, their assessments benefit from timely referral and input by the primary physician, who needs to know when revascularization deserves consideration. Rapid technical advances place extra reliance on the experience and judgment of the consulting cardiac interventionalist and cardiac surgeon because long-term outcomes data may not be available for the most recent innovations. That does not preclude the need for the primary physician to be familiar with the indications, contraindications, and key issues regarding revascularization versus medical therapy because referral is often tantamount to choosing a particular mode of therapy, given existing uncertainties and enthusiasm by the practitioners of each mode of treatment.

Coronary Artery Bypass Graft Surgery

Bypass graft surgery remains the predominant mode of revascularization for high-risk persons with stable angina. It not only improves symptoms and functional status, but it also reduces the risk of infarction and improves survival. Technical advances, particularly the advent of *off-pump CABG*, have lowered perioperative mortality, reduced recovery time, and reduced the risk of cognitive decline associated with bypass surgery.

Indications. The primary indication for CABG is *high-risk anatomy*, especially in the setting of *LV dysfunction*. CABG is the treatment of choice for persons with *left-main coronary* disease, significant (>70% stenosis) *three-vessel* disease with LV dysfunction (ejection fraction <50%), and two-vessel disease with proximal left-anterior-descending (LAD) artery involvement (*left-main equivalent* anatomy) plus reduced ejection fraction or significant amounts of myocardium at risk according to noninvasive testing. In these settings, CABG produces significant reductions in the rates of MI and cardiac death compared with medical therapy and with PCI.

CABG is also useful for improved anginal control in patients with less severe *multivessel disease*, who may not experience as great a survival benefit as those with high-risk coronary disease but do obtain better control of symptoms than that achieved by medical therapy alone. Included in this group are persons who have one- or two-vessel nonproximal LAD disease and a history of cardiac arrest or sustained VT, symptomatic restenosis after previous CABG or PCI, and symptomatic lesser-risk anatomy that is not amenable to angioplasty. CABG remains the preferred revascularization procedure for *diabetics*, although coated stents show promise in reducing restenosis rates in diabetics after angioplasty (see later discussion). Those who are reluctant to undergo a repeat revascularization procedure within the next 3 to 5 years should also be considered for CABG because the probability of needing a repeat procedure is much lower than with PCI.

Risks. In major centers, the perioperative complication rates for elective CABG in high-risk patients include *mortality* (0.8% to 1%), *infarction* (2.5%), *arrhythmia* (10%), major *bleeding* requiring reoperation (2%), *stroke* (1%), and *embolization* (1%). Higher complication rates are found in hospitals that do relatively fewer bypass procedures per year. *Cognitive changes*, sometimes referred to as *postpump syndrome*, are seen both early and late. The early changes occur in nearly two thirds of CHD patients and are believed to be related to the effects of general anesthesia because they are also seen in persons with CHD undergoing noncardiac surgery. However, the persistence of cognitive decline at 5 years is noted in up to one third of patients undergoing CABG. Risk factors for late decline include older age and early decline noted at the time of discharge. The cause(s) of cognitive decline are unknown, but purported mechanisms include preexisting cerebrovascular disease and microembolization from intraoperative manipulation of a diseased aorta. There is particular concern for microembolization occurring at the time the heart–lung bypass machine is removed from the aorta; no correlation has been found between time on heart–lung bypass and the risk of developing the early and late cognitive changes. Approaches to minimizing this risk include the development of filters and the use of non-bypass ("off-pump") surgery.

Off-pump surgery is an emerging "less invasive" surgical technology developed with the hope of lessening some of the risks attributed to the traditional on-pump approach to CABG. Eliminating the bypass pump produced encouraging early results, including a lower incidence of cognitive decline, fewer strokes, lower transfusion requirements, and shorter recovery time. However, long-term follow-up data from the original randomized trials show no differences in cognitive and cardiac outcomes at 5 years. The surgery is challenging because the heart is not stopped and the area of bypass must still be immobilized, putting some vessels out of reach or at least difficult to approach. Nonetheless, perioperative mortality and morbidity are equivalent to or better than those with traditional CABG. More data on long-term results should better help to define the role of this promising technology.

Minimizing Risk of Restenosis. Long-term patency rates are high, but by 10 years the risk of graft failure can approach 40%, especially in saphenous vein grafts, which are vulnerable to atherosclerotic change. Measures that lower restenosis risk include the use of internal thoracic (mammary) arteries (which are much less prone to atherosclerotic change; the 10-year patency rate is 90%) for grafting to critical vessels, such as the left main coronary artery or proximal LAD, and tight control of atherosclerotic risk factors, especially LDL cholesterol (see Chapter 27).

Contraindications. Most studies of surgical therapy for patients with *coronary spasm* show disappointing results (e.g., higher rates of mortality and nonfatal infarction). In such patients, surgical therapy should be considered only when medical therapy has failed and spasm has been documented in or about an area of fixed critical stenosis and not in other vessels or distally. Age per se is not a contraindication, although the risk of postpump syndrome is increased.

Identifying Candidates. *Exercise stress testing* and *echocardiography* are the best noninvasive means of screening and identifying the high-risk patient who would be a candidate for CABG (see Chapters 20 and 36). Those demonstrating a large amount of myocardium at risk and/or a reduced ejection fraction should be referred promptly for *angiography* and consideration of CABG. Persons without high-risk disease but in need of better symptom control and thus reasonable candidates for elective revascularization should be asked for their preferences, especially their willingness to undergo repeat revascularization in 3 to 5 years (a high likelihood with the use of PCI). Those wanting a more durable result might be considered for CABG, all other factors being equal.

Percutaneous Coronary Intervention (PCI)–Angioplasty and Stenting

Catheter-based revascularization has progressed dramatically over the last decade from a single-vessel balloon procedure (*percutaneous transluminal coronary angioplasty [PTCA]*) in patients with a low-risk discrete proximal stenosis to multivessel angioplasty accompanied by *stent* implantations in persons with complex coronary lesions (PCI). The high frequency of restenosis after angioplasty has been greatly mitigated by the advent and application of stent technology. More than 1 million stenting procedures are done annually in the United States, with the vast majority performed electively in persons with stable coronary disease, incurring billions of dollars in expenditures. Although recognized as effective for the relief of symptoms (angina, exercise intolerance), the widespread use of PCI has also generated concerns about cost-effectiveness and long-term safety, particularly with regard to reports of late-stage risks associated with the use of coated stents (see later discussion). Hoped-for improvements in rates of major cardiovascular events (e.g., nonfatal myocardial infarction, stroke, hospitalization, cardiac death) have yet to be definitively demonstrated; long-term randomized trials comparing medical therapy with PCI for the initial treatment of persons with stable coronary disease have found no significant differences in event rates.

Indications and Candidacy. In the setting of stable angina, the primary indications for PCI are relief of angina and improvement in exercise tolerance. The best candidates for PCI are those with *low-* or *moderate-risk* disease who remain symptomatic despite optimal medical therapy and lifestyle changes. PCI rivals CABG in providing symptomatic relief for persons with noncritical low- or moderate-risk coronary disease (see later discussion).

Originally, angioplasty was limited to a high-grade proximal stenosis in a noncritical vessel that was smooth, concentric, less than 0.5 cm in length, and noncalcified. Stenting was added to help preserve vessel patency after angioplasty; the FDA-approved indication for stenting is application to a single *de novo* coronary lesion of less than 30 mm in a native coronary artery of 2.5 to 3.5 mm in diameter. Advances in technique and materials (e.g., better introducers, thinner bare-metal stents, drug-eluting ["coated"] stents) have expanded the off-label use of angioplasty and stenting to more complex stenosis, multiple vessels, in-stent restenoses, patients with diabetes, and stenotic saphenous bypass grafts. These advances have contributed to offering revascularization procedures as an initial treatment to moderate-risk patients with considerable angina, based on the rationale that such intervention can be safely performed and provide better relief of anginal symptoms than medical therapy. However, a growing appreciation for the potential risks of these interventional procedures (see later discussion) and the failure to demonstrate a survival advantage in large-scale, randomized, controlled trials has tempered enthusiasm and reemphasized the central role of medical therapy both as initial treatment and as an essential part of any treatment program.

Risks. Experience and refinements in technology and technique have greatly limited the immediate procedural risks of angioplasty and stent implantation. Periprocedural risks include *bleeding* and *vascular injury* that require urgent surgical repair (1%), coronary *artery perforation* (<1%), *infection* (rare), and *contrast-induced nephropathy* (0% to 44%, depending on the presence of underlying kidney disease). Although the immediate success rate for angioplasty in patients with favorable lesions is greater than 85%, longer-term success is compromised by substantial rates of *restenosis* (e.g., 25% to 40% at 6 months with stand-alone angioplasty). The use of *antiplatelet therapy* (aspirin plus clopidogrel) and *stenting* at the time of angioplasty has markedly reduced restenosis rates but confers its own set of risks, including bleeding (see Chapter 83), thrombosis, and neointimal proliferation.

Thrombosis. Stent placement is associated with risks of *acute thrombosis* (heralded by angina) and *subacute thrombosis* (manifested by acute infarction or death; mortality rate, 25%). *Dual antiplatelet therapy* (aspirin plus *clopidogrel*) significantly reduces the absolute rates of stent-related acute and subacute thrombosis (e.g., to <0.5% and <1.5%, respectively). In persons receiving bare-metal stents, the risk of thrombosis becomes negligible beyond the first 30 to 60 days after placement. *Late thrombosis* (occurring up to >1 year after placement and potentially resulting in nonfatal MI or death) has been reported, especially in persons receiving *drug-eluting stents*, triggering concerns about the safety of PCI and its widespread application. The absolute late-thrombosis rate appears to be low (0.2%/yr to 0.5%/yr), and a significant increase in deaths and MI has yet to be documented, but cautions have been raised (especially with regard to enthusiasm for "off-label" applications of coated stents) and recommendations issued for extending dual antiplatelet therapy indefinitely pending more data and advances in stent technology. Patients being considered for stent placement, especially drug-eluting stents, need to be capable of long-term antiplatelet therapy.

Neointimal Proliferation. After 6 months of patency, the reappearance of angina in a patient treated with a bare-metal stent is about as likely to represent progression of another lesion that was not dilated as a late restenosis. Nonetheless, in-stent restenosis (>50% reduction in lumen diameter) remains a concern and can occur in up to 40% of patients by 1 year, often resulting from the *neointimal proliferation* of smooth muscle cells in the stented wall. Most patients remain asymptomatic, but those that do redevelop angina pose a difficult challenge because treatment is problematic. *Drug-eluting stents* (both *sirolimus coated* and *paclitaxel coated*) were developed to inhibit endothelial proliferation in vessels with bare-metal stents; 6- and 12-month rates of restenosis and adverse cardiac events were reduced by greater than 50%, but long-term follow-up studies of patients treated with such stents show increased rates of late thrombosis, raising concerns about their overall safety and proper role in the treatment of chronic stable angina.

Contraindications. Patients with *left-main disease, proximal LAD disease,* or *critical three-vessel disease* should not be treated with PCI; outcomes are better with CABG. As with bypass surgery, high rates of restenosis have occurred in patients with *variant angina,* making PCI ill advised in patients with vasospastic disease. *Diabetes mellitus* has been a relative contraindication to PCI due to a very high rate of restenosis; the use of coated stents in such patients reduces the restenosis rate, but the thrombosis risk remains substantial (4.5% at 1 year). Previous anatomic contraindications such stenosis near a branch point, diffuse occlusive disease of a vessel, and involvement of a smaller vessel are becoming less frequent barriers to successful PCI as technique and technology advance. Persons previously considered poor candidates for catheter revascularization, such as those with left ventricular dysfunction, are increasingly viewed by interventional cardiologists as reasonable candidates for PCI. Despite such enthusiasm and early technical successes, the reports of late-stage thrombosis with coated stents raise the question of whether the application of PCI has been overextended. The reader is urged to watch the literature for data from long-term outcomes studies.

PCI versus CABG

At issue is whether surgery or PCI is the preferred approach to revascularization in non–high-risk patients. Meta-analyses of randomized trials performed prior to the advent of coated stents found effects on symptoms and rates of survival and cardiac events in these groups to be similar (except for diabetics, who did better with CABG). Data from registries more indicative of everyday practice suggest an advantage in terms of cardiac outcomes for CABG in persons with multivessel disease. All studies find PCI patients significantly more likely to require a repeat revascularization procedure within 3 to 5 years. Whether coated stents will shift the balance in favor of angioplasty plus stenting in this patient population will have to await the arrival of data from randomized long-term trials. For now, the decision boils down to patient preference and candidacy.

"Alternative-Medicine" Therapies: Chelating (77)

Intravenous administration of the chelating agent *ethylenediaminetetraacetic acid* is widely performed in the United States by practitioners of alternative medicine. It is estimated that more than 100,000 persons are treated annually in the United States at a cost of approximately $4,000 each. In the only well-designed, randomized, controlled trial of chelation therapy among persons with stable angina, there was no difference in exercise capacity, quality of life, or exercise time to ischemia between patients treated with a full 3-month program of chelation or placebo. Chelation is not recommended.

PATIENT EDUCATION (78,79)

Patient education is critical, both to ensure proper compliance with what can be a rather complex medical regimen and to maximize functional status. An understanding of the rationale behind the medical regimen will facilitate its effective use. Counseling about prognosis and allowable activity can prevent unnecessary restriction of activity, relieve fear, and improve lifestyle. Of particular concern to many patients is the safety of engaging in *sexual activity*. The issue should be addressed openly and directly, even if the patient does not take the initiative to raise the subject. Failure to do so can lead to relationship problems, depression, and a worsening of symptoms. Guidelines for engaging in sexual activity are similar to those for any other form of physical exertion. The oxygen demands of intercourse among familiar middle-aged partners are about the same as those for climbing a flight of stairs. If intercourse takes place among unaccustomed partners, the physical and emotional stress may be considerably greater and the oxygen requirements increased substantially. If patients have serious concerns as to how much activity they can safely tolerate, an exercise test may be of value for reassurance, especially if they are needlessly limiting themselves.

With advances in medical therapy and revascularization technology, patients now have an expanded choice of treatment options. In circumstances in which outcomes are similar, the advantages and disadvantages of PCI versus CABG versus medical therapy need to be reviewed so that a treatment program well tailored to the patient's needs and preferences can be designed. Many of the racial differences noted in rates of revascularization among whites and blacks in the United States appear to be a function of familiarity rather than preference. Patient education is essential to ensuring that there is not inappropriate underutilization. Despite obtaining cardiac consultation, many patients will ask the independent opinion of their primary care physician, who they view as knowing them best. This role necessitates keeping well informed on the risks and benefits of treatment options for stable angina.

INDICATIONS FOR ADMISSION AND REFERRAL (78)

Admission is required when the anginal pattern is increasing in frequency or severity or is becoming harder to control. Episodes that are starting to last more than 15 minutes and beginning to occur at rest and with exertion suggest progression to *unstable angina*, with its attendant increase in the risk of acute infarction. Hospitalization may also be of benefit in the setting of exertional symptoms to judge the adequacy of a medical regimen and to check on compliance when a patient with stable angina reports insufficient relief of symptoms. Referral to a cardiologist for consideration of coronary angiography and angioplasty is indicated when maximum medical therapy has failed to control symptoms and when left-main or severe three-vessel disease is suspected. The same is true if tight aortic stenosis is a consideration (see Chapter 33).

THERAPEUTIC RECOMMENDATIONS (80,81)

Evidence to guide the selection of treatment modalities for patients with stable angina suffers from the tendency of investigators to concentrate their efforts on postinfarction populations. A number of recommendations for patients with stable angina are extrapolations from postinfarction studies (e.g., the mortality benefit of beta-blockers and ACE inhibitors in lower-risk patients). More long-term studies using cardiac events and mortality as outcomes are needed to validate these recommendations for anginal patients who have not infarcted. Pending such data, it seems reasonable to extrapolate the medical recommendations to this population, especially because most measures are well tolerated, relatively inexpensive, and safe. To withhold them might risk losing an opportunity to improve outcomes. The extrapolation of revascularization recommendations is another story because the risks associated with interventional therapy are much higher.

A management strategy supported by evidence assigns the patient as follows to initial medical therapy or revascularization on the basis of estimated risk and degree of incapacity as determined by stress testing, echocardiography, and severity of symptoms.

General Measures for All Patients (Including Those Undergoing Revascularization)

- Determine the patient's prognosis and degree of CHD risk by ascertaining the amount of myocardium at risk through stress testing (see Chapter 36), as well as by assessing LV function clinically and through echocardiography or radionuclide scanning, if needed (see Chapters 32 and 36). Use the resultant risk stratification to guide the design of the treatment program.
- Identify and aggressively treat all major CHD risk factors, particularly hypertension (see Chapter 26), hyperlipidemia (LDL cholesterol goal <70 mg/dL; see Chapter 27), smoking (see Chapter 54), and *diabetes* (see Chapter 102).
- Check for and correct any concurrent precipitating or aggravating factors, such as heart failure (see Chapter 32),

severe anemia (see Chapter 82), hyperthyroidism (see Chapter 104), hypoxemia (see Chapter 47), and critical aortic stenosis or hypertrophic cardiomyopathy (see Chapter 33).

■ Screen for and treat psychosocial factors that can adversely affect outcomes, including anxiety (see Chapter 226), depression (see Chapter 227), situational stress, and social isolation.

■ Begin low-dose enteric-coated aspirin (81 mg/d).

■ Begin beta-blockade with a generic formulation of a long-acting cardioselective agent (e.g., atenolol 25 to 50 mg/d or metoprolol 25 mg twice daily); adjust the dose to ensure adequate beta-blockade (heart rate <60 beats/min at rest, <100 beats/min with vigorous exertion). If beta-blockade must be terminated, do so only in a tapering fashion over 1 to 2 weeks; have the patient reduce activity during this time.

■ Begin ACE inhibitor therapy with a generic formulation (e.g., captopril 12.5 mg twice daily; lisinopril 10 mg/d; start with lower doses in the elderly); monitor blood pressure to minimize the risk of inducing postural hypotension; and give priority to ACE inhibition for patients with LV dysfunction or diabetes.

■ Thoroughly review with patient and family the rationale and proper use of therapies; encourage monitoring the response to treatment; and counsel on allowable activity, encourage exercise as tolerated, and help to avoid self-imposed unnecessary limits on activity.

■ Begin a gentle exercise program (e.g., walking 20 minutes three times a week) and a more intensive program for the highly motivated; obtain an exercise stress test first (see Chapter 31).

■ Promptly admit any patient with unstable angina or markedly worsening LV dysfunction and obtain cardiac consultation.

Low-Risk Patients (Mild to Moderate Angina, Normal Ejection Fraction, Small Amount of Myocardium at Risk, Probable Single-Vessel Disease)

■ Begin aspirin, beta-blockade, ACEI therapy, and aggressive treatment of CHD risk factors, especially LDL cholesterol (see prior discussion).

■ Prescribe as needed TNG, 0.4 mg, for the symptomatic relief of anginal episodes; instruct the patient to rest at the time of pain and to take a second and a third TNG if the pain does not resolve within 5 minutes of each TNG dose. Advise maintaining a fresh supply of TNG and discarding any bottle that has been open for more than 6 months or any tablets that fail to cause sublingual burning or head throbbing.

■ Prescribe the prophylactic use of sublingual TNG if angina is predictable and short-term (<30 minutes) protection will suffice (e.g., before carrying bundles, climbing stairs or a hill).

■ If anginal control is not sufficient with the foregoing measures but the patient responds well to TNG, then add a long-acting nitrate to the program (e.g., isosorbide dinitrate, beginning with 5 mg three times a day and advancing slowly over 1 to 2 weeks in increments of 5 mg per dose); dose in an asymmetric fashion (e.g., 8 a.m., 2 p.m., 8 p.m.) to minimize the risk of nitrate tolerance.

■ Consider a trial of long-acting calcium-channel blocker therapy (e.g., long-acting diltiazem 90 to 120 mg/d, amlodipine 5 mg/d) only if the patient continues to be unacceptably symptomatic despite full doses of nitrates and beta-blockers. Use only a long-acting formulation. Monitor LV function and check ECG for conduction defects, especially when used in combination with beta-blocker therapy. With the exception of amlodipine, do not use if there is underlying heart failure or clinically significant conduction-system disease.

■ Consider referral for angiography and possible revascularization only if the patient continues to be unacceptably limited by angina despite full compliance with the foregoing medical regimen plus aggressive treatment of CHD risk factors.

Moderate-Risk Patients (Moderate Angina, Moderate Amount of Myocardium at Risk, Probable Two-Vessel Disease, Normal Ejection Fraction)

■ Implement the full medical regimen (treatment of CHD risk factors, aspirin, beta-blockade, ACEI, with or without nitrates or calcium-channel blockers).

■ If symptoms are severe or exercise tolerance and functional status are impaired despite the implementation of the full medical program, then refer for angiography and consideration of revascularization.

■ If the patient is a candidate for revascularization, assess patient preferences and candidacy for PCI versus CABG (coronary anatomy, LV function, available expertise, willingness to undergo repeat PCI procedure, etc.).

High-Risk Patients (Moderate to Severe Angina; Large Amount of Myocardium at Risk; Suspected Three-Vessel, Left-Main, or Left-Main-Equivalent Disease; Reduced Ejection Fraction)

■ Refer immediately for angiography and consideration of CABG.

■ At the same time, implement aspirin, beta-blockade, ACEI, and aggressive control of CHD risk factors.

■ Recommend CABG for patients found to have left-main, left-main equivalent, or significant (>70% stenosis) three-vessel disease, especially if complicated by LV dysfunction.

A.H.G.

Annotated Bibliography

1. Cohn PF. Silent myocardial ischemia. Ann Intern Med 1988;109:312. (*An excellent succinct review, including a discussion of mechanisms, detection, prognosis, and treatment; 61 references.*)

2. Luchi RJ, Chahine RA, Raizner AE. Coronary artery spasm. Ann Intern Med 1979;91:441. (*An excellent review of pathophysiology and its clinical implications; 118 references.*)

3. Muller JE, Tofler GH, Stone PH. Circadian variation and triggers of onset of acute cardiovascular disease. Circulation 1989;79:733. (*The morning hours are the time of greatest risk.*)

4. Rozanski A, Bairey CN, Krantz DS, et al. Mental stress and the induction of silent myocardial ischemia in patients with coronary artery disease. N Engl J Med 1988;318:1005. (*A controlled study, finding*

that personally relevant stress was as potent an inducer of ischemia as exertion.)

5. Steg PG, Bhatt DL, Wilson PWF, et al. for the REACH Registry Investigators. One-year cardiovascular event rates in outpatients with atherothrombosis. JAMA 2007;297:1197. (*A cohort study involving >66,000 patients, documenting the high risk of significant events.*)

6. Bibbins-Domingo K, Gupta R, Na B, et al. N-terminal fragment of the prohormone brain-type natriuretic peptide (NT-proBNP), cardiovascular events, and mortality in patients with stable coronary heart disease. JAMA 2007;297:169. (*A prospective cohort study, showing that the predictive value of the serum level of this natriuretic peptide persisted even in the absence of diastolic dysfunction.*)

7. Hemingway H, McCallum A, Shipley M, et al. Incidence and prognostic implications of stable angina pectoris among women and men. JAMA 2006;295:1404. (*A prospective cohort study, showing that the implications were similar to those for men.*)

8. Kotler TS, Diamond GA. Exercise thallium-201 scintigraphy in the diagnosis and prognosis of coronary artery disease. Ann Intern Med 1990;113:684. (*Summary of the evidence for a consensus guideline; 193 references.*)

9. Kragelund C, Gronning D, Kober L, et al. N-terminal pro–B-type natriuretic peptide and long-term mortality in stable coronary heart disease. N Engl J Med 2005;352:666. (*A prospective cohort study, finding that serum levels were independently predictive of cardiovascular mortality in ambulatory patients.*)

10. Lee TH, Boucher CA. Noninvasive tests in patients with stable coronary artery disease. N Engl J Med 2001;344:1840. (*An excellent practical review.*)

11. Mark DB, Shaw L, Harrell FE Jr, et al. Prognostic value of a treadmill exercise score in outpatients with suspected coronary artery disease. N Engl J Med 1991;325:849. (*Demonstrates the ability of the electrocardiographic stress test to distinguish high- from low-risk patients.*)

12. Vidula H, Tian Lu, Liu K, et al. Biomarkers of inflammation and thrombosis as predictors of near-term mortality in patients with peripheral arterial disease: a cohort study. Ann Intern Med 2008;148:85. (*Finds that d-dimer, amyloid A, and highly sensitive C-reactive protein levels were predictive of cardiovascular events within 1 year.*)

13. Williams SV, Fihn SD, Gibbons RJ. Guidelines for the management of patients with chronic stable angina: diagnosis and risk stratification. Ann Intern Med 2001;135:530. (*Comprehensive evidence-based consensus guidelines.*)

14. Grobbee DE, Rimm EB, Giovannucci E, et al. Coffee, caffeine, and cardiovascular disease in men. N Engl J Med 1990;323:1026. (*An epidemiologic study of 45,000 men, finding no increase in the risk of coronary disease.*)

15. Nissen SE, Nicholls SJ, Sipahi I, et al. for the ASTEROID Investigators. Effect of very high-intensity statin therapy on regression of atherosclerosis: the ASTEROID Trial. JAMA 2006;295:1556. (*A major cohort study of intensive lipid lowering, demonstrating a reduction in coronary plaque.*)

16. Pitt B, Waters D, Brown WM, et al. Aggressive lipid-lowering therapy compared with angioplasty in stable coronary artery disease. N Engl J Med 1999;341:70. (*Finds that stable anginal patients randomized to high-dose atorvastatin had a 13% rate of ischemic events, compared with a 21% rate for those treated with angioplasty.*)

17. Sullivan MD, LaCroix AZ, Baum C, et al. Functional status in coronary artery disease: a one-year prospective study of the role of anxiety and depression. Am J Med 1997;103:348. (*Shows that anxiety and depression were important determinants of functional status.*)

18. Sytkowski PA, Kannel WB, D'Agostino RB. Changes in risk factors and the decline in mortality from cardiovascular disease: the Framingham Study. N Engl J Med 1990;322:1635. (*Documents a 40% decline in mortality, most of which was attributed to risk factor control.*)

19. Burris JF. β-Blockers, dyslipidemia, and coronary disease. Arch Intern Med 1993;153:2085. (*Addresses the question of adverse effect; finds no proof.*)

20. Bhatt AB, Stone PH. Current strategies for the management of angina in patients with stable coronary disease. Curr Opin Cardiol 2006;21:492. (*A summary of the state of the art.*)

21. DeCesare N, Bartorelli A, Fabbiocchi F, et al. Superior efficacy of propranolol versus nifedipine in double-component angina, as related to different influences on coronary vasomotility. Am J Med 1989;87:15. (*Finds that propranolol produced no important vasoconstriction, whereas nifedipine's effect was variable, ranging from vasodilation to vasoconstriction.*)

22. Dimsdale JE, Newton RP, Joist T. Neuropsychological side effects of beta-blockers. Arch Intern Med 1989;149:514. (*A review of 55 studies; concludes that there is little evidence for a difference in central nervous system effects between the lipophilic and lipophobic preparations.*)

23. Gottlieb SS, McCarter RJ, Vogel RA. Effect of beta-blockade on mortality among high-risk and low-risk patients after myocardial infarction. N Engl J Med 1998;339:489. (*A large-scale observational study of >200,000 patients, suggesting that high-risk patients benefit as much as, if not more than, low-risk patients.*)

24. Houston MC, Hodge R. Beta-adrenergic blocker withdrawal syndromes in hypertension and other cardiovascular diseases. Am Heart J 1988;116:515. (*Documents that withdrawal is usually mild, but of 338 patients developing withdrawal, 15 infarcted and 8 died.*)

25. Kendall MJ, Lynch KP, Hjalmarson A, et al. Beta-blockers and sudden cardiac death. Ann Intern Med 1995;123:358. (*A systematic review documenting the survival benefit of beta-blockade.*)

26. Ko DT, Hebert PR, Coffey CS, et al. Beta-blocker therapy and symptoms of depression, fatigue, and sexual dysfunction. JAMA 2002;288:351. (*A meta-analysis of randomized, controlled trials [RCTs], finding no support for the conventional view of significant impairment with the use of these agents; only small increases in risks of fatigue and sexual dysfunction were noted.*)

27. Sipahi I, Tuzcu M, Wolski KE, et al. β-Blockers and progression of coronary atherosclerosis: pooled analysis of 4 intravascular ultrasonography trials. Ann Intern Med 2007;147:10. (*A post hoc analysis of four major trials, finding that significant plaque regression was associated with beta-blocker use.*)

28. Skinner MH, Futterman A, Morrissette D, et al. Atenolol compared with nifedipine: effect on cognitive function and mood in elderly hypertensive patients. Ann Intern Med 1992;116:615. (*One of the few double-blinded, crossover, RCT studies on the central nervous system effects of a beta-blocker; no adverse effect was found on mood or cognitive function.*)

29. The Norwegian Multicenter Study Group. Timolol-induced reduction in mortality and reinfarction in patients surviving acute myocardial infarction. N Engl J Med 1981;304:801. (*A landmark trial, finding a 45% reduction in sudden death among post–myocardial infarction [MI] patients attributable to beta-blockade.*)

30. Viscoli CM, Horwitz RI, Singer BH. Beta-blockers after myocardial infarction: influence of first-year clinical course on long-term effectiveness. Ann Intern Med 1993;118:99. (*Finds that the benefit appears to be greatest in patients at greatest risk.*)

31. Francis GS. ACE inhibition in cardiovascular disease. N Engl J Med 2000;342:201. (*An editorial summarizing the mechanisms of action and clinical studies indicating a major role for angiotensin-converting-enzyme inhibitor use in coronary heart disease [CHD].*)

32. Fox KM. European Trial on Reduction of Cardiac Events with Perindopril in Stable Coronary Artery Disease Investigators. Efficacy of perindopril in reduction of cardiovascular events among patients with stable coronary artery disease: randomized, double-blind, placebo-controlled, multicentre trial (the EUROPA study). Lancet 2003;362:782. (*A major study, finding survival benefit in this group of moderate-risk patients; however, >60% had prior MI.*)

33. Yusuf S, Sleight P, Pogue J, et al. for The Heart Outcomes Prevention Evaluation (HOPE) Study Investigators. Effects of an angiotensin-converting-enzyme inhibitor, ramipril, on death from cardiovascular causes, myocardial infarction, and stroke in high-risk patients. N Engl J Med 2000;342:145. (*The oft-cited Heart Outcomes Prevention Evaluation [HOPE] study, a major RCT involving high-risk CHD patients with normal left ventricular function; found significant [20% to 30%] reductions in CHD morbidity and mortality.*)

34. The PEACE Trial Investigators. Angiotensin-converting-enzyme inhibition in stable coronary artery disease. N Engl J Med 2004;351:2058. (*A placebo-controlled RCT in persons with normal or minimally reduced left ventricular function and less risk than those in the HOPE study; failed to show improvement in outcomes.*)

35. Anand SS, Yusuf S. Oral anticoagulant therapy in patients with coronary artery disease: a meta-analysis. JAMA 1999;282:2058. (*Finds that high- and moderate-intensity anticoagulation reduces the rates of infarction and stroke to the same degree as aspirin but with increased bleeding risk.*)

36. Antithrombotic Trialists' Collaboration. Collaborative meta-analysis of randomised trials of antiplatelet therapy for prevention of death, myocardial infarction, and stroke in high risk patients. BMJ 2002;324:71. (*Finds benefit for aspirin in this high-risk group.*)

37. Chen W-H, Cheng X, Lee P-Y, et al. Aspirin resistance and adverse clinical events in patients with coronary artery disease. Am J Med 2007;120:631. (*Finds evidence for the existence of the phenomenon and its effect on outcomes.*)

38. Ridker PM, Manson JE, Gaziano JM, et al. Low-dose aspirin therapy for chronic stable angina: a randomized, placebo-controlled clinical trial. Ann Intern Med 1991;114:835. (*The original report from the Physicians' Health Study, showing that the risk of a first infarction was reduced by 87%; survival did not improve significantly, and the risk of stroke trended upward.*)

39. Willard JE, Lange RA, Hillis LD. Use of aspirin in ischemic heart disease. N Engl J Med 1992;327:175. (*A comprehensive review; 86 references.*)

40. Elkayam U. Tolerance to organic nitrates: evidence, mechanisms, clinical relevance, and strategies for prevention. Ann Intern Med 1991;114:667. (*Among the best reviews of nitrate tolerance; 134 references.*)

41. Parker JD, Parker JO. Nitrate therapy for stable angina pectoris. N Engl J Med 1998;338:520. (*A review by leading experts on nitrate use; 97 references.*)

42. Parker JO, Amies MH, Hawkinson RW, et al. Intermittent transdermal nitroglycerine therapy in angina pectoris: clinically effective without tolerance or rebound: Minitran Efficacy Study Group. Circulation 1995;91:1368. (*Data on the importance of a patch-free period.*)

43. Parker JO, Farrell B, Lahey KA, et al. Effect of intervals between doses on the development of tolerance to isosorbide dinitrate. N Engl J Med

1987;316:1440. (*Placebo-controlled RCT in patients with chronic stable angina; an onset of tolerance was found with around-the-clock dosing.*)

44. Parker JO, Van Koughnett KA, Farrell B. Nitroglycerin lingual spray: clinical efficacy and dose–response relation. Am J Cardiol 1986;57:1. (*Finds that efficacy and dosing were nearly identical to those of sublingual nitroglycerin.*)

45. Silber S, Vogler AC, Krause KH, et al. Induction and circumvention of nitrate tolerance applying different dosage intervals. Am J Med 1987;83:860. (*Finds that an eccentric schedule that allowed 10 to 12 hours of washout was most effective.*)

46. Abernethy DR, Schwartz JB. Calcium-antagonist drugs. N Engl J Med 1999;341:1447. (*A detailed review, including use in coronary disease; 102 references.*)

47. Packer M. Combined beta-adrenergic and calcium-entry blockade in angina pectoris. N Engl J Med 1989;320:709. (*A critical review of studies on this approach to anginal treatment, finding that the data support its use only in patients with preserved left ventricular function who fail full doses of single-agent therapy; 128 references.*)

48. Packer M, O'Connor CM, Ghali JK, et al. Effect of amlodipine on morbidity and mortality in severe chronic heart failure. N Engl J Med 1996;334:1107. (*A randomized, multicenter, controlled trial of 1,153 patients, finding no increase in the risk of cardiovascular morbidity or mortality with amlodipine use in patients with severe heart failure.*)

49. The Multicenter Diltiazem Postinfarction Trial Research Group. The effect of diltiazem on mortality and reinfarction after myocardial infarction. N Engl J Med 1988;319:385. (*A multicenter RCT, finding improved survival and lower rates of infarction in patients with normal left ventricular function but reduced survival and increased rates of infarction in those with reduced ejection fraction.*)

50. Yusuf S. Calcium antagonists in coronary artery disease and hypertension: time for reevaluation? Circulation 1995;92:1079. (*A retrospective review raising concern about safety.*)

51. Boden WE, O'Rourke RA, Teo KK, et al., for the Courage Trial Research Group. Optimal medical therapy with or without PCI for stable coronary disease. N Engl J Med 2007;356:2503. (*A major RCT, finding no reduction in death, MI, or other cardiovascular events with the initial addition of percutaneous coronary intervention[PCI] to optimal medical therapy.*)

52. Bravata DM, Dienger AL, McDonald KM, et al. Systematic review: the comparative effectiveness of percutaneous coronary interventions and coronary artery bypass graft surgery. Ann Intern Med 2007;147:703. (*A meta-analysis of 23 RCTs of patients with intermediate-severity coronary disease; early procedurally related death rates were similar, as were 5-year survival rates; coronary artery bypass graft [CABG] surgery provided better pain relief and fewer repeat revascularizations; surgery was associated with more periprocedural complications.*)

53. Bucher HC, Hangstler P, Schindler C, et al. Percutaneous transluminal coronary angioplasty versus medical treatment for non-acute coronary heart disease: meta-analysis of randomized controlled trials. BMJ 2000;321:73. (*Finds that angioplasty was superior for symptom relief.*)

54. Cameron A, Davis KB, Green G, et al. Coronary bypass surgery with internal-thoracic-artery grafts—effects on survival over a 15-year period. N Engl J Med 1996;334:216. (*Establishes a very low rate of graft failure and the importance of the use of this approach in CABG surgery.*)

55. CASS Principal Investigators. Myocardial infarction and mortality in the Coronary Artery Surgery Study (CASS) randomized trial. N Engl J Med 1984;310:750. (*One of the landmark randomized trials establishing the efficacy of and indications for coronary artery bypass.*)

56. van Dijk D, Spoor M, Hijman R, et al. for the Octopus Study Group. Cognitive and cardiac outcomes 5 years after off-pump vs on-pump coronary artery bypass graft surgery. JAMA 2007; 297: 701. (*Presents long-term follow-up data from an RCT involving low-risk patients, finding no differences in outcomes at 5 years.*)

57. Eisenstein EL, Anstrom KJ, Kong DF, et al. Clopidogrel use and long-term clinical outcomes after drug-eluting stent implantation. JAMA 2007;297:159. (*An observational study of a large Duke cohort, finding that extended use of clopidogrel was associated with better prognosis, suggesting the increased risk of clotting with drug-eluting stents.*)

58. Erbel R, Haude M, Hopp HW, et al. Coronary-artery stenting compared with balloon angioplasty for restenosis after initial balloon angioplasty. N Engl J Med 1998;339:1672. (*Finds that stenting reduced the rate of restenosis by about 40% and improved event-free survival at 250 days by about 12% but at a cost of increasing the rate of subacute thrombosis by 3.9%.*)

59. Gersh BJ, Kronmal RA, Schaff HV, et al. Comparison of coronary artery bypass surgery and medical therapy in patients 65 years of age or older. N Engl J Med 1985;313:217. (*A subgroup analysis of the Coronary Artery Surgery Study, demonstrating benefit in the elderly.*)

60. Guton RA. Coronary artery bypass is superior to drug-eluting stents in multivessel coronary disease. Ann Thoracic Surg. 2006;81:1949. (*A good summary of the evidence, with a slant toward the surgical perspective.*)

61. Hannan EL, Racz MJ, Walford G, et al. Long-term outcomes of coronary-artery bypass grafting versus stent implantation. N Engl J Med 2005;352:2174. (*A large cohort study, finding that for patients with two or more diseased vessels, CABG achieved the better long-term survival.*)

62. Hannan EL, Hasdai D, Lerman A, et al. Medical therapy after successful percutaneous coronary angioplasty. Ann Intern Med 1999;130:108. (*A retrospective cohort study, showing that the use of antianginal medication does not decrease after successful angioplasty.*)

63. Herman HC. Prevention of cardiovascular events after percutaneous coronary intervention. N Engl J Med 2004;350:2708. (*An editorial reviewing what works and what does not.*)

64. Hlatky MA, Boothroyd DB, Melsop KA, et al. Medical costs and quality of life 10 to 12 years after randomization to angioplasty or bypass surgery for multivessel coronary artery disease. Circulation 2004;110:1960. (*A long-term follow-up data, finding that CABG was cost-effective as compared with PCI for multivessel disease.*)

65. Hochman JS, Steg PG. Does preventive PCI work? N Engl J Med 2007;356:1572. (*An editorial summarizing the evidence and concluding that the answer is no for initial therapy of patients with stable angina.*)

66. Hodson JM, Stone GW, Lincoff M, et al. Society for Cardiovascular Angiography and Interventions. Late stent thrombosis: consideration and practical advice for the use of drug-eluting stents: a report from the Society for Cardiovascular Angiography and Interventions Drug-Eluting Task Force. Catheter Cardiovasc Interv 2007;69:327. (*Recommends long-term antiplatelet therapy for patients receiving coated stents.*)

67. Jeremias A, Kirtan A. Balancing efficacy and safety of drug-eluting stents in patients undergoing percutaneous coronary intervention. Ann Intern Med 2008;148:234. (*A very thoughtful review of the evidence, finding that benefits outweigh harms, but emphasizing the need for long-term antiplatelet therapy.*)

68. Machecourt J, Danchin N, Lablanche JM, et al. Risk factors for stent thrombosis after implantation of sirolimus-eluting stents in diabetic and nondiabetic patients: the EVASTENT Matched-Cohort Registry. J Am Coll Cardiol 2007;50:501. (*Finds no survival advantage and a 1- year thrombosis rate of 4.3%.*)

69. McFalls EO, Ward HB, Moritz TE, et al. Coronary-artery revascularization before elective major vascular surgery. N Engl J Med 2004;351:2975. (*RCT, showing no benefit in long-term outcomes.*)

70. Newman MF, Kirchner JL, Phillips-Bute B, et al. Longitudinal assessment of neurocognitive function after coronary-artery bypass surgery. N Engl J Med 2001;344:395. (*A prospective cohort study, finding a high rate of cognitive decline, both early and late; see also the accompanying editorial, Coronary-artery bypass surgery and the brain, N Engl J Med 2001;344:451.*)

71. Serruys PW, Unger F, Sousa JE, et al. Comparison of coronary-artery bypass surgery and stenting for the treatment of multivessel disease. N Engl J Med 2001;344:1117. (*RCT, finding that at 1 year, stenting for multivessel disease was associated with the same risks of cardiovascular morbidity and mortality as CABG, but that there was a greater need for repeated revascularization.*)

72. Smith PK, Califf RM, Tuttle RH, et al. Selection of surgical or percutaneous coronary intervention provides differential longevity benefits. Ann Thoracic Surg 2006;82:1420. (*A useful review of outcomes data, with a slant toward surgery.*)

73. Solomon AJ, Gersh BJ. Management of chronic stable angina: medical therapy, percutaneous transluminal coronary angioplasty, and coronary artery bypass graft surgery. Lessons from the randomized trials. Ann Intern Med 1998;128:216. (*A systematic review, finding that in low-risk patients, medical therapy was the preferred initial modality; in moderate-risk patients, revascularization was worth consideration; and in high-risk patients, CABG surgery was best.*)

74. Stone GW, Ellis SG, Cannon L, et al for the TAXUS Investigators. Comparison of a polymer-based, paclitaxel-eluting stent with a bare metal stent in patients with complex coronary artery disease. JAMA 2005;294:1215. (*RCT, finding that short-term rates of restenosis were better with coated stents in this population, but that rates of myocardial infarction and cardiac death were no different from those associated with the use of uncoated stents.*)

75. Varhaskas E. Twelve-year follow-up of survival in the randomized European coronary surgery study. N Engl J Med 1988;319:332. (*A late follow-up report of one of the three major randomized studies of bypass surgery, confirming survival benefit for patients with left-main, three-vessel, and "left-main equivalent" disease.*)

76. Veterans Administration Coronary Artery Bypass Surgery Cooperative Study Group. Eleven-year survival in the Veterans Administration randomized trial of coronary bypass surgery for stable angina. N Engl J Med 1984;311:1333. (*A landmark study, finding that only patients with high-risk disease demonstrated a benefit from surgery at 11 years of follow-up.*)

77. Knudtson ML, Wyse DG, Galbraith PD, et al. Chelation therapy for ischemic heart disease: a randomized controlled trial. JAMA 2002;287:481. (*Finds that this approach offers no benefit.*)

78. Peterson ED, Shaw LK, DeLong ER, et al. Racial variation in the use of coronary-revascularization procedures. N Engl J Med 1997;336:480. (*The rate of use was low among blacks, even after adjusting for clinical indications.*)

79. Whittle J, Conigliaro J, Good CB, et al. Do patient preferences contribute to racial differences in cardiovascular procedure use? J Gen Intern Med

1997;12:267. (*Shows that the answer was maybe, but not as much as familiarity with the procedure.*)

80. Gibbons RJ, Abrams J, Chatterjee K, et al. ACC/AHA 2002 guideline update for the management of patients with chronic stable angina—summary article: a report of the American College of Cardiology/American Heart Association Task Force on Practice Guidelines (Committee on the Management of Patients with Chronic Stable Angina). 2002. J Am Coll Cardiol 2003;41:159.

(*Evidence-based consensus guidelines and accompanying exhaustive review; >1,000 references.*)

81. Snow V, Fihn Stephen SD, Gibbons RJ, et al. Primary care management of chronic stable angina and asymptomatic suspected or known coronary artery disease: a clinical practice guideline from the American College of Physicians. Ann Intern Med 2004;141:562. (*Thoughtful, evidence-based consensus guidelines.*)

CHAPTER 31 ■ CARDIOVASCULAR REHABILITATION AND SECONDARY PREVENTION OF CORONARY HEART DISEASE

The risks of myocardial infarction (MI) and death from coronary heart disease (CHD) can be as high as 5%/yr to 10%/yr. When these are added to the disease's physical and psychological tolls, the importance of a comprehensive program of cardiac rehabilitation and secondary prevention becomes readily evident. The goals of such a program include (a) improvement of functional capacity and quality of life, (b) reduction in the risks of future cardiac events (e.g., MI, cardiac arrest, need for revascularization), and (c) prolongation of survival. The results of major long-term, randomized, controlled trials indicate that these goals can be achieved cost-effectively through the concerted application of preventive measures. Some components of the program focus on lifestyle changes, others include medical therapies and revascularization procedures; the control of atherosclerotic risk factors is paramount. Together, they make for an effective program that can save lives and improve quality of life. Despite substantial evidence for efficacy, there is a high prevalence of failure to implement these measures, particularly for patients at highest risk.

Although some elements of the secondary prevention program can be carried out by others, the primary physician has a major responsibility for program design, coordination, and compliance. One needs to know what interventions are effective and how to tailor a secondary prevention program to the needs and capabilities of the individual patient. On receiving a diagnosis of coronary artery disease or experiencing a myocardial infarction, most patients become highly motivated to live a healthier lifestyle, which provides an excellent opportunity to effect important changes in diet and exercise as part of a comprehensive program of risk reduction through secondary prevention.

EXERCISE (1–16)

Lifestyle modification is a key component of the comprehensive rehabilitation and secondary prevention program. Along with dietary modification (see later discussion), exercise is an essential element of the lifestyle-modification agenda and the centerpiece of rehabilitation programs.

Outcomes

Effects on Morbidity, Mortality, and Quality of Life

Cardiac rehabilitation programs for secondary prevention reduce all-cause mortality, cardiovascular mortality, and fatal reinfarction by 20% to 25%. The best effect is on sudden death, which declines by greater than 35%. Quality of life also increases as patients regain confidence and develop a better sense of physical well-being. Benefits accrue to the elderly as well as to younger patients. Because most data derive from comprehensive exercise rehabilitation programs that also incorporate such efforts as smoking cessation, dietary modification, and stress reduction, it is difficult to know the precise proportion of benefit due to exercise alone, but the training effect achieved contributes markedly to quality of life, and there are improvements in many important physiologic and biochemical parameters (see later discussion). Such programs are cost-effective, often achieving considerable savings through reductions in rates of rehospitalization, revascularization, length of stay, charges per hospitalization, and lost productivity.

Mechanisms of Benefit from Exercise

Increases in cardiac stroke volume and skeletal muscle oxygen extraction constitute a *training effect*. The trained subject is able to deliver a given quantity of oxygenated blood to the peripheral tissues at a lower heart rate and at lower systolic pressure. The decline in rate–pressure product (heart rate × systolic arterial pressure) corresponds to a reduction in *myocardial oxygen demand* for a particular level of exercise, allowing the trained patient to achieve a higher level of activity before demand outpaces blood supply.

Myocardial perfusion has been observed to increase by 25% to 50%, presumably through the *vasodilation of coronary arteries* and improvement of *collateral blood flow* to ischemic zones. There is an 8% to 25% rise in the concentration of *high-density-lipoprotein cholesterol*, a 22% reduction in *triglycerides*, improved *glycemic control* in diabetes, increase in *fibrinolytic response* to occlusive stimuli, and an increase in the *myocardial ventricular fibrillatory threshold*, rendering it less vulnerable.

Candidates, Goals, and Program Phases

Candidates

All persons with established coronary disease are candidates for a program of exercise and lifestyle modification. Those recovering from myocardial infarction often get the most attention and referrals to formal programs, but significant functional and survival benefits accrue to other persons with CHD, including those with chronic stable angina (see Chapter 30) and persons who have recently undergone revascularization. Benefits are not restricted to younger patients; the elderly also achieve reductions in cardiac morbidity and mortality.

Goals

Goals differ according to the clinical circumstances. For the post–myocardial infarction patient, prevention of physical deconditioning and psychological disability is the immediate priority, in addition to appreciation for the importance of vigorously controlling CHD risk factors. Shortly after discharge, the goal turns toward restoring former physical capacity, followed later by achieving an enhanced level of performance and lifelong adherence to good health habits. The ultimate goals for all CHD patients are improved functional capacity and quality of life, reduced risks of future cardiac events (e.g., infarction, cardiac arrest, need for revascularization), and prolonged survival.

Phase I: Early Rehabilitation

This phase begins *during hospitalization* for an acute coronary event. Physical deconditioning is avoided by initiating a program of low-level activity as soon as possible after clinical stability has been achieved (usually by day 3 post-MI or as soon as the patient who has undergone revascularization can walk). Before hospital discharge, most patients should be observed by their physician while climbing a *flight of stairs*. This will provide confidence that such tasks can be performed safely and will often uncover specific questions about what should and should not be done during the first weeks at home. Educational efforts emphasize risk-factor control (see later discussion).

Submaximal exercise testing (to a level of 5 metabolic equivalents [METs]) before hospital discharge can provide important prognostic information and help to restore patient confidence. A negative test predicts an excellent prognosis during the subsequent year, whereas a positive one with or without anginal symptoms indicates a poorer outcome and the need for consideration of revascularization. Serious ventricular dysrhythmias requiring attention may also be uncovered. Radionuclide scintigraphy or echocardiography is required for the stress test if the resting electrocardiogram is abnormal (see Chapter 36).

Phase II: Early Convalescence

This phase encompasses the time from hospital discharge to 3 to 6 weeks later. The prescribed activity level remains relatively low because high-level physical activity risks infarct expansion or possible ventricular aneurysm formation. Exercise intensity is regulated by monitoring the peak heart rate, which should not exceed the level achieved during the predischarge submaximal exercise test. If the predischarge exercise test discloses ischemic electrocardiographic changes, anginal symptoms, or ventricular dysrhythmias, then the heart rate during exercise training sessions should be maintained below the heart rate at which any of these pathologic events was observed. The exercise training modalities used during phase II, as in phase I, usually consist of *walking* and *stationary bicycling*. The process of educating the patient and the family about coronary risk factors continues and is reinforced (see later discussion).

Phase III: Late Convalescence/Physical Training

The program intensifies to increase the patient's level of physical conditioning. A *maximal exercise stress test* is performed at 3 to 6 weeks, quantifying the patient's heart rate and blood pressure responses to exercise and screening tests for latent myocardial ischemia and ventricular dysrhythmias. The exercise training modalities are broadened to establish a balanced exercise program of long-term patient appeal. Upper extremity conditioning may be added, especially in patients for whom upper extremity work is important to daily activity.

During phase III, efforts to modify risk factors continue and intensify. These include *dietary interventions* to correct lipid abnormalities and achieve ideal body weight (see later discussion and Chapters 27 and 233). *Hypertension control* (see Chapter 26) and *smoking cessation* (see Chapter 54) are critically important. *Management of psychological stress* and *depression* should also be addressed (see Chapters 226 and Chapters 227), particularly as the patient returns to work. A well-balanced cardiac rehabilitation program attends to all of these factors and should involve the patient's family as well.

Phase IV: Maintenance/Follow-Up

The goal is to encourage lifelong adherence to the healthy habits established during phase III. Follow-up visits at 6- to 12-month intervals are important. Blood pressure and pulse measurement, serum lipid levels, and even repeat maximal exercise tolerance tests can provide useful feedback to the patient and indicate areas that may require lifestyle changes to minimize coronary risk.

Program Design, Safety, and Compliance

Program Design: How Much and What Type of Exercise?

The *classic assumption* is that one must achieve a physiologic training effect to obtain health benefits; such a training effect requires *aerobic (endurance) exercise* (running, jogging, fast walking, cycling, rowing, cross-country skiing, swimming) performed at least *four times a week* for at least *30 minutes a session*, resulting in a heart rate of 70% to 85% of a predicted maximum. However, significant reductions in coronary risk do not require the attainment of maximum cardiopulmonary fitness. Moderate degrees of exercise may provide nearly equivalent results. Persons with low baseline levels of activity demonstrate the greatest improvement in outcomes with exercise training, even if they exercise with only moderate intensity (e.g., walking 3 to 4 miles/hr). Epidemiologic data suggest that simple informal exercise carried out as part of everyday life (e.g., walking, stair climbing, working in the yard) confers survival benefit. The current consensus recommendation for the inactive person is to *accumulate a total of 30 minutes* of moderate exertion over the course of the day rather than to put in 30 minutes of exercise at a single session.

The *traditional approach* to determining the proper intensity of exercise for a cardiac rehabilitation program is to *calculate 70% to 85% of a measured maximal heart rate* (usually as determined by exercise stress test using the form of exercise anticipated, e.g., treadmill testing for a walking/jogging program, bicycle ergometer testing for a cycling program). This exercise intensity translates to 60% to 80% of maximal oxygen consumption. Patients taking beta-blocker therapy require a formal graded exercise test under the influence of a beta-blocker to establish their proper intensity of exercise.

The *current consensus* regarding the approach to exercise is shifting from an emphasis on maximizing intensity to maximizing compliance. For previously inactive patients, this translates into a program of a *moderate degree of exercise*, usually prescribed as starting with *walking at a rate of 3 to 4 miles/hr* for 30 minutes each day. This more practical and sustainable approach to exercise training is designed to increase long-term compliance and extend participation in exercise programs beyond the meager 25% who currently engage in them for cardiac rehabilitation.

Program Safety

Rates of adverse coronary events are very low in supervised programs in post-MI patients. The reported rates for cardiac arrest and fatal myocardial infarction are 1 per 112,000 and 1 per 294,000 patient-hours, respectively. Home programs supplemented by occasional institutional visits and regular nurse follow-up can also be carried out safely, provided there is careful patient selection (e.g., no ischemia or dysrhythmias on stress testing, good functional capacity, frequent exercising, good reliability). Those at greatest risk, requiring close supervision, are persons who exercise infrequently and manifest poor functional capacity at baseline.

Exercise in unsupervised settings is associated with a small transient increase in the risk of sudden death during moderate to vigorous exercise, which is ameliorated by habitual exercise. In the Nurses' Health Study (which included women with prior MI), the rate of exercise-related sudden death was extremely low (1 per 36.5 million hours of exertion); the rate among men in the Physicians' Health Study was 19 times higher (1 per 1.5 million episodes of exercise).

Improving Compliance

It is estimated that only one fourth of CHD patients who would benefit from a well-designed exercise/rehabilitation program actually take part in one. Part of the reason is that many programs are institutionally based out of concern for safety. The increasing appreciation for the importance of maximizing patient compliance and the established safety of home programs for properly selected and supervised candidates have encouraged the use of home-based programs, which should facilitate participation. Physician enthusiasm, the provision of close supervision, and the adoption of a moderate exercise program rather than one that stresses more intensive exertion all help the patient to get started and continue. Most important to compliance is the design of a program that the patient likes to do and finds doable (see Chapter 18).

RISK-FACTOR REDUCTION
(4,17–57)

Aggressive risk-factor reduction is essential to a comprehensive program of secondary prevention. Significant reductions in cardiovascular morbidity and mortality are achievable. The magnitude of improvement in outcomes can be as large as or larger than interventions for the primary prevention of coronary disease.

Treating Established Risk Factors

The effective treatment of *hypertension* (systolic pressure <140 mm Hg; see Chapter 26), *hypercholesterolemia* (low-density-lipoprotein [LDL] cholesterol <70 mg/dL; see Chapter 27), and *smoking* (see Chapter 54) can each reduce cardiovascular morbidity and mortality significantly (by as much as 50%) in patients who have suffered myocardial infarction. With full cessation of smoking among post-MI patients, the risk of a recurrent coronary event falls to that of nonsmokers after 3 years. The treatment of *obesity* (see Chapter 233) and glycemic control in *diabetes* (see Chapter 102) are critical to the effective control of key CHD risk factors (e.g., lipids, blood pressure, hyperinsulinism) and may also have a direct effect on outcomes. The identification and treatment of underlying *chronic renal dysfunction* and *depression* are often overlooked.

Intensive Lipid Lowering

With aggressive lipid lowering (e.g., atorvastatin, 80 mg/d, to lower LDL cholesterol to <70 mg/dL), atherosclerotic plaque progression slows or halts and, in about 25% of cases, plaque regresses. Such intensive statin therapy significantly reduces the risk of new cardiovascular events (although no reduction in deaths has been noted) without increasing noncardiac risk (see Chapter 27); it also reduces stroke risk by 20% in persons with carotid disease (see Chapter 171).

Intensive Glycemic Control

Standard glycemic control in diabetes (hemoglobin A1c <7.0%) reduces microvascular risk and in some instances has been shown to reduce cardiovascular risk. More-intensive glycemic control (hemoglobin A1c <6.0% to 6.5%) shows promise for achieving enhanced reductions in macrovascular and microvascular outcomes, especially in high-risk persons such as those with a history of MI, but more study is required before it can be routinely recommended, because risk reduction has not been uniformly observed (in one study, risk actually increased). Of note, *rosiglitazone* use (which is popular in type 2 diabetes for reducing insulin resistance) has been associated with a significantly increased risk of MI and should probably be used very reservedly if at all in the treatment of diabetic post-MI patients.

Attention to Kidney Disease

Chronic renal dysfunction is a powerful determinant of cardiovascular complications and death, especially in post-MI patients. The risk correlates strongly with *glomerular filtration rate* (GFR); once it falls to less than 60 mL/min, the risk rises significantly. Even mild to moderate renal insufficiency confers significant risk. The risk is independent of other CHD risk factors. The early detection and treatment of renal dysfunction (see Chapter 142) hold considerable promise for improving CHD outcomes, yet such measures are often overlooked.

Concerted efforts to improve early detection of renal dysfunction are being implemented nationally. Many laboratories now routinely calculate and report GFR along with every serum *creatinine* determination. *Urine microalbumin* determinations are readily available and provide another means of early detection. Renal assessment in the elderly is especially important because of heightened CHD risk; however, advancing age and loss of muscle mass may reduce the sensitivity of creatinine-based GFR determinations. Serum measurement of *cystatin C* concentration (a circulating cysteine protease inhibitor freely filtered by the glomerulus) provides a promising alternative means of determining renal function and cardiovascular risk in the elderly; it is not affected by age, gender, or muscle mass, which reduce the sensitivity of serum creatinine–based GFR determinations in older patients.

Improved detection should facilitate more timely treatment. Observational studies of post-MI patients with renal dysfunction find inappropriately low prescribing rates for therapies of proven efficacy (e.g., angiotensin-converting-enzyme [ACE] inhibitors, beta-blockers, antiplatelet agents; see later discussion), suggesting ignorance of renal dysfunction's significance or an unnecessarily nihilistic approach to management. Even in post-MI patients with chronic kidney disease (in which there may be little that is renally reversible), attention to the preservation of existing kidney function and aggressive treatment of other major CHD risk factors holds considerable promise for improving cardiovascular outcomes.

Anxiety and Depression

Anxiety and situational stress play important roles in secondary prevention; stress management programs can help to reduce the number of cardiac events (see Appendix 226.1). *Depression* increases the risk of adverse CHD events in persons with coronary disease, and CHD events can precipitate or worsen depression, yet the majority of post-MI patients with depression go undetected and untreated. The use of semiselective serotonin reuptake inhibitor (SSRI) antidepressants is safe and effective for the treatment of major depression in persons with CHD; moreover, their use in the acute hospital setting has been found to reduce rates of ischemia and heart failure (at the cost of a small increase in risk of bleeding when taken in the setting of heparin/antiplatelet therapy). SSRIs are preferred in CHD over tricyclic antidepressants because of the arrhythmic potential of the latter (see Chapter 227). SSRI therapy can also be also useful for its anxiolytic effects (see Chapter 226). Referral for interpersonal psychotherapy appears to be no better than standard comprehensive care by one's personal physician.

Risk-Factor Reductions of Potential Benefit

There is considerable interest in treating some of the more recently discovered independent risk factors for CHD, including elevations in *homocysteine* and *C-reactive protein*.

Homocysteine

Excess levels of homocysteine may be injurious to vascular endothelium. Epidemiologic data indicate a dose-dependent association between plasma homocysteine and the risk of cardiovascular disease. The association appears to be independent of other cardiovascular risk factors and was initially believed to account for a substantial percentage of "idiopathic" cases, triggering enthusiastic efforts to lower homocysteine by prescribing folate and B-vitamin supplements. Subsequent studies suggest a more modest contribution to risk and fail to demonstrate a significant cardiovascular benefit from reducing elevations of the purported risk factor; in some instances, vitamin supplementation was paradoxically associated with an increased risk.

Measurement of Plasma Homocysteine. Homocysteine determinations are now widely available; accuracy is facilitated by fasting, and sensitivity is enhanced by methionine loading, which stresses the involved metabolic pathways.

Lowering Homocysteine Levels. Vitamin supplementation effectively lowers plasma homocysteine. Folic acid supplementation (0.4 to 0.8 mg/d) with or without vitamins B_6 (25 to 50 mg/d) and B_{12} (0.5 mg/d) lowers homocysteine levels by nearly 25% in 2 to 6 weeks, even in persons who are not deficient in these vitamins. The higher the pretreatment homocysteine level and the lower the folate stores, the greater is the reduction in homocysteine.

Impact on Cardiovascular Outcomes. Despite the enthusiasm that accompanied the discovery of an association between homocysteine levels and cardiovascular risk and the availability of practical means of measuring and lowering homocysteine, proof of benefit remains elusive, and some concern has emerged about possible harm from the use of folate and B-vitamin supplements. In randomized trials of homocysteine-lowering therapy in postangioplasty patients, rates of restenosis have actually increased.

Similarly, the lowering of homocysteine in post-MI patients by vitamin supplementation failed to reduce cardiovascular risk in a large-scale, placebo-controlled, randomized trial that found a trend toward an increase in adverse cardiovascular events. In another major randomized, controlled trial of vitamin supplementation therapy, no significant reduction in risk was found in persons with diabetes or known vascular disease despite the significant lowering of homocysteine.

There has been a view that vitamin supplementation therapy to lower homocysteine is of low risk, simple, inexpensive, potentially helpful, and therefore worth prescribing, especially in high-risk persons. However, with data emerging from large-scale, well-designed studies failing to confirm this view and even suggesting potential harm, it might be best to hold off recommending such treatment in persons with CHD and to withdraw it from the large number of persons already prescribed the program of folate and vitamins B_6 and B_{12}. More study is clearly needed to address the questions of lack of efficacy and potential harm before vitamin supplementation can be recommended for lowering homocysteine in patients with CHD.

C-Reactive Protein

C-reactive protein (CRP) is an acute-phase reactant that increases in the setting of inflammation. It activates both complement and endothelial cells. Recent interest in atherosclerosis as an inflammatory process has drawn attention to CRP as a possible marker/risk factor for CHD events. Initial observations suggested that CRP was a powerful independent predictor of CHD events, with an association similar to that for LDL cholesterol; subsequent studies found the association to be more moderate. Nonetheless, the relationship between CRP elevations and cardiovascular events in persons with CHD have led some to speculate that lowering CRP might improve outcomes. There are no randomized, prospective studies examining the effect of lowering CRP on CHD risk. In fact, the best means of lowering CRP levels is unclear. Of interest are the findings from retrospective analyses that statin drugs appear to lower CHD risk in persons with elevations in CRP and that the effect can be independent of the effect on lipids. Similar findings have been found with aspirin and beta-blockers. The literature should be watched closely for developments in this potentially promising area.

Dietary Risk Factors

High intakes of caffeine, alcohol, calories, and fat are implicated in CHD risk; green tea is purported to be protective.

Caffeine. Caffeine has long been suspected of being a CHD risk factor, but most studies fail to confirm the suspicion. A recent well-designed case-controlled study provided an interesting observation, namely that heavy coffee consumption (four or more cups per day) independently increased the risk of MI, but only in persons who metabolize caffeine slowly (those with the CYP1A2 genotype). Because it is not practical to measure caffeine metabolism or screen genetically, it might be reasonable, pending more definitive data, to advise limiting coffee and caffeinated beverage intake to less than four servings per day in persons at high cardiovascular risk.

Alcohol. Epidemiologic studies find a J-shaped curve for the association between alcohol consumption and cardiovascular risk. Low levels of consumption (one two drinks per day) are associated with reduced rates of CHD morbidity and mortality. Studies measuring atherosclerotic changes find an inverse correlation between them and moderate alcohol use. The relationships are strongest for wine consumption, but this may be biased by lifestyle differences between wine consumers and those of other alcoholic beverages.

Calories and Fat. Comparison of popular weight-loss diets (Atkins, Ornish, Weight Watchers, Zone) in randomized, short-term study of obese persons found similar reductions in cardiac risk factors despite differences in fat content. Studies in post-MI patients are limited; modest regression of atherosclerotic plaque has been found in patients adhering to the very low fat Ornish diet, but palatability and long-term compliance are difficult with such diets. Data from the Women's Health Study suggest that it is the type of fat and not total amount that matters most in cardiac risk reduction (see later discussion of dietary measures and also Chapter 233).

Green Tea for Prevention. Green tea demonstrates potentially cardioprotective effects in *in vitro* and in animal studies. In an observational Japanese population study, its degree of use was inversely correlated with cardiovascular mortality, especially in women. Although encouraging, these findings require confirmation by randomized, placebo-controlled trials in other racial groups and particularly in post-MI patients before green tea can be regularly recommended. Like the original findings for hormone replacement therapy, healthy behavior by users may be biasing the results.

Environmental Factors

Air pollution is becoming increasingly recognized as a CHD risk factor. Both short-term exposure to diesel exhaust and long-term exposure to air pollution have demonstrated independent associations with CHD morbidity and mortality. In men with coronary disease, brief exposure to diesel exhaust promoted myocardial ischemia and inhibited fibrinolytic activity. In postmenopausal women, chronic air pollution was associated with increased rates of cardiovascular disease and death.

Disproven or Unproven Risk-Factor Measures

Hormone Replacement Therapy

Because *menopause* is a risk factor for CHD, hormone replacement therapy (HRT) has been examined as a possible means of achieving primary and secondary prevention of CHD events in menopausal women. Although observational epidemiologic data suggested a strong association between HRT use in postmenopausal women having CHD and reduced cardiovascular risk, a prospective, randomized study of the question (the Heart and Estrogen/Progestin Replacement Study [HERS]) found worse rather than improved cardiovascular outcomes (see Chapter 118). Secondary analysis of the data found that HRT-associated CHD risk was greatest among women more distant from menopause and was minimal when used for short-term periods closer to menopause.

Treatment of Bacterial Infection

Bacterial antigens have been proposed as potential stimulants of the inflammatory process associated with atherosclerosis. *Chlamydia pneumoniae* is a leading candidate, being an intracellular pathogen found in persons with MI. Cytokines from infection have also been proposed as triggers of plaque rupture. In the largest randomized study of the question (the Weekly Intervention with Zithromax for Atherosclerosis and its Related Disorders trial), a 3-month course of azithromycin (Zithromax) in patients with prior MI did not reduce the rate of adverse cardiac events after 14 months. A weekly azithromycin dose for 1 year produced no improvement in CHD outcomes compared to placebo after nearly 4 years of follow-up. Such findings do not definitively rule out a role for infection, but more data are needed before the hypothesis can be considered sufficiently valid to warrant testing or treatment.

"Antioxidant" Vitamins and Amino Acid Supplements

Supplements are taken by nearly 40% of the population. The use of "antioxidant" vitamins is very popular and heavily promoted by commercial interests. In support of their use are the findings of (a) an association between oxidative change in plaque lipids (particularly in LDL cholesterol) and atherogenicity, and (b) low levels of CHD risk among those taking diets rich in fruits and vegetable containing "antioxidant" vitamins and minerals (e.g., vitamin C, vitamin E, beta-carotene, selenium). Nitric oxide is important for endothelial function, which declines with age; its availability can be enhanced by the intake of the amino acid L-arginine. These findings have led some to conclude that supplements containing high doses of these vitamins or L-arginine would be helpful and, being "natural" substances, would also be safe. Initial reports of supplement use were encouraging, but poor design and small sample sizes limited their validity. Data from well-designed, prospective, randomized trials have failed to show consistent benefit and, in some instances, have revealed potential harm. The U.S. Preventive Services Task Force concluded in 2003 that overall, there was insufficient evidence to recommend for or against the use of vitamins A, C, and E, multivitamins with folic acid, or antioxidant combinations. Subsequent well-designed studies suggested increased health risks associated with high-dose vitamin E supplements and B-vitamin/folate preparations (see earlier discussion and Chapters 27 and 30). A diet rich in fruits and vegetables appears to be a much better approach to CHD prophylaxis (see later discussion).

Vitamin E. Vitamin E has received the most attention and is widely used, stimulated by commercial promotion and an early randomized trial suggesting a reduction in the risk of MI (although increases in CHD-related and all-cause mortality were noted). Subsequent well-designed, placebo-controlled studies of vitamin E supplements have failed to confirm any significant benefit. Meta-analytic study not only failed to confirm any benefit, but also found that high-dose intake ($\geq$400 IU/day) increased all-cause mortality for its use. A major randomized study (the HDL-Atherosclerosis Treatment Study) found that the addition of vitamin E also blunted the beneficial effects of lipid-lowering therapy.

Vitamin C. Use of this "antioxidant" is also very popular. Again, randomized, controlled trials in persons with CHD found little or no benefit, countering preliminary data suggesting benefit.

Beta-Carotene. Supplement use not only failed to reduce the CHD risk in prospective, controlled trials, but it also increased the risk of lung cancer. When taken with vitamin A, beta-carotene increased the incidence of cardiovascular mortality and all-cause mortality.

l-Arginine. L-Arginine improves nitric oxide–related function in vascular endothelial cells and reduces vascular stiffness. Its 6-month daily use as a supplement to standard therapy in postinfarction patients failed in placebo-controlled trial to demonstrate improvements in vascular stiffness, ejection fraction, or mortality; there was an increase in postinfarction deaths, suggesting the survival may be compromised by its intake and arguing against it use.

PHARMACOLOGIC THERAPIES
(58–80)

Besides exercise and risk factor reduction, one needs to consider pharmacologic interventions that can enhance survival and the reduce rates of cardiac events. Evidence-based modalities include beta-blockade, ACE inhibition, and antiplatelet therapy. Some dietary interventions appear very promising. Failure to implement medical measures of proven efficacy is widespread and of great concern; the landmark HERS study of postmenopausal women found that only a minority were receiving beta-blockade and ACE inhibition.

Beta-Blockade

β-Adrenergic blockade significantly reduces the total mortality rate and the incidences of recurrent infarction and sudden death in patients who have had a recent MI. Both acute and chronic use are associated with improved outcomes. Rates of reduction in mortality range from 26% to 39%; reinfarction rates fall by 23% to 28%. Findings were initially confined to persons with ST-segment-elevation MI, but have been extended to those with non–ST-segment-elevation MI. Concerns for adverse effects often factor into prescribing decisions and probably contribute to the low rates of postinfarction beta-blocker utilization (30% to 60%) seen in community-based practice. Underutilization is especially common in elderly patients. The original major trials excluded individuals at increased risk for adverse effects of beta-blockade, such as patients with severe pulmonary disease, marked congestive heart failure, insulin-requiring diabetes mellitus, and the elderly. Subsequent studies found no increased risk from use in such "high-risk" patients and no compromise in benefit. In fact, high-risk groups actually demonstrate a higher absolute reduction in risk because of a higher baseline mortality rate. The mechanism of risk reduction extends beyond the lowering of blood pressure; significant in-

crease in plaque regression has been observed in persons taking beta-blockade.

Pending data from randomized, prospective studies, it is recommended that all postinfarction patients be given a trial of beta-blocker therapy soon after infarction and that those with relative contraindications to such therapy have the trial conducted under close supervision, starting at low doses (e.g., 12.5 to 25 mg/d of atenolol) and titrating upward as tolerated until beta-blockade is achieved. Because early morning and early evening are times of greatest adrenergic stimulation and cardiac risk, it is important that a beta-blocker program ensure adequate beta-blockade during these critical periods.

Persons at high cardiovascular risk (including those who have had an MI) are at increased risk of perioperative mortality when undergoing noncardiac surgery, especially when a high-risk surgical procedure (e.g., intrathoracic, intraabdominal, or major vascular) is undertaken. Large-scale observational data find a 10% to 40% reduction in in-hospital mortality associated with perioperative use of beta-blockade. Post-MI patients should be considered candidates for perioperative beta-blocker therapy if they are not already taking the drug, and beta-blocker treatment should be continued perioperatively if it was prescribed previously.

Angiotensin Blockade

Angiotensin blockade reduces CHD mortality and reinfarction risks in post-MI patients. Initially found to be effective in postinfarction patients with left ventricular dysfunction (ejection fraction <0.4), angiotensin blockade demonstrates clinically significant reductions (20% to 30%) in morbidity and mortality for CHD patients with preserved left ventricular function (Heart Outcomes Prevention Evaluation [HOPE] study), including those who have not suffered infarction. Not only is survival improved, but so are the rates of infarction, stroke, and need for revascularization. Proposed mechanisms of action include not only inhibition of the angiotensin–renin–aldosterone system, but also the ability to limit vascular smooth muscle proliferation, plaque rupture, and left ventricular hypertrophy and to improve vascular endothelial function and fibrinolysis. Efficacy is similar for both classes of angiotensin blockers.

ACE Inhibitors (see also Chapter 32)

All CHD patients should be considered for ACE-inhibitor therapy. The choice of ACE inhibitor and optimal dose have not been established, but there appears to be little difference among ACE inhibitors, suggesting that benefit may be attained with any drug in this class, starting at a modest dose (e.g., generic captopril 25 mg twice daily, generic lisinopril 10 mg/d; the HOPE study used ramipril 10 mg/d). About 10% of patients cannot tolerate the medication due to kinin-related cough or angioedema; they should be considered for therapy with angiotensin-receptor antagonists.

Angiotensin-Receptor Antagonists (ARB)

Patients who cannot tolerate ACE-inhibitor treatment are reasonable candidates for ARB therapy, which at full doses provides equivalent protection against cardiac death in post-MI patients with low ejection fraction (<0.30; see Chapters 30 and 32). Cost is considerably greater than for ACE-inhibitor therapy (no generic formulations are available until after 2010). Combined angiotensin-blockade therapy increases the risk of hypotension without improving outcomes.

Antiplatelet Agents and Oral Anticoagulants

A coronary thrombus contains a combination of platelet and thrombin elements, and its formation is mediated by both platelet and prothrombotic factors. Treatment with antiplatelet agents and anticoagulant agents has been applied to post-MI patients for secondary prevention.

Platelet Inhibitors

Platelet inhibition reduces mortality risk and rates of reinfarction. Significant reductions (20% to 30%) in death and reinfarction are achieved with long-term low-dose (81 mg/d) *aspirin* therapy in post-MI patients. Irreversible inhibition of platelet cyclooxygenase-1 (COX-1) halts the synthesis of prothrombotic substances such as thromboxane. The risk of bleeding is increased, but this is greatly outweighed by the benefits of therapy. *Clopidogrel* (Plavix; a thienopyridine derivative that inhibits platelet aggregation) is slightly more effective and adds another 20% improvement in risk reduction when used with aspirin, but it is much more costly, much less cost-effective, and associated with an increased risk of bleeding when it is used in combination with aspirin. It is reserved for instances in which aspirin cannot be tolerated or proves inadequate (see Chapter 30). *Platelet glycoprotein IIa/IIIb integrin blockade* at the time of stent implantation reduces the risk of short- and long-term ischemic complications associated with stent implantation. Chronic oral therapy shows no additional advantage.

The *nonsteroidal antiinflammatory drugs (NSAIDs)* may have short-term antithrombotic actions related to their COX-1 inhibition in platelets, but this action may interfere with the more durable protective effect of low-dose aspirin by blocking aspirin's access to the acetylation site on platelet cyclooxygenase-1. Moreover, these drugs also have potential prothrombotic actions, related to the degree to which they inhibit cyclooxygenase-2 (COX-2), which is necessary for the synthesis of vasodilatory prostaglandins. Evidence of increased cardiovascular morbidity and mortality have emerged with NSAID intake, particularly with extended use of the most potent of the selective COX-2 NSAIDs, leading to removal of some from the market (e.g., rofecoxib [Vioxx]) and making others poor choices for use in persons with CHD (see Chapter 157). Systematic review confirms the finding of a markedly increased cardiovascular risk with rofecoxib and less with celecoxib, and refutes the purported protective effects of naproxen and diclofenac.

Oral Anticoagulants

The importance of reducing thrombotic risk has stimulated major randomized, controlled trials involving the addition of oral anticoagulation with warfarin (e.g., Warfarin-Aspirin Reinfarction Study II). The addition of *high-intensity warfarin* (International Normalized Ratio [INR] 2.8 to 4.2) achieves a slightly better reduction in CHD risk than aspirin alone (the additional absolute risk reduction is 3.2%; the relative risk reduction is about 19%), but at a cost of increasing the risk of major bleeding by threefold. The addition of *intermediate-intensity warfarin* (INR 2.0 to 2.5) to low-dose aspirin (75 mg/d) lowers the absolute risk by 5% (nearly 29% in relative terms), but raises risk of nonfatal major bleeding by nearly fourfold (from 0.17%/yr to 0.67%/yr). *Low-intensity therapy* (INR 1.5) combined with low-dose aspirin is not much more effective than aspirin, but increases the risk of bleeding substantially. In most studies, warfarin's contributions to risk reduction are almost exclusively in rates of reinfarction and stroke but not of death.

Overall Approach

These findings argue for the use of low-dose aspirin as part of a prophylactic program of secondary prevention in CHD patients, with warfarin added in persons with increased thrombotic risk (e.g., antiphospholipid syndrome) or substituted in persons who are allergic to aspirin. There is some concern that aspirin may impair some of the non-ACE–related benefits of ACE-inhibitor therapy, but combination therapy still provides better prophylaxis than monotherapy—just not as much as might have been expected (see Chapter 30).

Antiarrhythmic Therapy (See Also Chapters 29 and 32)

Post-MI patients, especially those with left ventricular failure, are at increased risk of sudden death. *Beta-blockers* reduce the risk of cardiac sudden death in such patients. *Class I antiarrhythmics* can suppress induced ventricular tachycardia, but their proarrhythmic effects negate any survival benefit. Similarly, the class III antiarrhythmic *amiodarone* provides arrhythmia protection and has been used to reduce the number of disruptive defibrillator discharges in persons with an implantable defibrillator–cardioverter but without demonstrated reduction in mortality. Early placement of an *implantable defibrillator–cardioverter* (ICD) in post-MI patients with severe left ventricular dysfunction (ejection fraction <0.35) significantly reduces mortality from sudden death, but overall cardiac mortality is unchanged, suggesting that the net effect is to convert the means of death from arrhythmia to heart failure. Use in combination with ventricular resynchronization holds promise in persons with marked left ventricular dysfunction (see Chapter 32). More data are needed so that we can better identify candidates for ICD (see also Chapters 29 and 32).

DIETARY MEASURES AND SUPPLEMENTS (81–89)

Diet (See Also Chapters 27, 30, and 233)

The role of a *low-saturated-fat, low-cholesterol diet* is well established for CHD prevention. It remains an essential part of a lipid-control program essential to aggressive risk factor reduction (see Chapter 27). However, excessive substitution of carbohydrate for fat can lead to counterproductive serum lipid changes, with reductions in HDL cholesterol and increases in triglycerides and LDL cholesterol. Over the last decade, emphasis has shifted from the focus on the total amount of fat to the types of fat in the diet.

Low Fat

One area of debate is degree of fat restriction. Study of the Ornish diet, which is extremely low in total fat (especially saturated fat), in persons with CHD suggests an ability to halt plaque progression and achieve modest disease regression. A large-scale randomized study of the use of a low-fat diet (20% of calories) plus fruits and vegetables in postmenopausal women (the Women's Health Initiative Dietary Modification Study) failed to show an overall reduction in CHD risk, but there was a trend toward benefit in the subsets of women who had lower intakes of *trans* or saturated fats or higher consumptions of fruits and vegetables.

Polyunsaturated Fats—Omega-3 Fatty Acids

A more balanced approach has emerged with appreciation for the beneficial effects of *polyunsaturates* (PUFAs) and *monounsaturates* (see Chapter 27). PUFA intake reduces the risks of CHD morbidity and mortality by 20% to 30%. Sources rich in these beneficial fatty acids (e.g., plant oils, nuts, oily fish) should be regular parts of daily dietary intake.

Of particular interest among the PUFAs are the *omega-3 fatty acids*. Epidemiologic study finds a nearly 30% reduction in the risk of sudden death in MI survivors and apparently healthy men who consume fish rich in these fatty acids. In addition, serum levels of omega-3 fatty acids correlate strongly with the risk of cardiac sudden death. Purported mechanisms include beneficial effects on atherosclerosis, clotting, and fibrillatory threshold. A once- or twice-weekly serving of an oily fish, such as salmon, mackerel, fresh tuna, lake trout, sardines, or herring, is recommended.

Concerns over contamination of some of these fish species with methylmercury, *dioxin*, or *polychlorinated biphenyls (PCBs)* has caused some to hold back on increasing their fish consumption. However, the net benefit in reducing cardiovascular morbidity and mortality greatly outweighs the small theoretical risks from such contaminants in persons with CHD. Wild salmon offers very high omega-3 content with low levels of mercury, dioxins, and PCBs. Whether such benefit also derives from use of fish-oil tablets is unproven, and intake of such tablets may exacerbate the anticoagulant effect of warfarin; randomized, prospective trials are under way. Initial results of randomized trials of fish oil supplements in high-risk persons (e.g., those requiring an implantable defibrillator–cardioverter) suggest that the survival benefit is greatest in persons with recent MI.

Fiber

The role of *dietary fiber* in CHD risk is the subject of intense study. Epidemiologic studies of persons free of CHD find a modest but significant (approximately 20%) reduction in CHD risk associated with the intake of *cereal fiber* (as found in whole grains and bran); no such relation is found with fruit or vegetable fiber intake. Even the elderly seem to derive benefit. Prospective study and inclusion of persons with CHD will be needed better to define the benefit, which appears to require as little as two slices of whole wheat bread daily or a serving of bran cereal.

Fruits and Vegetables

The intake of *fruits* and *vegetables* has also been the subject of epidemiologic study for its effect on CHD risk. Data from the Nurses' Health Study and others showed that a high intake of green, leafy vegetables and vitamin C–rich fruits and vegetables was associated with a 20% reduction in CHD risk compared with that for low intake. Although such findings do not rule out confounding variables, they suggest little harm from recommending such fruit and vegetable consumption. Substituting vitamin supplements for such foods has proved to be disappointing (see prior discussions). *Garlic* shows minor, short-term beneficial effects on triglycerides, total and LDL cholesterols, and platelet aggregation but not on HDL cholesterol.

Mediterranean Diet

With the foregoing findings, it should come as no surprise that adherence to a traditional *Mediterranean diet* (rich in fruits, vegetables, legumes, nuts, unrefined cereals, and olive oil; moderate in fish and alcohol; and low in saturated fats) has been found to be associated with a 33% reduction in death due to CHD.

Supplements

See earlier discussion.

REVASCULARIZATION (2,90–97; See Also Chapter 30)

Revascularization by *coronary bypass graft (CABG)* surgery or *percutaneous coronary intervention (PCI*; also referred to as *percutaneous transluminal coronary angioplasty [PTCA])* in conjunction with *stent* placement offers the opportunity to improve exercise tolerance and control of angina and, in, selected instances, reduce the risks of adverse cardiac events and death. Proper application requires a careful determination of prognosis and risk stratification.

Initial Evaluation

Risk stratification is essential to determining the need for revascularization and the selection of the appropriate intervention. The combination of clinical and electrocardiographic (ECG) findings supplemented by stress testing and echocardiography is helpful for initial stratification to identify which patients require angiography for consideration of revascularization (see Chapters 20 and 30).

In the Setting of Acute Chest Pain

In the setting of acute chest pain, electrocardiographic ST-segment elevation is the prime indication for immediate angiography. Revascularization (usually *PTCA with stenting*) is preferred over *thrombolysis* if the necessary resources are available within 3 hours of the onset of symptoms (see Chapter 20). The patient with acute chest pain without ST-segment changes, even in the setting of acute non–Q-wave infarction, need not be studied urgently unless there is evidence of progressive ischemic injury or pump failure; such patients do just as well with medical therapy as with early revascularization, even after 2 years of follow-up.

After the Acute Phase

Submaximal stress testing at the time of discharge or maximal exercise testing performed 6 weeks into the early convalescence phase helps to estimate the prognosis. Patients with evidence of significant myocardium at risk and possible high-risk disease (see Chapters 30 and 36) need referral for angiography.

Treatment According to Risk Stratification

Of concern are the barriers limiting the referral of eligible persons for coronary angiography and the resultant underutilization of revascularization. Attention to risk stratification can help to overcome these barriers, ensure patient access to effective care, and also prevent overutilization. *Race* has emerged as an important barrier; African Americans have a lower rate of risk-adjusted referral and are less likely than whites to undergo revascularization. This observation holds even after controlling for payment mechanism, clinical presentation, age, gender, region of the country, and potential for overuse by whites. The reasons for this are unknown. Another barrier is *physician failure* to recognize indications for revascularization. Indications for revascularization are expressed in terms of risk categorization.

For High-Risk Patients

CABG revascularization produces long-term reductions in risks of reinfarction and CHD mortality that approach 40% in patients with high-risk disease (moderate to severe angina; large amount of myocardium at risk; three-vessel, left-main, or left-main-equivalent disease; reduced ejection fraction; see Chapter 30). High-risk disease still requires the consideration of CABG, but advances in PCI and stenting technology are making possible their application in patients with increasingly difficult anatomy. However, frequent off-label use of PCI plus stenting is not without concern as reports emerge of increased rates of adverse cardiac outcomes (see Chapter 30).

One high-risk group commonly treated with PCI plus stenting is made up of persons with persistent total occlusion of an infarct-related artery after acute phase treatment, particularly if the total occlusion involves the proximal portion of a major epicardial vessel or the ejection fraction is less than 50%. PCI plus stenting of such lesions within a month of infarction has been popular but in controlled trial, failed to achieve reductions in rates of death, reinfarction, or heart failure when added to optimal medical therapy; moreover, there was a trend toward an increased risk of reinfarction.

For Intermediate-Risk Patients

Both CABG and PCI plus stenting are reasonable considerations for patients with lesser-risk multivessel disease (preserved LV function, no left-main or proximal left anterior descending artery involvement) and medically refractory symptoms. Compared with optimal medical therapy in such patients, these revascularization procedures do not reduce mortality, but they similarly reduce the frequency of nonfatal events and improve functional status and quality of life.

PCI plus stenting has the advantage of obviating the risks associated with major bypass-pump surgery, but it requires significantly more repeat revascularizations. The advent of *drug-eluting stents* reduces the risk of endothelial proliferation and associated stent occlusions seen with use of bare-metal stents. However, reports of late stent thrombosis and associated adverse cardiac events have emerged, especially with the off-label use of coated stents. These findings call into question the purported advantage of drug-eluting stents and mandate the indefinite use of dual antiplatelet therapy with aspirin and clopidogrel (see Chapter 30).

CABG surgery is associated with a 5% to 30% risk of cognitive decline (often referred to as "postpump syndrome"), which is especially prevalent in elderly patients and believed to be due to microembolization. Off-pump techniques have been developed. Randomized, controlled trial in low-risk surgical candidates found little difference between the two CABG techniques in terms of cognitive or cardiac outcomes.

For Low-Risk Patients

Patients with symptomatically bothersome single-vessel disease inadequately controlled by medical therapy are reasonable candidates for PTCA with stenting. Medical therapy that improves prognosis (e.g., beta-blockers, aspirin, ACE inhibitors) needs to be continued, but drugs prescribed strictly for symptomatic relief (e.g., long-acting nitrates, calcium-channel blockers) can often be phased out after angioplasty.

Post-Revascularization Care

The most important element is continuation of the full range of cardiac rehabilitation and secondary preventive measures that improve survival and quality of life, including aggressive control of atherosclerotic risk factors (especially LDL cholesterol), use of medical therapies that improve survival (aspirin, beta-blockers, ACE inhibitors), and lifestyle modification (diet, exercise). In addition, the use of a drug-coated stents necessitates prolonged aspirin/clopidogrel therapy to counter late-thrombosis risk.

Intracoronary Stem Cell Infusion

Intracoronary infusion of stem cells from bone marrow or circulating blood continues to undergo testing and appears promising in patients with healed myocardial infarction. Improvement in ejection fraction has been demonstrated.

PATIENT EDUCATION (98)

The patient who has suffered an acute coronary event is among those in greatest need of health education and individualized lifestyle counseling. Patient and family are apt to be depressed and frightened by the diagnosis of "coronary disease," believing the prognosis to be grim and fearing invalidism, especially if an infarction has occurred. They need to be informed that in the vast majority of uncomplicated cases, a return to job and regular activity is the rule rather than the exception and that there is much that they can do to greatly improve the prognosis.

Communicating Prognosis

Prognosis is a major concern of the patient and family and should be reviewed, not only with the intent of being accurate and realistic, but also with an eye toward communicating the significant improvements in prognosis that are achievable by a comprehensive program of secondary prevention. Most published survival rates derive from prospective epidemiologic studies and do not reflect the effects of secondary-prevention programs. Average annual mortality in the Framingham Study was 5% for men and 7% for women. Patients at greatest risk for late cardiac death were those with persistent "malignant" ventricular irritability (see Chapter 29), azotemia, previous infarction, persistent congestive failure, angina, or advanced age. Once congestive heart failure ensued, 50% died within 5 years. The risk of postinfarction angina in the Framingham Study was 2.9% for men and 9.6% for women. The risk of heart failure was 2.3%. Many of the complications of infarction are a function of the degree of myocardial damage. This is consistent with the observation that prognosis correlates with the extensiveness of disease, a finding also supported by angiographic studies (see Chapter 30). As noted, 1-year survival can be estimated from a limited treadmill exercise test done before discharge.

In reviewing prognosis, it is essential to review the reductions in risk associated with the implementation of secondary preventive measures (Table 31.1). On average, each element of the program has the potential to reduce risk by 25% to 50%, providing a very substantial improvement in outcomes

TABLE 31.1

EFFECT OF SECONDARY PREVENTION MEASURES ON RISK OF CORONARY HEART DISEASE (CHD) EVENTS (NEW INFARCTION, CARDIAC ARREST, CARDIAC DEATH)

Measure	Reported Reduction in CHD Morbidity/ Mortality (%)
Lipid lowering	7–76
Exercise	20–25
Smoking cessation	50
Hypertension control	8–38
Stress management	10–65
Aspirin	25
Beta-blockade	20
Coronary artery bypass (in high-risk patients)	39
Angiotensin blockade	20–30
Angioplasty plus stenting	0–?

Adapted from Merz CNB, Rozanski A, Forrester JS. The secondary prevention of coronary artery disease. Am J Med 1997;102:572, with permission.

if implemented. This is a very important and highly motivating message that needs to be conveyed and goes far beyond the common perception that revascularization is the only thing that can be done. Although revascularization is essential for improving survival in high-risk patients, it makes little contribution (beyond improving quality of life) for the large majority of persons with lesser-risk disease.

Counseling

Counseling needs to begin in the predischarge period. Realistic concerns and excessive fears of incapacitation may dramatically alter self-image and diminish self-respect. The most effective way of dealing with such fears is specifically to elicit and address the patient's and the family's concerns and discuss the plan for recovery and rehabilitation and its effect on quality of life and survival. Specific statements concerning *exercise capacity* can be based on graded treadmill stress testing during the recovery period. Knowing what one should and should not do during various stages of the recovery process can help to reduce some of the anxiety that accompanies having heart disease.

Activity guidelines should be given. Unsupervised activities during the first month after an MI should require no more than 3 METs (see Chapter 18, Table 18.1). By the time 6 to 8 weeks have passed, tasks requiring up to 5 METs will be safe for most patients, provided a gradual increase in activity has not been interrupted by symptoms or complications. Specific guidelines, tailored to the patient's personal occupational and recreational interests, are essential. Some concerns may not always be verbalized by the patient. One such concern is the safety of resuming *sexual activity*. Often, there is fear of sudden death during intercourse. The safety of sexual activity should be routinely discussed with the patient and spouse, even if the topic is not initially raised by them. Sexual intercourse with a familiar partner requires about 3 to 5 METs. Thus, sexual activity can be safely resumed by most patients as early as 4 weeks post-MI. During the early return to full sexual activity, the patient should be advised to avoid coital positions that require sustained isometric exercise, such as upper torso weight-bearing with the arms.

The period after an acute coronary event is also a time when patients are particularly receptive to counseling about changes in *lifestyle* that reduce coronary risk, such as smoking cessation (see Chapter 54) and dietary change (see Chapter 27). The primary physician is ideally suited to take advantage of this opportunity. A balanced cardiac rehabilitation program offers a very positive response to a very frightening event. In many instances, the results are extremely gratifying, with a patient who is healthier and more fit than before the acute coronary event.

INDICATIONS FOR REFERRAL AND ADMISSION (99)

For *cardiac rehabilitation*, referral to a formal program is strongly urged because the effort will include not only attention to exercise, but also a comprehensive approach to all elements of rehabilitation and secondary prevention. Need for an institutionally based program is appropriate for elderly patients, those with considerable disability, and persons whose home environment or likelihood for compliance is poor.

For *revascularization*, the referral should be based on the findings from risk stratification, with cardiac surgery indicated for high-risk patients, a choice of CABG versus angioplasty for intermediate-risk individuals, and angioplasty for those at low risk bothered by refractory symptoms. Results are better at centers with large volumes and extensive experience, but performance at a community hospital or a rural center does not preclude obtaining a good outcome when teams are well trained and volume is greater than the necessary minimum to ensure safety and competence.

Patients who present with *acute chest pain* accompanied by *ST-segment elevation* should be transferred to a site that can perform angioplasty rather than undergo immediate thrombolysis if the PTCA can be performed within 3 hours of onset of symptoms (see Chapter 20). The onset of chest pain in a person who has previously undergone angioplasty suggests restenosis and requires admission for angiographic study.

A.H.G.

Annotated Bibliography

1. Ades PA. Cardiac rehabilitation and secondary prevention of coronary heart disease. N Engl J Med 2001;345:892. (*An excellent review, particularly of evidence related to exercise training and rehabilitation programs; 109 references.*)
2. American College of Physicians. Guidelines for risk stratification after myocardial infarction. Ann Intern Med 1997;126:556. (*An evidence-based consensus, focusing on risk assessment before discharge after acute myocardial infarction [MI].*)
3. Anderson RE, Blair SN, Cheskin LJ, et al. Encouraging patients to become more physically active: the physician's role. Ann Intern Med 1997;127:395. (*An excellent essay on getting patients started, designing the exercise prescription, and maintaining activity.*)

4. Blumenthal JA, Babyak MA, Krantz DS, et al. Stress management and exercise training in cardiac patients with myocardial ischemia. Arch Intern Med 1997;157:2213. (*A randomized trial, showing a marked reduction in cardiac events with a program of stress reduction and exercise.*)

5. Curfman GD. Shorter hospital stays for myocardial infarction. N Engl J Med 1988;318:1123. (*Presents evidence for shortened stays for patients with uncomplicated infarction.*)

6. Giri S, Thompson PD, Kiernan FJ, et al. Clinical and angiographic characteristics of exertion-related acute myocardial infarction. JAMA 1999;282:1731. (*Prospective observational cohort study finding that habitually inactive patients are at greatest risk for exertion-related MIs.*)

7. Hambrecht R, Wolf A, Gielen S, et al. Effect of exercise on coronary endothelial function in patients with coronary artery disease. N Engl J Med 2000;342:454. (*A randomized trial, finding improved vasodilation in both large and small vessels.*)

8. Kujala UM, Kaprio J, Sarna S, et al. Relationship of leisure-time physical activity and mortality. The Finnish Twin Cohort. JAMA 1998;279:440. (*Even leisure-time physical activity was associated with a significant reduction in mortality.*)

9. Lau J, Altman EM, Jimenez-Silva J, et al. Cumulative meta-analysis of therapeutic trials for myocardial infarction. N Engl J Med 1992;327:248. (*Summarizes data on the efficacy of comprehensive cardiac rehabilitation in secondary prevention after myocardial infarction.*)

10. Muller JE, Tofler GH, Stone PH. Circadian variation and triggers of onset of acute cardiovascular disease. Circulation 1989;79:733. (*The risk is greatest in the morning hours.*)

11. NIH Consensus Development Panel on Physical Activity and Cardiovascular Health. Physical activity and cardiovascular health. JAMA 1996;276:241. (*A useful summary of current knowledge presented in the form of answers to basic questions.*)

12. Taylor RS, Brown A, Ebrahim S, et al. Exercise-based rehabilitation for patients with coronary heart disease: systematic review and meta-analysis of randomized controlled trials. Am J Med 2004;116:682. (*An updated systematic review; confirms benefit in an extended population of patients; 75 references.*)

13. Theroux P, Waters DD, Halphen C, et al. Prognostic value of exercise testing soon after myocardial infarction. N Engl J Med 1979;301:341. (*Demonstrates both the safety and the usefulness of such testing.*)

14. Van Camp SP, Peterson RA. Cardiovascular complications of outpatient cardiac rehabilitation programs. JAMA 1986;256:1160. (*Documents the very low risk of cardiac events associated with supervised programs.*)

15. Wannamethee SG, Shaper AG, Walker M. Physical activity and mortality in older men with diagnosed coronary artery disease. Circulation 2000;102:1358. (*A prospective study of an exercise program in elderly men, finding that reductions in cardiac morbidity and mortality were achieved.*)

16. Whang W, Manson JE, Hu FB, et al. Physical exertion, exercise, and sudden cardiac death. JAMA 2006;295:1399. (*Data from the Nurses' Health Study, finding that the risk was extremely low and was reduced by regular exercise.*)

17. Anavekar NS, McMurray JJV, Velazquez EJ, et al. Relation between renal dysfunction and cardiovascular outcomes after myocardial infarction. N Engl J Med 2004;351:1285. (*Renal dysfunction was found to be a major risk factor for coronary heart disease [CHD] complications.*)

18. Bønaa KH, Njølstad I, Ueland PM, et al, for the NORVIT Trial Investigators. Homocysteine lowering and cardiovascular events after acute myocardial infarction. N Engl J Med 2006;354:1578. (*Finds that B vitamin supplementation reduced plasma homocysteine but with no reductions in adverse cardiovascular outcomes; a trend toward increased risk of adverse events was seen with folate/B_{12}/B_6.*)

19. Brown RG, Zhao XQ, Chait A, et al. Simvastatin and niacin, antioxidant vitamins, or the combination for the prevention of coronary disease. N Engl J Med 2001;345:1583. (*Not only was there no improvement in risk with the antioxidant program, but the agents blunted the benefit of statin therapy when used concurrently.*)

20. Cornelis MC, El-Sohemy A, Kagagambe EK, et al. Coffee, CYP1A2 genotype and risk of myocardial infarction. JAMA 2006;295:1135. (*A case-controlled study, finding an association between heavy coffee consumption and MI in slow metabolizers of caffeine.*)

21. Danesh J, Wheeler JG, Hirschfield GM, et al. C-reactive protein and other markers of inflammation in the prediction of coronary heart disease. N Engl J Med 2004;350:1387. (*An Icelandic prospective study, finding that C-reactive protein was only a moderate predictor of risk and less than originally suspected.*)

22. Di Castelnnuovo A, Rotondo S, Iacoviello L, et al. Meta-analysis of wine and beer consumption in relation to vascular risk. Circulation 2002;105:2836. (*Finds that low levels of consumption were associated with reduced atherosclerotic risk.*)

23. Eikelboom JW, Lonn E, Genest J Jr, et al. Homocyst(e)ine and cardiovascular disease: a critical review of the epidemiologic evidence. Ann Intern Med 1999;131:363. (*A systematic review, finding strong epidemiologic evidence for an association but no proof that this treatment lowers CHD risk.*)

24. Fairfiled KM, Fletcher RH. Vitamins for chronic disease prevention in adults: scientific review. JAMA 2002;287:3116. (*The best critical review of the evidence, including that for antioxidants in CHD; 152 references.*)

25. Frasure-Smith N, Lesperance F. Depression—a cardiac risk factor in search of a treatment. JAMA 2003;289:3171. (*An editorial summarizing the conflicting evidence on the cardiovascular benefit of treating depression.*)

26. Grayston JT, Kronmal RA, Jackson LA, et al. Azithromycin for the secondary prevention of coronary events. N Engl J Med 2005;352:1637. (*No benefit was noted after 4 years after 1 year of weekly treatment.*)

27. Grobbee DE, Rimm EB, Giovannucci E, et al. Coffee, caffeine, and cardiovascular disease in men. N Engl J Med 1990;323:1026. (*An epidemiologic study of 45,000 men, finding no increase in the risk of coronary disease.*)

28. Heart Protection Study Collaborative Group. MRC/BHF Heart Protection Study of cholesterol lowering with simvastatin in 20,536 high-risk individuals: a randomized placebo-controlled trail. Lancet 2002;360:7. (*A major randomized, controlled trial [RCT], finding a benefit of high-dose statin therapy in high-risk persons, regardless of low-density-lipoprotein–cholesterol level.*)

29. Howard BV, Van Horn L, Hsia J, et al. Low-fat dietary pattern and risk of cardiovascular disease: the Women's Health Initiative Randomized controlled dietary Modification Trial. JAMA 2006;295:655. (*Overall, there was no significant reduction in CHD risk, but there was a favorable trend in the subset with low trans or saturated fat intake or high intake of fruits and vegetables.*)

30. Hulley S, Grady D, Bush T, et al. Randomized trial of estrogen plus progestin for secondary prevention of coronary heart disease in postmenopausal women. Heart and Estrogen/Progestin Replacement Study (HERS) Research Group. JAMA 1998;280:605. (*A landmark RCT, the Heart and Estrogen/Progestin Replacement Study [HERS] trial failed to confirm observational reports that hormone replacement therapy is effective for the secondary prevention of CHD events.*)

31. Jenkins NP, Keevil BG, Hutchinson IV, et al. Beta-blockers are associated with lower C-reactive protein concentrations in patients with coronary artery disease. Am J Med 2002;112:269. (*An interesting observation that may help to explain the benefit independent of lipid lowering.*)

32. Kuriyama S, Shimazu T, Kikucki N, et al. Green tea consumption and mortality due to cardiovascular disease, cancer, and all causes in Japan: the Ohsaki study. JAMA 2006;296:1255. (*A prospective population study, finding that use was associated with reduced mortality due to cardiovascular disease.*)

33. Lesperance F, Frasure-Smith N, Koszycki D, et al. Effects of citalopram and interpersonal psychotherapy on depression in patients with coronary artery disease: the Canadian Cardiac Randomized Evaluation of Antidepressant and Psychotherapy Efficacy (CREATE) Trial. JAMA 2007;297:367. (*Selective serotonin reuptake inhibitor therapy was found to be effective; interpersonal psychotherapy provided no additional benefit.*)

34. Miller ER III, Pator-Barriuso R, Dalal D, et al. Meta-analysis: high-dosage vitamin E supplementation may increase all-cause mortality. Ann Intern Med 2005;142:37. (*A systematic analysis of the best evidence, finding an increase in all-cause mortality.*)

35. Miller KA, Siscovick DS, Sheppard L, et al. Long-term exposure to air pollution and incidence of cardiovascular events in women. N Engl J Med 2007;356:447. (*The degree of exposure correlated with CHD risk.*)

36. Mills NL, Tornqvist H, Gonzalez MC, et al. Ischemic and thrombotic effects of dilute diesel-exhaust inhalation in men with coronary disease. N Engl J Med 2007;357:1075. (*RCT, finding the inhibition of fibrinolytic activity and the promotion of myocardial ischemia.*)

37. Morris CD, Carson S. Routine vitamin supplementation to prevent cardiovascular disease: a summary of the evidence for the U.S. Preventive Services Task force. Ann Intern Med 2003;139:56. (*Finds a failure to confirm the initial suggestions of benefit.*)

38. Nissen SE. Halting the progression of atherosclerosis with intensive lipid lowering: results from the Reversal of Atherosclerosis with Aggressive Lipid Lowering (REVERSAL) trial. Am J Med 2005;118:22S. (*Intensive therapy with 80 mg/d of atorvastatin halted progression, whereas moderate therapy with 40 mg/d of pravastatin did not.*)

39. Nissen SE, Wolski K. Effect of rosiglitazone on the risk of myocardial infarction and death from cardiovascular causes. N Engl J Med 2007;356:2457. (*Presents evidence for a significant increase in the risk of MI associated with the use of the drug.*)

40. Nygard O, Nordrehaug JE, Refsum H, et al. Plasma homocysteine levels and mortality in patients with coronary artery disease. N Engl J Med 1997;337:230. (*One of the original epidemiologic reports suggesting that hyperhomocysteinemia was a potent and independent predictor of mortality.*)

41. O'Connor CM, Dunne MW, Pfeffer MA, et al. Azithromycin for the secondary prevention of coronary heart disease events: the WIZARD study: a randomized controlled trial. JAMA 2003;290:1459. (*No benefit was found despite 3 months of treatment and >1 year of follow-up.*)

42. Pedersen TR, Faergeman O, Kastelein JJ, et al. High-dose atorvastatin vs usual-dose simvastatin for secondary prevention after myocardial infarction: the IDEAL study: a randomized controlled trial. JAMA 2005;294:2437.

(*A large, multicenter Scandinavian study, showing modest but significant reductions in nonfatal cardiovascular events but no significant additional reductions in cardiac mortality or increases in noncardiac mortality*).

43. Rea TD, Heckbert SR, Kaplan RC, et al. Smoking status and risk for recurrent coronary events after myocardial infarction. Ann Intern Med 2002;137:494. (*A retrospective, population-based cohort study, finding that risk declined to that of nonsmokers after 3 years of cessation.*)

44. Rossouw JE, Prentice RL, Manson JoAnn E, et al. Postmenopausal hormone therapy and risk of cardiovascular disease by age and years since menopause. JAMA 2007;297:1465. (*A secondary analysis of data from the HERS study, finding that the risk was greatest for use in older women and minimal for perimenopausal women.*)

45. Schnyder G, Roffi M, Pin R, et al. Decreased rate of coronary restenosis after lowering of plasma homocysteine levels. N Engl J Med 2001;345:1593. (*An oft-quoted Swiss RCT; the rate of restenosis was reduced, but subsequent study failed to confirm the finding.*)

46. Shlipak MG, Sarnak MJ, Katz R, et al. Cystatin C and the risk of death and cardiovascular events among elderly persons. N Engl J Med 2005;352:2049. (*Finds that this marker of renal function was a strong predictor of cardiovascular risk and better than creatinine in elderly patients.*)

47. Shlipak MG, Heidenreich PA, Noguchi H, et al. Association of renal insufficiency with treatment and outcomes after myocardial infarction in elderly patients. Ann Intern Med 2002;137:555. (*A cohort study, finding increased mortality risk and undertreatment.*)

48. Siegel D, Grady D, Browner WS, et al. Risk factor modification after myocardial infarction. Ann Intern Med 1988;109:213. (*A substantial reduction in CHD risk can be achieved with a modest reduction in risk factors.*)

49. Stephens NG, Parsons A, Schofield PM, et al. Randomised controlled trial of vitamin E in patients with coronary disease. Cambridge heart antioxidant study. Lancet 1996;347:781. (*An often-quoted RCT, finding a reduction in nonfatal MI but increases in CHD and all-cause mortality.*)

50. The ACCORD Study Group. Effects of intensive glucose lowering in type 2 diabetes. N Engl J Med 2008;358:2545. (*This treatment failed to demonstrate a reduction in major cardiovascular events.*)

51. The ADVANCE Collaborative Group. Intensive blood glucose control and vascular outcomes in patients with type 2 diabetes. N Engl J Med 2008;358:2560. (*A major RCT, finding a 10% reduction in macrovascular and microvascular events; included patients with previous MI.*)

52. The Heart Outcomes Prevention Evaluation Study Investigators. Vitamin E supplementation and cardiovascular events in high-risk patients. N Engl J Med 2000;342:154. (*A major RCT, finding no effect on cardiovascular outcomes.*)

53. U.S. Preventive Services Task Force. Routine vitamin supplementation to prevent cancer and cardiovascular disease: recommendations and rationale. Ann Intern Med 2003;139:51. (*Finds evidence insufficient to recommend vitamins A, C, or E, multivitamins with folic acid, or antioxidant combinations.*)

54. Vittinghoff E, Shlipak MG, Varosy PD, et al. Risk factors and secondary prevention in women with heart disease: the Heart and Estrogen/Progestin Replacement Study. Ann Intern Med 2003;138:81. (*A secondary finding of the landmark HERS trial, finding poor implementation of proven preventive therapies among high-risk women.*)

55. The Heart Outcomes Prevention Evaluation (HOPE) 2 Investigators. Homocysteine lowering with folic acid and B vitamins in vascular disease. N Engl J Med 2006;354:1567. (*Folate/B_{12}/B_6 supplementation was found to reduce plasma homocysteine, but no benefit was seen in high-risk patients.*)

56. Wilson PWF. Homocysteine and coronary heart disease: how great is the hazard? JAMA. 2002;288:2042. (*An editorial summarizing the evidence and suggesting that the risk might be less than originally suspected.*)

57. Ziegelstein RC, Meuchel J, Kim TJ, et al. Selective serotonin reuptake inhibitor use by patients with acute coronary syndromes. Am J Med 2007;120:525. (*Use in the acute setting was found to be safe and effective; there was a small increase in bleeding risk.*)

58. Beta Blocker Heart Attack Trial Research Group. A randomized trial of propranolol in patients with acute myocardial infarction. JAMA 1982;247:1707. (*The first large-scale RCT to demonstrate reductions in total mortality and cardiovascular mortality in persons with MI.*)

59. Buresly K, Eisenberg MJ, Zhang X, et al. Bleeding complications associated with combinations of aspirin, thienopyridine derivatives, and warfarin in elderly patients following myocardial infarction. Arch Intern Med 2005;165:784. (*Risks are increased, but the overall risk remains small and manageable.*)

60. Echt DS, Liebson PR, Mitchell LB, et al. Mortality and morbidity in patients receiving encainide, flecainide, or placebo. The Cardiac Arrhythmia Suppression Trial. N Engl J Med 1991;324:781. (*In patients with asymptomatic ventricular arrhythmia after MI, antiarrhythmic therapy resulted in poorer survival.*)

61. Gaspoz JM, Coxson PG, Goldman PA, et al. Cost effectiveness of aspirin, clopidogrel, or both for secondary prevention of coronary heart disease. N Engl J Med 2002;346:1800. (*Aspirin was the most cost-effective.*)

62. Gottlieb SS, McCarter RJ, Vogel RA. Effect of beta-blockade on mortality among high-risk and low-risk patients after myocardial infarction. N Engl J Med 1998;339:489. (*A large-scale observational study, finding that high-risk patients benefit as much as, if not more than, others.*)

63. Hurlen M, Abdelnoor M, Smith P, et al. Warfarin, aspirin, or both after myocardial infarction. N Engl J Med 2002;347:969. (*RCT, finding that warfarin was slightly better than aspirin but that its use was associated with a significantly higher risk of bleeding.*)

64. Krumholz HM, Radford MJ, Wang Y, et al. Early beta-blocker therapy for acute myocardial infarction in elderly patients. Ann Intern Med 1999;131:648. (*Presents evidence for the underutilization of beta-blockade; 51% of patients did not receive this proven treatment.*)

65. Krumholz HM, Radford MJ, Ellerbeck EF, et al. Aspirin for secondary prevention after acute myocardial infarction in the elderly: prescribed use and outcomes. Ann Intern Med 1996;124:292. (*Despite the clear-cut evidence of benefit, 24% of patients were not prescribed aspirin.*)

66. Lewis HD, Davis JW, Archibald DG, et al. Protective effects of aspirin against acute myocardial infarction and death in men with unstable angina. N Engl J Med 1983;309;396. (*A classic study, finding that men treated for 12 weeks with buffered aspirin had a 51% lower incidence of death from acute infarction compared with placebo controls.*)

67. Lindenauer PK, Pekow P, Wang K, et al. Perioperative beta-blocker therapy and mortality after major noncardiac surgery. N Engl J Med 2005;353:349. (*A large-scale observational study, finding a 10% to 40% reduction in perioperative mortality with beta-blocker use in high-risk persons.*)

68. McGettigan P, Henry D. Cardiovascular risk and inhibition of cyclooxygenase: a systematic review of the observational studies of selective and nonselective inhibitors of cyclooxygenase 2. JAMA 2006;296:1633. (*Confirms the findings of increased cardiovascular risk with rofecoxib and less so with celecoxib; refutes the purported protective effects of naproxen and diclofenac.*)

69. Miller CD, Roe MT, Mulgund J, et al. Impact of acute beta-blocker therapy for patients with non–ST-segment elevation myocardial infarction. Am J Med 2007;120:685. (*Improved outcomes were demonstrated.*)

70. Moss AJ, Zareba W, Hall WJ, et al. Prophylactic implantation of a defibrillator in patients with myocardial infarction and reduced ejection fraction. N Engl J Med 2002;346:877. (*RCT, finding that the risk of death was reduced by 31% in this very high risk group.*)

71. Norwegian MultiCenter Study Group. Timolol-induced reduction in mortality and reinfarction in patients surviving acute myocardial infarction. N Engl J Med 1981;304:801. (*A landmark study of beta-blockade, demonstrating a 45% reduction in sudden death among post-MI patients.*)

72. O'Shea JC, Fuller CE, Cantor AB, et al. Long-term efficacy of platelet glycoprotein IIa/IIIb integrin blockade with eptifibatide in coronary stent intervention. JAMA 2002;287:618. (*A long-term follow-up of RCT, finding that late outcomes improved with early use.*)

73. Patrono C, Garcia-Rodriguez LA, Landolfi R, et al. Low-dose aspirin for the prevention of atherothrombosis. N Engl J Med 2005;353:2373. (*A comprehensive review, finding a 25% risk reduction in MI patients; 89 references.*)

74. Pfeffer MA, McMurray JJV, Velazquez EJ, et al. Valsartan, captopril, or both in myocardial infarction complicated by heart failure, left ventricular dysfunction, or both. N Engl J Med 2003;349:1893. (*A major RCT, Valsartan in Acute Myocardial Infarction [VALIANT], finding that the two drugs were equally effective but that combined therapy increased the frequency of adverse effects.*)

75. Pfeffer MA, Braunwald E, Moye LA, et al. Effect of captopril on mortality and morbidity in patients with left ventricular dysfunction after myocardial infarction. Results of the Survival and Ventricular Enlargements trial. N Engl J Med 1992;327:669. (*Compared with placebo, treatment with captopril improved long-term outcome.*)

76. Rasmussen JN, Chong A, Alter DA. Relationship between adherence to evidence-based pharmacotherapy and long-term mortality after acute myocardial infarction. JAMA 2007;297:177. (*Population-based, observational, long-term study, finding that survival was associated with adherence.*)

77. Sipahi I, Tuzcu M, Wolski KE, et al. β-Blockers and progression of coronary atherosclerosis: pooled analysis of 4 intravascular ultrasonography trials. Ann Intern Med 2007;147:10. (*A pooled analysis of major RCTs, showing that significant plaque regression was associated with the use of beta-blockers.*)

78. Smith P, Arnesen H, Holme I. The effect of warfarin on mortality and reinfarction after myocardial infarction. N Engl J Med 1990;323:147. (*Beneficial effects were noted, but the risk of bleeding increased.*)

79. The Heart Outcomes Prevention Evaluation Study Investigators. Effects of an angiotensin-converting-enzyme inhibitor, ramipril, on death from cardiovascular causes, myocardial infarction, and stroke in high-risk patients. N Engl J Med 2000;342:145. (*CHD patients with normal left ventricular function had significant reductions in CHD morbidity and mortality.*)

80. Viscoli CM, Horwitz RI, Singer BH. Beta-blockers after myocardial infarction: influence of first-year clinical course on long-term effectiveness. Ann Intern Med 1993;118:99. (*Benefit appeared to be greatest in patients whose clinical course was characterized by recurrent ischemic events, congestive heart failure, arrhythmias, or severe comorbidity.*)

81. Albert CM, Campos H, Stampfer MJ, et al. Blood levels of long-chain n-3 fatty acids and the risk of sudden death. N Engl J Med 2001;346:1113. (*A prospective, nested, case–control analysis of healthy men from the Physicians' Health Study, finding that levels correlated with a reduced risk of sudden death.*)

82. Albert CM, Hennekens CH, O'Donnell CJ, et al. Fish consumption and risk of sudden cardiac death. JAMA 1998;279:23. (*Epidemiologic data suggesting a relationship between omega-3 fatty acid intake and reduced rates of sudden death.*)

83. Brouwer IA, Zock PL, Camm AJ, et al., for the SOFA Study Group. Effect of fish oil on ventricular tachycardia and death in patients with implantable cardioverter defibrillators: the Study on Omega-3 Fatty Acids and Ventricular Arrhythmia (SOFA) randomized trial. JAMA 2006;295:2613. (*A large-scale, placebo-controlled, randomized trial, finding that overall protective benefit was only modest but was best in patients with recent MI.*)

84. Hu FB, Bronner L, Willett WC, et al. Fish and omega-3 fatty acid intake and risk of coronary heart disease in women. JAMA 2002;287:1815. (*A prospective observational study of participants in the Nurses' Health Study, showing that a higher consumption of fish and omega-3 fatty acids reduced the risk of CHD death.*)

85. Johipura KJ, Hu FB, Manson JE, et al. The effect of fruit and vegetable intake on risk for coronary heart disease. Ann Intern Med 2001;134:1106. (*Epidemiologic data from the Nurses' Health Study, showing an association between the consumption of fruits and vegetables and a reduction in CHD risk.*)

86. Lieber CS. Alcohol and health: a drink a day won't keep the doctor away. Cleve Clinic J Med 2003;70:2003. (*A critical review of the epidemiologic evidence for benefit, especially as it pertains to CHD, suggesting caution in extrapolating to individuals.*)

87. Mozaffarian D, Kumanyika SK, Lemaitre RN, et al. Cereal, fruit, and vegetable fiber intake and the risk of cardiovascular disease in elderly individuals. JAMA 2003;289:1659. (*A prospective cohort study, finding that cereal fiber intake was associated with a reduction in CHD risk.*)

88. Mozaffarian D, Rimm EB. Fish intake, contaminants, and human health: evaluating the risks and benefits. JAMA 2006;296:1885. (*A comprehensive review, finding that the benefits of eating fish greatly outweigh the risks.*)

89. Trichopoulou A, Costacou T, Barnia C, et al. Adherence to a Mediterranean diet and survival in a Greek population. N Engl J Med 2003;348:2599. (*An epidemiologic study confirming what Zorba always knew—you live longer.*)

90. Asmus B, Honold J, Schachinger V, et al. Transcoronary transplantation of progenitor cells after myocardial infarction. N Engl J Med 2006;355:1222. (*Early-phase study, demonstrating promising results.*)

91. Boden WE, O'Rourke RA, Crawford MH, et al. Outcomes in patients with acute non–Q-wave myocardial infarction randomly assigned to an invasive as compared with a conservative management strategy. N Engl J Med 1998;338:1785. (*Short-term worsening of outcomes and no long-term benefit were found from early angiography and revascularization.*)

92. Canto JG, Allison JJ, Kiefe CI, et al. Relation of race and sex to the use of reperfusion therapy in Medicare beneficiaries with acute myocardial infarction. N Engl J Med 2000;342:1094. (*Presents evidence of race as a limiting factor.*)

93. Hochman JS, Lamas GA, Buller CE, et al. Coronary intervention for persistent occlusion after myocardial infarction. N Engl J Med 2006;355:2395. (*RCT, finding that this procedure offered no benefit over medical therapy.*)

94. Stone GW, Moses JW, Ellis SG, et al. Safety and efficacy of sirolimus- and paclitaxel-eluting coronary stents. N Engl J Med 2007;356:998. (*A pooled analysis of four RCTs, finding evidence of an increased risk of late stent thrombosis.*)

95. van Dijk D, Spoor M, Hijman R, et al. Cognitive and cardiac outcomes 5 years after off-pump vs on-pump coronary artery bypass graft surgery. JAMA 2007;297:701. (*In low-risk patients, there was no difference in outcomes.*)

96. Win HK, Caldera AE, Maresh K, et al. Clinical outcomes and stent thrombosis following off-label use of drug-eluting stents. JAMA 2007;297:2001. (*A prospective multicenter registry study, noting higher rates of adverse outcomes and stent thromboses.*)

97. Yusuf S, Zucker D, Peduzzi P, et al. Effect of coronary artery bypass graft surgery on survival: overview of 10-year results from randomized trials by the Coronary Artery Bypass Graft Surgery Trialists Collaboration. Lancet 1994;334:563. (*A meta-analysis, demonstrating nearly a 40% reduction in mortality in high-risk patients at 10 years of follow-up.*)

98. Merz CNB, Rozanski A, Forrester JS. The secondary prevention of coronary artery disease. Am J Med 1997;102:572. (*A good summary of benefits.*)

99. Andersen HR, Nielson TT, Rasmussen K, et al. A comparison of coronary angioplasty with fibrinolytic therapy in acute myocardial infarction. N Engl J Med 2003;249:733. (*A randomized community trial, finding that angioplasty produced superior outcomes, despite the need to transfer patients to an invasive-therapy center.*)

CHAPTER 32 ■ APPROACH TO THE PATIENT WITH CHRONIC CONGESTIVE HEART FAILURE

Chronic congestive heart failure (CHF) ranks among the most prevalent and serious of cardiac problems encountered in office practice. The annual rate for the development of clinically overt CHF in the community setting is about 2.3 per 1,000 for men and 1.4 per 1,000 for women; the incidence is nearly twice these figures among persons older than the age of 50 years. Five-year survival rates, regardless of cause, average just about 50%, making the condition a greater threat to life expectancy than many malignancies.

The prevalence of heart failure has not changed in recent years, but the proportion of patients presenting with preserved ejection fraction has increased, necessitating an updated understanding of CHF pathophysiology, clinical presentation, diagnosis, and treatment.

Effective measures are available that improve quality of life, reduce hospitalizations, and prolong survival. Absolute survival rates have risen by greater than 10% in the last decade, coincident with the increased use of angiotensin-converting-enzyme (ACE) inhibitors and beta-blockers, which have emerged as cornerstones of treatment. Novel therapies with considerable promise (e.g., cardiac resynchronization, direct aldosterone inhibition, natriuretic peptide) are being tested and implemented.

The primary care physician is responsible for implementing a practical, cost-effective, evidence-based treatment program, designed in collaboration with cardiac consultation and maintained and monitored with the help of a strong patient-education program and community-based resources.

PATHOPHYSIOLOGY, CLINICAL PRESENTATION, AND COURSE (1–23)

Pathophysiology and Clinical Presentation

Congestive heart failure is the consequence of an index event that causes an injury to the left ventricle (LV). Compensatory cardiac and neurohumoral responses initially help to maintain cardiac output, but ultimately they prove to be dysfunctional and exacerbate the problem, leading to *left ventricular remodeling* and reduced LV function. The resultant LV impairment may include delayed myocardial activation and dyssynchronous contraction (*dyssynchrony*), leading to severe, persistent symptoms. Dysregulation of the renin–angiotensin–aldosterone system represents the principal neurohormonal mechanism, leading to fluid retention and volume overload. There may be racial differences in the mechanisms of heart failure. Blacks appear to be particularly responsive to therapies that improve nitric oxide bioavailability, which suggests that an impaired bioavailability of nitric oxide and increased oxidant stress are contributing factors.

Etiologies, Risk Factors, and Compensatory Responses

Any insult to the functional and/or structural integrity of the left ventricle may result in congestive heart failure. Important etiologies include *hypertension, myocardial infarction, aortic* and *mitral valvular diseases, dilated* and *hypertrophic cardiomyopathies,* and *myocarditis.*

Risk Factors. In the community setting, the leading independent risk factors for CHF are *hypertension, ischemic heart disease,* and *diabetes* (independent of ischemic disease). Elevations in *systolic blood pressure* and *pulse pressure* are important predictors, as is the presence of *valvular disease,* but alcohol consumption is not. Less-well-established independent risk factors include renal dysfunction in older patients (creatinine >1.4 mg/dL), *loss of diurnal variation in blood pressure, hyperinsulinism* (perhaps the underlying mechanism for diabetes), *subclinical hypothyroidism* (thyrotropin >7.0 mIU/L), and *excess salt* intake in obese persons. Drugs that cause salt and fluid retention (e.g., the *thiazolidinediones* ["glitazones"], which are widely prescribed in diabetes) may precipitate heart failure, especially in persons with other risk factors. A *parental history* of heart failure is associated with an increased prevalence of left ventricular dysfunction and heart failure in offspring, suggesting a strong influence of familial and genetic factors.

Cardiac Responses. The principal myocardial response is a *remodeling of the left ventricle.* At the microscopic level, there is cell dropout from accelerated programmed cell death (apoptosis), dissolution of the supporting collagenous matrix, and myocyte hypertrophy; myocyte "slippage" may ensue. If the precipitating insult produces abnormal loading conditions (as in myocardial infarction or valvular insufficiency), the left ventricle responds predominantly by dilating (some hypertrophy may also occur); over time, the LV becomes spherical. Hypertrophic responses may predominate when there is increased afterload. The permanently remodeled myocardium is fibrotic and dysfunctional.

Systemic Responses. The initial fall in cardiac output from the index event activates the *renin–angiotensin–aldosterone system* and triggers heightened *sympathetic activity,* resulting in sodium retention, vasoconstriction, and elevations in heart rate, preload, and afterload. In the failing heart, the result is pulmonary and systemic hypertension but no improvement in cardiac output. These cardiac and neurohormonal responses temporarily help to maintain cardiac output by way of the Frank–Starling mechanism but at the cost of inducing volume overload and stimulating progressive LV remodeling (α-adrenergic stimulation is a potent mediator of cardiac myocyte hypertrophy). The progressive decrease in cardiac output triggers further neurohumoral activity, and a vicious cycle is established. High serum levels of renin, angiotensin, and norepinephrine are associated with increased 5-year mortality rates.

Counterregulatory Responses. In response to volume overload, atrial and ventricular tissues release *natriuretic peptide,* which increases glomerular filtration and inhibits the secretion of renin and aldosterone, promoting vasodilation and the excretion of sodium and water. Sympathetic overactivity leads to *downregulation of β_1-adrenergic receptors* and *blunted β-receptor signaling. Prostaglandin* synthesis and *kinin* release promote vasodilation and renal sodium excretion. Although they are helpful, these counterregulatory changes are usually insufficient to overcome the powerful maladaptive neurohumoral responses triggered by heart failure.

Systolic and Diastolic Dysfunction

Both systolic and diastolic LV dysfunction are common in CHF.

Systolic Dysfunction. The traditional hallmark of CHF—systolic dysfunction—is the consequence of a myocardial insult that impairs *contractility* and is manifested by a *reduced ejection fraction* (EF) (<0.40) and a *dilated* left ventricle. The leading cause is prior myocardial infarction. About 60% of CHF cases in the community setting are due to systolic dysfunction, which also accounts for 60% of the mortality risk.

Diastolic Dysfunction. The finding in community-based settings of a normal ejection fraction in as many as 50% of patients presenting with CHF has led to a greater appreciation for the importance of diastolic dysfunction (*impaired LV filling*) in heart failure. Its increasing prevalence parallels the increase in important contributing factors, such as hypertension, atrial fibrillation, and diabetes. In addition, diastolic dysfunction has been demonstrated in the settings of valvular and cardiomyopathic conditions. Risk factors include advancing age, obesity, female gender, diabetes, and hypertension.

Diastolic dysfunction may occur either in the absence or presence of systolic dysfunction. Its presence markedly worsens prognosis (to the same degree that systolic function does). *Mechanisms* include defective diastolic myocardial relaxation (an active, energy-dependent process), valvular dysfunction, and loss of myocardial distensibility, as may occur in left ventricular hypertrophy or ischemia. Ventricular remodeling (with myocyte hypertrophy and myocardial fibrosis) contributes to the problem. Unlike systolic dysfunction, left ventricular wall thickness increases, whereas end-diastolic volume remains unchanged. The velocity of blood flow across the mitral valve becomes abnormal, reflecting poor diastolic relaxation and reduced ventricular distensibility.

Abnormal diastolic filling reduces cardiac output, especially during exercise, and raises pulmonary venous pressures, contributing to pulmonary venous congestion, dyspnea, and peripheral edema. Compensatory left atrial contractility may increase by as much as 50% to help preserve diastolic filling, but persistent elevations in atrial pressure lead to *atrial enlargement*, the substrate for *atrial tachycardias* and resultant compromise in diastolic filling time (which is so important to coronary perfusion and cardiac output).

Clinical Presentation

The classic "congestive" manifestations of established CHF—leg edema, orthopnea, paroxysmal nocturnal dyspnea, rales, jugular venous distention—are clinical features common to both systolic and diastolic dysfunction. However, some elements of the presentation differ according to stage of the disease and whether the predominant ventricular pathophysiology is systolic or diastolic.

Presentation by Stage of Disease. The evolving appreciation for the progressive nature of CHF has led to designation by the American College of Cardiology and American Heart Association of a staging system for CHF, with the implication that, like cancer, the disease progresses in irreversible although not necessarily inexorable fashion:

■ Stage A: at high risk, but no discernible structural abnormality
■ Stage B: structural abnormality, but no symptoms
■ Stage C: structural abnormality and symptoms of heart failure
■ Stage D: end-stage symptoms and refractory to standard treatment

Stage A patients typically have major risk factors for coronary disease or early valvular disease but no symptoms or manifestations of LV structural change. Nonetheless, they are at high risk, which can be ameliorated by tight control of the relevant CHF risk factors (e.g., see Chapters 26, 27, 33, and 102).

Stage B is characterized by the early evidence of structural change but little symptomatology. LV hypertrophy or dilation, reduced ejection fraction, or impaired diastolic filling may be noted on cardiac ultrasound. Here, too, timely intervention may prevent disease progression. It is estimated that nearly 50% of CHF patients are in stage B, but many of these go undetected.

Stage C represents further disease progression. Patients may initially complain of *fatigability*, *dyspnea on exertion*, or unexplained *weight gain*. At this early phase of stage C, there may be few overt physical signs of failure, but chest x-ray often shows *pulmonary congestion* (*redistribution* of pulmonary venous flow to the upper lung fields) and/or *cardiomegaly*. *Fatigue* becomes increasingly prominent as cardiac output falls. As pulmonary congestion increases, exertional dyspnea worsens and *orthopnea* is noted, and *rales* may become evident on auscultation of the lungs, but their absence does not rule out the presence of CHF. Mild ankle edema may be noted, but pedal edema is one of the least specific signs of CHF (see Chapter 22).

Stage D and the later phases of stage C are characterized by *paroxysmal nocturnal dyspnea*, *worsening ankle edema*, *jugular venous distention*, and *hepatojugular reflux*, all of which are indicative of markedly elevated pulmonary and systemic venous pressures (pulmonary capillary wedge pressure at least 15 mm Hg). As left ventricular dilation progresses, functional *mitral insufficiency* may become evident. An S_3 (third heart sound) *gallop* may be heard, indicative of advanced LV failure and predictive of poor prognosis (relative risk, 1.3). Sometimes, failure-induced *bronchospasm* dominates the pulmonary examination. The chest film will often show *interstitial pulmonary edema*; right-sided or bilateral *pleural effusions* are common.

Acute exacerbation requiring hospital admission is usually preceded by a period of *decompensation* characterized by *increasing dyspnea*, *worsening edema*, and *weight gain*. In many instances, the cause is dietary indiscretion or noncompliance with medication. The interval between the onset of clinical worsening and the need for hospitalization is about 1 week, allowing time for the detection and treatment of reversible factors and the avoidance of admission.

Presentation by Underlying Pathophysiology. Patients with *systolic dysfunction* tend to be male, aged 50 to 70 years, with a history of myocardial infarction, an audible S_3, signs of LV dilation, a chest x-ray showing cardiomegaly with congestion, and an ejection fraction of less than 0.40. Those with *diastolic dysfunction* are more likely to be older, female, obese, and with a history of diabetes and hypertension. Exercise intolerance is prominent, due to both shortness of breath from pulmonary venous hypertension and fatigue from poor cardiac output. There is often an audible fourth heart sound (S_4) and a left ventricular lift without evidence of dilation; venous congestion is prominent on chest x-ray without cardiomegaly. The ejection fraction is typically well preserved (>40%).

Atypical Presentations. The efficacy of potent diuretic therapy has created an atypical presentation sometimes referred to as *"cold and dry."* In this presentation, cardiac output remains low (the extremities feel cool), but characteristic congestive manifestations are absent. Complaints of *fatigue* might dominate the clinical picture, whereas dyspnea, orthopnea, leg edema, rales, and even radiologic signs of CHF (see later discussion) may be absent.

Clinical Course and Determinants of Prognosis

The clinical course tends to be progressive, determined in part by the rate and extent of LV remodeling. However, CHF is not a single disease, and, therefore, it does not have a uniform natural history. The clinical course and response to therapy vary considerably from person to person according to such determinants as *underlying etiology*, *state of the myocardium* at the time of presentation, *stage of illness*, and the patient's *functional capacity*. In addition, *renal function* plays a critical role in prognosis, which is significantly worsened by the onset of renal failure. Part of the variability in clinical course and response to therapy is due to genetic factors, which account for racial and familial differences. *Genetic polymorphism* (or sequence variation) in genes controlling both *renin–angiotensin* and *adrenergic signaling* (e.g., Del322–325 in the α_2 receptor and Arg389 in the β_1 receptor) has been linked to variations in disease progression and clinical responses to ACE inhibitors and beta-blockers.

Diastolic dysfunction contributes independently to all-cause mortality (hazard ratio of 8 to 10). Although its annual mortality rate (reported at 8%/yr to 17%/yr) is only half of that of *systolic dysfunction*, it makes a significant contribution to adverse cardiac outcomes and accounts for about 40% of CHF morbidity and mortality. The presence of a *third heart sound* and *hepatojugular reflux* increase the risk of an adverse cardiac event by nearly 30% each.

Similarly, an increase in *plasma norepinephrine* level correlates strongly with mortality risk, representing the autonomic compensatory response to a falling cardiac heart. *Anemia* has been linked to outcome, with each 1% fall in hematocrit correlating with a 2% rise in 1-year mortality.

DIAGNOSIS AND CLASSIFICATION
(1,5,10,12,14,24–32)

Clinical recognition of heart failure can be difficult. Early stages of the condition produce few symptoms or signs, and CHF can be hard to differentiate from other causes of acute dyspnea. Many of the symptoms of CHF (which are often the manifestations of compensatory mechanisms) are nonspecific and at times misleading, which results in both overdiagnosis and underdiagnosis. As many as 40% of patients being treated on clinical grounds for CHF do not fulfill the basic echocardiographic criteria for the condition, whereas more than half of CHF patients go undetected. Consequently, practical laboratory aids to clinical diagnosis have been sought.

Clinical Diagnosis

As noted, most symptoms and signs are individually neither very sensitive nor specific, but taken together, they can provide a reasonable estimate of pretest probability and aid in test selection and interpretation.

Clinical Criteria

Clinical features identified in the Framingham Heart Study as having the greatest predictive value and capable of serving as major criteria for the diagnosis of CHF include the following:

- Paroxysmal nocturnal dyspnea
- Orthopnea
- Elevated jugular venous pressure
- Presence of rales (crackles) on chest exam
- Third heart sound
- Cardiomegaly or pulmonary edema on chest x-ray
- Weight loss of 10 lb in 5 days in response to treatment for CHF

Other findings that make a lesser contribution to diagnosis (minor criteria) include *peripheral edema*, *nocturnal cough*, *exertional dyspnea*, *hepatomegaly*, *pleural effusion*, and *tachycardia* (heart rate >120 beats/min).

The earliest findings (*fatigability*, *dyspnea on exertion*, unexplained *weight gain*) are quite nonspecific. A story of *orthopnea* or *paroxysmal nocturnal dyspnea* is much more suggestive, as is the finding of *basilar rales* on pulmonary examination (although the absence of rales does not rule out CHF [negative predictive value, 35%]). The finding of S_3 is among the most specific of physical signs (the specificity for systolic dysfunction approaches 90%), but it is often difficult to elicit and may not be present in early or mild disease (sensitivity <35%); it also can occur in the absence of LV failure in elderly patients with hypertension and those with valvular mitral regurgitation. *Hepatojugular reflux* (sometimes referred to as *abdominojugular reflux*) has a specificity of almost 95% but a sensitivity of less than 25%. The presence of any three major criteria (e.g., S_3, cardiomegaly, basilar rales) constitutes reasonable presumptive evidence for the diagnosis.

The assessment of volume status can be difficult; orthostatic signs are sensitive for the detection of dehydration, but the detection of volume overload is more problematic unless it is marked. Blood pressure response to the *Valsalva maneuver* has been proposed as an improved means for assessing volume overload status. As volume increases, there is an exaggerated increase in the initial rise in blood pressure that occurs shortly after the onset of bearing down but a loss of the rebound increase in blood pressure that typically occurs after relaxation. This can be elicited by inflating the blood pressure cuff to 15 mm Hg above systolic pressure during normal respiration and listening for the return of Korotkoff sounds during and after the Valsalva maneuver.

Clinical Recognition of Systolic and Diastolic Dysfunction

Identifying the underlying pathophysiology can facilitate management, but making the distinction between systolic and diastolic dysfunction on clinical grounds can be difficult because the symptoms are similar in both forms of heart failure. Diastolic dysfunction is suggested by findings indicative of LV hypertrophy (i.e., a history of hypertension, S_4, LV lift, little displacement of the apical impulse). Systolic dysfunction is associated with causes and findings leading to LV dilation (i.e., a history of myocardial infarction, S_3, displaced apical impulse, mitral regurgitant murmur).

Laboratory Diagnosis

The absence of diagnostic clinical findings in early stages of CHF and the lack of diagnostic sensitivity and specificity for those manifestations that develop later lead to the need for considerable reliance on laboratory testing.

Chest X-Ray

The plain chest film remains an excellent, readily available test for the diagnosis of CHF. Characteristic findings include *upper zone flow redistribution* ("*cephalization*"), *cardiomegaly*, and signs of interstitial edema (*prominent interstitial markings*, *Kerley "B" lines*, and *perihilar haziness*). Patients who develop CHF only during exertion may not show characteristic interstitial edema changes on plain film, but cardiomegaly and upper zone redistribution may be present. The sensitivity of the chest film for cardiomegaly is about 80%.

Electrocardiogram

The electrocardiogram (ECG) is not particularly sensitive or specific, but its ready availability and capacity to detect atrial fibrillation, prior infarction, LV hypertrophy, left-bundle-branch block, and left atrial enlargement make it a useful addition to workup, with likelihood ratios in the range of 2 to 4. The absence of ECG abnormalities reduces the probability of heart failure (negative likelihood ratio, 0.65).

Cardiac Doppler-Ultrasound Study

Heart failure diagnosis and management benefit greatly from the use of cardiac ultrasound. When combined with Doppler study (for the determination of blood flow), ultrasound provides both measurement of ejection fraction and detection of diastolic dysfunction. It allows determinations of *ejection fraction*, *chamber size*, *wall thickness*, and *diastolic filling*, as well as detection of *valvular* and *wall motion abnormalities*, greatly extending the information obtained by clinical assessment and chest x-ray. It is the test of choice for the detection of diastolic dysfunction (EF >0.45, reduced diastolic filling) and can help to reveal its cause (e.g., left ventricular hypertrophy, ischemia). It is also an effective means of diagnosing systolic dysfunction (EF <0.45, LV dilation, mitral regurgitation). The test is the procedure of choice for the assessment of suspected CHF, both systolic and diastolic; it makes it possible to detect CHF in the preclinical stages of illness, when intervention may be the most efficacious. Despite its great utility, the test is underutilized in community practice.

Serum B-Type Natriuretic Peptide (BNP) Level

Natriuretic peptides are released by cardiac tissue in response to the vasoconstriction and sodium retention that accompany CHF. In the setting of acute dyspnea, elevations in B-type natriuretic peptide (>100 pg/mL) correlate strongly with the diagnosis, severity, and prognosis of CHF. Levels are greatest in systolic dysfunction, but they are also elevated in diastolic disease, although to a lesser extent. Test characteristics include a sensitivity of 90% and a specificity of 76%; the positive predictive value in the setting of suspected CHF is 79%, and the negative predictive value is 89%. Compared with other history, physical, and laboratory findings for CHF, its elevation is among the most predictive of CHF (odds ratio, 29.6). B-type natriuretic peptide or its prohormone (proBNP) can be measured conveniently with the use of a rapid assay. Serum levels do not correlate with ejection fraction, but the test's high sensitivity has been suggested as a means of determining who should undergo echocardiographic testing. A BNP of less than 100 pg/mL in a dyspneic patient virtually rules out heart failure (be it systolic or diastolic). The use of BNP has also been suggested as an improved means of determining volume status and response to diuretic therapy—physical examination is notoriously insensitive.

Classification

Congestive heart failure patients can be classified by functional status and stage of disease.

By Functional Status

The traditional approach to classification of CHF patients has been to use the *New York Heart Association* (NYHA) *functional classification* system: *Class I* patients are asymptomatic, *class II* patients have symptoms only with marked exertion, *class III* patients have symptoms with more modest activity, and *class IV* patients have symptoms at rest. Most studies of CHF select patients by functional class. Functional class is also a determinant of prognosis. In persons with a low ejection fraction, yearly mortality is 10% to 15% for class II patients, 15% to 25% for class III patients, and 30% to 50% for class IV patients.

By Stage of Disease

The recognition of the progressive nature of CHF has led to the classification by stage of disease (see prior discussion). As such, it is useful as a guide to management and is being referred to increasingly in the literature and in clinical guidelines.

PRINCIPLES OF MANAGEMENT

Overview of Strategy (1, 2,6,8–10,21, 22,29,33–36)

The basic elements of the management strategy are attending to risk factors, underlying etiologies, and precipitating factors

and treating etiologically and pathophysiologically as early and as often as possible. The realization that CHF is a progressive yet potentially preventable and reversible condition that can lead to irreversible remodeling underscores the importance of early diagnosis and treatment.

Screening for and Treating CHF Risk Factors and Underlying Etiologies

Heart failure is potentially preventable. There is ample evidence of the morbidity and mortality benefits associated with screening for and treating the major risk factors for CHF (e.g., *hypertension* [see Chapters 14, 19, and 26], *hyperlipidemia* [see Chapters 15 and Chapters 27], coronary artery disease [see Chapters 20, 30, and 31], diabetes mellitus [see Chapters 94 and 102], valvular heart disease [see Chapter 33], and atrial fibrillation [see Chapter 28]). For example, the treatment of hypertension with agents that achieve regression of left ventricular hypertrophy greatly improves the prognosis (see Chapter 26). Catheter ablation of atrial fibrillation that restores sinus rhythm enhances cardiac function, symptoms, exercise capacity, and quality of life. Similar benefits may accrue from eliminating high dietary *sodium* intake in obese persons as another independent risk factor that requires attention (see Chapters 26), as does hypothyroidism (see Chapter 104).

Identifying persons at high risk for CHF can be achieved by an office examination and a scoring system derived from the community-based Framingham Heart Study. Elements of the scoring system for estimating probability of CHF include age, systolic blood pressure, heart rate, LVH on ECG, evidence of coronary or valvular heart disease, diabetes, cardiomegaly on chest x-ray, and forced expiratory capacity (Tables 32.1 and 32.2). The use of such a system facilitates the identification of persons who require intensive medical therapy and helps overcome the underutilization of effective therapies.

Correction of Precipitating Factors

Attention to precipitating factors is another priority. Acute *ischemia* (see Chapter 30), severe anemia (see Chapter 82), high fever (see Chapter 11), atrial fibrillation and other supraventricular tachycardias (see Chapter 28), pneumonia (see Chapter 52), pulmonary embolization (see Chapter 35), thyroid disease (see Chapters 103 and 104), excess salt intake, marked obesity (see Chapter 233), and emotional stress (see Chapter 31) may worsen or precipitate failure in patients with decreased myocardial reserve. *Obstructive sleep apnea* may exacerbate the neurohumoral stimuli of heart failure, and therapy with continuous positive airway pressure can improve the ejection fraction, but its effects on CHF outcomes remain to be established. Although anemia may precipitate or worsen CHF, the use of recombinant *erythropoietin* does not reduce CHF morbidity or mortality and may increase the risk of thrombotic events. *Statin* therapy reduces the risk for death and hospitalization independent of the presence of underlying coronary disease. Acute intake of *alcohol* has no deleterious effect on cardiac function and may modestly reduce afterload.

Review of medications is also essential, especially the use of commonly prescribed, negatively inotropic cardiac drugs (e.g., *verapamil, disopyramide*), agents that cause sodium retention (e.g., *thiazolidinediones* [*glitazones*], which are used in diabetes), and medications that might depress prostaglandin-dependent vasodilatory responses (e.g., *nonsteroidal antiinflammatory drugs* [NSAIDs]). Many CHF patients may have been prescribed a *calcium-channel blocker* for the control of angina or hypertension. With the exception

TABLE 32.1

PROBABILITY OF CONGESTIVE HEART FAILURE WITHIN 4 YEARS FOR MEN AGED 45 TO 94 YEARS WITH CORONARY DISEASE, HYPERTENSION, OR VALVULAR DISEASE

Variables	Points									
	0	+1	+2	+3	+4	+5	+6	+7	+8	+9
Age, yr	45–49	50–54	55–59	60–64	65–69	70–74	75–79	80–84	85–89	90–94
Systolic blood pressure, mm Hg	<120	120–139	140–169	170–189	190–219	>219				
Heart rate, beats/min	<55	55–64	65–79	80–89	90–104	>104				
LVH on ECG	No				Yes					
Coronary heart disease	No									
Valve disease	No					Yes			Yes	
Diabetes	No	Yes								

Points	4-Year Probability of Congestive Heart Failure, %	Points	4-Year Probability of Congestive Heart Failure, %
5	1	24	30
10	2	25	34
12	3	26	39
14	5	27	44
16	8	28	49
18	11	29	54
20	16	30	59
22	22		

Excludes forced vital capacity and cardiomegaly.
ECG, electrocardiogram; LVH, left ventricular hypertrophy.
From Kannel WB, D'Agostino RB, Silbershatz H, et al. Arch Intern Med 1999;159:1197, with permission.

TABLE 32.2

PROBABILITY OF CONGESTIVE HEART FAILURE WITHIN 4 YEARS FOR WOMEN FOR AGED 45 TO 94 YEARS WITH CORONARY DISEASE, HYPERTENSION, OR VALVULAR DISEASES

Variables	Points									
	0	+1	+2	+3	+4	+5	+6	+7	+8	+9
Age, yr	45–49	50–54	55–59	60–64	65–69	70–74	75–79	80–84	85–89	90–94
Systolic blood pressure, mm Hg	<120	120–139	140–169	170–189	190–219	>219				
Heart rate, beats/min	<55	55–64	65–79	80–89	90–104	>104				
LVH on ECG	No				Yes					
Coronary heart disease	No								Yes	
Valve disease	No				Yes					
Diabetes	No	Yes								

Points	4-Year Probability of Congestive Heart Failure, %	Points	4-Year Probability of Congestive Heart Failure, %
5	1	24	30
10	2	25	34
12	3	26	39
14	5	27	44
16	8	28	49
18	11	29	54
20	16	30	59
22	22		

ECG electrocardiogram; LVH, left ventricular hypertrophy.
From Kannel WB, D'Agostino RB, Silbershatz H, et al. Arch Intern Med 1999;159:1197, with permission.

of amlodipine, calcium-channel blocker use in CHF is associated with a significant increase in the risks of worsening heart failure, life-threatening arrhythmias, myocardial infarction, and death. NSAID use is associated with CHF relapses.

Treating Pathophysiologically

Countering the major dysfunctional neurohumoral compensatory mechanisms of CHF can reduce symptoms, slow disease progression, and improve outcomes. *ACE inhibitors* and *angiotensin-receptor antagonists* block the heightened activity of the angiotensin–renin–aldosterone system, reducing both preload and afterload and extending survival. *Beta-blockers* blunt the excessive catecholamine response, slowing heart rate and reducing the stimulus to remodel. *Diuretics* correct volume overload. When applied in a timely fashion, such therapies have the potential to improve symptoms and outcomes across a wide range of patients. In advanced stages of heart failure, direct *aldosterone inhibition* and *cardiac glycoside* therapy can be helpful; mechanisms of action probably extend beyond diuresis and enhanced contractility to effects on remodeling and neurohumoral responses. Program design also benefits from attention to whether the predominant underlying pathophysiology is systolic or diastolic dysfunction.

Treatment of Systolic Dysfunction. Patients with systolic dysfunction achieve symptomatic relief and improved outcomes with a combination of *ACE inhibition, beta-blockade,* and *diuretic therapy.* Although the use of beta-blockade may seem paradoxical in the setting of a reduced ejection fraction, its use actually improves hemodynamics and outcomes by countering the heightened sympathetic stimulation of heart failure, even in the early stages of disease. *Cardiac glycosides* (e.g., *digoxin*) have been relegated to a supporting role, failing to show a survival benefit but being of symptomatic value in persons with a marked reduction in ejection fraction and persistent symptoms. Directly *inhibiting aldosterone* can provide an additional benefit in advanced heart failure. The *avoidance* of *NSAIDs* and *calcium-channel blockers* is essential because these drugs can precipitate fluid retention and cardiac decompensation.

Treatment of Diastolic Dysfunction. Standard combination medical therapy for heart failure improves diastolic function. Tight control of blood pressure, heart rate, and ischemia are top priorities, typically achieved with *ACE inhibitors* and *beta-blockers* early in the course of illness. Maintenance of a ventricular response rate that enables adequate time for diastolic filling and coronary perfusion is essential to ensuring diastolic relaxation. *Diuretics* can help to alleviate volume overload, but excessive diuretic use should be avoided because reduced preload can compromise the filling of a stiff ventricle.

Angiotensin-Converting-Enzyme Inhibitors (1,10,12,37–47)

Rationale for Use

Agents have long been sought that would act safely on both the arterial bed (to reduce impedance to the ejection of blood from the left ventricle) and on the venous bed (to decrease preload and reduce pulmonary and systemic venous congestion). With the advent of ACE inhibitors came the opportunity to achieve both goals with a single agent and in a more physiologically advantageous manner. Randomized trials comparing the combined use of hydralazine and nitrates with an ACE inhibitor

(e.g., the Vasodilator-Heart Failure Trial) found the latter to be superior, probably by virtue of less stimulation of adverse neurohumoral responses.

By acting on both the arterial and venous sides of the circulation, ACE inhibitors decrease left ventricular filling pressure and increasing cardiac output. They bind to a receptor on angiotensin-converting enzyme, preventing the formation of angiotensin II, a potent vasoconstrictor and stimulant of renin and aldosterone secretion. In addition, they inhibit bradykinin metabolism, leading to increases in vascular endothelial levels of this vasodilator. By inhibiting neurohumoral counterregulatory forces and increasing tissue bradykinins, they prevent remodeling and exert vasodilatory and natriuretic effects.

Unlike digitalis (the efficacy of which is confined to patients with significant systolic dysfunction), ACE inhibitors have been found to be effective in most CHF patients, whether they are suffering systolic or diastolic dysfunction and whether they have mild, moderate, or severe disease. Several landmark studies (e.g., the Cooperative North Scandinavian Enalapril Survival Study, the Studies Of Left Ventricular Dysfunction) have documented this broad spectrum of efficacy, demonstrating significant reductions in cardiac *mortality* and *morbidity*, as well as improvements in heart size, symptoms, and medication requirements.

Despite their proven efficacy, ACE inhibitors are still not sufficiently prescribed. Surveys of community practice show underutilization by primary care physicians for persons with CHF. This has prompted recommendations that ACE inhibitor use in CHF be considered a quality measure for primary care physicians.

Choice of Agent

Cost and convenience are the two major considerations because there is little evidence of other major differences among available agents. Generic captopril is the least expensive, but it has the disadvantage of requiring administration three times daily. Generic formulations of once-daily preparations (e.g., lisinopril) are available and much less expensive than brand-name preparations. In the few randomized, controlled studies directly comparing ACE inhibitors for the treatment of chronic CHF, both longer- and shorter-acting preparations proved to be similarly effective, although the longer-acting agents tended to have a greater propensity to cause prolonged hypotension, especially when used in high doses. With patent expiration pending for many of the proprietary ACE inhibitors, cost and choice of agent should improve.

Initiating Therapy and Minimizing Adverse Effects

ACE-inhibitor therapy should be prescribed as first-line treatment for CHF, starting with its use to treat risk factors such as diabetes, hypertension, and coronary disease (stage A) and continuing as evidence of structural change develops, even before symptoms ensue (stage B). As noted, early treatment produces significant reductions in morbidity and mortality and helps to prevent disease progression.

Hypotension. Because hypotension is common at the onset of therapy (especially in the elderly), it is recommended to start with *small doses* (e.g., as little as 6.25 mg of captopril, 2.5 to 5.0 mg of lisinopril) and *reduce any concurrent diuretic therapy.* The dose is then increased gradually to the doses associated with a survival benefit (e.g., captopril 50 mg three times a day, lisinopril 20 to 40 mg/d). Monitoring *blood pressure* is important not only to ensure adequate renal perfusion, but also to minimize dizziness and falls. Most CHF patients are elderly and can be very susceptible to even mild degrees of cerebral hypoperfusion. Continuous blood pressure monitoring is needed because the onset of hypotension may be delayed for a few weeks and yet persist.

Renal Dysfunction. Patients with preexisting bilateral renal artery stenosis and those receiving very large ACE-inhibitor doses are at greatest risk for renal impairment, limiting their use under such circumstances. Minor elevations in serum creatinine can be seen with the initiation of therapy due to changes in intrarenal hemodynamics, but these elevations are usually due to minor changes in intrarenal hemodynamics and are self-limited; they are not progressive. Monitoring of renal function (blood urea nitrogen [BUN], creatinine, urinalysis) is indicated. Any progressive deterioration in renal function requires dose reduction and close watching; rarely is the total discontinuation of therapy necessary unless there is renal artery stenosis or severe hypotension.

Hyperkalemia. Because ACE inhibitors reduce aldosterone levels, the *serum potassium* may rise and should be monitored, particularly in patients with preexisting renal dysfunction or those receiving potassium supplementation, a potassium-sparing diuretic, or an aldosterone inhibitor. In many instances, potassium supplementation or use of a potassium-sparing agent can be discontinued or at least reduced.

Cough and Angioedema. A dry, irritant nocturnal cough affects as many as 10% of users. It is believed to be triggered by increased levels of tissue kinins associated with the inhibition of kinin metabolism in slow metabolizers. The cough can interfere with sleep, causing the patient to stop the drug. Angioedema is less common but is believed to develop by a similar mechanism; persons prone to idiopathic angioedema should avoid taking ACE-inhibitor therapy. Those with unacceptable cough can consider a change in therapy.

Alternatives in Patients Intolerant to ACE-Inhibitor Therapy: Use of Angiotensin II Receptor Blockade and Other Vasodilators

A number of options are available for those who cannot tolerate ACE-inhibitor therapy or who have acute decompensation and require additional vasodilation.

Angiotensin II Receptor Blockade (ARB). These agents act at the receptor level to inhibit angiotensin II, which provides the vasodilating activity associated with angiotensin II blockade without increasing vascular endothelial kinins and triggering the bothersome cough and other kinin-attributed side effects associated with ACE-inhibitor therapy. Important clinical outcomes are similar to those achieved with ACE-inhibitors. A randomized trial comparing ARB treatment with ACE-inhibitor therapy (the Evaluation of Losartan in the Elderly study) showed similarly significant beneficial effects on morbidity and mortality but no particular survival or functional advantage of one class over the other. A meta-analysis of use in high-risk persons with chronic heart failure and systolic dysfunction found equal reductions in all-cause mortality and heart failure hospitalizations but no additional benefit when both agents were used together. Use in diastolic dysfunction is less well studied, but the data suggests similar efficacy. Because these drugs are expensive and not yet available generically, they should be reserved for persons who cannot tolerate ACE inhibitors.

Combination therapy with an *ACE inhibitor* for enhanced angiotensin blockade reduces the hospitalization rate for heart failure but not overall mortality; moreover, it markedly increases the rates of complications (e.g., hyperkalemia, worsening renal function, symptomatic hypotension).

Hydralazine/Isosorbide. Although largely replaced by ACE-inhibitor therapy, the combination vasodilator program of hydralazine and isosorbide has sufficient survival and hemodynamic benefits to warrant its consideration as an alternative in patients who cannot tolerate ACE inhibition or afford ARB therapy. Moreover, the use of a fixed-dose combination preparation (37.5 mg hydralazine/20 mg isosorbide) three times daily in blacks with stage III or IV systolic heart failure (EF <0.35) significantly increased survival and quality of life and reduced the rate of first hospitalization. These findings suggest that nitric oxide delivery is an important pathophysiologic factor in heart failure among blacks and that adding the combination to standard therapy is a reasonable consideration in those with advanced-stage disease. Cost is modest when these drugs are prescribed separately but are increased substantially with the use of the combination preparation. Disadvantages include postural hypotension, the need for frequent dosing, and reflex tachycardia. There is a small risk of lupus-like syndrome with prolonged hydralazine use.

Calcium-Channel Blockers. These coronary vasodilators are widely prescribed for use in coronary disease (see Chapter 30) and hypertension (see Chapter 26), and, consequently, many patients who develop CHF may already be taking one. Their safety for use in CHF has been put into question because of results of well-designed studies revealing significant increases in the rates of worsening heart failure, life-threatening arrhythmias, myocardial infarction, and death associated with their intake, particularly in patients with coronary disease and a low ejection fraction.

The mechanisms responsible for these cardiac complications are poorly understood. It was believed that the reflex tachycardia and negative inotropic effects of many of these agents were responsible, but the use of agents free of these effects does not lower the risk. Of the calcium-channel blockers, only *amlodipine* has been proven to be safe for use in anginal patients with severe chronic left ventricular dysfunction (EF <0.30). Of the drugs in its class, it appears to have the least effect on contractility, conductivity, and neurohumoral reflexes, but precisely why it is the best tolerated of the calcium-channel blockers in CHF is unclear. Despite its being better tolerated, amlodipine does not improve survival, carries a 5% risk of inducing pulmonary edema, and will remain expensive until generic formulations become available.

In sum, calcium-channel blockers should be avoided in patients with CHF; those who develop CHF while taking a calcium-channel blocker for angina or hypertension should be switched to agents whose benefits extend to CHF (e.g., ACE inhibitors, ARBs, beta-blockers). If calcium-channel–blocker therapy is deemed essential (e.g., persistent angina), one should consider amlodipine and obtain cardiac consultation.

Beta-Blockers (1,10,12,48–61)

Rationale for Use

Increased appreciation for the role of the sympathetic nervous system in the response to and perpetuation of CHF has led to the application of beta-blockade for treatment. As discussed earlier, sympathetic stimulation is one of the major dysfunctional neurohumoral responses to heart failure, increasing with severity of disease and serving as an independent predictor of mortality. By blocking catechol-mediated myocardial stimulation and its adverse contributions to ventricular remodeling and hemodynamics (e.g., increased heart rate, increased peripheral resistance, decreased contractility), beta-blockers can slow disease progression and enhance functional status and survival. Reverse remodeling has been observed with beta-blocker use. Both cardioselective and nonselective beta-blockers (e.g., *metoprolol-XL*, *bisoprolol*, *carvedilol*) have been shown to be effective. Use in combination with an ACE inhibitor achieves significant improvement in outcomes. Given their proven benefit, it is unfortunate that beta-blockers are underutilized in the treatment of CHF, probably as a consequence of concern about side effects and the seemingly paradoxical idea of using a negatively inotropic agent to improve cardiac performance.

Adverse Effects

At the outset of therapy, there may be *fluid retention* (manifested by an increase in weight) due to decreased renal perfusion. *Bradycardia* and *heart block* may occur with the use of high doses, especially in persons with underlying sinus node or conduction system disease; low doses may be tolerated. *Postural hypotension* can be problematic, especially on the initiation of therapy with carvedilol, due to its alpha-blocking action; the problem decreases with continued use. Separating the time of daily intake for beta-blocker and ACE-inhibitor administration can help to limit the risk of postural hypotension. The analysis of adverse effects and benefits associated with beta-blocker therapy finds, on balance, that the risks are well worth taking, given the likelihood of significant reductions in cardiac morbidity and mortality.

Choice of Agent and Patient Selection

The three beta-blockers studied to date (*metoprolol-XL*, *bisoprolol*, *carvedilol*) span the spectrum of agents in this class, suggesting that differences among beta-blockers are less important than their similarities. On a theoretical basis, blockade of the entire adrenergic system should be more favorable hemodynamically than blockade limited to cardiac beta receptors. In a large-scale, randomized, controlled study of this question (carvedilol vs. metoprolol, the Carvedilol or Metoprolol European Trial), carvedilol achieved a 15% greater reduction in mortality at 5 years but no significant difference in a combined endpoint of hospitalization and death. This survival advantage for carvedilol should be weighed against its greater tendency to cause orthostatic hypotension (see later discussion) and its high cost (about four times that of the branded long-acting formulation of metoprolol).

Benefit appears to accrue across the entire spectrum of disease stages and functional classes, although data on use in asymptomatic persons are more limited. Groups initially underrepresented in major studies (women, blacks, the very elderly) also appear to benefit. Persons with CHF related to hypertension and coronary artery disease do especially well with beta-blockade, but so do those with idiopathic dilated cardiomyopathy, with functional improvement related to changes in myocardial gene expression. Patients should be hemodynamically stable and relatively euvolemic at the time of initiating therapy. Contraindications to beta-blocker use in CHF include severe bronchospastic disease (although modest doses of a cardioselective beta-blocker may be tolerated), symptomatic bradycardia, and advanced heart block. Diabetes mellitus and a history of bronchospastic disease are not contraindications.

Initiating Therapy

Patients need to be warned that symptoms may worsen a bit during the first few weeks of beta-blocker treatment and that it may take several weeks for clinical benefit to become evident. To minimize adverse effects early on, doses at first should be small (e.g., metoprolol-XL 25 mg/d, carvedilol 3.25 mg/d) and titrated upward slowly. The immediate goal is a resting heart rate of 50 to 60 beats/min. Diuretic therapy may be necessary to counter the fluid retention that can develop early on.

Diuretics (1,10,12,23)

Rationale for Use

Diuretics are a key component of symptomatic therapy. They are directed at the volume overload that complicates heart failure. The degree of compensatory fluid retention in CHF is typically excessive, leading to pulmonary congestion and/or peripheral edema. In patients with mild to moderate CHF, symptoms of volume overload respond acutely to diuretic therapy. However, diuretic therapy alone is usually insufficient for the chronic treatment of CHF, in part because it stimulates the renin–angiotensin system and raises serum catecholamines, leading to increased afterload, reduced cardiac output, and further sodium retention. Consequently, concurrent ACE inhibition and beta-blockade are required.

Although diuretics may be effective in controlling peripheral edema and pulmonary congestion, most do little to prevent the progression of heart failure or improve prognosis. However, the selective inhibitors of aldosterone (although weak diuretics) improve survival when added to a disease-modifying program. There is suspicion that their effect on outcomes may be related as much to effects on remodeling as to improvements in volume status.

Overzealous use of diuretics can be counterproductive, producing prerenal azotemia or a dangerous fall in filling pressure (particularly important in diastolic dysfunction). Moreover, escalating diuretic therapy in mitral or aortic valve disease may inappropriately delay the timing of surgical therapy (see Chapter 33).

Preparations

Thiazides. These are sulfonamide derivatives, and are believed to inhibit sodium reabsorption in the cortical tubule. Although the number of thiazide preparations is large, they differ only in cost and duration of action. Most are very inexpensive and available generically (e.g., hydrochlorothiazide, chlorthalidone). Thiazides cause modest potassium depletion, which can be clinically important if there is underlying heart disease, especially in the setting of ventricular irritability, ischemia, or use of digitalis. Under such circumstances, careful monitoring for hypokalemia and assiduous potassium supplementation or use of a potassium-sparing diuretic may be needed. Mild hyperglycemia and hyperuricemia may result but are usually of little clinical significance (see Chapters 102 and 155). During the first 7 to 10 days of therapy, the serum calcium may rise, but it will stay elevated indefinitely only in patients with underlying hyperparathyroidism. Absorption from the gastrointestinal tract is rapid; the onset of action is 1 hour, and the half-life is 12 to 24 hours.

Metolazone. This sulfonamide diuretic is similar to the thiazides in site of action (cortical tubule) but possesses a longer half-life and is more effective in patients with impaired renal function. The effective half-life is 24 to 48 hours, compared with 12 to 24 hours for the thiazides. Because it is a sulfonamide, it shares many of the same side effects, such as hypokalemia, hyperglycemia, and hyperuricemia. The maximum daily dose is 10 to 20 mg. Metolazone can be combined with a loop diuretic for use in very refractory cases in which volume overload is a major problem.

Loop Diuretics. These potent agents act at the loop of Henle. Examples include *furosemide, ethacrynic acid, bumetanide,* and *torsemide.* With some of these drugs (e.g., furosemide) absorption can be erratic in CHF; torsemide absorption is more consistent than that of furosemide. For furosemide, the onset of action is 30 to 60 minutes; effects last 4 to 8 hours. Caution must be exercised with their use because serious volume depletion may occur. Frequent urination is a common complaint; evening doses should be avoided if possible. The starting dose of furosemide is 20 to 40 mg/d. Prerenal azotemia (manifested by a BUN–creatinine ratio of >20:1), postural hypotension, lightheadedness, and fatigue are clues to marked hypovolemia. Hypokalemia is the most serious metabolic consequence, necessitating careful monitoring of the serum potassium and supplementation should it fall to less than 3.5 mg/dL. Mild hyperglycemia and hyperuricemia may also occur. Ethacrynic acid is potentially ototoxic, especially when used in combination with an aminoglycoside antibiotic such as kanamycin. Audiograms should be obtained if ethacrynic acid is to be given for a prolonged period.

Aldosterone Blockers. The selective aldosterone-receptor antagonists (*spironolactone, eplerenone*) help to counter the excessive aldosterone secretion of advanced heart failure. Even with the use of ACE inhibition, aldosterone levels can reach 20 times normal, providing the rationale for adding a selective aldosterone blocker (survival benefit may also be linked to effects on remodeling that are additive to effects on volume status). Serious *hyperkalemia* may occur with the use of these agents, particularly in the setting of renal failure or treatment programs that include ACE inhibition, ARB therapy, or potassium supplementation. Frequent serum potassium determinations and discontinuation of potassium supplementation are essential. These drugs should not be used in renal failure, because life-threatening hyperkalemia may ensue. Spironolactone, but not eplerenone, can cause gynecomastia and breast pain in chronic users; there is also a question of increased risk of carcinogenesis with long-term use, but this is supported only by animal data.

Combination Preparations. Combinations containing a thiazide and a weak potassium-sparing diuretic (e.g., amiloride, triamterene) are heavily promoted. Although they are convenient to use and may facilitate compliance, they are expensive, and their fixed ratio limits dosing flexibility. Before prescribing such a preparation, the proper dose of each agent should be determined separately. The combination preparation is reasonable to use only if it can provide the exact doses desired. Many combinations contain subtherapeutic thiazide doses. Their onset of action is slow; the full effect may take up to 1 week to become evident. They should be used with caution, if at all, in persons taking ACE inhibitors, because of the risk of hyperkalemia.

Selection of Agent and Initiation of Therapy

When symptoms are slight (mild exertional dyspnea, minor ankle edema) or when the patient is asymptomatic but showing weight gain or x-ray findings indicative of early CHF, then diuretic therapy can be initiated with a *thiazide* (e.g., 25 to 50 mg/d of hydrochlorothiazide). The degree of dyspnea on exertion and weight change are the simplest clinical parameters to follow for gauging response to therapy in mild cases.

An increasing severity of symptoms is an indication for switching to a *loop diuretic* (e.g., *furosemide* or *ethacrynic acid*). Small doses of loop diuretics may also benefit patients with mild to moderate failure that cannot be adequately controlled by thiazides. Caution is warranted when treating a patient for the first time with a loop diuretic because a marked diuresis may be evoked, particularly with the use of a parenteral dose but sometimes with an oral dose. If a thiazide had been used previously, it should be stopped rather than continued in conjunction with the loop diuretic because the two agents are very potent when used together (see later discussion). If hypokalemia is a problem, potassium supplementation (see Appendix 32.1) or the use of a weak *potassium-sparing diuretic* (e.g., *amiloride, triamterene*) is indicated.

Use in Severe Congestive Heart Failure

In severe CHF, the absorption of oral loop diuretics declines, which accounts for the oft-noted reduction in efficacy during an exacerbation of heart failure. The maximal effect of a loop diuretic can be achieved by using a *large, single, daily dose* rather than divided doses. Parenteral administration of the drug or high-dose oral therapy is required to achieve diuresis. At times, supplementing oral therapy with an occasional *parenteral dose* in the office will suffice to counter worsening failure refractory to oral therapy. *Adding a thiazide* to the diuretic program may be useful in failure refractory to large doses of the loop diuretic alone. Alternatively, one can consider switching to *torsemide,* a loop diuretic with a more consistent absorption and bioavailability. For patients with renal impairment, *metolazone* can be useful as the adjunct. It is similar in potency to the thiazides but more effective in the setting of azotemia.

In the context of severe disease with high aldosterone secretion, an *aldosterone receptor antagonist* (e.g., *spironolactone, eplerenone*) can be considered. It enhances sodium excretion and improves outcomes (15% to 20% reductions in cardiac morbidity and mortality) when used in conjunction with ACE inhibition, beta-blockade, and loop diuretics. The mechanism of action may extend beyond diuresis to reducing collagen synthesis and cardiac remodeling. When small doses (e.g., 25 to 50 mg/d) of spironolactone or eplerenone are added to a program of maximal medical therapy, there are significant improvements in survival (Randomized Aldactone Evaluation Study [RALES], Epleronone Post-Acute Myocardial Infarction Heart Failure Efficacy and Survival Study [EPHESUS]). If an aldosterone antagonist is added to the standard maximal program, monitoring for hyperkalemia is essential, and potassium supplementation should be stopped or limited to persons who manifest a serum potassium of less than 3.5 mg/dL despite therapy.

Monitoring Diuretic Therapy

Monitoring *postural signs, BUN,* and *creatinine* is essential to avoid excess volume depletion and severe prerenal azotemia. When a potassium-wasting diuretic is being used in conjunction with digitalis therapy, it is critical carefully to monitor the *serum potassium* (see Appendix 32.1). The incidence of digitalis toxicity rises appreciably in the setting of hypokalemia. *Magnesium* depletion may also be triggered by diuretic therapy and contribute to digitalis sensitivity and refractory hypokalemia. Use of a potassium-sparing drug necessitates watching for hyperkalemia and discontinuing chronic potassium supplementation once any hypokalemia is corrected.

Digitalis (10,12,62–68)

Rationale

Once the centerpiece of treatment for CHF based on the view that the drug enhances contractility, cardiac glycosides now make a much more modest contribution to CHF management because major randomized, controlled studies (e.g., the Digitalis Investigation Group [DIG] trial) failed to find a survival benefit at therapeutic serum levels. The only significant benefit (aside from rate control in patients with atrial fibrillation; see Chapter 28) was a reduction in hospital admissions noted for severely symptomatic persons in sinus rhythm with marked systolic dysfunction (e.g., NYHA class III and IV disease, EF <0.25, audible S$_3$, marked left ventricular dilation). Post hoc analyses of the DIG trial data reveal increased mortality among patients with a serum digoxin level greater than 1.2 ng/mL (well within the traditional "therapeutic" range of 0.9 to 2.0 ng/mL for enhancing contractility) but a trend toward improved survival at lower digoxin levels (0.5 to 0.8). Such findings suggest that the benefit from cardiac glycosides might be more related to neurohumoral effects than improvements in contractility. Confirmation of the post hoc findings by prospective study is needed to test this hypothesis and more precisely define the contribution of cardiac glycosides to CHF management. For now, in patients in sinus rhythm, digitalis preparations are relegated to a secondary role.

Indications for Use

Pending new data, it appears prudent to limit the consideration of cardiac glycoside therapy to patients with marked systolic dysfunction who are already taking a full medical regimen of first-line agents (loop diuretic, ACE inhibitor, beta-blockade) and not achieving adequate symptomatic relief. Recent myocardial infarction is not a contraindication to digoxin use (there is no excess mortality). Other indications include heart failure induced by *rapid atrial fibrillation* (see Chapter 28), CHF resulting from uncontrolled hypertension, or severe aortic stenosis (but only for the short term and not as a substitute for blood pressure reduction [see Chapter 26] or valve surgery [see Chapter 33]). Efficacy in *cor pulmonale* is in question; the drug is occasionally beneficial, but the results are not impressive, and the risks of toxicity are increased in the setting of hypoxia.

Digitalis preparations are of little use in heart failure resulting from hypertrophic cardiomyopathies, whether they are idiopathic or due to longstanding hypertension (a common etiology among outpatients, especially women). Patients with idiopathic hypertrophic subaortic stenosis may develop worsening outflow tract obstruction with the use of digitalis. In addition, there is no proven benefit in cases of mitral stenosis (in the absence of atrial fibrillation) or during episodes of CHF due to transient ischemia.

Choice of Preparation and Pharmacokinetics

Digoxin is the preparation of choice. In the past, some variation in bioavailability was noted among different brands, but this has long been corrected. The half-life of digoxin is 36 hours; the onset of action is 1 to 2 hours when taken orally. *Absorption* from the gastrointestinal tract ranges from 50% to 75% complete and remains adequate in CHF but may fall in severe cases of malabsorption. *Excretion* is renal and decreases significantly with reduction in creatinine clearance.

Dose adjustments are sometimes necessary. Digoxin can be used safely in *renal failure* as long as renal function and serum levels are frequently checked and necessary dose adjustments made. Higher doses are not needed in obese patients because there is little lipid deposition. *Thyroid disease* can affect digitalis metabolism; hypothyroidism prolongs the half-life, and hyperthyroidism shortens it. The treatment of thyroid disease needs to be accompanied by an adjustment of digoxin dose. Similarly, *amiodarone* can increase serum digoxin levels both independently and as a consequence of effects on thyroid status.

Initiating and Maintaining Use

Initiation of therapy in clinically stable outpatients can commence with an oral maintenance dose and does not require loading doses. At a maintenance dose of 0.125 to 0.25 mg/d (determined by underlying renal function), one can attain a therapeutic serum level in 5 to 7 days (earlier, if the optimal therapeutic range suggested by the DIG study [0.5 to 0.8 ng/mL] is used). This has led to recommendations for a narrowing of the *therapeutic range* (0.5 to 0.8 ng/mL) and the use of smaller doses (e.g., 0.125 mg/day) both for loading and for maintenance.

Once initiated and if found to be of clinical benefit, digitalis should be continued chronically unless a reversible cause of pump failure has been fully corrected or there is no basis for using the drug in the first place. Patients who respond to digitalis clinically often deteriorate when the drug is withdrawn, even in the context of ACE-inhibitor use.

Monitoring Therapy

Digoxin levels require careful monitoring because of frequently changing renal clearance in CHF and the seriousness of digitalis toxicity. *Serum levels* should be measured at least three to four times per year, more frequently if there are changes in the patient's renal or volume status or if the patient is taking *amiodarone* (which can raise serum digoxin levels). As noted, the conventional target range of 0.9 to 2.0 ng/mL is being supplanted by recommendations for the lower, narrower range of 0.5 to 0.8 ng/mL. A serum sample should be drawn at least 6 hours after the last dose because there is a 4- to 6-hour rise in serum level after an oral dose. In most instances, it is best to have the patient omit the day's dose when coming to the office for a serum determination.

The physician needs to monitor factors that increase the "sensitivity" of the myocardium to the toxic effects of the drug. Such factors include *hypokalemia*, abnormalities in serum *calcium* and *magnesium*, organic heart disease, and pulmonary disease with acute *hypoxia*. Digitalis-induced ST-T–wave changes on the electrocardiogram have no correlation with optimal or toxic dose levels and cannot be used for such determinations. Serum drug levels are necessary.

Digitalis Toxicity

The serum level of digitalis is not in itself diagnostic of *toxicity* because there is considerable overlap in serum concentrations between patients with and patients without evidence of toxicity, but if the *digoxin level is greater than 2.0 ng/mL*, the probability of encountering toxicity increases considerably.

Symptoms of digitalis toxicity can be divided into noncardiac and cardiac manifestations. *Anorexia, nausea, vomiting, diarrhea*, *visual disturbances* including *yellow halos* around lights, and, in rare instances, delirium have been described since the time of William Withering, the British physician who introduced the use of digitalis in the late eighteenth century. *Arrhythmias* are the predominant cardiac manifestation of toxicity. Digitalis can cause any type of rhythm and/or conduction disturbance because it affects the automaticity of myocardial tissues and the conduction system. *Ventricular irritability* (especially bigeminy), *paroxysmal atrial tachycardia* with block, and *junctional tachycardia* are particularly characteristic features of digitalis excess.

The unexplained onset of an arrhythmia in a patient on digitalis raises the possibility of drug-related toxicity. The drug should be withheld; a serum level obtained; potassium, calcium, and magnesium levels checked; and serious consideration given to immediate hospitalization for monitoring and parenteral antiarrhythmic therapy. The high incidence and mortality rate of this preventable and often treatable condition call for vigilance.

If the findings from the DIG study are confirmed, then the definition of digitalis toxicity may need to be extended from the well-described clinical syndrome to the increased mortality risk associated with serum levels greater than 1.2 ng/mL.

Oral Anticoagulation and Antiplatelet Therapy (10,69)

Although CHF is not per se an indication for *warfarin* anticoagulant therapy, its presence can increase the risk for thromboembolic disease by reducing activity and causing leg edema (see Chapter 35). The same holds true for patients in atrial fibrillation who develop CHF (see Chapter 28). The initiation and monitoring of oral anticoagulant therapy require considerable attention to detail (see Chapter 83).

Aspirin use in persons with coronary artery disease complicated by heart failure is associated with a nearly 30% reduction in 1-year mortality. However, there is some concern that the inhibitory effect of aspirin on prostaglandin synthesis might counter some of the beneficial effects of ACE inhibitors in CHF, which appear to be prostaglandin mediated (see prior discussion). Prospective cohort study suggests a dose-related blunting by aspirin of the ACE-inhibitor survival benefit but no adverse effect with low aspirin doses (<160 mg/d).

Nonpharmacologic Measures (10,70,71)

Salt and Water Restrictions

Given the important contribution of excessive sodium intake to the development and exacerbation of CHF, it is essential that salt restriction be part of the basic management program. Many exacerbations are preventable. Patients are initially placed on a *no-added-salt diet* (4 g sodium/d). The patient and family are instructed to prepare and serve meals without the addition of salt and taught to avoid foods with inapparent but high salt content (e.g., cheese, cold cuts, canned soups, canned ham, bacon, catsup, and other processed foods). Rarely is extreme salt restriction (e.g., a 1- to 2-g-sodium diet) urged on the patient because it is often unrealistic, unpalatable, and demoralizing. Fluid restriction is reserved for severe cases that are complicated by hyponatremia.

Allowable Activity and Prescription of Exercise Training

The level of allowable activity needs to be tailored to the patient's medical status, lifestyle, and responsibilities. Patients with symptoms of failure on moderate exertion (NYHA class II disease) can continue to work, provided that reasonable limits are placed on emotional and physical demands. It may be more stressful psychologically (and consequently physically) to have to quit one's job than to continue working in a somewhat more limited capacity. In most instances, the amount of allowable activity can be determined from an office visit by a careful history that elicits the degree of exertion that precipitates symptoms. At times, the symptoms may be out of proportion to physical findings; taking a walk up a flight of stairs with the patient can provide helpful data regarding exercise tolerance. Treadmill testing is sometimes necessary to gauge exercise capacity, especially if the patient has coronary disease and it is unclear whether it is failure or ischemia that is limiting the patient. Regardless of etiology, a daily rest period and a reduction of psychological stress are key means of lessening myocardial work in the patient with failure.

If weight, orthopnea, and exertional dyspnea are increasing, then activity should be further restricted. A few days of bedrest are often beneficial and may obviate the need for hospitalization. The patient with failure who is put to bed should use a footboard or get out of bed periodically to avoid prolonged venous stasis and thrombus formation.

Exercise training has been shown to improve exercise tolerance and stroke volume, as well as reduce the number of hospitalizations, peripheral resistance, and cardiomegaly in patients with stable CHF. Long-term effects on survival are unknown, but the combined endpoint of shorter-term adverse cardiac events and mortality is reduced. Intermittent aerobic exercise with frequent rest breaks helps to maximize the training effect without inducing excessive cardiac stress. Although the ideal training regimen is yet to be defined, commonsense advice can be given for the activity prescription to be carried out at home.

Referral to a formal exercise program can be considered in highly motivated persons who are hemodynamically stable and eager to improve their level of activity. Group classes (e.g., in Tai chi mind–body movement) can be helpful, enhancing both quality of life and functional capacity.

Treatment of Psychological Factors (10,13,72,73)

Psychological factors are underappreciated and often overlooked. *Major depression* is common among CHF patients who require hospitalization and is independently associated with increased rates of readmission and death. It is also a major cause of poor compliance with treatment regimens; selective serotonin reuptake inhibitor (SSRI) antidepressants are well tolerated cardiovascularly (see Chapter 227), making antidepressant therapy a reasonable treatment option in CHF.

Anxiety is also common but less well studied in CHF. Its potential to impair quality of life (e.g., cause unnecessary restriction of activity) and exacerbate adrenergic stimulation argues for its consideration and treatment. There is little data to guide the use of specific pharmacologic therapy for anxiety in CHF (although beta-blockade can help with the catecholamine excess, and SSRIs have some anxiolytic activity), but nonpharmacologic stress reduction measures may help and deserve consideration (see Appendix 226.1).

Emotional and social supports are essential. Long-term study finds that a lack of such supports is associated with increase risks of fatal and nonfatal adverse cardiovascular outcomes. Involving the family and arranging for community resources are essential.

Treatment in the Context of Renal Failure (74)

Renal failure is a frequent accompaniment of CHF, either as a precipitant or as consequence. About one third of CHF patients have renal insufficiency, yet most studies exclude patients with significant azotemia, limiting evidence-based guidance. Nonetheless, some principles have emerged. They are expressed in term of the glomerular filtration rate (GFR), which can be estimated by the Cockcroft–Gault equation:

$$GFR = [(140 - age) \times body\ weight]/[72 \times serum\ creatinine]$$

where age is in years, body weight in kilograms, and serum creatinine in milligrams per deciliter. The equation as it stands is for men. For women, the weight is multiplied by 0.85.

As long as GFR remains greater than 60 mg/mL, all drugs used for CHF can be used with minimal concern. With the fall of GFR to the 30- to 60-mg/mL range, ACE inhibitors, ARBs, and beta-blockers can still be used reasonably safely without major concern, but in severe renal insufficiency (GFR <30 mg/mL), close monitoring of renal function and serum potassium is essential, and dose adjustment downward may be necessary. ARBs offer no advantage over ACE inhibitors in renal failure. Beta-blockers can be used safely in mild to moderate renal failure; those that are not renally excreted (e.g., metoprolol, carvedilol) are probably easier to use. Aldosterone inhibitors should be used cautiously with close monitoring of serum potassium when GFR falls to less than 60 mg/mL and avoided at a GFR of less than 30 mg/mL because of the high risk of severe hyperkalemia. Digoxin can be used in renal insufficiency but requires close monitoring of serum level and frequent dose adjustment.

Treatment of Acute Exacerbations (10,12,75–78)

The prevention of CHF exacerbations is often feasible because most of them are triggered by avoidable events (e.g., noncompliance, dietary indiscretion); moreover, most are heralded by up to 1 week of premonitory symptoms (e.g., weight gain, increasing exertional dyspnea). Continuous monitoring and prompt intervention can stave off an acute hospitalization. When the cause of the exacerbation is more serious (e.g., an acute ischemic event) or has not been detected and treated sufficiently, then the patient is likely to progress to frank pulmonary edema and require immediate hospitalization. Approaches to the inpatient treatment of acute decompensation are beyond the scope of this book, but drugs used for acute intravenous treatment of reversibly decompensated CHF are being promoted by some as outpatient therapy and deserve comment.

Nesiritide/B-Type Natriuretic Peptide

Nesiritide is a genetically formulated preparation of human B-type natriuretic peptide that, when given as an intravenous infusion, provides prompt, short-acting arterial and venous dilation presumably without the hemodynamic risks inherent in the use of conventional intravenous vasodilators such as dobutamine, nitroprusside, and nitroglycerin. Initial reports showed benefit in emergency room care of patients with an acute CHF decompensation. However, subsequent reports have emerged of higher rates of both renal dysfunction and death in placebo-controlled trials. Moreover, no evidence of benefit was found for intermittent outpatient infusion in end-stage disease.

Tolvaptan/Vasopressin-Receptor Antagonist

The use of an orally active *vasopressin-receptor antagonist* (e.g., *tolvaptan*) provides a promising approach to the treatment of acute decompensation and follow-up outpatient care. Patients with acute decompensation often present with hyponatremia, volume overload, and renal insufficiency poorly responsive to loop diuretics. This state is believed to reflect high *vasopressin* activity triggered by heart failure, leading to water retention and vasoconstriction. The *vasopressin-receptor antagonists ("vaptans")* have been developed and applied in this setting of acutely decompensated CHF. Among the short-term benefits noted are reduction in the symptoms and signs of CHF, diuretic requirements, and renal impairment, but there is no effect on long-term CHF morbidity or mortality. More study is needed to help define the spectrum of use for these orally active "aquarectics," especially with regard to use in the nonacute outpatient setting.

Milrinone, Phosphodiesterase Inhibitors

Like nesiritide, the phosphodiesterase inhibitor *milrinone* has been given as an intravenous infusion to persons with acutely decompensated CHF. The drug is a potent inotropic agent, but results have been marred by increased rates of hypotension, arrhythmias, and cardiac death associated with the use of phosphodiesterase inhibitors. Intermittent outpatient infusions to improve contractility and functional status are without established value in persons with advanced-stage disease. Such results underscore the importance of factors other than contractility in determining the outcome of CHF.

Treatment of Advanced Disease (10,12,23,79–85)

Patients with advanced disease (stage D, NYHA class III and IV) experience a very poor quality of life and increased risks of sudden death and death from progressive pump failure. Abnormal intraventricular activation (e.g., widening of the QRS, left-bundle-branch block on ECG) and electrical ventricular dyssynchronization are characteristic of this stage. Cardiac output declines, and life-threatening ventricular dysrhythmias may ensue. Although dire, this stage of illness is amenable to interventions short of transplantation that can improve quality of life, reduce the need for hospitalization, and perhaps prolong survival.

Atriobiventricular Pacemakers and Implantable Defibrillators

Cardiac dyssynchrony and life-threatening dysrhythmias constitute important risks of advanced heart failure, respectively leading to refractory symptoms and reduced survival. Implantation of an atriobiventricular pacemaker (also referred to as *cardiac resynchronization therapy* [CRT]) has been undertaken to counter dyssynchrony in patients with advanced disease

(EF <0.35, QRS >120 msec). Data from randomized, controlled trials reveal improved ejection fraction, exercise capacity, and quality of life and reduced hospitalizations and mortality (the 3-year survival improved by >30%). Resynchronization has no effect on rates of ventricular tachycardia, fibrillation, or ability to cardiovert.

Prophylactic implantation of a *cardioverter–defibrillator* (ICD) in both ischemic and nonischemic CHF patients with advanced systolic heart failure (EF <0.35) is increasingly being used in carefully selected patients. It reduces the risk of sudden cardiac death by 20% to 46%, particularly in patients with NYHA class II or III disease and those with a history of life-threatening ventricular dysrhythmias (see also Chapter 29). The postimplant complication rate is 1.4% for infection, lead placement problems, and device malfunction; 1.2% for death during implantation. The rate of inappropriate discharges is 19%. Compared to ICD, *amiodarone* shows no reduction in sudden death in CHF patients (see Chapter 29).

These encouraging results and Food and Drug Administration approval of these devices have generated considerable enthusiasm for CRT and ICD. Consideration of such therapy is reasonable in carefully selected patients, but questions of cost-effectiveness remain. Sex disparities in access to ICD implantation have been noted, with men significantly more likely to receive an ICD than women. It is important to keep in mind that CRT is technically demanding (requiring the implantation of a left ventricular pacing lead via the coronary sinus and coronary vein); complication rates in research centers are greater than 25%, with a reported frequency of coronary sinus dissection of about 3% and cardiac perforation of 1%. Adding ICD implantation increases cost and complexity. It remains to be determined whether combination CRT/ICD implantation (a popular approach among many cardiologists) gives better overall outcomes without significantly increasing the cost and risk of complications compared to CRT or ICD alone. Patients with comorbid illnesses that shorten life expectancy or end-stage CHF are not reasonable candidates. Cost is very high for CRT, and cost-effectiveness is a concern (>$100,000/ quality-adjusted life-year, similar to that of other invasive cardiac interventions). The literature should be followed closely.

Disease Management Programs

Patients with advanced disease who have had multiple hospitalizations for exacerbations have been proposed for disease management programs, ranging from telephonic monitoring by nurses to home visits by a nurse-specialists. The objectives are to maximize patient compliance, monitor disease parameters, and adjust medications in a timely fashion within preestablished parameters to reduce the rate of hospitalization and improve health status. Psychological support is also given. Results vary and appear to depend on how well the effort is coordinated with the patient's primary care practice. Disease management programs limited to telephone contact from centralized, nurse-staffed, monitoring services fail to reduce hospitalization rates. Those programs that include home visits and work closely with the primary care practice achieve much better results. Incorporating disease management into the primary care practice as part of a "medical home" reform of practice organization holds considerable promise.

Ventricular Assist Devices

Promising results have been obtained for patients with otherwise end-stage disease by implanting a ventricular assist device supplemented by β_2-agonist therapy. Regressions of pathologic left ventricular enlargement and remodeling have been achieved with such therapy in conjunction with improved functional status. Investigations are ongoing.

End-Stage Measures

With the exception of ventricular assist devices (which remain investigational) and transplantation (which is available to only 2,500 CHF patients per year in the United States), the management of end-stage disease is mostly supportive and guided by the same principles of terminal care that apply to most persons with end-stage diseases (see Chapter 90). Heroic measures that prolong survival without improving quality of life should cease. For example, persons who have implantable defibrillators should probably have them turned off because the frequency of disruptive overdrive pacing and defibrillatory discharges increases with the increasing frequency of serious ventricular dysrhythmias. There is no demonstrated value to intermittent outpatient intravenous infusions of vasodilators (e.g., B-type natriuretic peptide) or inotropic agents (e.g., milrinone), although they are promoted by some. Compassionate use of morphine for anxiety and dyspnea is perfectly reasonable and appropriate (see Chapter 90). Hospice care can be greatly comforting and improve quality of life.

Monitoring (10,12)

Close monitoring is essential, given the frequency of preventable decompensation due to poor compliance and dietary indiscretion. Simple measures often suffice, the most important being the use of *daily morning weights*. The importance of using daily weights cannot be overemphasized; weight gain typically precedes a worsening of symptoms. The degree of *exercise tolerance, vital signs, jugular venous pressure, rales, third heart sound, hepatojugular reflux,* and *peripheral edema* are also useful for monitoring and can be checked by the physician or visiting-nurse specialist. Key serum chemistries to follow include *potassium, BUN,* and *creatinine,* with *sodium* and *magnesium* also to be checked when intensive diuretic therapy is being undertaken. Measurement of *B-type natriuretic peptide* levels offers promise for monitoring the response to treatment (levels fall to <100 pg/mL with successful treatment) and predicting future decompensation; however, the cost-effectiveness will need to be established before this expensive test can be recommended for outpatient use. *Chest x-ray* and *echocardiography* are usually reserved for major reassessments done in the setting of acute decompensation.

PATIENT EDUCATION

Because the medical program is often complex and the need for compliance is great, the physician must take the time to discuss with the patient and family the rationale behind therapy and to set with them the guidelines for activity, diet, and use of medication. In this way they can become valuable partners in the treatment effort.

Patients should be instructed to weigh themselves each morning before breakfast and to keep a *weight record*. If their clinical status, weight, and medication program are stable, less frequent recordings are necessary. Patients are advised to call their physician if weight increases suddenly by more than

2 or 3 pounds because this may be the earliest sign of increasing CHF and a forerunner of more severe symptoms. Reliable patients with sufficient understanding may be instructed to adjust their diuretic doses according to weight. Debilitated or uncooperative individuals should have a family member or visiting nurse obtain weight recordings. Weight is among the most helpful parameters to follow in the outpatient management of failure.

Patients and their families must know the identity of the medication being used. It is easy for the patient to become confused because multiple-drug regimens are common and many of the pills are similar in appearance. Medication booklets are invaluable. Each tablet is taped to the page alongside its generic and brand names, dose schedule, indication for use, and warning signs of toxicity. For patients with poor eyesight, a family member or visiting nurse should set aside the pills to be taken each day.

INDICATIONS FOR REFERRAL AND ADMISSION

Patients with acutely worsening or refractory failure should be considered for hospital admission and cardiac consultation. For the patient with seemingly refractory disease, hospitalization provides the opportunity to observe the response to treatment under controlled conditions that ensure compliance with the medical regimen. Moreover, hospitalization helps to ensure the safe initiation of additional therapy and a search for a treatable underlying etiology that may have initially eluded detection. Cardiac consultation can be helpful when considering adjunctive pharmacologic therapy (e.g., aldosterone inhibition, digitalization) and is essential to exploring indications for pacemaker or defibrillator implantation. Relatively young patients failing maximal medical therapy may be appropriate for consideration of transplantation, provided renal, pulmonary, hepatic, and central nervous system functions are preserved. Other indications for admission include evidence of digitalis toxicity, renal failure, hypotension, and inadequate support and supervision at home.

THERAPEUTIC RECOMMENDATIONS (1,10)

Stage A, NYHA Class I Disease, High Risk/No Structural Change

- Screen for and treat risk factors and underlying etiologies, including *hypertension* (see Chapters 14, 19, and 26), coronary artery disease (see Chapters 20, 30, and 31), diabetes mellitus (see Chapters 94 and 102), high dietary sodium intake (especially in obese persons; see Chapters 26 and 233), hemodynamically significant valvular disease (see Chapter 33), thyroid disease (see Chapters 103 and 104), cardiomyopathy (see Appendix 33.1), and tachyarrhythmias (especially atrial fibrillation; see Chapter 28).
- Consider using the Framingham Heart Study scoring system (based on age, systolic blood pressure, heart rate, left ventricular hypertrophy on ECG, evidence of coronary or valvular heart disease, diabetes, cardiomegaly on chest x-ray, and forced expiratory capacity) to determine the risk for CHF and the appropriate level of aggressiveness of preventive measures.

- For high-risk persons (e.g., those with diabetes, hypertension, or coronary disease), begin ACE-inhibitor therapy or substitute ARB therapy if ACE inhibitors are not tolerated (see later discussion).

Stage B, NYHA Class I Disease, Asymptomatic/Initial Structural Change

The same as for stage A, plus:

- Prescribe and teach lifestyle changes, including moderation of sodium intake, regular exercise, and daily monitoring of weight.
- Regardless of pathophysiology, begin *ACE-inhibitor* therapy, starting at a low dose to minimize the risks of hypotension and hypoperfusion, especially in the elderly (e.g., 6.25 mg of *captopril* three times a day or 2.5 to 5.0 mg of *lisinopril* once daily). Monitor blood pressure, potassium, BUN, and creatinine.
- Gradually advance ACE-inhibitor therapy to improve exercise tolerance and relieve congestive symptoms while continuing to monitor blood pressure, potassium, and renal function. If tolerated, advance to doses associated with best outcomes (e.g., *captopril* 50 mg thrice daily; *lisinopril* 20 to 40 mg/d).
- Substitute an *angiotensin-receptor blocker* (e.g., *losartan* 50 to 100 mg/d, *valsartan* 80 to 160 mg/d) if ACE-inhibitor therapy is not tolerated due to cough or angioedema.
- Add a low dose of a *beta-blocker* (e.g., *carvedilol* 3.25 mg/d or *metoprolol-XL* 12.5 to 25 mg/d) if the patient has coronary disease, hypertension, or atrial fibrillation, provided the resting heart rate is greater than 70 beats/min and the systolic blood pressure is greater than 110 mm Hg. Titrate the dose slowly upward to achieve a resting heart rate of 50 to 60 beats/min and an exercise heart rate of no greater than 80 to 90 beats/min. During the first 8 weeks of treatment, monitor closely for fluid retention and clinical worsening; add diuretic therapy if volume overload develops.

Stage C, NYHA Class II to III Disease, Symptomatic with Mild to Moderate Exertion/Advancing Structural Change

The same as for stages A and B, plus:

- Initiate a *no-added-salt diet* (4 g sodium), but do not restrict water intake unless dilutional hyponatremia ensues.
- Check for and treat any exacerbating factors (e.g., noncompliance, fever, anemia, atrial fibrillation, infection, salt excess; treat these specifically if they are amenable to therapy rather than rely solely on symptomatic measures to ameliorate the CHF).
- Monitor weight and exercise tolerance closely; treat at the first sign of decompensation (e.g., weight gain, increase in exertional dyspnea).
- Begin *beta-blocker* therapy if it has not already been instituted (see prior discussion).
- Begin *diuretic* therapy if there is evidence of volume overload or pulmonary venous congestion. If symptoms are mild, begin with a *thiazide* (e.g., *hydrochlorothiazide* 25 to 50 mg/d). If thiazides do not suffice, switch to a *loop diuretic* (e.g., *furosemide* 20 to 40 mg once or twice daily). Be alert for a very brisk diuresis in patients who have never before

received a loop diuretic. Exercise particular caution with the use of potent diuretics in situations that require a high filling pressure (e.g., critical aortic stenosis). Divide the daily dose to minimize the inconvenience of a large diuresis in the morning or evening that might interfere with activity or sleep, but if the response is insufficient, give the entire loop diuretic dose in the morning (e.g., furosemide 80 to 120 mg every morning).

■ If the response to the initial choice of loop diuretic is erratic, consider switching to *torsemide* (50 mg once or twice daily); if the response is insufficient, add a thiazide (e.g., *hydrochlorothiazide* 25 mg before the loop diuretic dose) or *metolazone* (1.25 mg/d, $\frac{1}{2}$ hour before the loop diuretic) to the loop diuretic program. Monitor potassium, BUN, and creatinine.

■ Consider the addition of low-dose *aldosterone-inhibitor* therapy (e.g., *spironolactone* 25 mg/d) if the patient is still unacceptably symptomatic due to volume overload. Cease any potassium supplementation, and monitor potassium levels closely; use with extreme caution, if at all, in the setting of renal failure or worsening renal function (creatinine >2.5 mg/dL). If cosmetically unacceptable gynecomastia develops, consider switching to *eplerenone* (25 mg/d).

■ Consider the addition of *cardiac glycoside* therapy if the patient remains unacceptably symptomatic and has evidence of marked systolic dysfunction (third heart sound, marked LV dilation, EF <0.35). Use *digoxin* (beginning with 0.125 mg/d). Obtain a serum level after 3 to 5 days, and adjust the dose to achieve a level of 0.5 to 0.8 ng/mL. Monitor BUN, creatinine, potassium, and serum digoxin levels. Allow at least 6 hours since the last dose before drawing the levels. Monitor serum levels regularly and especially closely in the settings of amiodarone use and changing renal or thyroid function. Be prepared to reduce the dose.

■ Monitor closely and *hospitalize* for acute decompensation. Review for precipitants, aggravating factors, and noncompliance.

■ Consider instituting a *disease management program* if the patient requires repeated hospitalizations for acute decompensation due to poor compliance with the medical regimen.

■ Refer for consideration of *cardiac resynchronization therapy* if the patient is viable but unacceptably symptomatic despite a maximal medical regimen and has evidence of marked systolic dysfunction (EF <0.35) and intraventricular conduction delay (e.g., left-bundle-branch block, QRS >120 msec).

■ Refer for consideration of *implantable cardioverter-defibrillator* those heart failure patients with NYHA class II or III disease and LV systolic dysfunction (especially if there is a history of life-threatening ventricular dysrhythmias). (Use in class IV disease is less well established.)

Stage D, NYHA Class IV Disease, Symptomatic at Rest/End-Stage Disease Refractory to Standard Treatment

■ Continue the measures started in late stage C.
■ Refer for the consideration of transplantation or a left ventricular assist device if the patient is relatively young and has end-stage myocardial disease but preserved renal, hepatic, pulmonary, and neurologic functions.

■ If the patient is not a candidate, begin a hospice program, and disable the cardioverter–defibrillator if one has been implanted.

■ Consider a narcotic program (e.g., MS Contin 15 mg twice daily) for the management of severe anxiety and worsening dyspnea at the end stage of disease.

Monitoring and Adjusting Therapy

■ Advise the patient and family to check weight daily, measuring it before breakfast and calling the physician if there is an unexplained weight gain of more than 2 to 3 pounds since the last reading.

■ Monitor potassium, BUN, and creatinine regularly and closely.

■ If prerenal azotemia develops or worsens, adjust downward the doses of medical regimen components accordingly, especially ACE inhibitors, diuretics, ARBs, digoxin, and spironolactone.

■ Monitor heart rate and rhythm; if a cardiac dysrhythmia is noted, investigate promptly, especially in persons taking a digitalis preparation who manifest paroxysmal atrial tachycardia with block, ventricular irritability (especially bigeminy), junctional tachycardia, or severe bradycardia.

■ Use oral potassium supplements with care in patients taking an ACE inhibitor, ARB, or aldosterone inhibitor and only if the serum potassium falls to less than 3.5 mg/dL. If a potassium-sparing diuretic is used in conjunction with an ACE inhibitor or ARB, chronic oral potassium supplementation should be stopped.

■ Monitor serum magnesium in patients taking digitalis and those with refractory hypokalemia. Diuretic-induced hypomagnesemia is common and may impair potassium repletion; it also enhances the sensitivity to the toxic effects of digitalis.

Additional Measures and Precautions

■ Initiate oral anticoagulant therapy for CHF patients if prolonged bedrest, atrial fibrillation, or severe congestive cardiomyopathy ensue (see Chapter 83). Prescribe aspirin at 81 mg/d for persons with CHF due to coronary disease.

■ Avoid calcium-channel blockers in patients with chronic CHF, especially in persons with coronary heart disease and ejection fractions less than 0.35. If continued use is believed to be essential, consider the use of amlodipine, and obtain cardiac consultation.

■ Avoid, if possible, other cardiac drugs with negative inotropic effects and no proven benefit in CHF (e.g., disopyramide).

■ Provide the patient and the family with thorough instructions on the purpose and proper use of medications prescribed for CHF.

■ Check for and treat any underlying depression.

■ Advise bedrest for exacerbations of CHF, but discourage a major reorganization of the patient's lifestyle unless the symptoms are severe and refractory. A gentle exercise program may actually improve exercise tolerance once the exacerbation has cleared.

A.H.G.

Annotated Bibliography

1. Aurigemma GP, Gaasch WH. Diastolic heart failure. N Engl J Med 2004;351;1097. (*An excellent review of pathophysiology.*)
2. Bell DS. Heart failure: the frequent and often fatal complication of diabetes. Diabetes Care 2003;26:2433. (*A review of the evidence and implications of treatment of this often-overlooked cause.*)
3. Bhatia RS, Tu JV, Lee DS, et al. Outcome of heart failure with preserved ejection fraction in a population study. N Eng J Med 2006;355:260. (*The prognosis just a bad as for heart failure due to systolic dysfunction.*)
4. Bursi F, Weston SA, Redfield MM, et al. Systolic and diastolic heart failure in the community. JAMA 2006;296:2209. (*Finds a high prevalence of diastolic dysfunction, with poor prognosis, even in the setting of preserved ejection fraction.*)
5. Drazner MH, Rame JE, Stevenson LW, et al. Prognostic importance of elevated jugular venous pressure and a third heart sound in patients with heart failure. N Engl J Med 2001;345:574. (*A retrospective analysis of data from a major clinical treatment trial, finding that these features are predictive of poor outcome.*)
6. Feenstra J, Heerdink ER, Brobbee DE, et al. Association of nonsteroidal anti-inflammatory drugs with first occurrence of heart failure and with relapsing heart failure: the Rotterdam Study. Arch Intern Med 2002;162:265. (*A prospective cohort study, finding that nonsteroidal antiinflammatory drug use was associated with relapsing disease but not with its initial occurrence.*)
7. Haider AW, Larson MG, Franklin SS, et al. Systolic blood pressure, diastolic blood pressure, and pulse pressure as predictors of risk for congestive heart failure in the Framingham Heart Study. Ann Intern Med 2003;138:10. (*Data from the Framingham Heart Study, finding that pulse pressure and systolic pressure were the most powerful predictors.*)
8. He J, Ogden LG, Bazzano LA, et al. Risk factors for congestive heart failure in U.S. men and women. NHANES I epidemiologic follow-up study. Arch Intern Med 2001;161:996. (*A major epidemiologic study, finding that physical inactivity, smoking, overweight, diabetes, and coronary heart disease [CHD] were all predictors of poor outcome.*)
9. He J, Ogden LG, Bazzano LA, et al. Dietary sodium intake and incidence of congestive heart failure in overweight US men and women. Arch Intern Med 2002;162:1619. (*A high sodium intake in obese persons was found to be an independent risk factor.*)
10. Hunt SA, Abraham WT, Chin MH, et al. ACC/AHA 2005 guideline update for the diagnosis and management of heart failure in the adult. Circulation 2005;112:e154. (*Consensus practice guidelines.*)
11. Ingelsson E, Sundstrom J, Arnlov J, et al. Insulin resistance and risk of congestive heart failure. JAMA 2005;294:334. (*This factor was found to be an independent predictor of heart failure, and may be the mechanism for the role diabetes in heart failure.*)
12. Jessup M, Brozena S. Heart failure. N Engl J Med 2003;348:2007. (*A useful review, which includes many of the new concepts in pathophysiology, classification, and treatment; 89 references.*)
13. Jiang W, Alexander J, Christopher E, et al. Relationship of depression to increased risk of mortality and rehospitalization in patients with congestive heart failure. Arch Intern Med 2001;161:1849. (*A cohort study, finding that depression was independently associated with increased risk.*)
14. Kannel WB, D'Agostino RB, Silbershatz H, et al. Profile for estimating risk of heart failure. Arch Intern Med 1999;159:1197. (*Presents an approach for clinically identifying persons at risk based on predictors identified from an analysis of Framingham Heart Study data.*)
15. Lee DS, Pencina MJ, Benjamin EJ, et al. Association of parenteral heart failure with risk of heart failure in offspring. N Engl J Med 2006;355:138. (*A cross-sectional study, finding a strong association.*)
16. Levy D, Kenchaiah S, Larson MG, et al. Long-term trends in the incidence of and survival with heart failure. N Engl J Med 2002;347:1397. (*Updated epidemiologic community-based data from the Framingham Heart Study, showing a reduced incidence in women and a decreasing mortality in all patients.*)
17. Owan TE, Hodge DO, Herges RM, et al. Trends in prevalence and outcome of heart failure with preserved ejection fraction. N Engl J Med 2006;355:251. (*Documents a trend toward an increasing prevalence of diastolic dysfunction.*)
18. Redfield MM, Jacobsen SJ, Burnett JC, et al. Burden of systolic and diastolic ventricular dysfunction in the community: appreciating the scope of the heart failure epidemic. JAMA 2003;289:194. (*A cross-sectional, community-based echocardiographic study, revealing a high frequency of preclinical heart failure and diastolic dysfunction, with poor prognosis associated with the latter.*)
19. Schiff GD, Fung S, Speroff T, et al. Decompensated heart failure: symptoms, patterns of onset, and contributing factors. Am J Med 2003;114:625. (*A retrospective cohort study identifying clinical features suggestive of early decompensation that can be used to prevent the need for hospitalization.*)
20. Small KM, Wagoner LE, Levin AM, et al. Synergistic polymorphisms of β_1- and α_{2c}-adrenergic receptors and the risk of congestive heart failure. N Eng

J Med 2002;347:1135. (*Presents the evidence for a link between genetic polymorphisms and clinical outcomes.*)
21. Wang CH, Weisel RD, Liu PP, et al. Glitazones and heart failure: critical appraisal for the clinician. Circulation 2003;107:1350. (*Presents the evidence for its contribution to heart failure.*)
22. Wang J, Kurrelmeyer KM, Torre-Amione G, et al. Systolic and diastolic dyssynchrony in patients with diastolic heart failure and the effect of medical therapy. J Am Coll Cardiol 2007;49:88. (*Finds that dyssynchrony was common in both forms of heart failure and was responsive to medical therapy.*)
23. Weber KT. Aldosterone in congestive heart failure. N Engl J Med 2001;345:1689. (*A comprehensive review of this important component of congestive heart failure [CHF] pathophysiology; 86 references.*)
24. Chakko S, Woska D, Martinez H, et al. Clinical, radiographic, hemodynamic correlations in chronic congestive heart failure: conflicting results may lead to inappropriate care. Am J Med 1991;90:353. (*A critical look at methods for diagnosing CHF.*)
25. Felker GM, Cuculich PS, Gheorghiade M. The Valsalva maneuver: a beside "biomarker" for heart failure. Am J Med 2006;119:117. (*A review of its role in the assessment of volume overload.*)
26. Mogelvang R, Goetze MR, Schnohr P, et al. Discriminating between cardiac and pulmonary dysfunction in the general population with dyspnea by plasma pro-B-type natriuretic peptic. J Am Coll Cardiol 2007;50:1694. (*A community-based population study, documenting the ability of this approach to differentiate cardiac from pulmonary causes.*)
27. Kasner M, Westermann D, Steendijk P, et al. Utility of Doppler echocardiography and tissue Doppler imaging in the estimation of diastolic function in heart failure with normal ejection fraction: a comparative Doppler-conductance catheterization study. Circulation 2007;116:637. (*Confirms the validity of Doppler echocardiography as a diagnostic modality for the identification of diastolic dysfunction.*)
28. Maisel AS, Krishnaswamy P, Nowak RM, et al. Rapid measurement of B-type natriuretic peptide in the emergency diagnosis of heart failure. N Engl J Med 2002;347:161. (*A prospective cohort study, finding that the test was useful for the diagnosis and determination of severity in this setting.*)
29. Mueller C, Scholer A, Laule-Kilian K, et al. Use of B-type natriuretic peptide in the evaluation and management of acute dyspnea. N Engl J Med 2004;350:647. (*A randomized, controlled trial [RCT], finding that B-type natriuretic peptide measurement was useful in the emergency room setting.*)
30. Perloff JK. The jugular venous pulse and third heart sound in patients with heart failure. N Engl J Med 2001;345:612. (*A succinct discussion of how these are elicited, by a master of the exam.*)
31. Thomas JT, Kelley RF, Thomas SJ, et al. Utility of history, physical examination, electrocardiogram, and chest radiograph for differentiating normal from decreased systolic function in patients with heart failure. Am J Med 2002;112:4437. (*Presents the strengths and weaknesses of clinical assessment.*)
32. Wiese J. The abdominojugular reflux sign. Am J Med 2000;109:59. (*A literature review on the significance of this oft-mentioned finding.*)
33. Hsu L-F, Jais P, Sanders P, et al. Catheter ablation for atrial fibrillation in congestive heart failure. N Engl J Med 2004;351:2373. (*Significant improvements were noted in cardiac function, symptoms, exercise capacity, and quality of life.*)
34. Kaneko Y, Floras JS, Usui K, et al. Cardiovascular effects of continuous positive airway pressure in patients with heart failure and obstructive sleep apnea. N Engl J Med 2003;248:1233. (*An improvement was found in ejection fraction.*)
35. Nohria A, Lewis E, Stevenson LW. Medical management of advance heart failure. JAMA 2002;287:628. (*An outstanding practice review for the clinician; 99 references.*)
36. Okin PM, Devereux RB, Harris KE, et al. Regression of electrocardiographic left ventricular hypertrophy is associated with less hospitalization for heart failure in hypertensive patients. Ann Intern Med 2007;147:311. (*Presents evidence for a reduction in the risk of heart failure with treatment.*)
37. Braunwald E. ACE inhibitors—a cornerstone of the treatment of heart failure. N Engl J Med 1991;325:351. (*An editorial summarizing the evidence for the central role of these drugs in the treatment of CHF.*)
38. Cohn JN, Johnson G, Ziesche S, et al. A comparison of enalapril with hydralazine–isosorbide dinitrate in the treatment of chronic congestive heart failure. N Engl J Med 1991;325:303. (*Enalapril proved superior to hydralazine–isosorbide, although the mechanisms of action differed and suggested possible complementarity.*)
39. Guazzi M, Brambilla R, Reina G, et al. Aspirin–angiotensin-converting enzyme inhibitor coadministration and mortality in patients with heart failure: a dose-related adverse effect of aspirin. Arch Intern Med 2003;163:1574. (*A retrospective cohort study, finding that there was a dose-related reduction in survival with increased aspirin dose.*)
40. Lee VC, Rhew DC, Dylan M, et al. Meta-analysis: angiotensin-receptor blockers in chronic heart failure and high-risk acute myocardial infarction.

Ann Intern Med 2004;141:693. (*Presents evidence that angiotensin-receptor blockers are equivalent to angiotensin-converting-enzyme inhibitors in efficacy.*)

41. Packer M, O'Conner CM, Ghali JK, et al. Effect of amlodipine on morbidity and mortality in severe chronic heart failure. N Engl J Med 1996;335:1107. (*RCT in patients with ejection fraction <0.3, showing no association with worsening failure, life-threatening dysrhythmias, or sudden death.*)

42. Pfeffer MA, McMurray JJ, Velazquez EJ, et al. Valsartan, captopril, or both in myocardial infarction complicated by heart failure, left ventricular dysfunction, or both. N Engl J Med 2003;349:1893. (*RCT, finding reduced hospitalization rates but no survival benefit.*)

43. Phillips CO, Kashani A, Ko DK, et al. Adverse effects of combination angiotensin II receptor blockers plus angiotensin-converting enzyme inhibitors for left ventricular dysfunction: a quantitative review of data from randomized clinical trials. Arch Intern Med 2007;167:1930. (*Finds marked increases in risks of hyperkalemia, worsening renal function, and symptomatic hypotension.*)

44. Pitt B, Segal R, Martinez FA, et al. Randomised trial of losartan versus captopril in patients over 65 with heart failure. Evaluation of Losartan in the Elderly study (ELITE). Lancet 1997;349:747. (*Major RCT, showing similar morbidity and mortality benefits but no advantage for angiotensin-receptor blockers over angiotensin-converting-enzyme inhibitors.*)

45. Taylor AL, Ziesche S, Yancy C, et al. for the African-American Heart Failure Trial Investigators. Combination of isosorbide dinitrate and hydralazine in blacks with heart failure. N Engl J Med 2004;351:2049. (*RCT, finding that a fixed dose added to standard full medical therapy improved survival in blacks.*)

46. The CONSENSUS Trial Study Group. Effects of enalapril on mortality in severe congestive heart failure. N Engl J Med 1987;23:1429. (*A prospective, randomized, multicenter study of patients with severe heart failure, finding that adding enalapril to conventional therapy reduced mortality and improved symptoms.*)

47. The SOLVD Investigators. Effect of enalapril on survival in patients with reduced left ventricular ejection fractions and congestive heart failure. N Engl J Med 1991;325:293. (*An important randomized, prospective, multicenter trial of patients with mild to moderate heart failure, showing that enalapril reduced mortality and hospitalization.*)

48. Brophy JM, Joseph L, Rouleau JL. Beta-blockers in congestive heart failure: a Bayesian meta-analysis. Ann Intern Med 2001;134:550. (*Finds reductions in morbidity and mortality when beta-blockers were used in stable CHF.*)

49. Foody JM, Farrell MH, Krumholz HM. Beta-blocker therapy in heart failure: scientific review. JAMA 2002;287:883. (*A systematic review of RCTs, finding strong evidence for efficacy across a wide range of patients.*)

50. Gregory D, Udelson JE, Monstam MA. Economic analysis of beta blockade in heart failure. Am J Med 2001;110(7A):74S. (*Finds that all beta-blockers are cost-effective, but metoprolol is about one third the cost of carvedilol.*)

51. Hjalmarson A, Goldstein S, Fagerberg B, et al. Effects of controlled release metoprolol on total mortality, hospitalizations, and well-being in patients with heart failure: the Metoprolol CR/XL Randomized Intervention Trial in Congestive Heart Failure (MERIT-HF). JAMA 2000;283:1295. (*A major RCT, finding improvements in all outcome measures.*)

52. Ko DT, Hebert PR, Coffey CS, et al. Adverse effects of beta-blocker therapy for patients with heart failure: a quantitative overview of randomized trials. Arch Intern Med 2004;164:1389. (*The risks of hypotension, dizziness, and bradycardia were more than offset by reductions in cardiac morbidity and mortality.*)

53. MERIT-HF Study Group. Effect of metoprolol CR/XL in chronic heart failure: Metoprolol CR/XL Randomized Intervention Trial in Congestive Heart Failure (MERIT-HF). Lancet 1999;353:2001. (*One of the first large-scale studies to demonstrate a survival benefit with beta-blocker use in CHF; a nearly 50% reduction in mortality was seen in persons with mild to moderate heart failure.*)

54. Packer M, Coats AJS, Fowler MB, et al. Effect of carvedilol on survival in severe chronic heart failure. N Engl J Med 2001;344:1651. (*The Carvedilol Prospective Randomized Cumulative Survival [COPERNICUS] trial, showing benefit for patients with New York Heart Association class IV disease.*)

55. Packer M. Current role of beta-adrenergic blockers in the management of chronic heart failure. Am J Med 2001;110:81S. (*An excellent review of the evidence, combined with clinically relevant advice.*)

56. Poole-Wilson PA, Swedberg K, Cleland JFG, et al. Comparison of carvedilol and metoprolol on clinical outcomes in patients with chronic heart failure in the Carvedilol or Metoprolol European Trial (COMET): randomised controlled trial. Lancet 2003;362:7. (*A European RCT, finding no difference in outcomes.*)

57. Cohn JN. Optimal diuretic therapy for heart failure. Am J Med. 2001;111:577. (*An editorial that comments on new developments in diuretic therapy, especially the potential for the use of torsemide.*)

58. Palmer BF. Managing hyperkalemia caused by inhibitors of the renin–angiotensin–aldosterone system. N Engl J Med 2004;351:585. (*A useful review of a problem that takes on increasing importance with therapies for CHF.*)

59. Pitt B, Remme W, Zannad F, et al. Eplerenone, a selective aldosterone blocker, in patients with left ventricular dysfunction after myocardial infarction. N Engl J Med 2003;348:1309. (*A major RCT, the Eplerenone Post-Acute Myocardial Infarction Heart Failure Efficacy and Survival Study [EPHESUS] trial, finding a 17% reduction in the risk of cardiac death.*)

60. Pitt B, Zannad F, Remme WM, et al. The effect of spironolactone on morbidity and mortality in patients with severe heart failure. N Engl J Med 1999;341:709. (*RCT, the Randomized Aldactone Evaluation Study [RALES] trial, demonstrating significant reductions in mortality and morbidity.*)

61. Whang R. Magnesium deficiency: pathogenesis, prevalence, and clinical implications. Am J Med 1987;82(Suppl 3A):24. (*A succinct review of this important problem, especially in patients taking digitalis and diuretics.*)

62. Adams KF, Patterson JH, Gattis WA, et al. Relationship of serum digoxin concentration to mortality and morbidity in women in the Digitalis Investigation Group Trial. J Am Coll Cardiol 2005;46:497. (*Finds that morbidity and mortality are reduced at lower serum concentrations and increased at higher concentrations that are within in the old "therapeutic" range.*)

63. Bauman JL, DiDomenico RJ, Viana M, et al. A method of determining the dose of digoxin for heart failure in the modern era. Arch Intern Med 2006;166:2539. (*New dosing recommendations based on lower recommended serum levels.*)

64. Packer M, Gheorghiade M, Young JB, et al. Withdrawal of digoxin from patients with chronic heart failure treated with angiotensin-converting-enzyme inhibitors. N Engl J Med 1993;329:1. (*Withdrawal of digoxin was associated with an increased risk of worsening in patients with systolic dysfunction.*)

65. Rathore SS, Wang Y, Krumholz HM. Sex-based differences in the effect of digoxin for the treatment of heart failure. N Engl J Med 2002;347:1403. (*A post hoc analysis of data from the Digitalis Investigation Group [DIG] study, finding that there was a risk for women.*)

66. Rathore SS, Curtis JP, Wang Y, et al. Association of serum digoxin concentration and outcomes in patients with heart failure. JAMA 2003;289:871. (*Post hoc analysis of data from the DIG study, finding that risks and benefits were related to the serum digoxin level, with a level of 0.5 to 0.8 being best.*)

67. Slatton ML, Irani WN, Hall SA, et al. Does digoxin provide additional hemodynamic and autonomic benefit at higher doses in patients with mild to moderate heart failure and normal sinus rhythm? J Am Coll Cardiol 1997;29:1206. (*Presents evidence suggesting that most of the benefit is autonomic and is present at low doses.*)

68. The Digitalis Investigation Group. The effect of digoxin on mortality and morbidity in patients with heart failure. N Engl J Med 1997;336:525. (*A landmark RCT in persons with all levels of CHF, finding that there was a significant reduction in the rate of hospitalization for heart failure but no overall reduction in cardiovascular mortality; the best results were found in persons with severe left ventricular dysfunction.*)

69. Krumholz HM, Chen YT, Radford MJ. Aspirin and the treatment of heart failure in the elderly. Arch Intern Med 2001;161:577. (*A retrospective cohort study, finding that aspirin use was associated with lower mortality.*)

70. Hambrecht R, Gielen S, Link A, et al. Effects of exercise training on left ventricular function and peripheral resistance in patients with chronic heart failure: a randomized trial. JAMA 2000;283:3095. (*RCT, identifying improvements in clinical and physiologic parameters.*)

71. Smart N, Marwick TH. Exercise training for patients with heart failure: a systematic review of factors that improve mortality and morbidity. Am J Med 2004;116:693. (*An excellent review;108 references.*)

72. Krumholz HM, Butler J, Miller J, et al. Prognostic importance of emotional support for elderly patients hospitalized with heart failure. Circulation 1998;97:958. (*A cohort study, finding a significant effect on outcomes.*)

73. MacMahon KMA, Lip GYH. Psychological factors in heart failure. Arch Intern Med 2002;162:509. (*A superb review of the literature; 61 references.*)

74. Shlipak MG. Pharmacotherapy for heart failure in patients with renal insufficiency. Ann Intern Med 2003;138:917. (*A comprehensive review;119 references.*)

75. Colucci WS, Elkayam U, Horton DP, et al. Intravenous nesiritide, a natriuretic peptide, in the treatment of decompensated heart failure. N Engl J Med 2000;343:246. (*RCT, finding that hemodynamic and clinical improvements were achieved.*)

76. Sackner-Bernstein JD, Kowalski M, Fox M, et al. Short-term risk of death after treatment with nesiritide for decompensated heart failure. JAMA 2005;293:1900. (*Presents evidence suggesting worrisome adverse effects and tempering the initial enthusiasm for the drug.*)

77. Konstam MA, Gheorghiade M, Burnett JC, et al. for the EVEREST Investigators. Effects of oral tolvaptan in patients hospitalized for worsening heart failure: the EVEREST Outcome Trial. JAMA 2007;297:1319. (*A major RCT, noting that there was no effect on long-term mortality or heart failure–related morbidity.*)

78. Konstam MA, Gheorghiade M, Burnett JC, et al. Short-term clinical effects of tolvaptan, an oral vasopressin antagonist, in patients hospitalized for heart failure: the EVEREST Clinical Status Trials. JAMA 2007;297:1332. (*A major RCT, finding a short-term benefit for signs and symptoms.*)

79. Bardy GH, Lee KL, Mark DB, et al. for the SCD-HeFT Investigators. Amiodarone or an implantable cardioverter–defibrillator for congestive heart

failure. N Engl J Med 2005;352:225. (*RCT, finding a 23% reduction in the risk of death with an implantable cardioverter–defibrillator but none with amiodarone.*)

80. Birks EJ, Tansley PD, Hardy J, et al. Left ventricular assist device and drug therapy for the reversal of heart failure. N Engl J Med 2006;355:1873. (*Describes a promising approach in patients with end-stage disease that helps to slow disease progression and partially reverse the course of illness.*)

81. Cleland JGF, Daubert J-C, Erdmann E, et al. for the CARE-HF Study Investigators. The effects of cardiac resynchronization on morbidity and mortality in heart failure. N Engl J Med 2005;352:1539. (*A major RCT, demonstrating survival benefit, as well as improvements in quality of life, complications, and cardiac function.*)

82. Curtis LH, Al-Khatib SM, Shea AM, et al. Sex differences in the use of implantable cardioverter–defibrillators for primary and secondary preven-

tion of sudden cardiac death. JAMA 2007;298:1517. (*Men were significantly more likely to receive implantable cardioverter–defibrillators than were women.*)

83. Ezekowitz JA, Rowe BH, Dryden DM, et al. Systematic review: implantable cardioverter defibrillators for adults with left ventricular systolic dysfunction. Ann Intern Med 2007;147:251. (*Finds improvement in survival.*)

84. Laramee AS, Levinsky SK, Sargent J, et al. Case management in a heterogeneous congestive heart failure population. Arch Intern Med 2003;163:809. (*A study of the efficacy of this widely touted approach to improving outcomes and reducing costs; presents a helpful but complex picture.*)

85. McAlister FA, Ezekowitz J, Hooton N, et al. Cardiac resynchronization therapy for patients with left ventricular systolic dysfunction: a systematic review. JAMA 2007;297:2502. (*Cardiac resynchronization therapy reduced morbidity and mortality when combined with optimal medical therapy.*)

APPENDIX 32.1: MANAGING DISORDERS OF SERUM POTASSIUM IN CONGESTIVE HEART FAILURE (1–5)

Patients with heart failure have considerable underlying heart disease and, in conjunction with resultant LV remodeling and the use of digoxin, a markedly increased risk for serious cardiac dysrhythmias. This dysrhythmic potential is exacerbated by abnormalities of the serum potassium, which frequently occur in CHF as a consequence of potent diuretic programs and drugs that inhibit the angiotensin–aldosterone axis.

PATHOPHYSIOLOGY

The risk for a cardiac arrhythmia begins to rise as the serum potassium level falls to less than 4.0 mmol/L, particularly in the setting of digoxin use or underlying myocardial disease. Conduction-system dysfunction begins to appear with hyperkalemia, especially in persons with underlying heart disease, conduction-system abnormalities, or the use of drugs that slow conduction (e.g., beta-blockers, calcium-channel blockers).

Hypokalemia in Heart Failure

Both thiazides and loop diuretics block sodium reabsorption, which leads to increased presentation of sodium to the distal tubule, where absorption takes place in exchange for potassium. Thiazide-induced potassium loss is a function of thiazide dose and amount of sodium intake. Loop diuretics induce even greater potassium loss by presenting more sodium to the distal tubule for exchange with potassium. To counter these losses and to lower the risk for dysrhythmias, a strategy for maintaining, replacing, and monitoring potassium is essential to the management of CHF.

Hyperkalemia in Heart Failure

Normal potassium excretion requires the delivery of sodium to the distal nephron, the action of aldosterone, and the normal functioning of the cortical collecting tubule. In heart failure, all three components are commonly impaired, with severe proximal sodium retention, drug-induced aldosterone inhibition, and renal compromise. Since the addition of angiotensin blockade and aldosterone inhibition to CHF management, the frequency of serious hyperkalemia has markedly increased, es-

pecially in persons with underlying renal dysfunction. NSAID use may add to the problem by inhibiting renin secretion (via the inhibition of stimulatory prostaglandins).

PREVENTION AND TREATMENT OF HYPOKALEMIA

Several approaches are available for minimizing the risk of developing hypokalemia in persons taking diuretics for CHF. The simplest is to ensure an adequate potassium intake. Pharmacologic measures are also available.

Dietary Measures

Total body potassium stores average 3,500 mmol (mEq), of which 90% is intracellular. Normal serum levels range from 3.6 to 5.0 mmol/L but do not necessarily reflect total body stores. Minimum daily requirements are about 40 to 50 mmol (1,600 mg to 2,000 mg). Persons who consume large quantities of fruits and vegetables can take in more than 200 mmol/d. More commonly, the daily intake ranges from 62 mmol for urban whites to 25 mmol for urban blacks. Additional daily requirements to counter diuretic-induced losses are estimated at about 40 to 100 mmol.

Foods provide considerable opportunity for potassium replenishment. Those with the highest potassium content include *dried figs* (25 mmol/100 g); *dried dates* and *prunes*, *nuts*, *bran cereals*, *wheat germ*, and *lima beans* (25 mmol/100 g); and fresh *fruits* and *vegetables* (6.2 mmol/100 g). A 10-oz glass of *orange*, *pineapple*, or *grapefruit juice* has 15 mmol. Tomato juice is also high in potassium, but much salt is added to enhance its taste. Salt substitutes contain about 12 mmol of potassium per gram as potassium chloride.

An often overlooked measure is to *reduce excess sodium intake* (the more sodium that presents to the distal tubule, the more potassium is lost).

Concurrent Use of ACE Inhibitors and ARBs

Drugs that block the action of angiotensin II can achieve some blunting of aldosterone-induced sodium retention and potassium wasting. Response is quite variable, hard to predict, and often insufficient to obviate the need for potassium supplementation.

Use of Potassium-Sparing Diuretics

Triamterene and *amiloride* are weak diuretics, but when used in conjunction with a thiazide, they can preclude the need for potassium supplementation. When taken along with ACE inhibition or ARB therapy, they may cause the potassium level to rise. Direct aldosterone inhibition by *spironolactone* or *eplerenone* can also eliminate the need for potassium supplementation, even when loop diuretics are needed, but extreme caution is indicated when they are used in the context of declining renal function or diabetes; the risk of serious hyperkalemia is substantial. Caution is also warranted when they are used as an adjunct to ACE inhibition or ARB therapy (see later discussion). In all instances, renal function and serum potassium level require close monitoring.

Potassium Supplementation

Oral supplementation is recommended. The preferred potassium salt for replacement in CHF is the chloride because there is chloride loss with diuretic use, and volume-contraction alkalosis is also common. Trying to increase serum potassium by diet alone is usually insufficient and fails to provide the necessary chloride (most foods contain potassium as the phosphate salt).

Unless the serum level declines to dangerous levels (e.g., <2.5 mmol/L) or evidence of a worrisome dysrhythmia develops, replacement can be accomplished on an outpatient basis over days to weeks using oral supplementation. Long-term supplementation may be difficult to sustain due to inconvenience and gastrointestinal (GI) intolerance, necessitating the use of a potassium-sparing diuretic (see prior discussion). A crude rule of thumb in estimating the amount of replacement necessary is 100 mmol for every 0.3-mmol/L reduction in serum potassium below the normal range. A number of formulations are available; most come in 10- and 20-mmol doses, with 20 mmol usually the maximum dose at one time. Replacement should be gradual and measured; serum potassium levels need to be watched closely to avoid hyperkalemia, especially when these formulations are used in the context of potassium-sparing drugs.

Liquid, Powder, and Effervescent Formulations (e.g., KCL Elixir, K-Lyte, K-Lyte/CL)

Potassium chloride *elixir* is inexpensive, easy to swallow, and rapid acting, but its taste can be disagreeable, which compromises compliance. The 10% solution of the liquid contains 20 mEq per tablespoon (15 mL). Some find it unpalatable even when it is mixed in fruit juice. However, when faced with the high cost of alternatives, many patients who complain of its taste are willing to reconsider using it for a period of time. Its safety, chloride content, and ability to deliver more potassium per dose than many other preparations strongly recommend it. Citrus-flavored *effervescent tablets* and packets of *powder* are more convenient to use, also immediately acting, and may be slightly better tasting; cost is greater than for the elixir.

Wax-Matrix Extended-Release Tablets (e.g., Klotrix, Slow-K, Kaon-Cl, K-Tab)

The advantages of an extended-release tablet include no disagreeable taste, better convenience, and less GI upset, which all help to improve compliance. The wax-matrix tablets are relatively inexpensive and easy to swallow; however, the preparation is associated with mucosal injury in the upper small bowel, leading to upper GI bleeding, small-bowel ulcerations, and case reports of stricture and perforation.

Microencapsulated Tablets (e.g., Micro-K, K-Dur)

This expensive (the cost is >10 times that of the elixir) extended-release formulation is similar to wax-matrix tablets in advantages and has a significantly lower risk of causing GI tract erosions; it disintegrates well in the stomach. Encapsulated versions of the microencapsulated preparation have a tendency not to dissolve as well.

REFRACTORY HYPOKALEMIA

Causes include *hypomagnesemia* and *hyperaldosteronism*. Magnesium depletion can occur with the use of loop diuretics, and very high aldosterone states may occur as a response to severe heart failure. For prevention, many of the foods that are rich in potassium are also rich in magnesium and can be recommended, especially fresh green vegetables, legumes, nuts, and halibut. Magnesium supplements (e.g.,$MgCO_3$ or $MgCl_2$) can be prescribed; enteric-coated preparations usually have reduced bioavailability. Excess hyperaldosteronism, despite treatment with angiotensin blockade, can be countered by adding an aldosterone inhibitor to the medical program (e.g., spironolactone).

PREVENTION AND TREATMENT OF HYPERKALEMIA

Prevention

Care in design of the medical regimen for CHF and close monitoring of the serum potassium and renal function are the principal approaches to prevention. In CHF patients with underlying renal insufficiency, caution is needed in the use of angiotensin blockers; aldosterone antagonists may not be safe to use in persons with renal failure. Low doses of spironolactone (e.g. 25 mg/d) are safe to add to angiotensin blockade as long as the creatinine level is not elevated, but the risk of hyperkalemia increases substantially as the creatinine increases to greater than 1.8 mg/dL and as the spironolactone dose increases to greater than 25 mg/day. Repeated and careful reviews of the patient's entire medical regimen and the use of nonprescription drugs and supplements are essential. One needs to check for failure to discontinue a previously prescribed potassium supplementation program and use of NSAIDs and potassium-enhancing herbal preparations (e.g., noni juice, alfalfa, dandelion, ginseng, milkweed, hawthorn berries). Frequent determinations of serum BUN, creatinine, and potassium are essential during treatment for heart failure, especially when there are increases in the treatment regimen or a worsening of heart failure.

Treatment

All contributing drugs and supplements should be stopped or cut back. Modest elevations of serum potassium (up to 5.5 mg/dL) may be treated by a dose reduction of responsible agents and the correction of any underlying renal dysfunction from reversible causes such as excessive diuresis. An electrocardiogram should be obtained to check for conduction-system abnormalities, especially at higher levels of hyperkalemia and in persons with known conduction-system disease. Acutely, oral *Kayexalate* (15 to 30 mg) can be given every 4 to 6 hours as necessary. Chronic Kayexalate use is more problematic because it induces diarrhea and may cause mucosal injury to the GI tract.

A.H.G.

Annotated Bibliography

1. Cohn JN, Kowey PR, Whelton PK, et al. New guidelines for potassium replacement in clinical practice: a contemporary review by the National Council on Potassium in Clinical Practice. Arch Intern Med 2000;160:2429. (*Presents consensus guidelines and supporting evidence; 48 references.*)
2. Gennari FJ. Hypokalemia. N Engl J Med 1998;339:451. (*An excellent review; 57 references.*)
3. Palmer BF. Managing hyperkalemia caused by inhibitors of the renin–angiotensin–aldosterone system. N Engl J Med 2004;351:585. (*A practical review; 54 references.*)

4. Juurlink DN, Mamdani MM, Lee DS, et al. Rates of hyperkalemia after publication of the Randomized Aldactone Evaluation Study. N Engl J Med 2004;351:543. (*There has been a marked increase in rates since the publication of the Randomized Aldactone Evaluation Study [RALES], which encouraged the use of spironolactone.*)
5. Strom BL, Carson L, Schinnar R, et al. Upper gastrointestinal tract bleeding from oral potassium chloride. Comparative risk from microencapsulated vs wax-matrix formulations. Arch Intern Med 1987;147:954. (*A retrospective cohort study, finding that the relative risk was 0.67.*)

CHAPTER 33 ■ MANAGEMENT OF VALVULAR HEART DISEASE

RICHARD R. LIBERTHSON AND IGNACIO INGLESSIS

As a result of increased physician awareness and improvements in noninvasive diagnostic techniques, the diagnosis of valvular heart disease is being made earlier in the course of illness. Outpatient evaluation and management has become commonplace because symptoms are frequently absent or mild at the time the condition is discovered. Although consultation with a cardiologist is usually obtained, the responsibility for long-term care often falls on the primary physician. Proper management requires that the primary physician is familiar with the natural history of valvular disease, the early warning signs of hemodynamic deterioration, and the indications for medical and surgical therapies. Skill in the application of anticoagulation (see Chapter 83) and antibiotic prophylaxis (see Chapter 16) is essential, as is the ability to manage the early phases of heart failure (see Chapter 32) and atrial fibrillation (see Chapter 28). Of major importance is the proper timing of referral for consideration of valve repair.

NATURAL HISTORY (1–19)

Mitral Stenosis

Most cases of mitral stenosis are *rheumatic* in origin, even though as many as 50% of patients cannot give a history of rheumatic fever. In the elderly, there is an increasing incidence of mitral stenosis secondary to progressive annular calcification limiting leaflet mobility (see below). The symptom-free interval averages about 10 years (range, 3 to 25 years). In most instances, symptoms develop gradually over a decade, roughly paralleling the progression of stenosis; however, some people remain relatively free of complaints until stenosis becomes severe. Left atrial and pulmonary venous pressures increase substantially as the valve area falls to less than 1.5 cm^2, and at this point patients typically experience *dyspnea on exertion*. Any stimulus that rapidly increases blood flow or decreases the time available for diastolic filling can precipitate a sudden increase in pulmonary congestion and result in an acute shortness of breath. Strenuous activity, fever, emotion, and the onset of atrial fibrillation are often responsible for acute dyspnea.

Progressive narrowing of the valve orifice is accompanied by worsening exercise tolerance and increasing dyspnea. In patients with tight stenosis (valve area of <1.0 cm^2), the period from the onset of symptoms to incapacity averages 7 years, but the decline can be precipitous with the onset of atrial fibrillation or pneumonia. A chronic marked increase in pulmonary venous pressure often leads to *pulmonary hypertension*, with progressive vascular remodeling and a potentially irreversible elevation of pulmonary vascular resistance occurring in approximately 20% of patients. Cardiac output usually falls with the onset of severe pulmonary hypertension, and fatigue may become a prominent symptom. The right ventricle hypertrophies in response to the rise in pulmonary artery pressure, and *right-sided heart failure, tricuspid valve insufficiency*, and death ensue unless intervention occurs; deterioration may be rapid at this stage.

Atrial fibrillation complicates 40% to 50% of cases of symptomatic mitral stenosis. The correlation between the development of atrial fibrillation and the severity of stenosis is slight and is not due solely to the degree of left atrial enlargement. The loss of atrial systole and the increase in heart rate that characterize atrial fibrillation markedly reduce flow across the mitral valve and boost the left atrial pressure. Premature atrial contractions and paroxysmal atrial fibrillation often precede sustained atrial fibrillation due to mitral stenosis.

Systemic embolization occurs in 10% to 20% of patients with mitral stenosis. Age and the presence of atrial fibrillation are the major determinants of risk; the severity of stenosis is not a determinant. Embolization may be a presenting symptom of mitral stenosis.

In sum, there is typically a symptom-free period of about 10 years. Patients then begin to note dyspnea on exertion over the next 10 years, which progresses in many instances in the following decade. Once symptoms are present on minimal exertion, survival becomes markedly reduced. Patients with New York Heart Association class IV disease (symptoms at rest) have been found to have a 5-year mortality rate of 85%. Some patients have disease that may remain stable for many years; symptoms may not develop until late in the illness.

Mitral Regurgitation

Rheumatic Mitral Regurgitation

Rheumatic mitral regurgitation can remain asymptomatic for many years because the left ventricle dilates and adjusts well to the increase in volume load. Onset of dyspnea and fatigue may not occur for decades. Symptoms take an average of 10 years to progress to the point of disability and need for surgery. It is not until very *late* in the course of the disease that myocardial reserve falters. Once the left ventricle fails, patients note *progressive dyspnea* and *fatigue*; symptoms become present at rest (functional class IV disease). If pulmonary hypertension develops, signs of right-sided heart failure ensue. Prognosis is poor at this stage.

Atrial fibrillation is found in more than 75% of cases, but the abrupt episodes of pulmonary congestion that typify mitral stenosis complicated by atrial fibrillation are less frequent in mitral regurgitation, although rupture of one of the chordae tendineae can result in sudden deterioration.

Chronic Nonrheumatic Mitral Regurgitation

Chronic nonrheumatic mitral regurgitation is commonly encountered in the outpatient setting. In the Western world, the most common causes of chronic mitral regurgitation are ischemic heart disease and mitral valve prolapse secondary to myxomatous degeneration of the valve. Other etiologies include papillary muscle dysfunction and mitral annulus dilation secondary to cardiomyopathy, calcified mitral valve annulus, congenital disease, and drug-induced valve injury.

Mitral Valve Prolapse. Mitral valve prolapse (MVP) is one of the most common valvular disorders, with a community prevalence of 2.5%, which is less than the previous estimate of 5%, which resulted from data skewed by referral bias. Only patients with truly redundant and thickened mitral leaflets on B-mode (two-dimensional) cardiac ultrasound or those with a classic clinical examination should be considered to have MVP. These patients have myxomatous proliferation of the spongiosa and elongation of the chordae. Many patients with normal mitral valve leaflets that appear as bowed or saddle shaped on certain echocardiographic views have been mistakenly labeled as having MVP and approached as if they have its attendant risks.

Although patients with true MVP are at increased risk for valvular incompetence, endocarditis, systemic embolization, and dysrhythmias, the prognosis for most is excellent, and most are entirely asymptomatic and at only minimal risk. Many MVP patients do not experience hemodynamically significant regurgitation or an increase in regurgitant flow with time, but there is a subset that do, particularly those with an initial *left ventricular diastolic dimension greater than 60 mm.* The associated valvular insufficiency can cause *chronic volume overload,* leading to *left ventricular dysfunction* and necessitating mitral valve repair or replacement. The initial phases of left ventricular decline may not be accompanied by symptoms or a major

fall in ejection fraction, making early detection for timely intervention clinically problematic (see later discussion).

There is a slight increase in risk of *bacterial endocarditis,* especially in patients with clinically evident valvular incompetence (regurgitant murmur evident on examination) or a markedly redundant and thickened valve on echocardiogram. Although endocarditis prophylaxis has been recommended for patients with MVP who have evidence of mitral insufficiency, recent guidelines question its utility. Patients with normal variants have little or no increase in risk of endocarditis and do not require antibiotic prophylaxis (see Chapter 16).

Stroke risk is also much lower than previously estimated, due to stricter criteria and better precision in the diagnosis of MVP. Among younger persons with embolic stroke, there is no increase in the prevalence of MVP, suggesting that the risk is minimal in the absence of other embolic risk factors. A very small group of MVP patients have *malignant ventricular arrhythmias;* the overall risk of sudden death is extremely low in most patients with MVP but is heightened in those with a history of syncope, prior ventricular tachyarrhythmias, or a family history of sudden death. Risk appears related to the degree of myxomatous changes but not to the degree of valve incompetence or left ventricular dysfunction.

Some have raised the question of a relation between *panic disorder* and MVP because of panic-like symptoms occurring in a small percentage of patients with MVP. Indeed, a small percentage of MVP patients do suffer from *autonomic dysfunction* and complain of palpitations, atypical chest pain, orthostatic dizziness, near-syncope, cold extremities, throbbing headaches, and neurasthenia and manifest tachyarrhythmias, orthostatic hypotension, and peripheral vasoconstriction. However, careful studies have found no causal link between MVP and autonomic dysfunction or panic disorder.

Papillary Muscle Dysfunction. Papillary muscle dysfunction is responsible for as many as 10% of mitral regurgitation cases found clinically. Causes include ischemic injury, left ventricular dilation, and cardiomyopathy. Ischemic heart disease is the most frequent etiology, with 40% of posterior infarcts and 20% of anterior infarcts accompanied by the development of papillary muscle dysfunction. The amount of regurgitant flow is highly variable. Severe mitral regurgitation and marked pulmonary congestion can occur even in the context of only a minimal reduction in left ventricular ejection fraction. However, prognosis does depend on left ventricular systolic performance.

Calcification of the Mitral Annulus. Calcification of the mitral annulus occurs in older people, often in conjunction with calcification of the aortic valve. The mitral lesion is usually not of hemodynamic significance, but heart block can develop if calcification extends into the ventricular septum.

Congenital Mitral Insufficiency. Congenital mitral insufficiency develops secondary to the formation of mitral valve clefts and is associated with primum atrial septal defects. Varying degrees of insufficiency ensue.

Drug-Induced Disease. Use of the appetite suppressants *dexfenfluramine* and the combination *phentermine/fenfluramine* ("phen-fen") was popular in the mid- to late 1990s (see Chapter 234) before reports of new onset of valvular heart disease appeared. Aortic regurgitation was the most frequently noted problem (see later discussion), but mitral valve involvement was also seen. Risk appeared limited to use that exceeded 3 months. The precise magnitude of valve damage and the relative and absolute risks are somewhat less than originally feared (see subsection on nonrheumatic causes of aortic regurgitation).

Concern has arisen about the association between acquired valvular insufficiency and the use of *ergot-derived dopamine agonists* (e.g., *pergolide* and *cabergoline*), which are used in patients with Parkinson's disease, restless leg syndrome, and prolactinoma. Mitral leaflet thickening and "tenting" have been observed, leading to significant regurgitant flow. A frequency of nearly 25% and a relative risk of greater than 6.0 have been recorded in case–control study. At least 6 months of exposure were required for the changes to be seen and were greatest in those with higher daily doses (>3 mg of pergolide or cabergoline).

Mixed Mitral Disease

Mortality is increased when significant stenosis and regurgitation occur simultaneously. In one large series of patients managed medically, the 10-year survival rate from the time of diagnosis was 33%.

Aortic Stenosis

Because of the marked ability of the left ventricle to undergo hypertrophy and compensate for the pressure load, patients with aortic stenosis can remain symptom-free for many years, even with tight stenosis (valve area of <0.7 cm²). This is especially true in young patients. However, it must be remembered that sudden death can occur in previously asymptomatic individuals with critical aortic stenosis. The onset of *angina* and *effort syncope* suggests a hemodynamically critical lesion that is limiting cardiac output, although in as many as 30% to 60% of aortic stenosis patients with angina, there coexists significant occlusion of a coronary vessel. Survival averages 3 years from the onset of angina or effort syncope. The development of *congestive failure* is an ominous sign because it signals the inability of the myocardium to continue tolerating the severe pressure load; survival averages 2 years from the time that failure is first noted. More than half of patients with aortic stenosis die of congestive failure. Sudden death accounts for another 20%. The mean age of death for patients dying suddenly is 60 years; the mechanism of death in these cases is believed to be a dysrhythmia triggered by myocardial ischemia, although debate continues. The rate of stenosis is unpredictable, and stenosis can progress rapidly over a few years, especially as patients enter their 60s. Figures for survival are only averages; the range is wide, and many patients die soon after the onset of symptoms.

Congenital Aortic Stenosis

Age at clinical onset of aortic stenosis depends part on the underlying etiology. Significant aortic stenosis appearing in a patient younger than 30 years of age is congenital in origin, due most often to a *bicuspid* valve. In approximately 15% of such patients, obstruction is caused by a discrete *subaortic membrane*. Congenital bicuspid valve may be associated with aortic stenosis and/or incompetence as well as coarctation, dilation, and aneurysmal formation of the ascending aorta. Patients presenting between ages 30 and 70 years have either a bicuspid valve or a valve damaged by rheumatic fever. Bicuspid valves may calcify, worsening the degree of stenosis; affected patients may present in their early 60s with evidence of significant calcification and outflow tract obstruction.

Rheumatic Aortic Stenosis

Patients who present with significant aortic stenosis caused by rheumatic fever are on average 10 to 15 years older than patients who present with rheumatic mitral stenosis, due to the more gradual progression of the illness when it involves the aortic valve. Nevertheless, the course can be one of rapid deterioration.

Calcific Aortic Sclerosis and Aortic Stenosis

Aortic sclerosis in the elderly represents valve calcification and fibrosis in the absence of hemodynamically significant stenosis. By age 65 years, about 25% of the population has an audible systolic ejection murmur due to calcific aortic sclerosis, with 1% to 2% already having hemodynamically significant stenosis. By age 80 years, almost half of the population manifests evidence of valve calcification. Previously viewed as a degenerative condition of the aging heart, calcific aortic disease in the elderly is now recognized as having atherosclerotic-like features, with deposition of low-density lipoprotein, an inflammatory cell infiltrate, and eventual fibrosis and calcification. Even without significant stenosis, the condition is associated with a 50% increase in morbidity and mortality from coronary artery disease, underscoring the probable pathophysiologic link and serving as a marker for atherosclerotic disease.

Unlike the aortic stenosis of rheumatic disease, with its fusion of valve commissures, calcific disease aortic stenosis results in thickening of the valve leaflets and resultant loss of mobility and ability to open during systole. The degree of calcification and severity of stenosis may progress. The severity of stenosis parallels the *contractile state* of the left ventricle (LV) and the degree of *calcification*. The weaker the LV contraction, the less will the valve open and the greater is the outflow obstruction. A failing left ventricle may cause a rapid downhill course. The degree of calcification is an independent determinant of prognosis. Persons with severe calcification have a less than 20% chance of 4-year event-free survival.

Once symptoms develop (angina, syncope, heart failure), the 2-year survival rate falls to less than 50%. Whereas symptoms are an important indicator of prognosis, they may be absent in persons who harbor hemodynamically significant obstruction to left ventricular outflow. Besides valve calcification, other echocardiographic features that help to refine the prognosis in asymptomatic persons include *degree of valve calcification, aortic jet velocity*, and *valve area*. The presence of a high-velocity jet (>4.0 m/s) or a rapid rate of increase in velocity (>0.3 m/s per year) in a person with marked calcification reduces the 2-year probability of survival or surgery to 20%. A valve area of less than 1.0 cm² identifies severe stenosis in persons with calcific disease. Despite the poor prognosis of persons with severe stenosis, the risk of sudden death remains low (<1%/yr) in truly asymptomatic persons; however, once even mild symptoms develop, risk rises substantially.

Aortic Regurgitation

Rheumatic Fever

Most patients with severe aortic regurgitation live for decades with little incapacity because the left ventricle dilates to accommodate the extra volume load. The latent period from occurrence of rheumatic fever to the onset of clinical manifestations is about 10 years. During the next decade, symptoms appear and progress. The onset of symptoms is typically gradual, with *palpitations* being among the earliest changes noted by the patient, followed by *dyspnea on exertion* and *fatigability*. The appearance of *left ventricular hypertrophy* with strain and progressive *left ventricular dilation* are associated with a markedly increased risk of heart failure and death within 5 years. If exertional dyspnea worsens, other manifestations of congestive failure are likely to follow and signal the beginning of a rapidly declining phase of the disease due to left ventricular decompensation. At this stage, deterioration is rapid, with death occurring within 1 to 2 years of the onset of congestive failure. *Angina* is common, reported by almost 30% of patients; unlike the angina of aortic stenosis, it typically takes place *at rest* rather than on exertion. Angina becomes more frequent when there is worsening heart failure. *Sudden death* may also occur in patients with severe aortic regurgitation.

Nonrheumatic Causes

In the Western world, most cases of aortic insufficiency are nonrheumatic in origin. About 5% of persons with a *bicuspid aortic* valve also have aortic regurgitation. Other causes of aortic regurgitation include syphilis, myxomatous degeneration, bacterial endocarditis, and connective tissue disease. Aortic regurgitation secondary to untreated *syphilis* appears about 15 to 25 years after the initial infection and often has a more rapid downhill course than aortic regurgitation caused by rheumatic fever. *Myxomatous degeneration* has been found in 10% to 15% of cases of aortic regurgitation studied pathologically. The process is progressive and becomes clinically evident between the ages of 30 and 60 years. Patients with *Marfan's syndrome* may have significant dilation of the ascending aorta, effacing the sinus of Valsalva and impeding closure of the aortic valve. Severe, progressive valvular insufficiency may ensue. Although *bacterial endocarditis* can damage a tricuspid aortic valve, particularly one that is fibrotic or calcific, it is far more likely to occur with a bicuspid valve. Uncommon anomalies associated with aortic regurgitation include *ventricular septal defect* and *discrete subaortic membranes*.

Ankylosing spondylitis is complicated by aortic regurgitation in about 3% of cases. The severity of the lesion is highly variable, and conduction defects are frequent. Aortic regurgitation may appear before the onset of other symptoms, but in most instances it follows the appearance of arthritic symptoms by 10 to 20 years. The presence of severe aortic regurgitation shortens the otherwise normal life expectancy of patients with ankylosing spondylitis. *Reiter's syndrome* is associated with the development of aortic regurgitation in 5% of cases, typically in those with florid manifestations of the disease such as iritis, mucocutaneous changes, and extensive sacroiliac inflammation. The onset of aortic regurgitation occurs an average of 15 years after the disease is first noted, often preceded by conduction disturbances. The severity and course of the aortic regurgitation are highly variable.

Use of the diet-pill combination phen-fen or dexfenfluramine alone was very popular (see Chapter 234) before it was linked to valvular injury in the late 1990s. Fibrosis leading to incompetence of the aortic valve was the most common lesion, but mitral and tricuspid injury was also noted. At surgery, the fibrosis of the endocardial surface resembled that seen in carcinoid syndrome, leading some to link the pill's potent serotonergic effects with disturbance of valvular endocardial metabolism. Risk increased with dose and duration of treatment; a 1% to 5% risk was associated with a minimum of 3 months of use, rising to as high as 20% among those who took the pills for 18 months or more. With full cessation of use, stabilization and some improvement (particularly of aortic regurgitation) were noted and the risk of new disease ceased. In most instances, the degree of valve incompetence was mild, and patients remain asymptomatic. Whether asymptomatic persons will eventually become symptomatic remains to be determined, but because valve injury appears to be largely mild, the risk of developing symptomatic disease is probably low.

Mixed Aortic Valve Disease and Combined Aortic and Mitral Disease

Mixed Aortic Valve Disease

Many patients with aortic stenosis have some degree of aortic regurgitation, and vice versa. Whenever the gradient across the aortic valve is greater than 25 mm Hg in the context of significant regurgitation, there begins to develop a substantial pressure load and an increased volume load on the left ventricle. The clinical course is similar to that for isolated aortic stenosis of the same degree, although some clinicians believe that there is an earlier onset of symptoms. Connective tissue abnormalities in persons with a bicuspid aortic valve may result in clinically silent dilation of the ascending aorta and lead to dissection.

Combined Aortic and Mitral Disease

The etiology is mostly rheumatic; in fact, most cases of rheumatic fever produce some degree of multiple-valve damage, although disease of one valve often dominates the clinical picture. Mitral stenosis may be overlooked in the setting of concurrent heart failure, pneumonia, or aortic valvular disease. In a study of 152 patients with echocardiographically significant mitral stenosis, 15% of mitral stenosis cases were unrecognized before ultrasound examination, yet most had an audible murmur on reexamination. The most common combination is aortic regurgitation in conjunction with mitral disease. Atrial fibrillation and systemic embolization are more frequent than in isolated aortic regurgitation, as is the severity of pulmonary symptoms. Less common is the coexistence of aortic stenosis and mitral stenosis. Symptoms and signs of aortic stenosis are blunted by significant mitral stenosis, such that pulmonary symptoms, atrial fibrillation, and systemic embolization may dominate the presentation, but there may be more angina and syncope than expected from isolated mitral stenosis. Course is dictated by the severity of the individual lesions, but mitral stenosis can delay the appearance of some of the manifestations of advanced aortic stenosis.

ESTIMATING SEVERITY OF DISEASE (1–3,5–7,11–16,20–26)

Mitral Stenosis

Symptoms

Symptoms provide crude indications of the severity of stenosis. *Dyspnea* correlates with an increase in left atrial pressure and the development of *pulmonary venous congestion,* but the relationship between degree of stenosis and elevation of left atrial pressure is variable. *Fatigue* occurs most often in the context of *pulmonary hypertension,* but the nonspecific nature of the symptom lessens its utility in estimating severity. *Hemoptysis* is related to pulmonary *venous hypertension* but does not necessarily imply severe stenosis. Thus, history alone may fail to detect severe stenosis that is unaccompanied by marked pulmonary congestion; however, a worsening of dyspnea and a decline in exercise tolerance suggest hemodynamic deterioration and require further investigation.

Physical Examination

The interval between the second heart sound and the opening snap, referred to as the *S2 to OS interval*, and the duration and timing of the diastolic murmur provide additional clues of severity. The S2 to OS interval is a function of the elevation in left atrial pressure. The greater the pressure, the shorter is the interval. Unfortunately, the degree of mitral stenosis is not the only determinant of left atrial pressure; the interval can be affected by factors other than valve area, such as heart rate and left ventricular pressure. Moreover, the valve must be mobile to snap; in advanced disease, the valve may calcify, and the snap becomes inaudible. Nevertheless, the S2 to OS interval is useful because it can be determined at the bedside and does provide data that may help in judging severity when considered in the context of other findings. Perhaps the most precise use of the interval is in separating hemodynamically insignificant disease from moderate and severe mitral stenosis. An interval of greater than 0.11 second at rest with a heart rate of 70 to 80 beats/min argues against a significant lesion (although there are exceptions). Patients with moderate to tight stenosis usually demonstrate intervals of less than 0.08 second, which shorten with exercise. Proper estimation of the S2 to OS interval takes considerable practice.

The *intensity* of the *diastolic murmur* does not correlate with severity of stenosis, but its *duration* through diastole does. However, development of pulmonary hypertension may decrease cardiac output from the right side of the heart, result in a diminution of flow across the mitral valve, and consequently shorten the duration of the murmur.

Laboratory Studies

A few simple, carefully selected, noninvasive laboratory studies can be very helpful.

Chest X-Ray. Chest x-ray provides important evidence of severity. The earliest radiologic sign of mitral stenosis is dilation of the left atrium, which is best seen on a lateral view in conjunction with a barium swallow to outline the esophagus. Other signs include elevation of left-main-stem bronchus and a "double-shadow" right heart border. Overall, these findings are not very reliable manifestations of severity. A better sign is redistribution of the pulmonary venous blood flow, producing dilation of the upper-zone pulmonary veins. Upper-zone redistribution becomes prominent at a left atrial pressure of 25 mm Hg and parallels the severity of stenosis. This change in pulmonary venous flow is very sensitive to changes in left atrial pressure, but it is not unique to mitral stenosis. Radiologic evidence of pulmonary hypertension (dilation of the right pulmonary artery to 15 to 18 mm, rapid tapering of vessels, and right ventricular enlargement) strongly suggests advanced mitral stenosis, although again the findings are not specific for mitral stenosis. The presence of Kerley B lines, perihilar haze, and other manifestations of interstitial edema are seen in patients with severe dyspnea due to mitral stenosis; the absence of interstitial edema on chest film does not rule out tight mitral stenosis, but a patient with dyspnea at rest should always show these changes on chest x-ray; otherwise, one must question the etiology of the shortness of breath. In sum, no single radiologic finding is specific for severe mitral stenosis, but x-ray data can provide important supporting evidence.

Cardiac Ultrasound (Echocardiography). Cardiac ultrasound (echocardiography) is the most sensitive noninvasive method for evaluating mitral stenosis. *Two-dimensional (B-mode)* echocardiography provides definitive assessment by allowing direct visualization of the entire valve and its supporting apparatus, measurement of the valve orifice, left atrial and left ventricular chamber dimensions, and assessment of abnormality of other cardiac valves. The addition of *Doppler ultrasound* techniques—including *continuous-wave* Doppler and *color-flow* study—to the ultrasound examination provides detailed delineation of valve anatomy, blood flow, and magnitude of obstruction. A scoring system based on ultrasound estimates of valve mobility, degree of thickening, calcification, and anatomy of the subvalvular apparatus helps to identify candidates suitable for transcatheter balloon dilation of the stenotic valve.

Transesophageal ultrasound is useful when there is concern about intracavity thrombosis (as in atrial fibrillation; see Chapter 28) or valvular vegetations (as in endocarditis). *Cardiac catheterization* is indicated when symptoms are progressive and cardiac surgery or balloon valvuloplasty is being considered (see later discussion).

The Electrocardiogram. The electrocardiogram (ECG) is of limited utility for the estimation of severity. The best ECG sign appears to be the *QRS axis*; a *rightward shift* to greater than +60 is associated with a valve area of less than 1.3 cm^2 in more than 85% of cases. The absence of the rightward shift in axis means little. The greater the pulmonary artery pressure, the more likely it is that *right ventricular hypertrophy* will appear on the ECG.

Mitral Regurgitation

History and Physical Examination

A reasonable estimate of the severity of mitral insufficiency can be obtained by history and physical examination. *Dyspnea on exertion* and *fatigability* suggest hemodynamically significant regurgitation, although the absence of such symptoms does not rule out severe regurgitant disease (which can be asymptomatic until left ventricular decompensation begins to set in). On physical examination, severe mitral regurgitation produces *left ventricular enlargement* with a hyperdynamic, slightly diffuse, apical impulse displaced to the left but of normal timing and duration. In addition, there is a pansystolic murmur (its loudness does not correlate directly with severity), a loud *third heart sound* (S3), often a middiastolic rumble from increased flow across the mitral valve, and at times wide splitting of the second sound due to shortening of left ventricular systole and early aortic valve closure. In contrast to other forms of valvular disease, a third heart sound may sometimes be audible in a mitral regurgitation patient in the absence of other signs of severe mitral regurgitation and need not represent a failing left ventricle.

Laboratory Studies

In patients with advanced disease, cardiomegaly and left atrial enlargement are pronounced on *chest film*. A normal heart on chest x-ray and the absence of an apical pansystolic murmur rule out significant mitral regurgitation. The *ECG* reflects both left atrial and left ventricular enlargement but is hardly specific for mitral regurgitation.

Transthoracic cardiac ultrasound with *Doppler* is the test of choice for both estimation of severity and prognosis. As noted, some patients with severe mitral regurgitation, such as those with isolated mitral valve prolapse, may remain asymptomatic despite severe regurgitation, making ultrasound evaluation essential for the timely identification and treatment of persons who may be at high risk. By the time symptoms develop, left ventricular decompensation may already be underway. The severity of disease can be ascertained with the help of color-flow Doppler mapping. Prognostically important data provided by ultrasound include qualitative estimate of regurgitant flow, left atrial and left ventricular dimensions, ejection fraction, and, more recently, quantitative determination of regurgitant severity (i.e., regurgitant orifice). Echocardiographic parameters predictive of impending irreversible left ventricular dysfunction and clinical deterioration have been established to help time surgical correction; these include falling *ejection fraction* (<60%), *end-systolic dimension* (>40 to 45 mm), and *effective regurgitant orifice* (>40 mm^2).

Cardiac catheterization is indicated in patients with progressive symptoms and rapidly increasing heart size who are being considered for surgery. One needs to estimate the degree of regurgitation, assess ventricular function, and check for the presence and severity of associated valvular and coronary disease.

Evaluation of Mitral Valve Prolapse

In patients with mitral regurgitation due to MVP, the severity of regurgitation increases with *age, male gender, duration* of the murmur, degree of *valve leaflet thickening*, and degree of *posterior leaflet prolapse*. Only patients with truly redundant and thickened mitral leaflets are at risk for complications from MVP (e.g., valvular incompetence, endocarditis, systemic embolization, and dysrhythmias). Those with mild bowing and normal leaflets should be considered to have a variant of the normal mitral valve and not true MVP. Those with true MVP and associated valvular insufficiency are at risk for chronic volume overload leading to left ventricular dysfunction; there may be no premonitory symptoms or fall in the ejection fraction.

Aortic Stenosis

There are numerous pitfalls in the clinical estimation of the severity of aortic stenosis, especially in the elderly. Nevertheless, careful history and physical examination can provide important clues, supplemented by ultrasound examination.

History

Severe stenosis may be asymptomatic for quite some time, but the onset of effort *syncope, angina,* or symptoms of congestive *heart failure* point to advanced disease with markedly reduced chances of 5-year survival. At times, it is impossible to tell clinically whether these worrisome symptoms are due to critical aortic stenosis or to coexisting coronary disease; both need to be considered and thoroughly investigated (see later discussion). Hemodynamically significant disease may be also heralded by the onset of subtler complaints such as mild exercise intolerance or lightheadedness. Even if mild or dismissed by the patient, these symptoms should not be ignored because their onset is associated with a marked increase in the risk of an adverse cardiac event.

Physical Examination

Delay in carotid artery upstroke is one of the most helpful physical signs of significant aortic stenosis, especially in the young. A normal upstroke in a patient younger than 60 years of age is strong evidence against important stenosis; however, upstroke may appear normal in the elderly patient with severe stenosis because of a stiff noncompliant carotid artery. Particularly when there are prominent transmitted carotid thrills, the *brachial arteries* may better reflect the severity of aortic stenosis and should also be assessed by palpation. When coincidental aortic regurgitation is present, the upstroke may also appear normal in the presence of marked stenosis. A misleading delay in carotid upstroke can occur from the combination of systemic hypertension and congestive heart failure. The elevation of *systolic blood pressure* does not rule out hemodynamically significant aortic stenosis, although a pressure of greater than 200 mm Hg and a pulse pressure of greater than 80 mm Hg are unusual when stenosis is marked. *Lower-extremity pulse* and *blood pressure* should also be assessed to rule out coincident coarctation in persons suspected of having a bicuspid valve.

In young patients, the *intensity* of the *murmur* often correlates with severity; however, although it is generally true that critical aortic stenosis is unlikely in a young ambulating person who has less than a 3/6 systolic ejection murmur, rare exceptions do occur. In patients with far-advanced disease and a failing left ventricle, the murmur may decrease in intensity and appear insignificant as flow across the valve diminishes. In general, the longer the murmur takes to reach peak intensity, the greater is the stenosis. Unfortunately, the *timing of maximal intensity* may not be delayed in some cases of severe stenosis, but if the murmur does peak after midsystole, the stenosis is usually significant. Because the murmur of aortic stenosis in the elderly may lose its characteristic qualities, it is also best to judge severity on the basis of symptoms and other findings. Aortic stenosis in the elderly in the absence of evidence of significant outflow tract obstruction suggests *aortic sclerosis*.

A delay in the aortic component of the *second heart sound (S2)* is another sign of significant aortic stenosis. S2 may be single or paradoxically split. Calcification and increased rigidity of the valve will often diminish the intensity of the aortic closing sound; it may become inaudible. A forceful *left ventricular impulse* noted on palpation of the precordium is a reliable indication of secondary left ventricular hypertrophy due to significant outflow obstruction.

Laboratory Studies

The ECG and ultrasound are essential initial studies.

ECG. The ECG can contribute to the evaluation by showing signs of left ventricular *hypertrophy* (increased voltage and a strain pattern in the precordial leads V5 and V6). The likelihood of finding a strain pattern (i.e., ST- and T-wave depression in the apical and lateral leads) increases with the increase in gradient across the aortic valve. These ECG changes also identify patients at increased risk of sudden death because fewer than 10% of patients succumbing to sudden death demonstrate a normal ECG. In children, the ECG is less helpful; even severe aortic stenosis may not produce left ventricular hypertrophy and a strain pattern. *Exercise stress testing* is contraindicated for the workup of anginal chest pain in the setting of possible aortic stenosis (can result in sudden death in those with critical stenosis) and should not be attempted until hemodynamically significant aortic stenosis has been ruled out by ultrasound.

Cardiac Ultrasound. Cardiac ultrasound has become essential for the assessment of aortic stenosis and is capable of determining degree of calcification, valve anatomy, chamber size, and left ventricular contractility. In the elderly, the *degree of* *valvular calcification* correlates with the severity of stenosis. The absence of significant calcification in a patient older than 60 years of age greatly reduces the probability of important valvular stenosis. The findings of thickening and decreased mobility of the aortic valve leaflets suggest advancing disease, as does an increasing *aortic-jet velocity*, which correlates with increased risk in asymptomatic elderly persons. Poststenotic dilation of the aorta suggests aortic valvular stenosis but does not have quantitative meaning; however, it should be scrutinized to ensure that it does not achieve aneurysmal size and risk dissection, particularly in persons with a bicuspid valve and connective tissue defect.

Echocardiography can help to distinguish valvular from subvalvular stenosis and, if the stenosis subvalvular, whether it is secondary to a discrete membrane, a fibromuscular bar, or a hypertrophic myocardium as in *hypertrophic cardiomyopathy*. In the young patient with normal left ventricular function, the echocardiogram can provide an indirect estimate of the magnitude of the obstructive gradient. The echocardiogram also delineates the magnitude of left ventricular wall thickening and any associated valvular abnormality, particularly rheumatic valve disease. The addition of Doppler techniques to the echocardiographic evaluation provides an accurate determination of outflow tract pressure gradients (the mean gradient correlates best with the gradient found at catheterization) and helps to detect any accompanying aortic regurgitation. The finding of mitral regurgitation, especially if progressive on serial studies, correlates with the severity and progression of aortic stenosis.

Cardiac Catheterization. Cardiac catheterization is indicated in the young asymptomatic patient with evidence of severe stenosis, as well as in any patient with known aortic stenosis who begins to develop symptoms of angina, heart failure, or syncope. Elderly patients who are deemed healthy enough to be candidates for surgery should also have *coronary angiography* performed to identify significant occlusive disease that may be the source of symptoms or may limit chances of surviving surgery without correction at the time of valve replacement.

Aortic Regurgitation

History and Physical Examination

The severity of aortic regurgitation can usually be well assessed clinically in cases of isolated valvular insufficiency. Marked regurgitation that is longstanding produces dyspnea, a loud diastolic murmur that extends beyond middiastole, an S3, a bounding pulse, and a widened pulse pressure. The absence of a wide pulse pressure does not rule out hemodynamically significant aortic regurgitation, nor does the degree of widening necessarily correlate quantitatively with severity. Changes in peripheral resistance alone can cause large variations in pulse pressure. ECG and x-ray evidence of left ventricular hypertrophy and enlargement are indicative of longstanding significant regurgitation and suggest worsening left ventricular function if they progress.

Echocardiogram with Doppler

Echocardiogram with Doppler enhancement can determine left ventricular size and contractility and delineate the specific disease process in aortic regurgitation—be it rheumatic, annular dilation, or advanced luetic destruction. Signs of left ventricular dysfunction by ultrasound study often precede symptoms

and help to determine the optimal time for consideration of surgery (see later discussion). Doppler study has a sensitivity approaching 100% for the diagnosis of aortic regurgitation, especially when *color-flow* techniques are used, far superior to physical examination or B-mode echocardiography. Color-flow techniques can provide an excellent noninvasive estimate of regurgitant severity that is within 10% of that found at cardiac catheterization. *Transesophageal echocardiography* is worth considering when endocarditis is a concern.

Cardiac Catheterization

When aortic regurgitation occurs in the presence of coexisting aortic stenosis, mitral stenosis, or heart failure, the estimation of severity can be very difficult to perform on clinical grounds alone. Consultation with a cardiologist and *catheterization* are often needed.

PRINCIPLES OF MANAGEMENT (1–19,27–36)

Therapeutic Objectives and Timing of Intervention

The principal objectives are to preserve exercise capacity, lifestyle, and life expectancy and to minimize the chances of endocarditis and systemic embolization. The proper timing of intervention is essential to successful treatment. A common management error is inappropriately to delay surgery or valvuloplasty, allowing irreversible myocardial decompensation to develop; this increases the risk of operation and reduces the postoperative benefit. A physician can be lulled into a false sense of security by continuing to control symptoms through repetitive escalations of medical therapy. The need for progressive increases in medication suggests worsening ventricular function and the need for interventional therapy. By ignoring the significance of such developments, the physician may miss the optimal opportunity for the best possible surgical outcome, long-term improvement, and survival.

Roles of Medical and Surgical Interventions

Early in the course of illness, therapy is predominantly medical, directed at minimizing pulmonary venous congestion (see Chapter 32) and preventing potentially dangerous complications, such as arrhythmias (see Chapter 28 and 29), bacterial endocarditis (see Chapter 16), and systemic embolization (see Chapter 83). Most patients can be well managed on an outpatient basis for many years with a mild diuretic regimen supplemented by an angiotensin-converting-enzyme inhibitor or digitalis (see Chapter 32) before the need for interventional therapy. However, inappropriately escalating and prolonging medical therapy beyond the optimal time for surgery is a common mistake that must be avoided if the best surgical outcome is to be obtained.

More advanced stages of disease may require invasive intervention. Life expectancy and quality of life are clearly improved by properly timed intervention. Advances in valvuloplasty technique, prosthetic valve design, and operative technique have produced substantial reductions in interventional mortality. Mortality rates for patients undergoing valve surgery in major centers average less than 1% for mitral valvulotomy and less than 5% for mitral or aortic valve replacement. Operative mortality increases sharply when patients with advanced disease (e.g., functional class IV) undergo surgery. However, patients with severe disease should not be denied an operation if they have sufficient myocardial reserve and thus a chance for meaningful survival.

The 5-year life expectancy rate for patients with class IV disease who live through valve replacement is usually less than 50%, but this figure is much better than the rate of less than 5% for similar patients managed medically. Thus, even when surgery is inordinately delayed, it may still offer the patient some opportunity for prolonging survival. Contraindications to valve surgery include serious coexisting noncardiac illness that would compromise survival and the existence of end-stage myocardial decompensation, which would make surgery for naught. *Percutaneous balloon valvuloplasty* is being used effectively and safely for relief of severe mitral valvular stenosis in carefully selected patients. For young patients with valvular aortic stenosis, it has also proved to be efficacious, but in the elderly with severe aortic stenosis, results have been disappointing (a high restenosis rate and a small but definite risk for stroke, aortic insufficiency, and mortality). Balloon valvuloplasty has proven to be the most useful as a bridge to later surgery in patients with multiorgan failure and cardiogenic shock or as a palliative short-term measure for patients who are too ill to tolerate the risk of open heart surgery.

Postsurgical Management

It is important to emphasize that patients who undergo valve surgery still have a "cardiac problem" after surgical correction, whether a prosthetic valve with a variable and still unknown late course, a need for anticoagulation and endocarditis prophylaxis, or an associated cardiac abnormality such as coronary, myocardial, or conduction system disease. All too often this is forgotten after the patient undergoes valve repair. Such patients need continued close follow-up and always remain "cardiac patients."

PATIENT EDUCATION

Prophylaxis

Effective prevention of infectious and embolic complications requires thorough patient and family education. Of prime importance is teaching endocarditis prophylaxis (see Chapter 16). Patients with rheumatic heart disease need instruction in the prevention of group A β-hemolytic streptococcal infection (see Chapter 17). Persons with mechanical valves and those with valvular disease complicated by atrial fibrillation require detailed instruction on the proper use of warfarin anticoagulation (see Chapter 83). The chances of compliance are certain to improve if time is taken to explain the rationale for these prophylactic measures.

Activity and Self-Monitoring

Self-monitoring and prompt reporting of early symptoms of cardiac decompensation are essential. Patients and their families should also be fully briefed on allowable activity to avoid both unnecessary restriction and the risk of sudden death in the high-risk patient (e.g., the young asymptomatic person with critical aortic stenosis). If the safety of unlimited activity is in doubt, then a cardiac consultation can be helpful.

The patient's functional status and the proper timing of interventional therapy can be optimized by close, regularly scheduled follow-up and instructions to report promptly early symptoms of cardiac decompensation (e.g., the onset of exertional dyspnea or fatigue). Patient confidence and a sense of partnership care are fostered by such follow-up. It is helpful to note the treatability of valvular heart disease and its excellent prognosis when therapy is properly selected and timed. This provides the rationale for careful self-monitoring. If the patient cannot be depended on to relate symptoms accurately, then a family member or friend needs to be recruited to watch for early manifestations of worsening disease and monitor therapy. The importance of a detailed review of the medical program with all concerned cannot be overemphasized, given the very serious consequences from the misuse of diuretics, digitalis, and anticoagulants in valvular disease. Of particular importance is warning against unauthorized self-escalation of the medical program when symptoms worsen.

Choosing Type of Valve Surgery and Prosthesis

These decisions are usually the province of the surgeon in conversation with the patient and family, but patients or family members will often ask the opinion of the primary physician with whom they have a longstanding relation. A few principles and generalizations can be helpful to review but are not a substitute for a detailed discussion between cardiac surgeon and patient. Repairing a valve tends to be of lower risk and preferable to replacing it, provided repair is technically feasible and can be made sufficiently durable. Young persons who can undergo native valve repair might be spared the need for reoperation and long-term anticoagulation associated with bioprosthetic and mechanical valves. Catheter-based percutaneous approaches to valve repair are under development and hold promise for less invasive means of fixing damaged valves; these may prove especially useful in persons who are poor surgical risks and those reluctant to undergo surgery.

When valve repair is not feasible, a bioprosthesis or mechanical valve requires consideration. The durability of bioprosthetic valves increases with age at implantation but is usually less than 20 years. An advantage is that such valves do not require long-term anticoagulation. Good candidates for a bioprosthesis are older persons (>70 years of age for mitral valve and >65 years of age for aortic valve) and those who have a contraindication to warfarin anticoagulation (see Chapter 83). Mechanical valves are more durable (>20 years) and best for persons with a prolonged life expectancy, provided they can take warfarin on a long-term basis.

Advice to Patients Taking Medications Associated with Valvular Injury

Persons who took phen/fen diet pills in the late 1990s will benefit from a review of recent data on risk and natural history. Those who took the diet aids for less than 3 months and have no clinical evidence of valvular regurgitation can be reassured that they have no future risk and do not require ultrasound testing. Those who had longer-term exposure and clinical evidence of valvular incompetence, particularly of the aortic valve, should undergo color-flow Doppler ultrasound examination to determine severity of disease. They, too, can be reassured that in most instances the degree of damage is likely to be mild, nonprogressive (if not modestly reversible), and without a high risk of long-term hemodynamic consequences.

Persons taking ergot-derived dopamine agonists such as pergolide or cabergoline should be advised of the risk of heart-valve damage with extended use (>6 months) and at higher daily doses (>3 mg/d). All patients with a history of significant exposure should be advised to undergo cardiac ultrasound evaluation and follow-up if the initial study is abnormal. Persons with less than 6 months of use and low-dose intake can be reassured that the risk is very low, as can those taking nonergot dopaminergics. Alternative agents should be sought for the treatment of their underlying conditions.

THERAPEUTIC RECOMMENDATIONS AND INDICATIONS FOR REFERRAL AND ADMISSION (1–19,27–36)

- Monitor all patients by periodic assessment of exercise tolerance, cardiopulmonary examination, chest x-ray, and cardiac ultrasound examination (including Doppler study).
- All patients with any form of significant valvular heart disease should receive prophylaxis for bacterial endocarditis (see Chapter 16).
- Patients younger than 35 years of age with previous rheumatic fever should be considered for rheumatic fever prophylaxis (see Chapter 17), particularly if they have frequent β-streptococcal infections or exposure to young children.
- The onset of atrial fibrillation with a rapid ventricular response rate accompanied by acute hemodynamic deterioration is an indication for immediate hospital admission and treatment. Patients with slower rates who tolerate the atrial fibrillation can be treated on an outpatient basis (see Chapter 28).
- The occurrence of systemic embolization is an indication for urgent admission and intravenous anticoagulant therapy followed by long-term oral anticoagulant treatment (see Chapter 83). Some clinicians argue that valve surgery should be considered if embolization occurs; most concur that surgery is indicated if embolization happens repeatedly.
- The use of medications associated with valvular compromise (e.g., ergot-derived dopaminergic drugs [pergolide, cabergoline]) should be halted and cardiac ultrasound with Doppler obtained.

Mitral Stenosis

- Asymptomatic patients with mild to moderate stenosis need no restriction of activity. Those with evidence of tight stenosis and relatively few symptoms should be advised of the risk of precipitating symptoms by extreme exertion or pregnancy.
- Patients with mild dyspnea that occurs only on exertion can be started on a mild diuretic program (e.g., hydrochlorothiazide 50 to 100 mg/d) and advised to follow a no-added-salt diet. Digitalis is of no benefit in isolated mitral stenosis unless there is atrial fibrillation. Extremely vigorous exertion and emotional upset should be avoided to prevent precipitating symptoms.
- Chronic warfarin oral anticoagulation is indicated for the patient with mitral stenosis, particularly when there is atrial fibrillation (see Chapter 28).
- The development of tight mitral stenosis (as evidenced by a short S2 to OS interval, prolonged diastolic murmur, left atrial enlargement and upper-zone redistribution on chest x-ray, and narrowed valve orifice and reduced flow on ultrasound) necessitates referral to a cardiologist for the consideration of invasive intervention, either surgery or balloon angioplasty, even if few symptoms are reported. Consultation is also needed for worsening dyspnea that is inadequately controlled by a mild diuretic program and salt restriction.
- Young patients with evidence of isolated tight mitral stenosis with a pliable, noncalcified valve should be considered for interventional therapy early in the course of their illness, even before symptoms are disabling, because transcatheter or surgical valvulotomy can be performed. Both procedures provide long-lasting hemodynamic improvement.
- Early referral for cardiologic assessment is advisable because percutaneous balloon mitral valvulotomy is an increasingly attractive alternative to surgical mitral commissurotomy in appropriately selected patients.
- Older patients with fibrotic valves (absent opening snap, heavy valve calcification, and limited motion) must undergo valve replacement if surgery is needed. Because surgical mortality and complications are greater for valve replacement than for valvulotomy, surgery need not be advised until symptoms are more disabling. However, surgery should not be delayed until symptoms occur at rest or on minimal exertion because operative risk and long-term mortality increase substantially. A walk with the patient down a corridor or up a flight of stairs may be of great help in convincing both the physician and the patient that the time for surgery has arrived.
- Cardiac consultation for the consideration of catheterization is indicated in the patient being considered for surgery when there is a question of mixed mitral disease or the involvement of multiple valves or when symptoms are out of proportion to the objective evidence of disease.

Mitral Regurgitation

- Asymptomatic young patients need no restriction of aerobic activity; however, they should be advised against regular heavy isometric exercise such as weight lifting, which might increase the degree of regurgitation.
- Older asymptomatic persons should have periodic Doppler ultrasound examination to determine severity, estimate prognosis, and guide management.
- Asymptomatic persons with echocardiographic evidence of severe disease and poor prognosis (e.g., falling ejection fraction [<60%], increasing end-systolic dimension [>40 to 45 mm], and large effective regurgitant orifice [>40 mm^2]) should be referred for the consideration of value repair. (Despite their frequent use in clinical practice, systemic vasodilators have not been proven to modify the natural history of asymptomatic or minimally symptomatic severe mitral insufficiency.)
- The onset of fatigue and dyspnea in persons with mild to moderate disease and no evidence of left ventricular dysfunction can be treated with the initiation of a gentle diuretic program (e.g., 50 to 100 mg/d hydrochlorothiazide) in conjunction with a no-added-salt diet. A modest diuretic program that adequately controls symptoms may suffice for years in patients with mild to moderate mitral regurgitation and is not an indication for surgery.
- The development of any increase in dyspnea that requires the escalation of diuretic therapy is an indication for cardiac consultation concerning valve replacement. Progressive

deterioration in clinical status and increasing heart size suggest the presence of myocardial decompensation; prompt referral is indicated. Medical therapy is no substitute for valve surgery and does not delay the need for it.

- Refractory congestive failure due to mitral regurgitation is not a contraindication to surgery, although risk is increased. Before surgery, symptoms may be lessened by vasodilator therapy, particularly angiotensin-converting-enzyme inhibitors (e.g., captopril 25 to 50 mg three times daily; see Chapter 32), which can diminish the magnitude of regurgitant flow by decreasing afterload. The use of vasodilators can benefit the inoperable patient.
- Patients with incapacitating dyspnea and pulmonary congestion that is believed to be caused by papillary muscle dysfunction should be referred to the cardiologist for catheterization to determine whether valve replacement will be of benefit. In one series, patients with ejection fractions of greater than 0.35 had the best surgical survival. If there is coexisting coronary disease, it should be treated (see Chapter 30).
- Valve reconstruction is becoming an increasingly frequent option in mitral regurgitation, obviating the need for an artificial valve and its attendant risks in many cases; however, long-term durability remains to be established.
- Patients with a mildly prolapsed mitral valve rarely require treatment other than endocarditis prophylaxis when indicated (see Chapter 16). Dyspnea is uncommon, and digitalis, diuretics, and salt restriction are unnecessary because the magnitude of the regurgitation is usually insignificant and rarely progressive. However, patients with a dilated left ventricle and marked regurgitation should be followed with serial cardiac ultrasonography for the early detection of left ventricular dysfunction, a sign of poor prognosis and an indication for consideration of repair. The rare patient with a history of syncope or ventricular tachycardia or a family history of sudden death requires consideration of treatment for malignant ventricular dysrhythmias (see Chapter 29); patients with isolated palpitations do not. There is no evidence that prophylaxis for systemic embolization is needed in the absence of concurrent risk factors.
- Patients with calcification of the mitral valve annulus should be followed for the development of heart block. Regurgitant flow is usually small; consequently, dyspnea and pulmonary congestion are not major problems.
- Chronic anticoagulation is indicated in mitral regurgitation patients with atrial fibrillation, especially when it is accompanied by marked left atrial and left ventricular enlargement.

Aortic Stenosis

- Patients with aortic sclerosis are at no increased risk from their valvular disease, but the sclerosis is a marker of increased atherosclerotic risk, which should be attended to (see Chapters 26, 27, 30, and 31).
- Asymptomatic patients with mild aortic stenosis do not require restriction of activity.
- Young asymptomatic patients with evidence of tight stenosis should be advised against heavy physical exertion (e.g., competitive sports) and referred to a cardiologist for consideration of catheterization and valvuloplasty or valve replacement. Stress Doppler ultrasound evaluation can help in the difficult task of determining the timing of intervention. Cardiac catheterization may be needed.
- Many young patients with tight aortic stenosis may benefit from transcatheter aortic balloon valvuloplasty. Results in

appropriately selected young patients are comparable with those achieved with surgical valvuloplasty.

- In elderly patients, especially those with fibrotic, calcified valves and associated aortic incompetence, balloon valvuloplasty is appropriate only as a palliative measure in those unfit for surgery.
- The onset of angina, effort syncope, or congestive heart failure dictates prompt referral for the consideration of valve surgery. These are signs of critical stenosis and predict a poor prognosis unless definitive therapy is undertaken. Such patients are at risk for sudden death. Medical therapy is no substitute.
- Congestive failure can be treated symptomatically on a temporary basis by prescribing digitalis and a moderate diuretic program (e.g., the cautious use of furosemide 20 to 40 mg/d; see Chapter 32). Such therapy may help to reduce pulmonary congestion and sustain cardiac output temporarily, but the need for a high diastolic filling pressure must be kept in mind; overzealous diuretic therapy can cause a precipitous fall in cardiac output; afterload reduction may also be dangerous in severe aortic stenosis.
- Angina can be treated symptomatically but cautiously with nitrates pending surgery (see Chapter 30); β-blockers are contraindicated due to their negative inotropic effects. Coronary angiography is required at the time of cardiac catheterization to determine whether there is coexisting significant coronary artery disease and the need for a bypass procedure at the time of valve replacement.
- Advanced age is not an absolute contraindication to valve replacement. Survival from surgery is predominantly a function of the patient's myocardial reserve. Consequently, even patients in their 80s need not be denied surgery if they are otherwise reasonable surgical candidates and demonstrate an adequate ejection fraction, even in the setting of severe aortic stenosis.
- Because calcification of the aortic valve can progress rapidly over a few years, patients with aortic stenosis should have careful longitudinal care and regular follow-up, even when disease appears to be hemodynamically insignificant and the patient is asymptomatic.

Aortic Regurgitation

- No activity restrictions are necessary in young asymptomatic patients with mild regurgitation.
- Assess severity with an initial cardiac ultrasound examination that includes Doppler study and follow patients having evidence of severe regurgitation with serial ultrasound examinations in addition to regular office assessments.
- Asymptomatic patients with moderately severe disease may be treated with afterload reduction (e.g., lisinopril 10 mg twice daily), which appears to be capable of reducing left ventricular end-systolic and end-diastolic pressures and perhaps slowing disease progression.
- Patients with evidence of worsening left ventricular function (left ventricular hypertrophy) with a strain pattern on ECG, increasing cardiomegaly on chest film, falling ejection fraction, and increasing left ventricular end-systolic dimension on ultrasound examination) should be referred to a cardiologist for consideration of surgery, even in the absence of symptoms. Patients with a declining left ventricle have an increased risk of ventricular tachycardia and an increased 5-year mortality rate. The early identification of high-risk patients is suggested in the hope of correcting aortic

regurgitation before the development of irreversible myocardial decompensation, which may have already started by the time symptoms occur.

■ The onset of mild symptoms of pulmonary congestion (dyspnea on climbing more than one flight of stairs) in the absence of evidence of significant left ventricular dysfunction can be treated medically with digitalization, a mild diuretic (50 to 100 mg hydrochlorothiazide), or afterload reduction (e.g., lisinopril 10 mg twice daily), but close clinical follow-up and frequent serial ultrasound examinations are essential to prevent inappropriate delay of surgery. Progression of dyspnea to onset after climbing less than one flight of stairs or worsening of left ventricular function on follow-up ultrasound examination indicates the need for prompt cardiac consultation and consideration of surgery.

■ Patients with dyspnea prompted by minimal exertion, orthopnea, or paroxysmal nocturnal dyspnea require prompt referral for surgery because life expectancy is less than 1 year without surgery. Medical therapy with digitalis and diuretics may provide some symptomatic relief temporarily but must not be used in place of valve surgery at this stage of illness.

Annotated Bibliography

1. Brener SJ, Duffy CI, Thomas JD, et al. Progression of aortic stenosis in 394 patients. J Am Coll Cardiol 1995;25:305. (*A cohort ultrasound study, finding significant yearly progression; left ventricular hypertrophy and mitral regurgitation were major risk factors for increases in gradient; mitral regurgitation was associated with reduced left ventricular function.*)

2. Brinkner ME, Hillis LD, Lange RA. Congenital heart disease in adults. N Engl J Med 2000;342:256. (*A useful review for the generalist reader; 60 references.*)

3. Brunnen PL, Finlayson JD, Short D. Serious mitral stenosis with slight symptoms. Br Med J 1964;1:1958. (*A classic paper; symptoms may be slight, but young patients with tight stenosis are at risk for sudden deterioration; pregnancy was a major precipitant.*)

4. Enriquez-Sarano M, Tajik J. Aortic regurgitation. N Engl J Med 2004; 351:1539. (*An excellent clinical review; 42 references.*)

5. Freed LA, Levy D, Levine RA, et al. Prevalence and clinical outcome of mitral-valve prolapse. N Engl J Med 1999;341:1. (*The best available community-based data; a lower prevalence and a lower risk of adverse sequelae were found than in previous reports.*)

6. Ferencik M, Pape LA. Changes in size of ascending aorta and aortic valve function with time in patients with congenitally bicuspid aortic valves. Am J Cardiol 2004;93:525. (*Aneurysm may ensue.*)

7. Fukada N, Oki T, Iuchi A, et al. Predisposing factors for severe mitral regurgitation in idiopathic mitral valve prolapse. Am J Cardiol 1995;76:503. (*The severity of regurgitation correlated with age, male gender, duration of the murmur, degree of valve leaflet thickening, and presence of posterior leaflet prolapse.*)

8. Gardin JM, Weissman NJ, Leung C, et al. Clinical and echocardiographic follow-up of patients previously treated with dexfenfluramine or phenteramine/fenfluramine. JAMA 2001;286:2011. (*Long-term follow-up data on a large cohort; progression is unlikely.*)

9. Graboys TB, Cohn PF. Prevalence of angina and abnormal coronary arteriograms in severe aortic stenosis. Am Heart J 1977;93:683. (*Twenty percent had at least one significant luminal stenosis.*)

10. Jick H, Vasilakis C, Weinrauch LA, et al. A population-based study of appetite-suppressant drugs and the risk of cardiac valve regurgitation. N Engl J Med 1998;339:719. (*Documented a marked increased in risk, especially in those taking more than 4 months of treatment.*)

11. Liberthson RR. Sudden death from cardiac causes in children and young adults. N Engl J Med 1996;334:1039. (*A review of high-risk etiologies, including aortic stenosis and hypertrophic cardiomyopathy.*)

12. Nishimura RA, McGoon MD. Perspectives on mitral-valve prolapse. N Engl J Med 1999;341:48. (*An editorial providing an excellent summary of the case definition and the risk for complications.*)

13. Otto CM. Evaluation and management of chronic mitral regurgitation. N Engl J Med 2001;345:740. (*Practical review for clinicians; 25 references.*)

14. Otto CM, Lind BK, Kitzman DW, et al. Association of aortic-valve sclerosis with cardiovascular mortality and morbidity in the elderly. N Engl J Med 1999;341:142. (*There was a 50% increase in coronary morbidity and mortality even when there was no stenosis, suggesting a link with atherosclerotic disease.*)

15. Rosenhek R, Binder T, Porenta G, et al. Predictors of outcome in severe, asymptomatic aortic stenosis. N Engl J Med 2000;343:611. (*A prospective cohort study; the degree of calcification and increase in aortic-jet velocity predicted risk in this population.*)

16. Schade R, Anderson F, Suissa S, et al. Dopamine agonists and the risk of cardiac-valve regurgitation. N Engl J Med 2007;356:29. (*There was a marked increase in risk with ergot-derived preparations.*)

17. Selzer A. Changing aspects of the natural history of valvular aortic stenosis. N Engl J Med 1987;317:91. (*A clinically focused review; most cases were due to calcific disease of the elderly; offers an excellent discussion of how presentation differs from that of rheumatic aortic stenosis; 116 references.*)

18. Siemienczuk D, Greenberg B, Morris C, et al. Chronic aortic insufficiency: factors associated with progression to aortic valve replacement. Ann Intern Med 1989;110:587. (*Measurements of left ventricular size and function were predictive of the need for valve replacement.*)

19. Taylor AA, Davies AO, Mares A, et al. Spectrum of dysautonomia in mitral valvular prolapse. Am J Med 1989;86:287. (*Dysautonomic responses were unrelated to mitral valvular prolapse; refutes the purported etiologic link between these responses and mitral valve prolapse.*)

20. Vohra J, Sathe S, Warren R, et al. Malignant ventricular arrhythmias in patients with mitral valve prolapse and mild mitral regurgitation. Pacing Clin Electrophysiol 1993;16:387. (*Characteristics of patients at high risk for serious dysrhythmias.*)

21. Chen JTT, Beliar VS, Morris JJ, et al. Correlation of Roentgen findings with hemodynamic data in pure mitral stenosis. Am J Roentgenol 1968;102:280. (*A classic paper; prominent upper zone redistribution and pulmonary artery dilation were correlated closely with severity.*)

22. Choudhry NK, Etchells EE. Does this patient have aortic regurgitation? JAMA 1999;281:2231. (*Best review of the physical findings and the evidence supporting their significance.*)

23. Enriquez-Sarano M, Avierinos J-F, Messika-Zeitoun D, et al. Quantitative determinants of the outcome of asymptomatic mitral regurgitation. N Engl J Med 2005; 3512:875. (*Finds that a quantitative measure of regurgitant severity, i.e., regurgitant orifice, was the best predictor of left ventricular failure.*)

24. Folland ED, Kriegel BJ, Henderson WG, et al. Implications of third heart sounds in patients with valvular heart disease. N Engl J Med 1992;327:458. (*Indicative of failure in aortic stenosis but not in mitral regurgitation.*)

25. Marks AR, Choong CY, Sanfilippo AJ, et al. Identification of high-risk and low-risk subgroups of patients with mitral-valve prolapse. N Engl J Med 1989;320:1031. (*Patients with valve thickening and redundancy on ultrasound were at greatest risk of complications.*)

26. Oh JK, Taliercio CP, Holmes DR, et al. Prediction of the severity of aortic stenosis by Doppler aortic valve area determination. J Am Coll Cardiol 1988;11:1227. (*Prospective study; found an excellent correlation between Doppler findings and catheterization results.*)

27. Sherrid M, Goyal A, Delia E, et al. Unsuspected mitral stenosis. Am J Med 1991;90:189. (*Hemodynamically significant disease by ultrasound was missed clinically due to concurrent aortic stenosis, heart failure, pneumonia, or just a low index of suspicion; most cases had an audible mitral stenosis murmur on reexamination.*)

28. Biem HJ, Detsky AS, Armstrong PW. Management of asymptomatic chronic aortic regurgitation with left ventricular dysfunction: a decision analysis. J Gen Intern Med 1990;5:394. (*Strongly favors surgical intervention at the first signs of significant left ventricular dysfunction, even though the patient may remain asymptomatic.*)

29. Brady ST, Davis CA, Kussmal WG, et al. Percutaneous aortic balloon valvuloplasty in octogenarians: morbidity and mortality. Ann Intern Med 1989;110:761. (*Hemodynamics improved, but overall the short-term mortality was very high, 32%.*)

30. Hammermeister KE, Sethi GK, Henderson WG, et al. Comparison of outcomes in men 11 years after heart-valve replacement with a mechanical valve or bioprosthesis. N Engl J Med 1993;328:1289. (*Useful data for the selection of prosthesis.*)

31. Lieberman EB, Bashore TM, Hermiller JB, et al. Balloon aortic valvuloplasty in adults: failure of procedure to improve long-term survival. J Am Coll Cardiol 1995;26:1522. (*Found no improvement over the natural history of the disease; there was 6% event-free survival at 3 years.*)

32. Lin M, Chiang HT, Liu SL, et al. Vasodilator therapy in chronic asymptomatic aortic regurgitation: enalapril versus hydralazine therapy. J Am Coll Cardiol 1994;24:1046. (*Afterload reduction with enalapril was superior to vasodilator therapy with hydralazine.*)

33. Moreno PR, Jang IK, Newell JB, et al. The role of percutaneous aortic valvuloplasty in patients with cardiogenic shock and critical aortic stenosis. J Am Coll Cardiol 1994;23:1071. (*The procedure represented a less invasive option for poor surgical candidates.*)

34. Palacios IF. Farewell to surgical mitral commissurotomy for many patients. Circulation 1998;97:223. (*Update on the status of balloon dilation.*)

35. Reyes VP, Raju BS, Wynne J, et al. Percutaneous balloon valvuloplasty compared with open surgical commissurotomy for mitral stenosis. N Engl J Med 1994;331:961. (*In persons <30 years of age, percutaneous balloon valvuloplasty was superior.*)

36. Thamilarasan M, Griffin B. Choosing the most appropriate valve operation and prosthesis. Cleveland Clin J Med 2002;69:688. (*A useful review for the noncardiac physician; written from the perspective of the Cleveland Clinic experience; 53 references.*)

APPENDIX 33.1: APPROACH TO CONGENITAL AND HEREDITARY NONVALVULAR HEART DISEASE

HYPERTROPHIC CARDIOMYOPATHY (1–6)

Hypertrophic cardiomyopathy (HCM) is a common (prevalence 1 in 500) but heterogeneous genetic disorder of sarcomere development with a wide spectrum of clinical presentations, ranging from an incidental finding on cardiac ultrasound to an important cause of left ventricular outflow tract obstruction and sudden death. Because it sometimes produces a systolic ejection murmur, it may be confused with valvular aortic stenosis; however, it differs in terms of etiology, pathophysiology, and natural history, necessitating a separate consideration and customized approach to management.

Pathophysiology and Clinical Presentation

Genetics, Pathology, and Pathophysiology

HCM is actually a collection of autosomally dominant inherited disorders resulting from mutations in the genes that encode for proteins of the cardiac sarcomere. These mutations, which may be expressed at any time in life, lead to a spectrum of hypertrophic changes in the myocardium. The hypertrophy is typically asymmetric but distributed diffusely; in about one third of affected persons, it may be segmental. In the majority of patients, the degree and location of hypertrophy are insufficient to obstruct the ventricular outflow tract, but in about 25% of patients obstruction results (sometimes referred to as *idiopathic hypertrophic subaortic stenosis*). The underlying disease process may be progressive, but the rate and extent of progression are highly variable and in many instances of no clinical significance.

At the cellular level, there may be considerable *histologic disorganization* and disarray in conjunction with abnormal intramural coronary arteries. The *vascular abnormalities* may limit blood flow and result in a mismatch between oxygen supply and demand, leading to repeated episodes of ischemic injury and scarring of the myocardium.

Such disordered and damaged myocardium can lead to myocardial dysfunction and serious electrical instability in severely affected persons. Adverse electrophysiologic consequences include *ventricular tachycardia*, *ventricular fibrillation*, and increased risk of *syncope* and *sudden death*. In a subset of patients, hypertrophy results in *diastolic dysfunction* that compromises cardiac output and produces the characteristic picture of *heart failure* in the setting of a normal or supernormal ejection fraction. *Atrial fibrillation* is a consequence of the left atrial enlargement that ensues from a stiff left ventricle that is hard to fill.

Clinical Presentation and Course

Because it is an autosomally dominant genetic disease, there may be reports of recurrent syncope or premature sudden death among family members. Most persons with the condition are asymptomatic or report minimal exertional symptoms because severe myocardial involvement is the exception rather than the rule. The age of onset of symptoms is highly variable because the genetic expression of the hypertrophic process may occur at any time in life. The fraction of persons with severe disease may note lightheadedness, dyspnea, fatigue, or syncope; unfortunately, sudden death may be the initial presentation. An incidental systolic ejection murmur may be noted on physical examination in those with outflow tract obstruction. Paroxysmal or chronic atrial fibrillation may result as left atrial enlargement progresses.

As noted, onset may occur at any age, so that being asymptomatic and free of manifestations at one age does not rule out developing them later. The original estimates of prognosis were overly pessimistic (3% to 6% annual mortality) due to reliance on data from referral populations; community-based figures place the mortality risk at about 1%/yr. Again, because of the variable expression and progression of the underlying disease process, there is a wide spectrum of hypertrophic cardiomyopathic disease; generalizations are a bit misleading because those with mild disease may have no physical limitations and a normal life expectancy, whereas those with significant myocardial involvement have a much poorer prognosis and considerable limitation.

Workup

History

The history should be carefully reviewed for exertional symptoms (e.g., shortness of breath, fatigue, chest discomfort), which, even if mild, may be the first manifestations of significant underlying diastolic dysfunction and microvascular insufficiency. Complaints of lightheadedness, near-syncope, or syncope should be sought because they raise suspicion of serious ventricular dysrhythmias. Likewise, palpitations may herald ventricular instability or atrial fibrillation. The family history may suggest the diagnosis if there are reports of premature sudden death or recurrent syncope in close relatives.

Physical Examination

Most persons have no findings if their disease is mild. Manifestations of more serious disease should be sought. The pulse should be noted for an *irregular rhythm* indicative of atrial fibrillation occurring as a consequence of marked diastolic dysfunction. Those with left ventricular outflow tract obstruction may have a *systolic ejection murmur* that superficially resembles that of valvular aortic stenosis; however, the intensity of the murmur is maximal at the lower left sternal border and increases with Valsalva maneuver and decreases with leg elevation and other maneuvers that increase venous return. Moreover, there is no ejection sound in early systole, and the carotid pulse is bifid (*bisferiens*) in quality rather than *parvus et tardus*.

Laboratory Studies

The *ECG* may show increased voltage suggestive of left ventricular hypertrophy, although the relation between ECG voltage and degree of hypertrophy by ultrasound is not strong. The presence of marked repolarization abnormalities on the resting ECG of asymptomatic trained athletes (e.g., ST-wave depression, T-wave inversion) is associated with an increased risk of hypertrophic cardiomyopathy in later life and may be its initial clinical expression.

The test of choice for diagnosis is the two-dimensional transthoracic *cardiac ultrasound*. Minimum wall thickness indicative of hypertrophy is 13 to 15 mm; it may be as much as 30 mm. The diagnosis is made when the hypertrophy occurs in the absence of another explanation (e.g., hypertension, aortic stenosis). The ultrasound is also examined for evidence of left ventricular outflow tract obstruction. Again, because gene expression may occur at any time in life, a normal study at one time does not rule out the development of hypertrophy at a later date in persons with a positive family history. *Genetic* and *phenotypic testing* is being explored, looking for gene mutations and abnormal protein expressions (e.g., mutations in genes for troponin T and myosin-binding protein C).

Patients should undergo *Holter monitoring* if they report palpitations, lightheadedness, or near-syncope. *Exercise stress testing* can be informative if there is chest pain or other exercise-induced symptoms, but cardiac consultation should be obtained first, especially if there is evidence of outflow tract obstruction or suspicion of serious ventricular arrhythmias. The role of *electrophysiologic study* in the evaluation of HCM is not well established; the relation of findings to outcomes is unclear.

Management

The heterogeneous nature of hypertrophic cardiomyopathy necessitates risk stratification to help guide the selection of treatment modalities.

Risk Stratification

Sudden death represents the most feared outcome; heart failure is another serious consequence. Established independent predictors of *high risk* for poor outcome include the following:

- Prior cardiac arrest
- Spontaneous sustained ventricular tachycardia
- Multiple or prolonged episodes of nonsustained ventricular tachycardia on Holter monitoring
- Family history of premature cardiac death attributable to HCM
- Syncope or near-syncope, especially if it is exertional or recurrent in a young person and clearly not vasovagal in origin
- Hypotensive response to exercise
- Marked hypertrophy (wall thickness >30 mm)
- Outflow tract obstruction at rest (peak gradient >30 mm Hg)

Genotyping has been proposed as a means of identifying high-risk individuals, but correlations between specific mutations and outcomes are not yet well established. The role of electrophysiologic study in identifying those at risk for ventricular tachycardia is not well established.

Persons with HCM at lower risk may include those who have no symptoms, a wall thickness less than 45 mm, and none of the forgoing high-risk factors.

Endocarditis Prophylaxis and Prevention of Ventricular Tachycardia

Endocarditis prophylaxis (see Chapter 16) is required for those persons who have clinical or ultrasound evidence of outflow tract obstruction. The mitral valve is distorted by such obstruction, which increases endocarditis risk.

Pharmacologic measures (e.g., *β-blockers, verapamil, antiarrhythmics*) traditionally prescribed in an attempt to prevent ventricular tachycardia and reduce the risk of sudden death are generally ineffective. The use of an *implantable cardioverter-defibrillator* can reduce the risk of sudden death. Whether an asymptomatic high-risk person is a candidate for defibrillator implantation remains to be determined. Symptomatic persons who have evidence of ventricular tachycardia clearly benefit.

High-risk persons require a warning about engaging in strenuous exercise; such persons should be disqualified from engaging in competitive athletics, in which the risk of sudden death is considerable.

Heart Failure

The onset of exertional symptoms indicative of heart failure (e.g., dyspnea, fatigue) is an indication for pharmacologic intervention. *β-Blockers* (sometimes in conjunction with *disopyramide* when there is outflow tract obstruction) can improve functional status and relieve symptoms. For those with outflow tract obstruction, the decrease in contractility reduces the degree of interference with blood flow. *Verapamil* is an alternative to *β*-blockade, but only as a monotherapy and not in the setting of concurrent outflow tract obstruction. If heart failure progresses and systolic dysfunction develops, then standard treatment with diuretics, angiotensin-converting-enzyme inhibitors, and digitalis needs consideration (see Chapter 32).

Consideration of invasive intervention is indicated in patients with symptomatic drug-refractory disease. Options include the *Morrow procedure* (septal myomectomy), which in experienced centers has a less than 2% operative mortality, and catheter-applied *alcohol septal ablation*. The latter obviates the need for surgery, but evidence of efficacy is less compelling, and there is the potential risk of chronic electrical instability from scar formation. Dual-chamber pacing is being investigated.

Atrial Fibrillation

Patients who develop paroxysmal or chronic atrial fibrillation are at risk for systemic embolization and the need oral anticoagulation with *warfarin* (see Chapters 28 and 83). *β-Blockade* is recommended for rate control. *Amiodarone* may be of help in maintaining sinus rhythm when deemed desirable because of hemodynamic decompensation during paroxysmal atrial fibrillation (see Chapter 28).

PATENT FORAMEN OVALE (1,7,8)

Patent foramen ovale (PFO) is a very common developmental cardiac anomaly, demonstrated echocardiographically in greater than 25% of unselected adults and increasingly appreciated as a source of cryptogenic stroke.

Pathophysiology and Clinical Presentation

This vestigial remnant of fetal circulation results from failure of the primum and secundum septa to fuse after birth; a one-way flap valve over the persisting fossa ovalis allows right-to-left shunting. The potential for shunting provides a pathway for paradoxical thromboembolism. Although the structural anomaly is common, the risk of paradoxical embolization in otherwise healthy affected persons remains low (0.1%). The risk increases with foramen size (>4 mm), the presence of atrial septal aneurysm, increased right-to-left shunting (as with Valsalva maneuver, straining, or underlying cardiopulmonary disease), and risk factors for venous thromboembolism (e.g., inactivity, trauma, recent surgery, hypercoagulable state). Once considered a source of paradoxical embolism only in younger persons, PFO has also been confirmed as an independent stroke risk factor in persons older than the age of 55 years. Clinically, the condition is typically silent until systemic embolization occurs. The risk of stroke recurrence in a 55-year-old is estimated at 0.8%/yr.

Differential Diagnosis and Workup

Other important causes of cryptogenic stroke include *paroxysmal atrial fibrillation*, *aortic arch atheromata*, and *intracranial cerebrovascular disease*. Workup for PFO as the cause of cryptogenic stroke requires cardiac imaging; there are no suggestive or diagnostic cardiac history or physical examination findings, although checking for a prior history of thromboembolism and signs of deep vein thrombosis (see Chapter 22) can provide evidence of a potential source of thrombus. Cardiac imaging can begin with a *transthoracic echocardiogram* supplemented by *bubble study*. Greater sensitivity and more anatomic detail are provided by *transesophageal echocardiogram*, which also helps to rule out aortic arch atheromata as the source of systemic embolization. Patients should also be considered for a study of deep vein thrombosis and hypercoagulability (see Chapters 22 and 35).

Management

The goal in persons with paradoxical embolization is the prevention of recurrent stroke. Management decisions are problematic because data from randomized, controlled trials are lacking. Several well-designed trials comparing medical therapies (*aspirin* vs. *warfarin*) and medical therapy versus interventional procedures (*surgical* or *endovascular closure*) are underway. Current guidelines from professional societies emphasize the absence of evidence and remain vague; one organization suggests aspirin for persons with isolated patent foramen ovale, oral anticoagulation with warfarin for persons with concurrent or prior thromboembolism, and treatment of some form (although specific guidance lacking among available options) for persons with additional risk factors such as large orifice, septal aneurysm, or hypercoagulability. There are no guidelines or recommendations for the treatment of persons with an incidentally discovered patent foramen ovale.

Patient Education and Indications for Referral

Persons with a small, incidentally discovered PFO foramen ovale who are free of additional risk factors such as septal aneurysm or hypercoagulability can be reassured that the risk of stroke is very low and that no treatment needs to be undertaken. Those who are older and concerned might be offered low-dose aspirin for stroke prophylaxis. Patients with cryptogenic stroke and ultrasound-confirmed PFO should be referred for cardiac consultation for guidance as to treatment options.

A.H.G.

Annotated Bibliography

1. Brinkner ME, Hillis LD, Lange RA. Congenital heart disease in adults. N Engl J Med 2000;342:256. (*A useful review for the generalist reader; 60 references.*)
2. Maron BJ. Hypertrophic cardiomyopathy: a systematic review. JAMA 2002;287:1308. (*An outstanding review and the best summary of available evidence; 207 references.*)
3. Maron BJ, Casey SA, Poliac LC, et al. Clinical course of hypertrophic cardiomyopathy in a regional United States cohort. JAMA 1999;281:650. (*A retrospective cohort study; hypertrophic cardiomyopathy was found not to be a major risk factor for premature death or shortened life expectancy; the data help to put the condition in perspective.*)
4. Maron MS, Olivotto I, Betocchi S, et al. Effect of left ventricular outflow tract obstruction on clinical outcome in hypertrophic cardiomyopathy. N Engl J Med 2003;348:295. (*A cohort study, finding that significant obstruction at rest contributes independently to risk.*)
5. Pilliccia A, Di Paolo FM, Quattrinin FM, et al. Outcomes in athletes with marked ECG repolarization abnormalities. N Engl J Med 2008;358:152. (*A population study; abnormalities likely represent underlying cardiomyopathy that warrants further evaluation.*)
6. Spirito P, Bellone P, Harris KM, et al. Magnitude of left ventricular hypertrophy and risk of sudden death in hypertrophic cardiomyopathy. N Engl J Med 2000;342:1778. (*A cohort study; the degree of hypertrophy is an independent risk factor for sudden death.*)
7. Handke M, Harloff A, Olschewski M, et al. Patent foramen ovale and cryptogenic stroke in older patients. N Engl J Med 2007;357:2262. (*Patent foramen ovale was found to be an independent predictor of stroke risk in both younger and older patients.*)
8. Kizer JR, Devereus RB. Patent foramen ovale in young adults with unexplained stroke. N Engl J Med 2005;353:2361. (*A clinically oriented review; 45 references.*)

CHAPTER 34 ■ MANAGEMENT OF PERIPHERAL ARTERIAL DISEASE

DAVID C. BREWSTER

During the last decade, the treatment of peripheral arterial insufficiency has undergone substantial change and improvements. Plaque regression has now been demonstrated with aggressive lipid-lowering therapy (see Chapter 27), and in properly selected patients, percutaneous transluminal angioplasty (PTA) with and without intraluminal stenting may achieve results that approach those of bypass surgery. In addition, great progress has been made in arterial reconstructive surgery for severe cases, making possible the salvage of limbs that would have otherwise required amputation. The wealth of available therapeutic options and a relatively favorable natural history provide the symptomatic patient with substantial opportunity for improvement. The primary physician needs to know the natural history of arterial occlusive disease in order to optimize the timing and intensity of therapy. Also essential to ensuring proper selection, implementation, and coordination of care is knowledge of the techniques, efficacies, and indications for conservative therapy (including risk factor modification), angioplasty, and bypass surgery.

NATURAL HISTORY AND CLINICAL COURSE (1–9)

Prognosis for the Limb

The prognosis for the limb and for symptoms in patients presenting with claudication are quite favorable. Clinical course correlates well with the clinical severity of disease as measured by distance walked before onset of claudication and by physical findings; persons with the worst prognosis have ischemic ulcers or rest pain in the setting of longstanding diabetes mellitus or persistent smoking. In general, greater than 80% of patients with claudication alone remain stable or improve, and only approximately 5% progress to limb loss. Almost no patients who cease smoking require amputation, whereas in contrast, more than 10% who continue to smoke lose a limb. Observed outcomes at 5 years are stable symptoms in 70% to 80%, worsening claudication in 10 % to 20%, and progression to critical limb ischemia or limb loss in 1% to 2% of patients. Not surprisingly, most amputations occur in the high-risk group, but even in severe cases, nearly 70% stay the same or improve and only 15% come to amputation, underscoring the fact that progression to loss of limb is hardly inevitable.

Overall Prognosis

Although prognosis for the limb is generally favorable, *mortality* rates—both overall and cardiovascular—are high, reflecting the severity of underlying systemic atherosclerotic disease. The risk of dying from cardiovascular cause is sixfold greater in those with peripheral arterial disease than in those of similar age, sex, and lipid profile without it. All-cause mortality increases threefold, due almost entirely to the increase in cardiovascular risk. Combined mortality rates are in the range of 30%, 50%, and 70% at 5, 10, and 15 years after the onset of symptoms, respectively, which represent a relative risk about three times that for patients of similar age and gender. Concurrent disease of the coronary arteries, cerebral vasculature, or aorta accounts for most of the increased mortality, underscoring the systemic nature of atherosclerosis and its adverse effect on prognosis. The prevalence of systemic atherosclerosis in patients with peripheral arterial insufficiency should not be surprising, given that up to 80% of such patients give a history of smoking, 40% have hypertension, 30% have lipid abnormalities, and 20% have diabetes.

DIAGNOSIS AND WORKUP (1–4,7–9; See Also Chapter 23)

The underdiagnosis of peripheral artery disease in primary care practice is well documented. Not only does failure to recognize the condition lead to missed opportunities for symptomatic improvement, it also leads to failure to recognize and treat underlying systemic atherosclerotic disease that may compromise survival. A careful comprehensive cardiovascular history and physical examination in addition to a detailed look at the peripheral vasculature are essential. Patients who are clinically suspect can undergo noninvasive testing by Doppler ultrasound to confirm clinically significant disease, followed if necessary by noninvasive radiologic imaging (e.g., computed tomographic angiography [CTA], magnetic resonance angiography [MRA]) or formal angiography (see Chapter 23) if interventional therapy is being contemplated.

In the Patient with Suspected Atherosclerotic Disease

A full review of atherosclerotic risk factors is essential, as are a detailed history and physical examination for findings indicative of poor prognosis (e.g., rest pain, dependent rubor, cold extremity, painful ulceration, gangrenous or necrotic tissue). Patients with such evidence of more advanced disease should be referred promptly for noninvasive *Doppler ultrasound study* to identify candidates for angiography and surgical intervention (see Chapter 23). Because evidence of peripheral vascular disease is a strong predictor of concurrent cardiovascular disease with its attendant morbidity and mortality, a thorough cardiac assessment is essential (see Chapter 36), especially if surgical intervention is being contemplated (see later discussion).

In the Patient with Diabetes

A thorough history and physical examination, supplemented by a Doppler flow study, have been shown to be predictive of outcome and can help to direct management. Physicians encountering a diabetic with a foot ulcer should inquire into previous amputation and painful skin ulceration. Evaluation for superimposed infection is particularly important. If there has been previous amputation, the likelihood ratio for an adverse outcome is 4.0 and the patient should be considered for aggressive therapy (e.g., revascularization). If there is neither previous amputation nor findings to suggest more advanced limb-threatening ischemia, an initial conservative (medical) approach is reasonable.

PRINCIPLES OF MANAGEMENT (1–4,6–8,10–24)

Medical Management

The basic objectives of medical management are to control or limit disease progression, increase exercise tolerance, and minimize the risk of complications. The most important methods for achieving these objectives are cessation of cigarette smoking, regular daily exercise, and meticulous foot care.

Smoking Cessation (See Chapter 54)

Smoking hastens the progression of atherosclerosis and may further impair blood flow by inducing vasoconstriction. *Smoking cessation* ranks as a major priority for the patient with peripheral arterial disease. Cessation can reduce rest pain, claudication, risk of amputation, and need for bypass surgery. The risk of repeat occlusion after angioplasty or bypass falls by more than two thirds in those who quit. Moreover, quitting decreases overall cardiovascular morbidity and mortality. The chances of successfully quitting are greatest when a smoker becomes symptomatic from a complication of smoking; the physician's influence is considerable in this context.

The details of a comprehensive smoking cessation program are presented elsewhere (see Chapter 54), but a few considerations are relevant for persons with peripheral artery disease. Nicotine gum or transdermal patch can serve as a useful cessation aid by minimizing nicotine withdrawal; however, nicotine may induce vasospasm. Although nicotine therapy is probably not contraindicated in claudication because vasospasm usually does not play a major role, the gum or patch, if used, should be prescribed and monitored with care.

Exercise

Daily exercise, especially *walking*, remains a cornerstone of the treatment program, even though it now appears unlikely that it increases skeletal muscle blood flow or the development of collaterals in the ischemic limb. Suggested mechanisms include improvements in muscle metabolism, peak oxygen consumption, red cell movement, and pain threshold. Whatever the reason, physical training can significantly increase pain-free walking distance, which underscores the fact that claudication is not strictly a symptom of abnormal hemodynamics. The programs showing the best results are those that combine supervised *group* walking sessions with additional sessions performed daily at home. The best candidates are patients with stable intermittent claudication who are free of rest pain, ulceration, unstable angina, congestive heart failure, and severe lung disease or arthritis. Although group results are excellent, predicting outcome in an individual patient is difficult. Most patients who achieve benefit report it within 3 months of initiating an exercise program.

Regularity of exercise is more important than intensity or duration, although at least 30 min/d of continuous leg exercise appears to be necessary. Although walking is optimal, any form of dynamic exercise will suffice, including stationary bicycling, stair climbing, engaging in water aerobics, or using low-impact aerobic training equipment. An exercise program can also reduce cardiovascular risk (see Chapters 18 and 31).

Foot Care

Careful attention to foot care is vital to the prevention of limb loss. It has been estimated that up to 80% of amputations required in diabetics are attributable to poor foot care. Feet need to be inspected daily, especially in diabetics with peripheral neuropathy that limits protective sensation. As little as 1 hour of patient education has been shown to reduce the amputation and ulceration rate by two thirds.

Control of Atherosclerotic Risk Factors

The aggressive treatment of *hyperlipidemia* can reduce or halt atherosclerotic plaque progression in peripheral vessels; modest plaque regression has also been demonstrated with statin therapy. Some decrease in the risk and severity of symptomatic peripheral arterial disease can be expected, but the most important benefit stems from the marked reductions in cardiovascular morbidity and mortality. Because patients with peripheral arterial disease are at high risk for life-threatening cardiovascular complications, they stand to gain considerably from aggressive lipid-lowering therapy. Current consensus guidelines recommend a target low-density-lipoprotein cholesterol of less than 100 mg/dL in persons with peripheral arterial disease (see Chapter 27).

If *hypertension* is present, it too deserves attention (see Chapter 26). The effect of blood pressure reduction on the progression of peripheral vascular disease is unknown, but treatment clearly reduces morbidity and mortality from stroke and cardiovascular disease. Choosing an agent on the basis of its effect on peripheral vascular tone does not appear to be critical, although some patients complain of worsening symptoms on β-blockers. Controlled studies have failed to confirm an adverse effect with β-blockers. Antihypertensive agents with vasodilating potential (e.g., calcium-channel blockers) do not materially improve claudication symptoms. Angiotensin-converting-enzyme inhibitors are contraindicated if there is coexisting bilateral renal artery stenosis.

Weight reduction can be helpful by lessening work load and reducing metabolic demands of the extremities. In addition, weight reduction may also help to lower lipid levels, glucose intolerance, and cardiovascular risk (see Chapter 10).

The *control of diabetes* (see Chapter 102) is essential to limb preservation, mostly by reducing the risk of neuropathy and consequent foot injury and infection. There is also emerging evidence suggesting that "tight" control of diabetes may improve the clinical course of large-vessel peripheral arterial disease, but only if it is achieved early in the course of illness. Perhaps that is because diabetic peripheral vascular disease begins earlier and progresses more rapidly than in other patients.

Moreover, large vessels can remain relatively patent, whereas small vessels become occluded. Foot care is essential.

Hyperhomocysteinemia may be responsible in patients who present with extensive premature peripheral arterial disease (occurring before age 50 years); however, B-vitamin/folate treatment to lower homocysteine has been disappointing in its cardiovascular outcomes (see Chapter 31).

Pharmacologic Therapy

A host of pharmacologic therapies ranging from antiplatelet agents to vasodilators and chelating drugs has been applied with variable results.

Antiplatelet Agents and Oral Anticoagulants. There is no evidence that antiplatelet therapy improves claudication per se (although some angiographic evidence suggests an inhibitory effect on the progression of peripheral atherosclerosis). Antiplatelet therapy, principally with *aspirin*, is prescribed to reduce concomitant cardiovascular and stroke risks (see Chapters 30, 31, and 171). *Clopidogrel*, a similarly effective but expensive alternative, is useful in persons who cannot tolerate salicylates. The combined use of aspirin and clopidogrel adds no benefit and increases the risk of bleeding. The use of other antiplatelet agents is limited by their adverse effects (increased cardiovascular risk with *dipyridamole*; neutropenia and thrombotic thrombocytopenic purpura with *ticlopidine*).

Oral anticoagulants (e.g., *warfarin*) provide no benefit in the management of chronic peripheral arterial disease and increase the risk of life-threatening bleeding when added to antiplatelet therapy.

Cilostazol. This phosphodiesterase inhibitor possesses antiplatelet, antithrombic, and vasodilating properties. It is approved by the U.S. Food and Drug Administration for symptomatic treatment of intermittent claudication. Although the exact mechanism(s) of action responsible for benefit are uncertain, the drug does modestly increase walking distances (by 28% to 54%) in comparison with placebo and pentoxiphylline in patients with mild to moderate claudication. The onset of action can be slow, ranging from 2 to 12 weeks. Side effects include headache, which can be severe, and tachycardia; ventricular ectopy has been noted. The drug is contraindicated in persons with congestive heart failure. There is concern about long-term use, based on reports of cardiovascular injury in animals exposed to the drug for more than 52 weeks.

Pentoxifylline. Pentoxifylline, an agent that appears to increase erythrocyte deformability and blood viscosity and reduce platelet activity, has been promoted as a potentially useful drug for the treatment of symptomatic peripheral arterial disease. In placebo-controlled trials, benefit is nil to modest. Nausea and dizziness may further limit pentoxifylline's appeal; cost can be substantial.

Vasodilators. Vasodilators (e.g., papaverine) were the first pharmacologic agents tested, but they provide no demonstrable benefit to symptoms or clinical course when evaluated in placebo-controlled, double-blind, randomized trials. These agents may even worsen symptoms by producing a steal phenomenon. The failure of vasodilator therapy reinforces the view that vasoconstriction plays little role in claudication.

Vasoconstrictors (e.g., ergot derivatives) can be harmful and should be used with caution, if at all, in patients with severe disease, especially in those with ulcers or rest pain. *α-Blockers* also may aggravate ischemic symptoms and impede the healing of the skin lesions. *β-Blockers* do not compromise perfusion or worsen symptoms, despite anecdotal records.

Other Agents. Agents believed to block specific inducers of atherosclerosis (e.g., *vitamin E* and *omega-3 fatty acids*) have been under investigation. Vitamin E shows no benefit in controlled trials (see Chapter 31). *Levocarnitine* (which limits much buildup of acylcarnitines) has shown some promise but is not approved for use in the United States. *Chelation therapy* is of no benefit. *Gingko biloba* extract shows a modest benefit of questionable clinical significance.

Gene Therapy and Angiogenesis

These exciting areas are the subjects of intense investigation. Work is ongoing with growth factors for vascular endothelial cells and fibroblasts in an attempt to stimulate angiogenesis. The hope is to stimulate capillary proliferation and collateral blood vessel formation in ischemic tissues. Such arterial gene therapy holds promise, especially for patients with nonreconstructible disease by conventional angioplasty or surgery.

Interventional Therapies

When revascularization is required, options include percutaneous catheter-based interventional procedures and surgical methods such as endarterectomy and bypass. With the advent of angioplasty and stenting and improvements in the outcomes of surgical revascularization, the threshold for invasive therapy has been lowered, but the decision to consider such treatment should not be taken lightly or made prematurely. The relatively favorable natural history of peripheral vascular disease and the excellent responses to medical measures argue for resorting to interventional therapy only after other approaches have failed and the patient is incapacitated or a limb is at risk. Successful revascularization can improve the patient's perceived quality of life.

Candidacy

Patients who continue to have disabling symptoms despite the implementation of a full medical regimen (smoking cessation, exercise program, control of cardiovascular risk factors) are potential candidates for interventional therapy. Persisting *inability to walk two blocks* and *carry out activities of daily living* are typical functional criteria for the consideration of interventional therapy. *Rest pain* and a *nonhealing ulcer* are even more compelling reasons.

Interventional therapy is most appropriate in low-risk patients with lesions having a high likelihood of initial and long-term success. Before referring the patient for interventional therapy, a full set of noninvasive studies (including *Doppler ultrasound* scanning and *segmental blood pressures*) should be ordered to document more precisely the location and severity of disease (see Chapter 23). The best candidates for interventional measures are those with *proximal disease* and *preserved distal runoff*. Patients who prove to have predominantly small-vessel disease (e.g., diabetes) are much less likely to benefit from interventional therapy unless there is concurrent proximal disease that can be alleviated.

Angiography is often necessary to make the final determination. Significant advances in vascular imaging (e.g., *CTA* and *MRA*) often allow for noninvasive imaging of the peripheral vasculature and help to reduce the need for invasive angiographic study.

Percutaneous Transluminal Angioplasty and Stenting

Catheter-based endovascular revascularization using PTA and stenting has emerged as a cost-effective and less-invasive alternative to bypass surgery, especially for the patient with a segmental stenosis of a proximal vessel. In patients with lesions amenable to angioplasty, PTA and stenting can achieve short- and long-term results similar to those of surgery. The cost of PTA is one fifth that of surgery; however, durability of the result is moderately less, increasing the chances of needing a second procedure and reducing but not eliminating the cost differential. In addition, percutaneous methods may be combined with surgery (e.g., correcting a proximal iliac stenosis by balloon angioplasty and bypassing a more distal lesion with a femoropopliteal bypass graft). *Candidacy* for PTA is best for patients with *short segmental stenoses* in *proximal vessels* (e.g., aortoiliac or femoral arteries). About 30% of patients considered for interventional therapy have such lesions; the remainder tend to have more widespread or distal occlusive disease. Poor candidates for PTA include those with a complete occlusion, a stenotic lesion greater than 10 cm in length, multiple serial stenoses, calcified or eccentric plaque, or poor distal runoff. The percentage of patients treated initially with percutaneous interventions is increasing largely due to rapid technological improvements.

The procedure is typically performed at the time of angiography, using a balloon catheter inserted percutaneously at a remote site, usually the femoral artery, and manipulated fluoroscopically within the diseased segment of artery. With balloon inflation, the obstructing plaque is cracked and compressed and the vessel lumen enhanced. *Stenting* is used to improve the results of PTA when there is elastic recoil or localized plaque dissection that compromises the vessel lumen. Whether routine use of stents with PTA is a better overall strategy than selective use of stenting is under study. Data suggest that selective stenting is more cost-effective. Advances in stent technology are encouraging increasingly aggressive use of PTA to treat more extensively diseased arterial segments. The use of drug-eluting stents with the hope of reducing the incidence of recurrent disease, similar to coronary stents, is under active investigation.

Patency rates, both immediate and long term, are a function of location. Aortoiliac procedures average a 90% immediate success rate, and 80% are patent at 5 years; for a femoral lesion, the rates average 75% and 50%, respectively.

Risks include groin hematoma, dissection, renal ischemia, and distal embolization. The overall complication rate averages 10%, with about 2% to 5% being serious enough to warrant surgical intervention. Mortality is less than 0.5%. As expected, experienced teams in centers performing large numbers of PTAs have the best results and the fewest complications. PTA has a lower morbidity and mortality than standard surgery, making it an especially attractive option in patients who are bad surgical risks because of severe underlying comorbid disease.

Recanalization Techniques

Because angioplasty cannot be performed on a totally occluded vessel, there has been considerable interest in *recanalization techniques*. *Laser* methods and *mechanical arthrectomy* devices have been applied to allow percutaneous catheter-based opening of atherosclerotic arteries. The initial enthusiasm and commercial promotion of such devices have proven premature. These techniques are rarely used as sole therapy with available technology; they can sometimes serve as an adjunct to conventional balloon angioplasty, carving out a small channel in a limited area of total occlusion so that a standard PTA balloon catheter can traverse the lesion. Stenting is almost always required. The literature should be followed for well-designed studies of this emerging technology.

Surgical Therapy

Surgery remains an important option for the large number of patients who have disease that is not amenable to less invasive intervention. Key tasks are the identification of candidates and the proper timing of referral for consideration of surgery.

Candidacy and indications for surgical referral include advanced ischemia resulting in *ischemic rest pain*, *nonhealing ischemic ulcerations*, or *gangrene*. Such limbs are clearly at risk, and arterial reconstruction is indicated, if feasible, to maximize the chances of limb salvage. In such circumstances, patients should be referred for surgical investigation as soon as possible, before tissue necrosis or infection become too extensive. In patients with *claudication alone*, surgery should be considered only in those who are so severely disabled that their ability to earn a living is compromised, their desired lifestyle is intolerably limited, and their vascular lesions are not amenable to PTA. The role of arterial reconstruction for claudication alone remains controversial. In general, the physician must attempt to determine the significance of ischemic symptoms in each patient. The patient's age, work requirements, social circumstances, and general state of health must all be considered. When doubt exists, referral for a surgical opinion is often useful.

Risks of common revascularization procedures are often no greater and often less than the morbidity and mortality of major amputation. Many patients with significant arterial insufficiency that requires surgery also have underlying coronary disease that is hemodynamically critical. The coronary disease may be clinically silent due to the exercise restrictions stemming from severe claudication. Such patients have high rates of perioperative morbidity and mortality. *Stress testing* before surgery helps to identify high-risk patients who would benefit from coronary revascularization before peripheral vascular surgery (see Chapter 36).

The procedure usually involves harvesting the saphenous vein for use in bypass. If the saphenous vein is unavailable for use, a number of suitable alternative prosthetic grafts have been developed in recent years. With improvement of direct reconstructive methods, lumbar sympathectomy is rarely considered a primary mode of treatment. For poor-risk patients, various "extraanatomic" reconstructions are also available, which may be done with an even higher degree of safety.

Results have improved with advances in the surgical management of arterial insufficiency. With an experienced surgeon, careful preoperative cardiac evaluation, and good anesthetic and postoperative management, the patient may anticipate the successful correction of aortoiliac occlusive disease, with a mortality risk of only 1% to 2% and an excellent long-term patency of approximately 85% to 90% at 5 years. Femoropopliteal or tibial artery bypass may be done with an even greater degree of safety, although long-term patency is somewhat less, with approximately 70% to 75% of saphenous vein grafts still patent at 5 years.

PATIENT EDUCATION

Patient education is vital because a favorable outcome requires strong patient participation in the treatment program (cessation of smoking, daily exercise, foot care, risk factor reduction). Compliance is facilitated by the patient's understanding the atherosclerotic basis of the problem, the factors that may aggravate the severity of symptoms, and the rationale behind the measures recommended. Many patients come to the physician with a reluctance to walk and a fear of limb loss. The benefits of exercise, the likelihood of improvement, and the low risk of limb loss are usually of great comfort and reassurance to the patient and the family. The importance of foot care must be repeatedly emphasized, especially in the diabetic. A single hour of detailed foot care instruction can greatly reduce the risk of limb loss. Also important to stress is that even the most trivial foot injury or lesion requires prompt attention. Specific instructions for an appropriate exercise program are essential; recommending such a program can provide a considerable psychological boost.

The psychological management of the patient is essential in preventing depression and invalidism. Emphasis should be on the generally favorable prognosis and the patient's ability to improve his or her condition. Frequent follow-up in the early stages of the treatment program is reassuring and helps to maximize compliance. The patient with new claudication should be seen at least every 2 to 3 months to assess exercise tolerance and inspect the feet for potential pressure points and ulcers.

INDICATIONS FOR REFERRAL AND ADMISSION

Patients with disabling claudication who fail to respond to conservative therapy and have noninvasive evidence of proximal disease should be referred for consideration of revascularization. Patients needing immediate referral for consideration of bypass surgery are those with such severe disease (rest pain, nonhealing ulcers, early gangrene) that they are at risk for losing the limb. Urgent hospitalization is indicated for the patient with early gangrenous changes or signs of infection in an ischemic extremity. Those with refractory claudication whose lifestyle or livelihood are *intolerably* compromised by the inability to walk distances and who appear by noninvasive testing to have disease too distal or too diffuse for PTA are also potential candidates for surgery. The final determination regarding candidacy for angioplasty or surgery requires angiography, but noninvasive screening can maximize the appropriateness of the referral.

THERAPEUTIC RECOMMENDATIONS (1,17)

- *Cessation of smoking.* Total cessation is essential, both to limit disease progression and to prevent reocclusion after interventional therapy. The patient must be firmly told that he or she must stop smoking completely. Smoking as few as five cigarettes per day can compromise a limb. The physician must be unequivocal about this because patients often interpret half-hearted advice as only a suggestion (see Chapter 54).
- *Exercise.* In the patient with claudication, the best exercise is daily walking. Patients are advised to walk to the point of discomfort, stop briefly, and then resume walking. At least 30 minutes of relatively continuous walking each day is recommended. A weekly group session can be extremely useful. An exercise bicycle can be used as an alternative mode of exercise. It is important to emphasize to the patient that pain does not indicate harm or damage to the leg and that exercise can help rather than aggravate the condition. Any tendency

to restrict activity, sometimes to the point of invalidism or confinement to the home, should be avoided, unless severe ischemia is present. Consideration of the patient's cardiac status is important in the design of the exercise program (see Chapters 18 and 31).
- *Elevating the head of the bed.* Patients with advanced ischemia and rest pain at night may benefit from raising the head of the bed on 6- to 8-inch blocks so that the feet and legs are made slightly dependent; gravity may aid blood flow enough to allow more comfortable sleep.
- *Foot Care.* Emphasize foot care and teach it intensively, particularly in the diabetic patient, who often lacks protective sensation due to neuropathy and who may be more susceptible to infections. Because there is often a great deal of confusion about what is meant by "foot care," its components require elaboration:

  1. *Inspection.* The feet should be inspected daily for any scratches, cuts, fissures, blisters, or other lesions, particularly around the nail beds, between the toes, and on the heels.
  2. *Washing.* The feet should be washed daily with mild soap and lukewarm (never hot) water. They should be rinsed thoroughly and dried gently but completely, particularly between the toes. Excessive soaking, leading to maceration, should be avoided.
  3. *Lanolin.* A moisturizing cream such as lanolin or Eucerin should be applied to the skin of the foot and heel but not between the toes. A light film, well rubbed in, will prevent drying and cracking of the skin, which is often the genesis of a lesion, particularly on the heel. The cream should not be applied thickly or allowed to "cake" on the foot.
  4. *Lambs wool.* A small amount of lambaste or dry cotton or gauze may be placed between the toes to prevent lesions, which may occur if toes are allowed to rub together, particularly if orthopedic deformities of the toes are present.
  5. *Powder.* An antifungal powder, such as nystatin, should be applied between the toes if excessive moisture or maceration is a problem.
  6. *Proper footwear.* Properly fitting shoes with ample space in the forefoot are essential. Special shoes are rarely necessary.
  7. *Podiatry.* Nails should be cut with extreme care, in good light, and only if vision is normal. They should be cut straight across and even with the end of the toe, never close to the skin or into the corner of the nailbed. Any abnormality of the nails and any corns or calluses should be treated by the physician or podiatrist.
  8. *Avoidance of trauma.* Never use adhesive tape on the skin (paper tape is better) or any strong antiseptic solution. Avoid heating pads, hot packs, heat lamps, and scalding hot water. The patient should never walk barefoot.

- *Patient education.* Educate patients in detail regarding the key elements of self care, including, diet, exercise, and foot care; urge them to call at the first sign of difficulty; delay can lead to limb loss if gangrene and/or osteomyelitis ensues.
- *Weight reduction* (see Chapter 233).
- *Aggressive control of major atherosclerotic risk factors.* Aggressively treat hypertension (see Chapter 26), hyperlipidemia (see Chapter 27), smoking (see Chapter 54), and diabetes (see Chapter 102).
- *Medications.* Begin *aspirin* (or *clopidogrel* if aspirin is not tolerated) for its generally beneficial effects on cardiovascular risk (see Chapters 30 and 31). Consider a short course (<3 months) of *cilostazol* if symptoms are interfering with

the ability to engage in an exercise program (but avoid longer-term use and use in persons with heart failure or ventricular dysrhythmias).

■ *Referral for percutaneous intervention.* Consider referral for percutaneous intervention in patients with claudication alone if the pain is disabling and refractory to a full trial of medical therapy and noninvasive study suggests relatively focal proximal disease.

■ *Referral for consideration of surgery.* Consider only in patients who have failed medical therapy, have disease that appears amenable to surgery but not PTA, and are so sig-

nificantly disabled by claudication that their livelihood or lifestyle is intolerably compromised by their inability to walk distances. In patients with more severe disease (rest pain, nonhealing ulcers, or early gangrene) who have a limb that is in jeopardy, refer with some urgency. The final decision requires angiography, but noninvasive study to screen for appropriate candidates is essential.

■ *Preoperative stress testing.* Conduct preoperative cardiovascular risk stratification by stress testing to identify patients who might require cardiac revascularization prior to peripheral vascular surgery.

Annotated Bibliography

1. Hirsch, AT, Haskal ZJ, Hertzer NR, et al. ACC/AHA 2005 Practice guidelines for management of patients with peripheral arterial disease (lower extremity, renal, mesenteric, and abdominal aortic): a collaborative report from the American Association for Vascular Surgery/Society for Vascular Surgery, Society for Cardiovascular Angiography and Interventions, Society for Vascular Medicine and Biology, Society of Interventional Radiology, and the ACC/AHA Task Force on Practice Guidelines (Writing Committee to Develop Guidelines for the Management of Patients with Peripheral Arterial disease): endorsed by the American Association of Cardiovascular and Pulmonary Rehabilitation; National Heart, Lung, and Blood Institute; Society for Vascular Nursing; TransAtlantic Inter-Society Consensus; and Vascular Disease Foundation. Circulation 2006;113:e463. (*An excellent up-to-date consensus document on guidelines on peripheral arterial disease [PAD]*).

2. Oriel, K. Peripheral arterial disease. Lancet 2001;358:1257. (*A good overview of the natural history, diagnosis, and treatment of PAD.*)

3. American Diabetes Association. Peripheral arterial disease in people with diabetes. Diabetes Care 2003;25:3333. (*A summary of consensus conference and recommendations.*)

4. Coffman JD. Intermittent claudication—be conservative. N Eng J Med 1991;325:577. (*An editorial stressing the relatively good limb prognosis for mild to moderate disease.*)

5. Criqui MH, Langer RD, Fronek A, et al. Mortality over a period of 10 years in patients with peripheral arterial disease. N Engl J Med 1992;326:381. (*The relative risk of all-cause mortality was 3.0 due mostly to a sixfold increase in the risk of cardiovascular death.*)

6. Krupski WC. The peripheral vascular consequences of smoking. Ann Vasc Surg 1991;3:291. (*A thorough review of the vascular effects and possible mechanisms by which tobacco use causes or aggravates atherosclerotic disease.*)

7. Reiber GE, Pecoraro RE, Koepsell TD. Risk factors for amputation in patients with diabetes mellitus. Ann Intern Med 1992; 117:97. (*Identifies important clinical features that were predictive.*)

8. Hirsch AT, Criqui MH, Treat-Jacobson D, et al. Peripheral arterial disease detection, awareness, and treatment in primary care. JAMA 2001;286:1317. (*Evidence for underdiagnosis and undertreatment.*)

9. Koelemay MJ, Lijmer JG, Stoker J, et al. Magnetic resonance angiography for the evaluation of lower extremity arterial disease: a meta-analysis. JAMA 2001;285:1338. (*Magnetic resonance angiography was found to be highly accurate.*)

10. Brewster DC, Cambria RP, Darling RC, et al. Long-term results of combined iliac balloon angioplasty and distal surgical revascularization. Ann Surg 1989;210:324. (*Good long-term results were found for combined interventional therapy.*)

11. Byrne J, Darling RC, Change BB, et al. Infra-inguinal arterial reconstruction for claudication: is it worth the risk? An analysis of 409 procedures. J Vasc Surg 1999;29:259 (*Results emphasizing the benefit and safety of the procedure in most patients with claudication.*)

12. Clagett GP, Sobel M, Jackson MR, et al. Antithrombotic therapy in peripheral arterial occlusive disease; The Seventh ACCP Conference on Antithrombotic Therapy. Chest 2004;126:6095. (*An excellent summary of current rec-

ommendations for the use of antiplatelet and antithrombotic therapies in PAD.*)

13. Dawson DL, Cutler BS, Hiatt WR, et al. A comparison of cilostazol and pentoxifylline for treating intermittent claudication. Am J Med 2000;109:523. (*A large, multicenter, randomized, controlled trial [RCT], finding that cilostazol was superior to pentoxifylline and placebo, which were equal in effect; there was an increase in minor side effects with cilostazol.*)

14. Hiatt WR. Medical treatment of peripheral arterial disease and claudication. N. Engl J Med 2001; 344;1608. (*Excellent review of the data; 125 references.*)

15. McDermott, Kiu K, Ferrucci L, et al. Physical performance in peripheral arterial disease: a slower rate of decline in patients who walk more. Ann Intern Med 2006;144:10. (*A prospective cohort study; walking improved outcomes.*)

16. Mondillo S, Ballo P, Barbati R, et al. Effects of simvastatin on walking performance and symptoms of intermittent claudication in hypercholesterolemic patients with peripheral vascular disease. Am J Med 2003;114:359. (*A placebo-controlled RCT; significant improvement was found after 3 months of treatment.*)

17. Norgren L, Hiatt WR, Dormandy JA, et al. Inter-Society Consensus for the Management of Peripheral Arterial Disease (TASC II). J Vasc Surg 2007;45(Suppl S):S5. (*An updated, in-depth summary of interdisciplinary consensus recommendations for the medical and surgical management of patients with PAD.*)

18. Radack K, Wyderski RJ. Conservative management of intermittent claudication. Ann Intern Med 1990;113:135. (*Review of the evidence for the efficacy of walking, smoking cessation, and pentoxiphylline; 99 references.*)

19. Regensteiner, Hiatt WR. Current medical therapies for patients with peripheral arterial disease: a critical review. Am J Med 2002; 112:49. (*An evidence-based review; 75 references.*)

20. Schillinger M, Sabeti S, Loewe C, et al. Balloon angioplasty versus implantation of nitinol stents in the superficial femoral artery. N Engl J Med 2006;354:1879. (*RCT; an example of improved outcome with stent use.*)

21. Stewart KJ, Hiatt WR, Regensteiner JG, et al. Exercise training for claudication. N Engl J Med 2002;347:1941. (*The best review of exercise, including functional benefits and exercise prescriptions; 124 references.*)

22. Tetteroo E, van der Graaf Y, Bosch JL, et al. Randomized comparison of primary stent placement versus primary angioplasty followed by selective stent placement in patients with iliac-artery occlusive disease. Dutch Iliac Stent Trial Group. Lancet 1998; 351:1153. (*A study suggesting that routine stenting is not necessary or beneficial; selective stenting also saved expense.*)

23. The Warfarin Antiplatelet Vascular Evaluation Trial Investigators. Oral anticoagulant and antiplatelet therapy and peripheral arterial disease. N Engl J Med 2007;357:217. (*A major RCT, showing no additional benefit from combined therapy and an increased risk of major bleeding.*)

24. Wilson SE, Wolf GL, Cross AP. Percutaneous transluminal angioplasty versus operation for peripheral arteriosclerosis. Report of a prospective randomized trial in a selected group of patients. J Vasc Surg 1989;9:1. (*In a group of patients with lesions amenable to percutaneous transluminal angioplasty [PTA], short- and long-term success rates were similar for surgery and PTA.*)

CHAPTER 35 ■ MANAGEMENT OF PERIPHERAL VENOUS DISEASE

NANCY L. CANTELMO AND DAVID C. BREWSTER

The scope and prevalence of venous disease in ambulatory practice are considerable, ranging from superficial telangiectasias of cosmetic concern to deep vein thrombosis posing a risk of fatal pulmonary embolization. Early diagnosis is an important task for the primary physician (see Chapter 22); advances in treatment provide enhanced opportunities for outpatient management, both by the primary physician and the vascular specialist. A collaborative approach is often beneficial, necessitating knowledge of the range of treatment options and indications for referral.

PATHOPHYSIOLOGY AND CLINICAL PRESENTATION (1–15)

Normal Physiology

The high frequency of venous disorders of the lower extremities is unique to humans and reflects the consequences of gravity working on an upright posture. To return blood from the periphery to the right heart, the venous system in the legs must work against the force of gravity without the aid of organs specifically designed for this purpose. A number of factors work to lessen venous pressure in the leg and propel blood toward the heart. These include the *muscular pump* effect of the exercising calf musculature, the negative intrathoracic pressure created by the *bellows effect* of the chest wall with respiration, and the presence of multiple valves in both superficial and deep venous systems. The latter prevents reflux of blood and serves to reduce pressure in the veins that would otherwise equal the weight of an uninterrupted column of blood from the heart to the foot (approximately 100 mm Hg).

Although two venous systems, *superficial* and *deep*, are well known, a third system of *perforating* veins is less well recognized, directly connecting the superficial and deep systems. Valves exist in all three systems, maintaining flow from the superficial to the deep system and preventing retrograde flow. When functioning properly, these three systems work in coordinated fashion. The *deep intramuscular system*, composed of paired *anterior* and *posterior tibial* and *peroneal veins*, *popliteal veins*, and *femoral* and *deep femoral veins*, handles approximately 80% of venous return. The *superficial* system consists of the *great* and *small saphenous veins* and their tributaries. To clarify and standardize venous anatomy, a new nomenclature is now used (Table 35.1).

Clinical disorders of the venous system usually stem from *obstruction* to venous return due to thrombosis of the vein lumen or from *reflux* of blood due to incompetent venous valves that allow the retrograde flow of venous blood and persistent elevation of distal venous pressure in the leg and foot.

Varicose Veins

Pathophysiology

The superficial veins lie in the subcutaneous tissue and lack the support afforded by muscle and fascial compartments. Varicose veins are extremely common and affect from 10% to 20% of the adult population to some degree. Women are affected two times as often as men, and are also more likely to be symptomatic. A family history of varicosities is present in most patients and lends support to the concept of a hereditary or congenital etiology. *Family history*, *increased age*, and *female gender* are the strongest risk factors for varicose veins. It is unclear whether the primary problem is a congenital incompetence of valves or a weakness of the venous wall itself, which causes dilation of the vein lumen and subsequent valve inadequacy. Remodeling of the extracellular matrix and altered gene expression in response to venous distention and altered shear stress may lead to the disruption of venous architecture. Whatever the causes, a self-perpetuating cycle ensues of venous reflux leading to further vein dilation and valve failure.

In time, the poorly supported superficial veins widen, elongate, and become tortuous. In a smaller percentage of patients, the initial defect may be in the perforating veins, where poorly functioning valves allow abnormal flow toward the superficial system, causing eventual overdistention. In other patients, acquired factors such as *lower limb injury* or venous *thrombosis* may play a role. The increased incidence of varicose veins in women implicates hormonal factors, as does the relationship between the duration of hormone replacement therapy and varicose veins. Situations that raise intraluminal vein pressure, such as *multiparity*, *obesity*, and *prolonged standing*, are also important factors. The final common pathway remains valvular incompetence.

Clinical Presentation

Varicosities most commonly involve the veins of the greater saphenous system and its tributaries and therefore occur principally in the medial and anterior thigh, calf, and ankle regions. The small saphenous system may also be involved, producing varicosities of the posterior calf and lateral ankle region. In addition to location, veins are characterized by size. Varicose veins are defined as those greater than 4 mm in diameter and protruding. Reticular veins are smaller 2 to 4 mm and are usually nonprotruding. Spider veins or telangiectasias are less than 2 mm and red or purple in color.

Recurrent varices after surgery are a common and complex problem for patients and their physicians, occurring in from 20% to 80% of cases. Recognized causes are incomplete surgery with residual refluxing veins, the development of new varicosities from refluxing veins, and neovascularization—the

314

TABLE 35.1

CHANGES IN THE TERMINOLOGY OF VENOUS ANATOMY

Old Terminology	New Terminology
Femoral vein	Common femoral vein
Superficial femoral vein	Femoral vein
Hunterian perforator	Mid-thigh perforator
Cockett's perforators	Paratibial perforators
Long or greater saphenous vein	Great saphenous vein
Short or lesser saphenous vein	Small saphenous vein

From Caggiati A, Bergan JJ, Gloviczski P, et al. International Interdisciplinary Consensus Committee on Venous Anatomical Terminology. Nomenclature of veins of the lower limbs: an international interdisciplinary consensus statement. J Vasc Surg 2002;36:416, with permission.

TABLE 35.2

CLINICAL STAGING OF VENOUS DISEASE

Stage	Characteristics
C0	No visible palpable sign of venous disease
C1	Telangiectasias or reticular veins
C2	Varicose veins
C3	Edema
C4	Pigmentation, eczema, lipodermatosclerosis
C5	Healed venous ulcer
C6	Active venous ulcer

From Eklof B, Rutherford RB, Gergan JJ, et al. American Venous Forum International Ad Hoc Committee for Revision of the CZAP Classification. Revision of the CEAP Classification for chronic venous disorders: consensus statement. J Vasc Surg 2004;40:1248, with permission.

proliferation of blood vessels in tissues not normally containing them.

The presenting symptoms of varicose veins are extremely variable and sometimes bear little relationship to the apparent severity of the varicosities. Complaints are more frequent in women, particularly young women at the time of the menstrual period. *Aching* is the most commonly reported symptom. Other complaints include *cramping*, *"tired legs,"* and *heaviness*. Mild *swelling* is not uncommon, particularly in a leg with particularly severe varicosities, whereas significant swelling would be associated more commonly with deep system problems. *Itching* is reported particularly over distended veins or associated with an eczema-like rash. *Bleeding* or *ecchymosis* may occur, related to trauma or irritation, and may be difficult to control. *Phlebitis*, limited to the superficial system, presents as a warm, tender, firm, erythematous surface varicosity.

Chronic Venous Insufficiency

Pathophysiology

Chronic venous insufficiency (CVI) can be particularly disabling, causing suffering and significant economic impact. The concept and synonymous term "postphlebitic syndrome" were described by John Homans of Harvard University in 1916. CVI is found twice as often in men as in women. Although the superficial system often contributes to the pathophysiology, the deep and perforating systems assume greater significance in CVI. A documented history of *deep venous thrombosis* (DVT) can be obtained in fewer than one half of patients with chronic venous insufficiency, but it is believed to be the underlying etiology in most instances. The DVT can often be clinically silent. Despite subsequent recanalization of deep venous occlusions, the phlebitic inflammatory process deforms or destroys venous valves in the deep system, and their incompetence results in reflux and increased venous pressure. Perforating veins undergo similar changes through valvular damage or simply by exposure to chronically elevated pressure from the deep venous system.

In addition to the more common deep and perforator reflux, another, less-well-recognized cause for CVI also exists. Venous outflow obstruction in the *ileocaval veins* may be responsible for greater than 25% of CVI. The etiology of this obstruction

may be either persistent thrombosis or congenital anatomic obstruction.

In CVI, extravasation of macromolecules and red blood cells is caused by the high venous pressure on the dermal microcirculation, stimulating an inflammatory response that leads to tissue damage and impedes healing. In addition, reduced local capillary flow and tissue hypoxia further increase tissue breakdown and limit healing. Eventually these processes and accompanying infection lead to damage of the lymphatics, aggravating the problem.

Clinical Presentation

The hallmarks of chronic venous insufficiency are significant *edema* and *skin changes*. The edema of CVI is moderate to severe, as differentiated from the milder edema of superficial disease. The edema of CVI usually is improved by elevation, disappearing overnight, as distinguished from lymphedema, which does not resolve. The trophic changes of the skin associated with CVI are *hyperpigmentation*, *lipodermatosclerosis*, and active or healed *ulceration*.

In an effort to provide uniformity in both clinical and research situations, a classification has been developed, much like the TNM (tumor, nodes, metastases) system for cancer. The CEAP classification has four components: C (clinical), E (etiologic), A (anatomic), and P (pathologic). For clinical purposes, the C (clinical) component of the CEAP classification is widely used clearly to convey venous pathology. See Table 35.2.

Deep Vein Thrombophlebitis

Pathophysiology

The cause of acute thrombus formation in the venous system is often unclear, but in most instances factors contributing to *intimal damage*, *stasis*, and *hypercoagulability* (Virchow's triad) comprise the pathophysiologic determinants of venous thrombophlebitis. In about half of instances, the immediate cause is an identifiable self-limited event (e.g., recent *orthopedic surgery*, new onset of *paralysis*, concurrent *malignancy*, a prolonged *airplane flight*, *trauma*, *pregnancy*) or some other acquired factor. Risk is especially pronounced in persons undergoing *total knee replacement*, in which case the incidence

TABLE 35.3

CAUSES OF "IDIOPATHIC" DEEP VEIN THROMBOPHLEBITIS

Risk Factor	Risk[a]	Percentage of Cases of Idiopathic Disease
Hereditary Causes		
Factor V Leiden mutation	+	20% first DVT, up to 50% recurrent
Deficiency in protein S or C or antithrombin III	++	7% first DVT, up to 20% recurrent
Homocysteinemia	++	?
Prothrombin gene mutation	++	6% first DVT, up to 18% recurrent
Acquired Causes		
Adenocarcinoma	+++	8% first DVT, up to 17% recurrent
Antiphospholipid antibodies	+++	5% first DVT

DVT, deep vein thrombosis.
[a]The risk increases markedly when it is present in combination with factor V Leiden mutation.

can be as high as 40% to 80%. Prolonged airplane travel in cramped seating is an increasingly appreciated risk factor. Although the risk is minimal in healthy persons with no DVT risk factors, the observed incidence of new DVT in persons with a predisposition to DVT who take flights in excess of 6 hours ranges from 3% to 10%, leading to the moniker *coach-class thrombosis*. Although most cases are asymptomatic, and the majority manifest only distal clot, the condition can progress and lead to embolization.

In nearly half of cases, no clinical precipitant is evident, leading to the designation *idiopathic*. Many such cases are now appreciated to have a hereditary or acquired precipitant of DVT. A host of risk factors has been identified (Table 35.3). The emerging pathophysiologic view of idiopathic DVT is that many cases occur in the context of underlying chronic hypercoagulability (either hereditary or acquired) and that a supervening clinical or subclinical event exacerbates the hypercoagulability or causes venous stasis or endothelial injury, triggering acute thrombophlebitis. This view of idiopathic DVT as a chronic disease has important implications for therapy and is supported by the high frequency of recurrent disease, often occurring in a previously unaffected limb.

Hereditary Factors. An increasing number of hereditary risk factors are being identified. Among the most common is mutation in the gene controlling factor V synthesis, which leads to the production of *factor V Leiden*, which is resistant to inactivation by the endogenous anticoagulant activated protein C. The factor V variant can be found in 25% to 50% of persons with idiopathic DVT and is particularly prevalent among persons of European descent. Although not an extremely powerful risk factor by itself, factor V Leiden confers an independent degree of risk that may rise substantially in the context of other risk factors, such as estrogen use. The *prothrombin gene mutation* is found in only about 5% to 10% of cases, but its presence increases risk by about two to four times more than does factor V Leiden. Deficiencies in the production of proteins that limit clotting to the site of vascular injury (*proteins S and C and antithrombin III*) are found in about 20% of persons with recurrent DVT. Most patients are heterozygotes for the deficiency, which is a potent risk factor for DVT.

Acquired Factors. Major *trauma, recent surgery* (within 3 months), *pregnancy, estrogen use, immobilization,* and *congestive heart failure* are among the powerful, readily apparent precipitants of acquired causes of DVT (Table 35.3). Less

evident but no less important are *malignancy, heparin-induced thrombocytopenia,* and the production of *antiphospholipid antibodies*. There is also an association of less clear significance with *atherosclerotic disease. Malignancy,* especially adenocarcinoma originating in the lung, gastrointestinal tract, or urogenital system, substantially increases the risk of DVT (presumably by inducing hypercoagulability). Less appreciated is the relationship of *occult malignancy* to DVT. Among patients presenting with a first case of idiopathic DVT, more than 10% have been found to have an underlying occult malignancy. The risk of developing clinically evident cancer within 2 years of an episode of idiopathic DVT is estimated at about 8% for a first attack and 17% for recurrent DVT.

Antiphospholipid antibodies are believed to induce thrombosis by causing vascular injury or by interacting with other abnormal clotting factors to induce a hypercoagulable state. Two classes of antiphospholipid antibodies have been identified: *anticardiolipin* and *lupus anticoagulant*. Both appear to develop in response to prior infection. A *secondary antiphospholipid syndrome* is seen in persons with systemic lupus erythematosus. Low titers of antiphospholipid antibody can be found in a small proportion of normal persons and in up to 25% of pregnant woman by the end of the first trimester. A sevenfold increase in risk is associated with their production, especially the lupus anticoagulant variety, making this a potent acquired risk factor for DVT.

An important predictor of recurrent DVT is *residual venous thrombosis*. After an initial acute episode of DVT, there is a steady progression of clot organization and recanalization. At 6 months, nearly 40% of patients show no residual clot; by 1 year, the number rises to about 60%, and it peaks at about 75% at 3 years. Those with residual thrombus on ultrasound have $2^{1}/_{2}$ times the risk for recurrence of those without detectable clot.

Clinical Presentation

DVT is notoriously variable and often subtle in its clinical presentation. *Unilateral leg edema* may be the only finding; it stands out as the most sensitive indicator of DVT. Classically, the patient complains of *pain* in the limb that is worse with motion, walking, or dependency and better with rest or elevation of the extremity. Leg *edema* below the level of the clot, pain on compression of the knee, a *Homan's sign* (calf pain produced by dorsiflexion of the foot), and a palpable cord are cited as the classic physical findings but are extremely nonspecific.

With extensive DVT, a dusky *cyanosis* may appear. Unfortunately, most classic findings have proven to be disappointingly low in sensitivity and specificity. A patient reporting little or no pain and showing no calf tenderness may harbor extensive deep venous clots, whereas another with impressive pain, calf tenderness, and an apparently positive Homan's sign may be clot-free.

Postthrombotic/Postphlebitic Syndrome

Nearly 30% of persons with symptomatic proximal DVT will develop postthrombotic (postphlebitic) syndrome. Onset is usually within 1 year after DVT. Manifestations range from minor discomfort, swelling, skin discoloration, and venous ectasia to chronic pain, skin ulceration, and refractory edema. Symptoms can have a significant effect on quality of life. Timely initiation of proper anticoagulation might reduce the risk of development.

EVALUATION (16,17)

Varicose Veins

On physical examination the extent and location of varicosities in the standing patient should be noted, as well as the presence of edema or skin change. Significant trophic changes are unusual in patients with only superficial venous pathology but are commonly found in those with involvement of both superficial and deep systems. Complaints of leg pain should be carefully evaluated to rule out other possibilities, such as arterial insufficiency, musculoskeletal disorders, and neurologic problems. Severe varicosities occurring at a young age or varicosities after trauma may suggest an arteriovenous connection.

Venous Insufficiency

Venous insufficiency needs to be distinguished from other causes of leg edema such as lymphatic obstruction, hypoalbuminemia, and DVT (see Chapter 22). Any accompanying *leg ulcers* must be differentiated from those due to arterial insufficiency, which tend to be more "punched out" in appearance and localized to the dorsum or lateral aspect of the foot or ankle. A history of claudication, rest pain relieved by dependency, absent pulses, bruits, dependent rubor, and atrophic skin changes also helps to distinguish arterial disease from venous insufficiency.

Doppler (duplex) ultrasound has become a mainstay of diagnosis of venous disease, varicose veins, chronic venous insufficiency, and phlebitis after a thorough history and physical exam. If the patient is symptomatic and has significant signs and symptoms, a duplex exam is warranted.

Most ultrasound laboratories are able to perform adequate examination for DVT or superficial phlebitis; special expertise is needed to perform adequate duplex examination for reflux. If significant reflux is seen (>0.5 second), then a "mapping" is performed. This produces information on the location, size, and amount of reflux, which is essential for the treatment of the superficial or perforator reflux.

Superficial Thrombophlebitis

Physical examination should exclude other diagnoses that may be confused with superficial thrombophlebitis, such as cellulitis or lymphangitis. In the last two, there is an absence of a palpable thrombosed vein, widespread distribution of erythema and swelling beyond the course of a vein, and identification of a possible focus of infection. Musculoskeletal and neurologic causes of pain and tenderness should be sought, such as a Baker's cyst in the popliteal fossa (see Chapter 152) or radicular pain (see Chapter 147). Swelling of the extremity should also be carefully noted because isolated superficial phlebitis should not contribute to generalized edema. A duplex ultrasound examination is essential in a superficial phlebitis in the proximal great saphenous vein (GSV) and small saphenous vein (SSV) regions to ensure that its location is superficial and not close to or involving the deep system.

Deep Vein Thrombophlebitis

The initial evaluation of the patient who complains of *unilateral leg edema* (>3 cm difference in calf diameter) with or without calf pain must include consideration of DVT (see Chapter 22). Prompt detection of proximal deep vein thrombophlebitis is critical; undetected and untreated, it may lead to pulmonary embolization, with its substantial risk of major cardiopulmonary morbidity and mortality. Identification of DVT in the absence of obvious precipitants raises the question of underlying hypercoagulability and occult malignancy, which needs to be addressed because the results affect the approach to management.

History and Physical Examination

Truly unilateral swelling, particularly extending above the knee, makes deep venous thrombosis more likely, but cellulitis and lymphedema must also be considered. Pain alone is an unreliable symptom. The findings of calf tenderness and a "positive" Homan's sign are by no means conclusive. The relative inaccuracy of diagnosis by history and physical examination (which is incorrect in up to 50% of cases) necessitates laboratory testing, but a careful review of the history and physical examination for *DVT risk factors* (e.g., age, previous DVT, major trauma, recent surgery or pregnancy, current estrogen use, congestive heart failure, limb paralysis, concurrent adenocarcinoma, nephrotic syndrome, systemic lupus) helps to estimate the risk and pretest probability. History should also be reviewed for a *family history of recurrent DVT*, which if present suggests a hereditary hypercoagulable state such as factor V Leiden or deficiency in proteins S and C or antithrombin III.

Laboratory Studies for Suspected DVT

Combining pretest-probability estimates with *d-dimer testing* and *Doppler ultrasound* has made possible an efficient outpatient workup, obviating much of the need for hospitalization, empiric anticoagulation, and proceeding to invasive venous imaging. Most important, a negative D-dimer test in the setting of a low pretest probability obviates the need for further testing and effectively rules out DVT (see Chapter 22). Because it is sensitive but nonspecific, the D-dimer test may also give positive results in non-DVT settings, such as infection, inflammation, trauma, pregnancy, hemorrhage, and the postoperative state. Refinements in the test technology (e.g., use of a red blood cell agglutination D-dimer test in pregnancy) are being sought to reduce the false-alarm rate. In the meantime, proceeding to Doppler ultrasound when the condition cannot be ruled out by pretest probability and D-dimer test result is a reasonable next step. Duplex ultrasound has a high test sensitivity for the detection of DVT from the knee upward, which is the area most prone to spawning embolization.

Assessment for Hypercoagulability

Documented cases in which there is no apparent acute risk factor for DVT (so-called *idiopathic* DVT) manifest a high prevalence (approaching 40%) of underlying hypercoagulability (Table 35.3) and a high rate of recurrence (e.g., up to 27% per patient-year). Such figures argue for a careful consideration of *hereditary* and *acquired* causes of hypercoagulability.

Acquired Conditions. Among the important acquired etiologies of idiopathic disease is the *antiphospholipid antibody syndrome*, which is characterized by thrombosis and elevated titers of antiphospholipid antibody (i.e., *lupus anticoagulant* or *anticardiolipin antibody*). In less than half of such cases, the patient has clinically active systemic lupus or a lupus-like syndrome (*secondary antiphospholipid syndrome*); in the remainder, there is no evidence of active lupus, although the antinuclear antibody test may be positive (*primary antiphospholipid syndrome*). Some patients report a history of fetal loss. Those at greatest risk of thrombosis manifest high antibody titers, thrombocytopenia, Raynaud's phenomenon, and livedo reticularis.

The antiphospholipid antibody syndrome confers a significant risk of recurrent venous thrombosis, and arterial clot formation and should be considered in idiopathic and recurrent cases of DVT, especially if the patient has active lupus (see Chapter 146), a positive antinuclear antibody test, and a history of fetal loss. Identification of antiphospholipid antibodies is achieved by serologic testing that includes activated *partial thromboplastin time*, *Russell viper venom time*, and *dilutional studies*.

Assessment for occult malignancy becomes an issue in idiopathic cases, especially in the absence of other acquired or hereditary risk factors. The frequency of occult cancer in idiopathic disease is just high enough—about 10% in initial cases and close to 20% in recurrent idiopathic cases—to justify a malignancy workup. The workup should focus on the detection of potentially curable cancers (e.g., skin, breast, colon, prostate, bladder, lymph nodes, testes, uterus) and those that at least respond to treatment (e.g., small-cell cancer of the lung, ovarian carcinoma).

Standard screening procedures for curable malignancies are reasonable, but the routine ordering of computed tomography of the lung, abdomen, and pelvis in such cases has not proven to be particularly useful. The optimal laboratory investigation for underlying malignancy in patients with idiopathic DVT remains to be determined. The approach to testing should be based primarily on initial clinical findings. Patients not found to have cancer after an initial workup have a very low risk of presenting with cancer at a later date. Although such patients need to be followed closely, they require no special additional testing in the absence of new clinical findings.

Hereditary Conditions. Most hereditary hypercoagulable states (e.g., *factor V Leiden, deficiency in protein S or C,* and *antithrombin III*) represent gene mutations that by themselves confer only modest increases in hypercoagulability. However, when combined with an acquired risk factor for DVT, they appear greatly to increase the likelihood of thrombus formation. This could explain why some patients develop thrombophlebitis and others do not when exposed to the same external risk factors. Although some hereditary hypercoagulable states are rather common (e.g., factor V

Leiden can be found in 20% of whites with idiopathic DVT), it remains to be demonstrated that routine screening for these conditions is cost-effective. Testing should be considered when the results would substantively affect treatment decisions (e.g., duration of anticoagulation).

Hyperhomocysteinemia, which can lead to vessel wall injury and increased risks of venous thrombosis and premature atherosclerosis, may be hereditary (enzyme mutation, homozygous) or acquired (folate deficiency). Plasma homocysteine levels in excess of 18.5 nmol/mL (normal is 4 to 15 nmol/mL) confer a fourfold increase in the risk of DVT, leading many to screen for hyperhomocysteinemia in persons with recurrent idiopathic DVT, but evidence that homocysteine-lowering B-vitamin/folate therapy reduces DVT risk has yet to emerge.

MANAGEMENT (18–47)

Varicose Veins

Conservative Measures

The initial management of varicose veins (CEAP C2) is nonoperative, addressing valve incompetence and poor soft-tissue support. Untreated, most varicose veins will slowly worsen. All patients will benefit from proper *graduated compression hose* of medium weight, for example, 20 to 30 mm Hg, together with periodic *elevation* of the extremity at intervals during the day. Compression hose must be properly measured by trained personnel to be effective. The various stockings sold in department or drug stores are usually of too light a weight and improper fit. Ace wraps are cumbersome and often applied improperly, creating a "tourniquet" effect at the knee level. A below-the-knee stocking is usually most effective and better tolerated than thigh-high or pantyhose types.

Intervention

In patients with symptomatic varicose veins for whom conservative measures have failed, including compression, elevation, and medication, a duplex ultrasound should be performed. If no obstruction is seen in the deep system and no axial reflux is demonstrated (GSV, SSV), attention may then be directed at the symptomatic varicosities. Although *sclerotherapy* (the injection of a sclerosing solution into the vein in either liquid or foam form) is an option, bulging varicosities are usually best managed by *phlebectomy*. This involves microincision under local anesthesia to remove the varicosities. Transilluminated powered phlebectomy may also be performed under general anesthesia. The results are excellent, with the resolution of symptoms and a good cosmetic result.

For patients with reflux of the GSV, SSV, or a major tributary, removing this source of reflux is mandatory. *Stripping* and *ligating* of the refluxing vein used to be common, but less invasive *endoluminal ablation* (by laser or radiofrequency methods) is now the method of choice (endochemical ablation is under investigation). Some patients with very large and/or very superficial refluxing axial veins may still require stripping and ligating by modified techniques.

For patients with reticular or spider varicosities of a cosmetic nature (CEAP C1) without underlying varicose veins or reflux, a course of *sclerotherapy*, using a liquid or foam sclerosant, is the first line of treatment. *Cutaneous laser* is performed for residual, very small, red telangiectasias after sclerotherapy has eliminated the larger spider veins.

Short-term compression is mandatory for all patients after surgical or sclerotherapy treatment. Long-term compression is recommended for the possible prevention of recurrence.

Chronic Venous Insufficiency

Management before Ulceration (CEAP C3, 4)

Treatment of venous insufficiency is best initiated before the occurrence of venous ulceration, which may eventually occur if the condition is untreated. *Elastic support* and *periodic elevation* remain cornerstones of therapy. *Patient education* is essential because compliance is poor otherwise. A *knee-length or longer heavyweight elastic stocking*, for example, 30 to 40 mm Hg or greater—is prescribed and must be worn consistently from the moment the patient gets out of bed until he or she retires at night. Leg elevation is best accomplished with the patient supine and the leg on a pillow or by raising the entire foot of the bed at night. *Periodic elevation* during the day is recommended whenever possible. Good *skin care* with cleansing and the application of moisturizers is important to prevent dry, cracked skin and tissue breakdown. The chronic and incurable nature of the problem must be emphasized and the importance of these conservative measures understood by the patient.

Management after Ulceration (CEAP C6)

Aggressive wound care is the first priority. Wound centers are frequently helpful in this regard. There are many wound care products available, but data are insufficient to support a particular product. Compression wraps, garments, and pumps may help to reduce edema and promote healing. The mainstay of treatment has been *Unna's boot*, a two-layer dressing that exerts 20 to 30 mm Hg of pressure. A newer, four-layer dressing exerts 30 to 40 mm Hg of pressure.

Direct ulcer care involves wound cleansing, which is recommended to be done with a pressure device. Necrotic or devitalized tissue may be debrided mechanically or enzymatically. Infected wounds are treated with systemic antibiotics and/or local dressings, often using a silver-impregnated preparation. For clean but draining wounds, a moisture-absorbent foam or alginate dressing is recommended. For clean, dry wounds, moisture-donating dressings are recommended, such as saline-based hydrogels. Adjuvant therapies include skin grafting, bioengineered dermal equivalents, and nonliving dermal substitutes. In addition, negative-pressure wound devices may be helpful.

Recurrent ulceration is frequent in CEAP C5 patients (24% recurrence of ulceration in 1 year, 33% recurrence in 2 years, 49% recurrence in 3 years). Ultrasound examination can help to identify underlying pathology and facilitate determining what additional treatment might be helpful. Arterial and vena caval study may reveal important pathology.

Interventional therapy is a consideration in patients who are active, not morbidly obese, and of reasonable medical risk. Options include the treatment of superficial disease and/or perforator vessels (with the methods outlined previously) or direct intervention. Patients with deep system reflux should be advised to use lifelong compression hose. Active investigations are ongoing to develop procedures to restore deep system valvular competency.

For patients with ileocaval obstruction, evaluation is performed with contrast venography or intravenous ultrasound.

To relieve the obstruction and establish flow, intravenous balloon dilation and stenting are options.

Superficial Thrombophlebitis

Superficial thrombophlebitis in the lower leg is best managed by a combination of *local heat* and *compression* hose. *Anti-inflammatory agents* such as ibuprofen or other nonsteroidal drugs may be useful. Antibiotics have no role. Women taking birth control pills should consider discontinuing their use. Pain and inflammation usually resolve within 1 to 2 weeks.

Close follow-up is essential because there is an increased risk of thrombus extending into the deep system, especially if it reaches the saphenofemoral or saphenopopliteal junction. If superficial phlebitis extends close to the deep system, consideration should be given to anticoagulation and ligation of the saphenous vein at the level of the saphenofemoral or saphenopopliteal junction in the groin, particularly if the process has ascended while under treatment observation.

Deep Vein Thrombophlebitis /Venous Thromboembolism

Primary Prevention in the Outpatient Setting

In the outpatient setting, high-risk situations include prolonged airplane travel under cramped conditions and recovery from major hip or knee surgery.

For Airplane Travel. For persons with a preexisting risk factor for DVT, prolonged airplane travel (>5 to 6 hours) is associated with an increased risk of DVT (persons with no risk factors do not appear to be at risk). Prevention of such "coach-class thrombosis" can be facilitated by advising the at-risk traveler to get up and walk around during the flight, flex and stretch leg muscles periodically while seated, keep well hydrated (which also generates a trip to the lavatory), and avoid alcohol (which can lead to dehydration but usually also generates a trip to the lavatory). The use of compression stockings has proven to be effective in controlled trials with at-risk persons. A single preflight dose of low–molecular weight heparin for high-risk persons is under study. Aspirin is of no benefit.

For Recent Orthopedic Surgery. Persons who undergo major hip or knee surgery are at a very high risk for postoperative DVT and require prophylaxis. Prophylactic therapy is typically started after surgery because pre- or perioperative prophylaxis does not provide sufficiently added benefit to offset the increased risk of bleeding. *Low-dose heparin, low–molecular weight heparin*, and *warfarin* have all been used to reduce DVT risk in hip surgery to acceptable levels. Low–molecular weight heparin affords an increasingly popular approach to prophylaxis after hip surgery, given its ease of use, efficacy, and safety; the cost can be substantial, but savings are afforded by the lack of need for monitoring. Prolonged treatment (3 to 4 weeks) is superior to short-term (7 to 10 days) use.

Despite such measures, DVT risk is still 30% to 40% in persons undergoing total knee replacement, stimulating the search for more effective prophylactic therapies. Potent *synthetic antithrombotic agents* that selectively *inhibit activated factor X* appear to be promising for DVT prophylaxis in persons undergoing total knee replacement, reducing the DVT risk to about 10% at a cost of a tolerable increase in bleeding risk.

Initial Therapy: Heparinization (Unfractionated vs. Low–Molecular Weight Heparin)

DVT above the knee is associated with a high risk of *venous thromboembolization* and the need for anticoagulation.

Unfractionated Heparin Therapy. The traditional standard therapy of acute DVT/venous thromboembolism (VTE) involves prompt *hospitalization* for immediate intravenous treatment with *unfractionated heparin* and initiation of *oral anticoagulation* with *warfarin*. Heparin and warfarin are continued until the prothrombin time (as measured by the International Normalized Ratio (INR) has been in therapeutic range for 3 to 4 days (see Chapter 83), at which time heparin is stopped, warfarin is continued, and the patient is discharged. The advent of low–molecular weight heparin and the finding that it is of equal efficacy and easier to use in uncomplicated cases of DVT/VTE provide the opportunity for expanded outpatient treatment and a shortening of hospital stay.

Low–Molecular Weight Heparin. Its principal mechanism of action (accelerating the formation of irreversible complexes between antithrombin III and activated factor X) is the same as that of unfractionated heparin, but there is reduced interaction with platelets and thrombin, making possible equivalent efficacy with less risk for bleeding. Bioavailability is enhanced and half-life is longer because there is little binding to plasma proteins, red cells, or vascular endothelium. Prospective, randomized studies show low–molecular weight heparin to be at least as effective as unfractionated heparin in preventing thromboembolic events, as safe or safer with regard to major bleeding complications, and superior with respect to survival (reduced all-cause mortality at 6 months).

The efficacy, safety, and ease of use (standardized dose, twice-daily dosing, no need for partial thromboplastin time monitoring or intravenous access) enable anticoagulation to proceed much earlier on an outpatient basis. For patients with uncomplicated acute DVT, hospitalization has largely been eliminated. These features make low–molecular weight heparin the emerging treatment of choice for initial management of acute DVT uncomplicated by pulmonary embolization. Although low-molecular-weight heparin costs much more per dose than conventional heparin therapy, it is more cost-effective by virtue of its ability to eliminate hospital stay without increasing the risk of bleeding or thromboembolization.

Low-molecular-weight heparin preparations include *dalteparin, enoxaparin, nadroparin, reviparin,* and *tinzaparin*. Although they differ with respect to protein binding and other qualities, none stands out as clearly superior with regard to safety or efficacy. Dalteparin and enoxaparin are the most commonly prescribed preparations in the United States for outpatient use. They are administered twice daily by subcutaneous injection of a fixed weight-adjusted dose (e.g., dalteparin 100 units/kg twice daily or enoxaparin 1 mg/kg twice daily). The two drugs appear to be clinically equivalent, but dalteparin is about one third lower in cost.

Treatment is continued for approximately 1 week until oral anticoagulation with warfarin (started on day 1 or 2) is in therapeutic range (INR 2.0) for at least 2 days—the same as with unfractionated heparin. The patient must be medically stable and reliable and have a supportive home environment and available visiting-nurse services.

The major clinical contraindications to outpatient heparinization are preexisting bleeding difficulties and marked hypercoagulability (e.g., recent surgery, trauma, cancer). The patient should be medically and hemodynamically stable.

Monitoring requirements are minimal, but platelet counts and prothrombin times on days 3 and 7 are suggested to check for *heparin-induced thrombocytopenia* and to assess oral anticoagulation (see Chapter 83).

Initial Therapy: Thrombolysis

Thrombolytic therapy (e.g., *streptokinase, tissue plasminogen activator*) deserves consideration in patients with extensive and severe *proximal DVT*, especially of the *iliofemoral* system. The objective is to minimize the chances of developing postphlebitic syndrome by instituting clot-lysis therapy. The best results have been achieved in patients with proximal vein DVT of the femoral or iliac system treated within 3 days of the onset of symptoms; most studies have used streptokinase. Clot lysis occurs in about 50% of instances.

Because there is an increased risk of *major bleeding*, particularly cerebral hemorrhage, prompt referral to a vascular specialist is indicated to facilitate case selection. Contraindications include malignant hypertension, recent stroke or surgery, trauma, recent or active hemorrhage, any bleeding diathesis, pregnancy, and intracranial disease.

Initial Therapy: Vena Cava Filter

Despite the advent of retrievable filters, current recommendations are for the use of such filters only when there is a serious contraindication to anticoagulation in a person with documented DVT or venous thromboembolism. Data on safety and efficacy are minimal. In the only randomized, controlled study in the literature, there was a significant reduction in recurrent VTE at 12 days but not at 2 years; recurrent DVT was increased significantly at 2 years. The occurrence of postthrombotic syndrome was similar in both groups.

Subsequent Therapy: Oral Anticoagulation

Heparinization is continued while oral anticoagulation with *warfarin* is initiated (see Chapter 83). Heparin is stopped after the prothrombin time reaches an INR of greater than 2.0 for at least 24 to 48 hours (the time needed for previously synthesized prothrombin to clear the serum).

Duration. The duration of warfarin therapy for prophylaxis of recurrent DVT/VTE is a function of underlying etiology and number of episodes. For a first episode of DVT occurring in the setting of a clear-cut *self-limited precipitant* (e.g., surgery or trauma), a 3-month course usually suffices. For *pulmonary embolization* in the setting of a clear-cut precipitant, therapy is usually continued for 6 months. A first episode of *idiopathic VTE* is treated for a minimum of 6 to 12 months due to an increased risk of recurrence.

Chronic therapy is a consideration for patients at highest risk. Priority candidates include individuals with *idiopathic VTE* who have had *multiple recurrences* (the risk for recurrence can exceed 5%/yr), those who manifested a *severe degree of thrombosis* or had their DVT complicated by *pulmonary embolization*, and those subsequently found to have a circulating *lupus anticoagulant* (risk approaches 25%/yr). Other hypercoagulability risk factors do not appear to confer nearly as much risk, but even persons with uncomplicated idiopathic disease and no identifiable determinants of hypercoagulability manifest an increased risk of recurrent thrombosis and should be considered for chronic anticoagulation (see later discussion). Chronic anticoagulation is also indicated in other persons with a history of *recurrent DVT* or *DVT in the context of concurrent cancer.*

Intensity. The intensity of chronic oral anticoagulation that optimizes DVT/VTE prophylaxis while minimizing bleeding complications is an area of active study. The Prevention of Recurrent Venous Thromboembolism trial found low-intensity therapy (INR 1.5 to 2.0) to be superior to placebo, but the Evaluation of Losartan in the Elderly trial, comparing long-term, full-intensity warfarin therapy (INR 2 to 3) with low-intensity therapy (INR 1.5 to 2.0) in persons with idiopathic VTE, found that full-intensity therapy was superior with regard to death and recurrent VTE without any increase in risk of clinically important bleeding. Although these findings need confirmation, they suggest that full-intensity therapy is reasonably safe for chronic prophylaxis in appropriately selected candidates (see later discussion). It must be kept in mind that under study conditions, maintaining an INR between 2.0 and 3.0 dramatically reduces the risk of VTE recurrence while increasing the risk of major bleeding by only 3% per patient-year. Observational studies conducted in the community setting put the risk of major bleeding a bit higher, at 5% to 7% per patient-year. One option is to consider chronic low-intensity therapy for persons who might be at somewhat increased risk of bleeding.

In high-risk patients, there is concern about the need for more intensive prophylactic therapy. Persons with recurrent disease due to *antiphospholipid syndrome* show no additional benefit from more intensive oral anticoagulation; an INR goal of greater than 3.0 provides no better protection than does an INR of 2 to 3. However, *cancer* confers an especially high risk of recurrent VTE, which can be lessened by substituting *chronic low–molecular weight heparin* for standard-intensity warfarin therapy without any increase in the risk of hemorrhage.

Patient Selection. Optimizing the selection of patients for long-term warfarin prophylaxis requires a personalized approach that weighs individual risks and benefits and considers the patient's preferences and willingness to comply with the demands of treatment (Table 35.4; see also Chapter 83).

Subsequent Therapy: Low–Molecular Weight Heparin

The continuation of low–molecular weight heparin beyond the initial phase of anticoagulation in place of warfarin has demonstrated a reduction in the risk of recurrent VTE without an increase in the risk of major bleeding.

Subsequent Therapy: Long-Acting Activated Factor X Inhibition

A promising approach to DVT prophylaxis is the use of *idraparinux*, a long-acting inhibitor of activated factor X, in lieu of standard warfarin therapy. The drug is administered parenterally once weekly and does not require laboratory monitoring of clotting status. A randomized, controlled trial of 3 and 6 months' therapy in patients with DVT revealed an equivalent efficacy to warfarin but a decreased ability to prevent recurrent VTE in persons with prior pulmonary embolization. Extended use beyond 6 months was associated with an equal ability to prevent recurrent VTE but an increased risk of major hemorrhage. More study is needed before this approach can be recommended.

DVT below the Knee

DVT below the knee poses little risk of embolization so long as the clot does not propagate up into the thigh. The risk of propagation ranges from 10% to 30%. The risk of embolization from a clot that stays below the knee is small (short-term risk is 0.3% to 1.0%). Outpatients suspected of having DVT but without evidence of extension above the knee do not require immediate anticoagulation; however, they should be followed closely with serial evaluation for evidence of propagation. Those who require the closest monitoring are patients with multiple risk factors for DVT. Repeat noninvasive study, using Doppler ultrasound or plethysmography, is indicated (see prior discussion).

TABLE 35.4

AMERICAN COLLEGE OF CHEST PHYSICIANS RECOMMENDATIONS FOR THE DURATION OF ANTICOAGULATION FOR VENOUS THROMBOEMBOLISM

Clinical Subgroup	Treatment Duration
First episode DVT/transient risk	UH/LMWH followed by 3 mo VKA
First episode DVT/concurrent cancer	3–6 mo LMWH, indefinite anticoagulation until cancer resolves
First episode idiopathic DVT	UH/LMWH followed by 6–12 mo VKA (suggest indefinite)
First episode DVT/thrombophilia, antithrombin deficiency, factor V Leiden, prothrombin 20210 mutation, homocysteinemia, factor VIII elevation (>90th percentile)	UH or LMWH followed by 6–12 mo VKA (suggest indefinite if protein C and S deficiency, idiopathic)
First episode DVT/thrombophilia, antiphospholipid antibodies, two or more thrombophilias	UH or LMWH followed by 12 mo VKA (suggest indefinite)
Recurrent DVT	UH or LMWH followed by Indefinite VKA

DVT, deep vein thrombophlebitis; LMWH, low–molecular weight heparin; UH, unfractionated heparin; VKA, vitamin K antagonist (warfarin).
From Buller HR, Agnelli G, Hull RD, et al. Antithrombotic therapy for venous thromboembolic disease: the seventh ACCP conference on antithrombotic and thrombolytic therapy. Chest 2004;126:401S.

Postthrombotic Syndrome

The best measures are preventive, starting with timely initiation of appropriate anticoagulant therapy and compression. The use of custom-fitted compressive elastic stockings (providing 30 to 40 mm Hg of pressure at the ankle) starting early in the course of recovery reduces the risks of both mild and severe adverse sequelae by nearly 50%. Properly fitted stockings are expensive and difficult to put on, limiting their availability and use. Those who cannot put on such stockings (even with special donning devices) or find them too uncomfortable can try leg elevation and the avoidance of prolonged sitting or standing in conjunction with the use of lightweight support hose. If severe symptoms develop, the use of a full-length stocking may be required. Additional measures are similar to those for chronic venous insufficiency.

INDICATIONS FOR ADMISSION AND REFERRAL

Admission

Among patients with peripheral venous disease, those with DVT at or above the knee are at greatest risk acutely and most in need of immediate attention. Although urgent evaluation and prompt initiation of anticoagulation is definitely in order, hospitalization is no longer inevitable. As long as there is no evidence suggesting pulmonary embolization, iliofemoral extension, or hemodynamic instability (all indications for immediate admission) and as long as the patient is reliable and the home situation is supportive, heparinization can proceed safely and effectively at home with assisted or self-administered low–molecular weight heparin.

Referral

Surgical consultation is indicated for the patient with superficial phlebitis that extends close to the deep system for possible ligation of the GSV or SSV. For patients with DVT who have a *contraindication* for, *complication* of, or *failure* of anticoagulation, consideration should be given for an intracaval filter device. Surgical referral is also advisable for recurrent or nonhealing ulcerations due to chronic severe venous insufficiency. Consideration of surgery is reasonable for the patient with persistently symptomatic varicose veins (particularly if a conservative approach has failed), bleeding episodes, or recurrent bouts of superficial thrombophlebitis.

Annotated Bibliography

1. Caggiati A, Bergan JJ, Gloviczski P, et al. International Interdisciplinary Consensus Committee on Venous Anatomical Terminology. Nomenclature of veins of the lower limbs: an international interdisciplinary consensus statement. J Vasc Surg 2002;36:416. (*A description of the accepted venous anatomic nomenclature.*)
2. Criqui MH, Jasmosmos M, Frorek A, et al. Chronic venous disease in an ethnically diverse population. The San Diego Population Study. Am J Epidemiol 2003;158:448. (*Two population-based studies assessing signs, symptoms, and functional impairment of venous disease.*)
3. Crowther MA, Kelton JG. Congenital thrombophilic states associated with venous thrombosis: a qualitative overview and proposed classification system. Ann Intern Med 2003;138:128. (*An excellent review, which helps to summarize and apply current knowledge; 76 references.*)
4. Eklof B, Rutherford RB, Gergan JJ, et al. American Venous Forum International Ad Hoc Committee for Revision of the CZAP Classification. Revision of the CEAP Classification for chronic venous disorders: consensus statement. J Vasc Surg 2004;40:1248. (*Revision of the original CEAP [clinical, etiologic, anatomic, pathologic] classification, which is the one most commonly used.*)
5. Evans CJ, Allan PL, Lee AJ, et al. Prevalence of venous reflux in the general population on duplex scanning: the Edinburgh vein study. J Vasc Surg 1998;28:767. (*Epidemiologic evidence of prevalence.*)
6. Lapostolle F, Surget V, Borron SW, et al. Severe pulmonary embolism associated with air travel. N Engl J Med 2001;345:779. (*Provides evidence of the magnitude and severity of the risk.*)
7. McDaniel HB, Marston WP, Farber MA, et al. Recurrence of chronic venous ulcers on the basis of clinical, etiologic, anatomic and pathologic criteria and air plethysmography. Vasc Surg 2002; 35:723. (*Documents the high recurrence rate of ulcers over time.*)
8. Prandoni P, Filora F, Marchiori A, et al. An association between atherosclerosis and venous thrombosis. N Engl J Med 2003;348:1435. (*A significant association was found, but it was of unclear pathophysiologic and clinical significance.*)
9. Prandoni P, Lensing AWA, Cogo A, et al. The long-term clinical course of acute deep venous thrombosis. Ann Intern Med 1996;125:1. (*Nearly one third of patients with symptomatic proximal disease develop postthrombotic syndrome.*)
10. Prandoni P, Lensing AWA, Prins MH, et al. Residual venous thrombosis as a predictive factor of recurrent venous thromboembolism. Ann Intern Med 2002;137:955. (*A prospective cohort study; the risk was related to the presence of residual clot.*)
11. Price DT, Ridker PM. Factor V Leiden mutation and the risks for thromboembolic disease: a clinical perspective. Ann Intern Med 1997;1217:895. (*A good discussion of this very common mutation and its contribution to hypercoagulability.*)
12. Rodeghiero F, Tosetto A. Activated protein C resistance and factor V Leiden mutation are independent risk factors for venous thromboembolism. Ann Intern Med 1999;130:643. (*These hypercoagulable states account for up to 15% of cases of deep vein thrombosis [DVT], making attention to these states of potential importance in the evaluation of DVT, especially that which is recurrent.*)
13. Scurr JH, Machin SJ, Bailey-King S, et al. Frequency and prevention of symptomless deep-vein thrombosis in long-haul flights: a randomized trial. Lancet 2001;357:1485. (*Elastic compression stockings reduced the rate of DVT from 12% to 0% but increased the risk of superficial thrombophlebitis.*)
14. Simioni P, Prandoni P, Lensing AWA, et al. The risk of recurrent venous thromboembolism in patients with an Arg 506 to Gln mutation in the gene for factor V (factor V Leiden). N Engl J Med 1997;336:399. (*The original report identifying an increased risk of DVT in persons with this common gene mutation.*)
15. Strandness DE, Langlois Y, Kramer M, et al. Long-term sequelae of acute venous thrombosis. JAMA 1983;250:1289. (*Long-term sequelae including hyperpigmentation, pain, and swelling were not uncommon and were associated with occluded or incompetent distal deep veins.*)
16. Cornuz J, Pearson SD, Creager MA, et al. Importance of findings on the initial evaluation for cancer in patients with symptomatic idiopathic deep venous thrombosis. Ann Intern Med 1996;125:785. (*Of 142 patients presenting with DVT, 12% were found to have a cancer on comprehensive initial clinical evaluation; none of those who had no evidence on initial evaluation was found to have cancer later.*)
17. Labropoulos N, Leon LR Jr. Duplex evaluation of venous insufficiency. Semin Vasc Surg 2005;18:5. (*A description of the ultrasound exam for venous disease.*)
18. Agnelli G, Prandoni P, Santamaria MG, et al. Three months versus one year of oral anticoagulant therapy for idiopathic deep venous thrombosis. N Engl J Med 2001;345:165. (*A randomized, controlled trial; the risk of DVT was reduced only as long as oral anticoagulation continued; the risk returned to baseline when anticoagulation was terminated, irrespective of the duration of therapy.*)
19. Buller HR, Agnelli G, Hull RD, et al. Antithrombotic therapy for venous thromboembolic disease: the seventh ACCP conference on antithrombotic

and thrombolytic therapy. Chest 2004;126:401S. (*A consensus paper on therapeutic recommendations; see Table 35.4 in this chapter.*)

20. Crowther MA, Ginsberg JS, Julian J, et al. A comparison of two intensities of warfarin for the prevention of recurrent thrombosis in patients with the antiphospholipid antibody syndrome. N Engl J Med 2003;349:1133. (*A randomized, controlled trial [RCT], finding that moderate-intensity therapy [International Normalized Ratio of 2 to 3] was just a good as high-intensity therapy.*)

21. Crowther MA. Inferior vena cava filters in the management of venous thromboembolism. Am J Med 2007;120:S13. (*A review of the evidence, finding that the role of this approach is limited to persons with an absolute contraindication to anticoagulation and proven thromboembolism.*)

22. Dale JJ, Ruckley CV, Harper DR, et al. Randomised, double blind placebo-controlled trial of pentoxifylline in the treatment of venous leg ulcers. BMJ 1999;319:875. (*A modest but not statistically significant benefit was noted.*)

23. De Araujo T, Valencia I, Federman DG, et al. Managing the patient with venous ulcers. Ann Intern Med 2003;138:326. (*An evidence-based review for the clinician; 90 references.*)

24. Estrada CA, Mansfield CJ, Heudebert GR. Cost-effectiveness of low-molecular-weight heparin in the treatment of proximal deep vein thrombosis. J Gen Intern Med 2000;15:108. (*Finds savings and better outcomes.*)

25. Fletcher A, Cullum F, Sheldon TA. A systematic review of compression treatment for venous leg ulcers. BMJ 1997;315:576. (*The essential component is the application of 20 to 40 mm Hg of pressure at the ankle.*)

26. Ganz DA, Glynn RJ, Hogum H, et al. Adherence to guidelines for oral anticoagulation after venous thrombosis and pulmonary embolism. J Gen Intern Med 2000;15:776. (*Nearly 25% of patients failed to continue therapy, with rates of failure particularly high among African American patients.*)

27. Glynn RJ, Ridker PM, Goldhaber SZ, et al. Effect of low-dose aspirin on the occurrence of venous thromboembolism. Ann Intern Med 2007;147:525. (*Secondary analysis of RCT; no benefit was noted.*)

28. Gould MK, Dembitzer AD, Sanders GD, et al. Low-molecular-weight heparins compared with unfractionated heparin for treatment of acute deep venous thrombosis: a cost-effectiveness analysis. Ann Intern Med 1999;130:789. (*A decision-model study, finding low–molecular weight heparin to be highly cost-effective when used in inpatient care and to provide a cost saving when even a few patients can be treated on an outpatient basis.*)

29. Hull RD, Pineo GF, Brant RF, et al. Self-managed long-term low-molecular-weight heparin therapy: the balance of benefits and harms. Am J Med 2007;120:72. (*RCT; Effective and less risk of bleeding.*)

30. Hull RD, Pineo GF, Stein PF, et al. Extended out-of-hospital low-molecular weight heparin prophylaxis against deep venous thrombosis in patients after elective hip arthroplast: a systematic review. Ann Intern Med 2001;135:858. (*Concludes that the evidence supports extended out-of-hospital prophylaxis.*)

31. Hull RD, Raskob GE, Pineo GF, et al. Subcutaneous low-molecular-weight heparin compared with continuous intravenous heparin in the treatment of proximal vein thrombosis. N Engl J Med 1992;326:975. (*One of the original reports demonstrating safety and efficacy.*)

32. Kearon C, Fent M, Hirsh J, et al. A comparison of three months of anticoagulation with extended anticoagulation for a first episode of idiopathic venous thromboembolism. N Engl J Med 1999;340:901. (*RCT, finding a 95% reduction in the rate of recurrent DVT with prolonged anticoagulation and only a 3% per patient-year risk of major bleeding.*)

33. Kearon C, Ginsberg JS, Kovacs MJ, et al. Comparison of low-intensity warfarin therapy with conventional-intensity warfarin therapy for long-term prevention of recurrent venous thromboembolism. N Engl J Med 2003;349:631. (*A major randomized, multicenter trial, Evaluation of Losartan in the Elderly [ELITE]; unexpectedly found that conventional therapy was more effective and no less safe than low-intensity therapy.*)

34. Khamashta MA, Cuadrado MJ, Mujic F, et al. The management of thrombosis in the antiphospholipid-antibody syndrome. N Engl J Med 1995;332:993.

(*Long-term oral anticoagulation at an International Normalized Ratio of >3 proved to be most effective in this retrospective analysis.*)

35. Lee AYY, Levine MN, Baker RI, et al. Low-molecular-weight heparin versus a coumarin for the prevention of recurrent venous thrombolytic therapy in venous thrombosis. Arch Intern Med 1992;152:1265. (*A review concluding that although lytic therapy may have potential, its use is often limited by concomitant clinical contraindications.*)

36. Lurie F, Creton D, Eklof B, et al. Prospective, randomized of endovenous radiofrequency (Closure Procedure) versus ligation and stripping in a selected patient population (EVOLVeS Study). J Vasc Surg 2003; 38:207. (*A study that demonstrated the safety and efficacy of endothermal ablation with faster recovery and better cosmetic results compared with stripping.*)

37. Markel A, Manzo RA, Strandness DE. The potential role of thrombolytic therapy in venous thrombosis. Arch Intern Med 1992;152:1265. (*A review concluding that lytic therapy may have potential, with its use often limited by concomitant clinical contraindications.*)

38. Prandoni P, Lensing AWA, Prins MH, et al. Below-knee elastic compression stockings to prevent the post-phlebitic syndrome: a randomized controlled trial. Ann Intern Med 2004;141:249. (*This approach was found to be as effective as the use of customized stockings in preventing development of the syndrome; it reduced the risk of sequelae by nearly 50%.*)

39. Ray JG, Kearon C, Yi Q, et al. Homocysteine-lowering therapy and risk for venous thromboembolism: a randomized trial. Ann Intern Med 2007;146:761. (*No benefit was found.*)

40. Ridker PM, Goldhaber SZ, Danielson E, et al., for the PREVENT Investigators. Long-term, low intensity warfarin therapy for the prevention of recurrent venous thromboembolism. N Engl J Med 2003;348:1425. (*The landmark Prevention of Recurrent Venous Thromboembolism [PREVENT] trial, a placebo-controlled study in persons with idiopathic DVT, showing a significant reduction in the risk of recurrence; there was an 80% reduction in risk.*)

41. Rogers LQ, Lutcher CL. Streptokinase therapy for deep vein thrombosis: a comprehensive review of the English literature. Am J Med 1990;88:389. (*Concludes that streptokinase can be of value in properly selected patients, namely those with proximal DVT treated within 7 days of the onset of symptoms; 76 references.*)

42. Schulman S, Ganqvist S, Holmstrom M, et al. The duration of oral anticoagulant therapy after a second episode of venous thromboembolism. N Engl J Med 1997;336:393. (*The risk of recurrence was high and was markedly reduced by chronic anticoagulation in this prospective, randomized trial; a slight increase in the risk of major bleeding was noted.*)

43. Snow V, Qaseem A, Barry P, et al. Management of venous thromboembolism: a clinical practice guideline from the American College of Physicians and the American Academy of Family Physicians. Ann Intern Med 2007;146:204. (*Evidence-based recommendations on the treatment of venous thrombosis and embolism.*)

44. The Columbus Investigators. Low-molecular-weight heparin in the treatment of patients with venous thromboembolism. N Engl J Med 1997;337:657. (*A randomized, prospective study comparing low–molecular weight heparin with conventional heparin therapy; safety and efficacy were similar for both approaches to heparinization.*)

45. The van Gogh Investigators. Extended prophylaxis of venous thromboembolism with idraparinux. N Engl J Med 2007;357:1105. (*RCT; this approach was found to be as effective as standard therapy but had a higher risk of major hemorrhage.*)

46. The van Gogh Investigators. Idraparinux versus standard therapy for venous thromboembolic disease. N Engl J Med 2007;357:1094. (*RCT of this new long-acting factor X inhibitor; the results were comparable to standard therapy in persons with DVT but not in those with pulmonary embolism.*)

47. Vin F, Benigni JP. Compression therapy. International Consensus Document Guidelines according to scientific evidence. Int Angiol 2004; 23:317. (*A consensus statement supporting the value of compression.*)

CHAPTER 36 ■ STRESS TESTING AND OTHER NONINVASIVE STUDIES FOR DETECTION OF CORONARY DISEASE

The importance of diagnosing coronary heart disease (CHD) is underscored by its prevalence and serious consequences, as well as the availability of therapies that can improve quality of life and prolong survival. Exercise stress testing plays a central role in the evaluation of suspected and known CHD, providing a noninvasive means of detecting ischemia and helping to determine prognosis. Electrocardiographic (ECG), radionuclide, and echocardiographic approaches present the clinician with an array of study options, which include pharmacologic stressing for patients who cannot exercise. New imaging techniques (magnetic resonance imaging [MRI] angiography and computed tomography [CT]) further expand the choices for testing.

The variety of options and array of testing findings can be daunting. The design of an effective workup for CHD and proper test interpretation benefit from making a clinical estimate of the pretest probability for CHD (see Chapter 20) and paying attention to the performance characteristics, costs, advantages, and disadvantages of available testing modalities.

STRESS TESTING (1–37)

Physiologic Basis of the Test

Stress testing assesses the ability of the coronary circulation to meet the enhanced myocardial oxygen requirements of exercise- or drug-induced stress. Because the rate of oxygen extraction by the heart is relatively fixed, increased oxygen demand must be met by an increase in coronary blood flow. When coronary artery stenosis critically limits the blood supply, oxygen demand may so exceed supply that myocardial ischemia ensues, manifested by transient changes in ECG ST segments, ventricular wall motion, and radionuclide distribution. In addition, the patient may experience abnormal blood pressure and heart rate responses, angina, or an anginal equivalent such as severe dyspnea.

The demand placed on the coronary circulation can be quantified: The product of heart rate times systolic blood pressure closely parallels the measured myocardial oxygen consumption during isotonic exercise and is designated in *metabolic equivalents* (METS), where 1 MET = 3.5 mL of O_2 consumed/kg/min. Heart rate alone provides a good approximation of oxygen consumption. Because known quantities of work are being performed, the exercise stress test can also provide a measure of exercise capacity and aid in the detection, quantification, and localization of coronary disease.

Approaches to Stress Testing

The stress test may use exercise or pharmacologic measures to challenge the capacity of the coronary circulation. Exercise remains the simplest means, usually achieved by treadmill or stationary bicycle activity. Pharmacologic approaches stress the coronary circulation by inducing either reflex tachycardia or intracardiac vasodilation.

Exercise-Based Testing

Exercise testing for the detection of coronary disease uses dynamic (isotonic) rather than sustained-contraction (isometric) exercise. Isotonic exercise permits smooth increases in the rate–pressure product to be accomplished, allowing the patient's ischemic threshold to be approached gradually. Nevertheless, isometric exercise testing (e.g., by sustained handgrip) can be of use in special situations (e.g., assessing the safety of isometric activities in patients with known coronary disease).

Many different exercise protocols are available for the treadmill and the bicycle. Although the staged *Bruce protocol* is very popular and widely used, it has the disadvantages of unequal changes in work load between stages and a very abrupt increase in work load at stage IV, which is too vigorous for many cardiac patients. Walking protocols are generally preferred over protocols that require running for diagnostic purposes in unfit populations. *Bicycle ergometer protocols* usually consist of 2- to 3-minute stages in which workload is increased by 10 to 30 W per stage, depending on the level of physical conditioning of the subject. For both treadmill and bicycle tests, it is best to select a protocol that will allow the patient to reach maximal exertion within a 10- to 12-minute period. A longer test may be limited by the subject's endurance, and a shorter test usually increases the workload too rapidly.

The *testing protocols* for isotonic exercise testing are divided into *maximal* and *submaximal* types, depending on the level of exercise achieved during the test. *Testing methods* include ECG monitoring, echocardiographic imaging, and radionuclide imaging.

The Maximal Test. Maximal testing is defined as testing in which systemic oxygen consumption reaches a plateau before exercise is terminated. Maximal effort is usually approximated by exercising the individual to an age-adjusted predicted maximal heart rate. Values for maximal predicted heart rate can be obtained from standardized tables or regression formulas, but the values *220 minus age in years for men* and *210 minus age in years for women* provide reasonable approximations of the true maximal heart rate. Tests terminated before the maximum predicted heart rate has been achieved are less sensitive for diagnosis of CHD. In general, it is best to continue the test to the predicted maximum heart rate or to the maximum perceived effort or until angina, ischemia, arrhythmia, or hypotension occurs. If a patient is receiving a β-adrenergic blocking agent, the endpoint of heart rate is supplanted by having the patient exercise to exhaustion. If the perceived effort is "very hard" (19 or 20 on the Borg scale) at the termination of the test, it can be reasonably assumed that maximal exertion has been closely approximated.

The Submaximal Test. By definition, a submaximal test is one in which maximal systemic oxygen consumption is not achieved. The test may be terminated prematurely by design (at a certain percentage of predicted maximal heart rate or at a given level of systemic oxygen consumption), or it may be terminated because of the appearance of angina, marked ischemic ECG changes, cardiac arrhythmias, severe hypertension, or hypotension. Submaximal testing has been shown to be useful and safe for the early determination of prognosis soon *after myocardial infarction*. When conducted within 2 weeks of infarction, a submaximal exercise test to a 5-MET level identifies patients at increased risk for subsequent coronary events and death. Many cardiologists prefer to perform a symptom-limited exercise test 1 month after myocardial infarction in lieu of an earlier submaximal test.

Staged (Graded) Testing. Most exercise tests are *staged*, meaning that graded amounts of work are performed in a progressively increasing manner. The rationale for graded exercise is to obtain the greatest increase in heart rate before musculoskeletal fatigue limits the amount of exercise that the patient can perform. The onset of muscle fatigue before the achievement of maximum heart rate reduces test sensitivity. The *treadmill* and *bicycle ergometer* are the most popular devices for exercise testing. Slightly higher values for maximal oxygen consumption can usually be obtained on the treadmill than on the bicycle ergometer because a somewhat larger muscle mass is called on during treadmill exercise.

Electrocardiographic Monitoring. Continuous *ECG monitoring* is used during exercise testing, as is periodic determination of blood pressure and symptoms. Multilead systems have replaced the traditional single modified V5 ECG lead (CM5). Sensitivity is greatly enhanced by the use of multiple leads, especially for the detection of inferior ischemia. Twelve-lead monitoring is commonly performed multiple times during the test, and three to six leads are monitored continuously; adding another three leads over the right precordium appears to enhance the detection of ischemia due to right coronary or left circumflex disease (see later discussion). The ST segments are assessed for change with exercise. The depth, configuration, and extent of any ST-segment depressions correlate with the presence and severity of coronary disease (see later discussion and Fig. 36.1), as do blood pressure responses and time to development of symptoms. Because ischemic changes may not occur on the ECG until after exercise, monitoring is continued for at least 5 to 7 minutes into the recovery phase.

Radionuclide Imaging. Radioisotopes can be administered as part of exercise testing to help image myocardial perfusion. *Technetium sestamibi* and *thallium-201* are the two radionuclides in most widespread use. Their regional distribution in the myocardium is proportional to regional coronary blood flow; underperfused areas will take up less of the isotope and will appear as "cold" spots on the perfusion scan. Areas of viable but ischemic myocardium will appear underperfused during exercise but will "fill in" at rest. Therefore, sequential scanning during exercise and at rest is required to diagnose hemodynamically significant coronary stenoses and distinguish them from areas of previous infarction.

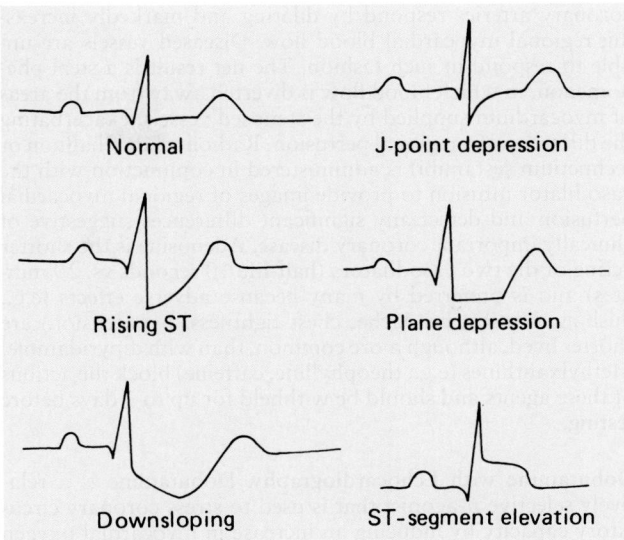

FIGURE 36.1. Exercise-induced ST-segment changes.

Sestamibi testing requires a 2-day protocol, with a 1-hour resting scan on day 1 and a 2-hour exercise and imaging session on day 2. Thallium study is done all in 1 day but requires 2 hours for exercise imaging and a 3-hour wait before a 1-hour imaging session at rest. Sestamibi administration allows for the determination of *ejection fraction*. Thallium provides images of pulmonary uptake, which parallel pulmonary capillary wedge pressure and correlate with prognosis. *Single-photon emission computed tomography* (SPECT) is replacing *planar scanning* technology for image production because it provides better sensitivity.

Echocardiographic Imaging. Stress echocardiographic study provides information on global ventricular function in response to exercise (by measuring the change in ejection fraction and end-systolic volume) and on segmental myocardial perfusion (by comparing regional ventricular wall motion at rest and during or just after maximal exercise). Ischemic manifestations include failure to increase ejection fraction with exercise and new regional wall-motion abnormalities. Compared with radionuclide testing, less time is required, there is no radiation exposure, and cost is lower; in addition, results are immediately available. Test sensitivity for ischemia is reduced by the presence of resting wall-motion abnormalities.

Pharmacologic Stress Testing

Patients who cannot exercise are potential candidates for pharmacologic approaches to testing the adequacy of the coronary circulation, whether by inducing reflex tachycardia or coronary vasodilation. Because the sensitivity of ST-segment changes associated with pharmacologic stress testing is low, cardiac imaging (either radionuclide or echocardiographic) is required. Although probably not as sensitive as exercise tress testing that achieves maximum predicted heart rate, pharmacologic stress testing does provide results that correlate with and help to predict long-term cardiac outcomes.

Adenosine or Dipyridamole with Radionuclide Scanning. These agents rapidly induce coronary vasodilation when given by intravenous infusion, usually over 4 to 6 minutes. Normal coronary arteries respond by dilating and markedly increasing regional myocardial blood flow. Diseased vessels are unable to respond in such fashion. The net result is a steal phenomenon, in which blood flow is diverted away from the areas of myocardium supplied by the stenosed vessels, exacerbating the differences in regional perfusion. Radionuclide (thallium or technetium sestamibi) is administered in conjunction with the vasodilator infusion to provide images of regional myocardial perfusion and detect any significant differences suggestive of clinically important coronary disease. Adenosine is the shorter acting of the two vasodilators (half-life 10 seconds vs. 20 minutes) and is preferred by many because adverse effects (e.g., flushing, nausea, headache, chest tightness, hypotension) are shorter lived, although more common, than with dipyridamole. Methylxanthines (e.g., theophylline, caffeine) block the actions of these agents and should be withheld for up to 3 days before testing.

Dobutamine with Echocardiography. Dobutamine is a relatively selective β-agonist that is used to stress coronary circulatory capacity by inducing an increase in myocardial oxygen demand through simulative effects on heart rate and myocardial contractility. Underperfused areas show up on ultrasound as thickened hypokinetic myocardium. Sometimes, the muscarinic blocking agent atropine is infused in addition to dobutamine if at least 85% of the maximum predicted heart rate is not achieved by dobutamine alone. Side effects of dobutamine include chest pain, palpitations, dysrhythmias, and blood pressure changes. They usually resolve quickly with cessation of the infusion. Test safety is similar to that for exercise.

Dipyridamole with Positron Emission Tomography. Positron emission tomography (PET) involves the administration of the vasodilator dipyridamole along with rubidium-82. The isotope's myocardial uptake is measured by PET, providing a very sensitive and specific, albeit expensive, means of imaging ischemia.

Stress Testing for Diagnosis of Coronary Heart Disease: Test Sensitivity, Specificity, and Predictive Value (1,7–18)

Gold Standard, Workup Bias, and Test Limitations

The gold standard for the diagnosis of CHD remains the *coronary angiogram*. A significant stenosis is defined as an angiographic narrowing of the vessel lumen by 50% or greater. Stress-test performance characteristics (sensitivity and specificity) are determined by comparing test results against angiographic findings. However, the figures cited in the literature for sensitivity and specificity may be subject to *workup bias* from the preferential enrollment of study patients likely to have coronary disease and therefore willing to undergo angiography. The consequence of such bias is an exaggeration of test sensitivity and an underestimation of test specificity. Workup bias always needs to be considered when interpreting published studies of sensitivity and specificity (see Chapter 2).

Another limitation of stress testing is that it does not identify lesions that may become the cause of sudden death; it only detects impaired blood flow. Most patients who die suddenly from coronary disease do not succumb from a chronic flow-limiting atherosclerotic plaque. Rather, they may die from the acute rupturing and thrombosis of a nonoccluding plaque. Exercise testing does not help to identify such non–flow-limiting

lesions, although it can provide an estimate of prognosis by determining the extent and severity of disease, which correlate with overall risk (see later discussion). Direct identification of dangerous plaques is an area of active investigation.

Importance of Pretest Probability in Patient Selection and Predictive Value

With an emphasis in the stress-test literature on test performance characteristics (i.e., sensitivity and specificity), it is easy to confuse them with predictive value (the probability of CHD, given a "positive" stress test). The latter is the relevant probability for the clinician caring for the patient with suspected coronary disease and necessitates considering not only test sensitivity and specificity, but also the patient's pretest probability for CHD. Figures for the predictive accuracy of the exercise stress test have varied greatly from series to series and between men and women, often because of wide differences in the prevalence of underlying coronary disease in the populations studied. The predictive accuracy of any diagnostic test is directly related to the *prevalence* of the disease in the population examined (see Chapter 2).

A stress test will have a low predictive accuracy when disease prevalence is low, regardless of how sensitive and specific the test is. Proper test interpretation necessitates knowing not only the sensitivity and specificity of the test, but also the patient's pretest likelihood of CHD. A positive test in a person with a low pretest probability is far more likely to be a false positive than a true positive. Careful estimation of the patient's pretest probability of CHD (see Chapter 20) is essential to proper stress-test interpretation. The prevalence of coronary disease has been found to be 16% in patients with nonanginal chest pain, 50% in those with atypical pain, and 89% when typical angina is present.

High Pretest Probability. The predictive value of a positive stress test for the diagnosis of CHD is mathematically greatest in patients with *typical angina* and *multiple coronary risk factors*; however, in such instances the history of classic angina (pretest probability for CHD about 90%) is about as good for diagnosis as the test's predictive value (about 90%). Thus, performing a stress test adds little to diagnosis beyond what is already known from the history. In such patients, the value of stress testing is confined to estimating prognosis and assessing the need for revascularization (see later discussion and Chapter 30).

Intermediate Pretest Probability. Stress testing may be of considerable diagnostic help in patients with *atypical chest pain*, as long as the criteria for atypical pain are rather rigid—for example, at least two characteristics of classic angina (see Chapter 20) must be present along with a risk factor or two. In this context, a positive exercise test would substantially increase the posttest likelihood of underlying coronary disease, and a negative test would substantially reduce it. In general, exercise testing makes its greatest diagnostic contribution for patients whose pretest likelihood of having coronary disease is intermediate.

Low Pretest Probability. In the setting of *noncardiac chest pain* and *no risk factors*, the stress test is not likely to perform well. Although a negative test can be very reassuring to the patient, the specificity of stress testing is not high enough to eliminate the risk of a false-positive result. The ratio of false positives to true positives in the setting of a low pretest probability is likely to be high, making it necessary to warn the patient that a positive test result in this setting is not tantamount to a diagnosis of coronary disease. In trying to reassure a nervous patient who does not have coronary disease by performing a stress test, one might actually make matters worse. Careful thought and patient preparation are needed before going ahead with stress testing in such patients. The same considerations and a high risk of false positives also limit the usefulness of stress testing as a screening procedure for the detection of CHD in *asymptomatic patients*.

Electrocardiographic Testing

Although not very sensitive for the detection of single-vessel coronary disease (sensitivity is 35% to 61%), the standard ECG study approaches other forms of stress testing for the detection of more serious anatomy such as left-main or three-vessel disease (sensitivity is 75% to 93%; see later discussion). Overall, the mean sensitivity for detection of coronary disease is about 68%, and specificity is 77%. When adjusted for workup bias, the figures are 45% and 85%, respectively. The wide ranges cited for ECG sensitivity and specificity have to do with differences in diagnostic criteria and approaches to testing and monitoring.

Diagnostic Criteria and Other Factors Affecting Test Sensitivity and Specificity. A major factor affecting sensitivity and specificity is the magnitude of *ST-segment depression* used as a diagnostic criterion for ischemia. Lowering the ST-segment criterion from at least 2.0 mm of ST depression to 1.0 mm increases sensitivity by nearly threefold but reduces specificity by 10 percentage points. The *configuration of the ST segment* (Fig. 36.1) is also important to specificity. A downsloping ST-segment criterion produces a specificity of 99%; horizontal or plane depression is associated with a specificity of 85%; and a slowly upsloping ST segment (at least 1.5-mm ST depression at 0.08 second after the J point) produces a specificity of 68%. Taking into account not only *ST-segment* changes but also any abnormal *blood pressure* or *heart rate* responses and any *angina* or severe *dyspnea* can raise the relative sensitivity by more than 20%. The occurrence of typical angina during exercise confers, by itself, a sensitivity of 51% and a specificity of 90%, about the same diagnostic significance as ST-segment changes.

The *type of exercise protocol* and the *number and location of ECG leads* affect sensitivity. Submaximal protocols are much less sensitive than maximal ones. A 12-lead study is more sensitive than one using fewer leads. The addition of 3 right-precordial leads to a standard 12-lead study markedly improves test sensitivity for single-vessel disease, particularly that involving either the right coronary artery or the left circumflex. With such multilead testing, sensitivity and specificity approach those of radionuclide scanning.

False Positives. The specificity of ST-segment changes is limited by the fact that ST-segment depression is not unique to coronary disease. Patients with *valvular* or *hypertensive* disease, nonischemic myocardial disease, and *preexcitation* syndromes may demonstrate ST-segment depression during exercise in the absence of ischemia. In addition, left ventricular *hypertrophy*, recent *glucose* ingestion, *hypokalemia*, and *sedatives* may produce false-positive results. *Digitalis* glycosides are notorious for their ability to cause deviations in ST segments. If possible, it is best to discontinue digitalis for at least 48 hours before testing. If this is not feasible, then exercise-associated ischemia should not be diagnosed until at least 2 minutes of ST-segment depression is observed. Studies have also suggested that false-positive

responses may be more common in middle-aged women than in men by a factor as high as three, but this may be more a reflection of the low pretest probability of CHD in this population than of a problem with the test. Simple *J-point depression* with a rapidly upsloping ST segment is a nonspecific finding and is not diagnostic of ischemia.

Asymptomatic patients with few or *no CHD risk factors* who are subjected to exercise testing and demonstrate "ischemic" changes are, as noted earlier, less likely to have underlying coronary disease and more likely to have a false-positive test. Therefore, asymptomatic patients with an abnormal stress test should be screened carefully for possible causes of a false-positive response. In asymptomatic populations, abnormal ST-segment responses should be viewed as a "risk factor" for coronary disease rather than as definite evidence of the disease. In these individuals, the incidence of coronary disease is modest (about 6%) but doubles by the sixth decade.

Radionuclide Scanning

Stress-test sensitivity is enhanced by radionuclide scanning. With the use of planar scanning, overall test sensitivity for the detection of coronary disease rises from 68% for ECG to 79% when planar scanning is used and to 88% with SPECT. Specificity is about the same as for ECG testing. Sensitivity for three-vessel and left-main disease rises from 86% for ECG to 93% and 98% for planar scanning and SPECT, respectively. Use of radionuclide scanning has been proved to be especially valuable in patients who have resting repolarization abnormalities on the ECG or left-bundle-branch block, both of which render interpretation of the standard exercise test difficult. Scanning is also useful in patients whose ECG stress-test results are suspected to be false positive or false negative. Test performance characteristics are about the same for exercise and pharmacologic methods of radionuclide stress testing. Test sensitivity is reduced by image attenuation due to obesity or large breasts.

Echocardiography

Echocardiographic assessment has a reported mean sensitivity of 76% for the detection of coronary disease and a specificity of 88% (Table 36.1). Mean sensitivity for three-vessel or left-main disease is 94%. Results are similar for exercise and dobutamine-stimulated testing, provided that the same increase in heart rate is achieved. Reported figures are from centers where there is major expertise in the performance of the study. Test performance is very operator dependent, and local results may be quite different from those reported in the literature if the operator is inexperienced. Obesity and emphysema may impair the performance of the test.

Positron Emission Tomography

Test sensitivity and specificity in research settings often exceed 95%, but when the test is applied in community settings, test performance drops into the 85% range.

Stress Testing for Assessment of Prognosis (1)

Stress testing represents a useful noninvasive means of screening for predictors of poor CHD prognosis, including left-main, three-vessel, and left-main-equivalent disease and left ventricular dysfunction. Treadmill exercise score and heart rate recovery are in themselves independent predictors of mortality. The assessment of prognosis of patients in the early postinfarction period also may be aided by exercise testing. In asymptomatic

TABLE 36.1

SENSITIVITY, SPECIFICITY, AND COSTS OF STRESS TESTS FOR THE DETECTION OF CORONARY DISEASE

Test Type	Sensitivity	Specificity	Sensitivity for Three-Vessel/Left-Main Disease	Relative Cost
Electrocardiographic	0.68	0.77	0.86	1.0
Echocardiographic	0.76	0.88	0.94	2.5
Thallium imaging, planar only	0.79	0.73	0.93	2.0
SPECT	0.88	0.77	0.98	4.0
PET[a]	0.91	0.82	?	14.0

PET, positron emission tomography; SPECT, single-photon emission computed tomography.
[a]Sensitivity and specificity as reported from non–research center settings.
Adapted from Garber AM, Solomon NA. Cost-effectiveness of alternative test strategies for the diagnosis of coronary artery disease. Ann Intern Med 1999;130:719, with permission.

women, heart rate recovery and exercise capacity have predictive value for long-term cardiovascular and all-cause mortality. In men, exercise capacity is a powerful predictor of mortality, equaling or exceeding other established risk factors. The use of exercise testing in the elderly for the determination of cardiovascular prognosis has been questioned because of a lack of correlation between ST-segment changes and cardiac outcomes; however, incremental prognostic information over that afforded by clinical data is provided by peak workload achieved.

Electrocardiographic Stress Test

Whereas ECG stress testing is relatively insensitive for the detection of single-vessel disease, it compares rather favorably with radionuclide and echocardiographic studies for the detection of high-risk anatomy (mean sensitivities 86%, 93% to 98%, and 94% respectively; Table 36.1) and poor prognosis. Stress-test findings indicative of worrisome disease include marked ST-segment depression, multilead ST-segment depression, early onset of ST changes, persistence of ST-segment depression past 8 minutes into the recovery period, downward-sloping ST configuration, hypotensive response at low workloads, impairment of heart rate response to exercise, and development of angina. The occurrence of both angina and ischemic changes during exercise predicts an increased likelihood of multivessel disease and poor prognosis; the same holds true for attenuated heart rate recovery after exercise. In the elderly, the principal determinant of prognosis on exercise testing is peak workload; other stress-test parameters offer little predictive value.

The Duke Exercise Treadmill Score. This widely used and well-validated prognostic formula incorporates easily measured stress-test parameters identified by multivariate analysis as independently predictive of CHD prognosis. It is calculated as follows: exercise time minus (five times the ST deviation in millimeters) minus (four times the treadmill angina index), where exercise time is in minutes of the Bruce treadmill protocol, ST deviation is the largest ST displacement in millimeters in any lead, and angina index is scored 0 for no angina, 1 for typical angina during the test, and 2 for angina that halts the test. A score of −11 or less indicates "high risk" (5-year mortality >25%), whereas a score of +5 or more predicts "low risk" (5-year mortality <6%). Patients at high and moderate to high risk require consideration of coronary angiography for

the identification of high-risk coronary disease and the determination of candidacy for bypass surgery (see Chapter 30). Even in the presence of resting ST-segment abnormalities, the ECG stress test retains its ability to risk-stratify patients with CHD by means of the Duke treadmill score.

Attenuated Heart Rate Recovery and Peak Exercise Capacity. Like the Duke treadmill exercise score, the attenuation of heart rate recovery after exercise is an independent predictor of mortality. Its presence adds to the predictive value of the Duke score, nearly doubling the hazard ratio. The peak exercise capacity as measured in METs is among the most powerful predictors of mortality among both normal individuals and those with coronary disease.

Stress-Related Ventricular Ectopy. Frequent ventricular ectopy in the recovery phase after stress testing modestly increases the predicted risk of death (hazard ratio, 1.5), but frequent ventricular ectopy during exercise does not.

Composite Predictive Model. An externally validated model adds other independent predictors of cardiovascular risk to the Duke score (i.e., heart rate recovery, stress-related ventricular ectopy in recovery, smoking, diabetes, hypertension, angina, age, and gender) to enhance and refine the prediction of cardiovascular risk. In initial validation study, it proved equally predictive as the Duke score, but reclassified some patients initially labeled as intermediate to high risk by the Duke score to the low-risk category. Further validation is necessary to see if the composite model warrants generalized use.

Submaximal Testing. Submaximal ECG stress testing is very helpful prognostically in the *postinfarction period*. The greater the workload tolerated, the better is the prognosis. Patients who develop angina on a limited exercise test conducted just before hospital discharge have twice the rate of postinfarction angina. Those with no ST-segment changes have a very low 1-year mortality (about 2%), compared with a 25% mortality for those who develop ST-segment depression during exercise testing.

Radionuclide Scanning

Unlike ECG testing, thallium and technetium images identify the location and extent of underperfused myocardium (sometimes referred to as the *amount of myocardium at risk*).

Diffuse ischemia suggests high-risk coronary disease (three-vessel or left-main stenosis) and the need to consider coronary revascularization (see Chapter 30). *Pulmonary uptake* of thallium is a sign of left ventricular dysfunction, another independent indicator of poor prognosis. First-pass resting sestamibi images provide an estimate of ejection fraction and aid in the assessment of left ventricular function.

Echocardiography

Stress echocardiography supplies information on the extent and the location of ischemia by its 16-segment analysis of left ventricular wall motion. The greater the number of segments manifesting wall-motion abnormalities, the greater is the probability of multivessel or left-main disease. Resting wall-motion abnormalities reduce predictive accuracy. Echocardiography provides an accurate estimate of left ventricular ejection fraction, an important prognostic determinant. In persons with left-bundle-branch block, pharmacologic stress echocardiography can provide strong prognostic information.

Other Roles for Stress Testing (1,31–33)

Determination of Exercise Capacity and Ensuring Safety of an Exercise Program

The patient is made to perform known quantities of work under direct observation and continuous ECG monitoring. This determination is essential for designing a safe cardiac rehabilitation program and may help to reassure the patient who is unnecessarily restricting activity out of fear of sudden death or infarction. The work level achieved during the test can be used to define the degree of incapacity (when it is in question) and provide guidelines for establishing safe levels of daily activity for the patient.

The use of stress testing before engaging in an exercise program is of established value to (a) sedentary persons with known or suspected cardiovascular disease who wish to engage in exercise programs of *moderate intensity* and (b) persons younger than the age of 40 years who plan on an exercise program of *vigorous intensity*. In the very elderly (age >75 years), the applicability of stress testing as a prerequisite for an exercise program has been called into question because the degree of exercise is likely to be very modest; monitoring blood pressure and other parameters may suffice, and the requirement for stress testing can be off-putting and discourage participation in even a very modest program.

Detection of Dysrhythmias

The assessment of atrial and ventricular rhythm disturbances can sometimes be facilitated by exercise testing, especially if the dysrhythmia is believed to be exercise induced. As noted, the development of ventricular ectopy in the recovery phase is predictive of increased mortality. If the objective is maximizing sensitivity for the detection of dysrhythmias, ambulatory monitoring should also be obtained and electrophysiologic study considered (see Chapters 25, 28, and 29).

Screening for Coronary Artery Disease

Use of the exercise treadmill test (ETT) has been proposed as a means of screening for CHD in asymptomatic persons. Although there is generalized agreement that the test is not useful in persons with a very low or very high estimate of pretest probability (see Appendix 26.1), there is debate regarding the use-

fulness of stress testing in persons at intermediate risk. Yields for the detection of significant silent coronary disease (>50% stenosis) range from 0.06% to 1.6% in asymptomatic populations at low to moderate risk and rise to only 9% in those at high risk (e.g., older men with multiple risk factors, diabetics). Although the prognostic value of an abnormal ETT (defined as ST-segment depression) can be expressed as a two- to five-fold increase in relative risk (which prompts some to recommend the test), the positive predictive value (true positives/total positives) remains inadequate in both men and women (range 2.2% to 46%). Similar findings are noted when other exercise test variables, such as frequent ventricular ectopy postexercise, are used (e.g., relative risk, 1.5; positive predictive value, 12%). After reviewing the literature, the U.S. Preventive Services Task Force concluded that evidence was lacking for a clear benefit from the use of ETT for CHD screening in asymptomatic persons and that the harms of false-positive tests (with subsequent catheterizations) outweighed any potential benefits.

Localization of Disease

By ECG. Although ECG stress testing can help to determine prognosis and guide the need for angiography, the study does not localize the site of ischemia. Most patients with a positive ECG stress test have ST-segment changes in the anteroapical leads irrespective of the location of their ischemia. More-diffuse involvement only indicates an increased probability of high-risk coronary anatomy. Coronary angiography is required when considering revascularization.

By Imaging Studies. In providing data on the localization of ischemia, imaging studies (echocardiographic and radionuclide) have the distinct advantage over ECG testing. Echocardiography also provides an additional physiologic look at myocardial function by being able to demonstrate wall-motion abnormalities at rest and with exercise.

Monitoring Persons Who Have Undergone Revascularization

There is no evidence that asymptomatic persons who have undergone revascularization benefit from routine follow-up stress testing. Those who develop angina after revascularization definitely require study, but persons who remain free of symptoms have an excellent prognosis and do not.

Safety and Contraindications

The reported mortality in a multicenter study involving 170,000 exercise tests was 0.01%. There was no relationship to the type of test or to exercise intensity. Morbidity requiring hospitalization was 0.2%. Safety is enhanced by a preexamination history, a physical examination, and a resting ECG. Patients with unstable angina, uncompensated congestive failure, severe anemia, high-grade heart block, severe aortic stenosis, cor pulmonale, or severe hypertension should not undergo testing. A physician should be present throughout, and a defibrillator and other resuscitation equipment should be in the room. The test should be terminated if blood pressure or heart rate falls suddenly during exercise or if exhaustion, angina, faintness, marked ST changes, severe hypertension, or serious arrhythmias (ventricular tachycardia, heart block, etc.) occur. When performed by experienced personnel, exercise testing is very safe and is one of the most useful noninvasive tests for evaluating cardiovascular function and disease.

The safety of pharmacologically induced stress testing is similar to that for exercise-induced studies. Contraindications to adenosine or dipyridamole stress testing include severe chronic obstructive pulmonary disease, asthma, and significant carotid or aortic stenosis. Contraindications to dobutamine stress testing include cardiac dysrhythmias and uncontrolled hypertension.

Stress Test Selection

The *ECG stress test* remains a very cost-effective diagnostic option for the patient with a normal resting ECG. Although the standard test is rather insensitive for the identification of single-vessel disease, its sensitivity for high-risk coronary disease and correlation with prognosis are very high, approaching those of the much more expensive radionuclide studies (Table 36.1). Moreover, the use of right-precordial leads holds promise for enhancing sensitivity for single-vessel disease. Even in the setting of nonspecific resting ECG abnormalities, the ECG stress test retains its prognostic utility when using the Duke treadmill score.

Echocardiographic stress testing represents another cost-effective option for CHD diagnosis. Sensitivity and specificity when performed by expert operators are similar to those for radionuclide scanning, and like the more expensive scans, information is provided on left ventricular function and regional perfusion.

Radionuclide scanning is very sensitive and specific for the diagnosis of coronary disease and extremely useful when resting ECG abnormalities preclude ECG stress testing for the identification of CHD. However, isotopic imaging is many times more expensive than ECG testing and only marginally better for the detection of high-risk disease and the determination of prognosis (Table 36.1). These factors limit its cost-effectiveness.

For patients who are unable to exercise, the infusion of a vasodilator (*adenosine* or *dipyridamole*) in conjunction with radionuclide scanning is a reasonable option; dobutamine echocardiography is another. PET cannot be recommending at this time because its cost is extremely high and test performance in the community setting is no better than that of radionuclide imaging.

NEW MODALITIES FOR NONINVASIVE DETECTION OF CORONARY HEART DISEASE (38–43)

A number of new imaging modalities have been developed in the hope of improving the noninvasive detection of coronary disease. As commercial ventures, some are being promoted rather prematurely directly to patients, but these technologies hold considerable promise and are the subject of serious study in major centers.

Computed Tomography of the Coronary Arteries

Two computed tomography (CT) approaches to noninvasive testing for coronary disease have been developed.

Electron Beam Computed Tomography

This technology provides the ability to detect and quantify coronary artery lesions without intravenous dye administration. It detects coronary vessel wall calcification, a sign of atherosclerotic change. Investigators of the technology have devised a *coronary artery calcium score* (CACS), which they find correlates with the degree of atherosclerosis, and have used it in conjunction with a clinical estimate of pretest probability (the *Framingham risk score* [FRS]; see Appendix 26.1) to determine the risk of coronary disease in asymptomatic persons. The CACS was found to enhance CHD risk prediction over the clinical risk assessment, but only in persons judged at intermediate risk by the FRS (i.e., FRS between 10 and 20). The net result was a 3% to 9% increase in predicted 10-year CHD risk. Unfortunately, the CT cannot rule out the presence of coronary disease; its false-negative rate is about 4% due to the presence of "soft" atherosclerotic plaque, which is not detectable by CT. Such soft plaque is less stable than calcified plaque and more likely to rupture and cause acute coronary thrombosis.

Although electron beam computed tomography (EBCT) shows some promise as a screening test in selected persons (e.g., those with intermediate pretest probability for CHD), it is certainly not yet ready to be applied for screening unselected populations. Any advantage over well-validated screening measures remains to be determined. The cost–benefit ratio is likely to be very low and has not been demonstrated. Because the prognostic value of the test is modest at best, the CACS should not be used as a basis for proceeding to invasive testing or for making major treatment decisions (although it might scare some patients into making healthy lifestyle changes). EBCT is likely to increase patient demand for stress testing because the patient with a "positive" CACS is certainly going to be worried and desirous of more definitive evaluation. Despite the claims of media advertising campaigns, the test cannot be recommended at present, but more testing of the technology is warranted and ongoing.

Multidetector Computed Tomography

This CT-based approach to noninvasive diagnosis is targeted more to diagnosis than screening, but it is of increasing interest with the advent of multidetector technology that improves test accuracy. The modality is being explored for use in persons with suspected coronary disease who are being considered for angiographic study. Although the radiation dose is substantial (about the same as a radionuclide stress test and two to three times that of angiography), it is hoped the technology can cut down on the number of unnecessary invasive studies by providing a sensitive noninvasive approach to the detection of hemodynamically significant plaques, especially in persons with equivocal stress test results. There are considerable challenges, not the least of which is accurately imaging a structure that is constantly in motion, limiting the study to persons in sinus rhythm. Other shortcomings include an inability to provide in-stent visualization, poor images in obese persons, and a high false-positive rate. With advances in multidetector technology, it is hoped that test accuracy will improve. Studies are ongoing to help determine the contribution of such testing to clinical decision making and outcomes. For now, it should be considered largely investigational.

Magnetic Resonance Angiography

Like multidetector CT, MRI angiography has the same objective, namely noninvasive imaging of the coronary vasculature.

It also affords the potential for the visualization of left ventricular structure and function. In studies comparing the technology with conventional angiography, it was less sensitive (74% vs. 92%) and equally specific (87% vs. 90%); sensitivity for detecting clinically significant disease was 54% versus 82%. Accuracy was best for the detection of lesions in the proximal and middle segments of the epicardial coronary arteries. Its principal use is likely to be similar to that for multidetector CT, namely noninvasively ruling out significant atherosclerotic disease to obviate the need for invasive angiographic study. It may also have a role in physiologic assessment of the left ventricle. Whether it can perform these tasks any better than available modalities remains the subject of ongoing study.

A.H.G.

Annotated Bibliography

1. Bartel AG, Behar US, Peter US, et al. Graded exercise stress tests in angiographically documented coronary artery disease. Circulation 1974;49:348. (*A classic paper demonstrating that the depth of ST-segment depression was correlated with the severity and extent of coronary disease.*)
2. Bruce RA. Methods of exercise testing. Am J Cardiol 1974;33:715. (*Another classic paper providing a concise and thorough discussion of the differences among various methods of stress testing by one of the pioneers in the field.*)
3. DeBusk RF. Specialized testing after recent myocardial infarction. Ann Intern Med 1989;110:470. (*Reviews exercise testing and other diagnostic tests for risk stratification after acute myocardial infarction.*)
4. Dewey M, Teige F, Schnapauff D, et al. Noninvasive detection of coronary artery stenoses with multislice computed tomography or magnetic resonance imaging. Ann Intern Med 2006;145:407. (*The best available comparison data.*)
5. Epstein SE, Quyyumi AA, Bonow RO. Sudden cardiac death without warning: possible mechanisms and implications for screening asymptomatic populations. N Engl J Med 1989;321:320. (*An interesting discussion of the pitfalls of using exercise testing to screen asymptomatic persons for coronary disease.*)
6. Fowler-Brown A, Pignone M, Pletcher M, et al. Exercise tolerance testing to screen for coronary heart disease: a systematic review for the technical support for the U.S. Preventive Services Task Force. Ann Intern Med 2004;140:W9. (*A systematic review for the U.S. Preventive Services Task Force; finds insufficient evidence to recommend the use of exercise tolerance testing for coronary heart disease [CHD] screening in asymptomatic persons.*)
7. Froelicher VF, Lehmann KG, Thomas R, et al. The electrocardiographic exercise test in a population with reduced workup bias: diagnostic performance, computerized interpretation, and multivariable prediction. Ann Intern Med 1998;128:965. (*A prospective multicenter study designed to minimize workup bias; found an increased specificity but a slightly reduced sensitivity for the detection of coronary disease.*)
8. Frolkis JP, Pothier CE, Blackstone EH, et al. Frequent ventricular ectopy after exercise as a predictor of death. N Engl J Med 2003;348:781. (*Frequent ectopy in the recovery phase predicts increased mortality risk.*)
9. Gibbons RJ, Balady GJ, Bricker JT, et al. ACC/AHA 2002 guideline update for exercise testing: summary article: a report of the American College of Cardiology/American Heart Association Task Force on Practice Guidelines. Circulation 2002;106:1883. (*Evidence-based consensus guidelines.*)
10. Gill JB, Ruddy TD, Newell JB, et al. Prognostic importance of thallium uptake by the lungs during exercise in coronary artery disease. N Engl J Med 1987;317:1485. (*Finds lung uptake to be an independent predictor of poor prognosis.*)
11. Gill TM, DiPietro L, Krumholz HM. Role of exercise stress testing and safety monitoring for older persons starting an exercise program. JAMA 2000;284:342. (*Argues that the requirement of stress testing in the very elderly may be counterproductive and not necessary to ensure safety.*)
12. Goraya TY, Jacobsen SJ, Pellikka PA, et al. Prognostic value of treadmill exercise testing in elderly persons. Ann Intern Med 2000;32:862. (*A prospective cohort study; workload was strongly predictive of outcome.*)
13. Kuntz KM, Fleischmann KE, Hunink MGM, et al. Cost-effectiveness of diagnostic strategies for patients with chest pain. Ann Intern Med 1999;130:709. (*A cost-effectiveness analysis finding exercise electrocardiography [ECG] and echocardiography to be cost-effective in patients with a mild to moderate risk of CHD.*)
14. Kwok JMF, Miller TD, Christian TF, et al. Prognostic value of a treadmill exercise score in symptomatic patients with nonspecific ST-T abnormalities on resting ECG. JAMA 1999;282:1047. (*An inception cohort study with 7 years of follow-up showing that the Duke treadmill score retains its prognostic value despite resting ECG abnormalities.*)
15. Kwok Y, Kim C, Grady D, et al. Meta-analysis of exercise testing to detect coronary disease in women. Am J Cardiol 1999;83:660. (*Finds that ECG, thallium, and stress echocardiography were only moderately sensitive and specific for the diagnosis of coronary disease in women.*)
16. Lauer MS, Pothier CE, Magid DJ, et al. An externally validated model for predicting long-term survival after exercise treadmill testing in patients with suspected coronary artery disease and a normal electrocardiogram. Ann Intern Med 2007;147:821. (*An attempt to improve on the Duke score by including additional validated risk factors.*)
17. Lee TA, Boucher CA. Noninvasive tests in patients with stable coronary artery disease. N Engl J Med 2001;344:1840. (*A succinct review, with a good summary of the evidence and guidelines, as well as practical clinical applications.*)
18. Leppo JA, Boucher CA, Okada RD, et al. Serial thallium-201 myocardial imaging following dipyridamole infusion. Circulation 1982;66:649. (*One of the original papers describing the utility of pharmacologic stress testing in lieu of exercise stress testing.*)
19. Mark DB, Hlatky MA, Harrell FE, et al. Exercise treadmill score for predicting prognosis in coronary artery disease. Ann Intern Med 1987;1106:793. (*The Duke treadmill scoring system; incorporates elements identified by multivariate analysis, such as exercise duration, ST-segment change, and the occurrence of angina, into a single predictive index.*)
20. Mark DB, Shaw L, Harrell FE Jr, et al. Prognostic value of a treadmill exercise score in outpatients with suspected coronary artery disease. N Engl J Med 1991;325:849. (*A prospective study validating the Duke criteria for risk stratification based on ECG stress-test findings.*)
21. Martin CM, McConahay DR. Maximum treadmill exercise electrocardiography. Circulation 1972;46:956. (*Provides data on the changes in test sensitivity and specificity with changes in ST-segment criteria.*)
22. Mayo Clinic Cardiovascular Working Group on Stress Testing. Cardiovascular stress testing: a description of the various types of stress tests and indications for their use. Mayo Clin Proc 1996;71:43. (*An excellent, succinct review for the generalist reader.*)
23. Michaellides AP, Psomadaki ZD, Dilaveris PE, et al. Improved detection of coronary artery disease by exercise electrocardiography with use of right precordial leads. N Engl J Med 1999;340:340. (*Sensitivity increased from 66% to 92% for the detection of coronary artery disease, a major advance for ECG stress testing if it can be confirmed.*)
24. Mora S, Redberg RF, Cui Y, et al. Ability of exercise testing to predict cardiovascular and all-cause death in asymptomatic women. A 20-year follow-up of the Lipid Research Clinics Prevalence Study. JAMA 2003;290:1600. (*A prospective cohort study; ECG findings were of little prognostic value, but exercise capacity and heart rate recovery did have predictive value.*)
25. Morrow K, Morris CK, Froelicher VF, et al. Prediction of cardiovascular death in men undergoing noninvasive evaluation for coronary artery disease. Ann Intern Med 1993;118:689. (*Data on the use of a predictive rule using clinical findings and results from exercise stress testing.*)
26. Myers J, Prakash M, Frelicher V, et al. Exercise capacity and mortality among men referred for exercise testing. N Engl J Med 2002;346:793. (*A large prospective cohort study; peak exercise capacity was the leading predictor of mortality risk.*)
27. Nallamothu N, Ghods M, Heo J, et al. Comparison of thallium-201 single-photon emission computed tomography and electrocardiographic response during exercise in patients with normal resting electrocardiographic results. J Am Coll Cardiol 1995;25:830. (*Single-photon emission computed tomography was found to be more sensitive than ECG for the detection of CHD.*)
28. Nishime EO, Cole CR, Blackstone EH, et al. Heart rate recovery and treadmill exercise score as predictors of mortality in patients referred for exercise ECG. JAMA 2000;284:1392. (*A prospective cohort study; heart rate recovery made an independent and significant contribution to prognosis.*)
29. Philbrick JT, Horowitz RW, Feinstein AR. Methodological problems of exercise testing for diagnosis of coronary artery disease: groups, analysis, and bias. Am J Cardiol 1987;106:793. (*The effect of "workup bias" on test performance is explored.*)
30. Picano E. Stress echocardiography: a historical perspective. Am J Med 2003;114:126. (*A very thoughtful discussion of the test and its contribution to evaluation, particularly in comparison to radionuclide imaging.*)
31. Rifkin RD, Hood WB. Bayesian analysis of electrocardiographic exercise stress testing. N Engl J Med 1977;297:681. (*Argues that the results of the stress test should be viewed as a probability statement rather than as a "positive" or "negative."*)
32. Schinkel AFL, Bax JJ, Elhendy A, et al. Long-term prognostic value of dobutamine stress echocardiography compared with myocardial perfusion scanning in patients unable to perform exercise tests. Am J Med 2004;117:117.

(A prospective cohort study; both tests provided comparable additional predictive value.)

33. Sox Jr HC, Littenberg B, Garber AM. The role of exercise testing in screening for coronary artery disease. Ann Intern Med 1989;110:456. (*A cost-effectiveness analysis of exercise testing as a screening test for coronary disease.*)

34. Tavel ME, Shaar C. Relation between the electrocardiographic stress test and degree and location of myocardial ischemia. Am J Cardiol 1999;84:119. (*The degree of ST depression and the extent of these changes were correlated with the extent of disease but did not localize it.*)

35. Theroux PT, Waters DD, Halphen C, et al. Prognostic value of exercise testing soon after myocardial infarction. N Engl J Med 1979;301:341. (*A classic study; the performance of a limited treadmill test just before hospital discharge provided useful prognostic information.*)

36. Weiner DA, McCabe C, Heuter DC, et al. The predictive value of anginal chest pain as an indicator of coronary disease during exercise testing. Am Heart J 1978;96:458. (*The occurrence of anginal pain during exercise was found to be as predictive as ischemic ECG changes.*)

37. Weiner DA, Ryan TJ, McCabe CH, et al. Exercise stress testing. N Engl J Med 1979;301:230. (*Data from the Coronary Artery Surgery Study examining the influence of the prevalence of coronary artery disease on the diagnostic accuracy of stress testing.*)

38. Einstein AJ, Hanzlova MJ, Rajagopalan S. Estimating risk of cancer associated with radiation exposure from 64-slice computed tomography coronary angiography. JAMA 2007;298:317. (*Documents a high level of radiation exposure and potential consequences, especially for use in young persons and women.*)

39. Garcia MJ, Lessick J, Hoffman MHK, et al. Accuracy of 16-row multidetector computer tomography for the assessment of coronary artery disease. JAMA 2006;296:403. (*Finds that the test as presently configured is limited by a high number of false positives and uninterpretable studies.*)

40. Greenland P, LaBree L, Azen SP, et al. Coronary artery calcium score combined with Framingham score for risk prediction in asymptomatic individuals. JAMA 2004;291:210. (*A prospective observational study; the test was found to be modestly additive to risk assessment in intermediate-risk persons only.*)

41. Greenland P, Gaziano M. Selecting asymptomatic patients for coronary computed tomography or electrocardiographic exercise testing. N Engl J Med 2003;349:465. (*Argues for screening intermediate-risk patients only.*)

42. Kim WY, Danias PG, Stuber M, et al. Coronary magnetic resonance angiography for the detection of coronary stenosis. N Engl J Med 2001;345:1863. (*A multicenter study showing good correlation with conventional angiography for the detection of this important disease; see also the accompanying editorial [Achenback S, Daniel WG. Noninvasive coronary angiography: an acceptable alternative? N Engl J Med 2001;345:1909] for a perspective on this technology.*)

43. Mozaffarian D. Electron-beam computer tomography for coronary calcium: a useful test to screen for coronary heart disease? JAMA 2005;294:2897. (*Finds that evidence for cost-effectiveness and a positive effect on important coronary outcomes is lacking; raises concerns about false-positive rate.*)

SECTION 4 ■ RESPIRATORY PROBLEMS

CHAPTER 37 ■ SCREENING FOR LUNG CANCER

Lung cancer is the most common fatal malignancy in the United States. Each year, it claims the lives of as many men and women as do tumors of the colon and rectum, breast, and prostate combined. The incidence of lung tumors in men has been rising dramatically since 1930. More recently, a dramatic increase among women has occurred. Approximately 10% of American men and 5% of American women alive today will have lung cancer during their lifetime; of these, >85% will die of the disease.

Most people are aware of the epidemic proportions of the lung cancer problem. Many have lost friends or relatives and know the grim prognosis of the disease based on that personal experience. As a result, there is screening for lung cancer to "catch it early." However, the screening of asymptomatic persons who are at high risk can offer little reassurance. Such efforts to improve the prognosis by early detection have been thwarted for decades by the limited sensitivity and specificity of available tests, poor compliance with screening programs among patients at highest risk, and, most important, the aggressive natural history of those lung tumors that progress to advanced disease and death. Although some see promise in the use of low-dose computed tomography (CT) adapted to lung cancer screening because of its greater sensitivity for detection of early-stage tumors, others argue that such optimism is based on the same false premise that explains the past disappointments in screening with chest radiography and sputum cytology. Furthermore, these critics point to evidence that CT scanning dramatically increases population-based rates of both lung cancer diagnosis and thoracotomy for lung resection without decreasing the incidence of advanced lung cancer or lung cancer mortality. We will not know whether the benefits of CT screening of asymptomatic patients at risk exceed the considerable harms of false-positive results and overdiagnosis until randomized trials now underway are completed. Nevertheless, CT screening for lung cancer has been widely promoted by some professional and policy enthusiasts, leading to both exaggerated fear and inappropriate reassurance among patients at risk. The primary care provider is in an ideal position to help patients to understand the controversy and the limits of current evidence and the potential for lung cancer screening to do more harm than good.

EPIDEMIOLOGY AND RISK FACTORS (1–3)

The epidemiology of lung cancer is dominated by its association with smoking. The historic decades-long increase in cancer death rates among men since the 1930s and the more recent increase among women can be explained by trends in cigarette consumption. A dose–response relationship between duration and intensity of cigarette smoking and risk for lung cancer has been documented in both men and women. In comparison with the risk for lung cancer among nonsmokers, the risk is increased 5, 10, and 20 times for men who smoke less than one-half a pack, one-half to one pack, and one to two packs per day, respectively. A decrease in risk has been demonstrated in smokers who are able to stop and in those who smoke filter-tipped cigarettes. Cigar and pipe smokers incur much less risk, but again a dose–response relationship has been documented (see Chapter 54).

The association between smoking and cancer is strongest for the epidermoid (squamous cell) and small-cell undifferentiated (oat cell) tumors. The relationship is less certain for adenocarcinoma (alveolar cell) and large-cell undifferentiated (anaplastic) histologic types.

As noted, the observation that lung cancer occurs in men far more often than in women can be explained for the most part by differences in historical smoking patterns. In fact, lung cancer without a smoking history is more common among women. A slight apparent excess of lung cancer cases also occurs in urban areas and among low-income groups. The presence of polycyclic organic matter in urban pollution and in some occupational environments (see Chapter 39) may provide a partial explanation. Exposure to asbestos, chromate, nickel, uranium, or radon gas has also been associated with significantly increased rates of lung cancer. The combined effect of such exposures and smoking is generally more than additive. For example, smokers exposed to asbestos have a 90-fold greater risk for lung cancer than do unexposed nonsmokers.

NATURAL HISTORY OF LUNG CANCER AND EFFECTIVENESS OF THERAPY (1–16)

Lung cancer's rapidly progressive and usually inexorable clinical course has frustrated clinicians for generations. The 5-year survival rate has been between 5% and 10%. At the time of symptomatic presentation, 75% of patients have lesions that are clearly unresectable. Of the remainder, 60% prove to be unresectable because of mediastinal involvement, discovered by further evaluation or at thoracotomy. Five-year survival rates after resection in the relatively few remaining patients vary from about 10% for patients with oat cell tumors to 30% for patients with squamous cell tumors.

Reports of 5-year survival rates based on the symptoms present at the time of diagnosis are relevant to the question of early detection. In a group of patients with an overall 5-year survival of 7%, the 6% with disease discovered before the appearance of symptoms had an 18% survival rate, compared with 10% to 15% for patients with local symptoms and 6% for those with systemic symptoms. Nearly one third of the patients had symptoms of metastatic disease; all of these people died within 5 years.

Higher survival rates have been reported in patients after resection of *in situ* lung cancer diagnosed by means of chest radiography or sputum cytology followed by bronchoscopy, but these may represent little more than selection of slow-growing or otherwise benign lesions. Some earlier, highly speculative estimates of growth rate suggested that squamous cell carcinomas and adenocarcinomas can take as long as 10 and 25 years, respectively, to reach a size likely to be detected by radiography. More recent analyses of volumetric doubling times of tumors detected by CT scans confirm that what used to be the preclin-

ical natural history of lung cancer is highly variable, and that any overestimation of the benefits of early detection are likely a consequence of lead time and time-linked bias sampling (see Chapter 3).

Such overestimation of the benefits of screening based on survival rates is an even greater potential problem when the more sensitive CT scan is used. For example, the International Early Action Lung Cancer Program (ELCAP) reported that low-dose CT screening produced an 88% 10-year survival rate for stage I disease and concluded that CT screening of high-risk individuals could prevent 80% of lung cancer deaths. Such a conclusion discounts the impact of lead time and time-linked sampling bias (see Chapter 3) and minimizes the potential role of overdiagnosis—the detection of indolent cancers that would not have presented clinically for many years, if ever.

A subsequent analysis of CT screening for lung cancer at three major cancer centers strongly contradicted the ELCAP conclusions. The actual outcomes for >3,000 asymptomatic current or former smokers screened by CT were compared with the outcomes that would have been expected in the absence of screening based on two well-validated predictive models (see Chapter 4). Over a median follow-up period of 3.9 years, the number of patients diagnosed with lung cancer and the number who had lung resections were 3 and 10 times larger than the numbers expected, respectively. However, there was no evidence for a decline in the number of diagnoses of advanced lung cancers or in the number of lung cancer deaths. At one of the three cancer centers, investigators demonstrated that the volumetric doubling time of the CT screen-detected tumors was more than five times that of lung cancers detected before the introduction of CT screening (518 days vs. 102 days), suggesting significant potential for overdiagnosis and the associated harms.

Two randomized trials of CT screening for lung cancer are underway: the National Lung Screening Trial in the United States, with a planned follow-up of 4.5 years, and the NELSON Trial in the Netherlands and Belgium, with a planned follow-up of 10 years. We will not know whether CT screening reduces the incidence of advanced lung cancer and lung cancer mortality rates until these trials are completed. In the meantime, all would agree that CT screening significantly increases the likelihood that lung cancer will be diagnosed and that patients with tumors so detected will incur the morbidity and risks of treatment with what is as yet an unproven benefit.

SCREENING AND DIAGNOSTIC TESTS (4–15,17–24)

Given the controversy about the value of low-dose CT screening for lung cancer, it is useful to understand the historical context, including the past enthusiasm for screening with chest radiography and/or cytologic examination. The trials of screening with these modalities also provide a critical understanding of their value and limitations as diagnostic studies when patients present with alarm symptoms or signs that raise concerns about lung cancer.

Chest Radiography

In a controlled British study of semiannual chest radiography in >29,000 men, 101 lung tumors were detected during a

3-year period. Seventy-six were detected in a control population of 25,000. The overall 5-year survival rates among cancer patients from the screened and control groups were 15% and 6%, respectively. Of the 101 cancers in the screened group, only 65 were detected by routine chest radiography; the remainder presented symptomatically during screening intervals.

The value of chest radiographic screening was also addressed by the Philadelphia Pulmonary Neoplasm Project, which attempted to screen >6,000 male volunteers >45 years with semiannual radiographic examinations. Lung cancer developed in 121 patients during a 10-year period, with an ultimate mortality rate of 92% at 5 years. The poor results were attributed to poor patient compliance with screening, patient and physician delay, advanced age or concomitant illness contraindicating surgical therapy, and inadequate sensitivity of the screening method.

Three additional randomized trials of lung cancer screening were conducted by members of the Cooperative Early Lung Cancer Group. Separate studies at the Mayo Clinic, Memorial Sloan–Kettering Cancer Center, and Johns Hopkins Hospital each enrolled >10,000 male smokers. In the Mayo study, those randomized to close surveillance were screened with both sputum cytology and chest radiographic examination every 4 months, whereas control patients were advised, but not reminded, to have such studies annually. At Memorial Sloan–Kettering and Johns Hopkins, patients were randomized to undergo either annual chest radiography and sputum cytology every 4 months or annual chest radiography alone. The findings of these studies indicate that screening, particularly sputum cytology, may advance the time of diagnosis, with more cancers detected in an earlier stage. However, no difference in survival was found between screening groups at Memorial Sloan–Kettering and at Johns Hopkins, which suggests that no benefit is derived from the addition of cytology to annual radiographic screening. Furthermore, in the Mayo study, no significant difference was noted in lung cancer mortality rates between the screened and control groups, despite the fact that more than twice as many postsurgical stage I lung cancers were found in the screened group as among controls. With extended follow-up of the Mayo study for a median duration of 20.5 years there was no difference in lung cancer mortality. In fact, there was a trend toward higher lung cancer mortality among those in the intervention arm, 4.4 (95% confidence interval [CI] = 3.9 to 4.9) deaths per 1,000 person-years compared with 3.9 (95% CI = 3.5 to 4.4) in the usual-care arm. In a detailed systematic review of the six completed randomized trials, a Cochrane Review Group found a relative increase of 11% in lung cancer mortality among those assigned to the intervention groups subjected to more chest x-rays than those in the control groups.

In addition to these questions about effect on mortality, it should be kept in mind that false-positive chest radiographic findings engender considerable fear and morbidity associated with confirmatory diagnostic tests. Although the specificity of radiographic screening has been shown to be in the range of 90% to 97%, it is still too low to provide an acceptable predictive value. A Veterans Administration study of lung cancer screens found 438 false-positive radiographic readings, compared with 97 true-positive readings, for suspected neoplasm. In the Memorial Sloan–Kettering study described earlier, 10,040 persons were screened with both chest radiography and cytology. Approximately 10% had abnormal chest radiographic findings that led to additional studies to rule out cancer. The predictive value of such a positive finding in this and other recent studies has been in the range of 1% to 5%.

Cytologic Screening

The sensitivity of cytologic screening varies with the cell type and location of the tumor and the methods of specimen collection. It used to be thought that a single cytologic specimen would detect about 70% of squamous cell lesions and that three specimens would increase sensitivity to 90%. However, data from more recent large, randomized trials indicate that cytologic examination is much less sensitive. Only 10% of cancers in the Memorial Sloan–Kettering study and 13% of those in the Mayo study were detected initially by cytology alone. Presumably, these disappointing findings can be explained by the spectrum problem, that is, decreased sensitivity for early- rather than late-stage tumors (see Chapter 3). The specificity of sputum cytologic examination is high, in the range of 98% to 99%. Although they are rare, false-positive findings are highly problematic and often require meticulous bronchoscopic examination to sixth- and seventh-generation bronchi.

It should be noted that as *diagnostic* tests, chest radiography and cytologic examination are complementary. In a Veterans Administration study, cytology alone had an overall screening sensitivity of 33% and a specificity of 98%; radiographic screening had a sensitivity of 42% and specificity of 98%; the sensitivity for combined radiographic and cytologic examination was 63%. Radiographic examination, including computed tomography, is more sensitive for peripheral lesions, whereas cytologic examination is more sensitive for central squamous cell tumors.

Low-Dose Computed Tomography

Computed tomography techniques were adapted in an effort to detect early lung cancer in the general population and among asymptomatic high-risk individuals more than a decade ago. Population-based screening in Japan and Germany, the prospective, uncontrolled Early Lung Cancer Action Project (ELCAP), and other studies have consistently demonstrated much greater sensitivity than chest radiography. Specificity, however, is problematic. More than 20% of prevalence screens were positive for lung nodules in the early stages of the ELCAP study program. These same prevalence screens among long-term smokers detected cancers among 2.7%, a rate four times higher than that detected with concurrent chest x-rays.

More recently, ELCAP prevalence screening detected nodules in 13% of a more heterogeneous population, including a minority of participants with occupational or passive smoking. Cancers were found in 1.3% of this larger, more diverse ELCAP study. Nearly all of the ELCAP detected cancers were resectable, and most were stage I. Estimated 10-year survival for all patients with ELCAP screening-detected cancers was 80%. Ten-year survival was 92% for those with resected stage I tumors. Despite these findings, the effect of computed tomographic screening on mortality awaits further study.

Randomized trials are underway in the United States and in the Netherlands and Belgium, but early answers will not be available for 5 years or more. In the meantime the U.S. Preventive Services Task Force has concluded that there is insufficient evidence to recommend for or against screening. The American Cancer Society recommends that individuals at risk for lung cancer who seek testing should be informed about possible benefits, risks, and limitations of testing for early lung cancer detection, as well as the associated diagnostic procedures and treatment, and that they should be encouraged to participate in trials.

SUMMARY AND CONCLUSIONS
(10,13,19,20)

- Lung cancer is a major cause of morbidity and mortality among men and women.
- Smoking is the overwhelming risk factor for lung cancer. Occupational exposures also are relevant.
- The presymptomatic natural history of lung cancer is highly variable. The 5-year survival despite all forms of therapy has historically been 5% to 10%. Survival is better when an asymptomatic lesion is detected, especially when an early-stage lesion is detected by CT scanning. However, analyses suggest that this improved survival among screen-detected cases is not associated with a decrease in lung cancer mortality in the population screened.

- Although some see promise in the use of low-dose computed tomography, high false-positive rates confer significant risk of morbidity and mortality, and there is concern about over-diagnosis of tumors that would not present for years, if ever, in the absence of screening and the associated overtreatment with significant morbidity. Randomized trials are underway to determine whether benefits outweigh harms.
- Cytologic examination of the sputum and chest radiography are complementary *diagnostic* tests. However, neither is sensitive nor specific enough to serve as a screening test.
- Individuals at risk for lung cancer who seek testing should be informed about possible benefits, risks, and limitations of testing for early lung cancer detection, as well as the associated diagnostic procedures and treatment, and they should be encouraged to participate in trials.

A.G.M.

Annotated Bibliography

Additional references concerning the relationship of lung cancer to smoking appear in the annotated bibliography in Chapter 54.

1. Mulshine JL, Sullivan DC. Clinical practice. Lung cancer screening. N Engl J Med 2005;352:2714. (*Well-reasoned analytic review of computed tomography screening, as well as other modalities; includes recommendations and points to be raised with patients who seek screening.*)
2. Hammond EC, Selikoff IJ, Seidman H. Asbestos exposure, cigarette smoking and death rates. Ann N Y Acad Sci 1979;330:473. (*Includes data from 18,000 insulation workers: relative risks are 90 and 50 for two-pack-a-day and half-pack-a-day smokers, respectively, in comparison with unexposed nonsmokers.*)
3. Patz EF Jr, Goodman PC, Bepler G. Screening for lung cancer. N Engl J Med 2000;343:1627. (*Review with a somewhat skeptical view of low-dose computed tomography.*)
4. Boucot KR, Weiss W. Is curable lung cancer detected by semiannual screening? JAMA 1973;224:1361. (*Reviews the data of the Philadelphia Pulmonary Neoplasm Project, in which the 5-year survival of men offered semiannual radiographic screening was only 8%.*)
5. Flehinger BJ, Kimmel M, Melamed MR. The effect of surgical treatment on survival from early lung cancer. Implications for screening. Chest 1992;101:1013. (*Analysis of the Hopkins, Mayo, and Sloan–Kettering data, with a focus on outcomes for patients with stage I cancer.*)
6. Fontana RS, Sanderson DR, Woolner LB, et al. Screening for lung cancer. A critique of the Mayo Lung Project. Cancer 1991;67:1155. (*A review of the Mayo Clinic trial, including the results of follow-up for 5 years beyond the 6-year study period.*)
7. Bach PB, Jett JR, Pastorino U, et al. Computed tomography screening and lung cancer outcomes. JAMA. 2007;297:953-961. (*Lung cancer diagnosis and lung resection increased 3-fold and 10-fold, respectively, with no decrease in diagnosis of advanced lung cancers or death.*)
8. Henschke CI, Naidich DP, Yankelevitz DF, et al. Early Lung Cancer Action Project: initial findings on repeat screenings. Cancer 2001;92:153. (*Prevalence screening results from the Early Lung Cancer Action Project; cancer was found in 2.7% of high-risk screenees.*)
9. The International Early Lung Cancer Action Program Investigators. Survival of patients with stage I lung cancer detected on CT screening. N Engl J Med 2006;355:1763-71. (*ELCAP results showing 13% prevalence of nodules and 1.3% prevalence of cancers; subsequent annual screening showed 5% nodules and 0.3% cancers; the 10-year survival for patients with screen-detected cases was 80%.*)
10. Humphrey L, Teutsch S, Johnson M. U.S. Preventive Services Task Force. Lung cancer screening with sputum cytologic examination, chest radiography, and computed tomography: an update for the U.S. Preventive Services Task Force. Ann Intern Med 2004;140:740. (*Background paper for the U.S. Preventive Services Task Force conclusion that current evidence does not support a recommendation for or against screening with low-dose computed tomography.*)
11. Black WC, Baron JA. CT screening for lung cancer: Spiraling into confusion? JAMA 2007;297:995. (*Illuminating analysis of the differences between the conclusions of ELCAP and Bach et al. [7] despite their not-dissimilar findings: increased survival among cases may well reflect nothing more than lead time and time-linked sample biases.*)

12. Mahadevia PJ, Fleisher LA, Frick KD, et al. Lung cancer screening with helical computed tomography in older adult smokers. JAMA 2003;289:313. (*Cost-effectiveness investigation concluding that helical computed tomography is not indicated until and unless ongoing trials provide evidence of benefit.*)
13. Manser RL, Irving LB, Stone C, et al. Screening for lung cancer (Cochrane Review). In: The Cochrane library, Issue 3. Oxford: Update Software, 2003. (*Excellent analysis of seven randomized, controlled trials concluding that frequent chest x-rays might be harmful, with an 11% higher risk of lung cancer mortality among those who received them.*)
14. Marcus PM, Bergstrahl EJ, Fagerstrom RM, et al. Lung cancer mortality in the Mayo Lung Project: impact of extended follow up. J Natl Cancer Inst 2000;92:1308. (*With a median follow-up time of 20.5 years, lung cancer mortality was 4.4 [95% confidence interval = 3.9 to 4.9] deaths per 1,000 person-years in the intervention arm and 3.9 [95% confidence interval = 3.5 to 4.4] in the usual-care arm.*)
15. Melamed MR, Flehinger BJ, Zaman MB, et al. Screening for lung cancer: results of the Memorial Sloan–Kettering study in New York. Chest 1984;86:44. (*The addition of sputum cytology to chest radiography was ineffective.*)
16. Bach PB, Cramer LD, Schrag D, et al. The influence of hospital volume on survival after resection for lung cancer. N Engl J Med. 2001;345:181. (*Patients at highest-volume hospitals had better rates of complications [20% vs. 44%], 30-day mortality [3% vs. 6%], and five-year survival [44% vs. 33%].*)
17. Sone S, Li F, Yang ZG, et al. Results of three-year mass screening programme for lung cancer using mobile low-dose spiral computed tomography scanner. Br J Cancer 2001;84:25. (*Japanese study with sensitivity and specificity of 55% and 88%, respectively, in prevalence screens.*)
18. Swensen SJ, Jett JR, Sloan JA, et al. Screening for lung cancer with low-dose spiral computed tomography. Am J Respir Crit Care Med 2002;165:508. (*Sensitivity of 91% and specificity of 49% in prevalence screens.*)
19. Smith RA, Cokkinides V, Eyre HJ. American Cancer Society guidelines for the early detection of cancer, 2003. CA Cancer J Clin 2003;53:27. (*Argues for informed decision making, with patients at risk for lung cancer fully informed about the limitations of screening and encouraged to participate in trials.*)
20. U.S. Preventive Services Task Force. Lung cancer screening: recommendation statement. Ann Intern Med 2004;140:738. (*Concludes that evidence does not support a recommendation for or against screening; available at http://www.ahrq.gov/clinic/gcpspu.htm.*)
21. New York Early Lung Cancer Action Project Investigators. CT screening for lung cancer: diagnoses resulting from the New York Early Lung Cancer Action Project. Radiology 2007;243:239. (*Initial computed tomography led to recommendations for further workup in 14.4% of baseline screens and 6% of annual repeat screens.*)
22. Black, C, de Verteuil R, Walker S, et al. Population screening for lung cancer using computed tomography, is there evidence for effectiveness? A systematic review of the literature. Thorax 2007;62:131. (*Meta-analysis of 12 studies concluding that evidence is insufficient to conclude that screening reduces lung cancer mortality.*)

23. van Iersel CA, de Koning HJ, Draisma G, et al. Risk-based selection from the general population in a screening trial: selection criteria, recruitment and power for the Dutch-Belgian randomised lung cancer multi-slice CT screening trial (NELSON). Int J Cancer 2007;120:868. (*Describes the population-based recruitment methods for this important trial.*)

24. National Cancer Institute Web site. National Lung Screening Trial. http://www.cancer.gov/nlst. Accessed August 23, 2007. (*A detailed description of this trial, which has enrolled nearly 50,000 current or former smokers at more than 30 sites and is slated to collect and analyze data to examine the risks and benefits of spiral computed tomography scans compared to chest x-ray, with results due in 2012.*)

CHAPTER 38 ■ TUBERCULOSIS SCREENING AND PROPHYLAXIS

BENJAMIN T. DAVIS

Active tuberculosis (TB) remains relatively uncommon in ambulatory practice, although its prevalence is beginning to increase again in some populations, especially patients infected with HIV, immigrants from countries where TB is endemic, and the urban poor. Because it is a contagious yet potentially treatable condition, TB is always an important consideration in patients presenting with hemoptysis (see Chapter 42), chronic cough (see Chapter 41), weight loss (see Chapter 9), or fever (see Chapter 11). Tuberculin reactivity remains prevalent. On a daily basis, the primary physician faces the questions of whether to test for reactivity and how to respond when it is present.

EPIDEMIOLOGY AND RISK FACTORS (1–7)

Until the mid-1980s, the number of reported TB cases in the United States was declining at an annual rate of about 6%, with most new cases occurring among the institutionalized elderly, who represented a remaining pool of latent endogenous infection. The prevalence of tuberculin skin test positivity in this population has been estimated at 20% and the prevalence of active disease at 2.4%. In 1985, the incidence of active TB began to grow for the first time in half a century, in part because of the HIV epidemic, but also because of cutbacks in funding for the public health clinics responsible for treating and preventing TB. Federal resources were returned to state and local TB-control programs in the early 1990s. Since 1992, the rates of TB have fallen annually, and the 2003 rate of 5.1 cases per 100,000 represents the lowest seen since national reporting began in 1953. TB remains a problem for patients infected with HIV, the foreign-born (23.4 cases per 100,000), and the urban poor. Compared with persons uninfected with HIV, whose risk for development of active TB after infection is *10% per lifetime*, HIV-infected persons have a risk for development of active disease of *10% per year*. Other population groups with a disproportionately high incidence of TB include alcoholics; intravenous drug users; patients with diabetes, malnutrition, end-stage renal disease, silicosis, or head and neck cancers; persons who have undergone gastrectomy; and patients who take immunosuppressive drugs, particularly tumor necrosis factor (TNF) inhibitors.

NATURAL HISTORY OF TUBERCULOSIS AND EFFECTIVENESS OF THERAPY (2–4,6–10)

Natural History

Mycobacterium tuberculosis is transmitted by way of fresh droplet nuclei expelled by a person with active pulmonary disease. It cannot be spread by hands, utensils, or other fomites, although organisms can be cultivated from room dust. Although inoculation can occur via the gastrointestinal tract, the vast majority of infections in the United States begin in the lung (see Chapter 49). Until the HIV epidemic, it was rare for primary infection to result in early progressive disease; young children were at greatest risk for this complication. However, among HIV-positive patients, the risk for rapid progression to active disease is substantial, with some studies showing a rate of 30% and a mean incubation period of only 80 days. Based on polymerase chain reaction and molecular epidemiology studies, it is now believed that 40% of all active TB cases in urban centers like New York City represent newly acquired infection rather than reactivation of latent disease.

Approximately 5% to 15% of new tuberculous infections eventually progress to serious disease. Risk is greatest during the years immediately following infection. Late reactivation occurs in only 3% to 5% of patients without clinical disease 5 years after infection.

Effectiveness of Therapy (10)

Three strategies may be used in the prevention of clinical tuberculosis: (a) biologic prophylaxis of uninfected persons with bacille Calmette–Guérin (BCG) vaccine; (b) chemoprophylaxis of newly or recently infected persons with isoniazid (INH); and

(c) INH chemoprophylaxis of selected persons with latent tuberculosis infection (LTBI).

Biologic Prophylaxis

Biologic prophylaxis with BCG vaccine is widely practiced in countries where TB is prevalent. The vaccine is used for prevention in uninfected persons; it is of no value in infected persons. BCG vaccine contains a live, attenuated strain of *Mycobacterium bovis*, which has little virulence in humans. It should not be administered to patients who react positively to the purified protein derivative (PPD) tuberculin skin test. BCG itself may cause a positive PPD test result in the first 2 to 3 years following vaccination. After this period, however, a positive PPD test result should not be ascribed to vaccination with BCG, nor should prior BCG vaccination be considered a reason not to perform skin testing, if it is otherwise indicated. The vaccine has been in clinical use since 1922, but its role remains controversial. Early trials demonstrated that BCG could prevent TB in up to 80% of recipients, but subsequent trials on the Indian subcontinent failed to demonstrate efficacy. The greatest benefit of BCG is likely to be the prevention of disseminated disease in infants and children. BCG is not recommended for routine use in the United States. The relatively low incidence of new tuberculous infections in the United States makes case finding and INH prophylaxis a more effective approach (see later discussion).

SCREENING AND DIAGNOSTIC TESTS (11–16)

The tuberculin skin test is the most useful test for the diagnosis of past or present tuberculous infection. The Mantoux test with use of an intradermal injection of Tween 80–stabilized *PPD* is more reliable than multiple-puncture tests, such as the tine test. PPD is available in three strengths: the *first strength* contains *1 tuberculin unit* (TU), the *intermediate strength contains 5 TU*, and the *second strength* contains *250 TU. Only the 5-TU strength should be used for screening.*

The tuberculin skin test result should be interpreted 48 to 72 hours after injection; the diameter of induration (not erythema) determines the interpretation. Until recently, a single standard was used to interpret the tuberculin skin test in all people: 0 to 4 mm was "negative," 5 to 9 mm was "doubtful," and 10 mm or greater was "positive." As noted earlier, authorities such as the Centers for Disease Control and Prevention (CDC) now recommend that different skin test criteria be applied to different population groups to provide a more accurate assessment of risk.

The current CDC *criteria for skin test positivity* include the following:

- Induration of *5 mm* for patients who are HIV positive, have undergone solid-organ transplantation, or who are receiving immunosuppressive therapy including TNF antagonists or the equivalent of 15 mg/d of prednisone for >1 month, and for patients who are *very likely to have TB*, such as close contacts of documented cases and patients with chest x-ray films that strongly suggest TB (see Chapter 49).
- Induration of *10 mm* for members of *high-incidence populations,* such as immigrants from countries where tuberculosis is endemic (particularly those who have immigrated within 5 years); injection-drug users; residents or employees of high-risk coaggregate settings (hospitals, nursing homes, homeless shelters, correctional facilities); patients with *medical conditions predisposing to active TB*, such as silicosis, diabetes, chronic renal insufficiency, leukemia or lymphoma, or cancer of the head or neck; persons who have undergone gastrectomy or jejunoileal bypass or whose weight is 10% or more below their ideal body weight; and children <4 years of age.
- Induration of *15 mm* for persons with no identifiable risk factors.

Repeated tuberculin skin tests can produce a *booster effect*, but only among patients already infected with TB. Among hospital employees or other populations who may undergo repeated skin testing, a booster effect can be mistaken for tuberculin conversion. Confusion can be avoided by repeated testing of persons with negative or doubtful skin test results 1 week later; any increase in the diameter of induration at 1 week can be attributed to the booster effect. In contrast, increased reactivity that occurs at 1 year but not at 1 week should be attributed to newly acquired infection.

False-negative reactions (*anergy*) have been documented in up to 20% of patients with TB, particularly those who are immunocompromised by HIV infection, overwhelming or advanced disease, malnutrition, or debility. Approximately 50% of patients with clinical AIDS may have false-negative PPD test results in the setting of active TB. The lowering of the criterion for a positive skin test result in HIV-positive patients to a 5-mm induration is an attempt to improve test sensitivity. The CDC no longer recommends the use of *Candida,* mumps, or tetanus toxoid antigens as controls for anergy because anergic HIV-positive patients do not benefit from INH chemoprophylaxis.

In addition to immunologic incompetence of the host, other causes of false-negative skin test results are mishandling of the antigen and faulty injection technique. Tuberculin should never be transferred from one container to another, and skin tests should be administered as soon as possible after the syringe is filled. Subcutaneous rather than intradermal injection may result in false-negative reactions. Because tuberculin sensitivity develops 2 to 10 weeks after initial infection, results of early skin tests may be negative in newly infected persons.

Although tuberculin skin testing is highly specific, false-positive reactions may also occur, usually because of cross-reactivity with atypical mycobacterial antigens acquired environmentally. This may cause intermediate skin test reactions in people who have not been exposed to *M. tuberculosis,* hence the requirement for larger areas of induration when a low-risk population is screened.

In 2005, the U.S. Food and Drug Administration (FDA) approved a whole-blood test for the diagnosis of latent TB infection, QuantiFERON-TB Gold. In this assay, blood samples are mixed *in vitro* with two peptides derived from *M. tuberculosis* and the amount of interferon-γ produced is measured. In patients infected with tuberculosis, white blood cells release interferon-γ in response to this exposure. Compared with the PPD, this whole-blood test offers greater specificity because receipt of BCG or infection with atypical mycobacteria will not result in a positive assay. The sensitivity, however, is not well established. Because the test involves a single blood draw, no follow-up visit is required. In addition, false-negative tests due to faulty administration or interpretation of PPDs are eliminated. The FDA has approved this test for use in any situation for which a PPD would be placed. A second whole-blood interferon-γ release assay, the enzyme-linked immunospot assay or its commercial variant T-SPOT.TB, shows similar promise.

CHEMOPROPHYLAXIS (17–21)

Chemoprophylaxis appears to reduce significantly the risk for progression from latent infection to active disease. In patients who have not received chemotherapy, a positive skin test result implies the presence of a few dormant but viable tubercle bacilli, which have the potential for reactivation. It has been demonstrated that the administration of *INH* daily for 6 to 12 months reduces the risk for reactivation by up to 80%. Because the risk for progressive disease is greatest soon after infection, recent converters to tuberculin reactivity are most likely to benefit from such therapy.

In 1999, the American Thoracic Society, the CDC, and the Infectious Disease Society of America revised the published guidelines for offering INH chemoprophylaxis of LTBI. This revision was intended to sharpen the focus of tuberculin screening and chemoprophylaxis to those populations most likely to progress from latent infection to active pulmonary tuberculosis and to deemphasize the routine screening and chemoprophylaxis of persons at low risk of active TB. A person's candidacy for INH chemoprophylaxis should *no longer depend on age*, provided that other risk factors for progression to active disease are present. Candidates for INH chemoprophylaxis (with the respective criterion for skin test positivity noted in parentheses) include the following:

- Patients with known or suspected HIV infection (5 mm).
- Close (especially household) contacts of patients with known active pulmonary TB (5 mm). Children and adolescent contacts of a person with TB should be offered INH regardless of PPD status until a PPD test can be repeated at 12 weeks.
- Patients with fibronodular disease on chest radiography compatible with old, healed TB (5 mm).
- Patients who have received solid-organ transplantation or who are receiving treatment with immunosuppressive drugs, particularly TNF inhibitors (5 mm).
- Recent immigrants (<5 years) from countries where tuberculosis is endemic (10 mm).
- Native-born patients from medically underserved low-income areas, especially if they are homeless (10 mm).
- Patients with documented PPD conversion within the preceding 2 years (10 mm).
- Injection-drug users uninfected with HIV (10 mm).
- Patients with medical conditions predisposing to active TB, such as silicosis, diabetes, chronic renal insufficiency, leukemia or lymphoma, or cancer of the head or neck; persons who have undergone gastrectomy or jejunoileal bypass or whose weight is 10% or more below their ideal body weight; and children <4 years of age.
- Patients residing in or employees working in long-term care facilities such as nursing homes, correctional facilities, and mental institutions (10 mm).
- Persons without risk factors for acquiring TB and without medical conditions predisposing to active TB should not be considered candidates for INH chemoprophylaxis.

When INH is used for prophylaxis, it should be administered *daily* for *9 months*. This recommendation applies to persons with or without HIV infection and with or without fibron-odular infiltrates on chest radiograph. INH may also be given twice weekly via directly observed therapy (DOT). Enthusiasm for INH prophylaxis must be tempered by the significant side effects of the drug, particularly hepatotoxicity. Liver injury is quite rare in patients <20 years and occurs in no more than 0.2% of those between ages 20 and 34 years. On the other hand, INH-induced liver disease may develop in >2% of patients >50 years (see Chapter 49). *INH alone should never be given to a patient with active TB.* A chest radiograph and a clinical encounter designed to uncover subtle signs and symptoms of active TB are mandatory before INH chemoprophylaxis is initiated. *If any doubt exists,* INH should be deferred pending the results of sputum cultures or the resolution of ambiguous symptoms.

In 1999, the CDC recommended that a *2-month regimen of rifampin* (RIF) and *pyrazinamide* (PZA) may be used as an alternative to chemoprophylaxis with INH alone. Between 2000 and 2003, the CDC received reports of 48 patients taking RIF/PZA with serious hepatotoxicity, including 11 patients who died. Through passive and active surveillance, the CDC estimated that the rates of hospitalization and death from hepatotoxicity due to RIF/PZA chemoprophylaxis for LTBI was 3.0 and 0.9 per 1,000 treatment initiations, respectively. Consequently, a 2-month regimen of rifampin and pyrazinamide is *no longer recommended for chemoprophylaxis of LTBI.*

RECOMMENDATIONS AND CONCLUSIONS

- As long as the tuberculin skin test and INH remain useful for case finding and prophylaxis, respectively, biologic prophylaxis with BCG for PPD-negative patients is not recommended.
- PPD testing should be performed *annually in all HIV-infected patients.* Other high-risk persons should also be tested, including household contacts of patients with active tuberculosis, injection-drug users, homeless persons, immigrants from countries with a high incidence of TB, prisoners, residents of long-term care facilities, and persons who are immunosuppressed or have chronic illnesses known to increase the risk for active TB.
- Healthy persons with a high risk for exposure to TB, such as those in the health care professions, should undergo tuberculin testing on an annual basis so long as they remain PPD negative.
- INH chemoprophylaxis should be considered for tuberculin-positive persons who are at risk for progressing from latent TB infection to active tuberculosis. INH should be given daily for 9 months. Care must be taken to ensure compliance to prevent the emergence of drug-resistant strains, and twice-weekly DOT may be appropriate. Active liver disease is a relative contraindication to INH chemoprophylaxis, and the recommendation for such patients should be individualized and may require expert consultation.
- Treatment with RIF and PZA for 2 months is *no longer recommended* for chemoprophylaxis of LTBI.
- Active TB must be excluded before INH chemoprophylaxis is begun.

Annotated Bibliography

1. Centers for Disease Control. Trends in tuberculosis—United States, 1998–2003. MMWR Morb Mortal Wkly Rep 2004;53:209. (*Documents falling rates during this time period.*)

2. Centers for Disease Control. Progress towards elimination of tuberculosis—United States, 1998. MMWR Morb Mortal Wkly Rep 1999;48:732. (*The 1998 rate of 6.8 cases per 100,000 population was 35% lower*

than the 1992 rate; this article also appears in JAMA 1999;282: 1125.)

3. Centers for Centers for Disease Control. Guidelines for preventing the transmission of tuberculosis in health-care settings, with special focus on HIV-related issues. MMWR Morb Mortal Wkly Rep 1990;39:RR-17. (*Important advice on preventing nosocomial infection; items germane to outpatient care are included.*)

4. Dye C, Scheele S, Dolin P, et al. Global burden of tuberculosis: estimated incidence, prevalence, and mortality by country. JAMA 1999;282:677. (*In 1997, there were 8 million new cases and nearly 2 million deaths.*)

5. Keane J, Gershon S, Wise RP, et al. Tuberculosis associated with infliximab, a tumor necrosis factor alpha–neutralizing agent. N Engl J Med 2001;345:1098. (*Report of 70 cases of tuberculosis after treatment with infliximab for median 12 weeks.*)

6. Selwyn PA, Hartel D, Lewis VA. A prospective study of the risk of tuberculosis among intravenous drug abusers with HIV infection. N Engl J Med 1989;320:545. (*Documents a very high risk for infection, even in those who are purified protein derivative negative.*)

7. Stead WW, Lofgren JP, Warren E, et al. Tuberculosis as an endemic and nosocomial infection among the elderly in nursing homes. N Engl J Med 1985;312:1483. (*A study of 25,000 elderly nursing home residents showed a high prevalence of tuberculin reactivity and active disease; the risk for new infection was great.*)

8. Dooley SW, Jarvis WR, Martone WJ, et al. Multidrug-resistant tuberculosis. Ann Intern Med 1992;117:257. (*A succinct summary of this worrisome condition and means of prevention.*)

9. Frieden TR, Sterling T, Pablos-Mendez A, et al. Emergence of drug-resistant tuberculosis in New York City. N Engl J Med 1993;328:521. (*High prevalence among HIV-positive persons, intravenous drug abusers, and those previously treated.*)

10. Centers for Disease Control, Advisory Committee for the Elimination of Tuberculosis. Use of BCG vaccines in the control of tuberculosis. MMWR Morb Mortal Wkly Rep 1989;37:663. (*Centers for Disease Control and Protection guidelines for bacille Calmette–Guérin prophylaxis.*)

11. American Thoracic Society/Centers for Disease Control. Diagnostic standards and classification of tuberculosis. Am Rev Respir Dis 1990;142:725. (*Standards for the administration and interpretation of the tuberculin skin test.*)

12. American Thoracic Society. Targeted tuberculin testing and treatment of latent tuberculosis infection. Am J Respir Crit Care Med 2000;161:S221. (*Current standards for tuberculin testing and the administration of isoniazid [INH] chemoprophylaxis.*)

13. Boyd JC, Marr JJ. Decreasing reliability of acid-fast smear techniques for detection of tuberculosis. Ann Intern Med 1975;82:849. (*Misleading title, but very useful article pointing out the high specificity of smears [99%] but their low predictive value [45%] because of low prevalence; sensitivity, 22%.*)

14. Centers for Disease Control. Anergy skin testing and preventive therapy for HIV-infected persons: revised recommendations. MMWR Morb Mortal Wkly Rep 1997;46:RR-15. (*Revised recommendations against the use of an "anergy panel" or control antigens for patients with or without HIV infection.*)

15. Thompson NJ, Glassrath JL, Snider DE Jr, et al. The booster phenomenon in serial tuberculin testing. Am Rev Respir Dis 1979;119:387. (*A good discussion of the booster phenomenon, with guidelines for serial skin testing in high-risk population groups.*)

16. Menzies D, Pai M, Comstock G. Meta-analysis: new tests for the diagnosis of latent tuberculosis infection: areas of uncertainty and recommendations for research. Ann Intern Med 2007;146:340. (*Concludes that both QuantiFERON and enzyme-linked immunospot assay show considerable promise.*)

17. Centers for Disease Control. Update: adverse event data and revised American Thoracic Society/CDC recommendations against the use of rifampin and pyrazinamide for treatment of latent tuberculosis infection—United States, 2003. MMWR Morb Mortal Wkly Rep 2003;52:735. (*A 2-month regimen of rifampin and pyrazinamide is no longer recommended for latest tuberculosis infection.*)

18. Centers for Disease Control, Advisory Committee for the Elimination of Tuberculosis. Screening for tuberculosis and tuberculous infection in high-risk populations, and the use of preventive therapy for tuberculous infection in the United States. MMWR Morb Mortal Wkly Rep 1990;39:RR-8. (*Recommends aggressive testing and treatment.*)

19. Gourevitch MN, Hartel D, Selwyn PA, et al. Effectiveness of isoniazid chemoprophylaxis for HIV-infected drug users at high risk for active tuberculosis. AIDS 1999;13:2009. (*Among tuberculin reactors, rates of active tuberculosis [TB] were 0.5/100 person-years and 2.0/100 person-years in those completing and not completing prophylaxis, respectively.*)

20. Centers for International Union against Tuberculosis Committee on Prophylaxis. Efficacy of various durations of isoniazid preventive therapy for tuberculosis: 5-year follow-up of the IUAT trial. Bull World Health Org 1982;60:555. (*In a cooperative European study of 27,830 tuberculin-positive adults with fibrotic pulmonary lesions, 52 weeks of INH therapy produced a 75% reduction in TB, and 24 weeks of treatment provided a 65% reduction; hepatitis occurred in 0.5% of the INH recipients and in 0.1% of the placebo recipients; for the 52-week regimen, the benefit–risk (TB averted–INH hepatitis induced) ratio was 2.1; for 24 weeks, the ratio was 2.6.*)

21. Wadhawan D, Hira S, Mwansa N, et al. Isoniazid prophylaxis among patients with HIV-1 infection (Abstract WB 2261). In: Proceedings of the Seventh International Conference on AIDS, Florence, Italy, 1991. (*INH prophylaxis reduced the risk for progression from infection to active disease in these high-risk patients.*)

CHAPTER 39 ■ EVALUATION AND PREVENTION OF OCCUPATIONAL AND ENVIRONMENTAL RESPIRATORY DISEASE

L. CHRISTINE OLIVER

Occupational lung disease is among the 10 leading causes of work-related health problems in the United States. Increasingly, environmental exposures are being recognized as an important cause of pulmonary disease. Causal factors include the inhalation of irritant chemical vapors and gases, organic and inorganic dusts, sensitizing agents, and toxic fumes, which adversely affect both the upper and lower respiratory tracts.

Prevention of exposure is key to reducing morbidity and mortality from occupational and environmental lung disease. Knowledge about and familiarity with these diseases is critically important for the primary care physician, who is often the first health care provider to see injured and ill individuals. Because respiratory symptoms caused by toxic exposures are nonspecific, recognizing their potential relationship to a toxic agent or agents is essential to proper diagnosis and treatment. Continued exposure often results in otherwise avoidable, irreversible functional abnormalities and the development of chronic and even fatal respiratory disease.

BACKGROUND (1–5)

In the United States and developed countries, work-related asthma is the leading form of occupational lung disease, having supplanted the pneumoconioses, or dust diseases of the lung. An estimated 15% to 26% of newly diagnosed cases of asthma in adults and 19% of reactivated cases are the consequence of occupational exposures. The most common cause of pneumoconiosis is asbestos. The National Occupational Respiratory Mortality System revealed a 20-fold increase in the number of deaths due to asbestosis in the United States from the 1960s to the late 1990s, with a plateau since 2000 at approximately 1,500 deaths per year. In contrast, deaths from byssinosis have fallen steadily since 1990. The number of coal miners compensated for coal workers' pneumoconiosis (CWP) under the Federal Black Lung Program has also declined, from 399,477 in 1980 to 98,777 in 1999. Approximately 10% of active coal miners and 20% of retired miners have CWP. The National Institute of Occupational Safety and Health (NIOSH) estimated that 1.7 million U.S. workers are potentially exposed to respirable silica, many at concentrations in excess of existing or recommended federal standards. With regard to malignancy, data from Surveillance, Epidemiology, and End Results indicate that >6,000 cases of asbestos-related malignant mesothelioma are diagnosed each year. Deaths from malignant mesothelioma numbered 2,485 in 1999 and increased gradually to 2,657 in 2004, without evidence of a plateau. The number of asbestos-related lung cancers has been estimated at a minimum of twice that of mesothelioma.

These figures underestimate the true occurrence of occupational lung disease. Because clinical findings in patients with work-related respiratory disease resemble those in persons with nonoccupational respiratory disease, the diagnosis is often missed. For pneumoconiosis and pulmonary beryllium disease (PBD), the latency period between exposure and manifestation of disease may be long, obscuring the causal relationship. The association is further obscured by the occurrence of "paraoccupational" disease among bystanders and household contacts and disease resulting from neighborhood exposure. For example, asbestos-related disease has been reported in family members of asbestos workers and in persons living in close proximity to shipyards and asbestos-manufacturing plants. PBD has resulted from residence in the neighborhood of beryllium plants, and asthma from residence near grain elevators.

Physicians underdiagnose occupational and environmental lung disease because of inadequate training in occupational medicine. Those who make the diagnosis do not always report it to regulatory agencies.

PATHOPHYSIOLOGY (1,6–10)

Inhaled vapors, gases, dusts, and fumes exert their effects on the respiratory tract in several ways. In the case of airways disease, there is *direct irritation* with *inflammation* and/or *an immunologic response with the development of hypersensitivity*. Inflammation causes cough and excessive mucus secretion. Alternatively, it may be associated with airways hyperreactivity, chest tightness, wheeze, and shortness of breath. Lower respiratory tract responses include chemical pneumonitis and pulmonary edema. Clinical manifestations may be immediate

or delayed, as after exposure to the irritant gases nitrogen dioxide and phosgene, when a delay of 12 to 24 hours may precede onset of pulmonary edema.

Mechanisms for immunologic responses include immunoglobulin E (IgE) and T cell mediation. For agents such as diisocyanates, mechanisms are not clearly defined. Sensitization is important etiologically in hypersensitivity pneumonitis, occupational asthma with latency, and PBD. In the case of diisocyanate-induced asthma and other work-related lung disorders, elevated toxin-specific IgE appears to correlate with disease, and IgG with exposure. Dusts such as silica and asbestos and metals such as beryllium are retained in the lungs over time and provoke a *fibrotic response* or, in the case of beryllium, *granuloma formation*. Particle size and dimensions determine distribution within the lung; particles with a diameter of 5 μm or less reach the lower respiratory tract. Larger particles impact the mucosa of the upper respiratory tract. Latency may be as long as 20 to 25 years and appears to be inversely related to the intensity of exposure. Elevated circulating levels of immunoglobulins, rheumatoid factor, antinuclear antibody, and α_1-antitrypsin have been observed in dust-induced lung diseases. Increased occurrence of rheumatoid arthritis and other connective tissue disorders has been reported in association with silica exposure.

Host factors such as cigarette smoking are important factors in the development of occupational lung disease. Asbestos acts synergistically with cigarette smoke to increase the risk for lung cancer. Cigarette smoking appears to increase the risk for the development of IgE-mediated occupational asthma in individuals exposed to platinum salts and tetrachlorophthalic anhydride. The prevalence of bronchitis and airways obstruction is increased in welders and coal miners who smoke in comparison with their nonsmoking coworkers.

Social and *economic factors* often determine the geographic proximity of home to industrial sources of air pollution, and *work practices* affect the likelihood that family members will bring workplace toxins home on their work clothes.

CLASSIFICATION OF OCCUPATIONAL LUNG DISEASE

Occupational respiratory disease can be classified clinically as follows: obstructive airway disease, interstitial lung disease, pneumonitis, cancer, and noncardiogenic pulmonary edema (Table 39.1).

Obstructive Airway Disease (1,6–12)

Work-related airways disease may be acute or chronic, and associated airways obstruction may be reversible or irreversible. The nature of the exposure and duration of exposure after onset of symptoms are important variables in determining outcome. Based on a comprehensive review of relevant epidemiologic literature, a Committee of the American Thoracic Society observed a median population attributable risk of 15% for both occupational asthma and chronic obstructive pulmonary disease (COPD).

Occupational Asthma

Occupational asthma is the most common occupational lung disease in developed countries, accounting for 9% to 15% of adult asthma. In the United States, a conservative estimate based on medical record review revealed that 21% of cases of

TABLE 39.1

CLASSIFICATION OF OCCUPATIONAL RESPIRATORY DISEASE

Airways Disease
Occupational Asthma
   Causal agents: toluene diisocyanate and other isocyanates, phthalic anhydride, nickel, chromium, platinum salts, formaldehyde, *Bacillus subtilis* proteolytic enzyme, grains, animal products, epoxy resins, Western red cedar, mahogany, oak, and irritant particulates, gases, vapors, and fumes
Byssinosis
   Causal agents: cotton, flax, and hemp
Industrial Bronchitis
   Causal agents: diesel emissions, construction dust, welding fume, coal dust, sulfur dioxide, and vanadium pentoxide
Building-Related Illness
   Causal agents: chemical irritants or sensitizers such as diisocyanates, formaldehyde, glutaraldehyde, ammonia, cleaning agents, paints, varnishes, floor-refinishing materials, entrained diesel emissions, mold, and construction dusts
Interstitial Lung Disease
   Causal agents: asbestos, silica, beryllium, cobalt, coal dust, talc, and nylon flock
Hypersensitivity Pneumonitis
   Causal agents: organic dusts such as thermophilic actinomycetes, fungal spores such as *Aspergillus* and *Penicillium*, and chemicals such as diisocyanates
Cancer
   Causal agents: asbestos, crystalline silica, diesel emissions, arsenic trioxide, hexavalent chromium, nickel, vinyl chloride monomer, uranium (radon daughter products), and radon
Noncardiogenic Pulmonary Edema
   Causal agents: oxides of nitrogen, phosgene, chlorine, ammonia, and sulfuric acid

new-onset adult asthma were work related. Occupation was determined to have caused significant aggravation of preexisting asthma in 9% of cases. Agents responsible included smoke from fire, cleaning agents, lacquers and epoxies, glues and adhesives, and welding fume.

At least 250 agents have been reported to cause occupational asthma, now classified as asthma with latency and asthma without latency. Both high– and low–molecular weight substances cause asthma with latency. High–molecular weight agents cause asthma that is IgE mediated and similar etiologically to "allergic" asthma unrelated to work. The mechanism in the case of low–molecular weight (<1,000 D) substances is less clear and may include an IgE-mediated response (e.g., diisocyanates).

Occupational asthma without latency is irritant induced. Reactive airways dysfunction syndrome is a form of irritant-induced asthma that is associated with a single high-level exposure to an irritant or exposure to irritants in poorly ventilated spaces. Irritants may take the form gases, vapors, fumes, or particulates. For example, the collapse of the World Trade Center (WTC) on September 11, 2001, resulted in the exposure of thousands of first responders and residents of nearby buildings to smoke and to particulates from crushed concrete and other structural and insulation materials. The subsequent development of "WTC" cough was widespread and related in part to irritant particulates; persistent airways hyperreactivity was demonstrated in those who were most heavily exposed.

One of the most common causes of occupational asthma is diisocyanates. In widespread use in the manufacture of rigid and flexible foams, in floor refinishing and sealant materials, in varnishes, and in packaging products, diisocyanates cause asthma by direct irritation of the bronchial mucosa and/or by sensitization through a not yet clearly defined immunologic mechanism. Dermal contact with isocyanates can cause respiratory sensitization. Once sensitized, individuals are at risk for severe and even fatal attacks of asthma on reexposure.

Unfortunately, there are no clinical tests for reliably determining whether sensitization has occurred.

Atopy and cigarette smoking affect the risk for IgE-mediated occupational asthma but not for IgE-independent asthma. Symptoms of occupational asthma are worse at work and generally improve with time away from the workplace. Some agents cause a delayed response, however, so that symptoms may develop at night after leaving work. It is important to look for patterns with regard to symptoms and work. Peak expiratory flow (PEF) diaries or pre- and postshift spirometry are useful in verifying reported temporal associations between asthma and work. For most patients, occupational asthma is a permanent condition. The longer the duration of exposure after the onset of symptoms, the more likely is the development of irreversible changes.

COPD

The National Institutes of Health/World Health Organization, in their Global Initiative for Chronic Obstructive Lung Disease, recognized the importance of occupational exposure to chemical vapors and gases and particulates in dust and fume in causing COPD, independent of cigarette smoking. The risk of disease is increased further in those who smoke.

Byssinosis

Byssinosis is a disease of textile mill workers characterized by chest tightness and/or shortness of breath, initially on the first day back at work (grade B1) and then on subsequent days (grade B2). Both acute cross-shift declines in forced expiratory volume in 1 second and the development of chronic irreversible airflow obstruction are observed. The etiologic agent(s) have not been clearly defined. Cotton bract has been implicated; epidemiologic studies have shown acute changes in lung function associated with endotoxin and chronic decline with cotton dust.

Microwave Popcorn Workers' Lung

Fixed obstructive lung disease has been observed among workers who manufacture microwave popcorn. The disease resembles bronchiolitis obliterans radiographically and microscopically; it is precipitous in onset and rapidly progressive. The etiologic agent is diacetyl, a chemical used in butter and other flavorings.

Industrial Bronchitis

Industrial bronchitis is a nonspecific manifestation of airway irritation and inflammation. It is characterized by cough and sputum and results from the inhalation of irritants. Acute bronchitis is self-limited. Chronic bronchitis is defined as cough and sputum production on most days for 3 months or more per year in two or more consecutive years. It may be associated with the development of irreversible airways obstruction. Causal agents include coal dust and silica, cement dust, diesel emissions, welding fume, and gases such as sulfur dioxide.

Interstitial Lung Disease (9,13–18)

Pneumoconiosis was at one time the most commonly recognized form of occupational lung disease. In 1950, the International Labor Organization (ILO) developed a system for classifying radiographic interstitial fibrosis of the lung that results from exposure to silica, coal dust, and asbestos. The most common of the pneumoconioses are described in what follows.

Asbestosis

Asbestosis is fibrosis of the lung parenchyma caused by asbestos exposure. Fibrosis of the pleura also occurs and takes the form of circumscribed pleural plaques, diffuse pleural thickening, or both. Pleural plaques may contain calcium. Asbestos-related pulmonary disease is related to total dose and latency. In epidemiologic studies, asbestosis is more closely associated with dose and pleural abnormalities with latency. For both, average latency is 20 or more years. Respiratory symptoms are nonspecific and depend on the extent of disease. Physical examination may reveal characteristic dry end-inspiratory crackles at the lung bases. Physiologic abnormalities include restrictive mechanics and impaired gas exchange. Small-airways dysfunction, probably resulting from peribronchiolar fibrosis, may be an early finding. Radiographic changes on posterior–anterior view of the chest include irregular, small opacities in the lower lung zones, pleural plaque, and blunting of the costophrenic angle consistent with diffuse pleural thickening. Lateral views of the chest are useful in detecting *calcified hemidiaphragmatic plaques*, a hallmark of asbestos exposure. High-resolution chest computed tomography (HRCT) scan is useful in determining the presence and extent of interstitial and pleural fibrosis. The presence of pleural plaques on chest x-ray has been associated with increased risk for subsequent development of lung cancer and malignant mesothelioma. The full effect of exposure to asbestos in asbestos-containing materials in schools and other public buildings remains to be determined. Asbestosis has been reported in school custodians and malignant mesothelioma in custodians and building occupants.

Silicosis

Silicosis results from exposure to crystalline silica, or silicon dioxide. Silica exposure occurs in a wide variety of occupational settings, including sandblasting and foundry and con-

struction work. Bystander exposure is important because it is often the case that sand blasters are provided with respiratory protection whereas workers around them are not. Silicosis occurs in a simple nodular form or in a "complicated" form with progressive massive fibrosis (PMF). Latency and severity of disease are directly related to the level of dust exposure. Fulminant silicosis may develop after 1 to 2 years of high-level exposure. With lower levels of exposure, latencies of 20 or more years are common. Silicosis may be complicated by mycobacterial or fungal infection. Radiographic abnormalities characteristically precede functional abnormalities and initially occur as small, rounded opacities involving the upper lung zones. Hilar lymph nodes may become enlarged with "eggshell" calcifications. At least 1 in 100 workers exposed to silica at exposure limits established by the Occupational Safety and Health Administration or recommended by NIOSH will develop radiographic evidence of silicosis. Physiologic abnormalities reflect the peribronchiolar location of the silicotic nodules and include small-airways dysfunction and impaired gas exchange in the early stages. With PMF, obstruction, restriction, or a mixed pattern may develop. Occupational exposure to silica also causes silicoproteinosis, a condition closely resembling pulmonary alveolar proteinosis.

Coal Workers' Pneumoconiosis

CWP results from the deposition of coal dust in peribronchial tissues, with the formation of dust macules and the distention of terminal bronchioles. The occurrence and extent of disease depend on both the level of dust exposure and the rank of the coal, with anthracite being more fibrogenic than bituminous coal. CWP occurs in two forms: "simple" pneumoconiosis, characterized by the presence of small dust nodules, usually <5 μm in diameter, and "complicated" pneumoconiosis, or PMF, characterized by large masses of dust and collagen tissue. The most prevalent respiratory symptom is chronic bronchitis, which is unrelated to the radiographic appearance of the lungs and is more common in miners who smoke. Other clinical manifestations generally appear after 10 or more years of exposure. Physiologic abnormalities are variable and, with the exception of the single-breath diffusing capacity for carbon monoxide (DLCO), are unrelated to the radiographic appearance in simple CWP. Reduced DLCO is associated with category p opacities (<1.5 mm in diameter) in simple CWP and with advanced PMF. Airway obstruction may occur in PMF and in association with chronic bronchitis.

Pulmonary Beryllium Disease (PBD)

PBD results from the inhalation of beryllium oxide. It is a T cell–mediated hypersensitivity disorder, with unpredictable latency and dose–response relationships. At risk are workers engaged in the manufacture of beryllium-containing products such as ceramics and computer parts, in work with dental amalgams, and in the nuclear, electronics, and aircraft industries. Acute disease follows the inhalation of relatively high concentrations of beryllium and may be associated with nasopharyngitis, tracheobronchitis, or chemical pneumonitis. Chronic beryllium disease is a systemic granulomatous disorder that is often confused with sarcoidosis. The chest radiograph typically reveals a diffuse reticulonodular infiltrate, with hilar lymphadenopathy in about 40% of patients. Lung function tests may reveal obstruction or restriction and impaired gas exchange.

Diagnosis depends on demonstrating that T cells from the patient's peripheral blood or lung recognize beryllium *in vitro*—the so-called beryllium lymphocyte proliferation test

(BeLPT). Beryllium *sensitization* is determined on the basis of the finding of two abnormal peripheral blood BeLPTs. PBD is diagnosed on the basis of noncaseating granulomas on lung biopsy and an abnormal BeLPT in either peripheral blood or lung lavage. Workers with beryllium sensitization are at increased risk for the development of PBD. Removal from exposure is the treatment of choice in either case. Effectiveness of corticosteroids in treating PBD is variable.

Hypersensitivity Pneumonitis

Hypersensitivity pneumonitis occurs following exposure to organic dusts, mold spores, and certain chemicals such as diisocyanates. Causal agents include thermophilic actinomycetes, *Aspergillus,* and serum and urine protein from animals and fish. Clinical disorders include farmer's lung, bird fancier's lung, bagassosis, humidifier fever, and animal handler's lung. Both acute and chronic reactions may occur. The chest radiograph may reveal miliary or larger discrete opacities in the middle and lower lung zones. Repeat exposure may result in recurrence of symptoms and ultimately in the development of chronic disease, with interstitial fibrosis on the chest radiograph and impaired lung function on physiologic testing. The acute phase may be mild and pass relatively unnoticed. Antigen-specific precipitins appear in about 90% of cases.

Other Work-Related Interstitial Lung Diseases (9)

Other work-related interstitial lung diseases are cobalt-induced "hard metals" disease observed in manufacturers and users of tungsten carbide, talcosis caused by excessive exposure to industrial- and cosmetic-grade talc, and nylon-flock workers' lung, observed in workers who manufacture nylon flock. The last-named is most likely caused by exposure to ultrafine respirable fragments of nylon.

So-called "benign" pneumoconioses occur following exposure to certain inert dusts. These include siderosis (iron oxide), stannosis (tin oxide), and baritosis (barium). The chest radiograph reveals interstitial opacities. Lung function generally remains intact.

Building-Related Illness (19,20)

Poor indoor air quality is often associated with respiratory symptoms and airways disease such as asthma. Potential causes are multiple and depend in part on the workplace setting. For example, health care workers are at risk for asthma induced by such agents as latex powder and formaldehyde and glutaraldehyde vapors. All three are sensitizers; the aldehydes are also strong irritants. Renovation of existing work spaces in any setting can be expected to generate particulates from construction work itself and toxic vapors/fumes from chemicals used in such activities as painting, varnishing, and floor refinishing. *Mold contamination* of buildings has been associated with respiratory symptoms and exacerbation of preexisting asthma, as well as with hypersensitivity pneumonitis.

Cancer (5,9,14,21,22)

Occupational and environmental exposures causally related to cancer of the lung include asbestos, silica, radon, diesel emissions, arsenic, chromium (hexavalent), nickel, vinyl chloride monomer, radiation, beryllium, and fumes from the welding of stainless steel. Of the environmental exposures, asbestos and radon are the two most closely linked to cancer.

Asbestos

Asbestos causes *bronchogenic carcinoma* and *malignant mesothelioma,* a tumor of mesothelial cells that most often involves the pleura. Neither asbestosis nor an asbestos-related pleural abnormality is a necessary prerequisite for the diagnosis of malignant mesothelioma or asbestos-induced lung cancer. Asbestos and cigarette smoke act synergistically to increase the risk for lung cancer. Smoking does not affect the risk for malignant mesothelioma. The risk for lung cancer appears to be greater with exposure to processed asbestos than to mined asbestos because processing breaks up the bundles into shorter, thinner fibers, which can reach the lung more readily.

Silica

In 1996 the International Agency for Research on Cancer declared crystalline silica a human lung carcinogen. Risk appears to be higher in those with 20 or more years of occupational exposure to silica and in those with silicosis.

Radon

Radon is a naturally occurring gas emanating from uranium-containing rock and soil, with higher emissions being found in certain geographic areas of the United States. Radon itself is harmless, but its daughter products emit α-particles, a potential source of radiation-induced injury to the tracheobronchial tree, particularly when attached to inhaled dust particles. It is estimated that up to 10% of homes in the United States are built on soils sufficiently radon-rich to produce indoor radon concentrations of concern (>4 pCi/L) as established by the Environmental Protection Agency (EPA). The EPA recommends that homes in radon-rich areas be tested and remediation efforts undertaken if the level exceeds 4 pCi/L.

DIAGNOSIS (1,6,7)

Eliciting the *occupational history* is the most important step in the diagnosis of occupational respiratory disease (Table 39.2). Although a chronologic lifetime work history is ideal, particularly for diseases with long latency, it is often unnecessary in the primary care setting. Specific information about the type, level, and duration of exposure is needed. Material safety data sheets for chemicals used in the workplace and the results of industrial hygiene surveys are useful sources of exposure information. It is important to characterize the temporal relationship of symptoms and disease to work and to inquire about similar illness in coworkers and family members.

Lung function tests and other laboratory tests provide valuable diagnostic information. A reduced DLCO may be the only abnormality in developing pulmonary fibrosis. Small-airways dysfunction may be an early sign of interstitial or obstructive lung disease. A PEF diary over a 2-week period is often useful in the diagnosis of occupational asthma. *Bronchial provocation* by inhalation under carefully controlled conditions is a useful tool in the diagnosis of occupational asthma.

If the history and clinical findings suggest a diagnosis of pneumoconiosis, then a *chest radiograph* should be interpreted according to the ILO system of classification, which was developed for purposes of standardization and more specific

TABLE 39.2

DIAGNOSIS OF OCCUPATIONAL RESPIRATORY DISEASE: THE OCCUPATIONAL HISTORY

Key Questions
  What is your present job?
  What was your previous job?
  What is the job you worked at the longest?

Risk Assessment
  Job title and description
  Exposures (chemical, gas, dust, fume): type and level (mild, moderate, heavy)
  Adequacy of workplace ventilation (good, fair, poor)
  Availability and use of personal respiratory protective equipment

Evaluation of Symptoms
  Temporal association of symptoms or symptom patterns with work
  Correlation with known health effects of exposures
  Occurrence of similar symptoms among coworkers

radiographic characterization and quantification of pneumoconiosis. HRCT may be indicated to verify radiographic findings and establish diagnosis. Thorough documentation of exposure–response associations is desirable, not only to design an effective treatment program, but also to determine disability and provide basis for workers' compensation benefits. These include health insurance for related medical costs and indemnity payments for time lost from work.

NATURAL HISTORY OF DISEASE AND EFFECTIVENESS OF CONTROL (1,6,7)

Occupational lung disease will progress in the face of continuing exposure and often even after exposure ceases. There are steps that can be taken to control exposures. These include substitution of nontoxic for more-toxic materials. Where that is not possible, engineering changes should be undertaken to improve ventilation in the workplace, both generally and at the site of toxin generation. Wet-down procedures reduce dust levels. Worker personal protection in the form of a respirator should be used as a last resort. If these measures are not effective, or if the exposure is to a substance to which the patient may be sensitized, removal of the patient from the worksite is the only therapeutic option.

RECOMMENDATIONS FOR PREVENTION

■ Include an occupational/environmental history as a routine part of the screening medical examination in all patients.
■ Recommend industrial hygiene testing of the workplace when toxic exposure is suggested by the history.
■ Obtain a chest radiograph or HRCT if pneumoconiosis is suspected and a PEF diary, supplemented by bronchial provocation testing, if occupational asthma is suspected.
■ If a diagnosis of occupational lung disease is confirmed, inform the patient and explain its possible relation to any occupational or environmental causes. Ascertaining patient understanding is important because of statutes of limitation associated with legal remedies, such as workers' compensation.
■ Work with the patient, the employer, and/or the community if possible to develop a reasonable approach to the reduction or elimination of the causal exposure.
■ Inform the employee and a regulatory agency, such as the Occupational Safety and Health Administration or state health department, of any serious or potentially life-threatening hazards to the patient, coworkers, or other citizens to facilitate an evaluation of the workplace.
■ Encourage patients to abstain from habits such as smoking that are inherently toxic to the lungs and exacerbate respiratory effects of workplace and environmental exposures.
■ Institute appropriate medical surveillance for the subsequent development of other exposure-related pulmonary disease, such as lung cancer.
■ Elimination of exposure through the use of rigorous engineering and environmental controls is the ultimate goal in prevention. Removal from the job or home should be a last resort.

Annotated Bibliography

1. Chan-Yeung M, Malo JL. Occupational asthma. N Engl J Med 1995;333:107. (*Very useful discussion for the general reader.*)
2. Milton DK, Solomon GM, Rosiello RA, et al. Risk and incidence of asthma attributable to occupational exposure among HMO members. Am J Ind Med 1998;33:1. (*Study of physician practices and patient understanding with regard to occupational asthma.*)
3. NIOSH National Institute for Occupational Safety and Health. Occupational respiratory disease surveillance. National statistics. National Occupational Respiratory Mortality System. Available at: http://webappa.cdc.gov/ords/norms.html. (*Current statistics.*)
4. NIOSH National Institute for Occupational Safety and Health. The work-related lung disease surveillance report, 2002. Available at: http://www.cdc.gov/niosh/docs/2003-111/2003-111.html. (*Current report of morbidity and mortality from occupational lung diseases, including asbestosis, coal worker's pneumoconiosis, silicosis, and malignant mesothelioma.*)
5. Lemen RA. Epidemiology of asbestos-related diseases and the knowledge that led to what is known today. In: Dodson RF, Hammar SP, eds. Asbestos. Risk assessment, epidemiology, and health effects. Boca Raton, FL: CRC Press, 2006:201. (*Comprehensive summary and historical overview of asbestos use and related diseases; extensive reference list.*)
6. Mapp CE, Boschetto P, Maestrelli P, et al. Occupational asthma. State of the art. Am J Respir Crit Care Med 2005;172:280. (*Up-to-date state-of-the-art review of occupational asthma.*)
7. American Thoracic Society Statement. Occupational contribution to the burden of airway disease. Am J Respir Crit Care Med 2003;167:787. (*Review of the literature regarding occupational exposures and asthma and chronic obstructive pulmonary disease.*)
8. Pauwels R, Anthonisen N, Bailey WC, et al. Global strategy for the diagnosis, management, and prevention of chronic obstructive pulmonary disease. NHLBI/WHO Workshop report. Update 2005. Available at: http://www.goldcopd.com. (*Includes discussion of the contribution of occupational exposures to vapors, gases, dusts, and fume to the development of chronic obstructive pulmonary disease.*)
9. Parkes WR. Occupational lung disorders. Boston: Butterworth-Heinemann, 1994. (*Chapters 12, 13, 20, and 21 provide a detailed discussion of silicosis, coal worker's pneumoconiosis, hypersensitivity pneumonitis, and occupational asthma; exceptional photographs.*)
10. Redlich CA, Karol MH. Diisocyanate asthma: clinical aspects and immunopathogenesis. Int Immunopharmacol 2002;2:213. (*Review of diisocyanate-related asthma, relevant to a broader understanding of sensitization and occupational asthma.*)

11. Anonymous. Fixed obstructive lung disease among workers in the flavor-manufacturing industry—California, 2004–2007. MMWR Morb Mortal Wkly Rep 2007;56:389. (*Up-to-date review of diacetyl-induced bronchiolitis obliterans.*)

12. Banach GI, Alleyne D, Sanchez R, et al. Persistent hyperreactivity and reactive airway dysfunction in firefighters at the World Trade Center. Am J Respir Crit Care Med 2003;168:54. (*Study of airway effects of irritant particulates and smoke.*)

13. NIOSH National Institute for Occupational Safety and Health. NIOSH hazard review. Health effects of occupational exposure to respirable crystalline silica. Available at: http://www.cdc.gov/niosh/02-129a.html. (*Comprehensive review of exposure variables and sources of exposure and human health effects, with an exhaustive list of references.*)

14. Becklake MR. Asbestos-related diseases of the lung and other organs: their epidemiology and implications for clinical practice. Am Rev Respir Dis 1976;114:55. (*Comprehensive review.*)

15. Oliver LC, Sprince N, Greene R. Asbestos-related disease in public school custodians. Am J Ind Med 1991;19:303. (*Reports an increased risk associated with building exposures.*)

16. Newman LS. Significance of the blood beryllium lymphocyte proliferation test. Environ Health Perspect 1996;104:953. (*Discussion of the test and its clinical significance.*)

17. Newman LS, Mroz MM, Balkissoon R, et al. Beryllium sensitization progresses to chronic beryllium disease. A longitudinal study of disease risk. Am J Respir Crit Care Med 2005;171:54. (*Informative study regarding the significance of beryllium sensitization to the future development of pulmonary beryllium disease.*)

18. Eschenbacher WL, Kreiss K, Lougheed MD, et al. Nylon-flock–associated interstitial lung disease. Clinical pathology workshop summary. Am J Respir Crit Care Med 1999:159:2003. (*Discussion of clinical features and pathology of nylon-flock workers' lung disease.*)

19. Oliver LC, Shackleton B. The indoor air we breathe: a public health problem for the '90s. Public Health Rep 1998;113:398409. (*A general discussion of the causes and health effects of poor indoor air quality.*)

20. Macher J, ed. Bioaerosols: assessment and control. Cincinnati, OH: American Conference of Government Industrial Hygienists, 1999. (*Good reference for the health effects of and evaluation for mold spores and other bioaerosols.*)

21. Hammond EC, Selikoff IJ, Seidman H. Asbestos exposure, cigarette smoking and death rates. Ann N Y Acad Sci 1979;330:473. (*Study of independent and interactive contributions of asbestos exposure and cigarette smoking to death from lung cancer in 17,800 asbestos insulation workers.*)

22. National Research Council. Health effects of exposure to radon. BEIR VI. Washington, DC: National Academy Press, 1999. (*Comprehensive and authoritative report on the risk associated with exposure to radon.*).

CHAPTER 40 ■ EVALUATION OF CHRONIC DYSPNEA

Dyspnea is the subjective sensation of difficult or uncomfortable breathing. Patients commonly complain of "shortness of breath" to describe their respiratory difficulty. *Acute dyspnea* is most often a manifestation of sudden left ventricular dysfunction (see Chapter 32), bronchospasm (see Chapter 48), pneumonia (see Chapter 52), pulmonary embolization (see Chapter 20), or anxiety (see Chapter 226). The patient often presents in the urgent care setting. Patients with chronic dyspnea, even when it is severe, are more likely to come to the office for care. Longstanding dyspnea can be evaluated safely in the outpatient setting.

The differentiation between heart and lung disease as the cause of dyspnea can be difficult; moreover, these causes often coexist. The reported prevalence of chronic obstructive pulmonary disease among patients with congestive heart failure ranges from 20% to 32%, depending on the clinical setting in which the study was conducted. In such instances, diagnosis requires determining which condition is predominant. In evaluating the chronically dyspneic patient, one needs to check for precipitants and reversible components in addition to ascertaining the cause. Also important are assessments of functional status and prognosis, which are often closely correlated.

PATHOPHYSIOLOGY AND CLINICAL PRESENTATION (1–5)

The pathophysiology of dyspnea is multifactorial and complex. In most instances, dyspnea results from cardiac or pulmonary decompensation and is provoked by the stimulation of receptors responsive to metabolic changes, pulmonary interstitial stretch, respiratory muscle tension, and central respiratory command. Shortness of breath is experienced when ventilatory demand exceeds the actual or perceived capacity of the lungs to respond. The work of breathing may be increased by altered chest wall mechanics, decreased lung compliance, airway obstruction, increased ventilatory requirements, or exogenous factors such as obesity.

Congestive Heart Failure (See also Chapter 32)

Congestive heart failure (CHF) can cause dyspnea as pulmonary capillary pressure rises and fluid accumulates in the interstitium, leading to a fall in pulmonary compliance and a sense of difficulty breathing. The earliest symptom is often dyspnea on exertion. More severe failure is manifested by orthopnea and finally paroxysmal nocturnal dyspnea. *Basilar crackles (rales)* and a *third heart sound (S_3)* are important signs of left-sided heart failure and pulmonary venous hypertension; the S_3 is one of the most specific signs of CHF; a documented S_3 has been reported to have a positive likelihood ratio (LR+) for heart failure of 24 (see Chapter 2). *Peripheral edema* and *jugular venous distention* are common manifestations of right-sided heart failure, but these findings, particularly leg edema, are very nonspecific (see Chapter 22). Jugular venous distention has LR+ of 8.5. Contributing and precipitating factors include fever, acute ischemia, excessive dietary sodium intake, dysrhythmias, concurrent use of agents that are negatively inotropic (e.g., beta-blockers, disopyramide, verapamil), and poor compliance with medical regimen (see Chapter 32).

Community studies have demonstrated a high prevalence of preclinical CHF, including approximately equal numbers of people with diastolic dysfunction and systolic dysfunction. Besides CHF, a number of other causes of pulmonary venous hypertension result in increased pulmonary capillary pressure and dyspnea. *Mitral stenosis* is the most important.

Airway Obstruction

Airway obstruction at any level of the respiratory tract can lead to difficulty breathing. *Tracheal stenosis* resulting from intrinsic disease or extrinsic compression is characterized by dyspnea in conjunction with stridor and inspiratory retraction of the supraclavicular space. *Chronic obstructive pulmonary disease* (COPD) (see Chapter 47) is the leading cause of airway obstruction. *Chronic bronchitis* is a subcategory of COPD that is defined as cough and sputum production persisting for 3 months or more in two consecutive years. Characteristically, these patients have a long history of smoking, productive cough, and a slowly progressive decline in exercise capacity. In advanced stages, they may become plethoric and cyanotic and cough incessantly; the term "blue bloater" has been applied to such patients. Tobacco-stained fingers, wheezes, coarse rales, rhonchi, and a prolonged expiratory phase of respiration are often present on examination. Signs of cor pulmonale (right ventricular heave, jugular venous distention, leg edema) are late findings indicative of severe, advanced disease.

Another group of COPD patients are those with *emphysema*. Sputum production is minimal compared with that in patients with bronchitis, and mismatching of ventilation and perfusion is less pronounced; consequently, hypoxia and cyanosis are less prominent. Gradual deterioration in exercise capacity takes place over many years. Patients with advanced emphysema appear thin and barrel-chested. They may purse their lips during expiration to keep their poorly supported airways from collapsing. The chest is hyperresonant, breath sounds are distant, and a few end-expiratory wheezes may be noted; expiration is prolonged.

Patients with COPD and *bronchiectasis* have a clinical presentation similar to that of patients with chronic bronchitis, except that their physical findings are more localized, the clinical course is punctuated by more frequent episodes of pneumonia, and their sputum tends to be more copious and sometimes bloody.

Asthma is another of the obstructive airway diseases. It usually produces attacks of acute dyspnea, but airway obstruction may persist for a prolonged period after an acute episode and result in more chronic respiratory complaints, including exercise intolerance, cough, and sputum production. At times, sputum production may be the predominant early symptom and mistaken for infection. Diffuse wheezes are commonly noted on examination; severe cases are characterized by the use of accessory muscles, retraction, and pulsus paradoxus. Exercise-induced asthma is common in young people and may contribute to recurrent dyspneic episodes (see Chapter 48).

Diffuse Interstitial Lung Disease

Diffuse *interstitial lung disease* alters pulmonary compliance and may lead to a disturbance in the balance between ventilation and perfusion. The process is usually very gradual, and often patients have few symptoms when pulmonary involvement is mild or even moderate; however, tachypnea and cyanosis ensue in severe cases. Diffuse, *"dry" midexpiratory crackles* are often heard on auscultation. As the interstitial process progresses, dyspnea and hypoxia worsen and exercise tolerance deteriorates (see Chapter 46).

Kyphoscoliosis

Kyphoscoliosis is the major chest wall deformity capable of seriously impairing pulmonary musculoskeletal mechanics. Advanced cases can even terminate in cor pulmonale and respiratory failure. With the increase in prevalence of obesity in the United States, it has become one of the more common causes of dyspnea even in the absence of pulmonary disease. Other extrapulmonary conditions hindering lung mechanics are marked *ascites* (see Chapter 71) and large *pleural effusions* (see Chapter 43). Dyspnea is often the chief complaint in such patients.

Pulmonary Hypertension

Pulmonary hypertension is a serious cause of chronic dyspnea and has a poor prognosis. It may be primary or secondary and is characterized by a fixed elevation in pulmonary artery pressure and resultant strain on the right side of the heart strain. Common physical findings include an accentuated pulmonic component of S_2, a right ventricular S_3, the murmur of tricuspid regurgitation, and peripheral edema.

Secondary pulmonary hypertension occurs with conditions that chronically elevate pulmonary artery pressure, such as recurrent pulmonary embolization, chronic hypoxemia, pulmonary parenchymal disease, and left-sided heart failure. Some forms of secondary disease have subtle presentations and can easily be mistaken for primary disease. For example, pulmonary hypertension resulting from recurrent pulmonary embolization typically occurs in patients with few symptoms of embolization. Except for recalling perhaps a single episode of pleuritic chest pain and acute dyspnea, most patients report few symptoms before the onset of pulmonary hypertension. In those with symptomatic, recurrent embolization, significant pulmonary hypertension rarely develops. The reason for this paradox is unclear. The source of emboli is believed to be the proximal deep veins of the legs.

Primary pulmonary hypertension is a diagnosis of exclusion. It occurs most commonly in women between the ages of 20 and 40 years. The mean age is about 35 years, and the ratio of women to men is 1.7:1. Dyspnea is the most frequently reported symptom, followed by fatigue, near-syncope, and Raynaud's phenomenon. An immunologic basis for the condition is suspected because of the high frequency of antinuclear antibody seropositivity in many of these patients, especially women. Immunologically mediated endothelial damage is postulated. Hyperventilation may result and be mistakenly attributed to anxiety.

Anxiety

Anxiety attacks are often confused with more serious conditions because the patient may appear to be in severe respiratory distress. Patients often report chest tightness or claim that they cannot take in enough air. The florid, acute case is represented by the hyperventilation syndrome (see Chapter 226), but more common is a less dramatic, chronic feeling of dyspnea and fatigue that is affected little by exertion. Frequent sighing, multiple bodily complaints, nervousness, and normal physical examination findings are typical of such patients.

Deconditioning

Patients with cardiopulmonary disease often limit their physical functioning, with the resulting sedentary state creating deconditioning and worsening the effects of dyspnea on exertion. Skeletal muscle atrophy is a common finding among patients with either COPD or CHF and has been linked to low-level systemic inflammation and oxidative stress. The muscle atrophy and sedentary behavior combine to create a vicious cycle of declining function in the setting of increasing dyspnea.

DIFFERENTIAL DIAGNOSIS (1,6–10)

The causes of chronic dyspnea encountered in the office setting are listed in Table 40.1.

WORKUP (11–28)

History

History remains the most useful diagnostic modality. In studies of dyspnea, the diagnosis is established by the history in about 75% of instances. However, differentiating dyspnea caused by cardiac disease from that caused by pulmonary pathology can be a challenge. For example, exertional dyspnea occurs in both cardiac and pulmonary disease. A frequent misconception is that paroxysmal nocturnal dyspnea is unique to heart failure. Excessive airway secretions from chronic obstructive lung disease often pool at night and lead to airway obstruction, causing dyspnea and forcing the patient to sit up to clear the airway.

TABLE 40.1

COMMON CAUSES OF CHRONIC DYSPNEA

Cardiac
Congestive heart failure
Other causes of pulmonary venous congestion (mitral stenosis, mitral regurgitation)

Pulmonary
Chronic obstructive pulmonary disease
Asthma
Pulmonary parenchymal disease (including interstitial diseases)
Pulmonary hypertension (including that caused by recurrent pulmonary embolization, sleep apnea, and mitral stenosis as well as primary disease)
Severe kyphoscoliosis
Exogenous mechanical factors (ascites, massive obesity, large pleural effusion)

Psychological
Anxiety

Other
Deconditioning
Severe chronic anemia

Wheezing is a nonspecific manifestation of large-airway bronchospasm, whether it is caused by heart failure or obstructive lung disease.

In general, a history dominated by chronic cough, sputum production, recurrent respiratory infection, occupational exposure, or heavy smoking suggests lung disease rather than a cardiac origin. However, unless a strong history of previous lung disease or substantial sputum production is present, it may be very hard to distinguish a cardiac from a pulmonary source on the basis of history alone. Moreover, as noted, both may coexist concurrently. Physical findings and laboratory studies are often necessary for a better differentiation (see later discussion).

Dyspnea that is a manifestation of a chronic anxiety state may superficially mimic cardiopulmonary disease and cause some confusion. Onset at rest in conjunction with a sense of chest tightness, suffocation, and inability to take in air are characteristic features of the history. In addition, little evidence of significant heart or lung disease is present, although the patient may fear it greatly. Multiple bodily complaints, a history of emotional difficulties, an absence of activity limitations, and a lack of exacerbation on exercising argue for a psychogenic cause. Unfortunately, patients with pulmonary hypertension may have episodes that can resemble anxiety-induced bouts of dyspnea; sometimes, a young patient with primary pulmonary hypertension is incorrectly labeled "neurotic."

It is helpful to define as precisely as possible the degree of activity that precipitates the sensation of dyspnea, estimate the severity of disease, determine the extent of disability, and detect changes over time. One means of achieving these objectives is to relate symptoms to the patient's daily activities and interpret the degree of restriction in terms of the expected endurance of a patient of similar age.

Factors that may contribute to the occurrence or worsening of dyspnea should be documented, including cigarette smoking, occupational exposure, excessive salt intake, weight gain, and increasing sputum production. The occupational history is particularly important because the relationships between exposures and lung disease are becoming increasingly evident (see Chapter 39).

The patient should be asked about hemoptysis; the symptom raises the possibilities of bronchiectasis, endobronchial malignancy, embolization with infarction, and pneumonia. If embolization is suspected, the physician must inquire about pleuritic chest pain, leg edema, and other symptoms of deep vein thrombosis (see Chapter 22) in addition to such risk factors as chronic venous insufficiency, inactivity, and—in young women—the use of oral contraceptives and pregnancy. Careful inquiry for historical evidence of recurrent pulmonary embolization is particularly important if pulmonary hypertension is encountered.

Physical Examination

Physical examination should begin with a check for tachycardia, tachypnea, fever, and hypertension. Weight increase must not be forgotten, for it may be an early sign of worsening CHF (see Chapter 32). The patient's respiratory efforts need to be observed carefully to obtain an estimate of the amount of work expended in breathing; contractions of the accessory muscles of respiration suggest severe difficulty. Retraction of the supraclavicular fossa implies tracheal stenosis that has become critical. Pursed-lip breathing and a prolonged expiratory phase are signs of significant outflow obstruction. The best way to observe air flow obstruction is to have the patient take a deep breath and blow out as hard and as fast as possible. The chest is examined for increased anterior–posterior diameter (suggestive of COPD) and deformity resulting from kyphoscoliosis or ankylosing spondylitis. Retraction of the intercostal muscles on inspiration is characteristic of emphysema.

The chest should be percussed for dullness and hyperresonance and auscultated for wheezes, crackles, and quality of breath sounds. Unfortunately, eliciting wheezing on maximal forced exhalation has proved neither sensitive nor specific for the diagnosis of asthma and cannot be recommended as a technique for uncovering underlying airway hyperreactivity. Crackles suggest fluid in the airway, as occurs with bronchitis, pneumonitis, and CHF. Normal findings on lung examination do not rule out pulmonary pathology but do lessen its probability and the likelihood that it is severe. The cardiac examination should focus on signs of left-sided heart failure (see Chapter 32), detection of left-sided heart murmurs (see Chapters 21 and 33), and signs of pulmonary hypertension and its consequences (accentuated and delayed pulmonic valve component of S_2, right ventricular heave, right ventricular S_3, right-sided systolic regurgitant murmur of tricuspid insufficiency, jugular venous distention, and peripheral edema). It is important to recognize that many of the signs of right-sided heart failure may be a consequence of longstanding pulmonary disease and therefore are not specific for a cardiac etiology. The abdomen is examined for ascites and hepatojugular reflux; the legs are checked for edema and other signs of phlebitis (see Chapters 16 and 30). Finally, the patient's mental status is checked for manifestations of an anxiety disorder; particularly germane is excessive sighing.

Laboratory Studies

Chest X-Ray

The chest radiograph is essential to evaluation and should be studied for pulmonary venous redistribution, effusions, interstitial changes, hyperinflation, infiltrates, enlargement of the pulmonary arteries (indicative of pulmonary hypertension), cardiac chamber enlargement, and valve calcification. Upper zone redistribution of pulmonary blood flow is among the earliest radiographic findings of CHF (see Chapter 32); however, redistribution may also occur in COPD because of destruction of vessels in the lower lung fields. The radiographic diagnosis can be made with a high degree of accuracy if any two of the following criteria are met: depression and flattening of the diaphragm with blunting of the costophrenic angles on posterior–anterior film; irregular lucency of the lung fields; abnormally enlarged retrosternal space; and diaphragmatic flattening or concavity on the lateral film. Chest radiography is sometimes useful for the detection of interstitial lung disease because physical findings may be minimal. However, radiographic findings may also be unimpressive, so further study is necessary (see later discussion).

High-Resolution Computed Tomography (CT)

Chest CT has no role in the evaluation of dyspnea in the early stages of evaluation for most patients but may be helpful when the etiology is unclear or when signs or symptoms point in the direction of interstitial lung disease, bronchiectasis, or pulmonary embolism.

Stains, Culture, and Cytology

When an infiltrate is present, *Gram's stains* of the sputum and culture are often informative, especially when the patient is febrile, is coughing more than usual, or reports a change in sputum.

Sputum cytology is indicated under similar circumstances, particularly if hemoptysis has developed. A *Ziehl–Neelsen stain* for acid-fast bacilli and *sputum culture for tuberculosis* are also important components of the workup when an infiltrate is detected (see Chapter 49).

Pulmonary Function Tests

Simple pulmonary function tests can be reliably performed in the office on an inexpensive spirometer. *Forced expiratory volume in 1 second* (FEV$_1$) and *vital capacity* are the most informative of these measurements for detecting obstructive and restrictive defects and determining their severity. The ratio of FEV$_1$ to vital capacity is markedly reduced in clinically important obstructive disease. In restrictive disease, the ratio is close to 1.0, but the vital capacity is significantly reduced. An FEV$_1$ determination can also provide prognostic information. A reading of <1.0 L/sec is associated with a poor 5-year survival rate among patients with COPD (see Chapter 47). Patients suspected of having tracheal stenosis may require *flow-volume studies* to identify the lesion and determine its severity; referral is indicated.

Arterial Blood Gas

Arterial blood gas determinations are not routinely available in most office settings, but they are worth obtaining when deteriorating ventilation is suspected. Hospitalization should be considered when the carbon dioxide tension (PCO$_2$) is inappropriately elevated for the respiratory rate and repeated determinations reveal further increases in PCO$_2$. Measuring arterial blood gases before and after exercise is helpful in assessing the severity of diffuse interstitial disease. A fall in oxygen tension is evidence of a significant degree of interstitial disease. When use of accessory muscles is noted and the patient's condition appears to be worsening, prompt hospital admission should be arranged without time taken to determine arterial blood gases in the office.

Pulse Oximetry

Pulse oximetry is a noninvasive alternative that provides estimates of arterial oxyhemoglobin saturation and of desaturation with exercise that can be useful in decision making. Accuracy of most oximeters is limited to ±4% of the actual oxygen saturation. Accuracy is especially a problem at levels below 88%. Accuracy may be lower in patients with darker skin or poor peripheral perfusion due to heart failure. Oximetry will overestimate oxygen saturation among heavy smokers with high carboxyhemoglobin levels. A significant desaturation during exercise measured with continuous pulse oximetry, defined as a decrease of >4%, should be confirmed with arterial blood gas determinations.

Diffusing Capacity

A reduction in *single-breath carbon monoxide diffusing capacity* may be the earliest sign of interstitial fibrosis. The test is particularly useful in the evaluation of dyspnea associated with suspected occupational interstitial disease (see Chapters 39 and 46). Abnormal rest oximetry and further desaturation with exercise would be expected.

Tests for Heart Failure

Sometimes, the combination of history, physical examination, chest radiography, and pulmonary function testing is not sufficient to determine the relative contributions of heart disease and lung disease to a case of dyspnea. When findings are equivocal, it may be helpful to order a *cardiac ultrasonographic* examination—a readily available, noninvasive means of determining chamber size, valvular anatomy, and left ventricular function. The ejection fraction will be reduced in the setting of left ventricular dysfunction and relatively preserved in patients with predominantly pulmonary disease. Cardiac ultrasonography in conjunction with *Doppler* study is an excellent means of detecting important treatable causes of pulmonary hypertension, such as tight mitral stenosis (see Chapter 33) and sometimes pulmonary embolization. *B-type natriuretic peptide (BNP)* effectively distinguishes between congestive heart failure and noncardiac causes of acute dyspnea in the emergency setting. In an early study, a cutoff level of 100 pg/mL had a sensitivity of 90% and a specificity of 76%, producing a positive predictive value in this population of roughly 80% and a negative predictive value of 90%. BNP levels have been shown to have prognostic as well as diagnostic significance. BNP measurements have been made in community settings to screen for preclinical systolic and diastolic dysfunction but have produced unacceptably high false-positive rates with need for further extensive evaluation. In some small studies it has effectively differentiated diastolic dysfunction from pulmonary disease as a cause of dyspnea. Neither the role of BNP testing in patients with subacute or chronic dyspnea nor the value of other uses of BNP testing in the nonacute primary care setting have been fully defined.

Exercise Testing

The neurotic patient with anxiety-induced dyspnea often benefits from undergoing chest radiography and simple pulmonary function testing; the confirmation of a well-functioning respiratory system may provide some reassurance and lessen concern over bodily symptoms. At times, a *walk with the patient* up and down a few flights of stairs is just as convincing for both physician and patient. Climbing stairs with a patient complaining of dyspnea is also useful if cardiopulmonary disease is suspected because exercise tolerance can be quantified in terms of the number of flights climbed and the heart and respiratory rates attained. The *6-minute walk test* is commonly used to assess exercise capacity in patients with COPD; simple distance is usually measured, although the product of distance times body weight has been advocated as having a more solid physiologic foundation. In the very rare cases in which there is no apparent cause after a thorough evaluation or when it is difficult to ascertain the contribution to symptoms made by more than one condition, cardiopulmonary exercise testing may be indicated. Measurement of blood pressure, heart rate, ventilation, oxygen saturation, oxygen uptake, and carbon dioxide output allow for the quantification of cardiac function, pulmonary gas exchange, and physical fitness.

Evaluation of Pulmonary Hypertension

Finding evidence suggestive of pulmonary hypertension (dyspnea, signs of right-sided heart strain on physical examination and electrocardiogram, prominent main pulmonary artery and hilar vessels in conjunction with decreased peripheral vessels on chest x-ray film) necessitates consideration of its treatable causes, such as recurrent pulmonary embolization, sleep apnea (see Chapter 46), and mitral stenosis (see Chapter 33). Although pulmonary hypertension is typically quite advanced by the time the diagnosis is made, efforts at earlier recognition and identification of treatable causes are imperative if the prognosis is to be improved.

Echocardiography has shown considerable promise in the noninvasive diagnosis of cor pulmonale and pulmonary hypertension and their antecedent conditions. The *perfusion lung scan* is a safe, noninvasive means of screening for recurrent pulmonary embolization and differentiating it from primary pulmonary hypertensive disease. In primary disease, the scan findings may be normal, or the scan may show a subsegmental or diffuse patchy, peripheral distribution of labeled albumin. In secondary disease resulting from recurrent pulmonary emboli, the scan shows multiple segmental or large subsegmental defects. More recently, use of *chest computed tomography* has replaced perfusion scanning in many settings, although it must be kept in mind that its sensitivity is limited for small peripheral emboli.

SYMPTOMATIC MANAGEMENT AND PATIENT EDUCATION (29–35)

The relief of dyspnea requires attention to *exacerbating factors* in addition to the underlying etiology. Symptomatic management begins with correcting reversible forms of airway obstruction (see Chapters 47 and 48) and precipitants of left ventricular dysfunction (see Chapter 32). Any concurrent respiratory tract infection requires treatment (see Chapter 52). If a large pleural effusion (see Chapter 43), a severe anemia (see Chapter 82), or an acute situational stress (see Chapter 226) is present, it too should receive prompt attention. Environmental irritants ought to be eliminated (see Chapter 39). All patients with dyspnea should be advised to stop smoking; often, the onset of even mild dyspnea is a sufficient stimulus to quit, especially when combined with the physician's urging (see Chapter 54).

Need for attention to the underlying cause cannot be overemphasized, whether it is heart disease (see Chapters 30, 32, and 33), lung disease (see Chapters 47, 48, and 52), a mechanical factor such as massive obesity (see Chapter 233), or an anxiety disorder (see Chapter 226). Dyspneic patients with such disorders greatly appreciate knowing the cause of their discomfort and its prognosis, especially when it differs from what their perception has been.

Many patients with chronic dyspnea request *home oxygen therapy*. Such requests are reasonable if the patient has a condition causing chronic hypoxemia, provided that no evidence of carbon dioxide retention, with its attendant risk of suppression of respiratory drive, is present. Patients without significant hypoxemia—even those with chronic emphysema—do not benefit from oxygen therapy.

Selected patients with lung or heart disease may benefit from an *exercise program*; exercise tolerance often improves with even modest reversals in deconditioning, although the effect on survival is unproven (see Chapters 18, 30, 31, and 47). It is important that patients be reminded to note the level of activity that they can tolerate and report any decrease. Precipitants of worsening exercise tolerance should also be monitored.

The use of *anxiolytics* is helpful only in patients whose dyspnea is a manifestation of a severe anxiety disorder. Even then, extreme caution must be exercised in the long-term use of such medications (see Chapter 226). Prescribing tranquilizers for a patient with heart or lung disease who is anxious because of trouble with breathing is more likely to exacerbate the respiratory problem than to help it.

Patients with end-stage disease who continue to experience breathlessness despite a clear diagnosis and maximum therapy of the underlying etiology are not uncommon. Depression and insomnia, as well as anxiety, become part of a vicious cycle that is difficult for family and caregivers as well as patients.

Opioids in low oral and parenteral doses have been shown to provide symptomatic improvement among patients for whom palliation has become the goal of care. The principal side effect is constipation. Nebulized opioids have not been found to be effective in systematic reviews.

INDICATIONS FOR REFERRAL AND ADMISSION

For patients with underlying heart or lung disease who experience a worsening of their chronic dyspnea, prompt hospital admission should be considered, especially if the change is rapid. It may represent acute left ventricular decompensation, ventilatory failure, or hypoxemia. Acute anxiety can superficially mimic cardiopulmonary decompensation and needs to be ruled out (see prior discussion) before hospitalization is authorized. Pulmonary consultation may be helpful in the patient with suspected pulmonary hypertension, both for design of the diagnostic assessment and for the selection of the treatment plan if a secondary cause is identified.

A.H.G./A.G.M.

Annotated Bibliography

1. Karnani NG, Reisfield GM, Wilson GR. Evaluation of chronic dyspnea. Am Fam Physician 2005;71:1529. (*Effective review of dyspnea attributable to cardiac, pulmonary, and other causes.*)
2. Tobin MJ. Dyspnea: pathophysiologic basis, clinical presentation, and management. Arch Intern Med 1990;150:1604. (*Useful review, with emphasis on pathophysiology; includes a good discussion of hyperventilation syndrome; 97 references.*)
3. Gelbach BK, Geppert E. The pulmonary manifestations of left heart failure. Chest 2004;125:669-682. (*A careful review of the pathophysiology relevant to the differential diagnostic challenges; 132 references.*)
4. Enright PL, McClelland RL, Newman AB, et al. Underdiagnosis and under-treatment of asthma in the elderly. Cardiovascular Health Study Research Group. Chest 1999;116:603. (*Asthma was both underdiagnosed and undertreated in this community-based sample of nearly 5,000 people of age 65 years or older.*)
5. Le Jemtel TH, Padeletti M, Jelic S. Diagnostic and therapeutic challenges in patients with coexistent chronic obstructive pulmonary disease and chronic heart failure. J Am Coll Cardiol 2007;49:171. (*Focuses on overlap in presentation, on chronic obstructive pulmonary disease [COPD] as a cardiovascular risk, and on the functional effect of skeletal muscle atrophy common to both conditions.*)
6. Redfield MM, Jacobsen SJ, Burnett Jr JC, et al. Burden of systolic and diastolic ventricular dysfunction in the community: appreciating the scope of the heart failure epidemic. JAMA 2003;289:194. (*Documents high prevalences of subclinical systolic and diastolic dysfunction, with the latter associated with marked increases in all-cause mortality.*)
7. Rich S, Levitsky S, Brundage BH. Pulmonary hypertension from chronic pulmonary embolism. Ann Intern Med 1988;108:425. (*A review exploring the often-confusing relationship between these two conditions; 87 references.*)
8. Rich S, Dantzker DR, Ayers SM, et al. Primary pulmonary hypertension: a national prospective study. Ann Intern Med 1987;107:216. (*Findings from a national registry; the best available data on clinical and epidemiologic features.*)
9. Sin DD, Jones RL, Man SF. Obesity is a risk factor for dyspnea but not for airflow obstruction. Arch Intern Med 2002;162:1477. (*Dyspnea without objective evidence of obstruction contributes to overdiagnosis of asthma and overuse of bronchodilators among the obese.*)
10. Wang TJ, Levy D, Benjamin EJ, et al. The epidemiology of "asymptomatic" left ventricular systolic dysfunction: implications for screening. Ann Intern Med 2003;138:907. (*Prevalence was 3% to 6%, but there was insufficient evidence to justify screening with echocardiography or β-type natriuretic peptide [BNP].*)
11. American Association for Respiratory Care. Exercise testing for evaluation of hypoxemia and/or desaturation: 2001 revision and update. Respir Care 2001;46:514. (*Guidelines for the use of exercise testing for diagnosing causes of dyspnea and monitoring oxygen therapy; 74 references.*)
12. Carter R, Holiday DB, Nwasuruba C, et al. 6-Minute walk work for assessment of functional capacity in patients with COPD. Chest 2003;123:1408. (*Simply suggests the use of distance multiplied by body weight rather that distance alone.*)
13. Baumstark A, Swensson RG, Hessel SJ, et al. Evaluating the radiographic assessment of pulmonary venous hypertension in chronic heart disease. Am J Radiol 1984;142:877. (*Suggests that the assessment can be quite accurate, with a sensitivity of 0.75 and a specificity of 0.88.*)
14. Boxt LM, Bettmann MA, Gomes AS, et al. Shortness of breath—suspected cardiac origin. American College of Radiology. ACR appropriateness criteria. Radiology 2000;215(Suppl):23. (*Rates the value of imaging tests, with standard chest x-ray coming out on top.*)
15. Come PC. Echocardiographic recognition of pulmonary arterial disease and determination of its cause. Am J Med 1988;84:384. (*Provides evidence for the utility of ultrasonography in the identification and differential diagnosis of pulmonary hypertension.*)
16. D'Alonzo GE, Bower JS, Dantzker DR. Differentiation of patients with primary and thromboembolic pulmonary hypertension. Chest 1984;85:457. (*The pattern on perfusion lung scan is different.*)
17. King DK, Thompson BT, Johnson DC. Wheezing on maximal forced exhalation in the diagnosis of atypical asthma. Ann Intern Med 1989;110;451. (*Wheezing proved neither sensitive nor specific.*)
18. Cabanes L, Richaud-Thiriez B, Fulla Y, et al. Brain natriuretic peptide blood levels in the differential diagnosis of dyspnea. Chest 2001;120:2047. (*BNP levels distinguished between patients with COPD and questionable diastolic dysfunction in this small study.*)
19. Evans SE, Scanlon PD. Current practice in pulmonary function testing. Mayo Clinic Proc 2003;78:758. (*Effective review.*)
20. Ferguson GT, Enright PL, Buist AS, et al. Office spirometry for lung health assessment in adults: a consensus statement from the National Lung Health Education Program. Chest 2000;117:1146. (*Recommends widespread use of office spirometry of smokers in the primary care office.*)
21. Hankinson JL, Odencrantz JR, Fedan KB. Spirometric reference values from a sample of the general U.S. population. Am J Respir Crit Care Med 1999;159:179. (*Major population study.*)
22. Jones NL. Exercise testing in pulmonary evaluation: clinical application. N Engl J Med 1975;293:647. (*Describes the use of exercise pulmonary function tests in evaluating dyspnea; the article on p. 341 of this issue details methods and physiology of exercise testing.*)
23. Maisel AS, Krishnaswamy P, Nowak RM, et al. Rapid measurement of B-type natriuretic peptide in the emergency diagnosis of heart failure. N Engl J Med 2002;347:61. (*In the emergency room, BNP with a cutoff of 100 pg/mL had a sensitivity of 90% and a specificity of 76% for congestive heart failure as etiology of acute dyspnea.*)
24. Mulrow CD, Lucey CR, Farnett LE. Discriminating causes of dyspnea through clinical examination. J Gen Intern Med 1993;8:383. (*The accuracy of clinical assessment was 70%.*)
25. Pratt PC. Role of conventional chest radiography in diagnosis and exclusion of emphysema. Am J Med 1987;82:998. (*A review arguing that a high degree of accuracy can be achieved if validated criteria are used; 40 references.*)
26. Raffin TA. Indications for arterial blood gas analysis. Ann Intern Med 1986;105:390. (*A critical review of uses of blood gas determinations; 76 references.*)
27. Schoepf UJ, Goldhaber SZ, Costello P. Spiral computed tomography for acute pulmonary embolism. Circulation 2004;109:2160. (*Detailed review of comparative advantages and disadvantages of computed tomography and older imaging approaches.*)
28. Vasan RS, Benjamin EJ, Larson MG, et al. Plasma natriuretic peptides for community screening for left ventricular hypertrophy and systolic dysfunction: the Framingham Heart Study. JAMA 2002;288:1252. (*Finds limited usefulness in screening.*)
29. Abernathy AP, Currow DC, Frith P, et al. Randomised, double blind, placebo controlled crossover trial of sustained release morphine for the management of refractory dyspnea. BMJ 2003;327:1. (*Significant palliation among COPD patients with 20 mg of sustained-release morphine per day.*)
30. Booth S, Kelly MJ, Cox NP, et al. Does oxygen help dyspnea in patients with cancer? Am J Respir Crit Care Med 1996;153:1515. (*Oxygen and air were equally effective in reducing dyspnea in this randomized, controlled trial.*)
31. Crockett AJ, Cranston JM, Moss JR, et al. Domiciliary oxygen for chronic obstructive pulmonary disease (Cochrane review). In: Cochrane library, Issue 4. Oxford: Update Software, 2003. (*Long-term oxygen therapy improved survival for patients with severe hypoxemia but not for those with moderate hypoxemia or with only arterial desaturation at night.*)
32. Crockett AJ, Cranston JM, Antic N. Domiciliary oxygen for interstitial lung disease (Cochrane review). In: The Cochrane library, Issue 4. Oxford: Update

Software, 2003. (*The single trial in this review did not show an effect on mortality.*)

33. Jennings AL, Davies AN, Higgins JPT, et al. Opioids for the palliation of breathlessness in terminal illness (Cochrane review). In: The Cochrane library, Issue 3. Oxford: Update Software, 2003. (*There was some evidence to support the use of oral or parenteral opioids but not nebulized forms.*)

34. Liss HP, Grant BJB. The effect of nasal flow on breathlessness in patients with chronic obstructive lung disease. Am Rev Respir Dis 1988;137:1285. (*Nasal cannular delivery of room air provided as much relief of dyspnea as did cannular delivery of oxygen.*)

35. Man GCW, Hsu K, Sproule BJ. Effect of alprazolam on exercise and dyspnea in patients with chronic obstructive lung disease. Chest 1986;90:832. (*No benefit was found in patients who had normal oxygen tension values.*)

CHAPTER 41 ■ EVALUATION OF SUBACUTE AND CHRONIC COUGH

Cough is one of the most common symptoms that patients bring to the attention of primary care clinicians. Cough can be designated as acute (<3 weeks in duration), subacute (3 to 8 weeks in duration), or chronic (>8 weeks in duration). Acute cough is most often due to infection, especially the common cold. When accompanied by other cold symptoms, including those associated with rhinitis or sinusitis, or with lower respiratory tract disease such as bronchitis or pneumonia, the diagnosis is often evident. Specific treatment and reassurance can be offered (see Chapters 50 and 52). When "acute" cough heralds the onset of previously unrecognized chronic disease such as asthma or congestive heart failure, diagnosis may require more probing. Again, effective management of the underlying condition relieves the cough (see Chapters 48 and 32). Persistent cough following upper respiratory infection and lasting more than 3 weeks is not uncommon. Termed "postinfectious cough," this syndrome accounts for a significant proportion of subacute coughs.

Both subacute cough that is not related to infection and chronic cough generally pose even more of a diagnostic challenge. The list of causes ranges from the trivial to the life threatening. Patients often fear that "something is wrong." Those who smoke and have chronic bronchitis generally recognize that smoking is the cause of the cough, but they also fear lung cancer. Others may have reason to be concerned about AIDS or tuberculosis (TB). The primary physician must keep in mind these more worrisome causes but be aware that the most common causes of persistent cough among patients without evident etiologies are asthma, gastroesophageal reflux, and postnasal drip syndrome. In all cases, the objective is to conduct an efficient evaluation that avoids both unnecessary testing and excessive delay in providing both reassurance and symptom relief.

PATHOPHYSIOLOGY AND CLINICAL PRESENTATION (1–17)

The physiologic function of cough is to remove foreign substances and mucus from the respiratory tract. It is a three-phase mechanical process that involves a deep inspiration, increasing lung volume, and muscular contraction against a closed glottis and sudden opening of the glottis. The maneuver produces and sustains a high linear air velocity to expel material from the respiratory tree.

Cough is a reflex response that is mediated by the medulla but is subject to voluntary control. The afferent limb may involve receptors in the larynx, respiratory tree, pleura, acoustic duct, nose, sinuses, pharynx, stomach, or diaphragm. The receptors respond to mechanical, inflammatory, or irritant stimuli. The trigeminal, glossopharyngeal, phrenic, and vagus nerves can carry the afferent signal. The efferent limb of the cough reflex involves the recurrent laryngeal, phrenic, and spinal motor nerves, which innervate the respiratory muscles.

Cigarette smoking is the most common cause of chronic cough; may trigger the cough reflex by direct bronchial irritation; alternatively, smoking may induce inflammatory changes and the production of mucus, which stimulates a self-propagating productive cough. Chronic bronchitis may ensue. Chronic cough and decreased flow rates have been observed in adolescents after only 3 to 5 years of smoking. Pipe and cigar smoking cause lesser degrees of difficulty.

Environmental irritants play a major role in the production of cough in patients living in industrialized urban areas. Pollutants that are frequently involved are heavy smog, sulfur dioxide, nitrous oxide, and industrial gases such as ammonia. In Great Britain, the relationship between air quality and the production of cough has been documented. The dusts and particulate matter that are capable of producing pneumoconioses contribute to the problem (see Chapter 39). The excessive drying of normal airway moisture that takes place in centrally heated homes (humidity may fall to less than 10% unless a humidifier is used) can result in a persistent dry cough during the winter months.

Inflammation anywhere along the upper or lower respiratory tract is capable of producing cough; receptors capable of transmitting impulses that stimulate cough are believed to be distributed throughout the respiratory system. The greater the inflammatory stimulus, the greater is the white cell response and the more purulent is the sputum. (The green coloration of very purulent sputum is caused by the degeneration of white cells.) A number of patients experience a dry, persistent cough after an upper respiratory infection; these postinfectious coughs commonly last more than 3 weeks and may last more than 8 weeks. The pathophysiology may be unrelated to postnasal drip or airway hyperactivity and is believed to be related to airway epithelial damage. In some populations, infection with *Bordetella* species has proven to be a relatively common explanation for highly prolonged cough associated with infection.

Asthma due to airway hyperreactivity may present as cough. Most patients with classical asthma complain of cough, and in some cases cough is the symptom that predominates in the clinical picture. Studies of asthmatic patients have emphasized that cough can occur in the absence of wheezing or abnormalities on routine pulmonary function testing. The cough is characteristically worse at night and can be triggered or exacerbated by exposure to environmental irritants, allergens, or cold. Exercise is a common stimulant. In such cases, the bronchorrheal component of asthma predominates, but methacholine or carbachol challenge will often unmask the obstructive manifestations (see Chapter 48).

Chronic bronchitis due to smoking is among the most common causes of chronic cough and sputum production. The condition is defined clinically as the presence of a productive cough that persists for at least 3 months for 2 consecutive years. A morning cough is often prominent, and bronchospasm is a frequent accompaniment (see Chapter 47). *Bronchiectasis* is also characterized by cough and sputum production, but it differs clinically from bronchitis in that repeated bouts of hemoptysis and pneumonia are more likely to occur. Copious amounts of purulent sputum are often produced. Chronic cough and sputum production commonly persist between episodes of pneumonia. Focal destruction of supporting lung tissue leads to dilation of bronchi and focal findings of rhonchi and wheezes on physical examination. A history of suppurative pneumonia in childhood is sometimes elicited. *Eosinophilic bronchitis* in the absence of asthma has also been associated with chronic cough in 10% to 15% of cases in both primary care and specialist clinics. Its pathophysiology is largely undefined, although the cough does respond to inhaled corticosteroids.

Carcinoma of the lung, more often than not in the smoker, may present with cough in its early stages, particularly when an endobronchial lesion is present. Often, the cigarette smoker notes a change in the pattern of a chronic "cigarette cough." *Hemoptysis* is noted in about 5% to 10% of early cases. Other clues are localized wheezing and purulent sputum suggestive of obstruction. In later stages, cough is present in conjunction with weight loss, anorexia, and dyspnea. In some instances, a systemic syndrome (e.g., inappropriate secretion of antidiuretic hormone, hypertrophic pulmonary osteoarthropathy, dermatomyositis, peripheral neuropathy) may precede the appearance of tumor.

Interstitial pathology including fibrosis and *pulmonary edema* may stimulate mechanical receptors and result in a nonproductive cough. *Congestive heart failure with chronic interstitial pulmonary edema* is associated with nocturnal cough because venous return is increased at night, which worsens heart failure (see Chapter 32). When failure is severe, frothy pink or blood-tinged sputum may be noted. *Extraluminal compression* of bronchi also stimulates mechanical receptors; examples of compressing lesions include hilar adenopathy, aortic aneurysm, and neoplasm.

Because receptors of the afferent limb of the cough reflex are found in the nose, pharynx, sinuses, and acoustic ducts, common afflictions in these areas have been found to be common causes of cough. *Chronic allergic rhinitis* (see Chapter 222) with resultant postnasal drip ranks as one of the leading causes of chronic cough in specialty clinic populations. The nasal mucosa may be edematous and the pharyngeal mucosal "cobblestoned" in appearance. Similarly, *sinusitis* (see Chapter 219) may be associated with a persistent cough and sputum production secondary to excessive retropharyngeal drainage of

mucus. It accounts for up to one third of patients with postnasal drip syndrome. Even impacted cerumen and external otitis have been implicated in stimulating the cough reflex (see Chapter 218).

Because there are afferent limb receptors for the cough reflex in the stomach and lower esophagus, it is not surprising that a condition as common as *gastroesophageal reflux* is associated with chronic cough. In fact, it is among the three most common causes identified in case series of patients with persistent chronic cough. Mechanisms include (a) esophageal irritation with stimulation of an esophageal–tracheobronchial reflex and (b) nocturnal aspiration of gastric juices. Cough may be the only presenting symptom.

The use of *angiotensin-converting-enzyme* (ACE) *inhibitors* has been associated with an unexpectedly high incidence of dry nocturnal cough, with reports of 10% to 15% of patients being affected, with the incidence higher among women than men. First reported with use of enalapril, the cough has been associated with most long-acting ACE inhibitor preparations. Patients complain of an irritated feeling. The cough usually does not respond to a switch to another ACE inhibitor, although reducing the dose may help. In about 50% of instances, the cough is so annoying that ACE inhibitor therapy must be terminated. The pathophysiology of ACE inhibitor–induced cough is not entirely understood, but it appears to be an increase in sensitivity to the cough reflex. Therefore, ACE inhibitors may be unmasking subclinical cough associated with one of the aforementioned mechanisms.

Psychogenic cough has been described as more prevalent in children, but it may occur in adults; characteristically, it is nonproductive, occurs at times of emotional stress, and ceases during the night. The prevalence of psychogenic cough in reported series varies inversely with the attention to systematic evaluation and the search for the foregoing mechanisms.

DIFFERENTIAL DIAGNOSIS (1–13,16,17)

The common causes of chronic cough are listed in Table 41.1. In an often-cited series of 139 consecutive cases of chronic cough encountered in the community setting, the cause was hyperactive airway disease in 21%, postnasal drip in 19%, postinfectious status in 9%, chronic bronchitis in 4%, gastroesophageal reflux in 4%, and, in a few cases, occupational lung disease and psychiatric illness. In one referral setting study, a postnasal drip syndrome accounted for 41% of cases, asthma for 24%, esophageal reflux for 21%, and chronic bronchitis for 5%. Cough was the sole presentation of asthma in 28% of asthmatic patients and of reflux in 43% of patients with reflux. In one fourth of cases, more than one cause was identified. Sinusitis accounted for 38% of cases of postnasal drip. Insight from a growing number of series of patients from specialty cough clinics using systematic approaches to diagnosis suggests that when a patient who is not a smoker and not taking ACE inhibitors presents with chronic cough and has a normal chest radiograph, it is highly likely that the etiology will be related to asthma, gastroesophageal reflux disease (GERD), a postnasal drip syndrome (recently designated more generally *upper airway cough syndrome [UACS]*), or some combination of these three entities. This has been termed the pathogenetic triad of chronic cough of relatively obscure origin. Nonasthmatic eosinophilic bronchitis is less common but noteworthy because of its ease of diagnosis in the referral settings that are the source of most published series and its responsiveness to therapy. Rare but noteworthy causes of chronic cough include irritation of the pleura, diaphragm, or pericardium. Osteophytes of the

TABLE 41.1

IMPORTANT CAUSES OF CHRONIC OR PERSISTENT COUGH

Environmental Irritants
Cigarette smoking (cigar and pipe smoking to a lesser degree)
Pollutants (sulfur dioxide, nitrous oxide, particulate matter)
Dusts (all agents capable of producing pneumoconioses)
Lack of humidity

Lower Respiratory Tract Problems
Lung cancer
Asthma (including cough-variant and eosinophilic bronchitis)
Chronic obstructive lung disease (especially bronchitis)
Interstitial lung disease
Congestive heart failure (chronic interstitial pulmonary edema)
Pneumonitis
Bronchiectasis

Upper Respiratory Tract Problems
Chronic rhinitis
Chronic sinusitis
Disease of the external auditory canal
Pharyngitis

Angiotensin-Converting-Enzyme Inhibitors

Gastrointestinal Problems
Gastroesophageal reflux

Extrinsic Compressive Lesions
Adenopathy
Malignancy
Aortic aneurysm

Psychogenic Factors

cervical spine and pacemaker malfunction have been reported as truly rare causes of cough.

WORKUP (6–11,16–26)

Although in some cases the cause of a chronic cough is readily apparent, presentations of even the common underlying conditions may be subtle, so that careful investigation is necessary. During the initial workup, the physician should consider serious causes (cancer, TB, heart failure) while checking for the much more common treatable causes (asthma, esophageal reflux, postnasal drip or UACS). In a detailed study of workup for chronic cough, history offered the highest yield, with 70% of patients having a true-positive finding; physical examination was second, with 49%; and laboratory studies were third, with an average of 22% of patients having true-positive findings.

History

A careful history and description of the cough, combined with a review of aggravating and alleviating factors and any associated symptoms, can provide useful information, although presentations overlap to a considerable degree. A cough that worsens when the patient lies down suggests postnasal drip, esophageal reflux, bronchiectasis, bronchitis, and heart failure. A cough accompanied by the production of clear sputum is consistent with a hypersensitivity mechanism, whereas persis-

tent purulence suggests chronic infection (e.g., chronic sinusitis, bronchiectasis, or TB), and bloody sputum raises the specter of cancer, TB, and bronchiectasis (see Chapter 42). Associated symptoms of orthopnea, dyspnea on exertion, and paroxysmal nocturnal dyspnea implicate heart failure; dyspnea may also reflect pneumonitis or asthma. Chronic bronchitis is diagnosed by the history of a chronic productive cough 3 months of the year for 2 consecutive years. The diagnosis is reinforced by a reduction in coughing with cessation of smoking or avoidance of environmental irritants.

Although postnasal drip, throat clearing, and nasal discharge are characteristic of conditions causing a postnasal drip syndrome, some of these symptoms may also occur in patients with asthma or even esophageal reflux. Chronic throat clearing is also consistent with a psychogenic etiology. Although heartburn or a sour taste in the mouth are reported by most patients whose cough is caused by reflux, as many as 40% of those whose cough proves to be linked to reflux do not report these symptoms. Hoarseness is usually indicative of tracheobronchial disease with laryngeal involvement but may represent a tumor impinging on the recurrent laryngeal nerve.

The history should also detail smoking habits, environmental and occupational exposures, and use of ACE inhibitors and should include a review for previous allergies, asthma, sinusitis, recent respiratory infection, and TB exposure.

Despite the importance of careful history taking, it does not suffice. For example, in one study, the positive predictive value of a history consistent with asthma (nocturnal cough, cold induced, exercise induced, aerosols) was 56%. The positive predictive value of a history consistent with postnasal drip syndrome (throat clearing, sensation of drip, nasal discharge, previous sinusitis) was 52%. A history consistent with GERD (dyspepsia, cough worse after meals) was least predictive, with a positive predictive value of 40%. This limited value of history taking for the common causes of cough without apparent etiology has led to an emphasis on trials of therapy addressing the possibilities of asthma, GERD, and postnasal drip or UACS.

Physical Examination

Physical examination should emphasize the upper respiratory tract, chest, and cardiovascular system. The physician needs to examine the skin for cyanosis and clubbing; the pharynx for postnasal discharge, mucosal edema, and tonsillar enlargement; the nose for polyps, discharge, and obstruction; the sinuses for tenderness; and the ears for impacted cerumen or otitis. The trachea is palpated for position and the neck for masses and adenopathy. Auscultation and percussion of the lungs (including the apices) are performed to detect wheezing, crackles, and signs of consolidation or effusion. Generalized wheezing is associated with obstruction from asthma or bronchitis, but localized wheezing may be a sign of tumor. Wheezing only on maximal forced exhalation was found to be neither sensitive nor specific for the diagnosis of variant asthma. During cardiac examination, the physician should evaluate the jugular venous pulse for elevated systemic venous pressure, palpate for chamber enlargement, and listen for a third heart sound, all indicative of heart failure.

Laboratory Studies

Testing can very often be held to a minimum when a careful history is taken and a thorough physical examination performed. For example, when the history is suggestive of chronic rhinitis causing a postnasal drip, one can proceed directly to a diagnostic trial of antihistamines and decongestants without resorting to laboratory testing. Alternatively, a topically active corticosteroid nasal spray may be used for the trial. Similarly, the patient with suspected asthma may be given a diagnostic trial of inhaled steroids (see Chapter 48). In most cases of chronic cough, only a few, well-chosen studies are usually necessary. *Chest radiography* is essential when historical or physical evidence raises the question of carcinoma, pneumonitis, tuberculosis, heart failure, or bronchiectasis. However, the test is overused and not necessary in the nonsmoker who presents with a persistent cough after a recent upper respiratory infection and whose physical examination findings are normal. The chest film may be used to provide reassurance, but a careful explanation and follow-up in 4 to 6 weeks should suffice. The search for pneumonitis should be reserved for patients with a history of disease related to HIV infection or findings suggestive of ongoing infection (persistent production of purulent sputum, night sweats, fever, respiratory rate >25/min, rales, asymmetric respirations, increased vocal fremitus).

High-resolution computed tomography (CT) *scan* may identify parenchymal disease not seen on chest x-ray such as bronchiectasis. However, even when CT is used highly selectively only in patients with abnormalities on chest x-ray or physical examination, it provides useful information in roughly 1 in 6 cases. It should not be used in the routine evaluation of cough.

Sinus films are usually unnecessary when the history is positive for postnasal drip. In fact, the correlation between the appearance on films and symptoms considered typical of sinusitis may be poor. In rare instances, a patient who has eluded diagnosis may have an occult sinusitis identified by sinus films, with mucosal thickening of more than 6 mm identified on radiographic study. However, routine sinus films are unnecessary.

When purulent sputum is present or an infiltrate has been identified on chest x-ray films, every effort should be made to obtain *sputum for examination*. Patients with a history of producing purulent sputum in conjunction with cough but who cannot raise sputum at the time of examination should be instructed to drink a few glasses of water and remain awhile to see if sputum can be raised. Inducing sputum by use of a saline spray may also be helpful. A surprisingly common omission in evaluating a cough productive of purulent sputum is failure to obtain and examine the sputum.

An important component of the sputum examination is the *Gram's stain*. In persons at high risk for TB (e.g., recent immigrants, immunocompromised hosts), an *acid-fast stain* for tubercle bacilli is needed. *Culturing* the sputum is also important, especially when TB is a possibility, because the acid-fast examination is not very sensitive and the diagnosis cannot be ruled out with certainty until three early-morning sputum samples have failed to produce growth by 4 to 6 weeks (see Chapters 38 and 49).

The recent description of *eosinophilic bronchitis* provides another reason to examine sputum. However, the capability to induce sputum and examine it to determine sputum eosinophilia (>3% eosinophils) is limited to referral settings.

Sputum cytology—in which three early-morning sputum samples are obtained—can be a useful screening test for pulmonary neoplasm (see Chapters 37, 42, and 53) when clinical findings raise suspicion (history of smoking, hemoptysis, nodule on chest x-ray film). Pulmonary histiocytes must be demonstrated on each specimen to prove that the sample of pulmonary secretions is adequate. A "negative" test result in the absence of histiocytes is the source of many false-negative readings.

Because sputum cytology is not a particularly sensitive test, it cannot be used to rule out lung cancer. When tumor remains

in the differential diagnosis, fiberoptic *bronchoscopy* should be considered. Bronchoscopy is also helpful in the evaluation of obstructing lesions and infiltrates that elude diagnosis because biopsy specimens, washings, and cultures can be taken. However, if the chest radiographic findings are normal and no hemoptysis or history of smoking is present, then the yield from bronchoscopy is very low, and further workup for cancer is unlikely to be productive.

Chronic Cough without Apparent Cause

When the cause remains elusive despite the extensive workup just described, *variant asthma, postnasal drip syndrome (or UACS)*, and *gastroesophageal reflux* should be considered. These conditions account for a substantial proportion of hard-to-diagnose cases of chronic cough. As noted earlier, the history and physical examination may not reveal the symptoms and signs typically associated with them. Starting empiric therapy with decongestants, first with bronchodilators and then histamine$_2$ antagonists, is a reasonable approach. If testing is to be effective and a false-positive diagnosis avoided, knowledge of test accuracy in identifying these conditions in patients with chronic cough is necessary. Traditional *spirometry* with *bronchodilator administration* was found in one study to have only a 50% positive predictive value in patients with chronic cough because of a high false-positive rate (33%), although its sensitivity was excellent (approaching 100%). *Methacholine challenge* to induce bronchospasm has a similarly high degree of sensitivity but a lower false-positive rate (22%), and so it has a slightly better positive predictive value (60%). Both tests rule out asthma if results are normal. A positive test result needs to be confirmed by a response to bronchodilator therapy.

The diagnosis of esophageal reflux is harder to make in the absence of typical symptoms. Whereas a history of retrosternal burning traveling upward has a predictive value of greater than 90% for gastroesophageal reflux, its absence does not rule it out. Prolonged *monitoring* of *esophageal pH* has proved to be the most effective test for esophageal reflux in patients with chronic cough. In the best study of its efficacy, the test had a positive predictive value of greater than 95%, with few false-positive and false-negative results. Monitoring of pH was far superior to barium swallow, which had a high false-negative rate. As noted, an alternative to pH monitoring is a *diagnostic trial of therapy with a histamine$_2$ blocker* (see Chapter 61). However, 1 to 2 months of therapy may be necessary to demonstrate a definitive reduction in cough. Thus, pH monitoring may be the most rapid means of diagnosis of reflux-induced cough. Patients with reflux symptoms do not need radiologic study or endoscopy unless cancer or obstruction is a concern (see Chapter 61).

SYMPTOMATIC THERAPY AND PATIENT EDUCATION (6–8,10,11,17,19,28–31)

The most effective means of stopping the cough is to identify and treat the underlying cause (see Chapters 47, 49, 61, and 222). An empiric trial of an etiologic therapy can be highly effective in providing a diagnosis as well as relief of symptoms (see prior discussion); however, certain etiologic therapies should not be used empirically, especially antibiotics in the absence of proven infection. Symptomatic management is distinguished from empiric etiologic therapy. It is directed at eliminating precipitants and suppressing the cough. The goal is to prevent the complications that may result from pro-longed forceful coughing, such as sleeplessness, musculoskeletal pain, rib fractures, pneumothorax, exhaustion, pneumomediastinum, posttussive syncope (see Chapter 24), and rupture of subconjunctival or nasal veins. The occurrence of any of these complications may be a reason for occasionally suppressing a cough that has not been completely diagnosed.

The first priority and simplest manipulation is to remove or reduce irritants. Of paramount importance is *cessation of smoking* and passive exposure to cigarette smoke; this alone eliminated cough in 77% and reduced it in another 17% of patients within 1 month. Second, an appropriate *humidity* should be maintained. If a humidifier is used, it should be kept clean because it can become colonized with bacteria or fungi and cause infection or hypersensitivity pneumonitis. Third, adequate internal *hydration* should be encouraged, with at least 1,500 mL of fluid consumed daily. These simple measures alone may abolish cough in many patients.

The patient with a chronic cough secondary to established underlying lung disease requires careful education. The patient must be informed that sputum should be expectorated when possible. Patients with chronic bronchitis or bronchiectasis can be taught how to cough with quiet, forceful expirations and how to perform *postural drainage* to promote the removal of mucus from the bronchioles. Postural drainage is best performed before meals and at bedtime. *Ipratropium* is sometimes helpful in reducing nighttime cough in the patient with chronic obstructive pulmonary disease (see Chapter 47).

Patients with chronic cough often request *temporary cough suppression* to allow uninterrupted sleep; such suppression is also required when complications of cough arise. A wide variety of agents have been used to treat cough. Agents that act peripherally are effective in acute or chronic bronchitis but are not available in the United States. The most effective agents that are available are the *narcotic antitussives*, which act centrally to suppress the medullary cough center. Other preparations are expectorants or mucolytic agents, which merely help to mobilize sputum. They can also have a placebo effect. When cough significantly interferes with sleeping or eating, a narcotic cough suppressant should be used. *Codeine* is usually considered the drug of choice. It should be given in relatively small doses of 8 to 15 mg at intervals of 3 to 4 hours, according to the patient's needs. In many instances, a dose before bedtime will suffice. Liquid and tablet preparations are equally effective. If a small dose does not suppress the cough, doses of up to 60 mg every 3 to 4 hours may be tried. It is worth noting that many patients expect to use a syrup for cough suppression; prescribing the drug in syrup form may provide some psychological benefit. Patients for whom a narcotic antitussive is prescribed should be given small quantities and followed closely to ensure that the cough resolves and excessive use does not result. The obvious exception to this precaution is the patient with incurable lung cancer or other terminal illness, who should receive the doses necessary to provide relief from the discomfort of persistent cough.

Nonnarcotic antitussives lack addiction potential but are not as effective as codeine. The most popular and effective over-the-counter cough suppressant is *dextromethorphan*, which has a mild suppressant effect. Many over-the-counter preparations contain *alcohol*, *sympathomimetics*, and *antihistamines*. The mucolytic effects of alcohol are minimal. The sympathomimetics are of little use except in patients whose cough derives from chronic vasomotor rhinitis (see Chapter 222). The antihistamines are most useful for patients with allergic upper airway disease (see Chapter 222) and are a helpful adjunct for inducing sleep when taken at bedtime. Some over-the-counter agents dull the peripheral sensory receptors; this is the rationale for putting mild topical anesthetics in sprays, syrups, and cough lozenges. They are of questionable utility.

Expectorants are heavily consumed. More than 60 preparations containing guaifenesin are available; terpin hydrate is another popular expectorant. These agents are often combined with an effective cough suppressant and, as such, produce a beneficial effect, but by themselves they have no proven effect and represent an unnecessary expense. They are given when the patient insists on something for cough but clear indications for cough suppression are lacking or when the patient believes that expectorants will help. Systematic review of randomized trials of over-the-counter remedies in the setting of acute cough suggests either no effect or an effect size small enough to be of doubtful clinical significance.

Patients with cough secondary to asthma respond to inhaled topically active *corticosteroids* and *bronchodilators* (see Chapter 48). Topical steroid therapy is effective for patients with eosinophilic bronchitis and may also help in allergic rhinitis (see Chapter 222). Patients with persistent cough after a recent respiratory tract infection and no signs of pneumonitis may benefit from a short course of inhaled steroid therapy, which presumably lessens residual inflammatory changes. Time is another effective therapy. If *Bordetella pertussis* infection is suspected, treatment with erythromycin or (if the patient is allergic) trimethoprim–sulfamethoxazole for 14 days should be considered.

Patients with suspected reflux should respond to a course of antireflux therapy with *antacids*, *histamine₂ blockers*, and *proton-pump inhibitors* (see Chapter 61), although, as noted, the benefits may not become apparent for several weeks.

INDICATIONS FOR REFERRAL

Although endobronchial cancer is feared, it is not a common cause of chronic cough in the absence of other findings, especially in the patient with normal chest radiographic findings. However, for the patient without a diagnosis who has risk factors for cancer (smoking, occupational exposure), a chest CT may be indicated. A consultation for consideration of bronchoscopy may also be warranted, particularly if the CT findings are abnormal. The patient without risk factors and normal chest radiographic findings, or the patient with risk factors and a normal chest CT, can be followed expectantly without resort to bronchoscopy because the likelihood of a positive study result is very small.

A.G.M./A.H.G.

Annotated Bibliography

1. Pratter MR. Overview of common causes of chronic cough. Chest 2006;129:59S. (*Upper airway cough syndrome [UACS] is the most common of the causes, which also include gastroesophageal reflux disease and asthma; among 31 papers in a special supplement covering all aspects of cough.*)

2. Bloustine S, Langston L, Miller T, et al. Ear cough (Arnold's reflex). Otol Rhinol Laryngol 1976;85:406. (*A clinical survey of 688 patients revealed an incidence of 1.74% for ear cough reflex, a reminder to examine the ear.*)

3. Corrao W, Braman SS, Irwin RS. Chronic cough as the sole presenting manifestation of bronchial asthma. N Engl J Med 1979;300:633. (*An important*

early paper presenting six patients with cough as the presenting symptom of asthma; they had no prior history of wheezing.)

4. Dicpinigaitis PV. Cough in asthma and eosinophilic bronchitis. Thorax 2004;59:71. (*An excellent succinct summary of the pathophysiology and treatment of cough-variant asthma and eosinophilic bronchitis.*)

5. Fontana GA, Pistolesi M. Chronic cough and gastro-esophageal reflux. Thorax 2003;58:1092. (*Reviews pathophysiology as well as diagnosis and treatment.*)

6. Pratter MR. Chronic upper airway cough syndrome secondary to rhinosinus diseases (previously referred to as postnatal drip syndrome). Chest 2006;129:63S. (*Introduces UACS and describes its differential diagnosis in detail; among 31 papers in a special supplement covering all aspects of cough.*)

7. Braman S. Chronic cough due to chronic bronchitis. Chest 2006;129104S. (*Cessation of smoking and exposure to other noxious stimuli is critical.*)

8. Pratter MR, Brightling CE, Boulet, et al. An empiric integrative approach to the management of cough. Chest 2006;129:222S. (*Offers algorithms for acute, subacute, and chronic cough; among 31 papers in a special supplement covering all aspects of cough.*)

9. Holmes RL, Fadden CT. Evaluation of the patient with chronic cough. Am Family Physician 2004;69:2159. (*A lucid review.*)

10. Irwin RS, Corrao WM, Pratter MR. Chronic persistent cough in the adult: the spectrum and frequency of causes and successful outcome of specific therapy. Am Rev Respir Dis 1981;123:413. (*An intensive study of a series of 49 patients revealed 12 with asthma; 14 with postnasal drip; 9 with asthma plus postnasal drip, usually following upper respiratory infection; 6 with bronchitis; 5 with esophagitis; and 1 each with cough of malignant, cardiac, or interstitial origin.*)

11. Irwin RS, Madison JM. Primary care: the diagnosis and treatment of cough. N Engl J Med 2000;343:1715. (*An excellent review including acute and subacute as well as chronic cough.*)

12. Irwin RS, Madison JM. Symptom research on chronic cough: a historical perspective. Ann Intern Med 2001;134:809. (*A thoughtful reflection on how we have come to know what we know about cough, together with arguments for the anatomic diagnostic approach.*)

13. Israeli ZH, Hall WD. Cough and angioneurotic edema associated with angiotensin-converting enzyme inhibitor therapy. Ann Intern Med 1992;117:234. (*A review of pathophysiology and clinical presentation.*)

14. Laudon RG. Smoking and cough frequency. Rev Respir Dis 1976;114:1033. (*Confirms that smokers cough more frequently than nonsmokers.*)

15. McFadden FR Jr. Exertional dyspnea and cough as preludes to acute attacks of asthma. N Engl J Med 1975;292:555. (*Wheezing may be absent as an early manifestation of an acute attack, and cough may dominate the clinical picture.*)

16. Morice AH, Kastelik JA. Chronic cough in adults. Thorax 2003;58:901. (*An excellent systematic review of the clinical experience of chronic cough.*)

17. Palombini BC, Villanova CA, Araujo E, et al. A pathogenic triad in chronic cough: asthma, postnasal drip syndrome, and gastroesophageal reflux disease. Chest 1999;116:279. (*The five most important causative factors were asthma, postnasal drip syndrome, gastroesophageal reflux disease, bronchiectasis, and tracheobronchial collapse.*)

18. Diehr P, Wood RW, Bushyhead J, et al. Prediction of pneumonia in outpatients with acute cough—a statistical approach. J Chron Dis 1984;37:215. (*A study of nearly 2,000 patients presenting with cough with or without radiographic evidence of pneumonia; presents a discriminate analysis scoring system.*)

19. Pratter MR, Bartter T, Akers S, et al. An algorithmic approach to chronic cough. Ann Intern Med 1993;119:977. (*Describes a sequential workup with the use of response to antihistamine–decongestant medication.*)

20. Thiadens HA, de Bock GH, Dekker FW, et al. Identifying asthma and chronic obstructive pulmonary disease in patients with persistent cough presenting to general practitioners: descriptive study. BMJ 1998;316:1286. (*Of those presenting with persistent cough, 39% were found to have asthma and 7% chronic obstructive pulmonary disease.*)

21. Irwin RS, French CT, Smyrnios NA, et al. Interpretation of positive results of a methacholine inhalation challenge and one week of inhaled bronchodilator use in diagnosing and treating cough-variant asthma. Arch Intern Med 1997;157:1981. (*The response to specific asthma therapy was not associated with the dose of methacholine required to reduce forced expiratory volume in 1 second.*)

22. King DK, Thompson BT, Johnson DC. Wheezing on maximal forced exhalation in the diagnosis of atypical asthma. Ann Intern Med 1989;110:451. (*The maneuver proved neither sensitive nor specific for the diagnosis of asthma.*)

23. McGarvey LP, Heaney LG, Lawson JT, et al. Evaluation and outcome of patients with chronic nonproductive cough using a comprehensive diagnostic protocol. Thorax 1998;53:738. (*Asthma, gastroesophageal reflux disease, and postnasal drip syndrome were equally common and responsive to therapy in this series.*)

24. McGarvey LPA. Which investigations are most useful in the diagnosis of chronic cough? Thorax 2004;59:342. (*A succinct but detailed and quantitative description of the anatomic diagnostic protocol.*)

25. Poe RH, Harder RV, Israel RH, et al. Chronic persistent cough: experience in diagnosis and outcome using an anatomic diagnostic protocol. Chest 1989;95:723. (*Irwin's protocol does not work as well in the community setting; in about 14% of cases, the underlying condition remains undiagnosed.*)

26. Smyrnios NA, Irwin RS, Curley FJ, et al. From a prospective study of chronic cough: diagnostic and therapeutic aspects in older adults. Arch Intern Med 1998;158:1222. (*Causes among older adults were the same as among younger adults: postnasal drip, gastroesophageal reflux disease, and asthma predominated.*)

27. Chang AB, Lasserson TJ, Kiljander TO, et al. Systematic review and meta-analysis of randomised controlled trials of gastro-oesophageal reflux interventions for chronic cough associated with gastrooesophageal reflux. BMJ 2006;332:11. (*Proton-pump inhibitors were effective but less universally so than guideline recommendations would suggest.*)

28. Morice AH, Menon MS, Mulrennan SA, et al. Opiate therapy in chronic cough. Am J Respir Crit Care Med 2007;175:312-315. (*A randomized, controlled trial, finding that morphine sulfate was effective as an antitussive in intractable chronic cough at doses of 5 to 10 mg.*)

29. Bolser DC. Cough suppressant and pharmacologic protussive therapy. Chest 2006;129:238S. (*A comprehensive review; among 31 papers in a special supplement covering all aspects of cough.*)

30. Metlay JP, Stafford RS, Singer DE. National trends in the use of antibiotics by primary care physicians for adult patients with cough. Arch Intern Med 1998;158:1813. (*Cough-related visits and the proportion of patients receiving antibiotics increased from 1980 to 1994; overall, 66% received antibiotics!*)

31. Schroeder K, Fahey T. Systematic review of randomized controlled trials of over the counter cough medicines for acute cough in adults. BMJ 2002;324:1. (*Reviews the conflicting evidence on the effectiveness of antitussives, expectorants, and histamine–decongestant combinations, at least for acute cough.*)

CHAPTER 42 ■ EVALUATION OF HEMOPTYSIS

Hemoptysis is the coughing up of either blood-tinged or grossly bloody sputum. Because of its well-known associations with cancer and tuberculosis, hemoptysis is an alarming symptom for both patient and physician. In the office, the primary physician is usually confronted with a patient who has noted sputum streaked with blood. Most patients prove to have inconsequential lesions, but a thorough evaluation is necessary because the seriousness of the underlying cause does not correlate with the amount of blood coughed up.

PATHOPHYSIOLOGY AND CLINICAL PRESENTATION (1–9)

Inflammation of the tracheobronchial mucosa accounts for many cases of hemoptysis. Minor mucosal erosions can result from *upper respiratory infections* and *bronchitis*; blood-streaked sputum is often noted, especially if coughing has been vigorous and prolonged. Patients with *bronchiectasis* are more subject to recurrent episodes of grossly bloody sputum because necrosis of the bronchial mucosa can be quite severe. Up to 50% of patients with bronchiectasis experience hemoptysis. In the United States, hemoptysis occurring with *tuberculosis* (TB) is usually caused by mucosal ulceration, although potentially fatal bleeding can occur when a blood vessel adjacent to a cavitary lesion ruptures. About 10% to 15% of patients with TB report some form of hemoptysis; most of these episodes are minor and involve sputum tinged with small amounts of blood. Endobronchial inflammatory injury from granuloma formation is the mechanism of hemoptysis associated with *sarcoidosis*; small amounts of blood-streaked sputum are occasionally noted.

Mucosal injury can also be a consequence of *bronchogenic carcinoma*. Disruption of endobronchial tissue may be minor and cause little more than minimal hemoptysis from time to time; hemorrhage is rare. Between 35% and 55% of patients with proven bronchogenic carcinoma report at least one episode of hemoptysis during the course of their illness; it is the presenting symptom in about 10% of cases. The amount of bleeding can vary considerably and need not be impressive. For example, in one study, malignancy was the cause in 25% of patients with minimal hemoptysis. However, most patients have a positive smoking history and abnormal chest radiographic findings. *Carcinoma metastatic to the lung* rarely results in hemoptysis. *Bronchial adenomas* are quite vascular, and they are commonly central and endobronchial in location; as a consequence, they frequently bleed, and recurrent episodes of hemoptysis are reported in about half of cases.

Injury to the pulmonary vasculature is an important source of hemoptysis. *Lung abscess* may result in damage to adjacent vessels and frequently presents with bloody and purulent sputum. *Necrotizing pneumonias*, such as those produced by *Klebsiella*, can cause substantial vascular disruption; 25% to 50% of patients cough up tenacious, bloody sputum referred to as "currant jelly." *Aspergillomas* are also capable of causing vascular injury; hemoptysis is the most common symptom of the condition. The patient with an aspergilloma is typically a compromised host with prior cavitary disease from TB, bronchiectasis, or the like. *Pulmonary infarction* secondary to embolization is characterized by the sudden onset of pleuritic pain in conjunction with hemoptysis; embolization without infarction does not cause hemoptysis. Pulmonary contusion resulting from blunt *chest trauma* may present with hemoptysis following a nonpenetrating blow to the thorax.

Marked elevations in pulmonary capillary pressure can cause vascular injury and extravasation of red cells. The pink, frothy sputum of *pulmonary edema* is a manifestation of this process. More grossly bloody sputum sometimes occurs in severe mitral stenosis when a dilated pulmonary–bronchial venous connection ruptures. Vasculitic injury is responsible for the hemoptysis found in *Wegener's granulomatosis* and *Goodpasture's syndrome*. Hematuria often accompanies both conditions. Hereditary vascular malformations are subject to recurrent bleeding. *Arteriovenous malformations* may be accompanied by an audible bruit on auscultation of the lung. In *hereditary hemorrhagic telangiectasia*, a family history of bleeding problems is often present, or prior episodes of bleeding from multiple sites have been noted; telangiectasia may be visible in the buccal cavity and on the skin. Bleeding into the interstitium characterizes *idiopathic pulmonary hemosiderosis*. This rare disease, uncommon in adults, is manifested by diffuse interstitial infiltrates, anemia, and hemoptysis.

Hemoptysis may be the first sign of a *bleeding disorder* or *excessive anticoagulant therapy*; however, an underlying bronchopulmonary lesion is usually also present.

DIFFERENTIAL DIAGNOSIS (1–11)

Acute and chronic bronchitis are the most common causes, followed by bronchogenic carcinoma, TB, pneumonia, and bronchiectasis. Most prevalence figures are obtained from chest clinics and inpatient units serving preselected populations of patients with either abnormal chest radiographic findings or unexplained hemoptysis; therefore, they cannot be readily extrapolated to the primary care setting. In everyday office practice, the nasal mucosa and oropharynx are more often the source of blood-tinged sputum than is the lower respiratory tract. The high incidence of pulmonary infections associated with HIV, the more widespread use of fiberoptic bronchoscopy, and increases in cigarette smoking and lung cancer in women also must be kept in mind when data from published clinical series that are >10 years old are being interpreted. In a fiberoptic bronchoscopy study performed in a general hospital setting that included both inpatients and outpatients, bronchitis accounted for 37% of cases, bronchogenic carcinoma for 19%, TB for 7%, and bronchiectasis for only 1%. The briskness of bleeding did not help in discriminating among causes. In primary care settings, the diagnosis of lung cancer following a first presentation with hemoptysis is much lower: 7.5% in men and 4.3% in women in a large study of alarm symptoms in the United Kingdom. This study included patients with abnormal chest x-rays at the time of presentation. In a review of studies comprising a total of nearly 1,000 patients with hemoptysis and normal chest radiographic findings, lung cancer was eventually diagnosed in 5.4%. Most cancers that cause hemoptysis are endobronchial, but about 15% are parenchymal. The more common and important causes of hemoptysis are listed in Table 42.1.

WORKUP (1–6,10,12–21)

As noted earlier, most cases of blood-tinged sputum encountered in the primary care setting, especially during the winter, originate in the upper respiratory tract. Such cases do not require further investigation. To avoid unnecessary workup for a pulmonary cause, the history and physical examination should first focus on the nasal and oropharyngeal mucosa. Only in the absence of an upper respiratory source of bleeding need further workup proceed in the manner detailed in the following paragraphs.

History

Evaluation of the patient with a suspected lower respiratory tract source of hemoptysis should begin with consideration of the epidemiology of the serious underlying causes. Concern about pulmonary neoplasm should be highest in the older man with a long history of heavy smoking or asbestos exposure. The elderly patient with evidence of old disease on chest x-ray

TABLE 42.1

IMPORTANT CAUSES OF HEMOPTYSIS

Gross Hemoptysis
Tuberculosis (with cavitary disease)
Bronchiectasis
Bronchial adenoma
Bronchogenic carcinoma (uncommon)
Aspergilloma
Necrotizing pneumonia
Lung abscess
Pulmonary contusion
Arteriovenous malformation
Hereditary hemorrhagic telangiectasia
Bleeding disorder or excessive anticoagulant therapy
Mitral stenosis (with rupture of a bronchial vessel)
Immune alveolar disease

Blood-Streaked Sputum
Any of the causes of gross hemoptysis
Upper respiratory tract infection
Chronic bronchitis
Sarcoidosis
Bronchogenic carcinoma
Tuberculosis
Pulmonary infarction
Pulmonary edema
Mitral stenosis
Idiopathic pulmonary hemosiderosis
Immune alveolar disease

films should be presumed to have reactivated TB infection. The adolescent with hemoptysis may have a new infection resulting from recent TB exposure. The compromised host with previous cavitary disease is at risk for an aspergilloma. TB is also a major concern among patients with HIV infection.

The patient's description of the sputum associated with hemoptysis can be of some diagnostic help. Pink sputum is suggestive of pulmonary edema fluid; putrid sputum is indicative of a lung abscess; material resembling currant jelly points to a necrotizing pneumonia; copious amounts of purulent sputum mixed with blood are consistent with bronchiectasis. The commonly described blood-streaked sputum is nonspecific.

The patient should be asked about previous episodes of bleeding, any family history of hemoptysis, hematuria, concurrent pleuritic chest pain, known heart murmur or history of rheumatic fever, lymph node enlargement, blunt chest trauma, symptoms of heart failure (see Chapter 32), and use of anticoagulant drugs. Determining the amount of blood produced is not particularly helpful for diagnostic purposes. As noted earlier, it is important to be certain that the patient has no history of a coexisting nasopharyngeal problem or a source of gastrointestinal bleeding that may be mistaken for true hemoptysis.

Physical Examination

Physical examination is directed at detecting nonpulmonary sources of bleeding in addition to evidence of chest and systemic disease. The vital signs should be checked for fever and tachypnea, the skin for ecchymoses and telangiectasia, and the nails for clubbing. Clubbing is associated with neoplasm, bronchiectasis, lung abscess, and other severe pulmonary disorders

(see Chapter 45). Nodes are examined for enlargement, which is suggestive of sarcoidosis, TB, and malignancy (see Chapters 12 and 51). The neck is noted for jugular venous distention, consistent with heart failure and severe mitral disease. Examination of the chest should include a search for bruits, signs of consolidation, wheezes, crackles, and chest wall contusion.

The history and physical findings can be used to determine the pace at which workup should proceed, in addition to the selection and sequence of laboratory tests. Patients with minimal hemoptysis may be evaluated on an outpatient basis as long as they are given explicit advice to return immediately if severe bleeding ensues. The patient with a suspected bleeding diathesis should not be sent home.

Laboratory Studies

Chest X-Ray

Chest radiography is essential to assessment. As noted earlier, the majority of patients with hemoptysis resulting from bronchogenic carcinoma have abnormal chest radiographic findings. In addition to uncovering a mass lesion, chest films may reveal an abscess, infiltrate, interstitial change (see Chapter 51), hilar adenopathy, signs of congestive failure (see Chapter 32), or evidence of significant mitral stenosis (see Chapter 33). Less common radiologic findings include peribronchial cuffing, indicative of bronchiectasis, and a crescentic radiolucency surrounding a coin lesion, characteristic of an aspergilloma. However, in most instances, the appearance of the chest film is normal, and consideration of further study is warranted.

Sputum Stains

A *sputum Gram's stain* is essential if the sputum appears grossly purulent or the patient is febrile. An *acid-fast stain* for tubercle bacilli is also essential, not only for diagnosis, but also for a rough assessment of infectivity (see Chapter 49). The sensitivity of the acid-fast smear depends on the diligence with which the search for pathogenic organisms is made. In one series, only 20% of culture-positive samples were identified in advance by acid-fast smear. It should be noted that despite the very high specificity of a positive smear, its predictive value may be as low as 50% when the sputum specimens of low-risk patients are examined. A *tuberculin skin test* should be performed if the patient's purified protein derivative reactivity status is not known. However, approximately 7% of all adults (25% of adults >50 years) will have positive reactions (see Chapters 38 and 49).

Sputum Cytologies

Sputum cytologies should be obtained in all patients without a clear diagnosis. It used to be thought that the sensitivity of a single sputum cytology examination was about 70% in the detection of squamous cell lesions and that three consecutive cytologic examinations increased the sensitivity to 90%. However, data from the large screening trials suggest a lower sensitivity, at least for early cancers. The specificity of sputum cytology is >99% when the specimen is reviewed by an experienced cytopathologist.

Fiberoptic Bronchoscopy

Fiberoptic bronchoscopy can be extremely helpful for diagnosis when used thoughtfully. Its most common indication is to exclude the possibility of tumor. However, the test should not be viewed as a routine part of the evaluation for hemoptysis because the yield is extremely low in situations in which the risk for malignancy is very low (e.g., a nonsmoker <50 years of age with normal chest radiographic findings). Bronchoscopy enhances the sensitivity of cytologic and bacteriologic studies when washings for specimens are obtained during the procedure, and the test has proved capable of detecting otherwise occult endobronchial cancers in patients at increased risk for lung malignancy (e.g., >50 years, male gender, history of smoking), even if the chest radiographic findings are nonlocalizing. Patients with a high-risk profile, "positive" or "suspect" cytology, or a radiologic abnormality are appropriate candidates for bronchoscopy. Subjecting low-risk patients to bronchoscopic examination is wasteful and unlikely to affect management or outcome. Moreover, the cost and morbidity associated with bronchoscopy are not trivial.

Serious complications are rare with fiberoptic bronchoscopy, but they do occur. In a review of 48,000 procedures, <100 life-threatening cardiovascular or respiratory complications were reported, most often in older persons with chronic obstructive pulmonary disease and coronary disease. Hypoxia occurs commonly following bronchoscopy.

Bronchoscopy is mandatory in all patients with massive hemoptysis who are being seriously considered for surgery, to localize the site of bleeding.

Chest Computed Tomography (CT)

Chest CT may better define a suspect lesion seen on chest x-ray films and may be indicated for some patients with normal chest radiographic findings to increase the sensitivity for parenchymal lesions. CT also identifies endobronchial tumors with a sensitivity of approximately 80%. However, the specificity of CT-visualized endobronchial lesions for cancer is somewhat limited (approximately 65%).

Bleeding Studies

The parameters of bleeding, such as the *prothrombin time*, *partial thromboplastin time*, *platelet count*, and *bleeding time*, should be considered if more than one site of bleeding is noted.

Cryptogenic Hemoptysis

Cryptogenic hemoptysis is hemoptysis occurring in patients with normal or nonlocalizing chest radiographic findings and nondiagnostic findings on fiberoptic bronchoscopy. What to do in such a situation can be perplexing. The prognosis appears to be favorable, with >90% of these patients experiencing resolution of their hemoptysis by 6 months and no cases of cancer, active TB, or other serious pathology emerging after the initial evaluation. A careful history and physical examination, in combination with chest radiography and the proper use of bronchoscopy, appear to exclude cancer, active TB, and other must-not-miss diseases effectively, so repeated bronchoscopy, pulmonary angiography, CT, and bronchography are of little use in these patients. In one study, bronchial inflammation (bronchitis) was the most common cause, followed by the sequelae of old tuberculous disease.

INDICATIONS FOR REFERRAL AND ADMISSION (1,12,16,19–21)

Patients with hemoptysis who are believed to be at increased risk for an underlying malignancy (abnormal chest radiographic findings, male sex, >50 years, smoking history) are candidates for bronchoscopy. Patients with brisk bleeding require urgent hospitalization.

A.G.M.

Annotated Bibliography

1. Bidwell JL, Pachner RW. Hemoptysis: diagnosis and management. Am Fam Physician 2005;72:1253. (*Lucid review highlighting diagnostic cues and offering an algorithm for efficient approach to diagnosis.*)
2. Jones R, Latinovic R, Charlton J, et al. Alarm symptoms in early diagnosis of cancer in primary care: cohort study using General Practice Research Database. BMJ 2007;334:1040. (*After 4,812 new episodes of hemoptysis, 220 diagnoses of respiratory tract cancer were made in men and 81 in women, for positive predictive values of 7.5% and 4.3%, respectively.*)
3. Barker AF. Medical progress: bronchiectasis. N Engl J Med 2002;346:1383. (*Excellent review.*)
4. Collard HR, Gruber MP. Anatomy of a diagnosis. N Engl J Med 2003;349:987. (*Clinical care demonstrates a logical approach to diagnosis, in this case leading to the urgent repair of aortobronchial fistula.*)
5. Hirshburg B, Biran I, Glazer M, et al. Hemoptysis: etiology, evaluation, and outcome in a tertiary referral hospital. Chest 1997;112:440. (*Retrospective analysis of 208 patients; bronchiectasis, cancer, bronchitis, and pneumonia each accounted for approximately 20% of cases.*)
6. Johnston H, Reisz G. Changing spectrum of hemoptysis. Arch Intern Med 1989;149:1666. (*A study of bronchoscopy in both inpatients and outpatients in the general hospital setting; emphasizes that bronchiectasis is waning as a cause of hemoptysis; bronchitis is first, followed by cancer and tuberculosis.*)
7. Leatherman J, Davies SF, Hoidal JR. Alveolar hemorrhage syndromes: diffuse microvascular lung hemorrhage in immune and idiopathic disorders. Medicine (Baltimore) 1984;63:343. (*Comprehensive review.*)
8. Weber F. Catamenial hemoptysis. Ann Thorac Surg 2001;72:1750. (*Describes this rare result of thoracic endometriosis.*)
9. Nelson JE, Forman M. Hemoptysis in HIV-infected patients. Chest 1996;110:737. (*Most cases are attributable to infection, usually bacterial.*)
10. Johnson JL. Manifestations of hemoptysis. How to manage minor, moderate, and massive bleeding. Postgrad Med 2002;112:101. (*Reviews differential diagnosis and treatment.*)
11. Santiago S, Tobias J, Williams AJ. A reappraisal of the causes of hemoptysis. Arch Intern Med 1991;151:2449. (*Bronchogenic carcinoma, bronchitis, and idiopathic disease were the leading causes.*)
12. Adelman M, Haponik EF, Bleecker ER, et al. Cryptogenic hemoptysis: clinical features, bronchoscopic findings, and natural history in 67 patients. Ann Intern Med 1985;102:829. (*Prognosis was excellent, and no cancer, tuberculosis, or other serious causes were missed by a careful history and physical examination combined with chest radiography and bronchoscopy.*)
13. Colice GL. Detecting lung cancers as a cause of hemoptysis in patients with a normal chest radiograph. Chest 1997;111:877. (*Review of the literature and decision analysis concluding that bronchoscopy, with or without initial sputum cytology, is the most efficient diagnostic strategy.*)
14. Fontana RS, Sanderson DR, Woolner LB, et al. Screening for lung cancer. A critique of the Mayo Lung Project. Cancer 1991;67:1155. (*Includes late follow-up of the Mayo trial with information about the sensitivity and specificity of chest radiography and sputum cytology.*)
15. Garvey CJ, Hanlon R. Computed tomography in clinical practice. BMJ 2002;324:1077. (*Describes advantages and disadvantages of conventional, spiral, and multislice computed tomography scanning and contrasts them with magnetic resonance imaging.*)
16. Herth F, Ernst A, Becker HD. Long-term outcome and lung cancer incidence in patients with hemoptysis of unknown origin. Chest 2001;120:1592. (*After workup, 19% of patients had hemoptysis of unknown origin; with observation for 6.6 years after initial presentation, lung cancer developed in 6%.*)
17. McGuinness G, Beacher JR, Harkin TJ, et al. Hemoptysis: prospective high-resolution CT/bronchoscopic correlation. Chest 1994;105:1155. (*Fifty-seven patients underwent both studies; computed tomography had a sensitivity of 84% and a specificity of 68%.*)

18. Millar AB, Boothroyd AE, Edwards D, et al. The role of computed tomography in the investigation of unexplained hemoptysis. Respir Med 1992;86:39. (*An unusually large proportion of parenchymal cancers was reported in this study.*)

19. O'Neil K, Lazarus AA. Hemoptysis: indications for bronchoscopy. Arch Intern Med 1991;151:171. (*Review of 119 cases; bronchogenic cancer was found in 2.5%.*)

20. Set PAK, Flower CDR, Smith IE, et al. Hemoptysis: comparative study of the role of CT and fiberoptic bronchoscopy. Radiology 1993;189: 677. (*Computed tomography had a low false-positive rate for endobronchial lesions.*)

21. Surratt PM, Smiddy JF, Gruber B. Deaths and complications associated with fiberoptic bronchoscopy. Chest 1976;69:747. (*In nearly 50,000 procedures, 52 severe respiratory complications and 27 severe cardiovascular complications were found.*)

CHAPTER 43 ■ EVALUATION OF PLEURAL EFFUSIONS

Most pleural effusions encountered in the physician's office are incidental findings, but they often pose a diagnostic challenge. Of major concern are the possibilities of exudative effusions caused by tumor or infection. More often, the effusion is a transudate, most commonly due to congestive heart failure. The primary physician should understand the indications for thoracentesis and be able to carry out the initial evaluation of a pleural effusion based on its findings. When the patient's respiratory status is satisfactory and there is no evidence of serious acute illness, the evaluation can be conducted safely without hospital admission.

PATHOPHYSIOLOGY AND CLINICAL PRESENTATION (1–8)

The pleural cavity normally contains a small volume of serous fluid, which serves as a lubricant. About 17 mL of such fluid is formed each day by transudation from the parietal pleural surface and is reabsorbed predominantly by the visceral pleura through lymphatic stomata into the lymphatic system. When the transudation of fluid is excessive or an exudative process involving the pleural surfaces is present, an effusion forms. Once >200 mL is formed, the effusion becomes visible radiographically. Effusions are classified pathophysiologically as transudates or exudates. Clinically, the distinction is based on pleural fluid protein and lactate dehydrogenase (LDH) concentrations. An effusion is *transudative* if any two of the following three criteria are met: (a) the ratio of pleural fluid protein to serum protein is <0.5, (b) the ratio of pleural fluid LDH concentration to serum LDH concentration is <0.6, and (c) the pleural fluid LDH concentration is less than two thirds of the upper limit of normal for the serum LDH concentration. If these ratios or levels are exceeded, the effusion is *exudative*.

Transudates

Increased hydrostatic pressure in the pulmonary interstitium and decreased colloid oncotic pressure produce transudates. Increased hydrostatic pressure below the diaphragm, as occurs in ascites or peritoneal dialysis, can also result in a transudative pleural effusion. Because transudates are rarely associated with pleural inflammation, they are usually not accompanied by pleuritic pain, but they may lead to shortness of breath if they are large enough to interfere with respiratory mechanics. They may be unilateral but are often bilateral. Physical examination of the lung reveals dullness and diminished breath sounds. If the effusion has produced some atelectasis, bronchial breath sounds and increased vocal fremitus above the effusion may be present. Most transudates have a protein concentration of <3.0 g/100 mL, but chronic transudates may show higher concentrations and mimic an exudative process.

Congestive Heart Failure

Congestive heart failure is among the most common causes of transudative effusions. Left-sided heart failure increases the pulmonary capillary pressure (see Chapter 32), which forces excess fluid into the interstitium. Right ventricular failure contributes by raising central venous pressure, which elevates the hydrostatic force in the capillaries of the parietal pleura and diminishes fluid reabsorption. Most effusions associated with congestive failure are *bilateral,* but at times an *isolated right-sided* effusion is seen. Isolated left-sided effusions resulting from congestive failure are rare. The reason for the right-sided preference is unknown. Symptoms and signs of congestive failure (see Chapter 32) are usually evident. In >85% of effusions resulting from heart failure, the protein concentration is <3.0 g/100 mL. The concentration may be greater if the effusion is chronic or the patient has recently been undergoing a brisk diuresis. The pleural fluid is usually clear, but it may be bloody with red cell counts in excess of 5,000/mL.

Pulmonary Embolism

Pulmonary embolism is accompanied by pleural effusion in approximately 40% of cases. The effusions are usually small, and about 20% of them are transudates, which can occur in the absence of pulmonary infarction. Cell count, differential, and protein concentration vary considerably. The transudative effusion associated with a pulmonary embolus may result from localized interstitial edema. Bilateral effusions can be seen when emboli affect both lungs. A small effusion on chest x-ray films in a patient with pleuritic chest pain can be an important clue (see Chapter 20). The effusions that result from infarction are more likely to be exudates and more likely to be bloody, as discussed later.

Other Causes of Transudation

In the *nephrotic syndrome*, a similar but more generalized interstitial edema may ensue and lead to effusion. *Overexpanded extracellular volume* as a consequence of severe *hypoalbuminemia* or *salt retention* can produce a transudative effusion, but edematous fluid first collects in parts of the body where hydrostatic pressures are greatest (e.g., lower extremities) before fluid appears in the pleural space. Cardiomegaly may be in evidence, but overt signs of congestive failure are usually absent. Generalized edema is rare before the serum albumin level falls below 2.0 to 2.5 g/100 mL.

Intraabdominal diseases are occasionally responsible for transudative effusions. A *right-sided* pleural effusion develops in between 5% and 10% of patients with *ascites* resulting from *cirrhosis*; the composition of the effusion resembles that of the ascitic fluid. In cases of *pancreatitis* or a *subphrenic abscess*, a *sympathetic effusion* with the characteristics of a transudate sometimes forms; it soon changes into an exudate.

Pleural effusions are common after *coronary bypass graft surgery* and do not imply serious pathology. The same holds for the postpartum patient. Transudates may form in the setting of *pericardial disease*, *myxedema*, and *sarcoidosis*; the mechanisms are unknown.

Exudates

Exudates result from inflammatory or infiltrative disease of the pleura and its adjacent structures; damage occurs to capillary membranes, and protein-rich material accumulates in the pleural space. Obstruction to lymphatic flow can also produce an exudative effusion. Because most exudates form as a consequence of pleural injury, they are often accompanied by pleuritic chest pain, especially in the acute phase, when a friction rub may be heard before much fluid accumulates. The fluid is initially free flowing but may become walled off and loculated when a marked inflammatory response develops. The protein content is usually >3.0 g/100 mL. The fluid is typically deep yellow or cloudy in appearance. The leukocyte count is often >1,000/mL; a count >10,000/mL is suggestive of an empyema, particularly if most of the cells are neutrophils.

Neoplasms

Malignant tumors are often responsible for the development of effusions. Most pleural fluid accumulations caused by malignancies have the characteristics of exudates, although at times the protein concentration is <3.0 g/100 mL. Mechanisms of exudate formation include pleural metastasis with increased permeability and obstruction of lymphatic outflow. The formation of a malignant effusion is often a poor prognostic sign, particularly if the pH of the fluid is <7.3 and the glucose level is <60 mg/dL, which indicates extensive pleural involvement with tumor.

Bronchogenic carcinoma is the tumor most frequently associated with a pleural effusion. Fluid collects in most instances as a direct result of pleural invasion; unilateral effusions are the rule. Patients report dyspnea when the effusion is large and occasionally complain of pleuritic chest pain. The pleural fluid is usually clear and straw-colored, but it may be bloody, and the glucose level may be very low. The white cell count is typically around 2,500/mL, with most cells being lymphocytes. Malig-

nant cells are found in about 60% of instances. Unfortunately, the disease and its effusions are progressive; thoracentesis is followed by rapid reaccumulation.

Pleural effusions caused by *metastatic carcinoma* are more likely to be bilateral than are those associated with bronchogenic carcinoma because they occur as a consequence of lymphatic obstruction or diffuse seeding of the pleura. When effusions are caused by seeding, results of cytologic examination of the pleural fluid are positive in up to 90% of cases. *Carcinoma of the breast* is the leading metastatic tumor producing pleural effusions, accounting for 25% of all malignant effusions. The characteristics of the pleural fluid are similar to those of effusions caused by bronchogenic carcinoma. *Lymphoma* is another major cause of malignant bilateral pleural effusions, responsible for up to 20% of cases. The formation of a large effusion is a sign of advanced disease; evidence of pleural, parenchymal, and lymph node involvement is often present by the time a significant effusion appears. The pleural fluid may be a transudate or an exudate; most of the cells are lymphocytes. Cough and dyspnea accompany parenchymal involvement, but pleuritic pain is rare.

Mesotheliomas have become an increasingly important source of effusion as the incidence of disease associated with *asbestos exposure* has increased. Only malignant mesotheliomas produce important pleural fluid accumulations. The latent period for mesothelioma formation ranges from 20 to 40 years after asbestos exposure; the degree of exposure may appear inconsequential (see Chapter 39). Chest pain, cough, and shortness of breath result from extensive pleural disease and large effusions. The fluid may be bloody and often contains malignant cells, but they are sometimes hard to identify cytologically, so chromosomal analysis is necessary. The fluid may be high in *hyaluronic acid*. Because the tumor is only locally invasive, no signs of extrathoracic disease are present.

Impressive effusions can form as a consequence of *benign ovarian neoplasms* (*Meigs' syndrome*). The tumor produces ascites, and fluid tracks across the diaphragm and into the thorax. The effusion is typically on the right but may be left-sided or even bilateral; it is exudative in quality, free of malignant cells, and similar in composition to the ascitic fluid from which it derives. Removal of the ovarian tumor results in prompt resolution of the effusion.

Infection

Pulmonary infections are an important source of exudative pleural effusions, but effusions are uncommonly associated with the *acute bacterial pneumonias* encountered in ambulatory patients. For example, an effusion develops in only about 5% of patients with *pneumococcal pneumonia*, and it is usually small and transient. Such effusions are termed *parapneumonic* to imply that bacteria need not have entered the pleural space to cause the effusion. The term *empyema* is reserved for cases in which organisms are recovered from the pleural fluid, either by Gram's stain or culture. Empyema is a rare but worrisome event, seen in <1% of the cases of pneumococcal pneumonia that present in the outpatient setting; most cases occur when proper antibiotic therapy is delayed. Cough, sputum production, fever, chills, and pleuritic pain may be prominent. Early, the pleural fluid appears serous and may be sterile, but it quickly turns purulent and positive for organisms when empyema develops. In some instances, the pleural fluid offers the only opportunity for recovery of the causative organism. Characteristics of the pleural empyema fluid include a white cell count in excess of 5,000 to 10,000/mL, with neutrophils predominating. The concentration of glucose is typically

<20 mg/100 mL. Pleural scarring may be substantial if the empyema fluid is allowed to remain.

Viral pneumonitis and *mycoplasmal pneumonia* are sometimes associated with pleural effusions in the course of illness, but the effusions are small, transient, and of little consequence (see Chapter 52).

The effusion caused by postprimary tuberculosis (TB) represents a delayed hypersensitivity reaction to spillage of organisms into the pleural space during early bacteremia or subclinical parenchymal disease (see Chapter 49). The effusion is almost always unilateral. The patient may be relatively free of symptoms or exhibit lethargy, fever, and weight loss; at times, the clinical picture is dominated by acute onset of pleuritic pain and fever. Cough and sputum are conspicuously absent. The chest radiograph may show little more than an isolated effusion, but the result of an intermediate-strength tuberculin skin test is usually positive. The pleural fluid has the qualities of an exudate; the glucose concentration may be low. The white cell count averages 1,000 to 2,000/mL; lymphocytes predominate; mesothelial cells are scarce (<2%). Neutrophils may be seen early in the course of the illness. Organisms are rarely found on acid-fast stain of the fluid and can be cultured from the fluid in only 25% of cases. Most of these effusions resolve spontaneously within a few months and leave little or no residual; however, symptomatic pulmonary parenchymal involvement eventually develops in more than half of such patients (see Chapter 47).

Autoimmune Disease

Connective tissue disease, particularly *systemic lupus erythematosus*, can produce transient pleuropericardial inflammation during its course, usually after other signs and symptoms have appeared. There may be a brief period of pleuritic pain. On occasion, pleural involvement may be the initial clinical presentation of the disease. In most instances, the pleural fluid has the characteristics of an exudate and may demonstrate low glucose and serum complement levels.

Rheumatoid arthritis is much less likely to produce a pleural effusion than is lupus, but the fluid often persists. Fewer than 5% of patients experience pleuropericardial involvement; these patients usually have a history of extraarticular manifestations and joint symptoms.

Occasionally, the effusion is the first manifestation of rheumatoid disease. The effusion is an exudate, with a predominance of lymphocytes and a very low (<20 mg/100 mL) glucose concentration. Although the fluid may contain rheumatoid factor, its presence is not unique to this disease.

Pulmonary Infarction

As noted earlier, pleural effusions are found in approximately 40% of pulmonary embolism cases. Of these, about 80% are exudates. In these cases, the fluid is likely to be bloody. Effusions due to embolism have no specific distinguishing features. A high index of clinical suspicion is essential.

Intraabdominal Pathology

Infection and other intraabdominal pathology can lead to the production of an exudative pleural effusion, particularly when recent abdominal surgery, intestinal perforation, or hepatobiliary disease is complicated by development of a *subdiaphragmatic abscess*. In addition to gastrointestinal symptoms, pleuritic pain, fever, weight loss, and malaise may be present. Often, the symptoms are nonspecific, so that patients put off the decision to seek medical help. The diaphragm on the involved side (which is the right in two thirds of the cases) is elevated and moves poorly on fluoroscopy. A pathognomonic subdiaphragmatic air–fluid level may be present on chest film. The pleural fluid is usually sterile, although it may have a high leukocyte count. If the diaphragm has been perforated, an empyema can form. The pleural effusion associated with *pancreatitis* may begin as a transudate but usually becomes exudative. The effusions are most often on the left, but may be bilateral or right sided. The fluid characteristically has a *high amylase* concentration and is blood tinged in one third of cases.

Drugs

Rarely, medications have been associated with otherwise unexplained exudative effusions. There have been >100 case reports each for amiodarone, nitrofurantoin, phenytoin, and methotrexate. Other drugs with fewer case reports include carbamazepine, procainamide, propylthiouracil, penicillamine, cyclophosphamide, and bromocriptine.

DIFFERENTIAL DIAGNOSIS (1,2,6–8)

Although the causes of pleural effusion can be conveniently divided into those conditions that produce transudates and those that result in exudates (Table 43.1), it is important to keep

---

TABLE 43.1

IMPORTANT CAUSES OF PLEURAL EFFUSIONS

Transudates
- Congestive heart failure
- Hypoalbuminemia, severe
- Salt-retention syndromes
- Ascites secondary to cirrhosis
- Early phases of a sympathetic effusion
- Neoplasm (on occasion)
- Peritoneal dialysis
- Postpartum
- Cardiac bypass graft surgery

Exudates
- Neoplasms
  - Bronchogenic carcinoma
  - Breast cancer
  - Lymphoma
  - Mesothelioma
  - Meigs' syndrome
- Infections
  - Tuberculosis (and atypical mycobacteria in AIDS patients)
  - Bacterial pneumonia (including empyema)
  - Viral pneumonitis
  - Mycoplasmal pneumonia
  - *Pneumocystis* pneumonia
- Pulmonary embolization
- Connective tissue disease
  - Rheumatoid arthritis
  - Systemic lupus erythematosus
- Intraabdominal disease
  - Subphrenic abscess
  - Pancreatitis
- Idiopathic

in mind that a number of conditions can cause both. In such conditions, the initial effusion is transudative but turns exudative as the disease process continues. Chronic congestive heart failure is the most frequently encountered such condition in the ambulatory population. Neoplasms account for the majority of cases seen in referral populations. In a series reported from the Mayo Clinic, bronchogenic carcinoma was the leading cause of malignant pleural effusion, accounting for 30% of cases, followed by breast carcinoma (25%) and lymphoma (20%). Infection is the third-most-common cause of accumulation of fluid in the pleural space, with TB still accounting for a substantial proportion of effusions subjected to full evaluation. Bloody effusions are most often caused by neoplasms but are also seen in congestive heart failure, pulmonary embolism with infarction, TB, and pancreatitis. About 15% of effusions are unexplained; most idiopathic effusions are exudates.

Among AIDS patients, infections cause more than two thirds of effusions, with bacterial, mycobacterial, and *Pneumocystis* pneumonias accounting for most. Hypoalbuminemia and Kaposi's sarcoma are the leading noninfectious causes of effusion among patients with advanced HIV disease.

WORKUP (9–23)

The presence of a pleural effusion is often noted as an incidental finding on chest x-ray or is suggested by the findings of dullness and diminished breath sounds upward from the lung base and confirmed by chest radiography. The first task after identifying the effusion is to assess the degree, if any, of respiratory compromise associated with the effusion. The vital signs should be checked for tachypnea and tachycardia, the skin should be checked for cyanosis, and the chest should be checked for use of accessory muscles of respiration. Patients with objective evidence of substantial respiratory compromise should be admitted to the hospital for further workup. Those who are comfortable can be assessed on an outpatient basis. Although radiographic features may suggest a diagnosis, the history and physical examination complemented by examination of the pleural fluid are essential to an accurate assessment.

History

The patient should be asked about the presence of fever, cough, sputum production, chest pain, dyspnea, edema, and abdominal pain; prior history of malignant, hepatic, renal, or HIV disease; exposure to TB or asbestos; and symptoms of rheumatoid disease (see Chapter 146). Cough, fever, and sputum production in conjunction with pleuritic chest pain suggest pneumonitis with pleural involvement. Pleuritic pain is also consistent with embolization, malignancy, and pleural inflammation with adjacent pericarditis resulting from connective tissue disease. Dyspnea may be induced by the effusion alone, but the symptom is indicative of congestive heart failure when accompanied by orthopnea and paroxysmal nocturnal dyspnea. A history of peripheral edema raises the possibilities of hypoalbuminemia, volume overload, and congestive failure. A history of alcohol abuse, recent abdominal surgery, or abdominal pain or distention points to a source below the diaphragm.

Physical Examination

In addition to the assessment for respiratory compromise, the vital signs are checked for fever and weight change. The integument is inspected for petechiae, purpura, spider angiomata, jaundice, clubbing (see Chapter 45), manifestations of rheumatoid disease (see Chapter 146), and rashes. The neck is noted for jugular venous distention and tracheal deviation, the lymph nodes are checked for enlargement, and the breasts are checked for masses. On lung examination, the level of the effusion and the extent of involvement are determined. It is worth noting any compression of adjacent lung, suggested by egophony and bronchial breath sounds heard above the effusion. A pleural friction rub may be audible but is usually lacking when a considerable amount of fluid has accumulated. The heart should be checked for a third sound, indicative of pump failure, and a three-component friction rub, suggestive of pericarditis. The abdomen is examined for signs of ascites, organomegaly, focal tenderness, and peritonitis (see Chapter 58). A pelvic examination is performed to rule out the presence of an ovarian mass, and the extremities are noted for edema, calf tenderness, and signs of joint inflammation.

Laboratory Evaluation

The centerpieces of the laboratory workup are the chest radiograph and pleural fluid analysis. The *chest radiograph* should be studied for pleura-based densities, infiltrates, signs of congestive heart failure (see Chapter 32), hilar adenopathy, coin lesions, and loculation of fluid, detection of which requires lateral decubitus views, ultrasound, or chest computed tomography. The elevation of a hemidiaphragm and the presence of a subdiaphragmatic air–fluid level are important radiographic signs of a subphrenic abscess. Again, ultrasound may be necessary. The location of the effusion may be helpful. Among transudative effusions caused by cardiac failure, unilateral effusions tend to be right sided, and bilateral effusions usually are asymmetric with more fluid on the right side. On the other hand, effusions associated with pericarditis or pancreatitis tend to be left sided.

When a cause is not readily evident from the history, physical examination, and chest film, then a *diagnostic thoracentesis* is indicated. In some instances, of course, a thoracentesis need not be performed on the first visit. Such instances include the afebrile patient with clinical evidence of congestive heart failure, the postpartum woman who is otherwise well, the patient who has undergone bypass graft surgery, and the young patient with a small effusion in conjunction with a viral or mycoplasmal pneumonia. These patients can be followed expectantly with repeated chest films; failure of the effusion to clear with resolution of the presumptive cause is an indication for thoracentesis.

A diagnostic thoracentesis can be performed safely and comfortably in the office on patients who have free-flowing effusions confirmed by lateral decubitus films. However, ultrasonography has been increasingly used to help guide thoracentesis, making referral for the procedure more the rule than the exception in many settings. Thoracentesis for loculated effusions is more difficult and is associated with a greater risk for pneumothorax; such effusions should not be tapped in the office. Ultrasound-guided aspiration should be used in these cases.

The *laboratory analysis* of pleural fluid should begin with determination of the *protein* and *LDH concentrations*. A simultaneous serum sample should also be sent for protein and LDH levels. As noted earlier, the three most useful findings for distinguishing a pleural exudate from a transudate are *pleural fluid LDH level* >200 U, *pleural-to-serum LDH ratio* >0.6, and *pleural-to-serum protein ratio* >0.5. Fulfillment of any two of these three criteria has sensitivity in excess of 90% and specificity of 99%. If this first step indicates that the effusion is a transudate, no further laboratory analysis of the fluid is indicated. In fact, because of the poor specificity of white and red blood cell counts, glucose and amylase levels, and even bacterial cultures (as a consequence of contamination), such tests performed on transudates may be misleading.

If any of the criteria for an exudate are met, the laboratory analysis should include a *differential cell count*, *bacterial culture* (including cultures for anaerobes and mycobacteria), and *cytologic examination*. Although a high white blood cell count may indicate infection, it is a nonspecific finding. Lymphocyte predominance is suggestive of TB or malignancy but does not help in distinguishing between the two. The sensitivity of cytologic examination depends on the mechanism of the malignant effusion and extent of disease; it may be as high as 95% in advanced disease with extensive pleural involvement but as low as 50% in early disease. However, a positive result of cytology is highly specific when reported by an experienced pathologist.

In certain circumstances, other tests may be useful. A *low pleural fluid glucose level* (<60 mg/dL) is associated with TB, other serious infections, and advanced pleural involvement with malignancy. A *low pleural fluid pH* (<7.30) has a similar meaning. Conversely, when the pleural fluid pH is low, the result of the pleural-fluid cytologic examination is likely to be positive if an underlying cancer is present. Very low glucose levels (<30 mg/dL) are most consistently associated with the effusion of rheumatoid arthritis. An elevated *amylase* level may point to pancreatitis as the cause of effusion, but it can also be seen in malignant effusion. Specific tumor markers have not proved useful, except in the case of *chromosomal analysis* for identifying malignant mesothelioma. Similarly, measurement of *complement levels* (CH50, C3, and C4) should be reserved for the rare instance when it is necessary to confirm that an exudative effusion in a patient with rheumatoid disease is caused by the underlying disorder and not another condition. Pleural-fluid antinuclear antibody measurement may be useful in further establishing the diagnosis of lupus pleuritis. Measurement of adenosine deaminase (ADA) and interferon-γ in the pleural fluid as well as polymerase chain reaction for *Mycobacterium tuberculosis* can be helpful in the diagnosis of TB pleural effusions. Estimates of sensitivity and specificity for ADA vary widely, most likely because of different methods of measurement. Interferon-γ has reported sensitivities ranging from 84% to 100%; specificities range from 95% to 100%. PCR findings are positive in 100% of culture-positive pleural fluids and 30% to 60% of those that are culture negative. False-positive results can be caused by DNA contamination or the presence of nonviable organisms.

In about 15% of cases, the cause of an exudative effusion is not evident after complete laboratory analysis of the pleural fluid from an initial thoracentesis. If malignancy is still suspected, repeated thoracentesis is indicated. Sensitivity approaches 90% with submission of fluid specimens from three separate pleural taps in patients with underlying malignancy. Test sensitivity is particularly high in cases of advanced pleural involvement by tumor, as suggested by pleural fluid pH <7.30 and glucose level <60 mg/dL.

Pleural biopsy alone may be less sensitive than cytologic examination of pleural fluid in detecting malignancy, but the two tests are complementary, with sensitivity in excess of 90% when used together. Pleural biopsy is most useful in detecting TB, having sensitivity of 60% to 80%. Again, the biopsy information is complementary; fluid culture or examination of pleural tissue (or both) will yield a diagnosis of TB in up to 95% of those with the disease. Both pleural tissue and pleural fluid should be submitted for mycobacterial culture. When biopsies are obtained from areas of focal nodularity seen on contrast computed tomography scans, image guidance should be used. Biopsy sites should be marked because local radiotherapy is indicated to prevent tumor seeding in the biopsy track when mesothelioma is diagnosed. When closed pleural biopsy does not establish a diagnosis, *thoroscopy* should be considered. It adds significantly to sensitivity of the workup for malignant disease. It also affords the opportunity for fluid drainage and talc pleurodesis in an effort to provide symptomatic relief (see later discussion.)

When a history of hemoptysis is present or a pulmonary abnormality is noted on chest radiography, *fiberoptic bronchoscopy* may prove useful. In the absence of such findings, routine bronchoscopy should not be used for undiagnosed pleural effusion.

Approximately 15% of pleural effusions remain undiagnosed after workup, including repeated cytologies and biopsy. In these cases, it is important carefully to reconsider those diagnoses that could be effectively treated with specific therapy, including mycobacterial and fungal infections and pulmonary embolism. Many undiagnosed exudates eventually prove to be due to malignancy after extended follow-up.

INDICATIONS FOR ADMISSION AND REFERRAL (9–11,15,22,24–27)

The patient with respiratory discomfort is best evaluated on an inpatient basis, especially if he or she is HIV positive; inpatient evaluation is also indicated when embolization, severe congestive failure, acute empyema, or an intraabdominal crisis is likely. Few of these patients present to the physician in the office; however, the patient with a chronic but enlarging collection of pleural fluid is apt to be encountered. The person who appears to be tolerating the effusion without much discomfort can be evaluated and managed on an outpatient basis as long as no evidence suggests an empyema or a subphrenic abscess, conditions that require surgical attention. Referral is appropriate when malignancy or TB is suspected and pleural biopsy or fiberoptic bronchoscopy is deemed necessary.

SYMPTOMATIC MANAGEMENT (24–27)

The patient can be made comfortable before a diagnosis is established. Pleuritic pain often responds to nonsteroidal antiinflammatory drugs, which have the advantage over narcotics of not producing a suppressive effect on respiration. Removal of fluid is indicated when the effusion is compromising respiratory efforts. Usually, no more than 1 L should be removed at one time to avoid intravascular volume depletion on reequilibration. Palliative management of malignant pleural effusions often includes the introduction of sclerosing agents to the pleural space after drainage. Talc has proved to be the most effective agent, and results are better with a thoroscopic approach. Malignant effusions are difficult to treat in the setting of advanced disease with marked pleural involvement (pleural fluid pH <7.30 and glucose level <60 mg/dL). Comfort measures are often preferable to repeated attempts at sclerosing therapy under such circumstances (see Chapter 92).

A.G.M.

Annotated Bibliography

1. Maskell NA, Butland RJA. BTS guidelines for the investigation of a unilateral pleural effusion in adults. Thorax 2003;58(Suppl II):ii8. (*Excellent review, including a detailed diagnostic algorithm and 116 references, followed by a series of equally effective reviews— including ref. 9—in a supplement dedicated to pleural effusion.*)

2. Fine NL, Smith LR, Sheedy PF. Frequency of pleural effusions in mycoplasma and viral pneumonias. N Engl J Med 1970;283:790. (*Small, transient effusions are common in these conditions, but large effusions are rare.*)

3. Sahn SA. The pleura. Am Rev Respir Dis 1988;138:184. (*An extensive review of pleural pathophysiology and pleural effusion.*)

4. Peek GJ, Morcos S, Cooper G. The pleural cavity. BMJ 2000;320:1318. (*A surgeon's perspective on pneumothorax as well as effusions.*)

5. Putnam Jr JB. Malignant pleural effusions. Surg Clin North Am 2002;82(4):867. (*Excellent review.*)

6. Weiss JM, Spodick DH. Association of left pleural effusion with pericardial disease. N Engl J Med 1983;308:696. (*Patients with pericarditis tend to have unilateral, left-sided pleural effusions or bilateral effusions that are larger on the left; this is in contrast to the right-sided dominance seen in congestive heart failure.*)

7. Hughson WG, Friedman PJ, Feigin DS, et al. Postpartum pleural effusion: a common radiologic finding. Ann Intern Med 1982;97:856. (*In a small prospective study, a majority of asymptomatic women had a pleural effusion within 24 hours after delivery.*)

8. Joseph J, Strange C, Sahn SA. Pleural effusions in hospitalized patients with AIDS. Ann Intern Med 1993;118:856. (*Although this was not a study of outpatients, the findings suggest causes to consider when an HIV-positive patient is encountered, especially one with AIDS.*)

9. Antunes G, Neville E, Duffy J, et al. BTS guidelines for the management of malignant pleural effusions. Thorax 2003;58(Suppl II): ii29. (*Superb review, which begins with pathophysiology, then summarizes management, with an algorithm that can keep the primary care provider in the decision-making role.*)

10. Rahman NM, Davies RJO, Gleeson FV. Investigating suspected malignant pleural effusion. BMJ 2007;334:206. (*Succinct case-based argument for rationale imaging.*)

11. Ferrer J, Roldan J, Teixidor J, et al. Predictors of pleural malignancy in patients with pleural effusion undergoing thoracoscopy. Chest 2005;127:1017. (*Thoracoscopy demonstrated 94% sensitivity and 100% specificity in the diagnosis of pleural malignancy; a symptomatic period >1 month, absence of fever, blood-tinged pleural fluid, and chest computed tomography findings were suggestive of malignancy.*)

12. Traill ZC, Davies RJO, Gleeson FV. Thoracic computed tomography in patients with suspected malignant effusions. Clin Radiol 2001;56:193. (*Pleural surfaces assessed at computed tomography showed features of malignancy with sensitivity 84% and specificity 100%.*)

13. Gopi A, Madhavan SM, Sharma SK, et al. Diagnosis and treatment of tuberculous pleural effusion in 2006. Chest 2007;131:880. (*Extensive review, including details of meta-analyses of adenosine deaminase, interferon-γ, and polymerase chain reaction.*)

14. Chang SC, Perng RP. The role of fiber optic bronchoscopy in evaluating the causes of pleural effusions. Arch Intern Med 1989;149:855. (*Useful in patients with hemoptysis or a pulmonary abnormality on chest radiography.*)

15. Frist B, Kahan AV, Koss LG. Comparison of the diagnostic value of biopsies of the pleura and cytologic evaluation of pleural fluids. Ann Intern Med 1972;77:507. (*Among 106 patients with malignant effusion, 97% had positive findings on fluid cytology and 38% had positive findings on pleural biopsy; together, the tests had a sensitivity approaching 100%.*)

16. Heffner JE, Brown LK, Barbieri CA. Diagnostic value of tests that discriminate between exudative and transudative pleural effusions. Primary Study Investigators. Chest 1997;111:970. (*Critical meta-analysis of studies of nearly 1,500 patients with pleural effusion.*)

17. Light RW. Useful tests on the pleural fluid in the management of patients with pleural effusions. Curr Opin Pulm Med 1999;5:245. (*Succinct expert review with a focus on excluding tuberculous pleuritis.*)

18. Light RW, Ball WC. Glucose and amylase in pleural effusion. JAMA 1973;225:259. (*Tuberculosis and malignant effusions were not universally associated with low glucose values.*)

19. Light RW, MacGregor MI, Ball Jr WC, et al. Cells in pleural fluid. Their value in differential diagnosis. Arch Intern Med 1973;132:854. (*In a review of the diagnostic significance of cell counts, the authors concluded that the finding of many mesothelial cells is incompatible with tuberculosis; red cell counts >10,000/mL suggest neoplasm, infarction, or trauma; a predominance of lymphocytes is consistent with tuberculosis and neoplasm.*)

20. Light RW, MacGregor MI, Luchsinger PC, et al. Pleural effusions: the diagnostic separation of transudate and exudate. Ann Intern Med 1972;77:507. (*A classic article, which details rigorous criteria for the separation of transudates from exudates.*)

21. Lossos IS, Breuer R, Intrator O, et al. Differential diagnosis of pleural effusion by lactate dehydrogenase isoenzyme analysis. Chest 1997;111:648. (*An algorithm based on lactate dehydrogenase isozyme alone had a positive predictive value of 83%.*)

22. Maskell NA, Gleeson FV, Davies RJO. Standard pleural biopsy versus CT-guided cutting-needle biopsy for diagnosis of malignant disease in pleural effusions: a randomised controlled trial. Lancet 2003;361:1326. (*Sensitivity increased from 47% to 87% with computed tomography guidance.*)

23. Sahn SA, Good Jr JT. Pleural fluid pH in malignant effusions. Ann Intern Med 1988;108:349. (*A pH <7.30 correlated with advanced pleural involvement by tumor and a very poor prognosis.*)

24. Colice GL, Curtis A, Deslauriers J, et al. Medical and surgical treatment of parapneumonic effusions: an evidence-based guideline. Chest 2000;118(4):1158. (*Reviews evidence for predicting the risk of complication of parapneumonic effusion, as well as treatments including no drainage, therapeutic thoracentesis, tube thoracostomy, fibrinolytics, video-assisted thoracoscopic surgery, and surgery.*)

25. Ferrer J, Roldan J, Teixidor J, et al. Predictors of pleural malignancy in patients with pleural effusion undergoing thoracoscopy. Chest 2005;127:1017. (*Thoracoscopy demonstrated 94% sensitivity and 100% specificity in the diagnosis of pleural malignancy; a symptomatic period >1 month, absence of fever, blood-tinged pleural fluid, and chest computed tomography findings were suggestive of malignancy.*)

26. Shaw P, Agarwal R. Pleurodesis for malignant pleural effusions (Cochrane review). In: The Cochrane library, Issue 3. Oxford: Update Software, 2003. (*Thoracoscopic pleurodesis with talc may be the optimal technique for pleurodesis in patients with malignant pleural effusions; see http://www.cochrane.org for updates.*)

27. Walker-Renard PB, Vaughan LM, Sahn SA. Chemical pleurodesis for malignant pleural effusions. Ann Intern Med 1994;120:56. (*Talc effectiveness was 93%, compared with 67% for tetracyclines and 54% for bleomycin.*)

CHAPTER 44 ■ EVALUATION OF THE SOLITARY PULMONARY NODULE

Solitary pulmonary nodules are incidental findings on chest x-ray or computed tomography (CT) images. They are defined as round lesions <3 cm in diameter and surrounded by pulmonary parenchyma and without other abnormal findings. Such nodules are found at a rate of 1 to 2 per 1,000 routine chest radiographs. They are found more frequently on chest CT images. The discovery is a worrisome finding because it raises the possibilities of primary lung cancer and solitary metastasis from a nonpulmonary source. The patient is usually asymptomatic and undergoing chest radiography for either an unrelated issue or screening. Granulomas and hamartomas account for the majority. Historically about 30% proved to be malignant, but with the identification of increasingly smaller nodules on CT images, that proportion may be declining.

Pulmonary malignancies with the greatest potential for cure present as solitary nodules. Consequently, thorough assessment is of the utmost importance. On the other hand, the majority of these lesions are not cancers, and to subject all patients to invasive studies and excision can lead to much unnecessary morbidity. The primary physician needs to determine the likelihood of malignancy on the basis of clinical and radiographic findings and identify the patient who requires referral for consideration of advanced imaging, transthoracic fine-needle aspiration biopsy, bronchoscopy, or surgery, which may be either thoracotomy or video-assisted thoracoscopic surgery. Workup can be performed on an outpatient basis.

PATHOPHYSIOLOGY AND CLINICAL PRESENTATION (1-4)

Solitary pulmonary nodules characteristically appear in the middle or lateral lung fields surrounded by normal lung and unaccompanied by satellite lesions. They have smooth contours and are usually round ("coin" lesions) or oval. Neoplastic, granulomatous, vascular, and cystic processes are the principal pathologic mechanisms responsible for nodule formation. The nodule displaces normal aerated lung parenchyma and does not cause symptoms unless airway obstruction, pleural invasion, interference with respiratory mechanics, or involvement of blood vessels or nerves occurs. Inflammatory lesions double in volume in <5 weeks, malignancies take between 1 and 18 months to double, and benign nodules take longer. A solitary nodule that does not change in size for 2 years has traditionally been considered benign, but some cancers, including bronchoalveolar-cell carcinomas, can appear stable for that long. In fact, one study suggested that the absence of appreciable growth over a 2-year period had a predictive value of only 65% for a benign lesion.

The older the patient, the greater are the chances that the nodule is malignant; the probability is <2% for patients younger than age 30 years and increases by 10% to 15% with each succeeding decade. A history of smoking greatly increases the probability that the nodule is malignant, as does concurrent weight loss, headache, or bone pain. The size of the nodule has also become increasingly important in discriminating benign from malignant lesions as use of chest CT for screening and diagnosis has increased and smaller-diameter lesions are discovered incidentally. More than 99% of noncalcified lesions <4 mm in diameter are benign, as are approximately 94% of noncalcified lesions between 4 and 8 mm in diameter. However, as many as 50% of lesions >8 mm in diameter prove to be malignant in some series.

Benign and malignant solitary lung nodules may have a similar appearance on chest x-ray films. However, the *distribution patterns of calcification* are different and of diagnostic utility. Benign lesions tend to have calcium deposited in central, peripheral, concentric, "popcorn," or homogeneous patterns, whereas eccentric patterns of calcification are more characteristic of malignancies (see later discussion and Fig. 44.1).

Among lung cancers, adenocarcinomas tend to be located peripherally; squamous- and small-cell cancers are usually more central in location. However, squamous-cell cancers that are located peripherally tend to show cavitation.

DIFFERENTIAL DIAGNOSIS (1–5)

Healed infectious granulomas account for the majority of solitary nodules. In most series, 20% to 40% of solitary pulmonary nodules prove to be cancers. Of these, >75% are *primary lung cancers*, and the remainder are *metastatic lesions*. Tumors of the *breast*, *colon*, and *testicles* are particularly prone to metastasize to the lung. Of the 60% to 80% of solitary pulmonary nodules that prove to be benign, 85% to 90% are granulomas; most are *tuberculous*, but in endemic areas, *histoplasmosis* and *coccidioidomycosis* are important considerations. Benign pulmonary tumors such as *hamartomas* account for about 5% of benign nodules. The remainder are *bronchogenic cysts*, *hydatid cysts*, *pseudolymphomas*, *arteriovenous malformations*, and *bronchopulmonary sequestrations*. Extrapulmonary lesions, such as skin lesions, moles, nipples, chest wall and rib lesions, and pleural plaques, may be confused with solitary lesions of lung parenchyma.

WORKUP (1–18)

The major issue posed by a solitary nodule is the chance of an early resectable lung cancer. Many surgeons argue that the risk of thoracotomy is small and the potential benefit considerable because resection of a nodule that proves to be an early primary lung cancer may provide the patient with a chance for cure. They note that for resected bronchogenic carcinomas and solitary lung metastases presenting as solitary nodules, average 5-year survivals are 60% and 35%, respectively. On the other hand, pulmonologists have argued that lesions that

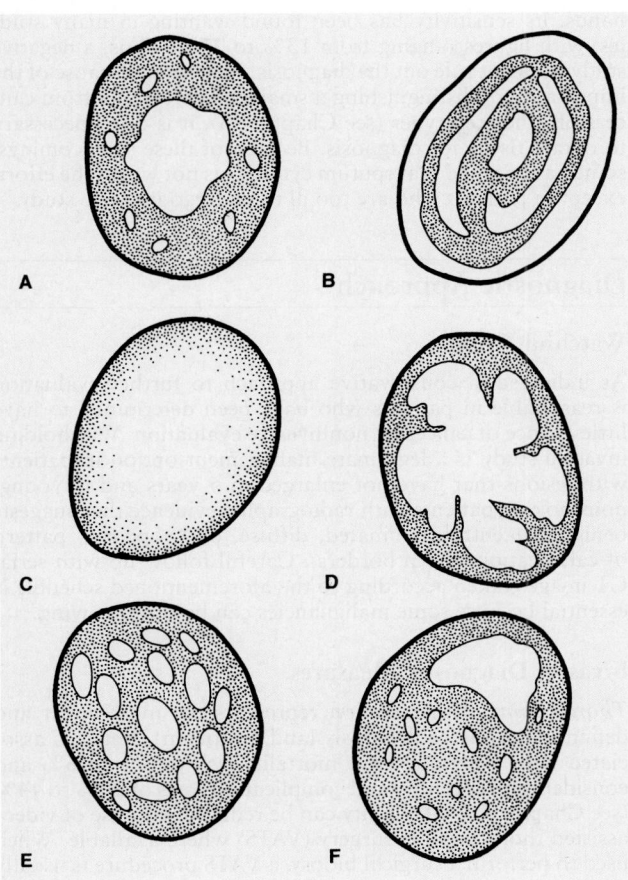

FIGURE 44.1. Patterns of calcification in solitary pulmonary nodules include central (A), laminated (B), diffuse (C), "popcorn" (D), stippled (E), and eccentric (F). Patterns A through D are virtually always benign; E and F may be benign or malignant.

possess many of the criteria of benignity can be managed conservatively, and that definitive tissue diagnosis can be approached by bronchoscopy or needle biopsy without resorting to early thoracotomy, which has a surgical mortality ranging from 3% to 6%. A review of the literature reveals passionate advocates on both sides. Conclusive data taking into account morbidity and mortality of both approaches are lacking.

The task of the primary care physician is to make the best possible clinical estimate of cancer risk based on history, physical examination, and appearance of the nodule on chest x-ray films and chest CT, with the possible addition of positron emission tomography (PET). Proper patient selection is the best means of maximizing the yield from invasive study and surgical intervention and minimizing the rate of false alarms and unnecessary morbid procedures.

History

The age of the patient and a history of smoking are important determinants of cancer risk. The likelihood ratio for malignancy in men increases markedly with age, estimated at 0.1 for those younger than age 35 years to 5.7 for those >70 years. Likelihood ratios for smoking range from 0.15 for those who have never smoked to 3.9 for those currently smoking more

than two packs per day. The probability of cancer is 50% for patients in their 60s but <2% for those <30 years. Although symptoms are often absent, it is worth inquiring into bone pain, headache, weight loss, and other symptoms suggestive of malignancy. A history of hemoptysis, even if minimal (see Chapter 42), and of known previous breast, bowel, or testicular cancer also increases the likelihood of malignancy. A history of exposure to tuberculosis (TB) or residence in an area in which histoplasmosis or coccidioidomycosis is endemic raises the possibility of a granulomatous etiology but does not rule out malignancy. A family history of hemorrhagic telangiectasia can be a valuable clue.

Physical Examination

The physical examination is generally unrevealing, but the presence of a breast or testicular mass, occult blood in the stool, clubbing (see Chapter 45), cutaneous or mucosal telangiectasia, or an audible bruit over the chest wall (suggestive of a vascular etiology) should be excluded. Perhaps the most important part of the physical examination is careful palpation of lymph nodes, particularly those in the supraclavicular and axillary regions. If enlarged, such nodes can be sampled by biopsy, which may eliminate the need for thoracotomy or other invasive procedures.

Laboratory Studies

Chest Radiography

Appearance of the lesion on chest x-ray and its *doubling time* are among the most useful data for determining the chances of malignancy. An assessment of doubling time—the period during which the tumor doubles in volume—can be especially helpful, but this is possible immediately only if *previous chest films* are available. It is important to keep in mind that doubling refers to volume, not diameter. In doubling, the diameter of the lesion need increase by only 28%, not 100%. A doubling time of >2 years or <30 days makes malignancy unlikely. Every effort should be made to locate old chest x-ray films to assess doubling time before further studies are undertaken. If previous films are unavailable, careful evaluation of the *radiologic appearance* of the nodule is indicated. This evaluation is markedly enhanced by obtaining a chest CT image. A most helpful sign is the presence of *calcification*. Laminated or concentric calcification is specific for granulomas. Central, diffuse, or homogeneous patterns of calcification are, with rare exceptions, also associated with benign lesions. However, radiographically visible calcium in stippled or eccentric patterns can occur in both malignant and benign lesions. Moreover, a primary cancer may engulf a preexisting calcified granuloma or scar; eccentricity of the calcium in the nodule should raise this possibility (Fig. 44.1).

The size of the nodule is not very helpful in distinguishing benign from malignant processes unless the diameter of the lesion is <8 mm, in which case malignancy is not likely. The *location* and the *shape* of the nodule on a chest x-ray film are also relatively poor discriminators. Both cancers and tuberculous granulomas are more common in the upper and middle lobes than in the lower lobes. Ill-defined borders suggest a primary malignancy, as does lobulation of the margin of the nodule. However, smooth borders are also seen with metastatic lesions. Cavitation occurs with nearly equal frequency in cancers and granulomas.

Computed Tomography

Chest CT has become the imaging technique of choice for evaluation of the solitary pulmonary nodule. It provides much better definition of the lesion and pattern of calcification than does chest radiography and reduces the false-negative rate associated with reliance on chest radiographic appearance alone. What appears to be a single nodule on plain film may actually be one of several lesions on CT and indicative of metastatic disease. Base-case estimates used in a rigorous cost-effectiveness analysis of sensitivity and specificity of CT for identifying malignancy were 96% and 56%, respectively. Serial CT images provide much more precise measures of growth and are usually obtained at 3, 6, 12, and 24 months during the process of watchful waiting. CT is also useful for guiding fine-needle aspiration biopsy and allows assessment of the mediastinum, which is useful in staging lesions suspected to be malignant (although its sensitivity and specificity for staging have been found wanting in patients with lesions <3 cm; see Chapter 53).

Taking thin sections (high-resolution CT) or using iodinated contrast can sometimes uncover calcification not visible by standard CT, can better confirm hamartomas and arteriovenous malformations, and can enhance the appearance of malignant nodules.

Positron Emission Tomography

Imaging with ^{18}F-2-fluoro-2-deoxy-D-glucose (FDG) has been shown to add useful discriminating information for nodules deemed indeterminate based on radiographic appearance. Studies suggest a sensitivity of 90% to 95% and a specificity of 85%. Decision analysis suggests that a CT plus an FDG-PET strategy may be most effective and may actually be cost-saving among patients for whom the probability of cancer is between 0.12 and 0.69. The clinical implication of these findings is that FDG-PET should be used selectively when the pretest probability of cancer based on patient history and appearance of the lesion on chest x-ray are discordant with the findings on CT scan. When pretest probability is low or intermediate and CT findings are benign, needle biopsy or watchful waiting without PET is appropriate. When pretest probability is high and CT findings are benign, FDG-PET can be helpful, leading to surgery or needle biopsy if positive and to needle biopsy or watchful waiting if negative. FDG-PET is much less helpful in smaller lesions (e.g., <8 mm in diameter) than in larger lesions.

Magnetic Resonance Imaging

Magnetic resonance imaging is inferior to CT for imaging solitary pulmonary nodules. It does not detect calcification well but reveals the mediastinum better than does CT, and it is useful for imaging chest wall invasion, aortopulmonic window adenopathy, and superior sulcus tremors.

Ancillary Studies

An intermediate-strength *tuberculin skin test* should be implanted (see Chapter 38). If sputum is available, it should be stained for *acid-fast organisms* and *cultured for TB*. In endemic areas, *fungal cultures* and histoplasmin complement fixation titers may important.

Sputum cytologic examination is the least invasive means of identifying a malignancy. Three first-morning samples should be obtained on consecutive days. Yield is highest when the sample contains pulmonary histiocytes (a sign of a deep sample) and the lesion is in the upper lobes, centrally located, communicating with a bronchus, or >2 cm in diameter (see Chapter 37). Although the specificity of the test is high in experienced

hands, its sensitivity has been found wanting in many studies, with figures ranging from 13% to 77%. Thus, a negative study does not rule out the diagnosis. Moreover, because of the importance of distinguishing a small-cell carcinoma from cancers of other cell types (see Chapter 53), it is often necessary to obtain tissue for diagnosis. Because of these shortcomings, some have argued that sputum cytology is not worth the effort, except in patients who are too ill to undergo invasive study.

Diagnostic Approach

Watchful Waiting

As indicated, a conservative approach to further evaluation is reasonable in patients who have been determined to have little chance of cancer by noninvasive evaluation. Withholding invasive study is a legitimate management option in patients with lesions that have not enlarged in 5 years and in young, nonsmoking patients with radiographic evidence that suggests benignity (central, laminated, diffuse, or "popcorn" pattern of calcification; sharp borders). Careful follow-up with serial CT images taken according to the aforementioned schedule is essential because some malignancies can be slow growing.

Invasive Diagnostic Measures

Thoracotomy with resection represents the most direct and definitive means of diagnosis (and treatment), but it is associated with a perioperative mortality risk of 3% to 6% and considerable morbidity and complication rates of 20% to 44% (see Chapter 53). Morbidity can be reduced with use of video-assisted thoracoscopic surgery (VATS) where available. When used to perform a surgical biopsy, a VATS procedure is usually converted to a thoracotomy with lobectomy if frozen section reveals malignancy.

Less-morbid but less-definitive options for a diagnosis include *transthoracic biopsy under CT guidance* including fine-needle aspiration. *Bronchoscopy with transbronchial biopsy* is another option, especially when the CT image reveals a bronchus leading to the lesion. Transthoracic biopsy is now the mainstay in the invasive diagnostic approach to the solitary pulmonary nodule. Sensitivity for detection of malignancy approaches 95% when the nodule is accessible to the transthoracic approach. Specific histologic types of malignant lesions can often be identified. The procedure fails to reveal a specific diagnosis in about 10% of patients with malignant lesions and in about 40% of those with benign lesions.

Fiberoptic bronchoscopic examination with bronchial brushing and biopsy may yield a diagnosis if a bronchus appears to enter the lesion on CT, but the sensitivity is substantially lower (10% to 30%) when nodules are small (<2 cm) and well circumscribed.

Mediastinoscopy and *thoracotomy* are indicated when the preprocedure probability of an early resectable primary lung cancer is high (see Chapter 53) and the patient is a good operative risk. Patients with severe obstructive or restrictive disease should first undergo formal pulmonary function testing.

Choice of Diagnostic Approach

Choice of diagnostic approach depends on the estimated probability of malignancy, location of the lesion, ability and willingness of the patient to tolerate the procedure (or the uncertainty, if watchful waiting is a consideration), and availability of the needed technical expertise.

The high-probability patient who can tolerate surgery and whose lesion has been determined to be resectable (see Chapter 53) should undergo thoracotomy and resection with or without video assistance. Patients with an intermediate probability of malignancy might be best approached by transthoracic fine-needle aspiration biopsy if it appears technically feasible. Patients with a very low risk are reasonable candidates for careful follow-up by serial CT study.

In sum, the optimal approach to evaluation of the patient with a solitary pulmonary nodule remains problematic because outcome data are lacking. It appears that a watchful waiting approach to evaluation is justified in patients judged to be at low risk for malignancy based on epidemiologic, historical, physical, and radiographic criteria. Patients at high risk for malignancy require a tissue diagnosis. Improvements in noninvasive evaluation techniques are reflected in the lower number of surgical procedures being performed for solitary nodules and the higher proportion of malignancies found among those that are sampled or resected. However, in a significant number of cases, substantial ambiguity remains after noninvasive evaluation. Formal clinical prediction rules have been developed based on elements of history (age, smoking behavior, and prior cancer) and radiologic appearance (nodule diameter, presence of spicules, and upper lobe location), but they do not yield better results than does a clinician who considers these and other factors. Patients for whom the probability of malignancy is neither low enough for them to be followed conservatively nor high enough for them to undergo surgery face a dilemma. The uncertainty and possible outcomes of alternative approaches should be shared with these patients so that a satisfactory plan can be devised.

PATIENT EDUCATION AND INDICATIONS FOR REFERRAL

Patients suspected on clinical and radiographic grounds of having a malignancy should be referred for tissue diagnosis. Decisions regarding the need for and type of invasive procedure should be made in conjunction with surgical and radiologic consultants. When the probability of malignancy is unclear, the patient needs to be informed about the lack of diagnostic certainty provided by noninvasive study and about the nature of further tests that might be undertaken.

Patients who cannot emotionally tolerate the uncertainty should be advised to undergo a definitive procedure to end the constant worry about the possibility of malignancy. The patient who can live with such uncertainty and is reluctant to undergo a thoracotomy or biopsy might be followed with serial chest films at 3- to 6-month intervals for 2 years.

A.G.M./A.H.G.

Annotated Bibliography

1. Winer-Muram HT. The solitary pulmonary nodule. Radiology 2006;239:34. (*Excellent review of diagnostic modalities, with a flow chart reflecting the interventional radiologist's approach.*)
2. Libby DM, Smith JP, Altorki NK, et al. Managing the small pulmonary nodule discovered by CT. Chest 2004;125:1522. (*Offers a diagnostic strategy for nodules detected on chest computed tomography [CT].*)
3. Ost D, Fein AM, Feinsilver SH. The solitary pulmonary nodule. N Engl J Med 2003;348:2535. (*Excellent review.*)
4. Rubins JB, Rubins HB. Temporal trends in the prevalence of malignancy in resected solitary pulmonary nodules. Chest 1996;109:100. (*An increasing proportion of procedures result in a diagnosis of malignancy, independent of age and lesion size, reflecting better noninvasive discrimination.*)
5. Toomes H, Delphendahl A, Manke HG, et al. The coin lesion of the lung: a review of 955 resected coin lesions. Cancer 1983;51:534. (*A useful series for statistics on types of lesions identified.*)
6. Becker GL, Whitlock WL, Schaefer PS, et al. The impact of thoracic computed tomography in clinically staged T1, N0, M0 chest lesions. Arch Intern Med 1990;150:557. (*Did not find CT to be helpful for staging the suspected lesion in patients with lung nodules <3 cm.*)
7. Cummings SR, Lillington GA, Richard RJ. Estimating the probability of malignancy in solitary pulmonary nodules. Am Rev Respir Dis 1986;134:449. (*Used prevalence, diameter of nodule, age, smoking history, calcification pattern, and type of edge; very useful.*)
8. Gould MK, Maclean CC, Kuschner WG, et al. Accuracy of positron emission tomography for diagnosis of pulmonary nodules and mass lesions: a meta-analysis. JAMA 2001;285:914. (*Sensitivity was 97%, and specificity was 78%.*)
9. Gould MK, Sanders GD, Barnett PG. Cost-effectiveness of alternative management strategies for patients with solitary pulmonary nodules. Ann Intern Med 2003;138:724. (*Positron emission tomography scans should be used only when pretest probability and CT findings are discordant or in patients with an intermediate pretest probability at high risk for surgical complications.*)
10. Gupta NC, Maloof J, Gunel E. Probability of malignancy in solitary pulmonary nodules using fluorine-18-FDG and PET. J Nucl Med 1996;37:943. (*Sensitivity and specificity were 93% and 88%, respectively, in this study.*)
11. Henschke CI, Yankelevitz DF, Naidich DP, et al. CT screening for lung cancer: suspiciousness of nodules according to size on baseline scans. Radiology 2004;231:164. (*Noncalcified nodules <0.5 mm do not justify immediate workup.*)
12. Khouri NF, Stitik FP, Erozan YS, et al. Transthoracic needle aspiration biopsy of benign and malignant lung lesions. Am J Roentgenol 1985;144:281. (*Diagnostic yield was well >80% and was helped by the use of a wide-aspiration needle, which facilitates the diagnosis of benign lesions.*)
13. MacDougall B, Weinerman B. The value of sputum cytology. J Gen Intern Med 1992;7:11. (*Sensitivity and specificity were found to be lacking, and the test was of limited use in the workup of suspected lung cancer.*)
14. Swenson SJ, Silverstein MD, Edell ES, et al. Solitary pulmonary nodules: clinical prediction model versus physicians. Mayo Clin Proc 1999;74:319. (*Clinicians performed as well as a prediction rule using three elements of history and three radiographic features.*)
15. Swenson SJ, Silverstein MD, Ilstrup DM, et al. The probability of malignancy in solitary nodules: application to small radiologically indeterminate nodules. Arch Intern Med 1997;157:849. (*Age, cigarette-smoking status, and history of cancer, as well as diameter, spiculation, and upper lobe location of the nodule, were independent predictors of malignancy.*)
16. Swenson SJ. Solitary pulmonary nodule: CT evaluation of enhancement with iodinated contrast material. Radiology 1992;182:343. (*Improved detection of malignancy was suggested.*)
17. Fulkerson WJ. Fiberoptic bronchoscopy. N Engl J Med 1984;311:511. (*Reviews the indications, contraindications, complications, and diagnostic yield of fiberoptic bronchoscopy and endobronchial biopsy.*)
18. Bach PB, Cramer LD, Schrag D, et al. The influence of hospital volume on survival after resection for lung cancer. N Engl J Med 2001;345:181-188. (*Patients at highest-volume hospitals had better rates of complications [20% vs. 44%], 30-day mortality [3% vs. 6%], and five-year survival [44% vs. 33%].*)

CHAPTER 45 ■ EVALUATION OF CLUBBING

The term *clubbing* refers to enlargement and sponginess of the nail beds of the fingers and toes and reduction in the angle created by the nail and the dorsum of the distal phalanx. It was described by Hippocrates in 400 BCE in a man with likely empyema. Clubbing is sometimes accompanied by a chronic subperiosteal osteitis—*hypertrophic osteoarthropathy*. Patients rarely complain of clubbed fingers; it is the physician who detects this abnormality as an incidental finding on physical examination. Because clubbing or hypertrophic osteoarthropathy may be the first clinical sign of a serious underlying condition, such as a pulmonary neoplasm, it is important for the primary physician to recognize these findings and investigate their possible causes.

PATHOPHYSIOLOGY AND CLINICAL PRESENTATION (1–4)

Hypotheses explaining the pathogenesis of clubbing and osteoarthropathy implicate autonomic influences, arteriovenous shunting, and blood-borne substances. The precise pathophysiology is uncertain, but it is known that intrathoracic vagotomy can abolish clubbing and osteoarthropathy, as can correction of an arteriovenous shunt or removal of a pulmonary tumor. A leading hypothesis holds that disruption of normal pulmonary circulation prevents megakaryocytes from being fragmented into platelets. The intact megakaryocytes then lodge in the fingertip circulation, where fragments are activated to release platelet-derived growth factor, which promotes growth and vascular permeability.

The pathologic examination of clubbed fingers reveals increased vascularity consistent with the megakaryocyte hypothesis. In hypertrophic osteoarthropathy, the periosteum is found to be edematous, hyperemic, and infiltrated by mononuclear cells. Periosteal elevation, new bone formation, and endosteal resorption in the distal ends of long bones, metacarpals, and metatarsals are all present. Soft-tissue swelling in the distal ends of the fingers and toes may lead to clubbing.

Clubbing is usually asymptomatic. Patients with hypertrophic osteoarthropathy may have pain in the wrists, ankles, hands, and feet; erythema and effusions are sometimes noted. Hypertrophic osteoarthropathy may precede clubbing or occur without it, but generally the two appear together. Clubbing often takes place in the absence of osteoarthropathy. Either finding may develop before the clinical presentation of one of the conditions associated with it.

Idiopathic hypertrophic osteoarthropathy, sometimes referred to as pachydermoperiostosis, is a benign condition that must be distinguished from hypertrophic osteoarthropathy secondary to systemic disease. These patients show periosteal new bone formation, swelling of the joints, and thickened and furred skin in addition to clubbing. The benign syndrome can be differentiated from secondary hypertrophic osteoarthropathy by its development in adolescence, slow growth, a paucity of joint symptoms, and the absence of concurrent hepatic, bowel, or pulmonary disease.

DIFFERENTIAL DIAGNOSIS (1,3–7)

Clubbing and hypertrophic osteoarthropathy occur in 2% to 12% of patients with *lung cancer*, developing with equal frequency in patients with large-cell cancer, squamous-cell cancer, or adenocarcinoma but rarely in the setting of small-cell cancer. Clubbing alone may be more frequent, and the prevalence depends on the sensitivity of the diagnostic criteria used to designate digits as "clubbed." A recently proposed sensitive, standardized measure identified clubbing in 37% of those with lung cancer and found no difference in prevalence among patients with squamous-cell cancer, adenocarcinoma, or small-cell cancer. Metastatic lung tumors are rarely responsible for such changes. In one series, 14% of patients with pleural tumors exhibited clubbing. With the decline in the incidence of *chronic pulmonary infectious* diseases (such as tuberculosis, lung abscess, and bronchiectasis), carcinoma of the lung has emerged as the leading cause of hypertrophic osteoarthropathy. Clubbing and osteoarthropathy are seen in patients with cyanotic congenital heart disease with *right-to-left shunts*, subacute bacterial *endocarditis*, and *cystic fibrosis*. Clubbing is a classic sign of chronic *hypoxemia* in patients with chronic obstructive lung disease. In addition, there are *hereditary* or idiopathic forms of clubbing and hypertrophic osteoarthropathy that have no clinical significance. Unilateral clubbing is associated with impairment of the vascular supply to the arm that occurs with aortic, subclavian, or innominate artery lesions. Clubbing may develop in jackhammer operators.

Clubbing has also been described in a number of nonpulmonary conditions, including inflammatory bowel disease (38% in Crohn's disease and 14% in ulcerative colitis) and chronic liver disease (24% to 29%). Case reports of clubbing in association with a myriad of diseases have been published. Some of these include esophageal cancer, early HIV infection, and anti-phospholipid antibody syndrome. Each of these reports includes disclaimers about the presence of comorbid pulmonary disease. Nonetheless, it is difficult to judge their significance.

Clubbing must be differentiated from a number of other phalangeal conditions that resemble it. In many normal people, particularly African Americans, curvature of the nails is increased. Infections of the terminal phalanges, such as felon and chronic paronychia, may be confused with clubbing, as may thyroid osteoarthropathy.

WORKUP (1,4,8–11)

The evaluation of clubbing should begin with confirmation of the characteristic physical findings: *loss of the angle* made by the nail and *increase* in the *ballotability* of the nail bed. The Schamroth sign results from both the loss of nail angle and an increase in soft tissue at the cuticle. When normal index fingers are placed in nail-to-nail opposition, there is a diamond-shaped window between the nails and cuticles. When clubbed fingers are placed in opposition, there is no such window, and the Schamroth sign is said to be present. Hypertrophic osteoarthropathy is identified by *radiography of the long bones*; the typical changes are increase in periosteal thickness and new bone formation at distal ends. Once it is clear that clubbing or hypertrophic osteoarthropathy is present, evaluation for an underlying cause can commence.

History

Before an elaborate search for a serious illness is undertaken, it should be established whether clubbing has been lifelong and is present in other family members, which would be indicative of the harmless familial variety. Symptoms such as cough, sputum production, hemoptysis, and dyspnea point to a respiratory problem and may have already triggered an evaluation of the lungs (see Chapters 40 through 42). The patient should be questioned about history of a heart murmur and exercise intolerance and about prior liver disease, cramping lower abdominal pain, diarrhea, bloody stools, and joint problems. Smoking and other risk factors related to the development of lung cancer (see Chapter 37) should be assessed. Exposure to tuberculosis also needs to be ascertained (see Chapter 38).

Physical Examination

Physical examination requires a check for fever, tachypnea, tachycardia, cyanosis, tobacco stains, jugular venous distention, barrel chest, wheezes, rhonchi, rales (crackles), signs of consolidation or effusion, heart murmur, skin lesions of hepatocellular disease, and signs of cirrhosis. Lymph nodes should be palpated for enlargement, and joints should be checked for hypertrophic changes and signs of inflammation.

Laboratory Studies

The only mandatory laboratory study is a *chest radiograph* because early pleural, pulmonary, or mediastinal neoplasm may be asymptomatic. A complete blood cell count and stool examination for occult blood may be of help. Further evaluation of the liver, thyroid, heart, or bowel should be undertaken only if symptoms or physical findings suggest disease in these areas. Patients with new onset of clubbing and a long history of smoking should be screened for the development of pulmonary neoplasm; periodic examinations including sputum cytology and chest computed tomography are appropriate.

Differentiating Osteoarthropathy from Rheumatoid Disease

Differentiating osteoarthropathy from rheumatoid disease can be difficult. An extensive review of patients with clubbing and lung cancer showed that the symptoms of osteoarthropathy were often mistaken for arthritis and predated the diagnosis of neoplasm by a mean of 4.9 months. Frequent complaints of bilateral joint discomfort in the small joints, such as the wrists and hands, and an adequate response to aspirin or nonsteroidal agents tended to persuade physicians that they were dealing with rheumatologic disease. Also noteworthy were the findings of acute elevation in acute-phase reactants and the presence of rheumatoid factor in 1 of 14 and antinuclear antibody in 5 of 12 cases. The symmetric involvement of small peripheral joints and the tendency to development of synovitis present a significant diagnostic dilemma, with some patients having a syndrome indistinguishable from that of an inflammatory arthritis.

SYMPTOMATIC MANAGEMENT AND PATIENT EDUCATION (12)

No symptomatic therapy is available for clubbing. It is an innocuous cosmetic disturbance. Discomfort in the bones and joints secondary to hypertrophic osteoarthropathy can be treated with aspirin and other nonsteroidal antiinflammatory drugs. Rarely, joint symptoms are disabling; these may require extreme therapies such as corticosteroids or intrathoracic vagotomy. Pamidronate has been tried when corticosteroids have failed to control pain in severe cases related to cystic fibrosis. Success has been reported, but evidence is fragmentary. When related to lung cancer, resection of the underlying tumor may reduce joint pain and swelling of the fingers. Such therapeutic options should be undertaken in consultation with a specialist familiar with the problem.

Patient education is important in any condition in which the physician discovers a potential sign of disease that is not obvious to the patient. It is likely that patients will be disturbed by the investigation and by the possibility of serious disease. The physician must take time to inform the patient that clubbing can be a harmless finding in addition to a helpful guide to the early diagnosis of disease. The patient who smokes should be strongly advised to quit (see Chapter 54).

A.H.G./A.G.M.

Annotated Bibliography

1. Spicknall KE, Zirwas MJ, English JC 3rd. Clubbing: an update on diagnosis, differential diagnosis, pathophysiology, and clinical relevance. J Am Acad Dermatol 2005;52:1020. (*Superb review of all aspects, including sensible algorithms for the evaluation of both unilateral and bilateral clubbing; 83 references.*)
2. Atkinson S, Fox SB. Vascular endothelial growth factor (VEGF)-A and platelet-derived growth factor (PDGF) play a central role in the pathogenesis of digital clubbing. J Pathol 2004;203:721. (*Vascular endothelial growth factor and platelet-derived growth factor are released after platelet trapping in the peripheral vasculature and may synergize in inducing the stromal and vascular changes present in digital clubbing.*)
3. Myers KA, Farquhar DRE. Does this patient have clubbing? JAMA 2001;286:341. (*Meticulous review of both the precision and the accuracy of clinical examination for clubbing and the accuracy of clubbing as a marker for disease.*)
4. Pineada CJ, Fonseca C, Martinez-Lavin M. The spectrum of soft tissue and skeletal abnormalities of hypertrophic osteoarthropathy. J Rheumatol 1990;17:626. (*Detailed description of characteristic findings.*)
5. Baughman RP, Gunther KL, Buchsbaum JA, et al. Prevalence of digital clubbing in bronchogenic carcinoma by a new digital index. Clin Exp Rheumatol 1998;16:21. (*A proposed new measure of clubbing yielded positive results in 37% of patients with cancer; no difference in prevalence was found among those with squamous-cell cancer, adenocarcinoma, or small-cell cancer.*)
6. Boonen A, Schrey G, Van der Linden S. Clubbing in human immunodeficiency virus infection. Br J Rheumatol 1996;35:292. (*Case reports of two patients in whom clubbing appeared soon after seroconversion.*)
7. Coutts II, Gilson JC, Kerr IH, et al. Significance of finger clubbing in asbestosis. Thorax 1987;42:117. (*Clubbing was not associated with the degree of asbestos exposure, but was with the severity of functional disease and fibrosis.*)

8. Kitis G, Thompson H, Allan RN. Finger clubbing in inflammatory bowel disease: its prevalence and pathogenesis. Br Med J 1979;2:825. (*Clubbing was found in 38% of patients with Crohn's disease and in 15% of those with ulcerative colitis.*)
9. Schamroth L. Personal experience. S Afr Med J 1976;50:297. (*Describes the loss of window between the nails and the cuticles when the nails of the index fingers are opposed.*)
10. Segal AN, Mackenzie AH. Hypertrophic osteoarthropathy: a ten-year retrospective analysis. Semin Arthritis Rheum 1985;12:220. (*Authoritative review with extensive study of 16 patients with hypertrophic osteoarthropathy; the differentiation from rheumatoid disease can sometimes be difficult.*)
11. Stenseth JH, Clagett OT, Woolner LB. Hypertrophic pulmonary osteoarthropathy. Dis Chest 1967;52:62. (*Review of 888 pulmonary neoplasms revealed a 9.2% incidence of hypertrophic osteoarthropathy.*)
12. Garske L, Bell SC. Pamidronate results in symptom control of hypertrophic pulmonary osteoarthropathy in cystic fibrosis. Chest 2002;121:1363. (*Case report of relief when nonsteroidal antiinflammatory drugs were contraindicated and after failure of corticosteroids.*)

CHAPTER 46 ■ APPROACH TO THE PATIENT WITH SLEEP APNEA

Transient episodes of breathing cessation (apnea) or a marked reduction in tidal volume (hypopnea) are common during sleep. Among adult men and women, 24% and 9%, respectively, have five or more episodes of apnea or hypopnea per hour of sleep. Despite the high prevalence, the condition is often overlooked because its symptoms (e.g., daytime tiredness, snoring) may be mistaken for normal phenomena of everyday life. Insufficient recognition in primary care practice continues despite the growing appreciation of the frequency and potentially serious consequences of this condition (e.g., motor vehicle accidents and deaths, cardiovascular morbidity and mortality, pulmonary hypertension). The primary care physician needs to be cognizant of the early and varied manifestations of sleep apnea and hypopnea so that a timely workup can commence and treatment can be instituted to reduce the risk of potentially life-threatening consequences.

PATHOPHYSIOLOGY AND CLINICAL PRESENTATION (1–16)

Definitions

Traditionally, *sleep apnea* has been defined by an apnea–hypopnea index (the total number of episodes of apnea or hypopnea per hour of sleep) of 5 or higher in association with excessive daytime somnolence. Use of this definition indicates that sleep apnea has a prevalence of 4% among men and 2% among women. However, as possible silent sequelae of sleep apnea including cardiovascular risk factors have been elucidated, many have extended the definition to include patients without manifest daytime somnolence. With or without somnolence, an apnea–hypopnea index of greater than 20 signifies clinically significant disease because it correlates with an increased risk for adverse outcomes. The apnea–hypopnea index can exceed 100 in some cases. It must be kept in mind, however, that the index does not correlate well with the severity of symptoms and effect on quality of life.

Sleep apnea may result from *central suppression* of respiration (as occurs with congestive heart failure and carbon dioxide retention) or from *upper airway obstruction*. In the former condition (*central sleep apnea*), air flow ceases because of the loss of central respiratory drive; in the latter (*obstructive sleep apnea*), air flow ceases because of obstruction despite chest and abdominal respiratory efforts during apnea. Obstructive sleep apnea is the most common form of sleep apnea encountered in the office setting. *Upper airway resistance syndrome* is an intermediate category, in which air flow is maintained by increased respiratory effort despite partial airway obstruction.

Mechanisms

Obstructive sleep apnea occurs when the patency of the nasopharyngeal airway becomes insufficient during sleep. Anatomic risk factors include nuchal obesity (cricothyroid neck circumference greater than 17 inches for men, greater than 16 inches for women), deviated septum, nasal polyps, enlarged uvula and soft palate, small chin with deep overbite, enlarged tonsils, and hypertrophy of the lateral pharyngeal musculature. Although obesity appears to be a major factor (causing fat deposition in the tongue and pharyngeal tissues), persons who are not obese are also at risk if they manifest other anatomic risk factors. Pharyngeal edema may mediate the increased risk of obstructive sleep apnea among patients with congestive heart failure. In addition to being anatomically predisposed, patients with obstructive sleep apnea appear to be unable to sustain sufficient oropharyngeal muscle dilator activity during sleep to prevent airway collapse during the negative pressure of inspiration. The suppressive effects of alcohol and sedatives on such neuromuscular function may explain their role in exacerbating obstructive sleep apnea. Hypothyroidism may be a risk factor.

When the obstruction is mild and not physiologically disturbing, *snoring* is the only manifestation, and sleep is not interrupted. With increasing degrees of obstruction, snoring becomes louder and compensatory respiratory efforts are triggered, causing electroencephalographically detectable *arousals from sleep*. Frequent arousals during the night disrupt normal sleep "architecture" and result in *daytime sleepiness*. In the upper airway resistance syndrome, near-normal air flow is maintained by compensatory respiratory efforts but at the cost of sleep arousals. More severe degrees of obstruction can lead to *hypopnea* (50% reduction in air flow with oxygen desaturation 4% or greater) or *apnea* (cessation of air flow for at least 10 seconds). The more severe and more prolonged the obstruction, the more likely and more severe are blood *oxygen desaturation* and *hypoxemia*, consequences of ventilation–perfusion mismatching as a result of the perfused lung not being adequately ventilated.

The adverse cardiovascular consequences of sleep apnea are related to hypoxemia. The decline in arterial oxygen increases pulmonary vascular resistance; when severe and chronic, it can lead to sustained *pulmonary hypertension* and ultimately *cor pulmonale*, particularly in persons with underlying chronic obstructive pulmonary disease or morbid obesity. Airway obstruction, episodes of apnea, and hypoxemia trigger compensatory increases not only in ventilatory effort, but also in sympathetic tone, which may explain the association between severe degrees of sleep apnea and *systemic hypertension*, *cardiac arrhythmias*, and increased *cardiovascular morbidity* and *mortality*. Sleep apnea is an independent risk factor for hypertension. Severe degrees of obstructive sleep apnea can also lead to hypercarbia and *central suppression* of respiration, as seen in persons with the *obesity–hypoventilation* (*Pickwickian*) *syndrome*. *Dysmenorrhea* and *amenorrhea* are consequences in women of reproductive age.

The disturbance in sleep caused by obstructive sleep apnea may impair *cognition* and *psychomotor performance*. In severe sleep apnea, hypersomnolence develops, markedly increasing the risk for injuries during work and driving. The risk ratio for *traffic accidents* increases to 6.3 and appears to be independent of other risk factors.

Clinical Presentations

Often, the patient presents at the insistence of a bed partner who is bothered or worried by *loud and intermittent snoring*, *disturbed* or *restless sleep*, periods of *irregular* or *halted breathing*, and *choking* or *gasping*. Patients presenting with obstructive sleep apnea typically complain of excessive *daytime sleepiness*; they may note falling asleep at work or at a meeting. Women are somewhat more likely to report *chronic fatigue*. Patients find that they awaken not feeling refreshed and may have a morning *headache*. Work performance may be suffering, and the history of a work-related or automobile *accident* resulting from sleepiness may be elicited. Family and friends may note a *personality change*. Obesity is common but is not a necessary part of the clinical presentation; approximately 70% of patients with sleep apnea are obese. Nearly half of premenopausal women with disordered nocturnal breathing are thin but have another contributing anatomic feature, such as a *severe overbite* or a *high hard palate*. A positive *family history* is noted, usually in persons with a contributing anatomic factor or obesity.

DIFFERENTIAL DIAGNOSIS (1–4,8–11,16)

Because obstructive sleep apnea may present as daytime tiredness, it must be differentiated from other causes of chronic fatigue (see Chapter 8). In patients who present with interrupted sleep, other sleep disturbances deserve consideration (see Chapter 232). In those whose presentation is predominantly one of

difficulty in breathing at night, heart failure (see Chapter 32), chronic obstructive lung disease (see Chapter 47), and other causes of snoring (see Chapter 223) should be considered. *Hypothyroidism* (see Chapter 104) and *acromegaly* have been associated with sleep apnea.

WORKUP (1–4,8–11,17–21)

History

A high index of suspicion is appropriate when a patient, whether obese or not, presents with symptoms of excessive daytime sleepiness, tiredness, or fatigue. A history of very loud intermittent snoring, irregular respiratory activity with spells of gasping or choking that interrupt sleep, or witnessed episodes of apnea is strongly suggestive. Also worth noting are any accidents, job performance difficulties, and personality changes or cognitive difficulties, especially if they occur in the context of daytime sleepiness. Risk factors that help in identifying patients with obstructive sleep apnea include marked obesity (body mass index >28 kg/m^2), increasing age, obstructive upper airway abnormalities, regular use of sedatives or alcohol, and hypothyroidism.

Physical Examination

The blood pressure should be checked for elevation and the integument noted for any cyanosis, clubbing, or signs of hypothyroidism (see Chapter 104). The upper airway is examined for overbite, a high hard palate, other potentially obstructing nasopharyngeal lesions (e.g., nasal polyps, tonsillar hypertrophy, large uvula), and nasopharyngeal narrowing. In persons with suspected severe obstructive sleep apnea, one should check for signs of pulmonary hypertension and cor pulmonale (e.g., right ventricular heave, loud pulmonic component of the second heart sound, jugular venous distention, leg edema).

The neck circumference should be measured to document any nuchal obesity. One clinical prediction rule is based on the adjustment of neck circumference in the presence of other risk factors: 4 cm is added to the actual measurement if hypertension is present, 3 cm is added if there is a history of habitual snoring, and 3 cm is added if the patient is reported to gasp or choke most nights. An adjusted neck circumference of less than 43 cm indicates a low probability of sleep apnea. An adjusted circumference of 43 to 48 cm indicates an intermediate probability with an odds ratio of 4 to 8; an adjusted circumference greater than 48 cm indicates a high probability with an odds ratio of 20.

Laboratory Studies

Sleep Study

The most definitive diagnostic procedure in symptomatic patients clinically suspected of obstructive sleep apnea is a formal *polysomnographic study*, which includes overnight monitoring of the electroencephalogram, eye movements, muscle activity, chest movements, air flow, and blood oxygen saturation. Although such testing is expensive, it is nevertheless cost-effective; the high sensitivity and specificity minimize both false-positive results (which generate unnecessary, expensive long-term therapy) and false-negative results (which can lead to the failure to treat disease and the risk for considerable morbidity and mortality).

Home Monitoring

Home-monitoring methods for diagnosis are improving, but they lack the sensitivity and specificity of polysomnography. Although the sensitivity and specificity of the most sophisticated home methods are reported to exceed 95%, and although the positive predictive value of a positive result can be high (approaching 99% in patients in whom obstructive sleep apnea is strongly suspected clinically), the negative predictive value and false-negative rate of these tests are disappointing (77% and 23%, respectively). Based on these performance characteristics, some health care systems recommend screening with a high-quality home-monitoring method (simple periodic oximetry is insufficient), with referral to formal polysomnography reserved for those in whom obstructive sleep apnea is strongly suspected clinically but whose home-monitoring test results are negative. A recent trial randomized patients with a high pretest probability of moderate to severe obstructive sleep apnea to either polysomnography or ambulatory titration using overnight oximetry. No advantage was found for polysomnography in these patients. The literature should be watched for confirmation of this approach and further definition of the appropriate population of patients.

Other Tests

Few routine laboratory studies are of value. A *thyroid-stimulating hormone* determination is indicated if clinical evidence of hypothyroidism is present. Unless the patient has very severe disease with signs of cor pulmonale, the measurement of *hematocrit, arterial blood gases*, and *pulse oximetry* in the office is likely to be of little value. Cardiac ultrasound is helpful when there is clinical suspicion of resultant pulmonary hypertension.

PRINCIPLES OF MANAGEMENT
(2–4,15,17,18,22–41)

Selection and Initiation of Therapy

Treatment can improve the survival and functional status of some patients with obstructive sleep apnea, but a proper matching of disease severity with treatment intensity is critical to achieving the best possible outcome. Unfortunately, few evidence-based criteria are available to guide patient selection and timing of therapy. *Positive findings on polysomnography*, demonstrating more than 20 apneic periods per hour in a symptomatic patient with arterial desaturation during sleep, provide the strongest grounds for the consideration of therapy; the risk for complications of obstructive sleep apnea is high in such persons, particularly those with underlying lung disease. A lesser frequency of apneic episodes (<20 per hour) is a more common finding and necessitates careful consideration of the overall clinical picture before treatment is recommended. No prospective data are available on outcomes in persons with milder disease (<20 episodes per hour) to help in treatment selection. Clinical judgment is required. Patients with preexisting lung disease plus sleep apnea have a worse prognosis than do those with no underlying lung disease, and they should be treated more aggressively. Minimally symptomatic patients with no concurrent pulmonary disease or evidence of impairment might first be prescribed a few potentially useful, noninva-

sive, simple measures (e.g., weight reduction if obese, changes in sleeping position) and followed expectantly. *Empiric therapy* based on clinical suspicion without reference to polysomnography is not recommended because clinical estimates lack the sensitivity and specificity required for a condition in which life-long therapy may be necessary.

Weight Reduction

A *weight reduction program* should be recommended for patients with mild disease who are obese. Weight reduction is also the centerpiece of the treatment program for obese patients with more symptomatic disease because it can greatly reduce or even cure sleep apnea. The implementation of a comprehensive, personalized program of weight reduction is essential to a successful weight loss effort (see Chapter 233).

Sleep Position

The position one assumes when sleeping can affect airway patency. Lying on one's back increases the risk for apneic episodes; sleeping on one's side reduces the risk. A trial of patient education to change sleeping position is worth a try, but most persons rotate at night during sleep. (One investigator suggested that patients try taping a tennis ball to their back at night to prevent lying in a supine position.)

Continuous Positive Airway Pressure

Nighttime nasal continuous positive airway pressure (CPAP) is becoming a mainstay in the treatment of obstructive sleep apnea. A sealed nasal mask is worn at night connected to a blower apparatus that pneumatically sustains sufficient airway pressure to maintain upper airway patency. Patient acceptance is steadily improving, and compliance now exceeds 80% in reported trials (probably closer to 50% in everyday practice), facilitated by advances in apparatus design. CPAP improves survival in persons with more than 20 episodes of apnea per hour. In a trial using subtherapeutic CPAP as a control intervention, therapeutic CPAP reduced daytime somnolence and improved self-reported health status. In another trial, CPAP improved blood pressure and left ventricular ejection fraction among patients with congestive heart failure. Because obstructive sleep apnea is associated with coronary heart disease, several studies have looked at the effect of CPAP on risk factors and measures of early atherosclerosis such as carotid intima–media thickness. Most of the reported studies have included patients with severe disease. Efficacy in patients with less severe disease remains to be established; at least one trial found no benefit for patients with objective apnea–hypopnea sleep disturbance but no daytime somnolence.

Surgery

Surgical approaches are worth considering only if symptoms are severe, more conservative measures have failed, and an obvious obstructing anatomic anomaly is identified. The surgical excision of obstructing tonsils, a nasal mass, or a pharyngeal tumor can be curative. Surgery has also been performed in patients with severe obstructive disease, even in the absence of a single, identifiable obstructing lesion. The procedure used most for this purpose has been the *uvulopalatopharyngoplasty*

(UPP). In performing the UPP, the surgeon excises the uvula, part of the soft palate, and any redundant pharyngeal tissue. The problem with recommending such surgery is that only about half of patients obtain a satisfactory result. Moreover, it has not been possible to predict in advance who will benefit from the surgery, and durable results are not always achieved. As a result, and with the improvements in CPAP therapy, UPP is becoming a less-used treatment option. Systematic review of the evidence concluded that a lack of standardization of surgical procedures and poor study design severely limited the available evidence.

Oral Appliances

Dental appliances that correct such precipitants as a deep overbite have been tried. Acceptance is variable; long-term efficacy remains to be established. Evidence indicates that they are not as effective as CPAP but are nonetheless preferred by most patients.

Pharmacologic Approaches

The most important pharmacologic intervention is avoidance of agents that might suppress respiration or neuromuscular function. Patients with sleep apnea should stop using alcohol and drugs with sedative activity. Sildenafil has also been reported to worsen respiratory and desaturation events in men with severe obstructive sleep apnea, presumably due to its effect on upper airway congestion and muscle relaxation. Because apneic episodes are most frequent during rapid eye movement (REM) sleep, the use of nonsedating agents that interfere with the REM phase of sleep, such as the nonsedating tricyclic antidepressant *protriptyline*, has been tried. Another approach is to administer drugs that might stimulate respiration, such as *medroxyprogesterone*. Neither approach has shown much promise and is not recommended. Systematic review of the evidence has found no beneficial effects for medroxyprogesterone, clonidine, buspirone, aminophylline, theophylline, or sabeluzole.

In contrast, treatment of underlying hypothyroidism with *thyroid hormone replacement* is effective in patients with documented hypothyroidism as the cause of sleep apnea. *Nocturnal oxygen supplementation* can reduce the desaturation caused by sleep apnea, and some suggest that it be used; however, it can also prolong an apneic episode and should not be administered except in carefully controlled circumstances when an underlying chronic hypoxemia is present (see Chapter 47). Its effect on long-term outcome remains to be established.

Other Approaches

In addition to modifications of existing approaches to sleep apnea syndrome, including improvements in oral appliances and CPAP devices to increase patient acceptance, other approaches are emerging. For example, atrial overdrive pacing has been shown to reduce significantly the number of episodes of both central and obstructive sleep apnea. Although this is of interest among patients with pacemakers inserted for other indications, its significance for the vast majority of patients with sleep apnea is yet to be determined.

INDICATIONS FOR REFERRAL

A patient with daytime tiredness and hypersomnolence should be considered a candidate for referral and consideration of a formal sleep study, especially if the patient's bed companion corroborates a history of loud snoring, disturbed sleep, abnormal respirations, and apneic periods. The presence of marked obesity and difficult-to-control hypertension should further raise the level of suspicion about an obstructive sleep disorder and prompt a consultation. Referral is best made to a pulmonary specialist experienced in the conduct and interpretation of polysomnography; however, it should be made clear that the purpose of the consultation is the assessment of the appropriateness of formal sleep testing and not the automatic performance of a polysomnographic study. Consultation with a pulmonary specialist experienced in the treatment of sleep disorders can also be very useful for a patient who fails to improve with weight loss and for whom CPAP and surgical approaches to therapy need to be considered.

PATIENT EDUCATION

A patient brought in by a spouse complaining of his or her excessive snoring must be given detailed information on the potential seriousness (accidents, cardiovascular morbidity and mortality) of this seemingly harmless condition. Unless they suffer from disabling daytime tiredness and excessive sleepiness, such patients are unlikely to appreciate the significance of their condition. Patient education is also essential regarding treatment. Because weight loss is so effective in alleviating upper airway soft-tissue obstruction in obese patients, instruction about a comprehensive approach to weight reduction (see Chapter 233) is an essential component of the office encounter. Also important is advice regarding the avoidance of sedatives and alcohol and, perhaps, sildenafil and other guanine monophosphate–specific phosphodiesterase-5 inhibitors.

A.G.M./A.H.G.

Annotated Bibliography

1. Patil SP, Schneider H, Schwartz AR, et al. Adult obstructive sleep apnea: pathophysiology and diagnosis. Chest 2007;132:325. (*An excellent review.*)
2. Eckert DJ, Jordan AS, Merchia P, et al. Central sleep apnea: pathophysiology and treatment. Chest 2007;131:595. (*Discusses the clinical implications of improved knowledge of central sleep apnea pathophysiology, as well as therapeutic treatment approaches.*)
3. Bradley TD, Floras JS. Sleep apnea and heart failure: Part 1. Obstructive sleep apnea, Part 2. Central sleep apnea. Circulation 2003;103:1671, 1822. (*An excellent two-part review focusing on physiology, prognostic implications, and therapy.*)
4. Flemons WW. Obstructive sleep apnea. N Engl J Med 2002;347:498. (*An excellent case-based review with a diagnostic algorithm.*)
5. Guilleminault C, Stoohs R, Kim YD, et al. Upper airway sleep-disordered breathing in women. Ann Intern Med 1995;122:493. (*A retrospective case–control study identifying features of the clinical presentation in women; many were thin and manifested craniofacial anomalies contributing to the obstruction of air flow.*)
6. He J, Kryger MH, Zorick FJ, et al. Mortality and apnea index in obstructive sleep apnea. Chest 1988;94:9. (*Increased mortality was seen in patients with >20 episodes of apnea per hour of sleep; continuous positive airway pressure [CPAP] improved survival.*)
7. Hla KM, Young T, Bidwell T, et al. Sleep apnea and hypertension: a population-based study. Ann Intern Med 1994;120:382. (*Sleep apnea was found to be an independent risk factor for hypertension.*)

8. Kohnlein T, Welte T, Tan LB, et al. Central sleep apnoea syndrome in patients with chronic heart disease: a critical review of the current literature. Thorax 2002;57:547. (*A comprehensive review of the prevalence, prognosis, clinical presentation, pathophysiology, diagnosis, and treatment of the central sleep apnea syndrome, as well as of its relationship to congestive heart failure.*)

9. Shamsuzzaman ASM, Gersh BJ, Somers VK. Obstructive sleep apnea. Implications for cardiac and vascular disease. JAMA 2003;290:1906. (*Reviews the relationship to hypertension, coronary disease, cerebrovascular disease, congestive heart failure, and arrhythmias; 154 references.*)

10. Kuna ST, Sant'Ambrogio G. Pathophysiology of upper airway closures during sleep. JAMA 1991;266:1384. (*An excellent review of the mechanisms of upper airway obstruction in sleep apnea.*)

11. Mooe T, Rabben T, Wiklund U, et al. Sleep-disordered breathing in women: occurrence and association with coronary artery disease. Am J Med 1996;101:251. (*A case–control study finding that sleep apnea is common in women with coronary artery disease and an independent predictor of coronary artery disease after correction for other risk factors.*)

12. Newman FJ, Nieto FJ, Guidry U, et al. Relation of sleep-disordered breathing to cardiovascular risk factors: the Sleep Heart Health Study. Am J Epidemiol 2001;154:50. (*Higher cardiovascular risk factors were found in those with higher sleep apnea measured by a respiratory disturbance index.*)

13. Peppard PE, Young T, Palta M, et al. Prospective study of the association between sleep-disordered breathing and hypertension. N Engl J Med 2000;342:1378. (*A study finding a dose–response relationship between the severity of sleep apnea and the risk of hypertension over 4 years.*)

14. Teran-Santos J, Jimenez-Gomez A, Codero-Guevara J, et al. The association between sleep apnea and the risk of traffic accidents. N Engl J Med 1999;340:847. (*The odds ratio was 6.3 in a comparison of persons having >10 episodes per hour with normal persons.*)

15. Wright J, Johns R, Watt I, et al. Health effects of obstructive sleep apnoea and the effectiveness of continuous positive airway pressure: a systematic review of the research evidence. BMJ 1997;314:851. (*Questions the evidence for the effect of sleep apnea on health, as opposed to daytime sleepiness, as well as the evidence for CPAP, concluding that small changes in daytime sleepiness are achieved but no improvements in morbidity, mortality, and quality-of-life indicators have been adequately assessed.*)

16. Young T, Palta M, Dempsey J, et al. The occurrence of sleep-disordered breathing among middle-aged adults. N Engl J Med 1993;328:1230. (*The prevalence was 24% among men and 9% among women, with sleep apnea found among 4% of men and 2% of women—much higher than previously estimated.*)

17. Mulgrew AT, Fox N, Ayas NT, et al. Diagnosis and initial management of obstructive sleep apnea without polysomnography: a randomized validation study. Ann Intern Med 2007;146:157. (*Polysomnography confers no advantage over the ambulatory approach in terms of diagnosis and CPAP titration.*)

18. Chervin RD, Murman DL, Malow BA, et al. Cost–utility of three approaches to the diagnosis of sleep apnea: polysomnography, home testing, and empirical therapy. Ann Intern Med 1999;130:496. (*A cost–utility analysis demonstrating that polysomnography provided the most quality-adjusted life-years.*)

19. Kramer NR, Cook TE, Carlisle CC, et al. The role of the primary care physician in recognizing obstructive sleep apnea. Arch Intern Med 1999;159:965. (*A retrospective chart audit showing that primary care physicians did recognize severely affected persons but that only a small fraction of patients at risk were identified.*)

20. Netzer NC, Stoohs RA, Netzer CM, et al. Using the Berlin Questionnaire to identify patients at risk for the sleep apnea syndrome. Ann Intern Med 1999;131:485. (*Identification as high risk predicted a respiratory disturbance index of >5 with a sensitivity of 0.86, a specificity of 0.77, and a likelihood ratio of 3.79.*)

21. Viner S, Szalai JP, Hoffstein V. Are history and physical examination a good screening test for sleep apnea? Ann Intern Med 1991;115:356. (*Age, body mass index, male gender, and snoring were predictive of sleep apnea in this logistic regression study, but sensitivity was not much better than that of a subjective clinical assessment.*)

22. Basner RC. Continuous positive airway pressure for obstructive sleep apnea. N Engl J Med 2007;356:1751. (*An excellent case-based review.*)

23. Barbe F, Mayorales LR, Duran J, et al. Treatment with continuous positive airway pressure is not effective in patients with sleep apnea but no daytime sleepiness. Ann Intern Med 2001;134:1015. (*Patients with objective apnea–hypopnea index abnormalities but no subjective sleepiness do not benefit from CPAP in this randomized, controlled trial of 55 patients.*)

24. Bridgman SA, Dunn KM. Surgery for obstructive sleep apnoea (Cochrane review). In: The Cochrane library, Issue 3. Oxford: Update Software, 2004.

(*There is a paucity of evidence, with poorly standardized procedures and no good trials; see* http://www.cochrane.org *for updates.*)

25. Engleman HM, Kingshott RN, Wraith PK, et al. Randomized placebo-controlled crossover trial of continuous positive airway pressure for mild sleep apnea/hypopnea syndrome. Am J Respir Crit Care Med 1999;159:461. (*Confirms benefits for daytime function after CPAP treatment for mild sleep apnea/hypopnea syndrome but highlights the unacceptability of CPAP in many such patients.*)

26. Garrigue S, Bordier P, Jais P, et al. Benefit of atrial pacing in sleep apnea syndrome. N Engl J Med 2002;346:404. (*Atrial overdrive pacing significantly reduced the number of episodes of central or obstructive sleep apnea without reducing the total sleep time.*)

27. George CF. Reduction in motor vehicle collisions following treatment of sleep apnoea with nasal CPAP. Thorax 2001;56:508. (*An observational study concluding that the risk of motor vehicle collisions due to obstructive sleep apnea is removed when patients are treated with CPAP.*)

28. Jenkinson C, Davies RJ, Mullins R, et al. Comparison of therapeutic and subtherapeutic nasal continuous positive airway pressure for obstructive sleep apnoea: a randomised prospective parallel trial. Lancet 1999;353:2100. (*Therapeutic nasal CPAP reduces excessive daytime sleepiness and improves self-reported health status compared with a subtherapeutic control.*)

29. Kaneko Y, Floras JS, Usui K, et al. Cardiovascular effects of continuous positive airway pressure in patients with heart failure and obstructive sleep apnea. N Engl J Med 2003;348:1233. (*In this small trial, CPAP improved blood pressure and left ventricular ejection fraction.*)

30. Steiropoulos P, Tsara V, Nena E, et al. Effect of continuous positive airway pressure treatment on serum cardiovascular risk factors in patients with obstructive sleep apnea-hypopnea syndrome. Chest 2007;132:843. (*With good CPAP compliance, lipid profile improved.*)

31. Drager LF, Bortolotto LA, Figueiredo AC, et al. Effects of continuous positive airway pressure on early signs of atherosclerosis in obstructive sleep apnea. Am J Respir Crit Care Med 2007;176:706. (*The treatment of obstructive sleep apnea significantly improved early signs of atherosclerosis.*)

32. Lim J, Lasserson TJ, Fleetham J, et al. Oral appliances for obstructive sleep apnoea (Cochrane review). In: The Cochrane library, Issue 3. Oxford: Update Software, 2004. (*This approach was not as effective as CPAP but was preferred by patients; see* http://www.cochrane.org *for updates.*)

33. Magalang UJ, Mador MJ. Behavioral and pharmacologic therapy of obstructive sleep apnea. Clin Chest Med 2003;24:343. (*The data do not support the use of any drug as an alternative to CPAP, but the studies have been of poor quality.*)

34. Mehta A, Qian J, Petocz P, et al. A randomized, controlled study of a mandibular advancement splint for obstructive sleep apnea. Am J Respir Crit Care Med 2001;163:1457. (*Effective for some but not others.*)

35. Chan ASL, Lee RWW, Cistulli PA. Dental appliance treatment for obstructive sleep apnea. Chest 2007;132:693. (*This approach was less efficacious than CPAP but was generally preferred by patients.*)

36. Patel SR, White DP, Malhotra A, et al. Continuous positive airway pressure therapy for treating sleepiness in a diverse population with obstructive sleep apnea. Arch Intern Med 2003;163:565. (*The procedure significantly improved subjective and objective measures of sleepiness.*)

37. Pillar G, Peled R, Lavie P. Recurrence of sleep apnea without concomitant weight increase 7.5 years after weight reduction surgery. Chest 1994;106:1702. (*Poor correlation was found between weight loss and apnea index in this study.*)

38. Shneerson J, Wright J. Lifestyle modification for obstructive sleep apnoea (Cochrane review). In: The Cochrane library, Issue 3. Oxford: Update Software, 2004. (*There was convincing evidence to support recommendations for weight loss, exercise, or improved sleep hygiene; see* http://www.cochrane.org *for updates.*)

39. Smith I, Lasserson T, Wright J. Drug treatments for obstructive sleep apnoea (Cochrane review). In: The Cochrane library, Issue 3. Oxford: Update Software, 2004. (*No beneficial effects were found for medroxyprogesterone, clonidine, buspirone, aminophylline, theophylline, or sabeluzole; see* http://www.cochrane.org *for updates.*)

40. White J, Cates C, Wright J. Continuous positive airways pressure for obstructive sleep apnoea (Cochrane review). In: The Cochrane library, Issue 3. Oxford: Update Software, 2004. (*CPAP was more effective than placebo; patients preferred CPAP to placebo but strongly preferred oral appliances to CPAP; see* http://www.cochrane.org *for updates.*)

41. Roizenblatt S, Guilleminault C, Poyares D, et al. A double-blind, placebo-controlled, crossover study of sildenafil in obstructive sleep apnea. Arch Inter Med 2006;166:1763. (*A single 50-mg dose of sildenafil at bedtime worsened respiratory and desaturation events.*)

CHAPTER 47 ■ MANAGEMENT OF CHRONIC OBSTRUCTIVE PULMONARY DISEASE

Chronic obstructive pulmonary disease (COPD) affects 5% of the adult population and is the fourth-leading cause of death and twelfth-leading cause of morbidity in the United States. It is the only major cause of death for which both morbidity and mortality rates are increasing. *Smoking* remains the principal risk factor for the development of COPD; nearly 90% of cases occur in the context of long-term heavy smoking, which increases the risk for COPD 30-fold. The marked increase in COPD prevalence, especially among women, noted since 1980 reflects the heavy smoking habits of the U.S. population in the decades after World War II.

Although COPD is essentially irreversible and is usually marked by a progressive decline in lung function, improvements in functional status and survival are possible with good care, most of which can be managed in the outpatient setting by the primary care physician. The primary physician needs to know the indications for bronchodilators, corticosteroids, oxygen supplementation, antibiotics, immunizations, and rehabilitative measures in addition to the potential value of surgical approaches. A positive attitude on the part of the physician regarding the impact of the patient's effective self-management is an important determinant of patient motivation and success in the doctor–patient collaboration that is essential to the effective management of COPD.

PATHOPHYSIOLOGY, CLINICAL PRESENTATION, AND COURSE (1–13)

Defining Chronic Obstructive Pulmonary Disease and Assessing Severity

COPD is a heterogeneous disorder marked by *obstruction* of airflow and a reduction in the expiratory flow rate. It is distinguished from asthma and other obstructive pulmonary diseases in that the airflow limitation is not fully reversible and is in most cases both progressive and associated with an abnormal inflammatory response of the lungs to noxious particles and gases such as those delivered in cigarette smoke. Spirometric measurement of airflow confirms the diagnosis when it documents *a reduction of the ratio of forced expiratory volume in 1 second* (FEV_1) *to forced vital capacity* (FVC) *to less than 70%*. Disease severity in COPD can then be assessed by the progressive decline in the post-bronchodilator FEV_1, as seen in Table 47.1.

Pathophysiology

Inflammation

Airway inflammation plays an important pathophysiologic role in obstructive pulmonary diseases. In stable COPD, the inflam-

mation appears to be predominantly *neutrophilic*. Of the cytokines measured in COPD, those that attract neutrophils (e.g., interleukin-8) are the most markedly elevated. Although lymphocytes are present in increased numbers, they are mainly type 1 helper CD8 T cells. In contrast, the predominant cells in asthma are eosinophils, mast cells, and type 2 helper CD4 T cells. During an acute exacerbation of COPD, the number of eosinophils found in bronchial biopsy specimens is increased 30-fold. These differences in inflammatory cell infiltrates may help to explain the disparate responses to corticosteroids seen in the two conditions and in different phases of COPD (see later discussion).

Despite the differences in inflammatory mechanisms between COPD and asthma, evidence is emerging that the inflammatory pathophysiology of *chronic asthma* might *predispose* patients to COPD, especially smokers. Asthmatic patients who smoke manifest an increased rate of deterioration in FEV_1 over time in comparison with nonasthmatic smokers and asthmatic patients who do not smoke. Moreover, bronchial hyperresponsiveness to methacholine challenge is a powerful independent predictor of progression of COPD in smokers. Perhaps the underlying inflammatory process in asthma is an important contributor to the development of COPD in smokers and may account for the steroid responsiveness seen in a subset of COPD patients.

Inflammation of the cells lining the bronchial wall leads to hyperplasia of the mucous glands and narrowing of the small airways. As noted, smoking or prolonged exposure to other bronchial irritants is the usual precipitant. However, even after withdrawal of such irritants, the inflammatory process often continues unabated. Airway edema, excess mucus production, and loss of ciliary transport result.

Alveolar Destruction

A second pathophysiologic process is *destruction of the alveolar walls* leading to pathologic enlargement of the air spaces distal to the terminal bronchioles. This is due to *imbalance between alveolar protease and antiprotease activity*. Alveolar tissue contains both proteases and antiproteases, with neutrophil-derived elastase being the most important protease and α_1-antitrypsin being the prime antiprotease. When antitrypsin activity is reduced or elastase levels are increased, alveolar wall destruction follows. Cigarette smoking may trigger the influx of elastase-rich neutrophils into the alveoli or the oxidative inactivation of antitrypsin. Patients who are homozygous for a hereditary deficiency of α_1-*antitrypsin* (<80 mg/L) are at greatly increased risk for the development of emphysema. They represent fewer than 2% of cases overall but account for many cases among nonsmokers without other environmental risk factors; they present with the onset of clinical disease before age 50 years and have a positive family history of early-onset emphysema.

TABLE 47.1

SPIROMETRIC CLASSIFICATION OF CHRONIC OBSTRUCTIVE PULMONARY DISEASE SEVERITY BASED ON POST-BRONCHODILATOR FEV$_1$

Stage I: mild	FEV$_1$/FVC <0.70 FEV$_1$ ≥80% predicted
Stage II: moderate	FEV$_1$/FVC <0.70 50% ≤ FEV$_1$ <80% predicted
Stage III: severe	FEV$_1$/FVC <0.70 30% ≤ FEV$_1$ <50% predicted
Stage IV: very severe	FEV$_1$/FVC <0.70 FEV$_1$ <30% predicted *or* FEV$_1$ <50% predicted plus chronic respiratory failure[a]

FEV$_1$, forced expiratory volume in 1 second; FVC, forced vital capacity.
[a]Respiratory failure: arterial partial pressure of oxygen (PaO$_2$) <8.0 kPa (60 mm Hg) with or without arterial partial pressure of CO$_2$ (PaCO$_2$) >6.7 kPa (50 mm Hg) while breathing air at sea level.
From Rabe KF, Hurd S, Anzueto A, et al. Am J Respir Crit Care Med 2007;176:532, and Global Initiative for Chronic Obstructive Lung Disease, available at http://www.goldcopd.com/ (accessed June 14, 2008); with permission.

The result of the imbalance between protease and antiprotease activity is fragmentation of the pulmonary elastic tissue, which leads to *destruction of the alveolar architecture* and the *capillary bed* that lies within the alveolar wall. Because both air space and the vascular bed are destroyed, ventilation and perfusion do not become markedly mismatched, and marked hypoxemia does not ensue. Expiratory flow rates decline with the loss of the normal elastic recoil of the lung and radial traction on airways; the poorly supported noncartilaginous airways collapse during expiration. Inspiratory flow rates can be normal because airway caliber is normal during inspiration. In many patients, a *reversible cholinergic component* of airway obstruction is also present that is responsive to muscarinic blockade. *Pulmonary compliance* increases with the decline in elasticity. As destruction of alveolar architecture progresses, the size of the pulmonary capillary bed is reduced, causing the *carbon monoxide diffusing capacity* to drop. Because the reduction in size of the vascular bed parallels the fall in alveolar surface area, ventilation still roughly matches perfusion, and significant hypoxemia does not ensue.

Oxidative Stress

Oxidative stress caused by inhaled cigarette smoke has been incriminated as a contributor to airway narrowing, both reversible and irreversible, and to alveolar destruction. This stress reflects an imbalance between oxidants and antioxidants similar to that between proteases and antiproteases. Increased levels of oxidation products such as hydrogen peroxide and nitric oxide are found in the breath condensates of patients with COPD. Oxidative stress can directly damage cells and the lung extracellular matrix. It also promotes inflammation through a number of mechanisms and exacerbates the protease/antiprotease imbalance by activating the former and deactivating the latter.

Clinical Presentation

Although smoking and other noxious stimuli precipitate both airway inflammation and alveolar destruction, one or the other process may predominate. Historically, the patient with airway inflammation producing a chronic cough and sputum production for 3 months of 2 consecutive years was characterized as suffering from *chronic bronchitis*. The patient with alveolar destruction evident on chest x-ray as hyperlucency of the pulmonary parenchyma and lung hyperinflation was given the diagnosis of *emphysema*. These diagnoses can best be thought of as extremes on the spectrum of COPD, with the clinical picture for any individual patient determined by the relative contribution of airway inflammation and alveolar destruction.

Chronic Bronchitis

For the patient at the chronic bronchitis end of the spectrum, obstruction to airflow occurs with both inspiration and expiration. Widespread bronchial narrowing and mucous plugging produce *hypoxemia* because of mismatching of ventilation and perfusion. *Hypercarbia* results from impeded ventilation. Chronic hypoxia and hypercarbia increase pulmonary arterial resistance and may lead to the development of *pulmonary hypertension* and eventually *cor pulmonale*. Sudden worsening may precipitate acute right-sided heart failure in severe chronic bronchitis. The patient may appear *plethoric* and *cyanotic*. *Secondary polycythemia* is common.

Emphysema

For the patient on the emphysema end of the spectrum, the clinical picture is dominated by *dyspnea*, particularly on exertion. Cough is only a minor complaint, and sputum production is scant. The patient with advanced disease is *thin* and *tachypneic*, often using accessory muscles of respiration and *pursed-lip breathing*. The latter helps to keep noncartilaginous airways from collapsing during expiration. Cyanosis is uncommon because the oxygen tension (PO$_2$) is only minimally reduced. The neck veins may seem distended, but only during expiration. The *anterior–posterior diameter* of the chest is *increased*, the *percussion note* is *hyperresonant*, and the *breath sounds* are *distant*. Usually, no signs of cor pulmonale are present, although the right ventricular impulse may be prominent because of displacement by hyperinflated lungs. As noted, hypoxemia is minimal, and little, if any, carbon dioxide retention occurs until the end stages of the disease. Chest radiography demonstrates hyperinflation and hyperlucency, especially at the apices, except in patients with antitrypsin deficiency, whose radiographic changes are greatest at the bases.

Clinical Course and Prognosis

The clinical course of COPD is generally *progressive*, although some patients seem to reach a plateau clinically, especially if they stop smoking. Early on, before the onset of symptoms, one can often detect an increase in the *closing volume* and a decrease in the *maximum midexpiratory flow rate* (sensitive measures of small-airway disease); measures of large-airway resistance are usually within normal limits during this phase of the illness. The presymptomatic, *small-airway stage* (stage 0) of COPD may represent a period of reversible disease; however, early fibrotic changes have been found in airways of such patients. It has not been resolved whether intervention at the time of early small-airway abnormalities will alter the course of disease and improve the prognosis.

Longitudinal studies of symptomatic patients have shown a *steady deterioration* in *pulmonary function* with time. When the FEV$_1$ is used as the measure of obstruction, an annual average decrease in flow rate of 50 to 70 mL/s has been noted. By the time the FEV_1 declines to 1 L/s, the mean annual mortality approaches 10%. The onset of resting tachycardia and signs of cor pulmonale are other indicators of a poor prognosis.

It remains difficult to predict survival in individual patients. Although the prognosis for patients with COPD is not very good, therapy does prolong survival (see later discussion). Cessation of smoking is critical. The rate of decline in FEV_1 can be reduced by 50% if the patient stops smoking and is able to sustain cessation. Intermittent quitters receive much less benefit.

WORKUP (7–15)

History

Description of symptoms should include any limitations of activity experienced in daily life, both at rest and during exercise. A detailed *history* of *smoking* and *environmental* or *work exposures* to pulmonary irritants is indicated. Estimates of *exercise capacity* (e.g., number of flights of stairs that can be climbed or distance that can be walked on level ground) are helpful, as is some indication of the progression of symptoms over time. The presence of *leg edema* and worsening exercise tolerance suggest the onset of right-sided heart failure in the patient with chronic bronchitis.

Physical Examination

It is important to note any tachypnea, tachycardia, prolongation of the expiratory phase, cyanosis, clubbing, use of accessory respiratory muscles, wheezes, signs of consolidation, diminution of breath sounds, and evidence of cor pulmonale (jugular venous distention, peripheral edema, right ventricular heave, loud pulmonic closure sound, and right ventricular third heart sound).

Laboratory Studies

Testing is necessary to confirm the diagnosis, assess severity, and identify comorbid conditions, thereby providing a basis for choosing therapy and estimating prognosis.

Spirometry

Spirometry is essential to confirm the diagnosis in patients with symptoms suggestive of COPD, including those with chronic cough and sputum production, as well as those who present with dyspnea. The most helpful measurement is the *ratio of FEV_1 to VC*. As noted, a reduction in this ratio to less than 70% is an indication of significant airflow limitation. Disease severity in COPD can then be assessed by the progressive decline in the post-bronchodilator FEV_1, with results compared with predicted values, as seen in Table 47.1. Crude estimates of obstruction can be provided by the FEV_1 alone. Should spirometry be unavailable, prolongation of the forced expiratory time beyond 6 seconds suggests an FEV_1/FVC ratio of less than 50%. Patients with a 50% reduction in FEV_1 are often dyspneic and hypoxemic on exertion; by the time the FEV_1 falls to 25% of the predicted value, they may note shortness of breath at rest.

Although determination of the FEV_1 *before and after* inhalation of a *bronchodilator* (e.g., albuterol) has been advocated to rule out asthma and provide a quick estimate of the benefit a patient may derive from bronchodilator therapy, the failure to obtain an improvement in flow rate does not rule out benefit. In fact, it has been shown that short-term changes in FEV_1 in response to bronchodilators are a poor predictor of symptomatic benefit over a 3- to 6-month period of treatment.

Evidence does not support the use of spirometry in asymptomatic patients; limited evidence suggests that subsequent interventions in such patients who do have abnormal results are not effective. Benefits of treatment are limited to patients with bothersome symptoms and with FEV_1 less than 60% of predicted. Modifying therapy based on spirometric results is generally not helpful.

Chest Radiography

Chest radiography is helpful, principally to rule out complications of COPD (e.g., pneumonia, pneumothorax) and other forms of chest disease that may present as dyspnea (e.g., heart failure, interstitial lung disease; see Chapter 40). Of the various forms of COPD, only severe emphysema is diagnosed radiologically; the criteria for radiologic diagnosis are the presence of two or more of the following findings: flattening of the diaphragm and blunting of the costophrenic angle on posterior–anterior view, irregularity of lung field lucency, enlargement of the retrosternal space, and flattening or concavity of the diaphragmatic contour on lateral view. High-resolution chest computed tomography (CT) has been shown to detect emphysema in heavy smokers who are asymptomatic and have normal chest x-rays, but evidence for clinical benefit for the use of CT in this situation is lacking. The degree and pattern of emphysema within the lungs can also be assessed more precisely with chest CT than chest x-ray. However, with the exception of assessment for lung volume reduction surgery, these findings have little effect on management decisions.

Measurement of Arterial Oxygen Saturation and Blood Gases

Measurement of arterial oxygen saturation and blood gases is worth considering in patients with an FEV_1 of less than 50% of the predicted value, a point at which hypoxemia is a possibility, especially in persons with chronic bronchitis. *Pulse oximetry* can be used as a screening test; it provides a measure of arterial oxygen saturation (SaO_2). If the SaO_2 is less than 92%, then measurement of the arterial blood gases is indicated to assess oxygenation and ventilation. Hypoxemia and hypercarbia are indications of severe chronic bronchitis. Blood gas measurement is particularly useful for documenting acute decompensation. In patients with severe chronic bronchitis (stages 3 and 4), baseline and serial studies of blood gases should be performed so that measurements of gases obtained at times of marked subjective worsening can be compared with baseline determinations.

Hematocrit and Hemoglobin Concentration

Hematocrit and hemoglobin concentration provide a rough indication of the severity and chronicity of hypoxemia and the possible need for phlebotomy. Measurement should be undertaken in persons with arterial oxygen pressure (PaO_2) of less than 50 mm Hg.

Electrocardiogram

Electrocardiogram should be studied for sinus tachycardia, multifocal atrial tachycardia, peaked P waves (P pulmonale), and signs of right ventricular hypertrophy (e.g., tall R wave in lead V1 and deep S wave in lead V6). The electrocardiographic abnormalities that appear in COPD generally reflect the severity of lung disease and the presence of cor pulmonale.

PRINCIPLES OF MANAGEMENT (11–64)

The prime goals of treatment are the slowing of disease progression, the improvement of respiratory health status and prolongation of survival through management of stable disease, and the prevention and management of exacerbations. The principal components of management for achieving these goals are risk factor avoidance and prophylaxis against preventable infection; stage-appropriate use of bronchodilators, corticosteroids, and oxygen; and pulmonary rehabilitation. Surgical approaches are a consideration for a minority of patients with severe emphysema. COPD is a progressive disease. As a result, treatment is generally marked by a stepwise increase in medications as severity increases (Fig. 47.1). To avoid treatment that is not beneficial, it is important that the clinician recognize the rationale for the recommended stepped care approach. As noted, there is no evidence that patients with mild to moderate airflow obstruction but without symptoms benefit from treatment with inhaled therapy. Similarly, patients with intermittent

symptoms and stage I airflow obstruction do not benefit from treatment with inhaled therapy in terms of frequency of exacerbations, health status, hospitalizations, or death. The strongest evidence for benefit is for patients with frequent exacerbations (stage III) or respiratory failure (stage IV).

There are now many inhaled agents for the treatment of COPD, including short- and long-acting β-agonist and anticholinergic agents, corticosteroids, and combinations. Table 47.2 lists inhaled agents and other preparations used in COPD management.

The success of treatment, especially as it becomes more complex and cumbersome for the patient as disease advances, is strongly influenced by the physician's interest in engaging the participation of patient and family members in self-management and collaborative care.

Risk Factor Avoidance and Prevention of Infection (1,6,12,15–23)

Smoking Cessation and Avoidance of Other Irritants

Regardless of the severity of their disease or the types of deficits present, all patients with COPD *must stop smoking* and should

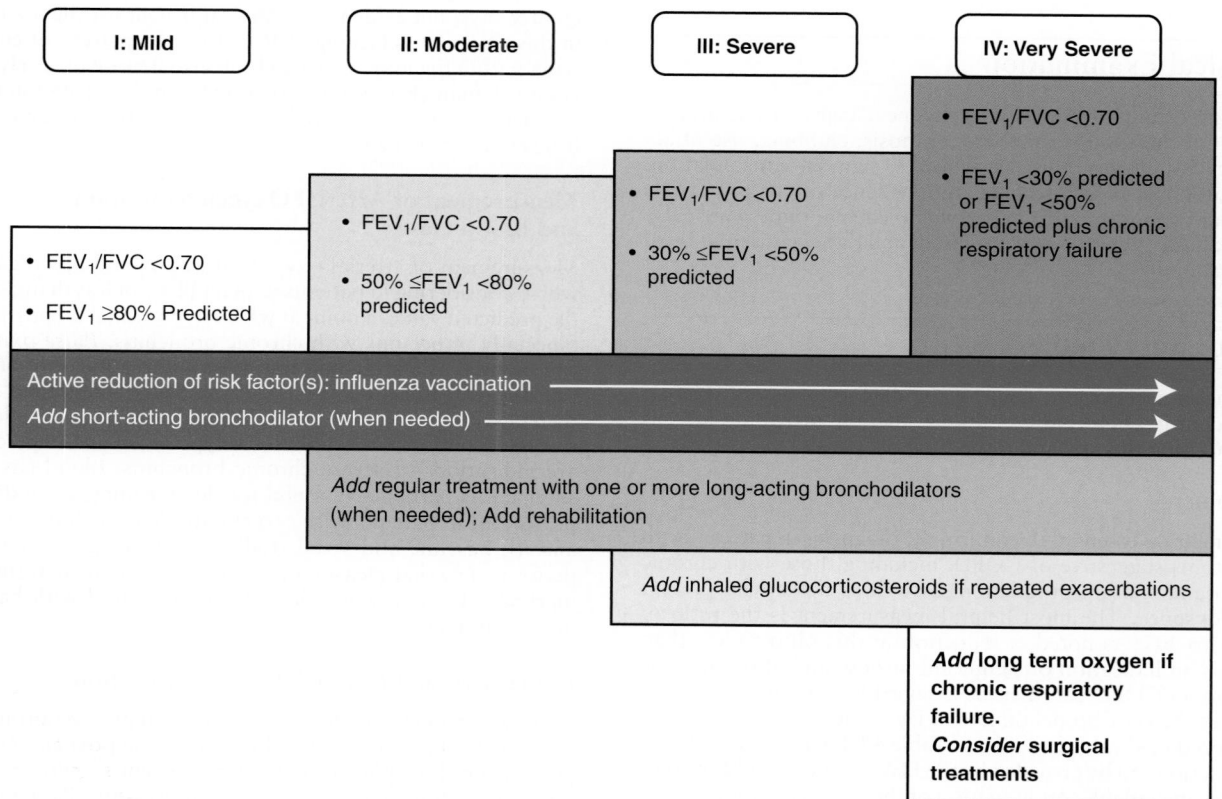

FIGURE 47.1. Therapies appropriate for consideration for stable chronic obstructive pulmonary disease by stages as defined in Table 47.1. Treatment should be determined by symptom intensity as well as stage, determined by decrease in forced expiratory volume in 1 second (FEV_1). Long-acting bronchodilators are generally added when the patient has persistent symptoms. Inhaled corticosteroids are generally added when the patient has regular exacerbations (e.g., three in a 2-year period). FVC, forced vital capacity. (From Rabe KF, Hurd S, Anzueto A, et al. Am J Respir Crit Care Med 2007;176:532, and Global Initiative for Chronic Obstructive Lung Disease, available at http://www.goldcopd.com/ [accessed June 14, 2008]; with permission.

TABLE 47.2

COMMONLY USED FORMULATIONS OF MEDICATIONS USED IN CHRONIC OBSTRUCTIVE PULMONARY DISEASE

Medication	Inhaler (μg)	Solution for Nebulizer (mg/mL)	Oral	Vials for Injection (mg)	Duration of Action (hr)
β_2-Agonists					
Short-acting					
Fenoterol	100–200 (MDI)	1	0.5% (syrup)		4–6
Salbutamol (albuterol)	100, 200 (MDI and DPI)	5	5 mg (pill) 0.24% (syrup)	0.1, 0.5	4–6
Terbutaline	400, 500 (DPI)			0.2, 0.25	4–6
Long-acting					
Formoterol	4.5–12 (MDI and DPI)				12+
Salmeterol	25–50 (MDI and DPI)				12+
Anticholinergics					
Short-acting					
Ipratropium bromide	20, 40 (MDI)	0.25–0.5			6–8
Oxitropium bromide	100 (MDI)	1.5			7–9
Long-acting					
Tiotropium	18 (DPI)				24+
Combination Short-Acting β_2-Agonists plus Anticholinergic in One Inhaler					
Fenoterol/ipratropium	200/80 (MDI)	1.25/0.5			6–8
Salbutamol/ipratropium	75/15 (MDI)	0.75/4.5			6–8
Methylxanthines					
Aminophylline			200–600 mg (pill)	240	Variable, up to 24
Theophylline (SR)			100–600 mg (pill)		Variable, up to 24
Inhaled glucocorticosteroids					
Beclomethasone	50–400 (MDI and DPI)	0.2-0.4			
Budesonide	100, 200, 400 (DPI)	0.20, 0.25, 0.5			
Fluticasone	50–500 (MDI and DPI)				
Triamcinolone	100 (MDI)	40		40	
Combination Long-Acting β_2-Agonists plus Glucocorticosteroids in One Inhaler					
Formoterol/budesonide	4.5/160, 9/320 (DPI)				
Salmeterol/fluticasone	50/100, 250, 500 (DPI) 25/50, 125, 250 (MDI)				
Systemic Glucocorticosteroids					
Prednisone			5–60 mg (pill)		
Methylprednisolone			4, 8, 16 mg (pill)		

DPI, dry powder inhaler; MDI, metered-dose inhaler; SR, slow release.
From Rabe KF, Hurd S, Anzueto A, et al. Am J Respir Crit Care Med 2007;176:532, and Global Initiative for Chronic Obstructive Lung Disease, available at http://www.goldcopd.com/ (accessed June 14, 2008); with permission.

be urged to do so in emphatic terms. As noted earlier, disease progression is accelerated by continued smoking and can be greatly slowed by its cessation. Nonetheless, a surprisingly large number of patients report receiving little or no warning about smoking from their physicians; studies indicate that the physician's urging can be critical to achieving cessation of smoking, especially for those who are symptomatic (see Chapter 54).

A reduction in exposure to other pulmonary irritants should be advised. Readily avoidable pulmonary irritants include aerosol deodorants, hairsprays, paint sprays, and insecticides. Occupational history should be reviewed (see Chapter 39) for important workplace irritants. A change in job or residence (for patients living in areas of severe air pollution) may be necessary but should be urged only when the relationship between exposure and disease is strong; otherwise, the advice might cause more harm than good.

Immunization against Influenza

Immunization against influenza is essential for all patients with COPD. Reductions in outpatient visits, hospitalization, and mortality in elderly persons with COPD have been demonstrated with administration of influenza vaccine. Trivalent influenza vaccine should be given each fall, at least 6 weeks before the onset of the influenza season. Serious reactions are rare unless the patient is allergic to egg protein. Mild fever and myalgias are sometimes noted. Because of ever-changing viral strains, vaccination must be performed yearly (see Chapter 6). Should an outbreak of influenza occur, protection for patients who were not immunized can still be provided (see Chapter 6).

Pneumococcal Vaccine

Pneumococcal vaccine is also important for patients with COPD. Available preparations incorporate the capsular antigens of 23 species that are responsible for 90% of the cases of pneumococcal pneumonia occurring in the United States. Mild erythema and pain at the injection site are the only common adverse reactions to the vaccine, which is administered as a single intramuscular injection of 0.5 mL. A repeated dose in 5 years may help to maximize antibody titers in the elderly (see Chapter 6). The antibody response is not blunted, nor is the frequency of adverse reactions increased, when the pneumococcal and influenza vaccines are given simultaneously. The only disadvantage is difficulty in determining the cause of hypersensitivity should a reaction occur.

The Question of Prophylactic Antibiotics

Patients with chronic bronchitis are typically *colonized* with *Haemophilus influenzae* and *Streptococcus pneumoniae*; *Moraxella* is also found. However, the role of *infection* in the genesis of acute exacerbations is unsettled. Although early studies suggested a benefit from the use of antibiotics during the winter months, several large-scale controlled trials refuted this finding. Prophylactic use of antibiotics does not reduce the frequency of exacerbations of COPD and should not be used. When administered to patients with acute exacerbation of COPD, antibiotic therapy produces a small improvement in outcome in comparison with placebo (see later discussion).

Bronchodilator Therapy: β-Agonists, Anticholinergics, and Methylxanthines (11–19,24–34)

Bronchodilators remain a mainstay of treatment, providing symptomatic relief of dyspnea in about 50% of patients. The mechanisms of action are diverse, complex, and not fully understood. In addition to bronchodilation, positive effects on mucociliary clearance, diaphragmatic action, cardiac contractility, and inflammatory mediator release have been described. It has been shown that an important mechanism of action is to improve lung emptying during expiration. The degree to which bronchodilators achieve this in individual patients is not readily predictable from the improvement in FEV_1 during an acute bronchodilator trial. As a result, many patients fail to show a response to a single exposure but demonstrate a significant improvement in symptoms after a clinical trial of 3 to 6 months. Furthermore, bronchodilation with β-agonists or anticholinergics has been shown not only to reduce exertional dyspnea and other symptoms, but also to reduce rates of acute exacerbation among patients with moderate or severe COPD. When side effects of bronchodilation are troubling, however, it should be kept in mind that there is not conclusive evidence that they have an effect on rate of decline in lung function or survival.

β-Agonists

Short-acting β-agonists constitute the first line of bronchodilator therapy; when used as needed they usually suffice for people with mild COPD. Their principal role is to provide prompt relief as necessary from acute dyspnea induced by bronchospasm. The metered-dose inhaler (MDI) formulations of the topically active, semiselective inhaled β_2-agonists (e.g., albuterol, metaproterenol) are preferred for their rapid onset of action, minimal systemic side effects (the drugs are relatively bronchoselective), and reasonable duration of action (2 to 4 hours). In patients with moderate disease and persistent symptoms, a long-acting β-agonist or anticholinergic (see later discussion) is likely to be easier for the patient and therefore more effective. The advent of long-acting β_2-agonist formulations (e.g., inhaled *salmeterol or formoterol*), with a duration of action of 12 hours, provides an important option for the prevention of exacerbations. Recent meta-analysis of multiple trials of salmeterol and formoterol indicate a 13% reduction in exacerbation rates. Combining either of these long-acting β_2-agonists with inhaled corticosteroid reduces exacerbations an additional 10%, but that difference was not statistically significant.

The use of inhaled β-agonists must be accompanied by thorough patient education. When used on an as-needed basis, their convenience and rapid onset of action sometimes lead to excessive use. Dosing may be inadequate with improper MDI technique (see Chapter 48). The purported advantage of administering β-agonist therapy by means of an *intermittent positive-pressure breathing* apparatus has not held up in trials even among patients with relatively severe disease, copious sputum, or severe emphysema. MDI administration is the delivery system of choice for short-acting β-agonists in the outpatient setting. Long-acting β-agonists are administered through dry powder inhalers (DPIs); again, patient education is necessary to assure proper technique.

Anticholinergic Agents

Muscarinic blockers provide longer-acting bronchodilation (≥6 hours) than short-acting β-agonists and work better for some patients as initial therapy in stage I disease either alone or complementing the shorter-acting β-agonists. An MDI formulation of the short-acting *ipratropium* is available alone or in combination with albuterol or metaproterenol. *Tiotropium* is another nonselective antagonist with similar binding affinity for muscarinic receptors, which dissociates from receptors much more slowly than ipratropium and therefore has a much longer duration of action. In placebo-controlled trials, the short-acting ipratropium has been shown not to reduce the frequency of exacerbations; the long-acting tiotropium reduces exacerbations by 16% compared with placebo. When it is compared with ipratropium rather than placebo, trials clearly indicate the superiority of the tiotropium. When compared with long-acting β-agonists alone or in combination with steroids there is no significant difference, although in the latter case, there is a trend favoring the β-agonist and corticosteroid combination. DPI application allows convenient delivery of tiotropium with a minimum of systemic side effects. The typical systemic anticholinergic side effects (e.g., blurred vision, urinary outflow obstruction, rapid heart rate) are rarely a problem when the drug is given in proper doses. Sputum volume can be reduced without increasing its viscosity.

Methylxanthines

Theophylline and its derivatives (e.g., aminophylline) have been relegated to *third-line* bronchodilator status in COPD, reserved for patients for whom β-agonists and muscarinic blockers do not suffice. Although these methylxanthines are inexpensive and symptomatically helpful, they have demonstrated an inconsistent ability to improve objective measures of airflow, a considerable number of cardiovascular side effects, and a narrow therapeutic range. Nonetheless, some patients report subjective benefit, perhaps related to effects other than bronchodilation (e.g., improved diaphragmatic and myocardial function, inhibition of inflammatory mediators). Patients who experience a worsening of airway hyperreactivity at night despite a β-agonist or muscarinic blocker may benefit from the addition of a long-acting, controlled-release theophylline formulation before bed.

The methylxanthines are available for outpatient use in oral and rectal formulations, but only the oral route should be used because rectal administration is associated with erratic absorption and a potential for dangerous sudden rises in serum concentrations. Absorption of an oral dose approaches 90%. Sustained-release preparations can provide therapeutic serum levels (8 to 12 μg/mL) for 12 to 24 hours. The wide variability in levels for a given dose is a consequence of individual differences in clearance, which is predominantly hepatic. Decreased clearance and increased serum levels occur with heart failure, hepatocellular disease, and drugs that inhibit the hepatic cytochrome oxidase system (e.g., cimetidine, macrolide antibiotics); smoking and intake of barbiturates increase clearance.

Serious side effects include *supraventricular* and *ventricular dysrhythmias* and *seizures*. Such adverse effects usually occur only when serum levels rise precipitously, but they can also occur while serum levels are in the "normal" range if concurrent heart failure or hypoxemia develops.

Choice of Bronchodilator Therapy

Although there is now a great deal of evidence about the effectiveness of bronchodilators in COPD, the choice of agent or agents for individual patients remains somewhat empiric; trial and error is usually necessary to arrive at an optimal program. With moderate disease without persistent symptoms, as-needed use of a short-acting inhaled β-agonist as rescue therapy is the first line of treatment; the addition of inhaled ipratropium at bedtime is still a reasonable second line of bronchodilator therapy in the absence of persistent symptoms. Alternatively, one can begin with ipratropium and add a short-acting β-agonist if necessary. When persistent symptoms do occur, they warrant treatment with either long-acting β-agonists or muscarinic blockers. In these circumstances, there is good evidence that tiotropium and the long-acting β-agonists (and inhaled corticosteroids; see later discussion), when used alone, have similar effectiveness in reducing exacerbations. However, there is also good evidence that these monotherapies do not reduce mortality.

Oral sustained-release theophylline is usually reserved for persons who continue to experience difficulty at night despite the optimal use of β-agonists or muscarinic blockers. The benefit of reduced-dose combination therapy over full-dose single-agent therapy is not fully established, but many patients appear to benefit from the convenience of combination formulations.

Antiinflammatory Therapy: Corticosteroids (11–19,35–44)

With the appreciation for the role of inflammation in COPD came a renewed interest in glucocorticosteroid therapy. In theory, steroid-induced antiinflammatory effects (e.g., suppression of cytokines, inhibition of eosinophils, stabilization of mast cells) have the potential to reduce the acute mucosal edema and bronchoconstriction of COPD flares and the subsequent airway remodeling and progressive loss of lung function of chronic active disease. However, early well-designed prospective clinical trials revealed marginal benefit at best for most patients. However, later trials against placebo controls demonstrated effectiveness in reducing exacerbation rates similar to those of either long-acting β-agonists or long-acting anticholinergic agents.

Other randomized trials indicate that the addition of inhaled corticosteroids to a long-acting β-agonist among patients with more severe (stages III and IV) COPD, with a history of frequent exacerbations (two or more per year), can reduce rates of exacerbation more than either treatment alone. Meta-analysis indicated that combining a long-acting β-agonist with inhaled corticosteroid provides a 20% to 25% relative risk reduction of exacerbation compared with placebo. The combination also produces greater improvement in symptoms and in lung function than either agent alone in some patients. The TORCH (TOwards a Revolution in COPD Health) trial suggested that this combination also decreases mortality but increases the risk of pneumonia. A subsequent meta-analysis estimated a 3-year number needed to treat of 36 to avert 1 death and of 12 to cause 1 case of pneumonia. The current recommended role for inhaled corticosteroids is in patients who have a demonstrated FEV_1 response or in those with stage III or IV disease ($FEV_1 < 50\%$ of predicted) with repeated exacerbations.

Another use for corticosteroids is during acute exacerbations of COPD. Here again, the effect has been generally disappointing. For example, in persons with an acute COPD flare requiring hospitalization, a 2-week course of systemic steroids was found to provide only a modest improvement in the rate of treatment failures, length of hospital stay, and pulmonary function. An 8-week course of therapy was no more efficacious than a 2-week course; at 6 months, no improvement in outcomes was demonstrated, and hyperglycemia severe enough to require treatment developed in many patients. However, in more recent studies, systemic glucocorticoids have been shown to shorten recovery time and restore lung function more quickly for some patients with more severe exacerbations of COPD. Oral prednisolone at 30 to 40 mg/d for 7 to 10 days, or the equivalent, appears to suffice for achievable benefit while minimizing side effects. Higher doses or longer periods of administration are unwarranted, given current evidence for benefit and potential harms.

Oxygen Therapy (11–19,45–49)

Long-term *continuous oxygen therapy* prolongs survival and reduces the risk for cor pulmonale when administered to patients with COPD who are chronically hypoxemic. Hypoxia seen as an indication for oxygen therapy has been a PaO_2 of 55 mm Hg or less (equivalent to an SaO_2 of $\leq 88\%$), but a comprehensive meta-analysis cites a PaO_2 cutoff of 60 mm Hg or less in estimating a 40% improved survival rate. In the presence of hypoxia, the more continuous the therapy, the better is the effect; around-the-clock oxygen therapy is superior to nocturnal oxygen administration. Measurable benefit requires continuous administration for at least *15 hours/d or more*. Administration for less than 12 hours/d is unlikely to be of any help. Although long-term *discontinuous oxygen therapy* at night or during activity is believed to be worthwhile for nonhypoxemic patients with COPD who manifest a drop in PaO_2 during sleep or low-level exertion, such therapy is not of proven benefit with regard to long-term survival or risk for pulmonary hypertension. Nonetheless, both forms of long-term oxygen therapy are reimbursable. Most COPD patients with profound nocturnal hypoxemia also are hypoxic during the day and require the continuous administration of oxygen. Concerns about the potential of continuous oxygen therapy to worsen carbon dioxide retention, especially during sleep, when carbon dioxide retention is at its worst, have not been borne out. Administration with nasal prongs usually suffices, and enough oxygen should be delivered to increase the resting PO_2 to 65 mm Hg and the exercise SaO_2 to greater than 90%. Some recommend adding an additional 1 L of flow per minute during sleep and exertion.

The need for *short-term supplemental oxygen* must be considered when *air travel* is planned. Prediction of the need for oxygen and tolerance of the cabin environment can be accomplished by preflight measurement of the arterial PO_2 and FEV_1. A formula has been derived based on these parameters to predict arterial oxygen levels at cruising altitude. Alternatively, one can have the patient inhale a hypoxic gas mixture (17.2% oxygen) that simulates the cabin environment of a jet aircraft at cruising altitude. Although no guidelines have been established for when to administer oxygen supplementation, a drop in PO_2 to below 50 mm Hg or the development of symptoms is a reasonable indication for oxygen supplementation during flights longer than 2 hours. Airlines will provide an oxygen supply if notified at least 48 hours in advance of travel; their units provide flows of 2 to 4 L of 25% or 30% oxygen per minute. Patients are usually not allowed to bring their own oxygen tanks into the cabin of domestic airlines.

Brief administration of oxygen has been advised to *improve exercise tolerance* in COPD patients. In unblinded studies, exercise tolerance improves, but in blinded, placebo-controlled study, little benefit has been demonstrated. Most hypoxemic COPD patients are chronically hypoxic and require continuous oxygen supplementation; brief administration is of no value to them. The small subset of patients who are hypoxemic and markedly dyspneic only with exercise might be candidates for a trial of short-term oxygen supplementation. A convenient means of identifying such patients is to measure their diffusing capacity during routine pulmonary function testing rather than try to measure arterial blood gases just after or during exercise. A diffusing capacity greater than 55% has been shown to be 100% specific in excluding arterial hypoxemia during exercise; sensitivity is 68%. If oxygen is to be tried, it should be limited to those who have a reduced diffusing capacity and demonstrate consistently better performance on oxygen than on air when both are administered in single-blind fashion. Pulse oximetry during exercise is another, less precise, albeit simpler, means of identifying patients who might benefit from oxygen supplementation. Arterial blood gas measurement is the preferred test for initiating oxygen therapy and adjusting it, particularly in patients who are at risk for retention of carbon dioxide with application of oxygen. Pulse oximetry is most useful when therapy is being adjusted, especially if impaired ventilation is not a concern and measurement of the partial pressure of CO_2 is not necessary.

Control of Secretions: Hydration, Mucolytics, and Expectorants (11–19,50,51)

Patients bothered by heavy, tenacious sputum may obtain benefit by maintaining good *fluid intake*, ensuring adequate *humidification* of the indoor environment (particularly in centrally heated homes), and practicing *postural drainage* when clearance of secretions is difficult and cough is incapacitating. The simplest method of postural drainage is to have the patient lean over the side of the bed, rest the elbows on a pillow placed on the floor, and cough as a family member or visiting nurse gently pounds on the chest. For hydration, ultrasonic nebulizers are no better than the simple maintenance of good systemic hydration, although the moisture they deliver does reach deep into the tracheobronchial tree. Occasionally, bronchospasm can be triggered by a nebulizer, and its reservoir can become contaminated and serve as a source of airway infection. Nebulized detergents are of no proven use, but *mucolytic agents* such as acetylcysteine are capable of thinning secretions; they are usually reserved for patients on respirators and not commonly used in outpatient practice. Oral *expectorants* are very popular with some bronchitic patients, who report improved ability to raise sputum; however, they are without proven clinical efficacy. These preparations need not be denied to the patient who feels that they are of benefit, but they should not be the mainstay of any therapeutic program. Glyceryl guaiacolate and potassium iodide are the most frequently prescribed expectorants; many are available without a prescription.

Exercise Training and Rehabilitation (11–19,52–54)

The main elements of a pulmonary rehabilitation program are exercise training, breathing retraining, chest physiotherapy, psychosocial support, and patient education. Often, the program is carried out as an intensive intervention at a rehabilitation center for patients with advanced disease who are functionally limited; however, some elements can be initiated at home in earlier phases of the illness (e.g., exercise). The evidence of benefit is strongest for exercise training and psychosocial interventions. The benefit derived from a program of comprehensive pulmonary rehabilitation appears to decline with time after completion of the program, especially after 1 year; no improvement in survival has been demonstrated.

Exercise Training

Among the simplest and most effective measures for improving exercise tolerance is an *exercise training program*. *Walking* has proved to be the best form of exercise for increasing duration and intensity of activity in COPD patients. Exercises that involve the arms and upper body appear to compromise respiratory mechanics. Three or four sessions per day of walking are recommended, ranging from 5 to 15 minutes each. The pace and duration of activity are matched to the patient's capabilities; most begin the program walking at a half-maximal pace and build gradually through a period of several weeks. Interval training is just as effective as continuous high-intensity training and is better tolerated by patients. At the end of the training period, heart and respiratory rates for a given level of activity are decreased; oxygen consumption also falls. Parameters of ventilatory function are not significantly changed, but increases of 25% are attained in maximum duration and intensity of exercise. Many patients enjoy marked improvement in the ability to carry out their daily activities. Although exercise training is often not implemented until patients become severely impaired, there is no reason that a walking program cannot be instituted earlier for most COPD patients.

Breathing Exercises

Breathing exercises may have some beneficial effect, especially psychologically, in those who readily panic and hyperventilate when they are dyspneic or show evidence of respiratory fatigue. Teaching the anxious patient to take slow, deep, relaxed breaths and exhale against pursed lips can lessen the work of moving air, provide a sense of control over breathing, and encourage a more relaxed respiratory pattern. Inspiratory muscle training is popular in some centers, with encouraging reports of improvement in exercise performance among patients who experience respiratory muscle fatigue. However, the importance of diaphragmatic dysfunction and the need for exercises continue to be debated.

Psychosocial Support

A comprehensive rehabilitation program entails group and individual meetings with a psychiatrist or other mental health professional in addition to sessions that include families or spouses to help them cope with the depression, anxiety, fear, and family dysfunction that COPD brings on a household. Behavioral approaches are sometimes taught to patients, such as the breathing relaxation techniques just noted.

Managing Acute Exacerbations (11–19,55–58)

Diagnosis and Assessment of Severity

An exacerbation of COPD is defined as a sustained worsening of the patient's condition, from the stable state and beyond normal day-to-day variations, that is acute in onset and requires change in regular medication or management. The severity and acuity of an exacerbation vary with the stage of stable COPD. In stage II or III disease, an exacerbation is marked by increased breathlessness and/or cough and sputum production and can usually be treated without hospitalization. An exacerbation in a patient with stage IV COPD usually means acute respiratory failure and admission to the hospital for intensive care.

Common causes include *tracheobronchial infection*, with bacteria accounting for about 40% of exacerbations and viruses and atypical organisms responsible for another 30%. Studies in urban areas suggest that seasonal increases in *atmospheric pollution* are responsible for 6% to 9% of exacerbations serious enough to lead to hospitalizations. Because so many patients with severe COPD have little respiratory reserve and have multiple chronic conditions, any pulmonary compromise can lead to exacerbation and respiratory failure. Pneumonia is often at the top of the list of concerns, followed by worsening congestive heart failure if the patient has a history of heart disease, but the clinician should also consider pulmonary embolism, pneumothorax, rib fractures leading to splinting and atelectasis, and inappropriate use of sedatives. In addition to a detailed history focusing on the time course of worsening symptoms and severity, laboratory investigations are in order, usually including arterial blood gases if pulse oximetry indicates a change in baseline SaO_2, chest x-ray, and electrocardiogram. The presence of purulent sputum during an exacerbation is sufficient indication for starting empirical antibiotic treatment, but *Gram's stain* and *culture* of sputum can be helpful when pneumonia is suspected, especially in patients exposed to multiple courses of antibiotics. Prior colonization with *S. pneumoniae*, *H. influenzae*, or *Moraxella* may make interpretation difficult.

Outpatient Management of Exacerbations

The benefit of *antibiotics* for COPD exacerbations has been the subject of debate. Meta-analysis of randomized trials of antibiotics for COPD flares find a benefit that is most likely to be of clinical significance in persons with severe disease, especially those who require hospitalization. Among the subset of patients whose exacerbations were characterized by increased cough and sputum production, antibiotics reduced the risk of short-term mortality by 75% and of treatment failure by 50%.

In exacerbations not complicated by comorbidity and a history of frequent past exacerbations with antibiotic use, the most likely bacterial organisms include *H. influenzae*, *S. pneumoniae*, and *Moraxella catarrhalis*. *Haemophilus parainfluenza*, *Mycoplasma pneumoniae*, and *Chlamydophila pneumoniae* are also common. Reasonable choices include a macrolide (e.g., azithromycin or clarithromycin), doxycycline, a second- or third-generation cephalosporin, or a respiratory quinolone. When the exacerbation is complicated by comorbidity and a history of frequent exacerbations with recent antibiotic exposure, a respiratory quinolone or amoxicillin–clavulanate is advised because of greater risk of gram-negative enteric pathogens and of increased β-lactam resistance. In patients at risk for *Pseudomonas aeruginosa* because of recurrent courses of antibiotics and/or steroids with bronchiectasis, the quinolone should be ciprofloxacin or levofloxacin. As noted, culturing the sputum can help to rationalize antibiotic choice.

Bronchodilator therapy is generally increased during COPD exacerbations. If not already used, an anticholinergic agent can be added to a β-agonist. *Systemic glucocorticoids* are beneficial in acute exacerbations, shortening recovery time, and should be considered for patients whose baseline FEV_1 is less than 50% of predicted. As noted, there is no need to treat with more than 30 to 40 mg of prednisolone per day for 7 to 10 days, or the equivalent.

Indications for *emergency room assessment* or *hospital admission* are discussed later.

Management of Cor Pulmonale (59)

Patients with chronic cor pulmonale can often be made more comfortable by careful attention to their volume status, degree of hypoxemia, and hematocrit. Reduction of excess intravascular volume can reduce edema; *diuretic therapy* (see Chapter 32) is an effective means of volume control. As noted earlier, continuous *low-flow oxygen therapy* is indicated in patients with cor pulmonale who are chronically hypoxic. Survival is improved, although the precise mechanism of improvement is unknown; pulmonary vascular resistance and secondary polycythemia are only modestly decreased. Whether oxygen therapy prevents the development or worsening of cor pulmonale is unsettled.

Cardiac output is a determinant of survival in patients with cor pulmonale. Augmented cardiac output is a normal response to a fall in PO_2. Many patients with cor pulmonale maintain a high cardiac index. It is suspected that a fall in cardiac output may be a determinant of poor prognosis. If this proves to be the case, then increased efforts at improving cardiac output may be indicated. However, attempts at inotropic therapy have produced equivocal results. *Digoxin* seems to help some patients but not uniformly or predictably. The incidence of digitalis toxicity, which is aggravated by hypoxemia, is high; the clinical response is often equivocal. The drug is worth a try in patients with reduced cardiac output, especially if concurrent left ventricular dysfunction is present (see Chapter 32), but it should be continued only in those who show objective improvement in addition to a subjective response to therapy. Patients who appear to improve with digitalis should be given a minimum maintenance dose and should be monitored closely for manifestations of digitalis toxicity (see Chapter 32).

Vasodilators (calcium-channel blockers, angiotensin-converting-enzyme inhibitors, and phosphodiesterase-5 inhibitors) have proved disappointing, with little improvement in cardiac output or pulmonary artery resistance noted during sustained use in most patients. In some instances, systemic hypotension and even hypoxemia may result.

Phlebotomy is indicated only for urgent treatment when secondary erythrocytosis is severe enough to cause a marked reduction in blood viscosity, significant impairment of oxygen delivery, and exacerbation of cor pulmonale. The risk for such decompensation is greatest when the hematocrit rises to greater than 55%.

Augmentation Therapy for α-Antitrypsin Deficiency

The rare patient with emphysema who has significant antitrypsin deficiency (<80 mg/dL) is a possible candidate for augmentation therapy (weekly or monthly infusions of α_1-antitrypsin). Only symptomatic patients with clinical evidence of emphysema and sufficiently low antitrypsin levels are considered appropriate for augmentation therapy because emphysema does not develop in all patients with low concentrations. A history of smoking rules out candidacy. Observational studies suggest that infusions of α_1-antitrypsin slow the deterioration of lung function. A randomized trial with follow-up over 3 years found no effect.

Surgical Interventions (11–19,60,61)

Bullectomy

Bullectomy is worth considering in the rare COPD patient with a few giant bullae unilaterally taking up more than one third of a hemithorax. Additional clinical criteria include being relatively free of severe emphysema and bullae in the contralateral lung, having chest computed tomographic evidence of bullae-compressing lung parenchyma, and having an FEV_1 less than 50% of the predicted value.

Lung Volume Reduction

This investigational surgical intervention for patients with late-stage nonbullous emphysema entails removing the most severely involved sections of emphysematous lung to improve pulmonary mechanics and gas exchange. Although initial reports were enthusiastic and encouraging, high early mortality among those randomized to surgery in large multicenter trials has forced reconsideration of indications and new approaches to preoperative risk stratification. Among those known to have high operative risk are those with FEV_1 less than 20% of predicted and those with a homogeneous pattern of emphysema on chest CT. The place of such surgery in the management of emphysema remains to be determined.

Lung Transplant

Although transplant of a single lung has a reasonable 3-year survival rate (up to 70%), most COPD patients are not candidates because of advanced age, continued smoking, or con-

current cardiovascular disease, not to mention the fact that available lungs are in very short supply.

Monitoring Therapy (11–19,62–64)

Functional status and *symptoms* remain among the most important measures of efficacy. Semiquantitative reports from the patient regarding such parameters as number of stairs climbed or distance walked can be useful. Important aspects of the physical examination to be monitored include the ratio of inspiration to expiration, respiratory rate, heart rate, jugular venous pressure, right ventricular impulse, and condition of extremities (edema). In a patient with known carbon dioxide retention, the presence of asterixis is an indication of worsening ventilatory status, further carbon dioxide retention, and encephalopathy. Serial determination of SaO_2, *arterial blood gases*, FEV_1, and *hematocrit* can help in objectively following the course of disease and detecting acute deterioration.

PATIENT EDUCATION (11–19,62–64)

The first priority is to stress the importance of *cessation of smoking*; this should be followed by the design of a specific program (see Chapter 54). Patients should be encouraged to maintain as much activity as possible and be provided with an exercise program if they can be motivated to comply. Patient, family, and physician should be involved in setting reasonable and realistic activity goals. They should also be aware that depression is common in this clinical setting and that it can be treated when recognized. Advice regarding adequate hydration and pulmonary toilet is basic to the care of patients with chronic bronchitis. Patients likely to panic and hyperventilate when they become dyspneic often benefit from being taught how to institute slow, relaxed, deep breathing in such circumstances.

Careful instructions regarding the indications and adverse effects of therapy can help the patient to carry out the prescribed program properly. Complex regimens should be written down and reviewed with both patient and family. It is essential to warn patients with carbon dioxide retention against unauthorized use of tranquilizers and sedatives because of the risk for further suppression of their respiratory drive. Patients for whom inhalers have been prescribed should be thoroughly instructed in their proper use (see Chapter 48); many treatment failures are a consequence of poor technique. Such patients also must be warned that excessive use of β_2-agonists can lead to tachyphylaxis and cardiac side effects; persistent overdoses of inhaled steroids (more than 20 puffs per day) can cause adrenal suppression.

Part of the patient education process should aim to restore as much self-confidence and self-reliance as possible. Instruction in self-adjustment of the medical regimen, in monitoring and reporting of functional status, and in implementation of a daily exercise program can have very positive effects on morale. The synergistic interaction of an involved patient and an interested and concerned physician has the potential to enhance the quality, if not the duration, of life for COPD patients.

INDICATIONS FOR ADMISSION AND REFERRAL

The patient with acute respiratory decompensation, especially if accompanied by signs of encephalopathy (e.g., asterixis, lethargy), should be urgently admitted to the hospital; no oxygen should be administered on the way to the hospital for fear of further suppressing the respiratory drive. Those with an acute exacerbation of cough, dyspnea, wheezing, and sputum production that is not immediately responsive to bronchodilator therapy might also require inpatient management and would possibly benefit from a pulmonary consultation. Pulmonary referral is also indicated when the patient remains chronically incapacitated despite a comprehensive program of standard medical therapy. Surgical consultation is not recommended without the prior recommendation of a pulmonary specialist.

THERAPEUTIC RECOMMENDATIONS (3,5,9,11,14)

Basic Measures for All Patients

- Review the entire treatment program thoroughly with the patient and family; encourage patient participation in setting goals and monitoring functional status.
- Insist on complete *cessation of smoking* and design a comprehensive smoking cessation program (see Chapter 54).
- Advise the patient to reduce exposure to known environmental irritants and allergens (see Chapters 39, 48, and 222).
- Administer trivalent influenza vaccine (0.5 mL intramuscularly) in the fall of each year, at least 6 weeks before the usual winter onset of the flu season, to all patients with COPD (except those having a known allergy to eggs). Consider administering antiviral therapy to unvaccinated COPD patients during an influenza epidemic (see Chapter 6).
- Administer *pneumococcal vaccine* to all COPD patients. The dose is 0.5 mL intramuscularly, and it can be given at the same time as the influenza vaccine. Repeated administration after 5 years may be needed in elderly persons (see Chapter 6).
- Advise patients bothered by heavy sputum production to keep well hydrated and to humidify the indoor environment (particularly patients living in centrally heated homes). Nebulized detergents and oral expectorants are of no proven benefit. Teach postural drainage techniques to patients bothered by difficulty in raising sputum.
- Perform pulmonary function testing on all patients with a peak flow rate less than 350 L/min, obvious bronchospasm, or dyspnea on exertion. Measure FEV_1 before and after the inhalation of a rapidly acting bronchodilator (e.g., albuterol).

Bronchodilators and Corticosteroids

- For stage I patients with mild, intermittent symptoms, begin with an MDI formulation of a short-acting bronchodilator on an as-needed basis. A β_2-*agonist* (e.g., one to two puffs of *albuterol* every 4 to 6 hours) is the usual first-line choice because of its rapid onset of action. Carefully instruct the patient in proper MDI use (see Chapter 48) and warn that the dose is not to exceed 12 puffs in 24 hours. A short-acting anticholinergic (e.g., ipratropium) or a short-acting combination agent (e.g., albuterol and ipratropium) are alternatives.
- For stage II patients with persistent symptoms, begin long-acting bronchodilator therapy while maintaining a short-

acting bronchodilator for as-needed rescue therapy. A regimen of tiotropium (one inhalation once daily) plus albuterol is a recommended approach. Salmeterol or formoterol (one inhalation twice daily) plus ipratropium, albuterol, or a combination is an alternative.
- Judge response to bronchodilator therapy on the basis of a change in symptoms, including exercise tolerance and expiratory flow rates, after about 4 weeks of therapy. If no response can be demonstrated, an alternative agent or combination therapy with a β-agonist and anticholinergic should be tried.
- If some bronchodilator response is noted but the control of symptoms remains inadequate, especially at nighttime, then consider adding a sustained-release oral *theophylline* preparation before bed (e.g., 200 to 400 mg of generic sustained-release theophylline daily at bedtime). Monitor symptoms closely for a response after about 4 weeks of therapy before deciding to continue therapy longer. Check the serum theophylline level and adjust the dose to achieve a therapeutic range of 8 to 12 $\mu g/mL$. Do not prescribe for patients with cardiac arrhythmias, and prescribe with caution for persons with underlying heart disease. Do not use anal suppository preparations.
- For stage III patients with frequent exacerbations on tiotropium, add salmeterol or formoterol. For those with frequent exacerbations on salmeterol or formoterol, add tiotropium.
- Consider the initiation of an empiric trial of *inhaled corticosteroid* in persons who respond inadequately to bronchodilator therapy and remain symptomatic. After 6 to 8 weeks, evaluate for sustained response; if no symptomatic or objective improvement is noted, then stop inhaled steroid therapy.
- For patients with severe or very severe COPD (stage III or IV) who have regular exacerbations (e.g., three in a 2-year period), begin a topically active *inhaled corticosteroid* MDI formulation (e.g., two puffs of *beclomethasone* four times daily or four puffs twice daily).
- Consider a 7- to 10-day course of *systemic corticosteroids* (e.g., oral *prednisolone* at 40 mg/d) for those with an acute exacerbation.

Additional Management for Stages II to IV Chronic Obstructive Pulmonary Disease

- For patients who are functionally limited by COPD, consider referral for a comprehensive program of *pulmonary rehabilitation*, which includes exercise training, breathing retraining, chest physiotherapy, psychosocial support, and patient education. Emphasis should be on those elements that have proved most beneficial (i.e., exercise training and psychosocial support).
- Teach slow, relaxed, deep breathing to patients likely to hyperventilate when dyspneic; consider targeted inspiratory muscle training in patients with severe (stages III and IV) COPD; a respiratory therapist may be of help in the teaching effort.
- Be sure that the program includes detailed patient and family education to help sustain the benefit of a rehabilitation program once it is completed.
- Begin long-term *continuous oxygen therapy* in patients who are chronically hypoxemic [resting PO_2 <55 mm Hg, or 56 to 59 mm Hg if evidence of concurrent right-sided heart failure or secondary polycythemia (hematocrit >55%) is present].

- Provide continuous administration for more than *15 hours/d*. Administration for less time is unlikely to improve long-term outcome and prognosis.
- Consider supplemental *noncontinuous oxygen therapy* during exertion to improve exercise capacity in nonhypoxemic patients only if they exhibit desaturation on pulse oximetry during exercise or a reduced diffusing capacity on routine pulmonary function testing; the patient should demonstrate consistently better performance on oxygen than on air when both are administered in a single-blind fashion.
- For patients with very severe (stage IV) disease with intractable breathlessness, for whom palliation is the principal goal, consider low-dose, oral, sustained-release morphine (e.g., 20 mg morphine sulfate per day). Treat constipation expectantly. Monitor for effectiveness and signs of respiratory depression.
- For patients with cor pulmonale, begin a diuretic program (e.g., 20 to 40 mg of *furosemide* daily) when peripheral edema begins to develop; increase the program as needed to control fluid accumulation caused by systemic venous hypertension. Phlebotomize the patient with secondary erythrocytosis (hematocrit >55%) when acute decompensation (worsening of right-sided heart failure or hypoxemia) is present.
- Consider a short-term trial of *cardiac glycoside* therapy (e.g., 0.25 mg of *digoxin* daily) in patients with severe right-sided heart failure; treat for 2 weeks, and check for objective signs of improvement (e.g., decreased edema, lower jugular venous pressure, reduced heart size). Use with care in the setting of hypoxemia, and check serum levels regularly. Monitor closely for evidence of digitalis toxicity (see Chapter 32).
- Refer for consideration of *surgical therapies* only severely emphysematous patients with incapacitating disease refractory to a comprehensive program of maximal medical therapy who could tolerate a major thoracic surgical procedure and who have ceased smoking.

Acute Exacerbation

- Initiate intensive MDI bronchodilator therapy with a rapidly acting *β-agonist* (e.g., six to eight puffs of *albuterol* immediately, then repeated every 30 to 60 minutes). If response is inadequate (e.g., the patient still manifests marked dyspnea and severe wheezing) or the drug is poorly tolerated (e.g., palpitations, chest pain), then hospitalize; if response is adequate, add four to eight puffs of *ipratropium* every 6 hours, reduce albuterol to two puffs four times daily, and follow closely.
- Consider initiating empiric *antibiotic* therapy, but only for patients with a new onset or marked increase of grossly purulent sputum in conjunction with other signs of infection (e.g., fever, elevated white cell count). Reasonable choices in uncomplicated cases include a macrolide (e.g., azithromycin or clarithromycin), doxycycline, a second- or third-generation cephalosporin, or a respiratory quinolone.
- When the exacerbation is complicated by comorbidity and a history of frequent exacerbations with recent antibiotic exposure, a respiratory quinolone or amoxicillin–clavulanate is advised because of the greater risk of gram-negative enteric pathogens and of increased β-lactam resistance. In patients at risk for *P. aeruginosa* because of recurrent courses of antibiotics and/or steroids or with bronchiectasis, the quinolone should be ciprofloxacin or levofloxacin. Culturing the sputum in such patients may help to rationalize antibiotic choice.
- Consider a 7- to 10-day course of *systemic corticosteroids* (e.g., oral *prednisolone* at 40 mg/d).

Indications for Consultation

- Obtain pulmonary consultation when the patient remains incapacitated despite a comprehensive, fully implemented program of medical therapy. Surgical consultation is not recommended without the prior recommendation of a pulmonary specialist.
- Refer patients with known α_1-antitrypsin deficiency for consideration of augmentation therapy with α_1-antitrypsin only if they do not smoke, show signs of emphysema, are symptomatic, and have an antitrypsin level less than 80 mg/dL.

A.G.M./A.H.G.

Annotated Bibliography

1. Anthonisen NR, Connett JE, Murray RP. Smoking and lung function of Lung Health Study participants after 11 years. Am J Respir Crit Care Med 2002; 166: 675. (*A study that found a reduction of 60 mL/yr in forced expiratory volume [FEV1] in patients with chronic obstructive pulmonary disease [COPD] compared with 30 mL/yr in those without it.*)
2. Burrows B, Blood JW, Traver GA, et al. The course and prognosis of different forms of chronic airways obstruction in a sample from the general population. N Engl J Med 1987;317:1309. (*Patients with emphysema had a 10-year mortality of 60%; those with asthmatic bronchitis had a lower mortality.*)
3. Hogg JC, Chu F, Utokaparch S, et al. The nature of small-airway obstruction in chronic obstructive pulmonary disease. N Engl J Med 2004;350:2645. (*An elegant documentation of the thickening of airway walls and the accumulation of inflammatory debris as the histologic correlates of lung function decline.*)
4. Silverman EK, Pierce JA, Province MA, et al. Variability of pulmonary function in alpha-1-antitrypsin deficiency: clinical correlates. Ann Intern Med 1989;111:982. (*Finds that many patients with the deficiency do not necessarily have pulmonary impairment attributable to the deficiency.*)
5. Donaldson GC, Seemungall TAR, Bhowmik A, et al. Relationship between exacerbation frequency and lung function decline in chronic obstructive pulmonary disease. Thorax 2002;57:847. (*Frequent exacerbations are associated with more rapid decline.*)
6. Anthonisen NR, Connet JE, Kiley JP, et al. Effects of smoking intervention and the use of an inhaled anticholinergic bronchodilator on the rate of decline in FEV₁. JAMA 1994;272:1497. (*Only smoking cessation reduced the rate of decline, and it made a major difference in outcome.*)
7. Niewoehner DE, Lokhnygina Y, Rice K, et al. Risk indexes for exacerbations and hospitalizations due to COPD. Chest 2007;131:20. (*Spirometry along with a few questions directed to the patient is strongly predictive of exacerbations and related hospitalizations over the ensuing 6 months.*)
8. Lange P, Parner J, Vestbo J, et al. A 15-year follow-up study of ventilatory function in adults with asthma. N Engl J Med 1998;339:1194. (*A marked decline was noted in asthmatic patients who continued to smoke, which was greater than that noted for smokers or other asthmatic patients, which suggests that asthma may predispose to COPD.*)
9. Badgett RG, Tanaka DJ, Hunt DK, et al. The clinical evaluation for diagnosing obstructive airway disease in high-risk patients. Chest 1994;106:1427. (*An excellent study showing how useful the history, physical examination, and simple office measures can be.*)
10. Pratt PC. Role of conventional chest radiography in diagnosis and exclusion of emphysema. Am J Med 1987;82:998. (*A detailed discussion of the use of the chest film in making and excluding the diagnosis of emphysema; the predictive value is very high when validated criteria are used.*)
11. GOLD Science Committee. Global Initiative for Chronic Obstructive Lung Disease. Global strategy for the diagnosis, management, and prevention

of chronic obstructive pulmonary disease. Executive summary. Bethesda, MD: National Heart, Lung and Blood Institute, January 2008. Available at http://www.goldcopd.com/. Accessed June 14, 2008. (*Consensus Statement.*)

12. Calverley PMA, Walker P. Chronic obstructive pulmonary disease. Lancet 2003;362:1053. (*A superb comprehensive review of COPD definitions, severity assessment, pathophysiology, and clinical assessment, as well as management; 128 references.*)

13. Wilt TJ, Niewoehner D, MacDonald R, et al. Management of stable chronic obstructive pulmonary disease: a systematic review for a clinical practice guideline. Ann Intern Med 2007;147:639. (*Long-acting inhaled therapies, supplemental oxygen, and pulmonary rehabilitation were found to be beneficial in adults who have bothersome respiratory symptoms, especially dyspnea, and FEV$_1$ <60% of the predicted value.*)

14. Qaseem A, Snow V, Shekelle P, et al. Diagnosis and management of stable chronic obstructive pulmonary disease: a clinical practice guideline from the American College of Physicians. Ann Intern Med 2007;147:633. (*Presents six recommendations and their rationale.*)

15. Rabe KF, Hurd S, Anzueto A, et al, GOLD Scientific Committee. Global strategy for the diagnosis, management, and prevention of chronic obstructive pulmonary disease. NHLBI/WHO Global Initiative for Chronic Obstructive Lung Disease (GOLD) Executive Summary. Am J Respir Crit Care Med 2007;176:532. (*A summary; see the full report and updates at http://www.goldcopd.com/ ; accessed June 14, 2008.*)

16. Sutherland ER, Cherniack RM. Management of chronic obstructive pulmonary disease. N Engl J Med 2004;350:2689. (*A review including a discussion of diagnosis and staging, as well as management.*)

17. Wise RA, Tashkin DP. Optimizing treatment of chronic obstructive pulmonary disease: an assessment of current therapies. Am J Med 2007;120:S4. (*Includes a treatment algorithm for pharmacologic and nonpharmacologic interventions, as well as the rationale for antibiotic selection for exacerbations.*)

18. MacNee W, Calverley PMA. Management of COPD. Thorax 2003;58:261. (*An excellent review of all aspects of management, including acute exacerbations; 99 references.*)

19. Sin DD, McAlister FA, Man SFP, et al. Contemporary management of chronic obstructive pulmonary disease. JAMA 2003;290:2301. (*A tour de force meta-analysis covering short-acting and long-acting bronchodilators, inhaled corticosteroids, inhaled glucocorticoids, domiciliary oxygen, and pulmonary rehabilitation;138 references.*)

20. Ferreira IM, Brooks D, Lacasse Y, et al. Nutritional supplementation for stable chronic obstructive pulmonary disease (Cochrane review). In: The Cochrane library, Issue 3. Oxford: Update Software, 2003. (*No effect was found; see http://www.cochrane.org for updates.*)

21. Nichol KL, Baken L, Nelson A. Relation between influenza vaccination and outpatients visits, hospitalizations, and mortality in elderly persons with chronic lung disease. Ann Intern Med 1999;130:397. (*Important evidence for the efficacy of influenza vaccination.*)

22. Saint S, Bent S, Vittinghoff E, et al. Antibiotics in chronic obstructive pulmonary disease exacerbations: a meta-analysis. JAMA 1995;273:957. (*A review of randomized trials finding a small but statistically significant improvement in outcome, particularly in persons with severe disease.*)

23. van der Meer RM, Wagena EJ, Ostelo RWJG. Cochrane Airways Group. Smoking cessation for chronic obstructive pulmonary disease (Cochrane review). In: The Cochrane library, Issue 3. Oxford: Update Software, Oxford, 2004. (*Combining pharmacologic and psychosocial interventions is most effective; see http://www.cochrane.org for updates.*)

24. Appleton S, Poole P, Smith B, et al. Long-acting beta2-agonists for chronic obstructive pulmonary disease (Cochrane review). In: The Cochrane library, Issue 3. Oxford: Update Software, 2004. (*Only a small increase was found in FEV$_1$; see http://www.cochrane.org for updates.*)

25. Sestini P, Renzoni E, Robinson S, et al. Cochrane Airways Group. Short-acting beta$_2$ agonists for stable chronic obstructive pulmonary disease (Cochrane review). In: The Cochrane library, Issue 3. Oxford: Update Software, 2003. (*There was good evidence for benefit; see http://www.cochrane.org for updates.*)

26. Niewoehner DE, Rice K, Cote C, et al. Prevention of exacerbations of chronic pulmonary disease with tiotropium, a once-daily inhaled anticholinergic bronchodilator. Ann Intern Med 2005;143:317. (*Tiotropium reduces COPD exacerbations and may reduce related health care utilization in patients with moderate to severe COPD.*)

27. Aaron SD, Vandemheen KL, Fergusson D, et al. Tiotropium in combination with placebo, salmeterol, or fluticasone–salmeterol for treatment of chronic obstructive pulmonary disease. A randomized trial. Ann Intern Med 2007;146:545. (*The addition of fluticasone–salmeterol to tiotropium therapy did not statistically influence rates of COPD exacerbation but did improve lung function, quality of life, and hospitalization rates in patients with moderate to severe COPD.*)

28. Brown CD, McCrory D, White J. Inhaled short-acting beta2-agonists versus ipratropium for acute exacerbations of chronic obstructive pulmonary disease (Cochrane review). In: The Cochrane library, Issue 3. Oxford: Update Software, 2004. (*There was insufficient evidence for superiority or for an additive effect; see http://www.cochrane.org for updates.*)

29. McCrory DC, Brown CD. Anti-cholinergic bronchodilators versus beta$_2$-sympathomimetic agents for acute exacerbations of chronic obstructive pulmonary disease (Cochrane review). In: The Cochrane library, Issue 3. Oxford: Update Software, 2004. (*There was insufficient evidence for superiority of either agent or for an additive effect; see http://www.cochrane.org for updates.*)

30. Barr RG, Rowe BH, Camargo CA Jr. Methylxanthines for exacerbations of chronic obstructive pulmonary disease: meta-analysis of randomised trials. BMJ 2003;327:643. (*This Cochrane Review did not find a benefit when used for acute exacerbations; see http://www.cochrane.org for updates.*)

31. Calverley P, Pauwels R, Vestbo J, et al. TRISTAN (TRial of Inhaled STeroids ANd long-acting beta2 agonists) Study Group. Combined salmeterol and fluticasone in the treatment of chronic obstructive pulmonary disease: a randomised controlled trial. Lancet 2003;361:449. (*The combination was superior to either alone in this study.*)

32. Calverley PMA, Anderson JA, Celli B, et al. Salmeterol and fluticasone propionate and survival in chronic obstructive pulmonary disease. N Engl J Med 2007;356:775. (*The reduction in death from all causes among patients with COPD in the combination-therapy group did not reach the predetermined level of statistical significance.*)

33. Nannini L, Cates CJ, Lasserson TJ, et al. Combined corticosteroid and long-acting beta-agonist in one inhaler versus placebo for chronic obstructive pulmonary disease. Cochrane Database Syst Rev 2007;(4);CD003794. DOI: 10.1002/14651858.CD003794.pub3. (*Compared with placebo, combination therapy led to a significant reduction of one fourth in exacerbation rates; there was a significant reduction in all-cause mortality; an increased risk of pneumonia is a concern.*)

34. Ram FS, Jones PW, Castro AA, et al. Oral theophylline for chronic obstructive pulmonary disease (Cochrane review). In: The Cochrane library, Issue 4. Oxford: Update Software, 2003. (*There was a modest effect; see http://www.cochrane.org for updates.*)

35. Boushey HA. Glucocorticoid therapy for chronic obstructive pulmonary disease. N Engl J Med 1999;340:1990. (*A very helpful pathophysiologic discussion correlating the observed modest effects of steroids with known and proposed disease mechanisms in COPD.*)

36. Highland KB, Strange C, Heffner JE. Long-term effects of inhaled corticosteroids on FEV1 in patients with chronic obstructive pulmonary disease. A meta-analysis. Ann Intern Med 2003;138:969. (*The use of inhaled corticosteroids was not associated with the rate of FEV$_1$ decline in 3,571 patients followed for 24 to 54 months.*)

37. Lung Health Study Research Group. Effect of inhaled triamcinolone on the decline in pulmonary function in chronic obstructive pulmonary disease. N Engl J Med 2000;343:1902. (*Steroids did not alter the rate of decline in lung function.*)

38. Niewoehner DE, Erbland ML, Deupree RH, et al. Effect of systemic glucocorticoids on exacerbations of chronic obstructive pulmonary disease. N Engl J Med 1999;340:1941. (*A major Veterans Administration study; only modest benefit was noted in this multicenter, randomized, placebo-controlled trial.*)

39. Paggiaro PL, Dahle RM, Bakran I, et al. Multicentre, randomized, placebo-controlled trial of inhaled fluticasone propionate in patients with chronic obstructive pulmonary disease. Lancet 1998;351:773. (*Evidence was noted for a modest degree of functional benefit.*)

40. Pauwels RA, Lofdahl CG, Laitinen LA, et al. Long-term treatment with inhaled budesonide in persons with mild chronic obstructive pulmonary disease who continue smoking. N Engl J Med 1999;340:1948. (*A major European trial failing to find any benefit from inhaled steroid therapy in slowing disease progression.*)

41. Singh JM, Palda VA, Stanbrook MB, et al. Corticosteroid therapy for patients with acute exacerbations of chronic obstructive pulmonary disease: a systematic review. Arch Intern Med 2002;162:2527. (*Short courses of systemic corticosteroids improved spirometric and clinical outcomes.*)

42. Sutherland ER, Allmers H, Ayas NT, et al. Inhaled corticosteroids reduce the progression of airflow limitation in chronic obstructive pulmonary disease: a meta-analysis. Thorax 2003;58:937. (*Treatment for >2 years at higher doses slowed the rate of lung function decline.*)

43. Callahan CM, Dittus RS, Katz BP. Oral corticosteroid therapy for patients with stable chronic obstructive pulmonary disease. Ann Intern Med 1991;114:216. (*A meta-analysis showing a modest benefit.*)

44. Wood-Baker R, Walters EH, Gibson P. Cochrane Airways Group. Oral corticosteroids for acute exacerbations of chronic obstructive pulmonary disease (Cochrane review). In: The Cochrane library, Issue 3. Oxford: Update Software, 2003. (*The treatment was found to improve outcomes over the first 72 hours; see http://www.cochrane.org for updates.*)

45. Crockett AJ, Cranston JM, Moss JR, et al. Domiciliary oxygen for chronic obstructive pulmonary disease (Cochrane review). In: The Cochrane library, Issue 3. Oxford: Update Software, 2004. (*The treatment was found to improve survival for patients with hypoxemia; see http://www.cochrane.org for updates.*)

46. Dillard TA, Berg BW, Rajagopal KR, et al. Hypoxemia during air travel in patients with chronic obstructive pulmonary disease. Ann Intern Med 1989;111:362. (*Arterial oxygen tension declined to significantly low levels;*

oxygen supplementation is urged for patients with severe COPD during air travel.)

47. Goldstein RS, Vivekanand R, Bowes G, et al. Effect of supplemental nocturnal oxygen on gas exchange in patients with severe obstructive lung disease. N Engl J Med 1984;310:425. (*Nocturnal oxygen therapy did not induce clinically worrisome increases in the partial pressure of CO_2.*)

48. Ram FS, Wedzicha JA. Ambulatory oxygen for chronic obstructive pulmonary disease (Cochrane review). The Cochrane library, Issue 3. Oxford: Update Software, 2004. (*Limited evidence allows no conclusions about short-term ambulatory oxygen; see http://www.cochrane.org for updates.*)

49. Timms RM, Khaja FU, Williams GW, et al. Hemodynamic response to oxygen therapy in chronic obstructive pulmonary disease. Ann Intern Med 1985;102:29. (*Detailed data showing a modest response; patients with the best response had the best prognosis.*)

50. Poole PJ, Black PN. Oral mucolytic drugs for exacerbations of chronic obstructive pulmonary disease: systematic review. BMJ 2001;322:1. (*This approach was found to reduce acute exacerbation and days of illness.*)

51. Jones AP, Rowe BH. Bronchopulmonary hygiene physical therapy for chronic obstructive pulmonary disease and bronchiectasis (Cochrane review). In: The Cochrane library, Issue 3. Oxford: Update Software, 2004. (*There was insufficient evidence for or against effectiveness; see http://www.cochrane.org for updates.*)

52. Lacasse Y, Brosseau L, Milne S, et al. Pulmonary rehabilitation for chronic obstructive pulmonary disease (Cochrane review). The Cochrane library, Issue 3. Oxford: Update Software, 2003. (*The procedure was found to relieve dyspnea and fatigue; see http://www.cochrane.org for updates.*)

53. Lacasse Y, Guyatt GH, Goldstein RS. The components of a respiratory rehabilitation program: a systematic review. Chest 1997;111:1077. (*The evidence is best for benefit from exercise training and psychosocial support.*)

54. Puhan MA, Büsching G, Holger PT, et al. Interval versus continuous high-intensity exercise in chronic obstructive pulmonary disease. Ann Intern Med 2006;145:816. (*Both groups experienced large improvements in health-related quality of life.*)

55. Bach PB, Brown C, Gelfand SE, et al. Management of acute exacerbations of chronic obstructive pulmonary disease: a summary and appraisal of published evidence. Ann Intern Med 2001;134:600. (*Reviews risk stratification and diagnostic assessment, as well as management; 129 references.*)

56. Keenan SP, Sinuff T, Cook DJ, et al. Which patients with acute exacerbation of chronic obstructive pulmonary disease benefit from noninvasive positive-pressure ventilation? A systematic review of the literature. Ann Intern Med. 2003;138:861. (*Patients with severe exacerbations of COPD benefit but not those with milder exacerbations.*)

57. Lightowler JV, Wedzicha JA, Elliott MW, et al. Non-invasive positive pressure ventilation to treat respiratory failure resulting from exacerbations of chronic obstructive pulmonary disease: Cochrane systematic review and meta-analysis. BMJ 2003;326:185. (*Noninvasive positive pressure ventilation as an adjunct to usual care was associated with a lower mortality; a relative risk of 0.41 was found; see http://www.cochrane.org for updates.*)

58. Ram FSF, Lightowler JV, Wedzicha JA. Cochrane Airways Group. Non-invasive positive pressure ventilation for treatment of respiratory failure due to exacerbations of chronic obstructive pulmonary disease (Cochrane review). In: The Cochrane library, Issue 3. Oxford: Update Software, 2004. (*There is good-quality evidence for benefit; the procedure should be considered early; see http://www.cochrane.org for updates.*)

59. Han MK, McLaughlin VV, Criner GJ, et al. Pulmonary diseases and the heart. Circulation 2007;116:2992. (*An excellent review of the pathophysiology.*)

60. National Emphysema Treatment Trial Research Group. A randomised trial comparing lung volume reduction surgery with medical therapy for severe emphysema. N Engl J Med 2003;348:2059. (*Improved exercise tolerance and survival were found among those with predominantly upper lobe disease.*)

61. National Emphysema Treatment Trial Research Group. Patients at high risk of death after lung-volume-reduction surgery. N Engl J Med 2001;345:1075. (*Among patients with severe physiologic impairment and homogeneous emphysema, mortality was higher in the surgery group.*)

62. Bourbeau J, Julien M, Maltais F, et al. Reduction of hospital utilization in patients with chronic obstructive pulmonary disease: a disease-specific self-management intervention. Arch Intern Med 2003;163:585. (*Hospital admissions were reduced by 40%.*)

63. Adams SG, Smith PK, Allan PF, et al. Systematic review of the chronic care model in chronic obstructive pulmonary disease prevention and management. Arch Intern Med 2007:167:551. (*A review finding lower rates of hospitalizations and emergency/unscheduled visits and a shorter length of stay compared with control groups.*)

64. Ng TP, Niti M, Tan WC, et al. Depressive symptoms and chronic obstructive pulmonary disease: effect on mortality, hospital readmission, symptom burden, functional status, and quality of life. Arch Intern Med 2007;167:60. (*Depressive symptoms in patients with COPD associated with poorer survival, longer hospitalizations, increased symptom burden and persistent smoking.*)

CHAPTER 48 ■ MANAGEMENT OF ASTHMA

Asthma is a chronic inflammatory disease of the airways that affects an estimated 5% to 7% of the population, with an increasing prevalence and mortality that are greatest among inner-city residents. A heightened appreciation for the underlying inflammatory pathophysiology of asthma has markedly altered the approach to therapy in the last two decades. Antiinflammatory agents have superseded bronchodilators as the mainstay of treatment.

Although there are no cures for asthma, effective outpatient management is achievable. Many exacerbations leading to emergency room visits are preventable, so much so that the frequency of emergency room visits for asthma has become a common outcome measure and proxy for the quality of primary care. The primary care physician needs to be skilled in asthma management and able to design a practical, cost-effective program that minimizes side effects, maximizes functional status, and reduces the frequency and severity of flares. Because patient involvement in asthma care is essential to a good outcome, the development of a strong patient–doctor collaborative relationship and the provision of detailed education tailored to the needs of the patient are extremely important. Neither doctor nor patient can manage asthma effectively alone.

PATHOPHYSIOLOGY, CLINICAL PRESENTATION, AND COURSE (1–7)

Pathophysiology (1,2,7)

Airway inflammation underlies the pathology and pathophysiology of asthma; characteristic features are mast cell degranulation, eosinophilic infiltration, endothelial activation, and recruitment and proliferation of T cells. The normal respiratory epithelium is denuded and replaced by proliferating goblet cells. The resulting edema, inflammatory exudate, and bronchial hyperresponsiveness lead to airway obstruction. Bronchial hyperresponsiveness is exacerbated by loss of the normal epithelial barrier and can be triggered by exposure to allergens, exercise, cold, and pharmacologic agents. Epidemiologically important allergens leading to *sensitization* include *dust mite* and *cockroach* antigens, which helps to explain the high prevalence of asthma among inner-city residents. Air pollutants and occupational exposures sensitize others.

Many precipitants and mediators of the bronchoconstriction, edema, and mucus production that characterize asthma have been identified; however, their precise roles and interrelationships remain to be elucidated. The list of mediators includes *prostaglandin D_2*, *leukotrienes* (slow-reacting substance of anaphylaxis), *eosinophilic chemotactic factor*, and *histamine*. Leukotrienes are emerging as particularly important mediators of inflammation. They increase the migration of eosinophils, production of mucus, airway wall edema, and bronchial hyperresponsiveness. They appear to be important triggers of bronchoconstriction on airway exposure to cold, dry air, as in exercise- and cold-induced asthma. There is growing evidence that the inflammatory cytokine tumor necrosis factor-α (TNFα) plays a critical role in airway inflammation among patients with asthma. TNFα is present in increased concentrations among patients with severe and refractory asthma, and early evidence suggests that TNFα antagonists can improve airway hyperresponsiveness.

Asthmatic reactions have early and late phases. The *acute bronchoconstrictive phase* involves the rapid development of reversible airway obstruction in response to stimuli that fail to affect normal persons. Stimuli include allergens (e.g., molds, sulfites, animal dander, pollens), aspirin, exercise, emotional stress, viral respiratory infections, and respiratory irritants such as perfumes and dusts.

In addition to the initial mediator-induced bronchospasm, asthmatic patients experience a second or *late-phase reaction* 6 to 12 hours later. This late-phase reaction is believed to be a manifestation of the inflammatory response that is more refractory to bronchodilator treatment than the initial one. Neutrophil chemotactic factor is believed to play a role. Even some patients with exercise-induced asthma experience a late reaction.

Elements of a *neurogenic pathway* have also been elucidated. Bronchial smooth muscle is responsive to autonomic influences; it has not been determined whether the effect is direct or by way of biochemical mediators. Vagal stimulation and cholinergic drugs cause bronchial constriction; β-adrenergic stimulation appears to be capable of countering the cholinergic influences. Bronchial irritants and emotional stress are believed to precipitate bronchospasm, in part, by way of triggering vagal reflexes. The nerve endings of asthmatic patients have been found to be devoid of the bronchodilator neuropeptide vasoactive intestinal polypeptide.

Traditionally, asthma has been divided clinically into "extrinsic" and "intrinsic" categories, with extrinsic disease believed to be a manifestation of immunologic reactivity to environmental antigens and intrinsic disease believed to be unrelated to allergen exposure. However, patients in both groups have demonstrated reactivity related to immunoglobulin E (IgE), which challenges the notion of separate allergen-related and non–allergen-related categories of asthma. Nonetheless, the categories are still used clinically (see the following discussion).

It used to be believed that asthma was not associated with any permanent sequelae, but *airway remodeling* has been detected pathologically. The full physiologic significance of this remodeling remains to be determined, but declines in pulmonary function over time have been identified in long-term epidemiologic studies.

Clinical Presentation (3–5)

Regardless of precipitant, the pathophysiologic final common pathway is airway inflammation, with bronchial edema, smooth-muscle contraction, and excessive mucus production. Clinical manifestations include *wheezing, dyspnea, cough,* and *sputum.* Presentations range from pure bronchospasm, with little cough and sputum production, to a predominance of bronchorrhea and coughing that mimics bronchitis or an upper respiratory tract infection. In fact, cough and sputum production may be the initial symptoms of an asthmatic attack. *Nocturnal exacerbation* of symptoms is common, linked to the diurnal variation in blood levels of catecholamines and vagal tone.

Extrinsic Asthma

Although classifying asthma according to allergen responsiveness may be an oversimplification, the extrinsic and intrinsic categories do describe two relatively distinct clinical presentations. Patients with *extrinsic asthma* typically give a history of atopy, onset of symptoms during childhood or adolescence, predictable seasonal occurrence, and response to environmental stimuli. However, the condition can occur at any age, and attacks may take place seasonally or year-round, precipitated by such common household allergens as dust mites, animal dander, and fungal spores. Anxiety, inhalation of airway irritants, and exposure to perfumes and strong household odors can also precipitate asthmatic episodes in these patients. The course of attacks is usually self-limited, although some patients have severe bouts requiring hospitalization. Prognosis is relatively good, with 70% found to be symptom-free 20 years after onset.

Intrinsic Asthma

Patients with *intrinsic asthma* usually begin having symptoms in the third or fourth decade. Although no identifiable extrinsic allergen is associated with attacks in these patients, they do demonstrate elevations in serum IgE, similar to those of patients with extrinsic disease. Sputum production can be considerable, so that differentiation from chronic bronchitis is sometimes difficult. Minor upper respiratory tract infections often precipitate attacks. Some patients present with exertional dyspnea or cough and no demonstrable wheezing, although expiratory flow rates are clearly reduced. Intrinsic asthma is sometimes more refractory to treatment than is extrinsic disease.

Postexertional Asthma

Postexertional asthma is a form of airway hyperreactivity most common in children and adolescents. The stimulus is believed to be a reduction in the temperature of inhaled air, which leads to mediator release (especially leukotrienes) in susceptible patients. Both initial and late-phase reactions have been identified. Vigorous exercise on a cold, dry day is particularly apt to trigger an attack; airway temperature can become quite low in such circumstances. Although bronchospasm does not occur during exercise, it becomes marked shortly after exercise ends and can last for up to 1 hour.

Occupational Asthma

Occupational asthma has gained increasing recognition as an important cause of work-related disability. True occupational asthma involves the development of sensitization through inhalation exposure to an occupationally related allergen. Exposure to irritant or toxic pollutants in the workplace can also trigger bronchospasm, especially in a person with pre-existing airway hyperresponsiveness. Cold air, sulfur dioxide in low concentrations, fluorocarbons, and inert dusts are common irritants that stimulate reflex bronchospasm. Toxic gases such as sulfur dioxide in high concentrations, halogens, ammonia, acid fumes, and solvent vapors cause inflammatory bronchoconstriction. Important allergens include animal proteins, enzymes, grain and cereal dusts, seeds, vegetable gums, and legumes. Other substances have pharmacologic activity; histamine-releasing compounds are present in cotton dust, organic acids are found in wood dust, and numerous chemicals have anticholinesterase activity. Some agents provoke asthma through multiple mechanisms; toluene diisocyanate has reflex, pharmacologic, β-blocking, and IgE effects.

Patients with occupational asthma caused by toxic or irritant substances characteristically report a direct relation between exposure and onset of symptoms. Those with allergen-induced disease note no symptoms at the time of the first exposure but marked wheezing after even minor repeated contact with the allergen (anamnestic response). Typically, patients with occupational asthma are symptom-free during days off from work, only to have a flare-up on returning (see Chapter 39).

Nasal Polyps and Aspirin Sensitivity

Nasal polyps and aspirin sensitivity comprise a curious but important familial asthma syndrome. The bronchospasm associated with aspirin intake may be marked. The finding of nasal polyps in a person with a history of asthma should lead to consideration of aspirin sensitivity. Aspirin sensitivity can be demonstrated with oral provocation testing among 21% of adults with asthma. Almost all patients with aspirin sensitivity have cross-reactivity with nonsteroidal antiinflammatory agents. Only 7% of those with aspirin sensitivity have cross-reactivity with acetaminophen.

Categories of Asthma

For management purposes (see later discussion), four categories of asthma have been defined:

- *Mild intermittent asthma:* Symptoms occur no more than twice weekly and nighttime symptoms no more than twice monthly; lung function (peak flow rate, forced expiratory volume in 1 second [FEV_1]) is reduced to no less than 80% of predicted; patient is asymptomatic between exacerbations; and peak expiratory flow rates are normal between attacks.
- *Mild persistent asthma:* Patient is symptomatic more than two times per week but less than once a day, and nighttime symptoms occur more than twice monthly; episodes may affect activity; pulmonary function is normal between episodes and decreases to no less than 80% of normal during episodes.
- *Moderate persistent asthma:* Daily symptoms occur, there is daily use of β_2-agonists, and nocturnal symptoms occur more than once a week; attacks limit activity; pulmonary function declines to 60% to 80% of normal and may not return to normal after an exacerbation.
- *Severe asthma:* Symptoms are continuous; there are frequent acute exacerbations and frequent nocturnal symptoms; activity is limited; pulmonary function is always abnormal and less than 60% of normal without treatment.

Clinical Course and Natural History (6)

Regardless of the type of asthma, subclinical but significant bronchospasm remains for days to weeks after the wheezing of an acute attack subsides. The continuing bronchial hyperresponsiveness is believed to be related to ongoing inflammation. Often, small airways may remain constricted even after large airways have relaxed. The clinical recurrences that commonly develop shortly after the apparent resolution of an acute attack are most often not new episodes but relapses.

The natural history of asthma and the consequences of airway remodeling that result from chronic airway inflammation remain to be fully established, but in population studies with long-term follow-up, asthmatic patients demonstrate a significant and steady decline in FEV_1 in comparison with those without asthma. This decline is exacerbated by smoking. Overall mortality for all forms of asthma is 0.1% annually; the rate increases markedly to 3.3% for patients with episodes of status asthmaticus. A disturbing increase in asthma mortality has occurred in the last two decades despite the availability of increasingly effective therapy. The cause for this increase is unclear, but much of it is localized to inner-city populations in New York City and Chicago, which suggests that increased exposure to potent allergens and air pollution may be contributing, in addition to inadequate access to proper health care.

PRINCIPLES OF MANAGEMENT (7–53)

Strategy (8,9)

The appreciation of the pivotal role of inflammation in the pathophysiology of asthma has led to a major restructuring of treatment, with *antiinflammatory therapy* emerging as the foundation of treatment for long-term control and *bronchodilators* relegated to a supporting role. The consensus view is that all patients with active disease should be started and maintained on continuous antiinflammatory therapy and that bronchodilators should be used as primary therapy only for those with infrequent, mild exacerbations and to prevent postexertional or cold-induced flares. The previous reliance on long-term bronchodilator therapy as first-line treatment has been largely abandoned because such therapy does not correct the underlying pathophysiology and is associated with poor outcomes, including higher rates of severe and life-threatening asthma exacerbations and asthma-related deaths (see later discussion). *Patient education* takes on heightened importance because of the need for constant monitoring, compliance, and timely adjustment of the treatment program.

As always, when confronted with an acute attack of bronchospasm and before initiating therapy for asthma, the physician should not forget to consider briefly the other acute causes of wheezing (e.g., pulmonary edema, pulmonary embolization, laryngeal edema, airway obstruction by tumor or foreign body, chronic obstructive lung disease flare; see Chapters 32 and 40 through 42).

Review of the patient's medication list is also indicated. Concurrent use of noncardioselective beta-blockers in asthmatics with underlying hypertension or cardiovascular disease can cause bronchospasm and blunt the bronchodilating effects of β_2-agonists. Concern about beta-blocker therapy has been reduced by the advent and judicious use of cardioselective (β_1) beta-blockers (e.g., atenolol, metoprolol). Meta-analytic work found only a 7.5% reduction in FEV_1 in mild to moderate asthmatic patients with the addition of a cardioselective beta-blocker and no impairment of the bronchodilating effects of beta-agonist therapy. Most asthmatic patients with a clear indication for beta-blockade (i.e., those with hypertension, coronary disease, or heart failure) need not forego or stop beta-blocker therapy as long as cardioselective preparations are used and doses are kept low. However, the safety of cardioselective beta-blockade in those with severe asthma is not well established.

Practice Guidelines

Recognizing the need to develop and promulgate a new treatment paradigm for asthma, the National Institutes of Health convened expert panels to develop *clinical practice guidelines* for asthma management and published them as the *National Asthma Education Program* (NAEP) (see later discussion). A stepped approach to care is used, based on the category of asthma manifested. The regular use of topically active *inhaled corticosteroids* is recommended, supplemented by the selective use of *inhaled β_2-agonist* bronchodilators. Oral steroids, other antiinflammatory agents, and other bronchodilators are used in adjunctive fashion. *Patient education* is a central feature of the guidelines because of the importance of compliance to successful management. Underuse of antiinflammatory therapy and failure to monitor peak flows correlate strongly with an increased number of emergency department visits and hospitalizations.

Implementation and Compliance

Like most practice guidelines, many of the NAEP recommendations are supported by the results of randomized, controlled trials (e.g., respective roles for inhaled steroids and bronchodilators), whereas others (e.g., approaches to monitoring and self-care) are based on expert opinion. Primary care physicians may need to customize for individual patients those elements that pertain to patient self-monitoring and self-treatment of an exacerbation. Surveys indicate that fewer than 50% of asthma patients who should take inhaled steroids daily do so, and fewer than 20% measure their peak flow regularly. Some have suggested that time pressures and staffing limitations in primary care practices may limit the teaching effort and contribute to inadequate outcomes. They propose *disease management* strategies, which emphasize the use of information technology to identify patients, customize the teaching intervention, monitor care, and control costs. The efficacy of the disease management approach is still being evaluated, but many studies have shown reductions in rates of emergency room visits and hospitalizations for both children and adults.

Treatment Guidelines (Incorporating the National Asthma Education Program Recommendations) (8–14)

Mild Intermittent Asthma

The treatment of choice is *bronchodilator* therapy as needed with a *short-acting β_2-agonist,* such as albuterol (Table 48.1). As-needed use is preferred to regular use, which is no more effective and may induce tachyphylaxis. *Patient education* includes instruction in proper inhaler use and technique, the role of medication, and avoidance of environmental precipitants. If

β_2-agonist therapy is needed more than twice weekly, therapy for mild persistent asthma should be considered.

These agents are also effective as *prophylaxis* for mild episodes of exercise- or cold-induced asthma when taken a few minutes before the inciting activity. If exercise is going to be very prolonged or prolonged protection against unexpected exercise is desired, then one might consider an as-needed dose of a *long-acting β_2-agonist* (e.g., *salmeterol*). The regular daily use of a long-acting β_2-agonist is not recommended because of the association of high-dose β_2-agonist therapy with adverse outcomes (see later discussion). Alternatives for the prophylaxis of mild exercise-induced asthma include the inhalation of *cromolyn* or *nedocromil* powder before activity and the once-daily oral use of *montelukast*. For the treatment of the rare severe exacerbation in patients with intermittent asthma, some recommend a short course of systemic corticosteroids.

Mild Persistent Asthma

Antiinflammatory therapy is added to the program to provide long-term control. A *low-dose inhaled glucocorticosteroid* is the treatment of choice (see Table 48.1). Alternatives include *cromolyn* and *nedocromil*. The use of a leukotriene-altering agent (e.g., *montelukast*) is another approach to antiinflammatory therapy for mild disease. Patient education should include the initiation of periodic self-monitoring with a *peak flow meter*. The treatment of acute symptoms with the as-needed use of a *short-acting β_2-agonist* continues as for mild intermittent disease; any requirement for daily or increased dosing should lead to the consideration of therapy for moderate asthma.

Moderate Asthma

Frequent exacerbations require increasing the dose of *inhaled steroids* to at least *moderate* levels or continuing low doses and *adding an inhaled long-acting β_2-agonist* (e.g., *salmeterol*) or a bedtime dose of *theophylline*, especially if nocturnal symptoms are present. Although *montelukast* is not as effective for maintenance as are inhaled glucocorticoids, adding this antiinflammatory agent may allow reduction of the steroid dose. Patient education should stress *daily* monitoring of *peak flow* and increasing the dose of inhaled steroid at the first indication of a decline in peak flow. Treatment of acute symptoms with as-needed use of a *short-acting β_2-agonist* is the same as for mild persistent disease; continued requirements for daily or increased dosing should lead to the consideration of therapy for severe asthma.

Severe Asthma

The foundation of therapy is *high-dose inhaled steroids*, supplemented during exacerbations by short courses of high-dose *systemic glucocorticosteroids* (e.g., oral prednisone). The prednisone program is rapidly tapered and discontinued after 5 to 10 days. Use of a *long-acting β_2-agonist* or *theophylline* can help to control symptoms (particularly nocturnal exacerbations) and may reduce steroid requirements. Daily patient *monitoring of peak flow* and the prompt initiation of maximal antiinflammatory therapy (e.g., high-dose prednisone) at the first sign of a marked decline in airway function are critical to avoiding severe exacerbations and emergency department visits. The use of a *short-acting inhaled β_2-agonist*, supplemented if necessary by inhaled *ipratropium*, can help to ease the symptoms of a severe bronchospastic attack, but these drugs are no substitute for maximum antiinflammatory

TABLE 48.1

DRUGS FOR ASTHMA

	Formulation and Average Dose
β_2-Agonists: Short Acting	
Albuterol (Ventolin, Proventil, ProAir)	MDI; 2 puffs prn
	MDI; 2 puffs prn
Bitolterol (Tornalate)	MDI; 2 puffs prn
Pirbuterol (Maxair)	MDI; 2 puffs prn
Pirbuterol (Maxair Autohaler)	Breath-actuated MDI; 2 puffs prn
Terbutaline	MDI; 2 puffs
β_2-Agonists: Long Acting	
Salmeterol (Serevent)	DPI; 1–2 puffs q12h
Formoterol (Foradil)	DPI; 1-2 puffs q12h
Anticholinergic: Short Acting	
Ipratropium (Atrovent)	MDI; 2-3 puffs qid
Anticholinergic: Long Acting	
Tiotropium (Spiriva)	DPI; 1 puff daily
Inhaled Corticosteroid/β_2-Agonists	
Budesonide/formoterol (Symbicort)	MDI: 2 puffs bid
Fluticasone/salmeterol (Advair)	DPI: 2 puffs bid
Inhaled Corticosteroids	
Beclomethasone (Vanceril Beclovent)	MDI; 4–8 puffs bid
Beclomethasone (Vanceril, Double Strength)	MDI; 2–4 puffs bid
Budesonide (Pulmicort Turbuhaler)	Breath-actuated; 1–2 inhalations bid
Flunisolide (AeroBid)	MDI; 2–4 puffs bid
Fluticasone (Flovent)	MDI; 2–4 puffs bid
Fluticasone (Flovent Rotadisk)	Breath actuated; 1 inhalation bid
Triamcinolone (Azmacort)	MDI; 2 puffs tid–qid
Inhaled Nonsteroidal Antiinflammatory Agents	
Cromolyn (Intal)	MDI; 2–4 puffs tid–qid or prn
Nedocromil (Tilade)	MDI; 2–4 puffs tid–qid or prn
Leukotriene Modifiers	
Montelukast (Singulair)	Oral 10 mg q am
Zafirlukast (Accolate)	Oral 20 mg bid
Zileuton (Zyflo)	Oral 600 mg qid
Theophylline	
Generic extended release	300 mg qhs
Slo-Bid Gyrocaps	300 mg qhs
Uni-Dur	200 mg qhs
Theo-Dur	400 mg qhs

bid, twice daily; DPI, dry powder inhaler; MDI, metered-dose inhaler; prn, as needed; q12h, every 12 hours; q am, every morning; qhs, at bedtime; qid, four times daily; tid, thrice daily.

therapy. The role of montelukast in severe disease remains to be defined.

Refractory cases require the consideration of exacerbating factors, such as exposure to offending allergens, gastroesophageal reflux, sleep apnea, and allergic bronchopulmonary aspergillosis (suggested by an eosinophil count of >1,000/mL). *Immunotherapy* is indicated if a responsible allergen is identified, and a trial of proton-pump inhibition can be helpful in persons with suspected reflux (see Chapter 61). The most common cause of refractory disease is *poor compliance* with the inhaled corticosteroid program and failure to monitor peak flows, which indicates a need for more patient education and counseling.

Treatment Modalities (in Order of Use in Stepped Care) (8–40)

β_2-Agonist Bronchodilators

As noted, bronchodilators have been relegated to a supporting role in the treatment of asthma. The inhaled semiselective *β_2-agonists* are the bronchodilators of choice; they produce prompt potent bronchodilation and little systemic adrenergic stimulation when used in moderation. Although β_2-agonists can provide effective symptomatic relief, their use is not without risk. It has been known for some time that the overuse of short-acting preparations during an acute flare can increase the risk of exacerbation and death. Similarly, recent evidence (see later discussion) indicates that long-acting preparations can also increase the risk of asthma exacerbations and asthma-related death. Careful prescribing and detailed patient education are essential to safe use. A common mistake of both physicians and patients is overreliance on bronchodilators and underuse of antiinflammatory therapy.

Preparations. Most preparations are available in aerosolized form dispensed from a *metered-dose inhaler* (MDI). A few are breath actuated, but most require breath–hand coordination. The onset of action is very rapid, and systemic absorption occurs. Some preparations are available as *nebulized solutions*. Nebulized delivery offers few advantages over MDI delivery and costs more, but patients unable to use pressurized aerosols (e.g., the very young, the elderly) may benefit; the doses delivered are higher, but the onset of action is slower than with MDIs, and the equipment is not portable.

Short-Acting Preparations. The short-acting preparations (e.g., *albuterol, pirbuterol, terbutaline, bitolterol*) have a rapid (2 to 5 minutes) onset of action that lasts 4 to 6 hours. Generic albuterol is well tolerated and among the least expensive. *Levalbuterol,* the L-isomer of albuterol, is available for delivery as a nebulized solution; it offers no particular advantages in safety or efficacy over racemic albuterol. Some of the short-acting inhaled agents are also available in longer-acting oral formulations; however, these formulations are not recommended because the onset of action is delayed, systemic adrenergic side effects can be considerable, and better-tolerated long-acting formulations are available.

Long-Acting Preparations. The inhaled *long-acting β_2-agonists* (e.g., *salmeterol* or *formoterol*) provide up to 12 hours of bronchodilation with a minimum of systemic side effects, so they are well suited for maintenance therapy. Compared with placebo, long-acting β_2-agonists reduce clinically relevant exacerbations by 25%; compared with regular use of *short-acting β_2-agonists*, the reduction in exacerbations with the long-acting β_2-agonists is 17%. Because their onset of action is delayed, they do not obviate the need for a short-acting β_2-agonist when acute bronchospasm arises. They are used only in conjunction with a program of corticosteroid therapy because concern persists (see later discussion) regarding an increase in airway hyperresponsiveness and adverse outcomes when β_2-agonists are used on a regular basis without antiinflammatory therapy. The cost per dose is about two times that of the short-acting preparations.

The modern β_2-agonists have largely replaced the *nonselective β-agonists* (e.g., *isoproterenol, ephedrine, metaproterenol, isoetharine*), which have a very short duration of action and can cause severe adrenergic side effects (palpitations, nervousness, cardiac dysrhythmias).

Adverse Effects. When used in high doses, all semiselective β_2-agents can trigger systemic adrenergic side effects (e.g., *palpitations, tremor, tachycardia*). High doses may also cause *hypokalemia*. For some time, it has been recognized that the overuse of inhaled β_2-agonists was associated with *worsening asthma control* and *increased asthma mortality*. Explanations for the observed findings range from delay in starting needed antiinflammatory treatment to direct toxic effects, such as exacerbation of *bronchial hyperresponsiveness*. In addition, regular β_2-agonist use leads to tolerance of the drug's effects, which contributes to a worsening of disease control.

After the introduction of the long-acting β_2-agonist salmeterol, postmarketing reports of asthma-related deaths were followed by the Salmeterol Multi-center Asthma Research Trial (SMART), which found a fourfold risk of asthma-related deaths with the drug's use. SMART was followed by a meta-analysis that documented a similar increased risk of death, as well as increased risks of severe exacerbations and hospitalization. These risks were associated with both salmeterol and the other long-acting drug, formoterol, and applied to adults and children. Based on these data, a U.S. Food and Drug Administration (FDA) panel considered withdrawing long-acting β_2-agonists, but instead issued a requirement for strong label warnings and recommended against use unless all other asthma drugs had failed.

The adverse effects of long-acting β_2-agonists raise important questions about heterogeneity in the biology of asthma with important clinical implications. Studies indicate that roughly 15% of the U.S. population shares the Arg/Arg genotype that results in a decline in airflow and worsening asthma control with the use of β_2-agonists. This genotype is disproportionately present in African-American populations, making β_2-agonist risk especially important.

Recommended Use. The use of *short-acting* inhaled preparations should be limited to providing prophylaxis for exercise- and cold-induced asthma and symptomatic relief of acute symptoms. These agents are to be taken only on an *as-needed basis*. Frequent bronchodilator use is an important sign of disease exacerbation and the need for additional antiinflammatory therapy. The regular use of a *long-acting* preparation may have a role in moderate and severe asthma but only as an *adjunct* to steroid therapy that has been increased to maximal doses before adding the long-acting β_2-agonist. Careful monitoring for a response is essential, and the long-acting β_2-agonist should be withdrawn if it fails to produce significant clinical improvement. At that point, substitution of an inhaled anticholinergic agent would be a reasonable step (see later discussion).

Inhaled Glucocorticosteroids

The *first-generation* inhaled glucocorticoids (e.g., *beclomethasone, triamcinolone, flunisolide*) were developed in an effort to achieve the advantages of long-term steroid therapy without the systemic side effects. With regular use, many of the histologic features of asthma disappear, airway hyperresponsiveness reverts to normal, and the number of exacerbations declines. These agents are topically active, bind to airway cell receptors, and inhibit the transcription and translation of cytokines and protein mediators. Airway eosinophilia is reduced but not entirely eliminated, which suggests that some degree of airway inflammation persists despite their use. The effect on lipoid inflammatory mediators is more variable, with leukotriene synthesis less consistently inhibited. Inhaled glucocorticoids reduce clinically relevant exacerbations by 55%.

The systemic absorption of inhaled steroid from the lung is limited, but some of the inhaled dose invariably is swallowed. Effective first-pass hepatic metabolism of drug absorbed from the gastrointestinal tract limits systemic effects, but such effects, including adrenal suppression, can increase with the use of very high doses (see later discussion). *Second-generation* formulations (e.g., *fluticasone, budesonide*) exhibit improved steroid-receptor binding in the lung and enhanced first-pass hepatic metabolism; however, any advantage in clinical outcomes remains to be determined.

Preparations. Most first-generation preparations are dispensed through *MDIs,* which require hand–breath coordination. At equivalent doses, they demonstrate similar efficacy and differ predominantly in the dose of steroid delivered per inhalation and cost per canister (see Table 48.1). To improve droplet delivery of drug to the lungs and reduce oropharyngeal deposition, a number of preparations come with a built-in *spacer,* which can also be purchased separately. For those who experience difficulty with hand–breath coordination, one of the *inhalation-triggered* dry-powder formulations (e.g., budesonide) may be worth considering (cost is also low). The risk for adverse systemic effects is greatest with preparations delivering the highest dose of inhaled steroid per puff because fewer puffs are needed to exceed the safe daily limit.

Adverse Effects. When used at moderate doses, the inhaled corticosteroids are well tolerated and produce few adverse systemic effects. The principal localized complaints—*sore throat* and *hoarseness*—are consequences of oropharyngeal deposition of the inhaled steroid and subsequent *oropharyngeal candidiasis* and *vocal cord muscle weakness.* They can be minimized by better inhaler technique (facilitated by the use of a spacer, as explained later), rinsing and gargling after MDI use, and use of nystatin mouthwash for established thrush. The risk for adverse systemic effects caused by the available preparations of inhaled glucocorticoids becomes a concern with sustained use at high doses (750 to 850 μg/d). *Hypothalamic–pituitary–adrenal suppression, decreased bone density, growth retardation in children,* and *glaucoma, cataracts,* and *dermal thinning in the elderly* have all been described. The risks associated with long-term therapy at lower doses remain to be defined.

Use. The topically active, inhaled preparations are preferable to systemic steroids in most instances because systemic adverse effects are limited at the usual doses, and so the risk for systemic steroid-related complications is greatly reduced. Although highly effective, the oral and parenteral preparations of systemic glucocorticoids (e.g., prednisone, methylprednisolone, hydrocortisone) should be reserved for severe exacerbations and refractory disease and used for as short a period as possible (see later discussion).

The original recommendations for inhaled steroids called for administration four times daily, but *twice-daily* regimens are nearly as effective and greatly facilitate compliance with maintenance therapy. Only during exacerbations might dosing four times daily be desirable. The onset of action is usually gradual, and it may take days for the patient to notice improvement—inadequately prepared patients may report that "the drug is not working." Full benefit may not be evident for several weeks. Response is generally dose related.

The use of *high-dose* inhaled steroids can reduce the need for systemic steroids in many cases of severe asthma, especially when supplemented by *β2-agonists* and other drugs. During severe acute exacerbations, a short course of high-dose systemic steroids is indicated because topical steroids may not penetrate obstructed airways, where need is greatest. Patients with extrinsic asthma may benefit from a topically active steroid also applied as a nasal spray during the ragweed season (see Chapter 222).

Oral Glucocorticosteroids

Systemic steroids remain the most effective treatment for asthma, especially the severe, acute exacerbations of this chronic inflammatory disorder. Limiting their use reduces the serious side effects associated with prolonged daily glucocorticosteroid intake (see Chapter 105). *Prednisone* is the most widely prescribed oral preparation; the cost is very low. Its half-life is 12 to 24 hours. The onset of action occurs clinically within 8 to 12 hours of intake.

Use and Adverse Effects. A *short-term course* (5 to 10 days) of high-dose prednisone (40 to 60 mg/d) begun at the earliest signs of an acute exacerbation can control an attack that does not respond promptly to maximum doses of inhaled steroids and bronchodilators. When combined with rapid tapering to full cessation within 5 to 10 days, a short course can obviate the need for emergency department treatment, reduce the risk for acute relapse, and avoid adrenal suppression.

Any *long-term* systemic steroid therapy should be confined to patients with chronic disabling symptoms refractory to maximal doses of all other forms of treatment. The adverse consequences of prolonged daily use of systemic glucocorticoids (osteoporotic fractures, adrenal suppression, skin changes, aseptic necrosis of bone, aggravation of diabetes mellitus) may outweigh the benefits in all but the most severe cases.

In most instances, the regular use of high-dose inhaled steroids supplemented by bronchodilator therapy and short courses of systemic steroids can obviate the need for long-term systemic steroid use. If it proves difficult to withdraw oral steroid therapy entirely, one can try an *alternate-day regimen* supplemented by full doses of inhaled steroid; this results in less adrenal suppression and fewer steroid-related adverse effects than does daily systemic therapy (see Chapter 105). Refractory cases require investigation for exacerbating factors (see prior discussion).

Although always desirable, a switch from long-term systemic steroids to an inhaled steroid program must be planned carefully to avoid triggering an exacerbation of asthma or precipitating adrenal insufficiency. Slow tapering of the daily dose, use of alternate-day steroid programs, and initiation of full doses of inhaled steroids and adjunctive therapies are essential. Before any long-term program of systemic steroids is discontinued, a Cortrosyn stimulation test (which assays the level of adrenal responsiveness) should be considered to help determine the speed of tapering (see Chapter 105).

Cromolyn Sodium and Nedocromil

Cromolyn sodium and nedocromil prevent the degranulation of mast cells, and so they are useful as prophylactic agents for *exercise-* or *allergen-induced asthma* and as substitutes for inhaled steroids in mild persistent disease. They have no direct bronchodilator activity but can decrease airway hyperresponsiveness through their action on mast cells. They are not as effective as inhaled *β2-agonists* for immediate use before exercise or exposure to cold air. Their regular use may avert the need for inhaled corticosteroids. A 4-week empiric trial is needed to assess efficacy; there is no way to predict response, and it may take weeks to emerge. Patients who fail a trial should be prescribed inhaled steroids, which are more effective. Because these drugs possess no direct bronchodilator activity, they should not be used to treat attacks.

Preparations and Use. Cromolyn is taken by the *inhaled* route. It is now available in an aqueous solution, and so the frequency of reactions to the often-irritating powdered formulation has been reduced. The dose schedule for patients with chronic asthma is one capsule four times daily. For prophylaxis of exercise-induced asthma, the patient inhales for several minutes before exercise or exposure to a known allergen (patients with exercise-induced asthma who cannot tolerate cromolyn can inhale a β_2-adrenergic aerosol a few times before engaging in activity). Cromolyn is expensive but is free of adverse side effects and should be considered a first-line drug in asthma prophylaxis. *Nedocromil* resembles cromolyn in action and effectiveness but is unrelated chemically. Use is similar to that of cromolyn. Side effects are minimal.

Leukotriene Modifiers

Appreciation of the role of inflammation in asthma has stimulated interest in inflammatory mediators and agents that inhibit them. The drugs of this class interfere with leukotriene activity, either by the inhibition of synthesis (*zileuton*) or receptor antagonism (*montelukast* and *zafirlukast*). They are less efficacious than inhaled steroids, reducing exacerbations by 40% when compared with placebo. However, they have proved useful for *prophylaxis* of mild exercise-induced asthma and for the *control* of mild to moderate persistent disease. Their role in the treatment of more severe categories of persistent disease, especially in combination with inhaled steroids, remains to be determined; it is hoped that they will have a steroid-sparing effect. Predictors of response have not been identified, so that a therapeutic trial is necessary. These drugs are especially effective in the treatment of aspirin-induced asthma. They are costly, and their long-term safety and efficacy, especially in persons with relatively severe disease requiring concurrent use of other drugs, has not been established. A vasculitis-like hypersensitivity reaction has been reported in association with leukotriene modifier therapy when concurrent steroid therapy is cut back.

Preparations. Of the available leukotriene modifiers, *montelukast* is the best tolerated and easiest to use. Its once-daily dosing schedule, reasonable efficacy (effective in two thirds of cases), and few adverse effects (it is the only drug in this class approved by the FDA for use in children younger than the age of 12 years) make it a practical although somewhat expensive choice for the prophylaxis of exercise-induced asthma. It also shows promise for the control of mild to moderate persistent asthma, allowing reductions in steroid and bronchodilator requirements. Drug absorption is not affected by food intake. The other agents in this class are of similar efficacy but are more difficult to use. *Zileuton* requires dosing four times daily and can cause hepatocellular injury, necessitating close monitoring of transaminases. *Zafirlukast* has the disadvantages of reduced bioavailability when taken with food and reduced efficacy when taken with other asthma drugs (e.g., theophylline). It also impairs warfarin metabolism, and transaminase monitoring is required.

Theophylline and Its Derivatives

The role of the methylxanthines *theophylline* and *aminophylline* (a derivative salt of theophylline) in asthma care has narrowed with the advent of faster, safer, more effective therapies (see prior discussion). Current use is limited to patients with moderate to severe asthma bothered by *nocturnal exacerbations* and to those with refractory, steroid-dependent disease. Although the methylxanthines became popular because they were the first oral active bronchodilators, their current usefulness as an adjunctive therapy may be a function of effects other than bronchodilation. They improve diaphragmatic function, myocardial contractility, and mucociliary transport and demonstrate such antiinflammatory effects as inhibition of anaphylactic mediator release and suppression of mast cell response. Their low cost and the availability of sustained-release preparations facilitate utilization.

Preparations. The preferred oral preparation is *aminophylline*. The half-life of oral theophylline or aminophylline averages 6 hours but can range from 4 to 8 hours; much individual variation is seen because of differences in clearance rates. Clearance occurs predominantly by hepatic biotransformation. Impairment of hepatic microsomal activity raises serum levels and prolongs the duration of action. Generic *sustained-release formulations* provide therapeutic serum levels for 12 to 24 hours at low cost and in convenient once- or twice-daily dosing regimens.

A number of formulations previously used for acute bronchodilation are no longer recommended, including *theophylline elixir* (expensive, very short-acting, erratic absorption), aminophylline *suppositories* (erratic absorption, unpredictable serum levels), and *combination preparations* (inability to titrate theophylline dose, irrational combinations of agents).

Adverse Effects. *Adverse effects* are proportional to the serum level. The therapeutic index of these drugs is narrow (10 to 20 μg/mL), and the monitoring of serum levels helps to ensure both safety and efficacy. Serum determinations are best obtained from blood drawn 4 to 6 hours after the last dose. The minor gastrointestinal side effects (*nausea, vomiting, reflux, diarrhea*) and the minor neurologic side effects (*agitation, tremor, insomnia*) are largely dose related but can occur even at subtherapeutic serum levels. The gastrointestinal side effects are not affected by the route of administration. Levels greater than 20 μg/mL are associated with a marked increase in risk for drug toxicity; at levels greater than 35 μg/mL, life-threatening *ventricular arrhythmias* can occur. *Seizures* refractory to standard anticonvulsant therapy have occurred without warning in patients with serum levels greater than 40 μg/mL.

Dose and Use. When used for bronchodilation, methylxanthines were always prescribed in doses sufficient to achieve the "therapeutic range" (i.e., 10 to 20 μg/mL), which bordered on toxicity. Smaller doses of the drug (producing serum levels of 8 to 10 μg/mL) appear to be less sufficient for reducing inhaled steroid requirements and improving nocturnal symptoms. Such supplementary *low-dose programs* are promising and may become the norm, providing a well-tolerated and inexpensive addition to current expensive treatment regimens.

Anticholinergic Therapy

Ipratropium, a topically active muscarinic blocking agent similar to atropine, is available as an MDI preparation. It is particularly useful in chronic obstructive pulmonary disease, in which its bronchodilator effects rival those of the β_2-agonists (see Chapter 47). Its efficacy is considerably less in asthma, although it may add some marginal bronchodilation to that provided by β_2-*agonist* therapy in severe bronchospasm. Compared with β_2-agonists, it is longer acting but slower to take effect. Unlike atropine, it is poorly absorbed, has little systemic effect, and can be used in patients with glaucoma and prostatism. However, care should be taken to avoid spray contact with the eyes in patients with narrow-angle glaucoma. It is the bronchodilator of choice for beta-blocker–induced bronchospasm and appears to be useful in the elderly. A combination preparation with albuterol is heavily promoted. *Tiotropium* is another nonselective antagonist with similar binding affinity for muscarinic receptors; it dissociates from receptors much more slowly than ipratropium and therefore has a much longer duration of action.

Other Agents

Methotrexate and *cyclosporine* have been studied as steroid-sparing agents for patients dependent on systemic steroid therapy. Although worth considering in refractory cases, this form of immunosuppressive therapy is not without its own serious toxic side effects (see Chapter 88). Other agents that have been tried to allow reduction in steroid use include chloroquine, colchicines, and dapsone. None have been proved effective.

Antibiotics have a limited role in prophylaxis. Although viral upper respiratory infections frequently precipitate attacks—making *influenza vaccination* a must—bacterial infections do not. Heavy sputum production has often been mistakenly attributed to infection when it was actually a manifestation of asthma. However, in cases in which bacterial infection is strongly suggested by a sputum Gram's stain, prompt treatment with an appropriate antibiotic (see Chapter 43) is important pending confirmation by culture.

Allergen Avoidance and Immunotherapy

Allergen identification is worthwhile, especially in patients with seemingly refractory disease, with incapacitating seasonal disease, or in occupational settings (see Chapter 39). Although history is helpful in suggesting allergens, *skin testing* helps to confirm them and also will identify additional allergens that are likely to be clinically important. The avoidance of exposure and desensitization are too often overlooked as important components of the prophylactic management program.

Desensitization therapy (with intradermal injections of offending allergens; see Chapter 222) has been shown in controlled study to reduce the frequency and severity of asthmatic episodes when a *single offending allergen* can be identified. It can reduce or eliminate the need for systemic steroid therapy. Patients with refractory extrinsic asthma should be considered for allergen testing and desensitization, especially when a single, well-defined, unavoidable seasonal allergen is suspected. The use of immunotherapy for perennial allergic asthma in which the patient is sensitive to multiple allergens has not proved effective.

Avoidance of the offending agent(s) can be an important component of therapy and limit exacerbations even when desensitization is not feasible. Detailed patient education can be very helpful, especially when simple effective measures are recommended (e.g., using air conditioning during periods of air pollution, covering mattresses and pillows with impermeable sheets and pillowcases, eliminating wall-to-wall carpets and heavy draperies to limit exposure to dust mite allergen). Unfortunately, avoidance is not always feasible, and pharmacologic methods of prophylaxis may have to be used.

Monoclonal Anti-IgE Antibody

A small proportion of patients with severe asthma and no evidence of atopy often require systemic steroids for control of their disease. Evidence suggests that IgE antibody produced locally in the airway tissue of such patients may be pathophysiologically important. Initial studies of the humanized monoclonal anti-IgE antibody omalizumab administered to block the action of airway IgE have been promising. Two randomized trials demonstrated that in the management of moderate to severe asthma, the addition of monthly subcutaneous injections of omalizumab to patients on optimized inhaled steroids has positive effects. Treatment with omalizumab in these circumstances produced larger reductions in inhaled corticosteroid dose, a greater likelihood of being able to discontinue inhaled corticosteroids, and fewer asthma exacerbations. In June 2003, the FDA approved omalizumab for subcutaneous use in moderate to severe asthmatics 12 years old and older with evidence of allergen sensitivity and poor symptom control with inhaled corticosteroids. Treatment generally consists of 150 to 375 μg every 2 to 4 weeks. Anaphylaxis occurs in approximately 1 in 1,000 patients. The cost is approximately $10,000 per year.

Monitoring Therapy (8,41–45)

The assessment of symptoms, signs, and expiratory flow rates (peak flow and FEV_1) is the basis of monitoring. The patient's subjective perceptions can be remarkably accurate and useful for monitoring. *Estimates by patients* of daily changes in airway obstruction and the severity of their condition correlate better with measurements of peak expiratory flow than do the clinical assessments of their physicians.

Physical Exam

Certain physical findings, such as the *ratio of inspiration to expiration*, help in judging the degree of bronchospasm semiquantitatively. However, wheezes and related physical findings are not sensitive indicators of airway obstruction. The absence of wheezes does not indicate the resolution of bronchospasm (see later discussion). *Pulsus paradoxus* and *sternocleidomastoid retraction* are signs of severe obstruction that suggest an FEV_1 of less than 1 L/s, but these findings are not inevitably present when expiratory flow rates are very low. Moreover, much variation is found between the degree of paradox and the severity of bronchospasm.

Spirometry

Spirometry provides additional sensitivity that helps to identify changes in airway function in the absence of symptoms and to categorize the severity of disease. If possible, the FEV_1 should be measured by the physician at each office visit and during exacerbations and the *peak expiratory flow rate* measured by the patient regularly and during exacerbations. The FEV_1 is still prolonged at the time wheezes disappear. Even after the FEV_1 has returned to normal, measures of small-airway obstruction (e.g., *maximum midexpiratory flow rate*) continue to indicate bronchospasm. The clearing of wheezes signifies little more than partial resolution of large-airway bronchospasm; small-airway bronchoconstriction may still be prominent and slower to resolve. Failure to continue therapy beyond the resolution of audible wheezes and the acute phase of bronchoconstriction is generally associated with a high rate of relapse.

Self-monitoring is made practical by the use of a *handheld peak expiratory flow meter*. In the NAEP guidelines, the monitoring of peak flow both periodically and during exacerbations is central to treatment decisions (see prior discussion).

Eosinophil Counts

Sputum and *blood eosinophil counts* correlate with the response to therapy in patients treated with steroids for an acute attack. Although blood eosinophilia is not an invariable feature of an acute exacerbation of asthma, it does decline with improvement of expiratory flow rate. The same holds true for sputum eosinophilia. The usefulness of the eosinophil count for predicting relapse and response to therapy is unsettled.

Blood Gases

Arterial blood gases provide important information in severe cases, particularly on the adequacy of ventilation. A carbon dioxide pressure (PCO_2) that is inappropriately high for the respiratory rate indicates ventilatory failure and an urgent need for hospitalization. However, because arterial blood gases are not readily available in most office settings, decisions usually must be made without them. *Chest radiography* rarely provides information of use in decision making.

Overall Approach

As shown, some of the most easily obtained parameters (the patient's subjective assessment of severity, the ratio of inspiration to expiration, pulsus paradoxus, sternocleidomastoid retraction, peak flow, and FEV_1) are among the more meaningful guides to clinical status and severity of illness.

The Seemingly Refractory Patient (7,46)

Patient noncompliance is often the cause of "refractoriness." Common shortcomings include *improper inhaler technique, underutilization of antiinflammatory medication,* and *overdependence on bronchodilators.* Poor hand–breath coordination, the slow onset of action of inhaled steroids, the fear of steroid side effects, and ignorance of the inflammatory nature of the illness contribute to such behavior. Other common patient mistakes include reliance on *nonprescription agents,* such as low-dose adrenergic inhalers, and *alternative medicine remedies* of no proven efficacy (e.g., acupuncture for asthma). Physician *inattention to allergen identification* is another common shortcoming; referral for allergen testing is indicated when the patient appears to be unresponsive to treatment.

Management of the Pregnant Patient (47)

Fetal morbidity and mortality are increased if asthma is uncontrolled during pregnancy. Most asthma drugs are safe to use during both pregnancy and breast-feeding, although in some instances data are lacking because of the difficulty in performing controlled studies. Epinephrine increases the risk for fetal malformations, and the safety of the β_2-agonists and cromolyn remains to be established; until safety is proven, they should be avoided if possible. The use of inhaled steroids at moderate doses appears to be without serious consequence, and even systemic steroids can be prescribed if necessary. Theophylline is safe, as is penicillin. Erythromycin is a reasonable alternative in penicillin-allergic patients; tetracycline is contraindicated because it damages fetal liver, bone, and teeth.

PATIENT EDUCATION
(41–44,48–56)

Patients need to be made partners in the management of their asthma. Successful outcomes depend on good compliance and proper use of medication. Instruction in *preventive measures* is always appreciated by patients. The bedroom environment deserves particular attention. Covering the mattress and pillows with impermeable materials limits exposure to dust mite allergen, a potential trigger of asthma and its exacerbations. Wall-to-wall carpets are another source of such allergens and should be avoided. Because asthma is a condition characterized by periodic exacerbations, every patient who is capable of understanding and carrying out a medication program should be given instructions for the initial self-treatment of an attack along with strong advice to call the physician promptly if relief

does not come quickly. Patients need to know that excessive delay may lead to refractory bronchospasm. Home use of a *handheld flow meter* has helped to encourage patient participation in monitoring and adjusting treatment in a timely fashion.

Addressing patient concerns and providing written information facilitates *compliance.* Many worry about becoming "dependent" on medication or "immune" to it. These fears need to be addressed openly. A medication booklet that lists prescribing information, side effects, and indications for use alongside a picture of the medication can be helpful to patient and family. Often, patients mistakenly stop the wrong medication or cease therapy altogether because they are fearful of or unfamiliar with the side effects of their medications.

Patients in whom bronchospasm is triggered by air pollution, pollens, or exercise need an *activity prescription.* Staying indoors, avoiding physical exertion, and using air conditioning on particularly bad days are helpful measures. Those with exercise-induced asthma need not restrict themselves so long as prophylactic measures suffice; however, very cold, dry days may be difficult.

Patients with asthma caused by occupational exposure or household factors need careful *counseling* when such difficult alternatives as leaving a job, giving up a favorite pet, or moving to a new location are being considered. Often, less extreme measures are adequate (see prior discussion). A number of patients with allergic asthma request advice about desensitization treatment. Allergen testing and the consideration of a trial of such therapy are reasonable if episodes are frequent and incapacitating and a single allergen can be identified (see prior discussion and Chapter 222).

Patients receiving steroids deserve an extra measure of instruction, particularly when switching from systemic to aerosol therapy. Writing out the tapering schedule and emphasizing the importance of taking systemic steroids at the time of an exacerbation or major stress will help to minimize the risk for adrenal insufficiency.

The *pregnant patient* with asthma will be reluctant to take medication. Detailed counseling about which medications can be used with safety and the importance of asthma control to the health of the fetus is needed to ensure compliance and alleviate concern.

Inhaler Technique

With the growing importance of MDI therapy, proper inhalation technique is essential. The delivery of drug to distal airways is facilitated by *increased duration of breath holding* and by *prolongation and moderation of inspiratory flow.* Rapid inspiration deposits drug in the upper airway; very deep inspiration is no better than moderate inspiration. During periods of respiratory distress, a greater number of inhales may be needed to deliver an adequate dose to the distal airways. Thus, patients need to be instructed to increase the number of inhales during a period of respiratory distress if benefit is not immediately forthcoming; however, they should also be reminded that rapid, deep inhales are neither necessary nor desirable. Extreme care is warranted when the β_2-agonist dose is increased because systemic absorption will occur when drug is deposited in the proximal airway.

Correct MDI use involves hand–breath coordination (i.e., coordinating inspiration with actuation of the MDI), a skill that takes some practice to master. Two recommended approaches are (a) placing the inhaler between closed lips, actuating the inhaler, breathing in, and holding the breath and (b) holding the mouthpiece 3 to 4 cm from open lips, releasing the medication at the beginning of a full 5-second inspiration, and holding the breath for 10 seconds. The latter technique is a bit more difficult but is preferred because less of a jet effect is created to deposit drug on the retropharynx; twice the dose is delivered to the lower respiratory tract if the inspiration is moderate, prolonged, and accompanied by breath holding.

Many patients make the mistake of inhaling first, then actuating the canister, holding their breath for 2 or 3 seconds more, and exhaling before taking the first inhale. Others inhale through the nose. Because many patients cannot perform aerosol inhalation correctly after a demonstration, they need to practice under observation. Moreover, about half forget how to do it when tested on follow-up. Repeated checks of technique are important.

Use of a Spacer

More than 40% of patients cannot master such techniques and need to use an inhalation chamber, often referred to as a "spacer." Commercially available spacers are aerosol-holding chambers that not only eliminate the need for hand–breath coordination but also cut down on oropharyngeal deposition of steroid. They improve delivery substantially, minimize adverse topical effects of inhaled steroids, and improve overall control. They should be considered for persons who cannot master MDI technique and for those who demonstrate inadequate disease control. The principal disadvantage of most spacers is their bulky size, although some inhalers come with spacers built in.

Breath-Actuated Systems

A few β_2-agonists and inhaled steroid preparations are available in *breath-actuated formulations*. These are triggered by inhalation and do not require as much hand–breath coordination as do MDIs.

INDICATIONS FOR ADMISSION AND REFERRAL (9)

Admission

One of the most difficult determinations is predicting the need for hospitalization at the time of initial presentation. The ability to make such predictions is particularly important for the care of patients with severe attacks who visit the office or emergency department. Some have argued that the response to maximum nonsteroidal therapy is a good predictor of immediate outcome and need for admission. Most studies provide little evidence that any one parameter is predictive, although one group noted that patients who sat bolt upright on admission to the emergency department had a strong likelihood of requiring admission. Another group developed an index of multiple clinical parameters selected by multivariate discriminant analysis to predict the need for hospitalization. A pulse rate of greater than 120/min, a respiratory rate of greater than 30/min, pulsus paradoxus of greater than 18 mm Hg, a peak expiratory flow rate of less than 120 L/min, moderate to severe dyspnea, accessory muscle use, and wheezing were the presenting clinical parameters used in the index. Although in the investigators' setting the index was capable of distinguishing between those who required admission and those who did not (sensitivity, 95%; specificity, 97%), it did not function nearly as well when applied prospectively by other investigators in their emergency department settings.

Without more definitive means of prediction, clinical status and response to therapy remain the most helpful guidelines for decision making. Consideration of hospital care is indicated for patients with an acute attack who manifest any one of the following:

1. Subjective report of severe difficulty breathing.
2. Failure to respond fully and promptly to inhaled β_2-agonist therapy followed promptly by full doses of prednisone.
3. Use of accessory muscles of respiration (sternocleidomastoid retraction).
4. Pulsus paradoxus of greater than 10 mm Hg.
5. FEV_1 of less than 1.0 L/sec; peak flow reduced by more than 50% and declining.
6. Arterial PCO_2 inappropriately high for respiratory rate.
7. Underlying cardiac condition.
8. Inadequate home situation or a history of poor compliance.

Referral

In certain instances, timely referral can be most helpful. Referral for patient *teaching* and *measurement of air flow* is essential if one's practice does not have the time, materials, equipment, or expertise available. *Identification of allergens* and *irritants* is another indication for referral and must be accomplished if the patient is to be advised regarding the avoidance of precipitants, even if desensitization is not indicated. *Failure to respond* to treatment, particularly if frequent severe exacerbations necessitate the use of systemic steroids, is yet another indication for referral.

THERAPEUTIC RECOMMENDATIONS (9,34)

Mild Intermittent Asthma

- Prescribe use as needed of an *inhaled semiselective β_2-agonist* (e.g., two to three puffs of *albuterol*, repeated in 20 minutes if necessary) for an episode of bronchospasm and for a few minutes before exercise or exposure to cold as prophylaxis for exercise- and cold-induced asthma. Avoid regular use.
- If an alternative to albuterol is desired for prophylaxis, consider a trial of *cromolyn* or *nedocromil* (two puffs inhaled a few minutes before activity or exposure to cold).
- If exercise is going to be very prolonged or prolonged prophylactic protection against unexpected exercise is desired, prescribe the use as needed of a *long-acting β_2-agonist* (e.g., one to three puffs of salmeterol twice daily taken at least half an hour before exercise) or a *leukotriene receptor antagonist* (e.g., 10 mg of *montelukast* every morning). Avoid the regular use of salmeterol.
- Teach the patient a self-management program, including proper inhaler technique, the importance of as-needed use only, and the avoidance of environmental precipitants.
- Consider advancing to treatment of mild persistent asthma if more than twice-weekly use of β_2-agonist therapy is required.

Mild Persistent Asthma

- Add daily *antiinflammatory* therapy; begin *low-dose* inhaled glucocorticosteroids (e.g., two to four puffs of *beclomethasone* twice daily); if it is desired to avoid corticosteroids, begin a 4-week trial of a *mast cell stabilizer* (e.g., two puffs of *cromolyn* or *nedocromil* two to four times daily) or consider *montelukast* (10 mg every morning).

- Teach the patient how to perform periodic self-monitoring with a *peak flow meter* and how to make a prompt adjustment in the steroid dose with any decline in air flow.
- Continue the treatment of acute symptoms with as-needed use of a *short-acting β_2-agonist*. Any requirement for *daily* or *increased* dosing should lead to consideration of therapy for moderate asthma.
- For patients whose asthma is well controlled with twice-daily inhaled corticosteroids, consider "step-down" alternatives based on the patient's preferences and relative concerns about long-term side effects of inhaled corticosteroids. Options include (a) as-needed use of inhaled corticosteroid and inhaled short-acting β_2-agonist together (e.g., beclomethasone and albuterol), (b) once-daily inhaled corticosteroid and long-acting β_2-agonist together (e.g., fluticasone and salmeterol), and (c) once-daily leukotriene-receptor antagonist (e.g., montelukast) with as-needed rescue albuterol.

Moderate Persistent Asthma

- Advance the antiinflammatory program to *intermediate-dose* inhaled *corticosteroids* (e.g., four to eight puffs of *beclomethasone* twice daily).
- If *nocturnal symptoms* are a problem or it is desired to limit steroid exposure, continue low-dose inhaled steroid therapy and add either a *long-acting β_2-agonist* (e.g., one to two puffs of *salmeterol* every 12 hours) or a methylxanthine (e.g., 300 mg of *extended-release theophylline* daily at bedtime) to the program. Never use a long-acting β_2-agonist bronchodilator in the absence of corticosteroid therapy; monitor response and withdraw if there is not significant improvement.
- Consider *montelukast* (10 mg every morning) as another alternative for limiting the steroid dose in persons with mild to moderate disease.
- Continue the treatment of acute symptoms with as-needed use of a *short-acting β_2-agonist*. Any requirement for *daily* or *increased* dosing should lead to the consideration of therapy for severe asthma.
- Emphasize the need for *daily* monitoring of *peak flow* and increasing the dose of inhaled steroid at the first sign of a decline in peak flow.
- Continue the as-needed use of a *short-acting β_2-agonist* for the treatment of acute symptoms; continued requirements for daily or increased dosing should lead to the consideration of therapy for severe asthma.

Severe Persistent Asthma

- Advance the antiinflammatory program to *high-dose* inhaled *corticosteroids* (e.g., four to six puffs of *beclomethasone* four times daily) and supplement with a *long-acting β_2-agonist* (e.g., two puffs of salmeterol every 12 hours)

or sustained-release theophylline (300 mg every 12 hours, with regular monitoring of the serum theophylline level). Never use a long-acting β_2-agonist bronchodilator in the absence of corticosteroid therapy; monitor response and withdraw if there is not significant improvement. Substitution of an inhaled anticholinergic agent (e.g., ipratropium or the longer-acting tiotropium) should be considered, especially for African American patients.

- For acute severe exacerbations, supplement inhaled steroids with a short course of high-dose *systemic glucocorticosteroids* (e.g., prednisone started at 40 to 60 mg/d and tapered to full cessation within 5 to 10 days).
- Emphasize to the patient the importance of regular daily *monitoring of peak flow* and prompt initiation of high-dose prednisone at the first sign of markedly declining airway function. Have the patient fill a prednisone prescription and keep it for the prompt initiation of therapy. Inform the patient that any delay in initiating steroid therapy and overreliance on short-acting bronchodilators can be dangerous.
- Continue as-needed use of a *short-acting β_2-agonist* for the treatment of acute symptoms and consider adding a trial of inhaled *ipratropium* (e.g., two puffs as needed) if β_2-agonist therapy alone does not suffice for an acute attack. Increase the number of puffs of short-acting bronchodilator and monitor the patient carefully if the exacerbation is marked (e.g., peak flow <60% of predicted). A short course of systemic steroids should be considered and started promptly if improvement is not rapid.
- Consider any persistent requirements for daily or increased dosing of bronchodilator therapy as indications to add daily systemic steroid therapy (e.g., 10 to 20 mg of prednisone every morning).
- Make repeated attempts to taper systemic steroids to the lowest dose sufficient to prevent attacks and, if possible, discontinue systemic steroids; if the discontinuation of systemic steroids is not possible, then consider switching to alternate-day therapy (e.g., 10 to 20 mg every other day). To facilitate tapering and maintain control, continue inhaled corticosteroid therapy at full doses in conjunction with a long-acting bronchodilator program.
- Taper systemic steroids slowly if the patient has been taking prednisone long enough to cause hypothalamic–pituitary–adrenal suppression (see Chapter 105). At times of stress and severe flares, be sure that inhaled steroid therapy is at maximum doses and consider resuming full doses of systemic steroid therapy (e.g., 40 to 60 mg of prednisone per day) until the episode passes.
- In *refractory cases*, check for and treat any exacerbating factors, such as exposure to an offending allergen, gastroesophageal reflux, sleep apnea, and allergic bronchopulmonary aspergillosis (suggested by an eosinophil count >1,000/mL). *Immunotherapy* is indicated if a single responsible allergen is identified. Check for *poor compliance* with the inhaled corticosteroid program and failure to monitor peak flows, which indicate the need for more patient education and counseling.

A.G.M./A.H.G.

Annotated Bibliography

1. Burrows B, Martinez FD, Halonen M, et al. Association of asthma with serum IgE levels and skin-test reactivity to allergens. N Engl J Med 1989;320:271. (*Prevalence is closely related to serum immunoglobulin E [IgE] levels; patients with both extrinsic and intrinsic asthma had evidence of immunologic hyperreactivity.*)

2. Rosenstreich DL, Eggleston P, Kattan M, et al. The role of cockroach allergy and exposure to cockroach allergen in causing morbidity among inner-city children with asthma. N Engl J Med 1997;336:1356. (*An important discovery that might explain the high prevalence of asthma among inner-city persons.*)

3. Jenkins C, Costello J, Hodge L. Systematic review of prevalence of aspirin induced asthma and its implications for clinical practice. BMJ 2004;328:432. (*Among adult asthmatics, prevalence was 21% by oral provocation testing and 3% by verbal history.*)

4. McFadden ER. Exertional dyspnea and cough as preludes to acute attacks of bronchial asthma. N Engl J Med 1975;292:555. (*A classic article documenting that intermittent episodes of cough and breathlessness represent variants of asthmatic attacks.*)

5. Beuther DA, Sutherland ER. Overweight, obesity, and incident asthma: a meta-analysis of prospective epidemiologic studies. Am J Respir Crit Care Med 2007;175:661. (*Overweight and obesity are associated with a dose-dependent increase in the odds of incident asthma in men and women.*)

6. Lange P, Parner J, Vestbo J, et al. A 15-year follow-up study of ventilatory function in adults with asthma. N Engl J Med 1998;339:1194. (*An important population-based natural history study from Copenhagen showing a clinically and statistically significant decline in forced expiratory volume in 1 second [FEV$_1$] over time among asthmatics in comparison with nonasthmatics.*)

7. Berry MA, Hargadon B, Shelley M, et al. Evidence of a role of tumor necrosis factor α in refractory asthma. N Engl J Med 2006;354:697. (*Patients with refractory asthma have evidence of upregulation of the TNF-α axis.*)

8. Hawkins G, McMahon AD, Twaddle S, et al. Stepping down inhaled corticosteroids in asthma: randomised controlled trial. BMJ 2003;326:1115. (*A step-down approach to the use of inhaled steroids at high doses in asthma can achieve a reduction in the dose without compromising asthma control.*)

9. National Asthma Education Program. Guidelines for the diagnosis and management of asthma II (U.S. Department of Health and Human Services Publication NIH 92-3091). Bethesda, MD: National Heart, Lung and Blood Institute, 1997. (*National consensus guidelines, which include an emphasis on prevention and self-monitoring; for updates, see http://www.nhlbi.nih.gov/guidelines/asthma/index.htm.*)

10. Legorretta AP, Christian-Herman J, O'Connor RD, et al. Compliance with National Asthma Management Guidelines and Specialty Care. Arch Intern Med 1998;158:457. (*Compliance with preventive guidelines was especially poor among primary care physicians and their patients; compliance was correlated with the frequency of emergency room visits and hospitalizations.*)

11. Papi A, Canonica GW, Maestrelli P, et al. Rescue use of beclomethasone and albuterol in a single inhaler for mild asthma. N Engl J Med 2007;356:2040. (*The symptom-driven use of inhaled beclomethasone [250 µg] and albuterol [100 µg] in a single inhaler is as effective as the regular use of inhaled beclomethasone [250 µg twice daily] and is associated with a lower 6-month cumulative dose of the inhaled corticosteroid.*)

12. The American Lung Association Asthma Clinical Research Centers. Randomized comparison of strategies for reducing treatment in mild persistent asthma. N Engl J Med 2007;356:3037. (*Patients with asthma that is well controlled with the use of twice-daily inhaled fluticasone can be switched to once-daily fluticasone plus salmeterol without increased rates of treatment failure.*)

13. Kraft M, Israel E, O'Connor GT. Treatment of mild persistent asthma. N Engl J Med 2007;356:2096. (*A case-based review, with each author advocating a different approach.*)

14. Grippi MA, Mulrow C. Trials that matter: minimizing treatment of mild, persistent asthma. Ann Intern Med 2007;147:344. (*A thoughtful review of recent trials and resulting new clinical options for patients and doctors to choose among.*)

15. Abramson MJ, Puy RM, Weiner JM. Allergen immunotherapy for asthma (Cochrane review). In: The Cochrane library, Issue 3. Oxford: Update Software, 2004. (*Immunotherapy reduces asthma symptoms and the use of asthma medications and improves bronchial hyperreactivity; see http://www.cochrane.org for updates.*)

16. Bjermer L, Bisgaard H, Bousquet J, et al. Montelukast and fluticasone compared with salmeterol and fluticasone in protecting against asthma exacerbation in adults: one year, double blind, randomised, comparative trial. BMJ 2003;327:891. (*The addition of montelukast in the treatment of patients whose symptoms remained uncontrolled by inhaled fluticasone could provide equivalent clinical control to salmeterol.*)

17. Corren J, Casale T, Deniz Y, et al. Omalizumab, a recombinant humanized anti-IgE antibody, reduces asthma-related emergency room visits and hospitalizations in patients with allergic asthma. J Allergy Clin Immunol 2003;111:87. (*This approach had a demonstrable clinical impact.*)

18. Dahlen SE, Malmstrom K, Nizankowska E, et al. Improvement of aspirin-intolerant asthma by montelukast, a leukotriene antagonist: a randomized, double-blind, placebo-controlled trial. Am J Respir Crit Care Med 2002;165:9. (*The addition of a leukotriene receptor antagonist such as montelukast improved asthma in aspirin-intolerant patients over and above what can be achieved by glucocorticosteroids.*)

19. Drazen JM, Israel E, Boushey HA, et al. Comparison of regularly scheduled with as-needed use of albuterol in mild asthma. N Engl J Med 1996;335:841. (*A multicenter, randomized, controlled, double-blinded trial, showing no additional benefit from regularly scheduled use of β-agonist therapy in comparison with as-needed use.*)

20. Ducharme FM. Inhaled glucocorticoids versus leukotriene receptor antagonists as single agent asthma treatment: systematic review of current evidence. BMJ 2003;326:621. (*Inhaled glucocorticoid doses equivalent to 400 µg/d of beclomethasone were found to be more effective than leukotriene-receptor antagonists in the treatment of adults with mild or moderate asthma in this Cochrane review; see http://www.cochrane.org for updates.*)

21. EH Walters, Walters JAE, Gibson MDP. Inhaled long acting beta agonists for stable chronic asthma (Cochrane review). In: The Cochrane library, Issue 3. Oxford: Update Software, 2004. (*Long-acting β_2-agonists are effective in the control of chronic asthma; see http://www.cochrane.org for updates.*)

22. Ernst P, Spitzer WD, Suisse S, et al. Risk of fatal and near-fatal asthma in relation to inhaled corticosteroid use. JAMA 1992;268:3462. (*The risk was markedly reduced by its use.*)

23. Evans DJ, Taylor DA, Zetterstrom O, et al. A comparison of low-dose inhaled budesonide plus theophylline and high-dose inhaled budesonide for moderate asthma. N Engl J Med 1997;337:1412. (*A double-blinded, placebo-controlled, randomized trial, finding that modest doses of theophylline reduced steroid requirements.*)

24. Garbe E, Suissa S, LeLorier J. Association of inhaled corticosteroid use with cataract extraction in elderly patients. JAMA 1998;280:539. (*A case–control epidemiologic study, finding a threefold increased risk for cataract extraction with the long-term use of high-dose inhaled steroids.*)

25. Holt S, Suder A, Weatherall M, et al. Dose–response relation of inhaled fluticasone propionate in adolescents and adults with asthma: meta-analysis. BMJ 2001;323:253. (*Most of the therapeutic benefit of inhaled fluticasone was achieved with a total daily dose of 100 to 250 µg, and the maximum effect was achieved with a dose of around 500 µg/d.*)

26. Lazarus SC, Boushey HA, Fahy JV, et al. Long-acting beta2-agonist monotherapy vs continued therapy with inhaled corticosteroids in patients with persistent asthma: a randomized controlled trial. JAMA 2001;285:2583. (*Patients with persistent asthma that is well controlled by low doses of triamcinolone cannot be switched to salmeterol monotherapy without the risk of a clinically significant loss of asthma control.*)

27. Leff JA, Busse WW, Pearlman D, et al. Montelukast, a leukotriene-receptor antagonist, for the treatment of mild asthma and exercise-induced bronchoconstriction. N Engl J Med 1998;339:147. (*A multicenter, double-blinded study sponsored by the manufacturer of this leukotriene-receptor antagonist, finding that it was safe and effective in persons with mild, exercise-induced asthma.*)

28. Lemanske RF Jr, Sorkness CA, Mauger EA, et al. Inhaled corticosteroid reduction and elimination in patients with persistent asthma receiving salmeterol: a randomized controlled trial. JAMA 2001;285:2594. (*After the addition of salmeterol, a substantial reduction [50%] in triamcinolone dose can occur without a significant loss of asthma control.*)

29. Malmstrom K, Rodriguez-Gomez G, Guerra J, et al. Oral montelukast, inhaled beclomethasone, and placebo for chronic asthma: a randomized, controlled trial. Ann Intern Med 1999;130:487. (*One of few well-designed comparison studies; oral montelukast was found to be more effective than placebo but not as effective as inhaled beclomethasone.*)

30. Nelson JA, Strauss L, Skowronski M, et al. Effect of long-term salmeterol treatment on exercise-induced asthma. N Engl J Med 1998;339:141. (*A small but well-designed placebo-controlled, random-order, double-blinded crossover trial, finding that long-term administration of salmeterol twice daily continued to provide protection, but the duration of the effect after each dose declined with time.*)

31. Pauwels RA, Lofdahl CG, Postma DS, et al. Effect of inhaled formoterol and budesonide on exacerbation of asthma. N Engl J Med 1997;337:1405. (*A randomized trial of asthma patients with exacerbations while on inhaled corticosteroid therapy, finding that the addition of long-acting inhaled β-agonist therapy was superior to high-dose inhaled steroids and without serious adverse effects.*)

32. Pauwels RA, Pedersen S, Busse WW, et al. START Investigators Group. Early intervention with budesonide in mild persistent asthma: a randomised, double-blind trial. Lancet 2003;361:1071. (*Long-term, once-daily treatment with low-dose budesonide decreased the risk of severe exacerbations and improved asthma control in patients with mild persistent asthma of recent onset.*)

33. Robinson DS, Campbell D, Barnes PJ. Addition of leukotriene antagonists to therapy in chronic persistent asthma: a randomised double-blind placebo-controlled trial. Lancet 2001;357:2007. (*Montelukast did not provide an additional benefit in patients with moderate or severe asthma.*)

34. Salpeter SR, Ormiston TM, Salpeter EE. Cardioselective beta-blockers in patients with reactive airway disease: a meta-analysis. Ann Intern Med 2002;137:715. (*A meta-analysis pooling data from 19 studies; the pooled effect of cardioselective beta-blockers on FEV$_1$ was minimal [7.5% decrease], and the FEV$_1$ increase after β_2-agonist administration was unchanged; argues for the safety of the judicious use of beta-blockade in asthma.*)

35. Spitzer WO, Siussa S, Ernst P, et al. The use of beta-agonists and the risk of death and near-death from asthma. N Engl J Med 1992;326:501. (*Provocative data from a study documenting the increased risk for treatment refractoriness and death associated with prolonged and excessive β-agonist use.*)

36. Nelson HS, Weiss ST, Bleecker ER, et al. The Salmeterol Multicenter Asthma Research Trial: a comparison of usual pharmacotherapy for asthma or usual pharmacotherapy plus salmeterol. Chest 2006;129:15. (*A study finding a twofold increase in asthma exacerbations and a fourfold increase in deaths with salmeterol, although numbers of events were small.*)

37. Salpeter SR, Buckley NS, Ormiston TM, et al. Meta-analysis: effect of long-acting β-agonists on severe asthma exacerbations and asthma-related deaths. Ann Intern Med 2006;144:904. (*A meta-analysis, finding that long-acting β-agonists increase severe and life-threatening asthma exacerbations, as well as asthma-related deaths.*)

38. Glassroth J. The role of long-acting β-agonists in the management of asthma: Analysis, meta-analysis, and more analysis. Ann Intern Med 2006;144:936. (*A good discussion of the clinical implications of a meta-analysis finding of increased risk, including the importance of understanding pharmacogenomic profiles.*)

39. Sin DD, Man J, Sharpe H, et al. Pharmacological management to reduce exacerbations in adults with asthma. JAMA 2004;292:367. (*A meta-analysis of randomized, controlled trials of inhaled corticosteroids, β-agonists, leukotriene modifiers, and anti-IgE therapy.*)

40. Walker S, Monteil M, Phelan K, et al. Anti-IgE for chronic asthma in adults and children (Cochrane review). In: The Cochrane library, Issue 3.Oxford: Update Software, 2004. (*Omalizumab was more effective than placebo at steroid sparing, but the mean steroid dose difference was of debatable clinical value; see* http://www.cochrane.org *for updates.*)

41. Gibson PG, Powell H, Coughlan J, et al. Self-management education and regular practitioner review for adults with asthma (Cochrane review). In: The Cochrane library, Issue 3. Oxford: Update Software, 2004. (*Self-monitoring by either peak expiratory flow or symptoms, coupled with regular medical review and a written action plan, improves health outcomes for adults with asthma; see* http://www.cochrane.org *for updates.*)

42. Pinnock H, Bawden R, Proctor S, et al. Accessibility, acceptability, and effectiveness in primary care of routine telephone review of asthma: pragmatic, randomised controlled trial. BMJ 2003;326:477. (*Compared with face-to-face consultations, telephone consultations enabled more people with asthma to be reviewed, without clinical disadvantage or loss of satisfaction.*)

43. Schatz M, Rodriguez E, Falkoff R, et al. The relationship of frequency of follow-up visits to asthma outcomes in patients with moderate persistent asthma. J Asthma 2003;40:49. (*These patients did not need routine follow-up visits more often than every 6 months.*)

44. Barr RG, Somers SC, Speizer FE, et al. Patient factors and medication guideline adherence among older women with asthma. Arch Intern Med 2002;162:1761. (*Asthma is undertreated among older women; women of advanced age with severe asthma were particularly at risk.*)

45. Rees J. Asthma control in adults. BMJ 2006;332:767. (*An excellent clinical review that emphasizes the need to tailor the approach.*)

46. Coughlan JL, Gibson PG, Henry RL. Medical treatment for reflux oesophagitis does not consistently improve asthma control: a systematic review. Thorax 2001;56:198. (*The published literature does not support the treatment of reflux esophagitis as a means of controlling asthma.*)

47. Blaiss MS. Management of rhinitis and asthma in pregnancy. Ann Allergy Asthma Immunol 2003;90:16. (*A useful review.*)

48. Rees J. Asthma control in adults. BMJ 2006;332:767. (*Different approaches to treatment and control may suit different patients, but simple, personalized management plans improve control.*)

49. Homer CJ. Asthma disease management. N Engl J Med 1997;337:1461. (*A detailed discussion of the possible contributions of disease management techniques in asthma care.*)

50. Ignacio-Garcia JM, Gonzalez-Santos P. Asthma self-management education program by home monitoring of peak expiratory flow. Am J Respir Crit Care Med 1995;151:353. (*Patient education and self-monitoring were found to be critical to effective control.*)

51. Janson SL, Fahy JV, Covington JK, et al. Effects of individual self-management education on clinical, biological, and adherence outcomes in asthma. Am J Med 2003;115:620. (*Education and training in self-management improve adherence with inhaled therapy, perceived control of asthma, and sputum eosinophilia.*)

52. Mickleborough TD, Gotshall RW, Cordain L, et al. Dietary salt alters pulmonary function during exercise in exercise-induced asthmatics. J Sports Sci 2001;19:865. (*A low-salt diet improved and a high-salt diet exacerbated pulmonary function during exercise in individuals with exercise-induced asthma.*)

53. Osman LM, Calder C, Godden DJ, et al. A randomised trial of self-management planning for adult patients admitted to hospital with acute asthma. Thorax 2002;57:869. (*A brief self-management program during hospital admission reduced postdischarge morbidity and readmission for adult asthma patients.*)

54. Ram FS, Wright J, Brocklebank D, et al. Systematic review of clinical effectiveness of pressurised metered dose inhalers versus other hand held inhaler devices for delivering beta 2 agonist bronchodilators in asthma. BMJ 2001;323:901. (*There was no evidence that alternative inhaler devices are more effective than standard pressurized metered dose inhalers for delivering β₂-agonist bronchodilators in asthma.*)

55. Stenius-Aarniala B, Poussa T, Kvarnstrom J, et al. Immediate and long term effects of weight reduction in obese people with asthma: randomised controlled study. BMJ 2000;320:827. (*Weight reduction in obese patients with asthma improves lung function, symptoms, morbidity, and health status.*)

56. Thoonen BP, Schermer TR, Van Den Boom G, et al. Self-management of asthma in general practice, asthma control and quality of life: a randomised controlled trial. Thorax 2003;58:30. (*Self-management lowers the burden of illness as perceived by patients with asthma.*)

CHAPTER 49 ■ MANAGEMENT OF TUBERCULOSIS

BENJAMIN T. DAVIS

The primary care physician most commonly encounters tuberculosis (TB) as a positive tuberculin skin test result in the absence of active infection. An estimated 7% of the U.S. population may fall into this category. However, the physician must remain vigilant for the signs and symptoms of active tuberculosis. The rapid diagnosis and treatment of TB may be impaired by several factors, including inadequate sensitivity of skin testing and sputum smears, a wide variety of clinical presentations, the several weeks required to obtain confirmatory cultures and antibiotic sensitivities, and the emergence of drug-resistant strains. There are two primary goals for the primary care physician caring for a patient with tuberculosis:

achieving safe and effective cure of the patient and minimizing the risk of transmission of tuberculosis to others. Consequently, collaboration with relevant departments of public health, clinical microbiology labs, and expert consultants when indicated is encouraged and expected.

PATHOPHYSIOLOGY AND EPIDEMIOLOGY (1–7)

Virtually all cases are acquired through *person-to-person aerosol* transmission of a nonmotile, acid-fast, gram-positive rod. People with active pulmonary infection shed infected droplets, which are then aerosolized into the environment. Because most infectious patients discharge relatively few organisms, casual contacts are at low risk for infection, and most secondary cases occur among household members, schoolmates, or other close contacts of the index case. TB is more common in immigrants and population groups in which crowding, poverty (especially homelessness), or a high risk for HIV infection is commonplace (see Chapter 38). Among HIV-infected patients, the risk for disease after infection is increased 1,000-fold. Serious outbreaks (with attack rates of 10%) have been reported among patients in hospital wards with a large concentration of AIDS patients.

Most persons harboring the tubercle bacillus mount an immune response sufficient to prevent progression from *primary infection* to clinical illness; they manifest a positive skin test result. About 5% of infected persons fail to contain the primary infection and progress to *active primary disease* within 2 years of initial infection. The proportion of infected persons who progress is much higher among AIDS patients. In the past, primary infection occurred almost entirely in childhood; however, as the epidemiology of tuberculosis has changed (see Chapter 38), primary tuberculosis is now also seen in adults, particularly among elderly nursing home residents and in patients coinfected with HIV.

Another 5% of infected patients (again, a higher proportion of AIDS patients) experience *reactivation of latent endogenous infection*, most often within 2 to 4 years of the initial infection or at times of lowered host resistance. However, reactivation can occur many decades after initial infection, as reported among elderly nursing home residents. More than one fifth of patients with reactivated disease have histories of inadequately treated clinical TB. In many instances, a discrete insult to host defenses, such as steroid therapy, alcoholism, malnutrition, neoplastic disease, HIV infection, or gastrectomy, can be implicated, but at times it is impossible to identify the reason for reactivation.

Until the advent of polymerase chain reaction technology and development of the techniques of molecular epidemiology, the vast majority of active TB cases in the United States were thought to represent reactivation of latent disease. Several recent studies, however, have suggested that in large metropolitan centers such as San Francisco and New York City, between 35% and 40% of active tuberculosis cases represent *newly acquired infection*. Although the AIDS epidemic accounts for some of this change in epidemiology, it is clear that clinical disease develops soon after infection in more immunologically "normal" persons than was previously thought.

CLINICAL PRESENTATION AND COURSE (1–3,5)

Primary Infection (1–2,5)

As noted, >90% of patients are entirely asymptomatic at the time of primary infection and can be identified only through conversion of the tuberculin skin test from negative to positive. The majority of these patients have normal findings on chest radiography. Among the 10% who progress directly to symptomatic disease, four broad syndromes can be identified: (a) *Atypical pneumonia* is the most common, characterized by fever and nonproductive cough. Chest x-ray films may show unilateral lower-lobe patchy parenchymal infiltrates or paratracheal or hilar adenopathy. Although such patients should receive full antituberculous chemotherapy when the disease is diagnosed (see later discussion), it usually resolves even without treatment. (b) *Tuberculous pleurisy* and effusion are accompanied by fever, cough, pleuritic chest pain, and occasionally dyspnea. Chest x-ray films reveal unilateral pleural effusions, often without identifiable parenchymal lesions. The tuberculin test result is almost always strongly positive. Diagnosis depends on examination and culture of the pleural fluid or on percutaneous needle biopsy of the pleura because sputum cultures are positive for organisms in only 30% of such cases. (c) *Direct progression* from primary disease to upper lobe involvement is another presentation. (d) Early *systemic dissemination*, which used to be seen exclusively in children, now occurs in HIV-infected patients.

Reactivation (Postprimary) Tuberculosis (1,2)

Notwithstanding our greater understanding of primary disease, this is still the most common clinical form of TB. Symptoms usually begin insidiously and progress during a period of many weeks or months before diagnosis. Constitutional symptoms are often prominent, including *anorexia, weight loss,* and *night sweats.* Most patients have *low-grade fever,* but higher temperatures and even chills may be seen occasionally when the disease progresses more rapidly. In addition, most patients present with pulmonary symptoms, including *cough* and *sputum production.* Dyspnea is relatively uncommon in the absence of underlying chronic lung disease. A frequent complaint is *hemoptysis,* often in the form of bright red streaks of blood caused by bronchial irritation. Although physical examination findings are usually nondiagnostic, chest x-ray films are highly suggestive of the diagnosis. Typical features include *infiltration* in the *posterior apical* pulmonary segments, which may be unilateral or bilateral and progresses to frank *cavitation.* Apical lordotic views and chest tomography may help to document cavitary disease. Occasionally, postprimary TB may involve the lower lung fields, and in rare instances the chest radiographic appearance may be normal. The tuberculin skin test result is positive in about 80% of patients with reactivation tuberculosis; patients with advanced disease are often malnourished and thus anergic.

Extrapulmonary Tuberculosis (1,3)

Approximately 20% of all newly recognized cases of TB in the United States are extrapulmonary. Although the frequency of pulmonary TB is constant, the incidence of extrapulmonary disease is increasing, largely among HIV-positive patients (see later discussion). Although the clinical features of extrapulmonary TB vary widely, certain generalizations are possible. Past history is not a reliable guide to the diagnosis. Only 25% of patients have a past history of TB; of these, virtually all have been inadequately treated. A long latent period between the first episode of infection and the extrapulmonary presentation is typical. Approximately 50% of patients with extrapulmonary disease have entirely normal chest radiographic findings; most of the others have stigmata of old, inactive pulmonary disease, and a minority have coexisting active pulmonary infection. Although extrapulmonary disease can involve all organ systems, either singly or in various combinations, the most commonly affected areas are the genitourinary tract, the musculoskeletal system, and the lymph nodes.

The most common type of extrapulmonary TB is infection of an individual organ system. The patient is most often afebrile and can be entirely free of constitutional complaints. The illness typically pursues an indolent course characterized by local organ dysfunction and eventual destruction rather than by progressive general decline. In fact, the clinical presentation in these persons more often suggests neoplastic disease than infection. The tuberculin skin test result is almost always positive. Clinical syndromes in this category include genitourinary tuberculosis, tuberculous arthritis and osteomyelitis, tuberculous lymphadenitis, and many others.

HIV-positive patients with TB may experience extrapulmonary disease and dissemination early on. When CD4 cell counts are well preserved (see Chapter 13), tuberculous infection usually causes pulmonary disease that resembles TB in HIV-negative persons. However, in more severely immunocompromised HIV patients, TB is often disseminated at presentation. A high incidence of tuberculous *meningitis* has been reported among HIV-positive patients, often in conjunction with *diffuse lymphadenopathy*. The occurrence of pulmonary or extrapulmonary TB in patients with HIV infection fulfills the criteria for the diagnosis of AIDS.

In HIV-infected patients with disseminated disease, the result of the purified protein derivative skin test is often negative. Chest radiographic findings are normal in >10% of patients. When infiltrates do occur, they are often nonspecific and involve the lower lobes. Despite these atypical features, the diagnosis can usually be established, if suspected, without much difficulty by visualizing or culturing the causative organism from the sputum or extrapulmonary sites.

DIAGNOSIS (1,8)

The tuberculin *skin test* is the most sensitive test for the diagnosis of infection with *Mycobacterium tuberculosis* (see Chapter 38); it is far more sensitive than chest radiography. A positive tuberculin test result does not by itself prove the presence of active disease, but it does indicate that infection has occurred. Negative tuberculin reactions have been documented in 20% of patients with TB, particularly those with overwhelming or advanced disease, malnutrition, and debility. In HIV-positive patients, especially those with low CD4 cell counts, the rate of false-negative skin test results has been as high as 50%. When active pulmonary disease is present, the diagnosis of pulmonary TB can usually be confirmed by examination of the *sputum*, with precautions taken to *avoid the spread of organisms during efforts to obtain sputum*. If patients are not able to produce sputum spontaneously, attempts should be made to *induce sputum* with the aid of hydration, pulmonary physiotherapy, intermittent positive-pressure breathing, and mucolytic agents. *Bronchoscopy* or *bronchoalveolar lavage* may be necessary for obtaining appropriate specimens. Although *cultures* are necessary for a positive diagnosis and are more sensitive than smears, sputum specimens should be examined microscopically either by the traditional *Ziehl–Neelsen (acid-fast) stain* or by the newer Truant *fluorescent stain*. Sputum or bronchoscopic washings should be examined both directly and after concentration by centrifugation and digestion. Carefully collected individual specimens are preferred to a 24-hour pool of sputum and saliva. Cultures of first morning–fasting *gastric aspirates* may also be helpful in children. Because gastric acid is toxic to mycobacteria, the collection bottles should contain a buffer such as sodium bicarbonate. Smears of gastric juice are misleading because of the potential presence of saprophytic mycobacteria, and they should not be performed.

Tissue biopsy is often required for the diagnosis of tuberculous pleurisy or extrapulmonary disease. *Whole-blood in-*

terferon γ-essay has shown high sensitivity and specificity in persons with active T.B., and lesser sensitivity in persons with latent T.B.

PRINCIPLES OF TREATMENT (1,9–21)

Prophylaxis in Uninfected Persons (16,21)

In many parts of the world where tuberculosis is common, bacille Calmette-Guérin (BCG) vaccine is used for the prevention of primary infection. It is intended only for prophylaxis and should not be given to patients with positive skin test results (see Chapter 38). Because the incidence of tuberculosis is relatively low in the United States, BCG vaccination is not recommended in this country. All close contacts of patients with active pulmonary tuberculosis should be considered for *isoniazid* (INH) chemoprophylaxis, particularly if they are children, adolescents, or immunocompromised adults (see Chapter 38).

Prophylaxis in Tuberculin Converters and Persons with Latent Disease (16,21)

Prevention of active TB can be achieved with INH (see Chapter 38 for detailed guidelines). Patients with a positive skin test result should be evaluated to exclude active infection. One needs to check for cough, fever, sputum production, pleuritic chest pain, lymphadenopathy, meningeal irritation, pleural effusion, pulmonary consolidation, and enlargement of the liver or spleen. Chest radiography is essential, and the results of complete blood cell count, differential, urinalysis, and liver function tests (particularly measurement of alkaline phosphatase) may provide clues of active disease (e.g., "sterile" pyuria or isolated elevation of alkaline phosphatase). If no active infection is identified, the patient should be reassured, and the potential risks and benefits of INH therapy should be explained so the patient can participate in therapeutic decisions.

Treatment of Patients with Active Tuberculosis (9–15,17,21)

Antituberculous drugs are the cornerstone of therapy. Because the patient will not be contagious shortly after starting therapy, most treatment can be administered on an outpatient basis after a brief period in the hospital. The chemotherapy of tuberculosis is different from other antimicrobial programs and proceeds according to a unique set of principles:

- Multidrug regimens and completion of a full course of therapy are necessary to prevent the emergence of drug-resistant organisms.
- Single daily dosing is preferred.
- Prolonged chemotherapy is necessary. Nearly all patients can be cured with regimens lasting 6 months. However, HIV-infected persons may require longer treatment. When INH and rifampin cannot be used simultaneously because of patient intolerance or drug resistance, older, more prolonged regimens of 18 to 24 months are necessary.
- Directly observed therapy (DOT) given twice or thrice weekly should be considered for all new patients.
- No matter what regimen is chosen, it is important to follow patients closely to ensure compliance and monitor for drug efficacy and toxicity.

- Because chemotherapy will control the organisms, surgery is reserved for the treatment of complications, such as restrictive pericardial scarring.
- Elaborate programs of rest and diet have no place in the modern treatment of tuberculosis.
- Prolonged surveillance beyond 1 year after completion of a full course of therapy is generally not necessary because of the efficacy of current chemotherapeutic regimens; however, immunosuppressed patients and those with drug-resistant organisms require more prolonged follow-up.

As little as 2 weeks of multidrug therapy will greatly decrease the infectiousness of patients with tuberculosis, although a few mycobacteria may still be present on sputum smears or cultures. The decision of whether to hospitalize patients with newly diagnosed TB should take into account the clinical status of the patient in addition to the health and ages of other people living at home. Certainly, the presence at home of children (especially infants), pregnant women, or persons infected with HIV or having debilitating medical conditions should prompt hospitalization until the index patient can be reliably considered noninfectious. Patients with extrapulmonary tuberculosis are much less infectious and can sometimes be managed entirely as outpatients.

Antituberculous Chemotherapeutic Agents

Isoniazid.

Introduced into clinical use in the early 1950s, INH remains the most important antituberculous drug. Of importance is the excellent tissue penetration of this small, water-soluble molecule. The distribution of INH includes the central nervous system, tuberculous abscesses, and intracellular sites. The major metabolism of INH is by hepatic acetylation. Although metabolites are excreted by the kidneys, it is not necessary to modify INH doses except in cases of advanced renal failure. INH is available both orally and parenterally. The usual dose is 5 mg/kg of body weight, not to exceed 300 mg/d for an adult.

The major adverse effects of INH include the following:

- *Neurotoxicity*, ranging from peripheral neuropathy (which can be prevented by administration of 50 mg of pyridoxine daily) to much less common manifestations, including encephalopathy, seizures, optic neuritis, and personality changes.
- *Hypersensitivity* reactions, including fever, rash, and rheumatic syndromes with or without the presence of antinuclear antibodies.
- *Hepatocellular injury*, including serious clinical hepatitis in <2% of cases, but a transient, clinically insignificant rise in transaminase levels in 10% to 20%. The risk for clinically significant hepatitis increases with age.

The U.S. Public Health Service does not recommend routine *transaminase* (aspartate aminotransferase and alanine aminotransferase) determinations in persons who are reliable and able to comply with directions for reporting symptoms of hepatitis. If transaminases are elevated before therapy is begun, however, it is prudent to monitor them at monthly intervals.

In symptomatic patients with an elevated transaminase, INH should be discontinued and liver function should be monitored. In asymptomatic persons with a mild elevation (up to 2.5 times normal), the drug can be continued, but the patient should be monitored weekly. If the transaminase level fails to return to normal in 3 to 4 weeks, it seems prudent to discontinue the INH. On the other hand, even if a patient is asymptomatic, a single, more substantial transaminase elevation may be grounds for discontinuing the agent. Again, it must be emphasized that these are rules of thumb rather than precise guidelines. INH treatment may be resumed cautiously in patients for whom it was stopped, with careful monitoring.

Rifampin

Rifampin is a major antituberculous drug and rivals INH in efficacy. Rifampin is a large, fat-soluble molecule that achieves excellent tissue penetration, including the central nervous system. The drug is excreted by the liver; modification of dose is not required in renal failure, but may be necessary in hepatic insufficiency. It is available in both oral and parenteral formulations. The average adult dose is 600 mg/d taken once daily. Patients should be cautioned to expect *orange discoloration of urine, sweat, tears,* and *saliva,* which is of no clinical significance.

Toxicities include *hypersensitivity* reactions (fever, rash, eosinophilia), *hematologic* toxicities (thrombocytopenia, leukopenia, hemolytic anemia), and *hepatitis* (including elevated transaminases in up to 10% of cases). Drug interactions occur; rifampin increases the metabolism of warfarin, quinidine, oral contraceptives, and methadone. Rifampin should not be used in high-dose intermittent therapy because toxic reactions (including hemolytic anemia, thrombocytopenia, and hepatic failure) occur frequently. However, intermittent therapy in doses of 600 mg given twice weekly appears to be well tolerated.

Pyrazinamide

Pyrazinamide, a derivative of nicotinic acid, was introduced in 1952 but was not widely used until its incorporation into short-course regimens in the 1980s. Like INH and rifampin, it is bactericidal, a major asset in short-course therapy. The drug is well absorbed from the gastrointestinal tract and is widely distributed in body tissues and fluids, including the cerebrospinal fluid. It is excreted by mixed hepatic and renal mechanisms. Major toxicities are hepatic dysfunction, hyperuricemia, and hypersensitivity. The usual dose is 15 to 30 mg/kg daily (maximum, 2 g).

Ethambutol

Ethambutol was introduced clinically in the United States in 1967 and represented a major advance in antituberculous chemotherapy. Although ethambutol penetrates tissues well—including the central nervous system when the meninges are inflamed—it is not bactericidal; it is only bacteriostatic. The drug is excreted by the kidneys. Dose modification in renal failure should be based on serum ethambutol levels (available through the manufacturer), and patients with renal failure who require the drug should be monitored. The major toxicities of ethambutol include hypersensitivity reactions, such as fever and rash, and optic neuritis, which is dose related and usually manifested first by a loss of color vision. Less common side effects include neuritis, gastrointestinal intolerance, headache, and hyperuricemia. The usual dose is 15 mg/kg daily; 25 mg/kg may be given daily for the first 2 months. Color vision and visual acuity should be monitored periodically because of a small risk for retinal injury; for this reason, the drug is usually not administered to young children.

Streptomycin

Streptomycin, the first effective antituberculous drug, remains useful. Like other aminoglycosides, streptomycin has only a fair tissue distribution, being inactive at an alkaline pH in an anaerobic milieu and penetrating the cerebrospinal fluid very poorly. It must be given parenterally. Streptomycin is excreted by the kidneys, and the dose should be reduced in patients with renal failure. Major toxicities include hypersensitivity reactions and *toxicity of the eighth nerve*, especially the vestibular division, which results in vertigo. The dose of streptomycin is 15 mg/kg, up to 1 g daily.

"Second-Line" Antituberculous Drugs

"Second-line" antituberculous drugs tend to be both less effective and more toxic than the standard agents, but occasionally they are of critical importance in patients with drug-resistant tuberculosis and in those who cannot tolerate the standard therapies. These drugs are cycloserine, ethionamide, amikacin, capreomycin, *para*-aminosalicylic acid, levofloxacin, moxifloxacin, and gatifloxacin.

Ensuring Adherence (18,20)

Poor adherence is the most important cause of treatment failure and the emergence of multidrug-resistant strains. Conversion to negative cultures takes four times longer in nonadherent patients; their risk for acquiring drug-resistant disease is five times greater, and the treatment time needed to achieve cure is nearly twice as long. However, adherence is a notoriously difficult thing to predict in an individual patient. Probably the most reliable predictors of poor adherence are prior poor adherence, adolescence, and heavy alcohol or intravenous drug use. Socioeconomic status, race, and ethnicity should not be used to predict adherence.

DOT coupled with a free supply of the necessary drugs appears to be one of the most successful adherence strategies for persons with active tuberculosis. The wide use of DOT has been a cornerstone of public health measures for tuberculosis control since the 1990s and has undeniably contributed to the reversal of the rising incidence in active disease seen in the 1980s. *DOT should be considered initially for all patients with newly diagnosed TB.*

CASE REPORTING AND PATIENT EDUCATION (21)

All cases of tuberculosis should be reported promptly to public health authorities so that contacts can be investigated and appropriate control measures instituted. However, it must be remembered that, particularly in elderly patients, the diagnosis of tuberculosis still carries a social stigma and dire prognostic implications. Reassurance and education are therefore of great importance. It should be stressed that tuberculosis occurs in all social and economic classes, that modern chemotherapy is truly curative, and that prolonged periods of hospitalization and isolation are no longer necessary.

Patients who are candidates for INH prophylaxis should understand the risks and benefits of INH therapy. If INH therapy is recommended and accepted, the patient should be instructed to discontinue the medication and report to the physician if adverse effects are noted, including skin rash, fever, fatigue, anorexia, abdominal distress, jaundice, and peripheral neuropathic symptoms. The importance of full compliance with the drug regimen, whether for prophylaxis or treatment of active disease, must be stressed.

THERAPEUTIC RECOMMENDATIONS (21)

Prophylaxis

- For more information, see Chapter 38.
- In the decision to use INH for prophylaxis, the risk for drug-induced hepatotoxicity (see next section, Antituberculous Chemotherapeutic Agents) must be weighed against the benefit of preventing active disease. The older the patient, the greater is the risk for hepatitis, although the benefit usually outweighs risk, especially in populations with a high incidence of infection and active disease (see Chapter 38 for detailed guidelines).
- Prompt diagnosis and institution of an effective, individualized treatment program are essential to preventing the spread of disease and emergence of resistant organisms. Of particular importance is the early recognition of TB in HIV-infected patients. A high index of suspicion and an awareness of the potentially atypical presentations of TB in these patients (e.g., disseminated disease, meningitis) are essential.

Active Disease

- Patients with active pulmonary or extrapulmonary tuberculosis should be treated for 2 months with INH, rifampin, and pyrazinamide, followed by INH and rifampin for 4 months, for a total duration of treatment of 6 months.
- Because nearly all centers in the United States currently report >4% resistance to one of the foregoing drugs and because of the now-recognized importance of newly acquired infection, ethambutol (or streptomycin) should be included in the initial regimen until the results of drug susceptibility tests are known, at which time it can be stopped if the presence of a sensitive organism is confirmed.
- The foregoing treatment regimen applies to patients with or without HIV infection. However, because relapse rates are higher in HIV-infected patients, careful clinical follow-up should be the rule. Many authorities advocate continuing INH and rifampin for 6 months following sputum conversion.
- If INH and rifampin cannot be administered simultaneously because of patient intolerance or drug resistance, multiple drug therapy should be continued for 18 to 24 months. Such patients should be referred to an infectious disease specialist or to the local public health authority for optimal management. For patients relapsing after a previous course of antituberculous chemotherapy or for patients in whom more widespread drug resistance is suspected, the initial therapy may involve six or more drugs and should be coordinated by an infectious disease specialist or public health authority.
- DOT should be considered initially for *all* patients in whom active TB is diagnosed. Twice- and thrice-weekly regimens have established efficacy when given as part of DOT.
- For use in *pregnancy*, INH, rifampin, and ethambutol all appear to be safe.
- After completion of therapy, all patients should be followed for 1 year, with monitoring for evidence of recurrence. Longer follow-up is appropriate for those with drug-resistant organisms, HIV infection, or poor adherence.
- *Hospitalization* should be considered in the *initial stages of active pulmonary disease* to minimize the risk for spread. Chemotherapy for 2 weeks usually suffices to render the patient noninfectious.

Annotated Bibliography

1. Frieden TR, Sterling TR, Munsiff SS, et al. Tuberculosis. Lancet 2003;362:887. (*Comprehensive review; 166 references.*)
2. Stead WW. Pathogenesis of the sporadic case of tuberculosis. N Engl J Med 1967;277:1008. (*Lucid and important overview of the "unitary concept" of the pathogenesis of tuberculosis [TB]; this excellent article clarifies the relationships among primary infection, inactive disease, and reactivated tuberculosis.*)
3. Berenguer J, Moreno S, Laguna F, et al. Tuberculous meningitis in patients infected with the human immunodeficiency virus. N Engl J Med 1992;326:668. (*HIV-infected patients are at increased risk for TB meningitis.*)
4. Frieden TR, Sterling T, Pablos-Mendez A, et al. Emergence of drug-resistant tuberculosis in New York City. N Engl J Med 1993;328:521. (*High prevalence was found among HIV-positive persons, intravenous drug abusers, and patients previously treated.*)
5. Stead WW, Kerby GR, Schlueter DP, et al. The clinical spectrum of primary tuberculosis in adults. Ann Intern Med 1968;68:73. (*Classic clinical study of primary TB, which includes an excellent summary of the wide spectrum of events that may occur after initial infection by Mycobacterium tuberculosis.*)
6. Stead WW, Lofgren JP, Warren E, et al. Tuberculosis as an endemic and nosocomial infection among the elderly in nursing homes. N Engl J Med 1985;312:1483. (*Exogenous infection can occur in the elderly, and nosocomial TB may be an important problem in nursing homes.*)
7. Horsburgh CR. *Mycobacterium avium* complex infection in the acquired immunodeficiency syndrome. N Engl J Med 1991;324:1332. (*Review of this important opportunistic mycobacterial infection in AIDS patients.*)
8. Kang WA, Lee HW, Yoon HI, et al. Descrepancy between tuberculosis skin tests and γ diagnosis of latent tuberculous infection. JAMA 2005;293:2756. (*Data on new testing modality.*)
9. Cohn DL, Catlin BJ, Peterson KL, et al. A 62-dose, 6-month therapy for pulmonary and extrapulmonary tuberculosis: a twice-weekly, directly observed, and cost-effective regimen. Ann Intern Med 1990;112:407. (*Demonstrates the efficacy of a strategy for poorly compliant patients.*)
10. Combs DL, O'Brien RJ, Geiter LJ. USPHS tuberculosis short-course chemotherapy trial 21: effectiveness, toxicity, and acceptability. Ann Intern Med 1990;112:397. (*Outcome measures for a 6-month regimen of isoniazid [INH] and rifampin plus pyrazinamide during the first 8 weeks were similar to those for a 9-month regimen of only INH and rifampin.*)
11. Dooley SW, Jarvis WR, Martone WJ, et al. Multidrug-resistant tuberculosis. Ann Intern Med 1992;117:3. (*Editorial summing up current knowledge of this serious condition and approaches to coping with it.*)
12. Gelband H. Regimens of less than six months for treating tuberculosis (Cochrane review). In: The Cochrane library, Issue 3. Oxford: Update Software, 2004. (*Longer periods of treatment [at least up to 6 months] result in higher success rates in patients with active TB, but the differences are small.*)
13. Goble M, Iseman MD, Madsen LA, et al. Treatment of 171 patients with pulmonary tuberculosis resistant to isoniazid and rifampin. N Engl J Med 1993;328:527. (*The overall response rate was only about 50%; the risk was proportional to the number of drugs received before current therapy.*)
14. Mukherjee JS, Rich ML, Socci AR, et al. Programmes and principles in treatment of multi-drug resistant tuberculosis. Lancet 2004;363:474. (*Further clinical and operational research is urgently needed to guide clinicians in the management of this disease.*)
15. Small PM, Schecter GF, Goodman PC, et al. Treatment of tuberculosis in patients with advanced human immunodeficiency virus infection. N Engl J Med 1991;324:289. (*Conventional therapy was effective in sterilizing the sputum, improving the chest radiographic pattern, and preventing relapse.*)
16. Stead WW, To T, Harrison RW, et al. Benefit–risk considerations in preventive treatment for tuberculosis in elderly persons. Ann Intern Med 1987;107:843. (*INH treatment of nursing home patients who had definite skin test conversions was beneficial, and benefits outweighed the risk for hepatitis.*)
17. Sterling TR, Alwood K, Gachuhi R, et al. Relapse rate after short-course (6-month) treatment of tuberculosis in HIV-infected and uninfected persons. AIDS 1999;13:1899. (*The relapse rate of 6.4% in HIV-infected persons was the same as that in HIV-seronegative persons.*)
18. Volmink J, Garner P. Directly observed therapy for treating tuberculosis (Cochrane review). In: The Cochrane library, Issue 3. Oxford: Update Software, 2004. (*Effects of direct observation on cure or treatment completion were similar to those of self-administered treatment.*)
19. Woldehanna S, Volmink J. Treatment of latent tuberculosis infection in HIV infected persons (Cochrane review). In: The Cochrane library, Issue 3. Oxford: Update Software, 2004. (*Treatment of latent tuberculosis infection reduces the risk of active tuberculosis in HIV-positive individuals with a positive tuberculin skin test.*)
20. Pablos-Mendez, Knirsch CA, Barr RG, et al. Nonadherence in tuberculosis: predictors and consequences in New York City. Am J Med 1997;102:164. (*One of the best epidemiologic studies; intravenous drug abuse and homelessness accounted for about 60% of cases of poor compliance, defined as >2 months of failure to take prescribed medications; nonadherence was associated with a fourfold increase in time required to convert to negative culture, a fivefold increase in risk for drug resistance, nearly a doubling of treatment time required to achieve cure, and twice the likelihood of failure to complete treatment.*)
21. American Thoracic Society/Centers for Disease Control and Prevention/Infectious Diseases Society of America. Treatment of tuberculosis. Am J Respir Crit Care Med 2003;167:603. (*Current standards for the treatment of tuberculosis.*)

CHAPTER 50 ■ MANAGEMENT OF THE COMMON COLD

WILLIAM A. KORMOS

The term *common cold* describes a self-limited catarrhal illness caused by a variety of respiratory viruses. It is indeed a common problem, with adults averaging two to four colds per year and with almost 7 days lost from work per person per year. Although most patients treat their symptoms at home, physicians are still frequently consulted for upper respiratory infections. The primary task for the physician is to distinguish the common cold from bacterial infections, allergic conditions, and epidemic diseases such as influenza. Once the common cold is diagnosed, reassurance about the self-limited nature of the disease and patient education about its predominantly viral cause is the next step. However, upper respiratory tract infections continue to be a great source of inappropriate use of antibiotics. A recent survey demonstrated that physicians prescribe antibiotics to half of patients labeled as having "colds." Instead, physicians should be knowledgeable about symptomatic therapies, including over-the-counter remedies. A targeted treatment plan aimed at the predominant symptoms is not only more effective, but also more responsible.

PATHOPHYSIOLOGY AND CLINICAL PRESENTATION (1–5)

The oropharynx and nasopharynx are lined by a stratified squamous epithelium and are normally teeming with a varied microbial flora. In addition, many potentially pathogenic bacteria can temporarily reside on these epithelial surfaces as "colonizers" without causing true infection. With a few exceptions, such as herpes simplex virus and Epstein–Barr virus, viruses are not usually long-term members of the normal flora of the respiratory tract.

Numerous host defenses protect the upper airway from infection. The first of these defenses are mechanical; particulate matter is expelled by the cough and sneeze reflexes, entrapped by viscous mucous secretions, and propelled outward by ciliary action. In addition, local immunologic defenses attempt to deal with organisms that have breached the mechanical barriers. These defenses include lymphoid tissue, respiratory secretions that contain immunoglobulin A antibodies, and a rich vasculature capable of rapidly delivering phagocytic leukocytes. Once in the nasal cavity, viruses gain access to the upper airway by binding to the intercellular adhesion molecule ICAM-1. Experimental trials are being conducted in which soluble ICAM-1 is used to block this step in the initiation of infection.

Mechanisms of transmission include *airborne transmission* of virus-laden respiratory secretions via small, aerosolized particles that remain suspended or large particles that travel only a few feet. However, the most efficient means of transmission is *direct mucous membrane contact* with virus, usually on contaminated hands. Self-inoculation of viruses surviving on the hands is accomplished by touching one's nose or eyes. Children are an important reservoir of these viruses. The timeless motherly warning that "you'll catch cold if you get wet or damp" has not been borne out by experimental studies, which have demonstrated equal susceptibility in chilled and nonchilled hosts. However, evidence from prospective, controlled studies suggests that *psychological stress*, especially chronic life stresses and poor social supports, can increase the risk for infection.

The common cold is caused by viral agents, mostly from five major families of viruses. *Rhinoviruses* are the most common viral agents associated with upper respiratory tract illness. Because there are more than 110 antigenic serotypes, cross-immunity does not exist, and reinfection with another serotype right after a recent cold is common. Coronavirus, parainfluenza virus, coxsackievirus, and respiratory syncytial virus account for the rest of the etiologic agents. *Influenza A* and *influenza B* produce a more severe syndrome, which overlaps with the common cold. Influenza infection typically occurs in the winter months (December to March) in the Northern Hemisphere. The clinical syndrome consists of fever and diffuse myalgia, often accompanied by a nonproductive cough and headache. Lack of fever significantly decreases the probability of influenza. Patients with underlying cardiopulmonary disease and the elderly are at a higher risk for the development of a secondary bacterial pneumonia following influenza infection.

Incubation periods for viral upper respiratory infections range from 1 to 5 days; virus shedding lasts up to 3 weeks. Typi-

cal symptoms include coryza, pharyngitis, laryngitis, headache, malaise, and fever, in various combinations. Experimental evidence suggests that these symptoms are more the results of the body's response to the infection (through mediators like bradykinin, prostaglandin, interleukin, and histamine) than the viral infection itself. Ear and sinus discomfort also are often present, frequently caused by mucosal edema that impairs drainage (see Chapters 218 and 219).

Whether known as the common cold, nasopharyngitis, or upper respiratory infection, these problems generally resolve spontaneously. Common viral upper respiratory infections rarely progress to pneumonia; most colds resolve spontaneously within 1 week, although symptoms may linger up to 2 weeks in one fourth of patients.

DIAGNOSIS (1)

The diagnosis of the "common cold" remains a clinical one, based on the typical presentation. Patients should be examined for localized bacterial infection, such as otitis media, sinusitis, or streptococcal pharyngitis (see Chapters 218 through 220). If the patient presents with symptoms typical of influenza, further diagnostic testing can be considered with *rapid testing*, in which antibodies to common influenza antigens are usually used. The sensitivity of these tests appears to be high and is even higher if nasopharyngeal washings rather than a swab are sent. Documentation of influenza has therapeutic implications and is useful for tracking the epidemiology of seasonal influenza infection. On the other hand, identification of the specific virus causing the "common cold" is neither practical nor important.

PRINCIPLES OF MANAGEMENT

Prevention (6–8)

The best things one can do to avoid "catching" a cold are to avoid aerosol exposure, wash hands, and keep hands away from mucous membranes (conjunctivae, nasal and oral mucosae). Gargling with "antiseptic" mouthwash is of no benefit. The use of "antibacterial soap" (compared with standard soap) showed no benefit in reducing viral diseases in a recent trial of urban families. The enthusiasm surrounding the use of high-dose vitamin C (ascorbic acid) for prophylaxis has waned as controlled studies have failed to demonstrate efficacy. Similarly, zinc lozenges and *Echinacea* extracts have proved no better for prevention than placebo in controlled trials.

Symptomatic Relief (1,6,8–21)

Therapeutic efforts are directed toward relieving nasal congestion, sneezing, rhinorrhea, headache, and grippe-like symptoms and preventing complications such as otitis, sinusitis, and lower respiratory tract infection. Targeted therapy aimed at the most bothersome symptoms is preferred to all-inclusive cold remedies, which often contain irrational mixtures or subtherapeutic doses of active ingredients. Sympathomimetics remain the mainstay of decongestant therapy. Data suggesting a cholinergic pathophysiology for rhinorrhea and sneezing have stimulated interest in new forms of anticholinergic therapy.

Decongestants

Decongestants can be helpful, not only for providing symptomatic relief, but also for preventing sinus and eustachian tube obstruction that can result in sinusitis and otitis media, respectively.

α-Adrenergic Agents. α-Adrenergic agents are the most commonly used decongestants. They work by causing generalized vasoconstriction, thereby reducing the formation of secretions. Because they produce systemic vasoconstriction, sympathomimetics may raise blood pressure when used in doses sufficient to alleviate nasal congestion. No oral adrenergic agent provides selective local vasoconstriction; sympathomimetic nasal sprays (e.g., Afrin) are more effective for this purpose but may be associated with rebound congestion after as little as 3 days of continuous use, leading to difficulty in discontinuing use and an increased risk of chronic abuse. According to most authorities, sympathomimetic nasal sprays are good for very short-term therapy, whereas oral preparations are better when treatment is to continue for longer than 3 to 4 days.

Anticholinergic Agents. Anticholinergic agents have been used for years in the treatment of the common cold, mostly in the form of over-the-counter *sedating first-generation antihistamines*, which exert an atropine-like drying effect. It is this effect, not antihistaminic activity, that probably accounts for the symptomatic usefulness of anticholinergics in patients bothered by profuse rhinorrhea and excessive sneezing. However, their marked drying effect can exacerbate symptoms of congestion and cause upper airway obstruction by impairing the flow of mucus. In addition, they cause drowsiness, a side effect that may impair daytime functioning, although it can provide some nighttime rest. These agents can also worsen symptomatic benign prostatic hyperplasia and glaucoma and should be avoided by patients with these conditions. Use of *second-generation, nonsedating antihistamines* is irrational and has *no place* in management of the common cold because these agents have little anticholinergic activity. Nonetheless, antihistamines continue to be widely consumed for use in colds, usually in combination with a sympathomimetic and other substances (see later discussion).

Ipratropium. Ipratropium, a topically active anticholinergic agent now available in a nasal spray preparation (0.6% twice daily), has been promoted for relief of nasal symptoms of the common cold. In a placebo-controlled, double-blind, randomized trial, the nasal spray preparation provided a significant reduction in subjective and objective measures of rhinorrhea and sneezing in comparison with saline placebo spray and with no treatment. Of note, significant benefit was also found with use of the saline control spray in comparison with no treatment. Global ratings by patients for overall effectiveness followed a similar pattern. Observed side effects included increased nasal dryness and blood-tinged mucus in approximately 10% to 15% of subjects. No cases of sinusitis or marked nasal obstruction were reported, which suggests that short-term use of the spray (up to 5 days) might be reasonably well tolerated.

Analgesics

Analgesics are useful for relief of the headache, fever, and aches that often accompany a cold. *Aspirin* and *acetaminophen* have similar analgesic and antipyretic effects and are key ingredients in the combination cold remedies. However, both have been found to be capable of delaying the immune response to experimental rhinovirus infection, although neither prolongs viral shedding. Nonprescription doses of *ibuprofen* showed similar effects, but prescription doses of *naproxen* did not alter viral shedding or antibody response in one trial. Salicylate derivatives such as salicylamide are sometimes used, although they are much less effective than aspirin. Due to its association with Reye's syndrome, aspirin should not be used for viral illnesses in children, but its use appears to be safe in adults.

Expectorants and Heated Humidification

Expectorants are included in many preparations in the belief that they stimulate the flow of mucus. There is no evidence to support this view, although these agents are widely prescribed and requested by patients. More important is adequate *hydration*, which helps loosen secretions and prevent upper airway obstruction and the complications that may ensue. *Warm fluids* (including tea and, yes, chicken soup) can increase the rate of mucous flow, providing some symptomatic relief, as can *inhaled steam* (another of grandmother's remedies) or the use of a dilute saline nasal spray.

Research suggesting that increasing the nasal mucosal temperature to 37°C could limit viral replication and decrease nasal congestion led to a renewed interest in the inhalation of warm, humidified air. A double-blinded study of steam inhalation through an *active device* showed *no significant benefit* over placebo therapy, although both were associated with considerable subjective improvement. Expensive heated nebulizer devices (such as "the Viralizer" and "Rhinotherm") have been heavily promoted as a means of promptly and completely relieving cold symptoms. Controlled studies have failed to confirm such excessive claims.

Cough Suppressants

Cough is often the presenting symptom that prompts the patient to seek medical care. However, trials of cough suppressants in the common cold have shown minimal benefit. Cough suppressants, such as *dextromethorphan*, appear to have some effect in reducing cough frequency and may help the patient to sleep uninterrupted by cough. Cough suppressants are commonly available in combination with expectorants, although they may be prescribed alone, which is more sensible therapy. Dextromethorphan is contraindicated in patients taking monoamine oxidase inhibitors, and it may cause serotonin syndrome (hypertension, hyperthermia, mental status changes) in patients using selective serotonin reuptake inhibitors. Although narcotic preparations are more potent cough suppressants, two trials of codeine preparations showed no significant benefit in the common cold. Hydrocodone has not been tested in this condition.

Zinc

Zinc is believed to inhibit viral attachment and replication and improve cellular immune function. Such effects have stimulated interest in its use as a treatment for the common cold. The results of well-designed, controlled studies using zinc gluconate lozenges have been equally divided between showing efficacy and showing no benefit. In the studies with positive findings, adequate blinding has been questioned because zinc lozenges have a distinct taste that may alert study subjects to their allotted treatment. The studies with negative findings have been criticized for subtherapeutic doses or ineffective preparations. One highly publicized study of 100 patients recruited from hospital employees demonstrated a significant reduction (nearly 40%) in the duration of illness and also in the duration of coughing, nasal drainage and congestion, hoarseness, headache, and sore throat. The lozenges in this study contained 13.3 mg of zinc, and patients were instructed to take them every 2 hours while awake (average of six per day). Side effects included nausea and a bad taste in the mouth, experienced by most of the patients. A second study of 50 patients demonstrated a similar reduction in cold symptoms (mean duration 8.1 vs. 4.5 days). Patients may be informed of the possible benefit of zinc lozenges but should be warned about the likely side effects (nausea, taste disturbance.) In addition, case reports have associated the use of intranasal zinc gel with the development of anosmia, so this particular zinc preparation should be avoided.

Echinacea

Extracts from plants of the genus *Echinacea* have gained widespread acceptance in Germany as a treatment for the common cold. These plant products are postulated to have immunomodulator activity, such as macrophage activation and interleukin production. Although many randomized trials have suggested a benefit in the reduction of symptoms, the interpretation of results is complicated by the variety of species used (*E. purpurea*, *E. pallida*, and *E. angustifolia*) and the different plant parts (root or herb) and formulations (tablets, liquid extracts, capsules). Two double-blinded, randomized, controlled trials conducted in the United States (enrolling >100 patients each) failed to show a reduction in the duration or severity of upper respiratory illnesses. In view of these negative trials and the lack of standardized herbal preparations, *Echinacea* should not be recommended for treatment of the common cold.

Other Agents and Combination Preparations

Americans spend nearly 1 billion dollars annually on over-the-counter cold remedies. Most contain a combination of ingredients, including first-generation sedating antihistamines, sympathomimetic amines, and analgesics. Some even contain more than one antihistamine or sympathomimetic. *Antitussives, atropine, caffeine, vitamin C, belladonna alkaloids,* and expectorants are other common additives. *Antacids, laxatives, quinine,* and *papaverine* are found occasionally. In general, these combination preparations should not be recommended as first-line therapy. As noted, the vitamin C included has not been shown to have any significant effect, even when given in gram doses.

Management of Influenza (22–24)

If the diagnosis of influenza is confirmed or highly suspected, several medications may be useful in decreasing the duration of symptoms if administered within the first 48 hours of the illness. Previously, *amantadine* and *rimantadine* were recommended as first-line therapy, although these agents were only active against influenza A. However, increasing resistance to these agents has occurred over the last decade, and in the 2005 to 2006 influenza season, the routine use of these agents was abandoned.

Neuraminidase Inhibitors

The *neuraminidase inhibitors zanamivir* and *oseltamivir* are newer agents for the treatment of influenza. These drugs are sialic acid analogues that inhibit the viral neuraminidase enzyme, which is essential to replication for both influenza A and influenza B. Early randomized trials of these agents showed a decrease in the duration of illness of 1 to 1.5 days if the drug is administered within 48 hours of symptom onset, similar to the effect seen with the older agents. Zanamivir is administered by an inhaler twice daily; oseltamivir is given as a pill (75 mg) twice daily. The advantage of these newer agents is their activity against both influenza A and influenza B; the development of resistance has been documented but is of uncertain clinical significance. In addition, because the average cost of these agents is at least 10 times greater than that of influenza vaccine, vaccination is clearly the more cost-effective method for avoiding flu symptoms.

PATIENT EDUCATION (25–27)

Among the most frustrating experiences in primary care practice is the request for *antibiotics* by patients suffering from a cold. Explaining that antibiotics have no role in an uncomplicated viral upper respiratory infection can be time-consuming at best and has the potential to develop into a power struggle. A proactive approach is to send educational materials to patients at the beginning of the upper respiratory infection season. Pamphlets and other informational materials are much appreciated by patients and can help cut down on unnecessary visits and telephone calls. They should include helpful hints at self-care and the indications for seeking medical attention (e.g., high fever; marked pain or tenderness in an ear or sinus; increasingly purulent sputum; dyspnea; pleuritic chest pain). The role of antibiotics in the treatment of viral upper respiratory infection should also be reviewed (i.e., only for complications such as otitis and sinusitis), in addition to the risks of unnecessary antibiotic therapy (e.g., allergic reactions, alteration of bacterial flora, emergence of resistant strains). Unnecessary office visits and telephone calls have been reduced by as much as 30% to 40% through well-designed educational efforts.

THERAPEUTIC RECOMMENDATIONS

Prevention is difficult, but *hand washing, keeping fingers away from mucous membranes,* and *avoiding droplet exposure* may help. Relief from cold symptoms and avoidance of complications are facilitated by rest, adequate fluid intake, analgesics, and, perhaps, inhalation of steam. Taking a *cough suppressant* before bed (e.g., dextromethorphan) and using a *sympathomimetic* nasal decongestant spray for a few days (e.g., phenylephrine; see Chapter 219) may aid in symptomatic management and are superior to expensive combination agents. Symptoms of incapacitating rhinorrhea and sneezing not well controlled by *first-generation antihistamines* may be treated with a short course of *ipratropium* nasal spray (two sprays of a 0.06% solution in each nostril four times daily). Proactive patient education just before the beginning of the cold season may help to reduce unnecessary office visits, telephone calls, and requests for antibiotics. Echinacea remains popular among patients, but its efficacy is uncertain. Zinc lozenges may shorten the duration of symptoms, but their use may result in nausea and dry mouth. Second-generation antihistamines and antibiotics are of no use in an uncomplicated viral upper respiratory infection.

Annotated Bibliography

1. Heikkinen T, Jarvinen A. The common cold. Lancet 2003;361:51. (*A detailed review of the common cold, with a discussion of pathogenesis, transmission, diagnosis, and treatment.*)

2. Cohen S, Tyrrell DAJ, Smith AP. Psychological stress and susceptibility to the common cold. N Engl J Med 1991;325:606. (*A careful controlled, prospective study showing a significant, although not particularly strong, relation between stress and the risk for getting a cold.*)

3. Douglas RG, Lindgren KM, Couch RB. Exposure to cold environment and rhinovirus common cold. N Engl J Med 1968;279:742. (*Your mother was wrong! Exposure to moisture and cold does not increase susceptibility to upper respiratory infections, at least not in this study of volunteers experimentally infected with rhinovirus.*)

4. Lane RS, Barsky AJ, Goodson JD. Discomfort and disability in upper respiratory tract infection. J Gen Intern Med 1988;3:540. (*The severity of symptoms was linked in part to the patient's emotional state.*)

5. Simon HB. The immunology of exercise: a brief review. JAMA 1984;252:2735. (*Your mother was wrong again! There is no evidence that exercise lowers "resistance" to respiratory or other infection, nor is it protective.*)

6. Coulehan JL, Eberhard S, Kapner L, et al. Vitamin C and acute illness in Navajo schoolchildren. N Engl J Med 1976;295:973. (*A double-blinded, placebo-controlled trial in 868 schoolchildren, failing to show prophylactic or therapeutic benefit.*)

7. Douglas RM, Hemila H, Chalker EB, et al. Vitamin C for preventing and treating the common cold (Cochrane review). In: The Cochrane library, Issue 1. Oxford: Update Software, 2008. (*Vitamin C had no apparent preventive effect, but it may shorten symptom duration by a small amount [8% relative reduction] when taken as prophylaxis; initiation after symptoms have appeared had no significant benefit; see http://www.cochrane.org for updates.*)

8. Graham NMH, Burrell CJ, Douglas RM, et al. Adverse effects of aspirin, acetaminophen, and ibuprofen on immune function, viral shedding, and clinical status in rhinovirus-infected volunteers. J Infect Dis 1990;162:1277. (*Documents modest reductions in immune function and slight increases in nasal symptoms; there was no effect on virus shedding.*)

9. Hayden FG, Diamond L, Wood PB, et al. Effectiveness and safety of intranasal ipratropium bromide in common colds. Ann Intern Med 1996;125:89. (*A randomized, double-blinded, placebo-controlled trial demonstrating a significant improvement in rhinorrhea and sneezing, in addition to a global benefit, with the use of this anticholinergic nasal spray; it was well tolerated overall, but nasal dryness and blood-tinged mucus were noted in about 15% of cases.*)

10. Macknin ML, Mathew S, Medendorp SVB. Effect of inhaling heated vapor on symptoms of the common cold. JAMA 1990;264:989. (*There was no benefit in comparison with the control group; both groups showed improvement.*)

11. De Sutter AIM, Lemiengre M, Campbell H, et al. Antihistamines for the common cold (Cochrane review). In: The Cochrane library, Issue 3. Oxford: Update Software, 2004. (*They were found to be not as effective as monotherapy; see http://www.cochrane.org for updates.*)

12. Taverner D, Latte J. Nasal decongestants for the common cold (Cochrane review). In: The Cochrane library, Issue 1. Oxford: Update Software, 2008. (*They were found to be moderately effective for short-term relief, but their safety was not tested in children younger than the age of 12 years; see http://www.cochrane.org for updates.*)

13. Over the counter (OTC) cough remedies. Med Lett 2001;43:24. (*An overview of common over-the-counter cold medicines; highlights the lack of well-designed studies that demonstrate symptom relief.*)

14. Caruso TJ, Prober CG, Gwaltney JM. Treatment of naturally acquired common colds with zinc: a structured review. Clin Infect Dis 2007; 45:569. (*A systematic review of 14 trials on the efficacy of zinc for the common cold; the trials were equally divided between benefit and no benefit, regardless of study quality.*)

15. Mossad SB, Macknin ML, Medendorp SV, et al. Zinc gluconate lozenges for treating the common cold: a randomized, double-blind, placebo-controlled study. Ann Intern Med 1996;125:81. (*Demonstrated a reduction in mean duration of cold symptoms from 7.6 days to 4.4 days in 100 employees of the Cleveland Clinic; the duration of cough, nasal congestion, headache, hoarse-*

ness, sore throat, and nasal drainage was significantly shortened; nausea and bad taste were common side effects.*)

16. Prasad AS, Fitzgerald JT, Bao, B et al. Duration of symptoms and plasma cytokine levels in patients with the common cold treated with zinc acetate. Ann Intern Med 2000;133:245. (*Another trial using zinc lozenges—this time zinc acetate—in 50 healthy individuals from Detroit; the mean duration of symptoms was reduced from 8.1 to 4.5 days; no change in cytokine levels was detected.*)

17. Alexander TH, Davidson TM. Intranasal zinc and anosmia: the zinc-induced anosmia syndrome. Laryngoscope 2006; 116: 217. (*A case series of 17 patients with anosmia following the use of intranasal zinc gel, which was associated with nasal burning; no structural explanations were identified after investigation, and 7 patients never developed an associated viral illness.*)

18. Barrett B, Vohmann M, Calabrese C. *Echinacea* for upper respiratory infection. J Family Pract 1999;48:628. (*A review of published trials of Echinacea in the prevention and treatment of upper respiratory infections; although the results appear to be positive, the methodologic quality has been questioned.*)

19. Linde K, Barrett B, Wolkart K, et al. *Echinacea* for preventing and treating the common cold (Cochrane review). In: The Cochrane library, Issue 1. Oxford: Update Software, 2008. (*Most studies are positive, but there is insufficient evidence to recommend a specific preparation; see http://www.cochrane.org for updates.*)

20. Yale SH, Liu K. *Echinacea purpurea* therapy for the treatment of the common cold. Arch Int Med 2004;164:1237. (*A randomized, double-blind trial of 128 patients treated with 100 mg of Echinacea extract three times daily or placebo; no difference in symptom duration or severity was found.*)

21. Turner RB, Bauer R, Woelkart K, et al. An evaluation of *Echinacea angustifolia* in experimental rhinovirus infections. N Engl J Med 2005; 353:341.(*A randomized, double-blinded, placebo-controlled study of three different preparations of E. angustifolia in 437 volunteers experimentally infected with rhinovirus; no benefit was seen in the prevention of infection or resolution of symptoms.*)

22. Bright RA, Shay DK, Shu B, et al. Adamantane resistance among influenza A viruses isolated early during the 2005–2006 influenza season in the United States. JAMA 2006; 295:891. (*A report from the Centers for Disease Control and Prevention, finding that 92% of influenza A [H3N2] viruses isolated contained a change in the M2 gene, which is known to be correlated with adamantine [amantadine and rimantadine] resistance.*)

23. Hayden FG, Osterhaus AD, Treanor JJ, et al. Efficacy and safety of the neuraminidase inhibitor zanamivir in the treatment of influenza virus infections. N Engl J Med 1997;337:874. (*A randomized, placebo-controlled trial of 262 patients with confirmed influenza infection, showing that the time to resolution of major symptoms decreased by 1 day in treated patients; in a subgroup analysis, no benefit was seen in patients treated 30 hours after the onset of symptoms.*)

24. Jefferson TO, Demicheli V, Di Pietrantonj C, et al. Neuraminidase inhibitors for preventing and treating influenza in healthy adults (Cochrane review). In: The Cochrane library, Issue 1. Oxford: Update Software, 2008. (*A systematic review of 13 treatment and 4 prophylaxis trials, finding that neuraminidase inhibitors were effective in treatment of symptomatic illness but not prevention; in addition, oseltamivir decreased lower respiratory tract complications [relative risk 0.32, 95% confidence interval 0.18 to 0.57]; see http://www.cochrane.orgfor updates.*)

25. Arroll B, Kenealy T. Antibiotics for the common cold and acute purulent rhinitis (Cochrane review). In: The Cochrane library, Issue 3. Oxford: Update Software, 2004. (*A detailed review of the harms of prescribing antibiotics, as well as lack of benefit; seehttp://www.cochrane.orgfor updates.*)

26. Gonzales R, Steiner JF, Sande MA. Antibiotic prescribing for adults with colds, upper respiratory tract infections, and bronchitis by ambulatory care physicians. JAMA 1997;278:901. (*A national survey of outpatient physicians, finding that antibiotics were prescribed for >50% of patients—a disturbing number—to treat conditions that were predominantly viral in origin.*)

27. Stergachis A, Newmann WE, Williams KJ, et al. The effect of self-care minimal intervention for colds and flu on the use of medical services. J Gen Intern Med 1990;5:23. (*A simple self-care pamphlet did not affect medical utilization, but the article includes an excellent discussion of other such interventions that did.*)

CHAPTER 51 ■ MANAGEMENT OF SARCOIDOSIS

Sarcoidosis is a disease characterized by the formation of noncaseating granulomas, particularly in the lungs, but also throughout the rest of the body. The etiology is unknown, but the activation of T cell lymphocytes in the lung plays an important role in the pathogenesis of granulomas. In the United States, sarcoidosis is has been reported to be up to 10 times more common in African Americans than in whites; in one study, age-adjusted annual incidence rates were 36 and 11 per 100,000, respectively. People of Scandinavian descent also have a high incidence of the disease. Women outnumber men. Onset is most often between the ages of 20 and 45 years, although recent data suggest a slight shift toward older persons, especially among women.

A large percentage of patients with sarcoidosis are asymptomatic. Autopsy studies suggest that the prevalence of subclinical disease may be 10-fold that of clinical cases. Nonetheless, sarcoidosis does produce a number of diverse clinical syndromes. Granuloma formation in the lung can be especially damaging, as can involvement in a number of other organ systems (e.g., eye, gastrointestinal tract). Once the diagnosis is established, the prime management decision regards the need for corticosteroid therapy. Improved methods of monitoring disease activity have enhanced the clinician's ability to treat sarcoidosis effectively while minimizing the risk for adverse effects from long-term steroid use. The primary physician should know the most efficacious means of establishing the diagnosis, determining disease activity, and deciding on whether therapy with systemic steroids is needed and, if so, for how long.

PATHOPHYSIOLOGY, CLINICAL PRESENTATION, AND COURSE (1–7)

Pathophysiology

The cause of sarcoidosis is unknown. A variety of infectious and exogenous agents have been suggested as inciting factors, but whether one or several agents are involved remains conjectural. It is suspected that the granulomas and inflammatory reactions of sarcoidosis are caused by an abnormal immunologic response to a provocative agent in susceptible hosts. Susceptibility is determined by specific genetic polymorphisms, which include variation of the major histocompatibility complex and cytokines such as tumor necrosis factor. Many potentially causative agents have been studied. The two that have at times seemed most probable are mycobacteria and propionibacteria. The former have been a candidate for decades because of the granulomatous nature of the inflammatory response in sarcoidosis. The latter are more recent suspects, identified as such because of high levels of propionibacteria DNA found with polymerase chain reaction amplification in biopsied thoracic lymph nodes of patients with sarcoidosis.

Although the specific cause of sarcoidosis is unknown, the pathogenesis of granulomatous inflammation has been well described. Bronchoalveolar lavage studies reveal that the early stage of pulmonary sarcoidosis consists of an alveolitis, with an increased number of T lymphocytes. Helper T cells predominate, and "activated" lymphocytes, capable of secreting various soluble mediators or lymphokines that may recruit monocytes and transform them into the macrophages of granulomas, are increased in number. The alveolitis of early disease and subsequent granulomatous inflammation are reversible, either spontaneously or with corticosteroid therapy, but the fibrosis that characterizes advanced chronic sarcoidosis is irreversible.

In contrast to the lungs, in which the number and activity of helper T cells are increased, the peripheral blood of patients with sarcoidosis may show a decreased number of T lymphocytes; this may account for the depressed cell-mediated immunity and cutaneous anergy observed in many such patients. However, the blood of patients with sarcoidosis often reflects an increased activity of B lymphocytes, which accounts for the hypergammaglobulinemia and elevated antibody levels and circulating immune complexes that are often observed.

The granulomas of pulmonary sarcoidosis often resolve spontaneously, leaving the lung morphologically unscathed. However, in about 20% of patients, the process is more destructive and is characterized by interstitial fibrosis, obliteration of capillaries, and destruction of the pulmonary architecture. The end stage is characterized by the formation of cystic spaces interspersed with bands of connective tissue.

Clinical Manifestations

Presentations of sarcoidosis vary with the sites of granulomatous inflammation. The most common presentation, especially in young adults, is *bilateral hilar adenopathy*, which occurs in 50% of patients with sarcoidosis and is often detected on routine chest radiography. About 25% of patients present with bilateral hilar adenopathy and *pulmonary infiltrates*, and 15% present with infiltrates alone. Disease in the hilum is not associated with invasion or compression of the bronchi or nodal calcification. *Erythema nodosum* may accompany bilateral hilar adenopathy. This combination is known as *Lofgren's syndrome*. Less common is *Heerfordt's syndrome*: parotid gland enlargement, fever, uveitis, and cranial nerve palsies.Some patients exhibit *cough, shortness of breath, wheezing,* or *chest discomfort* in addition to constitutional symptoms of *fever, malaise,* and *fatigue.* Although pulmonary symptoms are the most frequent, sarcoidosis may present with extrathoracic disease, including *hepatomegaly, splenomegaly,* or *uveitis* (manifested by red, watery eyes). Other presenting manifestations include *fever of unknown origin,* granulomatous *hepatitis, salivary* and *lacrimal gland enlargement, arthritis,* peripheral *adenopathy,* and *skin lesions.* Diagnosis is delayed longer among patients who present with nonspecific pulmonary symptoms than among those who present with skin findings.

Lofgren's syndrome is the combination of hilar adenopathy and erythema nodosum.

Hypercalcemia as a consequence of increased sensitivity to vitamin D is reported in 10% to 30% of patients but is sustained in only 2% to 3%. Recent data suggest that it is more frequent in white people and those older than 40 years of age. Cardiac conduction abnormalities, such as heart block, and neurologic abnormalities, including facial palsies, are each seen in about 5% of cases. In addition, many unusual presentations have been reported.

DIAGNOSIS (1–5, 8–13)

The diagnosis of sarcoidosis is sometimes a clinical challenge because the condition may be hard to distinguish from other interstitial lung diseases (see Appendix 51.1). However, *asymptomatic bilateral hilar adenopathy*, with or without erythema nodosum or uveitis, is likely to be a manifestation of sarcoidosis. In a retrospective series of 100 patients with bilateral hilar adenopathy conducted before the advent of AIDS, all 30 patients who were asymptomatic had biopsy-proven sarcoidosis. Moreover, 50 of 52 with bilateral hilar adenopathy and negative physical examination findings also had the disease. All 11 patients with neoplasms were symptomatic, and 9 had easily identifiable extrathoracic tumor on physical examination. Among symptomatic patients, all with erythema nodosum or uveitis had sarcoid. Thus, in the patient with bilateral hilar adenopathy who is asymptomatic and HIV-negative and who has negative physical examination findings or erythema nodosum or uveitis, a biopsy is not necessarily required to confirm the diagnosis of sarcoidosis. Nevertheless, some clinicians prefer to obtain a tissue diagnosis in all cases of sarcoidosis, including those with asymptomatic bilateral hilar adenopathy.

The use of imaging other than chest x-ray on a routine basis in sarcoidosis is controversial. There are findings on chest computed tomography (CT) that are characteristic of sarcoidosis, including hilar and mediastinal adenopathy, lung disease with upper lobe predominance, peribronchial irregularities, and subpleural micronodules. None of these findings, however, is specific enough to confirm a diagnosis. Abdominal adenopathy and hepatic and splenic nodules may be present on abdominal CT, but these findings too are nonspecific.

A decision to perform a *biopsy* must be made by viewing the potential for discovering treatable conditions and balancing this probability against the risks associated with the procedure. For the tissue diagnosis of hilar adenopathy, *mediastinoscopy* is the most direct approach and is usually well tolerated. For the documentation of pulmonary sarcoidosis, *fiberoptic bronchoscopy* with *transbronchial biopsy* is favored. This procedure has a reported sensitivity of 60% to 80%. In addition, bronchoscopy allows direct visualization of the bronchial tree, so it can be helpful in ruling out tumor and obtaining samples of secretions by *bronchoalveolar* lavage for laboratory study. The major complication of transbronchial lung biopsy is pneumothorax; this is infrequent when someone with experience performs the procedure.

In patients with extrathoracic sarcoidosis, accessible sites for biopsy include skin lesions and enlarged peripheral lymph nodes. Biopsy of conjunctivae, salivary glands, and liver may reveal noncaseating granulomas, even if clinical evidence of sarcoid in these tissues is absent. Because of the low morbidity associated with salivary gland and conjunctival biopsies, these may be particularly useful. It must be remembered that the histologic appearance of sarcoid granulomas is not etiologically specific. Therefore, the other known causes of noncaseating granulomas must be ruled out, including tuberculosis, syphilis, berylliosis, brucellosis, Q fever, biliary cirrhosis, Wegener's granulomatosis, drug reactions, and local sarcoid reactions in nodes draining solid tumors. Hodgkin's disease is particularly difficult to exclude with mediastinoscopy in patients presenting with unilateral or asymmetric hilar adenopathy.

The *Kveim test* has also been used in the diagnosis of sarcoidosis. The test requires the intracutaneous injection of heat-sterilized human sarcoid tissue, usually spleen. A positive reaction consists in the development of epithelioid granulomas detected on skin biopsy of the injection site at 4 to 6 weeks. The test has been shown to have limited usefulness, apart from concerns about the purity of the antigen, and has fallen out of favor. Other abnormalities that may be present in patients with sarcoidosis include cutaneous anergy, hyperglobulinemia, abnormal serum liver chemistries, and elevated levels of lysozyme; none of these findings is specific, but together they are supportive of the diagnosis. Similarly, films of the bones of the hands may reveal changes suggestive of sarcoidosis.

Serum levels of *angiotensin-converting enzyme* (ACE) are elevated in about 70% of patients with active sarcoidosis, but ACE determinations lack both sensitivity and specificity for establishing a diagnosis of sarcoidosis. ACE levels have been studied as markers of disease activity and therapeutic responsiveness, but results have proved disappointing in clinical practice (see later discussion). The same is true of *scanning with gallium-67*, although it has been helpful in identifying extrathoracic disease.

STAGING, NATURAL HISTORY, AND CLINICAL COURSE (1–5,14–22)

Staging

Intrathoracic sarcoidosis can be divided into *four stages*. In *stage 0*, the chest radiographic appearance is normal. In *stage I*, only bilateral hilar adenopathy is present; most patients are asymptomatic, the lung parenchyma appears normal on chest x-ray film, and pulmonary function tests show normal mechanics, although the carbon monoxide diffusion capacity may be impaired. In *stage II*, both hilar adenopathy and pulmonary infiltrates are present; pulmonary function tests show predominantly restrictive defects. In *stage III* disease, pulmonary infiltrates are present, accompanied by obstructive and restrictive defects; however, hilar adenopathy has resolved. *Stage IV* disease is marked by advanced fibrosis, bullae, and cysts.

Natural History

Patients with clear lungs and asymptomatic hilar adenopathy have an excellent prognosis. In one large series of untreated cases, complete remission occurred in more than 75% of patients within 5 years. In 50% of patients with untreated pulmonary parenchymal involvement, complete resolution was seen within 2 years. In one third of those in whom clearing did not occur, severe fibrosis developed. Overall, at 5 years, 87% were clinically well, 10% had died of respiratory failure, and 3% were disabled by pulmonary disease. Patients with Lofgren's syndrome also have a very favorable prognosis.

Most natural history data derive from referral centers. In a report from a nonreferral setting, 86 patients were followed for

10 years in a primary care practice; pulmonary fibrosis developed in 12, and none experienced respiratory failure or cor pulmonale. This latter study suggests that the course of sarcoidosis may be more benign than has been reported from referral centers, which are more likely to attract complicated cases. There is also a striking 10-fold difference in mortality rates derived from series of patients seen in referral centers (5% mortality) and those that are population based (0.5% mortality). One study raised the question of whether frequent and sustained use of corticosteroids in referral centers contributes to higher mortality.

In general, patients with stage I disease have an 80% chance of spontaneous remission, those with stage II disease have about a 50% remission rate, and those with stage III disease have about a 20% to 40% chance of spontaneous remission. Stage IV represents irreversible, advanced disease.

Extrathoracic Complications

Extrathoracic complications are infrequent. Hepatic granulomas are often present, but the development of clinically symptomatic *granulomatous hepatitis* is much less common; hepatic failure and portal hypertension are rare. Cranial and peripheral neuropathies tend to occur early in the disease and are usually transient; however, in some patients, significant neurologic damage is seen. *Uveitis* affects about 15% of patients, comes on acutely, and often resolves spontaneously. More worrisome is chronic iridocyclitis; it presents as pain and blurring of vision, and cataracts, secondary glaucoma, and blindness may eventually develop. As noted earlier, *hypercalcemia* persists in about 2% to 3% of cases, although it may be found transiently in up to 30%. Cardiac granulomas are found in 20% of sarcoidosis cases that come to autopsy, but fewer than 5% of patients experience difficulties with conduction or impulse formation. Rarely, infiltration of the myocardium produces pump failure.

The course of patients with sarcoidosis may occasionally be complicated by *infections* such as tuberculosis, aspergillar fungus balls, candidiasis, and cryptococcosis, attributable in part to the disease and in part to the use of long-term steroid therapy.

PRINCIPLES OF MANAGEMENT, THERAPEUTIC RECOMMENDATIONS, AND MONITORING (1–5,20–33)

The *goals* in the treatment of sarcoidosis include *relief of symptoms* and *prevention* of significant impairment of organ function. As noted earlier, the natural history of sarcoidosis is variable but often favorable. Hence, the indications for therapy are frequently unclear. Patients who present with stage I disease (asymptomatic bilateral hilar adenopathy or erythema nodosum) usually have a benign course, so that no treatment is indicated unless symptoms develop. Even patients with stage II or III disease may undergo spontaneous remission, and it is not possible to identify whose disease will progress and whose will remit. No evidence is available to indicate that treatment in the early phases of pulmonary sarcoidosis prevents progression to pulmonary fibrosis.

The view that emerges from studies is that treatment should be reserved for patients who are symptomatic and have evidence of active pulmonary disease (dyspnea on exertion, abnormal results of pulmonary function studies, infiltrate on chest x-ray films). Gallium scanning and ACE determinations have also been used to provide evidence of disease activity, but in clinical practice they have not proved to be particularly accurate. Newer measures of disease activity, including serum levels of interleukin 2 (IL-2), a cytokine, and bronchoalveolar lavage levels of macrophage inflammatory protein 1, a chemokine, have been shown to correlate with stage of disease, but clinical utility is undetermined. Additional indications for treatment include important extrathoracic disease, such as uveitis, conduction abnormalities, hypercalcemia, neuropathy, and severe skin involvement (see later discussion).

The principal treatment for sarcoidosis is *systemic corticosteroid therapy*. The great variability in the clinical course of the disease and the previous lack of sensitive indicators of disease activity have made it difficult rigorously to document the efficacy of steroid therapy. Older studies relied on such crude measures as symptoms, radiographic findings, and pulmonary function test values. Recent evaluations examining the effect of corticosteroids on more direct indicators of the disease process (see later discussion) have found marked suppression of the alveolitis but little influence on anatomic abnormalities present before the initiation of steroid therapy.

Most authorities recommend commencing with large doses of steroids (e.g., 40 to 60 mg prednisone), given on a daily basis for from 6 weeks to 6 months, then tapering or switching to alternate-day therapy if measures of disease activity indicate response. Improvement is usually evident by 2 to 3 weeks. Steroid therapy is most effective if it is instituted before the development of pulmonary fibrosis. However, there is no evidence that prophylactic treatment is worth the adverse effects of long-term steroid use (see Chapter 105).

Steroids consistently produce subjective improvement in dyspneic patients with early sarcoidosis and may even reduce pulmonary infiltrates when they are secondary to alveolitis or granulomatous changes. Lung volumes usually improve, but not necessarily the diffusion capacity, which may be permanently altered by destructive changes. Relapses after cessation of therapy are frequent, so close monitoring is necessary for at least 12 months after discontinuation of treatment. *Alternate-day steroid therapy* (e.g., 15 to 25 mg every other day) has proved successful as a maintenance program in some patients, controlling disease when given after an initial course of daily steroids; this approach minimizes the adverse effects of long-term steroid therapy (see Chapter 105). Nevertheless, it must be kept in mind that it remains unproven that the long-term outcomes of sarcoidosis are improved by corticosteroid treatment.

Adrenal corticosteroids are also indicated for active ocular disease. Every patient with sarcoidosis should have an ophthalmologic examination, especially if visual symptoms develop. Topical steroids may be used, but systemic therapy is usually added. Treatment is also indicated in the presence of significant or progressive involvement of any other organ. The onset of hepatitis, facial nerve palsies, meningitis, myocardial conduction defects, hypercalcemia, and persistent constitutional symptoms (fever, fatigue) are all indications for treatment.

In an effort to improve treatment outcomes or to avoid or minimize the toxic effects of prolonged steroid therapy, other approaches have been tried. Inhaled steroids have been used in several randomized trials, either alone or after a course of systemic steroids. The evidence does not support a role for inhaled steroids in achieving improvement in lung function. There may be a reduction in symptoms, but clear evidence is lacking. Because of its ability to complement systemic steroid therapy in rheumatoid arthritis, methotrexate has been used by some investigators. Case series suggest a modest improvement with a regimen that is well tolerated and able to decrease dependence on steroids, but this has not been documented in a randomized study. A small, randomized trial suggests that chloroquine may be effective. A randomized trial of cyclosporin A does not support its use. Azathioprine and infliximab have also been used. Evidence for effectiveness is lacking.

Monitoring

Whenever steroid therapy is undertaken, an objective documentation of the response to treatment is essential. Because the predominant pathologic process in sarcoidosis is an alveolitis leading to granuloma formation, and because corticosteroids work by suppressing the alveolitis, the optimal means of monitoring disease activity and response to therapy would be to follow measures of the alveolitis. It has not been possible to distinguish between the extent of alveolitis and anatomic derangement by means of *chest radiography* and *determination of lung volumes* and *diffusion capacity*. Although these parameters are certainly useful for assessing the severity of disease, they are relatively insensitive measures of disease activity and suboptimal for judging the adequacy of therapy and the need for continued treatment. Even the sensitivity of the diffusion capacity for measuring disease extent has come under question. In one study, the diffusion capacity was well preserved, whereas lung volumes and measures of oxygenation (e.g., alveolar–arterial oxygen gradient and oxygen saturation) showed declines.

Attempts to improve on such crude measures of disease activity have been discouraging. Parameters generally reflective of inflammation, such as the erythrocyte sedimentation rate and serum globulin levels, have proved inadequate. Initial studies of *determination of ACE levels*, *gallium scanning*, and serial *bronchoalveolar lymphocyte counts* were encouraging, but a later controlled study found that these tests were no more sensitive for monitoring and managing steroid therapy than the combination of serial chest radiography and measurement of the diffusion capacity and lung volumes. Some authorities still argue that following the levels of ACE (which is believed to be produced by epithelioid cells within the sarcoid granuloma) can be useful in patients with very high levels before therapy, a situation most common in stage II disease.

As noted previously, serum levels of IL-2 and bronchoalveolar lavage levels of macrophage inflammatory protein 1, a chemokine, have been shown to correlate with stage of disease, but their clinical utility for monitoring disease and response to therapy is undetermined. Until better tests are devised, the best approach to monitoring appears to be either serial determinations of the diffusion capacity and lung volumes together with chest radiography, or serial determinations of the ACE levels if the initial serum ACE level is markedly elevated.

PATIENT EDUCATION

Serious consequences of sarcoidosis are relatively infrequent. The nature of the disease should be carefully explained, with emphasis on its relatively benign, self-limited nature in the asymptomatic patient. Patients who are treated with steroids should be counseled about side effects and the risks inherent in such treatment (see Chapter 105). Careful follow-up must be emphasized in both the asymptomatic patient (to detect the development of functional abnormalities) and the patient with symptoms (to document objective benefits of treatment). Patients should be instructed about early signs of important complications, such as red eyes, blurred vision, eye pain, and dyspnea on exertion, so that therapy is not unnecessarily delayed.

A.G.M.

Annotated Bibliography

1. Baughman RP, Lower EE, du Bois RM. Sarcoidosis. Lancet 2003; 361:1111. (*A comprehensive review, with a detailed summary of genetic susceptibility and immunologic response, as well as of diagnosis and treatment.*)
2. Martin WJ, Ianuzzi MC, Gail DB, et al. Future directions in sarcoidosis research. Am J Respir Crit Care Med 2004;170:567-571. (*An excellent discussion, pointing out all that we do not know about pathogenesis, infectious etiology hypotheses, genetics, and diagnosis and treatment.*)
3. Hunninghake GW, Costabel U, Ando M, et al. ATS statement on sarcoidosis. Am J Respir Crit Care Med 1999;160:736. (*What we do and do not know about sarcoidosis according to the American Thoracic Society.*)
4. Newman LS, Rose CS, Maier LA. Sarcoidosis. N Engl J Med 1997;336:1224. (*A comprehensive review; 159 references.*)
5. Thomas KW, Hunninghake GW. Sarcoidosis. JAMA 2003;289: 3300. (*A succinct review; 34 references.*)
6. Rossman MD, Kreider ME. Lessons learned from ACCESS (A Case Controlled Etiologic Study of Sarcoidosis). Proc Am Thorac Soc 2007;4:453-456. (*Reviews key findings of the multiple studies derived from this trial.*)
7. Kreider ME, Christie JD, Thompson B, et al. ACCESS Research Group. Relationship of environmental exposures to the clinical phenotype of sarcoidosis. Chest 2005;128:207. (*Several exposures were associated with significantly less likelihood of extrapulmonary disease; the effects were significantly different in patients of different self-defined race.*)
8. James DG. Kveim revisited, reassessed. N Engl J Med 1975;292: 859. (*Reviews the test and its sensitivity and specificity; now of historical interest.*)
9. Judson MA, Thompson BW, Rabin DL, et al. The diagnostic pathway to sarcoidosis. Chest 2003;123:406. (*Diagnosis is often delayed, more so when the presentation includes pulmonary symptoms and less so when skin lesions are present.*)
10. Koontz CH, Joyner LR, Nelson RA. Transbronchial lung biopsy via the fiberoptic bronchoscope in sarcoidosis. Ann Intern Med 1976;85:64. (*Test sensitivity was 63%, with a higher probability of a positive biopsy result in symptomatic patients.*)
11. Lower EE, Broderick JP, Brott TG, et al. Diagnosis and management of neurological sarcoidosis. Arch Intern Med 1997;157:1864. (*Facial nerve paralysis was most common but was self-limiting; other neurologic signs and symptoms were more chronic.*)
12. Rybicki BA, Maliarik MJ, Major M, et al. Epidemiology, demographics, and genetics of sarcoidosis. Semin Respir Infect 1998;13:166. (*African Americans and women were found to be at greater risk.*)
13. Winterbauer RH, Belic N, Moores KD. Clinical interpretation of bilateral hilar adenopathy. Ann Intern Med 1973;78:65. (*A classic article from the pre-HIV era, providing evidence that asymptomatic patients with only bilateral adenopathy need not undergo biopsy for definitive diagnosis.*)
14. Baughman RP, Teirstein AS, Judson MA, et al. Clinical characteristics of patients in a case control study of sarcoidosis. Am J Respir Crit Care Med 2001;164:1885. (*Women were more likely to have eye and neurologic involvement and erythema nodosum and to be age 40 years or older; men were more likely to be hypercalcemic; African Americans were more likely to have skin involvement other than erythema.*)
15. Cox CE, Donohue JF, Brown CD, et al. Health-related quality of life of persons with sarcoidosis. Chest 2004;125:997. (*Experienced physicians based their assessments of sarcoidosis symptoms on measures that were not related to issues of importance to patients.*)
16. Gottlieb JE, Israel HL, Steiner RM, et al. Outcome in sarcoidosis. The relationship of relapse to corticosteroid therapy. Chest 1997;111:623. (*A 74% relapse rate was found in the steroid-induced remission group but only an 8% relapse rate in the spontaneous remission group.*)
17. Mana J, Gomez-Vaquero C, Montero A, et al. Lofgren's syndrome revisited: a study of 186 patients. Am J Med 1999;107:240. (*Confirms the favorable prognosis and concludes that histologic diagnosis is unnecessary.*)
18. **Warshauer DM, Lee JKT.** Imaging manifestations of abdominal sarcoidosis. AJR Am J Roentgenol 2004;182:15. (*A superb review with >40 images; 68 references.*)
19. Reich JM. Mortality of intrathoracic sarcoidosis in referral vs population-based settings. Chest 2002;121:32. (*Mortality was 5% in the referral setting*

and 0.5% in population-based analysis; raises the issue of a lower threshold for sustained treatment with systemic corticosteroids as a factor in higher referral-setting mortality.)

20. Baltzan M, Mehta S, Kirkham TH, et al. Randomized trial of prolonged chloroquine therapy in advanced pulmonary sarcoidosis. Am J Respir Crit Care Med 1999;160:192. *(This small study found a significant improvement.)*

21. Gibson GJ, Prescott RJ, Muers MF, et al. British Thoracic Society sarcoidosis study: effects of long-term corticosteroid treatment. Thorax 1996;51:238. *(Improvements were found in symptoms, respiratory function, and radiographic appearance with long-term steroids.)*

22. Grutters JC, Fellrath J, Mulder L, et al. Serum soluble interleukin-2 receptor measurement in patients with sarcoidosis: A clinical evaluation. Chest 2003;124:186. *(No relation was found between soluble interleukin-2 receptor level and response to treatment, nor was an association found with radiographic evolution and lung function outcome.)*

23. Harkleroad LE, Young RL, Savage PJ, et al. Pulmonary sarcoidosis: long-term follow-up of the effects of steroid therapy. Chest 1982;82:84. *(Although only 25 patients were entered into this alternate-case steroid trial, a 15-year follow-up was available; no discernible benefit was found from early steroid therapy.)*

24. Lawrence EC, Teague RB, Gottlieb MS, et al. Serial changes in markers of disease activity with corticosteroid treatment in sarcoidosis. Am J Med 1983;74:747. *(There were initially encouraging data on the value of the gallium scan and the determination of angiotensin-converting-enzyme levels for monitoring the response to steroid therapy; see ref. 28 for a less sanguine view.)*

25. Lieberman J, Schleissner LA, Nosal A, et al. Clinical correlations of serum angiotensin-converting enzyme (ACE) in sarcoidosis. A longitudinal study of serum ACE, gallium 67 scans, chest roentgenograms and pulmonary function. Chest 1983;84:522. *(Another enthusiastic early report.)*

26. Lower EE, Baughman RP. Prolonged use of methotrexate for sarcoidosis. Arch Intern Med 1995;155:846. *(Found an improvement in two thirds of this series of 50 patients who completed at least 2 years of methotrexate therapy.)*

27. Milman N. Oral and inhaled corticosteroids in the treatment of pulmonary sarcoidosis—a critical reappraisal. Sarcoidosis Vasc Diffuse Lung Dis 1998;15:150. *(Concludes that evidence does not support the use of inhaled agents.)*

28. Paramothayan NS, Jones PW. Corticosteroid therapy in pulmonary sarcoidosis. JAMA 2002;287:1301. *(This approach was found to improve chest x-ray and vital capacity and diffusing capacity; there was no evidence for an effect on long-term disease progression; see http://www.cochrane.org for updates.)*

29. Paramothayan S, Lasserson T, Walters EH. Immunosuppressive and cytotoxic therapy for pulmonary sarcoidosis (Cochrane review). In: The Cochrane library, Issue 3. Oxford: Update Software, 2004. *(There is little randomized, controlled trial evidence that cytotoxic and immunosuppressive agents are beneficial in pulmonary sarcoidosis; see http://www.cochrane.org for updates.)*

30. Pietinalho A, Tukiainen P, Haahtela T, et al. Oral prednisolone followed by inhaled budesonide in newly diagnosed pulmonary sarcoidosis: a double-blind, placebo-controlled multicenter study. Finnish Pulmonary Sarcoidosis Study Group. Chest 1999;116:424. *(An early radiographic response was not sustained; no change was found in forced vital capacity.)*

31. Turner-Warwick M, McAllister W, Lawrence R, et al. Corticosteroid treatment and pulmonary sarcoidosis: do serial lavage lymphocyte counts, serum converting enzyme measurements, and gallium 67 scans help management? Thorax 1986;41:903. *(These studies proved no more sensitive than chest radiography and pulmonary function tests.)*

32. Wyser CP, van Schalkwyk EM, Alheit B, et al. Treatment of progressive pulmonary sarcoidosis with cyclosporin A. A randomized controlled trial. Am J Respir Crit Care Med 1997;156:1371. *(Higher complication rates were not justified by modest improvements in this trial.)*

33. Baughman RP, Drent M, Kavuru M, et al. Infliximab therapy in patients with chronic sarcoidosis and pulmonary involvement. Am J Respir Crit Care Med 2006;174:795. *(Found a statistically significant improvement in percentage of predicted forced vital capacity at week 24, but clinical importance is not clear.)*

APPENDIX 51.1: EVALUATION OF INTERSTITIAL LUNG DISEASE

A diffuse infiltrative pattern that is labeled "interstitial" in appearance may be noted on a chest radiograph ordered during the workup of dyspnea. Alternatively, findings consistent with interstitial lung disease might be noted incidentally on a chest x-ray or CT ordered for another indication. In either case, a wide variety of diagnostic possibilities emerge, including (a) systemic diseases such as sarcoidosis and connective tissue diseases and (b) diseases limited to the lungs, such as occupational lung diseases and the idiopathic interstitial pneumonias, including idiopathic pulmonary fibrosis. There are more than 200 different conditions that can lead to interstitial lung disease. With such a large number of diagnostic possibilities at hand, an efficient approach to workup is a challenge. The primary physician's role is to narrow the differential by careful attention to important elements of the history and physical examination, supplemented by a few well-chosen initial laboratory studies.

PATHOPHYSIOLOGY (1–9)

The pulmonary interstitium is defined to include the alveolar walls consisting of epithelial cells and capillaries as well as the septae and perivascular, perilymphatic, and peribronchiolar connective tissue. Interstitial lung diseases are disorders affecting the interstitium that have been grouped together because of similar radiographic, clinical, and pathophysiologic characteristics. The taxonomy of these conditions has evolved as environmental and occupational exposures and drugs have been recognized for their etiologic roles, and as sarcoidosis, connective tissue diseases and inherited conditions have been

recognized as distinct entities. The remaining "idiopathic" or "cryptogenic" cases have been variously labeled over the years with terms like Hamman-rich syndrome, fibrosing alveolitis, or idiopathic pulmonary fibrosis. The classification of these idiopathic interstitial pneumonias continues to evolve as we learn more about the relationship between different clinical findings—including findings on high-resolution computed tomography (HRCT)—and histologic patterns on one hand and prognosis and responsiveness to treatment with corticosteroids or immunomodulary therapy on the other.

Most interstitial lung diseases involve chronic inflammation that leads to progressive fibrosis of the interstitium. Some diseases that cause an interstitial pattern on chest x-ray and computed tomography examinations, however, are invasive or infiltrative rather than inflammatory. Others include alveolar filling with blood or exudative fluid. The physiologic consequence of the alveolar compromise that is the hallmark of interstitial lung diseases is the development of a *restrictive defect*; this is manifested by a reduction in forced vital capacity and a *ventilation–perfusion mismatch* that is created when inflammation and fibrosis of the gas-exchanging surfaces cause a reduction in carbon monoxide diffusing capacity and oxygen tension (PO_2). Symptoms may be minimal, although progressive dyspnea is the rule, at times accompanied by a dry, paroxysmal cough. The lungs may be clear to auscultation, or basilar crackles may predominate.

Among patients with idiopathic interstitial pneumonias, it was once assumed that all subgroups were characterized by chronic inflammation leading to progressive fibrosis of the interstitium. However, it is now recognized that the histologic subgroup termed "usual interstitial pneumonia" (UIP) since 1969 is a disease of minimal inflammation and chronic fibroproliferation caused by abnormal wound healing. The term idiopathic pulmonary fibrosis is reserved for those cases characterized by progressive dyspnea, restrictive physiology, and the UIP histologic pattern. This newer understanding of the heterogeneity of pathophysiologic mechanisms is consistent with the heterogeneity of the prognoses and responsiveness to therapy of the different subgroups, including the lack of steroid responsiveness that distinguishes idiopathic pulmonary fibrosis.

DIFFERENTIAL DIAGNOSIS (1–6,10–12)

The conditions responsible for interstitial lung disease can be grouped according to their underlying pathophysiology: Those with a known etiology include occupational lung diseases and drug-induced or radiation-induced inflammatory responses leading to fibrosis. More common in most settings are the idiopathic interstitial pneumonias, sarcoidosis, and connective tissue disorders. Rarer causes include other primary lung diseases and alveolar filling diseases (Table 51.1).

Except in industrial settings, where the pneumoconioses predominate, sarcoidosis and idiopathic pulmonary fibrosis are the most common ultimate diagnoses. Idiopathic pulmonary fibrosis was referred to as "cryptogenic fibrosing alveolitis" in Europe. Its histologic pattern is that of UIP. It is the most common of the interstitial pneumonias, accounting for 47% to 64% of interstitial pneumonias. Other interstitial pneumonias are classified as either nonspecific interstitial pneumonia (14% to 36% of interstitial pneumonias), cryptogenic organizing pneumonia (4% to 12%), acute interstitial pneumonia (<2%), respiratory bronchiolitis and desquamative interstitial pneumonia (10% to 17%), and lymphoid interstitial pneumonia (rare). Among the interstitial pneumonias, the distinction between idiopathic pulmonary fibrosis and nonspecific interstitial pneumonia is the most common and important diagnostic challenge because of their similar clinical pictures despite dramatically different responsiveness to therapy and prognoses. Idiopathic pulmonary fibrosis responds poorly to corticosteroid or cytotoxic therapy and has a 5-year mortality of 50% to 80%. Nonspecific interstitial pneumonia does respond to corticosteroids and has a 5-year mortality of less than 10%.

WORKUP (1–6,12–18)

History

History should focus on the duration of symptoms, speed of progression, and presence of fever, hemoptysis, pleuritic chest pain, and symptoms of extrathoracic disease (e.g., joint pain, lymphadenopathy, skin changes). Most conditions have a chronic, progressive course, but acute onset with *fever* and a rapidly progressive course suggest a hypersensitivity pneumonitis, usually a consequence of exposure to organic antigens (ranging from cocaine to bird droppings). Fever, bothersome dry cough, and a subacute course (2 to 10 weeks) accompanied by a patchy, bilateral air space process characterize bronchiolitis obliterans organizing pneumonia, in which a lymphocytic infiltrate and granulation tissue occupy the distal airways and alveoli. *Productive cough* is rare in interstitial lung disease, but its presence indicates fluid-filled alveoli, as can occur in diffuse alveolar cell carcinoma. *Hemoptysis* suggests conditions that cause diffuse alveolar bleeding (e.g., Goodpasture's syndrome, lupus, severe mitral stenosis, idiopathic pulmonary hemosiderosis). Bleeding that originates from or occurs in the context of upper airway disease is a

TABLE 51.1

DIFFERENTIAL DIAGNOSIS OF INTERSTITIAL LUNG DISEASE

Idiopathic Interstitial Pneumonias
  Idiopathic pulmonary fibrosis
  Nonspecific interstitial pneumonia
  Cryptogenic organizing pneumonia
  Acute interstitial pneumonia
  Respiratory branchiolitis
  Desquamative interstitial pneumonia
  Lymphoid interstitial pneumonia

Sarcoidosis
Occupational Lung Diseases
  Silicosis
  Asbestosis
  Coal worker's pneumoconiosis
  Berylliosis
  Organic dusts (pigeon, turkey, duck, chicken, humidifier)

Connective Tissue Disease
  Systemic lupus erythematosis
  Rheumatoid arthritis
  Scleroderma
  Polymyositis

Drugs and Radiation
  Chemotherapeutic agents (busulfan, bleomycin, methotrexate)
  Antibiotics (nitrofurantoin, sulfonamides, isoniazid)
  Gold
  Amiodarone
  Penicillamine
  Lupus-like reactions (hydralazine, procainamide)
  Radiation

Primary Lung Disease
  Histiocytosis X
  Lymphangiomyomatosis
  Lymphangiectatic carcinomatosis
  Lipoidosis

Alveolar Filling Disease
  Diffuse alveolar bleeding (Goodpasture's syndrome, lupus, mitral stenosis, idiopathic pulmonary hemosiderosis)
  Alveolar proteinosis
  Alveolar cell carcinoma
  Eosinophilic pneumonia
  Lipoid pneumonia

hallmark of Wegener's granulomatosis. *Pleuritic pain* indicates that an inflammatory process has spread to involve the pleura, which is characteristic of the connective tissue diseases and some drug-induced conditions. Sudden, severe pleuritic pain and acute dyspnea raise the question of a spontaneous pneumothorax, which occurs with many of the primary lung diseases, such as histiocytosis X and lymphangiomyomatosis.

The presence of extrapulmonary symptoms—especially if they predate the development of lung findings—can be diagnostic. *Polyarticular symptoms* and *skin changes* characterize the connective tissue/rheumatoid diseases and sarcoidosis; the latter is often associated with *lymph node enlargement*. Patients with idiopathic pulmonary fibrosis may have arthralgias, but symptoms of joint inflammation are absent. A history of renal disease, especially *nephritis*, can be a clue for Goodpasture's syndrome and lupus, although in the former, pulmonary disease usually predates renal involvement.

The *drug* and *occupational history* is one of the most important parts of the clinical assessment. Long-term use of such chemotherapeutic agents as methotrexate, busulfan, bleomycin, and cyclophosphamide may result in interstitial lung changes, as may prolonged use of nitrofurantoin, gold, amiodarone, or penicillamine. High-dose procainamide can lead to a lupus-like serositis syndrome. Radiation therapy may trigger a diffuse pneumonitis 6 to 12 weeks after treatment, followed by fibrosis. Occupational exposures, including distant ones, to inorganic dusts such as silicone, asbestos, talc, beryllium, and coal deserve careful review. Patients with a hypersensitivity pneumonitis should be queried about exposure to organic dusts on the job; typically, symptoms are worse at work. They should also be asked about nasal inhalation of cocaine, which has been reported as a cause of hypersensitivity pneumonitis. A *smoking* history is always pertinent. It is uncommon for lung disease to develop in non-smoking patients with Goodpasture's syndrome. Among patients with idiopathic pulmonary fibrosis, 75% have a smoking history.

Physical Examination

Physical examination is particularly useful for signs of extrathoracic disease; the pulmonary findings are usually nonspecific. The skin is checked for signs of connective tissue disease (rheumatoid nodules, malar flush, changes of scleroderma) and sarcoidosis (see prior discussion), and the lymph nodes are checked for sarcoid-related enlargement. Patients with hemoptysis should undergo a careful upper airway examination that includes a search for the signs of necrotizing changes in the nasal passages and sinuses that typify Wegener's granulomatosis. The joints are examined for evidence of inflammation (swelling, warmth, redness, effusion), which is indicative of rheumatoid disease but also occurs with sarcoidosis and Wegener's granulomatosis. Enlargement of the liver and spleen are oft-noted features of sarcoidosis and occasional findings in advanced connective tissue disease and histiocytosis X.

As noted earlier, the pulmonary findings are typically nonspecific and may even be grossly normal. Bilateral basilar rales are common in many forms of interstitial lung disease, especially the drug-related, idiopathic, connective tissue, and pneumoconiosis varieties. In those conditions associated with alveolar filling, the rales are likely to be "wet" in quality, whereas those without fluid in the alveoli produce "dry" crackles (sometimes referred to as "Velcro" rales) on end-inspiration. The heart is checked for mitral stenosis if a history of hemoptysis is present and for signs of cor pulmonale and right-sided heart failure (right ventricular heave or third heart sound, increased intensity of second heart sound, jugular venous distention, peripheral edema) resulting from chronic hypoxemia-induced pulmonary hypertension.

Chest Radiographic Findings

Chest radiographic findings are usually nonspecific but can be helpful. Radiologic adjectives describing the diffuse changes associated with interstitial disease include such terms as *reticular (linear)*, *reticulonodular*, *nodular*, and *ground glass*. The lower lobes tend to be more involved than the upper ones, and a "honeycomb" or cystic appearance to the lung fields develops

as fibrous tissue replaces normal alveoli. Exceptions to these generalizations are the upper lobe predilection and nodular infiltrates of silicosis, berylliosis, chronic hypersensitivity pneumonitis, and histiocytosis X.

Unfortunately, no particular radiographic pattern is diagnostic, although a few emerge as useful. The alveolar filling diseases tend to produce alveolar densities in an ill-defined or "fluffy" nodular pattern; an air bronchogram might ensue as involved alveoli become silhouetted by uninvolved airway. The development of such a pattern in a patient with previously known interstitial disease suggests a superimposed process, such as alveolar cell carcinoma or active inflammation. Frankly nodular infiltrates are seen with sarcoidosis and Wegener's granulomatosis as a result of granuloma formation; nodular infiltrates may even occur with the pneumoconioses and hypersensitivity pneumonitis.

Radiographic findings outside of the lung parenchyma are important and worth noting. The concurrent appearance of pleural involvement suggests connective tissue disease, asbestosis, and occasionally sarcoidosis. Bilateral hilar adenopathy can be pathognomonic of sarcoidosis (see earlier discussion). Diffuse infiltrates, hilar adenopathy, and pneumothorax point to histiocytosis X. A thin rim of calcium in the hilar nodes is characteristic of silicosis.

High-Resolution Chest Computed Tomography Findings

High-resolution chest CT (HRCT) has greatly facilitated the diagnosis of interstitial lung, increasing spatial resolution with visualization of parenchymal detail at the level of the pulmonary lobule. Findings include patchy peripheral reticular abnormalities, intralobular linear opacities, irregular septal thickening, and subpleural honeycombing. Such findings are usually most prominent in the lower lobes. Expert interpretation of CT findings, in the context of accompanying history and physical examination findings, as consistent with idiopathic pulmonary fibrosis is correct in more than 80% of cases. However, as many as one half of cases that are eventually proven to be idiopathic pulmonary fibrosis require biopsy to distinguish it from non-specific interstitial pneumonia. Use of HCRT to select biopsy sites increases diagnostic yield in such situations.

Pulmonary Function Tests

Pulmonary function tests help to confirm the interstitial nature of the disease (particularly when radiographic findings are minimal) and provide a baseline with which to judge disease course, although they correlate poorly with degree of pathologic change. The ratio of *forced expiratory volume in 1 second* (FEV_1) to *forced vital capacity* (FVC) increases and demonstrates a restrictive pattern secondary to a steady reduction in FVC. Some interstitial conditions (e.g., lymphangiomyomatosis, histiocytosis X) can also cause airway obstruction and may reduce FEV_1. The diffusion capacity is typically reduced, although it may be preserved until rather late in the course of illness, when mismatching of ventilation and perfusion becomes prominent. *Arterial blood gases* are initially normal, but with disease progression, hypoxemia, hypocarbia, and a respiratory alkalosis ensue. The hypocarbia is a manifestation of tachypnea, triggered predominantly by the increased work of breathing as the lung stiffens during progression of the fibrotic process.

Laboratory Studies

Few routine noninvasive laboratory studies are of diagnostic value. A simple yet often overlooked test is *urinalysis*, which can provide important evidence of glomerular injury (red cells, casts, albuminuria) suggestive of connective tissue disease, Wegener's granulomatosis, and Goodpasture's syndrome. Most other tests should be ordered only when the history, physical examination, and chest radiograph indicate a reasonable pretest probability of the condition in question. Unselective testing is associated with a high rate of false-positive results (see Chapter 2). If connective tissue disease is suspected, then *rheumatoid factor*, *antinuclear antibody*, and *DNA-binding* studies (see Chapter 146) and a urinalysis should be considered. Hypersensitivity pneumonitis, especially if it is drug induced, may produce a finding of 10% to 20% eosinophils on the *peripheral smear* examination, but test sensitivity is low (20%). The ACE level is useful for gauging disease activity but lacks sensitivity for the diagnosis of sarcoidosis. The measurement of *precipitating antibodies* is frequently ordered when inhalation of a potentially sensitizing organic dust is suspected, but the test does not distinguish between an etiologic role and exposure. Patients suspected of having Goodpasture's syndrome are usually positive for *anti–glomerular basement membrane antibody*. Patients with Wegener's granulomatosis test positive for *anti–neutrophil cytoplasmic autoantibodies* in only 60% of cases, but specificity is high (up to 95%).

Fiberoptic bronchoscopy with *bronchoalveolar lavage* provides an opportunity to sample the cellular and fluid contents of the distal airways (counts of total white cells, macrophages, lymphocytes and lymphocyte subsets, neutrophils, and eosinophils; malignant cells; antibodies). Alterations in the normal cellular profile may aid the diagnosis, as can the discovery of malignant cells. However, because of the considerable overlap among causes, the findings are usually nonspecific. Lavage data sometimes help to stage illness and predict the response to therapy.

Lung Biopsy

Except for patients with connective tissue disease, pneumoconiosis, or drug- or radiation-induced disease, lung biopsy is a consideration for many patients with interstitial lung disease.

The morbidity of *transbronchial biopsy*, a means of obtaining tissue during bronchoscopy, is low. Unfortunately, however, it rarely establishes a definitive tissue diagnosis. Most forms of interstitial disease that necessitate a tissue diagnosis require more tissue than can be obtained by the transbronchial approach. However, when sarcoidosis, lymphangitic carcinomatosis, or an alveolar filling disease is suspected, a transbronchial biopsy may suffice. In most other instances, an *open-lung biopsy* or, when an experienced operator is available, a *video-assisted thoracic lung biopsy* is required. Open or video-assisted biopsies should be taken from at least two sites chosen based on HRCT results. Areas of "honeycombing" represent end-stage changes that are often of little diagnostic value and should be avoided. Sites most likely to provide definitive diagnostic findings are those at the interface between involved and less involved lung tissue as indicated by HRCT findings.

Recent consensus recommendations of the American Thoracic Society and the European Respiratory Society included criteria for the diagnosis of idiopathic pulmonary fibrosis in the absence of surgical lung biopsy. Major criteria include exclusion of other known causes of interstitial lung disease; pulmonary function tests that confirm a restrictive defect and impaired gas exchange; bibasilar reticular abnormalities with minimal ground-glass opacities on HRCT; and transbronchial biopsy or bronchoalvelolar lavage showing no evidence of an alternative diagnosis. Minor criteria include age greater than 50 years, insidious onset, duration of illness greater than 3 months, and bibasilar inspiratory crackles. All major criteria and three of four minor criteria obviate the need for biopsy in most cases.

INDICATIONS FOR REFERRAL AND ADMISSION (1,4,6,9,18–23)

Referral to a pulmonary medical specialist is indicated when the diagnosis remains elusive after completion of the noninvasive segment of the evaluation and the need for lavage or a tissue diagnosis is being considered. A thoughtful consultation may save the patient an unnecessary procedure and help to select those patients most likely to warrant an invasive evaluation. Hospitalization is indicated when severe ventilation–perfusion mismatching leads to clinically significant hypoxemia (PO_2 <55 mm Hg).

A.G.M./A.H.G.

Annotated Bibliography

1. American Thoracic Society. Idiopathic pulmonary fibrosis: diagnosis and treatment. International Consensus Statement. Am J Respir Crit Care Med 2000;161:646. (*Reviews the basis for a new classification, as well as diagnosis and treatment.*)
2. King TE Jr. Clinical advances in the diagnosis and therapy of the interstitial lung diseases. Am J Respir Crit Care Med 2005;172:268. (*An excellent review of epidemiology, etiology, diagnosis, prognosis, and treatment with a very insightful historical perspective; 92 references.*)
3. Green FHY. Overview of pulmonary fibrosis. Chest 2002;122:334S. (*An overview of interstitial lung disease with a focus on idiopathic forms.*)
4. Gross TJ, Hunninghake GW. Medical progress: idiopathic pulmonary fibrosis. N Engl J Med 2001;345:517. (*An excellent review of pathogenesis, diagnosis, and therapy; 92 references.*)
5. Khalil N, O'Connor R. Idiopathic pulmonary fibrosis: current understanding of the pathogenesis and the status of treatment. Can Med Assoc J 2004;171:153. (*A superb review of diagnosis, as well as pathogenesis and treatment; 93 references.*)
6. Martinez FJ. Idiopathic interstitial pneumonias: usual interstitial pneumonia versus nonspecific interstitial pneumonia. Proc Am Thorac Soc 2006;3:81. (*A superb review with focus on recent advances in diagnosis and therapy; 127 references.*)
7. Yang IV, Burch LH, Steele MP, et al. Gene expression profiling of familial and sporadic interstitial pneumonia. Am J Respir Crit Care Med 2007;175:45. (*Differences in gene expression profiles between familial and sporadic idiopathic interstitial pneumonias [IIPs] may provide clues to their etiology and pathogenesis.*)
8. Raghu G, Weycker D, Edelsberg J, et al. Incidence and prevalence of idiopathic pulmonary fibrosis. Am J Respir Crit Care Med 2006;174:810. (*Prevalence and incidence were estimated to be 42.7 and 16.3 per 100,000, respectively, using broad criteria, and 14.0 and 6.8 per 100,000, respectively, with narrow criteria.*)
9. Martinez FJ, Safrin S, Weycker D, et al.; IPF Study Group. The clinical course of patients with idiopathic pulmonary fibrosis. Ann Intern Med 2005;142:963. (*Idiopathic pulmonary fibrosis [IPF] was the primary cause*

of death in 89% of patients who died; acute clinical deterioration preceded death in 47% of these patients.)

10. Copper JA Jr. Drug-induced lung disease. Adv Intern Med 1997;42:231. (*An exhaustive review.*)

11. Gibson PG, Bryant DH, Morgan GW, et al. Radiation-induced lung injury: a hypersensitivity pneumonitis. Ann Intern Med 1988; 109:288. (*Interesting data regarding mechanism, and a review of clinical presentation.*)

12. Hunninghake GW, Fauci AS. Pulmonary involvement in the collagen vascular diseases. Am Rev Respir Dis 1979;119:471. (*A classic and comprehensive review.*)

13. Nolle B, Specks U, Ludemann J, et al. Anticytoplasmic antibodies: their immunodiagnostic value in Wegener's granulomatosis. Ann Intern Med 1989; 111:28. (*Sensitivity averaged 63% during active disease; specificity was 95%.*)

14. Egan JJ, Martinez FJ, Wells AU, et al. Lung function estimates in idiopathic pulmonary fibrosis: the potential for a simple classification. Thorax 2005;60:270. (*An excellent review of lung function studies and the implication of changes in function for prognosis.*)

15. Lynch DA, David Godwin J, Safrin S, et al. High-resolution computed tomography in idiopathic pulmonary fibrosis: diagnosis and prognosis. Am J Respir Crit Care Med 2005;172:488. (*The extent of reticulation and honeycombing on high-resolution computed tomography [HRCT] was found to be an important independent predictor of mortality in patients with IPF.*)

16. Reynolds HY. Bronchoalveolar lavage. Am Rev Respir Dis 1987;135:250. (*An excellent review of the procedure and its findings and diagnostic utility.*)

17. McLoud T. Role of high-resolution computed tomography in idiopathic pulmonary fibrosis. Am J Respir Crit Care Med 2005;172:408. (*Reviews evidence that surgical biopsy is not required in patients with classic features of reticulation and honeycombing, which are diagnostic of IPF, and that HRCT findings provide an independent predictor of survival.*)

18. Ferson PF, Landreneau RJ. Thoracoscopic lung biopsy or open lung biopsy for interstitial lung disease. Chest Surg Clin North Am 1998;8:749. (*A detailed review of advantages and disadvantages of these alternatives for different indications.*)

19. Davies HR, Richeldi L, Walters EH. Immunomodulatory agents for idiopathic pulmonary fibrosis. Cochrane Database Syst Rev 2003;3:CD003134. (*There is evidence little to justify the routine use of any noncorticosteroid agent in the management of IPF/usual interstitial pneumonia [UIP].*)

20. Richeldi L, Davies HR, Ferrara G, et al. Corticosteroids for idiopathic pulmonary fibrosis. Cochrane Database Syst Rev 2003;3:CD002880. (*There is no evidence for an effect of corticosteroid treatment in patients with IPF/UIP.*)

21. Demedts M, Behr J, Buhl R, et al. High-dose acetylcysteine in idiopathic pulmonary fibrosis. N Engl J Med 2005;353:2229. (*Acetylcysteine added to prednisone and azathioprine preserved vital capacity and carbon monoxide diffusion capacity better than standard therapy alone.*)

22. Hunninghake GW. Antioxidant therapy for idiopathic pulmonary fibrosis. N Engl J Med 2005;353:2285. (*An important editorial commenting on ref. 21 and raising questions about why recommendations for steroids and immunomodulary therapy persist.*)

23. Noth I, Martinez FJ. Recent advances in idiopathic pulmonary fibrosis. Chest 2007;132:637. (*An excellent review, with emphasis on management from investigational drugs to lung transplant.*)

CHAPTER 52 ■ APPROACH TO THE PATIENT WITH ACUTE BRONCHITIS OR PNEUMONIA IN THE AMBULATORY SETTING

WILLIAM A. KORMOS

Although most respiratory tract infections seen in the office setting are limited to the upper airway (see Chapters 50 and 218 through 220), the differential diagnosis should include lower respiratory tract infection in patients who present with a productive cough, dyspnea, and pleuritic chest pain. In such patients, four questions need to be addressed: (a) Is the process limited to the trachea and the bronchi, or is pneumonia present? (b) Is a diagnostic workup indicated, or can empiric treatment be started? (c) Are antibiotics indicated, and, if so, which ones? (d) Can the patient be safely treated as an outpatient, or is hospital admission necessary? These basic questions are becoming increasingly germane as new strategies emerge for cost-effective management and concerns grow about the rising frequency of antibiotic-resistant organisms. The assessment and decision-making processes become considerably more complicated if the patient is HIV-positive (see Chapter 13) or immunosuppressed for other reasons.

PATHOPHYSIOLOGY AND CLINICAL PRESENTATION (1–12)

Mechanisms

Microorganisms gain access to the lower respiratory tract through inhalation or aspiration. Generally, normal defense mechanisms in the upper and lower respiratory tract protect against infection. Organisms are entrapped by the mucus-producing cells and ciliated epithelium that line the nasal mucosa and oropharynx. Local production of immunoglobulin A in the nasal mucosa prevents bacterial adherence. The cough reflex removes large particles from the lower airways, and ciliated epithelium and mucus in the bronchial tree capture particles too small to be removed by coughing. Alveolar fluid contains complement and immunoglobulin, which act as opsonins, and pulmonary macrophages then eliminate bacteria. If the burden is high, macrophages may produce cytokines, including tumor necrosis factor and interleukin-1, to recruit neutrophils to the area.

Infection of the lower respiratory tract occurs when the inoculum or the virulence of a microorganism overwhelms the host defenses. Cigarette smoke interferes with ciliary function and macrophage activity, and alcohol use may increase aspiration (by interfering with the cough reflex) and promote colonization in the upper airway by gram-negative bacteria. Deficiencies in humoral immunity occur in adults with common variable immunodeficiency, hematologic malignancies, or splenectomies. These people are more susceptible to infection with encapsulated organisms such as *Streptococcus pneumoniae* and *Haemophilus influenzae*. Patients with HIV infection have deficiencies in both cell-mediated and humoral immunity, which predisposes them to infection by numerous organisms.

The presentations of bronchitis and pneumonia are similar. Cough may be productive or nonproductive of sputum, and associated symptoms, including fever, chest discomfort, and fatigue, may be present in both entities. Pleurisy or dyspnea tends to suggest more extensive involvement, as seen in pneumonia. "Classic" community-acquired pneumonia presents with a sudden chill followed by fever, pleuritic pain, and productive cough. The "atypical pneumonia" syndrome, associated with *Mycoplasma* or *Chlamydophila* infection, often begins with a sore throat and headache, followed by a nonproductive cough and dyspnea. Physical examination findings may be misleading, especially in the patient with underlying lung disease. Evidence of consolidation on the lung examination (bronchial breath sounds, egophony) is indicative of pneumonia but is present in few outpatients. The chest x-ray film in acute bronchitis usually reveals no infiltrate or signs of consolidation, in contrast to the x-ray film in pneumonia. However, even this most clear-cut distinction between bronchitis and pneumonia can be misleading because changes of chronic lung disease can simulate new infiltrates in some patients with bronchitis, whereas dehydration can minimize radiographic abnormalities in patients with pneumonia. The clinical presentations are, in part, a function of the causative organism.

Gram-Positive Organisms (3–7)

Streptococcus Pneumoniae

Streptococcus pneumoniae is the most common cause of pneumonia, accounting for 30% to 50% of all cases of bacterial pneumonia. It is especially likely to be the agent infecting healthy young ambulatory patients, but it may affect all age groups. It is also responsible for acute exacerbations in patients with chronic bronchitis, but its role in acute bronchitis in healthy persons is unclear. Classic clinical features of pneumococcal pneumonia include abrupt onset of fever with a single rigor, cough with rusty sputum, and pleuritic chest pain. Radiologic evidence of lobar consolidation is typical, but infiltrates can be patchy, especially in patients with chronic lung disease. The sputum Gram's stain reveals abundant polymorphonuclear leukocytes and gram-positive diplococci (classically lancet shaped) in pairs or short chains.

The most common complication of pneumococcal pneumonia is bacteremia, which occurs in about one third of patients. Blood-borne distant sepsis (e.g., septic arthritis, peritonitis, meningitis) is much less common. Sterile pleural effusions are common, whereas empyema is less frequent.

Staphylococcus Aureus

Staphylococcus aureus is the etiologic agent in up to 10% of cases of bacterial pneumonia. Except in infancy, when it can be a primary infection, staphylococcal pneumonia most commonly follows a viral respiratory tract infection, particularly *influenza*. It may also occur as a nosocomial infection or as a result of bacteremic seeding of the lungs, especially in patients who have staphylococcal endocarditis or are intravenous drug users. Patients with staphylococcal pneumonia of respiratory or bloodstream origin are usually extremely ill. *S. aureus* produces tissue necrosis, and the distinctive feature of staphylococcal pneumonia is the tendency to produce multiple small lung abscesses. Healing usually leaves some degree of residual fibrosis. Abundant polymorphonuclear leukocytes and gram-positive cocci in pairs, clumps, and clusters are found on the sputum Gram's stain. Local suppurative complications, including lung abscess, empyema, and pneumothorax, are relatively common. Bacteremia with metastatic seeding of distant sites, such as endocardium, bone, joints, liver, and meninges, may occur.

Group A Streptococci

Group A streptococci are a rather uncommon cause of infection, but this type of pneumonia has occurred in epidemics, especially in closed groups such as military units. Occasionally, streptococcal pneumonia can occur after primary influenza pneumonia. Streptococcal pneumonia usually begins abruptly with fever, cough, and severe debility. Chest pain is prominent in most patients. The distinctive clinical and radiologic feature is rapid spread in the lung, with resultant early empyema formation. Initially, the empyema fluid may be thin, possibly because of the many enzymes elaborated by group A streptococci, but later frank purulence occurs. Other complications, such as lung abscess, bacteremia, metastatic infection, and poststreptococcal glomerulonephritis, are uncommon. In patients with streptococcal pneumonia, the sputum Gram's stain reveals numerous polymorphonuclear leukocytes and gram-positive cocci in pairs and short to long chains.

Gram-Negative Organisms (4–5,8)

Haemophilus Influenzae

Haemophilus influenzae has long been recognized as a common cause of bronchitis in adults with chronic lung disease; however, recognition of this organism as a cause of frank pneumonias, sometimes with bacteremia, is increasing. Most cases of bronchitis are caused by untypeable strains of *H. influenzae*, but pneumonias are often caused by the more invasive encapsulated strains, especially type b. Radiographically, a bronchopneumonia pattern is typical. Abundant polymorphonuclear leukocytes and small, pleomorphic, gram-negative coccobacillary organisms are the characteristic findings in the sputum of patients with pneumonia or bronchitis cased by *H. influenzae*. Complications of *H. influenzae* pneumonia in adults are uncommon, but in patients with underlying chronic lung disease, the illness may be particularly severe, with development of hypoxia and respiratory failure.

Klebsiella Pneumoniae

Klebsiella pneumoniae typically produces pulmonary infection in debilitated patients, especially *alcoholics*, and *Klebsiella* pneumonia is one of the few gram-negative bacillary pneumonias seen commonly in ambulatory patients. It usually presents as an acute illness; rarely, it may cause chronic pneumonitis. The organism has a high propensity to produce tissue necrosis, which accounts for the hemoptysis, dense lobar consolidation, and high incidence of abscess formation seen in this illness. Sputum may appear dark red and mucoid ("currant jelly" sputum). Abundant polymorphonuclear leukocytes and large gram-negative bacilli, occasionally with thick capsules, are characteristically seen on sputum Gram's stain. Lung abscess and empyema may occur.

Other Gram-Negative Bacillary Pneumonias

Other gram-negative bacillary pneumonias were once rare but have increased during the last 15 years and now account for up to 15% of cases of bacterial pneumonia. They are principally hospital-acquired infections and remain rare in the ambulatory population. Patients with gram-negative bacillary pneumonia are typically debilitated from other illnesses or elderly and frequently have received antibiotic therapy during which their normal respiratory flora are replaced with these otherwise unusual pathogens. Abundant polymorphonuclear leukocytes and gram-negative bacilli are seen on sputum Gram's stain. Complications, including lung abscess, empyema, and bacteremia with metastatic spread of infection, may occur.

Moraxella (Branhamella) Catarrhalis

Moraxella (Branhamella) catarrhalis is a gram-negative coccus that morphologically resembles organisms of the *Neisseria* family but differs in biochemical and DNA characteristics. It is found in the oropharynx of normal hosts and was not considered pathogenic until the 1980s, when it was established as the cause of lower respiratory tract infection in some patients with chronic obstructive pulmonary disease. In more than 80% of *M. catarrhalis* infections, an *underlying pulmonary disease* is present. Diabetes, alcoholism, malignancy, and steroid use are other known risk factors. Cases appear to be concentrated in the *winter* months, perhaps indicating a relation to preceding viral infection. The typical lower respiratory tract infection that ensues is mild and sometimes even self-limited. The organism is readily identified by Gram's stain, and almost all sputum cultures are positive for organisms. Chest radiography shows an interstitial or interstitial–air space infiltrate. Bacteremia is rare, and full recovery with prompt response to antibiotics is the rule, although almost all isolates are positive for β-lactamase.

Bordetella Pertussis

Bordetella pertussis, a gram-negative pleomorphic bacillus, is a frequently overlooked cause of acute bronchitis. Acquired immunity from childhood wanes after 15 to 20 years, so young adults are rendered susceptible to pertussis. Several studies have shown that pertussis accounts for up to 25% of patients with acute bronchitis lasting 2 or more weeks. The disease typically has three phases. The *catarrhal phase* is indistinguishable from an upper respiratory infection, with rhinorrhea, low-grade fever, and mild congestion lasting 1 to 2 weeks. Patients are contagious in this stage and early into the next stage, the *paroxysmal phase*, which lasts for 2 to 4 weeks and is characterized by severe paroxysms of nonproductive coughing, with 10 to 30 coughs in a row. Posttussive syncope and vomiting are not uncommon; the characteristic "whoop" is absent in adults because of their larger airways. Finally, the symptoms gradually resolve during the next 1 to 3 months in the *convalescent phase*. The nasopharyngeal culture, which is used in children to establish the diagnosis, is often negative for organisms by the time adults seek medical attention. A single elevated pertussis serology has been advocated as a rapid means of diagnosing pertussis.

Legionnaires' Disease (9,10)

First identified in a 1976 Philadelphia hotel outbreak, Legionnaires' disease is now recognized as an important cause of community-acquired pneumonia. *Legionella pneumophila*, an aerobic, fastidious, small, gram-negative bacillus, has been reported as the causative agent in 5% to 10% of all cases of community-acquired pneumonia and in up to 30% of cases of severe community-acquired pneumonia. The organism survives in water and, to a lesser extent, soil; infection is acquired by inhalation of contaminated aerosols or microaspiration of contaminated water. Epidemics have been traced to contaminated cooling systems, whirlpool baths, and potable water; nosocomial infections have occurred through contaminated hospital water supplies. Risk factors for *Legionella* infection include cigarette smoking, chronic lung disease, and immunosuppression. *L. pneumophila* is responsible for more than 90% of all cases; of the 14 serotypes of *L. pneumophila* identified, serogroup 1 is responsible for the majority of these cases. The next most common *Legionella* species is *L. micdadei* (the Pittsburgh pneumonia agent), which can cause cavitary lung disease in immunosuppressed patients.

The spectrum of clinical illness resulting from *Legionella* infection ranges from mild upper respiratory disease (Pontiac fever) and self-limited atypical pneumonia to multifocal pneumonia and respiratory failure. After a short prodrome, the full-blown form of Legionnaires' disease begins acutely with high fever, nonproductive cough, and dyspnea. *Pleuritic chest pain* occurs in about one third of cases. Systemic manifestations such as *diarrhea* or *confusion* are often seen but are not specific to legionellosis.

Relative bradycardia occurs in a few patients, but in most cases the physical examination findings are nonspecific. Chest radiography shows interstitial infiltrates or areas of patchy consolidation with characteristic rapid progression. Extrapulmonary findings are uncommon but include myocarditis, pericarditis, rhabdomyolysis, and renal dysfunction. Sputum is typically absent or scant. The sputum Gram's stain fails to reveal pathogens, but *L. pneumophila* can be cultured on a specialized buffered charcoal yeast extract agar. *Legionella* urinary antigen is very sensitive for disease caused by *L. pneumophila* serogroup 1 (about 80% of all cases) and is easy to obtain.

Mixed Flora

Aspiration Pneumonias

Aspiration pneumonias are usually mixed infections caused by aerobic and anaerobic streptococci, *Bacteroides*, and *Fusobacterium*. These organisms are normal flora of the upper airway that cause pneumonia if they attain a foothold in the lung parenchyma. Predisposing factors include alteration of consciousness (drugs, anesthesia, alcohol, head trauma) and diminution of the gag reflex, which permits aspiration to occur. Patients usually are mildly to moderately ill but can be toxic, especially if lung abscess or empyema occurs. Hospitalized patients, ambulatory patients receiving antibiotics, and edentulous patients have altered respiratory flora and fewer anaerobic organisms, if any. Aspiration of mouth organisms in such persons may result in staphylococcal or gram-negative bacillary pneumonia, as discussed previously, rather than the mixed aerobic–anaerobic infection considered here. The sputum from patients with aspiration pneumonia may be malodorous and characteristically shows abundant polymorphonuclear leukocytes and mixed flora, including gram-positive cocci in pairs and chains and pleomorphic gram-negative rods on Gram's stain. Lung abscess and empyema are fairly common complications of aspiration pneumonia, especially if therapy is delayed.

Nonbacterial Organisms (11,12)

Mycoplasma Pneumoniae

Mycoplasma pneumoniae is a cell wall–deficient organism that accounts for 10% to 20% of cases of community-acquired pneumonia. It is a leading cause of the *atypical pneumonia syndrome* (fever, dry cough, nonspecific infiltrate on chest film) and also a cause of acute bronchitis in otherwise healthy adults. The organism spreads by way of respiratory droplets and appears to have a long incubation period; onset of illness tends to be insidious. The disease often begins with headache, sore throat, and malaise and then progresses to a nonproductive cough. The physical examination findings are usually unimpressive in comparison with the *patchy peribronchial infiltrates* seen on chest x-ray films. Bullous myringitis has been reported in *Mycoplasma* pneumonia, but it is actually uncommon in clinical practice. Skin examination may show *erythema multiforme*, which is highly correlated with *Mycoplasma* infection in the patient with pneumonia. Laboratory studies reveal a normal white blood cell count and differential in most cases. The sputum is scant, with a predominance of mononuclear cells and no organisms. Sputum culture is not practical because a special medium is required and results do not become available for 2 weeks. Testing for the organism by polymerase chain reaction is a new technique with high sensitivity and specificity, although it is not widely available. *Cold agglutinins* are present in approximately 50% of cases. *Mycoplasma* pneumonia is usually a mild, self-limited illness, but it can produce severe pneumonia in children with sickle cell anemia, in immunosuppressed hosts, and in the elderly. Uncommon complications include hemolytic anemia, aseptic meningitis, Guillain–Barré syndrome, and myopericarditis.

Chlamydophila Pneumoniae

Chlamydophila pneumoniae (formerly known as *Chlamydia pneumoniae*, or *TWAR*) is an obligate intracellular organism that causes an atypical pneumonia or acute bronchitis. It appears to account for 5% to 15% of cases of community-acquired pneumonia, with higher rates in young adults. *C. pneumoniae* appears to spread from person to person by respiratory droplets. The prodrome resembles that of *Mycoplasma* pneumonia, with headache and sore throat followed by a dry cough, but the chest radiograph shows less extensive involvement. The diagnosis is difficult because culture requires tissue culture techniques that are not routinely performed. Serology (acute and convalescent titers) has been used to establish the diagnosis, and, as in *Mycoplasma* pneumonia, polymerase chain reaction is an upcoming (but not proven) new technology. The infection is usually self-limited; rare fatalities have been reported in debilitated patients.

Viruses, Intracellular Parasites, and Fungi

Viruses are the most common cause of acute bronchitis, accounting for more than 80% of all cases. Viral pneumonia resembles an atypical pneumonia and is clinically indistinguishable except when it is part of a distinctive systemic viral illness, such as rubeola in children or varicella in adults. Many viruses are capable of producing lower respiratory tract infections, including influenza virus, adenoviruses, respiratory syncytial virus, and parainfluenza virus. Cytomegalovirus is a common cause of viral pneumonia in transplant recipients. The most important cause of viral pneumonia is influenza, which can be recognized by its epidemic spread and marked systemic symptoms, such as fever and myalgia. Influenza pneumonia may be mild or a fulminant illness capable of causing lethal respiratory failure. Bacterial pneumonia, especially of the pneumococcal, staphylococcal, or streptococcal variety, is a frequent complication.

Severe Acute Respiratory Syndrome

In late 2002, an outbreak of severe pneumonia occurred in Southeast Asia that was not responsive to the usual therapies. Named the severe acute respiratory syndrome (SARS), this disease spread to more than 20 countries, including a sizable outbreak in Toronto, Canada. The causative agent was quickly identified as a novel coronavirus. SARS presents with a viral syndrome of fever, myalgias, and cough and then progresses with worsening respiratory distress. Chest x-ray demonstrates multilobar infiltrates, predominantly in the lower lobes. Common laboratory findings include lymphopenia, thrombocytopenia, and elevated creatinine kinase. Treatment remains supportive because no effective antiviral therapy has been identified. The illness was fatal in 10% to 15% of patients.

Psittacosis

Psittacosis is caused by a member of the *Chlamydia* group of obligate intracellular parasites, which are also responsible for lymphogranuloma venereum and trachoma. The disease is transmitted from parrots or other birds (including pigeons and turkeys) to humans. The clinical features of psittacosis are indistinguishable from those of other nonbacterial pneumonias, with prominent headache, nonproductive cough, and fever. Occasionally, a faint macular rash or splenomegaly develops.

Q Fever

Q fever, caused by *Coxiella burnetii*, is unique among rickettsial infections in that pneumonia is prominent, no rash is associated, and spread is through the inhalation of infected dust particles rather than by way of the bite of an insect vector. The organisms reside principally in animals; human contact with cattle, sheep, goats, or infected animal hides or hide products is the most important epidemiologic factor and is often the only clue to diagnosis. The clinical features of Q fever are similar to those of the other nonbacterial pneumonias, except that hepatitis occurs in up to one third of patients.

Fungi and Other Opportunistic Organisms

Immunosuppressed patients (e.g., those taking corticosteroids or HIV-positive patients) are at heightened risk for a community-acquired opportunistic infection (e.g., *Aspergillus*, *Candida*, or *Pneumocystis*; see Chapter 13). HIV-positive patients are also at increased risk for *primary tuberculosis* (see Chapter 49). However, some fungal infections may occur in immunocompetent hosts. For example, exposure to spore-containing dusts may lead to *histoplasmosis* (in the Midwest) or *coccidioidomycosis* (in the Southwest), characterized in the initial phases by a nonproductive cough, flulike illness, liver or splenic enlargement, alveolar infiltrates, and sometimes hilar adenopathy; however, most often the chest radiographic findings are normal.

DIFFERENTIAL DIAGNOSIS

The differential diagnosis of community-acquired pneumonia is listed in Table 52.1. In most epidemiologic studies, *S. pneumoniae* is the most common cause, followed by *H. influenzae*, influenza virus, and *Legionella*.

In addition to the conditions listed in Table 52.1 and detailed earlier, noninfectious diseases can occasionally mimic infectious processes. Bronchial asthma (see Chapter 48) and hypersensitivity pneumonitis (see Chapter 51) are common examples. The radiologic findings associated with chronic pulmonary diseases, especially chronic bronchitis (see Chapter 47) and bronchiectasis (see Chapter 41), may be misleading if previous x-ray films are not available. Atelectasis, pulmonary infarction, pulmonary edema (see Chapter 32), and lung tumors may also be confused with pneumonia.

Workup (1,2,10,13,14)

The first task is to differentiate lower respiratory tract infection from the other causes of cough (see Chapters 32, 41, 42, and 51) and from upper respiratory infection (see Chapters 50, 219, and 220). The predominant symptom of a patient presenting with a lower respiratory tract infection is usually cough, either productive or nonproductive of sputum. A predominant symptom of nasal discharge, sore throat, or ear pain can direct the workup away from the lower respiratory tract. Once a lower tract infection is suspected, the focus quickly shifts to the task of diagnosing pneumonia or bronchitis. Unfortunately, the distinction cannot be made reliably on the basis of any single element of the history or physical examination. A search for a specific cause is important if the presentation is unusual, unique exposures are present, or the patient is immunosuppressed.

TABLE 52.1
DIFFERENTIAL DIAGNOSIS OF PNEUMONIA IN AMBULATORY PATIENTS

Bacterial
Streptococcus pneumoniae
Haemophilus influenzae
Legionella species (most often *L. pneumophila*)
Staphylococcus aureus
Klebsiella pneumoniae (and other Enterobacteriaceae)
Moraxella catarrhalis
Streptococcus pyogenes
Mixed aerobic/anaerobic organisms (aspiration)

Nonbacterial
Mycoplasma pneumoniae
Chlamydophila pneumoniae
Chlamydia psittaci
Mycobacterium tuberculosis
Coxiella burnetti (Q fever)
Viral (influenza, adenovirus)
Pneumocystis carinii
Fungi

History

Symptoms of pneumonia were previously classified as "typical" (productive cough, rigors, pleurisy) or "atypical" (nonproductive cough with a prodrome of headache and sore throat). These classifications originally were developed to discriminate pneumococcal pneumonia from pneumonia caused by "atypical" organisms such as *Mycoplasma* and *Chlamydophila*. However, the overlap in symptoms of pneumonia of different causes is substantial, so this classification is unreliable. As stated, the type of cough and the presence of dyspnea and fever are also unreliable for differentiating bronchitis from pneumonia.

The history is most useful for determining additional *comorbid conditions* that may influence prognosis or clarify etiology. Advanced age, congestive heart failure, cerebrovascular disease, active malignancy, and renal or liver disease all predict a poorer outcome in patients with pneumonia. In addition, patient characteristics may increase the likelihood of particular organisms. Risk factors for drug-resistant *S. pneumoniae* include age greater than 65 years, alcoholism, immunosuppressed state, and use of β-lactam antibiotics in the last 3 months. Alcoholics also have a higher incidence of infection with gram-negative organisms, especially *K. pneumoniae*, and patients with chronic lung disease are often colonized with *H. influenzae* and *M. catarrhalis*. Nosocomial pathogens, including resistant organisms and *Pseudomonas*, should be considered in nursing home residents. HIV-positive patients are at risk for infection with a number of opportunistic pathogens, such as *Pneumocystis (carinii) jiroveci* and *Mycobacterium tuberculosis*.

The history may also be useful in *identifying unusual exposures* or epidemiologic associations to raise the possibility of specific causes. Patients should be assessed for close contact with birds (psittacosis), livestock (Q fever), or rabbits (tularemia). A patient residing in or traveling to the southwestern United States (coccidioidomycosis) or the Midwest (histoplasmosis) may acquire an acute fungal pneumonia, which is usually self-limited without treatment except in immunocompromised hosts. A history of recent travel in hotels or on cruise ships in the previous 2 weeks raises the suspicion for *Legionella* infection. Patients who are at high risk for tuberculosis exposure (immunosuppressed, homeless, exposed to known contact) should be assessed for mycobacterial infection.

Physical Examination

No single physical examination finding can definitively diagnose pneumonia, although the clinician should focus on the vital signs and pulmonary examination to assist diagnosis and prognosis. High fever (>104°F), hypothermia, tachypnea, and tachycardia are all associated with an increased 30-day mortality. Conversely, several studies have demonstrated that the presence of entirely normal vital signs decreases the probability of pneumonia in outpatients to less than 1%. The pulmonary examination in pneumonia often demonstrates crackles, although patients with bronchitis may have similar findings. The classic findings of lung consolidation (dullness to percussion, egophony, bronchial breath sounds) are more specific for pneumonia but are found in fewer than 25% of patients with radiographic evidence of pneumonia. Some physical findings may have etiologic significance. Erythema multiforme is associated with *Mycoplasma* pneumonia, and confusion is seen more often in *Legionella* infection.

Laboratory Studies

In the patient with acute bronchitis, laboratory testing is often unnecessary. Inflammatory markers, such as C-reactive protein, are increased in patients with pneumonia but do not appear to be additive to the current diagnostic plan, which focuses on history and physical examination. However, if pneumonia is suspected, posteroanterior and lateral *chest radiography* is required to confirm the diagnosis. In addition to indicating the extent of disease, the chest x-ray film may also show a pleural effusion, which is associated with a poorer outcome. Unless the pleural effusion is minimal, *thoracentesis* should be performed to assess for the presence of an empyema or complicated parapneumonic effusion. Pleural fluid is sent for Gram's stain, culture, cell count, and determination of glucose, protein, and lactate dehydrogenase levels and pH (see Chapter 43).

The value of routine sputum collection for *Gram's stain* and *culture* is controversial. In acute bronchitis, the predominance of viral and atypical bacterial organisms makes these tests unlikely to influence treatment decisions. For the patient with pneumonia, a recent joint guideline from the Infectious Disease Society of America and the American Thoracic Society advocates performing sputum Gram's stain and culture in all patients hospitalized with community-acquired pneumonia. This recommendation recognizes the limitations of Gram's stain and culture but also argues for the importance of detecting resistant or atypical organisms and tailoring antibiotic treatment according to culture results. With the increasing presence of resistant organisms, it is reasonable to obtain a specimen for Gram's stain and culture if the patient is producing sputum.

If a sputum sample is obtained, it is essential to ensure that it is adequate. In a large cohort study of 1,669 patients with community-acquired pneumonia, a good-quality sputum specimen was obtained in only 532 patients (32%). The specimen should be obtained from a deep cough, with the use of nebulized saline solution if necessary. For a causative organism to be predicted accurately, the Gram's stain should show fewer than 10 epithelial cells and more than 25 polymorphonuclear cells per low-power field. Interpretation needs to be performed by an experienced observer. Small gram-negative rods may be overlooked by an inexperienced observer, and inadequate decolorization results in misclassification of gram-negative organisms as gram-positive. *Pneumococcal* infections show gram-positive, lancet-shaped diplococci; gram-negative cocci suggest *Moraxella*, and gram-negative coccobacillary forms are indicative of *H. influenzae*. Identification of a predominant organism on Gram's stain has been shown to be specific for infection with that organism and can help in interpreting a subsequent sputum culture. Despite attempts to obtain an adequate specimen, upper respiratory contamination, fastidious pathogens, and delay in transportation all limit the utility of the sputum culture, which is negative in about 50% of cases. However, when a predominant organism is seen on Gram's stain, the yield increases to about 85%. Ideally, all cultures should be obtained and sent before antibiotics are started, but failure to obtain a sputum specimen should not delay antibiotic treatment.

In hospitalized patients, additional tests, including a complete blood count, the assessment of renal function, and the determination of electrolytes, are obtained. Hyponatremia may be caused by dehydration or the syndrome of inappropriate antidiuretic hormone and is more frequently associated with legionellosis. Serum liver enzymes are frequently elevated in patients with pneumonia, regardless of the cause. An *arterial blood gas* may be obtained if the patient has an underlying pulmonary disease or the clinical picture warrants the test. *Blood cultures* are positive in about 5% to 15% of patients and may be the only accurate method of identifying the causative organisms. Pneumococcus is the most frequent organism identified by blood cultures, and penicillin sensitivity can be determined on these isolates. Blood for two sets of cultures should be drawn from different sites before the initiation of antibiotic therapy in hospitalized patients.

The detection of *Legionella urinary antigen* is an accessible and rapid method for diagnosing Legionnaires' disease. The test is very sensitive for *L. pneumophila* serogroup 1, which accounts for more than 80% of cases of pneumonia in humans. The antigen persists in the urine even after antibiotics have been started and may persist for months after infection. A *Legionella* urinary antigen test should be performed in all patients with a clinical picture suggestive of legionellosis. Legionnaires' disease can also be diagnosed in 3 to 5 days by culture of the organism on special media. Serology may also be used to detect infection, but the delay in results makes this a less useful test. A single *antibody titer* of 1:256 is presumptive evidence, but confirmation requires demonstration of a fourfold rise in titer between acute and convalescent specimens.

A nasal swab should be sent for influenza antigen if influenza is suspected. Diagnosis of influenza will change treatment, as well as raise the possibility of prophylactic treatment with oseltamivir for close contacts of the patient. Pneumococcal antigen tests are also available and are 50% to 80% sensitive for pneumococcal pneumonia. Because empiric treatment regimens must always cover pneumococcal infection, the need for confirmation of this diagnosis by urine antigen testing is less essential.

Additional testing in patients with community-acquired pneumonia is usually unnecessary. Measurement of acute and convalescent serologic titers can confirm infection with *Mycoplasma*, *Chlamydophila*, *Coxiella burnetii*, or viral agents. In the HIV-infected patient with pneumonia, an induced sputum sample or bronchoalveolar lavage is stained for *Pneumocystis* and *M. tuberculosis* (see Chapter 13).

PRINCIPLES OF MANAGEMENT (1,15–24)

General Measures (15,16)

Admission versus Outpatient Management

Many patients with community-acquired lower respiratory tract infections can be managed on an outpatient basis, provided that they are alert, reliable, have help available to them, and have no signs of serious compromise (see Indications for Admission). In the Pneumonia Patient Outcomes Research Trial (PORT), about 50% of patients were identified to be at low risk for complications and appropriate for outpatient treatment. These patients had a 30-day mortality of less than 1%. Therapeutic serum levels can be achieved with oral antibiotic regimens for patients treated at home. See Therapeutic Recommendations.

Symptomatic and Supportive Measures

Patients with bronchitis or pneumonia often ask for medication to relieve the cough that prompted them to seek medical care. Suppression is not encouraged in patients with acute cough because the cough reflex remains an important defense mechanism. Adequate *hydration* is essential to help clear secretions; this can be achieved by fluid intake and local airway humidification. *Expectorants* such as guaifenesin may be helpful to some patients in loosening the sputum, although they have not been proven to make a significant difference in outcome. *Pulmonary physical therapy* may help to mobilize secretions, but prospective trials have failed to demonstrate that this time-honored intervention improves outcome (see Chapters 41 and 47).

Cough Suppressants. In some patients, persistent coughing results in severe musculoskeletal chest pain or respiratory fatigue. Nocturnal cough may interfere with sleep and prevent the patient from getting adequate rest. In these cases, several treatments may be offered. In two small trials of patients with acute bronchitis, β_2-agonists, such as albuterol, have decreased the duration of cough. Expiratory flow rates can be decreased in these patients, as in those with reactive airway disease. Because the persistent cough in bronchitis appears to be related to bronchial irritation, not to continuing infection, this treatment makes physiologic sense. However, its use is limited by the lack of large studies, side effects of the medication, and time required to teach inexperienced patients how to use inhalers. Cough suppressants, which directly diminish the cough reflex, include dextromethorphan and codeine. These medicines may provide temporary relief, especially when taken before bed (see Chapter 41). Although the tablet form is equally effective, patients may prefer a syrup formulation for cough suppression. Fever, another bothersome symptom, can be controlled with aspirin or acetaminophen (see Chapter 11).

Antibiotic Therapy. Antibiotics are a cornerstone of initial management of *pneumonia*. Because most etiologic testing requires 24 to 48 hours, initial treatment decisions are usually empiric, based on the best estimate of specific underlying pathogen(s). Therapy is then modified in response to diagnostic test results and the patient's response to therapy. For most bacterial infections, continued treatment for 10 to 14 days is recommended. In *acute bronchitis* (which is usually of viral origin in otherwise healthy persons), the empiric use of antibiotics does not improve outcomes. Nonetheless, the inappropriate prescribing of antibiotics for acute bronchitis remains a common practice, particularly in response to patient demand.

Oxygen Therapy. Oxygen therapy may be required in hospitalized patients with pneumonia. In general, treatment should be titrated to the patient's respiratory status and not be focused on a specific oxygen saturation or concentration. Lung consolidation in pneumonia functions as a shunt, and an increase in oxygen may not result in improved arterial oxygenation. In addition, patients with severe chronic lung disease may experience hypercapnia with excessive oxygen therapy (see Chapter 47).

Specific Conditions (1,17–24)

Acute Bronchitis

At least eight randomized, placebo-controlled trials involving the use of doxycycline, trimethoprim/sulfamethoxazole, and erythromycin have failed to show a benefit of empiric antibiotic therapy in healthy patients with acute bronchitis. In most studies, cough resolved at 1 week regardless of treatment, and persistence of cough for 2 weeks was not unusual. These smaller trials have been combined in two separate systematic reviews that have confirmed minimal benefit of antibiotics in these patients. Newer, more potent antibiotics, such as azithromycin, have fared no better in randomized, controlled trials. Despite this evidence, several studies have suggested that physicians prescribe antibiotics for more than 60% of outpatients with acute cough and no underlying lung disease. Epidemiologic studies show that relatively few of these patients actually have pneumonia as the cause of their cough. Healthy patients with acute bronchitis should be treated with conservative measures for cough and counseled about the natural history of the disease. Emphasizing the predominantly viral etiology of the prob-

lem can help to alleviate patient expectations for antibiotics. One study demonstrated that labeling the problem a "chest cold" helped to communicate this issue to patients.

The one exception to this approach is the patient with *pertussis*. Early antibiotic therapy with erythromycin can effectively treat *B. pertussis* infection, but most adults who seek medical attention are in the paroxysmal phase, when tracheal damage has already occurred. However, they may still be infectious in the early paroxysmal phase, and treatment can decrease the transmission of *B. pertussis*. Therefore, the patient with documented or suspected pertussis is treated with 500 mg of *erythromycin* four times daily for 7 to 14 days. Prophylactic treatment with the same regimen (adjusted for weight in children) is recommended for household members and close contacts, especially unvaccinated infants. Because many patients cannot tolerate this dose of erythromycin, a second-generation macrolide (e.g., azithromycin, clarithromycin) may be substituted for 5 to 10 days (the optimum duration for these newer agents is unknown). In the patient intolerant of macrolides, trimethoprim/sulfamethoxazole (160/800 mg twice daily for 14 days) may be used.

Acute Exacerbation of Chronic Bronchitis

Antibiotics are effective in relieving symptoms and preventing the deterioration of lung function in patients with established chronic bronchitis. *S. pneumoniae*, *H. influenzae*, and *M. catarrhalis* are the common pathogens in these patients. A second-generation β-lactam, such as cefuroxime, is the treatment of choice. Alternatives include a second-generation macrolide, a respiratory fluoroquinolone, or trimethoprim/sulfamethoxazole. Additional treatment depends on the patient's condition and underlying lung function (see Chapter 47).

Community-Acquired Pneumonia

Antibiotics are clearly indicated for the treatment of community-acquired pneumonia, although no randomized trials have been completed. Evidence consists in the significant decrease in pneumonia mortality since the introduction of antibiotics and the adverse outcomes associated with delayed or inappropriate antibiotic therapy in patients with pneumonia. Increasing drug resistance, notably penicillin resistance in *S. pneumoniae*, has complicated the empiric selection of antibiotics. The initial treatment is directed at the most common pathogens, and patients are classified by age, comorbidities, and severity of pneumonia.

Healthy Young Adults. In persons less than 60 years old, the most common organisms are *S. pneumoniae*, *Mycoplasma*, *Chlamydophila*, and *Legionella*. All of these organisms are covered adequately with *erythromycin* (500 mg four times daily), which is the first-line treatment. Although macrolide resistance is increasing in *S. pneumoniae*, observational studies have validated this approach as an effective, inexpensive strategy. Penicillins or cephalosporins will not cover the atypical organisms in this age group. Because multiple daily doses and gastrointestinal symptoms will limit the tolerability of erythromycin, the second-generation macrolides (azithromycin 500 mg on day 1, followed by 250 mg daily for 4 days, or clarithromycin 500 mg twice daily for 10 days) are commonly substituted. Second-line therapy remains *doxycycline* (100 mg twice daily). Respiratory fluoroquinolones, such as levofloxacin, moxifloxacin, and gemifloxacin, have adequate activity against the pathogens and are well tolerated. However, indiscriminate use will certainly translate into resistant strains.

Older fluoroquinolones (e.g., ciprofloxacin) have less activity against the pneumococcus and are not recommended.

Older Adults and Patients with Comorbidities. *S. pneumoniae* remains the most common cause of pneumonia, but *H. influenzae*, *M. catarrhalis*, and other gram-negative organisms are alternative possibilities. The atypical organisms such as *Mycoplasma* and *Chlamydophila* were believed to be unusual in this population, but more recently studies have documented their importance. Therefore, the recommended first-line treatment is a *second-generation macrolide (azithromycin or clarithromycin) plus a β-lactam (high-dose amoxicillin, 1 g three times daily, or amoxicillin-clavulanate, 2 g twice daily)*. Due to concern for pneumococcal resistance, this regimen should also be used in patients with recent (within 3 months) exposure to antibiotics. Alternative therapy for the two-drug combination is a *respiratory fluoroquinolone*, which has adequate pneumococcal coverage.

Patients who are ill enough to be hospitalized for pneumonia often require *parenteral antibiotic therapy*. The causative organisms are similar to those described previously, but the potential for worsening respiratory status is higher in these sicker patients. Empiric treatment may be selected based on the patient characteristics described for the first two groups, but therapy is often broadened in sicker patients to cover potentially resistant organisms and a wider spectrum of organisms. For hospitalized patients, the first-line treatment is a *third-generation cephalosporin (e.g., 1 g of ceftriaxone daily) plus a second-generation macrolide* in a dose sufficient for *Legionella* infection (e.g., azithromycin 500 mg daily or clarithromycin 500 mg twice daily). This combination therapy has been associated with better outcomes in observational studies and provides additional coverage in the presence of resistant *S. pneumoniae*. Therapy can then be narrowed after the results of diagnostic tests, such as *Legionella* urinary antigen and blood cultures, become available. Focused therapy may also be initiated on presentation when an adequate Gram's stain is highly suggestive of a particular pathogen (see Table 52.3), although observational studies suggest that this approach is not followed. The alternative empiric treatment is a *respiratory fluoroquinolone*.

This alternative offers the advantage of single-agent therapy, but, once again, concern about emerging resistance and overuse of these agents has tempered the enthusiasm for broadly recommending fluoroquinolones as first-line therapy.

Antibiotic Resistance in *S. pneumoniae*

Previously, *S. pneumoniae* was almost universally susceptible to penicillin. However, resistance to penicillin, mediated by mutations in penicillin-binding proteins, was first reported in the 1960s in Australia. During the last decade, these resistant organisms have become an increasing concern in the United States. Approximately 30% of pneumococci in the United States have intermediate penicillin resistance (mean inhibitory concentration [MIC] of 0.1 to 1.0 μg/mL), and up to 10% are highly penicillin resistant (MIC >2.0 μg/mL). These highly resistant organisms are often cross-resistant to multiple antibiotics, including trimethoprim/sulfamethoxazole and erythromycin. Fortunately, parenteral penicillin appears to achieve adequate levels in the tissues for the effective treatment of pneumococci with intermediate resistance. For highly resistant organisms, alternative agents are recommended. Fluoroquinolone resistance has been very low in *S. pneumoniae* ($<2\%$); however, as these agents are being used more frequently, resistant strains are increasing. The increasing prevalence of pneumococcal resistance to antibiotics serves to emphasize the need to vaccinate high-risk patients (see later discussion); more than 85% of resistant organisms are serotypes contained in the 23-valent vaccine. In addition, penicillin resistance has decreased since the introduction of the pediatric conjugate vaccine (which contains serotypes responsible for almost 80% of resistant organisms) in 2000.

THERAPEUTIC RECOMMENDATIONS (1)

Treatment for lower respiratory tract infections is tailored to the clinical syndrome and likely pathogens. Table 52.2 summarizes the empiric antibiotic recommendations for the various

---

TABLE 52.2

EMPIRIC TREATMENT FOR LOWER RESPIRATORY TRACT INFECTIONS

Clinical Syndrome	Preferred Empiric Treatment	Alternative Treatment
Acute bronchitis	None	Doxycycline, erythromycin
Acute exacerbation of chronic bronchitis	Second-generation cephalosporin	Second-generation macrolide,[a] trimethoprim/sulfamethoxazole
Community-acquired pneumonia		
Healthy young adults	Macrolide	Doxycycline, respiratory fluoroquinolone[b]
Elderly (age >60 yr) or comorbid disease	Second-generation macrolide[a] plus β-lactam[c]	Respiratory fluoroquinolone
Hospitalized patient (non–intensive care unit)	Third-generation cephalosporin plus second-generation macrolide	Respiratory fluoroquinolone

[a]Second-generation macrolides include clarithromycin and azithromycin.
[b]Respiratory fluoroquinolones are agents with adequate pneumococcal activity, including levofloxacin, moxifloxacin, and gemifloxacin.
[c]β-Lactams with adequate activity against potentially resistant pneumococci include amoxicillin 1 g three times daily and amoxicillin–clavulanate 2 g twice daily.

TABLE 52.3

PATHOGEN-SPECIFIC THERAPY FOR LOWER RESPIRATORY TRACT INFECTIONS

Organism	First-Line Agent	Alternative Agents
Streptococcus pneumoniae		
Penicillin sensitive (MIC <0.1 μg/mL)	Penicillin or amoxicillin	Erythromycin, respiratory fluoroquinolone
Intermediate penicillin resistance (MIC 0.1–2.0 μg/mL)	Parenteral penicillin or ceftriaxone	Respiratory fluoroquinolone
Highly penicillin resistant (MIC >2.0 μg/mL)	Ceftriaxone, cefotaxime (based on susceptibilities)	Vancomycin, respiratory fluoroquinolone
Legionellosis	Erythromycin or second-generation macrolide	Respiratory fluoroquinolone
Haemophilus influenzae, Moraxella catarrhalis	Second-generation cephalosporin	Second-generation macrolide, trimethoprim/sulfamethoxazole
Chlamydophila pneumoniae, Chlamydia psittaci, Mycoplasma pneumoniae	Doxycycline or erythromycin	Second-generation macrolide, respiratory fluoroquinolone
Staphylococcus aureus	Nafcillin	Vancomycin (if methicillin resistant); cefazolin
Klebsiella pneumoniae	Second- or third-generation cephalosporin	β-Lactam/β-lactamase inhibitor, fluoroquinolone
Streptococcus pyogenes	Penicillin	Cephalosporin, erythromycin
Coxiella burnetti (Q fever)	Doxycycline	Chloramphenicol
Mixed anaerobic/aerobic infection (aspiration)	Clindamycin	Penicillin plus metronidazole
Bordetella pertussis	Erythromycin or second-generation macrolide	Trimethoprim/sulfamethoxazole
Influenza A	Oseltamivir	Zanamivir

MIC, minimum inhibitory concentration.

clinical syndromes, and Table 52.3 describes the recommendations for specific pathogens.

Monitoring Therapy (6,25)

Clinical improvement is best indicated by improved vital signs. The PORT study validated temperature, respiratory rate, heart rate, and blood pressure as reliable measures of stability. On average, patients achieved "normal" vital signs at a median of 3 days after hospitalization. However, patients were often not completely "afebrile" (temperature <99°F) until day 6. Once patients reached clinical stability, indicated by normal vital signs along with a normal mental status and an ability to take oral medication, deterioration in clinical status was rare (<1%). Patients may be switched from intravenous to oral antibiotics when improvement is seen and may be safely discharged without further inpatient observation.

Repeating chest radiography at frequent intervals is wasteful if the patient is progressing well clinically. The clearing of radiologic findings often lags far behind clinical resolution; the continued presence of a slowly resolving infiltrate is neither a sign of poor response to therapy nor indicative of a serious prognosis. This is particularly true of pneumococcal or *Legionella* pneumonia, in which radiography may still show an infiltrate months later. However, when the patient's condition is worsening or fever is not resolving, radiographic examination is important for the detection of complications such as lung abscess and empyema. In addition, the possibility of unusual or resistant organisms should be considered in these patients and antibiotic therapy appropriately adjusted.

PATIENT EDUCATION (26–28)

Patients with lower respiratory tract infections need to be educated about their natural history. As stated, patients with acute bronchitis often have a persistent cough for 1 to 2 weeks. However, these patients usually show an overall improvement by the end of the first week. In patients with pneumonia, the recovery period is much longer. More than 50% of patients with pneumonia continue to report fatigue and cough 1 month after diagnosis. Patients with persistent symptoms often require more outpatient visits during follow-up.

Patients can monitor their temperature at home if they are being treated in the outpatient setting. Persistent fever, worsening respiratory status, and increasing confusion are reasons to seek medical attention. Patients who smoke should be strongly urged to quit if they have not already done so. In fact, this is an excellent opportunity to encourage patients to quit because many do at this time (see Chapter 54).

Patients who recover from community-acquired pneumonia are eligible to receive pneumococcal and influenza vaccinations. Patients who are elderly (older than 65 years), have congestive heart failure or obstructive lung disease, are immunosuppressed, or have undergone splenectomy are also candidates for vaccination (see Chapters 6 and 47). The *polyvalent pneumococcal vaccine* incorporates 23 capsular types of pneumococci, which together account for about 90% of cases of pneumococcal pneumonia in the United States. One-time revaccination after 5 years is recommended for immunosuppressed persons, patients with functional asplenia, and elderly persons who received the initial vaccination before age 65 years. The influenza vaccine, composed of a purified inactivated virus, is modified each year to include prevalent strains of influenza A and influenza B. Influenza vaccine should be offered to all patients older than age 50, pregnant women, and the high-risk groups mentioned previously. Hypersensitivity to eggs is a contraindication to influenza vaccination. The vaccines may be given at the same time without an increase in side effects or decrease in immunogenicity.

INDICATIONS FOR ADMISSION (29–31)

As mentioned previously, one of the most important decisions in the care of the patient with a community-acquired lower respiratory infection is selecting the proper setting for care. The decision is obvious in the case of a healthy young patient with an acute bronchitis or a seriously ill patient with overt respiratory compromise. In between are the many patients who are elderly or have underlying cardiopulmonary disease and present in the ambulatory setting with a lower respiratory tract infection; they are a source of concern.

Many studies have examined large numbers of patients with community-acquired pneumonia to determine predictors of poor outcome. Common predictors of worse outcome in these studies include advanced age, comorbidities, and abnormal vital signs. It is important to note that these trials often excluded immunosuppressed patients, who have an overall worse prognosis and are likely to require hospitalization. A useful prediction rule, known as the Pneumonia Severity Index (PSI), has been validated on more than 38,000 inpatients with pneumonia and the more than 2,200 patients of the PORT study (Fig. 52.1 and Table 52.4). Patients with none of the comorbidities or vital sign abnormalities indicated in Fig. 52.1 are assigned to class 1 (low risk). The remaining patients are assigned a point score based on the system given in Table 52.4. Patients with a PSI of less than 90 have a low mortality (<1%) and a low risk for deterioration (<6%) and may be considered for outpatient therapy. Another prediction rule is the CURB-65 rule. This acronym stands for confusion, uremia (blood urea nitrogen >20 mg/dL), respiratory rate greater than 30 per minute, blood pressure less than 90 mm Hg systolic or 60 mm Hg diastolic, and age 65 years or older. Mortality was low for patients with no or one risk factor (0.7% and 2.1%, respectively). Of course, any prediction rule does not replace clinical judgment; these rules perform poorly in extreme or unusual circumstances. For example, a 20-year-old man with hypotension,

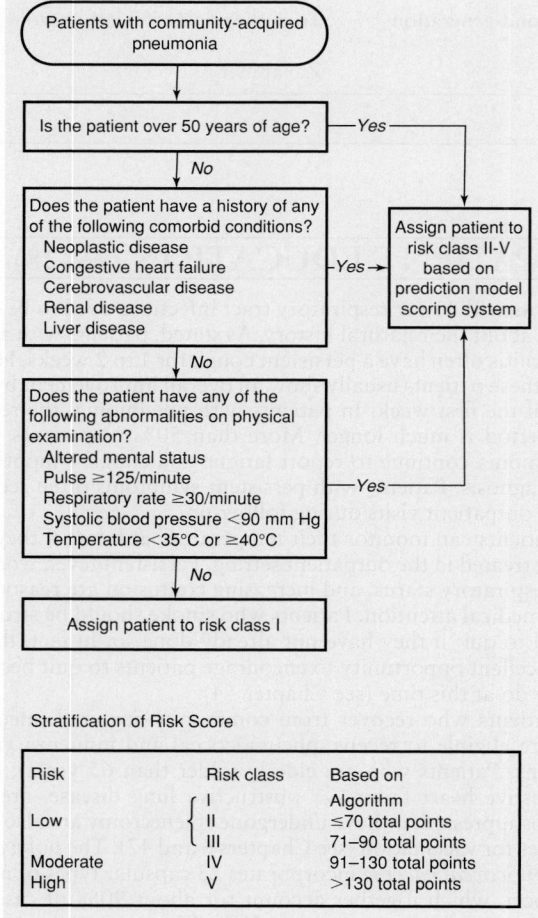

FIGURE 52.1. An algorithm for triage in patients with community-acquired pneumonia. (From Fine MJ, Auble TE, Yealy DM, et al. A prediction rule to identify low-risk patients with community-acquired pneumonia. N Engl J Med 1997;336:243, with permission.

TABLE 52.4

PNEUMONIA PORT SCORING

Patient Characteristic	Points Assigned[a]
Demographic Factors	
Age: male	Age (yr)
Age: female	Age (yr) − 10
Nursing home resident	+10
Comorbid Illnesses	
Neoplastic disease	+30
Liver disease	+20
Congestive heart failure	+10
Cerebrovascular disease	+10
Renal disease	+10
Physical Examination Findings	
Altered mental status	+20
Respiratory rate >30/min	+20
Systolic blood pressure <90 mm Hg	+20
Temperature <35°C or >40°C	+15
Pulse >125/min	+10
Laboratory Findings	
pH <7.35	+30
Blood urea nitrogen >10.7 mmol/L	+20
Sodium <130 mEq/L	+20
Glucose >13.9 mmol/L	+10
Hematocrit <30%	+10
Oxygen tension <60 mm Hg[b]	+10
Pleural effusion	+10

PORT, Patient Outcomes Research Trial.
[a]A risk score (total point score) for a given patient is obtained by summing the patient age in years (age minus 10 years for a female patient) and the points for each applicable patient characteristic.
[b]Oxygen saturation <90% also was considered abnormal.
Adapted from Fine MJ, Auble TE, Yealy DM, et al. A prediction rule to identify low-risk patients with community-acquired pneumonia, N Engl J Med 1997;336:243, with permission.

tachycardia, and hypoxia could have a low score but clearly requires hospitalization, if not intensive care.

In addition, the decision for hospitalization depends on the *quality of the home environment* and the *ability to tolerate* *oral therapy*. Alternative options, such as home intravenous therapy and subacute care facilities, have become increasingly practical and cost-effective, especially in the era of managed care.

Annotated Bibliography

1. Mandell LA, Winderlink RG, Anzueto A, et al. Infectious Diseases Society of America/American Thoracic Society consensus guidelines on the management of community-acquired pneumonia in adults. Clin Infect Dis 2007;44: S27. (*Joint guidelines from leading subspecialty societies.*)

2. Metlay JP, Fine MJ. Testing strategies in the initial management of patients with community-acquired pneumonia. Ann Intern Med 2003;138:109. (*A discussion of the predictive value of history, physical examination, and laboratory testing for diagnosis and prognosis in pneumonia.*)

3. Austrian R, Gold J. Pneumococcal bacteremia with special reference to bacteremic pneumococcal pneumonia. Ann Intern Med 1964;60:759. (*A classic study of clinical features and prognostic indicators in bacteremic pneumococcal pneumonia.*)

4. Fang GD, Fine M, Orloff J, et al. New and emerging etiologies for community-acquired pneumonia with implications for therapy. Medicine (Baltimore) 1990;69:307. (*Despite aggressive diagnostic workup, only 59% of patients with community-acquired pneumonia had an identifiable cause; Legionella was the third-most-common pathogen.*)

5. Woodhead MA, MacFarlane JT, McCracken JS, et al. Prospective study of the aetiology and outcome of pneumonia in the community. Lancet 1987;1:671. (*A British study, finding that Pneumococcus was the most frequent pathogen, identified in 36% of cases; Haemophilus influenzae accounted for 10% of cases; no cause was identified in 45% of cases; mortality was 3%.*)

6. Jay SJ, Johannson WG, Pierce AK. The radiographic resolution of Streptococcus pneumoniae pneumonia. N Engl J Med 1975;293:798. (*A classic study showing that delayed resolution of radiographic abnormalities is typical.*)

7. Ruiz-Gonzalez, A, Falguera M, Nogues A, et al. Is Streptococcus pneumoniae the leading cause of pneumonia of unknown etiology? A microbiologic study of lung aspirates in consecutive patients with community-acquired pneumonia. Am J Med 1999;106:385. (*This organism accounted for 25% of all cases and for 33% of cases of otherwise unknown cause.*)

8. Wright SW, Edwards KM, Decker MD, et al. Pertussis infection in adults with a persistent cough. JAMA 1995;273:1044. (*An emergency department–based study, finding that 21% of patients with cough lasting >2 weeks had evidence of pertussis infection.*)

9. Mayer RD. Legionella infections: a review of 5 years of research. Rev Infect Dis 1983;5:258. (*An excellent overview of the epidemiology, pathogenesis, diagnosis, and management of this important infection.*)

10. Plouffe JF, File TM, Breiman RF, et al. Reevaluation of the definition of Legionnaires' disease: use of the urinary antigen assay. Clin Infect Dis 1995;20:1286. (*Urinary antigen was detected in 56% of all cases and was highly specific.*)

11. Mansel JK, Rosenow EC, Smith TE, et al. Mycoplasma pneumoniae pneumonia. Chest 1989;95:639. (*An excellent review of this important cause of atypical pneumonia.*)

12. Marrie TJ, Grayston JT, Wang SP, et al. Pneumonia associated with the TWAR strain of Chlamydia. Ann Intern Med 1987;106:507. (*A study showing that TWAR can cause serious pneumonia in older patients in addition to mild acute respiratory disease in younger ones.*)

13. Metersky ML, Ma A, Bratzler DW, et al. Predicting bacteremia in patients with community-acquired pneumonia. Am J Respir Crit Care Med 2004;169:342. (*A prediction rule was developed in a large Medicare database; predictive factors include vital sign abnormalities, liver disease, hyponatremia, and high or low white blood cell count.*)

14. Garcia-Vazquez E, Angeles Marcos M, Mensa J, et al. Assessment of the usefulness of sputum culture for diagnosis of community-acquired pneumonia using the PORT predictive scoring system. Arch Intern Med 2004; 164:1807. (*A study from Barcelona of 1,669 patients with pneumonia; adequate sputum sample was obtained from 32%, and the specificity of Gram's stain for Streptococcus pneumoniae or H. influenzae was excellent; the severity of pneumonia did not influence yield.*)

15. Hueston WJ. Albuterol delivered by metered-dose inhaler to treat acute bronchitis. J Family Pract 1994;39:437. (*A small, blinded, placebo-controlled trial showed a significant resolution of cough at 7 days.*)

16. Smucny J, Becker L, Glazier R. Beta2-agonists for acute bronchitis (Cochrane review). In: The Cochrane library, Issue 4. Oxford: Update Software, 2007. (*A systematic review of five trials, suggesting that any benefit is limited to patients with evidence of airway obstruction; no benefit was found in most; see http://www.cochrane.org for updates.*)

17. Evans AT, Husain S, Durairaj L, et al. Azithromycin for acute bronchitis: a randomized, double-blind controlled trial. Lancet 2002;359:1648. (*No benefit was demonstrated.*)

18. Bent S, Saint S, Vittinghoff E, et al. Antibiotics in acute bronchitis: a meta-analysis. Am J Med 1999;107:62. (*A meta-analysis finding a small benefit, insufficient to justify use.*)

19. Fahey T, Stocks N, Thomas T. Quantitative systematic review of randomised controlled trials comparing antibiotic with placebo for acute cough in adults. BMJ 1998;316:906. (*Another meta-analysis, examining many of the same studies as in ref. 18; finds no effect of antibiotics on cough or course of illness.*)

20. Gonzales R, Steiner JF, Sande MA. Antibiotic prescribing for adults with colds, upper respiratory tract infections, and bronchitis by ambulatory care physicians. JAMA 1997;278:901. (*Antibiotics were prescribed to 51% of patients with a cold, 52% with upper respiratory infection, and 66% with acute bronchitis; rates were higher among women and lower among African Americans.*)

21. Fahey T, Smucny J, Becker L, et al. Antibiotics for acute bronchitis (Cochrane review). In: The Cochrane library, Issue 4. Oxford: Update Software, 2007. (*A systematic review of nine trials with >750 patients, showing a modest benefit in symptom relief and duration, but potential harms of treatment may negate this; see http://www.cochrane.org for updates.*)

22. Whitney CG, Farley MM, Hadler J, et al. Increasing prevalence of multidrug-resistant Streptococcus pneumoniae in the United States. N Engl J Med 2000;343:1917. (*A national database of invasive pneumococcal strains, showing a 24% prevalence of penicillin resistance and increasing multidrug resistance.*)

23. Dimopoulos G, Siempos II, Korbila IP, et al. Comparison of first-line with second-line antibiotics for acute exacerbations of chronic bronchitis: a meta-analysis of randomized controlled trials. Chest 2007;132:447. (*A meta-analysis of 12 randomized, controlled trials, showing a lower success rate [odds ratio, 0.51] with first-line agents [ampicillin, trimethoprim-sulfamethoxazole, doxycycline] than with second-line agents [amoxicillin/clavulanic acid, second-generation macrolides, second-generation or third-generation cephalosporins, and quinolones].*)

24. Kyaw MH, Lynfield R, Schaffner W, et al. Effect of introduction of the pneumococcal conjugate vaccine on drug-resistant Streptococcus pneumoniae. N Engl J Med 2006;354:1455. (*Rates of invasive pneumococcal infection decreased by 57% following introduction of the vaccine, and a decrease in penicillin resistance was seen as well.*)

25. Halm EA, Fine MJ, Marrie TJ, et al. Time to clinical stability in patients hospitalized with community-acquired pneumonia: implications for practice guidelines. JAMA 1998;279:1452. (*Most patients reached clinical "stability" by day 3 of hospitalization, and normalized vital signs were a valid basis for a discharge decision.*)

26. Gonzales R, Steiner JF, Lum A, et al. Decreasing antibiotic use in ambulatory practice: impact of a multidimensional intervention on the treatment of uncomplicated acute bronchitis in adults. JAMA 1999;281:1512. (*Patient education and academic detailing reduced prescription rates from 74% to 48%.*)

27. Anonymous. Prevention of pneumococcal disease: recommendations of the Advisory Committee on Immunization Practices (ACIP). MMWR Morb Mortal Wkly Rep 1997;46(RR-8):1. (*Guideline for pneumococcal vaccination, with a new emphasis on revaccination.*)

28. Sims RV, Steinmann WC, McConville JH, et al. The clinical effectiveness of pneumococcal vaccine in the elderly. Ann Intern Med 1988;108:653. (*Documents a 70% efficacy in the elderly.*)

29. Fine MJ, Auble TE, Yealy DM, et al. A prediction rule to identify low-risk patients with community-acquired pneumonia. N Engl J Med 1997;336:243. (*A prediction rule, prospectively validated on >40,000 patients, accurately predicted a low-risk group with a 30-day mortality of <1%.*)

30. Lim WS, van der Eerden MM, Laing R, et al. Defining community-acquired pneumonia severity on presentation to the hospital: an international derivation study. Thorax 2003; 58:377. (*A study of >1,000 inpatients with community-acquired pneumonia, developed and validated the CURB-65 rule; a low score [0 or 1] predicted a 30-day mortality of 1.5%.*)

31. Aujesky D, Auble TE, Yealy DM et al. Prospective comparison of three validated prediction rules for prognosis in community-acquired pneumonia. Am J Med 2005; 118:384. (*A prospective, multicenter study that compared the Pneumonia Severity Index and the CURB-65 prediction rules; both rules accurately identified low-risk patients suitable for outpatient treatment.*)

CHAPTER 53 ■ APPROACH TO THE PATIENT WITH LUNG CANCER

JEFFREY W. CLARK

Lung cancer is the leading cause of cancer deaths world wide. It is the most common cause of cancer death among both men and women in the United States, with more than 160,000 deaths per year. It is estimated that cigarette smoking accounts for greater than 85% of lung cancers (see Chapter 54). Once it has metastasized, lung cancer has a poor prognosis. Overall, only approximately 15% of lung cancer patients are alive after 5 years. Thus it is critical that the primary physician be skilled in prevention, especially in informing individuals of the grave dangers of tobacco use (see Chapter 54). The physician should also be alert to early signs of lung cancer (see Chapters 41, 42, and 44), capable of conducting the workup, staging, and monitoring of the disease, and knowledgeable about treatment options and their effects on survival and quality of life.

PATHOLOGY, CLINICAL PRESENTATION, AND COURSE (1–4)

The common types of bronchogenic carcinoma are designated as squamous cell, adenocarcinoma, large cell, and small cell. Each has its own epidemiologic and clinical characteristics. With the exception of small-cell disease, they share a similar natural history and response to therapy, although several recent studies suggest some differences in response to therapy that are important especially in considering adjuvant treatment. Given the overall similar clinical behavior of non–small-cell lung cancers, lung cancers are often classified as small-cell lung cancer (SCLC) and non–small-cell lung cancer (NSCLC).

Small-Cell Lung Cancer

Small-cell lung cancer accounts for less than 20% of cases. It is typically central in location. Growth is rapid, with 50% to 75% of patients manifesting evidence of metastatic disease beyond the chest at the time of clinical presentation and initial staging. These tumors derive from endocrine cells of the bronchial mucosa and can produce a variety of paraneoplastic syndromes (see Chapter 92). Untreated, the course of illness is rapid, with a median survival of only a few months. However, these tumors tend to be very responsive to chemotherapy (see later discussion).

Non–Small-Cell Lung Cancer

One fourth to one third of patients with NSCLC present with localized disease (stages I and II). Another one fourth to one third have locally or regionally advanced disease (stages IIIa and IIIb), and one third to one half present with advanced disease and distant metastases (stage IV). Survival is a function of stage at the time of presentation, with nearly 40% of the first group surviving 5 years, 7% of the second group, and fewer than 1% of patients in the last group (Table 53.1). Overall survival for all patients is approximately 13%.

Adenocarcinomas have become the most common lung cancers and make up a higher percentage of the carcinomas in women. Many present peripherally. They sometimes arise in areas of fibrosis secondary to prior pulmonary parenchymal damage. Cancers of this cell type are less closely associated with smoking than others.

Squamous cell (*epidermoid*) *carcinoma* is the second-most-common lung cancer. Like most other bronchogenic carcinomas, it is strongly associated with smoking. Most of these tumors occur centrally and can produce bronchial obstruction. They tend to ulcerate and may cause bleeding.

Undifferentiated large-cell carcinomas are, in most instances, probably a form of adenocarcinoma. Unlike well-differentiated adenocarcinomas, they are often centrally located and bronchoscopically visible as an endobronchial mass lesion. These cancers tend to metastasize hematogenously relatively early, leading to disease in the bones, liver, and brain.

Clinical Presentation

Clinical presentation is partially a function of tumor location; *central endobronchial* lesions may produce symptoms early in the course of illness. *Hemoptysis, cough, sputum production*, and a *localized wheeze* are among the symptoms reported in early phases; however, the frequency with which these symptoms are noted in early stages of disease is low. Hemoptysis occurs as a presenting symptom in only 7% to 10% of patients with lung cancer, although up to 40% will report hemoptysis at some time in their illness. Rarely, a systemic syndrome, such as hypertrophic osteoarthropathy (see Chapter 45), peripheral neuropathy, or inappropriate secretion of antidiuretic hormone, may precede other evidence of disease (see Chapter 92). Symptoms of *advanced disease* include *anorexia, weight loss, nausea* and *vomiting, hoarseness* (recurrent laryngeal nerve involvement), *pleuritic chest pain, bone pain*, and *neurologic deficits*.

In patients who present with metastasis or in whom metastasis later develops, the most frequently involved sites include local or regional *lymph nodes* within the chest (25% to 45%), liver (30% to 45%), *bone* and *bone marrow* (20% to 40%), and *central nervous system* (20% to 35%).

TABLE 53.1

STAGING AND SURVIVAL IN NON–SMALL-CELL LUNG CANCER

Stage	Tumor	Nodes	Metastases	Five-Year Survival
I	T1 or T2	N0	M0	50%
II	T1 or T2	N1	M0	30%
IIIa	T1-2 or T3	N1 or N0	M0	15%
IIIb	Any T	Any N	M0	<5%
IV	Any T	Any N	M1	0%

Staging for small-cell lung cancer is designed as either "limited disease" (confined to the thorax) or "extensive disease" (metastasis outside the thorax).
T1, lesions ≤3 cm in diameter; T2, lesions >3 cm; T3, invasion of mediastinum, diaphragm, or chest wall; T4, invasion of heart, great vessels, or malignant pleural effusion; N0, no nodal involvement; N1, tracheobronchial or hilar node involvement; N2, ipsilateral mediastinal nodes; N3, contralateral or supraclavicular nodes; M0, no metastasis; M1, systemic metastasis.
Adapted from Mountain CF. A new international staging system for lung cancer. Chest 1986;89(Suppl 4): 225S, with permission.

Clinical Course and Prognosis

Overall 5-year survival remains less than 15%. The poor prognosis is related in large part to the advanced stage of disease at the time of diagnosis. Unfortunately, local and regional disease is most often asymptomatic. The median overall survival for patients with lung cancer is less than 12 months. Important exceptions to these dim statistics exist, however—in particular, the improved survival for patients with SCLC with systemic therapy and those with NSCLC whose tumors are surgically resectable.

As noted earlier, the clinical course is different for SCLC and NSCLC. For NSCLC, clinical course and survival are a function of the surgical pathologic stage. The staging scheme for *NSCLC* utilizes the tumor–node–metastasis (TNM) system to reflect prognostic subgroups (see Table 53.1 and Chapter 86). A new staging system that better defines specific subsets of patients has been developed with plans to introduce it in 2009. Survival improves markedly with surgical resectability. For example, patients whose disease is confined to the lung (stage I) have a 5-year survival approaching 50%. With involvement of the hilar and mediastinal lymph nodes, survival rates decrease significantly but less so than was previously believed if complete tumor resection is achieved. Unfortunately, only a small minority of patients present with surgically curable disease. Screening efforts have failed to provide satisfactory early detection (see Chapter 37). Ongoing studies are reevaluating the potential role of spiral computed tomography (CT) or chest x-ray in the screening of high-risk individuals.

SCLC differs substantially from NSCLC in how it is staged, being divided into *localized* and *extensive* groups. This is because treatment is defined based on these two subgroups. Before the advent of contemporary chemotherapy, median survival was 1 to 3 months; it has increased severalfold to 10 to 24 months, depending on the extent of disease, with a median of 16–24 months for those with localized disease and 10–14 months for those with extensive disease. Five-year survival remains poor (5% to 10%) because of the high probability of metastasis, even among those who present with limited disease.

WORKUP AND STAGING (4,5)

The basic approach to diagnosis and staging is to begin with noninvasive studies and proceed to increasingly invasive studies only as necessary. Staging is performed to determine prognosis and treatment and, in particular, to assess the resectability of the tumor. Computed tomography and positron emission tomography (PET) have greatly facilitated the noninvasive assessment of hilar and mediastinal node involvement. Invasive studies should be considered only if the results will alter treatment plans. Many patients with lung cancer have concurrent chronic lung disease and may be seriously compromised by a complication of an invasive study. The histopathologic diagnosis of lung cancer may be obtained with a variety of procedures, ranging from sputum cytology to thoracotomy (see Chapters 37 and 44).

DIAGNOSIS (4)

Chest radiography is usually the initial diagnostic modality, although increasingly lesions are initially diagnosed by CT scans; the appearance of the lesion and its doubling time are helpful in distinguishing benign from malignant disease. Although the detection of lesions as small as 3 mm has been reported, most lesions are not visible until they are at least 5 mm or more in diameter. The finding of a calcified nodule can be helpful, especially if the pattern of calcification is eccentric (see Chapter 44).

Chest CT aids diagnosis by confirming the presence of a suspected lung lesion. As CT procedures have improved, the ability to detect smaller lesions has increased. CT has become critical to staging by determining the presence and extent of hilar and mediastinal node involvement (see later discussion).

PET scans can further aid in defining the nature of primary lung lesions and in defining the extent of disease to better plan therapy.

Sputum cytology may provide evidence of lung cancer and even cell type. Test sensitivity ranges from 25% to 75%, depending on the site of the tumor. Optimal collection requires obtaining three deep, first-morning samples. The presence of pulmonary histiocytes indicates an adequate specimen. A negative cytologic examination result does not rule out cancer, especially in patients with peripheral lesions.

The yield of cytologic testing can be greatly enhanced by the use of *fiberoptic bronchoscopy* complemented by *washings*, *brushings*, or *forceps biopsy*. With centrally located, visualized lesions, washings provide a diagnosis in nearly 80% of instances; for brushings, the yield is 92%, and for forceps biopsy, it is 93%. The yield falls in the case of peripheral lesions; it is 20% to 30% for peripheral lesions less than 3 cm in diameter and about 40% to 70% for those larger than 3 cm. The complication rate is low in experienced hands, with hypoxemia, hemorrhage, pneumothorax, or laryngospasm occurring in 0.1% to 0.3% of cases. On occasion, *transbronchial biopsy* is deemed the best means of establishing the diagnosis (e.g., in suspected alveolar cell carcinoma; see Chapter 51). The risk for pneumothorax rises to 5%.

With peripheral lesions, *percutaneous transthoracic fine-needle biopsy*—usually guided by CT—has proved to be accurate in the diagnosis of lung cancers. Reports on the diagnostic accuracy of these radiologically guided procedures quote sensitivity of greater than 90% and specificity of greater than 95% when they are performed by skilled radiologists using "fine-needle" techniques that allow not only aspiration, but also the removal of a tiny core of material. However, sensitivity and specificity may be compromised by the occasional inadequacy of the specimen obtained, which is sometimes an aspirate of cytologic material rather than a solid core of tissue; in such instances, the architectural relationships may be obscured or unavailable in cytologic specimens. Pneumothorax ensues in close to 30%, but it is usually small, of little clinical consequence, and resolves spontaneously without the need for a chest tube. Hemorrhage is rare unless a vascular lesion is sampled. For patients with limited pulmonary reserve, who may be unable to tolerate any degree of pneumothorax, a video-assisted thoracotomy procedure to obtain tissue may be preferable to needle aspiration. Video-assisted thoracotomy is also useful for lesions that may be difficult to sample percutaneously.

The biopsy of suspected metastatic lesions, such as Scalene nodes, is indicated when these lesions are readily accessible for biopsy; it can save the patient extensive testing for both diagnosis and staging.

STAGING (5)

Staging is performed to determine the prognosis and select therapy. For NSCLC, the principal challenge is to assess surgical candidacy, which requires an accurate evaluation of hilar and mediastinal lymph nodes. The challenge is to evaluate the regional nodes accurately. This usually requires a combination of CT-PET (or CT + PET) and mediastinoscopy (see later discussion). For small-cell lung cancer, staging is necessary to separate patients with localized disease and therefore candidates for combined modality therapy with both radiation and chemotherapy with a small chance for long-term survival from those with extensive disease who should be treated with chemotherapy alone (see latter for discussion of prophylactic cranial irradiation). It is important that, whenever possible, the evaluation of patients is done by consultation with a multidisciplinary team including medical oncologist, thoracic surgeon, radiation oncologist, and pulmonologist.

Chest radiography has largely been replaced by *chest CT* for evaluation of patients with NSCLC.

Chest CT with contrast has been used extensively to improve the sensitivity of radiologic staging. Although the sensitivity and specificity of CT in the diagnosis of mediastinal disease appear to be reasonable for patients with clinical stage I disease who have a lung lesion larger than 3 cm (T2, N0, M0; see Table 53.1 for staging terminology), results for those with earlier stage I disease (T1, N0, M0; lung nodule <3 cm) have been disappointing. False-positive and false-negative rates of 5% to 10% have been reported for the diagnosis of contralat-

eral mediastinal node involvement in such patients. Potential surgical candidacy should not be based solely on the basis of a result of CT. For patients with a pulmonary lesion larger than 3 cm, CT with contrast continues to be a useful noninvasive step for assessing the hilum and mediastinum, but a negative CT result does not rule out microscopic spread from central or late peripheral lesions.

CT is sensitive for the detection of metastasis below the diaphragm (to the liver and adrenals), and upper abdominal views should always be obtained at the time of chest CT. Positive findings, confirmed by needle biopsy, would indicate stage IV disease, for which surgery is inappropriate.

For judging tumor involvement of the chest wall, magnetic resonance imaging (MRI) is superior to CT. MRI is also better for assessing disease in the superior sulcus and defining subcarinal nodal involvement, and it should be part of the staging in this setting.

PET scanning, and, more recently, combined *CT-PET scans,* can show metastatic disease not detected by CT. This is helpful in determining patients who might not be surgical candidates because of distant metastases. The role of CT-PET in mediastinal staging continues to evolve as technological improvements enhance its sensitivity and specificity.

Symptomatic metastasis to the head is relatively common for patients with more advanced disease, and *brain MRI* is usually part of the staging for patients with stage IIA disease with nonsquamous histology and all stage IIB or higher patients (see Chapter 86). Although metastases can also occur to bone, *bone scan* is usually only indicated in the setting of evaluations of symptoms.

Pulmonary function tests are important in evaluating the potential ability of the patient to tolerate surgery.

More-invasive staging techniques are indicated when the patient's surgical candidacy remains in question after CT-PET or CT + PET. In general, all patients (except potentially those with small [T1] peripheral lesions who have a very small likelihood of having positive mediastinal lymph nodes) should undergo *mediastinoscopy* for the evaluation of the mediastinum and hilum before thoracotomy because the presence of microscopic tumor is important in determining the specific treatment approach. In general, patients with involvement of contralateral lymph nodes are not surgical candidates. Under general anesthesia, a cervical incision is made and mediastinal node biopsy is carried out under direct visualization. Efforts to improve mediastinal staging, such as by technological improvements in CT and PET scanning, continue.

Advances in the techniques of needle biopsy and fiberoptic endoscopy have enhanced the roles of *transthoracic* and *transbronchial needle aspiration biopsy* in the staging of lung cancer. These techniques offer a less morbid alternative to mediastinoscopy for the tissue-based assessment of mediastinal spread. They do not require general anesthesia or a formal surgical procedure and can be performed under CT guidance.

The rest of staging is determined by the tumor cell type. For patients with inoperable *NSCLC,* further staging is guided by the presence of symptoms that might necessitate therapy for a specific lesion (e.g., radiation therapy for a symptomatic bone metastasis).

Staging is considerably different for patients with *SCLC.* The issue is extent of disease rather than resectability. The goal is to distinguish between limited and extensive disease (the latter implies spread beyond the hemithorax of origin and regional nodes). Given the frequency of systemic disease at presentation, *CT scans, bone scans,* and *head MRI* are all components of initial staging. Patients who have evidence of possible bone marrow invasion (e.g., thrombocytopenia, neutropenia, or nucleated red blood cells on peripheral smear) should have a bone marrow biopsy. Diagnostic thoracentesis should be done if a pleural effusion is present.

PRINCIPLES OF MANAGEMENT (6–35)

Small-Cell Disease (6–16)

Small-cell disease is biologically unique among bronchogenic cancers in that the cells are much more sensitive to chemotherapy and radiation, probably in part because of their rapid rate of proliferation. Surgical treatment is usually not possible because 85% of patients have extensive disease at the time of presentation. For patients with very early disease (stage I, clinically T1-2, N0) surgical resection should be considered. For these patients, preoperative mediastinal staging is required. These patients should then receive postoperative adjuvant chemotherapy or combined chemotherapy and mediastinal radiation therapy as appropriate, depending on nodal status. For all other patients, irrespective of whether disease is limited to the chest or disseminated, the treatment of choice is *combination chemotherapy*. For patients with limited disease, concurrent *radiation* is given as adjunctive therapy. As noted previously, survival irrespective of stage has been prolonged fourfold to fivefold by chemotherapy. However, cure rates remain low. Only about 10% of limited-stage patients survive 5 years, and those who survive 2 years have a greater than two thirds chance of relapse. The majority of patients with extensive disease die within 2 years.

Chemotherapy

Since the introduction of combination chemotherapy in the 1970s, survival rates have improved modestly, and considerable progress has been made in reducing treatment morbidity, complexity, and duration. The use of *etoposide* plus *cisplatin* (or *carboplatin*) has improved survival. Shorter courses of therapy (no more than 4 to 6 months) are standard; longer courses are without additional benefit. The combination of irinotecan and cisplatin is also active and an option for patients with extensive stage disease.

Radiation

Patients with limited disease show a high response rate to irradiation. Survival appears to improve when concurrent radiation is used as an adjunct to chemotherapy, although toxicity increases. Prophylactic cranial radiation (PCI) decreases the risk for clinical brain metastases. Cranial irradiation among patients in complete remission has been shown to produce a modest reduction in the relative risk for death and for recurrence. A recent study suggested that PCI is also beneficial in decreasing the incidence of brain metastasis and improving failure-free and overall survival in patients with extensive stage SCLC who have responded to systemic chemotherapy.

Surgery

Surgery has a very limited role in SCLC for only those patients detected with very early stage disease (see prior discussion) because of the nearly universal occurrence of occult disease beyond the initial lesion.

Non–Small-Cell Disease (6–8,16–30)

Surgery

Surgery offers the only possibility for cure. About 35% to 45% of patients presenting with NSCLC have potentially resectable disease, but only 60% of this group have a successful resection. For the latter group, the 5-year survival or cure rate ranges from 25% to 40%. Thus, at best, fewer than 15% of patients who present with NSCLC can expect a cure. Patients with localized disease are being treated with less radical, more conservative surgery, often utilizing video-assisted thoracotomies. The goal is to preserve as much functional lung tissue as possible, especially in patients with underlying lung disease. Previously, pneumonectomy was performed in more than 70% of patients and included hilar in addition to mediastinal lymph nodes. A regional excision that employs wedge or segmental resection for stage I peripheral lobe lesions is now preferred. The general surgical dictum is to employ the minimal degree of surgery necessary to remove all macroscopic evidence of tumor with clear negative margins. Patients with more extensive disease (e.g., stage IIIA and the subset of IIIB patients who are resectable) require more extensive surgery including mediastinal lymph node dissection. These patients may be treated with preoperative "neoadjuvant" chemotherapy and radiation therapy. Decisions on the most appropriate sequencing of therapy requires close cooperation of a multidisciplinary team approach to these patients. Surgical excision is particularly indicated for nodules with long doubling times or long disease-free intervals, especially if the nodules are solitary and are not associated with extrathoracic disease.

Radiation Therapy

Radiation therapy is used for both curative intent and palliation. Preoperative radiation therapy (in combination with chemotherapy; see later discussion) may promote the resectability of tumors and probably increases survival rates for patients with stage IIIA or IIIB disease. In patients with tumors of the superior sulcus, preoperative radiation therapy has improved the likelihood of cure despite the contiguous extension of such tumors to bone or the chest wall. In general, when surgery is used in combination with prior radiation, the resection must usually be a pneumonectomy, and, in principle, all sites that were diseased before the radiation therapy must be resected.

When radiation is used as sole therapy with a *curative intent*, results have been disappointing. In general, patients with NSCLC respond poorly to irradiation as a curative therapy, but good intrathoracic control of tumor, even eradication, can be achieved. In a major randomized trial of definitive radiation therapy for patients with unresectable stage III cancer, higher rates of regression and better disease control in the chest were observed with the use of high-dose therapy (60 Gy). However, no improvement was noted in baseline 5-year survival, which remained at 5%. Although radiation may achieve local control, it does not prevent subsequent progression of distant metastases. This has led to attempts to combine chemotherapy with irradiation (see later discussion).

Chemotherapy

Although chemotherapy produces lower response rates in NSCLC than in SCLC, studies over the last decade have established the importance of chemotherapy in both the adjuvant (or neoadjuvant) and metastatic disease settings. It has been used as neoadjuvant therapy before surgery in patients with extensive but surgically resectable disease (e.g., stage III), adjuvantly after surgery, and in patients with inoperable disease, either alone or in combination with radiation therapy. The goals are to improve local control and decrease the risk for distant metastasis. Overall results have been modest, but improvements in survival are seen with platinum-based chemotherapy compounds. Combination chemotherapy regimens, most commonly *cisplatin-* or carboplatin-based therapy, usually in combination with a taxane (paclitaxel or docetaxel), have provided a modest survival advantage as compared with single-agent therapy, and when possible, combination chemotherapy approaches are generally preferred (see Chapter 88). A meta-analysis of trials comparing surgery with surgery plus chemotherapy showed a relative reduction in short-term mortality risk of 13%, which produced an absolute mortality reduction of 5% at 5 years. The same meta-analysis included trials comparing radical radiotherapy with radical radiotherapy plus chemotherapy. Again, the relative reduction in short-term mortality risk was 13%; this produced an absolute mortality reduction of 4% at 2 years. Cisplatin-based (or carboplatin-based) chemotherapy regimens have also produced some improvement in survival (improvements of median survival measured in months) for patients with stage IV disease. A number of other chemotherapeutic agents, including navelbine, gemcitabine, and camptothecin analogues (e.g., irinotecan) have meaningful activity against NSCLC and may also be used in treatment. Overall, approximately 30% to 40% of patients with metastatic disease treated with combination chemotherapy are alive at 1 year. Like all decisions in medicine, the benefits in the improvement in survival have to be weighed against the risks of drug-induced morbidity. Patients with poor performance status (e.g., 3 to 4) are often not candidates for chemotherapy. Further refinement of chemotherapy and its use in combined-modality programs offers promise, but much work remains to be done. As discussed later for epidermal growth factor receptor inhibitors (such as erlotinib), as more is learned about the biology of specific tumors, there is an extensive ongoing effort to tailor therapy for patients with specific subsets of tumors that are likely to benefit while not exposing the majority of patients that will not benefit to the toxicity of the agent(s).

Molecularly targeted agents are now approved for the treatment of patients with NSCLC. The first of these to be approved were the epidermal growth factor receptor (EGFR) inhibitors gefitinib (Iressa) and erlotinib (Tarceva). Although overall response rates are relatively low for metastatic disease (approximately 11%), a growing body of evidence suggests that individuals who have a mutation in the EGFR gene are significantly more likely to respond than are those without mutations, allowing for the selection of patients who are likely to respond. This has led to ongoing trials of initial therapy with EGFR inhibitors in patients with mutations as a potential approach to therapy that might provide enhanced efficacy while sparing them the potential toxicities of chemotherapeutic agents. This raises the potential that therapy can be tailored for individuals based on the specific genetic makeup of their tumor, which has been one of the long-sought objectives of medical oncology. Studies are evaluating this approach in newly diagnosed patients. It appears that patients with bronchiolar alveolar carcinoma and adenocarcinoma, both of which are more common in women, are more likely to have the mutation than those with other histologic types of NSCLC. The major toxicity of this class of agents is an acneiform rash, which can be extensive and require aggressive treatment. The monoclonal antibody ECFR inhibitor, cefuximab, used in combination with chemotherapy, improves survival of patients whose tumors do not have k-ras mutations and is being considered by the FDA for approval for

this purpose. The second class of molecularly targeted agent that has been approved for use in the treatment of patients with metastatic NSCLC in combination with chemotherapy is the vascular endothelial growth factor inhibitor bevacizumab. Although it has limited activity as a single agent, it enhances the effectiveness of at least certain chemotherapy combinations and has been approved based on phase III study showing a survival advantage for patients who received chemotherapy combined with bevacizumab over those receiving the chemotherapy alone.

Management of Stage III Disease

The management of stage III disease deserves special comment because the majority of patients with NSCLC present with advanced disease, and there is some debate about the best sequencing of therapies in specific patients with stage III disease. Although the overall prognosis remains guarded for these patients, there is improved survival associated with multimodality therapy (neoadjuvant chemotherapy and radiation therapy followed by surgical resection) of stage IIIA and a subset of patients with IIIB disease and with the concurrent administration of cisplatin-based chemotherapy and radiotherapy for those patients with stage III disease who are not surgical candidates. It is especially important that these patients be seen by a multidisciplinary team early in their evaluation so that the most appropriate treatment approach can be determined.

MONITORING

The potential benefit of monitoring of patients with surgically resectable and potentially curable lung cancer for sites of metastatic disease is somewhat limited because of the generally poor prognosis if metastasis occurs. Therefore, monitoring is primarily directed at searching for either isolated metastatic lesions that might be potentially resectable or new primary tumors that might be potentially curable if detected early in this population at high risk for the development of additional cancers. Chest radiography is indicated at regular intervals, ranging from every 4 months during the first 2 years and then every 12 months subsequently. Current National Comprehensive Cancer Network guidelines recommend spiral chest CT scans at 4 to 6 months postoperatively and then at 1 year and yearly after that. Routine monitoring for recurrent disease outside of the chest is unnecessary in the absence of specific symptoms suggesting bone, liver, or brain metastasis.

The monitoring of patients with extensive disease is directed at assessing the efficacy of therapy. One needs to select objective measures of tumor burden (see Chapter 86) that can be followed conveniently to gauge the response to treatment. CT scans of areas of known disease are most commonly used.

MANAGEMENT OF COMPLICATIONS (4,31–34)

Superior Vena Cava Syndrome

Obstruction of the superior vena cava by lung tumor produces the classic clinical syndrome of facial edema, proptosis, suffusion of the conjunctivae, and dilation of the veins of the upper thorax and neck. Asymptomatic neck vein distention is an early manifestation. In late stages, the patient may have relentless headache. In patients with lung cancer, the syndrome is invariably caused by tumor extending into the right side of the mediastinum and compressing the venous system adjacent to the mediastinal lymph nodes. The secondary effects of compression are thrombosis and tumor invasion; without treatment, neurologic function may be compromised. The histopathologic types of lung cancer that lead to the syndrome are variable, but most commonly the culprit is undifferentiated SCLC (see Chapter 92). Because superior vena cava syndrome may be the initial presentation of lung cancer, the issue of the need for tissue diagnosis is frequently encountered in this setting. When the result will change the mode of therapy, tissue diagnosis should be attempted, with care taken to minimize risk to the patient.

Even when a tissue diagnosis is not obtained, the response to radiotherapy is rather good; in unselected series, more than 70% of patients demonstrate a response. Although patients with superior vena cava syndrome secondary to lung cancer have an inoperable tumor, their prognosis is no worse than that of other patients with unresectable stage III lung cancer.

Malignant Pleural Effusion

Malignant pleural effusion is another important complication. It occurs in 10% to 15% of patients with carcinoma of the lung and may be secondary to direct pleural implantation or a consequence of mediastinal obstruction to lymphatic drainage of the pleural surface. Only 20% to 30% of pleural effusions that develop as a consequence of bronchogenic carcinoma are cytologically confirmed, and many are transudates. Pleural biopsy is often required for definitive diagnosis.

The effusion should be treated locally when it causes significant respiratory discomfort or pain. Radiation therapy to the mediastinum or to the pleura has been of limited effectiveness. Surgical drainage with an intrathoracic tube for 2 to 3 days may result in a secondary inflammatory response adequate to seal the pleural space. However, usually the use of intrapleural chemotherapeutic agents (e.g., bleomycin) or chemical irritants (e.g., doxycycline or talcum powder) is necessary and may be effective in 50% to 60% of patients. There is not a significant difference in efficacy between these agents.

Tumor Humoral Syndromes

Tumor humoral syndromes are associated with SCLC. Because the tumor is derived from endocrine cells of the bronchial mucosa, it is capable of producing adrenocorticotropic hormone, antidiuretic hormone, and even, on occasion, serotonin. The clinical pictures that may result are Cushing's syndrome, inappropriate secretion of antidiuretic hormone, and carcinoid syndrome, respectively.

Complications of Surgical Therapy

Complications of surgical therapy include prolonged air leakage from a bronchopleural fistula and postoperative intrapleural infection with development of empyema. Both are potentially serious and require prompt surgical attention. Pulmonary insufficiency is uncommon, thanks to the careful preoperative pulmonary evaluation of candidates for resection; however, pneumonia in the remaining lung can lead to respiratory compromise.

Complications of Chemotherapy

Complications of chemotherapy are related to the use of such agents as cisplatin or carboplatin, taxanes (paclitaxel or docetaxel), navelbine, irinotecan, gemcitabine, and erlotinib (see Chapter 88).

Complications of Radiation Therapy

Complications of radiation therapy include radiation pneumonitis, esophageal stricture, pericardial and myocardial fibrosis, rib fractures secondary to radiation-induced osteonecrosis, and radiation fibrosis, which can produce a long-term decrease in pulmonary function.

PATIENT EDUCATION (35)

Most lay persons believe that lung cancer is fatal. Although the prognosis and efficacy of treatment still require significant improvement for most types of lung cancer, the patient with a newly discovered, suspect pulmonary nodule needs to know that differences in prognosis can be significant, according to tissue type and stage of disease at the time of presentation. During the workup and staging, this background information can help to sustain patient and family through a worrisome period of uncertainty and provide a rationale for the procedures that need to be carried out.

Once the diagnosis and extent of disease are known, the prognosis and treatment options should be shared with the patient and family. When surgical cure is a genuine possibility and the patient can tolerate the surgery, it should be urged. However, in lung cancer, in which the prognosis is often poor, the treatment plans should be formulated jointly, and the patient's preferences and willingness to undergo treatment should be elicited and respected. A realistic assessment for the patient and family of prognosis and the pros and cons of treatment are essential for effective decision making. All too often, inappropriately aggressive forms of therapy are rushed into, mostly for the sake of "doing something." Clearly, these discussions should occur in collaboration with a medical oncologist and the rest of the multidisciplinary team.

Patients with incurable disease need to know their prognosis, which is best explained at a level of detail consistent with their desire to know. The news of lung cancer in a loved one is very upsetting to family members, who will try to shield the patient from the information. Facilitating communication among family, patient, and care givers is essential to preserving the patient's quality of life and helping the family to cope (see Chapter 87).

Annotated Bibliography

1. de la Monte SM, Hutchins GM, Moore GW. Paraneoplastic syndromes and constitutional symptoms in prediction of metastatic behavior of small cell carcinoma of the lung. Am J Med 1984;77:851. (*An autopsy series of 85 patients, indicating that patients with paraneoplastic syndromes had a more benign clinical course and less metastasis to the central nervous system.*)

2. Stupp R, Monnerat C, Turrisi AT 3rd, et al. Small cell lung cancer: state of the art and future perspectives. Lung Cancer 2004;45:105. (*An effective review.*)

3. Perez CA, Pajak TF, Rubin P, et al. Long-term observations of the pattern of failure in patients with unresectable non–oat-cell cancer of the lung treated with definitive radiotherapy: report by the Radiation Oncology Group.

Cancer 1987;59:1874. (*A major study, showing that disease control was good but survival was unaffected because of metastatic disease.*)

4. Beckles MA, Spiro SG, Colice GL, et al. Initial evaluation of the patient with lung cancer: symptoms, signs, laboratory tests, and paraneoplastic syndromes. Chest 2003;123(Suppl):97S. (*An effective review; the entire supplement of 29 articles and nearly 350 pages is devoted to all aspects of lung cancer.*)

5. Toloza EM, Harpole L, McCrory DC. Noninvasive staging of non–small cell lung cancer. Chest 2003;123(Suppl):137S. (*An effective review.*)

6. Greenberg ER, Chute CG, Stukel T, et al. Social and economic factors in the choice of lung cancer treatment. N Engl J Med 1988;318:612. (*When stage of illness was controlled for, patients of higher socioeconomic status tended to undergo more-aggressive therapy without evidence of improved survival.*)

7. Lin AY, Ihde DC. Recent developments in the treatment of lung cancer. JAMA 1992;267:1661. (*An excellent, authoritative, yet succinct review for the general reader; a good guide to the plethora of data from clinical trials; 33 references.*)

8. Montazeri A, Gillis CR, McEwan J. Quality of life in patients with lung cancer: a review of literature from 1970 to 1995. Chest 1998;113:467. (*Finds that the palliation of symptoms, psychosocial interventions, and the understanding of patients' feelings and concerns contribute to an improved quality of life.*)

9. Adjei AA, Marks RS, Bonner JA. Current guidelines for the management of small-cell lung cancer. Mayo Clin Proc 1999;74:809. (*An effective review.*)

10. Auperin A, Arrigada R, Pignon JP, et al. Prophylactic cranial irradiation for patients with small-cell lung cancer in complete remission. Prophylactic Cranial Irradiation Overview Collaborative Group. N Engl J Med 1999;341:476. (*The relative risk for recurrence or death was 0.75 among those in remission when treated with irradiation.*)

11. Turrisi AT 3rd, Kim K, Blum R, et al. Twice-daily compared with once-daily thoracic radiotherapy in limited small-cell lung cancer treated concurrently with cisplatin and etoposide. N Engl J Med 1999;340:265. (*Twice-daily dosing was associated with longer median survival than once-daily treatment— 23 vs. 19 months.*)

12. Johnson BE, Grayson J, Makuch RW, et al. Ten-year survival of patients with small-cell lung cancer treated with combination chemotherapy with or without irradiation. J Clin Oncol 1990;8:396. (*Presents the long-term experience of the National Cancer Institute in the treatment of small-cell lung cancer with chemotherapy.*)

13. Pignon JP, Arriagada R, Ihde DC, et al. A meta-analysis of thoracic radiotherapy for small-cell lung cancer. N Engl J Med 1992;327:1618. (*A modest improvement in survival was found among patients with limited disease treated with chemotherapy.*)

14. Agra Y, Pelayo M, Sacristan M, et al. Chemotherapy versus best supportive care for extensive small cell lung cancer (Cochrane review). In: The Cochrane library, Issue 3. Oxford: Update Software, 2004. (*Chemotherapy prolongs survival even in extensive disease; see* http://www.cochrane.org *for updates.*)

15. Slotman B, Faivre-Finn C, Kramer G, et al., for the EORTC Radiation Oncology Group and Lung Cancer Group. Prophylactic cranial irradiation in extensive small-cell lung cancer. N Engl J Med 2007;357(7):664. (*Prophylactic cranial irradiation reduces the incidence of symptomatic brain metastases and prolongs disease-free and overall survival.*)

16. Sun S, Schiller JH, Spinola M, et al. New molecularly targeted therapies for lung cancer. J Clin Invest 2007;117:2740. (*Reviews the clinical implications of the molecular pathogenesis of lung cancer.*)

17. Albain KS, Crowley JJ, Turrisi AT 3rd, et al. Concurrent cisplatin, etoposide, and chest radiotherapy in pathologic stage IIIB non–small-cell lung cancer: a Southwest Oncology Group phase II study, SWOG 9019. J Clin Oncol 2002;20:3454. (*The 5-year survival of 15% suggests the efficacy of the combined therapy approach.*)

18. Bunn PA, Vokes EE, Langer CJ, et al. An update on North American randomized studies in non–small cell lung cancer. Semin Oncol 1998;25:2. (*An effective update.*)

19. Mathur PN, Edell E, Sutedja T, et al. Treatment of early stage non–small cell lung cancer. Chest 2003;123(1 Suppl):176S. (*An effective review.*)

20. Robinson LA, Wagner H Jr, Ruckdeschel JC. Treatment of stage IIIA non–small cell lung cancer. Chest 2003;123(1 Suppl):202S. (*An effective review, pointing out that although significant controversy remains on the optimal therapy of stage IIIA disease, evidence from the review of multiple trials argues for multimodality therapy.*)

21. Errett LE, Wilson J, Chiu RCJ, et al. Wedge resection as an alternative procedure for peripheral bronchogenic carcinoma in poor-risk patients. J Thorac Cardiovasc Surg 1985;90:656. (*An example of the trend toward less-radical surgery in selected patients.*)

22. PORT Meta-analysis Trialists Group. Postoperative radiotherapy for non–small cell lung cancer (Cochrane review). In: The Cochrane library, Issue 3. Oxford: Update Software, 2004. (*Presents evidence of a detrimental effect on the survival of stage I and II non–small-cell lung cancer patients; there was no clear evidence that it was detrimental or beneficial in those with stage III, N2 disease; see* http://www.cochrane.org *for updates.*)

23. Rowell NP, Williams CJ. Radical radiotherapy for stage I/II non–small cell lung cancer in patients not sufficiently fit for or declining surgery (medically inoperable) (Cochrane review). In: The Cochrane library, Issue 3. Oxford: Update Software, 2004. (*The evidence is poor, but the suggestion is made that radical radiation early produces better results than later palliative radiation when surgery is contraindicated in early-stage disease; see* http://www.cochrane.org *for updates.*)

24. Hotta K, Matsuo K, Ueoka H, et al. Role of adjuvant chemotherapy in patients with resected non–small-cell lung cancer: reappraisal with a meta-analysis of randomized controlled trials. J Clin Oncol 2004;22:3860. (*A meta-analysis of 11 trials, showing a mortality hazard ratio of 0.87 for those who received adjuvant chemotherapy with surgery.*)

25. Keller SM, Adak S, Wagner H, et al. A randomized trial of postoperative adjuvant therapy in patients with completely resected stage II or IIIA non–small-cell lung cancer. Eastern Cooperative Oncology Group. N Engl J Med 2000;343:1217. (*The addition of chemotherapy to radiation did not improve overall survival.*)

26. Lynch T, Bell D, Sordella R, et al. Activating mutations in the epidermal growth factor receptor underlying responsiveness of non–small cell lung cancer to gefitinib. N Engl J Med 2004;350:2129. (*Mutations in epidermal growth factor receptor [EGFR] occur in a subset of lung cancer patients with adenocarcinoma or bronchoalveolar carcinoma and are associated with response to gefitinib therapy.*)

27. Non–small Cell Lung Cancer Collaborative Group. Chemotherapy for non–small cell lung cancer (Cochrane review). In: The Cochrane library, Issue 3. Oxford: Update Software, 2004. (*A meta-analysis of 52 trials with 9,387 patients, showing a relative risk reduction of death of 13% for chemotherapy plus external radiation therapy [XRT] vs. XRT alone, and a 27% relative risk reduction for chemotherapy vs. supportive care; see* http://www.cochrane.org *for updates.*)

28. Non–small Cell Lung Cancer Collaborative Group. Chemotherapy in non–small cell lung cancer: a meta-analysis using updated data on individual patients from 52 randomised clinical trials. BMJ 1995;311:899. (*The addition of chemotherapy to either surgery or radiotherapy afforded a modest benefit, with the relative risk for death consistently at 0.87.*)

29. Paez J, Janne P, Lee J, et al. EGFR mutations in lung cancer: correlation with clinical response to gefitinib therapy. Science 2004;3041:1497. (*Mutations in EGFR occur in a subset of lung cancer patients with adenocarcinoma or bronchoalveolar carcinoma and are associated with response to gefitinib therapy.*)

30. Pritchard RS, Anthony SP. Chemotherapy plus radiotherapy compared with radiotherapy alone in the treatment of locally advanced, unresectable, non–small-cell lung cancer. A meta-analysis. Ann Intern Med 1996;125:723. (*A modest reduction in relative mortality risk was found with chemotherapy added to radiotherapy.*)

31. Wilson LD, Detterbeck FC, Yahalom J. Superior vena cava syndrome with malignant causes. N Engl J Med 2007;356:1862. (*An effective review.*)

32. Shaw P, Agarwal R. Pleurodesis for malignant pleural effusions (Cochrane review). In: The Cochrane library, Issue 3. Oxford: Update Software, 2003. (*Thoracoscopic pleurodesis with talc may be the optimal technique for pleurodesis in patients with malignant pleural effusions; see* http://www.cochrane.org *for updates.*)

33. Walker-Renard PB, Vaughan LM, Sahn SA. Chemical pleurodesis for malignant pleural effusions. Ann Intern Med 1994;120:56. (*Talc effectiveness was 93%, compared with 67% for tetracyclines and 54% for bleomycin.*)

34. Heffner JE, Klein JS. Mayo Clin Proc 2008; 83:235. (*An extensive summary of pathogenesis, diagnosis, and management.*)

35. Silvestri G, Pritchard R, Welch G. Preferences for chemotherapy in patients with advanced non–small cell lung cancer: descriptive study based on scripted interviews. BMJ 1998;317:771. (*Overall, 78% of the patients undergoing chemotherapy would opt for supportive care; the wide variation in survival benefit was perceived as justifying the toxicity.*)

CHAPTER 54 ■ SMOKING CESSATION

NANCY A. RIGOTTI

Cigarette smoking is the major preventable cause of death in the United States. Smoking cessation has benefits for almost every smoker, even those who have smoked for many years, those who are elderly, or those who already have a chronic tobacco-related disease. Although the health risks of smoking are widely recognized and the prevalence of smoking has fallen dramatically in the last four decades, millions of Americans continue to smoke. Nevertheless, most smokers say that they want to quit. Multiple studies have shown that a physician's actions can help a patient to stop smoking and have identified effective smoking cessation therapies. Addressing tobacco use in primary care is highly cost-effective and is acceptable to smokers, even those who are not ready to quit. The primary care physician needs routinely to identify patients' smoking status and motivate smokers to quit, advise them about treatment options, refer them as needed to additional resources, and monitor their progress. This requires knowledge about smoking cessation techniques and an appreciation of how and when to use them.

EPIDEMIOLOGY OF SMOKING AND QUITTING (1–5)

Since 1964, when the Surgeon General's Report first publicized the health risks of smoking, the prevalence of cigarette smoking by adults in the United States has decreased from >40% to 21%, and the male predominance in smoking prevalence has narrowed, so that at present 23% of men and 19% of women smoke. Smoking is now most prevalent in populations that have less education and a lower socioeconomic status.

Most smokers know that cigarette smoking is harmful to health, although they may not be aware of the full range of smoking-related illnesses and may not be convinced that these apply to them. Nonetheless, 70% of smokers state in surveys that they would like to quit, and 40% of smokers make an attempt to quit each year, but the majority do not succeed. Although the success rate for any single attempt at quitting is low, smokers who repeatedly try to quit increase their likelihood of success, especially if they learn from their past experience. Lighter smokers are more successful than heavier smokers. Smokers most likely to quit are those who have confidence that their attempt will succeed, have a strong belief in their personal control over events, and have strong social support for nonsmoking, such as a nonsmoking spouse and friends. Smokers with depression or alcohol or other substance abuse have a lower success rate than smokers without these problems and require more-intensive interventions.

Health concerns are the most common reasons given by former smokers for quitting. However, a smoker is less likely to cite the future risk of lung cancer and heart disease than to cite a current smoking-related symptom, such as cough or dyspnea. Actual symptoms may successfully motivate a smoker to quit by making personally salient the more serious health risks of smoking. The likelihood that a smoker will quit increases with the severity of the symptom or diagnosis. Although <5% of smokers in the general population quit each year, approximately one third of smokers quit after a first myocardial infarction. Between 25% and 40% of pregnant women smokers quit during pregnancy, but 70% of them resume smoking in the year after delivery. Other reasons for quitting cited by former smokers include a desire to exert self-control over one's life, concern about the cost and social unacceptability of smoking, aesthetic objections to the smoking habit, and fear of setting a bad example for others.

Approximately 80% of smokers who try to quit do so without assistance from physicians, medications, or formal treatment programs. Fewer than 5% of these quit attempts succeed. In contrast, long-term cessation rates with state-of-the-art treatment programs that combine medication and psychosocial counseling are ~30%. Many more smokers entering a program will quit initially, but many of those who attain short-term cessation resume smoking before 1 year has passed. Reducing cigarette consumption and switching to a different brand can be part of a smoker's preparation for quitting—being especially helpful in building a sense of confidence and control—but are no substitute for setting a definite date for abrupt and total cessation. Smokers sometimes switch to a cigarette brand that is lower in tar and nicotine delivery in the hope of reducing their health risk, but doing so provides no actual risk reduction and is not an acceptable alternative to cessation.

WHY PEOPLE SMOKE (6–8)

Smoking is a complex behavior that is initiated and maintained for different reasons. External factors such as the influence of peers, parents, and the media appear to be most important in the initiation of smoking. Adolescents whose parents and friends smoke are more likely to begin smoking. Once the smoking habit is established, it is sustained by both biologic and psychosocial factors.

Nicotine is the constituent of tobacco smoke that is responsible for causing physiological dependence on cigarettes. Chronic nicotine exposure produces changes in the brain, such as the upregulation of nicotinic acetylcholine receptors, which lead to tolerance and a craving for cigarettes when smoking stops. Smokers smoke to maintain a constant level of nicotine to avert the *nicotine withdrawal syndrome*, symptoms of which include restlessness, irritability, impatience, difficulty concentrating, an anxious or depressed mood, and an increased appetite. Nicotine withdrawal symptoms begin within a few hours of smoking cessation, peak 48 to 72 hours later, and gradually wane over weeks. The duration and the severity of nicotine withdrawal are highly variable, representing different degrees of nicotine addiction among smokers. No biochemical test can measure nicotine addiction, but heavily addicted smokers tend to have their first cigarette shortly after arising (i.e., within 30 minutes), smoke more cigarettes per day, and have difficulty when forced to abstain from cigarettes for even a few hours. This model of pharmacologic dependence can explain the initial difficulties that smokers have when they stop smoking but cannot alone explain why smokers have difficulty remaining abstinent after the first few weeks.

Cigarette smoking is also a habit, a learned behavior that continues because it is rewarding to the smoker. Certain repeated situations, such as finishing a meal, become strongly associated with smoking and trigger the urge to smoke. Cravings for cigarettes, which are produced by a combination of learned associations and physical changes in the brain, last longer than nicotine withdrawal symptoms and can trigger both early and late relapses in smokers who stop smoking. Smokers also use cigarettes to handle environmental stress and regulate emotions, especially strong negative emotions like anger or frustration. There is a strong epidemiologic association between depression and smoking. Smokers are much more likely than nonsmokers to have a current or past history of depression. Nicotine withdrawal symptoms are more intense in smokers with comorbid depression or depressive symptoms, and stopping smoking can trigger or worsen depressive symptoms in smokers with a depression history. This may explain the observation that smokers with depression are less likely to succeed at quitting.

TECHNIQUES FOR SMOKING CESSATION (1–4,9–23)

The evidence in support of smoking cessation therapies was reviewed systematically for the U.S. Public Health Service's (USPHS) clinical practice guideline Treatment of Tobacco Use and Dependence, which was updated in 2008. This document concluded that two methods had the strongest evidence of efficacy: psychosocial counseling and pharmacotherapy. Combinations of the two were more effective than either method alone, as might be expected because they target different factors that maintain smoking behavior (e.g., psychological dependence and physiologic nicotine addiction). Maintaining long-term tobacco abstinence remains the challenge in smoking cessation treatment. Short-term cessation rates of 60% to 70% are common after a treatment program. However, a predictable and rapid return to smoking follows initial cessation, such that about half of individuals who initially quit resume smoking within 1 year. An effective smoking cessation program should have a 1-year cessation rate of 30%.

Pharmacotherapy (2–4,9–22)

Meta-analyses conducted for the 2008 USPHS guideline panel identified several drugs with efficacy for smoking cessation. Using any of them makes quitting less difficult and increases smoking cessation rates compared to placebo, but these products do not obviate the commitment and effort needed to stop smoking. The cessation rates achieved by all of them are higher when they are used in combination with smoking cessation counseling.

Three of these drugs—nicotine replacement, the antidepressant bupropion, and varenicline, a partial agonist at the $\alpha_4\beta_2$ nicotine receptor, were designated as first-line treatment. Each of them at least doubles the success rate of a quit attempt compared to placebo, and all are approved by

the U.S. Food and Drug Administration (FDA) for this indication. Two other agents—the tricyclic antidepressant nortriptyline and the antihypertensive clonidine—were designated as second-line agents because a smaller body of clinical evidence supported their efficacy. Neither second-line drug is FDA approved for smoking cessation. Because of the demonstrated efficacy of pharmacotherapy, the USPHS guideline panel recommended that all smokers willing to quit be offered one of these drugs, unless they are medically contraindicated (Table 54.1).

Nicotine Replacement Therapy

Five nicotine replacement products are sold in the United States (transdermal patch, gum, lozenge, oral inhaler, and nasal spray). Three are sold without a prescription (patch, gum, and lozenge), and two are available by prescription only (inhaler and nasal spray). To use any of these products, smokers are instructed to pick a day to stop smoking cigarettes and immediately begin using the nicotine replacement product. All of them relieve the symptoms of nicotine withdrawal by delivering nicotine to the bloodstream, but none of them produces the rapid peaks of blood nicotine produced by inhaling tobacco smoke. With nicotine withdrawal relieved, the smoker can focus on breaking the behavioral or "habit" aspects of tobacco use. Smokers often worry that that they will remain dependent on nicotine if they use these products when stopping smoking. This rarely occurs because the dose of nicotine delivered and the pattern of nicotine delivery differ so much from inhaled tobacco smoke that a smoker using nicotine replacement is already being weaned from nicotine dependence. The smoker using nicotine replacement also avoids exposure to other harmful constituents of tobacco smoke, such as carbon monoxide and cancer-causing tars.

Nicotine can be delivered transdermally with a nicotine patch, through the oral mucosa with a nicotine chewing gum, lozenge, or inhaler, or via the nasal mucosa with a nasal spray. All nicotine replacement products have been shown to be superior to placebos in randomized, controlled trials, but they have rarely been compared with one another. One study that compared the patch, gum, inhaler, and nasal spray found no difference in efficacy among methods. All products produce higher cessation rates when used in combination with a behavioral smoking counseling program. The drugs can be combined safely, largely because each agent produces lower blood nicotine levels than smoking and because smokers can control the dosing of these agents and do not use them at levels that produce nicotine toxicity. In several trials, the nicotine patch combined with the gum, inhaler, or nasal spray produced better results than a single product. Combining nicotine replacement products is an option for patients who do not succeed with a single agent.

Transdermal Nicotine

The nicotine transdermal patch provides the most continuous delivery of nicotine of all nicotine replacement products and it is easiest for a smoker to use, but it does not offer a smoker the option of adjusting nicotine exposure over the course of the day. It approximately doubles the success of a quit attempt compared to a placebo patch. Nicotine patches are sold without prescription in the United States.

Starting on the quit day, a nicotine patch is applied each morning to any nonhairy skin site on the upper torso. It is removed and replaced the next morning. The patch site should be rotated daily to avoid skin irritation, the most common side effect. Insomnia and vivid dreams are also reported and

TABLE 54.1

DRUGS USED TO TREAT TOBACCO USE

Product	Daily Dose	Treatment Duration	Common Side Effects
Nicotine Replacement Therapy			
Transdermal patch[a,b] (e.g., Nicoderm CQ)	7-, 14-, 21-mg patch worn for 24 hr[c]	8 wk	Skin irritation Insomnia, vivid dreams
Nicotine polacrilex gum[a,b] (Nicorette) 2 mg (<25 cigarettes/d) 4 mg (>25 cigarettes/d)	1 piece/hr[d] (<24 pieces/d)	8-12 wk	Mouth irritation Sore jaw Dyspepsia Hiccups
Nicotine polacrilex lozenge[a,b] (Commit) 2 mg (first cigarette >30 min after waking) 4 mg (first cigarette within 30 min of waking)	7-9 lozenges/d (max 20/d)	12 wk	Mouth irritation Dyspepsia Hiccups
Oral inhaler[a,b] (Nicotrol inhaler)	6-16 cartridges/d (delivered dose, 4 mg/cartridge)	3-6 mo	Mouth and throat irritation
Nasal spray[a,b] (Nicotrol NS)	1-2 doses/hr (max 40/d)	3-6 mo	Nasal irritation Sneezing Cough Teary eyes
Nonnicotine Therapy			
Bupropion SR[a,b] (Zyban, Wellbutrin SR)	150 mg daily for 3 d, then 150 mg twice daily[e]	7-12 wk (up to 6 mo to maintain abstinence)	Insomnia Dry mouth
Nortriptyline[f]	75-100 mg once daily[g]	12 wk	Dry mouth Sedation Dizziness
Clonidine[f]	0.1-0.3 mg twice daily	3-10 wk	Dry mouth Sedation Dizziness
Varenicline (Chantix)[a,b]	0.5 mg daily for 3d, 0.5 mg twice daily for 4 d, then 1 mg twice daily	12 weeks (up to 6 mo to maintain abstinence	Nausea Vivid dreams

[a]Approved by the U.S. Food and Drug Administration as a smoking cessation aid.
[b]Recommended as a first-line drug for tobacco treatment by U.S. Public Health Service clinical guideline.
[c]User can remove the patch at bedtime if he or she is troubled by insomnia.
[d]The user should chew the gum slowly until a distinct taste indicates that nicotine is being released. The user should then place the gum between the cheek and gum until the taste disappears to allow the nicotine to be absorbed through the oral mucosa. The sequence should be repeated for 30 min before the gum is discarded. Acidic beverages (such as coffee and soft drinks) reduce nicotine absorption and should be avoided for 30 min before chewing.
[e]Start 1 wk before quit date.
[f]Not approved by the U.S. Food and Drug Administration as a smoking cessation aid. Recommended as a second-line drug by the U.S. Public Health Service clinical guideline.
[g]Start 10 to 28 d before quit date with 25 mg daily and increase as tolerated.

can be managed by removing the patch at bedtime. An 8-week course of the patch is sufficient. Most smokers should start with the strongest dose (21 mg/d) for 4 to 6 weeks, then gradually taper to lower-dose patches (14 and 7 mg/d) over 2 to 4 weeks. Those who weigh <100 lb or smoke <10 cigarettes (one-half pack) per day are advised to begin with the 14-mg/d strength. The nicotine patch has been shown to be safe for use in patients with stable angina. Because of the vasoconstrictive action of nicotine, the risks and benefits of patch use must be weighed carefully in patients with unstable angina, recent (e.g., last 2 weeks) myocardial infarction, or serious ventricular arrhythmia. No data about safety in these situations is available, but the nicotine patch, unlike cigarette smoking, is not thrombogenic and therefore has little theoretical risk of triggering acute cardiovascular events. The benefits of nicotine replacement likely outweigh potential risks even in smokers

with acute coronary syndromes who are having nicotine withdrawal. A similar argument can be made for its use in pregnant or breast-feeding women who cannot quit with nonpharmacologic methods.

Nicotine Chewing Gum

Nicotine chewing gum, available without prescription in 2- and 4-mg doses, replaces nicotine from cigarettes and also provides the smoker with an oral substitute for cigarettes. The nicotine in the gum is released by chewing and absorbed through the oral mucosa, resulting in blood levels that peak 20 minutes after use starts. However, if the gum is chewed too rapidly, the nicotine is released faster than it can be absorbed by the buccal mucosa. Nicotine that is swallowed does not enter the bloodstream but can cause side effects of heartburn and dyspepsia. For this reason, careful chewing technique is important.

Smokers who smoke 25 or more cigarettes per day have a better result with the 4-mg gum, whereas the 2-mg gum is recommended for lighter smokers. Using the gum allows the smoker to have more control over nicotine dosing than using the patch, but the gum is more difficult to use properly and results in more variable blood nicotine levels and therefore less constant suppression of withdrawal symptoms.

Smokers are instructed to chew the gum whenever they have an urge to smoke, continuing for 3 months. Dependence develops in <5% of users, who have difficulty stopping. A "chew and park" pattern of gum use is recommended. A piece of gum is chewed until the nicotine taste appears, then parked in the buccal mucosa until the taste disappears, whereupon it is chewed a few more times to release more nicotine. This cycle is repeated for 30 minutes, at which point the gum is discarded. Nicotine absorption may be compromised by the consumption of acidic beverages (e.g., coffee, carbonated drinks). By lowering the pH of saliva, they block nicotine absorption when ingested during or immediately before gum use. Not drinking acidic beverages around the time of gum use solves the problem.

Side effects are mostly a consequence of overly vigorous chewing and release of excess nicotine—sore jaw, mouth irritation or ulcers, nausea, vomiting, hiccups, intestinal distress, headache, and excess salivation.

Nicotine Lozenge

The nicotine lozenge, sold without prescription, resembles the nicotine gum, in that it is also an oral product with similar pharmacokinetics to the gum. The lozenge is placed in the mouth and allowed to dissolve over 20 to 30 minutes, making it easier to use properly than the gum. Like the gum, the lozenge is sold in 2- and 4-mg doses. The selection of dose is based on how soon after awakening a person smokes his or her first cigarette. Those who smoke within 30 minutes of awakening (a measure of nicotine dependence) are directed to use the 4-mg dose, whereas others should use the 2-mg dose. The dosing schedule is similar to that of the gum—one to two lozenges per hour for the first 6 weeks and then tapering down over the final 6 weeks. The lozenge can be used by smokers who cannot use nicotine gum because the gum adheres to dentures and can damage dental restorations.

Nicotine Inhaler

The nicotine inhaler, available only by prescription in the United States, is a hollow plastic cylinder containing a nicotine-impregnated plug. When the smoker inhales through this device, nicotine vapor (not smoke) is delivered to the mouth and throat, where it is absorbed. The nicotine vapor does not reach the lungs. Consequently, the inhaler's pharmacokinetics resembles that of nicotine gum. The inhaler addresses not only physical dependence, but also the behavioral and sensory aspects of smoking. The recommended dose is 6 to 16 cartridges per day for the first 6 to 12 weeks, followed by gradual reduction of dose over the next 6 to 12 weeks.

Nicotine Nasal Spray

Nicotine nasal spray was developed to provide more rapid delivery of nicotine and thereby mimic more closely the effect of smoking a cigarette. The delivery device is similar to a nasal antihistamine spray, and one or two doses are taken per hour for a period of about 3 months. As with gum and transder-

mal patches, the quit rates with the device are about twice those attained with placebo. Nasal and throat irritation, rhinitis, sneezing, and tearing are common side effects and result in poor compliance by smokers.

Bupropion

Bupropion, an atypical antidepressant with dopaminergic and noradrenergic activity in the brain, is the second drug with strong evidence of efficacy for smoking cessation. In a series of randomized, controlled clinical trials, sustained-release (SR) bupropion (*Zyban or Wellbutrin SR*) consistently doubled long-term smoking cessation rates compared with placebo. Its effect on smoking cessation is independent of its antidepressant effect, given that the trials establishing its efficacy excluded patients with depression. It is equally effective among persons with and without a history of depression. The drug appears to work on the neurochemistry of addiction by increasing dopamine release in brain pathways known to be involved in reward.

Because bupropion SR takes 5 to 7 days to reach steady-state blood levels, it is started 1 week before a smoker's target quit date. The recommended dose is 150 mg/d for 3 days, then 150 mg twice a day. In one dose–response trial, a 150-mg/d dose was as effective as the 300-mg/d dose, and thus is an alternative for smokers who cannot tolerate the full dose. Recommended duration of treatment is 7 to 12 weeks, although if a smoker is successful in quitting, the drug is approved for use of up to 6 months to prevent relapse to tobacco. The drug is well tolerated, with the most common side effects being insomnia, agitation, and dry mouth. The most serious side effect is seizure because bupropion reduces the seizure threshold. In clinical trials, the risk of seizure was 0.1%, and the drug is contraindicated in patients with a seizure disorder or predisposition to seizure.

One randomized trial that directly compared bupropion and nicotine replacement found bupropion to be superior to the nicotine patch and to placebo. In that trial the combination of nicotine patch and bupropion was safe and produced slightly higher cessation rates than bupropion alone, but the difference was not statistically significant. The superiority of bupropion over nicotine replacement therapy was not demonstrated in another clinical trial that compared the two. A review of the entire body of evidence by the USPHS smoking cessation guideline panel led them to designate bupropion and nicotine replacement as equally effective first-line agents for smoking cessation. The choice of drug is to be based on other considerations, such as medical contraindications and patient preference.

Varenicline

Varenicline, approved by the FDA for smoking cessation in 2006, is a selective partial agonist at the $\alpha 4 \beta 2$ nicotinic acetylcholine receptor, the nicotine receptor subtype that appears to mediate nicotine dependence. As a partial agonist, it has both agonist and antagonist properties at this receptor. As a partial agonist, it relieves nicotine withdrawal symptoms. In addition, when varenicline binds to the nicotine receptor, it prevents nicotine from cigarette smoke from binding, thereby blocking the usual rewarding effect of smoking a cigarette. Two large randomized, controlled trials compared varenicline with placebo and with bupropion. In each, varenicline produced a higher long-term cessation rate than both placebo and bupropion. It nearly tripled the cessation rate compared to placebo, appearing to represent an improvement over the doubling of quit rates observed in placebo-controlled trials of nicotine replacement and bupropion. How it compares to nicotine replacement has not been tested directly. Its efficacy when accompanied with the lower level of behavioral support usually provided in the physician office setting is also not yet known. The most common side effect is nausea, but it is usually well tolerated. Varenicline is used for 12 weeks at a dose of 1 mg twice daily, with a lower initial dose titrated to full dose over the first week to minimize nausea. Treatment starts 1 week before the smoker's quit date to allow for blood levels to stabilize before a smoker quits. Because it is not nicotine and does not bind to the subtype of nicotinic receptors that mediate nicotine's cardiovascular effects (increases in heart rate and blood pressure), varenicline is expected to be safe to use in patients with cardiovascular disease. A clinical trial of the drug in this setting is underway.

Nortriptyline

Like bupropion, nortriptyline, a tricyclic antidepressant, has demonstrated efficacy for smoking cessation in randomized, placebo-controlled clinical trials. In these trials, nortriptyline was started 2 weeks before the smoker's target quit date and given for 12 weeks. The initial dose of 25 mg was increased to 75 mg over 1 to 2 weeks. Nortriptyline is categorized as a second-line agent in the USPHS clinical guideline because it has less extensive evidence of efficacy than bupropion or nicotine replacement. Since the release of those guideline, several additional clinical trials have shown that the drug is effective for smoking cessation. Nortriptyline is not approved for smoking cessation by the U.S. Food and Drug Administration.

Clonidine

Clonidine, a centrally acting adrenergic blocker, is best known as an antihypertensive agent, but it also reduces symptoms of withdrawal from drugs of abuse, including nicotine. Meta-analyses of several clinical trials demonstrated that clonidine has efficacy for smoking cessation, but its use is limited by the side effects of sedation, hypotension, and dry mouth. The USPHS guideline classifies it as a second-line agent that is an alternative when first-line agents are not effective or are contraindicated.

Other Pharmacologic Agents

Although bupropion and nortriptyline have efficacy for smoking cessation, there is no evidence for the efficacy of any selective serotonin reuptake inhibitor antidepressant for this indication. Minor tranquilizers such as benzodiazepines have been prescribed as a means of blunting the anxiety and irritability of nicotine withdrawal, but they are no better than placebo. Smokers who complain of irritability are more appropriately treated with drugs that reduce nicotine withdrawal symptoms directly.

Smoking Cessation Counseling (9–11,23)

Counseling strategies have been developed to address the psychological dependency or "habit" aspect of tobacco use. These can be delivered in person, by telephone, or through the Internet and form the content of most formal smoking cessation programs. They can also be adapted for use in brief interventions delivered by physicians and other clinicians or delivered in written form via self-help booklets. The evidence review done by the USPHS guideline task force found that counseling delivered in person or by telephone is effective for smoking cessation. Trials of the efficacy of Web-based counseling are underway.

These techniques have a smoker identify and then alter the environmental stimuli that trigger smoking. Cues to smoke are identified by *self-monitoring techniques*. Smokers might be asked to record in a daily log all cigarettes smoked, the circumstances that preceded each cigarette, and the importance of that cigarette to the smoker. Environmental cues to smoke, identified from this daily log, are progressively avoided or modified so that they no longer trigger smoking. At a point in the relearning process, smoking stops altogether. Counseling techniques also teach smokers how to use cognitive and behavioral methods to manage withdrawal symptoms, cigarette cravings, or negative emotions such as anger or frustration. Counseling also aims to increase a smoker's confidence in his or her ability to quit smoking, in part by mobilizing social support for nonsmoking in the smoker's environment.

Both nonprofit and commercial organizations offer group and individual counseling programs for smoking cessation that employ these cognitive–behavioral techniques. *Self-help manuals* containing these techniques have low efficacy rates by themselves but can be effective when used in conjunction with other counseling, such as that provided in a physician's office. Self-help manuals are available at minimal cost from nonprofit organizations like the American Cancer Society, the American Lung Association, and the National Cancer Institute. Most state public health departments sponsor free *telephone counseling services* that assist a smoker to stop and prevent relapse to smoking. A uniform toll-free telephone number (1-800-QUIT-NOW) connects any smoker to the appropriate state telephone counseling program. These programs generally do an initial assessment, provide general information about quitting, and ask the smoker to set a quit date in the near future. They then call the smokers proactively several times after the quit date. A number of Web-based counseling programs have also been developed and are available. Both telephone and Web-based counseling programs provide smokers with social support as well as practical information about the quitting process. Some telephone and Web programs also offer to mail over-the-counter forms of nicotine replacement to smokers.

Hypnosis

Hypnosis is marketed for smoking cessation and is of interest to many smokers who hope that it offers an effortless way to stop smoking. Most studies evaluating hypnosis have been uncontrolled, with small samples and brief follow-up, and the USPHS review of the evidence found no convincing evidence to support the efficacy of hypnosis for smoking cessation.

Acupuncture

Acupuncture, like hypnosis, is used for smoking cessation, and smokers often ask about its efficacy. However, acupuncture has not proved to be effective in randomized, placebo-controlled trials, and the USPHS guideline panel did not find it to be an efficacious smoking cessation method.

ROLE OF THE PHYSICIAN (1–4,9,10,24–26)

A physician is in an excellent position to encourage smoking cessation because 70% of smokers see a physician each year, and health concerns are the most common reason why smokers quit. A physician's advice and assistance doubles the chance that a smoker will make an attempt to quit. Providing all patients with no more than brief advice to stop smoking has been shown to be more effective than doing nothing to promote cessation, and it is a cost-effective medical practice. Doing more (i.e., brief smoking cessation counseling) has, in randomized, controlled trials, increased patients' attempts to stop smoking and, in most trials, increased long-term smoking cessation rates as well. Surveys indicate that physicians are not taking advantage of their opportunity to alter their patients' smoking habits. Only 60% of current smokers recall ever being told to quit smoking by a physician. In fact, a physician's advice can make a difference. Physicians who devote more time to counseling smokers can expect to be even more effective.

The USPHS clinical practice guideline outlined an evidence-based, cost-effective, five-step strategy, known as the 5A's, for physicians to use in ambulatory care. Its components include systematically identifying the smoking status of all patients seen in a practice, advising every smoker to quit, assessing each smoker's readiness to attempt cessation, assisting smokers who are ready to quit, and monitoring their progress in follow-up. A team approach in which staff members routinely assess a patient's smoking status, remind the physician to counsel each smoker identified, and provide more in-depth counseling and follow-up after the physician's introduction to cessation can enhance outcomes and reduce the expenditure of the physician's time. Follow-up is critical.

RECOMMENDATIONS
(1–4,9,10,27,28)

The five-step smoking cessation strategy for office practice is summarized in Table 54.2.

1. *Ask about smoking habits at every visit.* Smoking habits should be assessed as a part of every patient encounter in ambulatory practice. All smokers should be asked about their level of interest in quitting and what, if anything, they have done in the past to try to quit. The assessment should estimate the smokers' level of nicotine dependence (e.g., the number of cigarettes per day and the time between awakening and the first morning cigarette). The smoker's prior cessation efforts, degree of social support for quitting smoking, and confidence in his or her ability to quit, along with any medical problems, help to guide treatment recommendations.
2. *Advise every smoker to stop smoking.* Clear advice to stop smoking should be made to all smokers at every visit. Total cessation is the goal. Switching to low-tar, low-nicotine cigarettes does not reduce health risks and is not an alternative to cessation. Advice to quit should be tailored to the individual's clinical situation. The contribution of smoking to any of the patient's current symptoms should be emphasized. A positive focus is recommended on the benefits of cessation, including short-term benefits, such as increased exercise tolerance or improved taste and smell, rather than on the harms of continuing to smoke.
3. *Assess a smoker's readiness to quit smoking.* The asymptomatic smoker may be the most difficult one to motivate. Most smokers do have minor smoking-related symptoms that would improve with cessation, such as morning cough or limited exercise tolerance. Smokers unable to quit for their own sake may do so for their children's health.

   Smokers with an *acute respiratory illness* commonly stop smoking for a few days on their own. The physician can suggest that the smoker take advantage of the period of reduced desire to stop smoking permanently. For the smoker with a *chronic disease* associated with smoking, the physician should point out the potential for reduced symptoms, improved function, and slowed progression of disease. Ra-

diologic or pulmonary function tests are not recommended for asymptomatic smokers because they do not detect early disease and have not been shown to increase cessation rates. Normal results may falsely reassure smokers that their health is not being jeopardized.

Smokers reluctant to attempt cessation often harbor a specific concern, such as a fear of failure, weight gain, withdrawal symptoms, or the loss of a pleasurable habit or way to handle life stresses. Helping the smoker to clarify this concern and develop arguments to the contrary can be useful. Smokers may not be aware that effective treatments are available to them. Even smokers who are reluctant to quit should be told that treatment is available and asked if they would be willing to try it. If the smoker remains unwilling to consider cessation, the physician should simply make a strong antismoking recommendation and address the patients' tobacco use at subsequent visits.

4. *Assist the smoker to quit* by asking for a commitment to quit and helping the smoker to identify a program that will work for him or her. Encourage smokers to set a date on which they will stop smoking, preferably within 4 weeks so that they do not forget it. The physician should record the date in the medical record, as a reminder to follow the patient's progress. The physician should then work with the smoker to develop a personalized cessation program that will build the smoker's confidence that he or she can quit and maximize the patient's chances of success. A program generally includes pharmacotherapy plus behavioral counseling that is provided by a booklet, by telephone, or by a formal in-person cessation program. Providing booklets and specific information about community smoking-cessation resources such as groups or telephone quitlines facilitates patient follow through with referral. Smokers concerned about weight gain should be advised to begin a concurrent exercise program. Smokers in whom cough and sputum production increase immediately after cessation should be reassured that this is temporary and common and represents a return of ciliary clearance activities in the respiratory tract. Smokers with concomitant alcohol or other substance abuse or clinical depression are unlikely to succeed in quitting smoking unless these other conditions are addressed at the same time by appropriate referral for substance abuse or mental health care (see Chapters 227 and 235).

   Weight gain may need to be addressed. Most smokers gain some weight after they stop smoking, with men averaging 2.8 kg and women 3.8 kg. The risk for large weight gain (>13 kg) is low; it occurs in about 10% of men and 13.5% of women. African Americans and heavy smokers (>15 cigarettes per day) are also at increased risk. However, weight gain does not cancel the health benefits of smoking cessation. Prescribing a program of *exercise* (see Chapters 18 and 233) can help to control weight and may enhance the likelihood of cessation. Trying to diet and stop smoking at the same time leads to less success in smoking cessation and is not recommended.
5. *Arrange follow-up.* Continued monitoring of the smoking habit is essential. Including smoking as a problem in the patient's medical record will remind the physician to manage it as part of the patient's continuing care. One or more return visits for follow-up will increase patients' success rates and should be done to monitor the response to pharmacotherapy. The first follow-up should be scheduled shortly after the quit date. At follow-up, smokers who quit should be congratulated but cautioned of the need to maintain vigilance against relapse. Former smokers should be monitored

TABLE 54.2

SMOKING CESSATION STRATEGY FOR OFFICE PRACTICE. U.S. PUBLIC HEALTH SERVICE GUIDELINE PANEL—5A'S

Ask about smoking at every visit: "Do you smoke?"
- Should be done by office staff

Advise every smoker to stop smoking
- Make advice firm and clear: "Quitting smoking is the most important thing you can do to stay healthy"
- Tailor advice to patient's clinical condition
- Be positive: Stress benefits of cessation, not harms of smoking

Assess readiness to quit: "Are you interested in quitting at this time?"
- Stages of readiness to quit:
  - Stage 1: Precontemplator ("I don't plan to quit")
  - Stage 2: Contemplator ("I'm worried but not ready to quit now")
  - Stage 3: Preparation ("I'm ready to quit. What should I do?")

Assist the smoker in stopping smoking
- **For smokers who are ready to set a quit date (preparation stage)**
  - Help the smoker to make a plan
  - Offer pharmacotherapy
  - Provide behavioral treatment
    (a) Booklet
    (b) Refer to telephone counseling (1-800-QUITNOW) or web-based resources (http://www.quitnet.com, http://www.smokefree.gov)
    (c) Consider referral to a formal program of the smoker has:
        Past or current depression
        Alcohol or substance abuse
        Poor social support for nonsmoking
        Low confidence in ability to quit
    (d) Give support: express confidence in the smokers' ability to quit

- **For smokers not ready to set a quit date (contemplation stage)**
  - Address patient's barriers to trying to quit
    (a) Fear of failure
    (b) Nicotine withdrawal
    (c) Weight gain
    (d) Loss of a coping tool
- **For smokers not ready to quit (precontemplation stage)**
  - Elicit *patient's* view of benefits and harms of continuing to smoke; correct knowledge gaps, challenge smokers' denial of smoking harms
  - Identify barriers to quitting smoking
  - Advice: Avoid exposing family to passive smoke
  - Invite smoker to return when ready to quit
  - Ask again at the next visit

Arrange follow-up: See soon after quit date; monitor on later visits
- *If the patient was able to quit smoking*
  - Congratulate
  - Anticipate high-risk situations: "What times have been difficult for you to avoid smoking?"
  - Rehearse coping strategies
  - Assess withdrawal symptoms, need for treatment
- *If patient was not able to quit smoking*: Be positive
  - Redefine "failure" as "partial success"
  - Ask: "Tell me about the first cigarette..."
  - "Looking back, what could you have done differently?" "What did you learn from the experience?"
  - Ask for another quit date

Adapted from Fiore MC, Bailey WC, Cohen SJ, et al. A clinical practice guideline for treating tobacco use and dependence. Rockville, MD: U.S. Department of Health and Human Services, Public Health Service, 2000, and The Tobacco Use and Dependence Clinical Practice Guideline Update Panel and Staff. A clinical practice guideline for treating tobacco use and dependence: a US Public Health Service report [consensus statement]. JAMA 2000;283:3244, with permission.

carefully during the first year after cessation, which is when most relapses occur. For smokers whose attempts to quit have been unsuccessful, the physician should focus on positive aspects, such as the length of time the smoker was abstinent, and encourage another attempt. Through care-

ful questioning, the physician can help the patient to determine what circumstances caused the effort to fail and then encourage the patient to learn from the experience so as to increase the chance of success in the next attempt to quit.

Annotated Bibliography

1. Rigotti NA. Clinical crossroads: a 36-year-old woman who smokes cigarettes. JAMA 2000;284:741. (*Reviews smoking patterns and cessation methods in the context of a case of a smoker who is having difficulty quitting.*)
2. Rigotti NA. Treatment of tobacco use and dependence. N Engl J Med 2002;346:506. (*A concise review of the U.S. Public Health Service [USPHS] clinical guideline and current evidence regarding the efficacy of treatment methods.*)
3. Schroeder SA. What to do with a patient who smokes. JAMA 2005;294:482. (*Clinical review of smoking cessation methods in the context of a case of a smoker who needs treatment.*)
4. Wilson JF. In the clinic: smoking cessation. Ann Intern Med 2007;146:ITC2 (*Clinically oriented summary of tobacco treatment methods using material derived from the American College of Physicians' educational resources.*)
5. Ayanian JZ, Cleary PD. Perceived risks of heart disease and cancer among cigarette smokers. JAMA 1999;281:1019. (*Most smokers in a national sample did not perceive themselves to be at excess risk of cancer and heart disease, despite broad public awareness that smoking is harmful to smokers in general.*)
6. Jarvis M. Why people smoke. BMJ 2004;328:277. (*Brief description of current theories that explain the maintenance of smoking.*)
7. Lasser K, Boyd JW, Woolhandler S, et al. Smoking and mental illness: a population-based prevalence study. JAMA 2000;284:2606. (*Smoking is more common among individuals with psychiatric disorders, including depression, anxiety, and schizophrenia.*)
8. West R. ABC of smoking cessation: assessment of dependence and motivation to stop smoking. BMJ 2004; 328:338. (*A short, clinically oriented summary of how to use a few simple questions to determine a smoker's level of nicotine dependence and motivation to quit.*)
9. Fiore MC, Bailey WC, Cohen SJ, et al. A clinical practice guideline for treating tobacco use and dependence: a US Public Health Service report. JAMA 2000;283:3244. (*The evidence-based clinical practice guideline for treating tobacco use in medical practice, released in 2000 by the USPHS; update expected in 2008.*)
10. Aveyard P, West R. Managing smoking cessation. BMJ 2007; 335: 37. (*A practical clinical review of treatment methods and suggested strategies for use by primary care clinicians, and approaches for light smokers, pregnant women, and adolescents.*)
11. Cochrane Tobacco Addiction Group. Available at: www.cochrane.org/reviews/en/topics/94.html. (*Source of regularly updated systematic reviews and meta-analyses that cover a wide range of issues in the treatment of smokers.*)
12. Jorenby DE, Hays JT, Rigotti NA, et al. Efficacy of varenicline, an alpha4beta2 nicotine acetylcholine receptor partial agonist, vs placebo or sustained-release bupropion for smoking cessation: a randomized controlled trial. JAMA 2006;296:56. (*This treatment was found to be more effective than bupropion in this three-arm, randomized trial.*)
13. Gonzales D, Rennard SI, Nides M, et al. Varenicline, an alpha4beta2 nicotine acetylcholine receptor partial agonist, vs sustained-release bupropion and placebo for smoking cessation: a randomized controlled trial. JAMA 2006;296:47. (*Varenicline was superior to both placebo and bupropion at 1 year follow-up.*)
14. Tonstad S, Tonnesen P, Hajek P, et al. Effect of maintenance therapy with varenicline on smoking cessation: a randomized controlled trial. JAMA 2006; 296: 64. (*A randomized, controlled trial of relapse prevention with varenicline; smokers who quit smoking after 12 weeks of varenicline did better long term if they were given an additional 3 months of treatment vs. placebo.*)
15. Hall SM, Humfleet GL, Reus VI, et al. Psychological intervention and antidepressant treatment in smoking cessation. Arch Gen Psychiatry 2002;59:930. (*Randomized, controlled trial showing that both nortriptyline and bupropion produced better results at 1 year than placebo and did not differ from one another.*)
16. Hajek P, West R, Foulds J, et al. Randomized comparative trial of nicotine polacrilex, a transdermal patch, nasal spray, and an inhaler. Arch Intern Med 1999;159:2033. (*A direct comparison of four nicotine replacement products found that all had similar efficacy for smoking cessation.*)
17. Shiffman S, Dressler CM, Hajek P, et al. Efficacy of a nicotine lozenge for smoking cessation. Arch Intern Med 2002;162:1267. (*One of several studies demonstrating the efficacy of the newest form of nicotine replacement in the United States.*)
18. Hurt RD, Sachs DPL, Glover ED, et al. A comparison of sustained-release bupropion and placebo for smoking cessation. N Engl J Med 1997;337:1195. (*The 1-year quit rate was 23%, compared with 12% for placebo; weight gain was also significantly reduced.*)
19. Ahluwalia JS, Harris KJ, Catley D, et al. Sustained-release bupropion for smoking cessation in African Americans: a randomized controlled trial. JAMA 2002;288:468. (*Bupropion was effective for smoking cessation in African American smokers, as it was previously shown to be in populations that are largely white.*)
20. Hays JT, Hurt RD, Rigotti NA, et al. Sustained-release bupropion for pharmacologic relapse prevention after smoking cessation: a randomized, controlled trial. Ann Intern Med 2001;135:423. (*Among smokers who achieved abstinence with 7 weeks of bupropion, an additional year of the drug delayed the time to smoking relapse but did not produce more cessation at long-term follow-up.*)
21. Jorenby DE, Leischow SJ, Nides MA, et al. A controlled trial of sustained-release bupropion, a nicotine patch, or both for smoking cessation. N Engl J Med 1999;340:685. (*One-year quit rates were 16% in patch-alone and placebo groups, 30% in the bupropion group, and 36% in the patch-plus-bupropion group.*)
22. Prochazka AV, Weaver MJ, Keller RT, et al. A randomized trial of nortriptyline for smoking cessation. Arch Intern Med 1998;158:2035. (*The 6-month quit rate was 14%, compared to 3% with placebo.*)
23. Zhu SH, Anderson CM, Tedescko GJ, et al. Evidence of real-world effectiveness of a telephone quitline for smokers. N Engl J Med 2002;347:1087. (*A randomized, controlled trial: at 1 month, significantly more smokers offered immediate and repeated telephone counseling were abstinent compared with controls [23.7% vs. 16.5%]; at 1 year, the rates were still significantly different, but decreased [9.1% vs. 6.9%].*)
24. Russell MAH, Wilson C, Taylor C, et al. Effect of general practitioners' advice against smoking. BMJ 1979;2:231. (*Careful randomized, controlled study in which routine advice to stop smoking resulted in a significant increase in cessation that was sustained during 1 year.*)
25. Katz DA, Muehlenbruch DR, Brown RL, et al. Effectiveness of implementing the Agency for Healthcare Research and Quality smoking cessation clinical practice guideline: a randomized, controlled trial. J Natl Cancer Inst 2004;96:594. (*A randomized, controlled trial demonstrating that implementing the USPHS guideline in primary care practices produces higher patient quit rates at 2- and 6-month follow-up than usual care.*)
26. Thorndike AN, Rigotti NA, Stafford RS, et al. National patterns in the treatment of smokers by physicians. JAMA 1998;279:604. (*Analysis of the national survey found that physicians identified patient smoking status at two thirds of outpatient visits but only counseled about smoking at 21% to 29% of visits; primary care physicians did better than specialists; counseling was more likely to occur if the patient had a smoking-related diagnosis.*)
27. Williamson DF, Madans J, Anda RF, et al. Smoking cessation and severity of weight gain in a national cohort. N Engl J Med 1991;324:739. (*The average weight gain was 3.8 kg in women and 2.8 kg in men; there was a major weight gain of >13 kg in 9.8% of men and 13.4% of women.*)
28. Marcus BH, Albrecht AE, King TK, et al. The efficacy of exercise as an aid for smoking cessation in women. Arch Intern Med 1999;159:1229. (*A program of vigorous physical activity reduced postcessation weight gain and increased smoking cessation rates compared with an educational program.*)

CHAPTER 55 ■ SCREENING FOR GASTRIC CANCER

Gastric cancer is among the most common malignancies and is the second-leading cause of cancer-related death worldwide. It is the leading cause of cancer death in Japan, with an annual death rate nearly 20 times that in the Unites States. Given this difference, it is not surprising that population-based screening programs have been sponsored for many years in Japan. The incidence of gastric cancer in the United States has been decreasing at a rate of 2% to 4% annually for decades. During the 1930s, the death rate for gastric cancer was greater than 30 in 100,000; during the 1970s, the rate was approximately 10 in 100,000; at the turn of the last century, it was approximately 5 in 100,000. At present, Americans have approximately a 1% chance of acquiring a gastric malignancy during their lifetime. Case-fatality rates remain high; approximately 75% of the 25,000 Americans in whom gastric cancer develops each year eventually die of the disease. *Helicobacter pylori* infection has been classified as a carcinogen because of its association with an increased risk for gastric cancer, so new prevention strategies have become possible by screening for the risk associated with infection.

The usual insidious onset of the disease and the lack of suitable screening tests have heretofore thwarted preventive measures. Advances in endoscopic instrumentation, allowing more complete visualization of the stomach, have raised questions about unmet potential in preventing gastric cancer deaths among high-risk populations. Some have used cost-effectiveness analyses to argue for screening people at high risk of gastric cancer for *H. pylori* infection in the hopes that antibiotic treatment could reduce cancer risk. The primary care physician must understand the etiology and natural history of gastric cancer, as well as the limitations of diagnostic tools in the detection of early disease.

EPIDEMIOLOGY AND RISK FACTORS (1–8)

The international variation in the incidence of gastric cancer is marked. Among the countries with the highest incidence are Japan, China, Chile, Finland, and Iceland. Much of the international variation can be explained by variation in the prevalence of *H. pylori* infection, which is high in Asia and eastern Europe and, for the most part, low in western and northern Europe as well as North America. Incidence also varies, predictably, with age and gender. Gastric cancer is twice as likely to develop in men in most countries. More than 60% of cases occur in people older than age 65 years. Fewer than 10% of cases occur in people younger than age 30 years. The incidence among nonwhites and people in low socioeconomic groups in the United States is twice that among whites and the more well-to-do. It has long been recognized that migrants from areas of high risk

(e.g., Japan) eventually acquire the lower rates of their new home (e.g., the United States). Nonetheless, genetic factors do play a role in determining the risk for gastric cancer. Germ-line mutations of the *CDH1* gene, which encodes an epithelial cell adhesion molecule, have been identified in some families with apparent hereditary gastric cancer. The greater impact of genetic factors, however, is in determining the host response to *H. pylori* infection. Some infected patients develop gastritis of the antrum with only low-grade gastritis of the corpus of the stomach. They retain normal or high acid secretion and may suffer from duodenal ulcer, but they rarely develop gastric cancer. It is those who develop extensive corpus gastritis followed by hypochlorhydria and gastric atrophy who are at risk for cancer. Gene cluster polymorphisms that enhance production of interleukin-1 have been incriminated in promoting this sequence of events. Blood group, as a long-recognized minor risk factor for gastric cancer, has also been connected to the host response to *H. pylori* infection. The A and B phenotypes, compared with group O individuals, have a slightly higher risk of gastric cancer because of a greater likelihood of colonization of gastric mucosa with *H. pylori*.

Before *H. pylori* was recognized as a potent carcinogen, a number of environmental factors had been suggested as explanations for the geographic variability of gastric cancer incidence. Phenol, present in all smoked foods, and the high salt concentration in salted fish and meat products were linked to the high incidence of gastric cancer in Finland, Iceland, and Japan. Talc-treated rice had been implicated in Japan and northern China. Provinces in Chile with high gastric cancer rates are agricultural, with high concentrations of nitrate present in the soil and drinking water. Nitrosamines, derived from nitrates and secondary amines, are suspected causes of gastric cancer in Chile and, to a lesser extent, in the United States, where nitrates and nitrites are used as food additives in meat and fish. In addition, *H. pylori* impairs the bioavailability of vitamin C, potentially increasing the risk for gastric cancer and other diseases associated with antioxidant deficiency.

The association between atrophic gastritis and gastric cancer had been long recognized. An annual incidence of gastric cancer of 1% among patients with known atrophic gastritis was demonstrated in one study with yearly radiographic examination. The atrophic gastritis associated with pernicious anemia is also a risk factor for gastric cancer. Evidence indicates that patients with pernicious anemia have at least a fourfold increase in risk. Some studies found even higher rates.

Prior gastric surgery for benign ulcer disease has long been considered a risk factor for subsequent gastric cancer. Increased risk was not evident early after surgery, but several Scandinavian studies suggested that those who lived more than 10 to 15 years after surgery faced a twofold to threefold increase in gastric cancer risk. Recommendations for annual endoscopic examination followed. More recently, a large, population-based study conducted in Olmstead County, Minnesota, found gastric cancer to be no more common among patients with prior gastric surgery than among the population at large.

NATURAL HISTORY OF GASTRIC CANCER AND EFFECTIVENESS OF THERAPY (3,6,9–10)

Gastric cancer typically has an insidious presentation. Gastric cancer develops over decades from normal stomach tissue progressing through chronic atrophic gastritis, intestinal metaplasia, dysplasia, and, finally, cancer. The most common initial symptom is epigastric discomfort. Later symptoms include early satiety, indigestion, weight loss, and other systemic symptoms. The percentage of patients who survive 5 years has not improved significantly in recent years; it remains at 20% of unselected cases. The patients who are operated on early in the course of their disease have a 60% to 90% 5-year survival rate. Some population-based studies from Japan confirm that 5-year survival rates of 70% can be achieved among patients with gastric cancer detected by screening. Furthermore, follow-up for 15 years suggests that the cancer death hazard rate decreases rapidly for 7 years after the detection and treatment of cancer and then remains very low. Other studies from Japan question the value of screening, especially among people younger than 50 years of age.

Among highly selected patients with "early gastric cancer," defined as gastric cancer confined to the mucosa or submucosa but not extending to the muscularis propria, resection may be curative for as many as 95%. Intensive screening efforts in Japan have increased the proportion of gastric cancers detected in this early stage from approximately 5% to 30%. Efforts have not been as successful elsewhere, where fewer than 10% of cases meet the criteria for early gastric cancer. The duration of the asymptomatic detectable period is unknown, but early gastric cancer has been found as long as 3 years after biopsy specimens were originally misread as benign. The natural history of early gastric cancer appears to include protracted cycles of healing and ulceration.

SCREENING AND DIAGNOSTIC TESTS (6,11–16)

None of the tests generally used in the United States for the *diagnosis* of gastric carcinoma are suitable for wide screening efforts.

Gastric Cytology

The collection and examination of specimens for gastric cytopathologic analysis, unlike that for cervical cytopathology, is a laborious process. Samples must be obtained either by endoscopic scraping or by gastric lavage. Examination of the resulting slides usually takes 2 to 3 hours rather than the several minutes sufficient for the screening examination of cervical Papanicolaou smears. Many studies have demonstrated the sensitivity of gastric cytopathology studies to be approximately 90%. It is not known how much this figure is influenced by the spectrum of disease, that is, how sensitive cytology can be for the early, curable cancer. Specificity in

a laboratory with experienced personnel should be approximately 97% to 98%. False-positive results are often found in association with healing gastric ulcer and other gastric pathology. Although cytopathology is useful for further diagnosis in documented cases of abnormality of gastric mucosa, it cannot be recommended for indiscriminate screening.

Endoscopy

Similarly, endoscopy must be considered a diagnostic rather than a screening procedure. Its sensitivity in making the diagnosis of gastric cancer is 90%. However, recent evidence suggests that endoscopic visualization is much less sensitive for early cancers, with a visual diagnosis being made in fewer than 50% of cases in some series. Multiple biopsies of any and all suspected lesions can increase the sensitivity to 90%. Attempts have been made to increase the recognition of early cancers with indigo-carmine staining of the mucosa applied locally via the endoscope or fluorescein given intravenously.

Diagnostic Radiology

The sensitivity of contrast studies in the diagnosis of gastric cancer has been reported to be as high as 95%. Obviously, however, it is least sensitive in cases of early disease and is too expensive and time-consuming to be considered a screening test in asymptomatic patients. In Japan, where gastric cancer is the leading cause of cancer death, radiographic techniques have been adapted to mass screening. These modifications in the standard contrast studies have been shown to have a sensitivity and specificity of 90%. Recently, endoscopic ultrasonography has proved be more effective than conventional computed tomographic scanning for the local staging of early gastric cancer, but neither has a role in screening.

Screening for Occult Blood

Stool analysis for occult blood (described in detail in Chapter 56) is an appropriate screening procedure for all gastrointestinal malignancies. Yearly guaiac testing has been recommended as part of the general screening for all adult patients. This is especially important for patients with an identified increased risk for gastric cancer, such as those with a history of pernicious anemia or documented atrophic gastritis.

Screening for and Eradicating *H. pylori* Infection

H. pylori infection can be readily detected and treated, especially in the clinical setting (see Chapter 68). Consensus conferences have recommended against mass screening, but some authorities have indicated that patients with a high risk of cancer (known preneoplastic conditions, prior treatment for gastric cancer, or a strong family history) should be offered testing and, if positive, treatment. When patients with infection and preneoplastic lesions are treated effectively for *H. pylori*, those lesions regress over time. A population-based trial of eradication therapy among infected people produced nearly a 40% reduction in cancer incidence compared with untreated controls but was underpowered, and that result was not statistically significant. The same trial indicated a much greater reduction in risk for the subset of patients known to have no cancer precursor lesions before the initiation of treatment. Nonetheless, too little is known about the effect of screening for and eradicating *H. pylori* infection to justify recommendations for or against its use.

CONCLUSIONS AND RECOMMENDATIONS

- Despite a significant downward trend in incidence, gastric cancer remains a disease of high morbidity and mortality.
- The yearly analysis of stool for occult blood is indicated in all adult patients. This is especially important for those with a history of pernicious anemia, atrophic gastritis, *H. pylori* infection, or other gastric pathology.
- The value of gastric cytology, endoscopy, and contrast studies as routine procedures in high-risk patients is unproven. They are diagnostic procedures and should generally be reserved for symptomatic patients or patients with occult blood demonstrated by stool analysis.
- The value of screening asymptomatic patients for *H. pylori* infection in the clinical setting is unproven. Further study is necessary to determine the effect of finding and eradicating infection on gastric cancer risk. Screening of high-risk patients for infection should be undertaken only after discussion about the clinical uncertainty.

A.G.M.

Annotated Bibliography

1. Calam J, Baron JH. Pathophysiology of duodenal and gastric ulcer and gastric cancer. BMJ 2001;323:980. (*A simple and elegant exposition of the pathophysiology of Helicobacter pylori gastritis and its role in carcinogenesis.*)
2. Correa P. *Helicobacter pylori* and gastric carcinogenesis. Am J Surg Pathol 1995;19S:S37. (*Describes a multifocal atrophic gastritis associated with H. pylori infection in populations at high risk for gastric cancer.*)
3. Mera R, Fontham ETH, Bravo JC, et al. Long term follow up of patients treated for *Helicobacter pylori* infection. Gut 2005;54:1536. (*A follow-up over 12 years showed a regression of preneoplastic lesions among patients for whom treatment eradicated infection.*)
4. *Helicobacter* and Cancer Collaborative. Gastric cancer and *Helicobacter pylori*: a combined analysis of 12 case control studies nested within prospective cohorts. Gut 2001;49:347. (*Estimates the relative risk of noncardia cancer at 5.9; there was no increase in cardia cancer.*)
5. Hitchcock CR, MacLean LD, Sullivan WA. Secretory and clinical aspects of achlorhydria and gastric atrophy as precursors of gastric cancer. J Natl Cancer Inst 1957;18:795. (*An early review of data, indicating that the risk was increased 4.5 and 21.9 times among patients with achlorhydria and pernicious anemia, respectively; recommends frequent radiographic studies.*)
6. Hohenberger P, Gretschel S. Gastric cancer. Lancet 2003;362: 305. (*A comprehensive review of all aspects; 117 references.*)
7. Schafer LW, Larson DE, Melton LJ, et al. The risk of gastric carcinoma after surgical treatment for benign ulcer disease. N Engl J Med 1983;309:1210. (*The finding that no evident increase was found in the risk for gastric cancer after surgical treatment for benign peptic ulcer disease led the authors to conclude that endoscopic surveillance is not indicated in this population.*)
8. Scheiman JM, Cutler AF. *Helicobacter pylori* and gastric cancer. Am J Med 1999;106:222. (*A succinct review of association, pathophysiology, and clinical policy implications.*)
9. Bedikian AY, Chen TT, Khankhanian N, et al. The natural history of gastric cancer and prognostic factors influencing survival. J Clin Oncol 1984;2:305. (*A useful review of natural history, with an emphasis on clinical determinants of survival.*)
10. Correa P, Fontham ET, Bravo JC, et al. Chemoprevention of gastric dysplasia: randomized trial of antioxidant supplements and anti–*Helicobacter pylori* therapy. J Natl Cancer Inst 2000;92:1881. (*Notes the decades-long progression from normal stomach tissue through chronic atrophic gastritis, intestinal metaplasia, dysplasia, and, finally, cancer.*)
11. Kurihara M, Shirakabe H, Yarita T, et al. Diagnosis of small early gastric cancer by x-ray, endoscopy, and biopsy. Cancer Detect Prev 1981;4:377. (*The sensitivity of double-contrast radiography was 75%; that of endoscopy plus biopsy was >95%.*)
12. Muramaki R, Tsukuma H, Ubukata T, et al. Estimation of validity of mass screening program for gastric cancer in Japan. Cancer 1990;65:1255. (*Radiographic techniques adapted for mass screening for gastric cancer in Japan achieved sensitivity and specificity of 90%.*)
13. Parsonnet J, Harris RA, Hack HM, et al. Modeling cost-effectiveness of *Helicobacter pylori* screening to prevent gastric cancer: a mandate for clinical trials. Lancet 1996;348:150. (*Based on the assumption that H. pylori treatment would prevent 30% of attributable gastric cancers, this approach would have a reasonable cost-effectiveness ratio.*)
14. Wong BC, Lam SK, Wong WM, et al. *Helicobacter pylori* eradication to prevent gastric cancer in a high-risk region of China. JAMA 2004;291:187. (*There was no effect overall on gastric cancer incidence over 7.5 years; however, among patients infected without precancerous lesions, eradication was associated with cancer prevention.*)
15. Yamazaki H, Oshima A, Muramaki R, et al. A long-term follow-up study of patients with gastric cancer detected by mass screening. Cancer 1989;63:613. (*Includes survival curves and hazard rates for >1,000 patients with gastric cancer detected by mass screening in Japan.*)
16. Logan RFA, Langman MJS. Screening for gastric cancer after gastric surgery. Lancet 1983;2:667. (*Accepts the evidence for increased risk but nevertheless does not favor endoscopic screening.*)

CHAPTER 56 ■ SCREENING FOR COLORECTAL CANCER

MICHAEL J. BARRY

Colorectal cancer (CRC) is a common malignancy in both men and women, accounting for about 10% of cancer deaths. Americans face a lifetime risk of colorectal cancer of approximately 1 in 17. The majority of colorectal cancers that present with signs or symptoms have already spread beyond the intestinal wall, resulting in a poor 5-year survival. However, cancers detected and removed while they are still localized are associated with a 5-year survival greater than 80%. The long asymptomatic period, the availability of tests that can identify localized disease, and the improved outcomes with early therapy have long suggested that screening for colorectal cancer might be effective. Evidence from multiple randomized trials, primarily of fecal occult blood testing, has confirmed that screening can reduce not only colorectal cancer mortality, but, through the removal of precancerous polyps, its incidence as well.

EPIDEMIOLOGY AND RISK FACTORS (1–14)

The incidence of colorectal cancer is greater in economically developed societies. The high-fat, low-fiber *diet* prevalent in Western societies has been implicated in the etiology of these cancers. Whether intake of dietary fiber, fruits and vegetables, or red or processed meats among Americans is associated with the risk for colorectal cancer has been harder to prove.

Advancing *age* is an important risk factor, with the incidence of colorectal cancer rising from about 75 in 100,000 in the sixth decade to 300 in 100,000 in the eighth decade.

Family history is also a risk factor. Having a first-degree relative with colorectal cancer raises personal risk about twofold, with a greater risk when the cancer has been diagnosed before age 50 years and when more than one first-degree relative has been affected. Newer evidence suggests that a first-degree relative with a larger adenomatous polyp also increases the risk for colorectal cancer. Autosomal dominant familial adenomatous polyposis confers a risk for colorectal cancer of about 50% by age 40 years, and a number of other familial cancer syndromes also increase risk greatly. Genetic testing is available for familial adenomatous polyposis and hereditary nonpolyposis colon cancer.

Ulcerative colitis, particularly pancolitis of more than 10 years' duration, increases a patient's risk for colorectal cancer 5- to 10-fold, although isolated ulcerative proctitis probably confers substantially less or no additional risk. Patients with extensive Crohn's colitis also appear to have a significant increase in risk.

In some observational studies, the use of aspirin or nonsteroidal antiinflammatory drugs has appeared to be associated with a lower risk for colorectal cancer. Regular aspirin use, especially at doses higher than generally used for cardiovascular prevention and for prolonged durations, is associated with a 22% reduction of colorectal cancer incidence in cohort studies. The gastrointestinal toxicities of these agents at higher doses reduce their utility in colorectal cancer chemoprevention.

Almost all colorectal cancers are believed to arise from *adenomatous polyps*. The prevalence of adenomatous polyps increases with age, occurring in 30% of 50-year-olds (3% of which are >1 cm), 40% of 60-year-olds (4% of which are >1 cm), and 50% of 70-year-olds (5% of which are >1 cm). Once a person has had an adenomatous polyp removed, it has been suggested that his or her future risk for colorectal cancer is higher. However, the magnitude of future risk, if any, is uncertain, especially if the index polyp is small (<1 cm).

Patients with *resected colorectal cancers* have a threefold increase in risk for developing metachronous cancer in other locations of the colon. Recurrences of index cancers are usually extraluminal and not amenable to detection by endoscopic screening.

The prevalence of *synchronous colonic neoplasia* is high and important to consider in the evaluation of the patient with a positive screening test result. Synchronous adenomas occur in 40% to 50% of patients with an index polyp; 3% to 5% with a carcinoma harbor a second one.

NATURAL HISTORY OF COLORECTAL CANCER AND EFFECTIVENESS OF THERAPY (4,8,10,13–17)

Sporadic polyps are common lesions, with the most common being small, hyperplastic outcroppings of the colonic mucosa that do not have malignant potential. Adenomas are truly neoplastic and may include malignant foci. The risk for malignancy increases with the size of the adenoma, ranging from 0.5% of colonoscopically removed polyps from 0.5 to 0.9 cm in diameter to 25% or more of polyps greater than 3 cm in diameter. Histology also affects cancer risk. Villous adenomas are the polyps with the highest malignant potential, and they tend to be larger and more sessile than tubular or mixed tubulovillous adenomas, which are associated with less risk (Table 56.1). About 10% of polyps have villous histology, tubular adenomas account for 70%, and the remainder are of mixed histology. The probability and time frame for the development of a nonmalignant polyp into an invasive cancer are not well defined, although the time frame is probably around 10 years. Of interest, although the prevalence of polyps increases with age (see prior discussion), average polyp size does not, which suggests that most polyps do not progressively enlarge.

TABLE 56.1

POLYPOID LESIONS OF THE COLON AND RECTUM: RELATION OF SIZE TO CANCER (1,116 POLYPOID LESIONS, MASSACHUSETTS GENERAL HOSPITAL, 1954–1963)

Diameter (CM)	Percentage Cancerous
<0.5	0.5
0.5–0.9	1
1.0–1.4	1.8
1.5–1.9	6
2.0–2.4	10
2.5–3.4	23
≥ 3.5	29

From Behringer GE. Changing concepts in the histopathologic diagnosis of polypoidlesions of the colon. Dis Colon Rectum 1970;13:116, with permission.

Symptoms occur late in the course of colorectal cancer growth. The duration of the asymptomatic detectable period is estimated to be several years. When cancers are found after symptomatic presentation, 60% have already disseminated to regional nodes or distant organs. Five-year survival rates vary dramatically with the stage of disease at the time of diagnosis. Patients whose tumors are confined locally to the bowel wall (Dukes stage A) or pericolic fat (Dukes B) have an 80% 5-year survival, whereas those whose tumors exhibit regional lymph node metastases (Dukes C) have a 46% 5-year survival; this probability drops to 5% with distant metastases (Dukes D).

SCREENING TESTS

Digital Rectal Examination (8–13)

Only about 10% of colorectal cancers are within reach of the examining finger. Although many U.S. physicians perform this time-honored examination annually among patients who are older than 40 years, there is little evidence to support the practice to screen for colorectal cancer.

Fecal Occult Blood Testing
(6,8,9,11–13,16,18–26)

Intermittent occult bleeding occurs with some asymptomatic colorectal cancers and large polyps. Serial sampling of stools for occult blood can be performed to identify this bleeding. Guaiac-impregnated filter paper slides (Hemoccult II and others) are capable of detecting small amounts of fecal blood, which is present in some patients with colorectal cancer. The fact that colonic tumors selectively enrich the stool surface with blood enhances the sensitivity of guaiac testing of stool samples. Stool sampling is best performed serially because of the intermittent nature of the bleeding (e.g., two samples from a stool on each of 3 days).

Sensitivity, Specificity, and Yield

A six-test guaiac stool sequence has a sensitivity of 15% to 50% for CRC. The lower figure is probably more accurate for early cancers in asymptomatic patients. Sensitivity falls when prepared slides are stored for more than 4 days before being developed. *Rehydration* of the sample before application of developer can increase sensitivity, at the cost of a loss in specificity. Some guaiac cards, such as Hemoccult II SENSA, appear to have operating characteristics more like rehydrated Hemoccult II cards. False-positive test results may occur with nonmalignant lesions, aspirin (at doses >325 mg daily) and nonsteroidal antiinflammatory drugs, rare red meat, or foods with high peroxidase activity. Studies on the ability of iron supplements to cause false-positive guaiac results have been conflicting. A specificity of 97% to 98% can be attained by omitting rare red meat, horseradish, cantaloupe, and uncooked fresh vegetables (especially broccoli, turnip, radish, and cauliflower) 2 days before the first sample is collected. However, such dietary restrictions may decrease patient compliance. High doses of vitamin C increase the false-negative rate. Guaiac testing of single stool samples obtained on office-based digital rectal exams in truly asymptomatic patients, although widely performed, is not a recommended screening strategy.

Although a single set of guaiac cards has limited sensitivity for colorectal cancer, a program of annual testing may have sensitivity as high as 80% to 90%.

Based on screening results in population studies and randomized trials, the clinician should expect 2% to 5% of persons older than the age of 50 years to have a positive fecal occult blood test (FOBT) result (Hemoccult II). Of these, about 10% will have colorectal cancer and 40% either cancer or polyps. Most of these polyps are too small to cause detectable bleeding but are found serendipitously when follow-up studies are performed after a positive occult blood test result. When rehydration is used, the positivity rate is about 10%. Of these, about 2% will have colorectal cancers and 30% either cancers or adenomas.

Individuals with a positive FOBT result require a thorough evaluation for colorectal neoplasia. Smaller polyps produce guaiac positivity only on occasion, but their high prevalence makes them the most common lesions found during the evaluation of patients with occult bleeding. *Colonoscopy*, which is preferable, and the combination of *sigmoidoscopy* and *air-contrast barium enema* are acceptable alternatives for follow-up evaluation of the patient with a positive test for occult blood. Colonoscopy offers the advantage of allowing a biopsy or polypectomy to be performed during the same examination and is more sensitive for detecting smaller polyps.

Outcomes

The best outcome measure of screening efficacy is *reduced colorectal cancer mortality*, as judged from prospective, randomized, controlled clinical trials with a long period of follow-up. One such study, the Minnesota Colon Cancer Study, demonstrated a 33% reduction in cumulative colorectal cancer mortality (from 8.3 in 1,000 to 5.9 in 1,000 over 13 years) as a result of annual occult blood screening. This trial used a six-sample annual testing protocol, followed by colonoscopy for persons with positive test results. The guaiac cards were rehydrated, which increased the sensitivity of testing from 81% to 92% but increased the false-positive rate from 2% to 10%. As a result of this decrease in specificity, 38% of screenees underwent colonoscopy during the study. Compared with the control group, screened patients demonstrated a shift to detection of earlier cancers. Despite the large relative benefit in terms of mortality, the absolute risk that any one man or woman will die of colorectal cancer is quite low. As a result, data from this trial indicate that about 300 men would need to be screened annually for 13 years to prevent 1 colorectal cancer death. In a subsequent publication, reporting 18 years of follow-up, the Minnesota investigators reported that even biennial screening reduced colorectal cancer mortality by 21%.

As seen from the Minnesota study, rehydration of the guaiac card increases its sensitivity, but it also increases the number of colonoscopies needed, the cost of screening, and the false-positive rate. Two other trials, conducted in Denmark and the United Kingdom, respectively, used guaiac cards without hydration and conducted screening biennially rather than annually. Population-based samples of patients were randomized without their knowledge, so it is likely that the persons screened were representative of actual practice. Only 4% of persons screened in these studies underwent colonoscopy. Even under these circumstances, the trials demonstrated 18% and 15% reductions in colorectal cancer mortality, respectively. A Cochrane meta-analysis of four randomized trials showed an overall 16% reduction in the risk of colorectal cancer mortality.

Sigmoidoscopy (6,8,9,11–13,16,27–30)

About 25% of colon cancers are within the range of the *rigid sigmoidoscope*, whereas the longer (65 cm) *flexible sigmoidoscope* can potentially detect about 50% of cancers. The risk for a bowel perforation—the major complication of sigmoidoscopy—is low, about 1 in 1,000 flexible sigmoidoscopic examinations. The number of cancers found per 1,000 examinations ranges from 1.5 for the rigid scope to 3 for the 65-cm flexible scope. Adenomatous polyps are found in up to 20% of persons screened. When polyps are detected at sigmoidoscopy, the patient then usually undergoes colonoscopy for polyp removal and histologic examination, as well as examination of the rest of the colon.

Outcomes

Sigmoidoscopy can clearly find localized cancers and polyps for removal, but the key question is the effect of the procedure on colorectal cancer mortality rates when used for periodic screening. Data from randomized trials are pending, but a retrospective, case–control study of periodic rigid sigmoidoscopy for colorectal cancer screening suggested a 60% to 70% reduction in colorectal cancer mortality risk. As would be expected, the protective association appeared to be specific for cancers within reach of the sigmoidoscope; the exposure odds were not reduced for more proximal cancers. The marginal value, in terms of mortality reduction, of adding sigmoidoscopic screening to regular guaiac testing is undefined. The right frequency for sigmoidoscopy screening is unclear. On one hand, the protective effect of sigmoidoscopy on mortality from colorectal cancer within its reach appears to last for 10 years or more. On the other hand, a repeat exam 3 years after a negative sigmoidoscopy reveals larger adenomas or cancer in about 1% of patients.

Colonoscopy (6,8,9,11–13,16,27,31–35)

Primary colonoscopic screening is growing in popularity because all colorectal cancers are theoretically within the reach of the colonoscope (incomplete insertion or suboptimal preparation will limit sensitivity to some degree). The risk of perforation is about 1 in 500 exams. In a major Veterans Administration study comparing colonoscopy with sigmoidoscopy and one-time fecal occult blood testing, colonoscopic screening of men ages 50 to 75 years revealed large or dysplastic polyps in 10% and cancer in 1%. Approximately 70% of these

lesions would have been discovered by a sigmoidoscopic exam (with follow-up colonoscopy for any distal polyps). A one-time set of six stool cards detected 24% of the neoplastic lesions, but because of poor sensitivity of the stool blood tests for proximal neoplasia, the combined sensitivity of sigmoidoscopy and one-time fecal occult blood testing was only 76% relative to colonoscopy. Presumably, however, serial annual fecal occult blood testing combined with sigmoidoscopy would have an even better combined sensitivity relative to colonoscopy. As with sigmoidoscopy, the protective effect of a negative colonoscopy appears to last for at least 10 years, although long-term protection is less robust for cancers in the ascending colon.

Outcomes

There is no direct evidence of the magnitude of reduction in colorectal cancer mortality that can be expected from a strategy of periodic colonoscopy. However, given that studies of fecal occult blood testing and sigmoidoscopy have demonstrated that early detection of colorectal cancer reduces mortality, it is not unreasonable to assume that colonoscopy, which maximizes sensitivity for detection of colorectal cancer and adenomas, would have an even greater mortality benefit than these other screening strategies. A modeling exercise has suggested that the benefits of colorectal cancer screening among persons age 80 years and older are much smaller than for younger individuals.

EMERGING TESTS (6,22,36–40)

Computed Tomography Colonography

Computed tomography (CT) colonography requires similar colon preparation as for colonoscopy and must be followed by colonoscopy for individuals with suspicious findings. CT colonography appears to have a lower sensitivity for smaller adenomas, which may be an advantage or a disadvantage, given the costs generated by follow-up of these lesions and their lower malignant potential. One recent study in which patients underwent both CT colonography and colonoscopy found that the positive predictive value for polyps greater than 5 mm identified by CT colonography with three-dimensional reconstruction was only 41%, whereas the negative predictive value was 88%. If techniques for CT colonography evolve to allow less-intensive colon preparation (which some patients find more objectionable than colonoscopy), this test may make colorectal cancer screening more acceptable for some people. However, at present, people who undergo both CT colonography and colonoscopy generally prefer the latter.

Immunochemical Fecal Occult Blood Tests

Immunochemical FOBT uses antibodies to detect human hemoglobin in stool. Early results suggest that these tests may be more sensitive, although no more (and perhaps less) specific, than guaiac-based FOBT.

Stool DNA Mutations

Tests are becoming available to screen single stool samples for DNA mutations associated with colorectal neoplasms, both cancers and advanced polyps. Comparisons of the performance of these tests to traditional fecal occult blood testing have suggested higher sensitivity but similar specificity. At present, testing for stool DNA mutations is expensive. Whether this newer strategy for screening could obviate even infrequent colonoscopy in some patients remains to be seen.

OVERALL SCREENING STRATEGY
(6,12,13,41)

A recent guideline from the American Cancer Society and several professional societies emphasizes the importance of polyp detection, recommending colonoscopy every 10 years; or flexible sigmoidoscopy, double contrast barium enema, or CT colography every 5 years beginning at age 50 for average risk patients. The U.S. preventive Services Task force recently recommended high sensitivity FOBT annually, flexible sigmoidoscopy every 5 years combined with FOBT every 3 years, or colonoscopy every 10 years for average risk patients age 50–75. Combined annual FOBT and periodic colonoscopy is not a recommended screening strategy.

Despite good evidence of effectiveness, colorectal cancer screening is underused, and strategies to increase physician and patient compliance with screening recommendations are needed.

CONCLUSION AND RECOMMENDATIONS

Conclusion

- The relatively high prevalence of colorectal cancer, the slow evolution from an adenomatous polyp to a cancer, and the accumulating evidence that screening reduces mortality from this disease suggest that an aggressive approach to screening is reasonable and appropriate. Although the impact of annual FOBT plus periodic sigmoidoscopy or periodic colonoscopy on colorectal cancer mortality has not been directly measured, it is likely to be higher than the effect of annual fecal occult blood testing or periodic sigmoidoscopy alone.

Recommendations: Test Selection and Frequency of Screening

- All patients at average risk should be offered some form of colorectal cancer screening beginning at age 50 years. Two practical strategies with the highest sensitivity are annual FOBT plus flexible sigmoidoscopy every 5 years or colonoscopy alone every 10 years. However, FOBT alone or sigmoidoscopy alone is also an effective screening strategy. Patient preference, local availability of high-quality endoscopy, and the patient's insurance coverage need to be considered in negotiating an optimal screening program with an individual patient.
- Patients at higher risk for colorectal cancer, such as persons with a family history of colorectal cancer or larger (>1 cm) adenomas in first-degree relatives before age 60 years, may especially benefit from the higher-sensitivity screening strategies. Screening might be started at age 40 years or at 10 years before the youngest affected relative was diagnosed.
- Patients at the highest risk, such as persons with a past personal history of colorectal cancer or larger adenomas, long-standing ulcerative colitis with pancolonic involvement, familial adenomatous polyposis, or nonpolyposis colon cancer should have a strategy of periodic colonoscopy worked out with an endoscopist.

Recommendations: Test Performance

- Perform guaiac-based FOBT by instructing the patient to obtain two samples on each of 3 days, restricting dietary peroxidases and rare red meat according to the test instructions. Do not rely on a single guaiac test on stool obtained from a digital rectal exam.
- Follow any positive FOBT result with colonoscopy.
- Proceed to colonoscopy for patients with suspicious lesions or polyps found on screening sigmoidoscopy.
- For average-risk, asymptomatic persons being screened with periodic colonoscopy, interim fecal occult blood tests are not necessary.

Annotated Bibliography

1. Butterworth AS, Higgins JPT, Pharoah P. Relative and absolute risk of colorectal cancer for individuals with a family history. Eur J Cancer 2006;42:216. (*Provides estimates of the relative and absolute risks of colorectal cancer depending on family history.*)
2. Calver PM, Frucht HF. The genetics of colorectal cancer. Ann Intern Med 2002;137:603. (*Excellent summary of the genetic and clinical applications, including counseling high-risk individuals; 57 references.*)
3. Dube C, Rostom A, Lewin G, et al. The use of aspirin for primary prevention of colorectal cancer: a systematic review prepared for the U.S. Preventive Services Task Force. Ann Intern Med 2007;146:365. (*A systematic literature review and meta-analysis of the evidence associating aspirin use with colorectal neoplasia risk.*)
4. Hawk ET, Umar A, Viner JL. Colorectal cancer chemoprevention—an overview of the science. Gastroenterology 2004;126:1423. (*Comprehensive review of the science and ongoing trials; 287 references.*)
5. Imperiale TF, Wagner DR, Lin CY, et al. Risk of advanced proximal neoplasms in asymptomatic adults according to distal colorectal findings. N Engl J Med 2000;343:169. (*Quantifies the higher risk of proximal neoplasms with distal lesions, including hyperplastic polyps.*)
6. Lieberman D. Screening for colorectal cancer in average-risk populations. Am J Med 2006;119:728. (*A thorough review of screening by a leading investigator; 47 references.*)
7. Marques-Vidal P, Ravasco P, Camilo ME. Foodstuffs and colorectal cancer risk: a review. Clin Nutr 2006;25:14. (*Reviews the epidemiologic evidence for the relationship between diet and colorectal cancer risk.*)
8. Pignone M, Rich M, Teutsch SM, et al. Screening for colorectal cancer in adults at average risk: a summary of the evidence for the U.S. Preventive Services Task Force. Ann Intern Med 2002;137:132. (*Succinct review of the evidence used by the task force to inform its recommendations.*)
9. Pignone M, Saha S, Hoerger T, et al. Cost-effectiveness analyses of colorectal cancer screening: a systematic review for the U.S. Preventive Services Task Force. Ann Intern Med 2002;137:96. (*A formal systematic review of the best economic studies.*)
10. Ransohoff DF, Lang CA. Small adenomas detected during fecal occult blood test screening for colorectal cancer: the impact of serendipity. JAMA 1990;264:76. (*The high predictive value of occult blood tests for polyps is the result of their high prevalence rather than that they bleed.*)
11. Ransohoff DF, Sandler RS. Screening for colorectal cancer. N Engl J Med 2002;346:40. (*Brief but thorough review of screening issues.*)
12. Levin B, Lieberman DA, McFarland B, et al. Screening and surveillance for the early detection of colorectal cancer and adenomatous polyps, 2008: A joint guideline from the American Cancer Society, the US multi-society task force on colorectal cancer, and the American College of radiology. Gastroenterology 2008;134:1570–1595. (*2008 guideline emphasizes the importance of polyp detection and removal to prevent colorectal cancer.*)
13. U.S. Preventive Services Task Force. Screening for colorectal cancer: U.S. Preventive Services Task Force Recommendations Statement. Ann Intern Med 2008;149 October 6 [epub ahead of print]. (*2008 update of the USPSTF recommendations on colorectal screening. The new recommendations are backed by a detailed decision model.*)

14. Wallace MB, Kemp JA, Trnka YM, et al. Is colonoscopy indicated for small adenomas found by screening flexible sigmoidoscopy? Ann Intern Med 1998;129:273. (*Data from this prospective cohort study suggest that the answer is no for a single distal tubular adenoma <5 mm but yes for multiple small adenomas or advanced histology.*)

15. Ahlquist DA, McGill DB, Fleming JL, et al. Pattern of occult bleeding in asymptomatic colorectal cancer. Cancer 1989;63:1826. (*Documents the relatively low sensitivity of guaiac tests for asymptomatic cancers.*)

16. Davila RE, Rajan E, Baron TH. ASGE guideline: colorectal cancer screening and surveillance. Gastrointest Endosc 2006;63:546. (*Guidelines from the American Society for Gastrointestinal Endoscopy emphasize colonoscopy in cancer screening and follow-up surveillance.*)

17. Winawer SJ, Zauber AG, O'Brien MJ, et al. Randomized comparison of surveillance intervals after colonoscopic removal of newly diagnosed adenomatous polyps. N Engl J Med 1993;328:901. (*A longer interval is just as effective as a shorter one.*)

18. Allison JE, Tekawa IS, Ransom LJ, et al. A comparison of fecal occult blood tests for colorectal cancer screening. N Engl J Med 1996;334:155. (*A comparison of three different screening tests and one combination of two tests suggests that improvement over Hemoccult II sensitivity is possible with only modest loss of specificity.*)

19. American College of Physicians. Suggested technique for fecal occult blood testing and interpretation in colorectal cancer screening. Ann Intern Med 1997;126:808. (*American College of Physicians guidelines for performing fecal occult blood testing and following up on suspected results.*)

20. Hardcastle JD, Chamberlain JO, Robinson MHE, et al. Randomised trial of faecal-occult-blood screening for colorectal cancer. Lancet 1996;348:1472. (*A population-based trial with a 15% mortality reduction attributable to biennial Hemoccult tests without rehydration.*)

21. Hewitson P, Glasziou P, Irwig L, et al. Screening for colorectal cancer using the faecal occult blood test. Cochrane Database Syst Rev 2007(Jan 24/1):CD001216. (*A Cochrane meta-analysis of four randomized, controlled trials of fecal occult blood [FOBC] testing.*)

22. Imperiale TF, Ransohoff DF, Itzkowitz SH, et al. Fecal DNA versus fecal occult blood for colorectal-cancer screening in an average-risk population. N Engl J Med 2004;351:2704. (*Compares the operating characteristics of fecal DNA and FOBC testing in an average-risk population using colonoscopy as the gold standard.*)

23. Kronborg O, Fenger C, Olsen J, et al. Randomised study of screening for colorectal cancer with faecal-occult-blood test. Lancet 1996;348:1467. (*In this population-based trial, an 18% mortality reduction was achieved with biennial screening and without the rehydration of Hemoccult II tests.*)

24. Lieberman DA, Weiss DG. One-time screening for colorectal cancer with combined fecal occult-blood testing and examination of the distal colon. N Engl J Med 2001;345:555. (*Describes the joint sensitivity of one-time fecal occult blood testing and sigmoidoscopy relative to colonoscopy.*)

25. Mandel JS, Bond JH, Church TR, et al. Reducing mortality from colorectal cancer by screening for fecal occult blood. N Engl J Med 1993;328:1365. (*Randomized, prospective study showing a 33% relative reduction in colorectal cancer [CRC] mortality risk with annual screening for 13 years and the use of rehydrated cards.*)

26. Mandel JS, Church TR, Ederer F, et al. Colorectal cancer mortality: effectiveness of biennial screening for fecal occult blood. J Natl Cancer Inst 1999;91:434. (*In an update of the trial cited in ref. 25, after 18 years, annual screening reduced CRC mortality 33%, and biennial screening reduced CRC mortality 21%.*)

27. Gatto NM, Frucht H, Sundararajan V, et al. Risk of perforation after colonoscopy and sigmoidoscopy: a population-based study. J Natl Cancer Inst 2003;95:230. (*The most precise and generalizable estimates of perforation risks.*)

28. Schoen RE, Pinsky PF, Weissfeld JL, et al. Results of repeat sigmoidoscopy 3 years after a negative examination. JAMA 2003;290:41. (*An early report from the important Prostate, Lung, Colorectal and Ovarian [PLCO] cancer screening trial demonstrates a modest yield for colorectal neoplasia when a screening sigmoidoscopy is repeated over the short term.*)

29. Selby JV, Friedman GD, Quesenberry CP, et al. A case–control study of screening sigmoidoscopy and mortality from colorectal cancer. N Engl J Med 1992;326:653. (*Exposure to sigmoidoscopic screening was associated with a substantial reduction in the risk of dying of CRC within the reach of the scope.*)

30. Weissfeld JL, Schoen RE, Pinsky PF, et al. Flexible sigmoidoscopy in the PLCO cancer screening trial: results from the baseline screening examination of a randomized trial. J Natl Cancer Inst 2005;97:989. (*Detailed account of the yield of flexible sigmoidoscopic screening in about 75,000 participants in the PLCO trial.*)

31. Imperiale TF, Wagner DR, Lin CY, et al. Results of screening colonoscopy among persons 40 to 49 years of age. N Engl J Med 2002;346:1781. (*Prospective cohort study finding no increase in yield or other important outcomes from early colonoscopy in normal-risk persons.*)

32. Lieberman AD, Weiss DG, Bond JH, et al. Use of colonoscopy to screen asymptomatic adults for colorectal cancer. N Engl J Med 2000;343:162. (*Describes the relative sensitivity of sigmoidoscopy to colonoscopy.*)

33. Lin OS, Kozarek RA, Schembre DB, et al. Screening colonoscopy in very elderly patients: prevalence of neoplasia and estimated impact on life expectancy. JAMA 2006;295:2357. (*Study examining the yield and estimated benefits of colorectal cancer screening according to age.*)

34. Lindsay DC, Freeman JG, Cobden I, et al. Should colonoscopy be the first investigation for colonic disease? BMJ 1988;296:167. (*Randomized trial of colonoscopy vs. rigid sigmoidoscopy and air-contrast barium enema in the workup of colonic disease.*)

35. Singh H, Turner D, Xue L, et al. Risk of developing colorectal cancer following a negative colonoscopy examination: evidence for a 10-year interval between colonoscopies. JAMA 2006;295:2366. (*A population-based study from Manitoba examining the incidence of colorectal cancer after a negative colonoscopy compared to controls.*)

36. Bosworth B, Rockey DC, Paulson EK, et al. Prospective comparison of patient experience with colon imaging tests. Am J Med 2006;119:791. (*More than 600 patients underwent air-contrast barium enema, computed tomography colonography, and colonoscopy; they generally preferred colonoscopy.*)

37. Levi Z, Rozen P, Hazazi R, et al. A quantitative immunochemical fecal occult blood test for colorectal neoplasia. Ann Intern Med 2007;146:244. (*The operating characteristics of an immunochemical FOBT with colonoscopy as a gold standard, although without concurrent comparison to guaiac FOBT.*)

38. Mulhall BP, Veerappan GR, Jackson JL. Meta-analysis: computed tomographic colonography. Ann Intern Med 2005;142:635. (*A meta-analysis of the sensitivity and specificity of computed tomography colonography for detecting polyps of different sizes.*)

39. Pickhardt PJ, Choi R, Hwang I, et al. Computed tomographic virtual colonoscopy to screen for colorectal neoplasia in asymptomatic adults. N Engl J Med 2003;349:2191. (*In a well-designed study in which participants had both tests, computed tomography colonography had a sensitivity for polyps of size >5 mm similar to colonoscopy but poor specificity, so most apparent polyps were false positives.*)

40. Regueiro CR. AGA Future Trends Committee report: colorectal cancer screening: a qualitative review of emerging screening and diagnostic technologies. Gastroenterol 2005;129:1083. (*A thorough review of the many emerging tests for CRC screening;150 references.*)

41. Rabeneck L. What can we do about low colorectal cancer screening rates? Am J Gastroenterol 2007;102:1736. (*Discusses the reasons and potential solutions for the fact that CRC screening rates are <50% in North America.*)

APPENDIX 56.1: EXAMINATION OF THE ANORECTUM AND SIGMOID COLON WITH DIGITAL RECTAL EXAMINATION, ANOSCOPY, AND SIGMOIDOSCOPY

PATRICK S. YACHIMSKI AND LAWRENCE S. FRIEDMAN

Careful, competent examinations of the anorectal area and distal colon are essential for evaluation of complaints referable to these structures and continue to play a role in colorectal cancer screening. The anorectal examination is indicated in all patients who are to undergo sigmoidoscopy and should be incorporated into all complete physical examinations in adults.

ANORECTAL EXAMINATION (1,2)

Digital Rectal Examination

The physician must establish rapport with the patient by taking a history and performing other parts of the physical examination before rectal examination. Apprehension and embarrassment may be minimized by explaining each step, describing the anticipated sensations, and draping the patient to expose only the perineum. In selected instances, it may be advisable for a medical assistant or suitable chaperone to be present during rectal examination.

Inspection

The patient may be examined in either the knee-chest or left lateral decubitus position. After retraction of the buttocks, the perianal skin and anal orifice are inspected for fecal material (reflecting poor hygiene, painful lesions that make cleansing difficult, or incontinence), drainage, dermatoses, scars, prolapsed hemorrhoids, fistulas, fissures, abscesses, hematomas, condylomata, and carcinomas. Lesions are described anatomically (e.g., anterior, right-sided), not with reference to the face of a clock. By asking the patient to strain or perform a Valsalva maneuver, the physician may assess perineal descent. Perineal and sacrococcygeal tissues should be palpated with the gloved but unlubricated index finger for tenderness, induration, fluctuance, or masses.

Palpation

Digital examination of the rectum is then performed by placing the gloved, lubricated index finger at the anal orifice and gently inserting as the patient bears down. The small finger may be used in patients with painful or stenotic anal lesions. Anesthetic ointment may be helpful if a tender lesion is present. Digital rectal examination may be exquisitely painful for patients with anal fissure. If an anal fissure is suspected, consideration should be given to deferring examination until healing has occurred or arranging for examination under anesthesia.

The anal sphincter tone and strength of contraction are noted, and the finger is swept circumferentially as it is advanced into the rectum. Abnormalities sought include fissures, fistulous tracts, abscesses, polyps, and cancers. Internal hemorrhoids are not palpable unless they are thrombosed. In inflammatory bowel disease, the mucosa may feel gritty. Stool in the rectum is deformable, which distinguishes it from other rectal masses. The rectal ampulla should be checked carefully (Fig. 56.1); it is often overlooked and may harbor a neoplasm. To evaluate dyssynergic defecation in a patient who reports constipation or incomplete evacuation, the physician may ask the patient to attempt to expel the examining finger to simulate defecation.

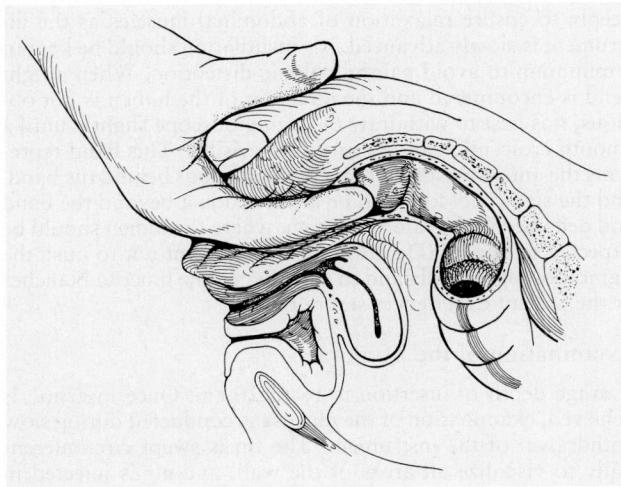

FIGURE 56.1. Digital examination.

The average effective depth of insertion of the index finger is 7.5 cm. In women, care must be taken not to mistake the cervix (or a tampon) for a rectal "tumor" along the anterior rectal wall; the cervix is smooth and symmetric. In men, the prostate and, if possible, the seminal vesicles should be examined. Finally, on withdrawal, the examining finger should be inspected for the character of feces and the presence of blood, pus, or mucus. A test for occult blood should be performed unless gross blood is evident.

Anoscopy

Anoscopy may be a useful adjunct to the anorectal examination, particularly in the evaluation of bright-red rectal bleeding, perianal pain, or suspected hemorrhoids. The yield of anoscopy is superior to that of sigmoidoscopy for detecting lesions within the anal canal. Some have suggested screening anoscopy for evidence of human papillomavirus infection in patients with a history of receptive anal intercourse.

Anoscopes are disposable plastic tubes with a diameter of 2 cm at the tip and a length of 7 cm. An external light source is required unless there is a built-in light source. With the patient in the same position as for the anorectal examination, the lubricated anoscope is held in the right hand with the thumb pressing the obturator as the instrument is introduced with slow, gentle pressure. The instrument is first directed along the longitudinal axis of the anal canal toward the umbilicus and then pointed more posteriorly at the anorectal angle. It is inserted the full length and held in the left hand so that the flange rests against the anus. The obturator is removed, and the anoscope is slowly withdrawn as the mucosa is examined.

The normal rectal mucosa is pink, with a visible delicate network of submucosal vessels. In patients with proctitis, the vascular pattern is obliterated and the mucosa may be friable. On withdrawal, the anal mucosa is red. Hemorrhoids appear as purple bulges into the lumen; occasionally, blood may be seen to issue from a hemorrhoid. Fissures may be identified at the anal verge.

SIGMOIDOSCOPY (2–17)

Indications

Screening for Colorectal Cancer (See Also Above)

About 50% of CRCs are within reach of the flexible sigmoidoscope. Screening by flexible sigmoidoscopy has been shown to reduce mortality from CRC, and, in combination with FOBT, is cost-effective. Moreover, detection of polyps on flexible sigmoidoscopy also leads to reduced mortality from CRC by permitting their removal before they undergo malignant transformation. Polyps larger than 1 cm in diameter or with villous features on histology are considered at high risk for malignant transformation and are markers of additional high-risk polyps in the proximal colon.

Evaluation of Complaints Referable to the Distal Colon

Sigmoidoscopy permits direct visualization of the colonic mucosa. As such, it as an essential part of the evaluation of patients presenting with a host of complaints or problems referable to the large bowel (Table 56.2). In addition, sigmoidoscopy can permit direct visualization of abnormalities detected by digital rectal examination or radiologic imaging, such as polyps and suspected mass lesions. In patients with inflammatory

TABLE 56.2

INDICATIONS FOR SIGMOIDOSCOPY

Symptoms
   Rectal pain
   Rectal discharge
   Bright-red bleeding per rectum
   Hematochezia
   Persistent or recurrent diarrhea
   Change in bowel habits
   Chronic constipation
   Unexplained weight loss

Signs
   Rectal mass
   Enlarged sentinel lymph node[a]
   Positive fecal occult blood test result[a]
   Unexplained hepatic nodule or enlargement or other signs
      of metastatic cancer[a]

Laboratory Abnormalities
   Unexplained iron-deficiency anemia[a]
   Mass or polyp in distal colon on barium enema
   Other laboratory manifestation of metastatic disease from
      unknown primary lesion[a]

Screening
   Patients at average risk of colon cancer

[a] Colonoscopy is preferred, but sigmoidoscopy in combination with
barium enema is an alternative approach.

bowel disease involving the rectum or descending colon, sigmoidoscopy is useful for monitoring disease activity and response to therapy.

Preparation

Satisfactory cleansing of the bowel can be achieved in most patients with a single tap water or sodium phosphate *enema* administered 45 minutes before examination. If the examination has been scheduled in advance, the patient can be instructed to self-administer one or two enemas at home on the morning of examination. After the preparation, the patient should take nothing by mouth. Adequate preparation is particularly advisable in older persons, who often have large amounts of retained stool in the rectal vault.

For patients with diarrhea or suspected inflammatory bowel disease, it is acceptable to forego enema before sigmoidoscopy. These patients can often achieve adequate preparation by having a *bowel movement* just before the examination. Moreover, because enemas may induce edema and erythema of the mucosa, enema administration may make it difficult for the practitioner to distinguish subtle mucosal changes caused by proctitis from those induced by the enema.

The risk of endocarditis associated with sigmoidoscopy is negligible. Therefore, routine antibiotic prophylaxis is not recommended for patients undergoing sigmoidoscopy yet is considered optional for patients with prosthetic valves, a history of endocarditis, congenital heart disease, or other high-risk conditions. Sedation and analgesia are seldom necessary but may be used in patients with painful anal lesions.

Contraindications

Contraindications to sigmoidoscopy include acute peritonitis, suspected bowel perforation or infarction, suspected acute diverticulitis, a severely uncooperative patient, and inability to obtain informed patient consent. Sigmoidoscopy is not contraindicated in pregnancy.

Rigid Sigmoidoscopy

Once a procedure performed routinely by primary care physicians, rigid sigmoidoscopy is performed less frequently since the advent of flexible sigmoidoscopes. Still, rigid sigmoidoscopy is easy to learn, requires inexpensive equipment, and can be readily performed in the office to evaluate a patient with anorectal complaints.

Instrument

The rigid sigmoidoscope is a metal or disposable plastic tube, 25 cm long and approximately 1.5 cm in diameter, usually with distal fiberoptic lighting, a proximal magnifying lens, and a connection for air insufflation. Additional standard equipment includes cotton swabs, suctioning apparatus, and biopsy and grasping forceps.

Patient Position

The patient is examined in the same position as for the rectal and anoscopic examinations. The left lateral decubitus position is better tolerated than the knee-chest position by older and debilitated patients and may be less embarrassing to patients in general. However, the knee-chest position permits a greater range of scope motion.

Insertion

The lubricated instrument is inserted with the right hand holding the obturator firmly in place and with gentle pressure against the anal sphincter as the patient bears down. The sigmoidoscope is initially directed toward the umbilicus and then posteriorly at the anorectal junction (Fig. 56.2).

Once past the anorectal ring, the obturator is withdrawn, and the sigmoidoscope is advanced with the lumen in view at all times. It is important to note whether the sigmoidoscope is advancing up the lumen or merely pushing the rectal mucosa. The rectosigmoid junction is reached at about 12 to 15 cm from the anus, at which point the lumen bends sharply forward and to the left. The patient may experience painful spasm and should be reassured and instructed to breathe slowly and deeply to ensure relaxation of abdominal muscles as the instrument is slowly advanced. Air insufflation should be kept to a minimum to avoid painful colonic distention. When a tight bend is encountered and the direction of the lumen is not obvious, it is best to withdraw the sigmoidoscope slightly until a smooth crescentic band of mucosa is visible. This band represents the anterior aspect of mucosa as it bends behind the band, and the sigmoidoscope can be advanced just beyond the band and deflected in the same direction, where the lumen should be expected to appear (Fig. 56.3). It is important not to push the sigmoidoscope blindly and to desist when the mucosa blanches or the patient experiences severe pain.

Examination of the Mucosa

Average depth of insertion is 16 to 20 cm. Once insertion is achieved, examination of the mucosa is conducted during slow withdrawal of the instrument. The tip is swept circumferentially to visualize all areas of the wall, and air is injected in small amounts to flatten folds and allow adequate inspection. The mucosa should be examined and described; any lesions should be noted, and the distance from the anal verge should be recorded.

Biopsy Specimens

Biopsy of suspected lesions and abnormal mucosa may be obtained with angled forceps. Mucosal biopsies should be shallow and taken from the posterior rectal wall, where the risk for perforation is small. Because of the risk for perforation, barium enema examination should be avoided for at least 5 days after a rigid sigmoidoscopic biopsy.

Flexible Sigmoidoscopy

Instrument

Flexible sigmoidoscopes are 60 to 65 cm in length with large-caliber suction, as well as controls for air and water installation. Two hand dials permit four-quadrant tip deflection for enhanced visualization and maneuverability. Biopsy forceps and other devices may be passed through a dedicated instrument channel. The diameter of the shaft is 11 mm, making the instrument narrower and longer than the rigid sigmoidoscope. Visualization of the lumen and mucosa is achieved either through an eyepiece on the instrument or through image transmission to a video monitor. Video endoscopes are standard in modern endoscopy suites; however, fiberoptic sigmoidoscopes with an eyepiece remain in use in office-based practices, where video equipment may be either too expensive or impractical.

Insertion

The average depth of insertion of the flexible instrument in the hands of experienced endoscopists is approximately 50 cm. This is typically sufficient to allow examination of the descending colon to the level of the splenic flexure. The control dials and button are managed with the left hand as the right hand grasps the shaft of the sigmoidoscope and advances the instrument up the colon. Acute angulations are traversed by various combinations of tip deflection, shaft twisting, and repetitive back-and-forth motions. However, even accomplished endoscopists may encounter difficulty in advancing the instrument through sharp angles in a tortuous sigmoid colon or in a patient with multiple large-mouthed diverticula.

Examination of the Mucosa

The mucosa may be examined during both the insertion and withdrawal phases of examination. The irrigation and suction channels may be used to remove small amounts of remnant fecal material and permit more complete mucosal visualization. Tip deflection allows a wide range of view. Full 180-degree tip deflection (retroflexion) within the rectum allows a retroflexed view of the rectal ampulla, including evaluation for internal hemorrhoids and polyps.

Biopsy specimens

Biopsy specimens may be obtained using disposable biopsy forceps passed through the instrument channel of the sigmoidoscope.

Complications

Perforations are rare, occurring in fewer than 1 in 10,000 sigmoidoscopies. They are more likely to occur if the examiner

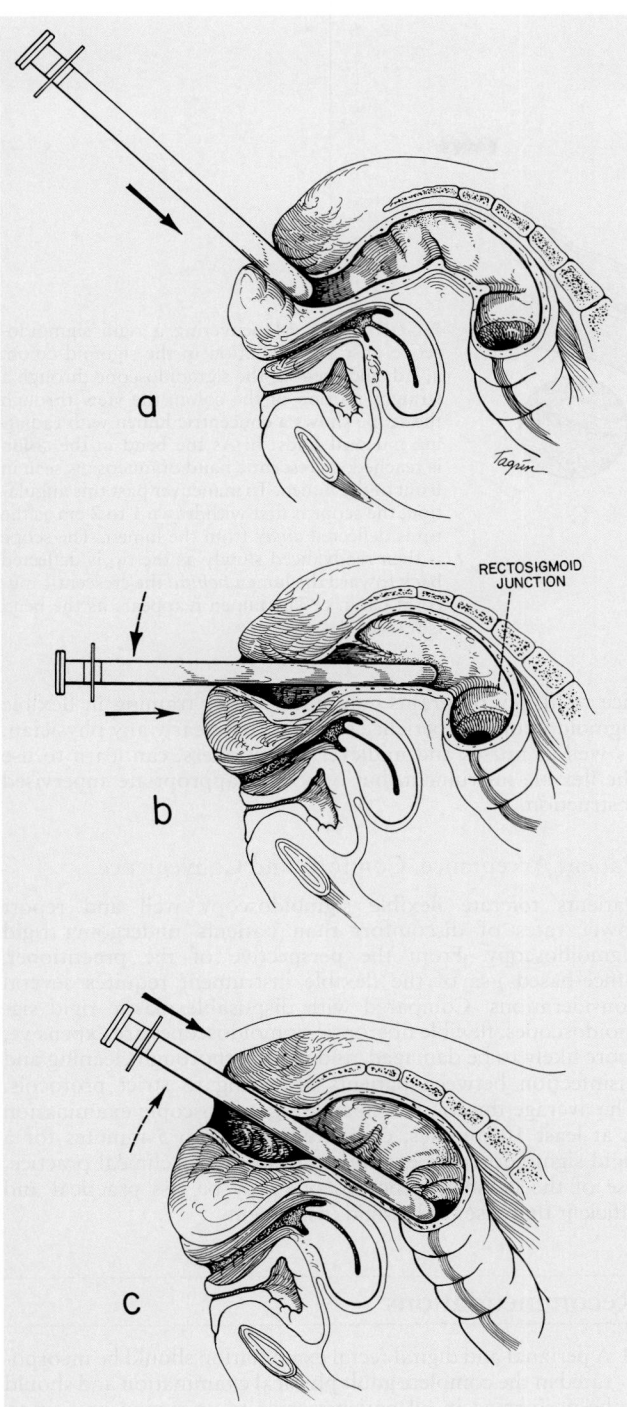

FIGURE 56.2. Overview of rigid sigmoidoscopic examination. a: The tip of the sigmoidoscope is inserted into the anal canal in the direction of the umbilicus. b: At the anorectal junction (about 3 cm from anus), the tip is deflected toward the sacrum. c: At the rectosigmoid junction (about 12 to 15 cm from anus), the tip is deflected anteriorly and to the left.

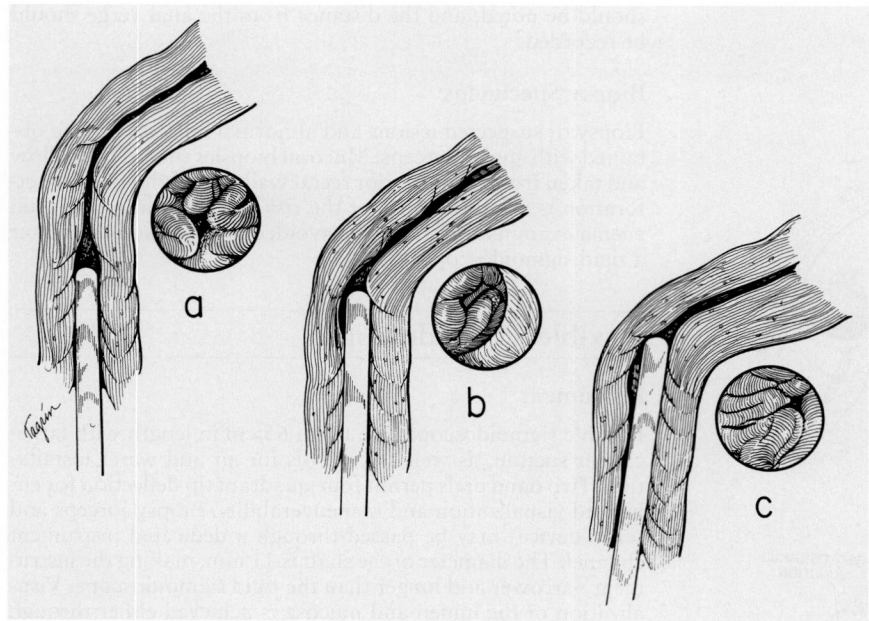

FIGURE 56.3. Maneuvering a rigid sigmoidoscope past an angulation in the sigmoid colon. a: Advancement of the sigmoidoscope through a straight portion of the colon; the view through the scope shows a concentric lumen with radiating mucosal folds. b: As the bend in the colon is reached, a crescentic band of mucosa is seen in front of the lumen. To maneuver past this angulation, the scope is first withdrawn 1 to 2 cm as the tip is deflected *away* from the lumen. The scope is then readvanced slowly as the tip is deflected back toward the lumen *behind* the crescentic mucosal band. c: The lumen reappears as the bend is traversed.

persists in pushing the sigmoidoscope forward in a bowel that is fixed at any point, as by tumor, or in situations in which the integrity of the bowel is compromised, as in acute colitis or diverticulitis. Bleeding from biopsy sites is infrequent and self-limited, even in the setting of therapeutic coagulopathy. Warfarin and aspirin do not need to be interrupted for sigmoidoscopy with biopsy. Cardiopulmonary complications are rare, and when they occur, are typically encountered in sigmoidoscopies performed under sedation and analgesia. Informed consent should be obtained before the procedure.

Choice of Procedure

Diagnostic Yield

The yield of flexible sigmoidoscopy is greater than that of rigid sigmoidoscopy. Whereas the average depth of insertion of the rigid instrument is no more than 20 cm, the average depth of insertion for the flexible instrument in the hands of an experienced endoscopist is about 50 cm. In addition, retroflexion of the flexible sigmoidoscope within the rectum allows identification of rectal lesions that may be missed by rigid sigmoidoscopy. In comparative studies, the flexible instrument identified two to six times as many neoplasms and detected some abnormalities, such as diverticula, not generally within reach of the rigid sigmoidoscope. The yield of the flexible sigmoidoscope when used for CRC screening by primary care physicians appears to be acceptable in comparison with the yield by experienced endoscopists. However, as a screening test, flexible sigmoidoscopy detects only about half of colorectal polyps and cancers, and patients undergoing sigmoidoscopy for gastrointestinal symptoms may still require additional tests, such as a colonoscopy, to complete the evaluation.

Competency

Competency in flexible sigmoidoscopy is usually achieved after performance of 25 examinations under the supervision of a qualified mentor. Many internal medicine and family prac-

tice residency programs continue to offer training in flexible sigmoidoscopy. Experience suggests that nearly any physician, as well as nurses and midlevel practitioners, can learn to use the flexible instrument, but only with appropriate supervised instruction.

Patient Acceptance, Comfort, and Convenience

Patients tolerate flexible sigmoidoscopy well and report lower rates of discomfort than patients undergoing rigid sigmoidoscopy. From the perspective of the practitioner, office-based use of the flexible instrument requires several considerations. Compared with disposable plastic rigid sigmoidoscopes, flexible fiberoptic sigmoidoscopes are expensive, more likely to be damaged, and require thorough cleaning and disinfection between patients according to strict protocols. The average duration of flexible sigmoidoscopic examination is at least 10 minutes, compared with 2 to 5 minutes for a rigid sigmoidoscopic examination. In a busy clinical practice, use of the flexible sigmoidoscope may be less practical and efficient than use of the rigid instrument.

Recommendations

- A perianal and digital rectal examination should be incorporated in the complete adult physical examination and should be performed in all patients prior to anoscopy or sigmoidoscopy.
- Anoscopy is safe, simple to perform, and well tolerated by patients. Anoscopy should be considered the procedure of choice for evaluation of anal pathology.
- Either rigid or flexible sigmoidoscopy may be performed in an office setting. Factors influencing the choice between these two options include diagnostic considerations and anticipated diagnostic yield, desired depth of insertion, and patient comfort. Rigid sigmoidoscopy is acceptable when a careful examination for rectal pathology is desired. Flexible sigmoidoscopy is preferred over rigid sigmoidoscopy for

determining the source of rectal bleeding, evaluating a radiologically detected lesion in the sigmoid colon, or evaluating suspected colitis.

- Although colonoscopy is now commonly performed for colorectal cancer screening, flexible sigmoidoscopy (in combination with FOBT) remains a viable screening option. Rigid sigmoidoscopy lacks sensitivity as a screening test for colorectal cancer.

- It is reasonable for primary care physicians to master the technique of rigid sigmoidoscopy and to consider learning the technique of flexible sigmoidoscopy only if they are willing to commit sufficient time and ensure adequate procedure volume to develop and maintain true proficiency. Unless expertise has been achieved, the primary care physician should refer patients in need of flexible sigmoidoscopy to a gastroenterologist or surgeon skilled in performing the examination.

Annotated Bibliography

1. Kelly SM, Sonowski RA, Foutch PG et al. A prospective comparison of anoscopy and fiberendoscopy in detecting anal lesions. J Clin Gastroenterol 1986;8:658. (*In 115 patients with anal pathology, anoscopy detected 99% of lesions, compared with 84% detected by the combination of straight withdrawal and retroflexed fiberoptic examination.*)

2. Hull TL. Diseases of the anorectum. In: Feldman M, Friedman LS, Brandt LJ, eds. Sleisenger and Fordtran's gastrointestinal and liver disease: pathophysiology/diagnosis/management, 8th ed. Philadelphia: Elsevier Saunders, 2006:2833. (*Comprehensive discussion of indications for and techniques of rigid and flexible sigmoidoscopy, in addition to the anorectal examination and management of common anorectal disorders.*)

3. Ahlquist DA. Triage by flexible sigmoidoscopy: inevitably "short-sighted." Gastroenterology 1998;115:777. (*Editorial discussing the limitations of flexible sigmoidoscopy as a screening tool for colorectal cancer because of its inability to detect or predict the presence of proximal colonic neoplasms.*)

4. Ashley OS, Nadel M, Ransohoff DF. Achieving quality in flexible sigmoidoscopy screening for colorectal cancer. Am J Med 2001;111:643. (*Evidence-based review of technique and competencies.*)

5. Bohlman TW, Katon RM, Lipshutz GR, et al. Fiberoptic pansigmoidoscopy: an evaluation and comparison with rigid sigmoidoscopy. Gastroenterology 1977;72:644. (*In 120 patients, the flexible instrument was inserted nearly three times as far—55 cm vs. 20 cm—and identified pathologic lesions three times more often—39% vs. 13%.*)

6. Lehman GA, Buchner DM, Lappas JC. Anatomical extent of fiberoptic sigmoidoscopy. Gastroenterology 1983;84:803. (*A 60-cm examination, achieved in 50% of those examined, viewed the entire sigmoid colon 80% of the time.*)

7. Lewis JD, Ng K, Hung KE, et al. Detection of proximal adenomatous polyps with screening sigmoidoscopy: a systematic review and meta-analysis of screening colonoscopy. Arch Intern Med 2003;163:413. (*Distal adenomatous polyps were associated with an increased prevalence of synchronous proximal neoplasia; 2% to 5% of patients undergoing screening colonoscopy may have isolated advanced proximal neoplasia.*)

8. McCarthy BD, Moskowitz MA. Screening flexible sigmoidoscopy: patient attitudes and compliance. J Gen Intern Med 1993;8:120. (*Seventy-five percent of patients agreed to the procedure; only 14% said they would not do it again.*)

9. Nivatvongs S, Fryd DS. How far does the proctosigmoidoscope reach? A prospective study of 1,000 patients. N Engl J Med 1980;303:380. (*The average depth of insertion of the rigid sigmoidoscope was 19.5 to 20.3 cm in male patients and 18.6 cm in female patients.*)

10. Selby JV, Friedman GD, Quesenberry CP, et al. A case–control study of screening sigmoidoscopy and mortality from colorectal cancer. N Engl J Med 1992;326:653. (*A retrospective study indicating a survival benefit with screening by proctosigmoidoscopy.*)

11. Guidelines for antibiotic prophylaxis for gastrointestinal endoscopy. Gastrointest Endosc 2003;58:475. (*Standards of practice published by the American Society for Gastrointestinal Endoscopy concerning endoscopic procedures, including sigmoidoscopy.*)

12. Guidelines on the management of anticoagulation and antiplatelet therapy for endoscopic procedures. Gastrointest Endosc 2002;55:755. (*Standards of practice published by the American Society for Gastrointestinal Endoscopy concerning endoscopic procedures, including sigmoidoscopy.*)

13. Hanson JM, Atkin WS, Cunliffe WJ, et al. Rectal retroflexion: an essential part of lower gastrointestinal endoscopic examination. Dis Colon Rectum 2001;44:1706. (*Prospective evaluation of 480 patients, 2.5% of whom were found to have rectal polyps during retroflexion that had not been detected on digital rectal examination or routine sigmoidoscopic exam.*)

14. Rao VS, Ahmad N, Al-Mukhtar A, et al. Comparison of rigid versus flexible sigmoidoscopy in detection of significant anorectal lesions. Colorectal Dis 2005;7:61. (*Among 115 patients with a normal rigid sigmoidoscopy, 39 (34%) had lesions within 20 cm of the anal verge detected by flexible sigmoidoscopy.*)

15. Winawar SJ, Miller C, Lightdale C, et al. Patient response to sigmoidoscopy: a randomized, controlled trial of rigid and flexible sigmoidoscopy. Cancer 1987;60:1905. (*Patients randomized to flexible sigmoidoscopy reported less discomfort, anxiety, and embarrassment than those randomized to rigid sigmoidoscopy.*)

16. Levin TR, Conell C, Shapiro JA, et al. Complications of screening flexible sigmoidoscopy. Gastroenterology 2002;123:1786. (*There were 7 serious complications, including 2 perforations, reported in a series of 109,534 screening flexible sigmoidoscopies.*)

17. Shapero TF, Hoover J, Paszat LF et al. Colorectal cancer screening with nurse-performed flexible sigmoidoscopy: results from a Canadian community-based program. Gastrointest Endosc 2007;65:640. (*Referral to colonoscopy for 13% of patients and cancer detection rate of 2.8 per 1000 screened.*)

CHAPTER 57 ■ PREVENTION OF VIRAL HEPATITIS

JULES L. DIENSTAG

Viral hepatitis is an infectious disease of the liver that is estimated to afflict more than 5 million people and to cause several thousand deaths in the United States each year. Although the majority of those infected are either asymptomatic or minimally symptomatic, chronic viral hepatitis is associated with substantial morbidity, and fulminant hepatitis, which is often fatal, may develop in a small proportion of acutely infected patients.

Prevention of infection and prophylaxis against clinical disease are prime objectives in the management of viral hepatitis. The primary physician has the major responsibility for these tasks because patients and their contacts often present at a time during acute infection when infectivity is high. Prevention of viral hepatitis requires knowledge of the common modes of viral transmission, the periods of maximal communicability, and the efficacy of globulin preparations and vaccines.

EPIDEMIOLOGY AND RISK FACTORS

Viral Types

Five distinct types of viral hepatitis are recognized: A through E. Although other types of hepatitis viruses (e.g., "hepatitis G") have been described, none has proved to be a true hepatitis virus or to account for the small proportion of cases that cannot be linked serologically to hepatitis viruses A through E.

Sources of Outbreaks (1,2,4–10,13–16,24,30,34)

In general, outbreaks of hepatitis are often traced to a source of hepatitis A virus (HAV) or, in developing countries, to hepatitis E virus (HEV). Occasionally, clusters of hepatitis B follow exposure of several persons to contaminated needles or blood products. Among urban adults presenting to a primary care physician with sporadic cases of acute hepatitis, hepatitis B accounts for approximately 50% of cases, hepatitis C for 15%, and hepatitis A for the remainder. More than 95% of transfusion-associated cases were attributable to hepatitis C; however, the frequency of transfusion-related cases has been reduced dramatically to negligible levels by excluding blood donors with risk factors for viral hepatitis as well as the use of sensitive screening tests for hepatitis C (see later discussion). Hepatitis D is caused by a defective virus that infects only in the presence of infection with hepatitis B virus. Chronic infection with hepatitis B virus (HBV) is prevalent in 0.1% to 0.5% (1 million persons), and chronic infection with hepatitis C virus (HCV) is prevalent in 1.6% (4 million persons) of the U.S. population.

Hepatitis A (1,2,16,17,24,34)

HAV is shed in the feces, and transmission occurs predominantly by the *fecal–oral* route (e.g., ingestion of contaminated food, water, shellfish). Prior exposure to hepatitis A is manifested by the presence of antibody to HAV (anti-HAV), which confers lifelong immunity. Many patients older than the age of 60 years test positive for anti-HAV, but acute infection is rare in this age group. Because children and adolescents are least likely to have had previous exposure to the virus, they are the most susceptible to infection. Spread of infection is greatest where poor sanitary conditions and crowding exist, with prevalences as high as 75% among low-income people, compared with 20% to 30% for residents in middle- to upper-income neighborhoods. In developed countries, the prevalence of anti-HAV and of immunity to the virus has fallen by approximately 10% per decade since the 1970s. The down side of this declining prevalence of anti-HAV is the growing prevalence of susceptibility to infection in population subgroups that heretofore had been immune. The resulting shift in acute cases from the very young, in whom the disease tends to be subclinical, to adults, in whom the disease tends to be associated with jaundice and is relatively severe, has translated into an increased frequency of clinically apparent, severe hepatitis A in adults. Acute hepatitis A does not progress to chronic infection.

Hepatitis B (4,5,8,10,21)

Hepatitis B can be transmitted both by *percutaneous* and *nonpercutaneous* modes of spread. The application of sensitive screening methods for the detection of HBV has essentially eliminated posttransfusion hepatitis type B. Reliance on blood obtained from volunteer donors, which is less likely to contain the virus, in addition to blood donor exclusion practices and screening tests to prevent transfusion-transmitted HIV infection and hepatitis C has also contributed to reducing the frequency of hepatitis B after transfusion. Injection-drug use remains a common route of exposure. Perinatal transmission from mother to offspring accounts for most HBV infections in the Far East and Africa, whereas sexual transmission is an important and efficient mode of spread in the United States and other Western countries. About 0.1% of healthy blood donors, reflective of the general population, are infected; the percentages increase markedly for injection-drug users and patients exposed to blood, such as hemophiliacs and patients in hemodialysis units. Surgeons, laboratory technicians, oral surgeons, and other medical personnel exposed to blood and body fluids are at increased risk for contracting hepatitis B. Spread of infection from health care personnel who are infected with HBV is a rare event.

Hepatitis C (6,7,10–13,15,19,20,23,26–29)

Hepatitis C, initially labeled "non-A, non-B hepatitis," was first recognized in *transfusion* recipients and found to be the predominant type of hepatitis after transfusion. In the 1970s, it occurred in up to 10% of transfusion recipients, usually within 1 to 3 months after they had received blood from volunteer donors. The frequency of infection fell with the exclusion of blood donors at risk for HIV infection and was further reduced by the use of screening tests for HIV (see Chapter 7), surrogate tests for hepatitis C (e.g., alanine aminotransferase, antibodies to hepatitis B core antigen), and, finally, direct testing for antibodies to HCV and then for HCV RNA. Currently, the risk for hepatitis C after transfusion is barely measurable, and transfusion-associated infections are almost never encountered. Hepatitis C can be spread by *any percutaneous route*, such as needlestick inoculation (3% to 10% risk of infection) or self-injection among drug users. The risk for hepatitis C resulting from sexual or perinatal transmission is believed to be very low, on the order of 1% to 5%. In about one third of patients with acute hepatitis C and in almost all volunteer blood donors with hepatitis C, risk factors are not readily apparent; however, in most such cases, remote or less obvious percutaneous exposures—predominantly long-forgotten, transient injection-drug use— can be identified or inferred. Although acute hepatitis C is a rare event nowadays in the general population, chronic hepatitis C is encountered regularly, primarily among persons infected decades ago, during the 1960s and 1970s, when experimentation with injection-drug use was common.

Hepatitis D (Delta Hepatitis) (14,30)

Hepatitis D, or delta hepatitis, is caused by a defective RNA virus that requires *coinfection with HBV* (a DNA virus) to support its replication. Infection with this agent occurs either simultaneously with acute hepatitis B infection or is superimposed on chronic hepatitis B. Like hepatitis B, hepatitis D is transmitted by *percutaneous inoculation* and *intimate contact*. In nonendemic areas, such as the United States and western Europe, hepatitis D is confined primarily to populations with frequent percutaneous exposures, such as injection-drug users and hemophiliacs. In endemic areas, such as the Mediterranean countries, hepatitis D is transmitted primarily through intimate contact. Hepatitis D tends to be rare in the United States.

Hepatitis E (3)

Hepatitis E, prevalent in India, Asia, Central America, and developing countries, is transmitted by the *fecal–oral* route. Similar epidemiologically and clinically to hepatitis A, hepatitis E tends to be recognized clinically in a population cohort somewhat older than that for, and almost invariably immune to, hepatitis A and is more likely to cause severe, even fatal hepatitis, especially in pregnant women. Rarely encountered in the United States except for imported cases from endemic countries, hepatitis E does not cause chronic infection.

NATURAL HISTORY

Both hepatitis A and hepatitis E are self-limited and do not lead to chronic liver disease; however, hepatitis B, C, and D can cause chronic hepatitis and cirrhosis; longstanding chronic hepatitis B and C can be complicated by hepatocellular carcinoma.

Hepatitis A (1,2,9,16,17)

Hepatitis A has an average incubation period of 30 days (range, 15 to 45 days) from the time of exposure to the onset of symptoms. An early manifestation of disease is elevation of serum aminotransferase levels, which occurs about 1 week before the onset of flulike symptoms. Fecal shedding of HAV occurs well before the rise in aminotransferase levels and up to 2 weeks before the development of symptoms. HAV can be detected in serum for no more than a few days, and the virus disappears from stool within 2 to 3 weeks, usually at the same time as the onset of jaundice and resolution of prodromal symptoms. A fall in virus levels parallels a rise in the titer of anti-HAV, which persists indefinitely. Initially, *anti-HAV* is of the *immunoglobulin M* (IgM) class; during convalescence, anti-HAV of the *immunoglobulin G* (IgG) class becomes predominant. Therefore, a diagnosis of acute hepatitis A can be made by detecting IgM anti-HAV in a single serum sample. No episodes of chronic hepatitis or a carrier state result from hepatitis A infection. Fatalities are rare; fewer than 5% of cases of fulminant hepatitis result from HAV infection, but cases of increased clinical severity are becoming more common (see prior discussion).

Hepatitis B (4,5,8,21–23)

Hepatitis B is a much more variable disease. The incubation period averages 12 weeks, with a range of 4 weeks to 6 months.

Acute Infection

About 2 to 4 weeks before the onset of symptoms, the viral envelope protein, *hepatitis B surface antigen (HBsAg)*, appears in the serum, followed by a rise in aminotransferase levels and symptoms. This viral antigen usually is cleared from the serum by 4 to 6 months; persistence of HBsAg in serum beyond 6 months is considered chronic infection. Symptoms of acute hepatitis B typically last 4 to 6 weeks, but the clinical expression of acute hepatitis B is very variable, ranging from clinically inapparent disease to fulminant hepatitis (in 0.1% of acute cases) with hepatocellular failure and death. Determinants of disease severity include age, immunologic competence, undefined host factors, viral genotype, and virulence of the virus.

Chronic Infection

Approximately 1% to 2% of patients with *clinically apparent* disease progress to having *chronic infection* and continue to harbor circulating HBsAg. A much larger number of cases of chronic hepatitis B do not originate as clinically apparent acute illness; thus, the number of chronic cases is much larger than anticipated based on the number of recorded acute cases. Among patients with chronic hepatitis B, some have detectable serologic markers of high-level virus replication and some remain *inactive carriers*. Those with high-level replication tend to be highly infectious for contacts and to have chronic hepatitis that is progressive and of at least moderate severity, whereas inactive carriers lack evidence of high-level virus replication, infectivity, and liver injury (see later discussion). The fatality rate for acute hepatitis B is about 0.1%; however, among those requiring hospitalization, the mortality rate is 1%. Although hepatocellular carcinoma is rare in immunocompetent patients who become chronically infected following adulthood acute infection, this dreaded complication of chronic HBV infection is common among those who become chronically infected after perinatally acquired acute infection. In Asia, where perinatal infection is the most common route of exposure, the lifetime risk of death from cirrhosis and hepatocellular carcinoma has been reported to be as high as 40%.

Serology

Antibody to HBsAg (anti-HBs) is produced early during infection but becomes detectable with commercially available serologic assays only as HBsAg disappears. Almost all patients with self-limited acute hepatitis B acquire detectable levels of anti-HBs, which persist indefinitely and correlate with subsequent immunity.

Antibody to the nucleocapsid core of HBV (anti-HBc) appears in the circulation within 1 week or so after HBsAg becomes detectable and persists indefinitely. Occasionally, during late acute infection, an interval occurs in which HBsAg has already disappeared and anti-HBs has not yet become detectable. This so-called "window period" can be identified by the presence of isolated anti-HBc; however, now that tests for HBsAg and anti-HBs are so sensitive, this window period is rarely encountered among patients with acute hepatitis B. Most cases in which anti-HBc occurs in the absence of HBsAg and anti-HBs represent HBV infection in the remote past. In rare instances, isolated anti-HBc represents a false-positive test result, whereas in patients at high risk for blood-borne infections (e.g., injection-drug users), isolated anti-HBc may represent low-level HBV infection in which the level of HBsAg does not exceed the detection threshold. On the other hand, isolated anti-HBc can be detected in a proportion of injection-drug users with chronic hepatitis C, and, in this setting, the presence of low-level HBV infection cannot be demonstrated in serum or liver, even with sensitive amplification assays.

A test for anti-HBc of the IgM class (IgM anti-HBc) can distinguish between acute or relatively recent acute hepatitis

B (IgM positive) and infection in the remote past or current chronic infection (IgM negative), in which anti-HBc is of the IgG class. In a small proportion of cases of acute hepatitis B, HBsAg does not reach the threshold for detection; in such cases, a diagnosis of acute hepatitis B can be established by detecting IgM anti-HBc.

Hepatitis Be antigen (HBeAg) is a second product of the gene that codes for the nucleocapsid core; its presence signifies *high-level virus replication*. As such, patients with HBeAg have a high level of circulating virions and infectivity and substantial liver injury. HBeAg becomes detectable in *all* patients early during acute hepatitis B, and therefore this test has no clinical utility during early acute hepatitis B; however, if circulating HBeAg persists beyond the first 3 months of acute hepatitis, the likelihood of chronic infection is increased.

Testing for HBeAg is more important during chronic infection because the presence of HBeAg denotes a more highly replicative chronic infection, associated with increased infectivity (e.g., 20% to 30% infectivity of a needlestick) and liver injury (chronic hepatitis). When *anti-HBe* can be detected in the absence of HBeAg during chronic infection, the patient can be classified as having a less replicative infection, with *limited infectivity* (e.g., 0.1% infectivity of a needlestick) and liver injury (inactive carrier).

Complicating this simple distinction between highly replicative and relatively nonreplicative chronic hepatitis B are patients with *"pre-core" HBV mutations*. For HBeAg to be produced, the pre-core region of the gene encoding the nucleocapsid core protein must be operative; one of a number of mutations in the pre-core gene (pre-core and core-promoter mutations) precludes elaboration of HBeAg, but this mutation does not prevent production of complete virions or high-level HBV replication. Common in Mediterranean and Asian countries and still rare in the United States but growing in frequency, patients with pre-core mutant HBV have all the virologic (i.e., detectable HBV DNA; see later discussion) and clinical hallmarks of highly replicative HBV infection in the absence of HBeAg. This category of patients has been labeled "HBeAg-negative chronic hepatitis B."

At least eight different genotypes of HBV have been identified, and genotype A is most prevalent in the United States and Europe. Preliminary observations suggest that progression and complications of hepatitis B are more common in patients with certain genotypes than in those with others; however, these distinctions remain to be validated, and HBV genotyping has not become a part of routine diagnostic testing.

Quantitative Markers of Hepatitis B Viral Replication

HBV DNA is a quantitative marker of HBV replication and is helpful in following patients with chronic disease and in monitoring the success of antiviral therapy (see Chapter 70). Insensitive hybridization assays identify circulating HBV DNA down to a threshold of approximately 10^5 to 10^6 virions per milliliter, below which infectivity and liver injury are less common. Clinical assays for HBV DNA have shifted to ultrasensitive amplification techniques such as *polymerase chain reaction*, which can detect HBV DNA in serum down to thresholds of 100 to 1,000 virions per milliliter, well below the level associated with infectivity and liver injury. In HBeAg-positive chronic hepatitis B, levels of HBV DNA tend to exceed 10^6 virions per milliliter and can reach 10^9 virions per milliliter or even higher. Among patients who lack HBeAg but have circulating anti-HBe, inactive hepatitis B carriers have HBV DNA levels of less than 10^3 to 10^4 virions per milliliter, whereas those with pre-core–mutant HBV infection (HBeAg-negative chronic hepatitis B)

have high levels of HBV DNA, usually on the order of, but rarely greater than, 10^5 to 10^6 virions per milliliter.

Hepatitis C (6,7,10–13,20,23,26–29,34)

Hepatitis C has a mean incubation period of 7 weeks (range, 2 to 15 weeks), with most cases occurring after 5 to 10 weeks of incubation. Only one fourth of patients with acute, transfusion-associated hepatitis C become icteric, compared with two thirds of those with transfusion-induced hepatitis B. After acute HCV infection, however, more than 50% of patients have chronic elevation of aminotransferase levels, and *chronic infection* (with or without liver injury) occurs in 85% of all acutely infected patients. Contributing to this high rate of chronic infection is the common failure to mount an effective, neutralizing immunologic response to HCV.

Progression to Cirrhosis and Hepatocellular Carcinoma

Among patients with chronic hepatitis following acute hepatitis C, 20% may progress to cirrhosis during the first one to two decades of illness, even patients with mild liver disease. On the other hand, morbidity within the first 20 years after acute hepatitis C is limited. Although certain hepatitis C genotypes (e.g., *genotype 1*, occurring in 70% to 80% of U.S. patients) may be associated with more-severe liver disease, perhaps the best predictor of progression to cirrhosis is *liver histology*. Patients with moderate to severe necrosis, inflammation, or fibrosis almost always progress to cirrhosis during the following 10 years (in severe cases) to 20 years (in moderate cases), whereas 80% of those with negligible or mild histologic features do not progress to cirrhosis during this interval. In addition, because most patients with chronic hepatitis C are identified in their 40s and 50s after having acquired the infection in their late teens and 20s, a liver biopsy obtained at the time of diagnosis provides information on histologic grade (necroinflammatory activity) and stage (fibrosis) associated with the decades preceding the biopsy. After approximately 30 years of infection, patients with chronic hepatitis C have an increased risk for hepatocellular carcinoma. Almost all such patients are already cirrhotic, and the risk for hepatocellular carcinoma in cirrhotic patients with chronic hepatitis C ranges from 1% to 4% annually.

Serology and Markers of Viral Replication

Highly sensitive assays for *antibody to hepatitis C (anti-HCV)* yield positive results during acute infection, and results remain positive indefinitely in most patients. Thus, assays for anti-HCV can be used for routine diagnostic purposes during acute hepatitis C. Because of occasional nonspecificity of immunoassays for anti-HCV, a supplemental confirmatory test is needed when a positive result is encountered in a patient at very low risk for blood-borne infection (e.g., an asymptomatic blood donor with no risk factors). For such circumstances, a *recombinant immunoblot assay (RIBA)* was developed to identify the viral or nonviral proteins responsible for the positive test result.

Such RIBA tests, however, have been supplanted in routine clinical practice by assays for *HCV RNA*, the most sensitive test for hepatitis C infection. Tests for HCV RNA include a *branched-chain complementary DNA test*, in which the detection molecule is amplified, with a sensitivity threshold of 2×10^5 virion equivalents per milliliter, and a *polymerase chain reaction assay (PCR)* and *transcription-mediated amplification (TMA) assay*, with a sensitivity threshold of 5 to 100 virion equivalents per milliliter, and results are now reported as international units per milliliter (IU/mL). Quantitative PCR and

TMA assays are available that have a broad dynamic range and a sensitivity as low as approximately 5 IU/mL; these assays can be used to confirm the presence of HCV infection in anti-HCV–reactive patients, to document resolution of infection after antiviral therapy, and to monitor HCV RNA levels prior to and during antiviral therapy (see Chapter 70).

Hepatitis D (Delta Hepatitis) (14,30,31)

Hepatitis D (delta hepatitis) has an incubation period similar to that for hepatitis B; when hepatitis B and hepatitis D infections are acquired simultaneously, a single clinically apparent episode of hepatitis may ensue. When the two infections occur simultaneously, the risk for *fulminant hepatitis* is increased to 5%, but, in general, the outcome of simultaneous acute hepatitis B and D is no different from the outcome of hepatitis B alone. In contrast, among patients with chronic hepatitis B infection, superimposed hepatitis D may lead to severe, fulminant hepatitis in up to 20% of cases, convert mild or inactive chronic hepatitis into severe chronic hepatitis, or accelerate the course of chronic hepatitis. On the other hand, some patients who have had HBV/HDV coinfection for several years may have clinically and histologically inactive, indolent disease. A diagnosis of delta hepatitis is made by demonstrating the appearance of *antibody to hepatitis D (anti-HDV)*. Immunohistochemical detection of HDV in liver biopsy specimens and assays for *HDV RNA* in serum are available in specialized research laboratories but have not found their way into routine practice.

Hepatitis E (3)

Hepatitis E has a mean incubation period of about 40 days, slightly longer than that for hepatitis A. Its clinical course is similar to that of hepatitis A, except that more patients experience a *cholestatic illness* and the likelihood of fulminant disease is higher (1% to 2% overall and 10% to 20% in pregnant women). The disease is *self-limited* and does not progress to chronic infection. The virus is excreted in stool early, and antibodies to HEV become detectable during acute illness. Serologic tests are available routinely in endemic areas and in specialized laboratories in the United States.

PRINCIPLES OF PROPHYLAXIS

The principal means of prophylaxis, *minimizing exposure* to hepatitis viruses and use of *immunoglobulin* preparations (passive immunoprophylaxis) and *vaccines* (active immunoprophylaxis), vary for each of the hepatitis viruses. Antiviral therapy is available with which to treat hepatitis B and hepatitis C, as reviewed in Chapter 70.

Hepatitis A (2,17,24,31–34)

Precautions against contact with a patient who has hepatitis A are most appropriate during the prodromal stage of illness, when the patient sheds virus most substantially.

Minimizing Exposure

During the early phase of clinical hepatitis A, when jaundice first appears, some shedding of virus may persist; precautions such as avoiding intimate contact and carefully washing hands after contact are probably reasonable for 1 or 2 weeks longer. The patient should not serve food to others and can minimize transmission of virus by using disposable dishes and utensils and through meticulous personal hygiene. If a patient is sufficiently ill to require hospital admission, by that time during clinical illness, viral shedding will have subsided, and additional precautions, beyond universal precautions in practice nowadays, are not indicated.

Passive Immunoprophylaxis

Passive immunoprophylaxis for hepatitis A can be accomplished by the use of standard *immune globulin* (IG) or formalin-inactivated hepatitis A vaccine. IG preparations contain high titers of anti-HAV and are about 80% effective in preventing clinical disease. IG was believed to protect by passive–active immunization (passively administered antibody acts to minimize clinical illness but does not prevent infection and the durable immunity that follows natural infection). Newer analyses suggest that IG more often prevents infection entirely. IG is currently used exclusively for *postexposure prophylaxis* and must be administered within 1 to 2 weeks of exposure to be most effective. Patients with a prior history of serologically documented hepatitis A need not receive IG because they are already protected by their own anti-HAV. Household contacts and small groups experiencing a common-source outbreak should be given IG prophylaxis if the outbreak is identified early enough. Routine immunoprophylaxis is not necessary for casual contacts at work or school.

Active Immunoprophylaxis

For *preexposure prophylaxis, hepatitis A vaccine* has supplanted IG. Two "killed" hepatitis A vaccines are available, and both are safe, immunogenic, and highly effective in preventing hepatitis A. Doses of the two vaccines vary slightly, and regimens for the two vaccines vary with age of the vaccinee, but both require at least two injections spaced 6 to 12 months apart. Universal childhood hepatitis A vaccination is recommended. Vaccination also is recommended for those who travel to areas of the world where hepatitis A is endemic. (In cases of imminent travel to endemic areas, when inadequate time remains [<4 weeks] before travel to achieve vaccine-induced protection, IG should be given along with the first dose of hepatitis A vaccine.) Hepatitis A vaccine also is recommended for military personnel, populations and communities with cyclical outbreaks or high frequencies of hepatitis A, laboratory workers exposed to fecal specimens, day care center employees, primate handlers, patients with chronic hepatitis C and other chronic liver diseases, men who have sex with men, injection-drug users, and patients with clotting disorders who require frequent clotting factor concentrates. Vaccine-induced immunity is projected to last 20 years or longer.

Hepatitis B (4,18,19,33,35,36)

Reducing the spread of hepatitis B has been aided by screening *blood donors* for HBsAg. People discovered to be *inactive carriers* are still potential sources of infection for others, although their infectivity is limited. Health care workers with hepatitis B need not be removed from work unless proven to be a source of infection for their patients; however, health care workers and professionals with highly replicative HBV infection (HBeAg-reactive and/or HBV DNA $>10^5$ to 10^6 virions/mL) who perform "exposure-prone" invasive procedures are advised to have their privileges evaluated by an expert review panel. *Food handlers* have not been implicated in the transmission of hepatitis B, and HBsAg-positive persons need not be restricted from food preparation or serving.

Minimizing Exposure

Minimizing exposure is facilitated by having the patient use a separate razor, toothbrush, and other personal items. During acute hepatitis B, avoidance of intimate contact should be recommended, but confinement to home is unnecessary. Ensure that any materials containing HBsAg are handled carefully, particularly blood samples and other body fluids; use of gloves is required. If universal precautions are followed in the handling of clinical materials, additional precautions are unnecessary. Hands should be washed thoroughly after direct contact with the patient or with the patient's blood or body fluids.

Passive Immunoprophylaxis

Passive immunoprophylaxis of hepatitis B is achieved by providing the susceptible person with protective antibody—anti-HBs. This can be accomplished by passive immunization with IG containing anti-HBs. *Hepatitis B immune globulin* (HBIG) is prepared from the plasma of persons with high-titer anti-HBs and contains anti-HBs at titers in the range of 1:100,000 or higher. HBIG, which appears to attenuate clinical illness rather than prevent infection, is recommended in conjunction with vaccine for *postexposure prophylaxis* (see later discussion).

Active Immunization

Active immunization with recombinant *hepatitis B vaccines*, derived from recombinant yeast into which the gene for HBsAg has been inserted, have replaced earlier-generation, plasma-derived vaccines in the United States. Hepatitis B vaccine has been recommended as *preexposure prophylaxis*, primarily for population subgroups considered to be at high risk for exposure to HBV (e.g., health care and laboratory workers exposed to blood, hemodialysis staff and patients, residents and staff of custodial institutions, sexually promiscuous persons, injection-drug users, incarcerated prisoners, patients requiring repeated administration of blood products or clotting factors, household and sexual contacts of persons with chronic hepatitis B, travelers to endemic areas, unvaccinated children younger than the age of 18 years, and residents in the households of immigrants from endemic areas).

Universal Vaccination

Although these groups remain targets for vaccination, attempts to vaccinate them have not been successful in limiting the spread of HBV within the general population of developed countries. Therefore, the U.S. Public Health Service has recommended *universal vaccination in childhood* and also vaccination of adolescents born before universal vaccination was implemented and who were not vaccinated at birth. Three deltoid injections of the vaccine are recommended, the first two given 1 month apart and the third given at 6 months. Doses vary according to age group and vaccine manufacturer.

Postexposure Prophylaxis

Postexposure prophylaxis in susceptible persons is best provided by a combination of *HBIG* and *hepatitis B vaccine*. Babies born to mothers with chronic hepatitis B (or acute hepatitis B during the third trimester of pregnancy), sexual contacts of patients with acute hepatitis B, and individuals who sustain HBsAg-positive needlesticks should receive HBIG plus hepatitis B vaccine. The HBIG provides immediate, high-level, passively acquired anti-HBs, and the vaccine adds long-lasting immunity and probably attenuation of clinical illness in the postexposure setting. HBIG should be administered as soon as possible after exposure (e.g., as soon as possible but no later than 48 hours after a needlestick, in the delivery room for babies). The first dose of vaccine can be given simultaneously or within a few hours in newborns, simultaneously and up to within 1 week in those sustaining needlestick exposures, or within 2 weeks in those with sexual exposure. Because early prophylaxis is paramount after an HBsAg needlestick, HBIG should be administered immediately and without a delay to wait for the results of susceptibility (antibody) testing. Hepatitis B vaccine and HBIG do not interfere with each other, even when administered simultaneously. Although determination of the HBeAg status of the contact case or inoculum source may provide information about relative infectivity, HBeAg status should not be a criterion for providing prophylaxis to contacts. The delay necessitated by waiting for HBeAg testing may limit the efficacy of efforts at prophylaxis, and infectivity can occur in the absence of HBeAg, although the likelihood is reduced. Nonintimate household contacts do not require prophylaxis, nor do casual contacts at work or school.

Durability of Protection. The duration of protection after hepatitis B vaccination is not known definitively but appears to be at least 10 years. Even after anti-HBs falls below detectable levels, new exposures are likely to be accompanied by an anamnestic immune response, and adequate immunity against clinically apparent infection and chronic infection appears to be maintained. Based on these observations, authorities have not recommended routine booster vaccination in immunocompetent persons. Booster doses are recommended for hemodialysis patients who lose protective levels of anti-HBs after vaccination.

Differentiating between Infection and Immunization. Hepatitis B vaccine consists entirely of HBsAg protein (no core proteins are included); making the distinction between immunization and infection is therefore possible by assaying for the presence of antibody to core protein (anti-HBc).

Hepatitis D (Delta Hepatitis) (14)

Prevention of delta hepatitis in persons susceptible to HBV infection can be achieved by administering *hepatitis B vaccine*. Once immune to HBV, a person is immune to hepatitis D also. For those with chronic hepatitis B, immunoprophylaxis against hepatitis D is not available, and prevention of delta hepatitis requires limitation of percutaneous and intimate contacts with persons known to be infected with hepatitis D virus.

Hepatitis C (7,10–13,19,20,25)

The annual incidence of posttransfusion hepatitis C has been reduced dramatically by excluding commercially donated blood and persons highly likely to transmit blood-borne disease and also by screening prospective donors for anti-HCV and donor blood for HCV RNA. Barrier sexual precautions with latex condoms are recommended for persons with multiple sexual partners or with sexually transmitted diseases; however, no such precautions are recommended for stable, monogamous sexual partners. Persons with hepatitis C, however, should avoid sharing razors, toothbrushes, and other such implements with sexual partners and family members. Special precautions are not recommended for babies born to mothers with chronic hepatitis C; breast-feeding is not restricted.

Immune globulin and HBIG are of no proven benefit in preventing hepatitis C, and IG is no longer recommended for needlestick, sexual, or perinatal exposure to hepatitis C. Efforts to develop a protective vaccine based on immunization with envelope proteins have been pursued but have not been fruitful; therefore, no vaccine is available to prevent hepatitis C, and the acquisition of durable immunity after naturally acquired hepatitis C is rare.

Hepatitis E (3)

Whether globulins prepared in developed countries, where hepatitis E is rare, protect against HEV infection in Asia and other parts of the world where hepatitis E is common is not known. Effective recombinant vaccines have been developed and are available in endemic areas.

RECOMMENDATIONS AND PATIENT EDUCATION

Hepatitis A Precautions (To Be Continued until 1 Week after Onset of Jaundice)

- Advise the patient to wash hands thoroughly after toilet use.
- There is no need to confine the patient to home, but the patient should avoid intimate contact.
- Prohibit the patient from handling and serving food to others.
- Advise others to avoid contact with the patient's fecal material and to wash hands thoroughly if contact is made.

Hepatitis A Prophylaxis

- For postexposure prophylaxis, administer IG to household contacts within 2 weeks of exposure; the dose is 0.02 mL/kg, with an average adult dose of 2 mL intramuscularly.
- For preexposure prophylaxis, administer two intramuscular injections of hepatitis A vaccine at least 6 months apart (dose recommendations vary between the two vaccine manufacturers). For imminent travel to endemic areas, when time is too short to achieve vaccine-induced immunization, IG should be administered, at the same dose as for household contacts, along with the first dose of vaccine

Hepatitis B Precautions (To Be Continued until HBsAg Clears from the Serum)

- Screen all blood donors for HBsAg.
- Use volunteer blood rather than blood from commercial donors.
- Use disposable syringes and needles; do not recap used needles and/or use safety needles.
- Have the patient use a separate razor, toothbrush, and other personal items.
- Have any materials containing HBsAg handled carefully, particularly blood samples and other body fluids; use of gloves is required. Following universal precautions when handling clinical materials makes additional precautions unnecessary.
- Recommend avoidance of unprotected intimate contact, but confinement to home is unnecessary.
- Wash hands thoroughly after direct contact with the patient or with the patient's blood or body fluids.

Hepatitis B Prophylaxis

Preexposure

- Administer three 1-mL intramuscular injections of hepatitis B vaccine at 0, 1, and 6 months to persons in high-risk groups. (Doses for specific age groups may vary according to manufacturer.) High-risk groups include health care workers exposed to blood, residents and staff of custodial institutions, household and sexual contacts of persons with chronic hepatitis B, promiscuous men who have sex with men and promiscuous heterosexuals, patients with hereditary hemoglobinopathies and clotting disorders who require long-term therapy with blood products, and hemodialysis patients.
- Universal vaccination of all children, in conjunction with routine vaccinations of childhood, is recommended. For children born after the implementation of universal hepatitis B vaccination, vaccination during adolescence is recommended.

Postexposure

- Administer 0.06 mL of HBIG intramuscularly per kilogram of body weight (approximately 5 mL) to those who sustain an accidental percutaneous or transmucosal exposure to HBsAg-positive blood or body secretions or needles and instruments contaminated with HBsAg-positive material. This globulin injection should be administered as soon after exposure as possible; although globulin injections are recommended up to 7 days after inoculation, their efficacy is probably nil beyond 2 days. Passive immunoprophylaxis with HBIG should be followed by a complete, three-injection course of hepatitis B vaccine; these injections can be started at the same time as HBIG or within the first few days to 1 week after exposure.
- Administer HBIG, at the dose cited earlier, to sexual contacts of patients with acute hepatitis B as soon after exposure as is practical. Because recognition of hepatitis in a sexual contact is often delayed, early prophylaxis is usually impossible. In one study, prophylaxis within 30 days of recognized exposure was effective, but recommendations call for prophylaxis within 14 days of exposure. HBIG should be followed by a complete three-injection course of hepatitis B vaccine in all sexual contacts of patients with acute hepatitis B.
- Administer 0.5 mL of HBIG intramuscularly to newborns of HBsAg-positive mothers immediately after birth, preferably in the delivery room. This should be followed by a complete three-injection course of hepatitis B vaccine, 0.5 mL per dose, preferably to be started simultaneously but no later than within 7 days of birth (dose may vary according to manufacturer).
- No prophylaxis is necessary for casual contacts or nonintimate household contacts.

Hepatitis D Prophylaxis

- Vaccination against hepatitis B prevents hepatitis D in individuals susceptible to hepatitis B.

- For individuals already infected with hepatitis B, prevention of hepatitis D relies on limiting percutaneous and intimate contact with persons known to harbor hepatitis D virus infection.

Hepatitis C Precautions and Prophylaxis

- Precautions are the same as those for hepatitis B (i.e., limitation of exposure to the blood and body fluids of infected patients).
- The best means of limiting transfusion-associated hepatitis C is to rely exclusively on volunteer rather than commercial blood donors and to screen donors for anti-HCV and blood products for HCV RNA.

- IG, which has not been shown to be effective in preventing hepatitis C, is not recommended for individuals who sustain a needlestick injury, sexual contacts of acute cases of hepatitis C, or babies born to mothers with hepatitis C.
- An effective hepatitis C vaccine has not been developed.

Hepatitis E Prophylaxis

- Approaches to preventing exposure to enteric agents apply to the prevention of hepatitis E (see hepatitis A).
- A recombinant vaccine is available routinely in endemic areas but not in the United States for the prevention of hepatitis E. The efficacy of IG is not known.

Annotated Bibliography

1. Wheeler C, Vogt TM, Armstrong GL, et al. An outbreak of hepatitis A associated with green onion. N Engl J Med 2005;353:890. (*Outbreaks of acute hepatitis A continue to occur; this report describes a large outbreak involving persons who ate at a single Pennsylvania restaurant; the offending contaminated food was green onions imported from Mexico. Because of the persistence of such outbreaks, despite targeted hepatitis A vaccination of persons at high risk, the U.S. Public Health Service recommended universal vaccination of children.*)
2. Martin A, Lemon A. Hepatitis A virus: from discovery to vaccines. Hepatology 2006;43:S164. (*A comprehensive review of hepatitis A.*)
3. Shrestha MP, Scott RM, Joshi DM, et al. Safety and efficacy of a recombinant hepatitis E vaccine. N Engl J Med 2007;356:895. (*Demonstration of the efficacy of a recombinant hepatitis E vaccine in a large phase II study conducted in an endemic area.*)
4. Alter MJ, Hadler SC, Margolies HS, et al. The changing epidemiology of hepatitis B in the United States: need for alternative vaccination strategies. JAMA 1990;263:1218. (*Argument for a policy of universal hepatitis B vaccination in childhood.*)
5. Alter MJ. Epidemiology of hepatitis B in Europe and worldwide. J Hepatol 2003;39(Suppl 1):S64. (*Concise review of modes of spread and distribution of hepatitis B.*)
6. Dienstag JL, McHutchison JG. American Gastroenterological Association technical review on the management of hepatitis C. Gastroenterology 2006;130:231. (*This review contains information on the clinical and epidemiologic features of hepatitis C, as well as background data on which management recommendations are based.*)
7. Strader DB, Wright T, Thomas DL, et al. Diagnosis, management and treatment of hepatitis C (AASLD practice guidelines). Hepatology 2004;39: 1147. (*A comprehensive review of the clinical and management features of hepatitis C.*)
8. Hoofnagle JH, Doo E, Liang TJ, et al. Management of hepatitis B: summary of a clinical research workshop. Hepatology 2007;45:1056. (*Summary of a workshop held at the National Institutes of Health and covering the clinical and epidemiologic features of hepatitis B and its and management.*)
9. Purcell RH. Hepatitis viruses. Changing patterns of human disease. Proc Natl Acad Sci USA 1994;91:2401. (*A concise but compelling summary of changes in the clinical and epidemiologic expression of hepatitis viruses, some resulting from changes in human behavior and population shifts.*)
10. Schreiber GB, Busch MP, Kleinman SH, et al. The risk of transfusion-transmitted viral infection. N Engl J Med 1996;334:1685. (*Improvements in blood donor screening, including virus-nonspecific measures and specific viral screening tests, have reduced the frequency of transfusion-associated hepatitis B and C and HIV infection to negligible levels.*)
11. National Institutes of Health Consensus Development Conference. Management of hepatitis C. Hepatology 1997;6(Suppl 1):1S. (*A comprehensive overview of all aspects of hepatitis C, including excellent sections on diagnosis, diagnostic test methods, epidemiology, and management.*)
12. National Institutes of Health Consensus Development Conference. Management of hepatitis C. Hepatology 2002;36(Suppl 1):1S. (*A updated comprehensive overview of all aspects of hepatitis C.*)
13. Lauer GM, Walker BD. Medical progress: hepatitis C virus infection. N Engl J Med 2001;345:41. (*A review of virology, immunology, pathophysiology, clinical features, and management.*)
14. Farci P. Delta hepatitis: an update. J Hepatol 2003;39(Suppl 1):S212. (*Brief but authoritative review.*)
15. Armstrong GL, Wasley A, Simard EP, et al. The prevalence of hepatitis C virus infection in the United States, 1999 through 2002. Ann Intern Med 2006;144:705. (*Results of a national survey involving 10,000 persons; demonstrated that 1.6% of the population have antibodies to hepatitis C virus and that the prevalence is higher in African Americans and Americans of Mexican descent than in whites; compared to a similar survey conducted during the previous decade, the peak prevalence of hepatitis C virus infection had shifted from the fourth to the fifth decade, reflecting the aging of a cohort infected primarily during the 1960s and 1970s.*)
16. Wilner IR, Uhl MD, Howard SD, et al. Serious hepatitis A: an analysis of patients hospitalized during an urban epidemic in the United States. Ann Intern Med 1998;128:111. (*This report buttresses the general observation that with a reduction in the frequency of acute hepatitis A in young children, more-severe cases are being recognized among adults.*)
17. Centers for Disease Control and Prevention. Prevention of hepatitis A through active or passive immunization: recommendations of the Advisory Committee on Immunization Practices (ACIP). MMWR Morb Mortal Wkly Rep 2006;55:1. (*Official recommendations of the U.S. Public Health Service for administration of immune globulin and hepatitis A vaccine to prevent hepatitis A; this update contains the new recommendation for universal childhood hepatitis A vaccination.*)
18. Centers for Disease Control and Prevention. A comprehensive immunization strategy to eliminate transmission of hepatitis B virus in the United States: recommendations of the Immunization Practices Advisory Committee (ACIP); Part 1: Immunization of infants, children, and adolescents. MMWR Morb Mortal Wkly Rep 2005;54:1. Part 2: Immunization of adults. MMWR Morb Mortal Wkly Rep 2006;55:1 (*Official recommendations of the U.S. Public Health Service, including universal hepatitis B vaccination in childhood and catch-up vaccination in adolescents who missed childhood vaccination.*)
19. Centers for Disease Control and Prevention. Updated U.S. Public Health Service guidelines for the management of occupational exposures to HBV, HCV, and HIV and recommendations for postexposure prophylaxis. MMWR Morb Mortal Wkly Rep 2001;50(RR-11):1. (*Recommendations for minimizing and undertaking prophylaxis against the spread of these blood-borne infections among health care workers.*)
20. Centers for Centers for Disease Control and Prevention. Recommendations for prevention and control of hepatitis C virus (HCV) infection and HCV-related chronic disease. MMWR Morb Mortal Wkly Rep 1998;47:1. (*Official recommendations of the U.S. Public Health Service for approaches to limiting the spread of hepatitis C virus infection.*)
21. Lok AS, McMahon BJ. Chronic hepatitis B. Hepatology 2007;45:507. (*A comprehensive overview of the clinical and epidemiologic features of hepatitis B, as well as recommendations for management.*)
22. Chu CJ, Lok ASK. Clinical significance of hepatitis B virus genotypes. Hepatology 2002;35:1274. (*Discusses the distribution of hepatitis B genotypes around the world and observations suggesting that progression and complications of hepatitis B vary among genotypes, i.e., a virus-related, rather than a host-related determinant of outcome.*)
23. Pawlotsky JM. Molecular diagnosis of viral hepatitis. Gastroenterology 2002;122:1554. (*Valuable review of methods for detecting hepatitis B virus DNA and hepatitis C virus RNA, including comparisons of relative sensitivity, dynamic ranges, and performance.*)
24. Wasley A, Samandari T, Bell BP. The incidence of hepatitis A in the United States in the era of vaccination. JAMA 2005;294:194. (*Following the adoption of childhood hepatitis A vaccination, hepatitis A rates have declined to historic lows; between the 1990s and the early 2000s, the overall yearly*

incidence of hepatitis A rates declined 76% to 2.6/100,000; declines were greater among children; rates are now higher in adults than in children, peaking in men aged 25 to 39 years.)

25. Farci P, Alter HJ, Govindarajan S, et al. Lack of protective immunity against reinfection with hepatitis C virus. Science 1992;258:135. (*This report summarizes virologic reassessment of earlier cross-challenge studies in experimentally infected chimpanzees and shows that neither heterologous nor homologous immunity develops after hepatitis C infection.*)

26. Seeff LB. Natural history of chronic hepatitis C. Hepatology 2002;36 (Suppl 1):S35. (*A comprehensive review of data on the natural history of chronic hepatitis B; among transfusion recipients who acquire hepatitis C virus infection, overall mortality does not exceed that in control groups of transfused patients in whom hepatitis C did not develop; however, liver morbidity and mortality are greater in the hepatitis C group; generally, hepatitis C is a slowly insidious disease, progressing to cirrhosis in one fourth of patients within 20 years.*)

27. Yano M, Kumada H, Kage M, et al. The long-term pathological evolution of chronic hepatitis C. Hepatology 1996;23:1334. (*Serial liver biopsies over 20 years in this group of Japanese patients with chronic hepatitis C showed that the rate of progression to cirrhosis was related to baseline histology; milder histologic grade and stage predicted limited progression, whereas moderate and severe histologic features predicted eventual progression to cirrhosis over 20 years for moderate hepatitis and over 10 years for severe hepatitis.*)

28. Tong MJ, El-Farra NS, Reikes AR, et al. Clinical outcomes after transfusion-associated hepatitis C. N Engl J Med 1995;332:1463. (*In a tertiary referral center, patients encountered with chronic hepatitis C have progressive disease, including cirrhosis and hepatocellular carcinoma: progression is more pronounced among those who acquire the disease later in life.*)

29. Major ME, Feinstone SM. The molecular virology of hepatitis C. Hepatology 1997;25:1527. (*A review of hepatitis C virology, including genotypes and quasi-species diversity.*)

30. Rosina F, Conoscitore P, Cuppone R, et al. Changing pattern of chronic hepatitis D in southern Europe. Gastroenterology 1999;117:161. (*Although hepatitis D tends to be a severe and progressive disease, this study showed that the disease can become clinically indolent after several years of severe hepatitis.*)

31. Lemon SM, Thomas DL. Vaccines to prevent viral hepatitis. N Engl J Med 1997;336:196. (*An excellent review of the development, features, and application of hepatitis B and A vaccines.*)

32. Sagliocca L, Amoroso P, Stroffolini T, et al. Efficacy of hepatitis A vaccine in prevention of secondary hepatitis A infection: a randomized trial. Lancet 1999;353:1136. (*Although hepatitis A vaccination cannot always be given in a timely fashion to household contacts of patients with acute hepatitis A, it does prevent secondary cases and should be recommended.*)

33. Centers for Disease Control and Prevention. General recommendations on immunization: recommendations of the Advisory Committee on Immunization Practices and the American Academy of Family Physicians. MMWR Morb Mortal Week Rep 2002;51(RR-2):1. (*U.S. Public Health Service recommendations for vaccination to prevent hepatitis virus infection.*)

34. Vento S, Garofano T, Renzini C, et al. Fulminant hepatitis associated with hepatitis A virus superinfection in patients with chronic hepatitis C. N Engl J Med 1998;338:286. (*The only report to suggest a high frequency of fulminant hepatitis A in patients with chronic hepatitis C; although this experience has not been confirmed and has actually been challenged by other observers, hepatitis A vaccination has been recommended in patients with chronic hepatitis C.*)

35. Chang MH, Chen CJ, Lai MS, et al. Universal hepatitis B vaccination in Taiwan and the incidence of hepatocellular carcinoma in children. N Engl J Med 1997;336:1855. (*Hepatitis B vaccination of infants in China has reduced the incidence of hepatocellular carcinoma in children; thus, hepatitis B vaccine can prevent hepatocellular carcinoma in a population in which hepatitis B is endemic; in essence, hepatitis B vaccine, in addition to preventing acute and chronic hepatitis, is a "cancer vaccine."*)

36. Margolis HS, Coleman PJ, Brown RE, et al. Prevention of hepatitis B virus transmission by immunization: an economic analysis of current recommendations. JAMA 1995;274:1201. (*This analysis indicates that vaccination of infants, and also vaccination of adolescents not vaccinated at birth, is cost-effective.*)

CHAPTER 58 ■ EVALUATION OF ABDOMINAL PAIN

JAMES M. RICHTER

One of primary care's most daunting challenges is the outpatient assessment of abdominal pain. When the pain is acute in onset, triage decisions have to be made regarding the need for hospital admission and surgical intervention. If the pain is chronic or recurrent, the challenge is to design a safe, cost-effective plan for workup that will efficiently distinguish among a myriad of possible etiologies. In instances in which the exact cause of pain is not immediately evident, an empiric trial of therapy or a thoughtful test selection may help to suggest the underlying pathophysiology, narrow the differential diagnosis, and guide further assessment and treatment. Also important are the need to decide on the proper speed and extent of evaluation and to keep in mind nondigestive etiologies, such as ovarian carcinoma (see Chapter 116) and myocardial ischemia (see Chapter 20), that may present as abdominal discomfort.

PATHOPHYSIOLOGY AND CLINICAL PRESENTATION (1–11)

The major mechanisms of abdominal pain include distension of a hollow viscus from obstruction, peritoneal irritation, vascular insufficiency, mucosal ulceration, altered bowel motility, capsular distention, metabolic disorder, nerve injury, abdominal wall injury, and referral from an extraabdominal site.

Obstruction

Pain receptors in the bowel, biliary tree, and ureters respond to *distention* and increased wall tension. The severity of the pain is a function of the speed of onset as well as the degree of distention. Obstruction that develops slowly during weeks to months may be relatively subtle in presentation in comparison with acute obstruction, which produces a more dramatic picture. In acute obstruction, the pain is severe and "colicky" or wavelike in nature; it makes the patient restless.

Small Bowel

The pain of acute *small-bowel* obstruction is greatest when the obstruction is jejunal. The patient is often comfortable between bouts of pain. Severity decreases with time as bowel motility diminishes. Complete strangulation of the small bowel is associated with steady pain from secondary vascular insufficiency or peritoneal irritation. Vomiting is common, particularly in proximal obstruction; when the problem is distal, vomiting is less frequent. Flatus and passage of small amounts of stool may occur at the outset, but they soon cease if the obstruction is complete. Diarrhea is noted in some cases of partial obstruction. On examination, the patient appears restless during bouts of pain. The temperature is typically normal or only mildly elevated. The abdomen may be distended, especially when the obstruction is distal. High-pitched, hyperactive bowel sounds are characteristic but not always present. Tenderness to palpation is not impressive unless ischemia or leakage of bowel contents has occurred and caused peritonitis. The stool is usually negative for occult blood.

Large Bowel

Obstruction of the large bowel is, in most instances, less painful and associated with less vomiting than is obstruction of the small intestine. Constipation or a change in bowel habits often precedes complete obstruction. Diarrhea may occur with partial obstruction. Distention is greater than that seen in small-bowel obstruction. Stools are frequently positive for occult blood.

In cases of bowel obstruction, the white blood cell count may be normal, even in association with a strangulating obstruction (i.e., with compromise of the intestinal blood supply in addition to blockage of the lumen). A plain *radiograph of the abdomen* (supine and upright) in patients with small-bowel obstruction often shows distention of loops of small bowel with high air–fluid levels. This, together with an absence of gas in the large bowel (distal to the obstruction), is characteristic of small-bowel obstruction. The radiographic appearance of colonic obstruction varies with the competency (or incompetency) of the ileocecal valve. If the valve is competent, less small-bowel dilation ensues.

Cystic Duct

Sudden obstruction of the cystic duct by a stone produces acute pain, sometimes referred to as biliary *"colic."* Unlike the cramping pain of acute intestinal obstruction, the pain of acute cystic duct obstruction is mostly steady, lasting more than 1 hour after sudden onset. *Acute cholecystitis* is associated with localized peritonitis in addition to obstruction. Pain is typically maximal in the right upper quadrant or epigastrium, radiates to the scapular region, and is accompanied by nausea, vomiting, and fever without jaundice; at times only mild epigastric discomfort is present (see Chapter 69). *Murphy's sign* (inspiratory arrest in response to right upper quadrant palpation) may be seen, and right upper quadrant tenderness to percussion or pressure over the gallbladder is also a suggestive finding. Laboratory investigation usually reveals a leukocytosis and sometimes a modest alkaline phosphatase elevation; bilirubin levels are usually not elevated. *Gallstones* in the absence of ductal obstruction or gallbladder wall inflammation are often asymptomatic (see Chapter 69).

Common Bile Duct

Acute common bile duct obstruction produces *epigastric pain*, often accompanied by marked *nausea* and *vomiting*; *jaundice* ensues. Obstruction and dilation that occur more gradually are often *painless*. Physical examination may reveal a tender right upper quadrant, but in comparison with that of acute cholecystitis, tenderness may be less focal and deeper. A palpable gallbladder suggests gradual progressive development of ductal obstruction, typically caused by malignancy. Alkaline phosphatase is markedly elevated, as is serum bilirubin.

Urinary Tract

Obstruction within the urinary tract can present as abdominal pain. Acute ureteral blockade by a stone is extremely uncomfortable. Onset is sudden and the pain is cramping, beginning in the back and flank and radiating into the lower abdomen and groin. If acute pyelonephritis develops, upper abdominal pain, fever, and chills may ensue. Acute bladder outflow obstruction presents as lower abdominal distention and suprapubic pain. Symptoms of prostatism (see Chapter 134) may precede the episode.

Peritoneal Irritation

Peritoneal irritation causes a severe continuous pain because of the rich innervation of the parietal peritoneum. Focal injury results in well-localized discomfort that is described as sharp, aching, or burning. Spread of the irritant process leads to more-generalized abdominal pain. Severity is related to the nature of the irritant and the speed with which the noxious exposure occurs. Reflex spasm of the overlying abdominal wall musculature can produce involuntary guarding. Rebound tenderness is prominent on physical examination. Most important, the pain is accentuated by pressure changes in the peritoneum; thus, palpation, coughing, or movement may increase the pain, leading the patient to lie still, in contrast to the restlessness of patients with "colicky" pain.

Focal Peritonitis

Focal peritonitis of the retroperitoneum, which is characteristic of *early appendicitis*, may be tested by having the patient lie on the left side and extend the right hip (*psoas sign*). Bowel sounds are often reduced or absent, especially when the irritation is generalized. The origin of the peritoneal irritant need not be digestive; it can originate from other systems (e.g., from *ovarian carcinoma*).

Familial Mediterranean Fever

Familial Mediterranean fever, an infrequent autosomal recessive disorder most prevalent among Sephardic Jews, Turks, Arabs, and Armenians, causes recurrent attacks of serositis and fever. Any serosal surface may be involved, accounting for its protean manifestations, including fever, peritoneal irritation, pleuritis, and arthritis. Self-limited attacks lasting days to weeks typically begin during childhood or early adulthood. Presentations may mimic peritonitis, juvenile rheumatoid arthritis (monoarticular or oligoarticular joint involvement), or pleurisy. The brief but severe attacks are accompanied by marked elevations in sedimentation rate and acute-phase reactants. A serious consequence is *amyloidosis*, sometimes resulting in renal impairment. Colchicine provides dramatic relief from the pain of an acute attack and also prevents amyloid deposition and renal impairment.

Vascular Disease

Vascular disease of the abdomen can result in a host of abdominal pain presentations, many of which simulate those of other etiologies.

Acute Arterial Insufficiency

Acute arterial insufficiency (resulting from atherosclerosis, embolus, or sickle cell crisis) may present with severe abdominal pain, but sometimes the early presentation is subtler, with mild constant pain the only symptom for several days in the absence of tenderness or rigidity. The diagnosis may not become apparent until ischemic necrosis, bowel perforation, and peritoneal soilage set in, leading to peritonitis, lactic acidosis, and shock.

Chronic Mesenteric Insufficiency

Chronic mesenteric insufficiency characteristically produces dull or aching postprandial pain ("*abdominal angina*") localized to the epigastrium or midabdomen when the increased oxygen demand of digesting a meal outpaces the available blood supply. Onset is usually within an hour of eating, peaking at the time of maximal oxygen demand; severity is proportional to the size and fat composition of the meal as well as the degree of obstruction to blood flow. Symptoms can persist for 2 to 3 hours.

Symptoms vary with the vascular territory involved and may herald acute infarction in cases of critical stenosis. Nausea, vomiting, and bloating characterize celiac artery ischemia. In midgut ischemia due to superior mesenteric artery disease, the predominant complaints are pain and weight loss. Constipation accompanied by occult blood loss characterizes chronic inferior mesenteric artery insufficiency. Some patients lose considerable amounts of weight because of the fear that eating will induce pain. Abdominal bruits are reported in 20% to 60% of cases; extraabdominal signs of atherosclerotic vascular disease (e.g., carotid or femoral bruits) are often detectable.

Aortic Dissection

Aortic dissection or rupture of an *abdominal aortic aneurysm* produces severe acute abdominal pain that often radiates to the back or genitalia. Before dissection, aneurysms are usually silent, but physical examination may reveal an increase in aortic diameter (>3.0 cm). The greater the increase in aortic diameter on examination, the more likely it is that an aneurysm is present. Clinically silent abdominal aneurysms are often discovered serendipitously during workup for other causes of abdominal pain. Risk of catastrophic rupture is minimal as long as aneurysm diameter remains less than 5.0 cm. However, the probability over time of continued growth in diameter is substantial, necessitating careful follow-up (see later discussion). Aneurysms may also compromise arterial flow to the gut and result in ischemia.

Mesenteric Venous Thrombosis

Mesenteric venous thrombosis is a less common cause of intestinal ischemia than is arterial occlusion. It may present similarly, although it often has a more slowly progressive course. Both aortic dissection and mesenteric thrombosis typically result in pain complaints that are in excess of those elicited by physical examination.

Mucosal Injury

Ulceration or inflammation of the gastrointestinal tract is often accompanied by pain.

Peptic Ulcer Disease

Although the exact mechanism of pain in peptic ulcer disease is incompletely understood, it is believed that acid inflaming submucosal tissue and nerves plays a major role. This hypothesis is supported by the observation that neutralization of acid often provides immediate relief. The pain pattern of duodenal ulcer disease usually parallels the acid–peptic cycle (see Chapter 68). Unless perforation or penetration into the pancreas is present, the pain is mostly confined to the epigastrium. Patients use such terms as *gnawing*, *aching*, and *burning* to describe their discomfort. Radiation of pain into the back in patients with duodenal ulcer suggests perforation into the pancreas.

Inflammation

Inflammation of the middle or lower intestine, as seen with acute *gastroenteritis* and acute flares of *inflammatory bowel disease* (see Chapter 73), can disturb motility and absorption. In most instances, the pain is diffuse, but occasionally it is focal and can simulate appendicitis or other surgical conditions. Fever, nausea, and vomiting are often prominent in the early stages of gastroenteritis; bowel sounds are usually hyperactive.

Immune-Mediated Injury (Adult Celiac Disease [Sprue]; see also Chapter 64)

A genetically predisposed inappropriate T cell response to ingested gluten causes immune-mediated damage to the small-bowel mucosa. Presenting symptoms can be subtle and nonspecific, including episodic or nocturnal *diarrhea*, *flatulence*, and *weight loss* along with *iron deficiency*. Steatorrhea may be absent if disease is limited to the proximal small bowel. *Bloating*, *fatigue*, and *vague abdominal discomfort* are common and may be mistaken for symptoms of irritable bowel syndrome. *Iron-deficiency anemia* may be the only manifestation.

Altered Bowel Motility

This mechanism predominates in functional bowel disturbances, of which irritable bowel syndrome and psychophysiologic disturbances are the best examples.

Irritable Bowel Syndrome

Spasmodic, nonpropulsive, segmental contractions of large bowel result in high intraluminal pressures, manifested by cramping lower abdominal pain and bloating. In addition, there is a component of perceptive (nociceptive) dysfunction contributing to feelings of abdominal discomfort (see Chapter 74). Constipation alternating with diarrhea and mucous stools are typical findings, as are pain relieved by defecation, more frequent and loose stools with the onset of pain, and a feeling of incomplete evacuation. Altered motility and chronically increased intraluminal pressures may lead to *diverticular disease* (see Chapter 75).

Functional Dyspepsia

This condition is characterized by chronic or recurrent upper abdominal discomfort or pain, often in conjunction with food-related dysmotility symptoms (e.g., bloating, fullness, nausea, early satiety). Many patients have concurrent esophageal reflux and irritable bowel syndrome, supporting the concept of "irritable gut syndrome" (see Chapter 74).

Psychiatric Disturbances

Psychiatric disturbances, especially *anxiety* and *mood disorders*, are common in persons with irritable bowel syndrome who seek medical attention. Symptoms may arise from any area of the intestinal tract—esophagus, stomach, small intestine, and biliary tree, as well as the colon. The result is a broad spectrum of presentations, which includes nausea, vomiting, dyspepsia, and flatulence in addition to cramping abdominal pain.

Acute Ileus

Causes include *peritonitis* (resulting from a variety of causes), systemic *infections*, bowel *ischemia*, abdominal *surgery* (a common etiology), abdominal *trauma*, *pharmacologic agents* (especially *anticholinergics* and *narcotics*), and *metabolic disturbances* (particularly *hypokalemia*).

Intestinal Pseudoobstruction

Clinical features mimic those of intestinal obstruction. Symptoms may be chronic (recurrent or persistent) or occur acutely (so-called acute ileus). Symptoms can include vomiting and abdominal distention; diarrhea or constipation may also be seen. Plain films of the abdomen demonstrate intestinal dilation, suggestive of partial obstruction. It is noteworthy that the syndrome of chronic pseudoobstruction may precede the recognition of associated systemic diseases by many years (see later discussion). *Chronic intestinal pseudoobstruction* is often idiopathic, although it may occur in the setting of scleroderma, Parkinson's disease, drug use (opiates, phenothiazines, tricyclic antidepressants, or antiparkinsonian medications), hypercalcemia, diabetes, myxedema, amyloidosis, radiation enteritis, and chronic laxative abuse.

Capsular Distention

Distention of the well-innervated capsule surrounding digestive organs is a potential source of constant, *aching* abdominal pain. *Hepatic* capsular distention leading to right upper quadrant pain occurs in hepatitis, congestive heart failure, fatty infiltration (hepatic steatosis), and subcapsular hematoma. The pain of *splenic* capsular distention, as may occur secondary to blunt trauma (e.g., in a motor vehicle accident), localizes to the left upper quadrant. With subdiaphragmatic peritoneal irritation, the patient may experience pain radiating to the ipsilateral shoulder. With splenic trauma, a deceptive period of many hours may pass before peritoneal signs develop if a subcapsular hematoma temporarily retards the spilling of blood into the peritoneum.

Metabolic Disturbances

Metabolic disturbances may mimic intraabdominal etiologies or sometimes result from them and exacerbate the clinical presentation.

Ketoacidosis

Ketoacidosis presents with severe abdominal pain in 8% of instances and may be accompanied by emesis and an elevated white blood cell count. Symptoms are caused, at least in part, by accompanying gastroparesis. An acute intraabdominal event such as cholecystitis in a diabetic may be the precipitant.

Porphyria

Porphyria sometimes simulates bowel obstruction because of the cramping abdominal pain and hyperperistalsis that may occur. *Acute intermittent porphyria* presents with moderate to severe colicky abdominal pain, which may be localized or generalized. Abdominal symptoms may be the result of intestinal dysmotility; vomiting and diarrhea are also common complaints. Fever and leukocytosis may be present, but on examination the abdomen is found to be soft. Proximal muscle pain and a range of neuropsychiatric symptoms accompany the abdominal pain. The clinical features of *hereditary coproporphyria* and *variegate porphyria* are similar to those described for acute intermittent porphyria; skin lesions may be prominent.

Lead Poisoning

Lead poisoning may also present with abdominal pain. Such pain is typically wandering, poorly localized, colicky, and accompanied by a rigid abdomen. Encephalopathy, peripheral neuropathy, and anemia are associated features. The *urine coproporphyrin* test is a more reliable indicator of this entity than is a serum lead level, which can be normal.

Angioneurotic Edema

Angioneurotic edema, caused by C′ *esterase inhibitor deficiency*, may result in episodic and severe abdominal pain. If this diagnosis is suspected, it is useful to check the serum level of C4, which is low in cases of C′ esterase inhibitor deficiency.

Nerve Injury

Nerve injury from encroachment or irritation is an important mechanism of abdominal pain. The source of pain may be intraabdominal, as occurs when a pancreatic cancer or pancreatitis damages or inflames adjacent splanchnic nerves, or it may be extraabdominal, as occurs when a nerve root supplying an abdominal wall dermatome becomes irritated in herpes zoster. Abdominal pain occurs in about 75% of patients with *cancer of the pancreas*; it is usually epigastric and most common in patients with tumor involving the body or tail of the pancreas. Sometimes, the pain radiates to the back or is confined to it. Nerve root irritation from *herpes zoster* may be mistaken for an intraabdominal process, especially before the rash appears. Often, the patient complains of a severe, lancinating pain resembling that from an intraabdominal source. An associated rectus muscle spasm may simulate peritonitis, but there is no effect on bowel function, as there is with peritoneal irritation, and palpation may actually alleviate the rectus muscle spasm. The pain of herpes infection often precedes the rash by several days and may persist after the skin clears, particularly in the elderly (see Chapter 193).

Abdominal Wall Pathology

Abdominal wall pathology can also be mistaken for disease inside the abdominal cavity. Traumatic injury to the musculature of the wall produces pain that is constant, aching, and exacerbated by movement or pressure on the abdomen. The muscles may be in spasm, simulating the involuntary guarding of peritonitis. When a generalized myositis is responsible for the muscle pain, discomfort occurs in the limbs, as well as in the abdomen. Occasionally, a tender mass in the wall, such as a rectus sheath hematoma, is found to be the source of difficulty.

Referred Pain

Chest Sources

Referred pain from a process originating in the chest is sometimes an etiology of abdominal complaints. *Pulmonary infarction* and *pneumonia* of the lower lobes are among the chest problems that may present as pain in the upper abdomen; at times, reflex muscle spasm accompanies the pain. Upper abdominal pain, nausea, and vomiting may be the principal manifestations of an acute *inferior myocardial infarction*. However, symptoms and signs of cardiac or pulmonary disease accompany most intrathoracic sources of abdominal pain.

Ovarian Cancer and Other Pelvic Sources

Both benign and malignant ovarian masses, even those still confined to the pelvis, are frequent sources of abdominal complaints. In addition to causing pelvic pain and urinary urgency, such pelvic pathology is significantly associated with increasing abdominal girth and bloating. Even though such symptoms are nonspecific and common in primary care practice, they take on added meaning when new in onset or more frequent (20 to 30 times per month vs. 2 to 3 times per month) or more severe than usual. Almost half of women with ovarian cancer experience the combination of bloating, increased abdominal size, and urinary symptoms, compared with 8% of those without such cancer presenting to primary care clinics.

DIFFERENTIAL DIAGNOSIS (11)

Because the number of possible causes of abdominal pain is large, it is helpful to consider the differential diagnosis in terms of pathophysiologic mechanisms (Table 58.1). The nature of the pain can sometimes be more discriminating than location and suggest a pathophysiology that can narrow the differential. Etiologies causing obstruction, peritoneal irritation, and vascular insufficiency are among the most dangerous. In about 70% of cases, adhesions or external hernias cause mechanical small-bowel obstruction; 90% of cases of large-bowel obstruction are attributable to diverticular disease and carcinoma. Acute arterial insufficiency results most often from systemic embolization secondary to atrial fibrillation, severe atherosclerotic occlusive disease, and hypoperfusional states. Pelvic pathology is a common extraabdominal source of peritoneal irritation.

Other pathophysiologic mechanisms, such as nerve injury, metabolic imbalance, abdominal wall disease, and disordered motility, may produce symptoms that superficially mimic those of a more worrisome etiology; however, conditions associated with these mechanisms are usually more annoying than dangerous (an important exception is diabetic ketoacidosis). Pain referred from an extraabdominal site is more of a problem; significant cardiac disease (e.g., inferior myocardial infarction) or pulmonary pathology (e.g., lower lobe pneumonia) may present as abdominal pain.

WORKUP (1–31)

The first priority is to determine the likelihood of serious pathophysiology and the pace and extent of workup. Patients with acute pain need to be examined promptly for evidence of obstruction, peritoneal irritation, vascular compromise, and cardiopulmonary disease. The presence of fever, jaundice,

---

TABLE 58.1

PRINCIPAL MECHANISMS OF ABDOMINAL PAIN

Obstruction
  Gastric outlet
  Small bowel
  Large bowel
  Biliary tract
  Urinary tract

Peritoneal Irritation
  Infection
  Chemical irritation (blood, bile, gastric acid)
  Systemic inflammatory process
  Spread from a local inflammatory process

Vascular Insufficiency
  Embolization
  Atherosclerotic narrowing
  Hypotension
  Aortic aneurysm dissection

Mucosal Ulceration
  Peptic ulcer disease
  Gastric cancer

Altered Motility
  Gastroenteritis
  Inflammatory bowel disease
  Irritable bowel syndrome
  Diverticular disease

Metabolic Disturbance
  Diabetic ketoacidosis
  Porphyria
  Lead poisoning

Nerve Injury
  Herpes zoster
  Root compression
  Nerve invasion

Muscle Wall Disease
  Trauma
  Myositis
  Hematoma

Referred Pain
  Pneumonia (lower lobes)
  Inferior myocardial infarction
  Pulmonary infarction

Psychopathology
  Depression
  Anxiety
  Neuroses

---

dehydration, or bleeding requires expedited evaluation. The evaluation of chronic pain can proceed at a more gradual pace, with time allowed to get to know the patient and the problem before undertaking extensive testing.

History

A complete description of the pain should be obtained, including localization, characterization, area of referral, time course of onset and resolution, and precipitating and alleviating factors. The chronologic sequence of symptom occurrence should be clearly outlined.

Checking for Serious Underlying Pathology

In addition to obtaining a complete description of the patient's pain, one needs to inquire into symptoms and historical factors indicative of pathology requiring urgent attention, including prior abdominal surgery; previous episodes of obstruction; known gallbladder or kidney stones; family history of sprue or history of chronic diarrhea; emesis; rectal bleeding or melenotic stools; absence of flatus; obstipation; fever and rigors; distention; difficulties in urination; presence of atherosclerotic risk factors (especially smoking); known systemic vascular disease; and any cardiac or pulmonary symptoms. Inquiry into pregnancy, strong family history of ovarian or breast carcinoma, and symptoms of pelvic pathology, such as pain, dyspareunia, abnormal vaginal discharge, or irregular menstrual bleeding, are essential in women presenting with abdominal discomfort. Women who present with increasing abdominal girth and bloating, especially when of new onset or much more frequent or severe than usual, especially if accompanied by pelvic discomfort or urinary symptoms, should undergo investigation for ovarian neoplasm.

Taking into Account Potentially Confounding Variables

The physician must learn to interpret accurately the "true" quality and quantity of the patient's experience, especially in cases of chronic abdominal pain, in which a host of nonmedical factors can alter pain perception and affect daily living. A thorough psychosocial history helps to elucidate the psychological and ethnic factors that might contribute. Exploring patient fears, concerns, and expectations is also critical to understanding the patient, designing an effective treatment plan, and communicating a sense of caring and understanding.

Clinical Diagnosis of Functional Disease

The symptoms of functional bowel disease may mimic those of more serious pathology, which makes it necessary first to rule out the latter. Compounding the diagnostic challenge is the fact that the recognition of functional disease relies heavily on the history because there are no characteristic physical or laboratory findings. Clinical criteria predictive of functional disease have been identified to enable a "positive" diagnosis of functional disease to be made, rather than just an exclusionary one.

Irritable Bowel Syndrome. The widely used *Manning criteria* (visible abdominal distention, pain relief with defecation, more frequent stools with onset of pain, looser stools with onset of pain, passage of mucus per rectum, and feeling of incomplete evacuation) were developed to differentiate irritable bowel syndrome from other gastrointestinal disorders. Predictive value rises with the number of criteria that the patient fulfills and with the exclusion of findings suggestive of underlying bowel pathology. With all six criteria present, the predictive value can be as high as 80% to 90%, although it is lower in the elderly (70% to 80%) because of the increased risk for colon cancer (which can mimic some of the findings). The *Rome criteria* (see Chapter 74) are a refined iteration of the Manning criteria with the following features:

At least 3 months of continuous or recurrent symptoms of abdominal pain or discomfort associated with any or all of the following:

- Relief with defecation
- Change in stool frequency
- Change in stool consistency plus two or more of the following:
    - Altered stool frequency (more than three bowel movements per day or fewer than three per week)
    - Altered stool form (lumpy and hard or loose and watery)
    - Altered stool passage (straining, urgency, or incomplete evacuation)
    - Passage of mucus
    - Bloating or feeling of abdominal distention

Functional Dyspepsia. The *Rome criteria* for this condition identify two forms: ulcer like and dysmotility like. For the ulcer-like variant (in which abdominal pain dominates), the principal criterion is 3 months or more of upper abdominal pain with no evidence of organic disease, plus three or more of the following:

- Very well localized pain
- Pain relieved by food (>25% of the time)
- Pain relieved by antacids or histamine$_2$ blockers
- Pain that awakens patient from sleep
- Periods of remission and relapse (at least 2 weeks of remission)

Physical Examination

Particular attention should be paid to the patient's *general appearance*. The patient who appears reluctant to change position and keeps still is likely to have peritoneal irritation, whereas the patient with obstruction is often restless. It is important to check the *vital signs* for postural changes in the blood pressure or heart rate because obstruction, peritonitis, and bowel infarction can produce large losses of intravascular volume. Any hypotension, atrial fibrillation, or fever should be noted; however, absence of fever does not rule out serious pathology, especially in the elderly or chronically ill patient. The *skin* is examined for jaundice, other stigmata of chronic liver disease, clubbing or spooning of the fingernails, signs of trauma, excoriations, prior surgical scars, and evidence of dehydration, edema, or dermatomal rash. In addition, the sclerae are noted for icterus. The *chest* is checked for splinting, a pleural friction rub, and signs of consolidation (particularly in the lower lobes), and the *heart* is checked for murmurs, chamber enlargement, and signs of heart failure (see Chapter 32).

Abdominal Examination

The abdominal examination should be performed with care to avoid unnecessary discomfort. A sharp increase in pain with coughing demonstrates rebound tenderness without the need for palpation and release. Examination of the abdomen includes checking for distention, ascites, altered bowel sounds (increased or absent), hepatic rub, vascular bruit, tenderness, guarding, rebound, hepatosplenomegaly, inguinal hernia, and masses (including a dilated aorta, loops of bowel, stool, distended bladder or uterus). An increased abdominal venous pattern suggests portal hypertension; periumbilical adenopathy suggests pancreatic or ovarian cancer. In a person with risk factors for vascular disease, the abdominal aorta should be palpated to determine its diameter. The index fingers are placed along the lateral margins of the aorta a few centimeters above the umbilicus and the distance between them measured, with the estimated thickness of the skin subtracted. Any diameter larger than 3 to 4 cm raises the possibility of aneurysm and necessitates proceeding to imaging (ultrasonography or computed tomography).

Pelvic and Rectal Examinations

These are essential parts of the evaluation, with checks for masses and tenderness, and are more revealing if done gently. The fecal occult blood test is also mandatory.

Abdominal Wall and Nerve

Examining for nerve and muscle wall injury is often overlooked in the urgency of searching for more worrisome pathology. Two important signs of nerve involvement are pain in a dermatomal distribution and hyperesthesia. Both occur with nerve injury from herpes zoster or nerve root impingement; however, hyperesthesia is also seen with focal peritoneal irritation. Testing is performed by gentle stroking of the skin overlying the area of pain. The rash of herpes may not appear until the time of the follow-up assessment. Abdominal wall pathology may be discovered by careful palpation of the wall for masses and muscle tenderness and by noting any exacerbation of pain when the muscles are contracted, as occurs with sitting up. Any pain on sitting up should not be confused with that secondary to involuntary muscle spasm associated with peritoneal irritation. The limbs should also be checked for muscle tenderness, which is suggestive of a generalized muscle disorder.

Physical Findings in the Elderly

The usual physical findings of acute peritoneal irritation may be absent in the elderly, especially at the outset. The only manifestations may be unexplained mild fever, tachycardia, reduction in bowel sounds, and vague abdominal discomfort without frank rebound or guarding. A high index of suspicion is required. Acute abdominal pain out of proportion to tenderness on physical examination in a person with known atherosclerotic disease should raise suspicion of vascular compromise.

Examining the Patient with Suspected Psychogenic Pain

Use of deep palpation while the patient is distracted can provide helpful evidence when psychogenically amplified pain or a major degree of psychocultural overlay is suspected. A lack of tenderness is characteristic. A widely used approach is to push down slowly, firmly, and deeply with a stethoscope, distracting the patient by appearing to auscultate. Such a maneuver should be performed only after more serious pathology has been ruled out by history and physical examination.

Laboratory Studies: Initial Office Testing for Serious Acute Etiologies

Relatively few laboratory tests are needed for an initial assessment in the office setting. Studies are aimed at determining the likelihood of obstruction, peritonitis, acute vascular insufficiency, metabolic abnormality, and cardiac or pulmonary disease.

Complete Blood Cell Count and Differential

Although very nonspecific, the complete blood cell count and differential are reasonably sensitive for confirming the presence of an acute inflammatory process. Unfortunately, the complete blood cell count may show little change in the elderly or chronically ill patient, even in an acute intraabdominal emergency. When there is concern about an inflammatory etiology, the differential should be ordered, even if the white cell count is "normal," particularly in the elderly, because a shift to immature forms sometimes occurs without a significant elevation in the white cell count. At times, a relatively benign condition such as viral gastroenteritis may produce an impressive elevation in the white cell count (as high as 20,000 cells/mL) accompanied by a marked shift to immature forms, which simulates the peripheral blood picture of a patient with more worrisome disease. The complete blood cell count and differential must be carefully interpreted in the context of the entire clinical picture and not used alone to decide whether to admit the patient.

Pregnancy Testing

Because of the seriousness of an ectopic pregnancy, every woman of reproductive age who presents with lower abdominal pain in the office setting should have pregnancy ruled out early in the assessment and usually before a radiologic study is performed. A *serum human chorionic gonadotropin β subunit* is the most sensitive test; kit-based urine testing is less sensitive (see Chapter 112).

Plain Films of the Abdomen

Supine and upright films are essential if one suspects bowel obstruction or perforation. *Multiple (i.e., three) air–fluid levels,* distention of the small bowel, and absence of gas in the large bowel are characteristic of complete small-bowel obstruction; however, such findings are present in fewer than 50% of cases of bowel strangulation, especially in the early stages of obstruction. *Partial mechanical obstruction* may produce some loops of bowel with air–fluid levels, but there is also gas in the colon; the same findings are found in patients with adynamic ileus. In colonic obstruction with a competent ileocecal valve, only the large bowel appears distended, but if the valve is not competent, both the large and small bowel demonstrate distention and gas, mimicking the findings of adynamic ileus. Distinguishing partial small-bowel obstruction from ileus requires repeated films or a barium study and correlation with the physical examination. Suspected obstruction of the large bowel is an indication for a barium enema or colonoscopy. On the plain film, *free air* under the diaphragm indicates perforation of a viscus; *absent psoas shadows* suggest retroperitoneal bleeding, abscess, or mass; and displaced stomach or bowel (determined by gas patterns) may be caused by compression from a tumor. Plain films detect *calcifications,* such as those representing a biliary or renal stone, abdominal aortic disease, or pancreatitis. Calcification of the aortic wall has been found on plain films of the abdomen in more than 60% of abdominal aneurysms; a cross-table lateral view best demonstrates the finding.

Plain films of the abdomen are commonly overinterpreted in evaluating abdominal pain. Limiting the study to patients who have moderate to severe tenderness or who are strongly suspected of having bowel obstruction, urinary tract calculi, trauma, ischemia, or gallbladder disease (regardless of degree of tenderness) can reduce use by more than 50% without compromising the detection of clinically important pathology. Plain films reveal little unsuspected pathology, especially in patients with mild tenderness on examination. Using plain films to "rule out" serious pathology is possible only with bowel obstruction and perforation, for which the sensitivity of the plain film approaches 100%. Its sensitivity for the detection of other conditions is much lower.

Urinalysis and Serum Chemistries

A *urine specimen* should be checked for pyuria, hematuria, bacteria, sugar, and ketones. Mild to moderate ketonuria is common when the patient has not eaten, and is unrelated to diabetes; the diagnosis of ketoacidosis requires urine ketones in large concentrations (see Chapter 102). Red cells in the urine of a patient with flank pain suggest a stone in the ureter (see Chapter 135).

The *blood urea nitrogen*, *glucose*, *electrolyte*, and *amylase* levels should be measured. Elevation of the serum amylase occurs not only in pancreatitis, but also in intestinal obstruction, perforated ulcer, and biliary tract disease (see Chapter 72). Although not especially specific, the serum amylase is sensitive. Serum electrolytes can be helpful in cases of vomiting, diarrhea, or adynamic ileus; tests of renal and liver function should also be performed and blood sugar determined when clinical findings are suggestive.

Chest Film and Electrocardiogram

The initial investigation of acute upper abdominal pain should also include a *chest film* and *electrocardiogram* to look for pleuropulmonary disease in the lower lobes and acute ischemic changes in the inferior myocardium. Moreover, an upright chest film often provides the best view of air under the diaphragm.

Testing for Familial Mediterranean Fever

Patients presenting with fever and peritoneal signs accompanied by oligoarthritis and/or pleuritis should be evaluated for familial Mediterranean fever, especially if they are of Sephardic, Turkish, Arabic, or Armenian descent and have a prior history of similar self-limited attacks dating to early adulthood and/or a positive family history. Use of a *DNA amplification assay* for rapid detection of the responsible *genetic mutation* is available at centers in areas where the condition is common. Detecting *C5a inhibitor deficiency* in serosal or synovial fluid is diagnostic but not practical.

Emergent Testing

Patients with evidence of acute obstruction, peritonitis, bowel ischemia, or worrisome metabolic or cardiopulmonary disease need emergency admission and testing.

Abdominal computed tomography (CT) with Gastrografin oral contrast is the test of choice in patients with suspected *diverticulitis*, especially if there is concern on clinical grounds for abscess formation. CT with intravenous contrast is indicated for suspected *dissecting aortic aneurysm*. When *appendicitis* is the concern, helical or multidetector *CT of the appendix* (with Gastrografin contrast) should be performed in the emergency department. CT maximizes diagnostic accuracy (95% to 98%) and, in doing so, shortens time to surgery for those with a positive test result and spares hospitalization and unnecessary surgery in persons with a negative result. The net impact is an improvement in outcomes and a reduction in costs.

Abdominal ultrasound examination of the biliary tree is the test of choice for suspected *acute cholecystitis* and *choledocholithiasis*. The test can also detect *aortic aneurysm*. Ultrasonographic examination of the kidneys is needed when *hydronephrosis* from urinary tract obstruction secondary to *ureterolithiasis* is suspected.

Laboratory Studies: Subsequent Outpatient Evaluation

The workup of patients without sufficient evidence of serious acute pathology necessitating immediate hospitalization can be continued on an outpatient basis. Any patient sent home with undiagnosed acute abdominal pain requires careful follow-up and reexamination because several serious etiologies (e.g., bowel ischemia, cholecystitis) may initially present with an indolent picture, particularly in the elderly.

Despite the abundance of available tests, a repeated history and physical examination remain among the most productive of diagnostic measures. Additional testing is most productive when directed at working hypotheses suggested by the clinical findings and initial testing. Test selection should be judicious and based on the need to confirm or rule out specific diagnoses. Blind searches that involve "running the bowel" in the absence of suggestive clinical evidence are not only wasteful but also potentially misleading and may subject the patient to unnecessary risk. Test selection can be considered in terms of pain location, as follows.

Epigastric Pain

Epigastric pain that parallels the acid–peptic cycle or responds to food or antacids suggests peptic ulcer disease. If the patient is younger than the age of 40 years and little clinical evidence for malignancy is present (e.g., no dysphagia, weight loss, melena, hematemesis), then *serologic testing* for *Helicobacter pylori* and symptomatic treatment for presumed acid-mediated disease (see Chapter 68) can be started without first documenting the lesion. However, failure to respond to a 4- to 8-week course of empiric therapy or the development of worrisome symptoms, especially in older patients (who are at increased risk for esophageal and gastric cancers), necessitates direct visualization with *esophagogastroduodenoscopy*, which provides an opportunity for biopsy if there is serious concern for gastric cancer.

Recurrent bouts of epigastric or right upper quadrant pain are an indication for *abdominal ultrasonography*, which is the test of choice for suspected cholecystitis (see Chapter 69) and useful for the detection of biliary and ureteral obstructions (see Chapters 62 and 135, respectively). It can help to identify ascites and aortic aneurysm and sometimes localize an intraabdominal abscess.

Recurrent postprandial symptoms in a person with known atherosclerotic disease or risk factors (especially smoking) raises the question of mesenteric ischemia. *Duplex scanning* (the combination of *Doppler* with *B-mode ultrasonography*) can provide a sensitive (87% to 96%), noninvasive approach to initial assessment of celiac and superior mesenteric blood flow in thin persons, but the increasing prevalence of obesity, overlying bowel gas, and need for a skilled operator make the test less practical as an initial screening test in everyday clinical practice. *CT angiography* or *magnetic resonance angiography* should be considered as alternatives; renal function needs to be taken into account because of the dye load required.

Periumbilical Pain

Periumbilical pain is not a very discriminating symptom, but it suggests small-bowel pathology, which can be assessed by an *upper gastrointestinal series* with *small-bowel follow-through* or *video capsule* study. A lymphoma or carcinoid tumor may cause an intermittent partial obstruction. Postprandial periumbilical pain in a person with atherosclerotic risk factors raises the question of mesenteric ischemia, which can be explored noninvasively by *CT* or *magnetic resonance angiography* (see prior discussion). Bloating, diarrhea, and iron deficiency may be manifestations of sprue, best screened for with serum determinations of IgA *antibodies to endomesium and transglutaminase*.

Lower Abdominal Pain

All patients with lower abdominal pain accompanied by signs of rectal bleeding (either gross or occult) should be evaluated by *colonoscopy* or the combination of *barium enema* and *sigmoidoscopy* to identify the source (see Chapter 63). However, a young patient (<40 years) with constipation, obvious hemorrhoidal bleeding, and no risk factors for colorectal cancer need undergo only a sigmoidoscopy to rule out associated rectosigmoid pathology, such as that of inflammatory bowel disease. Sigmoidoscopy is ideal for the assessment of suspected rectosigmoid masses or mucosal abnormalities. A full colonoscopy is needed when the source of lower gastrointestinal bleeding is unknown, as in cases of hematochezia or positive fecal occult blood testing. Barium enema or computed colonography are reasonable alternatives to colonoscopy for investigating the cause of pain. Endoscopic study makes possible not only direct visualization, but also biopsy of suspected lesions, polypectomy, and an assessment of the extent of disease in patients with inflammatory bowel disease.

Patients with lower abdominal pain in the absence of bleeding, weight loss, or a change in bowel habits are less likely to benefit from radiologic or endoscopic evaluation unless their symptoms are particularly severe or chronic. Likely etiologies include diverticulosis and mild diverticulitis, the former associated with functional motility disorders and cramping pain and the later causing episodes of pain that are more constant and associated with signs of localized peritoneal irritation.

At times, the patient insists on having a study for reassurance purposes. This is particularly common among women who have been alerted to the possibility of ovarian cancer presenting initially as vague abdominal symptoms (e.g., bloating, increased abdominal girth; see earlier discussion). A *transvaginal pelvic ultrasound* may be worth considering, especially when symptoms are new in onset, frequent, and accompanied by urinary and pelvic complaints. The contribution of a normal test result to the patient's peace of mind has to be taken into account in any decision regarding whether to test. Carrying out age-appropriate screening for colorectal cancer (see Chapter 56) helps to provide appropriate reassurance without excessive testing.

Flank and Adnexal Pains

The patient with flank pain, hematuria, or pyuria may have a renal source of abdominal pain. *Renal ultrasonography* can reveal a stone, tumor, or ureteral dilation. *Abdominal CT* with renal protocol has largely replaced *intravenous pyelogram* in detecting disease in the kidneys or ureters or displacement of a ureter by an abdominal or retroperitoneal mass. *Transvaginal pelvic ultrasonography* is indicated when the patient with adnexal pain has tenderness or a mass noted on bimanual examination or has concurrent abdominal bloating and increased abdominal girth.

Suspected Pancreatic Cancer

The sensitivity and specificity of *multidetector abdominal CT* for the detection of pancreatic cancer now exceeds that of *transabdominal ultrasonography*, and the frequency of indeterminate readings is lower (e.g., 4% vs. 23%). CT is less dependent on the skill of the operator, but it is more expensive and involves radiation exposure, a particularly important consideration in children. In addition to imaging the pancreas, it provides excellent views of the liver, retroperitoneum, and spine. Both ultrasonography and CT visualize the common bile duct, portal vein, and hepatic artery and detect any displacement, encroach-

ment, or encasement of the major intraabdominal vessels and organs; diagnostic yield can be greatly enhanced by adding *needle biopsy* of any suspected lesion.

Endoscopic ultrasound is even more sensitive and more specific for detecting pancreatic cancer than multidetector CT, with endoscopic ultrasound having a sensitivity of 98%, compared to 86% for multidetector CT; however, success is very dependent on the skill of the endoscopist. If a mass is found, needle aspiration biopsy is usually needed to confirm a diagnosis of malignancy. Although much progress has been made in identifying pancreatic masses in symptomatic patients, early detection in the asymptomatic period remains an elusive goal.

Testing for Lead Poisoning and Porphyria

The patient with acute colicky pain but no signs of obstruction or inflammation may have lead poisoning and should have urine samples checked for *coproporphyrin*. Serum lead levels are unreliable. The person with acute intermittent porphyria may also present with colicky pain. Often, such persons are believed to be psychiatrically disturbed because of abnormal behavior during an attack. The diagnosis is suggested by periodic attacks of cramping pain, constipation, nausea and vomiting, and neuromuscular symptoms in conjunction with the altered psychological state. The *Watson–Schwartz test* for *urinary porphobilinogen* is a reliable screening test for acute intermittent porphyria in patients who are symptomatic.

Suspected Functional Disease

The diagnosis of functional bowel disease is a clinical one, facilitated by careful attention to the history and the physical examination. In the absence of history or physical examination evidence (e.g., significant weight loss, positive stool test for occult blood or iron-deficiency anemia) suggesting a more serious medical condition, the initial diagnostic evaluation can be relatively limited.

Irritable Bowel Syndrome. Because of the considerable overlap between the symptoms of this disease and those of inflammatory bowel disease in younger persons and colorectal cancer in older patients, the most useful test is *flexible sigmoidoscopy* or *colonoscopy*, depending on the patient's age and clinical presentation. The routine ordering of chemistry profiles, thyroid indices, urinalyses, and tests for ova and parasites appears to add little to the assessment or to decision making.

Before settling on a diagnosis of irritable bowel disease, final consideration of other mimicking conditions is indicated. New onset of persistent bloating and abdominal distention in a woman with other vague pelvic or urinary symptoms raises the question of *ovarian cancer* and the need for *transvaginal ultrasound*. Similarly, screening for *adult celiac disease* by obtaining serum for *antiendomesial* and *antitransglutaminase antibodies* (see Chapter 64) should also be considered, especially if there is concurrent diarrhea and iron deficiency or a positive family history of sprue.

Functional Dyspepsia. An empiric trial of treatment for peptic ulcer disease or gastroesophageal reflux disease is one approach. Another is to consider *serologic testing* for *H. pylori* infection, which is etiologic in peptic ulcer disease but not associated with functional dyspepsia. The decision to order upper gastrointestinal endoscopy is more difficult. The rationale is early detection of gastroesophageal malignancy. Because of the expense, discomfort, and potential morbidity associated with the procedure and a lack of evidence for any significant alteration in outcomes, early upper gastrointestinal endoscopy cannot be recommended in persons with little clinical or epidemiologic evidence of risk for malignancy. Suggested criteria for its use include onset of symptoms after the age of 40 years, especially in persons whose symptoms persist without remission for longer than 8 weeks.

Evaluation of Undiagnosed Abdominal Pain

A most vexing problem arises when the cause of abdominal pain remains undetermined despite a careful initial medical evaluation. There may be pressure from patient and family to look still harder for a serious cause and a tendency, from frustration, to order progressively more invasive studies in search of such an etiology. Certainly, further anatomic study is indicated in patients with a strongly positive family history of bowel malignancy (see Chapter 56), significant weight loss, presence of a mass, unexplained iron-deficiency anemia, or a stool test that is positive for occult blood. However, the cause of undiagnosed abdominal pain is often an underlying psychological disturbance or sometimes a condition that can mimic it (e.g., lead poisoning or porphyria) and requires positive identification to facilitate treatment. At other times, no cause can be uncovered, and a plan for observation and follow-up is required.

Identification of Contributory Psychopathology

Abnormal illness behaviors characterize patients with psychosocial problems that present as a bodily complaint such as abdominal pain (see Chapter 230). Such behaviors include an exaggerated presentation with disability out of proportion to the degree of detectable disease, chronic complaints that defy precise diagnosis, persistent attempts to validate suffering, excessive dependence on the physician and others for care, avoidance of health-promoting behaviors, and attempts to maintain the sick role.

Include a history of *multiple bodily complaints*, a *chronic nonprogressive* clinical course that may span many years, *lack of relation* between symptoms and physiologic stimuli, inconsistent or *distractible* physical findings, and presence of the *somatic symptoms of depression* (e.g., early-morning awakening, fatigue, decreased libido, altered appetite). Such behaviors and presentations of pain divert attention from the patient's psychosocial suffering and root causes unless they are recognized, understood, and responded to appropriately (see Chapters 226, 227, and 230). In the absence of worrisome objective findings, one can avoid exhaustive testing of these patients and concentrate more on their underlying psychosocial problems.

Eliciting the Patient's Perspective

Of particular importance is eliciting the patient's concerns, beliefs, and expectations. Responding to them directly during the initial history and physical examination can help to direct the evaluation (often obviating unnecessary testing) and provide meaningful reassurance. Also pertinent are the patient's daily functioning at work and at home, social supports, and psychological state. If elicited early, these elements can speed recognition of psychosocial distress. The abdominal pain may be only a symptom of psychosocial suffering. Although the patient, family, or friends may be pressing for a medical diagnosis, the real need is for care rather than a diagnostic label. The risk of a missed anatomic diagnosis is less than 3% when the initial evaluation findings are normal and evidence of abnormal illness behavior and clinical features of psychological disturbance are present.

Patients with a clinical picture suggestive of functional disease may also benefit from inquiry into psychosocial issues, such as concurrent stresses, losses, and the effect of the pain on the patient's life and daily activities. However, a suggestion at the outset that the problem is probably psychogenic is inaccurate (about half of patients with functional disease have no etiologic psychopathology), and it also invites resistance and hostility if proclaimed before a careful evaluation is completed.

Avoiding an Adversarial Stance

Care must be taken neither to deny the reality of the patient's pain and suffering nor to emphasize the psychosocial nature of the problem any more than the patient is willing to accept. A detailed and pertinent history and physical examination that address patient concerns along with simple screening laboratory tests should suffice. Any requests for aggressive testing can be postponed as long as a plan for careful longitudinal follow-up is in place and available data show no evidence for dangerous underlying pathology. A caring response and an open-minded attitude help to forge a working partnership and avoid triggering an adversarial relationship. In patients with neurotic complaints presenting with irritable bowel syndrome, thorough reassurance that specifically addresses patient concerns can be most effective, especially when delivered in a sympathetic and respectful fashion.

Observation and Follow-Up

When the diagnosis remains unclear, close follow-up is essential.

Acute Pain. If urgent admission does not seem warranted, close follow-up is mandatory. Repeated histories and examinations may yield additional information and lead to the diagnosis and proper treatment. Such factors as the degree of distress manifested by the patient, any elevation in temperature or white blood cell count, other laboratory abnormalities, and the ability of the patient to eat and drink all need to be reassessed. Judgment also must be made as to whether a patient with undiagnosed abdominal pain should undergo more invasive testing. In general, patients with unexplained abdominal pain in conjunction with recurrent nausea and vomiting, jaundice, fever, weight loss of more than 10% of body weight, or blood in the stool require more extensive evaluation.

Chronic Pain. The patient with chronic or recurrent abdominal pain that defies explanation poses one of the most difficult problems in clinical medicine. In a study of 64 patients with abdominal pain of unknown etiology despite extensive assessment, the younger the age and the shorter the duration of the symptoms, the better were the chances for improvement. Older women with pain for more than 3 months were least likely to improve or be given a diagnosis. Of those subjected to *exploratory laparotomy*, a diagnosis was obtained in only 10%; the rate of improvement was the same as for those who did not undergo exploration. In 15% of the total study population, a cause for the patient's abdominal pain was found, but in only 6% did the condition require surgery. Thus, very few patients with abdominal pain of unknown etiology are endangered by continued observation, as long as signs of serious pathophysiology are absent. The morbidity of exploratory laparotomy in such patients greatly exceeds the benefit. Unexplained pain that is present for less than 2 weeks is likely to resolve spontaneously, but such improvement is unlikely when pain has persisted for more than 3 months.

Clinically Silent Abdominal Aortic Aneurysm. Patients with a clinically silent abdominal aortic aneurysm found

Chapter 58: Evaluation of Abdominal Pain   **477**

serendipitously during workup for abdominal pain require close attention and follow-up. Those with aneurysm diameters of less than 5.0 cm are at little risk for rupture and can be followed expectantly; however, careful monitoring of aneurysm diameter is essential, as is achievement of smoking cessation. Obtaining an *abdominal ultrasound* at 6-month intervals provides a convenient noninvasive approach to monitoring. Referral for consideration of elective interventional repair (endovascular vs. conventional) is indicated once diameter exceeds 5.0 to 5.5 cm. Choice of therapy depends on overall clinical assessment; surgery carries a substantial perioperative risk, but survival rates at 2 years are comparable.

INDICATIONS FOR ADMISSION AND REFERRAL

Admission

Any evidence suggestive of peritoneal irritation, obstruction, or acute vascular compromise is an indication for immediate hospitalization and surgical consultation. Sometimes, further observations made in the hospital can save the patient a surgical procedure, but no patient with the possibility of a condition that might require urgent surgery should be sent home from the office. Elderly patients are especially prone to subtle presentations. The patient with unexplained pain that has defied outpatient diagnostic attempts may benefit from further assessment in the hospital, especially if a need for large amounts of pain medication has developed. Admission provides an opportunity for 24-hour observation, specialty consultation, and assessment of the need for further study.

Referral

Consideration of invasive study is an indication for consultation with the gastroenterologist or surgeon before plans are made to proceed. Conversely, the internist can feel comfortable following the patient who appears well and has an otherwise normal history, physical examination findings, and screening laboratory results. For the overly anxious patient, a session with the gastroenterologist to talk over concerns and review the workup to date can be useful and may obviate need for further testing. Psychiatric consultation is indicated for patients with evidence of serious depression (see Chapter 227) or excessive somatization (see Chapter 230).

SYMPTOMATIC THERAPY
(12,16,21,32–36)

Symptomatic relief may be a high priority in some instances, even before a definitive diagnosis is achieved. Analgesics and therapeutic trials are the principal means used, but selective use is essential to ensure patient safety. Behavioral methods can be useful in persons with suspected psychopathology whose symptoms appear refractory.

Analgesics

In the Setting of Acute Pain

Although analgesics (particularly opiates) have traditionally been considered inappropriate for most patients with acute abdominal pain of unknown etiology (out of concern that important diagnostic findings may be obscured), their compassionate use is undergoing reconsideration. In patients with terminal cancer, the use of narcotics must not be denied, even if the cause of abdominal pain is not fully defined (see Chapter 90). Opiate use in other acute abdominal pain settings has been found potentially to blunt physical findings such as guarding but not substantially to alter clinical decision making so as to cause errors in management.

In the Setting of Chronic Pain

Patients with undiagnosed chronic pain who request pain medication represent the opposite situation. Many such patients have underlying psychopathology and a strong potential for narcotic abuse. Narcotic analgesics are to be avoided in such instances, even if the request is for "just a few pills."

Therapeutic Trials

Thoughtfully applied empiric therapy can provide relief as well as diagnostically useful information.

Suspected Peptic Ulcer Disease

Patients with suspected peptic ulcer disease and no evidence of malignancy are reasonable candidates for a 4-week course of *antacids*, *histamine$_2$ blockers*, or *proton pump inhibitors* (see Chapter 68); they may begin to feel better within days. The use of empiric antibiotics for *H. pylori* infection to relieve symptoms empirically is not cost-effective and exposes many patients to unnecessary antibiotic therapy because many of these patients actually have functional dyspepsia (which is unrelated to *H. pylori* infection) rather than true peptic ulcer disease.

Suspected Irritable Bowel Syndrome (see also Chapter 74)

Patients with probable *irritable bowel syndrome* can be tried on a *high-fiber* program, such as a tablespoon of psyllium in 8 oz of water two to three times daily (psyllium is preferred to high-fiber cereal because of the need for milk intake with the latter and the associated risk for lactose intolerance in susceptible persons, which can simulate irritable bowel syndrome and confuse the diagnosis; see Chapter 64). As noted earlier, a trial of *antidepressant therapy* (with an agent low in anticholinergic activity) may be useful.

Patients with refractory functional disease linked to underlying psychosocial distress are among the hardest to help, especially when illness behavior is greatly distorted. Although formal psychiatric care may be necessary, simple behavioral methods that can be initiated by the primary physician can help to modify illness behavior. One is to provide the patient with techniques to increase control over the illness. Useful approaches include *participating* in treatment decisions, learning *relaxation* techniques, and beginning an *exercise* program. Even keeping a *symptom diary* can help to provide a sense of control.

Equally important for such patients is the reinforcement of positive behaviors and removal of rewards for symptoms. Follow-up should be scheduled at regular intervals rather than as needed for symptoms. However, *setting limits* to time and availability is appropriate, with no more than 20 minutes necessary for a visit and unscheduled visits discouraged. During the visit, the focus should be on *accomplishments* ("What have you been able to do?") rather than on symptoms ("How do you feel?"). Reports of accomplishments are best received with positive reinforcement and requests for elaboration, whereas complaints of suffering and symptoms should be accorded a neutral stance and no request for elaboration unless worrisome new symptoms are reported. Setting *realistic treatment goals* is critical, with emphasis on improving quality of life and not on removing symptoms. Cognitive-behavioral therapy may be helpful (see Chapter 74).

Annotated Bibliography

1. Anuras S, Shirazi S. Chronic pseudoobstruction. Am J Gastroenterol 1984;79:525. (*The syndromes of acute and chronic colonic pseudoobstruction are differentiated; 99 references.*)
2. Brandt LJ, Boley SJ. AGA technical review on intestinal ischemia. American Gastrointestinal Association. Gastroenterology 2000;118:954. (*Authoritative review.*)
3. Bytzer P, Talley NJ. Dyspepsia. Ann Intern Med 2001;134:822. (*A clinical review for a general audience.*)
4. Goff BA, Mandel LS, Melancon CH, et al. Frequency of symptoms of ovarian cancer in women presenting to primary care clinics. JAMA 2004;291:2705. (*Large-scale case–control study; finds that the recent onset or increased frequency of bloating, abdominal distention, or pelvic pain is more likely to be associated with ovarian masses.*)
5. Jorgensen T. Abdominal symptoms and gallstone disease: an epidemiological investigation. Hepatology 1989;9:856. (*No symptoms identifiable as predictive of gallstones were found in this Danish population study.*)
6. Moawad J, Gewertz BL. Chronic mesenteric ischemia: clinical presentation and diagnosis. Surg Clin North Am 1997:77:357. (*Useful, succinct review; 35 references.*)
7. Lederle FA, Simel DL. Does this patient have abdominal aortic aneurysm? JAMA 1999;281:77. (*A systematic review to determine the sensitivity, specificity, and positive predictive value of abdominal palpation, the maneuver of choice for detection by physical examination.*)
8. Paulson EK, Kalady MF, Pappas TN. Suspected appendicitis. N Engl J Med 2003;348:236. (*Excellent clinical review; 53 references.*)
9. Powell JT, Greenhalgh RM. Small abdominal aortic aneurysms. N Engl J Med 2003;348:1895. (*A review that addresses natural history and management; 48 references.*)
10. Shatila AH, Chamberlain BE, Webb WR, et al. Current status of diagnosis and management of strangulation obstruction of the small bowel. Am J Surg 1976;132:299. (*Still useful for its comparison of presentations of simple obstruction and strangulation; clinical differentiation is often not reliable.*)
11. Silen W. Cope's early diagnosis of the acute abdomen, 18th ed. Oxford: Oxford University Press, 1991. (*Classic text; concise, systematic approach to the diagnosis of acute abdominal problems; emphasis is on history and physical findings; required reading for the primary physician.*)
12. Arrents NLA, Thijs JC, van Zwet AA, et al. Approach to the treatment of dyspepsia in primary care: a randomized trial comparing "test-and-treat" with prompt endoscopy. Arch Intern Med 2003;163:1606. (*The test-and-treat approach is as effective and safe as prompt endoscopy, with fewer endoscopies required.*)
13. Derlet RW, Kinser D, Ray L, et al. Prospective identification and triage of nonemergency patients out of an emergency department: a 5-year study. Ann Emerg Med 1995;25:215. (*Rapid identification of less dangerous causes of abdominal pain.*)
14. Dewitt J, Devereaux B, Chriswell M, et al. Comparison of endoscopic ultrasonography and multidetector computed tomography for detecting and staging pancreatic cancer. Ann Intern Med 2004;141:753. (*Endoscopic ultrasound proved to be superior.*)
15. Donaldson RM, Joyce CM, Feinstein AR. Effect of restraints on diagnostic approaches to abdominal pain and weight loss. Am J Med 1986;81:641. (*A provocative study examining test utilization when quests for economy and "team" approaches to ordering tests are initiated.*)
16. Drossman DA. Diagnosing and treating patients with refractory functional gastrointestinal disorders. Ann Intern Med 1995;123:688. (*Includes an excellent and detailed discussion of approaches to the diagnosis of irritable bowel syndrome.*)
17. Eisenberg RL, Heineken P, Hedgcock MW, et al. Evaluation of plain abdominal radiographs in the diagnosis of abdominal pain. Ann Intern Med 1982;97:257. (*Effort to develop criteria for ordering abdominal films in patients with abdominal pain.*)
18. Eisenberg S, Aksentijevich I, Deng Z, et al. Diagnosis of familial Mediterranean fever by molecular genetics methods. Ann Intern Med 1998;129:539. (*Evidence supporting a DNA amplification method for rapid, cost-effective, accurate diagnosis.*)
19. Hadithi M, von Blomberg BME, Crusius JBA, et al. Accuracy of serologic tests and HLA-DQ typing for diagnosing celiac disease. Ann Intern Med 2007;147:294. (*Testing for immunoglobulin A antibodies to tissue transglutaminase and endomesium had the highest sensitivity and specificity.*)
20. Lederle FA. Ultrasonographic screening for abdominal aortic aneurysms. Ann Intern Med 2003;139:516. (*Systematic review; recommends one-timing screening for older male smokers; 73 references.*)
21. Lederle FA, Wilson SE, Johnson GR, et al. Immediate repair compared with surveillance of small abdominal aortic aneurysms. N Engl J Med 2002;346:1437. (*Veterans Administration Cooperative Study; 569 men with aneurysms of <5.5 cm were randomized to immediate repair vs. surveillance; death rates were similar in both groups, as were survival trends and death from aneurysm rupture.*)
22. Moneta GL, Lee RW, Yeager RA, et al. Mesenteric duplex scanning: a blinded prospective study. J Vasc Surg 1993;17:79. (*Sensitivity study of the detection of significant celiac and superior mesenteric artery disease; values ranged from 87% to 96%.*)
23. Rao PM, Rhea JT, Novelline RA, et al. Effect of computed tomography of the appendix on treatment of patients and use of hospital resources. N Engl J Med 1998;338:141. (*Computed tomography findings resulted in a change in management in 58% of cases and reduced rates of unnecessary surgery and hospital days and saved $447 per patient.*)
24. Richter JM, Christensen MR, Simeone JH, et al. Chronic cholecystitis: an analysis of diagnostic strategies. Invest Radiol 1987;22:111. (*Analysis of the clinical utility of ultrasonography and other studies in the evaluation of abdominal pain.*)
25. Sarfeh IJ. Abdominal pain of unknown etiology. Am J Surg 1976;132:22. (*An old but still informative study; spontaneous improvement was most likely in younger patients with symptoms of <2 weeks' duration; laparotomy did not influence the rate of improvement; it established the diagnosis in only 1 of 23 patients explored.*)
26. Shih MC, Hagspiel KD. CTA and MRA in mesenteric ischemia: part 1, Role in diagnosis and differential diagnosis. Am J Roentgenol 2007;188:452. (*Evidence for the use of computed tomography and magnetic resonance angiography for the noninvasive diagnosis of intestinal ischemia.*)
27. Stefansson T, Nyman R, Nilsson S, et al. Diverticulitis of the sigmoid colon: a comparison of CT, colonic enema, and laparoscopy. Acta Radiol 1997;38:313. (*Prospective study finding that computed tomography was best for detection, especially if abscess is suspected.*)
28. Teraswa T, Blackmore CC, Bent S, et al. Systematic review: computer tomography and ultrasonography to detect acute appendicitis in adults and adolescents. Ann Intern Med 2004;141:537. (*Computed tomography was found to be more the accurate test.*)
29. Tolliver BA, Herrera JL, DiPalma JA. Evaluation of patients who meet clinical criteria for irritable bowel syndrome. Am J Gastroenterol 1994;89:176. (*Prospective study of 196 patients with clinically suspected disease to determine the yield of a wide range of tests.*)
30. Trowbridge RL, Rutowski NK, Shojania KG. Does this patient have acute cholecystitis? JAMA 2003;289:80. (*An attempt to identify those elements that have greatest diagnostic utility.*)
31. The United Kingdom Small Aneurysm Trial Participants. Long-term outcomes of immediate repair compared with surveillance of small abdominal aortic aneurysms. N Engl J Med 2002;346:1445. (*Randomized trial; no difference was found in mean survival, although a late survival benefit was associated with smoking cessation.*)
32. Allison JE, Hurley LB, Hiatt RA, et al. A randomized controlled trial of test-and-treat strategy for *Helicobacter pylori*. Arch Intern Med 2003;163:1165. (*Open-label, randomized, controlled trial in a managed care setting in persons taking long-term acid suppression therapy for presumed peptic ulcer disease.*)
33. Blankensteijn JD, de Jong S, Prinssen M, et al. Two-year outcomes after conventional or endovascular repair of abdominal aortic aneurysms. N Engl J Med 2005;352:2398. (*Randomized, controlled trial; survival at 2 years was the same; the perioperative survival advantage with endovascular repair was not sustained after the first year.*)
34. Calvert EL, Houghton LA, Cooper P, et al. Long-term improvement in functional dyspepsia using hypnotherapy. Gastroenterology 2002;123:1778. (*Hypnotherapy was highly effective in a prospective randomized trial, improving symptoms and costs.*)
35. Ranji SR, Goldman LE, Simel DL, et al. Do opiates affect the clinical evaluation of patients with acute abdominal pain. JAMA 2006;296:1764. (*A literature review finding that although some physical findings may be blunted, no significant increase in management errors was found.*)
36. Soll AH. Medical treatment of peptic ulcer disease. JAMA 1996;275:622. (*American College of Gastroenterology guidelines for the treatment of peptic ulcer.*)

CHAPTER 59 ■ EVALUATION OF NAUSEA AND VOMITING

Nausea and vomiting are extremely common presenting complaints; in one study of primary care practice they ranked second only to symptoms of upper respiratory tract infection. Although in most instances the symptoms are caused by self-limited disease, they may be a manifestation of a more serious underlying illness. The primary care physician needs to recognize the more worrisome causes of nausea and vomiting, provide relief from these debilitating symptoms, and correct any important fluid and electrolyte disturbances.

PATHOPHYSIOLOGY AND CLINICAL PRESENTATION (1–8)

Mechanisms

Two major central nervous system centers are involved in the vomiting reflex—the vomiting center and the chemoreceptor trigger zone. Irritation of vagal and sympathetic afferents in the pharynx, heart, peritoneum, mesentery, bile ducts, stomach, and bowel triggers impulses to the vomiting center in the medullary reticular formation. Gastric irritation, the distention of a hollow viscus, myocardial ischemia, increased intracranial pressure, metabolic disturbances, drugs, pharyngeal stimulation, and emotional upset are important noxious stimuli that act through this pathway. Vestibular disturbances, centrally acting drugs, and metabolic derangements stimulate the chemoreceptor trigger zone in the floor of the fourth ventricle, which in turn activates the vomiting center. A cortical pathway to the vomiting center has been postulated to account for some forms of psychogenic vomiting. Neurotransmitters serotonin, histamine, and substance P (neurokinin-1) play important roles in mediating emesis. In chemotherapy-induced disease, blocking of the 5-HT$_3$ serotonin and substance P receptors can prevent both immediate and delayed emesis (see later discussion).

Clinical Presentations

The act of vomiting is a stereotyped response that varies little regardless of cause. Even so-called *projectile vomiting* (which is characterized by forceful emesis without prior nausea or retching), which is supposedly limited to cases of increased intracranial pressure, occurs in other conditions. Moreover, nausea, retching, and nonprojectile vomiting are seen with increased intracranial pressure.

Nausea and vomiting may be only one part of a symptom complex or may dominate the clinical picture (as in psychogenic vomiting, early pregnancy, digitalis toxicity, and metabolic disturbances). Considerable overlap exists among presentations. With some causes of nausea and vomiting, symptoms are more likely to occur independent of meals, whereas in others, they are characteristically associated with food intake.

Metabolic Etiologies

Early-morning nausea and vomiting are typical of *metabolic causes*. Up to 75% of cases of diabetic ketoacidosis are accompanied by nausea and vomiting. Emesis and nausea are found among as many as 90% of patients in addisonian crisis. Uremia may be heralded by similar symptoms; nausea often improves with the correction of any associated hyponatremia, but it can be refractory. *Binge drinkers* experience early-morning nausea and dry heaves from excessive alcohol intake.

Early Pregnancy

Early-morning nausea and vomiting are characteristic of early pregnancy, occurring in more than 50% of instances. The problem is severe in fewer than 1% of cases but can lead to electrolyte abnormalities, dehydration, and weight loss. Most cases are mild; symptoms begin after the first missed period and terminate by the fourth month. Women with severe cases often have a history of vomiting in response to psychosocial stress. Disturbed motility is also noted in many cases. The diagnosis of pregnancy is sometimes overlooked.

Psychogenic Disease

In contrast to the causes of early-morning vomiting, conditions such as psychoneurotic illness, acid or bile reflux, peptic ulcer disease, and gastritis can trigger symptoms soon after food is ingested. Psychogenic vomiting is characterized by years of recurrent emesis. It can often be traced back to childhood and is more common when a family history of vomiting is present. Patients report that symptoms appear just after the intake of food and can be sufficiently controlled voluntarily to avoid vomiting in public. Some patients admit to inducing emesis; most are surprisingly untroubled by the problem. Nausea accompanies almost all episodes. A study of 20 patients with psychogenic vomiting revealed a marked predominance of women engaged in hostile relationships; abdominal pain and depression were uncommon. *Bulimia* is a form of psychogenic emesis in which vomiting is self-induced, often after a period of binge eating. A preoccupation with being thin and a poor self-image in a young woman are characteristic. Laxative abuse frequently complicates the clinical picture (see Chapter 234).

Peptic Ulcer Disease and Gastritis

A pyloric channel ulcer or acute gastritis may be associated with marked postprandial emesis. The vomiting in ulcer disease is believed to be in part a consequence of irritation, edema, and spasm of the pyloric sphincter mechanism. Concurrent bleeding can lead to vomiting of "coffee grounds." Patients who undergo surgery for peptic ulcer may be troubled by recurrent *bilious vomiting*, which is believed to be caused by reflux of bile into the stomach or gastric remnant. Patients vomit bile within 15 minutes of eating; little food is present. Nausea and a bad taste in the mouth are present on awakening in the morning.

Gastric Retention

Gastric retention results in vomiting of food eaten more than 6 hours previously. A succussion splash is detectable on examination, and food is seen in the stomach on upper gastrointestinal series. In chronic cases, gastric outflow obstruction or atony may be secondary to diabetic neuropathy, anticholinergic use, or gastric malignancy. Transient gastric dilation is a frequent concomitant of pancreatitis, peritonitis, gallbladder disease, and hypokalemia. A *cyclic idiopathic* form of nausea and vomiting has been described with gastric hypomotility demonstrated.

Gastroesophageal Reflux Disease

Gastroesophageal reflux disease usually does not present with nausea as the predominant symptom (see Chapter 61), but a subset of patients with otherwise unexplained intractable nausea may suffer from reflux. Treatment of their reflux results in resolution of the nausea.

Acute Gastroenteritis

Acute episodes of vomiting accompany a host of conditions, which range from the self-limited to life threatening. The most common is *viral gastroenteritis*. After many years of attributing this illness to viral infection, investigators have finally isolated and identified the responsible viruses. Explosive bouts of nausea and vomiting in conjunction with watery diarrhea, cramping abdominal pain, myalgias, headache, and fever are typical. Recovery is rapid in most instances, but symptoms may linger for 7 to 10 days. Similarly, anorexia, nausea, and vomiting often dominate the prodromal stage of *acute viral hepatitis* (see Chapter 70).

Acute gastroenteritis that results from *food poisoning* secondary to *Salmonella* or *Shigella* infection has a similar clinical presentation and course; onset is 24 to 48 hours after exposure to the contaminated food. Domestic fowl and their eggs represent the largest single reservoir of *Salmonella* infection. Inadequate cooking is often responsible for human infection. Intake of pastries and similar items containing *staphylococcal enterotoxin* causes symptoms indistinguishable from those of viral gastroenteritis, except that onset is within 1 to 6 hours after ingestion of the spoiled food, fever is rare, and complete clearing takes place by 24 to 48 hours. *Clostridial* food poisoning rarely produces prominent nausea and vomiting.

Cholera

Persons who travel to an epidemic area are at risk for contracting *cholera*, especially if they have eaten raw or undercooked seafood or have had drinks chilled with contaminated ice. South America is the latest area to experience an epidemic. High U.S. sanitary standards for the handling of sewage, water, and food have so far prevented outbreaks from spreading to this country. The causative organism is a toxigenic strain of *Vibrio cholerae*, which elaborates an enterotoxin that induces the secretion of water and electrolytes from the intestinal mucosa. Mild infection is characterized by a nonspecific diarrheal illness. In 3% to 5% of cases, the disease is much more severe (*cholera gravis*) and presents as profuse, watery diarrhea with flecks of whitish mucus ("rice water stools"), vomiting, and

dehydration. Vomiting is exacerbated by the acidosis that results from bowel bicarbonate loss. Circulatory collapse, altered consciousness, renal failure, and death are possible outcomes.

Peritoneal Irritation and Acute Obstruction

Peritoneal irritation and acute obstruction may precipitate acute emesis, usually in the context of severe abdominal pain (see Chapter 58). *Intestinal obstruction*, especially of the proximal small bowel, produces marked nausea and vomiting of bilious material. Distention may be lacking, but intermittent cramping abdominal pain is characteristic. Feculent emesis is found in distal small-bowel obstruction. In *acute pancreatitis*, emesis is seen in 85% of patients; however, upper abdominal pain radiating into the back is the cardinal symptom, occurring in 95% of patients (see Chapter 72). Anorexia, nausea, and vomiting are early symptoms in more than 90% of patients with *acute appendicitis*; usually emesis clears early. As with pancreatitis, pain typically precedes other symptoms. *Acute pyelonephritis* may mimic a gastrointestinal etiology by causing nausea, vomiting, and abdominal pain. *Acute cholecystitis* sometimes triggers acute emesis, but it does so less regularly than does *acute cholangitis* resulting from sudden obstruction of the common duct.

Myocardial Infarction

Myocardial infarction may activate vagal afferents and produce nausea, vomiting, and epigastric discomfort, simulating intraabdominal disease. A prospective series of 62 patients with acute infarction revealed nausea and vomiting at the outset in 69% of those with inferior infarctions and 27% of those with anterior infarctions.

Neurologic Emergencies

Neurologic emergencies can provoke severe bouts of acute emesis. In *midline cerebellar hemorrhage*, nausea and vomiting are profuse, in association with severe gait ataxia; meningeal signs and headache are also seen. Within a few hours, the patient may become comatose and die unless the condition is promptly diagnosed and treated (see Chapter 165). One third of patients with *increased intracranial pressure* experience vomiting. When it is sudden, forceful, and not preceded by nausea, it is described as *projectile*, but this presentation is not specific. Concurrent bilateral frontal or occipital headache is the rule. *Migraine headaches* and *vestibular disease* are less worrisome neurologic causes of acute emesis (see Chapters 165 and 166). The former is suggested by photophobia and throbbing unilateral headache, the latter by vertigo.

Drugs

Of the many causes of drug-induced vomiting, *digitalis intoxication* is among the most serious. Anorexia is an early sign, followed by nausea and vomiting resulting from stimulation of the chemoreceptor trigger zone. Visual disturbances, such as seeing colored halos, are suggestive of the diagnosis (see Chapter 32). Hypokalemia and dehydration induced by vomiting may precipitate or worsen digitalis toxicity.

Cancer Chemotherapies and Radiation Therapy

Cancer chemotherapies and radiation therapy produce substantial nausea and vomiting, with cisplatin being among the most problematic of chemotherapy agents. The mechanism of nausea and vomiting is believed to involve drug-induced release of serotonin from enterochromaffin cells, which leads to the activation of serotonin receptors on visceral afferent fibers and the stimulation of the vomiting center and chemoreceptor trigger zone. Drugs that block such serotonin and substance P receptors have proved to be uniquely effective (see later discussion and Chapter 90).

Drug Withdrawal and Substance Abuse

Drug withdrawal and substance abuse may trigger emesis. Nausea, dry heaves, and retching beginning at about 36 hours are characteristic features of opiate withdrawal syndrome. Sweats, chills, and restlessness precede other symptoms; the vomiting peaks by 72 hours and then subsides (see Chapter 235).

DIFFERENTIAL DIAGNOSIS

Table 59.1 lists some of the more common and important conditions associated with prominent nausea and vomiting. Causes

TABLE 59.1

SOME IMPORTANT CAUSES OF NAUSEA AND VOMITING

Nausea/Vomiting as Predominant or Initial Symptom
Acute
   Digitalis toxicity
   Ketoacidosis[a]
   Opiate use
   Cancer chemotherapeutic agents
   Early pregnancy
   Inferior myocardial infarction[a]
   Drug withdrawal
   Binge drinking
   Hepatitis
Recurrent or Chronic
   Psychogenic vomiting
   Metabolic disturbances (uremia, adrenal insufficiency)
   Gastric retention (gastroparesis, outlet obstruction)
   Bile reflux after gastric surgery
   Pregnancy
Nausea/Vomiting in Association with Abdominal Pain[b]
   Viral gastroenteritis
   Acute gastritis
   Food poisoning
   Peptic ulcer disease
   Acute pancreatitis
   Small-bowel obstruction and pseudoobstruction
   Acute appendicitis
   Acute cholecystitis
   Acute cholangitis
   Acute pyelonephritis
   Inferior myocardial infarction
Nausea/Vomiting in Association with Neurologic Symptoms
   Increased intracranial pressure
   Midline cerebellar hemorrhage
   Vestibular disturbances
   Migraine headaches
   Autonomic dysfunction

[a]Abdominal pain is sometimes present.
[b]Abdominal pain is sometimes absent.

of simple regurgitation are omitted from the list because they are usually manifestations of esophageal difficulties (see Chapter 61) and unaccompanied by emesis. For convenience, the etiologies are listed according to clinical presentation; however, it is important to keep in mind that overlap and variation in the clinical picture can be considerable. For example, some causes listed as being accompanied by abdominal pain may present with just isolated emesis.

WORKUP (1,2,4,7–10)

The history and physical examination, supplemented by a few well-chosen laboratory studies, are sufficient for diagnosis in most cases.

History

History should focus on such details as timing of symptoms, their relation to meals, characteristics of the vomitus, and associated complaints.

Timing and Relation to Meals

An early-morning onset points to metabolic disturbances, alcoholic binge, and early pregnancy. Emesis precipitated by meals suggests psychogenic vomiting, pyloric channel ulcer, and gastritis. Onset a few hours after eating raises the possibility of obstruction of the gastric outflow tract, gastric atony, or bowel obstruction. Emesis of food that was ingested more than 12 hours earlier strongly suggests gastric stasis and an organic etiology, as does vomiting of large volumes (>1,500 mL daily). However, the absence of such features hardly rules out organic disease.

Nature of the Vomitus

Vomiting blood or "coffee ground" material is indicative of gastritis and ulcer disease. Bilious vomitus means that the pyloric channel is open. When the material vomited is pure gastric juice, peptic ulcer disease and Zollinger–Ellison syndrome are suggested. Lack of acid suggests gastric cancer. Feculent material is a sign of distal small-bowel obstruction and blind-loop syndrome.

Associated Symptoms, Past Medical History, Psychosocial History

The history needs to include inquiry into abdominal pain, fever, jaundice, weight loss, abdominal surgery, external hernias, family history of emesis, symptoms of diabetes, prior renal disease, ischemic heart disease, drug use (e.g., digitalis, narcotics), visual disturbances, headache, ataxia, vertigo, last menstrual period, and concurrent emotional stresses and conflicts. Gentle questioning about self-image, binge eating, and self-induced emesis is indicated when the patient is a young woman suspected of bulimia.

Epidemiologic Data

Epidemiologic data need to be obtained, particularly any exposure to commonly contaminated foods (e.g., raw shellfish, pastries, poultry) or hepatitis and any travel to an area with poor sanitation and outbreaks of cholera. Vomiting in conjunction with diarrhea sufficient to cause severe dehydration in an adult suggests cholera, especially if there are supportive epidemiologic data.

Physical Examination

One checks for *postural hypotension* (indicative of marked volume depletion or circulatory collapse). Other findings to check for include blood pressure elevation, irregularities of rate and rhythm, Kussmaul's respiration, pallor, hyperpigmentation, jaundice, papilledema, retinopathy, nystagmus, stiff neck, abdominal distention, visible peristalsis, abnormal bowel sounds, succussion splash, peritoneal signs, focal tenderness, organomegaly, masses, flank tenderness, muscle weakness, ataxia of gait, and asterixis. If there is a history of vertigo in conjunction with nausea, then Báranáy's maneuver (see Chapter 166) might reproduce symptoms and confirm the diagnosis of a vestibular etiology.

Patients suspected of having a "functional" disorder should be checked carefully for signs of autonomic insufficiency. A finding of postural hypotension, lack of sweat, or blunted pulse and blood pressure responses to Valsalva's maneuver suggests autonomic dysfunction and a bowel motility problem as the underlying etiology of the nausea and vomiting.

Laboratory Studies

Test ordering should be a function of the clinical presentation and is best conducted as a means of testing clinically generated hypotheses rather than as a routine request for "nausea and vomiting studies."

Acute Emesis with Concurrent Abdominal Pain

In patients with emesis accompanied by acute abdominal pain, the first priority is to rule out an acute surgical cause such as bowel obstruction, peritonitis, or blockage of a hollow viscus. *Plain and upright films of the abdomen* are indicated when such causes are suspected (see Chapter 58). The onset of pancreatitis may be dominated by emesis in addition to abdominal pain, and if pancreatitis is suspected, a serum *amylase* determination is indicated. For suspected acute cholecystitis and choledocholithiasis, liver function studies (e.g., *alkaline phosphatase, aspartate aminotransferase*) and prompt consideration of *abdominal ultrasonography* are required.

Acute Nausea and Vomiting without Associated Abdominal Pain

The absence of abdominal pain does not rule out serious underlying pathology. The acute onset of nausea and vomiting in conjunction with ataxia of gait and a stiff neck is very suggestive of a midline cerebellar hemorrhage; emergency *computed tomography* of the posterior fossa is needed (see Chapter 165). If the patient is a known diabetic, ketoacidosis should be suspected and *urine* and *serum ketones* and blood *glucose* should be checked (see Chapter 102). In a patient with risk factors for coronary artery disease, an *electrocardiogram* should be obtained; inferior ischemia may present as gastrointestinal upset (see Chapter 20). Hepatitis may present like acute gastroenteritis, with anorexia, nausea, and vomiting; a *transaminase* determination can be diagnostic. If the patient is taking a medication that potentially causes nausea and vomiting, a *serum drug level* might be informative. If a *digitalis* preparation is being taken, the drug should be withheld, an electrocardiogram obtained, a serum level ordered, and a potassium supplement prescribed if the potassium level is less than 4.0 mg/100 mL (see Chapter 32).

Recurrent Vomiting

Recurrent vomiting raises the question of a psychogenic cause, but before coming to such a conclusion, the physician should consider pregnancy, metabolic derangements, and chronic gastroesophageal disease. Metabolic disease and pregnancy are suggested by vomiting that occurs in the early morning. A *urinalysis* and determinations of the serum *blood urea nitrogen, creatinine, electrolytes, glucose,* and, in a woman of childbearing age, *human chorionic gonadotropin β subunit* should be obtained (see Chapter 112).

Gastroesophageal causes are suggested by postprandial symptoms and best investigated by *upper gastrointestinal series* if there is concern about gastric outlet obstruction or retention and by *endoscopy* if mucosal injury is a possibility (see Chapters 62 and 68).

Psychogenic vomiting is suggested by the characteristic history of chronic emesis, with vomiting around mealtime, partial suppressibility, and a conflict-ridden social situation. The need for additional studies in such cases is best individualized; some patients may insist on further testing, whereas others will be comforted by knowing that extensive studies are not necessary.

Therapeutic Trials

A therapeutic trial may have diagnostic utility and provide symptomatic relief. When a gastroesophageal motility disorder is suspected, a short course of a prokinetic agent such as *metoclopramide* (e.g., 10 mg, 1/2 hour before meals) supplemented by a *proton-pump inhibitor* (e.g., 20 mg of omeprazole daily) can be useful. Patients suspected of having an underlying affective disorder sometimes respond to a 4- to 8-week trial of *antidepressant medication*; an agent with minimal anticholinergic activity (e.g., trazodone, desipramine, or fluoxetine) is preferred to minimize the chances of gastrointestinal side effects.

INDICATIONS FOR REFERRAL AND ADMISSION

Hospital admission for parenteral fluid and electrolyte replacement and additional workup is indicated if postural hypotension is present, especially if the patient is elderly. Prompt hospitalization also is needed for a patient with evidence of bowel obstruction, increased intracranial pressure, or any other gastrointestinal, neurologic, or metabolic emergency. In the case of a patient whose condition remains undiagnosed after extensive evaluation and is unresponsive to therapeutic trials and for whom evidence of an underlying psychiatric disturbance is lacking, gastric emptying and motility studies should be considered. These studies are performed at only a few specialty centers; referral should be made in consultation with a gastroenterologist. Patients suspected of psychogenic vomiting require psychiatric consultation because they may be seriously disturbed. Suicidal attempts are not uncommon among bulimic patients and others with psychogenic emesis. Referral to a mental health professional skilled and experienced in the treatment of patients with eating disorders is optimal for those suffering from bulimia (see Chapter 234).

SYMPTOMATIC RELIEF (5,6,11–16)

When a cause has been identified but treatment of the underlying condition does not adequately control the symptoms, antiemetic drug therapy may help to provide symptomatic relief (see also Chapters 88 and 91). The available agents work by suppressing the vomiting center, the chemoreceptor trigger zone, or peripheral receptors. Symptomatic therapy must not be used in lieu of making a diagnosis.

Phenothiazines

Phenothiazines and other centrally acting agents are indicated for initial symptomatic treatment of vomiting caused by drugs, metabolic disorders, and gastroenteritis. They suppress the chemoreceptor trigger zone and probably the vomiting center and peripheral receptors also. *Prochlorperazine* (*Compazine*) and *promethazine* (*Phenergan*) are the phenothiazines used most often for vomiting. Prochlorperazine can be given orally in doses of 5 to 10 mg every 6 hours or rectally in a dose of 25 mg three times daily. The oral dose of promethazine is 12.5 to 25.0 mg every 6 to 8 hours; the rectal dose is 25 mg three times daily. This class of drugs is not effective for motion sickness or vestibular disease. *Trimethobenzamide* (*Tigan*) is a centrally acting, nonphenothiazine antiemetic useful for emesis of central causes. The oral dose is 250 mg three times daily. Rectal suppositories are given three times daily. Like all centrally acting agents, it can cause drowsiness, especially in the elderly. In *hepatitis*, nausea and vomiting may respond to very cautious use of phenothiazines. However, because they are metabolized by the liver and in rare instances can cause cholestasis, they should be used only in limited doses for short periods of time (see Chapter 70).

Antihistamines

For symptomatic relief from the nausea and vomiting of *vestibular disturbances*, the antihistamine *meclizine* (*Antivert*) has proved to be useful; it acts on the vestibular system and the chemoreceptor trigger zone and helps to control the nausea and vomiting associated with vestibular dysfunction. Because meclizine can suppress or blunt important clues of vestibular disease, it should not be used unless a diagnosis has been established. Other antihistamines are quite popular for the treatment or prevention of motion sickness because, in comparison with meclizine, they provide either a more rapid onset of action (e.g., *dimenhydrinate* [*Dramamine*]) or a more prolonged effect (e.g., *transdermal scopolamine*). The average dose of meclizine is 25 mg four times daily for vestibular disease. A single transdermal scopolamine patch applied behind the ear several hours before a trip will provide prophylaxis for up to 3 days. Anticholinergic side effects (constipation, dry mouth, giddiness) are common. Meclizine is teratogenic in animals and is not indicated for vomiting resulting from pregnancy. All antihistamines can cause drowsiness and should not be used before driving or use of machinery.

Prokinetic Agents (Metoclopramide)

Metoclopramide blocks both dopaminergic and serotonin receptors, which accounts for its antiemetic action and its side effects. For patients with emesis resulting from gastroparesis (as in advanced diabetes mellitus), its dopaminergic blocking effect promotes gastric emptying and gastroesophageal sphincter closure. In highly emetogenic chemotherapy, it augments other antiemetics and helps to prevent delayed emesis. It is usually given orally (10 mg before each meal and before bed), although it can be administered intravenously. The drug's dopaminergic side effects can lead to dystonia in young patients and mental confusion in older patients. Because metoclopramide is often used to augment the antiemetic effects of other serotonergic drugs (see later discussion and Chapter 91) or taken concurrently with selective serotonin reuptake inhibitor antidepressants, it must be used carefully, keeping in mind the potential for inducing the *serotonin syndrome*, a predictable consequence of excess central and peripheral serotonergic stimulation. The onset of the syndrome can be rapid and include a confusing picture of agitation, fever, tachycardia shivering, diaphoresis, mydriasis, intermittent tremor or myoclonus, and hyperreflexia; circulatory collapse may ensue. Early tip-offs to the syndrome include the recent use of serotonergic drugs and the presence of tremor, hyperreflexia, clonus, or inner restlessness (akathisia) in the absence of other extrapyramidal signs.

Antiemetics in Cancer and Cancer Chemotherapy

The nausea and vomiting associated with advanced cancer or highly emetic cancer chemotherapy can be especially disturbing and demoralizing, as well as exhausting and a therapy-limiting factor (see also Chapter 91). The control of nausea and vomiting due to advanced disease ranks as a top priority in palliative care. In the setting of chemotherapy, even a single episode of emesis can lead to disabling anticipatory symptoms.

The prevention of both immediate and delayed chemotherapy-induced emesis is now achievable with agents that block receptors of key neurotransmitters involved in the vomiting reflex. Similar approaches can be used for the treatment of emesis due to advanced disease. The advent of *selective serotonin S3 receptor* ($5\text{-}HT_3$) *antagonists* (e.g., *ondansetron*, *granisetron*) represented a major advance in preventing emesis due to highly emetogenic agents such as cisplatin, which induce serotonin release from enterochromaffin cells. This class of antiemetics is also helpful in palliative care and effective orally as a single dose for severe gastroenteritis. *Substance P receptor inhibitors* (e.g., *aprepitant*) are also highly effective in chemotherapy-induced emesis. Combining $5\text{-}HT_3$ and substance P blockade with dexamethasone provides excellent prevention of both immediate and delayed emesis and represents a major improvement in the approach to this dreaded chemotherapy side effect. The principal disadvantage is high cost.

A host of other agents and substances has been tried, ranging from *phenothiazines* to *tetrahydrocannabinol* (as found in marijuana); few provide truly satisfactory control, particularly when highly emetogenic chemotherapy agents are used. High-dose *metoclopramide* can provide additional benefit when added to a program of steroids and neurotransmitter blockade (see Chapter 91). *Benzodiazepines* are often added as a supplement to antiemetic programs, especially when anxiety is high and sleep is poor.

Drugs for Morning Sickness

Morning sickness is best treated with small morning feedings and support; the goal is to try to avoid the use of antiemetics. No antiemetic is approved for use in pregnancy. The more prolonged, severe form of nausea and vomiting in pregnancy (hyperemesis gravidarum) may remit with hypnosis or supportive psychotherapy, but drug therapy is sometimes necessary.

Although a large number of agents has been studied, none has proven uniquely effective, and fetal safety is a top concern. Among those worth considering are the *antihistamines*, which may provide some benefit and are nonteratogenic. *Vitamin B₆ (25 mg/d)* has proved useful in controlled trials, mostly for reducing nausea; it too appears to be safe. *Vitamin B₁₂* has also shown benefit in placebo-controlled trials. *Metoclopramide* has also been used for years in severe cases without reports of fetal injury. Approval for *Bendectin* has been withdrawn because of concern for teratogenic effects. *Ginger* is a herbal therapy supported by one randomized trial. There is some suggestion of benefit from *P6 acupuncture*, but data are limited. *Corticos-*teroids, *phenothiazines*, and *diazepam* have not proven useful, and all have potentially adverse consequences.

Treatment of Psychogenic Vomiting

The best approach involves attention to the issues troubling the patient. No controlled studies have been performed of the effectiveness of antiemetics; fortunately, patients often do not request medication for symptomatic relief.

A.H.G.

Annotated Bibliography

1. Abell TL, Kim CH, Malageldα JR. Idiopathic cyclic nausea and vomiting—a disorder of gastrointestinal motility? Mayo Clin Proc 1988;63:1169. (*Gastrointestinal motor disturbances are found.*)
2. Ahmed S, Gupta R, Brancato R. Significance of nausea and vomiting during acute myocardial infarction. Am Heart J 1977;95:671. (*Nausea and vomiting occurred in 69% of patients with inferior infarctions, compared with 27% of those with anterior infarctions.*)
3. Baron TH, Ramirez R, Richter JE. Gastrointestinal motility disorders during pregnancy. Ann Intern Med 1993;118:366. (*Discusses the pathophysiology of vomiting in pregnancy.*)
4. Brzana RJ, Koch KL. Gastroesophageal reflux disease presenting with intractable nausea. Ann Intern Med 1997;126:704. (*A case series of 10 outpatients with intractable nausea, demonstrating that all had reflux and that nausea resolved with treatment of the underlying reflux.*)
5. Cubeddu LX, Hoffman IS, Fuenmayor NT, et al. Efficacy of ondansetron (GR 38032F) and the role of serotonin in cisplatin-induced nausea and vomiting. N Engl J Med 1990;322:810. (*A randomized, placebo-controlled study, demonstrating that ondansetron is effective and safe.*)
6. Hesketh PJ, Grunberg SM, Gralla RJ, et al. The oral neurokinin-1 antagonist aprepitant for the prevention of chemotherapy-induced nausea and vomiting: a multinational, randomized, double-blind, placebo-controlled trial in patients receiving high-dose cisplatin—The Aprepitant Protocol 052 Study Group. J Clin Oncol 2003;21:4112. (*Presents evidence for the efficacy of the first substance P inhibitor, confirming the important mechanistic role of substance P.*)
7. Hill OW. Psychogenic vomiting. Gut 1968;9:348. (*A classic study, showing a high frequency of hostile living situations and symptoms developing at mealtime.*)
8. Swerdlow DL, Ries AA. Cholera in the Americas. JAMA 1992;267:1495. (*A succinct and excellent review of the epidemiology, clinical presentation, diagnosis, and treatment of this condition; 42 references.*)
9. Bothe F, Beardwood J. Evaluation of abdominal symptoms in the diabetic. Ann Surg 1937;105:516. (*A classic study, finding that 75% of patients in ketoacidosis had nausea and vomiting and 8% had severe abdominal pain and elevated white blood cell counts simulating an acute abdomen; intraabdominal disease can precipitate ketoacidosis.*)
10. Malageldα JR, Camillieri M. Unexplained vomiting: a diagnostic challenge. Ann Intern Med 1984;101:211. (*A useful review of approaches to this difficult situation; details the neuromuscular disorders that may present as unexplained emesis; 61 references.*)
11. Freedman SB, Adler M, Seshadri R, et al. Oral ondansetron for gastroenteritis in a pediatric emergency department. N Engl J Med 2006;354:1698. (*A single dose was found to be safe and effective in children presenting with severe gastroenteritis.*)
12. Kris MG. Why do we need another antiemetic? Just ask. J Clin Oncol 2003;21:4007. (*An editorial nicely summarizing the evidence of efficacy for existing and new treatments.*)
13. Richards RD, Valenzuela GA, Davenport KG, et al. Objective and subjective results of a randomized, double-blind, placebo-controlled trial using cisapride to treat gastroparesis. Dig Dis Sci 1993;38:811. (*The agent was found to be effective.*)
14. Sahakian V, Rouse D, Sipes S, et al. Vitamin B6 is effective for nausea and vomiting of pregnancy. Obstet Gynecol 1991;78:33. (*A randomized, placebo-controlled, double-blind trial.*)
15. Schwartzberg LS. Chemotherapy-induced nausea and vomiting: clinician and patient perspectives. J Support Oncol 2007;5(2 Suppl 1):5. (*A thoughtful and practical discussion.*)
16. Boyer ES, Shannon M. The serotonin syndrome. N Engl J Med 2005;352:1112. (*The best review of this important dose-related complication of serotonergic therapy.*)

CHAPTER 60 ■ EVALUATION OF DYSPHAGIA AND SUSPECTED ESOPHAGEAL CHEST PAIN

Dysphagia is the unpleasant sensation of difficulty in swallowing as a consequence of neuromuscular or anatomic pathology involving the esophagus (and sometimes the oropharynx). Such pathology may also trigger substernal chest pain and simulate angina (see Chapter 20). *Odynophagia* refers to painful swallowing, which usually results from serious mucosal inflammation. Because esophageal dysfunction and pain may be a manifestation of or mimic important pathology, it deserves to be assessed fully and not dismissed as a trivial problem or glibly invoked to account for symptoms.

PATHOPHYSIOLOGY AND CLINICAL PRESENTATION (1–15)

Dysphagia

Dysphagia implies an abnormality in swallowing and arises from either a loss of coordinated motor activity or mechanical obstruction, be it intrinsic narrowing or extrinsic compression of the esophagus.

Transfer Dysphagia

Transfer dysphagia (also referred to as *oropharyngeal dysphagia*) usually occurs as a consequence of neurologic or neuromuscular disease and presents as choking or difficulty in initiating swallowing. The patient reports the symptom as beginning immediately on trying to swallow. In many instances, other neurologic symptoms dominate the clinical picture, but at times, difficulty in swallowing is the major complaint, with aspiration and regurgitation of fluid into the nose. The problem is particularly common among the very old. Cortical and brainstem lesions resulting from stroke, tumor, and degenerative disease are important causes. In addition, medications with central effects (e.g., benzodiazepines, L-dopa, phenothiazines) may blunt the swallowing mechanism. Unlike esophageal disease, oropharyngeal dysphagia is accurately localized to the suprasternal area. Patients with neuromuscular etiologies report more difficulty in swallowing liquids than solids, nasal regurgitation, coughing, and aspiration. Patients with anatomic narrowing and mechanical obstruction of the pharynx or upper esophagus have more difficulty with solids than liquids.

Achalasia

Achalasia, the most common cause of motor dysphagia, is a slowly progressive motility disorder with a chronic course. The pathologic hallmark is a loss of cells in the myenteric ganglia. Lesions in the dorsal vagal nucleus and vagal trunks have also been described. It has been speculated that these changes represent damage caused by a neurotropic virus. As a consequence of a loss of smooth-muscle ganglion cells, the esophagus functions poorly, exhibits episodes of aperistalsis, and demonstrates exquisite sensitivity to gastrin and cholinergic agents. The gastroesophageal sphincter fails to relax properly, leading to functional obstruction at the gastroesophageal junction. In addition, a *loss of peristaltic activity* occurs in the distal esophagus. Dysphagia and substernal chest pain ensue. The resting pressure at the lower esophageal sphincter (LES) rises, and barium study shows an absence of peristalsis and delay in esophageal emptying. Paradoxically, vigorous nonpropulsive (tertiary) esophageal contractions resulting in chest pain may be observed early in the disease in young patients. Swallowing liquids and solids is equally difficult, yet by eating slowly and drinking small amounts, the patient may be able to consume a full meal. Pain is reported by 70% to 80% of patients, especially if they eat or drink rapidly, but pain is not an invariable accompaniment, and only 2% of patients with chest pain caused by esophageal disease have achalasia. Very cold liquids or emotion may provoke symptoms. Patients find that repeated swallowing or performing a rapid Valsalva maneuver can help to pass material into the stomach. Regurgitation is common and can be provoked by changes in position or physical exercise; pulmonary aspiration sometimes results. Patients may have foul breath because of retained esophageal material. Squamous cell carcinoma of the esophagus is sometimes a complication of achalasia; it occurs in 5% to 10% of patients.

Carcinoma-induced achalasia is seen with tumors at the gastroesophageal junction. Adenocarcinoma of the stomach is the most common of these neoplasms. The mechanism by which tumor induces achalasia is unclear, but manometric findings are identical to those of primary achalasia. Patients are typically older than the age of 50 years and complain of marked weight loss and symptoms of dysphagia of less than 1 year's duration.

Scleroderma

Scleroderma can impair neuromuscular function and result in a decrease in LES tone in addition to a lack of propulsive motor activity. *Reflux* is more of a problem than is dysphagia (helping to distinguish scleroderma from other motility disorders), but as many as 20% of patients may have some difficulty in swallowing. About 75% of patients with scleroderma have esophageal involvement as part of the CREST syndrome (calcinosis, Raynaud's phenomenon, esophageal dysmotility, sclerodactyly, and telangiectasia).

Diffuse Esophageal Spasm

Diffuse esophageal spasm is characterized clinically by nonprogressive dysphagia and substernal chest pain that may mimic angina (see later discussion and Chapter 20). Radiologically and manometrically, patients manifest nonpropulsive *simultaneous contractions* (tertiary contractions) throughout the entire esophagus (especially the distal portion) in more than 10% of wet swallows. Such contractions are also observed in normal persons under conditions of emotional stress and dry swallows, which leads some to view this condition as little more than a transient abnormality in motor function induced by stress. However, as noted earlier, the condition may also be an early manifestation of neuromuscular disease that progresses to achalasia. Unlike achalasia, diffuse esophageal spasm is intermixed with periods of normal peristaltic activity. Dysphagia is noted with both liquids and solids. Diffuse esophageal spasm accounts for about 10% of cases of noncardiac chest pain caused by abnormal esophageal motility. Some asymptomatic patients manifest the radiologic and manometric criteria for esophageal spasm but rarely experience discomfort.

"Nutcracker" Esophagus

"Nutcracker" esophagus is a picturesque radiologic description applied to the condition of patients experiencing *very high amplitude contractions* in the distal esophagus. Some view the condition as a severe variant of diffuse esophageal spasm, where the resultant pressures exceed the mean by more than two standard deviations. These peristaltic contractions are not only of exceptionally high amplitude but also of long duration. There are no simultaneous contractions, as there are in diffuse esophageal spasm, and only occasionally does impairment of esophageal function lead to dysphagia. The principal symptom is *chest pain* (see later discussion), with nutcracker esophagus accounting for about half of all cases of noncardiac chest pain associated with an esophageal motility disturbance. In many instances, reflux precipitates the contractile abnormalities and may contribute to the chest pain. At issue is whether the condition might be considered a component or consequence of *gastroesophageal reflux disease*. Achalasia develops in about 3% to 5% of patients, and degenerative changes are noted in ganglia and nerves, suggesting to some a possible link to achalasia. Supersensitivity to gastrin and cholinergic agents can be demonstrated.

Hypertensive Lower Esophageal Sphincter

Hypertensive LES is characterized by increased resting LES pressure but normal relaxation and peristalsis, with no impediment to bolus passage. About half of the patients have high-amplitude contractions, consistent with nutcracker esophagus.

Nonspecific Esophageal Motility Disorder

Nonspecific esophageal motility disorder designates persons who manifest abnormal esophageal manometry results but fail to meet specific diagnostic criteria for one of the preceding conditions. Contractions may be nontransmitted, retrograde, of high or low amplitude, prolonged, spontaneous, or even retrograde. In addition, the lower esophageal sphincter may fail to relax.

Mechanical Obstruction

Mechanical obstruction differs clinically from motor dysfunction, in that the patient has more difficulty with solids than with liquids. The duration of symptoms is shorter (<1 year) for patients with malignancy than it is for those with benign causes of obstruction; progression is often rapid. Most patients with tumor are older than the age of 50 years and report marked weight loss. The location of discomfort does not necessarily correlate with the site of obstruction because the pain may be referred. Spontaneous pain is not a common feature of neoplasm involving the esophagus. Patients with stricture caused by severe esophagitis usually have a long history of reflux.

Inflammatory Lesions

Inflammatory lesions of the pharynx or esophagus may cause *odynophagia* (pain on swallowing). Esophageal motility is not disturbed, but swallowing is made difficult by the pain. Even saliva may be irritating. *Radiation therapy*, *tablet ingestion*, *malignancy*, and *infection* are important causes of this severe esophageal irritation. Tetracycline, quinidine, potassium tablets, nonsteroidal antiinflammatory drugs, and iron preparations have been implicated. The elderly are at greatest risk because they are likely to consume more tablets with less water, and saliva production decreases with age. The discomfort is often associated with ingestion of the tablets and generally decreases during a period of a few days.

Infectious esophagitis caused by *Candida*, *herpes simplex virus*, or *cytomegalovirus* is being increasingly recognized in immunocompromised patients, including the growing number with AIDS, and in patients taking broad-spectrum antibiotics on a long-term basis. Onset may be rapid and accompanied by fever, chills, nausea, vomiting, and epigastric pain. Viral or fungal esophagitis rarely occurs in immunologically intact persons; when it does, it is usually short-lived and self-limited.

Conditions Confused with Dysphagia

Sometimes, *globus hystericus*, a condition seen in anxiety disorders, is confused with dysphagia. The patient complains of a constant "lump in the throat" and has a perception of obstruction, although he or she has no actual difficulty in swallowing food. An involuntary tightening of the cricopharyngeal muscle has been observed in some patients with this condition and may account for the symptoms. Symptoms are unrelated to swallowing, and esophageal function is normal.

Esophageal Chest Pain

Esophageal chest pain mechanisms include acid stimulation of chemoreceptors, prolonged or severe contractile waves, and distention of stretch receptors; multiple mechanisms may be operative concurrently (e.g., acid reflux stimulation of abnormal contractile waves). In patients undergoing cardiac catheterization for the evaluation of chest pain, nearly 50% of those with normal studies are found to have esophageal abnormalities by endoscopy or 24-hour pH monitoring; evidence of *gastroesophageal reflux disease* (GERD) is common.

The chest pain in GERD patients typically occurs after meals or at night (awakening one from sleep), stays localized to the retrosternal area or radiates through to the back, lasts hours, and may be associated with classic heartburn, but not necessarily. Esophageal motor abnormalities may ensue.

Motor dysfunction is also noted in esophageal chest pain without GERD. Some patients subject to attacks of esophageal chest pain are suspected of having an esophageal version of irritable bowel syndrome, with motor dysfunction and increased sensitivity to distention and chemical stimuli. Researchers have considered whether there might be an *"irritable gut syndrome,"* with a common pathophysiology extending from the esophagus to the rectosigmoid. They note that many patients with esophageal chest pain also report symptoms of irritable bowel syndrome.

Chest pain is particularly prevalent in patients with *nutcracker esophagus*. The chest pain associated with esophageal motor disorders can mimic that of angina in terms of location (substernal), quality (tightness), radiation (into the arm or back), and response to nitroglycerine (prompt relief).

Adding to the confusion with coronary pain is the fact that esophageal chest pain need not be accompanied by dysphagia, although heartburn is frequently reported as a preceding symptom. Sometimes, the chest discomfort is triggered by drinking very hot or very cold liquids, but it need not occur in relation to swallowing.

DIFFERENTIAL DIAGNOSIS

The causes of dysphagia can be divided into motor and obstructive categories, and these are often subdivided according to whether they affect the upper or lower esophagus (Table 60.1). Most esophageal cancers are of the squamous cell variety, although half of those in the distal half of the esophagus are adenocarcinomas, which suggests that they arise in the cardia of the stomach. True dysphagia must be distinguished from conditions that may produce esophageal pain without interfering with the mechanics of swallowing, such as most forms of esophagitis and motor disorders with propulsive but high-amplitude contractions (e.g., nutcracker esophagus). The patient with globus hystericus reports a constant sensation of having something in the throat, but swallows normally.

No detailed population studies have been performed on the prevalence of dysphagia and the relative frequencies of its causes. However, in a study of 910 patients with noncardiac chest pain, 28% were found to have abnormal esophageal motility. Of these 28%, 48% had nutcracker disease, 36% had nonspecific esophageal motility dysfunction, 10% had diffuse esophageal spasm, and 2% had achalasia.

TABLE 60.1

DIFFERENTIAL DIAGNOSIS OF DYSPHAGIA

Motor Disease
   Pharyngeal (transfer dysphagia)
      Pseudobulbar palsy
      Myasthenia gravis
      Multiple sclerosis
      Amyotrophic lateral sclerosis
      Parkinson's disease
   Transesophageal
      Achalasia
      Scleroderma
      Diffuse esophageal spasm
   Distal
      "Nutcracker" esophagus
      Hypertensive lower esophageal sphincter

Obstructing Lesions
   Upper esophageal
      Tumor
      Zenker's webs (Plummer–Vinson syndrome)
      Goiter
      Enlarged lymph nodes
      Cervical spine osteophytes
   Lower esophageal
      Carcinoma
      Stricture (chronic reflux, corrosive agents, intubation)
      Webs and rings
      Foreign bodies
      Food impaction
      Mediastinal tumors
      Aortic aneurysm

Odynophagia
   Opportunistic esophageal infection (cytomegalovirus,
      herpesvirus, *Candida*)
   Tablet-induced irritation
   Severe reflux esophagitis
   Malignancy

throwing back the head and shoulders. Mechanical obstruction is characterized by a more rapid onset and progressive course, more difficulty with solids than with liquids, no aggravation with cold foods, and regurgitation on trying to swallow a bolus. As noted, the location of discomfort helps to locate the lesion only if it is very high or very low in the esophagus; with a distal lesion, pain may be referred to the neck. Hiccups point to difficulty in the terminal portion of the esophagus. Intermittent dysphagia that occurs only with solid food is indicative of a lower esophageal (Schatzki's) ring.

Other historical features with some discriminative value include the presence of painful swallowing and neurologic defects. Pain in conjunction with dysphagia suggests spasm or achalasia (although pain may occur in these conditions without concurrent difficulty in swallowing). Pain on swallowing saliva alone is characteristic of serious mucosal inflammation. Dysphagia that comes on only after activity and is associated with motor aphasia, diplopia, or dysphonia is indicative of myasthenia. Tremor or difficulty in initiating movement suggests Parkinson's disease (see Chapter 174). Other historical facts to note are recent use of topical upper respiratory or inhaled steroid aerosols or broad-spectrum antibiotics and concurrent immunodeficiency (e.g., AIDS).

The pace of illness deserves attention. Very acute dysphagia suggests infection, irritation, or food impaction. Rapid progression is caused by tumor until proven otherwise, whereas slow progression is most consistent with a motor disorder. Weight loss may occur with any etiology but is more predictive of obstruction.

Physical Examination

The skin is noted for pallor, signs of scleroderma (sclerodactyly, telangiectasia, calcinosis), and hyperkeratotic palms and soles (a rare finding suggestive of esophageal carcinoma). The mouth should be examined carefully for inflammatory lesions, ill-fitting dentures, and pharyngeal masses. The HIV-positive patient with oral candidiasis is at increased risk for esophageal involvement. Lymph nodes are palpated in the neck and elsewhere to detect enlargement suggestive of neoplasm or infection (see Chapter 12), and the thyroid is palpated for a goiter that might extrinsically compress the esophagus. The abdomen is checked for masses, tenderness, and organomegaly and the stool for occult blood (suggestive of neoplasm and esophagitis). The neurologic examination should be thorough and include testing for motor dysfunction, with a search for tremor, rigidity, and fatigability in addition to cranial nerve deficits, abnormal Babinski's response, and abnormal gag reflex.

Laboratory Studies

The history and physical examination usually provide sufficient evidence to distinguish oropharyngeal from esophageal dysphagia and a mechanical form of esophageal dysphagia from a neuromuscular one. Making such a determination before laboratory testing helps to focus the laboratory workup, interpret the results, and avoid unnecessary studies.

Upper Gastrointestinal Endoscopy and Biopsy

Upper gastrointestinal endoscopy and biopsy have largely supplanted the barium swallow for the initial assessment of dysphagia, especially in the setting of longstanding *gastroesophageal reflux disease* and concern about premalignant or

WORKUP (1,16–26)

History

History alone can provide a tentative diagnosis in nearly 80% of cases. Diagnostically useful inquiries include checking for the presence of reflux (retrosternal burning moving upward) and correlation of discomfort/pain with the reflux's precipitants (e.g., meals, recumbency). A history of heartburn in conjunction with difficulty in swallowing solids may herald a stricture secondary to chronic reflux esophagitis, especially if the problem is chronic. Scleroderma is suggested when symptoms of reflux and dysphagia occur in the context of sclerodactyl skin changes and symptoms of Raynaud's phenomenon (distal blanching and cyanosis in response to cold).

Also useful diagnostically are inquiries into the duration and progression of symptoms, the relation of symptoms to the ingestion of solids or liquids, the effect of cold on swallowing, and the response to swallowing a bolus. Motor disease is suggested by gradual onset, slow progression, chronic course, equal difficulty with liquids and solids, aggravation of symptoms on swallowing cold substances, and passage of a bolus by repeated swallowing, forceful drinking, Valsalva maneuver, or malignant mucosal transformation (see Chapter 61) or when obstruction is suspected clinically. On occasion, even the patient with achalasia may require endoscopy, particularly when contraction of the LES is so persistent that stenosis cannot be ruled out by barium study alone. Stretching of the sphincter can be accomplished at the same time. However, endoscopy for radiographically negative dysphagia is generally of low yield and should not be the initial test in a person with transfer dysphagia.

Acute onset of *odynophagia* suggests severe esophageal inflammation and, in an immunocompromised host, raises the possibility of an infectious etiology. *Endoscopic examination* is needed to examine for plaques, vesicles, and pseudomembranes. Brushings and biopsy specimens are obtained as needed and prepared appropriately to detect fungi, giant cells, intranuclear inclusion bodies, and malignant cells. All patients with new-onset odynophagia require endoscopic evaluation.

Barium Swallow

Barium swallow is the test of choice in the assessment of *transfer dysphagia*. Its sensitivity is also excellent for determining the location and severity of an obstructing mass lesion or stenosis, but it often lacks precision in identifying the nature of the lesion, particularly in distinguishing cancer from postinflammatory scarring and stenosis. When an obstructing lesion is suspected, endoscopy with biopsy is required, especially when the history suggests malignancy (e.g., rapid progression, marked weight loss, solids more problematic than liquids).

By providing fluoroscopic evidence of esophageal function, the barium swallow can sometimes help in documenting motor disorders, although test sensitivity is not high. Early achalasia and esophageal spasm may produce few findings on a routine barium swallow, especially when symptoms are infrequent. The characteristic radiologic features of achalasia include dilation of the distal two thirds of the esophagus, segmental contractions, and termination of the distal esophagus into a narrowed segment (often referred to as a "break"), caused by the tonically contracted LES. When the patient is upright, an air–fluid level may be present on the barium esophagram. If diffuse esophageal spasm occurs during barium examination, it produces multiple tertiary contractions and differs from achalasia, in that no break is observed. The functional assessment of dysphagia is facilitated by performing all barium studies with the patient in the supine position to cancel the effect of gravity and by dipping a piece of bread into barium to trace better the movement of solid food. *Video studies of the oropharyngeal phase* of swallowing are essential in the evaluation of suspected oropharyngeal dysphagia, not only for diagnosis, but also to determine the risk for aspiration. Radiologic expertise is required for the interpretation of such films.

Manometry

Strong clinical suspicion of motor dysfunction and failure of endoscopy and barium swallow to reveal a probable etiology raise the question of proceeding to manometry. The diagnosis of nutcracker esophagus is especially dependent on manometric data. For many other conditions, a single manometry often gives indeterminate data. Many patients suspected of achalasia or esophageal spasm fail to show typical manometric findings at the time of testing. Furthermore, others who are symptom-free may demonstrate abnormalities when tested. Still others end up being placed in a category of nonspecific motility disease. The use of 24-hour pressure monitoring can help to overcome some of these limitations (see later discussion). Many

authorities insist on manometric data before concluding that a patient has esophageal spasm or a related motor disorder.

Provocative Testing

Provocative testing is most useful and worth serious consideration when the physician is confronted with a patient who complains of *atypical chest pain*. Once cardiac disease is ruled out (see Chapter 20), an esophageal problem is high on the list of possible explanations. Provocative testing provides a ready means in the office of identifying an esophageal origin for an atypical pain, although it does not specify a mechanism, and it is of less use in the evaluation of dysphagia. The objective of provocative testing is to reproduce the patient's exact symptoms. Two tests have proved most useful: the Bernstein or acid perfusion test and edrophonium (Tensilon) infusion.

The Bernstein Test. The Bernstein test was initially used to confirm symptoms caused by reflux, but a positive test result has also proved specific for esophageal chest pain, even in the absence of documented reflux. In 7% to 27% of cases, noncardiac chest pain has been associated with a positive Bernstein test result and deemed to be of definite esophageal origin, although evidence of acid reflux may not be found on 24-hour pH monitoring. The test consists in instilling a small amount of acid through a nasogastric tube placed in the esophagus.

Edrophonium Testing. Edrophonium testing grew out of a desire to find a safe and well-tolerated means of stimulating esophageal contractions. Ergonovine was originally tried, and although it was successful in reproducing symptoms, its risks of serious cardiac side effects negated its usefulness. Edrophonium (a relatively gentle muscarinic agonist) has proved superior to acid perfusion, bethanechol, and pentagastrin in reproducing atypical chest pain, with 24% to 34% of patients having a positive test result (reproduction of pain during wet swallows). Like the Bernstein test, edrophonium identifies an esophageal origin for the pain but does not specify the mechanism (correlation between response to edrophonium and manometric findings is poor). Side effects of a rapid bolus of intravenous edrophonium (80 μg/kg of body weight) include mild degrees of lightheadedness, nausea, and abdominal cramps but not the tachycardia, hypertension, or coronary vasoconstriction seen with ergonovine.

Ambulatory pH Monitoring

Ambulatory pH monitoring of both *intraesophageal pH* and *pressures* for 24 hours can be useful, especially in cases that defy explanation despite comprehensive testing. Such monitoring provides an opportunity to correlate acid reflux with the occurrence of symptoms. Compared to traditional esophageal tests (single manometry study, Bernstein and edrophonium tests), 24-hour pH monitoring provides an explanatory correlation more frequently in persons with noncardiac chest pain (e.g., in 46% of instances vs. 19% for both edrophonium and the Bernstein tests and even less for a single manometric study). Abnormal motor activity may be difficult to detect at the time of a single manometric study or may be induced by the study itself and have little to do with the patient's problem. Around-the-clock monitoring opens new avenues of evaluation.

Therapeutic Trial of Proton-Pump Inhibition for Diagnosis

Using a short course of proton-pump inhibitor therapy (e.g., omeprazole 40 mg twice daily for a week) as a diagnostic test of reflux-induced noncardiac chest pain has a reported sensitivity of 78% and a specificity of 86%. Such a trial can spare more-expensive and more-invasive workup.

SYMPTOMATIC RELIEF AND PATIENT EDUCATION (2,4,9–11,20,26,27)

Motility Disorders

A conservative approach sometimes suffices for patients with mild motor disease. The dysphagic person with achalasia is often able to manage reasonably well by *eating slowly*, *drinking small quantities* at a time, and *avoiding cold foods*. A trial of *sublingual nitrates* or *calcium-channel blockers* before eating may sufficiently relax spastic smooth muscle in patients with mild to moderate dysfunction to provide relief.

Patients with *atypical chest pain* caused by esophageal disease benefit greatly from knowing definitively that their pain is not indicative of heart disease. A thorough explanation after a careful evaluation can greatly reduce morbidity and even the frequency of symptoms. Given the presumed relation of atypical chest pain to esophageal spasm, nitrates and calcium-channel blockers have been used. The results have been variable, which is not surprising because the relation of spasm to pain is variable; however, benefit does accrue for some patients, which makes a trial of these agents worthwhile. *Antireflux therapy* (e.g., use of proton-pump inhibition; see Chapter 61) can be an important component of the treatment program when the workup suggests acid reflux as a triggering factor. *Antidepressants* with little anticholinergic activity, such as trazodone, have proved effective in patients suspected of having a psychiatric precipitant of esophageal motor dysfunction. *Relaxation techniques* and other *behavioral methods* are worth a try in those with stress-induced esophageal motor dysfunction (see Chapter 226).

Anticholinergic therapy has been disappointing. When *odynophagia* is present and an inflammatory lesion is suspected as the precipitant, especially when opportunistic infection might be the cause (e.g., patients with HIV disease), antifungal or antiviral therapy may be needed (see Chapter 13).

Patients with severe achalasia get little relief from dietary or drug manipulations; *esophageal dilation* or *myotomy* is needed. Myotomy is more effective but requires major surgery and often produces severe reflux that does not respond to antireflux surgery. Consequently, pneumatic esophageal dilation is usually the most effective invasive procedure for the treatment of severe motor disease. Dysphagia is relieved immediately, and sufficient LES pressure remains to prevent bothersome reflux.

Obstructing Lesions

Regardless of etiology and pending definitive diagnosis, all patients suspected of having obstruction should be advised to take predominantly liquids or soft solids. The goal is to provide an adequate caloric intake that can be swallowed with a minimum of discomfort. Patients with mechanical obstruction often require dilation or surgery, but there are many exceptions. The best management for a person with a lower esophageal ring is to advise slow intake of small amounts; dilation does not work very well. Restoration of adequate iron intake will reverse the pathologic changes of sideropenic dysphagia unless a carcinoma has developed in the pharynx. Carcinoma of the upper or middle one third of the esophagus is often unresectable and best treated by radiation therapy; considerable palliation is sometimes achieved. Oropharyngeal dysphagia caused by obstruction is treated surgically (e.g., removal of a Zenker's diverticulum or large goiter), whereas attention to the underlying neurologic deficit is necessary in cases caused by motor dysfunction, although myotomy may help as well. The patient with globus hystericus can be given thorough reassurance, although symptoms are not likely to resolve easily.

Reflux

See Chapter 61.

INDICATIONS FOR REFERRAL

Patients with oropharyngeal dysphagia who aspirate more than 10% of a barium test bolus and show barium residue in the oropharynx with subsequent swallows are at great risk for aspiration and should be referred for consideration of a nonoral means of nutrition. In addition, those with evidence of neuromuscular disease severe enough to cause oropharyngeal dysphagia might benefit from a neurologic consultation. The patient with an obstructing lesion requires endoscopic evaluation and referral to a gastroenterologist or surgeon for consideration of endoscopic biopsy. The patient who is referred for further evaluation and therapy should still be followed closely by the primary care physician, especially to monitor nutritional status.

A.H.G.

Annotated Bibliography

1. Achem SR, Kotts BE, Wears R, et al. Chest pain associated with nutcracker esophagus: a preliminary study of the role of gastroesophageal reflux. Am J Gastroenterol 1993;88:187. (*Reflux may play a role in up to one third of patients.*)
2. Adler DG, Romero Y. Primary esophageal motility disorders. Mayo Clin Proc 2001;76:195. (*A succinct review; 22 references.*)
3. Bernstein LM, Baker LA. A clinical test for esophagitis. Gastroenterology 1958;34:760. (*The original description of the acid perfusion test.*)
4. Clouse RE, Lustman PJ. Psychiatric illness and contraction abnormalities of the esophagus. N Engl J Med 1983;309:1337. (*Documents the association between psychiatric conditions, including depression and anxiety states, and symptomatic esophageal motility disorders, many presenting as chest pain.*)
5. Cohen S. Esophageal motility disorders and their response to calcium channel antagonists: the sphinx revisited. Gastroenterology 1987;93:201.

(*Poor response to these muscle relaxants challenges the view of a simple etiologic association.*)
6. Cooke RA, Anggiansah A, Chambers JB, et al. A prospective study of oesophageal function in patients with normal coronary angiograms and controls with angina. Gut 1998;42:323. (*The frequency of abnormalities and the correlation of pH events with chest pain was the same among patients with normal coronary angiograms as in controls with angina.*)
7. Dalton CB, Castell DO, Richter JE. The changing face of the nutcracker esophagus. Am J Gastroenterology 1988;83:358. (*Detailed characterization of the condition in view of accumulating data.*)
8. Domenech E, Kelly J. Swallowing disorders. Med Clin North Am 1999;83:97. (*A useful review of causes of transfer dysphagia.*)
9. Goff JS. Infectious causes of esophagitis. Annu Rev Med 1988;39:163. (*An excellent review of these important causes of odynophagia.*)

10. Kahrilas PJ. Esophageal motility disorders: current concepts of pathogenesis and treatment. Can J Gastroenterol 2000;14:221. (*A comprehensive review for both specialist and generalist, which includes a discussion of underlying pathophysiology.*)

11. Kahrilas PJ. Gastroesophageal reflux disease. JAMA 1996;276:983. (*A systematic review of the management of gastroesophageal reflux disease with esophageal and extraesophageal complications.*)

12. Rao SS, Gregersen H, Hayek B, et al. Unexplained chest pain: the hypersensitive, hyperreactive, and poorly compliant esophagus. Ann Intern Med 1996;124:950. (*Lower thresholds for pain and reactive contractions are revealed by impedance planimetry after otherwise normal cardiac and esophageal evaluations.*)

13. Richter JE, Castell DO. Diffuse esophageal spasm: a reappraisal. Ann Intern Med 1984;100:242. (*Argues for a manometric diagnosis of spasm; a critical review of diagnostic criteria.*)

14. Wilcox CM. Esophageal disease in the acquired immunodeficiency syndrome: etiology, diagnosis, and management. Am J Med 1992;92:412. (*A thorough review.*)

15. Young LD, Richter JE, Anderson KO, et al. Effects of psychological and environmental stressors on peristaltic esophageal contractions in healthy volunteers. Psychology 1987;24:132. (*Presents data suggesting that stress can induce esophageal motor dysfunction.*)

16. Browning TH. Diagnosis of chest pain of esophageal origin: a guideline of the Patient Care Committee of the American Gastroenterological Association. Dig Dis Sci 1990;35:289. (*A consensus statement offering evaluation guidelines.*)

17. Edwards DAW. Discriminative information in the diagnosis of dysphagia. J R Coll Physicians Lond 1975;9:257. (*A critical discussion of important historical data; diagnostic accuracy by history alone is close to 80%.*)

18. Fass R, Fennerty MB, Ofman JJ, et al. The clinical and economic value of a short course of omeprazole in patients with non-cardiac chest pain. Gastroenterology 1998;115:42. (*Reasonable testing characteristics were found and cost savings were achieved in diagnostic evaluation.*)

19. Hewson EG, Sinclair JW, Dalton CB, et al. Twenty-four-hour esophageal monitoring: the most useful test for evaluating noncardiac chest pain. Am J Med 1991;90:576. (*The test identified an esophageal etiology in 46% of instances.*)

20. Janssens J, Vantrappen G, Ghillebert G. Twenty-four-hour recording of esophageal pressure and pH in patients with noncardiac chest pain. Gastroenterology 1986;90:1978. (*Correlations among pressure, pH, and chest pain were often variable.*)

21. Katz PO, Dalton CB, Richter JE, et al. Esophageal testing of patients with noncardiac chest pain or dysphagia. Ann Intern Med 1987;106:593. (*Provocative testing proved best in patients with chest pain; manometric studies were superior in patients with dysphagia.*)

22. Kim CH, Weaver AL, Hsu JJ, et al. Discriminant value of esophageal symptoms. Mayo Clin Proc 1993;68:948. (*Presents further evidence of the value of a careful history; the authors develop a discriminant model, but not one based on a primary care population.*)

23. Nord HJ. Extraesophageal symptoms: what role for the proton pump inhibitors. Am J Med 2004;11(5A):56S. (*Reviews the evidence for proton-pump inhibitor therapy as a diagnostic test in atypical chest pain.*)

24. Rose S, Achkar E, Easley KA. Follow-up of patients with noncardiac chest pain. Value of esophageal testing. Dig Dis Sci 1994;39:2063. (*Many patients continue to blame the esophagus even when tests results are normal.*)

25. Tavitian A, Raufman JP, Rosenthal L. Oral candidiasis as a marker for esophageal candidiasis in the acquired immunodeficiency syndrome. Ann Intern Med 1986;104:54. (*A useful clinical marker.*)

26. Ward BW, Wu WC, Richter JE, et al. Long-term follow-up of symptomatic status of patients with noncardiac chest pain: is diagnosis of esophageal etiology helpful? Am J Gastroenterol 1987;82:215. (*The reassurance provided reduced morbidity and even the frequency of episodes.*)

27. Richter JE, Dalton CB, Bradley LA, et al. Oral nifedipine in the treatment of noncardiac chest pain in patients with the nutcracker esophagus. Gastroenterology 1987;93:21. (*Found disappointing results, although these agents show an ability to decrease pressure.*)

CHAPTER 61 ■ APPROACH TO THE PATIENT WITH HEARTBURN AND REFLUX (GASTROESOPHAGEAL REFLUX DISEASE)

FRANCIS X. CAMPION AND JAMES M. RICHTER

"*Heartburn,*" a nearly universal experience of retrosternal burning that radiates upward as a consequence of gastric acid reflux into the esophagus, may be a harmless transient phenomenon as well as a manifestation of gastroesophageal reflux disease (GERD). In Western nations, the prevalence of GERD ranges from 10% to 20%; in Asian nations, approximately 5% of persons report GERD, but the incidence appears to be growing. When recurrent heartburn is encountered, key tasks include selecting the most cost-effective approach to controlling symptoms, deciding who requires endoscopic assessment, and preventing stricture and cancer.

PATHOPHYSIOLOGY AND CLINICAL PRESENTATION (1–11)

Normal Esophageal Physiology

The physiologic action of the *lower esophageal sphincter* (LES) is critical to maintaining a pressure barrier between the stomach and the esophagus. The LES is a complicated region of smooth muscle modulated by the interaction of hormonal, neural, and dietary factors. Gastrin increases its resting tone; estrogens, progesterone, glucagon, secretin, and cholecystokinin all decrease sphincter pressure. Vagus nerve input helps to maintain resting tone, as does α-adrenergic stimulation. Pharmacologic agents that increase sphincter tone include bethanechol, metoclopramide, pentobarbital, histamine, edrophonium, and antacids. Anticholinergics, theophylline, meperidine, and the calcium-channel blockers all decrease resting tone. Saliva may add an important protective mechanism, inducing peristalsis in addition to aiding in washout, dilution, and neutralization of acid refluxed into the esophagus.

Mechanisms of Reflux

GERD is a multifactorial problem, involving *reduction in resting LES tone*, transient episodes of *inappropriate relaxation* of the LES, irritant action of *gastric acid* and *digestive enzymes*, *decreased secondary peristalsis*, and *defective mucosal resistance* to caustic liquids. Also implicated are *impaired esophageal clearance* of acid from the esophagus and *delayed gastric emptying*.

LES pressures in normal persons and those with symptomatic reflux vary considerably and frequently overlap. Pressures between 6 and 20 mm Hg are found in both patients and controls. Normal pressure ranges from 12 to 30 mm Hg; pressures below 6 mm Hg are apt to allow reflux, and those above 20 mm Hg usually prevent it. In many patients, reflux occurs as a result of transient episodes of inappropriate sphincter relaxation rather than low basal tone. *Anatomic factors*, such as the presence of a *hiatus hernia*, are not as important as they once were believed to be, but patients with hiatus hernia may be modestly predisposed to reflux disease. A portion of the esophagus must be situated intraabdominally for optimal esophageal function and sphincter competence; moreover, peristaltic clearing of acid is impaired in patients with a hiatus hernia. *Obesity* increases the risk of symptomatic GERD, particularly in premenopausal women and those taking estrogen, which suggests a contributing role for estrogen.

Contributing factors include *tobacco, ethanol, chocolate,* and foods with high concentrations of *fat* or *carbohydrate,* all of which decrease LES pressure and increase heartburn. *Citrus fruits* and fruit juices may exacerbate symptoms; the mechanism by which they cause heartburn is not clear. Although *pregnancy* may cause reflux because of increased intraabdominal pressure, the primary reason for heartburn in pregnancy is reduced sphincter pressure as a consequence of increased circulating levels of progesterone and estrogen. Reflux can be precipitated in normal persons by *exercise*, with jogging after meals the most common cause. There is no clear etiologic link between *Helicobacter pylori infection* and GERD; in fact, the frequency of *H. pylori* in GERD populations appears to be lower than in those without GERD.

Clinical Features

Heartburn

Heartburn often accompanies gastroesophageal reflux. Exacerbating factors include large meals, supine posture, and bending over; food and antacids provide temporary relief. Severity ranges from an occasional episode of postprandial discomfort without sequelae to a syndrome of marked esophageal inflammation that can lead to bleeding, stricture, and malignant transformation. The patient characteristically complains of retrosternal ache or burning within 30 to 60 minutes of eating, especially after large meals. Many patients learn to avoid lying down after meals. Reflux may trigger esophageal *chest pain* that can mimic cardiac angina, with some patients describing chest heaviness or pressure that, like angina, may radiate to the neck, jaw, or shoulders (see Chapters 20 and 60); pain may also radiate interscapularly, mimicking aortic dissection.

Regurgitation

Regurgitation of fluid or food particles may occur, particularly at night. The patient may describe soiling of the pillow with gastric contents or may awake because of coughing or a strangling sensation. *Nocturnal aspiration* is occasionally associated with gastroesophageal reflux and can cause recurrent pneumonias, bronchospasm, and chronic cough. Patients with reflux sometimes describe a reflex salivary hypersecretion or *"water brash."* Water brash is especially common in children, but direct questioning is often required to determine its occurrence.

Hoarseness, *sore throat*, and the feeling of a *lump in the throat* are other common otolaryngologic manifestations of reflux.

Painful or Difficult Swallowing (Odynophagia, Dysphagia)

Painful or difficult swallowing usually suggests longstanding reflux disease with active inflammation, stricture, or both. Solid food may stick in the distal esophagus (with or without stricture formation), although food usually passes into the stomach after repeated swallowing or drinking liquids unless a fairly tight obstruction is present (see Chapter 60). Odynophagia is seen in cases complicated by severe erosion and may be a symptom of malignancy or infection.

Barrett's Esophagus and Adenocarcinoma

A strong, severity-related risk for *adenocarcinoma of the esophagus* is conferred by symptomatic reflux. In a substantial number of patients with longstanding severe reflux, a premalignant change develops that is referred to as *Barrett's esophagus,* which denotes metaplastic columnar epithelialization of the distal esophagus (annual incidence, 0.6%; prevalence, 10% among those with reflux lasting >20 years). Barrett's esophagus is believed to represent a reparative response to tissue injury from chronic exposure to gastric acid, pepsin, and bile. Histologically, the normal stratified squamous epithelium of the mucosa is replaced by columnar epithelium. Dysplastic transformation may ensue and eventually lead to adenocarcinoma. The risk for the development of adenocarcinoma with onset of Barrett's esophagus is less than 1% annually but rises 5-fold with the onset of low-grade dysplasia and 10-fold in persons with high-grade dysplasia. Symptoms are those of reflux and its complications.

Esophageal Ulcers, Strictures, and Hemorrhage

Esophageal ulcers, strictures, and *hemorrhage* may also develop as a consequence of chronic severe esophagitis. *Bleeding* may be slow and chronic, resulting in iron-deficiency anemia, or brisk, resulting in hematemesis.

Dental Erosions

Dental erosions occur in a substantial proportion of patients with marked reflux as a consequence of the effects of acid and bile on tooth enamel. Patients with teeth erosions of unknown etiology are often found to have reflux on evaluation.

Reflux-Induced Asthma and Laryngitis

Reflux-induced asthma and laryngitis are among the airway consequences of chronic GERD. Unexplained wheezing, voice change, chronic cough, and lump in the throat are among the symptoms reported; reflux must be considered when such complaints develop in the absence of a known cause.

DIFFERENTIAL DIAGNOSIS (1)

The diagnosis of gastroesophageal reflux disease is secure when the patient describes heartburn and experiences regurgitation of stomach contents. However, many patients report only a dull substernal discomfort or ache, and in such circumstances, the physician must consider *myocardial ischemia*, esophageal *spasm* or high-amplitude *esophageal peristalsis, cholelithiasis,* and *mediastinal inflammation*. Gastroesophageal reflux may accompany *peptic ulcer disease* (particularly in gastric hypersecretory conditions) and *cancer* of the gastroesophageal junction. Esophageal *infections* with opportunistic organisms such as cytomegalovirus, herpes virus, and *Candida albicans* can cause heartburn in the immunocompromised host. Reflux esophagitis may also accompany intestinal dysmotility syndromes, including intestinal pseudoobstruction and scleroderma. *Diabetic gastroparesis* may predispose a patient to reflux and heartburn because of retarded emptying of gastric contents.

WORKUP (1,12–15)

History

The characteristic history of a retrosternal burning sensation radiating upward, associated with large meals and supine posture, is virtually diagnostic of reflux disease. An attempt should be made to identify any aggravating factors, such as intake of fatty foods, concentrated sweets, chocolate, alcohol, peppermint, coffee, tea, anticholinergics, calcium-channel blockers, and theophylline compounds. The use of drugs capable of causing esophageal injury (nonsteroidal antiinflammatory drugs, quinidine, wax-matrix potassium chloride tablets, tetracycline, and bisphosphonates) should also be elicited. Inquiry should be made regarding response to food or antacids. Surgery near the gastroesophageal junction (e.g., antireflux surgery or vagotomy) may predispose the patient to reflux disease. A history of Raynaud's phenomenon raises the possibility of scleroderma. Consideration of achalasia, malignancy, esophagitis, and stricture is indicated if dysphagia is part of the clinical presentation (see Chapter 60).

Physical Examination

The physical examination is generally unrevealing, but several points are worth special attention. Sclerodactyly, calcinosis, and telangiectasia suggest underlying scleroderma (see Chapter 146). The epigastrium should be carefully examined for the presence of a mass lesion, and the stool should be examined for occult blood. Dental erosions, hoarseness of voice, and wheezing may be observed.

Diagnostic Studies and Empiric Trials

No single test is accepted as the standard for the diagnosis of reflux disease. Fortunately, a careful history is sufficient to establish the diagnosis in the majority of patients, and laboratory tests are needed only in atypical or severe cases. When a classic reflux story is elicited, initial therapy can be instituted on the basis of history alone for simple heartburn in a young patient. A brief trial of high-dose proton pump inhibitor therapy is a reasonably sensitive (75%) and cost-effective confirmatory test in patients with classic GERD symptoms.

Esophageal pH Monitoring and Physiologic Testing

Esophageal pH monitoring for 24 hours is the most sensitive and specific test for reflux, but it is usually unnecessary for common cases of GERD. However, it does allow correlation of distal esophageal pH with symptoms, and can be of help in confusing situations, such as atypical chest pain, ear, nose, and throat symptoms, and pulmonary symptoms (see Chapter 60). Two-channel pH monitoring includes a second probe near the proximal esophagus and may identify acid reflux causing airway irritation. Two other tests, *esophageal manometry* and *esophageal impedance studies*, can be even more sensitive than the pH probe by giving some inference of the volume of refluxant.

Esophagoscopy and Barium Swallow

Dysphagia, painful swallowing, significant weight loss, or occult blood loss necessitates ruling out neoplasm and stricture, best assessed by *endoscopy* in conjunction with *biopsy*. *Barium swallow* may also reveal signs of neoplasm or stricture, but it does not obviate the need for biopsy; the test remains widely used for the diagnosis of reflux, but its sensitivity may be as low as 25%, and it is far less accurate than a careful history.

MANAGEMENT (1,16–29)

A stepwise approach is recommended in the latest national consensus guidelines for the diagnosis and management of GERD. Otherwise, healthy patients with a classic history of uncomplicated reflux can be treated empirically, first with simple *nonpharmacologic measures* and then the addition of *pharmacologic intervention* as needed (Table 61.1). For many patients, lifestyle modifications, changes in food selection, and antacids as needed will suffice. For those patients who do not achieve symptomatic control with these measures, a *"step-up"* or *"step-down"* approach may be used for advancing medication. The step-up approach begins with a histamine$_2$ blocker (H$_2$-blocker) with change to a proton pump inhibitor (PPI) and then the addition of prokinetic agents. A step-down approach begins with a PPI and then tapers to H$_2$-blocker therapy. The goals are similar: to heal injury, relieve symptoms, and achieve maintenance with the least amount of medication necessary.

The small subgroup of "functional heartburn" patients who do not respond to standard-dose treatment should be given a trial of more intensive PPI therapy and, if unsuccessful, referred for consideration of additional workup (see prior discussion), especially if a patient fails to respond or manifests dysphagia, weight loss, anemia, or a stool test positive for occult bleeding. A detailed evaluation is especially important in older patients, in whom the risk for malignancy is increased.

Step 1: Lifestyle Modification

The first and most important steps are *dietary intervention*, *lifestyle modification*, and *antacids* (Table 61.1, step 1, and Chapter 68, Tables 68.1 and 68.2). Attention to these measures is essential to a good outcome; they often suffice. Even if additional therapy is needed; these conservative measures constitute the foundation of all treatment programs and must not be omitted. They represent the most cost-effective approach to therapy for the majority of patients.

Step 2: Suppression of Gastric Acid Production

A major objective of symptomatic therapy is a reduction in esophageal exposure to gastric acid. When step 1 measures fail to suffice, suppression of gastric acid production can be implemented with either an H$_2$-blocker or a PPI. In the United States, both classes of drug are available in low-dose preparations without a prescription. Many patients present only after their trial of nonprescription treatment has failed. For low-risk

TABLE 61.1

TREATMENT OF ESOPHAGEAL REFLUX

Step 1: Lifestyle Modification
  a. Dietary manipulations: avoidance of foods high in fat or carbohydrate (chocolate can be particularly problematic, being high in both)
  b. Weight reduction if obese
  c. Avoidance of large evening meals near bedtime or before exercise
  d. Elevation of the head of the bed with 6-in. blocks under the bedposts or a foam wedge between the mattress and the box spring (pillows under the head are not adequate)
  e. Avoidance, if possible, of medications that decrease sphincter tone, including theophylline compounds, calcium-channel blockers, meperidine, and anticholinergics
  f. Avoidance, if possible, of drugs that may injure the esophageal mucosa (tetracycline, quinidine, wax-matrix potassium chloride tablets, nonsteroidal antiinflammatory drugs)
  g. Avoidance of cigarettes, alcohol, and coffee

Step 2: Suppression of Gastric Acid Production
  a. Antacids after meals and at bedtime
  b. Oral histamine$_2$ blocker (twice-daily regimen is best, e.g., ranitidine 150 mg, cimetidine 800 mg, famotidine 20 mg)
  c. Proton pump inhibitor (e.g., omeprazole 20–40 mg/d or lansoprazole 15–30 mg/d), treatment of choice for erosive esophagitis and Barrett's esophagus

Step 3: Promotility Therapy
  a. Metoclopramide (a dopamine antagonist) 10–15 mg four times daily
  b. Bethanechol (a cholinergic agent) 25 mg four times daily

Step 4: Antireflux Surgery
  a. Discuss surgery for severe, difficult-to-control, or persistent symptoms
  b. Nissen fundoplication, laparoscopy
  c. Endoscopic procedures: "EndoCinch" (endoscopic sewing); "Stretta procedure" (radiofrequency energy applied to the cardia and distal esophagus)
  d. Other procedures await clinical trials and U.S. Food and Drug Administration approval

Adapted from De Vault K, Castell D. Updated guidelines for the diagnosis and treatment of gastroesophageal reflux disease. Am J Gastroenterol 2005;100:190, with permission.

patients, the goal is to use as little medication as necessary and use symptom-relief as the measure of efficacy.

Histamine$_2$-Blocker Treatment

H$_2$-blocker treatment (Table 61.1, step 2) can be used in place of or in combination with antacid therapy (antacid contributing to the immediate neutralizing of postprandial acid, and H$_2$-blocker providing more-sustained acid suppression). Because H$_2$-blocker absorption may by reduced by up to 20% when an H$_2$-blocker is taken with antacids, the two agents should not be taken at the same time. H$_2$-blockers are more convenient to use than a high-dose antacid program and provide better around-the-clock symptom relief and esophageal healing. A twice-daily, full-dose regimen achieves best results (e.g., 800 mg of cimetidine twice daily, 150 mg of ranitidine twice

daily, or 20 mg of famotidine twice daily). In milder cases of reflux, a once-daily dose at the time of maximal symptoms often suffices, supplemented when necessary by an antacid for prompt relief of any breakthrough heartburn.

Proton Pump Inhibitors

Proton pump inhibitors afford the most rapid relief of symptoms and the greatest degree of mucosal healing compared to other pharmacologic measures, such as H$_2$-blockers and antacids. A single daily dose of a PPI achieves nearly complete suppression of gastric acid production. It has demonstrated efficacy in healing erosive lesions and controlling refractory symptoms. However, relapses after completion of therapy are common, so long-term maintenance therapy must be considered, especially in persons with erosive esophagitis (see later discussion). Patients with GERD-associated asthma and chronic cough may need double the standard dose of PPI to achieve improvement in these symptoms. *Choice of PPI should be based on cost and interactions with other medications; side effects are similar* (see Chapter 68). PPIs, especially branded formulations, can be very costly; the increasing availability of generics (e.g., omeprazole) has helped to lower cost. The need to take PPIs with meals, differences in bioavailability, and genetic variation in enzyme capacity lead to variable responses among patients. Choosing between PPI therapy and H$_2$-blocker treatment is a matter of how much the extra cost is worth in terms of effect on the quality of life in persons with mild to moderate disease.

Step 3: Promotility Therapy

Some patients will report persistent symptoms despite the foregoing measures. In such situations, prokinetic drugs have been used in an attempt to increase LES pressure and halt reflux (Table 61.1, step 3).

Metoclopramide

Metoclopramide, a dopamine-receptor antagonist, is the leading choice for prokinetic therapy. The drug augments gastric emptying and raises LES tone. It is most useful for patients who have reflux without severe heartburn and those with gastroparesis. However, up to one third of patients may not tolerate the drug because of its central nervous system side effects. *Cisapride*, a dopamine antagonist that had been useful for treatment of reflux, has been removed from general availability in the United States due to reports of serious cardiac arrhythmias (torsades de pointes) associated with its prolongation of the QT interval.

Bethanechol

Bethanechol, a potent cholinergic agonist, raises LES pressure, increases salivary flow, and improves acid clearance by the esophagus. However, because of its cholinergic side effects, it is not particularly well tolerated. The drug is contraindicated in patients with asthma and other conditions in which cholinergic therapy may aggravate symptoms.

Step 4: Antireflux Surgery and Endoscopic Procedures

Antireflux surgery is best reserved for patients who experience severe or persistent reflux symptoms. *Nissen laparoscopic fundoplication* has become the standard for surgical intervention in GERD, involving fundoplication, crural tightening, and return of the esophagogastric junction to below the diaphragm. It can be as effective as PPI therapy in carefully selected patients, particularly those who are young, have typical GERD symptoms, have an abnormal pH study, and have a good response to PPI therapy; however, durability of the repair varies among patients as reported in clinical trials. Normal gastric emptying should be demonstrated before a patient is subjected to surgery. For most patients, preoperative assessment should include upper endoscopy, esophageal manometry, and a 24-hour pH monitor test.

Approximately 65% of patients are able to discontinue PPI therapy after antireflux surgery; however, laparoscopic antireflux surgery has yet to demonstrate better cost-effectiveness than maintenance medical therapy with PPIs; moreover, many patients who undergo surgery still require some antisecretory therapy for control of symptoms. There is no advantage over PPI therapy in terms of developing Barrett's esophagus, stricture, or malignancy. A major complication of surgery is difficulty with gastric emptying, which can lead to chronic bloating. Additional risks include dysphagia and decreased ability to belch, which can exacerbate bloating and flatulence.

Endoscopic procedures are showing promise in improving reflux symptoms, but failure to document normalization with ambulatory pH testing and the frequent need for continued PPI therapy suggest limits to their efficacy. The "*EndoCinch*" *device* is used for endoscopic sewing; the "*Stretta procedure*" uses radiofrequency treatment of the cardia and distal esophagus. *Full-thickness plication* and injection of a nonresorbable substance into the lower esophageal sphincter have become available. Physicians are encouraged to await proper scientific studies and assessment of longer-term outcomes before adopting these newer therapies.

Maintenance Therapy

Management of gastroesophageal reflux disease can be a challenge because of its chronicity and frequent symptomatic relapses. Lifestyle and pharmacologic measures may need to be continued indefinitely, especially in the setting of severe disease. Patients have been maintained on *H2-blockers* and *PPIs* for years with a good safety profiles.

Indications

Persons with endoscopically documented erosive esophagitis should be considered candidates for long-term maintenance PPI therapy, but only after a symptomatic recurrence and only if that recurrence has taken place in the context of full implementation of dietary and other nonpharmacologic measures. Immediate implementation of PPI maintenance therapy before a symptomatic recurrence should be reserved for those with a severe erosion (grade 4) and those in whom symptoms cause a reduction in quality of life (>25%). The ability of PPI therapy to reduce the risk for development of Barrett's esophagus remains to be determined.

Safety

Initial concerns about the safety of long-term PPI therapy (e.g., risk for gastrin-stimulated carcinoid stomach tumors, as noted in mice) have not materialized in clinical practice, so most authorities prescribe long-term PPI treatment when necessary. The possibility of the development of atrophic gastritis (a risk factor for gastric carcinoma) as a consequence of long-term PPI therapy in persons with concurrent *H. pylori* infection should be kept in mind, and any *Helicobacter* infection should be eradicated (see Chapter 68). Because of their safety, several of these agents are available for purchase without a prescription. Long-term safety studies are ongoing for these drugs.

If prolonged PPI use is a concern, then one can consider a maintenance program of long-term *H2-blocker* therapy. Sometimes, reduced doses suffice (e.g., 150 mg of ranitidine daily at bedtime). Although H_2-blockers are not as effective as PPIs in healing and preventing recurrences of erosive esophagitis, they may suffice for controlling symptoms.

Screening for and Management of Barrett's Esophagus

Barrett's esophagus represents a serious complication of chronic reflux disease due to its association with esophageal cancer, necessitating consideration of screening and aggressive treatment.

Screening and Surveillance

Although GERD-related cancer risk is low and the value of screening has not yet been proven in randomized trial, current consensus guidelines favor endoscopic screening for Barrett's esophagus in persons who have had chronic severe GERD symptoms. Current guidelines acknowledge that although the age threshold for initial endoscopy is not established, those with more than 5 years of severe symptoms, particularly older white men, are at greatest risk and the best candidates for at least a single screening. Those persons found to have Barrett's esophagus changes are candidates for *endoscopic surveillance* and biopsy, with the surveillance interval a function of presence and grade of dysplasia. Those with Barrett's histology but no dysplasia on two consecutive annual biopsies can have their surveillance interval extended to every 3 years. The finding of low-grade dysplasia requires more frequent surveillance (e.g., every 6 months); the finding of high-grade dysplasia is an indication for consideration of *surgery*. Surveillance is offered only to persons sufficiently fit and willing to undergo surgery should severe dysplasia or early cancer be found. Results from randomized trials are needed. Improved means for detecting dysplasia are under investigation.

Treatment

Medical therapy for Barrett's esophagus is similar to that for erosive disease (e.g., long-term *PPI* therapy; see earlier discussion). The immediate goal is to eliminate symptoms of heartburn and regurgitation. Although Barrett's esophagus is not known to be reversible by medical therapy, it is hoped that long-term PPI therapy will reduce the risk for progression to dysplasia and cancer by minimizing further esophageal injury. Attempts to reverse the histologic changes associated with Barrett's esophagus are under study and include a variety of *ablative approaches* based on *laser* and other techniques in combination with PPI therapy. The hope is that by removing the metaplastic epithelial tissue and providing a reduced acid environment, the esophagus will heal by laying down normal squamous mucosa. *Surgical therapy* that restores the integrity of the gastroesophageal junction appears no better than PPI therapy for prevention or reversal of Barrett's changes or for reducing the risk of cancer.

Chronic Cough

In some patients, chronic reflux has resulted in respiratory problems, particularly chronic cough, believed to be caused by nocturnal reflux and subsequent aspiration (see Chapter 41). Pharyngitis, nocturnal coughing and choking spells, and wheezing have also been described. A trial of high-dose antireflux therapy is indicated when a patient with chronic pulmonary complaints reports symptoms of reflux. Several weeks of treatment may be needed to allow for airway healing before symptom resolution is noted. Any use of theophylline for pulmonary complaints in patients with reflux should be stopped because it can aggravate the problem by reducing LES pressure (see Chapter 48).

PATIENT EDUCATION AND INDICATIONS FOR REFERRAL

Successful management depends on the patient's compliance with medications, diet, and postural measures. A thorough explanation of the mechanisms of reflux and its aggravating factors helps to provide a rational basis for the patient's action. Patients need to realize that no single measure will alleviate the discomfort of reflux, but when all are performed together, relief is extremely likely. The lack of direct connection between hiatus hernia and reflux also deserves mention because this is commonly misunderstood, often leading to a belief that surgery is required for treatment.

The chief indication for referral is consideration of endoscopy, indicated in persons with chronic symptomatic disease of at least 5 years' duration, dysphagia, odynophagia, unexplained weight loss, or iron-deficiency anemia. Patients who are pregnant or have supraesophageal symptoms such as persistent cough, laryngeal symptoms, or aspiration should be considered for specialty referral. The increased awareness of the association between severe chronic GERD and adenocarcinoma of the esophagus has stimulated interest in early diagnosis, especially in detection of premalignant change such as Barrett's esophagus. Surgical referral is worth considering in persons who remain symptomatic despite maximal medical therapy. Modern laparoscopic techniques provide minimally invasive approaches to surgical correction; however, some questions remain regarding the durability of such corrections.

Annotated Bibliography

1. DeVault K, Castell D. Updated guidelines for the diagnosis and treatment of gastroesophageal reflux disease. Am J Gastroenterol 2005;100:190. (*Consensus statement of the Practice Parameters Committee of the American College of Gastroenterology.*)
2. El-Serag HB, Time trends of gastroesophageal reflux disease: a systematic review. Clin Gastroenterol Hepatol 2007:5:17.(*A careful review of 17 studies tracking gastroesophageal reflux disease [GERD] in 10 countries.*)
3. Lagergren J, Bergstrom A, Lindgren A, et al. Symptomatic gastroesophageal reflux as a risk factor for esophageal adenocarcinoma. N Engl J Med 1999;340:825. (*A population study demonstrating a strong, dose-related, independent risk for adenocarcinoma of the esophagus conferred by symptomatic reflux.*)
4. Karamanolis G, Sifrim D. Developments in pathogenesis and diagnosis of gastroesophageal reflux disease. Curr Opin Gastroenterol 2007;24(4):428.(*An excellent review including options for physiologic testing to differentiate manifestations of GERD including cough and non-acid reflux.*)
5. Mittal RK, Balaban DH. The esophagogastric junction. N Engl J Med 1997;336:924. (*Excellent review of pathophysiology; 54 references.*)
6. Nilsson M, Johnsen R, Ye W, et al. Obesity and estrogen as risk factors for gastroesophageal reflux. JAMA 2003;290:66. (*A population-based, cross-sectional, case–control study that found significant association between body mass index and reflux, especially in premenopausal women and those taking estrogens.*)
7. Raghunath A, Hungin AP, Wooff D, et al. Prevalence of *Helicobacter pylori* in patients with gastro-oesophageal reflux disease: systematic review. BMJ 2003;326:1460. (*In pooled results of 20 studies, Helicobacter pylori was actually less common in persons with GERD.*)
8. Shaheen N, Ransohoff DF. Gastroesophageal reflux, Barrett esophagus, and esophageal cancer: scientific review. JAMA 2002;287:1972. (*A systematic review that found insufficient evidence to support the routine endoscopic screening of GERD patients; 43 references.*)
9. Shay S, Richter J. Direct comparison of impedance, manometry, and pH probe in detecting reflux before and after a meal. Dig Dis Sci 2005;50:1584. (*Impedance monitoring can be more sensitive then 24 pH probe studies and manometry before and after a meal but is not yet widely available.*)
10. Splecher SJ. Barrett's esophagus. N Engl J Med 2002;346:836. (*Excellent review; especially helpful in pointing out areas where no evidence exists on critical issues; 57 references.*)
11. Weaver EM. Association between gastroesophageal reflux and sinusitis, otitis media, and laryngeal malignancy: a systematic review of the evidence. Am J Med Sci 2003;115 (Suppl 3A):81S. (*A literature review that found evidence for a positive association between GERD and sinusitis and laryngeal malignancy, but none with otitis media.*)
12. Chang AB, Lasserson TJ, Connor FL, et al. Systematic review and meta-analysis of randomized controlled trials of gastro-esophageal reflux interventions for chronic cough associated with gastroesophageal reflux. BMJ 2006;32:11. (*A meta-analysis that found that proton pump inhibitors [PPIs] were more effective than placebo in treating chronic cough related to GERD*).
13. Fennerty MB. Use of antisecretory agents as a trial of therapy. Gut 2002;50(Suppl 4):iv63. (*Evidence for using PPI therapy as a cost-effective means for diagnosing GERD and achieving symptom control.*)
14. Richter JE. Diagnostic tests for gastroesophageal reflux disease. Am J Med Sci 2003;326:300. (*Review of tests for diagnosis and management of routine cases and patients with refractory symptoms.*)
15. Sampliner RE. The Practice Parameters Committee of the American College of Gastroenterology. Practice guidelines on the diagnosis, surveillance and therapy of Barrett's esophagus. Am J Gastroenterol 2002;97:1888. (*Consensus statement.*)
16. Feldman M. Comparison of the effects of over-the-counter famotidine and calcium carbonate antacid on postprandial gastric acid: a randomized controlled trial. JAMA 1996;275:1428. (*Effects on gastric acidity were similar, but the antacid had a more rapid onset and a shorter duration of action.*)
17. Galmiche JP, Bruley des Varannes S. Endoluminal therapies for gastro-oesophageal reflux disease. Lancet 2003;361:1119. (*Review of endoscopic suturing, radiofrequency energy, and other therapies, with a good discussion of procedural morbidity and cost-effectiveness.*)
18. Harris RA, Kupperman M, Richter JE. Prevention of recurrences of erosive reflux esophagitis: a cost-effectiveness analysis of maintenance proton pump inhibition. Am J Med 1997;102:78. (*A decision analysis; maintenance therapy is cost-effective after a recurrence and at the outset only for those who have grade 4 disease or a marked decline in quality of life.*)
19. Heudebert GR, Centor RM, Klapow JC, et al. What is heartburn worth? A cost–utility analysis of management strategies. J Gen Intern Med 2000;15:175. (*Choice was based on the effect of reflux symptoms on the quality of life in persons with uncomplicated disease.*)
20. Howden CW, Castell DO, Cohen S, et al. The rationale for continuous maintenance treatment of reflux esophagitis. Arch Intern Med 1995;155:1465. (*A review supporting the long-term prophylactic use of acid neutralization in patients with severe esophagitis.*)
21. Inadomi JM, Sampliner R, Lagergren J, et al. Screening and surveillance for Barrett esophagus in high-risk groups: a cost–utility analysis. Ann Intern Med 2003;138:176. (*A cost-effectiveness study that found that one-time screening endoscopy followed by surveillance for those with Barrett's esophagus complicated by dysplasia was cost-effective.*)
22. Kiljander TO. The role of proton pump inhibitors in the management of gastroesophageal reflux disease related asthma and chronic cough. Gastroenterology 2003;115(Suppl 3A):65S. (*Detailed discussion of GERD-related asthma and management recommendations.*)
23. Klinkenberg-Knol EC, Festen HPM, Jansen JBMJ, et al. Long-term treatment with omeprazole for refractory reflux esophagitis: efficacy and safety. Ann

Intern Med 1994;121:161. (*Treatment of 5 years or more was effective but was associated with an increased frequency of atrophic gastritis.*)

24. Kuipers EJ, Lundell L, Klinkenberg-Knol EC, et al. Atrophic gastritis and *Helicobacter pylori* infection in patients with reflux esophagitis treated with omeprazole or fundoplication. N Engl J Med 1996;334:1018. (*Potentially important consequence of this infection and long-term use of PPI therapy.*)
25. Vigneri S, Termini R, Leandro G, et al. A comparison of five maintenance therapies for reflux esophagitis. N Engl J Med 1995;333:1106. (*PPIs are more effective than histamine$_2$ blockers.*)
26. Oleynikov D, Oelschlager B. New alternatives in the management of gastroesophageal reflux disease. Am J Surg 2003;186:106. (*Review of the surgical literature on laparoscopic and endoscopic therapies.*)
27. Richter JE. Let the patient beware: the evolving truth about laparoscopic antireflux surgery. Am J Med 2003;114:71. (*An editorial expertly summarizing available data and advantages and disadvantages of the surgical approach.*)
28. Richter JE. Medical management of patients with esophageal or supraesophageal gastroesophageal reflux disease. Am J Med Sci 2003;115(Suppl 3A):179S. (*Review of medical and surgical management, with details on the use of PPI therapy.*)
29. Robinson M, Lanza F, Avner D, et al. Effective maintenance treatment of reflux esophagitis with low-dose lansoprazole: a randomized, double-blind, placebo-controlled trial. Ann Intern Med 1996;124:859. (*Low-dose therapy is as effective as a full-dose program in persons with erosive esophagitis during the course of 1 year.*)

CHAPTER 62 ■ EVALUATION OF JAUNDICE

JAMES M. RICHTER

The onset of jaundice or dark urine usually prompts the patient or the patient's family to seek medical attention. When associated symptoms are minimal, the patient is likely to present on an ambulatory basis, concerned about hepatitis or cancer. The primary physician needs to distinguish jaundice caused by hepatocellular dysfunction (which can be managed medically) from that caused by biliary tract obstruction (which usually requires an anatomic intervention). More-specific determination of etiology is a secondary task that is less important to initial decision making. Effective clinical assessment necessitates familiarity with the mechanisms and clinical presentations of jaundice in addition to the indications for and limitations of the noninvasive diagnostic studies available in the outpatient setting.

PATHOPHYSIOLOGY AND CLINICAL PRESENTATION (1–3)

The mechanisms responsible for jaundice include excess bilirubin production, decreased hepatic uptake, impaired conjugation, intrahepatic cholestasis, extrahepatic obstruction, and hepatocellular injury. Clinically, jaundice becomes noticeable when the serum bilirubin level reaches 2.0 to 2.5 mg/100 mL. The yellow hue may be mimicked by carotenemia, but in the latter, no scleral icterus is present. Deeply jaundiced patients often demonstrate a greenish tinge resulting from the oxidation of bilirubin to biliverdin.

Excess Bilirubin Production

Excess bilirubin production results from accelerated red cell destruction. Occasionally, markedly ineffective erythropoiesis may be responsible. The excessive amounts of hemoglobin and resultant bilirubin released into the bloodstream overwhelm the normal hepatic capacity for uptake, and an unconjugated hyperbilirubinemia ensues. Total bilirubin rises as a result of the increased indirect fraction. The results of all tests of hepatocellular function are normal (as are urine and stool appearances). Symptoms, signs, and laboratory test findings point to hemolysis or ineffective erythropoiesis (see Chapter 79).

Decreased Uptake and Conjugation

Decreased uptake and conjugation are other mechanisms of unconjugated hyperbilirubinemia. The only evidence of hepatocellular dysfunction is an increase in unconjugated bilirubin. Frequently the cause is a concurrent acquired illness, such as an infection, cardiac disease, or cancer in a patient with a hereditary predisposition to decreased uptake and conjugation (*Gilbert's syndrome*). This benign disorder produces recurrent, self-limited episodes of mild jaundice; typically, the unconjugated fraction rises to no more than 1.5 to 3.0 mg/100 mL. Fasting and minor illness can also precipitate mild jaundice.

Intrahepatic Cholestasis

Intrahepatic cholestasis may occur at a number of levels: intracellularly (e.g., hepatitis), at the canalicular level (when estrogen induced), at the ductule (phenothiazine exposure), at the septal ducts (primary biliary cirrhosis), and at the intralobular ducts (cholangiocarcinoma). Regardless of site, there are similarities in presentation. Jaundice begins gradually; pruritus is common. The liver is large, smooth, and nontender; it may be firm but not rock-hard. Splenomegaly is unlikely except in primary biliary cirrhosis. Stools are pale, and steatorrhea develops in severe cases. A hyperbilirubinemia is present, predominantly of the conjugated fraction, with marked alkaline phosphatase elevation, mild transaminase rise, and normal serum albumin. Urine is dark and positive for bilirubin. The prothrombin time may be prolonged because of malabsorption, but the prolongation is reversible by vitamin K injection.

Extrahepatic Obstruction

Extrahepatic obstruction occurs when stone, stricture, or tumor block the flow of bile within the extrahepatic biliary tree.

A history of gallstones, biliary tract surgery, or prior malignancy may be elicited. The gallbladder is sometimes palpable, especially when cancer produces obstruction gradually, allowing time for painless dilation of the biliary tree. Sudden onset with pain results from passage of a stone that becomes wedged into the common duct; fever and sepsis may follow shortly thereafter, indicating cholangitis. Weight loss is a nonspecific finding, but when it is marked and accompanied by jaundice, it suggests carcinoma of the head of the pancreas or metastatic disease obstructing the common duct. Extrahepatic obstruction and intrahepatic cholestasis may be identical in presentation. The liver is usually enlarged; tenderness is minimal unless cholangitis or rapid distention occurs. A rock-hard mass strongly points to malignancy. As in intrahepatic cholestasis, conjugated bilirubin exhibits the greatest rise in association with a high serum alkaline phosphatase level and a mild to moderate increase in the transaminase level. Any prolongation of the prothrombin time is at least partially reversible with parenteral vitamin K. Urine is dark because of the conjugated bilirubinuria. Stools may be pale from absence of bile.

Hepatocellular Disease

Hepatocellular disease is typified by hepatitis, with prodromal symptoms of anorexia, nausea, abdominal pain, and malaise preceding jaundice (see Chapters 52 and 70). Hepatic tenderness and some hepatomegaly are common. Ecchymoses may be present. Transaminases may reach dramatic levels, except in cases of hepatitis C and alcoholic hepatitis, in which the rise is no more than five times normal. The alkaline phosphatase rises modestly to two to four times above the baseline. Urine is dark, and stools are pale. There may be evidence of decreased protein synthesis. The prothrombin time is the first measure of synthetic function to become abnormal because the half-lives of the clotting factors made in the liver are less than 7 days. If synthetic function remains depressed beyond 2 weeks, the serum albumin begins to fall. Chronic hepatocellular disease may lead to fibrosis and cirrhosis with portal hypertension, peripheral edema, ascites, gynecomastia, testicular atrophy, bleeding, and encephalopathy (see Chapter 71).

DIFFERENTIAL DIAGNOSIS (1)

The causes of jaundice are extensive but can be grouped according to major pathophysiologic mechanisms and type of hyperbilirubinemia (conjugated or unconjugated; Table 62.1). It is important to recognize that more than one mechanism can

---

TABLE 62.1

DIFFERENTIAL DIAGNOSIS OF JAUNDICE BY PATHOPHYSIOLOGIC MECHANISMS

> **Unconjugated Hyperbilirubinemias (Urine Negative for Bilirubin)**
> Increased bilirubin production
> Decreased hepatic uptake of bilirubin
> Decreased conjugation
> **Conjugated Hyperbilirubinemias (Urine Positive for Bilirubin)**
> Hepatocellular disease
> Intrahepatic cholestasis
> Extrahepatic obstruction

---

be operating in a given case. The vast majority of cases are caused by obstruction, intrahepatic cholestasis, or hepatocellular injury. In young patients, hepatitis predominates. In the elderly, stones and tumor are often responsible. Drugs account for many cases of intrahepatic cholestasis, with symptoms often mimicking those of extrahepatic etiologies.

WORKUP (1,4–18)

Overall Approach

The *history* and *physical examination* often provide a diagnosis or at least indicate whether the underlying pathophysiology is hepatocellular injury or biliary obstruction. In a study of 61 cases of jaundice documented by liver biopsy, history and physical examination alone correctly identified 70% of viral hepatitis cases, 80% of cirrhosis cases, and 77% of those with obstructive jaundice. The working pathophysiologic hypothesis (or hypotheses) can be tested and confirmed by a few basic laboratory studies.

History

Key historical items found useful for discriminating among etiologies include the presence of abdominal pain (indicative of obstruction) and a history of alcoholism, exposure to hepatitis, and flulike onset (all suggestive of a hepatocellular etiology). Of little discriminant value are a history of weight loss, pruritus, nausea, vomiting, and distaste for tobacco. Dark urine and pale stools confirm a conjugated hyperbilirubinemia but do not distinguish between hepatic and obstructive disease. Absence of abdominal pain does not rule out obstruction, especially that which develops slowly from tumor growth or primary biliary cirrhosis. The history should also be checked for other hepatocellular disease risk factors (e.g., previous blood transfusion, travel to an area endemic for hepatitis, consumption of raw shellfish, intravenous drug abuse, high-risk sexual practices, and use of potentially hepatotoxic drugs, especially acetaminophen). A history of gallstones, previous biliary tract surgery, and high fever points to an obstructive cause. A family history of episodic jaundice in the setting of an intercurrent illness is consistent with Gilbert's disease. Intrahepatic cholestasis is a consideration if the patient reports use of estrogens, phenothiazines, and other drugs that can cause cholestasis.

Physical Examination

Findings that favor a diagnosis of advanced hepatocellular disease include a small liver, signs of portal hypertension (ascites, splenomegaly, prominent abdominal venous pattern), asterixis, peripheral edema (from hypoalbuminemia), spider angiomata, gynecomastia, and palmar erythema. Mild to moderate hepatic enlargement and mild tenderness to punch are also consistent with early or mild hepatocellular disease, especially that caused by acute viral hepatitis. A palpable gallbladder (Courvoisier's sign) suggests malignant obstruction of the common bile duct. Marked hepatic enlargement (≥ 6 cm below the inferior costal margin) occurs in some instances of extrahepatic obstruction and also in advanced hepatic infiltration, severe passive hepatic congestion, and metastatic cancer to the liver. If obstruction is acute in onset, there may be some associated guarding, rebound tenderness, and fever. The finding of ecchymoses is consistent with both obstructive and hepatocellular mechanisms. The same is true for the detection of pale stools and dark urine.

Laboratory Investigation

Laboratory investigation is used to identify the predominant pathophysiology and to assess severity, especially when the history and physical examination findings are nondiagnostic. Testing may begin with a check of the urine for bilirubin, a simple, inexpensive, yet often overlooked test that can be performed quickly in the office. Because only conjugated bilirubin appears in the urine, its presence indicates a conjugated hyperbilirubinemia and the possibility of cholestasis, obstruction, or hepatocellular injury; its absence argues for excess bilirubin production, decreased uptake, and impaired conjugation. Determinations of direct and indirect serum bilirubin levels quantitatively confirm urinary findings and indicate disease severity.

Unconjugated Hyperbilirubinemia

An elevation predominantly of the unconjugated bilirubin fraction and urine negative for bilirubin should initiate a search for hemolysis (see Chapter 79), ineffective erythropoiesis, hereditary causes of jaundice, and concurrent systemic illness. Standard "liver function tests" add little to the assessment of unconjugated hyperbilirubinemia; results are normal or very mildly and nonspecifically elevated.

Conjugated Hyperbilirubinemia: Differentiating Hepatocellular Injury from Intrahepatic and Extrahepatic Cholestasis

The finding of bilirubin in the urine should focus attention on the liver and biliary tree. Testing needs to include determinations of serum transaminases (serum glutamic–oxaloacetic transaminase [SGOT], serum glutamic–pyruvic transaminase [SGPT]); the newer nomenclature refers to them as aminotransferases (aspartate aminotransferase [AST], alanine aminotransferase [ALT]). Alkaline phosphatase, prothrombin time, and serum albumin must also be determined. Mechanical obstruction and intrahepatic cholestasis are characterized by marked rises in alkaline phosphatase (four to five times normal) and modest elevations in transaminases (two to three times normal). The 5'-nucleotidase level rises similarly to the alkaline phosphatase level but more specifically. Hepatocellular disease characteristically causes a proportionately far greater rise in serum transaminase levels than in alkaline phosphatase concentrations. As noted earlier, two exceptions are hepatitis C and alcoholic hepatitis, in which transaminases may be only mildly elevated (no more than two to three times the upper limits of normal). SGPT (ALT) elevations are more specific for liver disease; SGOT (AST) also rises with myocardial or skeletal muscle injury.

The differentiation of hepatocellular disease from cholestatic and obstructive conditions can be attempted by studying measures of liver synthetic function and, if need be, their response to vitamin K. A prolonged prothrombin time unresponsive to parenteral vitamin K (intramuscular or subcutaneous administration is preferred because of reports of anaphylaxis with intravenous administration) is strongly suggestive of hepatocellular failure. Cholestasis and obstruction may also produce prolongation of the prothrombin time, but it can be reversed by vitamin K. Serum albumin levels fall when substantial hepatocellular injury has occurred and synthetic capacity has been suppressed for a few weeks. Interpretation of the albumin level requires consideration of dietary intake and sources of possible protein loss.

Liver biopsy is sometimes needed to determine the cause of hepatocellular injury (see also Chapters 70 and 71) but is contraindicated in the setting of suspected obstructive jaundice because bile peritonitis can ensue if there is ductal dilation. Once obstruction is ruled out or relieved, biopsy can proceed, especially when evidence of hepatic failure, portal hypertension, or encephalopathy is present or when jaundice persists longer than 3 months.

Marked Elevation in Alkaline Phosphatase: Differentiating Extrahepatic Obstruction from Intrahepatic Cholestasis

A marked elevation in alkaline phosphatase occurs in the setting of obstructive pathophysiology, as well as intrahepatic cholestasis. The latter occasionally occurs in some cases of hepatocellular injury, such as viral, alcoholic, and drug-induced forms of hepatitis. However, a low alkaline phosphatase level (<50 IU/100 mL) is rarely seen in the presence of extrahepatic obstruction. Elevations in alkaline phosphatase also occur in settings of increased bone metabolism. Bony causes can be distinguished from hepatobiliary causes by measuring the heat-stable fraction of the enzyme or the 5'-nucleotidase (these are of hepatobiliary tract origin).

Although hepatocellular disease can usually be distinguished from cholestasis and extrahepatic obstruction on the basis of clinical data and results of liver function tests (including response to vitamin K), cholestasis and obstruction may be indistinguishable without further testing. Clinical evaluation and liver function tests have a sensitivity of 90% for detection of obstruction, but they have a predictive value of only 75%; 25% of patients suspected on clinical grounds of having obstruction turn out to have intrahepatic cholestasis. The distinction is critical to management because mechanical obstruction requires direct surgical, endoscopic, or radiologic intervention to restore bile flow.

Thus, the clinical impression of obstruction must be confirmed by imaging techniques. Only when the clinical likelihood of obstruction is very low is imaging of the biliary tree unnecessary for differentiating intrahepatic cholestasis from extrahepatic obstruction. Available imaging modalities include the following.

Ultrasonography provides a low-cost, noninvasive approach to imaging the biliary tree in the evaluation of jaundice. Specificity is better than 90%. Sensitivity ranges from 47% to 90%, depending on the duration and degree of bile duct obstruction. Cases of early, acute, or intermittent obstruction may be missed unless ultrasonographic study is repeated after the ducts have had a few days to dilate. False-positive results may occur when ductal dilation persists after cholecystectomy or relief of obstruction. In about half of cases, ultrasonography cannot indicate the level of obstruction, nor is it particularly good at detecting the cause of the obstruction unless it is a mass in the head of the pancreas. Stones in the common duct are frequently missed (sensitivity of 50% if the duct is not dilated, 75% if the duct is dilated). Ultrasonographic studies in patients with overlying bowel gas or marked obesity are often of inadequate technical quality, so a repeated study or computed tomography is required.

Computed tomography is similar to ultrasonography in sensitivity, specificity, and predictive value for the diagnosis of obstructive jaundice. Unlike ultrasound, results are not obscured by overlying bowel gas or fat, and the test can detect the level of obstruction and provide anatomic detail better than ultrasound, which are helpful if surgical intervention is planned; however, radiation dose is significant. Cholangiography is usually still necessary.

Magnetic resonance cholangiopancreatography (MRCP) is an MR-based approach that provides enhanced detection of stones and other pathology in the common bile duct; sensitivity approaches that of invasive imaging modalities. The cost is high, but less than that of *endoscopic retrograde cholangiopancreatography* (ERCP), and safety is greater than other modalities because no radiation exposure or invasive procedure is required. MRCP is increasingly accurate and can be used to screen patients for ERCP candidacy.

Percutaneous transhepatic cholangiography or *ERCP* with retrograde cannulation of the common bile duct should be considered if common duct obstruction is strongly suspected on clinical grounds (even if ultrasonography or computed tomography is nondiagnostic) or if additional anatomic detail is required for planning treatment. Both invasive procedures are relatively safe, have similar complication rates and rates of visualization, and provide equally diagnostic information. The predictive value of a positive test result is very high, but occasionally stones are missed in dilated ductal systems.

Transhepatic cholangiography is technically simple in patients with dilated intrahepatic ducts; however, 3% to 10% of patients experience cholangitis, hemorrhage, or bile leakage. Endoscopic retrograde cholangiopancreatography and the newer *endoscopic ultrasonography* also allow examination of the ampulla and pancreas and have slightly lower incidences of serious complications. For patients who may have a retained common duct stone after cholecystectomy, the opportunity to perform an endoscopic papillotomy makes the retrograde cholangiogram advantageous. Techniques have been developed for draining an obstructed biliary tract either endoscopically or transhepatically. Overall, both procedures are valuable diagnostically and also have therapeutic uses; final selection is based on the clinical circumstance in addition to local availability and expertise. Selection should be made in consultation with a surgeon, radiologist, or gastroenterologist experienced in evaluating obstructive jaundice.

Ancillary Testing

Other studies deserve comment, more for their limited usefulness than because they are indicated in evaluation of jaundice.

Plain films of the abdomen and *upper gastrointestinal series* rarely provide diagnostic information. *Hepatobiliary scintigraphy* is better suited for the diagnosis of cholecystitis; it provides poor anatomic resolution and often cannot aid in distinguishing between intrahepatic cholestasis and extrahepatic obstruction. *Cholescintigraphy* has no value in the evaluation of jaundice and can be misleading.

INDICATIONS FOR ADMISSION, CONSULTATION, AND REFERRAL

Most patients with jaundice turn out to have acute viral hepatitis and can be managed on an ambulatory basis, unless they are unable to maintain their hydration or begin to show evidence of severe hepatocellular failure such as a prolonged prothrombin time (see Chapter 71). Admission is mandatory when jaundice is complicated by fever and peritoneal signs indicative of *cholangitis.* Intravenous antibiotics and prompt surgical consultation are required.

As noted earlier, if extrahepatic obstruction is suspected clinically, consultation with a gastroenterologist, surgeon, or radiologist experienced in the evaluation of jaundice can be very useful, especially when it is difficult to differentiate between intrahepatic cholestasis and extrahepatic obstruction.

When hepatocellular disease is suspected and evidence of hepatic failure, portal hypertension, or encephalopathy is present or when jaundice persists for longer than 3 months, liver biopsy may be indicated for definitive diagnosis. Consultation should be sought with a gastroenterologist familiar with liver disease and needle-biopsy techniques.

SYMPTOMATIC RELIEF

Mild jaundice in itself is innocuous, but more marked elevations in bilirubin may produce considerable pruritus. Presumably, the mechanism involves the deposition of bile salts in the skin, although recent evidence refutes this view. Cholestyramine has been used successfully to treat pruritus and is worth a try in patients who are uncomfortable. One 9-g packet of the powder containing 4 g of cholestyramine resin is mixed in orange juice or apple sauce and taken three times a day. Absorption of fat-soluble vitamins may be impaired by cholestyramine, and oral or parenteral supplements of vitamins A, D, and K can be prescribed. Cholestyramine may also interfere with the absorption of drugs; they should be taken at least 1 hour before cholestyramine. Constipation or diarrhea is a minor common side effect.

Annotated Bibliography

1. Frank BB, Members of the Patient Care Committee of the American Gastroenterological Association. Clinical evaluation of jaundice. JAMA 1989;262:3031. (*Comprehensive yet succinct overview of the approach to the jaundiced patient.*)
2. Felsher B, Rickard D, Redeker A. The reciprocal relation between caloric intake and the degree of hyperbilirubinemia in Gilbert's syndrome. N Engl J Med 1970;283:170. (*Increase in unconjugated bilirubin occurred with fasting or very low caloric intake.*)
3. Ostapowicz G, Fontana RJ, Schiodt FV, et al. Results of a prospective study of acute liver failure at 17 tertiary care centers in the United States. Ann Intern Med 2002;137:947. (*Acetaminophen overdose and idiopathic drug reactions are now more common than viral hepatitis as a cause of hepatic failure.*)
4. Trauner M, Meier PJ, Boyer JL. Molecular pathogenesis of cholestasis. N Eng J Med 1998;339:1217. (*A comprehensive review of recent developments in molecular and cellular biology.*)
5. Barish MA, Yucel EK, Ferrucci JT. Magnetic resonance cholangiopancreatography. N Engl J Med 1999;341:258. (*A review of this new, noninvasive alternative to endoscopic retrograde cholangiopancreatography for imaging the pancreaticobiliary tree.*)

6. Chan YL, Chan ACW, Lam WWM, et al. Choledocholithiasis: comparison of MR cholangiography and endoscopic retrograde cholangiopancreatography. Radiology 1996;200:85. (*Promising results for magnetic resonance imaging; sensitivity is in excess of 90%.*)

7. Datta D, Sherlock S. Cholestyramine for long-term relief of the pruritus complicating intrahepatic cholestasis. Gastroenterology 1966;50:323. (*Cholestyramine is effective; 4 to 7 days of therapy is required before relief is obtained.*)

8. Fregia A, Jensen DM. Evaluation of abnormal liver function tests. Comprehens Ther 1994;20:50. (*Assessment of abnormal liver function tests from a cost-conscious perspective.*)

9. Matzen P, Malchow-Moller A, Brun B. Ultrasound, computed tomography, and cholescintigraphy in suspected obstructive jaundice. Gastroenterology 1983;84:1492. (*Presents data on test sensitivity and specificity.*)

10. Mueller PR, van Sonnenberg E, Simenone JF. Fine needle trans-hepatic cholangiography. Ann Intern Med 1982;97:567. (*Discussion of this technique and its central role in the evaluation of biliary obstruction from the radiologist's perspective.*)

11. O'Connor KW, Snodgrass PJ, Swonder JE, et al. A blinded prospective study comparing four current noninvasive approaches in the differential diagnosis of medical versus surgical jaundice. Gastroenterology 1983;84:1498. (*Demonstrates the importance and accuracy of clinical evaluation.*)

12. Prati D, Taioli E, Zanella A, et al. Updated definitions of health ranges for serum alanine aminotransferase levels. Ann Intern Med 2002;137:1. (*A reconsideration of the definition of normal.*)

13. Pratt DS, Kaplan MM. Laboratory tests. In: Schiff's diseases of the liver, 8th ed. Schiff ER, Sorrell MF, Moddrey WC, eds. Philadelphia: Lippincott, 1999. (*A clinically useful review of the interpretation of liver function tests.*)

14. Richter JM, Silverstein MD, Schapiro RH. Suspected obstructive jaundice: a decision analysis of diagnostic strategies. Ann Intern Med 1983;99:46. (*Comparison of comprehensive diagnostic strategies for the investigation of suspected obstructive jaundice.*)

15. Saini S. Imaging of the hepatobiliary tract. N Engl J Med 1997;336:1889. (*Succinct, practical review with data on the sensitivity and the specificity of imaging studies; a good guide to test selection.*)

16. Scharschmidt BF, Goldberg HI, Schmid R. Approach to the patient with cholestatic jaundice. N Engl J Med 1983;308:1515. (*Good review of tests available for the workup of obstructive jaundice.*)

17. Sherman KE. Alanine aminotransferase in clinical practice. Arch Intern Med 1991;151:260. (*Review of this increasingly used aminotransferase for the detection of hepatocellular injury.*)

18. Shanmugam V, Beattie GC, Yule SR, et al. Is magnetic resonance cholangiopancreatography the new gold standard in biliary imaging? Br J Radiol 2005;78:888. (*Accuracy was similar to that of endoscopic retrograde cholangiopancreatography; it was less invasive and had fewer complications.*)

APPENDIX 62.1: EVALUATION OF THE PATIENT WITH AN INCIDENTAL ASYMPTOMATIC ELEVATION IN SERUM AMINOTRANSFERASE (TRANSAMINASE) LEVELS (1–3)

The incidental finding of an asymptomatic elevation in serum hepatic aminotransferase (transaminase) raises the question of underlying liver disease. Proper interpretation of an abnormal result and determination of when to initiate a workup for liver disease necessitate an understanding of the test and the differential diagnosis of asymptomatic elevations.

TESTING FOR SUBCLINICAL LIVER INJURY (1–3)

The serum ALT (SGPT) is widely used to screen for hepatocellular injury. The traditional upper limit of normal (40 U/L in men, 30 U/L in women) was established prior to appreciation for chronic hepatitis C and nonalcoholic steatohepatitis, resulting in asymptomatic persons with such conditions being included among "normals." When these individuals are excluded, the test's upper limit of normal requires downward revision (from 40 U/L to 30 U/L in men and from 30 U/L to 19 U/L in women). Doing so improves its sensitivity for the detection of liver disease without major compromise in specificity (e.g., sensitivity for the detection of asymptomatic chronic hepatitis C rises from 0.55 to 0.76, whereas specificity declines from 0.97 to 0.89).

In situations in which the pretest probability of underlying hepatocellular disease is very low (no risk factors for hepatitis C or nonalcoholic steatohepatitis), the probability of underlying liver disease is likely to be low. A positive result in such circumstances might warrant only a repeated determination in 4 weeks and cessation of intake of alcohol and any potentially offending drugs. However, before the finding is dismissed, it is important to assess for risk factors and subtle manifestations of conditions associated with long-term subclinical hepatocellular injury.

DIFFERENTIAL DIAGNOSIS (3–6)

The causes of such low-grade, subclinical hepatocellular injury include mild chronic *hepatitis C*, *hepatitis B*, and hepatitis associated with *autoimmune* disease (including *primary biliary cirrhosis*). Chronic occult liver injury may also occur in *hereditary hemochromatosis*, the most common genetic disorder among white Americans. Fatty liver is an important cause, resulting in half of the instances from surreptitious *alcohol* abuse; *nonalcoholic steatohepatitis* (NASH) accounts for the remainder of cases. About half of cases of NASH are a consequence of *obesity*, *hyperlipidemia*, or *diabetes*, but for another 40% to 50% of cases, no clear precipitant can be found. A rare cause of isolated aminotransferase elevation is *Wilson's disease*.

WORKUP (1–6)

Before an extensive workup is undertaken, the serum aminotransferase level should be repeated, usually at 4 weeks, after the patient has refrained from alcohol and any noncritical drugs with potential to cause hepatocellular injury. Once the elevation is confirmed, a focused workup should ensue.

History

History is reviewed for risk factors for viral hepatitis (see Chapter 57) and alcohol abuse (see Chapter 228), for symptoms of autoimmune disease (see Chapter 146), and for a family history of hemochromatosis or its complications (cirrhosis, heart failure, diabetes, arthritis) not explained by other causes. More commonly, persons with hereditary hemochromatosis may first note fatigue and arthralgias. Medications need to be reviewed in detail. In addition, a review of symptoms pertinent to estimating the severity of hepatocellular injury (fatigue, easy bruising, jaundice) should be included. A history of obesity, glucose intolerance, and hyperlipidemia may contribute to nonalcoholic steatosis.

Physical Examination

Physical examination should be noted for any etiologic clues or risk factors for liver disease, such as obesity (body mass index >25), hyperpigmentation, arthritis, and liver enlargement. Examining for signs of hepatocellular injury (jaundice, ecchymoses, spider angiomata) is also warranted.

Laboratory Studies

Laboratory studies can begin with an assessment of the type and severity of hepatocellular injury. Measuring the *alkaline phosphatase* level helps to determine whether the problem has a cholestatic component (see previous discussion). The *serum albumin* and *prothrombin time* are the best parameters of hepatocellular synthetic function and are helpful in determining degree of injury. Potentially useful diagnostic tests should be selected on the basis of clinical suspicion and not simply ordered uncritically as a standard panel for assessment of an isolated SGOT elevation.

If alcohol abuse is suspected, the diagnosis might be supported by a determination of the *SGPT* (ALT) and *SGOT* (AST); an SGPT-to-SGOT ratio of 2:1 is characteristic of alcoholic liver injury. *Hepatitis serologies* should be measured (e.g., antibodies to hepatitis B surface antigen, hepatitis C virus, and the hepatitis B surface antigen; see Chapter 57). Any suspicion of autoimmune disease is an indication for an *antismooth muscle antibody* determination (see Chapter 146) in addition to an *antimitochondrial antibody* determination. *Ultrasonography* is helpful to for assessing suspected fatty liver and the cholestatic pattern on liver function tests (see earlier discussion).

If the patient has a family history of idiopathic cirrhosis or other features of suggestive of hemochromatosis (fatigue, arthralgias, poor libido, diabetes), the serum *iron*, *transferrin* (total iron-binding capacity), and *ferritin* should be measured. A transferrin saturation (ratio of serum iron to total iron-binding capacity) greater than 45% is the screening threshold used by most authorities to diagnose hemochromatosis. The ferritin concentration helps to determine the degree of iron overload; treatment is usually indicated when it is greater than 300 ng/L in men and greater than 200 ng/L in women. The young patient with concurrent neuropsychiatric disease should be considered for a serum *ceruloplasmin* determination to check for Wilson's disease.

A key question is the utility of *liver biopsy* in persons who present with incidental aminotransferase elevation. Biopsy is certainly useful for determining disease extent and severity when a particular condition has been identified before biopsy (e.g., hepatitis C), but the contribution of biopsy to diagnosis in idiopathic cases is less clear. In a review of biopsies performed in such cases, steatosis was found in the vast majority of cases, and chronic hepatitis plus cirrhosis accounted only for about one fourth. One needs to ask whether the result will change management of the patient; if so, then biopsy for diagnosis is worth considering. Given the high frequency of occult steatosis, one might take an alternative approach to biopsy in the obese or diabetic person and recommend exercise, diet, and weight loss followed by a repetition of liver function tests.

A.H.G

Annotated Bibliography

1. Prati D, Taioli E, Zanella A, et al. Updated definitions of health ranges for serum alanine aminotransferase levels. Ann Intern Med 2002;137:1. (*A reconsideration of the definition of normal.*)
2. Pratt DS, Kaplan MM. Laboratory tests. In: Schiff's diseases of liver, 8th ed. ER Schiff, MF Sorrell, & WC Moddrey, eds. Philadelphia: Lippincott, 1999. (*A clinically useful review of the interpretation of liver function tests.*)
3. Sherman KE. Alanine aminotransferase in clinical practice. Arch Intern Med 1991;151:260. (*Review of this increasingly used aminotransferase for the detection of hepatocellular injury.*)
4. Kumar KS, Malet PF. Nonalcoholic steatohepatitis. Mayo Clin Proc 2000;75:733. (*Concise review; 38 references.*)
5. Powell LW, George DK, McDonnell SM, et al. Diagnosis of hemochromatosis. Ann Intern Med 1998;129:925. (*Best review of this important, often missed cause of incidental aminotransferase elevation; 41 references.*)
6. Sheth SG, Gordon FD, Chopra S. Nonalcoholic steatohepatitis. Ann Intern Med 1997;126:137. (*Detailed review.*)

CHAPTER 63 ■ EVALUATION OF GASTROINTESTINAL BLEEDING

JAMES M. RICHTER

Ambulatory patients frequently report gastrointestinal bleeding to the primary physician. They may complain of *melena* (tarry black stools), *hematochezia* (bright red or maroon blood per rectum), or *hematemesis* (vomiting fresh or changed blood). Sometimes, gastrointestinal bleeding may be occult and evident only as a *positive result on a screening test for fecal occult blood* or as *iron-deficiency anemia*. Decisions regarding the nature and pace of the evaluation of gastrointestinal bleeding depend on the characteristics, severity, and acuteness of the problem. Optimal decision making requires knowledge of the probability of a serious underlying lesion and of the sensitivity and specificity of radiographic studies, endoscopy, and stool guaiac testing.

PATHOPHYSIOLOGY AND CLINICAL PRESENTATION (1–10)

Hematemesis and Melena

Hematemesis usually represents bleeding proximal to the ligament of Treitz, although the site of blood loss may on rare occasions be in the jejunum. The absence of hematemesis does not, however, exclude the possibility of active upper gastrointestinal bleeding. *Melena* is typically seen with blood loss proximal to the ileocecal valve, where hemoglobin is converted into hematin, which gives the stool its tarry appearance. Right-sided colonic bleeding may also cause melena when transit is slow.

Representative prevalence figures from studies of outpatients and those seen in emergency departments presenting with melena or hematemesis find that about 35% have ulcer disease, 10% Mallory–Weiss tears, 10% esophageal varices, 5% gastritis, and 1% gastric cancer. In 20%, no cause is found, usually because endoscopy is not performed; in 5%, multiple lesions are detected.

Patients with chronic renal failure are at increased risk for bleeding, with vascular malformations and esophagitis being the most common causes.

Hematochezia

Hematochezia most often originates in the left side of the colon or anorectal region, although very brisk movement of blood from the right side of the colon, small bowel, or even stomach can lead to a similar presentation. *Occult gastrointestinal bleeding* may be indicated by a positive result on a test for fecal occult blood or may be suggested by the presence of iron-deficiency anemia without apparent cause. The source of occult bleeding may be anywhere in the gastrointestinal tract. In a study of anemic competitive runners, an increase in fecal hemoglobin was detected.

In the setting of *severe hematochezia,* age has a major influence on the differential diagnosis. In young adults, Meckel's diverticulum, inflammatory bowel disease, and polyps lead the list of causes. In adults to age 60 years, diverticulosis, inflammatory bowel disease, and polyps are the predominant etiologies, followed by malignancy and vascular malformations. In persons older than the age of 60 years, vascular malformations, diverticulosis, malignancy, and polyps are responsible for most cases.

Most patients who present with *mild to moderate anorectal bleeding* have lesions of the anal canal, about 15% have colorectal disease, and about 5% have perianal skin problems. Leading causes include hemorrhoids (about 50%) fissure-in-ano (20%), neoplasm (5%), and inflammatory bowel disease (5%). In close to 10% of cases, no cause is found at the time of the examination. The majority of neoplasms are more than 10 cm above the anus, beyond the reach of digital examination.

In patients with *undiagnosed rectal bleeding* subjected to colonoscopy, almost half have significant lesions; polyps, inflammatory bowel disease, cancer, diverticular disease, and vascular malformations are the leading findings.

Manifestations and Predictors of Blood Loss

Clinical manifestations are a function of the rate and duration of bleeding. *Postural hypotension* (an orthostatic fall in blood pressure of <10 mm Hg or an increase in heart rate of >10 beats/min on moving from a supine position to standing) in the setting of known bleeding suggests intravascular volume depletion and serious acute hemorrhage. *Fatigue* and *exertional dyspnea* are typical presenting symptoms of anemia resulting from slow, chronic blood loss. Patient descriptions of the volume of bleeding are frequently unreliable. Early predictors of severity of acute lower intestinal tract bleeding include heart rate greater than 100 beats/min, systolic blood pressure less than 115 mm Hg, syncope, nontender abdominal examination, early recurrent rectal bleeding, aspirin use, and two active comorbid conditions.

Gastrointestinal Bleeding in the Context of Therapeutic Oral Anticoagulation

Patients with gastrointestinal bleeding while taking anticoagulant medication *in the therapeutic range* are likely to have an underlying lesion and warrant thorough evaluation. In a study examining 3,800 courses of anticoagulant therapy, gastrointestinal bleeding occurred in 45 patients. In 32 patients, a source was determined; 13 had hemorrhoids, 9 had peptic ulcers, 7 had neoplasms, and 3 had other lesions. Risk of severe upper gastrointestinal hemorrhage is significantly increased by concurrent nonsteroidal antiinflammatory drug (NSAID) use, especially in the elderly.

DIFFERENTIAL DIAGNOSIS

The chief causes of gastrointestinal bleeding can be conveniently grouped by clinical presentation (Table 63.1). Hematemesis prompts consideration of important upper gastrointestinal etiologies. Melena requires consideration of upper gastrointestinal causes and of small-intestinal and right-sided colonic sources. Hematochezia raises the question of anorectal or colonic disease and, if brisk, a small-bowel or even upper gastrointestinal lesion. The prevalence of specific disorders varies with the population studied, diagnostic methods employed, and time of investigation in relation to bleeding. *Nosebleeds* and *respiratory tract bleeding* must be considered in the differential diagnosis of melena and guaiac-positive stools.

WORKUP (11–20)

The history and physical examination may provide information regarding the location and severity of bleeding, but additional investigations are usually necessary to determine the exact cause. In the previously mentioned series of 311 cases of anorectal bleeding, history and physical examination alone yielded a definite diagnosis in 28%. Nevertheless, history and physical examination have important roles that help in determining the pace of workup and the selection and ordering of tests.

Screening for Major Acute Blood Loss and Risk Stratification

Whenever active bleeding is suspected in a person presenting to the physician's office, the first priority is to determine the

TABLE 63.1

DIFFERENTIAL DIAGNOSIS OF GASTROINTESTINAL BLEEDING

Hematemesis
  Esophageal varices
  Esophagitis
  Esophageal ulceration
  Mallory–Weiss tear
  Esophageal cancer
  Gastritis or duodenitis
  Gastric or duodenal ulcer
  Gastric neoplasm (carcinoma, lymphoma, or rarely
    leiomyoma/sarcoma)
  Telangiectasia
  Angiodysplasia, especially in patients with renal failure

Melena
  All causes of hematemesis plus:
  Meckel's diverticulum
  Crohn's disease
  Small-bowel neoplasms (rare)

Hematochezia
  Hemorrhoid
  Anal fissure
  Colonic polyp
  Colorectal carcinoma
  Angiodysplasia
  Diverticular disease
  Inflammatory bowel disease
  Any upper gastrointestinal or small-bowel lesion if bleeding
    is brisk

severity and rate of blood loss. The patient should be asked about any *postural light-headedness*. The precise volume lost is not reliably determined by the history, but reports of very large amounts should be taken seriously. When the patient complains of voluminous blood loss or light-headedness, an immediate check of vital signs for *postural hypotension* is indicated. Immediate hospital admission should be considered if the systolic blood pressure falls more than 10 to 15 mm Hg or the heart rate increases by more than 10 to 15 beats/min when the patient stands up from a supine position. In acute lower intestinal tract bleeding, a heart rate of greater than 100 beats/min, a systolic blood pressure of less than 115 mm Hg, syncope, nontender abdominal examination, early recurrent rectal bleeding, concurrent aspirin use, or two active comorbid conditions suggest increased risk of severe bleeding.

Risk stratification helps to determine the need for admission and early endoscopic evaluation and treatment. Clinical predictors of poor prognosis include age older than 65 years, comorbid illness or poor overall health status, fresh blood on rectal examination or in the emesis, hypotension, and continued bleeding. A low hemoglobin level is also predictive of increased risk, but decline in hemoglobin or hematocrit in the acute phase of blood loss may be deceptively small if sufficient time for reequilibration of intravascular volume has not elapsed.

History

Once it is clear that the speed or volume of blood loss does not pose an immediate hazard, the office evaluation can proceed.

Clarifying the nature of the bleeding (melena, hematemesis, or hematochezia) helps not only to assess severity, but also to identify the approximate site of bleeding. Obtaining an accurate description is essential, as is checking for potentially confounding factors. Dark stools must not be mistaken for genuine melena, and one should check for intake of substances that may turn stool black, such as bismuth (Pepto-Bismol), iron, charcoal, or spinach. Red stools can occur after large quantities of beets have been eaten. Factors that can produce a false-positive result on the stool Hemoccult test should be considered (e.g., use of cough syrup containing glycerol guaiacolate, a recent meal of rare red meat), but a positive test result should not be dismissed lightly.

When hematemesis is reported, sources of esophageal, gastric, and duodenal bleeding must be sought. A history of cirrhosis, chronic liver disease, or alcoholism raises suspicion of esophageal varices. Use of aspirin, alcohol, or NSAIDs suggests bleeding caused by ulceration or gastritis. A history of peptic ulcer or the presence of epigastric pain responsive to antacids or related to food intake raises the possibility of bleeding from a gastric or duodenal ulcer, as does known *Helicobacter pylori* infection, especially in the setting of NSAID use. Another explanation for bleeding needs to be kept in mind in patients with a history typical of ulcer disease; more than one potential site of bleeding may be discovered (e.g., esophageal varices). Even if no hematemesis is noted, the source may still be above the ligament of Treitz; however, small-bowel and colonic lesions become more likely. Diarrhea, urgency, tenesmus, and lower abdominal cramping suggest inflammatory bowel disease (see Chapter 73). With ulcerative colitis, diverticulosis, and other forms of rectosigmoid disease, some frank rectal bleeding is often present. Brisk rectal bleeding in the absence of abdominal pain is particularly common with diverticular disease. Weight loss or change in bowel habits raises suspicion of colonic cancer. A history of diverticular disease may be a clue to the cause of blood loss, but a coincident carcinoma must be ruled out. Many patients with rectal bleeding admit to past or present hemorrhoidal problems, but in almost half of the cases, another lesion is found to be the cause of blood loss.

Physical Examination

As noted previously, when evidence of acute bleeding is present, the evaluation should begin with a check for *postural signs* and a cardiopulmonary examination to assess the severity of volume loss and the presence of any hemodynamic compromise. Next, the skin is inspected for pallor, ecchymoses, petechiae, telangiectases, and stigmata of chronic liver disease (e.g., jaundice, palmar erythema, spider angiomata). The nose and pharynx are examined for sources of bleeding. Lymph nodes are palpated for enlargement (e.g., left supraclavicular adenopathy suggests an intraabdominal malignancy), and the abdomen is palpated for organomegaly, ascites, and masses. Anorectal lesions are sought on inspection and digital examination; the stool is checked for color and the presence of occult blood (see Chapter 56). Anoscopy is an essential part of the examination for patients who complain of anal symptoms.

If the patient convincingly describes hematemesis, one may assume that the bleeding is from the upper gastrointestinal tract, but if there is evidence of recent significant bleeding of uncertain origin, a nasogastric tube should be passed to aspirate gastric contents and examined for the presence of blood.

Laboratory Studies

Laboratory studies should be performed to determine the chronicity and magnitude of blood loss and the presence of coincident disease. The hemoglobin concentration should be measured in all patients; however, if blood loss is acute, the hemoglobin concentration may not yet accurately reflect the severity of blood loss. A low mean corpuscular volume suggests the possibility of iron deficiency resulting from chronic gastrointestinal blood loss. Studies of coagulation (platelet count, prothrombin time, and partial thromboplastin time) and tests of liver and renal function are useful in checking for factors that may exacerbate bleeding.

Hematochezia

In stable patients, the main concern is the possibility of colon cancer; risk increases with age. Fewer than 5% of such cancers occur in patients younger than age 40 years, and fewer than 1% in those younger than age 30 years. Thus, if the physical examination or anoscopy reveals a bleeding hemorrhoid or other cause of local anal pathology in a young patient, it may not be necessary to proceed with further tests. The finding on sigmoidoscopy of stool negative for occult blood from above the point of bleeding also provides reassurance. On the other hand, 80% of colorectal malignancies are found in patients older than the age of 50 years. When a person older than 50 years old presents with rectal bleeding, a thorough search for tumor is required, even if a local lesion such as a hemorrhoid is discovered. Twenty-seven percent of patients with carcinoma of the rectum and 10% of those with carcinoma of the sigmoid have been noted to have coincidental hemorrhoids.

Colonoscopy is the diagnostic procedure of choice for patients with hematochezia who are at risk for colon cancer and whose bleeding is not entirely explained by documented anorectal pathology. Most patients older than the age of 40 years with rectal bleeding are candidates for colonoscopy, which is indicated for all patients whose bleeding is not clearly anorectal and whose source is beyond the range of the sigmoidoscope. There is increasing interest in *computed colonography*, but data are insufficient to establish its role in the assessment.

Hematemesis

Endoscopy has proved diagnostically superior to barium studies and offers the possibility of tissue biopsy for *H. pylori*. The sensitivity of the upper gastrointestinal series is around 60%, compared with 95% for endoscopy. Esophagitis, Mallory–Weiss tears, and gastritis, which are often undetectable radiologically, are readily seen by endoscopy. Moreover, barium obscures mucosal detail and interferes with endoscopy for 24 to 48 hours. Thus, for suspected acute brisk upper gastrointestinal bleeding, endoscopy is the procedure of first choice, with barium study reserved as a supplementary procedure for patients with inactive bleeding, unexplained chronic blood loss, or suspected small-bowel disease.

Early endoscopy (within the first 24 hours) is indicated in persons who manifest hemodynamic signs of severe bleeding or are deemed to be at high risk. In most hemodynamically stable patients, early endoscopy probably does not result in improved outcome for patients with hematemesis, but it does provide a clear diagnosis and helps to predict the risk for further bleeding.

Patients with small bleeds who are hemodynamically stable and do not have liver disease or a significant risk for gastric cancer may be presumed to have peptic ulcer disease and can be treated for *Helicobacter-* or NSAID-induced peptic ulcer (see Chapter 68). Patients at high risk for recurrent bleeding (such as those with evidence of chronic liver disease or an initial bleed that requires a transfusion) and those with persistent bleeding despite medical therapy should undergo early endoscopy. In addition, it may be useful to perform upper gastrointestinal endoscopy to exclude esophageal and gastric mucosal features indicative of a high risk for rebleeding (e.g., a "visible vessel" in an ulcer crater).

Melena

Because melena may have an upper or lower gastrointestinal source, one needs to decide which part of the gastrointestinal tract to evaluate first. The decision must be individualized to the patient, although, in general, an upper gastrointestinal source of bleeding is more likely.

Occult Bleeding

The evaluation of occult gastrointestinal bleeding is generally aimed at detecting asymptomatic neoplasms at a curable stage. Because colonic adenomas and carcinomas are the most common gastrointestinal neoplasms, evaluation of the colon has greatest utility in this setting. A cost-effectiveness analysis comparing different strategies for evaluating a positive result on testing for fecal occult blood suggested that *colonoscopy* would save more lives at lower cost than the combined use of *barium enema* and *flexible sigmoidoscopy*. The orally passed *video capsule* is emerging as a valuable tool for the evaluation of occult bleeding, especially of the small bowel. If no cause of occult bleeding is identified within the colon, evaluation of the upper gastrointestinal tract and small bowel may be considered, although the yield for detection of cancer is likely to be low. In a study of 26 patients followed for 2 to 8 years after a negative result on colonoscopy or barium enema/sigmoidoscopy, only 1 patient was later found to have a gastric cancer. In 5 others, a nonmalignant upper gastrointestinal source emerged as the cause of the occult bleeding. A prospective study of patients with iron-deficiency anemia found that site-specific symptoms predicted the location of the source of bleeding. Upper gastrointestinal sources were common. Synchronous sources of blood loss were rare, so further evaluation was unnecessary when an obvious source was found.

PROPHYLACTIC AND SYMPTOMATIC MANAGEMENT (21–29)

Patients at high risk for upper gastrointestinal bleeding (such as those with varices or a prior history of upper gastrointestinal bleeding, especially if exposed to anticoagulants, NSAIDs, or *H. pylori* infection) are candidates for prophylactic measures (see Chapters 68 and 71).

For patients with varices, *beta blockade* has been used successfully to prevent a first bleed in patients with known varices (see Chapter 71). *Endoscopic ligation* may also be used for primary prophylaxis in patients with varices but is less cost-effective than other measures; the procedure may also be considered for secondary prophylaxis.

For patients with a history of bleeding from an ulcer or gastritis, *histamine2 blockers* and *proton-pump inhibitors (PPIs)* are worth consideration in selected patients, especially those requiring chronic NSAID or aspirin therapy. Controlled trial finds that patients on aspirin therapy for cardiovascular prophylaxis who had a gastrointestinal bleed have less recurrent bleeding by adding the PPI esomeprazole to their aspirin program than by switching to clopidogrel. Any concurrent *Helicobacter* infection should be identified and fully treated (see Chapter 68). The prostaglandin analogue *misoprostol* might be an adjunct to acid suppression for patients who continue to require NSAID therapy. Patients taking steroids do not appear to require such prophylaxis unless an additional risk factor for bleeding is present.

Modest falls in hematocrit that accompany chronic low-grade gastrointestinal blood loss can be treated with *oral iron* (300 mg of ferrous sulfate three times daily) to make up for the resulting iron deficiency (see Chapter 82). Marked but gradual decreases in hematocrit are usually well tolerated unless the patient has cardiopulmonary disease. Most patients do not need transfusion unless they are symptomatic. Oral iron usually produces a prompt reticulocytosis and at least partial correction of the anemia (see Chapter 82). Patients with presumed anal bleeding can be given fiber supplements or stool softeners to decrease mechanical trauma to the lesion (see Chapter 65).

INDICATIONS FOR ADMISSION AND REFERRAL

The patient with a story of recent or ongoing brisk bleeding, especially if it is accompanied by orthostatic hypotension or other symptoms or signs of hemodynamic compromise, requires emergency department evaluation. Prompt hospitalization is indicated for the person with a profound anemia, even in the absence of evidence for dramatic blood loss. Some patients who are hemodynamically stable may be expeditiously evaluated in a short stay with endoscopy. Hospitalization should be considered for patients with a lower tract source disease or less severe or perhaps even chronic gastrointestinal blood loss if they have a concurrent condition that might be aggravated by anemia (e.g., ischemic heart disease). For most others, evaluation can proceed safely on an ambulatory basis if the patient does not have serious cardiopulmonary disease and is responsible enough to recognize and promptly report signs of worsening blood loss or volume depletion. Referral to a gastroenterologist should be considered for patients who are potential candidates for endoscopy and also for patients whose source of bleeding remains elusive after initial evaluation.

Annotated Bibliography

1. Battistella M, Mamdami MM, Juurlink DN, et al. Risk of upper gastrointestinal hemorrhage in warfarin users treated with nonselective NSAIDS or COX-2 inhibitors. Arch Intern Med 2005;165:189. (*Case–control study; the risk nearly doubles and is similar for both classes of nonsteroidal antiinflammatory drugs [NSAIDs].*)
2. Carson JL, Strom BL, Schinnar R, et al. The low risk of upper gastrointestinal bleeding in patients dispensed corticosteroids. Am J Med 1991;91:223. (*The risk was 2.8 cases per 10,000 person-months, arguing against prophylactic therapy unless other risk factors are present.*)
3. Graham DY. Aspirin and the stomach. Ann Intern Med 1986;104:390. (*Comprehensive review noting that the degree of mucosal injury seen by endoscopy does not predict the risk for or the degree of bleeding.*)
4. Papatheodoridis GV, Papdelli D, Cholongitas E, et al. Effect of *Helicobacter pylori* infection of the risk of upper gastrointestinal bleeding in users of nonsteroidal anti-inflammatory drugs. Am J Med 2004;116:601. (*The risk is doubled by the presence of the infection.*)
5. Sharara AI, Rockey DC. Gastroesophageal variceal hemorrhage. N Engl J Med 2001;345:669. (*Detailed review; 118 references.*)
6. Stewart JG, Ahlquist DA, McGill DB, et al. Gastrointestinal blood loss and anemia in runners. Ann Intern Med 1984;100:843. (*Documents an increase in fecal hemoglobin.*)
7. Wilcox CM, Alexander LN, Cotsonis G. A prospective characterization of upper gastrointestinal bleeding with hematochezia. Am J Gastroenterol 1997;92:231. (*Duodenal ulcer is a common cause of upper tract bleeding presenting as hematochezia.*)
8. Wilcox CM, Truss CD. Gastrointestinal bleeding in patients receiving long-term anticoagulant therapy. Am J Med 1988;84:683. (*Half of episodes were upper gastrointestinal in origin; a lower gastrointestinal origin was noted in 33%.*)
9. Yuan Y, Tsoi K, Hunt RH. Selective serotonin reuptake inhibitors and risk of upper GI bleeding: confusion or confounding? Am J Med 2006;119:719. (*A systematic review finding that the evidence was weak for the association but was strongest in those taking NSAIDs or aspirin concurrently*).
10. Zuckerman GR. Upper gastrointestinal bleeding in patients with chronic renal failure. Ann Intern Med 1985;102:588. (*Upper gastrointestinal angiodysplasia was the most common source; esophagitis was also prevalent.*)
11. Barkun A, Bardou M, Marshall JK, et al. Consensus recommendations for managing patients with nonvariceal upper gastrointestinal bleeding. Ann Intern Med 2003;139:843. (*Sections on risk stratification and the need for early endoscopy are especially useful for the primary physician.*)
12. Barry MJ, Mulley AG, Richter JM. Effect of workup strategy on the cost-effectiveness of fecal occult blood screening for colorectal cancer. Gastroenterology 1987;93:301. (*Comparative analysis of seven potential strategies for evaluating the colon in asymptomatic patients with guaiac-positive stool.*)
13. Cave DR. Obscure gastrointestinal bleeding: the role of the tagged red blood cell scan, enteroscopy, and capsule endoscopy. Clin Gastroenterol Hepatol 2005;10:959. (*A current review of new techniques to examine the small bowel and investigate obscure bleeding sources.*)
14. Farrell JJ, Friedman LS. Review article: the management of lower gastrointestinal bleeding. Aliment Pharmacol Ther 2005;21:1281. (*An updated review of the approach to lower intestinal bleeding.*)
15. Griffiths WJ, Neumann DA, Welsh JD. The visible vessel as an indicator of uncontrolled or recurrent gastrointestinal hemorrhage. N Engl J Med 1979;300:1411. (*Classic paper; identifies an important sign of high risk for repeat hemorrhage.*)
16. Harewood GC, McConnell JP, Harrington JJ, et al. Detection of occult upper gastrointestinal bleeding: performance differences in fecal occult blood tests. Mayo Clin Proc 2002;77:23. (*Cross-sectional study with useful data.*)
17. Jensen DM, Machicado GA, Jutabha R, et al. Urgent colonoscopy for the diagnosis and treatment of severe diverticular hemorrhage. N Engl J Med 2000;342:78. (*Prospective cohort study; early scoping and treatment improved outcomes.*)
18. Rockey DC. Occult gastrointestinal bleeding. N Engl J Med 1999;341:38. (*A comprehensive review of testing for occult bleeding.*)
19. Rockey DC, Cello JP. Evaluation of the gastrointestinal tract in patients with iron-deficiency anemia. N Engl J Med 1993;329:1691. (*Lesions are frequently found; site-specific symptoms help to predict location and direct workup.*)
20. Simon JB. Fecal occult blood testing: clinical value and limitations. Gastroenterologist 1998;6:66. (*Detailed review of the test, with a good discussion of its limitations.*)
21. Barkin JS, Ross BS. Medical therapy of chronic gastrointestinal bleeding of obscure origin. Am J Gastroenterol 1998;93:1250. (*Patients who had chronic occult bleeding, often elderly persons with suspected vascular ectasia, improved with combination estrogen and progesterone therapy.*)
22. Chan FKL, Chung SCS, Suen BY, et al. Preventing recurrent upper gastrointestinal bleeding in patients with *Helicobacter pylori* infection who are taking low-dose aspirin or naproxen. N Engl J Med 2001;344:967. (*Randomized trial; eradication of infection and use of omeprazole were found to be helpful when NSAIDs were resumed.*)
23. Chan KLC, Ching SYL, Hung LCT, et al. Clopidogrel versus aspirin and esomeprazole to prevent recurrent ulcer bleeding. N Engl J Med 2005;352:238. (*A randomized, controlled trial; aspirin plus proton pump inhibitor therapy was superior to clopidogrel in the prevention of recurrent ulcer bleeding.*)
24. Laine L, El Newihi HM, Migikovsky B, et al. Endoscopic ligation compared with sclerotherapy for the treatment of bleeding esophageal varices. Ann Intern Med 1993;119:1. (*Endoscopic ligation caused fewer local complications and eradicated varices more rapidly.*)
25. Lau JYW, Sung JJY, Lam YH, et al. Endoscopic retreatment compared with recurrent bleeding after initial endoscopic control of bleeding ulcers. N Engl J Med 1999;340:751. (*Endoscopic retreatment is more cost-effective than emergency surgery.*)

26. Longstreth GF, Feitelberg SP. Outpatient care of selected patients with acute non-variceal upper gastrointestinal haemorrhage. Lancet 345;1995:108. (*A substantial proportion of selected patients with nonvariceal bleeding can be safely treated without hospital admission.*)

27. Rokkas T, Karameris A, Mavrogeorgis A, et al. Eradication of *Helicobacter pylori* reduces the possibility of rebleeding in peptic ulcer disease. Gastrointest Endosc 1995;41:1. (*Patients with duodenal ulcer disease had fewer episodes of bleeding if they were successfully treated for Helicobacter pylori.*)

28. Strate LL, Orav EJ, Syngal S. Early predictors of severity in acute lower intestinal tract bleeding. Arch Intern Med 2003;163:838. (*A prospective cohort study; identified tachycardia, hypotension, syncope, nontender abdomen, and recurrent bleeding per rectum as independent predictors.*)

29. Sung JJY, Chan FKL, Lau JYW, et al. The effect of endoscopic therapy in patients receiving omeprazole for bleeding ulcers with nonbleeding visible vessels or adherent clots: a randomized comparison. Ann Intern Med 2003;139:237. (*Adding endoscopic therapy was better than using omeprazole alone.*)

CHAPTER 64 ■ EVALUATION AND MANAGEMENT OF DIARRHEA

JAMES M. RICHTER

Diarrhea is clinically characterized by the frequent passage of unformed stools. Episodes that are brief, self-limited, and well tolerated do not require medical attention, but when diarrhea becomes severe or chronic, a thoughtful evaluation is needed to ensure proper management. The primary care physician needs to know how to conduct an expeditious assessment of acute or severe diarrhea and coordinate a cost-effective approach to the evaluation of chronic diarrhea.

PATHOPHYSIOLOGY AND CLINICAL PRESENTATIONS (1–24)

Pathophysiology

The pathophysiologic common denominator is increased stool water content, which may be a consequence of increased fluid secretion, decreased absorption, or altered bowel motility. At times, several mechanisms are operative. *Increased fluid secretion* can result from inflammation, hormones, or enterotoxins. The resulting secretory diarrhea has a stool volume that remains in excess of 250 mL/24 hr despite fasting, a low stool osmolality, and a normal stool electrolyte concentration. *Decreased reabsorption of fluid* occurs with abnormalities of the bowel mucosa, loss of reabsorptive surface, or the presence of unabsorbable, osmotically active materials in the bowel lumen, such as lactose in patients with lactase deficiency. Patients with diarrhea resulting from decreased reabsorption typically respond to fasting with a decrease in stool volume to less than 250 mL/24 hr, an increase in stool osmolality, and low stool concentrations of sodium and potassium. *Increased bowel motility* decreases the contact time with the bowel mucosa, limiting fluid reabsorption. It can ensue after vagotomy or may be chemically stimulated, as in hypergastrinemia or with the use of laxatives.

Acute Diarrheas

A diarrhea is categorized as "acute" if its duration is less than 2 weeks. Infectious causes dominate and include viral, bacterial, and parasitic agents. Bacteria may cause diarrhea by producing a toxin in contaminated food or after ingestion or by invading the bowel mucosa. Some parasites invade the bowel wall, whereas others cling to it and alter the absorptive surface.

Viruses

Viruses causing acute gastroenteritis have long been the most common source of acute diarrhea in the United States, although it was not until the late 1970s that the responsible organisms were finally isolated and identified. Epidemics of viral gastroenteritis are particularly common. More than 70% of outbreaks of nonbacterial gastroenteritis investigated by the Centers for Disease Control and Prevention (CDC) are linked to the *noroviruses*. In children, *rotavirus* infection is a common cause. Outbreaks have been found to occur during all seasons and involve water-borne, food-borne, and person-to-person modes of transmission.

Symptoms last about 1 week. The prominent symptom in children is vomiting, and in adults it is diarrhea. After an incubation period of 48 to 72 hours, symptoms usually begin abruptly with diarrhea, nausea, vomiting, headache, low-grade fever, abdominal cramps, and malaise; they resolve spontaneously within 24 to 96 hours. The diarrhea tends to be predominantly secretory in quality. Abdominal examination reveals diffuse tenderness (without guarding) and hyperactive bowel sounds. The white blood cell count is usually normal but may be elevated.

Staphylococcus aureus

Staphylococcus aureus is a common contaminant of custard-filled pastries and processed meats. The organism produces an enterotoxin that causes nausea, vomiting, abdominal cramps, and diarrhea within 2 to 8 hours after contaminated food has been eaten. Symptoms usually last less than 12 hours. A common-source pattern and lack of fever are typical.

Clostridium perfringens

Clostridium perfringens is another common food contaminant, especially of foods that have been warmed on steam tables. The organism releases an enterotoxin in the intestine. Consequently, the incubation period of 8 to 24 hours is a bit longer than that for staphylococcal food poisoning. It too has a common-source epidemiology; fever is absent. Symptoms include diarrhea, abdominal cramps, and occasionally some vomiting.

Bacillus cereus

Bacillus cereus is a toxin-producing bacterial contaminant of rice and bean sprouts. One form of toxin-induced illness leads to vomiting but no diarrhea; severe abdominal cramping and diarrhea characterize another. The incubation period is 8 to 16 hours after the ingestion of contaminated food. The symptoms are self-limited.

Escherichia coli 0157:H7

Escherichia coli 0157:H7 is increasingly being recognized as responsible for much food-borne diarrhea. It accounts for up to 2.5% of all cases of acute diarrhea and up to one third of cases of bloody acute diarrhea. Transmission to humans is usually by the ingestion of contaminated meat (typically hamburger) that is undercooked. Person-to-person transmission also occurs. Peak incidence is in the summer months. The organism does not directly invade the bowel wall, but the two Shiga-like toxins it produces cause mucosal edema, ulceration, and hemorrhage. The mean incubation period is 3 days (range, 1 to 9 days). Among individuals who become symptomatic, the clinical presentation ranges from mild, crampy, nonbloody diarrhea to life-threatening hemorrhagic colitis complicated by hemolytic–uremic syndrome or thrombotic thrombocytopenic purpura. The typical presentation starts with crampy abdominal pain, followed within hours by watery diarrhea that progresses to grossly bloody stools. Children, the elderly, and compromised hosts are at greatest risk.

Salmonella

Salmonella species cause diarrhea by invading the bowel wall. Achlorhydric patients who lack the antibacterial action of normal gastric acidity are at increased risk. The most common form of *Salmonella* infection is a self-limited diarrheal illness resulting from the ingestion of contaminated food (eggs and poultry are the major sources). Children are at greatest risk; late summer and fall are the times of peak incidence. Although most episodes of salmonellosis are mild, debilitated patients are at risk for serious bacteremia. In the typical outpatient case, symptoms begin 12 to 36 hours after ingestion and resolve within 5 days, although diarrhea may persist for up to 2 weeks. The initial presentation is rather nonspecific, with watery diarrhea, cramps, nausea, vomiting, and fever. In addition to colonization, an enterotoxin is released that stimulates the secretory diarrhea. In later stages, invasion spreads to the large bowel, and leukocytes may be noted in the stool. A distinguishing feature of salmonellosis is that the leukocytes are often mononuclear cells. In severe cases, dysentery can develop.

Typhoid fever, a rare but "must-not-miss" form of *Salmonella* disease, is caused by infection with *Salmonella typhi.* About 500 cases occur in the United States each year, mostly among young people. Infections are both water-borne and food-borne. Although diarrhea develops in only a small percentage of patients with typhoid fever, it does occur. The classic and most severe form is a *"pea soup" diarrhea* developing in the third week of illness. Early symptoms suggestive of the condition are progressive fever, relative *bradycardia*, evanescent rash on the trunk ("*rose spots*"), *splenomegaly*, cough, headache, and right lower quadrant abdominal pain.

Shigella

Shigella infection produces an invasive diarrheal illness. Transmission is by the fecal–oral route, and stubborn reservoirs include day care centers, Native American reservations, urban ghettos, and rural villages in developing countries. Young children are at greatest risk and often the source of infection within a family. The illness proceeds in two stages. First, colonization takes place in the small bowel, resulting in a *watery diarrhea* and periumbilical pain, followed in a few days by invasion of the large bowel, associated with frequent small stools, tenesmus, and polymorphonuclear leukocytes on smear. In florid cases, the patient has fever, toxicity, *bloody diarrhea*, nausea, vomiting, and cramps. Most often, the disease is subtler and may be difficult to distinguish from other diarrheal illnesses accompanied by fever.

Campylobacter jejuni

Campylobacter jejuni infection is responsible for more cases of diarrhea in the United States than is either *Salmonella* or *Shigella*. Infection derives most often from animal sources, such as poultry and household pets; fecal transmission between people also occurs. The incubation period is 2 to 7 days. Clinically, the illness resembles that caused by *Salmonella* or *Shigella*; however, symptoms may persist longer. Although the illness is usually self-limited and resolves within 1 week, the relapse rate is as high as 20%. In half of all cases, a Gram's stain of the stool shows characteristic curved, gram-negative rods arranged in "seagull-wing" fashion.

Yersinia enterocolitica

Yersinia enterocolitica also causes an illness that resembles salmonellosis. It is acquired by eating contaminated meat or dairy products. The incubation period is 12 hours to 3 days. An intense, regional lymphoid reaction may arise in the terminal ileum (the portal of entry for the organism) and result in a clinical picture of fever, *right lower quadrant abdominal pain*, and diarrhea that can simulate the onset of Crohn's disease. In 10% to 40% of patients, fever, arthralgias, polyarthritis, or erythema nodosum develops. The illness is usually self-limited.

Vibrio parahaemolyticus and Non–Toxin-Producing Vibrio Cholerae

Vibrio parahaemolyticus and non–toxin-producing *Vibrio cholerae* are pathogenic species that have caused outbreaks of diarrheal disease among people eating raw seafood, particularly oysters and sushi-style red snapper and salmon. The incubation period is measured in hours to several days. The illness that ensues is usually mild and self-limited, although an occasional patient may present with fever, nausea, vomiting, and crampy diarrhea.

Listeria monocytogenes

Listeria monocytogenes is another of the food-borne pathogens found in tainted processed meats and poultry products and also in unpasteurized milk products. Person-to-person transfer does not occur. About 2,000 cases per year occur in the United States. Deaths are common, with mortality rates of 20% to 30% reported. The elderly and the immunocompromised are at greatest risk, but even immunocompetent persons can develop a febrile diarrhea. The onset of symptoms is typically 1 to 2 days after exposure. The initial symptoms resemble those of a viral gastroenteritis (fever, cramps, myalgias, diarrhea, headache). Days to weeks later, meningitis and bacteremia may ensue, especially in the immunocompromised host.

Vibrio cholerae

Vibrio cholerae causes the prototypical toxin-mediated secretory diarrheal disease that results from drinking water contaminated with the organism. Most outbreaks are pandemic in the Indian subcontinent, Southeast Asia, Africa, and the Middle East. Isolated outbreaks have been reported in Mediterranean countries. In the United States, rare individual cases sometimes occur along the Gulf Coast. The disease ranges in severity from a mild illness to fulminant, life-threatening diarrhea with copious production of gray, watery, mucoid ("rice water") stool. In severe cases, fluid losses may exceed 1 L/hr and are accompanied by vomiting, muscle cramps, and severe thirst. Dehydration, serious volume depletion, and a metabolic acidosis may ensue. In mild cases, the patient reports painless, nonbloody diarrhea of abrupt onset.

Entamoeba histolytica

Entamoeba histolytica usually exists in a commensal relationship with its host, and most patients harboring the protozoan are asymptomatic carriers. Occasionally, this relationship breaks down and the ameba invades the colonic wall; an acute bloody diarrhea is the result. The clinical presentation ranges from mild to fulminant illness. Occasionally, the illness is mistaken for inflammatory bowel disease (see Chapter 73), and it may have a protracted course with exacerbations and remissions. Asymptomatic carriers such as returning tourists and immigrants are often the source of infection in developed countries. Because the organism does not have a soil phase, amebiasis is not restricted to warmer climates. Well-documented outbreaks have occurred in the United States and Europe, in addition to those that originate in developing countries.

Giardia lamblia

Giardia lamblia is a leading parasitic cause of diarrhea, especially overseas but also in the United States. Infection with the flagellated protozoan is particularly common where water supplies are contaminated by human sewage, but the organism is also endemic to such areas as the Rocky Mountains and St. Petersburg, Russia. The exact means by which Giardia causes diarrhea is unsettled, although heavy infestations can lead to malabsorption by coating large areas of the small bowel, particularly the lower duodenum and upper jejunum. The majority of patients with giardiasis are asymptomatic, but the organism is being recognized more frequently as an important cause of acute, intermittent, and chronic diarrheas in the United States. The ensuing loose stools may be watery or greasy; mucus is often present, but blood is rare. The patient may complain of epigastric or periumbilical discomfort. Mild steatorrhea and malabsorption occur with heavy parasite burdens.

Cryptosporidium, Microsporidia, and Other Protozoans

Cryptosporidium, Microsporidia, and other protozoans are increasingly recognized causes of acute watery diarrhea (and sometimes of chronic disease). Point-source outbreaks occur in addition to sporadic cases. Transmission is by person-to-person contact through stool or by water or food contaminated with the spore or oocyst forms of the organism. Intestinal inflammation may develop. Children and immunocompromised adults are at the greatest risk for severe and prolonged illness. A profuse, watery diarrhea can develop, with stool volumes that may exceed 3 L daily. Although the illness is usually self-limited, it may persist in immunocompromised hosts. A mild illness develops in otherwise healthy, immunocompetent patients; they may become infected during occupational contact (e.g., with animal dung). For such patients, symptoms resolve spontaneously within 5 to 21 days.

Diarrhea in HIV-Infected Patients

Diarrhea in HIV-infected patients is a major problem, with a host of possible etiologies (see Chapter 13). In HIV-infected persons who engage in receptive anal intercourse, the presentation may be one of diarrhea, tenesmus, and rectal pain. In this setting, polymicrobial etiologies are not uncommon and may include Neisseria, Giardia, E. histolytica, Campylobacter, Chlamydia, Shigella, Salmonella, and protozoans.

Traveler's Diarrheas

Patients traveling from industrialized to developing nations are at considerable risk for the development of diarrhea. Etiologic agents include E. coli, Salmonella, Shigella, E. histolytica, G. lamblia, S. typhi, and V. cholerae. Invasive E. coli strains can also cause a dysentery syndrome. Toxigenic E. coli are responsible for a large proportion of cases labeled as "traveler's diarrhea" or "turista." Poor food-handling practices and contaminated water transmit the agent. With enterotoxin production, a watery diarrhea ensues because the toxin promotes fluid secretion in the small bowel.

Brainerd Diarrhea

Brainerd diarrhea remains an unexplained, probably infectious, self-limited diarrheal disease that often occurs in point-source outbreaks.

Drug-Induced Diarrheas

Drugs are an important cause of both acute and chronic diarrheas (Table 64.1).

Acute Diarrhea. Mechanisms of acute diarrhea include excessive fluid secretion (alcohol, phenolphthalein, and castor oil), reduction of fluid absorption (magnesium-containing antacids), and stimulation of bowel motility (caffeine-containing beverages and herbal teas). An osmotic diarrhea with crampy pain and watery stools may follow oral or parenteral use of broad-spectrum antibiotics, which disrupt the salvage of unabsorbed carbohydrate by killing normal colonic flora.

Persistent Diarrhea: Pseudomembranous Colitis. Broad-spectrum antibiotics can cause chronic diarrhea by promoting growth and toxin-producing production by Clostridium difficile. The antibiotics most often responsible are ampicillin and clindamycin, but other broad-spectrum agents have also

TABLE 64.1

DIFFERENTIAL DIAGNOSIS OF DIARRHEA

Acute Diarrhea	Chronic or Recurrent Diarrhea
Viruses	**Protozoa**
Noroviruses and Rotaviruses	*Giardia lamblia*
Bacterial Toxins	*Entamoeba histolytica*
Staphylococcus	*Cryptosporidium*
Clostridium	**Inflammation**
Bacteria	Ulcerative colitis
Salmonella	Crohn's disease
Shigella	Ischemic colitis
Escherichia coli (including 0157:H7)	Pseudomembranous colitis
Campylobacter	Collagenous colitis
Yersinia	Lymphocytic colitis
Bacillus cereus	**Drugs**
Vibrio parahaemolyticus	Laxatives
Vibrio cholerae	Antibiotics
Listeria	Quinidine
Protozoa	Guanethidine; other antihypertensive
Giardia lamblia	agents
Entamoeba histolytica	Caffeine
Cryptosporidium	Digitalis
Microsporidia	**Functional**
Drugs	Irritable bowel syndrome
Laxatives	Diverticulosis
Antibiotics	**Tumors**
Caffeine	Bowel carcinoma
Alcohol	Villous adenoma
Antacids	Islet cell tumors
Functional	Carcinoid syndrome
Anxiety	Medullary carcinoma of thyroid
Acute presentations of chronic or	**Malabsorption**
recurrent diarrhea (see next column)	Sprue
	Intestinal lymphoma
	Bile salt malabsorption
	Whipple's disease
	Pancreatic insufficiency
	Lactase deficiency
	Other disaccharidase deficiencies
	Alpha-beta lipoproteinemia
	Postsurgical
	Postgastrectomy dumping syndrome
	Enteroenteric fistulas
	Blind loops
	Parasympathetic denervation
	Short-bowel syndrome
	Bile and diarrhea
	Other
	Cirrhosis
	Diabetes mellitus
	Heavy metal intoxication
	Other neurogenic diarrheas
	Hyperthyroidism
	Addison's disease
	Pellagra
	Scleroderma
	Amyloidosis

been implicated. Immunocompromised patients, the elderly, and those with underlying bowel disease are most susceptible. Fever, abdominal pain, and profuse watery stools that can become bloody characterize pseudomembranous colitis. Symptoms range from mild to severe, usually starting after the initiation of a course of antibiotics, but onset can be delayed for as much as 4 to 8 weeks after the cessation of antibiotics and persist for months, mimicking inflammatory bowel disease. The sigmoidoscopic finding of nodular, inflammatory ulcers or yellow-white mucosal plaques is characteristic.

Chronic and Recurrent Diarrheas

Although the number of etiologies is vast, consideration of a few exemplary conditions provides a good sense of the range and types of presentations. In addition, a number of the causes of acute diarrhea may account for chronic or recurrent disease.

Irritable Bowel Syndrome

Irritable bowel syndrome is the most common of the motility disorders responsible for chronic diarrhea or hyperdefecation (see Chapter 74). It can present as diarrhea alternating with constipation or as chronic, recurrent diarrhea. In addition to diarrhea and constipation, patients may complain of distention, cramping, and mucus-laden stools. The condition waxes and wanes over many years. Neither fever nor blood is present. Any rectal bleeding that may occur is secondary to anal trauma resulting from straining and passage of hard stool.

Inflammatory Bowel Diseases

Inflammatory bowel diseases are typical of the diarrheas that result from inflammatory destruction of the bowel wall (see Chapter 73). Abdominal pain, bloody stools, purulent discharge, and fever are seen in patients with active disease affecting the large bowel. Extraintestinal manifestations may involve the skin, joints, liver, and heart. Microscopic examination of the stool reveals red cells, leukocytes and no pathogens.

Diabetic Enteropathy

Diabetic enteropathy results from diabetes-induced autonomic neuropathy (see Chapter 102). When the small bowel is involved, the ensuing stasis allows bacterial overgrowth. The bacteria deconjugate bile acids, which may also lead to fat malabsorption. With involvement of the large bowel, the patient experiences distressing nocturnal diarrhea. Postural hypotension, impotence, and other symptoms and signs of autonomic insufficiency may accompany the diarrhea and suggest the diagnosis.

Dumping Syndrome

Dumping syndrome is another motility disorder and is seen most commonly in patients who have undergone vagotomy and gastroenterostomy. Patients complain of sweating, postural lightheadedness, tachycardia, and diarrhea following meals. Concentrated carbohydrates are most likely to trigger symptoms. Lying down minimizes symptoms, as does the avoidance of concentrated sweets. The onset of the syndrome is soon after surgery, and symptoms usually subside within 12 months, although they may persist. Besides dysmotility, osmotic factors may contribute, but their precise role is unclear.

Villous Adenoma

Villous adenoma of the rectosigmoid causes a secretory, non-inflammatory chronic diarrhea. Watery diarrhea, independent of food and fluid intake, is typical; severe potassium depletion can result. In some patients with this tumor, excessive secretion of mucus occurs, with the loss of sufficient protein to produce hypoalbuminemia and a protein-losing enteropathy syndrome.

Malabsorption of Fat or Carbohydrate

Malabsorption of fat or carbohydrate can lead to an osmotic diarrhea, as occurs in patients with *pancreatic insufficiency*, *sprue*, and *short-bowel* syndrome. Some of the osmotically active substances may also stimulate increased bowel secretion of fluids and electrolytes. Malabsorption of fat characteristically presents as *steatorrhea* (foul, bulky, greasy stools). Patients may note that the stools seem to be "sticky" and difficult to flush down the toilet. Steatorrheic stools "float," not because of their fat content, but because of an increase in trapped gas. Associated symptoms are a function of the severity of the caloric and vitamin deficiencies that ensue and may include weight loss, ecchymoses, bone pain, glossitis, muscle tenderness, and peripheral neuropathy. Cramping lower abdominal pain typically precedes bowel movements. Early concerns about severe diarrhea and abdominal pain associated with the regular use of *Olestra*, a nonabsorbable sucrose ester fat substitute used in snack foods, have not been confirmed in randomized, prospective, controlled trials.

Celiac Sprue. Of the malabsorptive causes, celiac sprue is the most common and most underrecognized. Prevalence estimates have increased with improved methods of diagnosis and range from 0.3% to 0.8%. A genetically predisposed inappropriate T cell response to ingested gluten causes immune-mediated damage to the small-bowel mucosa. Although classically described as a disease of children, sprue may have its onset in adulthood, with almost one fifth of cases beginning in the sixth decade. Onset may occur during pregnancy or in the postpartum period. Presenting symptoms can be subtle and nonspecific; they may include episodic or nocturnal *diarrhea*, *flatulence*, and *weight loss* along with *iron deficiency*. Steatorrhea may be absent if disease is limited to the proximal small bowel. *Bloating*, *fatigue*, and *vague abdominal discomfort* are common and may be mistaken for symptoms of irritable bowel syndrome. *Iron-deficiency anemia* may be the only manifestation. Extraintestinal manifestations include neurologic problems (peripheral neuropathy, ataxia, psychiatric disturbances), fractures (from vitamin D deficiency), and infertility. Screening can be achieved by checking serum for *antiendomesial* and *antitransglutaminase immunoglobulin A (IgA)* antibodies, whose sensitivity exceeds 81%, with a specificity of greater than 99%.

Lactase Deficiency (Milk Intolerance)

Lactase deficiency (milk intolerance) leads to the malabsorption of lactose and an osmotic diarrhea. It is particularly common among African Americans, Native Americans, Asians, and Jews. Onset is typically in adulthood. A secondary form of the disease may develop in patients with extensive disease of the small bowel. Patients report nausea, bloating, cramps, and diarrhea after ingesting more than their customary intake of milk products. Weight loss and steatorrhea are absent or mild; appetite remains good. Avoidance of milk products (except for yogurt containing live cultures, which provide lactase) terminates symptoms. Diagnosis may be confirmed by a trial of abstinence and by abnormal results on lactose tolerance testing or hydrogen breath testing (which detects excessive hydrogen production resulting from the bacterial metabolism of undigested lactose).

Laxative Abuse

Laxative abuse is an important etiology of chronic diarrhea. Patients with eating disorders (see Chapter 234) tend to use laxatives constantly and surreptitiously in a relentless attempt to lose weight. Depending on the type of agent used, either a secretory or an osmotic diarrhea may develop. Agents associated with secretory diarrheas include castor oil and phenolphthalein preparations. Osmotic diarrheas occur when the patient takes a preparation that contains magnesium (e.g., milk of magnesia) or another poorly absorbable substance. These substances appear in the stool and can be tested for if laxative abuse is suspected. Patients who abuse laxatives may present with unexplained dehydration, electrolyte depletion, or preoccupation with weight loss.

Lymphocytic Colitis and Collagenous Colitis

These two recently described conditions are associated with chronic diarrhea. They occur predominantly in women and cause chronic watery diarrhea, often complicated by steatorrhea and malabsorption. The colonic appearance is grossly normal, but biopsy reveals collagenous or lymphocytic infiltrates. The small bowel usually is normal but may show spruelike changes in patients with lymphocytic disease, and persons with the condition may present with spruelike malabsorption unresponsive to a gluten-free diet.

Bile Acid Diarrhea

Bile acid diarrhea is seen after cholecystectomy and ileal resection. It is an irritant diarrhea caused by the action of excessive bile acids on the bowel and responds to bile acid sequestrants (e.g., cholestyramine).

Incontinence

A number of patients who complain of "diarrhea" actually suffer from incontinence. Typically, their stool volumes are normal (<2.5 mL/d), although their stools may be soft; poor sphincter tone and evidence of stool incontinence are found on physical examination (see Chapter 66).

DIFFERENTIAL DIAGNOSIS
(23,25,26,31)

Acute Diarrhea

Infectious agents (see Table 64.1) dominate the differential diagnosis for acute diarrhea. Viruses are the most important frequent cause. Staphylococcal toxin, clostridial toxin, and ingestion of *Campylobacter, Salmonella, Shigella,* and enteropathogenic *E. coli* are common bacterial etiologies. Of increasing importance are the potentially life-threatening outbreaks of food-borne disease caused by toxin-producing *E. coli* 0157:H7 and *Listeria*. Protozoans such as *Cryptosporidium. Giardia* and ameba are less frequent sources of acute diarrhea in the United States. Drug-induced acute disease is associated with the use of antibiotics, laxatives, magnesium-containing antacids, and agents such as quinidine. Alcohol and caffeine-containing beverages should be considered. Most causes of chronic diarrhea are also capable of causing acute presenta-

tions. In more than 50% of cases of acute traveler's diarrhea, the cause is enterotoxigenic *E. coli* or *Salmonella*; *Shigella, Giardia,* and *Campylobacter* account for most of the remainder.

Chronic Diarrhea

The differential diagnosis is even more extensive (see Table 64.1) and includes causes of acute disease that may become chronic (e.g., laxative abuse, pseudomembranous colitis, protozoan infections, amebic infestations) in addition to a host of intrinsic bowel diseases. A *malabsorption* picture may be the consequence of celiac sprue, bile salts, lactase deficiency, intestinal lymphoma, Whipple's disease, or pancreatic insufficiency. *Postsurgical* diarrhea may reflect postgastrectomy dumping syndrome, fistulas, blind loops, loss of parasympathetic enervation, extensive bowel resection, or excessive bile acid. Diarrhea with *bleeding* may herald neoplasia, ischemia, or inflammatory bowel disease. Irritable bowel syndrome, Crohn's disease, or diverticular disease of the bowel may cause diarrhea alternating with constipation. A variety of *extraintestinal conditions* may be responsible, including cirrhosis, alcoholism, pellagra, and heavy metal intoxication from lead, mercury, or arsenic. Endocrinopathies also must be considered (e.g., diabetes mellitus, Addison's disease, hyperthyroidism).

Diarrhea of Unknown Etiology

In studies of patients referred for chronic diarrhea of unknown etiology, the vast majority turn out to be abusing laxatives or to have a subtle form of inflammatory bowel disease (including collagenous or lymphocytic varieties) or irritable bowel syndrome. Most of the remainder have a more readily diagnosed condition that was overlooked on initial evaluation.

Diarrhea in the HIV-Infected Patient

The common infectious causes are frequently seen, but such uncommon causes as *Cryptosporidium, Mycobacterium avium–intracellulare,* herpes simplex virus, cytomegalovirus, *Neisseria gonorrhoeae, Giardia,* and *Chlamydia trachomatis* must also be considered (see Chapter 13).

WORKUP
(1,3,4,6,7,9,10,14,16,18,20,21,25–31)

Before embarking on a workup, one needs to confirm that the problem is indeed diarrhea and not simply an occasional loose stool or frequent defecation of formed stools. Stool volume, frequency, and water content should all be increased.

Acute and Traveler's Diarrheas

History

The *nature of the bowel movements* should be determined, including their frequency, consistency, and volume and the presence of gross blood, pus, or mucus (Tables 64.2 and 64.3), as well as the presence of any *associated symptoms*, such as fever, rash, and abdominal pain. Symptoms of postural hypotension (e.g., postural lightheadedness) should be noted early because they suggest significant volume depletion and the possible need for hospitalization for rehydration.

Onset can be diagnostically meaningful. Diarrhea occurring within hours of ingestion of a potentially contaminated food is

TABLE 64.2

IMPORTANT FEATURES OF SOME ACUTE DIARRHEAS

Etiology	Nature of Diarrhea W/S	OB	GB	Associated Symptoms and Signs	Epidemiologic Data	Laboratory Results
Viral	+/+	–	–	n, v, fever, myalgias, abdominal cramps, HA	Occurs in short-lived epidemics	WBC: nl or elevated; stool: usually no WBC
Staphylococcus aureus	–/+	–	–	n, v, no fever	Custards; incubation: 2–8 hr	WBC: nl; stool: no WBC
Clostridium perfringens	+/+	–	–	n, v, no fever	Steam tables; incubation: 8–24 hr	WBC: nl; stool: no WBC
Bacillus cereus	+/+	–	–	n, v, no fever	Rice, sprouts	WBC: nl, stool: no WBC
Salmonella	+/–	+	+	n, v, fever, in some cases dysentery	Eggs, turtles, poultry	Stool: WBC+, culture+
Salmonella typhi	+/+ "Pea soup"	+	–	Rose spots, HA, splenomegaly, bradycardia, fever, toxic	Water, food	Stool: mono, culture+
Shigella	+/– Dysentery	+	–	n, v, fever, toxic in severe cases	High-poverty areas; day care centers; Native American reservations	Stool: WBC+, culture+
Escherichia coli 0157:H7	+/–	+	+	Crampy abdominal pain without fever followed by bloody diarrhea, hemolytic uremic syndrome, thrombotic thrombocytopenic purpura	Undercooked, contaminated processed meat and poultry	Stool: WBC+, culture+, toxin+
Campylobacter	+/– Dysentery	+	+	n, v, fever	Poultry, pets	Stool: WBC+, culture+
Yersinia	+/+	+	–	Simulates Crohn's disease and appendicitis; joint complaints	Dairy products, meat	Stool: WBC+, culture+
Vibrio species	+/+	–	–	n, v, cramps, occasionally fever	Raw seafood; 2-d course	Stool: culture+
Cryptosporidium	+/–	–	–	Occasionally n, v, cramps, dehydration	AIDS patients, immunosuppressed	Stool for o & p+ (spores, oocytes)
Giardia	See Table 64.3					
Entamoeba histolytica	See Table 64.3					

+, present; –, absent; GB, gross blood; HA, headache; n, nausea; nl, normal; o & p, ova and parasites; OB, occult blood; v, vomiting; WBC, white blood cells; W/S, watery/soft.

suggestive of food poisoning, which is confirmed if others have been similarly affected. Food-borne illness with a short incubation period and no fever indicates the ingestion of a preformed enterotoxin. Fever and a slightly longer incubation period are characteristic of an infectious etiology (see Table 64.3). Some toxin-producing organisms (e.g., *E. coli* 0157:H7) require a few days of incubation.

In addition to onset, a review of *epidemiologic information* is critical because the clinical presentation is often nonspecific. Reviews of travel (both international and domestic), personal contacts, and food intake are all essential. Among the foods to consider are custard-filled pastries, undercooked

processed meats, foods warmed on steam tables, eggs, poultry, raw seafood, unpasteurized milk and fruit juices, rice, and bean sprouts. Important contacts include children who attend day care centers because they may contract rotavirus, *Giardia*, *Shigella*, *Cryptosporidium*, or *Campylobacter*. A sexual history is also indicated.

Drug history needs review, particularly the use of laxatives, magnesium-containing antacids, excess alcohol, caffeine-containing beverages, herbal teas, antibiotics, digitalis, quinidine, loop diuretics (furosemide, ethacrynic acid), and antihypertensive agents and the excessive intake of sorbitol-containing "sugar-free" gums and mints.

TABLE 64.3

IMPORTANT FEATURES OF TRAVELER'S DIARRHEAS

Etiology	Nature of Diarrhea			Associated Symptoms and Signs	Epidemiologic Data	Laboratory Results
	W/S	OB	GB			
Escherichia coli	+/–	–	–	Usually no fever, although occasionally toxicity	Contamination of water, food	Stool: WBC –; can also be +
Entamoeba histolytica	+/+ Dysentery			Can simulate inflammatory bowel disease; asymptomatic carriers	Returning tourists, immigrants	Stool for o & p+; serology+
Giardia	–/+	+/–	+/–	Upper abdominal pain	Contamination of water supply	Stool for o & p+
Vibrio cholerae	+/– "Rice water"	–	–	Marked dehydration, cramps, vomiting	Contamination of water supply	Stool: WBC –
Shigella	See Table 64.2					
Salmonella	See Table 64.2					

+, present; –, absent; GB, gross blood; o & p, ova and parasites; OB, occult blood; WBC, white blood cells; W/S, watery/soft.

Physical Examination

Vital signs must be checked. Postural signs of significant volume depletion are an indication for prompt intravenous repletion. Any elevation in temperature or loss of weight also needs to be noted. The patient who appears to be markedly dehydrated or toxic is a candidate for hospital admission. The skin is examined for manifestations of sepsis; the macular "rose spot" rash on the trunk is an important clue for typhoid. The lymph nodes are checked for enlargement and the abdomen for tenderness, guarding, rebound, abnormal bowel sounds, organomegaly, and masses. A rectal examination and fecal occult blood test complete the physical evaluation.

Laboratory Studies: Initial Evaluation

The laboratory workup should be individualized. The patient who feels well except for frequent loose stools requires no immediate laboratory testing. On the other hand, the patient who is ill with fever, nausea, abdominal cramps, or other systemic symptoms requires more extensive evaluation.

Stool Testing for Leukocytes. Finding large numbers of white cells suggests an inflammatory or invasive diarrhea, such as occurs with *Shigella*, *Salmonella*, *Campylobacter*, invasive or certain toxigenic *E. coli*, and *Entamoeba*, but testing for leukocytes has largely been abandoned. Some advocate *fecal lactoferrin* as a marker of white blood cells and inflammatory disease.

Gram's Stain of the Stool. Gram's stain of the stool will provide etiologic information in selected instances, such as suspected *Campylobacter* infection. In about half of such cases, the Gram's stain will demonstrate gram-negative rods arranged in a characteristic seagull-wing configuration.

Stool Cultures. Stool cultures are usually not necessary in acute diarrhea because most cases are self-limited. However, if the patient appears to be ill with significant fever, blood in the stool, or immunocompromise, then *bacterial cultures* should be obtained. The laboratory should be notified when *E. coli* 0157:H7 is a consideration because special growth media and other procedures are required to identify the pathogen.

Sigmoidoscopy. Severely ill patients with gross blood or purulent mucus in the stool should undergo sigmoidoscopy to examine the appearance of the colonic mucosa; samples of the mucosa and cultures can also be obtained (for details, see the later section on the workup for chronic diarrhea). Preparatory enemas and cathartics should be avoided so as not to distort the appearance of the bowel wall (see Chapter 56).

Laboratory Studies: Subsequent Evaluation

If the diarrhea persists for 2 weeks or more, a secondary evaluation is indicated. *Stools* should once again be examined for *blood*, sent for bacterial *culture*, and examined for ova and parasites.

Stool Examination for Ova and Parasites. Ova and parasite examinations are fraught with limitations that must be kept in mind. If *giardiasis* is a consideration, at least three stool samples are necessary because the excretion of the organism is intermittent. Many primary care physicians use a therapeutic trial of metronidazole when they strongly suspect giardiasis. Identifying *E. histolytica* trophozoites by stool examination can be difficult; their visualization is easily impaired by the presence of barium, bismuth, and kaolin compounds. An *enzyme immunoassay test for Giardia* is now available and is useful as a screening test.

Other Studies. If symptoms persist and the diagnosis remains uncertain, the patient requires further assessment for a chronic or recurrent diarrheal syndrome (see later discussion). Persons in whom neurologic deficits or meningeal signs develop after a diarrheal illness require culturing of the *blood* and *cerebrospinal fluid* for *Listeria*.

Chronic or Recurrent Diarrhea

History

Diarrhea lasting 4 weeks or more or a pattern of recurrent diarrhea requires an etiologic assessment (see Table 64.1). As in acute diarrhea, *characterization of the diarrhea* and elicitation of any *associated symptoms* are important (Table 64.4).

TABLE 64.4

FEATURES OF REPRESENTATIVE CHRONIC DIARRHEAS

Etiology	Nature of Diarrhea			Associated Symptoms and Signs	Laboratory Results
	W/S	OB	GB		
Irritable bowel syndrome	–/+ Mucus prominent	–	–	Bloating, intermittent alternating constipation	Stool: WBC/RBC–
Ulcerative colitis	+/+	+	+	Fever, abdominal pain, extraintestinal disease, bowel ulcers/inflammation	Stool: WBC/RBC+; endoscopy+
Crohn's disease	–/+	+/–	+/–	Abdominal pain, obstruction, skip areas	Proctoscopy+/–; WBC+; o & p–
Pseudomembranous colitis	+/+	+/–	+/–	Simulates inflammatory bowel disease clinically; bowel ulcers/plaques	Stool: + for Clostridium difficile toxin/WBC/RBC
Diabetic enteropathy	+/+	–	–	Signs of autonomic insufficiency; occasionally malabsorption	Stool: fat+ (in small-bowel type)
Dumping syndrome	+/+	–	–	Gastric surgery; occurs with meals; sweats, tachycardia	Normal
Malabsorption of fat	–/+ Steatorrhea	–	–	Weight loss, vitamin deficiency, sprue, pancreatic disease	Stool: fat+
Stools: + for fat actase deficiency	+/+	–	–	Associated with milk products, cramping, bloating	Abnormal lactose tolerance test result
Laxative abuse	+/+	–	–	Wasting, bulimia, dehydration	Stool: laxatives+
Villous adenoma	+/– Secretory, mucus	+	–	Protein wasting, no relation to meals	Hypokalemia, low albumin
Colon cancer	+/+	+	+	Change in bowel habits	Iron deficiency

+, present; –, absent; GB, gross blood; o & p, ova and parasites; OB, occult blood; RBC, red blood cells; WBC, white blood cells; W/S, watery/soft.

Suggestive Patterns. A few patterns are suggestive. Frequent passage of *small volumes* of loose stools in association with left lower quadrant crampy abdominal pain or tenesmus points to rectosigmoid pathology. *Large volumes* of loose stools in conjunction with periumbilical or right lower quadrant pain indicate disease of the small bowel, as does diarrhea occurring *shortly after a meal* or ingestion of certain foods. Diarrhea following meals should also lead to a search for malabsorption, an osmotic etiology, the dumping syndrome, or a fistula. The presence of *foul, bulky, greasy* stools further supports the diagnosis of fat malabsorption. *Bloody stools* require investigation for neoplasm, invasive infection, ischemia, and inflammatory bowel disease. The presence of *fever* has similar diagnostic implications. *Frothy stools* and *excessive flatus* are signs of fermentation of unabsorbed carbohydrates, as occurs in lactase deficiency and giardiasis. *Alternating diarrhea* and *constipation* is the classic pattern for irritable bowel syndrome, especially when accompanied by mucoid stools, but Crohn's disease may present in similar fashion. Similarly, *bloating, abdominal discomfort,* and *fatigue* in conjunction with intermittent diarrhea are characteristic of functional bowel disease but may also be the presentation of celiac sprue.

Travel. Travel in conjunction with diarrhea that persists for more than 2 weeks raises the possibilities of giardiasis and amebiasis; pseudomembranous colitis is a consideration if the traveler has recently taken antibiotics. The slow resolution of traveler's diarrhea suggests postdysentery lactase deficiency and postdysentery irritable bowel syndrome.

Drugs. A thorough review of drug intake is mandatory; especially important is a check for *antibiotic use,* even if it was a few months before the onset of symptoms. A history of surreptitious *laxative abuse* may be hard to elicit, but inquiring gently and nonjudgmentally may elicit suggestive information.

Prior Surgery. Previous abdominal surgery should be specified, with any procedures that may have produced blind loops and allowed for bacterial overgrowth noted.

Physical Examination

Any fever, dehydration, postural hypotension, or cachexia should be noted. The skin should be inspected for jaundice, pallor, rash, and manifestations of inflammatory bowel disease. The abdomen is examined for distention, ascites, hepatosplenomegaly, tenderness, rebound, and masses. Rectal examination may reveal fecal impaction, perirectal fistula, or a patulous anal sphincter. Stool is tested for occult blood.

Laboratory

Blood tests are helpful but rarely diagnostic. They should include a *complete blood cell count* for evidence of anemia and leukocytosis. The finding of a microcytic anemia should suggest anemias due to iron deficiency and chronic disease and raise the index of suspicion for inflammatory bowel disease and celiac sprue. *Serum electrolytes* detect serious losses and imbalances. Determinations of *amylase* for pancreatic disease, *liver function tests* and *prothrombin time* for hepatobiliary disease, and *serum calcium* and *glucose* may detect metabolic conditions that can lead to diarrhea. Eosinophil counts are normal in most parasitic infections that cause diarrhea—the only gastrointestinal parasites that stimulate peripheral eosinophilia are worms.

Examination of Stool for White and Red Blood Cells. A *Wright's stain* of the stool for leukocytes provides a relatively simple means of distinguishing invasive from noninvasive etiologies of diarrhea, but the test has dropped from use as the means for its performance have become less available in the office. The presence of blood can be assayed by guaiac testing.

Other Stool Tests. Additional stool testing can be helpful in selected instances. For suspected laxative abuse, one *alkalinizes the stool*; if it contains phenolphthalein (a common ingredient of many over-the-counter laxatives), it will turn pink. For suspected fat malabsorption, a stool sample is subjected to Sudan stain for the *qualitative detection of fat*. Patients with a positive result on qualitative study are candidates for a *72-hour quantitative stool fat determination*. Normally, stool fat should not exceed 6% of the daily fat intake. Stool fat in excess of 6 g/d while the patient is on a test diet of 100 g of fat per 24 hours indicates fat malabsorption.

Sigmoidoscopy or Colonoscopy. Sigmoidoscopy performed without cleansing enemas is a potentially definitive procedure in persons suspected of having inflammatory bowel disease and amebiasis and helps to differentiate such conditions from irritable bowel syndrome (see Appendix 56.1). The presence of mucosal ulceration, plaques, friability, and bleeding should be noted. Nodular inflammatory ulcers and yellow-white mucosal plaques are characteristic of pseudomembranous colitis. Ulceration is also noted with inflammatory bowel disease and amebic colitis. If Crohn's disease, ischemia, or colonic neoplasia is suspected, *colonoscopy* should be substituted for sigmoidoscopy. Pseudomembranous colitis and amebic disease may produce an endoscopic appearance similar to that of inflammatory bowel disease, and so biopsies are necessary (see later discussion).

Barium Enema and Upper Gastrointestinal Series. Barium enema and upper gastrointestinal series have a narrow, specific role in demonstrating anatomic abnormalities (blind loops and fistulas). Because barium obscures the identification of ova and parasites, stool collections must be complete before a barium study is obtained.

Stool for *C. difficile* Toxin. Patients with recent antibiotic exposure or inflammatory exudates on sigmoidoscopy require evaluation for pseudomembranous colitis. Up to three stool samples should be assayed for *C. difficile* toxin to maximize sensitivity, although it must be understood that some patients without disease harbor the organism and might show detectable amounts of toxin in the stool.

Tests for Ova and Parasites. When epidemiologic data are suggestive (e.g., travel to an endemic area, HIV/AIDS), multiple *stool samples* should be sent for ova-and-parasite examination; false-negative examinations for trophozoites are common and are associated with the administration of preparatory enemas, recent exposure to antibiotics, and the concurrent use of barium, bismuth, or kaolin. Fresh, loose stools are needed for the identification of trophozoites; less fresh specimens can be used for the detection of ova.

When amebic disease is seriously suspected clinically and epidemiologically, yet results of examinations for ova and parasites are negative, *serologic testing* is indicated. The standard test is an indirect hemagglutination assay. A positive titer is greater than 1:128. It takes 2 to 4 weeks for seroconversion to occur. By the time most patients with amebic disease present with diarrhea, they are seropositive. The test is 85% sensitive in the setting of intestinal disease and 95% sensitive with extraintestinal spread. The test works best in nonendemic areas, where most people are seronegative.

Sometimes, *small-bowel aspiration* or even *biopsy* may be necessary to establish the diagnosis of giardiasis or cryptosporidiosis. *Immunologic assay of the stool* based on enzyme-linked immunosorbent assay (ELISA) technology can identify *Giardia* antigen with high sensitivity and specificity (92% and 98%, respectively); the test is rapidly obviating the need for biopsy and aspiration.

Testing for Celiac Sprue. Advances in serologic testing have greatly facilitated the diagnosis of celiac sprue. Serologic testing can help to differentiate patients who need biopsy (the definitive test) from those who do not. The presence of *antiendomesial* and *antitransglutaminase antibodies* is associated with a sensitivity of just greater than 80% and a specificity of 99%; their absence gives a negative predictive value of 99%, making these IgA serologic tests useful for screening. A negative serum test rules out the diagnosis and usually obviates the need for biopsy. *HLA-DQ genotyping* helps to identify persons at risk for sprue (sensitivity, 100%), but the predictive value of HLA testing is insufficient for diagnosis due to low specificity (56%) resulting from incomplete penetrance of the genetic defect (i.e., a substantial number of persons with the genotype never develop clinically significant disease). *Antigliadin antibodies* are useful for monitoring disease activity but are inadequate for use in screening.

Persons who test positive serologically still need confirmatory *small-bowel biopsy* because of the lifelong dietary consequences of the diagnosis. Response to an *empiric trial of a gluten-free diet* is insufficient for diagnosis. Those with anemia should have serum *iron* and *folate* checked. Testing for vitamin D malabsorption can be achieved by serum determinations of *vitamin D*, *calcium*, and *alkaline phosphatase*.

Therapeutic Trials

Therapeutic trials can sometime substitute as diagnostic measures. For example, the cessation of diarrhea in response to *restriction of milk products* strongly supports the diagnosis of lactose intolerance. Other recognized empiric trials include a course of *antibiotic therapy* in patients suspected of blind-loop syndrome and the use of *pancreatic enzymes* in patients believed to have pancreatic insufficiency. The once-common trial of *metronidazole* for patients with suspected giardiasis is being deferred in favor of sensitive ELISA stool testing for *Giardia* antigen. As noted earlier, some patients with suspected sprue are given empiric trials of a gluten-free diet, but serologic testing and small-bowel biopsy are preferred for diagnosis.

Diarrhea in the AIDS Patient

Often, patients with AIDS experience acute or chronic diarrhea. They especially are susceptible not only to the common pathogens, but also to such uncommon ones as *Cryptosporidium*, *M. avium–intracellulare*, herpes simplex virus, cytomegalovirus, *Neisseria gonorrhoeae*, and *C. trachomatis*. Evaluation should focus on finding the pathogen and may require sigmoidoscopic biopsy to obtain tissue for viral or mycobacterial culture (see Chapter 13).

Chronic Diarrhea of Unknown Etiology

The leading possibilities are *surreptitious laxative abuse*, subtle forms of *inflammatory bowel disease*, *sprue*, and *irritable*

bowel syndrome. Laxative abuse should be considered in young women who are preoccupied with their weight and have low self-esteem and a poor body image (see Chapter 234). An otherwise unexplained *hypokalemia* is also suggestive. Collagenous and lymphocytic forms of colitis must be considered in *women* who present with *chronic watery diarrhea* complicated by *steatorrhea* and malabsorption, especially those who are believed to have sprue but fail to respond to a gluten-free diet. Irritable bowel syndrome is suggested by the presence of *abdominal pain* in addition to diarrhea. Tip-offs to sprue include *positive family history*, episodes of diarrhea beginning in *adolescence* or *early adulthood*, and *unexplained iron-deficiency anemia*.

One attempts to characterize the type of diarrhea further by determining *stool volume, osmolality,* and *electrolyte content*. A stool volume of less than 200 mL/d is strongly suggestive of irritable bowel syndrome. Osmotic diarrheas show increased stool osmolality and low sodium and potassium concentrations. The differential diagnosis of osmotic diarrhea includes ingestion of nonabsorbable solutes (magnesium, bran), maldigestion of food, and malabsorption of osmotically active substances (e.g., carbohydrates). Stool volumes of greater than 1 L/d indicate a secretory diarrhea, such as may occur with surreptitious laxative abuse (see Chapter 234), villous adenoma (see Chapter 56), carcinoid syndrome, and pancreatic cholera (from the secretion of vasoactive intestinal peptide).

If there is a clinical suspicion of sprue, serum should be sent for *antiendomesial* and *antitransglutaminase antibody* determinations; persons who test positive can proceed to *small-bowel biopsy*. *Colonoscopy with biopsy* should be considered in women with unexplained watery diarrhea, especially if it is complicated by steatorrhea and malabsorption, because the endoscopic appearance of the bowel is grossly normal in collagenous and lymphocytic forms of colitis.

Inpatient Study

The next step for patients whose condition remains undiagnosed is inpatient evaluation with the imposition of a 24- to 72-hour fast and intravenous hydration. The fast helps to differentiate between osmotic and secretory causes; with the former, diarrhea ceases or is markedly reduced during fasting. Stool analysis is repeated under conditions of fasting and standardized diets.

PRINCIPLES OF MANAGEMENT
(1,3,4,6,7,9,10,14,16,18,20, 21,25,26,28,31–47)

Acute Diarrheas

Because most causes are self-limited, the principal therapeutic measures are supportive. The most important is hydration, supplemented when necessary by the use of absorbent preparations and motility inhibitors and occasionally by antibiotics.

Hydration

The vast majority of cases of acute diarrheal illness should be managed by *maintaining hydration* and waiting for the spontaneous resolution of symptoms. Often, hydration can be maintained with oral fluids, even in cases of profuse diarrhea. Solutions rich in electrolytes and sugar facilitate the absorption of water. An 8-oz glass of *fruit juice* to which is added a pinch of table salt and half a teaspoon of honey or a teaspoon of table sugar makes a well-tolerated replacement solution. Nondiet

cola drinks that have been allowed to stand and lose their carbonation are a reasonable substitute. Either can be taken along with a similarly sized glass of water containing a fourth of a teaspoon of baking soda to replenish losses in stool electrolytes, which in acute infectious diarrhea are sodium (125 mEq/L), potassium (20 mEq/L), bicarbonate (45 mEq/L), and chlorine (90 mEq/L). If adequate hydration cannot be maintained orally, intravenous therapy is necessary.

Absorbent

Absorbent preparations are commonly used for the symptomatic therapy of simple acute diarrhea. Solutions of kaolin and pectin have no proven benefit but seem to be harmless; however, they should not be relied on for the treatment of severe diarrhea. Doses of *bismuth subsalicylate (Pepto-Bismol)* in excess of those recommended on the bottle (e.g., 2 to 3 tablespoons every 3 hours) are sometimes effective (see later discussion).

Inhibition of Motility

Opiates such as *diphenoxylate* (dispensed as a combination with small amounts of atropine [Lomotil] to discourage abuse) and *loperamide* (Imodium) are effective in the symptomatic treatment of diarrhea by directly inhibiting the motility of the intestinal smooth muscle. Diphenoxylate and loperamide are derived from meperidine but have less effect on the central nervous system. They should be used cautiously, if at all, in conditions in which toxic megacolon is possible (e.g., inflammatory bowel disease). Their use should also be restricted in certain bacterial diarrheas, such as shigellosis, to avoid prolonging the clinical course. There is also concern for their use in outbreaks of *E. coli* 0157:H7 infection, in which an increased risk for complications has been noted.

The usual dose of diphenoxylate is 2.5 to 5 mg every 4 hours, up to 20 mg daily. Loperamide is given as 2 or 4 mg every 4 hours, up to 16 mg daily. Lower maintenance doses are often sufficient after initial control has been achieved. Other opiates are potent antidiarrheal agents but carry a higher risk for addiction; they are useful when their coincident analgesic activity is needed. Deodorized tincture of opium (0.5 to 1 mL), paregoric (4 mL), or codeine (30 to 60 mg) can be given orally every 4 hours. *Anticholinergics* are useful only for irritable bowel syndrome (see Chapter 74).

Antibiotics

The *empiric use* of antibiotics is not recommended routinely for acute bacterial diarrheas because most infections are self-limited. Empiric antibiotics have a minimal effect on the course of illness (with the exception of shigellosis outbreaks) and may prolong the asymptomatic bacterial carrier state (especially with *Salmonella* infection) and promote the emergence of resistant organisms. Moreover, one risks triggering an antibiotic-induced diarrhea and inducing antibiotic resistance (e.g., in *Campylobacter*). Antibiotics may also be counterproductive in *E. coli* 0157:H7 infection, in which case their use has been associated in some instances with an increased risk for complications.

Antibiotics are best reserved for very ill patients with positive stool cultures or other evidence for a specific bacterial etiology (e.g., typhoid fever, salmonellosis, shigellosis, pseudomembranous colitis, *Campylobacter* infection, and *Yersinia* infection).

Salmonella. Elderly patients and others who would be endangered by a *Salmonella* bacteremia (persons with vascular prostheses or sickle cell anemia) should receive a course of antibiotics to limit metastatic infection. *Bacteremia* and *typhoid fever* can be treated with parenteral *ampicillin* or oral *chloramphenicol*; in milder cases, oral *trimethoprim/sulfamethoxazole* (TMS; one double-strength tablet twice daily for 2 weeks) suffices.

Shigella. Patients with severe dysentery caused by shigellosis can be treated with a *quinolone* or oral *amoxicillin* (500 mg three times daily for 3 to 5 days), but antibiotic sensitivity testing is needed because amoxicillin-resistant strains are common. *TMS* (one double-strength tablet twice daily for 3 to 5 days) is an excellent alternative. Pending stool culture results, providing a few days of empiric therapy for shigellosis is reasonable if the epidemiologic history is suggestive and the patient is experiencing severe bloody diarrhea. Antiperistaltic drugs are contraindicated.

Campylobacter. *Campylobacter* is sensitive to oral *erythromycin* (500 mg four times daily for 7 days). Most patients with *Yersinia* infection have a self-limited illness, but toxic patients are candidates for oral *chloramphenicol* (50 mg/kg daily in four divided doses for 7 days) or parenteral therapy.

Pseudomembranous Colitis. *Pseudomembranous colitis* usually resolves without antibiotic treatment, but oral *vancomycin* in a liquid suspension (as little as 125 mg four times daily for 7 to 10 days) and *metronidazole* (250 mg three times daily for 5 to 10 days) have proved equally capable of controlling the disease. Relapses occur in 10% to 20% of cases, and so retreatment is necessary. Metronidazole is preferred for initial use because it is far less expensive. *Cholestyramine* (one packet in water three times daily) is used in conjunction with antibiotics to help bind the enterotoxin; it has proved useful in protracted cases. *Probiotics* may have a role in treating mild or chronic symptoms.

Parasitic Infection. Symptomatic patients with diarrhea caused by parasitic infection also benefit from definitive antimicrobial therapy. *E. histolytica* responds to *metronidazole* (750 mg three times daily for 5 to 10 days) for the treatment of trophozoites and *diiodohydroxyquin* (650 mg three times daily for 21 days) for the elimination of cysts. *Giardiasis* is treated with quinacrine (100 mg three times daily for 7 days) or metronidazole (250 mg three times daily for 7 to 10 days). Retreatment is often necessary.

Traveler's Diarrhea

Prevention

Although much attention has been given to pharmacologic agents for prophylaxis, care in what one eats and drinks remains the most important means of preventing traveler's diarrhea. The use of local water supplies should be avoided when they are in question. This includes foregoing fresh vegetables, which may have been washed in such water, and even ice cubes. Drinking bottled water is preferable.

Chemoprophylaxis. Because the majority of "turista" cases are caused by enterotoxigenic *E. coli*, chemoprophylaxis has been directed at this organism. TMS (one double-strength tablet daily) and *ciprofloxacin* (500 mg daily) can reduce the risk for diarrhea, which ranges from 20% to 30%. For the symptomatic relief of acute diarrhea, ciprofloxacin (500 mg twice daily for 3 days) is effective, as is TMS (one double-strength tablet twice daily). Some resistance to TMS is emerging, making ciprofloxacin the preferred agent. *Doxycycline*, a tetracycline derivative, taken on the day of travel (200 mg) and daily (100 mg) while away has also proved to be useful, although as many as 40% of the toxigenic *E. coli* strains are resistant to the drug, and the drug often causes gastrointestinal upset and photosensitivity. Another approach under study is the use of the nonabsorbable antibiotic *rifaximin*, which, when taken at 200 mg twice daily for 2 weeks, significantly reduces the risk of toxigenic *E. coli*–related traveler's diarrhea without markedly altering normal fecal flora. The efficacy of rifaximin in Asia and other areas where *Shigella* is the more likely pathogen remains to be demonstrated.

The prophylactic use of antibiotics has been in vogue, but the growing awareness of antibiotic-induced diarrhea, the high frequency of bacterial resistance to some agents, and the efficacy of *bismuth subsalicylate* is leading to less reliance on antimicrobials.

Treatment

Although antibiotics are sometimes used, their disadvantages (see prior discussion) suggest the use of other measures first, if possible.

Bismuth Subsalicylate. Bismuth subsalicylate (Pepto-Bismol) has proved effective as both prophylaxis and treatment for traveler's diarrhea when given in large doses (60 mL four times daily). Unlike antibiotics, it has the advantage of not altering the normal bowel flora. Its mechanism of action is believed to involve the inhibition of colonization by toxigenic bacterial strains. Bismuth turns the stools black; it is useful to alert patients to this side effect so that its occurrence does not cause alarm.

Diphenoxylate or Loperamide. Diphenoxylate or loperamide is often more convenient for symptomatic relief of traveler's diarrhea than are other measures. In most instances, these agents can be used for brief periods with safety, except when *Shigella* or *Salmonella* infection is a serious consideration (i.e., when fever or rectal bleeding is present). Loperamide has also been a useful adjunct to the antibiotic treatment of symptomatic disease.

Antibiotics. Antibiotics are indicated in severe cases of acute traveler's diarrhea. *Ciprofloxacin* (500 mg twice daily) or TMS (one double-strength tablet twice daily) is effective, especially when used with *loperamide* (2 mg after each loose stool, up to 16 mg/d). A 3-day course of antibiotics usually suffices. Giving travelers a 3-day antibiotic supply plus loperamide to carry with them is reasonable and appreciated. Ciprofloxacin is probably preferred because of the emergence of TMS-resistant strains of *E. coli*.

Chronic Diarrhea

Unlike the treatment of acute diarrhea, in which many cases are self-limited and nonspecific measures aimed at symptomatic relief are appropriate, the effective management of chronic diarrhea requires an etiologic diagnosis and specific therapy. Simply suppressing symptoms without identifying a cause may delay the identification of a serious underlying condition (e.g., colon cancer or inflammatory bowel disease). Empiric trials are limited to use in diagnosis (see prior discussion).

Many causes are treatable. For example, exacerbations of *inflammatory bowel disease* have effective treatments (see Chapter 73). Malabsorption associated with *pancreatic insufficiency* improves with the use of enzyme supplements (see

Chapter 72). Steatorrhea caused by *sprue* responds to a gluten-free diet, but not all patients respond to the dietary change because often a concurrent contributing factor is present. *Lactase deficiency* requires the limitation of milk products or the use of exogenous lactase. The *dumping syndrome* can be controlled with small feedings. Persistent pseudomembranous colitis is an indication for antibiotic therapy (see earlier discussion). Cessation of surreptitious *laxative abuse* cures the diarrhea that accompanies it (see Chapter 234). In the setting of *irritable bowel syndrome*, a high-fiber diet is indicated if the clinical picture is predominantly one of constipation interspersed with brief episodes of diarrhea, but if diarrhea predominates, there are other options for symptomatic relief (see Chapter 74).

Chronic Diarrhea of Unknown Etiology

For patients whose condition remains undiagnosed after an extensive workup yet who appear otherwise well, a trial of therapy for irritable bowel syndrome is reasonable (see Chapter 74). Many such patients with unexplained diarrhea turn out to have a bowel motility disorder and associated psychosocial stresses. Clues to the diagnosis include an absence of weight loss, normal findings on laboratory studies, and a suggestive psychosocial history. Failure to respond after 4 weeks of management should lead to a gastroenterological consultation. One should not resort to nonspecific antidiarrheal agents to treat patients who have not been given a diagnosis.

INDICATIONS FOR ADMISSION AND REFERRAL

Admission

Most patients with diarrhea can be managed on an outpatient basis. However, for those who are unable to maintain their hydration orally and become significantly volume depleted (with postural hypotension), hospital admission and parenteral fluid replacement must be seriously considered. Sometimes, several hours of intravenous fluids given in the emergency department will suffice and obviate an admission. Infants, elderly persons, and persons with chronic or debilitating illnesses such as diabetic renal failure are particularly vulnerable to the complications of volume depletion and warrant close monitoring. Patients with inflammatory diarrhea manifested by bloody, purulent stools and fever are also candidates for admission, as are those with neurologic deficits and meningeal signs following a diarrheal illness, who require assessment for listeriosis. Patients with undiagnosed chronic diarrhea may benefit from the observation and testing possible only during hospitalization.

Referral to a Gastroenterologist

Referral to a gastroenterologist is indicated for patients who have complicated acute disease (e.g., hemorrhagic diarrhea),

poorly controlled inflammatory bowel disease, or undiagnosed chronic diarrhea or who require colonoscopy or intestinal biopsy.

PATIENT EDUCATION

Because most cases of acute diarrhea are self-limited, the patient with no evidence of serious underlying pathology can be reassured and advised to concentrate on maintaining hydration. The sugar and electrolyte preparations described in this chapter are easy to take and should be encouraged. Many people believe that taking fluids will seriously worsen their diarrhea, and they request opiates or antibiotics; the proper role for such agents needs to be reviewed, and their unrestricted use should be limited. Many patients ask whether kaolin and pectin preparations are helpful; there is no evidence that they alter symptoms or the course of the illness, but neither is harmful. Although antibiotics have been in vogue for prophylaxis of traveler's diarrhea, patients should be informed of the emergence of resistant strains, the potential complications of antibiotic use, and the efficacy of bismuth preparations. A few bottles of a bismuth preparation (e.g., Pepto-Bismol), a few tablets of diphenoxylate for "emergencies," and advice to use bottled water and avoid foods likely to be contaminated (e.g., raw vegetables washed with local water) represent reasonable alternatives to antibiotic prophylaxis. Patients with chronic undiagnosed diarrhea need to be prepared for a potentially extensive evaluation. In the meantime, advice on perianal care is much appreciated and should not be overlooked while the investigation proceeds.

Perianal Hygiene

Much can be done to relieve the perianal discomfort that accompanies severe, unrelenting diarrhea. *Sitz baths* for about 10 minutes two or three times a day can be soothing, followed by gentle drying with *absorbent cotton* (not toilet paper or towels). Washing with warm water on absorbent cotton after each bowel movement is also helpful in lieu of using toilet paper, which can be irritating. Also important is the avoidance of soap. Desitin may be effective, and a short course of *hydrocortisone cream* may be useful when considerable anal inflammation is present. Some patients report that cleaning gently with cotton pads soaked in *witch hazel* (Tucks) provides considerable relief. Ointments containing topical anesthetics should be avoided; they can be irritating in themselves.

Recovery Phase

After the resolution of diarrhea, it is best to avoid milk and dairy products for approximately another 7 to 10 days because mild lactose intolerance commonly accompanies many cases. The best foods to begin eating are easily digested, high-carbohydrate substances such as bananas, rice, baked potatoes, and apple sauce. Continued repletion of fluid is important.

Annotated Bibliography

1. Afzalpurkar RG, Schiller LR, Little KH, et al. Self-limited nature of chronic idiopathic diarrhea. N Engl J Med 1992;327:1849. (*Presents clinically useful data on this difficult problem.*)
2. Aureli P, Fiorucci GC, Caroli D, et al. An outbreak of febrile gastroenteritis associated with corn contaminated by *Listeria monocytogenes*. N Engl J Med 2000;342:1236. (*An important report of food-borne infection with this organism in immunologically competent persons.*)
3. Bartlett JG. Narrative review: the new epidemic of *Clostridium difficile*–associated enteric disease. Ann Intern Med 2006;145:758. (*A succinct, practical update from a leading authority; 77 references.*)

4. Bayless TM, Rothfeld TM, Massa C, et al. Lactose and milk intolerance: clinical implications. N Engl J Med 1975;292:1156. (*A classic paper on the prevalence, characteristics, and diagnosis of this condition.*)

5. Blaser MJ, McDermott KT, Little JR, et al. *Campylobacter* enteritis in the United States: a multicenter study. Ann Intern Med 1983;98:360. (*Campylobacter was more frequently isolated than Salmonella and Shigella combined.*)

6. Cover TL, Aber RC. *Yersinia* enterocolitica. N Engl J Med 1989;321:16. (*A comprehensive review of this pathogen; 201 references.*)

7. Dolin R N. Noroviruses; challenges to clinical control. N Engl J Med 2007 357:1072. (*A succinct discussion of virology, epidemiology, prophylaxis, and treatment.*)

8. DuBois R, Lazenby AJ, Yardley JH, et al. Lymphocytic enterocolitis in patients with "refractory sprue." JAMA 1989;262:935. (*A description of this now-recognized cause of chronic, watery diarrhea and steatorrhea.*)

9. Farrell RJ, Kelly C. Celiac sprue. N Engl J Med 2002;346:180. (*An excellent review, with emphasis on enhanced clinical recognition and appreciation for its prevalence; 43 references.*)

10. Farthing MJG. Giardiasis. Gastroenterol Clin North Am 1996;25:493. (*A comprehensive review of a very common and often difficult clinical problem.*)

11. Fine KD, Meyer RL, Lee EL. The prevalence and causes of chronic diarrhea in patients with celiac sprue treated with gluten-free diet. Gastroenterology 1997;112:1830. (*A host of reasons other than noncompliance was detected.*)

12. Goodgame RW. Understanding intestinal spore-forming protozoa: *Cryptosporidium, Microsporidia, Isospora,* and *Cyclospora.* Ann Intern Med 1996;124:429. (*Everything you ever wanted to know; 170 references.*)

13. Glynn MK, Bopp C, Dewitt W, et al. Emergence of multidrug-resistant *Salmonella enteritidis* serotype typhimurium DT 104 infections in the United States. N Engl J Med 1998;338:1333. (*Documents the widespread nature of this increasingly important pathogen.*)

14. Haque R, Huston CD, Hughes M, et al. Amebiasis. N Engl J Med 2003;348:1565. (*A comprehensive review of an important cause of chronic diarrhea; 50 references.*)

15. Kelly CP, LaMont JT. *Clostridium difficile* infection. Annu Rev Med 1998;49:375. (*A comprehensive clinical review of Clostridium difficile infection.*)

16. Musher DM, Musher BL "Contagious acute gastrointestinal infections" N Engl J Med 2004, 351:2417. (*A comprehensive review; 127 references.*)

17. Sandler RS, Zorich NL, Filloon TG, et al. Gastrointestinal symptoms in 3,181 volunteers ingesting snack foods containing Olestra or triglycerides: a 6-week randomized, placebo-controlled trial. Ann Intern Med 1999;130:253. (*No clinically significant increase was found in gastrointestinal side effects.*)

18. Simon D, Brandt LJ. Diarrhea in patients with acquired immunodeficiency syndrome. Gastroenterology 1993;105:1238. (*A comprehensive review of pathogens in AIDS.*)

19. Slutsker L, Ries AA, Greene KC, et al. *Escherichia coli* 0157:H7 diarrhea in the United States: clinical and epidemiologic features. Ann Intern Med 1997;126:505. (*A population prevalence study that includes clinical features of infection with this increasingly important pathogen.*)

20. Su C, Brandt LJ. *Escherichia coli* 0157:H7 infection in humans. Ann Intern Med 1995;123:698. (*A systematic review; 217 references.*)

21. Valdovinos MA, Camilleri M, Zimmerman BR. Chronic diarrhea in diabetes mellitus: mechanisms and approach to diagnosis and treatment. Mayo Clin Proc 1993;68:691. (*A detailed consideration of the consequences of autonomic neuropathy.*)

22. Vugia DJ, Abbott S, Mintz ED, et al. A restaurant-associated outbreak of Brainerd diarrhea in California. Clin Infect Dis 2006;43:55. (*Brainerd diarrhea remains an unexplained, probably infectious diarrheal disease.*)

23. Weber R, Ledergerber B, Zbinden R, et al. Enteric infections and diarrhea in human immunodeficiency virus–infected persons. Arch Intern Med 1999;159:1473. (*Data from the Swiss HIV Cohort study on the frequency and causes of acute and chronic diarrhea in this population.*)

24. White DG, Zhao S, Sudler R, et al. The isolation of antibiotic-resistant *Salmonella* from retail ground meats. N Engl J Med 2001;345:1147. (*Documents the commonality of such organisms.*)

25. AGA technical review on the evaluation and management of chronic diarrhea. Gastroenterology 1999;116:1464. (*An extensive review of the literature and clinical recommendations.*)

26. American Gastroenterological Association medical position statement: guidelines for the evaluation and management of chronic diarrhea. Gastroenterology 1999;116:1461. (*The American Gastroenterological Association's summary guidelines.*)

27. Donowitz M, Kokke FT, Saidi R. Evaluation of patients with chronic diarrhea. N Engl J Med 1995;332:725. (*A review, together with a practical, stepped approach to assessment; 42 references.*)

28. Fekety R. Guidelines for the diagnosis and management of *Clostridium difficile*–associated diarrhea and colitis. Am J Gastroenterol 1997;92:739. (*American College of Gastroenterology guidelines.*)

29. Phillips S, Donaldson L, Geisler K, et al. Stool composition in factitious diarrhea: a 6-year experience with stool analysis. Ann Intern Med 1995;123:97. (*The utility of stool analysis is documented in cases of chronic diarrhea, with laxative abuse detected.*)

30. Raoult D, Birg ML, La Scola B, et al. Cultivation of the bacillus of Whipple's disease. N Engl J Med 2000;342:620. (*A major accomplishment, which should lead to a serologic test.*)

31. Thielman NM, Guerrant RL. Acute infectious diarrhea. New Engl J Med 2004;350:38. (*A succinct, clinical review of the management of acute diarrhea.*)

32. Ericson CD, DuPont HL, Mathewson JJ, et al. Treatment of traveler's diarrhea with sulfamethoxazole and trimethoprim and loperamide. JAMA 1990;263:257. (*A randomized, double-blind study, finding that combination therapy was the most effective.*)

33. Taylor DN, Sanchez JL, Candler W, et al. Treatment of traveler's diarrhea: ciprofloxacin plus loperamide compared with ciprofloxacin alone. Ann Intern Med 1991;114:731. (*The addition of loperamide was helpful, especially during the first 24 hours.*)

34. Duggan C, Lasche J, McCarty M, et al. Oral rehydration solution for acute diarrhea prevents subsequent unscheduled follow-up visits. Pediatrics 1999;104:29. (*A simple, effective therapy.*)

35. DuPont HL, Jiang Z-D, Okhuysen PC, et al. A randomized, double-blind, placebo-controlled trial of rifaximin to prevent traveler's diarrhea. Ann Intern Med 2005;142:805. (*Presents evidence of its efficacy in the context of travel to Mexico.*)

36. DuPont HL, Ericson CD. Prevention and treatment of traveler's diarrhea. N Engl J Med 1993;328:1821. (*An excellent review.*)

37. DuPont HL, Hornick RB. Adverse effect of Lomotil therapy in shigellosis. JAMA 1973;260:1525. (*An older but important finding: the use of Lomotil may exacerbate and prolong illness in patients with shigellosis.*)

38. DuPont HL. The Practice Parameters Committee of the American College of Gastroenterology. Guidelines on acute infectious diarrhea in adults. Am J Gastroenterol 1997;92:1962. (*Consensus guidelines.*)

39. Goodman LJ, Trenholme GM, Kaplan RL, et al. Empiric antimicrobial therapy of domestically acquired acute diarrhea in urban adults. Arch Intern Med 1990;150:541. (*A randomized, controlled trial; empiric ciprofloxacin was effective for suspected acute bacterial diarrhea; trimethoprim/sulfamethoxazole was not.*)

40. Graham DY, Estes NK, Gentry LO. Double-blind comparison of bismuth subsalicylate and placebo in the prevention and treatment of enterotoxigenic *E. coli*–induced diarrhea in volunteers. Gastroenterology 1983;85:1017. (*A study of 32 volunteers, confirming the effectiveness of bismuth subsalicylate in preventing diarrhea.*)

41. Molina J, Tourneur M, Sarfati C, et al. Fumagillin treatment of intestinal microsporidiosis. N Engl J Med 2002;346:1963. (*Presents a new, orally effective treatment for this cause of chronic diarrhea in immunocompromised patients.*)

42. Murphy GS, Bodhidatta L, Echeverria P, et al. Ciprofloxacin and loperamide in the treatment of bacillary dysentery. Ann Intern Med 1993;118:582. (*This approach was found to be effective.*)

43. Palmer DL, Koster KT, Islam AF, et al. Comparison of sucrose and glucose in the oral electrolyte therapy of cholera and other severe diarrhea. N Engl J Med 1977;292:1107. (*A discussion of the uses and limitations of oral fluid and electrolyte therapy.*)

44. Palmer KR, Corbett CL, Holdsworth CD. Double-blind, crossover study comparing loperamide, codeine, and diphenoxylate in the treatment of chronic diarrhea. Gastroenterology 1980;79:1272. (*Loperamide was more effective than diphenoxylate and as effective as codeine, and it caused fewer side effects than either agent.*)

45. Wistrom J, Jertborn M, Ekwall E, et al. Empiric treatment of acute diarrheal disease with norfloxacin: a randomized, placebo-controlled study. Ann Intern Med 1992;117:202. (*Efficacy was demonstrated, but the benefit was limited mostly to the very ill and those with positive cultures.*)

46. Kane SV, Sandborn WJ, Rufo PA, et al. Fecal lactoferrin is a sensitive and specific marker in identifying intestinal inflammation. Am J Gastroenterol 2003;98:1309. (*Fecal lactoferrin is more predictive and reproducible than microscopic examination of stool for leukocytes in identifying patients with inflammatory disease.*)

47. Yan F, Polk DB. Probiotics as functional food in the treatment of diarrhea. Curr Opin Clin Nutr Metab Care 2006;9:717. (*A review discussing the data indicating that probiotics have some role in the treatment of diarrheal disease.*)

CHAPTER 65 ■ APPROACH TO THE PATIENT WITH CONSTIPATION

JAMES M. RICHTER

Constipation is a common experience of persons living in industrialized and postindustrialized societies. Chronic constipation affects 15% of adults, accounts for more than 2.5 million physician visits a year, and ranks among the most frequent reasons for self-medication, particularly in the elderly. For patients, there is no uniform definition of constipation. To some, it means movements that are too infrequent or stools that are too hard. Others complain of incomplete or difficult evacuation. Consensus criteria help to identify those with functional etiologies (Table 65.1). Bowel habits vary widely among normal people, and perceptions of what constitutes normal function are diverse. Population studies show that most people have more than three bowel movements per week, with men likely to have at least five.

The primary physician must be able to detect any underlying pathology and provide symptomatic relief and reassurance to those with functional etiologies. The prevalence of excessive laxative use and inadequate dietary fiber intake make it imperative that the physician be knowledgeable about the actions and adverse effects of available laxative preparations in addition to dietary alternatives to their use.

PATHOPHYSIOLOGY AND CLINICAL PRESENTATION (1–14)

The process of elimination of fecal waste requires two processes: enteric transit and rectal evacuation of stool. Constipation may arise secondary to interference with either of these processes.

Impaired Colonic Transport

Colonic transport can be impaired by inadequate dietary fiber, metabolic factors, mechanical obstruction, motor disorders, drugs, psychiatric conditions, and neurologic disease.

Inadequate Dietary Fiber

The time it takes food to reach the anus is partially a function of the amount of fiber in the diet. Normal people placed on a diet containing 15 g of bran fiber per day have twice the number of movements per week as those on an uncontrolled or low-fiber diet. Patients with constipation solely on the basis of low dietary fiber usually have intermittent complaints that fully resolve with alteration of diet alone.

Inactivity

Exercise has an important positive effect on the propulsion of bowel contents. Colonic transit is significantly greater in physically active people than in those who get little exercise. Previously active persons often become constipated when confined to bed due to illness. Less dramatic, but probably no less important, is the effect of a sedentary lifestyle; constipation is common in inactive people.

Metabolic and Endocrine Disturbances

Metabolic and endocrine disturbances can slow colonic transport. Hypokalemia, hypercalcemia, hypothyroidism, and diabetes are the most important of these in terms of frequency or potential reversibility. *Hypokalemia* can produce a generalized ileus and is most often seen in patients who take diuretics. *Chronic laxative abuse* may also produce hypokalemia; surreptitious use of laxatives and diuretics, self-induced vomiting, a pathologic desire to lose weight, and personality disorder are characteristic of such patients, who present with fatigue and electrolyte disturbances. When constipation is caused by *hypothyroidism*, other manifestations of the disease are usually present, although sluggish bowel movements may be the presenting complaint. Constipation is a bothersome problem in some patients with *diabetes*; 20% of those with neuropathy report severe difficulty. Significant *hypercalcemia* (serum calcium level >12 mg/100 mL) can slow bowel motility.

Mechanical Obstruction

Mechanical obstruction from tumor, stricture, or volvulus may be responsible for the new onset of constipation. Cramping abdominal pain and distention in conjunction with a marked change in bowel habits are characteristic. Many patients with *colorectal cancer* report constipation, which is often a symptom of advanced disease. Constipation is a more common presentation of *Crohn's disease* than is diarrhea because transmural involvement predisposes to scarring and obstruction (see Chapter 73).

Motor Dysfunction

Constipation is the most frequent symptom of *irritable bowel syndrome,* a common motility disorder of unknown etiology (see Chapter 74). Patients complain of chronic abdominal discomfort related to alterations in bowel habits and relieved by defecation. They report irregular bowel movements, often diarrhea alternating with constipation (although one may predominate). Passage of mucus, a sense of incomplete evacuation, and bloating or distention add to the clinical picture.

Drug Use

Drug use may precipitate constipation. *Opiates* and agents with anticholinergic activity such as *antidepressants* are frequently implicated. *Calcium-channel blockers* may slow down

TABLE 65.1

ROME DIAGNOSTIC CRITERIA FOR FUNCTIONAL CONSTIPATION (12)

1. Must include two or more of the following:
   a. Straining during at least 25% of defecations
   b. Lumpy or hard stools in at least 25% of defecations
   c. Sensation of incomplete evacuation for at least 25% of defecations
   d. Sensation of anorectal obstruction/blockage for at least 25% of defecations
   e. Manuel maneuvers to facilitate at least 25% of defecations
   f. Fewer that three defecations per week
2. Loose stools are rarely present without the use of laxatives
3. There are insufficient criteria for irritable bowel syndrome

Criteria should be fulfilled for the last 3 months with symptom onset at least 6 months prior to the diagnosis.

bowel motility, and cholestyramine may induce constipation by binding bile salts. *Aluminum hydroxide* and *calcium carbonate* antacids are constipating. The habitual use of *laxatives* is associated with impaired motor activity. The typical clinical picture is a long history of chronic constipation or a desire to feel "well cleaned out," followed by increasing laxative dependence, decreasing response, and, ultimately, a sluggish, poorly contracting bowel. The question of whether a prior underlying motor disorder or actual damage from laxative use is the cause remains unsettled.

Psychiatric Disease and Psychosocial Distress

Psychiatric disease and psychosocial distress can play important roles. An underlying depression is often contributory, and bowel complaints may be one of many somatic symptoms (see Chapter 227). Patients with irritable bowel syndrome have an increased prevalence of somatization, anxiety, and phobias. Disturbances in bowel motility and visceral perception have been documented. Constipation develops in the presence of an excessive degree of nonpropulsive contractions and segmentation of bowel contents. At other times, excessive propulsive activity is noted, typically after meals, resulting in diarrhea.

Neurologic Impairment

Constipation may be a presenting symptom of neurologic disease. *Spinal cord injury* that leads to compression of the cauda equina can halt bowel motility and also cause urinary retention and incontinence. *Multiple sclerosis* may compromise bowel function, as can ganglionic abnormalities. In most instances, other neurologic deficits are present. Disease limited to loss of neurons in the bowel wall typically presents as chronic, refractory constipation; it may date from childhood or, as noted previously, be associated with longstanding laxative use. A permanently damaged neuromotor apparatus may also occur as a consequence of *scleroderma*.

Impaired Evacuation

Among the mechanisms of compromised evacuation are inhibition of the normal defecation reflex, dehydration, and pelvic floor dysfunction.

Inhibition of the Rectal Defecation Reflex

Inhibition of the rectal defecation reflex has been documented in cases of painful local anal pathology, neurogenic disease (e.g., Parkinson's disease, multiple sclerosis), long-term use of laxatives, and voluntary suppression. Patients with this problem are found to have stool packed into the rectal ampulla. *Voluntary suppression* of the urge to defecate may be a concomitant of a hectic daily pace or traveling. The resulting intermittent constipation may lead to excessive use of laxatives and enemas and damage to the reflex emptying mechanism.

Pelvic Floor Dysfunction

Pelvic floor dysfunction accounts for some cases of intractable constipation of unknown etiology. It may be a consequence of inadequate relaxation or inappropriate contraction of the puborectalis and anal sphincter muscles, pelvic floor dyssynergy, or both. Patients complain of the need to strain despite a strong urge to defecate. They may also report a persistent uncomfortable sense of rectal fullness and the need to remove stool digitally from the rectum to obtain relief. With pelvic floor dyssynergy, patients find that supporting the perineum helps during a bowel movement.

Other Purported Mechanisms

Inadequate fluid intake is commonly believed to play a role, but confirmatory evidence is lacking. Water is known to be an effective means of distending the stomach, which can stimulate intestinal activity.

DIFFERENTIAL DIAGNOSIS (4,8,10,12,15,16)

The causes of constipation can be grouped according to pathophysiology: impaired motility, rectal dyssynergy neurologic disorders, obstruction, and local anorectal pathology (Table 65.2). Many cases remain undiagnosed after initial assessment but respond to empiric therapy. Slow colonic transit and pelvic floor dysfunction often play etiologic roles in such cases, especially in middle-aged and older women with chronic intractable constipation.

WORKUP (3,4,6,8,10,12)

History

Evaluation begins with a definition of the size, character, and frequency of bowel movements, followed by a determination of the chronicity of the problem. Acute constipation is more often associated with organic disease than is a longstanding problem. Chronic complaints that wax and wane for months and years point to a functional disturbance, perhaps compounded by habitual laxative use. The patient must be asked about symptoms that suggest an underlying significant gastrointestinal disease, such as abdominal pain, nausea, cramping, vomiting, weight loss, melena, rectal bleeding, rectal pain, and fever. Anorexia, bloating, belching, flatus, mucus in the stool, headache, depression, and anxiety should also be recorded; these symptoms may be associated with constipation of any etiology but often accompany functional disorders.

It is helpful at the first visit to take a history of working, eating, and bowel habits. Inquiry into dietary fiber intake and physical activity is essential. Use of medications, including

TABLE 65.2

IMPORTANT CAUSES OF CONSTIPATION

Mechanism	Etiology
Impaired motility	Inadequate dietary fiber
	Inactivity
	Laxative abuse
	Irritable colon syndrome
	Diverticulitis
	Hypothyroidism
	Hypokalemia
	Diabetes
	Hypercalcemia
	Pregnancy
	Scleroderma
	Drugs (opiates, anticholinergics, tricyclic antidepressants, ganglionic blockers, calcium- and aluminum-containing antacids, sucralfate, disopyramide, calcium-channel blockers, antihistamines)
Neurological dysfunction	Multiple sclerosis
	Spinal cord injury
	Neurogangliomatosis
Psychosocial dysfunction	Depression
	Situational stress
	Anxiety
	Somatization
	Phobias

anticholinergic agents and nonprescription drugs (especially laxatives and antacids), needs to be detailed. The patient's perspective and concerns should be elicited, and a careful psychosocial history obtained, with attention to situational stresses, anxieties, patient's interpretation of the symptoms, and methods of coping.

History can be especially helpful in identifying defecatory disorders. It should be checked for straining; use of unusual postures, intrarectal or intravaginal finger, or perineal pressure to expel stool; and inability to expel a liquid enema.

Physical Examination

One begins by recording the patient's weight and noting overall nutritional status. Skin is checked for pallor and signs of hypothyroidism (see Chapter 104). The abdomen is examined for masses, distention, tenderness, and high-pitched or absent bowel sounds. Rectal examination includes careful inspection and palpation for masses, fissures, inflammation, and hard stool in the ampulla. The last finding rules out significant obstruction and poor colonic motility and suggests that the problem is in part inadequate rectal emptying. The stool is noted for color and consistency and tested for occult blood. Anal and perineal anatomy, sphincter tone, sensitivity, and reflexes are noted. Disordered enervation of the anus is indicated if the anal canal opens wide when the puborectalis muscle is pulled posterior. Anoscopy or endoscopy is needed to identify internal hemorrhoids, fissures, tumors, and other local pathology. A neurologic examination should be performed to search for focal deficits and a delayed relaxation phase of the ankle jerks, suggestive of hypothyroidism. A mental status exami-

nation includes checking for signs of depression (see Chapter 227), anxiety (see Chapter 226), and somatization (see Chapter 230).

Laboratory Studies

Laboratory investigation should be tailored to the suspected underlying pathophysiology. The first priority is investigation for bowel obstruction when suggested by history and/or physical examination. If obstruction is either ruled out or not a concern in the first place, it can be treated empirically and followed expectantly. Failure to respond necessitates consideration of further diagnostic study.

Suspected Bowel Obstruction, Ileus, or Malignancy

The acute onset of constipation requires ruling out obstruction and ileus, especially when accompanied by abdominal discomfort. Radiologic investigation is indicated, starting with plain *supine* and *upright films* of the abdomen, plus measurements of serum *potassium* and *calcium* levels. More chronic or recurrent forms of constipation should be assessed with a check of the serum *glucose* level for diabetes (see Chapter 93) and of the serum *thyroid-stimulating hormone* for hypothyroidism (see Chapter 104).

If colonic obstruction is suspected (especially if Crohn's disease or cancer is a possibility), *colonoscopy* or *sigmoidoscopy* plus *barium enema* is required. Colonoscopy is the test of choice in a case with occult fecal blood, rectal bleeding, anemia, or weight loss in an older patient, all of which suggest the possibility of colorectal cancer (see Chapters 56 and 63). More than 25% of patients with colorectal carcinomas have constipation. The finding of pigmented colonic mucosa (melanosis coli) on direct visualization of the bowel lumen suggests abuse of anthraquinone laxatives such as castor oil or senna.

No Evidence of Obstruction or Malignancy

The elderly person presenting with no evidence of obstruction, anemia, or occult blood loss can probably be managed for a few weeks with an empiric program that includes stopping any suspected medications and increasing dietary fiber, fluids, and exercise. A trial of gentle laxative use (see later discussion) may also be helpful. Such a patient should be monitored with stool occult blood tests before making a decision to subject him or her to colonoscopy or barium enema. If symptoms resolve and no other risk factors or findings suggestive of colorectal cancer are present, then the patient can forego bowel visualization at least for the time being. A return visit for repeated assessment of the situation should be scheduled within 4 to 8 weeks.

Failure to Respond to Empiric Measures

When the cause of constipation is obscure, it is helpful to re-review medications, stop all that can be held, and consider colonic transit time testing. A repeat check of medications, both prescription and nonprescription, is essential. The *codeine* in a cough suppressant, the *anticholinergic* activity of a drug for incontinence or depression, the *calcium* in an over-the-counter antacid or calcium supplement, and the *iron* in a multiple vitamin may be responsible for an otherwise puzzling diagnostic problem.

When clinical findings are insufficient to differentiate impaired transit from impaired defecation, a *colonic transit time* can be helpful. The test involves swallowing a gelatin capsule containing radiopaque markers. A film of the abdomen is obtained 120 hours after intake, noting percentage and location of retention. Greater than 20% retention suggests delayed transit; localization to the distal colon and rectum indicates a defecatory mechanism.

Suspected Impairment of Defecation

Most primary care physicians will want to refer these patients to a gastroenterologist or colorectal surgeon for full assessment including *anorectal manometry* and *balloon expulsion*, office-based procedures that can help identify and refine definition of the defecatory problem. High resting pressure and pain on manometry suggests fissure; hyposensitivity to balloon distention suggests a neurologic disorder. Inability to expel a 50-cc water-filled latex balloon within 2 minutes indicates a defect in defecation. A barium-based fluoroscopic *defecogram* provides information on emptying, structural abnormalities, and anal and perineal action during evacuation.

SYMPTOMATIC MANAGEMENT AND PATIENT EDUCATION
(3,4,6,8,10,12,15–26)

Empiric symptomatic management is appropriate for the patient with a suspected functional etiology, but only after obstruction and other forms of serious organic pathology have been ruled out.

Basic First Steps

The first intervention after a careful workup is *reassurance* that no evidence for a serious underlying illness has been found. Cancer is a common fear, especially in elderly patients with new onset of constipation. Detailed and personalized *patient education* about diet, exercise, and use of laxatives is the next priority. Explanation is needed to reassure the patient that a daily bowel movement is not essential to good health and that comfortable patterns of elimination depend on good living and eating habits. *Daily exercise* should be prescribed, based on the patient's physical capacity (see Chapter 18). Adequate *fluid intake* (1.5 to 2 L daily; six to eight glasses of water) is also essential, especially if a high-fiber diet is prescribed.

The patient should *stop taking stimulant laxatives*, enemas, *and nonessential drugs* that may suppress colonic motility. Trying to establish a convenient, uninterrupted *time for defecation* each day may be useful; 15 to 20 minutes after breakfast provides a good opportunity because spontaneous colonic motility is greatest during that period. Continuing this routine each day regardless of travel or situational distractions should be encouraged. Although no controlled studies are available to prove the efficacy of this approach, it seems to help some people, although days or weeks can pass before success is noted.

In general, these first steps can relieve constipation, but in chronic cases, it may take weeks to months for more satisfactory bowel function to return. Often, immediate results are expected; when they do not appear, the patient becomes frustrated, stops the program, and returns to laxative and enema use.

Dietary Fiber and Fiber Supplements

The use of fiber and bulk laxatives can help to alleviate symptoms by softening stools and reducing abdominal discomfort.

Most clinicians prefer to start with dietary fiber before resorting to bulk laxatives; data on relative efficacy and safety are limited. One begins to increase the fiber content of the diet by adding bran, fruits, green vegetables, and whole-grain cereals and breads. Most studies show that 15 g of fiber per day is needed for the best effects, but the amount can be individualized. A large breakfast including bran cereal, juice, milk or coffee, and whole-grain bread is helpful.

Some patients refuse to eat bran because it makes them feel bloated and gassy. The patient can be reassured that these side effects usually resolve within 1 month of continued use. If dietary and exercise efforts fail or the patient insists on medication, a *nondigestible fiber residue* such as ground *psyllium* seed (Metamucil), *methylcellulose* (Citrucel), or *polycarbophil* can be beneficial. It acts to increase bulk by means of its hydrophilic properties, but it is best taken with plenty of fluids. The usual dose is one teaspoon in 8 oz of liquid three times a day. Placebo-controlled studies show significant improvement in symptoms with use, but the placebo groups also show improvement, which suggests that explanation, reassurance, and increased attention are also important to improved bowel function.

Laxatives of First Choice

Some elderly patients remain refractory to the basic first steps and press for prescription of a laxative. A few classes are relatively safe and worth considering when simpler measures have failed. Efficacy in controlled trials is similar to that of fiber.

Nonabsorbable Saccharide/Bulk Laxatives

Nonabsorbable saccharide/bulk laxatives (e.g., *lactulose*, *sorbitol*, or *polyethylene glycol* solutions [*MiraLAX*]) have been shown to be safe and effective when used on a long-term basis in the elderly. These agents induce a potent osmotic effect, retaining fluid in the bowel lumen and softening the stool. Polyethylene glycol solutions are a useful adjuvant to fiber supplements and are available without a prescription. Sorbitol (30 to 60 mL daily at bedtime) costs about one tenth the cost of lactulose yet equals or exceeds it in efficacy and tolerability. Side effects include excessive flatulence, bloating, and cramping.

Magnesium-Containing Laxatives

Magnesium-containing laxatives (e.g., milk of magnesia, magnesium citrate) are also osmotically active, but they should be used more cautiously because they may induce magnesium and sodium overload in older persons with renal dysfunction. They are less expensive than sorbitol.

Surfactant Laxatives

Surfactant laxatives such as *docusate* soften stool by promoting the mixing of water and fat. They maybe helpful in patients reporting hard stools, but data supporting their efficacy are limited (see later discussion), and their cost is high.

Other Laxative Preparations

Most other laxatives are probably worth avoiding for regular use because of the potential for adverse effects (although definitive data documenting adverse effects are limited).

Stimulant/Irritant Laxatives

Stimulant/irritant laxatives include the derivatives of diphenylmethane (*bisacodyl*), anthraquinone (*senna*), and cascara. These irritants trigger colonic contraction acutely; long-term use is associated with an increased risk for bowel refractoriness and worsening constipation (*laxative abuse syndrome*).

Enemas

When *fecal impaction* is present, a *hypertonic enema* (e.g., Fleet) will often relieve the situation. *Soapsuds enemas* should be avoided because colitis has been reported with their use. The patient is instructed to squat over the toilet by standing on a chair in front of the bowl, providing a more favorable position for evacuation. Only infrequently does one need to resort to disempaction.

Prevention

Prevention of constipation during an illness that requires bed rest can be achieved with a high-fiber diet, bulk agents, and use of a commode in preference to a bedpan. Correction of any coincident hypokalemia is important (see Chapter 32). There is no evidence that prophylactic use of laxatives or stool softeners is effective. A randomized, controlled study of docusate sodium (Colace), a popular and expensive stool softener, failed to demonstrate any effect on the quality or frequency of stools. Use of minor tranquilizers in overly anxious patients has little direct effect on constipation. When severe depression requires use of antidepressants, the least constipating agent should be selected (i.e., one with minimal anticholinergic activity). All tricyclic antidepressants have at least some anticholinergic activity, but desipramine, nortriptyline, and trazodone seem to have the least. Alternatively, a nontricyclic antidepressant such as sertraline might be a reasonable choice (see Chapter 227).

Management of Defecatory Problems

Biofeedback, botulinum toxin, and surgery have been applied to defecatory problems. *Biofeedback* has a reported overall success rate of about 65%, especially in persons with inability appropriately to relax pelvic musculature. Persons who fail biofeedback and remain unable to relax the pelvic floor may benefit from *botulinum type A toxin* injection into the puborectalis muscle; the effect is long acting, but efficacy is not established by data from controlled trials. *Surgery* is a consideration in persons with a rectocoele and in women who must use digital vaginal pressure to achieve defecation.

The Patient–Doctor Relationship

The importance of establishing a trusting, therapeutic patient–doctor relationship cannot be overemphasized, especially when the probability of underlying psychosocial distress is high. One facilitates the establishment of trust by eliciting concerns and perspective and taking time to explain and answer questions. A patient who has used a particular agent for decades needs to be told why it is being removed from the program; otherwise, chances of compliance are low. Long-term laxative users should be warned that it might take 4 to 6 weeks before spontaneous bowel movements return. Patience and sympathetic support can be rewarding, but expectations of quick results must not be raised (see also Chapter 74).

Annotated Bibliography

1. Sonnenberg A, Koch TR. Epidemiology of constipation in the United States. Dis Colon Rectum 1989;32:1. (*Constipation accounts for >2.5 million physician visits per year.*)
2. Baron TH, Ramirez B, Richter JE. Gastrointestinal motility disorders in pregnancy. Ann Intern Med 1993;118:366. (*Constipation is common; mechanisms are reviewed.*)
3. Burkitt D, Walker A, Paintner N. Effect of dietary fibre on stools and transit times and its role in causation of disease. Lancet 1972;2:1408. (*Classic article on fiber and its link to constipation and other bowel problems.*)
4. DeLillo AR, Rose S. Functional bowel disorders in the geriatric patient: constipation, fecal impaction, and fecal incontinence. Am J Gastroenterol 2000;95:902. (*A practical review of common and frustrating clinical issues.*)
5. Everhart JE, Go VLW, Johannes RS, et al. A longitudinal survey of self-reported bowel habits in the United States. Dig Dis Sci 1989;34:1153. (*A report of a large sample of people's bowel habits over 10 years.*)
6. Graham DY, Moser SE, Estes MK. The effect of bran on bowel function and constipation. Am J Gastroenterol 1982;77:599. (*Twenty grams of wheat or corn bran reduced transit time by 50% and improved constipation clinically in 6 of 10 constipated women.*)
7. Holdstock D, Misiewicz JJ, Smith T, et al. Propulsion in the human colon and its relationship to meals and somatic activity. Gut 1970;11:91. (*Physical activity was found to stimulate mass movements and inactivity reduced them.*)
8. Kam MA. Clinical case: chronic constipation. Gastroenterol 2006:131:233. (*A clinical discussion of a case of constipation and an approach to management.*)
9. Katz L, Spiro H. Gastrointestinal manifestations of diabetes. N Engl J Med 1966;275:1350. (*A classic review; constipation is a frequent gastrointestinal complaint of diabetics.*)
10. Lembo A, Camilleri M. Chronic constipation. New Engl J Med 2003;349:1360. (*A succinct clinical review covering both evaluation and management; 57 references.*)
11. Locke GR, Pemberton JH, Phillips SF. AGA Technical review on constipation. Gastroenterology 2000;119:1766. (*Detailed review of the pathophysiology of constipation.*)
12. Longstreth GF, Thompson GW, Chey WD, et al. Functional disorders. Gastroenterology 2006;130:1480. (*The symptom-based Rome consensus criteria for functional disease.*)
13. Oster JR, Materson BJ, Rogers AI. Laxative abuse syndrome. Am J Gastroenterol 1980;74:451. (*Classic article outlining this important cause of chronic constipation.*)
14. Pare P, Ferrazzi S, Thompson WG, et al. An epidemiological survey of constipation in Canada: definitions, rates, demographics, and predictors of health care seeking. Am J Gastroenterol 2001;96:3130. (*A major epidemiologic study that found 27% prevalence.*)
15. Brandt LJ, Prather CM, Quigley EMM, et al. Systematic review on the management of chronic constipation in North America. Am J Gastroenterol 2005;100:S5. (*The American College of Gastroenterology systematic review and consensus recommendations.*)
16. Camileri M, Thompson WG, Fleshman JW, et al. Clinical management of intractable constipation. Ann Intern Med 1994;121:520. (*A review of both the basic approach and the tertiary center's protocol for patients who fail standard therapy.*)
17. Cann PA, Read NW, Holdsworth CD. What is the benefit of coarse wheat bran in patients with irritable bowel syndrome? Gut 1984;25:168. (*Double-blind, placebo-controlled study demonstrating efficacy.*)
18. Chiarioni G, Whitehead WE, Pezza V, et al. Biofeedback is superior to laxatives for normal transit constipation due to pelvic floor dyssynergy.

Gastroenterology 2006;130:657. (*Biofeedback is superior to laxatives for normal transit constipation due to pelvic floor dyssynergy.*)

19. Enck P. Biofeedback training in disorganized defecation: a critical review. Dig Dis Sci 1993;38:1953. (*Finds an overall success rate of 67%, but no data from controlled trials.*)

20. Goodman J, Pang J, Bessman A. Dioctyl sodium sulfosuccinate: an ineffective prophylactic laxative. J Chronic Dis 1976;29:59. (*Randomized, prospective study of patients admitted to the hospital; the drug made no difference in quality or frequency of stools.*)

21. Hull C, Greco RS, Brooks DL. Alleviation of constipation in the elderly by dietary fiber supplementation. J Am Geriatr Soc 1980;28:410. (*In an institutional geriatric population, adding bran prevented constipation and reduced laxative use.*)

22. Kirwn WO, Smith AN. Colonic propulsion in diverticular disease, idiopathic constipation and the irritable bowel syndrome. Scand J Gastroenterol 1974;12:331. (*Transit time is prolonged in all three diseases and can be significantly reduced by bran.*)

23. Lederle FA, Busch DL, Mattox BS, et al. Cost-effective treatment of constipation in the elderly: a randomized double-blind comparison of sorbitol and lactulose. Am J Med 1990;89:597. (*Demonstrates efficacy and comparability; useful in elderly patients with refractory functional disease.*)

24. Locke GR, Pemberton JH, Phillips SF. Clinical practice guidelines on constipation. Gastroenterology 2000;119:1763. (*Authoritative review of constipation management for the specialist.*)

25. Longstreth GF, Fox DD, Youkeles MS, et al. Psyllium in irritable bowel syndrome: a double-blind study. Ann Intern Med 1981;95:53. (*Both treatment and control groups showed equally impressive degrees of improvement, which suggests that other factors are also operative.*)

26. Matthews DA, Suchman AL, Branch WT Jr. Making "connections": enhancing the therapeutic potential of patient–clinician relationships. Ann Intern Med 1993;118:973. (*Important insights into the treatment of patients with functional bowel disease.*)

CHAPTER 66 ■ APPROACH TO THE PATIENT WITH ANORECTAL COMPLAINTS

Anorectal complaints often go incompletely evaluated. Although they are usually a result of minor conditions such as hemorrhoids or fissures, causes range beyond the trivial to inflammatory bowel disease, cancer, and infection. In addition, anorectal problems generate a substantial amount of worry and discomfort and can be socially disabling. As a result, they deserve careful consideration by the primary care physician. Challenges include the renewed prevalence of unsafe anal sexual practices in younger persons and the consequences of such behavior, and the management of fecal incontinence in the elderly.

PATHOPHYSIOLOGY AND CLINICAL PRESENTATION (1–13)

Anorectal complaints result from traumatic, vascular, infectious, inflammatory, neurologic, and malignant causes. Symptoms include pain, discharge, itching, mass, and fecal incontinence. *Pain* is most often a manifestation of anal pathology; anal and perianal skin are richly innervated with pain-sensitive nerve fibers; rectal tissue is relatively insensitive to pain. A fissure, distention by abscess or hemorrhoid, invasion by tumor, or marked inflammation can lead to considerable discomfort. Secondary anal sphincter spasm may ensue, prolonging and intensifying the pain. *Discharge* results from inflammation of the rectal mucosa or drainage of an abscess. Cancer, abscess, and thrombosed hemorrhoids can produce an anorectal *mass*; condylomata acuminata may also cause anal skin nodularity. *Itching* represents a minor form of skin irritation that occurs with a variety of mechanical and inflammatory lesions; it is intensified by moisture in the perianal area. Chronic itching leads to excoriation, edema, thickening, fissuring, and lichenification of the perianal skin. *Bleeding* is a common and important manifestation of anorectal pathology; its causes range from hemorrhoids and fissures to carcinoma and inflammatory bowel disease (see Chapter 63).

Hemorrhoids

The most common of all anorectal problems, hemorrhoids affect about half of patients older than the age of 50 years. They represent dilations of the anorectal vascular network. Epidemiologically, they are associated with diets high in fat and low in fiber. Theories explaining the development of hemorrhoids invoke a number of mechanisms, including increased venous pressure secondary to upright posture and straining at stool, arteriovenous communications in rectal tissue, and prolapsed cushions of tissue secondary to the loss of support. Clinically, hemorrhoids are associated with pregnancy, portal hypertension, and constipation. The relative absence of hemorrhoids in African populations that have high-residue diets has led to the suggestion that an increase in dietary fiber might prevent the development of hemorrhoids.

Although the traditional view is that hemorrhoids are venous varicosities resulting from straining at stool, they do not always present in a fashion consistent with this postulate. For example, hemorrhoids appear in early pregnancy in many young women, long before the development of significant intraabdominal pressure from a large fetus. Moreover, hemorrhoidal blood is characteristically arterial in quality (bright red) rather than the dark variety that would be expected from a strictly venous source. Nonetheless, many patients with hemorrhoids have been found to have increased resting anal sphincter pressures, which supports the hypothesis that increased anal pressure causes straining at stool. The straining stresses and compromises the supporting fibrous tissue of the rectal mucosa, allowing the now poorly supported mucosa to slide down and become entrapped by the sphincter. Venous engorgement is a consequence of the entrapment.

Classification

Hemorrhoids may be classified by presentation as *first degree* when they merely bleed, *second degree* if they prolapse on high pressure but return spontaneously, and *third degree* when the anal suspensory ligament is stretched to the point of permanent prolapse. Hemorrhoids are considered to be *internal* when they are derived from the superior hemorrhoidal plexus above the dentate line and *external* when they are located below the dentate line and covered by squamous epithelium. External hemorrhoids are covered by pain-sensitive anal skin and arise from the inferior hemorrhoidal plexus. Internal hemorrhoids are covered by the much less pain-sensitive rectal mucosa and represent dilations of the superior hemorrhoidal plexus.

Clinical Presentation

Pain, incomplete defecation, constipation, excessive moisture, rectal itching, bleeding, and a prolapsed mass are the common presentations. Clinical presentation depends in part on the location of the hemorrhoid and the presence of complications. External hemorrhoids that have thrombosed present as tender, bluish swellings. Internal hemorrhoids often bleed, but only when they prolapse do they present as a mass; when irreducible, they are subject to thrombosis. Recurrent bleeding may be seen with either type; sudden rupture may cause rather dramatic, although relatively harmless, bright-red bleeding. Hemorrhoids are regularly encountered as incidental findings on physical examination. Skin tags are evidence of previous hemorrhoids that have thrombosed, leaving connective tissue. The most bothersome complications of hemorrhoids include bleeding, prolapse, and thrombosis.

Fistula-in-Ano

Fistula-in-ano is a communication between the anal canal and the perianal skin. It is usually nontender. The external opening may be single or multiple, with a granulation tissue bud and chronic seropurulent drainage. Occasionally, an indurated cord of tissue may be palpable, extending from the external fistulous opening toward the anal canal. The fistula may result from rupture or surgical drainage of a perirectal abscess; other causes include Crohn's disease, carcinoma, tuberculosis, radiation therapy, lymphogranuloma venereum, and anal fissure. Patients complain of persistent and irritating drainage of blood, pus, or mucus.

Perirectal Abscess

Perirectal abscess and fistula-in-ano are two stages of the same disease process, beginning as an infection in the anal glands, which empty into the anal crypts at the mucocutaneous junction, and subsequently spreading into the adjacent tissue. The abscess thus formed often drains through the perianal skin. Symptoms and signs are a function of the size and the location of the abscess. The first manifestation is rectal pain, which may occur before any mass becomes palpable. Patients characteristically complain of constant, throbbing pain in the perianal region or in the rectum. A mass may be identified externally on examination of the anus or internally during palpation the rectum. The formation of perirectal abscesses is a particularly important problem in patients with Crohn's disease, immunodeficiency states, and hematologic disorders.

Infected Pilonidal Cyst or Sinus

Infected pilonidal cyst or sinus is most common in boys and young men between the ages of 16 and 30 years. These are midline, in the area of the natal cleft. Multiple sinuses may be present. Recurrent secondary infections are frequent.

Carcinoma of the Anus

Carcinoma involving the perianal skin or anorectal tract typically does not cause pain until relatively late in its clinical course, often in the setting of a large, ulcerated, bleeding lesion. Earlier lesions present as painless nodules or plaques. Pruritus, mucoid drainage, and changes in bowel habits are more subtle manifestations that sometimes occur. Patients who are HIV-positive and engaging in receptive anal intercourse are at markedly increased risk for both squamous cell carcinoma of the anus and intraepithelial neoplasia.

Proctalgia Fugax

Proctalgia fugax, as the term implies, is fleeting but severe rectal pain believed to be related to spasm of the levator ani and coccygeal muscles. Although usually brief, symptoms can last for more than 30 minutes. Suspected precipitants include chronic trauma from poor posture; psychogenic factors may also be operative. No associated physical findings are present, except for muscle tenderness on digital examination.

Proctitis

Proctitis—inflammatory disease of the rectum—is associated with a wide variety of conditions, ranging from infection and trauma to radiation and inflammatory bowel disease. Regardless of the cause, the presentation is usually one of mucopurulent discharge, rectal bleeding, and, in severe cases, rectal pain and tenesmus. Patients with *ulcerative proctitis* demonstrate on sigmoidoscopy an inflamed rectal mucosa and a clearly demarcated upper border, above which the mucosa is normal. Systemic symptoms and extraintestinal manifestations are rare when the disease is limited to the rectum. The risk for carcinoma is low, and diffuse colitis develops in fewer than 10% to 15% of patients.

Infectious Proctitis

Infectious proctitis occurs mostly among *men having sex with men (MSM)* who engage in frequent rectal intercourse with multiple partners. Gonorrhea, amebic disease, chlamydial infection, and herpes simplex infection are prominent in this population (see later discussion). *Gonococcal proctitis* is especially common. The rate of asymptomatic carriage of gonorrhea among promiscuous male homosexuals is reportedly as high as 60% to 70%. Symptomatic gonococcal proctitis presents with discharge and rectal discomfort (see later discussion). Diarrhea is the hallmark of symptomatic *amebic infection*, *shigellosis*, and *Campylobacter* infection (see Chapter 64). *Herpes simplex proctitis* can be a very painful condition, accompanied by tenesmus, constipation, rectal ulceration, and discharge. Involvement of the sacral nerve roots can lead to bladder and erectile difficulties, paresthesias, and pain in the thighs and buttocks.

Solitary Rectal Ulcer

Solitary rectal ulcer is a rare condition of unknown cause associated with rectal discharge, bleeding, and, occasionally, dull pain. The characteristic finding on sigmoidoscopy is a single shallow ulcer 7 to 10 cm from the anus; its borders may be heaped or nodular. Chronicity is the rule; complications are rare. These lesions must be distinguished from cancer and lymphogranuloma venereum by biopsy.

Pruritus Ani

Pruritus ani (chronic perianal itching) is not a diagnosis but rather a syndrome that results from a variety of mechanical and inflammatory lesions. Anatomic lesions that produce chronic discharge (such as *fistulas*, *fissures*, and *hemorrhoids* with intermittent mucosal eversion) can result in pruritus ani. Infectious causes are numerous. *Anogenital warts* (*condylomata acuminata*) are viral in origin and generally transmitted by sexual contact. They may be confined to the perianal region or also involve the penis, vulva, and anal canal. Multiple, soft, filiform excrescences characterize these lesions, which may enlarge, become confluent, and even bleed. *Gonococcal proctitis* can lead to anal soreness, burning, and purulent discharge. Infestations with *pinworm* (*Enterobius vermicularis*) typically cause nocturnal anal itchiness, especially among children, but sometimes spread to involve adult family members. Nocturnal symptoms are caused by the daily evening migration of the female pinworm downward to deposit eggs on the perianal skin. Anal involvement is characteristic of some systemic dermatologic diseases, such as *psoriasis* and *scabies*. *Contact dermatitis* or *eczema* resulting from the use of a topical agent is common and can complicate the diagnosis of the original cause of pruritus. Applied initially as a remedy for itching, the agent may only aggravate the problem by causing skin sensitization. Itching is intensified by moisture in the perianal area and often aggravated by the use of topical agents applied in an attempt to quell symptoms. The passage of *alkaline stools* (as occurs in severe diarrhea) can have an irritant effect on the anal skin. Persistent anal itching may be a form of *neurodermatitis*; such patients characteristically present with multiple excoriations. *Candida infection* is found among diabetics, male homosexuals, and patients recently taking broad-spectrum antibiotics; perianal erythema and itching are presenting manifestations.

Fecal Impaction

Fecal impaction ranks as one of the major sources of anorectal discomfort among the elderly and the bedridden. Chronic incomplete evacuation leads to the formation of an obstructing bolus of desiccated hard stool in the rectum. Symptoms of anal discomfort and constipation are typical, but anorexia, malaise, or nonspecific lower abdominal fullness may be all that is reported. Paradoxically, diarrhea rather than constipation is sometimes the only complaint; this is caused by the collection of liquid stool, which distends the proximal colon and passes around the obstructing bolus. Unless this problem is corrected by disimpaction, complications such as intestinal obstruction, rectal prolapse, and even bowel perforation may ensue.

Fecal Incontinence

Fecal incontinence follows damage to the normal anal sphincter mechanism. Perianal disease, anal surgery, colorectal mucosal damage, and neurologic disease can have devastating psychosocial consequences when the anal sphincter becomes compromised.

Sphincter Injury

Sphincter injury can occur from anorectal surgery, from tears and excessive straining associated with childbearing, and from years of straining at stool (causing stretch injury to the pudendal nerve). In addition, prolapse of rectal mucosa and large internal hemorrhoids can prevent sphincter closure.

Rectal Inflammation

Rectal inflammation, either from inflammatory bowel disease or radiation therapy, can cause extreme urgency resulting in fecal incontinence. The sphincter remains competent, but the urgency is so severe that it may be uncontrollable if the person is unable to reach a toilet immediately.

Neurologic Compromise

Neurologic compromise of either motor or sensory function may be found, as occurs with demyelinating disease, diabetes, and spinal cord injury. Besides sphincter weakness, there might be a loss of the ability to differentiate among formed stool, gas, and liquid in the rectal ampulla.

Overflow Incontinence

Overflow incontinence is seen when there is retained hard stool in the ampulla and liquid stool passes around the inspissated mass. In the opposite circumstance of profuse diarrhea, the volume of liquid stool overwhelms the sphincter mechanism.

Anorectal Problems Associated with Receptive Anal Intercourse

Anorectal problems associated with receptive anal intercourse can be complex in etiology and presentation. In a major study, more than 80% of homosexual men presenting to a venereal disease clinic with anorectal or intestinal symptoms were infected with one or more sexually transmissible anorectal or enteric pathogens. Three principal syndromes were noted: a *proctitis* characterized by anorectal pain, lesions, and discharge but no evidence of disease above the rectum; a *proctocolitis*, which, in addition to manifestations of proctitis, included diarrhea, tenesmus, and inflammation extending into the sigmoid mucosa; and an *enteritis* (see Chapter 64), which consisted of diarrhea and abdominal pain but no anorectal symptoms or signs.

TABLE 66.1

DIFFERENTIAL DIAGNOSIS OF ANORECTAL PROBLEMS

Problem	Differential Diagnosis
Anal discomfort	Hemorrhoids Fissure-in-ano (hard bowel movement, cancer, venereal disease) Fistula-in-ano (perirectal abscess, Crohn's disease, carcinoma, radiation, tuberculosis lymphogranuloma venereum) Perirectal abscess (Crohn's disease, immunodeficiency, hematologic disorders) Infected pilonidal cyst Carcinoma of the anal epidermis Infections (syphilis, candidiasis, condylomata acuminata)
Rectal discomfort	Proctitis (ulcerative, gonococcal, amebic, herpetic), often accompanied by discharge and bleeding Perirectal abscess Impaction Proctalgia fugax Solitary rectal ulcer
Pruritus ani	Excess moisture (poor hygiene), pinworms, eczema, scabies, diabetes, liver failure, irritants (topical agents, alkaline stools), fissure, early cancer, neurodermatitis, and infections (see above)
Incontinence	Rectal surgery, neurologic disease, perianal disease

As noted, gonococcal, herpetic, chlamydial, and syphilitic forms of proctitis occur with increased frequency among these patients. *Gonorrhea* occurs in about one third of patients; *herpes simplex type 2 virus* is cultured from about one fifth, who also manifest rectal mucosal ulcerations. About 3% of symptomatic persons have anal syphilitic chancres, and another 3% show evidence of secondary anorectal syphilitic disease (erythematous nodular or indurated rectal mucosal lesions from which biopsy specimens test positive).

A clinical and sigmoidoscopic picture of *proctocolitis* occurs in about 15% of cases. Such patients complain of anorectal discomfort, tenesmus, diarrhea, constipation, and abdominal cramps. On sigmoidoscopy, inflammatory changes start at the rectum and extend beyond 15 cm into the sigmoid colon. *Campylobacter*, *Entamoeba histolytica*, *Chlamydia*, and *Clostridium difficile* are significantly correlated with the enterocolitis; often, more than one organism is recovered. Polymicrobial infection is commonplace among symptomatic male homosexuals with many sexual partners.

Although much of the proctitis in this population is infectious in origin, *culture-negative proctitis* occurs with some frequency and has been linked to exposure to the *coloring agents* and *scents* found in some of the lubricants used for anal intercourse. Manifestations of several causes may present simultaneously. The patient complaining of hemorrhoidal pain may actually have concurrent gonorrhea, allergic proctitis, and chlamydial infection. Traumatic complications of rectal intercourse include prolapsed hemorrhoids, anal fistulas and fissures, perirectal abscesses, rectal ulcers, and anal tears. Foreign bodies are sometimes recovered.

DIFFERENTIAL DIAGNOSIS

The differential diagnosis of anorectal problems can best be considered in anatomic terms, depending on whether symptoms and signs are predominantly anal, anorectal, or rectocolonic (Table 66.1). This is particularly true when the causes of anorectal disease in MSM are considered (Table 66.2).

WORKUP (1–14)

History

Although a careful physical examination is the most important part of the evaluation, the history can provide important epidemiologic and etiologic information. Determining whether the condition is predominantly anal (local pain only), anorectal (local anal pain plus rectal discomfort, tenesmus, rectal discharge, constipation), or rectocolonic (rectal discomfort, tenesmus, and rectal discharge plus diarrhea, abdominal pain, bloating, nausea) helps to focus the evaluation.

Also important is creating a supportive, nonjudgmental environment for the evaluation of *men who have sex with men (MSM)*. Because the risk for sexually transmitted anorectal disease is very high in this population of men (necessitating screening and thorough evaluation of anorectal complaints), it is essential that the office environment be conducive for their care. If that is not possible, then referral to a practice that can provide care in such as manner is indicated.

Patients with anal complaints should be questioned about masses, nodules, focal tenderness, history of hemorrhoids, psoriasis, passage of hard stool, bleeding, discharge, generalized itching, nocturnal pattern, and recent trauma. Detailed inquiry into the use of topical medications (many of which are sensitizing), involvement of other household members or sexual partners, and hygienic practices should also be made.

For patients with anorectal involvement, the physician should check into symptoms of inflammatory bowel disease (see Chapter 73), obtain a careful and detailed sexual history focusing on the number of partners and practice of receptive rectal intercourse, and note any reports of inguinal adenopathy

TABLE 66.2

DIFFERENTIAL DIAGNOSIS OF ANORECTAL PROBLEMS IN MEN HAVING SEX WITH MEN

Syndrome	Etiology
Proctitis	*Neisseria gonorrhoeae*
	Herpes simplex
	Chlamydia (nonlymphogranuloma strains)
	Syphilis
	Condylomata acuminata
	Trauma
	Chemical irritants
Proctocolitis	*Campylobacter*
	Shigella
	Entamoeba histolytica
	Chlamydia (lymphogranuloma strains)
Enteritis	*Giardia lamblia*

(seen with herpes and lymphogranuloma), sacral root paresthesias, and difficulty with micturition (other telltale symptoms of herpes simplex infection). Patients with rectocolonic symptoms are likely to have either inflammatory bowel disease or a polymicrobial infection from rectal intercourse; the consideration of associated symptoms and risk factors is indicated.

Physical Examination

Having the patient in the lateral decubitus position with one knee tucked into the chest provides the best position for the anal examination, even for obese persons. Thorough and gentle inspection of the anus and perianal region is the sine qua non for a successful diagnosis of anorectal problems. One examines the anal skin for erythema, eczema, psoriatic patches, ulcerations, vesicles, fistulas, fissures, condylomata, nodules, hemorrhoids, and inflammatory changes. The presence of perianal or rectal ulcers in association with proctitis in a male homosexual is indicative of syphilis or herpes simplex. If the lesions appear as scaling plaques, a look at the skin of the extensor surfaces of the extremities might provide additional evidence for a diagnosis of psoriasis. In a very anxious patient with multiple excoriations over other parts of the body, neurodermatitis should be suspected as the cause of pruritus ani. If an inflamed anorectal mucosa is encountered, gonorrhea needs to be considered and inquiry into rectal intercourse needs to be pursued.

Gently spreading the buttocks and observing for gaping of the anal sphincter and exposure of the rectal mucosa provides evidence of sphincter injury. Stretching the perianal skin will reveal fissures, which come into view at the anal verge, most often in the posterior midline but occasionally in the anterior midline. With chronic fissures, scarring and induration are seen in addition to an associated hypertrophied anal papilla at the pectinate line; a skin tag marks the external limit. Crohn's disease is likely in patients with multiple fissures, recurrent fistulas, or perirectal abscesses. A painless hard nodule or plaque in the anal region may represent carcinoma. When the lesion is ulcerated, the diagnosis is more obvious and the disease is more advanced.

Digital rectal examination is almost always an essential component of the examination. Sphincter tone is assessed. Resting tone, an indication of internal sphincter function, is assessed; voluntary squeezing helps to determine the state of the external sphincter. However, in the presence of a painful fissure, this can be an extremely painful procedure that is likely to alienate the patient and cause such pain as to make adequate examination impossible. The same applies to the use of anoscopy in such patients. On the other hand, rectal examination should never be deferred in patients who are not acutely and severely uncomfortable.

One needs to check for masses (both fluctuant and firm), discharges, ulcerations, and other mucosal changes and also to test the stool for occult blood. Ascribing anorectal symptoms to hemorrhoids without performing as complete an examination as possible is a common reason for delay in the diagnosis of carcinoma.

Observing the patient in the upright position can also be helpful, especially for the detection of prolapsed internal hemorrhoids and rectal tissue. The patient is asked to sit on a commode, lean forward and strain, with the observer standing behind.

Palpation for enlarged lymph nodes should not be overlooked. Prominent inguinal adenopathy is characteristic of herpetic and chlamydial infections (lymphogranuloma venereum species).

Diagnostic Studies

Unless the patient has a very painful lesion, *anoscopy* needs to be performed (see Appendix 56.1) to visualize the canal and mucosa adequately and obtain samples of any discharge. One inspects for mucosal inflammation, fissure, fistula, mass, plaque, ulcer, and discharge. Patients with rectal inflammation, fistula formation, nonhealing fissures, bleeding, or diarrhea are candidates for *sigmoidoscopy*. Hematochezia in the presence of hemorrhoids in a person with risk factors for colorectal cancer or age greater than 50 years necessitates colonoscopy because the presence of hemorrhoids does not rule out cancer. In fact, persons with colorectal cancer have an increased incidence of hemorrhoidal disease (see Chapter 63). Involvement of the sigmoid mucosa suggests inflammatory bowel disease (see Chapter 73) and infectious forms of colitis (see Chapter 64). Patients with atypical fissures (especially those that fail to heal), painless hard anorectal nodules, and mucosal ulcerations are candidates for *biopsy* to rule out malignancy, inflammatory bowel disease, and chronic infection (syphilis, tuberculosis). Children with nocturnal pruritus ani can be evaluated for pinworm infestation by taking a cellophane tape impression of the anus and microscopically examining it under low power for the characteristic eggs.

MSM patients engaging in receptive anal intercourse with many sexual partners should undergo *anoscopy* to determine the nature of rectal involvement and to obtain samples of mucus for *Gram's stain* and culture on *Thayer–Martin plates*. A positive smear with Gram's stain is excellent presumptive evidence of gonorrhea, although a negative smear does not rule out the diagnosis. Any chancre-like lesions should be subjected to *dark-field* examination for spirochetes. *A serologic test for syphilis* is also obtained. Those who are *HIV-positive* should be screened by *Papanicolaou smear* of the anal canal and of any suspicious lesions for evidence of human papillomavirus–related anal squamous intraepithelial neoplasia and anal squamous cell carcinoma.

MSM patients with evidence of rectal pathology on anoscopy require *sigmoidoscopy*; establishing the extent of mucosal involvement helps to narrow the list of possible causes. Those with a *proctocolitis* picture of mucosal involvement extending greater than 15 cm or symptoms of colitis (diarrhea, nausea, abdominal cramping) should have specimens *cultured* for *Campylobacter*, *Chlamydia* (lymphogranuloma strains), and *Shigella* and have their stools examined for the *ova* and *trophozoites* of *Entamoeba histolytica*. Those with *proctitis* only (no mucosal disease >15 cm) are more likely to have gonorrhea, herpes simplex, or chlamydial infection (nonlymphogranuloma strains), and specimens can be cultured accordingly. Viral cultures are not necessary because the diagnosis of herpes simplex proctitis can usually be made on the basis of its characteristic clinical presentation (severe anorectal pain, multiple perianal ulcers, rectal ulceration, inguinal adenopathy, difficult micturition, impotence, and paresthesias in the S-4 and S-5 distributions).

SYMPTOMATIC MANAGEMENT AND INDICATIONS FOR REFERRAL (1–19; See Also Chapters 137 and 141)

Acute Anal Fissure

Patients with anal pain caused by fissure should initially be treated symptomatically. Lubricants, such as mineral oil, and agents providing a soft, bulky stool, such as methylcellulose, will decrease trauma and counteract the attendant sphincter spasm. Frequent warm sitz baths provide intermittent relief of pain and spasm. Topical analgesics are of limited use and may result in skin sensitization. Systemic analgesics are sometimes necessary, but if narcotics are used, constipation may be aggravated.

Chronic Anal Fissure

If the pain has not improved with conservative measures in several days to weeks, the patient should be referred for the consideration of surgical treatment, which has a high success rate. In general, chronic or recurrent fissures will require surgery more often than acute or superficial fissures. In patients in whom the pain of fissure precludes digital or instrumental examination at the first visit, these may be performed at the time of surgical treatment under adequate anesthesia. *Sphincterotomy* is used to counter the internal sphincter spasm that maintains the tear, but because the procedure permanently weakens the sphincter, it may be followed by incontinence. Up to 30% of patients undergoing sphincterotomy may be so affected. Less invasive alternatives include one to two injections of *botulinum toxin* into the internal anal sphincter (95% healing rate) and daily application of *topical nitroglycerin* ointment for 2 to 6 weeks (60% healing rate). Botulinum toxin injection appears to heal fissures with a frequency equal to that of surgery without inducing long-term incontinence.

Perirectal Abscess

Perirectal abscess will not resolve on antibiotics alone; the proper treatment is surgical drainage. Antibiotic therapy should be reserved for patients with extensive cellulitis, signs of systemic infection, immunosuppression, valvular heart disease, or intravascular prostheses. Incision and drainage of a perirectal abscess usually requires anesthesia and is not often an office procedure. Similarly, the treatment for an infected pilonidal sinus is surgical drainage, which is accomplished satisfactorily under local anesthesia.

Fistula-in-Ano

The only successful treatment is surgical. However, patients with inflammatory bowel disease should not undergo surgery for fistula because this will usually fail as long as any active proximal disease is present. Surgery is reserved for palliation of the complications of fistula (i.e., drainage of recurrent perirectal abscess).

Suspected Carcinoma

Suspected carcinoma and the need for biopsy require surgical consultation, as does the patient with severe recurrent discomfort from *hemorrhoids* (see Appendix 66.1).

Pruritus Ani

Specific therapy is related to the identification of a specific cause (e.g., diabetes in the patient with candidiasis). Identification of the cause may be a challenging exercise for the primary physician. Pruritus resulting from anatomic lesions generally remits after the correction of the underlying problem. *Anogenital warts* are effectively treated with a topical application of 25% podophyllin in tincture of benzoin repeated every 1 to 2 weeks. The patient is instructed to bathe between 6 and 12 hours after the application. Care should be taken to avoid applying the compound to intact skin. If anoscopy reveals intraanal warts at the initial examination, curettage and electrocoagulation under anesthesia will be necessary.

Pinworms

All family members should be treated simultaneously. Pyrantel pamoate (Antiminth) is the drug of choice; a one-time oral dose of 11 mg/kg of body weight usually suffices. Preventive measures are difficult to enforce, except for hand washing before meals and after bowel movements. The best prevention is simultaneous treatment of all members of the household.

Idiopathic

No specific cause is found. Pruritus appears to be a form of neurodermatitis affecting the perianal skin. However, the symptoms are often relieved by careful attention to *perianal hygiene* after bowel movements; the perianal skin is kept dry with the application of witch hazel, and topical steroid ointments (0.25% hydrocortisone ointment) are used for several weeks to break the cycle of itching and skin changes caused by scratching. When contact dermatitis is believed to be caused by topical agents, the offending medication should be discontinued.

Anorectal Sexually Transmitted Diseases (See Chapters 136, 137, 141, and 192)

Pending the results of cultures, patients with a nonspecific *proctitis* (inflammation limited to the lower 15 cm of the bowel and no ulcers) should be treated empirically by covering for gonorrhea and *Chlamydia* (see Chapters 136 and 137). Both infections may be present simultaneously. The presence of ulceration suggests syphilis and herpes simplex but does not rule out concurrent gonorrhea and chlamydial infection; polymicrobial infection is found in about 25% of patients (see Chapters 137, 141, and 192).

Fecal Incontinence

The best results are obtained when treatment is etiologic. For inflammatory disease, topical and systemic steroids and sulfasalazine may provide symptomatic relief (see Chapter 73). Bulking agents such as psyllium or synthetic analogues can enhance sphincter performance. Patients bothered by voluminous diarrhea might require an antidiarrheal agent such as *loperamide* or *diphenoxylate* (see Chapter 64), with the former also able to increase sphincter tone. *Biofeedback* with a sphincter probe that measures voluntary contractions helps to support a supervised program of sphincter exercises in persons who have sustained sphincter injury. However, only those who retain some degree of rectal sensation are candidates for biofeedback. The technique requires responding to the feeling of rectal fullness. Formal manometry is sometimes helpful in retraining the anal sphincter response to rectal distention. Persons with incomplete evacuation as the cause of incontinence can benefit from a daily enema or suppository. Failure to respond to these measures is an indication for referral, as is suspected malignancy.

PATIENT EDUCATION AND INDICATIONS FOR REFERRAL

Patient Education

When poor or excessive personal hygiene, application of irritating agents, or neurotic behavior is responsible for symptoms, the relationship between rectal discomfort and precipitants should be explained so that the patient can take appropriate corrective action. Patients who obtain temporary relief of symptoms by applying a topical sensitizing agent may be reluctant to halt their medication if no other therapy is advised. Daily sitz baths can be prescribed in its place. Prevention through counseling is an important component of therapy in male homosexuals. Patients need to know that receptive anal sex with multiple partners carries a very high risk for intestinal infection and that they should certainly refrain from sexual activity if they become symptomatic.

As noted, creating an environment conducive to care is critical for the effective communication and management of MSM patients. If such a setting cannot be provide, referral is indicated.

Indications for Referral

Persons with refractory cases or suspected malignancy require proctologic consultation. Endoscopic evaluation, ultrasound, or manometry may be indicated, as might consideration of surgery. Sphincter injury may necessitate sphincteroplasty or direct repair. Success rates as high as 80% are common unless there is pudendal nerve injury, in which case the success rate falls to 20% to 30%. Symptomatic prolapsed internal hemorrhoids benefit from hemorrhoidectomy. Rectal prolapse also requires surgical correction—the sooner the better. Sacral nerve root stimulation is being tried in some persons with neurologic impairment. In very elderly patients, a colostomy represents an option when all else fails.

A.H.G.

Annotated Bibliography

1. Alexander-Williams J. Causes and managements of anal irritation. Br Med J 1983;287:1528. (*A classic review of the British approach.*)
2. Goodell SE, Quinn TC, Mkrtichian PA, et al. Herpes simplex virus proctitis in homosexual men. N Engl J Med 1983;308:868. (*One of the original major papers documenting the high frequency and distinctive clinical presentation of this infection.*)
3. Lebedeff DA, Hochman EB. Rectal gonorrhea in men: diagnosis and treatment. Ann Intern Med 1980;92:463. (*Although its treatment recommendations are outdated, this is still a useful study for its documentation of the clinical presentation and the utility of Gram's stain and culture.*)
4. Lieberman DA. Common anorectal disorders. Ann Intern Med 1984;101:837. (*Still one of the best reviews; 107 references.*)
5. Owen WF. Sexually transmitted disease and traumatic problems in homosexual men. Ann Intern Med 1980;92:805. (*An old review but still clinically relevant; 60 references.*)
6. Palefsky JM, Holly EA, Ralston ML, et al. High incidence of anal high-grade squamous intraepithelial lesions among HIV-positive and HIV-negative homosexual/bisexual men. *AIDS*. 1998;12:495. (*HIV-positive patients are at high risk.*)
7. Quinn TC, Goodell SE, Fennell C, et al. Infections with *Campylobacter jejuni* and *Campylobacter*-like organisms in homosexual men. Ann Intern Med 1984;101:187. (*The original description of the clinical presentation of infection with this class of organisms; about 25% of symptomatic patients were infected.*)
8. Quinn TC, Goodell SE, Mkrtichian E. *Chlamydia trachomatis* proctitis. N Engl J Med 1981;305:195. (*Chlamydia trachomatis of lymphogranuloma venereum immunotypes is associated with severe acute proctitis that mimics Crohn's disease.*)
9. Quinn TC, Stamm WE, Goodell SE, et al. The polymicrobial origin of intestinal infections in homosexual men. N Engl J Med 1983;309:576. (*An important article, documenting the polymicrobial nature of intestinal infection in this population.*)
10. Ramanujam PS, Prasad ML, Abcarian H, et al. Perianal abscesses and fistulas: a study of 10,023 patients. Dis Colon Rectum 1984;27:595. (*A classic overview of the problem.*)
11. Rudolph W, Galandiuk S. A practical guide to the diagnosis and management of fecal incontinence. Mayo Clin Proc 2002;77:271. (*A succinct but very useful review for primary physicians.*)
12. Jensen SL. Lignocaine ointment versus hydrocortisone ointment or warm sitz baths plus bran intake in the treatment of first episode acute anal fissures: a prospective randomised study. Br Med J 1986;292:1167. (*Sitz baths and bran worked best.*)
13. Smith LE, Henrich SD, McCullah RD. Etiology and treatment of pruritus ani. Dis Colon Rectum 1982;25:358. (*A practical article on this mundane but important issue.*)
14. Goldie SJ, Kuntz KM, Weinstein MC, et al. The clinical effectiveness and cost-effectiveness of screening for anal squamous intraepithelial lesions in homosexual and bisexual HIV-positive men. JAMA 1999;281:1822. (*Finds that screening by an anal Pap test is cost-effective.*)
15. Brisinda G, Maria G, Bentivoglio AR, et al. A comparison of injections of botulinum toxin and topical nitroglycerin ointment for the treatment of chronic anal fissure. N Engl J Med 1999;341:65. (*Botulinum toxin was superior to nitroglycerin ointment in this randomized trial of nonsurgical therapies.*)
16. Centers for Disease Control and Prevention. Sexually transmitted diseases treatment guidelines, 2006. MMWR Morb Mortal Wkly Rep. 2006;55:1. (*Current guidelines, including those related to receptive anal intercourse and resulting local infections.*)
17. Enck P. Biofeedback training in disordered defecation: a critical review. Dig Dis Sci 1993;38:1953. (*Finds that biofeedback is especially useful in persons who have had anorectal procedures.*)
18. Makadon HJ, Mayer KH, Garofalo R. Optimizing care for men who have sex with me. JAMA 2006;296:2362. (*A thoughtful essay on the importance of creating a comfortable setting for care.*)
19. Maria G, Cassetta E, Guid D, et al. A comparison of botulinum toxin and saline for the treatment of chronic anal fissure. N Engl J Med 1998;338:217. (*A double-blind, placebo-controlled trial demonstrating efficacy for botulinum toxin healing chronic fissures.*)

APPENDIX 66.1: MANAGEMENT OF HEMORRHOIDS

Hemorrhoids are a source of much misery, although they are of no consequence unless they become thrombosed, prolapse, or bleed. Therapy is directed toward the relief of symptoms and should be accomplished with a minimum of discomfort, cost, and time lost from work. Simple approaches to pain relief and sensible modification in bowel habits to prevent progression constitute the essentials of medical therapy. The primary physician must be certain that symptoms are attributable to hemorrhoids, alleviate any anxiety about neoplasm, provide conservative medical therapy, and decide on the need for and timing of surgery.

PRINCIPLES OF MANAGEMENT (1–7)

In most cases, it is not necessary to remove hemorrhoids to treat them effectively. Symptomatic relief and a halt to progression can usually be achieved by the use of simple local measures and minor changes in diet. For a painful attack, a *cold pack* applied for the first few hours offers considerable relief. Hot *sitz baths* (with a little salt added to the water to make it a more isotonic solution) are soothing and effective when they are used at least once or twice daily for about 20 to 30 minutes. Softening the stool helps to minimize straining and can be accomplished by increasing *dietary fiber* and making short-term use of *stool softeners* (e.g., dioctyl sodium sulfosuccinate). Irritant laxatives should be avoided. Patients should set aside a regular time each day to have an unhurried bowel movement and avoid vigorous wiping. Stubborn itching and inflammation respond well to *topical corticosteroids*; *hydrocortisone cream* and suppositories are adequate and relatively inexpensive. Topical hydrocortisone cream (1%), which can be purchased without a prescription, provides good relief from itching caused by the mild inflammation of anal tissue. It has been added to many of the popular over-the-counter preparations, although generic hydrocortisone is the least expensive formulation.

A host of *over-the-counter preparations* are heavily promoted. Many contain a topical anesthetic, such as benzocaine or pramoxine. *Benzocaine* may produce some temporary pain relief, but it is quite sensitizing; the resultant allergic response may actually worsen symptoms. *Pramoxine* is another topical anesthetic found in popular over-the-counter preparations (e.g., Anusol, Tronolane anesthetic hemorrhoid cream). It is similar in efficacy to benzocaine but is less sensitizing; it acts within 3 to 5 minutes of application, and effects last several hours. However, the cream formulation can still be irritating because of the presence of paraben preservatives. *Preparation H* is among the best-selling and most widely advertised over-the-counter hemorrhoidal therapies. It contains shark liver oil, live yeast cell derivatives, and phenyl mercuric nitrate; none of these agents, singly or in combination, has been shown to have any beneficial effect on hemorrhoids, although they are promoted as being able to shrink hemorrhoids and reduce inflammation.

Hemorrhoids that bleed repeatedly, prolapse, produce intractable pain, or become thrombosed deserve surgical evaluation. Internal hemorrhoids that have been bleeding persistently or have prolapsed can be removed in the surgeon's office with the use of *rubber band ligation*. A rubber band is placed at the base of the hemorrhoid; within a week the lesion sloughs. Mul-

tiple attempts are sometimes necessary. *Injection of sclerosing agents* (e.g., 5% phenol in oil) into the upper pole of internal hemorrhoids is another means of dealing with them; the procedure has fallen out of favor because of its association with scarring of the anal canal. *Cryosurgery* is relatively painless and does not require anesthesia, but a foul-smelling discharge is produced for about 1 week after the procedure, and stricture is occasionally a late occurrence. Excruciatingly painful external hemorrhoids that have become thrombosed can be excised under local anesthesia and the *clot removed*. Excellent nonsurgical results have been reported with the use of heat delivered through an infrared *photocoagulation probe* to treat first- and second-degree hemorrhoids. The heat is directed to the root of the hemorrhoid to interrupt its vascular supply, which causes it to contract.

Definitive *hemorrhoidectomy* is the treatment of last resort. In contrast with the other surgical therapies mentioned, it requires hospitalization, and the recovery period can last several weeks. Moreover, there is a risk for compromising the competence of the anal sphincter. Nevertheless, it does represent a serious treatment option for patients with disabling, refractory disease.

THERAPEUTIC RECOMMENDATIONS (1–7)

- Advise frequent hot sitz baths for the relief of pain. At the initial recognition of pain, the patient can apply a cold pack for the first few hours, then take hot baths three or four times a day.
- If inflammation and itching are present, prescribe a suppository preparation containing a steroid (e.g., hydrocortisone). If symptoms are predominantly external, prescribe 1% or 2.5% hydrocortisone cream.
- Topical anesthetics may be useful for the acute relief of severe pain. If this form of therapy is to be used, an agent that is minimally sensitizing (e.g., pramoxine) should be chosen.
- Treat constipation by having the patient increase dietary fiber and use a stool softener, such as 100 mg of dioctyl sodium sulfosuccinate three times daily. After the resolution of acute symptoms, the high-fiber diet should be continued.
- For thrombosed hemorrhoids, the following measures may be helpful:
  1. Instruct the patient to lie prone with ice applied to the thrombosed hemorrhoid.
  2. Prescribe oral analgesics; codeine may be required.
  3. Prescribe stool softeners.
  4. Conservative therapy should be successful in 3 to 5 days; otherwise, refer the patient for surgical removal of the clot, which will relieve the pain promptly.
- Intractable symptoms require surgical therapy. The specific method chosen depends on the surgical expertise available in the community.

PATIENT EDUCATION AND PREVENTION (1–7)

Instruction concerning proper diet and bowel habits is extremely helpful.

- Advise the patient to increase the intake of dietary fiber; suggest bran, carrots, green vegetables, and fruits with skin.

Consider use of a psyllium preparation. Some people find foods such as chili, onions, and alcohol irritating. If this applies to your patient, suggest that they be avoided.

■ Emphasize the importance of providing a regular time to have bowel movements. After bowel movements, the patient should avoid vigorous wiping; patting should suffice, and it minimizes irritation.

■ Instruct the patient not to linger on the toilet or strain at stool. Long periods of standing should be avoided.
■ Caution the patient against the use of irritant laxatives.
■ At the first sign of recurrent symptoms, institute frequent hot sitz baths.
■ Instruct the patient to pat dry rather than wipe or rub.

A.H.G.

Annotated Bibliography

1. FDA Advisory Review Panel on OTC Hemorrhoidal Drug Products. Fed Reg 1980;45:35576. (*Concludes that it is unclear whether topical anesthetics are effective for the treatment of hemorrhoids.*)
2. Johnson JF, Sonnenberg A. The prevalence of hemorrhoids and chronic constipation. Gastroenterology 1990;98:380. (*The best data, with divergent patterns noted.*)
3. Lieberman DA. Common anorectal disorders. Ann Intern Med 1984;101:837. (*An extensive review of the anatomy and physiology of the anus and rectum, with special attention to hemorrhoids, fissure-in-ano, pruritus ani, and fecal incontinence; required reading for all primary physicians.*)
4. Murie JA, Sim AJ, MacKenzie I. Rubber band ligation versus haemorrhoidec-tomy for prolapsing haemorrhoids. Br J Surg 1982;69:536. (*A long-term, prospective clinical trial showing that ligation is effective, except for permanently prolapsed painful lesions.*)
5. Prasad GC, Prakash V, Tandon AK, et al. Studies on etiopathogenesis of hemorrhoids. Am J Proctol 1976;27:33. (*An excellent review of the pathogenesis of hemorrhoids.*)
6. Stern H, McLeod R, Cohen Z, et al. Ambulatory procedures in anorectal surgery. Adv Surg 1987;20:217. (*Includes a discussion of hemorrhoid treatments offered by the surgeon in the office setting.*)
7. To tie; to stab; to stretch, perchance to freeze [Editorial]. Lancet 1975;2:645. (*Concludes that hemorrhoidectomy should be reserved for cases in which other methods fail.*)

CHAPTER 67 ■ APPROACH TO THE PATIENT WITH AN EXTERNAL HERNIA

Abdominal hernias are exceedingly common; they often cause occupational disabilities and pose a risk for incarceration and strangulation of bowel. Fortunately, adequate evaluation can usually be performed in the office by means of history and physical examination. The primary physician must distinguish between patients who require surgical referral and those who may be managed expectantly.

PATHOPHYSIOLOGY AND CLINICAL PRESENTATION (1,2)

Pathophysiology

A hernia is a defect in the normal musculofascial continuity of the abdominal wall that permits the egress of structures not normally passing through the parietes. In general, the significant feature of a hernia is not the size of the protrusion or the sac, but the size and rigidity of the defect in the abdominal wall. The fixation and rigidity of the hernial ring are the features that lead to incarceration and strangulation. The distinction between congenital and acquired hernia is not often clear because many hernias that appear after trauma or straining represent a congenital predisposition, such as indirect inguinal hernia in the adult. This distinction has little bearing on management, although it can make a considerable difference to the patient, who may be compensated if the hernia can be attributed to trauma at work. Some of these hernias are incidental to, and antedate, the perceived injury.

Disorders resulting in increased intraabdominal pressure may contribute to the appearance of a hernia and also affect the postoperative management. For example, chronic cough resulting from cigarette smoking or bronchitis can precipitate or worsen herniation; the same is true of symptomatic prostatism.

Clinical Presentations

Reducible Hernia

The symptoms of an uncomplicated or reducible external hernia are related not to its size but to the degree of pressure on its contents. Patients with large scrotal hernias containing much intestine may have few symptoms other than a dragging sensation. A mass appears on standing, which reduces when the patient is supine. Pain may be intermittent, disappearing when the hernia is reduced. Patients with small hernias containing an entrapped knuckle of bowel may have rather severe pain and nausea. Many patients with femoral, umbilical, or epigastric hernias may be entirely unaware of their existence.

Irreducible or Incarcerated Hernia

Irreducible or incarcerated hernia is one in which the contents cannot be replaced into the abdomen. Here, the mass remains palpable with the patient relaxed and in the supine position. A strangulated hernia is an irreducible hernia in which the blood supply to the entrapped bowel loop has been compromised, resulting in small-bowel obstruction and infarction. These patients complain of colicky abdominal pain, nausea, and vomiting and show signs of small-bowel obstruction with distention, tympany, and hyperperistalsis. In addition, careful examination demonstrates a tender, irreducible groin or ventral hernia.

Inguinal Hernias

Indirect inguinal hernias, which account for one half of all hernias in adults, pass through the internal abdominal inguinal ring along the spermatic cord through the inguinal canal and exit through the external inguinal ring. In male patients, these can descend into the scrotum. Direct inguinal hernias pass through the posterior inguinal wall medial to the inferior epigastric vessels, through Hesselbach's triangle. Femoral hernias pass through the femoral canal inferior to the inguinal ligament and become subcutaneous in the fossa ovalis. It is often difficult to distinguish among these three forms, especially when incarceration is present and the sac is large.

Indirect inguinal hernias are eight to ten times more common in men than in women, whereas femoral hernias are three to five times more common in women than in men. Nevertheless, the most common hernia in women is the indirect inguinal type. The diagnosis is less often made in women because physical examination of the external inguinal ring is more difficult. Direct hernias increase in incidence with advancing age and are the least likely of the external hernias to become incarcerated or strangulated.

Strangulation is common in femoral hernias. The majority of patients with strangulated inguinal hernias are aware of the hernia before strangulation. In contrast, nearly half of those with strangulated femoral hernias are unaware of the hernia before strangulation. In addition, groin pain and tenderness are absent in a significant percentage of cases of strangulated femoral hernia.

Ventral Hernias

The commonly encountered ventral hernias include umbilical, epigastric, and incisional varieties. Ventral hernias are often more obvious when the patient is standing. Umbilical hernias pass through the umbilical ring and represent a failure of the ring to be obliterated after birth. In the infant, these often close spontaneously within the first 2 years of life. In the adult, they are more common in women and are associated with obesity, multiparity, and cirrhosis with ascites. Umbilical hernias are often missed because they are obscured by subcutaneous fat. They are associated with a high risk for incarceration and strangulation, and mortality rates are higher than with inguinal hernias because the large bowel is frequently entrapped.

Incisional Hernias

Incisional hernias are those that develop in the scar of a previous laparotomy or in a drain site. They are associated with a previous postoperative wound infection, dehiscence, malnutrition, obesity, and smoking. They are more common in vertical than in transverse scars. Incisional hernias often have multiple defects and several rings. They are frequently irreducible or only partially reducible because of adhesions within the sac. Patients with very large incisional hernias may be remarkably free of symptoms of intestinal obstruction, although incarceration is not uncommon (6% to 15%); strangulation is relatively uncommon (2%) because of the usually large size of the defects.

Epigastric Hernias

Epigastric hernias occur through the linea alba between the xiphoid process and the umbilicus. They may be difficult to detect in the obese patient and must be looked for in patients with epigastric pain. Incarcerated epigastric hernia may produce symptoms that mimic those of peptic ulcer disease or biliary colic.

DIFFERENTIAL DIAGNOSIS (1)

Recognizing a hernia usually presents little difficulty, although distinguishing one type of inguinal hernia from another can sometimes be complicated. The differential diagnosis of an entrapped femoral hernia includes not only inguinal hernia but also femoral lymphadenopathy, saphenous varix, psoas abscess, and hydrocele. On occasion, it is impossible to differentiate an incarcerated femoral hernia from a single enlarged femoral lymph node (the lymph node of Cloquet). Other causes of groin pain or swelling include muscle strain, hip arthritis, inguinal adenopathy, and undescended testicle.

WORKUP (1,2)

The diagnosis and evaluation of external hernias require no more than a brief history and careful physical examination; laboratory and radiologic studies are unnecessary unless major complications have resulted.

History

The patient is questioned about groin pain, swelling, the ability to reduce the hernia, the circumstances of onset, and aggravating and alleviating factors, such as exacerbation on standing, straining, or coughing. The acute onset of colicky abdominal pain, nausea, and vomiting suggest entrapment and strangulation in a patient with a known hernia.

Physical Examination

Physical examination is directed toward differentiating herniation from other causes of inguinal swelling or pain and distinguishing among (a) hernias that are uncomplicated and require no therapy, (b) those that can be repaired electively, and (c) those in which emergency surgery is the safest course. The physical examination is also important in distinguishing the anatomic type of hernia; the prognosis and likelihood of incarceration and strangulation differ among the various types.

Inspection

The patient should be examined in both the supine and standing positions. Inspection is often as important as palpation for detection. Examination should include Valsalva's maneuver to increase intraabdominal pressure. In male patients, small inguinal hernias are looked for by invaginating the scrotal skin while the patient is standing. To detect ventral hernias, patients should be supine and then asked to lift their head from the examining table and bear down to tense the abdominal wall.

Palpation

Palpation follows and is best performed with the patient standing. In male patients, one inserts the index finger into the inguinal canal by following the spermatic cord. Distinguishing a direct from an indirect hernia can be difficult. An indirect hernia projects more inferiorly, and protrusion into the scrotum is almost always a sign. To detect a femoral hernia, one palpates the fossa ovalis, inferior to the inguinal canal. If a groin hernia is detected, one should gently attempt reduction of the hernia while the patient relaxes the abdominal muscles.

Examination of the Irreducible Hernia

If a hernia is irreducible, the physician should look for local tenderness, discoloration, edema, fever, and signs of small-bowel obstruction. It is often difficult to distinguish a simple incarceration from early strangulation; for this reason, these two lesions are managed identically by immediate referral to a surgeon. Surgical exploration is the only way to be certain that no compromised bowel is trapped in the hernia sac. Conversely, when signs of small-bowel obstruction are present, it is essential to examine thoroughly for a strangulated femoral hernia because groin pain and tenderness may be absent.

Additional Groin Examination

The groin area also is checked for lymphadenopathy and other masses that do not change with position or Valsalva's maneuver. If groin pain is present but no mass, then a musculoskeletal cause is suggested, and a careful examination of hip movement is indicated.

Checking for Associated Conditions

A few conditions are believed to have more than a chance association with hernias, and some researchers argue that they should be screened for. Whether the adult patient with a recent hernia is more likely to have an occult carcinoma of the colon remains a source of controversy. It has been suggested that patients undergo screening for colorectal cancer (see Chapter 56). However, if the patient reports no change in bowel habits and the stools are repeatedly negative for blood on guaiac testing, it is unnecessary to submit the patient to more-extensive investigation for occult malignancy. Symptoms and signs of prostatism are frequently present in elderly men with hernia and may require relief before herniorrhaphy. The entire abdomen should be examined for masses, hepatomegaly, and ascites, which are sometimes associated with hernia formation.

PRINCIPLES OF MANAGEMENT AND INDICATIONS FOR REFERRAL (1–7)

Conservative Therapy versus Surgery

The key determination is the need for surgery, which can be based on the findings at physical examination.

Reducible Inguinal Hernia

Patients with minimally symptomatic reducible inguinal hernia have a choice. They can undergo elective surgical repair or be managed expectantly; the outcomes are not statistically different. Elective surgery is very safe and effective. Surgical repair can be performed under local anesthesia in the high-risk patient, and newer laparoscopic techniques (see later discussion) make for less perioperative morbidity. Watchful waiting is also a reasonable alternative; the risk of incarceration for those managed expectantly is very small (reported rate, 1.8 per 1,000 patient-years). Any plan for watchful waiting should be accompanied by careful patient education regarding the symptoms of strangulation and specific instructions promptly to report such symptoms. Reduction by means of a truss may be unsatisfactory, even in patients with relative medical contraindications to surgery.

Nontender Incarcerated Inguinal Hernia

If the hernia is of recent onset and signs of inflammation or bowel obstruction are absent, it may be safe to attempt gentle reduction ("taxis"). This is best accomplished with the patient supine and the hips and knees flexed. If gentle pressure over the hernial sac fails to reduce the mass further, efforts should be abandoned, and the patient should be referred for surgery forthwith. Often, patients have more experience in reducing their hernia than does the physician. Patients with evidence of strangulated groin hernias should be subjected to immediate operation regardless of medical contraindications; if they are not treated, death will result from bowel necrosis.

Reducible Femoral Hernias

Reducible femoral hernias should undergo prompt elective repair because of the high incidence of strangulation. Whenever there is a question of an incarcerated femoral hernia, it is safest to proceed immediately with surgical exploration.

Umbilical Hernias

Surgery is unnecessary if physical examination reveals a small, asymptomatic fascial defect without protrusion. When herniation is detected, however, umbilical defects should be repaired because the risk for incarceration and strangulation is high. The danger of strangulation is compounded by the greater likelihood of colonic entrapment, which is associated with a higher mortality rate than is strangulation of small intestine. Therefore, all incarcerated umbilical hernias should be managed as if they were strangulated. Elective umbilical herniorrhaphy should be avoided in patients with ascites; instead, efforts should be directed toward reducing the ascites (see Chapter 71). The problem in patients with cirrhosis and ascites is made more difficult when the skin overlying the sac thins out and poses the risk of rupture.

Small-Neck Incisional Hernias or Tender Incarceration

Small-neck incisional hernias or tender incarceration should undergo repair on an urgent basis. Patients who have trophic changes or ulceration in the skin overlying incisional hernias are also candidates for urgent surgery. In some instances, cellulitis of the skin overlying the hernia sac develops and is difficult to distinguish from strangulation of the contents of the sac. Using mesh in the repair reduces the recurrence rate by nearly 50%, even for small hernias.

Large Incisional Hernias

Large incisional hernias can pose a management problem because durable repair is difficult to achieve. Recurrence rates after initial repair range from 25% to 50% and remain at nearly 50% for repair of repeated herniation. The management of large incarcerated incisional hernias that occur in the abdomen in very obese patients is a particular problem. Major efforts should be directed toward weight reduction before repair if it is possible to delay. If, however, the presence of intestinal obstruction is a possibility or the viability of the contents of the sac is doubtful, the advice of a surgeon should be sought promptly. Both polypropylene mesh and suture repair are available; mesh reduces the recurrence rate by nearly 50% in persons with a midline incisional hernia, regardless of hernia size. With the use of mesh, care needs to be taken to avoid its contact with the underlying viscera.

Treatment of Contributing Factors

Factors contributing to hernia formation should be corrected if possible. Prostatism that leads to straining at urination needs attention, be it medical or surgical (see Chapter 138). Patients with chronic cough secondary to chronic obstructive pulmonary disease, cigarette smoking, asthma, or esophageal reflux should have the underlying condition addressed promptly (see Chapter 41) to diminish symptoms caused by the hernia and to decrease the possibility of postoperative complications.

Conventional versus Laparoscopic Hernia Repair

The effective application of laparoscopic techniques to the repair of inguinal hernias provides an alternative surgical approach for patients. In the largest multicenter, randomized prospective study, laparoscopic repair proved superior to open repair in terms of time required for recovery from surgery (1 vs. 2 weeks), return to work (2 vs. 3 weeks), and the resumption of athletic activities (3 vs. 5 weeks). In addition, the risk for recurrence was reduced by 50%, and fewer wound infections were noted. Most recurrences that did follow laparoscopic surgery were traceable to errors in surgical technique. The duration of surgery was similar for both procedures. The time to discharge was less, as was the degree of postoperative pain, with laparoscopic surgery. Disadvantages include the higher cost of surgery, the need for general anesthesia, and the additional surgical skill required. (A clear and prolonged learning curve is associated with laparoscopic surgery, with the potential for inexperienced operators to cause serious complications, such as viscus perforation, when unsupervised.) If the requisite surgical skill is available, then patients capable of undergoing general anesthesia and desiring a more rapid return to activity can be offered laparoscopic repair.

PATIENT EDUCATION

Patients who are to be managed conservatively must be taught to watch for signs of complications. It is the responsibility of the physician to instruct the patient in the symptoms of incarceration and strangulation and in the urgency of seeking help should they occur. If the patient is deemed incompetent to make such observations and promptly to obtain help, a strong case can be made for proceeding with surgery. Patients scheduled for elective surgery also require instruction because incarceration occasionally occurs before the planned operation.

Many patients with asymptomatic or mildly symptomatic reducible hernias will be reluctant to undergo surgery because their symptoms are minimal. If they fall into the high-risk group (e.g., femoral or small-neck incisional hernias), they should be informed of the strong likelihood of strangulation and the minuscule morbidity and mortality associated with surgery.

Patients who are advised to have surgery appreciate estimates of time to walking (same day for local anesthesia and general anesthesia in the morning), time to return to physically undemanding work (2 to 3 weeks), time to resumption of unlimited activity (3 to 6 weeks), risk for recurrence (10%), and effect on sexual function (none). A discussion of the advantages and disadvantages of open versus laparoscopic repair is also worthwhile in the context of a review of the patient's surgical candidacy.

A.H.G.

Annotated Bibliography

1. Gilbert AI. An anatomic and functional classification for the diagnosis and treatment of inguinal hernia. Am J Surg 1989;157:331. (*A useful, succinct summary.*)
2. Mudge M, Hughes LE. Incisional hernia: a 10-year prospective study of incidence and attitudes. Br J Surg 1985;72:70. (*The occurrence rate was 10% to 20% after laparotomy.*)
3. Barry MK, Donohue JH, Harmsen WS, et al. Transabdominal preperitoneal laparoscopic inguinal herniorrhaphy: assessment of initial experience. Mayo Clin Proc 1998;73:717. (*The Mayo Clinic initial experience, showing the importance of the learning curve in achieving optimal outcomes.*)
4. Fitzgibbons RJ Jr, Giobbie-Harder A, Gibbs JO, et al. Watchful waiting vs repair of inguinal hernia in minimally symptomatic men: a randomized clinical trial. JAMA 2006;295:285. (*No significant difference was found in outcomes.*)
5. Flanagan L Jr, Bascom JV. Repair of the groin hernia: outpatient approach with local anesthesia. Surg Clin North Am 1984;64:257. (*An increasingly common approach, which reduces cost considerably.*)
6. Liem MSL, van der Graaf Y, van Steensel CJ, et al. Comparison of conventional anterior surgery and laparoscopic surgery for inguinal hernia repair. N Engl J Med 1997;336:1541. (*A multicenter, randomized, controlled trial, showing significant advantages for laparoscopic surgery.*)
7. Luijendijk RW, Hop WCJ, van den Tol P, et al. A comparison of suture repair with mesh repair for incisional hernia. N Engl J Med 2000;343:392. (*A randomized trial, finding that mesh repair was superior for patients with midline hernia.*)

CHAPTER 68 ■ MANAGEMENT OF PEPTIC ULCER DISEASE

Peptic ulcer disease is a major source of morbidity, affecting up to 2.0% of the U.S. population at any one time. Male patients outnumber female patients by two to one. The peak prevalence for duodenal ulcer (which accounts for 80% of cases) is between ages 45 and 54 years; gastric ulcer peaks between the ages of 55 and 64 years. Advances in understanding the pathogenesis of peptic ulcer have revolutionized treatment and markedly improved outcomes. The primary care physician must be capable of designing and implementing a cost-effective program that alleviates pain, promotes healing, limits complications, and prevents recurrences. Other tasks include the timely identification of patients who require endoscopy or consideration of surgery. The management of nonulcer dyspepsia, which may mimic peptic ulcer disease, shares aspects of peptic ulcer treatment (see Chapter 74).

PATHOPHYSIOLOGY, CLINICAL PRESENTATION, AND COURSE (1–22)

Peptic ulcers arise principally in the stomach and the duodenum—areas exposed to gastric acid and pepsin. Although the precise mechanisms of ulcer formation are incompletely understood, the process appears to involve the interplay of acid production, pepsin secretion, *Helicobacter pylori* infection, and mucosal defense mechanisms.

Gastric Acid Production, Pepsin Secretion, and Mucosal Defenses

Acid Production and Pepsin Secretion

Excess acid production is the hallmark of duodenal ulcer disease, with significant increases noted in basal and peak acid outputs, parietal and chief cell masses, and responses to food and hormonal stimulation. Zollinger–Ellison syndrome (with its associated hypergastrinemia and parietal cell overproduction) is the prototypical acid hypersecretory condition resulting in ulcer formation. Some patients with duodenal ulcer demonstrate *rapid gastric emptying*, which raises the acid exposure of the proximal duodenum. Pepsin secretion is also elevated in duodenal ulcer disease. Gastric acid production is relatively normal in patients with gastric ulcers.

Mucosal Defense

Peptic ulcer disease results from compromise of the major determinants of gastric mucosal integrity, namely the secretion of *mucus*, the *production of bicarbonate*, and *cellular repair*. The mucous barrier may become compromised by increased degradation of mucus, decreased secretion, or the production of defective mucus. Bile acids, pepsin, pancreatic enzymes, and mechanical forces contribute to the degradation of mucus. *Gastric prostaglandin production* appears to be important to sustaining the production of mucus, the secretion of bicarbonate, and mucosal repair. By helping to maintain a neutral pH and aqueous environment at the surface of the gastric epithelium, mucus and bicarbonate protect the mucosa from acid, pepsin, and other potentially injurious agents (see later discussion).

Role of Nonsteroidal Antiinflammatory Drugs

Mechanisms

Aspirin and other nonsteroidal antiinflammatory drugs (NSAIDs) impair the principal mechanisms of mucosal protection and account for a major portion of peptic ulcer disease in modern societies. By inhibiting cyclooxygenases (COX) 1 and 2 and their conversion of arachidonic acid to prostaglandins, aspirin and the so-called *nonselective NSAIDs* block production not only of the COX-2–dependent prostaglandins important to inflammation, fever, and pain, but also the COX-1–derived prostaglandins involved in mucosal protection, platelet aggregation, and renal function. The selective NSAIDs that block only COX-2 (so-called *COX-2 drugs*) avoid much of the mucosal injury associated with the use of nonselective preparations.

With long-term use, all nonselective NSAIDs (including enteric-coated and nonaspirin salicylates and NSAID prodrugs) are capable of producing solitary deep *gastric ulcers*. Established risk factors include advanced age, concurrent use of corticosteroids, prior history of ulcer, high NSAID doses, and possibly concurrent *H. pylori* infection, alcohol use, and smoking. Despite some relative *in vitro* differences in COX selectivity among the nonselective agents, the clinical risks of major gastrointestinal injury and clinically important ulceration are similar, estimated by the U.S. Food and Drug Administration (FDA) to be 2% per patient-year of NSAID use. NSAID-associated risk generally increases with dose and duration of therapy. A higher risk with increasing dose is also seen with aspirin, but low doses (e.g., 81 mg/d) are not risk-free. About 15% of long-term NSAID users demonstrate gastric ulceration at endoscopy; up to one fourth of complications have been observed within the first month of therapy. The *elderly* are at greatest risk (reported relative risk, about 4.0).

In addition to inhibiting prostaglandin synthesis, many NSAID preparations produce acute diffuse mucosal injury by means of a *direct erosive effect*. Endoscopic study has shown that significant mucosal injury results from both plain and tablet forms of buffered aspirin, although not with enteric-coated aspirin preparations, unless gastric emptying is delayed. Similar acute erosions occur with uncoated NSAIDs, but not with enteric-coated preparations or prodrug formulations. Such diffuse acute injury is rarely associated with symptoms or clinically significant ulceration, although minor occult bleeding may ensue. Concurrent *H. pylori* infection, smoking, alcohol use, alcohol-related disease, and preexisting peptic ulcer disease greatly increase the risk for ulcer and ulcer complications in NSAID-treated patients.

Gastric versus Duodenal Disease

NSAID use is associated primarily with gastric ulceration and not with new *duodenal ulceration*, but preexisting duodenal ulceration may be exacerbated and complicated by NSAID use. It is estimated that more than half of ulcer complications associated with NSAID use occur in patients with preexisting duodenal ulcers. Much of the ulcer morbidity associated with NSAID use may be related to preexisting, subclinical disease.

Role of *Helicobacter Pylori* Infection

Infection with *H. pylori* has emerged as a major, if not the major, precipitant of peptic ulcer disease. The organism's flagellated anatomy and urea-splitting capability make it well suited to survive in the acidic mucoid environment of the gastric mucosa. It attaches to epithelial cells and, without invading, induces apoptosis and an inflammatory response. These reactions lead to cell death and ulcer formation. *H. pylori* infection is associated with 95% to 99% of cases of *duodenal ulcer* and ulcer recurrence and with more than 90% of *gastric ulcers* unrelated to NSAID use. *Helicobacter* infection also is strongly associated with antral *gastritis* and is a major risk factor for *gastric carcinoma* and *mucosa-associated lymphoid tissue lymphoma* of the stomach; its eradication results in remission of the latter. Cancer risk appears to increase when *H. pylori* is present in the setting of atrophic gastritis.

Cure of *Helicobacter* infection can speed ulcer healing and greatly reduce rates of recurrence. The organism does not appear to cause ulcers per se, but rather seems to enhance mucosal susceptibility to the injurious actions of acid and pepsin. Acid hypersecretors may be particularly vulnerable to ulcer formation in the context of *Helicobacter* infection and subject to slow healing and a high rate of recurrence. The prevalence of *H. pylori* infection increases with age, approaching 90% in ulcer patients older than age 65 years. The mode of transmission is unclear, although person-to-person fecal–oral spread is suspected because clusters occur in families.

Other Precipitants

A host of psychological, dietary, pharmacologic, and hereditary factors have been implicated in the cause or aggravation of ulcer disease.

Stress

Stress has long been considered a key precipitant, a view supported by a higher incidence of chronic stress in ulcer patients than in controls, increased acid production in response to stress, and a more prolonged course and poorer prognosis in patients with chronic severe anxiety. Patients in whom ulcers develop view life stresses more negatively than do controls. Acid hypersecretion and ulcer formation have been observed in small-scale studies of patients undergoing severe emotional stress; with the subsidence of stress, acid secretion falls and ulcers heal. Confirmation of these small-scale observations will strengthen the association between stress and ulcer disease.

Smoking

Smoking is an important risk factor identified by epidemiologic studies. For example, ulcers are twice as likely to develop in cigarette smokers as in nonsmokers. The risk for gastric ulcer correlates with the number of cigarettes smoked, and patients with ulcers have increased rates of smoking. The rates of recurrence are dramatically increased in patients who smoke, and healing is markedly slowed. Impaired prostaglandin production has been demonstrated in the gastric mucosa of smokers.

Alcohol and Coffee

Alcohol and coffee have also been implicated. Coffee, including decaffeinated forms, stimulates acid secretion, as do other caffeine-containing beverages, but evidence proving ulcer causation is lacking. *Ethanol* can compromise the mucosal barrier and cause gastritis, and beer is almost as potent a stimulant of acid secretion as is gastrin. Nonetheless, the data on the link between alcohol use and ulcer disease are conflicting. However, patients with alcohol-related cirrhosis are at an increased risk for ulcer formation and complications.

Glucocorticosteroids

Their contribution has been debated ever since these agents first became available, with randomized, controlled trials and meta-analyses producing conflicting results. Discrepancies are related in part to a failure to control for concurrent NSAID use. The risk appears to be nil if the patient is not taking NSAIDs concurrently and the dose is less than 30 mg/d. However, high-dose steroid therapy (>30 mg/d) may confer an increment of risk, as might the underlying disease for which the prednisone is being taken. In the absence of concurrent NSAID use, the overall risk appears to be very modest.

Heredity

Heredity plays some role. The incidence of ulcer in the parents, siblings, and children of ulcer patients is increased, and studies of twins show a greater concordance (e.g., both twins affected) among identical than among fraternal twins. Increased meal-stimulated gastrin release and pepsin secretion have been found to be hereditary traits among ulcer patients and their families.

Clinical Presentation

Peptic ulcers usually occur at or near mucosal transition zones, areas that believed to be particularly vulnerable to the effects of acid, pepsin, bile, and pancreatic enzymes. Gastric ulcers are found in the *antrum* at the *lesser curvature*, near the junction of the acid-secreting parietal cells and the antral mucosa. Duodenal ulcers arise mostly at the *junction* of the *antrum* and *duodenum*.

The clinical presentations of gastric and duodenal peptic ulcers often overlap and may be nonspecific. Patients can present with pain, bleeding, or obstruction, or they may be symptom-free. Epigastric pain, relieved by antacids and occurring as clusters of daily symptoms for a few weeks separated by pain-free periods of months, is characteristic of peptic disease. Duodenal ulcer pain is classically relieved by food, absent before breakfast, and responsible for awakening the patient at night; it starts 2 to 3 hours after a meal. However, careful studies of patients with documented duodenal ulcers have shown that in some of them pain is often worsened by meals, present before breakfast, and continuous rather than periodic. Gastric ulcer pain is more likely to be precipitated by food and often radiates from the epigastrium to the back or substernal region. It, too, can awaken the patient and be relieved by food. In both conditions, the pain may be dull, aching, gnawing, or burning in quality, consistent with its visceral quality.

Symptoms may be absent and dissociated from mucosal changes. Silent disease is particularly common among the elderly and in patients using NSAIDs. A complication is the first clinical manifestation of ulcer disease in about 25% of persons with ulcer disease unrelated to NSAID use; the figure is considerably higher in the setting of NSAID use.

Clinical Course

Natural History and Clinical Course

The clinical course prior to treatment of *H. pylori* was characterized by the majority of patients becoming pain-free within the first 4 weeks and their ulcers healing completely by 4 to 12 weeks (depending on the size of the lesion). Of interest, there was little correlation between the cessation of pain and objective healing. The 5-year recurrence rates were high (30% to 90%). Although it was rare for a patient to have more than two or three recurrent gastric ulcers, multiple recurrences were not unusual for those with duodenal ulcers. No correlation was found between the recurrence rate and ulcer size, duration of symptoms, or location. Recurrent ulcers healed just as rapidly and completely as original lesions. The rate of development of a major complication, such as hemorrhage, perforation, or obstruction, was less than 1% annually. Bleeding was slightly more common from duodenal than from gastric ulcers and two to three times more common than perforation.

With the application of therapies to eradicate *H. pylori* infection and markedly suppress acid production, the clinical course of peptic ulcer disease has improved substantially. Complete healing is now achieved in up to 95% of cases within 4 to 6 weeks of initiation of treatment, and the 1-year risk for relapse is now about 5% with the eradication of *Helicobacter* (but >50% when acid suppression is the only form of initial therapy).

Workup (23–29)

A presumptive diagnosis of acid-peptic disease can often be made on *clinical grounds* alone (see Chapter 58). Aside from testing all patients for *H. pylori* infection (see later discussion), the initial workup of uncomplicated peptic ulcer disease need not include confirmation by barium study or endoscopy. Cost-effectiveness studies demonstrate that the *commencement of empiric therapy* is superior to prior confirmation of the diagnosis by endoscopy or upper gastrointestinal series. The only time confirmatory studies are needed initially is when clinical findings suggest a complication of peptic ulcer disease or gastric cancer (e.g., weight loss, dysphagia, recurrent nausea and vomiting, iron-deficiency anemia, and stool test positive for occult blood, especially in a person >40 years of age).

Testing for Helicobacter Infection

There is no gold standard, but the reference method remains endoscopic antral mucosal *biopsy* with *special staining* (Warthin–Starry [silver] stain, with a sensitivity of 90% and a specificity of 100%). The *Campylobacter-like organism (CLO) test* provides a more rapid means of endoscopic diagnosis (sensitivity 90%, specificity 96%). Noninvasive testing is possible with the ^{13}C-urea breath test (sensitivity 91%, specificity 91%), by *serologic testing*, which measures immunoglobulin G and immunoglobulin A antibodies to *Helicobacter* (sensitivity 71%, specificity 85%), and by *stool antigen testing* (sensitivity 97%, specificity 94% for the monoclonal antibody version). Because no statistically significant difference between these test performances has been found in head-to-head study, noninvasive testing is preferred in persons who do not need to undergo initial endoscopy.

Serologic Testing

Serologic testing is used by many primary care physicians in lieu of endoscopic examination or breath testing because it is readily available, convenient, reasonably sensitive and specific, and inexpensive. Sensitivity and specificity for regionally adjusted testing (there is some geographic variation in strains) approach those for breath testing. This approach has been found to be cost-effective for the detection of infection in persons who have never been treated, but it cannot be used definitively to determine cure or recurrence of infection because the test result often remains positive (although antibody titers do decline) for years after the eradication of the organism. Positivity means only prior exposure to the organism. Testing for eradication can be achieved noninvasively by performing a ^{13}C urea breath test or a *stool antigen test*.

^{13}C Urea Breath Testing

Based on the use of ^{13}C- or ^{14}C-labeled carbon dioxide, breath testing takes advantage of urea splitting by live organisms and, unlike serology, provides direct evidence of active infection. Consequently, breath testing is very useful as a noninvasive method for determining *eradication* of infection, which becomes important in the settings of relapse, recurrence, and disease complicated by bleeding. Test sensitivity and specificity approach those of endoscopic measures and can be used in lieu of invasive testing. The test is costly and not widely available, limiting it is use in primary care practice, both for diagnosis and for the determination of eradication, but its use can obviate the need for invasive testing. Testing for cure or relapse requires waiting 4 weeks after treatment.

Stool Antigen Testing

The detection of *H. pylori* antigen in the stool provides a convenient alternative to other modes of testing, especially for determining the eradication of infection. Under study conditions, the sensitivity and specificity of the monoclonal antibody stool antigen test were 97% and 94%, respectively. Negative and positive predictive values were 97% and 95%, respectively. The diagnostic accuracy was 96%; the likelihood ratio for a positive test was 17 and for a negative test was 0. Although the ^{13}C-urea breath test is the most accurate among the noninvasive tests for the determination of cure, this test offers a reasonable alternative.

Endoscopy versus Upper Gastrointestinal Series

At the time of *initial presentation*, patients older than 40 years of age who have any clinical findings that raise concern about gastric cancer or complicated ulcer disease (see prior discussion) should promptly undergo visualization of the stomach and the duodenum. The most cost-effective approach to initial testing remains a subject of debate. Endoscopists correctly argue that gastroscopy is superior to barium study for the detection of gastric ulcer, malignancy, and *H. pylori* because *brushings*, *biopsy*, *CLO test*, and *cultures* can be performed at the same time. However, radiologists counter that with the use of air-contrast techniques, the sensitivity of endoscopy for detecting malignancy can be approached with a procedure that entails one third of the cost and is safer and more comfortable for the patient. The debate continues; test selection should be individualized. Later in the course of illness, the patient with refractory or recurrent disease in the absence of evidence for persistent *H. pylori* infection should undergo endoscopy to check for gastric malignancy, as should the person with an ulcer that appears suspect on barium study.

About 4% of all gastric ulcers prove malignant. The sensitivity of barium study for the detection of gastric malignancy is in the range of 80% to 85%, compared with 95% for endoscopy with biopsy and brushing. Most malignant ulcers manifest radiologic signs of cancer, including irregular shape, nodular base, absence of radiating gastric folds, folds that are blunted or stop before the ulcer, and rigidity of adjacent stomach. Ulcers in the fundus are more likely to be malignant; those within 1 cm of the pylorus are almost always benign. Ulcers that appear malignant by any of these criteria require biopsy.

Subjecting all patients with benign-appearing ulcers on barium study to endoscopy is likely to be of low yield and add little to survival. For persons presenting with an ulcerated gastric carcinoma, the 5-year survival is only 25% to 35%. A more productive alternative might be to refer for endoscopy and biopsy only those patients with a radiologically suspect gastric ulcer and those with an ulcer that fails to heal fully despite documented eradication of *Helicobacter* infection (see later discussion). The literature should be followed for further cost–benefit studies.

Principles of Therapy

The major objectives of therapy are to speed healing, reduce pain, and prevent complications and recurrences while minimizing the costs and side effects of therapy. Although peptic ulcer disease represents a heterogeneous set of disorders, the overall approach to medical therapy is similar and centers on (a) limiting precipitants such as NSAIDs, stress, and smoking, (b) eradicating *Helicobacter* infection, (c) reducing gastric acidity, and (d) protecting the mucosal barrier. Combination programs are often used, particularly in instances of *Helicobacter*-induced disease. Antibiotics are prescribed to treat the underlying infection, and acid suppression is given to speed ulcer healing and promote the relief of symptoms.

Limiting Precipitants (1–8,11,12,16,17,19,22,30)

Avoidance of Agents Injurious to the Mucosal Barrier

Any program to speed healing, limit recurrences, and prevent complications must address both the short-term and prolonged use of agents injurious to the mucosal barrier.

Aspirin and NSAIDs. If possible, these drugs should be avoided because they greatly increase risk and refractoriness to therapy. Using *enteric-coated* and *prodrug* NSAID formulations and taking them with meals might mitigate superficial erosive injury but do little to prevent the deep ulcers that ensue with long-term use of these potent prostaglandin inhibitors. Prescribing a proton-pump inhibitor (e.g., omeprazole, lansoprazole) in conjunction with NSAID use can markedly reduce the

risk of ulcer disease (see later discussion) but drives up cost and involves taking additional medication.

COX-2 inhibitor use has been another popular approach to NSAID therapy in persons with gastrointestinal (GI) intolerance to nonselective NSAIDS or a history of peptic ulcer disease. The risks of peptic ulceration and GI bleeding are markedly reduced; however, emerging evidence of significant cardiovascular risk with the long-term use (>18 months) of rofecoxib has led to its recall and concern about use of other drugs in this class. Whether the adverse cardiovascular effects seen with rofecoxib (which is the most COX-2 selective of the COX-2 agents) are unique to it or a class effect remains to be determined (see also Chapter 156).

Alcohol and Steroids. Although it is not an independent risk factor, *alcohol* should probably be restricted because it may impair healing and cause complications. *Glucocorticosteroids* may exacerbate the chance of an ulcer developing in the context of NSAID therapy but pose little direct risk, and a concurrent prophylactic regimen is not required unless other risk factors are present or large doses (e.g., >30 mg/d of prednisone) are going to be used for prolonged periods.

Alleviating Emotional Stress

Persons with difficult home or work situations may benefit from counseling. Treatment begins with a careful history that elicits pertinent psychosocial information. The very act of discussing these issues and the opportunity to ventilate one's feelings to a supportive listener may lessen tension and help to point the way to solutions. A brief course of minor tranquilizer therapy is sometimes helpful in augmenting supportive psychotherapy and enabling the patient to cope with the combination of stress and illness (see Chapter 226). Before the days of cost containment, very stressed patients were hospitalized to facilitate ulcer healing; however, only stays greater than 4 weeks were shown to be effective.

Smoking Cessation

Smoking impedes the healing of peptic ulcers and may interfere with the action of histamine$_2$ (H$_2$)-receptor antagonists (gastric ulcer patients who continue to smoke have blunted responses to cimetidine therapy). Cessation should be urged during recovery from an ulcer. Although the role of smoking as a causative factor in ulcer disease is less well established, there is ample medical justification for advising its discontinuation (see Chapter 54).

Dietary Measures

Contrary to common belief, evidence is lacking that any particular dietary manipulation promotes healing or reduces acidity. The one exception is the avoidance of eating before bedtime, which reduces nocturnal and postprandial stimuli to acid secretion. Otherwise, bland diets, frequent feedings, small feedings, and avoidance of spices, fruit juices, and acidic foods have never been shown to affect the course of ulcer disease. Milk is also without specific benefit; in fact, its high content of protein and calcium stimulates gastric acid secretion. Some patients claim that certain foods "disagree" with them; these can be avoided, but not for the sake of altering acid production. The intake of *coffee* (including decaffeinated forms) and other caffeinated beverages should be limited but need not be eliminated entirely; their link with ulcer disease is not especially strong.

Eradicating *Helicobacter* Infection (13,21,23,28,30–41)

The eradication of *Helicobacter* infection is critical to the effective treatment of peptic ulcer disease in infected persons. Antibiotic therapy promotes ulcer healing, prevents relapse, and reduces the need for long-term acid suppression/inhibition therapy. Combination antibiotic programs are required because of the high frequency of antibiotic resistance to single agents. There has always been a high frequency of resistance to metronidazole, but more recently, resistance to clarithromycin (especially in persons with prior repeated exposure to macrolide antibiotics) has become increasingly responsible for treatment failures (see later discussion). Acid suppression is also necessary because gastric acidity limits the efficacy of some antibiotics needed for eradication. The list of regimens that meet the minimum criteria for approval continues to grow (see Table 68.1).

Drugs and Drug Regimens

Most FDA-approved programs are triple-drug regimens composed of two antibiotics and an antisecretory agent. The principal antibiotics used in first-line therapy programs include *amoxicillin, clarithromycin, metronidazole tetracycline*, and *bismuth. Proton-pump inhibitors* (PPIs) and *ranitidine bismuth citrate* are used for acid suppression. The most commonly prescribed regimens (e.g., *PPI/amoxicillin/clarithromycin, PPI/ amoxicillin/metronidazole*, and *PPI/clarithromycin/metronidazole*) are of equivalent efficacy (approximately 80% cure rates on an intention-to-treat basis). Treatment is for 7 to 14 days. Meta-analysis found that 7-day triple-drug regimens achieved 95% of the eradication rate of 14-day regimens.

Antibiotic resistance is a growing concern. Antibiotic resistance is increased in persons with prior exposure to macrolide or nitroimidazole antibiotics. Resistance to clarithromycin is found in about 10% of isolates and is increasing. The A2143G point mutation appears to confer most of the resistance to standard clarithromycin-based regimens. About 20% to 30% of *H. pylori* isolates are resistant to metronidazole. There is little primary resistance to amoxicillin or tetracycline. Increasing the duration of treatment from 7 to 14 days increases the cure rate by 5% to 10%, as does increasing the daily dose of clarithromycin from 1.0 to 1.5 g/d.

Sequential therapy offers one approach to overcoming clarithromycin resistance. The rationale is based on evidence that cell-wall efflux channels in resistant organisms help to remove clarithromycin and that giving amoxicillin before clarithromycin allows attack of the cell wall prior to administration of clarithromycin. Initial study confirmed the enhanced efficacy of a sequential approach *(e.g., PPI/amoxicillin for 5 days, followed by PPI/clarithromycin/metronidazole for 5 days)*, which achieved a 15% improvement in cure rates compared to standard therapy when used as initial therapy in settings in which clarithromycin resistance was prevalent. Cure rates approached 90% with very few dropouts and minimal side effects. Sequential therapy appears to be very promising, but more confirmatory study is needed before this program can be recommended as the standard approach to treatment. In the future, testing for the A2143G mutation may help to inform the selection of an antibiotic regimen.

For the acid-suppression component of the program, all proton-pump inhibitors appear to be equally effective. Comparable results have been obtained with *bismuth ranitidine citrate*–based regimens, and they appear to be less affected by antibiotic resistance. The most affordable but least convenient program entails the use of *bismuth subsalicylate*

TABLE 68.1

U.S. FOOD AND DRUG ADMINISTRATION–APPROVED TREATMENT OPTIONS FOR *Helicobacter Pylori* ERADICATION (see text above for preferred regimens)

Omeprazole (40 mg daily) plus clarithromycin (500 mg three times daily) for 2 wk, then omeprazole (20 mg daily) for 2 wk

Omeprazole (20 mg twice daily) plus clarithromycin (500 mg twice daily) plus amoxicillin (1 g twice daily) for 10 d

Lansoprazole (30 mg twice daily) plus clarithromycin (500 mg twice daily) plus amoxicillin (1 g twice daily) for 10 d

Lansoprazole (30 mg twice daily) plus amoxicillin (1 g twice daily) plus clarithromycin (500 mg three times daily) for 10 d

Lansoprazole (30 mg three times daily) plus amoxicillin (1 g three times daily) for 2 wk[a]

Esomeprazole (40 mg daily) plus clarithromycin (500 mg twice daily) plus amoxicillin (1 g twice daily) for 10 d

Ranitidine bismuth citrate (400 mg twice daily) plus clarithromycin (500 mg three times daily) for 2 wk, then ranitidine bismuth citrate (400 mg twice daily) for 2 wk

Ranitidine bismuth citrate (400 mg twice daily) plus clarithromycin (500 mg twice daily) for 2 wk, then ranitidine bismuth citrate (400 mg twice daily) for 2 wk

Bismuth subsalicylate (525 mg four times daily) plus metronidazole (250 mg four times daily) plus tetracycline (500 mg four times daily)[b] for 2 wk plus histamine$_2$-receptor antagonist therapy as directed for 4 wk

---

[a]This dual-therapy regimen has restrictive labeling. It is indicated for patients who are either allergic to or intolerant of clarithromycin or for infections with known or suspected resistance to clarithromycin.

[b]Although it is not approved by the Food and Drug Administration for this indication, amoxicillin has been substituted for tetracycline in patients for whom tetracycline is not recommended.

From Suerbaum S, Michetti P. *Helicobacter pylori* infection. N Engl J Med 2002;347:1175, with permission.

(Pepto-Bismol), *tetracycline, and metronidazole* in conjunction with *ranitidine*. A lack of compliance (multiple daily doses are required) and antibiotic-induced diarrhea are common problems with this regimen and limit its efficacy. For persons who fail the first course of therapy, an empiric approach to retreatment is a four-drug regimen, consisting of a PPI (or ranitidine) plus a bismuth-based, three-drug program with high-dose metronidazole. Another is a three-drug, PPI-based program that avoids the use of metronidazole or clarithromycin if it was used in the first treatment cycle.

Cost-Effectiveness

The efficacy, safety, and low cost of antibiotic therapy have made the eradication of *Helicobacter* infection the mainstay of cost-effective management for peptic ulcer disease; antibiotic therapy usually obviates the need for the long-term or recurrent use of expensive acid-suppression therapy. Even with the cost of endoscopy figured in, antibiotic treatment for *Helicobacter* is a far more cost-effective approach to peptic ulcer disease than is maintenance acid suppression. Cost-effectiveness data strongly favor the treatment of *Helicobacter* over traditional acid-suppression therapy. Once infection is eradicated, the rate of recurrence falls not only dramatically but also often permanently.

The finding that 7-day, triple-drug regimens achieve up to 95% of the *Helicobacter* eradication rates of 14-day regimens suggests that it might be more cost-effective to treat most patients for 7 days and reserve 14-day programs for severe cases and those that prove refractory; prospective trials are needed to test this hypothesis. The sequential 10-day program (in which clarithromycin is given only for the last 5 days) also offers a potentially cost-effective alternative.

Neutralizing and Suppressing Gastric Acid (42–57)

Options include H_2-blockers and proton-pump inhibitors. Antacids used to be a mainstay of therapy but have been largely supplanted by nonprescription and generic forms of H_2-blockers and proton-pump inhibitors.

Histamine$_2$-Receptor Antagonists

These drugs block the H_2-receptors of parietal cells, resulting in a 50% to 80% reduction in basal, postprandial, and vagally stimulated acid production. The available preparations include cimetidine, ranitidine, famotidine, and nizatidine; cimetidine and ranitidine are widely available without prescription. Despite advertising claims of major differences among these agents, they are remarkably similar in efficacy. No clinically significant differences have been found in rates of ulcer healing or prevention of relapse. About 75% of duodenal ulcers are healed by 4 weeks and 84% to 97% by 8 weeks; 55% to 65% of gastric ulcers are healed by 4 weeks and 80% to 90% by 8 weeks. Recurrence rates after the completion of therapy range from 45% to 70% at 3 months to 75% to 90% at 1 year and are no different from those noted with other treatments. Rarely is maintenance therapy necessary if *Helicobacter* infection has been eradicated. The cost of treatment is low with the use of generic and over-the-counter formulations of cimetidine and ranitidine. When prescribed in therapeutic doses, these agents are similar in efficacy and very well tolerated. All are effective in twice-daily dosing regimens.

Adverse Effects. These drugs are very well tolerated; adverse effects are usually mild and occur in less than 1% of patients. Frequency and severity are usually of concern only with their use in the elderly (e.g., *confusion*) or at very high doses (e.g., *gynecomastia* with cimetidine). *Drug–drug interactions* are more common, especially with cimetidine due to *inhibition of hepatic microsomal enzymes* even at lower doses, necessitating caution and dose adjustment in persons taking hepatically metabolized or excreted drugs (e.g., warfarin, benzodiazepines, phenytoin, theophylline compounds, carbamazepine, propranolol). The effect can last for up to 2 weeks after discontinuation. The absorption of ketoconazole may be impaired. These agents do cross the placenta and are present in breast milk.

Cost-Effectiveness. In most instances, the use of generic H_2-blocker therapy (e.g., cimetidine or ranitidine) can achieve effective ulcer healing at a fraction of the cost of PPI therapy (even generic formulations); it should be considered when affordability is of paramount concern and essential to compliance. Although efficacy in controlled studies is less than that for PPI therapy, the difference is often clinically insignificant in uncomplicated cases.

Proton-Pump Inhibitors

The gastric H^+/K^+-ATPase ("proton pump") inhibitors are the most potent of the acid-inhibiting drugs, reducing 24-hour acid production by more than 90% with a single daily dose and effectively halting food-stimulated acid production when taken before a major meal. In comparison, standard doses of H_2-blockers reduce acid production by 50% to 80%. With higher PPI doses, acid production is almost completely stopped. The speed of ulcer healing and pain reduction (40% to 80% at 2 weeks and 80% to 95% at 4 weeks) is greater with these agents than with standard doses of H_2-blockers. Ulcers refractory to high doses of H_2-blockers can be healed by PPI therapy. However, in the absence of eradicating *H. pylori* infection, rates of relapse are similar to those with other forms of acid-suppression therapy. Of interest, these agents appear to have some antibacterial effect on *Helicobacter* and are useful in regimens used to eradicate *Helicobacter* infection (see prior discussion). The PPIs are the drugs of choice for *Zollinger–Ellison syndrome*. When used in conjunction with nonselective NSAIDs, they can reduce the risk of ulcer formation (see later discussion).

Adverse Effects. Side effects are infrequent and mild (e.g., gastrointestinal upset). Overall, these agents are well tolerated. *Drug–drug interactions* are possible due to microsomal displacement and potentiation of hepatically metabolized drugs (e.g., benzodiazepines, phenytoin, and warfarin); careful monitoring and dose adjustment are indicated. They can also increase the absorption of digoxin and decrease prednisone efficacy. Lansoprazole increases the clearance of theophylline.

Hypergastrinemia may ensue with long-term use; in rats, hyperplasia of enterochromaffin cells and development of carcinoid tumors have been observed at high PPI doses. No such tumors have been observed with prolong PPI use in humans (see Chapter 61). Moreover, there is no reported increase in colorectal cancer associated with hypergastrinemia. Although PPI therapy per se does not appear to increase the cancer risk, there is concern about its contribution in the setting of *Helicobacter* infection. *Atrophic gastritis* and *bacterial* overgrowth seen in the context of high-dose, long-term PPI therapy may exacerbate the risk of gastric cancer in persons with *H. pylori* infection. All persons requiring long-term, high-dose PPI therapy should be tested and treated for *H. pylori* infection (see Chapter 61).

Concern has arisen over the potential of PPI therapy to reduce calcium absorption by virtue of its inhibition of acid production, which is necessary for solubilizing calcium salts and calcium absorption. Observational study suggests a modest increase in the risk of hip fracture (odds ratio, 1.44) that is dose and duration dependent. To minimize risk, it might be reasonable to prescribe the lowest PPI dose possible for the shortest period of time and recommend increased dietary low-fat dairy products (high in calcium), the intake of calcium supplements with meals (improves absorption), the use of vitamin D supplements (800 IU/day; enhances calcium absorption), and the consideration of citrated calcium for supplement use (requires less acid for absorption). Long-term acid suppression might also reduce *vitamin B$_{12}$ absorption*; serum levels should be monitored yearly.

The marked PPI reduction in gastric acidity (a protective factor against bacterial infection) has raised concerns about an increased *susceptibility to infection*. Increases in the risk of *community-acquired pneumonia* and *community-acquired Clostridium difficile infection* have been documented. The amount of risk conferred appears to be small (4% to 5%).

Cost-Effective Prescribing. Despite marketing blitzes to the public, there is no benefit to brand-name formulations of PPIs or H$_2$-blockers compared with generics; slightly modified brand-name preparations (e.g., esomeprazole [Nexium]) are no more effective than generic racemic ones (e.g., omeprazole). When a generic H$_2$-blocker might suffice, it can be used in preference to PPI therapy, but for severe or refractory disease, generic PPI therapy is likely to give better results. The increasing availability of generic formulations (e.g., omeprazole, ranitidine) makes possible major cost savings that can be passed on to patients. Over-the-counter brand-name formulations of these drugs are available; cost to the patient may be higher than generic prescription formulations; comparison shopping should be advised.

Prostaglandin Analogues (Misoprostol)

Misoprostol, a prostaglandin analogue, counters the prostaglandin inhibition associated with NSAID use. The drug reduces the risk for ulcer formation associated with NSAID therapy and prevents the recurrence of NSAID-induced gastric ulceration and bleeding. Although more effective than placebo, misoprostol is less effective than H$_2$-blockers or PPIs for the treatment of non-NSAID–induced peptic ulcers and not as well tolerated (see later discussion). Its major contribution is toward the prevention and treatment of *NSAID-induced* peptic ulcers, offering protection against gastric ulceration and its complications among long-term NSAID users (see later discussion) and achieving full healing in more than 70% of NSAID-induced ulcers at 8 weeks.

Adverse Effects. The most common and bothersome side effects are *nausea* and *diarrhea*, which are common at full therapeutic doses. Taking the drug with meals and decreasing the dose can help to limit GI upset. The drug is an *abortifacient* and contraindicated in women who are pregnant; use of an alternative agent should be considered in sexually active women of childbearing age.

Cost-Effective Use. The drug is very expensive and less effective than PPI therapy for the healing of non-NSAID–induced

ulcers. Evidence for its efficacy in preventing GI complications of long-term NSAID therapy is stronger for this drug than for PPI therapy (due largely to a dearth of PPI data), making this an expensive but effective option for the prophylaxis of NSAID-induced disease in high-risk patients (see later discussion).

Antacids

Because they are reasonably effective, inexpensive, and safe, antacids remain a treatment option. When taken in four-times-daily regimens, antacids have been shown endoscopically to be more effective than placebo and comparable with H$_2$-blockers and sucralfate in promoting the healing of duodenal ulcers. Their effectiveness in gastric ulcer disease and in preventing recurrences of gastric and duodenal ulcers is less well established. These agents are no more effective than placebo for the relief of pain from duodenal ulcer, although they are better than placebo for symptoms attributable to gastric ulcer. Substantial doses and proper timing are required, especially for the healing of duodenal ulcers.

Preparations, Doses, and Timing. The preferred preparations are those containing magnesium hydroxide, aluminum hydroxide, or a combination of the two. Calcium carbonate antacids (e.g., Tums, Rolaids) have considerable acid-neutralizing capacity and are inexpensive, convenient, and well tolerated; concern about rebound acid hypersecretion was never confirmed to be clinically important.

About 140 mEq at a time is necessary to bring the gastric pH into the range of 3.5 to 5.0. Typical 30-mL doses of many popular antacids provide only 60 mEq. If given with a meal, the antacid is wasted because food is a perfectly adequate buffer. When an antacid is given 1 hour after eating, gastric acidity is minimized for another 1 to 2 hours, countering the food-induced stimulation of acid secretion. A second dose 3 hours after a meal provides another hour of acid neutralization and tides the patient over to the next meal.

Adverse Effects and Drug Interactions. *Diarrhea* is common and a result of the cathartic effect of insoluble magnesium salts; alternating with an aluminum hydroxide antacid can help. *Phosphate depletion* is possible in patients using an aluminum-containing antacid; insoluble aluminum phosphate forms. In renal failure, hypercalcemia, hypermagnesemia, and excess accumulation of aluminum are possible due to an inability to excrete the small amounts that may get absorbed with the use of antacid preparations. Excess sodium absorption may occur with the use of sodium-containing antacids. The absorption of warfarin and L-dopa increase and that of H$_2$-blockers, phenothiazines, sulfonamides, isoniazid, and penicillin decrease, making separation of medication intake and antacid use advisable. Potent antacids can cause the premature release of aspirin from enteric-coated tablets when they are taken simultaneously.

Cost-Effectiveness and Convenience. Although antacids are safe, effective, and low in cost per dose, their cost and inconvenience can mount when they must be taken multiple times a day in large amounts. Trying to achieve adequate acid neutralization with antacid tablets alone can become difficult; at least eight tablets must be taken just to obtain 140 mEq of acid-neutralizing capacity. For the treatment of gastric ulcer, acid neutralization is less of an issue, and much smaller doses may suffice (e.g., two to three extra-strength tablets of an aluminum-containing antacid).

Anticholinergic Agents

Anticholinergic therapy can suppress the parasympathetic muscarinic activity that triggers gastric acid secretion, especially the nocturnal surge. These agents are not nearly as potent as H_2-receptor antagonists in suppressing acid production. The frequency and severity of anticholinergic side effects make therapy intolerable for many patients. Because more effective and better tolerated therapies are available, anticholinergics are now rarely prescribed.

Protecting the Mucosa (58)

Sucralfate

Sucralfate, an aluminum hydroxide/sulfated sucrose formulation, acts locally to form a presumably cytoprotective coating over the injured mucosa, perhaps also absorbing pepsin and binding bile acids. It has no acid-neutralizing activity per se (making it useful in intensive care unit settings in which neutralizing gastric acid increases the risks of gastric bacterial overgrowth and pneumonia) and little is absorbed (although aluminum salts are released and some aluminum is absorbed). It is comparable with H_2-receptor blockers in the healing of duodenal ulcers of all etiologies and in the healing of non-NSAID–related gastric ulcers; it is slightly less effective than H_2-blockers for preventing recurrences and has no proven benefit in the treatment or prevention of NSAID-related gastric ulcers. It is commonly used to help *facilitate ulcer healing* in persons with large ulcers, especially those that are slow to heal. Disadvantages include high cost, need for frequent dosing (usually four times daily, although twice-daily, double-dose programs can be used), and gastrointestinal upset. The claim that sucralfate preferentially heals ulcers in smokers has not been substantiated. Sucralfate is most effective when taken 1 hour before meals and at bedtime, although twice-daily administration of double-strength doses has been found to be adequate for the treatment of duodenal ulcer.

Adverse Effects. The most bothersome side effect is *constipation*. Sucralfate may also interfere with the gastrointestinal *absorption* of *tetracycline*, *fluoroquinolone* antibiotics (e.g., ciprofloxacin, norfloxacin), *digoxin*, *phenytoin*, and, to a clinically insignificant degree, H_2-blockers. No data are available regarding safety in patients who are pregnant, nursing, or of advanced age. The drug binds phosphate and has been reported to cause *hypophosphatemia* and *aluminum toxicity* in patients with chronic renal failure.

Cost-Effective Use. The cost is about the same as that of brand-name formulations of PPIs, and efficacy is comparable to that of H_2-blockers, which argue on a cost-effectiveness basis for a supplementary rather than a primary role for sucralfate in the outpatient management of peptic ulcer disease.

Antacids

There is some speculation that the "coating effect" of antacids may account for some of the symptomatic relief associated with their use (see prior discussion).

Prevention (40,59–66)

Although the eradication of *H. pylori* infection has greatly reduced the need for chronic acid suppression, prophylaxis remains an important consideration in the large number of persons requiring long-term NSAID therapy.

Prevention of NSAID-Induced Ulcer Disease and Its Complications

The prevalence and severity of NSAID-induced peptic ulcer disease and its complications, such as GI bleeding, necessitate attention to prevention. Several approaches to prophylaxis have been suggested, including the use of nonselective NSAIDs that disproportionately inhibit COX-2, a switch to a selective *COX-2 inhibitor*, and the concurrent use of a *PPI, misoprostol,* or an *H_2-blocker*. Adding a PPI twice daily to a nonselective NSAID significantly reduces the rates of ulcers and complications, achieving about the same degree of reduction as switching to a COX-2 agent; however, substantial risk remains. Adding a PPI twice daily to COX-2 therapy further reduces the risk but does not eliminate it entirely, especially in persons with prior NSAID-induced ulcer bleeding. Concurrent therapy with a PPI appears to be superior to adding an H_2-blocker or misoprostol. *Sucralfate* does not protect against NSAID-induced disease.

Besides an inability fully to reduce risk, there are a number of additional shortcomings for these prophylactic measures, including the cardiovascular risk associated with COX-2 agents (see Chapter 156), the GI upset associated with misoprostol use, and the loss of COX-2 semiselectivity with increasing doses of non–COX-2 NSAIDS that preferentially block COX-2 at low doses (e.g., nabumetone [Relafen] and etodolac [Lodine]); only meloxicam (Mobic) remains relatively COX-2 selective at full doses. The best way to avoid NSAID-induced ulcer risk is to avoid unnecessary NSAID therapy (see Chapter 157).

Prevention of Recurrence and Relapse

The standard duration for an initial acid suppression regimen is 4 weeks to achieve full healing in 90% of patients. Up to 12 weeks of such treatment may be necessary for very large benign ulcers. The eradication of *Helicobacter* infection is essential; it reduces relapse and recurrence rates by more than 90% in infected persons and eliminates the need for chronic acid-suppression therapy. However, without the eradication of *H. pylori* infection, the risk for ulcer recurrence within 1 year is greater than 50%. Using 2 weeks of triple antibiotic therapy compared with 1 week of treatment improves outcomes by 10%. The resolution of pain cannot be used as a therapeutic endpoint because the cessation of pain correlates poorly with the completion of healing or the eradication of infection. Unfortunately, patients commonly terminate treatment when their symptoms resolve, which increases their risk for relapse.

Follow-Up (23–26)

Monitoring Response: Gastric Ulcer

If a *gastric* lesion has been detected initially by radiography and has all the hallmarks of a benign lesion (see prior discussion), if symptoms resolve fully, and if no clinical findings suggestive of cancer or complicated disease are present (see prior discussion), then follow-up barium study or endoscopy can probably be foregone. Although some authorities advocate routine endoscopic or radiologic *documentation of healing*, no studies show this to be cost-effective in uncomplicated cases in which symptoms resolve within 4 to 6 weeks and do not recur. However, if a refractory gastric ulcer is suspected (e.g., persistent pain after 8 weeks despite a full medical regimen), then *endoscopic examination* and *biopsy* are needed, especially in patients older than age 40 years, who are at an increased risk for gastric cancer. Barium study is not sufficient because even malignant ulcers may shrink in size in response to therapy. Earlier endoscopic evaluation is indicated if evidence of bleeding or obstruction or another reason for concern about gastric carcinoma is present (see prior discussion).

Monitoring Response: Duodenal Ulcer

In the case of a *duodenal* ulcer (in which cancer risk is nil), follow-up radiologic or endoscopic evaluation should be restricted to patients with the persistence or recurrence of pain, symptoms of gastric outlet obstruction, or evidence of bleeding. Periodic repetition of studies is unnecessary and expensive, even when typical symptoms recur, unless a different course of therapy, such as surgery, is contemplated. Following the results of stool guaiac tests and blood cell counts can help to detect bleeding, as can careful questioning of the patient.

Refractory or Recurrent Disease (23–25,28,41,67,68)

The persistence of pain 4 weeks after the initiation of proper therapy suggests an unhealed ulcer. If endoscopic evaluation was carried out initially to rule out a malignant lesion and a large ulcer was found, then acid-suppression therapy can be continued, with high-dose PPI therapy used to speed healing. Eight to 12 weeks of treatment may be necessary. If *H. pylori* infection was not tested for and treated initially, then this should be done at this time. If testing was performed initially and the test-positive patient complied fully with the anti-*Helicobacter* treatment regimen and is a nonsmoker (smoking doubles the treatment failure rate), then testing for the eradication of infection can help to guide further action. If, despite the eradication of *Helicobacter* infection, symptoms persist beyond 4 to 8 weeks, then endoscopic evaluation is needed (if it was not performed initially) to rule out malignancy or complicated disease. Recurrent disease raises the question of resistant *Helicobacter* infection, repeated NSAID exposure, Zollinger–Ellison syndrome, and malignancy.

Testing for and Treating Persistent *Helicobacter* Infection

Testing. The potential contribution of *Helicobacter* infection to persistent or recurrent disease necessitates testing for active infection. *Serologic testing* for the persistence of *H. pylori* infection is problematic because even with the full eradication of infection, antibody titers usually decline slowly over time. Seroconversion from positive to negative is highly specific but not sensitive. Much more sensitive noninvasive options are the *stool antigen test* and the ^{14}C or ^{13}C *breath test* (see prior discussion). If these tests are unavailable and concern persists, endoscopic evaluation can be performed, with biopsy, CLO testing, and drug-sensitivity determinations performed. Several weeks should be allowed to elapse after treatment before testing for eradication.

Treating. The optimal approach to *Helicobacter* treatment failure has not yet been defined, but a number of options are available based on the high probability of antibiotic resistance when noncompliance and smoking have been ruled out. Resistance to metronidazole is well established; resistance to clar-

ithromycin (mediated by the A2143G mutation) is becoming increasingly prevalent (especially where exposure to macrolide antibiotics is high).

If drug-sensitivity data are available, the new regimen can be customized accordingly. In most instances, antibiotic sensitivity data are not available, and an empiric approach is required. A number of second-line regimens have been proposed, all to be taken for 10 to 14 days. Because resistance to metronidazole and/or clarithromycin is common, either agent might best be avoided in the new antibiotic program if it was contained in the original one; one should also avoid less effective agents such as amoxicillin and tetracycline. One recommended program is to repeat the first-line regimen, substituting a new first-line drug for the likely resisted one. Another is a bismuth-based, triple-drug regimen *that includes high-dose metronidazole supplemented by a PPI or H$_2$-blocker*. Although not validated for use in initial treatment failure, a course of sequential therapy might provide a means of overcoming macrolide resistance (see earlier discussion).

Checking for Noncompliance and Aggravating Factors

In addition to checking for *Helicobacter*, it is crucial to check for noncompliance and aggravating factors such as *smoking*, *stress*, and the use of nonprescription *NSAIDs* or *aspirin*. Many instances of refractory disease and recurrence are closely linked to these factors.

Strengthening the Acid-Suppression Regimen

When an ulcer is slow to heal, it may be worthwhile to increase the dose of acid-suppression therapy or switch to a more potent agent. Patients who genuinely fail H$_2$-blocker treatment may achieve a more rapid and complete response with PPI therapy, but it is more important to eradicate *Helicobacter* infection (see prior discussion) and check for malignancy and Zollinger–Ellison syndrome (see the following discussion).

Assessing for Malignancy and Zollinger–Ellison Syndrome

Truly refractory cases (i.e., those in which *Helicobacter* infection, aggravating factors, and noncompliance have been addressed) should be evaluated endoscopically for malignancy and studied biochemically for *Zollinger–Ellison syndrome*, especially if multiple ulcers, occurrences in unusual places, marked abdominal pain, or a secretory diarrhea (resulting from hypergastrinemia) is present. Patients with Zollinger–Ellison syndrome often manifest evidence of *multiple endocrine adenomatosis* (e.g., concurrent hyperparathyroidism and pituitary adenomas). A fasting serum *gastrin* level greater than 500 pg/mL in the presence of acid hypersecretion is diagnostic.

Surgery

With advances in medical therapy, surgery for peptic ulcer disease is becoming increasingly rare. The most compelling *indications for surgery* include brisk bleeding of 6 to 8 U of blood in 24 hours (see Chapter 63), recurrent episodes of bleeding, perforation, gastric outlet obstruction refractory to medical therapy, and failure of a benign gastric ulcer to heal after 15 weeks. Operations are most often performed on patients who fail to respond to medical therapy and have disabling symptoms.

For Duodenal Ulcer Disease. The *proximal gastric vagotomy* effectively limits recurrences without producing the disabling side effects associated with earlier forms of surgery for duodenal ulcer disease. The operation involves selective severing of the nerve supply to the acid-secreting fundus; the nerves to the antrum are left intact, so control of gastric emptying is preserved. The incidence of ulcer recurrences is slightly higher (10%) than with vagotomy and antrectomy (5%) but similar to that with vagotomy and pyloroplasty (12%). Surgical mortality is lower, and such potentially disabling postsurgical side effects as the dumping syndrome and diarrhea are much less common. Because the operation is technically demanding, it should be considered only by surgeons specifically trained to perform it. The procedure should not be carried out in patients with delayed gastric emptying.

For Gastric Ulcer Disease. The procedure of choice for gastric ulcer is *distal gastrectomy* with excision of the ulcer.

PATIENT EDUCATION

Enlisting the patient's active involvement and overcoming much of the mythology surrounding ulcer disease are prime objectives of the patient education effort.

Basic Advice on Diet and Aggravating Factors

Patients appreciate dietary instruction, such as knowing what foods they can eat and what substances to avoid. Many ulcer patients unnecessarily put themselves on a "bland diet" and increase their intake of milk products, hoping that these actions will help their ulcers to heal. Others take aspirin or over-the-counter NSAIDs for the relief of ulcer pain. The use of coffee, alcohol, and tobacco also needs to be reviewed. Many physicians insist that coffee drinking be stopped, although this may cause more difficulty than is warranted by its role in pathogenesis. Switching to decaffeinated coffee offers little advantage. On the other hand, the cessation of smoking is essential, and detailed cessation counseling is critical (see Chapter 54) because continuation of the habit greatly impedes healing. Alcohol intake should also be discouraged.

Maximizing Compliance

Even when an effective medical program has been designed, inadequate compliance can be a problem. Full compliance with the multidrug antibiotic regimens used to treat *Helicobacter* infection can be especially problematic, particularly when a 2-week, thrice-daily or four-times-daily dosing regimen is required. The more expensive twice-daily regimens may be worth the extra initial expense for patients whose ability fully to comply is questionable. Alternatively, a 1-week, thrice-daily program can be considered, which is almost as effective.

Other common compliance errors that need to be addressed include stopping medication as soon as symptoms disappear, taking antacids with meals (which wastes the antacid), and taking cimetidine at the same time as antacids (which partially impairs cimetidine absorption).

Counseling

The patient with marked situational stress contributing to the ulcer problem often benefits from counseling; however, any suggestion to change jobs or family situations because of an ulcer is like to be counterproductive. There is no evidence that such extreme solutions contribute to healing, and they may actually heighten stress. One useful supplement to counseling is teaching simple *relaxation techniques*; these are especially useful for patients bothered by multiple somatic manifestations of stress (see Chapter 226).

Self-Monitoring

The patient needs to be taught to watch for complications of ulcer disease. In particular, the manifestations of gastrointestinal bleeding (see Chapter 63) should be well understood so that the patient does not delay in seeking help.

Shared Decision Making

If the question of elective surgery arises, the patient should be made a full partner in the decision because few definite guidelines for operation are available. A value judgment is necessary, and the costs and benefits of surgery versus continued medical therapy need to be discussed.

INDICATIONS FOR REFERRAL AND ADMISSION

Refractoriness to therapy is an indication for referral to a gastroenterologist for review of the program and consideration of endoscopy. Admission is mandatory when symptoms of *hemorrhage*, *peritoneal irritation*, *or gastric outlet obstruction* are present; both surgeon and gastroenterologist need to be consulted.

A most difficult issue is when and whom to select for *elective surgery*. Much has to do with the patient's preferences; gross generalizations are meaningless. Clearly, those with recurrent major bleeds, gastric outlet obstruction, or evidence of malignancy need to be seen by the surgeon. Seventy-five percent of patients with intractable pain obtain relief when treated surgically, but subgroups with alcohol abuse, character disorders, or severe neuroses do poorly after surgery. The decision to resort to elective surgery for recurrent disease should be made in conjunction with the patient, and the small risk for operative mortality and the morbidity of postgastrectomy syndrome should be weighed against the morbidity and cost of recurrent pain, time lost from work, and the need for long-term drug therapy.

THERAPEUTIC RECOMMENDATIONS (69)

Nonpharmacologic Interventions and Initial Testing

- Avoid, or at least limit to the extent medically possible, the use of agents potentially injurious to the mucosa, including aspirin, excess alcohol, NSAIDs, and perhaps long-term, high-dose glucocorticosteroids.
- Insist on the total cessation of smoking (see Chapter 54).

- Suggest a decreased intake of coffee (including decaffeinated forms) and other caffeine-containing beverages; however, complete cessation of intake is unnecessary.
- Do not restrict any foods or insist on a bland or milk-laden diet. Frequent small feedings are unnecessary, and a bedtime snack may stimulate nocturnal acid secretion. The patient should avoid only foods that cause discomfort.
- Attend to stress-related issues, but avoid recommending a major job or geographic change.
- Test for *Helicobacter* infection. For initial noninvasive testing, obtain quantitative serology, and use a reference laboratory; alternatively and if available, order a ^{13}C breath test or stool test for *H. pylori* antigen. If endoscopy is required (see later discussion), have a rapid urease test (e.g., CLO test) performed at the same time.
- Order upper gastrointestinal endoscopy or barium study before initiating therapy if clinical findings suggest malignancy or complicated disease (e.g., the patient manifests weight loss, gastrointestinal bleeding, or persistent nausea and vomiting).

Initial Pharmacologic Therapy

- For ulcer patients who test positive for *H. pylori*, begin a three-drug regimen of a *PPI* (e.g., *omeprazole* 20 to 40 mg twice daily) plus *clarithromycin* (500 mg twice daily) and either *metronidazole* (500 mg twice daily) or *amoxicillin* (1 g twice daily); continue for 1 week for most patients; consider a 2-week course for those with severe disease who are on an amoxicillin-containing program.
- In areas where *Helicobacter* resistance to macrolide antibiotics is high or in patients with multiple prior exposures to macrolide antibiotics, consider *sequential therapy* with 5 days of a *PPI* (omeprazole 20 to 40 mg twice daily) and *amoxicillin* (1 g twice daily), followed by 5 days of *PPI*, plus *clarithromycin* (500 mg twice daily) and *metronidazole* (500 mg twice daily).
- For patients with an NSAID-induced ulcer, begin treatment with either a *PPI* (e.g., 20 to 40 mg of *omeprazole* twice daily) or *misoprostol* (200 mg with each meal and before bed); continue for 4 to 8 weeks, depending on severity at the time of presentation.
- For all patients, continue full acid-suppression therapy for at least 4 weeks, using either a PPI (e.g., 20 to 40 mg of *omeprazole* twice daily or 30 mg of *lansoprazole* daily) or an H$_2$-receptor antagonist (e.g., 400 mg of *cimetidine* twice daily). Base selection on affordability, severity of disease, capacity for compliance, and potential for interaction with other medications.
- Consider addition of *sucralfate* (1 g at 1 hour before each meal and at bedtime) to aid the healing of large, non–NSAID-induced ulcers if the ulcer is large and resolution is slow.

Prophylaxis of NSAID-Induced Disease

- For patients with a prior history of NSAID-induced peptic ulceration or upper gastrointestinal bleeding who absolutely require continuous NSAID therapy for the maintenance of daily functioning (see Chapters 156 and 157):
  - Add a *PPI* (e.g., 20 to 40 mg of omeprazole twice daily); or
  - *Misoprostol* (200 mg with breakfast and supper); or
  - Switch to a *selective COX-2 agent* (e.g., celecoxib 100 mg twice daily) and add PPI therapy; use only after a full assessment of the patient's total cardiovascular risk and full disclosure to the patient of the possible cardiovascular complications of COX-2 therapy.

Refractory or Recurrent Disease

- Check for failure to eradicate *H. pylori* infection, either by biopsy and CLO test if undergoing endoscopy or noninvasively by *stool antigen* testing or *breath test* (if available); alternatively and less ideally, repeat quantitative *serology* and compare pretreatment titers with current titers; consider endoscopic examination and CLO testing, and obtain antibiotic sensitivities if possible.
- For persons testing positive for continued infection, consider:
  - Represcribing a first-line regimen (see Table 68.1), but substitute metronidazole for clarithromycin if metronidazole was used in the original program; substitute clarithromycin if metronidazole was used in the first program; treat for 10 to 14 days; or
  - Starting a bismuth-based, triple-drug regimen (see prior discussion) with high-dose metronidazole (e.g., 500 mg four times daily) plus a PPI or an H$_2$-blocker, or
  - Instituting a course of sequential therapy (see prior discussion).
- Reemphasize the importance of compliance, smoking cessation, and avoidance of NSAIDs.
- Consider prophylactic therapy if the disease is NSAID related (see prior discussion).
- For persistent or recurrent disease unresponsive to treatment, refer for endoscopic examination and biopsy to rule out malignancy and complicated disease, especially if endoscopy was not performed initially.
- Refer the patient with refractory multiple ulcers, frequent recurrences, or associated secretory diarrhea for consideration of Zollinger–Ellison syndrome when symptoms are accompanied by marked hypergastrinemia in the context of acid hypersecretion.
- Admit patients with evidence of bleeding, gastric outlet obstruction, or perforation and obtain surgical consultation.

A.H.G.

Annotated Bibliography

1. Anda RF, Williamson DF, Escobedo LG, et al. Smoking and the risk of peptic ulcer disease among women in the U.S. Arch Intern Med 1990;150:1437. (*The first National Health and Nutrition Examination Survey, finding that the relative risk was 1.8 overall and increased with the amount smoked, and that an estimated 20% of all ulcers in women were a consequence of smoking.*)
2. Bombardier C, Lanine L, Reicin A, et al. Comparison of upper gastrointestinal toxicity of rofecoxib and naproxen in patients with rheumatoid arthritis. N Engl J Med 2000;343:1520. (*The oft-quoted Vioxx GI Outcomes Research [VIGOR] study, finding that gastrointestinal [GI] toxicity was reduced with the long-term use of a cyclooxygenase-2 [COX-2] agent, although there was a suggestion of increased cardiovascular risk.*)
3. Conn HO, Blitzer BL. Nonassociation of adrenocorticosteroid therapy and peptic ulcer. N Engl J Med 1976;294:473. (*The first of two studies examining pooled data, concluding that there is little association between steroids and the risk for ulcer.*)

4. Curatolo PW, Robertson D. The health consequences of caffeine. Ann Intern Med 1983;98:641. (*A thorough review, examining the evidence linking caffeine with ulcer disease and acid secretion; 281 references.*)

5. Friedman DG, Siegelaub AB, Seltzer C. Cigarettes, alcohol, coffee and peptic ulcer. N Engl J Med 1974;290:469. (*There was an increased prevalence of ulcer disease in smokers; coffee consumption and alcohol were not independent predictors of ulcer disease.*)

6. Gabriel SE, Jaakkimainen L, Bombardier C. Risk for serious gastrointestinal complications related to use of nonsteroidal antiinflammatory drugs. Ann Intern Med 1991;115:787. (*The relative risk increased about three times; other risk factors include age >60 years and prior ulcer disease.*)

7. Graham DY, Smith JL. Aspirin and the stomach. Ann Intern Med 1986;104:390. (*An excellent review, emphasizing the differences between acute and chronic effects; 98 references.*)

8. Griffin MR, Piper JM, Daugherty JR, et al. Nonsteroidal antiinflammatory drug use and increased risk for peptic ulcer disease in elderly persons. Ann Intern Med 1991;114:257. (*The risk is substantial and increases with dose.*)

9. Hansson LE, Nyren O, Hsing AW, et al. The risk of stomach cancer in patients with gastric or duodenal ulcer disease. N Engl J Med 1996;335:242. (*A Swedish population study, finding an increased risk in patients with gastric ulcer.*)

10. Huang JQ. H. pylori, NSAID use and risk of peptic ulcer disease: meta-analysis of 5 case–control studies. Am J Gastroenterol 2000;95:A146. (*The risk was increased in the setting of Helicobacter infection.*)

11. Mahl GF. Anxiety, HCl secretion and peptic ulcer etiology. Psychosom Med 1950;12:158. (*A classic study, showing that acute anxiety raises acid secretion.*)

12. Messer J, Reitman D, Sacks HS, et al. Association of adrenocorticosteroid therapy and peptic ulcer disease. N Engl J Med 1983;309:21. (*A secondary analysis of pooled data, finding an increased risk for ulcer disease, although the absolute risk is small.*)

13. Ohkusa T, Fujiki K, Takashimizu I, et al. Improvement in atrophic gastritis and intestinal metaplasia in patients in whom Helicobacter pylori was eradicated. Ann Intern Med 2003;134:380. (*An uncontrolled, prospective trial, observing a reduction in precancerous changes.*)

14. Piper JM, Ray WA, Daugherty MS, et al. Corticosteroid use and peptic ulcer disease: role of nonsteroidal antiinflammatory drugs. Ann Intern Med 1991;114:735. (*Corticosteroid use was associated with an increased risk for ulcer only in the context of concurrent nonsteroidal antiinflammatory drug [NSAID] use.*)

15. Pounder R. Silent peptic ulceration: deadly silence or golden silence? Gastroenterology 1988;96(Suppl):626. (*Symptoms and ulceration are frequently dissociated.*)

16. Rutter M. Psychological factors in short-term prognosis of physical disease. 1. Peptic ulcer. J Psychosom Res 1963;7:45. (*Another classic paper, finding that severe anxiety prolongs recovery and makes relapse more likely.*)

17. Singh G. Recent considerations in nonsteroidal anti-inflammatory drug gastropathy. Am J Med 1998;195:31S. (*Data from the Angiotensin II Receptor Antagonist Micardis in Isolated Systolic hypertension [ARAMIS] study, finding no major difference in the risk of GI toxicity among 12 NSAIDs.*)

18. Sogtag S, Graham DY, Belisto A, et al. Cimetidine, cigarette smoking, and recurrence of duodenal ulcer. N Engl J Med 1984;311:689. (*Smoking is a major factor in the recurrence of duodenal ulcer.*)

19. Sorensen HT, Mellemkjaer L, Blot WJ, et al. Risk of upper gastrointestinal bleeding associated with use of low-dose aspirin. Am J Gastroenterol 2000;95:2218. (*Risk is increased even at the low dose of 75 mg/d.*)

20. Spiro HM. Is the steroid ulcer a myth? N Engl J Med 1983;309:45. (*Editorial examining the contradictory data on this topic.*)

21. Suerbaum S, Michetti P. Helicobacter pylori infection. N Engl J Med 2002;347:1175. (*Definitive review; 107 references.*)

22. Wolfe MM, Lichtenstein DR, Singh G. Gastrointestinal toxicity of nonsteroidal antiinflammatory drugs. N Engl J Med 1999;340:1888. (*A comprehensive review; 113 references.*)

23. Cutler AF, Prasad VM, Santogade P. Four-year trends in Helicobacter pylori IgG serology following successful eradication. Am J Med 1998;105:18. (*Even with the full eradication of infection, antibody titers plateaued and persisted in >70% of cases.*)

24. Cutler AF, Havstad S, Ma CK, et al. Accuracy of invasive and noninvasive tests to diagnose Helicobacter pylori infection. Gastroenterology 1995;109:136. (*The ^{13}C-urea breath test and serology were as accurate as biopsy and the Campylobacter-like organism [CLO] test for diagnosis.*)

25. Dooley CP, Larson AW, Stace NH, et al. Double-contrast barium meal and upper gastrointestinal endoscopy. Ann Intern Med 1984;101:538. (*A randomized study, indicating superior sensitivity and specificity for endoscopy but admitting that a cost–benefit relationship is not established.*)

26. Feldman M, Cryer B, Lee E, et al. Role of seroconversion in confirming cure of Helicobacter pylori infection. JAMA 1998;280:363. (*Seroconversion had a sensitivity of 60% and a specificity of 100%, which suggests its possible usefulness as an initial test for a cure, but many patients with a cure still had detectable antibody.*)

27. Fendick AM, Chernew ME, Hirth RA, et al. Alternative management strategies for patients with suspected peptic ulcer disease. Ann Intern Med 1995;123:260. (*Noninvasive management strategies were more cost-effective than immediate endoscopy.*)

28. Javier P, Gisbert JP, de la Morena F, et al. Accuracy of monoclonal stool antigen test for the diagnosis of H. pylori infection: a systematic review and meta-analysis. Am J Gastroenterol 2006;101:1921. (*The sensitivity and specificity were >95%.*)

29. Wolfe MM. Diagnosis of gastrinoma: much ado about nothing? Ann Intern Med 1989;111:697. (*An editorial suggesting that a screening serum gastrin level might be warranted in patients with duodenal ulcer.*)

30. Buchman E, Kaung DT, Dolank D, et al. Unrestricted diet in treatment of duodenal ulcer. Gastroenterology 1969;56:1016. (*A classic study, finding that dietary restrictions made little or no difference.*)

31. De Francesco V, Margiotta M, Zullo A, et al. Clarithromycin-resistant genotypes and eradication of Helicobacter pylori. Ann Intern Med 2006;144:94. (*A post hoc analysis, finding that a high frequency of the A2143G mutation was responsible for treatment failures and that a sequential treatment program was more effective in eradication than was standard triple therapy.*)

32. Dore MP, Leandro G, Realdi G, et al. Effect of pretreatment antibiotic resistance to metronidazole and clarithromycin on outcome of Helicobacter pylori therapy: a meta-analytic approach. Dig Dis Sci 2000;45:68. (*Cure rates fell by 35% to 50%.*)

33. Fuccio L, Minardi E, Zagari RM, et al. Meta-analysis: duration of first-line proton-pump inhibitor-based therapy for Helicobacter pylori eradication. Ann Intern Med 2007;147:553. (*Seven-day regimens achieved 95% of the eradication rate of 14-day regimens.*)

34. Graham DY, Lew GM, Klein PD, et al. Effect of treatment of Helicobacter pylori infection on the long-term recurrence of gastric and duodenal ulcer. Ann Intern Med 1992;116:705. (*A randomized, controlled trial [RCT], showing that the eradication of the organism can lead to cure.*)

35. Hentschel E, Brandstatter G, Dragosics B, et al. Effect of ranitidine and amoxicillin plus metronidazole on the eradication of Helicobacter pylori and the recurrence of duodenal ulcer. N Engl J Med 1993;328:308. (*RCT, showing that eradication of Helicobacter pylori infection significantly speeds healing and prevents recurrences.*)

36. Howden CW, Hunt RH. Guidelines for the management of Helicobacter pylori infection. Am J Gastroenterol 1998;93:2330. (*Consensus guidelines, but a bit dated.*)

37. Kuipers EJ, Lundell L, Klinkinberg-Knol EC, et al. Atrophic gastritis and Helicobacter pylori infection in patients with reflux esophagitis treated with omeprazole or fundoplication. N Engl J Med 1996;334:1018. (*There was an increased risk for this premalignant gastric change in persons with complete acid suppression and concurrent Helicobacter infection.*)

38. McMahon BJ, Hennessay TW, Bensler JM, et al. The relationship among previous antimicrobial use, antimicrobial resistance, and treatment outcomes for Helicobacter pylori infections. Ann Intern Med 2003;139:463. (*A retrospective cohort study, finding that the previous use of macrolides or metronidazole was associated with a greater risk for failure due to clarithromycin-resistant H. pylori.*)

39. Sonnenberg A, Townsend WF. Costs of duodenal ulcer therapy with antibiotics. Arch Intern Med 1995;155:922. (*A cost-effectiveness analysis, finding that antibiotics plus short-term acid suppression was the most cost-effective by a wide margin.*)

40. Sung SJY, Chung SCS, Ling TKW, et al. Antibacterial treatment of gastric ulcers associated with Helicobacter pylori. N Engl J Med 1995;332:139. (*Early RCT, finding that the recurrence rate at 1 year was 52.3% with omeprazole alone and 4.5% with antibiotics.*)

41. Vaira D, Zullo A, Vakil N, et al. Sequential therapy versus standard triple-drug therapy for Helicobacter pylori eradication. Ann Intern Med 2007;146:556. (*RCT, showing significantly better cure rates for the sequential program.*)

42. Cantu TG, Korek JS. Central nervous system reactions to histamine$_2$-receptor blockers. Ann Intern Med 1991;114:1027. (*All H$_2$-blockers are capable of causing central nervous system effects, not just cimetidine.*)

43. Drake D, Hollander D. Neutralizing capacity and cost-effectiveness of antacids. Ann Intern Med 1981;94:215. (*Excellent reference data on the comparative characteristics of available antacids.*)

44. Hade JE, Spiro HM. Calcium and acid rebound: a reappraisal. J Clin Gastroenterol 1992;15:37. (*A review, with no evidence that the original laboratory findings of acid rebound are clinically significant.*)

45. Hawkey CJ, Karrasch JA, Szczepanski L, et al., for the OMNIUM Study Group. Omeprazole compared with misoprostol for ulcers associated with nonsteroidal antiinflammatory drugs. N Engl J Med 1998;338:727. (*RCT, showing that both agents were effective for healing NSAID-induced injury, but that omeprazole was better tolerated and superior for maintenance therapy.*)

46. Ippolitto A, Elashoff J, Valenzuela J, et al. Recurrent ulcer after successful treatment with cimetidine or antacid. Gastroenterology 1983;85:875. (*Recurrence rates after antacid therapy were 29% at 3 months and 56% at 6 months, compared with 36% and 55%, respectively, after cimetidine.*)

47. Isenberg JI, Peterson WL, Elashoff JD, et al. Healing of benign gastric ulcer with low-dose antacid or cimetidine. N Engl J Med 1983;308:1319. (*Demonstrates the efficacy for both cimetidine and low-dose antacids, although cimetidine was superior.*)

48. Klinkenberg-Knol EC, Nelis F, Dent J. Long-term omeprazole treatment in resistant gastroesophageal reflux disease: efficacy, safety, and influence on gastric mucosa. Gastroenterology 2000;118:661. (*There was no evidence of increased cancer risk.*)

49. Laheij RJ, Sturkenboom HC, Hassing RJ, et al. Risk of community-acquired pneumonia and use of gastric acid-suppressive drugs. JAMA 2004;292:1955. (*Finds an increased risk.*)

50. Lipsy RJ, Fennerty B, Fagan TC. Clinical review of histamine₂-receptor antagonists. Arch Intern Med 1990;150:745. (*A comparison of cimetidine, ranitidine, famotidine, and nizatidine, finding that the differences were subtler than was previously believed; 99 references.*)

51. Peterson WL, Cook DJ. Antisecretory therapy for bleeding peptic ulcer. JAMA 1998;280:877. (*A critical review of the evidence, concluding that proton-pump-inhibitor [PPI] therapy is worthwhile.*)

52. Peterson WL, Sturdevant RA, Frankl HD, et al. Healing of duodenal ulcer with an antacid regimen. N Engl J Med 1977;297:341. (*A classic RCT, documenting the efficacy of high-dose therapy at 1,000 mEq daily, a surprisingly high rate of pain relief by placebo, and a delayed healing in cigarette smokers.*)

53. Steinberg WM, Lewis JH, Katz DM. Antacids inhibit absorption of cimetidine. N Engl J Med 1982;307:400. (*The original U.S. report of this interaction; the degree of inhibition was modest, at 10% to 20%.*)

54. Termanini B, Gibril F, Sutliff VE, et al. Effect of long-term gastric acid suppressive therapy on serum vitamin B12 levels in patients with Zollinger–Ellison syndrome. Am J Med 1998;104:422. (*A 30% reduction in serum B₁₂ was found in persons on long-term, high-dose omeprazole therapy.*)

55. Walan A, Bader JP, Classen M, et al. Effect of omeprazole and ranitidine on ulcer healing and relapse rates in patients with benign gastric ulcer. N Engl J Med 1989;320:69. (*A major European study, showing that omeprazole was superior to H₂-blocker therapy.*)

56. Yang Y-X, Lewis JD, Metz DC. Long-term proton pump inhibitor therapy and risk of hip fracture. JAMA 2006;296:2947. (*An observational case–control study, finding a significant relation between PPI therapy and the risk of osteoporotic fracture; the degree of risk was dose and time dependent.*)

57. Yeomans ND, Tulassay Z, Juhasz L, et al., for the ASTRONAUT Study Group. A comparison of omeprazole with ranitidine for ulcers associated with nonsteroidal antiinflammatory drugs. N Engl J Med 1998;338:719. (*RCT, finding that omeprazole was superior to ranitidine for healing and prophylaxis.*)

58. McCarthy DM. Sucralfate. N Engl J Med 1991;325:1017. (*A comprehensive review; 159 references.*)

59. Graham DY, Agrawal NM, Campbell DR, et al. Ulcer prevention in long-term users of nonsteroidal anti-inflammatory drugs: results of a double-blind, randomized, multicenter, active and placebo-controlled study of misoprostol vs lansoprazole. Arch Intern Med 2002;162:169. (*PPI therapy was superior to placebo and misoprostol.*)

60. Graham DY, White RH, Moreland LW, et al. Duodenal and gastric ulcer prevention with misoprostol in arthritis patients taking NSAIDs. Ann Intern Med 1993;119:257. (*RCT, showing a reduction by misoprostol in the rate of ulcer development.*)

61. Lai KC, Lam SK, Chu KM, et al. Lansoprazole use for the prevention of recurrences of ulcer complications from long-term low-dose aspirin use. N Engl J Med 2002;346:2033. (*RCT, finding that there was a significant reduction in recurrence rate.*)

62. Lee Hooper L, Brown TJ, Elliott R, et al. The effectiveness of five strategies for the prevention of gastrointestinal toxicity induced by non-steroidal anti-inflammatory drugs: systematic review. BMJ 2004;329:948. (*The best review of the question, finding that although the data are limited, misoprostol and the concurrent use of PPI offered some protection.*)

63. Lisse JR, Perlman M, Johansson G, et al. Gastrointestinal tolerability and effectiveness of rofecoxib versus naproxen in the treatment of osteoarthritis: a randomized, controlled trial. Ann Intern Med 2003;139:539. (*The COX-2 drug was found to be better tolerated in terms of GI adverse effects.*)

64. Mukherjee D, Nissen S, Topol EJ. Risk of cardiovascular events associated with selective COX-2 inhibitors. JAMA 2001;286:954. (*Calls attention to possible cardiovascular risk.*)

65. Raskin JB, White RH, Jackson JE, et al. Misoprostol dosage in the prevention of nonsteroidal anti-inflammatory drug-induced gastric and duodenal ulcers: a comparison of three regimens. Ann Intern Med 1995;123:344. (*A multicenter RCT, finding that twice-daily and thrice-daily regimens are better tolerated than four-times-daily programs and yet retain efficacy and reduce cost.*)

66. Simon LS, Weaver AL, Graham DY, et al. Anti-inflammatory and upper gastrointestinal effects of celecoxib in rheumatoid arthritis. A randomized controlled trial. JAMA 1999;282:1921. (*A significant reduction in ulcer and bleeding risks was found with this COX-2 drug.*)

67. Suzuki T, Matuso K, Ito H, et al. Smoking increases the treatment failure for Helicobacter pylori eradication. Am J Med 2006;119:217. (*A meta-analysis, finding a pooled odds ratio of 1.95*).

68. Thompson JC. The role of surgery in peptic ulcer disease. N Engl J Med 1982;307:550. (*An editorial that nicely summarizes the indications for surgery.*)

69. Soll AH, for the Practice Parameters Committee of the American College of Gastroenterology. Medical treatment of peptic ulcer disease: practice guidelines. JAMA 1996;275:622. (*Slightly dated, but underscores the importance of eradicating Helicobacter pylori infection and eliminating NSAID use.*)

CHAPTER 69 ■ MANAGEMENT OF ASYMPTOMATIC AND SYMPTOMATIC GALLSTONES

Gallbladder disease afflicts more than 20 million Americans, with more than 500,000 undergoing cholecystectomy each year. Prevalence is particularly high among middle-aged, obese women. Most patients with gallstones are asymptomatic, and only a few suffer from recurrent bouts of abdominal discomfort. Occasionally, a complication such as acute cholecystitis, pancreatitis, or choledocholithiasis may ensue. The primary physician needs to know when treatment is necessary and how to help the patient choose among elective surgery, medical therapy, and expectant management.

PATHOPHYSIOLOGY, CLINICAL PRESENTATION, AND COURSE (1–18)

Pathophysiology and Risk Factors

Most gallstones are cholesterol laden, and develop as a consequence of bile becoming supersaturated with cholesterol.

Hereditary factors play a strong role, as do female gender and obesity, due, respectively, to the lithogenic effects of estrogen and the increased risk associated with even moderate degrees of weight gain and caloric excess (relative risk, 2 to 3). Rapid weight loss is also an important risk factor. In men, regular exercise protects against developing symptomatic disease (the effect is unknown in women).

Biliary sludge is a microprecipitate mixture of bile, cholesterol crystals, and calcium bilirubinate that forms when bile becomes supersaturated. Pathogenesis is believed to be similar to that of gallstones and may represent a transitional state. Its existence was revealed with the advent of ultrasound imaging of the biliary tree. Factors associated with its formation include rapid weight loss, pregnancy, transplantation, and treatment with drugs such as ceftriaxone or octreotide.

Presentation

Gallbladder disease may be asymptomatic or manifested by recurrent pain. Characteristically, *biliary colic* is rather sudden in onset, builds to a maximum within 1 hour, is steady, is localized to the right upper quadrant or epigastrium, lasts 2 to 4 hours, and occasionally radiates to the left or the right scapula. There is often nausea and vomiting. *Dyspeptic symptoms*, fatty food intolerance, belching, and bloating have also been attributed to chronic gallbladder disease, but the association is probably coincidental. Prospective studies have shown that such symptoms are just as common in middle-aged women without gallstones as in those with them. When patients with these symptoms are operated on, the dyspepsia often persists after cholecystectomy.

The clinical presentation of choledocholithiasis may be highly variable, ranging from acute nausea, vomiting, fever, upper abdominal pain, and jaundice to mild recurrent episodes of biliary colic. In many instances, the patient may be asymptomatic for years before an attack develops, occurring when a stone blocks the distal end of the common duct.

The rare patient with true biliary colic but a normal gallbladder study on ultrasound may have *acalculous gallbladder disease* (an uncommon condition) or *multiple small stones*, which are detected by observing delayed gallbladder emptying in response to a fatty meal or cholecystokinin. *Biliary sludge* is usually an incidental finding or can be found in the context of biliary colic, acute pancreatitis, or acute cholecystitis, especially if it is obscuring the presence of small stones.

Clinical Course

The clinical course of untreated gallbladder disease depends on whether the patient has been asymptomatic. Overall, asymptomatic patients appear to have a relatively favorable prognosis, but symptomatic individuals with episodes of true biliary colic have twice the rate of complications.

Among *symptomatic patients* with at least one bout of pain requiring a hospitalization, about one third have *recurrent pain* and one fifth experience complications such as *jaundice*, *cholangitis*, or *pancreatitis* over 5 to 20 years of follow-up; one half remain *asymptomatic*. Among symptomatic persons with small stones (diameter <5 mm), there is a fourfold increase in the risk of pancreatitis. In men, increased physical activity correlates inversely with the risk of symptomatic disease. Although there is no certainty that the onset of complications will be preceded by episodes of biliary pain, greater than 90% of patients who suffer a complication of gallbladder disease have prior warning symptoms of biliary colic, although they

are often mild and are ignored. Most patients with pain on presentation have similar patterns of pain on follow-up.

In *asymptomatic* people (with *silent gallstones*) followed expectantly for up to 20 years, there is a cumulative probability of biliary colic of about 20%, a 27% rate of dyspepsia, a 4.5% rate of transient jaundice, and no deaths from the delay of surgery. The increased risk in asymptomatic patients is associated with *very large stones* (>2.5 cm), *age greater than 60 years*, and *diabetes*.

Carcinoma of the gallbladder occurs mostly in older women with gallstone disease. The initial association with stone formation was based on circumstantial autopsy data. Community-based study has shown a much weaker association, pertaining only to men.

Biliary sludge follows a variable clinical course, ranging from complete resolution, to waxing and waning, to the formation of gallstones. In cases of acute abdominal pain associated with the presence of sludge, there is a disappearance of sludge and symptoms in 50% of cases, and another 20% remain asymptomatic with sludge persisting. In the remainder, stones may develop, and/or symptoms may persist.

DIAGNOSIS (19–22)

Asymptomatic Gallstones

Asymptomatic disease is usually detected as an incidental finding during a radiologic or ultrasound investigation that encompasses the upper abdomen for a reason other than suspected gallbladder disease. With the advent and widespread application of ultrasound and computed tomography techniques, the frequency of detection of asymptomatic disease has been increasing.

Acute Cholecystitis

The occurrence of classic biliary colic provides strong presumptive evidence for the diagnosis of cholecystitis; dyspepsia and fatty food intolerance do not. Real-time *ultrasound* of the gallbladder and biliary tree is the test of choice for the evaluation of symptomatic patients with suspected acute cholecystitis. The only preparation necessary is 6 hours or more of fasting. The test takes about 15 minutes. Adequate images are obtained in about 98% of instances, although obesity can reduce visualization. Ultrasound can be performed rapidly, provides anatomic information, is low in cost, and allows the examination of other potentially causative abdominal structures. Major criteria for a positive study are the presence of stones or nonvisualization of the gallbladder (no fluid-filled lumen). Minor criteria include tenderness of the gallbladder during ultrasound examination, thickening of the gallbladder wall, and a rounded shape. Sensitivity and specificity are greater than 95%.

Patients with a nondiagnostic ultrasound but still strongly suspected of having acute cholecystitis (e.g., presence of biliary colic, mild elevations in liver function tests), should have the test repeated. The stone may have passed from the gallbladder into the common bile duct (see later discussion). Besides the presence of stone, other findings correlate with the presence of cholecystitis, including localized tenderness over the gallbladder ("*sonographic Murphy's sign*") and gallbladder wall thickening.

An alternative to ultrasound for the detection of acute cholecystitis is *scintigraphy* with the radionuclide ^{99m}Tc hepatobiliary iminodiacetic acid scan. The isotope is taken up by the liver and excreted into the bile. Images are obtained after 1 hour. The patient needs to be fasting (but no longer than 2 to 4 hours) and free of underlying hepatocellular disease and alcoholism (which cause false-positive tests). The gallbladder, cystic duct, common bile duct, and duodenum are visualized by 60 minutes in the normal person. Nonvisualization of the gallbladder after 1 hour is characteristic of acute cholecystitis (the common bile duct and duodenum remain visualized). Sensitivity and specificity approach those of ultrasound, but the cost is greater, and the test takes more time. Scintigraphy can help to determine the patency of the cystic duct.

Ultrasound has largely replaced the *oral cholecystogram* for the diagnosis of acute cholecystitis because it is more sensitive, is equally specific, and provides results much faster and with none of the gastrointestinal upset and allergic reactions that are associated with oral cholecystography. Computed tomography of the gallbladder is not sufficiently sensitive to warrant its use for detection of stones; gallstones and bile can have the same density.

Choledocholithiasis

Symptomatic patients with recurrent pain plus persistent mild elevations in liver function tests, a dilated common bile duct, jaundice, or signs of acute pancreatitis require further evaluation for a stone in the common bile duct. As noted, *ultrasound* may be nondiagnostic because the sensitivity of a single study for detecting stones in the duct is only 50% when there is no ductal dilation and 75% when ductal dilation is present. Overlying bowel gas can obscure visualization of a common duct stone. If clinical suspicion remains high, a repeat ultrasound study is indicated. *Computed tomography* has about the same sensitivity (75%) as ultrasound for the detection of a common duct stone. *Magnetic resonance cholangiopancreatography* has a sensitivity of greater than 90% and represents a major advance in the noninvasive imaging of the biliary tree for the detection of stones; it requires no iodinated contrast or invasive procedure, and its high sensitivity can obviate the need for invasive study. If noninvasive testing is nondiagnostic in the setting of suspected common duct stone, then *endoscopic retrograde cholangiopancreatography* (ERCP) deserves consideration. Sensitivity exceeds 90%, and therapeutic sphincterotomy can be performed at the same time.

Chronic Cholecystitis

Ultrasound is the diagnostic test of choice in patients with recurrent episodes of biliary colic. The *oral cholecystogram* has come back into use in patients who are being considered for gallstone dissolution because the test can provide information on gallbladder function and stone composition (see later discussion).

PRINCIPLES OF MANAGEMENT
(3,7–9,12,14,17,23–33)

Given the rather benign natural history of asymptomatic gallstone disease, watchful waiting usually suffices in most patients, but one still needs to identify high-risk patients who require closer follow-up and possible consideration of elective cholecystectomy. Symptomatic patients want advice on treatment options, which include open cholecystectomy, laparoscopic cholecystectomy, and gallstone dissolution. There have yet to be randomized, controlled clinical trials comparing treatment options, which necessitates that management be based on extrapolation from available data on the natural history of the disease and on the risks and outcomes of interventions.

Asymptomatic Gallstones

There is no evidence that the vast number of patients with asymptomatic gallstones would benefit from surgery or stone dissolution. Although surgical mortality is only 0.5%, only 20% of asymptomatic patients will ever develop biliary colic and acute cholecystitis, and only a small fraction of these people will experience a complication such as pancreatitis. In most patients, the risks of conservative management are not much different from those of surgery and involve far less expense, morbidity, and time lost from work. A substantial fraction of the 500,000 cholecystectomies done each year for asymptomatic gallstones and stones accompanied by dyspeptic symptoms (but not true biliary colic) could probably be avoided. Many such patients continue to have symptoms after surgery. Similarly, there is no evidence that stone dissolution therapy improves outcomes in patients with asymptomatic stones, although data on this issue are sparse. Patients at high risk for gallbladder cancer might be reasonable candidates for prophylactic cholecystectomy, but few risk factors have been identified (other than calcified gallbladder and stones >3 cm in diameter).

Similarly, for asymptomatic persons found to have *biliary sludge*, clinical observation and expectant management are appropriate. Should biliary colic or other complications develop, then cholecystectomy deserves consideration. Nonetheless, up to 30% of patients with a single episode of biliary colic may have no further symptoms or complications, making watchful waiting an option, as long as close follow-up is assured.

Acute Cholecystitis

Patients presenting with symptoms of acute cholecystitis require hospitalization for prompt diagnosis, intravenous fluids, and surgical consultation. The elderly, diabetics, and other debilitated persons are at particularly high risk of a complication from cholecystitis. Although *immediate surgery* may not be necessary, inpatient care for assessment and initial supportive care is warranted. There is considerable debate among surgeons as to whether urgent surgery is indicated. Analyses suggest little risk to delaying surgery until the acute inflammatory phase of the illness has receded, provided there are no acute complications such as choledocholithiasis or pancreatitis. Performing *nonelective open cholecystectomy* raises the mortality risk fourfold (i.e., up to 10% in the elderly). Long-term outcomes are similar for *open* and *laparoscopic cholecystectomy* (see later discussion). In general, laparoscopic surgery shortens the length of hospital stay and the time required for return to work but also increases risks of injury to the common bile duct and retained stones.

Symptomatic Gallstones

Symptomatic patients with recurrent attacks of biliary colic and confirmed gallstones or persistent biliary sludge and suspected gall stones should be advised to undergo *elective cholecystectomy*, provided they are reasonable surgical candidates.

Before the advent of laparoscopic surgery, it was unclear which form of therapy was best for such patients, and several analytic studies found little difference between medical and traditional surgical approaches. However, with the development of minimally invasive laparoscopic surgical techniques, the decision has shifted in favor of gallbladder removal by laparoscopic cholecystectomy (see later discussion). Here, the risk of complications from gallbladder disease (although relatively low) exceeds the risk of surgery.

Patients unwilling or too frail to undergo general anesthesia and surgery are candidates for medical therapy, which aims at stone dissolution by the use of bile acids. Some patients will refuse all forms of treatment, preferring to "see how it goes." Such patients subject themselves to a small increase in mortality risk, but recent studies suggest that the risk is actually modest and that the real issue is the patient's willingness to risk future attacks of pain and possible morbid complications (e.g., pancreatitis). Patients with only a single episode of biliary colic and no risk factors for complications of gallstone disease (i.e., diabetes, age >60 years, stones >2.5 cm or <0.5 cm) are probably the best symptomatic candidates for an expectant approach to treatment, having a reasonable chance of remaining symptom-free into the future. Similarly, persons with a single episode of biliary colic associated with sludge have a 30% chance of no recurrences or complications and could be followed expectantly.

Surgery

Surgery is the most definitive means of achieving a long-term solution. *Conventional open cholecystectomy* remains one of the most commonly performed of all surgical procedures, although laparoscopic cholecystectomy has become very popular and has replaced the traditional cholecystectomy in many settings (see later discussion). Mortality rates for conventional open cholecystectomy range from 0.3% to 0.5% in patients younger than the age of 50 years and rise to 1.4% to 2.7% in those older than age 70 years. The complication rate from traditional elective surgery is 5% and doubles for nonelective surgery. Conventional surgery is successful; only about 4% of patients experience chronic postoperative pain, with a retained stone often the cause. Surgery is sometimes undertaken to relieve dyspeptic symptoms, although results are inconsistent and usually disappointing. This is not surprising, given the poor correlation between stones and dyspepsia.

Laparoscopic cholecystectomy provides the opportunity for a much less invasive procedure, with the length of hospital stay reduced from an average of 6 days to 1.2 days. More than three fourths of patients return to work within 10 days, compared with 1 month for conventional gallbladder surgery. The procedure takes about 30 minutes longer to perform than an open cholecystectomy. The reported complication rate among surgeons experienced in the technique is 5%, similar to that for open surgery in such patients, but the proportion of serious complications is reduced. The overall rate of bile duct injury is slightly higher (0.5% vs. 0.2%), but it falls with experience (to 0.1%). Only one case of trocar-induced bowel perforation was reported in more than 1,500 procedures, and no deaths were attributable to surgery or a postoperative complication. The most common problem is superficial infection at the site of the insertion of the umbilical trocar. About 5% of cases have to be converted to open procedures, mostly due to poor visualization of the gallbladder.

The laparoscopic approach represents an excellent option in patients with uncomplicated symptomatic gallstone disease. Suspicion of a common duct stone necessitates consideration of an open procedure; however, common duct exploration is possible with laparoscopic surgery. If a common duct stone is found, the procedure needs to be converted to an open cholecystectomy or followed postoperatively by ERCP to achieve stone removal. With increasing availability and surgical skill, this procedure is likely to become the treatment of choice for uncomplicated symptomatic gallbladder disease. Although the cost per patient has declined markedly with the advent of laparoscopic surgery, total costs have not fallen because more patients are undergoing surgery.

Medical Therapy

Medical therapy is an option for patients who are poor surgical candidates or reluctant to undergo elective cholecystectomy. The objective is stone dissolution by biochemical.

Bile Acids. Up to 80% of gallstones have cholesterol as the major constituent, making them potentially dissolvable in the presence of increased bile acid. Only the naturally occurring bile acid *ursodeoxycholic acid* (*ursodiol*) has been proven to be both effective in dissolving stones and free of the serious gastrointestinal side effects that accompanied trials of other bile acids (e.g., *chenodiol*, which causes liver injury, diarrhea, and low-density-lipoprotein–cholesterol elevations). Ursodiol is safe for long-term use. The agent not only dissolves stones directly, but also desaturates the cholesterol content of the bile by suppressing hepatic cholesterol synthesis and biliary cholesterol secretion. It is the only bile acid approved by the U.S. Food and Drug Administration for stone dissolution, replacing chenodiol.

Gallstone dissolution is achievable in patients with small (2 cm) *cholesterol stones*, especially if there is a *functioning gallbladder* (as determined by oral cholecystogram). The overall stone dissolution rate is just less than 50% and higher for those with pure cholesterol stones (as determined by the oral cholecystogram findings of floating radiolucent stones in a functioning gallbladder). Results are best in patients with a few small stones. Many patients become pain-free even before full stone dissolution is achieved, and 40% become stone-free after 2 years of continuous bile acid therapy. Patients with larger (>10 mm) or calcified stones fail to achieve complete stone dissolution.

The effects of therapy can be well documented by periodic oral cholecystogram or gallbladder ultrasound. Therapy is contraindicated in patients with inflammatory bowel disease or peptic ulcer because the drug increases bile acids, which may be harmful to colonic and gastric mucosa. Stones recur at the rate of 15%/yr. This high recurrence rate suggests a role for chronic suppressive therapy. Continued symptoms despite dissolution occur in about 4% of cases.

Ursodiol is expensive, with the costing upward of $2 to $3 per day. However, a major cost-to-benefit analysis showed that ursodiol treatment is a reasonable alternative to surgery in patients deemed poor surgical risks (although comparisons with laparoscopic surgery have not been performed). Some authorities have even advocated using ursodiol initially in all symptomatic patients and operating only on those who fail medical therapy. However, the excellent results reported with laparoscopic surgery, particularly the marked reductions in recovery time and perioperative morbidity, have probably tilted the decision back in favor of surgery for most patients who can tolerate general anesthesia.

Choledocholithiasis

Stones in the common duct are associated with increased risks of complications and death. Consequently, they need to be removed. Endoscopic sphincterotomy and the retrieval of stones by balloon catheter or basket can performed during ERCP. Stones too large to be extracted can be broken up by lithotripsy or dissolved with the use of ursodiol.

Prevention

Diet and Exercise

Obesity and caloric excess are major risk factors for gallstone formation in women, and some gallstone patients with dyspeptic symptoms feel better if they avoid fatty foods; however, the relationship between stones and fatty food intolerance is tenuous at best (see Chapter 74). Major population studies found that an isocaloric diet high in polyunsaturated fat and low in *trans* fats was associated with an 18% reduced risk of gallstone disease in men, and one rich in fruits and vegetables was associated with a 25% reduction in women. Multivariate analysis showed that it is the number of calories consumed rather than the proportion of calories coming from saturated fat or cholesterol intake that seems to correlate best with risk. Although obesity and caloric excess can lead to stone formation, rapid weight loss through fasting, starvation diets, and gastric bypass cause bile to become very lithogenic, triggering stone formation. Perhaps modest weight reduction achieved in a gradual fashion might be of some prophylactic value in high-risk patients such as obese women. Prospective study of dietary factors is sorely needed. Exercise appears to be protective of symptomatic disease in men; it has not been studied in women.

Alcohol and Tobacco

The daily consumption of small amounts of alcohol (about 1 oz/d) has been found in retrospective studies of women to correlate with a 20% reduction in the risk of symptomatic gallstone disease. This closely parallels the 20% lower bile cholesterol saturation found among modest drinkers compared with control subjects. Smoking also appears to reduce the risk in women, probably by its adverse effects on estrogen production and degradation.

Avoidance of Lithogenic Medications

The risk of gallstone formation rises markedly with the use of *estrogen* and *clofibrate*. The use of estrogens in postmenopausal women increases the risk by 75%. Patients with known gallstones should not take them, and those taking such drugs should be monitored for gallstone formation, particularly if there is a strongly positive family history of stone disease. *Thiazide* use, either past or current, is associated with a modest increase in the relative risk of gallstones (relative risk, 1.16 and 1.39, respectively).

PATIENT EDUCATION

The truly asymptomatic gallstone patient can be reassured of the low probability of becoming symptomatic or suffering a complication. Such patients can be followed expectantly and should not be pushed into surgery, medical therapy, or unnecessary dietary restriction. Previously, asymptomatic patients with large stones, diabetes, or advanced age were considered candidates for prophylactic stone removal because they had an increased mortality risk from a complication. However, improvements in medical and surgical therapy of symptomatic patients have greatly reduced the risk for such patients, making prophylactic surgical or stone-dissolution therapy unnecessary.

Because symptomatic patients have a slightly increased mortality risk and a modest chance of a complication, they need to be informed of the therapeutic options so that patient preferences and treatment modality can be matched. The principal therapeutic benefit is a reduction in the frequency of symptoms and in the risk of complications; the mortality benefit is small and almost clinically insignificant. The wish to refuse therapy can be respected, so long as the patient understands the risks of choosing expectant therapy. However, the short hospital stay, low morbidity, and speedy recovery afforded by laparoscopic cholecystectomy may be particularly appealing to previously reluctant symptomatic patients. Ursodiol is also well tolerated and may be an attractive option for qualifying patients fearful of any surgery.

Any dyspepsia should be clearly differentiated from biliary colic. Patients need to know that the link between dyspepsia and gallstones is not well founded and that the presence of dyspeptic symptoms is not an indication for surgery or medical therapy, although other measures might help (see Chapter 74).

INDICATIONS FOR REFERRAL AND ADMISSION

Patients with evidence of acute cholecystitis should be admitted to the hospital for evaluation, surgical consultation, and supportive measures. Consultation with a surgeon regarding elective cholecystectomy is also indicated for patients with recurrent biliary colic. Referral for consideration of laparoscopic cholecystectomy should be made exclusively to a surgeon skilled and experienced in performing the procedure. High levels of morbidity (e.g., bile duct injury, perforation) and mortality have resulted from performance of the procedure by inadequately trained personnel. Referral may be useful for symptomatic patients who are deemed too frail to undergo elective surgery, as well those with a suspected common duct stone who may require ERCP.

THERAPEUTIC RECOMMENDATIONS (2,3,13,18–33)

- Patients with asymptomatic cholelithiasis can be managed expectantly because the risk of developing symptomatic disease or a complication is only 1%/yr.
- Patients with a single episode of biliary colic are also reasonable candidates for expectant management, as long as they continue to be free of recurrent pain.
- Patients with documented gallstones and recurrent biliary colic or a history of a complication of gallstone disease (cholecystitis, pancreatitis) should be advised to undergo elective cholecystectomy, provided they can tolerate general anesthesia and surgery. *Laparoscopic cholecystectomy* has become the surgical procedure of choice, reducing perioperative morbidity and shortening the recovery period when performed by a surgeon skilled in the procedure.
- Symptomatic nonsurgical patients with a functioning gallbladder and radiolucent (i.e., cholesterol) gallstones can be given a trial of bile acid therapy with *ursodiol* (10 to 15 mg/kg per day). Therapy is continued for at least 12 months and often for 24 months. Results are best in those with stones that are less than 2 cm in diameter and fewer than three in number. The presence of calcification rules out bile acid therapy. The effects of therapy should be monitored with a gallbladder ultrasound every 6 months. The risk of recurrence is high after bile acid therapy is stopped.

■ Estrogen preparations, clofibrate, and other drugs that may trigger stone formation should be stopped, or doses should be decreased in persons with gallstones or a high risk of developing them.

■ Restricting *saturated fat* and *cholesterol* is of little or no benefit in altering the clinical course of gallstone disease. However, obesity and caloric excess are major risk factors, and gradual weight reduction through modest caloric restriction might be helpful. Fasting and starvation diets are to be avoided because they make the bile even more lithogenic.

Modest *alcohol* consumption (<1 oz/d) is not harmful. *Exercise* can be recommended as a preventive measure, as can diets rich in *fruits* and *vegetables* and nonhydrogenated *polyunsaturates*.

■ Dyspeptic symptoms should not be considered grounds for medical or surgical treatment because their relation to gallstone disease is tenuous at best. Dyspeptic symptoms are likely to respond better to other measures (see Chapter 74).

A.H.G.

Annotated Bibliography

1. Barbara, L, Sama L, Morselli Labate AM, et al. A population study on the prevalence of gall stone disease: the Sirmione Study. Hepatology 1987;7:913. (*The prevalence of gallstones is high, and the relative prevalence of symptoms is low.*)

2. Carveth SW, Priestley JT, Gage R. Size and number of gallstones in acute and chronic cholecystitis. Mayo Clin Proc 1959;34:371. (*A classic observation; stones >2.5 cm are more likely to precipitate attacks of cholecystitis than are smaller stones.*)

3. Cirillo DJ, Wallace RB, Rodabough RJ, et al. Effect of estrogen therapy on gallbladder disease. JAMA 2005;293:330. (*There was an increased risk of biliary tract disease in postmenopausal women using estrogen therapy.*)

4. Gracie WA, Ransohoff R. The natural history of silent gallstones. N Engl J Med 1982;307:798. (*A retrospective cohort study, identifying no mortality associated with asymptomatic gallstones and finding a 15-year accumulative probability of biliary pain of only 18%.*)

5. Ko CK, Sekimima JH, Lee SP, et al. Biliary sludge. Ann Intern Med 1999;130:301. (*A review; 118 references.*)

6. Lee SP, Maher K, Nicholls JF. Origin and fate of biliary sludge. Gastroenterology 1988;95:508. (*The best natural history study.*)

7. Leitzmann MF, Tsai C-J, Stampfer MJ, et al. Thiazide diuretics and the risk of gallbladder disease requiring surgery in women. Arch Intern med 2005;165:567. (*Population data from the Women's Health Study, showing that thiazide use was associated with a 39% increase in the risk for current users and a 19% increase in past users.*)

8. Leitzmann MF, Giovannucci EL, Rimm EB, et al. The relation of physical activity to risk for symptomatic gallstone disease in men. Ann Intern Med 1998;128:417. (*A prospective cohort study of male health professionals, showing that physical activity was inversely correlated with the risk of symptomatic gallstone disease.*)

9. Maclure KM, Hayes KC, Colditz GA, et al. Weight, diet, and the risk of symptomatic gallstones in middle-aged women. N Engl J Med 1989;321:563. (*Prospective data, confirming the strong association between obesity and symptomatic gallstones; moderate overweight increased risk; alcohol decreased it.*)

10. Maringhini A, Moreau JA, Melton J, et al. Gallstones, gallbladder cancer, and other gastrointestinal malignancies. Ann Intern Med 1987;107:30. (*A community study, finding that there was only a minor increase in risk and much less risk than previously reported from autopsy studies.*)

11. McSherry CK, Ferstenberg H, Calhoun WF, et al. The natural history of diagnosed gallstone disease in symptomatic and asymptomatic patients. Ann Surg 1985;202:59. (*Documents a very favorable prognosis in 691 patients followed for an average of 5 years.*)

12. Pastides H, Tzonou A, Trichopoulos D, et al. A case–control study of the relationship between smoking, diet, and gallbladder disease. Arch Intern Med 1990;150:1409. (*One of the few studies examining the relationship of these factors to symptomatic gallbladder disease.*)

13. Price WH. Gallbladder dyspepsia. Br Med J 1963;3:138. (*Classic observations, showing that the frequency and the severity of dyspeptic complaints are unrelated to the presence or absence of gallstones.*)

14. Schein CJ. Acute cholecystitis in the diabetic. Am J Gastroenterol 1969;51:511. (*There is an increased mortality risk from cholecystitis in diabetics; later studies showed the risk to be lower than reported here.*)

15. Shiffman ML, Sugarman HJ, Kellum JM, et al. Gall stone formation after rapid weight loss: a prospective study in patients undergoing gastric by pass for morbid obesity. Br Med J 1983;286:763. (*Gallstones frequently develop after gastric bypass.*)

16. Thistle JL, Cleary PA, Lachin JM, et al. The natural history of cholelithiasis: the National Cooperative Gallstone Study. Ann Intern Med 1984;101:171. (*The most important predictor of biliary tract pain was a history of pain; only 4% required elective cholecystectomy in 2 years of follow-up.*)

17. Tsai C-J, Leitzmann MF, Willett WC, et al. The effect of long-term intake of *cis* unsaturated fats on the risk for gallstone disease in men. Ann Intern Med 2004;1412:514. (*A prospective population cohort study, showing that a high intake of polyunsaturated fats in a balanced diet was associated with a decreased risk of gallstone disease.*)

18. Tsai C-J, Leitzmann MF, Willett WC, et al. Fruit and vegetable consumption and risk of cholecystectomy in women. Am J Med 2006;119:760. (*Data from the Women's Health Study, noting a reduced risk with increased fruit and vegetable consumption.*)

19. Chan YL, Chan ACW, Lam WWM, et al. Choledocholithiasis: comparison of MR cholangiography and endoscopic retrograde cholangiopancreatography. Radiology 1996;200:85. (*Results were promising for magnetic resonance imaging; sensitivity was >90%.*)

20. Cooperberg PL, Burhenne HJ. Real time ultrasonography in calculus gallbladder disease. N Engl J Med 1980;302:1277. (*One of the original studies establishing ultrasound as the test of choice; sensitivity was 98%, and specificity was 95%; a comparison with oral cholecystography in a subsample showed greater sensitivity and similar specificity.*)

21. Dolgin SM, Schwartz JS, Kressel HY, et al. Identification of patients with cholesterol or pigment gallstones by discriminant analysis of radiographic features. N Engl J Med 1981;304:808. (*Describes oral cholecystogram findings that help to identify patients with cholesterol stones; buoyancy was highly predictive of cholesterol composition.*)

22. Health and Policy Committee, American College of Physicians. How to study the gallbladder. Ann Intern Med 1988;109:752. (*A still-relevant consensus statement on recommended approaches to imaging the gallbladder.*)

23. Bates T, Mercer JC, Harrison M. Symptomatic gallstone disease: before and after cholecystectomy. Gut 1984;25:579. (*One year after surgery, nearly half of patients complained of digestive symptoms.*)

24. Broomfield PH, Chopra R, Sheinbaum RC, et al. Effects of ursodeoxycholic acid and aspirin on the formation of lithogenic bile and gallstones during loss of weight. N Engl J Med 1988;319:1567. (*Ursodiol prevented lithogenic changes in bile.*)

25. Fullarton GM, Bell G, and the West of Scotland Laparoscopic Cholecystomy Audit Group. Prospective audit of the introduction of laparoscopic cholecystectomy in the west of Scotland. Gut 1994;35:1121. (*Total costs did not go down because more patients chose to have surgery.*)

26. Kane RL, Lurie N, Borbas C, et al. The outcomes of elective laparoscopic and open cholecystectomies. J Am Coll Surg 1995;180:136. (*The length of stay was reduced by 3 days and return to work by 2 weeks.*)

27. Kowdley KV. Ursodeoxycholic acid therapy in hepatobiliary disease. Am J Med 2000;108:481. (*A succinct recent review for the generalist reader; 48 references.*)

28. NIH Consensus Development Panel on Gallstones and Laparoscopic Cholecystectomy. JAMA 1993;269:1018. (*A consensus view on the indications for laparoscopic gallbladder surgery.*)

29. Ransohoff DF, Gracie WM. Management of patients with symptomatic gallstones: a quantitative analysis. Am J Med 1990;88:154. (*A decision-analysis study, finding that the survival benefit from surgery or medical therapy was modest at best; management decisions were best based on considerations other than mortality.*)

30. Ransohoff DF, Gracie WA. Treatment of gallstones. Ann Intern Med 1993;119:606. (*An authoritative review of the risks and benefits of available treatment strategies; 92 references.*)

31. Ransohoff DF, Gracie WA, Wolfenson LB, et al. Prophylactic cholecystectomy or expectant management for silent gallstones. Ann Intern Med 1983;99:199. (*A decision-analysis study; there is a small survival benefit for prophylactic cholecystectomy, which may well be offset by financial costs, morbidity, and time preferences.*)

32. Rubin RA, Kowalskin TE, Khandelwal M, et al. Ursodiol for hepatobiliary disorders. Ann Intern Med 1994;121:207. (*The best review of bile acid therapy; 142 references.*)

33. Weinstein MC, Coley CM, Richter JM. Medical management of gallstones: a cost-effectiveness analysis. J Gen Intern Med 1990;5:277. (*Finds that medical therapy with ursodiol was a cost-effective alternative to conventional surgery, especially in the elderly.*)

CHAPTER 70 ■ MANAGEMENT OF HEPATITIS

JULES L. DIENSTAG

Viral and nonviral forms of hepatitis are more common than generally thought. More than 50,000 cases of viral hepatitis in the United States are reported to the Centers for Disease Control and Prevention each year, although the actual number is estimated to be 10 times as high. Hepatitis B accounts for 30% to 35% of cases of acute viral hepatitis, hepatitis A for 45% to 50%, and hepatitis C for 15% to 20%; both hepatitis D and especially E are very rare in the United States, and a few percent of cases cannot be attributed to any known hepatitis virus. In addition, a proportion of patients with acute types B, C, and D progress to chronic infection. Some become inactive carriers; others have chronic hepatitis, which is associated with an increased risk of cirrhosis and death. Approximately 25% to 40% of chronic liver disease in the United States and Europe derives from chronic hepatitis C infection and 10% to 15% from hepatitis B. Other important causes include alcohol-associated liver injury, hemochromatosis, autoimmune hepatitis, and nonalcoholic steatohepatitis (NASH). In about 15% to 20% of cases, the cause is unknown ("cryptogenic").

The primary physician needs to be skilled in the management of both viral and nonviral forms of hepatitis because these are illnesses usually encountered in the outpatient setting. Effective outpatient management requires knowledge of diagnosis (see Chapters 57 and 62), natural history, and treatment options. Immunosuppressive therapy for nonviral disease, interferon and nucleoside analogues for viral disease, and transplantation for end-stage forms have widened the therapeutic options substantially. Although many treatment decisions require subspecialty consultation, especially in persons with advanced disease, the primary physician retains responsibility for long-term management and follow-up, working in conjunction with the liver specialist. This charge requires knowing the indications and contraindications for the various treatment options and the best means of monitoring clinical course and therapeutic interventions.

CLINICAL PRESENTATION AND NATURAL HISTORY (1–13)

Acute Viral Hepatitis

In most instances, acute viral hepatitis is a self-limited illness; on the order of 85% of hospitalized patients and more than 95% of outpatients recover completely and uneventfully within 3 months (except in the case of hepatitis C; see later discussion). Most persons with acute viral hepatitis never become jaundiced; their illness is labeled mistakenly as a nonspecific viral syndrome unless liver biochemical tests, such as aminotransferase levels, are ordered. A large proportion of patients remain asymptomatic, especially children. In elderly or immunologically compromised patients, the prognosis is more guarded, with an increased risk of severe and protracted disease.

Prodromal symptoms occur after an *incubation period* of 2 to 4 (rarely 6) weeks for hepatitis A, 2 to 8 weeks for hepatitis E, 4 to 24 weeks for hepatitis B (with or without simultaneous acute delta hepatitis infection), and 3 to 15 weeks (80% within 5 to 10 weeks) for hepatitis C. Characteristically, prodromal symptoms consist of 1 to 2 weeks of malaise, anorexia, nausea, vomiting, change in senses of taste and smell, low-grade fever, right upper quadrant or midepigastric abdominal discomfort, and fatigue. Aminotransferase elevations may precede or coincide with the onset of prodromal symptoms.

If jaundice develops, it usually does so as the prodromal complaints begin to subside, although the persistence of prodromal symptoms is observed in more severe cases. By the time 6 to 8 weeks have elapsed, most patients are well on their way to full recovery. Occasionally, isolated mild aminotransferase elevations persist after clinical recovery. If these biochemical abnormalities resolve within 3 to 6 months, the mild elevations have no prognostic significance.

Fulminant Acute Hepatitis

This is the most ominous form of acute hepatitis, characterized by overwhelming hepatocellular necrosis and signs of liver failure—encephalopathy, ascites, progressive jaundice, and coagulopathy. This complication is seen more often in cases of hepatitis B (especially with simultaneous delta hepatitis infection) than in those of hepatitis A or C, although the frequency is particularly high among pregnant women with hepatitis E (see Chapter 57). Before the availability of liver transplantation, the mortality of fulminant hepatitis approached 80%, despite the best intensive medical care.

Other Variants of Acute Hepatitis

In 5% to 10% of cases of acute hepatitis B, the prodromal phase of the illness may be characterized as a *serum sickness–like syndrome,* with urticaria, arthralgias, fever, and polyarticular arthritis. Some patients with acute viral hepatitis, especially those with hepatitis A or E, have a *cholestatic* illness, with marked jaundice, elevation of serum alkaline phosphatase activity, and pruritus lasting 1 to several months.

Approximately 5% to 10% of patients with viral hepatitis experience mild clinical and biochemical *relapses* during convalescence. These occur in approximately 10% of patients with acute hepatitis A and are associated with a return of virus excretion in stools and infectivity. In patients with acute hepatitis B, what appears clinically as a relapse may represent the clinical expression of simultaneous delta hepatitis infection. Episodic swings in aminotransferase levels are common during acute and chronic hepatitis C, attributable to the emergence of viral variants ("quasispecies") that evade host immunologic containment; in some instances, these recurrent aminotransferase elevations are accompanied by clinical "relapses."

Progression to Chronic Hepatitis

The risk of progression varies among the several types of viral hepatitis. Although an occasional case of hepatitis A may be slow to resolve and last more than 6 months, no cases of chronic hepatitis have been linked to hepatitis A infection. Similarly, hepatitis E does not progress to chronic infection. In patients with hepatitis B, the persistence of *hepatitis B surface antigen* (HBsAg) and *hepatitis B e antigen* (HBeAg) increases the risk of chronic hepatitis, although the early presence of either has no predictive value. In fact, no reliable predictors of chronicity have been identified in patients with acute hepatitis B or C. Clinical manifestations of progression to chronic viral hepatitis may be subtle, with little more than a persistence of mild symptoms and biochemical abnormalities for 6 or more months. Many patients remain asymptomatic, and almost all remain anicteric.

Hepatitis B. Hepatitis B can progress to chronic hepatitis but usually at a very low rate (approximately 1%) when clinically apparent acute infection occurs among immunocompetent adults. When accompanied by high levels of hepatitis B virus (HBV) replication, chronic hepatitis B can be categorized as mild, moderate, or severe, based on liver histologic grade (necroinflammatory activity) and stage (fibrosis). Patients with negligible virus replication—HBV DNA levels less than or equal to 10^3 to 10^4 virions per milliliter—are inactive HBsAg carriers.

The likelihood of chronic HBV infection is higher, approaching 90%, when acute infection occurs at birth or in *early childhood* or when acute infection occurs in an *immunocompromised host*. Most patients who present with chronic hepatitis B have no history of having experienced an acute hepatitis-like clinical illness, acquiring their infection subclinically. In patients with simultaneous acute *hepatitis B and D* (delta hepatitis), the likelihood of *chronicity* is not increased, but the *severity* of acute and chronic hepatitis is amplified.

Although most inactive hepatitis B carriers are asymptomatic and have a nonprogressive course, a small proportion may actually have subtle and insidious progression to chronic liver disease. Rarely, acute hepatitis-like exacerbations can occur. Such events may represent superimposed infection with another hepatitis virus (A, C, D) or reactivation of hepatitis B. Occasionally, an acute hepatitis-like elevation of aminotransferase activity represents a successful spontaneous seroconversion from highly replicative, HBeAg-positive, high-level HBV DNA infection to relatively nonreplicative, anti-HBe–positive, low-level HBV DNA infection; when such seroconversions occur, chronic liver injury gives way to an inactive carrier state. With early-generation clinical assays for HBV DNA, the level of HBV DNA in "nonreplicative" carriers fell below the detection threshold, but with exquisitely sensitive amplification techniques such as polymerase chain reaction assays, HBV DNA can be detected in inactive carriers, albeit at a threshold of less than 10^3 to 10^4 virions per milliliter.

Another important category of chronic hepatitis B has been recognized, *HBeAg-negative chronic hepatitis B*. Such patients have either precore or core-promoter mutations in the C gene of HBV. The C gene, which codes for the nucleocapsid core protein (HBcAg), also codes for HBeAg protein; HBeAg production requires an intact precore gene sequence. When one of several mutations in the precore region prevents elaboration of HBeAg, HBcAg and intact virus particles can still be synthesized, leading to highly replicative hepatitis B, despite the absence of HBeAg. Patients with such mutations in the precore region have levels of HBV DNA greater than or equal

to 10^5 virions per milliliter (but lower than levels observed in HBeAg-positive patients, 10^6 to 10^9 virions per milliliter) and substantial liver injury despite the absence of HBeAg, the conventional marker for high-level HBV replication and infectivity. Also characteristic in this subset of patients are fluctuating, even intermittently normal, aminotransferase levels. Often, these HBeAg-negative variants emerge after many years of HBeAg-reactive chronic hepatitis B. HBeAg-negative chronic hepatitis B does respond to antiviral therapy, but virologic relapse is the rule after discontinuation of therapy.

Patients with chronic hepatitis B, especially those with infection acquired early in life, are at a markedly increased risk of progression to *cirrhosis* and *hepatocellular carcinoma*.

Hepatitis C. In hepatitis C, 50% to 60% of patients experience elevations in aminotransferase that persist for more than 1 year after acute infection, and almost all of these go on to have longstanding chronic hepatitis. Moreover, even among patients in whom aminotransferase elevations appear to resolve within the first 6 months, chronic viremia persists in almost all. Between the 50% to 60% with chronic hepatitis after acute hepatitis C virus (HCV) infection and the remainder with *chronic viremia*, chronicity of HCV infection occurs in more than 85% of acutely infected persons. What is more, patients with chronic viremia remain at risk for the development of chronic hepatitis.

Among patients with chronic hepatitis C, *cirrhosis* develops in 20% of cases within 10 to 20 years after the onset of acute infection. Most have little clinically apparent effect of their disease for many decades, but in patients with moderate to severe chronic hepatitis on liver biopsy, the risk of progression to cirrhosis over 10 to 20 years is high. Among those with compensated cirrhosis, 10-year survival is very good, approximately 80%; once hepatic decompensation begins, the 10-year survival is diminished to less than 50%; in compensated cirrhotic patients with chronic hepatitis C, hepatic *decompensation* occurs in approximately 4% to 5% per year; the risk of *hepatocellular carcinoma* (rare during the first three decades of infection and in the absence of advanced fibrosis) increases at a rate of 1% to 4% per year.

Toxic and Drug-Induced Hepatitis

Drugs can trigger hepatocellular injury through a direct toxic effect or by means of an idiosyncratic reaction. Some agents are associated with a cholestatic reaction, either as part of an idiosyncratic process or independent of it. The severity of drug-induced hepatitis can range from an asymptomatic increase in liver enzymes to life-threatening illness. Prompt cessation of the drug is essential to limiting further hepatic injury; rechallenge may lead to an exaggerated reaction. Most cases are self-limited, provided that severe injury has not already occurred. Acetaminophen hepatotoxicity, one of the more commonly encountered forms of drug-induced hepatitis, is managed by the administration of *N*-acetylcysteine (see later discussion).

Direct Toxins

Directly toxic reactions are dose related and predictable in all patients treated and cause characteristic and reproducible histologic patterns of liver injury. The latency period is short, and manifestations suggestive of a hypersensitivity reaction are absent. *Acetaminophen* is the most commonly used drug that is directly hepatotoxic, although only when taken in massive doses.

Idiosyncratic Reactions

Idiosyncratic drug reactions, once believed to be immunologically mediated but now recognized to result primarily from the hepatotoxic effects of drug metabolites, are less predictable than those from direct toxins. They occur in only a small proportion of treated persons and cause variable histologic patterns of liver injury. Susceptibility to this type of drug hepatotoxicity may result from idiosyncratic, probably genetic, differences from person to person in the generation of toxic drug metabolites. In the idiosyncratic type of drug hepatotoxicity, latency is variable, and liver injury is not dose dependent. In about 25% of patients, extrahepatic manifestations suggestive of a hypersensitivity reaction (e.g., fever, rash, arthralgias, eosinophilia) occur. Hepatitis resulting from *halothane, isoniazid, methyl dopa, valproic acid,* and *trimethoprim/sulfamethoxazole* follows an idiosyncratic pattern.

Cholestatic Reactions

Two predominant types of cholestatic reactions occur: *bland cholestasis,* with little evidence of hepatitis, and *inflammatory cholestasis.* As is the case for other types of drug hepatotoxicity, some categories of cholestatic drug injury appear to represent predictable, dose-dependent, direct toxicity and others unpredictable, non–dose-dependent, idiosyncratic reactions. Oral contraceptives cause bland cholestasis, and the reaction is dose dependent and variable in onset. *Erythromycin* (especially the estolate preparation, but also other forms) and *chlorpromazine* are capable of causing idiosyncratic cholestasis with hepatitis, as are other phenothiazines, amoxicillin–clavulanic acid, and oxacillin. *Anabolic steroids* (17α-substituted androgens) also can cause cholestasis, often accompanied by a mild degree of hepatocellular injury. Other drugs cause a clinical picture reminiscent of sclerosing cholangitis, with inflammatory destruction of intrahepatic bile ducts (e.g., the chemotherapeutic agent floxuridine), whereas others (e.g., carbamazepine, chlorpromazine, tricyclic antidepressant agents) can result in the disappearance of bile ducts—"ductopenic" cholestasis—reminiscent of chronic rejection after liver transplantation.

Drug-Induced Steatosis

Macrovesicular or microvesicular steatosis or fatty infiltration with accompanying hepatitis (steatohepatitis) complicates therapy with several drugs. Among patients treated with antiretroviral drugs for HIV infection, severe steatohepatitis, a reflection of mitochondrial toxicity, has been observed in association with the use of reverse transcriptase inhibitors such as zidovudine and didanosine and with protease inhibitors such as indinavir and ritonavir.

Chronic Hepatitis

Classification by Grade and Stage

The distinctions between what used to be labeled "chronic persistent" and "chronic active" hepatitis are no longer recognized as valid and have been phased out of clinical use. Chronic persistent hepatitis, which now is called *minimal* or *mild chronic hepatitis,* referred to more indolent disease, whereas chronic active hepatitis was the designation for more progressive disease that is now labeled *as moderate to severe chronic hepatitis.* The obsolete distinctions have been replaced by assessments of relative inflammatory activity (grade) and fibrosis (stage). In clinical trials of chronic hepatitis, especially of chronic viral hepatitis, a numerical histologic index is used to assess severity (grade) and progression (stage). The *histologic activity index* includes numeric scores for periportal necrosis (including piecemeal and bridging necrosis), intralobular necrosis (focal and confluent), portal inflammation, and fibrosis.

Mild Chronic Hepatitis. In mild chronic hepatitis, mononuclear-cell inflammation is confined to the portal tract, the limiting plate of periportal hepatocytes is not eroded, hepatocellular necrosis and inflammation do not extend into the lobule, and fibrosis is absent or very limited. This mild category of chronic hepatitis was believed in the past to be predictive of a good prognosis and limited progression; however, although the benignity of mild chronic hepatitis tends to persist, the prognostic value of this designation is now recognized to be more limited and does not preclude progression to more severe chronic hepatitis or even cirrhosis.

Moderate to Severe Chronic Hepatitis. Moderate to severe chronic hepatitis is characterized histologically by a mononuclear-cell portal infiltrate that not only expands portal zones, but also extends beyond the portal tract into the adjacent periportal lobular area with erosion of the limiting plate of periportal hepatocytes (*piecemeal necrosis* or *interface hepatitis*). Fibrous septa extending into the lobule are also characteristic, fibrosis can range from mild to severe, and a proportion of such patients may have cirrhosis on their initial liver biopsies. A more severe form of this lesion includes *bridging necrosis,* in which confluent necrosis and cell dropout span lobules (bridging portal tract to portal tract or portal tract to central vein).

Chronic Viral Hepatitis

In the chronic forms of viral hepatitis, the *level of virus replication* and the *histologic pattern* appear to be the most important determinants of progression. In patients with chronic hepatitis B, one fourth of patients with mild chronic hepatitis B can still become cirrhotic. Similarly, in patients with histologically mild chronic hepatitis C, 20% can progress to cirrhosis over one to two decades. Superinfection with *hepatitis D* can cause progression to more severe liver disease among persons with chronic mild hepatitis B.

Hepatitis B. The 15-year survival of histologically mild chronic hepatitis B exceeds 95%, that of moderately severe chronic hepatitis B is about 85%, and that of the most histologically severe forms of chronic hepatitis B *with* cirrhosis is about 40%. Progression to cirrhosis has been noted in 13% of patients with mild chronic hepatitis B, in 16% of patients with moderate chronic hepatitis B (without bridging necrosis), and in 88% of those with severe chronic hepatitis B (with bridging necrosis).

The determinant of prognosis that underlies histology in chronic hepatitis B is virus replication. *Level of virus replication* (as measured by serum concentration of HBV DNA and the presence of HBeAg) is probably the most important determinant of progression to cirrhosis in patients with chronic hepatitis B. For example, in one study, cirrhosis developed in 53% of those with persistent, high-level HBV DNA but in none of those with HBV DNA undetectable by hybridization assays ($\leq 10^5$ to 10^6 virions per milliliter). In patients with chronic hepatitis B, *conversion from HBeAg to anti-HBe* may signal an improvement in liver histology, whereas superinfection with hepatitis D is usually associated with deterioration in histology in up to one third of patients and an acceleration of the disease process.

In sum, although histologic appearance is important, liver biopsy provides only a measure of disease at one point in time. In chronic hepatitis B, the degree of virus replication activity may be the best predictor of prognosis. *Lifelong infection* with HBV, such as occurs primarily among those infected at or shortly after birth, is associated with an increased risk of *hepatocellular carcinoma*, whether cirrhosis is present or not.

Hepatitis C. Episodic bursts of inflammatory activity often punctuate the clinical course of patients whose liver biopsies show mild chronic hepatitis C. As with hepatitis B, histologic features of chronic hepatitis C can change, and even patients with clinically and histologically mild chronic hepatitis C can progress insidiously and slowly to cirrhosis. Chronic hepatitis C is commonly associated with erosion of the limiting plate of periportal hepatocytes (piecemeal necrosis) but rarely with clinical or histologic criteria for severe chronic hepatitis (10-fold elevation of aminotransferase activity, disabling symptoms, multilobular collapse). Still, despite this apparent relative benignity, chronic hepatitis C may progress insidiously, even in the absence of symptoms or marked elevations in aminotransferase activity, and it may lead to cirrhosis in 20% of cases within 10 to 20 years. Although a wide range of frequencies of progression to cirrhosis has been reported, and although most patients with chronic hepatitis C do very well with limited clinical consequences over several decades, patients with longstanding chronic infection often demonstrate histologic progression. Although a correlation exists between HBV replication and disease progression, a similar correlation between HCV replication and disease progression cannot be demonstrated invariably. Among the several variables associated with progression in chronic hepatitis C, duration of infection is important; however, the best clinical predictor of progression may be histologic stage and grade. Mild inflammation and necrosis and mild fibrosis characterize a cohort of patients with an excellent prognosis and limited progression to cirrhosis over time, whereas moderate to severe necrosis/inflammation and/or fibrosis in the absence of successful therapeutic intervention (see later discussion) portend progression to cirrhosis almost invariably over one to two decades.

Nonviral (Autoimmune, Idiopathic) Chronic Hepatitis

An autoimmune mechanism is believed to account for many cases of nonviral chronic hepatitis. The severity of histologic change may have a degree of prognostic value. Like other autoimmune diseases, the condition predominates in women between the ages of 20 and 40 years. An acute form with severe fatigue, jaundice, fever, amenorrhea, and anorexia sometimes occurs, but many patients present asymptomatically. Extrahepatic manifestations, including arthritis, rash, and thyroiditis, are common, whereas others, such as glomerulonephritis and pleuropericarditis, occur only rarely. Asymptomatic patients are typically discovered when an incidental modest elevation in aminotransferase levels is noted on routine testing. Marked elevation in *gamma globulin* (more than two times normal) is characteristic, as are high titers of *antinuclear antibody* and *antibody to smooth muscle*. Enzyme immunoassays for antibody to hepatitis C may yield false-positive readings in such patients; therefore, in patients with what appears to be autoimmune hepatitis, if screening tests for anti-HCV are reactive, a confirmatory test, such as a test for HCV RNA, should be done. The bilirubin may be higher than in viral hepatitis. Histology and disease activity are important determinants of prognosis for nonviral chronic hepatitis.

Untreated severe autoimmune hepatitis (defined by disabling symptoms, sustained aminotransferase elevations more than 10 times normal, gamma globulin levels twice normal, and bridging or multilobular collapse on biopsy) may progress to cirrhosis and eventual death. The 6-month fatality rate in the absence of therapy is 40% in patients with these findings. Bridging or multilobular necrosis on liver biopsy is associated with cirrhosis in 40% and death in 20% of patients after 5 years. In contrast, patients with less severe disease (piecemeal necrosis alone, minimal symptoms) are usually not at substantial risk for death, and progression to cirrhosis is rare (3% to 10%).

Mild autoimmune chronic hepatitis has a good prognosis in most cases but is not uniformly benign. This lesion has been documented to deteriorate to more severe chronic hepatitis and to progress to cirrhosis in certain patients, such as those with an initial histologic diagnosis of severe hepatitis whose liver biopsies improve with therapy and in immunosuppressed patients with a histologic diagnosis of mild chronic hepatitis.

Nonalcoholic Fatty Liver Disease

Fatty liver accounts for approximately 20% of patients referred to specialists for the evaluation of abnormal liver biochemical tests. Among this group, a large majority have simple *fatty infiltration* of the liver, but a small proportion have fatty infiltration accompanied by necrosis and inflammation (nonalcoholic steatohepatitis [NASH]) including neutrophilic infiltration, and the presence of Mallory's hyaline, reminiscent of alcohol-associated liver injury. Simple fatty infiltration tends to be entirely benign and even responds to weight reduction; however, NASH can be progressive and accompanied by fibrosis. According to current estimates, NASH culminates in cirrhosis in approximately 15% of cases, and NASH is believed to be the most common cause of so-called "cryptogenic" cirrhosis. Nonalcoholic steatohepatitis is associated with insulin resistance and the "metabolic syndrome" and occurs in as many as 50% of patients with diabetes mellitus and of obese persons and is almost universal in the morbidly obese; however, steatosis can occur in the absence of obesity. Liver biopsy is the only reliable method for establishing a diagnosis of nonalcoholic fatty liver disease and for distinguishing between simple fatty infiltration and NASH. The likelihood of NASH is increased in patients with a body mass index exceeding 30, type 2 diabetes, age greater than 45 years, and a ratio of aspartate aminotransferase to alanine aminotransferase exceeding 1.

PRINCIPLES OF MANAGEMENT
(1–4,9–35)

Acute Viral Hepatitis

Because it is a generally benign and self-limited illness, acute viral hepatitis can be managed in most cases on an outpatient basis. Hospitalization should be reserved for high-risk patients (e.g., elderly or immunocompromised patients, patients with difficult-to-manage underlying chronic diseases) and those with signs of severe hepatocellular injury (e.g., marked prothrombin time prolongation, encephalopathy, ascites and edema, hypoglycemia, or hypoalbuminemia) and/or with inability to maintain oral intake. Other than specific antiviral therapy (see later discussion), specific therapy for acute viral hepatitis is not available or necessary to accelerate convalescence or prevent sequelae. The usual goals of care are to maintain *adequate nutrition* and *patient comfort*, to *avoid* additional *hepatocellular insults* from hepatotoxic medications and alcohol, and to *prevent the spread* of infection to others.

Neither *specific dietary manipulations, corticosteroids,* nor strict *bedrest* has any beneficial effect on the course or prognosis of acute uncomplicated or acute severe viral hepatitis. *Oral contraceptives* do not necessarily need to be stopped, but *alcohol* intake should cease, and the use of other drugs known to cause liver injury should be discontinued or monitored carefully. *Exercise* does not interfere with recovery; patients should be encouraged to engage in as much physical activity as they can tolerate without discomfort or undue fatigue.

Symptoms may be incapacitating. Nausea and vomiting can be controlled by the cautious use of antiemetics; however, because phenothiazines cause cholestatic hepatitis in approximately 1% of patients, *nonphenothiazine antiemetics,* such as *trimethobenzamide,* should be used. Small *frequent feedings,* especially in the morning when nausea is at a low ebb, can ensure adequate calorie intake. No specific foods need to be restricted, although some patients with acute hepatitis cannot tolerate fatty foods. In patients with cholestasis and pruritus, the bile-sequestering resin *cholestyramine* usually provides relief. The identification of a patient with acute viral hepatitis should prompt consideration of prophylactic measures to limit the spread of infection to contacts (see Chapter 57).

Hepatitis A and E

Therapy for acute hepatitis A and E is not available; instead, management relies on the nonspecific measures reviewed previously.

Hepatitis B

Because patients with clinically apparent acute hepatitis B almost always recover, specific antiviral therapy is not indicated. For the unfortunate 1% to 2% of immunologically competent patients with clinically apparent acute hepatitis who remain chronically infected, antiviral therapy can be instituted once chronicity has been documented. In patients with severe, rapidly progressive, or fulminant acute hepatitis B, anecdotal reports support the use of one of the oral polymerase inhibitors (see later discussion).

Hepatitis C

For patients with acute hepatitis C, antiviral therapy during early acute hepatitis has been shown to reduce the frequency of chronicity and is recommended (see later discussion). Most authorities recommend treatment for at least 6 months with standard doses of pegylated interferon once a week plus ribavirin daily in patients with acute hepatitis C; however, the optimal doses and duration of therapy have not been determined. In clinical practice, such acute cases are encountered primarily among health workers who sustain accidental needle sticks or other percutaneous exposures and among injection-drug users.

Monitoring and Follow-Up

The patient is monitored clinically by observing symptoms and checking liver biochemical tests, especially those that reflect hepatocellular function. An *aminotransferase* level obtained weekly at the outset and then monthly is useful for judging the presence of ongoing disease, although the absolute level is not a particularly sensitive determinant of disease severity in the acute phase of illness. *Prothrombin time* is a good measure of hepatocellular synthetic function and should be checked when the patient presents initially and when worsening is suspected. *Serum bilirubin,* a marker of hepatic excretory function, also correlates with severity. A fall in *serum albumin* indicates reduced hepatocellular synthetic function, but because its half-life is 28 days, this change does not become apparent until late in the acute illness.

An office visit 1 to 2 weeks after the first presentation is often helpful to be sure that worsening has not occurred and that the patient is managing satisfactorily. Thereafter, follow-up depends on how well the patient feels. At 3 months, a repeat aminotransferase, bilirubin, albumin, prothrombin time, and, in cases of hepatitis B, *HBsAg* and *HBeAg* determinations should be performed to ascertain disease activity, severity, and viral antigen status.

If symptoms and laboratory evidence of activity persist after 3 months, repeat evaluations at monthly intervals are indicated. *Liver biopsy* is not indicated in patients with acute viral hepatitis unless clinical suspicion of chronic hepatitis is present and/or the information obtained has the potential to influence management decisions.

Fulminant Acute Hepatitis

In those rare instances when follow-up reveals the rapid development of fulminant acute viral hepatitis, corticosteroid therapy has been shown not only to be ineffective but also to be detrimental and should not be used. In most cases, specific medical therapy has not been shown to be effective. The best approach involves meticulous attention to the details of the multisystem dysfunction that accompanies acute liver failure. Such patients should be admitted to an intensive care unit and considered for early referral to a transplantation center. *Liver transplantation* is the only intervention that has truly life-saving potential. With timely transplantation, survival rates exceeding 60% are possible. Recurrent viral hepatitis may occur in the new liver, but not invariably, and antiviral therapy for hepatitis B and C can be used after transplantation to reduce the impact of reinfection. Experimental trials have been done to assess a variety of hepatic assist devices, but none has been proven effective. As noted, reversal of acute fulminant hepatitis B has been observed anecdotally with the early administration of a nucleoside analogue polymerase inhibitor, as reported with the use of lamivudine (see later discussion).

Drug-Induced Hepatitis

Treatment is largely supportive. All possible offending agents should be stopped; immunosuppressive and antiinflammatory drugs are of no benefit. Acetaminophen hepatotoxicity is treated with oral *N*-acetylcysteine begun as soon as possible after exposure to toxic doses, preferably within 8 hours, but it is effective even after 24 to 36 hours. After an initial loading dose, the treatment is continued every 4 hours until a total of 15 to 20 doses has been administered.

Chronic Viral Hepatitis

Treatment of chronic viral hepatitis depends on the cause and the severity of disease. Therapy focuses on the termination of viral replication. Immunosuppression, which is useful in nonviral hepatitis (see later discussion), has no place and may even be detrimental, resulting as it does in an increase in viral replication. Therapeutic decisions may be made independent of histologic severity, but *liver biopsy* is indicated to establish the presence of necroinflammatory liver disease, to assess the stage and the grade of the disease, and to exclude other causes for abnormal liver chemistry tests (e.g., infiltration with fat or iron). In patients considered for antiviral therapy, a brief period of observation before instituting treatment may be helpful to ensure that the patient is not in the process of spontaneous improvement.

Hepatitis B

Antiviral therapy is the cornerstone of treatment, and two categories of agents are available: parenteral preparations of *interferon alfa* and oral inhibitors of viral replication, including the nucleoside analogues (*lamivudine, entecavir,* and *telbivudine*) and the nucleotide analogues (*adefovir* and *tenofovir*).

Candidates for Therapy. Criteria for therapy include the following:

- HBV DNA exceeding 10^4 copies/mL
- Elevated alanine aminotransferase (ALT) levels
- Histologic evidence of hepatitis

Both those patients with HBeAg-reactive disease (associated with high HBV DNA levels [10^6 to 10^9 copies/mL]) and those who are HBeAg-negative (associated with lower levels [10^4 to 10^6 copies/mL]) are candidates for antiviral therapy. All available agents (interferon, pegylated interferon, lamivudine, adefovir, entecavir, telbivudine, tenofovir) can be used as first-line therapy.

Antiviral therapy is recommended for patients with detectable HBV DNA at a level of greater than 2×10^4 IU/mL if ALT levels are elevated (more than twice the upper limit of normal) in both HBeAg-reactive and HBeAg-negative patients. If ALT levels are normal, even in the presence of high-level hepatitis B viremia, therapy is not begun. For inactive carriers, no therapy is indicated. For patients with high-level viremia but with modest ALT levels (one to two times the upper limit of normal), a liver biopsy to assess the degree of fibrosis and inflammatory activity may be useful to help in decision making about beginning therapy. For patients with cirrhosis and detectable HBV DNA, antiviral therapy is advised to prevent or delay decompensation; referral to a transplantation center (see later discussion) should be initiated for patients with decompensated chronic hepatitis B.

Interferon. Interferon alfa was the first antiviral drug to be approved for the treatment of chronic hepatitis B. Treatment consists of a 16-week course of either daily subcutaneous injections of 5 million units or thrice-weekly injections of 10 million units.

Efficacy. When given to patients with compensated replicative chronic hepatitis B (i.e., with circulating HBV DNA at levels $\geq 10^5$ to 10^6 virions/mL and HBeAg), approximately 30% experience seroconversion to nonreplicative infection (loss of HBeAg and reduction in HBV DNA). About one fourth of responders in early trials (just <10% of the total) also lost detectable HBsAg. Improvements in serum aminotransferase activity and liver histology also occur in those with sustained reductions in viral replication. Among patients who respond, improvement in the natural history of the disease (80% clearing of HBsAg over the decade after therapy), improved survival without decompensation, and reduced risk of hepatocellular carcinoma have been documented.

Candidacy. Interferon is effective in patients with *compensated replicative chronic hepatitis B* (modest levels of HBV replication, elevated aminotransferase activity, HBeAg). HBeAg-negative patients may also respond if treatment is extended for 1 year or longer (up to 20% achieve a durable suppression of HBV replication and the maintenance of normal ALT activity).

Interferon is ineffective in those with very high levels of HBV replication and in those with normal or near-normal aminotransferase activity. Others not responding well include immunosuppressed patients and persons infected in early childhood. In decompensated patients, the acute hepatitis-like exacerbation ("hepatitis flare") that can accompany successful interferon therapy may precipitate liver failure, rendering them poor candidates for routine interferon treatment.

Adverse Effects. Major adverse effects of interferon include *flulike symptoms, fatigue, marrow suppression, irritability* (and other emotional disturbances, including *depression* and anxiety), and autoimmune *thyroiditis* (rarely, other autoimmune disorders). Successful interferon therapy is often accompanied by a transient, acute, hepatitis-like *elevation in aminotransferase* activity, which is believed to represent an enhancement of cell-mediated immune cytolysis of HBV-infected hepatocytes. *Transient hair loss*, rashes, and gastrointestinal disturbances occur in some patients. Almost all interferon-associated adverse effects, with the notable exception of autoimmune thyroiditis, are reversible, resolving when therapy is discontinued.

Pegylated Interferon. Sustained response rates are achieved by binding interferons to polyethylene glycol (pegylating). Pegylated interferon (PEG IFN) preparations have supplanted standard interferon due to their longer half-lives and slower elimination, allowing once-a-week subcutaneous administration and achieving a prolonged concentration plateau. Long-acting, once-weekly *pegylated interferon* is now an approved treatment for chronic hepatitis B. Easier to tolerate and administer and more effective than standard interferon, PEG IFN has supplanted interferon as therapy for hepatitis B.

Efficacy. Compared with lamivudine in HBeAg-positive patients, PEG IFN is not as potent in suppressing HBV DNA during therapy; however, 24 weeks after the completion of therapy it achieves durable HBeAg seroconversion in 32% compared to only 19% of patients treated with lamivudine, and it suppresses HBV DNA to undetectable levels in 14% versus 5% of cases. The combination PEG IFN–lamivudine suppresses HBV DNA more profoundly than either drug alone during treatment but is inferior to PEG IFN monotherapy in HBeAg seroconversion. HBsAg seroconversion does not occur during treatment but can emerge at 24 weeks posttreatment in a small number of patients. In HBeAg-negative patients, combination therapy suppresses HBV DNA more profoundly than either drug alone; however, combination therapy shows no advantage in maintaining HBV DNA suppression over PEG IFN monotherapy, which is superior to lamivudine at 24 weeks after treatment in (19% vs. 7%).

Adverse Effects. PEG IFN is associated with the usual interferon side effects, as enumerated above, but not with antiviral drug resistance.

Lamivudine. Lamivudine, a potent inhibitor of HBV and HIV reverse transcriptase, was the first nucleoside analogue approved for routine use in patients with chronic hepatitis B. Lamivudine does not require injections, has no appreciable side effects, and is at least as effective as, if not more effective than, standard interferon. It established oral polymerase inhibition as a viable approach to antiviral therapy for patients with chronic hepatitis B and serves as the standard against which newer agents were evaluated. Newer oral antiviral agents (see later discussion) either are more effective or are associated with reduced resistance, relegating lamivudine monotherapy to increasing obsolescence, but its low cost and well-established safety record (including during late pregnancy) make it useful when resources are limited. In addition, many patients with hepatitis B who began therapy with lamivudine are currently being treated effectively with a combination of lamivudine and one of the newer agents.

Efficacy. Daily doses of 100 mg (one third of the dose for HIV infection) suppress HBV DNA by a median of $5.5 \log_{10}$ copies/mL in HBeAg-positive chronic hepatitis B and $4.5 \log_{10}$ copies/mL in HBeAg-negative chronic hepatitis B and are equally effective in patients who have failed interferon therapy and in treatment-naive patients. A 12-month course of therapy results in HBeAg loss in approximately 30% of cases, seroconversion from HBeAg to anti-HBe in approximately 16% to 20%, normalization of alanine aminotransferase in 40% to 80%, and histologic improvement in more than one half to two thirds of patients. Among the histologic changes are a reduction in necroinflammatory activity in 60% and a halting of progression to fibrosis in 20% of patients. Compared with placebo recipients, patients treated with lamivudine are less likely during 1 year of therapy to progress to cirrhosis. Among those with HBeAg responses (loss or seroconversion), the antiviral response is durable in approximately 80%; a durable HBeAg response lasting at least 6 months (preferably longer in Asian patients, who are more likely to reactivate) can be used as a milestone for discontinuing therapy. In the absence of an HBeAg response, however, continued therapy is required.

Although lamivudine suppresses HBV replication substantially in almost all patients (to undetectable levels in 40% to 70% of cases), a sustained response is less likely in patients with normal aminotransferase activity and in patients with precore HBV variants (HBeAg-negative chronic hepatitis B), who nevertheless do benefit histologically and biochemically. After discontinuation of therapy, however, in the absence of an HBeAg response, aminotransferase elevations (acute hepatitis-like flares) occur in 20% to 30% of patients, but these flares are transient and clinically mild in most cases.

Close monitoring after discontinuing therapy is essential for identifying and retreating severe posttreatment exacerbations. Losses of HBsAg are uncommon during lamivudine therapy but are observed after therapy in patients with HBeAg loss. Among those who are treated for several years, fibrosis, even cirrhosis, can be reversed, and maintenance therapy in compensated cirrhotic patients has been shown to reduce the occurrence of hepatic decompensation, eligibility for liver transplantation, and even hepatocellular carcinoma. Lamivudine, unlike interferon, can be used in patients with decompensated cirrhosis; it can reverse decompensation in a substantial proportion of patients and may delay or avoid the need for liver transplantation.

Resistance. The frequency of HBeAg responses increases with each year of lamivudine therapy (up to 50% after 5 years), but the downside of long-term therapy is the emergence of viral *resistance*. In one fourth of patients treated for 1 year and in up to 70% of those treated for 5 years, a viral mutation emerges in the tyrosine-methionine, aspartate-aspartate ("YMDD") motif of the HBV DNA polymerase. Although YMDD mutants are less responsive to lamivudine than is wild-type HBV, measures of disease activity remain well below baseline levels, perhaps because, initially and until other compensatory mutations emerge, mutants tend to replicate less effectively than wild-type

HBV. The withdrawal of lamivudine results invariably in a return of wild-type HBV and more severe liver injury.

Eventually, in YMDD-mutant chronic hepatitis B, liver histology tends to deteriorate and clinical response is lost; fortunately, lamivudine-resistant chronic hepatitis B can be managed effectively with adefovir or tenofovir (see later discussion), and such treatment is instituted when lamivudine resistance is recognized. Although specialized assays have been developed to detect YMDD mutations, lamivudine resistance can be identified reliably by the detection of reproducible increases in HBV DNA among patients in whom virus replication had been suppressed effectively. In patients with hepatitis B, beginning with monotherapy has proven effective, an approach that would not work for other viral diseases, such as HIV/AIDS. In the future, however, multidrug regimens that preempt the emergence of viral resistance are likely to be introduced.

Adverse Effects. Lamivudine has no recognized side effects or effects on nonhepatic laboratory values; transient elevations in aminotransferase activity occur in about one fourth of patients but no more frequently than in placebo recipients. Posttreatment flares may follow the cessation of therapy; therefore, patients should be monitored closely for several months after discontinuing lamivudine therapy, and therapy should be reinstituted if severe hepatitis B reactivation occurs.

Adefovir Dipivoxil. Adefovir dipivoxil, a nucleotide analogue inhibitor of HBV DNA polymerase administered orally at a daily dose of 10 mg, reduces HBV DNA by 3.5 to $4 \log_{10}$ copies/mL. Like lamivudine, adefovir suppresses HBV DNA both in interferon nonresponders and treatment-naive patients and both in HBeAg-reactive and HBeAg-negative chronic hepatitis B. Likewise, adefovir is going to become progressively less attractive as an antiviral agent for hepatitis B because of late resistance, relatively late and inferior suppression of HBV DNA, low rate of HBeAg seroconversion, and high proportion of primary nonresponders compared to newer oral agents (especially tenofovir; see later discussion). Still, because adefovir had been used extensively for more than 5 years, many patients in whom it was effective, either as initial therapy or as rescue therapy for patients with lamivudine resistance, continue to be treated with this antiviral drug.

Efficacy. In placebo-controlled clinical trials of 48 weeks of therapy, adefovir was shown to result in histologic improvement and the normalization of alanine aminotransferase activity in approximately 50% of patients with HBeAg-positive chronic hepatitis B and in more than two thirds of patients with HBeAg-negative chronic hepatitis B, HBeAg loss in 24%, HBeAg seroconversion in 12%, and suppression of HBV DNA to levels undetectable by polymerase chain reaction amplification (fewer than 10^2 to 10^3 copies/mL) in 21% of HBeAg-reactive and 51% of HBeAg-negative patients. Like lamivudine, adefovir retards the progression of fibrosis. Like interferon and lamivudine, adefovir is more likely to achieve HBeAg seroconversion in patients with elevated aminotransferase levels. The durability of HBeAg responses is similar to that achieved after lamivudine therapy; as is true for lamivudine, adefovir needs to be continued, perhaps indefinitely, in HBeAg-reactive patients who fail to achieve an HBeAg response and in virtually all patients with HBeAg-negative chronic hepatitis B.

Resistance. Resistance to adefovir has not been encountered among immunocompetent patients during the first year of therapy; thereafter, the frequency of resistance is negligible initially, 2.5% at the end of year 2, but increases to approximately 30% at the end of year 4. This level of resistance compares very favorably against the approximately 25%-year-1 and approximately 70%-year-5 resistance encountered during lamivudine therapy. Moreover, adefovir is effective in patients with lamivudine-resistant, YMDD-mutant chronic hepatitis B, reducing HBV DNA levels by approximately 4 $\log_{10}$ copies/mL and restoring responsiveness to antiviral therapy. When adefovir is used to treat patients with lamivudine resistance, adefovir should be *added* to lamivudine because the presence of lamivudine is likely to prevent the emergence of future adefovir resistance.

Adverse Effects. When used at higher doses than the 10 mg recommended for chronic hepatitis B, adefovir can cause reversible renal tubular injury, reflected clinically by the elevation of serum creatinine; however, at daily doses of 10 mg, creatinine elevations exceeding 0.5 mg/dL are rarely encountered. Nevertheless, creatinine monitoring is recommended (see later discussion). The frequency of adefovir dosing is reduced for patients with underlying renal insufficiency. Otherwise, adefovir is very well tolerated and is indistinguishable from placebo in causing side effects. Like lamivudine, adefovir can be associated with elevations of alanine aminotransferase levels during therapy, as HBV DNA falls, and after the discontinuation of therapy, as HBV DNA returns to pretreatment baseline.

Entecavir. Entecavir, a guanosine nucleoside analogue, appears to be the most potent of the available agents in suppressing HBV DNA.

Efficacy. In HBeAg-positive patients taking a daily dose of 0.5 mg, entecavir markedly suppressed HBV DNA (by 6.9 $\log_{10}$ copies/mL). In a major study, therapy suppressed HBV DNA to undetectable levels in 67% of cases, resulted in histologic improvement in 72%, and led to a return to normal of alanine aminotransferase activity in 68%, but HBeAg seroconversion occurred in only 21%. For those who had not achieved an HBeAg seroconversion and who were treated longer, the benefit of therapy continued; HBV DNA was undetectable at years 2 and 3 of therapy in 81% and 87%, respectively. Cumulative HBeAg seroconversion increased to 31% at 96 weeks and 39% at 144 weeks. The durability and predictors of HBeAg responses are similar to those for lamivudine. Moreover, among patients with HBeAg treated for 2 years, HBsAg loss occurred in 5%. In patients with HBeAg-negative chronic hepatitis B, 48 weeks of entecavir therapy resulted in histologic improvement in 70%, undetectable HBV DNA in 90%, and a return to normal of alanine aminotransferase in 78%.

Resistance. The barrier to entecavir resistance is high; in registration trials, no antiviral resistance was encountered during years 1 and 2 of entecavir therapy, and, when therapy was extended for up to 4 years in the subset who continued and were monitored for that long, the frequency of resistance was less than 1%. At a higher daily dose of 1.0 mg, entecavir is also effective against (and has been approved for) lamivudine-resistant chronic hepatitis B; however, in lamivudine-resistant patients, entecavir resistance has been encountered in 7% during year 1, another 9% during year 2, and up to approximately 40% at the end of 4 years. Therefore, most authorities do not recommend entecavir for lamivudine-resistant chronic hepatitis B.

Adverse Effects. Flares of alanine aminotransferase during and after treatment are less likely and lower in amplitude during

and after entecavir treatment than with lamivudine. In clinical trials, entecavir was comparable in tolerability to lamivudine.

Telbivudine. A cytosine analogue, telbivudine is almost as potent as entecavir, but its usefulness is reduced by the emergence of resistance in a substantial proportion of patients, making the drug less useful than more potent agents with a higher barrier to resistance, for example, entecavir.

Efficacy. Telbivudine suppresses of HBV DNA at 1 year by 6.5 $\log_{10}$ copies/mL in HBeAg-reactive and 5.2 $\log_{10}$ copies/mL in HBeAg-negative chronic hepatitis B. When tested against a lamivudine control, it was superior suppressing HBV DNA both at the end of 1 and 2 years but not in achieving histologic and biochemical improvement or HBeAg seroconversion (in the HBeAg-reactive group). The durability of HBeAg responses is similar to that for the other oral agents, approximately 80%.

Resistance. Telbivudine and lamivudine are cross-resistant; therefore, telbivudine cannot be used to treat lamivudine resistance. The frequency of resistance is lower than that for lamivudine, especially during the first year of therapy, but resistance emerged in clinical trials among 22% of HBeAg-reactive and 9% of HBeAg-negative patients. Some have suggested assessing the rapidity of HBV DNA suppression at 6 months during telbivudine therapy and making a determination then to continue therapy if suppression is profound (which is associated with a very low rate of resistance through 1 year of therapy).

Adverse Effects. Telbivudine appears to be comparably safe to lamivudine, although asymptomatic elevations of creatine kinase are more common, and rare reports of myopathy have appeared.

Tenofovir. Tenofovir is a nucleotide analogue that was approved in 2001 to treat HIV/AIDS and that has proven to be more potent than adefovir in suppressing HBV DNA, both in patients with HIV/HBV coinfection and those with HBV infection alone. The drug was approved for hepatitis B in 2008 and is likely to supplant adefovir for use in hepatitis B. Preliminary evidence suggests that it is effective in lamivudine-resistant chronic hepatitis B; it has been used "off-label" for this indication since its initial release in 2001.

Efficacy. Under study conditions in HBeAg-negative patients, 1 year of tenofovir achieved the suppression of HBV DNA (<400 copies/mL) and histologic improvement in 71%, compared to 49% in the adefovir group. In a similar study among HBeAg-positive patients, this composite endpoint was observed in 67%, compared to 12% for adefovir. The profundity of HBV DNA suppression was impressive, and in the HBeAg-positive group, 3% experienced HBsAg seroconversions. Tenofovir was not superior in histologic response or in HBeAg seroconversion.

Resistance and Adverse Effects. No resistance was encountered to tenofovir during a 1-year trial. The drug has an excellent safety profile, but creatinine monitoring is advisable during therapy.

Monitoring and Follow-Up. For all patients undergoing treatment, monitoring of liver tests and HBeAg status helps to detect resistance to treatment, especially for oral-agent therapy. *Aminotransferase levels* are checked once a month during the early months of therapy and subsequently at 3-month intervals; *bilirubin* and *albumin* are checked periodically. At a minimum,

HBeAg status is tested at the end of therapy, but interval testing (every 3 to 6 months) during therapy can be helpful.

For patients treated with interferon or PEG IFN, the monitoring of *white blood cell* and *platelet counts* is indicated at 1- to 3-month intervals to detect marrow suppression. The testing of thyroid function (*thyroid-stimulating hormone*) at 1- to 3-month intervals identifies patients with thyroiditis who are candidates for the reduction or cessation of treatment or initiation of thyroid hormone–replacement therapy.

Patients treated with adefovir or tenofovir should have a baseline *creatinine* determination followed by periodic creatinine monitoring beginning 6 to 8 months after the onset of therapy.

Choice of Antiviral Therapy. Because 1 year of finite PEG IFN therapy is superior to 1 year of finite lamivudine therapy, some authorities prefer PEG IFN as first-line therapy over lamivudine or, for that matter, any other oral agent. On the other hand, PEG IFN and oral agents are not used the same way. Whereas weekly injections of PEG IFN are used for 1 year, oral agents are continued until after HBeAg seroconversion or indefinitely (in HBeAg-reactive patients without an HBeAg response and in virtually all HBeAg-negative patients). Moreover, the HBeAg responses that are achieved after 1 year of PEG IFN, with its associated weekly injections, often distracting side effects, and requirement for physician attention, can be achieved after an additional 6 to 12 months of oral agent therapy with virtually no side effects and with limited physician supervision. Even HBsAg responses occur in patients treated with oral agents, again, after a longer period of treatment. Similarly, the absence of resistance, another advantage for PEG IFN, is less of an issue with the newer generation of potent oral agents, entecavir and tenofovir.

Generally, consensus statements from recommending bodies and agencies support PEG IFN and oral agents equally, especially the new generation of potent oral drugs with limited resistance, but oral agents are more popular, especially in the United States. Patients with decompensated chronic hepatitis B are not candidates for interferon-based therapy but may respond to oral agents, sometimes with a reversal of clinical signs of decompensation. Similarly, patients with compensated cirrhosis are candidates for maintenance oral-agent, but not interferon-based, therapy to prevent decompensation.

Liver Transplantation. Patients with decompensated chronic hepatitis B or with acute fulminant hepatitis B are candidates for liver transplantation. The success of liver transplantation for chronic hepatitis B is approximately 75% now that antiviral regimens are offered routinely. The most common approach is a combination of high-dose hepatitis B immune globulin plus a potent oral agent with a high barrier to resistance.

Hepatitis D

Interferon achieves reductions in hepatitis D virus RNA and a fall in aminotransferase activity, but the cessation of therapy is followed commonly by a return of these markers to pretreatment levels. Long-term, high-dose interferon or PEG IFN therapy continued for a full year may produce more durable results, and multiyear therapy may be required to control the disease. Corticosteroid therapy is ineffective. Currently approved oral agents are not effective for hepatitis D. *Liver transplantation* has been successful in patients with end-stage disease, with an outcome better than that for hepatitis B alone.

Hepatitis C

Major advances in the treatment of chronic hepatitis C have been made possible with the availability of interferons and the nucleoside analogue ribavirin. Candidates for antiviral therapy include those with *compensated chronic hepatitis C* and *moderate to severe chronic hepatitis on liver biopsy*. Patients with normal and near-normal aminotransferase activity and histologically *mild disease* tend to do reasonably well without therapy, but combination therapy with PEG IFN and ribavirin is now recommended, having been shown to be just as effective as in those with more severe disease. Decompensated patients are unlikely to respond. Cirrhosis per se is not a contraindication to antiviral therapy, but maintenance therapy in cirrhotic patients does not prevent hepatocellular carcinoma or other complications of cirrhosis. Corticosteroids have never proven useful in the treatment of chronic viral hepatitis.

Quantitative testing for *HCV RNA* level should be determined before therapy as a baseline against which to monitor virologic response during therapy. Similarly, *HCV genotype* should be evaluated prior to therapy to determine the duration of treatment (24 weeks for patients with genotypes 2 and 3; 48 weeks for patients with genotype 1).

Interferon Alfa. Interferon alfa at a subcutaneous dose of 3 million units three times a week for 6 months normalizes aminotransferase levels (biochemical response) in 50% of patients and reduces HCV RNA to undetectable levels in 25% (virologic response). Histologic improvement occurs in up to 75% by the end of therapy. However, relapse is high, yielding a sustained virologic response rate (measured at least 6 months after the completion of therapy) of less than 10%. The frequency of sustained virologic responses can be doubled by increasing the duration therapy to 12 months; neither dose escalation, switching from one nonpegylated interferon preparation to another, nor induction therapy with initial high-dose intensive regimens enhances responsiveness. Standard interferon alfa has been supplemented by pegylated interferon.

Pegylated Interferons (PEG IFN). Pegylated interferon preparations (interferons bound to polyethylene glycol) have a longer half-life and slower elimination, offering once-a-week subcutaneous administration, a prolonged concentration plateau, and sustained response rates twice those of nonpegylated preparations.

Two PEG IFNs are available: 12-kD PEG IFN alfa-2b (administered at a weight-based dose of 1.5 µg/kg) and 40-kD PEG IFN alfa-2a (administered at a weight-independent dose of 180 µg). The likelihood of a response to interferon is increased in patients with *low-level HCV RNA* (<2 million copies/mL or 800 IU/mL) and in those with HCV *genotypes 2 and 3*. Long-term virologic and biochemical monitoring after sustained virologic responses have shown that a sustained virologic response is almost always durable for many years and is tantamount to a "cure."

Combination Pegylated Interferon plus Ribavirin Therapy. Although ribavirin monotherapy is ineffective, ribavirin in combination with PEG IFN reduces the occurrence of posttreatment relapse, yielding sustained overall virologic response rates of approximately 55%. Combination PEG IFN plus the oral nucleoside analogue ribavirin represents first-line therapy for chronic hepatitis C and is the *treatment of choice*.

Efficacy. For patients with hepatitis C genotype 1, responsiveness to treatment is less than that with genotypes 2 and 3; a full 48-week course of combination therapy is warranted and ribavirin doses of 1,000-1,200 mg daily are required. Sustained response rates of 42% to 51% have been reported. For patients with hepatitis C genotypes 2 and 3, 24 weeks of combination therapy suffice to achieve sustained response rates of approximately 80%; moreover, only daily ribavirin doses of 800 mg are required. Contraindications include coronary artery disease, cerebrovascular disease, anemia, pregnancy, and renal failure (see later discussion).

The rapidity of antiviral suppression is predictive of the ultimate likelihood of a sustained virologic response. Patients who manifest a *rapid virologic response* (HCV RNA suppressed to undetectable within 4 weeks) have a very high likelihood of a sustained virologic response. In the absence of an *early virologic response* (≥ 2-$\log_{10}$ reduction in HCV RNA at 12 weeks of therapy), almost no patient will achieve a sustained response. Whether to continue treatment after failure to achieve an early virologic response is debated.

In patients with genotype 1, especially those with a low baseline level of HCV RNA, as many as 90% with a rapid virologic response will achieve a sustained virologic response, even if therapy is contracted from 48 to 24 weeks. In the absence of a rapid virologic response, the likelihood of a sustained virologic response with only 48 weeks of therapy is low but can be improved by extending therapy for another 24 weeks. In patients with genotypes 2 and 3, some studies suggested that a full 24-week course of therapy may be shortened from 24 weeks to 12 to 16 weeks if a rapid response is achieved; however, a 24-week course of therapy is best, even in the presence of a rapid virologic response.

Besides genotype 1 and high HCV RNA level, other factors that predict reduced responsiveness to PEG IFN–ribavirin therapy include African American ethnicity, obesity, the presence of hepatic steatosis, age greater than 40 years, male gender, advanced histologic fibrosis, and poor adherence to the treatment regimen.

Pegylated interferon–ribavirin combination therapy is also effective in patients who relapsed after a course of interferon monotherapy, achieving sustained virologic responses in at least 50%. Combination therapy, however, has been less effective in nonresponders to a prior course of interferon (with or without ribavirin) therapy, resulting in a sustained virologic response in fewer than 20% of patients. In refractory nonresponders to optimal therapy, novel interferon preparations have not performed any better than PEG IFN–based therapy.

Side Effects. Most side effects of combination PEG IFN–ribavirin therapy are similar to those for interferon alone (see hepatitis B, prior discussion), but ribavirin can cause *hemolysis*, which is mild in most cases but severe and brisk (hemoglobin levels <10 g/dL) in approximately one fourth of patients. Therefore, combination therapy is contraindicated in patients who cannot tolerate anemia, including patients who are already anemic and those with, or with risk factors for, coronary artery disease or cerebrovascular disease, in whom anemia can result in a life-threatening ischemic event. Because ribavirin is renally excreted and teratogenic, the drug is *contraindicated* in patients with *renal insufficiency* and during *pregnancy* (birth control must be used in fertile patients who take ribavirin). Ribavirin can also cause *pruritus*, chest *congestion*, and *rashes* and can precipitate *gout* in susceptible patients. For patients with neutropenia or thrombocytopenia, PEG IFN dose reduction may be required; for those with ribavirin-associated anemia, the ribavirin dose may be reduced or exogenous erythropoietin added. Erythropoietin has been shown to improve patient quality of life but has not been proven to increase the rate of sustained virologic response.

Monitoring and Follow-Up. In patients taking ribavirin, monitoring for hemolysis is carried out by frequent monitoring of the *complete blood count*. During treatment, quantitative *HCV RNA* should be checked periodically; a reduction in HCV RNA of at least 2 $\log_{10}$ at 12 weeks is considered an early virologic response. Similarly, as noted previously, the level of HCV RNA should be checked at treatment week 4; if such a rapid virologic response occurs, the likelihood of a sustained virologic response is predictably very high. Finally, HCV RNA should be repeated at the end of therapy to document a complete end-treatment response, and in those with an end-treatment response, HCV RNA testing should be repeated intermittently over the next 6 months to document a sustained virologic response. Most authorities in the United States (but not in Europe) recommend a pretreatment liver biopsy to document that histologic necrosis/inflammation and fibrosis justify the initiation of treatment.

Novel Antiviral Agents. Several orally administered direct inhibitors of HCV polymerase and protease have been developed, and, in early trials, several of these, when combined with standard-of-care therapy (PEG IFN and ribavirin) have been found to inhibit HCV RNA profoundly and to result in a sustained virologic response after treatment courses as short as 12 to 24 weeks. The results of ongoing clinical trials are awaited.

Liver Transplantation. Liver transplantation is indicated for those with *end-stage decompensated chronic hepatitis C*. Although *reinfection* of the allograft is universal, its clinical effect on the new liver is negligible in most cases over the early years after transplantation; however, the rate of histologic progression is increased, and, eventually, patient survival is affected adversely. Contemporary antiviral therapy, even with the most optimal regimen of PEG IFN plus ribavirin, whether administered preemptively after transplantation or reflexively after the onset of recurrent HCV-associated liver injury, has met with limited success and a high frequency of intolerability in liver allograft recipients.

Nonviral (Autoimmune or Idiopathic) Chronic Hepatitis

Approaches to the therapy of nonviral and viral types of chronic hepatitis are distinctly different. In nonviral disease, histology plays a predominant role in determining prognosis, and immunosuppression is an important treatment modality in severe cases.

Mild Disease. In mild asymptomatic autoimmune and idiopathic forms of chronic hepatitis, the prognosis is excellent. *No treatment* beyond simple symptomatic relief is indicated. Long-term, high-dose immunosuppressive therapy (e.g., with prednisone) is not indicated because the high probability of adverse effects (see Chapter 105) outweighs any potential benefit. Additional randomized, controlled trials are needed better to define the efficacy of other forms of immunosuppressive therapy in such patients.

Moderate to Severe Disease. Moderate-to-severe chronic nonviral hepatitis tends to be a more serious and progressive disease. Severe cases have been shown to respond to *immunosuppressive–antiinflammatory* therapy (*prednisone-azathioprine*); however, only 15% to 20% of patients with autoimmune or idiopathic chronic hepatitis fulfill criteria for severe disease. The need for and efficacy of immunosuppressive therapy in symptomatic patients with less severe disease remains unknown.

Prednisone–Azathioprine. Immunosuppressive/antiinflammatory therapy with high-dose prednisone alone or the combination of reduced-dose prednisone plus azathioprine produces clinical, biochemical, and histologic remission in 80% of persons with severe disease and reduces mortality significantly. Histologic remission to mild hepatitis or to normal occurs within 6 to 36 months. In the prednisone-only regimen, treatment begins at 60 mg daily, and the dose is reduced over the course of 1 month to a maintenance level of 20 mg daily. Promising results have been obtained with lower-dose corticosteroid-only regimens in which the high-dose phase is omitted. The combination regimen is initiated with 30 mg daily of prednisone combined with 50 mg daily of azathioprine. The azathioprine dose remains constant, whereas the prednisone dose is reduced over the course of the first month to a daily maintenance level of 10 mg. Neither azathioprine alone nor alternate-day prednisone therapy has been found to be effective as an alternative regimen.

Adverse Effects. About two thirds of patients treated with high-dose corticosteroids alone experience severe steroid complications (see Chapter 105), compared with fewer than 20% of those treated with prednisone plus azathioprine. Azathioprine-induced bone marrow suppression may occur in patients receiving the combination-therapy regimen, necessitating close monitoring. Occasionally, unacceptable drug toxicity, intolerable gastrointestinal upset, compression fractures, or failure to respond necessitates the premature cessation of therapy.

Duration of Therapy. Therapy is continued until objective evidence of remission occurs (i.e., a fall in aminotransferase activity to a level below twice normal and improvement in morphologic features of chronic hepatitis). Although aminotransferase levels do not always reflect histologic activity absolutely faithfully, such biochemical monitoring has been documented to be valuable and a satisfactory substitute for repeat invasive biopsies. In responsive cases, symptoms improve within 6 months, aminotransferase levels within 12 months, and histology within 24 months. Rarely, treatment for more than 36 months is necessary to achieve remission. After 4 years, the likelihood of drug-induced complications becomes greater than the likelihood of beneficial drug effect. Nevertheless, many patients cannot be weaned from maintenance treatment and require the indefinite continuation of therapy.

Once remission is achieved, therapy is discontinued by a gradual tapering of prednisone over 6 weeks. Patients are monitored closely for signs of relapse, which occurs in 50% of patients. Relapse is especially common in patients with cirrhosis, often necessitating prolonged therapy for many years or multiple courses of treatment. Approximately 20% of patients fail to respond to conventional doses but may respond to higher doses. Relapses usually occur early. If remission lasts for more than 6 months after the cessation of therapy, relapse is less likely. Most cases of relapse are accompanied by symptoms and biochemical abnormalities, but in 10% of cases, the only sign of relapse is a change in histology. After relapse, 80% of patients respond again to the reinitiation of therapy. After the cessation of therapy, again, the relapse rate is 50%. The likelihood of relapse after combination prednisone–azathioprine therapy may be reduced by long-term maintenance azathioprine monotherapy after steroid withdrawal.

Monitoring and Follow-Up. In nonviral disease, patients with mild chronic hepatitis may be followed casually, but those who are symptomatic require careful monitoring and periodic reassessment to be sure that signs of progression do not materialize. When severe chronic disease has been identified, very close follow-up monitoring is vital. If prednisone and azathioprine are used, frequent periodic platelet and white blood cell counts are required. Aminotransferase, bilirubin, and gamma globulin levels should be obtained every 1 to 3 months to monitor response and to identify treatment failure. Patients with mild to moderate chronic disease who do not receive therapy should be monitored in similar fashion and biopsied again if symptoms or biochemical tests worsen.

Liver Transplantation. For patients with end-stage disease who have sustained a life-threatening complication, referral to a liver transplantation center is an appropriate consideration (see later discussion).

Nonalcoholic Fatty Liver Disease

For patients with simple fatty infiltration of the liver, weight reduction can result in improvement in hepatic steatosis; however, for patients with NASH, therapy has not been defined. Among the approaches considered are weight reduction, treatment of hyperlipidemia and diabetes mellitus, the use of antioxidants such as vitamin E, and treatment of insulin resistance (see Chapter 102); however, none of these treatments has been shown definitively to be effective in controlled trials. Because therapy for NASH has not been established, liver biopsy may be of only limited value for patient management, other than to provide relative prognostic information.

INDICATIONS FOR REFERRAL AND ADMISSION

Referral

Prompt consultation is indicated in most patients with fulminant or severe forms of hepatitis, whether viral or nonviral, because treatment decisions are difficult, and increasingly effective antiviral and immunosuppressive therapies are available.

Viral Hepatitis

Referral is indicated for consideration of liver biopsy when prognostic information or confirmation of disease severity is needed. Examples include patients with acute viral hepatitis B or C who fail to show signs of recovery within 6 months and who were not treated at the time of initial diagnosis and those with progressive or severe cases of chronic hepatitis B or C who might be candidates for antiviral therapy. Of particular importance is obtaining help from a hepatologist, gastroenterologist, or pathologist experienced in interpreting biopsy material from patients with chronic hepatitis. Antiviral therapy is evolving so rapidly, and the approach to antiviral therapy is sufficiently nuanced, that, generally, antiviral therapy is accomplished optimally by specialists; therefore, any patient who is a candidate for antiviral therapy should be referred.

Autoimmune and Idiopathic Chronic Hepatitis

Referral for biopsy to confirm the diagnosis is indicated for patients with suspected autoimmune or idiopathic chronic hepatitis (e.g., hyperglobulinemia, autoantibodies). Generally, immunosuppressive therapy should be initiated by a specialist, but, once initiated, therapy can be monitored by the patient's primary care physician with periodic review by the specialist.

Admission

Admission to the hospital is indicated for *worsening mental status*, *gastrointestinal bleeding*, *refractory ascites*, *coagulopathy*, or *poor home environment*. When decompensation does not respond readily to medical therapy, then referral to a *liver transplantation center* is indicated. Spontaneous or recurrent hepatic encephalopathy, wasting, refractory ascites and/or hepatic hydrothorax, variceal bleeding, and spontaneous bacterial peritonitis are among the indications for transplantation in patients with chronic liver disease. Given the long waiting time for a donor liver, patients should be referred as early as possible to be evaluated for transplantation candidacy.

PATIENT EDUCATION

Hepatitis often affects previously vigorous people accustomed to full activity. The prolonged course and magnitude of malaise may precipitate a reactive depression. Thorough explanation of the disease's course, design of a sensible treatment program that actively involves the patient and the family, and close follow-up can maximize compliance and minimize depression.

Instruction concerning diet and activity is central to a comprehensive treatment program. In particular, preventing the unnecessary restriction of activity is important, as is ensuring adequate nutrition. Patients can be told to do as much as they feel like doing, as long as they avoid overtiring themselves. Small, frequent meals, especially in the morning, are tolerated best. Foods do not need to be restricted, but carbohydrates seem to be the best-tolerated food when nausea is pronounced. Alcohol should be proscribed. Many patients with hepatitis take "alternative" therapies of no proven benefit. Most of these preparations are harmless, but some can actually injure the liver. Although patients should be discouraged from taking these substances, such warnings often fall on deaf ears.

Patients and household members have many questions regarding the transmissibility of viral hepatitis. Explicit instructions regarding preventive measures are greatly appreciated (see Chapter 57). Of particular concern is sexual activity, especially for young persons who might want to have children. In hepatitis B, the risk of transmission by sexual intercourse is high, but prophylaxis with hepatitis B immune globulin and especially vaccine reduces the risk in the patient's sexual partner. In hepatitis C, the risk of sexual transmission is negligible, especially between monogamous, stable sexual partners, rendering allowable unprotected intercourse.

THERAPEUTIC RECOMMENDATIONS
(5,7–16,19–35)

See Chapter 57 for prophylactic measures.

Acute Viral Hepatitis

- Maintain adequate caloric intake and a balanced diet. Small feedings are tolerated best, especially in the morning. No foods need to be restricted.
- Ensure adequate rest, but activity does not need to be restricted if the patient feels capable of remaining active.
- Omit potentially hepatotoxic agents, especially alcohol.

- Treat severe pruritus with cholestyramine.
- Treat severe nausea and vomiting with a nonphenothiazine antiemetic, such as trimethobenzamide (Tigan) suppositories.
- Admit the patient to the hospital if signs of marked worsening of hepatocellular function occur (e.g., encephalopathy, bleeding, prolongation of prothrombin time). Also consider admission for maintaining adequate caloric and fluid intake when symptoms are severe or for managing complicated underlying diseases.
- Refer patients with fulminant hepatitis for consideration of liver transplantation. In cases of hepatitis B, a trial of one of the oral antiviral agents may be considered but should not interfere with the evaluation for transplantation.
- For patients with acute hepatitis C, therapy with pegylated interferon plus ribavirin should be initiated as soon as possible.
- Check aminotransferase, prothrombin time, bilirubin, albumin, and globulin at onset and periodically during the acute illness; aminotransferase levels should be monitored at 1- to 4-week intervals during acute illness. In patients with acute hepatitis B, repeat HBsAg testing can be done at 12 to 24 weeks to document viral clearance or to demonstrate persistent infection. Retest any patient with evidence of persistent symptoms or laboratory abnormalities every 4 weeks. Refer for liver biopsy and potential antiviral therapy those with a combination of failure to resolve infection and inflammation by 6 to 12 months and persistence of disabling symptoms.

Drug-Induced Hepatitis

- Stop all drugs that might be responsible, and institute supportive measures.
- Avoid rechallenging the patient with the same agent. Acetaminophen hepatotoxicity should be treated with *N*-acetylcysteine.

Nonviral Chronic Hepatitis

- Follow patients with *mild* chronic hepatitis at regular intervals and rebiopsy for signs of marked worsening. Otherwise, treat symptomatically. Steroids are not indicated.
- For patients with *severe* chronic hepatitis (multilobular or bridging necrosis, disabling symptoms, and marked aminotransferase and globulin elevations), begin high-dose *prednisone* (60 mg daily) or combination prednisone (30 mg daily) plus *azathioprine* (50 mg daily). Combination therapy is preferred for the elderly, diabetics, and others who cannot tolerate long-term, high-dose steroids. Because of the effect of azathioprine on fertility, this drug should be avoided, if possible, in young adults who are planning to raise families.
- Taper prednisone by 5 to 10 mg at a time over the course of 1 month until a maintenance dose of 10 mg daily (with 50 mg daily azathioprine) or 20 mg daily is established.
- Monitor aminotransferase, bilirubin, and globulins at 2 weeks and then every 1 to 3 months. If the patient is taking azathioprine, obtain platelet and white cell counts monthly during the initial course of therapy and at periodic intervals thereafter.
- Continue maintenance therapy for at least 24 to 36 months, and then consider attempting discontinuation of therapy with a 6-week period of tapering medication.

- Initiate reconsultation if clinical improvement fails to occur within 2 to 8 months of initiating therapy; high-dose treatment may be indicated.
- Treat relapses in the same manner as new cases.

Chronic Viral Hepatitis

- Avoid immunosuppressive therapy in patients with chronic viral hepatitis.
- Consider *pegylated interferon* alfa-2a, 180 μg daily for 48 weeks, in patients with compensated chronic hepatitis B who demonstrate a sustained presence of HBV DNA and elevated aminotransferase levels.
- Most authorities would choose, instead of pegylated interferon, to consider one of the oral nucleoside or nucleotide analogues, such as lamivudine (100 mg/d for 52 weeks), adefovir (10 mg/d for 48 weeks), entecavir (0.5 mg/d for 48 weeks), telbivudine (600 mg/d for 48 weeks), or tenofovir (300 mg/d for 48 weeks) for chronic "replicative" hepatitis B. Because of the frequency of resistance to lamivudine and to telbivudine, and because tenofovir is superior to adefovir, the optimal agents to choose between are entecavir and tenofovir. Therapy can be stopped in patients who achieve HBeAg seroconversion; in those who retain HBeAg, therapy should be continued. For patients with HBeAg-negative chronic hepatitis B, who almost invariably require prolonged therapy, adefovir, entecavir, or tenofovir is preferable because resistance is less likely, and tenofovir should be favored over adefovir because of its superiority.
- Treat patients with compensated chronic *hepatitis C, genotype 1,* who manifest sustained elevations of aminotransferase and detectable HCV RNA with *pegylated interferon* (pegylated interferon alfa-2b, 1.5 μg/kg; or pegylated interferon alfa-2a, 180 μg) subcutaneously once a week plus oral ribavirin at a daily dose of 1,000 mg (for those weighing <75 kg) or 1,200 mg (for those weighing $\geq$75 kg) for 48 weeks. In patients with genotypes 2 and 3, a 24-week course of therapy may suffice, and only 800 mg/d of ribavirin is required. For patients who relapse after therapy with pegylated interferon and ribavirin is completed, retreating with the same medications will recapitulate the original response. For nonresponders to a course of pegylated interferon and ribavirin, long-term maintenance therapy had been considered but has been shown in a large prospective, controlled trial to be ineffective. For relapsers and nonresponders to current state-of-the art therapy, newer antiviral agents may be required to achieve responsiveness. For patients with maintained normal aminotransferase levels, histologic progression tends not to occur, and some choose not to be treated, but treatment is as effective as in patients with elevated aminotransferase levels.
- Consider once-a-week *pegylated interferon* for patients with *hepatitis D.* Long-term therapy for at least 1 year, preferably longer, is required. Some patients may benefit from several years of therapy.
- Monitor patients receiving pegylated interferon by checking leukocyte, granulocyte, and platelet counts at 1- to 3-month intervals. Check aminotransferase levels and thyroid-stimulating hormone every 1 to 3 months. In patients treated for hepatitis B, monitor HBV DNA monthly to every few months and measure HBeAg periodically and at the end of therapy. In patients being treated for hepatitis C, monitor HCV RNA at 4 weeks and then at approximate intervals of 3 months. Those receiving ribavirin need close monitoring of hematocrit/hemoglobin.
- Admit the patient to the hospital when there is evidence of marked worsening of hepatocellular function. Consider early referral for liver transplantation in patients with hepatic decompensation.

Annotated Bibliography

1. Niederau C, Heintges T, Lange S, et al. Long-term follow-up of HBeAg-positive patients treated with interferon alfa for chronic hepatitis B. N Engl J Med 1996;334:1422. (*A study finding that responders experienced a marked improvement in survival and in survival without hepatic decompensation.*)
2. Lau DTY, Everhart J, Kleiner DE, et al. Long-term follow up of patients with chronic hepatitis B treated with interferon alfa. Gastroenterology 1997;113:1660. (*The loss of detectable hepatitis B e antigen [HBeAg] during interferon therapy was associated with an 80% chance of losing hepatitis B surface antigen [HBsAg] and normalizing alanine aminotransferase levels over the ensuing decade.*)
3. van Zonneveld M, Honkoop P, Hansen B, et al. Viral hepatitis: long-term follow-up of α-interferon treatment of patients with chronic hepatitis B. Hepatology 2004;33:804. (*Retrospective data, revealing that clinical outcomes in treated patients were better in those without cirrhosis than in those with cirrhosis.*)
4. Lin SM, Sheen IS, Chien RN, et al. Long-term beneficial effect of interferon therapy in patients with chronic hepatitis B virus infection. Hepatology 1999;29:971. (*Presents evidence for an improved clinical course and a reduced risk of hepatocellular carcinoma.*)
5. EASL Jury. EASL International Consensus Conference on Hepatitis B, 13–14 September, 2002, Geneva, Switzerland. J Hepatol 2003;39(Suppl 1):S3. (*An international consensus conference on hepatitis B, including brief articles on every important aspect of hepatitis B and its management.*)
6. Dienstag JL Goldin RD, Heathcote EJ, et al. Histologic outcome during long-term lamivudine therapy. Gastroenterology 2003;124:105. (*Histologic improvement, including the reversal of cirrhosis, was documented in patients with chronic hepatitis B treated cumulatively for a total of 3 years with lamivudine.*)
7. Liaw Y-F Sung JJ, Chow WC, et al. Lamivudine for patients with chronic hepatitis B and advanced liver disease. N Engl J Med 2004;351:1521. (*A landmark randomized, controlled trial [RCT], demonstrating that antiviral therapy prevented hepatic decompensation in patients with chronic hepatitis B and advanced fibrosis/cirrhosis.*)
8. Marcellin P, Chang TT, Lim SG, et al. Adefovir dipivoxil for the treatment of hepatitis B e antigen–positive chronic hepatitis B. N Engl J Med 2003;348:808. (*A placebo-controlled RCT, showing that the treatment was effective in improving histology, biochemical features, and virologic markers.*)
9. Hadziyannis SJ, Tassopoulos NC, Heathcote EJ, et al. Adefovir dipivoxil for the treatment of hepatitis B e antigen–negative chronic hepatitis B. N Engl J Med 2003;348:800. (*A prospective, placebo-controlled, RCT, demonstrating the efficacy of adefovir for HBeAg-negative chronic hepatitis B.*)
10. Peters MG, Hann HW, Martin P, et al. Adefovir dipivoxil alone or in combination with lamivudine in patients with lamivudine-resistant chronic hepatitis B. Gastroenterology 2004;126:91. (*RCT, finding that adefovir was highly effective in patients with lamivudine-resistant chronic hepatitis B.*)
11. Chang TT, Gish RG, de Man R, et al. A comparison of entecavir and lamivudine for HBeAg-positive chronic hepatitis B. N Engl J Med 2006:354;1001. (*RCT, demonstrating the efficacy of entecavir and its superiority over lamivudine in HBeAg-reactive chronic hepatitis B.*)
12. Lai CL, Shouval D, Lok AS, et al. Entecavir versus lamivudine for patients with HBeAg-negative chronic hepatitis B. N Engl J Med 2006;354:1011. (*Prospective, lamivudine-controlled, RCT demonstrating the efficacy of entecavir and superiority over lamivudine in HBeAg-negative chronic hepatitis B.*)
13. Marcellin P, Lau GK, Bonino F, et al. Peginterferon alfa-2a alone, lamivudine alone, and the two in combination in patients with HBeAg-negative chronic hepatitis B. N Engl J Med 2004;351:1206. (*RCT, demonstrating the efficacy of 48 weeks of pegylated interferon therapy in patients with HBeAg-negative chronic hepatitis B; when pegylated interferon, lamivudine, and a combination of the two were compared, pegylated interferon monotherapy achieved a higher frequency than lamivudine monotherapy of hepatitis B virus [HBV]*)

DNA suppression measured 24 weeks after the end of therapy; combination therapy offered no advantage over pegylated interferon monotherapy.)

14. Lau GK, Piratvisuth T, Luo KX, et al. Peginterferon alfa-2a, lamivudine, and the combination for HBeAg-positive chronic hepatitis B. N Engl J Med 2005;352:2682. (*RCT, demonstrating the efficacy of 48 weeks of pegylated interferon therapy in patients with HBeAg-positive chronic hepatitis B; when pegylated interferon, lamivudine, and a combination of the two were compared, pegylated interferon monotherapy achieved a higher frequency than lamivudine monotherapy or combination therapy of HBeAg seroconversion and HBV DNA suppression measured 24 weeks after the end of therapy.*)

15. Lok SFL, McMahon BJ. AASLD practice guidelines: chronic hepatitis B. Hepatology 2007;45:507. (*A comprehensive overview of the clinical and epidemiologic features of hepatitis B, as well as updated management guidelines.*)

16. Samuel D, Muller R, Alexander G, et al. Liver transplantation in European patients with the hepatitis B surface antigen. N Engl J Med 1993;329:1842. (*A retrospective European analysis, showing that a marked improvement was provided by long-term hepatitis B immune globulin infusions after liver transplantation.*)

17. Farci P, Roskams T, Chessa L, et al. Long-term benefit of interferon a therapy of chronic hepatitis D: regression of advanced hepatic fibrosis. Gastroenterology 2004;126:1740. (*A long-term follow-up, finding that histologic improvement was seen in patients treated successfully with interferon for chronic hepatitis D.*)

18. Fattovich G, Giustina G, Degos F, et al. Morbidity and mortality in compensated cirrhosis type C: a retrospective follow-up study of 384 patients. Gastroenterology 1997;112:463. (*A European retrospective natural history study, finding a 10-year survival of 80%; an annual mortality of 1.9%; an annual decompensation of 3.9%; and an annual rate of hepatocellular carcinoma of 1.4%.*)

19. Yano M, Kumada H, Kage M, et al. The long-term pathological evolution of chronic hepatitis C. Hepatology 1996;23:1334. (*A unique Japanese study, examining serial liver biopsies over 20 years and finding that the severity of histologic grade and stage at baseline were predictive of clinical course.*)

20. National Institutes of Health Consensus Development Conference. Management of hepatitis C. Hepatology 1997;26(Suppl 1):1S. (*Consensus guidelines on every aspect of hepatitis C evaluation and management; all recommendations are evidence based.*)

21. Manns MP, McHutchison JG, Gordon SC, et al. Peginterferon alfa-2b plus ribavirin compared with interferon alfa-2b plus ribavirin for initial treatment of chronic hepatitis C: a randomised trial. Lancet 2001;358:958. (*RCT, finding that sustained virologic response was achieved in 54% of patients treated with pegylated interferon and ribavirin for 1 year.*)

22. Fried MV, Shiffman ML, Reddy KR, et al. Peginterferon alfa-2a plus ribavirin for chronic hepatitis C virus infection. N Engl J Med 2002;347:975. (*RCT, finding that in the pegylated interferon/ribavirin arm, 56% of patients achieved a sustained virologic response after 1 year of therapy.*)

23. Hadziyannis SJ, Sette H, Morgan T, et al. Peginterferon alfa-2a (40 kilodaltons) and ribavirin combination therapy in chronic hepatitis C: randomized study of treatment duration and ribavirin dose. Ann Intern Med 2004;140:346. (*RCT, finding that for genotype 1, 48 weeks of pegylated interferon therapy and 1,000 to 1,200 mg of ribavirin were necessary; however, for genotypes 2 and 3, 24 weeks of therapy with only 800 mg of ribavirin sufficed.*)

24. National Institutes of Health Consensus Development Conference. Management of hepatitis C: 2002. Hepatology 2002;36(Suppl 1):1S. (*Updated*

National Institutes of Health consensus guidelines, incorporating advances associated with the introduction of pegylated interferon plus ribavirin, the new standard in management.*)

25. Strader DB, Wright T, Thomas DL, et al. Diagnosis, management, and treatment of hepatitis C (AASLD Practice Guideline). Hepatology 2004;39:1147. (*A comprehensive review of the management of hepatitis C and guidelines issued by the American Association for the Study of Liver Diseases.*)

26. Pearlman BL. Chronic hepatitis C therapy: Changing the rules of duration. Clin Gastroenterol Hepatol 2006;4:963. (*A review of new data suggesting that, for therapy to be optimally effective, the duration of hepatitis C virus suppression is important.*)

27. Dienstag JL, McHutchison JG. American Gastroenterological Association medical position statement on the management of hepatitis C. Gastroenterology 2006;130:225. American Gastroenterological Association technical review on the management of hepatitis C. Gastroenterology 2006;130:231. (*A comprehensive review of the clinical and epidemiologic features of hepatitis C, as well as background data to support management recommendations.*)

28. Shiffman ML, Di Bisceglie AM, Lindsay KL, et al. Peginterferon alfa-2a and ribavirin in patients with chronic hepatitis C who have failed prior treatment. Gastroenterology 2004;126:1015. (*RCT; although previous reports suggested that shorter durations of therapy were sufficient in patients with genotypes 2 and 3 who achieved a rapid virologic response, this more definitive trial demonstrated that a full 24 weeks of therapy was superior in patients with these more treatment-responsive genotypes, even when a rapid virologic response was achieved.*)

29. Muir AJ, Bornstein JD, Killenberg PG, et al. Peginterferon alfa-2b and ribavirin for the treatment of chronic hepatitis C in blacks and non-Hispanic whites. N Engl J Med 2004;350:2265. (*RCT, finding that standard-of-care therapy with pegylated interferon and ribavirin was significantly less efficacious in African American patients than in white patients.*)

30. Forman LM, Lewis JD, Berlin JA, et al. The association between hepatitis C infection and survival after orthotopic liver transplantation. Gastroenterology 2002;122:889. (*Despite the early apparent clinical benignity of recurrent hepatitis C after liver transplantation, ultimately recurrent hepatitis C takes a toll.*)

31. Lee WM. Drug-induced hepatotoxicity. N Engl J Med 2003;349:474. (*An up-to-date review of the pathogenesis, categorization, and management of drug-associated hepatotoxicity.*)

32. Summerskill WHJ, Korman MG, Ammon HV, et al. Prednisone for chronic active liver disease: dose titration, standard dose, and combination with azathioprine compared. Gut 1975;16:876. (*The classic study that established prednisone or prednisone plus azathioprine as superior to placebo and azathioprine alone in autoimmune hepatitis; this landmark study continues to guide therapy >30 years later.*)

33. Czaja AJ, Freese DK. Diagnosis and treatment of autoimmune hepatitis. Hepatology 2002;36:479. (*An American Association for the Study of Liver Disease practice guideline; an authoritative review of contemporary approaches to the diagnosis and management of autoimmune hepatitis.*)

34. Krawitt EL. Autoimmune hepatitis. N Engl J Med 2006;354:54. (*A concise, contemporary review of the management of autoimmune hepatitis.*)

35. Sanyal AJ. American Gastroenterological Association technical review on nonalcoholic fatty liver disease. Gastroenterology 2002;123:1705. American Gastroenterological Association medical position statement: nonalcoholic fatty liver disease. Gastroenterology 2002;123:1702. (*Evidence-based, comprehensive, authoritative review of nonalcoholic fatty liver disease, supporting a position paper on the clinical approach to this disease.*)

CHAPTER 71 ■ MANAGEMENT OF CIRRHOSIS AND CHRONIC LIVER FAILURE

Cirrhosis represents an irreversible state of chronic liver injury. The best treatment is *prevention*, based on detecting and addressing treatable causes such as *chronic hepatitis*, *chronic alcohol abuse*, *hemochromatosis*, and *primary biliary cirrhosis* (see also Chapters 57, 70, and 228). Even after its onset, the patient can be kept comfortable, active, and independent if precipitants of further hepatocellular injury are eliminated and complications are prevented or treated promptly. Although consultative help from specialists is often necessary, responsibility for long-term management usually rests with the primary care physician, who needs to be capable of treating etiologies and dealing with such complications as ascites, peripheral edema, encephalopathy, infection, bleeding, renal dysfunction, and electrolyte imbalances. With the advent of liver transplantation, prognosis has improved markedly for appropriately referred persons with end-stage disease.

CLINICAL PRESENTATION AND COURSE (1–16)

Clinical Presentation

Onset may be rather dramatic if the initial presentation is a late-stage complication such as brisk *variceal bleeding* or *encephalopathy*. In the office setting, the patient may present more subtly with complaints of *fatigue*, easy *bruising*, mild abdominal *swelling*, or new onset of bilateral *ankle edema*. With the development of portal hypertension, the presentation is characterized by *splenomegaly*, abdominal *distention* with *shifting dullness*, and a prominent *abdominal venous pattern*. Signs of chronic hepatic dysfunction may be evident, including *palmar erythema, Dupuytren's contractures, spider angiomata, parotid and lacrimal gland hypertrophy, gynecomastia, testicular atrophy*, loss of *axillary* and *pubic hair*, and *clubbing*. Although nonspecific abnormalities in routine liver function tests are common, the best measures of hepatocellular synthetic impairment are prolongation of the *prothrombin time* (PT) and decline in the *serum albumin*. PT prolongation occurs first because of the short serum half-lives of the hepatically synthesized clotting factors (e.g., 7 days) that determine it. The decline in serum albumin follows later because of the longer serum half-life of albumin (28 days).

Most presentations of cirrhosis and chronic hepatic failure are nonspecific, but the initial manifestations of a few treatable etiologies are worth noting because of the potential benefit of early recognition and treatment.

Hemochromatosis

Hereditary (primary) hemochromatosis is among the most common of autosomal hereditary conditions, having an estimated prevalence of 1 in 250 among people of European ancestry. Mutations in the *HFE gene* (such as C282Y, which accounts for about 90% of cases) cause excessive iron absorption and iron overload. Decades of chronic iron deposition can injure parenchymal cells of the liver, heart, pancreas, joints, and gonads and can lead to fibrosis and organ failure. Homozygotes are at greatest risk for clinical liver disease, but the degree of penetrance and the risk of organ damage are highly variable; heterozygous individuals rarely develop overt liver disease unless they have another risk factor for cirrhosis. Consequently, although the prevalence of the gene mutation is high, the risk of clinical liver disease is much lower, although not fully established. The risk can be increased by the use of supplements containing iron or vitamin C (which enhances iron absorption). Patients who develop cirrhosis are at increased risk of hepatocellular carcinoma.

For many years the patient is asymptomatic; the only hepatic manifestation may be incidentally noted minor elevations in serum transaminases (aminotransferases; see Appendix 62.1). Initial symptoms are nonspecific and include mild *fatigue* or *arthralgias*. By the fifth or sixth decade, manifestations of organ failure may begin to appear, heralded by *dyspnea, glucose intolerance, arthritis*, and *gonadal dysfunction* and by mani-

festations of *cirrhosis* and chronic hepatocellular dysfunction. The skin might appear slate gray or *bronzelike* from the chronic iron deposition. Films of involved joints (e.g., metacarpophalangeal joints, knees) may show *chondrocalcinosis*. Elevations in serum *transferrin saturation* and *ferritin* are indicative of iron overload.

Workup. The best initial tests are serum transferrin saturation (ratio of iron to the total iron-binding capacity) and ferritin; a percentage saturation of greater than 55% and a ferritin level of greater than 300 μg/L (200 μg/L in women) are considered strongly suggestive of the diagnosis. Candidates for workup include those with unexplained conditions that may be a consequence of underlying hemochromatosis, such as isolated transaminase elevations, unexplained liver disease, cardiomyopathy, gonadal failure, type 2 diabetes, or hyperpigmentation. Testing for the C282Y mutation will be positive in 90% of patients with characteristic elevations in transferrin saturation and ferritin, but the absence of the mutation does not rule out the condition. Liver biopsy is indicated when the serum ferritin exceeds 1,000 μg/L; the risk of hepatic fibrosis appears to be minimal at lower levels.

Screening. Despite the frequency and potential seriousness of the condition, genetic screening for hemochromatosis (testing for the C282Y mutation) is not recommended by the U.S. Preventive Services Task Force because penetrance of the gene mutation is incomplete and the benefits of treatment (phlebotomy) are uncertain; more data are needed. Phenotypic screening by determination of *serum ferritin* and *transferrin saturation* offers the best yield in case finding, but the evidence is insufficient to recommend for or against its general application. Screening high-risk subgroups, such as first-degree relatives of patients with clinical hemochromatosis, is left to clinical judgment and the discussion of risks and benefits with individual family members.

Primary Biliary Cirrhosis

This autoimmune condition targets the intrahepatic bile ducts. The resultant inflammatory process leads to cholestasis and, if unchecked, fibrosis terminating in cirrhosis. The cause is unknown, but molecular mimicry in genetically predisposed persons is believed to be responsible. Unlike many other autoimmune conditions, no specific histocompatibility complex allele has been associated with the condition, but first-degree family members are at increased risk. Suspected causative agents include bacteria, viruses, and environmental chemicals (e.g., halogenated hydrocarbons). The hallmark of the condition is the presence of *antimitochondrial antibodies*, which target dehydrogenases, predominantly of cells in the biliary tree. Other autoimmune diseases may coexist with the condition (e.g., *Sjögren's syndrome, Hashimoto's thyroiditis*).

The condition is predominantly one of middle-aged women (peak incidence occurs in the fifth decade). *Fatigue* (often marked) and *itching* (often severe) are typically the initial complaints. *Hepatomegaly* may be the first physical finding, and a markedly *elevated alkaline phosphatase* is the principal laboratory abnormality noted before the onset of manifestations associated with *cirrhosis*. *Jaundice* with skin excoriations accounts for the initial presentation in about one fourth of patients. The sedimentation rate is markedly elevated; liver function tests reveal a cholestatic pattern. *Hyperlipidemia* is common; *steatorrhea* may ensue, compromising the absorption of fat-soluble vitamins. *Antimitochondrial antibody* is found in about 90% of cases, and *immunoglobulin M antibody titers* are elevated.

Diagnosis is made by *liver biopsy* with staining for copper, which reveals characteristic asymmetric interlobular ductal inflammation and fibrosis.

Alcoholic Liver Disease

Early hepatic injury may be manifested by mild elevations in aminotransferase levels. A *ratio of alanine aminotransferase (ALT) to aspartate aminotransferase (AST) of greater than 2:1* is characteristic of alcoholic liver injury. A palpable liver from *fatty infiltration* is another early presentation. Risk factors for the development of cirrhosis include prolonged consumption of *excess alcohol* (e.g., more than 16 oz/d for 10 years or more), *female gender*, and concurrent *viral hepatitis C* infection. The simultaneous use of *acetaminophen* (even at normal doses) and excess alcohol increases the risk of liver injury, especially when the patient is fasting. *Gastritis* and *upper gastrointestinal* (GI) bleeding are common consequences of alcohol excess and may be presenting manifestations.

Nonalcoholic Steatohepatitis (NASH)

This increasingly appreciated condition may account for a substantial proportion of patients who present with so-called *cryptogenic cirrhosis*. Estimates for the prevalence of nonalcoholic fatty liver disease range as high as 10% to 25% of the adult population, rising to greater than 50% among obese persons. The condition appears to originate with insulin resistance and an excess in the uptake of fat by hepatocytes. In some persons (perhaps those who are genetically predisposed), oxidative injury ensues, leading to steatohepatitis, fibrosis, and possible cirrhosis. Because obesity is the leading cause of insulin resistance, the number of persons potentially at risk is large.

Clinical Presentation. Other than an enlarged liver, there are no early signs or symptoms at the time of diagnosis, which is usually made after the incidental encounter of minor elevations in *aminotransferases* or an *enlarged fatty liver* on abdominal imaging. A major proportion of asymptomatic elevations in liver enzymes (in the absence of substantial alcohol intake) are attributable to nonalcoholic fatty liver disease.

Diagnosis and Prognosis. Definitive diagnosis requires the exclusion of a daily intake of alcohol sufficient to cause alcoholic liver disease (two beers, 8 oz of wine, 3.0 oz of hard liquor); liver biopsy is needed for confirmation. Risk factors for cirrhosis and thus indications for liver biopsy include age older than 45 years, obesity or type 2 diabetes, and an ALT/AST ratio of greater than 1.0. The severity of liver damage found on biopsy correlates with the prognosis: Patients with steatosis and no cellular damage have little risk of cirrhosis, but persons with evidence of steatohepatitis are at considerably greater risk, particularly if there are concurrent risk factors such as hepatitis C. The precise degree of risk for cirrhosis is not established, but among those coming to biopsy (a selected population), about one fourth experience progressive liver damage. Given the number of persons potentially at risk, recognition and treatment are important.

Chronic Hepatitis

See Chapter 70.

Clinical Course and Complications

Portal hypertension, fluid retention, and shunting lead to a host of problems, including ascites, peripheral edema, varices,

encephalopathy, and hepatorenal syndrome. The principal causes of death in patients with cirrhosis are variceal bleeding, encephalopathy, and infection. In addition, patients with cirrhosis, especially those with chronic hepatitis B infection, are at increased risk for hepatocellular carcinoma.

Ascites

Ascites is the consequence of a complex set of interacting and incompletely understood forces. Portal hypertension has long been recognized as a key factor, but increasingly appreciated is the role of locally produced nitric oxide, a potent vasodilator that acts on the splanchnic arterial bed lowering splanchnic artery pressure. As cirrhosis and portal hypertension advance, the increasing degree of splanchnic vasodilation is sufficient to lower systemic blood pressure, triggering sodium retention. The combination of portal hypertension, fluid retention, and splanchnic arterial vasodilation raises capillary transudation pressure in the intestinal vascular bed, leading to the accumulation of ascetic fluid.

Stages of ascites can be categorized according to degree of discomfort, effect on daily activity, and response to diuretic therapy.

Moderate-Volume Ascites. Patients with moderate-volume ascites may have mild to moderate discomfort but do not suffer rapid increases in ascites or major interference with daily activity. There is some sodium retention, but free water excretion and renal function are usually well preserved, so serum sodium and creatinine levels remain normal. Response to diuretic therapy is good.

Large-Volume Ascites. The further accumulation of ascetic fluid causing marked discomfort and interference with daily activities characterizes large-volume ascites. Sodium excretion is low (urinary sodium <10Meq/L), and ascetic fluid accumulation can be rapid. Renal function and free-water excretion remain preserved, but the response to diuretics is reduced, necessitating high-dose diuretic therapy (see later discussion).

Refractory Ascites. At this stage, there is no response to high-dose diuretic therapy, or, if there is a response, it is associated with encephalopathy, hyponatremia, or hepatorenal syndrome. Rapid reaccumulation after paracentesis is characteristic, as are hyponatremia, hyperkalemia, or azotemia in response to diuretics.

Encephalopathy

Hepatic encephalopathy is believed to be a consequence of intestinally derived toxic substances that escape hepatic detoxification as a result of portosystemic shunting and hepatocellular dysfunction. Candidates include ammonia, benzodiazepine-like substances, mercaptans, phenol, neuroinhibitors, false neurotransmitters, and short-chain fatty acids.

There are no pathognomonic clinical findings, and so the diagnosis requires ruling out other causes of altered mental status (e.g., medications, intracranial bleed, renal failure). Elevated *ammonia levels* correlate reasonably well with the severity of hepatic encephalopathy. *Venous* levels are adequate for monitoring and useful in following the clinical state of individual patients but can be falsely elevated when a tourniquet is left on too long at the time of blood drawing. *Arterial* sampling for the determination of the partial pressure of ammonia offers no advantage over venous sampling. Patients can be assessed and followed by checking for asterixis and performing routine mental status examinations that include tracing a five-point star and signature testing.

Spontaneous Bacterial Peritonitis (SBP)

This complication develops in about 10% of ascitic patients per year as bacteria spread from the bowel lumen to regional nodes, blood stream, and ascitic fluid. The most common pathogen is *Escherichia coli*. A *leukocyte count* of greater than 250 cells/mL is considered diagnostic; Gram's stain is usually negative. Prognosis is poor with the onset of SBP, which also increases the risk of hepatorenal syndrome; the recurrence rate within 1 year is 70%.

Variceal Bleeding and Coagulopathy

Esophageal varices are a consequence of portal hypertension leading to portosystemic shunting. Bleeding from esophageal varices occurs in 20% to 30% of cirrhotic patients: One third may die during the initial hospitalization, one third rebleed within 6 weeks, and one third survive for 1 year or more. The bleeding may be exacerbated by coagulopathy, resulting from reductions in vitamin K–dependent clotting factors (II, VII, IX, and X) secondary to decreased hepatic protein synthesis and increased plasma proteolytic activity. In addition, bile-salt deficiency, neomycin therapy, and malnutrition may contribute to the malabsorption of *vitamin K,* and hypersplenism may account for thrombocytopenia.

Hepatorenal Syndrome

The hepatorenal syndrome occurs in the context of advanced liver disease and results from severe renal vasoconstriction, a consequence of systemic hypoperfusion. The condition is characterized by *elevated serum creatinine*, urinary sodium *less than 10 mEq/L*, and a *hyperosmolar urine*. Its onset heralds a poor prognosis (median survival <1 month), often precipitated by an attack of spontaneous bacterial peritonitis. Type 1 hepatorenal syndrome is associated with a rapid rise in serum creatinine and progressive oliguria; type 2 disease manifests a more indolent clinical course.

Hepatocellular Carcinoma

Patients with cirrhosis are at increased risk for hepatocellular carcinoma, especially those with underlying chronic hepatitis B and C and hemochromatosis. The determination of serum α-*fetoprotein* (AFP) is commonly ordered as a screening test, but sensitivity and specificity are low, and there are scant data to support its routine use. *Abdominal ultrasound* is widely used and more sensitive; AFP as a confirmatory test may add some specificity. The cost-effectiveness of screening and the ability of screening to prolong survival are not well established, but screening is commonly conducted.

Determinants of Prognosis

The principal causes of death in patients with cirrhosis are variceal bleeding, encephalopathy, and infection. In addition, patients with cirrhosis, especially those with chronic hepatitis B infection, are at increased risk for hepatocellular carcinoma. Irrespective of etiology, the development of *ascites, encephalopathy, hyperbilirubinemia, variceal bleeding, hepatorenal syndrome, hypergammaglobulinemia* (from bypass of the hepatic reticuloendothelial system), and *hypoalbuminemia* are poor prognostic signs, as is decreased liver size. The onset of ascites is associated with a 50% 2-year mortality rate, and variceal bleeding has a 35% short-term mortality rate. The

---

TABLE 71.1

CLASSIFICATION SYSTEMS OF LIVER FAILURE: CHILD–PUGH CLASSIFICATION OF HEPATIC DECOMPENSATION

Clinical Feature	Class		
	1	2	3
Encephalopathy grade	0	1–2	3
Ascites	None	Slight	Moderate
Bilirubin (mg/dL)	1–2	2–3	>3
Albumin (g/dL)	>3.5	2.8–3.5	<2.8
Prothrombin time prolongation (sec)	1–4	5–6	>6

Adapted from Pugh RN, Murray-Lyon IM, Dawson JL, et al. Transection of the oesophagus for bleeding oesophageal varices. Br J Surg 1973;60:646–649, with permission.

2-year mortality for worsening renal function is 33%. Specific etiologies are subject to additional factors.

In the context of alcoholic liver disease, *continued alcohol consumption* is associated with an 80% chance of developing cirrhosis, whereas complete abstinence lowers the risk to 15%. Even after alcoholic cirrhosis has developed, survival continues to be affected by alcohol ingestion. Five-year survival is 60% to 85% in patients who abstain, compared with 40% to 60% for those who continue to drink. The onset of jaundice or ascites further decreases 5-year survival (to 30% in drinkers). The concurrent presence of hepatitis C worsens prognosis in persons with other forms of liver disease.

In symptomatic primary biliary cirrhosis, the average length of survival from the onset of symptoms is about 12 years, whereas the survival of asymptomatic patients approaches normal. The prognosis of patients with postnecrotic cirrhosis is difficult to assess because it is hard to date its onset; the cirrhosis develops insidiously over years from subclinical chronic active hepatitis.

Estimating Prognosis

Prognosis is determined by the nature, severity, and activity of the underlying illness (Table 71.1). The traditional prognostic indicator, the *Pugh modification* of the *Child–Turcotte prognostic classification*, uses encephalopathy grade, degree of ascites, bilirubin, serum albumin, and prothrombin time. It has been supplanted for purposes of determining candidacy for liver transplantation by the better-validated *Model for End-Stage Liver Disease (MELD)*, which predicts 3-month mortality and assigns a priority score for transplantation based on serum bilirubin, creatinine, and International Normalized Ratio (INR) (Table 71.2).

TABLE 71.2

MODEL FOR END-STAGE LIVER DISEASE (MELD)

MELD score = 6.43 + 9.57 × log(creatinine) + 3.78 × log(bilirubin) + 11.2 × log(INR)

The score is expressed as a rounded integer between 6 and 40; the higher the score, the worse is the 3-month mortality rate.
INR, International Normalized Ratio.
Adapted from Wiesner R, Edwards E, Freeman R, et al. Model for end-stage liver disease (MELD) and allocation of donor livers. Gastroenterology 2003;124:91.

PRINCIPLES OF MANAGEMENT

Treatment of the underlying etiology and the manifestations and complications of cirrhosis and chronic hepatic failure constitute the basic elements of management. Outcomes can be improved when all elements are addressed in the treatment program.

Treatment of the Underlying Etiology
(1,4,7,10,14,17,18)

Alcoholic Cirrhosis

Complete *abstinence* is the mainstay of treatment (see Chapter 228); prognosis is markedly worsened by continued drinking (see prior discussion). Attention to good nutrition, daily multiple-vitamin supplements (including 1 mg of folic acid), and correction of any iron deficiency or electrolyte deficits are important supportive measures. The search continues for agents that might halt hepatic fibrosis and promote hepatocyte regeneration. Concern about hepatic injury associated with the consumption of therapeutic doses of *acetaminophen* (<4 g/d) in persons with alcoholic liver disease derives from findings of retrospective studies but has not been confirmed in short-term prospective, randomized trials. Glucocorticosteroids and portacaval shunting have failed to demonstrate an improvement in survival, although corticosteroids do improve short-term survival in patients with acute alcoholic hepatitis. A randomized, placebo-controlled, long-term study of *colchicine* revealed a doubling of 5- and 10-year survival. The drug is an inhibitor of collagen deposition. However, confirmatory data are needed before it or other drugs found experimentally to improve survival (e.g., propylthiouracil) can be recommended. *Liver transplantation* is sometimes considered in patients who have become totally and permanently abstinent.

Hemochromatosis

Iron removal by *phlebotomy* might reduce the risk of cirrhosis and improve survival, but data from controlled trials are lacking. Uncontrolled observational studies suggest that phlebotomy might achieve normal life expectancy if it is started before the onset of cirrhosis or diabetes; fatigue, glucose intolerance, and liver function abnormalities also seem to improve. Based on such observations, weekly phlebotomies of 500 mL are recommended to patients, performed early in the course of illness until the serum iron and ferritin levels fall to normal; then phlebotomies are performed as needed according to the results of periodic serum ferritin determinations. Limiting the intake of iron-rich foods (red meat, iron-fortified cereals and other foods), iron and vitamin C supplements, and other mineral supplements (e.g., zinc and manganese) is also recommended.

Nonalcoholic Fatty Liver Disease

Weight reduction improves liver function tests in nonalcoholic fatty liver disease. Gradual weight reduction (no more than 2 lb/wk) appears to improve histologic appearance, but more rapid weight reduction may actually worsen it. Preliminary short-term studies suggest a possible benefit from pharmacologic intervention, but controlled, prospective trials remain to be conducted. Promising results have been associated with the use of gemfibrozil, vitamin E, and metformin (improvements in liver function studies) and with glitazones and ursodiol (histologic improvement). Tightening the control of diabetes and hyperlipidemia is recommended but not always effective.

Primary Biliary Cirrhosis

Medical therapy is capable of altering prognosis when applied in the early stages of disease. The treatment of pruritus and disorders of fat malabsorption is another priority.

Ursodiol. Ursodiol (ursodeoxycholic acid), a choleretic agent, can improve biochemical manifestations, slow disease progression, reduce the risk of cirrhosis, and improve survival. Most patients have at least a partial response, and nearly 30% benefit greatly. The risk of death and the need for liver transplantation are significantly reduced after 4 years of use. In daily doses of 12 to 15 mg/kg of body weight, the drug has proven to be both safe and effective; it is the only drug approved by the U.S. Food and Drug Administration for the condition. Benefit is limited once cirrhosis sets in. Side effects are minor and include hair loss, weight gain, diarrhea, and flatulence.

Colchicine, Methotrexate, and Other Agents. For patients who do not respond sufficiently to ursodiol alone, *colchicine* (0.6 mg twice daily) is typically added to the treatment program. Although it is not as effective as ursodiol, it can reduce the risk of major complications and the need for transplantation when it is added to the medical regimen. *Methotrexate* represents the next step treatment for disease inadequately controlled by ursodiol and colchicine. It achieves histologic, biochemical, and clinical remissions in a substantial fraction of patients, but improved survival remains to be established. The dose is 0.25 mg/kg weekly. Adverse effects include interstitial pneumonia and hepatic fibrosis after 3.0 g of total accumulated dose (see Chapter 156).

A host of other immunomodulatory agents have been tried (e.g., prednisone, penicillamine, azathioprine, thalidomide) but without evidence of sufficient efficacy to warrant the use and risks of associated adverse effects. *Liver transplantation* markedly improves survival (82% at 5 years); disease recurs in 30% of cases at 10 years.

Treatment of Pruritus. Severe pruritus associated with this condition can be relieved by *cholestyramine* in a dose of 4 g orally with meals. *Rifampin* (150 mg twice daily) is used in persons who do not respond to cholestyramine. Refractory pruritus responds to opiate antagonists (e.g., *naltrexone*).

Complications of Fat *Malabsorption*. Because of decreased fat absorption from low intestinal bile-salt concentrations, these patients are particularly prone to develop deficiencies of the fat-soluble vitamins. They may require supplemental *vitamin K* (10 mg subcutaneously every 4 weeks), *vitamin D* (50,000 U orally two to three times a week or 100,000 U intramuscularly every 4 weeks) with oral *calcium* (1 g daily), and *vitamin A* (25,000 U orally per day). Night blindness unresponsive to vitamin A may be due to zinc deficiency, which is treated with oral *zinc sulfate* (220 mg/d). For patients with steatorrhea, *medium-chain triglyceride* preparations often help.

Secondary Biliary Cirrhosis

This condition can be halted by relieving or bypassing the obstruction to bile flow (see Chapter 62).

Chronic Hepatitis

Nonviral chronic hepatitis may benefit from *corticosteroid/ azathioprine* therapy; viral hepatitis responds to *interferon alfa* plus *ribavirin* (see Chapter 70).

Wilson's Disease

The condition responds to *d-penicillamine* therapy, which should be administered in cooperation with a hepatologist experienced in using the drug because of its potential for serious side effects.

Treatment of Complications (19–42)

Ascites and Edema

Increased portal pressure, hypoalbuminemia, secondary hyperaldosteronism, and impaired free-water clearance lead to ascites and peripheral edema, manifested by a *fluid wave, shifting dullness*, and *peripheral edema*. Abdominal ultrasound can be used for confirmation and to rule out venoocclusive disease involving the hepatic veins or the hepatic region of the inferior vena cava (*Budd–Chiari syndrome*). Although ascites is not a hazard per se, gross ascites can cause abdominal discomfort and respiratory compromise; under such circumstances, it should be treated. The development of refractory ascites is a very poor prognostic sign and an indication for the consideration of transplantation.

Evaluation before Onset of Treatment. *Diagnostic paracentesis* is needed to exclude infection and malignancy in patients with new onset of ascites, worsening hepatic function, fever, or increasing encephalopathy. The *serum-to-ascites albumin gradient* (serum albumin concentration minus the ascites albumin concentration) can help to differentiate portal hypertension from other causes, especially when the ascitic protein concentration is high. A gradient of greater than 1.1 mg/dL is indicative of portal hypertension. Ascitic fluid should also be sent for cytologic examination, cell count, and culture. Blood pressure, renal function (*blood urea nitrogen, creatinine*), serum *electrolytes*, and *urinary sodium* should be measured before the initiation of therapy.

Moderate-Volume Ascites. Patients typically can be managed on an ambulatory basis. Sodium restriction and a diuretic program often suffice to keep the ascites under control.

Sodium and Fluid Restriction. A reduction in daily *dietary sodium* intake is the first priority. One begins with a *2-g sodium diet*, a reasonable compromise between maximizing sodium restriction and dietary palatability. Greater reductions in salt are usually not dietarily tolerable. Adequate nutrition is critical. In the absence of encephalopathy, a daily protein intake of at least 50 g is recommended. Excessive water intake should be prohibited and *free water* should be restricted to 1,000 to 1,500 mL/d if hyponatremia ensues. An effective program of salt and water restriction requires a cooperative patient and a conscientious family. A dietitian can provide invaluable assistance. The patient should be instructed to check weight daily. Measuring abdominal girth is an unreliable index of fluid loss because of variations due to gaseous distention of the GI tract. About 15% of patients will respond to sodium and fluid restrictions alone. Bedrest is of no added benefit.

Diuretics. Diuretics may be needed if a diuresis has not occurred spontaneously after a full week of salt restriction. Urinary sodium determination can help to guide diuretic selection, especially when there is no weight loss. In persons with moderate-volume ascites, treatment can be conducted on an outpatient basis, provided renal function is normal.

Spironolactone (an aldosterone inhibitor) is the agent of first choice, especially when the initial urinary sodium concentration is greater than 30 mEq/L. Spironolactone inhibits the hyperaldosteronism of portal hypertension and counters the hypokalemic alkalosis commonly seen in cirrhotic patients with ascites. Its diuretic action is mild and unlikely to cause rapid intravascular volume depletion. The initial dose of spironolactone is 100 mg/d orally in divided doses. If diuresis does not follow within 1 week, the daily dose may be increased by 100 mg every 4 or 5 days to a maximum of 200 to 400 mg daily (higher doses may cause hyperkalemic acidosis).

The treatment target is a weight loss of no more than 2 lb/d in the setting of peripheral edema and 1 lb/d if peripheral edema has resolved. If adequate diuresis and weight loss do not occur on a maximal dose of spironolactone and the volume of ascites remains moderately large, then a loop diuretic such as *furosemide* (starting at 20 to 40 mg/d) may be added, especially if urinary sodium is less than 30 mEq/L but greater than 10 mEq/L. As long as the urinary sodium does not fall below 10 mEq/L, loop-diuretic doses can be advanced (e.g., furosemide to 80 to 160 mg/d). Weight is monitored closely, as is urinary sodium.

Large-Volume Ascites. If ascitic volumes become large, then options include high-dose diuretic therapy (400 mg/d spironolactone and 160 mg/d of furosemide) and large-volume paracentesis. In randomized trials, large-volume paracentesis has been shown to be superior.

Large-Volume Paracentesis. By intravenously infusing *albumin* (8 g/L of ascitic fluid removed) at the time of paracentesis, one can remove several liters of ascitic fluid without precipitating serious intravascular volume depletion, hyponatremia, and hepatorenal syndrome. Albumin is superior to other plasma expanders. Results are comparable to shunting, but the cost is much less, despite the need for readmissions to remove reaccumulated fluid every 10 to 30 days. Persons with peripheral edema may not always require albumin infusion. Although expensive, the use of albumin can obviate more expensive interventions, but there is no evidence that it confers a survival advantage. Risks of bowel perforation and infection are very rare when performed properly, and the risk of bleeding is small as long as INR does not exceed 1.6.

High-Dose Diuretic Therapy. When using high-dose diuretic therapy, extreme care is needed to avoid precipitating renal failure, hypokalemia, hyponatremia, and encephalopathy. The maximum amount of ascitic fluid that can be safely mobilized in 24 hours is about 700 to 900 mL, although peripheral edema can be mobilized at a faster rate. This translates to a daily weight loss of 0.5 kg in patients with ascites alone and of 1 kg in those with both ascites and peripheral edema. Daily weight loss in excess of these amounts suggests overdiuresis, with its attendant risk of intravascular volume depletion leading to hepatorenal syndrome and encephalopathy. If urinary sodium falls to less than 10 mEq/L, then continued advancing of loop diuretic therapy is unlikely to be helpful and may prove harmful.

Refractory Ascites. Treatment options include large-volume paracentesis in conjunction with albumin infusion and the insertion of a portosystemic shunt.

Transjugular Intrahepatic Portosystemic Shunting (TIPS). This expensive, more invasive alternative to large-volume paracentesis had been believed to improve response and survival, but initially promising results have not been confirmed by others. Advantages do include the elimination of the need for repeated paracentesis, but the risk of shunt stenosis approaches 75% at 6 to 12 months. TIPS is reserved for persons who cannot undergo large-volume paracentesis.

Monitoring. Monitoring of *blood urea nitrogen*, *creatinine*, *serum electrolytes*, and *urinary sodium* helps to guide treatment. However, some cirrhotic patients with renal impairment do not manifest an elevated serum creatinine (believed to be related to reduced creatine synthesis by the liver). This reduces the sensitivity of the serum creatinine in some cirrhotic patients and can complicate the monitoring of their renal status. Other measures of renal function may be required. Measurement of *urinary sodium* helps to guide the use of loop diuretics, especially in persons who fail to diurese easily. *Daily weights* are essential. *Urine output* is a helpful measure but can be hard to obtain in the outpatient setting. A falling urine output accompanied by *orthostatic signs* (rise in pulse and fall in blood pressure on change from supine to standing position) suggests inadequate intravascular volume. An oral fluid challenge of several hundred milliliters of isotonic fluid can confirm the presence of hypovolemia by inducing a temporary increase in urine output.

Spontaneous Bacterial Peritonitis

Hospital admission is indicated for intravenous antibiotic therapy with a *third-generation cephalosporin*. Because of the high risk of associated hepatorenal syndrome, *albumin* is often infused as well. Rates of recurrence and mortality are very high, making long-term fluoroquinolone prophylaxis a reasonable consideration (e.g., *norfloxacin*, 400 mg/d). Survival is improved, but fluoroquinolone-resistant spontaneous bacterial peritonitis is an emerging concern. *Trimethoprim/sulfamethoxazole* (one double-strength tablet every 5 of 7 days/wk) is sometimes used as an alternative as well as for primary antibiotic prophylaxis.

Hepatic Encephalopathy

The key elements of treatment are removing precipitants, reducing ammonia production, improving ammonia metabolism, lowering false transmitters, and inhibiting γ-aminobutyric acid (GABA)–benzodiazepine receptors.

Removal of Precipitants. Important precipitating factors include GI bleeding; excessive dietary protein intake; hypokalemic alkalosis; infection; constipation; the use of sedative, opiate, or hypnotic drugs; surgical procedures; and volume depletion resulting from diuresis or paracentesis. Precipitants are identified in about 50% of patients; the prognosis is usually better in those with an identifiable contributory factor than in those in whom the onset of encephalopathy is associated only with worsening hepatocellular function.

Reducing Ammonia Production. A mainstay of therapy is the restriction of dietary protein intake. Limiting intake to 0.8 to 1.0 g/kg is recommended but may need to be relaxed a bit over time if it is hard to maintain adequate nutrition. Controlled trials support dietary protein restriction and the substitution of animal protein with vegetable sources (their metabolism produces less ammonia). Sometimes, oral *amino acid supplements* (high in branched-chain varieties and low in aromatic amines) are added; they have no proven effect on encephalopathy, but they can help to prevent negative nitrogen balance.

Simple *gut cleansing* with enemas or cathartics is effective when bleeding, constipation, or a large dietary protein intake has led to encephalopathy. *Lactulose* (a synthetic, nonabsorbable disaccharide metabolized to organic acids by enteric bacteria) causes an osmotic catharsis and also suppresses the growth of ammonia-forming, urease-producing bacteria in favor of lactose-fermenting organisms. The initial dosage for patients with mild encephalopathy is 15 to 30 mL orally every 4 to 6 hours, with adjustments thereafter to produce two to three loose stools a day. Side effects of oral lactulose include diarrhea and abdominal distress, which usually resolve after a reduction in dose.

The use of poorly absorbed antibiotics, such as the aminoglycoside *neomycin*, decreases the intestinal concentration of ammonia-forming bacteria; efficacy is comparable to that of lactulose. Combination therapy can be used. Adverse effects of neomycin include oto- and nephrotoxicity when excessive doses are used or there is concurrent renal insufficiency; the drug also causes malabsorption. *Metronidazole* (800 mg/d for 1 week) may be used instead of neomycin; when used for short periods, it is less toxic. The eradication of *Helicobacter pylori* is meeting with some initial success in uncontrolled studies, presumably because of its contribution to ammonia production (it is a urea splitter). Repopulating the colon with non–urease-producing organisms, such as *Lactobacillus acidophilus*, has been tried with variable success; *Enterococcus faecium* use has been more promising.

Improving Ammonia Metabolism. Dietary supplements of *ornithine aspartate*, *benzoate*, and *phenylacetate* are believed to increase ammonia metabolism, and studies are encouraging, with benefits approaching those seen with lactulose in persons with mild encephalopathy. *Zinc*, a required cofactor of several enzymes of the urea cycle, is often deficient in cirrhotic patients. The treatment of zinc deficiency with 600 mg/d of zinc supplement has been helpful in some but not all controlled trials of this element.

Reducing False Transmitters. The restriction of aromatic amino acids and the use of preparations rich in branched-chain amino acids are based on the hypothesis that such an approach reduces the production of false neurotransmitters. The results of controlled trials are equivocal at best. Nitrogen balance may improve, but improvement in encephalopathy may be hard to come by.

Inhibition of GABA-Benzodiazepine Receptors. The binding of ligands to this receptor is believed to be pathophysiologically important in hepatic encephalopathy. The receptor antagonist *flumazenil* shows some promise in preliminary studies of persons with advanced encephalopathy.

Variceal Bleeding

Primary and secondary prophylaxis against bleeding is the principal concern of the primary care physician. In patients with known varices, the risk of bleeding is high (e.g., 65% in the first year).

Identification of Persons at Risk. Independent risk factors include marked hepatocellular dysfunction, ascites, encephalopathy, large varices, and the presence of dilated venules on the varices. Because clinical and endoscopic risk factors are independent and therefore not predictive of one another, some authorities recommend the endoscopic assessment of all cirrhotic patients to determine the risk and candidacy for treatment. Others use a Child–Pugh score combined with a low platelet count as a means for identifying persons who would benefit from endoscopic screening.

Medical Prophylaxis. *Nonselective beta-blockers* (e.g., *nadolol, propranolol*) are useful in patients at high risk for variceal bleeding (e.g., those with large varices on endoscopic examination). The resultant beta-blockade and unopposed α-adrenergic stimulation reduce splenic blood flow and portal pressure. When prescribed in doses that produce a 25% reduction in resting heart rate, these agents can decrease the risk of variceal bleeding by about 50%. The rate of death from hemorrhage is also reduced but all-cause mortality is not. Persons with Child class A and B disease respond best. Efficacy is less in secondary prevention. Use to prevent the development of varices in unselected cirrhotic patients who were initially varices-free has not been successful, but the identification of certain subgroups that might benefit (e.g., those with low baseline hepatic venous pressure gradient) is ongoing.

The addition of a long-acting nitrate (*isosorbide mononitrate*) to beta-blockade provides enhanced secondary prophylaxis, improving survival by 20% and reducing the risk of recurrent bleeding by 70% over that achieved by endoscopic ligation of varices.

Endoscopic Therapy. *Endoscopic band ligation* of varices has emerged as the preferred endoscopic approach to *primary prevention*, superseding sclerotherapy (better outcomes, fewer treatments and complications). Results are superior to those for beta-blockade and are enhanced when both are used. For *secondary prevention*, band ligation is a reasonable alternative to combination medical therapy (beta-blockade/long-acting nitrates) but is not as effective.

Shunting. Shunting is reserved as a secondary prophylaxis measure of last resort for persons who fail endoscopic and medical therapies. *TIPS* is the best tolerated of shunt procedures, involving angiographic placement of a stent from a branch of the hepatic vein through the liver parenchyma and into a branch of the portal vein. Portal pressure and the risk of bleeding are reduced, but stent failure occurs in up to 50% of cases, and encephalopathy often worsens or develops. The procedure has a 5% mortality risk. For patients awaiting liver transplantation, TIPS can be used to bide time. *Portosystemic shunt surgery* remains the final treatment option. Although it reduces the risk of hemorrhage, shunt surgery increases the risk of encephalopathy, and operative mortality rates are high. There is no survival benefit.

Hepatorenal Syndrome

Prevention is key because there is no effective treatment other than liver transplantation. Careful avoidance of volume depletion and prompt volume replacement are essential measures (see earlier discussion), as are prevention and prompt treatment of spontaneous bacterial peritonitis, a major precipitant (see earlier discussion). The avoidance of nephrotoxic agents is also essential, including nonsteroidal antiinflammatory drugs, aminoglycoside antibiotics, and iodinated contrast agents for imaging procedures.

The development of the hepatorenal syndrome requires hospital admission for treatment. Vasoconstrictor therapy (e.g., intravenous norepinephrine or terlipressin or oral midodrine in combination with subcutaneous octreotide) in conjunction with albumin infusion has been used successfully, reducing serum creatinine to below 1.5 mg/dL over 5 to 15 days of treatment.

Coagulopathy

If a patient with cirrhosis is discovered to have a prolonged PT, a trial of *vitamin K*, 10 mg subcutaneously daily for 3 days, will correct hypoprothrombinemia caused by bile-salt deficiency, neomycin, or malnutrition but not hypoprothrombinemia related only to hepatocellular disease. In the absence of bleeding, measures to correct abnormal coagulation parameters are generally not indicated.

Liver Transplantation (15,43)

In the face of terminal hepatocellular failure, liver transplantation becomes an important consideration. In properly selected patients, 5-year survival may be as high as 85%.

Candidates

The best candidates are those who are highly motivated, emotionally stable, and willing to comply with a medical program. Postnecrotic cirrhosis, primary biliary cirrhosis, and primary sclerosing cholangitis are among the primary indications, as are refractory ascites, recurrent spontaneous bacterial peritonitis, recurrent variceal bleeding, and encephalopathy. Alcohol-induced liver disease associated with continued drinking is a strong relative contraindication, as are hepatitis B liver disease, hepatocellular carcinoma, and renal failure. Absolute contraindications are AIDS, extrahepatic sepsis, metastatic cancer, and severe cardiopulmonary disease. Advanced age is not a poor prognostic factor, nor is alcoholic liver disease in a person who abstains from drinking for 6 months before transplantation.

Evaluation and Indications for Liver Transplantation

The development of *refractory ascites* is an indication for the consideration of liver transplantation; the 5-year survival rate (30% to 40%) compared with that for patients with transplantation (70% to 80%). Other indicators of poor prognosis and the need for transplantation include *spontaneous bacterial peritonitis* and *hepatorenal syndrome*. As noted earlier, the *MELD score* (based on serum bilirubin, INR, and creatinine and expressed as the nearest integer between 6 and 40) provides a validated estimate of the relative 3-month survival and serves to designate priority for transplantation. Despite international consensus on MELD implementation, waiting times for persons with the same MELD score differ among transplant centers; those doing the largest volume of transplants have had the shortest waiting times and perform more transplants on less sick patients.

THERAPEUTIC RECOMMENDATIONS AND MONITORING

General Measures

- Instruct patients to maintain a caloric intake of at least 2,000 to 3,000 kcal/d.
- Prohibit the use of alcohol or other hepatotoxic agents.

- Instruct patients to avoid tranquilizers and sedatives.
- Monitor PT, serum albumin, and bilirubin to assess the severity and progression of hepatocellular dysfunction.
- Have the patient keep a record of daily weights.
- Check stools at each visit for evidence of occult bleeding.
- Check for asterixis and other signs of encephalopathy at each visit.
- Check the abdomen for evidence of ascites (shifting dullness, fluid wave, bulging flanks) and, if it is suspected, obtain a ultrasound to confirm the presence of ascites and rule out venooclusive disease.

Management of Ascites

- Perform a diagnostic paracentesis in patients with the new onset of ascites or clinical deterioration in the setting of pre-existing ascites. Send fluid for cell count and differential, total protein and albumin concentrations, culture, and cytologic examination.
- Restrict daily sodium intake to no more than 2 g/d and maintain protein intake at a minimum of 50 g/d. Consult with a dietitian, and provide the patient and family with specific menus and food lists.
- Restrict fluid intake to 1,500 mL when there is marked hyponatremia (serum sodium concentration <125 mEq/L).
- If salt restriction does not result in diuresis, begin spironolactone 100 mg daily in divided doses. If natriuresis and diuresis do not occur after 1 week, increase the daily dose of spironolactone by 100 mg every 4 to 5 days to a maximum of 400 mg/d.
- If spironolactone alone is ineffective in causing diuresis, add furosemide 20 to 40 mg/d to the regimen and cautiously increase the dose as necessary. Monitor urinary sodium and continue furosemide as long as urinary sodium is greater than 10 mEq/L.
- Adjust the diuretic dose so that no more than 0.5 kg of fluid (approximately 1 lb) is lost per day in patients with ascites alone and no more than 1 kg/d (2 lb) in those with both ascites and peripheral edema. Halt diuretics at the first sign of intravascular volume depletion.
- Consider daily potassium supplementation (20 to 40 mEq of KCl elixir) in patients receiving furosemide; administer cautiously, if at all, to patients concurrently taking a potassium-sparing diuretic such as spironolactone.
- Monitor serum potassium, blood urea nitrogen, creatinine, urinary sodium, daily weight, and postural signs to avoid inducing intravascular volume depletion, renal failure, hypokalemia, and encephalopathy. Be aware that in some patients the serum creatinine may be falsely normal and remain within normal limits despite worsening renal function.
- Consider large-volume paracentesis (5 to 6 L) with concurrent intravenous albumin infusion (6 to 8 g/L of fluid removed) for patients with refractory ascites, especially if urinary sodium is less than 10 mEq/L. Admit for the procedure.

Encephalopathy

- At the first sign of encephalopathy, *restrict dietary protein* intake to 0.8 to 1.0 gm/kg. Obtain dietary consultation to construct a diet emphasizing plant protein over animal protein. Consider the use of an oral supplement rich in branched-chain amino acids if protein intake is insufficient.
- Monitor mental status and check for asterixis; use five-point star or signature testing. Monitoring venous ammonia levels is less useful; in drawing blood for a determination, avoid prolonged tourniquet application.
- When protein restriction fails to control encephalopathy, begin oral *lactulose*, 15 to 30 mL every 4 to 6 hours, with subsequent adjustments in the dosage to allow two to three soft stools a day. Add oral *neomycin* 1 g twice daily or *metronidazole* 250 mg three times daily if lactulose alone does not suffice. Metronidazole is probably the better tolerated for short-term use.
- Consider dietary supplementation with *ornithine aspartate*, *benzoate*, or *phenylacetate* in patients with mild encephalopathy.

Prevention of Variceal Bleeding and Bleeding Due to Clotting Factor Deficiency

- Begin a nonselective, long-acting beta-blocker (e.g., extended-release *propranolol* 60 mg/d; or *nadolol* 20 mg/d) for *primary prevention* in patients with risk factors for variceal bleeding (marked hepatocellular dysfunction, ascites, encephalopathy, large varices, and the presence of dilated venules on the varices). Advance dose as tolerated to achieve 25% reduction in the resting heart rate (hold for a rate <55 beats/min).
- Consider *endoscopic band ligation* for primary prevention in those who cannot tolerate beta-blockade—band ligation is preferable to and has superseded sclerotherapy.
- Add a long-acting nitrate (e.g., *isosorbide mononitrate*, starting at 20 mg/d) to beta-blockade for secondary prophylaxis. Advance the nitrate to 40 mg twice daily.
- Consider *endoscopic band ligation* for persons who fail secondary prophylaxis with medical therapy. Reserve shunting procedures such as TIPS for refractory recurrent bleeding and a transition to transplantation.
- Monitor PT and platelet count. Administer vitamin K (10 mg subcutaneously daily for 3 days) if there is a prolongation of PT due to drug-induced bile-salt malabsorption, neomycin, or malnutrition. Platelet transfusions are unwarranted unless there is active bleeding in the context of a very low platelet count (see Chapter 81).

INDICATIONS FOR REFERRAL AND ADMISSION (15,43)

Prompt hospitalization is required for patients with GI bleeding, worsening encephalopathy, increasing azotemia, signs of peritoneal irritation, or unexplained fever. Intractable ascites may respond to elective admission for large-volume paracentesis. Decisions about the management of refractory ascites, encephalopathy, variceal bleeding, and uncommon etiologies of cirrhosis (e.g., primary biliary cirrhosis, Wilson's disease, hemochromatosis) are best made in consultation with a gastroenterologist skilled in treating liver disease. The same pertains to candidacy for liver transplantation. When urine output falls in the absence of a clear-cut explanation, a nephrologic consultation may be of considerable help, especially because creatinine level may not adequately reflect renal function.

Patients with a poor prognosis (e.g., hepatorenal syndrome, refractory ascites, variceal bleeding) should be referred for the consideration of transplantation. Determination of the MELD score should be performed to help to stratify risk and ascertain priority for receiving a liver transplant.

PATIENT EDUCATION AND SUPPORT

It should be emphasized to the patient and the family that prognosis can often be greatly improved and symptoms lessened by careful adherence to the prescribed medical program. In particular, dietary discipline and the omission of alcohol are central

to a successful outcome and should be stressed. Many of these patients are chronic alcoholics with low self-esteem. A nonjudgmental, sympathetic physician can be instrumental in providing support, raising self-esteem, and improving the chances of compliance (see Chapter 228). Depression is a frequent accompaniment of the later stages of chronic liver disease and is manifested by failure to comply with the medical regimen and outright expressions of wanting to die. Treatment is very difficult. Antidepressant drugs may cause oversedation and thus are risky. There are no simple measures, but the physician's concern and support can help enormously (see Chapter 227).

A.H.G.

Annotated Bibliography

1. Angulo P. Nonalcoholic fatty liver disease. N Engl J Med 2002;346:1221. (*A Comprehensive review; 95 references.*)
2. Arroyo V, Gines P, Gerbes AL, et al. Definition and diagnostic criteria of refractory ascites and hepatorenal syndrome in cirrhosis. Hepatology 1996;23:164. (*Finds a lack of response to high-dose diuretics.*)
3. Black M, Friedman AC. Ultrasound examination in the patient with ascites. Ann Intern Med 1989;110:253. (*An editorial urging the routine use of ultrasound in patients with new onset of ascites, both for its confirmation and to rule out a venoocclusive etiology.*)
4. Borowsky SA, Strome S, Lott E. Continued heavy drinking and survival in alcoholic cirrhotics. Gastroenterology 1981;80:1405. (*Eighty percent of those who continued to drink heavily died an average of 7.2 months after discharge; 95% of abstainers were still alive at 14 months.*)
5. Giannini E, Risso D, Botta F, et al. Validity and clinical utility of the aspartate aminotransferase–alanine aminotransferase ratio in assessing disease severity and prognosis in patients with hepatitis C virus–related chronic liver disease. Arch Intern Med 2003;163:218. (*The ratio correlates with disease stage and prognosis; it is suggested that it is a convenient marker.*)
6. Kamath PS, Wiesner RH, Malinchoc M, et al. A model to predict survival in patients with end-stage liver disease. Hepatology 2001;33:464. (*A validation study of the Model for End-Stage Liver Disease.*)
7. Kaplan MM, Gershwin ME. Primary biliary cirrhosis. N Engl J Med 2005;353:1261. (*An excellent review by leading authorities; 98 references.*)
8. Morrison ED, Brandhagen DJ, Phatak PD, et al. Serum ferritin level predicts advanced hepatic fibrosis among U.S. patients with phenotypic hemochromatosis. Ann Intern Med 2003;138:627. (*A cross-sectional study, finding that the risk of advanced fibrosis is low when ferritin is <1,000 μg/L.*)
9. Powell LW, George K, McDonnell SM, et al. Diagnosis of hemochromatosis. Ann Intern Med 1998;129:925. (*A useful review of screening and workup; 41 references.*)
10. Powell WJ Jr, Klatskin G. Duration of survival in patients with Laennec's cirrhosis. Am J Med 1968;44:406. (*A classic paper, showing that survival is improved in cirrhotic patients who abstained from alcohol compared with those who continued to drink heavily.*)
11. Qaseem A, Aronson M, Fitterman N, et al. Screening for hereditary hemochromatosis: a clinical practice guideline from the American College of Physicians. Ann Intern Med 2005;143:517. (*Consensus recommendations, including the use of serum ferritin and transferrin saturation.*)
12. Schmitt B, Golub RM, Green R. Screening primary care patients for hereditary hemochromatosis with transferrin saturation and serum ferritin level: systematic review of the American College of Physicians. Ann Intern Med 2005;143:522. (*Finds that the benefits of screening do not outweigh the risks.*)
13. U.S. Preventive Services Task Force. Screening for hemochromatosis: recommendation statement. Ann Intern Med 2006;145:204. (*Recommends against genetic screening of the general population.*)
14. Whitlock EP, Barlitz BA, Harris EL, et al. Screening for hereditary hemochromatosis: a systematic review for the U.S. Preventive Services Task Force. Ann Intern Med 2006;145:209. (*The evidence base for the U.S. Public Health Service Task Force recommendations.*)
15. Wiesner R, Edwards E, Freeman R, et al. Model for end-stage liver disease (MELD) and allocation of donor livers. Gastroenterology 2003;124:91. (*Presents a prognostic scoring system for recipient selection.*)
16. Williams JW, Simel DL. Does this patient have ascites? How to divine fluid in the abdomen. JAMA 1992;267:2645. (*The best review of the diagnostic utility of history and physical examination methods.*)
17. Lindor K. Ursodeoxycholic acid for the treatment of primary biliary cirrhosis. N Engl J Med 2007;357:1524. (*A clinically focused review; 59 references.*)
18. Niderau C, Fischer R, Purschel A, et al. Long-term survival in patients with hereditary hemochromatosis. Gastroenterology 1996;110:1107. (*Presents evidence of a survival benefit from phlebotomy, but the study was uncontrolled.*)
19. Cello JP, Ring EJ, Olcott EW, et al. Endoscopic sclerotherapy compared with percutaneous transjugular intrahepatic portosystemic shunts after initial sclerotherapy in patients with acute variceal hemorrhage. A randomized controlled trial. Ann Intern Med 1997;126:858. (*Shunt use was associated with a lower rate of rebleeding but an increased risk of encephalopathy.*)
20. Conn HO, Levy CM, Vlahcevic ZR, et al. Comparison of lactulose and neomycin in the treatment of chronic portal systemic encephalopathy; a double-blind controlled trial. Gastroenterology 1977;72:573. (*A classic study, finding that the treatments were equally effective and free of significant toxicity at the doses used.*)
21. Duvoux C, Zanditenas D, Hezode C, et al. Effects of noradrenalin and albumin in patients with type 1 hepatorenal syndrome: a pilot study. Hepatology 2002;36:374. (*Presents evidence of efficacy.*)
22. Ginès P, Arroyo V, Vargas V, et al. Paracentesis with intravenous infusion of albumin as compared with peritoneovenous shunting in cirrhosis with refractory ascites. N Engl J Med 1991;325:829. (*A randomized comparison showing equal effectiveness and similar total hospital days.*)
23. Ginès P, Cárdenas A, Arroyo V, et al. Management of cirrhosis and ascites. N Engl J Med 2004;350:1646. (*The best review of major studies, providing a thoughtful overall approach; 64 references.*)
24. Groszmann RJ, Garcia-Tsao G, Borsch J, et al, for the Portal Hypertension Study Collaborative Group. Beta-blockers to prevent gastroesophageal varices in patients with cirrhosis. N Engl J Med 2005;353:2254. (*A randomized, controlled trial [RCT], finding no benefit in unselected patients, but benefit in those with a low hepatic venous pressure gradient; there was an increase in the risk of adverse effects.*)
25. Gupta S, Bent S, Kohlwes J. Test characteristics of α-fetoprotein for detecting hepatocellular carcinoma in patients with hepatitis C: a systematic review and critical analysis. Ann Intern Med 2003;139:46. (*Notes the scarcity of data; the existing data suggest low sensitivity and specificity.*)
26. Laine L, Cook D. Endoscopic ligation compared with sclerotherapy for treatment of esophageal variceal bleeding: a meta-analysis. Ann Intern Med 1995;123:280. (*Ligation was found to be superior for the treatment of recurrent bleeding.*)
27. Lucey MR, Carr K, Beresford TP, et al. Alcoholic liver disease is not a contraindication to liver transplantation. Hepatology 1997;25:1223. (*The prognosis is good; up to two thirds of patients who abstain for 6 months prior to transplantation never drink again.*)
28. Niederau C, Fischer R, Purschel A, et al. Long-term survival in patients with hereditary hemochromatosis. Gastroenterology 1996;110:1107. (*Observational data, showing that iron removal by phlebotomy improves survival and decreases morbidity and may lead to a normal life expectancy if it is started before the onset of cirrhosis or diabetes.*)
29. North Italian Endoscopic Club. Prediction of the first variceal hemorrhage in patients with cirrhosis of the liver and esophageal varices. N Engl J Med 1988;319:983. (*A multivariate analysis, identifying risk factors predictive of bleeding.*)
30. Ong JP, Affarwal A, Krieger D, et al. Correlation between ammonia levels and the severity of hepatic encephalopathy. Am J Med 2003;114:188. (*Ammonia levels correlate with the severity of encephalopathy; venous sampling suffices.*)
31. Pagliaro L, D'Amico G, Sorensen TIA, et al. Prevention of first bleeding in cirrhosis: a meta-analysis of randomized trials of nonsurgical treatment. Ann Intern Med 1992;117:59. (*Beta-blockers prevent first bleeding in high-risk patients; sclerotherapy is of unproven efficacy for primary prophylaxis.*)
32. Papadakis MA, Arieff AI. Unpredictability of clinical evaluation of renal function in cirrhosis. Am J Med 1987;82:945. (*Some cirrhotic patients with reduced glomerular filtration have normal serum creatinine levels, which may remain within normal limits despite a worsening renal function.*)
33. Poynard T, Cales P, Pasta L, et al. Beta-adrenergic antagonist drugs in the prevention of gastrointestinal bleeding in patients with cirrhosis and esophageal varices. N Engl J Med 1991;324:1532. (*An analysis of pooled*

data, showing a reduction in the risk of first bleeding and mortality from hemorrhage.)

34. Rector WG Jr, Reynolds TB. Superiority of serum ascites–albumin differences in "exudative" ascites. Am J Med 1984;77:83. (*Finds that this measure was better than the total protein for differential diagnosis.*)

35. Riordan SM, Williams R. Treatment of hepatic encephalopathy. N Engl J Med 1997;337:473. (*A very useful pathophysiologic approach to the treatment adopted for this chapter.*)

36. Rossle M, Ochs A, Gulberg V, et al. A comparison of paracentesis and transjugular intrahepatic portosystemic shunting in patients with ascites. N Engl J Med 2000;342:1701. (*RCT, finding that transjugular intrahepatic portosystemic shunting [TIPS] improved the chances of survival without an increased risk of encephalopathy.*)

37. Sanyal AJ, Genning C, Reddy KR, et al. The North American Study for the Treatment of Refractory Ascites. Gastroenterology 2003;124:634. (*Finds that large-volume paracentesis is superior to TIPS.*)

38. Sarin SK, Lamba GS, Kumar M, et al. Comparison of endoscopic ligation and propranolol for the primary prevention of variceal bleeding. N Engl J Med 1999;340:988. (*RCT, finding that this approach was better than beta-blockade.*)

39. Shear L, Ching S, Gabuzda GJ. Compartmentalization of ascites and edema in patients with hepatic cirrhosis. N Engl J Med 1970;282:1391. (*An elegant, classic study, finding that the maximum rate at which ascites can be absorbed is 930 mL per 24 hours, and concluding that the therapeutic aim in patients with ascites should be a weight loss of no more than 0.5 kg/d.*)

40. Stigmann GV, Goff JS, Michaletz-Onody PA, et al. Endoscopic sclerotherapy as compared with endoscopic ligation for bleeding esophageal varices. N Engl J Med 1992;326:1527. (*RCT, finding that ligation was superior and safer.*)

41. Villanueva C, Minana J, Ortiz J, et al. Endoscopic ligation compared with combined treatment with nadolol and isosorbide mononitrate to prevent recurrent variceal bleeding. N Engl J Med 2001;345:647. (*RCT, finding that combination medical therapy was superior to ligation for prevention.*)

42. Zaman A, Becker T, Lapidus J, et al. Risk factors for the presence of varices in cirrhotic patients without a history of variceal hemorrhage. Arch Intern Med 2001;161:2564. (*Child–Pugh class and platelet count identified persons with varices.*)

43. Ahmad J, Bryce CL, Cacciarelli T, et al. Differences in access to liver transplantation: disease severity, waiting time, and transplantation center volume. Ann Intern Med 2007;146:707. (*Meld score and waiting time differ by transplant center volume.*)

CHAPTER 72 ■ MANAGEMENT OF PANCREATITIS

JAMES M. RICHTER

The primary physician encounters pancreatitis in three forms that lend themselves to ambulatory management: (a) the recovery phase of acute pancreatitis, (b) chronic or chronic relapsing pancreatitis presenting as recurrent abdominal pain, and (c) pancreatic insufficiency, with steatorrhea and weight loss. The primary physician must be able to distinguish acute pancreatitis from other causes of acute upper abdominal pain (see Chapter 58), distinguish chronic abdominal pain due to pancreatitis from that due to pancreatic carcinoma and other important etiologies (see Chapters 58 and 76), and recognize and manage pancreatic insufficiency and other causes of steatorrhea (see Chapter 64). The objectives of management include relief of pain, removal of precipitants, and assurance of adequate nutrition.

PATHOPHYSIOLOGY, CLINICAL PRESENTATION, AND COURSE (1–16)

Pathophysiology

In the United States, most cases of pancreatitis are a result of excess ethanol ingestion or biliary tract disease, chiefly among middle-aged alcoholic men and elderly women with gallstones, respectively. Autoimmune disease, penetrating duodenal ulcer, trauma, hypercalcemia, hypertriglyceridemia, vascular insufficiency, tumor, heredity, ampullary stenosis, and drugs such as thiazide diuretics, glucocorticosteroids, azathioprine, and sulfasalazine are also associated with pancreatitis. Often a specific cause of pancreatitis is not found. In patients with AIDS, the risk of acute pancreatitis increases by 35 to 500 times, due in part to some of the drugs used to treat the condition and to increased risk of infection. Mutations in the cystic fibrosis gene are found in persons with chronic pancreatitis, suggesting a genetic predisposition.

The manifestations of acute pancreatic disease are produced by inflammatory breakdown of pancreatic architecture, with release of digestive enzymes into the interstitium of the gland, leading to autolysis. Chronic pancreatitis is characterized by recurrences of acute inflammation and the adverse consequences of destruction, scarring, and distortion of the pancreatic ductal and glandular tissue (e.g., pseudocyst formation and pancreatic insufficiency).

Clinical Presentation and Course

Acute Pancreatitis

Typically, acute pancreatitis produces constant epigastric, periumbilical, or left or right upper abdominal pain radiating to the back, often increased by food and decreased by upright posture. Vomiting can be persistent. Examination reveals abdominal tenderness and may include decreased bowel sounds, distention, and fever. The clinical presentation in HIV-infected patients is similar to that in immunocompetent patients but is often obscured by concurrent illnesses.

The course of acute pancreatitis depends on the severity of the disease and the underlying etiology. Patients with HIV infection or frank AIDS have particularly poor prognoses. In a patient recovering from acute pancreatitis, symptoms, principally pain, are reliable indicators of disease activity. There are grading systems that predict very severe disease but none that predict mild disease appropriate for ambulatory management. Elevated enzymes in an otherwise asymptomatic patient are usually of no significance. The serum amylase routinely falls to normal within several days but may remain elevated for weeks after an uncomplicated illness. In other instances, persistently elevated enzymes in an asymptomatic person may be a clue to the presence of a silent pseudocyst. Pseudocysts arise in about half of patients with severe pancreatitis, mostly in those with alcohol-induced disease or AIDS. Spontaneous resolution occurs over 3 months in about 50% of patients; those with persistent lesions greater than 5 cm usually require surgical drainage.

Chronic Pancreatitis

Chronic pancreatitis characteristically presents and proceeds as bouts of mild to severe recurrent epigastric pain, often occurring in *alcoholic patients* after years of excessive drinking. Sometimes chronic pancreatitis is heralded by a severe attack of acute pancreatitis. At other times, there may be mild pain or simply the painless insidious onset of exocrine insufficiency and diabetes. The pain of chronic pancreatitis is not entirely constant, and often varies in intensity over days to weeks. There may be exacerbations of pain, nausea, and vomiting after eating or drinking alcohol.

The clinical course of chronic pancreatitis is variable and depends on elimination of precipitating factors. Gallstones, particularly common bile duct stones, should be promptly removed, either surgically or endoscopically. Successful and early removal greatly reduces the risk of recurrent or chronic pancreatitis. With recurrent disease, *pancreatic insufficiency* may gradually develop over years, manifested by weight loss and steatorrhea. Although mild glucose intolerance may occur early in the disease process, the onset of clinical *diabetes* is a late complication and a sign of advanced disease. There appears to be an increased risk of pancreatic cancer.

Pancreatic Insufficiency

Patients with pancreatic exocrine insufficiency complain of *weight loss* and frequent greasy bowel movements (i.e., steatorrhea). Weight loss is often striking but nonspecific in these patients, who tend to substitute alcohol for other forms of nourishment. Steatorrhea is a late development, not seen until more than 80% of pancreatic exocrine function has been lost.

DIAGNOSIS (4,11,13,14,16–25)

Acute Pancreatitis

The diagnosis of acute pancreatitis is supported by increases in the serum amylase and serum lipase. The *serum amylase* is elevated principally in pancreatic disease but may also be high in renal insufficiency, salivary gland disease, biliary tract obstruction, aortic dissection, and such other intraabdominal conditions as perforated peptic ulcer, mesenteric infarction, and small-bowel obstruction without detectable pancreatitis. Patients with AIDS may have hyperamylasemia from salivary gland pathology or macroamylasemia. Macroamylasemia is also seen in connective tissue diseases, lymphoma, and liver disease. The *serum lipase* is more specific but less sensitive and is a good confirmatory test. Assays of *amylase isozymes* have also been developed as confirmatory tests and are especially useful when nonpancreatic sources of hyperamylasemia need to be ruled out (e.g., as in AIDS).

Improved rapid screening methods for diagnosis acute pancreatitis continue to be sought. *Trypsinogen-2 dipstick testing* of the urine is being studied as a means of quickly ruling out acute pancreatitis in the urgent care/emergency room setting. The qualitative version of the test has a sensitivity of 94% and a specificity of 95% for acute pancreatitis. When applied to patients with acute abdominal pain, a negative result effectively rules out acute pancreatitis; a positive result needs confirmation because the test has a 5% false-positive rate.

The serum amylase is the best initial diagnostic study. At times *ultrasonography* can be used for diagnostic purposes; it shows edema of the gland and any biliary tract pathology. Contrast-enhanced *computed tomography* (CT) of the abdomen also can be used to detect such findings and provide an estimate of severity. Intraglandular necrosis, surrounding edema, and fluid collections can also be detected. The test is considered the gold standard for severe cases of acute pancreatitis but is less sensitive for mild disease. *Endoscopic ultrasonography* and *magnetic resonance cholangiopancreatography* are emerging technologies for pancreatic and biliary tree imaging. Provide enhanced sensitivity and specificity compared to transabdominal ultrasound for detection of gallstones and pancreatic pathology because they are not affected by overlying bowel gas. Unlike CT, they require no iodinated dye load. They are worth considering in persons who appear to have "idiopathic" disease after standard diagnostic testing and imaging. If a mass is palpable or pain recurs, a *pseudocyst* should be ruled out by ultrasonography or CT scan of the upper abdomen.

Chronic Pancreatitis

Individuals who present with chronic recurrent abdominal pain and a history of relapsing pancreatitis usually do not present difficult diagnostic problems, but the patient without such a history requires more extensive assessment. Elevated serum *amylase* and *lipase* levels are helpful, but the sensitivity of these tests is lower than in acute pancreatitis. A *plain film of the abdomen* may reveal *pancreatic calcification*, which is a late finding in alcoholic pancreatitis. *Ultrasonography* may demonstrate a diffusely enlarged gland, local mass, or pseudocyst. If ultrasound evaluation is normal and pancreatic disease is strongly suspected on clinical grounds, *CT* of the upper abdomen should be performed. If uncertainty about cancer or the cause of chronic pancreatitis persists, *endoscopic retrograde cholangiopancreatography* (ERCP) or magnetic resonance *cholangiopancreatography* should be considered. Disadvantages of ERCP include risk of inducing an attack of acute pancreatitis. *Endoscopic ultrasound* offers much of the diagnostic detail of ERCP with less risk, proving excellent visualization of the pancreas and biliary tree. The test is unimpeded by overlying bowel gas, which can substantially lower the sensitivity and specificity of conventional transabdominal ultrasound. If a solitary pancreatic mass suggestive of malignancy is found by an imaging study, it should be followed by consideration of *needle biopsy*.

Pancreatic Insufficiency

Objective evidence of maldigestion may be obtained by a *qualitative examination for stool fat* with Sudan stain. Where this is not available, a 72-hour *quantitative stool fat analysis* can also be used to establish the presence of steatorrhea and a *d-xylose test* can be used to exclude small-bowel mucosal disease. The *bentiromide test* is a simple outpatient study for detecting pancreatic exocrine insufficiency. When bentiromide (500 mg) is given orally, it normally is acted on by pancreatic chymotrypsin to produce *para*-aminobenzoic acid, which is absorbed by the small bowel and excreted in the urine. In normal persons, greater than 50% is excreted in 6 hours. This test appears to have a sensitivity of 80% and a specificity of 90% for exocrine insufficiency. A trial of pancreatic enzyme replacement may be valuable diagnostically. When significant uncertainty persists, direct pancreatic function tests, such as secretin stimulation, may be needed objectively to demonstrate exocrine insufficiency. A small group of patients with pancreatic insufficiency who do not give a history of alcoholism or recurrent abdominal pain should be evaluated for hemochromatosis and cystic fibrosis.

PRINCIPLES OF MANAGEMENT
(1–4,6,8–10,13–16,18,26–31)

Acute Pancreatitis

About 50% of patients have mild self-limited disease and will recover spontaneously. Such patients with mild pain and no vomiting may be treated on an ambulatory basis with restriction of fat and protein and careful monitoring. Patients with more severe disease who require hospitalization generally benefit from a *diet moderately restricted in fat* to lessen the degree of pancreatic stimulation. *Histamine₂-receptor antagonists, proton pump inhibitors,* and *anticholinergics* are frequently given with the hope of reducing the stimulus to pancreatic secretion but are of no proven benefit. A patient who returns with severe pain and vomiting should be readmitted.

Identification and treatment or removal of precipitants, such as alcohol abuse, hypercalcemia, gallstones, and hypertriglyceridemia, are essential to successful therapy. Of the conditions associated with pancreatitis, alcoholism is the most difficult. Even the pain of pancreatitis often does not dissuade the dedicated drinker from abusing alcohol. Nevertheless, the *treatment of alcoholism* should be undertaken with considerable effort (see Chapter 228) because there is much to gain by the cessation of drinking. Total cessation appears necessary.

A check for drugs associated with pancreatitis is indicated (thiazides, corticosteroids, estrogens, azathioprine). In the *HIV-infected patient,* treatment of potentially etiologic opportunistic infections (e.g., toxoplasmosis, cytomegalovirus) and elimination of inciting medications (e.g., didanosine, pentamidine, sulfonamides, corticosteroids) are priorities in addition to the standard approaches to treatment.

All patients should undergo evaluation of the biliary tract by *ultrasonography* to rule out gallstone disease, a treatable cause of pancreatitis. In acute pancreatitis, removal of stones obstructing the common bile duct by *ERCP* may diminish the severity of the disease. After an acute episode, the serum calcium should be repeated because *hypercalcemia* can be masked by the decrease in calcium that may result from an attack. Repeatedly marked elevations in *fasting triglyceride* concentration suggest the diagnosis of hypertriglyceridemia, which responds to gemfibrozil (see Chapter 27).

Chronic Pancreatitis

Patients with chronic pancreatitis may develop recurrent bouts of pain and vomiting indistinguishable from the effects of acute pancreatitis. Those with severe pain and inability to maintain

hydration orally should be admitted. Others with less severe exacerbations may be managed on an outpatient basis. Many are bothered by chronic pain.

Initial treatment consists in eliminating causative factors (see earlier discussion) and attempting to control the often disabling pain. Most important is the continued total cessation of alcohol intake. Even in persons with idiopathic disease, continued use of alcohol is associated with more frequent bouts of severe pain, pancreatic calcification, and complications. In such persons, even small amounts of alcohol (<50 g/d) can lead to such adverse consequences, necessitating total cessation.

For *pain control,* pancreatic enzymes and low-fat diets may decrease pancreatic secretion but do not reliably lessen the pain. Nonnarcotic analgesics (aspirin, ibuprofen, acetaminophen) should be tried but are usually inadequate, necessitating the use of more-potent agents. *Methadone, sustained-release morphine* or *oxycodone (OxyContin)* are the narcotics best suited for long-term outpatient use. Sometimes, *antidepressants* are useful adjuncts for pain control (see Chapter 227). The establishment of a *supportive doctor–patient relationship* complements pharmacologic pain control efforts.

Numerous *surgical procedures* have been designed to alleviate the pain of chronic pancreatitis; none is totally effective. Patients with persistent pain in the absence of gallbladder disease or alcoholism should have an endoscopic *retrograde pancreatogram* to search for a surgically treatable anatomic abnormality, such as a dilated or obstructed duct. If a markedly dilated duct is found, a modified *Puestow sphincteroplasty procedure* can be performed or *stent* placed to improve drainage of pancreatic juices into the small bowel. The operation may provide reasonable pain relief without removal of pancreatic tissue. Large, persistent pseudocysts should be drained internally; however, reduction in pain is not consistently achieved. Sometimes partial or even subtotal pancreatectomies are attempted for control of pain; at best, results are equivocal.

In patients with severe active disease, the pancreas is progressively destroyed, and eventually the pain subsides as the disease "burns" itself out. Then the management priority shifts to treatment of pancreatic insufficiency.

Pancreatic Insufficiency

Management of pancreatic insufficiency begins with a therapeutic trial of oral pancreatic enzymes to judge the efficacy of therapy. The patient who benefits from use of exogenous enzymes will tolerate the unpleasant taste and mild discomfort they cause. *Pancreatin* contains trypsin, amylase, and some lipase, whereas *pancrealipase* contains trypsin, amylase, and extra amounts of lipase. The usual dose is 0.5 to 2.5 g with each meal. Because enzyme preparations are partially inactivated by gastric acid or require increased alkalinity in the duodenum, they may work better when given with antacids, bicarbonate, histamine₂-receptor antagonists, or proton pump inhibitors. *Medium-chain triglycerides* are often helpful because they can be absorbed in the absence of lipase. Therapy can be assessed by monitoring symptoms, weight, and qualitative stool fat determinations. Clinically significant fat-soluble vitamin deficiencies are uncommon, perhaps because intact bile secretion prevents complete fat malabsorption.

Most patients with chronic pancreatitis have abnormal glucose tolerance tests. Mild glucose intolerance can be watched, but insulin dependence may occur. Hypoglycemia may be a problem because loss of glucagon secretion leads to a "brittle" diabetic state, but ketoacidosis is rare. The vascular complications of diabetes are infrequent but eventually occur if severe pancreatic insufficiency persists.

PATIENT EDUCATION

Most patients know little about the pancreas and its role in digestion. Moreover, few are aware of the connection between alcohol abuse and pancreatitis. Patient cooperation regarding diet, alcohol intake, and use of enzyme extracts may be facilitated by a better understanding of the function of the pancreas and the nature of pancreatitis. In addition, patients with acute pancreatitis who are making good recoveries can be comforted by the fact that recurrence is not common when the underlying cause is treated.

The patient with intractable pain and narcotic dependence poses one of the most difficult problems encountered in clinical medicine. A major pitfall is the development of an adversarial relationship between patient and physician concerning the need for narcotics. Although there are no simple solutions, it is essential to elicit, understand, and respond to patient concerns, fears, and needs at the outset. A well-informed patient who has confidence in the physician and in himself or herself requires less pain medication than one who is scared, feels abandoned, and is in conflict with the physician.

INDICATIONS FOR ADMISSION AND REFERRAL

Some patients present with rather mild symptoms but later develop a fulminant illness. Patients older than the age of 55 years are at risk for a serious progression, as are those who manifest fever, tachycardia, hyperglycemia, serum calcium less than 8.0 mg/dL, or amylase greater than 1,000 mg/dL at the time of initial presentation. Such individuals deserve admission for careful monitoring, even if they do not appear seriously ill at the outset. Patients who cannot maintain oral hydration also require admission. Patients with refractory pain might benefit from evaluation by a gastroenterologist skilled in endoscopic retrograde pancreatography or endoscopic ultrasonography. Surgical consultation is indicated if an anatomic abnormality, pseudocyst, or obstructive lesion is detected on workup of the pancreas and biliary tract. Patients with chronic refractory pain may benefit from a psychiatric or pain management assessment, supplemented by antidepressant therapy.

MANAGEMENT RECOMMENDATIONS
(4,6,10,13–16,18,26–31)

Recovery Phase of Acute Pancreatitis

- Begin feedings with foods rich in carbohydrates and low in protein and fat. Gradually increase the amount of protein in the diet as tolerated, followed by slow resumption of fat intake.
- Check for and treat any underlying alcohol abuse (see Chapter 228), hypertriglyceridemia (see Chapter 27), or hypercalcemia (see Chapter 96).
- Eliminate, if possible, use of drugs associated with pancreatitis (azathioprine, estrogens, thiazides, corticosteroids). In the HIV-infected patient, check for and treat any toxoplasmosis or cytomegalovirus infection, and eliminate any potentially inciting medication (e.g., didanosine, pentamidine, sulfonamides, corticosteroids).
- Obtain ultrasound examination of the gallbladder and biliary tract; refer the patient for consideration of surgery if stones are found.

Chronic Pancreatitis

- Check for and treat any inciting cause, such as alcoholism, biliary tract disease, hypercalcemia, or hyperlipidemia (see previous discussion). Advise total cessation of alcohol.
- Readmit the patient if severe recurrent acute pancreatitis develops.
- Temporarily limit fat intake during flare-ups.
- Begin with mild analgesics for pain control, such as aspirin or acetaminophen 600 mg every 4 hours.
- Pain unrelieved by mild analgesia is an indication for a course of narcotic analgesics, such as methadone 5 or 10 mg every 6 or 8 hours.
- Further evaluation is needed to rule out carcinoma, pseudocyst, and biliary tract disease. Begin with ultrasonography and proceed to CT, ERCP, or endoscopic ultrasonography if clinical questions remain.
- Refer the patient for surgery or radiology if a treatable lesion is found.
- Aggressive surgical procedures other than sphincteroplasty aimed at relieving ductal obstruction do not reliably relieve pain.
- Consider a trial of antidepressant therapy (see Chapter 227) for patients with refractory pain. Psychiatric or pain management consultation may also help.

Pancreatic Insufficiency

- Give an oral pancreatic extract with each feeding in doses of 0.5 to 2.5 g (two to eight tablets) with full meals and 0.5 g with snacks. Lack of effect may require the addition of a histamine$_2$-receptor antagonist (e.g., ranitidine, 150 mg twice daily) or a proton pump inhibitor to neutralize gastric acid and prevent enzymes from becoming inactivated.
- Provide a high-calorie diet rich in carbohydrate and protein.
- Supplement the diet with a medium-chain triglyceride preparation. Restrict fat in symptomatic steatorrhea.
- Monitor glucose tolerance and treat clinical diabetes, if present, with insulin, cautiously; these patients often exhibit brittle disease.

Annotated Bibliography

1. Ammann RW, Akobintz A, Largiader F, et al. Course and outcome of chronic pancreatitis: a longitudinal study of a mixed medical–surgical series of 245 patients. Gastroenterology 1984;86:820. (*Excellent clinical course/natural history study.*)

2. Bank S, Marks IN, Vinik AI. Clinical and hormonal aspects of pancreatic diabetes. Am J Gastroenterol 1975;64:13. (*Classic clinical description of pancreatic diabetes, its therapy, and its distinctive properties.*)

3. Dassopoulos T, Ehrenpreis ED. Acute pancreatitis in human immunodeficiency virus–infected patients: a review. Am J Med 1999;107:78. (*A detailed review for the generalist; 102 references.*)

4. Draganov P, Forsmark CE. Idiopathic pancreatitis. Gastroenterology 2005;128:756. (*Excellent review of this difficult condition.*)

5. Etemad B, Whitcomb DC. Chronic pancreatitis: diagnosis, classification, and new genetic developments. Gastroenterology 2001;120:682. (*An extensive review of recent observations of genetic and diagnostic approaches.*)

6. Finkelberg D, Sahani D, Deshpande V, et al. Autoimmune pancreatitis. N Engl J Med 2006;355:2670. (*Best review of the subject; 42 references.*)

7. Lankish MR, Layer P, DiMagno EP. The effect of small amounts of alcohol on the clinical course of chronic pancreatitis. Mayo Clin Proc 2001;76:242. (*Retrospective analysis followed by a prospective cohort study of persons with idiopathic disease; even small amounts of alcohol induced symptomatic recurrences.*)

8. Lowenfels AB, Maisonneuve D, Cavallini G, et al. Pancreatitis and the risk of pancreatic cancer. N Engl J Med 1993;328:1433. (*An association is found.*)

9. Lowenfels AB, Maisonneuve P, Cavallini G, et al. Prognosis of chronic pancreatitis: an international multicenter study. Am J Gastroenterol 1994;89:1467. (*Age at diagnosis, smoking, and continued drinking were the key prognostic factors.*)

10. Mallory A, Kern F Jr. Drug-induced pancreatitis: a critical review. Gastroenterology 1980;78:813. (*Still a useful paper, which includes a discussion of how to separate the presumptive from the definite.*)

11. Pitchumoni CS, Agarwal N, Jain NK. Systemic complications of acute pancreatitis. Am J Gastroenterol 1988;83:597. (*Still a useful review.*)

12. Sachdeva CK, Bank S, Greenberg R, et al. Fluctuations in serum amylase in patients with macroamylasemia. Am J Gastroenterol 1995;90:800. (*An important cause of hyperamylasemia in the absence of pancreatitis.*)

13. Sharer N, Schwarz M, Malone G, et al. Mutations of the cystic fibrosis gene in patients with chronic pancreatitis. N Engl J Med 1998;339:645. (*Evidence for a genetic basis for so-called idiopathic disease.*)

14. Steer ML, Waxman I, Freedman S. Chronic pancreatitis. N Engl J Med 1995;332:1482. (*Comprehensive review.*)

15. Toskes PP. Alcohol consumption and chronic pancreatitis. Mayo Clin Proc 2001;76:241. (*Editorial; hypothesizes that idiopathic disease might be genetic in origin, exacerbated by environmental factors such as alcohol.*)

16. Whitcomb DC. Acute pancreatitis. N Engl J Med 2006;354:2142. (*A clinically focused review;54 references.*)

17. Agarwal N, Pitchumoni CS, Sivaprasad AV. Evaluating tests for acute pancreatitis. Am J Gastroenterol 1990;85:356. (*Analysis of serologic and imaging studies.*)

18. Arvanitakis M, Delhaye M, De Maertelaere V, et al. Computed tomography and magnetic resonance imaging in the assessment of acute pancreatitis. Gastroenterology 2004;126:715. (*A review of the use of imaging for acute pancreatitis*).

19. Baron TH, Morgan DE. The diagnosis and management of fluid collections associated with pancreatitis. Am J Med 1997;102:555. (*Useful review of a difficult problem.*)

20. Forsmark CE. The diagnosis of chronic pancreatitis. Gastrointest Endosc 2000;52:293. (*Reviews difficulties in diagnosing chronic pancreatitis and the evolving role of endoscopic ultrasound.*)

21. Frossard JL, Sosa-Valencia L, Amouyal G, et al. Usefulness of endoscopic ultrasound in patients with "idiopathic" acute pancreatitis. Am J Med 2000;109:196. (*Cohort study, with an 80% yield found for the test in persons with previously undiagnosed disease.*)

22. Kemppainen EA, Hedstrom JI, Puolakkainen PA, et al. Rapid measurement of urinary trypsinogen-2 as a screening test for acute pancreatitis. N Engl J Med 1997;336:1788. (*A negative test had a high negative-predictive value; a positive test required further confirmation.*)

23. Romagnuolo J, Currie G. Noninvasive vs selective biliary imaging for acute biliary pancreatitis: an economic evaluation by using decision-tree analysis. Gastrointest Endosc 2005;61:86. (*Finds that endoscopic ultrasound is the best test for ruling out a biliary cause.*)

24. Steinberg WM, Goldstein SS, Davis SS, et al. Diagnostic assays in acute pancreatitis. Ann Intern Med 1985;102:576. (*Compares sensitivity and specificity of amylase, lipase, trypsinogen, and amylase isozymes; recommends the use of amylase as the initial study.*)

25. Toskes P. Bentiromide as a test of exocrine function in adults with pancreatic exocrine insufficiency. Determination of appropriate dose of urinary collection interval. Gastroenterology 1983;85:565. (*Standardization of the bentiromide test as a simple outpatient test for pancreatic insufficiency.*)

26. Cahen DL, Gouma DJ, Nio Y, et al. Endoscopic versus surgical drainage of the pancreatic duct in chronic pancreatitis. N Engl J Med 2007;356:676. (*A randomized, controlled trial; surgical drainage was more effective when there was obstruction of the pancreatic duct.*)

27. Folsch UR, Nitsche R, Ludtke R, et al. Early ERCP and papillototomy compared with conservative treatment for acute biliary pancreatitis. N Engl J Med 1997;336:237. (*In patients without obstructive jaundice, conservative treatment was better.*)

28. Gress F, Schmitt C, Sherman S, et al. A prospective randomized comparison of endoscopic ultrasound- and computed tomography–guided celiac plexus block for managing chronic pancreatitis pain. Am J Gastroenterol 1999;94:900. (*Celiac block can be helpful in some patients with severe chronic pain.*)

29. Richter JM, Schapiro RH, Mulley AG, et al. Association of pancreatitis and its treatment by sphincteroplasty of the accessory ampulla. Gastroenterology 1981;81:1104. (*Patients with pancreas divisum develop recurrent acute pancreatitis more frequently than do people with normal anatomy.*)

30. Twersky Y, Bank S. Nutritional deficiencies in chronic pancreatitis. Gastroenterol Clin North Am 1989;18:543. (*A thorough and useful approach to this important problem.*)

31. Warshaw AL, Banks PA, Fernandez-Del Castillo C. AGA technical review: treatment of pain in chronic pancreatitis. Gastroenterology 1998;115:765. (*Evidence-based review and recommendations.*)

CHAPTER 73 ■ MANAGEMENT OF INFLAMMATORY BOWEL DISEASE

DEANNA NGUYEN AND JAMES M. RICHTER

Ulcerative colitis and Crohn's disease account for most of the inflammatory bowel disease seen in primary care practice. Abdominal pain, diarrhea, and bleeding are the principal presenting manifestations. The first priority is to distinguish inflammatory bowel disease from other causes of diarrhea (see Chapter 64). The chronicity, potentially disabling symptoms, risk of malignancy (in the case of ulcerative colitis or Crohn's colitis), potency and serious adverse effects of medications, and

occasional refractoriness to medical therapy make management a major challenge. The primary care physician needs to know how to treat exacerbations, maintain remissions, and psychologically sustain these patients through difficult times. Competent care is based on a thorough understanding of the roles for medical and surgical therapy, skill in providing psychological support, and a good working relationship with consultants. Although patients with severe or refractory disease may need to be referred to the gastroenterologist, most of the others can be well managed by the primary care physician.

PATHOPHYSIOLOGY, CLINICAL PRESENTATION, AND COURSE (1–17)

Ulcerative Colitis

Ulcerative colitis is an idiopathic diffuse inflammatory disease of the colonic mucosa. Although pathogenesis is poorly understood, there is growing evidence of a dysregulated immune response to colonic flora. The disease typically begins in adolescence or young adulthood but may occur at almost any age. Whites are affected more often than African Americans. Prevalence is highest among Jews of eastern European descent, and among first-degree relatives of patients there is a 10-fold increase in risk for having the disease.

Clinical Presentation

The cardinal symptoms are *urgency*, *tenesmus*, and *bloody diarrhea*; in severe cases, *fever*, *anorexia*, and *weight loss* are also present. Patients may present with constipation due to proctitis or complain of abdominal cramping with bowel movements. The variability of presentations is remarkable, ranging from malaise and no symptoms referable to the colon, to fever, prostration, abdominal distention, and passage of large volumes of liquid stool. The disease need not be confined to the bowel; extracolonic manifestations include *arthritis*, *uveitis*, *jaundice*, and *skin lesions*. The course is characteristically chronic, recurrent, and unpredictable. An insidious presentation does not predict a benign course, and a fulminant onset may be followed by long, relatively asymptomatic periods.

Ulcerative colitis almost always involves the distal colon and rectum, making diagnosis possible by sigmoidoscopy. The mucosa becomes edematous, obscuring the fine network of submucosal vessels. The moist, glistening mucosal surface is lost, and a granular appearance develops. The bowel wall is friable, bleeding spontaneously or when touched with a swab. In advanced cases, pseudopolyps and discrete ulcers may be seen. Smears of mucus from the bowel wall show polymorphonuclear leukocytes. Radiologic findings range from mucosal denudation to frank ulceration, with a loss of haustral markings and a tubular appearance. There are no skip areas.

Liver involvement occurs in the form of pericholangitis and fatty infiltration, which are common histologic findings in ulcerative colitis but are seldom symptomatic. Much less frequently, *chronic active hepatitis*, *cirrhosis*, or *sclerosing cholangitis* is seen. A *migratory pauciarticular arthritis* affecting principally the large joints develops in 10% of patients. This arthritis often coincides with an exacerbation of colitis and resolves with control of the underlying disease. *Ankylosing spondylitis* also occurs but runs a course independent of the colitis. *Uveitis* may be seen at any time during the course of the disease, whereas *episcleritis* or *scleritis* usually mirrors bowel symptoms. *Erythema nodosum*, *oral aphthous ulcerations*, and *pyoderma gangrenosum* are found in about 5% of patients; the first two usually during active colitis, whereas the last may occur independent of bowel inflammation.

Course

The prognosis for patients with ulcerative colitis seen in the primary care setting is far better than that for patients studied in referral centers, who are likely to have more severe disease. Long-term, community-based studies find that nearly 90% of patients go into complete remission after the first attack and less than 10% develop chronic persistent disease. Among those with chronic disease, nearly three fourths have disease limited to the distal bowel (rectum or rectosigmoid). Overall mortality in community-based populations of ulcerative colitis patients is no different from that of the general population, although it is increased in patients with severe first attacks or extensive disease.

There is an increased risk of cancer, which correlates with the extent and duration of disease and age at diagnosis. Risk begins to increase substantially after 8 years of illness. A meta-analysis showed a risk of 2% at 10 years after diagnosis, 8% after 20 years, and 18% after 30 years. However, more recent data suggest that the risk may be lower due to better management of the disease.

Ulcerative Proctitis

Ulcerative proctitis is a variant of ulcerative colitis, distinguished by the limited extent of inflammation, its good prognosis, and the paucity of serious complications. Typically, the patient with ulcerative proctitis is a young adult who presents with *rectal bleeding* and *tenesmus*. The bleeding is usually not severe; it is sometimes mistakenly attributed to hemorrhoids. *Diarrhea* or *constipation* may accompany the bleeding, but often there are only small, frequent bowel movements associated with a small amount of mucus. On sigmoidoscopy, an edematous friable rectal mucosa is observed; the bowel above the rectosigmoid is uninvolved. On barium enema or colonoscopy, the remainder of the large bowel is normal.

The clinical presentation of ulcerative proctitis is not pathognomonic; the condition must be distinguished from infectious forms of proctocolitis, including AIDS-related etiologies (see Chapters 13 and 66). Although prognosis is good, relapses are common. Fewer than 15% of cases progress to generalized ulcerative colitis. The distant complications of ulcerative colitis are rare, and the risk of carcinoma of the rectum is only slightly, if even at all, increased compared to unaffected individuals.

Crohn's Disease

Pathophysiology

Crohn's disease is a chronic relapsing inflammatory disorder of the alimentary tract. Purported mechanisms include an *autoimmune-like* response, as well as a dysregulated response to intestinal microbial flora. There are high levels of selected T cell populations, with mucosal T helper cells producing increased amounts of tumor necrosis factor-α. The infusion of monoclonal antibodies directed against this cytokine can produce remission of otherwise refractory disease (see Management). There may also be inadequate production of counterregulatory substances.

Pathologically, the distribution of bowel inflammation may be *discontinuous*, with diseased segments of bowel separated by normal areas. Because the granulomatous inflammatory process may extend *transmurally* through all layers of the bowel wall, it has a tendency to cause *perforation*, *strictures*, *fistulas*, and *abscesses*.

Clinical Presentation

Peak onset is in the second and third decades, but the condition may begin late in life. It often affects the distal ileum and right colon but frequently involves only the small bowel or colon. It may occur in any portion of the alimentary tract, from the buccal mucosa to the anus. Symptoms vary, depending on the location and extent of disease. *Diarrhea* and *abdominal pain* (particularly in the right lower quadrant) are cardinal symptoms, occurring in almost 80% of patients. *Weight loss, vomiting, fever, perianal discomfort,* and *bleeding* are also common complaints. *Constipation* may be an early manifestation of obstruction. Symptoms can develop subtly or can present in fulminant fashion with the patient systemically toxic. Extraintestinal involvement occurs in 15% to 20% of cases, with *arthritis, ankylosing spondylitis, uveitis, erythema nodosum, aphthous oral ulcers,* and *pyoderma gangrenosum* being the predominant manifestations of disease outside the bowel. In addition, *cholelithiasis* and *nephrolithiasis* have a higher incidence in these patients than in the general population.

Physical examination may reveal a discrete abdominal mass, especially in the right lower quadrant, but usually a normal abdomen or doughy loops of bowel are found. Abdominal or perianal fistulous tracts are noted on examination in up to 10% of patients. Extraintestinal findings include inflamed joints, spinal deformities, erythema nodosum, pyoderma gangrenosum, uveitis, and aphthous ulcers.

Sigmoidoscopy is abnormal in fewer than 20% of cases; fistulous tracts and discrete inflammatory ulcers are sometimes encountered in the rectosigmoid. Imaging studies show segmental involvement of large and small bowel, often with strictures, fistulas, and ulcers. Because there are typically "skip" areas and cecal involvement, definitive diagnosis usually requires colonoscopy with ileal intubation (see Workup).

Prognosis

Although it is difficult to extrapolate from referral center data to patients seen in primary care settings, a pattern emerges of disease activity that waxes and wanes over many years. Disease-free intervals may last as long as several years or even decades, but recurrences are the rule. Several years of relief from symptoms may be afforded by surgical resection, but there is no evidence that any medical and surgical therapy alters the ultimate course of the illness. In referral center series, as many as 70% of patients ultimately require surgical resection.

WORKUP (2,13,18,19)

Proper management requires establishing a working diagnosis and determining the extent of disease.

Ulcerative Colitis

Diagnosis

Clinical presentation and sigmoidoscopic demonstration of mucosal inflammation usually suggest the diagnosis; stool culture and examination for ova and parasites help to exclude potentially mimicking bacterial and parasitic infections (see Chapter 64). Because the disease almost invariably affects the distal colon and rectum, *sigmoidoscopy* or *colonoscopy* is an essential component of the workup. The procedure is best performed without cleansing preparations, so as not to distort the appearance of the bowel mucosa (see Appendix 56.1). In

acute phases of the illness, the mucosa appears friable and inflamed; there is loss of the normal vascular pattern. As the disease progresses, a *purulent exudate* and *discrete small ulcers* may form. With severe colitis, there may be pus, spontaneous bleeding, and large ulcers. A *granular mucosa* and inflammatory *pseudopolyps* (tags of damaged mucosa and granulation tissue) characterize chronic phases of the disease. One should *culture the stool* for *Entamoeba histolytica, Campylobacter, Shigella, Salmonella, Escherichia coli 0157, Yersinia,* and *Neisseria gonorrhea* and *test for Clostridium difficile* toxin(s) (see Chapters 64 and 66). *Rectal biopsy* helps to confirm the diagnosis and exclude conditions such as *Crohn's disease of the rectosigmoid,* amoebic colitis, pseudomembranous colitis, cytomegalovirus infection, and herpetic pancolitis. *Barium enema* or *colonoscopy* can be used to provide supportive evidence when the diagnosis is in doubt and helps to document the extent of disease. There is a small risk of *perforation* when the procedure is performed on an acutely and severely inflamed bowel; under such circumstances, it is safer to delay full colonoscopic exam for determining the extent of disease until there has been clinical improvement.

Estimating Disease Activity and Severity

The appearance of the bowel mucosa on *colonoscopy* remains the mainstay of assessment of disease activity. Scoring systems based on clinical parameters are sometimes used in research settings but have little utility in clinical practice. Disease severity is defined more clinically. *Mild* disease is defined as fewer than four bowel movements a day and no signs of toxicity (i.e., fever, tachycardia, anemia, or elevation of sedimentation rate). *Moderate* disease is characterized by four to six bowel movements a day plus minimal toxicity. *Severe* disease is manifested by six or more bowel movements a day and/or signs of toxicity.

Crohn's Disease

Diagnosis

Crohn's disease of the colon may mimic ulcerative colitis clinically. Differentiating features include *skip areas* in the colon, significant *small bowel involvement, fistulas, strictures, perianal disease, oral apthous ulcers,* and *granulomas* on biopsy. The diagnosis is suggested by a history of recurrent lower abdominal pain and diarrhea, especially with nocturnal bowel movements; it is reinforced by finding on physical examination a mass or tenderness in the right lower quadrant.

Small bowel involvement can be demonstrated by both noninvasive and invasive study. *Upper gastrointestinal series* with *small bowel followthrough* (SBFT) may show *segmental narrowing,* areas with loss of the normal mucosal pattern interspersed with areas of normal mucosa, fistula formation, and the *"string sign"* (a narrow band of barium flowing through an inflamed or scarred area) in the terminal ileum. The advent of *video capsule endoscopy* and computed tomographic (CT) *enterography* provides improved noninvasive imaging compared to SBFT and a noninvasive alternative to *colonoscopy,* which requires terminal ileum intubation for the detection of small bowel involvement. CT enterography also enables the detection of other intraabdominal abnormalities, such as mesenteric adenopathy and intestinal fistulas. One risk of video capsule endoscopy is capsule impaction, which necessitates surgical removal.

Colonic disease may be documented noninvasively by *air-contrast barium enema,* with asymmetric segmental changes distinguishing Crohn's disease of the large bowel from ulcerative colitis. Disease of the terminal ileum can often be detected on barium enema; however, involvement of the terminal ileum is not unique to Crohn's disease; some ulcerative colitis patients also demonstrate inflammatory changes in the terminal ileum ("*backwash ileitis*"), but they lack the skip pattern characteristic of Crohn's disease.

Invasive study by *sigmoidoscopy* demonstrates rectosigmoid inflammation in the 20% to 50% of patients with disease in this area; however, the findings may be nonspecific (mild erythema). *Colonoscopy* may be needed in difficult cases and helps in judging the extent and severity of disease, especially documenting the presence of absence of disease in the terminal ileum. *Biopsy* should always be done as part of the endoscopic examination; findings of chronic inflammation help to confirm inflammatory bowel disease and differentiate it from acute intestinal inflammatory conditions.

Estimating Disease Activity and Severity

Disease activity in the colon is best assessed by *colonoscopy* and in the small bowel by colonoscopy with ileal intubation and/or *barium enema or CT enterography*. Disease severity is categorized clinically. *Mild to moderate* disease is defined as having symptoms but functioning adequately on an ambulatory basis, maintaining oral intake of food and fluids, and showing no signs of toxicity or complications. In *moderate to severe* disease, symptoms are more severe, sometimes interfering with daily activity and not responding fully to treatment. In severe disease, there may be toxicity, complications, and failure to respond to full doses of oral corticosteroids.

Differentiation between Crohn's Disease and Ulcerative Colitis

It is not always possible to distinguish these two entities. In the instances of indeterminate colitis, it may be helpful to test for presence of *perinuclear anti–neutrophil cytoplasmic antibodies* (found in about half of patients with ulcerative colitis) and anti–*Saccharomyces cerevisiae antibodies* (associated with Crohn's disease). However, the sensitivity and specificity of such antibody testing are too limited for these studies to be useful in differentiating between inflammatory bowel disease and other colonic conditions. Use should be limited to distinguishing between Crohn's disease and ulcerative colitis and only in conjunction with a consideration of all other clinical findings.

PRINCIPLES OF MANAGEMENT (2,4–8,10,12,14,15,19–42)

The inflammatory bowel diseases are chronic illnesses and require long-term comprehensive management. Such management entails attention to the patient's medical, psychological, and nutritional needs and support for the family. For the most part, treatment is empirical and directed at providing symptomatic relief; however, advances in the understanding of inflammatory bowel disease pathophysiology are leading to a host of new treatments with the potential to improve treatment outcomes.

Ulcerative Colitis

Because the disease typically follows a relapsing course with acute exacerbations and intervals of remission, the approach to treatment depends on the patient's current clinical status. During remission, treatment is prophylactic; during flare-ups, the goal is control of the inflammatory process. Surgery is a consideration for those with refractory disease, especially when the entire colon is involved.

Dietary and Nutritional Measures

No specific diet improves or exacerbates ulcerative colitis. However, a *reduction in dietary fiber* may be of some benefit during periods of active disease. In patients with inactive disease, 1 or 2 teaspoons of *psyllium hydrophilic colloid* (Metamucil) in water daily often helps to bind the stool. There is an increased incidence of lactase deficiency in these patients; an empirical trial of a *milk-free diet* is reasonable when diarrhea persists despite other evidence of clinical remission. Those who are anemic from blood loss need oral or *parenteral iron supplementation* (see Chapter 82). Oral iron may be poorly tolerated, necessitating parenteral administration. Anemia may also be due to folic acid deficiency. *Folic acid supplementation* is indicated when the intake of leafy vegetables and fresh fruits is poor or when sulfasalazine or methotrexate is being taken (see later discussion). Anemia may also be due to chronic disease and may not respond to dietary and nutritional measures.

Sulfasalazine and Sulfapyridine-Free 5-Aminosalicylate Agents (5-ASAs)

This group of medications continues to be the recommended initial treatment for mild to moderate disease and for the prevention of relapses. The precise mechanism of action of 5-ASA compounds remains speculative. Hypotheses include effects on prostaglandin synthesis (particularly arachidonic acid metabolism) and the inhibition of polymorphonuclear leukocyte migration.

Preparations. *Sulfasalazine* was the first of these agents. After oral administration, about 70% of reaches the colon, where it is metabolized by intestinal bacteria, locally releasing *sulfapyridine* and the salicylate analogue *5-aminosalicylate (5-ASA)*, the presumed active moiety. The sulfa component facilitates transport to the colon, but it is also the source of allergic reactions and gastrointestinal upset (see later discussion). *Sulfapyridine-free 5-aminosalicylates* have been developed to overcome sulfa-related problems and are now in widespread use.

Olsalazine was the first of the sulfa-free 5-ASA agents. It consists of two 5-ASA molecules bound by an azo bond, which is cleaved by bacteria in the colon, releasing the active 5-ASA moiety. It is useful for achieving control of mild to moderate disease and for maintaining remissions. *Mesalamine* is 5-ASA specially coated to produce delayed release. The oral tablet formulation (Asacol) dissolves at a pH of 7, the luminal pH of the terminal ileum and colon. The methylcellulose capsule formulation (Pentasa) releases 5-ASA into the small bowel and the colon. In controlled trials, oral 5-ASA agents perform at least as well as sulfasalazine in the treatment of active mild to moderate ulcerative colitis and in maintaining remissions. Patients with very active disease should take mesalamine with meals if they note that the coated tablet is being passed undissolved; taking the pill with food can slow transit and allow more time for dissolution. *Balsalazide*, a formulation of 5-ASA linked to an inert carrier molecule via a diazo bond, releases in the colon, where bacterial enzymes break the diazo bond.

Although these oral 5-ASA agents appear to be better tolerated than sulfasalazine, they are considerably more expensive and require a large number of pills daily, threatening compliance. The latter problem is addressed with use of a once-daily, high-concentration *Multi Matrix System (MMX) mesalamine* formulation.

Efficacy. Randomized, controlled studies have shown sulfasalazine to be effective as initial treatment for patients with mild to moderate symptoms when given in doses of 4 g/d for 2 to 4 weeks. About 80% of patients respond. Because sulfasalazine is less effective than corticosteroid therapy, it is reserved for relatively mild cases; however, combined use with steroids has been suggested for the early treatment of severe disease.

Controlled studies have also documented sulfasalazine's efficacy for maintaining remissions. In one major study, more than 65% of patients given maintenance doses of 2 g/d remained symptom-free for at least 1 year, compared with 25% of patients given placebo. The prophylactic effect of maintenance therapy persists when the drug is continued beyond 1 year. The optimum dose is 2 g/d (4 g/d provides even better protection, but the frequency of side effects is markedly increased). The sulfapyridine-free 5-ASA compounds have been shown to be equivalent in efficacy in inducing and maintaining remission in mild to moderate ulcerative colitis. Asacol is commonly used at doses ranging from 2.4 to 4.8 g/d.

Adverse Effects. *Sulfasalazine* is usually well tolerated in non–sulfa-allergic persons (being safe enough to use during pregnancy and when breast-feeding), but up to 20% of patients experience adverse effects with sulfasalazine, mostly due to the sulfapyridine moiety. These range from common forms of dose-related *gastrointestinal upset* (nausea, vomiting, anorexia, heartburn) and *mild hypersensitivity reactions* (rash, fever) to uncommon but potentially serious idiosyncratic reactions such as *agranulocytosis, hepatocellular injury,* and *lupus-like phenomena.* Other potential hematopoietic effects include *anemia* (from folic acid deficiency, hemolysis, or marrow suppression), *granulocytopenia,* and *thrombocytopenia. Low sperm counts* and qualitative sperm abnormalities have been noted in men taking the drug, usually after about 2 months of therapy; these conditions reverse when the medication is stopped.

The non–sulfa-containing 5-ASA compounds are much better tolerated. The most common side effect of *olsalazine* is a dose-related *diarrhea* that can be minimized by increasing the dose gradually and taking the drug with meals. Side effects of *mesalamine* are minimal, with *headache* being the most common, but 5-ASA–related *interstitial nephritis* (seen in animal studies and case reports) is a concern with long-term, high-dose use. Idiosyncratic reactions include *pleuropericarditis, pancreatitis,* and *nephrotic syndrome. MMX mesalamine* appears to have a similar safety profile as standard mesalamine.

Of note, the use of any 5-ASA agent is associated with a potential for an *idiosyncratic reaction* of worsening *abdominal pain* and *diarrhea,* a possibility that should be considered in the differential in worsening diarrhea.

Drug Interactions. Drug interactions associated with sulfasalazine include the inhibition of *folic acid* absorption (usually not clinically significant) and a 25% reduction in *digoxin* bioavailability. Sulfasalazine's metabolism is slowed when *cholestyramine* or broad-spectrum *antibiotics* are used concurrently, an effect of uncertain clinical significance. *Ferrous sulfate* appears to have a similar effect on sulfasalazine, although iron absorption is not appreciably hindered; these drugs should not be taken at the same time. Because of the risk of neutropenia, any concurrent use with *azathioprine* or *6-mercaptopurine (6-MP)* requires extreme caution and close monitoring.

Of note, there is a potential interaction in the absorption of anticoagulants such as warfarin, enoxaparin, and similar compounds.

Topical 5-Aminosalicylate Agents

5-Aminosalicylate enemas represent a reasonable option in patients with distal colitis. At maximum dose, they are more effective than hydrocortisone enemas and are useful for persons with mild to moderate disease limited to the distal large bowel. During an acute flare, the use of both oral and topical 5-ASA formulations has been shown to be more effective than the use of either one alone. Once in remission, patients should be prescribed a maintenance program of daily topical therapy (two or three times a week) or switched to an oral formulation because of relapse risk. The safety profile is excellent; adverse effects are nil, other than idiosyncratic reactions, and the only common side effects are local itching and mild rectal irritation. The cost is considerably higher than that of a hydrocortisone enema. However, unlike steroid enemas, there is no concern about systemic steroid absorption.

Glucocorticosteroids

Steroids suppress the inflammatory process of ulcerative colitis and have important roles both as systemic agents in severe disease and as topical agents in disease confined to the rectosigmoid. When uveitis and colitis flare simultaneously, oral steroids are often effective for both. (In the absence of active colitis, the uveitis may be treated with topical steroids and mydriatics.) The best means of treating other systemic manifestations (e.g., erythema nodosum, oral aphthous ulcerations) is to control the underlying disease with systemic steroids. Patients with severe disease requiring daily steroids should receive, in addition to standard measures (see Chapter 105), calcium and vitamin D supplementation because absorption may be impaired.

Systemic Preparations. Systemic preparations are used in moderate to severe and severe disease, especially in markedly symptomatic patients with extensive bowel involvement. Those without systemic toxicity can be treated on an outpatient basis starting with the equivalent of 40 to 60 mg/d of *prednisone*. Patients who are too ill for oral therapy (i.e., those with vomiting, high fever, or signs of bowel distention) should be admitted to the hospital for intravenous treatment. Once symptoms lessen, steroids are gradually tapered over 6 to 12 weeks to the lowest dose that maintains control. Every effort should be made to taper and terminate systemic steroid therapy, both because only some ulcerative colitis patients benefit from chronic steroid use and because the adverse effects of chronic steroid therapy can be disabling (see Chapter 105). Occasionally, *alternate-day steroid* administration may suffice after a flare-up has been brought under control and poses less risk of steroid side effects.

Topical Preparations. Topical preparations are useful for disease confined to the rectosigmoid area, especially in a *foam* formulation, which is often well tolerated and may be used initially in conjunction with mesalamine *enema* to decrease the severity of inflammation. *Hydrocortisone enemas* are widely prescribed and effective, but prolonged high-dose use can lead to systemic steroid side effects (some hydrocortisone does get absorbed). The topically active steroids *beclomethasone* and *budesonide* have been found to be equally efficacious to topical hydrocortisone but with less systemic absorption and no effect on serum cortisol levels; however, the cost is considerably greater.

Immunomodulators

Patients who require chronic steroid therapy, particularly at high doses, are candidates for a trial of steroid-sparing immunomodulator therapy with *6-MP* or *azathioprine*. Because the onset of action can be slow (up to 6 months), concurrent therapy with a second agent is necessary until the drug's effect sets it. Side effects are less frequent than with systemic steroids, but these can be serious (see later discussion). The intravenous administration of *cyclosporine* is sometimes used in very ill patients not responding to intravenous steroids in an attempt to avoid or delay surgery. Results from controlled trials are variable, and the risk of toxicity is high. Cyclosporine should be used only as a bridge to longer-term agents, such as 6-MP and azathioprine.

Humanized antibodies to tumor necrosis factor (TNF) provide an encouraging, albeit very expensive new avenue of treatment. *Infliximab*, a partially humanized mouse antibody against TNF-α, has been proven beneficial in steroid-refractory or steroid-dependent ulcerative colitis and can be used as induction and maintenance therapy for moderate to severe disease. *Adalimumab*, a fully humanized antibody to TNF-α currently used in severe Crohn's disease unresponsive to infliximab, is likely to be applied to refractory cases of ulcerative colitis in the near future.

Antidiarrheal Agents

Opiates are useful for providing symptomatic relief of diarrhea, mostly during chronic active colitis. They must be used with caution in acutely ill patients because of the risk of precipitating *toxic bowel dilation*. *Diphenoxylate*, *codeine*, *tincture of opium*, *paregoric*, and *loperamide* all limit the number of bowel movements. They are given before meals and at bedtime. Loperamide is among the most effective and least addicting but is considerably more expensive. Codeine is excellent for short-term use and superior to diphenoxylate in efficacy. Tincture of belladonna and other anticholinergics help to control cramps.

Psychological Support

Although psychological disturbances are more prevalent in patients with inflammatory bowel disease than in control subjects, there is little evidence that psychiatric disease is etiologically linked to the development of ulcerative colitis. Formal psychotherapy has not proven useful, but a close, supportive, and empathetic patient–doctor relationship is invaluable to psychologically sustaining the patient through this illness (see later discussion). Fears and worries about debility, surgery, colostomy, and body image contribute markedly to the psychosocial impairment and disability associated with this illness.

Surgery

Total colectomy offers the potential for the complete cure of bowel disease, the remission of most peripheral manifestations, and the prevention of colon cancer. As such, it represents an important therapeutic consideration, albeit a difficult one. Indications include dysplasia, suspected cancer, and unresponsiveness of bowel or systemic symptoms to maximal medical management. Multifocal low-grade dysplasia in a flat lesion and dysplasia-associated lesion or mass (DALM) are increasingly appreciated premalignant lesions that should prompt consideration for colectomy. Patients with severe persistent disease requiring continuous high-dose corticosteroids that cannot be tapered after 6 to 12 months and who are unresponsive to or intolerant of 6-MP, azathioprine, or anti TNF therapy also warrant serious consideration for surgery, as do those with frequent severe relapses or complications from prolonged exposure to systemic steroids.

The traditional procedure is *proctocolectomy* with *Brooke ileostomy*. It has the advantage of being the fastest and safest procedure. The disadvantages of an ileostomy include incontinence, the need to frequently empty an external ileostomy appliance, skin excoriations, and potential need for stomal revision (in about 10% to 20% of cases). Total *proctocolectomy* with *continent ileostomy (Koch pouch)* creates a continent ileostomy that does not require wearing an appliance; it is best suited for those who desire the control of stomal output but is not without problems.

The most commonly performed procedure is *ileal pouch–anal anastomosis* (total colectomy, with or without rectal mucosectomy, ileal reservoir, and ileoanal anastomosis), which provides the opportunity to retain continence and avoid a stoma. Although there is likely to be some incontinence initially, this usually passes. About four to eight bowel movements per day are common, helped by the chronic use of low-dose antidiarrheal therapy (e.g., loperamide). Potential complications include pelvic infection, strictures, and small-bowel obstruction. In addition, "pouchitis" can occur in up to 60% of patients, and decreased fecundity has been noted in women of childbearing age.

Regardless of the surgical procedure chosen, the morbidity of active disease and the threat of cancer must be weighed against the risks of major surgery. The mortality of elective colectomy can be as high as 1% to 3%, with most patients having no postoperative complications. Stoma revision is necessary in 10% to 20% of cases.

Screening for Cancer

All patients with pancolitis of 8 or more years (when cancer risk begins to rise) should be considered for colon cancer screening. Because bowel cancer is often multicentric, the best method of screening is *colonoscopy* with multiple *biopsies*. Cancer screening should begin at 8 to 10 years with 1- to 2-year intervals.

Patients with high-grade dysplasia, multifocal low-grade dysplasia, or adenoma-like DALM should undergo colectomy if they are deemed good surgical candidates, but it is controversial whether patients with unifocal low-grade dysplasia in a flat polyp may be followed by frequent colonoscopies or be advised to undergo colectomy.

Crohn's Disease

Most patients can be treated on an outpatient basis by the judicious use of medications and careful follow-up. A strong working alliance between the patient and the primary physician is essential because the disease is chronic, relapsing, and incurable.

Diet

Adequate nutrition is critical to the promotion of healing. Sufficient protein and calories must be provided but in a manner that limits the stress put on an inflamed and often strictured bowel. Patients with cramps and diarrhea should have the *fiber* content of their diet reduced; those with steatorrhea will benefit from a decrease in *fat* intake to less than 80 g/d. An empiric trial of restricting *milk products* may terminate diarrhea due to lactase deficiency, which often accompanies the illness. More severely ill patients require *partial bowel rest*, which removes the stimulus that food has on bowel motility and secretion. *Elemental and semielemental diet preparations* (e.g., Magnacal,

Ensure, Sustacal, Isocal, Peptamen, Vivonex) have been found to induce remission, improve symptoms, and decrease disease activity in patients with acute disease. They are convenient and usually well-tolerated sources of the extra nutrition needed during exacerbations. *Total parenteral nutrition* should be used in patients whose oral intake is not adequate or in whom surgery is indicated.

Vitamin and mineral deficiencies are common and must be corrected for proper healing and the avoidance of such complications as anemia and bone disease. *Folic acid* supplementation is particularly important in patients taking sulfasalazine or methotrexate, which impairs its absorption. Patients who have ileal disease or have had ileal surgery may need extra *vitamin B₁₂*. *Vitamin D* levels are likely to be low when intake is poor or steatorrhea is a problem. An oral supplement of 4,000 IU or more usually suffices. Most vitamin and mineral deficiencies can be overcome by taking a multiple vitamin containing about five times the normal daily vitamin requirements and such minerals as iron, calcium, magnesium, and zinc.

Smoking Cessation

Smoking cessation (Chapter 54) is a top priority. Patients with Crohn's disease who quit smoking have fewer flare-ups, less frequent need for potent immunosuppressants, and fewer postoperative recurrences than those who continue to smoke.

Antidiarrheal Agents

The use of these agents in Crohn's disease is similar to that in ulcerative colitis (see earlier discussion). The risks include addiction and the exacerbation of obstructive symptoms.

Sulfasalazine and Other 5-Aminosalicylate Preparations

The National Cooperative Crohn's Disease Study demonstrated a modest efficacy of *sulfasalazine* in patients with disease of the colon but no benefit in those with disease limited to the small bowel. Doses of 4 to 6 g/d are used to treat acute exacerbations of abdominal pain and diarrhea in patients with colonic involvement. Improvement typically occurs within 4 to 8 weeks; however, the drug does not sustain remissions, except after surgery. Nonetheless, it may reduce the risk of recurrence by up to 40%, with the benefit most notable for disease of the small bowel. The combination of sulfasalazine with *corticosteroids* has not been shown to have a steroid-sparing effect or allow more rapid tapering of steroids once a remission has been induced.

Because of potential sulfa-related adverse effects of sulfasalazine, sulfa-free 5-ASA preparations (e.g., *mesalamine, olsalazine, or balsalazide*) are now more commonly used. Olsalazine and balsalazide deliver 5-ASA exclusively to the colon, making them useful for those with disease confined to the large bowel. Mesalamine tablets (Asacol) are formulated to deliver 5-ASA to the terminal ileum and large bowel; mesalamine capsules (Pentasa) release 5-ASA to the entire small bowel and colon. A meta-analysis failed to show a treatment benefit for Pentasa, and the efficacy of routine long-term prophylactic use is not established. Although 5-ASA compounds do not appear to be as obviously effective in Crohn's disease as they are in ulcerative colitis, they are often tried, given their safety profile and the lack of safe and effective treatment for mild Crohn's disease.

Adverse Effects. See this section under Ulcerative Colitis.

Antibiotics: Metronidazole and Ciprofloxacin

Both of these agents have been shown to be effective in Crohn's colitis. *Metronidazole*, in doses of approximately 20 mg/kg per day, is effective in the treatment of patients with Crohn's ileocolitis or colitis and is a reasonable next step in patients who fail to respond adequately to a 5-ASA agent. In addition, uncontrolled studies have demonstrated healing of rectovaginal fistulas, abscesses, and proctocolectomy wounds. It appears that maintenance therapy at a lower dose can minimize the recurrence of perineal disease. *Gastrointestinal upset, metallic taste*, and *paresthesias* (a manifestation of peripheral neuropathy associated with chronic use) sometimes limit patient acceptability. There is a small risk (1% to 2%) of an *Antabuse-like reaction* occurring with concurrent alcohol use. Persons on long-term therapy who would like to have an occasional drink can conduct a trial of modest alcohol intake at home (where any vomiting will not be embarrassing) to see if they are at risk.

Ciprofloxacin demonstrates efficacy at 1-g/d dosing in patients with mild to moderate disease and appears to be better tolerated than metronidazole, making it an increasingly popular antibiotic choice. It is often used in combination with metronidazole. A new antibiotic agent, *rifaximin*, shows promise.

Glucocorticosteroids

If a patient is acutely ill or has moderate to severe disease not responding to 5-ASA therapy or antibiotic therapy, then systemic steroids are indicated. High doses (e.g., the equivalent of 40 to 60 mg/d *prednisone*) should be used initially.

As acute disease activity subsides, the steroid dose should be empirically tapered to the minimum necessary to control symptoms. Occasionally, *alternate-day regimens* suffice to control disease activity; they have the advantage of minimizing the steroid side effects (see Chapter 105). As long as 4 months of steroid therapy may be necessary to treat an exacerbation.

Newer oral steroid preparations are now available, such as controlled-release *budesonide*, which is topically active in the terminal ileum and proximal colon yet much less likely to cause systemic side effects because it is 90% inactivated after the first pass through the liver. It has proven to be more effective than mesalamine in persons with active mild to moderate disease and as effective as systemic corticosteroids in patients with mild disease, yet it is relatively free of adverse systemic effects.

Although steroids occupy a central place in the treatment of Crohn's disease, they are ineffective for maintaining remissions, preventing exacerbations, or healing fistulas. Prophylactic steroids are not indicated in Crohn's disease. Moreover, some extraintestinal manifestations and perianal disease do not respond well to glucocorticoids. An important goal of treatment is the discontinuation of steroids, necessitating the consideration of maintenance mesalamine tablets, antibiotics, and other immunomodulatory/antiinflammatory agents.

Thiopurines: 6-Mercaptopurine and Azathioprine

These closely related immunomodulators are especially useful for their *steroid-sparing* effects, providing an option for maintenance therapy that is considerably less toxic than chronic steroids. In controlled studies, these agents achieve or maintain control and allow a reduction or discontinuation of steroids in two thirds to three fourths of patients. There can be a delay in onset of effect of up to 6 weeks to months, necessitating the continuation of concurrent therapy until the effect sets in. The optimal duration of treatment is unknown; treatment may need to be continued indefinitely as long as no adverse effects are observed. Unlike other forms of medical treatment for Crohn's disease, chronic immunosuppressive immunomodulatory therapy has been shown to be capable of *maintaining remission*, especially in patients with fistulas or frequent relapses.

Limitations to immunomodulator therapy include a slow onset of action and potentially serious side effects. The onset of action may take as long as 3 to 6 months in some patients. In addition, immunomodulator therapy may induce serious *infection*, *pancreatitis*, *bone marrow suppression*, or *drug-induced hepatitis*, or even *lymphoma*. The monitoring of blood counts is essential. Despite the potential for such adverse effects, 6-MP and azathioprine have a good safety profile. Safe thiopurine dosing is facilitated by testing for drug-metabolism genotype or enzymatic activity. Patients with normal thiopurine methyltransferase enzymatic activity or homozygous wild-type alleles can be started at higher doses of medications. If they have intermediate activity or are heterozygous for the low-metabolizing allele, they should be started on a low dose and titrate up as tolerated. If enzymatic activity is low or absent or if they are homozygous for the low-metabolizing allele, it is safest to avoid thiopurines. The optimal daily dose of 6-MP should be 1 to 1.5 mg/kg and that for azathioprine 2 to 2.5 mg/kg. The initiation of immunomodulator therapy should not be done without first consulting a gastroenterologist familiar with the use of these agents.

Methotrexate and Other Immunomodulating/Antiinflammatory Agents

Many other agents have been examined for use as steroid-sparing therapy. They should be used only in consultation with a gastroenterologist familiar with their use in inflammatory bowel disease.

Methotrexate. Methotrexate, the folic acid antagonist with antiinflammatory effects, reduces steroid needs and improves disease control in patients requiring chronic steroid therapy. Required doses range from 15 to 25 mg once weekly. Factors limiting its use include stomatitis, nausea, transaminitis, and potential for hepatic fibrosis; the drug is also strongly teratogenic (an important consideration in women of childbearing age). Some side effects can be minimized with the concurrent use of folic acid 1 to 2 mg/d.

Biologics. Inhibition of Tumor Necrosis Factor with Monoclonal Antibodies. The infusion of monoclonal antibody cA2 (*infliximab*) directed against TNF-α helps to induce and maintain remission in patients with moderate to severe disease resistant to other forms of therapy. Patients with refractory fistulas achieve a marked clinical response, with some fistulas healing completely; however, over time, patients may become less responsive, necessitating an increase in dose (from 5 mg/kg to 10 mg/kg) and/or a shortening of the dosing interval (<8 weeks). Even after such attempts, a total loss of response may require a switch to a fully humanized antibody to TNF-α, *adalimumab*, which theoretically should induce less antidrug antibody formation. *Serum sickness*–like and lupus-like reactions have occurred with repeat infusions, and *lymphoma* and *antinuclear antibody positivity* have been noted in patients receiving cA2 therapy. The long-term immunogenicity of infliximab appears to limit its efficacy, making concurrent administration of antimetabolite immunomodulators advisable at least for the first 6 months, although this is still controversial, given the potentially increased risk, although minimally, of

hepatosplenic T cell lymphoma with concurrent therapy. The cost is very high (in the thousands of dollars) even for a single infusion. Consultation is required for the cA2 use of biologics. The important advantage of adalimumab over infliximab is the convenience of being able to self-administer the medication versus having to come to the clinic for periodic intravenous infusions.

Omega-3 Fatty Acids. Omega-3 fatty acids, which are found in fish oil and are believed to suppress inflammatory mediators such as the leukotrienes and prostaglandins, have produced modest improvements in acute disease and in the maintenance of remission.

Cyclosporin A. Cyclosporin A, an immunomodulator with a faster onset of action than that of azathioprine and 6-MP, has produced promising results in uncontrolled studies but unimpressive findings in placebo-controlled trials. The risk of toxicity is high.

Experimental Approaches. Advances in the understanding of the interaction of bowel flora, gut epithelium, and the immune system are leading to a host of very promising new approaches to therapy. In addition to infliximab for the inhibition of tumor necrosis factor (see earlier discussion), there have been encouraging results with monoclonal antibodies directed against integrins (e.g., *natalizumab*), with agents that stimulate regulatory T cells, and with microbes that can inhibit inflammatory and immune responses. The literature should be followed closely because these approaches have the potential to enhance treatment options.

Surgery

Unlike ulcerative colitis, surgery in Crohn's disease does not cure the patient. It is therefore best reserved for patients who have intractable disease, perforation, obstruction, severe bleeding, or fistulous disease. It has been estimated that the probability of surgery is 78% at 20 years and 90% at 30 years from the onset of Crohn's disease symptoms. The objective of surgery is to remove grossly involved bowel and spare as much normal-appearing bowel as possible. Postoperative recurrence rates have been estimated to be 30% to 50% per decade and are inversely related to preoperative disease duration. The most common operation is removal of a diseased portion of the terminal ileum with an *ileocolonic anastomosis*. For patients with colonic involvement, *colectomy* with an internal anastomosis connecting the ileum to the sigmoid colon or total *proctocolectomy* with *Brooke ileostomy* is the procedure of choice. Ileostomy is necessary in patients with marked rectosigmoid disease. From 20% to 40% of ileostomies need revision within 5 years because of disease in the stomal area.

Surgical treatment is undertaken with reluctance and only in the setting of severely disabling disease or serious complications. The patient presenting with obstruction may respond sufficiently to bowel rest, nasogastric suction, steroids, and other conservative measures, avoiding the need for immediate surgery, unless the obstruction persists or recurs quickly. In lieu of bowel resection, *stricturoplasty* should be considered if the length of stricture is appropriate for the more limited procedure. All attempts should be made to use a conservative surgical approach that preserves functional bowel. The loss of bowel, especially the right colon, can lead to disabling postsurgical diarrhea.

Perianal fistulous disease often requires a combination of medical and surgical therapy. Surgery is required for the drainage of perianal abscesses and can also be of help in conjunction with antibiotic therapy for superficial and low fistulas. High and extrasphincteric fistulas may benefit from a combination of surgical measures, antibiotics, and immunomodulator therapy.

Screening for Cancer

Patients with Crohn's colitis are at an increased risk for colon cancer; they should undergo cancer screening according to guidelines similar to those for ulcerative colitis (see earlier discussion).

Management of the Pregnant or Nursing Patient with Inflammatory Bowel Disease

For patients with a flare-up of inflammatory bowel disease during nursing or pregnancy, both 5-ASA and steroids are safe and effective. To maintain remission throughout pregnancy in ulcerative colitis, 5-ASA compounds should be continued. Metronidazole should be avoided. It is controversial whether immunomodulatory agents are injurious to the fetus or nursing child; if possible, they should be avoided; if are used, they should be continued with careful monitoring and only after thorough discussion with the patient about the potential risks. The risk of a bad outcome during pregnancy from halting immunomodulator therapy is probably higher than the risk from the medications themselves. Women with ulcerative colitis are prone to suffer new attacks or exacerbation during the first trimester of pregnancy and have a spontaneous abortion rate of about 10%. Pregnancy seems to inhibit relapses during later trimesters. If conception occurs during remission, the risks of complications of the pregnancy appear to be no greater than average.

PATIENT EDUCATION

The education and support of the patient and the family are essential. Fears abound when patients are told they have ulcerative colitis or Crohn's disease. These diagnoses conjure up images of colostomy, recurrent hospitalizations, invalidism, and social isolation. It is important to emphasize that the vast majority of patients lead fully functional lives, and many obtain satisfactory control of their disease through medical therapy.

Because these are chronic diseases that affect young adults, questions of conception, pregnancy, and childbearing arise. Although there is some familial pattern to the occurrences of the inflammatory bowel diseases, transmission is not purely genetic, and there is ample evidence that when the disease is in remission, fertility is essentially normal, and healthy, full-term infants can be delivered. However, conception might be a problem when a male patient is taking sulfasalazine (see earlier discussion) or when a woman has undergone colectomy with J pouch reconstruction (see earlier discussion).

The issue of cancer risk in patients with longstanding and extensive ulcerative colitis or Crohn's colitis can be addressed directly and clearly, reassuring those with minimal disease that their risk is no greater than that of the general population. Even those with extensive disease appreciate knowing the magnitude of the risk.

The primary physician can do much to prepare the patient who requires colectomy and subsequent ileostomy. Thorough patient education combined with a caring approach that includes a willingness to listen to concerns and fears is invaluable and greatly appreciated. Many patients have fears and anxieties that they will not discuss unless the physician broaches them. Also helpful in preparation for ileostomy is to have an ileostomy patient of the same age and sex discuss the procedure and its consequences with the surgical candidate. Seeing that one can go on to lead a fully active life is comforting. Where available, a local association of ostomates is a valuable resource. Finally, the more widespread use of ileoanal anastomosis in carefully selected patients may increase the acceptability of surgery.

Many patients can be taught to adjust their medication within a prearranged set of guidelines and limits. Dosages of 5-ASA to be used for mild exacerbations can be specified and extra supplies of oral and topical medication can be provided, allowing the patient to play an active role in his or her care and ensuring prompt treatment of a flare-up. Antidiarrheal agents can also be provided for as-needed use, but only to reliable patients who are not likely to abuse them. Patients should be instructed to call if fever develops, diarrhea worsens, bleeding occurs, or abdominal pain becomes marked.

The need for a steady exchange of information with the patient, including careful explanation of procedures and therapies, and the importance of close follow-up and availability cannot be overemphasized. Attentiveness and responsiveness alleviate much of the fear and worry that accompany inflammatory bowel disease and support the development of an effective therapeutic alliance. Additional information and support is available to the patient from local chapters of the National Crohn's and Colitis Foundation of American.

INDICATIONS FOR REFERRAL AND ADMISSION

Referral for gastroenterologic consultation is indicated when full doses of 5-ASA in combination with oral corticosteroids (with or without antibiotics in patients with Crohn's disease) fail to control symptoms. Most patients treated with immunomodulators are managed in conjunction with a gastroenterologist. In addition, Crohn's disease and ulcerative colitis patients who require recurrent high doses of chronic daily steroid therapy should be referred for the consideration of immunomodulators (6-MP, azathioprine, methotrexate) or biologics (infliximab or adalimumab). Ulcerative colitis patients with disabling, chronic, refractory disease should have a surgical consultation. Patients with longstanding colonic disease are at an increased risk for cancer and therefore need referral for periodic colonoscopy and biopsy. Patients with extraintestinal disease may need specialty consultation, especially an ophthalmologic slit-lamp examination to check for uveitis.

Prompt hospitalization for parenteral management is indicated for patients who are toxic, bleeding heavily, in severe pain, or too sick to obtain adequate nutrition orally. Bowel rest, nasogastric feeding of elemental diets, and parenteral steroids are prescribed, and surgical consultation is obtained, especially if there is severe bleeding, toxicity, distention, or evidence of peritoneal irritation. Home nasoenteric feeding has been demonstrated for carefully selected patients with malabsorption and weight loss refractory to conventional outpatient therapy. Nocturnal tube feedings of a low-fat elemental diet can correct such nutritional problems, but the program requires patients who can insert their feeding tubes at night.

MANAGEMENT RECOMMENDATIONS (10–34)

Ulcerative Colitis

General Measures

- Document mucosal inflammation with colonoscopy or sigmoidoscopy.
- Reduce dietary fiber during an exacerbation.
- Advise adequate rest and sleep.
- Prescribe a folic acid supplement (1 mg/d) when leafy vegetables are restricted or sulfasalazine is being used.
- Add oral *iron* supplementation (300 mg ferrous sulfate three times daily) when there is considerable rectal bleeding and documented iron-deficiency anemia.
- Schedule visits frequently in the early phases of the illness to provide psychological support and close monitoring. Phone checks are helpful.
- Consider antidiarrheal agents (e.g., *loperamide* 2 to 4 mg) for temporary symptomatic control of troublesome diarrhea in patients with mild to moderate disease. Avoid prolonged use and use in patients with severe disease (high risk of toxic dilation).
- If mild diarrhea persists during remissions, initiate a trial of *psyllium hydrophilic colloid* (1 teaspoon in 8 oz of water once or twice daily); if this is unsuccessful, try restricting milk products.
- Begin periodic colorectal cancer screening in those patients who have had disease lasting more than 8 years; refer for consideration of periodic colonoscopy and biopsy every 1 to 2 years.
- Screen for osteoporosis in patients who have had frequent use of steroids. If patients are on immunomodulators or biologics, make sure that their vaccinations (e.g., influenza, etc.) are up to date. Advise the concurrent intake of calcium and vitamin D with steroid use.

Mild to Moderate Disease

- Begin *sulfasalazine*, 500 mg four times a day with meals, and increase the dose as tolerated over several days to 4 g/d, or a nonsulfa 5-ASA preparation (e.g., *olsalazine* 500 mg twice a day; *mesalamine* 2.4 to 4.8 g/d total). Continue this dose for 2 to 4 weeks until symptoms abate, and then decrease it to the smallest dose that maintains the control of symptoms.
- If a 5-ASA preparation fails to achieve control within a few weeks, begin oral *prednisone*, starting with a dose of 40 mg/d. Initially, give in divided doses for patients who are having symptoms around the clock, but change to an every-morning program as soon as possible to limit the degree of adrenal suppression. Continue this dose for 7 to 10 days.
- If control is achieved, begin tapering prednisone by 5 to 10 mg every 2 weeks until 20 mg, after which, taper by 5 mg/wk. If the patient has been on prednisone for an extended period of time, consider tapering by 2.5 mg/wk once patient gets to 10 mg/d; taper to the lowest dose necessary to suppress disease activity.
- Once steroids are tapered off and disease activity ceases, decrease the 5-ASA dose to a maintenance dose of 2 g/d of sulfasalazine, 2.4 g/d of mesalamine, or 1 g/d of olsalazine.

Moderate to Severe Disease

- Start with *prednisone*, 60 mg/d in divided doses; consider holding 5-ASA compounds, given the potential for idiosyncratic worsening of symptoms. Once the symptoms come under control, give the entire prednisone dose in the morning, and begin tapering empirically by 5 mg/kg as previously described; resume 5-ASA indefinitely to maintain remission (sulfasalazine at 4 g/d or mesalamine at 2.4 to 4.8 g/d).
- If food intake is inadequate over time because of nausea or abdominal pain, consider supplementing the diet with a nutritionally balanced low-residue *liquid dietary preparation* (e.g., Magnacal, Ensure, Sustacal, Isocal).
- Monitor carefully for marked blood loss, volume depletion, severe abdominal pain, distention, and peritoneal signs; any of these is an indication for prompt hospital admission, parenteral therapy, and urgent surgical consultation.
- Refer for consideration of steroid-sparing immunomodulator therapy (6-MP, *azathioprine*) or biologics (e.g., *infliximab*) for those patients requiring repeated courses of steroids, unable to be weaned off of steroids, or refractory to steroids.
- Refer for consideration of elective surgery those patients refractory to maximal medical therapy, those requiring daily steroids for prolonged periods (>6 months), and those found on cancer screening to have a stricture or dysplasia.

Ulcerative Proctocolitis

- If disease is limited to the rectosigmoid, begin treatment with oral *5-ASA* (as noted earlier) and/or a topical agent. *Enemas* of *hydrocortisone* or *5-ASA* are both effective topically, the latter being slightly more efficacious in inducing remission. During a flare, consider using both oral and topical formulations of 5-ASA. During remission, patients can be maintained on one or the other.
- Prescribe hydrocortisone as a 100-mg retention enema taken once nightly, a 25-mg suppository once or twice daily, or a 90-mg foam preparation once or twice daily. The selection of a preparation can be based on patient preference and empirical results.
- Prescribe a mesalamine enema in doses of 1 to 4 g/d for acute symptoms and 1 g/d for maintenance.
- If disease is limited to only the rectum, patients may respond to mesalamine suppositories 1,000 mg at bedtime.
- Continue therapy until symptoms clear; continue oral 5-ASA (or topical, if the patient prefers) for prophylaxis.

Crohn's Disease

General Measures

- Document the extent of disease by barium studies, colonoscopy, CT enterography, and/or capsule endoscopy.
- Limit the *fiber* content of the diet in patients with obstructive symptoms.
- Decrease the *fat* intake to less than 80 mg/d when there is steatorrhea.
- Conduct a trial of restricting *milk products* from the diet of patients with diarrhea; if the diarrhea promptly improves, continue with a lactose-restricted diet.
- Supplement the diet with a *multivitamin* preparation that contains five times the normal daily vitamin requirements plus iron, calcium, magnesium, and zinc. Check for a deficiency of vitamin B_{12} in patients with ileal disease, and supplement if necessary.
- Consider antidiarrheal therapy (e.g., *loperamide* 2 to 4 g or *codeine* 15 mg with meals and before bed) for symptomatic

relief of diarrhea; use caution—obstruction may be aggravated, and prolonged use can lead to narcotic dependence.

■ Advise partial *bowel rest* and the use of elemental *low-residue* dietary preparations when cramps and diarrhea are severe.

■ Admit for refractory disease, severe bleeding, toxicity, abdominal pain, abscess formation, or evidence of obstruction. Such patients need surgical consultation.

■ Screen for osteoporosis in patients who have had frequent use of steroids. If patients are on immunomodulators or biologics, make sure that their vaccinations (e.g., influenza, etc.) are up to date. Advise the concurrent intake of calcium and vitamin D with steroid use.

Colonic Disease

■ Begin *sulfasalazine* (500 mg four times a day) and quickly increase the dose to 1 g four times a day over several days or *mesalamine* (up to 4.8 g/d).

■ If there is a response to a 5-ASA preparation, consider the common practice of continuing treatment indefinitely even though available data have yet to show benefit in maintaining remission.

■ If there is no response to a 5-ASA agent, switch to antibiotic therapy with *ciprofloxacin* 1 g/d and/or *metronidazole* in doses of 10 to 20 mg/kg per day (e.g., 250 to 500 mg three times a day); continue for a 4-week trial. If there is a satisfactory response, continue for 4 to 6 months, then stop if symptoms have ceased. If there is no response, consider *rifaximin*.

■ If there is inadequate response to these antibiotics, switch to *prednisone* 40 to 60 mg/d. As disease activity subsides, give the entire dose in the morning and begin tapering to the lowest dose that controls the symptoms (often as little as 5 mg/d).

■ Refer patients with refractory disease, especially if steroid dependent, for consideration of immunomodulatory therapy with *6-MP*, *azathioprine*, or *methotrexate* or therapy with biologics (*infliximab* or *adalimumab*).

Perianal Disease

■ Prescribe *ciprofloxacin* (1 g/d) or *metronidazole* (750 to 1,500 mg/d) for persistent perianal disease; a prolonged course of treatment may be necessary.

■ Consider *surgical referral* if a perianal abscess develops or if perianal fistulous disease is refractory to antibiotics alone.

■ Consider gastroenterology referral for the consideration of *immunomodulatory* and *monoclonal antibody* therapies in conjunction with surgical intervention for refractory fistulous disease.

Ileal Disease

■ *Mesalamine* capsules (up to 4.8 g/d) are worth a 4- to 6-week trial.

■ If there is no response, or if ileal symptoms are severe, then prescribe *budesonide* (9 mg/d for 4 weeks, then 6 mg/d for 2 weeks, then 3 mg/d for 2 weeks).

■ Consider the use of *6-MP, azathioprine, infliximab, or methotrexate* for patients with refractory symptoms, a recurrent need for steroids, or persistent requirements for steroids. The first three options are also effective for fistula closure. A trial of immunomodulators for several months is often necessary and may need to be continued indefinitely, as long as no adverse effects are detected. Because immunomodulator therapy can cause marrow suppression and carcinogenesis, gastroenterologic consultation is essential.

Annotated Bibliography

1. Bamias G, Nyce MR, De La Rue SA, et al. New concepts in the pathophysiology of inflammatory bowel disease. Ann Intern Med 2005;143:895. (*A thorough review of recent hypotheses on the pathogenesis of inflammatory bowel disease [IBD].*)

2. Baumgart D, Sandborn W. Inflammatory bowel disease: clinical aspects and established and evolving treatments. Lancet 2007;369:1641. (*A comprehensive update on all aspects of IBD.*)

3. Baumgart D, Garding S. Inflammatory bowel disease: cause and immunobiology. Lancet 2007;369:1627. (*A review of hypotheses regarding the pathogenesis of IBD.*)

4. Bernstein CM, Blanchard JF, Leslie W, et al. The incidence of fracture among patients with inflammatory bowel disease. Ann Intern Med 2000;133:795. (*The incidence of fracture was 40% greater than in the general population.*)

5. Comminelli F. Cytokine-based therapies for Crohn's disease. N Engl J Med 2004;351:2045. (*A review of potential therapeutic agents that target different cytokines that are believed to be essential to disease pathogenesis.*)

6. Cosnes J, Beaugerie L, Carbonnel F, et al. Smoking cessation and the course of Crohn's disease: an intervention study. Gastroenterology 2001;120:1093. (*Smoking cessation decreases the number of flare-ups and the need for immunosuppressive medications.*)

7. Drossman DA. Psychosocial aspects of inflammatory bowel disease. Stress Med 1986;2:119. (*A good review of the psychological and psychosocial dimensions of this condition.*)

8. Dworken HJ. Ulcerative colitis. A clearer picture. Ann Intern Med 1983;99:717. (*Reviews the data on prognosis derived from community-based studies, arguing for a more optimistic view of the illness.*)

9. Eaden J, Abrams K, Mayberry J. The risk of colorectal cancer in ulcerative colitis: a meta-analysis. Gut 2001;48:526. (*The cancer risk was increased in ulcerative colitis.*)

10. Elson CO. Genes, microbes, and T cells—new therapeutic targets in Crohn's disease. N Engl J Med 2003;346:614. (*A brief but very useful summary of advances in pathophysiology and implications for treatment.*)

11. Farmer RG, Whelan G, Fazio VW. Long-term follow up of patients with Crohn's disease. Gastroenterology 1985;88:818. (*Discusses the relationship between clinical pattern and prognosis.*)

12. Garrett JW, Drossman DA. Health status in inflammatory bowel disease; review of biologic and behavioral considerations. Gastroenterology 1990;99:90. (*Outcomes appear to be a function of both the disease and quality-of-life factors.*)

13. Glotzer DJ, Gardner RC, Goldman H, et al. Comparative features and course of ulcerative and granulomatous colitis. N Engl J Med 1970;282:582. (*A classic review, comparing and contrasting the two conditions.*)

14. Kane S. Inflammatory bowel disease in pregnancy. Gastroenterol Clin North Am 2003;32:323. (*Reviews issues regarding IBD and pregnancy.*)

15. Lichtenstein G, Hanauer SB, Kane SV, et al. Crohn's is not a 6-week disease: lifelong management of mild to moderate Crohn's disease. Inflamm Bowel Dis 2004;10(Suppl 2):S2. (*A review of the natural history and management strategies for mild to moderate disease.*)

16. Robertson DAF, Ray J, Diamond I, et al. Personality profile and affective states of patients with inflammatory bowel disease. Gut 1989;30:623. (*Personality disturbances were frequent and correlated with the duration of the disease; many patients reported stress preceding the onset of symptoms.*)

17. Schwartz DA, Loftus EV, Tremaine WJ, et al. The natural history of fistulizing Crohn's disease in Olmsted County. Gastroenterology 2002;122:875. (*Fistulas in Crohn's disease were common in the community, but only 34% of patients developed recurrent fistulas; surgery was often required.*)

18. Hara A, Leighton J, Heigh R, et al. Crohn disease of the small bowel: preliminary comparison among CT enterography, capsule endoscopy, small-bowel follow-through, and ileoscopy. Radiology 2006;238:128. (*Capsule endoscopy and computed tomographic enterography had similar rates of detection of small bowel disease compared to standard ileoscopy.*)

19. Schwartz DA, Pemberton JH, Sandborn WJ. Diagnosis and treatment of perianal fistulas in Crohn disease. Ann Intern Med 2001;135:906. (*An authoritative review; 125 references.*)

20. Colombe J, Lemann M, Cassagnou M, et al. A controlled trial comparing ciprofloxacin with mesalamine for the treatment for active Crohn's disease. Am J Gastroenterol 1999;94:674. (*Ciprofloxacin was equally efficacious to mesalamine 4g/d in achieving remission in mild to moderate Crohn's disease.*)

21. Disanayake AS, Truelove SC. A controlled therapeutic trial of long-term maintenance treatment of ulcerative colitis with sulfasalazine. Gut 1973;14:923. (*Original data documenting the efficacy of sulfasalazine for prophylaxis; the recurrence rate was one fourth that of the control group.*)

22. Donaldson RM. Management of medical problems in pregnancy: inflammatory bowel disease. N Engl J Med 1985;312:1616. (*A practical approach to this important management issue.*)

23. Feagan BG, Fedorak RN, Irvine EJ, et al. A comparison of methotrexate with placebo for the maintenance of remission in Crohn's disease. N Engl J Med 2000;342:1627. (*In patients with Crohn's disease who enter remission with methotrexate, a low dose maintains the remission.*)

24. Feagan BG, Rochon J, Fedorak RN, et al. Methotrexate for the treatment of Crohn's disease. N Engl J Med 1995;332:292. (*A multicenter randomized, controlled trial in patients with chronically active disease; the drug was superior to placebo in improving symptoms and reducing steroid requirements.*)

25. Greenberg GR, Feagan BG, Martin F, et al. Oral budesonide as maintenance treatment for Crohn's disease: a placebo-controlled dose-ranging study. Gastroenterology 1996;110:45. (*The treatment achieved a more prolonged remission, but it was not sustainable beyond 1 year.*)

26. Hanauer S, et al. Maintenance infliximab for Crohn's disease: ACCENT I randomised trial. Lancet 2002;359:1541. (*Infliximab was an effective maintenance therapy for moderate to severe Crohn's disease.*)

27. Hanauer S, Stromberg U. Oral Pentasa in the treatment of active Crohn's disease: a meta-analysis of double-blind, placebo-controlled trials. Clin Gastroenterol Hepatol 2004;2:379. (*A meta-analysis of the three largest trials failed to show a treatment benefit of Pentasa.*)

28. Kamm MA, Sandborn WJ, Gassull M, et al. Once-daily, high-concentration MMX mesalamine in active ulcerative colitis. Gastroenterol 2007;132:66. (*Once-daily Multi Matrix System [MMX] mesalamine was effective and safe for the induction of remission in mild to moderate ulcerative colitis.*)

29. Kane SV, Schoenfeld P, Sandborn WJ, et al. The effectiveness of budesonide therapy for Crohn's disease. Aliment Pharmacol Ther 2002;16:1509. (*Budesonide was more effective than mesalamine at inducing remission in patients with mild to moderate Crohn's disease.*)

30. Klotz UK, Maier K, Fischer C, et al. Therapeutic efficacy of sulfasalazine and its metabolites in patients with ulcerative colitis and Crohn's disease. N Engl J Med 1980;303:1499. (*A classic paper, establishing that 5-aminosalicylate is the active moiety of sulfasalazine.*)

31. Kornbluth A, Sachar DB. Ulcerative colitis practice guidelines in adults (update): American College of Gastroenterology, Practice Parameters Committee. Am J Gastroenterol 2004;99:1371. (*Current consensus practice guidelines.*)

32. National Cooperative Crohn's Disease Study. Gastroenterology 1979;77:825. (*A landmark randomized, controlled trial [RCT], showing the efficacy of sulfasalazine in acute colonic disease; no improvement was found in patients with disease confined to the small bowel.*)

33. Pearson DC, May GR, Fick GH, et al. Azathioprine and 6-mercapto-purine in Crohn's disease: a meta-analysis. Ann Intern Med 1995;122:132. (*These agents are effective in treating active disease and in maintaining remission; however, adverse effects requiring withdrawal are common.*)

34. Present DH, Meltzer SJ, Krumholz MD, et al. 6-Mercaptopurine in the management of inflammatory bowel disease: short- and long-term toxicity. Ann Intern Med 1989;111:641. (*Reports an 18-year experience.*)

35. Provenzale D, Shearn M, Phillips-Bute BG, et al. Health related quality of life after ileoanal pull through: Evaluation and assessment of new health status measures. Gastroenterology 1997;113:7. (*Quality of life for these operated patients is excellent.*)

36. Rijk MC, van Hogezand RA, van Lier HJ, et al. Sulfasalazine and prednisone compared with sulfasalazine for treating active Crohn disease. Ann Intern Med 1991;114:445. (*A multicenter RCT; prednisone helped only in speeding initial improvement.*)

37. Rutgeerts P, Sandborn WJ, Feagan BG, et al. Infliximab for induction and maintenance therapy in ulcerative colitis. N Engl J Med 2005, 353:2464. (*Infliximab was effective in inducing and maintaining remission in moderate to severe ulcerative colitis.*)

38. Sandborn WJ, Rutgeerts P, Enns R, et al. Adalimumab induction therapy for Crohn disease previously treated with infliximab: a randomized trial. Ann Intern Med. 2007;146:829. (*Patients who had lost previous response to or were intolerant of infliximab responded to adalimumab.*)

39. Sands BE, Anderson FH, Bernstein CN, et al. Infliximab maintenance therapy for fistulizing Crohn's disease. N Engl J Med 2004; 350:876. (*Patients with fistulizing disease who responded to infliximab induction therapy had a higher likelihood of sustained response.*)

40. Thomsen OO, Cortot A, Jewell D, et al. A comparison of budesonide and mesalamine for active Crohn's disease. N Engl J Med 1998;339:370. (*A double-blind, multicenter trial in persons with active mild to moderate Crohn's disease, showing that budesonide was superior to slow-release mesalamine and did not suppress adrenal function.*)

41. Ursing B, Almy T, Barney F, et al. A comparative study of metronidazole and sulfasalazine for active Crohn's disease. A Cooperative Crohn's Disease Study in Sweden. II. Results. Gastroenterology 1982;83:550. (*Metronidazole produced results comparable with those of sulfasalazine; moreover, the drug worked in some patients who failed to respond to sulfasalazine.*)

42. Whelan G, Farmer RG, Fazio VW. Recurrence after surgery in Crohn's disease, relationship to location and disease. Clinical pattern and surgical indication. Gastroenterology 1985;88:1826. (*A prospective long-term cohort study from the Cleveland Clinic, reporting the frequency of recurrence after operation.*)

CHAPTER 74 ■ APPROACH TO THE PATIENT WITH FUNCTIONAL GASTROINTESTINAL DISEASE

Functional gastrointestinal (GI) disease accounts for a large proportion of the GI complaints seen in office practice, not only in the primary care setting, but also in the referral practices of gastroenterologists. The International Working Group consensus definition of functional GI disease refers to "a variable combination of chronic or recurrent GI symptoms not explained by structural or biochemical abnormalities." Symptoms may be attributed to dysfunction of the pharynx, esophagus, stomach, biliary tree, small and large intestine or anorectum." Included under the rubric of functional GI disease are two common, often-troubling syndromes: *irritable bowel syndrome* (IBS) and *nonulcer dyspepsia*. The former is associated with large-bowel discomfort or pain, disturbed defecation, and distention, often with predominant constipation, diarrhea, or gaseousness. The latter is characterized by upper abdominal discomfort, bloating, distension, and nausea, which is often, but not necessarily, exacerbated or triggered by eating. Another increasingly appreciated functional malady is *irritable esophagus* (sometimes referred to as esophageal spasm; see Chapter 61). In many cases of functional disease, there is a strong interplay biopsychosocial factors and gut physiology.

The primary care physician needs to be expert in the recognition and management of these conditions not only because they can mimic more serious disease (sometimes leading to unnecessary testing and treatment), but also because they are the source of much worry, functional impairment, and substantial health care expenditures.

IRRITABLE BOWEL SYNDROME

IBS is a functional disturbance of intestinal motility and visceral perception, which is strongly influenced by emotional factors. It accounts for about half of GI complaints seen by physicians. Epidemiologic studies suggest that nearly 20% of adults suffer from some form of the condition, although only a fraction seek medical attention. "*Spastic bowel*," "*mucous colitis*," and "*spastic colitis*" are less accurate terms sometimes used to refer to the syndrome. Because there are no definitive diagnostic tests, the identification of the condition requires taking a careful history to avoid misdiagnosis. A comprehensive biopsychosocial approach to management (including a strong patient–doctor relationship) is essential to optimizing patient outcomes.

Pathophysiology and Clinical Presentation (1–17)

Pathophysiology

The pathophysiology of IBS appears to involve a complex interplay of functional disturbances in motor and sensory activity and visceral perception (nociception), which are triggered and/or exacerbated by psychological distress and luminal irritants.

Abnormal motor function is a hallmark of this syndrome, which is capable of producing both diarrhea and constipation. *Neurotransmitter imbalance* (especially dysfunctional *serotonin* release) appears to play an important role. The GI tract contains the highest concentration of serotonin-secreting cells, which are capable of stimulating vagal activity and potent motor and secretory responses. The altered motility produces nonpropulsive colonic contractions and abnormal slow-wave myoelectric patterns. When excessive, these contractions may impede propulsion of stool, prolong transit time, and cause constipation. Diarrhea occurs when the increase in contractility is localized to the small bowel and proximal colon. A pressure gradient develops, causing accelerated movement of intestinal contents. Meals normally cause an increase in colonic contractions, but controlled study has shown that patients with irritable colon syndrome have a significantly exaggerated increase in motor response to food. Patients with diarrhea-predominant disease have more jejunal, fast, and high-amplitude contractions postprandially than do healthy individuals, resulting in reduced colonic transit time. In some patients, the diarrhea appears to be responsive to drug therapy that targets serotonin receptors (see later discussion).

Visceral hypersensitivity also plays an important role, particularly in the *abdominal pain* and *anorectal discomfort* experienced. *Abnormal nociception* has been demonstrated in balloon manometry studies of IBS patients, who manifest excessive sensitivity to balloon distention in the ileum, rectosigmoid, and anorectum. In persons who suffer predominantly from diarrhea, there are reduced thresholds for the initiation of reflex motor activity and discomfort; urgency is precipitated at abnormally small volumes of balloon distention. In patients with constipation, the threshold for reflex motor activity is abnormally high, and emptying is delayed. Fecal material collects and hardens, and the bowel becomes distended; pain ensues. Excessive afferent sensory activity and differences in its central processing have also been detected, probably contributing to the nociceptive dysfunction. Serotonergic and noradrenergic neurotransmission are believed to be active in central and peripheral components of IBS pathophysiology and serve as a possible link between the two.

The combination of abnormal motor, sensory, and cortical functioning has the potential to cause the patient much discomfort. For example, increased sensitivity can trigger excessive reflex motor activity, leading to a cycle of anorectal discomfort or pain before a bowel movement, a sense of incomplete evacuation after one, and increased frequency of movements, perhaps as a result of learned behavior or underlying psychopathology.

Psychosocial stress and *psychopathology* not only result from IBS, but they also may contribute to it. *Situational stress* has long been recognized as an important precipitating factor. Hypermotility in response to stress has been documented in both healthy persons and patients with IBS, but the latter show a significantly higher frequency of life stress. In addition, there is a high prevalence of psychopathology among IBS patients presenting for care. *Somatization*, *personality disturbances*, *anxiety*, and *depression* are frequently identified. Such psychopathology appears to be more a predictor of illness behavior than a direct cause of bowel dysfunction. Psychiatric symptoms and poor coping skills usually predate bowel complaints. Disturbances in bowel function can be especially troubling to patients with preexisting psychopathology and more likely to precipitate medical encounters than might similar symptoms in otherwise well-adjusted persons. *Hypervigilance* is characteristic. This finding has been invoked to explain why only a fraction of patients with IBS ever present for medical care. Patients with IBS who do not consult physicians have been found to be psychologically similar to control subjects. Those who come for care evidence greater degrees of serious situational stresses, psychopathology, and perhaps learned visceral responses to bowel discomfort and threatening situations. Such factors in turn may modify the underlying pathophysiology and illness behavior, determining the severity of symptoms, frequency of episodes, and thresholds for seeking and continuing with medical care.

Intraluminal factors can alter bowel motor function and cause it to behave in an "irritable" manner. *Selective malabsorption* of certain sugars, such as *lactose* (the common dairy-product sugar), *fructose* (the common citrus-fruit sugar), and *sorbitol* (often found in "sugar-free" candy) can be responsible. Sorbitol is a common sweetener in candies and chewing gum and is capable of causing bloating and diarrhea if taken in large amounts, as are milk products in patients with lactose intolerance. *Food allergies* may play a role in some patients. *Bile acid* malabsorption has been detected in up to 10% of patients with diarrhea-predominant IBS. The resulting large quantities of fatty acids descending on the colon can trigger painful rapid contractions, leading to marked discomfort and diarrhea. Such factors might help to explain the observed onset of IBS-like symptoms in up to 10% of persons after recent bacterial or viral *gastroenteritis*, especially in those with concurrent psychosocial stress.

Clinical Presentation and Course

Most patients experience the onset of symptoms well before age 40 years; about one half are younger than 30 years, and one fourth are younger than 20 years. The combination of abdominal pain and diarrhea and/or constipation helps to differentiate IBS from other forms of functional GI disease, in which only one feature is present. In about two thirds of IBS patients, either diarrhea or constipation may predominate.

Abdominal pain or *discomfort* is almost universal. In two thirds of patients, abdominal pain is reported most often in the left lower quadrant or lower abdomen; one third note upper abdominal pain, and one fourth experience it in multiple sites. The pain is typically achy rather than crampy, and is often relieved by a bowel movement or the passage of flatus, and it usually does not disturb sleep. Pain radiation is variable and can extend into the left chest and arm when gas is trapped in the splenic flexure.

Constipation is a prominent complaint, characterized by small, hard, infrequent stools and an empty rectal ampulla. Prolonged retention of stool allows the full absorption of intestinal water content. About one third of patients report *mucous* stools, *pellet-like stools,* and/or excessive *flatus.* A constipation-predominant form of IBS occurs in about one third of patients, more commonly in men.

Diarrhea characteristically alternates with constipation; in about 10% of patients, *diarrhea* is the sole manifestation. The diarrhea is typically small in volume, associated with visible amounts of mucus, and may follow a hard movement by a few hours. There may be urgency. In about one third of patients, a diarrhea-predominant form of IBS is noted, more frequently in women.

Dyspepsia and excessive eructation are also reported, supporting the view of a process that involves the entire GI tract. Weight loss is rare. As noted, symptoms usually parallel situational stresses; an intercurrent infectious gastroenteritis may trigger an exacerbation. Fifty percent of patients consider their symptoms to be related to stress, whereas one third deny it. Two thirds manifest symptoms of anxiety or depression. Rectal bleeding is absent unless there is coincident hemorrhoidal disease.

Chronicity is the rule, with little change in symptoms over time, except for waxing and waning. Duration is measured in years. There is no evidence of significant morbidity or mortality. Severity waxes and wanes, but the constellation of symptoms remains remarkably constant. In natural history studies, about 50% of patients are unchanged at 1 year, about 30% to 35% are improved (10% symptom-free), and 15% to 20% are worse. The symptom-free period is usually less than a few months. One third of employed IBS patients lose time from work. At 2 years of follow-up, a similar pattern is found. Persons with symptoms triggered by a major life stress enjoy long symptom-free periods after the acute problem abates, whereas those with continuous intestinal complaints in response to daily living rarely became asymptomatic.

Diagnosis and Initial Evaluation (4,18–25)

Clinical Criteria for Diagnosis of IBS

The lack of an objective laboratory marker for IBS necessitates clinical criteria for diagnosis. The two most widely used and best-validated sets of criteria are those specified by *Manning* and colleagues in the late 1970s and the subsequently developed *Rome Diagnostic Criteria* (Table 74.1). These symptom-based criteria have been largely validated and are widely used for suggesting the diagnosis of IBS.

Although the sensitivity and specificity of the Manning criteria have, for the most part, been confirmed, there are some questions regarding the discriminant value of individual items.

TABLE 74.1

DIAGNOSTIC CRITERIA FOR IRRITABLE BOWEL SYNDROME

Manning Criteria
- Continuous or recurrent symptoms during several months of abdominal pain or discomfort relieved with defecation or associated with a change in frequency or consistency of stool; and/or:
- An irregular or varying pattern of disturbed defecation at least 25% of the time, consisting of two or more of the following: altered frequency; altered consistency; straining, urgency, or feeling of incomplete evacuation; passage with mucus; and bloating or feeling of distention.

Rome Criteria
- Recurrent abdominal pain or discomfort at least 3 d/mo for the past 3 mo and onset at least 6 mo before diagnosis, associated with two or more of the following:
  - Improvement with defecation
  - Onset associated with a change in frequency of stool
  - Onset associated with a change in form (appearance) of stool

Manning criteria: From Manning AP, Thompson WG, Heaton KW, et al. Towards positive diagnosis of the irritable bowel syndrome. BMJ 1978;2:653.
Rome criteria: Adapted from Mayer EA. N Engl J Med 2008;358:1692, based on Longstreth GF, Thompson WG, Chey WD, et al. Functional bowel disorders. In Drossman DA, Corazziari E, Spiller R, et al., eds. Rome III: the functional gastrointestinal disorders, 3rd ed. McLean, VA: Degnon, 2006:487, with permission.

Consequently, the *Rome Diagnostic Criteria* were developed to overcome some of the shortcomings of the Manning criteria and are often used for patient selection in clinical studies.

Some clinical situations require ruling out organic pathology that might resemble and be mistaken for IBS (see later discussion). Detailed history taking and careful physical examination, combined with selective parsimonious testing and a few diagnostic trials of therapeutic measures, will usually provide the best combination of completeness and cost efficacy.

Subgroups

Based on clinical presentation, subgroups are designated: *IBS with diarrhea predominant (IBS-D), IBS with constipation predominant (IBS-C),* and *IBS with mixed bowel habits.*

Differential Diagnosis and Overall Approach to Workup

Colon cancer, inflammatory bowel disease, celiac sprue, and ovarian cancer are the principal "must-not-miss" conditions that may mimic the presentation of IBS. Concern about such etiologies often precipitates the patient's coming for evaluation. A detailed initial history and careful physical examination supplemented by a few simple laboratory studies (e.g., complete blood count) can address the diagnostic criteria for IBS and check for warning signs of more serious disease, helping to differentiate the IBS patient from one who needs more extensive workup for a mimicking must-not-miss condition. Colonoscopy and other expensive testing are not required for diagnosis unless symptoms and signs of worrisome pathology are elicited. Prospective studies with up to 30 years of follow-up for such an approach to IBS workup have shown only a 1% rate of missing the must-not-miss conditions.

Alarm Symptoms. Attention to so-called "alarm symptoms" (*weight loss, evidence of GI blood loss, anemia, fever, frequent nocturnal symptoms, positive family history of colon cancer, onset after age 50 years, sudden change in symptoms*) helps to screen for the must-not-miss conditions. Persons with IBS-like symptoms manifesting one of the alarm "symptoms" should not be labeled as having IBS until more extensive testing is conducted (see later discussion and also Chapters 58, 64, and 65).

When Constipation Predominates. In this setting, it may be necessary to rule out a malignancy and Crohn's disease, particularly in patients older than the age of 40 years who have an alarm symptom such as weight loss or a family history of colon cancer. In such patients, one needs to consider *colonoscopy* (see Chapter 65). In young persons, a *stool test for occult blood* and a *complete blood count* (for microcytic anemia) should suffice. The absence of evidence for GI blood loss helps to exclude organic disease. A test of *thyroid-stimulating hormone* is indicated to rule out hypothyroidism, which also may present as constipation. Patients taking diuretics should have a serum *potassium* checked because hypokalemia may reduce bowel contractility and produce an ileus. A clinical trial of *increased dietary fiber*, *stool softeners* (dioctyl sodium sulfosuccinate), or an *osmotic laxative* (psyllium) complements the diagnostic assessment.

When Diarrhea Predominates. Here, it is important to be sure that there are no symptoms suggestive of celiac sprue, inflammatory disease, and other important causes of chronic diarrhea (see Chapter 64). Once completed, a *dietary review* can be helpful, especially for evidence of intolerance to lactose or sorbitol. A check of *blood sugar* is needed to rule out diabetes mellitus (which may present as diarrhea due to diabetic gastroenteropathy; see Chapter 102), as is a check of the *stool for ova and parasites*. A diagnostic trial of eliminating sorbitol-containing candies and restricting lactose-containing milk products (yogurt containing live cultures is relatively lactose-free) helps to rule out contributions from intraluminal factors. A *lactose-hydrogen breath test* is an alternative means of testing for lactose intolerance. A trial of the bile acid-binding resin *cholestyramine* serves as a simple test for bile acid malabsorption.

If diarrhea persists undiagnosed, a *colonoscopy with or without mucosal biopsy* might be reasonable to exclude inflammatory bowel disease and collagenous and lymphocytic forms of colitis (see Chapter 64). Because the clinical presentation can be mimicked by celiac sprue, testing for *antiendomesial* and/or *tissue transglutaminase antibodies* (see Chapter 64) is indicated when the possibility cannot be ruled out clinically; sensitivity is greater than 90% for these immunoglobulin A antibodies (see Chapter 64).

When Abdominal Pain, Distention, and Bloating Predominate. In this setting, intermittent bowel obstruction, inflammatory bowel disease, celiac sprue, and pelvic pathology (especially ovarian carcinoma and endometriosis) require consideration. A *plain film of the abdomen* during an attack of severe pain should suffice to rule out obstruction. A complete blood count also helps to check for significant underlying bowel pathology. A negative serum determination for *antiendomesial antibodies* eliminates concern for celiac disease, especially when there is concurrent anemia. *Transvaginal ultrasound* is indicated when

symptoms are of new onset or of increased frequency (almost daily) or severity, especially if they are accompanied by urinary tract or pelvic complaints (see Chapter 58). Such bloating and discomfort may also occur with lactose, fructose, or sorbitol intolerance, which can be tested for as detailed.

Psychological Assessment

Because the prevalence of underlying psychopathology is very high in patients with IBS, definitive therapy often requires identifying and addressing the patient's psychological difficulties. In the context of conducting a thorough workup, the clinician needs sensitively to elicit details of the patient's life situation, aspirations, accomplishments, frustrations, and losses. Concerns, fears, expectations, and responses to previous life stresses can also be very informative, as can the mental status of the patient on examination. *Anxiety disorders* are commonly identified (see Chapter 226), but *depression* (see Chapter 227) and *somatization* (see Chapter 230) often go unrecognized.

Principles of Management
(3,4,6,9,11–13,17,22,26–41)

Establishing a strong patient–doctor relationship, treating important underlying psychopathology, modifying diet, and supplementing these efforts with the judicious use of medication constitute the basic approaches to the management of the patient with IBS. No single treatment modality has been proven successful in randomized, placebo-controlled studies, but patient confidence in the diagnosis and a strong patient–doctor relationship are central to effective management. Such a relationship helps to minimize the unnecessary repetition of diagnostic evaluations, the dependence on drugs for provision of symptomatic relief, and the excessive use of ambulatory medical services.

Establishing a Strong Patient–Doctor Relationship

The first rule in the care of patients with IBS is to *take their symptoms seriously* and not dismiss them as inconsequential. Such an approach communicates a sense of caring and is essential to the formation of an effective patient–doctor relationship, the sine qua non of IBS management. As noted earlier, it begins with a careful history and physical examination that addresses potentially serious etiologies, especially those of concern to the patient (e.g., cancer, inflammatory bowel disease). One cannot overemphasize the therapeutic importance of such an initial evaluation.

Once IBS has been identified (usually by the end of the initial or second office visit), the physician needs to *review the diagnosis* with the patient. Anxious, emotionally troubled patients, such as those who present with IBS, often believe that there is something seriously awry and will not accept a simplistic "there's nothing wrong with your bowels." They appreciate knowing the basis for their diagnosis and how more-worrisome conditions were ruled out. In this way, the patient does not leave frustrated and feeling that the "doctor cannot find what is wrong."

The establishment of a supportive doctor–patient relationship in conjunction with providing reassurance, explanation, and advice can have an important effect on outcome. When such care was given to patients in the prospective British study cited earlier, most reported feeling better, less concerned about their bowels, and better able to cope with their symptoms and the stresses of daily life. Although relapses were frequent, these seemed to be less important when they occurred in the context of close medical support. The failure of many physicians to provide adequate support is suggested by the 20% rate of self-referral to alternative medicine practitioners noted in patients with IBS. Developing a positive doctor–patient relationship has been found to be a key determinant in reducing the use of ambulatory health services by IBS patients.

Management of Underlying Psychosocial Stress and Psychopathology

A distinguishing characteristic of patients who present to physicians with IBS is their high probability of underlying psychopathology. Often this is manifested by an exaggerated emotional response to bowel symptoms. Sometimes, the best intervention is withdrawing all previously prescribed medications and simply listening empathically to the patient's problems, helping the patient to cope with his or her life situation. Additional considerations are cognitive–behavioral therapy and targeted psychopharmacologic interventions when specific psychopathology is identified. In the absence of identified psychopathology, the casual use of psychopharmacologic agents as "bowel relaxants" (e.g., benzodiazepine/antispasmodic combination preparations) is ineffective and should be avoided.

Cognitive–behavioral therapy is proving to be an important nonpharmacologic component of IBS management, achieving marked improvements in symptoms in controlled trials (with an odds ratio of 12 for attaining 50% reductions). It entails a combination of efforts to change maladaptive thinking patterns and modify dysfunctional behaviors. The focus is on identifying stressors and thoughts that precipitate symptoms and behavioral approaches to dealing with them (see Chapter 230). Typically, cognitive–behavioral therapy is administered over several weeks by a specially trained therapist working in a group or individual setting, but self-administered approaches are being explored to facilitate more widespread application; initial results in IBS patients are promising.

Emphasis on behavioral approaches is useful in highly motivated patients who seek a sense of control over their symptoms. *Relaxation techniques* help those with exaggerated sympathetic responses to stress. Patients are taught how to blunt such responses and relax skeletal muscles. *Biofeedback* is used predominantly for the treatment of fecal incontinence, aiming for improved control over internal sphincter activity; the method is expensive but promising. *Hypnosis* has also been found to be useful.

Psychotherapy represents an important treatment option for patients who want to deal with their illness through better understanding. To be successful, the therapy has to be viewed as personally relevant. The goal is learning to understand and cope with psychosocial stresses.

A *multifaceted approach* seems to be the best strategy. In a study of combined therapy that included medication, psychotherapy, and behavioral techniques, results were best when the treatment program encompassed a combination of approaches. Predictors of a good response included the presence of overt anxiety or depression, a short duration of bowel symptoms, and the absence of constant or diffuse pain.

Treatment of Concurrent Depression (see also Chapter 227). Patients with IBS who manifest evidence of depression and receive antidepressant therapy have a high rate of improvement. Modest doses of tricyclic antidepressants (e.g., *amitriptyline* 25 to 75 mg at bedtime) have been found to be particularly effective in depressed IBS patients with diarrhea, probably due in part to the effect of their anticholinergic activity in reducing bowel hyperactivity (see further discussion). Higher doses are helpful in treating the underlying depression, which also helps to alleviate bowel complaints. However, in patients with constipation, a tricyclic antidepressant with strong anticholinergic effects such as amitriptyline may actually worsen symptoms; the use of one with little anticholinergic activity might be a better choice (e.g., a *selective serotonin receptor inhibitor* [SSRI] or a *tricyclic antidepressant* with minimal anticholinergic activity, e.g., *desipramine* or nortriptyline). Low doses may suffice, especially for the relief of abdominal pain.

Treatment of Concurrent Chronic Anxiety (see Chapter 226). Many patients with IBS suffer from chronic anxiety, but one must be careful not to prescribe anxiolytics chronically because of their strong potential for inducing addiction and causing withdrawal syndromes (see Chapter 226). An *antidepressant with anxiolytic properties* may be a reasonable substitute (e.g., *doxepin, nortriptyline, trazodone,* or an *SSRI;* see Chapter 227).

Treatment of Concurrent Somatization Disorder. Treatment of patients with somatization disorders first requires withdrawing the vast array of medications prescribed by the multitude of physicians they have visited over the years and then setting up regularly scheduled visits for them to talk about their symptoms and personal problems. Such supportive measures by the primary physician complemented by *cognitive–behavioral therapy* often help to reduce complaints and the demand for medication (see Chapter 230).

Dietary Measures

Although a major part of the therapeutic effort in IBS involves redirecting the patient's attention away from his or her bowels, it is often necessary to provide patients with symptomatic relief before they are willing to turn their attention to the factors precipitating their symptoms. Dietary manipulations are sometimes helpful in this regard.

Foods that might exacerbate IBS should be avoided, including caffeinated beverages, alcohol, sorbitol-containing candies and gums, citrus fruits for those with fructose intolerance, and milk products for those who prove to be lactose intolerant. Reducing the intake of such poorly digestible carbohydrates as beans and cabbage may help patients suffering from bloating, gas, and abdominal pain.

Many IBS patients insist they have *food allergies* as the cause of their symptoms. Although recent study suggests an increased incidence of food allergies in IBS, true food allergies are rare and typically cause acute hypersensitivity reactions, not chronic GI complaints. No changes in colonic motor activity have been found to occur in such patients on intake of the offending food. However, food intolerance (as noted earlier) is often seen in patients with IBS, and it may be worthwhile trying to avoid foods that seem to be poorly tolerated. Some food intolerance is mislabeled as IBS. For example, patients with gluten intolerance (adult celiac disease, nontropical sprue) may present with abdominal discomfort and diarrhea. Persistent diarrhea, bloating, cramping, and excessive flatus may be manifestations of underlying lactose intolerance. A 1- to 2-week trial of restricting a suspected offending food or substance is reasonable when clinical suspicion is high. On the other hand, patients who present having already restricted an unnecessarily large number of foods can have them added back. Rechallenging them with the purported offending agent rebuilds their confidence and avoids nutritional deficiency.

Increasing dietary fiber can in theory help to restore propulsive colonic motor activity. However, some patients report a worsening of bloating and gaseousness with the initiation of a high-fiber diet due to bacterial metabolism of nondigestible fiber, although this tends to subside with time. Controlled clinical trials examining bran and high-fiber diets in IBS have produced variable results, sometimes showing improvement in both groups. There is no harm in prescribing a high-fiber diet, especially in persons with constipation-predominant disease, and it may have other health benefits. It is best to start with the equivalent of about 1 tablespoon of bran daily and build up to 3 tablespoons per day as tolerated.

An alternative is to use *bulking agents,* such as the hydrophilic colloid *psyllium* (Metamucil). A total daily dose of 15 to 25 g is necessary to achieve benefit and is most helpful in IBS patients bothered predominantly by constipation. *Low-residue diets* have been tried. There is no evidence that they are of any use.

Pharmacologic Therapy

Pharmacologic intervention should proceed only in the context of a balanced program that includes patient education, cognitive–behavioral measures, and psychosocial support. Precipitously or prematurely resorting to pharmacologic measures in a hasty attempt to suppress symptoms completely can lead to frustration and excessive, even dangerous, escalation of drug intake. In fact, at the outset of therapy, it is often useful to *stop all nonessential medicines* that may affect bowel function, especially irritant laxatives, anticholinergics, and narcotics in persons with constipation-predominant disease. Nevertheless, there is a role for carefully selected applications of medication when some symptomatic relief is deemed necessary. Advances in understanding the physiology of bowel motility have led to promising pharmacologic approaches to symptomatic relief.

Diarrhea. Patients suffering from disabling diarrhea may benefit from the use of an *opiate derivative.* Transit time is prolonged, water and ion absorption are enhanced, and anal sphincter tone is strengthened. These effects result in less diarrhea, rectal urgency, and fecal soiling. *Loperamide* (*Imodium,* available without prescription in doses of 2 to 4 mg four times a day) is the preferred opiate derivative, having low habituation potential and being less likely to exert central nervous system effects than other derivatives, such as *tincture of opium* or *diphenoxylate* (Lomotil).

As noted earlier, persons with an underlying depression and a predominance of diarrhea may benefit from the use of a low dose of tricyclic antidepressant therapy (e.g., *amitriptyline* 25 to 50 mg/d), but the anticholinergic side effects can exacerbate constipation. Patients with diarrhea due to bile acid malabsorption experience improvement with *cholestyramine,* which is often given on an empirical basis to those with refractory symptoms.

Alosetron (*Lotronex,* 0.5 mg twice daily), *a 5-hydroxytryptamine (5-HT₃)–receptor antagonist,* has been shown to be useful in the treatment of refractory, disabling diarrhea by blocking excess serotonergic activity, which diminishes visceral sensitivity to rectal distention and reduces diarrhea. Initial results showed benefit only in women, but subsequent study found that men also probably responded. Constipation is a common side effect. Serious but rare adverse effects (incidence, 0.10%) have been observed with use, including *ischemic colitis, bowel obstruction, fecal impaction,* and *bowel perforation;* U.S. Food and Drug Administration (FDA) approval limits prescribing to women with at least 6 months

of refractory disease and only by physicians experienced in the drug's use.

Constipation. As noted, *fiber* is worth a try as initial treatment, but it may exacerbate bloating. *Osmotic laxatives* such as *milk of magnesia, magnesium citrate,* nonabsorbable sugars (e.g., *lactulose, sorbitol*), and *polyethylene glycol* (MiraLAX) solutions are often given with some benefit. *Senna* and *cascara* preparations are potent anthraquinone-derivative laxatives used when all else fails, but tachyphylaxis and long-term safety (enteric nerve damage) are concerns. Drugs with anticholinergic activity should be avoided because they are likely to worsen constipation. As noted earlier, if antidepressants are needed, it is best to select a preparation without anticholinergic activity (e.g., *trazodone* or an *SSRI*).

Tegaserod (Zelnorm), a 5-HT₄ agonist, has demonstrated moderate efficacy (20% reduction of symptoms) in women with refractory constipation, shortening transit time and increasing the frequency of bowel movements. Side effects include diarrhea and abdominal pain. The drug was temporarily withdrawn due to worrisome reports of an increased risk of adverse cardiovascular events (e.g., myocardial ischemia, stroke, unstable angina; frequency about 0.1%) and reinstituted on an investigational basis limited to women without cardiovascular disease younger than the age of 55 years.

Lubiprostone (Amitiza), a chloride-channel opener that purportedly works by increasing fluid secretion into the bowel lumen, was recently approved by the FDA for the treatment of IBS with chronic constipation in women. It appears to reduce symptoms in women and represents the only FDA-approved medical therapy for IBS with constipation; however, experience with the drug is limited, and no efficacy in men has been demonstrated. More experience with the agent will be necessary to better define its role in IBS therapy. Cost is high.

Abdominal Pain and Distention. Patients suffering from postprandial pain and distention often request symptomatic relief. *Anticholinergics* such as dicyclomine (Bentyl) and hyoscyamine (Levsin) are often used to reduce the cholinergic stimulation of colonic activity that occurs in response to a meal. Although such agents have been shown to inhibit the postprandial increase in nonpropulsive colonic contractions, their clinical effectiveness is unproven. Chronic use should be avoided because of the risk of worsening constipation and pain. Combination preparations containing an anticholinergic with a *tranquilizer* (e.g., a benzodiazepine or a barbiturate) are promoted as "bowel relaxants" or "antispasmodics" but have no proven benefit and are best avoided because of their habituation potential and poor efficacy. Whether newer anxiolytics that are less sedating and free of habituation potential (e.g., *buspirone* 15 to 30 mg/d), will prove beneficial remains to be proven.

Antidepressants are effective and better tolerated. They appear to raise the threshold for somatic pain and reduce anxiety. Both *tricyclics* and *SSRIs* are especially useful in persons with concurrent depression, but even low doses of antidepressants, especially those *tricyclics* with lesser degrees of anticholinergic activity (e.g., desipramine, nortriptyline), can provide relief of pain; the best candidates include patients who suffer from generalized somatic pain and poor sleep. *SSRI therapy* improves overall sense of well-being and provides some improvement in pain, despite the purported role of serotonin in IBS pathophysiology. The serotonin-norepinephrine reuptake inhibitors, which are useful in neuropathic pain, have not been studied in IBS.

In refractory cases, *analgesics* are sometimes resorted to, but efficacy is limited. A better option is to redouble nonpharmacologic efforts, especially cognitive–behavioral therapies, which approach pharmacologic interventions in ability to provide symptomatic relief. Referral may be useful as well. Research is ongoing in the use of *kappa-opioid agonists* for pain, as well as *5-HT$_3$-receptor antagonists*, which are purportedly active in visceral nociception.

Herbal Therapy

Herbal therapies have become very popular among patients who suffer from chronic functional conditions that resist a simple approach to cure. Chinese herbal preparations have been applied for centuries for the treatment of GI symptoms, but data from well-designed studies of their use in IBS patients are too limited to determine their place in IBS management.

Patient Education

Because IBS is a condition characterized by an exaggerated response to symptoms, patient education is central to effective management. As noted earlier, the basic elements of the patient education effort include addressing patient fears, providing a specific diagnosis, and explaining the pathophysiologic basis of symptoms. In patients with symptoms triggered by psychosocial stress, an explanation (perhaps aided by diagrams) of how such stress can lead to functional alterations in bowel motility helps patients better to understand their condition and cope with it.

When important situational stress or psychopathology is uncovered, it needs to be discussed openly so that the patient can begin to focus on the underlying issues rather than on bowel symptoms. Sometimes, having the patient keep a diary of symptoms, stresses, and feelings can help to reveal connections that have otherwise eluded the patient. The major lesson to be mastered by patients with IBS is the relationship between their psychological state and symptoms, a message that often takes patience, sensitivity, and skill to communicate effectively. It is important not to push the discussion and treatment of psychological issues beyond what the patient is prepared to accept. Patients initially unwilling to consider such issues should be respected, but once a supportive relationship is established, they often begin to cope better and spend less time obsessing about their bowels and more on the underlying issues triggering their "disease."

Patients who are not psychologically minded can still be helped greatly by changing the focus of their care from the cure of symptoms to improvement in functional status. At each office visit, instead of asking for an in-depth recitation of bowel complaints, the physician should spend more time inquiring into how the patient is dealing with the demands of daily life and helping the patient to cope with them. The visit agenda shifts from eliminating symptoms to solving problems. Such a shift is often remarkably refreshing and revealing; it helps to improve functional capacity and reduces the intensity of bodily complaints.

Indications for Referral and Admission

This is a condition in which a continuous relationship is essential, and any perceived need for referral should be acted on only after thorough discussion with the patient. In general, referral is helpful when there are refractory disabling symptoms, such as uncontrollable diarrhea, intractable constipation, or incapacitating pain, or when serious psychopathology is encountered. Motivated patients may also benefit from referral for cognitive–behavioral therapy or, if insight is desired, psychotherapy. A hospital admission may, in rare circumstances, be appropriate and very beneficial in helping the patient to learn new means of coping with stress and providing a respite from an intolerable living situation.

Management Recommendations (2,4,25–35)

- Take the patient's bowel complaints seriously; do not minimize their importance or deny their reality.
- Elicit a full psychosocial database and a complete history of the patient's bodily symptoms.
- Conduct a thorough workup that includes a detailed history and physical looking for "alarm symptoms," and consider the full range of diagnostic possibilities, both organic and psychological (see also Chapters 58, 64, and 65).
- Obtain a detailed psychosocial history that includes current stresses and worries and how the patient copes with them.
- Provide a thorough explanation of the diagnosis, and directly address the patient's concerns and fears.
- Establish a supportive relationship, and begin supportive psychotherapy for patients with underlying situational or psychosocial stresses.
- Identify, discuss, and treat specifically any underlying depression (see Chapter 227), anxiety disorder (see Chapter 226), somatization (see Chapter 230), or other psychiatric condition.
- When treating a depressed patient with antidepressant medication, consider its degree of anticholinergic activity, and match it appropriately to bowel symptoms (e.g., amitriptyline 25 to 50 mg at bedtime is helpful for the patient with diarrhea; an SSRI, e.g., fluoxetine 20 mg/d, might be considered if constipation is problematic; see Chapter 227).
- Stop all nonessential medicines that may affect bowel function, especially irritant laxatives.
- For *constipation*, increase dietary fiber and recommend regular exercise. Add a bulking agent such as *psyllium* (Metamucil), 1 rounded teaspoon in 8 oz of water three times a day, if constipation is still troublesome. A stool softener (e.g., *dioctyl sodium sulfosuccinate* 300 mg, thrice a day) is sometimes helpful. Follow with a nonabsorbable osmotic laxative such as milk of magnesia (2 tablespoons at bedtime to thrice daily). Supplement with *lactulose* (10 mg/15 mL of syrup; 15 to 30 mL/d) or *polyethylene glycol solution* (e.g., MiraLAX, 17 g dissolved in 8 oz of water taken once daily) if need be. Avoid the long-term use of irritant laxatives such as senna and cascara preparations. If symptoms prove refractory, consider referral for 5-HT$_4$-agonist therapy (tegaserod), but only if the patient is female, younger than 55 years of age, and free of cardiovascular disease.
- For *abdominal pain* and *distention*, begin pharmacotherapy with a low dose of a tricyclic antidepressant with anticholinergic activity (e.g., *amitriptyline* 25 to 50 mg at bedtime); reduce the dose or cease if constipation becomes bothersome and switch to a less constipating antidepressant (e.g., nortriptyline 25 mg at bedtime, desipramine 25 mg at bedtime, or an SSRI, e.g., fluoxetine 20 mg in the morning). Avoid the use of anticholinergics and tranquilizers.
- For diarrhea, limit the intake of potentially contributing substances such as caffeine, sorbitol-containing candies and chewing gums, alcohol, and lactose-containing dairy products (yogurt preparations excluded). Major dietary restrictions are usually unnecessary. However, if there is a strongly suggestive history of intolerance to a food or substance, consider a 1- or 2-week trial of omitting its intake. When

short-term symptomatic relief is essential, prescribe *loperamide* (*Imodium*), 4 mg twice daily, as needed. For more sustained control, consider treating with a tricyclic antidepressant having anticholinergic activity (e.g., *amitriptyline* 25 mg daily). For more refractory diarrhea, consider a diagnostic trial of *cholestyramine* (a 9-g packet in water twice daily), which will counter any concurrent bile acid malabsorption. Refer for consideration of a *5-HT₃–receptor antagonist* (e.g., alosetron) if all else fails to control diarrhea.

- Despite the presence of chronic anxiety, avoid the use of sedatives, tranquilizers, and combination preparations containing anticholinergics plus a benzodiazepine or barbiturate; the risks of habituation and withdrawal outweigh any benefit. Antidepressants with anxiolytic activity (e.g., amitriptyline, trazodone, doxepin, fluoxetine) are reasonable alternatives, as might be the nonaddicting azaperone anxiolytics (e.g., buspirone).
- Help redirect the patient's attention away from bowel symptoms and endless searches for cure and toward better coping with daily stresses; focus on accomplishments rather than symptoms, and on taking control through exercise, good eating habits, and behavioral changes rather than on repeated recitation of symptoms. Consider referral for cognitive–behavioral therapy.
- For motivated patients with well-identified psychosocial stressors, consider referral for a combination of behavioral techniques and psychotherapy.
- At this time, there is insufficient evidence to recommend a trial of Chinese herbal medicine.
- See the patient at regular intervals, and be available for help at times of increased stress.

NONULCER DYSPEPSIA

Nonulcer dyspepsia is a poorly defined condition characterized by recurrent upper abdominal pain and discomfort that frequently, but not exclusively, occurs with eating. The discomfort may encompass bloating, nausea, distention, early satiety, and anorexia. The term *dyspepsia* literally means "bad digestion," although it is not meant to be synonymous with or inclusive of other symptoms of "indigestion" (such as heartburn, eructation, or regurgitation). Rather, the emphasis is on the abdominal pain, which may resemble the discomfort of peptic ulcer disease, thus the term *nonulcer*. Older terms for this condition also alluded to its ulcer-negative status, including *x-ray–negative dyspepsia* and *functional dyspepsia*.

Nonulcer dyspepsia is twice as prevalent as ulcer-related dyspeptic disease and is one of several GI conditions that can cause upper abdominal pain in the absence of an ulcer (see Chapter 58). Billions of dollars are spent annually on its evaluation and treatment, yet remarkably little is known about its pathogenesis. However, new data are emerging, and the primary care physician needs to understand the relative importance of diet, smoking, acid secretion, gastric motility, stress, and *Helicobacter pylori* infection to fashion a rational and cost-effective treatment plan.

Pathophysiology, Clinical Presentation, and Course (1–6)

Mechanisms

The pathophysiology of nonulcer dyspepsia is largely unknown. A number of factors have been proposed, and, as in many other functional disorders, the etiology is probably multifactorial.

Dysmotility. Among the most consistent abnormalities is disordered upper GI motility. Gastric emptying is delayed, and gas transit is slowed in about half of dyspeptic patients. Distention and bloating are common and believed to be manifestations of this slowing.

Altered Nociception (Visceral Perception). Altered nociception is suggested by the increase in pain reported by about half of dyspeptic patients to intragastric balloon inflation at volumes that do not cause pain in normal persons.

Psychological Factors. Patients who present with dyspepsia have higher frequencies of anxiety, depression, and neuroticism, and exacerbations of symptoms often coincide with increases in situational stress. However, investigators cannot determine whether this pattern is because of the role of psychological factors in dyspepsia or because of the role of such factors in health-seeking behavior. It is noteworthy that persons with dyspepsia report greater stress in their lives.

Excessive Acid Production. Although excess acid production may play some role in nonulcer dyspepsia (especially in patients who go on to develop a peptic ulcer), it does not appear to be the predominant pathogenic factor. Patients and control subjects show little difference in gastric acid secretion. Histamine₂-blocker therapy and antacids are little better than placebo in providing relief, but combination therapy and the use of proton-pump inhibitors does provide relief for some patients, probably those with an underlying ulcer "diathesis" or concurrent esophageal reflux.

Helicobacter pylori Infection. Of great interest has been the contribution of *H. pylori* infection because it can cause gastritis. *H. pylori* infection is present in about 60% of cases of nonulcer dyspepsia, but this high frequency is not much greater than that for the population at large. Large-scale, randomized, placebo-controlled studies of eradicating *H. pylori* infection have shown only modest benefit (e.g., 25% long-term cure rates, compared with rates of 7% to 21% in omeprazole-treated control subjects; the odds ratio is 1.9 for improvement in persons referred to gastroenterologists). These results indicate that although *H. pylori* infection may be important in a small subset of patients or have a minor effect in others, it is not the major causative factor that it was hypothesized to be.

Maldigestion/Malabsorption of Carbohydrates. Dyspeptic symptoms are common in persons with lactase deficiency and those who take in large amounts of nonabsorbable sugars through heavy use of chewing gum, diet foods, and related products with sorbitol, fructose, or mannitol.

Other Factors. A number of other potential precipitants have been examined. *Smoking, alcohol, coffee,* and *tea* were not found to have any relation to nonulcer dyspepsia. Although *fatty-food intolerance* is a common complaint in dyspeptic patients, controlled studies using disguised meals failed to confirm fatty foods as precipitants. *Bile reflux* has been proposed and when found can cause dyspepsia-like symptoms, but no increase in bile concentrations have been found in dyspeptic patients who have not undergone prior surgery. *Nonsteroidal antiinflammatory drugs* and *aspirin* are well-recognized gastric irritants, but in case-controlled studies, no relation was found between their use and nonulcer dyspepsia.

Clinical Presentation and Course

Recurrent upper abdominal pain and discomfort are the hallmarks. In about half of instances, symptoms are associated with meals. Bloating and gaseous distention may accompany the pain. Acid reflux, biliary colic, painful or altered defecation, and chronic pain are not considered part of its presentation but rather as features of other forms of nonulcer upper abdominal pain; however, they often coexist with dyspepsia (e.g., 25% of dyspeptic patients also report reflux symptoms).

The clinical course is benign, with little evidence that the condition ultimately leads to peptic ulceration or other forms of upper GI pathology. Previously, nonulcer dyspepsia was seen as part of a continuum that progressed to duodenitis and frank peptic ulceration, but this suspicion has not been confirmed (although a small subset of patients go on to develop a peptic ulcer). Typically, the condition is chronic. Although it may wax and wane, it usually does not worsen substantially.

Workup (7–9)

Because the symptoms of nonulcer dyspepsia are nonspecific and may mimic more serious pathology, the diagnostic task includes ruling out the must-not-miss etiologies (gastric and esophageal cancers, erosive gastritis; see Chapter 60). The presence of "alarm symptoms" (see later discussion) helps to identify patients at increased risk and in need of more extensive workup beyond a careful history and physical exam.

Upper Endoscopy

Selectivity is necessary for cost-effective workup. If everyone was studied endoscopically at the time of initial presentation, the yield would be extremely low and the testing would be wasteful because most patients will have nonulcer dyspepsia and a normal study. Most authorities recommend a workup strategy based on risk stratification for the serious pathology noted earlier. Consensus criteria cite age older than 45 years (or any other demographic risk factor for gastric cancer) and unexplained weight loss, persistent nausea and vomiting, dysphagia, odynophagia, jaundice, iron-deficiency anemia, or a positive guaiac stool test as indicative of having "alarm symptoms" and being at increased risk of serious underlying pathology. Although a relatively low threshold is set for endoscopy by using a cutoff age of 45 years (some use older than 50 years, others older than 55 years), the cost of endoscopy can be quickly surpassed by indefinite unnecessary use of commonly used empiric therapies (e.g., acid suppression, prokinetic agents), not to mention the cost of delay in the diagnosis of a more serious, potentially treatable condition and the persistent worry about cancer by the patient.

These recommendations are based on cost-effectiveness analyses; they need to be validated by prospective study. Nonetheless, patients who are deemed low risk can skip endoscopy and proceed to consideration of *H. pylori* testing, a so-called "*test-and-treat strategy*" (see further discussion). Subsequent endoscopic investigation of low-risk patients deserves consideration in those who fail to respond to a trial of empiric therapy or later develop any of the manifestations suggestive of more serious disease.

Testing for *H. pylori* Infection

Low-risk patients benefit from testing for *H. pylori* infection because eradication cures symptoms in the 20% of *H. pylori*–positive dyspeptic patients who prove to have a peptic ulcer or a peptic ulcer "diathesis" and the 20% of *H. pylori*–positive dyspeptic patients with nonulcer dyspepsia who respond to eradication of the infection. Serologic study for *H. pylori* antibodies (see Chapter 68) usually suffices for this purpose; a stool sample for antigen testing is more specific (92% vs. 50% for serum antibody testing).

Other Studies

The clinical presentation can also determine the need for other investigations. Patients with heartburn are likely to have gastroesophageal reflux and should be worked up accordingly (see Chapter 61). Patients reporting paroxysmal attacks of constant epigastric or right upper quadrant pain lasting a few hours and radiating into the back require the consideration of biliary tract disease and *abdominal ultrasound* and *liver function testing* (see Chapter 69). Unrelenting upper abdominal pain radiating into the back, especially if it is alcohol related, suggests chronic pancreatitis; serum *amylase* and abdominal ultrasound are indicated (see Chapter 72). Altered bowel habits in conjunction with upper abdominal pain argue for IBS involving the transverse colon; other possibilities include inflammatory bowel disease, colon cancer, and celiac sprue, necessitating colonoscopy and serologic study, respectively (see IBS discussion).

Principles of Management (10–18)

Given the poor understanding of the precise pathophysiology of nonulcer dyspepsia, its likely multifactorial nature, and the lack of tight correlation between clinical presentation and response to treatment, it should not be surprising that there is little consensus on how best to treat the condition. Options include a test-and-treat strategy (serologic testing for and eradication of *H. pylori* infection), chronic acid suppression, prokinetic therapy, dietary manipulations, and psychotherapy.

Eradication of *H. pylori* Infection

In the *test-and-treat strategy*, patients who test serologically positive for *H. pylori* infection are considered reasonable candidates for its eradication (see Chapter 68). Even though the majority of antibody-positive nonulcer dyspeptic patients do not experience marked improvement, there appears to be a sufficient proportion who do get some benefit to justify the expense and risks of antibiotic exposure. Moreover, the other advantages to *H. pylori* eradication besides the cure of dyspeptic symptoms (see Chapter 68) help to support the test-and-treat approach.

Acid Suppression

Contrary to common belief, there is little evidence that acid-inhibiting or acid-neutralizing treatment significantly improves symptoms in patients with documented nonulcer dyspepsia. Much of the confusion about the efficacy of such antiulcer therapy seems to result from a substantial placebo effect, the heterogeneous nature of patients with dyspepsia, and the poor characterization of patients in many studies. Randomized, controlled trials have failed to demonstrate consistent benefit from the use of antiulcer therapy in patients with carefully documented nonulcer dyspepsia. This correlates with data showing little excess acid production in most of these patients. Those who respond to empiric therapy may be the subset with an underlying peptic ulcer diathesis. Some interpret response to empiric proton-pump inhibition as a sign of underlying gastroesophageal reflux or peptic ulcer disease. More and better data are required to clarify the use of these very expensive drugs in dyspepsia. In the meantime, physicians are likely to continue prescribing acid-suppression antiulcer therapy empirically because there is little else to offer patients. If such therapy is to be offered, it should be given for a limited time and not continued if symptoms fail to resolve.

Enhancing Gastric Motility

If indeed nonulcer dyspepsia is a disease of altered upper GI motility, then drugs that facilitate such motility would be expected to be beneficial. *Metoclopramide*, the original dopaminergic blocking agent available for stimulating gastric motility, provides some benefit as short-term therapy. Long-term administration of the drug is associated with a risk of tardive dyskinesia, making it inappropriate for prolonged use.

Itopride (a dopamine D_2 agonist with anticholinesterase activity combining purportedly to improve gastric accommodation, secretion, and emptying) has shown considerable promise. In placebo-controlled, randomized trial, it achieved significant symptomatic improvement for dyspeptic patients. More data are needed to help determine efficacy and the optimal duration of treatment.

Diet, Alcohol, Smoking

No data indicate that a low-fat diet, restriction of alcohol, cessation of smoking, or reduction of stress has any consistently positive effect on nonulcer dyspepsia. The lack of effect may be as much a function of the heterogeneous nature of the dyspeptic population as it is an indication of a true absence of benefit. Patients with concurrent IBS-like symptoms should be treated accordingly (see prior discussion).

Addressing Psychosocial Stresses

Most authorities recommend taking a careful history to identify any psychosocial precipitants and responding to them. In otherwise-refractory cases in which there is a clear-cut association between dyspepsia and psychosocial factors, the latter should be addressed thoroughly. Any underlying anxiety disorder or depression should be treated specifically (see Chapters 226 and 227). Low-dose *tricyclic antidepressant* therapy (e.g., nortriptyline starting at 12.5 mg at bedtime and titrating upward) has even been recommended as empiric therapy in the absence of contraindications, given its ability to alter pain sensory thresholds.

Patient Education and Indications for Referral

Patients who present with recurrent upper abdominal pain are fearful of cancer and other serious forms of GI pathology. For many, the first priority is knowing that they do not have a life-threatening illness. As with any disorder that can mimic more worrisome illness, the patient's concerns should be taken seriously and addressed directly (the approach to patient reassurance with regard to IBS also applies here).

Referral to a gastroenterologist is indicated when endoscopy is considered. The most appropriate candidates are those at increased risk of gastric malignancy and other serious upper GI pathology (see earlier discussion). At times, a consultation with the gastroenterologist will help to reassure the low-risk but overly concerned patient, although the need for such referrals can be kept to a minimum by thorough patient education and support.

A.H.G.

Annotated Bibliography

Irritable Bowel Syndrome

1. Almy T. Experimental studies on the irritable colon. Am J Med 1951;10:60. (*A classic paper on the relation of stress to bowel activity.*)
2. Drossman DA, McKee DC, Sandler RS, et al. Psychosocial factors in the irritable bowel syndrome. A multivariate study of patients and nonpatients with irritable bowel syndrome. Gastroenterology 1988;95:701. (*Underlying psychopathology is a major predictor of a person's becoming a patient.*)
3. Drossman DA, Thompson WG. The irritable bowel syndrome: review and a graduated multicomponent treatment approach. Ann Intern Med 1992;116:1009. (*An outstanding review, and the best discussion of psychosocial factors and their management; 117 references.*)
4. Horwitz BJ, Fisher RS. The irritable bowel syndrome. N Engl J Med 2001;344:1846. (*A succinct review, with particularly good sections on pathophysiology and treatment; 50 references.*)
5. Jones AV, McLaughlan P, Shorthouse M, et al. Food intolerance: a major factor in the pathogenesis of the irritable bowel syndrome. Lancet 1982;2:115. (*Presents the evidence for intolerance to wheat, corn, dairy products, coffee, tea, and citrus fruits.*)
6. Merrick MV, Eastwood MA, Ford MJ. Is bile acid malabsorption underdiagnosed? An evaluation of accuracy of diagnosis by measurement of SeHCAT retention. BMJ 1985;290:665. (*Discusses the role of bile acid malabsorption.*)
7. Mertz H, Fullerton S, Naliboff B, et al. Symptoms and visceral perception in severe functional and organic dyspepsia. Gut 1998;42:814. (*Half of dyspeptic patients have pain on intragastric balloon inflation at volumes too low to cause pain in normal individuals.*)
8. Miura M, Lawson DC, Clary EM, et al. Central modulation of rectal distention-induced blood pressure changes by alosetron, a 5-HT₃ receptor antagonist. Dig Dis Sci 1999;44:20. (*Presents evidence of a central role for serotonin.*)
9. Nanda R, James R, Smith H, et al. Food intolerance and the irritable bowel syndrome. Gut 1989;30:1099. (*Reviews the evidence for the role of food intolerance.*)
10. Newcomer AD, McGill DB. Clinical importance of lactose deficiency. N Engl J Med 1984;310:42. (*An editorial summarizing the data on lactose deficiency in clinical syndromes, including its role in irritable bowel syndrome [IBS].*)
11. Owens DM, Nelson DK, Talley NJ. The irritable bowel syndrome: long-term prognosis and the physician–patient interaction. Ann Intern Med 1995;122:107. (*The Olmstead County, Minnesota, experience, finding that prognosis was good, and the initial diagnosis was unlikely to change; the use of health services was reduced by a strong patient–doctor relationship.*)
12. Rumessen JJ, Gudmand-Hoyer E. Functional bowel disease: malabsorption and abdominal distress after ingestion of fructose, sorbitol, and fructose–sorbitol mixtures. Gastroenterology 1988;95:694. (*Presents the evidence for the role of these agents in some cases of IBS.*)
13. Smith RC, Greenbaum DS, Vancouver JB, et al. Psychosocial factors are associated with health care seeking rather than diagnosis in irritable bowel syndrome. Gastroenterology 1990;98:293. (*The title says it all.*)
14. Spiller R, Campbell E. Post-infectious irritable bowel syndrome. Curr Opin Gastroenterol 2006;22:13. (*Notes a 10% incidence of IBS-like symptoms after gastroenteritis.*)
15. Sullivan M, Cohen S, Snape W. Colonic myoelectric activity in irritable bowel syndrome. N Engl J Med 1978;298:878. (*Patients with IBS had an abnormally prolonged increase in postprandial motor activity, which was reduced by an anticholinergic agent.*)
16. Whitehead WE, Holtkotter B, Enck P, et al. Tolerance for rectosigmoid distention in irritable bowel syndrome. Gastroenterology 1990;98:1187. (*Sensation thresholds are altered.*)
17. Zwetchkenbaum JF, Burakoff R. Food allergy and the irritable bowel syndrome. Am J Gastroenterol 1988;83:901. (*Disputes the role of food allergy.*)
18. Fass R, Longstreth GF, Pimentel M, et al. Evidence- and consensus-based practice guidelines for the diagnosis of irritable bowel disease. Arch Intern Med 2001;161:2081. (*Points out the dearth of evidence available to guide workup; provides a consensus approach.*)
19. Green PHR, Cellier C. Celiac disease. N Engl J Med 2007;357:1731. (*An excellent review of this must-not-miss mimicker of IBS.*)

20. Kruis W, Thieme C, Weinzierl M, et al. A diagnostic score for the irritable bowel syndrome, its value in the exclusion of organic disease. Gastroenterology 1984;87:1. (*An elaborate regression study, providing a weighted score with high specificity and sensitivity; blood in the stool rules out the diagnosis.*)

21. Manning AP, Thompson WG, Heaton KW, et al. Towards positive diagnosis of the irritable bowel syndrome. BMJ 1978;2:653. (*Classic diagnostic criteria; still widely used.*)

22. Mayer EA. Irritable bowel syndrome. N Engl J Med 2008;358:1692. (*A clinically focused, evidence-based review, with emphasis on diagnosis and treatment; 40 references.*).

23. Suleiman S, Sonneberg A. Cost-effectiveness of endoscopy in irritable bowel syndrome. Arch Intern Med 2001;161:369. (*Finds that the procedure is useful if clinical evidence is suggestive of serious underlying pathology.*)

24. Svendsen JH, Munck LK, Andersen JR. Irritable bowel syndrome—prognosis and diagnostic safety. Scand J Gastroenterol 1985;20:415. (*Disease waxes and wanes; only rarely—0% to 3% of cases—is there a missed diagnosis of organic disease, even after 5 years of follow-up.*)

25. Talley NJ, Thieme C, Weinzierl M, et al. Diagnostic value of the Manning criteria in irritable bowel syndrome. Gut 1990;31:77. (*The best critique of these diagnostic criteria.*)

26. Bensoussan A, Talley NJ, Hing M, et al. Treatment of irritable bowel syndrome with Chinese herbal medicine. JAMA 1998;280:1585. (*The only randomized, double-blind, placebo-controlled trial; improvements were noted in symptom score and quality of life; benefit ceased with the cessation of therapy, except in patients given a customized program.*)

27. Camilleri M, Northcutt AR, Kong S, et al. Efficacy and safety of alosetron in women with irritable bowel syndrome: a randomized controlled trial. Lancet 2000;355:1035. (*An important report on the efficacy of 5-HT$_3$-receptor–antagonist therapy in women with severe IBS-related diarrhea.*)

28. Cann PA, Read NW, Holdsworth CD. What is the benefit of coarse wheat bran in patients with irritable bowel syndrome? Gut 1984;25:168. (*Bran did help pain, constipation, diarrhea, and urgency, as did placebo, except for constipation, which responded better with bran.*)

29. Cann PA, Read NW, Holdsworth CD, et al. Role of loperamide and placebo in management of irritable bowel syndrome. Dig Dis Sci 1984;29:239. (*Loperamide proved superior to placebo in patients with diarrhea, urgency, and incontinence.*)

30. Chang. L, Ameen VZ, Dukes GE, et al. A dose-ranging, phase II study of the efficacy and safety of alosetron in men with diarrhea-predominant IBS. Am J Gastroenterol 2005:100:115. (*Presents the evidence of efficacy in men as well.*)

31. Chang. L, Chey WD, Harris L, et al. Incidence of ischemic colitis and serious complications of constipation among patients using alosetron: systematic review of clinical trials and post-marketing surveillance data. Am J Gastroenterol 2006;101:1069. (*Finds a very small but significant increase in the risk of serious gastrointestinal complications.*)

32. Deutsch E. Relief of anxiety and related emotions in patients with gastrointestinal disorders. Am J Dig Dis 1971;16:1091. (*Diazepam relieved anxiety but did not improve bowel symptoms any better than did placebo.*)

33. Drossman DA, Toner BB, Whitehead WE, et al. Cognitive–behavioral therapy versus education and desipramine versus placebo for moderate to severe functional bowel disorders. Gastroenterology 2003;125:19. (*Both cognitive–behavioral therapy and desipramine were found to be effective.*)

34. Jackson JL, O'Malley PG, Tomkins G, et al. Treatment of functional gastrointestinal disorders with antidepressant medications: a meta-analysis. Am J Med 2000;108:65. (*Finds evidence of efficacy but cannot determine whether the benefit was independent of the effect on depression.*)

35. Lackner JM, Mesmer C, Morely S, et al. Psychological treatments for irritable bowel syndrome: a systematic review and meta-analysis. J Consult Clin Psychol 2004;72:1100. (*Finds that cognitive–behavioral therapy was very effective and the best performing of all psychological measures.*)

36. Lackner JM, Jaccard J, Krasner SS, et al. Self-administered cognitive behavioral therapy for moderate to severe IBS: clinical efficacy, tolerability, feasibility. Clin Gastroenterol Hepatol 2008;6:899. (*Presents promising results for self-administered cognitive–behavioral therapy.*)

37. Longstreth GF, Fox DD, Youkeles MS, et al. Psyllium therapy in the irritable bowel syndrome. Ann Intern Med 1981;95:53. (*A randomized, controlled trial, finding that both treatment and control groups improved significantly, suggesting a strong psychological overlay of symptoms and the efficacy of supportive measures.*)

38. Prior A, Colgan SM, Whorwell PJ. Changes in rectal sensitivity after hypnotherapy in patients with irritable bowel syndrome. Gut 1990;31:896. (*Pain threshold was raised, suggesting a mechanism and role for hypnotherapy in IBS.*)

39. Schwarz SP, Taylor AE, Scharff L, et al. Behaviorally treated irritable bowel syndrome patients: a four-year follow-up. Behav Res Ther 1990;28:331. (*Lasting response was demonstrated.*)

40. Smart HL, Mayberry JF, Atkinson M. Alternative medicine consultations and remedies in patients with irritable bowel syndrome. Gut 1986;27:826.

(*Up to 20% of patients use alternative treatment; this suggests that needs are not being met by their physicians.*)

41. Tack J, Fried M, Houghton LA, et al. Systematic review: the efficacy of treatments for irritable bowel syndrome—a European perspective. Aliment Pharmacol Ther 2006;24:183. (*Findings include considerable bloating from the use of fiber, limiting its usefulness.*)

Nonulcer Dyspepsia

1. Friedman LS. *Helicobacter pylori* and nonulcer dyspepsia. N Engl J Med 1998;339:1928. (*An editorial summarizing the best evidence available and making very reasonable recommendations.*)

2. Johannessen T, Petersen H, Kristensen P, et al. Cimetidine for symptomatic relief of dyspepsia. Scand J Gastroenterol 1992;27:189. (*Presents evidence for benefit with histamine$_2$-blocker therapy.*)

3. Nyren O, Adami HO, Bates S, et al. Absence of therapeutic benefit from antacids or cimetidine in nonulcer dyspepsia. N Engl J Med 1986;314:339. (*Presents evidence against benefit from antiulcer therapy.*)

4. Talley NJ, Boyce P, Jones M. Dyspepsia and health care seeking in a community: how important are psychological factors? Dig Dis Sci 1998;43:1016. (*Finds an increased incidence of psychological factors among patients—a pathophysiologic mechanism or a cause of health seeking?*)

5. Talley NJ, McNeil D, Piper DW. Environmental factors and chronic unexplained dyspepsia: association with acetaminophen but not other analgesics, alcohol, coffee, tea, or smoking. Dig Dis Sci 1988;33:641. (*Surprising but well-documented findings.*)

6. Talley NJ, Phillips SF. Nonulcer dyspepsia: potential causes and pathophysiology. Ann Intern Med 1988;108:865. (*An exhaustive, slightly dated, but still-useful review with excellent discussions of disease mechanisms, possible precipitants, and workup, all with practical implications; 268 references.*)

7. Health and Public Policy Committee, American College of Physicians. Endoscopy in the evaluation of dyspepsia. Ann Intern Med 1986;102:266. (*Recommends a 6- to 8-week course of empiric antiulcer therapy in low-risk patients before considering endoscopic evaluation.*)

8. Talley NJ, Silverstein MD, Agreus L, et al. AGA technical review: evaluation of dyspepsia. Gastroenterology 1998;114:582. (*A consensus guideline.*)

9. Zell SC, Budhraja M. An approach to dyspepsia in the ambulatory care setting: evaluation based on risk stratification. J Gen Intern Med 1989;4:144. (*Argues for a diagnostic approach that assigns low-risk patients to empiric antiulcer treatment rather than endoscopic study.*)

10. Arents NLA, Thijs JC, van Zwet AA, et al. Approach to treatment of dyspepsia in primary care: a randomized trial comparing "test-and-treat" with prompt endoscopy. Arch Intern Med 2003;163:1606. (*Confirms in the primary care setting the safety of the test-and-treat approach.*)

11. Blum AL, Talley NJ, O'Morain C, et al. Lack of effect of treating *Helicobacter pylori* infection in patients with nonulcer dyspepsia. N Engl J Med 1998;339:1875. (*A well-designed randomized, placebo-controlled study, showing no difference in symptoms at 12 months despite the documented eradication of infection.*)

12. Fisher RS, Parkman HP. Management of nonulcer dyspepsia. N Engl J Med 1998;339:1376. (*A useful review of management, most notable for its excellent discussion of theories of pathogenesis; 59 references.*)

13. Greenberg PD, Cello JP. Lack of effect of treatment for *Helicobacter pylori* on symptoms of nonulcer dyspepsia. Arch Intern Med 1999;159:2283. (*A randomized, controlled trial, finding that the eradication of Helicobacter pylori failed to show a benefit in most patients.*)

14. Holtmann G, Talley NJ, Liebregts T, et al. A placebo-controlled trial of itopride in functional dyspepsia. N Engl J Med 2006;354:832. (*Presents evidence of efficacy for this example of a new class of agents.*)

15. Jaakkimainen RL, Boyle E, Tudiver F. Is *Helicobacter pylori* associated with non-ulcer dyspepsia and will eradication improve symptoms? A meta-analysis. BMJ 1999;319:1040. (*The odds ratio for improvement was 1.9 in patients referred to gastroenterologists; suggests that the role and benefit of treatment are modest.*)

16. Johnson AF. Controlled trial of metoclopramide in the treatment of flatulent dyspepsia. BMJ 1971;2:25. (*Nausea and pain were relieved.*)

17. McColl K, Murray L, El-Omar E, et al. Symptomatic benefit from eradicating *Helicobacter pylori* infection in patients with nonulcer dyspepsia. N Engl J Med 1998;339:1869. (*A placebo-controlled study, showing a modest long-term benefit—21% vs. 7%—from antibiotic therapy in patients positive for H. pylori.*)

18. Ofman JJ, Etchason J, Fullerton S, et al. Management strategies for *Helicobacter pylori*–seropositive patients with dyspepsia: clinical and economic consequences. Ann Intern Med 1997;126:280. (*A decision-analysis study, supporting the cost-effectiveness of serologic testing and treatment for H. pylori infection.*)

CHAPTER 75 ■ MANAGEMENT OF DIVERTICULAR DISEASE

Diverticula—abnormal herniations of colonic mucosa through the muscularis—are extremely common, and their prevalence increases with age. Autopsy studies estimate their presence in 20% of people older than 40 year, which increases to nearly 70% by age 70 years. About 15% of people with the condition develop attacks of *diverticulitis*, in which the diverticula become plugged and inflamed. It is possible that the recent emphasis on increasing the fiber content of the diet will reduce the incidences of diverticula and their complications in Western countries. The primary physician encounters many elderly patients with gastrointestinal (GI) complaints referable to diverticular disease. The physician must effectively and economically recognize and treat mild manifestations of disease, reduce the chances of complications, and decide when admission and surgical intervention are necessary.

PATHOPHYSIOLOGY, CLINICAL PRESENTATION, AND COURSE (1–13)

Pathophysiology

Increased intracolonic pressure causes herniation of colonic mucosa. Consequently, diverticula occur most frequently in the sigmoid colon, where the colon is narrowest and pressure is greatest; however, diverticula can occur anywhere within the colon, including the ascending portion, which makes for atypical clinical presentations. In Western populations, about 85% of diverticula are found in the distal colon, with 15% located in the right side of the large bowel; in Asia, right-sided involvement is more common. Diverticula show a predilection for points of relative weakness in the muscularis, especially where branches of the marginal artery penetrate the colonic wall. The possibility of muscular degeneration has been suggested but is unproven. Research indicates that the *low fiber content* of modern diets has an important causal role, resulting in the production of less-bulky stool and increased intracolonic pressure. *Irritable bowel syndrome*, with its abnormal colonic motor activity and segmentation, might contribute to diverticular formation by way of increased intraluminal pressures.

The diverticular sac that ensues is a thin, purely mucosal structure. Obstruction of the sac's neck by undigested food residues or a fecalith leads to distention and *microabscess* formation as mucous secretions accumulate and bacteria proliferate. If the blood supply to the sac becomes mechanically compromised, the sac may perforate. *Microperforations* commonly occur, producing peridiverticular and pericolonic inflammation and abscess formation. Walling off is the rule because these perforations typically occur adjacent to mesocolon. The bowel lumen is typically uninvolved. Even if a peridiverticular abscess ruptures into the peritoneal cavity, gross peritonitis from fecal soilage usually does not occur because the diverticular neck is sealed by obstructing material. The bacteriology of the abscesses is predominated by *anaerobes*, *Escherichia coli*, and *streptococci*.

A less common but potentially catastrophic complication of diverticulosis is *free colonic perforation*, which occurs from the rupture of an uninflamed diverticulum. Fecal soilage follows because there is no plug in the diverticular neck to prevent leakage of bowel contents. Frank peritonitis is the consequence.

Clinical Presentation and Course

Diverticulosis

Diverticulosis is usually asymptomatic and often discovered incidentally on screening colonoscopy, abdominal computed tomography (CT), or barium enema. However, colonic motor activity is sometimes disturbed, and intermittent left lower quadrant pain may result. Constipation is common, as is constipation alternating with diarrhea, and occasionally there is tenderness.

Complications from diverticulosis include hemorrhage, microperforation (diverticulitis), perforation, and obstruction. The estimated complication rate is about 1%/yr. *Bleeding* is a particularly important concern. Diverticular disease is one of the most common causes of lower GI bleeding (see Chapter 63); erosion into a blood vessel may result in brisk rectal hemorrhage. *Perforation* in the absence of diverticulitis is rare, but it is potentially catastrophic due to the high risk of fecal soilage. Diverticulitis is the consequence of microperforation and may lead to obstruction.

Diverticulitis

Diverticulitis is characterized clinically by left lower quadrant pain, tenderness, fever, and leukocytosis in a patient with known diverticulosis. Frequently, a tender mass is noted. Right-sided presentations are possible, especially in Asian populations, and may mimic appendicitis or Crohn's disease. In rare instances, there are extraintestinal manifestations (arthritis, pyoderma gangrenosum) that may simulate those of Crohn's disease and lead to misdiagnosis. Bladder symptoms (dysuria, urgency, frequency) may occur if the process occurs adjacent to the bladder or bladder nerves.

Complicated diverticulitis refers to the development of abscess, fistula, stricture, bowel obstruction, or peritonitis. Frank *perforations* may lead to abscess formation. The abscesses may spontaneously drain into the bowel or erode into an adjacent organ, such as the ureter, bladder, or vagina, forming *fistulas*. Perforations that fail to become walled off may cause peritonitis. Those that enter the vagina result in vaginal gas or feces;

those that erode into the urinary tract lead to dysuria or pneumaturia. Chronic inflammation can thicken the bowel wall and cause *obstruction*.

Clinical presentation and course can be defined in terms of stages (Hinchey classification) as follows:

Stage 1: abscess less than 4 cm, confined to the pericolic area or mesentery

Stage 2: abscess greater than 4 cm, confined to the pelvis

Stage 3: rupture of peridiverticular abscess with peritonitis

Stage 4: rupture of uninflamed bowel into free peritoneal space

The risk of death is 5% for stages 1 and 2; 13% for stage 3, and 43% for stage 4. Persons with stage 1 disease can often be managed on an outpatient basis (see later discussion). Recurrences are not uncommon, but mild recurrences do not increase the risk of complicated disease.

DIAGNOSIS (6,8,10,11,14–16)

Diverticulosis

As noted earlier, diverticulosis is usually an incidental finding in a patient undergoing a *colonoscopy*, *sigmoidoscopy*, or *barium enema* for another reason. However, the diagnosis should also be considered in a patient presenting with relatively painless but brisk rectal bleeding. If the bleeding is not too severe, *proctosigmoidoscopy* can be performed to confirm the diagnosis and site of blood loss. A high rate of diagnostic errors has been found when barium enema is obtained in symptomatic persons, leading some to recommend that colonoscopy follow the barium enema. There is no contraindication to colonoscopy in asymptomatic persons with suspected diverticulosis; in the absence of inflammation, risk of perforation is small.

Diverticulitis

The diagnosis of acute diverticulitis should be suspected in an older patient who presents with new onset of left lower quadrant abdominal pain, low-grade fever, focal tenderness with or without guarding, and an elevated white blood cell count. Some elderly patients may not demonstrate much fever, abdominal pain, or peritoneal signs; a markedly elevated white blood cell count may be the only clue to a deteriorating situation. In rare instances, the pain may be suprapubic or localized to the right lower quadrant if there is a redundant sigmoid or a right-sided diverticulum. Nausea, vomiting, and diarrhea or constipation may accompany the bowel complaints and simulate gastroenteritis. The absence of bowel sounds, marked rebound, and guarding indicate significant peritoneal inflammation. In many instances, the diagnosis of diverticulitis can be made on clinical grounds, but in situations of diagnostic uncertainty, confirmatory testing should be obtained.

Computed tomography of the abdomen has become the test of choice for the immediate confirmation of acute diverticulitis, supplanting barium enema. Although more expensive than barium enema, CT has proven to be more cost-effective and does not require the insufflation of air-contrast barium enema with its associated risk of perforation. In addition, it can help to identify other causes of mimicking lower abdominal pain such as appendicitis, Crohn's disease, and pelvic pathology.

Diagnostic findings for diverticulitis include inflammation of pericolic fat, peridiverticular abscess, thickening of the bowel wall more than 4 mm, and the presence of diverticula. The test can be used to differentiate cancer from diverticulitis and provides the opportunity for guiding needle aspiration and drainage of large abscesses (>4 cm). Reported test sensitivity often exceeds 95%, but false negatives can occur due in part to the inability to detect small abscesses and to differentiate tumor from diverticulitis when there is marked bowel-wall thickening. For this reason, follow-up colonoscopy is recommended after the acute inflammatory phase of illness has passed.

Barium enema is now largely relegated to a secondary role. If there is an urgent need to differentiate between diverticulitis and cancer in the acute setting, a single-contrast study (substituting water-soluble contrast media for barium and omitting air insufflation) can be performed, but differentiation is best postponed to later. The finding of contrast outside of the bowel lumen outlining an abscess cavity or showing an intramural sinus tract or fistula helps to make the diagnosis of diverticulitis.

Ultrasound offers low-cost, noninvasive, readily available study of the area in question, but it appears to lack the sensitivity and specificity of CT (reported range 84% to 95%, and 80% to 95%, respectively). The detection of bowel-wall thickening and abscess is possible with ultrasound. The test is very operator dependent, suggesting that the impressive test performance characteristics reported in research studies from academic centers might be considerably more difficult to achieve in community settings. The test is a reasonable first choice for imaging in situations in which a pelvic etiology is also under consideration.

Colonoscopy is usually performed 6 weeks later (after acute inflammatory symptoms have cleared) to rule out malignancy and inflammatory bowel disease, which may present in similar fashion. It allows for direct visualization and biopsy if tumor is present. When deemed essential in the acute phase to rule out other serious causes (e.g., inflammatory bowel disease, ischemia, cancer), it can be attempted if bowel preparation and air insufflation are kept to a minimum and the inability to pass the scope beyond the rectosigmoid junction is respected as indicative of acute diverticulitis.

PRINCIPLES OF MANAGEMENT (1,2,4,6,8,10–14,16–21)

Diverticulosis

The goals of therapy are the prevention of symptoms, the relief of pain, and the avoidance of complications. Because diverticular disease is believed to be, in part, a manifestation of a low-fiber diet, diets rich in *insoluble fiber* have been recommended and studied. The most palatable approach is encouragement of diets rich in insoluble fiber from daily intake of *fruits* and *vegetables;* these show a 37% reduction in the risk of symptomatic diverticular disease. *Physical activity* adds to risk reduction. *Bran* has been tried as a source of insoluble fiber, with a reversal of abnormal bowel physiology and a reduction in symptoms noted in more than 90% of cases when intake averages about 15 g/d. This can cause flatulence and bloating during the first 2 to 3 weeks in many people, but these usually resolve with continued bran intake. Patients unable to tolerate bran may be treated with a bulk agent such as *psyllium* (Metamucil).

Irritant laxatives should be avoided. The efficacy of *anticholinergics* is controversial; painful spasm may be lessened, but the risk of constipation is increased, raising the likelihood of inspissation of fecal material. Indigestible materials (e.g., seeds) that may block the mouth of a diverticulum should be omitted from the diet.

Acute Diverticulitis

Outpatient versus Inpatient Management

Immunocompetent patients can be treated at home when symptoms are mild, reliability is good, the ability to take in fluids is preserved, and the home situation is conducive. Patients should manifest minimal peritoneal signs and only mild fever. Those who appear more toxic require inpatient management. A key requirement for outpatient management is the ability to maintain good oral intake of fluids.

Outpatient Management of Acute Phase

Initial priorities are to maintain hydration and reduce bowel activity, lessening the chances of volume depletion and perforation. *Rest* and *clear liquids* usually suffice. Strong analgesics and antipyretics should not be prescribed because they may mask signs of worsening inflammation. A course of *broad-spectrum oral antibiotic therapy* directed against both anaerobes and facultative aerobes is recommended (e.g., *trimethoprim/sulfamethoxazole* or *ciprofloxacin* plus *metronidazole*; alternatively, *amoxicillin/clavulanate*. The oral antibiotic regimen is continued typically for 7 to 10 days (3 to 5 days beyond the resolution of fever). Patients who improve can be advanced to a *low-residue liquid diet* that does not contain indigestible fiber (note that some liquid supplements are high in indigestible fiber). Persons who fail to respond or respond slowly may have a complication such as abscess formation and should undergo CT imaging and consideration for hospital admission (see later discussion).

Subsequent Management

Although controlled data are lacking, most authorities recommend treatment with a high-fiber diet as for diverticulosis (see prior discussion) after acute symptoms have ceased. An important decision in the subsequent management of the patient with diverticulitis is whether to opt for *elective surgical resection* of the involved bowel after the initial resolution of symptoms. Proponents of elective surgical therapy argue that the frequency of complications warrants prophylactic operation once a patient experiences an attack of diverticulitis. However, rates of recurrence of medically and surgically treated persons are nearly identical. Moreover, most patients never have another attack, and those that do have mild recurrences appear to be at no increased risk for complications.

INDICATIONS FOR ADMISSION AND REFERRAL (8)

The onset of brisk rectal bleeding from diverticulosis requires prompt hospital admission (see Chapter 63). In suspected diverticulitis, the development of a temperature greater than 101°F on oral antibiotic therapy, inability to take fluids orally, or worsening or persistence of pain or peritoneal signs indicate the need for hospital admission, intravenous antibiotics, and CT scanning. The CT finding of an *abscess greater than 4 cm* in diameter (stage 2 disease) necessitates consultation for the consideration of imaging-guided percutaneous needle drainage of the abscess, which helps to speed healing. The presence of generalized peritoneal signs is an indication for urgent surgical consultation.

THERAPEUTIC RECOMMENDATIONS AND PATIENT EDUCATION (8,16,18,20)

Diverticulosis

For the patient with known diverticula and occasional pain or constipation, the following recommendations should be observed:

- Increase the fiber content of the diet. The best sources are bran, root vegetables (particularly raw carrots), and fruits with skin. Bulk laxatives such as psyllium hydrophilic mucilloid (Metamucil) can be used in patients who cannot tolerate bran, but these are relatively expensive. Inform patients that any bloating or flatulence due to bran intake usually resolves with continued use.
- Prescribe regular aerobic exercise.
- Have patients avoid foods with seeds or indigestible material that may block the neck of a diverticulum, such as nuts, corn, popcorn, cucumbers, tomatoes, figs, strawberries, and caraway seeds.
- Have patients avoid laxatives, enemas, and opiates because they are potent constipating agents; consider anticholinergic therapy for refractory cramping, but use with care and for short periods only.
- Instruct patients to report fever, tenderness, or bleeding without delay.

Diverticulitis

- Consider outpatient management for patients with mild diverticulitis (mild to moderate abdominal pain, minimal peritoneal signs, temperature <101°F, ability to take oral fluids, modestly elevated white count) who have a conducive home environment.
- Prescribe bedrest and a clear liquid diet.
- Use only mild nonopiate analgesics for pain.
- Monitor temperature, pain level, abdominal examination for signs of peritonitis, and white blood cell count for elevation.
- Begin a broad-spectrum oral antibiotic program (*trimethoprim/sulfamethoxazole* 160/800 mg twice daily or *ciprofloxacin* 500 mg twice daily, plus *metronidazole* 500 mg four times daily, and continue for 7 to 10 days (until the patient is afebrile for 3 to 5 days); alternatively, prescribe *amoxicillin/clavulanate* 875/125 mg twice daily).
- Arrange for prompt hospitalization for intravenous antibiotics and CT scanning if temperature goes above 101°F despite antibiotics, pain worsens, frank peritoneal signs develop, or white cell count rises; obtain consultation for the consideration of percutaneous drainage if there is a peridiverticular abscess on CT scan greater than 4 cm; obtain urgent surgical consultation if there is evidence of more-generalized peritonitis.

A.H.G.

Annotated Bibliography

1. Aldoori WH, Giovannucci WL, Rochett HRH, et al. A study of dietary fiber types and symptomatic diverticular disease in men. J Nutr 1998;128:714. (*A major prospective study, finding an inverse relation between the intake of insoluble dietary fiber—fruits and vegetables—and the risk of symptomatic diverticular disease.*)
2. Aldoori WH, Giovannucci WL, Rimm EB, et al. Prospective study of physical activity and risk of symptomatic diverticular disease in men. Gut 1995;36:276. (*Finds that activity decreases risk.*)
3. Almy T, Howell DA. Diverticular disease of the colon. N Engl J Med 1980;302:324. (*A classic review; 119 references.*)
4. Boles R, Jordan S. Clinical significance of diverticulosis. Gastroenterology 1958;35:579. (*A classic natural history study, with a mean duration of follow-up of 15 years, finding that the frequency of hemorrhage, obstruction, or perforation was 15%.*)
5. Chapman JR, Dozois EJ, Wolff BG, et al. Diverticulitis: a progressive disease? Do multiple recurrences predict less favorable outcome? Ann Surg 2006;243:876. (*Presents evidence suggesting that the answer is no*).
6. Ferzoco LB, Raptopoulos V, Silen W. Acute diverticulitis. N Engl J Med 1998;338:1521. (*A succinct, thoughtful review; 51 references.*)
7. Horner JL. Natural history of diverticulosis of the colon. Am J Dig Dis 1958;3:343. (*A study of 503 patients followed in the ambulatory setting for a mean of 8 years, finding that the incidence of diverticulitis was 15%.*)
8. Jacobs DO. Diverticulitis. N Engl J Med 2007;357:2057. (*An excellent, clinically focused review, with emphasis on key decisions and supporting evidence; 49 references.*)
9. Klein S, Mayer L, Present DH, et al. Extraintestinal manifestations in patients with diverticulitis. Ann Intern Med 1988;108:700. (*A report of three cases of pyoderma gangrenosum and arthritis in patients with carefully documented diverticulitis.*)
10. Markham NI, Li KC. Diverticulitis of the right colon—experience from Hong Kong. Gut 1992;33:547. (*A good description of this uncommon but important variant.*)
11. McGuire HH. Bleeding colonic diverticula: a reappraisal of natural history and management. Ann Surg 1994;220:653. (*Much of the bleeding occurs from lesions in the proximal colon.*)
12. Munson KD, Hensien MA, Jacob LN, et al. Diverticulitis: a comprehensive follow-up. Dis Colon Rectum 1996;39:318. (*Modern data on the risk of recurrence, including that after surgery.*)
13. Wilcox CM, Alexander LN, Cotsonis GA, et al. Nonsteroidal antiinflammatory drugs are associated with upper and lower gastrointestinal bleeding. Dig Dis Sci 1997;42:990. (*Finds an increased risk for diverticular bleeding with the use of nonsteroidal antiinflammatory drugs.*)
14. Ambrosetti P, Grossholz M, Becker C, et al. Computed tomography in acute left colonic diverticulitis. Br J Surg 1997;84:532. (*A large, prospective study, reporting a sensitivity of 97%.*)
15. Eggesbo HB, Jacobsen T, Kolmannskog F, et al. Diagnosis of acute left-sided colonic diverticulitis by three radiological modalities. Acta Radiol 1998;39:315. (*Finds that computed tomography was superior to ultrasound.*)
16. Stollman NH, Raskin JB. Diagnosis and management of diverticular disease of the colon in adults. Am J Gastroenterol 1999;94:3111. (*Practice guidelines from the American College of Gastroenterology.*)
17. Larson D, Masters S, Spiro H. Medical and surgical therapy in diverticular disease. Gastroenterology 1976;71:734. (*Patients were followed for a mean of 9.8 years; no difference in outcome was found, and in about 75% of instances, no further problems occurred among those in either group.*)
18. Mazuski JE, Sawyer RG, Nathens AB, et al. The Surgical Infection Society guidelines for antimicrobial therapy for intra-abdominal infections: an executive summary. Surg Infect (Larchmt) 2002;3:161.(*Consensus recommendations for antibiotic therapy.*)
19. Painter N, Almeida A, Colebourne K. Unprocessed bran in treatment of diverticular disease of the colon. Br Med J 1972;2:137. (*Seventy patients were treated with bran in a prospective but uncontrolled study; >90% showed marked improvement in symptoms.*)
20. Rafferty J, Shellito P, Hyman NH, et al. Practice parameters for sigmoid diverticulitis. Dis Colon Rectum 2006;49:939. (*Concensus recommendation.*)
21. Taylor I, Duthie H. Bran tablets and diverticular disease. Br Med J 1976;2:988. (*A crossover trial of bran tablets, high-roughage diet, and a bulk agent plus an antispasmodic, finding that each improved bowel function, but that bran was the most effective in relieving symptoms and normalizing colonic motor activity.*)

CHAPTER 76 ■ MANAGEMENT OF GASTROINTESTINAL CANCERS

JEFFREY W. CLARK

Gastrointestinal malignancies are among the most common tumors found in adults worldwide. The primary treatment of local disease is surgical, although increasingly adjuvant or neoadjuvant chemotherapy and radiation therapy play important roles in the management of patients with resectable disease. The care of advanced disease is a responsibility often shared by the primary physician in close conjunction with oncologic colleagues. It is important for the primary physician to know the indications, limitations, efficacy, and side effects of available treatment modalities to help counsel the cancer patient and make the best use of therapies offered by the surgeon, radiation therapist, and oncologist.

Advances in treatment leading to improved outcomes include combining chemotherapy and radiation therapy with surgery and applying new biologic therapies involving mon-

oclonal antibodies directed against tumor growth factors. Prevention remains a critical component because overall mortality remains high (50% to 80%), although rates vary by specific disease. Continued improvements in the management of the gastrointestinal complications of cancer, such as obstruction, ascites, and cachexia, have improved the quality of life for these patients (see Chapter 91).

ESOPHAGEAL CANCER

As is true of many malignancies, carcinoma of the esophagus is difficult to diagnose and treat because symptoms usually do not occur until late in the course of illness. As a result, by the time patients become symptomatic, palliation is often the only therapeutic option. Of the approximately 14,000 new cases of esophageal cancer diagnosed annually in the United States, less than 10% of patients survive 5 years. Thus, improvements in prevention and early detection are necessary to have a significant effect on the overall mortality from this disease.

There are two major histologic types: *epidermoid* (squamous cell carcinoma) and *adenocarcinoma*. Worldwide, squamous cell carcinoma is the most common histologic type. However, in the United States, the incidence of squamous cell carcinoma continues to decline, and adenocarcinoma is increasing in frequency.

Risk Factors (1,2)

Risk factors for squamous cell carcinoma include heavy *smoking*, excessive *alcohol* use, *achalasia*, chronic ingestion of very *hot drinks or foods*, chronic intake of foods high in *nitrosamines*, and distant *lye* ingestion. The risk factors for adenocarcinoma are less well established, but chronic severe *gastroesophageal reflux* and the development of *Barrett's esophagus* are principal etiologic factors; both duration and severity contribute to risk. *Obesity* may also be a risk factor for adenocarcinoma.

Clinical Presentation

Adenocarcinoma often appears in the setting of Barrett's esophagus, a premalignant metaplastic change that is the consequence of prolonged severe acid reflux disease. Barrett's esophagus has a significant potential for dysplastic transformation leading to malignancy (see Chapter 61). Aside from heartburn, such patients are usually asymptomatic at the time of malignant transformation.

The first symptoms of esophageal cancer may go unnoticed because they are usually nonspecific. One warning symptom is pain on swallowing (*odynophagia*), which may begin as mild burning pain on swallowing. By the time there is frank difficulty with swallowing (*dysphagia*) and *inanition*, disease is usually advanced. Dysphagia usually indicates a markedly narrowed esophageal lumen and a substantial tumor burden.

These tumors begin as superficial mucosal lesions. They tend to spread silently under the mucosa and extend readily into the mediastinum because the esophagus has no serosal surface barrier. Tumor may extend regionally into the trachea and regional lymph nodes and vertically up and down the esophageal mucosa and submucosa. Distant metastases most commonly occur in the liver and intraabdominal node-bearing areas. The next-most-frequent sites include lung, bone, and brain. At the time of diagnosis, less than one third of patients have cancer confined to the esophageal wall, the stage in which cure is most likely to occur with surgical resection.

Diagnosis (1,3,4)

Next to prevention, early diagnosis is the next best means for improving outcome. Patients with a longstanding history of severe heartburn should be considered for endoscopy and biopsy because they have an increased risk of Barrett's esophagus and adenocarcinoma. Those found to have metaplastic change indicative of Barrett's esophagus are candidates for a program of regular *surveillance endoscopy* and biopsy (see Chapter 61). Those who show dysplastic change need referral for possible surgical resection. New onset of odynophagia

in a heavy smoker or drinker should also trigger consideration of endoscopy. Although the presence of small nodules, minor erosions, thickened folds, or mucosal depressions is suggestive of early cancer, mucosal biopsy is required for definitive diagnosis.

Staging (1,3,4)

Besides biopsy to determine the depth of tumor penetration (the primary determinant of staging), there are a number noninvasive means useful to the staging evaluation. Physical examination should include a check for supraclavicular adenopathy and hepatomegaly. *Computed tomography (CT)* of the chest and upper abdomen should be performed to check for mediastinal invasion. *Magnetic resonance imaging (MRI)* can also be used for this purpose, providing a similar degree of sensitivity for the detection of invasion without radiation exposure but at greater cost. *Positron emission tomography (PET scanning)* may also be useful in evaluation, especially to rule out metastatic disease not detectable on CT. *Endoscopic ultrasound (EUS)* is proving useful in determining the depth of invasion and may be superior to CT for this purpose. However, each of these modalities continues to evolve, and so the optimal use of the combinations of these approaches needs to be evaluated on an ongoing basis. Although imaging of the brain (with either CT or MRI) is not universally recommended, it should be considered, given the relatively high frequency of brain metastases seen.

From a staging standpoint, the most important distinction is between patients with potentially resectable disease and those who are not surgical candidates. As stated earlier, the most curable lesions are those confined to the mucosa. Unfortunately, nearly 75% of patients who present with dysphagia have at least locally advanced disease.

Principles of Management (1,5–12)

Surgery remains the modality of choice for initial therapy and is usually done with curative intent. However, only a relatively small percentage of patients have potentially curable disease at the time of detection. In addition, even after surgical resection, the rates of local recurrence and distant metastasis remain high. Combination regimens of chemotherapy and radiation, especially preoperatively in combination with surgery, continue to be explored to reduce the risk of recurrence. Some trials have shown a statistically significant survival benefit, whereas others have not; this remains an area of ongoing investigation. At the present time, many oncologists lean toward such neoadjuvant therapy for patients with potentially respectable disease that is clinically stage IIB or III. Surgery alone is usually used for earlier-stage disease. Unfortunately, most patients have unresectable disease at the time of presentation, so that therapy remains palliative.

Nutrition

Nutrition is a top priority for these patients. The morbidity of esophageal carcinoma is due largely to the severe dysphagia, odynophagia, and inanition that characterize advanced disease. Many patients are unable to swallow even their own saliva. Even partial obstruction leads to weight loss and cachexia. A weight loss of more than 10% at the time of presentation is a poor prognostic sign. Good nutrition is essential for the tolerance of surgery, chemotherapy, and radiation therapy. Blenderized diets and liquid diet supplements are helpful, and hyperalimentation is used as a temporary support during treatment for patients with the potential for meaningful survival.

Surgery

Surgery is the primary treatment modality for *cure*, achieving cure in the approximately 10% of cases found to have early-stage disease and for those with severe dysplasia or carcinoma *in situ* found during surveillance biopsy of Barrett's esophagus (see Chapter 61). The type of esophagectomy performed is determined by the location of the tumor. Achieving tumor-free margins of at least 2 cm is required. Except for very early disease picked up by surveillance (which might allow for a more localized resection), most cases usually require the resection of at least a substantial portion of the esophagus, necessitating a major thoracoabdominal procedure.

Perioperative morbidity and mortality historically have been high in such surgeries, although they have declined in the last decade. Death rates in most recent series are less than 5% to 10%, and major nonfatal complications occur in 30%. Median survival for patients undergoing surgery for cure is about 2 years, although it is considerably higher for those with very early disease confined to a small area of mucosa. Three-year survival is in the range of 25%. Preoperative irradiation does not appear to add much benefit, but when it is combined with preoperative chemotherapy, the results are more promising (see later discussion).

Surgery may also be performed for *palliation*, reestablishing the ability to swallow. Palliative surgical resection is most successful in patients with disease confined to the distal esophagus. However, even partial esophagectomy is a major procedure, with a high risk of major postoperative complications and surgical mortality. Increasingly, stents are being used to try to maintain patency of the esophagus for patients who are not candidates for surgery.

In recent years, the placement of *stents* for patients who cannot be resected has been increasingly utilized. As both the structure of the stents and procedures for placing them endoscopically have improved, they have had an increasingly important role in the palliation of patients. However, there is room for significant improvement.

Radiation Therapy

Radiation therapy is a consideration in persons with locally advanced disease not amenable to surgical resection. However, their central intrathoracic location adjacent to such key structures as the heart, lungs, and spinal cord makes the delivery of curative doses difficult without causing radiation injury. A program of chemotherapy (see later discussion) added to radiation enables the use of lower radiation doses and provides superior survival compared with radiation alone in patients with localized disease, be it adenocarcinoma or squamous cell cancer. Local-regional persistence of disease is the principal cause of treatment failure, suggesting to some that, when it becomes feasible, surgery after chemoradiation might be worthwhile (see later discussion).

Chemotherapy

The high risk of distant and local failures with surgery and radiation has prompted trials of chemotherapeutic regimens for use in combination with curative-intent surgery or radiation. The addition of *cisplatin* and *fluorouracil* improves outcomes in patients treated with radiation therapy; results have been equivocal when used as an adjuvant to surgery. Better chemotherapeutic regimens are being sought. Various combinations including agents such as *paclitaxel, irinotecan, 5-fluorouracil, epirubicin*, and platinum agents (*cisplatin* and *oxaliplatin*) have been shown to be active against esophageal cancers. In addition, biologic agents (e.g., *anti–epidermal growth factor receptor* agents such as cetuximab and *anti–vascular endothelial growth factor* agents such as *bevacizumab*) are being explored in combination with chemotherapeutic agents. Ongoing studies are evaluating which combinations of these agents either alone or in combination with radiation therapy provide the greatest benefit to patients while having acceptable toxicity.

Multimodality Therapy

The combination of all three modalities appears to be promising, particularly when chemoradiation is delivered neoadjuvantly before surgery. However, this remains an area of controversy because there are randomized, phase III studies that have shown survival benefit for combined modality therapy, whereas other studies have not shown a statistically significant benefit for combined therapy over surgery alone. At the present time in the United States, neoadjuvant chemotherapy and radiation therapy followed by surgical resection is the most common approach for patients with potentially resectable disease that is stage IIB or higher. Patients with earlier-stage disease usually undergo surgical resection alone.

Laser Therapy

Laser therapy is available for palliation in patients too ill to undergo surgery or radiation. Adverse effects are few, and therapy can be performed on an outpatient basis after an initial 2- to 3-day hospitalization. However, even when relief can be achieved, there is no change in survival rate.

Stenting and Dilation

For dysphagic patients too ill for surgery, palliation can be provided by endoscopic placement of a stent. Esophageal dilation is useful for temporary relief. Gastrostomy may be of help for nutrition but provides no symptomatic relief from disabling dysphagia.

Prevention (13,14)

Prevention remains the most effective means of dealing with this devastating cancer. Efforts to achieve cessation of smoking and alcohol abuse (see Chapters 54 and 228) are essential to reduce the risk of squamous cell cancers. Surveillance endoscopy plus biopsy of high-risk patients (e.g., those with Barrett's esophagus) offers the potential to identify dysplastic transformation and early adenocarcinoma, leading, it is hoped, to marked improvements in survival. The optimal approach to surveillance remains to be determined (see Chapter 61). Similarly, the identification of chronic symptomatic reflux as a risk factor for adenocarcinoma raises the possibility that acid-suppression therapy (e.g., by proton-pump inhibition) might reduce the chances of malignant transformation of esophageal mucosa (see Chapter 61). Prospective, randomized study is needed.

GASTRIC CANCER

There are approximately 23,000 new cases of gastric cancer in the United States each year and 14,000 deaths attributable to it annually. Over the last century, the incidence has decreased markedly in the United States, although this cancer remains one of the most common worldwide. Overall mortality has been relatively unchanged over the last 20 years, although there has been a small improvement in survival for patients whose disease can be resected who receive adjuvant therapy. Overall 5-year survival is approximately 78% for early-stage disease but declines rapidly to 20% for those with stage IIIA disease and less than 10% for those with stage IIIB or IV disease. Onset is uncommon before the age of 40 years, but incidence increases markedly thereafter. Improvement in outcome has been linked to advances in early diagnosis. Unfortunately, because of the absence of early symptoms and the nonspecific nature of symptoms when they do occur, most patients are still not diagnosed until they have advanced disease.

About 90% of gastric malignancies are adenocarcinomas, with those that are well differentiated and circumscribed having a much better prognosis than those that are poorly differentiated and infiltrative. Lymphomas are the second-most-common histology, although leiomyosarcomas, gastrointestinal stromal tumors, neuroendocrine tumors, and metastatic disease are also seen.

Risk Factors (1–3)

Throughout the world, dietary factors appear to play a major role, linked at least in part by the contribution of *Helicobacter pylori* infection to pathogenesis. Large-scale epidemiologic studies find a strong independent association between *Helicobacter* infection and the risk of gastric carcinoma. *H. pylori* infection is most prevalent among populations with inadequate means of food preservation and a high risk of food spoilage, populations with the highest prevalences of gastric cancer. The decline in gastric cancer in the United States over the last century may be related to improvements in food handling. Infection of the gastric mucosa by *H. pylori* leads to chronic inflammation and the development of *atrophic gastritis*, a recognized premalignant change. Infection during childhood is believed to be especially harmful. It is estimated that up to 70% of cases are causally related to *Helicobacter* infection, but only a small number of persons with the infection develop gastric carcinoma, suggesting additional causative factors.

In countries where the risk is high, research suggests that *dietary nitrate* sources are important risk factors. Foods associated with an increased risk of gastric cancer include dried salted fish, which are rich in nitrates. The nitrates may be converted to carcinogenic nitrites and nitroso compounds by bacteria found in unrefrigerated, partially decomposed food. This may account for the high rates of gastric cancer among lower socioeconomic groups. (Well-refrigerated and carefully handled raw fish popular in Japan and more recently in the United States as served in sushi bars does not appear to carry a nitrite risk.) In the United States, nitrate sources include hot dogs and other processed meats such as cold cuts. Other dietary risk factors that may be important include a low consumption of vegetables and fruits, fiber, and antioxidants (such as garlic and vitamins A and C) and high salt intake.

Other identified risk factors include *smoking, previous gastric surgery* (usually Billroth II anastomosis), and *chronic atrophic gastritis*. Increased prevalence also occurs among Native Americans, Asians, Hispanics, and Scandinavians. *Genetic factors* include blood type A, hereditary nonpolyposis colorectal cancer, familial adenomatous polyposis, Li–Fraumeni syndrome, and families with gastric cancer history but in which a genetic abnormality has not been defined.

Clinical Presentation and Course (1–3)

Clinical presentation can be subtle, making early diagnosis difficult. Unexplained iron-deficiency anemia or asymptomatic guaiac stool test positivity may be the only manifestation. Nonspecific abdominal pain, gastric ulceration with or without bleeding, weight loss, nausea, decreased appetite, early satiety, dysphagia, melena, and obstructive symptoms are the major patterns of clinical presentation, but most are manifestations of advanced disease. About 75% of patients with early disease have epigastric pain as the initial complaint; however, it may be subtle and resemble dyspepsia. Most are free of the nausea, vomiting, anorexia, and weight loss that characterize more advanced disease. Gastric ulcer is an important presentation, characterized by a suspicious appearance on barium study or endoscopy or a more benign-appearing radiologic defect that fails to heal completely or quickly recurs after 6 weeks of ulcer therapy (see Chapter 68).

The disease often progresses silently until signs or symptoms of metastatic disease, such as weight loss, anorexia, early satiety, abdominal pain, or ascites, become evident and cause the patient to seek medical attention. Spread occurs by direct extension and by seeding of the lymphatics, blood vessels, and peritoneal surface. Metastases develop locally and at distant sites, most frequently the liver (40%), lung (15%), and bone (15%). Among patients who come to surgery, approximately 80% are found to have lymph node metastases, whereas 40% have peritoneal involvement and 35% show spread to the liver or lung.

Diagnosis (2,4,5)

A high index of suspicion is warranted; early diagnosis provides the best chance for survival. Patients older than the age of 40 years presenting with any of the manifestations noted earlier should undergo testing as soon as possible. Endoscopy with brushings and biopsy is the preferred method for definitive diagnosis. In the absence of an ulcer, all atypical areas of mucosa should be biopsied. Endoscopy has largely replaced upper gastrointestinal series for diagnosis, in part because it permits the obtaining of biopsy specimens.

Principles of Management (2,6–9)

Surgery is the treatment of choice, but the ability to achieve cure is limited by the finding of metastatic disease at surgery in 80% of cases. Adjuvant chemotherapy in combination with radiation therapy has been shown to improve survival, although overall survival remains poor. Prevention and early detection are the best hopes for improving outcomes.

Surgery

Surgery is the primary mode of treatment, for both cure and palliation. The median survival for patients managed by complete surgical resection is greater than 3 years. The 5-year survival rate varies according to the location of the tumor: It is 25% in patients with distal lesions and 10% for those with proximal ones. When lymph node involvement is found, survival falls by 50%. The surgical loss of the stomach's food-reservoir function necessitates small, frequent feedings. Without careful patient education and the use of high-calorie supplements, total gastrectomy can lead to malnutrition.

Subtotal or total gastrectomy is optimal for the management of bleeding or obstruction related to tumors at the gastroesophageal junction. Linitis plastica or total wall involvement of the stomach is incurable and is not manageable by surgery.

Chemotherapy

Adjuvant chemotherapy (perioperative without radiation or postoperative in combination with radiation) can improve the survival of patients with resected gastric cancer at high risk for recurrence or development of metastatic disease. Chemotherapy (such as combinations of 5-fluorouracil [5-FU], epirubicin, and cisplatin; or irinotecan and cisplatin) for the treatment of patients with metastatic disease produces responses in 40% to 50% of patients. The average duration of response is 6 to 9 months, and there are short-term improvements in survival, although there is no improvement in long-term survival. Complete responses are rare. Clinical research is continuing to attempt to identify the most active combinations and the potential role of newer agents, such as targeted therapy.

Radiation

Radiation, in conjunction with chemotherapy, is an important component of postoperative adjuvant treatment of patients with resected stage IB to IV gastric adenocarcinoma. It may also be useful in the palliation of patients with bleeding or obstruction, who are not candidates for resection. However, surgery remains the modality of choice for palliation of these symptoms when feasible.

Patient Monitoring

Patient monitoring should be guided by symptoms and not by routine testing for potential metastatic sites because only palliative therapeutic options exist for patients with advanced disease.

Prevention and Early Detection (10)

As for many cancers, *smoking cessation* (see Chapter 54) is an important step in trying to decrease the incidence of this often deadly cancer. Although the relationship between *Helicobacter* infection and gastric carcinoma is becoming increasingly well established, it remains to be proven that eradication or prevention of *Helicobacter* infection will reduce risk (see Chapter 68). Nonetheless, treatment of symptomatic *H. pylori* infection (see Chapter 68) is often recommended. Improving food handling and preservation and making sure that young children are not exposed to spoiled food seem like reasonable public health measures. Other dietary measures worth undertaking include increasing vegetable and fruit intake, increasing the intake of antioxidants (olive oil, vitamins A and E, and garlic), increasing fiber in the diet, decreasing salt intake, and decreasing the intake of high-nitrite-containing foods (e.g., nitrate-preserved meats [hot dogs, cold cuts] and salted fish). Early detection through endoscopic or radiologic screening has been carried out in populations where risk is very high (e.g., Japan). Such measures would not be cost-effective in the United States, where disease prevalence is relatively low and declining.

Gastric Lymphoma (11)

Unlike adenocarcinoma, gastric lymphomas have a much higher cure rate. The management of these lymphomas is reviewed in Chapter 84. Of special note are the patients with mucosa-associated lymphoid tissue lymphomas limited to the stomach that are associated with *H. pylori* infection. Although these make up only an estimated 10% of gastric lymphomas, they are important to recognize because 50% to 80% of these lymphomas can regress after treatment with antibiotic therapy against *H. pylori*.

PANCREATIC CANCER

Carcinoma of the pancreas is the fourth-leading cause of cancer death in the United States. Mortality is high (close to 98% at 5 years); fewer than 20% of patients survive 1 year. High death rates are due partially to difficulties in early detection, which stem from the tumor's retroperitoneal location. For decades, pancreatic cancer had been gradually increasing in frequency, although incidence may have plateaued over the last 30 years. There are about 33,000 new cases annually. The disease is rare before age 40 years, but incidence rises rapidly thereafter. Overall, there is an approximately equal distribution by gender.

Risk Factors (1–7)

Hypotheses regarding pathogenesis include the concentration and excretion of carcinogens by acinar cells, inducing neoplastic transformation among ductal cells. Lifestyle factors are appearing increasingly important in determining the risk of pancreatic cancer. *Smoking* is one of the most clearly established risk factors. Emerging data also suggest that obesity and inactivity may play important roles; diabetes increases risk. Other risk factors include *chronic pancreatitis* (especially when related to genetic mutation) and history of *radiation therapy* to the retroperitoneum. Chronic exposure to potential *environmental toxins*, such as dry-cleaning chemicals and gasoline-related compounds, are associated with increased risk.

Clinical Presentation (5,8)

In most instances, the tumor remains silent until late in the course of disease, with presentation determined largely by the tumor's location. In about two thirds of cases, the cancer begins in the head of the pancreas; in the remainder, it occurs in the body or tail. Disease that originates in the pancreatic head near the pancreaticobiliary junction may extend locally to obstruct bile flow and cause painless jaundice—one of the few potentially early symptomatic presentations of pancreatic cancer. *Jaundice*, with or without pain, is an eventual manifestation in about 50% of patients, although in many it is due to metastasis or late extension. More often than not, symptoms are late in onset and nonspecific. Disease of the body or tail of the pancreas may present with vague upper *abdominal or back pain* or discomfort, unexplained *weight loss*, unexplained *depression*, unexplained onset of *diabetes* or *pancreatitis*, or even migratory *thrombophlebitis*. Persistent nausea and vomiting suggest invasion and obstruction of the upper gastrointestinal tract. Carcinomas of the tail may not cause symptoms until they metastasize. Endocrine or neuroendocrine pancreatic cancers are also an important cause of ectopic hormone production (e.g., insulin, glucagon, gastrin, vasointestinal polypeptide, corticotropin).

The clinical course of pancreatic carcinoma is dominated by regional extension into the retroperitoneum and liver. The tumor tends to spread perineurally and lymphatically. The median survival for patients with extrapancreatic adenocarcinoma is 12 weeks from the time of presentation to 19 to 42 weeks for those with tumor confined to the pancreas.

Diagnosis (5,9–11)

The workup begins with imaging the pancreas; *abdominal CT* is the study of choice, and is able to detect lesions as small as 1 cm (occasionally smaller) and provide detailed images of the biliary tree and pancreatic ducts. It provides better definition of the tumor and adjacent structures than *transabdominal ultrasound*, helping to determine anatomy and detect metastasis to the liver and draining lymph nodes. *Abdominal MRI* offers no advantages over CT and costs more, but technical improvements in ultrasound, CT, and MRI continue to be made, making the optimal approach to imaging a dynamic issue that needs to be assessed continually. The potential role for CT combined with *positron emission tomography (PET-CT)* to detect metastatic disease not seen with CT alone is being investigated.

Tissue is still needed to confirm the diagnosis, because symptoms, signs, and appearances on imaging studies may be nonspecific, and there are no definitive blood tests; however, diagnosis no longer requires laparotomy. When a distinct pancreatic mass is identified in the absence of clearly identifiable metastatic disease, *fine-needle aspiration biopsy* can be performed. Where available, this can be done effectively with guidance by *EUS*, which can optimally define the best site for obtaining tissue. Alternatively, biopsy can be done *percutaneously*, guided by direct *ultrasound* or *CT* visualization, especially when there is metastatic or clearly unresectable disease. Limiting the yield from percutaneous needle biopsy and causing a substantial false-negative rate is the large zone of fibrosis and inflammation that typically surrounds the tumor; other drawbacks include the risk of seeding along the needle tract. Patients with a mass at the pancreaticobiliary junction are excellent candidates for *endoscopic retrograde cholangiopancreatography (ERCP)*. Early ampullary lesions causing jaundice can be visualized and biopsied directly, leading to prompt diagnosis, definitive treatment, and improved 5-year survival (as high as 50%). A *pancreatogram* is taken during ERCP, with ductal narrowing, obstruction, and extravasation of dye comprising additional signs of malignancy (although they also can occur in chronic pancreatitis). An irregular stricture longer than 10 mm is characteristic of cancer. Cytologic sampling, especially that obtained by brushing, has a reported sensitivity approaching 85%, although results vary.

Staging (5,9–11)

Pancreatic-protocol CT with contrast (or equivalently MRI) with careful evaluation of the critical vascular structures and their relationship to the cancer is the staging procedure of choice for visualizing the tumor and determining resectability. The presence of metastases beyond the immediate peripancreatic area rule outs operable disease. Microscopic nodal disease in the peripancreatic region may not be visible by CT, but neither is it considered a contraindication to surgery. Data regarding vascular involvement (either by careful *CT* or *MRI* imaging) are essential because involvement of critical vessels (e.g., SMA) rules out surgical cure. *EUS with transendoscopic fine-needle aspiration* allows the determination of spread beyond the pancreatic capsule and local nodal involvement.

Principles of Management (5,12–18)

The chance for cure is limited because it depends on surgically removing the entire tumor, which is usually well advanced by the time it is detected. Careful staging is critical. One needs to distinguish among tumors that are localized and resectable, localized and not resectable, and metastatic. In addition, patients with duodenal obstruction need to be identified because they require either stenting (if possible) or an operation to palliate symptoms.

At a number of institutions, patients being considered for surgery are asked to undergo *staging laparoscopy* because up to 20% are found at laparoscopy to have previously undetected peritoneal or omental metastases, ruling out resectability. Other studies have shown a lower frequency of undetected metastases, especially in patients with small lesions. Current CT and MRI imaging cannot detect very small peritoneal lesions.

Surgery

In general, only patients with lesions that do not have involvement of critical vasculature (e.g., the superior mesenteric artery) are candidates for curative surgery. This accounts for no more than 5% to 22% of patients who present with the disease. Although operative mortality has declined significantly over the last 20 years and in most major centers is now less than 5%, the risks of surgery remain significant. The operations are difficult, and postoperative complications can be serious. The decision to subject a patient with pancreatic cancer to a major operation with a high degree of operative morbidity and only modest chances for curative resection must be made individually.

For the majority of lesions that are in the head of the pancreas, the operation of choice is the *Whipple procedure* (pancreatoduodenectomy), which is a major surgical undertaking and should attempted only by surgeons able to perform it with less than 5% mortality. Five-year survival rates are best in patients with a small (2 cm or less) tumor, approaching 30% at centers with surgical expertise in performing the operation. Survival increases to as high as 57% for small lesions with negative lymph nodes (unfortunately, an uncommon occurrence). Overall 5-year survival for patients who can undergo a resection is 15% to 25%. *Regional pancreatectomy* or *total pancreatectomy* provides no survival benefit over a Whipple procedure and are reserved for the situation in which this is necessary to obtain clear margins.

Surgery is also recommended for palliation. Patients with biliary obstruction are candidates for biliary bypass or endoscopic stent placement, which can relieve jaundice and lower the risk of cholangitis. Surgical or percutaneous ablation of the celiac ganglion can provide relief from intractable pain.

Radiation Therapy

Radiation therapy is often used for patients with localized but unresectable disease; in conjunction with 5-FU, it modestly prolongs survival. It can also help to control intractable retroperitoneal pain for up to 6 months. The role of intraoperative radiation remains to be defined, as does that of the concurrent administration of gemcitabine (a potent radiation sensitizer).

The role of adjuvant chemoradiation therapy after surgical resection is controversial. Most institutions in the United States continue to utilize adjuvant chemoradiation as the standard approach, whereas in Europe, adjuvant chemotherapy is often used without radiation therapy. Trials are ongoing, including the evaluation of preoperative radiation and chemotherapy (neoadjuvant therapy) to determine whether there is any additional benefit to this approach.

Chemotherapy

Chemotherapy had traditionally offered little to persons with unresectable disease. The standard chemotherapeutic agent, 5-FU, has a poor response rate and minimally prolongs survival. *Gemcitabine*, a nucleoside analogue, is slightly more effective than 5-FU, and is able to reduce pain, improve functional status, and slightly improve survival. There is a suggestion that longer infusions of gemcitabine may be more active. In addition, there is a slight additional prolongation of survival when *erlotinib* (a small molecular inhibitor of the tyrosine kinase activity of the epidermal growth factor receptor [EGFR]) is added to gemcitabine. *Capecitabine* (an oral precursor of 5-FU) combined with gemcitabine might improve survival over gemcitabine alone. To date, combinations of gemcitabine with other chemotherapeutic agents (such as Alimta, bevacizumab, or cetuximab) have not offered any survival advantage as compared with gemcitabine alone. However, various combinations, as well as new agents, continue to be explored.

Supportive Measures

Supportive measures are essential, not only to patients who are dying of their disease (see Chapter 90), but also to those who have undergone pancreatectomy. In the latter group, insulin therapy and pancreatic enzyme preparations are needed. Insulin requirements are in the range of 20 to 30 units per day. The ongoing management of pain can be challenging; neurolytic celiac plexus block can reduce pain but has not shown improvement in quality of life or survival (see Chapter 90). Treatment of anorexia, nausea, malabsorption (often with associated diarrhea), and depression are very important components to support quality of life (see Chapter 91).

Monitoring

CA 19-9, a tumor marker developed with monoclonal antibody technology, is useful for monitoring, and is sensitive in the setting of advanced disease. It is best applied for surveillance after surgery (provided levels were high before surgery and fall immediately afterward) and as a marker of response to chemotherapy. *Carcinoembryonic antigen (CEA)* is elevated in some patients who have normal CA 19-9 levels and can be similarly used.

Prevention and Screening (1,2,10)

Smoking cessation should be urged, as well as lifestyle modifications. Exposure to potentially contributing environmental factors such as ionizing radiation to the retroperitoneum, dry-cleaning chemicals, and gasoline should be limited.

The hope for better outcomes through screening and early diagnosis remains unrealized. The tumor marker *CA 19-9*, although useful for monitoring disease progression and response to treatment, is often normal in early stages, which limits its usefulness for screening. In addition, specificity has been disappointing (high levels have been reported in other gastrointestinal cancers, e.g., bile duct or gastric). The same holds for the tumor marker CEA. No marker has been proven to be sufficiently sensitive or specific to warrant its use in routine screening or diagnosis.

GALLBLADDER CANCERS (1)

Gallbladder cancer is an uncommon malignancy in the United States, with an estimated 5,000 to 7,500 new cases per year. Histologically, most of these tumors are adenocarcinomas, with a small percentage being squamous cell cancers or of mixed histology. Other types of cancer (e.g., sarcomas, small-cell cancers, lymphomas) can rarely arise in the gallbladder. The only curative therapy is surgery, and the 5-year survival rate for patients that cannot have surgery is less than 5%. Thus, improvements in prevention and early detection will be necessary to reduce mortality from this disease.

Risk Factors

Most gallbladder cancers arise in the setting of underlying chronic gallbladder inflammation. The most common risk factor for gallbladder cancer is the presence of *gallstones*. However, because gallstones are very common, most individuals with gallstones do not develop gallbladder cancer. Other risk factors include chronic infection with *Salmonella* (cause of typhoid), *porcelain gallbladder* (wall of the gallbladder lined with calcium deposits), congenital abnormalities (e.g., choledochal cysts, bile duct abnormalities), *polyps*, certain chemicals used in industrial processes (e.g., *polychlorinated biphenyls*), *inflammatory bowel disease*, *obesity*, and ethnicity (e.g., *Native Americans* from the southwestern United States, Hispanics). It is more common in women than men. The median age is approximately 65 years.

Clinical Presentation

Patients are usually asymptomatic until they present with symptoms indicating advanced disease. The exception to this is the uncommon situation in which gallbladder cancer is found incidentally at the time of cholecystectomy for presumed gallbladder inflammation. For those who present with symptoms, similarly to many other GI malignancies, these symptoms are often nonspecific. These include pain, decreased appetite, nausea, vomiting, weight loss, fatigue, weakness, abdominal swelling (from ascites), fever, and jaundice.

Diagnosis

The provisional diagnosis of gallbladder cancer is usually made by imaging study (ultrasound or CT). Preoperative needle biopsy is not performed because the gallbladder is going to be removed regardless of findings, and omitting the procedure eliminates the potential risk of seeding. When metastatic disease is a concern, suspicious lesions can be biopsied percutaneously under ultrasound or CT (or less commonly MRI) guidance; some lesions are more readily accessible by ERCP or EUS. The diagnosis is sometimes made intraoperatively at the time of gallbladder resection for suspected cholecystitis (see later discussion under Surgery).

Staging

There are a number of noninvasive approaches to staging. Physical examination provides a check for jaundice, right upper quadrant abdominal tenderness, and evidence of distant spread (supraclavicular lymphadenopathy, ascites). Laboratory testing of liver function (including albumin and prothrombin time) and tumor markers (CA 19-9 is usually the most sensitive marker, but when it is negative, CEA should be checked) facilitates the assessment. Ultrasound can be used to evaluate the extent of local disease and any metastasis to regional lymph nodes and liver. CT of the chest and upper abdomen should be performed to check for tumor involvement of adjacent structures and distant metastases; MRI is an alternative. The potential role for PET scanning in evaluating gallbladder cancer has not been determined. Imaging of the brain and bones is not recommended in the absence of symptoms or signs suggesting metastasis to these locations.

From a staging standpoint, the most important distinction is between patients with disease that can be resected and those who are not surgical candidates, because surgery is the only known curative therapy. The most curable lesions are those that are small and solitary. Unfortunately, the vast majority of patients have unresectable disease at the time of presentation.

Principles of Management

Surgery remains the modality of choice for initial therapy and is usually done with curative intent. However, only a relatively small percentage of patients have potentially curable disease at the time of detection. In addition, even after surgical resection, the rates of local recurrence and distant metastasis remain high. Unfortunately, given the relative rarity of this tumor, trials have not evaluated the potential benefit of adding adjuvant chemotherapy and radiation therapy to surgery, so that usually information is derived from single-institutional experiences.

Surgery

Surgery is the modality of choice for primary therapy. It provides the potential for cure in the minority of cases found to have disease at sufficiently early stage that a surgical approach might be of benefit. Patients with porcelain gallbladders should have open cholecystectomies, given the high risk for gallbladder cancer. Patients who have cancer incidentally found at the time of cholecystectomy and have any invasion beyond the lamina propria (T1B or greater) and do not have evidence of metastatic disease need to have re-resection to include resection of adjacent liver and lymph nodes.

Radiation Therapy

Radiation therapy may be useful in patients with localized disease not amenable to surgical resection, especially those with significant pain. Although no prospective, randomized trials have been done (because this is an uncommon tumor and the trials are therefore difficult to complete), retrospective series suggest that radiation therapy alone or, more commonly, the combination of 5-FU chemotherapy and radiation therapy postoperatively, may decrease recurrence rates for those with stage T2 or higher lesions.

Chemotherapy

Historically, systemic chemotherapy has not been very effective in treating patients with unresectable disease. *Gemcitabine*-based chemotherapy in combination with a platinum-containing regimen and/or 5-FU (or capecitabine, an oral precursor of 5-FU) has shown some promise.

Supportive Measures

See Chapters 87, 90, and 91.

Prevention

Internationally, decreasing the incidence of *Salmonella typhi* infection through public health measures and treatment is important. Treating patients who have chronic inflammatory bowel or biliary tract disease might also decrease the risk of subsequent gallbladder cancer. Removing the gallbladder of a patient with asymptomatic gallstones remains without proven benefit.

CHOLANGIOCARCINOMA (1)

Cholangiocarcinomas are cancers of the bile ducts. Histologically, most of these tumors are adenocarcinomas, with a small percentage being squamous cell cancers or of mixed histology. Cancer can arise anywhere in the biliary system. Anatomically, there are three important areas that should be distinguished: intrahepatic, perihilar (at the junction of external bile ducts and the liver), and lesions close to the ampulla. This is an uncommon malignancy in the United States, with an estimated 2,500 to 3,000 new cases per year. The only curative therapy is surgery, and the 5-year survival rate for patients that cannot have surgery is less than 5%. Thus, improvements in prevention and early detection are necessary to make a significant impact on the overall mortality from this disease.

Risk Factors

Most cholangiocarcinomas arise in the setting of underlying biliary tract inflammation. The major risk factors for cholangiocarcinoma include chronic infection with parasites (e.g., the liver flukes *Clonorchis sinensis and Opisthorchis viverrini*), chronic typhoid, hepatolithiasis, biliary cirrhosis, ulcerative colitis, primary sclerosing cholangitis (usually in the setting of ulcerative colitis), toxic substances (e.g., Thoratrast), and genetic or congenital abnormalities (e.g., choledochal cysts, bile duct abnormalities).

Clinical Presentation

Patients usually present with symptoms that primarily occur in the setting of advanced disease. Similar to many other GI malignancies, these symptoms are often nonspecific. These include decreased appetite, nausea, weight loss, fatigue, weakness, abdominal or back pain, abdominal swelling (from ascites), fever, and jaundice.

Diagnosis

Diagnosis can be suspected based on the appearance of lesions on imaging studies. However, except in situations in which the lesion is going to be resected regardless of what the biopsy shows or when the decision is made not to pursue further therapeutic options, the biopsy of a lesion is required to establish the diagnosis. Biopsies are usually done percutaneously under ultrasound, CT, or, if necessary, MRI guidance. Alternatively, some of these lesions are more readily accessible at the time of upper endoscopic evaluation, either by ERCP or by EUS.

As with all other malignancies, it is important to consider the issue of potential early diagnosis. Next to prevention, early diagnosis is most likely to be the next best means for improving outcome. Unfortunately, studies have not convincingly shown that screening high-risk populations improves survival because available testing methodologies lack the necessary sensitivity and specificity.

Staging

From a staging standpoint, the most important distinction is between patients with disease that can be resected and those who are not surgical candidates, because surgery is the only known curative therapy. The most curable lesions are those that are small and solitary with no evidence of vascular involvement.

Beginning with the physical examination, one should check for jaundice, liver and spleen enlargement, and evidence of ascites. Laboratory studies include liver function tests, albumin, clotting parameters, and tumor markers (CA 19-9 and CEA, with the former being more sensitive, but if it is not elevated, it is worth checking CEA). CT of the chest and upper abdomen should be performed to gauge the extent of local disease, distant metastases, and vascular involvement (especially important in persons considered to be potential surgical candidates). MRI scanning is an alternative. A role for PET scanning has not been established. Ultrasound offers a simple, less expensive means of evaluating lesions, but its performance is more operator dependent. The choice of test should take into account local imaging capabilities. Imaging of the brain and bones is unnecessary in the absence of symptoms suggesting metastases to these locations.

Principles of Management

Surgery remains the modality of choice for initial therapy and is usually done with curative intent. However, only a relatively small percentage of patients have potentially curable disease at the time of detection. In addition, even after surgical resection, the rates of local recurrence and distant metastasis remain high. Unfortunately, given the relative rarity of this tumor, trials have not evaluated the potential benefit of adding adjuvant chemotherapy and radiation therapy to surgery; extrapolations are usually made from experience with pancreatic cancer.

Surgery and Stenting

As noted, surgery is the modality of choice for primary therapy, providing the potential for cure in the occasional case of early-stage disease. Stenting of the bile ducts (usually done endoscopically, but sometimes percutaneously) can relieve biliary obstruction in patients who are not surgical candidates.

Ablative Measures and Radiation

Radiofrequency ablation, cryoablation, and stereotactic radiation therapy approaches may be useful in patients with localized disease not amenable to surgical resection; however, there are no data from prospective, randomized trials to guide decision making. Transarterial chemoembolization (TACE) may be useful for patients with localized disease not amenable to one of the foregoing approaches (see further discussion of TACE under Hepatocellular Cancer).

Chemotherapy

Historically, systemic chemotherapy has not been very effective in treating patients with unresectable disease, but combinations involving gemcitabine and platinum agents (cisplatin or oxaliplatin) with or without 5-FU may be more effective than previous approaches. In addition, cetuximab—the monoclonal antibody against EGFR (which is expressed on a high percentage of cholangiocarcinomas)—is being evaluated for use.

Supportive Measures

See Chapters 87, 90, and 91.

Prevention

In endemic areas, public health measures to decrease the incidence of liver fluke infection are very important. Treating sclerosing cholangitis, primary biliary cirrhosis, and ulcerative colitis might also decrease the risk of subsequent cholangiocarcinoma.

HEPATOCELLULAR CARCINOMA

The majority of primary liver cancers are either *hepatocellular carcinomas* arising from hepatocytes (most common) or cancers of the biliary system (*cholangiocarcinomas*, discussed previously). Less common tumors include *sarcomas* (angiosarcomas or hemangiosarcomas, which are approached similarly to other sarcomas) and *hepatoblastomas*, which occur primarily in childhood.

Hepatocellular cancer is one of the most common malignancies worldwide and is increasingly frequent in the United States, with an estimated 13,000 to 19,000 new cases per year. Fewer than 20% of newly diagnosed patients survive for 5 years. Resection and liver transplantation offer the hope of cure, but prevention and early detection are necessary to achieve a reduction in overall mortality from this disease.

Risk Factors (1–4)

Most hepatocellular cancers arise in the context of underlying liver inflammation and especially in the setting of cirrhosis, in which there is progression from cirrhosis to dysplastic nodule to early cancer. Worldwide, the major risk factors for hepatocellular carcinoma include *chronic hepatitis B* and *C*. In the United States, *cirrhosis* in the setting of excessive alcohol intake is a significant risk factor. The hepatitis C epidemic appears to be responsible for much of the increase in hepatocellular cancer in the United States. In certain regions of the world, prolonged exposure to *aflatoxins* (especially aflatoxin B1) is a major risk factor. Other causes of prolonged inflammation, such as *hereditary hemochromatosis*, *primary biliary cirrhosis*, and *nonalcoholic steatohepatitis*, are also associated with an increased risk of hepatocellular cancer. Longstanding *diabetes* may contribute.

Clinical Presentation (1–3)

Patients usually present with nonspecific symptoms that develop in the setting of advanced disease, for example, decreased appetite, nausea, weight loss, fatigue, weakness, vague abdominal or back pain, abdominal swelling (from ascites), and jaundice.

Multifocality of the cancer in the liver is common. Distant metastases most commonly occur in the lung, abdominal lymph node–bearing areas, and bone and may be the source of accompanying symptoms.

Diagnosis (3,6)

Diagnosis can be suspected based on the appearance of lesions on imaging studies; tissue *biopsy* is usually needed for confirmation, except in situations in which the liver lesion is going to be resected regardless of what the biopsy shows or when the decision is made not to pursue further therapeutic options. Biopsies are usually done percutaneously under ultrasound, CT, or MRI guidance.

Staging (3,6)

From a staging standpoint, the most important distinction is between patients with disease that can either be resected or who are candidates for liver transplantation and those who are not surgical candidates. The most curable lesions are those that are small and solitary; vascular invasion (a contraindication to surgery) usually does not occur until growth exceeds 2 cm. Unfortunately, the vast majority of patients have unresectable disease at the time of presentation.

Assessment begins with physical examination, checking for jaundice, hepatomegaly, splenomegaly, ascites, and other potential findings of chronic alcohol abuse and cirrhosis (see Chapter 70). Laboratory testing should include liver function studies, albumin, clotting parameters, and α-fetoprotein (which is elevated in approximately 75% of patients).

Computed tomography (CT) of the chest and upper abdomen should be performed to check for the local extent of disease as well as metastases; *MRI* is an alternative. The assessment of vascular involvement is important in making decisions about surgery and can be done by CT or MRI. The role of PET scanning has not been determined. *Ultrasound* is a potentially less expensive means of evaluating the liver but is highly operator dependent. The choice of imaging study should take into account local expertise. Imaging of the brain or bones is not recommended in the absence of suggestive symptoms.

Principles of Management (3,5,6)

Surgery and liver transplant represent potentially curative treatment modalities. Ablative measures help to prevent tumor growth in persons awaiting transplant. Trials of adjuvant therapies are ongoing, including combined-modality treatment and therapies directed against tumor and vascular growth factors.

Surgery and Transplantation

Surgery (either resection or liver transplantation) offers the best chance for cure in the 5% of cases found to have early disease. As noted, a single lesion less than 2 cm in size represents a potentially surgically curable disease. Transplant is the preferred surgical treatment because even after surgical resection, the rates of local recurrence and distant metastasis remain high. Patients meeting the *Milan criteria* for liver transplant candidacy (tumor size <5 cm for a single lesion and <3 cm for two or three lesions) have survival rates after orthotopic liver transplantation that approach those for patients with advanced liver disease without cancer.

Ablation

Radiofrequency ablation, cryoablation, alcohol injection, and stereotactic radiation therapy have been most useful as a means of limiting disease in patients with localized disease awaiting transplantation. These measure have also been used in those who are not candidates for transplant; however, only a small percentage of tumors are amenable to this approach (i.e., those <5 cm in diameter).

Transarterial chemoembolization may be useful for patients with localized disease not amenable to other ablative approaches; it affords a small survival advantage in selected patients. The procedure involves delivery via the hepatic artery of chemotherapy along with an embolizing agent, repeated every 3 to 6 months as long as the patient remains an appropriate candidate. Eligible patients need to have sufficient underlying residual liver function to tolerate the procedure; those with thrombosis of the portal vein, biliary obstruction, or encephalopathy are not candidates.

Chemotherapy and Kinase Inhibitors

Historically, systemic chemotherapy has not been very effective in treating patients with unresectable disease. Newer therapies such as the use of *sorafenib* (Nexavar), an oral kinase inhibitor with activity against vascular endothelial growth factor receptors, can increase median survival by about 2.8 months over placebo. Side effects include potential blood pressure elevations and skin rash, which need to be managed carefully. Studies are ongoing of this approach and others.

Prevention and Screening (3,6)

Prevention is the best means for improving outcome. Clearly, decreasing the incidence of hepatitis B and C infection through vaccination programs (for hepatitis B), public health measures, and education about high-risk behavior are all important (see Chapter 57). Treating patients who have chronic infection with hepatitis B or C, although only moderately effective, may also decrease the risk of subsequent development of cirrhosis hepatocellular cancer (see Chapter 70). The treatment of primary biliary cirrhosis might reduce the risk of hepatocellular cancer (see Chapter 71); there is no direct evidence that the treatment of hemochromatosis reduces the risk of liver cancer, but it can reduce the risk of cirrhosis (see Chapter 71).

Early detection through screening might help to reduce mortality. Some authorities recommend liver imaging in cirrhotic patients every 6 months; α-fetoprotein monitoring may contribute to early detection.

COLORECTAL CANCER

Colorectal cancer is one of the most common malignancies and, although it is one of the more potentially curable cancers, it results in approximately 57,000 deaths annually. More than 150,000 new cases develop each year.

Risk Factors (1–5)

Polyp formation usually precedes the development of colon cancer. Adenomatous polyps, villoglandular polyps, and villous

TABLE 76.1

STAGING FOR COLORECTAL CANCER

Stage	Description	5-Year Survival (%)
A	Lesion confined to submucosa; nodes negative	>90%
B1[a]	Muscularis involved but not serosa; nodes negative	80–85
B2[a]	Lesion extends through serosa; nodes negative	70–75
C1[a]	Lesion extends into muscularis only; nodes positive	70–75
C1[a]	Lesion extends through serosa; 1–4 nodes positive	60–65
C2[a]	Lesion extends through serosa; >4 nodes positive	30–40

[a]Gastrointestinal Tumor Study Group modification of the Dukes staging system.
Adapted from Steel G, Mayer RJ, Podolsky DK, et al. In: Osteen, R., ed. *Cancer manual*, 9th ed. Boston: American Cancer Society, Massachusetts Division, 1996:402, with permission.

adenomas represent premalignant lesions that may also harbor early cancers. Those with villous histology pose the greatest risk of malignant transformation. "Hyperplastic" polyps may also be associated with an increased risk of cancer (see later discussion and Chapter 56).

Both familial/genetic factors and environmental precipitants have been identified and postulated. High-risk patients are those with a *first-degree relative* with colorectal cancer (especially if cancer developed at an early age), longstanding *pancolitis, familial polyposis, Gardner's syndrome* (polyps, osteomas, epidermoid cysts, and soft tissue tumors), and *hereditary nonpolyposis colorectal cancer (HNPCC)*. A number of genetic mutations, including a relatively high frequency of mutation of the *ras gene* and loss of the *tumor suppressor gene p53*, have been found in colorectal tumors. Mutations in the *cyclooxygenase-2 (COX-2) gene* may predispose to polyp formation. Epidemiologic evidence supports this link, finding a reduction in polyp risk among persons chronically taking drugs that inhibit COX-2 activity such as *aspirin* and other *nonsteroidal inflammatory drugs (NSAIDs)*.

A number of dietary factors have been suggested by epidemiologic study, including diets low in *fiber* and high in *fat*, as well as deficiencies in *folic acid, vitamin D*, and *calcium* intake, but confirmation by demonstrating reduced risk in randomized trials of dietary changes and use of supplements remains elusive (see later discussion).

Clinical Presentation

The clinical presentation of colorectal cancer is related to the site of the tumor. Tumors of the ascending colon may be asymptomatic until late stages, producing little more than mild iron-deficiency anemia or intermittently guaiac-positive stools. Tumors of the descending colon and rectosigmoid can cause symptoms earlier in the course of illness, presenting as rectal bleeding or change in bowel habits (diarrhea and constipation). At the time of surgery, a significant percentage of patients have tumors that have penetrated the bowel wall or have metastases in regional lymph nodes.

Rectal cancers commonly present with occult or frank rectal bleeding, with or without an alteration in bowel habits. Tenesmus is usually a late symptom representing extension of the tumor beyond the bowel wall. Rectal or perianal pain is a consequence of the invasion of the perirectal structures in the sacral plexus. Tumors can arise on the posterior wall, making it particularly important to examine the rectal ampulla on routine rectal examination.

Prognosis and Clinical Course (6–9)

Prognosis depends on the extent of penetration and local spread. The TNM (tumor, nodes, metastases) classification is the primary staging system used, although a modification of the standard Dukes classification often is used interchangeably with TNM (Table 76.1). Stage I (Dukes A) patients have tumor limited to the submucosa and a 5-year survival of greater than 90%. Those with stage II (Dukes B) disease have a 5-year survival ranging from approximately 65% to 80%. Once the lymph nodes are involved, representing stage III (Dukes C), 5-year survival falls to approximately 35% to 65%. To determine lymph node status accurately, at least 12 lymph nodes should be removed and sampled. Prognosis is also adversely affected by preoperative elevation of serum CEA level (≥ 5 ng/mL), local extent of disease (especially the presence of serosal involvement), lymphovascular invasion, and the presence of residual disease. Patients with metastatic disease (stage IV, Dukes D) have a 5-year survival of 4% .

In addition to lymph nodes, the most common sites of metastasis are the liver (60% overall and 30% of metastases to a single organ site) due to portal blood flow draining the intestines, the peritoneal surface (30%), and the lung (20%). Rectal cancers tend to invade locally and to recur in the pelvis alone or in association with distant metastases to the liver or lung, bypassing the intraabdominal cavity.

Diagnosis

Diagnosis in a patient suspected of colorectal cancer (e.g., because of guaiac-positive stools, rectal bleeding, unexplained iron-deficiency anemia, or change in bowel habits) is best accomplished by *colonoscopy* that extends to the cecum, supplanting flexible *sigmoidoscopy* plus *barium enema* in most instances (see also Chapters 63, 65, and 79). Barium study does not allow for biopsy, and the false-negative rate can be as high as 40% for single-contrast studies; sensitivity is improved with use of air-contrast techniques, but elderly patients find such barium studies uncomfortable. Patients who cannot undergo colonoscopy can be screened by *CT colonography*, which under study conditions approaches colonoscopy in sensitivity for the detection of lesions with advanced histology; a positive study needs to be confirmed by biopsy via colonoscopy.

For patients in whom a cancer is detected in the rectosigmoid, a preoperative examination of the entire colon and cecum is required because synchronous tumors are present in up to 5% of patients. Similarly, colonoscopy is needed when a benign adenomatous polyp is found on sigmoidoscopic examination of the rectosigmoid (see Chapter 56).

Staging (6–9)

Staging for colon cancer is based predominantly on findings at *surgery* and *pathologic examination* (see Table 76.1). At the time of surgery, adequate *lymph node sampling* and detailed examination of draining lymph nodes is especially important. Very careful analysis of the nodes is required to ensure that there is no evidence of tumor micrometastasis that is associated with a significantly worse prognosis and the need for potential adjustment of treatment decisions.

Because accurate knowledge of tumor location might affect treatment decisions and potentially the extent of surgery, *CT scanning* prior to surgery has become more common. PET in combination with CT (PET-CT) shows considerable promise for enhanced staging prior to surgery. A preoperative *CEA* level provides a baseline for postoperative monitoring and helps to assess prognosis.

For rectal cancers, *endorectal ultrasound* or *coil magnetic resonance* is very important to determine the extent of disease and should always be obtained preoperatively.

Treatment (10–19)

Patients with disease detected in the early stages have an excellent prognosis and are candidates for surgical cure, emphasizing the importance of early diagnosis and treatment, including the removal of polyps that may represent premalignant disease (see Chapter 56). Patients presenting with late-stage disease have a much worse prognosis, but rapid advances in treatment are providing significant improvements in survival.

Surgery

Surgery is the primary modality of therapy, both for cure and for palliation (e.g., to prevent or relieve bowel obstruction). For colon cancer, colectomy is the procedure of choice. Because the tumor spreads lymphatically, adequate amounts of bowel on both sides of the lesion must be removed to ensure adequate removal of all tissue that may contain cancerous cells. Patients presenting with obstruction may benefit from a temporary diverting colostomy followed at a later date by reanastomosis. Salvage surgery, often with curative intent for resectable recurrences of tumor (e.g., in the abdomen, lung, or liver), is being increasingly performed, given the low perioperative mortality risk and the roughly 25% 5-year disease-free survival rate.

Surgical management of rectal cancer consists in either a low anterior resection with reanastomosis or, if that is not possible, an abdominoperineal resection with colostomy. When possible, an effort should be made to preserve the anal sphincter. In either case, a total mesorectal excision with sharp dissection should be used. Local excision is reserved for very early lesions.

The appreciation that adenomatous polyps, villoglandular polyps, and villous adenomas may harbor cancers or be premalignant has led to the recommendation of polypectomy when detected, aided greatly by fiberoptic colonoscopy and sigmoidoscopy. Cancer confined to the polyp is considered carcinoma *in situ*; detectable invasion of the stalk or muscu-

laris necessitates surgical resection of the tumor with partial colectomy.

Radiation Therapy

In rectal cancer, radiation therapy plays an important role, especially in the treatment of lesions that have either penetrated through the bowel wall (e.g., T3 or T4 disease) or metastasized to the perirectal lymph nodes (e.g., stage III disease). The tendency of rectal cancers that have penetrated the bowel wall to recur locally is relatively high. The adjunctive use of radiation therapy in such patients significantly reduces the risk of local recurrence. In the United States, patients with clinical T3, T4, or stage III disease are given combined chemotherapy and radiation therapy preoperatively (neoadjuvant). In certain countries in Europe, a shorter course of radiation therapy alone is often used in the preoperative setting. It is hoped that ongoing studies will help to define the optimal approach. In either case, preoperative treatment is, in general, associated with less toxicity than postoperative therapy and enhances the ability to perform subsequent resection in certain patients. Postoperative chemoradiotherapy is reserved for those not treated preoperatively whose findings at surgery suggest a high risk of recurrence (i.e., those with stage IIB and III disease).

Radiation therapy does not have an established role for colon cancer. It may be useful for the small percentage of patients with T4 lesions that invade adjacent structures or perforate, but there is no consensus.

Adjuvant Chemotherapy and Other Systemic Therapies

Adjuvant chemotherapy can significantly reduce the risk of recurrence in persons with resected stage III disease. The standard program consists of postoperative intravenous *5-FU* plus *leucovorin*. The advent of *capecitabine* (*Xeloda*; a precursor of 5-FU) provides an orally administered alternative to intravenous 5-FU plus leucovorin; it is better tolerated and as effective. The addition of *oxaliplatin* to the 5-FU/leucovorin program (*FOLFOX: fluorouracil, leucovorin,* and *oxaliplatin*) enhances the response and survival of candidate patients. Typically, treatment is begun as soon as possible after surgery, usually some time between 3 and 8 weeks.

Meta-analysis of available studies suggests that patients with *late stage II* disease, especially those at high risk for developing metastatic disease (i.e., presenting with perforation, obstruction, poorly differentiated histology, or high preoperative CEA), also benefit from adjuvant chemotherapy. The potential role for adjuvant chemotherapy in less advanced stage II disease is being explored, helped by genetic and molecular analyses of tumors (e.g., to determine the presence of gene mutations) to better identify those most likely to benefit from adjuvant therapy and spare those who are not.

Promising new additions to the adjuvant systemic-therapy adjuvant program include the chemotherapy agent *irinotecan* and *monoclonal antibody* preparations directed against either *vascular endothelial growth factor* (e.g., *bevacizumab* [*Avastin*]) or *EGFR* (e.g., *cetuximab* [*Erbitux*], *panitumumab* [*ABX-EGF*]). Their use has increased initial response rates to 40% to 50% when used in combination and have improved median survival from approximately 1 year (with 5-FU and leucovorin alone) to approximately 20 to 24 months in the metastatic disease setting. They have received U.S. Food and Drug Administration approval for use in patients with advanced disease. These new agents are very expensive, and their cost-effectiveness from a societal perspective has been questioned. At the present time, the choice of adjuvant program in an individual patient is based on clinical factors.

Other Therapies

No benefit has been found for *immunotherapy*, although a number of vaccine trials are ongoing.

Monitoring (6)

Attentive follow-up is essential because of the risk of a second bowel cancer (occurring in up to 15% of patients) and the appearance of new polyps. Moreover, a new primary in the bowel can be resected with a high cure rate if it is detected early through surveillance. Limited metastatic disease to the lung or liver is also potentially amenable to curative resection, with an approximately 25% chance of disease-free survival at 5 years.

Colonoscopy

Regularly scheduled *colonoscopy* should begin 6 months after surgery and take place every 24 to 36 months if no polyps are found and every 6 to 12 months if they are. Any encountered polyps are removed. If colonoscopy is unavailable or cannot reach the cecum, *CT colonography* or *air-contrast barium enema* in conjunction with *sigmoidoscopy* is a possible substitute.

CEA

Monitoring the tumor marker CEA (see Chapter 86) helps to provide early detection of potentially resectable recurrent or metastatic disease. The serum CEA level roughly correlates with tumor burden in colorectal cancer, which makes it useful in the detection of disease recurrence and in monitoring after initial resection. The recommended interval for CEA determinations is every 3 months for the first 2 years, provided that the CEA was elevated before surgery and fell to low levels within 2 to 4 weeks after it. If the CEA rises by 30% or more per month from its postoperative level, then a search for curable recurrent disease should be undertaken. However, sensitivity and specificity have been found wanting, especially for the early detection of liver metastases, and evidence that CEA surveillance is cost-effective and saves a significant number of lives remains to be obtained.

CT Scan

Some authorities recommend the addition of periodic CT scanning of the abdomen and chest for the early detection of resectable metastatic disease. Typically, the patient undergoes yearly scanning once adjuvant therapy has been completed. Technology continues to evolve, and the most cost-effective approach to monitoring remains to be established.

Other Measures

One should also monitor *symptoms* (weight loss, fatigue, change in bowel habits), the *physical examination* (especially chest and abdomen), and *alkaline phosphatase* (rises with infiltration of the liver) to help detect recurrent but curable disease.

Supportive Therapy
(See Also Chapters 87, 90, and 91)

Patients who have undergone abdominoperineal resection with permanent or temporary colostomy need careful counseling pre- and postoperatively to help them to adapt to their situation. Becoming comfortable with the details of ostomy care and having an opportunity to discuss their fears and concerns (sexual function, odor, appearance, bag changes, recurrence of cancer) are essential components of the rehabilitation effort. Ostomy groups and stoma nurses are important resources for the patient, but there is no substitute for a supportive understanding patient–doctor relationship.

Patients presenting with nonresectable disease benefit from a comprehensive review of prognosis, available treatment modalities, and patient and family preferences. A meeting set up by the physician to include the patient and family can be most helpful in facilitating communication, addressing the obvious but difficult questions regarding prognosis and treatment, and formulating a personalized plan that aims to maximize the patient's quality of life, comfort, and dignity. It helps to assure the patient and family of close follow-up and a program of support that makes sense to all. Such a meeting may also be an opportune time to address the elements necessary to complete an advance directive (see Chapter 1).

Prevention (20–32)

A host of approaches are available, ranging from screening for polyps to genetic testing, lifestyle modifications, and medications to prevent polyp formation.

Screening

The best approach to primary prevention is a screening program. Screening programs that use fecal occult blood testing, sigmoidoscopy, or colonoscopy are capable of saving lives; screening recommendations and intervals are based on estimated risk (see Chapter 56). All polyps detected need to be removed and subjected to pathologic examination. Flat and depressed lesions also need to be addressed because they have an even higher risk of high-grade histology.

Genetic Testing

Genetic testing can contribute significantly to prevention in familial forms of colorectal cancer. HNPCC, the most common of the familial colorectal cancer syndromes, is due to deleterious mutations in *mismatched repair genes*, most commonly *hMSH2* or *hMLH1*. These mutations confer a significantly increased risk of cancer and warrant heightened surveillance and preventive measures. New colorectal cancer patients who should be evaluated for hereditary nonpolyposis include those with a family history of a first-degree relative with colorectal or endometrial cancer, age less than 50 years at the time of diagnosis of colorectal cancer, or a history of multiple cancers. There are other genetic predispositions for developing colorectal cancer, including *FAP* due to mutations in the *APC gene*, which is associated with the development of multiple polyps in the colon. Screening for this or other genetic syndromes should be performed when appropriate.

Aspirin and Other NSAIDs

The suggestion that COX-2 activity might be related to polyp formation and the epidemiologic observation that chronic users of NSAIDs appear to have a lower risk of developing colonic polyps has stimulated prospective trials of aspirin and other NSAIDs for the prevention of colorectal cancer. Both the Men's Health Study and the Women's Health Study randomized trials failed to show a benefit from low-dose aspirin use. Trials involving the use of COX-2–inhibiting NSAIDs had to be stopped before completion because of an increased incidence of cardiovascular complications (see Chapter 156). The U.S. Preventive Services Task Force does not recommend aspirin or NSAID use for the prevention of colorectal cancer in individuals at average risk; the risks appear to outweigh the potential benefits of treatment. However, given evidence of benefit in individuals at high risk, it should be evaluated and discussed on an individual basis in that setting.

Dietary and Lifestyle Factors

Based on epidemiologic data, dietary factors (*low-fat* diet, intake of *fiber*, *calcium*, and *vitamin D*) might lower colorectal cancer risk, but randomized trials have failed to demonstrate a significant improvement in outcomes. One possible explanation for the disappointing results may be the long lead time necessary for the development of colorectal cancer (nearly a decade), which could obscure an eventual benefit because most studies are of shorter duration. Because these interventions are relatively harmless, they can be suggested, pending results from trials with a longer duration of follow-up.

Epidemiologic data suggest a benefit from physical activity, which can be recommended not only for its effect on colorectal cancer, but also for its well-established cardiovascular benefits (see Chapter 18).

Hormone Replacement

Hormone replacement therapy in postmenopausal women has been shown in some studies to decrease the risk of colorectal cancer and large adenomas, but the association is not well established by prospective study, and the benefit disappears quickly with the cessation of hormone therapy. The potential benefits seen do not justify hormonal replacement therapy, especially given the other adverse health consequences that have been noted (see Chapter 118).

Management of Colorectal Polyps (29,33,34)

The finding of a sporadic polyp on screening colonoscopy is a common event. Polyps representing true neoplasia with the potential for malignant transformation include *villous adenomas*, *tubular adenomas*, and mixed *tubulovillous adenomas*, although there is some evidence that the presence of even *hyperplastic polyps* is associated with some increased risk of the subsequent development of cancer. Greater appreciation for the enhanced malignant potential of *nonpolypoid colorectal neoplasms* (flat and depressed lesions) has directed renewed attention to the importance of their detection and removal.

Villous adenomas have the highest malignant potential and tend to be larger and more sessile than tubular or mixed tubulovillous adenomas (see Chapter 56, Table 56.1). With adenomatous polyps, the risk of malignancy increases with polyp diameter. Lesions less than 1 cm in size have a 0.5% chance of harboring malignancy; for polyps greater than 3.0 cm, the risk increases to greater than 15%. Small tubular adenomas account for nearly 70% of the polyps found. Polypectomy reduces the risk of new colon cancers by 70% to 90%.

All polypoid lesions found should be excised and sent for histologic categorization. Neoplastic lesions found at sigmoidoscopy are an indication for colonoscopy because of the increased risk of synchronous premalignant polyps or even cancer-containing lesions proximal to the reach of the sigmoidoscope.

The optimal frequency for repeat colonoscopy is unsettled. The best determinant of frequency is individual risk. Current consensus guidelines recommend performing the first follow-up study 1 year after removal of a high-risk lesion (e.g., one with villous histology; there is a longer interval for a lesser-risk lesion, and 3 to 6 months if there was not a complete colonoscopy before removal), followed by one every 3 years if the first study is normal and 1 to 3 years if a new polyp is found (see Chapter 56).

Patients with *FAP* are at very high risk of developing colorectal cancer (approximately 50% by age 40 years). Prophylactic colectomy is often recommended for such persons. Vigilant colonoscopic surveillance (every 1 to 3 years beginning at age 20 to 25 years) is an alternative to prophylactic colectomy in persons with *HNPCC* discovered through genetic screening. The benefits both for screening and prophylactic surgery in HNPCC are less well defined than for FAP, so that there has to be careful discussion of the pros and cons of each of the approaches with each individual at risk.

CARCINOMA OF THE ANAL CANAL (1,2)

Carcinoma of the anal canal is an increasing concern, especially in persons engaging in receptive anal intercourse, because of the condition's link to sexually transmitted human papillomavirus infection. HIV-positive men having sex with men are at greatest risk. There are an estimated 3,500 new case per year in the United States, accounting for about 1.5% of gastrointestinal tract cancers. Emphasis on public education, safe sexual practices, and cytologic screening, especially of HIV-positive men engaging in unprotected receptive rectal intercourse, should help to reduce the incidence of this condition. Concurrent chemotherapy and radiation therapy provide a high probability of cure without the need for surgery.

Annotated Bibliography

Esophageal Cancer

1. Enzinger PC, Mayer RJ. Esophageal Cancer. N Engl J Med 2003;349:2241. (*An excellent review*).
2. Lagergren J, Bergstrom A, Lindgren A, et al. Symptomatic gastroesophageal reflux as a risk factor for esophageal adenocarcinoma. N Engl J Med 1999;340:825. (*A population study, demonstrating a strong, dose-related, independent risk of adenocarcinoma of the esophagus conferred by symptomatic reflux.*)
3. Lehr L, Rupp N, Siewert JR. Assessment of resectability of esophageal cancer by computed tomography and magnetic resonance imaging. Surgery 1988;103:344. (*Roughly equivalent results were found with each approach; there was still some difficulty in detecting penetration into the mediastinum.*)
4. Tio TL, Coene LO, Luiken HM, et al. Endosonography in the clinical staging of esophagogastric cancer. Gastrointest Endosc 1990;35:S2. (*The overall accuracy [89%] was much better than that available from computed tomography [CT]; overstaging was 6%, understaging was 5%.*)
5. Al-Sarraf M, Martz K, Herskovic A, et al. Progress report of combined chemoradiotherapy versus radiotherapy alone in patients with esophageal cancer: an intergroup study. J Clin Oncol 1997;15:277; Erratum, J Clin Oncol 1997;15:866. (*Combined chemotherapy and radiation therapy prolonged survival compared with radiotherapy alone.*)
6. Cooper JS, Guo MD, MacDonald JS, et al. Chemoradiotherapy of locally advanced esophageal cancer: long-term follow-up of a prospective randomized trial (RTOG 85-01). JAMA 1999;281:1623. (*The results were found to be durable; the 5-year survival was 26%.*)

7. Cunningham D, Starling N, Rao S, et al. for the Upper Gastrointestinal Clinical Studies Group of the National Cancer Research Institute of the United Kingdom. Acpecitabine and oxaliplatin for advanced esophagogastric cancer. N Engl J Med 2008;358:36. (*Oral regimens were found to give results comparable to that of standard intravenous chemotherapy.*)

8. MacDonald JS, Smalley SR, Benedetti J, et al. Chemoradiotherapy after surgery compared with surgery alone for adenocarcinoma of the stomach or gastroesophageal junction. N Engl J Med 2001;345:725. (*The procedure can prolong survival in properly selected persons.*)

9. Schattenkerk ME, Obertop H, Mud HJ, et al. Survival after resection for carcinoma of the oesophagus. Br J Surg 1987;74:165. (*Presents useful outcome statistics for surgical therapy.*)

10. Urba SG, Oprringer MB, Turrisi A, et al. Randomized trial of preoperative chemoradiation versus surgery alone in patients with locoregional esophageal carcinoma. J Clin Oncol 2001;19:305. (*There was no statistically significant survival difference with the addition of preoperative chemoradiation.*)

11. Walsh TN, Noonan N, Hollywood D, et al. A comparison of multimodal therapy and surgery for esophageal adenocarcinoma. N Engl J Med 1996;335:462. (*Reports promising early results for the combination of radiation and chemotherapy followed by surgery.*)

12. Sampliner RE, The Practice Parameters Committee of the American College of Gastroenterology. Practice guidelines on the diagnosis, surveillance and therapy of Barrett's esophagus. Am J Gastroenterol 1998;93:1028. (*A consensus statement on the diagnosis and management of Barrett's esophagus.*)

13. Sharma P. Barrett esophagus: will effective treatment prevent the risk of progression to esophageal adenocarcinoma? Am J Med 2004;117:79S. (*A review of the evidence.*)

14. Wright TA, Gray MR, Morris AI, et al. Cost effectiveness of detecting Barrett's esophagus. Gut 1996;39:574. (*Finds that was detection cost-effective.*)

Gastric Cancer

1. Eckardt VF, Giebler W, Kanzler G, et al. Clinical and morphological characteristics of early gastric cancer. Gastroenterology 1990;98:708. (*Provides very useful data on the presentation, diagnosis, clinical course, and outcome of early gastric cancer in the community setting.*)

2. Hohenberger P, Gretschel S. Gastric cancer. Lancet 2003;362:305. (*A good overview of etiology and prognosis.*)

3. Uemura N, Okimoto S, Yamamoto S, et al. *Helicobacter pylori* infection and the development of gastric cancer. N Engl J Med 2001;345:784. (*Presents evidence of a relationship.*)

4. Cutler AF, Havstad S, Ma CK, et al. Accuracy of invasive and noninvasive tests to diagnose *Helicobacter pylori* infection. Gastroenterology 1995;109:136. (*The ^{13}C-urea breath test and serology were found to be as accurate as biopsy and the Campylobacter-like organism test for diagnosis.*)

5. Van de Velde CJH. Gastric cancer: staging and surgery. Ann Oncol 2002;13:3. (*A good overview of current surgical management.*)

6. MacDonald JS, Smalley SR, Benedetti J, et al. Chemoradiotherapy after surgery compared with surgery alone for adenocarcinoma of the stomach or gastroesophageal junction. N Engl J Med 2001;345:725. (*Finds a survival benefit for adjuvant combined chemotherapy and radiation therapy after the surgical resection of gastric cancer.*)

7. Parsonnet J, Friedman GD, Wandersteen DP, et al. *Helicobacter pylori* infection and the risk of gastric carcinoma. N Engl J Med 1991;325:1127. (*An important case–control study, providing strong epidemiologic evidence for a link between the two conditions.*)

8. Sakurmoto S, Sasako M, Yamaguchi T, et al. for the ACTS-GC Group. Adjuvant chemotherapy for gastric cancer with S-1, an oral fluoropyramide. N Engl J Med 2007;357:1810. (*An example of oral therapy compared to surgery alone, found to be effective in East Asian patients.*)

9. Webb A, Cunningham D, Scarffle JH, et al. Randomized trial comparing epirubicin, cisplatin and fluorouracil versus fluorouracil, doxorubicin and methotrexate in advanced esophagogastric cancer. J Clin Oncol 1997;15:261. (*Evidence of enhanced efficacy.*)

10. Hunt RH. Will eradication of *Helicobacter pylori* infection influence the risk of gastric cancer? Am J Med 2004;117(5A):86S. (*A thoughtful discussion of the issue.*)

11. Bertoni F, Conconi A, Capella C, et al. Molecular follow-up in gastric mucosa-associated lymphoid tissue lymphomas: early analysis of the LY03 cooperative trial. Blood 2002;99:2541. (*A proportion of patients with mucosa-associated lymphoid tissue lymphomas of the stomach will have molecular complete remissions with antibiotic treatment [triple therapy], and even those with residual disease may have prolonged benefit clinically.*)

Pancreatic Cancer

1. Ahlgren JD. Epidemiology and risk factors in pancreatic cancer. Semin Oncol 1996;23:241. (*A good review of both genetic and external risk factors for pancreatic cancer.*)

2. Michaud DS, Giovannucci E, Willett WC, et al. Physical activity, obesity, height, and the risk of pancreatic cancer. JAMA 2001;286:921. (*Presents evidence that lifestyle factors play an important role.*)

3. Cameron JL, Crist DW, Sitzmann JV, et al. Factors influencing survival after pancreaticoduodenectomy for pancreatic cancer. Am J Surg 1991;161:120. (*Small tumor size, negative nodes, and lack of vessel involvement predict good results.*)

4. Gordis L. Consumption of methylxanthine-containing beverages and risk of pancreatic cancer. Cancer Lett 1990;52:1. (*Coffee drinking does not cause pancreatic cancer.*)

5. Li D, Xie K, Wolff R, et al. Pancreatic cancer. Lancet 2004;363:1049. (*An excellent overview of the current understanding of pancreatic cancer and its treatment.*)

6. Lowenfels AB, Maisonneuve P, Cavallini G, et al. Pancreatitis and the risk of pancreatic cancer. N Engl J Med 1993;328:1433. (*A positive association was found.*)

7. MacMahon B, Trichopoulos D, Warren K, et al. Coffee and cancer of the pancreas. N Engl J Med 1981;304:630. (*The study that started the controversy.*)

8. Kalser MH, Barkin J, MacIntyre JM. Pancreatic cancer: assessment of prognosis by clinical presentation. Cancer 1985;56:397. (*Classic clinical presentation data, indicating that the onset of symptoms is usually a sign of advanced disease, although jaundice may be an early manifestation in some patients.*)

9. McMahon PM, Halpern EF, Fernandez-del Castillo C, et al. Pancreatic cancer: cost-effectiveness of imaging technologies for assessing resectability. Radiology 2001;221:93. (*Overview of the cost-effectiveness of current imaging techniques for determining whether pancreatic cancers are resectable.*)

10. Steinberg W. The clinical utility of the CA 19-9 tumor-associated antigen. Am J Gastroenterol 1990;85:350. (*The antigen was found to be useful for monitoring but not for screening or early diagnosis.*)

11. Venu RP, Geenen JE, Kini M, et al. Endoscopic retrograde brush cytology: a new technique. Gastroenterology 1990;99:1475. (*The approach greatly enhances the diagnostic yield from endoscopic retrograde cholangiopancreatography.*)

12. Neoptolemos JP, Stocken DD, Friess H, et al. A randomized trial of chemoradiotherapy and chemotherapy after resection of pancreatic cancer. N Engl J Med 2004;350:1200. (*Shows a possible benefit of chemotherapy, but does not demonstrate a benefit of radiation.*)

13. Oettle H, Post S, Neuhaus P, et al. Adjuvant chemotherapy with gemcitabine vs observation in patients undergoing curative-intent resection of pancreatic cancer: a randomized controlled trial. JAMA 2007;297:267. (*Finds promising results with gemcitabine adjuvant therapy.*)

14. Regine WF, Winter KA, Abrams RA, et al. Fluorouracil vs gemcitabine chemotherapy before and after fluorouracil-based chemoradiation following resection of pancreatic adenocarcinoma: a randomized controlled trial. JAMA 2008;299:1019. (*An example of current approaches to adjuvant therapy.*)

15. Warshaw AL, Fernandez del Castillo C. Pancreatic carcinoma. N Engl J Med 1992;326:455. (*A classic review, with a focus on surgical therapy; 186 references.*)

16. Willett CG, Fernandez del Castillo C, Shih HA, et al. Long term results of intraoperative electron beam irradiation (IOERT) for patients with unresectable pancreatic cancer. Ann Surg 2005; 241:295. (*A small number of patients with early but unresectable disease achieved 5-year survival.*)

17. Zhu AX, Clark JW, Willett CG. Adjuvant therapy for pancreatic cancer: an evolving paradigm. Surg Oncol Clin N Am 2004;13(4):605. (*Reviews the current status of adjuvant therapy in pancreatic cancer treatment and ongoing studies evaluating its role.*)

18. Gilbert Y. Wong GY, Schroeder DR, et al. Effect of neurolytic celiac plexus block on pain relief, quality of life, and survival in patients with unresectable pancreatic cancer: a randomized controlled trial. JAMA 2004; 291:1092. (*Pain was reduced but not sufficiently to improve quality of life.*)

Gallbladder and Biliary Tract Cancers

1. de Groen PC, Gores GJ, LaRusso NF, et al. Biliary tract cancers. N Engl J Med 1999;341:1368. (*A comprehensive review; 126 references*).

Hepatic Cancer

1. Hassan MM, Hwang LY, Hatten CJ, et al. Risk factors for hepatocellular carcinoma: synergism of alcohol with viral hepatitis and diabetes mellitus Hepatology 2002;36:1206. (*A good discussion of risk factors.*)

2. Hashem B, El-Serag HB, Davila JA, et al. The continuing increase in the incidence of hepatocellular carcinoma in the United States: an update. Ann Intern Med 2003;139:817. (*Presents important epidemiologic data.*)

3. Llovet JM, Burroughs A, Bruix J. Hepatocellular carcinoma. Lancet 2003;362:1907. (*A comprehensive review.*)

4. Tanabe KK, Lemoine A, Finkelstein DM, et al. Epidermal growth factor gene functional polymorphism and the risk of hepatocellular carcinoma in patients with cirrhosis. JAMA 2008;299:53. (*Finds that epidermal growth factor gene polymorphism genotype is associated with risk.*)

5. Shu AX, Abou-Alfa GK. Expanding the treatment options for hepatocellular carcinoma: combining transarterial chemoembolization with radiofrequency ablation. JAMA 2008;299:1716. (*A promising ablation measure.*)

6. Schwartz M, Roayaie S, Konstadoulakis M. Strategies for the management of hepatocellular carcinoma. Nat Clin Pract Oncol 2007;4:424. (*A useful overview, with emphasis on transplantation.*)

Colorectal Cancer and Polyps

1. Atkin WS, Morson BC, Cuzick J. Long-term risk of colorectal cancer after excision of rectosigmoid adenomas. N Engl J Med 1992;326:658. (*The risk was increased in patients with villous, tubulovillous, and large adenomas.*)

2. Beresford SA, Johnson KC, Ritenbaugh C, et al. Low-fat dietary pattern and risk of colorectal cancer: The Women's Health Initiative Randomized Controlled Dietary Modification Trial. JAMA 2006;295:643. (*Finds no benefit after 8 years of use.*)

3. Bingham SA, Day NE, Luben R, et al. Dietary fibre in food and protection against colorectal cancer in the European Prospective Investigation into Cancer and Nutrition (EPIC): an observational study. Lancet 2003;361:1496. (*The amount of dietary fiber in foods was inversely related to colorectal cancer risk.*)

4. Fuchs CS, Giovannucci EL, Colditz GA, et al. Dietary fiber and the risk of colorectal cancer and adenoma in women. N Engl J Med 1999;340:169. (*Data from the Nurses' Health Study failing to confirm a protective effect for dietary fiber.*)

5. Giovannucci E, Ascherio A, Rimm EB, et al. Physical activity, obesity, and risk for colon cancer and adenoma in men. Ann Intern Med 1995;122:327. (*A prospective cohort study, finding that physical activity was associated with reduced risk, and abdominal adiposity with increased risk.*)

6. Fletcher RH. Carcinoembryonic antigen. Ann Intern Med 1986;104:66. (*A thoughtful review of its use for staging and surveillance.*)

7. Steel G, Mayer RJ, Podolsky DK, et al. In: Osteen, R., ed. *Cancer manual*, 9th ed. Boston: American Cancer Society, Massachusetts Division, 1996:399. (*The Dukes classification system.*)

8. Liefers G-J, Cleton-Jansen A-M, de Velde CJH, et al. Micrometastases and survival in stage II colorectal cancer. N Engl J Med 1998;339:223. (*The presence of micrometastases was associated with an adverse prognosis.*)

9. Veit-Haibach P, Kuehle CA, Beyer T, et al. Diagnostic accuracy of colorectal cancer staging with whole-body PET/CT colonography. JAMA. 2006;296:2590. (*The procedure was found to be useful for the detection of otherwise unrecognized disease.*)

10. Bosset J-F, Collette L, Calais G, et al., for EORTC Radiotherapy Group Trial 22921. Chemotherapy with preoperative radiotherapy in rectal cancer. N Engl J Med 2006;355:1114. (*Finds that chemotherapy with 5-fluorouracil [5-FU] improves local control but not overall survival.*)

11. Goldberg RM, Fleming TR, Tangen CM, et al. Surgery for recurrent colon cancer: strategies for identifying resectable recurrence and success rates after resection. Ann Intern Med 1998;129:27. (*Presents evidence suggesting that monitoring for and removing surgically resectable recurrences improves outcomes.*)

12. Hurwitz H, Fehrenbacher L, Novotny W, et al. Bevacizumab plus irinotecan, fluorouracil, and leucovorin for metastatic colorectal cancer. N Engl J Med 2004;350:2335. (*A randomized, controlled trial of an example of current approaches to multimodality therapy including antibodies directed against epidermal growth factor [EGF]; the approach improved survival.*)

13. Jonker DJ, O'Callaghan CJ, Karapetis CS, et al. Cetuximab for the treatment of colorectal cancer. N Engl J Med 2007;357:2040. (*RCT of this EGF antagonist, finding that it improved overall and progression-free survival and preserved quality of life in advanced disease.*)

14. Meyerhardt JA, Niedzwiecki D, Hollis D, et al. Association of dietary patterns with cancer recurrence and survival in patients with stage III colon cancer. JAMA 2007;298:754. (*A higher intake of a Western diet was associated with a higher risk of recurrence.*)

15. Meyerhardt JA, Mayer RJ. Systemic therapy for colorectal cancer. N Engl J Med 2007;352:476.(*An authoritative review, including a good discussion of new modalities.*)

16. Schrag D. The price tag on progress—chemotherapy for colorectal cancer. N Engl J Med 2004;351:317. (*Argues that the aggressive treatment of late-stage disease might not be very cost-effective from a societal perspective.*)

17. Swedish Rectal Cancer Trial. Improved survival with preoperative radiotherapy in resectable rectal cancer. N Engl J Med 1997;336:980. (*RCT, finding that long-term survival improved by 15%.*)

18. Twelves C, Wong A, Nowacki MP, et al. Capecitabine as adjuvant treatment for stage III colon cancer. N Engl J Med 2005;352:2696. (*Presents evidence of efficacy and better tolerability from this new oral chemotherapy agent, which can be used in place of 5-FU and leucovorin as first-line therapy.*)

19. Weeks JC, Nelson H, Gelber S, et al. Short-term quality-of-life outcomes following laparoscopic-assisted colectomy vs open colectomy for colon cancer: a randomized trial. JAMA 2002;287:321. (*Finds only minimal short-term benefits.*)

20. Baron JA, Beach M, Mandel JS, et al. Calcium supplements for the prevention of colorectal adenomas. N Engl J Med 1999;340:101. (*RCT, finding a significant but only moderate reduction in the rate of recurrence in persons who had a previous adenoma.*)

21. Chan AT, Ogino S, Fuchs CS. Aspirin and the risk of colorectal cancer in relation to the expression of COX-2. N Engl J Med 2007;356:2131. (*Reduces the risk, but only for colorectal cancers that overexpress cyclooxygenase-2.*)

22. Cook NR, Lee I-M, Gaziano M, et al. Low-dose aspirin in the primary prevention of cancer: the Women's Health Study: a randomized controlled trial. JAMA 2005;294:47. (*RCT, observing no protective effect.*)

23. Creagan ET, Moertel CG, O'Fallon JR, et al. Failure of high-dose vitamin C therapy to benefit patients with advanced cancer. N Engl J Med 1979;301:1189. (*RCT, finding that high-dose vitamin C is no more effective than placebo.*)

24. Giovannucci E, Stampfer MJ, Colditz GA, et al. Multivitamin use, folate, and colon cancer in women in the Nurses Health Study. Ann Intern Med 1998;129:524. (*A prospective cohort study, showing that long-term use, especially for folate, was associated with reduced risk.*)

25. Goldstein F, Martinez E, Platz EA, et al. Postmenopausal hormone use and risk for colorectal cancer and adenoma. Ann Intern Med 1998;128:705. (*A prospective cohort study, finding benefit while the patient was taking replacement therapy, but that benefit persisted only if treatment continued.*)

26. Ivanovich JL, Read TE, Ciske DJ, et al. A practical approach to familial and hereditary colorectal cancer. Am J Med 1999;107:68. (*A review, stressing the importance of a detailed family history followed by more intensified screening, cancer risk assessment, genetic testing, and consideration of prophylactic surgery.*)

27. Peters U, Sinha R, Chatterjee N, et al. Dietary fibre and colorectal adenoma in a colorectal cancer early detection program. Lancet 2003;361:1491. (*Increased dietary fibre was associated with a lower risk of colonic adenomas*).

28. Rostom A, Dubé C, Lewin G, et al. Nonsteroidal anti-inflammatory drugs and cyclooxygenase-2 inhibitors for primary prevention of colorectal cancer: a systematic review prepared for the U.S. Preventive Services Task Force. Ann Intern Med 2007;146:376. (*Evidence-based concensus recommendation.*)

29. Syngal S, Weeks JC, Schrag D, et al. Benefits of colonoscopic surveillance and prophylactic colectomy in patients with hereditary nonpolyposis colorectal cancer mutations. Ann Intern Med 1998;129:787. (*A decision-analysis study of the options for patients with a high genetic risk of malignancy.*)

30. Syngal S, Fox EA, Li C, et al. Interpretation of genetic test results for hereditary nonpolyposis colorectal cancer. JAMA 1999;282:247. (*A helpful discussion of genetic data; the finding of deleterious mutations was found to be useful to management in 25% of families examined.*)

31. U.S. Preventive Services Task Force. Screening for colorectal cancer: recommendation and rationale. Ann Intern Med 2002;137:129. (*The most recent U.S. Preventive Services Task Force recommendations, concluding that screening reduces mortality and recommending that all persons of average risk older than age 50 years be screened; notes that data are insufficient to identify the best screening strategy, but that all methods appear to be reasonably cost-effective, and suggests that the choice be determined by patient preference.*)

32. Wactawski-Wende J, Kotchen JM, Anderson GL, et al. Calcium plus vitamin D supplementation and the risk of colorectal cancer. N Engl J Med 2006;354:684. (*RCT, finding no benefit after 7 years of treatment.*)

33. Soetikno RM, Kaltenbach T, Rouse RV, et al. Prevalence of nonpolypoid (flat and depressed) colorectal neoplasms in asymptomatic and symptomatic adults. JAMA 2008;299:1027. (*Finds that the risk of advanced histology was greater with raised lesions.*)

34. Winawer SJ, Zauber AG, Ho MN, et al. Prevention of colorectal cancer by colonoscopic polypectomy. N Engl J Med 1993;321:1977. (*Presents original evidence of benefit.*)

Anal Cancer

1. Goldie SJ, Kuntz KM, Weinstein MC, et al. The clinical effectiveness and cost-effectiveness of screening for anal squamous intraepithelial lesions in homosexual and bisexual HIV-positive men. JAMA 1999;281:1822. (*Finds that screening by anal Papanicolaou test was cost-effective.*)

2. Ryan DP, Compton CC, Mayer RL. Carcinoma of the anal canal. N Engl J Med 2000;342:792. (*The best available review.*)

CHAPTER 77 ■ SCREENING FOR ANEMIA

Anemia is a sign of illness rather than a diagnosis in itself. The incidental finding of a low hematocrit or hemoglobin level suggests a host of underlying conditions that range from the trivial to the life threatening. Patients with fatigue or other subjective symptoms often ask about their "blood count." The absence of anemia in such instances is reassuring. However, is the patient who is otherwise well likely to benefit from either the identification or the treatment of asymptomatic anemia? The answer to this question depends on the prevalence and the nature of the conditions most likely to cause asymptomatic anemia and on the relationship between the hemoglobin level and those symptoms attributed to lower levels.

EPIDEMIOLOGY AND RISK FACTORS (1–7)

By far the most common cause of asymptomatic anemia is *iron deficiency* resulting from the inadequate dietary replacement of iron lost from the body. Daily iron requirements for men and postmenopausal women are between 0.5 and 1 mg. Because additional iron is needed by menstruating and pregnant women, their daily requirements are 2 and 2.5 mg, respectively. Because only 5% to 10% of the 10 to 20 mg of the iron contained in the average adult diet is absorbed, it is not surprising that iron deficiency is common in women of childbearing age. Population studies have found that 10% to 20% of menstruating women have abnormally low concentrations of hemoglobin (usually <12 g/100 mL). Between 20% and 60% of pregnant women have hemoglobin levels less than 11 g/100 mL. Anemia is less likely to occur in women taking birth control pills and more likely to occur in women with intrauterine devices. Iron deficiency is rare in male adults; if present, it is a clear indication for diligent investigation of the gastrointestinal tract. Absorption of iron may be decreased after gastrectomy or in the presence of achlorhydria.

Sideroblastic and megaloblastic anemias are much less common. The prevalence of *pernicious anemia*, the most common form of vitamin B_{12} deficiency, is 0.1% in persons of northern European extraction. Pernicious anemia is much less common among other ethnic and racial groups. *Folate deficiency* is common during pregnancy and in patients with alcoholic liver disease, in whom it is often accompanied by sideroblastic anemia. Anticonvulsant drugs, including phenytoin, primidone, and phenobarbital, may interfere with folate absorption, so megaloblastic anemia results. *Thalassemia minor* is a common cause of mild anemia in patients of Mediterranean or east Asian or southeast Asian extraction. *Sickle cell disease* and trait, by far the most common forms of hemoglobinopathy, are discussed separately (see Chapter 78).

NATURAL HISTORY OF ANEMIA AND EFFECTIVENESS OF THERAPY (2,4–9)

Obviously, the natural history of anemia depends on the underlying cause. What symptoms can mild or moderate anemia be expected to produce? The hyperkinetic symptoms that follow compensatory increases in cardiac stroke volume and heart rate are rarely present before hemoglobin levels have fallen to 7.5 g/100 mL. Other highly subjective symptoms, including irritability, fatigue, and headache, have been attributed to milder degrees of anemia. A British survey, however, found no relationship between the frequency of such symptoms and the level of hemoglobin (ranging from 8 to 12 g/100 mL) among women found to have iron-deficiency anemia during a screening program. Indirect evidence showed that levels of less than 8 g/100 mL were associated with symptoms severe enough to prompt presentation to a physician. Among the asymptomatic women identified by screening, no benefits of treatment were detected. It has been noted by some investigators that symptoms associated with vitamin B_{12} deficiency may predate the onset of anemia (see Chapters 79 and 82).

It is particularly important that clinicians understand the lack of demonstrated association between mild and moderate levels of anemia and symptoms. Direct-to-consumer advertising and physician-directed efforts by pharmaceutical companies generally portray a stronger relationship that is not supported by the evidence.

Most studies of screening for anemia have been conducted in the preoperative or inpatient setting. For example, in an assessment of hematocrit in more than 300,000 veterans aged 65 years and older facing noncardiac surgery, 43% had levels below 39%. Although 30-day postoperative mortality rates increased monotonically with the degree of anemia in this study, it is not clear whether anemia was a marker for comorbid chronic disease or a modifiable risk factor for death.

The few studies that have been performed on outpatients have shown little benefit from screening for anemia. In a Swiss study of the utility of the complete blood cell count in 595 outpatients attending a university-based clinic, 34 (5.8%) had a low hemoglobin level, and a new diagnosis (iron deficiency without serious underlying pathology) was made in only 3 of them (0.5%). A report from Great Britain demonstrated a 10% prevalence of anemia among screened women. The absence of treatable underlying conditions other than iron deficiency was noteworthy, and, again, no benefits of treatment could be demonstrated.

Iron-deficiency anemia is not uncommon among pregnant women and has been associated with a two- to threefold increased risk for low birth weight, preterm delivery, and perinatal mortality. Screening for anemia is generally recommended as part of the first prenatal evaluation. The results of randomized trials of iron supplementation for pregnant women without anemia or with mild anemia have been mixed. When iron supplementation is prescribed for women who already have children, they should be reminded of the risk of overdose among toddlers; 30% of fatal pediatric overdoses can be attributed to iron supplements.

SCREENING AND DIAGNOSTIC TESTS (4–7,10)

The laboratory measurements of *hematocrit* and *hemoglobin concentration* are straightforward. Automated methods are reliable and reproducible when specimens are properly handled. The mean hematocrit for adult men at sea level is 46%, with a range of 41% to 51%; for women, the mean is 42% and the range is 37% to 47%. Slight differences may be noted when automated techniques are used to measure the hematocrit. The normal mean hemoglobin concentration is approximately 16 g/100 mL for men, with a range of 14 to 18 g/100 mL; for women, the mean is 14 g/100 mL and the range is 12 to 16 g/100 mL. In men older than 65 years, the mean falls to 13.5 g/100 mL, and in women older than 65 years, it falls to 13.1 g/100 mL. It must be remembered, as with all continuous laboratory variables, that the choice of a reference value for defining normality is arbitrary. This is particularly true in light of the unclear relationship between significant symptoms and mild "anemia."

CONCLUSIONS AND RECOMMENDATIONS

- Anemia is a common condition. It may be secondary to serious underlying disease or a simple dietary deficiency. Determination of the hemoglobin concentration or hematocrit is recommended as an important part of the evaluation of a variety of presenting complaints, including fatigue, weight loss, abdominal pain, and gastrointestinal bleeding (see Chapters 8, 9, 58, and 63).
- Although determination of the complete blood cell count may provide clues in asymptomatic patients to the presence of early treatable disease, such as gastrointestinal malignancy, more sensitive and more specific screening methods are available and preferred (e.g., stool guaiac testing and sigmoidoscopy for early detection of colorectal cancer; see Chapter 56).
- Preoperative anemia has been associated with increased 30-day postoperative mortality in older men. Although it is not clear whether anemia is a marker for comorbid chronic disease that increases risk or an independent and modifiable risk factor for death, assessment of hematocrit and characterization of any anemia found are warranted elements of preoperative assessment, especially in the presence of known chronic disease (see Chapter 79).
- No clear relationship has been found between mild to moderate degrees of anemia and significant symptoms. No clearly measurable benefits after the treatment of mild anemia have been identified in screening studies.
- Thus, routine screening for anemia in nonpregnant, asymptomatic patients is not recommended.
- Iron-deficiency anemia is common among pregnant women and is associated with poorer outcomes of pregnancy. Screening for anemia at the time of the first prenatal visit is recommended.

A.G.M.

Annotated Bibliography

1. Beghe C, Wilson A, Ershler WB. Prevalence and outcomes of anemia in geriatrics: a systematic review of the literature. Am J Med 2004;116:3S. (*Part of an extensive series of papers defining the prevalence of anemia in different chronic conditions, funded by Amgen; found that the prevalence of anemia rises with age, especially after age 85 years.*)
2. Wu WC, Schifftner TL, Henderson WG, et al. Preoperative hematocrit levels and postoperative outcomes in older patients undergoing noncardiac surgery. JAMA 2007;297:2481. (*In this retrospective cohort of >300,000 veterans 65 years and older facing noncardiac surgery, 43% had a hematocrit <39%.*)
3. Elwood PC, Shinton NK, Wilson IL, et al. Haemoglobin, vitamin B12 and folate levels in the elderly. Br J Haematol 1971;21:557. (*In 10% of elderly men, hemoglobin levels are <13 g/100 mL; in 10% of elderly women, they are <12.5 g/100 mL; no megaloblastic anemia was found.*)
4. Elwood PC, Waters WE, Greene WJ, et al. Evaluation of a screening survey for anemia in adult nonpregnant women. Br Med J 1967;4:714. (*Not a very extensive follow-up, but no serious underlying disease was detected among anemic women.*)
5. Institute of Medicine. Iron-deficiency anemia: recommended guidelines for the prevention, detection, and management among U.S. children and women of childbearing age. Washington, DC: National Academy Press, 1993. (*Authoritative review and recommendations.*)
6. U.S. Preventive Services Task Force. Guide to clinical preventive services, 2nd ed. Baltimore: Williams & Wilkins, 1996. (*Screening for anemia is recommended for pregnant women at their first prenatal visit and for high-risk infants.*)
7. U.S. Preventive Services Task Force. Guide to clinical preventive services, 2007. Rockville, MD: Agency for Healthcare Research and Quality. Available at: http://www.ahrq.gov/clinic/pocketgd07/gcp2d.htm#anemia. (*Recommendation updates.*)
8. Elwood PC, Waters WE, Greene WJW, et al. Symptoms and circulating haemoglobin level. J Chron Dis 1969;21:615. (*Symptoms were not correlated with hemoglobin level in those found to be anemic on screening.*)
9. Murphy JF, O'Riordan J, Newcombe RG, et al. Relation of haemoglobin levels in first and second trimester to outcome of pregnancy. Lancet 1986;1:992. (*There was an association with an increased risk for low birth weight, preterm delivery, and perinatal mortality.*)
10. Ruttman S, Clemencon D, Dubach UC. Usefulness of complete blood counts as a case-finding tool in medical outpatients. Ann Intern Med 1992;116:44. (*One of the few studies performed in the outpatient setting; the yield was 5.8%, but no significant pathology was found in this middle-aged population.*)

CHAPTER 78 ■ SCREENING FOR SICKLE CELL DISEASE AND SICKLE CELL TRAIT

Sickle cell disease is the most common of the clinically significant hemoglobinopathies. In the United States, the disease and trait occur almost exclusively among African Americans. Sickle cell disease afflicts 1 in 375 African Americans and 1 in 60,000 whites. During the late 1960s and early 1970s, sickle cell disease received a great deal of attention in the medical and lay press. The importance of screening for the disease and trait was stressed. Some states legislated mandatory adult screening programs. All but a few states have focused screening efforts on newborns. As a result, sickle cell disease (the hemoglobin SS homozygous state) is now usually identified through state-sponsored universal screening programs. Children in whom anemia is not identified by screening present later with impaired growth, increased susceptibility to infection, or painful crisis. Screening of adults is aimed at the identification of asymptomatic carriers of sickle cell trait (the hemoglobin AS heterozygous state). The principal objective is to reduce the prevalence of the homozygous condition by means of genetic counseling. Whether screening benefits the people screened has been debated. Screening can be harmful without subsequent effective education and counseling that allows for informed decisions to be made about pregnancy and prenatal diagnosis. An understanding of the natural history of sickle cell trait and disease, sensitivity to the concerns of affected patients, and selective use of screening tests are all necessary if such harmful effects are to be avoided.

EPIDEMIOLOGY AND RISK FACTORS (1–6)

Sickle cell disease has a prevalence of less than 0.35% among African American children in the United States. Double heterozygotes, including those with hemoglobin SC or S-β-thalassemia, are even less common. The prevalence of sickling disease is lower among adults because the life span of SS homozygotes and double heterozygotes is decreased.

Screening surveys have documented a prevalence of sickle trait of 7.4% among African American veterans and 8.7% in the African American community of San Francisco. Some studies have shown regional differences in prevalence. Prevalence does not decrease with age. Sickle cell trait is present with a low frequency in southern Italy and with a higher frequency in parts of Greece. It remains a rare finding in Americans of Mediterranean extraction.

NATURAL HISTORY OF SICKLE CELL DISEASE AND EFFECTIVENESS OF THERAPY (1,7–13)

The natural history of sickle cell disease is variable. Most children exhibit failure to thrive and have frequent infections.

Anemia is usually moderate but can become severe, often as a result of infection or folate deficiency. The course is punctuated by painful crises precipitated by infection, dehydration, or hypoxia. Organ infarction, congestive heart failure, cholelithiasis, and skin ulcers are some of the complications of chronic disease. Because supportive care has improved, the life expectancy of patients with sickle cell disease has increased; however, it still remains significantly shortened by 25 to 30 years in comparison with that of African Americans who do not have sickle cell disease. Comprehensive care including preventive measures such as prophylactic penicillin and immunization has been shown to reduce morbidity and mortality for children with sickle cell disease. This is the basis for state-sponsored universal neonatal screening in most states. Other elements of supportive care such as preoperative transfusion have led to other opportunistic screening strategies as well.

In contrast to sickle cell disease, life expectancy is not affected by sickle cell trait. AS red blood cells sickle at a much lower oxygen tension than do SS cells. The only clinical abnormality that occurs with any frequency among patients with sickle cell trait is painless hematuria, presumably the result of small infarcts of the renal medulla, where red cells are particularly susceptible to sickling.

Concern about a risk for sudden death during extreme physical exertion in patients with sickle trait has been raised by case reports and population studies of military recruits. Indeed, the presence of sickle cell trait was associated with an increased risk for otherwise unexplained sudden death among military recruits who were engaged in extreme exertion during basic training. This led to a suggestion that African American recruits and athletes be screened for sickle trait. However, although the relative risk for sudden death may be elevated, the absolute risk still appears to be very small (about 1 in 3,000 in the Army recruit study) and practically nil for physically well-conditioned persons during exercise (no episodes of sudden death were attributable to sickle trait among Olympic or professional athletes, even when they performed at high elevations).

Thus, for untrained persons with sickle trait, a small increase in risk may indeed exist, especially at extremes of exertion and altitude, but under most other circumstances, sickle trait appears to be a benign condition. Some data even suggest that the reason for an occasional sudden death in patients with what appears to be ordinary sickle trait is the undetected presence of an electrophoretically silent hemoglobin variant migrating like hemoglobin A but causing significant sickling in patients heterozygous for hemoglobin S.

If sickle trait is a generally benign condition, then the principal reason for screening adults is to provide genetic counseling. It is important to consider the effectiveness of such counseling. Evidence suggests that the identification and counseling of heterozygotes do not alter marriage and parenthood decisions. The person who does not wish to make such decisions on the basis of carrier status is not likely to benefit from screening. Some families have been traumatized by questions of paternity raised by indiscriminate screening. Because of the confusion among patients and physicians about differences between sickle cell disease and trait, unnecessary anxiety may be the most common result. Surveys have demonstrated that many internists and general practitioners do not sufficiently understand the implications of screening test results to be able to counsel patients properly.

SCREENING AND DIAGNOSTIC TESTS (14–16)

A number of techniques have been developed to diagnose sickle cell disease during early gestation of fetuses at risk. Chorionic villus sampling for fetal DNA has been used successfully to identify sickle cell disease at 8 weeks of pregnancy and thereby permits earlier diagnosis than amniocentesis. Some reproductive centers are developing techniques for diagnosis preimplantation by using small amounts of DNA from single cells. The availability of prenatal diagnosis should be explained before screening the prospective parents. Careful counseling must also precede the responsible application of any prenatal diagnostic method. Risks of the procedure to mother and fetus, risks of false-positive and false-negative test results, and the acceptability of therapeutic abortion should be discussed.

Newborn screening is usually accomplished with blood samples spotted on to filter paper after a heel stick with subsequent electrophoresis or thin-layer isoelectric focusing. Polymerase chain reaction techniques may be used in the future to detect sickle cell genes directly. In older children and adults, the "sickle cell prep" using 2% metabisulfite solution is now rarely used. Instead, current practice generally includes the combination of cellulose acetate electrophoresis together with either agar electrophoresis or a commercial solubility test (e.g., Sickledex), or the combination of thin-layer isoelectric focusing and a solubility test. Combinations are necessary because the solubility tests are positive in the presence of hemoglobin S but do not distinguish among homozygotes, heterozygotes, and double heterozygotes (hemoglobin S combined with thalassemia or hemoglobin C). Hemoglobin electrophoresis does not suffice alone because some nonsickling hemoglobin variants travel in the same electrophoretic band as hemoglobin S (e.g., hemoglobin Lepore). Examining a peripheral blood smear and checking a reticulocyte count provide supportive data for diagnosis of sickle cell disease (see Chapter 79).

CONCLUSIONS AND RECOMMENDATIONS (15,16)

■ Sickle cell disease is a serious health hazard that usually presents during early childhood. Screening of newborn infants permits appropriate prophylaxis, and immunization is recommended. It is now provided for all infants in most states.

■ Sickle cell trait is generally a benign condition. Although there is some question of an increased relative risk for sudden death in untrained persons required to exert extreme physical effort at very high altitude, the absolute risk is extremely low and nil in trained persons.

■ Thus, the principal reason for screening adults for the presence of sickle trait is to facilitate genetic counseling. Screening of high-risk pregnant women at their first prenatal visit should be preceded by counseling about the subsequent need for paternal testing and the availability of prenatal diagnosis. Indiscriminate screening followed by inadequate counseling may be harmful and is not likely to provide benefits to those persons who will not revise marriage and parenthood decisions on the basis of test results.

■ Screening for sickle trait should be offered to African American adults in reproductive age groups. The implications of test results should be fully explained before testing is performed.

A.G.M./A.H.G.

Annotated Bibliography

1. Agency for Health Care Policy and Research. Sickle cell disease: screening, diagnosis, management and counseling in newborns and infants. Clinical practice guideline no. 6 (AHCPR Publication no. 93-0562). Rockville, MD: Agency for Health Care Policy and Research, U.S. Department of Health and Human Services, Public Health Service, 1993. (*Guidelines based on a critical synthesis of the evidence.*)
2. Ashley-Koch A, Yang Q, Olney RS. Sickle hemoglobin (HbS) allele and sickle cell disease. Am J Epidemiol 2000;151:839. (*An extensive review of epidemiology.*)
3. Davies SC, Cronin E, Gill M, et al. Screening for sickle cell disease and thalassemia—a systematic review with supplementary research. Health Technol Assess 2000;4:1. (*Identifies prevalence thresholds that make screening cost-effective.*)
4. Motulsky AG. Frequency of sickling disorders in U.S. blacks. N Engl J Med 1973;288:31. (*Estimates the prevalence of double heterozygosity and of SS disease in newborns [1 in 625 with SS, 1 in 833 with SC, and 1 in 1,667 with S-β-thalassemia] and in the population.*)
5. Murphy JR. Sickle cell hemoglobin in black football players. JAMA 1973;225:981. (*The rate of hemoglobin AS among African American football players in the National Football League was 6.7%.*)
6. Pemberton PL, Down JF, Porter JB, et al. A retrospective observational study of preoperative sickle cell screening. Anaesthesia 2002;57:334. (*Rates of screening and prevalences for different ethnicities in London.*)
7. Charache S. Sudden death in sickle trait. Am J Med 1988;84:459. (*Editorial summarizing the evidence; concludes that the risk is very small and clinically unimportant under most circumstances.*)
8. Gaston MH, Verter JI, Woods G, et al. Prophylaxis with oral penicillin in children with sickle cell anemia. A randomized trial. N Engl J Med 1986;314:1593. (*The incidence of infection was reduced by >80%.*)
9. Kark JA, Posey DM, Schumacher HR, et al. Sickle-cell trait as a risk factor for sudden death in physical training. N Engl J Med 1987;317:781. (*An increased risk for sudden death was found among recruits with sickle cell trait.*)
10. Martin TW, Weisman IM, Zeballos RJ, et al. Exercise and hypoxia increase sickling in venous blood from an exercising limb in individuals with sickle cell trait. Am J Med 1989;87:48. (*At 4,000 m, sickling increased significantly in venous blood, but not in arterial blood; oxygen consumption and exercise performance were the same as for controls.*)
11. Platt OS, Brambilla DJ, Rosse WF, et al. Mortality in sickle cell disease: life expectancy and risk factors for early death. N Engl J Med 1994;330:1639. (*The life expectancy of African Americans with sickle cell disease is on average 25 to 30 years less than that of other African Americans.*)
12. Sears DA. The morbidity of sickle cell trait. Am J Med 1978;64:1021. (*Extensive review; although certain abnormalities do occur with increased frequency in sickle cell trait, survival is not impaired; 296 references.*)

13. Vichinsky E. New therapies in sickle cell disease. Lancet 2002;360:629. (*Reviews new approaches, including nitric oxide and l-arginine, as well as stem-cell transplantation, and concludes that greater access to multidisciplinary specialty care is a critical need.*)
14. Goossens M, Dumez Y, Kaplan L, et al. Prenatal diagnosis of sickle-cell anemia in the first trimester of pregnancy. N Engl J Med 1983;309:831. (*Earlier diagnosis of sickle cell disease is possible through chorionic biopsy techniques.*)
15. Farfel MR, Holtzman NA. Education, consent, and counseling in sickle cell screening programs: report of a survey. Am J Public Health 1984;74:373. (*Of 52,000 persons screened in Maryland during a 1-year period, 25% were screened without informed consent.*)
16. Kellon DB, Beutler E. Physician attitudes about sickle cell disease and sickle cell trait. JAMA 1974;227:71. (*Finds that many primary care practitioners misunderstood the implications of sickle cell screening; there is little reason to believe that this has changed since.*)

CHAPTER 79 ■ EVALUATION OF ANEMIA

In most instances, the office presentation of anemia is incidental, with no obvious cause and no hemodynamic compromise. Because anemia is not a diagnosis, its appearance necessitates identification of the underlying cause, especially in men, women who are neither menstruating nor pregnant, and the elderly; in all these groups, the probability of disease is high. In more than 50% of cases, a clinically important cause is discovered. The task for the primary physician is to design a cost-effective assessment that concentrates on testing for causes of prognostic significance.

DEFINITION, PATHOPHYSIOLOGY, AND CLINICAL PRESENTATION (1–20)

Definition

Anemia is defined as a reduction in the hematocrit or hemoglobin concentration. The widely accepted World Health Organization definition is expressed in terms of hemoglobin concentration: for male adults, less than 13 g/dL; for nonpregnant women, less than 12 g/dL; for pregnant women, less than 11 g/dL. Although the cutoff points are somewhat arbitrary, derived statistically from population data, these numbers can have meaning for individual patients because they tend to correlate with health status and prognosis, particularly in the elderly. Although the mean hemoglobin concentration tends to decline with age, the significance of anemia does not, and consequently the diagnostic criteria are not adjusted downward for age. Because anemia is defined in terms of red cell mass and hemoglobin concentration, a spurious diagnosis of anemia may be made when the plasma volume is expanded. Similarly, if the plasma volume is contracted, a true anemia may be masked.

Pathophysiology

Anemia may result from *bleeding, inadequate red cell production,* or *excessive red cell destruction*; often, two or more mechanisms operate simultaneously. Production is decreased when defects in stem cell proliferation or differentiation, DNA synthesis, hemoglobin synthesis, or a combination of these deficiencies is present. Excessive destruction can result from membrane disorders, abnormal hemoglobins, enzyme deficiencies, and a host of extrinsic problems, such as mechanical disruption or antibody-mediated injury.

The development of symptoms and signs depends on the abruptness and severity of onset, age of the patient, and ability of the cardiopulmonary system to compensate for the decrease in blood volume and oxygen-carrying capacity. When onset is gradual, symptoms may be minimal because there is adequate time for compensatory adjustments to occur. Important responses include an increase in 2,3-diphosphoglycerate, which facilitates oxygen delivery to tissues, and an expansion of the plasma volume.

Clinical Presentation

Symptoms are a function of the severity and the speed of onset of the anemia. Patients experiencing a rapid onset of anemia, with little time for compensatory mechanisms to act, are likely to have the most symptoms. Those who have a hematocrit greater 30% and a gradual onset and are otherwise in good health rarely note symptoms. However, if the hematocrit falls further, *exertional dyspnea* and *fatigue* may begin to appear after strenuous activity. Greater reductions in the hematocrit result in cardiopulmonary symptoms that come with less activity. Age and cardiopulmonary reserve are also important determinants of symptoms. A potpourri of nonspecific complaints frequently accompanies anemia, including headache, tinnitus, poor concentration, palpitations, vague abdominal discomfort, anorexia, nausea, and diarrhea or constipation. *Tachycardia* and diminished peripheral resistance occur as the hemoglobin falls to less than 7.5 g/100 mL; a *systolic flow murmur* resulting from high output is common. *Pallor* is an obvious finding, best seen in the conjunctiva, but it is of little help as an indicator of severity. More-specific clinical findings depend on the underlying cause, which can best be classified on the basis of red cell morphology (determined by the appearance on a Wright-stained peripheral smear, the mean corpuscular volume calculated by an autoanalyzer, and the degree of anisocytosis).

Microcytic Anemias

Iron Deficiency

Inadequate dietary intake, inadequate absorption, and *excessive blood loss* may result in iron-deficiency anemia. Most patients with mild disease are asymptomatic and manifest only a low-grade microcytic anemia. In otherwise healthy menstruating women, iron deficiency is often blamed for a host of symptoms, including *fatigue, headache, paresthesias,* and *irritability*. Although fatigue may certainly be a manifestation of severe anemia, the correlation between these symptoms and hemoglobin concentration has been poor in women with mild anemia. In placebo-controlled, double-blinded studies, they fail to show consistent symptomatic benefit with iron therapy. Some investigators attribute *Menorrhagia* to instances of iron deficiency, but others dispute this. *Pica* and *dysphagia* (caused by an esophageal web) are classic, although rare, features today.

The physical findings that occur in iron deficiency are a bit more specific. *Atrophic glossitis* and *cheilitis* are common features; *koilonychia*, with spooning, ridging, and thinning, is rare. Other physical findings and symptoms are manifestations of the underlying cause. The earliest laboratory changes are *depletion of marrow iron stores* and a corresponding *fall in serum ferritin*. These are followed by a *decrease in serum iron* and an *increase in transferrin*, which in many cases produce a reduction in the *transferrin saturation* to *less than 16%*. The first change in the peripheral blood is a drop in the *hematocrit* and *hemoglobin concentration*. An *anisocytosis* develops, manifested by an elevation in the *red cell distribution width* (RDW). Later, with increasing severity of anemia (hemoglobin concentration <9 g/dL), red cells become *microcytic* and eventually *hypochromic*.

Thalassemia Minor (Thalassemia Trait)

This condition is typically detected in asymptomatic patients undergoing an evaluation for a microcytic hypochromic anemia that does not respond to iron. A gene defect leads to impaired red cell maturation by causing an excess of either α or β chains of hemoglobin to accumulate. The most prevalent form is β-thalassemia trait, common among persons of Mediterranean ancestry. It is associated with an increase in *hemoglobin A2*. There are no characteristic physical findings. The red cell count is elevated, and the smear may reveal *target cells, basophilic stippling, polychromatophilia, poikilocytosis,* and *anisocytosis* in addition to microcytosis. α-Thalassemia trait is seen among African Americans. The hemoglobin A2 level is normal, but a mild anemia, hypochromia, and microcytosis are present.

Sideroblastic Anemias

Sideroblastic anemias form a heterogeneous set of disorders, which include a *primary* type, which may be a preleukemic state; a *congenital* pyridoxine-responsive variant; and *secondary* variants associated with rheumatoid arthritis, polyarteritis, malabsorption, chronic alcoholism, cancer, porphyria, lead poisoning, and true pyridoxine deficiency. These, too, are conditions of abnormal red cell maturation. They can lead to significant anemia requiring the repeated transfusion of red cells. Their hallmark is the accumulation of nonheme iron within the mitochondria of red cells. When stained for iron, immature red cells demonstrate a ring of stain around the nucleus (*ringed sideroblasts*). In the primary type, patients are typically older than 60 years of age and may have *primary myelodys-*

plasia, a proliferative disease of the bone marrow in which a clone of stem cells suppresses production of other cell lines. A *secondary myelodysplastic syndrome* occurs as a consequence of cancer chemotherapy. The spleen is usually not enlarged, as it is in myeloproliferative disorders. The smear is classically microcytic but may be macrocytic or dimorphic, especially in acquired forms. Cells can be hypochromic, which leads to confusion with iron deficiency. Anisocytosis and poikilocytosis are pronounced. The *serum iron* is *elevated*, as is *transferrin saturation*. Marrow iron stains show many abnormal ringed sideroblasts. The anemia may be refractory, sometimes followed by marrow failure and acute myeloid leukemia.

Anemia of Chronic Disease

Although it is usually normochromic–normocytic, this anemia can mimic that of iron deficiency in having a low serum iron and sometimes presenting as a microcytic anemia (see later discussion).

Macrocytic Anemias

Vitamin B$_{12}$ Deficiency

A classic cause is reduced gastric production of intrinsic factor, as occurs in *pernicious anemia* and after subtotal *gastrectomy*. The association of pernicious anemia with *Hashimoto's thyroiditis* and *vitiligo* suggest an autoimmune mechanism, which is confirmed by the identification of autoantibodies to intrinsic factor and parietal cells. Dietary lack is rare because vitamin B$_{12}$ is available in everyday foods, and body stores can hold up to a 3-year reserve. However, patients with achlorhydria or hypochlorhydria resulting from atrophic gastritis or gastric surgery may fail to split cobalamin from food, resulting in so-called *food-cobalamin malabsorption*, which is believed to be responsible for much of the vitamin B$_{12}$ deficiency seen in the elderly and in patients with prior gastric surgery. Population studies find a prevalence of vitamin B$_{12}$ deficiency of 1.9% in persons older than the age of 60 years. *Blind-loop syndrome* and *terminal ileal disease* are other causes.

Onset is gradual. In pernicious anemia, symptoms usually become evident in the sixth decade. Gastrointestinal problems such as *anorexia* and *diarrhea* may predominate. *Sore tongue* resulting from *atrophic glossitis* is a classic presentation, as is *numbness* and *tingling* in the extremities associated with peripheral neuropathy. The neurologic deficits result from defects in the maintenance of myelin integrity. Besides peripheral neuropathy, injury to the posterior columns and corticospinal tracts of the spinal cord (i.e., *subacute combined degeneration*) may be present, manifested by disturbances of *position* and *vibratory sense* and *incoordination, spasticity,* and *upturned toes*. Cerebral dysfunction may also ensue, leading to *memory loss, depression,* and *irritability*. If vitamin B$_{12}$ deficiency is uncorrected, demyelination can progress to axonal degeneration and irreversible neuronal death. Nerve damage can occur in the absence of anemia.

By the time the anemia is discovered, it may be severe. *Hypersegmented polymorphonuclear leukocytes* are an early finding on peripheral blood smears that is specific for the megaloblastic anemias. *Oval macrocytes* are also characteristic, although poikilocytosis is considerable. Classically, the mean corpuscular volume rises to greater than 100 μm^3 and the serum vitamin B$_{12}$ level falls to less than 100 pg/mL, but in up to one third of cases macrocytosis may be absent or the vitamin B$_{12}$ level may be greater than 100 pg/mL. The serum concentration of *holotranscobalamin II* (the vitamin B$_{12}$ carrier protein) begins to decline before the vitamin B$_{12}$ level does. Macrocytosis may be absent if concurrent iron deficiency is present, but the hypersegmented polymorphonuclear leukocytes persist. In pernicious anemia, *achlorhydria* is found on stimulation testing. Serum *homocysteine* levels frequently become elevated, which may predispose to vascular disease (see Chapter 31); levels of the metabolite *methylmalonic acid* increase.

Folate Deficiency

Inadequate dietary intake is the usual cause of folate deficiency because body stores are limited to a 3-month reserve. Chronic alcohol abuse is the classic cause. Increased demand sometimes occurs, as in pregnancy, hemolysis, malignancy, or severe psoriasis. Decreased uptake resulting from malabsorption or drugs (e.g., phenytoin, other anticonvulsants) also can trigger the anemia. The same is true for folate antagonists such as methotrexate, trimethoprim, and triamterene. Hematologic features resemble those of vitamin B$_{12}$ deficiency; no neurologic deficits are present. Folate deficiency is an important cause of *hyperhomocysteinemia*, which is associated with an increased risk for arterial and venous thrombosis (see Chapter 31).

Liver Disease

Hepatocellular disease is responsible for a host of anemias, especially when accompanied by alcoholism and poor diet. It accounts for many cases of macrocytic anemia. Folate deficiency, marrow suppression, hypersplenism, bleeding, and bile salt alteration of the red cell membrane all contribute. The smear shows considerable poikilocytosis with *spiculated red cells* and some *macrocytes;* if folate deficiency occurs, a megaloblastic picture is superimposed.

Sideroblastic Anemia

See prior discussion.

Normochromic–Normocytic Anemias

Anemia of Chronic Disease

A common accompaniment of chronic inflammatory diseases, malignancy, and renal failure, the anemia of chronic disease involves the *trapping of iron* by activated macrophages of the reticuloendothelial system, rendering it unavailable for erythropoiesis. *Hepcidin*, a recently discovered acute-phase protein, is believed to play a role in diverting iron to macrophages. In addition, some suppression of erythropoiesis by humoral substances (interleukins, tumor necrosis factor, prostaglandins) elaborated in the course of the underlying chronic disease process often occurs. Of interest, erythropoietin is inappropriately low in almost all cases.

The anemia is usually moderate, with hemoglobin levels in the range of 7 to 11 g/dL. Both serum iron and iron-binding capacity are reduced. The smear is most often *normocytic*, but it can be *hypochromic* and even *microcytic*, mimicking iron deficiency. The *serum iron falls* before anemia sets in; *transferrin saturation* may be less than 16%, again simulating iron deficiency. However, *marrow iron stores* are *normal* or *increased*, and serum *ferritin* levels are usually *elevated* due to increased uptake and deposition of iron into the reticuloendothelial system. The *reticulocyte count* is low, indicating the underproduction of red cells.

Another important anemia of chronic disease is that associated with *HIV infection*, which affects the bone marrow. Myelofibrosis occurs. Anemia is seen in about 15% of asymptomatic HIV-positive persons, 45% of those with AIDS-related complex, and 75% of those with untreated AIDS. For unknown reasons, *erythropoietin* is inappropriately *low*. The smear in most cases is *normochromic–normocytic*. *Rouleaux* formation resulting from circulating immune complexes sometimes develops, but hemolysis is uncommon. The anemia can be exacerbated by *medications* used in the treatment of HIV infection (zidovudine, pentamidine, trimethoprim, sulfonamides). Zidovudine is especially toxic to marrow, causing anemia in about 30% of instances. *Neutropenia* and *thrombocytopenia* occur to a lesser extent. Patients most susceptible to the adverse hematologic effects of zidovudine are those with a low CD4 cell count, preexisting anemia, concurrent vitamin B$_{12}$ deficiency, or neutropenia.

Hemolytic Anemias

Hemolytic anemias constitute a diverse group. Inherited forms are caused by intrinsic red cell defects; acquired types depend primarily on extrinsic mechanisms, such as immunologic or mechanical injury. Clinical presentations vary according to the rate of destruction, compensatory adaptations, and underlying cause. Jaundice sets in when the capacity of the liver to conjugate excess bilirubin from hemoglobin breakdown is exceeded; the serum level of unconjugated bilirubin climbs. *Splenomegaly* evolves as the trapping of damaged red cells progresses. Sudden fever, chills, headache, back and abdominal pain, and *hemoglobinuria* characterize severe acute hemolysis.

The reticulocyte count is elevated unless an accompanying marrow defect is present. The peripheral smear usually appears normochromic–normocytic but may be macrocytic because of the release of immature forms during rapid red cell destruction and regeneration. Polychromatophilia is common, and *nucleated red cells, stippling, schistocytes,* and *Howell–Jolly bodies* may be noted. *Spherocytes* occur in *hereditary spherocytosis*, a condition of reduced cell membrane area resulting from a defect in the synthesis of the membrane protein spectrin. *Spherocytosis* is also seen in *immune hemolytic anemia* as a consequence of membrane loss.

Sickle Cell Disease.   Sickle cell disease is the most prevalent hemolytic condition in the African American population. *Sickle cell trait* is asymptomatic and anemia is absent, although mild hematuria caused by sickling in the hypertonic renal medulla sometimes occurs. The peripheral smear is normal except for an occasional *target cell*. Hemoglobin electrophoresis reveals less than 50% of total hemoglobin to be of the S variety. Patients homozygous for the sickle cell gene have *sickle cell anemia*, a much more serious condition in which painful crises are precipitated by stress (especially infection). Intravascular sickling ensues, the red cells become rigid, and vascular occlusion may result, leading to arterial desaturation, hemolysis, and organ damage. *Leg ulcers, hepatomegaly, hematuria, renal concentrating defects,* and mild *jaundice* commonly occur. Patients report acute, severe *pain* in the lower extremities, back, or abdomen. *Fever* and *leukocytosis* may also be present. Attacks typically last from a few hours to a few days and then resolve spontaneously. Aplastic crises develop when a concurrent illness suppresses erythropoiesis. The smear is normochromic; *sickled cells* may be noted in addition to target forms. Hemoglobin electrophoresis reveals a predominance of *hemoglobin S*. The addition of a reducing agent, such as metabisulfite, to a drop of blood causes the cells to sickle within a few minutes and confirms the diagnosis.

Glucose-6-Phosphate Dehydrogenase Deficiency.   Glucose-6-phosphate dehydrogenase deficiency is a sex-linked red cell defect compromising the enzyme that maintains hemoglobin in an unoxidized state. In its episodic form, which is seen in African Americans, the condition causes hemolysis after exposure to oxidant compounds (sulfonamides, antimalarials) or infection. A chronic variety occurs in persons of Mediterranean ancestry.

Drug-Induced Hemolytic Anemias. Drug-induced hemolytic anemias usually manifest an immune mechanism, such as adsorption to the red cell of drug–antibody complexes (quinidine); adsorption to the red cell of drug to form a hapten, followed by the binding of antidrug antibody (high-dose penicillin); or induction of a red cell "autoantibody" (long-term methyldopa). The hallmark of most drug-related hemolytic episodes is a positive *direct Coombs' test* result. Withdrawal of the offending agent ends the process.

Autoimmune Hemolytic Anemias. Autoimmune hemolytic anemias result when patients produce antibodies against their own red cells. They are classified according to the type of antibody produced (immunoglobulin G [IgG] or immunoglobulin M). Those of the *IgG class* are directed against the Rh antigen. Most are *"warm" autoantibodies,* although many are idiopathic; about 50% occur in the context of lymphoma, lupus, ulcerative colitis, or chronic lymphocytic leukemia. The diagnosis is made by detecting IgG and C3d proteins on the red cell surface. Macrophages that can detect these proteins bind the involved red cells. Hemolysis is mostly extravascular. The red cells are cleared by the spleen. The *IgM* form of autoimmune hemolytic anemia is a *cold hemagglutinin* condition. These antibodies are seen in mycoplasmal, Epstein–Barr virus, or cytomegalovirus infection and in lymphoproliferative conditions. *Cold agglutinin* titers are markedly elevated in the setting of hemolysis (>1:1,000).

Aplastic Anemias

Aplastic anemias are usually idiopathic but may be linked to a marrow toxin (cytotoxic drugs, radiation), an idiosyncratic drug reaction (chloramphenicol, gold, sulfur compounds, carbamazepine), or a viral infection (hepatitis B virus, hepatitis C virus, cytomegalovirus, HIV, parvovirus). Onset is gradual, with fatigue and bleeding noted first; infection is a later problem. No organomegaly occurs. The smear appears normochromic–normocytic, but the number of platelets is diminished. There are no signs of increased red cell production. The reticulocyte count is zero, and a pancytopenia is present.

Renal Failure

The anemia of chronic renal failure is caused by a reduction in both production and survival of red cells. Lack of erythropoietin and metabolic injury to erythrocytes are postulated mechanisms. The severity of the anemia parallels the degree of azotemia. The smear is normochromic–normocytic; burr cells are sometimes prominent. Anemia is common once the glomerular filtration rate falls to less than 60 mL/min.

Hypothyroidism

Hypothyroidism is associated with a number of anemic states. The most common is a mild normochromic–normocytic anemia. Iron deficiency may occur secondary to heavy menstrual bleeding. In addition, a macrocytic picture that clears after the administration of exogenous thyroid hormone is sometimes encountered. A true megaloblastic anemia caused by vitamin B_{12} deficiency occurs in about 10% of hypothyroid patients with a macrocytic smear; the relation between hypothyroidism and pernicious anemia is unresolved, but an autoimmune mechanism is postulated.

DIFFERENTIAL DIAGNOSIS (21)

A practical method for organizing the many causes of anemia is to group them according to (a) the appearance of the Wright-stained smear of the peripheral blood and (b) the electronically determined red cell indices. This widely used approach allows causes to be classified into normochromic–normocytic, hypochromic, microcytic, and macrocytic categories (Table 79.1) and facilitates workup.

Iron deficiency accounts for most of the anemias seen in the office setting. In community-based primary care practices, iron deficiency is the underlying cause in 95% of anemic women and 50% of anemic men. In male patients and the elderly, the source is typically occult bleeding from an underlying gastrointestinal lesion, which is identified in about half of cases. The prevalence of iron-deficiency anemia among premenopausal women is conservatively estimated to be 15%, rising to well over 30% during pregnancy. Even in menstruating women with iron deficiency, an underlying gastrointestinal lesion is not uncommon. Iron deficiency resulting from malabsorption may be the initial presentation of adult celiac disease. Among immigrants from impoverished countries, hookworm infestation is a leading malabsorptive cause of iron deficiency.

TABLE 79.1

DIFFERENTIAL DIAGNOSIS OF ANEMIA (REPRESENTATIVE ETIOLOGIES)

Microcytic (MCV <80 fL)
Iron deficiency
Anemia of chronic disease
Thalassemia trait
Sideroblastic anemia

Normocytic (MCV 80–100 fL)
Hemolysis
  Drug induced
  Autoimmune (idiopathic, collagen disease, lymphoma)
  Cold agglutinin induced (viral infection, lymphoma)
  Hemoglobinopathy (sickle cell disease, G-6-PD deficiency)
  Hereditary spherocytosis
  Microangiopathy (heart valve, jogging, vasculitis, DIC)
Anemia of chronic disease, including HIV infection
Renal failure
Hypothyroidism
Myelofibrosis
Early stage of iron deficiency
Sideroblastic anemia
Mixed anemia (e.g., iron and vitamin B_{12} deficiencies)

Macrocytic (MCV >100 fL)
Vitamin B_{12} deficiency
Folate deficiency
Aplastic anemia
Acute hemolysis or hemorrhage with brisk reticulocytosis
Chronic liver disease
Myelodysplastic syndromes
Hypothyroidism, severe

MCV, mean corpuscular volume; G-6-PD, glucose-6-phosphate dehydrogenase; DIC, dissented intravascular coagulation.

TABLE 79.2

CLASSIFICATION OF ANEMIAS BY USE OF DATA FROM AUTOMATED CYTOMETRY

MCV <80 fL: Microcytosis	MCV 80–100 fL: Normocytosis	MCV >100 fL: Macrocytosis
Low RDW		
Anemia of chronic disease	Hypoproliferation (e.g., renal failure)	Aplastic anemias
Most thalassemias	Hereditary spherocytosis	Myelodysplastic syndromes
	Anemia of chronic disease	
High RDW		
Iron deficiency	Sickle cell disease	Megaloblastic anemias
Sideroblastic anemia	Early iron deficiency	Acute hemolysis or hemorrhage
Hemoglobin H	Marrow infiltration	Liver disease
	Chronic hemolysis	

MCV, mean corpuscular volume; RDW, red cell distribution width.

Other common causes of anemia include vitamin B_{12} deficiency (nearly 10% of cases) and chronic disease (at least 5% of cases). Among the elderly, vitamin deficiencies are common, with folate deficiency accounting for about 15% of cases and vitamin B_{12} deficiency for about 10%.

WORKUP (1,2,4,7,9–14,16–18, 20,22–35)

Diagnosis and Morphologic Categorization of Anemia

The diagnosis of anemia is based on measurement of the *hematocrit* or the *hemoglobin concentration* of venous blood. Any abnormal test result needs to be repeated for confirmation before further evaluation is undertaken. Proper interpretation requires consideration of the patient's *intravascular volume status*. An overly expanded plasma volume will dilute the red cell mass and lead to a false-positive diagnosis. Conversely, dehydration can mask an underlying anemia.

Morphologic categorization helps to focus the subsequent evaluation, which proceeds according to whether the anemia is microcytic, macrocytic, or normocytic. Examination of the Wright-stained *peripheral blood smear* and determination of the *red cell indices* (mean corpuscular volume [MCV] and mean corpuscular hemoglobin concentration [MCHC]) with an autoanalyzer are the time-tested means of classifying anemias morphologically. Recent advances in flow cytometry have made possible an automated means of determining the degree of variability in size of a patient's red cells. This measure of anisocytosis is referred to as the *red cell distribution width*. Technically, the RDW is the coefficient of variation of cell volume; it serves as a means of detecting red cell heterogeneity, which could previously be done only by examination of the peripheral smear. Although examination of the Wright-stained smear still provides morphologic information unattainable from other sources, the combined use of the MCV and RDW for the initial classification of anemias markedly enhances interpretation (Table 79.2).

The peripheral smear and red cell indices should be analyzed together; they provide complementary information. Overdependence on machine-generated indices can lead to errors in diagnosis. For example, anemia resulting from deficiencies of both iron and vitamin B_{12} often produces a dimorphic population of microcytic and macrocytic red cells readily observed on peripheral smear, yet the electronically determined MCV will calculate the average size and erroneously suggest a normocytic type of anemia. Moreover, some vitamin B_{12}–deficient patients with normal ferritin levels have normocytic indices.

The Wright-stained smear can also mislead when used alone, and it often lacks sensitivity. Cells that are easily flattened out (as in liver disease) may appear larger on smear than they actually are; the MCV will give a more correct determination of size. The sensitivity of the smear in the detection of iron deficiency has been found to be as low as 49%.

The determination of red cell size on the peripheral smear is facilitated by using the nucleus of the mature small lymphocyte as a good reference standard for normal red cell diameter. One can also prepare a control smear of known blood to help judge abnormalities. Use of the MCV and appearance on peripheral smear serves to classify the anemia morphologically and facilitate evaluation.

Not all automatically determined cell indices have been found to be valuable. Careful studies suggest that the MCHC and the mean corpuscular hemoglobin add little to the evaluation of anemia, although the MCHC is still used as a means of quantifying the degree of hypochromia.

Workup by Morphologic Category: Microcytic Anemia

The basis for the classification of microcytosis is the presence of small red blood cells on smear and an *MCV of less than 80 fL*. A prime consideration should be iron deficiency and the important underlying conditions that might precipitate it, but thalassemia and anemia of chronic disease are also important to consider, as are sometimes sideroblastic anemias.

History and Physical Examination.

History should focus on any abnormal blood loss, change in bowel habits, melena, heavy use of aspirin or nonsteroidal antiinflammatory drugs, family history of anemia (especially in patients of Mediterranean descent), concurrent malignancy, HIV infection, symptoms of other chronic infections or chronic inflammatory disorders, number of pregnancies, pica, dysphagia, history of lead exposure, dietary iron intake, quantity of menstrual blood loss, gastric resection, changes in nails, and soreness of the tongue.

Physical examination includes checking for glossitis, cheilitis, koilonychia, lymphadenopathy, hepatosplenomegaly, rectal mass, stool positive for occult blood, pelvic mass, and other signs of chronic infectious, inflammatory, and neoplastic disorders.

Laboratory Studies

Laboratory studies usually allow one to differentiate iron-deficiency anemia, thalassemia, sideroblastic anemia, and anemia of chronic disease, although some overlap does occur and may cause confusion and wasteful expenditures if tests are not thoughtfully selected.

Testing for Iron Deficiency and Differentiating It from Anemia of Chronic Disease.   The definitive test is bone marrow iron stores, but because the test is invasive and painful, serum tests are used whenever possible.

Serum Ferritin.   The test of choice for the screening and diagnosis of iron deficiency is the serum *ferritin*. Ferritin is the storage protein for iron, which correlates best with marrow iron stores. Levels are somewhat higher in men than in women and increase gradually with advancing age. The test is highly sensitive and specific for the diagnosis of iron deficiency. For example, a serum concentration of less than 15 μg/L has a predictive value for iron deficiency of greater than 90% when the pretest probability is only 50%. A level greater than 100 μg/L virtually rules out the diagnosis.

There are some settings in which the sensitivity of the ferritin level may be compromised. Ferritin is an acute-phase reactant that increases in response to inflammatory disease or hepatocellular dysfunction, which potentially limits the sensitivity of this test. In addition, the test may be less sensitive in the elderly because ferritin levels increase with age and also with concurrent chronic and malignant disease (which are more common in this population). However, when the serum ferritin level is less than 50 μg/L in the setting of inflammatory or liver disease, the test retains much of its predictive value for iron deficiency. Levels between 50 and 100 μg/L constitute a diagnostic "gray zone," in which case careful attention to other clinical and laboratory data is required to obtain an accurate diagnosis.

Serum Iron, Total Iron-Binding Capacity, and Transferrin Saturation.   Serum iron, total iron-binding capacity (TIBC), and transferrin saturation (calculated as a percentage: [Fe/TIBC] × 100) have been traditional components of the workup for iron deficiency, but under most circumstances, they add little information beyond that obtained from the ferritin determination, and they lack its sensitivity or specificity. These tests need not be ordered routinely in patients with microcytic anemia. Nonetheless, a transferrin saturation of less than 16% has been used as a criterion for iron deficiency and to help to distinguish iron deficiency from anemia of chronic disease, both of which may cause a low serum iron. However, the specificity of the figure is limited because some patients with the anemia of chronic disease manifest similar reductions in transferrin saturation. Nonetheless, the more typical pattern for the anemia of chronic disease is a low iron level and low TIBC, in contrast to the low iron level and increased TIBC characteristic of iron deficiency. The RDW is almost always increased.

Therapeutic Trial of Iron.   A therapeutic trial of oral iron therapy can also be used in uncomplicated cases as a simple alternative to the determination of the ferritin level or an examination of the marrow. The reticulocyte count is monitored during a 7- to 10-day period. A significant increase in the reticulocyte count is strong evidence for the diagnosis of iron deficiency.

Transferrin Receptor Level.   Methods that overcome the limitations of standard blood tests have been sought. Serum levels of the *transferrin receptor* (a glycoprotein on cells requiring high levels of iron) correlate inversely with bone marrow iron stores. A *transferrin receptor–ferritin index* (transferrin receptor level/log of ferritin level) performed well in an experimental assessment of anemic elderly patients, demonstrating a sensitivity of 88% and a specificity of 93%, compared with a sensitivity of 16% and a specificity of 100% for standard tests.

Bone Marrow Aspiration.   Direct examination of a sample stained for *iron stores* remains the gold standard for the diagnosis of iron deficiency, but up to 20% of aspirates are unsatisfactory, yielding insufficient marrow stroma. Ferritin testing has all but eliminated the need for marrow aspiration in the diagnosis of iron deficiency, but the test is sometimes necessary in confusing cases.

Workup for the Underlying Etiology of Iron Deficiency.   When the cause of the iron deficiency is not evident, a workup for *gastrointestinal blood loss* is indicated. Idiopathic iron-deficiency anemia is associated with a gastrointestinal tract lesion in about one half to two thirds of cases. The most common upper gastrointestinal lesion is peptic ulcer; colon cancer is the leading colonic lesion in this setting. Site-specific symptoms are predictive of the location of the lesion, but patients may be asymptomatic. In asymptomatic patients, there is a high frequency of atrophic gastritis and *Helicobacter pylori* infection in those with no evidence of gastrointestinal blood loss, and colon cancer and peptic ulcer disease in those with guaiac-positive stools. Concomitant lesions are present in fewer than 1% of cases, so it is unnecessary to study both the upper and lower gastrointestinal tract if a likely source is found on the first examination.

Endoscopy is the test methodology of choice (see Chapter 63). Barium studies are considerably less sensitive, and their yield is nil in the setting of a negative endoscopic evaluation. The vast majority of patients with no detectable lesion on upper and lower gastrointestinal endoscopy have a favorable prognosis; most respond to iron therapy. Those who do not are likely to have an underlying medical illness. Menstruating women require workup just as do other patients; screening for occult gastrointestinal blood loss is particularly important. A positive fecal occult blood test result, hemoglobin less than 10 g/dL, and abdominal symptoms are predictive of the endoscopic finding of a gastrointestinal lesion in an anemic menstruating woman.

When iron *malabsorption* is suspected clinically (concurrent chronic diarrhea, guaiac-negative stools), consideration should be given to testing for *adult celiac disease (antiendomysial IgA antibodies, small-bowel biopsy;* see Chapter 64), *H. pylori infection,* and *atrophic gastritis (endoscopy;* see Chapter 68). If the patient is from an undeveloped country, checking the *stool* for evidence of hookworm *ova* and *parasites* is in order.

Testing for Thalassemia.   Once iron deficiency has been ruled out as the cause of microcytic anemia, the focus shifts to differentiating among anemia of chronic disease, thalassemia, and sideroblastic anemia. History is very important in this regard. A person of Mediterranean extraction without underlying chronic illness is likely to have thalassemia trait, which necessitates a look at the *peripheral smear* for abnormalities of red cell morphology (e.g., *target cells, poikilocytosis*) and a check of the *red cell indices* for *reduced MCHC* and *increased red cell count*. Determination of the *hemoglobin A2* level can confirm the diagnosis, but it may not be elevated if concurrent iron deficiency is present. A *hemoglobin electrophoresis* may be needed when thalassemia trait is suspected in an African American patient because hemoglobin A2 is not increased in α disease.

Differentiating Anemia of Chronic Disease from Sideroblastic Anemia. Once iron deficiency and thalassemia trait are deemed to be of low probability, then the task shifts to differentiating anemia of chronic disease from sideroblastic anemia. Here, the *serum iron* level and *TIBC* may help. In the anemia of chronic disease, the *serum iron* level and *transferrin saturation* are likely to be low normal or reduced, but *ferritin* is normal to increased. In sideroblastic anemia, high-normal to increased levels of iron, transferrin saturation, and ferritin are characteristic, suggesting a sideroblastic state in the absence of another reason for iron overload and the need for a bone marrow aspirate to search for ringed sideroblasts.

Workup by Morphologic Category: Macrocytic Anemia

The criteria for inclusion in this group are an MCV of greater than 100 fL, a normal MCHC, and the presence of macrocytes on smear. Often, the latter are hard to detect in mild cases. Marked macrocytosis (MCV >115 fL) identified electronically is associated with a high probability of folate or vitamin B_{12} deficiency, liver disease, or alcoholism accompanied by liver disease.

Megaloblastic versus Nonmegaloblastic

The first objective is to distinguish megaloblastic from nonmegaloblastic causes. The *peripheral smear* is the most helpful test. The presence of *hypersegmented polymorphonuclear leukocytes* (having nuclei with five or more lobes) is among the earliest and most specific signs of a megaloblastic anemia and is seen in more than 65% of cases. *Oval macrocytes* are also an early and characteristic finding but may be absent in the setting of concurrent iron deficiency. An increase in hypersegmented polymorphonuclear leukocytes can be screened for by counting the number of neutrophils with five or more lobes in a routine 100-cell differential. Finding three neutrophils with five lobes or even one with six is strong presumptive evidence for megaloblastic anemia.

Bone marrow aspiration may be needed in confusing situations (such as differentiating a sideroblastic anemia from a truly megaloblastic type, or searching for megaloblastic changes in a patient with a low-normal vitamin B_{12} level), but a peripheral smear suffices in most instances. It must be remembered that megaloblastic marrow changes can revert to normal within 12 to 24 hours of therapy, and thus treatment should be delayed if marrow examination is anticipated. However, neutrophil hypersegmentation may persist for up to 2 weeks after the initiation of vitamin replacement.

Folate versus Vitamin B_{12} Deficiency

Once a megaloblastic anemia has been identified, the focus shifts to folate versus vitamin B_{12} deficiency. History and physical examination can give important clues. A history of gastric surgery, inflammatory bowel disease, Hashimoto's thyroiditis, vitiligo, or raw-fish intake (fish tapeworm) may provide the substrate for vitamin B_{12} deficiency. Neuropsychiatric symptoms and signs in addition to those of subacute combined system disease further suggest vitamin B_{12} deficiency, as do the findings of glossitis and diarrhea. Alcoholism, poor nutrition, pregnancy, blood dyscrasias, sprue, severe psoriasis, and anticonvulsant intake suggest folate lack. Antimetabolite therapy with folate antagonists such as methotrexate can cause a megaloblastic picture with normal serum folate levels.

Serum Vitamin B_{12}. Vitamin B_{12} determination can be very helpful, but a number of pitfalls are encountered in interpreting the results. The bioassay for vitamin B_{12} is affected by recent antibiotic intake. Assays in which radioactive cobalt or immunologic techniques are used are not affected. However, up to one third of patients with documented pernicious anemia will have vitamin B_{12} levels greater than 100 ng/L (the often-cited cutoff for diagnosis). Persistence in pursuing the diagnosis is necessary when clinical suspicion is high. Vitamin B_{12} levels may be artificially low in patients with folate deficiency alone; folate and vitamin B_{12} levels must always be measured together.

Methylmalonic Acid and Total Homocysteine. Serum measurements of methylmalonic acid and total homocysteine enhance the sensitivity of diagnostic testing for vitamin B_{12} deficiency and are helpful in cases in which the serum vitamin B_{12} or folate result is confusing. Both folate and vitamin B_{12} are needed for the conversion of homocysteine to methionine. In both folate and vitamin B_{12} deficiency, homocysteine is increased, but only in vitamin B_{12} deficiency is methylmalonate increased; however, renal insufficiency can also increase methylmalonic acid levels.

Folic Acid Determination. The *serum folate* level provides a seemingly straightforward means of detecting folate deficiency. However, even in deficiency states, the recent intake of green vegetables can cause a false rise in the serum folate level and compromise test sensitivity. Falsely low levels can occur after a few days of low dietary folate intake, intermittent heavy alcohol intake, or the use of anticonvulsant or antineoplastic agents. Concomitant measurement of serum and *red cell folate* can help to establish the diagnosis of a true folate deficiency because erythrocyte folate levels are better indicators of total body folic acid stores. However, erythrocyte folate may be normal in early folate deficiency, concomitant iron deficiency, and thalassemia. An alternative to serum testing is a therapeutic trial of folate replacement (provided there is no concurrent B_{12} deficiency, which could be masked and exacerbated by the folate replacement and harm the patient; see next paragraph).

Empiric Trial of Replacement Therapy. An empiric means of determining vitamin B_{12} or folate deficiency is to conduct a *therapeutic trial* of replacement therapy. Such a trial is appropriate when serum assays are unavailable or the results are equivocal. The hematocrit and reticulocyte counts are measured twice before administration, then followed every few days for up to 10 days after a small but effective dose of vitamin B_{12} (e.g., 100 μg intramuscularly [IM]) or folate (1 mg IM) has been given. The trial result is positive if a significant rise in reticulocyte count occurs within 10 days. It is important to use only small folate doses in such trials. Large folate doses can transiently and nonspecifically improve the hematologic picture in a patient with vitamin B_{12} deficiency and lead to its progression by increasing the demand for folate, obscuring the diagnosis and delaying detection and treatment. Thus, a trial of folate replacement for diagnosis should only occur after it is established that there is no concurrent B_{12} deficiency.

Determining the Cause of Vitamin B_{12} Deficiency

To distinguish vitamin B_{12} deficiency caused by malabsorption from that caused by lack of intrinsic factor, an *oral Schilling test* with and without intrinsic factor is used. An unlabeled IM dose of 1,000 μg of vitamin B_{12} is given to saturate binding sites. Then an oral dose of radioactive vitamin B_{12} without intrinsic factor is given, and both urine and plasma samples are taken to determine the amount of vitamin B_{12} absorbed. The test is repeated with the addition of intrinsic factor. In malabsorptive states, no improvement will occur with intrinsic factor, whereas it will in pernicious anemia. One difficulty with the test is that vitamin B_{12} deficiency can cause malabsorption, which confuses test interpretation. Thus, the test should be postponed until the deficiency is corrected. In addition, sensitivity is not very high; false-negative results occur in up to 40% of cases. The commonly used double-isotope method of performing the Schilling test (labeled free cobalamin and labeled cobalamin bound to intrinsic factor are administered at the same time) often produces false-negative results. The Schilling test is not helpful for detecting food-cobalamin malabsorption. Such patients have a normal test result because the test uses free cobalamin and does not assay the ability to split cobalamin from food.

Two other tests can improve the diagnostic accuracy and yield in cases of suspected pernicious anemia. Testing for *anti-intrinsic factor antibody* provides a highly specific approach to diagnosis. The test helps to confirm the presence of pernicious anemia; specificity is high so long as no vitamin B_{12} is injected within 48 hours of testing; sensitivity is only modest (60% to 70%). Determination of the *serum gastrin* level may also be helpful because it is elevated in more than 80% of cases. *Antiparietal cell antibodies* are present in more than 90% of cases, but the false-positive rate can be as high as 10% to 30%.

If pernicious anemia is found, *endoscopic examination* of the stomach is indicated because of the increased risk for gastric cancer and carcinoid tumors; thyroid function needs to be assayed by the determination of the thyroid-stimulating hormone level.

Nonmegaloblastic Macrocytic Anemias

These can be divided into subgroups according to whether marrow activity is increased, normal, or decreased. To make this determination, a *reticulocyte count* is obtained. (A normal value is 0.8% to 2.5% in male patients and 0.8% to 4.1% in female patients; correction for anemia is made by multiplying the reticulocyte count by the hematocrit and dividing the result by 0.45.) Reticulocytes are increased by hemorrhage or hemolysis; in the absence of overt bleeding, a workup for hemolysis is indicated (see later discussion). Low-normal or decreased counts occur in myxedema and chronic liver disease and are indications for performing thyroid and liver function studies (see Chapters 71 and 104). Marked reductions may occur in myelophthisic states and sideroblastic anemia. The patient should be questioned and examined carefully for symptoms of any of these conditions, and the smear should be studied again for teardrop and fragmented forms and for sideroblasts, respectively. A *bone marrow biopsy* is indicated when a sideroblastic anemia or a myelophthisic process is a concern; aspiration of the marrow may yield only a dry tap and is insufficient.

Workup by Morphologic Category: Normochromic–Normocytic Anemia

This category encompasses a diverse group of conditions that can be classified according to the marrow response, manifested by the *reticulocyte count*.

Elevated Reticulocyte Count: Workup for Hemolysis

If no evidence of recent brisk bleeding is present, then hemolysis and its precipitants require consideration. The history is reviewed thoroughly for medications (e.g., penicillins, cephalosporins, macrolides, tetracyclines, sulfa drugs, quinidine, methyldopa); symptoms of sickle cell disease (e.g., fever and attacks of chest, musculoskeletal, and abdominal pain); a family history of anemia; symptoms of a viral infection (mononucleosis, cytomegalovirus infection, viral hepatitis); lymphoproliferative disease; and systemic lupus. During the physical examination, the patient is checked for splenomegaly and signs of an underlying viral, lymphoproliferative, or connective tissue disease (see Chapters 12, 84, and 146).

The laboratory assessment includes a check of hemolytic indices: *bilirubin, haptoglobin,* and *lactic dehydrogenase.* Haptoglobin is the most sensitive but least specific because it is an acute-phase reactant. Lactic dehydrogenase and unconjugated bilirubin are less sensitive but more specific for significant hemolysis. In a patient taking a potentially offending drug, a *direct Coombs' test* should be undertaken to assess the possibility of drug-related hemolysis. A drug-related or infection-related episode in an African American patient should also raise the question of glucose-6-phosphatase deficiency, especially when the drug is a sulfonamide or an antimalarial. An African American patient presenting with painful episodes of hemolysis should have a smear examined and a *hemoglobin electrophoresis* obtained, and a *metabisulfite test* for sickling of red cells should be performed. If an underlying lymphoproliferative disorder or connective tissue disease is detected, then consideration of an immune hemolytic anemia is appropriate, and a sampling of the blood for *IgG autoantibodies* is indicated. Concurrent viral infection or lymphoproliferative disease raises the question of an IgM-based hemolytic process and the need to check *cold hemagglutinin* levels. Bone marrow examination in cases of suspected hemolysis is unnecessary.

Reticulocyte Count Reduced or Not Appropriately Elevated: Workup for Metabolic Disease and Anemia of Chronic Disease

A metabolic basis of marrow suppression is suggested by this presentation. Causes that require consideration include *renal failure, myxedema, Addison's disease,* and *alcoholic liver disease.* Even early forms of *vitamin B_{12} deficiency* and *iron deficiency* may present with relatively normal red cell indices, as can *the anemia of chronic disease,* so they also must be checked for (see prior discussions).

Reticulocyte Count Nil: Workup for Aplastic Anemia

A very low or absent reticulocyte count suggests an aplastic anemia, especially if it is accompanied by evidence of pancytopenia on the peripheral smear and cell counts. A history of drug use (e.g., chloramphenicol, phenylbutazone, antimetabolites, gold, zidovudine, pentamidine), toxin exposure (benzene, insecticides), or recent viral illness may provide a clue to the cause. In the majority of instances, the history is unrevealing. *Bone marrow biopsy* is indicated if the condition persists after all drugs are halted. The finding of fatty marrow on biopsy strongly suggests marrow aplasia. The causes of the marrow hypocellularity range from aplastic anemia to a host of other conditions that need to be considered, including paroxysmal nocturnal hemoglobinuria, myelodysplasia, preleukemia phases of acute myelogenous leukemia, and lymphocytic leukemia. *Cytogenetic testing* is often performed to help in the differentiation when it is difficult to do so morphologically (e.g., chromosomes are typically normal in aplastic anemia and abnormal in myelodysplastic syndromes).

SYMPTOMATIC THERAPY (12)

Few patients who present with an anemia of gradual onset require immediate correction of the anemia, but anemia can have an adverse impact on quality of life and does deserve treatment. The one exception to the lack of need for immediate treatment is the patient with significant cardiopulmonary disease, who may be compromised by a decrease in oxygen-carrying capacity (i.e., hematocrit <30%). In almost all other instances, evaluation should proceed in an orderly manner, and therapy should be withheld until a specific diagnosis can be made and a specific therapy can be implemented (see Chapter 82). The exception to this rule is the use of therapy as a diagnostic trial (e.g., vitamin B_{12} replacement). All too common is the practice of simultaneously prescribing multiple hematinics, which obscures important findings and the detection of serious underlying disease. The elderly and other patients with limited cardiopulmonary reserve should be admitted for inpatient evaluation and consideration of transfusion therapy when they are experiencing dyspnea, angina, or marked fatigue because of their anemia.

PATIENT EDUCATION

Many patients believe that anemia is caused by a vitamin deficiency or iron deficiency and consequently attempt self-treatment before they see a physician. Others request vitamin therapy. A common error among both patients and physicians is to attribute symptoms of depression, such as fatigue and listlessness, to an underlying anemia. Unless the hematocrit is well less than 30% or the patient has very little cardiopulmonary reserve, this attribution is unjustified (see Chapter 8). Finally, the patient needs to be told to what extent the anemia accounts for symptoms, what the possible causes are, and what the appropriate workup will be.

RECOMMENDATIONS

All Cases

- Classify the anemia, and conduct the workup on the basis of a peripheral smear and MCV: The anemia is microcytic if MCV is less than 82 fL and red cells are small, macrocytic if MCV is greater than 95 fL and red cells are large, and normocytic if MCV is between 82 and 95 fL and red cells are normal in size.

Microcytic Anemia

- Test first for iron deficiency. Obtain a serum ferritin—the test of choice for iron deficiency. One need not order a serum iron or TIBC for a diagnosis of iron deficiency unless there is reason to suspect that the ferritin may be elevated as a con-

sequence of acute inflammation. If iron deficiency is found but its cause is not evident, begin a search of the gastrointestinal tract for a source of occult blood loss (see Chapter 63).
- If iron deficiency is ruled out, assess for thalassemia. Check for Mediterranean extraction and family history of anemia or thalassemia. Examine the peripheral smear and red cell indices for characteristic manifestations (e.g., target cells, teardrops, increased red cell count, reduced MCHC), and consider testing for hemoglobin A2 level.
- If iron deficiency and thalassemia have been ruled out, obtain a transferrin saturation and ferritin level to help to differentiate anemia of chronic disease from sideroblastic anemia. If both are elevated, then consider a bone marrow aspirate to check for ringed sideroblasts. If the transferrin saturation is low and ferritin is increased, then this suggests anemia of chronic disease and no need for bone marrow study.

Macrocytic Anemia

- Examine the peripheral smear for hypersegmented polymorphonuclear leukocytes and oval macrocytes. If they are present, obtain serum vitamin B_{12} and folate levels.
- If the serum vitamin levels are not diagnostic, serum homocysteine and methylmalonate levels enhance diagnostic sensitivity; alternatively, perform a diagnostic trial with a small dose of vitamin B_{12} or folate, monitoring the reticulocyte count. If a folate trial is contemplated, be sure that the patient does not have concurrent B_{12} deficiency before giving folate.
- If vitamin B_{12} deficiency is detected, consider a Schilling test to differentiate lack of intrinsic factor from malabsorption.
- If the macrocytic anemia is nonmegaloblastic, obtain a reticulocyte count, and examine the peripheral smear to determine whether marrow activity is increased, normal, or decreased.
- If the reticulocyte count is high in the absence of hemorrhage, check for hemolysis; if it is normal or slightly reduced, consider hepatic and thyroid dysfunction; if it is markedly reduced, review the peripheral smear for teardrops and ringed sideroblasts, and consider bone marrow biopsy.

Normocytic Anemia

- Check the reticulocyte count, and determine whether it is elevated, inappropriately normal or low, or nil. If the count is elevated, evaluate for evidence of recent hemorrhage; if none, confirm hemolysis with haptoglobin, bilirubin, and lactate dehydrogenase determinations.
- If hemolysis is confirmed, check for a drug-induced cause (direct Coombs' test), an autoimmune type (IgG or cold agglutinins), or a hemoglobinopathy (sickle cell disease, glucose-6-phosphatase deficiency).
- If the reticulocyte count is low or not appropriately elevated, search for underlying hepatocellular, endocrine, and renal failure (see Chapters 71, 104, and 142, respectively) and for early iron-deficiency anemia and anemia of chronic disease (see prior discussions).
  If the reticulocyte count is nil in the setting of pancytopenia, teardrop forms, and fragmented cells, then halt all potentially offending medications; if that does not result in a prompt restoration of marrow function, order a bone marrow biopsy.

A.H.G.

Annotated Bibliography

1. Annibale B, Capurso G, Chistolini A, et al. Gastrointestinal causes of refractory iron deficiency anemia in patients without gastrointestinal symptoms. Am J Med 2001;111:439. (*A cohort study of asymptomatic patients, finding a high frequency of atrophic gastritis and Helicobacter pylori infection in those with no evidence of gastrointestinal blood loss, and colon cancer and peptic ulcer disease in those with gastrointestinal blood loss.*)

2. Astor BC, Muntner P, Levin A, et al. Association of kidney function with anemia: the Third National Health and Nutrition Examination survey (1988–1994). Arch Intern Med 2002;162:1401. (*An epidemiologic study, finding that there was a high prevalence of anemia when the glomerular filtration rate fell to <60 mL/min.*)

3. Beghe C, Wilson A, Ershler WB. Prevalence and outcomes of anemia in geriatrics: a systematic review of the literature. Am J Med 2004;116(7A):3S. (*A review, finding that the incidence increases with age and there is an association with heart failure, weakness, falls, and depression; 43 references.*)

4. Beutler E. Glucose-6-phosphate dehydrogenase deficiency. N Engl J Med 1991;324:169. (*An authoritative review; 85 references.*)

5. Bunn HF. Pathogenesis and treatment of sickle cell disease. N Engl J Med 1997;337:762. (*One in a series of excellent reviews of basic mechanisms and their implications for treatment.*)

6. Carmel R. Prevalence of undiagnosed pernicious anemia in the elderly. Arch Intern Med 1996;156:1097. (*The prevalence was found to be nearly 3% in the diverse sample studied.*)

7. Carmel R. Pernicious anemia. The expected findings of very low serum cobalamin levels, anemia, and macrocytosis are often lacking. Arch Intern Med 1988;148:1712. (*The title says it all.*)

8. Committee on Iron Deficiency. Iron deficiency in the United States. JAMA 1968;203:407. (*A classic paper on natural history and epidemiology that is still useful.*)

9. Corazza GR, Valentini RA, Andreani ML, et al. Subclinical coeliac disease is a frequent cause of iron-deficiency anemia. Scand J Gastroenterol 1995;30:153. (*The condition was found in 5% of patients in this population presenting with iron deficiency; makes the point that this may be the presenting manifestation.*)

10. Forman SJ. Myelodysplastic syndrome. Curr Opin Hematol 1996;3:297. (*A useful review of classification and diagnosis.*)

11. Izaks GJ, Westendorp RGJ, Knook DL. The definition of anemia in older persons. JAMA 1999;281:1714. (*A community-based study, finding that a reduced hemoglobin concentration is predictive of underlying illness.*)

12. Nissenson AR, Goodnough LT. Anemia: not just an innocent bystander? Arch Intern Med 2003;163:1400. (*A review of the prevalence and consequences of anemia.*)

13. Olivieri NF. The beta-thalassemias. N Engl J Med 1999;341:99. (*A definitive review; 120 references.*)

14. Scadden DT, Zon LI, Groopman JE, et al. Pathophysiology and management of HIV-associated hematologic disorders. Blood 1989;74:1455. (*An excellent review of this increasingly important cause of anemia.*)

15. Serjeant GR, Ceulaer CD, Lethbridge R, et al. The painful crisis of homozygous sickle cell disease: clinical features. Br J Haematol 1994;87:568. (*One of the best systematic studies of the condition, finding that skin cooling was a perceived precipitant, and that low-grade fever was common.*)

16. Toh B-H, van Driel IR, Gleeson PA. Pernicious anemia. N Engl J Med 1997;337:1441. (*An authoritative review of pathophysiology.*)

17. Tudhope G, Wilson G. Anemia in hypothyroidism. Q J Med 1960;29:513. (*A classic study of 116 cases of hypothyroidism, finding anemia in >30%; pernicious anemia occurred in 7%.*)

18. Weiss G, Goodnough LT. Anemia of chronic disease. N Engl J Med 2005;352:1011. (*A comprehensive review of pathophysiology, diagnosis, and treatment; 96 references.*)

19. Wood M, Elwood P. Symptoms of iron deficiency anemia: a community survey. Br J Prev Soc Med 1966;20:117. (*In the 295 patients studied, little correlation was found between symptoms and serum hemoglobin concentration.*)

20. Young NS. Acquired aplastic anemia. Ann Intern Med 2002;136:534. (*A comprehensive review; 62 references.*)

21. Tefferi A. Anemia in adults: a contemporary approach to diagnosis. Mayo Clin Proc 2003;78:1274. (*An updated look at classification and differential diagnosis.*)

22. Bini EJ, Micale PL, Weinshel EH. Evaluation of the gastrointestinal tract in premenopausal women with iron deficiency anemia. Am J Med 1998;105:281. (*A positive fecal occult blood test result, a hemoglobin level <10 g/dL, and the presence of abdominal symptoms were predictive of finding a gastrointestinal lesion endoscopically.*)

23. Crosby WH. Reticulocyte count. Arch Intern Med 1981;141:1747. (*A detailed discussion of this important test and its clinical significance.*)

24. Edwin E. The segmentation of polymorphonuclear neutrophils in hypovitaminosis B12. Acta Med Scand 1967;182:401. (*A classic article, finding that 64% of patients exhibited hypersegmentation on smear; presents a good discussion of errors in counting lobes.*)

25. Gulati FL, Hyun BH. The automated CBC. A current perspective. Hematol Oncol Clin North Am 1994;8:593. (*A review of the technical and performance characteristics of these measurements, with implications for their clinical use.*)

26. Guyatt GH, Oxman AD, Ali M, et al. Laboratory diagnosis of iron-deficiency anemia. J Gen Intern Med 1992;7:145. (*A detailed literature review, concluding that ferritin is the test of choice; 73 references.*)

27. Kis AM, Carnes M. Detecting iron deficiency in anemic patients with concomitant medical problems. J Gen Intern Med 1998;13:455. (*A ferritin level of <100 μg/L is best for detection in the context of inflammation, infection, or malignancy.*)

28. Old JM. Screening and genetic diagnosis of haemoglobin disorders. Blood Rev 2003;17:43. (*A useful review of the details of workup.*)

29. Rimon E, Levy S, Sapir A, et al. Diagnosis of iron deficiency anemia in the elderly by transferring receptor–ferritin index. Arch Intern Med 2002;162:445. (*A proposed index for improving the diagnosis of iron deficiency in the elderly.*)

30. Robinson AR, Mladenovic J. Lack of clinical utility of folate levels in the evaluation of macrocytosis or anemia. Am J Med 2001;110:88. (*A provocative retrospective study, finding low sensitivity and little impact on care; the authors suggest an empiric trial of folate as a better approach to diagnosis.*)

31. Rockey DC, Cello JP. Evaluation of the gastrointestinal tract in patients with iron-deficiency anemia. N Engl J Med 1993;320:1691. (*A prospective study, finding that there was a high prevalence of gastrointestinal lesions, site-specific symptoms were predictive of location, and concomitant lesions were rare.*)

32. Stabler SP, Marcell PD, Podell ER, et al. Elevation of total homocysteine in the serum of patients with cobalamin or folate deficiency detected by chromatography–mass spectrometry. J Clin Invest 1988;81:466. (*Discusses the utility of measuring homocysteine levels.*)

33. Thompson WG, Babitz L, Cassino C, et al. Evaluation of current criteria used to measure vitamin B12 levels. Am J Med 1987;82:291. (*The use of a mean corpuscular volume >95 fL or a vitamin B12 level <100 pg/mL may lead to false-negative results.*)

34. Van der Weyden M, Rother M, Firkin B. Metabolic significance of reduced B12 in folate deficiency. Blood 1972;40:23. (*A classic report, showing that low B12 levels are found in folate deficiency, and that the level is moderately reduced and improves with folate replacement, which can mask B12 deficiency.*)

35. Wilcox CM, Alexander LN, Clark WS. Prospective evaluation of the gastrointestinal tract in patients with iron deficiency and no systemic or gastrointestinal symptoms or signs. Am J Med 1997;103:405. (*Half of the patients were found to have an underlying lesion; prognosis was good if none were found.*)

CHAPTER 80 ■ EVALUATION OF ERYTHROCYTOSIS (POLYCYTHEMIA)

When an elevated red cell count, hemoglobin concentration, or hematocrit occurs unexpectedly, it raises the question of *polycythemia*, a term used to denote an absolute increase in circulating red cell mass (some use the term *erythrocytosis* for all increases in red cell mass except those with an autonomous etiology). The upper limit of normal for a hematocrit is 52% for men and 47% for women. In the context of marked dehydration or severe chronic lung disease, the elevation may come as no surprise. In the absence of obvious concurrent disease, a search for an important underlying illness (e.g., polycythemia vera, occult malignancy, right-to-left shunt, hemoglobinopathy) is warranted. The finding may even be spurious because of volume contraction. In most instances, the primary physician should be able to distinguish among the variety of causes on clinical grounds, aided by a few simple laboratory studies.

PATHOPHYSIOLOGY AND CLINICAL PRESENTATION (1–12)

An absolute increase in red cell mass may represent abnormal stem cell proliferation (as in polycythemia vera), a response to chronic hypoxemia (as in chronic lung disease), or a manifestation of renal disease or extrarenal malignancy.

Polycythemia Vera

Pathophysiology and Genetics

Polycythemia vera is one of the *chronic myeloproliferative disorders* (the others being *essential thrombocythemia* and *myelofibrosis* with myeloid metaplasia). It affects all marrow elements as a consequence of clonal proliferation of a multipotent hematopoietic stem cell. Genetic mutations in chromosome 9p have been observed. The majority of patients exhibit the V617F somatic mutation in the Janus kinase (JAK) gene, producing a cytoplasmic kinase causing cytokine-independent proliferation of marrow cell lines. The affected stem cells can proliferate in the absence of erythropoietin, but they also demonstrate hypersensitivity to it and other growth factors. Not only is red cell mass increased, but so are leukocyte and platelet counts; however, thrombopoietin levels are normal or increased despite the increase in platelets, due to an error in the normal feedback mechanism. Besides increases in numbers of all three marrow elements, other hematologic manifestations include *extramedullary hematopoiesis*, *splenomegaly*, *hyperuricemia*, a *hypercellular bone marrow*, an increased risk of *thrombosis*, and progression to *myelofibrosis* with *myeloid metaplasia*.

The V617F mutation is also found in persons with other myeloproliferative disorders, including acute myeloid leukemia. Most homozygous patients exhibit polycythemia vera or myelofibrosis; those with essential thrombocythemia usually do not, but a subset with JAK 12 exon mutations may develop V617F-negative polycythemia.

Clinical Presentation and Course

Population-based studies found an incidence in the United States of 2.3 per 100,000. The prevalence is higher because survival is prolonged in the majority of patients. The peak age at onset is 50 to 60 years. Some patients have a relatively benign course, with red cell volume controlled by occasional phlebotomy, but others experience a much more malignant illness characterized by recurrent thrombosis and evolution toward *myeloid metaplasia*, *myelofibrosis*, and *acute leukemia*. Population-based study suggested that the risks of progression and hematologic complications are low. Prior exposure to myelosuppressive therapy (see later discussion) is a risk factor for malignant transformation.

It is not surprising that the presence of true polycythemia is often unsuspected because symptoms develop gradually and are frequently vague and rather nonspecific. In early stages, the patient may be entirely asymptomatic, with an elevated hematocrit as the only manifestation. As the disease progresses, the white blood cell (WBC) and platelet counts also increase, and symptoms and signs ensue as the red cell volume expands. Most symptoms are attributable to *hyperviscosity*, *hypervolemia*, and the resultant sluggish blood flow, which develop when the hematocrit increases to greater than 55%. Disturbed hemostasis ensues, exacerbated by defective platelet function.

Patients may present with either *thrombosis* (often in uncommon sites, such as hepatic, mesenteric, or retinal veins) or *bleeding* in the form of epistaxis, menorrhagia, easy bruisability, or oozing from the gums. The patient with advancing disease has a deep red appearance; peripheral cyanosis and ecchymoses may be noted. Blood pressure is usually normal, but *neurologic symptoms* are common (e.g., headache, dizziness, vertigo, tinnitus, "fullness" of the head, and blurred vision). Patients may complain of angina pectoris or claudication when coexisting atherosclerotic disease is present. Generalized *weakness*, fatigue, sweating, and lassitude are frequently reported. Gastrointestinal complaints may predominate (e.g., fullness, belching, epigastric or left upper quadrant discomfort); hepatomegaly is present in 40% of cases and *splenomegaly* in 70%. A classic symptom is *pruritus* after bathing, believed to be caused by abnormal histamine release. In addition, gouty joint symptoms occur in the context of marked secondary hyperuricemia caused by increased cell turnover.

Typically, the serum hemoglobin concentration is greater than 18.5 g/dL in men and greater than 16.5 g/dL in women, or an unexplained increase in hemoglobin concentration of 2 g/dL is present. In about 60% to 70% of cases, the WBC count increases to greater than 12,000/mm^3. More than half of patients experience an increased platelet count. The red cells appear normochromic and normocytic unless iron deficiency develops, in which case the red cells may appear microcytic and hypochromic. The erythrocyte sedimentation rate is frequently very low. *Erythropoietin* levels are never elevated (in contrast to erythropoietin levels in other forms of polycythemia) and are often low. Leukocyte alkaline phosphatase concentrations are increased in 80% of cases, as are vitamin B_{12} levels, a consequence of an increase in vitamin B_{12}-binding proteins.

Reactive Erythrocytosis (Secondary Polycythemia)

Chronic hypoxemia triggers *erythropoietin* production, which in turn stimulates the marrow production of red cells. The increase is usually an appropriate physiologic response to tissue hypoxia and occurs when the arterial oxygen tension (PaO_2) continually decreases to less than 55 mm Hg or, more precisely, when the arterial oxygen saturation (SaO_2) decreases to less than 92%. Residence at a *high altitude* and *severe pulmonary disease* are common causes of chronic hypoxemia. Other etiologies include *cyanotic heart disease* with right-to-left shunt, heavy cigarette *smoking* (associated with excessive levels of carboxyhemoglobin), and a *hemoglobin variant* that poorly releases oxygen to tissues.

Pathologic Secondary Erythrocytosis

When *erythropoietin* production is increased in the absence of tissue hypoxemia, then pathologic secondary polycythemia may ensue. Renal disease and a host of extrarenal malignancies have been implicated. Such instances of inappropriate erythropoietin production are unusual, but their occurrence can be an early clue of underlying disease. In about 1% to 3% of *renal cell carcinomas*, erythrocytosis is a manifestation, occurring at a time when cure is possible. *Focal glomerulonephritis*, *hydronephrosis*, *renal artery stenosis*, and *polycystic kidney diseases* are occasionally associated with elevations in erythropoietin and erythrocytosis. The mechanism is believed to involve a reduction in blood flow to renal tissue involved in erythropoietin production. Huge *uterine myomas*, *cerebellar hemangiomas*, and *hepatomas* are also causes, although the mechanisms are unclear; up to 10% of patients with hepatoma in one series had erythrocytosis. In rare instances, an increase in circulating *androgens* is associated with polycythemia.

Relative (Spurious) Erythrocytosis

Relative spurious erythrocytosis is a term that denotes a heterogeneous set of conditions, characterized by an increase in hematocrit without an increase in red cell mass. The most common and usually self-evident cause is *dehydration*. The situation is more controversial with regard to a group of patients who appear to have a normal to increased erythrocyte mass and a low to normal plasma volume (also referred to as *Gaisböck's syndrome* or *stress erythrocytosis*). There is some debate on the actual existence of such a state, but it has been reported in obese, tobacco-smoking, middle-aged, hypertensive men. Such men manifest an increased risk for thromboembolization.

DIFFERENTIAL DIAGNOSIS (2,12)

Patients with erythrocytosis can be separated on the basis of their underlying pathophysiology into three diagnostic categories: (a) polycythemia vera, (b) secondary erythrocytosis, and (c) relative (spurious) erythrocytosis. Secondary erythrocyto-

TABLE 80.1

DIFFERENTIAL DIAGNOSIS OF POLYCYTHEMIA

Polycythemia Vera
  Secondary polycythemia
    Physiologic (systemic hypoxia)
      High altitude
      Right-to-left shunt
      Heavy smoking
      Severe pulmonary disease
      Abnormal hemoglobin with high O_2 affinity
    Pathologic (no systemic hypoxia)
      Renal cell carcinoma
      Uterine myoma
      Cerebellar hemangioma
      Hepatoma
      Hydronephrosis
      Cystic kidney disease
      Renal artery stenosis
Relative Polycythemia
  Marked volume depletion
    Protracted vomiting
    Persistent diarrhea
    Excessive diuretic use
    Renal
  High to normal erythrocyte mass, low to normal volume: hypertensive, obese, middle-aged, male smoker

sis can be subdivided into physiologic and pathologic varieties (Table 80.1).

WORKUP (2,4,7,8,12–15)

The cause of erythrocytosis can usually be identified clinically with the aid of a few well-selected laboratory tests. The first task is to rule out decreased plasma volume and then to determine whether the true increase in hematocrit is a physiologic response or a pathologic process.

History

The history should first be checked for risk factors for volume depletion (e.g., diuretic use, vomiting, diarrhea) and for precipitants of chronic hypoxemia (e.g., residence at a high altitude, known cyanotic heart disease, smoking more than two packs per day, chronic lung disease). Inquiry into a familial occurrence of polycythemia helps to identify an abnormal hemoglobin, and a history of renal disease is also useful for the recognition of pathologic secondary erythrocytosis. Important clues for polycythemia vera are easy bruising, bleeding, and thrombosis, especially if the clotting involves an unusual site (e.g., retina, hepatic or portal vein, mesenteric vasculature). Symptoms of hyperviscosity should be reviewed, although most are nonspecific (e.g., lassitude, headache, sweating). It is common to ask about pruritus worsened by bathing, a classic symptom of polycythemia vera. Any report of abdominal discomfort should be noted because it might be a manifestation of the organomegaly associated with polycythemia vera.

Physical Examination

Postural signs should be checked for evidence of volume depletion (see Chapter 24). The integument is noted for plethora, cyanosis, clubbing, and ecchymoses. A comprehensive cardiopulmonary examination is essential and should include a search for signs of chronic lung disease (see Chapter 40), structural heart disease with a right-to-left shunt (see Chapter 21), hepatic enlargement, splenomegaly, and abdominal and pelvic masses. Splenomegaly can be an important clue for polycythemia vera because it is not found in most other forms of erythrocytosis; however, its absence does not rule out the diagnosis, particularly in the early phases of the disease.

Laboratory Evaluation

Testing should begin with a *complete blood cell count*, *platelet count*, and *peripheral blood smear examination* because two thirds of patients with polycythemia vera have an elevated WBC count (usually to 12,000 to 25,000/mm^3 and occasionally 50,000 to 100,000/mm^3), with increased numbers of immature forms and basophils; moreover, half have elevated platelet counts in the range of 450,000 to 1 million/mm^3. Large, bizarre platelets and megakaryocytic fragments may be seen on the blood smear. In polycythemia vera, cell morphology becomes abnormal with the progression of disease. For example, in the setting of myeloid metaplasia, anisocytosis and poikilocytosis with teardrop forms, ovalocytes, elliptocytes, and nucleated red blood cells may be seen. A microcytic, hypochromic smear may be noted if concurrent iron deficiency is present (found in about 10% of cases and sometimes obscuring the diagnosis). In secondary and spurious forms of erythrocytosis, the WBC count, platelet count, and blood smear are normal, which helps to differentiate these conditions from polycythemia vera.

Distinguishing Polycythemia Vera from Pathologic Secondary Erythrocytosis

The *traditional consensus diagnostic criteria* for polycythemia vera were (a) an elevated total red cell volume, a normal arterial oxygen saturation, and splenomegaly; or (b) in the absence of splenomegaly, an elevation in at least two of the following: *platelet count* (>400,000/mm^3), *WBC count* (>12,000/mm^3), *leukocyte alkaline phosphatase level*, *serum B$_{12}$ level*, or unbound *B$_{12}$-binding capacity*. However, the lack of specificity of these criteria has led to the development of additional diagnostic tests to confirm the diagnosis. Such testing can be expensive and should be limited to patients with a reasonable pretest probability of having the disease (e.g., manifesting at least one or two of the characteristic features in addition to an elevated hematocrit, such as generalized pruritus after bathing, splenomegaly, persistent leukocytosis, persistent thrombocytosis, or atypical thrombosis).

Traditionally, either direct measurement of *red cell mass* or an estimation based on *red cell volume* was considered necessary for diagnosis; however, this measurement is expensive and often not readily available, and it does not distinguish between polycythemia vera and pathologic secondary erythrocytosis, the most important differentiation that needs to be made. The determination of serum *erythropoietin* is invaluable in helping to make the distinction. A high erythropoietin level virtually rules out polycythemia vera and suggests secondary erythrocytosis because erythropoietin production should be suppressed in polycythemia vera. A low erythropoietin level strongly supports the diagnosis of polycythemia vera while ruling out pathologic secondary erythrocytosis (which is driven by excess erythropoietin production).

If the erythropoietin level is normal (which can occur in mild disease, after phlebotomy, and with secondary disease), then a *bone marrow biopsy* is indicated. If the histology is characteristic of polycythemia vera (hypercellularity, increased number of megakaryocytes, giant megakaryocytes, mild reticulin fibrosis, decreased marrow iron stores), then the diagnosis can be considered confirmed. In the few instances in which diagnosis remains elusive, platelets can be tested for the expression of *thrombopoietin receptor protein*, which is deficient in polycythemia vera. Testing granulocytes for the *polycythemia vera-1 gene*, which appears to be unique to the condition, is another option available in some centers. Others perform *in vitro* testing of *erythroid stem cells*, which manifest colony growth in the absence of exogenous erythropoietin.

Testing for Secondary Polycythemia (Reactive Erythrocytosis)

Although history and physical examination often suffice, an *arterial blood gas* or *arterial oxygen saturation* determination can be important in the assessment of less obvious cases. A PaO$_2$ of less than 55 mm Hg and an SaO$_2$ of less than 92% indicate significant hypoxemia. The SaO$_2$ should be measured directly rather than calculated from the PaO$_2$ because false negatives occur in smokers. When a strong family history of polycythemia is present, one should obtain a *hemoglobin electrophoresis* in search of a mutant hemoglobin with an abnormally high oxygen affinity. *Cardiac ultrasonography with Doppler* (and *bubble study*, if available) is indicated when structural heart disease with right-to-left shunt is suspected.

Testing for Causes of Pathologic Secondary Erythrocytosis

One should look for signs and symptoms of renal lesions and tumors, especially renal cell carcinoma. *Renal ultrasonography* or *computed tomography* is a reasonable screening test for such lesions; a positive study result is followed by contrast-enhanced *computed tomography* of the abdomen. *Abdominal ultrasonography* is a useful screening test for hepatoma, and *pelvic ultrasonography* can help to confirm a large uterine myoma when one is suspected on physical examination.

Testing for Relative Erythrocytosis

A *postural decline in blood pressure* and *increase in pulse* usually suffice for a diagnosis of dehydration, but a ratio of *blood urea nitrogen* to *creatinine* greater than 20 can provide supporting evidence, if desired. Only when the clinical evidence is insufficient to distinguish relative erythrocytosis from other forms should a *determination of red cell mass* be ordered. The calculation of red cell mass is rather elaborate and requires a laboratory experienced in the test. A radioisotope label (chromium-51) is administered to tag the red cells so that the mass can be calculated. The patient's body habitus needs to be taken into account when the result is interpreted. Tall, muscular persons have a greater red cell mass than short, fat persons because blood volume is greater in muscle than in fat. A normal red cell mass is diagnostic of relative erythrocytosis.

SYMPTOMATIC THERAPY
(8,12,16–22)

When possible, treatment should be directed at the underlying cause, but regardless of cause, the increased red cell mass may require reduction if becomes too great, causes symptoms, and threatens the well-being of the patient. Phlebotomy becomes the treatment of choice.

Reducing Red Cell Mass

The risks associated with erythrocytosis (hyperviscosity, thrombosis, impaired hemostasis) begin to increase substantially as the hematocrit moves into the 55% to 60% range. When the condition cannot be treated etiologically in prompt fashion, phlebotomy should be performed. Phlebotomy improves oxygen delivery, relieves hyperviscosity symptoms, and prevents the thromboembolic and hemorrhagic complications of polycythemia. The target hematocrit is in the low to middle 40s, the level at which tissue oxygenation is optimal in normovolemic patients. Phlebotomy is especially useful in patients with polycythemia vera and pathologic secondary erythrocytosis. Even in cases in which the increase in red cell mass represents a physiologic accommodation to chronic hypoxemia, phlebotomy may be indicated if the erythrocytosis becomes excessive (hematocrit >60%) and threatens oxygen delivery. Reducing the hematocrit to less than 55% improves exercise tolerance in patients with severe chronic obstructive pulmonary disease.

Phlebotomy is conducted by removing up to 500 mL of blood as often as every 2 to 3 days to achieve a hematocrit of less than 55%. For patients who cannot tolerate such large losses of volume (e.g., the elderly), phlebotomy is limited to removal of no more than 250 mL once or twice a week. Iron deficiency may ensue but should not be corrected in cases of polycythemia vera or pathologic secondary erythrocytosis because such treatment may stimulate a fulminant recurrence of red cell production. In patients with cardiopulmonary disease, a modest amount of iron replacement to correct microcytosis is probably beneficial because microcytic erythrocytes increase blood viscosity and decrease oxygen delivery. The severely erythrocytic patient who is to undergo surgery requires phlebotomy to prevent compromised hemostasis. Preoperative phlebotomy should be followed by the administration of a volume expander to correct volume depletion.

Treating Secondary Polycythemia

For the person with a right-to-left shunt or erythropoietin-secreting tumor, surgical intervention is often required. *Cessation of cigarette smoking* (see Chapter 54) is always an important goal in polycythemia; in patients with relative erythrocytosis or reactive polycythemia resulting from heavy smoking and high carboxyhemoglobin levels, the hematocrit will begin to decrease within 1 week and return to normal 3 to 4 months after smoking is terminated. For selected patients with severe chronic obstructive pulmonary disease, *long-term oxygen therapy* may help to normalize the arterial oxygen saturation (see Chapter 47).

Treating Polycythemia Vera

The control of polycythemia vera with *phlebotomy* alone is usually possible in cases in which the platelet count and WBC count remain relatively normal. Phlebotomy has been shown to increase median survival from 2 to 12 years by reducing the risk for thrombosis. The frequency of treatments is a function of the hematocrit and symptoms. Most symptoms can be alleviated by reducing the hematocrit to approximately 50%; however, continued frequent phlebotomy is recommended until a normal hematocrit is achieved (middle 40s in men, low 40s in women).

A maintenance schedule can then be set up based on monthly monitoring.

Myelosuppression

Myelosuppressive therapy deserves consideration when phlebotomy proves inadequate, thrombocytosis develops, or extramedullary hematopoiesis ensues. The optimal treatment has not been identified; a longitudinal investigation by the Polycythemia Vera Study Group compared *radioactive phosphorus* (*P32*), *alkylating agents*, and *hydroxyurea*. Although P32 and alkylating agents (e.g., chlorambucil) are effective, they are also leukemogenic over time; thus, they are reserved for elderly patients. Hydroxyurea appears to be preferred because it is less likely to cause malignant transformation but can suppress the disease. Its disadvantages include the need for frequent administration and the ingestion of a large number of pills; in addition, remissions are far less sustained than with P32. Patients who fail hydroxyurea therapy can be given a treatment of P32, especially if they are elderly; it will induce a 6- to 24-month remission and is less leukemogenic than alkylating agents.

Pruritus

Although the response to antihistamines is quite variable and the role of mast cells in causing pruritus is not well established, a trial of antihistamine therapy for bothersome pruritus can be attempted. The combination of a histamine$_1$ blocker (e.g., 60 mg of *fexofenadine* every morning; 4 mg of *chlorpheniramine* daily at bedtime) and a histamine$_2$ blocker (e.g., 400 mg of *cimetidine* thrice daily) may suffice. Reports of response to low doses of *aspirin* and selective serotonin reuptake inhibitor therapy (e.g., *paroxetine*) suggest additional modalities that can be tried. In persons requiring myelosuppressive therapy, interferon-α has been used with benefit.

Hyperuricemia

Secondary hyperuricemia occurs in this disease and can lead to acute gout; *allopurinol* (300 mg administered once daily) prevents gouty attacks and should be considered when the uric acid level increases to greater than 9 to 10 mg/dL.

Thrombosis and Bleeding

Thrombosis and bleeding are the most important complications of polycythemia vera. The most effective approach to limiting such risk appears to be phlebotomy with volume expansion. Prophylactic therapy with high-dose *aspirin* (900 mg/d) plus dipyridamole fails to halt thrombosis and increases the risk of gastrointestinal bleeding; randomized studies involving low-dose aspirin are ongoing, supported by the rationale that low doses can suppress thromboxane biosynthesis, which is increased in polycythemia vera and may be related to the increased risk of clotting. The development of thrombosis is an indication for *oral anticoagulation*, but the risk for bleeding is increased in patients with polycythemia vera who are taking warfarin.

Late-Stage Complications

In the later stages of the illness, painful *splenic infarction* or *congestive splenomegaly* may necessitate *splenectomy*. Transitions to *myelofibrosis* with *myeloid metaplasia* and *leukemia* are associated with a lack of responsiveness to chemotherapy and a very poor prognosis. The risk of transformation to leukemia in the first decade after myelosuppressive treatment is 5%; the risk of transformation to myelofibrosis with myeloid metaplasia is 10%.

PATIENT EDUCATION AND INDICATIONS FOR REFERRAL

Patient education is essential to encouraging smokers to give up cigarettes (see Chapter 54) and patients with chronic obstructive lung disease to follow a maximal program for improving oxygenation (see Chapter 47). The patient's understanding of the basis of the disease and its prognosis should help in achieving compliance (see Chapter 1). When polycythemia vera is a strong diagnostic consideration, the patient should be referred to a hematologist for confirmatory testing and the design of a treatment program. Referral is also appropriate when the diagnosis is difficult and the measurement of red cell mass or bone marrow biopsy is being considered.

A.H.G.

Annotated Bibliography

1. Balcerzak SP, Bromberg PA. Secondary polycythemia. Semin Hematol 1975;12:353. (*An excellent review of the pulmonary physiology related to tissue hypoxia-induced polycythemia and other classes of secondary polycythemia.*)
2. Berlin NI. Diagnosis and classification of the polycythemias. Semin Hematol 1975;12:339. (*Traditional consensus criteria.*)
3. Birgegard G, Wide L. Serum erythropoietin in the diagnosis of polycythemia vera and after phlebotomy treatment. Br J Haematol 1992;81:603. (*The level was found to be useful, but phlebotomy can induce false-negative results.*)
4. Brown SM. Spurious (relative) polycythemia: a nonexistent disease. Am J Med 1971;50:200. (*A classic paper; patients with this condition were men with high-normal red cell masses and low-normal plasma volumes.*)
5. Editorial. Polycythemia due to hypoxemia: advantage or disadvantage? Lancet 1989;2:20. (*A fresh look at the pathophysiology.*)
6. Gruppo Italiano Studio Policitemia. Polycythemia vera: the natural history of 1,213 patients followed for 20 years. Ann Intern Med 1995;123:656. (*Prognosis is poorer in patients treated with myelosuppressive therapy.*)
7. Kralovics R, Passamonti F, Buser AS, et al. A gain-of-function mutation of JAK2 in myeloproliferative disorders. N Engl J Med 2005;352:1779. (*Presents evidence for a gene mutation that triggers the stem-cell proliferation.*)
8. Lamy T, Devillers A, Bernard M, et al. Inapparent polycythemia vera: an unrecognized diagnosis. Am J Med 1997;102:14. (*Emphasizes the importance of clinical features for diagnosis.*)
9. Lederle FA. Relative erythrocytosis: an approach to the patient. J Gen Intern Med 1987;2:128. (*A useful review; 31 references.*)
10. Ruggeri M, Tosetto A, Frezzato M, et al. The rate of progression to polycythemia era or essential thrombocythemia in patients with erythrocytosis or thrombocytosis. Ann Intern Med 2003;139:470. (*A population-based study, finding that the risks of progression and development of complications were low.*)
11. Smith JR, Landaw SA. Smokers' polycythemia. N Engl J Med 1978;298:6. (*The condition occurs in heavy smokers and resolves when smoking is stopped.*)
12. Tefferi A. Polycythemia vera: a comprehensive review and clinical recommendations. Mayo Clin Proc 2003;78:174. (*An exhaustive but also very clinically useful review; 340 references.*)
13. Fairbanks VF, Klee GG, Wiseman GA, et al. Measurement of blood volume and red cell mass: re-examination of 51Cr and 125I methods. Blood Cells Mol Dis 1996;22:169. (*A critical look at the utility of testing for red cell mass and plasma volume.*)
14. Moliterno AR, Hankins WD, Spivalk JL. Impaired expression of the thrombopoietin receptor by platelets from patients with polycythemia vera. N Engl J Med 1998;338:572. (*An observation with implications for improved diagnosis.*)
15. Weinberg RS. In vitro erythropoiesis in polycythemia vera and other myeloproliferative disorders. Semin Hematol 1997;34:64. (*Discusses the use of the in vitro growth of stem cells as a diagnostic test for polycythemia vera.*)
16. Berk PD, Goldberg JD, Donovan PD, et al. Therapeutic recommendations in polycythemia vera based on Polycythemia Vera Study Group protocols. Semin Hematol 1986;23:132. (*Consensus recommendations based on the best prospective trials.*)
17. Berk PD, Goldberg JD, Silverstein MN, et al. Increased incidence of acute leukemia in polycythemia vera associated with chlorambucil therapy. N Engl J Med 1981;304:441. (*The incidence of acute leukemia was 13 times that of patients treated with phlebotomy and 2.3 times that of patients given radioactive phosphorus.*)
18. Chetty KG, Brown SE, Light RW. Improved exercise tolerance of the polycythemic lung patient following phlebotomy. Am J Med 1983;74:415. (*The exercise tolerance of patients with chronic obstructive pulmonary disease improves when the hematocrit is lowered by phlebotomy to <55%.*)
19. Diehn F, Terreri A. Pruritus in polycythemia vera: prevalence, laboratory correlates, and management. Br J Haematol 2001;115:619. (*A large-scale study, presenting useful data on responses to a host of treatments.*)
20. Fruchtman SM, Mack K, Kaplan ME, et al. From efficacy to safety: a Polycythemia Vera Study Group report on hydroxyurea in patients with polycythemia vera. Semin Hematol 1997;34:17. (*A compilation of the best evidence and a discussion of the evolution of use of the drug.*)
21. Gruppo Italiano Studio Policitemia. Low-dose aspirin in polycythemia vera: a pilot study. Br J Haematol 1997;97:453. (*An encouraging finding that needs confirmation.*)
22. Perloff JK, Rosove MH, Child JS. Adults with cyanotic congenital heart disease: hematologic management. Ann Intern Med 1988;109:406. (*A very useful article about an often-overlooked issue.*)

CHAPTER 81 ■ EVALUATION OF BLEEDING PROBLEMS AND ABNORMAL BLEEDING STUDIES

The problems of bleeding encountered in the office setting range from abnormal results on screening studies to easy bruising, petechial rashes, and recurrent episodes of unexplained frank blood loss. Sometimes, the only manifestation is a low platelet count, prolonged prothrombin time (PT), or a delay in the bleeding time. When the volume of blood loss is small, the rate of bleeding is slow, and the risk for serious hemorrhage is low, evaluation may take place in the outpatient setting. The workup involves examination of the intrinsic and extrinsic clotting systems in addition to an evaluation of blood vessels, platelet function, and platelet quantity to identify which part of the hemostatic apparatus is at fault. Often, a careful history and physical examination, supplemented by a few simple laboratory studies, can yield a clinically meaningful answer and guide therapy. An important objective is to determine whether the problem is inherited or acquired. At times, an anatomic lesion coexists with a bleeding diathesis; the clinician always needs to address this possibility, especially when the bleeding originates from the lung, gastrointestinal tract, vagina, or urinary tract (see Chapters 42, 63, 111, and 129, respectively).

PATHOPHYSIOLOGY AND CLINICAL PRESENTATION (1–11)

Overview

Hemostasis is achieved by the interplay of the coagulation cascade, platelets, and vessel wall. The platelets provide the initial primary hemostatic plug in response to vascular injury, followed secondarily by the generation of fibrin at the site of damage. Blood coagulation is a carefully controlled process, limited by endogenous anticoagulants. Normal hemostasis represents a delicate balance between coagulant and anticoagulant factors. Any upset in this system of checks and balances may result in bleeding or thrombosis.

Disorders of Primary Hemostasis

These involve *platelets* and/or the *vessel wall* and present as spontaneous bleeding or bleeding into *superficial tissues* (skin and mucous membranes, including the lining of the bowel and the genitourinary tract). The appearance of *petechiae* and *slow oozing* after trauma, rather than brisk bleeding, is typical. *Menorrhagia* or *epistaxis* may be a presenting complaint.

Disorders of Secondary Hemostasis

These involve the *clotting factors* or the *fibrinolytic system* and lead to bleeding that is characteristically deep and *visceral*, causing such problems as *hemarthrosis*, *retroperitoneal hemorrhage*, and *deep hematomas*.

Disorders of Primary Hemostasis: Qualitative Platelet Disorders

Platelet function defects can be classified according to the step in platelet activity that is affected: adhesion, aggregation, activation, secretion, or acceleration of coagulation. Patients with isolated qualitative platelet defects have a prolonged bleeding time in conjunction with normal-appearing platelets that are adequate in number.

Defective Adhesion

The most important cause of impaired adhesion is *von Willebrand's disease*; acquired forms are seen in the setting of malignancy and connective tissue disease or with high-dose antibiotic administration.

von Willebrand's Disease. This is inherited in an autosomal-dominant pattern and is associated with decreased secretion or abnormal synthesis of a glycoprotein polymer (*von Willebrand's factor*) needed for platelet adherence to a site of vascular endothelial injury. The release of von Willebrand's factor in the classic form of the disease can be stimulated by *desmopressin (DDAVP)*. Rarer forms of the disease are not corrected by DDAVP. In addition, because of a *deficiency of factor VIII procoagulant*, the partial thromboplastin time (PTT) is prolonged. Platelet agglutination fails to occur in the presence of the antibiotic *ristocetin*, a laboratory characteristic of this disease that is useful for its detection. Mucous membrane bleeding is a frequent manifestation. The severity of bleeding is variable and most severe among homozygous persons, who may bleed from the gastrointestinal tract; hemarthrosis is rare. Cryoprecipitate can also correct the problem.

Acquired Forms. Acquired forms of von Willebrand's disease are seen in *lymphoma*, other malignancies, and *connective tissue disease*. High doses of *semisynthetic penicillins* or *cephalosporins* can produce an acquired adhesion defect by coating the platelet surface and reducing binding to glycoprotein.

Defective Activation and Release

Patients with activation problems have an impaired production or an impaired response to prostaglandin-dependent activators such as *thromboxane A2*, which attracts platelets and constricts vessels. Nonselective *nonsteroidal antiinflammatory drugs* (NSAIDs) affect platelet activation and secretion by *inhibiting cyclooxygenase-2* (COX-2), which helps to convert arachidonic acid to thromboxane. In addition, such NSAIDs inhibit the release of *adenosine diphosphate*, which is needed for platelet aggregation. (Some of the more selective NSAIDs that inhibit COX-2 do not impair thromboxane formation, a feature that may contribute to their suspected prothombotic potential.)

Aspirin, unlike NSAIDs, produces irreversible inhibition of cyclooxygenase even with single small doses; the effect persists for the life span of the platelet (7 days). Reversible inhibition is seen with the use of NSAIDs and *omega-3 fatty acids* (found in oily fish). Severe bleeding does not result, but an underlying bleeding diathesis may be aggravated.

In patients with *storage pool disease*, the adenosine diphosphate and serotonin contents of platelet granules are reduced or released prematurely, as occurs in patients who have undergone *cardiopulmonary bypass*. Bleeding is typically mild, and the bleeding time is only mildly prolonged.

Defective Aggregation

Patients with a rare hereditary defect in platelet aggregation, *Glanzmann's thrombasthenia*, are missing a bridging protein called glycoprotein IIb/IIIa. The platelets of such persons cannot bind to fibrinogen and thus fail to aggregate by way of fibrinogen cross-links. *Clot retraction is abnormal*; the bleeding time is markedly prolonged. Serious bleeding can occur. Patients taking high doses of *semisynthetic penicillins* or *cephalosporins* also demonstrate reduced binding to fibrinogen.

Defective Acceleration of Coagulation

When platelets bind factors V and X on their surface, the rate of prothrombin conversion is greatly accelerated. Patients whose platelets cannot bind these clotting factors have a *mildly prolonged PT*, *normal bleeding time*, and *normal platelet aggregation*.

Mixed or Unknown Defects in Function

A number of conditions are associated with poorly defined but potentially important qualitative defects in platelet function. Uremia is the most important and is believed to be related to a dialyzable toxin. In addition to dialysis, the correction of anemia and administration of DDAVP, conjugated estrogens, and cryoprecipitate can reduce the prolongation in bleeding time. *Dysproteinemias* and *myeloproliferative* diseases also produce complex defects in platelet function, as can high parenteral doses of β-lactam antibiotics.

Disorders of Primary Hemostasis: Quantitative Platelet Defects

A normal platelet count ranges from 150,000/mm^3 to 300,000/mm^3. The presence of too many or too few platelets can impair primary hemostasis.

Thrombocytosis

Thrombocyte counts greater than 400,000/mm^3 may interfere with platelet function; thrombosis is the more likely consequence, but occasionally mucous membrane bleeding or hemorrhage may occur, especially following trauma or surgery. In most instances, the bleeding is inconsequential, but it is more likely when there is underlying myeloproliferative disease. Thrombocytosis may be primary or secondary.

Essential thrombocythemia is the primary myeloproliferative form of thrombocytosis. Like polycythemia, there is evidence of autonomous clonal hematopoiesis due to an acquired clonal somatic mutation. Thrombopoietin levels are inappropriately normal or elevated. Although the mean age of onset is 60 years, young women may develop the condition, which can cause miscarriage. Overall, the clinical course in the first 10 years after diagnosis is relatively indolent. The risk of thrombosis is about 15% to 25%; risk factors include age at diagnosis greater than 60 years, leukocytosis, and history of thrombosis. The risk of bleeding is considerably less. Transformation to polycythemia, myelofibrosis, or leukemia is rare in the first decade after diagnosis (1.4%) and is seen mostly in persons with mutations in the JAK2 gene; the risk increases over time to 24% after three decades. Vasoocclusive symptoms due to transient excessive platelet aggregation include migraine headache, dysesthesias, and redness in the hands and feet.

Secondary thrombocytosis occurs in the context of inflammatory disease, infection, or malignancy.

Thrombocytopenia

A platelet count of less than 100,000/mm^3 is associated with a prolonged bleeding time. The diagnosis requires confirmation with a peripheral smear because spurious forms occur caused by *in vitro* clumping of platelets in response to citrate or small amounts of circulating cold agglutinin. The risk for serious bleeding from true thrombocytopenia does not occur until the platelet count falls to well less than 50,000/mm^3. Easy bruising is seen with counts of 30,000/mm^3 to 50,000/mm^3; spontaneous bruising, menorrhagia, and prolonged bleeding with trauma arise as the count drops to less than 20,000/mm^3. At less than 10,000/mm^3, spontaneous epistaxis, gastrointestinal and genitourinary bleeding, and an increased risk for central nervous system hemorrhage occur. A petechial rash of the lower legs may be an initial manifestation. The lesions differ from those of vasculitis in that they are painless, flat, nonpruritic, and without an erythematous blush. Hemorrhagic bullae in the buccal mucosa are another characteristic finding. Bleeding may begin from the gastrointestinal or urinary tract. Thrombocytopenia develops when platelet destruction is increased (trauma, immune injury, disseminated intravascular coagulation, thrombotic thrombocytopenic purpura), production is decreased (marrow failure), or abnormal pooling occurs (hypersplenism).

Increased Destruction

Accelerated destruction is the most common cause of thrombocytopenia. The primary mechanism is immunologic, occurring in association with drugs, viruses, lymphoproliferative disorders, and connective tissue diseases, as well as idiopathically.

Immune (Idiopathic) Thrombocytopenic Purpura. Immune (idiopathic) thrombocytopenic purpura (ITP) is a major cause of platelet destruction, mediated by the production of immunoglobulin G (IgG) autoantibodies directed against platelets. The idiopathic form is most common in young adults, children, and women. In adults, the condition is more chronic, characterized by a waxing and waning course with few spontaneous remissions. It may present as bleeding in the context of aspirin or NSAID use, as an incidental finding on routine blood count, or as menorrhagia, epistaxis, or purpuric rash following a viral infection. The physical examination findings are otherwise normal, and the spleen usually is not palpable, although it may be slightly enlarged. No lymphadenopathy, hepatomegaly, or sternal tenderness is present, which helps to distinguish the condition form secondary forms. Mild fever is sometimes noted.

Secondary Immune Thrombocytopenias. Immune-mediated thrombocytopenia can occur in the context of *lymphoproliferative disorders*, *systemic lupus erythematosus*, and HIV and hepatitis C infections and with *drugs*. The clinical picture follows a pattern similar to that for ITP, except that there might also be findings indicative of the underlying cause (e.g., recent new drug exposure or lymphadenopathy, hepatomegaly, splenomegaly, arthritis, arthralgias, skin rash, renal dysfunction). Platelet counts drop to less than 100,000/mm^3 in about 15% of cases. The prevalence of thrombocytopenia is 10% among asymptomatic HIV patients and up to 30% in those with symptomatic disease.

Drug-induced immune thrombocytopenia is idiosyncratic. *Heparin* (less likely with the low-molecular-weight preparations), *histamine$_2$ blockers*, *quinidine*, *sulfonamides*, and *anticonvulsants* are common precipitants, although *any* drug may be responsible, as may *herbal remedies* and over-the-counter medications (e.g., *acetaminophen*, *NSAIDs*). Usually 5 to 7 days of use are needed to allow time for sensitization if there is no prior exposure. A rapid fall in the platelet count to less than 20,000//mm^3 is characteristic, and acute hemorrhage may ensue. A prompt return of the count to safe levels is typical as soon as the responsible drug is withheld. In *heparin-induced thrombocytopenia*, the PF-4-heparin antibodies are almost always present; platelet counts usually do not drop to less than 10,000//mm^3, and recovery typically occurs within 4 to 10 days of stopping therapy. The problem is much less common with low-molecular-weight heparin. Bleeding is uncommon, but thrombotic complications often occur even after the platelet count returns to normal.

Thrombotic Thrombocytopenic Purpura. Thrombotic thrombocytopenic purpura (TTP) causes *platelet consumption*, rather than outright destruction, as hyaline–platelet complexes form in small vessels, trapping platelets. Microangiopathic hemolytic anemia ensues, fever develops, and microvascular damage to the kidneys and the central nervous system may become manifest, producing the findings of *hemolytic–uremic syndrome*, which is considered a component of TTP and not a separate condition. Unlike disseminated intravascular coagulation, there is no consumption of clotting factors.

The precise mechanism is unknown, but vascular endothelial damage appears to be pathophysiologically important. Precipitants include *food poisoning* due to a Shiga toxin–producing organism (e.g., *Escherichia coli* 0157:H7 or *Shigella* species), *adverse drug response* (quinine, ticlopidine, clopidogrel, mitomycin C), *autoimmune disorders*, and *pregnancy* or *postpartum* state. The combination of *anemia*, a peripheral smear showing *schistocytes*, and *thrombocytopenia* in conjunction with *fever, neurologic symptoms*, and *renal dysfunction* constitute the clinical syndrome. Serum lactic dehydrogenase can rise markedly. Patients with the acute fulminant form of the disease are unlikely to present in the outpatient setting, but those with the chronic relapsing form may do so.

Decreased Production

The bone marrow may be suppressed by drugs, depressed after a viral infection, or replaced by tumor. Thrombocytopenias associated with conditions causing *marrow failure* or a *myelophthisic process* usually occur in the context of a generalized pancytopenia (see Chapter 80). On occasion, individual *drugs* cause selective *inhibition of platelet production*. Chlorothiazide, tolbutamide, and ethanol are among the best documented. Megakaryocyte production is reduced in *megaloblastic anemia*, and quick recovery is noted with replacement therapy. *Transient thrombocytopenia* may follow influenza, hepatitis, rubella, and other viral diseases. The thrombocytopenia of *HIV disease* involves viral invasion of megakaryocytes in addition to increased peripheral destruction.

Increased Pooling

Pooling may occur in disorders associated with an abnormally enlarged spleen. Splenomegaly results in excessive trapping and a decrease in the number of circulating platelets.

Disorders of Secondary Hemostasis: Defects of the Intrinsic Pathway

These conditions prolong the PTT (the PT remains normal) by impairing the synthesis or functioning of intrinsic pathway clotting factors. Detection may be difficult because the PTT will not become prolonged until the reduction in the concentration of a functioning intrinsic clotting factor exceeds 75%. Fortunately, many clotting factor deficiencies do not cause serious bleeding, but the most common ones—the hemophilias—do.

Deficiencies of Factors VIII and IX. Hemophilias A and B

Hemophilias A and B represent deficiencies of factors VIII and IX, respectively. They account for more than 80% of patients with an inherited bleeding diathesis and, because they are X linked, affect only male individuals. The risk for bleeding depends on the degree of factor deficiency. Patients with concentrations as low as 5% of normal experience little bleeding, except after surgery or major trauma; those with concentrations that are 1% to 5% of normal may bleed after minor trauma; those with concentrations that are less than 1% of normal

undergo spontaneous hemorrhage, typically into muscle and weight-bearing joints. Bleeding can also occur into the central nervous system, genitourinary tract, and retroperitoneum. As noted, detection may be difficult if factor levels are greater than 25% of normal because the PTT will be normal. Chromosomal mapping is being developed to help to detect female carriers. Relatively early prenatal detection is available by DNA analysis of chorionic villi tissue, provided that tissue is also available from other affected family members. Fetal blood may be sampled for the determination of antihemophilic factor levels later in pregnancy by ultrasonographically guided aspiration.

Factor Xi Deficiency

Factor Xi deficiency occurs mostly among Ashkenazi Jews, and is inherited as an autosomal-recessive disorder. A severe insult such as major trauma or surgery is needed to precipitate bleeding.

Other Deficiencies

Other deficiencies of intrinsic pathway factors may cause a prolongation of the PTT but do not lead to clinical bleeding, even in the setting of major surgery or serious trauma.

Inhibitors

The *lupus anticoagulant* is an IgG antibody elicited in the setting of connective tissue disease and phenothiazine use. Bleeding complications are rare, but a hypercoagulable state is sometimes seen in patients with this anticoagulant that leads to an increased risk for venous thrombosis and spontaneous abortion (see Chapter 22). Both the PTT and the PT are prolonged because the antibody is directed against the phospholipids used in both assays. Hemophiliacs who have had multiple transfusions of antihemophilic factor have close to a 15% risk for the development of antihemophilic factor inhibitors, IgG antibodies against the replaced factors. Such antibodies are also noted in patients with connective tissue or lymphoproliferative disease, those who are pregnant, and persons of advanced age.

Disorders of Secondary Hemostasis: Defects of the Extrinsic Pathway

The major clotting factors of the extrinsic pathway (II, VII, X) depend for their synthesis and modification on a healthy liver and an adequate dietary intake of vitamin K. Some vitamin K also derives from bacterial production by gut flora. Hereditary deficiencies of extrinsic pathway factors are rare. Most bleeding traced to the extrinsic pathway is the consequence of impaired vitamin K production or liver disease. Causes include *hepatocellular insufficiency, cholestasis* (which impairs absorption of lipid-soluble vitamin K), *poor dietary intake*, and the use of *broad-spectrum antibiotics* that kill normal gut flora. The characteristic laboratory finding is a prolongation of the PT. Prolongation of the PT also occurs with *warfarin* anticoagulant therapy. Warfarin inhibits the vitamin K–dependent postsynthetic modification of factors II, VII, IX, and X; this prevents them from being able to bind calcium and achieve biologic activity (see Chapter 83).

Vascular Defects

Vascular defects are characterized by *purpuric bleeding* into the skin and mucous membranes in the absence of a detectable clotting factor or platelet abnormality. Ecchymoses and petechiae are the predominant manifestations. The most common form occurs as a result of aging—so-called *senile purpura*. Atrophy of connective and fatty tissues makes the vessels fragile and subject to ecchymotic bleeding, especially in areas of constant sun exposure (face, neck, dorsum of hands, forearms). The skin fragility and easy bruising seen with *Cushing's syndrome* are believed to have a similar basis, the catabolic effects of prolonged corticosteroid excess. *Scurvy* causes defective collagen synthesis; affected patients may present with gingival bleeding or hemorrhage into subcutaneous tissue and muscle. Perifollicular bleeding is characteristic. *Purpura simplex* is a mild condition seen in otherwise healthy women; they experience ecchymoses mostly in the lower extremities (sometimes colorfully referred to as "devil's pinches"), especially during menstrual periods. Most cases are believed to be acquired, and some have been linked to the use of NSAIDs.

Hereditary Disorders

Diseases of connective tissue formation, such as *Marfan's syndrome* and *Ehlers–Danlos syndrome*, produce structural defects in supporting connective tissue and major vessels. Bleeding ranges from easy bruising to serious hemorrhage. In *Rendu–Weber–Osler disease*, the developmental anomaly is *telangiectasis* formation because of a lack of vessel support and contractility. Bleeding from these thin, convoluted networks of venules and capillaries can result from minor trauma or occur spontaneously. The telangiectatic lesions are violaceous, flat, and usually no larger than a few millimeters, and they range in shape from pinpoint to spidery. They occur on the mucous membranes, face, trunk, and palmar and plantar surfaces. Lesions also arise in major viscera, which leads to a risk for serious hemorrhage. The clinical course is often one of repeated hemorrhagic episodes.

Pharmacologic Agents

Purpuric bleeding in the absence of demonstrable platelet or clotting factor abnormalities is characteristic. *Drug-induced vascular purpura* is believed to have an autoimmune mechanism, with antibodies directed at the endothelial surface, although the responsible antibodies are often difficult to detect. Drugs in this category include *procaine penicillin*, *thiazides*, *quinine*, *iodides*, *sulfa drugs*, and *coumarins*. The bleeding ceases when the drug is withdrawn.

Immune Complex Formation

Minor purpuric bleeding is sometimes seen in the setting of *systemic lupus*, *rheumatoid arthritis*, and *Sjögren's syndrome* and is believed to be linked to immune complex deposition. In *amyloidosis*, deposition of amyloid protein in the skin and subcutaneous tissue leads to vascular fragility, especially about the orbits and upper torso. The "raccoon eyes" appearance of such patients is characteristic.

Mixed Defects

A number of conditions impair the hemostatic apparatus at multiple levels. Chronic *renal failure*, *dysproteinemias*, *chronic liver disease*, and *consumption coagulopathies* are the most important examples.

Uremia

Renal failure impairs platelet function and causes deficiencies in the production of clotting factors. Prolonged oozing from arterial and venipuncture sites is common. Dialysis and the correction of the anemia help to reduce the bleeding tendency, which ranges from purpura and mucous membrane bleeding to gastrointestinal hemorrhage.

Dysproteinemias

Cryoglobulinemia, *macroglobulinemia*, and *myeloma* can lead to damage of the endothelial surface as immune complexes and paraproteins precipitate from the serum. The sludging and hyperviscosity commonly associated with these conditions also result in capillary anoxia. Impaired clotting factor and platelet activity and endothelial damage cause a multifactorial bleeding diathesis.

Chronic Liver Disease

Hepatocellular failure precipitates bleeding by a number of routes. Patients with severe failure can no longer make adequate amounts of vitamin K–dependent clotting factors, even with the administration of vitamin K. In addition, fibrinogen production suffers, and the fibrinogen that is made is defective. Patients with portal hypertension may become thrombocytopenic from platelet sequestration in the spleen, although in itself this rarely causes bleeding. However, varices are common in such patients, which increases the risk for gastrointestinal hemorrhage (see Chapter 63).

Disseminated Intravascular Coagulation

This consumption coagulopathy takes place in the setting of illness that causes exposure of blood to tissue thromboplastin (e.g., snake bite, extensive burn, serious infection, cancer). Activation of the extrinsic pathway in the microcirculation consumes clotting factors and platelets; it leads to bleeding that ranges from minor petechiae to hemorrhage. The condition is rarely encountered in the office setting.

DIFFERENTIAL DIAGNOSIS

The causes of a bleeding diathesis can be organized according to the subdivisions of the hemostatic apparatus: platelet function, platelet number, intrinsic pathway, extrinsic pathway, and vessels (Table 81.1). Differential diagnosis proceeds by identifying which segment of the clotting system is at fault.

WORKUP (1–3,12–20)

When a patient presents with easy bruising or bleeding, the clinician needs to ascertain the likelihood of an underlying defect in hemostasis. Bleeding from multiple sites, easy bruising, spontaneous bleeding, the presence of ecchymoses greater than 3 cm in diameter, or prolonged bleeding after a surgical or dental procedure strongly suggests a bleeding diathesis. Before embarking on a detailed evaluation in the office, one should be sure that no serious hemorrhage or major volume depletion is present. Inquiry is required into dyspnea, lightheadedness, marked postural fatigue, and observed quantity of blood loss. A quick check of postural signs, skin color, and skin temperature will provide added objective evidence of intravascular volume status and degree of anemia. Once the presence of or

TABLE 81.1

DIFFERENTIAL DIAGNOSIS OF BLEEDING BY MECHANISM

Qualitative Platelet Disorders	
Defective adhesion	von Willebrand's disease: high doses of semisynthetic penicillins and cephalosporins
Defective aggregation	Glanzmann's thrombasthenia; high doses of semisynthetic penicillins and cephalosporins
Defective activation	Nonsteroidal antiinflammatory drugs; dipyridamole; cardiopulmonary bypass
Defective acceleration	Factor V deficiency
Quantitative Platelet Disorders	
Thrombocytosis	Myeloproliferative disease
Thrombocytopenia	
Decreased production	Thiazides, alcohol, viral infection, marrow failure, megaloblastic anemia, myelophthisic process
Increased destruction	Drugs: quinidine, quinine, methyldopa, sulfonamide antibiotics, phenytoin, valproate, carbamazepine, barbiturates, gold salts, abciximab, vancomycin, acetaminophen, nonsteroidal antiinflammatory drugs, H_2-blockers, heparin
	Diseases: systemic lupus, sepsis, idiopathic thrombocytopenic purpura, chronic lymphocytic leukemia
Increased sequestration	Hypersplenism
Intrinsic Pathway Defects	
Factor VIII deficiency	Hemophilia A
Factor IX deficiency	Hemophilia B
Factor XI deficiency	Ashkenazi Jewish descent
Extrinsic Pathway Defects	
Vitamin K–dependent factor deficiency	Poor diet, cholestasis, hepatocellular failure, coumarin, broad-spectrum antibiotics
Vascular Defects	
Connective tissue fragility	Age, Cushing's syndrome, scurvy, purpura simplex
Hereditary defect	Marfan's syndrome, Rendu–Weber–Osler disease
Drug induced	Procaine penicillin, sulfonamides, thiazides, quinine, iodides, coumarins,
Paraproteinemia	Myeloma, macroglobulinemia, cryoglobulinemia
Connective tissue disease	upus, rheumatoid arthritis, Sjögren's syndrome
Multiple Defects	
Uremia	
Chronic hepatocellular failure	
Disseminated intravascular coagulation	
HIV infection	

risk for severe hemorrhage has been ruled out, the outpatient evaluation can commence.

The next task is to ascertain which segment(s) of the hemostatic system are at fault. This determination, along with an assessment of whether the condition is acquired or hereditary, can greatly help to focus the evaluation (Table 81.2).

History

One needs a detailed history of the bleeding problem, including its onset, precipitants, location, clinical course, prior history, associated family history, and drug history. Inquiry into past surgery, childbirth, menstruation, nosebleed (both nostrils), dental extraction, trauma, laceration, and injection can provide important information. Especially important is the history of a transfusion requirement after minor trauma or surgery when such transfusion would ordinarily not be required.

On the other hand, not all patients with a history of easy bruising have a bleeding diathesis. Easy bruising is common and often occurs in otherwise normal patients. Bruises that occur on the limbs and are less than 3 cm in diameter are likely to be harmless and caused by inapparent trauma in the ab-

sence of recalled injury. Similarly, minor bleeding up to 2 days after a molar extraction is within normal limits. However, ecchymoses occurring spontaneously on the trunk or measuring greater than 3 cm in diameter on the limbs are more worrisome.

As noted earlier, bleeding that is transient, superficial (confined to the skin and mucous membranes), and spontaneous or immediately posttraumatic suggests a platelet problem or vascular fragility. In contrast, patients with serious clotting factor problems characteristically report bleeding that is deep (into tissues or viscera), delayed, and prolonged. A past medical history or family history of abnormal bleeding is strong presumptive evidence of a hereditary disorder, but its absence does not rule it out. For example, 30% of hemophiliacs give no family history of bleeding. In a patient with a suspected hereditary cause, gender should be noted because many hereditary bleeding disorders are sex linked, especially those involving clotting factors.

A thorough review of *medications* is essential. The use of medications capable of interfering with platelet function (aspirin, NSAIDs, semisynthetic penicillins, cephalosporins, dipyridamole, clopidogrel), platelet number (thiazides, quinine, quinidine, methyldopa, sulfonamides, other antimicrobials, anticonvulsants, barbiturates, heparin; see Table 81.2),

TABLE 81.2

DIFFERENTIATING PLATELET, COAGULATION, AND VASCULAR DISORDERS

Clinical Features	Platelet	Coagulation	Vascular
Onset	Immediate	Delayed	Immediate
Duration	Short	Prolonged	Variable
Precipitant	Trauma	Often spontaneous	Variable
Site	Skin, mucous membranes, gastrointestinal tract	Joints, muscle, viscera	Skin, gastrointestinal tract
Family history	Absent	Usually present	Usually absent
Drug related	Often	Rarely	Sometimes
Gender predominance	Often female	Usually male	Usually female
Response to focal pressure	Usually effective	Ineffective	Effective
Platelet count	Normal, low, or excessive	Normal	Normal
Prothrombin time	Normal	Abnormal in cases of factor II, VII, IX, and X deficiency	Normal
Partial thromboplastin time	Normal	Abnormal with factor VIII or IX deficiency	Normal

or coagulation factor synthesis (e.g., warfarin) should be noted. Checking for the duration of drug exposure can be informative. Most drug-induced immune thrombocytopenias require at least 5 to 7 days of use if the patient had not been previously exposed; onset is much more rapid if there had been prior exposure.

The presence of a recent or *concurrent illness* that might affect hemostasis should be given particular attention, including chronic liver disease, uremia, viral infection, connective tissue disease, myeloproliferative states, and paraproteinemias.

Physical Examination

After taking the vital signs and checking for significant volume depletion, one can proceed with a systematic examination. The general appearance is noted for cushingoid habitus and marfanoid appearance. On examination of the skin, the size, number, and location of any *purpuric lesions* should be recorded, and note should be made of whether they are *petechial* (<3 mm) or *ecchymotic* (>3 mm). Purpura represents bleeding into the skin, usually as the result of vessel breakage or leakage. Petechial lesions occur with thrombocytopenia, qualitative platelet disorders, and vascular defects. Petechial rashes are also a hallmark of vasculitis, but the lesions in vasculitic cases are characteristically palpable, tender, and pruritic and are surrounded by an erythematous flush. One can readily distinguish petechiae from nonpurpuric erythematous skin lesions by noting their failure to blanch when compressed with a glass slide. *Blanching* lesions must not be dismissed too hastily because they may be *telangiectases*, which are an important clue to Rendu–Weber–Osler syndrome. Ecchymoses occurring in areas subject to trauma are a common finding in normal individuals; however, ecchymotic lesions greater than 6 cm in the absence of major trauma are likely to represent an underlying bleeding abnormality. The skin is also noted for signs of chronic liver disease (spider angiomas, jaundice).

The mucous membranes are examined for bleeding, the lymph nodes for enlargement, the abdomen for hepatosplenomegaly, and the joints and muscles for hematomas and hemarthroses. Rectal and pelvic examinations are conducted for evidence of bleeding. In a patient with thrombocytopenia, careful examination for splenomegaly is important because it may be the only clue of sequestration. Percussion of the Traube space (the area of resonance over the stomach) for dullness, combined with splenic palpation with the patient in the right lateral decubitus position, is the best means of detecting splenomegaly by physical examination (sensitivity of 46%, specificity of 97%).

Laboratory Studies

Although the history and physical examination often provide important clues regarding etiology, laboratory investigation helps to classify the cause of the bleeding more definitively. Primary hemostasis is assessed by *platelet count* and *bleeding time*. The *PT* best assays the extrinsic clotting system, and the *PTT* best assays the intrinsic one.

Platelet Count

The count is routinely performed by an automated particle-counting machine on a sample of blood collected into a tube containing the anticoagulant ethylenediaminetetraacetic acid (EDTA). Falsely low counts occur when platelets clump on exposure to EDTA, a common phenomenon when blood is processed at low temperatures. It can be prevented by warming the blood slightly before processing, using another anticoagulant, or performing a finger-stick platelet count. The presence of a cold agglutinin in the blood will also cause clumping and a falsely low level, as will antibody that produces rosettes of platelets about white cells. A confirmatory look at the peripheral smear is always helpful. Finding platelets on examination of a peripheral smear is good presumptive evidence of adequate quantity.

Bleeding Time

The bleeding time is a sensitive but nonspecific test of qualitative platelet function; values are also abnormal in thrombocytopenia, uremia, von Willebrand's disease, and afibrinogenemia. Even anemia may produce a prolonged bleeding time, which is correctable by the transfusion of red cells alone. The test often gives false-positive readings, as demonstrated by the high rate of normal findings on follow-up platelet aggregation studies.

The Ivy method is the standard technique for performance of the test. A cut is made in a relatively avascular area of the forearm, with the use of a template to ensure an incision of 1 cm in length and 1 mm in depth, while venous return is obstructed with a blood pressure cuff inflated to 40 mm Hg. Blotting paper is applied to the edge of the incision; a normal result is cessation of blotter-detected oozing by 9 minutes. Recent aspirin or current NSAID use will produce a modest prolongation in the bleeding time, although this usually does not represent a significant risk for bleeding unless a preexisting bleeding diathesis is present.

Prothrombin Time and Partial Thromboplastin Time

The PT and PTT assay extrinsic and intrinsic clotting factor cascades, respectively, in addition to the common pathway. The PT assesses factor VII and common pathway factors X and V, prothrombin, and fibrinogen. The PTT reflects levels of kininogen, prekallikrein, and factors VIII, IX, XI, and XII, in addition to those of the common pathway. Its sensitivity is limited; a clotting factor deficiency of greater than 75% is needed to prolong the PTT. The PT is slightly more sensitive, becoming prolonged when factor VII falls by 55% to 65%. However, bleeding is rare in the absence of such reductions. PTT prolongations not associated with bleeding include those caused by deficiencies of factor XII, kininogen, or prekallikrein and the presence of an inhibitor.

Screening for an inhibitor is carried out by mixing equal volumes of the patient's plasma and normal donor plasma. If the prolongation in PT or PTT is corrected, then no inhibitor is present and the workup proceeds to determine the missing clotting factor. If it is not corrected, then this is strong suggestive evidence of the presence of an inhibitor, and identifying it is the next step. The PT and the PTT do not assess the final factor XIII–dependent cross-linking of fibrin; *urea clot solubility testing* is required. Testing for *fibrinolysis* also must be performed separately.

Testing for a Qualitative Platelet Defect

In the setting of bleeding consistent with defective initial hemostasis (see prior discussion) and a normal platelet count, normal PT, and normal PTT, one should consider determining the bleeding time, provided that no explanation is readily evident (e.g., recent aspirin or NSAID use, uremia, and so forth). An abnormal study is followed by *in vitro* testing of platelet function. *Aggregation testing* is conducted by adding an aggregating substance such as adenosine diphosphate, epinephrine, collagen, or thrombin to a platelet-rich plasma sample. If the bleeding time and the PTT are prolonged, then *ristocetin-induced agglutination* of platelets can be performed to check for von Willebrand's disease. Aggregation is normal in von Willebrand's disease, but the platelets fail to agglutinate. Aggregation and ristocetin studies are best ordered in consultation with a hematologist.

Testing for the Cause of Thrombocytopenia

First, pseudothrombocytopenia must be ruled out. Then the task turns to differentiating increased destruction from decreased production and sequestration. Examination of the *peripheral blood smear* is helpful in this regard.

In the Setting of Pancytopenia. Pancytopenia strongly suggests a marrow problem. A myelophthisic picture on peripheral smear suggests marrow invasion due to a myeloproliferative disorder, indicating the need for *bone marrow examination*. Marrow biopsy may also show a hypocellular marrow indica-

tive of marrow failure; an increase in megakaryocytes argues for increased destruction.

Isolated Thrombocytopenia. Isolated thrombocytopenia is almost always caused by increased destruction or sequestration. The presence of large, immature platelets on the peripheral smear in a patient with an isolated thrombocytopenia points to increased destruction. Sequestration is best determined on physical examination by checking for an enlarged spleen or obtaining an abdominal ultrasound to help make the determination.

In the workup for the cause of increased destruction, one should consider a few preliminary investigations to check for obvious, readily detectible secondary causes that may obviate the need for more sophisticated anti–platelet antibody studies. For example, simply *withdrawing* all potentially offending drugs and monitoring the platelet count may suffice for the diagnosis of a medication-induced etiology. For confirmation, *rechallenging* with a very small dose and monitoring platelet count closely for rapid decline can help with confirmation.

Serologic studies can be helpful for causative viral infections and connective tissue diseases (e.g., enzyme-linked immunosorbent assay and Western blot for HIV, anti–hepatitis C antibody, antinuclear antibody) when there are suggestive clinical findings. In most instances, *antibody testing for drug-induced thrombocytopenia* is not particularly useful or practical. Although such antibodies can often be detected under research conditions, they may be undetectable in clinical settings or present in the absence thrombocytopenia. The exception is serologic testing for *PF-4-heparin antibodies*; the antibody is almost always present. Serologic assays have a sensitivity of 97% and a specificity of 74% to 86%. Negative results help to rule out the condition in persons with an intermediate to high pretest probability. Testing is not recommended in persons with low pretest probability due to the modest specificity of the test. In those with intermediate pretest probability, *functional assay* testing can provide supportive evidence of the diagnosis.

In the absence of evidence for other etiologies and in the presence of a normal complete blood cell count (mild lymphocytosis included), one should consider *idiopathic thrombocytopenic purpura*. Officially, diagnosis of the condition remains one of exclusion. Attempts to identify discriminating laboratory findings suggest that the combination of normal red and white cell counts, increase in anti–GPIIb/IIIa antibody–producing B cells, increased platelet-associated anti–GPIIb/IIIa antibody, elevated reticulocyte count, and normal or slightly increased thrombopoietin predict ITP in persons presenting with thrombocytopenia. Whole blood is required to test for the presence of platelet-bound IgG autoantibodies (serum may contain little of the antibody). Detection is complex, and controversies abound concerning the meaning of findings.

Testing for Consumption of Platelets. The consumption of platelets is suggested by the presence of red cell *schistocytes* on *peripheral smear*, which is indicative of a microangiopathic condition, such as occurs with thrombotic thrombocytopenic purpura and disseminated intravascular coagulation. The PTT is normal in the former and abnormal in the latter. Because of the urgency of timely diagnosis of thrombotic thrombocytopenic purpura, it is important to check for the other readily obtainable diagnostic criteria for the condition, which include a *platelet count of less than 30,000/mm³*, evidence of *red cell hemolysis* (see Chapter 79), *hematuria, proteinuria, increased serum creatinine, mental status changes*, and *fever*. Not all features may be present on initial testing (e.g., renal function may still be in the normal range), but if the clinical context is right (e.g., bloody diarrhea in a child or an elderly patient suspected of having been exposed to *E. coli* 0157:H7) and multiple laboratory features are present, then the diagnosis should be considered possible and appropriate action taken (see later discussion).

Preoperative Screening for a Bleeding Disorder

The most important component of preoperative screening is the history. The absence of abnormal bleeding during a previous surgical procedure or trauma is strong evidence of normal hemostasis. Current medication use also needs to be carefully reviewed, especially NSAIDs, salicylates, and drugs known to precipitate thrombocytopenia. Although the platelet count, PT, PTT, and bleeding time are frequently determined, the yield is low in patients with unsuspected deficits. In particular, little if any correlation is found between bleeding time and the risk for surgical bleeding. Routinely obtaining a preoperative bleeding time in a patient with no known or suspected bleeding abnormality is of no proven value.

The PTT, PT, and platelet count continue to be ordered routinely, but their value in the absence of a condition known to compromise hemostasis is unproven. In a study of 829 consecutive and otherwise healthy patients undergoing PT and PTT screening before orthopedic surgery, unexpected abnormalities were found in about 8%; none had an impact on patient management.

SYMPTOMATIC MANAGEMENT AND PATIENT EDUCATION (1–3,21–31)

Patients with a clinically insignificant laboratory abnormality deserve detailed reassurance that their hemostasis is adequate. For example, the patient with a minor prolongation of bleeding time on preoperative testing yet no prior history of abnormal bleeding is unlikely to have anything more serious than recent salicylate exposure. Functional hemostasis will usually be preserved, and no special precautions or further action (other than repeating the bleeding time) need be taken. However, the patient with a clinically important bleeding diathesis requires some basic advice, even as evaluation proceeds. The nature of the advice depends on the type of bleeding abnormality at hand.

Platelet Disorders

General Measures

Patients with a known qualitative platelet disorder and a history of bleeding should be counseled to avoid salicylates and NSAIDs. Patients with no history of abnormal bleeding before NSAID use can probably continue on the agent, provided the bleeding is clinically unimportant and the indication for drug use is compelling. However, the drug should be stopped in anticipation of a major surgical procedure.

Patients with platelet counts of less than 50,000/mm³ are at risk for posttraumatic bleeding and should be advised to put off surgery, dental extraction, and contact sports until the problem is corrected. The use of stool softeners and a soft toothbrush is recommended. Those with counts of less than 20,000/mm³ are at risk for serious spontaneous bleeding and require hospitalization. Although workup is in progress to identify a cause, all but the most essential medications should be halted, with substance exposures (solvents, insecticides, alcohol) limited and NSAIDs and salicylates prohibited.

Etiologic Therapy

In most instances, treatment of thrombocytopenia should be etiologic and carried out in consultation with a hematologist. A few exceptions are worth noting:

Drug-induced thrombocytopenia should be treated by *halting the suspected medication* immediately. Usually no other treatment is necessary.

HIV infection with thrombocytopenia is an indication for prompt initiation of *antiretroviral therapy* (see Chapter 13).

Idiopathic thrombocytopenic purpura is an indication for immediately starting *high-dose corticosteroid therapy* (e.g., 1 mg of *prednisone* per kilogram per day), especially if the patient is symptomatic. Prednisone can be tapered after 1 to 2 weeks if the platelet count normalizes; if it does not, then splenectomy may be needed. In both instances, hematologic consultation is still warranted, but it should not delay the implementation of initial therapy. A program of very high dose dexamethasone (40 mg/d) given for just for 4 days has shown promise as an effective alternative but needs confirmation before it can be recommended. Eradication of concurrent *Helicobacter pylori* infection appears to have a modest effect in increasing the platelet count, but is insufficient for other than mild disease. *Rituximab* produces response rates of greater than 60% but with a very high incidence of serious side effects and a 2.9% death rate; use is problematic, and it should not be prescribed without hematologic consultation. Studies examining the use of a thrombopoiesis-stimulating protein are ongoing.

Thrombocythemia is best treated with low-dose *aspirin* and *hydroxyurea* when platelet counts get high enough to threaten thrombosis and bleeding. High-risk patients are those older than the age of 60 years with platelet counts of greater than 1 million/mm³ and a history of thrombosis, hemorrhage, hypertension, or diabetes.

Clotting Factor Problems

Excessive Anticoagulation

Most patients on warfarin who exhibit bleeding from excessive anticoagulation need to hold their dose for only a few days to allow the PT to drift back into a safe therapeutic range (see Chapter 83). Large doses of vitamin K should not be used to correct the PT unless anticoagulation is no longer desired because it is difficult to resume anticoagulation quickly in a patient who has recently received large doses; smaller doses are less problematic. An urgent need to correct the PT without impairing future anticoagulation efforts can be met by administering fresh-frozen plasma.

Vitamin K Deficiency

Patients with a poor intake or malabsorption of vitamin K can be given oral vitamin K supplements (2.5 to 10 mg/d) or parenteral doses (10 to 25 mg intramuscularly); in addition, the underlying cause of the malabsorption should be treated (see Chapter 64). Patients with severe hepatocellular failure will not respond to vitamin K because synthetic function has been compromised (see Chapter 71).

Hemophilia

The patient with hemophilia and the patient's family face life-long problems. A detailed discussion of the management of such patients is beyond the scope of this chapter, but basic management includes specifying guidelines for permissible physical activity and teaching proper first aid. If the degree of bleeding has been only mild to moderate, then one can encourage participation in noncontact sports and other activities that entail little risk for injury. The goal is to allow as much normal activity as possible. First-aid treatment of an acute hemarthrosis should be learned by the family. One immobilizes the joint and applies ice packs to reduce pain and swelling. The use of splinting and elastic bandages can help to ensure that a position of good joint function is maintained.

Pain control is important. Aspirin and related nonsteroidal agents must be avoided. Acetaminophen and codeine work well when given in adequate doses for short periods of time. The primary physician should not try to aspirate a hemarthrosis; the risk for causing further bleeding and introducing infection is high.

The administration of *factor VIII concentrate* has been the mainstay of therapy and is used for episodes of acute bleeding and before surgery and dental work. Carefully obtained and elaborately treated concentrate preparations have greatly reduced the risk for transfusion-related HIV infection, and *recombinant preparations* are now available, although they are more expensive. *Desmopressin* is useful in mild disease and as prophylaxis, by increasing the production of factor VIII and von Willebrand factor.

Genetic counseling is an important component of hemophiliac care. Definitive identification of women who are carriers of the hemophilia gene has been difficult, but DNA analysis techniques offer hope of improved identification to facilitate genetic counseling. Early prenatal diagnosis is also available (see prior discussion).

von Willebrand's Disease

In patients with von Willebrand's disease, *DDAVP* is the treatment of choice because it enhances the production of both von Willebrand factor and factor VIII, increasing levels three- to fivefold. It is effective both for episodes of acute bleeding and prophylaxis. For prophylaxis, the drug can be given by subcutaneously at 0.3 μg/kg or by nasal inhalation (300 μg/puff). *Plasma concentrates* containing von Willebrand factor and factor VIII can be given for active bleeding. Platelet concentrates and estrogen–progesterone are used as adjuvants.

Vascular Defects

Patients with *purpura simplex* and *senile purpura* can be reassured. Occasionally, these patients take large doses of vitamins C and K in the hope of lessening their easy bruising; such self-treatment measures are without proven efficacy and only add unnecessary expense. NSAIDs may exacerbate the cosmetic problem and can be withheld if the easy bruising disturbs the patient, but they should not be avoided if there is an important indication for their use. Patients with recurrent bleeding from more serious vascular disease (e.g., hereditary hemorrhagic telangiectasia) should be advised to avoid any agent that might compromise hemostasis. Episodes of bleeding respond to compression if the rest of the hemostatic system is kept intact. Patients with vascular defects often have an iron deficiency from recurrent bleeding; the resulting anemia responds well to oral iron (see Chapter 82).

INDICATIONS FOR ADMISSION AND REFERRAL

Bleeding problems carry the potential for serious harm and call for very careful evaluation and monitoring. If the severity of the condition is in doubt, prompt hospital admission should be considered, especially if a potentially serious but treatable condition is suspected (e.g., TTP, in which timely plasma exchange can have an important effect on outcome). Patients who manifest volume depletion, gross bleeding, bleeding from multiple sites, or a change in mental status require emergency admission. The person who otherwise appears well but has a dangerously low platelet count ($<20,000/mm^3$), an absence of platelets on smear, or a markedly prolonged bleeding time is best evaluated and monitored in the hospital. Hemophiliacs with acute bleeding require emergency transfusion of factor VIII.

Referral or consultation with a hematologist can be helpful when a patient with clinical bleeding is suspected of having a qualitative platelet disorder. Proper test selection and interpretation will be facilitated. Referral is also indicated for patients with unexplained, clinically significant clotting factor deficiencies, severe thrombocytopenia, or suspected hemophilia or von Willebrand's disease.

A.H.G.

Annotated Bibliography

1. Arepally GM, Ortel TL. Heparin-induced thrombocytopenia. N Engl J Med 2006;355:809. (*A clinically oriented review; 49 references.*)
2. Aster RH, Bougie DW. Drug-induced immune thrombocytopenia. N Engl J Med 2007;357:580. (*The best review to date; 57 references.*)
3. Cines DB, Blanchette VS. Immune thrombocytopenic purpura. N Engl J Med 2001;346:995. (*A comprehensive review; 103 references.*)
4. Dojouri K, Vesely SK, George JN. Quinine-associated thrombotic thrombocytopenic purpura–hemolytic uremic syndrome: frequency, clinical features, and long-term outcomes. Ann Intern Med 2001;135:1047. (*Documents the role and the features of quinine as a cause.*)
5. Furie B, Furie BC. Molecular and cellular biology of blood coagulation. N Engl J Med 1992;326:800. (*An excellent short review of basic mechanisms.*)
6. George JN, Vesely SK. Thrombotic thrombocytopenic purpura–hemolytic uremic syndrome: diagnosis and treatment. Cleveland Clinic J Med 2001;68:857. (*A very practical review for the nonhematologist by a leading authority; 29 references.*)
7. Mannucci PM, Tuddenham EGD. The hemophiliac—from royal genes to gene therapy. N Engl J Med 2001;344:1773. (*A useful discussion of genetic mechanisms and management.*)
8. Terreri A, Fonseca R, Pereira DL, et al. A long-term retrospective study of young women with essential thrombocythemia. Mayo Clin Proc 2001;76:22. (*The Mayo Clinic experience, demonstrating long survival and a low risk of life-threatening hemorrhagic complications, as well as an increased incidence of first-trimester miscarriages.*)
9. Warkentin TE, Kelton JG. Temporal aspects of heparin-induced thrombocytopenia. N Engl J Med 2001;344:1286. (*A natural history study, finding that a fall in platelet count can occur over hours in persons with previous heparin exposure.*)
10. Warkentin TE, Levine MN, Hirsh J, et al. Heparin-induced thrombocytopenia in patients treated with low-molecular-weight heparin or unfractionated heparin. N Engl J Med 1995;332:1330. (*The risks for thrombocytopenia and thrombotic events are significantly less with low-molecular-weight heparin.*)

11. Wolanskyj AP, Schwager SM, McClure RF, et al. Essential thrombocythemia beyond the first decade: life-expectancy, long-term complications, and prognostic factors. Mayo Clin Proc 2006;81:159. (*A cohort longitudinal observation study, finding that life expectancy was worse and leukocytosis was predictive of thrombosis and reduced survival.*)

12. Barber A, Green D, Galluzzo T, et al. The bleeding time as a preoperative screening test. Am J Med 1985;78:761. (*This measure was not found to be of value for routine use.*)

13. Barkun AN, Camus M, Green L, et al. Bedside assessment of splenic enlargement. Am J Med 1991;91:512. (*Recommends percussion of the Traube space followed by palpation.*)

14. British Committee for Standards in Haematology General Haematology Task Force. Guidelines for the investigation and management of idiopathic thrombocytopenic purpura. Br J Haematol 2003;120:574. (*Current standards that emphasize ruling out other conditions.*)

15. Bushick JB, Eisenberg JM, Kinman J, et al. Pursuit of abnormal coagulation screening tests generates modest hidden preoperative costs. J Gen Intern Med 1989;4:493. (*Routine prothrombin time [PT] and partial thromboplastin time [TPP] added little additional cost, but the impact of abnormal results was nil.*)

16. Kuwana M, Okazaki Y, Satoh T, et al. Initial laboratory findings useful for predicting the diagnosis of idiopathic thrombocytopenic purpura. Am J Med 2005;1026. (*Finds that the absence of anemia and leukocytopenia, an increase in anti–GPIIb/IIa antibody–producing B cells, an increase in platelet-associated anti–GPIIb/IIa antibody, an elevated reticulocyte count, and a normal or slightly increased thrombopoietin were predictive of idiopathic thrombocytopenic purpura in persons presenting with thrombocytopenia.*)

17. Lind SE. The bleeding time does not predict surgical bleeding. Blood 1991;77:2547. (*A review of the data, finding little predictive value for this measure.*)

18. Mannucci PM. Thrombotic thrombocytopenic purpura: a simpler diagnosis at last? Thromb Haemost 1999;82:1380. (*A discussion of better means of diagnosis.*)

19. Rodgers RPC, Levin J. A critical appraisal of the bleeding time. Semin Thromb Hemost 1990;16:1. (*A detailed review of the utility and shortcomings of this measure.*)

20. Suchman AL, Griner PF. Diagnostic uses of the activated partial thromboplastin time and prothrombin time. Ann Intern Med 1986;104:810. (*Screening with the PT and PTT adds little in the absence of a history of bleeding; normal PT and PTT values rule out a clotting factor abnormality in the patient with a bleeding problem.*)

21. Arnold DM, Dentali F, Crowther MA, et al. Systematic review: efficacy and safety of rituximab for adults with idiopathic immune thrombocytopenia. Ann Intern Med 2007;146:25. (*Finds few randomized studies, an overall response rate of nearly 63%, but a high frequency of significant toxicities and a 2.9% death rate.*)

22. Bussel JB, Kuter DJ, George JN, et al. AMG 531, a thrombopoiesis-stimulating protein for chronic ITP. N Engl J Med 2006;355:1672. (*A phase 2 study of a promising therapy for idiopathic thrombocytopenic purpura.*)

23. Cheng Y, Wong RSM, Soo YOY, et al. Initial treatment of immune thrombocytopenic purpura with high-dose dexamethasone. N Engl J Med 2003;349:831. (*A prospective cohort study, finding that 40 mg/d for 4 days was effective.*)

24. Cohen AJ, Kessler CM. Treatment of inherited coagulation disorders. Am J Med 1995;99:675. (*A useful review for the generalist reader, especially the section on von Willebrand's disease.*)

25. Gernsheimer T, Stratton J, Ballem PJ, et al. Mechanisms of response to treatment in autoimmune thrombocytopenic purpura. N Engl J Med 1989;320:974. (*Prednisone stimulated platelet production; splenectomy prolonged survival.*)

26. Harrison CN, Campbell PJ, Buck G, et al. Hydroxyurea compared with anagrelide in high-risk essential thrombocythemia. N Engl J Med 2005;353:33. (*A randomized, controlled trial, finding that hydroxyurea plus low-dose aspirin was superior.*)

27. Lusher JM, Arkin S, Abildgaard CF, et al. Recombinant factor VIII for the treatment of previously untreated patients with hemophilia A. N Engl J Med 1993;328:453. (*A major multicenter report of the safety and efficacy of this treatment, including the development of inhibitors.*)

28. Mannucci PM. Treatment of von Willebrand's disease. N Engl J Med 2004;351:683. (*A comprehensive review; 103 references.*)

29. Mannucci PM. Hemostatic drugs. N Engl J Med 1998;339:245. (*A succinct general overview.*)

30. McMillan R. Therapy for adults with refractory chronic immune thrombocytopenic purpura. Ann Intern Med 1997;126:307. (*An excellent summary of first-line therapy that can be administered by the primary physician, in addition to indications for referral.*)

31. Stasi R, Rossi Z, Stipa E, et al. *Helicobacter pylori* eradication in the management of patients with idiopathic thrombocytopenic purpura. Am J Med 2004;118:414. (*A cohort study, finding that eradication was beneficial.*)

CHAPTER 82 ■ MANAGEMENT OF COMMON ANEMIAS

Anemia is prevalent throughout the population and occurs in all age groups, but it is especially common in the elderly (11% in noninstitutionalized persons greater than the age of 65 years), in whom it is both a risk factor for reduced survival and independently associated with impaired cognition and reduced functional status (1).

Most of the anemias encountered in the outpatient setting are sufficiently mild or chronic to allow time for the careful design of a cost-effective treatment program. The ease with which a number of anemias (e.g., deficiencies of iron, folate, and vitamin B$_{12}$) can be corrected sometimes leads to empiric therapy or self-treatment without adequate workup for the underlying cause. The skillful application of appropriate treatment is based on a thorough etiologic evaluation (see Chapter 79). Once the cause is understood, attention can be turned to treatment modalities. Increasingly prominent among treatment options is erythropoietin therapy, with an expanding list of indications, but also with emerging concerns that necessitate caution in prescribing. Those caring for patients with sickle cell anemia (who are subject to painful crises) also need to be familiar with the first line of treatment so as to prevent such disabling episodes.

IRON-DEFICIENCY ANEMIA (2–6)

Iron-deficiency anemia is extremely common, occurring in about 10% to 15% of premenopausal women and frequently seen in persons with chronic gastrointestinal blood loss or poor iron absorption. Proper management necessitates identifying the underlying cause (see Chapter 79). Ascribing the anemia to a trivial cause (e.g., menstruation, hemorrhoids) and treating it empirically without a thorough workup for more serious disease (e.g., bowel malignancy) can seriously compromise outcome. A response to iron replacement should not be taken as a sign of a benign cause. The physician must determine whether inadequate intake, poor absorption, increased loss, or a combination of factors is responsible for the anemia. Knowing the most economical, effective, and best-tolerated forms of supplemental iron facilitates the design of an optimal replacement therapy program.

Clinical Presentation and Course

In menstruating women, the balance between dietary iron intake (1 mg/d) and loss (15 mg/mo) is precarious. Low-grade anemia, especially when losses from pregnancy (approximately 500 mg) are not made up, is common. However, the many vague symptoms in otherwise healthy menstruating women that are attributed to "low iron" have not been found to correlate with the degree of anemia or respond to the correction of anemia in controlled studies (see Chapter 79).

Iron-deficiency anemia is usually slow in onset, so that compensatory changes, such as increases in 2,3-diphosphoglycerate and cardiac output, minimize symptoms. When blood loss has been rapid or the anemia is severe (hemoglobin level <7 g/dL), patients are likely to become symptomatic, especially if cardiopulmonary reserve is limited. Replacement therapy is required in such cases, regardless of the underlying cause. The degree of anemia does not correlate with the seriousness of the cause.

Pica (defined as a craving for ice, starch, clay, or any other substance) is particularly common in patients with severe iron deficiency but often goes unreported. Up to 50% of iron-deficient patients may exhibit pica, with *pagophagia* (the craving for ice) accounting for the vast majority of cases. No correlation has been found between the presence of pica and the cause of iron deficiency. Symptoms resolve with treatment.

The occasional patient with severe iron deficiency who presents with *glossitis, angular stomatitis, koilonychia,* or *esophageal web* improves after correction of the deficiency. Whether the *menorrhagia* sometimes seen with iron deficiency is corrected by iron is a subject of debate. Patients who have undergone *subtotal gastrectomy* and gastrojejunostomy have up to a 60% chance of incurring iron deficit because of a loss of acid-secreting capacity, rapid gastric emptying, and bypass of the duodenum. *Pregnancy* is almost certain to produce iron deficiency because a net loss of more than 500 mg of iron occurs. Iron deficiency from chronic gastrointestinal blood loss has been documented in *long-distance runners.*

Unless the cause of the iron deficiency is removed, recurrence rates are high, even when treatment is prescribed. In a series of 100 cases, 29 relapses were noted: In 24 instances, inadequate iron was being taken; in 12, blood loss continued in excess of iron therapy; and in 4 patients, malabsorption was documented.

Principles of Management

As noted, the importance of identifying and treating the underlying cause cannot be overemphasized, especially when the anemia is found in male patients or the elderly. Even in menstruating women, the probability of finding silent but important gastrointestinal disease is substantial. Correcting iron deficiency without attending to the underlying cause can mask an important clue to treatable disease and compromise timely treatment.

Indications

Symptoms are often minimal, and the morbidity from a mild anemia is low, so that treatment in such situations is less important than the discovery of the underlying cause. Moreover, as noted previously, correction of the iron deficit is not certain to alleviate the host of vague symptoms often attributed to it. Nevertheless, replacement therapy makes sense when (a) the patient is symptomatic and has a limited cardiopulmonary reserve, (b) the anemia has become moderately severe (hemoglobin level of 8 to 9 g/dL), (c) the patient is pregnant, (d) the patient has undergone a subtotal gastrectomy and gastrojejunostomy, (e) continued heavy blood loss is anticipated, or (f) the patient is recovering from megaloblastic anemia.

Absorption

Oral iron absorption occurs best under conditions of low pH in the proximal small bowel, such as 1 to 2 hours before a meal or at bedtime. Antacid use reduces absorption, as does food intake; the phytates and phosphates in food bind iron. When iron tablets are taken with meals, absorption drops by more than 50%. Absorption also varies according to the severity of the deficit. About 20% of an oral dose is taken up initially, but absorption falls to 5% after 1 month of replacement therapy, even though the anemia remains incompletely corrected. Ascorbic acid improves absorption in achlorhydric patients.

Side Effects

Upper and lower gastrointestinal symptoms are the principal side effects of oral iron therapy; they can be severe enough to interfere with treatment. The upper gastrointestinal effects are especially troublesome and include *nausea, vomiting, epigastric cramping,* and *acid reflux.* Onset is usually within 1 hour of iron intake. Upper gastrointestinal symptoms are proportional to the amount of ionized iron delivered to the stomach and the proximal small bowel, and they decrease with a reduction in dose. Many patients mistakenly attribute their symptoms to the type of iron preparation used and switch to another; however, most often it is the amount of iron released in the upper digestive tract that accounts for symptoms. Dose reduction is all that is required and frequently suffices. In the very elderly (age >80 years), low-dose therapy can be as effective as normal dosing, minimizing adverse gastrointestinal side effects and improving compliance. The lower gastrointestinal side effects of *constipation* and *diarrhea* are reported by about 25% of users, but these are less a function of the amount of iron available for absorption than are upper gastrointestinal side effects. Constipation usually responds to dietary fiber or a stool softener.

The intramuscular administration of iron has been associated with the development of *sarcomas* at injection sites and should be avoided. Fatal *anaphylactic reactions* and *asthma* have been associated with all parenteral forms of iron administration. If parenteral iron must be given, it should be administered by the intravenous route—first a very small test dose and then a slow drip; a syringe with epinephrine should be drawn up at the same time and kept on hand.

Preparations

Ferrous iron is required for oral use; *ferric* iron is poorly absorbed. The most cost-effective approach to oral iron replacement is use of generic *ferrous sulfate*. It is the least expensive (as little as 10% of the cost of other preparations) and provides the most elemental iron. Its absorption does not require gastric acid, making the preparation useful even in the setting of *Helicobacter pylori* infection and achlorhydria. All commonly used ferrous salts (i.e., *sulfate, gluconate, citrate*) have equivalent rates of absorption, differing principally in the amount of elemental iron released. Choice is a matter of cost and side effects. The severity of gastrointestinal upset is predominantly a function of the amount of iron released rather than the type of ferrous salt used. This is the reason for the increased frequency of gastrointestinal upset associated with the use of ferrous sulfate, which releases the most elemental iron. Some preparations contain ascorbic acid to facilitate absorption, but ferrous sulfate provides sufficient iron to make absorption-enhancing measures unnecessary in most instances. *Slow-release* and *enteric-coated* preparations have been touted as producing fewer side effects and requiring only once-daily administration. However, they dissolve slowly and can bypass the proximal small bowel (where most absorption takes place) before dissolving to a significant degree. There is *no* evidence they are worth the extra cost, which can be several times that of unadulterated ferrous sulfate. An ingenious but expensive ferrous sulfate formulation uses a *gastric delivery system* that is activated by stomach secretions; as a result, the capsule floats and remains within the stomach for a few hours after food has passed. The capsule slowly releases iron during this period, so that iron absorption is enhanced by two to three times, gastrointestinal upset is minimized, and the necessary frequency of dosing is reduced.

Parenteral iron has a very limited role. It should be used only in patients who have had an adequate trial of oral iron and have shown a genuine intolerance to all available preparations. Patients with inflammatory bowel disease may require parenteral iron because of the irritant effect of oral iron and the need to take large doses to keep up with blood loss. Parenteral iron has also been suggested for patients with malabsorption, but most patients are able to absorb a sufficient amount of oral iron. Parenteral iron is best given by the intravenous route (see prior discussion).

Dosing

The *recommended oral dose* for iron deficiency is 300 mg of ferrous sulfate three times daily. As noted, absorption is maximized by dosing 1 to 2 hours before a meal or at bedtime. Although taking iron with a meal reduces absorption, it also lessens disagreeable gastrointestinal symptoms, such as nausea and epigastric discomfort. For the alleviation of gastrointestinal side effects, reducing frequency of dosing is less effective than reducing the dose taken. As noted, low-dose therapy may be as effective in the very elderly as full doses by reducing gastrointestinal upset and enhancing compliance.

Drug–Drug Interactions

The *effect of iron on absorption* of other drugs needs to be kept in mind. When iron is ingested simultaneously, the absorption of *levodopa, methyldopa, tetracycline,* and *fluoroquinolone antibiotics* is reduced by up to 90%. A similar but more variable effect on L-*thyroxine* has been noted. Iron intake should be delayed for several hours after the intake of these other medications, and monitoring of their efficacy should be stepped up during iron therapy.

Drugs that neutralize or inhibit acid secretion (e.g., *antacids, histamine₂ blockers, proton-pump inhibitors*) may reduce iron absorption because a low pH is required in the proximal small bowel for optimal uptake. Taking iron with orange juice (rich in ascorbic acid) or using an ascorbic acid–containing preparation can help in situations in which the suppression of gastric acid is needed.

Duration of Therapy

The response to iron is apparent within 10 days of initiation of therapy; a reticulocytosis is first noted, followed by a rise in the hemoglobin concentration of 0.1 to 0.2 g/dL daily. Therapy for several weeks is required to bring the hemoglobin level back up to normal, and replenishing iron stores may take months. However, speed is not an issue unless blood loss is rapid, in which case blood transfusion rather than iron therapy is the treatment of choice. The response to parenteral iron therapy is no more rapid than that seen with oral preparations.

Patient Education and Prevention of Iron Deficiency

To maximize compliance, patients need to be instructed about the best means of minimizing gastrointestinal side effects. Starting with a small dose of ferrous sulfate (e.g., 300 mg/d) and building to 900 mg/d avoids initial intolerance. Taking iron just after eating may also help. It needs to be made clear that therapy has to be continued on a regular basis for weeks and often months.

The prevention of iron deficiency is most important in individuals with increased needs (i.e., pregnant women and young children). The average U.S. diet contains 12 mg of iron per 2,000 calories. Twenty percent is absorbed by markedly iron-deficient patients and 5% to 10% by others; thus, about 0.6 to 1.2 mg is taken up under normal circumstances each day. The daily requirement for men and postmenopausal women is 0.5 to 1.0 mg, so that dietary intake should suffice. However, the requirement for menstruating women is 1.5 mg/d, and that for pregnant women is 2.5 mg/d. Iron-rich foods can be added to the diet to avoid the need for iron supplements. Liver, oysters, and heavily iron-enriched cereals (containing >45% of the recommended daily iron allowance) are the best dietary sources, providing more than 5 mg of iron per serving. Lean beef, veal, moderately iron-fortified cereals (containing >25% of the daily allowance), and beans are good sources, providing 3 to 5 mg of iron per serving. Fish, chicken, egg yolks, raisins, and fortified breads and pasta are fair sources, providing 1 to 3 mg per serving. Green vegetables are rich in iron, but the iron is less readily available for absorption because it is bound to the phosphates and phytates present in these foods.

When diet alone seems to be inadequate and needs are very high, as in pregnancy, a once-daily dose of 150 to 300 mg of ferrous sulfate is recommended to avoid significant iron deficiency. It must be emphasized that most people who eat a balanced diet do not require iron supplements. Taking widely promoted supplements that contain iron, vitamins, and minerals is expensive and unnecessary in most instances. Excessive iron is associated with increased risks for malignancy and atherosclerotic disease. Patients taking expensive vitamin preparations should be advised that much simpler, less costly, yet equally efficacious preparations are available.

VITAMIN B₁₂ DEFICIENCY (7–13)

Vitamin B₁₂ deficiency can result from inadequate intake, impaired absorption, increased requirements, or faulty utilization. Poor intake is distinctly rare, occurring mostly in ultrastrict vegetarians who refrain from eating eggs and dairy products as well as meat. Many cases of vitamin B₁₂ deficiency are secondary to pernicious anemia; the lack of intrinsic factor compromises absorption. Absorption can also be impaired by achlorhydria, disease of the terminal ileum, bacterial overgrowth resulting from stasis, and gastrectomy. Faulty utilization is uncommon; it occurs with genetic defects in the synthesis of transcobalamin, the plasma protein that transports vitamin B_{12}.

Clinical Presentation and Course

Irrespective of cause, vitamin B_{12} deficiency may lead to slowly evolving *megaloblastic anemia, glossitis,* and *neuropathy*. Macrocytosis is usually the first hematologic manifestation and can precede anemia by as much as 1 to 2 years. Hypersegmentation of neutrophils is another early hematologic finding. Because of the body's large vitamin B_{12} storage capacity, the onset of clinical manifestations may take months to years. Although megaloblastic anemia and glossitis also occur with folic acid deficiency, the neuropathy is distinctive. Traditionally, neurologic symptoms were believed to be a late development, associated with a vitamin B_{12} level of less than 100 pg/mL. However, careful studies have documented vitamin B_{12}–responsive neuropsychiatric deficits in the absence of such marked vitamin B_{12} deficiency, anemia, or machine-determined macrocytosis (although hypersegmentation and macrocytosis were often noted on examination of the peripheral smear).

Classically, the neurologic syndromes include those of peripheral neuropathy and subacute combined degeneration (symmetric paresthesias in the hands and feet, and progression to ataxia resulting from loss of vibratory and position sense as the posterior columns of the spinal cord become involved). However, cortical involvement is also prevalent and may present as memory loss (simulating dementia), disorientation, depression, hallucinations, agitation, personality change, perversions of taste and smell, irritability, or central visual scotomas. If left untreated, many neurologic deficits can become permanent.

In pernicious anemia, coincident thyroid disease, rheumatoid arthritis, vitiligo, or gastric cancer may be present. *Achlorhydria* after histamine stimulation is characteristic. The diagnosis is usually made by the Schilling test, with the use of exogenous intrinsic factor to help to document its absence (see Chapter 79).

Principles of Management

Prompt recognition and treatment are essential to minimize the risk for permanent neurologic damage. Early disease produces reversible demyelination; if uncorrected, it progresses to nerve death and permanent neurologic dysfunction. Thus, in a patient with neurologic symptoms suggestive of vitamin B_{12} deficiency, prompt diagnosis (see Chapters 79, 167, and 169) and treatment are paramount. Parenteral therapy is preferred (except in the rare patient with poor intake) because most vitamin B_{12} deficiency is secondary to impaired absorption. However, the use of large oral doses (>100 μg/d) may result in sufficient absorption of vitamin B_{12} in some cases. *Cyanocobalamin* is the most commonly used parenteral formulation, although *hydroxycobalamin* is better bound to serum proteins and less rapidly excreted, so that less frequent administration is possible. In practice, either form of vitamin B_{12} suffices.

Replacement Regimens

Many initial replacement regimens are recommended. A commonly used program is 1,000 μg/wk of an intramuscular cobalamin preparation for several weeks, followed by monthly doses. Although this regimen probably provides more B_{12} than can be initially used, it helps to reconstitute depleted B_{12} stores. If neurologic symptoms are present, a twice-monthly follow-up dose is recommended for 6 months. Some argue that 1,000-μg doses are unnecessary because only 100 μg can be effectively metabolized at one time, with the remainder promptly excreted in the urine. However, because of their low cost and safety, maintenance doses of 1,000 μg are often given. Others note that monthly injections after initial replacement are unnecessary, finding that an injection once every 3 to 4 months suffices for many patients. The optimal program can be individualized, although it is probably best to continue with a monthly regimen in patients with neurologic sequelae. More important than the interval of therapy is its indefinite continuation, which must be ensured. Relapse of symptoms is common in the absence of continued therapy. Compliance with a monthly injection program is often poor; having the visiting nurse or family member give the injection is helpful and far less inconvenient than a monthly office visit.

Vitamin B_{12} deficiency can be prevented in the elderly, in whom gastric atrophy, hypochlorhydria, and food-cobalamin malabsorption (see Chapter 79) are frequent findings, with a daily oral intake of 25 to 1,000 μg of cyanocobalamin. About 1% is absorbed.

Response to Treatment

The response can be dramatic, with marked reticulocytosis noted within 72 hours and a rapid improvement in neurologic deficits, especially those that are mild or of short duration. However, neurologic problems that have been present longer may take 6 to 12 months to improve, and deficits that persist after 12 to 18 months of therapy are probably permanent, which underscores the importance of a timely diagnosis for successful therapy.

During recovery, serious *hypokalemia* can develop in patients who have had a severe depletion of vitamin B_{12} as potassium is taken up by new red cells. The serum potassium level should be monitored, and supplements should be provided if it falls to less than normal. Concurrent folic acid supplementation is not needed. In fact, the inappropriate use of a large pharmacologic dose of oral folate (e.g., 5 mg) alone may partially and nonspecifically correct the anemia and mask an underlying vitamin B_{12} deficiency, which puts the patient at risk for an acute, marked deterioration of neurologic function if vitamin B_{12} is not given. There is no harm in having the patient take folate in addition to vitamin B_{12}, but this is rarely necessary unless the diet is extremely poor.

Other Treatment Modalities

Patients with a vitamin B_{12} deficiency caused by bacterial overgrowth or disease of the terminal ileum require treatment directed at the underlying bowel problem. Oral *antibiotic therapy* with tetracycline or amoxicillin provides temporary relief from bacterial overgrowth. More-definitive treatment of inflammatory bowel disease may be indicated (see Chapter 73).

Unnecessary Vitamin B_{12} Therapy

Many well-intentioned physicians have used parenteral vitamin B_{12} as a nonspecific therapy for patients bothered by fatigue or other vague symptoms. In one study of a rural health clinic, 10% of all patients attending the clinic were found to be receiving such treatment regularly, 6% in the absence of appropriate indications for its use. Many persons without a vitamin B_{12} deficiency report symptomatic benefit from monthly injections, probably as a consequence of a strong placebo effect. Even after being told that it is unnecessary, a large proportion remain reluctant to halt such therapy or stop temporarily, only to seek out a physician willing to restart it. Although giving vitamin B_{12} entails little direct risk, its use can be misleading and should be abandoned in favor of a more comprehensive and etiologic approach to the patient's underlying problems, whether they are those of anxiety, depression, somatization, or an underlying medical problem (see Chapters 8, 226, 227, and 230). Patients taking vitamin B_{12} injections unnecessarily should be counseled on the need to explore the underlying cause of their symptoms.

FOLIC ACID DEFICIENCY (14)

Causes

Most folic acid deficiency results from inadequate intake, although occasionally increased need or impairment of absorption or utilization is encountered. *Dietary deficiency* is in part a consequence of the limited capacity to store folate; within 3 months of initiation of an inadequate diet, megaloblastic changes and anemia can develop. Foods rich in folate include green vegetables (asparagus, lettuce, spinach, broccoli), liver, yeast, and mushrooms. The excessive boiling of vegetables in water can remove a substantial amount of available folic acid. *Alcoholism* is responsible for many cases of inadequate intake.

Impaired absorption is seen in the context of ileal disease (e.g., tropical and nontropical sprue, heavy infestation with *Giardia*), short-bowel syndrome, and phenytoin use. *Increased demand* takes place in the setting of pregnancy, severe hyperthyroidism, hemolytic anemia, malignancy, and florid psoriasis. *Utilization* is *hindered* by the use of methotrexate; triamterene and trimethoprim have similar although less marked effects on dihydrofolate reductase. Patients undergoing hemodialysis experience substantial folic acid *loss*, so that replacement therapy is necessary.

Clinical Presentation

Folate deficiency is one of the megaloblastic anemias. It is sometimes accompanied by glossitis. Anemia occurs within 3 to 4 months of the onset of deficiency. Diagnostic features include a low serum folate level (<15 ng/mL) and a marked reticulocytosis in response to physiologic doses (200 μg) of folic acid. The response to treatment with folic acid is prompt. No neurologic deficits are associated with folic acid deficiency, but elevations in serum *homocysteine* occur, which are associated with premature atherosclerotic disease and a heightened risk for venous thrombosis (see Chapters 30, 31, and 35).

Treatment

Treatment for most patients involves orally administered pharmacologic doses of folic acid (1 to 2 mg/d). Most forms of folic acid deficiency, even malabsorptive types, can be overcome by oral therapy. Four to five weeks of treatment usually reverses the anemia and replenishes body stores. When the underlying cause persists (e.g., malabsorption, malignancy, psoriasis, hemodialysis), long-term therapy is indicated. Patients taking methotrexate can be given folinic acid, which bypasses the inhibition of dihydrofolate reductase. As noted, the nonspecific use of folic acid to treat a megaloblastic anemia is ill advised

because it may mask an underlying vitamin B_{12} deficiency, delay diagnosis and treatment, and precipitate neurologic symptoms. If alcoholism is the basis of the folate deficiency, then the drinking problem requires careful attention in its own right (see Chapter 228). Patients with folate deficiency will benefit from dietary counseling and perhaps a referral to the nutritionist.

ERYTHROPOIETIN-RESPONSIVE ANEMIAS (15–19)

End-Stage Renal Disease

Anemias secondary to erythropoietin-deficiency states such as end-stage renal disease have previously been among the most refractory to treatment. Erythropoietin-replacement therapy, made possible by the advent of *recombinant human erythropoietin* (e.g., *darbepoetin* [Aranesp], *epoetin alfa* [Procrit]—also referred to as *erythropoietic-stimulating agents* [ESAs]), represents a major advance in the management of such anemias.

Indications and Target Hemoglobin

Randomized, controlled trials have established the cost-effectiveness of erythropoietin use in dialysis patients with regular transfusion requirements, achieving an almost universal elimination of such requirements, a normalization of the hematocrit, and an improved quality of life. The currently recommended target hemoglobin is 12 mg/dL.

Adverse Effects

Side effects are modest (e.g., *iron deficiency* necessitating iron replacement, mild increases in *blood pressure*) when the target hemoglobin is limited to a goal of 12 gm/dL, but overtreatment (driven in part by strong financial incentives) is common. Meta-analytic data revealed that treatment to a hemoglobin level greater than 12 gm/dL increased the risk of *all-cause mortality* (relative risk [RR] 1.17), poorly controlled *hypertension* (RR, 1.27), and *arteriovenous access thrombosis* (RR, 1.34). The mechanism(s) responsible for these serious adverse effects are unclear, but suspicion is strong that the principal factor is the high dose of erythropoietin and not the hemoglobin level per se. Consequently, doses should be kept low. In addition, pure *red cell aphasia* due to antibody formation against erythropoietin has been noted with the chronic use of some recombinant erythropoietin preparations, predominantly in persons with chronic renal failure.

Preoperative Anemia

A reduced requirement for allogeneic transfusions has become a major objective for patients undergoing elective surgery. The donation of autologous blood has become a standard practice in many settings. The presence of anemia before surgery is a major predictor of the need for intraoperative or postoperative transfusion. The increasing desire to reduce exposure to allogeneic blood has stimulated a demand for autologous transfusion and an interest in the contribution of erythropoietin therapy. Work is ongoing on better methods for procuring autologous blood to bring the costs of this approach down to the range of that for allogeneic transfusion.

Weekly preoperative use of recombinant erythropoietin therapy can limit transfusion requirements (and so the need for allogeneic blood) and facilitate the donation of autologous blood. A preoperative program of two to four weekly subcutaneous doses of erythropoietin plus autologous blood donation appears to limit the risk for exposure to allogeneic blood significantly. Although the preoperative use of erythropoietin to facilitate autologous transfusion appears to be a relatively safe and effective alternative to allogeneic transfusion, it is important to keep in mind that allogeneic transfusion is safer than ever due to improvements in education and behavioral risk-factor screening of donors and better laboratory testing. The estimated risk for viral transmission is about 1 in 700,000 units for transfusion-transmitted HIV; for hepatitis C, about 1 in 100,000; and for hepatitis B, 1 in 63,000.

Indications

The best candidates for preoperative erythropoietin to support autologous transfusion appear to be patients with a preoperative hematocrit in the range of 33% to 39% who are to undergo surgery entailing an expected large blood loss (2 to 6 units). Once-weekly erythropoietin administration is the most cost-effective mode of administration in this setting. Due to concerns about the increased risk of death, hypertension, and thrombosis seen in other settings of erythropoietin use, it probably wise to limit erythropoietin use, avoid high-dose therapy, and keep to a target hemoglobin goal of no more than 12 mg/dL.

Cancer and Cancer Chemotherapy

Erythropoietin has also proved to be cost-effective in the setting of cancer chemotherapy, in which severe anemia and reduced serum erythropoietin levels are common; treatment makes possible more-aggressive cancer therapy and markedly reduced transfusion requirements. Nonetheless, there is no evidence of improved survival, and reductions in transfusion benefit and improvement in quality of life occur only in patients with hemoglobin levels less than 10 g/dL. Emerging evidence of increased risks of new malignancy, more rapid tumor growth, thromboembolic events, and all-cause mortality have greatly tempered enthusiasm for erythropoietin use in cancer, limiting it to persons undergoing chemotherapy and triggering revised treatment recommendations and black-box warnings from the U.S. Food and Drug Administration.

Indications for Use

Due to the risks noted previously, ESA therapy is currently limited to patients with chemotherapy-associated anemia. The most recent American Society of Hematology and American Society of Clinical Oncology clinical practice guidelines recommend the following:

■ Initiating ESA therapy only as hemoglobin approaches or falls to less than 10 g/dL.
■ Continuing therapy beyond 6 to 8 weeks only if there has been response.
■ Monitoring iron stores and supplementing iron intake.
■ Prescribing very cautiously in clinical settings associated with an elevated risk for thromboembolic complications.

■ Avoiding use in patients with cancer who are not receiving chemotherapy.

SICKLE CELL DISEASE (20–22)

The need to treat sickle cell disease is especially pressing in patients with painful crises. Vascular occlusion may result from hemolytic episodes induced by sickling; this leads in turn to the chest pain syndrome and stroke, which can be life threatening, and to asplenia. Transfusion requirements can be high. Theoretically, the ideal approach to therapy would be to block sickling (hemoglobin S polymerization), reduce the intracellular hemoglobin concentration, and induce the formation of hemoglobin F.

Direct Inhibition of Sickling and Reduction of Intracellular Hemoglobin Concentration

No sufficiently safe and effective drugs are available that directly inhibit sickling. Reducing the intracellular hemoglobin concentration is a less direct means of inhibiting sickling; the rate of sickling is proportional to the concentration of hemoglobin S. To achieve a lower intracellular concentration, efforts have focused on increasing intracellular water. This is accomplished through the inhibition of potassium loss with low-dose *clotrimazole* therapy, which blocks one set of potassium channels. The results of initial studies are promising, but confirmation and safety of long-term use remain to be demonstrated. *Magnesium* supplements have been shown to block other modes of potassium egress from red cells and are being studied in sickle cell disease.

Increasing Hemoglobin F

Hemoglobin F inhibits the polymerization and sickling of hemoglobin S. Efforts to encourage the synthesis of hemoglobin F have led to the use of the myelosuppressive drug *hydroxyurea* in the treatment of sickle cell disease. Although the mechanism by which hydroxyurea increases hemoglobin S synthesis is unknown, it has proved to be effective in national prospective, randomized trials in reducing hemolysis, which necessitates transfusion, and the number and severity of painful crises and episodes of chest pain syndrome. Paradoxically, the increase in hemoglobin F is only short lived, yet the effect of the drug persists, which correlates with its suppression of neutrophil and reticulocyte counts. The major concern with the long-term use of hydroxyurea is that it is associated with the induction of malignancy. This concern has stimulated searches for alternatives. Results with *erythropoietin* are mixed; *butyric acid* and its analogues are also being studied for their effects on hemoglobin F synthesis. *Gene therapy* is likely to be applied in the future to manage this classic genetic disease.

A.H.G.

Annotated Bibliography

1. Denny SD, Kuchibhatia MN, Cohen HJ. Impact of anemia on mortality, cognition, and function in community-dwelling elderly. Am J Med 2006;119:327. (*A cross-sectional community-based cohort study, finding that there was a significant effect of anemia on survival, cognition, and functional status.*)
2. Boggs DR. Fate of a ferrous sulfate prescription. Am J Med 1987;82:124.

(*Most patients received a more expensive, less effective enteric-coated or slow-release form, even when it was not ordered.*)
3. Campbell NR, Hasinoff BB. Iron supplements: a common cause of drug interactions. Br J Clin Pharmacol 1991;31:251. (*A good summary of these important interactions; most occur when tablets are taken simultaneously.*)

4. Crosby W. Who needs iron? N Engl J Med 1977;297:543. (*A succinct and still pertinent review of iron requirements and the need for supplementation.*)
5. Rector WG. Pica—its frequency and significance in patients with iron-deficiency anemia due to chronic gastrointestinal blood loss. J Gen Intern Med 1989;4:512. (*The condition was found to be frequent and resolved with therapy; there was no relation to etiology.*)
6. Rimon E, Kagansky N, Kagansky M, et al. Are we giving too much iron? Low-dose iron therapy is effective in octogenarians. Am J Med 2005;118:1142. (*A randomized, controlled trial, finding that lower-dose therapy usually sufficed.*)
7. Carmel R. Prevalence of undiagnosed pernicious anemia in the elderly. Arch Intern Med 1996;156:1097. (*Mild deficiency was common and unrecognized but responded to treatment, with improved neurologic function.*)
8. Kuzminski AM, Del Giacco EJ, Allen RH, et al. Effective treatment of cobalamin deficiency with oral cobalamin. Blood 1998;92:1191. (*The best initial treatment remains parenteral intramuscular administration.*)
9. Lawhorne L, Ringdahl D. Cyanocobalamin injections for patients without documented deficiency: reasons for administration and patient responses to proposed discontinuation. JAMA 1989;261:1920. (*A well-documented example of unwarranted empiric use.*)
10. Lindenbaum J, Healton EB, Savage DG, et al. Neuropsychiatric disorders caused by cobalamin deficiency in the absence of anemia or macrocytosis. N Engl J Med 1988;318:1720. (*Emphasizes the need for a high index of suspicion and early treatment.*)
11. Savage D, Lindenbaum J. Relapses after interruption of cyanocobalamin therapy in patients with pernicious anemia. Am J Med 1983;74:765. (*Emphasizes the importance of ensuring an indefinite provision of therapy.*)
12. Teunisse S, Bollen AE, van Gool WA, et al. Dementia and subnormal levels of vitamin B12: effects of replacement therapy. J Neurol 1996;243:522. (*A prolonged duration of vitamin B_{12} deficiency was associated with a poor neurologic response.*)
13. Toh BH, van Driel IR, Gleeson PA. Pernicious anemia. N Engl J Med 1997;337:1441. (*An authoritative review of pathophysiology, diagnosis, and treatment.*)
14. Malinow MR, Duell PB, Hess PB, et al. Reduction of plasma homocyst(e)ine levels by breakfast cereal fortified with folic acid in patients with coronary disease. N Engl J Med 1998;338:1009. (*Fortified breakfast cereal can reduce plasma homocysteine modestly, a purported risk factor for coronary mortality.*)
15. Casadevall N, Nataf J, Viron B, et al. Pure red-cell aplasia and antierythropoietin antibodies in patients treated with recombinant erythropoietin. N Engl J Med 2002;346:469. (*This rare adverse immune response was found in persons taking the agent chronically for anemia of chronic renal failure, but the result bears keeping in mind with all use.*)
16. Glynn SA, Kleinman SH, Schreiber GB, et al. Trends in incidence and prevalence of major transfusion-transmissible viral infections in US blood donors, 1991 to 1996. JAMA 2000;284:229. (*Important data on viral risk from transfusion and means to lower it.*)
17. Kaushansky K. Lineage-specific hematopoietic growth factors. N Engl J Med 2006;354:2034. (*An excellent review for the generalist reader, including sections on mechanisms and use; 78 references.*)
18. Phrommintikul A, Haas SJ, Elsik M, et al. Mortality and target haemoglobin concentrations in anemic patients with chronic kidney disease treated with erythropoietin: a meta-analysis. Lancet 2007;369:38. (*There was an increased risk of death, hypertension, and arteriovenous access thrombosis when hemoglobin increased to >12 mg/dL.*)
19. Rizzo JD, Somerfield MR, Hagerty KL, et al. Use of epoetin and darbepoetin in patients with cancer: 2007 American Society of Hematology/American Society of Clinical Oncology clinical practice guideline update. Blood 2008;111:25. (*Current guidelines for use, incorporating new data on enhanced neoplasia risk in some settings.*)
20. Ballas SK. Management of sickle cell pain. Curr Opin Hematol 1997;4:104. (*A good review of modalities for painful episodes.*)
21. Bunn HF. Pathogenesis and treatment of sickle cell disease. N Engl J Med 1997;337:762. (*An excellent review of basic mechanisms and implications for treatment.*)
22. Charache S, Terrin ML, Moore RD, et al. Effect of hydroxyurea on the frequency of painful crises in sickle cell anemia. N Engl J Med 1995;332:1317. (*A major national randomized trial, demonstrating efficacy.*)

CHAPTER 83 ■ OUTPATIENT ORAL ANTICOAGULANT THERAPY

ELAINE M. HYLEK

Oral anticoagulant therapy with coumarin derivatives effectively prevents thromboembolism in a variety of conditions, ranging from venous thrombosis to atrial fibrillation. Oral platelet inhibitors help to prevent thrombosis and restenosis of coronary arteries. This expanded range of applications for oral anticoagulants makes their proper use an important responsibility of the primary care physician. To optimize patient care, physicians must know (a) the indications for warfarin and antiplatelet therapy, (b) how to initiate and maintain patients on oral anticoagulants in the outpatient setting, (c) common complications, and (d) the drugs and conditions that interfere with or potentiate the anticoagulant effect. This chapter focuses primarily on coumarin derivatives and aspirin (see Chapter 30 for a discussion of the use of other antiplatelet agents).

WARFARIN

Mechanisms of Action

Warfarin and other coumarin derivatives act by inhibiting the action of vitamin K in the γ-carboxylation of glutamic acid residues on coagulation factors II, VII, IX, and X. Without γ-carboxylation, these proteins cannot participate in coagulation. The warfarin-induced decline in active, carboxylated coagulation factors is a function of the half-life of each factor, which varies from 5 hours for factor VII to 72 hours for factor II. The prothrombin time (PT) may be prolonged after only 2 to 3 days of therapy, but this represents primarily the depression of factor VII. The full antithrombotic effect of warfarin is achieved only after 5 to 7 days, with the depletion of factor II.

Indications (1–10)

Therapy is indicated in conditions associated with a high risk for thrombus formation and subsequent embolization. These include the following:

- Atrial fibrillation (see Chapters 28 and 33)
- Valvular heart disease and prosthetic heart valves (see Chapter 33)
- Systemic embolization (see Chapter 171)
- Deep venous thrombosis (see Chapter 35)
- Pulmonary embolization (see Chapter 35)
- Dilated cardiomyopathy and left ventricular thrombus (see Chapter 32)
- Following myocardial infarction in selected patients (see Chapter 31)

Atrial Fibrillation

Atrial fibrillation is highly prevalent, and is found in 5% of people older than 60 years and nearly 10% of people older than 80 years. It increases the risk for stroke more than fivefold; the patient in atrial fibrillation has a 5% average annual risk for stroke. Patients with atrial fibrillation secondary to valvular heart disease are at even greater risk (see also Chapters 28 and 32).

Prosthetic Heart Valves

Prosthetic heart valves increase the risk for systemic emboli, especially stroke. The risk is higher with caged-ball and tilting-disk valves and with valves in the mitral rather than the aortic position. Anticoagulation is continued indefinitely. Patients with bioprosthetic valves need only short-term (e.g., for 3 months) anticoagulation unless another indication, such as atrial fibrillation or a history of systemic embolism, is present (see also Chapter 33).

Deep Venous Thrombosis and Pulmonary Embolism

Deep venous thrombosis and pulmonary embolism are indications for anticoagulation. A 3- to 6-month course may suffice when risk factors are reversible or time limited, such as surgery, temporary immobilization, or estrogen use. Patients with a first episode of idiopathic deep venous thrombosis or deep venous thrombosis in the presence of an inherited thrombophilia should be treated for at least 6 months. In patients with recurrent deep venous thrombosis or pulmonary embolism, a known hypercoagulable state, or homozygosity for factor V Leiden, anticoagulation should be continued indefinitely (see also Chapter 35).

Dilated Cardiomyopathy

Dilated cardiomyopathy puts patients at risk for embolization. When this condition was accompanied by atrial fibrillation, the annual risk for embolic events in the absence of anticoagulation exceeded 15% in one cohort study. Without atrial fibrillation, the risk is in the 1% to 5% range. The absence of randomized trials demonstrating risk reduction with anticoagulation precludes definitive recommendations. Potential benefits and risks must be weighed for individual patients (see also Appendix 33.1).

TABLE 83.1
CONTRAINDICATIONS TO ANTICOAGULANT THERAPY WITH WARFARIN
Absolute Contraindications Previous central nervous system bleeding Recent neurosurgery Active frank bleeding Early pregnancy and delivery **Relative Contraindications** Active peptic ulcer disease Chronic alcoholism Bleeding diathesis Severe hypertension

Myocardial Infarction

Some patients may benefit from anticoagulation following myocardial infarction. Anterior Q-wave infarction, particularly with evidence of mural thrombosis, or atrial fibrillation warrants anticoagulation. Otherwise, there is no evident advantage for warfarin over aspirin in chronic stable angina or in the secondary prevention of myocardial infarction (see also Chapter 31).

Contraindications

Contraindications to the use of oral anticoagulants need to be considered in the context of urgency of anticoagulation, risk and seriousness of potential complications, and duration of therapy (Table 83.1). Patients with previous *central nervous system bleeding*, *recent neurosurgery*, or *frank bleeding* should not receive warfarin. Important relative contraindications include active *peptic ulcer disease*, *chronic alcoholism*, *blindness* (unless in supervised situations), *bleeding diathesis*, and *severe hypertension*. When taken in early *pregnancy*, coumarins may cause birth defects; when they are used at delivery, fetal hemorrhage can occur. Heparin should be used in place of warfarin during early pregnancy and childbirth. Embarking on oral anticoagulant therapy is unwise when follow-up cannot be readily maintained, when laboratory facilities for accurately measuring the PT are inadequate, or when the patient is not adherent to the treatment plan.

Initiating and Monitoring Therapy (11–17)

Initiation for Acute Pulmonary Embolization and Systemic Thromboembolization

Patients with acute pulmonary embolization or acute systemic thrombosis should be admitted to the hospital for immediate administration of *heparin* to halt clot propagation. Intravenous *unfractionated heparin* has been the standard initial anticoagulant treatment. Evidence suggests that *low-molecular-weight heparin* (which can be administered subcutaneously twice daily and does not require continuous monitoring of the PT time) is at least as safe and effective and may be a more convenient alternative to conventional therapy in stable patients. Low-molecular-weight-heparin should not be used in patients with significant renal impairment. Physicians should refer to the package insert for detailed dosing information.

Warfarin should be started on the first day of heparin therapy and overlapped with heparin for at least 4 days to ensure adequate reduction in prothrombin levels. Initiating warfarin therapy with 5-mg daily dose is recommended. Starting doses less than 5 mg are advised for elderly women and malnourished patients. Initiation with a 10-mg dose should be reserved for young, healthy patients. Once the International Normalized Ratio (INR) is greater than 2.0 on at least 2 consecutive days, heparin can be discontinued.

Initiation for Acute Deep Venous Thrombosis

For patients with deep venous thrombosis, subcutaneous administration of *low-molecular-weight heparin* is an effective alternative to intravenous (IV) administration of unfractionated heparin for initial anticoagulation (see Chapter 35). It allows for a shortened hospital stay or an entirely at-home anticoagulant treatment program, which reduces costs. Warfarin therapy is instituted in the same fashion as for IV heparin therapy.

Initiation for Chronic Atrial Fibrillation and Other Nonacute Indications

Patients who are in less urgent need of immediate full anticoagulation (e.g., chronic stable atrial fibrillation) can be safely started on warfarin alone as outpatients. A generally accepted approach to initiating outpatient warfarin therapy is to give 5 mg daily, measure the INR on the fourth day, and adjust the dose accordingly. The starting dose should be set at 2.5 mg daily in patients who weigh less than 110 lb, are older than 75 years, or are at increased risk for bleeding. Warfarin is best taken on an empty stomach at a specific time each day. Administration at bedtime allows for changes to be made in the dose on the same day that the INR is measured. The U.S. Food and Drug Administration has approved several generic warfarins; the same generic or brand formulation should be used consistently to avoid patient confusion and INR fluctuation.

Monitoring

The intensity of anticoagulation is measured with the PT test and expressed as the prothrombin time ratio (PTR), which is the ratio of the patient's PT to the control PT of the laboratory. Standardization of the PTR across laboratories is necessary to account for the different sensitivities of the various thromboplastin reagents used in the assay. The INR has replaced the PTR as the universally accepted measure of anticoagulation intensity. To calculate the INR, the PTR is raised to the power of the International Sensitivity Index (ISI) of the specific reagent used (i.e., PTR^{ISI}).

It can take up to 3 months to achieve a stable warfarin dose. Once stabilized, the INR can be checked every 3 to 4 weeks. The variability in the warfarin dose response mandates frequent monitoring. Changes in the warfarin requirement may be precipitated by a change in diet, particularly the intake of foods with a high content of vitamin K (e.g., most leafy vegetables) or by medications that interfere with the hepatic clearance of warfarin. Many commonly used drugs potentiate the anticoagulant effect of warfarin and should prompt close monitoring (see later discussion). Patients with lupus anticoagulants (among the antiphospholipid antibodies that can cause hypercoagulability and thrombosis; see Chapter 35) may pose a particular problem in monitoring because these antibodies can interfere with the PT assay. Both overestimation and underestimation of the degree of anticoagulation can result. Consultation with a hematologist is needed to design the anticoagulation monitoring program for such a patient.

Technologic advances have made finger-stick *home monitoring* an increasingly practical option. In studies of home monitoring with properly trained patients or family members, control was equal to that achieved with an anticoagulation clinic, and rates of major and minor complications were lower.

Intensity and Duration of Therapy and Adjustment of Dose (18–22)

Recommended Intensity of Therapy

After the initiation of therapy, the dose should be adjusted to maintain the therapeutic range. Extensive study supports the use of lower ranges of anticoagulation intensity (INR target range of 2.0 to 3.0) for most groups of patients. Efficacy is maintained while the risk for hemorrhagic complications is reduced. Only those patients at highest risk for thromboembolism (e.g., mechanical prosthetic heart valves) should receive *high-intensity anticoagulation* (INR range of 2.5 to 3.5). *Low-intensity therapy* (INR target of 1.5 to 2.0) has been tried for deep vein thrombosis but has been proved to be less effective and no safer than standard-intensity therapy (see Chapter 35).

Adjustment of Dose

There is wide variability in patient response to warfarin, determined in part by genetic variants of the hepatic microsomal enzyme *CYP2C9*, which is the principal enzyme responsible for warfarin metabolism. Genetic variants have been identified (e.g., *CYP2C9*2* and *CYP2C9*3*) that are associated with increased risks of overanticoagulation and bleeding; however, these mutations appear to be rare. More commonly, differences in the *warfarin target gene*, which encodes for the vitamin K epoxide reductase complex 1 (*VKORC1*) appear to predict response to warfarin therapy. Whether gene typing will become a routine part of warfarin therapy remains to be established, but the mechanisms for personal differences in response to warfarin are becoming much better understood and underscore the need for dose adjustment.

The warfarin dose can be adjusted in numerous ways when the INR is out of range. One method designed to maximize safety and avoid wide swings in the INR is based on making 10% changes in the weekly dose unless the INR is grossly out of range. For example, if the patient is taking 7.5 mg/d, the weekly dose is 52.5 mg. If the INR is too low, the weekly dose is increased by 10%, so the patient takes 10 mg on 2 days of the week and 7.5 mg on the other 5 days. The INR is then measured weekly for the next 2 weeks, with continued adjustment in dose if necessary.

Outpatient anticoagulation requires facilities for accurate INR measurement and reliable collection of blood samples and the ability to contact patients promptly. Careful monitoring and follow-up are essential for a safe and successful outpatient anticoagulation program. At the beginning of therapy, patients should attend an educational session with a nurse who can instruct them in the use of warfarin, answer questions, test their understanding, and provide informative booklets for them to take home. Patients who fail to keep an appointment for an INR test should be promptly contacted. A computer system can provide reminders so that no patient is lost to follow-up. Commercial laboratory services are sometimes used to draw samples at home for patients who have difficulty coming to the office. Home monitoring devices are another option for selective patients.

Duration of Therapy

In the absence of hemorrhagic complications, anticoagulation should be continued indefinitely in patients with atrial fibrillation, valvular heart disease, or mechanical prosthetic heart valves. Patients with recurrent deep venous thrombosis, recurrent pulmonary embolism, or a known hypercoagulable state should also receive anticoagulants indefinitely. Those with a single episode of deep venous thrombosis caused by a self-limited risk factor and no known hypercoagulable state can stop their warfarin after 3 to 6 months (see Chapter 35).

D-*Dimer testing* has been explored as a means of better determining the duration of therapy. In persons with idiopathic deep venous thrombosis, those with an elevated D-dimer level 1 month after discontinuation of anticoagulant therapy have been found to have a significant risk of recurrence that can be reduced by the resumption of warfarin. These findings require confirmation before routine D-dimer testing can be recommended in this setting, but the results are encouraging for this difficult determination.

Complications (23–28)

Reports of the incidence of hemorrhagic complications in patients on long-term anticoagulant therapy have varied widely, depending on the patient population, the definition of bleeding used, and the INR target under study. Several series have demonstrated that hemorrhage severe enough to require hospitalization or transfusion should occur in fewer than 2% of patients who are carefully monitored. The rate of *intracranial hemorrhage* among patients managed in a structured setting is approximately 0.6%/yr. Risk factors for hemorrhagic complications include an INR higher than 4.0, the recent initiation of

anticoagulation, and a wide fluctuation in the INR. A history of gastrointestinal bleeding is a risk factor; peptic ulcer disease per se is not. Older patients generally experience a higher incidence of complications, but this may be partly mediated through other risk factors more common among the elderly.

Patients experiencing urinary, gastrointestinal, or gynecologic bleeding while on anticoagulant therapy should undergo a diagnostic evaluation to identify any underlying pathologic lesion.

Hemorrhagic necrosis of the skin (more common among women) and cyanotic toes (more common among men) occur rarely, even with INRs in the therapeutic range. The mechanism may be a transient inhibition of endothelial vitamin K–dependent antithrombotic proteins (proteins S and C) in patients congenitally deficient in such factors.

Effects of Drugs and Concurrent Illnesses on Anticoagulation (29–33)

Potentiation

Drugs that potentiate the effect of warfarin may do so by preventing the synthesis or absorption of vitamin K, displacing warfarin from binding sites, inhibiting microsomal degradative enzyme activity, increasing the catabolism of clotting factors, or impairing platelet function (Table 83.2). The risk for bleeding is particularly high with concurrent use of nonsteroidal

TABLE 83.2

COMMON DRUGS THAT INTERACT WITH ORAL ANTICOAGULANTS

Effect	Mechanism	Drug
Prolongation of PT	Inhibits clearance	Amiodarone
		Metronidazole
		Trimethoprim/sulfamethoxazole
		Cimetidine[a]
		Omeprazole[a]
		Sulfinpyrazone[a]
		Disulfiram
		Anabolic steroids
	Inhibits vitamin K	Cephalosporins; second, third generation
		Acetaminophen
	Increases metabolism of clotting factors	L-Thyroxine
	Unknown	Erythromycin
		Tamoxifen
		Phenytoin
		Isoniazid
		Ketoconazole
		Piroxicam
Reduction of PT	Increases warfarin clearance	Barbiturates
		Carbamazepine
		Rifampin
	Reduces warfarin absorption	Cholestyramine
	Increases synthesis of clotting factors	Estrogens
	Unknown	Penicillins

PT, prothrombin time.
[a]Causes only a minimal prolongation of PT.
Adapted from Hirsh J. Oral anticoagulant drugs. N Engl J Med 1991;324:1865, with permission.

antiinflammatory drugs (NSAIDs). In the elderly, a 13-fold increase in hemorrhagic peptic ulcer disease results from taking NSAIDs plus warfarin. The substitution of daily acetaminophen for NSAIDs reduces the risk for bleeding from gastric injury, but it raises the risk for excessive anticoagulation by potentiating the effects of warfarin; close INR monitoring and warfarin dose adjustment are advised with new daily use of acetaminophen.

Hepatocellular failure results in impaired synthesis of clotting factors and albumin; cholestasis makes for less efficient absorption of vitamin K. Both conditions are capable of prolonging the INR and potentiating the effects of warfarin.

Inhibition

Anticoagulant effects are decreased by agents that induce microsomal enzymes, decrease the absorption of warfarin, or increase the synthesis of clotting factors or binding proteins (see Table 83.2). Moreover, coumarins cause a decrease in the metabolism of tolbutamide and phenytoin by competing for the same degradative enzymes. The INR should be measured when any change in a drug program is made, and it should be followed closely thereafter until stability has been achieved.

Reversal of Anticoagulation and Elective Interruptions in Therapy (34–37)

Rapid Reversal

Serious bleeding, a dangerously high INR (>20), and a need for urgent surgery are among the circumstances in which rapid reversal of oral anticoagulation is indicated. The administration of *fresh-frozen plasma* provides a rapid correction of the INR but involves exposure to blood products and a large colloid load. Reversal with *recombinant human factor VIIa concentrate* has shown promise as an alternative to fresh-frozen plasma that is free of exposure risk and the need for a large colloid load. However, as reported with prothrombin complex concentrates, there is a prothrombotic risk with *recombinant factor VIIa*. Due to its expense, its use requires parsimonious application. Alternatively, the administration of *vitamin K* (which stimulates the hepatic synthesis of the clotting factors inhibited by warfarin) is also effective but somewhat slower, taking 12 to 48 hours to reduce the INR to a safe level. Intravenous, subcutaneous, and oral preparations are available. The high-dose IV preparation of vitamin K (1 to 10 mg) is the most potent and most rapidly acting of the various formulations, but it may overshoot and impair repeated anticoagulation. In less urgent settings, subcutaneous vitamin K (1 to 3 mg) can be used, but systemic absorption can be erratic, leading to treatment failure. Oral vitamin K (1.0 to 2.5 mg) can reverse INRs of less than 10 more rapidly than subcutaneous vitamin K and nearly as quickly as intravenous vitamin K.

Interruptions

The decision to discontinue anticoagulant therapy in the context of nonemergent bleeding or elective surgery needs to be individualized. The risk for thrombosis must be balanced against the risk for hemorrhage. The risk for embolization is substantial and greatest for persons with acute deep venous thrombosis or acute arterial embolization who have been taking warfarin for less than 1 month. A somewhat lesser risk is associated with recurrent deep venous thrombosis, nonvalvular atrial fibrillation, placement of a mechanical heart valve, and deep venous thrombosis after more than 1 month of warfarin. The risk for postoperative bleeding can be minimized by withholding anti-

coagulation for about 4 days before elective surgery to allow the INR to drift to less than 1.5, the level at which most surgery can be carried out with little risk for serious hemorrhage.

When patients are at high risk for thromboembolization, perioperative heparin must be considered. Full-dose, low-molecular-weight heparin can be instituted in the outpatient setting as the INR starts to decrease. The patient can be transitioned to IV unfractionated heparin approximately 24 hours before surgery and the infusion stopped 5 hours prior to the procedure. Postoperative heparinization, begun 12 hours after surgery (without a loading bolus), is associated with a 3% daily risk for major hemorrhage and should be reserved for those patients at highest thromboembolic risk whose risk for postoperative bleeding is acceptable. If the risk for bleeding is unacceptably high in such persons, then a vena cava filter should be considered preoperatively.

Patient Education (38–41)

Before the initiation of outpatient anticoagulant therapy, the patient and designated family member(s) need to (a) understand the risks and benefits of warfarin, (b) become familiar with the requirements for taking warfarin responsibly (e.g., avoidance of NSAIDs and excessive amounts of alcohol), (c) be able to recognize signs of abnormal bleeding (e.g., melena), and (d) be versed in the triage protocol for hemorrhagic complications. Instruction of the patient by a nurse trained in anticoagulation management, supplemented by an information booklet appropriate to the patient's educational level, is essential to the patient education effort. Any patient who is incapable of understanding the instructions or is deemed unreliable should not be placed on therapy because the risks for hemorrhage probably outweigh any possible benefits. The one exception is the patient who can be closely supervised by family members or health care professionals.

The physician should know the tablet color coding of the warfarin brand that the patient is using. This helps to ensure that proper doses are being taken. Constancy of brand should be advised, both to minimize dosing errors and to ensure the consistency of anticoagulant effect.

Foods and Supplements

A very important component of patient education is a review of foods and nonprescription substances (including herbal preparations and other "natural" supplements) that can affect warfarin anticoagulation (Table 83.3). Eating *avocados* and *green vegetables* rich in folate (e.g., spinach, broccoli) can inhibit

---

TABLE 83.3

EFFECTS OF FOODS AND HERBAL PREPARATIONS ON WARFARIN ANTICOAGULATION

Potentiates Warfarin Effect
Ginkgo
Inhibits Warfarin Effect
Avocado
Green vegetables (e.g., broccoli, spinach) if >250 g/d is consumed
Garlic
St. John's Wort
Ginseng

warfarin, but only if large amounts are eaten (>250 g) on a single occasion. Patients should be encouraged to maintain a *stable* diet that is rich in these nutrients; patients may mistakenly believe that they need to forego green vegetables. *Ginkgo* potentiates warfarin and can cause bleeding, whereas St. Johns Wort, garlic, and ginseng may accelerate its metabolism and impair its anticoagulant action.

Purchasing a Brand versus a Generic Preparation of Warfarin.

Generic warfarin can be safely substituted for Coumadin-brand warfarin; however, the INR should be closely monitored during any change in warfarin preparation, and consistency of use of a particular generic preparation is recommended.

Direct Thrombin Inhibitors and Factor Xa Antagonists (42)

These agents represent promising avenues of exploration as alternatives to warfarin therapy. They are characterized by oral administration, minimal interference with food and drugs, a wide therapeutic index, and no requirement for routine monitoring of coagulation parameters. Indications for use are the subject of ongoing studies.

ANTIPLATELET THERAPY (43–49)

Aspirin and clopidogrel represent the major antiplatelet agents useful in clinical medicine. they have a wide spectrum of applications in the prevention of artherothrombotic complications and differ markedly in cost and more modestly in side effects and efficacy. Combination antiplatelet therapy has been explored, as has use in conjunction with oral anticoagulation.

Aspirin

Aspirin inhibits platelet aggregation by irreversibly acetylating and inactivating platelet prostaglandin H synthetase, inhibiting cyclooxygenase-1 (COX-1) activity. This direct inhibition of the COX-1 pathway makes the drug effective in the treatment and prevention of platelet-related arterial atherothrombotic complications.

Efficacy

Aspirin significantly reduces the risk of arterial atherothrombotic events compared to placebo, especially in high-risk persons, and is comparable to clopidogrel and superior to warfarin for this indication. Differences in benefit from low-dose aspirin have been observed between men and women for the primary prevention of myocardial infarction (see Chapter 31), but the differences are not due to differences in the suppression of COX-1 platelet function, which is complete in both sexes. Aspirin performs comparably to clopidogrel in persons with multiple cardiac risk factors and slightly less well in persons with symptomatic atherosclerotic disease or in those undergoing angioplasty and coronary stent implantation (see Chapters 30 and 31). It is only 20% as effective as warfarin for the prevention of systemic embolization due to atrial fibrillation (see Chapter 28).

Combination therapy with clopidogrel reduces the risk of restenosis after stenting, and combination with warfarin modestly reduces the risk of reinfarction in very high risk coronary disease (myocardial infarction with ST elevation), but the bene-

fits are modest and the increase in the risk of major hemorrhage is greatly increased. Overall, the risk-to-benefit ratio of combination therapy is not particularly favorable; such treatment should be reserved for persons at very high risk. In most settings in which oral anticoagulation with warfarin is indicated, aspirin has been found to be either ineffective or equivocally effective. Among patients with atrial fibrillation, only those for whom warfarin is contraindicated are appropriate candidates for aspirin therapy (see Chapters 28 and 33).

Adverse Effects

Peptic ulceration and upper gastrointestinal bleeding are the principal adverse effects, resulting from the inhibition of prostaglandin E2 (necessary for the maintenance of the gastric mucosal barrier) and contact injury to the gastric mucosa. The risk of major gastrointestinal (GI) bleeding is increased markedly (relative risk, 2.07 vs. placebo; absolute annual increase in risk, 0.12%/yr). The risk of major intracranial bleeding increases, but to a lesser extent (relative risk, 1.65; absolute annual increase in risk, 0.03%). Bleeding risks increases when aspirin is used in conjunction with clopidogrel (relative risk, 1.25) or warfarin (relative risk 3.41).

A significant reduction in GI bleeding risk can be achieved by the concurrent administration of a proton-pump inhibitor during aspirin therapy. Such combination therapy is superior to switching to clopidogrel for reducing risk of recurrent ulcer bleeding in persons with a prior history of a bleeding complication (8%/yr with clopidogrel vs. 0.7%/yr with aspirin plus esomeprazole).

Dosing and Preparations

The minimum effective dose of aspirin for these indications ranges from 75 to 160 mg/d. Doses up to 325 mg/day are prescribed, with the higher doses used in stroke prophylaxis. Once-daily dosing suffices in most instances. Enteric coating reduces direct gastric mucosal injury and resultant GI upset but does not markedly reduce ulcer and bleeding risks, which are due to systemic prostaglandin inhibition.

Indications

The drug provides effective primary and secondary prophylaxis for atherothrombotic events, including unstable angina (see Chapter 20), myocardial infarction (see Chapters 30 and 31), transient ischemic attack and stroke (see Chapter 171), and coronary restenosis after angioplasty and stent implantation (see Chapter 30). It can be used in conjunction with clopidogrel in persons with symptomatic atherothrombotic disease (see later discussion) and after coronary artery stenting; use with warfarin should be limited to very high risk settings in which thromboembolism is a major concern (e.g., caged-ball or caged-disk prosthetic heart valves; ST-segment elevation; transmural myocardial infarction).

Inhibition of ADP-Induced Platelet Aggregation (Clopidogrel)

Clopidogrel is most commonly used inhibitor of adenosine diphosphate–induced platelet aggregation. Ticlodipine, the other available drug in this class, is much less frequently prescribed due to its risk of agranulocytosis. These drugs do not interfere with the prostaglandin synthesis, thus providing antiplatelet activity without the adverse upper gastrointestinal side effects of aspirin. However, cost is high compared to that of aspirin, and benefits are modest.

Efficacy

A major trial comparing aspirin with clopidogrel in persons with high-risk cardiovascular disease found an 8.7% reduction in the relative risk of combined cardiovascular endpoints (stroke, myocardial infarction, vascular death) for clopidogrel compared to aspirin, predominantly in persons with symptomatic peripheral vascular disease, with lesser benefit noted in stroke and little in the setting of recent myocardial infarction. Outside of post–angioplasty/stenting situations, cost-effectiveness analysis found that clopidogrel use is most compelling in persons with peripheral vascular disease. Persons with symptomatic atherothrombosis have a small benefit with combination therapy over aspirin alone, but not if they are high risk but asymptomatic.

Side Effects

Although the risk of major GI bleeding from the use of clopidogrel is smaller than with aspirin (relative risk, 0.55), it is still increased but small in comparison to placebo (absolute increase in risk, 0.12%/yr). Aside from gastrointestinal bleeding, *bleeding* risks are similar for aspirin and clopidogrel. *Thrombotic thrombocytopenic purpura* is a rare complication of use.

Indications

Aspirin remains the preferred agent for primary and secondary prophylaxis of cardiovascular disease and its complications. Adding clopidogrel to aspirin is indicated in persons with symptomatic atherothrombotic disease and in the setting of angioplasty and stenting (see Chapters 30 and 31).

Although current methods of outpatient anticoagulation are effective and safe when applied carefully, they have not precluded the search for safer, more convenient outpatient approaches to anticoagulation.

CONCLUSIONS AND RECOMMENDATIONS

Warfarin

- Warfarin is highly effective in preventing thromboembolism. The recommended intensity of anticoagulation for most indications is an INR of 2.0 to 3.0. Patients with metallic prosthetic heart valves should be given aspirin in addition to warfarin, with a target INR of 2.5 to 3.5.
- Only patients who are believed to be at low risk for stroke or those in whom anticoagulant therapy is contraindi-

cated should be treated with aspirin for prophylaxis against thromboembolic stroke in atrial fibrillation (see Chapter 28).
- When initiating warfarin therapy, one should begin with 5 mg/d; initiation with 10-mg doses may be used for young patients with few comorbid illnesses. Older women and malnourished patients are particularly sensitive to warfarin. A starting dose of 3 mg/d is advised in these groups.
- Patients with temporal risk factor–related deep venous thrombosis or pulmonary embolism should be treated with warfarin for 3 to 6 months. Patients with idiopathic deep venous thrombosis or pulmonary embolism should be treated for at least 6 months. Patients with recurrent thrombosis or an ongoing hypercoagulable state or who are homozygous for activated protein C resistance should be treated indefinitely with warfarin. The role of D-dimer measurement for use in determining the need for prolonged anticoagulation remains to be established.
- The rapid reversal of anticoagulation therapy is indicated for severe bleeding, an INR of greater than 20, and urgent surgery. The administration of fresh-frozen plasma achieves reversal within hours. Vitamin K accomplishes the same in 6 to 48 hours, depending on dose and route of administration.
- The decision to discontinue anticoagulant therapy in the context of nonemergent bleeding or elective surgery needs to be individualized. The risk for embolization must be balanced against the risk for hemorrhage.
- The reversal of oral anticoagulation for elective surgery can be accomplished simply by withholding warfarin for 4 days or until the INR is less than 1.5, the level at which the risk for hemorrhage becomes minimal in most forms of surgery. For high-risk patients, perioperative heparinization must be considered.
- Anticoagulant therapy mandates frequent monitoring, lifestyle changes, and commitment by the patient and health care team to optimize its safety and efficacy.

Aspirin and Clopidogrel

- Aspirin should be used by all persons at risk for atherothrombosis. Aspirin can reduce the risk for vascular events, including myocardial infarction, stroke, and transient ischemic attack.
- Adding clopidogrel provides enhanced prophylaxis only in very high risk situations such as angioplasty with stenting and symptomatic atherothrombotic disease.
- Substituting clopidogrel for aspirin in patients with a history of upper GI bleeding is not as effective as adding a proton-pump inhibitor to aspirin therapy.
- Aspirin should not be added to warfarin therapy, except in the rare instances in which thromboembolic risk is extremely high.

Annotated Bibliography

1. Boston Area Anticoagulation Trial for Atrial Fibrillation Investigators. The effect of low-dose warfarin on the risk of stroke in patients with nonrheumatic atrial fibrillation. N Engl J Med 1990;323:1505. (*One of several randomized trials demonstrating benefit in patients with chronic or paroxysmal atrial fibrillation; also shows the efficacy of low-intensity therapy.*)
2. European Atrial Fibrillation Trial Study Group. Optimal oral anticoagulant therapy in patients with nonrheumatic atrial fibrillation and recent cerebral ischemia. N Engl J Med 1995;333:5. (*Recommends a target international normalized ratio [INR] of 3.0.*)
3. Ezekowitz MD, Bridgers SL, James KE, et al. Warfarin in the prevention of stroke associated with nonrheumatic atrial fibrillation. N Engl J Med 1992;327:1406. (*A Veterans Administration study, further confirming that low-intensity therapy reduces the risk in patients older than 70 years.*)
4. Stroke Prevention in Atrial Fibrillation Investigators. Predictors of thromboembolism in atrial fibrillation. Ann Intern Med 1992;116:1,6. (*A two-part study, finding that recent congestive heart failure, hypertension, previous embolism, left ventricular dysfunction, and left atrial enlargement were independent predictors of stroke risk.*)

5. Cannegieter SC, Rosendaal FR, Wintzen AR, et al. Optimal oral anticoagulant therapy in patients with mechanical heart valves. N Engl J Med 1995;333:11. (*Recommends a target INR of 3.0 to 4.0.*)

6. Ridker PM, Goldhaber SZ, Danielson E, et al., for the PREVENT Investigators. Long-term, low intensity warfarin therapy for the prevention of recurrent venous thromboembolism. N Engl J Med 2003;348:1425. (*The Prevention of Recurrent Venous Thromboembolism [PREVENT] trial, a placebo-controlled study in persons with idiopathic deep venous thrombosis [DVT], showing an 80% reduction in risk.*)

7. Kearon C, Ginsberg JS, Kovacs MJ, et al. Comparison of low-intensity warfarin therapy with conventional-intensity warfarin therapy for long-term prevention of recurrent venous thromboembolism. N Engl J Med 2003;349:631. (*A major randomized, multicenter trial, finding unexpectedly that conventional therapy was more effective and no less safe than low-intensity therapy.*)

8. Meltzer RS, Visser CA, Fuster V. Intracardiac thrombi and systemic embolization. Ann Intern Med 1986;104:689. (*An excellent review of data justifying oral anticoagulation.*)

9. Smith P, Arneson H, Holme I. The effect of warfarin on mortality and reinfarction after myocardial infarction. N Engl J Med 1990;323:147. (*Intriguing data from Europe, suggesting that warfarin may reduce the rate of reinfarction.*)

10. The Matisse Investigators. Subcutaneous fondaparinux versus intravenous unfractionated heparin in the initial treatment of pulmonary embolism. N Engl J Med 2003;349:1695. (*A randomized, controlled trial [RCT], finding that the inhibition of factor Xa was at least as safe and effective for the initial treatment of pulmonary embolism.*)

11. Gurwitz JH, Avorn J, Ross-Degnan D, et al. Aging and the anticoagulant response to warfarin therapy. Ann Intern Med 1992;116:901. (*The response increased with age, so that close monitoring is particularly important in the elderly.*)

12. Harrison L, Johnston M, Massicotte MP, et al. Comparison of 5-mg and 10-mg loading doses in initiation of warfarin therapy. Ann Intern Med 1997;126:133. (*The 5-mg dose takes effect nearly as rapidly but with less risk of complications.*)

13. Koopman MMW, Prandoni P, Piovella F, et al. Treatment of venous thrombosis with intravenous unfractionated heparin administered in the hospital as compared with subcutaneous low-molecular-weight heparin administered at home. N Engl J Med 1996;334:682. (*The safety and efficacy of low-molecular-weight heparin [LMWH] were found to be as good as if not better than those for unfractionated heparin.*)

14. Kovacs MJ, Rodger M, Anderson DR, et al. Comparison of 10-mg and 5-mg warfarin initiation nomograms together with low-molecular-weight heparin for outpatient treatment of acute venous thromboembolism: a randomized, double-blind, controlled trial. Ann Intern Med 2003;138:714. (*Among younger patients, the 10-mg starting program was superior for acute oral anticoagulation in the setting of thromboembolism.*)

15. Levine M, Gent M, Hirsh J, et al. A comparison of low molecular weight heparin administered primarily at home with unfractionated heparin administered in the hospital for proximal deep vein thrombosis. N Engl J Med 1996;334:677. (*A randomized trial, finding evidence for the efficacy and safety of LMWH.*)

16. Menendez-Jandula B, Souto JC, Oliver A, et al. Comparing self-management of oral anticoagulant therapy with clinic management: a randomized trial. Ann Intern Med 2005;142:142. (*The degree of control was the same, and the complication rates were lower.*)

17. Moll S, Ortel TL. Monitoring warfarin therapy in patients with lupus anticoagulants. Ann Intern Med 1997;127:177. (*A prospective case series, demonstrating overestimation and underestimation of anticoagulation by prothrombin time [PT] assay in such persons.*)

18. Agnelli G, Prandoni P, Becattini C, et al. Extended oral anticoagulant therapy after a first episode of pulmonary embolization. Ann Intern Med 2003; 139:19. (*The risk of recurrence was independent of the duration of therapy.*)

19. Azar AJ, Cannegieter SC, Deckers JW, et al. Optimal intensity of oral anticoagulant therapy after myocardial infarction. J Am Coll Cardiol 1996;27:1349. (*Assuming an equal harm of thrombotic and hemorrhagic complications, an INR of 2.0 to 4.0 was considered to be optimal.*)

20. Hirsh J, Levin MN. The optimal intensity of oral anticoagulant therapy. JAMA 1987;258:2723. (*Argues that an INR of 2 to 3 is best for most indications.*)

21. Hylek EM, Skates SJ, Sheehan MA, et al. An analysis of the lowest effective intensity of prophylactic anticoagulation for patients with nonrheumatic atrial fibrillation. N Engl J Med 1996;335:540. (*The odds of stroke rose sharply as the INR fell to <2.0.*)

22. Palareti G, Cosmi B, Legnani C, et al, for the PROLONG Investigators. D-Dimer testing to determine the duration of anticoagulation therapy. N Engl J Med 2006;355:1780. (*RCT, finding that patients with elevations 1 month after the cessation of therapy had an increased risk of recurrence that could be reduced by the resumption of anticoagulation.*)

23. Feder W, Auerback R. Purple toes: an uncommon sequela of oral coumarin drug therapy. Ann Intern Med 1961;55:911. (*The original report of this complication, seen in 1% of patients, known to be caused by a congenital deficiency of factor S or C and to be worsened by warfarin therapy.*)

24. Fihn SD, McDonell M, Martin D, et al. Risk factors for complications of chronic anticoagulation. Ann Intern Med 1993;118:511. (*High-intensity anticoagulation, wide fluctuations in PT, recent initiation of therapy, and poor patient selection were major risk factors.*)

25. Hylek EM, Singer DE. Risk factors for intracranial hemorrhage in outpatients taking warfarin. Ann Intern Med 1994;120:897. (*The odds of hemorrhage increased sharply as the PT ratio exceeded 2.0 or the INR exceeded 3.7 to 4.3.*)

26. Landefeld CS, Goldman L. Major bleeding in outpatients treated with warfarin: incidence and prediction by factors known at the start of outpatient therapy. Am J Med 1989;87:144. (*Age older than 65 years, history of stroke or gastrointestinal bleeding, serious comorbid condition, and atrial fibrillation were predictors of risk.*)

27. Landefeld CS, Rosenblatt MW, Goldman L. Bleeding in outpatients treated with warfarin: relation to the prothrombin time and important remediable lesions. Am J Med 1989;87:153. (*A companion study, confirming that the risk for bleeding increased with the intensity of anticoagulation; confirmed the value of checking for underlying lesions.*)

28. Petty GW, Brown RD Jr, Whisnant JP, et al. Frequency of major complications of aspirin, warfarin, and intravenous heparin for secondary stroke prevention: a population-based study. Ann Intern Med 1999;130:14. (*Provides rates from "real-world" practice.*)

29. Franco V, Polanczyk CA, Clausell N, et al. Role of dietary vitamin K intake in chronic oral anticoagulation: prospective evidence from observational and randomized protocols. Am J Med 2004;116:651. (*Presents evidence that dietary vitamin K intake can affect the level of anticoagulation.*)

30. Higashi MK, Veenstra DL, Kondo LM, et al. Association between CYP2C9 genetic variants and anticoagulation-related outcomes during warfarin therapy. JAMA 2002;287:1690. (*A retrospective cohort study, identifying variants with a reduced hepatic microsomal degradation of warfarin and finding them to be associated with increased risks of overanticoagulation and bleeding.*)

31. Hylek EM, Heiman H, Skates SJ, et al. Acetaminophen and other risk factors for excessive warfarin anticoagulation. JAMA 1998;279:657. (*A case–control study, finding that acetaminophen was independently associated with excessive anticoagulation.*)

32. Rieder MJ, Reiner AP, Gage BF, et al. Effect of VKORC1 haplotypes on transcriptional regulation and warfarin dose. N Engl J Med 2005;352:2285. (*Identifies haplotypes that affect an enzyme controlling vitamin K metabolism, and suggests that haplotype identification can predict the response to warfarin.*)

33. Shorr RI, Ray WA, Dougherty JR, et al. Concurrent use of nonsteroidal antiinflammatory drugs and oral anticoagulants places elderly persons at high risk of hemorrhagic peptic ulcer. Arch Intern Med 1993;153:1665. (*The risk increases 13-fold.*)

34. Crowther MA, Douketis JD, Schnurr T, et al. Oral vitamin K lowers the International Normalized Ratio more than subcutaneous vitamin K in the treatment of warfarin-associated coagulopathy: a randomized controlled trial. Ann Intern Med 2002;137:251. (*The title says it all.*)

35. Deveras RAE, Kessler CM. Reversal of warfarin-induced excessive anticoagulation with recombinant human factor VIIa concentrate. Ann Intern Med 2002;137:884. (*A case series, identifying a promising alternative to fresh-frozen plasma.*)

36. Lubestsky A, Yonath H, Olchovsky D, et al. Comparison of oral vs intravenous phytonadione (vitamin K1) in patients with excessive anticoagulation: a prospective randomized controlled study. Arch Intern Med 2003;163:2469. (*In patients without excessive bleeding, oral therapy was comparable in safety and efficacy and less likely to overshoot.*)

37. Whitling AM, Bussey HI, Lyons RM. Comparing different routes and doses of phytonadione for reversing excessive anticoagulation. Arch Intern Med 1998;158:2136. (*A retrospective study, but provides useful data on the efficacy and safety of various vitamin K preparations.*)

38. Kearon C, Hirsh J. Management of anticoagulation before and after elective surgery. N Engl J Med 1997;336:1506. (*A critical review that provides practical recommendations.*)

39. Izzo AA, Ernst E. Interactions between herbal medicines and prescribed drugs: a systematic review. Drugs 2001;61:2163. (*A good review, including a discussion of the effects on warfarin.*)

40. Karlson B, Keijd B, Hellstrom K. On the influence of vitamin K–rich vegetables and wine on the effectiveness of warfarin treatment. Acta Med Scand 1986;220:347. (*Large amounts can inhibit vitamin K, but not smaller-sized portions.*)

41. Milligan PE, Banet GA, Waterman AD, et al. Substitution of generic warfarin for Coumadin in an HMO setting. Ann Pharmacother 2002;36:764. (*Substitution is safe, but the INR should be monitored when making the change.*)

42. Di Nisio M, Middeldorp S, Buller HR. direct thrombin inhibitors. N Engl J Med 2005;353:1028. (*An excellent review of the uses and the evidence supporting them; 63 references.*)

43. Becker DM, Segal J, Vaidya D, et al. Sex differences in platelet reactivity and response to low-dose aspirin therapy. JAMA 2006;295:1420. (*No aspirin*

resistance was found to account for the observed differences in response to prophylaxis.)

44. Bhatt DL, Fox KAA, Hacke W, et al for the CHARISMA Investigators. Clopidogrel and aspirin versus aspirin alone for the prevention of atherothrombotic events. N Engl J Med 2006;354:1706. (*Overall, combination therapy was no better than aspirin alone.*)

45. CARIE Steering Committee. A randomised, blinded, trial of clopidogrel versus aspirin in patients at risk of ischemic events (CARIE). Lancet 1996; 348:1329. (*Finds at best a modest increase in benefit compared to aspirin.*)

46. Chan FKL, Ching JYL, Hung LCT, et al. Clopidogrel versus aspirin and esomeprazole to prevent recurrent ulcer bleeding. N Engl J Med 2005;352:238. (*RCT, finding that aspirin plus proton-pump inhibitor therapy was significantly better at reducing risk than switching to clopidogrel.*)

47. Dutch TIA Trial Study Group. Comparison of two doses of aspirin (30 mg versus 383 mg per day) in patients after a transient ischemic attack or minor ischemic stroke. N Engl J Med 1991;325:1261. (*Low-dose aspirin was as effective as higher doses in preventing stroke recurrence.*)

48. McQuaid KR, Lanie L. Systematic review and meta-analysis of adverse events of low-dose aspirin and clopidogrel in randomized controlled trials. AM J Med 2006;119:624. (*The absolute increase in the risk of major bleeding for aspirin compared to clopidogrel was statistically significant but clinically modest except for bleeding from the upper gastrointestinal tract.*)

49. Schleinitz MD, Weiss JP, Owens DK. Clopidogrel versus aspirin for secondary prophylaxis of vascular events: a cost-effectiveness analysis. Am J Med 2004;116:797. (*Cost-effectiveness was shown in the setting of peripheral vascular disease.*)

CHAPTER 84 ■ APPROACH TO THE PATIENT WITH LYMPHOMA

JEREMY S. ABRAMSON

The lymphomas are a diverse group of malignancies arising from B and T lymphocytes and are generally categorized as either Hodgkin's lymphoma (HL) or non-Hodgkin's lymphoma (NHL). NHL is significantly more common, accounting for approximately 65,000 new cases annually in the United States, compared to 8,000 new cases of HL. Multiple subtypes are identified within NHL and HL, each with distinct biology, clinical presentation, natural history, and therapies.

Although the treatment of these conditions is the province of the oncologist, the primary care physician has an important role in diagnosing and staging the disease, coordinating plans for management, delivering follow-up care on an outpatient basis, and monitoring for late systemic side effects of chemotherapy and radiation. Because they are likely to conduct the initial evaluation, it is essential that primary physicians be prepared to discuss with patients and their families the meaning of findings. Even after referral, the primary physician often encounters requests for advice, as the physician the patient knows best. Consequently, a serious working knowledge of the clinical presentation, prognosis, staging methods, and treatment options is important for the primary physician if the patient is to be well served.

HODGKIN'S LYMPHOMA

Pathology and Clinical Presentation (1,2)

HL is a malignant lymphoid disease that most commonly occurs within lymph nodes but may also involve the spleen, bone marrow, and other extranodal sites. Thomas Hodgkin first described this entity in 1832, although the lymphoid derivation remained elusive until 1994, when molecular techniques defined the germinal center B cell as the cell of origin, thus changing "Hodgkin's disease" to "Hodgkin's lymphoma." The World Health Organization (WHO) recognizes two distinct categories within Hodgkin's lymphoma: *classical Hodgkin's lymphoma (CHL)* and *nodular lymphocyte predominance Hodgkin's lymphoma (NLPHL)* (Table 84.1).

Classical Hodgkin's Lymphoma

This category accounts for 95% of Hodgkin's lymphoma cases and encompasses the following histologic subtypes: *nodular sclerosis (NSHL), mixed cellularity (MCHL), lymphocyte-rich (LRHL),* and *lymphocyte-depleted (LDHL)* Hodgkin's lymphoma. Pathologically, CHL is characterized by the presence of few neoplastic *Reed–Sternberg (RS) cells* surrounded by a dominant population of nonmalignant polyclonal host inflammatory cells. RS cells are usually *CD15 positive* and *CD30 positive* but negative for CD45 and traditional B cell and T cell markers.

Nodular sclerosis disease is the most common subtype, particularly among younger patients, and accounts for approximately 70% of cases, with a slight female predominance. It usually presents clinically as early-stage disease (I or II) in the mediastinum or cervical lymph nodes, but it may be locally aggressive, compressing local structures and causing pleural or pericardial effusion. Systemic *"B" symptoms (fever >38°C,* drenching *night sweats,* or unintentional *weight loss* of >10% of body weight over the preceding 6 months) are present in approximately one third of patients at diagnosis.

Mixed cellularity disease accounts for approximately 20% to 25% of cases; it is the most common subtype in the elderly, in HIV-infected patients, and in persons living in developing countries. It has a male predominance and commonly presents at advanced stages with "B" symptoms. Peripheral lymph nodes are most frequently involved; mediastinal disease is uncommon, in contrast to NSHL.

Lymphocyte-rich disease is an uncommon variant, accounting for 5% of cases. Like MCHL, it occurs predominantly in

TABLE 84.1

WORLD HEALTH ORGANIZATION CLASSIFICATION OF LYMPHOMAS (2)

Hodgkin's Lymphomas
  Classical Hodgkin's lymphoma
    Nodular sclerosis
    Mixed cellularity
    Lymphocyte rich
    Lymphocyte depleted
  Nodular lymphocyte-predominant Hodgkin's lymphoma
Non-Hodgkin's Lymphomas
  Indolent non-Hodgkin's lymphomas
    B cell diseases
      Follicular lymphoma (grades I–II)
      Small lymphocytic lymphoma/chronic lymphocytic leukemia
      Marginal zone lymphomas
      Lymphoplasmacytic lymphoma (+/− Waldenström's macroglobulinemia)
      Hairy-cell leukemia
    T cell diseases
      Large granular lymphocyte leukemia
      Mycosis fungoides
  Aggressive non-Hodgkin's lymphomas
    B cell diseases
      Diffuse large B cell lymphomas
      Follicular lymphoma (grade III)
      Mantle cell lymphoma
      B cell prolymphocytic leukemia
    T cell diseases
      Peripheral T cell lymphomas
      Anaplastic large-cell lymphoma
      Adult T cell leukemia/lymphoma
      T cell prolymphocytic leukemia
  Highly aggressive non-Hodgkin's lymphomas
    B cell diseases
      Burkitt's lymphoma
      Precursor B cell lymphoblastic lymphoma
    T cell diseases
      Precursor T cell lymphoblastic lymphoma

peripheral lymph nodes without mediastinal involvement, but presentation is usually at limited stage and without symptoms. There is a male predominance.

Lymphocyte-depleted disease is a very rare variant, notable pathologically for a dominant RS cell population with few of the infiltrating host inflammatory cells. Many cases previously diagnosed as LDHL would now likely be classified as variants of non-Hodgkin's lymphoma.

Nodular Lymphocyte Predominant Hodgkin's Lymphoma

Nodular lymphocyte predominant Hodgkin's lymphoma accounts for only 5% of HL overall and is distinguished from the classical HL subtypes by distinct biology, natural history, and approach to therapy. NLPHL occurs at a slightly older median age than classical HL (median age in the fourth decade) and has a strong male predominance. The disease is limited in stage (I to II) in 75% of cases, in contrast to CHL, which occurs roughly equally at limited and advanced stages. It presents most often in peripheral nodes that are palpable on physical

examination but rarely within the mediastinum, abdomen, or extranodal sites. Systemic "B" symptoms are rarely present. Unlike CHL, NLPHL follows a distinctly indolent natural history, with an excellent overall prognosis of approximately 80% to 90% of patients alive 10 years after diagnosis, regardless of treatment.

Pathologically, NLPHL is similar to CHL, in that there is a paucity of malignant cells surrounded by a rich inflammatory infiltrate. Unlike CHL, however, the pattern of infiltration is *nodular* rather than diffuse, and the reactive cells are predominantly *small lymphocytes*. The tumor cells of NLPHL, known as *lymphocytic and histiocytic "L&H" cells*, are distinguished from classical RS cells by immunohistochemistry. They strongly express *CD45* and the B cell marker CD20 and do not express the traditional RS cell markers CD15 and CD30.

Clinical Presentation

Hodgkin's lymphoma presents most commonly with *painless lymphadenopathy* or less commonly with symptoms of *cough, chest pain, shortness of breath*, or the radiographic finding of *mediastinal lymphadenopathy* or a prominent *mediastinal mass*. Involved nodes are typically firm, mobile, and nontender and may be discrete or matted. Extranodal involvement most commonly involves the *spleen*, with involvement of the lung, *liver*, and *bone marrow* being less frequent. Involvement of other extranodal sites is uncommon. Systemic "B" symptoms (*fever* >38°C, drenching *night sweats*, or unintentional *weight loss* of >10% of body weight over the preceding 6 months) may be present, as may rare findings of *pruritus* or alcohol-induced pain in involved nodal sites.

Diagnosis

The differential diagnosis of Hodgkin's lymphoma includes *non-Hodgkin's lymphoma, infectious mononucleosis, HIV infection*, other *nonbacterial adenopathies* in the young, and *drug reactions* and *autoimmune diseases* (see Chapter 12). In the elderly, *other malignancies* are a common diagnostic consideration. In patients younger than the age of 30 years, benign entities account for approximately 80% of lymphadenopathies, with the majority of malignant causes being lymphoma. The likelihood of lymphadenopathy being malignant increases with patient age, duration (particularly >30 days), lymph node size, and number of involved sites (see Chapter 12). Malignant adenopathy also tends to be painless, whereas inflammatory or infectious adenopathy is likelier to be painful and accompanied by overlying erythema.

Laboratory workup for lymphadenopathy of unclear etiology begins with *complete blood count, peripheral smear, chest x-ray, HIV testing*, and consideration of *antinuclear antibody testing* (see Chapter 12). Definitive diagnosis for HL is best performed with either *excisional biopsy* or *core needle biopsy*, which preserves the tissue architecture necessary for definitive diagnosis in both HL and NHL. Successful diagnosis with *fine needle aspiration (FNA)* in lymphoma can only be made in a small minority of cases, and concordance between FNA and subsequent excisional biopsy findings is quite poor, so FNA should not be routinely incorporated into the initial diagnostic workup of lymphadenopathy when lymphoma is suspected. Sampling of few cells via FNA is particularly insensitive for the detection of HL, in which less than 1% of the overall cellularity may comprise malignant RS cells, with the majority of sampled

TABLE 84.2

HODGKIN'S DISEASE: STAGES, RELATIVE INCIDENCES, AND PROGNOSIS

Stage	Definition	Relative Incidence (%)	Therapy	Cure (%)
I	Confined to single node-bearing area	30	Chemotherapy ± radiation	70–90
II	Confined to two contiguous node-bearing areas on one side of diaphragm	25		
III	In nodal areas on both sides of diaphragm	25	Chemotherapy	50–60
IV	Visceral lesions (liver, lung) *not* in contiguity with nodes	20		
Special Categories				
E	Visceral extranodal disease in continuity with nodes (e.g., lung mass extending out from hilum)			
B	Symptoms of fever, weight loss, or sweats			
S	Splenic involvement			
X	Bulky disease (greater than 10 cm or greater than 1/3 the width of the maximal intrathoracic diameter			

cells being benign reactive host inflammatory cells, leading to frequent false-negative results.

Staging and Prognosis (3–5)

Staging

The prognosis and treatment of Hodgkin's lymphoma depend on the extent of disease, making classification by stage an important part of HL management (Table 84.2). Staging in HL uses the so-called Ann Arbor staging system:

Stage I: Disease confined to a single nodal area or localized involvement of a single extranodal site.

Stage II: Two or more contiguous nodal areas on the same side of the diaphragm or more than one nodal region in conjunction with localized involvement of an extralymphatic organ on the same side of the diaphragm.

Stage III: Nodal involvement on both sides of the diaphragm, with or without involvement of the spleen or a local extranodal organ or site.

Stage IV: Diffuse extranodal disease (liver, lung parenchyma, bone marrow, etc.).

Designation "E" (for extranodal): Involvement of an organ contiguous with a lymph node–bearing area (distinctly better prognosis than hematogenous visceral spread).

Designation "S" (for spleen): Disease in the spleen.

Designation "X": The presence of bulky disease (>10 cm on diameter or mediastinal disease or greater than one third of the maximal thoracic diameter on chest radiograph).

Designation "B": Fever (>38°C), drenching night sweats, or significant weight loss (>10%) in the previous 6 months.

Symptoms are incorporated into the staging system because they are important determinants of prognosis, particularly in limited-stage disease. Approximately 20% of patients present with at least one "B" symptom. When they are absent, the designation is "A"; when any of the three is present, the designation is "B." Pruritus is no longer considered a "B" symptom due to minimal influence on prognosis.

Clinical staging begins with ascertaining important findings in the history and physical examination. *Physical exam* concentrates on careful palpation of all peripheral lymph nodes and the assessment of liver and spleen size (although organ enlargement or its absence is not necessarily a definitive indicator).

Imaging studies provide important staging information and often start with a plain *chest x-ray* for the initial workup of symptoms. Whole-body computed tomographic (CT) scanning with *neck/chest* and *abdominal/pelvic* CT scanning offers markedly increased sensitivity and should be performed in all patients. *Positron emission tomographic (PET) scanning* enhances test sensitivity for nodal and extranodal disease, either as a separate test or combined with CT (PET-CT); it is becoming a routine staging procedure in Hodgkin's lymphoma. (PET scanning is also used during and after treatment to assess the response to therapy; see later discussion). *Magnetic resonance imaging (MRI)* offers no advantage over CT and is relegated to staging patients who are unable to undergo CT imaging (e.g., patients who are pregnant at diagnosis).

Bone marrow biopsy is indicated only in select circumstances in which it would change the treatment approach, such as in patients being considered for an abbreviated course of systemic therapy who possess risk factors for marrow involvement. Pathologic staging with *laparotomy* is no longer routinely performed due to the sensitivity of modern radiographic techniques, as well as the incorporation of systemic therapy in limited-stage disease.

Prognostic Scoring

As important as staging is to the determination of prognosis, it is not sufficient fully to predict the outcome of treatment, especially in persons presenting with advanced disease. Prognostic risk factors have been identified, but the validity of modifying treatment based on these risks remains to be proven and is the subject of ongoing randomized clinical trials. The ultimate goal is to decrease treatment intensity and treatment-related toxicities in low-risk patients and increase the dose intensity and the cure rate in high-risk patients.

Risk Factors in Advanced-Stage (III and IV) Disease. Predictors of worse prognosis include *serum albumin less than 4.0 g/dL*, a *hemoglobin concentration less than 10.5 g/dL*, *male gender*, *age older than 45 years*, *stage IV disease*, *white cell count greater than 15,000/mm³*, and *lymphocytopenia*

(<600 cells/mL or <8% of white cells). Patients with no risk factors have a nearly 85% chance of being free of disease progression at 5 years, compared to only 40% in patients with five or more risk factors.

Risk Factors in Early-Stage (I and II) Disease. Predictors of worse prognosis include *age greater than 50 years, large mediastinal mass, involvement of more than three nodal areas, "B" symptoms,* and *elevation of the erythrocyte sedimentation rate.*

Prognosis

The prognosis of HL has improved dramatically with the advent of careful staging and improved radiation technology and chemotherapy programs. The overall 5-year survival is 80% when all stages of disease are combined. Although it is a highly treatable and curable disease, many patients experience disease recurrence and some prove refractory. Prognosis in NLPHL is generally more favorable than that in classical HL, owing to a significantly more indolent natural history. Although late relapses are more common than in classical subtypes of HL, very few patients die from NLPHL.

Principles of Management (5–11)

Overall Approach

Combination chemotherapy is the mainstay of the treatment of late-stage disease, as well as in early-stage disease where it may be combined with local/regional irradiation. Although the selection of a treatment regimen is the responsibility of the oncologist, it is important for the primary physician to be cognizant of the major treatment regimens and their outcomes. The treatment of classical HL is a function of disease stage and associated prognostic factors but not of histologic subtype. The treatment of NLPHL is approached differently from that for classical HL. Therapy for all Hodgkin lymphoma achieves a substantial cure rate in all stages.

Stages I and II Classical Hodgkin's Lymphoma

Radiation therapy achieves a substantial cure rate in persons with localized early-stage disease; however, adverse late effects (especially when applied to young persons; see later discussion) and recurrences outside the field of irradiation have stimulated the development of chemotherapy programs for use with radiation. The resultant significant decreases in recurrence rates have led to combined-modality therapy becoming the standard approach to limited-stage HL. Treatment with four monthly cycles of ABVD chemotherapy (doxorubicin [Adriamycin], bleomycin, vinblastine, and dacarbazine) followed by radiation therapy to all involved sites of disease represents the best standard of care in most patients with limited-stage classical HL.

Patients with a very low risk disease may be treated with as few as two cycles of chemotherapy followed by radiation. Randomized trials have demonstrated no incremental benefit favoring additional radiation beyond the involved fields (i.e., extended field or subtotal nodal irradiation) or increased cycles of chemotherapy beyond four. Given the late risks of radiation treatment in young patients with HL (see later discussion), treatment with chemotherapy alone in low-risk patients is being studied. The initial results of randomized trials show no difference in overall survival, suggesting a similar efficacy with the omission of radiotherapy. Long-term follow-up is needed, but based on these trials, chemotherapy alone with six cycles of

ABVD is being considered for patients with nonbulky, limited-stage, classical HL.

Adverse Effects. The side effects of radiation therapy can be significant and continue to develop decades after the completion of therapy. Most feared is the incidence of *secondary malignancy,* which steadily increases in the years following treatment, reaching a sobering 25% incidence at 25 years postradiation. Common secondary cancers include breast cancer and lung cancer, followed by cancers of the skin, soft tissues, digestive tract, thyroid gland, urogenital tract, myelodysplasia, acute leukemia, and non-Hodgkin's lymphomas. Nonmalignant complications include *premature coronary artery disease, valvular heart disease, radiation pneumonitis* and *fibrosis, hypothyroidism,* and dental problems due to *decreased salivation.* Chemotherapy has its own set of complications (see later discussion and Chapter 88). Cardiac evaluation with an echocardiogram or multiple gated acquisition scan and pulmonary function tests for diffusing capacity for carbon monoxide should be obtained prior to and during treatment with anthracycline and bleomycin, respectively.

Stages III and IV Classical Hodgkin's Lymphoma

Combination chemotherapy is the cornerstone of treatment, offering long-term survival to nearly three fourths of patients. *ABVD* is the most widely used regimen based on improved efficacy and tolerability over its predecessor, MOPP (mechlorethamine, Oncovin, procarbazine, and prednisone). ABVD offers a complete remission rate of greater than 80% and 5-year failure-free and overall survival rates of approximately 65% to 80% and 75% to 90%, respectively. ABVD is administered on an outpatient basis every 2 weeks for a total of 6 months. There is no role for *radiation therapy* in advanced-stage patients who are in complete remission after chemotherapy alone, but radiation is used for patients in a partial remission following the completion of chemotherapy.

Other combination regimens, such as the intensified BEACOPP (bleomycin, etoposide, doxorubicin [Adriamycin], cyclophosphamide, vincristine [Oncovin], procarbazine, and prednisone) and Stanford V (doxorubicin, vinblastine, mechlorethamine, vincristine, bleomycin, etoposide, prednisone) regimens, continue to be evaluated for potential improvement over ABVD. The intensified BEACOPP regimen has demonstrated a modest improvement in disease control over ABVD but at the cost of significantly increased toxicity, including infections, sterility, and secondary leukemia. The choice of program is a subject of much debate among oncologists worldwide. Clinical trials are seeking to identify high-risk patients who might benefit from early intensified therapy, an approach that has not yet been prospectively validated as effective. In the absence of a single treatment program offering higher efficacy and decreased toxicity versus competing regimens, the choice of therapy requires balancing efficacy with treatment-related adverse effects and remains an art requiring an oncologist experienced in the treatment of Hodgkin's lymphoma.

Adverse Effects (See Also Chapter 88). Combination chemotherapy with ABVD is associated with *fatigue, bone marrow suppression, increased susceptibility to infection, gastrointestinal upset, constipation, neuropathy, and mouth sores,* among others. Doxorubicin carries a unique but low risk of *myocardial injury* and *congestive heart failure,* and bleomycin carries a risk of lung injury, including *pneumonitis* and *fibrosis,* which may be life threatening. Risks of sterility and secondary leukemia, which were common with the MOPP regimen, are rare with modern ABVD.

Treatment of Nodular Lymphocyte-Predominant Hodgkin's Lymphoma

Given its distinctly indolent natural history, NLPHL is generally treated less aggressively than its classical HL counterparts. Limited-stage disease, which accounts for the vast majority of cases, may be cured with *local radiotherapy* or even *surgery* alone. Uncommon cases of advanced-stage disease may be treated with combination *chemotherapy* with excellent response rates. Single-agent *rituximab*, the monoclonal antibody directed at the CD20 protein, which is expressed on the malignant L&H cells, has been shown to be highly effective and tolerable. Unlike classical HL, late relapses in this disease are common after initial therapy, and second-line treatment may be required. Death from relapsed NLPHL is quite rare.

Special Circumstances

Specific consideration of treatment options is needed in children (for whom the limitation of potential long-term toxicities is important); in young women (for whom limiting breast and ovarian radiation is important); in pregnant patients (who may not be candidates for chemotherapy or radiation); in HIV-positive individuals (who have suppressed immune function and are at greater risk for serious infectious complications); and in older individuals (who have the potential for increased toxicities from systemic chemotherapy).

Treatment of Relapsed Disease

Relapse occurs in 15% to 40% of patients, depending on stage, and may be as high as 60% in high-risk advanced-stage patients. The probability of responding to "salvage" chemotherapy is approximately 70% to 90% and is a function of the length of the initial remission. Unlike most malignancies, relapsed Hodgkin's lymphoma may be cured with second-line treatment. Patients who enjoyed an initial remission of greater than 1 year, as well as patients who relapse without extranodal disease or "B" symptoms, have a higher chance of cure with salvage therapy. Multiple combination regimens are available for salvage therapy and generally include chemotherapy agents with different mechanisms of action from those of the initial therapy.

Long-term disease-free survival with standard-dose salvage chemotherapy alone is low, and so most eligible patients have salvage chemotherapy followed by *high-dose chemotherapy* with *autologous stem cell transplantation*; the cure rate approaches 50%. Modern autologous stem cell transplantation is very safe, with a treatment-related mortality of less than 5%. Potential risks of autologous stem cell transplantation include *infection*, *organ injury*, and secondary *myelodysplasia* or *acute leukemia*, among others. Patients who relapse after autologous stem cell transplantation may yet achieve long-term disease control with an *allogeneic stem cell transplant* from a matched related or unrelated donor but with a high potential risk of transplant-related morbidity and mortality.

Monitoring

Periodic *examination of involved nodes* is the simplest means of judging the response to therapy. *CT* and *PET scanning* have been found to be useful for assessing the response to therapy during and immediately after treatment. PET scanning after two cycles of chemotherapy carries prognostic significance; patients achieving a complete response by PET scan enjoy a significantly lower recurrence rate than those patients with persistent PET positivity, even if they achieve a complete response at the conclusion of treatment. *Early PET negativity* appears to be the most important prognostic factor. The incorporation of PET scan with CT scan at the conclusion of treatment also enhances response assessment, particularly in the evaluation of residual masses that are common following treatment of Hodgkin's lymphoma, usually representing scar tissue and debris rather than active lymphoma.

After the completion of therapy, patients in remission are generally evaluated with full-body CT scans every 3 to 6 months for the first 3 years and then every 6 to 12 months to complete 5 years of radiographic surveillance. There is no clear role for the incorporation of PET scans in the routine surveillance of Hodgkin's lymphoma patients, given the high rate of false-positive findings and the excellent sensitivity of CT scans alone. The risk of relapse of classical Hodgkin's lymphoma is sufficiently low after 5 years from completion of therapy that routine scanning is no longer required, but careful periodic history and physical examination continue for the life of the patient. Patients should be watched for the potential development of toxicities, including heart disease and secondary malignancies, as outlined previously.

Patient Education and Indications for Consultation and Referral

Many patients will greet the diagnosis of Hodgkin lymphoma with dread, equating it with a fatal outcome. Without raising false hopes, the physician can point to the excellent 5-year survival rates and the high percentage of patients who are disease-free after 10 years. Although the risk of sterility with modern chemotherapy is very low, it is important to review this prospect with the patient before treatment is begun. Pretherapy sperm storage has been advocated for young men, whereas young women can be counseled in encouraging terms because they are most likely to be capable of bearing healthy children after treatment. The use of oral contraceptive therapy or gonadal hormone–releasing hormone agonists during chemotherapy may afford ovarian protection and should be discussed with the oncologist. Interested patients may also be referred to a specialist in reproductive endocrinology to be sure that all of their issues concerning potential future childbearing can be addressed.

Once the diagnosis is confirmed, referral to the oncologist for a discussion of staging and design of a treatment program is indicated. During the period of initial treatment, the patient is followed closely by the oncologist, but the primary physician can and should help to coordinate care and provide support to the patient and family as necessary. The role of the primary care physician in the lifelong monitoring of the patient for disease recurrence and late consequences of therapy is critical and should be performed in collaboration with the patient's oncologist.

NON-HODGKIN'S LYMPHOMAS

The NHLs represent a heterogeneous group of malignancies arising from lymphocytes. There are approximately 65,000 cases of NHL each year in the United States, occurring primarily in patients older than the age of 60 years and roughly equally in men and women, although there is variability across histologic subsets. The World Health Organization defines approximately three dozen subtypes of NHL, based on cellular origin, microscopic appearance, immunophenotype, and genetic characteristics (see Table 84.1). These entities originate from distinct stages of lymphocyte development and differentiation and are characterized by unique biologic and clinical features.

About 85% of NHLs arise from B cells, with the remainder deriving from T cells. The etiology of NHL in most patients is unknown, although a minority of patients have risk factors, including immunodeficiency states, certain oncogenic infections, autoimmune diseases, and exposure to certain toxins or radiation. The NHLs may be broadly grouped based on clinical behavior, with indolent, aggressive, and highly aggressive NHLs carrying an untreated natural history roughly measured in years, months, and weeks, respectively.

Clinical Presentation and Course (1,2)

Indolent Non-Hodgkin's Lymphomas

Indolent NHLs frequently present with *painless lymphadenopathy* in *multiple nodal sites*. The majority of patients with indolent lymphoma present at an advanced stage with frequent involvement of the *bone marrow* and *spleen*. *Extranodal visceral sites* and peripheral blood may be involved. Systemic "B" symptoms are uncommon. These diseases usually progress slowly over many months to years and may spontaneously regress over time. Despite the fact that they often exhibit long natural histories and are highly responsive to chemotherapy and radiation, they are rarely curable with conventional therapies.

The most common example of such an indolent NHL is *follicular lymphoma (grades I to II)*, which represents approximately 22% of NHLs in the United States and is typified pathologically by the t(14;18) chromosomal translocation, resulting in the constitutive expression of BCL2, a potent antiapoptotic protein. Follicular lymphoma grade III follows a more aggressive course and is classified and treated as with the aggressive B-cell lymphomas (see later discussion).

Other indolent NHLs include *marginal-zone lymphomas* (10%), *small lymphocytic lymphoma/chronic lymphocytic leukemia* (7%), and *lymphoplasmacytic lymphoma* (1%). All indolent lymphomas carry a low risk of transformation into a high-grade lymphoma over the lifetime of the disease. Marginal zone lymphomas (MZLs) derive from mature B cells and may occur in either nodal or extranodal sites; extranodal marginal zone lymphoma and splenic marginal zone lymphoma are subtypes that warrant special attention due to their special features. MZLs are commonly antigen-driven diseases that are frequently associated with specific infectious pathogens. All marginal zone lymphomas have been associated with paraprotein production, usually immunoglobulin M (IgM) or IgG, and with concomitant autoimmune cytopenias.

Extranodal marginal zone lymphoma, also known as *mucosa-associated lymphoid tissue (MALT) lymphoma*, is the most common MZL, accounting for almost 8% of NHLs. MALT lymphomas present in an *extranodal mucosal location* and are most commonly limited in stage. The *stomach* is the most common location, where it is associated with *Helicobacter pylori* infection in the majority of cases. Antibiotic treatment of *H. pylori* in such circumstances usually results in a complete remission of the lymphoma. Other sites of MALT involvement include the rest of the *gastrointestinal tract, the* *bronchi* and *lungs, periocular tissue, skin, thyroid gland*, and *breast*, among others.

Splenic marginal zone lymphoma, as the name implies, presents with dominant disease in the spleen, often causing massive splenomegaly and anemia. Presentation is often at stage IV, owing to subtle bone marrow infiltration, and may involve the peripheral blood with *villous lymphocytes*. Lymph node involvement is uncommon, and the disease carries a highly indolent natural history that can most commonly be managed with splenectomy alone. This disease has been associated with *hepatitis C virus infection*, which should be checked for in all affected patients with this diagnosis.

Small lymphocytic lymphoma (SLL) and *chronic lymphocytic leukemia (CLL)* are synonymous indolent pathologic diseases often grouped together as CLL/SLL. The leukemia name applies to cases with involvement of peripheral blood and/or bone marrow, whereas the lymphoma name is reserved for those cases that are limited to solid tissues without a circulating phase. This disease may be associated with a clonal paraprotein and autoimmune cytopenias. *Lymphoplasmacytic lymphoma* is an indolent mature B cell neoplasm, which frequently produces an *IgM paraprotein* leading to the syndrome of *Waldenström's macroglobulinemia*. Symptoms of the condition may be referable to the tumor infiltration itself or to the circulating paraprotein, resulting in hyperviscosity, neuropathy, autoimmune cytopenias, and coagulopathy, among other problems.

Aggressive Non-Hodgkin's Lymphomas

Aggressive NHLs present most commonly with a *rapidly growing lymph node* and/or *extranodal mass*. Greater than half of patients will have extranodal disease at diagnosis, and virtually any site may be involved. The most common extranodal site of involvement is the *gastrointestinal tract*, with other frequently involved sites being the lungs, bone, central nervous system, urogenital tract, liver, kidneys, salivary glands, Waldeyer's ring, bone marrow, and spleen. Systemic "B" symptoms are present in about one third of patients, and *lactate dehydrogenase (LDH)* is elevated at diagnosis in about half. Although the disease is rapidly growing and potentially fatal without treatment, approximately half of these patients are cured with conventional therapies, with some variation across disease subtypes.

Diffuse large B-cell lymphoma (DLBCL) is the prototypical aggressive NHL and is the most common lymphoid malignancy in adults, accounting for approximately one third of all NHLs. The median age of DLBCL is in the 60s, but it may occur at any age. Half of patients present with limited-stage disease and the rest with advanced-stage disease. The disease is curable, even at the advanced stage, in greater than half of patients. There are several uncommon variants of DLBCL recognized by distinct histopathologic features and their proclivity for certain anatomic sites, including primary mediastinal B cell lymphoma, intravascular B cell lymphoma, and primary effusion lymphoma. Follicular lymphoma grade III, unlike lower-grade follicular lymphomas, follows an aggressive clinical course akin to that of DLBCL.

Mantle cell lymphoma (MCL) is a B cell lymphoma representing 6% of all NHLs. It is uniquely characterized by the t(11;14) chromosomal translocation, resulting in constitutive expression of *cyclin D1*, a critical cell cycle regulatory protein. Unlike the other aggressive B cell lymphomas, MCL is not curable with conventional therapy. Although a small subset of MCLs follow an indolent natural history, the vast majority behaves aggressively and carries a poor overall survival of 3 to 5 years. Some patients may enjoy prolonged disease free survivals through use of intensive chemotherapy strategies. The disease usually presents at advanced stage, with frequent involvement of both nodal and extranodal sites, spleen, bone marrow, and peripheral blood. The most common extranodal site of disease is the gastrointestinal tract, where it may be discovered endoscopically as multiple lymphomatous polyposis. Unlike other aggressive B cell lymphomas, which present roughly equally in men and women, MCL has a marked male predominance.

T cell lymphomas are significantly less common than B cell lymphomas, tend to follow an aggressive clinical course, and are generally less responsive to chemotherapy than their B cell counterparts. *Peripheral T cell lymphomas (PTCLs)* represent approximately 8% of all NHLs, or approximately 5,000 new cases annually in the United States. Approximately half of PTCLs can be classified as discrete subtypes, although half fall into a category of peripheral T cell lymphoma, unspecified (PTCLu). These uncommon subtypes of PTCL include anaplastic large-cell lymphoma, extranodal NK/T cell lymphoma, angioimmunoblastic T cell lymphoma, enteropathy-type T cell lymphoma, hepatosplenic T cell lymphoma, subcutaneous panniculitis-like T cell lymphoma, and the HTLV-1–related adult T cell leukemia/lymphoma. These diseases tends to present at an advanced stage, although there is variation across subtypes, and the prognosis is poor, with a 5-year overall survival of 25% to 40%.

Anaplastic large-cell lymphoma (also known as *T/null cell lymphoma*) represents only 3% of adult NHLs but is the most common NHL of childhood. In adults, this disease presents with advanced-stage disease and "B" symptoms, as well as a striking male predominance, in the third and fourth decades of life. The key determinant of prognosis is expression of the *anaplastic lymphoma kinase (ALK) protein*, the product of the t(2;5) chromosomal translocation. ALK expression denotes a significantly better cure rate with standard therapy compared to that for ALK-negative patients.

Highly Aggressive Non-Hodgkin's Lymphoma

Highly aggressive NHLs include *Burkitt's lymphoma* and *precursor T cell or B cell lymphoblastic lymphoma/leukemia.* Burkitt's lymphoma is a mature B cell lymphoma accounting for 3% of NHLs in adults. The disease has endemic and sporadic variants. *Endemic Burkitt's lymphoma* is predominantly a disease of children in equatorial Africa and Papua New Guinea, corresponding to the distribution of *malaria.* It presents commonly as rapidly growing tumors of the jaw, is uniformly positive for *Epstein–Barr virus (EBV)*, and is highly treatable. *Sporadic Burkitt's lymphoma* occurs in the United States and may occur in either healthy or immunodeficient hosts; *HIV infection* is a prominent risk factor. EBV is usually negative in immunocompetent hosts with sporadic disease but is present in 30% to 40% of HIV-related Burkitt's lymphoma, although it does not affect prognosis or choice of therapy. The biologic sine qua non of Burkitt's lymphoma's is the *t(8;14)*, or occasionally t(2;8) or t(8;22), *chromosomal translocation*, resulting in constitutive activity of the cMYC oncogene. Burkitt's lymphoma proliferates rapidly, with nearly 100% of tumor cells in cell cycle and a doubling time as fast as 24 hours. Nodal as well as extranodal sites are usually involved, and central nervous system infiltration is common. Tumor lysis syndrome may occur spontaneously in this disease and is particularly common once therapy is initiated, which warrants careful monitoring and prophylaxis. This disease is curable in approximately 60% of adults with intensive combination chemotherapy.

Precursor T cell and B cell lymphoblastic lymphoma/leukemias (T-ALL/LBL and B-ALL/LBL, respectively) usually present as *acute leukemias* with involvement of bone marrow and peripheral blood. When it presents with a dominant *tissue phase* as lymphoblastic lymphoma, T cell LBL accounts for the vast majority of cases and presents with a mediastinal mass in half of patients. The disease presents most commonly in adolescents and young adults, with a strong male predominance. Lymphoblastic lymphoma may be cured with the same intensive induction chemotherapy programs used for acute lymphoblastic leukemias.

Staging and Risk Stratification for Prognosis (3–6)

Staging

The Ann Arbor staging system for NHL is identical to that used for Hodgkin's lymphoma (Table 84.3). The Ann Arbor system was originally created for Hodgkin's lymphoma based on the tendency of that disease to spread predictably to contiguous nodal sites. NHLs disseminate less predictably and may skip nodal regions entirely, making this staging system less well suited for prognostication in these diseases, although stage continues to be valuable in the selection of therapy.

Although the approach to staging is in part determined by tumor histology (see later discussion), some generalizations are appropriate. A thorough *physical examination* of all *peripheral nodal areas* is essential, as is visualization of *Waldeyer's ring.* The *liver* and *spleen* should be carefully checked. *Full-body CT scanning* is required for adequate staging. In aggressive lymphomas, as with Hodgkin's lymphoma, this is best performed with *PET-CT* scanning, which increases the sensitivity over CT scan alone. PET scans have not yet proven useful when added to CT scans in the routine staging and management of indolent NHLs, and so they should only be included in select circumstances.

TABLE 84.3

TREATMENT OF NON-HODGKIN'S LYMPHOMAS

Grade and Stage	Treatment
Indolent	
Early stage	Radiation
Late stage	Treatment only if indicated (single or multiagent chemotherapy, radiation, watchful waiting)
Aggresive	
Early stage	Multiagent chemotherapy +/– radiation
Late stage	Multiagent chemotherapy
Highly Aggressive	
All stages	High-dose multiagent chemotherapy

Laboratory assessment should include *complete blood count*, *renal* and *hepatic function tests*, *LDH*, and *peripheral blood smear* examination. Patients with aggressive and highly aggressive histologies should be assessed for spontaneous tumor lysis with tests for *uric acid*, *phosphorus*, *calcium*, *potassium*, and kidney function. Anemia is common in lymphoma patients and warrants further evaluation (see Chapter 79); mechanisms include immune-mediated hemolysis, hypersplenism, marrow infiltration, and inflammation. Patients with aggressive or highly aggressive B cell lymphomas should be checked for the *HIV antibody*, which is a risk factor for the development of these diseases. *Hepatitis serologies (B and C)* should be checked in all patients. Patients with gastric lymphoma should have *H. pylori serology* and consideration of more definitive testing (see Chapter 68).

In certain subtypes, circulating lymphoma cells may be detected by automated cell count or peripheral blood smear examination. Such cells may be further classified by *peripheral blood flow cytometry*, which can confirm and quantify circulating clonal lymphoid populations in the bloodstream. Immune dysfunction occurs in many patients, which should not be surprising, given that most lymphomas are B cell disorders. Certain NHL subsets, such as SLL/CLL, MZL, and lymphoplasmacytic lymphoma, are frequently associated with a monoclonal gammopathy, which may be detected by checking *quantitative immunoglobulins* and a *serum protein electrophoresis*. Immunoglobulins are also valuable to check in patients presenting with frequent infections because they may have a defect in humoral immunity due to a paucity of healthy antibody-producing cells.

Routine staging in all aggressive lymphomas should include *bone marrow aspiration and biopsy*. In the indolent NHLs, marrow examination should only be performed if it will change the approach to management, which is usually not the case.

Lumbar puncture should be considered in patients at risk for central nervous system spread (i.e., those with highly aggressive histology, neurologic signs and symptoms, HIV infection, or involvement of high-risk locations such as bone marrow, testes, epidural space or paranasal sinuses).

Risk Stratification

Prognostic models have been developed for both aggressive and indolent lymphomas to help to identify patients at high risk for relapse after therapy and in need of more intensive therapy.

For aggressive lymphoma, the *International Prognostic Index (IPI)* uses pretreatment variables independently predictive of relapse after standard anthracycline-based chemotherapy. These consist of *advanced age, poor performance status, elevated LDH, advanced Ann Arbor stage,* and involvement of *multiple extranodal sites*. Risk groups can be generated by summing the aforementioned risk factors present at diagnosis to predict long-term survival ranging from approximately 25% in the highest risk group to 75% in the lowest. Recent advances incorporating the monoclonal antibody rituximab for aggressive B cell lymphomas suggest that long-term overall survival in DLBCL has been improved to 55% in the poorest-risk cohort to over 90% in the most favorable one.

For indolent NHLs, a similar model has been developed, known as the *Follicular Lymphoma International Prognostic Index (FLIPI)*. Its prognostic variables include *advanced age, Ann Arbor stage III or IV, anemia, more than five involved nodal regions,* and *elevated LDH*. Risk groups are generated that predict respective 5- and 10-year overall survival of 90% and 70% in the lowest-risk group and 50% and 35% in the highest-risk group. These numbers are based on historical data

and are likely improved today with the incorporation of rituximab into the therapy of low-grade B cell lymphomas.

Principles of Management (7–18)

Overall Approach

Histology, staging, and risk stratification inform the design of the treatment program; *chemotherapy* is the predominant mode of treatment (see Table 84.3); most patients already have widespread disease at the time of initial clinical presentation, rendering localized treatment ineffective. Chemotherapy may be administered as a single agent or as a multidrug regimen. For patients with B cell lymphomas expressing CD20, the monoclonal *antibody rituximab* may be used alone or in combination, depending on the underlying disease. *Radiation* plays a role in the management of localized disease as well as in the palliation of symptomatic sites of advanced-stage disease. All aggressive NHL (independent of stage) and localized (stage I/II) indolent lymphomas should have the initiation of treatment early with the goal of treating for cure.

Indolent Non-Hodgkin's Lymphoma

The vast majority of cases present at advanced stages and, although highly treatable, are incurable with systemic therapy; consequently, treatment is directed at decreasing symptoms and prolonging length and quality of life. However, the few cases that present at limited stage are potentially curable with *radiation therapy* alone, which highlights the need for careful staging. Most forms of therapy produce responses and remissions, but relapses are the rule. Studies have demonstrated no improvement in overall survival with an earlier introduction of therapy, and so treatment is indicated only if the disease itself is causing adverse effects. Certain low-risk cases may never progress sufficiently to require therapy, and nearly 25% of cases undergo spontaneous regression during the course of the disease.

Indications for Treatment. Bulky or rapidly growing disease, symptomatic disease, disease interfering with organ function, bone marrow infiltration resulting in cytopenias, hypogammaglobulinemia with infections, autoimmune cytopenias, high-grade transformation, and patient preference constitute indications for therapy. In the absence of indications for treatment, patients may be followed closely by their oncologist in partnership with their primary care physician, customarily with clinical and laboratory evaluation every 3 to 6 months and restaging CT scans every 6 to 12 months, depending on the patient and the disease.

Treatment Modalities. At such time as treatment is indicated, *local low-dose radiotherapy* to a single focus of problematic disease may be employed to avoid the use of systemic therapies. Should systemic therapy be required, options range from *single-agent therapy* with an oral alkylating agent or the monoclonal CD20-directed antibody *rituximab*, to *combination* approaches. Higher response rates and improved progression-free survival may be achieved with chemotherapy combinations, although at the cost of increased treatment-related toxicity. Ultimately, the choice of therapy is a personal decision to be made collaboratively between the patient and their physicians, carefully balancing efficacy and tolerability of available treatments.

Treatment of Relapse and Disease Progression. Patients progressing after initial treatment can be *retreated*, often with *similar regimens*, with the goal of inducing a second remission. There is an emerging role of *rituximab* given intermittently as a single agent for *maintenance therapy*, which has been shown to prolong survival in certain patients after cytoreduction with combination chemotherapy. *High-dose chemotherapy* with *autologous stem cell rescue* may improve overall survival versus routine chemotherapy alone and should be considered in selected younger patients with progressive disease. There is no role for high-dose therapy in the initial treatment of these diseases. *Radioimmunotherapy*, in which a monoclonal antibody is covalently bound to a radiation-emitting isotope, has emerged as an effective option in select patients with relapsed indolent B cell NHL. Overall, median survival is about 8 to 10 years, regardless of type of therapy used, though this may be an underestimate of results achieved with modern therapy.

Patients with lymphomas related to either *H. pylori* or hepatitis C virus infection often experience a response with the use of *antibiotics* (see Chapter 68) or *antiviral therapy* (see Chapter 70) alone, which should be attempted first in all such patients before proceeding to chemotherapy or radiation.

Aggressive Non-Hodgkin's Lymphoma

The cure of patients with aggressive lymphoma using *combination chemotherapy* was first reported in 1972. The *CHOP regimen* (*cyclophosphamide, hydroxydaunomycin [doxorubicin], Oncovin [vincristine], and prednisone*) subsequently emerged as an enduring standard of care based on phase II and phase III studies demonstrating equivalent efficacy and improved safety compared to competing regimens.

Indications for Treatment. *Limited-stage aggressive lymphoma* is treated with Rituximab-CHOP with or without *local radiation*, providing a 5-year overall survival of approximately 85%. Involved-field radiotherapy after chemotherapy offers a modest protective benefit against local recurrence but without benefit in terms of overall survival, likely due to the ability to salvage patients at relapse and the risks of radiotherapy itself. The IPI risk score can predict patients who are likelier to be cured or not with standard therapy.

Advanced-stage aggressive lymphomas are treated with six to eight cycles of anthracycline-based chemotherapy, most commonly Rituximab-CHOP, with up to 65% of patients alive at 5 years posttreatment. Radiation therapy is included only in patients who fail to achieve a complete response to chemotherapy alone. As with limited-stage disease, the IPI risk score predicts patients who are likelier to do better or worse with anthracycline-containing chemotherapy. Patients with HIV infection are generally given concomitant antiretroviral therapy, as well as prophylaxis against opportunistic infection, which has significantly improved outcome in this high-risk patient population.

Treatment of Relapse and Disease Progression. In patients with either limited- or advanced-stage aggressive lymphoma who relapse after initial chemotherapy, salvage therapy is used, consisting of an *alternative combination chemotherapy* regimen followed by *high-dose chemotherapy with autologous stem cell transplantation*, which results in cure of nearly half of patients with relapsed or refractory disease. Many patients will undergo high dose chemotherapy due to lack of response to salvage treatment, or due to advanced age or comorbid disease. The duration of initial remission and response to salvage chemotherapy are the most important predictors of success after autologous stem cell transplantation.

Treatment of Mantle Cell Lymphoma. MCL is an aggressive and generally incurable B cell lymphoma that is approached uniquely. Intensive treatment strategies are designed to prolong progression-free survival but without clear benefit in lengthening overall survival. Strategies include *rituximab* plus *CHOP* followed immediately by *high-dose chemotherapy* and *autologous stem cell transplantation* or other intensive combination chemoimmunotherapy approaches. Selected patients may be offered *allogeneic stem cell transplantation* with the goal of cure, although broader application of this approach is limited by the older age of the patient population and the high attendant significant risks of morbidity and mortality. Recently, novel therapies have shown encouraging benefits in patients with relapsed MCL, including the proteasome inhibitor *bortezomib*, the immunomodulator *lenalidomide*, and the mammalian target of rapamycin (mTOR) pathway inhibitor *temsirolimus*.

Highly Aggressive Non-Hodgkin's Lymphoma

Intensive chemotherapy using multidrug regimens is indicated for all patients with highly aggressive histologies who are capable of tolerating such therapy. Age, tumor burden, advanced-stage disease, and increased LDH correlate with prognosis. Despite their aggressive natural history, these tumors are highly sensitive to chemotherapy, with response rates exceeding 90%. Regimens are similar to those used in the treatment of acute lymphoblastic leukemia and cure approximately 60% of patients with Burkitt's lymphoma and 40% of patients with lymphoblastic lymphoma.

These patients are at extremely high risk for *tumor lysis syndrome* owing to the rapid proliferative rate and exquisite chemosensitivity, so *prophylaxis* and frequent laboratory monitoring is mandatory. Lumbar *puncture* should be performed at baseline to evaluate for central nervous system involvement, given the high risk of leptomeningeal lymphomatosis in these diseases. Systemic and *intrathecal chemotherapy* directed at the central nervous system is included for all patients. Burkitt's lymphoma patients with HIV infection may be treated similarly to their non-HIV–infected counterparts, but *antiretroviral therapy*, prophylaxis against opportunistic infections, and white cell growth factor support are required.

Investigational Therapies for Non-Hodgkin's Lymphoma

Investigational therapies being explored for the treatment of lymphoma include improved *anti-CD20 molecules* as well as novel *monoclonal antibodies* directed against additional B cell and T cell antigens. As the biologic underpinnings of lymphomas are better understood, novel small molecules are being developed specifically to interfere with oncogenic pathways in discrete subsets of disease. The role of *allogeneic stem cell transplantation*, particularly with the better-tolerated, reduced-intensity conditioning regimens, continue to be explored for diseases that are not curable with traditional therapies.

Monitoring Therapy

Monitoring patients on chemotherapy requires close surveillance of *blood counts* (see Chapter 88). *Bone marrow suppression* is the leading complication. *White cell growth factor* can be used as secondary prophylaxis against infection in patients who develop neutropenic fever or as primary prophylaxis in high-risk patients. Relapse typically occurs within the first

3 years after treatment and nearly all within 5 years, and so close surveillance with *clinical exams*, laboratory testing, and *CT scans* is performed during this time period. Watching for the development of neurologic symptoms is particularly important in patients with a predisposition to central nervous system recurrence (see prior discussion).

Patient Education

The encouraging results of chemotherapy, particularly in patients with aggressive advanced disease, provide hope for all newly diagnosed patients. As with Hodgkin's lymphoma, the patient can be given a fairly accurate assessment of the prognosis after careful histologic study and staging have been carried out. Often, the prognosis is far better than the patient's fearful expectations and can be shared profitably. Even elderly patients may tolerate therapy and be cured of their life-threatening disease.

A detailed review of the possible adverse effects of therapy (e.g., sterility, infection; see Chapter 88) must be made, as must

that of the experimental nature of those therapies for which data on long-term outcomes are lacking. Novel therapies are being rapidly developed for all lymphomas, and so consultation with an oncologist specializing in the care of lymphoma is advised.

Indications for Referral

These malignancies are potentially curable. Referral to the oncologist should be made early, when the diagnosis is first suspected. Management of the patient with Hodgkin's and non-Hodgkin's lymphomas needs to be a cooperative venture from the start, with the primary physician working closely with the oncologist experienced in lymphoma care. Selection of a treatment modality requires the judgment of an oncologist who is knowledgeable about available protocols, which are constantly undergoing revision. The primary physician monitors response and adverse effects, maintains continuity, provides psychological support, and follows the patient for lifelong risks of recurrence and late toxicities of therapy.

Annotated Bibliography

Hodgkin Lymphoma

1. Hasenclever D, Diehl V. A prognostic score for advanced Hodgkin's disease. N Engl J Med 1998;339:1506. (*Presents a clinical prognostic model for advanced-stage disease*).
2. Jaffe ES, Harris NL, Stein H, et al. Tumours of haematopoietic and lymphoid tissues. World Health Organization. Classification of tumours: pathology and genetics. Lyon, France: IARC Press, 2001. (*The World Health Organization consensus classification system.*)
3. Lister TA, Crowther D, Sutcliffe SB, et al. Report of a committee convened to discuss the evaluation and staging of patients with Hodgkin's disease: Cotswolds meeting. J Clin Oncol 1989;7:1630. (*The Ann Arbor staging system.*)
4. Hehn ST, Grogan TM, Miller TP. Utility of fine-needle aspiration as a diagnostic technique in lymphoma. J Clin Oncol 2004;22(15):3046. (*Finds that fine-needle aspiration was inadequately sensitive for diagnosis.*)
5. Juweid ME, Cheson BD. Positron-emission tomography and assessment of cancer therapy. N Engl J Med 2006;354:496. (*A thorough review for the generalist reader of this important imaging technology for staging and monitoring.*)
6. Canellos GP, Anderson JR, Propert KJ, et al. Chemotherapy of advanced Hodgkin's disease with MOPP, ABVD, or MOPP alternating with ABVD. N Engl J Med 1992;19:1478. (*A landmark trial, establishing ABVD [Adriamycin, bleomycin, vinblastine, and dacarbazine] as the primary treatment of advanced-stage disease.*)
7. Diehl V, Franklin J, Pfreundschuh M, et al. Standard and increased-dose BEACOPP chemotherapy compared with COPP-ABVD for advanced Hodgkin's disease. N Engl J Med 2003;348:2386. (*An intensive regimen offers benefit over ABVD at the cost of additional toxicity.*)
8. Ferme C, Eghbali H, Meerwaldt JH, et al. Chemotherapy plus involved-field radiation in early-stage Hodgkin's disease. N Engl J Med 2007;357:1916. (*Presents evidence of the efficacy of this fundamental change in approach.*)
9. Meyer RM, Gospodarowicz MK, Connors JM, et al. A randomized comparison of ABVD chemotherapy with a strategy that includes radiation therapy in patients with limited-stage Hodgkin's lymphoma. J Clin Oncol 2005;23:4634. (*Presents evidence that radiation can be safely omitted in limited-stage disease.*)
10. Phillips GL, Wolff SN, Herzig RH, et al. Treatment of progressive Hodgkin's disease with intensive chemoradiotherapy and autologous bone marrow transplantation in refractory Hodgkin's disease. Blood 1989;73:2086. (*An initial report of autologous stem cell transplantation for relapsed/refractory disease.*)

11. Travis LB, Hill DA, Dores GM, et al. Breast cancer following radiotherapy and chemotherapy among young women with Hodgkin disease. JAMA 2003;290:465. (*A matched case–control study, finding a significantly increased risk of breast cancer associated with radiation therapy.*)

Non-Hodgkin's Lymphoma

1. Armitage JO, Weisenburger DD. New approach to classifying non-Hodgkin's lymphomas: clinical features of the major histologic subtypes. Non-Hodgkin's Lymphoma Classification Project. J Clin Oncol 1998;16:2780. (*A nice clinical summary of major lymphoma subtypes.*)
2. Jaffe ES, Harris NL, Stein H, et al. World Health Organization classification of tumours. Pathology and genetics of hematopoietic and lymphoid tissues. Lyon, France: IARC Press; 2001. (*The "bible" of lymphoma classification.*)
3. Gascoyne RD, Aoun P, Wu D, et al. Prognostic significance of anaplastic lymphoma kinase (ALK) protein expression in adults with anaplastic large cell lymphoma. Blood 1999;93:3913. (*Presents the prognostic significance of anaplastic lymphoma kinase protein expression in anaplastic large-cell lymphoma.*)
4. Horning SJ, Rosenberg SA. The natural history of initially untreated low-grade non-Hodgkin's lymphomas. N Engl J Med 1984;311:1471. (*Indolent lymphomas may enjoy a long natural history with observation alone.*)
5. The International Non-Hodgkin's Lymphoma Prognostic Factors Project. A predictive model for aggressive non-Hodgkin's lymphoma. N Engl J Med 1993;329:987. (*Defines a clinical risk model in aggressive non-Hodgkin's lymphoma [NHL].*)
6. Solal-Céligny P, Roy P, Colombat P, et al. Follicular lymphoma International Prognostic Index. Blood 2004;104:1258. (*Defines a clinical risk model in indolent NHL.*)
7. Aleman BP, Raemaekers JM, Tirelli U, et al. Involved-field radiotherapy for advanced Hodgkin's lymphoma. N Engl J Med 2003;348:2396. (*Radiation therapy does not improve survival over chemotherapy alone.*)
8. Ardeshna KM, Smith P, Norton A, et al. Long-term effect of a watch and wait policy versus immediate systemic treatment for asymptomatic advanced-stage non-Hodgkin lymphoma: a randomised controlled trial. Lancet 2003;362:516. (*A randomized, controlled trial, finding that early treatment in indolent NHL does not improve survival over watchful waiting.*)
9. Coiffier B, Lepage E, Briere J, et al. CHOP chemotherapy plus rituximab compared with CHOP alone in elderly patients with diffuse large-B-cell lymphoma. N Engl J Med 2002;346:235. (*A landmark trial, demonstrating the benefit of rituximab combined with CHOP [cyclophosphamide,*

hydroxydaunomycin (doxorubicin), Oncovin (vincristine), and prednisone] for aggressive B cell lymphoma.)

10. Fisher RI, Gaynor ER, Dahlberg S, et al. Comparison of a standard regimen (CHOP) with three intensive chemotherapy regimens for advanced non-Hodgkin's lymphoma. N Engl J Med 1993;328:1002. (*Establishes CHOP as standard therapy for aggressive NHL.*)
11. Horning SJ, Weller E, Kim K, et al. Chemotherapy with or without radiotherapy in limited-stage diffuse aggressive non-Hodgkin's lymphoma: Eastern Cooperative Oncology Group study 1484. J Clin Oncol 2004;22:3032. (*Radiation after standard chemotherapy decreased local recurrence but did not improve survival.*)
12. MacManus MP, Hoppe RT. Is radiotherapy curative for stage I and II low-grade follicular lymphoma? Results of a long-term follow-up study of patients treated at Stanford University. J Clin Oncol 1996;14(4):1282. (*Local radiotherapy may cure limited-stage indolent NHL.*)
13. Marcus R, Imrie K, Belch A, et al. CVP chemotherapy plus rituximab compared with CVP as first-line treatment for advanced follicular lymphoma. Blood 2005;105(4):1417. (*Rituximab improved survival in indolent B cell lymphoma when added to combination chemotherapy.*)
14. Mead GM, Sydes MR, Walewski J, et al. An international evaluation of CODOX-M and CODOX-M alternating with IVAC in adult Burkitt's lymphoma: results of United Kingdom Lymphoma Group LY06 study. Ann Oncol 2002;13:1961. (*Adult Burkitt's lymphoma can be cured with intensive chemotherapy.*)
15. Miller TP, Dahlberg S, Cassady JR, et al. Chemotherapy alone compared with chemotherapy plus radiotherapy for localized intermediate- and high-grade non-Hodgkin's lymphoma. N Engl J Med 1998;339:21. (*Short-course chemotherapy followed by radiation was effective in limited-stage, nonbulky, aggressive lymphoma.*)
16. Phillip T, Guglielmi C, Hagenbeek A, et al. Autologous bone marrow transplantation compared with salvage chemotherapy in relapses of chemotherapy-sensitive non-Hodgkin's lymphoma. N Engl J Med 1995;333:1540. (*Survival improved with autologous stem cell transplantation for relapsed aggressive lymphoma.*)
17. Schouten HC, Qian W, Kvaloy S, et al. High-dose therapy improves progression-free survival and survival in relapsed follicular non-Hodgkin's lymphoma: results from the randomized European CUP trial. J Clin Oncol 2003;21:3918. (*Finds benefit for autologous stem cell transplantation in relapsed indolent lymphoma.*)
18. van Oers MH, Klasa R, Marcus RE, et al. Rituximab maintenance improves clinical outcome of relapsed/resistant follicular non-Hodgkin lymphoma in patients both with and without rituximab during induction: results of a prospective randomized phase 3 intergroup trial. Blood 2006;108:3295. (*Maintenance rituximab improved survival after second-line chemotherapy in indolent B cell lymphoma.*)

CHAPTER 85 ■ APPROACH TO THE PATIENT WITH METASTATIC TUMOR OF UNKNOWN ORIGIN

JEFFREY W. CLARK

A malignancy is designated as a tumor of unknown origin (TUO) when it satisfies several criteria: (a) the tissue is histologically confirmed to be malignant, and a primary tumor of any specific organ cannot be identified; (b) routine screening fails to identify the primary source; and (c) a very late metastasis (as occurs in breast cancer, melanoma, and renal cell carcinoma) is also ruled out. Less than 3% of all carcinomas in patients fall into this category, and this percentage is likely to continue to decline as more sensitive diagnostic techniques are developed.

A TUO poses several problems, ranging from the utility of pursuing further workup to the efficacy of empiric therapy for disease that is already widely metastatic. Any decision to conduct a more extensive evaluation or treat empirically must include a consideration of the low probability that a treatable cancer is present. Moreover, the evaluation of a TUO can prove expensive and uncomfortable. However, within this very heterogeneous group are a few very responsive malignancies that can be effectively treated if recognized.

Guided by the principle of looking for the most treatable disease, the primary physician should be able to conduct the major part of an effective workup in the outpatient setting and work closely with the oncologist in presenting thoughtful treatment options to the patient.

CLINICAL PRESENTATION AND NATURAL HISTORY OF DISEASE (1–6)

Clinical Presentation

Common sites of metastatic presentation are the lung, mediastinum, liver, bone, and lymph nodes. Others include the bone marrow, brain, spinal cord, peritoneum, and retroperitoneum.

Lung

A TUO may present as a solitary nodule, multiple nodules, or recurrent pleural effusion (see Chapters 43 and 44). When a TUO presents in the *mediastinum*, it may do so as a catastrophic secondary complication, such as dysphagia, stridor, or respiratory difficulty, or superior vena cava syndrome.

Bone

A TUO may appear as a lytic or blastic lesion of the axial skeleton, long bones, or skull. Sometimes, the patient reports bone pain or has a pathologic fracture. Often, a TUO is discovered as an incidental radiographic finding. Bone marrow invasion may be heralded by pancytopenia or a myelophthisic picture.

Lymph Node

Asymmetric cervical, axillary, or inguinal disease is characteristic. Axillary nodes that histologically manifest adenocarcinoma are most commonly associated with ipsilateral breast cancer, even in the presence of normal findings on a breast examination and mammogram. The presence of malignancy in an inguinal node may represent local spread from carcinoma of the vulva, prostate, perineum, endometrium, or ovary, or it may represent systemic involvement by lymphoma. Metastasis from testicular cancer usually does not present as inguinal adenopathy except in cases of previous pelvic and retroperitoneal node dissection.

Liver

Involvement is usually discovered when the results of liver function tests are abnormal (e.g., isolated elevation of alkaline phosphatase), a hepatic nodule is detected on physical examination, or a focal defect is noted on abdominal ultrasonography or computed tomography scan. When a primary is discovered, the most frequent sites of origin prove to be the pancreas, liver, bowel, and stomach. Tumor that has spread to the peritoneum can lead to malignant ascites. Involvement of the retroperitoneum is usually a silent consequence of spread. Brain metastasis may be asymptomatic, but the new onset of a focal neurologic deficit or headache is suggestive. Spinal cord involvement may present urgently with symptoms of cord compression (see Chapter 167).

Treatment-Responsive Cancers

A number of treatment-responsive tumors that often present as TUOs have been defined. Most manifest a poorly differentiated or undifferentiated histologic appearance. *Extragonadal germ-cell cancers* are a subset of poorly differentiated neoplasms that may be potentially curable. They frequently manifest as disease of the *mediastinum*, *retroperitoneum*, or *lymph nodes*. Other features are patient *age less than 50 years* and elevations in serum *human chorionic gonadotropin (HCG)* or *α-fetoprotein (AFP)* levels. *Poorly differentiated carcinoma of neuroendocrine origin* (determined by electron microscopy) may also be responsive to treatment.

Ovarian carcinoma may present as adenocarcinoma of the peritoneum, with *malignant ascites* in a woman with no known primary, and may respond to treatment, even when no ovarian disease can be found, with a longer median survival than would be expected for most other metastatic carcinomas. *Prostate cancer* may have a number of atypical presentations, such as *bony metastasis* and poorly differentiated or undifferentiated histology and little clinical evidence of a primary lesion.

Natural History and Clinical Course

Because a TUO represents metastatic disease, it is not surprising that overall median survival is usually relatively short. Overall, long-term survival is not improved by treatment when all TUO patients are considered as a group, although the outcomes for responsive clinical and histopathologic subgroups can be improved considerably with treatment (see later discussion).

TABLE 85.1

TREATABLE MALIGNANCIES THAT MAY PRESENT AS A TUMOR OF UNKNOWN ORIGIN

Potentially Curable, Even When Metastatic
Gestational trophoblastic tumors
Germ-cell cancer, gonadal (e.g., testicular carcinoma)
Hodgkin's disease
Non-Hodgkin's lymphoma
Squamous cell carcinoma of the oropharynx
? Poorly differentiated carcinoma of neuroendocrine type[a]
? Poorly differentiated carcinoma of extragonadal germ-cell origin

Very Responsive to Treatment, Although Not Curable When Metastatic
Prostate cancer
Breast cancer
Small-cell carcinoma of the lung
Ovarian carcinoma
Endometrial cancer
Thyroid cancer
Poorly differentiated carcinoma of neuroendocrine type[a]
Poorly differentiated carcinoma of extragonadal germ cell origin[a]
Peritoneal carcinomatosis[a]

[a]Presents as tumor of unknown origin with poorly differentiated or undifferentiated histology.

DIFFERENTIAL DIAGNOSIS (1,6)

Based on data from autopsy studies, *pancreatic carcinoma* leads the list of causes of cancer of unknown origin, accounting for approximately 25% of cases. *Cancers* of the *lung, kidney, colorectum,* and *prostate* together account for another 30%. From the perspective of workup and management, a consideration of potentially treatable cancers is most important (Table 85.1); this is aided by a differential diagnosis according to the region of presentation (Table 85.2).

In older men, the most common treatable malignancy is *prostate cancer*; in *younger men*, it is *germ-cell carcinoma*. In *women*, *breast* and *ovarian* cancers lead the list of treatable cancers. Other important causes are cancers of the *nasopharynx, oropharynx,* and *lung (small-cell type).* As noted, even patients with a poorly differentiated or undifferentiated histology may have a *treatable* cancer, such as *lymphoma, neuroendocrine carcinoma, extragonadal germ-cell cancer, primary peritoneal carcinoma,* or *carcinoma of the prostate.*

WORKUP (1,3,6–10)

Searching for Treatable Disease

When faced with a TUO, the priority is to search for treatable disease. Conducting the workup on the basis of probability rather than on responsiveness to therapy (Table 85.3) may lead to searches that have less effect on outcome. The expense and discomfort incurred by the many diagnostic studies ordered in search of likely but poorly responsive disease can be avoided if the physician adopts the discipline of searching for malignancies that respond to treatment (see Tables 85.1

TABLE 85.2

TREATABLE CAUSES OF METASTATIC DISEASE BY SITE OF PRESENTATION

Site of Presentation	Source of Primary
Lung and Mediastinum	Lung (small cell)
	Breast
	Hodgkin's disease
	Extragonadal germ cell
	Neuroendocrine
	Germ cell (testicular)
Bone	
Osteoblastic lesions	Prostate
	Lung (small-cell)
	Hodgkin's disease
Osteolytic or mixed lesions	Breast
Liver	Breast
	Lung (small-cell)
Brain	Breast
	Lung (small-cell)
	Lymphoma
Bone Marrow	Breast
	Lung (small-cell)
	Prostate
Lymph Nodes	
High cervical	Squamous cell cancer
	Hodgkin's disease, lymphoma
	Neuroendocrine
Axillary	Breast (ipsilateral)
	Lymphoma
	Lung (small-cell)
Inguinal	Prostate
	Ovary
	Endometrium
	Lymphoma
Retroperitoneal	Lymphoma
	Hodgkin's disease
	Testes
	Prostate
	Ovarian
	Neuroendocrine
	Extragonadal germ cell

TABLE 85.3

COMMON CANCERS AND THEIR RESPONSIVENESS TO THERAPY

Tumor	Response Rate (%)
More Responsive	
Breast	40–60
Ovary	60–70
Prostate	60–70
Head, neck	50–70
Testicular	80–100
Lymphoma	80
Lung (small-cell)	80
Less Responsive	
Neurosecretory	30–50
Sarcoma	30
Colon	40–50
Melanoma	10–15
Hepatoma	20
Renal	25–40
Lung (non–small-cell)	30–50
Brain	20–35

chitectural information, which can be critical for diagnosis. Moreover, cytologic preparation may misrepresent nuclear and cytoplasmic abnormalities, which can be induced by inflammation or drugs. Therefore the *cytologic diagnosis* should be confirmed by *tissue diagnosis* whenever feasible.

Histologic Assessment. Evaluation begins with histologic diagnosis of the tumor by *cell type* (adenocarcinoma, lymphoma, small-cell carcinoma of the lung, sarcoma, squamous cell carcinoma, melanoma, undifferentiated). Special stains may be used (see later discussion). The histologic designation of adenocarcinoma does not definitively establish the primary source of the tumor. A glandular malignancy can develop in multiple organs. The histologic distinction among adenocarcinoma of the ovary, stomach, lung, or breast is sometimes possible by pathology laboratory methods, but other approaches may be needed to assist in establishing the most likely primary site, including clinical assessment (see later discussion).

Immunohistochemical Staining. Receptor analysis and staining for specific protein markers (e.g., leukocyte common antigen, cytokeratins, S-100, and TTF-1) are becoming increasingly helpful and the approach of choice when one encounters a histologic designation of "undifferentiated carcinoma." Often, sufficient information is provided to guide therapeutic decisions, such as detecting substances useful in differentiating a carcinoma from a lymphoma, melanoma, or germ-cell tumor. Other important markers include *prostate-specific antigen* and *prostatic acid phosphatase*, which are suggestive of prostate cancer, and *AFP* and *HCG* for germ-cell tumors. Increase in knowledge about specific tumor markers should further enhance the ability to identify tumors by their molecular characterestics in the future.

Electron microscopy can sometimes be useful when immunohistochemistry is inconclusive. Subcellular structures are examined for evidence of differentiation, from which one can infer the cell line of origin (i.e., its histogenesis). Such a review of ultrastructure can help to classify a cell as epithelial, mesenchymal, mesothelial, or melanocytic in origin and subclassify within each category according to characteristic ultrastructural

to 85.4). Treatment in patients with cancer is determined first and foremost by stage of disease, but if the presentation is that of metastatic disease, the tumor is usually sufficiently staged. An exception to this would be malignancies, such as colorectal cancer, in which resection of certain metastatic sites (e.g., liver or lung) can sometimes be associated with long-term survival.

Tissue Diagnosis

The importance of biopsy and histologic diagnosis cannot be overstated; the pathologist plays a central role in the workup of an unknown primary cancer. Before other investigations are initiated, an adequate *tissue biopsy* sample from the metastatic site is essential to enable thorough histologic examination and performance of *immunohistochemical studies* and, when appropriate, *electron microscopy*. Careful communication and close collaboration with both those doing the biopsy and pathologist are critical to ensure that this is properly done. *Cytologic sampling* is usually insufficient because it does not provide ar-

TABLE 85.4

DIAGNOSIS OF SOME TREATABLE CANCERS PRESENTING AS TUMOR OF UNKNOWN ORIGIN

Malignancy	Diagnostic Features, Relevant Studies
Squamous cell, nasopharynx, oropharynx	PE (nodule, plaque), CT or MRI, blind biopsy
Lymphoma	PE (adenopathy), immunohistochemical stains
Ovarian cancer	PE (ascites or mass), pelvic CT or MRI, AFP, HCG, peritoneal implants
Prostate cancer	PE (nodule), PSA, prostate ultrasonography, immunohistochemical stains
Breast cancer	PE (breast nodule), receptor studies
Testicular cancer	PE (testicular nodule), ultrasonography, serum AFP, HCG
Extragonadal germ-cell cancer	PE (adenopathy), CT (lung nodules, mediastinal mass, retroperitoneal mass), immunohistochemical studies, serum AFP, HCG
Neuroendocrine carcinoma	PE (adenopathy), CT (retroperitoneal nodes, mediastinal nodes), EM

AFP, α-fetoprotein; CT, computed tomography; EM, electron microscopy; HCG, human chorionic gonadotropin; MRI, magnetic resonance imaging; PE, physical examination; PSA, prostate-specific antigen.

features (e.g., melanosomes, membrane-bound secretory granules, elongated microvilli, lysosomes, large bundles of tonofilaments, membrane-bound mucin vacuoles). However, because of problems with sampling and cell preservation, the sensitivity and specificity of electron microscopy are not high. The sample must be cut into very small cubes (which makes for sampling errors) and preserved in glutaraldehyde promptly (any delay in processing or use of a fixative other than glutaraldehyde can distort cell architecture).

Receptor Studies and Cytogenetics. Testing for the presence of *estrogen* and *progesterone receptors* helps to identify *breast* cancer if receptor levels are high; however, these receptors are also found in a number of other malignancies, including *ovarian* and *endometrial* cancers, reducing specificity if levels are not high. *Cytogenetic studies* are a promising diagnostic technique and likely to enhance tumor identification as the methodology matures. For example, testing for *i(12p) marker chromosome* may be useful in identifying patients with suspected midline germ-cell tumors. Advances in the technology for detecting nucleic acid sequences and other molecular markers continue, offering more extensive profiling of the genetic and protein makeup of tumors.

Clinical Assessment

All patients should undergo a careful *physical examination* with special emphasis on the detection of the most treatable malignant disease (i.e., cancer of the breast, uterus, or ovaries in women; cancer of the prostate or testicles in men; lymphoma and head and neck cancer in all patients). Certainly a careful examination of *skin, lymph nodes,* and *rectum* should be performed in all patients. Depending on the site of metastasis, other elements of the physical examination may also prove useful (see later discussion and Table 85.4).

Other Laboratory Studies and Imaging

Most routine blood chemistries are not helpful, although a few serologic markers (e.g., prostate-specific antigen, AFP, β-HCG

subunit) can aid in searching for treatable disease (see Table 85.4). Imaging studies are guided by the same principle of looking for treatable cancer rather than conducting an extensive workup for all possible primary tumors (e.g., *mammography* for breast cancer; *ultrasonography* for a testicular or prostatic cancer; *pelvic CT, MRI, or ultrasound* for ovarian disease). *PET or PET-CT* is increasingly being used to identify potential sites of disease, which may aid in defining the most appropriate areas for biopsy.

Workup by Site of Presentation

The clinical presentation (see Table 85.2 and later discussion) in conjunction with pathologic data can help to guide the workup.

Pulmonary Nodules, Pleural Effusions, and Mediastinal Masses

An *open biopsy* procedure may be necessary to obtain sufficient tissue for detailed histopathologic study and definitive diagnosis because needle aspiration may provide insufficient material. Of particular importance is the identification of lymphoma and extragonadal germ-cell, small-cell, and neuroendocrine cancers, which are among the more treatable malignancies that present as mediastinal or rapidly growing pulmonary mass lesions. Also worth considering is colorectal cancer because treatment has improved over the last 5 years with new chemotherapeutic regimens and the potential benefit for resection of metastatic lesions in the appropriate setting (see Chapter 76). Detailed study by the pathologist can be very useful. Immunohistochemical studies are essential, complemented by electron microscopy if necessary and serologic testing for AFP and β-HCG subunit.

Pleural effusions caused by malignancy can be identified cytologically. When this is not sufficiently diagnostic, a pleural biopsy in conjunction with aspiration may be more informative (see Chapter 43). A diagnosis of adenocarcinoma in cytologic fluids does not identify the primary source; one must look specifically for the source by immunohistochemical, receptor, and mammographic studies.

Mediastinal disease that produces symptoms of dysphagia, respiratory difficulty, or superior vena cava syndrome is usually a consequence of primary lung cancer, metastatic breast cancer, or lymphoma. These can be rather well managed by radiation therapy, chemotherapy, or a combined approach as appropriate. Although it is important to distinguish among these (especially to determine whether the condition is a lymphoma), once that distinction has been made, prompt treatment of the tumor is important to relieve symptoms and prevent potentially serious complications. More silent mediastinal disease may be caused by neuroendocrine or extragonadal germ-cell cancer, which can be identified by the methods noted earlier.

Osseous Metastases

The identification of an isolated bony lesion that is radiographically characteristic of neoplasia should be followed by a *biopsy* if tissue is not obtainable elsewhere. The appearance of the lesion on plain film should be noted to determine whether it is *lytic*, *blastic*, or *mixed*, which can help to limit the differential diagnosis (see Table 85.2) and focus the evaluation. If the bony lesion is difficult to sample, one can obtain a bone scan to identify other sites of tumor that may be more easily accessible to biopsy. Having established a histologic diagnosis of malignancy in the bone, the search for the primary should, as always, be confined to treatable disease. Tumors of the lung and kidney are among the most common sources of skeletal metastases of unknown cause.

Liver Metastases

Liver metastases are usually diagnosed by *ultrasonography* or *CT* and confirmed by *CT-guided needle biopsy*. Most are adenocarcinomas with gastrointestinal sources, although breast and lung are other important origins. Histologic evaluation can be helpful in trying to distinguish among these. Symptomatic patients with hepatic metastases from a TUO have a median life expectancy of less than 6 months, but asymptomatic persons may have a significantly longer survival. As mentioned, one exception to this would be potentially resectable lesions due to colorectal cancer, in which the resection of metastatic lesions can be associated with long-term survival and the chemotherapeutic choices are different from the usual empiric regimens used for TUOs.

Ascites

Although malignant ascites can occur from a wide variety of malignancies, it is most commonly derived from metastatic cancer of the ovaries, pancreas, stomach, or colon involving the peritoneal surface. Given differences in the treatment approach, it is worth ruling out ovarian or primary peritoneal cancer in women. *Pelvic ultrasonography*, *CT*, or *MRI* and testing for the tumor marker serum *CA-125* are indicated. Peritoneal implants have been noted in patients without detectable ovarian disease, so it is worth considering the diagnosis without a detectable ovarian lesion.

High Cervical Lymphadenopathy

Because enlargement of a high cervical node may result from a contiguous primary tumor in the nasopharynx or oropharynx or a lymphoma (two treatable cancers), intensive assessment is warranted. A careful examination of the nasopharynx, oral cavity (including base of the tongue), and larynx is essential, as is detailed examination of all lymph nodes. *CT* or *MRI* is helpful in the examination of the deeper lymph nodes and submucosal and neck structures. If *node biopsy* reveals squamous cell or epidermoid histology, but no primary is evident, then blind biopsies of areas likely to harbor nasopharyngeal tumor (base of the tongue, nasopharynx) are conducted. If the histopathology is adenocarcinoma, then sinuses or the salivary glands may be the primary source. Again, careful *physical examination* supplemented by *CT* or *MRI* may help to reveal the primary. If histologic studies indicate a lymphoma or Hodgkin's disease, then the evaluation shifts to staging activities (see Chapter 84).

Axillary Adenopathy

Axillary adenopathy necessitates a careful *breast examination*, *mammography*, and possibly *breast MRI*. The diagnosis of breast cancer may be assisted by performing estrogen and progesterone receptor assays on nodal tissue obtained from the axilla. Immunohistochemical study for markers of lymphoma is also indicated. Chest CT may be warranted if small-cell histology is suggested.

Inguinal Adenopathy

Inguinal adenopathy is approached diagnostically in much the same manner as cervical adenopathy, with an emphasis on local disease and lymphoma, because they are potentially quite responsive to treatment (see Table 85.3). Detailed pathologic study is essential and should include immunohistochemical and receptor studies of the tissue obtained at biopsy. Careful pelvic and anorectal examinations are performed, complemented by ultrasonographic or MRI scans of the pelvis. If inguinal node biopsy identifies a lymphoma, then workup proceeds for staging (see Chapter 84).

Retroperitoneal Mass

An incidentally discovered retroperitoneal mass is likely to represent advanced-stage lymphoma, sarcoma, or metastatic prostate, germ-cell, or ovarian cancer. Many of these are responsive to therapy and thus important to identify. Because it is difficult to obtain samples from this site, a search for a more accessible site is indicated. Careful physical examination of the peripheral nodes, prostate and testicles in men, and pelvic organs in women is indicated. Ultrasonographic examination may help to detect a small prostatic or testicular lesion. Ultrasonography may also help to identify an ovarian tumor. MRI may also be helpful in evaluating for a pelvic primary. Serum marker studies (e.g., AFP, β-HCG subunit, prostate-specific antigen, or CA-125 as appropriate) aid in the diagnostic effort.

Brain

Once a primary brain tumor has been ruled out, the most common sites of primary lesions for metastasis are lung (including small-cell carcinoma) breast, kidney (renal cell cancer), and melanoma (see prior discussion). However, it is important to also consider more treatable disease such as lymphoma. If no tissue is available peripherally, then there should be consideration of brain biopsy. If a brain biopsy is performed, detailed immunohistochemical and receptor studies should be conducted.

Bone Marrow Invasion

When pancytopenia or a myelophthisic picture with leukoerythroblastic changes is encountered, marrow invasion should be considered and confirmed by *bone marrow biopsy* (see Chapter 79). The marrow examination includes a search for clusters of malignant cells, which may help in identification. Once their presence is confirmed, a search for the several treatable tumors can commence (see Table 85.1).

TREATMENT (3,5,7,10–14)

As emphasized earlier, the workup focuses intensively on the identification of the most treatable cancers (see Tables 85.1 and 85.3). However, when the primary remains unknown (as in a substantial proportion of cases), the options for treatment become more problematic, with a choice between empiric treatment for most-treatable possible tumor and watchful waiting. Data on the efficacy and cost–benefit ratio of both approaches are limited. The interpretation of published outcomes data is often hindered by the absence of a careful, detailed characterization of patients and their tumors. Only a few prospective, randomized, controlled trials have been performed, and although responses have been documented, median long-term survival remains uncommon. Consequently, any discussion with the patient and family must address the uncertain benefit of empiric treatment and its potential adverse effects. When patients with germ-cell and neuroendocrine TUOs are excluded, response rates are in the range of 25% to 30%. Therefore, the decision about proceeding with empiric treatment in this setting needs to be carefully weighed in discussions among the patient, the primary care physician, and the oncologist.

Empiric Therapy

Both chemotherapy and radiation are used empirically. *Chemotherapy* options involve two basic approaches. "*Broad-spectrum*" *approaches* use a platinum-containing agent, a taxane, and/or etoposide and monitor for marrow suppression. Treatment is halted if no evidence of benefit is noted after two cycles. The *most-likely-treatable-tumor* approach takes into account cell type, age, sex, and site (see Tables 85.1, 85.2, and 85.4). If the pathologic type is undifferentiated, treatment is directed toward the most responsive tumors in this class—namely, lymphoma and germ-cell neoplasms. Metastatic adenocarcinoma in men can be treated as metastatic prostate cancer and in women as metastatic ovarian or breast cancer because these are the most treatable malignancies. Metastatic prostate cancer may respond to hormonal therapy, which has significantly less morbidity than chemotherapy. Carcinoma of the breast shows a similar response rate to therapy; modalities include hormonal treatment for patients with estrogen receptor– or progesterone receptor–positive tumors and chemotherapy for others (see Chapter 122).

Empiric *radiation therapy* includes *radiation with or without node dissection* in patients who have high cervical adenopathy and epidermoid or squamous cell histology. Treatment is conducted on the ipsilateral side, with cure rates of 20% to 35% reported. Radiation may also provide reasonable *palliation* for patients with localized symptomatic disease, especially disease that involves bone, mediastinum, or lymph nodes. Symptomatic *bony metastases* can be treated palliatively with local radiation therapy and, if necessary, stabilized orthopedically. In the absence of symptoms, a bony metastasis may be monitored unless a definitively responsive tumor, such as prostate or breast cancer, can be identified.

As always, patients with suspected oncologic emergencies (e.g., spinal cord compression, hypercalcemia, superior vena cava syndrome) should be treated expeditiously while the workup is ongoing (see Chapter 92).

PATIENT EDUCATION AND INDICATIONS FOR REFERRAL

The finding of metastatic cancer is always very upsetting news, and it is even more perplexing when a source is hard to identify. However, an intelligently designed, selective search for the most treatable disease can provide considerable reassurance and hope. Such a diagnostic strategy should be shared with the patient and family, both to provide hope and a sense of control over a difficult situation and to reduce irrational pressure to "find the cause" at all costs.

A search that proves unrevealing poses the issue of empiric therapy. Here, a thoughtful and frank consultation with the oncologist is indicated to review the options. The lack of adequate data on cost and benefit often make counseling difficult, but an experienced and wise oncologist can be of great help to the patient and family.

Annotated Bibliography

1. Abbruzzese JL, Abbruzzese MC, Lenzi R, et al. Analysis of a diagnostic strategy for patients with suspected tumors of unknown origin. J Clin Oncol 1995;13:2094. (*A predefined limited diagnostic study was evaluated in an attempt to define a cost-effective approach to workup.*)
2. Copeland EM, McBride CM. Axillary metastases from unknown primary sites. Ann Surg 1972;178:25. (*The breast is the most common primary source in women with an undifferentiated axillary lesion.*)
3. Gentile PS, Carloss HW, Huang T-Y, et al. Disseminated prostatic carcinoma simulating primary lung cancer. Cancer 1988;62:711. (*The presentation of this very treatable malignancy may be quite atypical.*)
4. Greco FA, Vaughn WK, Hainsworth JD. Advanced poorly differentiated carcinoma of unknown primary site: recognition of a treatable syndrome. Ann Intern Med 1986;104:547. (*Patients with poorly differentiated histology and tumor in the mediastinum, retroperitoneum, and lymph nodes responded well to cisplatin-based chemotherapy.*)
5. Hainsworth JD, Johnson DH, Greco FA. Poorly differentiated neuroendocrine carcinoma of unknown primary site. Ann Intern Med 1988;1090:364. (*Identifies a very treatable subgroup; electron microscopy was found to be useful.*)
6. Le Chevalier TL, Cvitkovic E, Caille P, et al. Early metastatic cancer of unknown primary origin at presentation. Arch Intern Med 1988;148:2035. (*In an autopsy study, pancreas, lung, kidney, and colon were the most common primary sites; the authors recommend a workup strategy.*)
7. Levine MN, Drummond MF, LaBelle RJ. Cost-effectiveness in the diagnosis and treatment of carcinoma of unknown primary origin. Can Med Assoc J 1985;133:977. (*Argues that much diagnostic work is wasteful and treatment ineffective.*)
8. Pentheroudakis G, Golfinopoulos V, Pavlidis N. Switching benchmarks in cancer of unknown primary: from autopsy to microarray. Eur J Cancer 2007;43:2026. (*A discussion of a change in the approach to diagnosis.*)
9. Pentheroudakis G, Briasoulis E, Pavlidis N. Cancer of unknown primary site: missing primary or missing biology? Oncologist. 2007;12:418. (*A thoughtful review.*)
10. Schapira DV, Jarrett AR. The need to consider survival, outcome, and expense when evaluating and treating patients with unknown primary carcinoma. Arch Intern Med 1995;155:2050. (*A retrospective look, revealing high costs, very low yield, and poor survival when these issues were not taken into account in planning the workup and treatment.*)
11. Bataini JP, Rodriquez J, Jaulerry C, et al. Treatment of metastatic neck nodes secondary to an occult epidermoid carcinoma of the head and neck. Laryngoscope 1987;97:1080. (*Finds very high rates of response and some cures.*)
12. Freudenberg LS, Rosenbaum-Krumme SJ, Bockisch A, et al. Cancer of unknown primary. Recent Results Cancer Res. 2008;170:193. (*A good overview of the efficacy of workup and treatment.*)
13. Hainsworth JD, Greco FA. Treatment of patients with cancer of an unknown primary site. N Engl J Med 1993;329:257. (*A review of treatment options.*)
14. Sporn JR, Greenberg BR. Empiric chemotherapy in patients with carcinoma of unknown primary site. Am J Med 1990;88:49. (*A thoughtful review, including the identification of patients with responsive disease; 43 references.*)

CHAPTER 86 ■ APPROACH TO STAGING AND MONITORING

JEFFREY W. CLARK

Staging and monitoring are essential components of cancer management. Staging is performed to assess the extent of disease, and it is used to help determine prognosis and choice of therapy. Monitoring serves to detect the reappearance or progression of cancer and contributes significantly to updating prognosis and revising treatment plans. Staging and monitoring strategies are determined by tumor type, natural history, response to therapy, and characteristic pattern of spread. The frequency and duration of monitoring depend on the rate of disease recurrence.

The primary physician is in an ideal position to conduct much of the noninvasive staging and monitoring needed in the care of the cancer patient. To do so effectively requires an understanding of the limitations of the many available laboratory tests and radiologic procedures so that important decisions about test and procedure selection can be made effectively and unnecessary expense and discomfort can be avoided.

STAGING (1–3)

Terminology and Principles

Cancer stage is defined by the anatomic distribution of disease. The task of staging is to identify the amount and distribution of tumor. Several staging systems are used to express the extent of disease. Most incorporate designations for *local disease* (confined to a visceral site), *regional extension* (with or without involvement of contiguous lymph nodes), and *distant metastasis*. By far the most commonly used one for solid tumors is the TNM system (see later discussion). Hematologic malignancies incorporate other factors (e.g., bone marrow involvement) that necessitate different staging systems.

The TNM System

To standardize staging, the TNM system is being used with increasing frequency. The T refers to tumor, the N to nodes, and the M to metastases. Numbers are added to designate subcategories, reflecting the size of the tumor (T1 to T5), the degree of nodal involvement (N0 to N3), and the absence or presence of distant metastases (M0 or M1).

Although varying slightly among tumors, the various subcategory designations have specific meaning. For the T categories, *Tis* indicates carcinoma *in situ*; *T*1, the smallest measurable tumor mass or tumor confined to mucosa or submucosa; *T*2, larger tumor mass or tumor extending directly to adjacent structures; *T*3, very large tumor or still further direct extension; and *T*4, tumor of any size with local tissue invasion and direct extension into adjacent structures. With regard to N categories, *N*0 designates no nodal metastasis; *N*1, ipsilateral or regional involvement or movable regional nodes; *N*2, more extensive regional disease or fixed, matted nodes; *N*3, contralateral or distant nodal metastasis.

The TNM staging classification is increasingly preferred because of its consistency, comparability, and precision. Other staging systems commonly used for particular cancers have direct correlates to the TNM system and can be expressed in its terms (Table 86.1).

Staging Principles

A well-designed staging evaluation reflects the characteristic pattern of a malignancy and the speed of local and metastatic spread. Staging is performed both clinically (by means of history, physical examination, imaging procedures, and serum markers) and pathologically (by direct sampling of tissue). The two are complementary.

History and Physical Examination

Although much emphasis is placed on laboratory and radiologic procedures in clinical staging, the history and physical examination continue to play central roles in the determination of tumor mass, local spread, and metastasis. In almost every cancer workup, historical and physical data are required for intelligent staging and determination of the need for additional study. The failure to conduct a careful history and physical examination risks subjecting the patient to unnecessary or misguided studies.

Imaging Procedures

If, after a detailed history has been taken and a physical examination performed, it is deemed necessary to obtain further information noninvasively regarding the anatomic extent of disease, then one usually considers imaging studies. Among the most frequently ordered are computed tomography (CT), magnetic resonance imaging (MRI), ultrasonography, and radionuclide scanning (particularly PET scans). Even the plain film of the chest or bone can sometimes provide diagnostic information. Limitations include lack of specificity and inability to detect very early lesions.

Computed Tomography and Magnetic Resonance Imaging

Computed tomography and magnetic resonance imaging represent important advances over older contrast and radionuclide studies. They provide not only improved detection of tumor, but also better quantification of tumor burden. CT is the less expensive and more readily available of the two technologies, but MRI provides enhanced resolution in some areas,

TABLE 86.1

TNM STAGING AND CORRELATION WITH CONVENTIONAL STAGING SYSTEMS FOR CANCERS OF THE LUNG, BREAST, AND COLON

Tumor		Conventional Stage/ TNM Designation	Comments
Lung	0	Tis, N0, M0	Carcinoma *in situ*
	1	T1–2, N0, M0	Local tumor ± visceral pleura involved
	2	T1–2, N1, M0	Ipsilateral hilar, peribronchial nodes
	3a	T3, N0–1, M0	Extension to chest wall, diaphragm
	3b	T1–3, N2, M0	Ipsilateral mediastinal nodes involved
	4	Any T, any N, M1	
Breast	0	Tis, N0, M0	Paget's disease of the nipple, no palpable tumor, carcinoma *in situ*
	1	T1, N0–1a, M0	Tumor <2 cm, nodes feel normal
	2	T0 or T1, N1b, M0	Nodes feel diseased
	3	T2, N1a or b, M0	Tumor 2–5 cm in diameter
	3	T3, N1–2, M0	Tumor >5 cm in diameter
	4	T4, any N, any M	Direct involvement of chest wall and skin
		Any T, N3, any M	Supraclavicular nodes
		Any T, any N, M1	
Colon	0	Tis, N0, M0	
	A	T1, N0, M0	Confined to mucosa, submucosa
	B1	T2, N0, M0	Transmural disease, no extension
	B2	T3–5, N0, M0	Transmural disease plus extension
	C1	T1–2, N1, M0	Regional nodes, no direct extension
	C2	T3–4, N1, M0	Regional nodes, plus extension
	D	Any T, any N, M1	

Adapted from American Joint Committee on Cancer. Manual for staging of cancer, 2nd ed. Philadelphia: JB Lippincott, 1983, with permission.

particularly the central nervous system. *Chest CT* has been found to be superior to conventional full-lung tomography for the detection of pleural, mediastinal, and parenchymal lesions. The test is particularly useful for staging patients with lung cancer and those with malignancies with high rates of metastasis to the lung and mediastinum (e.g., sarcomas, melanomas, and testicular cancers). *CT of the abdomen* enhances evaluation of the retroperitoneum by identifying enlarged lymph nodes that are difficult to detect noninvasively. A positive scan result, confirmed by biopsy if appropriate, can obviate the need for surgical exploration. CT has also improved the detection, sampling, and quantification of tumor in the pancreas, liver, adrenal gland, and kidney. Results of pelvic CT for the detection and staging of early ovarian and prostate cancers have been variable; the test often lacks sensitivity in the detection of early disease or early spread to pelvic nodes. MRI (see later discussion) or *CT of the head* has virtually eliminated invasive and radionuclide staging studies of the central nervous system. Conducting the study with contrast agents (as appropriate) can further improve sensitivity of both CT and MRI.

Particularly in the central nervous system, *MRI* has contributed to the staging and monitoring of cancer. Compared with CT, it is more sensitive and offers a better assessment of the posterior fossa and spinal cord. Its increased cost is justified when enhanced sensitivity is required. MRI can sometimes be useful in helping to evaluate lesions within an organ (e.g., liver) seen on CT scan that need additional characterization. In addition, MRI continues to be investigated as a means of staging of pelvic malignancies because this can be an area of decreased sensitivity for CT imaging. Ultrasound also contin-

ues to be evaluated as a better means of imaging the pelvis (see under ultrasound).

PET Scanning and Other Radionuclide Imaging

PET scanning, especially in combination with CT (PET/CT), represents a major advance in staging and restaging by providing simultaneous metabolic as well as anatomic information, helping to identify metastatic disease and distinguish active tumor from areas of necrosis and scarring (findings important to decision making). Usefulness in initial staging and restaging after treatment have been considerable in Hodgkin's disease and non-Hodgkin's lymphoma (see Chapter 84), as well as in solid tumors, including non–small-cell lung, esophageal, colorectal, breast, cervical, and head and neck cancers. Radiation dose is modest, but the addition of whole-body CT to the procedure adds to it substantially.

Radionuclide bone scanning remains the most sensitive means of detecting metastasis to *bone*. It is far superior to plain films, except in cases of myeloma. However, bone scan results can be nonspecific, so that confirmation by other means is sometimes necessary. In cancers with a high propensity for spread to bone (prostate, breast, small-cell cancers), the bone scan serves an integral role in the initial evaluation. In other instances, it is used late in the course of disease to evaluate bone pain.

Ultrasound

Ultrasonography has been found to be extremely useful for assessment of the prostate, ovaries, testes, kidneys, and thyroid, accurately distinguishing solid from cystic masses, an important advantage in the evaluation of pelvic, testicular, renal, and thyroid masses. It is also used extensively to help guide needle biopsy. Resolution for transabdominal studies wanes for lesions less than 1 cm in diameter. The results of about 20% of such studies are inadequate because of overlying bowel gas. Transrectal ultrasonographic techniques have improved the detection and staging of early rectal and prostate cancers, providing results comparable to those of MRI for the staging of these cancers. Another important use of ultrasound is for use in conjunction with endoscopic evaluation, particularly for pancreatic and biliary cancers.

Standard Radiographs

The advent of CT, MRI, PET, and ultrasound technologies have relegated standard radiographs and associated imaging studies to lesser roles in cancer staging and monitoring due to their reduced sensitivity.

Serum Chemistries and Markers

Most serum chemistries and tumor markers are more useful for monitoring than for staging, being too insensitive and nonspecific. Exceptions include a *prostate-specific antigen* level greater than 10, which is associated with an increased risk of bone metastasis, but even this finding is nonspecific enough to require confirmation by other means (see Chapter 126). An isolated elevation in serum *alkaline phosphatase* level suggests liver involvement, but the finding is too nonspecific to be useful without confirmatory studies.

Surgical Staging and Other Invasive Procedures

Surgical staging is indicated when the results will alter therapeutic decision making. Clinical staging may underestimate the extent of disease by virtue of its limited ability to detect microscopic spread. However, invasive study should be conducted only when the choice of therapy will be affected; otherwise, the morbidity and risks incurred may not be justifiable.

Lymph Node Dissection

Lymph node dissection (or lymphadenectomy) at the time of surgery for the primary lesion serves as a prognostic and therapeutic determinant for many cancers, including prostate, breast, melanoma, and colorectal cancer. *Sentinel node biopsy* with the use of radionuclide markers for nodal identification is being applied in malignant melanoma and breast cancer as an alternative to standard node dissections. This approach involves performing intraoperative lymph node mapping to allow selective lymphadenectomy. More extensive lymphadenectomy is then reserved for patients with a positive sentinel lymph node.

Mediastinoscopy

This procedure helps to determine operability for patients with lung cancer; the more invasive *Chamberlain procedure* is sometimes necessary.

Bone Marrow Biopsy

Marrow biopsy provides an efficient means of pathologic staging in cancers that frequently metastasize to bone marrow (e.g., lymphoma or small-cell carcinoma of the lung).

MONITORING (3–11)

Principles

Monitoring for disease recurrence is appropriate for asymptomatic patients who have undergone curative cancer therapy. It provides the opportunity for diagnosing recurrence or new metastatic disease at a time when it may be potentially curable. However, even in this setting, defining the appropriate tests to use for optimizing the detection of potentially curable disease while minimizing potential cost and morbidity of testing procedures remains a difficult task.

Monitoring is primarily used in the care of patients with incurable disease, when it is used to evaluate tumor response to palliative treatment to know how long to continue current therapy or whether to consider alternative approaches. Monitoring activities that can affect decision making and improve outcomes are the only ones that should be undertaken. All others just add expense and may even cause harm in the case of a false-positive result. The cost-effectiveness of many routine programs of monitoring has been called into question by some, and this is an area of ongoing evaluation. In an attempt to get some standardization in the approach to monitoring patients, national organizations, such as the National Comprehensive Cancer Network, have developed guidelines for monitoring patients in specific settings. As technology evolves and provides greater sensitivity and specificity in detecting malignant lesions, it is possible that specific additional roles for certain types of monitoring will be defined. However, each of these has to be carefully evaluated for the value added before it can become a routine component of monitoring.

Monitoring Techniques

Many of the techniques useful for staging are pertinent to monitoring. Checking for residual disease or a new primary is the objective when curative therapy is employed; monitoring for reduction in tumor burden is the goal when palliation is undertaken. The frequency and duration of monitoring depend on the rate of disease recurrence. Tumor type, response to therapy, stage of disease, and pattern of metastasis also influence the selection of monitoring activities. Test sensitivity and specificity are important considerations. As noted, the emphasis should be on monitoring activities that will affect decision making and outcomes. Aggressive routine follow-up is pointless when the findings will not influence management or improve results.

Tumor Markers

Tumor markers have been sought with the hope of obtaining a means of tumor detection more sensitive than those provided by other clinical methods. Although initially developed to aid in early diagnosis, most markers have actually been found to be better suited for monitoring disease recurrence or progression after curative or palliative therapy. Baseline and posttreatment levels are obtained and follow-up readings repeated at regular intervals.

Carcinoembryonic Antigen.   Carcinoembryonic antigen is present in both normal and malignant tissue; serum levels in excess of the upper normal limit (this may vary by laboratory) are suggestive of tumor, but the test is too insensitive and nonspecific for screening. Its most useful application is in early detection of recurrence, especially for cancers of the colon and rectum, breast, and lung. Serial determinations of carcinoembryonic antigen are among the noninvasive means for identifying recurrent colorectal cancer after surgery.

α-Fetoprotein. α-Fetoprotein has been found in high serum concentrations in association with hepatomas, testicular carcinomas, and extragonadal germ cell tumors. Although lacking sufficient specificity for diagnostic purposes, repeated determinations of the α-fetoprotein level can be used to monitor for disease recurrence and assess adequacy of treatment.

β-Human Chorionic Gonadotropin Subunit. β-Human chorionic gonadotropin subunit is another useful tumor marker for germ cell tumors of the testes and ovaries. Monitoring of the β subunit provides information similar to that obtained from the α-fetoprotein level, although it is important to obtain both because one or the other may be more sensitive for a given patient.

Prostate-Specific Antigen. Prostate-specific antigen is unique to prostate tissue and is found in both malignant and normal cells. A concentration in excess of 10 ng/mL is strongly suggestive of cancer and is found in fewer than 2% of patients with benign prostatic hypertrophy. Levels increase with the tumor burden and rise briefly after needle biopsy or with prostatitis but not after a prostate examination. False-negatives occur with the use of finasteride.

Levels of Cancer Antigen (CA) 125. Levels of CA 125, produced by 80% of epithelial ovarian cancers, correlate with the clinical course and are useful for monitoring. The specificity is reasonably high, although false positives do occur in the setting of a number of other malignancies.

CA 15-3 and CA 19-9. These tumor markers are undergoing assessment for monitoring of breast and pancreatic/biliary cancers, respectively. Serum CA 15-3 levels have been found to correlate with response to treatment in nearly 80% of patients, but upward of 15% of persons with benign breast disease also manifest elevations, compromising the specificity of the test. Ongoing evaluation of markers that may provide greater sensitivity and specificity is an active area of research.

Monitoring Local or Regional Disease

Patients with local or regional disease who have undergone curative therapy should be monitored at regular intervals. The periodic evaluation should be directed at (a) *finding new primary tumors* in the involved organ and (b) detecting the presence of isolated (i.e., one to three) *asymptomatic metastases* in those sites where resection for cure is still possible (e.g., lung or liver in colorectal cancer).

In general, for most solid tumors, in the absence of symptoms or signs of recurrence, monitoring is conducted at 3-month intervals for the first 2 years after initial curative therapy. Thereafter, follow-up may be accomplished at 6-month intervals for a minimum of 5 years. In general, most tumors recur at a maximum rate during the first 2 years after the initial operation—if in fact they are destined to recur. Three malignancies are notorious for late recurrence: breast carcinoma, melanoma, and renal cell carcinoma. In some patients with these tumors, the lag period before the development of detectable metastases may extend beyond 10 years after initial diagnosis.

Monitoring Metastatic Disease

Follow-up examinations for patients with metastatic disease who receive systemic therapy should be performed at intervals determined by the *time expected for an objective clinical response*. For hormonal therapy of breast cancer, clinical evidence of response may take as long as 3 months to appear. The effects of cytotoxic chemotherapy may be seen rapidly—for example, within two courses of treatment or 4 to 6 weeks. This is particularly true for more responsive tumors such as breast, testicular, ovarian, and small-cell lung carcinomas.

Patients with metastatic disease receiving palliative systemic therapy should be examined for evidence of new disease. Unnecessary chemotherapy-induced morbidity can be avoided if ineffective palliative systemic therapy is discontinued at the first signs of new disease. Response to therapy may be objectively demonstrated after a predictable interval, but new growth or spread may be noted on earlier examination.

An important corollary to the monitoring of patients with metastatic disease on systemic therapeutic regimens is to define the *most objective site of disease* to be followed and to avoid additional staging procedures if they do not alter the therapeutic plan. For example, a patient with hepatic metastases from a primary breast cancer need not undergo a bone scan unless bone pain or a fracture occurs. The tumor is already established as being incurable, and therapy is determined by the presence of liver metastases. Alternatively, the patient with bony metastases that are difficult to monitor may undergo selective staging to identify a more measurable marker of metastatic disease, such as plasma CA 15-3. The National Comprehensive Cancer Network has developed guidelines for monitoring for different malignancies, and these are useful tools for specific situations.

Annotated Bibliography

1. American Joint Committee on Cancer. Manual for staging of cancer, 2nd ed. Philadelphia: JB Lippincott, 1983. (*Basic outline of the TNM staging scheme.*)
2. Harris MN, Shapiro RL, Roses DF. Malignant melanoma: primary surgical management (excision and node dissection) based on pathology and staging. Cancer 1995;75:715. (*A review of the role of lymph node dissection and of intraoperative lymph node mapping in allowing selective lymphadenectomy.*)
3. Juweid ME, Cheson BD. Positron-emission tomography and assessment of cancer therapy. N Engl J Med 2006;354:496. (*Thorough review for the generalist reader of this important imaging technology for staging and monitoring.*)
4. American Society of Clinical Oncology. Clinical practice guidelines for the use of tumor markers in breast and colorectal cancer. J Clin Oncol 1996;14:2843. (*Evidence-based expert panel recommendations.*)
5. American Society of Clinical Oncology. Recommended breast cancer surveillance guidelines. J Clin Oncol 1997;15:2149. (*An example of evidence-based consensus guidelines for follow-up.*)
6. Bast RC Jr, Klug TL, St John E, et al. Radioimmunoassay using a monoclonal antibody to monitor the course of epithelial ovarian cancer. N Engl J Med 1983;309:883. (*The development of the CA-125 test.*)
7. Beard DB, Haskell CM. Carcinoembryonic antigen in breast cancer. Am J Med 1986;80:241. (*A review of the role of carcinoembryonic antigen in breast cancer; it is especially useful in patients with advanced disease.*)

8. Edelman MJ, Meyers FJ, Siegel D. The utility of follow-up testing after curative cancer therapy. A critical review and economic analysis. J Gen Intern Med 1997;12:318. (*Reviews most follow-up strategies for common treatable malignancies and finds aggressive routine follow-up to be of questionable value in most cancers.*)

9. Fletcher RH. Carcinoembryonic antigen. Ann Intern Med 1986;104:66. (*A critical review pointing out the limitations of its usefulness.*)

10. Stamy TA, Yang N, Hay AR, et al. Prostate-specific antigen as a serum marker for adenocarcinoma of the prostate. N Engl J Med 1987;317:909. (*The original report; prostate-specific antigen was found to be more sensitive than acid phosphatase; both were elevated in benign prostatic hypertrophy.*)

11. Stieber P, Molina R, Chan DW, et al. Clinical evaluation of the Elecsys CA 15-3 test in breast cancer patients. Clin Lab 2003;49:15. (*Predictive of response to treatment, but elevations also found in benign disease.*)

CHAPTER 87 ■ COMPREHENSIVE CARE OF THE CANCER PATIENT

JEFFREY W. CLARK

The treatment of cancer is multifaceted, involving the interdigitation of physician support and treatment with surgery, radiation, cytotoxic agents, biologic response modifiers, and, more recently, targeted agents. Comprehensive care requires a team approach in which the primary physician plays a central role in coordinating the effort. To succeed in this role, the primary physician needs to understand the major issues of cancer management and be capable of interacting effectively with cancer specialists. The patient and family are likely to request the opinion of the primary physician, so that an ability to explain and assess management recommendations is necessary. Most cancer patients can remain at home with their families and receive optimal therapy on an outpatient basis when a primary physician is able to work closely with a cancer center or a local specialist in cancer management.

For most solid tumors, curative treatment that focuses on the primary tumor site has traditionally been the province of surgery, with radiation and chemotherapy relegated to palliative roles. More recently, radiation and chemotherapy have been employed as adjuvants in the treatment of local disease, enhancing the capability of surgery to cure. Certain malignancies (e.g., leukemia, lymphomas, germ cell tumors) may be curable with chemotherapy alone. Advances in radiation therapy have effected cures of some cancers in early stages. Biologic response modifiers and targeted agents hold promise for achieving further improvements in outcome.

Effective care of the cancer patient begins with communicating the diagnosis and strengthening the relationship between patient and physician. It also requires the establishment of a close working partnership with the cancer specialist, whose job will be to design and implement the treatment program. The primary physician can and should maintain a central role in the care of the cancer patient, but to do so requires a thorough understanding of the natural history of the tumor, its staging and monitoring (see Chapter 86), and its responsiveness to treatment. In addition, the patient will call on the primary physician for relief from symptoms related to the tumor or its treatment. This necessitates a thorough knowledge of measures to control pain (see Chapter 90), emesis (see Chapter 91), and related side effects of cancer therapy (see Chapters 88 and 89).

SUPPORTING THE PATIENT AND FAMILY THROUGH DIAGNOSIS AND TREATMENT (1–8)

For many patients, the diagnosis of cancer evokes images of pain, suffering, mutilation, and certain death. These basic fears are so intertwined with the word "cancer" that confirmation of the diagnosis places extreme emotional stress on both patient and family. It is in managing this anguish that the primary physician plays a most important role as the person to whom the patient and family can turn. The primary physician must be not only the source of scientific and medical expertise, but also the provider of emotional support and understanding.

Giving Bad News

It is always difficult to give bad news. Physicians sometimes avoid telling the patient the diagnosis in accurate and specific terms at the outset, resorting to such euphemisms as "lump," "mass," and "lesion." Further inhibiting communication may be the ill-advised, although well-intentioned, insistence of family members that the diagnosis be kept from the patient out of fear of precipitating a severe depression. Such concerns are usually ill conceived. It is rare that ignorance of the diagnosis or prognosis is helpful for the patient or family. Quite the contrary, patients and their families deal better with cancer when they are well informed.

The *goal* in communicating the diagnosis and prognosis is to be accurate without destroying all hope. First and foremost, the words "cancer" and "malignant tumor" should be used at the outset of the interview and not avoided, although constant repetition of the terms is usually unnecessary. The term "fatal" ought to be omitted in discussions of the prognosis because it implies little hope of control. When informed of an incurable malignancy, the patient and family want to know, "How much time is left?" A rough estimate may be necessary when patients must arrange their affairs, but, if possible, the physician should avoid indicating a specific period of time because it is apt to be inaccurate. Preferably, the physician should direct the patient toward realistic therapeutic approaches and reinforce the role of living as fully as possible with the highest quality of life that can be maintained instead of dying.

The *candor* expressed by telling the diagnosis "as it is" facilitates the development of trust among patient, family, and medical staff and breaks down the barrier that often isolates cancer patients from their families. Being well informed also helps to alleviate the sense of hopelessness and loss of control that can be one of the most frightening aspects of living with a malignant disease. Families are especially grateful for full and frequent reports of the patient's status and prognosis.

The *consequences* of not fully informing the patient and family can be considerable. The patient who is unaware of the diagnosis and prognosis may fail to put affairs in order and continue to have unrealistic plans or uncomfortable relationships with other members of the family, which might otherwise be resolved if all were to understand the prognosis. Similarly, the uninformed family is unable to grieve gradually over time, and death may appear to be sudden. The resulting unresolved grief may profoundly affect the surviving family members (see Chapter 227). Both patient and family may need to grieve and resolve their own fears and anxieties. By virtue of having a long-standing relationship with the patient and family, the primary physician is in an ideal position to provide effective support and guidance.

The Patient's Response

Cancer patients have been observed to pass through a series of emotional states. These include periods of denial, hostility, anger, hope, depression, and finally acceptance. The physician can help to alleviate the more dysfunctional reactions and facilitate the patient's coping. The reactions of patients at the time of presentation of the diagnosis depend on preconceived ideas about cancer and what the specter of cancer suggests to them. Common misconceptions include the certainty of death, intractable pain, and erosive, disfiguring disease. To avoid needless worry, it is essential at the outset to address these common concerns directly, even if the patient does not express them. Nonetheless, a good number of patients will respond with denial, hostility, and rejection of loved ones, regression, or even withdrawal. It is important to recognize such reactions as psychological defense mechanisms and respond to them in an understanding and patient manner.

Denial

Denial of the diagnosis is generally a transient reaction. When denial is mild, physicians may need only to reinforce their remarks with a repeated presentation of the facts or a provision of objective and tangible evidence. However, in some patients, denial is extreme and functions as a crude psychological defense mechanism, necessary for sustaining the psyche. A constant onslaught of evidence and reinforcement of the diagnosis or prognosis may be counterproductive and is not justified.

Hostility

Hostility is occasionally an early reaction to the diagnosis. Anger may be directed against the medical team for delay in diagnosis or for inadequate attention and also toward family members, who may be viewed as not particularly upset and happy to finally "get their way." This phase is generally transient, receding as the patient comes to recognize the reality of the situation and the need for family and physician. Hostility is difficult for both patient and doctor and may be intense enough to lead the physician and family to reject the patient emotionally. If recognized, this reaction should be allowed to run a natural course without withdrawal of support.

Regression

Regression is an accentuated response commonly occurring in the patient with a dependent personality who may have appeared overly independent before illness. If it is more than transient, the regression may turn infantile and must be mitigated by providing a parental figure who will be, on one hand, supportive and, on the other hand, stern and demanding. Infantile regression places an inordinate burden on the family, who are called on to provide extraordinary amounts of support.

Withdrawal

Withdrawal is an extreme form of regression, often tinged with elements of hostility. Direct confrontation is essential for the patient who withdraws; constant encouragement and the setting up of goals to be achieved (e.g., ambulation, planning trips, visiting friends) are critical.

Family Reactions to the Diagnosis

Reactions of the family are critical to the patient's well-being and to aiding the health care team in providing maximum support. Thus, the physician must be concerned with the family's responses to the patient and the diagnosis. The physician is frequently obliged to deal with many members of the family, often with differing levels of need for information and support. Not uncommonly, complete families—wives, husbands, and children—may be alienated by the patient, who disallows them the opportunity to resolve their confusion. Such alienation, which may approach pathologic proportions, can be understood with the help of the physician. A frequent family reaction is to provide smothering protection in compensation for guilt over previous misunderstandings with the patient and the need to resolve such differences. Again, the physician can help to alleviate such pathologic reactions.

Psychological Reactions to Cancer Treatment

The patient who enters treatment for cancer is subjected to a reinforcement of the diagnosis and a rekindling of the fears regarding threats to self-esteem and self-image. The latter may be particularly demoralizing if the cancer treatment involves bodily disfigurement or a physical limitation that is either cosmetically mutilating or functionally disabling. Thus, the patient who requires a mastectomy, jaw resection, amputation, or colostomy faces a significant and frightening change in self-image. The distortions that are incorporated into the patient's unconscious, perhaps as a result of real or imagined experiences with friends, are potentially devastating. Often, these distortions are unrealistic and unsubstantiated, but, more important, they may not be expressed. The physician must inquire into the patient's concerns and offer a realistic appraisal to minimize unnecessary anguish (see Chapter 1.1).

Patient education is a most important component of the approach to dealing with the stress of therapy. It additionally serves to cushion the stress by allowing the patient to intellectualize about the disease and its treatment. In this "demythologizing process," patient fears are identified and dealt with openly. Often, the result is a more acceptable view of one's illness and treatment. Educational materials available from the American Cancer Society and the National Cancer Institute can complement the educational effort by addressing common questions that patients have about cancer therapy. Detailed explanation of the therapy in terms of its effect on the tumor and its potential side effects allows the patient to approach treatment realistically. The use of support groups and meditation techniques can facilitate the patient's coping with the stresses of cancer therapy.

Such supportive efforts are designed to strengthen the patient psychologically and improve quality of life. Whether they affect survival or immune function is uncertain, but they certainly can help morale and coping with illness.

APPROACHES TO TREATMENT (9-15)

The approach to treatment is determined by tumor type and stage (see Chapter 86). In the earliest stages of disease, the malignancy is localized and cure is possible through locally or regionally applied therapy. Regional spread reflects more advanced disease, and the chances of cure are lessened but not eliminated. More systemic forms of therapy are added to local measures. With important exceptions (e.g., testicular cancer), distant metastasis indicates that cure is unlikely, and the goal is palliation through the use of systemic therapies.

Local Tumor Control: Surgery and Radiation

Surgery

Surgery has traditionally played the dominant role in the management of localized cancer. The diagnosis is established and confirmed by surgical biopsy, and cure may be effected by operation. Nonetheless, the emphasis has shifted recently toward minimizing surgical procedures, particularly when the prognosis is determined by factors such as distant metastases and when salvage by secondary local modalities can be accomplished. For example, lymph node dissection for malignant melanoma, limb amputation for osteogenic sarcoma, ostomy and abdominoperineal resection for rectal cancer, and radical mastectomy for breast cancer have been scaled down in many cases to lesser procedures so that morbidity is reduced without a compromise in survival. The surgical approach to these lesions may be modified by the addition of local therapy (e.g., radiation) or systemic therapy (e.g., cytotoxic agents).

Radiation Therapy

Radiation therapy has become more effective through the development of high-energy linear accelerators and technical improvements in delivery, which have lowered rates of morbidity and increased rates of survival and local control. For example, radiation has is an important component of treatment for localized breast cancer after lumpectomy (see Chapter 122). Radiation in conjunction with surgery and often chemotherapy may be curative in some tumors when administered preoperatively or postoperatively. In other malignancies, the combined application of radiation and either surgery or chemotherapy may promote palliation and chances for long-term survival, although it rarely achieves cure (see Chapter 89).

Regional Cancer: Surgery Plus Adjuvant or Combined Therapy

Adjuvant therapy involves the addition of chemotherapy and or radiation to surgical procedures. The rationale for adding radiation therapy is primarily to promote the local control of presumed residual microscopic tumor. In theory, chemotherapy functions as an adjuvant modality because it affects micrometastases at a time when they are rapidly proliferating and likely to be quite drug sensitive.

Adjuvant therapy has been proposed or is part of ongoing trials of treatments for a number of regional cancers and is a proven and established therapy for others. For example, in breast cancer, premenopausal women with positive lymph nodes and pathologic stage II disease have benefited from the addition of chemotherapy. It has reduced the incidence of recurrence and prolonged disease-free survival. In patients with rectal cancer extending beyond the bowel wall (so-called Dukes stage B2 or C lesions), the use of radiation therapy has reduced local recurrence rates and in combination with chemotherapy increased median survival. In certain situations, (e.g., rectal cancer) preoperative radiation therapy and chemotherapy may offer advantages over postoperative radiation therapy and chemotherapy.

With the vast majority of tumors, regional disease is incurable despite the use of adjuvant modalities, and some have a particularly poor prognosis. Long-term survival is seen in fewer than 5% of patients with pancreatic cancers that are regionally advanced and therefore unresectable. Because of the potential of selection bias in phase II trials, it is important to refer to results from randomized phase III studies for a determination of efficacy whenever these are available. For some tumors (e.g., testicular cancer, osteogenic sarcoma, Hodgkin's disease), the role of chemotherapy and/or radiation therapy is important in extending survival time and limiting the morbidity of regional disease.

The advent of a host of advances in treatment (e.g., more effective cytotoxic drugs, *dose-intensified or dose-dense* therapy, *marrow transplantation*, hematologic *growth factors*, *biologic response modifiers*, targeted agents, and local *radiation* for site sterilization (see Chapters 88 and 89) should improve approaches to local, regional, and even advanced cancers and become an increasing part of standard management. The optimal application of such forms of therapy will require reference to data from well-designed randomized trials.

Metastatic Cancer: Cytotoxic Drugs, Biologic Response Modifiers, Targeted Therapy

The management of advanced disease is largely palliative and involves systemic therapy usually provided by cytotoxic drugs. Targeted agents (e.g., monoclonal antibodies are small molecules targeted to specific mutated proteins in malignant cells) are likely to play an increasingly active role as research into their efficacy advances.

Chemotherapeutic Regimens

Chemotherapeutic regimens have become increasingly sophisticated and complex, but they are also more effective because of the development of new agents and multiple-drug regimens (see Chapter 88). Decisions concerning the use and timing of cytotoxic therapy in advanced disease are difficult because of the potential morbidity associated with such therapy and the frequent lack of established benefit in promoting cure or even in prolonging survival. The decision to use chemotherapy in advanced disease is often a philosophical and psychological one, based on the feelings of patient, family, and physician.

Any decision to employ chemotherapy should involve an analysis of host tolerance in addition to potential tumor responsiveness. Most important, the use of chemotherapy must be preceded by informed consent of the patient, who should be aware of the side effects as well as the potential for response. A common misconception is that the drugs invariably create morbidity and prolong life only at the cost of agonizing discomfort. In fact, when effective, chemotherapy can improve the quality of life as well as prolong it, and when it is ineffective, it does not necessarily induce more than transient morbidity. Some of the newer chemotherapy regimens for this phase of illness use weekly administrations of drugs that are well tolerated at modest doses (e.g., paclitaxel, gemcitabine).

In addition to these considerations, the indications for the use of chemotherapy in advanced, incurable disease include the following:

- A probability of clinical benefit for chemotherapy that exceeds the potential toxicity associated with the combination of agents used.
- Progressive tumor growth during a period of observation.
- Symptomatic metastatic disease (e.g., pleural effusion, ascites, significant pain).

Within these guidelines, cytotoxic therapy can be administered with a reasonable risk–benefit balance.

Participation in early phase I trials of *experimental drug therapy* should be reserved for the following:

- Patients who have failed with use of known effective drugs.
- Patients who wish to have a new form of treatment, fully comprehend the investigational nature of the treatment, and are willing to participate in the investigational approach.

Participation in later-phase trials (phase II or phase III) is appropriate for many individuals even as initial treatment approach for their disease. However, in these situations as well, it is essential that patients fully understand the investigational nature of the trial in which they are considering participation.

Targeted Agents

As more knowledge is gained about specific molecular changes in malignant cells, including mutations, agents that target these specific features of the malignant cells are becoming increasingly important components of the treatment for various cancers. At the present time, there are two broad groups of targeted agents. The first of these are monoclonal antibodies. A number of monoclonal antibodies have been approved to treat a number of cancers as single agents, as part of combined treatment regimens, or both. Four of the more commonly used monoclonal antibodies are rituximab (targeting the CD20 antigen expressed frequently on B cell malignancies), herceptin (targeting the Her2 receptor overexpressed on 20% to 25% of breast cancers), bevacizumab (targeting the vascular endothelial growth factor molecule that is important in tumor angiogenesis), and cetuximab (targeting the epidermal growth factor receptor on colorectal cancer cells) (see also Chapter 89). The second class of targeted agents now approved for cancer therapy are the *small molecules* targeting specific protein targets in certain malignancies. A number of these have been approved, including *imatinib* (chronic myeloid leukemia and gastrointestinal stromal tumors), *dastatanib* (chronic myeloid leukemia), *sunitinib* (gastrointestinal stromal tumors and renal

cell carcinoma), *sorafenib* (hepatocellular carcinoma and renal cell carcinoma), *toricel* (renal cell carcinoma), *erlotinib* (lung and pancreas), *bortezomib* (multiple myeloma), *lapatinib* (breast cancer), and *lenalidomide* (myelodysplastic syndromes).

One of the attractive features for targeted agents is their relative lack of overlapping toxicities with chemotherapeutic agents and therefore the ability to combine essentially full-dose chemotherapy regimens with full doses of the targeted agent. One exception to the absence of overlapping toxicities is the potential for cardiac toxicity seen with Herceptin, which can enhance cardiac toxicity seen with chemotherapeutic agents. So, although as a general principle overlapping toxicities do not appear to be as big an issue when combining these different types of agents, as always it is important to be cognizant of situations in which overlapping toxicities might occur and carefully to monitor for these.

MANAGEMENT OF THE PRETERMINAL PHASE (16–18; See Also Chapter 90)

"Terminal cancer" is an expression commonly employed by both patients and physicians but with distinctly different definitions. Strictly defined, "terminal cancer" means that death will ensue within a 4-week period. The physician should avoid using the term "terminal" in talking with the patient or family. Not infrequently, patients may absorb the label and yet live for months or even years. The term imposes on both family and patient a tremendous stress that often results in withdrawal.

The physician's role in the terminal phase is a crucial one. It is essential to remain sensitive to all the patient's needs and, specifically, to the patient's need to know that the physician is always available. If the patient is at home, frequent home visits may be enormously appreciated. It may be helpful to allow the patient to come to the office once or twice a week, even though no specific medications are to be administered.

It is not incumbent on the physician to reinforce the inevitability of death to patients who have entered a preterminal or terminal state and are sustaining hope for a reversal of the tumor. More important, however, the family must be apprised precisely during this period to allow them to pass through the grieving process successfully.

The best approach to the management of the preterminal patient is to initiate *hospice care*, a comprehensive program of physical and psychological comfort measures delivered by skilled health care professionals either at home or in an inpatient facility. Hospital routines, laboratory studies, and life-sustaining therapies are omitted in favor of psychological and symptomatic support. Priorities include relief of pain (see Chapter 90) and psychological support of the patient and the family.

Psychotropic Drugs

Antidepressant therapy (e.g., use of an selective serotonin reuptake inhibitor, such as sertraline, at a dose of 25 to 50 mg each morning) can help with the somatic symptoms of depression, such as marked fatigue and awakening in the early morning (see Chapter 227). Pain control may also be enhanced. Unless a contraindication is present, antidepressants should not be withheld on the basis of the common clinical misconception that "the patient is appropriately depressed, considering the diagnosis and prognosis." Checking for suicidal ideation is important because overdose can be fatal. Asking about suicide does not suggest the act to the patient; rather, it conveys an understanding of how profoundly the patient is suffering.

Benzodiazepines (e.g., 2 mg of diazepam daily at bedtime) given for short periods can facilitate coping with particularly stressful situations and the resultant difficulty in falling asleep. Patients with panic disorder may require more prolonged therapy with anxiolytics (see Chapter 226).

Nutrition and Pain Control

See Chapters 90 and 91.

Alternative or Complementary Approaches to Care

So-called "alternative" or "complementary" approaches to standard modern oncologic care are frequently sought by patients and their families, more as "natural" or "holistic" supplements to standard care than as substitutes. Subsumed under the rubric of "alternative medicine" are *meditation*, *relaxation* techniques, *mental imagery*, *massage*, *herbal remedies*, *megavitamins*, *chiropractic manipulation*, and *acupuncture*. Few data from randomized, controlled trials are available on which to base their use (although this is likely to change as U.S. government support for such trials emerges). Most claims of efficacy are based on anecdotal reports at best. Many patients view these measures as "natural" and therefore harmless and thus worth a try. Sociodemographic factors correlating with the use of alternative therapies include upper levels of income, younger age, and higher levels of education. Other triggers of use identified in cohort studies of cancer patients include depression, fear of recurrence of cancer, and psychosocial distress.

The primary care physician needs to be cognizant of the highly frequent use of alternative medicine among cancer patients and of the increased likelihood of underlying fear and psychosocial distress that may be driving the patient to seek such therapy. Eliciting and effectively addressing such fear and distress may be one of the most therapeutic responses one can make to the patient's use of or request for alternative medicine. Valuing informed medical opinions, patients hope their physicians will be knowledgeable about the safety and efficacy of such practices. The scientific literature should be followed closely and patients provided with the best of available information when it is desired. In this manner, patient safety and satisfaction can be maximized and unnecessary expense avoided.

APPROACH TO THE CARE OF CANCER SURVIVORS (19,20)

Patients who survive cancer are increasing in number and are more commonly encountered than ever before in primary care practice. They present challenges in management that reflect both the psychological and physiologic consequences of the disease and its therapy. An expanding appreciation of their needs is essential to helping them to return to full and productive lives.

Psychological Consequences

Although surviving cancer may be expected to be a cause for joy, studies show that considerable anxiety persists. Having had cancer appears to produce a heightened *sense of vulnera-*bility and fear of death and a decreased feeling of control and mastery over one's life. Fear of death wanes as the duration of survival increases, but *anxiety about recurrence* may persist and result in hypochondriasis or avoidance of follow-up health care. Contact with patients having active disease can be very stressful, rekindling feelings of fear and vulnerability. Conversely, some patients demonstrate marked anxiety over the loss of close contact with the health care team that characterized the active phase of their illness. Frank *separation anxiety* has been reported. Others begin to express feelings of anger over perceived shortcomings in diagnosis and care.

Physical disabilities resulting from cancer or its treatment can have a profound psychological impact, with *depression* being the most common and important. If not appreciated, it may present as fatigue or other physical complaints that generate concern in both patient and physician.

Preoccupation with bodily sensations is another common manifestation of depression (see Chapter 227) that might be encountered in the surviving cancer patient. When not appreciated, symptoms of depression can be mistaken for more serious disease.

Interpersonal and Social Consequences

The psychosocial effects of having had cancer are equally important to keep in mind in helping the patient to adjust to survivorship. Some will miss the privileges that the *sick role* provided and may have difficulty in returning to the responsibilities of normal life. Family members and work colleagues may find it awkward to relate to the survivor, not knowing whether to treat the him or her as still partially incapacitated or back to normal. A return to sexual activity may be a source of concern for the patient. Most patients with a close supportive marital relationship and no permanent loss of sexual capacity appear to do reasonably well, but preexisting marital problems or the absence of a close relationship can lead to considerable *sexual dysfunction*. Such dysfunction may result in depression. Sexual dysfunction may also be a symptom of an underlying depression unrelated to sexual issues. Of course, patients who have sustained gonadal injury or bodily mutilation are prime candidates for sexual dysfunction and its interpersonal consequences. Overall, psychological distress appears to be highest in patients lacking a close, supportive relationship. Single patients are most vulnerable.

Elements of *interpersonal isolation* have been reported, especially among those who are single and reluctant to share information about their cancerous past with a potential mate. Feelings of isolation may also be triggered by difficulty in discussing the cancer experience with friends, family, or coworkers. *Work difficulties* are often encountered. Survivors have fears, real or imagined, of losing their job. Prolonged absence and a perceived inability to perform may compromise their previous position and lead to long-term job insecurity. With job insecurity comes concern about maintaining adequate and affordable *health insurance*, especially in light of a past history of major illness and the tendency of insurance companies to "cherry pick" those whom it will insure. It is hoped that insurance reform with community rating will alleviate this major worry of surviving cancer patients.

Physiologic Consequences

See Chapters 88 and 89 and the chapters on specific cancers for a detailed discussion of physiologic consequences.

Supportive Therapy and Preparing the Patient

An understanding of the difficulties that cancer survivors may encounter helps the physician to prepare the patient for life after cancer therapy. Counseling the patient and family about the challenges and potential difficulties likely to be experienced can go a long way toward ensuring an effective return to daily life. The counseling is carried out in the same honest, open, and supportive manner that characterized discussions in earlier phases of the illness. The issues can be every bit as difficult for the patient and require that physician support continue unabated. Regularly scheduled office visits for a check of symptoms, physical findings, and progress in returning to normal life are greatly appreciated and extremely therapeutic. Studies suggest that it takes as long as 3 years after the time of successful treatment for survivors to regain the confidence and social functioning that was lost as a result of having had cancer. Many survivors also exhibit a wisdom and sense of value and proportion that comes from having faced death, an appreciation of life that benefits all whom they encounter.

Annotated Bibliography

1. Burstein HJ, Gelber S, Guadagnoli E, et al. Use of alternative medicine by women with early-stage breast cancer. N Engl J Med 1999;340:1733. (*A cohort study finding that the use of alternative medicine is a marker for psychosocial stress and poor quality of life.*)
2. Cassileth BE, Walsh WP, Lusk EJ. Psychosocial correlates of cancer survival. J Clin Oncol 1988;6:1753. (*A long-term study with practical implications.*)
3. Cassileth BE, Zupkis RV, Sutton-Smith K, et al. Information and participation preferences among cancer patients. Ann Intern Med 1980;92:832. (*Most patients prefer maximum amounts of information; those who are more hopeful want to participate in treatment decisions.*)
4. Lieberman M. The role of self-help groups for helping patients and families cope with cancer. CA Cancer J Clin 1988;38:162. (*Reviews the many plusses and some minuses.*)
5. Reiser SJ. Words as scalpels: transmitting evidence in the clinical dialogue. Ann Intern Med 1980;92:837. (*A very thoughtful article on communicating the diagnosis, with an interesting historical perspective.*)
6. Rodin G, Lloyd N, Katz M, et al.; Supportive Care Guidelines Group of Cancer Care Ontario Program in Evidence-Based Care. The treatment of depression in cancer patients: a systematic review. Support Care Cancer 2007;15:123. (*Important reading for all who care for cancer patients.*)
7. Silberfarb PS. Psychiatric treatment of the patient during cancer therapy. CA Cancer J Clin 1988;38:133. (*Very practical advice.*)
8. Weeks JC, Cook EF, O'Day SJ, et al. Relationship between cancer patients' predictions of prognosis and their treatment preferences. JAMA 1998;279:1709. (*Overestimation of prognosis was found to drive the desire for life-extending therapy.*)
9. American Society of Clinical Oncology. Recommendations for the use of hematopoietic colony-stimulating factors: evidence-based clinical practice guidelines. J Clin Oncol 1997;15:3288. (*Example of an evidence-based approach to effective implementation.*)
10. Murdoch D, Sager J. Will targeted therapy hold its promise? An evidence-based review. Curr Opin Oncol 2008;20:104. (*A superb summary of the evidence.*)
11. Garcia-Carbonero R, Hidalgo H, Pax-Ares L, et al. Patient selection in high-dose chemotherapy trials: relevance in high-risk breast cancer. J Clin Oncol 1997;15:178. (*Documents a great deal of selection bias, which can compromise results in nonrandomized trials.*)
12. Goldie JH, Goldman AJ, Gudauskas GA. Rationale for the use of alternating non–cross-resistant chemotherapy. Cancer Treat Rep 1982;66:439. (*The theoretical basis for modern multiple-drug regimens.*)
13. Hartmann O, Le Corroller AG, Blaise D, et al. Peripheral blood stem cell and bone marrow transplantation for solid tumors and lymphomas: hematologic recovery and costs. A randomized trial. Ann Intern Med 1997;126:600. (*An example of hematologic support of aggressive chemotherapy; the use of peripheral blood stem cells was associated with more rapid recovery at lower cost.*)
14. Rose PG, Bundy BN, Watkins EB, et al. Concurrent cisplatin-based radiotherapy and chemotherapy for locally advanced cervical cancer. N Engl J Med 1999;340:1144. (*An important example of combined-modality therapy prolonging survival in locally advanced disease.*)
15. Thomas LR. Does bone marrow transplantation confer a normal life span? N Engl J Med 1999;341:50. (*An editorial that considers benefits and risks.*)
16. Lynn J, Teno JM, Phillips RS, et al. Perceptions by family members of the dying experience of older and seriously ill patients. Ann Intern Med 1997;126:97. (*A prospective cohort study finding that although families often think the goal is comfort, life-sustaining measures are often used.*)
17. Papper S. Care of patients with incurable, chronic neoplasm: one patient's perspective. Am J Med 1985;78:271. (*A deeply moving essay written by a leading clinician while dying of myeloma.*)
18. Christakis NA, Escarge JJ. Survival of Medicare patients after enrollment in hospice programs. N Engl J Med 1996;335:172. (*An outcomes-based study of hospice care; there was some selection bias, but one of the best studies of benefits and limitations.*)
19. Anderson BL. Sexual functioning morbidity among cancer survivors. Cancer 1985;55:1835. (*Differentiates between dysfunction secondary to physiologic and psychological factors.*)
20. Welch-McCaffrey D, Hoffman B, Leigh SA, et al. Surviving adult cancers. Part 2: psychosocial implications. Ann Intern Med 1989;111:517. (*An excellent and useful discussion of key issues; 58 references.*)

CHAPTER 88 ■ PRINCIPLES OF CANCER DRUG THERAPY

JEFFREY W. CLARK

Drug therapy (including targeted and biologic agents) is an important component of cancer management, aiming to prolong life, improve its quality, and in some instances effect cure. However, many drug therapies lack selectivity and adversely effect normal tissue, offsetting their antitumor benefit. Targeted drug therapies offer the promise of greater treatment specificity. A well-constructed program attempts to strike an effective balance between beneficial and adverse effects and requires the expertise of the oncologist. Carefully weighing the risks and potential benefits and thoroughly discussing them with the patient and family are critical to an informed approach to treatment.

Although design of the treatment program rests with the oncologist, the primary care physician has an important collaborative role, which is increasing as more cancer chemotherapy is conducted on an outpatient basis and away from cancer centers. Working closely with the oncologist, the primary physician may be called on to monitor the effects of therapy and provide initial care for the wide range of medical and emotional problems that may arise (see Chapter 87). These responsibilities necessitate knowledge of the general indications for chemotherapy, including targeted and biologic agents, and an awareness of the major toxic and adverse side effects of commonly used agents. The primary care physician must also know how to evaluate the response to treatment and alleviate side effects.

PRINCIPLES OF THERAPY (1–22)

Types of Regimens and Their Indications

Chemotherapy may be given as preoperative (neoadjuvant) therapy, as postoperative (adjuvant) therapy, for curative intent (e.g., testicular cancer, Hodgkins, Non-Hodgkins) or as palliative (occasionally curative) therapy for advanced disease.

Neoadjuvant Chemotherapy

Neoadjuvant chemotherapy is used for the preoperative treatment of *locally invasive tumors* that are moderately sensitive and responsive to drugs (e.g., stage III non–small-cell lung cancer, stage III breast cancer, and stage II and III rectal cancer, and potentially resectable gastric cancer; see Chapters 53, 76, and 122). The goals are to decrease tumor bulk, make possible a more conservative surgical approach, and reduce the risk for systemic disease via macrometastasis. For patients with locally invasive disease, an early consultation with the medical oncologist may be helpful and even precede the surgical referral.

Postoperative Adjuvant Therapy

Postoperative adjuvant therapy has been established as standard treatment for several cancers, including breast cancer (see Chapter 122), stage II and III rectal cancer (see Chapter 76), stage III colon cancer (see Chapter 76), and resected gastric cancer, stages Ib to IV (see Chapter 76). The rationale behind giving chemotherapy to patients who have undergone what appears to be curative surgery is the frequency of distant micrometastases and local recurrences. Chemotherapy applied just after surgery has been more successful in prolonging survival than therapy delayed until clinical evidence arises of recurrence or spread.

Chemotherapy of Advanced Disease

Chemotherapy of advanced disease has evolved in some instances from a strictly palliative modality to a *curative* one (e.g., lymphoma, and germ- cell tumors such as testicular cancer; see Chapters 84 and 143). This change has resulted from the discovery of increasingly effective chemotherapeutic agents and the development of *multiple-drug regimens* that have increased not only response rates, but also the duration of response and the rates of complete clinical remission and cure.

Nonetheless, much of chemotherapy in advanced disease remains *palliative*, designed to reduce morbidity and prolong survival without placing too heavy a burden on the patient. This is not always possible; it takes good judgment to decide what and when to offer and when to withhold palliative therapy. When patients fail to demonstrate a clinically meaningful response, their chemotherapy regimen should be stopped or at least changed to an alternative program.

Basic Chemotherapy Strategies

Designing combination programs and applying dose-intensified therapy through the use of marrow transplantation and marrow growth factors are important chemotherapy strategies that maximize outcomes while helping to minimize risk.

Combination Chemotherapy

The use of regimens with different modes of cellular action increases the effectiveness of therapy without greatly increasing toxicity. The best choices for such regimens are agents with nonadditive side effects. Synergistic or additional effects are achieved while adverse effects are minimized. A meaningful response to cytotoxic chemotherapy is usually expected within two courses of treatment.

Dose-Intensification and Dose-Dense Approaches

Using the highest possible doses without causing intolerable toxicities over a defined time period is essential to ensuring the effectiveness of therapy, especially when treating with curative intent. The use of too small a dose produces inferior outcomes. When cure is being attempted, it is best to try to maintain maximal doses and treat drug side effects by means other than dose reduction. Reductions in dose are among the most common causes of drug failure. Dose intensity and consequent long-term survival can be increased substantially by complementing chemotherapy with marrow-supportive efforts that include bone marrow transplantation and the use of hematopoietic growth factors.

Bone Marrow Transplantation

Efficacy is best established for use in lymphomas, myelomas, and leukemias. Investigational use is ongoing; studies have failed to demonstrate a defined role for breast cancer or other solid tumors (e.g., ovarian, renal cell). For leukemias at high risk for recurrence, the *allogeneic transplantation* of HLA-matched donor marrow cells has produced the best outcomes once cancerous marrow cells are eliminated by dose-intensified chemotherapy. *Autologous transplantation* and the use of *peripheral stem cells* have also produced meaningful results in patients with lymphomas or myeloma, extending the use of high-dose chemotherapy and reducing the costs and risks of marrow reconstitution.

Risks are substantial. Acutely, the most serious are *life-threatening infection* and *acute graft-versus-host reactions*. Within a few years, *lymphomas* and *hematopoietic disorders* may emerge as a consequence of compromised immune function and Epstein–Barr virus infection. Later in life, solid tumors may appear, especially in patients also receiving radiation therapy. *Chronic graft-versus-host disease* may also compromise late outcomes. Such risks underscore the importance of careful patient selection, follow-up, and attention to cancer risk factors such as smoking. Although risk–reward ratios often favor proceeding to transplantation, the decision to proceed should be informed by data from well-designed randomized, controlled trials with long-term follow-up.

Growth Factors

Granulocyte colony–stimulating factor (either a short-acting formulation such as *Neupogen* or a longer-acting one such as

Neulasta) or *granulocyte/macrophage colony–stimulating factor* can provide support to the neutrophilic cell line and lessen the risks for infection that can result from intensive chemotherapy in cancer patients. These agents are expensive but cost-effective when used prophylactically in situations in which febrile neutropenia is highly likely. They are not used routinely to treat episodes of neutropenia, but they do have a role in supporting dose-dense chemotherapy in appropriate settings (e.g., adjuvant therapy for breast cancer), allogeneic and autologous marrow transplantation, and the use of peripheral stem cells.

Erythropoietin (delivered weekly or every other week using *Aranesp*) is useful for treating the anemia associated with cancer chemotherapy. However, its use should primarily be limited to patients treated with palliative chemotherapy. Effective therapy for reducing the risks from thrombocytopenia are not yet available; *interleukin-1 (IL-1)* is approved for this indication, but efficacy is limited, and the drug is not routinely used.

Followup

Follow-up assessment for response and determination of further chemotherapy is usually conducted within 2 to 3 months of initiation of the treatment program. Continued treatment is unwarranted in the presence of disease progression, with the exception of drug regimens (such as those containing irinotecan) in which there may be a delayed response.

Cytotoxic Chemotherapeutic Agents

Cytotoxic drugs have been grouped into categories based on their mechanism of action or the chemical derivation of the drug (Table 88.1). Most currently used cytotoxic agents work by inhibiting the replication of cells, primarily by interfering with DNA synthesis or function or by inhibiting mitosis.

Alkylating Agents

In general, the alkylating agents have a broad spectrum of antitumor activity, chemically interacting directly with DNA. Secondary malignancy is a concern associated with their use. The most commonly used drugs in this class are *cyclophosphamide*, *chlorambucil*, *melphalan*, and *ifosfamide*. Tumor types treated with these agents include non-Hodgkin's lymphoma, Hodgkin's lymphoma, multiple myeloma, small-cell lung cancer, sarcomas, breast cancer, and germ-cell tumors.

Antimetabolites

These drugs interfere with the synthesis of DNA by blocking the action of important metabolic precursors and cofactors. Their greatest effect is on rapidly growing cells. The most commonly used agents in this class are *fluorouracil (5-FU)*, *gemcitabine*, and *methotrexate*. Other examples include *cytarabine*, *6-mercaptopurine*, and the newer agents in this class, such as *fludarabine*, *deoxycoformycin*, *2-chlorodeoxyadenosine*, and the multitargeted antifolate *Alimta*, which has activity against mesothelioma and non-squamous non-small cell lung cancer.

In general, the antimetabolites are rapidly metabolized and excreted in the urine. However, methotrexate and Alimta are distributed throughout total body water and accumulate in pleural effusions and ascitic fluid, which can serve as drug reservoirs and increase the risk of drug toxicity.

Topoisomerase Inhibitors

Etoposide and the anthracycline antibiotics *doxorubicin*, *epirubicin*, *daunorubicin*, and *mitoxantrone* cause DNA intercalation and impair the action of the topoisomerase II enzyme needed for DNA replication. Doxorubicin and epirubicin have a relatively broad spectrum of activity and are usually used in combination with other agents for a variety of malignancies. *Cardiotoxicity* is a major limiting factor with use of the anthracyclines (see later discussion).

Topoisomerase I inhibitors (e.g., *irinotecan* and *topotecan*) inhibit the enzyme involved in the winding and unwinding of DNA strands during replication. Inhibition leads to DNA breaks. Irinotecan is most commonly used for colorectal cancer, esophageal cancer, and small-cell lung cancer. Topotecan is primarily used in the treatment of ovarian cancer.

Mitotic Spindle Inhibitors

These agents inhibit mitosis. *Paclitaxel*, *docetaxel*, *vincristine*, *vinblastine*, and *vinorelbine* are the best-known examples. Paclitaxel and docetaxel are among the most commonly used agents in cancer therapy and are active in a broad range of cancers, including breast, lung, ovarian, head and neck, bladder, esophageal, and gastric cancers. Vincristine and Vinblastine are primarily used for Hodgkins and non-Hodgkins lymphomas. Vinblastine is also useful for germ-cell tumors and Ewing's sarcoma. Vinorelbine is primarily used in lung and breast cancers.

Inorganic Ions (Platinum Compounds)

Platinum-containing compounds (*cisplatin*, *carboplatin*, and *oxaliplatin*) work primarily by forming inter- and intrastrand cross-links between DNA, leading to DNA damage and ultimately cell death. The platinum compounds, usually used in combination with other agents and/or radiation therapy, are effective in the treatment of a wide variety of tumors, including germ-cell tumors and ovarian, lung, head and neck, esophagus, stomach, and bladder cancers. In combination with 5-FU and leucovorin, oxaliplatin has activity against colorectal cancer.

Adverse Effects of Chemotherapeutic Agents

The principal factor limiting the usefulness of chemotherapeutic agents is their relative *lack of selectivity* for the tumor cell (Table 88.2). Cytotoxic drugs adversely affect normal cells, especially those populations with a rapid turnover (bone marrow, hair follicles, gastrointestinal mucosa). This leads to the development of *bone marrow suppression*, *alopecia*, and *gastroenteritis* shortly after the initiation of chemotherapy.

Acute Marrow Suppression

Typically, acute marrow suppression begins 7 to 10 days after the administration of chemotherapy and may last for about 1 week. Continuous cytotoxic therapy may cause a longer-lasting *cumulative suppression*, but most forms of adjuvant chemotherapy are usually not associated with persistent suppression, although a transient fall in cellular constituents may occur.

The most serious risks of chemotherapy are *leukopenia*, leading to overwhelming sepsis, and *thrombocytopenia*, putting the patient at risk for hemorrhage. In most instances, leukopenia and thrombocytopenia are dose related and may be prevented or lessened by dose adjustment in patients with marginal marrow reserve because of marrow invasion, advanced age, or prior therapy. Nonetheless, most chemotherapeutic

TABLE 88.1

CYTOTOXIC CHEMOTHERAPEUTIC AGENTS

Class/Agents	Dose Frequency	Acute Toxicity			Other Toxicity	Elimination	Plasma Half-Life (hr)
		Leukocyte	Platelet	Nausea/Vomiting			
Plant Derivatives							
Paclitaxel	q3wk	Moderate	Moderate	Mild	Anaphylactoid response, sensory neuropathy, alopecia	M	6–8
Vincristine	qwk	Mild	Mild	Mild	Distal neuropathy, inappropriate ADH	M	2.6
Vinblastine	qwk	Marked	Marked	Mild	Mucositis	M	3.1
VP-16 (etoposide)	qd × 3–5	Moderate	Mild	Mild	Distal neuropathy	M, R	6
Antibiotics							
Dactinomycin	qd × 5	Marked	Marked	Moderate	Alopecia, mucositis	M, R	?
Doxorubicin	q3wk	Marked	Marked	Moderate	Alopecia, cardiomyopathy	M	3–25
Daunorubicin	3 d, q3wk	Marked	Marked	Moderate	Alopecia, cardiomyopathy	M	3–?
Mitomycin C	qd × 3, q3wk	Marked	Marked	Moderate	Renal, pulmonary	M	?
Bleomycin	qwk	Rare	Rare	Mild	Skin, pulmonary, fibrosis, fever, allergic reactions	R	0.4–2
Antimetabolites							
Methotrexate (high dose with leucovorin	q3wk q6hr × 7 doses	Mild	Mild	Moderate	Hepatic dysfunction, renal failure	R, M	2–8
Methotrexate	Twice weekly	Moderate to marked	Moderate to marked	Mild	Stomatitis	R	2–8
5-Fluorouracil	qwk or qd × 5, q4wk	Moderate to marked	Moderate to marked	Mild	Cerebellar, conjunctivitis	M	0.3
5-Fluorouracil with leucovorin	qwk × 6, qd × 5, q4wk	Marked	Marked	Mild	Diarrhea, stomatitis	M	0.3
6-Mercaptopurine	qd × 5	Moderate to marked	Moderate to marked	Mild	Cholestasis	M	0.3–0.6
Cytarabine (cytosine arabinoside)	q12hr × 5–10 d	Marked	Marked	Moderate	Cholestasis, mucositis	R, M	0.15
Hydroxyurea	qd × 5	Marked	Moderate	Moderate	None	R, M	1.7
Fludarabine	qd × 5	Moderate	Mild	Mild	Pneumonitis, neurotoxicity	R, M	9.3
Pemetrexed (almita)	q3 wk	Moderate	Mild	Moderate	Dyspnea	R	3.5

(*continued*)

TABLE 88.1

CYTOTOXIC CHEMOTHERAPEUTIC AGENTS (*Continued*)

Class/Agents	Dose Frequency	Acute Toxicity			Other Toxicity	Elimination	Plasma Half-Life (hr)
		Leukocyte	Platelet	Nausea/ Vomiting			
Alkylating Agents							
Cyclophosphamide	qd × 5	Marked	Mild	Moderate	Cystitis, water retention, alopecia	M	1–4
Ifosfamide	qd × 5	Moderate	Moderate	Mild	Neurotoxicity, urothelial neurotoxicity	M	5–6
and mesna	qd × 5.5	None	None	None	None	M	?
Melphalan	qd	Moderate	Moderate	Mild	Leukemia	M	2
Busulfan	qd	Marked	Marked	Mild	Pulmonary fibrosis	M	?
CCNU (lomustine)	q6wk	Marked	Marked	Moderate	Leukemia, pulmonary fibrosis, renal failure	M	?
BCNU (carmustine)	q6wk	Marked	Marked	Marked	Leukemia, pulmonary fibrosis, renal failure	M	1.0
Streptozocin	qd × 5, q3–4wk	Mild	Mild	Moderate-marked	Renal failure, hyperglycemia, hepatic enzyme elevation	R	0.25
Chlorambucil	qd	Moderate	Moderate	Mild	Leukemia	M	1.5
(*cis*-diaminedichloroplatinum)	q3–4wk	Moderate	Moderate	Severe	Renal failure, Mg^{2+} wasting, peripheral neuropathy, ototoxicity	R, M	0.3
Carboplatin	q3–4wk	Marked	Marked	Mild		R	
Topisomerase I Inhibitors							
Irinotecan	q1–3wk	Moderate	Mild	Moderate	Diarrhea	M	10–20
Topotecan	qd × 3–5	Moderate	Moderate	Moderate	None	M	2–3
Miscellaneous							
Dacarbazine	qd × 5	Mild	Mild	Marked	Flulike syndrome, venoocclusion	M	0.65
Procarbazine	qd × 10–14 d	Moderate	Moderate	Mild	Sensitivity to amines	M	?
Mitoxantrone	q3wk	Moderate	Moderate	Mild	Cholestasis, cardiac	M	0.25–37

ADH, antidiuretic hormone; M, metabolized in the liver; q, every; qd, daily; R, renally.
Adapted from Chabner BA. Anticancer drugs. In: DeVita VT, Hellman S, Rosenberg SA, eds. Cancer: principles and practice of oncology, 4th ed. Philadelphia: Lippincott, 1993:325, with permission.

TABLE 88.2

SIDE EFFECTS OF SOME COMMONLY USED AND IMPORTANT NEW CHEMOTHERAPEUTIC AGENTS

Class and Agent	Side Effects
Alkylating Agents	
Cyclophosphamide	Early: n/v, facial burning, metallic taste, blurred vision, hypersensitivity
	Delayed: bone marrow depression, alopecia, hemorrhagic cystitis, bladder cancer, pulmonary infiltrates and fibrosis, SIADH, leukemia
Ifosfamide	Early: n/v, confusion, nephrotoxicity, metabolic acidosis, cardiotoxicity
	Delayed: bone marrow depression, hemorrhagic cystitis, alopecia, SIADH, renal failure, neurotoxicity
Antimetabolites	
Methotrexate	Early: n/v, diarrhea, hepatic injury, hypersensitivity
	Delayed: oral and GI ulceration with possible perforation, bone marrow depression, hepatotoxicity with cirrhosis late; renal toxicity; pulmonary infiltrates and fibrosis, osteoporosis, alopecia, conjunctivitis, depigmentation, menstrual dysfunction, infertility, encephalopathy, lymphoma
5-Fluorouracil	Early: n/v, diarrhea, hypersensitivity rarely
	Delayed: oral and GI ulcers, bone marrow depression; diarrhea, cerebellar neurologic defects, arrhythmias, angina, alopecia, hyperpigmentation, conjunctivitis, palmar–plantar dysesthesias, heart failure, seizures
6-Mercaptopurine	Early: n/v, diarrhea
	Delayed: bone marrow depression, cholestasis, oral and intestinal ulcers, pancreatitis
Cytarabine	Early: n/v, diarrhea, anaphylaxis, acute respiratory distress (high doses)
	Delayed: bone marrow depression, conjunctivitis, megaloblastic anemia, oral ulceration, liver injury, fever, pulmonary edema, neuropathy (high doses), rhabdomyolysis, pancreatitis, rash
Gemcitabine	Early: fatigue, n/v
	Delayed: bone marrow depression, edema, pulmonary toxicity, anal pruritis
Fludarabine	Early: n/v, diarrhea, hypersensitivity
	Delayed: bone marrow depression, immunosuppression, CNS effects, visual disturbances, renal injury at high doses, pulmonary infiltrates
Topoisomerase Inhibitors	
Etoposide	Early: n/v, diarrhea, fever, hypotension, local phlebitis, hypersensitivity
	Delayed: bone marrow depression, alopecia, rash, peripheral neuropathy, leukemia, mucositis and liver injury with high doses.
Doxorubicin	Early: n/v, red urine, local tissue damage, diarrhea, fever, ECG changes, ventricular irritability, anaphylaxis
	Delayed: bone marrow depression, cardiotoxicity (very late), alopecia, stomatitis, anorexia, conjunctivitis, acral pigmentation, dermatitis, acral erythrodysesthesia, hyperuricemia
Bleomycin	Early: n/v, rarely diarrhea
	Delayed: bone marrow depression, pulmonary infiltrates and fibrosis, alopecia, gynecomastia, ovarian failure, hyperpigmentation, azoospermia, leukemia, cataracts, hepatitis, seizures, secondary malignancy with prolonged use
Irinotecan	Early: n/v, diarrhea, fever
	Delayed: diarrhea, anorexia, stomatitis, bone marrow depression, asthenia, alopecia, abdominal cramping and pain
Topotecan	Early: n/v, diarrhea, headache, flulike illness
	Delayed: bone marrow depression, asthenia, stomatitis, alopecia, abdominal pain
Mitotic Spindle Inhibitors	
Vinblastine	Early: n/v, local tissue injury from extravasation
	Delayed: bone marrow depression, alopecia, peripheral neuropathy, stomatitis, jaw pain, paralytic ileus
Vincristine	Early: local tissue injury from extravasation
	Delayed: peripheral neuropathy, alopecia, mild bone marrow depression, constipation, ileus, jaw pain, SIADH, optic atrophy
Paclitaxel, Docetaxel	Early: hypersensitivity reactions
	Delayed: bone marrow depression, peripheral neuropathy, alopecia, myalgias, cardiac toxicity, mucositis
Platinum Compounds	
Cisplatin	Early: n/v
	Delayed: bone marrow depression, peripheral neuropathy, decreased hearing accuracy
Carboplatin	Early: n/v, hypersensitivity reaction
	Delayed: bone marrow depression
Oxaliplatin	Early: n/v, oral cold sensitivity, hypersensitivity reaction
	Delayed: bone marrow depression, peripheral neuropathy

CNS, central nervous system; ECG, electrocardiographic; GI, gastrointestinal; n/v, nausea and vomiting; SIADH, syndrome of inappropriate secretion of antidiuretic hormone.
Adapted from the Medical Letter. Drugs of choice, rev. ed. New Rochelle, NY: Author, 1999:39.

regimens induce some degree of leukopenia, which can serve as a measure of the cytotoxic effect and a guideline to dosing.

Gastrointestinal Toxicity

Nausea, vomiting, mucosal injury (stomatitis), and diarrhea can be disabling. Although not as life threatening as leukopenia and thrombocytopenia, gastrointestinal side effects can significantly compromise quality of life, morale, and willingness to undergo further chemotherapy.

Alopecia

Hair loss occurs with most forms of chemotherapy. It can be partial, but with certain agents (e.g., *doxorubicin* or *irinotecan*) hair loss is generally total. It begins approximately 2 weeks after the initiation of treatment and becomes complete by 4 to 6 weeks. Hair loss is almost always transient, and often some hair grows during the course of treatment; however, total restitution does not take place until chemotherapy is stopped. When hair growth returns, darker, finer, more curly hair is usually produced, but with time, the normal texture and color return.

Secondary Malignancy

Of concern for younger patients, especially those undergoing curative-intent therapy for a leukemia or a lymphoma, is the significant risk for *acute leukemia*, which usually arises within the first decade after chemotherapy for lymphoma, especially when alkylating agents have been used. *Breast cancer* is the principal solid tumor seen years later in women who underwent radiation therapy for Hodgkin's disease earlier in life. Although the evidence for risk is compelling, the benefits of treatment continue to outweigh the risks.

Cardiotoxicity

Free radical injury to myocytes and the release of cardiotoxic cytokines can lead to *cardiomyopathy*, a treatment-limiting, dose-related effect of the *anthracycline* chemotherapeutic agents (e.g., *doxorubicin*). Cardiomyopathy can occur relatively early in treatment (within 1 year) and at therapeutic doses; however, symptoms of ventricular dysfunction may not appear until years later. The best means of detection is through monitoring of cardiac ejection fraction, either by transthoracic *ultrasound* or radionuclide *multiple gated acquisition scan*, which is more sensitive for the detection of early contractile dysfunction.

The best treatment is prevention by careful regular monitoring of the ejection fraction. Once damage has occurred and symptoms ensue, the only treatment is conventional management for heart failure (e.g., angiotensin-converting-enzyme inhibitors, beta-blockade; see Chapter 32). Methods to counter the cardiotoxicity continue to be sought.

New Cytotoxic Therapies: The Biologic Agents

Interleukins

Naturally occurring cytokines such as the interleukins are produced by activated T cells and demonstrate immunostimulatory and antineoplastic effects. *IL-2* triggers peripheral mononuclear cells to release a host of biologically active cytokines that in turn modulate the activity of natural killer cells, B cells, and suppressor cells, with the eventual lysis of cancer cells. The best antitumor effects have been observed in patients with metastatic renal cell carcinoma, for which IL-2 treatment is approved by the U.S. Food and Drug Administration.

Adverse effects are caused by the release of tumor necrosis factor and IL-1 and include *fever, chills, lethargy, diarrhea, thrombocytopenia, liver dysfunction,* and *myocarditis.* *Vascular leakage* is a major side effect. Adverse effects are dose related.

Interferons

Interferons are proteins with antiproliferative and immunomodulatory properties. *Interferon alfa*, an interferon with antitumor activity, is produced by leukocytes, often in response to viral infection. It induces lymphocyte activation and has demonstrated antitumor effects clinically. Although interferon alfa can exert antitumor effects when used as monotherapy, it can also produce responses in combination with chemotherapeutic agents (e.g., with cytarabine in chronic myelogenous leukemia).

Adverse effects are dose dependent and can be troublesome, frequently causing therapy to be stopped. The most common is a *flulike syndrome* of fevers, sweats, fatigue, and myalgias, which is experienced by most patients during the first several weeks of therapy. The flulike symptoms are often transient and likely to resolve unless the dose is increased, but a host of even more disabling symptoms may follow. These include marked *anorexia, depression, anxiety, emotional lability, hair loss, tinnitus, reversible hearing loss,* and *thyroid dysfunction.* An increased susceptibility to bacterial *infection* and *cardiotoxicity* may also develop.

Targeted Therapies

With increased knowledge of tumor biology comes the ability to target specific mutations and other factors that are unique or relatively unique to cancerous cells. This allows for a significantly enhanced therapeutic index (the ratio of cytotoxic effects against malignant cells to the toxic effects on normal cells). There are two broad groups of targeted therapies in use for cancer treatment: (a) monoclonal antibodies directed against specific antigens on proteins, and (b) small molecules that target specific mutations or functions of overexpressed proteins found in malignant cells.

Monoclonal Antibodies

Monoclonal antibodies directed against tumor growth factors (especially *epidermal growth factor* and *vascular endothelial growth factor*) have been noteworthy for their contribution to cancer drug therapy. They have enhanced the treatment of a wide range of hematologic and solid tumors (Table 88.3) Monoclonal antibodies directed against cell surface proteins and used either uncoupled or conjugated to cytotoxic agents (e.g., radioactive yttrium) have been applied to treatment of lymphomas and leukemias. Many monoclonal antibody agents are under development.

A useful property of monoclonal antibodies is that, in general, their toxicities do not overlap with those of chemotherapy, allowing full doses in combination therapy. An exception is Herceptin, which has overlapping cardiotoxicity with anthracyclines and taxanes (although with careful monitoring, this toxicity is usually manageable).

Targeted Small Molecules

When targeting a mutant protein, these agents can be highly specific for malignant cells. To date the most commonly developed agents inhibit the tyrosine kinase function of the targeted

TABLE 88.3

MONOCLONAL ANTIBODIES FOR CANCER TREATMENT

Antibody	Target	Use
Rituximab (Rituxan)	B cell CD20 antigen	B cell lymphomas
Trastuzumab (Herceptin)	Her2 receptor	20%–25% of breast cancers
Bevacizumab (Avastin)	Vascular endothelial growth factor	Colorectal, lung cancers
Cetuximab (Erbitux)	Epidermal growth factor receptor	Colorectal, lung, head and neck cancers
Panitumumab (Vectibix)	Epidermal growth factor receptor	Colorectal cancer

protein. Two targeted small molecules, *Gleevec* (for chronic myeloid leukemia and gastrointestinal stromal tumor tumors) and *Iressa* (for non–small-cell lung cancer), have shown sufficient activity to be approved for the treatment of patients with specific cancers. Both of these inhibit the tyrosine kinase activity of the specific target protein. These mutations are more commonly seen in women with adenocarcinomas or bronchioalveolar carcinomas and may be more frequent in the Japanese population. Many of these agents are not entirely selective and may inhibit a number of kinases. Although this multitargeting increases the potential for side effects, it may also allow for the treatment of more than one malignancy. For most malignancies, targeted agents are only effective against a subset of cancers that manifest the mutant or overexpressed protein. The hope is that, as the specific patients are defined who might respond to any given agent, tailored individual therapy will become a reality.

PRACTICAL ISSUES (23–27)

Administration of Chemotherapy

It is important to be aware of several acute side effects that can occur during chemotherapy administration so they can be dealt with expeditiously.

Allergic Reactions

Occurring with almost any agent, acute allergic reactions are most commonly seen with the *taxanes* (due to use of *chemophore* as a delivery vehicle). Pretreatment with steroids and antihistamines is important in taxane use to decrease the incidence and severity of allergic reactions. *Oxaliplatin* and *carboplatin* can cause both *allergic-like reactions* (which can usually be controlled by slowing the rate of infusion) and *true allergic reactions* (much less common) that require discontinuation of the drug or if it is necessary to continue the drug, desensitization.

Extravasation and Vascular Injury

Extravasation is a concern with drugs that need to be administered intravenously. Extravasation of vesicant drugs (e.g., *doxorubicin, epirubicin, paclitaxel, docetaxel, vincristine, vinblastine, dacarbazine*) can cause marked tissue irritation and secondary inflammation leading to ulceration and necrosis. Surgical grafting and debridement are sometimes necessary. The best treatment is prevention, with proper venous access being the most important element, facilitated by the placement of a central venous access device for individuals with poor venous access. In the event of extravasation, the infusions should be stopped immediately and either warm or cold compresses applied as per specific guidelines (excessive pressure should be avoided in the application of compresses). Any accumulation of drug should be removed by aspiration. The actual inflammation and necrosis may not occur for 3 to 10 days following the injection, although pain is generally present early on. Corticosteroids have been used, but definitive evidence of efficacy has not been demonstrated.

Even without extravasation, the repeated use of irritating intravenous chemotherapy drugs can lead to endothelial deterioration and vein sclerosis, particularly when small-caliber veins are used for infusion. Devices for venous access facilitate administration, and their use is now routine and widespread.

Suppression of Nausea and Vomiting (See Also Chapter 91)

The drugs most likely to induce severe nausea and vomiting include *cisplatin, dacarbazine, doxorubicin,* and *high doses of cyclophosphamide.* Some agents cause vomiting that begins approximately 30 to 45 minutes after injection; with others, particularly cyclophosphamide and doxorubicin, the vomiting begins 4 to 5 hours after injection. Recent advances in understanding the mechanisms of chemotherapy-induced nausea and vomiting have led to the development of effective multifaceted programs (see Chapter 91).

Management of Bone Marrow Suppression

Generalized marrow suppression is common. The pattern of suppression is a function of the type of drug, dose, and schedule of administration (Table 88.4). Standard approaches to this problem include making adjustments in the dose and timing of chemotherapy. Dose adjustments for subsequent courses of therapy are based on the nadir levels observed, as well as the duration of neutropenia. In monitoring patients on chemotherapeutic regimens, the anticipated *nadir days* for blood counts are the most crucial times to obtain *follow-up complete blood cell counts* with differentials. For patients in whom neutropenia develops, the observation period should be intensified, depending on the level of the count and the presence of associated fever or sepsis. The advent of marrow growth factors (see prior discussion) has enhanced the ability to administer the optimal doses of chemotherapy, which ordinarily might be limited by the onset of marrow suppression. Growth factors work best when given prophylactically rather than after marrow suppression has set in. They are expensive but can prevent hospitalizations and limit complications.

Evaluation of Response to Therapy

See Chapter 86.

TABLE 88.4

CHRONOLOGIC PATTERNS OF MARROW SUPPRESSION SECONDARY TO CHEMOTHERAPY

Agent	Nadir Day	Operation
Nonsuppressive Drugs		
Bleomycin		
Vincristine		
Streptozotocin		
Corticosteroids		
Dacarbazine		
Marrow-Suppressive Drugs		
Alkylating drugs		
Cyclophosphamide		
Nitrogen mustard	5–8	Variable
Mitomycin C	Delayed	Cumulative
Antibiotics		
Doxorubicin	12–14	5 d
Dactinomycin		
Antimetabolites		
5-Fluorouracil	5–10	<5 d
Cytosine arabinoside		
Methotrexate		
Gemcitabine		
Natural products		
Vinblastine	8–12	3 d
Paclitaxel	7–14	5 d
Topoisomerase I and II Inhibitors		
Etoposide	7–14	7 d
Irinotecan	7–14	5 d
Topotecan	10–14	7 d
Others		
Nitrosoureas	14–28	Cumulative
Hydroxyurea	Variable	
Procarbazine	Variable	

PATIENT EDUCATION

The ability to tolerate the challenges posed by chemotherapy is enhanced by a strong and trusting patient–doctor relationship, detailed patient education, and frequent communication. Fully educating patients and families about diagnosis, prognosis, treatment rationale, and side effects of planned therapy can greatly facilitate the development of trust and confidence. Concerns about alopecia, sterility, gastrointestinal upset, and other side effects should be elicited and directly addressed. The probability of response also deserves review. A comprehensive educational effort appropriate for the patient's level of understanding allows the patient to participate meaningfully in decision making and encourages a sense of partnership in the undertaking, an attitude that can help to sustain the patient through this often difficult time.

INDICATIONS FOR ADMISSION AND REFERRAL

The onset of *febrile neutropenia* (absolute neutrophil counts <500/mm³) requires immediate hospitalization and empiric antibiotic therapy after cultures obtained. The development of *bleeding* in the setting of thrombocytopenia is an indication for urgent hospitalization and consideration of platelet transfusion. The asymptomatic patient with *severe thrombocytopenia* (platelet count <10,000/mm³) also deserves consideration for admission and platelet transfusion. Counts of 10,000/mm³ to 50,000/mm³ are an indication for close observation and a warning to the patient to avoid trauma.

Referral to the oncologist should be made at the time of diagnosis for the consideration and design of a drug treatment regimen. Chemotherapy programs are in a constant state of revision as new combinations are tried and new agents developed. Each patient's treatment program must be designed in conjunction with an oncologist. When such expertise is not locally available, patients may need referral to a regional center for consultation and program design. Referral back to the oncologist is indicated when there is evidence of disease progression despite treatment or the development of a serious complication requiring hospital admission.

Annotated Bibliography

1. Duell T, van Lint MT, Ljungman P, et al. Health and functional status of long-term survivors of bone marrow transplantation. Ann Intern Med 1997;126:184. (*A retrospective multicenter study, finding that most patients were in good health after 5 years, but late cancers and chronic graft-versus-host disease were problematic for some.*)
2. Fojo AT, Ueda K, Slamon DJ, et al. Expression of a multidrug-resistant gene in human tumors and tissues. Proc Natl Acad Sci USA 1987;84:265. (*Reports on the mechanism of multiple-drug resistance.*)
3. Garcia-Carbonero R, Hidalgo M, Paz-Ares L, et al. Patient selection in high-dose chemotherapy trials: relevance in high-risk breast cancer. J Clin Oncol 1997;15:3178. (*Study inclusion criteria were actually found to be an independent predictor of good outcome, which underscores the importance of reading studies carefully for sources of bias.*)
4. Goldie JH, Goldman AJ, Gudauskas GA. Rationale for the use of alternating non–cross-resistant chemotherapy. Cancer Treat Rep 1982;66:439. (*The early theoretical basis for combination chemotherapy.*)
5. Guilhot F, Chastang C, Michallet M, et al. Interferon alfa-2b combined with cytarabine versus interferon alone in chronic myelogenous leukemia. N Engl J Med 1997;337:223. (*A major study, providing an example of interferon efficacy, especially when combined with conventional chemotherapy.*)
6. Hartmann O, Le Corroller AG, Blaise D, et al. Peripheral blood stem cell and bone marrow transplantation for solid tumors and lymphomas: hema-tologic recovery and cost. A randomized, controlled trial. Ann Intern Med 1997;126:600. (*The use of peripheral blood stem cells produced more rapid marrow recovery at lower cost.*)
7. Imrie K, Esmail R, Meyer RM, et al. The role of high-dose chemotherapy and stem-cell transplantation in patients with multiple myeloma: a practice guideline of the Cancer Care Ontario Practice Guidelines Initiative. Ann Intern Med 2002;136:619. (*Consensus guidelines on the use of stem cell transplantation.*)
8. Pui C-H, Boyett JM, Hughes WT, et al. Human granulocyte colony-stimulating factor after induction chemotherapy in children with acute lymphoblastic leukemia. N Engl J Med 1997;336:1781. (*An example of the application of granulocyte colony-stimulating factor [G-CSF] in the setting of intensive chemotherapy.*)
9. Sung L, Dror Y. Clinical applications of granulocyte-colony stimulating factor. Front Biosci 2007;12:1988. (*A review of the use of G-CSF.*)
10. Livingston DM, Shivdasani R. Toward mechanism-based cancer care. JAMA 2001;285:588. (*A useful review of cancer molecular biology for the clinician and treatments based on it.*)
11. Rai KR, Peterson BL, Appelbaum FR, et al. Fludarabine compared with chlorambucil as primary therapy for chronic lymphocytic leukemia. N Engl J Med 2001;343:1750. (*A randomized, controlled trial [RCT] of this important new antimetabolite, demonstrating enhanced response.*)

12. Rowinsky EK, Donehower RC. Paclitaxel (Taxol). N Engl J Med 1995;332: 1004. (*An excellent review of this increasingly important chemotherapeutic agent.*)
13. Shan K, Lincoff M, Young JB. Anthracycline-induced cardiotoxicity. Ann Intern Med 1996;125:47. (*A systematic review of this important adverse effect; 146 references.*)
14. Singal PK, Iliskovic N. Doxorubicin-induced cardiomyopathy. N Engl J Med 1998;339:900. (*Reviews the major dose-related complication of this commonly used chemotherapeutic agent.*)
15. Stadtmauer EA, O'Neill A, Goldstein LJ, et al. Conventional-dose chemotherapy compared with high-dose chemotherapy plus autologous hematopoietic stem-cell transplantation for metastatic breast cancer. N Engl J Med 2000;342:1069. (*A major RCT, failing to demonstrate improved survival; illustrates the importance of prospective, systematic study of a modality before widespread application.*)
16. Green MR. Targeting targeted therapy. N Engl J Med 2004;350:2191. (*A useful editorial summarizing the status of targeted therapy.*)
17. Savage DG, Antman KH. Imatinib mesylate—a new oral targeted therapy. N Engl J Med 2002;346:683. (*A review of this targeted therapy; 118 references.*)
18. Kwak EL, Clark JW, Chabner B. Targeted agents: the rules of combination. Clin Cancer Res 2007;13(18 Pt 1):5232. (*A review.*)
19. Lièvre A, Bachet JB, Boige V, et al. KRAS mutations as an independent prognostic factor in patients with advanced colorectal cancer treated with cetuximab. J Clin Oncol 2008;26:374. (*An example of targeted therapy directed at a specific mutant protein.*)
20. Murdoch D, Sager J. Will targeted therapy hold its promise? An evidence-based review. Curr Opin Oncol 2008;20(1):104. (*An editorial with a thoughtful critique.*)
21. Press MF, Lenz HJ. EGFR, HER2 and VEGF pathways: validated targets for cancer treatment. Drugs 2007;67:2045. (*A review of monoclonal antibody therapy.*)
22. Sirikantaramas S, Asano T, Sudo H, et al. Topoisomerase I inhibitors: camptothecins and beyond. Nat Rev Cancer 2006;6:789. (*A review of agents directed at this target.*)
23. Gralla RJ, Osoba D, Kris MG, et al. Recommendations for the use of antiemetics: evidence-based, clinical practice guidelines. J Clin Oncol 1999;17:2971. (*Consensus recommendations.*)
24. Kuizon D, Gordon SM, Dolmatch BKL. Single-lumen subcutaneous ports inserted by interventional radiologists in patients undergoing chemotherapy: incidence of infection and outcome of attempted catheter salvage. Arch Intern Med 2001;161:406. (*A retrospective study, finding that there was a low complication rate, but that infection remained the leading cause of catheter loss and required catheter removal.*)
25. Rodríguez Sánchez CA. Recommendation of the scientific societies on the treatment of anaemia in cancer patients. Clin Trans Oncol 2007;9:582. (*A review of hematopoietic growth factor support.*)
26. Stieber P, Molina R, Chan DW, et al. Clinical evaluation of the Elecsys CA 15-3 test in breast cancer patients. Clin Lab 2003;49:15. (*An example of the use of this tumor marker in clinical practice for monitoring the therapy of breast cancer; it was found to be helpful, but there was some lack of specificity.*)
27. Wirth A, Seymour JF, Hicks RJ, et al. Fluorine-18 fluorodeoxyglucose positron emission tomography, gallium-67 scintigraphy, and conventional staging for Hodgkin's disease and non-Hodgkin's lymphoma. Am J Med 2002;112:262. (*Presents evidence for the utility of positron emission tomography scanning and its superiority to gallium scanning for staging.*)

CHAPTER 89 ■ PRINCIPLES OF RADIATION THERAPY

THEODORE HONG AND THOMAS DELANEY

Modern radiation therapy represents an important means of achieving local and regional control of malignancy in addition to providing palliation. When given with the intent of controlling disease and attempting cure, it is termed *radical or curative*; when given for symptomatic relief, it is designated *palliative*. Although the design and implementation of such therapy is the responsibility of the radiation oncologist, the primary physician shares in the decision to use the modality, monitors and supports the patient while it is being administered, and watches for and treats late complications. The primary care physician needs to be familiar with basic aspects of radiation therapy, its applications, and its side effects.

PRINCIPLES OF MANAGEMENT

Response to Irradiation (1–5)

Determinants of Radiosensitivity

Exponential killing of both tumor and normal cells occurs after an initial, sublethal accumulation of radiation damage. The ability of cells to accumulate some radiation damage before the manifestation of cell death is believed to be linked to *repair capacity*. The general shapes of the radiation response curves of cells in culture are remarkably similar, with most of the difference in *radiosensitivity* a consequence of subtle differences in the ability of cells to accumulate and repair radiation damage. Cells in the S phase of the cell cycle (when DNA synthesis is taking place, but no mitosis) are the least sensitive to radiation, probably because of the enhanced capacity for repair in this phase. In response to radiation injury, normal cells initially stop proliferating because of "checkpoints" in the cell cycle designed to allow the cell to repair DNA damage before cell division is attempted. Malignant cells often have mutations in these critical cell-cycle regulatory genes (such as *p53*) that perturb the checkpoint function, so progress through the cell cycle is uninterrupted despite the presence of radiation-damaged DNA; as a consequence, cell death occurs during mitosis.

The response to irradiation is also affected by the *volume* of the tumor. Except for uniquely radiosensitive tumors (lymphomas and seminomas), larger tumors are more difficult to eradicate with any given dose of irradiation. This is in part related to the larger number of tumor cells that must be killed. Another part of the reason for this resistance, however, is *tissue hypoxia*. Oxygen facilitates the cytotoxic effect of x-rays, which is mediated in part by oxygen free radicals. Hypoxic cells are about three times more refractory to irradiation than are cells treated in the presence of oxygen. Interior areas of large tumors can become hypoxic and relatively refractory to radiation. However, as the tumor shrinks, the access of its hypoxic cells to oxygen increases, and they become more susceptible to radiation if doses are given in sequential fractionated fashion (see later discussion). Nevertheless, the presence of anemia (hemoglobin levels <10 to 12.5 g/dL) has been shown to have a negative effect on radiotherapy treatment outcome in multiple anatomic sites, which has led to the clinical practice of administering red blood cell transfusions to maintain hemoglobin levels during a course of radiotherapy.

Strategies for Improving Response

Effective approaches include the use of *particle beams*, concurrent *chemotherapy*, and compounds that *sensitize hypoxic tumor cells*. Particle beams such as neutrons are less dependent on oxygen for their cytotoxic action than are x-rays and represent another means of treating large, poorly vascularized tumors. Other particles, such as protons, have significantly better dose distribution properties than conventional x-rays, so the dose to the tumor can be increased substantially while adjacent normal tissue is spared. Many chemotherapy compounds, such as cis-platinum, 5-fluorouracil, and paclitaxel, enhance radiation cytotoxicity, which results in simultaneous improvement in local and distant control of tumor. Compounds that sensitize hypoxic tumor cells and improve their response to radiation therapy are under investigation.

The *dose* of irradiation that can be safely directed at a malignancy is limited by the tolerance of the organs surrounding it. Although the energy (i.e., voltage) of the radiation determines its ability to penetrate tissue, it is the amount of radiation actually absorbed that determines the biologic effects. *High-energy* megavoltage beams spare the skin, with better cosmetic results. Focusing beams on a tumor from multiple directions concentrates the dose in the tumor and avoids excessive irradiation of critical adjacent normal structures. Damage can be particularly injurious when radiation is absorbed by cells of the heart, liver, brain, intestines, bone marrow, kidneys, or lung (see later discussion). These structures have defined radiation tolerances that are related to the volume irradiated and the dose received. Usually, tradeoffs must be made between therapeutic benefits and adverse effects.

Minimizing Adverse Effects

The probability of radiation-induced complications depends on how narrow the difference is between the dose needed for control of the tumor and the dose that causes injury to normal tissue. (The ratio of the two doses is termed the *therapeutic ratio*.) The greater the difference in doses, the better is the result. Dose fractionation, shielding of normal tissue, and use of imaging techniques to define tumor volume and location precisely have helped to limit the adverse effects of radiation therapy.

Fractionating the dose helps to widen the margin of safety and improve the selective killing of tumor cells. Normal cells repair sublethal radiation damage more effectively than do tumor cells. Traditional fractionation programs provide about 200 centigray (cGy) or rads per treatment, applied five times per week. Newer fractionation schemes hyperfractionate radiation with two to three treatments per day to exploit differences in radiation repair capacity between tumor and normal tissue maximally and accelerate the treatment to overcome the repopulation of tumor cells that occurs during the conventional treatment of some tumors.

Shielding helps to protect vital organs adjacent to the portal from radiation exposure. Often, custom-fabricated lead shields or analogous, automated blocking devices in the head of the treatment machine (multileaf collimators) are used to prevent the irradiation of normal tissue abutting the tumor. *Computed tomography* (CT), *magnetic resonance imaging* (MRI), and *positron emission tomography* (PET) scans have improved the delineation of tumor volume and the surrounding anatomic structures so that the target can be more precisely defined. *Simulation* reproduces the geometry of the actual radiation portal and helps to ensure that only the desired tissue is irradiated. CT-based simulation is increasingly used for this purpose; patients are scanned in the treatment position with markers on the skin or other structures to allow the tumor to be referenced to a reproducible spatial coordinate system. The CT data set is transferred electronically to a three-dimensional treatment system that allows the tumor, normal tissues, and doses to be displayed in three dimensions. This technology permits the radiation dose to the tumor to be escalated, so the tumor control rate is increased while normal tissue is simultaneously protected; as a result, fewer side effects to normal tissue are produced.

Specific applications of this technology include *stereotactic radiosurgery* and intensity-modulated radiation therapy (IMRT). For stereotactic radiosurgery, the patient is rigidly immobilized in a head or body frame for CT stimulation and radiation treatment. IMRT employs sophisticated, computer-controlled radiation planning and treatment delivery to target the tumor with heterogeneous beams from multiple angles, resulting in better conformation of the high-dose radiation region to the tumor and lower radiation doses to selected normal tissues. In addition, amifostine is the first compound to be shown to be a clinically useful and preferential protector of normal tissue from radiation damage.

Clinical Applications (6–13)

Three basic *delivery modes* are used. External sources (teletherapy or external beam) are the most frequently applied. Brachytherapy, in which encapsulated sources are placed directly into the body at tumor sites, has selective advantages in the treatment of very localized disease. Improvements in imaging and radiation treatment planning have resulted in a resurgence of interest in brachytherapy at such sites as the prostate, where the therapeutic ratio for this technique is high. Systemic delivery via radionuclides is the third mode. Recently, intravenous administration of radionuclide-labeled monoclonal antibodies has found utility for effective and selective treatment of some lymphomas. The theoretical attractiveness of the latter two methods is closer proximity of the radiation source to the tumor and the limited exposure of normal tissue to radiotherapy.

Radiation is applied to achieve cure and control in addition to palliation. It may be the sole treatment or an alternative therapy, or it may be combined with other modalities (Table 89.1).

As Sole or Alternative Therapy

Like surgery, radiation therapy is primarily a method of treating local or regional disease. The goal is to "sterilize" both the primary site and likely areas of local and regional spread. In some instances, such as stage I *Hodgkin's disease* or early low-grade *non-Hodgkin's lymphoma* (see Chapter 84), radiation therapy is the treatment of choice. When preservation of function and appearance can be achieved with comparable survival outcome, radiation may be preferred by some patients over surgery (as in localized *breast cancer*, localized *prostate cancer*, or early *head* and *neck cancers*). When surgery and radiation provide similar rates of cure and control, the choice depends largely on the effect of treatment on the patient.

As Combination Therapy

Several characteristics of radiation therapy make it a good complement to *surgery*. Surgery is the more effective of the

TABLE 89.1

APPLICATIONS OF RADIOTHERAPY

Tumor	Comments
Radiation Therapy Alone Curative	
Hodgkin's disease	Stage IA–IIA; 90% 10-yr survival
Lymphoma (indolent)	Stage I–II; 50% 10-yr survival
Cervical cancer	Curative for early-stage disease; stage IB–IIA 85% 5-yr disease-free survival
Testicular cancer	Seminomas; cure rates for early stage disease >95%
Head and neck cancer	Early stage disease (T1, T2); results are comparable with those of surgery with less functional and cosmetic loss
Prostate cancer	External beam or brachytherapy are excellent alternatives to surgery for organ-confined disease; external beam and hormonal therapy for locally advanced disease
Radiation Combined with Another Modality Potentially Curative	
Uterine cancer	With surgery ± chemotherapy, good results for stages I, II, and III; 60%–90% 5-yr survival
Head and neck cancer	With surgery and/or chemotherapy in locally advanced cases
Soft-tissue sarcomas	In combination with surgery, often function or limb sparing
Breast cancer	In combination with surgery and chemotherapy/hormonal therapy, breast preservation with survival equivalent to that of mastectomy possible for tumors ≤5 cm
Esophagus	Chemoradiation cures 25% of patients with localized disease
Lung	Chemoradiation cures 15% of patients with locally advanced non–small-cell and 20%–25% of patients with limited small-cell carcinoma
Bladder	Chemoradiation is an organ-sparing option with similar treatment outcome as cystectomy
Rectum	Addition of chemoradiation to radical surgery improves outcome in patients with node-positive or transmural tumors
Anus	Chemoradiation has replaced surgery as the primary treatment, curing 75% of patients
Radiation Therapy Palliative	
Bony metastases	For pain not controlled by analgesics, chemotherapy, or hormonal therapy
Brain metastases	Stereotactic radiosurgery an alternative to craniotomy for patients with one or two lesions
Spinal cord compression	Treat emergently with steroids especially when there is a single focal obstructing lesion; patients with myeloma, lymphoma, and small-cell cancers respond especially well to radiation

two modalities in the management of bulky disease, whereas radiation appears to be more effective in the treatment of small-volume, locally invasive disease, which is the basis for the sequence of surgery for local disease followed by radiation as adjunctive therapy. Radiation can also reduce tumor bulk and destroy microscopic disease, thereby facilitating surgical removal and local control. By allowing the use of lower doses of radiation and less-radical surgery, combination therapy minimizes side effects and has become the cornerstone of the organ-preservation treatments for cancer. Such combination therapy often also includes chemotherapy (see later discussion).

With Surgery. Whether to administer radiation before, during, or after surgery depends on several practical and theoretical issues. Favoring *preoperative treatment* are the need to reduce tumor size for easier resection and the desirability of sterilizing tumor cells that might be spread during surgery. Moreover, *postoperative irradiation* may be less effective if the vascular bed is surgically reduced and oxygen delivery impaired. Factors favoring postoperative treatment include prompt performance of surgery, ability to determine the need for radiotherapy based on a pathologic review of the resected specimen, avoidance of radiation effects on wound healing, and destruction of any remaining microscopic disease. *Intraoperative treatment* allows one to displace normal thoracic, abdominal, or pelvic organs (which are quite intolerant of the high radiation doses necessary to sterilize gross tumor) and target diseased tissue more precisely.

With Chemotherapy. The application of radiation in combination with chemotherapy to achieve cure is established for selected stages of *Hodgkin's* and *non-Hodgkin's lymphomas*, and the combination has been demonstrated to result in improved outcome in locally advanced cancers of the *head and neck, lung, esophagus, bladder, rectum, anus,* and *uterine cervix* in comparison with radiotherapy alone. The rationale is to treat local disease with radiation and administer chemotherapeutic agents that both increase the efficacy of radiation against the primary tumor and target occult systemic metastases. Radiation can also be used to treat areas not readily accessible to chemotherapy, such as the brain in patients with small-cell lung cancer. Although improved survival has been demonstrated, acute and late toxicities can be additive. Marrow suppression can be the limiting problem. Other instances of additive adverse effects include the following: cyclophosphamide (Cytoxan) and radiation produce acute hemorrhagic cystitis; 5-fluorouracil and radiotherapy cause acute mucositis of the oral cavity and acute radiation enteritis; cis-platinum, etoposide, and taxanes combined with thoracic radiotherapy produce acute esophagitis; and combination chemotherapy with radiation increases the risk for leukemia. Some drugs enhance radiation reactions in normal tissues, even when given up to 1 year after radiotherapy. Adriamycin is the most prominent example of a drug producing this *recall phenomenon.*

With Targeted Therapy. As noted, targeted therapies seek selectively to target a certain biologic pathway that may be different in cancers as opposed to normal tissues. Because these therapies exhibit different, nonoverlapping toxicities when compared to cytotoxic chemotherapy, there has been considerable interest in exploring their potential as *radiosensitizers.*

Under trial conditions, the addition of the targeted therapy cetuximab (Erbitux) improved overall survival and locoregional control of head and neck cancer treatment. Most impressive, this study showed that this benefit was obtained without significant additional side effects. The combination of radiation therapy with targeted therapy is one of the most active areas of clinical investigation in radiation oncology.

The optimal strategies for the application of combined-modality therapy are continuing to evolve. The literature should be followed for the results of studies now ongoing.

As Palliative Therapy

Radiation serves an important function in providing symptomatic relief to some patients with incurable disease. For those tumors that respond to chemotherapy or hormonal therapy, radiation should be held in reserve. However, if localized tumor is not sensitive to other modalities, palliative radiation may be an effective means of providing symptomatic relief. In most instances, the treatment of asymptomatic lesions yields little benefit, although prophylactic brain irradiation appears to be useful in patients with small-cell lung cancer. One of the best examples of palliative therapy is for painful *bony metastases* from such tumors as those of breast and prostate. Within 2 to 3 weeks of the start of a relatively short course of radiotherapy (2 weeks), many patients experience relief from bone pain. Analgesics including narcotics can play a very important role in pain control in the interval before onset of pain relief; if narcotics are used, an appropriate bowel regimen to prevent constipation must be prescribed. Radiation to bony metastases has also been used to stabilize a weight-bearing bone, but if cortical involvement is present, then surgical stabilization of the bone may be necessary. Radiation plays an important role in the urgent treatment of certain oncologic emergencies, including *spinal cord compression* and *superior vena cava syndrome* (see Chapter 92).

Adverse Effects and Their Prevention and Management (2,4,14–17)

As noted previously, many normal cells tolerate radiation better than do malignant cells. However, the degree of *tolerance* varies greatly (Table 89.2). Tissues with high rates of turnover

TABLE 89.2

SERIOUS ADVERSE EFFECTS OF RADIOTHERAPY

Tissue	Adverse Effect	Dose Limit [cGy (rads); ≤5% toxicity]
Bone marrow	Marrow suppression	250
Kidney	Nephrosclerosis	2,000
Lungs	Pneumonitis	2,000
Liver	Hepatitis	3,000
Heart	Pericarditis	4,500
Spinal cord	Myelitis	4,500
Small intestine	Ulceration, fibrosis	4,500
Skin	Dermatitis, sclerosis	5,500
Brain	Necrosis	6,000

Modified from Chabner BA. Principles of cancer therapy. In: Wyngaarden JB, Smith LH, eds. Cecil's textbook of medicine, 16th ed. Philadelphia: Saunders, 1982:1034, with permission.

and large stem cell populations are among the most vulnerable. Even organs with almost no proliferative capacity are at risk by virtue of the vulnerability of their vascular endothelium. Much radiation-induced injury is vascular in nature. Toxicity may be acute or chronic. Acute toxicity is noted in tissues with the highest rates of turnover (e.g., marrow, skin, gastrointestinal mucosa). *Acute radiation toxicity* is often defined as that appearing within 90 days after the start of radiotherapy. It usually resolves with supportive care in the majority of patients without significant late consequences. *Toxicity appearing later*, however, is usually more serious and clinically significant because it may involve irreversible injury to the involved normal tissue.

Tolerance to radiotherapy decreases as the dose is increased. The *dose limit* for a tissue can be expressed as the cumulative dose that produces a 5% incidence of toxicity when radiation is delivered in 200-cGy fractions for 5 days per week. Beyond the dose limit, the incidence of toxicity rises quickly.

Bone Marrow Suppression

The bone marrow is the most radiosensitive tissue, with marrow suppression developing when exposure exceeds 250 cGy. Suppression is usually transient and reversible, unless large marrow volumes are irradiated. Skin, gastrointestinal mucosa, and lung are of intermediate sensitivity.

Radiation Pneumonitis

Radiation pneumonitis starts to appear when the dose to a large volume of the lung surpasses 2,000 cGy; the incidence reaches 100% at doses of 4,000 cGy. The onset, usually within 6 to 12 weeks, is characterized by dyspnea, cough, low-grade fever, hypoxemia, and a "ground glass" appearance on chest x-ray films. CT may show straight lines that match the radiotherapy field. In cases of radiation injury, restrictive defects and chronic hypoxemia can follow if fibrosis sets in, which typically takes place during the ensuing 6 to 24 months.

Infectious and other causes of dyspnea such as pulmonary embolus and cardiac failure, however, must be excluded before attributing respiratory symptoms to radiation therapy. It is important for the primary care physician to discuss the patient's symptoms with the treating radiation oncologist, especially because today's computerized radiation treatment planning systems provide very precise visual displays with quantitative information on the dose delivered to individual lobes, which can be very helpful in deciding whether radiotherapy might have contributed to the observed symptoms.

Treatment is mainly supportive. High-dose steroids (1 mg of prednisone per kilogram initially with gradual taper as tolerated) and oxygen can alleviate symptoms during the acute phase; once fibrosis occurs, no treatment is available. The best approach is prevention through careful limitation by the treating radiation oncologist of the volume of lung irradiated to a significant dose.

Other Radiation-Induced Organ Injury

Nephrosclerosis is the renal response to doses in excess of 2,000 cGy. *Hepatitis* is a consequence of doses to the liver greater than 3,000 cGy. Gastrointestinal *ulceration* followed by perforation or fibrosis is a complication of bowel doses exceeding 4,500 cGy. *Pericarditis* and *spinal cord injury (myelitis)* are risks of 4,500-cGy doses to the heart and spinal cord, respectively. With mediastinal irradiation, pericarditis can become constrictive, and valvular injury has also been noted.

Skin injury has been declining with application of modern techniques for minimizing damage. Although acute reactions are common, the skin can tolerate as much as 5,500 cGy given over time; *dermatitis* becomes a problem at higher doses. The brain (except the brainstem) can withstand up to 6,000 cGy before the risk for *necrosis* begins to rise. Radiation can also induce cataracts and retinal damage and can lead to blindness. Gonadal radiation is likely to induce permanent *sterility*, and pelvic irradiation during the first trimester of pregnancy is *teratogenic*. The issue of sperm banking or oocyte preservation should be raised with patients of childbearing age interested in future childbearing if the gonads are to receive damaging radiation doses as part of treatment.

Risk for Secondary Malignancy

There is a small but finite risk for secondary malignancy in the irradiated tissues; it is approximately 0.2% at 10 years in most adult patients, but in some instances can be considerably higher (e.g., 1%/yr for development of breast cancer in women who underwent thoracic radiation therapy for cure of Hodgkin's disease as adolescents; see Chapter 84). Similarly, in children with bilateral retinoblastoma and mutations of the tumor suppressor gene, this risk may also approach 1%/yr.

Minor and Temporary Side Effects

Minor and temporary side effects can be quite disabling unless anticipated and dealt with. The most common and problematic are the gastrointestinal and the dermatologic ones.

Gastrointestinal Side Effects. Nausea occurs with abdominal irradiation; onset can be as soon as 1 to 2 hours after treatment. Prior administration of prochlorperazine, ondansetron, or granisetron helps to lessen gastrointestinal upset. Some patients with refractory symptoms may respond to a regimen employing more than one class of antiemetic drug (see Chapter 91). Small, frequent feedings are better tolerated than large ones. If nausea and vomiting become problems, the daily radiation dose can be scaled back or treatment temporarily halted. Head and neck irradiation may cause dryness in the mouth and difficulty with mastication and swallowing. Initiation of pilocarpine (Salagen) and amifostine treatment with the start of radiotherapy can help to maintain salivary function. The use of blenderized meals or liquid dietary supplements can help to maintain adequate caloric intake. Diarrhea resulting from bowel radiation responds to diphenoxylate (Lomotil) and loperamide.

Dermatologic Side Effects. Skin care is often overlooked. Although the use of megavoltage machines has reduced skin exposure to 30% of the total dose delivered, avoidance of heat, abrasion, and excessive sun exposure helps to preserve the integrity of irradiated skin.

PATIENT EDUCATION

Patients undergoing radiation therapy need plenty of emotional support. The fears associated with cancer are compounded by the awesome machinery and concerns about exposure to radiation. Patients who are well informed tolerate therapy better than those who are not. Answering questions and addressing concerns about the rationale for radiation therapy, the side effects to be expected, and how they will be controlled are essential to the successful conduct of a radiation therapy program. Printed and online information about radiation treatment can be very useful for the patient. In particular, one needs to review the risk for sterility with patients of reproductive age and the chances of a second malignancy in patients considering curative radiotherapy. Such cost–benefit discussions are critical to helping the patient make an informed choice. Knowing that treatment can be adjusted to one's tolerance to therapy is also reassuring. Patient support groups are often available to help the patient and the family cope with the diagnosis and treatment.

COORDINATION OF CARE

Conducting a radiotherapy program is in the province of the radiation oncologist, carried out in the context of an overall treatment plan developed by the surgeon, medical oncologist, and radiation oncologist in consultation with the primary care physician. The primary physician can ensure that the therapeutic program is well suited to the patient's needs and carefully monitored. A multidisciplinary team approach works best when one member has been designated as the person to whom the patient can always turn for advice and help; in many instances, this important role can be best carried out by the primary care physician.

Annotated Bibliography

1. Fletcher GH. The evolution of the basic concepts underlying the practice of radiotherapy. Radiology 1978;127:3. (*Classic discussion of the development of combination therapy with radiation as one component.*)
2. Lichter AS, Lawrence TS. Recent advances in radiation oncology. N Engl J Med 1995;332:371. (*A review emphasizing technical advances and treatment results, in addition to providing an overview of the basic principles of radiation therapy; 115 references.*)
3. Tannock IF. Treatment of cancer with radiation and drugs. J Clin Oncol 1996;14:3156. (*Critical review of the status of combined chemotherapy and radiation.*)
4. Thames HD, Ang KK. Altered fractionation: radiobiological principles, clinical results, and potential for dose escalation. Cancer Treat Res 1998;93:101. (*A discussion of fractionation.*)
5. Auchter RM, Lamond JP, Alexander E, et al. A multiinstitutional outcome and prognostic factor analysis of radiosurgery for resectable single brain metastasis. Int J Radiat Oncol Biol Phys 1996;35:27. (*Results of radiosurgery were similar to those of resection for single brain metastases.*)
6. Gunderson LL, Willett CG, Harrison L, et al. Intraoperative irradiation: current and future status. Semin Oncol 1997;24:715. (*Details rationale and results.*)
7. Morris AD, Morris RD, Wilson JF, et al. Breast-conserving therapy vs. mastectomy in early-stage breast cancer: a meta-analysis of 10-years. Cancer J Sci Am 1997;3:6. (*An example of curative radiotherapy.*)
8. Press OW, Eary JF, Appelbaum FR, et al. Phase II trial of ^{131}I-B1 (anti-CD20) antibody therapy with autologous stem cell transplantation for relapsed B-cell lymphomas. Lancet 1995;346:336. (*A promising report of systemic radiotherapy in which a radionuclide is coupled to a monoclonal antibody.*)
9. Ragde H, Blasko JC, Grimm PD, et al. Interstitial iodine 125 radiation without adjuvant therapy in the treatment of clinically localized prostate carcinoma. Cancer 1997;80:442. (*Template-guided brachytherapy under real-time ultrasonographic visualization yields excellent treatment results at 7 years.*)
10. Shipley WU, Winter KA, Kaufman DS, et al. Phase III trial of neoadjuvant chemotherapy in patients with invasive bladder cancer treated with selective bladder preservation by combined radiation therapy and chemotherapy:

initial results of Radiation Therapy Oncology Group 89-03. J Clin Oncol 1998;16:3576. (*Excellent example of the use of conservative surgery, chemotherapy, and radiotherapy as a paradigm for organ-preserving approaches to cancer treatment.*)

11. Zelefsky MJ, Fuks Z, Hunt M, et al. High-dose intensity modulated radiation therapy for prostate cancer: early toxicity and biochemical outcome in 772 patients. Int J Radiat Oncol Biol Phys 2002;53:1111. (*Sophisticated computerized treatment planning and control of delivery allows further dose escalation with fewer toxicities.*)

12. Zelefsky MJ, Leibel SA, Gaudin PB, et al. Dose escalation with three-dimensional conformal radiation therapy affects the outcome in prostate cancer. Int J Radiat Oncol Biol Phys 1998;41:491. (*Technical innovations allow escalation of radiation dose and improve outcome.*)

13. Bonner JA, Harari PM, Giralt J, et al. Radiotherapy plus cetuximab for squamous cell carcinoma of the head and neck. N Engl J Med 2006;354:567.

(*The first study to show that the addition of a targeted therapy to definitive radiation therapy can improve survival.*)

14. Stewart JR, Fajardo LF, Gillette SM, et al. Radiation injury to the heart. Int J Radiat Oncol Biol Phys 1995;31:1205. (*Constrictive pericarditis, valvular thickening, and infarction may occur.*)

15. Taghian A, de Vathaire F, Terrier P, et al. Long-term risk of sarcoma following radiation treatment for breast cancer. Int J Radiat Oncol Biol Phys 1991;21:361. (*The cumulative incidence of sarcoma was 0.2% at 10 years.*)

16. Travis LB, Hill DA, Dores GM, et al. Breast cancer following radiotherapy and chemotherapy among young women with Hodgkin disease. JAMA 2003;290:465. (*A matched case–control study that found that a significantly increased risk of breast cancer was associated with radiation therapy.*)

17. Tucker MA, Coleman CN, Cox RS, et al. Risk of second cancers after treatment for Hodgkin's disease. N Engl J Med 1988;318:76. (*The risk was found to be 1% annually for patients undergoing curative therapy.*)

CHAPTER 90 ■ MANAGEMENT OF CHRONIC CANCER PAIN AND PALLIATIVE CARE

PART 1: MANAGEMENT OF CHRONIC CANCER PAIN

LINDA A. KING AND J. ANDREW BILLINGS

The relief of pain is an essential objective in the treatment of the cancer patient at all phases of the illness. Unrelieved pain interferes with a patient's ability to work, enjoy life, and function maximally in family and society. Effective amelioration of pain can almost always be achieved with the proper use of analgesics. Unfortunately, the undertreatment of pain is frequent. Common barriers to effective pain management reflect problems with health care professionals, patients, and the health care system, and they need to be explored actively and addressed (Table 90.1).

Fear of unrelieved cancer pain is widespread. The primary care physician must know the appropriate treatments and their limitations and must also be able to support the cancer patient and minimize the emotional suffering that is invariably intertwined with the perception of pain.

Pathophysiology and Clinical Presentation (1–3)

Pain in cancer patients may result from direct effects of the tumor (e.g., infiltration into bone, viscera, nerves), from treatments directed at the cancer (e.g., chemotherapy, radiation, surgery), or from causes unrelated to the cancer (e.g., arthritis, migraines). Three broad physiologic categories describe the major underlying pathophysiology: somatic, visceral, and neu-

ropathic. Multiple pain complaints caused by multiple mechanisms are the rule.

Somatic pain arises from the activation of nociceptors in cutaneous or deep musculoskeletal tissues. This pain is usually well localized and often described as dull or aching. Examples include pain from bone metastases, surgical incision, and radiation burns.

Visceral pain results from infiltration, compression, or distention of thoracic or abdominal viscera. It is usually poorly localized and often described as deep, squeezing, or as if caused by pressure. Referral of the pain to overlying or distant cutaneous sites is common. Causes of visceral pain include hepatic metastases that distend the liver capsule and metastases that obstruct the biliary tree, bowel, or urinary tract.

Neuropathic pain results from direct injury to the peripheral or central nervous system. Pain from nerve injury may be described as constant, aching, or squeezing (and thus may be similar to somatic pain); paroxysms of sharp, burning, or shocklike pain may be superimposed and are pathognomonic. The pain may follow a nerve distribution and can be associated with sensory or motor (including sphincter) disturbances that indicate a neurologic injury. Allodynia is pathognomonic. Causes of neuropathic pain include spinal nerve root compression, radiation-induced plexopathy, and chemotherapy-associated neuropathy.

Common Pain Syndromes

Bone Pain

Metastases to the bony skeleton are a common cause of cancer pain. The development of pain in a bony site is invariably secondary to the interruption of the cortex, which may or may not be observed radiographically. Common sites are vertebrae, long bones, pelvis, and skull. Any tumor type can involve bone;

BARRIERS TO CANCER PAIN MANAGEMENT

Problems Related to Health Care Professionals
Inadequate knowledge of pain management
Poor assessment of pain
Concern about the regulation of controlled substances
Fear of patient addiction
Concern about side effects of analgesics
Concern about patients becoming tolerant to analgesics

Problems Related to Patients
Reluctance to report pain
Concern about distracting the physician from the treatment
  of underlying disease
Fear that pain means the disease is worse
Concern about not being a "good patient"
Reluctance to take pain medications
Fear of addiction or of being thought of as an addict
Worries about unmanageable side effects
Concern about becoming tolerant to pain medications

Problems Related to the Health Care System
Low priority given to cancer pain treatment
Inadequate reimbursement and prohibitive costs
Restrictive regulation of controlled substances
Problems of availability of treatment or access to it

From Jacox A, Carr DB, Payne R, et al. Management of cancer pain. Clinical practice guideline No. 9 (AHCPR publication No. 94-0592). Rockville, MD: Agency for Health Care Policy and Research, U.S. Department of Health and Human Services, Public Health Service, March 1994.

the most common are metastatic *lung*, *breast*, and *prostate cancers* and *multiple myeloma*. Some tumors produce either lytic or blastic lesions alone, but most produce mixed lesions. Bone pain is typically somatic unless the tumor or a fracture disrupts a nerve.

Back Pain

Back pain in patients with cancer usually signifies bone or epidural metastasis. Untreated *metastases* may destabilize the spine and encroach on the spinal cord or cauda equina. Rapid progression of back pain in a patient with cancer is an oncologic emergency and requires prompt evaluation to rule out *spinal cord compression* and irreversible neurologic compromise. *Leptomeningeal carcinomatosis* may cause back pain in the absence of vertebral disease. *Thoracic pain* may be a consequence of local invasion of the intercostal nerves. Pleuritic pain may develop if a malignancy spreads to involve the pleura. Direct invasion of a contiguous bony structure may result in local or referred pain.

Abdominal and Pelvic Pain

Abdominal and pelvic pain from cancer is typically visceral in nature and therefore poorly localized and possibly referred to distant sites. Anorexia, nausea, and vomiting are common accompaniments. Crampy pain is characteristic of intestinal obstruction (see Chapter 58). Ascites can be uncomfortable because of associated abdominal distention. Hepatic metastases may cause pain by distending the liver capsule or irritating the peritoneal surface.

Peripheral Nerve Compression

Peripheral nerve compression syndromes result in pain in the shoulder or arm (*brachial plexus*), buttocks and perineum (*sacral plexus*), lumbar area (*paraspinal nerves*), and mouth or face (*trigeminal nerve*). All are secondary to nerve entrapment and, occasionally, to nerve invasion by tumor growth.

WORKUP (4,5)

Prompt, careful assessment of the cancer patient's pain is essential to the timely design and implementation of a rational treatment plan. Assessment should be carried out at the time of the initial report of pain, at regular intervals thereafter, and with any treatment changes. Cancer patients commonly report multiple types of pain. Each complaint should be individually assessed and prioritized. Because pain is a subjective phenomenon, the patient's report of pain must be taken seriously. The focus of the workup includes an assessment of the underlying mechanism(s) of pain in addition to their impact on the patient's quality of life (especially sleep) and ability to carry out the activities of daily living.

History

A careful pain history will characterize the location, intensity, temporal pattern, and quality of the pain, as well as aggravating and alleviating factors (including medication) and associated symptoms. Well-localized pain suggests a somatic mechanism; more-diffuse pain is indicative of a visceral source; and a nerve distribution points to a neuropathic cause. Pain that is somatic in quality suggests bony metastasis. If the pain is more diffuse and visceral in quality, one needs to consider capsular distention and also the obstruction of a viscus, whether bowel, biliary tree, or urinary tract. A neuropathic distribution should lead to a check for sensory and motor disturbances (including those involving sphincters).

A numeric rating scale (Fig. 90.1) helps to quantify pain intensity, follow it over time, and standardize assessment among

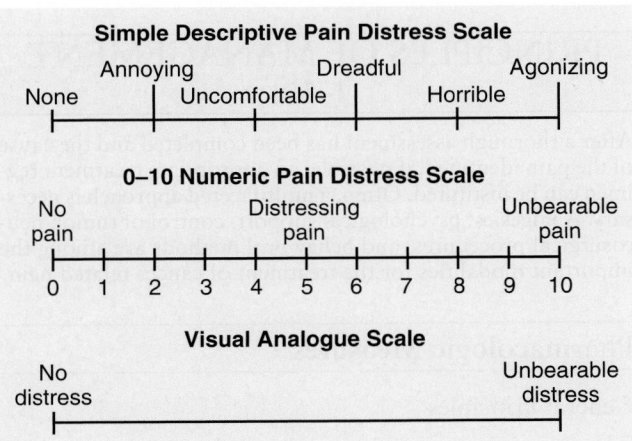

FIGURE 90.1. Pain assessment intensity scales. (From Jacox A, Carr DB, Payne R, et al. Management of cancer pain. Clinical practice guideline No. 9 [AHCPR publication No. 94-0592]. Rockville, MD: Agency for Health Care Policy and Research, U.S. Department of Health and Human Services, Public Health Service, March 1994.)

clinicians. Exploring the past use of analgesic therapies, their effectiveness, and their side effects helps in the design of the treatment program.

Another important component of the history is elucidating the effect of the pain on the patient's psychosocial state (mood, relationships with others) and on activities of daily living (especially sleeping, dressing, eating, and moving around). A numeric rating scale (see Fig. 90.1) helps to quantify pain intensity and follow it over time. Exploring the past use of analgesic therapies, their effectiveness, and their side effects helps in the design of the treatment program. Identifying how the patient interprets the meaning of the pain provides an opportunity to understand and ease the worry that contributes to the pain.

Physical Examination

A focused physical examination can provide essential corroborating evidence for the underlying mechanism(s) and site(s) of pain suggested by the history. A careful neurologic examination can confirm the neuronal distribution of the pain. Examining for motor and sensory deficits and sphincter incompetence is critical. Similarly, somatic pain may be confirmed by the finding of focal tenderness. If the pain is poorly localized, then examination for an obstructed viscus or distended organ capsule is in order.

Laboratory Studies

Imaging studies and other laboratory means of confirming the cause of pain are especially important to management when a surgical, chemotherapeutic, or radiotherapeutic approach to pain control is being considered. Determining the specific cause of the pain (e.g., bone metastases, bowel obstruction, spinal cord compression) allows appropriate, disease-specific therapy to be instituted. Patients with advanced disease who are not candidates for such aggressive therapeutic measures need not undergo extensive testing unless the results will affect clinical decision making. In such patients, the decision to initiate or escalate an analgesic program may require little more than a good clinical assessment. In any event, while the workup is proceeding, troublesome pain should be treated empirically.

PRINCIPLES OF MANAGEMENT (1–10)

After a thorough assessment has been completed and the cause of the pain identified, if possible, an appropriate treatment regimen can be instituted. Often, a multifaceted approach is necessary. Analgesics, psychological support, control of tumor, neurosurgical procedures, and behavioral methods are among the important modalities for the treatment of cancer-related pain.

Pharmacologic Measures

General Principles

Selection of the appropriate analgesic therapy must be individualized for each patient. The World Health Organization's analgesic ladder (Fig. 90.2) provides a standard initial approach to drug selection for cancer pain, based on pain severity and previous analgesic use. The ladder begins with the use of acetaminophen, aspirin, or nonsteroidal antiinflammatory drugs (NSAIDs) for mild to moderate pain. When pain persists or increases, a weak opioid or a stronger opioid at a low dose is added. Pain that is moderate to severe at presentation or more persistent should be treated with opioids at higher doses or with a stronger opioid preparation. The simplest route and dosage schedule and the least invasive pain management measures are preferred for initial use. Chronic cancer pain requires around-the-clock or basal (not as-needed) dosing, supplemented by as-needed (PRN) "rescue" doses for breakthrough pain.

Acetaminophen, Aspirin, and Nonsteroidal Antiinflammatory Drugs

These nonopioid drugs comprise the analgesics useful as initial therapy for mild pain (Table 90.2). Except for acetaminophen (which has no antiinflammatory action), they have analgesic, antipyretic, and antiinflammatory effects. Adding aspirin or acetaminophen to an oral opioid regimen can boost the analgesic effect, which may allow the use of lower opioid doses and reduce opioid side effects. Unlike opioids, none of these drugs produces tolerance or physical dependence, but they do have a ceiling to their analgesic effects, beyond which no additional analgesia is achieved. The long-term use of oral NSAIDs for pain control in cancer has not been well studied, but the evidence suggests reasonable efficacy, especially for bone pain or pain with an inflammatory component.

The analgesia provided by NSAIDs is equivalent to that of aspirin, acetaminophen, and opioids at low doses. NSAIDs are available in various oral formulations, including tablets, capsules, and liquids. Ketorolac, the only parenteral NSAID preparation, is recommended for short-term (<5 days) use only. Because responses to individual NSAIDs vary, titration of the dose and trials of different preparations are occasionally necessary to achieve the best response. (For a discussion of adverse effects, see Chapters 68 and 156.)

Cyclooxygenase-2 Inhibitors

The selective cyclooxygenase-2 (COX-2) inhibitors block both isoforms of cyclooxygenase to inhibit prostaglandin synthesis. The COX-1 isoform is found in abundance in platelets, and its inhibition by NSAIDs is responsible for many of the side effects of these drugs. COX-2 inhibitors are believed to cause fewer gastrointestinal and platelet side effects than do the traditional NSAIDs, but they are significantly more expensive and have been associated with an increased risk of thrombotic complications (see Chapter 156). Celecoxib (Celebrex) has relatively lower COX-2 selectivity than preparations that were withdrawn from the market and is still available.

Opioids

Opioids are the preferred analgesics for the management of moderate to severe cancer pain. They are highly effective, easily titrated, and generally well tolerated.

Titration and Dosing. Opioid doses are titrated in each patient to maximize pain relief promptly and minimize side effects. Dose requirements vary greatly among patients and with time, so that careful and ongoing titration is necessary to achieve and maintain adequate analgesia. The degree of analgesia that can be provided by increasing the dose of opioids is not limited, as it is with nonopioid analgesics.

To provide optimal *chronic pain control*, opioids should be prescribed on a *regularly scheduled (around-the-clock) basis* rather than on a PRN basis. This regimen actually reduces the

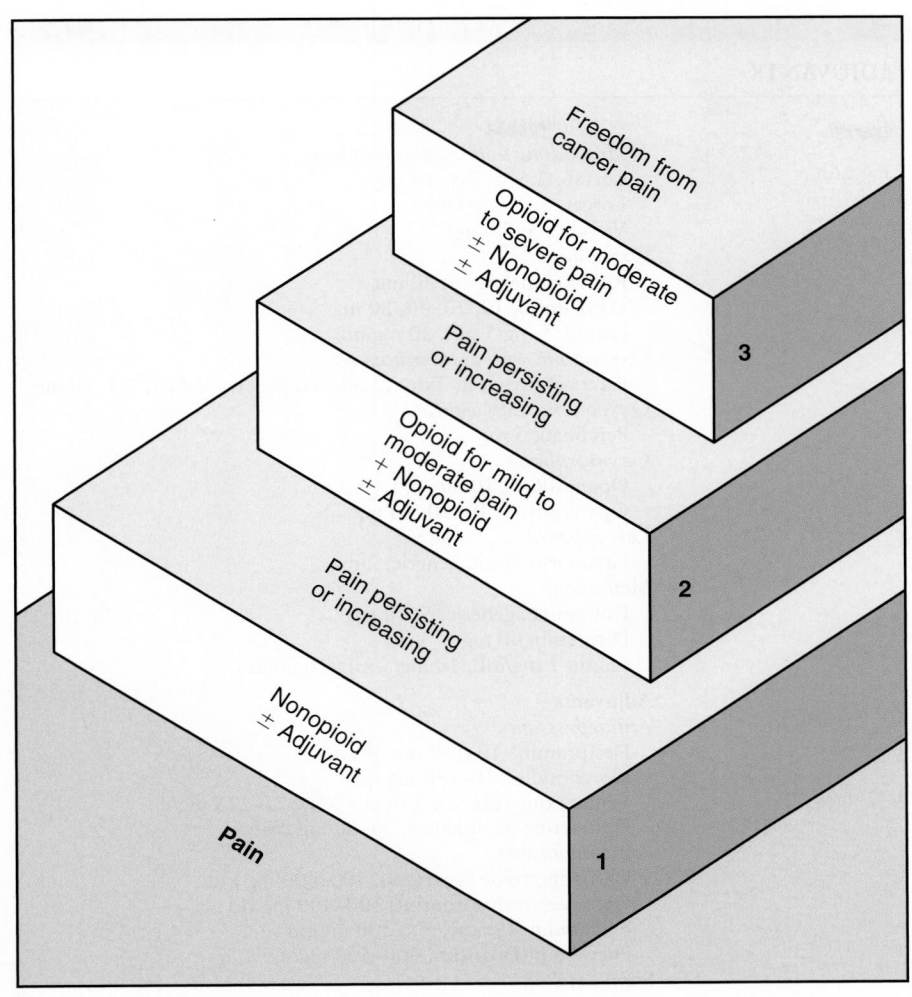

FIGURE 90.2. The World Health Organization's three-step analgesic ladder. (From world Health Organization. Cancer pain relief: with a guide to opioid availability, 2nd ed. Geneva: Author, 1996:15, with permission.)

total daily amount of opioid required to control pain, as compared to a purely PRN regimen.

Dose titration is best accomplished by using a *short-acting preparation* and rapidly increasing the dose until pain resolves. The dose is increased by about 25% if pain persists; 50% increases are appropriate for severe pain. The goal is rapid implementation of effective pain control, accomplished by going "fast and high." Once the necessary daily opioid dose is established, a *long-acting oral preparation* that is taken two or three times daily or transdermal fentanyl can be substituted at an equianalgesic total daily dose.

For *breakthrough pain*, concomitant *shorter-acting oral opioids* should always be prescribed. Breakthrough doses should be approximately equivalent to 10% to 25% of the total 24-hour dose and should be used every 1 to 4 hours as needed. In patients with acute worsening of pain who require frequent doses of breakthrough medication, or when pain is difficult to control or sedation is problematic, *patient-controlled intravenous analgesia* can be useful. The patient's use of bolus doses becomes a guide to establishing an appropriate basal infusion (typically increased 25% during the night).

Routes of Administration. The oral route of opioid administration (Table 90.2) is ideal for patient convenience, but other routes (Table 90.3) are available for patients who cannot take their medication by mouth. The intravenous (IV) route allows for the continuous administration of opioids in addition to that of rapidly acting intermittent boluses as needed, although at a greater cost than that of other routes. Intramuscular (IM) dosing should generally be avoided because of the discomfort associated with injection and the availability of other, equally effective routes of delivery. Clinicians must understand equianalgesic dose guidelines and the duration of action when switching between opioids or routes of administration. In general, the same opioid doses are required for oral, sublingual, buccal, and rectal administration. Similarly, roughly the same doses are required for IM, IV, and subcutaneous (SC) administration.

Side Effects. The most common side effects of opioids include *constipation, nausea, vomiting,* and *sedation*; less commonly, these agents produce *psychosis* and *delirium, pruritus, myoclonus, dry mouth,* and *urinary retention.* Significant *respiratory depression,* a dreaded side effect in the treatment of acute pain, is extremely rare and not a concern in the carefully conducted management of chronic pain.

Constipation (and, occasionally, nausea and vomiting) should be treated prophylactically while monitoring carefully for other side effects. Although tolerance to many side effects (including nausea, sedation, and respiratory depression)

TABLE 90.2

COMMONLY USED ANALGESICS AND ADJUVANTS

Nonopioid Analgesics
Acetaminophen and Salicylates
    Acetaminophen, up to 650 mg q4h or 975 mg q6h
    Aspirin, up to 650 mg q4h or 975 mg q6h
    Choline magnesium trisalicylate (Trilisate),
       750–1,500 mg tid
Nonsteroidal Antiinflammatory Drugs
    Ibuprofen (Motrin, Advil), 600 mg q6h
    Naproxen (Naprosyn, Aleve), 250–500 mg bid
    Ketorolac (Toradol), 30 mg IM or IV q6h
       (up to 5 d)
    Celecoxib (Celebrex), 100–200 mg bid

Opioid Analgesics
Morphine
    MSIR tablets or capsules, 15, 30 mg
    MSIR "soluble" tablets, 10, 15, 30 mg
    Roxanol (elixir), 10 mg/5 mL, 20 mg/5 mL,
       100 mg/5 mL
    MS Contin, 15, 30, 60, 100, 200 mg
    Oramorph SR, 15, 30, 60, 100 mg
    Avinza, 30, 60, 90, 120 mg
    Kadian, 20, 30, 50, 60, 80, 100, 200 mg
Fentanyl
    Duragesic transdermal patches, 12.5, 25, 50, 75, 100 μg
    Actiq transmucosal lozenges, 200, 400, 600, 800,
       1,200, 1,600 μg
    Fentora buccal tablets, 100, 200, 400, 600, 800 μg
Hydromorphone
    Dilaudid, generic, 2, 4, 8 mg
    Liquid 5 mg/5 mL
    Suppository, 3 mg
Codeine
    Codeine sulfate tablets, 15, 30, 60 mg
    Elixir and solution, 15 mg/mL
Codeine with acetaminophen
    Tylenol No. 2, No. 3, No. 4 (15, 30, 60 mg,
       respectively)
Codeine with aspirin
    Empirin No. 3, No. 4, 30, 60 mg, respectively
               (continued)

(Continued)
Hydrocodone with acetaminophen
    Lortab, 2.5, 5, 7.5, 10 mg
    Lorcet, 5, 7.5, 10 mg
    Vicodin, 5, 7.5 mg
Oxycodone
    Roxicodone, 5, 15, 30 mg
    OxyContin, 10, 20, 40, 80 mg
    Liquid, 5 mg/5 mL, 20 mg/mL
Oxycodone with acetaminophen
    Percocet, Roxicet, Tylox, Endocet, generic, 2.5, 5, 7.5, 10 mg
Oxycodone with aspirin
    Percodan, 5 mg
Oxymorphone
    Opana IR, 5, 10 mg
    Opana ER, 5, 10, 20, 40 mg
Levorphanol
    Levo-Dromoran, generic, 2 mg
Methadone
    Dolophine, generic, 5, 10 mg
    Dispertab, 40 mg
    Liquid 1 mg/mL, 10 mg/5 mL, 10 mg/mL

Adjuvants
Antidepressants
    Desipramine 10–150 mg qhs
    Nortriptyline 10–150 mg qhs
    Venlafaxine (Effexor, Effexor XR), 75–225 mg/d
    Duloxetine (Cymbalta), 30–60 mg daily
Anticonvulsants
    Carbamazepine (Tegretol), 100–800 mg bid
    Gabapentin (Neurontin), 100–400 mg tid
    Pregabalin (Lyrica), 50 –200 mg tid
    Phenytoin (Dilantin), 300–500 mg/d
Stimulants
    Dextroamphetamine (Dexedrine), 5–10 mg/d bid
    Methylphenidate (Ritalin), 2.5–15.0 mg qd–bid
    Modafinil (Provigil), 200–400 mg daily
Corticosteroids
    Dexamethasone (Decadron), 4–96 mg bid–qid
    Prednisone, 10–100 mg/d bid

bid, twice daily; q4h, every 4 hours; q6h; every 6 hours; qd, daily; qhs, at bedtime; qid, four times a day; tid, three times a day; PO, orally;
IM, intramuscularly.
Adapted from Jacox A, Carr DB, Payne R, et al. Management of cancer pain. Clinical practice guideline No. 9 (AHCPR publication No. 94-0592).
Rockville, MD: Agency for Health Care Policy and Research, U.S. Department of Health and Human Services, Public Health Service, March 1994; and
Fowler B, Lynch M, Abrahm J. *Pain management tables and guidelines.* Boston:Dana Farber Cancer Institute Pain and Palliative Care Program, 2004;
with permission.

typically occurs over 1 to 5 days, constipation persists and should be managed with regularly scheduled laxative regimens (see Chapter 91).

Tolerance. Opioid tolerance is defined as the need for an increasing amount of drug to achieve the same analgesic effect. Tolerance develops with regular opioid use and is manifested by a shortened duration of pain control and an overall increase in the perception of pain. *The addition of a nonopioid analgesic* (see prior discussion) *or an adjuvant drug* (see later discussion) can compensate for tolerance, but the simplest means of overcoming tolerance is to *increase dose or dose frequency.* *Cross-tolerance* among opioids is common but not complete after prolonged opioid administration, so that it may be

possible to boost analgesia by switching to another opioid, starting at as low as 1/10 of the equianalgesic dose.

Dependence. *Physiologic dependence* presents as the development of opioid *withdrawal* symptoms if opioids are abruptly discontinued or if opioid antagonists are administered. A withdrawal syndrome, although usually mild in patients with cancer pain, can be easily avoided by tapering the opioid dose by roughly 25%/d over a few days to a week.

Psychological dependence (*addiction*) is an abnormal behavior pattern in which a person becomes *overwhelmingly involved in the acquisition and use of a drug.* Addiction is very uncommon in cancer patients who take opioids for pain relief. Patients and their families should be counseled about the

TABLE 90.3

APPROXIMATE EQUIANALGESIC DOSES OF SHORT-ACTING OPIOIDS FOR CHRONIC PAIN[a,b]

Oral Dose (mg)	Usual Oral Dosing Interval	Analgesic	Parenteral Dose (mg)	Usual Parenteral Dosing Interval
200	q3–4h	Codeine	130	q3–4h
30	q3–4h	Hydrocodone (Vicodin, Zydone)		
20–30		Oxycodone (Percodan, Percocet, Tylox, Roxicet, Roxicodone, Roxiprin)[c,d]		
30	q4h	Morphine[c,e,f]	10	q3–4h
20	q4–12h	Methadone (Dolophine)[g]	10	q4–8h
7.5	q3–4h	Hydromorphone (Dilaudid)[e]	1.5	q3–4h
4	q4–6h	Levorphanol (Levo-Dromoran)	2	q4–6h

h, hours; q, every.

Fentanyl (Duragesic) patch or other long-acting opioid preparations should be considered for patients with a relatively stable basal dose and relatively well controlled pain. According to the manufacturer, a 10-mg intramuscular (IM) or subcutaneous (SC) or intravenous (IV) dose or 60-mg oral dose of morphine every 4 hr for 24 hr (total 60 mg/d IM/SC/IV or 360 mg/d oral) is approximately equivalent to transdermal fentanyl 100 μg/hr. Palliative care clinicians generally divide the 24-hr oral morphine dosage by 3.8 to get the roughly equivalent dose per hour of fentanyl. Patches should be replaced every 48–72 hr.

[a]All doses and intervals are approximate and should be adjusted according to the patient's response. When a patient has been on a particular opioid for weeks or months, conversion to a relatively lower dose of another opioid is often adequate, especially with methadone, which has occasionally been reported to be 5–30 times as potent as predicted by this kind of table when used after prolonged or high-dose treatment with other opioids.

[b]This table does not include meperidine (Demerol) or pentazocine (Talwin), which generally should not be used for chronic cancer pain.

[c]Oxycodone is available as a long-acting preparation (OxyContin). Morphine is also available in long-acting preparations—MS Contin or Oramorph SR, lasting 8–12 hr, or Avinza or Kadian, lasting 24 hours. Sustained-action tablets should not be crushed or chewed, but Kadian and Avinza capsules can be broken and suspended in a liquid.

[d]Some oxycodone preparations are compounded with acetaminophen or aspirin. Acetaminophen should not exceed 4,000 mg/d for prolonged periods.

[e]Morphine and hydromorphone (Dilaudid) are available as suppositories. Rectal dose and intervals are generally the same as with oral administration.

[f]Liquid morphine preparations can be administered by the sublingual or buccal route. Dose and intervals are similar to those for oral administration.

[g]Methadone's long half-life may be associated with an accumulation of opioid and the delayed development of toxicity and may allow for longer dosing intervals. When switching to methadone from high doses or prolonged administration of other opioids, a pain or palliative care specialist should be consulted.

rarity of addiction when opioids are prescribed for cancer pain because misconceptions often result in the avoidance of pain medications or the underreporting of pain. Similarly, health care professionals often inappropriately withhold opioids from patients who could benefit from these analgesics.

Pseudo-addiction describes the development of *drug-seeking behaviors* that resemble psychological dependence but that occur with *inadequate* and *inappropriate pain regimens*, such as "only-as-needed" dosing for continuous pain, dosing intervals longer than the duration of action of the medication, or inadequate doses. The drug-seeking behaviors are eliminated if an appropriate analgesic regimen is prescribed.

Choice of Opioid Agent. Choice should coincide with the patient's needs. For patients with *mild to moderate pain* that is becoming persistent, a *low-potency opioid* such as *codeine* is a reasonable initial choice. As one of the least potent opioids, starting doses (15 to 30 mg) provide pain control comparable to that achieved with full analgesic doses of aspirin, acetaminophen, or an NSAID. Codeine in *combination with acetaminophen* provides effective analgesia at low cost for patients with mild to moderate pain.

For *more severe pain*, the related compounds *oxycodone* and *hydrocodone* are about eight times more potent than codeine and are similar in potency to morphine. These opioids are also available in combination with aspirin and acetaminophen. The potential for toxicity at higher daily doses of the nonopioids in these formulations may limit the overall dose of the preparation that can be administered daily. Oxycodone is available in a long-acting, *slow-release formulation* (e.g., OxyContin) with an effect lasting 8 to 12 hours. *Morphine* is the prototype opioid analgesic for severe cancer pain.

It is effective both orally and parenterally and has a duration of action of approximately 3 to 4 hours. The use of *sustained-release preparations* (e.g., MS Contin, Oramorph SR, Kadian, Avinza) provides prolonged analgesia (8 to 24 hours) with less frequent dosing, but the cost can be substantial. These long-acting formulations cannot be crushed or chewed, but Kadian and Avinza capsules can be broken open and the contents sprinkled into food or liquid for patients who cannot swallow pills easily or are receiving tube feedings.

Hydromorphone (Dilaudid) is *more potent than morphine*, although its duration of action is briefer and it is also more costly. The duration of action and strength are reduced considerably when it is taken orally rather than parenterally. Because hydromorphone is more potent and more soluble than morphine, a smaller injected volume can be used in patients requiring parenteral opioid infusions.

Oxymorphone, a metabolite of oxycodone, is now available in both short-acting and long-acting oral formulations (Opana, Opana ER). Oral oxymorphone is *three times more potent than oral morphine*. Taking oxymorphone with food or alcohol increases its peak concentration and should be avoided.

Methadone and levorphanol have proved useful because of their *longer duration of action*. The cost of methadone is low, which makes it an attractive alternative to long-acting morphine preparations. With repeated dosing, excessive central nervous system depression can result because of the sustained half-life of these agents. Careful dose titration is required for proper use. Recent reports describe a risk of *QT-interval prolongation* and *torsades de pointes* with high-dose methadone.

Meperidine (Demerol) is available for both oral and parenteral use but is not recommended for chronic cancer pain because of the *short duration of action* plus potentially serious side effects. Its metabolite, normeperidine, causes *dysphoria*, *tremors*, and *irritability*, especially in patients with impaired renal function. In patients taking monoamine oxidase inhibitors, meperidine can cause serious and sometimes lethal side effects.

Fentanyl, a potent opioid, is available for parenteral administration but also as a *transdermal* preparation for long-acting analgesia and as an *oral transmucosal system* for acute or incident pain. The transdermal preparation (Duragesic patch) provides 2 to 3 days of continuous analgesia but is generally more expensive than oral opioids and requires careful titration to avoid excessive sedation. The use of transdermal fentanyl should generally be reserved for patients who are already receiving opioid therapy. The starting dose should be based on the patient's previous morphine requirement or determined empirically by starting with the lowest-strength patch.

There are several oral transmucosal formulations of fentanyl. Actiq contains fentanyl in a cherry-flavored "lollipop" matrix that is absorbed across the buccal mucosa when applied to the inside of the cheek for 10 to 20 minutes. Although it is available in various strengths, all patients should be started with the lowest (200 μg) strength, with further titration based on efficacy and side effects. Fentora is fentanyl in an effervescent buccal tablet. Doses of Fentora are lower than those for Actiq because of its greater absorption.

Pentazocine (Talwin) and butorphanol tartrate (Stadol) are opioid agonists–antagonists available orally and as a nasal spray, respectively. The opioid-antagonist qualities of these drugs can precipitate withdrawal in a patient already taking an opioid agonist; therefore, they are not optimal drugs for cancer patients with longstanding opioid requirements.

Adjuvant Agents

Various agents can be used to enhance the effectiveness of the analgesics discussed previously and sometimes may be effective as sole agents (see Table 90.2), especially when rapidly escalating opioid doses lead to sedation.

Tricyclic Antidepressants. (see Chapter 227). These antidepressants are effective for *neuropathic pain, concurrent depression*, and *sleep disturbance* related to ongoing pain. The analgesic effects may occur at lower doses and may develop more quickly than the antidepressant effects. Starting doses of desipramine or nortriptyline (as low as 10 to 25 mg at bedtime) can reduce pain, with upward dose adjustment as necessary. Anticholinergic side effects and sedation may limit titration, especially in the elderly.

Serotonin and Norepinephrine Reuptake Inhibitors. *Venlafaxine (Effexor)* and *duloxetine (Cymbalta)* have shown some benefit for neuropathic pain, as well as depression. Side effects are typically less than seen with the tricyclic antidepressants, but their cost is greater, and efficacy is less well established. *Selective serotonin reuptake inhibitors* appear to be minimally effective for neuropathic pain.

Anticonvulsants and Local Anesthetics. *Gabapentin* (Neurontin), *carbamazepine* (Tegretol), and *phenytoin* (Dilantin), as well as newer anticonvulsant drugs such as *pregabalin* (Lyrica), *topiramate* (Topamax), and *lamotrigine* (Lamictal), show some activity in relieving neuropathic pain. Doses should be started low and titrated to effect. Local anesthetics such as IV *lidocaine* and oral *mexiletine* have also been used effectively on occasion for neuropathic pain. A transdermal lidocaine patch (Lidoderm) has shown efficacy for postherpetic neuralgia.

Stimulants. *Dextroamphetamine* (Dexedrine) and *methylphenidate*(Ritalin) are sometimes used to counter the somnolence associated with opioid use, and they may improve analgesia. They can also have the beneficial effects of increasing energy and appetite and are effective, quick-acting antidepressants. The narcolepsy drug *modafinil* (Provigil) also appears to be beneficial in managing opioid-induced sedation.

Glucocorticoids. These agents may lessen the pain associated with tumor-associated inflammation or infiltration while improving appetite and providing a stimulant effect with an enhanced sense of well-being. The anticipated side effects of ongoing corticosteroid use (hyperglycemia, edema, infection, gastrointestinal bleeding; see Chapter 105) may limit their long-term use.

Benzodiazepines. These agents are helpful on an intermittent basis if a patient reports situational stress or anxiety or increased pain with resultant difficulty in falling asleep. They can also assist in the management of nausea and vomiting (see Chapter 92). However, delirium may be aggravated by benzodiazepines (except in the case of sedative–hypnotic withdrawal); agitation caused by depression should be treated with an antidepressant.

Bisphosphonates and Calcitonin. Monthly bisphosphonate therapy has been shown to reduce bone pain and the incidence of pathologic fractures in certain cancers by inhibiting osteoclast activity. Calcitonin can reduce pain in the setting of pathologic fracture (see Chapter 164).

Nonpharmacologic Measures: Physical and Psychological Modalities

These interventions represent an important component of a multifaceted approach to pain management. Such interventions should be used with, not instead of, appropriate analgesic regimens.

Physical Modalities

Cutaneous stimulation by the application of *cold* or *hot* packs or by the use of *massage, vibration, transcutaneous electrical stimulation*, or *acupuncture* helps to manage pain when employed in conjunction with appropriate analgesics. These modalities are easy to use and relatively inexpensive, and they cause minimal morbidity.

Psychosocial Interventions

Relaxation techniques (focused-breathing exercises, meditation, music therapy), *guided imagery, biofeedback*, and *hypnosis* can be very helpful, especially for episodic pain and pain related to specific activities. These easily learned techniques enable patients to gain a sense of control over the pain. Belief in the validity of the underlying method strongly correlates with a positive outcome.

Psychological Support

The importance of psychological support from both physician and family cannot be overemphasized. The active involvement of the primary physician is vital to the successful control of pain. The empathy and confidence expressed, with attention to the patient's concerns (including fears of tolerance and addiction), are as central to effective pain relief as are tumor control and the proper use of analgesics (see Chapter 87).

Nonpharmacologic Measures: Invasive Modalities

Anesthetic Procedures

Patients in whom adequate pain control is not achieved with application of any the aforementioned measures or who experience intolerable side effects may be candidates for invasive anesthetic or neurosurgical procedures. Before such an invasive measure is used, a multidisciplinary team including oncologists, pain specialists, and neurosurgeons should review the situation to ensure appropriate patient selection. The pain must be characterized as precisely as possible to target the planned interventions appropriately. A number of approaches are available.

Epidural or intrathecal injection of opioids and local anesthetics can be used for either short-term or long-term control of intractable pain. Operator expertise is essential to ensure proper catheter placement and manage potential complications, including respiratory depression, hypotension, and infection. An *implanted programmable pump* can deliver opioids and other drugs into the intrathecal space of patients who have benefited from an initial trial of neuraxial analgesics. These devices can be refilled percutaneously and are most appropriate for patients with at least a 3-month prognosis.

Nerve blocks use the application of a local anesthetic, corticosteroid, or neurolytic agent to control intractable pain related to an identifiable nerve structure. The application of a short-acting local anesthetic provides useful diagnostic and management information by confirming the specific source of pain and predicting likely side effects of the procedure. Once an appropriate site has been identified by diagnostic block, a neurolytic agent such as ethanol or phenol is injected to destroy the involved nerve and provide long-term pain relief. Neurolytic blocks can relieve pain related to tumor infiltration of the upper abdominal organs (celiac block), pelvic organs (hypogastric block), head and neck (stellate ganglion block), and legs (lumbar sympathetic block). Precise technique is required for the successful implementation of a nerve block and to prevent damage to surrounding tissue and other nerves.

Neurosurgical procedures for pain control are used infrequently because of the development of more advanced, radiologically guided techniques for anesthetic blocks. Pituitary ablation (hypophysectomy) has been used successfully in rare patients with refractory disseminated pain.

INDICATIONS FOR REFERRAL AND ADMISSION

The successful management of cancer pain requires a team approach. The primary physician plays a major role in the design and implementation of an effective analgesic program and in monitoring the patient for painful complications of the malignancy. When such complications arise, prompt consultation with the oncologist, radiation therapist, or surgeon is often indicated because of the potential need for further systemic treatment or additional local measures. Patients with refractory pain in the absence of evident, focally approachable disease may benefit from consultation with a pain or palliative care specialist. The patient with new onset of pain suggestive of spinal cord compression or pathologic fracture requires prompt consultation and hospital admission.

PATIENT AND FAMILY EDUCATION

Patients endure their condition much better when they know that additional pain relief is available. Educational effort should take into account any cultural or language barriers that might contribute to undertreatment, a phenomenon noted with greater frequency among minority patients with cancer. To avoid underdosing, all family and health care team members need to be informed of the patient's analgesic needs and the minimal risk for true addiction. The issues of drug tolerance and physiologic dependence should be reviewed and their significance discussed. Few patients should have to endure disabling pain, given the array of effective treatment modalities available. Many patients do best when they maintain an active role in their care. Enlisting their help in the design, implementation, and monitoring of the pain management program can be of considerable psychological benefit. Effective pain control is central to sustaining a reasonable quality of life and is one of the most basic requests of cancer patients.

RECOMMENDATIONS (4,5)

- Carefully assess each complaint of pain. Patients may have multiple pains with multiple origins and mechanisms.
- Attempt to diagnose each underlying cause because specific causes respond best to specific treatments. In particular, be alert for bone pain, neuropathic pain, and cord compression.
- Treat the worry in addition to the discomfort. Psychological support contributes greatly to effective pain control.
- Use the stepped approach for analgesic use as outlined by the World Health Organization's analgesic ladder, while recognizing that analgesic therapy must be individualized for each patient.
  1. For *mild-to-moderate pain*, begin with acetaminophen, aspirin, or NSAIDs.
  2. When pain *persists* or *increases*, add a weak opioid or a stronger opioid at a low dose.
  3. For pain that is *moderate to severe*, treat with higher doses of opioids or a stronger opioid preparation.
  4. Add in adjuvants promptly when neuropathic pain is problematic or the side effects of analgesics are limiting effectiveness.
  5. Treat *chronic cancer pain* with around-the-clock (*not as-needed*) dosing, supplemented by as-needed ("rescue") doses for breakthrough pain.
- Initiate opioid therapy by quickly establishing the necessary opioid dose. Do this by titrating with a short-acting preparation, increasing each dose by 25% to 50% until satisfactory pain control is achieved. Use as high a dose of opioid as is necessary to achieve effective pain relief. Once the effective dose is established, switch to a long-acting preparation along with a short-acting rescue or breakthrough agent.
- Treat "*breakthrough*" *pain* with doses of a short-acting opioid equal to 10% to 25% of the total 24-hour opioid dose and give every 2 to 4 hours as needed.
- Use the simplest route of administration, the most convenient dosage schedule, and the least invasive pain management measures. Oral therapy is preferred.
- Address common misunderstandings about addiction to minimize underdosing.
- Consider adding simple nonpharmacologic modalities, such as the application of heat or cold, massage, relaxation

techniques, and guided imagery, which can complement appropriate analgesic regimens.

- If *tolerance* to one opioid makes the analgesic regimen problematic, consider switching to another opioid.
- Use equianalgesic doses when switching between different opioids and routes.
- To help control severe *neuropathic* or *bone pain*, consider an adjuvant agent (e.g., tricyclic antidepressant or anticonvulsant for neuropathic pain, NSAIDs or bisphosphonate for bone pain).

- Minimize the adverse effects of opioid use by periodically adjusting the dose and always prescribing laxatives to prevent severe constipation.
- For *pain caused by severe localized disease*, consider tumor-specific therapy (e.g., radiation, surgery, chemotherapy).
- Reassess frequently and at regular intervals, especially when pain worsens and after medication changes have been made.
- When pain is not responding well to treatment, reevaluate the role of psychosocial factors, consider whether pain is neuropathic, and seek help from pain or palliative care specialists.

Annotated Bibliography

1. American Pain Society. Principles of analgesic use, 5th ed. Skokie, IL: Author, 2003. (*An excellent resource on pain medications and their proper use.*)
2. Bernabei R, Gabmassi G, Lapane K, et al. Management of pain in elderly patients with cancer. JAMA 1998;279:1877. (*Highlights populations at particular risk for inadequate pain management.*)
3. Bruera E, Kim HK. Cancer pain. JAMA 2003; 290:2476. (*A recent summary of strategies to manage cancer pain.*)
4. National Comprehensive Cancer Network. NCCN Clinical Practice Guidelines in Oncology. Adult cancer pain. Version 1.2008. Available at: http://www.nccn.org/professionals/physician_gls/PDF/pain.pdf. (*A consensus statement by the National Comprehensive Cancer Network experts on cancer pain management.*)
5. Miaskowski C, Cleary J, Burney R, et al. Guideline for the management of cancer pain in adults and children. Glenview, IL: American Pain Society, 2005. (*A comprehensive clinical practice guideline from the American Pain Society, accompanied by a guide for patients.*)
6. Bruera E, Sweeney C. Methadone use in cancer patients with pain: a review. J Palliative Med 2002;5:127. (*A thoughtful review of the benefits and challenges of using methadone for pain control in cancer patients.*)
7. Markman JD, Philip A. Interventional approaches to pain management. Med Clin North Am. 2007;91:271. (*A review of the most commonly used procedures for pain management.*)
8. McNicol E, Horowicz-Mehler N, Fisk RA, et al. Management of opioid side effects in cancer-related and chronic noncancer pain: a systematic review. J Pain 2003;4(5):231. (*A systematic review of the incidence and treatment of various opioid side effects.*)
9. Drugs for pain. Treatment Guidelines from the Medical Letter. 2007;56:23. (*A succinct overview, providing a very useful comparisons of drugs.*)
10. Ross J, Saunders Y, Edmonds P, et al. Systematic review of role of bisphosphonates on skeletal morbidity in metastatic cancer. BMJ. 2003;237:469. (*A systematic review of the use of bisphosphonates for bone pain and complications in cancer.*)

PART 2: PALLIATIVE CARE

ERIC L. KRAKAUER

Palliative care is comprehensive care focused on alleviating suffering and optimizing the quality of life of patients living with a life-threatening or terminal illness. Major concerns are pain and symptom relief, information sharing and advance care planning, psychosocial and spiritual support of both the patient and family, and the coordination of care, including arranging for services in the community. The orchestration and provision of palliative care is part of the purview of any primary physician who cares for a dying patient. It may be provided in an acute care hospital, a skilled nursing facility, an inpatient hospice, or the home. Community hospice organizations can assist in arranging palliative care outside of the hospital.

PRINCIPLES OF PALLIATIVE CARE (1–10)

Transition to Palliative Care

Although attention to palliation and comfort should be part of the care plan for all patients, including those receiving disease-modifying or life-sustaining treatments, many patients reach a point at which they want the primary focus of care to shift to comfort and achievement of the best possible quality of life. Helping patients and surrogates to determine the timing of this

shift often requires (a) an assessment of their understanding of the diagnosis and prognosis; (b) the communication of information about the illness—what is wrong, the likely outcomes, the potential benefits and burdens of each potential treatment plan; and (c) an understanding of the patients' goals and values. Previously executed advance directives such as a living will, health care proxy, or durable power of attorney for health care can be useful in these discussions. Factors that may impede a patient's ability to make treatment decisions, such as delirium, dementia, or denial, should be taken into account. When the patient's capacity to understand medical information is questionable, a psychiatric consultation may be useful. Efforts should be made to discern and respect cultural and familial factors that may inform a patient's decisions.

Nonabandonment

As the goal of care shifts from cure or life support to comfort, it is important to reassure patients, surrogates, and families through words and deeds that they will not be ignored or abandoned and that attentive palliative care will be provided. A decision to forego disease-modifying or life-sustaining interventions or to request a "Do Not Resuscitate" or "Comfort Measures Only" order should never lead to a diminution of attention to the patient's well-being. Phoning a patient or making a home visit can be very comforting.

Proportionality

When deliberating with patients or surrogates about specific treatments, it is important to weigh the potential benefits against the potential or certain burdens. If a treatment seems likely to be more burdensome than beneficial by the patient's criteria, the physician should suggest that it not be used.

Withholding and Withdrawing Treatments

It sometimes can be emotionally more difficult for surrogates and families to withdraw life-sustaining treatments that have been initiated than to withhold them. However, it is widely accepted that no ethical or legal distinction should be made between withdrawing and withholding such treatments if the patient would not want them or if their burdens to the patient would outweigh the benefits by the patient's criteria. When discussing with surrogates or families the withdrawing or withholding of artificial nutrition and artificial hydration, it may be helpful to allay the common misconception that lack of nutrition or dehydration is necessarily uncomfortable or inhumane (see the later sections on the management of anorexia and of dry mouth, respectively).

Comprehensive Care

Palliative care is best provided by a team, directed by the physician, that may include nurses, social workers, chaplains, hospice workers, health aides, and specialists in oncology, radiation therapy, psychiatry, surgery, interventional radiology, or palliative care. Regular case review with team members is necessary to ensure coordinated, high-quality care. Although the patient is the focus of care, the family's emotional, social, and spiritual needs also require attention, both for their well-being and for the patient's. After the patient's death, grieving families may benefit from bereavement care.

Maximizing Dignity and a Sense of Control

Patients may fear the loss of dignity and control as much as any physical symptom. "Dignity-conserving care" entails treating even the most debilitated, dependent, and vulnerable patient with kindness and respect. The care plan should be developed so as to maximize the patient's personal sense of dignity and to give the patient as great a sense of control as possible.

Double Effect

It is important to make clear to patients, surrogates, families, and clinicians that palliative care or a shift of focus to comfort is not euthanasia or physician-assisted suicide. Rather, palliative care is standard, appropriate medical care that can be provided along with curative, disease-modifying or life-sustaining treatment and that becomes essential when such treatment is no longer beneficial or desired. It is particularly important to make this clear when control of the patient's symptoms may require the administration of opioids, benzodiazepines, or other medications in doses high enough to cause serious side effects. In this situation, the principle of double effect can help to guide provision of optimum palliative care.

The principle of double effect states that "an action with two possible effects, one good and one bad, is morally permitted if the action (a) is not in itself immoral; (b) is undertaken only with the *intention* of achieving the possible good effect, without *intending* the possible bad effect even though it may be *foreseen*; (c) does not bring about the possible good effect by means of the possible bad effect; and (d) is undertaken for a proportionately grave reason." For example, a patient with advanced metastatic lung cancer and intractable pain may be given opioids even at the risk of side effects including sedation, hypotension, respiratory depression, respiratory arrest, and death as long as the action (giving opioids to relieve pain) (a) is not in itself immoral (giving opioids for pain is not); (b) is intended only to relieve pain and suffering and to ensure comfort; (c) does not intend to achieve relief and comfort by means of the possible side effect (death); and (d) is undertaken for the purpose of relieving the pain and suffering of a dying patient.

When a terminally ill patient wishes to be made comfortable, the intention of treatment should be to use the minimum doses of medications necessary for comfort—no more but also no less. When it is anticipated that adequate symptom control may risk unintentionally hastening the patient's death, the patient or surrogate should be advised of this and reassured that this is medically appropriate and ethically legitimate, as well as compassionate.

PALLIATIVE CARE ASSESSMENT (1–3,10)

A thorough palliative care assessment includes a comprehensive history and a physical examination. It should address not just the medical issues of the patient, but also the psychosocial and spiritual issues and the needs of the family and significant others. Certain aspects of the palliative care assessment require particular attention.

Review of Symptoms

The palliative care assessment replaces the standard review of systems with a review of *symptoms* that is designed to explore typical causes of suffering at the end of life. It generally should cover pain, shortness of breath, nausea, vomiting, constipation, anorexia, dry mouth, odynophagia, insomnia, anxiety, and depression. Further review of symptoms should be tailored to the patient's illness.

Functional Status

The patient's performance status currently and during the prior 2 weeks should be assessed. Categories might include the following: fully active, restricted strenuous activities, ambulatory/not able to work, limited self-care, and confined to bed or chair/no self-care.

Awareness of Illness and Preferences for Care

The patient's and family's understanding of the diagnosis and prognosis should be explored along with any associated fears. Patients should be asked whether they would like to receive all diagnostic and prognostic information and make all necessary decisions. Some patients may prefer that a surrogate receive this information and make these decisions or that decisions be made by the physician. The existence of any advance directive such as a living will or health care proxy form (durable power of attorney) should be established. The physician particularly needs to know whom the patient wishes to serve as surrogate in the case of decisional incapacity. The patient's hopes and goals for care should be explored and discussed. Helpful questions include the following: "Are there important tasks that would require your immediate attention if you knew that you would be unable to function well in the future?" "If time were limited, what would be your priorities?" "Are there any upcoming events, such as births, weddings, or graduations, that are especially meaningful to you?" The patient's preferred location of care—home or hospital—should be explored. If possible without upsetting the patient, the preferred location of death also should be explored. Two principles are useful guides for discussions about preferences for care: (a) The patient (or surrogate) is the expert on the patient's values, goals, and wishes, and it behooves the physician to try to explore, understand, and respect them. (b) The physician is the expert on the medical means to achieve the patient's goals and to honor the patient's values and wishes. Suboptimal care can result when physicians fail to confirm the patient's values and goals. It also can result when patients or surrogates begin practicing medicine as occurs, for example, when they are offered a menu of life-sustaining treatments from which to choose rather than an informed recommendation, or when they determine opioid doses. These situations should be avoided.

Social History

The social history should probe for sources of social suffering and identify psychosocial supports for both the patient and family. It should include the patient's living situation, names of all immediate and close family members and friends, work history, religion and degree of participation in organized religion, major sources of joy, major losses and stresses including deaths in the family, and the patient's and family's history of coping with these losses.

Medications

When the focus of care is shifted to palliation, the medication list should be reviewed and irrelevant medications discontinued.

Physical Examination

Physical examination should focus on evaluating current symptoms and anticipating future symptoms. Care should be taken to minimize the discomfort of the examination itself.

Laboratory and Imaging Studies

Diagnostic tests not needed for comfort care should not be performed. Occasionally, studies are indicated to help determine the prognosis, plan optimal palliative care, or maximize the patient's quality of life.

Impression

This should include a list of the major medical problems, a determination of prognosis, and a list of actual and potential causes of discomfort. A differential diagnosis of an uncomfortable symptom should be performed whenever the cause is not obvious.

Plan

The treatment plan should be organized primarily by *symptom* rather than by organ system or disease. The list of symptoms should be exhaustive and should include anticipated symptoms. For example, three actual or potential symptoms—abdominal pain, delirium, and acute respiratory distress—may be caused by the same underlying disease, but management of each symptom should be addressed separately. The preferred location of care should be identified and contingency plans made for major changes in the patient's condition. Psychosocial and spiritual supports (family, friends, social worker, clergy, visiting nurses, home health aides, hospice volunteers) should be identified. If relevant, financial or insurance problems should be addressed. Plans should be made to facilitate communication between the physician and the primary caregiver, nurses, and other physicians involved in the patient's care. If the patient wishes to forego resuscitation in the event of cardiac arrest or respiratory failure, a plan should be made to protect the patient from unwanted resuscitation in the event 911 is called. Many states have established protocols for this purpose.

MANAGEMENT OF MAJOR SYMPTOMS IN PALLIATIVE CARE (11–15)

Dyspnea

Dyspnea is a common symptom among terminally ill patients with primary or secondary lung neoplasms, pneumonias, cardiogenic or noncardiogenic pulmonary edema, chronic obstructive pulmonary disease, pulmonary embolism, and other conditions frequently seen at the end of life. The cause (or causes) of dyspnea should be identified and treated as aggressively as is compatible with the overall goals of care. Chest radiography, computed tomography, antibiotics for pneumonia, or thoracentesis, chest tubes, and pleurodesis for large pleural effusions may or may not be appropriate, depending on the patient's wishes and the plan of care. Occasional patients are maintained at home on positive inotropic agents for end-stage congestive heart failure. Workup for pulmonary embolism is rarely indicated for a patient whose care is focused on comfort.

When air hunger persists despite maximal appropriate treatment of the underlying condition, palliative treatment with a strong opioid such as *morphine* is indicated. Mild symptoms can be treated with morphine 5 to 10 mg orally (PO) or sublingually every 4 hours as needed (or around the clock if the symptoms are constant), and the dose can be titrated upward (e.g., to 15, 20, 30 mg) to achieve the desired effect. The regimen for patients who persistently require frequent doses should be changed to a long-acting opioid (e.g., MS Contin) at the equianalgesic dose, with a short-acting rescue dose available as needed for breakthrough dyspnea (see Part 1 of this chapter). For sudden, severe, or rapidly progressing dyspnea that is typical of massive pulmonary embolism, septic shock, or intrapulmonary lymphangitic spread of tumor, SC or IV morphine often is necessary. Even at home, a constant SC or IV infusion can be administered by means of a small infusion device and titrated to comfort. The starting dose depends on the previous dose of opioids and the severity of symptoms. When a change is made from oral to parenteral morphine, the total daily parenteral dose should equal one third of the total daily oral dose.

An opioid-naive patient can be started on an infusion of 1 to 2 mg/hr. Rescue doses of 5% to 10% of the total 24-hour dose can be given for breakthrough dyspnea. If more than one rescue dose is needed in any 2-hour period, the infusion rate can be increased by 25%. In the setting of severe respiratory distress, opioid doses necessary to achieve comfort may have the unintended but foreseeable side effect of hastening death (see preceding discussion of the principle of double effect).

Dyspnea frequently is associated with anxiety. *Benzodiazepines* can be helpful adjuncts to opioids if anxiety persists after the dyspnea is relieved. Troublesome respiratory secretions causing choking, coughing, or respiratory distress can be treated with *scopolamine* transdermal patches (most patients need at least 1 mg/d) or glycopyrrolate via a nebulizer (0.8 mg every 6 hours), orally (1 to 2 mg three times daily), or parenterally (0.1 to 0.2 mg IV or SC every 6 hours). Secretions are often reduced or absent in patients whose artificial nutrition and hydration are discontinued before the terminal phase. Oxygen sometimes reduces dyspnea even in patients who are not hypoxic, as does a cool breeze from a fan.

Anorexia

Anorexia can be the consequence of any of the causes of chronic nausea. In the absence of nausea, it also occurs in association with malignancy, chronic infections such as HIV/AIDS or tuberculosis, end-stage congestive heart failure or cirrhosis, and depression. Treatable underlying causes should be addressed if appropriate. Medications that enhance the appetite for some patients include *megestrol acetate* (Megace; 160 to 800 mg PO daily), a corticosteroid (e.g., *dexamethasone* 4 to 20 mg PO each morning or twice daily in divided doses), or *dronabinol* (Marinol; 2.5 to 5 mg PO twice daily before meals). Artificial nutrition by means of nasogastric, gastrostomy, or jejunostomy tubes or parenteral nutrition often is not appropriate in patients for whom the goal of care is comfort; these interventions may be more burdensome than beneficial by prolonging the dying process and worsening terminal respiratory distress.

Dry Mouth

Xerostomia, a very common symptom among dying patients, may be caused by dehydration, mouth breathing, or opioids and other medications with anticholinergic side effects, or it may follow head and neck surgery or radiation. Patients may take sips or ice chips if they wish. In severe cases, or when patients are unable to sip fluids, a saliva substitute (several commercial brands are available) should be applied every 4 hours around the clock and as needed. Petroleum jelly may be applied to the lips three times a day. Patients and families worried about discontinuing artificial hydration for fear of discomfort from dehydration may be assured that dry mouth is usually the only uncomfortable symptom of dehydration and that careful oral care is effective in preventing it.

Thrush

Candidal infection of the oropharynx and esophagus is common in patients who are immunosuppressed because of cancer, cancer therapy, AIDS, or the use of immunosuppressive medications such as corticosteroids. Oropharyngeal disease in non-AIDS patients may be treated with *fluconazole*, 200 mg single dose PO or IV, or with *nystatin* (5-mL Swish and Swallow four times daily) or *clotrimazole* (10-mg troche five times daily) for 14 days. Patients with AIDS should be given nystatin or clotrimazole as stated or *fluconazole* (100 mg PO or IV daily) for 7 to 14 days.

Constipation

This very common symptom can cause serious distress in terminally ill patients, who frequently are immobile, dehydrated, and taking constipating medications such as opioids. Opioid regimens should virtually always be accompanied by a bowel regimen. Patients should be advised to make sure that they move their bowels at least every 2 to 3 days. A typical starting regimen is *senna* (Senokot, two tablets PO once or twice daily; hold as needed in case of loose stools) and/or *polyethylene glycol* (17 gm in 4 to 8 oz of water or juice PO daily) (see also Chapter 65).

Bowel Obstruction

Bowel obstruction causing abdominal pain or vomiting often can be managed medically even when the obstruction is proximal. *Dexamethasone* (16 mg IV each morning or twice daily in divided doses) has multiple antiemetic effects and may help to reduce a malignant obstruction from complete to partial. *Octreotide* (100 to 200 μg SC or IV every 8 hours or 10 to 50 μg/hr IV drip) can markedly reduce gastrointestinal secretions and bilious vomiting. Depo dosing once per month also is available. With long-term use, biliary sludging and gallstones can occur. IV *morphine* and *scopolamine* can relieve crampy abdominal pain associated with obstruction. If vomiting is refractory, *decompression* may be required with a nasogastric tube. If the obstruction persists and the patient's estimated survival is longer than 1 week, permanent decompression with a venting gastrostomy tube may be considered.

Delirium and Agitation

The myriad possible causes of delirium and agitation in dying patients include side effects of medications, metabolic derangements (e.g., electrolyte abnormalities, uremia, liver failure), pain, infection, and central nervous system disease. Underlying causes should be addressed if this can be done in keeping with the patient's goals. Among medications, common offenders are benzodiazepines, opioids, antihistamines, and anticholinergics. When an opioid is believed to be the offending agent, an alternate opioid can tried. Because of incomplete cross-tolerance to opioids, pain relief is often adequate with two thirds of the equianalgesic dose of the alternate agent. Because of the risk for delirium and paradoxical agitation, *benzodiazepines* such as *lorazepam* (Ativan) should be used cautiously in elderly or debilitated patients. Often, haloperidol (0.5 to 1 mg PO at bedtime or two or three times daily) is all that is needed to promote sleep or relieve agitation.

Depression

For the rapid treatment of depression in a patient with a short prognosis, psychostimulants such as *dextroamphetamine* (Dexedrine) or *methylphenidate* (Ritalin) are the treatments of choice. The dosage for either is 2.5 to 5 mg PO each morning, titrated upward to the desired effect with a maximum of 30 mg PO twice daily, at 8 a.m. and noon (see also Chapter 227). Anxiety and agitation are contraindications and possible side effects (see also Chapter 226).

Sedation

Sedation is a common side effect of opioids and other medications used frequently in palliative care. It can be treated with dextroamphetamine or methylphenidate as stated previously.

Myoclonus

Myoclonus is a common side effect of opioid analgesics, particularly when given in high doses. Its appearance is idiosyncratic and may resolve with a switch to an alternate opioid. Again, adequate analgesia often can be maintained with less than the equianalgesic dose of the alternate agent because of incomplete cross-tolerance. Mild myoclonus may cause no discomfort. If myoclonus is severe or clearly uncomfortable and not controlled by switching to an alternate opioid, *lorazepam* (Ativan; started at 0.5 to 1 mg PO or IV every 6 hours) or *diazepam* (Valium; started at 2 to 5 mg PO or IV every 8 hours) may be effective.

Hemorrhage

Sudden massive hemorrhage can be very distressing to the patient and family members. However, some highly motivated patients and families may remain at home during hemorrhage if they are properly prepared by the primary care physician and if adequate home hospice care or nursing is available to ensure comfort. If massive hemorrhage is a likely scenario, the physician should explore the patient's desire to remain at home and the family's willingness to do whatever is necessary to keep the patient at home. The physician should reconfirm that the goal of care is comfort, that no resuscitation is to be performed, and that no blood products are to be given. The physician also should ascertain that a hospice or visiting nurse is available around the clock and able to get to the home in less than 1 hour. The physician should discuss the possibility of massive hemorrhage with the primary nurse and review the management plan. The physician then should explain to the patient and family what might happen, what the patient might feel, and exactly what measures would be taken to ensure comfort.

When hemorrhaging occurs, several simple steps are appropriate. First, the patient and family should be calmed and reassured that the situation can be handled. The nurse or other clinician on the scene should cover the blood or melena and remove it frequently. A strong opioid like morphine and/or a benzodiazepine such as lorazepam should be given IV or SC to calm the patient. A constant IV or SC infusion of the opioid should be started. As the patient exsanguinates, additional symptoms may arise, such as shortness of breath, chest pain from ischemia, lightheadedness, and anxiety. Rescue doses (IV or SC boluses) of the opioid and sometimes also of the benzodiazepine should be given to control these symptoms quickly.

Pain

See Part 1 of this chapter.

Ascites

See Chapters 71, 91, and 92.

Hiccups

See Chapter 221.

Nausea and Vomiting

See Chapters 59 and 91.

Dysphagia, Odynophagia

See Chapter 60.

Insomnia

See Chapter 232.

Seizure

See Chapter 170.

Pressure Ulcers

See Chapter 197.

Pruritus

See Chapter 178.

Terminal Distress

See section on dyspnea.

OTHER ISSUES AND INDICATIONS FOR ADMISSION

Hospice and Home Services

Hospice services are available in inpatient hospices, in some nursing homes, and at home through home hospice organizations or visiting nurse associations. The primary care physician may choose to remain in charge of the patient's care in all settings. Most hospices accept patients only when the patient and family are aware of the terminal diagnosis and prognosis and accept care focused primarily on comfort.

Psychosocial and Spiritual Support

Emotional and spiritual support and counseling can be extremely important for dying patients and their loved ones. All accredited hospice organizations have a social worker, chaplain, and volunteers available. They can assist with the search for meaning in the dying process, religious and spiritual issues, anticipatory grieving, life review, preparation of a legacy, and financial issues.

Bereavement

Hospices also make available some form of support for bereaved family members and loved ones. A note of condolence from the physician with an offer to be available by phone to answer any lingering questions can be very comforting. The physician also might call the family to provide support, answer questions, and assess the need for a referral for formal bereavement counseling.

Indications for Admission

In some situations, it is necessary to admit a patient to the hospital to protect the patient from end-of-life suffering. For example, a patient with severe or refractory pain, dyspnea, or seizures may require treatments not available at home. In other cases, adequate home nursing care may not be available, or the family may be overwhelmed. Patients who are near death may be admitted for terminal care. Others are admitted just long enough to control symptoms and arrange appropriate end-of-life care in a skilled nursing facility, inpatient hospice, or the home.

CONCLUSIONS AND RECOMMENDATIONS

- Patients with chronic life-threatening illnesses and their families need reassurance that attentive comfort care can be provided if desired in lieu of aggressive, life-sustaining treatment.
- The benefits and burdens of all diagnostic and therapeutic measures should be weighed, and the physician should suggest that predominately burdensome measures not be used.
- Ethical or legal distinctions usually are not made between withdrawing and withholding a treatment that is more burdensome than beneficial or not desired by the patient.
- Artificial nutrition and hydration are medical treatments that may be provided or not provided, like any other intervention, depending on the benefit-to-burden ratio and the patient's or surrogate's wishes.
- Treatments intended only to relieve serious refractory symptoms in a terminally ill patient often may be provided even at the risk of unintended but foreseeable side effects, including a hastening of death.
- Sources of physical and psychosocial suffering should be thoroughly explored, along with the patient's awareness of the diagnosis and prognosis and preferences for end-of-life care.
- A differential diagnosis of uncomfortable symptoms should be performed and the underlying cause treated to the fullest extent consistent with the goals of care.
- The physician should anticipate sources of terminal distress and make treatment plans in advance.
- Dyspnea can be treated with a strong opioid such as morphine administered PO, sublingually, IV, or SC.
- Troublesome respiratory secretions can be treated with anticholinergics such as scopolamine or glycopyrrolate.
- Xerostomia should be treated with a saliva substitute around the clock, particularly in dehydrated patients.
- Inpatient and outpatient hospice services are available to help manage symptoms and psychosocial problems under the direction of the physician. Hospice teams include nurses, social workers, chaplains, health aides, and volunteers.
- Dying patients sometimes must be admitted to the hospital to control refractory symptoms.

Annotated Bibliography

1. Block SD. Assessing and managing depression in the terminally ill patient. Ann Intern Med 2000;132:209. (*A superb review of grief and clinical depression in the terminally ill patient, with an overview of treatment recommendations.*)
2. Block SD, Billings JA. Patient requests to hasten death: evaluation and management in terminal care. Arch Intern Med 1994;154:2039. (*An excellent discussion of ways to understand and manage patients' requests to hasten death.*)
3. Chochonov HM. Dignity and the essence of medicine: the A, B, C, and D of dignity conserving care. BMJ 2007;335:184. (*An inspiring examination of the simple, yet often neglected ways for physicians to fulfill their fundamental obligation to care for the patient.*)
4. Covinsky KE, Goldman L, Cook EF, et al. The impact of serious illness on patients' families. JAMA 1994;272:1839. (*A good analysis of the often severe social and economic burdens on family members of terminally ill patients.*)
5. Dunn PM, Levinson W. Discussing futility with patients and families. J Gen Intern Med 1996;11:689. (*A nice analysis of pitfalls encountered in discussing end-of-life care with patients and families.*)
6. Ebell MH, Becker LA, Barry HC, et al. Survival after in-hospital cardiopulmonary resuscitation: a meta-analysis. J Gen Intern Med 1998;13:805. (*A very useful meta-analysis of data on cardiopulmonary resuscitation outcomes in patients with various underlying conditions.*)
7. Krakauer EL, Crenner C, Fox K. Barriers to optimum end-of-life care for minority patients. J Am Geriatr Soc 2002;50:182. (*A review of institutional, cultural, and individual barriers to optimum end-of-life care for minority patients; includes suggestions for providing culturally sensitive care.*)
8. Sepulveda C, Marlin A, Yoshida T, et al. Palliative care: the World Organization's global perspective. J Pain Symptom Manage 2002;24:91. (*The World Health Organization's definition of palliative care and an overview of available guidelines.*)
9. Sulmasy DP, Pellegrino ED. The rule of double effect. Arch Intern Med 1999;159:545. (*A good overview of the principle of double effect and its critical importance to palliative care.*)
10. SUPPORT Investigators. A controlled trial to improve care for seriously ill hospitalized patients. JAMA 1995;274:1591. (*A summary of the most comprehensive study of end-of-life care.*)
11. Ganzini L. Artificial nutrition and hydration at the end of life: ethics and evidence. Palliat Support Care 2006;4:135. (*A review of the evidence supporting and not supporting a beneficial effect of artificial nutrition and hydration at the end of life, together with a review of the ethical and legal principles governing decisions about artificial nutrition and hydration at the end of life.*)
12. Krakauer EL, Penson RT, Truog RD, et al. Sedation for intractable distress of a dying patient: acute palliative care and the principle of double effect. Oncologist 2000;5:53. (*A discussion of medical and ethical issues involved in sedating dying patients with intractable distress.*)
13. Mercadante S, Casuccio A, Mangione S. Medical treatment for inoperable malignant bowel obstruction: a qualitative systematic review. J Pain Symptom Manage 2007;33:217. (*A systematic review of randomized trials of the most commonly used drugs in the medical management of inoperable malignant bowel obstruction, assessing the effectiveness of these treatments.*)
14. Qaseem A, Snow V, Shekelle P, et al. Evidence-based interventions to improve the palliative care of pain, dyspnea, and depression at the end of life: a clinical practice guideline from the American College of Physicians. Ann Intern Med 2008;148:141. (*Recommendations for effective palliative interventions based on a systematic review of the literature.*)
15. Weil JV, McCullough RE, Kline JS, et al. Diminished ventilatory response to hypoxia and hypercapnia after morphine in normal man. N Engl J Med 1975;292:1103. (*A classic study demonstrating a physiologic reason for the effectiveness of morphine in treating air hunger resulting from hypoxia or hypercapnia.*)

CHAPTER 91 ■ MANAGING THE GASTROINTESTINAL COMPLICATIONS OF CANCER AND CANCER TREATMENT

JEFFREY W. CLARK

The gastrointestinal symptoms that accompany cancer and cancer therapy are among the most difficult for the patient to bear, often compromising nutritional status and quality of life. Problems may arise from primary disease, metastases, side effects of therapy, or metabolic disturbances. Successful primary care of the cancer patient necessitates attending to the anorexia, nausea, vomiting, weight loss, abdominal pain, ascites, diarrhea, and related gastrointestinal problems that often worsen their lives.

NAUSEA AND VOMITING (1–13)

Cancer therapies are far and away the leading cause of nausea and vomiting in patients with malignancy. The prevention and control of nausea and vomiting is very important, not only for patient comfort, but also for to ensure the ongoing delivery of a full course of treatment. The presentation of emesis may precede, follow soon after, or follow after a delay from the time of delivery of cancer therapy; it may also become persistent.

Pathophysiology and Clinical Presentation

There are both peripheral and central components of therapy-induced nausea and vomiting. The peripheral pathway involves acute injury to the rapidly dividing cells of the gastric mucosa. The resultant cellular damage and accompanying inflammation cause the release of serotonin from gastric enterochromaffin cells into the gastric lumen, with subsequent activation of *serotonin S3-receptors* in the gut wall and centrally in the brainstem vomiting center. Central stimulation of the vomiting center is also believed to occur when chemotherapy drugs directly stimulate the chemoreceptor trigger zone. A number of central receptors effecting emesis have been identified, including those responsive to *dopamine, endorphin, serotonin,* and *substance P.*

Most treatments produce *acute,* self-limited emesis that lasts only a few hours; however, the experience can be very uncomfortable, exhausting, and demoralizing. A milder, *delayed* emesis that can occur 1 to 5 days after therapy is most commonly seen with cisplatin therapy and is believed to be related to the development of gastritis and the persistence of active drug metabolites. Although less severe, it is discouraging and can impede nutrition. *Anticipatory* vomiting is a psychogenic behavioral phenomenon derived from the association of severe emesis with the administration of cancer treatment. Nausea and vomiting can be brought on just by the anticipation of chemotherapy. *Refractory emesis* suggests a metabolic or

anatomic complication of cancer or cancer therapy (see later discussion).

Antiemetic Agents

Serotonin S3-Receptor Blockers (Ondansetron, Granisetron, Dolasetron)

Serotonin S3-receptor blockers (5-HT3 antagonists) (Ondansetron, Granisetron, Dolasetron) have been found to be effective in the prevention of both acute and delayed chemotherapy-induced nausea and vomiting. When the drugs are used alone, complete prevention of acute nausea and vomiting is achieved in about 40% to 50% of patients; more than 70% have no vomiting but some nausea. When they are combined with a program of acute glucocorticoid therapy (e.g., *dexamethasone*), their prophylactic efficacy increases to 90% for prevention of emesis and to 70% for prevention of both nausea and vomiting. All three available serotonin blockers are similar with regard to efficacy and side effects, which include constipation, headache (occasionally severe), mild dizziness, and a transient, clinically insignificant prolongation of electrocardiographic intervals. These drugs can be administered intravenously (IV) or orally.

Ondansetron is the most commonly used of the oral preparations (one to four 8-mg doses are administered orally prior to chemotherapy [or the equivalent IV dose can be given as appropriate], and then one 8-mg dose can be given every 8 hours as needed). The use of one or the other of these agents depends on the familiarity of oncologist with the agent(s) and cost issues. As new 5-HT3 antagonists with different properties are introduced, it is important to consider the potential value of these properties in making decisions about using one agent or another in a specific situation.

Glucocorticoids

Glucocorticoids have been found to be effective, especially in the prevention of delayed nausea and vomiting (perhaps because of their antiinflammatory effects). In controlled trials, they have outperformed phenothiazines in the prevention of acute emesis and work well in combination with 5-HT3 antagonists, which make them particularly attractive. They also do not have the sedative effects seen with most other antinausea medications (except the 5-HT3 antagonists). However, they can cause restlessness or difficulty with sleep. A typical program is a 4- to 10-mg oral dose of dexamethasone given just before chemotherapy, followed by three more doses given every 6 hours.

Metoclopramide

Metoclopramide blocks both dopaminergic and serotonin receptors, which accounts for its antiemetic action and its side effects. Given parenterally in high doses just before chemotherapy, it too can suppress emesis, but to a considerably lesser degree than the serotonin-receptor blockers (42% complete suppression vs. 75%). It is frequently used at lower doses given more frequently in combination with other agents, especially to prevent delayed emesis. Its dopaminergic blocking effect promotes gastric emptying and gastroesophageal sphincter closure but also leads to dystonia in young patients and mental confusion in older patients. It is usually given orally, although it can also be administered IV.

Substance P Blockade (Neurokinin-1–Receptor Antagonists; Aprepitant [Emend])

The identification of substance P receptors in the central sites triggering emesis has led to the investigation of agents that block such receptors and inhibit substance P–mediated effects. Substance P blockers in combination with 5-HT$_3$ blockers and dexamethasone have significant additional benefit, especially in the prevention of delayed emesis. This improves the prevention of delayed emesis especially for highly emetogenic regimens, such as those containing high-dose cisplatin. It is given orally for 3 days beginning the day that chemotherapy is started.

Benzodiazepines

Benzodiazepines potentiate the activities of the central inhibitory neurotransmitter γ-aminobutyric acid and can enhance the antiemetic effects of other agents. They also cause a desirable degree of mild amnesia. A short-acting preparation such as *lorazepam* is commonly given both before chemotherapy and then on an ongoing basis. It too is best used as part of a combination program. Some prescribe an *antihistamine* (e.g., diphenhydramine) in place of a benzodiazepine. *Psychogenic vomiting* that occurs in anticipation of chemotherapy responds to sublingual, oral, or IV lorazepam or oral alprazolam in conjunction with behavioral *desensitization* therapy; however, the best treatment is prevention of emesis at the outset of chemotherapy. This point cannot be emphasized to strongly.

Phenothiazines

Phenothiazines, such as *prochlorperazine* (Compazine), are well established as a treatment for mild nausea and vomiting associated with other conditions, but they are less effective in chemotherapy if used alone. However, when combined with other antiemetic agents, they may help to provide additional prophylaxis. Phenothiazines act centrally, blocking serotonin and dopamine receptors in the chemoreceptor trigger zone. Sedation accompanies their use and is often desired, but extrapyramidal symptoms may also ensue. They are available in oral, suppository, and parenteral forms. The route of administration has little influence on effectiveness. On the day of treatment, a prochlorperazine capsule or suppository is given 4 to 8 hours before the administration of chemotherapy and again on a regularly scheduled basis for the next 24 hours. The main drawback to phenothiazine therapy is the precipitation of extrapyramidal symptoms, which are most likely to occur when daily doses exceed 50 mg. Their onset necessitates discontinuation of therapy. Under such circumstances, the mild antiemetic *trimethobenzamide* (Tigan) is worth a try, although it is less effective than prochlorperazine. *Haloperidol*, a major tranquilizer that is not a phenothiazine, is similar to prochlorperazine in antiemetic and extrapyramidal effects. It blocks dopaminergic receptors. Side effects are similar to those of metoclopramide.

Cannabinoids and Marijuana

Cannabinoids and marijuana were transiently popular, but they were found to be little better than phenothiazines and have been supplanted by more effective regimens with fewer side effects. Evidence suggests that there are some antinausea and appetite-stimulant effects with the use of purified tetrahydrocannabinol (Marinol), which can be used in combination with other agents to prevent or decrease nausea or vomiting. Side effects include somnolence and confusion (which is usually mild but can be bothersome, especially in older patients). There is no evidence that smoking crude marijuana is required to achieve these effects.

Design of a Comprehensive Prophylactic Program

The optimal goal of antiemetic therapy is to prevent the nausea and vomiting associated with cancer therapy. This eliminates the dread of undergoing therapy and prevents any behaviorally triggered emesis. To design an effective prophylactic program, the physician must be familiar with the propensity of various agents to cause emesis (Table 91.1) and the mechanisms and synergistic effects of available antiemetic drugs (Table 91.2).

A combination strategy takes advantage of the mechanistic synergistic effects afforded by administering effective drugs with different modes of action. More complete and extended prophylaxis, the use of lower doses of individual agents, and therefore a reduction in side effects become possible. For example, to treat a patient with anticipatory, acute, and delayed forms of emesis, an effective program might include a benzodiazepine (lorazepam), a serotonin-receptor blocker (e.g., ondansetron), and a corticosteroid (dexamethasone). For highly emetogenic chemotherapeutic agents, the neurokinin-1–receptor antagonist Emend can be added. A small amount of light food intake before chemotherapy is encouraged because it minimizes retching on an empty stomach, which produces muscle cramps and pain.

Refractory Emesis

A few treatable causes need to be considered when a patient presents with refractory emesis. Persistent vomiting can be a manifestation of *bowel obstruction* or severe *ileus*, which respond to decompression by *nasogastric suctioning*. *Hypercalcemia* and *hypokalemia* may be causes, as well as consequences, of vomiting; the monitoring of electrolytes and the correction of any imbalances can help to lessen the anorexia, nausea, and vomiting that sometimes accompany them.

ANOREXIA AND WEIGHT LOSS (13)

The cachexia of cancer is one of its hallmark manifestations, characterized by anorexia, early satiety, profound weight loss, and inanition. Maintaining adequate nutrition becomes very difficult in this situation. However, it is important to encourage and help this in whatever manner is possible.

TABLE 91.1

CHEMOTHERAPEUTIC AGENTS AND THEIR EMETIC POTENTIAL

Agent	Emetic Potential	Agent	Emetic Potential	Agent	Emetic Potential
Cisplatin	High	5-Fluorouracil	Low	Lomustine	Moderate
Dacarbazine	High	Methotrexate	Low	Doxorubicin	Moderate
Dactinomycin	High	Vincristine	Low	Procarbazine	Moderate
Mechlorethamine	High	Vinblastine	Low	Daunorubicin	Moderate
Cyclophosphamide	High	Chlorambucil	Low	Cytosine arabinoside	Moderate
Carboplatin	Moderate				
Docetaxel	Low				
Paclitaxel	Low				
Gemcitabine	Low				
Etoposide	Low	Carmustine	Moderate		
Bleomycin	Low				
Mitomycin C	Low				

Adapted from Gralla RJ. In: DeVita VT, Hellman S, Rosenberg SA, eds. Cancer: principles and practice of oncology, 3rd ed. Philadelphia: Lippincott, 1989:2138, with permission.

Pathophysiology

Although multifactorial, *cachexia* has been strongly linked to elaboration of the macrophage-derived protein *cachectin* (also referred to as *tumor necrosis factor*), which is capable of inducing a wasting syndrome in animals and mediating adverse metabolic changes in human malignancy. Increased gluconeogenesis, excessive catabolism of body protein (especially muscle), abnormal fat metabolism, and abnormal substrate use have all been observed. In addition to cachectin, tumor-induced tissue breakdown, caloric wasting, and sequestration of protein-rich ascitic fluid in the abdomen may also contribute. Further aggravating the situation are disorders of digestion and absorption that are associated with malnutrition, obstructive lesions, and surgical therapies such as gastrectomy or intestinal bypass procedures. Abnormal caloric utilization is a consequence of tumor-related changes of metabolism, with food intake and lean body mass being channeled to support the caloric demands of the tumor.

The mechanisms behind *anorexia* are incompletely understood. A paraneoplastic syndrome has been postulated, linked to a tumor-induced polypeptide that can affect the satiety center in the brain. In addition, radiation and chemotherapeutic agents may contribute by distorting taste, causing stomatitis, and injuring the gastrointestinal mucosa and liver.

Management

The most effective means of overcoming anorexia and cachexia is to achieve control of the underlying malignancy. In the interim, patients need practical suggestions that can be put to immediate use.

Dietary Measures

Small, frequent feedings (about six per day) of foods high in protein and calories should be advised. *Liquid dietary supplements* in the form of milk shakes and commercial preparations are excellent if tolerated. If nausea is prominent, the patient should be advised to try foods that are salty, beverages that are cool and clear, and desserts such as gelatin and popsicles. Dry foods such as toast and crackers also help. Dietians recommend that the food be served in a relaxed family or group setting, attractively prepared and readily available. When altered taste makes food unpalatable, meat should be avoided and dairy products substituted as the main source of protein. Acidic foods may stimulate the appetite when taste acuity seems to wane, as may extra seasoning and spicy foods. The use of zinc to treat dysgeusia has been reported, but the results are not very impressive. Foods best to avoid when nausea is prominent include those that are overly sweet, greasy, or high in fat.

Medications

Tricyclic antidepressants (e.g., amitriptyline) have a nonspecific appetite-stimulating effect that is sometimes helpful and often independent of the antidepressant effect. Corticosteroids have sometimes been used to stimulate appetite, but their effect is transient and not worth the major side effects associated with the high doses and prolonged administration needed to achieve

TABLE 91.2

COMBINATION APPROACH TO PROPHYLAXIS OF CHEMOTHERAPY-INDUCED EMESIS

Select

Neurotransmitter Blocking Agent
   Ondansetron (blocks serotonin S_3-receptors, peripheral
      and central)
   Metoclopramide (blocks dopamine ± serotonin receptors)
   Phenothiazine (blocks central dopamine ± receptors)

Plus

Benzodiazepine or Antihistamine
   orazepam (increases central inhibitory transmission; mild
      amnesia)
   Diphenhydramine (sedates)

Plus

Corticosteroid
   Dexamethasone (mechanism unknown; ?
      antiinflammatory role)
   Methylprednisolone (same)

a sustained increase in appetite. *Megastrol* has been administered as an anabolic steroid with some success. *Marijuana* and Δ-9-tetrahydrocannabinol (*Marinol*) can be effective in stimulating appetite in some patients.

Treatment of Stomatitis

Stomatitis is an often overlooked cause of poor intake and weight loss. The management of chemotherapy-induced stomatitis includes the avoidance of smoking, alcohol, and foods that are very hot, cold, spicy, or salty. Rinsing the mouth out with either bicarbonate or salt in water several times a day can be helpful in decreasing the severity of stomatitis. A mixture of *Benadryl elixir* and *Kaopectate* used as a mouthwash is often helpful and well tolerated. *Chlorhexidine gluconate* is an antimicrobial oral rinse that can be used as a preventative, but a non–alcohol-based mouthwash is better once sores occur. *Viscous Xylocaine* preparations are not very helpful because they wash away quickly and thus provide only very transient relief; paste preparations last considerably longer. Unfortunately, taste can be distorted as a consequence of the topical anesthetic effect.

When radiation therapy to the head and neck results in *xerostomia* and *mucositis*, the dryness and thick secretions can be lessened by chewing gum or sucking on hard candy, which helps to stimulate salivation. The use of gravies and the avoidance of dry foods helps deglutition in patients whose salivary glands are damaged by radiation. In refractory situations, artificial saliva preparations can be used.

MALNUTRITION (14,15)

One of the most serious consequences of nausea, vomiting, and cachexia is malnutrition. A self-perpetuating and debilitating cycle of food rejection and malnutrition weakens host immune defenses and permits further tumor growth. Moreover, host tolerance to radiation and chemotherapy is compromised, so that the ability to tolerate therapeutic doses of either form of treatment is restricted. The goals and methods of nutritional therapy vary according to the patient's clinical situation. In most instances in which gastrointestinal function remains intact, minor dietary alterations and oral dietary supplements are sufficient. More elaborate means of nutritional support are sometimes necessary and appropriate on a temporary basis to tide the patient over a difficult period. Such therapy is rarely indicated in the very late stages of cancer.

Detection

Recognition of mild to moderate malnutrition is important. Manifestations include a 10% weight loss, a serum albumin level of less than 3.5 g/dL, a total lymphocyte count of less than 1,500/mm³, and a serum creatinine level that is low for the patient's size. More-severe malnutrition is characterized by further weight loss, a serum albumin level of less than 3.0 g/dL, and a lymphocyte count of less than 1,000/ mm³.

Use of Supplements

For patients who have upper alimentary discomfort but can still swallow liquids, a *nutritionally complete liquid preparation* may offer a more comfortable and palatable means of keeping well nourished. These preparations are available commercially and are reasonably well tolerated. Most contain all the necessary vitamins and minerals. Lactose-free formulations are available for patients who may have acquired lactose intolerance. Blenderized meals are another alternative.

Hyperalimentation

More-intensive temporary nutritional support is worth considering during difficult phases of cancer therapy, although the evidence of cost-effectiveness is often lacking, and indiscriminate use can be counterproductive and increase morbidity. Most controlled studies of hyperalimentation and other nutritional therapies have failed to demonstrate any significant improvement in response to chemotherapy or radiation, lessening of side effects of these treatment modalities, prolongation of survival, or improved tolerance to higher doses or longer periods of treatment. However, the selective use of hyperalimentation may be of benefit in some instances.

Enteral Hyperalimentation

Enteral hyperalimentaiton is used for the nutritional support of malnourished patients with an *obstructed or injured upper alimentary tract*, provided that the remainder of the gastrointestinal tract is intact. Such hyperalimentation is particularly well suited to patients recovering from radiation or surgery in the upper alimentary tract. A feeding tube is either passed or surgically placed beyond the point of obstruction or injury. An enteral hyperalimentation program can then commence. The use of long (43-in.), flexible silicon nasal feeding tubes makes it possible to administer feedings directly into the distal duodenum or proximal jejunum, so that the risks for aspiration and reflux that occur with gastrostomy feedings are avoided. When a feeding tube cannot be passed nasally, feedings can be administered through a jejunostomy.

Enteral hyperalimentation ues milk-based and soy-based formulas in addition to less viscous formulations, although sometimes a pump is needed. The formulas are quite hypertonic and must be started at less than full strength (usually at half-strength) and increased during several days, as tolerated. Cramps, symptoms of dumping syndrome (flushing, tachycardia, sweating), and diarrhea are the major manifestations of intolerance. The goal is a daily intake of 2,000 to 3,000 calories.

Total Parenteral Nutrition

This alternative form of nutritional support is reserved for short-term use in persons whose oral or enteral intake is likely to be inadequate for more than 10 to 14 days. The best evidence for its efficacy is in severely *malnourished cancer patients about to undergo surgery*; morbidity and mortality are reduced with preoperative administration of total parenteral nutrition. It can be carried out *at home* so long as the patient and family are capable of mastering the procedures necessary to ensure the sterility of the line and the integrity of the infusion apparatus. Visits by a hyperalimentation nurse are also helpful. The access site can be maintained as a heparin lock, which allows the patient to disconnect easily from the infusion. About 12 to 14 hours are needed for infusions daily, which are administered as solutions containing 4.2% or 5.2% amino acids and 20% to 25% glucose. The infusion schedule provides the patient with 10 to 12 hours of independence each day and an opportunity to ambulate. Careful monitoring of metabolic parameters, including glucose, calcium, phosphate, magnesium, blood urea nitrogen, and creatinine levels, is essential, as is close coordination with a hyperalimentation consultant.

DIARRHEA AND CONSTIPATION

Diarrhea

Diarrhea is another gastrointestinal nemesis familiar to cancer patients (see also Chapter 64). When it ensues from radiation- or chemotherapy-induced enteritis, the problem is usually self-limited, resolving within the 1 to 2 weeks needed for the mucosal surface to reconstitute itself. If it is persistent or troublesome, low doses of *diphenoxylate* (Lomotil) or nonprescription *loperamide* (Imodium) can be prescribed for symptomatic relief (see Chapter 64). The use of loperamide aggressively to control diarrhea is especially important for irinotecan-containing chemotherapy. *Steatorrhea* is experienced by patients who have undergone pancreatectomy or who have pancreatic insufficiency; the intake of several *pancreatic enzyme* tablets with each meal (see Chapter 72) usually alleviates the problem. The postgastrectomy patient is at risk for the symptoms of the *dumping syndrome*. Avoidance of sweets and large *fluid volumes* (especially those rich in sugar) helps to prevent attacks, as does lying down after a meal (see Chapter 64).

Constipation

Constipation can be a very troublesome and often unavoidable consequence of *narcotic use* for pain control (see also Chapter 65). However, the prophylactic institution of some simple measures can help to prevent disabling symptoms and fecal impaction. These include a *high-fiber diet*, good *fluid intake* (at least 2 L/d), the use of *stool softeners* (e.g., dioctyl sodium sulfosuccinate), and, if necessary, the administration of a gentle *laxative* before bed (e.g., 15 mL of milk of magnesia). Constipation may also be a sign of *obstruction* in the lower intestinal tract or ileus, conditions that need to be ruled out before laxative therapy is escalated. *Hypokalemia* and *hypercalcemia* are two other important causes that deserve attention.

MALIGNANT ASCITES (16)

Ascites may occur as a complication of diffuse peritoneal implantation or the combination of portal venous hypertension and hypoalbuminemia. When it is caused by peritoneal implants and the primary is unknown, one should consider treatable malignancies such as ovarian cancer. Occasionally, the ascites will cause disabling symptoms such as marked abdominal distention and pain. Only in debilitating circumstances should it be treated. The most direct means is *therapeutic paracentesis*. Recent experience with large-volume paracentesis suggests that it can be performed with safety so long as care is taken to preserve intravascular volume. About 4 to 6 L of ascitic fluid are removed slowly during 60 to 90 minutes. (An infusion of albumin is administered simultaneously in severely hypoalbuminemic patients.)

Large-volume therapeutic paracentesis has reduced the need for *peritoneal venous shunting*, which is associated with a high rate of complications, including encephalopathy, disseminated intravascular coagulation, peritonitis, sepsis, and superior vena cava syndrome (see Chapter 71). Shunting should be considered only in the most refractory and disabling of cases. The use of surgical drainage for ascites is not as effective as it is for effusions of the pleural space. Similarly, the intraabdominal instillation of chemotherapeutic agents and radioisotopes has been relatively ineffective. Sclerosing drugs

and irritants to seal the peritoneal space are not recommended because an irritant effect on the bowel may result in necrosis, perforation, or secondary fibrosis and adhesions leading to obstruction. In particular, refractory cases, semipermanant or permanent paracentesis drainage catheters may be considered.

PERITONEAL IMPLANTS, BOWEL OBSTRUCTION, AND FISTULAS

Peritoneal implants within the abdominal cavity may develop in a diffuse miliary pattern or coalesce into large mass lesions capable of causing obstruction. A surgical *bypass* procedure or regional surgical resection ("*debulking*") is indicated under such circumstances for palliation when there is some hope of prolonging meaningful survival. For patients with an indolent malignancy, particularly those with a localized point of obstruction, an aggressive surgical approach is worthy of consideration. When implants are centered in the pelvic area, fistulas communicating with the bladder or skin may form; local *surgical excision* or *radiation therapy* can help to control the problem.

OBSTRUCTIVE JAUNDICE

Endoscopic placement of a *stent* in the common bile duct has largely replaced surgery for the palliative treatment of obstructive jaundice. Stenting requires expertise and should not be attempted by persons unfamiliar with the procedure because major complications can occur, particularly *recurrent cholangitis* (which must be carefully watched for and treated promptly if it occurs). The procedure can be uncomfortable, and the stents can become dislodged. However, if the procedure is successful, significant palliation and an improved quality of life can result. Continued improvements in stent technology and techniques of stent placement make this an increasingly important approach for palliation. For patients who cannot have their stents placed endoscopically, *percutaneous stent* placement by interventional radiology can sometimes be effective in relieving biliary obstruction.

Radiation therapy has also been used to treat obstructive jaundice caused by tumor in the porta hepatis. It is particularly useful in patients with radiosensitive neoplasms (e.g., breast cancer, lymphoma).

GASTROINTESTINAL COMPLICATIONS OF RADIATION THERAPY (1,17,18)

Radiation therapy can lead to a number of gastrointestinal complications, both acute and chronic.

Acute Complications

In the short term, radiation enteritis may ensue due to direct mucosal-cell injury, manifested by *nausea* and *vomiting*, which usually respond to the standard approaches (see prior discussion). In more severe cases, *diarrhea* and *abdominal cramps* may develop, which are best treated with IV hydration, electrolyte replacement as appropriate, and antidiarrheal agents as needed (e.g., Imodium, Lomotil, Kaopectate). Altering the diet to decrease the intake of high-fiber foods (e.g., nuts, fresh vegetables, and fruit), alcohol, fatty foods, milk products, and spicy foods can also be beneficial in improving symptoms. Depending on the severity of symptoms, the radiation oncologist may decide to have a break in the radiation therapy.

Long-Term Complications

Symptoms due to chronic effects of radiation on the intestine and other organs in the abdomen occur less commonly. These can include *altered anal sphincter control* (for a subset of patients requiring anal, rectal, or pelvic radiation),*chronic diarrhea*,*lactose intolerance*, *fistula formation, stenoses, adhesions*, and *bladder irritation*. Many of the symptomatic management approaches discussed earlier for acute enteritis apply here as well. Total parenteral nutrition may be necessary for severe cases. In addition, surgical management may be required for severe cases. It is important for the primary care physician to be aware of these potential long-term complications so that they can be dealt with promptly and appropriately if they arise.

Annotated Bibliography

1. Abdelsayed GG. Management of radiation-induced nausea and vomiting. Exp Hematol 2007;35(4 Suppl 1):34. (*A discussion of the most recent approaches.*)
2. Beck TM, Ciociola A, Jones SE, et al. Efficacy of oral ondansetron in the prevention of emesis in outpatients receiving cyclophosphamide-based chemotherapy. Ann Intern Med 1993;118:407. (*The agent was demonstrated to be safe and effective, with 66% of patients experiencing no emetic episodes.*)
3. Cubeddu LX, Hoffmann IS, Fuenmayor NT, et al. Efficacy of ondansetron (GR 38032F) and the role of serotonin in cisplatin-induced nausea and vomiting. N Engl J Med 1990;322:810. (*Major initial evidence of efficacy and the importance of serotonin S$_3$-receptors.*)
4. Feeney K, Cain M, Nowak AK. Chemotherapy induced nausea and vomiting—prevention and treatment. Aust Family Physician 2007;36:702. (*Very practical discussion and recommendations.*)
5. Gralla RJ, Itri LM, Pisko SE, et al. Antiemetic efficacy of high-dose metoclopramide. N Engl J Med 1981;305:905. (*A randomized, controlled study, establishing efficacy in cisplatin-induced vomiting.*)
6. Kris MG, Gralla RJ, Clark RA, et al. Consecutive dose-finding trials: adding lorazepam to the combination of metoclopramide plus dexamethasone. Cancer Treat Rep 1985;69:1257. (*Presents evidence for the efficacy of multiple-drug, multiple-mechanism therapy.*)
7. Kris MG, Gralla RJ, Clark RA, et al. Incidence, course, and severity of delayed nausea and vomiting following the administration of high-dose cisplatin. J Clin Oncol 1985;3:1379. (*Cisplatin is the major cause.*)
8. Marty M, Pouillart P, Scholl S, et al. Comparison of the 5-hydroxytryptamine (serotonin) antagonist ondansetron (GR38032) with high-dose metoclopramide in the control of cisplatin-induced emesis. N Engl J Med 1990;322:816. (*Ondansetron was found to be far superior.*)
9. Morrow GR, Morrell C. Behavioral treatment for the anticipatory nausea and vomiting induced by cancer chemotherapy. N Engl J Med 1982;307:1476. (*Describes the phenomenon and details behavioral approaches to treatment.*)
10. Navari RM, Reinhardt RR, Gralla RJ, et al. Reduction of cisplatin-induced emesis by a selective neurokinin-1–receptor antagonist. N Engl J Med 1999;340:190. (*A randomized, placebo-controlled trial of a new class of antiemetic, finding it to enhance the control of delayed emesis markedly and to add some prevention of acute emesis to that provided by dexamethasone and granisetron.*)
11. Schwartzberg LS. Chemotherapy-induced nausea and vomiting: clinician and patient perspectives. J Support Oncol 2007;5(2 Suppl 1):5. (*A thoughtful and practical discussion.*)
12. The Italian Group for Antiemetic Research. Dexamethasone, granisetron, or both for the prevention of nausea and vomiting during chemotherapy for cancer. N Engl J Med 1995;332:1. (*The combination program provided the best results.*)
13. Voth EA, Schwartz RH. Medical applications of delta-9-tetrahydrocannabinol and marijuana. Ann Intern Med 1997;126:791. (*A literature review, concluding that a modest benefit may be derived from the use of pure tetrahydrocannabinol for chemotherapy-induced nausea and anorexia, but that the use of crude marijuana adds little and entails many disadvantages.*)
14. Klein S, Koretz RL. Nutritional support in patients with cancer: what do the data really show? Nutr Clin Pract 1994;9:91. (*A good review of the evidence.*)
15. Rivadeneira DE, Evoy E, Fahey TJ III, et al. Nutritional support of the cancer patient. CA Cancer J Clin 1998;48:69. (*A very practical, fully documented discussion of the best approaches to nutritional support, giving supporting evidence.*)
16. Epstein M. Refractory ascites. N Engl J Med 1989;321:1675. (*An editorial summarizing methods of treatment.*)
17. Bismar MM, Sinicrope FA. Radiation enteritis. Curr Gastroenterol Rep 2002;4:361. (*A useful review.*)
18. Turina M, Mulhall AM, Mahid SS, et al. Frequency and surgical management of chronic complications related to pelvic radiation. Arch Surg 2008 143:46. (*Useful overview.*)

CHAPTER 92 ■ COMPLICATIONS OF CANCER: ONCOLOGIC EMERGENCIES AND PARANEOPLASTIC SYNDROMES

JEFFREY W. CLARK

The complications of cancer are great in number and variable in degree of urgency. They range from commonly experienced gastrointestinal difficulties and pain syndromes (see Chapters 90.1 and 91) to true emergencies, stubborn malignant effusions, and the uncommon but important paraneoplastic phenomena.

Most oncologic emergencies and malignant effusions are consequences of anatomic spread. Paraneoplastic syndromes result from hormonal and immunologic disturbances. The primary care physician's important role in monitoring the cancer patient requires familiarity with the early presentations of these complications, many of which are amenable to intervention. In most instances, hospital admission for inpatient treatment is necessary, so the emphasis is on early detection.

ONCOLOGIC EMERGENCIES AND URGENCIES (1–12)

The anatomic spread of tumor is capable of causing emergent complications, including spinal cord compression, cardiac tamponade, and hypercoagulability with acute bleeding or clotting. Urgent adversities associated with malignancy ensue from a combination of tumor invasion and metabolic/immunologic effects (e.g., superior vena cava syndrome, hypercalcemia, fever, infection).

Spinal Cord Compression

Extradural or epidural cord compression occurs in approximately 5% of patients with cancer. It is a *true emergency*, with early diagnosis and treatment essential to preventing serious, permanent neurologic damage. The majority of cases of epidural compression result from bony metastases in the vertebral bodies extending into the epidural space. Less frequently, metastatic tumor reaches the epidural space hematogenously or by direct extension through the intervertebral foramina. Malignancies with a propensity to spread to bone (e.g., myeloma, lymphoma, melanoma, renal cell carcinoma, and tumors of lung, breast, and prostate) are associated with the greatest risk for cord compression. Lymphoma may metastasize directly to the epidural space and not produce any bony changes. In more than 90% of cases, the initial symptom is *back pain*, often radicular in nature. The course is progressive; weakness and sensory deficits in the extremities follow. Sphincter incontinence is a late development, unless the cauda equina is the initial site of compression.

Diagnosis

Plain films of the spine should be obtained in all cancer patients with back pain. If the radiographic findings are normal in the area of pain, the pain is not progressive, the patient does not have lymphoma, and no neurologic deficits are present, no further workup need be carried out immediately, but the patient should be followed closely. However, any persistent or progressive back pain over time requires additional workup (usually magnetic resonance imaging [MRI]; see later discussion) because plain x-rays are not particularly sensitive for diagnosing the presence of malignant lesions. A high index of suspicion for malignancy is always warranted. If the radiographic findings are abnormal or if any neurologic deficits are noted, then immediate hospital admission and prompt neurologic and oncologic consultations are needed.

Magnetic resonance imaging is the diagnostic procedure of choice, being the most sensitive and least invasive of the imaging procedures, especially when gadolinium enhancement is used. It allows identification of all affected areas without the need for injection of contrast into the spinal canal.

Treatment

High-dose corticosteroids (e.g., 4 mg of dexamethasone every 6 hours) and *radiation therapy* are the mainstays of treatment, with *surgical decompression* indicated when neurologic function deteriorates rapidly. Patients with myeloma, lymphoma,

or small-cell cancers respond well to irradiation. Chemotherapy is worth considering in those with multifocal obstructing disease and may also be used initially for very responsive tumors (e.g., lymphomas or myeloma) when the findings do not suggest immediate need for decompression. The prognosis depends on the extent of neurologic damage at the time of presentation. Patients who are ambulatory have a 60% to 80% chance of leaving the hospital able to walk; those with paraplegia have less than a 20% chance of regaining their ability to walk. This underlines the absolute urgency required in evaluating and treating these patients.

Meningeal Carcinomatosis

Diffuse seeding of the meninges with malignant cells is a serious complication of a number of solid tumors (lymphoma, melanoma, cancers of breast, lung, and stomach) and leukemias. Even if true cord compression is not present, the entire neuraxis may become involved, with the development of meningeal, cranial nerve, and root symptoms. The diagnosis is confirmed by lumbar puncture, which typically reveals malignant cells in the cerebrospinal fluid. Corticosteroids, irradiation, and intrathecal administration of cytotoxic agents are the treatment modalities of choice.

Cardiac Tamponade

Life-threatening tamponade may arise as a complication of malignancy, either indolently or rapidly, depending on the progression of the underlying tumor. Compression may be caused by tumorous encasement, malignant effusion, or scarring from radiation-induced pericarditis. Cancers associated with tamponade include tumors of the breast and lung, lymphoma, leukemia, and melanoma. In some instances, symptoms and signs of pericarditis (see Chapter 20) precede those of tamponade. The presence of *pulsus paradoxus* strongly suggests significant tamponade.

Unexplained elevation of neck veins, narrowed pulse pressure, inspiratory distention of neck veins, and a pericardial friction rub should raise suspicion. Unfortunately, a pericardial friction rub is often absent in cases of tamponade caused by a malignant pericardial effusion. The usual accompanying symptoms (dyspnea, weakness, chest discomfort, cough) are nonspecific. More definitive diagnosis is best made by *cardiac ultrasonography*, the most sensitive and specific noninvasive test for documenting the problem and its physiologic significance.

A strong clinical suspicion of tamponade necessitates urgent hospitalization for prompt sonography and cardiac consultation. Sometimes a right-sided heart catheterization is performed when the degree of tamponade is unclear or the diagnosis is still questionable. *Pericardiocentesis* is the treatment of choice for urgent tamponade and may also yield positive cytology.

Hypercoagulability

A number of the natural inhibitors of clotting, many of which are endothelial in origin (protein C, protein S, tissue plasminogen factor, antithrombin III), are disrupted directly by tumor invasion or indirectly by substances elaborated by cancers. Patients with adenocarcinomas appear particularly susceptible to recurrent or migratory *thrombophlebitis* or even thrombotic arterial occlusions. A more disseminated consumption coagulopathy (*disseminated intravascular coagulation* [DIC]) sometimes develops and can present acutely as a generalized bleeding diathesis. Acute DIC is a true medical emergency. Suggestive laboratory findings include prolongations in the prothrombin time, partial thromboplastin time, and thrombin time, a low platelet count, and elevated concentrations of fibrin split products. The peripheral smear shows a microangiopathic picture (schistocytes). Chronic DIC is subtler in presentation, with thrombotic end-organ damage and thrombosis being the principal manifestations. Acute DIC requires immediate hospitalization to stop the bleeding. Once the consumptive process has been slowed, platelet and plasma transfusions are given to replace those blood elements that have been consumed. More definitive therapy requires treatment of the underlying malignancy.

Superior Vena Cava Syndrome

Obstruction of the superior vena cava is usually caused by extrinsic compression. The majority of cases are associated with bronchogenic carcinoma (especially small-cell carcinoma), lymphoma, and metastatic disease.

Diagnosis

The earliest manifestation is asymptomatic, unexplained *distention of the neck veins*. Late signs include swelling of the face, neck, and upper extremities, plethora, shortness of breath, and persistent headache. Although the condition is rarely fatal, increased intracranial pressure and thrombosis leading to neurologic deficits may ensue. The clinical diagnosis is reinforced by the finding of a mass on chest radiography in the right superior mediastinum or hilar area. *Chest computed tomography* with careful evaluation of the vasculature should be performed.

Treatment

At one time, it was considered essential to treat the mass immediately with emergency *radiotherapy*. Now, the view is one of *urgency* rather than emergency. The first task is to consider whether a *tissue diagnosis* should be obtained before radiotherapy is instituted (see Chapter 44) because a host of tumors with different degrees of radiosensitivity may be responsible for the condition. Although many malignancies respond within 1 week to radiation, some may respond better to chemotherapy, and occasionally a nonmalignant process that would not benefit from radiation is the cause (e.g., tuberculous adenopathy, substernal goiter). When a tissue diagnosis will alter therapy, invasive study to obtain tissue should proceed. If a small-cell carcinoma or lymphoma is found, *chemotherapy* might be placed ahead of radiation as the treatment of choice (see Chapters 53 and 84).

Optimal therapy depends on the underlying diagnosis, prior treatment, and overall clinical status of the patient. Diuretics and corticosteroids can occasionally diminish local symptoms, but the effect is transient, and these agents are no substitute for more definitive therapy. The use of heparin provides no benefit. The occurrence of superior vena cava syndrome does not worsen the prognosis (if adjusted for stage of disease), particularly in cases of small-cell lung cancer.

Hypercalcemia

Hypercalcemia is an accompaniment of advanced carcinomas with extensive *lytic bony involvement* (breast cancer, myeloma, hematologic malignancies) and also a complication of epidermoid cancers (renal cell, ovarian, bladder, head and neck, and epidermoid and squamous cell lung cancers) with little or no bony metastasis. In the latter case, hypercalcemia has been linked to tumor elaboration of a protein with some parathyroid hormone–like activity (*parathyroid hormone–related protein* [PTHRP]). Cancers that invade bone and trigger a blastic response (e.g., prostate, oat cell cancers) are rarely associated with hypercalcemia.

Diagnosis

Monitoring the serum calcium level provides the simplest means of early detection. Initially, the patient is asymptomatic. Later, such nonspecific symptoms as weakness, fatigue, lethargy, nausea, and constipation ensue. If the hypercalcemia progresses, it leads to an osmotic diuresis manifested by thirst and polyuria. The electrocardiogram may undergo change, with prolongation of the PR interval, shortening of the QT interval, and widening of the T wave. Dysrhythmias become a risk at very high calcium levels. Calcium potentiates the effects of digitalis and can trigger digitalis toxicity.

Treatment

Hospitalization is needed if a decision is made to treat the hypercalcemia. (When it occurs in the setting of terminal illness, therapy may not be indicated.) One begins vigorous rehydration with *intravenous saline solution*, followed by *furosemide* to accelerate saline diuresis. *Calcitonin* also rapidly reduces serum calcium levels, but daily injections are required, and tachyphylaxis may be induced. *Corticosteroids* are useful for acute–subacute management, especially in cases of myeloma, lymphoma, and metastatic breast cancer. Long-term control can be achieved with the use of *bisphosphonates*; (e.g., pamidronate or zoledronic acid). Treatment of the underlying tumor remains the most definitive measure. Even with control of hypercalcemia and relief of symptoms, prognosis is poor and life expectancy limited.

Febrile Neutropenia

Infection ranks as the leading cause of death in patients with leukemia and the cause of death in half of those with lymphoma and solid tumors. Malnutrition, immune dysfunction, mechanical compromise, and a lowered neutrophil count (mostly caused by cytotoxic therapy) all contribute to the high risk of mortality from infection.

Diagnosis

Neutropenia is defined in cancer patients as *granulocyte counts of less than 500/mL*, the minimum needed to counter infection. Patients in whom fever develops during periods of neutropenia should be considered infected until proven otherwise. The majority of neutropenic cancer patients with fever will have a bacterial infection (often caused by a gram-negative organism). The possibility of viral, fungal, or parasitic infection is increased in patients who have leukemia or who are on long-term steroid therapy or prolonged broad-spectrum antibiotic coverage.

Often, neutropenic patients lack the usual signs of inflammation, which makes it hard to determine the site of infection at the time of presentation. Bacteremia without an identifiable primary site and pneumonitis lead the list of presentations. Onset of fever in the neutropenic patient is an indication for *prompt hospitalization*, regardless of whether any additional signs of infection are present. The mortality in such patients ranges from 18% to 40% within the first 48 hours. Once the patient is admitted, *cultures of urine, sputum*, and *blood* samples are needed, as are samples of material from any suspected site (e.g., *cerebrospinal fluid*).

Treatment

In the absence of an identified pathogen, broad-spectrum antibiotic therapy is initiated, often with a *third-generation cephalosporin* (e.g., *ceftazidime* or *cefepime*) or a fluoroquinolone (e.g., levofloxacin); an *aminoglycoside* is added when *Pseudomonas* infection is a concern; and vancomycin is added when gram-positive organisms (e.g., the presence of a portacath) might be important causes of infection. The short-term prognosis for patients treated early and aggressively is good. With the aggressive use of antibiotics, 60% to 90% of neutropenic, febrile cancer patients recover from their infection. (Consideration should be given for GCSF (or GMCSF) prophylaxis after the next cycle of chemotherapy.

Malignant Ascites

Malignant ascites can lead to marked abdominal distention and respiratory compromise; treatment is supportive in most instances because the finding is a sign of end-stage disease. No randomized trials have compared treatment options, which range from peritoneal–venous shunt to intermittent drainage to medical management. Also largely unknown is the benefit of intracavitary versus systemic antitumor therapy. A wide range of agents has been tried intraperitoneally, but results are modest at best. Although peritoneal–venous shunting was at first applied with enthusiasm, an increased recognition of its risks (infection, DIC, venous thrombosis) and disappointing performance (frequent shunt clogging and failure) have limited its application. Only a small subset of patients (life expectancy >3 months; nonloculated, nonbloody, viscous ascitic fluid; uncomfortably rapid reaccumulation of fluid despite repeated paracentesis and medical therapy) should be considered for shunting (see Chapter 91).

Malignant Pleural Effusions

Malignant pleural effusions resulting from pleural implants or lymphatic obstruction can impair respiration. Lung, breast, and ovarian cancers are important causes of pleural implants; lymphomas lead to lymphatic obstruction. The optimal therapy is systemic treatment of the underlying malignancy. Repeated thoracentesis is ineffective and associated with considerable morbidity. Definitive local therapy requires placement of an indwelling chest tube for several days to allow thorough drainage and closure of the third space. Instillation of a sclerosing agent (e.g., tetracycline) after drainage promotes the scarring process and helps to limit reaccumulation of exudate.

Thrombocytopenia and Bleeding

See Chapter 81.

Paraneoplastic Syndromes (6–9,13–17)

Ectopic Hormone Syndromes

Small-cell (oat cell) carcinoma of the lung is the archetypal tumor capable of ectopic hormone production. A variety of other tumors may behave in similar fashion. One or more polypep-tides may issue from the tumor and lead to such complications as Cushing's syndrome and inappropriate secretion of antidiuretic hormone (ADH).

Cushing's Syndrome. Cushing's syndrome develops in approximately 5% of patients with small-cell carcinoma of the lung because of the ectopic production of *adrenocorticotropic hormone* (ACTH), although some degree of ectopic ACTH synthesis may take place in as many as 80% of patients with the tumor. The clinical syndrome can be subtle and is usually not manifested by the typical cushingoid appearance; instead, it is characterized by *increased pigmentation* and metabolic and immunosuppressive effects, such as severe, recalcitrant *hypokalemia* and *impaired resistance* to infection. The hypokalemia requires extraordinary doses of supplemental potassium and the use of spironolactone. Serum and urinary ketosteroids are especially abundant, with some patients demonstrating virilization. Metabolic inhibitors of adrenal hormone synthesis (metyrapone, mitotane, aminoglutethimide) have been tried; success has been variable. The prognosis is very poor; median survival is less than 2 months.

Syndrome of Inappropriate Secretion of Antidiuretic Hormone. Syndrome of inappropriate secretion of antidiuretic hormone is not unique to cancers, but small-cell carcinomas (about 10% of cases) and a host of other cancers are capable of elaborating a polypeptide with ADH activity. The earliest manifestations are *hyponatremia* and renal sodium wasting. *Urine osmolality is inappropriately elevated.* If the serum sodium falls to very low levels, confusion and disorientation may ensue. Treatment includes the use of *lithium carbonate* or *demeclocycline*, two agents that counter the action of ADH. A *restricted intake of free water* also helps to restore the serum sodium level. Infusions of hypertonic saline solution are to be avoided because these patients, although not edematous, tend to be volume overloaded. However, diuretics are contraindicated because of sodium depletion. Inappropriate secretion of ADH is rapidly reversible with effective *treatment of the underlying tumor*.

Hypercalcemia. Hypercalcemia associated with epidermoid cancers is, as noted previously, caused by the ectopic production of PTHRP, a protein with *parathyroid hormone–like activity*. Unlike the hypercalcemia of osteolytic disease, the hypercalcemia associated with epidermoid cancers is characterized by elevations in urinary cyclic adenosine monophosphate and serum PTHRP. Because symptoms may not develop until the serum calcium becomes markedly elevated, routine monitoring of the serum calcium is the best means of early detection and is worthwhile in patients with malignancies that frequently lead to this complication (multiple myeloma, squamous cell cancers of the head, neck, and lung; ovarian cancer; bladder cancer; hypernephroma). The diagnosis requires a high index of suspicion and direct testing for PTHRP; the protein is too different structurally from parathyroid hormone (PTH) to be detected by standard assays for PTH. Symptomatic relief can be achieved acutely by lowering the serum calcium (see prior discussion and Chapter 96). Treatment of the underlying cancer is more definitive.

Hyperthyroidism and Acute Thyrotoxicosis. Hyperthyroidism and acute thyrotoxicosis have resulted from ectopic production of chorionic gonadotropin (which functions like thyroid-stimulating hormone). Choriocarcinomas are the main source of the overproduction. Patients can present with all the typical hypermetabolic manifestations of thyrotoxicosis.

Beta-blockers are only modestly effective; primary treatment must be directed at the tumor.

Others. The ectopic production of *human chorionic gonadotropin* by testicular and lung cancers is sometimes sufficient to cause *gynecomastia*. *Fasting hypoglycemia* is a classic manifestation of insulinoma and a rare complication of sarcoma.

Immunologically Mediated Paraneoplastic Syndromes

A series of syndromes, mostly neurologic in nature, have been linked to aberrations in immune function such as production of antibodies that cross-react with specific antigens expressed on nerve cells. The precise identification of the mediator or immune complex has not been possible in all instances; at times, the link to an immune mechanism is merely speculative.

Myasthenic (Eaton-Lambert) Syndrome

Myasthenic (Eaton-Lambert) syndrome occurs most commonly in patients with small-cell carcinoma of the lung and characteristically results in *proximal muscle weakness* of the limbs. Its electromyographic pattern is distinct from that of true myasthenia, being characterized by facilitation and an increasing evoked muscle potential. Clinical management includes the administration of *guanidine*; the anticholinesterases used to treat myasthenia do not work.

Subacute Cerebellar Degeneration

Subacute cerebellar degeneration is another remote neurologic syndrome, characterized by injury to the Purkinje cells of the cerebellum. Ataxia, dysarthria, dysphagia, and even dementia may comprise the clinical picture. It has been associated most commonly with small-cell carcinoma of the lung and with ovarian and breast cancers.

Peripheral Neuropathy

Peripheral neuropathy is the most common form of neurologic deficit in cancer. The mechanism(s) are poorly defined but likely to be multifactorial. The most typical is a symmetric sensory neuropathy seen in patients with advanced malignant disease. Motor and mixed sensory and motor neuropathies have also been described.

Paraneoplastic Syndromes of Unknown Etiology

A host of other purportedly paraneoplastic syndromes have been described, linked to malignancy by the fact that symptoms recede with effective treatment of the underlying tumor. A tumor secretory product or other mechanism has not yet been identified.

Hypertrophic Pulmonary Osteoarthropathy

Hypertrophic pulmonary osteoarthropathy presents with the findings of digital clubbing and tenderness along the distal long bones. Most commonly, the syndrome occurs in the setting of *primary or metastatic lung tumors*. Radiography of the long bones shows an *elevated periosteum*, and radionuclide scanning demonstrates a distinctive pattern of *increased uptake along the cortical margins*. The exquisite pain accompanying these changes is relieved by removal of the tumor. The mechanism of the syndrome is unknown.

Hyperpyrexia and Tumor-Related Fever

Hyperpyrexia and tumor-related fever have been observed in patients with hepatic metastases, typically from colon cancer, and also as a manifestation of the "B" syndrome associated with Hodgkin's disease or non-Hodgkin's lymphoma. The release of pyrogens from tumor has been proposed as the cause of fever, but other possibilities include the inability to detoxify endogenous endotoxin and an alteration in the metabolism of fever-producing steroids. The fever can be controlled with the administration of *nonsteroidal antiinflammatory drugs*, which can also serve as a diagnostic test for the condition. As with other paraneoplastic syndromes, the best control is obtained by treating the underlying malignancy.

Nephrotic Syndrome

In some patients with Hodgkin's disease or non-Hodgkin's lymphoma, massive edema with proteinuria and hypoalbuminemia develops. The renal lesion appears as an accumulation of immune complexes along the basement membrane. The nature of the antigen is unknown. The problem does not respond to steroid therapy but does regress with control of the malignancy.

Cachexia

See Chapter 91.

Cutaneous Paraneoplastic Syndromes

Cutaneous paraneoplastic syndromes are quite rare, but they are important to recognize as clues to the presence of internal malignancy. They may be a consequence of hormone secretion, such as the hyperpigmentation or *melanosis* associated with ACTH-producing tumors or the *necrotizing erythema* seen with glucagon-secreting malignancies of the pancreas. The proliferation of *seborrheic keratoses* can be a sign of internal malignancy; *acanthosis nigricans* or freckling and hyperpigmentation in the axillary folds suggest neurofibromatosis and intestinal cancer. *Acquired ichthyosis* is associated with lymphomas and several other tumors.

Annotated Bibliography

1. Abrahm JL. Management of pain and spinal cord compression in patients with advanced cancer. Ann Intern Med 1999;131:37. (*A thoughtful, case-based discussion.*)
2. Ahmann FR. A reassessment of the clinical implications of the superior vena cava syndrome. J Clin Oncol 1984;2:961. (*Argues that taking the time and effort to make a tissue diagnosis helps in selecting treatment properly.*)
3. Baker WF Jr. Clinical aspects of disseminated intravascular coagulation. Semin Thromb Hemost 1989;15:1. (*A comprehensive review that includes a discussion of disseminated intravascular coagulation in cancer.*)
4. Byrne TN. Spinal cord compression from epidural metastases. N Engl J Med 1992;327:614. (*One of the best reviews of the subject.*)

5. Callahan JA, Seward JB, Nishimura RA, et al. Two-dimensional echocardiographically guided pericardiocentesis. Am J Cardiol 1985;55:476. (*This ultrasonographic technique is useful for diagnosis and treatment.*)

6. Gucalp R, Ritch P, Wiernik PH, et al. Comparative study of pamidronate disodium and etidronate disodium in the treatment of cancer-related hypercalcemia. J Clin Oncol 1992;10:134. (*The second-generation bisphosphonate pamidronate was superior.*)

7. Nussbaum SR, Younger J, VanderPol CJ, et al. Single-dose intravenous therapy with pamidronate for the treatment of hypercalcemia of malignancy. Am J Med 1993;95:297. (*Evidence for the efficacy of second-generation bisphosphonates.*)

8. Portenoy RK, Lipton RB, Foley KM. Back pain in the cancer patient: an algorithm for evaluation and management. Neurology 1987;37:134. (*Emphasizes the importance of a high index of suspicion for spinal metastasis and cord compression.*)

9. Ralston SH, Gallacher SJ, Patel U, et al. Cancer-associated hypercalcemia: morbidity and mortality. Ann Intern Med 1990;112:499. (*The prognosis poor even if the condition is corrected, but morbidity can be reduced.*)

10. Sarpel S, Sarpel C, Yu E, et al. Early diagnosis of spinal-epidural metastasis by magnetic resonance imaging. Cancer 1987;59:1112. (*Shows enhanced capacity for the detection of early lesions.*)

11. Wilkes JB, Fidios P, Vaickur L, et al. Malignancy-related pericardial effusion: 127 cases from Roswell Park Cancer Institute. Cancer 1995;76:1377. (*A large series providing details of presentation, clinical course, and treatment.*)

12. Worschmidt F, Bunemann H, Geilmann HP, et al. Small-cell lung cancer with and without superior vena cava syndrome: a multivariate analysis of prognostic factors in 408 cases. Int J Radiol Oncol Biol Phys 1995;33:77. (*Superior vena cava syndrome was actually associated with a favorable prognosis.*)

13. Burtis WJ, Brady TG, Orloff JJ, et al. Immunochemical characterization of circulating parathyroid hormone–related protein in patients with humoral hypercalcemia of cancer. N Engl J Med 1990;322:1106. (*Identifies parathyroid hormone–related protein and links it convincingly to humoral hypercalcemia.*)

14. Hainsworth JD, Workman R, Greco A. Management of the syndrome of inappropriate antidiuretic hormone secretion in small-cell lung cancer. Cancer 1983;51:161. (*Antitumor chemotherapy resulted in the resolution of the syndrome of inappropriate secretion of antidiuretic hormone.*)

15. Martinez-Lavin M, Matucci-Cerinic M, Jajic I, et al. Hypertrophic osteoarthropathy: consensus conference on its definition, classification, assessment, and diagnostic criteria. J Rheumatol 1993;20:1386. (*Comprehensive consideration of the condition.*)

16. Posner PB. Paraneoplastic syndromes. Neurol Clin 1991;9:919. (*Slightly dated but still excellent review by a leading authority.*)

17. Wysolmerski JJ, Broadus AE. Hypercalcemia of malignancy: the central role of parathyroid hormone–related protein. Annu Rev Med 1994;45:189. (*Review of the causes of hypercalemia and the important role of parathyroid hormone–related protein.*)

SECTION 7 ■ ENDOCRINOLOGIC PROBLEMS

CHAPTER 93 ■ SCREENING FOR DIABETES MELLITUS

Diabetes is, after obesity and thyroid disease, the most common metabolic disorder seen by the primary care physician. Patients' concerns about the possible need for insulin injections and about such well-known complications as blindness, kidney disease, premature vascular disease, and erectile dysfunction make diabetes one of the most feared diagnoses. Detection campaigns and advertising have further heightened public awareness. Patients commonly request diabetes screening, even in the absence of symptoms or risk factors. There is no question that treatment effectively reduces symptoms associated with the metabolic derangements induced by diabetes. Results of the Diabetes Control and Complications Trial (DCCT) have definitively answered long-standing questions about the reduction in complication rates that can be achieved with intensive efforts to control glucose level, at least for type 1 disease. Less definitive but consistent results are also available for type 2 disease from the United Kingdom Prospective Diabetes Study (UKPDS). Nevertheless, the benefits of treatment initiated in the asymptomatic phase have not been demonstrated. Furthermore, the proven risk-reduction effect of glucose control is largely limited to microvascular disease, which manifests as retinopathy, nephropathy, and lower limb amputation. Because coronary disease, cerebrovascular disease, and peripheral vascular disease confer greater disease burden among diabetics, the screening question must be considered in the context of other risk factors for macrovascular disease.

EPIDEMIOLOGY AND RISK FACTORS (1–9)

Diabetes mellitus is heterogeneous. The destruction of β-cells in the islets of Langerhans through a number of pathophysiologic mechanisms is responsible for the clinical syndrome of type 1 diabetes mellitus, previously referred to as *insulin-dependent diabetes mellitus*. The etiology and pathogenesis of type 2 diabetes, previously called *non–insulin-dependent diabetes mellitus*, may be even more heterogeneous; multiple lesions include a blunted β-cell response to glucose, a defect at the insulin receptor, and a defect in hepatic uptake of glucose that contributes to glucose intolerance. Depending on the diagnostic criteria used, the prevalence of all types of diabetes in the United States is between 3% and 7%; type 2 diabetes is nearly 10 times more common than type 1 diabetes.

Type 1 Diabetes

Type 1 diabetes is generally manifested in childhood or early adulthood. Only 20% of patients with type 1 diabetes have a first-degree relative with diabetes. However, a predisposition to type 1 diabetes, apparently mediated through the immune system, is inherited. This pathologic predisposition to autoimmune destruction of the β-cells has been linked to the presence of certain HLA antigens, some of which are also associated with other autoimmune diseases, including Hashimoto's thyroiditis and Addison's disease. Overall, the risk for the eventual development of diabetes in a sibling of a patient with type 1 disease is between 3% and 6%. The role of the autoimmune destruction of β-cells in many patients with type 1 diabetes is attested to by the presence of islet cell antibodies in a large proportion of newly diagnosed cases. Islet cell antibodies can also be detected in nondiabetic relatives of patients with type 1 disease.

At least in some cases, islet cell destruction is triggered by a viral infection, which perhaps initiates the autoimmune response. The role of viral infection has been linked to a seasonal variation in the incidence of type 1 disease and has raised questions about a relationship between socioeconomic status and the risk for type 1 diabetes, but the evidence is equivocal. Environmental toxins (e.g., nitrosamines) and foods have also been incriminated as triggers for autoimmune islet cell destruction.

Type 2 Diabetes

Type 2 diabetes has a much stronger *genetic component* than does type 1 diabetes; concordance in identical twins is greater than 90%. The genetic link is not related to HLA antigens, and islet cell antigens are no more prevalent than in the general population.

The overwhelming risk factor for type 2 diabetes is overnutrition and resulting *obesity*. Eighty percent of diabetic adults are obese or have a history of obesity. Among adults who are at least 25% greater than their ideal body weight, one of every five has elevated fasting blood sugar levels, and three of every five have abnormal results on glucose tolerance tests. Obesity increases insulin levels and decreases the concentration of insulin receptors in tissue, including skeletal muscle and fat. The relationship between the concentration of insulin receptors and glucose tolerance is modified, however, by intracellular sequences following insulin binding that are poorly understood. Exercise increases the concentration of insulin receptors, and a *sedentary lifestyle* is associated with glucose intolerance. Regular exercise has been shown to be associated with a decreased incidence of type 2 diabetes after adjustments for body mass index.

Steroids reduce receptor affinity for insulin, as do uremia and hepatic failure. Other drugs can impair glucose tolerance by further diminishing the sluggish response of β-cells to glucose. These include *thiazide* diuretics, β-adrenergic blockers, α-adrenergic stimulants, and phenytoin. Prostaglandin inhibitors, including indomethacin and salicylate, may increase β-cell release of insulin.

Persons with *impaired glucose tolerance* are also at greater risk for frank type 2 diabetes (see later discussion). Although long-term follow-up studies indicate that as many as half of those with impaired glucose tolerance will have normal glucose tolerance test results 5 to 10 years later, somewhere between 1% and 5% of these patients become diabetic each year.

In approximately 3% of previously euglycemic women, glucose intolerance develops during pregnancy. The fetal hyperglycemia and hyperinsulinemia that accompany maternal diabetes result in increased neonatal morbidity and mortality and the increased birth weight common in infants of diabetic mothers. *Gestational diabetes* in the mother resolves after delivery in 90% of cases, but type 2 diabetes eventually develops in more than half of these women.

NATURAL HISTORY OF DIABETES AND EFFECTIVENESS OF THERAPY (1,5–21)

The natural history of diabetes mellitus has been difficult to define because the condition is so heterogeneous. This problem has historically been confounded by studies that have defined diabetes according to varying degrees of glucose intolerance.

The natural history of asymptomatic impaired glucose intolerance is variable; only 15% to 30% of these patients progress to frank diabetes during 10 to 15 years. Patients with impaired glucose tolerance are at increased risk for the development of the macrovascular complications that result from accelerated atherogenesis. However, unless glucose intolerance progresses to frank diabetes, characteristic diabetic microangiopathy does not develop in these patients. Intensive lifestyle and drug interventions in people with impaired fasting glucose or impaired glucose tolerance have been shown to reduce the rate of progression to frank diabetes by 42% to 58%.

The *asymptomatic detectable period* for type 2 diabetes has been estimated to have a mean duration between 10 and 12 years, but the true mean and the distribution of durations are unknown. The asymptomatic detectable period seems to be much shorter for type 1 diabetes than it is for type 2 diabetes. The markedly lower prevalence of asymptomatic type 1 diabetes in comparison with type 2 disease makes such patients a very small target for screening efforts.

The incidence of *vascular* and *neurologic complications* clearly tends to increase with the duration of clinical diabetes. However, some long-term studies of patients followed for as long as 40 years have indicated that clinical evidence of microvascular disease, atherosclerosis, or neuropathy may occur in only 20% to 40% of type 1 patients.

The increased risk for vascular and neurologic complications is reflected in the relative mortality rates of diabetics. The relative risk for death of diabetic patients, in comparison with that of age-matched nondiabetic persons, increases with the duration of known disease. In one study of patients followed for up to 25 years, the increase in mortality risk with increased duration was greater after age 40 years and among women. Progress has been made in reducing mortality among persons with diabetes, more so in men than in women. *Coronary artery disease* is the most common cause of death among diabetics. Autopsy studies indicate that coronary disease is two to three times more common among diabetics than among nondiabetics. Peripheral vascular disease is also very common among diabetics; clinical studies have indicated a prevalence of about 60%. Diabetics in the Framingham Study were shown to be four to five times more likely to have *intermittent claudication* and two to three times more likely to suffer the morbid consequences of stroke than were nondiabetics. On the other hand, the presence of peripheral vascular disease in a nondiabetic person increases the risk for the eventual development of type 2 diabetes.

Retinopathy is the most common specific complication of diabetes. In general, the incidence of retinopathy increases with the duration of diabetes, regardless of age at onset. Prevalence ranging from 40% to 80% has been reported among patients with known diabetes lasting 20 to 30 years. In one study of patients whose diabetes began before age 30 years, nearly all had retinopathy 25 to 30 years later, and about 50% had proliferative changes. Retinopathy was less prevalent among those whose diabetes began later in life and those not receiving insulin. Laser photocoagulation has been shown to decrease the progression of diabetic retinopathy. However, this does not provide a basis for recommending screening for diabetes; retinopathy that warrants treatment is very rare early in the course of disease. (Once diabetes is diagnosed, screening for retinopathy is indicated.)

Renal disease has been reported in 15% to 80% of diabetic patients at autopsy. Renal failure is the cause of death in 6% to 12% of diabetic patients. Prevalence estimates vary widely from study to study, but it is clear that the risk for glomerulosclerosis with clinically evident functional impairment increases dramatically with the duration of disease.

Although the *duration of glucose intolerance* and associated metabolic abnormalities can be related to many of the complications of diabetes, the variability of the natural history must be kept in mind. It has been argued that all complications, including specific microangiopathic changes, have been identified in patients without evident glucose intolerance. The DCCT provided compelling evidence that rates of microvascular complications and other consequences of diabetes could be reduced with intensive efforts to control glucose levels among patients with type 1 diabetes. Intensive therapy was associated with an increased frequency of hypoglycemic episodes and considerable inconvenience and cost. Among type 2 diabetics, the UKPDS and two smaller trials showed that tight glycemic control can reduce the progression of albuminuria and retinopathy. However, the trials were not large enough or long enough to confirm an effect on end-stage renal disease or blindness. The UKPDS found a nonsignificant trend toward reduction in myocardial infarction with tight control but no difference in other cardiovascular outcomes. Given these findings, it is unlikely that tight control initiated earlier because screening advanced the time of diagnosis would lead to clinically significant risk reduction over a period of 10 to 20 years after diagnosis. These considerations led the U.S. Preventive Services Task Force (USPSTF) to conclude that there is insufficient evidence to recommend for or against routinely screening asymptomatic adults for type 2 diabetes, impaired glucose tolerance, or impaired fasting glucose.

Despite the tenuous relationship between early detection of diabetes and reduced risk of microvascular and macrovascular disease, *diabetes as a potent cardiovascular risk factor* raises other arguments for screening. Cardiovascular risk is increased at least twofold among people with undiagnosed diabetes. Earlier knowledge of diabetes could alter the approach to treatment of other risk factors, including hypertension and lipid disorders. Diabetics randomized to a lower blood pressure treatment target of 80 mm Hg were shown to have lower cardiovascular and all-cause mortality. Furthermore, diabetic patients might be afforded better protection against cardiovascular events by the selective use of angiotensin-converting-enzyme inhibitors or angiotensin-receptor blockers rather than other antihypertensive agents, although conclusive evidence for this advantage is lacking. These agents do slow the development of diabetic nephropathy compared to other antihypertensive agents. Diabetics do not have higher total cholesterol and low-density-lipoprotein cholesterol levels, and treatment with statins or fibrates provides the same relative risk reduction of cardiovascular disease for both diabetics and nondiabetics. However, diabetics do have higher triglyceride levels and lower high-density-lipoprotein (HDL) cholesterol levels, leading to speculation that initial fibrate treatment, with its positive effect on HDL cholesterol, might be more appropriate for diabetics. Furthermore, behavioral interventions to reduce cardiovascular risk are likely to have a greater absolute risk reduction among diabetics than among nondiabetics because of greater baseline risk. These considerations led the USPSTF to recommend screening for type 2 diabetes in adults with hypertension or hyperlidemia.

Prevention of diabetes among patients with impaired glucose tolerance is also an area of great interest. Interventions designed to prevent or delay diabetes have included pharmacologic and lifestyle approaches. In the Diabetes Prevention Program trial, intensive lifestyle intervention reduced diabetes incidence by 58%, whereas metformin reduced the incidence by 31%. A meta-analysis of 17 trials with more than 8,000 participants concluded that both lifestyle and pharmacologic interventions reduced the rate of progression to diabetes, with the former at least as effective as the latter. The number needed to treat for benefit was 6.4 for lifestyle interventions and 10.2 for oral diabetes drugs. An extensive cost-effectiveness model of such interventions found that lifestyle modification is likely to have important effects on morbidity and mortality and should be recommended to all high-risk people.

Gestational diabetes is a special case. As noted, it occurs in 3% of pregnancies, although considerable variation is noted in different populations. It is associated with perinatal morbidity, including macrosomia and the associated increased risk for serious birth trauma and cesarean section. Evidence from observational studies and randomized trials supports the contention that the identification of gestational diabetes, followed by management with diet, insulin, or both, can reduce the incidence of macrosomia. However, these same trials did not show a reduction in other important maternal or perinatal outcomes such as cesarean section rates, birth trauma, or perinatal mortality. As a result, the USPSTF concluded that evidence is insufficient to recommend for or against routine screening for gestational diabetes.

SCREENING AND DIAGNOSTIC TESTS (5,7,9,19,22–25)

In 1979, the National Diabetes Data Group published criteria for the diagnosis of diabetes. In 1997, these criteria were updated by a committee of the American Diabetes Association. According to these revised criteria, at least one of the following conditions must be met to establish the diagnosis of diabetes in the nonpregnant adult:

1. Symptoms of diabetes plus a *casual glucose* concentration of 200 mg/dL (11.1 mmol/L) or more. Casual is defined as any time of day without regard to time since last meal. The classic symptoms of diabetes include polyuria, polydipsia, and unexplained weight loss.
2. A *fasting plasma glucose* concentration of 126 mg/dL (7.0 mmol/L) or more (fasting defined as no caloric intake for at least 8 hours).
3. A 2-hour postprandial level of 200 mg/dL or more during an *oral glucose tolerance test* (OGTT), performed as described by the World Health Organization (glucose load equivalent to 75 g of anhydrous glucose dissolved in water).

To confirm a diagnosis of diabetes, any one of the criteria must also be met on a subsequent day. It is worth noting that capillary blood glucose levels are lower than plasma levels by approximately 10 mg/dL during fasting but are equal to or higher than plasma levels after a glucose load.

In addition to defining these diagnostic criteria, which have since been widely accepted in the United States, the group suggested new designations for persons with glucose intolerance who do not meet the criteria for frank diabetes. The term *impaired glucose tolerance* is reserved for patients with a glucose tolerance between normal and that of frank diabetes (e.g., fasting plasma glucose from 110 to 125 mg/dL).

It should be remembered that any criteria for the diagnosis of diabetes based on glucose levels are, by necessity, arbitrary.

The sensitivity and specificity of the tests depend on the arbitrary levels chosen. At the time of their publication, the principal effect of the revised criteria, which require higher levels than were commonly used previously, was to increase the specificity of the criteria at the expense of sensitivity. This tradeoff reflected the judgment that little benefit can be expected from aggressive identification and treatment of early or mild degrees of glucose intolerance and that the label *diabetes* can engender substantial anxiety and morbidity. The recommendations made in 1997 increase sensitivity at the expense of specificity, reflecting an implicit judgment that more benefit than harm will result from identifying and labeling patients with less severe levels of glucose intolerance as diabetic.

Despite the widespread acceptance of these diagnostic tests, the indications for performing oral glucose tolerance tests and any blood glucose measurements to screen asymptomatic persons remain controversial. The American Diabetes Association (ADA) advocates the use of a fasting glucose level to screen for diabetes among people older than age 45 years. They recommend earlier screening for those at higher risk for diabetes because of racial background, family history, obesity, or prior evidence of impaired glucose tolerance. However, the ADA acknowledges that no evidence from a prospective, randomized trial is available to support such recommendations. As already noted, the USPSTF concluded that evidence is insufficient to recommend for or against routine screening for diabetes in asymptomatic adults.

The detection of autoantibodies as predictors of type 1 diabetes among asymptomatic persons with a strong family history of type 1 disease has also received considerable attention. However, because no interventions have been proved to slow or prevent the onset of disease, this approach is not recommended in the general population.

Screening for gestational diabetes is generally accomplished between 24 and 28 weeks of gestation by administering 50 g of glucose orally and measuring the glucose level 1 hour later. A level greater than 140 mg/dL prompts further evaluation with an oral glucose tolerance test (see Chapter 102). This policy is recommended by the ADA and is generally accepted. However, it is not supported by conclusive evidence from randomized trials. For this reason, both the USPSTF and the Canadian Task Force on the Periodic Health Examination recommended neither for nor against this practice. Selective screening on the basis of age (>35 years), body mass index, and race has been advocated.

Some have advocated the use of hemoglobin A1c measurements to screen for and diagnose diabetes. However, in population-based studies, fasting glucose levels have been found to be more sensitive and more specific.

Some studies have shown that screening for diabetes may induce short-term increases in anxiety among screened persons, and people who screen positive subsequently report poorer health than those who screen negative. However, screening for type 2 diabetes has been shown to have limited psychological impact on patients.

CONCLUSIONS AND RECOMMENDATIONS (5,7,21,24,25)

- Diabetes mellitus is a common but heterogeneous condition. The most important risk factor for type 1 diabetes is a family history of diabetes in a twin, a sibling, or a parent. Family history is even more predictive for type 2 diabetes, but the most important risk factor is obesity. Persons with a history of gestational diabetes or with impaired glucose tolerance also are at greater risk for the development of frank diabetes.

- The natural history of diabetes and the incidence of complications are highly variable. The incidence of diabetic complications increases with the duration of disease. Close control of glucose levels in patients with type 1 diabetes has been shown to reduce the incidence of microvascular diabetic complications, at the expense of increased rates of hypoglycemia and substantial inconvenience and cost. Consistent but less conclusive evidence exists for type 2 diabetes, but there is no conclusive evidence for an effect on the macrovascular complications that confer much higher burdens of morbidity and mortality. It is unlikely that earlier glucose control made possible by screening would result in significant risk reduction benefit for 10 to 20 years after the diagnosis of diabetes. Therefore, evidence is insufficient to recommend for or against screening the asymptomatic adult patient for diabetes, impaired glucose tolerance, or impaired fasting glucose.

- Undiagnosed diabetes increases the risk of cardiovascular disease. Patients with diabetes and hypertension have been shown to benefit from more-aggressive blood pressure treatment targets. Patients with diabetes and lipid disorders may also benefit from different approaches to treatment than nondiabetic patients. It is likely that these different approaches to the treatment of hypertension and hyperlidemia, as well as other cardiovascular risk factors, would result in significant reduction in cardiovascular risk within 10 years of the diagnosis of diabetes. Patients with hypertension or hyperlipidemia should therefore be screened for type 2 diabetes.

- Treatment of gestational diabetes does reduce the incidence of macrosomia but has not been shown to affect other perinatal outcomes. Therefore, evidence is insufficient to recommend for or against screening for gestational diabetes. If screening is performed, it should be done with a 50-g, 1-hour glucose challenge test (GCT) at 24 to 28 weeks of gestation followed by an OGTT for women who screen positive on the GCT.

- All patients should be encouraged to exercise, eat a healthy diet, and maintain a healthy weight to reduce the risk of developing type 2 diabetes.

A.G.M.

Annotated Bibliography

1. Danema D. Type 1 diabetes. Lancet 2006;367:847. (*Major challenges remain in the development of approaches to the prevention and management of type 1 diabetes and its complications.*)
2. Harris MI, Hadden WC, Knowler WC, et al. Prevalence of diabetes and impaired glucose tolerance and plasma glucose levels in U.S. population ages 20 to 74 years. Diabetes 1987;36:523. (*An extrapolation of survey results provides a prevalence estimate of 6.6% to 3.4% previously diagnosed and 3.2% undiagnosed.*)
3. Norris SL, Kansagara D, Bougatos C, et al. Screening adults for type 2 diabetes: a review of the evidence for the U.S. Preventive Services Task Force. Ann Intern Med 2008;148:855. (*Critical look at best evidence; finds benefit in screening those at increased cardiovascular risk.*)
4. Manson JE, Nathan DM, Krolewski AS, et al. A prospective study of exercise and incidence of diabetes among U.S. male physicians. JAMA 1992;268:63. (*The relative risk was 0.77 for those who exercised once a week and 0.58 for those who exercised five or more times weekly.*)

5. Harris R, Donahue K, Rathore SS, et al. Screening adults for type 2 diabetes: a review of the evidence for the U.S. Preventive Services Task Force. Ann Intern Med. 2003;138:215. (*Presents the evidence and rationale behind the conclusion that there is insufficient evidence for routine screening of asymptomatic adults but sufficient evidence to recommend screening adults with either hypertension or hyperlidemia.*)

6. Stranges S, Marshall JR, Natarajan R, et al. Effects of long-term selenium supplementation on the incidence of type 2 diabetes. A randomized trial. Ann Intern Med 2007;147:217. (*Selenium supplementation did not seem to prevent type 2 diabetes, and it may increase the risk for the disease.*)

7. U.S. Preventive Services Task Force. Screening for type 2 diabetes. U.S. Preventive Services Task Force recommendation statement. Ann Intern Med 2008;148:846. (*Evidence-based consensus recommendations.*)

8. Hanley, AJG, Karter AJ, Williams K, et al. Prediction of type 2 diabetes mellitus with alternative definitions of the metabolic syndrome. The Insulin Resistance Atherosclerosis Study. Circulation 2005;112:3713. (*The International Diabetes Federation and National Cholesterol Education Program metabolic syndrome definitions predicted diabetes mellitus at least as well as the World Health Organization definition, despite the fact that did not require the use of oral glucose tolerance testing or measures of insulin resistance or microalbuminuria.*)

9. Pradhan AD, Rifai N, Buring JE, et al. Hemoglobin A1c predicts diabetes but not cardiovascular disease in nondiabetic women. Am J Med 2007;120:720. (*Presents findings suggesting that hemoglobin A1c levels are elevated well in advance of the clinical development of type 2 diabetes.*)

10. Diabetes Control and Complications Trial Research Group. The effect of intensive treatment of diabetes on the development and progression of long-term complications in insulin-dependent diabetes mellitus. N Engl J Med 1993;329:977. (*Intensive therapy reduced retinopathy, proteinuria, and neuropathy in symptomatic patients.*)

11. UK Prospective Diabetes Study Group. Efficacy of atenolol and captopril in reducing risk of macrovascular and microvascular complications in type 2 diabetes: UKPDS 39. BMJ 1998;317:713. (*No evidence was found that either drug had any specific beneficial or deleterious effect, suggesting that blood pressure reduction in itself may be more important than the treatment used.*)

12. UK Prospective Diabetes Study Group. Intensive blood glucose control with sulphonylureas or insulin compared with conventional treatment and risk of complications in patients with type 2 diabetes. Lancet 1998;352:837. (*Intensive therapy reduced the risk for microvascular complications by 25%, but no evident effect on macrovascular disease was noted.*)

13. Diabetes Prevention Program Research Group. Reduction in the incidence of type 2 diabetes with lifestyle intervention or metformin. N Engl J Med 2002;346:393. (*Intensive lifestyle intervention reduced the incidence by 58%, and metformin reduced the incidence by 31%.*)

14. Gillies CL, Abrams KR, Lambert PC, et al. Pharmacological and lifestyle interventions to prevent or delay type 2 diabetes in people with impaired glucose tolerance: systematic review and meta-analysis. BMJ 2007;334:299. (*Lifestyle interventions seem to be at least as effective as drug treatment.*)

15. Hansson L, Zanchetti A, Carruthers SG, et al. Effects of intensive blood-pressure lowering and low-dose aspirin in patients with hypertension: principal results of the Hypertension Optimal Treatment (HOT) randomised trial. Lancet 1998;351:1755. (*In patients with diabetes, there was a 51% reduction in major cardiovascular events in the target group for 80 mm Hg compared with the target group for ≤90 mm Hg.*)

16. Nathan DM, Singer DE, Godine JE, et al. Retinopathy in older type II diabetics: association with glucose control. Diabetes 1986;35:797. (*The duration of diabetes and level of hemoglobin A1c were major predictors of retinopathy among 185 patients with type 2 diabetes of ages 55 to 75 years.*)

17. Parving HH, Lehnert H, Brochner-Mortensen J, et al. The effect of irbesartan on the development of diabetic nephropathy in patients with type 2 diabetes. N Engl J Med 2001;345:870. (*Irbesartan is renoprotective independent of its blood pressure–lowering effect in patients with type 2 diabetes and microalbuminuria.*)

18. Sacks FM, Tonkin AM, Craven T, et al. Coronary heart disease in patients with low LDL-cholesterol: benefit of pravastatin in diabetics and enhanced role for HDL-cholesterol and triglycerides as risk factors. Circulation 2002;105:1424. (*Among patients with coronary heart disease [CHD] who have low low-density-lipoprotein cholesterol, diabetics have much higher subsequent CHD risk than nondiabetics; pravastatin reduced the event rate in diabetics to that of nondiabetic participants.*)

19. Singer DE, Nathan DM, Fogel HA, et al. Screening for diabetic retinopathy. Ann Intern Med 1992;116:660. (*Reviews the natural history of diabetic retinopathy and makes the case for screening patients with diagnosed diabetes.*)

20. Tuomilehto J, Lindstrom J, Eriksson JG, et al. Prevention of type 2 diabetes mellitus by changes in lifestyle among subjects with impaired glucose tolerance. N Engl J Med 2001;344:1343. (*The cumulative incidence of diabetes after 4 years was 11% in the intervention group and 23% in the control group.*)

21. Eddy DM, Schlessinger L, Kahn R. Clinical outcomes and cost-effectiveness of strategies for managing people at high risk for diabetes. Ann Intern Med 2005;143:251. (*The most important potentially controllable factor is the cost of the lifestyle program; compared with no program, lifestyle modification for high-risk people can be made cost-effective over 30 years if the annual cost of the intervention can be reduced to about $100.*)

22. Eborall HC, Griffin SJ, Kinmonth AL, et al. Psychological impact of screening for type 2 diabetes: controlled trial and comparative study embedded in the ADDITION (Cambridge) randomised controlled trial. BMJ 2007;335:486. (*Screening for type 2 diabetes has limited psychological effect on patients.*)

23. Eborall H, Davies R, Kinmonth L, et al. Patients' experiences of screening for type 2 diabetes: prospective qualitative study embedded in the ADDITION (Cambridge) randomised controlled trial. BMJ 2007;335:490. (*There was limited psychological effect of screening for type 2 diabetes.*)

24. Expert Committee on the Diagnosis and Classification of Diabetes Mellitus. Report of the Expert Committee on the Diagnosis and Classification of Diabetes Mellitus. Diabetes Care 1997;20:1183. (*Recommends revised criteria for diagnosis and screening.*)

25. Naylor CD, Sermer M, Chen E, et al. Selective screening for gestational diabetes mellitus. N Engl J Med 1997;337:1591. (*Selecting women for screening based on age, race, and body mass index can reduce the number of screening tests by one third without a loss in sensitivity.*)

CHAPTER 94 ■ SCREENING FOR THYROID CANCER

Cancer of the thyroid is a relatively rare disease with a low mortality rate. It accounts for 1% of all new malignant disease and only 0.2% of cancer deaths. The primary physician should be aware of the iatrogenic relationship between childhood irradiation of the head and neck and thyroid cancer and also appreciate the indications for genetic screening for inherited medullary carcinoma of the thyroid.

EPIDEMIOLOGY AND RISK FACTORS (1–12)

Generally, the incidence of thyroid cancer increases with age. This is particularly true of tumors with an anaplastic or follicular histopathologic pattern and of the medullary carcinomas.

The most common tumors, with a papillary histopathologic pattern, have a bimodal, age-specific incidence, peaking in the 30s and late in life. Thyroid tumors occur more than twice as frequently in women than men. In the United States, African Americans seem to be at lower risk than others. Wide variations in thyroid cancer prevalence at autopsy have been reported internationally, from 3% to more than 10% of thyroids that have not been exposed to radiation, with the highest rates reported in Japan. Approximately 25% of medullary carcinomas, which make up 5% to 10% of thyroid cancers, are familial.

The major identifiable risk factor for the development of thyroid cancer has been a history of *external irradiation of the head and neck*. External irradiation was used as early as 1907 to shrink an enlarged thymus in infancy. During the 1920s and subsequently until the 1950s, it was used extensively to treat enlarged tonsils and adenoids, cervical adenitis, mastoiditis, sinusitis, hemangiomas, tinea capitis, and acne. Concern about ill effects began to mount in 1950, when a history of neck irradiation was noted in 9 of 28 cases of childhood thyroid cancer, with a latency period of 5 or more years. Further documentation followed, and radiation to the neck was discontinued. In 1973, attention focused on the issue again when 40% of a series of adults with thyroid cancer were found to have a history of irradiation. Large studies indicated that more than 25% of exposed persons had detectable thyroid abnormalities; the prevalence of cancer was estimated at 7% to 9%. Some radiation-exposed persons were at greater risk than others. Radiation during infancy appeared to be most carcinogenic, with cancer risk decreasing as age at the time of radiation increased. Although the threshold dose for cancer risk was low, the risk seemed to be greatly increased for persons who received multiple treatments. The exposed population at risk was substantial—estimates ranged from 1 million to 2 million persons. With the aging of that cohort, the prevalence of iatrogenic risk for thyroid cancer and the incidence of irradiation-induced cancers have decreased substantially.

Medullary thyroid cancer arises from neuroendocrine C cells of the thyroid gland. Approximately 25% of cases are associated with inherited tumor syndromes such as multiple endocrine neoplasia (MEN) 2A (medullary thyroid cancer, parathyroid tumors, and pheochromocytoma), MEN 2B (medullary thyroid cancer, mucosal neuromas, pheochromocytoma, and marfanoid habitus), or familial medullary carcinoma. All familial forms are inherited with the pattern of autosomal dominance, with mutations in the tyrosine kinase protooncogene *RET* identifiable in 98% of cases. Medullary thyroid cancer has been the most common cause of death in patients with MEN 2. There is great potential for genetic testing, followed by prophylactic thyroidectomy of young children shown to be carriers of predisposing RET protooncogene mutations, to reduce mortality and morbidity for these patients.

NATURAL HISTORY OF THYROID CANCER AND EFFECTIVENESS OF THERAPY (10,12–15)

The prevalence of occult carcinoma of the thyroid is not well defined. Autopsy studies have indicated that the prevalence ranges from 5% to 13%. An often-quoted study showing an overall prevalence of 5.7% found the highest age-specific rates in the fifth and sixth decades.

A high prevalence of asymptomatic thyroid cancer is not surprising, considering the benign clinical course of most thyroid tumors after diagnosis. Follow-up studies have determined that the probability of survival depends on the tissue type and age of the patient. For localized papillary carcinoma, survival approximates that of age-matched controls; in one large study, no deaths occurred among patients younger than 40 years of age during 10 to 15 years of follow-up. The course of follicular cancer is only slightly more aggressive. Anaplastic tumors, on the other hand, run a rapid clinical course to death.

The relatively high prevalence of occult thyroid cancer presumed to be present in general raises a number of questions about the significance of tumors found during the evaluation of patients with radiation exposure. In the largest cohort study of irradiated patients, 47% of the tumors were incidental findings identified after surgery was recommended because of palpable or scan abnormalities. No evidence indicates that tumors found in patients with past radiation exposure are more likely to result in morbidity or mortality than are occult tumors found in the general population. However, they do have a high frequency of recurrence.

Medullary thyroid carcinoma has a prognosis worse than that of papillary or follicular tumors. Patients with MEN syndromes often present with symptoms associated with other elements of the syndrome. Historically when patients were found to have medullary cancers, about 50% were found to have lymph node involvement. Recent follow-up of patients identified by DNA analysis as carriers of RET mutations and subjected to prophylactic thyroidectomy have been encouraging. In one study of 50 patients 19 years of age or younger with the RET mutation characteristic MEN 2A who underwent prophylactic thyroidectomy, there was no evidence of persistent or recurrent medullary thyroid cancer 5 or more years after surgery.

SCREENING AND DIAGNOSTIC TESTS (14,10,16–19)

The sensitivity of *history taking* in identifying persons at risk is not known. Many who were irradiated during early childhood may be unaware of their exposure. *Physical examination* of the thyroid gland is often difficult, and the palpable nodule is a nonspecific finding that can be found in 4% to 7% of the adult population. *Thyroid scan* is more sensitive in detecting thyroid abnormalities, but because it fails to distinguish between benign and malignant disease, it is even less specific. A number of studies have indicated that physical examination itself becomes more sensitive after scanning has been performed and the physician is aware of scan results.

Large studies using both multiple examinations and technetium (^{99m}Tc) scanning indicate that 60% of thyroid abnormalities (identified by either or both modalities) will be identified by palpation alone. Scanning alone will be more than 95% sensitive. However, palpable abnormalities appear to be more specific for cancer. In one study of patients with palpable nodules who ultimately underwent thyroidectomy, the prevalence of cancer was 34%; it was 19% among patients who went to surgery on the basis of scan abnormalities alone. Physical examination was nearly 80% sensitive in identifying thyroid glands containing cancers. Cancers found in glands with scan abnormalities alone were often incidental, unrelated to the scan abnormality.

The availability of high-resolution *ultrasonography* has increased the ability to identify small thyroid nodules. Ultrasonography has been shown to be better than physical examination, isotope scanning, magnetic resonance imaging, and computed tomography in detecting nodules. However, no specific sonographic criteria distinguish between benign and malignant nodules. In one study, 14% of cystic thyroid lesions were cancers, compared with 23% of solid lesions.

Attempts to use measurements of serum thyroglobulin as a screening test for thyroid cancer have not been successful. Despite poor specificity, thyroglobulin abnormalities are disappointingly insensitive.

When abnormalities are detected on examination or on scan, additional diagnostic steps are indicated. The refinement of *fine-needle aspiration biopsy* with *cytologic examination* has made this the first-line diagnostic test in many centers (see Chapter 95).

In cases of questionable physical examination or scan findings, some physicians have suppressed the thyroid for 3 to 6 months in an effort to shrink normal thyroid tissue and thereby increase the sensitivity of the examination for autonomous nodules. Although this remains a reasonable approach when cancer risk is low, it must be kept in mind that regression following thyroid hormone suppression is neither perfectly sensitive nor highly specific for thyroid cancer. Cases have been reported of confirmed carcinomas that apparently responded to suppression therapy; only a minority of nodules that do not respond prove to be malignant.

On the basis of animal experiments, long-term thyroid suppression as prophylaxis for thyroid cancer has also been advocated for all patients with a history of irradiation exposure or, more selectively, those with questionable scan findings.

The penetrance of inherited medullary thyroid carcinoma is as high as 95%, warranting prospective family screening to identify gene carriers. Screening is recommended by age 5 years in familial medullary carcinoma and MEN type 2A and by age 6 months in MEN 2B. Genetic testing should also be offered to patients with apparent sporadic medullary cancer. Prophylactic thyroidectomy is recommended for family members who are found to be carriers of a familial *RET* mutation.

CONCLUSIONS AND RECOMMENDATIONS

- Childhood irradiation was an important risk factor for thyroid carcinoma, which may be diagnosed decades after exposure.
- The prevalence of thyroid abnormalities among the estimated 1 to 2 million patients with a history of exposure was about 25%. The prevalence of thyroid cancer was estimated to be 7% to 9%.
- The significance of occult thyroid cancer in exposed patients is not known. The prevalence of occult tumors in the general population appears to be high.
- Patients at risk because of an exposure history should be carefully examined yearly or at least every 2 years.
- Needle biopsy may be preferred in cases in which a single nodule has been identified. Multiple examinations by experienced examiners may be necessary. Thyroid suppression may increase the sensitivity of thyroid palpation. The examination of patients with normal examination but abnormal scan findings should be repeated yearly.
- Patients in known kindreds with inherited medullary thyroid carcinoma should be screened from early childhood. Genetic testing should be offered to patients with sporadic medullary tumors. Prophylactic thyroidectomy should be offered to carriers of a familial *RET* mutation.

A.G.M.

Annotated Bibliography

1. Boikos SA, Strakis CA. Molecular mechanism of medullary thyroid carcinoma: current approaches in diagnosis and treatment. Histol Histopathol 2008;23:109. (*A review from the National Institutes of Health, focusing on clinical issues in the relationship between multiple endocrine neoplasia 2 and medullary thyroid cancer.*)
2. Moore SW, Appfelstaedt J, Zaahl MG. Familial medullary carcinoma prevention, risk evaluation, and RET in children of families with MEN 2. J Pediatr Surg 2007;42:326. (*Describes an active screening program and its impact.*)
3. Gonzalez-Villalpando C, Frohman LA, Bekerman C, et al. Scintigraphic thyroid abnormalities after radiation. Ann Intern Med 1982;97:55. (*Palpable and nonpalpable thyroid nodules were much more common among patients with prior radiation exposure than among controls.*)
4. Kim WB, Han S, Kim TY, et al. Ultrasonographic screening for detection of thyroid cancer in patients with Graves' disease. Clin Endocrinol 2004;60:719. (*The prevalence of cancer was 3.3% in Graves' patients.*)
5. McTiernan AM, Weiss NS, Daling JR. Incidence of thyroid cancer in women in relation to previous exposure to radiation therapy and history of thyroid disease. J Natl Cancer Inst 1984;73:575. (*The relative risk for exposed women was 16.5.*)
6. McTiernan AM, Weiss NS, Daling JR. Incidence of thyroid cancer in women in relation to reproductive and hormonal factors. Am J Epidemiol 1984;120:423. (*Despite the effect on the production of thyroid-stimulating hormone, pregnancy and the use of exogenous estrogens had little or no effect on the risk for thyroid carcinoma in this case–control study.*)
7. Negri E, Ron E, DalMaso L, et al. A pooled analysis of case–control studies of thyroid cancer. Cancer Causes Control 1999;10:143. (*Any associations between thyroid cancer and menstrual or reproductive factors are weak.*)
8. Sampson RJ, Woolner LB, Bahn RC, et al. Occult thyroid carcinoma in Olmstead County, Minnesota: prevalence of autopsy compared with that in Hiroshima and Nagasaki, Japan. Cancer 1974;34:2072. (*Prevalence was 5.6% among 157 autopsies of patients with clinically occult thyroid cancer; the highest age-specific prevalence was between 40 and 60 years.*)
9. Schneider AB, Recant W, Pinsky SM. Radiation-induced thyroid carcinoma. Ann Intern Med 1986;105:405. (*Describes the clinical course of the Michael Reese Hospital cohort at a mean follow-up of 10 years, noting a high frequency of recurrent disease; small nodules were managed conservatively.*)
10. Sherman SI. Thyroid carcinoma. Lancet 2003;361:501. (*An excellent review of all aspects of thyroid cancer, including screening for inherited medullary thyroid carcinoma; 168 references.*)
11. VanHerle AJ, Rich P, Ljung BE, et al. The thyroid nodule. Ann Intern Med 1982;96:221. (*An extensive review of the diagnostic value of fine-needle aspiration, thyroid scanning, and ultrasonography, including an analysis of alternative sequencing strategies; recommends fine-needle aspiration followed by scanning in patients with cytologically suspect lesions.*)
12. Bucci A, Shore-Freedman E, Gierlowski T, et al. Behavior of small thyroid cancers found by screening radiation-exposed individuals. J Clin Endocrinol Metab 2001;86:3711. (*The increased risk of recurrence for small tumors found on screening was associated with short latency, lymph node involvement, multifocality, and higher radiation dose.*)
13. De los Santos ET, Keyhani-Rofagha S, Cunningham JJ, et al. Cystic thyroid nodules. The dilemma of malignant lesions. Arch Intern Med 1990;150:1422. (*Of 71 cystic lesions, 14% were malignant, compared with 23% of 150 solid lesions; sensitivity and specificity of fine-needle aspiration cytology were 88% and 52%, respectively, for cystic lesions, and 100% and 55%, respectively, for solid lesions.*)
14. Gagel RF, Tashjian AH, Cummings T, et al. The clinical outcome of prospective screening for multiple endocrine neoplasia type 2a. N Engl J Med 1988;318:478. (*Reports an 86% disease-free survival in 22 patients followed for a mean of 11 years after being given a screening diagnosis of medullary thyroid carcinoma.*)
15. Skinner MA, Moley JA, Dilley WG, et al. Prophylactic thyroidectomy in multiple endocrine neoplasia type 2A. N Engl J Med. 2005;353:1105-13. (*No evidence was found for persistence or recurrence in 50 patients 5 or more years after surgery.*)

16. Friedman M, Toriumi DM, Mafee MF. Diagnostic imaging techniques in thyroid cancer. Am J Surg 1988;155:215. (*Argues that refinement of fine-needle aspiration cytology has made radionuclide scanning and other imaging studies second-line diagnostic tools for thyroid cancer.*)

17. Gharib H, Goeller JR. Fine-needle aspiration biopsy of the thyroid: an appraisal. Ann Intern Med 1993;118:282. (*Advocates fine-needle aspiration as the first step in diagnosis.*)

18. Miki H, Inoue H, Komaki K, et al. Value of mass screening for thyroid cancer. World J Surg 1998;22:99. (*Only 36 cancers were found among 18,619 screenees in Japan.*)

19. Ravetto C, Colombo DS, Dottorini ME. Usefulness of fine-needle aspiration in the diagnosis of thyroid carcinoma: a retrospective study in 37,895 patients. Cancer 2000;90:357. (*Documents its role as an appropriate initial procedure.*)

CHAPTER 95 ■ EVALUATION OF THYROID NODULES

DAVID M. SLOVIK

Thyroid nodules are extremely common, both clinically and on imaging studies of the neck. A palpable thyroid nodule can be detected in 4% to 7% of the adult population (10 to 20 million people in the United States). The prevalence of nodules in autopsy series approaches 50%, a figure that is approximated by patients undergoing modern high-resolution, real-time ultrasonography of the thyroid. The incidence of thyroid nodules increases with age and head or neck irradiation; it is more common in women than in men. In patients with thyroid nodules, the rate of carcinoma is twice as high in men than women and highest in those older than age 60 years or younger than age 30 years.

The principal objective in evaluating thyroid nodules is to differentiate malignant from benign lesions. Most thyroid nodules are benign. About 70% of nodules subjected to fine-needle biopsy prove to be benign; 4% to 5% are malignant; in the remainder, the cytologic findings are either inadequate or indeterminate. Additional tasks are to determine the functional status of a nodule and assess any adverse effect on neighboring structures.

Because of the high frequency and potential importance of thyroid nodules, the primary care physician must be able to coordinate a cost-effective evaluation; to that end, familiarity with the indications for and utilities of scanning, ultrasonography, and fine-needle aspiration is necessary. In addition, an understanding of the respective roles of surgery, suppressive therapy, and watchful waiting facilitate the formulation of an appropriate program of symptomatic management.

PATHOPHYSIOLOGY AND CLINICAL PRESENTATION (1–15)

Thyroid nodules may be single or multiple, with or without underlying disturbances of hormonal homeostasis. A solitary nodule is usually more worrisome because it may represent a malignancy, although on occasion a multinodular gland may harbor a cancer, especially if there is a dominant nodule. Thyroid nodules are usually asymptomatic and discovered incidentally by the patient or examining physician or as a consequence of a radiologic procedure (e.g., neck computed tomography or carotid ultrasonography). Large nodules may cause a cosmetic problem or compress an adjacent structure. The nodules are usually painless unless rapid growth, inflammation, or hemorrhage occurs, and they may then produce significant discomfort.

Solitary Nodule

Solitary thyroid nodules represent benign adenomas, carcinomas, or multinodular conditions in which only a single nodule is palpable.

Benign Adenomas

Benign adenomas account for most nonmalignant, truly solitary nodules. The majority, designated as *follicular* (*macrofollicular* or *microfollicular*), have a fibrous capsule and a histologic appearance characteristic of thyroid tissue; the remainder, labeled *colloid* or *adenomatous nodules*, are not well encapsulated and are usually found in a multinodular goiter. They behave similarly. Growth is typically slow, extending over many years. Follicular adenomas rarely become large enough to encroach on the trachea or esophagus. Thyroid adenomas are usually monoclonal in origin. Thyroid-stimulating–hormone (TSH) receptors are present in most, making them hormonally responsive. Most do not produce much thyroid hormone, and their limited radioiodine uptake on scan sometimes gives the appearance of a "cold" nodule.

Benign adenomas that outgrow their blood supply may undergo necrosis, degenerate, become filled with fluid, and appear on ultrasonography as nodules with solid and cystic elements. Adenomas make up a significant proportion of such "cystic" lesions.

A few follicular adenomas produce such large quantities of thyroid hormone that the patient presents with thyrotoxicosis (see Chapter 103). This is particularly true of so-called "*toxic*" *adenomas* exceeding 3 cm in diameter. They function autonomously, suppress TSH (which renders the rest of the gland atrophic), and appear as "*hot*" *nodules* on thyroid scan. Patients with a smaller hot nodule may remain euthyroid, although enough thyroid hormone is produced to suppress the rest of the gland and render it atrophic.

Thyroid Carcinomas

Thyroid carcinomas are uncommon; they account for approximately 1% of all malignant neoplasia. The current incidence is 5 to 10 per 100,000 persons annually, although it is higher in areas with radiation exposure. They are more frequent in women than in men (3:1). The prevalence is higher in children, adults younger than 30 years or older than 60 years, and patients with a history of prior head or neck irradiation or a family history of thyroid cancer. On radioiodine scan, most thyroid carcinomas present as *"cold" nodules*, failing to take up iodine, although on technetium scan, a rare malignant nodule will take up the radionuclide. On ultrasonography, most cancers are solid, although a mixed cystic–solid appearance is encountered in about 20%, and even a purely cystic-appearing lesion may occasionally be malignant.

Papillary and Mixed Papillary–Follicular Carcinomas. Papillary and mixed papillary–follicular carcinomas are the most common and account for 70% of all thyroid malignancies. Up to 15% to 20% of all autopsies show microscopic foci of papillary carcinoma. A tumor that contains any papillary element is considered papillary even if it contains follicular components. The lesions tend to be very slow growing, spreading locally to adjacent cervical lymph nodes but not metastasizing distantly until very late and then in only 5% of cases. Consequently, the prognosis is good even after local spread has occurred. Although most are solid, some may present as mixed cystic–solid lesions because of necrosis and liquefaction.

Follicular Carcinomas. Follicular carcinomas, which make up another 10% to 20% of thyroid cancers, are also slow growing. Local spread to regional nodes may occur without invasion of the thyroid capsule, but this does not alter the prognosis. Hematogenous spread can develop early, and the initial presentation is often a metastasis to lung or bone. Follicular carcinomas represent a wide spectrum of disease. Prognosis depends on the degree of vascular invasion and metastases.

Anaplastic Carcinomas. Anaplastic carcinomas make up another 10% to 12% of cases. These show a high degree of cellular undifferentiation and are among the most aggressive of human cancers, being very invasive, usually inoperable, and fatal within 1 year. They often present as a rapidly growing thyroid mass, with hoarseness, dyspnea, and dysphagia.

Medullary Carcinomas. Medullary carcinomas, derived from the parafollicular cells of the thyroid, represent 10% of thyroid cancers. Sporadic and familial forms of the disease are seen; among the latter are familial medullary cancers unaccompanied by other conditions and *multiple endocrine neoplasia* (MEN) types IIA and IIB (which occur in conjunction with pheochromocytoma and hyperparathyroidism). Mutations in the *HRPT2 gene* have been found with sporadic disease, and mutations in the *RET protooncogene* have been strongly associated with familial medullary thyroid carcinoma and MEN 2A and 2B. Timing of malignant transformation and clinical onset of hereditary forms varies by specific mutation. The malignancy often presents as a nodule located in the upper half of the thyroid gland. It can be multicentric, especially in the familial forms. Approximately 70% of medullary carcinomas of the thyroid occur sporadically. *Calcitonin,* produced by the parafollicular or "C" cells, is a unique tumor marker for medullary carcinoma, yet these patients remain eucalcemic.

The prognosis is highly variable but similar to that of follicular carcinoma. Tumor spread is often to the lymph nodes of the neck and mediastinum, but distant spread to the lungs, bone, and liver may also occur.

Lymphoma. Lymphoma may sometimes develop as a primary lesion within the thyroid; it makes up 1% to 4% of thyroid malignancies. Up to 70% arise in patients with chronic lymphocytic thyroiditis. Its clinical course is a function of tissue type and stage at time of presentation (see Chapter 84). Spread to local nodes is common and prominent.

Multiple Nodules

Hashimoto's Thyroiditis

Hashimoto's thyroiditis, an autoimmune condition, is the leading cause of a multinodular gland in the United States. Evidence of the condition can be found in about 4% of the general population and up to 15% of women older than the age of 65 years. Women patients outnumber men by a ratio of 3:1. Pathologically, there is a marked lymphocytic infiltration, formation of germinal centers, atrophy of thyroid follicles, absent colloid, fibrosis, and oxyphilic or eosinophilic changes involving follicular epithelial cells. Although not unique to this condition, *antimicrosomal antibodies* are found in 70% to 95% of patients. About one third of patients manifest a multinodular goiter, although euthyroid goiter is actually the most common presentation. The immunologically mediated injury impairs thyroxine synthesis and increases leakage of hormone into the circulation. One third of patients experience progressive loss of glandular function and eventually become hypothyroid. Hyperthyroidism in uncommon but can occur in patients with a prominent lymphocytic infiltrate.

Multinodular Goiter

Multinodular goiter is the second-most-common cause of a multinodular gland in adults. It represents an advanced stage of focal autonomous hyperplasia, which initially presents as a diffusely enlarged gland but then progresses to multinodularity as areas of focal hyperplasia undergo degenerative changes. Nodules may also develop when colloid accumulates in hyperplastic cells (*colloid cysts*). Uptake of radioiodine on scan is heterogeneous; some areas may not take up iodine and appear "cold." The thyroid gland feels less firm than it does in Hashimoto's disease. The TSH level may be slightly reduced, reflecting the autonomous nature of the thyroxine output of the gland, but free thyroxine levels are usually within normal limits.

Cancers

Cancers may arise in a multinodular gland, although this is very uncommon. Thyroid cancer and lymphoma are the leading causes. Cervical adenopathy, hoarseness (resulting from recurrent laryngeal nerve compression), and the continued enlargement of a "cold" nodule on thyroid scan are distinguishing features of the clinical presentation. A history of head and neck irradiation or family history of thyroid cancer (suggestive of hereditary disease) are risk factors. The nodule may be tender if the tumor is rapidly growing (as with lymphoma), a finding atypical of other multinodular goiters. Occasionally metastases to the thyroid occur, primarily from breast and renal cell carcinoma.

Incidentalomas

The term incidentalomas is used to refer to nonpalpable thyroid nodules detected incidentally in the course of imaging of the neck area by ultrasonography or other sensitive diagnostic modalities. The risk for malignancy is low when the diameter of the lesion is less than 1.5 cm. Even if some incidentalomas represent early papillary cancers, the rate of growth is likely to be very slow for lesions smaller than 1.5 cm.

DIFFERENTIAL DIAGNOSIS

The vast majority of solitary nodules are benign, even those that fail to take up radionuclide on thyroid scan (see later discussion). In the United States, Hashimoto's thyroiditis accounts for the majority of cases of multinodular goiter. Cancers account for about 10% to 20% of solitary thyroid nodules; the prevalence is lower in patients with multinodular glands (Table 95.1).

WORKUP (4–9,16–21)

As noted earlier, the main objective is to differentiate a carcinoma from benign causes of nodularity. Although a definitive assessment cannot be made by history and physical examination alone, these elements provide important information regarding risk and need for biopsy or excision. Other tasks include identification of autonomous function and compression of adjacent structures.

History

The history is reviewed not only for the clinical presentation of the nodule and associated symptoms, but also for important cancer risk factors, such as a history of head and neck irradiation in childhood, exposure to excessive environmental radiation, and a positive family history of thyroid cancer. Age and gender are also relevant. Patients younger than 30 years and older than 60 years and male patients are at increased risk for a malignant thyroid nodule. Symptoms suggestive of local compression or invasion (e.g., *hoarseness, dysphagia,* and *tracheal wheezing*) should be noted, as should the new appearance of a nodule or the rapid growth of an existing one. However, bleeding into a benign cyst or subacute thyroiditis may cause a similarly abrupt change and new onset of symptoms. Moreover, most benign cystic and solid nodules tend to grow over time, making reports of increase in size an unreliable predictor of malignancy. Conversely, many thyroid cancers are slow growing and may have been present for years; duration is not particularly useful for distinguishing benign from malignant disease. Such factors as residence in an iodine-deficient area, presence of goiter, or intake of goitrogens (e.g., lithium, turnips, beets) favor a benign thyroid lesion, as does a family history of goiter (as opposed to thyroid cancer). Symptoms of hypothyroidism or hyperthyroidism argue against malignancy.

Physical Examination

The physical examination focuses on the gland and adjacent lymph nodes. The gland is noted for its overall size, consistency, and number and size of nodules. A solitary hard nodule that is irregular and fixed (fails to move with swallowing) is suggestive of malignancy, as is the rapid growth of a large, solid thyroid mass. However, finding a soft nodule does not rule out the diagnosis of cancer because a papillary carcinoma that has undergone cystic degeneration can be soft to the touch. Finding a single nodule increases the chances of cancer; few multinodular goiters harbor a cancer.

The adjacent lymph nodes, especially those on the same side as the nodule, require detailed examination. A thyroid nodule with associated cervical adenopathy should be viewed with marked suspicion. A single node may represent metastasis

---

TABLE 95.1

DIFFERENTIAL DIAGNOSIS OF THYROID NODULARITY

Cause	Distinguishing Characteristics
Solitary Nodule	
Benign adenoma	Solid or mixed cystic and solid; most euthyroid and responsive to TSH; those >3 cm may become autonomous and present as a "hot" nodule on scan
Cancer	
Papillary or mixed	Single hard nodule; local adenopathy; "cold" on scan; slow growing; metastasizes very late
Follicular	Same, although metastasizes earlier; some cystic
Medullary	May be familial; multiple endocrine neoplasia; calcitonin elevated; "cold" nodule
Lymphoma	Primary cancer arises in patients with chronic lymphocytic thyroiditis; prominent regional nodes
Multinodular	
Hashimoto's thyroiditis	Multinodular, rubbery gland; antithyroid antibodies; one third are hypothyroid; heterogeneous uptake; TSH responsive
Multinodular goiter	Multiple nodules, enlarged gland; heterogeneous uptake on scan with some areas of decreased or absent uptake; clinically euthyroid, although some with mild decrease in TSH; autonomous gland
Cancer	
Thyroid	Same as preceding
Lymphoma	May arise in a Hashimoto's gland

TSH, thyroid-stimulating hormone.

from the thyroid, whereas multiple nodes in a young person with a thyroid nodule raise the possibility of lymphoma. The vocal cords should be viewed in patients with hoarseness as vocal cord paralysis suggests cancer.

Laboratory Studies

Thyroid-Stimulating Hormone

In any patient with a thyroid nodule, a TSH level should be initially obtained because it will direct further diagnostic studies. A low TSH, suggestive of overt or subclinical hyperthyroidism, should be followed by a *radioisotope scan*. If the nodule is hot, then therapy should be considered for hyperthyroidism. If the TSH is normal, then a *fine needle aspiration* should be performed.

Fine-Needle Aspiration Biopsy

Fine-needle aspiration biopsy (with or without ultrasound guidance) has become the test of choice for the initial evaluation of most euthyroid patients with a thyroid nodule, having supplanted the radionuclide thyroid scan and ultrasonography in determining which patients need surgical excision. The fine needle (usually 25 to 27 gauge) is inserted into the nodule and its contents are aspirated and then smeared directly on slides, fixed, stained, and then analyzed. In skilled hands, the sensitivity of fine-needle biopsy exceeds 95%. Although radionuclide scanning and ultrasonography also provide high sensitivity, their specificity is poor. The specificity of fine-needle biopsy ranges from 70% when patients with "suspicious" readings are included in the group in need of surgery to greater than 90% when they are not. In comparison with ultrasonography and radionuclide scan, fine-needle biopsy has reduced by half the number of patients who undergo operations needlessly, doubled the incidence of malignancy in surgically excised nodules, and reduced costs by greater than 25%. The procedure is safe, inexpensive, and readily performed in the office setting. A skilled physician is needed to perform the procedure and an experienced pathologist to interpret the results so that errors in sampling and interpretation are minimized.

Failure to drain a cystic lesion completely and obtain samples from the residual mass is an important source of false-negative results. With cytologic information provided by aspiration biopsy only, it can be difficult for even experienced pathologists to differentiate benign Hürthle cell and follicular adenomas from their malignant counterparts. Patients with lesions labeled "suspicious" or "indeterminate" usually must undergo surgical excision of the nodule, although sometimes malignancy can be ruled out by radionuclide scanning.

The cytologic results are generally divided into four categories: (a) nondiagnostic; (b) benign, including macrofollicular or colloid adenomas and lymphocytic thyroiditis; (c) suspicious or indeterminate, including microfollicular or cellular adenomas and Hürthle cell; and (d) malignant.

Radionuclide Scanning

As noted previously, radionuclide scanning has been supplanted by fine-needle aspiration biopsy as the initial test of choice in patients with a euthyroid nodule, but by imaging using one of the radioisotopes of iodine or technetium, it provides a measure of the iodine-trapping function in a nodule compared with the surrounding thyroid tissue. Nodules are classified as *hypofunctioning* ("*cold*"), 80% to 85% of all nodules; *indeterminate* ("*warm*"), 10%; or *hyperfunctioning* ("*hot*"), less than 5%. Although it is true that most malignant disease has the appearance of a "cold" nodule on scan, only 5% to 15% of all cold nodules are malignant. Moreover, uptake in a nodule ("warm" nodule) does not entirely rule out malignancy. Thus, radionuclide scanning is best relegated to a supplemental role performed after fine-needle biopsy in patients with "suspicious" cytologic findings. A "hot" nodule on the scan of such patients indicates an autonomously hyperfunctioning nodule, which is associated with a very low risk for cancer. A "suspicious" nodule that is "warm" or "cold" on scan is more likely to be cancerous, so surgical excision must be considered. A radionuclide scan can also be of help in detecting multinodularity, although thyroid ultrasonography is even more sensitive.

Thyroid Ultrasonography

Thyroid ultrasonography provides high sensitivity in the detection of nodules (down to 1 mm), and a unique ability to differentiate solid from cystic lesions. As such, it is very helpful in localizing lesions for biopsy. However, even with the development of new, high-resolution ultrasonographic technology to detect ever-smaller lesions, the test lacks diagnostic specificity because no clearly defined architectural criteria are available for differentiating benign from malignant lesions. Combined data show that 21% of solid lesions, 12% of mixed lesions, and 7% of purely cystic lesions are malignant. Now that "cystic" is no longer considered synonymous with "benign," the test has fallen into disuse as a means of determining risk for malignancy. It is excellent for determining multinodularity, but the meaning of such multinodularity is unclear because up to 40% of all patients with a solitary nodule clinically are found by modern ultrasonography to have multiple nodules.

Ancillary Laboratory Studies

Most such studies are usually of little direct help in deciding who should undergo biopsy, but they occasionally provide supportive information. An abnormal *TSH level* is uncommon in malignant disease, as are high titers of *anti–thyroid peroxidase antibodies* (useful in suspected cases of Hashimoto's and subacute lymphocytic thyroiditis). Routine use of plain films is not cost-effective. A very high *erythrocyte sedimentation rate* in the setting of an acutely tender gland is very suggestive of subacute granulomatous thyroiditis. A serum *calcitonin* determination is indicated when the patient has a strong family history of thyroid cancer. No other markers are known for thyroid cancers. *Thyroglobulin* is a normal thyroid tissue component and is most useful as a tumor marker after total thyroid ablation; elevations do occur with cancer, but they also occur with benign nodular thyroid disease. The response to *TSH suppression* (by administration of thyroid hormone) is not reliable for differentiating cancer from benign disease because both may either shrink or not in response to exogenous hormone. In rare instances, a plain film of the chest or neck may incidentally reveal punctate calcifications characteristic of the psammoma bodies of papillary carcinoma or the shell-like calcification characteristic of a benign lesion, but routinely obtaining such films is of low diagnostic yield.

Genetic testing for diagnosis and management of medullary thyroid cancer is still in the developmental stage but is likely to play an increasingly important role as more data are collected on the significance of particular gene mutations. For example, in families with hereditary forms of medullary thyroid cancer, identifying the responsible RET gene mutation may help to determine the need for and timing of prophylactic thyroidectomy.

Testing Sequence

The most cost-effective testing sequence for the euthyroid patient with a single thyroid nodule on physical examination and without a low TSH is to begin with *fine-needle aspiration biopsy*. If the cytology is "malignant," then surgery is indicated. If the reading is "benign," then observation for 1 year and *follow-up ultrasonography* are reasonable. If the reading is "suspicious," then *radionuclide scan* for determination of nodule uptake is indicated. A "hot" nodule indicates autonomous function, with a very low risk for cancer, and requires only clinical follow-up with or without treatment, depending on whether the patient is euthyroid or thyrotoxic. A "warm" or "cold" nodule in a patient with "suspicious" cytology indicating nonfunction of the nodule raises the question of cancer and necessitates surgical excision.

If after 1 year of observation the follow-up thyroid ultrasonography indicates an increase in nodule size, then repeated biopsy is indicated. An enlarging nodule that continues to appear benign on repeated biopsy can be treated with levothyroxine suppressive therapy (see later discussion) and restudied by ultrasonography in another year's time. If the nodule has stopped enlarging on suppressive therapy, then suppressive therapy can be continued and the patient reassessed annually. If the size is increasing, then surgical removal is undertaken. Malignant or suspect pathologic findings are always an indication for surgery.

Patients with Multinodular Glands

Biopsy is usually not required unless the concern for cancer is increased because of neck irradiation, cervical adenopathy, rapid growth of a single nodule in an otherwise stable gland, onset of recurrent laryngeal nerve palsy, or a dominant nodule. Most cases represent Hashimoto's thyroiditis, and a diagnosis can be made by obtaining antithyroid antibody determinations. High titers of *antiperoxidase antibodies* correlate best with biopsy-proven disease. Antithyroglobulin titers are less useful. The risk for *lymphoma* of the thyroid is increased in patients with Hashimoto's disease, so *needle biopsy* of the gland is mandated in the presence of an enlarging tender goiter, cervical adenopathy, or a goiter markedly enlarging on thyroid hormone–suppressive therapy (which should cause the nodule size to decrease in Hashimoto's disease).

Further Evaluation of the Benign Adenoma

When a lesion is found to be a benign adenoma, the question arises of whether it is functioning autonomously and thus posing a risk for toxicity. Adenomas smaller than 2 cm rarely change much in size or function and can be followed. Those larger than 3 cm are at risk for progressing to toxicity within a few years. Autonomous function is determined by performing *serial radionuclide scans*. Observation rather than ablation is now preferred for the smaller, low-risk lesions. Annual determination of the nodular size and hormonal output usually suffices. Periodic scanning (e.g., every 5 years) can be repeated to see whether suppression of extranodular tissue function is increasing, a sign of impending toxicity. Other signs include size greater than 3 cm, a rise in serum triiodothyronine to the upper limits of normal, and decreasing responsiveness to stimulation or suppression.

Incidentalomas

Controversy exists as to whether incidentally discovered thyroid nodules less than 1.5 cm and in the absence of known risk factors (e.g., head and neck irradiation) require evaluation. However, studies have shown some of these incidentally found nodules to be cancer. Patients with lesions larger than 1.5 cm, prior head or neck irradiation, a strongly positive family history of thyroid cancer, or ultrasonographic findings suggestive of malignancy require biopsy at the outset.

SYMPTOMATIC THERAPY AND FOLLOW-UP (5,6,9,15,22–32)

Euthyroid Patients with a Benign Solitary Nodule

The best approach to management is unclear because no definitive data from prospective, randomized studies are available. Small, asymptomatic, solitary nodules can be followed without therapy unless they enlarge. Optimal management of larger nodules is less clear. *Low-dose suppressive therapy* (sufficient to reduce the TSH level to low but not undetectable levels) with *levothyroxine* is advocated by some as a relatively safe means of reducing the risk for nodule growth and decreasing the nodule size. In approximately 10% to 30% of patients with a nontoxic solitary nodule, the nodule size decreases when doses of levothyroxine sufficient to suppress TSH are given, although such treatment does not appear to work in patients with colloid nodules. The rationale for suppressive therapy is that reducing TSH stimulation should diminish the size of lesions that are TSH responsive (e.g., follicular adenomas, Hashimoto's thyroiditis). Critics of suppressive therapy argue that the risk for nodule growth is small and the ability of suppressive therapy to reduce nodule size is modest at best. Moreover, even partially suppressive doses of levothyroxine are associated with a risk for osteoporosis, especially in postmenopausal women, who are the majority of patients.

The required dose of levothyroxine for suppressive therapy is in the range of 0.1 to 0.15 mg daily, with small doses (e.g., 0.05 mg/d) given first and increased gradually until the TSH level declines to about 0.3 mU/L. Further suppression markedly increases the risk for thyroxine-induced osteoporosis (see Chapter 103). Suppressive therapy is relatively contraindicated in the elderly and those with underlying coronary disease (see Chapter 103).

Pending better data, one suggested approach is to observe the nodule for 1 year after the initial biopsy, recheck its size by ultrasonography, perform another biopsy on any nodule that appears to be enlarging, and, if the nodule is benign, institute modest suppressive therapy in an attempt to halt enlargement and achieve some reduction in size. If the nodule continues to enlarge, then *surgical removal* is recommended; otherwise, levothyroxine is continued and the nodule size is checked at regular intervals.

Nontoxic Multinodular Goiter

Such nodular glands often do not shrink much because they are composed of a great deal of fibrous tissue. Dominant nodules caused by bothersome *large cysts* may require *surgical removal*, but smaller ones can be aspirated as necessary, both to rule out malignancy (incidence about 1%) and to increase comfort and improve appearance. Hormone therapy has no effect on the recurrence of thyroid cysts after aspiration or on nodular disease because glandular function typically becomes increasingly autonomous with age. *Radioiodine* is sometimes used, but high doses are required, which increases the chances of precipitating Graves' disease (5%) and possibly late malignancy.

Toxic Nodules and Autonomously Functioning Solitary Adenomas

Patients with these lesions are at high risk for overt or subclinical thyrotoxicosis, especially if the nodule is larger than 3 cm in diameter, the serum triiodothyronine level is at the upper limit of normal, and the nodule is increasingly unresponsive to thyroxine suppression. Such patients should be considered for *ablative therapy*. Ablation is mandatory for those with autonomous nodules that have already become toxic. One needs to choose between surgery and radioiodine. *Surgery* represents a definitive approach with low risk if performed by a skilled thyroid surgeon. Young patients are the best candidates. *Radioiodine* is simpler and usually the treatment of choice in the elderly. The theoretical risk of inducing cancer in the remaining thyroid tissue makes radioiodine a less attractive option for young people, although no increase in the incidence of malignancy has been reported. A palpable nodule often remains after irradiation; it is of no consequence except for the cosmetic effect. The patient needs to be monitored for the development of posttreatment hypothyroidism (see Chapter 104).

PATIENT EDUCATION

The primary care physician should counsel and closely follow patients who have undergone previous head or neck radiation (see Chapter 94). Regular follow-up is important for any patient with a nodule, and the patient should be instructed to call if a change in size, development of lymphadenopathy, pain, dysphagia, or hoarseness is noted.

The patient with an autonomous nodule or a multinodular goiter should be advised to avoid substances containing high concentrations of iodine (medications, kelp, radiographic contrast media) because they may precipitate thyrotoxicosis. If a contrast study is necessary, the patient should be started on a β-blocking agent 10 days before the study.

INDICATIONS FOR REFERRAL

Detection of a solitary thyroid nodule in a clinically euthyroid patient should prompt a referral to a consultant skilled in performing fine-needle biopsy of the thyroid. Finding a worrisome nodule (see earlier discussion) in a patient with a multinodular gland represents another indication for consideration of biopsy. Patients with a toxic or large (>3 cm), autonomously functioning adenoma require consultation for discussion of ablative therapy. Those with goiters that are unresponsive to thyroid hormone and are causing obstruction or unpleasant cosmetic effects may be surgical candidates.

Annotated Bibliography

1. Alexander EK, Hurwitz S, Heering JP, et al. Natural history of benign solid and cystic thyroid nodules. Ann Intern Med 2003;138:315. (*Retrospective case series; most lesions increase in size, making growth an unreliable predictor of malignancy.*)
2. Belfiore A, La Rosa GL, La Porta GA, et al. Cancer risk in patients with cold nodules: relevance of iodine intake, sex, age and multinodularity. Am J Med 1992;93:363. (*Male sex and age <30 or >60 years were predictors of cancer, but multinodularity was not.*)
3. Belfiore A, Russo D, Vigneri R, et al. Graves' disease, thyroid nodules and thyroid cancer. Clin Endocrinol 2001;55:711. (*Review; a nodule diagnosed in Graves' disease patients indicates a higher risk for malignancy than one diagnosed in euthyroid patients.*)
4. De los Santos ET, Keyhani-Rofagha S, Cunningham JJ, et al. Cystic thyroid nodules: the dilemma of malignant lesions. Arch Intern Med 1990;150:1422. (*A retrospective study; 20% of cystic lesions were malignancies.*)
5. Hamburger JI. Lymphoma of the thyroid. Ann Intern Med 1983;99:685. (*A clinical review noting a relation between lymphoma and Hashimoto's thyroiditis.*)
6. Hegedus L. The thyroid nodule. N Engl J Med 2004;351:1764. (*Nice review with emphasis on the clinical approach.*)
7. Knudson N, Laurberg P, Perrild H, et al. Risk factors for goiter and thyroid nodules. Thyroid 2004;12:879. (*Identifies iodine status and tobacco smoking.*)
8. Machens A, Niccoli-Sire P, Hoegel J, et al. Early malignant progression of hereditary medullary thyroid cancer. N Engl J Med 2003;349:1517. (*Timing of transformation is closely linked to a specific gene mutation.*)
9. Pearce EN, Farwell AP, Braverman LF. Thyroiditis. N Engl J Med 2003;348:2646. (*Excellent updated review; 76 references.*)
10. Rallison ML, Dobyns BM, Meikle AW, et al. Natural history of thyroid abnormalities: prevalence, incidence, and regression of thyroid diseases in adolescents and young adults. Am J Med 1991;91:363. (*Data from a population exposed to high levels of environmental radiation; emphasizes the dynamic nature of these conditions.*)
11. Rojeski MT, Gharib H. Nodular thyroid disease. N Engl J Med 1985;313:428. (*Useful review, especially of evaluation methods; 115 references.*)
12. Ross DS. Nonpalpable thyroid nodules. J Clin Endocrinol Metab 2002;87:1938. (*Discussion of nonpalpable thyroid nodules, which are usually found incidentally during radiologic study of the head and neck.*)
13. Shattuck TM, Valimaki S, Obara T, et al. Somatic and germ-line mutations of the HRPT2 gene in sporadic parathyroid carcinoma. N Engl J Med 2003;349:18. (*Evidence for pathogenetic significance.*)
14. Simpson WJ, McKinney SE, Carruthers JS, et al. Papillary and follicular thyroid cancer. Am J Med 1987;83:479. (*Extrathyroidal extension, poor differentiation, and older age were most predictive of reduced survival.*)
15. Tan GH, Gharib H. Thyroid incidentalomas: management approaches to nonpalpable nodules discovered incidentally on thyroid imaging. Ann Intern Med 1997;126:226. (*Review finding that prognosis is good for nodules <1.5 cm and no thyroid cancer risk factors; close follow-up is critical, but biopsy is not necessary initially.*)
16. Asp AA, Georgitis W, Waldron EJ, et al. Fine needle aspiration of the thyroid: use in an average health care facility. Am J Med 1987;83:489. (*Excellent sensitivity and specificity demonstrated.*)
17. Baker BA, Gharib H. Correlation of thyroid antibodies and cytologic features in suspected autoimmune thyroid disease. Am J Med 1983;74:941. (*Establishes that antimicrosomal antibodies are the antibody test of choice for Hashimoto's disease.*)
18. Frates MC, Benson CB, Doubilet PM et al. Prevalence and distribution of carcinoma in patients with solitary and multiple thyroid nodules on sonography. J Clin Endocrinol Metab 2006;91:3411. (*For exclusion of cancer in a thyroid with multiple nodules >10 mm, up to four nodules should be considered for fine-needle aspiration.*)
19. Gharib H, Goellner JR, Zinsmeister AR, et al. Fine-needle aspiration biopsy of the thyroid. Ann Intern Med 1984;101:25. (*Addresses the difficult issue of what to do with the "suspicious" finding.*)
20. Marqusee E, Frates M, Doubilet PM, et al. Usefulness of ultrasonography in the management of nodular thyroid disease. Ann Intern Med 2000;133:696. (*Retrospective chart review; altered care in 63% of patients.*)
21. Papini E, Guglielmi R, Bianchini A, et al. Risk of malignancy in nonpalpable thyroid nodules: predictive value of ultrasound and color Doppler features. J Clin Endocrinol Metab 2002;87:1938. (*Identifies sonographic features predictive of malignancy.*)
22. Bennedbaek FN, Hegedus L. Management of the solitary thyroid nodule: results of a North American survey. J Clin Endocrinol Metab 2000;85:2493. (*A survey study showing more frequent use of fine-needle aspiration biopsy and less use of imaging compared to European counterparts; suppression therapy with levothyroxine was used in >40%, despite controversies regarding its effects*).

23. Bonnema SJ, Bennedbaek FN, Ladenson PW, et al. Management of the non-toxic multinodular goiter: a North American survey. J Clin Endocrinol Metab 2002;87:112. Questionnaire to clinicians of American Thyroid Association. (*Thyroid-stimulating hormone level and thyroid antibodies were measured by 100% and 74% of respondents, respectively.*)

24. Fogelfeld L, Wiviott MBT, Shore-Freedman E, et al. Recurrence of thyroid nodules after surgical removal in patients irradiated in childhood for benign conditions. N Engl J Med 1989;320:835. (*A study of the utility of treatment with exogenous thyroid hormone; the rate of recurrence was reduced, but not the risk for cancer.*)

25. Gharib H, James EM, Charboneau JW, et al. Suppressive therapy with levothyroxine for solitary thyroid nodules. N Engl J Med 1987;317:70. (*A double-blinded, randomized study of patients with colloid nodules; no benefit was found.*)

26. Gharib H, Mazzaferri EL. Thyroxine suppressive therapy in patients with nodular thyroid disease. Ann Intern Med 1998;128:386. (*A review of published evidence concludes that most patients with benign findings on cytology are best followed without suppressive therapy because most nodules do not continue to enlarge.*)

27. Hermus AR, Huysmans DA. Treatment of benign nodular thyroid disease. N Engl J Med 1998;338:1438. (*Excellent general review; 77 references.*)

28. Mandel SJ, Brent GA, Larsen PR. Levothyroxine therapy in patients with thyroid disease. Ann Intern Med 1993;119:429. (*Includes discussion of the use of thyroxine to reduce the size of solitary nodules.*)

29. McCowen KD, Reed JW, Fariss BL. The role of thyroid therapy in patients with thyroid cysts. Am J Med 1980;68:853. (*Treatment with hormones did not prevent the recurrence of cysts after aspiration.*)

30. Ridgway EC. Medical treatment of benign thyroid nodules: have we defined a benefit? Ann Intern Med 1998;128:403. (*Editorial on the management of benign thyroid nodules; argues for follow-up and the selective use of suppressive therapy; the algorithm is incorporated into the assessment and follow-up strategy presented in this chapter.*)

31. Ross DS, Ridgway EC, Daniels GH. Successful treatment of solitary toxic thyroid nodules with relatively low-dose iodine 131, with low prevalence of hypothyroidism. Ann Intern Med 1984;101:488. (*Reports excellent results with no induction of hypothyroidism.*)

32. Zelmanowitz F, Genro S, Gross JL, et al. Suppressive therapy with levothyroxine for solitary thyroid nodules: a double-blind controlled clinical study and cumulative meta-analysis. J Clin Endocrinol Metab 1998;83:3881. (*Evidence in support of suppressive therapy; the degree of benefit is clinically modest but statistically significant.*)

CHAPTER 96 ■ APPROACH TO THE PATIENT WITH HYPERCALCEMIA

DAVID M. SLOVIK

The advent of automated laboratory screening has led to an increased recognition of asymptomatic persons with hypercalcemia, with an estimated annual incidence of 51/100,000. In addition, outpatients with nonspecific complaints, such as fatigue, weakness, abdominal discomfort, or constipation, may have hypercalcemia discovered during biochemical testing. Mild hyperparathyroidism is usually the explanation for these often inadvertently recognized elevations in calcium levels. Hypercalcemia may also herald other important underlying diseases, such as malignancy or sarcoidosis. Asymptomatic hyperparathyroidism is not necessarily a benign condition. The effect of excessive levels of parathyroid hormone for prolonged periods on target organs, such as bone and the kidney, may lead to skeletal loss and impaired renal function. Primary hyperparathyroidism and malignancy account for more than 90% of cases of hypercalcemia.

The primary physician must be able to interpret an abnormal calcium value and diagnose its cause. If hyperparathyroidism is present, one must decide between surgery and medical therapy. The treatment of hypercalcemia resulting from malignancy can improve quality of life and deserves consideration.

PATHOPHYSIOLOGY AND CLINICAL PRESENTATION (1–12)

The serum calcium concentration is maintained within narrow limits by parathyroid hormone. Precise calcium homeostasis is necessary because of the vital role of calcium in membrane function, hormonal secretion and action, and neuromuscular function. The free or ionized portion of serum calcium is responsible for its physiologic actions. Slightly less than 50% of serum calcium is in the form of free calcium ions; the remainder is bound to plasma proteins, mostly albumin. Globulins can also bind serum calcium. Calcium binding by serum proteins is pH dependent. Increased binding at alkaline pH explains the common symptom of paresthesias that occur in conjunction with hyperventilation. The normal range for serum calcium is generally 8.5 to 10.4 mg/dL, or 2.1 to 2.6 mmol/L. The normal range for ionized serum calcium is 1.1 to 1.3 mmol/L. True hypercalcemia requires an increase in the ionized fraction of serum calcium. A rough convenient correction factor to apply to the total serum calcium is the subtraction or addition of 0.8 mg/dL for the calcium concentration for every 1.0 g/dL of serum albumin greater or less than 4.0 g/dL, respectively.

Hyperparathyroidism

In the ambulatory setting, primary hyperparathyroidism is the most common cause of hypercalcemia. It is caused by an increase in osteoclastic bone resorption, mediated by the binding of excess parathyroid hormone (PTH) to receptors on osteoblasts, in addition to an increase in gut calcium absorption. PTH also increases renal tubular reabsorption of calcium and decreases renal tubular phosphate reabsorption, which results in phosphate wasting. Pathologically, approximately 80%

to 85% of patients are found to have a single parathyroid adenoma, whereas 15% to 20% have four-gland hyperplasia; the latter is more common in younger patients and is often associated with the syndrome of multiple endocrine neoplasia. Parathyroid cancer accounts for less than 1% of all cases of hypercalcemia attributed to excess parathyroid hormone secretion.

The incidence of hyperparathyroidism increases with age, peaking in the fifth and sixth decades of life, and hyperparathyroidism occurs more commonly in women than men by approximately a 2:1 ratio. It is not certain whether the increased recognition of the disease relates to multiphasic biochemical screening or the number of cases of the disease has increased, possibly as a result of head and neck irradiation in infancy or other environmental factors that affect parathyroid cell proliferation.

The majority of patients with hyperparathyroidism do not have symptoms. The "classic" presentation of "stones, bones, abdominal groans, and psychic moans" has been replaced by a more subtle and nonspecific presentation. *Fatigue, weakness,* mild gastrointestinal symptoms (*constipation, abdominal pain*), changes in *intellectual performance,* and *depression* may all be manifestations of hypercalcemia or excessive PTH. Often, such nonspecific symptoms are recognized only after successful parathyroid surgery has been performed, when the patient describes an improved sense of well-being.

The resultant hypercalcemia of hyperparathyroidism can lead to a renal concentrating defect and *increased urination.* Hyperparathyroidism is also associated with an increase in *calcium oxalate stones,* particularly in patients with elevated levels of 1,25-dihydroxyvitamin D_3 and urinary calcium excretion in excess of 300 to 350 mg/24 hr. Bone pain results from skeletal fracture and osteitis fibrosa cystica. A possible but somewhat controversial increase in peptic ulcer disease and pancreatitis has been noted, as well as a spectrum of psychiatric disease. In persons with mild disease, survival appears to be unaffected.

Hyperparathyroidism may be observed in familial settings, such as the autosomal dominant syndromes of *multiple endocrine neoplasia* (MEN) types 1 and 2. In MEN 1, parathyroid hyperplasia occurs in conjunction with adenomas of the pituitary and pancreas. In MEN 2, parathyroid hyperplasia may occur with medullary cancer of the thyroid and bilateral adrenal pheochromocytoma. Both MEN 1 and MEN 2 are associated with mutations in the RET protooncogene.

Patients with "*normocalcemic hyperparathyroidism*" often have serum calcium levels at the upper limit of normal, which on repeated determinations fluctuate into the frankly elevated range. *Thiazide diuretics* may transiently elevate serum calcium by reducing urinary calcium excretion. More sustained elevations suggest mild underlying hyperparathyroidism, which is unmasked by thiazide therapy.

Malignancy

Malignancy is the other major cause of hypercalcemia and the most common cause of hypercalcemia among hospitalized patients. Cancers of the *breast, lung,* and *kidney* lead the list of malignant causes, accounting for 50% to 60% of such cases. The incidence of hypercalcemia during the course of breast cancer ranges from 18% to 42%, and that in lung cancer ranges from 6% to 16%. Other malignancies associated with hypercalcemia include *multiple myeloma* (incidence of 30% to 100%), *squamous cell carcinomas* of the head and neck (2%), *lymphoma* and *leukemia* (1%), and *genitourinary cancer* (1%).

Several *mechanisms* for the hypercalcemia of malignancy have been identified, with a common theme being increased osteoclastic bone resorption. Such resorption and resultant hypercalcemia can occur with or without bony metastasis, and many tumors that commonly metastasize to bone do not cause hypercalcemia. Squamous cell cancers produce a parathyroid hormone–related protein (PTHRP), a *PTH-like peptide* with an amino-terminal structure similar to that of PTH and a nearly identical effect on mineral ion homeostasis. Myeloma cells produce *interleukin-1β* and *interleukin-6,* which stimulate osteoclast-mediated bone resorption. In some patients with lymphoma and leukemia, an increase in *1,25-dihydroxyvitamin D_3* is implicated.

Hypercalcemia is rarely the sole presenting manifestation of an underlying malignancy. The presence of hypercalcemia in association with malignancy indicates a grim prognosis; the median survival is approximately 2 months. Very high levels of serum calcium (>14 mg/dL) are most often associated with malignancy, but levels up to 20 mg/dL may be seen in acute primary hyperparathyroidism caused by large parathyroid adenomas.

Familial Hypocalciuric Hypercalcemia

Familial hypocalciuric hypercalcemia is an autosomal dominant disorder characterized by mild hypercalcemia, hypocalciuria, normal-to-elevated serum magnesium concentrations, and normal or slightly increased PTH levels. The primary defect is a loss-of-function mutation in the calcium-sensing receptor in the parathyroid glands and kidney, so that higher-than-normal serum calcium concentrations are needed to suppress PTH. Urinary calcium excretion is often less than 100 mg/24 hr.

Other Causes

Sarcoidosis

In *sarcoidosis,* enhanced conversion of inactive vitamin D to its active 1,25-dihydroxy form by granulomatous tissue increases absorption of calcium from the gut and resorption of bone. Hypercalcemia from *vitamin D intoxication* can result from ingesting very high doses of vitamin D, 25-hydroxyvitamin D, or 1,25-dihydroxyvitamin D. Hypercalcemia may occur when an excess of 50,000 U of vitamin D is consumed daily along with high doses of calcium supplements.

The Milk-Alkali Syndrome

The milk-alkali syndrome is the third-highest cause of hypercalcemia because of the high intake of calcium carbonate preparations for osteoporosis treatment. High intakes, often greater than 3 to 4 g of calcium, can lead to hypercalcemia, metabolic alkalosis, and renal insufficiency.

Medications

Thiazide diuretics cause a transient, mild increase in serum calcium, generally within the normal range. As noted earlier, a sustained increase in serum calcium beyond 10 days implies underlying metabolic bone disease, usually hyperparathyroidism. Mild hypercalcemia may be seen in the osteoporotic hypertensive patient on *high-dose calcium* along with *high-dose vitamin D* for osteoporosis and a thiazide diuretic for hypertension. *Theophylline excess* is another pharmacologic cause of hypercalcemia.

Hyperthyroidism

Hyperthyroidism is associated with mild elevations in serum calcium in approximately 15% to 20% of patients because of increased skeletal turnover. *Immobilization* in young persons who have not completed skeletal growth and in patients with Paget's disease may cause severe hypercalcemia due to a high-bone-turnover state. *Lithium* therapy for manic–depressive illness is sometimes associated with hypercalcemia. Persons taking lithium may have an altered calcium set-point for PTH secretion. *Addison's disease* and hypervitaminosis A may cause hypercalcemia.

DIFFERENTIAL DIAGNOSIS (2,6,8)

Hyperparathyroidism is overwhelmingly the most likely cause of hypercalcemia in the medically well, asymptomatic patient. In a Swedish population survey that yielded 95 persons with hypercalcemia, hyperparathyroidism was suspected in 88 patients and confirmed surgically in 57 of the 59 who underwent neck exploration for cure of hyperparathyroidism. Primary hyperparathyroidism accounts for more than 60% of hypercalcemic patients and is extremely likely to be the explanation for hypercalcemia in patients with an elevation of serum calcium dating back several years. *Malignancy, granulomatous disease, hyperthyroidism, Addison's disease*, and *excess ingestion* of *vitamin D* and *calcium* are the causes of most other cases. Occasionally, an underlying *MEN syndrome* or *hypocalciuric hypercalcemia* is present.

WORKUP (5,10,13-18)

Before a more extensive laboratory evaluation is undertaken, a *repeated calcium determination* is indicated to confirm the elevation. Measuring serum albumin and globulin levels helps to confirm that the calcium elevation is not an artifactual result of elevated protein binding of calcium. Obtaining a serum ionized calcium, if available, can help to confirm the hypercalcemia.

Hypercalcemia that appears ephemeral may be spurious, caused by prolonged application of the tourniquet at the time of blood drawing. Should hypercalcemia be confirmed, then evaluation can proceed.

History

In the "asymptomatic" patient, subtle manifestations of hyperparathyroidism, such as fatigue, weakness, lethargy, arthralgias, nonspecific gastrointestinal complaints, impairment of intellectual performance, and depression, should be specifically sought. Associated conditions such as hypertension, gout, pseudogout, and nephrolithiasis should be recognized. A history of increased urination may indicate calcium-related defects in urine-concentrating ability. Symptoms of underlying malignancy, particularly of breast, lung, and hematologic origin, should be pursued. Review of intake of antacids, food additives, and over-the-counter and health food–store preparations may uncover excessive ingestion of vitamin D or calcium. Symptoms of hyperthyroidism (see Chapter 103) also need to be considered.

Physical Examination

Physical examination in the totally asymptomatic patient is generally unrevealing. However, a careful search for signs of malignancy (breast mass, lymphadenopathy, bone tenderness) and sarcoidosis (lymph node enlargement, abnormalities on lung examination) should be undertaken. Signs of hyperparathyroidism are not readily apparent; band keratopathy is rarely visible without the slit lamp.

Laboratory Studies

After confirmation of hypercalcemia, a *serum PTH determination* should follow. Despite the occasional usefulness of other tests to exclude the myriad causes of hypercalcemia, the most direct and efficient approach to workup in the ambulatory setting (where hyperparathyroidism accounts for most cases) is to proceed directly to PTH testing for hyperparathyroidism.

Testing for Hyperparathyroidism

With widespread availability of the sensitive, specific *PTH immunoradiometric assay*, it is possible quickly and accurately to determine whether hyperparathyroidism is responsible for the hypercalcemia. In virtually all patients with hyperparathyroidism, PTH 1–84 is either frankly elevated or at the upper limit of the normal range (10 to 60 pg/mL). An elevated PTH concentration or an inappropriately "normal" level as measured by the modern assay in the setting of hypercalcemia confirms hyperparathyroidism. In hypercalcemia associated with malignancy, PTH is either undetectable or below normal in most patients. A single PTH determination can confirm the diagnosis of hyperparathyroidism.

Improvements in the sensitivity and specificity of immunoradiometric assays for the intact PTH molecule have proved to be a great advance in differentiating patients with hyperparathyroidism from those with other causes of hypercalcemia. Older carboxyl-terminal and midregion radioimmunoassays for PTH recognized PTH-like factors present in the serum in some patients with hypercalcemia of malignancy. The elevation noted by such PTH assays was minimal for the degree of hypercalcemia present. These older assays did not test for PTHRP, which is detected by more modern assays.

When hyperparathyroidism is under consideration, serum *electrolytes* and *phosphate* concentrations can provide indirect evidence of the diagnosis. Fasting hypophosphatemia, hyperchloremia, and mild metabolic acidosis suggest the diagnosis. This is because PTH induces renal phosphate and bicarbonate wasting. A normal serum phosphate level does not exclude the diagnosis of hyperparathyroidism, and hypophosphatemia can be observed in malignancy. Furthermore, phosphate must be measured in the fasting state because food causes phosphate to shift into cells as glucose is phosphorylated. *Alkaline phosphatase* elevation implies increased osteoblastic activity and can be seen in malignancy, hyperparathyroidism with PTH bone disease, and Paget's disease.

Testing for Other Etiologies

Although *anemia* and an *elevated erythrocyte sedimentation rate* can be seen in severe hyperparathyroidism with osteitis fibrosa cystica, these laboratory findings are more suggestive of multiple myeloma, the diagnosis of which requires a serum *immunoelectrophoresis* or, occasionally, a urine immunoelectrophoresis for light-chain excretion. *Chest radiographic findings* of hilar adenopathy or pulmonary parenchymal abnormalities, in conjunction with an elevated *angiotensin-converting enzyme*, are indicative of sarcoidosis. The hypercalcemia of sarcoidosis may be more severe after an interval of sun exposure, so more sophisticated diagnostic studies may be required, including diffusing capacity, a hydrocortisone-suppression study in which orally administered hydrocortisone (40 mg three times daily for 10 days) normalizes the hypercalcemia of sarcoidosis, and even bronchoscopy or mediastinoscopy with biopsy for histologic confirmation (see Chapters 12 and 51).

A *bone scan* will detect the skeletal metastases of breast cancer. *Skeletal radiography* may show lytic or metastatic lesions. Radiographic findings are frequently normal in hyperparathyroidism, but the finding of *subperiosteal bone resorption* is specific for and diagnostic of hyperparathyroidism. Cortical bone is lost preferentially in hyperparathyroidism. Therefore, it is important that noninvasive measurements of skeletal mass include cortical bone, which predominates at sites such as the forearm diaphyses (in contrast to trabecular bone, which predominates in the spine and is lost earliest following menopause). In cases of hypercalcemia with low PTH levels, suggesting a non-PTH cause, a search for an occult malignancy may be necessary by obtaining a computed tomography scan of the neck, chest, abdomen and pelvis.

Familial hypocalciuric hypercalcemia can be considered and excluded in patients without frankly elevated serum PTH by the finding of a 24-hour *urinary calcium excretion* of 80 to 100 mg.

Thyroid hormone determinations, TSH, and, if low, then T4 and T3 levels (see Chapter 103), as well as measurements of serum cortisol after administration of Cortrosyn, should be performed if the patient has a history suggestive of hyperthyroidism or Addison's disease, respectively. A measurement of *25-hydroxyvitamin D* (to assess vitamin D stores) and *1,25-dihydroxyvitamin D$_3$* will unequivocally allay concerns of excessive vitamin D intake.

MANAGEMENT (5,9,11,13,19-31)

Hyperparathyroidism

Medical versus Surgical Therapy

A basic decision in the management of hyperparathyroidism is whether to treat definitively with surgery or follow expectantly and consider medical modalities. The decision must take into account the degree of symptomatology and the natural history of the disease. Prospective studies have attempted to ascertain the natural history of disease in asymptomatic patients. Only in rare instances does recurrent nephrolithiasis, pancreatitis, or hypercalcemic crisis develop. The major consequence of untreated disease appears to be a decrease in skeletal mass, which may predispose to fracture. There is no way to predict who will suffer these effects; monitoring is required. Routine skeletal radiography and alkaline phosphatase measurements are insufficient for long-term follow-up of bone demineralization. *Bone densitometry* is required (see Chapter 144). Because cortical bone loss is most prominent, measurements are made in the proximal wrist. Marked elevation of *urinary calcium* may predict the development of nephrolithiasis.

Candidacy for Surgical Cure

Most authorities agree that the symptomatic patient with recurrent kidney stones or parathyroid bone disease or serum calcium greater than 12.5 to 13.0 mg/dL is a candidate for surgery. Less clear are the indications for surgery in asymp-

TABLE 96.1

INDICATIONS FOR SURGICAL TREATMENT OF HYPERPARATHYROIDISM

Serum calcium 1 mg/dL above the upper limit of normal
History of an episode of life-threatening hypercalcemia
Reduced creatinine clearance
Presence of kidney stones detected by radiography
A 24-hr urine calcium excretion >400 mg
Substantially reduced bone mass determined by direct measurement
(T-score below −2.5 at any site)
Medical surveillance neither desirable nor suitable
  Patient is young (<50 yr old)
  Patient requests surgery
  Consistent follow-up is unlikely
  Coexistent illness complicates management

Adapted from Bilezikian JP, Potts JT Jr, Fuleihan Gel-H, et al. Summary statement from a workshop on asymptomatic primary hyperparathyroidism: a perspective for the 21st century. J Bone Miner Res 2002;17(Suppl 2):N2, with permission.

tomatic or minimally or nonspecifically symptomatic patients with mild hypercalcemia. A 1990 National Institutes of Health consensus conference to establish guidelines for the management of hyperparathyroidism in asymptomatic persons formulated a set of criteria for surgical intervention that was updated at another conference in 2002 (Table 96.1). Surgical cure is warranted for all persons younger than age 50 years and for those who have a bone density T-score that is less than −2.5 at any site, 30% reduction in creatinine clearance, and a urinary calcium excretion greater than 400 mg in 24 hours, which implies, on a restricted calcium intake, that a negative calcium balance is occurring. Cure rates for the initial neck exploration in experienced surgical centers are better than 90%.

As just noted, curative surgical treatment should be a serious consideration for persons with asymptomatic hyperparathyroidism who are young or middle-aged because of the likelihood of progression of skeletal disease, particularly in women, who must anticipate the synergistic effects of menopausal bone loss. The cost of medical surveillance, which includes yearly or biannual assessment of renal function and skeletal mass, may surpass the cost of surgical cure after 5 to 10 years of follow-up studies. Some now recommend parathyroidectomy for nearly all patients, especially with the development of safer, minimally invasive surgical techniques. Long-term follow-up study finds that surgery results in normalization of biochemical abnormalities and an increase in bone density. However, three fourths of asymptomatic patients who do not undergo surgery experience no progression of their disease within 10 years, which suggests that for truly asymptomatic patients, an alternative to surgery is close follow-up. For such patients, biannual serum calcium determinations and annual measurements of urinary calcium excretion and bone mineral density allow timely recognition of the need for operative cure. Nonetheless, asymptomatic patients at high risk for disease progression, especially women as they enter menopause, should be advised about a surgical option.

Before surgery, localization of the parathyroid adenoma is helpful, even to the skilled surgeon. Neck ultrasonography and technetium-99m sestamibi scanning with computer programs that subtract thyroidal uptake of technetium have localized parathyroid adenomas in approximately 70% of patients preoperatively. Anatomic localization by selective angiography or, less commonly, by venous sampling is generally reserved for patients in whom neck exploration by an experienced parathyroid surgeon fails to cure the disease.

Medical Therapy

For patients who do not undergo surgical cure for hyperparathyroidism, several medical alternatives exist. These alternatives may help to limit nonspecific symptoms of hypercalcemic hyperparathyroidism and, more important, may prevent skeletal loss.

Estrogen and progestogen therapy given to postmenopausal women may lower or even normalize serum calcium, reduce bone resorption, and increase skeletal mass. It represents a reasonable therapeutic option in older women without any contraindications for estrogen therapy. In women with a family or personal history of breast cancer, *tamoxifen* treatment has a beneficial effect on the skeleton and may be of therapeutic value.

Oral phosphate therapy, particularly for patients with moderate hypophosphatemia, may lessen fatigue and weakness and reduce urinary calcium excretion, thereby reducing the likelihood of renal stones. Serum calcium is lowered by the oral administration of phosphate, given as 250 to 500 mg of neutral phosphate four times daily. The most common side effect of this therapy is dose-related frequent bowel movements, which are often preferred to the constipation of hyperparathyroidism. Phosphate should be very cautiously administered in cases of renal insufficiency because the calcium phosphate solubility product of 65 might be exceeded and calcium be deposited in skeletal and extraskeletal sites. Phosphate therapy has a potential drawback: It increases PTH secretion and, theoretically, can accelerate bone resorption.

Diuretics such as *furosemide* or *bumetanide* increase renal calcium excretion. *Thiazides* may actually decrease PTH secretion and urinary calcium excretion and worsen hypercalcemia. However, the risk for dehydration requires caution in the use of diuretic agents.

Calcitonin has *not* proved useful on a long-term basis in hyperparathyroidism. Tachyphylaxis develops with calcitonin therapy. Because hyperparathyroidism is characterized by high bone turnover, the *bisphosphonates* may be helpful. In small studies, alendronate produced increases in spinal bone density but without any significant change in parathyroid hormone or serum calcium levels.

Cinacalcet, a calcimimetic that alters the calcium-sensing receptor, is approved for the management of hyperparathyroidism associated with renal failure and parathyroid carcinoma. Its potential role in primary hyperparathyroidism is being evaluated.

Most physicians limit *dietary calcium* in patients with hyperparathyroidism. However, this restriction of dietary calcium may result in accelerated bone resorption as the body responds by maintaining the set-point elevation of serum calcium with increased PTH secretion. It is prudent to increase the dietary calcium intake to 1 to 1.5 g daily in patients with hyperparathyroidism but no associated nephrolithiasis or increased levels of 1,25-dihydroxyvitamin D_3. Patients with vitamin D deficiency may with caution receive a low dose of vitamin D supplements (e.g., 400 to 1,000 IU), but high doses of vitamin D should be avoided because of the potential of worsening hypercalcemia and hypercalciuria.

Patients who are taking phosphate or estrogen therapy or are being followed expectantly for hypercalcemia and the development of skeletal or renal disease should be instructed to maintain a *fluid intake* of at least 2 L daily and report any illness that might lead to dehydration and worsening hypercalcemia.

Management of Hypercalcemia of Malignancy

See Chapter 92.

INDICATIONS FOR REFERRAL AND HOSPITALIZATION

Because one cannot predict in which patients with asymptomatic hyperparathyroidism the progressive complications of disease will develop, recommendations for who should be referred for surgical cure cannot be rigidly applied. The decision to refer for surgery should take into account the patient's preferences and willingness to cooperate with the demands of long-term surveillance and the availability of skilled surgical care. As noted earlier, the patients who should be urged to consider surgery are those who are younger than age 40 years, have a cortical bone density two standard deviations below normal, or have a urinary calcium excretion greater than 350 to 400 mg/24 hr (which, on a restricted calcium intake, implies a negative calcium balance). Patients for whom surgical cure is being planned should be referred to surgeons experienced in the complexities of parathyroid surgery, not only for cure of potential hyperplasia and discovery of a parathyroid adenoma in an unusual location, but also for prevention of the complications of recurrent laryngeal nerve injury and hypoparathyroidism. Minimally invasive surgical techniques lessen the operative time, recuperative time, and likelihood of complications from surgery.

Hospitalization is necessary for patients with severe hypercalcemia. Hydration and intravenous bisphosphonates such as pamidronate that limit osteoclastic resorption of bone are helpful.

PATIENT EDUCATION

Several recommendations will prevent the likelihood of more-severe hypercalcemia in patients with mild hyperparathyroidism. Adequacy of fluid intake and prevention of dehydration that might occur during an acute gastrointestinal illness should be encouraged. Although the administration of thiazide diuretics and calcium has been discouraged, thiazides may actually limit hypercalciuria and renal stone disease, and dietary calcium may decrease PTH secretion and limit negative calcium balance. Patients should be encouraged to remain active and avoid immobilization. The necessity of surveillance for PTH-induced skeletal disease and the delineation of symptoms that might represent manifestations of hyperparathyroidism (e.g., symptoms of nephrolithiasis and pancreatitis) should be carefully reviewed.

Sharing information with patients on the clinical course of hyperparathyroidism helps them choose among treatment options. The truly asymptomatic patient with mild disease needs to know that without surgery there is only a 25% chance of disease progression. Symptomatic patients are at greater risk.

Annotated Bibliography

1. Broadus AD, Horst RL, Lang R, et al. The importance of circulating 1,25-dihydroxyvitamin D in the pathogenesis of hypercalciuria and renal stone formation in primary hyperparathyroidism. N Engl J Med 1980;302:421. (*Elevated 1,25-dihydroxyvitamin D_3 levels were found to increase gut absorption of calcium and produce marked hypercalciuria.*)

2. Christensson T, Hellstrom K, Wengle B, et al. Prevalence of hypercalcemia in a health screening in Stockholm. Acta Med Scand 1976;200:131. (*In a population of >15,000, hypercalcemia was confirmed in 95 patients, with probable hyperparathyroidism in 88.*)

3. Deftos LJ. Hypercalcemia in malignant and inflammatory diseases. Endocrinol Metab Clin North Am 2002;31:141. (*Review of the causes of hypercalcemia, with a discussion of pathophysiologic mechanisms.*)

4. Heath III H, Hodgson SF, Kennedy MA. Primary hyperparathyroidism: incidence, morbidity, and potential economic impact in a community. N Engl J Med 1980;302:189. (*There has been increased case finding with the advent of multiphasic biochemical screening, as well as an increase recognition of the disease in older women.*)

5. Marx SJ. Hyperparathyroidism and hypoparathyroid disorders. N Engl J Med 2000;343:1863. (*Comprehensive review; 109 references.*)

6. Marx SJ, Attie MF, Levine M, et al. The hypocalciuric or benign variant of familial hypercalcemia: clinical and biochemical features in 15 kindreds. Medicine (Baltimore) 1981;60:397. (*A genetic, clinical, and physiologic review of familial hypocalciuric hypercalcemia.*)

7. Maruani G, Hertig A, Paillard M, et al. Normocalcemic primary hyperparathyroidism: evidence for a generalized target-tissue resistance to parathyroid hormone. J Clin Endocrinol Metab 2003;88:4641. (*There may be some target organ resistance at the bone and kidney in a subset of patients with primary hyperparathyroidism who are normocalcemic.*)

8. McPherson ML, Prince SR, Atamer ER, et al. Theophylline-induced hypercalcemia. Ann Intern Med 1986;105:52. (*Documents elevations in the settings of both excess and therapeutic theophylline levels.*)

9. Nussbaum SR. Pathophysiology and management of severe hypercalcemia. Endocrinol Metab Clin North Am 1993;22:343. (*A review of mechanisms of hypercalcemia, with an emphasis on the newer inhibitors of osteoclastic bone resorption, especially bisphosphonates.*)

10. Silverberg SJ, Bilezikian JP. "Incipient" primary hyperparathyroidism: a "forme fruste" of an old disease. J Clin Endocrinol Metab 2003;88:5348. (*Postulates that elevated parathyroid hormone levels and normal serum calcium may represent the earliest manifestation of primary hyperparathyroidism.*)

11. Stewart AF. Hypercalcemia associated with cancer. N Engl J Med 2005;352:373. (*Excellent review for the generalist; 46 references.*)

12. Strewler GJ. The physiology of parathyroid hormone–related protein. N Engl J Med 2000;342:177. (*Basic science review of this protein, which mediates the hypercalcemia of cancer.*)

13. NIH Consensus Development Conference on Diagnosis and Management of Asymptomatic Primary Hyperparathyroidism. Proceedings of the Conference. J Bone Miner Res 1991;Suppl 1–2:S1. (*A scholarly compendium on the clinical spectrum and treatment options for hyperparathyroidism, especially asymptomatic disease.*)

14. Nussbaum SR, Zahradnik R, Lavigne J. Highly sensitive two-site immunoradiometric assay for parathyrin and its clinical utility in evaluating patients with hypercalcemia. Clin Chem 1987;33:1364. (*Immunoradiometric assay for intact parathyroid hormone can distinguish hypercalcemic patients with hyperparathyroidism from those with malignancy, providing an advantage over earlier, region-specific assays.*)

15. Parisien M, Silverberg SJ, Shane E, et al. The histomorphometry of bone in primary hyperparathyroidism: preservation of cancellous bone structure. J Clin Endocrinol Metab 1990;70:930. (*There is a disproportionate loss of cortical bone in hyperparathyroidism; a skeletal study must assess cortical bone.*)

16. Simeone JF, Mueller PR, Ferucci JT, et al. High-resolution real-time sonography of the parathyroid. Radiology 1981;141:745. (*Ultrasonography may demonstrate the location of a parathyroid adenoma in 70% to 80% of patients.*)

17. Stewart AF, Horst R, Deftos LJ, et al. Biochemical evaluation of patients with cancer-associated hypercalcemia. Evidence for humoral and non-humoral groups. N Engl J Med 1980;303:1377. (*The "classic" study segregating cancer patients with humoral hypercalcemia, often without bone metastases, from patients with metastatic disease.*)

18. Taillefer R, Boucher Y, Potvin C, et al. Detection and localization of parathyroid adenomas in patients with hyperparathyroidism using a single radionuclide imaging procedure with technetium 99-sestamibi (double-phase study). J Nucl Med 1992;33:1801. (*This technique reliably detects parathyroid adenomas and greatly simplifies surgery.*)

19. Bilezikian JP, Silverberg SJ. Asymptomatic primary hyperparathyroidism. N Engl J Med 2004;350:1746. (*Discussion of the approach to patients with primary hyperparathyroidism.*)

20. Bilezikian JP. Management of acute hypercalcemia. N Engl J Med 1992;326:1196. (*A review of treatment options.*)

21. Bilezikian JP, Potts JT Jr, Fuleihan Gel-H, et al. Summary statement from a workshop on asymptomatic primary hyperparathyroidism: a perspective for the 21st century. J Clin Endocrinol Metab 2002;87:5353. (*A detailed review by a panel of experts on multiple issues and questions relative to this disorder.*)

22. Gartenberg F, Silverberg SJ, Bilezikian JP. Optimal dietary calcium intake in primary hyperparathyroidism. Am J Med 1997;102:543. (*Intake can be liberalized as long as 1,25-dihydroxyvitamin D_3 levels are not elevated.*)

23. Grey A, Lucas J. Horne A et al. Vitamin D repletion in patients with primary hyperparathyroidism and coexistent vitamin D insufficiency. J Clin Endocrinol Metal 2005;90:2122. (*Vitamin D repletion did not exacerbate hypercalcemia.*)

24. Irvin GL, Carneiro DM. Management changes in primary hyperparathyroidism. JAMA 2000;284:934. (*Evidence for the approach of watchful waiting, close monitoring, and minimally invasive surgery.*)

25. Marcus R, Madvig P, Crim M, et al. Conjugated estrogens in the treatment of post-menopausal women with hyperparathyroidism. Ann Intern Med 1984;100:633. (*Estrogen therapy normalized serum calcium and decreased bone turnover in 10 women with hyperparathyroidism for up to 2 years.*)

26. Palmer M, Adami HO, Bergstrom R. Survival and renal function in persons with untreated hypercalcemia: a population-based cohort study with 13 years of follow-up. Lancet 1987;1:59. (*Decreased survival was largely explained by cardiovascular deaths.*)

27. Peacock M, Bilezikian JP, Klassen PS, et al. Cinacalcet hydrochloride maintains long-term normocalcemia in patients with primary hyperparathyroidism. J Clin Endocrinol Metab 2005;90:135. (*Cinacalcet, a calcimimetic, rapidly normalized serum calcium and parathyroid hormone in patients with primary hyperparathyroidism.*)

28. Silverberg SJ, Shane E, Jacobs TP, et al. A 10-year prospective study of primary hyperparathyroidism with or without parathyroid surgery. N Engl J Med 1999;341:1249. (*A long-term follow-up study demonstrating the risks and benefits of curing the condition in asymptomatic persons.*)

29. Silverberg SJ, Brown I, Bilezikian JP. Age as a criterion for surgery in primary hyperparathyroidism. Am J Med 2002;113:681. (*Relative youthfulness—age <50 years—was regarded as an indication for parathyroidectomy.*)

30. Utiger RD. Treatment of primary hyperparathyroidism. N Engl J Med 1999;341:1301. (*An editorial recommending surgery for nearly all patients, arguing that almost all are symptomatic.*)

31. Wermers RA, Khosla S, Atkinson EJ, et al. Survival after the diagnosis of hyperparathyroidism: a population-based study. Am J Med 1998;104:115. (*Survival is normal in persons with mild disease.*)

CHAPTER 97 ■ EVALUATION OF HYPOGLYCEMIA

DAVID M. SLOVIK

Except in cases of diabetes, the workup for hypoglycemia is most often an exercise in ruling out underlying pathology triggered by nonspecific symptoms (e.g., irritability, fatigue, sweats, confusion, palpitations, tremulousness) that are attributed to a "low blood sugar." At other times, the assessment is precipitated by the chance finding of a low blood glucose level. In the setting of diabetes, tight glucose control leading to hypoglycemic episodes is common and readily confirmed (see Chapter 102). In patients who do not have diabetes, confirmation may be more problematic, made so by a lack of glucose measurements taken during symptomatic periods and the nonspecific nature of the hypoglycemic symptoms. Compounding the diagnostic problem are unaddressed manifestations of psychopathology, which the patient may prefer to attribute to "hypoglycemia." Although true hypoglycemia in the absence of diabetes is rarely encountered in the office setting, its causes include serious, treatable conditions that must not be missed. These factors make the workup of hypoglycemia challenging. The primary care physician needs to know how to differentiate suspected from true hypoglycemia and, in the nondiabetic patient, how to identify the rare case that requires an in-depth search for serious underlying disease. A cost-efficient strategy for assessment is needed because the question of hypoglycemia comes up so often.

PATHOPHYSIOLOGY AND CLINICAL PRESENTATION (1–15)

Mechanisms

Hypoglycemia can result from increased insulin secretion, enhanced glucose utilization, or inadequate functioning of one or more compensatory regulatory mechanisms (e.g., glucagons, epinephrine, growth hormone, and cortisol). When hypoglycemia occurs, the liver responds with increased glycogenolysis and gluconeogenesis, stimulated by glucagon and epinephrine, which activate hepatic phosphorylase. In addition, the pituitary secretes growth hormone, which inhibits the utilization of glucose by muscle and enhances lipolysis, and adrenocorticotropic hormone (ACTH), which promotes cortisol production. The increased cortisol acts to stimulate gluconeogenesis and diminish muscle uptake of glucose.

No single threshold of glucose concentration invariably triggers hypoglycemic symptoms or characterizes patients with a disorder of glucose homeostasis. Glucose levels lower than 45 mg/dL (2.5 mmol/L) have been documented in metabolically normal men during prolonged exercise and in healthy, asymptomatic women. More than 20% of normal patients demonstrate serum sugar levels less than 50 mg/dL during glucose tolerance testing. Conversely, hypoglycemic thresholds may rise in poorly controlled diabetes, in which levels as high as 75 mg/dL (4.3 mmol/L) may trigger symptoms. This has led to the view

that the onset of hypoglycemic symptoms is related to the robustness of counterregulatory responses in addition to the rate of fall in serum glucose and the absolute serum glucose concentration. In patients with tightly controlled insulin-dependent diabetes, the catecholamine response is blunted, and they may exhibit few symptoms until their glucose concentration falls to a very low level.

Clinical Manifestations of Hypoglycemia and Its Etiologies

Hypoglycemic symptoms are typically categorized as *neuroglycopenic* (fatigue, drowsiness, lethargy, visual disturbances, behavioral changes, impaired performance of routine tasks, confusion, loss of consciousness) or *catecholamine mediated* (sweating, anxiety, tremulousness, headache, palpitations, tachycardia). Adrenergic symptoms characteristically accompany acute, rapid falls in blood sugar, especially if levels drop to concentrations below 40 mg/dL. Neuroglycopenic symptoms can develop in the absence of premonitory adrenergic complaints. Symptoms suggestive of hypoglycemia can be ascribed to hypoglycemia only if they occur at a time of documented hypoglycemia and are relieved by the administration of glucose.

In the outpatient setting, most cases of true hypoglycemia occur among persons who look well. Their condition is a consequence of insulin excess, and they may have no apparent symptoms indicative of the underlying cause. Those cases resulting from a failure of counterregulatory mechanisms usually occur in very ill patients, who are typically hospitalized with end-stage disease.

Exogenous Insulin or Oral Hypoglycemic Agents

Exogenous insulin or oral hypoglycemic agents account for most of the cases of hypoglycemia seen in clinical practice, which develops in persons attempting tight control of their diabetes. Although the hypoglycemia associated with diabetic therapy may occur at any time in relation to meals, it tends to be most severe in the fasting state or when meals are delayed or missed. The hypoglycemia associated with the use of potent, long-acting oral agents can be particularly severe and prolonged (see Chapter 102). Surreptitious administration of insulin or oral hypoglycemic agents is seen among self-destructive persons, typically nurses with access to diabetic medications and syringes. Patients injecting insulin secretly may have high levels of immunoreactive insulin but very low serum levels of proinsulin and C-peptide (formed as part of proinsulin and split during endogenous synthesis) because they produce little endogenous insulin. However, those taking excessive doses of oral hypoglycemic agents have high levels of insulin and C-peptide because the drugs stimulate endogenous insulin secretion. The diagnosis requires finding excessive amounts of oral agent and oral-agent metabolites in the plasma or urine.

Early Adult-Onset Diabetes

Postprandial hypoglycemia may occur 3 to 5 hours after meals as a consequence of delayed insulin release, a characteristic feature of type 2 diabetes. Insulin levels may be inappropriately high for the level of serum glucose at hand. In most type 2 diabetic patients, the mismatching of insulin and serum glucose levels is not sufficient to cause true symptomatic hypoglycemia, but on occasion it may be noted.

Insulinomas

These rare but important causes of uncontrolled insulin production account for the large majority of patients with truly endogenous hyperinsulinemia. More than 85% of insulinomas are benign islet cell tumors. Many occur in the setting of multiple endocrine neoplasia type 1 (MEN 1), which also includes parathyroid hyperplasia and pituitary adenoma. The clinical presentation of insulinomas can be confusing and highly variable in timing and severity. The only valid generalizations are that fasting and exercise may precipitate symptoms, and that profound degrees of hypoglycemia may ensue (leading to seizures in 10% of cases). Levels of serum glucose are not always low after an overnight fast. In a series of 39 patients with proven islet cell tumors, about half still had glucose levels greater than 60 mg/dL after 10 hours of fasting. Another series found symptoms to occur with equal frequency early in the morning, late in the afternoon, and several hours after a meal. Nonetheless, evidence of hyperinsulinism is evident in more than 75% of patients after 24 hours of fasting, and 80% report a combination of neuroglycopenic and adrenergic symptoms. Serum levels of insulin and C-peptide are high.

Non–Islet Cell Tumors

Some large mesenchymal tumors, hepatomas, gastric cancers, and adrenocortical carcinomas synthesize and release large amounts of the prohormone form of insulin-like growth factor II ("big" IGF-II). IGF-II inhibits the uptake of glucose by the liver and increases glucose uptake by the tumor itself and by insulin-responsive tissues (e.g., muscle and fat); hypoglycemia is the result. Insulin secretion is suppressed, so levels of immunoreactive insulin in the serum become very low. The presentation is that of hypoglycemia in the setting of a known malignancy. Rarely, the tumor may be silent, but usually its presence dominates the clinical picture. Serum insulin and C-peptide levels are low. IGF-II may be detected in the serum in elevated quantities. Reduction in tumor bulk alleviates the hypoglycemia.

Defects in Glycogenolysis or Gluconeogenesis

Such defects are uncommon in the office setting; they are seen predominantly among very sick and often hospitalized patients with advanced pituitary or adrenal insufficiency, end-stage liver or renal disease, or severe HIV infection. The common pathophysiologic denominator is failure of glucose counterregulatory mechanisms to maintain glucose homeostasis. Symptoms may be exacerbated by poor nutritional intake and substance abuse. For example, symptomatic hypoglycemia may be noted after severe alcoholic binge drinking in the absence of food intake. Ill patients are particularly sensitive to the hypoglycemic effects of drugs, including pentamidine when given for *Pneumocystis* pneumonia, trimethoprim/sulfamethoxazole in the setting of renal failure, quinine or quinidine in the setting of malaria, and propoxyphene in renal failure. Salicylates, beta-blockers, and haloperidol can also cause non–insulin-related hypoglycemia.

True Reactive Hypoglycemia (after Gastric Surgery)

Onset of true hypoglycemia 1 to 2 hours after eating characterizes the reactive hypoglycemia of patients who have undergone gastric surgery. About 5% to 10% of such patients experience a reactive hypoglycemia, which is believed to be related to pyloric sphincter incompetence and the excessively rapid entry of concentrated carbohydrates into the small bowel. Unidentified gut factors are stimulated, causing the release of excessive insulin. Symptoms should not be confused with those of the dumping syndrome (see Chapter 64), which consist of nausea, fullness, and weakness developing within an hour after eating. An occasional patient with a functional defect in gastric emptying may present in similar fashion.

Functional Reactive "Hypoglycemia."

This common postprandial syndrome is characterized by autonomic hypoglycemia-like symptoms occurring within 2 to 4 hours after a meal and relieved or prevented by a snack. Patients may report that symptoms are especially likely to occur with the intake of concentrated sweets. Some authorities argue that the designation of "functional reactive hypoglycemia" is inappropriate because the serum glucose is usually normal at the time symptoms occur, so the criteria of Whipple's triad are not met. Insulin secretion is normal, and no relation between glucose levels and symptoms can be demonstrated. The pathophysiology of this alimentary variant is unknown, but it may respond to a high-protein, low-carbohydrate diet. The "functional reactive hypoglycemia" label is also sometimes applied inappropriately to asymptomatic patients who manifest a low serum glucose during a 5-hour glucose tolerance test, a normal occurrence in 10% to 20% of healthy persons.

DIFFERENTIAL DIAGNOSIS
(2–4,8,12,14)

The main differential diagnostic issue for the primary care physician is less about distinguishing among the causes of true hypoglycemia than about confirming its presence because "hypoglycemic" symptoms are quite nonspecific and more often due to etiologies other than true hypoglycemia. Two important groups of nonhypoglycemic patients must be differentiated from patients who manifest genuine falls in glucose in conjunction with symptoms: (a) The first group comprises persons with *anxiety* or *depression* who have multiple bodily complaints of a functional or psychophysiologic nature (see Chapters 226 and 227). Such patients commonly complain of fatigue, headache, muscle spasms, palpitations, numbness, sweating, and mental dullness and often show manifestations of a somatization disorder (see Chapter 230). They may attribute their symptoms to "hypoglycemia," which conveniently explains their difficulties but promotes avoidance of the psychosocial issues at hand. Requests for glucose tolerance testing are frequent. (b) The second group is bothered by *postprandial* symptoms in the context of normal serum glucose levels, experiencing symptoms that are very similar to those experienced by patients with truly reactive hypoglycemia.

Once true hypoglycemia is identified, attention turns to its causes. The traditional classification of etiologies for hypoglycemia ("fasting" vs. "reactive") is fading from use because truly reactive hypoglycemia does not occur except in patients who have undergone gastric surgery, and fasting hypoglycemia can also occur postprandially. More-modern etiologic classifications use pathogenetic and clinical categories such as "insulin

TABLE 97.1

SOME IMPORTANT CAUSES OF TRUE HYPOGLYCEMIA SEEN IN THE OFFICE SETTING

Patient Looks Healthy/Insulin-Related
Excessively tight diabetic control with insulin or sulfonylurea therapy
Factitious hypoglycemia induced by surreptitious insulin administration
Sulfonylurea overdose
Insulinoma
Intense exercise
Prior gastric surgery
Early type 2 diabetes

Patient Looks Sick/Non–Insulin-Related
End-stage renal disease
End-stage liver disease
Severe infection/sepsis
Pituitary failure
Alcohol binge, severe, with little food intake
Hepatic dysfunction secondary to severe congestive heart failure, sepsis, infiltrative disease
Insulin-like growth factor II production by malignancy (most patients are ill)

Patient Looks Sick/Drug-Related
Pentamidine for *Pneumocystis* pneumonia
Salicylates in renal failure
Propoxyphene in renal failure
Trimethoprim/sulfamethoxazole in renal failure
Quinine in cerebral malaria
Gatifloxacin in infection

related versus non–insulin related" and "healthy versus ill appearing" (Table 97.1).

WORKUP (2,16–21)

The first task is to confirm that the patient with low blood glucose or "hypoglycemic" symptoms actually has true hypoglycemia. Complicating the evaluation is the difficulty of documenting the relationship between symptoms and blood glucose level. As noted, many persons have "hypoglycemic" symptoms in the context of normal blood glucose levels, and low blood glucose levels are found in many asymptomatic persons. Diagnostic criteria (Whipple's triad) have been proposed to facilitate the identification of the truly hypoglycemic symptomatic patient.

Once the criteria of Whipple's triad have been met, then the focus shifts to detecting important treatable disease, which may sometimes be obvious; however, in other cases, a search for occult disease, substance abuse, or other surreptitious patient behavior may be necessary.

Identifying True Hypoglycemia

Diagnostic Criteria (Whipple's Triad)

The diagnostic criteria include (a) *symptoms* consistent with neuroglycopenia (blurred or double vision, confusion, odd behavior, lethargy) or adrenergic stimulation (anxiety, tremulousness, headache, palpitations, sweats); (b) a *low serum glucose* concentration (<50 mg/dL, 2.8 mmol/L) at the time of symptoms; and (c) *relief of symptoms with the administration of glucose.* These criteria are sometimes referred to as *Whipple's triad,* named for the physician who first suggested them as a means of distinguishing normal persons from those with underlying disease. Simply having adrenergic symptoms or a low serum glucose level in the absence of symptoms does not suffice because many healthy persons may have an isolated glucose level below 50 mg/dL. The objective is to document the correlation between symptoms and a low serum glucose concentration. Without such documentation, one cannot make a diagnosis of physiologically significant hypoglycemia. The occurrence of symptoms in the presence of a normal blood glucose level rules out true hypoglycemia.

Testing and Confirming True Hypoglycemia

Determination of the *serum glucose at the time of symptoms* is essential for diagnosis and helps to eliminate from consideration the large number of cases with symptoms that are not caused by hypoglycemia. In a study of patients referred with a presumptive diagnosis of reactive hypoglycemia, fewer than 20% actually had a serum glucose level less than 50 mg/dL during symptoms, a finding that emphasizes the importance of a blood sugar determination at the time of symptoms. If the blood glucose level is greater than 50 mg/dL at the time of symptoms, then true hypoglycemia is ruled out, and no further evaluation is needed. The traditional 5-hour oral *glucose tolerance test* is not indicated because it provides no useful information. Even if a low blood glucose level is detected during glucose tolerance testing (which occurs in up to 20% of normal persons), the number is meaningless in the absence of a correlation with symptoms. Thus, the glucose tolerance test can be skipped. More important is a determination of the glucose level at the time of symptoms.

Finger-stick methods have improved the ability to sample blood sugar at the time of symptoms, although reagent strip techniques may be inaccurate at low glucose concentrations, and self-testing may be poorly performed, especially when patients are symptomatic. Venipuncture is more accurate but less convenient. However, a sample is worth obtaining as long as symptoms are present.

Patients not fulfilling criteria for hypoglycemia should be evaluated for other conditions. It is essential that one avoid mislabeling them as hypoglycemic, even if symptoms follow meals. Patients with no correlation between their symptoms and serum glucose levels are unlikely to have an underlying disturbance in glucose homeostasis. For them, an alternative explanation for symptoms should be sought. Symptoms of *anxiety disorders,* *depression,* and *hyperthyroidism* may mimic those of hypoglycemia. A story of early-morning awakening, chronic fatigue, and disturbed appetite and libido in conjunction with a history of personally significant losses provides strong presumptive evidence for depression (see Chapter 227). Paroxysms of anxiety, palpitations, difficulty in breathing, and chest tightness unrelated to meals suggest a panic attack disorder (see Chapter 226). The presence of heat intolerance, weight loss despite normal food intake, constant nervousness unrelated to meals, and skin and hair changes point to hyperthyroidism (see Chapter 103).

Evaluating True Hypoglycemia

History

Once hypoglycemia has been established, the evaluation proceeds to determine whether the condition is insulin related or not. In diabetics, the use of *insulin* and *sulfonylurea agents* needs to be reviewed (biguanides and thiazolidinediones do not in themselves confer a risk for hypoglycemia; see Chapter 102). As noted earlier, intensive insulin therapy may reduce the counterregulatory responses to hypoglycemia and lower the glucose level at which symptoms occur, so a high index of suspicion is necessary. A person using such drugs surreptitiously is likely to deny any intake, but a *vocational history* of medical or paramedical work should raise one's index of suspicion. If *postprandial* symptoms develop, then one should check for a history of *type 2 diabetes* or *gastric surgery*. In a patient with a history of gastric surgery, onset within 1 to 2 hours after eating is very strong evidence for rapid emptying as the underlying pathophysiology. The appearance of symptoms beginning 3 to 5 hours after eating in a patient with a family history of diabetes or recent development of polyuria/polydipsia argues for early type 2 diabetes.

The physician should check for non–insulin-related causes by inquiring into recent binge drinking in the absence of food intake, end-stage liver or kidney disease, adrenal insufficiency, hypopituitarism, and a history of malignancy. Such persons are ill, and the cause is usually evident, with symptoms of the underlying condition dominating the clinical presentation (see Chapters 71, 101, and 142). All medications should be reviewed, looking for those that might be contributory, especially in persons with underlying illness (e.g., pentamidine, trimethoprim/sulfamethoxazole, quinine, quinidine, propoxyphene, salicylates, beta-blockers, and haloperidol).

Patients with *insulinomas* report few symptoms other than those related to their hypoglycemia, which typically worsen *after exercise* or in the *absence of food intake* (e.g., just before breakfast or late in the afternoon, especially with exercise). The occurrence of neuroglycopenic symptoms (blurred vision, diplopia, sweats, confusion, changes in behavior, poor memory) during these periods should raise suspicion of the diagnosis. Because insulinomas often develop in the context of multiple endocrine neoplasia type 1, with primary hyperparathyroidism, symptoms of hypercalcemia may be evident (see Chapter 96).

Physical Examination

In most cases of reactive hypoglycemia, few etiologically suggestive physical findings are noted. The exception is the upper abdominal surgical scar in a patient who has undergone gastric surgery. Patients with fasting hypoglycemia should be checked for postural hypotension, alcohol on the breath, needle marks at common insulin injection sites, jaundice, ecchymoses, hyperpigmentation, visual field defects, abdominal mass, ascites, and other signs of hepatocellular failure (see Chapter 71). A careful neurologic examination is essential to rule out focal neurologic injury, which would indicate a cause of symptoms other than hypoglycemia.

Laboratory Studies

Laboratory studies can help in the differentiation between insulin-related and non–insulin-related causes. Concurrent measurements of plasma *insulin*, *C-peptide*, *proinsulin*, and *glucose* at the time of symptoms are key to the differentiation. Often, an *overnight fast* is sufficient to elicit hypoglycemia and make possible these simultaneous determinations. Because exercise promotes a fall in serum glucose, it may be used in conjunction with fasting to elicit hypoglycemia and precipitate symptoms. In two thirds of patients with insulinomas, hypo-

glycemia develops within 24 hours; fewer than 5% have to fast for 72 hours (which requires an inpatient admission).

Inappropriately high levels of insulin in the presence of a low glucose level suggest an insulin-related cause (insulinoma); low or normal insulin levels are indicative of a cause other than insulin. An insulin-to-glucose ratio in excess of 0.3 is consistent with insulinoma and characteristically increases as fasting progresses. An insulin level greater than 6 to 10 μg/mL and a C-peptide level greater than 0.2 to 0.4 nmol/mL strongly suggest insulinoma but may also occur with surreptitious sulfonylurea use, which can be identified by testing a urine or plasma sample for the presence of *sulfonylurea*. A high insulin level in the setting of a low C-peptide level indicates an exogenous insulin source. When insulinoma is a concern, a 72-hour fast may be warranted, which would require hospitalization. Testing to locate an insulinoma can be difficult. In most settings, preoperative assessment by *ultrasonography* or *computed tomography* is adequate for lesions larger than 1.5 cm in diameter but insufficient for smaller lesions. A host of modalities for improved preoperative localization are being developed, but palpation by the surgeon with the aid of intraoperative ultrasonography remains the best means of localization.

The need for additional studies in patients with non–insulin-dependent hypoglycemia depends on the clinical context. *Cortisol* and *ACTH* determinations are indicated if hypopituitarism or adrenal insufficiency is suspected (see Chapter 105). Liver and renal function testing should be obtained to look for severe liver disease and chronic renal failure. When tumor-induced hypoglycemia is suspected, an *IGF-II* determination can be considered; usually, the tumor burden is significant and has been identified earlier; if not, radiologic investigation may be warranted.

SYMPTOMATIC MANAGEMENT AND PREVENTION (3,22,23; See Also Chapter 102)

Acutely, symptomatic management during a hypoglycemic episode involves either the administration of *oral sugar* preparations or, if necessary, *intravenous glucose*; on occasion, *parenteral glucagons* can be administered. Longer term, hypoglycemia is best treated by attending to the underlying cause (e.g., removing the insulinoma, debulking a tumor producing IGF-II, arranging for psychotherapy for self-destructive behavior, adjusting the diabetes treatment regimen; see Chapter 102).

Patients with *postprandial hypoglycemia* (e.g., after gastric surgery) may respond to dietary interventions, such as *frequent feedings* (six per day) and diets *high in protein* and *low in concentrated carbohydrate*. In addition, treatment with anticholinergic agents (e.g., 7.5 mg of propantheline before meals) delays gastric emptying; results are fair at best. Other approaches include administration a β-blocking agent before meals (e.g., 10 mg of propranolol), reversal of a 10-cm segment of the jejunum, and administration of pectin. Patients who have *postprandial symptoms without hypoglycemia* (i.e., those previously labeled as having *functional reactive hypoglycemia*) may benefit from similar dietary measures, although no controlled studies have established the efficacy of any of these dietary manipulations. Some patients note that avoidance of concentrated sweets helps, but the mechanisms of symptom production and reduction are unclear.

Prevention of hypoglycemia is one of the principal challenges of diabetes management (see Chapter 102).

PATIENT EDUCATION (22,23)

The patient who seeks medical attention because of a fear of hypoglycemia should be taken seriously, but once the diagnosis has been ruled out, reassurance and refocusing attention to other possible causes of symptoms should follow. Patients with underlying psychopathology may initially refuse to accept the fact that hypoglycemia is not responsible for their symptoms because the attribution serves as a psychologically comfortable explanation. One needs to explore their concerns sympathetically while redirecting further evaluation to an exploration of anxiety, depression, and somatization disorders (see Chapters 226, 227, and 230). The patient with "functional reactive hypoglycemia" whose glucose levels are normal during the occurrence of symptoms can be reassured that although the symptoms are "real," they are not related to low blood glucose or disturbances in glucose homeostasis, and that simple dietary recommendations (see prior discussion) may help. Requests for glucose tolerance testing are common, but they are readily withdrawn when the lack of specificity of the test is explained. Patients with a suspected insulinoma appreciate being told that almost all cases are benign, and that removal of the tumor cures their condition, with little risk for relapse or recurrence.

INDICATIONS FOR ADMISSION AND REFERRAL

Patients with suspected insulinoma are at risk for a profound fall in serum glucose and should be referred promptly to an endocrinologist and surgeon familiar with the management of this rare condition. Although the initial hours of a 72-hour fast may be performed as an outpatient, the continuation of the fast should be under supervision in the hospital. Patients with severe symptoms (seizure, mental confusion) should be admitted immediately to the hospital for glucose infusion and detailed evaluation. Routine referral of patients with postprandial symptoms for glucose tolerance testing is no longer considered appropriate.

Annotated Bibliography

1. Boyle PJ, Schwartz NS, Shah SD, et al. Plasma glucose concentrations at the outset of hypoglycemic symptoms in patients with poorly controlled diabetes and in nondiabetics. N Engl J Med 1988;318:1487. (*Symptoms occur at higher glucose levels when the diabetes is poorly controlled.*)
2. Cryer PE. Diverse causes of hypoglycemia-associated autonomic failure in diabetes. N Engl J Med 2004;350:2272. (*A review of hypoglycemia in diabetes from the perspective of pathophysiology.*)
3. Cryer PE, Davis SN, Shamoon H. Hypoglycemia in diabetes. Diabetes Care 2003;26:1902. (*Nice discussion, including pathophysiology and prevention*).
4. Fajans SS, Floyd JC. Fasting hypoglycemia in adults. N Engl J Med 1976;294:766. (*A physiologically oriented review of fasting hypoglycemia, with a table of causes organized around pathophysiologic mechanisms.*)
5. Felig P, Cherif A, Minagawa A, et al. Hypoglycemia during prolonged exercise in normal men. N Engl J Med 1982;306:895. (*Hypoglycemia is a normal event during maximal exertion.*)
6. Gastineau CF. Is reactive hypoglycemia a clinical entity? Mayo Clin Proc 1983;58:545. (*An example of the debate surrounding the issue.*)
7. LeRoith D. Insulin-like growth factors. N Engl J Med 1997;338:633. (*Detailed summary for the generalist reader, including mechanisms of hypoglycemia in patients with tumors.*)
8. Lev-Ran A, Anderson RW. The diagnosis of postprandial hypoglycemia. Diabetes 1981;30:996. (*Data substantiating a diagnosis of reactive hypoglycemia, with a discussion focusing on what constitutes a "low" glucose level.*)
9. Merimee TJ, Tyson JE. Stabilization of plasma glucose during fasting—normal variations in two separate studies. N Engl J Med 1974;291:1275. (*Fasting blood sugar levels in normal women may be as low as 40 mg/dL.*)
10. Oberg K, Skogseid B, Eriksson B. Multiple endocrine neoplasia type I: clinical, biochemical, and genetic investigations. Acta Oncol 1989;28:383. (*Comprehensive review of this syndrome, which can include insulinoma.*)
11. Park-Wyllie LY, Juurlink DN, Kopp A, et al. Outpatient gatifloxacin therapy and dysglycemia in older adults. N Engl J Med 2006;354:1352. (*Population-based study; both hypo- and hyperglycemia are associated with the use of this particular fluoroquinolone.*)
12. Seltzer HS. Drug-induced hypoglycemia: a review of 1418 cases. Endocrinol Metab Clin North Am 1989;18:163. (*Sulfonylureas are the major cause of drug-related hypoglycemia.*)
13. Service FJ, McMahon MM, O'Brien PC et al. Functioning insulinoma—incidence, recurrence, and long-term survival of patients: a 60-year study. Mayo Clin Proc 1991;66:711. (*Recurrence was highest in those with multiple endocrine neoplasia type 1; long-term survival was normal in patients with benign disease.*)
14. Service FJ. Hypoglycemia and the postprandial syndrome. N Engl J Med 1989;321:1472. (*An editorial emphasizing that most patients with postprandial syndrome do not have hypoglycemia.*)
15. Simonson DC, Tamborlane WV, DeFronzo RA, et al. Intensive insulin therapy reduces counterregulatory hormone responses to hypoglycemia in patients with type I diabetes. Ann Intern Med 1985;103:184. (*Documents the risk for profound hypoglycemia in such patients.*)
16. Charles MA, Hofeldt F, Shackelford A, et al. Comparison of oral glucose tolerance tests and mixed meals in patients with apparent idiopathic postabsorptive hypoglycemia. Diabetes 1981;30:465. (*Mixed meals did not cause hypoglycemia, but a glucose load did; provides a rationale for treatment.*)
17. Cox DJ, Gonder-Frederick L, Ritterband L, et al. Prediction of severe hypoglycemia. Diabetes Care 2007;30:1370. (*Episodes of significant hypoglycemia are often preceded by patterns in glucose fluctuations that increase the risk for imminent hypoglycemia.*)
18. Kioschinsky T, Dannehl K, Gries FA. New approach to technical and clinical evaluation of devices for self-monitoring of blood glucose. Diabetes Care 1988;11:619. (*A still useful critique of self-monitoring techniques.*)
19. Palardy J, Havrankova J, LePage R, et al. Blood glucose measurements during symptomatic episodes in patients with suspected postprandial hypoglycemia. N Engl J Med 1989;321:1421. (*Study of a referral population indicating that postprandial hypoglycemia is infrequent and that glucose tolerance testing is of little diagnostic utility.*)
20. Scarlett JA, Mako ME, Rubenstein AH, et al. Factitious hypoglycemia: diagnosis by measurement of serum C-peptide and insulin-binding antibodies. N Engl J Med 1977;297:1029. (*Documents the usefulness of these measures in patients who self-administer insulin surreptitiously.*)
21. Service FJ, Natt N. The prolonged fast. J Clin Endocrinol Metab 2000;85:3973. (*Argument for continuing the fast for 72 rather than 48 hours because 14% did not develop hypoglycemia until after 48 hours.*)
22. Ritholz MD, Jacobson AM. Living with hypoglycemia. J Gen Intern Med 1998;13:799. (*Qualitative study underscoring the experiential dimension of the problem.*)
23. Yeager J, Young RT. Nonhypoglycemia as an epidemic condition. N Engl J Med 1974;291:907. (*A succinct discussion of how to manage patients with self-diagnosed "hypoglycemia."*)

CHAPTER 98 ■ EVALUATION OF HIRSUTISM

DAVID M. SLOVIK

Hirsutism is the development in women of androgen-dependent terminal body hair in a male pattern. It is present in 5% to 10% of women of reproductive age and results from increased androgenic activity. Excessive growth occurs of hormone-dependent pubic, axillary, abdominal, chest, back, and facial hair. Women commonly present for evaluation when such hair growth is viewed as exceeding that of others in their societal, geographic, or racial environment. For those living in a society preoccupied with stereotypical perceptions of beauty, hirsutism may be extremely upsetting and connote loss of femininity and sexuality. For the primary physician, hirsutism raises the question of an underlying endocrinopathy, ranging in severity from minor changes in androgen metabolism to the development of a hormonally active neoplasm.

When confronted with a complaint of excessive hair growth, the primary care physician must decide when to begin evaluating for endocrine disease and when to reassure and treat symptomatically if at all. Women with signs of virilization, progressive hair growth beginning after age 25 years, or concurrent amenorrhea should undergo endocrine evaluation (see later discussion).

PATHOPHYSIOLOGY AND CLINICAL PRESENTATION (1–11)

Pathophysiology

Hirsutism is a manifestation of excessive androgenic effect, either from increased androgen levels or increased end-organ sensitivity. The hormonal stimulus for hair growth is *5-α-dihydrotestosterone,* a potent testosterone metabolite derived from the peripheral conversion at the hair follicle of testosterone by 5-α-reductase. *δ-4-Androstenedione* and *dehydroepiandrosterone* (DHEA), produced by the ovaries and adrenal glands, are the *precursors* for 50% to 70% of circulating testosterone in women; the remainder of the testosterone is secreted directly by the ovaries or occasionally by the adrenals.

Hirsute women generally have *increased production rates of DHEA and δ-4-androstenedione,* which are relatively weak androgens, or of *testosterone,* a more potent androgen. Serum measurements of the total concentrations of androgens reflect the binding of sex steroid hormones to sex hormone–binding globulin; however, only the free fraction, which in the case of testosterone is 1% of total testosterone, is biologically active. The source of enhanced androgen production may be the ovary, the adrenal gland, or both. Testosterone excess is usually of ovarian origin, dehydroepiandrosterone sulfate (DHEA-S) excess is of adrenal origin, and androstenedione excess can be of either adrenal or ovarian origin. *Hyperinsulinism* resulting from insulin resistance has been noted to trigger excess ovarian androgen production, providing a possible link between *obesity* and hirsutism, a common association. In addition, obesity leads to a reduction in the concentration of sex hormone–binding globulin.

Virilization (temporal hair recession, acne, deepening voice, increased muscle mass, and clitoromegaly) develops with extremely high levels of circulating androgens.

Clinical Presentation

Hair follicles are located over the entire body except for the palms and soles. Hair growth is of two types: (a) *lanugo (neonatal)* or *vellus,* which is androgen independent, soft, unpigmented, and rarely more than 2 cm long; and (b) *terminal,* which is coarse, stiff, and pigmented and grows in excess of 2 cm. A survey of college women revealed that one fourth had easily noticeable facial hair, one third reported hair extending along the linea alba from the pubic area (male escutcheon), and 17% had periareolar hair. Three fourths of women older than age 60 years have a measurable growth of facial hair. Hirsutism has familial, ethnic, and racial patterns. Eastern European women are more hirsute than Scandinavian women; white women are more hirsute than black women, who have more body hair than Asian women. The *Ferriman–Gallwey scale* is used to define and grade hirsutism. Hair growth in each of nine androgen-dependent areas of the body is graded from 0 (no hair growth) to 4 (frankly virile growth). A score of 8 or greater is generally accepted as indicative of hirsutism. There are some limitations in using this scale, principally its reliance on subjective assessment; intraobserver reproducibility is good, but not interobserver reproducibility.

Ovarian Sources

Polycystic Ovary Syndrome. Polycystic ovary syndrome (PCOS) is the most common cause of androgen excess in women (65% to 85%). It is characterized by menstrual irregularity (*oligomenorrhea* or *amenorrhea*) and *hyperandrogenism* (either clinical or with elevated androgen levels). Androgen excess is usually evident at the time of puberty or shortly thereafter, and the symptoms gradually worsen with age. Gonadotropin dynamics are abnormal, with a loss of pulsatile secretion of luteinizing hormone (LH), an increased ratio of LH to follicle-stimulating hormone (FSH), and elevated levels of LH. Concurrent *obesity* and *insulin resistance* are noted in many patients, which contribute to androgen excess. Both LH and insulin stimulate excessive secretion of ovarian testosterone and androstenedione. *Acanthosis nigricans, precocious puberty,* and the *metabolic syndrome* may occur. Large numbers of small ovarian follicles form, but follicular growth is abnormal, and no preovulatory follicles develop. Menstrual abnormalities and *infertility* are the consequence (see Chapter 112). The ovaries may be of normal size or enlarged, and they characteristically contain multiple follicular cysts.

Ovarian Hyperthecosis. *Ovarian hyperthecosis* is a nonmalignant condition, characterized by increased testosterone production by luteinized theca cells in the stroma. It may be part of the spectrum of polycystic ovary syndrome.

Ovarian Tumors. Ovarian tumors, including arrhenoblastomas and hilar cell tumors, are capable of causing *virilization* through an excess production of testosterone. The virilized patient often has testosterone levels exceeding 150 to 200 ng/dL. Hirsutism caused by these tumors is most likely to occur later in life with more rapid progression of symptoms compared with polycystic ovary syndrome.

Adrenal Sources

Late-onset congenital adrenal hyperplasia (nonclassical congenital adrenal hyperplasia) designates a heterogeneous group of mild disorders of cortisol biosynthesis that are increasingly recognized as an important cause of adult-onset hirsutism. They are most commonly due to a deficiency in the activity of 21-hydroxylase, which leads to increased production of both 17-hydroxyprogesterone (substrate for 21-hydroxylase) and androstenedione with resultant hyperandrogenicity. These patients are not cortisol deficient due to an increase in adrenocorticotropic hormone (ACTH) secretion. Their condition is inherited as an autosomal-recessive trait closely linked to the HLA gene.

Adrenal Tumors. Adrenal neoplasms may cause androgen excess. *Cushing's syndrome*, especially if the underlying cause is an *adrenocortical carcinoma*, may produce virilization. Other causes of Cushing's syndrome are more likely to produce excess hair growth and typical cushingoid features without true virilization.

Other Causes

Hyperprolactinemia. Androgen excess may accompany *hyperprolactinemia* because prolactin stimulates androgen production, particularly DHEA. Characteristic features are amenorrhea and galactorrhea (see Chapter 112). Many of these women have polycystic ovary syndrome and the hyperandro-genism related to it, especially because DHEA-S is such a weak androgen.

Idiopathic Hirsutism. This etiology appears to involve *enhanced peripheral conversion of testosterone* to dihydrotestosterone by increased 5-α-reductase activity in hair follicles and skin. It initially was believed to result from overproduction of testosterone, but serum androgen concentrations are more often within the normal range; ovulatory cycles and the appearance of ovaries on ultrasound are also normal.

Idiopathic Hyperandrogenism. Idiopathic hyperandrogenism is characterized by clinical hyperandrogenism, increased serum androgen levels, normal ovulatory cycles, and normal ovaries on ultrasound.

Drugs. Drugs are another important cause of hirsutism. Most potent are the *anabolic steroids* (methyltestosterone, oxandrolone), used surreptitiously by some women engaged in competitive body building or athletics. The sex steroid precursor *androstenedione* is available without prescription and is very popular among adolescents; it is estimated that 2.5% of all adolescent girls take the drug regularly, especially those engaged in competitive athletics. When used in doses of 300 mg/d by young men, it results in increased levels of testosterone and estradiol. Similar increases in sex hormones are likely in young women, although they are not yet documented.

   Danazol, used to treat endometriosis, may also bring on hirsutism. In an occasional patient, *oral contraceptives* containing androgenic progestogens may stimulate hair growth (see Chapter 119), although this is not a frequent side effect. *Phenytoin, glucocorticoids, cyclosporine, diazoxide,* and *minoxidil* stimulate hair growth by poorly understood, nonandrogenic mechanisms.

DIFFERENTIAL DIAGNOSIS (1,5,9)

The causes of hirsutism can be divided into those that do and those that do not cause virilization and categorized according to adrenal and ovarian sources of androgen excess (Table 98.1). Among 950 hirsute patients presenting to an

TABLE 98.1

DIFFERENTIAL DIAGNOSIS OF HIRSUTISM

Cause	Mechanism
Hirsutism without Virilization	
Idiopathic	Increased peripheral conversion of androgens
Late-onset congenital adrenal hyperplasia	Adrenal androgen overproduction
Cushing's syndrome (ACTH induced)	Adrenal androgen overproduction
Polycystic ovary disease	Ovarian androgen overproduction
Insulin resistance/obesity	Ovarian androgen overproduction
Drugs: anabolic steroids, danazol, minoxidil, phenytoin, diazoxide, glucocorticoids	Varies, ranging from direct androgenic activity to nonandrogenic effects
Hirsutism with Virilization	
Ovarian hyperthecosis	Autonomous ovarian androgen production
Ovarian neoplasms	Autonomous ovarian androgen production
Adrenal neoplasms, especially adrenal carcinoma	Autonomous adrenal androgen production

ACTH, adrenocorticotropic hormone.

endocrine clinic with evidence of androgen excess, PCOS accounted for 72.1% (classic anovulatory 56.6%, mild ovulatory 15.5%), idiopathic hyperandrogenism for 15.8%, idiopathic hirsutism for 7.6%, 21-hydroxylase-deficient, nonclassic adrenal hyperplasia for 4.3%, and androgen-secreting tumor for 0.2%.

Some patients with anorexia nervosa report an increase in body hair (see Chapter 234), and excessive tweezing (hypertrichosis) may traumatize the hair follicle and cause coarse hair to grow at the site of repeated injury.

WORKUP (1,3,9,10,12-14)

The paramount objective in the evaluation of hirsutism is to identify the women who are likely to have important underlying endocrine disease.

History

The history should include information about menstrual history, time course of symptoms, other clinical features of androgen excess, medication history, and family history. Features suggestive of serious endocrine disease include *virilization* (voice change, temporal hair recession, increased muscle mass, acne); *rapid progression*, particularly a sudden increase in hair growth after age 25 years; *amenorrhea* or menstrual changes; and *galactorrhea*. The new onset of *hypertension* in the setting of hirsutism should also raise suspicion. A peripubertal onset of hirsutism is generally reassuring. A detailed *drug history* (anabolic steroids, androgens, oral contraceptives, danazol, phenytoin, corticosteroids, minoxidil, cyclosporine, diazoxide) is essential. Inquiry into any daily or regular use of nonprescription sex hormone precursors, such as *androstenedione*, is essential because the substance is popular among adolescent competitive athletes, who take it to enhance their performance (as noted earlier, the estimated prevalence of regular use among adolescent women is 2.5%). *Southern European* or *Mediterranean ancestry* in conjunction with hirsutism of a similar degree in a mother, grandmothers, aunts, and sisters reduces the probability of serious disease. However, a positive family history may also be found in some patients with polycystic ovary disease and partial congenital adrenal hyperplasia.

Physical Examination

Terminal hair on the face, about the areolae, and on the lower abdomen is normal, but new growth, especially on the lip, chin, upper abdomen, sternum, upper back, and shoulders, suggests *androgen excess* and *hirsutism*. The Ferriman–Gallwey score is helpful to assess the location and quantity of terminal hair. *Virilization* is indicated by temporal and vertical scalp hair loss, a deep voice, acne, an increase in muscle mass, and clitoromegaly. *Acanthosis nigricans* suggests insulin resistance. *Cushing's syndrome* should be suspected when centripetal obesity, muscle wasting with myopathy, and violaceous striae are encountered. Patients with *oligomenorrhea* require a pelvic examination to detect bilaterally enlarged cystic ovaries; however, a significant number of women with polycystic ovary physiology do not have palpable ovarian abnormalities. Women with virilization and amenorrhea should be examined carefully for a palpable adrenal or ovarian neoplasm. Most of these tumors

are inefficient producers of androgens and do not result in high levels of circulating androgens until they become quite large.

Laboratory Studies

An abundance of costly endocrinologic hormonal assays may be performed in the evaluation of hirsutism. To avoid the expense of unnecessary testing, it is important to define the likely diagnostic considerations and the goals of therapy for hirsutism so that appropriate hormonal evaluation may be obtained, rather than the indiscriminate measurement of all ovarian and androgen sex steroids and pituitary hormones. On the basis of the history and physical examination findings, patients can be categorized as likely to have idiopathic or familial, oligomenorrheic/amenorrheic, cushingoid, or virilizing forms of disease.

Idiopathic and Familial Forms of Hirsutism

A young woman with a minor increase in facial hair beginning in the peripubertal period but with perfectly regular ovulatory menses is most likely free of serious underlying disease and need not undergo detailed testing. The same pertains to the normally menstruating woman of southern European ancestry whose female relatives have similar amounts of facial and body hair. In idiopathic hirsutism, serum *free testosterone* levels may be high but serum *total testosterone* levels normal.

Oligomenorrheic/Amenorrheic Disease

When amenorrhea or oligomenorrhea, obesity, and hirsutism occur, especially in the context of infertility, polycystic ovary disease needs to be considered, as well as late-onset congenital adrenal hyperplasia and other causes of hyperprolactinemia.

Polycystic Ovary Disease. Because pelvic examination may not reveal bilaterally enlarged cystic ovaries, *pelvic ultrasonography* and laboratory testing can help to confirm the clinical suspicions. The *serum testosterone* concentration (either total or free hormone) provides the best estimate of androgen production in hirsute women. In women with polycystic ovary syndrome, serum testosterone levels are usually elevated but may be normal. Most women with polycystic ovary syndrome have levels less than 150 mg/dL. *Free (unbound) testosterone* and *ratios of LH to FSH* are also increased. Because an increase in androgens suppresses sex hormone-binding globulin, measurement of the *free serum testosterone* is a more sensitive indicator of androgen excess (but more expensive) than measurement of the total testosterone. Free testosterone correlates best with testosterone production rates. In many patients, a single random measurement of testosterone should suffice. However, because testosterone secretion is episodic, three serum samples taken 15 minutes apart, in the early morning, if possible, may be pooled for immunoassay. *Prolactin* should be measured in all women with oligomenorrhea or amenorrhea, especially if galactorrhea is also present.

Congenital Adrenal Hyperplasia. Patients with menstrual irregularities but no evidence of polycystic disease should be evaluated for a late-onset congenital adrenal hyperplasia (most often 21-hydroxylase deficiency). This condition can be identified by performing an *ACTH stimulation test* and measuring the *plasma 17-hydroxyprogesterone* 30 to 60 minutes after the intravenous administration of one ampule (25 μg) of cosyntropin (synthetic ACTH). A pretest level of

17-hydroxyprogesterone greater than 300 ng/dL is suggestive, but many patients have normal levels, so ACTH stimulation testing is necessary. A posttest level greater than 1,200 ng/dL at 30 minutes is diagnostic. Although these patients represent a minority of hirsute women, no distinguishing clinical features of this entity set it apart from the more common polycystic ovary syndromes.

Cushingoid Appearance. Patients with clinical features of Cushing's syndrome should be screened with either a *24-hour urinary free cortisol determination* or an *overnight dexamethasone-suppression test*. The 24-hour urinary free cortisol determination, which is the more specific study, is greater than 100 μg in Cushing's syndrome. *Urinary 17-ketosteroids* are elevated in adrenocortical carcinoma. For overnight dexamethasone suppression, the patient is given 1 mg of dexamethasone at midnight, and the plasma cortisol is measured at approximately 8:00 a.m. the next day. Cortisol should be suppressed to less than 5 μg/dL. If the 24-hour urinary free cortisol is elevated or an elevated cortisol is not suppressed by dexamethasone, more-extensive dexamethasone testing to determine the likelihood and cause of Cushing's syndrome needs to be pursued.

Virilization

When virilization is present, *serum testosterone, DHEA-S,* and *urinary 17-ketosteroids* should be measured. Serum testosterone levels less than 150 ng/dL usually exclude androgen-secreting ovarian and adrenal-secreting tumors in most women. Measurement of 17-ketosteroids detects elevated adrenal androgens, such as androstenedione and DHEA in adrenal cortical carcinoma. Although both the adrenals and the ovaries can synthesize all of the androgenic steroids, adrenal hormonal production is best assessed by measuring *DHEA-S* because more than 90% is formed in the adrenal gland. In women with rapid-progressing hirsutism or virilization, DHEA-S should be obtained. A serum level greater than 500 μg/dL suggests an adrenal tumor. Androstenedione is synthesized equally by the adrenal and the ovary glands. When the presence of a tumor is suspected in one of these glands, *ultrasonography* or *computed tomography* is required. Before a search for tumor is begun, the history should again be checked for the regular use of exogenous androstenedione, as in competitive athletes, especially adolescent girls, for body building.

SYMPTOMATIC MANAGEMENT AND PATIENT EDUCATION (1,2,4,9,10,15–20)

The approach to the management of hirsutism is based on the extent and the severity of the hirsutism, both physically and psychologically, and on the underlying pathophysiology. Options include (a) supportive reassurance that no important underlying endocrine disease is present; (b) cosmetic manipulations, such as bleaching, waxing, use of depilatories, and electrolysis; (c) medical therapy with estrogens or glucocorticoids directed at suppressing ovarian and adrenal hormone overproduction; (d) medical therapy directed at antagonizing the action of androgens at the receptor level; and (e) definitive curative therapy of underlying diseases such as Cushing's syndrome or masculinizing adrenal and ovarian neoplasms.

Supportive Measures and Cosmetic Manipulations

Patients free of significant endocrine disease can be effectively managed with *reassurance* that hirsutism does not impair sexuality or fertility. Adolescents taking exogenous sex hormone precursors such as androstenedione to enhance their athletic performance will benefit from a nonjudgmental review of the cosmetic and developmental consequences of taking these "natural" supplements.

If a woman is concerned about her appearance, cosmetic manipulation or medical therapy is appropriate. Hair may be bleached with a 6% *hydrogen peroxide* solution or commercially available cream bleaches. *Shaving* removes unwanted hair; however, because hair grows at the rate of 1 mm/d, "stubble" appears within several days. *Epilation* with tweezers or hot wax may retard hair growth for several months but may cause low-grade folliculitis. *Chemical depilation* may require the use of low-concentration hydrocortisone topically to prevent irritation. *Electrolysis*, the only permanent method of hair removal, involves electrocoagulation and destruction of the hair root. It is a costly and time-consuming process and should be performed only by a licensed electrologist. *Laser* treatment may be used or *eflornithine hydrochloride cream* (13.9%; Vaniqa), a Food and Drug Administration–approved topical drug that inhibits unwanted hair growth in women. The latter is modestly effective but expensive and requires indefinite use.

Weight reduction should be part of any program for the obese hirsute woman. Normalization of weight limits the peripheral conversion of androstenedione to testosterone by fatty tissue and reduces the hyperinsulinism that may contribute to ovarian production of androgens. Impressive results can be achieved.

Suppression of Ovarian and Adrenal Androgen Overproduction

Oral Contraceptives

Those containing estrogen and progestin slow hair growth in greater than 60% of hyperandrogenic women. They suppress ovarian androgen production by decreasing levels of FSH and LH and inhibit adrenal androgen secretion. In addition, estrogen increases sex hormone–binding globulin levels, thus decreasing levels of free testosterone, and also competes with the cytosolic receptor for dihydrotestosterone. Oral contraceptives also work well for patients with *idiopathic disease* by reducing the amount of available androgenic substrate.

Preparations containing at least 35 μg of ethinyl estradiol or 50 μg of mestranol are needed to reduce androgen levels; those with lower amounts of estrogen are less effective. Progestins with nonandrogenic properties are preferred. Preparations such as norgestrel and levonorgestrel should be avoided because of their androgenic effects. The least androgenic progestins, such as norethindrone (0.5 to 1 mg) or ethynodiol diacetate in combination with ethinyl estradiol or mestranol, are preferred. If the hormonal and clinical responses to these therapies, determined at 3 months, are inadequate, an oral contraceptive containing larger amounts of estrogen may be used. Side effects of these drugs, including an increased risk for thromboembolism in smokers (see Chapter 119), must be reviewed. A decrease in hirsutism is usually not evident for 3 to 6 months;

a decrease in the rate of hair growth is noted initially, followed by a transformation to lighter, finer hair.

Glucocorticoids

These agents may reduce hirsutism and induce ovulation in partial *congenital adrenal hyperplasia*, where androgens are of adrenal origin. However, glucocorticoid therapy is otherwise not generally indicated in the treatment of hirsutism because of the serious side effects. Prednisone 5 to 7.5 mg daily or dexamethasone 1 mg at bedtime may be enough to suppress androgen production. Potential concerns with this form of therapy are suppression of the hypothalamic–pituitary–adrenal axis and induction of a cushingoid appearance. Alternate-day corticosteroid therapy may suffice and reduce the risk for such adverse effects. Following the changes in the 17-hydroxyprogesterone concentration is an effective means of monitoring therapy.

Metformin

This diabetes drug reduces insulin resistance and may help to treat the hirsutism associated with polycystic ovary disease; although the mechanism is not clear, reduction in hyperinsulinism is believed to play a role.

Antagonizing Testosterone at the Target Tissue

Spironolactone

This antihypertensive drug decreases androgen levels by decreasing testosterone biosynthesis and antagonizing its peripheral action on the hair follicle. Doses as high as 100 mg twice daily diminish hirsutism over 3 months but may cause menstrual disturbances. One might begin therapy with 50 mg twice daily taken from day 4 through day 22 of each menstrual cycle. The drug is *teratogenic* and should not be used in large doses by women of childbearing age. It is often given as an adjunct to oral contraceptives in patients with severe polycystic ovary disease.

Cimetidine

As a histamine$_2$-receptor antagonist, cimetidine competes with androgens for target-tissue binding; it appears to be less effective than spironolactone.

Flutamide and Finasteride

Flutamide, a selective androgen receptor antagonist, and *finasteride*, a 5-α-reductase inhibitor, offer improved blockade of testosterone action at the target tissue. Studies are ongoing.

Ketoconazole

This antifungal agents also inhibits testosterone production.

Antagonizing Central Stimulation of Androgen Production

Gonadotropin-Releasing Hormone Agonists

These agents when taken daily suppress gonadotropin secretion and therefore androgen production.

INDICATIONS FOR REFERRAL

Patients with virilization and elevated testosterone levels require evaluation by an endocrinologist and a gynecologist because a virilizing tumor may be present. If polycystic ovary syndrome is present and if infertility is an issue, referral for clomiphene therapy and evaluation for endometrial hyperplasia with endometrial biopsy are appropriate. Hyperprolactinemia necessitates coronal computed tomography or magnetic resonance imaging to recognize a prolactinoma or pathologic process interrupting the dopaminergic inhibition of prolactin. Patients with Cushing's syndrome should be referred for endocrinologic evaluation of a pituitary, adrenal, or ectopic origin.

Annotated Bibliography

1. Azziz R, Carmina E, Sawaya ME. Idiopathic hirsutism. Endocrine Rev 2000;21:347. (*Useful review of this difficult problem.*)
2. Azziz R, Sanchez LA, Knochenhauer ES, et al. Androgen excess in women: experience with over 1000 consecutive patients. J Clin Endocrinol Metab 2004;89:453. (*Cohort study; polycystic ovary syndrome accounted for most cases; the therapeutic success rate was high in those willing to stay with treatment.*)
3. Azziz R, Dewailly D, Dwerbach D. Nonclassic adrenal hyperplasia: current concepts. J Clin Endocrinol Metab 1994;78:810. (*A clinically focused discussion.*)
4. Barnes R, Rosenfield RL. The polycystic ovary syndrome: pathogenesis and treatment. Ann Intern Med 1989;110:386. (*A still-useful comprehensive discussion of disease mechanisms, including the loss of luteinizing hormone pulsatility.*)
5. Carmina E, Rosato F, Janni A, et al. Relative prevalence of different androgen excess disorders in 950 women referred because of clinical hyperandrogenism. J Clin Endocrinol Metab 2006;91:2. (*Classic polycystic ovary syndrome was the most common cause.*)
6. Ehrmann DA, Rosenfield RL. Hirsutism—beyond the steroidogenic block. N Engl J Med 1990;323:909. (*Editorial focusing on late-onset congenital adrenal hyperplasia.*)
7. Eldar-Geva T, Hurwitz A, Vecsei P, et al. Secondary biosynthetic defects in women with late-onset congenital adrenal hyperplasia. N Engl J Med 1990;323:855. (*A high incidence was found among women with hirsutism, menstrual disorders, and unexplained infertility; mechanisms are examined.*)
8. Leder BZ, Longcope C, Catlin DH, et al. Oral androstenedione administration and serum testosterone in young men. JAMA 2000;283:779. (*Increases in both testosterone and estradiol were found; suggests that prolonged use could cause hirsutism and even virilization.*)
9. Rosenfield RL. Hirsutism. N Engl J Med 2005;353:2578.(*Excellent review; 55 references.*)
10. Setji TL, Brown AJ. Polycystic ovary syndrome: diagnosis and treatment. Am J Med 2007;120:128. (*A more recent general review with updated treatment recommendations.*)
11. Yesalis CE, Barsukiewicz CK, Kopstien AN, et al. Trends in anabolic–androgenic steroid use among adolescents. Arch Pediatr Adolesc Med 1997;151:1197. (*Use among female adolescents is estimated to be 2.5%.*)
12. Derksen J, Nagesser SK, Meinders AE, et al. Identification of virilizing adrenal tumors in hirsute women. N Engl J Med. 1994;331:968. (*Use of serum testosterone and dehydroepiandrosterone sulfate as screening tests.*)
13. Siegel SF, Finegold DN, Lanes R, et al. ACTH stimulation tests and plasma dehydroepiandrosterone sulfate levels in women with hirsutism. N Engl J Med 1990;323:849. (*Basal levels were unrevealing, but levels measured after adrenocorticotropic hormone stimulation differed between normal subjects and many patients with hirsutism.*)
14. Wild RA, Vesely S, Beebe L, et al. Ferriman Gallwey self-scoring I: performance assessment in women with polycystic ovary syndrome. J Clin Endocrinol Metab 2005;90:4112. (*Questions the usefulness of the scale because there is a great deal of discordance.*)

15. Harbone L, Fleming R, Lyall H, et al. Metformin or antiandrogen in the treatment of hirsutism in polycystic ovary syndrome. J Clin Endocrinol Metab 2003;88:4116. (*Metformin and perhaps other antihyperglycemic agents that reduce hyperinsulinemia and insulin resistance may be helpful.*)
16. Rittmaster RS. Medical treatment of androgen-dependent hirsutism. J Clin Endocrinal Metab 1995;80:2555. (*Helpful review of agents used to treat hirsutism.*)
17. Wagner RF Jr. Physical methods for the management of hirsutism. Cutis 1990;45:319. (*Useful information to give to patients.*)
18. Cumming D, Yang JC, Rebar RW, et al. Treatment of hirsutism with spironolactone. JAMA 1984;247:1295. (*An early report of efficacy in 39 patients; responses were observed as early as 2 months; side effects were limited.*)
19. Diamanti-Kandarakis E, Baillargeon JP, Ivorno MJ, et al. A modern medical quandary: polycystic ovary syndrome, insulin resistance, and oral contraceptive pills. J Clin Endocrinal Metab 2003;88:1927. (*Critical discussion of the use of oral contraceptive pills and insulin-sensitizing drugs in polycystic ovary syndrome.*)
20. Vigersky RA, Hehlman I, Glass AR, et al. Treatment of hirsute women with cimetidine. N Engl J Med 1980;303:1042. (*An early report rate of hair growth that decreased without a decrease in serum androgen.*)

APPENDIX 98.1: APPROACH TO AN INCIDENTALLY ENCOUNTERED ADRENAL MASS

Most adrenal masses are clinically silent and discovered incidentally during imaging studies conducted for other reasons. The prevalence of such lesions is about 0.4% in series based on imaging studies and 2.1% in autopsy series. Adrenal masses discovered in the context of evaluation for hirsutism, virilization, Cushing's syndrome, hypertension, and refractory hypokalemia pose the possibility of a functioning adrenal neoplasm and require aggressive evaluation (see Chapter 19 and the preceding part of this chapter). At issue is what to do about clinically silent adrenal "incidentalomas" because of the small but real risk of important underlying pathology.

DIFFERENTIAL DIAGNOSIS (1,2)

In persons without malignancy, about two thirds of these lesions prove to be benign, nonfunctioning neoplasms (Table 98.2). In persons with known cancer, about three fourths represent clinically silent metastases from an extraadrenal primary site. Among large adrenal neoplasms (>6 cm), adrenal cortical carcinoma accounts for about 25%, but the figure drops to about 2% for smaller lesions (<4 cm).

CLINICAL COURSE (1,2)

Most nonfunctioning adrenal neoplasms do not grow substantially in size, and the risk of transformation of small, nonfunctioning nodules (<3 cm) to functioning nodules is low. Adrenal cortical carcinomas are the exception to this rule, growing very rapidly, and are associated with very poor survival (e.g., 50% mortality at 2 years).

WORKUP (1,2)

History and Physical Examination

The history should include inquiry into any changes in skin, hair, menses, or libido, as well as paroxysms of palpitations, hypertension, persistent hypokalemia, and glucose intolerance. Past medical history should be reviewed for prior malignancy (especially of the lung, breast, or kidney) and family history for multiple endocrine neoplasia. The physical examination should take note of any elevations in blood pressure or pulse, cushingoid appearance, hirsutism, or virilization and include a check for signs of primary and metastatic cancer.

Laboratory

The radiologic appearance alone may be diagnostic (e.g., myelolipoma, adrenal cyst). Radiologic signs of a benign adenoma on computed tomography include homogeneity, low attenuation, and smooth borders. Lesions less than 4 cm have a less than 2% chance of being malignant. Initial biochemical assessment for a functioning neoplasm should include a *1-mg dexamethasone-suppression test* for detection of subclinical hypercortisolism and a *plasma free metanephrines* determination to screen for pheochromocytoma (see Chapter 26). In persons with hypertension, a serum *potassium* should also be checked for hypokalemia, suggestive of an aldosterone-producing adenoma; consideration should also be given to obtaining an *aldosterone/plasma renin ratio* (see Chapter 26) for enhanced detection. Computed tomography–*guided skinny-needle biopsy* is worth considering when the appearance of the lesion is suspicious for malignancy (irregular border, high attenuation, large size) and there are no other biopsy sites evident; however, hemangioma and pheochromocytoma must be ruled out first because of the risks of precipitating hemorrhage and hypertensive crisis, respectively.

MANAGEMENT (1,2)

Biochemically Active Neoplasms

Adrenalectomy is often recommended for hormonally active adrenal neoplasms, even if they are clinically silent. Aldosterone-secreting lesions can be treated medically with aldosterone inhibition (e.g., spironolactone).

TABLE 98.2

CAUSES OF ADRENAL "INCIDENTALOMAS"

Malignant
  Adrenal cortical carcinoma
  Metastases from other cancers

Benign
  Adenoma (functioning or nonfunctioning)
  Cyst
  Hemangioma
  Ganglioneuroma
  Pheochromocytoma
  Myelolipoma

Nonfunctioning Neoplasms

Watchful waiting after initial evaluation and careful follow-up are reasonable, especially if the mass is less than 4 cm and without evidence of biochemical function or radiologic signs of malignancy. The optimal interval and duration of monitoring are unknown, but repeat computed tomography scan and biochemical testing in 6 to 12 months appear reasonable. If the mass is radiologically unchanged, less than 3 cm, and hormonally inactive, there is little further risk of change, and monitoring can cease after 12 months. For lesions between 4 and 6 cm, options include adrenalectomy and annual radiologic and biochemical monitoring for 3 to 4 more years. For lesions greater than 6 cm, adrenalectomy is recommended due to the high frequency of adrenal cortical carcinoma.

Metastatic Cancer

Treatment is directed at the underlying malignancy; there is no proven benefit from resecting the adrenal metastasis, even if it is the only metastasis evident.

Annotated Bibliography

1. Grumbach MM, Biller BMK, Braunstein GD, et al. Management of the clinically inapparent adrenal mass ("incidentaloma"). Ann Intern Med 2003;138:424. (*National Institutes of Health consensus statement, which includes commentary on the adequacy of underlying evidence; serves as the basis for recommendations in this appendix.*)

2. Mansmann G, Lau J, Balk E, et al. The clinically inapparent adrenal mass: update in diagnosis and management. Endocrine Rev 2004;25:309. (*Comprehensive review and exhaustive reference list.*)

CHAPTER 99 ■ EVALUATION OF GYNECOMASTIA

DAVID M. SLOVIK

Gynecomastia is defined as enlargement of the male breast as the result of an increase in glandular tissue, which distinguishes it from pseudogynecomastia with fat deposition but no glandular proliferation, which is often seen in obese men. Clinically a rubbery or firm mass extends concentrically from the nipples. Some patients present out of fear of loss of masculinity or onset of breast cancer. Others may not have recognized the change and come to the physician at the suggestion of friends or family. Gynecomastia is a normal transient physiologic event in up to 70% of pubertal boys; its prevalence in adults is less than 1%, although men older than age 50 years have a higher prevalence.

The primary physician must be able to recognize gynecomastia, differentiate it from malignancy, and initiate an evaluation to rule out important underlying medical causes that range from hormonally active neoplasms to cirrhosis and hyperthyroidism. In most instances, the cause is benign and the tasks are to allay fears and help the patient to decide about treatment.

PATHOPHYSIOLOGY AND CLINICAL PRESENTATION (1–8)

Pathophysiology

Estradiol is the growth hormone of the breast. Gynecomastia represents a phenomenon of relative *estradiol excess* leading to the proliferation of breast tissue. Under normal circumstances, most estradiol in men is derived from the peripheral conversion of testosterone and adrenal estrone. The basic mechanisms of gynecomastia are a decrease in androgen production, an absolute increase in estrogen production, and an increased availability of estrogen precursors for peripheral conversion to estradiol. Blocking of androgen receptors and increased binding of androgen are additional modes of reduced androgen effect.

Reduced Androgen Production, Availability, and Receptor Blockade

A decrease in androgen production accounts for many cases seen in older men, those with testicular endocrine failure due to *cancer therapy*, and those taking the antifungal agent *ketoconazole*. Androgen availability is reduced in both *hyperthyroidism* and *cirrhosis* through an increase in sex hormone–binding globulin, which enhances the binding of testosterone relative to estradiol and decreases free testosterone. Blockade of androgen receptors accounts for the gynecomastia associated with use of *spironolactone, cimetidine, flutamide,* and perhaps *marijuana*. *Cocaine* use is also associated with gynecomastia, but the mechanism is unclear.

Increased Estrogen Production

Age-related increases in *adipose tissue* increase extraglandular aromatization of testosterone to estradiol and androstenedione to estrone. Increased estrogen production may also be seen with *Klinefelter's syndrome, adrenal carcinomas, tumors producing ectopic human chorionic gonadotropin (hCG),* and *Leydig cell tumors* of the testes. Tumors that produce hCG stimulate the testicular production of estradiol. Teratomas of the testes and carcinomas of the *lung, pancreas,* and *colon* are known sources of ectopic hCG. The transient gynecomastia of *puberty* represents a brief physiologic increase in testicular estrogen secretion and lasts 1 to 2 years before receding. Gynecomastia seen with *malnutrition* and *starvation* is probably due to reduced gonadotropin and testosterone levels relative to estrogen and may worsen with refeeding due to a rise in estradiol production that outpaces the increases in gonadotropin and testosterone.

Increased Estrogen Precursor Availability

Increased estrogen precursor availability is the mechanism of gynecomastia in patients who have *androgen-secreting tumors* or *congestive heart failure* or who use *exogenous androgen* (which leads to an increased conversion of testosterone and androstenedione to estradiol and estrone). This effect has also been documented with the use of *androstenedione,* the popular "natural" sex hormone precursor supplement taken by body builders and adolescents. *Hyperthyroidism* causes an increased peripheral conversion of testosterone to estrogen precursors. Much of the conversion takes place in fatty tissue. An exogenous estrogen effect is seen with the use of *digitalis* and *synthetic estrogens. Ketoconazole* and *spironolactone* cause a release of free estrogen by displacement from sex hormone–binding globulin.

Clinical Presentations

The most noticeable feature is an increase in breast tissue. Although usually *bilateral,* gynecomastia is *unilateral* in one third of cases. Idiopathic and drug-induced gynecomastia is typically unilateral, whereas in pubertal and hormonal cases the changes are often bilateral. It may be that asymmetry is a more accurate description than unilateral enlargement, based on the prevalence of bilaterally histologic but not clinically evident gynecomastia in autopsy series. *Tenderness* may also be noted in one third of patients, but actual pain is less frequent. Enlargement is usually central and symmetric, although it is occasionally eccentric.

A few distinctive clinical presentations are worth noting: In *Klinefelter's syndrome,* gynecomastia develops around puberty in a patient with long limbs, small and firm testes, infertility, and normal or deficient secondary sex features. In cirrhosis, patients present with loss of libido, loss of body hair, and testicular atrophy (see Chapter 71).

Recovery from *malnutrition* or *serious chronic illnesses* (severe heart failure, renal failure, liver failure) leads to a picture resembling a second puberty, with development of transient gynecomastia.

Carcinoma of the male breast is distinct from gynecomastia; it is characterized by a unilateral, eccentrically located firm mass that may be fixed. Male breast cancer is rare; it is generally not more frequent in patients with gynecomastia, although the incidence in patients with Klinefelter's syndrome is higher.

DIFFERENTIAL DIAGNOSIS (1,2,8)

The differential diagnosis can be organized by underlying pathophysiology (Table 99.1). It can also be considered in terms of age of presentation. In healthy pubertal boys, transient physiologic gynecomastia is the most likely explanation. Testicular or adrenal tumors are rare in this age group, but Klinefelter's syndrome may account for a number of cases. In adult men, alcohol-related liver disease and drugs predominate, with the list including estrogens, androgens, androstene-

TABLE 99.1

DIFFERENTIAL DIAGNOSIS OF GYNECOMASTIA

Inhibition of Androgen Effect
  Spironolactone (at high doses only)
  Cimetidine (common at high doses)
  Flutamide

Decreased Androgen Availability Secondary to Increased Binding or Conversion
  Cirrhosis (very common)
  Hyperthyroidism (uncommon, except with thyrotoxicosis)

Decreased Androgen Synthesis
  Testicular failure, primary (Klinefelter's syndrome) or secondary (orchiectomy, cancer drugs, ketoconazole)

Increased Estrogen Synthesis or Estrogen Effect
  Estrogen-secreting tumor of the testis or adrenal gland (very rare)
  Klinefelter's syndrome (about 15% of pubertal cases)
  Ectopic human chorionic gonadotropin–secreting tumor of testis, lung, colon, pancreas (rare)
  Digitalis (uncommon)
  Exogenous estrogen (dose related)

Increased Availability of Estrogen Substrate
  Androgen-producing tumor (rare)
  Exogenous androgen (common)
  Congestive heart failure (common)

Physiologic
  Puberty
  Recovery from chronic illness or starvation
  Old age

dione, spironolactone, digitalis preparations, flutamide, ketoconazole, cimetidine, and marijuana. The association also exists but is more tenuous with use of phenothiazines, amphetamines, reserpine, methyldopa, isoniazid, tricyclic antidepressants, phenytoin, and heroin. In one series, 22% of patients had a history of taking a drug associated with gynecomastia and 26% had alcoholic liver disease.

Less common causes include recovery from malnutrition or a serious chronic illness. Much rarer forms are tumor-related ectopic hCG production and feminizing adrenal, testicular, and pituitary tumors. In just less than 10% of cases, a probable cause is not identified. Gynecomastia must be distinguished from carcinoma of the male breast.

WORKUP (1–9)

History

Notice should be taken of onset, location, associated symptoms, and course over time. Most important is a detailed inquiry into drug and substance use, including alcohol, exogenous estrogens, anabolic steroids, and prescription medications (e.g., cimetidine, spironolactone, flutamide, digitalis, ketoconazole). The use of androstenedione by adolescents and body builders is common and needs to be checked for, as does anabolic steroid use in competitive athletes. Any symptoms of hyperthyroidism (see Chapter 103), heart failure (see Chapter 32), or hepatocellular failure (see Chapter 71) should be noted, as should the resolution of a chronic illness. In addition, note should be made of any changes suggesting hypogonadism (decreased libido, impotence, change in testicular size, and change in skin, voice, and hair quality and distribution). Weight loss, chronic cough, hemoptysis, change in bowel habits, headaches, or visual field disturbances can be important etiologic clues.

Physical Examination

Onset at puberty should trigger an examination for features of Klinefelter's syndrome (arm span greater than height, small and firm testes, absence of secondary sex characteristics). If an adolescent has a normal general physical and genital examination, then pubertal gynecomastia is the likely explanation. In adults, one needs to look for signs of hepatocellular failure (jaundice, spider angiomas, pallor, palmar erythema) and hyperthyroidism (warm, sweaty skin; tremor; exophthalmos; and goiter).

During the breast examination, the glandular texture of true gynecomastia must be distinguished from the fatty consistency of breast enlargement related to obesity and the firmness and nodularity of a carcinoma. The question of malignancy in the breast tissue must always be considered in gynecomastia. Asymmetry and nodules deserve special note, and careful palpation of the axillary nodes is necessary. If the enlargement is unilateral and eccentric, the breast is particularly firm, a nodule is palpated (a nodule under the nipple is particularly worrisome), or axillary adenopathy is present, then a biopsy should be performed. Galactorrhea should be looked for.

On cardiopulmonary examination, one checks for signs of heart failure (see Chapter 32), and on abdominal examination, for signs of cirrhosis (see Chapter 71). The abdomen is palpated for a deep mass suggestive of adrenocortical carcinoma and the stool tested for occult blood. The testicles are examined for atrophy and masses, the latter suggesting neoplasm and the need for a carcinoma workup (see Chapter 131).

Laboratory Studies

Gynecomastia not associated with puberty, drugs, hyperthyroidism, hepatocellular failure, or another obvious cause requires further evaluation. Laboratory testing should begin with measurement of *serum luteinizing hormone* and may be supplemented by determinations of testosterone, estradiol, β-hCG, dehydroepiandrosterone sulfate, and prolactin. The necessary laboratory workup can proceed according to luteinizing hormone concentration.

High Luteinizing Hormone Concentrations

High luteinizing hormone concentrations are consistent with testicular failure, Klinefelter's syndrome, and hCG-secreting tumors. Ectopic hCG production can be identified by finding elevated *serum β-hCG subunit levels*. This should trigger a search for testicular tumors or ectopic production (see Chapter 92). To check for Klinefelter's syndrome, a buccal smear is obtained and examined for chromatin positivity (Barr bodies). If the smear is negative, the diagnosis is most likely primary testicular failure or a chromatin-negative variant of Klinefelter's syndrome.

Low Luteinizing Hormone Concentrations

Low luteinizing hormone concentrations are more worrisome because they raise the question of autonomous androgen or estrogen production (in addition to exogenous sex steroid use). Repeated questioning of the patient regarding exogenous steroid use, including regular use of popular precursor preparations such as *androstenedione* and other anabolic steroid preparations, is critical. If the patient's responses are convincingly negative, then levels of *free testosterone* and *estradiol* should be measured, but with full cognizance of the pitfalls involved in interpreting the results. For example, total testosterone may be affected by the concentration of sex hormone–binding protein and not reflect the free testosterone concentration. Consequently, free testosterone should be measured. However, testosterone secretion can fluctuate greatly, so that three samples obtained during 15 minutes should be pooled for best results. The estradiol concentration measured may correlate poorly with the rate of estrogen production because of vagaries in peripheral uptake. Thus, normal levels do not necessarily rule out an estrogen-secreting tumor, although marked elevations are very suggestive, provided exogenous use has been ruled out. If serum estrogens are elevated, then adrenal cancer and Leydig cell tumor of the testes should be ruled out.

Normal Luteinizing Hormone Concentration, Normal Sex Hormone Levels

Normal luteinizing hormone concentration with normal sex hormone levels makes serious underlying endocrinopathy unlikely, and such patients can be followed expectantly with periodic reevaluation. It is important to keep in mind that gynecomastia may resolve after the condition that caused it resolves. The search for an underlying cause may yield few clues if the cause was transient and self-limited.

SYMPTOMATIC MANAGEMENT, PATIENT EDUCATION, AND INDICATIONS FOR REFERRAL (2,10,11)

The duration of gynecomastia and presence of tenderness, pain, or adverse psychosocial consequences affect the approach and response to symptomatic management.

Gynecomastia of Recent Onset and Reversible Etiology

Most gynecomastias of recent onset regress spontaneously. Thus, watchful waiting with reevaluation is reasonable for adolescents with pubertal gynecomastia and for patients after stopping medications for treating underlying medical conditions known to cause gynecomastia. Removal of the offending drug usually produces regression of breast enlargement within several months. Counseling adolescents who are using androstenedione on a daily basis for body building is especially important because it may help to prevent adverse developmental consequences (see Chapter 238). The gynecomastia that accompanies puberty or refeeding after starvation is a transient phenomenon that can be managed by providing reassurance. Resolution of gynecomastia usually follows treatment of hyperthyroidism. When hCG-secreting tumors are discovered, resection of the tumor is indicated if possible.

When a benign condition such as drug-induced gynecomastia is discovered, the patient can be reassured that the condition is not a reflection of loss of maleness or a carcinomatous process. It must be remembered that some conditions that produce gynecomastia may reduce potency; this situation must be confronted and discussed with the patient. No evidence of carcinomatous degeneration in gynecomastia has been found except in Klinefelter's syndrome. Pain, irritation, or social problems that may arise should be dealt with symptomatically and sympathetically.

Persistent Gynecomastia, Tenderness, or Adverse Psychosocial Consequences

Medical therapies with androgens, antiestrogens, and aromatase inhibitors can be considered in those patients with persistent gynecomastia, severe pain, tenderness, or embarrassment that interferes with normal activities. A 3-month trial of *tamoxifen*, a generally well tolerated antiestrogen, can be tried initially to reduce breast size in patients with painful

gynecomastia. *Surgical therapy* should be considered for those patients who do not respond to medical therapy, have long-standing gynecomastia, and are considerably bothered by the cosmetic problems of breast enlargement.

Consultation

Consultation with an endocrinologist is essential when a case of Klinefelter's syndrome is suspected, and also when ectopic hCG production is a concern or autonomous sex hormone production is under consideration (low gonadotropin levels). Referral is also indicated when treatment of gynecomastia is being considered, be it medical therapy or surgery.

Annotated Bibliography

1. Bannagan GA, Hajdu SI. Gynecomastia: clinicopathologic study of 351 cases. Am J Clin Pathol 1972;57:431. (*Idiopathic and drug-induced cases of gynecomastia are usually discrete and unilateral, whereas endocrine and pubertal cases are bilateral.*)
2. Braunstein GD. Gynecomastia. N Engl J Med 1993;328:490. (*Comprehensive review of pathogenesis and clinical issues.*)
3. Braunstein GD, Vaitukaitis JL, Carbone PP, et al. Ectopic production of human chorionic gonadotropin by neoplasms. Ann Intern Med 1973;78:39. (*One of the original reports of ectopic production of human chorionic gonadotropin.*)
4. Cavanaugh J, Niewoehner CB, Nutall FQ. Gynecomastia and cirrhosis of the liver. Arch Intern Med 1990;150:563. (*Factors other than the ratio of estrogen to testosterone are operative.*)
5. Feldman D. Ketoconazole and other imidazole derivatives as inhibitors of steroidogenesis. Endocrine Rev 1986;7:409. (*Detailed discussion of the effects of this important class of drugs on testosterone production.*)
6. Jensen RT, Collen MJ, Pandol HD. Cimetidine-induced impotence and breast changes in patients with gastric hypersecretory states. N Engl J Med 1983;308:883. (*A side effect of high-dose, long-term therapy; resolves with cessation of cimetidine therapy.*)
7. Leder BZ, Longcope C, Catlin DH, et al. Oral androstenedione administration and serum testosterone in young men. JAMA 2000;283:779. (*Increases in both testosterone and estradiol were found when androstenedione was taken.*)
8. Yesalis CE, Barsukiewicz CK, Kopstien AN, et al. Trends in anabolic–androgenic steroid use among adolescents. Arch Pediatr Adolesc Med 1997;151:1197. (*Rate of use among male adolescents is estimated to be 4.9%.*)
9. Wilson JD. Gynecomastia: a continuing diagnostic dilemma. N Engl J Med 1991;324:334. (*An editorial emphasizing the difficulties encountered in evaluating this condition.*)
10. Courtiss EH. Gynecomastia: analysis of 159 patients and current recommendations for treatment. Plast Reconstr Surg 1987;79:740. (*The plastic surgeon's perspective.*)
11. Parker LN, Gray DR, Lai MK, et al. Treatment of gynecomastia with tamoxifen: a double-blind, crossover study. Metabolism 1986;35:705. (*Medical therapy with an antiestrogen proved beneficial for patients with painful gynecomastia.*)

CHAPTER 100 ■ EVALUATION OF GALACTORRHEA AND HYPERPROLACTINEMIA

DAVID M. SLOVIK

Discharge of milk or colostrum from the breast in the absence of nursing is referred to as *galactorrhea*. When it is accompanied by disturbed menses or infertility, it suggests the possibility of hyperprolactinemia and the associated risk for pituitary neoplasm. When a patient presents with galactorrhea, underlying pituitary disease must be carefully considered.

PATHOPHYSIOLOGY AND CLINICAL PRESENTATION (1–9)

Galactorrhea

Normal milk production involves the interplay of prolactin and breast tissue primed by estrogen and progestin. Prolactin is a

polypeptide hormone that is secreted by the lactotroph cells of the pituitary gland under tonic inhibitory control, predominantly by dopamine. During pregnancy and lactation, the prolactin content of the pituitary increases 10- to 20-fold. Galactorrhea can occur in the setting of a normal or elevated serum prolactin level. The upper normal value for serum prolactin in most laboratories is 20 ng/mL.

Normoprolactinemic Galactorrhea

Normoprolactinemic galactorrhea is believed to be a consequence of local breast stimulation or irritation in women with hormonally primed breast tissue. It is hypothesized that stimulation of the breast may cause a mild, transient elevation in prolactin secretion, although this is not sustained. Many cases are associated with a distant pregnancy or the use of oral contraceptives. Gonadal function is preserved, with menses and fertility remaining normal. Galactorrhea in the absence of sustained hyperprolactinemia is usually noted as an isolated symptom or an incidental finding on breast examination.

Hyperprolactinemic Galactorrhea

Hyperprolactinemic galactorrhea develops as a consequence of excessive prolactin production, caused either by a loss of hypothalamic inhibition of lactotrophs in the anterior pituitary or by the development of an autonomously functioning pituitary adenoma. In rare instances, hyperprolactinemia results from a decreased clearance of prolactin (as in renal failure). Even in the context of high prolactin levels, galactorrhea does not occur unless the breast is primed by estrogen, which accounts for the rarity of the condition in men. The most common symptoms of hyperprolactinemia in premenopausal women are amenorrhea and infertility; galactorrhea occurs in 80% of such women.

Hyperprolactinemia

Elevations in prolactin may be a consequence of physiologic stimulation, medications, pituitary/hypothalamic disease, and prolactinoma.

Physiologic and Drug-Induced Hyperprolactinemia

Pregnancy and lactation are the most important physiologic causes of hyperprolactinemia. Because the secretion and release of prolactin are under tonic inhibition by dopamine, any process that interferes with dopamine secretion and release will cause hyperprolactinemia. Prolactin levels rise after exercise, meals, chest wall stimulation, and physical and psychological stress, but under such physiologic circumstances the levels are rarely higher than 40 ng/mL.

Higher levels (up to 100 ng/mL) are seen with medications that affect dopaminergic activity, including phenothiazines, thioxanthenes, butyrophenones, tricyclic antidepressants, monoamine oxidase inhibitors, selective serotonin reuptake inhibitors, reserpine, methyldopa, verapamil, metoclopramide, cimetidine, estrogen, opiates, and cocaine.

Hypothalamic/Pituitary Disease

Prolactin elevations may result from pituitary or hypothalamic pathology. Examples include infiltration by granulomatous disease, compression of the pituitary stalk by nonsecreting pituitary tumors and craniopharyngiomas, acromegaly, and primary hypothyroidism (owing to thyroid-releasing hormone stimulation of lactotrophs). Prolactin levels also may be elevated in patients with chronic renal failure due to decreased clearance.

Prolactinomas

Very high serum concentrations of prolactin are associated with autonomously functioning *prolactinomas* derived from lactotrophs in the anterior pituitary. The degree of hyperprolactinemia tends to correlate with tumor size. Prolactinomas larger than 10 mm in diameter ("macroadenomas") are typically associated with prolactin levels greater than 250 ng/mL and sometimes greater than 1,000 ng/mL. Except in pregnancy, serum prolactin in excess of 250 to 300 ng/mL is almost always the result of a prolactinoma. Microadenomas (<10 mm in diameter) may produce less impressive elevations. They typically have a benign course and undergo little additional enlargement.

Associated Symptoms

Because patients with hyperprolactinemia are at risk for hypogonadism, they may experience, in addition to galactorrhea, disturbed menses, *amenorrhea*, *infertility*, and *osteoporosis*. In premenopausal women, symptoms of hyperprolactinemia correlate with its severity. Prolactin elevations greater than 100 ng/mL are typically associated with findings of hypogonadism with estrogen deficiency due to inhibition of the release of gonadotropin-releasing hormone and subsequent inhibition of luteinizing hormone and follicular-stimulating hormone. Moderate elevations of 50 to 100 ng/mL may cause a short luteal phase of the menstrual cycle due to insufficient progesterone secretion, but even mild hyperprolactinemia can cause infertility.

Men with hyperprolactinemia commonly have hypogonadism and report *impotence*, *infertility*, *decreased libido*, *gynecomastia*, and, rarely, galactorrhea. The pituitary tumors tend to be large. Men and women with a substantially enlarging sellar mass may complain of *headache* or a *visual field cut*.

DIFFERENTIAL DIAGNOSIS
(4,6,7,10)

The differential diagnosis of galactorrhea can be organized according to whether prolactin is elevated and whether an elevation in prolactin is the result of a decrease in hypothalamic inhibition or overproduction by a functioning adenoma (Table 100.1). Only 20% of patients with galactorrhea have hyperprolactinemia. Prolactinoma is a leading cause in patients with galactorrhea, amenorrhea, and hyperprolactinemia. Pregnancy should be ruled out in women of childbearing age with

---

TABLE 100.1

DIFFERENTIAL DIAGNOSIS OF GALACTORRHEA

Normoprolactinemic Galactorrhea
Local breast stimulation/irritation (suckling, trauma, inflammation)
Oral contraceptive use
Recent pregnancy
Idiopathic (? transient elevation in prolactin from stress, breast stimulation)

Hyperprolactinemic Galactorrhea
Impairment of hypothalamic pituitary inhibition
  Drugs (phenothiazines, thioxanthenes, butyrophenones, tricyclic antidepressants, monoamine oxidase inhibitors, selective serotonin reuptake inhibitors, metoclopramide, cimetidine, heroin, cocaine, opiates, reserpine, methyldopa)
  Lesions of the pituitary stalk (nonfunctioning sellar tumors, infarction)
  Hypothalamic disease (craniopharyngioma, infiltrative disease, infarction)
Overproduction by a pituitary adenoma
  Prolactinoma
  Hypothyroidism (simulates adenoma by thyrotropin-releasing hormone stimulation of lactotrope cells)
Idiopathic
  ? Microadenoma not detectable by neuroimaging
  ? Stress, trauma, breast stimulation

hyperprolactinemia. Other causes originating in the region of the pituitary include empty-sella syndrome, craniopharyngioma, pinealoma, and parasellar sarcoidosis. Nonprolactinomic disease about and within the pituitary accounts for about one third of cases of galactorrhea and amenorrhea. Persistent galactorrhea after childbirth accounts for just less than 10% of cases. Drugs associated with galactorrhea include oral contraceptives and agents with central dopaminergic-blocking activity (phenothiazines, haloperidol, metoclopramide) and, less commonly, reserpine, methyldopa, isoniazid, and tricyclic antidepressants.

WORKUP (7,10,11–13)

History and Physical Examination

The history for workup of galactorrhea should include careful questioning about menstrual pattern (e.g., oligomenorrhea, amenorrhea), recent pregnancy, infertility, medications, change in libido, symptoms of hypothyroidism (see Chapter 104), breast stimulation, chest trauma, and the presence of headache or visual complaints. A thorough review of medications and substance use is essential, particularly oral contraceptives and drugs that block central dopaminergic transmission (see earlier discussion).

The physical examination should include a detailed examination of the breasts to be sure the discharge is indeed milky and not caused by local breast disease, although no increased risk for breast cancer has been found in patients with true galactorrhea. Confrontation testing of the visual fields and fundoscopy examination are important, although the findings are usually normal. Any signs of hypothyroidism (see Chapter 104) should be noted and then confirmed by measuring the thyroid-stimulating hormone level.

In men, hyperprolactinemia may cause hypogonadotropic hypogonadism with findings of impotence, decreased libido, infertility, gynecomastia, and, rarely, galactorrhea (due to less estrogen priming of breast tissue compared with women).

Laboratory Testing

Testing begins with a prolactin determination.

Prolactin Testing

The development of accurate prolactin assays and the association of galactorrhea with high prolactin levels and pituitary tumors have made determination of the *serum prolactin concentration* an essential part of the diagnostic evaluation. A single measurement is usually adequate to document hyperprolactinemia. However, the prolactin level may be transiently elevated by stress, time of day, sleep, meals, or breast stimulation, but usually no higher than 40 ng/mL. In this circumstance, repeat elevated levels are needed to confirm hyperprolactinemia. Prolactin levels between 20 and 200 ng/mL can be found with any cause of hyperprolactinemia. However, values greater than 200 ng/mL usually indicate a prolactinoma. The patient with galactorrhea and amenorrhea is at increased risk for a pituitary neoplasm, and her prolactin concentration must be measured unless the explanation for both is apparent (e.g., recent pregnancy, medication). In up to 10% of patients with hyperprolactinemia, an elevation of *macroprolactin* is seen. The macroprolactin results from the binding of monomeric prolactin to an endogenous antiprolactin autoantibody. These patients present with varied clinical symptoms, with many having normal menses and fertility.

Additional Testing and Neuroimaging

Based on the clinical circumstances, it might be necessary to rule out hypothyroidism (*thyroid-stimulating hormone, serum thyroxine*), renal failure (*creatinine*), and pregnancy (*β-human chorionic gonadotropin*).

Patients with galactorrhea, menstrual irregularities, and an otherwise unexplained elevation in serum prolactin should undergo neuroimaging of the sellar region. *Magnetic resonance imaging* (MRI) *with gadolinium enhancement* is the procedure of choice, although *computed tomography* is a reasonable alternative if MRI is unavailable. Gadolinium enhancement of MRI of the sellar structures is based on differences in vascularity between normal pituitary tissue and adenomas. Nonetheless, microadenomas can be difficult to detect, although the absence of a visible lesion rules out an anatomically threatening neoplasm. Even patients with mild unexplained elevations of prolactin (<200 ng/mL) should undergo neuroimaging of the pituitary region. A sellar or parasellar mass can be responsible for a mild prolactin elevation due to compression of the pituitary stalk, and some pituitary tumors are poorly functioning. Finding a lesion of greater than 10 mm in a patient with a modest rise in prolactin necessitates consideration of other types of pituitary tumors. *Formal visual field testing* should be performed in all patients with a sellar mass or visual symptoms.

SYMPTOMATIC MANAGEMENT (7,11,12–21)

No Evidence of a Mass Lesion

From a practical standpoint, regular menses and a normal prolactin level in a patient with galactorrhea make the likelihood of a clinically important pituitary tumor unlikely. Patients in whom the likelihood of tumor is low can be followed carefully with periodic determinations of prolactin, usually at 1-year intervals; if prolactin levels become elevated, neuroimaging of the sella can be pursued.

For patients with galactorrhea secondary to the use of a dopaminergic-blocking agent, a reduced dose of the drug can be tried, although full cessation may be necessary to terminate symptoms. Prolactin levels begin to fall within days of stopping medications that cause hyperprolactinemia. If hypothyroidism is the contributing factor, it should be corrected (see Chapter 104). Symptomatic patients with *idiopathic disease* (galactorrhea, abnormal periods, elevated prolactin, normal MRI findings, no other evident disease) who want relief from their symptoms can be treated as if they have a microadenoma (see later discussion); many of these patients may have lactotroph microadenomas that are too small to detect.

Prolactinoma

The treatment approach depends on the size of the lesion and its natural history.

Microadenomas

Microadenomas (<10 mm in diameter) have an excellent prognosis. Long-term studies of untreated patients demonstrate that in 80% to 90% of cases, the size of a microadenoma remains the same or the tumor regresses with time; only 10% to 20% continue to grow. Prolactin levels follow a similar pattern. However, with microadenomas that grow, the correlation between tumor size and prolactin level may not be close, so close monitoring of both parameters is necessary.

Despite the favorable prognosis, many patients with stable microadenomas may require treatment because of menstrual irregularities, gonadal dysfunction, severe galactorrhea, or infertility. Osteoporosis is also a risk. The treatment of choice for prolactinomas is a dopaminergic agonist, either *bromocriptine* or *cabergoline*. These drugs inhibit prolactin synthesis, secretion, and cellular proliferation.

In many instances, dopaminergic agonist therapy results in rapidly falling prolactin levels that return to normal; galactorrhea ceases within several weeks, tumor size decreases, menses resume within 2 months as gonadal function returns, and osteoporosis slowly recedes. For control of symptoms, continuous administration is required, although in some patients the tumor undergoes spontaneous regression. A 2-year course of treatment followed by a trial of cessation is a common approach to bromocriptine therapy for patients with a symptomatic microadenoma.

Bromocriptine. *Bromocriptine,* an ergot derivative, has been used for two decades. The doses needed to control symptoms range from 2.5 to 10 mg/d, although smaller doses often suffice for maintenance. The most common side effects are nausea, orthostatic hypotension, and dizziness, which can be minimized by administering the drug at bedtime with a snack. Therapy is initiated at a dose of 0.625 to 1.25 mg and slowly increased at weekly intervals until prolactin is normal. The usual dose is 5 to 7.5 mg/d. Barrier contraception should be used until regular menses are established and stopped when one menstrual cycle has been missed.

Cabergoline. *Cabergoline,* a nonergot agonist, is a long-acting dopamine agonist with a high affinity for lactotroph dopamine receptors. It can be administered twice a week in a dose of 0.25 mg. It has fewer side effects than bromocriptine but is more expensive. Long-term remission may sometimes be seen after withdrawing dopamine agonist therapy. Experience with use during pregnancy is limited; bromocriptine should be used if fertility is the goal. Reports have emerged of cardiac valve regurgitation in patients treated with high-dose cabergoline for Parkinson's disease or movement disorders. The dose of cabergoline associated with these problems was 3 mg/d, more than 20 times the dose used in hyperprolactinemic patients.

Oral Contraceptives. An alternative to dopamine-agonist therapy when pregnancy is not desired is the use of oral contraceptives, the benefits of which include regular periods, birth control, and the prevention of osteoporosis.

Macroadenomas

Macroadenomas are also treated initially with *bromocriptine* or *cabergoline*. In many instances, the drug suffices to control symptoms and shrink the adenoma. The usual dose needed to establish control with bromocriptine is 7.5 to 10 mg/d and with cabergoline is 0.5 to 1.5 mg twice weekly. Tumor size and prolactin concentration decline substantially. Lower doses may be effective for maintenance, but whether to continue therapy indefinitely or at some point discontinue treatment is uncertain.

Surgery is reserved for patients with very large tumors, patients in whom fertility is desired (the tumor may grow during pregnancy), and patients with rapidly progressing visual loss or symptoms refractory to medical therapy. *Radiation therapy* is sometimes considered, especially in persons who poorly tolerate dopamine-agonist therapy or desire definitive treatment.

PATIENT EDUCATION AND INDICATIONS FOR REFERRAL

Patients with pituitary adenomas understandably worry about further tumor growth. Concern can be lessened by explaining the very favorable prognosis for the vast majority of microadenomas and the excellent response of most prolactinomas to medical therapy. The patient with galactorrhea and amenorrhea should be informed that numerous options for induction of fertility are available and that these may be pursued according to the patient's wishes. By providing accurate information, moral support, and close follow-up, the primary physician can spare the patient a great deal of unnecessary concern.

Although the basic evaluation of galactorrhea and hyperprolactinemia can be effectively carried out by the primary physician, a consultation with the endocrinologist is indicated in a number of situations (e.g., macroadenoma, suspected pituitary neoplasm other than prolactinoma, failure to respond to bromocriptine or cabergoline, visual loss, desire to become pregnant).

Annotated Bibliography

1. Fish LH, Mariash CN. Hyperprolactinemia, infertility, and hypothyroidism. A case report and review of the literature. Arch Intern Med 1988;148:709. (*Makes the important observation that hypothyroidism may mimic prolactinoma.*)
2. Gibney J, Smith TP, McKenna TJ. Clinical relevance of macroprolactin. Clin Endocrinol 2005;62:633. (*A useful discussion of the subject.*)
3. Hooper JH, Welsh VC, Shackleford RT. Abnormal lactation associated with tranquilizing drug therapy. JAMA 1961;178:506. (*Abnormal lactation occurred in 26 of 100 women receiving major tranquilizers; the effect was dose dependent.*)
4. Kleinberg DL, Noel GL, Frantz AA. Galactorrhea: a study of 235 cases, including 48 pituitary tumors. N Engl J Med 1977;296:589. (*In one of the largest reported series, 34% of cases had concurrent amenorrhea and 32% had idiopathic galactorrhea without amenorrhea.*)
5. Klibanski A, Biller BMK, Rosenthal DI, et al. Effects of prolactin and estrogen deficiency in amenorrheic bone loss. J Clin Endocrinol Metab 1988;67:124. (*Bone loss results from prolactin-induced hypogonadism.*)
6. Molitch ME. Medication-induced hyperprolactinemia. Mayo Clin Proc 2005;80:1050. (*Extensive review with 119 references.*)
7. Schlechte JA. Prolactinoma. N Engl J Med 2003;349:2035. (*Excellent clinical review; 55 references.*)
8. Schlechte JA, Dolan K, Sherman B, et al. The natural history of untreated hyperprolactinemia: a prospective analysis. J Clin Endocrinol Metab 1989;68:412. (*Resumption of normal periods, normal prolactin levels, and resolution of the prolactinoma was noted in 6 of 30 patients.*)
9. Vallette-Kasic S, Morange-Ramos E, Selim, et al. Macroprolactinemia revisited: a study of 106 patients. J Clin Endocrinol Metab 2002;87:581. (*The incidence was at least 10% of those who had prolactinemia.*)
10. Biller DM. Diagnostic evaluation of hyperprolactinemia. J Reprod Med 1999;44(12 Suppl):1095. (*Good review of testing modalities.*)
11. Casanueva FF, Molitch ME, Schlechte JA, et al. Guidelines of the pituitary society for the diagnosis and management of prolactinomas. Clin Endocrinol 2006;65:265. (*Current recommendations for diagnosis and management put together by an expert committee.*)

12. Molitch ME. Diagnosis and treatment of prolactinomas. Adv Intern Med 1999;44:117. (*Comprehensive review with exhaustive reference list.*)
13. Newton DR, Dillon WP, Norman D, et al. Gd-DTPA–enhanced MR imaging of pituitary adenoma. Am J Neuroradiol 1989;10:949. (*Data on the efficacy of gadolinium-enhanced magnetic resonance imaging of pituitary adenomas.*)
14. Biswas M,, Smith J, Jadon D, et al. Long-term remission following withdrawal of dopamine agonist therapy in subjects with microprolactinomas. Clin Endocrinol 2005;63:26. (*In 30% to 40% of cases, the abrupt withdrawal of chronic agonist therapy was followed by long-term remission.*)
15. Colao A, Vitale G, Cappabianca P, et al. Outcome of cabergoline treatment in men with prolactinoma: effects of a 24-month treatment on prolactin levels, tumor mass, recovery of pituitary function, and semen analysis. J Clin Endocrinol Metab 2004;89:1704. (*The treatment was found to be as effective and safe in men as in women.*)
16. Colao A, DiSarno A, Cappabianca P, et al. Withdrawal of long-term cabergoline therapy for tumoral and non-tumoral hyperprolactinemia. N Engl J Med 2003;349:2023. (*The therapy can be safely withdrawn in patients with normalized prolactin levels and no evidence of tumor, but monitoring is required.*)
17. Dalkin AC, Marshall JC. Medical therapy of hyperprolactinemia. Endocrinol Metab Clin North Am 1989;18:259. (*Comprehensive review, with a particularly detailed and useful section on the use of bromocriptine.*)
18. Koppelman MC, Jaffe MJ, Rieth KG, et al. Hyperprolactinemia, amenorrhea and galactorrhea. Ann Intern Med 1984;100:115. (*Most untreated patients experienced either no growth or spontaneous regression, with resumption of menses in some.*)
19. Liuzzi A, Dallabonzana D, Oppizzi G, et al. Low doses of dopamine agonists in the long-term treatment of macroprolactinomas. N Engl J Med 1985;313:656. (*The efficacy of low maintenance doses was demonstrated, but therapy could not be halted.*)
20. Pellegrini I, Rasolonjanahary R, Gunz G, et al. Resistance to bromocriptine in prolactinoma. J Clin Endocrinol Metab 1989;69:500. (*Reviews the mechanisms of resistance, carefully emphasizing the need to monitor therapy.*)
21. Schade R, Andersohn F, Suissa S, et al. Dopamine agonists and the risk of cardiac-valve regurgitation. N Engl J Med 2007;356:29. (*High-dose pergolide and cabergoline were associated with increased risk of cardiac valve regurgitation.*)

CHAPTER 101 ■ POLYURIA AND POLYDIPSIA: EVALUATION OF SUSPECTED DIABETES INSIPIDUS

DAVID M. SLOVIK

When a patient presents with polyuria and polydipsia, the primary care physician needs to include diabetes insipidus (DI) in the differential diagnosis. DI is characterized clinically by the excretion of large volumes of inappropriately dilute urine. Although uncommon, DI may be a manifestation of important hypothalamic–pituitary disease or renal tubular dysfunction. The primary care physician needs to know how to screen for DI in a patient with polyuria and polydipsia and how to proceed with the basic elements of the diagnostic investigation.

PATHOPHYSIOLOGY AND CLINICAL PRESENTATION (1–10)

Plasma osmolality is carefully regulated to maintain each individual's normal value at a level between 285 and 290 mOsm/kg. When water is lost, even a 1% increase in plasma osmolality stimulates hypothalamic osmoreceptors to release *antidiuretic hormone (ADH, vasopressin, AVP)* from the posterior pituitary. This in turn stimulates water retention by the kidney. Osmoreceptor stimulation also triggers central thirst mechanisms. These actions serve to reestablish normal serum osmolality. The ability of ADH to stimulate water reabsorption is mediated by kidney *aquaporins*, which are ADH-responsive water channels; aquaporin-2 is the major one.

A lesion in any portion of this osmoregulatory system can result in DI and its attendant *water diuresis*. *Dehydration* and *hypertonicity* may ensue unless the thirst mechanism remains intact and access to water is adequate. Clinically, DI is characterized by the excretion of large volumes of dilute urine in conjunction with *excessive thirst* and *polydipsia*. Urinary frequency must be distinguished from true polyuria, which is generally defined as the excretion of more than 3 L/day or 50 ml/kg per day. Some patients may excrete as much as 15 to 20 L/day. *Craving for ice water* is common (especially with central DI) due to stimulation of osmoreceptors in the back of the throat. Nocturia is common.

The urine is almost always colorless, even in the morning, because of its dilute nature. *Urine osmolality* is inappropriately *low* (<250 mOsm/kg). *Serum osmolality* may be *increased*, especially if the thirst mechanism is impaired.

Central or Neurogenic Diabetes Insipidus

Central or neurogenic diabetes insipidus is the most common form of DI and is associated with deficient secretion of ADH. It can be due to *complete* or *partial ADH deficiency* and occurs in the context of an injury to the hypothalamus or posterior pituitary. Mechanisms for acquired central DI include trauma, destruction by malignant or granulomatous disease, autoimmune inflammatory processes, vascular insult, and pituitary surgery. Because the thirst center is situated near the hypothalamic osmoreceptors, it, too, may be involved, although in many cases the thirst mechanism is preserved and dehydration avoided. Anterior pituitary adenomas usually do not cause

DI unless they are large and extend posteriorly or beyond the sella. Onset of polyuria is typically abrupt. *Familial central diabetes insipidus* is an autosomal dominant disease caused by mutation in the *arginine vasopressin gene*.

Nephrogenic Diabetes Insipidus

Nephrogenic diabetes insipidus is characterized by *normal ADH secretion* but *impaired renal response* to ADH. Acquired forms of nephrogenic DI result from conditions or medications that damage renal tubulointerstitial function and concentrating ability (most commonly hypercalcemia, hypokalemia, sickle cell disease, lithium use). Onset of polydipsia is usually gradual. *Hereditary nephrogenic DI* is primarily an X-linked disorder.

Primary Polydipsia

Primary polydipsia also produces polyuria, but unlike DI, this condition appears to originate with an *altered perception of thirst* and a primary increase in water intake. It is particularly prevalent among patients with chronic psychiatric disturbances (especially schizophrenia) but is also seen with organic brain disease (e.g., multiple sclerosis). Detailed study of such patients has revealed multiple defects in the regulation of osmolality, including problems with urinary dilution, regulation of water intake, and ADH secretion. Increased thirst and fluid intake are followed by polyuria, although some patients may hide this behavior. A fall in serum osmolality (<285 mOsm/kg) may be accompanied by hyponatremia. Symptoms tend to be episodic and onset of polydipsia gradual.

DIFFERENTIAL DIAGNOSIS (8,10,11)

The differential diagnosis for patients with polyuria and polydipsia in the outpatient setting includes *diabetes mellitus* (see Chapter 102), *diuretic use*, DI, and *primary polydipsia*. The differential can be organized as follows: (a) whether the diuresis is related to water or solute; (b) if related to water, whether it is a manifestation of DI or primary polydipsia; and (c) if DI, whether it is central or nephrogenic (Table 101.1). Other causes of urinary frequency unaccompanied by polydipsia (e.g., *urinary tract infection*, *bladder dysfunction*) need to be ruled out (see Chapters 133, 134, and 140).

WORKUP (1,2,8,11–13)

The initial diagnostic evaluation of the patient with polyuria can proceed logically and efficiently by addressing a set of basic questions as follows.

Is This True Polyuria or Just Urinary Frequency?

A history of frequently voiding large volumes of dilute (colorless or pale) urine, both day and night, suggests true polyuria, whereas frequent voiding of small volumes of concentrated urine is indicative of bladder dysfunction caused by infection or other local disease. A *24-hour urine collection* provides

TABLE 101.1

DIFFERENTIAL DIAGNOSIS OF POLYURIA/POLYDIPSIA IN THE OUTPATIENT SETTING

Solute Diuresis
  Diabetes mellitus
  Diuretics

Water Diuresis
  Diabetes insipidus
    Central
      Idiopathic
      Trauma
      Tumor (local or metastatic to the sellar region)
      Granulomatous disease (sarcoidosis, tuberculosis)
      Postsurgical (removal of pituitary adenoma)
      Vascular (Sheehan's syndrome, old stroke)
    Nephrogenic
      Drugs (lithium, demeclocycline, amphotericin)
      Tubulointerstitial disease (pyelonephritis, polycystic kidney disease, sickle cell disease, obstructive uropathy)
    Metabolic (hypercalcemia, hypokalemia)
    Primary polydipsia
      Psychogenic (schizophrenia)
      Central nervous system disease (multiple sclerosis)
      Idiopathic

objective confirmation of true polyuria when the volume exceeds 3 L or 50 mL/kg.

If True Polyuria, Is This a Water Diuresis or a Solute Diuresis?

Measurement of the Urine Osmolality and Total Solute Excretion

Measurements of the urine osmolality and total solute excretion are very helpful. Patients with a concentrated urine (*>350 mOsm/L*) have a condition causing a solute diuresis. Those with a dilute urine (*<250 mOsm/L*) have a water diuresis. Patients with a urine osmolality between these levels may have either. To differentiate, one calculates the *total solute excretion* (calculated on a 24-hour urine collection) from the product of the urine output and urine osmolality. If it is less than 1,200 mOsm/d, then a water diuresis is likely. If a solute diuresis is suspected, checking the urine for glucose and electrolytes can be confirmatory.

If a Water Diuresis, Is This Diabetes Insipidus or Primary Polydipsia?

Measurement of the Serum Osmolality

Measurement of the serum osmolality can be helpful. A clearly elevated serum osmolality (>290 mOsm/L) in the context of inappropriately dilute urine (osmolality <275 mOsm/L) suggests DI, although many patients with DI and an intact thirst mechanism and access to water have a serum osmolality close to normal. A low serum osmolality suggests primary polydipsia.

Direct Measurement of the Serum ADH

Direct measurement of the serum ADH can help to clarify the situation, but reliable assays are not widely available. Very low levels occur with central DI; very high levels indicate renal DI; inappropriately elevated levels suggest primary polydipsia.

Clinical Context

The clinical context may help suggest the cause of the water diuresis. When it occurs in the setting of known renal tubulointerstitial disease or drug use, nephrogenic DI is likely. A central mechanism is suggested when the patient presents with other manifestations of pituitary disease or has a condition that may damage the central nervous system (e.g., trauma, cancer, granulomatous disease). Onset in a patient with mental illness raises the probability of primary polydipsia. Knowing the rate of onset of the polyuria may be helpful. Abrupt onset suggests central DI, whereas gradual onset suggests nephrogenic DI and primary polydipsia.

Water Deprivation and Desmovasopressin Testing

When the cause remains uncertain and in the absence of a reliable measure of ADH, it may be necessary to perform a water-deprivation test and administer *desmovasopressin* (DDAVP), an ADH analogue. The response to DDAVP helps to clarify the underlying mechanism of the water diuresis. By raising plasma osmolality, either by water deprivation or less commonly by infusing hypertonic saline, one can distinguish between DI and other causes of polyuria. The plasma ADH level can further help to distinguish between these causes. The water-deprivation test needs to be done in a supervised (i.e., inpatient) setting with close monitoring.

In central DI, after DDAVP administration, the urine osmolality increases greater than 50% (often greater than 100%) with a comparable 50% decrease in urine volume. Smaller increases in urine osmolality can be seen with partial central DI (15% to 50%). An unequivocal absence of change in urine concentration (<10%) strongly suggests nephrogenic DI or primary polydipsia. In primary polydipsia, the urine output falls and urine osmolality rises; in the setting of continued polydipsia, hyponatremia may occur.

Pituitary–Hypothalamic Imaging

Biochemical evidence of central DI is an indication for neuroimaging to determine whether a mass lesion or other disease is compromising the integrity of the pituitary. *Magnetic resonance imaging* (MRI) with *gadolinium* enhancement is the procedure of choice, although *computed tomography* is a reasonable alternative if MRI is unavailable or cost is a major issue. Gadolinium enhancement of MRI of the sellar structures is based on differences in vascularity between normal and abnormal tissues.

Is This Definitely Primary Polydipsia?

When primary polydipsia is suspected (low-normal or low serum osmolality, polyuria, low urine osmolality, concurrent psychiatric disease), an inpatient *water-restriction test* (as previously described) can be confirmatory; all parameters return to normal when water is restricted. Because such dehydration testing can be very dangerous for patients with other causes of a water diuresis, it is necessary to conduct this test in a carefully supervised inpatient setting. Supervised water restriction is also necessary because patients with primary polydipsia tend to be psychotic and drink surreptitiously.

SYMPTOMATIC RELIEF (1,3,8,14,15)

Treatment of Central DI

Desmopressin is the treatment of choice for central DI. It is a synthetic V2R (ADH receptor) agonist administered intranasally, orally, or parenterally. Significant individual variations occur in response and duration of action, especially with the oral preparation. The intranasal ADH is taken before bed to eliminate nocturnal polyuria. An initial dose of 5 μg at bedtime is used, and the dose is adjusted to allow normal amounts of daytime urination. The usual maintenance dose is 5 to 20 μg once or twice a day. Excessive doses can lead to a DDAVP-induced fluid retention and hyponatremia. The oral preparation is one tenth of the potency of the nasal spray due to poor gastrointestinal absorption. The initial dose is 0.05 mg at bedtime, and the usual maintenance is 0.1 to 0.8 mg in divided doses.

Drugs that enhance ADH secretion (*clofibrate*, *chlorpropamide*, *carbamazepine*) are also helpful. Somewhat paradoxically, *thiazide diuretics* and *amiloride* relieve the symptoms of central DI and can be used in nephrogenic DI.

Treatment of Nephrogenic DI

Because the kidneys are poorly responsive to ADH, the best treatment is volume contraction. As just noted, *thiazides* and *amiloride* can also be helpful in nephrogenic DI. By inducing a mild sodium diuresis, they enhance the proximal resorption of sodium and water, so the amount of water that reaches the distal tubule is reduced. *Nonsteroidal antiinflammatory drugs* (e.g., indomethacin) are sometimes helpful in nephrogenic DI. By inhibiting renal prostaglandins (which are active in settings of renal disease), they reduce water delivery to the distal tubule.

Treatment of Primary Polydipsia

Treatment of the underlying psychiatric disturbance is the only current treatment for primary polydipsia.

INDICATIONS FOR ADMISSION AND REFERRAL

As noted, patients requiring DDAVP testing or a trial of water restriction need to either be admitted to have the test done or have it performed under close medical supervision in the office or clinic. An endocrinologic consultation can be helpful in further planning the diagnostic evaluation and in interpreting its results. Patients in whom central DI is suspected should have neuroimaging of the sella region (MRI is best) and endocrinologic consultation for further testing of the hypothalamic–pituitary axis. Renal DI suggests extensive renal tubulointerstitial disease and the need for further investigation and consultation. The patient with primary polydipsia should undergo a careful psychiatric workup to search for an underlying thought disorder.

Annotated Bibliography

1. Berl T. Psychosis and water balance. N Engl J Med 1988;318:441. (*An editorial summarizing disturbances of regulation of osmolality in psychotic persons.*)
2. Bichet DG. Nephrogenic diabetes insipidus. Am J Med 1998;105:431. (*Discussion of basic science aspects of vasopressin, including genetics, cellular action, receptor function, and clinical correlations.*)
3. Boton R, Gaviria M, Batlle DC. Prevalence, pathologies, and treatment of renal dysfunction associated with chronic lithium therapy. Am J Kidney Dis 1987;10:329. (*The most prevalent effect of lithium on the kidney is impairment of concentrating ability; overt polyuria was present in 19% of cases; amiloride was helpful in treating nephrogenic diabetes insipidus.*)
4. Goldman MB, Luchins DJ, Robertson GL. Mechanisms of altered water metabolism in psychotic patients with polydipsia and hyponatremia. N Engl J Med 1988;318:397. (*Defects in regulation of osmolality and secretion of antidiuretic hormone were found.*)
5. Kim GH, Lee JW, Oh YK, et al. Antidiuretic effect of hydrochlorothiazide in lithium-induced nephrogenic diabetes insipidus is associated with upregulation of aquaporin-2 Na-Cl co-transporter and epithelial sodium channel. J Am Soc Nephrol 2004;15:2836. (*A good example of aquaporin pathophysiology.*)
6. Maghnie M, Cosi G, Genovese E, et al. Central diabetes insipidus in children and young adults. N Engl J Med 2000;343:998. (*Children and young adults with acquired central diabetes insipidus are prone to develop anterior pituitary hormonal deficiency, especially that of growth hormone.*)
7. Pivonello R, DeBellis A, Faggiano A, et al. Central diabetes insipidus and autoimmunity; relationship between the occurrence of antibodies to arginine vasopressin-secreting cells and clinical, immunological and radiological features in a large cohort of patients with central diabetes insipidus of known and unknown etiology. J Clin Endocrinol Metab 2003;88:1629. (*Evidence for an autoimmune mechanism.*)
8. Robertson GL. Diabetes insipidus. Endocrinol Metab Clin North Am 1995;24:549. (*Authoritative review.*)
9. Vokes TJ, Robertson GL. Disorders of antidiuretic hormone. Endocrinol Metab Clin North Am 1988;17:281. (*Authoritative review, with a good section on inadequate production.*)
10. Garofeanu CG, Weir M, Rosas-Arellano P, et al. Causes of reversible nephrogenic diabetes insipidus: a systemic review. Am J Kidney Dis 2005;45:626. (*A meta-analysis showing that most risk factors for reversible nephrogenic diabetes insipidus were medications; 110 references.*)
11. Robertson GL. Differential diagnosis of polyuria. Annu Rev Med 1988;39:425. (*Comprehensive discussion of causes and workup.*)
12. Halperin M, Skorecki KL. Interpretation of the urine electrolytes and osmolality in the regulation of body fluid tonicity. Am J Nephrol 1986;6:241. (*Written for the subspecialist, but there are some very useful sections for the generalist reader.*)
13. Zeerbe RL, Robertson GL. A comparison of plasma vasopressin measurements with a standard indirect test in the differential diagnosis of polyuria. N Engl J Med 1981;305:1539. (*Use of the assay improves the workup for polyuria.*)
14. Batlle DC, VonRiotte AB, Gaviria M, et al. Amelioration of polyuria by amiloride in patients receiving long-term lithium therapy. N Engl J Med 1985;312:408. (*Amiloride mitigated lithium-induced polyuria by blunting the inhibitory effect of lithium on water transport in the renal collecting tubule.*)
15. Tetiker T, Sert M, Kocak M. Efficacy of indapamide in central diabetes insipidus. Arch Intern Med 1999;159:2085. (*An example of the efficacy of a thiazide-like diuretic; there was a 40% reduction in urinary volume.*)

CHAPTER 102 ■ APPROACH TO THE PATIENT WITH DIABETES MELLITUS

DAVID M. SLOVIK

Diabetes mellitus, the most prevalent endocrinologic problem encountered in primary care practice, is characterized by hyperglycemia, a relative or absolute deficiency of insulin, insulin resistance, and a propensity for the development of long-term microvascular and macrovascular complications. If recent trends showing a dramatic increase in prevalence (believed to be a consequence of a decline in physical activity and excessive caloric intake) continue, then the condition will soon affect nearly 20 million people in the United States. It is estimated that greater than 7% of adults in the United States have diabetes mellitus. The primary physician is in the unique position to provide comprehensive care to the diabetic patient. The ultimate goals of therapy are the prevention of microvascular and macrovascular complications, consequences of diabetes that make the condition a major risk factor for cardiovascular disease, stroke, visual impairment, renal failure, impotence, peripheral neuropathy, foot ulcers, limb loss, and death.

Effective management requires care that is thoughtful and meticulous, incorporating intensive patient education involving the entire health care team. Euglycemic control, with the level of hemoglobin A_{1c} (HbA$_{1c}$) kept less than 7.0%, has emerged as a major treatment objective because of its association with a marked reduction in the risk for microvascular complications. The challenge for the primary care physician is to design a therapeutic program that is safe, practical, and acceptable to the patient. Important decisions include lifestyle adjustments (exercise, weight reduction) and determining when to initiate pharmacologic therapy, selecting among available agents, and setting an achievable goal for glycemic control. Practical tasks include creation of an effective means for diabetic surveillance and provision of education and encouragement that enable the patient to become a partner in management.

PATHOPHYSIOLOGY, CLINICAL PRESENTATION, AND COURSE (1–17)

Diagnostic Criteria

The increasing appreciation of the pathologic significance of hyperglycemia and the importance of early diagnosis has resulted in a revision of diagnostic criteria by the Expert Committee on the Diagnosis and Classification of Diabetes Mellitus. The threshold for diagnosis based on the *fasting plasma glucose level* has been revised downward from 140 mg/dL to 126 mg/dL to increase the sensitivity of this determination. The 2-hour-postprandial glucose determination conducted as part of a glucose tolerance test is more sensitive for the diagnosis of diabetes than the fasting glucose level, but it is poorly reproducible and less convenient to perform. The fasting plasma glucose level is now deemed the preferred test to diagnose diabetes in children and nonpregnant adults. Use of HbA$_{1c}$ levels for the diagnosis of diabetes is not recommended. For individuals, the diagnosis can be made based on the presence of any one of three glucose abnormalities found on two separate days:

- Fasting plasma glucose 126 mg/dL or greater.
- Random plasma glucose 200 mg/dL or greater in a person with diabetic symptoms (polyuria, polydipsia, or weight loss).
- Two-hour-postprandial plasma glucose level 200 mg/dL or greater after administration of the equivalent of a 75-g oral glucose load (oral glucose tolerance test).

In addition, the diagnostic criteria for a *normal fasting glucose* and *impaired fasting glucose* (IFG) have been updated by the American Diabetes Association. The normal fasting plasma glucose was lowered to less than 100 mg/dL and *impaired fasting glucose* was reset to 100 to 125 mg/dL. Similarly, *impaired glucose tolerance (IGT)* was redefined as a fasting glucose less than 126 mg/dL and a 2-hour PG of 140 to 199 mg/dL. IFG and IGT are "pre-diabetes" and are risk factors for the development of future diabetes and cardiovascular disease.

Classification

The preferred approach to classification, as issued by the American Diabetes Association, is according to underlying pathophysiology. Consequently, the preferred terms for diabetes classification are *type 1* and *type 2*. Older classification terms, such as *insulin-dependent* and *non–insulin-dependent diabetes*, are discouraged because exogenous insulin may be needed to treat either form of the disease. Similarly, *juvenile-onset, maturity-onset, adult-onset,* and *maturity-onset diabetes of the young* are discouraged because age of onset is not always pathophysiologically meaningful. No distinction is made between primary and secondary causes of diabetes.

Type 1 Diabetes

Type 1 diabetes is characterized by autoimmune destruction of the pancreatic beta cells leading to an absolute deficiency of insulin. Patients are *ketosis prone* and require insulin to live. Onset is typically in youth, but it may occur at any age. Patients may have detectable serum *autoantibodies* to such pancreatic antigens as islet cells and glutamic acid dehydrogenase. Peripheral *insulin resistance* is less of a factor in type 1 disease than in type 2 disease, but recent data suggest that it plays an important contributing role.

Type 2 Diabetes

Type 2 diabetes is characterized by variable degrees of insulin secretory deficiency and resistance. Insulin is present but in amounts insufficient to meet metabolic needs in a timely fashion. Because they have some insulin, these patients are *not ketosis prone* (except under severe stress, e.g., infections or surgery).

They exhibit *impaired insulin* secretion at any plasma glucose concentration and *insulin resistance* (impaired insulin action at the level of the insulin receptor). *Obesity*, which is present in 60% to 80% of patients with type 2 diabetes, is believed to play a major role in insulin resistance. Type 2 diabetes is the most common type of diabetes.

Impaired Glucose Tolerance

Patients are identified on the basis of a *fasting glucose less than 126 mg/dL* and a *2-hour glucose* level of *140 to 199 mg/dL*. The risk for the development of overt type 2 diabetes is increased (1% to 5% annually), as is the risk for cardiovascular disease. Microvascular complications do not develop in those who do not progress to frank diabetes.

Gestational Diabetes

In pregnancy, even minor degrees of glucose intolerance can be important (see later discussion). Risk assessment should occur at the first prenatal visit. Screening is suggested at 24 to 28 weeks of gestation, although earlier if there is a high degree of suspicion. A plasma or serum *glucose 140 mg/dL or greater at 1 hour* after oral administration of a 50-g glucose load is abnormal.

Other Types

Other types include *genetic defects* of beta-cell function or in insulin action, *injury* to pancreatic exocrine tissue (e.g., pancreatitis, pancreatectomy), *endocrinopathies* (e.g., Cushing's syndrome, hyperthyroidism, acromegaly), *drugs* (e.g., glucocorticoids, thiazide diuretics), *infections* (congenital rubella, cytomegalovirus), *uncommon forms of immune-mediated diabetes* (e.g., stiff-man syndrome and anti–insulin receptor antibodies), and *other genetic syndromes* associated with diabetes (e.g., Down's syndrome and the diabetes insipidus, diabetes mellitus, optic atrophy, and deafness syndrome).

Pathogenesis

The basic pathogenesis of diabetes is incompletely understood; genetic and acquired factors have been identified. As noted, the principal lesion in type 1 disease is pancreatic *beta-cell failure*, usually due to *autoimmune destruction* of the beta cells, which leads to a loss of insulin production. Type 2 disease is characterized by *impaired insulin secretion* and *insulin resistance*. *Inappropriate hepatic glucose production* and *decreased muscle glucose uptake* are the pathophysiologic hallmarks of insulin resistance; they occur despite the secretion of insulin.

Metabolic syndrome is a term used to denote the broader metabolic perturbations common in type 2 diabetes and often preceding it. Associated with caloric excess and inactivity, the syndrome's features include insulin resistance, obesity, dyslipidemia, hypertension, and a strongly increased risk for macrovascular atherosclerotic disease (coronary risk increased two- to fourfold).

Weight gain is an important contributor to type 2 disease, exacerbating insulin resistance. Glucose intolerance in diabetic patients may also be worsened by infection, stress, thiazides, glucocorticoids, and pregnancy. Excess secretion of growth hormone, cortisol, catecholamines, or glucagon may contribute to glucose intolerance, as can diseases that destroy a substantial portion of the pancreas (e.g., chronic pancreatitis, hemochromatosis, cystic fibrosis).

Clinical Presentation and Course

Type 1 disease may present emergently as ketoacidosis or less dramatically with the classic triad of polyuria, polydipsia, and polyphagia. Onset is usually in the first two decades of life but may occur later. In contrast, type 2 diabetes typically becomes evident later in life (incidence rises significantly starting in the fourth decade), often discovered as an incidental finding on screening urinalysis or blood sugar measurement. Sometimes, fatigue is the predominant symptom. In patients with more significant hyperglycemia, polyuria, polydipsia, and polyphagia with weight loss are encountered. Occasionally, the diagnosis is made during an evaluation for cardiovascular, renal, neurologic, or infectious disease. A complication such as myocardial ischemia, stroke, intermittent claudication, impotence, peripheral neuropathy, proteinuria, or retinopathy may be the initial manifestation. Erectile dysfunction is a common initial complaint in men.

The overall clinical course of untreated diabetes is one of progressive worsening of glycemic control due to the combination of pancreatic endocrine failure and peripheral insulin resistance. The rate of clinical decline in glycemic control may wax and wane, affected by the interplay of these two pathophysiologic factors. The rate of clinical failure is typically rapid and progressive in type 1 disease, following years of silent immune-mediated islet-cell destruction; however, early on, there may be a transient *"honeymoon period"* before beta-cell exhaustion sets in. In untreated type 2 disease, the overall clinical course is also progressive, but it is usually more indolent and more heavily influenced by the state of insulin resistance. Early clinical type 2 disease is characterized by impaired timing of insulin release producing postprandial hyperglycemia and the potential for episodes of hypoglycemia; total insulin production may actually rise. As the disease progresses and beta-cell reserve declines, hyperglycemia worsens. Initially, drugs that increase insulin production and release improve glucose tolerance, but with further beta-cell decline, hyperglycemia worsens and eventually becomes unresponsive to such agents. Complications set in over time at a rate and intensity related to the severity and duration of glucose intolerance.

Complications

Complications of diabetes occur with a very high frequency. Most correlate with the magnitude and duration of hyperglycemia; there does not appear to be any glycemic threshold for the development of such complications. The major complications of diabetes can be categorized as microvascular (retinopathy, neuropathy, nephropathy) or macrovascular disease causing large-vessel atherosclerosis.

Macrovascular Disease

Premature atherosclerosis may develop in large and medium vessels, leading to coronary ischemia, stroke, and peripheral arterial insufficiency. The effects of smoking, hypertension, and other risk factors for vascular disease appear to be synergistic with those of hyperglycemia. Purported mechanisms include hyperglycemic *alteration of lipid deposits* to make them more atherogenic and insulin resistance resulting in *increased blood pressure*, *reduced levels of high-density-lipoprotein* (HDL) *cholesterol*, and *increased levels of very low density–lipoprotein* (VLDL) *cholesterol,* an atherogenic phenotype termed *syndrome X.* It is suspected but remains to

be proven that tight control reduces the risk for large-vessel atherosclerosis. However, major reductions in the risk for coronary events and stroke can be achieved by correcting other major cardiovascular risk factors, such as smoking, hypertension, and hyperlipidemia. Effective treatment of such risk factors appears more important than normalization of glucose per se in the prevention and limitation of cardiovascular complications (see later discussion).

Microvascular Disease

Microvascular disease accounts for much of the morbidity of diabetes, causing nephropathy, retinopathy, and neuropathy. The risk for these microvascular complications can be markedly reduced by achieving tight glucose control (see later discussion).

Diabetic Nephropathy. Diabetic nephropathy is one of the leading causes of end-stage renal failure in adults, accounting for 25% of cases (see Chapter 142). Characteristic renal changes include glomerular basement membrane thickening and mesangial proliferation. Mesangial proliferation correlates strongly with the onset of proteinuria and hypertension. Subclinical and histologic findings for diabetic nephropathy are present long before the stage of clinical proteinuria. An elevated glomerular filtration rate (hyperfiltration), genetic determinants, and hypertension contribute to the progression of renal impairment. With persistent proteinuria, hypertension becomes established and glomerular filtration begins to decline at the rate of 1 mL/min per month.

The risk for the development of nephropathy correlates with the duration of disease and the degree of hyperglycemia. Renal failure eventually develops in 30% to 50% of type 1 diabetics and 6% to 9% of type 2 patients. Tight control of the blood glucose can reduce the risk for renal failure, particularly as primary prevention and if instituted early. It can reverse mild proteinuria in type 1 diabetics who do not yet have renal insufficiency. In the presence of significant proteinuria (greater than 500 mg/d), near-normalization of the plasma glucose may not slow the rate of renal deterioration. Bladder dysfunction and resultant urinary tract infections can also contribute to renal impairment in patients with diabetic neuropathy.

Retinopathy. The risk for retinopathic changes (see Chapter 209) is related to the duration and degree of hyperglycemia. After 20 years of diabetes, all age groups show a 75% to 80% prevalence of retinopathy. The cumulative incidence of retinopathy can be reduced by more than 50% with intensive insulin therapy. The greatest effect is in primary prevention and in those with mild to moderate nonproliferative retinopathy. Strict glycemic control is of little benefit in advanced retinopathy. Reversible changes in the lens configuration occur with wide fluctuations in plasma glucose and may cause transiently blurred vision. In addition, cataracts and glaucoma occur with increased frequency (see Chapters 207 and 208).

Neuropathy. Neuropathy may develop in approximately 50% of diabetic patients and lead to a peripheral sensory deficit, autonomic dysfunction, or a mononeuritis. Mechanisms include *myo-inositol depletion* in nerve cell membranes (which prolongs conduction time) and hyperglycemia-induced *sorbitol accumulation* in nerve tissues that have a polyol pathway for glucose metabolism (e.g., Schwann cells). *Microangiopathic changes* that decrease the blood supply to the myelin sheaths are believed to be responsible for the mononeuropathy. Independent risk factors include duration of diabetes, current level of glycosylated hemoglobin, body mass index (BMI), smoking, hypertension, and presence of cardiovascular disease.

The *peripheral neuropathy* is predominantly sensory; sensation is reduced in the lower extremities, and the condition may progress to cause pain and dysesthesias. *Autonomic neuropathy* most commonly presents as impotence. Gastrointestinal motility disturbances (delayed gastric emptying), orthostatic hypotension, and urinary retention are other potential manifestations. Autonomic neuropathy is almost always seen in association with distal polyneuropathy. Its presence is an important predictor of foot and other infections.

Diabetic *mononeuropathy* involves discrete cranial or peripheral nerves, singly or as a *mononeuritis multiplex*. Cranial nerves III and VI are most commonly affected. In contrast to other diabetic neuropathies, mononeuropathies resolve almost completely within 1 year of onset.

Increased Susceptibility to Infection

Increased susceptibility to infection in diabetics appears to result from impaired leukocyte function, compromised vascular supply, and neuropathy. Cellulitis and candidiasis occur, with infections of ischemic foot lesions especially serious because they may lead to osteomyelitis and may require amputation. Overall, the occurrence of perioperative infections correlates with end-organ involvement by diabetes and marked degrees of hyperglycemia. Recent studies show a sixfold increase in all perioperative complications (stroke, infection, and renal insufficiency) in patients with end-organ disease. Urinary tract infections are common in patients with an autonomic bladder (see Chapter 134). Risk of infection is reduced by improved glycemic control; daily multivitamin supplementation might also be helpful.

WORKUP

See Chapter 93.

PRINCIPLES OF MANAGEMENT (16,18–76)

Screening

Screening to detect pre-diabetes (IFG or IGT) and diabetes should be considered in individuals 45 years of age and older, especially if their BMI is 25 kg/m^{2}or greater (see Chapter 93). Screening of individuals less than age 45 years should be considered if they are overweight and have other risk factors for diabetes. Testing should be repeated at 3-year intervals.

Prevention

Prevention of type 2 disease is an achievable and important consequence of improved screening for diabetes. The importance of *diet, exercise,* and *weight* in the genesis, prevention, and treatment of type 2 disease was highlighted by the landmark Diabetes Prevention Program trial. High-risk obese persons (mean BMI 34) with fasting and postprandial glucose levels approaching those of frank diabetes mellitus achieved a marked improvement in glycemic control and prevention or at least delay in onset of frank type 2 disease when they implemented lifestyle modifications. A supervised program of modest weight reduction (sustained 7% weight loss), regular aerobic exercise (2.5 hours/wk of moderately brisk walking), and a low-fat, low-calorie diet can prevent onset when fully implemented and maintained. *Metformin* also proved effective, but less so than lifestyle modification, underscoring the importance of diet, exercise, and weight in the genesis, prevention, and treatment of type 2 disease.

Treatment Goals and Strategy

Treatment Goals

The principal goal of diabetes therapy is *normalization of blood glucose* to prevent the multisystem complications that may result from hyperglycemia. The landmark Diabetes Control and Complication Trial (DCCT) and the U.K. Prospective Diabetes Study (UKPDS) convincingly demonstrated that maintaining blood glucose concentrations close to the normal range (e.g., HbA$_{1c}$ <7.0%) delays the onset and limits the progression of the long-term microvascular complications of diabetes—retinopathy, nephropathy, and neuropathy. In addition, a strong trend was noted in the UKPDS toward a reduction in coronary events.

Based on these data, the American Diabetes Association recommends a *treatment goal* of *HbA$_{1c}$ less than 7.0%* and as close to normal as possible without significant hypoglycemia. Because HbA$_{1c}$ reflects mean glycemia over the preceding 2 to 3 months, it should be measured two times a year or more frequently in patients whose therapy has changed or who are not meeting glycemic goals. Although tight glucose control can markedly decrease the morbidity associated with small-vessel disease, it remains to be proven whether it can reduce the serious large-vessel consequences of diabetes (which cause death in the majority of patients with type 2 disease). Nonetheless, normalization of carbohydrate metabolism stands as a major treatment objective for all diabetics. The challenge is how to accomplish normalization and reduce risk, given the imperfect treatment modalities and monitoring methods available. Strong patient motivation and close support are essential. Advances in treatment promise to facilitate achievement of control.

Normalization of blood sugars to nondiabetic postprandial and fasting levels is an ideal objective that is not without risk. The risk for hypoglycemia with intensive insulin therapy is a serious concern; it can be especially dangerous in patients who have underlying coronary or cerebrovascular disease. However, the goal of safe and convenient glucose normalization is becoming easier to achieve. Until implantable glucose sensors and insulin delivery systems automate the control process, the maintenance of normoglycemia will still require attention to the details of diet, exercise, weight control, and the many facets of medical therapy to achieve the best possible outcome.

Overall Treatment Strategy

The approach is pathophysiologically based, with a focus on the importance of establishing euglycemia as quickly as possible because diabetic complications are mostly a function of the degree and duration of hyperglycemia. Because the fasting glucose level is the most important determinant of daily glycemia, efforts to normalize it are given top priority. A reduction in postprandial glucose is also important, but the postprandial glucose level is a lesser determinant of overall control.

In type 1 disease, the emphasis is on intensive *insulin* therapy to make up for the loss of insulin production. *Diet* and *exercise* also play key roles because there is an increasing appreciation for the contribution of insulin resistance to poor glycemic control in type 1 disease.

In type 2 disease, insulin resistance is treated with *diet, weight reduction, exercise,* and, if necessary, *drug therapy* that improves insulin responsiveness. Impaired insulin secretion is countered by pharmacologic measures that increase endogenous insulin secretion or provide it exogenously. Combination programs are often necessary to attain the treatment goals, especially as the disease advances. Lifestyle modification (diet and exercise) remains the cornerstone of management. Traditionally, it has been initiated before starting drug therapy in type 2 cases, but recent expert consensus calls for more aggressive early intervention in hyperglycemic type 2 patients. Recommendations include treating with metformin in combination with lifestyle modification as the initial approach, followed by the early addition of other oral drugs or insulin if glycemic control is not readily achieved. Early drug therapy is also indicated if it is unlikely that the patient can lose weight or if the patient is pregnant.

Insulin remains the agent of first choice in persons with severe hyperglycemia (fasting glucose >240 mg/dL), whether from type 1 or type 2 disease. Other agents—the sulfonylureas, biguanides (e.g., metformin), thiazolidinediones (e.g., the glitazones), α-glucosidase inhibitors (e.g., acarbose), meglitinides (e.g. repaglinide, nateglinide), amylin analogues (pramlintide), glucagon-like peptide-1 (GLP-1) analogues (exenatide), and dipeptidyl peptidase-4 inhibitors (sitagliptin)—are effective in type 2 disease with moderate hyperglycemia (fasting glucose between 140 and 240 mg/dL). Compared to the newer and more expensive agents, metformin and the second-generation sulfonylureas demonstrate equivalent or superior efficacy at lower cost in control of hyperglycemia, lipids, and other intermediate treatment endpoints.

Coordination of care is essential because successful diabetes care requires a multifaceted collaborative approach involving the complementary inputs of many health care professionals (e.g., primary physician, nurse, dietician, podiatrist, ophthalmologist, endocrinologist). The ability to deliver and coordinate this care (whether orchestrated by a well-organized primary care practice, a diabetes specialty practice, or a commercial managed care program) demonstrably improves outcomes. Enhanced communication between patients and health care professionals reduces the need for avoidable hospitalizations and improves glycemic control.

Lifestyle Modification—Diet and Exercise

The cornerstone of therapy for all overweight patients with type 2 diabetes is weight reduction through calorie restriction and exercise. Achieving ideal body weight is the most important goal for the physician to encourage and advance to achieve metabolic control. However, even modest weight loss can improve hyperglycemia. A substantial reduction in blood glucose can be seen even within several days of instituting a low-calorie diet.

Weight loss has been shown to enhance the sensitivity of peripheral insulin receptors to endogenous insulin and reduce the requirements for administered insulin. Hepatic glycogen stores are depleted rapidly with caloric restriction. It is not possible to predict the exact improvement in glucose control from each pound lost, but a reduction of body weight may lead to an improvement in glucose tolerance. The glycemic response to weight loss is related to the initial fasting blood glucose. Patients who start off with lower fasting blood glucose levels will tend to normalize their blood glucose with less weight loss than those who start off with higher values.

The hyperglycemia of most type 2 diabetics can be controlled by achieving an ideal body weight; however, such weight reduction is often difficult to maintain because a permanent restriction in caloric intake is required. Rigidly developed and prescribed diets should be avoided in favor of diets adapted to the patient's lifestyle. The goal is gradual, sustained weight reduction of approximately 1 to 2 lb each week (see Chapter 233). Consultation with a registered dietitian may be very helpful.

An effective *exercise program* (see Chapter 18) is another cornerstone of treatment. Exercise enhances weight loss by increasing caloric consumption, which is important in obese persons, who may require fewer calories to maintain their body weight. In addition, aerobic exercise facilitates glycemic control independent of its effect on weight, reducing insulin resistance in liver and muscle in patients with type 2 disease.

Diet Composition. Diet composition for type 2 diabetics is controversial and less critical than achieving an ideal body weight. The American Diabetes Association recommends diets *low in calories, low in fat,* and *liberal in complex carbohydrates,* with as much as 60% of total calories allowed from carbohydrates. Simple carbohydrates are discouraged due to their adverse effects on glycemic control. Eating of potatoes causes greater increases in blood glucose than does eating beans or wheat, yet even inclusion of sucrose or ice cream in mixed meals does not necessarily adversely affect glucose control. Nonetheless, there is a trend toward tightening carbohydrate allowances in type 2 diabetics due to studies showing worsening glycemic control and increases in VLDL triglyceride and total cholesterol when carbohydrate intake is high. Type 2 patients may benefit from a diet that is lower in total carbohydrates and higher in unsaturated fat and fiber. Hypertriglyceridemia secondary to the increase in carbohydrates has not been a problem, and in several studies, triglycerides and cholesterol levels have fallen substantially.

Increasing *fiber* content, which occurs with a higher intake of complex carbohydrates and a decreased intake of refined carbohydrates and animal fats, is associated with a low prevalence of diabetes mellitus. Increased intake of unprocessed foods (e.g., cereals, grains, fruits, and vegetables) improves glucose tolerance in type 2 diabetics and decreases insulin requirements in type 1 diabetics. Improved glycemic control through delayed absorption is suspected. *Vitamin supplements*, particularly those with purported antioxidant action (see Chapter 31), have not demonstrated benefit in randomized, controlled trials; however, simple multivitamin supplementation does appear to reduce the risk of infection.

Low-carbohydrate diets (see also Chapter 233) have become popular among obese persons. When studied in a research setting in obese persons with type 2 disease, a diet limiting carbohydrate to 21 g/d for 2 weeks achieves weight loss and improvements in glycemic control, triglycerides, and total cholesterol. Whether such short-term benefits are sustainable and any better than those associated with conventional dietary approaches to weight loss and diabetes management remain to be determined.

Special Dietary Considerations for Patients on Insulin. For *type 1 insulin-requiring diabetics* who are at ideal body weight, the essential aspect of dietary therapy is the *regularity of caloric intake* and the spacing of meals. Three meals, supplemented by snacks midmorning, midafternoon, and before bed, are needed to provide a source of glucose during the sustained presence of exogenously administered insulin. The commonly used American Diabetic Association diets recommend 2/9 of calories at breakfast, 2/9 at lunch, 4/9 at dinner, and 1/9 as snacks. The timing of meals must match peak insulin effects and activity schedules; increased activity requires increased food intake or a decrease in insulin dose to prevent hypoglycemia. Simple sugars are generally restricted because they worsen postprandial hyperglycemia; however, patients should carry a source of simple sugar, such as fruit juice or sugar candy, to limit an insulin reaction. Patients who are not taking insulin do not require elaborate exchange systems, careful timing of meals, or other special dietary accommodations.

Exercise. Exercise has important effects on glucose control in diabetes. It increases glucose consumption and reduces insulin resistance. As noted, its benefits extend beyond those attributable to weight loss alone. All forms of *aerobic* exercise, even walking and other forms of nonvigorous activity, improve insulin sensitivity. Significant improvement in glycemic control has been demonstrated from a program of moderate aerobic exercise performed three times per week for 30 to 60 minutes.

A few *precautions* are worth noting in those who may engage in more vigorous activity. The increased absorption of insulin in an exercising limb may precipitate hypoglycemia in patients on insulin; therefore, the abdomen should be used as the site for insulin injection. Because of the possibility of underlying ischemic heart disease, an exercise electrocardiogram should be considered before a rigorous exercise program is undertaken by a sedentary person with longstanding diabetes or other atherosclerotic risk factors (see Chapters 18 and 36).

Drug Therapy: Oral Agents

Biguanides (e.g., Metformin)

Metformin is becoming a cornerstone of drug treatment for type 2 disease because of its proven efficacy not only in controlling glucose intolerance, but also in improving important macro- and microvascular outcomes. It differs from the traditional oral hypoglycemics (i.e., the sulfonylureas) in that it does not stimulate endogenous insulin secretion; rather, drugs of this class enhance tissue responsiveness to insulin. Consequently, biguanides are less likely to induce hypoglycemia and are effective in the treatment of patients with tissue resistance to insulin, such as obese persons.

Mechanism of Action. These drugs facilitate insulin uptake by peripheral tissue, especially muscle and liver, and decrease hepatic gluconeogenesis and basal glucose output, thereby helping to lower fasting glucose levels. Glucose utilization also improves in adipose and intestinal tissues. The net result is an improvement in fasting and postprandial hyperglycemia. Insulin demand declines as glucose utilization improves. Serum lipid abnormalities also improve.

Preparations. *Metformin* is the only biguanide approved in the United States for the treatment of type 2 diabetes. The drug is rapidly and well absorbed in the small intestine, with peak plasma concentrations in 2 hours. It is rapidly excreted unchanged by the kidneys. Impaired renal function (creatinine >1.5 mg/dL in men and >1.4 mg/dL in women) is a contraindication for use. The drug is not metabolized by the liver. Its cost is about two to three times that of the oral hypoglycemics. The original biguanide, phenformin, is no longer marketed because of its associated risk for lactic acidosis and an excess cardiovascular mortality (see later discussion).

Dosing. The starting dose of metformin is 500 mg once daily with dinner. After 1 week, the dose is increased to twice daily, given with the two largest meals of the day (usually breakfast and dinner) to minimize gastrointestinal upset. The dose can be increased by 500 mg every 1 to 2 weeks until treatment goals are met (the usual effective dose is 850 mg twice daily) or the maximum dose of 2,000 to 2,500 mg/d is reached. An extended-release formulation is also available, which can help to improve compliance, although at increased cost. Use of generic metformin helps to minimize expense.

Efficacy. The efficacy of metformin is about the same as that of a second-generation sulfonylurea when used as monotherapy in an obese person with moderate glucose intolerance; it lowers fasting glucose and glycosylated hemoglobin levels to the same degree. At 5 years, incidence of monotherapy failure is less for metformin than for glyburide (21% vs. 34%). Metformin has a synergistic effect when combined with sulfonylurea therapy in patients who do not respond well to monotherapy. Unlike the sulfonylureas, metformin is effective even in severe fasting hyperglycemia (>300 mg/dL), indicative of poor beta-cell responsiveness. In the landmark UKPDS trial, obese diabetics who attained tight control with metformin treatment exhibited a reduction in *microvascular disease*, and they were also the only group to show a reduced risk for *macrovascular* complications (i.e., myocardial infarction, stroke, and cardiovascular death). Plasma triglycerides and low-density-lipoprotein (LDL) cholesterol levels were decreased.

Adverse Effects. The most common side effect of biguanide therapy is dose-related *gastrointestinal upset* (*nausea, diarrhea, bloating, abdominal discomfort*). The risk for serious prolonged *hypoglycemia* is minimal. *Lactic acidosis* represents the most potentially serious adverse effect. One of the original biguanides—phenformin—was taken off the market by the U.S. Food and Drug Administration (FDA) in 1977 because of its association with fatal episodes of lactic acidosis. The risk for lactic acidosis associated with metformin is greatest in the setting of hypoxemia, hypovolemia, and states with decreased tissue perfusion and in renal insufficiency (creatinine >1.5 mg/dL). Accumulation of the drug secondary to reduced excretion results in impaired hepatic metabolism of lactate. Other risk factors include binge drinking, use of intravenous radiologic contrast agents, hepatic failure (lactate is metabolized by the liver), and serious underlying illness, particularly heart failure. Long-term data on safety have yet to be accumulated. Because insulin secretion is not increased with metformin use, weight gain does not occur; some patients may even lose weight. Patients who are to undergo a radiologic procedure that requires intravenous iodinated contrast should have their metformin therapy held for a few days prior to the procedure and remain well hydrated.

Patient Selection. Obese patients are particularly good candidates for metformin therapy because the drug helps to reverse their insulin resistance. Peripheral responsiveness to insulin improves and insulin needs decrease, so hyperinsulinism and its adverse effects, including weight gain, are minimized. The typical candidate is a *moderately obese person with type 2 diabetes* who has persistent moderate hyperglycemia (fasting glucose between 140 and 240 mg/dL, glycosylated hemoglobin >7.0%) despite a full program of diet and exercise. Early addition of metformin is suggested. Other candidates for metformin include obese patients who do not achieve tight control while taking a sulfonylurea at maximal doses. In this setting, metformin is *added to the oral hypoglycemic program* to improve control through its complementary mode of action. The sulfonylurea dose is reduced to lessen the risk for hypoglycemia. Combination therapy is most effective when initiated before the onset of symptomatic hyperglycemia (fasting glucose >250 mg/dL). Nonobese patients are also reasonable candidates for metformin. Typically, metformin lowers fasting blood glucose by approximately 20%.

Patients who started drug therapy with a sulfonylurea and become unresponsive to maximal doses have likely exhausted their beta-cell reserve and can be *switched to metformin* or considered for exogenous insulin therapy (sometimes in conjunction with metformin). The same pertains to the severely hyperglycemic obese patient (fasting glucose >300 mg/dL). Some diabetologists use metformin to *supplement an insulin* program in obese type 2 diabetics who require large insulin doses and have difficulty losing weight. The combined program helps to reduce insulin requirements and the appetite stimulation and weight gain that accompany hyperinsulinism. Caution and careful patient monitoring are required when a patient taking exogenous insulin is started on metformin; the insulin requirement may drop considerably, putting the patient at risk for hypoglycemia.

Sulfonylureas

The sulfonylureas have been around for almost 50 years. With the advent of potent, long-acting, second-generation preparations and increasing evidence of their efficacy and safety, the sulfonylureas have become a mainstay of treatment for *mild to moderately severe type 2 disease (fasting glucose between 140 and 240 mg/dL)*. From 80% to 90% of newly treated type 2 diabetics respond to therapy. An absolute average reduction in HbA$_{1c}$ of 1.5 to 2.0 percentage points, along with a reduction in fasting glucose of 60 to 70 mg/dL, is achieved in most cases. However, the secondary failure rate is high, and with time, despite continued therapy, glucose control worsens and a second oral agent or insulin is required.

Mechanism of Action. The sulfonylureas acutely increase the sensitivity of beta cells to glucose and stimulate endogenous insulin release, probably by binding to a specific beta-cell receptor. This action can lead to hypoglycemia—hence the term *oral hypoglycemic agents*. These agents are effective in persons who require additional insulin secretion and have an adequate beta-cell reserve; they are ineffective in patients with type 1 diabetes. Enhancement of basal insulin secretion inhibits basal hepatic glucose production and improves the fasting glucose level. Efficacy declines with time as beta-cell function deteriorates; glycemic control worsens despite the use of maximum doses. Although these agents also increase insulin receptor binding and enhance tissue sensitivity to insulin, such effects are minor compared with the stimulation of insulin release and are insufficient to sustain glycemic control when insulin release declines.

Preparations. The *first-generation sulfonylureas* (e.g., *chlorpropamide, tolbutamide, tolazamide*) have given way to *second-generation agents*, such as *glyburide* (Micronase, DiaBeta), *glipizide* (Glucotrol), and *glimepiride* (Amaryl), in the treatment of type 2 diabetes. *Second-generation drugs* are more potent and longer acting. All are of equal efficacy. Although they cost 5 to 10 times more than first-generation drugs, they remain the least costly of the oral agents; all are similarly priced. These drugs are nonionically bound to plasma proteins and are less variable in their bioavailability than the earlier oral agents. They are metabolized by the liver and consequently should be used with caution in reduced doses in patients with liver disease. Glipizide releases insulin slightly more rapidly than the others, but this feature provides no special long-term advantage. In contrast to chlorpropamide, the second-generation agents do not cause inappropriate secretion of antidiuretic hormone, and only rarely cause disulfiram (Antabuse)-like effects. Like those of their predecessors, the effects of these agents may be potentiated by sulfonamides, salicylates, and clofibrate or inhibited by warfarin.

Dosing Schedules. Dosing schedules for these agents are convenient because the duration of action is 12 to 24 hours. A sustained-release glipizide preparation allows for once-daily dosing, which is a marginal convenience benefit but a means of reducing the cost of therapy if used in place of a twice-daily program. The duration of action of glimepiride is slightly longer than that of other preparations (16 to 24 hours), so once-a-day dosing is also possible. A lower-dose formulation is available for glimepiride than for sustained-release glipizide, which facilitates its use in the elderly and those with mild hyperglycemia. The starting doses of the second-generation agents are 2.5 mg for glyburide, 5.0 mg for glipizide, and 1 mg for glimepiride, taken once daily in the morning. Treatment is started at low doses and increased every 1 to 2 weeks, with monitoring of fasting and postprandial sugars. Failure to demonstrate any reduction in glucose early on suggests that oral-agent therapy will probably fail, even at increased doses. The maximum daily dose is 15 to 20 mg/d for glipizide and glyburide, usually given on a twice-daily schedule for optimal effectiveness. For glimepiride, the maximum dose is 8 mg given once daily. Monitoring of blood sugars and HbA$_{1c}$ is required (see later discussion).

Efficacy. In about 25% of patients, treatment goals are achieved with sulfonylurea therapy alone. In another 50% to 60% of patients, the initial response is good, but an additional agent is required over time to achieve treatment goals. The 15% who fail to exhibit a primary response probably have more-advanced disease or slowly progressive type 1 diabetes. Predictors of a good response include newly diagnosed diabetes, mild to moderate disease, good beta-cell function (high levels of C-peptide), and no history of prior insulin therapy or presence of islet cell antibodies. In the UKPDS, when the goals of intensive therapy were reached, reductions in long-term microvascular complications could be demonstrated, although no decreases in the risk for macrovascular disease were noted. In head-to-head randomized comparison of monotherapy with metformin or rosiglitazone, glyburide had a higher rate of treatment failure than the other two drugs.

Second-generation sulfonylureas can achieve results comparable with those of single-dose neutral protein Hagedorn (NPH) insulin in lowering HbA$_{1c}$. However, as beta-cell function declines with time, pharmacologic coaxing of further insulin output is less likely to succeed. In the UKPDS, only 24% of patients on sulfonylurea monotherapy had adequate control 9 years after diagnosis. Addition of a second agent is usually necessary, either one that reduces peripheral resistance to endogenous insulin (e.g., metformin) or one that provides exogenous hormone (see later discussion).

Adverse Effects. The principal risk of sulfonylurea use is *hypoglycemia* (a result of increased insulin release). Hypoglycemia (which tends to be prolonged) occurs at a frequency of 4% with the use of glyburide and 2% to 4% with glipizide. Occasionally, patients whose diabetes has become refractory to a first-generation sulfonylurea may benefit from substitution with a second-generation agent. Doses in excess of 15 to 20 mg/d provide little additional control. The risk for hypoglycemia is greatest with potent, long-acting sulfonylureas, which can cause sustained, severe hypoglycemia. Under study conditions, about 5% of patients experience hypoglycemia with sulfonylurea use. Outside study settings, the risk is likely to be higher.

Concern about an increase in *cardiovascular risk* was suggested by data from the University Group Diabetes Project (UGDP), which revealed a small but significant increase in the rate of cardiovascular death in patients on long-term tolbutamide therapy. Questions about the UGDP study design and the veracity of the finding triggered an extensive controversy. Oral-agent use declined for several years because of concern about this observation, and a new generation of sulfonylureas was developed. The controversy appears to have been put to rest by new long-term data from the UKPDS, which found, after 10 years of follow-up, no increase in the incidence of coronary events associated with the prolonged use of oral agents.

The effect on cardiovascular risk factors is important to note. *Weight gain* is an important consequence of the enhanced insulin secretion stimulated by oral-agent therapy. Weight gain may be on the order of 5 to 10 lb with most agents, although there is some suggestion that it may be less with long-acting glipizide. *Triglycerides* decrease modestly, but overall effects on *lipids* are minimal.

In head-to-head comparison with metformin and rosiglitazone, glyburide demonstrated a lower risk of cardiovascular events and heart failure compared to rosiglitazone but a greater risk of hypoglycemia than with the other two agents.

Patient Selection. These agents are commonly prescribed as initial pharmacologic therapy for patients who remain moderately hyperglycemic (fasting glucose between 140 and 240 mg/dL) despite dietary and exercise measures. The insulin requirements of such patients may be increased, especially if they are obese, and they initially benefit from the increased release of endogenous insulin. The best results are achieved in patients who are not obese. The sulfonylurea drugs are a first choice for oral-agent therapy and the least costly. Their convenience of use in comparison with insulin and their minimal side effects make them a popular choice for patients with type 2 diabetes. In the very elderly, they should be prescribed with care because of the increased vulnerability of these patients to the adverse consequences of hypoglycemia.

Thiazolidinediones

In the United States, two thiazolidinediones, *pioglitazone* (Actos) and *rosiglitazone* (Avandia), are approved for treatment of type 2 diabetes. These agents appear to work predominantly by decreasing insulin resistance in peripheral tissues, including fat, muscle, and liver, thus increasing glucose utilization and decreasing glucose production. They have become very popular because they are generally well tolerated, do not cause hypoglycemia, and can enhance glycemic control when used in conjunction with other oral agents or insulin. The major past concern surrounding their use has been idiosyncratic hepatocellular injury (see later discussion) and, more recently, cardiovascular toxicity.

Mechanism of Action. The main sites of action are muscle, fat, and liver, with improved sensitivity to insulin. These agents differ from metformin and the sulfonylureas in decreasing hepatic fat content and increasing insulin sensitivity in muscle. Compared with metformin, there is less of an effect on hepatic responsiveness, which might account for the reduced efficacy.

Adipocytes proliferate, possibly accounting for the observed increase in weight.

Efficacy. Although these drugs can be used as monotherapy for type 2 diabetes, they are not as effective as metformin and second-generation sulfonylureas in lowering HbA$_{1c}$ (usually <1%). However, because these drugs are relatively well tolerated by most patients, they demonstrate superior cumulative performance in head-to-head comparison with metformin and glyburide in incidence of monotherapy failure at 5 years. Nonetheless, concerns over their adverse effects (see later discussion) have relegated them to a second-line role, complementing other hypoglycemic therapies. Onset of action may be evident by 7 days, manifested by a drop in fasting blood sugar, but the full effect may take 4 to 6 weeks. About 25% of patients manifest no benefit; most have a low fasting C-peptide level.

Adverse Effects. The initial drug in this class, troglitazone (Rezulin), had to be removed from the market because of idiopathic reactions causing *hepatocellular injury* severe enough to result in death or need for liver transplantation. Subsequent thiazolidinediones have not demonstrated this degree of hepatocellular risk, but long-term data are incomplete. Careful, regular monitoring of hepatocellular enzymes is recommended. Any increase in alanine aminotransferase (ALT) level beyond 1.5 to 2.0 times the upper limit of normal is an indication for weekly ALT monitoring and consideration of ceasing therapy. *Weight gain* occurs, especially when used in combination with sulfonylureas.

A significant increase in the risk of *myocardial infarction* and a borderline significant increase in the risk of *cardiovascular death* have emerged from meta-analytic data on rosiglitazone use. Pioglitazone data suggest less risk of myocardial infarction, but both agents can cause *fluid retention, edema,* and *congestive heart failure.*

Preparations, Dosing, and Patient Selection. *Pioglitazone* is begun at 15 mg/d and *rosiglitazone* at 2 mg/d. Treatment is advanced on a monthly basis until maximum doses are reached (45 mg/d for pioglitazone and 8 mg/d for rosiglitazone).

These agents have been used as *monotherapy* and in *combination* with insulin, the sulfonylureas, or metformin to reduce insulin resistance and improve glycemic control. Until hepatocellular and cardiovascular risk are more firmly established, it is recommended that marked caution be used in their application and that they be reserved for second- or third-line use in patients who have not achieved glycemic control by other means. Only patients without underlying liver disease who are willing to have their liver function monitored regularly should be considered candidates. Risks and benefits of use in persons with high cardiovascular risk or heart failure should be weighed very carefully, with preference given to alternative drug choices pending better definition of cardiac risk.

α-Glucosidase Inhibitors

Acarbose (Precose) is a poorly absorbed complex oligosaccharide of bacterial origin with the ability to inhibit α-glucosidase. When taken at the beginning of a meal, it interferes with the pancreatic enzymatic hydrolysis of dietary carbohydrates (particularly disaccharide and complex carbohydrates), thereby inhibiting conversion to monosaccharides and slowing absorption of glucose. Less than 1% of the drug is absorbed.

Efficacy and Patient Selection. Significant additional reductions in levels of postprandial glucose and glycosylated hemoglobin have been noted when acarbose is used in conjunction with diet, oral agents, or insulin. Its efficacy is about midway between that of diet alone and that of oral agents. Few data are available regarding its use in type 1 disease. Although acarbose can improve glycemic control in persons with type 2 disease and complement other forms of therapy, its gastrointestinal side effects (see later discussion) limit its clinical acceptability for long-term use. Nonetheless, it represents an additional treatment option that can be useful in selected cases.

Adverse Effects. The principal side effects are gastrointestinal (*abdominal cramping*, *distention*, *flatulence*, and *diarrhea*) and are caused by the fermentation of unabsorbed carbohydrate by colonic bacteria. The effect is dose related and seems to decrease with time. Occasional *impairment of iron absorption* may lead to microcytic anemia. Use with oral hypoglycemics or insulin may increase the risk for *hypoglycemia*, which must be treated with glucose because the drug interferes with the absorption of sucrose and other sugars. Concurrent use with metformin is problematic because acarbose potentiates the bioavailability of metformin and exacerbates its gastrointestinal side effects. The drug does not cause significant weight loss.

Dosing. The starting dose is 25 mg three times daily, taken at the beginning of meals. The maximum is 50 to 100 mg three times daily, depending on weight. The cost is about two to three times that of the oral hypoglycemics and similar to that of metformin.

Meglitinides

Members of this new class of hypoglycemic agents act like a rapid sulfonylurea by *increasing beta-cell secretion of insulin.* Onset of action is rapid and duration short; consequently, they are taken just before a meal. The two meglitinides available are *repaglinide* (Prandin) and *nateglinide* (Starlix). The starting dose for repaglinide is 0.5 mg three times daily and for nateglinide is 120 mg three times daily; doses are taken 15 minutes before meals. *Hypoglycemia* can occur but tends to be slightly less frequent and severe than in sulfonylurea therapy and is uncommon in general. *Weight gain* is noted; effects on lipids are minimal. The cost is two- to sixfold more than that of brand-name sulfonylureas and nearly an order of magnitude greater than that of generic formulations of these agents. Clearance is rapid and unaffected by renal function, making them useful in the setting of renal insufficiency.

Drug Therapy: Injectable Peptides

Amylin Analogues

Pramlintide (Symlin) is a synthetic analogue of *amylin*, a pancreatic neuroendocrine hormone contributing to glucose control during the postprandial period by decreasing gastrointestinal motility and *blunting the absorption of carbohydrates*. Best candidates are *insulin-treated patients* with type 1 and type 2 diabetes, who take the drug at mealtimes by subcutaneous injection. Modest falls in HbA_{1c} are produced. A particularly desirable effect is *weight loss*, which helps to counter the weight gain associated with insulin therapy. Severe *hypoglycemia* may develop when it is used in combination with insulin. It should not be given to patients with hypoglycemia unawareness.

Glucagon-Like Peptide-1 Analogues

Exenatide (Byetta) is a 39–amino acid mimetic of incretin, a GLP-1 analogue. The incretins are part of an endogenous system involved in regulating glucose homeostasis. They *stimulate insulin secretion*, *suppress glucagons*, and *delay gastric emptying*. Exenatide is used as adjunctive therapy to improve glycemic control in patients with type 2 diabetes who are taking metformin, a sulfonylurea, or a combination of both. Side effects are primarily gastrointestinal (nausea is most common). It is administered as a subcutaneous injection twice daily before the morning and evening meals. Its place in the treatment of type 2 disease remains to be fully established. Cost is high, and degree of glucose lowering is modest. An advantage associated with its use is a small degree of *weight loss*. In a large randomized trial comparing exenatide to insulin glargine in patients with suboptimally controlled type 2 diabetes, improvements in glycemic control were similar, but persons taking exenatide also achieved weight loss; however, the incidence of adverse gastrointestinal side effects was also greater. Exenatide is not approved for use with insulin.

Dipeptidyl Peptidase-4 Inhibitors

Sitagliptin (Januvia) and *vildagliptin (Glavus)* inhibit the inactivation of incretin hormones such as GLP-1, thus prolonging their action. These agents are used as an adjunct to diet and exercise to improve glycemic control in type 2 diabetes. They may be prescribed as monotherapy, but the degree of glycemic lowering is modest and less than that for metformin, with which they may be used in conjunction. Unlike exenatide, they cause a persistent elevation in GLP-1 levels rather than a prandial elevation. The recommended dose of sitagliptin is 100 mg once daily. Adjustment in the dose is necessary in moderate to severe renal insufficiency. Their precise role in type 2 disease management remains to be determined; cost is high.

Drug Therapy: Insulin

Insulin is the drug therapy of choice for type 1 diabetes, for patients with symptomatic type 2 diabetes whose disease cannot be controlled by diet alone with or without a program of oral-agent therapy, and for diabetics in whom near-normalization of blood sugar is a goal of therapy.

Preparations

Insulin therapy should be initiated with a *human recombinant insulin* preparation. All standard insulin preparations are available as human recombinant formulations. Human insulin has largely replaced *highly purified animal insulins*, being comparable in cost yet less likely to produce local reactions, insulin allergy, immune resistance, or lipoatrophy. In some patients, human insulin may be absorbed more rapidly than animal insulins and have a shorter duration of action. Newly developed insulin analogues, although more costly, provide improved performance characteristics that can be important in selected patients. Insulin is available in rapid-, short-, intermediate-, and long-acting preparations, as well as in mixtures of the preparations. An inhaled preparation is available.

Short- and Rapid-Acting Insulins. These preparations are intended for *prandial glycemic control*. The standard short-acting preparation is *regular insulin,* which has an onset of 30 to 45 minutes, a peak at 2 to 4 hours, and a duration of 5 to 8 hours. In comparison, the rapid-acting *insulin analogues* (*insulin lispro*, *insulin aspart*, and *insulin glulisine*) have an on-set of only 5 to 15 minutes, a peak at 45 to75 minutes, and a duration of 2 to 4 hours. Because they need not be taken until just before a meal, the rapid-acting preparations allow for a better match between insulin administration and food intake, helping to improve compliance and reducing the risk of hypo-glycemic reactions. Their very short duration of action means that they make little contribution to daily basal insulin require-ments, necessitating combined use with a longer-acting insulin preparation.

Candidates for short- or rapid-acting insulin include persons taking intensive insulin therapy who require tight control but are at high risk for hypoglycemia from high doses of long-acting preparations. Other potential users include those with a recent onset of type 1 disease who retain some basal insulin secretion. The availability of some rapid-acting preparations as an injection pen enhances convenience and compliance, albeit at some increase in cost.

Intermediate-Acting Insulin. *NPH* has an onset of action of 2 hours, a peak at 6 to 10 hours, and a duration of 8 to 24 hours, making it useful for *basal glycemic control*. In type 2 patients, a starting insulin regimen might be a single injection of NPH before bed to raise basal insulin levels and improve fasting glycemic control. Split daily doses are also used as the disease progresses; cost is low, and mixtures can be made with other insulins, allowing a single injection each time.

Long-Acting Insulin Analogues. *Insulin glargine (Lantus)* and *insulin detemir (Levemir)* have a steady absorption pattern over 24 hours, producing less risk of nocturnal hypoglycemia than intermediate-acting insulin. For *insulin glargine*, onset of action is about 2 hours, there is no peak, but serum levels plateau at 4 to 6 hours and last 20 to 24 hours. *Insulin detemir* has a similar onset, no peak, and a duration of 6 to 20 hours; it can be administered once or twice daily.

Long-acting insulins provide a useful source of basal in-sulin in type 1 patients undertaking intensive insulin therapy who are bothered by nocturnal hypoglycemia (see later discus-sion). They are similarly effective in type 2 disease. A typical in-tensive insulin program with this long-acting insulin analogue involves its administration at bedtime, supplemented by rapid-acting insulin taken before meals (see later discussion). One disadvantage is adsorption to other insulins when mixed in the same syringe (necessitating the use of a separate syringe and an extra injection).

Mixtures of Intermediate and Short- or Rapid-Acting Insulins. *Fixed-mixture preparations* of NPH and a rapid-acting or short-acting insulin are available commercially (e.g., 70/30 intermediate/short acting and 75/25 intermediate/rapid act-ing). Although they provide increased convenience for patients who require only twice-daily insulin administration and pre-sumably facilitate compliance by reducing the number of in-jections, these preparations do not afford flexibility of dose adjustment and, like most fixed drug-mixture preparations, should be considered only after optimal doses of intermediate- and short/rapid-acting insulin have been established indepen-dently. Moreover, most patients taking insulin before meals also require an injection before lunch, which should not be the mixture preparation. The cost of the mixture preparations is increased. Customized mixtures can be made up by the patient or family member, accomplishing the same goals but better suited to the needs of the individual patient. A mixture con-taining regular insulin necessitates administration at least 30 to 45 minutes before breakfast and dinner to ensure that the peak action of regular insulin is properly timed and not too late, which is not an issue with mixtures containing a rapid-acting insulin. As noted, long-acting insulin analogues cannot be mixed in a syringe with other insulins.

Inhaled Insulin (Exubera). A short-acting, inhaled insulin preparation has been approved by the FDA for use in non-smoking adult patients with type 1 or type 2 diabetes who are free of underlying pulmonary disease. The inhaled prepara-tion is intended for use before meals as an alternative to rapid- and short-acting subcutaneously administered insulin prepara-tions. It is taken 10 minutes before meals with the aid of a pulmonary inhaler and dispenses a dry powder. Improvement in glycemic control is slightly less than that associated with parenterally administered insulin, but patient acceptability is better, particularly in persons reluctant to inject insulin. Mild weight gain and episodes of hypoglycemia can occur, as with any insulin. In the short-term, pulmonary function appears to be unaffected, but data on long-term use are not yet available, and there is the theoretical concern about chronic inhalation of an immunogenic, growth-promoting substance. Mild to mod-erate cough may be experienced. Long-term safety has not been established, nor has use in pregnancy. Efficacy does not appear to be compromised by upper respiratory infection, but experi-ence in persons with lower respiratory infection is limited. Cost is substantial; cost-effectiveness is unknown.

Insulin Programs

Insulin is the treatment of choice for type 1 disease and an option for type 2 diabetes. Because of the increasingly recog-nized value of tight glycemic control, traditional insulin reg-imens are being reexamined and new programs of intensive therapy are being designed to provide better control (Table 102.1). The ideal goal is to enhance control without increas-ing the frequency and severity of hypoglycemic episodes. Both basal and prandial components of the insulin regimen must be considered.

Basal Insulin Programs. The basal program is essential be-cause it influences the fasting glucose level, the principal de-terminant of overall glycemic control. Typically, *twice-daily* (*"split"*) doses of an intermediate-acting insulin (*NPH*) or a single dose of a *long-acting insulin* is administered to maintain normoglycemia during the fasting state.

An important shortcoming of traditional basal regimens (twice-daily NPH) is the increased risk of *hypoglycemia* asso-ciated with efforts to tighten control. The peak action of these standard insulin preparations often occurs at times of fasting (e.g., afternoon or early morning) rather than at times of food intake. A typical twice-daily split-dose program of NPH insulin taken before breakfast or dinner produces peak insulin effects between 4 to 10 hours after injection, depending on whether the patient is an early (*type A*), normal (*type B*), or late (*type C*) reactor to insulin. Unless the timing of dosing or food intake is changed, the likelihood of hypoglycemia increases as con-trol is tightened. Solutions to this problem include changing the timing of the evening NPH administration to bedtime and switching to a more constantly absorbed, long-acting insulin preparation (e.g., insulin glargine).

The opposite problem with basal regimens occurs when dos-ing is inadequate. If the basal insulin level is insufficient to suppress morning hepatic glucose production, then *fasting hy-perglycemia* occurs, the so-called *dawn phenomenon*. This is not to be confused with the rebound fasting hyperglycemia

TABLE 102.1

COMMON INSULIN REGIMENS

	Regimen
Standard Regimens: Response to Insulin	
Early (type A)	Two-thirds dose of intermediate insulin before breakfast
	One-third dose of intermediate insulin before dinner
Normal (type B)	Full dose of intermediate insulin before breakfast
Late (type C)	Reduced dose of intermediate insulin plus a short-acting insulin before breakfast
	Small dose of short-acting insulin before dinner if postprandial evening hyperglycemia occurs
More Intensive Insulin Regimens: Degree of Control	
Tight	Long-acting insulin at night
	Divide total daily intermediate insulin dose into injections before breakfast and before dinner
	Add a small dose of rapid-acting or short-acting insulin before meals
Very tight	ong-acting insulin at night
	Rapid-acting or short-acting insulins before each meal or more frequently based on self-monitored glucose measurements to achieve preprandial glucose between 70 and 120 mg/dL, postprandial glucose of <180 mg/dL, and normal hemoglobin A_{1c} of <6.05%
	Pump therapy

that occurs as a response to nocturnal hypoglycemia (i.e., the *Somogyi effect*; see later discussion).

Prandial Insulin Programs. Although prandial control does not have the same importance as basal glucose control to overall glycemic management, it remains an important objective. In traditional single- or split-dose programs, *regular insulin* is often used in conjunction with a basal insulin program to lower postprandial glucose. Timing before meals is determined by whether a short-acting or rapid-acting insulin is used. For persons whose mealtimes are irregular or unpredictable, a *rapid-acting insulin* is preferred over regular insulin because the injection can be administered just before eating (within 5 to 15 minutes), obviating the 30- to 45-minute premeal requirement of regular insulin and the poor compliance and postprandial hyperglycemia or hypoglycemia that may ensue. Use of a rapid-acting insulin provides a better matching of insulin administration with meals and reduces the hypoglycemic risk associated with intensifying a standard prandial regimen; the cost is slightly increased over that with the use of regular insulin.

In many instances, regular insulin or a rapid-acting preparation is mixed with NPH and administered as a single injection to minimize the number of daily injections (*note*: long-acting insulin analogues such as insulin glargine cannot be mixed in a syringe with other insulins; see earlier discussion). The before-dinner timing of the mixed-insulin regimens may increase the risk of nocturnal hypoglycemia due to an early-morning peaking of insulin activity from the basal program. The net result can be a wide daily fluctuation in blood sugars, with periods of hypoglycemia, hyperglycemia, and suboptimal overall control.

Intensive Insulin Therapy. Intensive insulin therapy attempts to overcome the limitations of basal and prandial control associated with typical mixed and split standard insulin regimens. An intensive regimen is based on frequent home glucose monitoring, multiple daily injections of rapid- or short-acting insulin before meals to provide better prandial control, and use of a long-acting insulin preparation for basal control.

Prandial control traditionally relied on the use of *regular insulin*, but its required lead time of 30 to 45 minutes before a meal is inconvenient for those with erratic meal schedules and may compromise compliance. Moreover, its 4- to 6-hour duration of action increases the risk for hypoglycemia. When problematic, these disadvantages can be overcome with use of *the rapid-onset insulins (lispro, aspart, glulisine)*; its fast onset and short duration of action make it well suited for prandial control in an intensive regimen, although cost is increased. In addition, basal insulin requirements may increase because the short duration of action makes for little contribution to basal insulin levels.

Basal control requires use of a long-acting insulin. Preparations such as NPH can be given twice a day (two thirds of the total dose in the morning and one third in the afternoon) along with rapid- or short-acting insulin. The advantages of NPH include low cost and ability to be mixed with regular insulin, minimizing the number of daily injections needed. The principal disadvantage derives from difficulty in achieving constant basal insulin levels, leading to periods of hypo- or hyperglycemia.

Safe basal control requires achieving a constant basal insulin level. One approach to the problem of erratic glycemic control is to postpone the evening NPH dose until bedtime (requires the patient making an additional daily injection). If basal glycemic control remains erratic, switching from NPH to a *long-acting insulin* (e.g., insulin glargine) is worth consideration. The latter's steadier rate of absorption can provide more constant basal insulin levels and less risk of hypoglycemia. Glargine's disadvantages include increased cost and inability to be mixed with other insulins, necessitating a separate daily injection.

Self-monitoring is an essential component of intensive insulin therapy, helping to ensure proper dosing, scheduling, and safety (see later discussion). The major complication of intensive insulin therapy is frequent and relatively severe *hypoglycemia*. Testing before breakfast and dinner is essential. Patients who adjust their prandial insulin dose regularly may test more frequently. A 3 a.m. blood glucose determination is occasionally added to ensure that nocturnal hypoglycemia is not occurring. *Indications* for intensive therapy include type 1 diabetes and type 2 disease in younger, sophisticated, motivated patients without established complications. Intensive therapy is also indicated in pregnancy because of the proven benefit of glucose control in limiting fetal morbidity and mortality and the potential for preventing congenital malformations, which are increased in children of diabetic mothers (see later discussion).

Combined Oral-Agent and Insulin Programs. In type 2 disease, with its multiple mechanisms of glucose intolerance, combination programs using agents with different mechanisms of action are a logical consideration when maximal doses of insulin or oral agents prove insufficient. In patients with type 2 disease who require very large insulin doses and experience unacceptable weight gain, the addition of *metformin* can improve glycemic control and reduce insulin requirements by countering insulin resistance in liver and muscle. Weight gain and other adverse effects of hyperinsulinism can be minimized. Similarly, a patient whose oral-agent program is ineffective may benefit substantially from supplementation with a single modest dose of *NPH insulin* administered before bed. The small amount of insulin suppresses early-morning hepatic glucose production (the dawn phenomenon), thereby reducing morning hyperglycemia without inducing hypoglycemia; overall glycemic control improves significantly.

Open-Loop Pump Therapy. Pump therapy represents an attempt to duplicate the normal physiologic pattern of insulin release. Insulin infusion devices (worn externally and connected to an indwelling catheter) and multiple daily injections are being widely applied in gestational diabetes and in patients with type 1 diabetes that is difficult to control. This therapeutic approach requires patient motivation and sophistication, close monitoring, and careful supervision to be safe and effective. Comparable control of glycemia can be achieved by the use of an insulin pump and conventional intensive therapy. The major advantage of insulin pumps is that they facilitate frequent insulin administration. Complications include catheter infection, inadvertent catheter displacement from the skin, and cost.

Islet Transplantation. Despite the array of treatment options, some patients with type 1 disease are disabled by recurrent, refractory hypoglycemia associated with insulin therapy. Use of the Edmonton protocol (glucocorticoid-free immunosuppressive therapy and infusions of freshly prepared islets from two or more pancreases) has been reported to restore long-term, endogenous insulin production and glycemic control.

Initiation of Therapy

Insulin therapy can be started safely on an ambulatory basis as long as the patient is reliable, nonketotic, and not severely hyperglycemic with intercurrent illness. Treatment can be initiated with either an intermediate-acting or long-acting insulin along with a rapid-or short-acting preparation as needed.

Type 1 Disease .If a type 1 patient has fasting and postprandial hyperglycemia, then insulin glargine plus a rapid-acting insulin is the best choice. Otherwise insulin NPH or detemir twice a day along with pre-meal rapid- or short-acting insulin can be used.

Type 2 Disease. For type 2 diabetics with both fasting and postprandial hyperglycemia, the best initial program is NPH twice a day or the combination of insulin glargine at night-

time (or insulin detemir twice a day) along with premeal rapid-acting insulin as needed. If fasting hyperglycemia is the only problem, then NPH or insulin detemir before bed should suffice. If postprandial hyperglycemia is the only difficulty, then one can start with a morning dose of NPH or insulin detemir.

Technique and Storage

Insulin is injected subcutaneously and is absorbed directly into the circulation. The abdomen and limbs are convenient injection sites; rotation among sites minimizes discomfort and, rarely, lipoatrophy. Insulin is absorbed fastest from the abdominal wall. Rotation among multiple abdominal *injection sites* is preferable to limb injections especially in athletically active diabetic patients because of the possibility of more rapid insulin absorption from an exercising limb. Insulin, best *stored* in the refrigerator, may be left at room temperature for up to 12 hours without loss of biopotency.

Degree of Control

As noted earlier, the large-scale, long-term, randomized, controlled DCCT (for type 1 disease) and UKPDS (for type 2 diabetes) firmly established that normalization of glycemia (HbA$_{1c}$ <7.0%) significantly reduces the risks for microvascular complications. Very tight control (HbA$_{1c}$ between 6.0% and 7.0%) is the objective of intensive insulin regimens. Whether and under what conditions such control can also reduce the risk for macrovascular complications remain to be determined. So far, only obese patients achieving tight glycemic control with metformin have experienced significant reductions in cardiovascular and stroke risk. That the weight gain seen with intensive insulin therapy might be a manifestation of the insulin resistance syndrome, which includes hypertension and an increased coronary risk, is a concern. Efforts to counter such insulin resistance may be necessary to achieve a reduction in coronary risk. More study is needed.

The practical issue is whether such tight control can be accomplished safely in a given patient and whether the means of therapy available are compatible with the patient's lifestyle and personal choice for therapy. In type 1 disease, an intelligent, well-motivated, reliable person can be taught to regulate daily insulin doses, but less capable patients risk hypoglycemic reactions when tight control is attempted. In type 2 diabetes, the advent of well-tolerated agents that turn off hepatic gluconeogenesis and peripheral insulin resistance has made it possible to improve control with a lesser risk for hypoglycemia.

Worsening Hyperglycemia during Insulin Therapy

In a patient taking a previously adequate dose of insulin, hyperglycemia requires prompt attention (Table 102.2). Although important changes in caloric intake or failure to take insulin properly may be the explanation for worsening hyperglycemia, occult infection (especially in the urinary tract), coronary ischemia, severe emotional stress, and the Somogyi phenomenon (rebound hyperglycemia) must be investigated. A recently recognized phenomenon, worsening hyperglycemia in the early-morning hours is caused by the surges in growth hormone levels that occur during sleep. An intermediate-acting insulin given at bedtime can provide excellent coverage for such early-morning hyperglycemia.

The Somogyi Phenomenon. The Somogyi phenomenon, in which rebound hyperglycemia and possibly ketosis occur after insulin-induced hypoglycemia, may be mistaken for inadequate control. The hypoglycemia usually goes unnoticed

TABLE 102.2

IMPORTANT CAUSES OF WORSENING HYPERGLYCEMIA DURING INSULIN THERAPY

Inadequate dose
Increased caloric intake
Failure to take insulin properly
Occult infection (especially urinary tract)
Coronary ischemia
Severe emotional stress
Use of corticosteroids
Somogyi phenomenon
Insulin resistance
Growth hormone surge in early morning

because it occurs at night or in a patient with severe autonomic neuropathy. Hypoglycemia is followed by several days of poor control. Clues to recognizing nocturnal hypoglycemia include night sweats, poor sleep, nightmares, and morning headaches. The best way to recognize the Somogyi effect is to be cognizant of its potential existence and to measure blood glucose at a time of suspected hypoglycemia.

If detection is impractical, a diagnostic trial of reduced insulin may be used to confirm the clinical suspicion. Doses of insulin should be decreased slowly each day rather than precipitously because a dramatic decrease in insulin dose will cause hyperglycemia to worsen. In diabetics using NPH as part of a program of intensive insulin therapy, simply switching the evening NPH administration from dinnertime to bedtime may resolve the nocturnal hypoglycemia problem and result in a reduction in fasting glucose levels. Similarly, switching from NPH to insulin glargine may reduce nocturnal hypoglycemia (see later discussion).

Insulin Resistance. Insulin resistance is occasionally the cause of poor control. It is arbitrarily defined as the requirement for *more than 200 U of insulin* daily. Most cases of insulin resistance result from obesity; restoring normal weight is the best treatment. As noted earlier, the hepatic and muscle refractoriness to insulin seen in type 2 disease may respond to therapy with metformin or a thiazolidinedione. More-classic insulin resistance is immunologically mediated by antibodies directed at bovine or porcine insulin or against protamine or protamine–insulin complexes. There appears to be no increased frequency of antibody production against insulin lispro.

For patients with immunologic insulin resistance, switching therapy to a different source of insulin or to human recombinant insulin may be advantageous. At times, high-dose glucocorticoids (80 to 100 mg of prednisone daily) may be necessary. Most patients respond, and steroid therapy can often be rapidly tapered. Immunologic insulin resistance is commonly seen in patients who have been receiving insulin in intermittent-treatment programs. In patients who receive insulin for limited intervals only (e.g., during myocardial infarction or weight reduction for obesity), human insulin represents the best choice of therapy for limiting antibody development.

Hypoglycemia and Insulin Reactions

When food intake is delayed or diminished, physical activity is increased, or the insulin dose is excessive or poorly timed, hypoglycemia may ensue. Risk of hypoglycemia is especially great in persons taking an intensive insulin regimen. Profound hypoglycemia may lead to loss of consciousness. If autonomic neuropathy is present or if a patient is taking a β-adrenergic blocker, many hypoglycemic symptoms will be masked and mental confusion may be the paramount symptom. Autonomic symptoms may become blunted in patients who experience frequent hypoglycemic episodes, necessitating careful home glucose monitoring, especially when patients engage in a program of intensive insulin therapy. Patient and family education and the availability of a syringe containing *glucagon* are essential measures to ensure patient safety. Also critical are considerations of adjustments in the dose, timing, and types of insulin preparations used. Despite the adverse short-term consequences of hypoglycemia on cognitive function, no decline in cognitive function has been found among long-term insulin users with type 1 disease and many episodes of transient hypoglycemia.

Postprandial hypoglycemia necessitates review of the prandial insulin program. Attention to timing of insulin administration and dose are the first steps, informed by data from increased finger-stick monitoring. Persistence of episodes necessitates consideration of switching from a standard short-acting preparation to a rapid-acting insulin such as *insulin lispro*, which might help to better match insulin administration with intake of food.

Fasting hypoglycemia, especially nocturnal hypoglycemia, mandates a review of the basal insulin program. In those using twice-daily *NPH* for the basal insulin component, simply changing the evening dose from dinnertime to *bedtime* may resolve the nocturnal hypoglycemia problem, as may considering *insulin glargine* for the basal program. Insulin glargine's steadier rate of absorption may avoid the peaks sometimes associated with other insulin. *Insulin pump* therapy is another approach to basal insulin administration.

Insulin Allergy

Insulin allergy, manifested as cutaneous reactions to insulin, occurs in approximately 5% of patients. Urticaria, angioedema, or anaphylaxis is rare. Insulin allergy may be treated by a change to human insulin administered with antihistamines. Desensitization may be necessary if systemic allergic manifestations have occurred. Lispro insulin has not been associated with an increased risk for insulin allergy.

Preoperative Insulin Management

In the preoperative management of the diabetic patient taking insulin, medical evaluation is critical because most perioperative complications relate not to hyperglycemia or hypoglycemia, but rather to coexisting cardiac or renal disease. It is important that the potential for infection be considered carefully and sources of fever, such as pulmonary, skin, and urinary tract infection, be investigated.

Many insulin programs for perioperative management have been advanced. For patients scheduled to undergo same-day surgery and instructed to take nothing by mouth after midnight, their dose of basal insulin should be reduced by one third to one half on the morning of surgery and carbohydrate supplied as intravenous 5% dextrose at the rate of 150 mL/hr. If possible, surgery should be performed early in the day and regular insulin given in the postoperative period as needed for marked hyperglycemia.

Control of Associated Cardiovascular Risk Factors

As noted earlier, control of hyperglycemia prevents or limits the microvascular, neurologic, and renal complications of diabetes. Except in obese patients with type 2 diabetes who achieve tight control with metformin, it has not yet been proved that the risk for macrovascular disease is similarly reduced by tight control. Consequently, it is most important that all associated risk factors for the development of coronary artery disease be meticulously controlled. Diabetes confers a degree of coronary risk similar to that associated with prior myocardial infarction. In diabetics, aggressive efforts to control hypertension, reduce hypercholesterolemia, and cease smoking (see Chapters 26, 27, and 54) result in marked reductions in the risk for coronary events and stroke and in all-cause mortality. With 75% of deaths in diabetic patients caused by cardiovascular problems, the importance of *reducing atherosclerotic risk factors* cannot be overemphasized. These efforts are even more productive than attempts at tight control of blood sugar and must not be overlooked.

Hypertension

The treatment of hypertension in diabetics requires attention not only to the degree of control achieved, but also to its effects on metabolic control, recognition of hypoglycemia, and "renal hyperfiltration." The drugs of choice inhibit the angiotensin system and include the *angiotensin-converting-enzyme* (ACE) *inhibitors* and *angiotensin-receptor blockers* (ARBs). They appear to limit hyperfiltration and preserve renal function (see later discussion). Patients must be monitored for hyperkalemia. The *thiazide* diuretics may modestly compromise glucose intolerance, which makes them less desirable as first-line agents than angiotensin blockade, especially in full doses. In smaller doses, they have few adverse effects on blood glucose and may facilitate blood pressure control. *Beta-blockers* are effective but can mask the sympathomimetic warning symptoms of hypoglycemia. They should be used with care in patients undergoing intensive insulin therapy. Impotence and postural hypotension are features of diabetes that may affect the choice of antihypertensive therapy (see Chapter 26).

Lipid Disorders

Lipid abnormalities are a consequence of diabetes and sometimes also of treatments for diabetes. HDL cholesterol is often low and VLDL and LDL cholesterols and triglycerides increased. Effective control of hyperglycemia often improves the lipid profile by reducing triglycerides and raising HDL cholesterol, but intensive insulin therapy that causes weight gain may actually increase LDL cholesterol and lower HDL cholesterol. Metformin use is associated with reductions in triglycerides and LDL cholesterol and slight increases in HDL cholesterol. The thiazolidinediones decrease triglycerides and raise HDL cholesterol, but they also increase LDL cholesterol. The sulfonylureas and acarbose have no effects on lipids.

The drugs used to treat lipid disorders are usually well tolerated in diabetes. The *statins* can very effectively lower LDL cholesterol and modestly raise HDL cholesterol. The *fibrates* are effective for reducing triglycerides and raising HDL cholesterol (see Chapter 27), but they should not be used with statins. *Niacin* is effective for raising low HDL cholesterol but can exacerbate glucose intolerance (see Chapter 27).

Renal Failure

Renal failure is a potent yet often underappreciated risk factor for cardiovascular disease. Essential preventive measures including tight control of blood sugar and blood pressure, regular monitoring of urine for microalbinuria, and prompt initiation of angiotensin blockade (with ACE inhibitor or ARB)

at the earliest sign of nephropathy. Initiation of angiotensin blockade may be appropriate for all diabetic patients even before there is evidence of nephropathy, particularly in persons with concurrent hypertension (see later discussion).

Management of Complications

Renal Failure

ACE inhibitors and *ARBs* reduce proteinuria and significantly slow the progression of azotemia. The beneficial effect on nephropathy occurs even in normotensive patients and is independent of reduction in blood pressure. Benefit is believed to be related to afferent arteriolar dilation and reduced hyperfiltration. Control of hypertension is essential, particularly as renal function declines (see Chapter 26). Studies suggest that treating all diabetic patients prophylactically with an ACE inhibitor or generic ARB may be cost-effective, irrespective of renal sediment findings. *Protein restriction* (0.5 mg/kg) may also reduce hyperfiltration in early nephropathy, but ACE-inhibitor or ARB therapy is likely to be more acceptable.

The progression to renal failure may be inexorable once heavy proteinuria (>3 g/d) develops. However, the primary care physician may still be able to prevent some forms of late renal insufficiency, such as that associated with bladder dysfunction, pyelonephritis, and acute papillary necrosis and the contrast-induced acute renal failure that occurs in diabetics with moderate to advanced renal insufficiency. Prompt and aggressive *treatment of urinary tract infections* (see Chapters 133 and 140), therapy to *limit urinary retention*, which increases the risk for infection (see Chapter 134), and avoidance of unnecessary contrast studies all help to prevent renal insults.

If *contrast studies* are necessary, it is essential to assure full *hydration* and limit the dye load to the smallest amount possible. Nephrotoxic antibiotics and *nonsteroidal antiinflammatory drugs* (which can inhibit renal prostaglandin activity) should be avoided prior to the dye study.

Metformin use needs to be restricted in the setting of renal insufficiency (creatinine >1.5 mg/dL in men and >1.4 mg/dL in women) because it is excreted by the kidneys and high doses increase the risk for lactic acidosis.

During the last decade, the outlook for the diabetic patient undergoing hemodialysis or renal transplantation has improved, although the mortality rate for diabetics on these treatment modalities remains higher than that of nondiabetics. Continuous ambulatory *peritoneal dialysis* has been offered to diabetic patients because of concerns that the heparin used in hemodialysis may worsen diabetic retinopathy. However, early information suggests that infection rates are higher in diabetic patients on continuous peritoneal dialysis.

Peripheral Vascular Disease

The microvascular and macrovascular complications of diabetes are readily evident in the limbs. Ischemic skin ulcers, claudication, and limb loss are common complications. Amputation of a lower extremity is often the consequence of peripheral vascular disease and neuropathy in patients with diabetes. In comparison with a control diabetic population, diabetic amputees had more severe neuropathy and vascular impairment and lower HDL cholesterol levels, and they had received less outpatient diabetic education. Management includes tightening glycemic control, reducing atherosclerotic risk factors, exercising, quitting smoking, and maintaining meticulous foot care (see Chapter 34).

Foot Problems

Because of vascular insufficiency and neuropathy, diabetic patients have unique foot care problems. Early detection of diminished sensation is facilitated by testing with a standardized monofilament, which is superior to the conventional physical examination for detecting protective foot sensation. Meticulous foot care is essential to preventing cellulitis, osteomyelitis, and the potential need for amputation. Feet must be kept clean, interdigital spaces dry, calluses pared down, and toenails carefully trimmed. Frequent inspection for skin breakdown and cellulitis by the patient needs to be stressed, as does the importance of wearing properly fitting shoes. Before bathing, diabetic patients should use their hands to test the water temperature so that scalding injuries that may occur because of a loss of temperature sensation in the lower extremities can be prevented. Regular podiatric care is a well-considered preventive measure for all diabetics, especially those who are elderly or have poor eyesight, a history of foot infection, or a significant loss of sensation.

Neuropathy

Prevention through tight glycemic control remains the best approach to diabetic neuropathy. However, if symptoms emerge and become problematic, then consideration of pharmacologic intervention is warranted.

Distal Sensory Neuropathy. Pain due to a *distal sensory neuropathy* can be disabling. Multiple agents have been tried for symptomatic relief, but no singularly effective treatment program has emerged. Traditionally, the *tricyclic antidepressants* (e.g., *amitriptyline, nortriptyline*; usually 25 to 50 mg at bedtime) were the first line of treatment. However, their anticholinergic side effects (e.g., dry mouth, urinary retention, constipation, orthostatic hypotension) and tendency to trigger cardiac dysrhythmias (see Chapter 227) make them suboptimal choices, especially in the elderly.

Duloxetine (Cymbalta), an antidepressant and reuptake inhibitor of both serotonin and norepinephrine, has been approved by the FDA for the treatment of diabetic neuropathic pain. Benefit may be seen shortly after initiation of therapy. Side effects include nausea, dizziness, fatigue, drowsiness, and constipation. The usual dose is 60 mg/d; higher doses are of little benefit. Dose adjustment is necessary in renal insufficiency; it should not be given to patients with hepatic insufficiency.

Pregabalin (Lyrica), a γ-aminobutyric acid (GABA) analogue similar to gabapentin (see Chapter 170), is also FDA approved for painful diabetic neuropathy. Side effects include dizziness, somnolence, dry mouth, and peripheral edema. The maximum recommended dose is 100 mg three times a day. The dose should be adjusted for renal insufficiency. Cost is very high.

Gabapentin (Neurontin), a GABA analogue approved for treatment of postherpetic neuralgia and epilepsy (see Chapter 170), helps to control neuropathic pain but is not approved for diabetic neuropathy. Side effects include dizziness, somnolence, and confusion. A low dose should be used initially and can then be titrated upward over several weeks.

Autonomic Insufficiency. *Postural hypotension, impotence,* and *urinary retention* associated with autonomic neuropathy are usually permanent. Postural hypotension may respond to volume expansion, *midodrine* (an α1 selective adrenergic agonist) and to the synthetic mineralocorticoid *fludrocortisone* (Florinef). *Erectile dysfunction* is a reasonable indication for consideration of *sildenafil* (Viagra) or similar agents, which

can be moderately effective in diabetic men (see Chapter 132). However, these should not be taken by patients who are concurrently on nitrates for the treatment of cardiovascular disease. Anxiety and depression, which are often superimposed on neurologic dysfunction, must be excluded (see Chapters 132 and 229).

Enteropathy

Gastrointestinal motility problems, which include esophageal motility dysfunction, gastroparesis, and diabetic diarrhea, can be difficult to treat. Small, frequent feedings may be helpful. *Metoclopramide* (Reglan), a dopamine agonist, may lessen the symptoms of gastroparesis. It is usually administered in a 10-mg dose 30 minutes before meals and at bedtime. In addition to the pill formulation, an oral liquid and intravenous preparation are available. Patients with diarrhea caused by bacterial overgrowth of the bowel can be treated with a trial of a *broad-spectrum antibiotic* (e.g., *neomycin* or tetracycline). *Cholestyramine* may be beneficial in controlling the diarrhea of diabetic autonomic neuropathy. Fortunately, refractory nocturnal diarrhea often resolves spontaneously.

Regular dental examinations are a necessity because of the higher incidence in diabetic patients of *pyorrhea* and abscesses, which may also reduce diabetic control.

Ophthalmopathy

Diabetic *retinopathy* is the most important systemic disease causing blindness. Proliferative retinopathy accounts for the majority of cases of blindness among type 1 diabetics, whereas *macular edema* resulting from nonproliferative retinopathy accounts for most cases of blindness in type 2 diabetes. Prevention is the best treatment, achieved by a reduction in hyperglycemia. Even partial normalization of glucose levels is helpful. Photocoagulation with laser therapy can retard visual loss by 50% (see Chapter 209). Cataracts and glaucoma are also important complications (see Chapters 207 and 208 for discussions of management).

Glucose Intolerance in Pregnancy

Fetal hyperglycemia contributes to excessive fetal growth, which increases the risks for birth trauma, asphyxia, neonatal respiratory distress syndrome, and death *in utero*. In addition, the need for cesarean section is increased. Maintenance of blood sugars in the physiologic range (60 to 120 mg/dL) takes on added importance during pregnancy because the complications of fetal hyperglycemia can be prevented and perinatal mortality reduced to the rate seen in nondiabetics. Even in nondiabetic pregnant women in whom an otherwise insignificant degree of hyperglycemia develops (2-hour-postprandial blood sugars in the range of 140 to 160 mg/dL), the risk for macrosomia and its complications is increased. Women with postprandial readings in excess of 165 mg/dL have an increased incidence of diabetes in later life.

Screening and *diagnosis* are critical. The importance of glucose intolerance during pregnancy has led to the recommendation by the American Diabetic Association that all pregnant women be screened for glucose intolerance by weeks 24 to 28 of gestation. Diabetic risk assessment should occur at the first prenatal visit. Those with clinical characteristics consistent with a high risk of gestational diabetes (e.g., marked obesity, personal history of gestational diabetes or delivery of a previous large-for-gestation-age infant, glycosuria, polycystic ovary syndrome, strong history of diabetes) should undergo glucose testing as soon as possible. Data from the Nurses' Health Study showed that advanced maternal age, family history, nonwhite ethnicity, higher body mass index, weight gain in early adulthood, and cigarette smoking are independent risk factors.

Screening is conducted with a *1-hour, 50-g oral glucose load,* which can be given at any time of day. Patients with a 1-hour serum glucose level in excess of 140 mg/dL need confirmatory testing. *Diagnosis* can be established by a *3-hour, 100-g glucose tolerance test.* Two or more abnormal values for serum glucose during the test (in excess of 95 mg/dL fasting, 180 mg/dL at 1 hour, 155 mg/dL at 2 hours, and 140 mg/dL at 3 hours) establish the diagnosis.

Dietary measures are the foundation of prevention and treatment, just as in other forms of diabetes. All patients with gestational diabetes should have *nutritional counseling,* with emphasis on caloric and carbohydrate intake. The diets should limit simple sugars and total calories (based on ideal weight). Guidelines for caloric distribution aim for 10% of calories for breakfast, 30% for lunch, 30% for dinner, and 30% for snacks.

Monitoring of blood sugar is essential. Fasting and postprandial determinations are preferred. Patients with fasting sugars in excess of 95 mg/dL or 2-hour-postprandial levels greater than 120 mg/dL may need insulin therapy and consideration of consultation with a diabetologist. More frequent monitoring is required of persons under treatment with insulin.

Treatment centers on *insulin* therapy for those who do not achieve normalization of glycemic control by dietary measures. Dose is determined and adjusted according to results from finger-stick testing. For diabetic patients already on insulin, adjustments in dose may be necessary. During the first trimester, the insulin dose of a patient with type 1 diabetes should be reduced because insulin requirements decrease and the risk for hypoglycemia is increased. In the second trimester, the type 1 diabetic requires more insulin as the diabetes becomes more labile and the chances for the development of ketoacidosis (with its associated risk for fetal death) rise. Third-trimester dose requirements usually do not change, but the increase in the glomerular filtration rate can lower the tubular threshold for glucose and make urine testing unreliable.

Within a few hours of delivery, insulin requirements fall considerably, returning completely to prepregnancy levels within 1 to 2 weeks. Optimal control is facilitated by the use of home glucose monitoring (see later discussion).

Infection

Diabetes increases the risk of infection, particularly that associated with foot ulcers and the urinary tract. Fungal infections are more commonly seen than in nondiabetic patients. Purported mechanisms include impairment of neutrophil function and compromise of antioxidant-dependent systems. An increased frequency of micronutrient (vitamin and mineral) deficiency is hypothesized to contribute to this increased risk. Use of a daily multivitamin supplement has been found in diabetics to significantly reduce the risk of infection. Diabetic patients in whom a dietary history reveals a likelihood of micronutrient deficiency are reasonable candidates for a vitamin and mineral supplement containing 100% of recommended daily allowances.

Monitoring

Monitoring must address three parameters: glycemic control, diabetic complications, and adverse drug effects.

For Glycemic Control

Home monitoring of *capillary blood glucose* by the *finger-stick method* represents a marked improvement in monitoring over previous methods, such as urine glucose testing, and should be used whenever possible. The patient obtains a finger-stick sample of capillary blood, which is tested for glucose concentration by colorimetric reading of a reagent strip to which a drop of blood is applied. More-sophisticated meters and color charts are available for the glucose determination. Insurance companies are increasingly covering the costs. Measurements are most useful for patients on insulin therapy; hour-to-hour and day-to-day adjustments can be made based on the results of blood sugar monitoring. Frequent measurements, both in the fasting state and at several intervals before meals and at bedtime, are valuable when an insulin program is being started or adjusted and also during periods of illness or worsening control. Most patients can be taught the method. Numerous devices automatically perform the finger-stick. Once a stable insulin dose has been achieved, a single measurement need be taken only once every several days, typically before breakfast. Patients who are capable of adjusting their insulin doses can use home monitoring to keep their sugars in the mid-100 range after a meal. Home monitoring does not obviate the need to inform the patient carefully about symptoms of hyperglycemia and hypoglycemia (see later discussion).

Hemoglobin A_{1c} determination provides an estimate of overall glycemic control for the preceding 2 to 3 months. The degree of glycosylation of hemoglobin in the red blood cell reflects the glucose concentration in the red blood cell environment during the cell's life span. The level correlates well with the results of frequent blood glucose determinations. The goal for HbA_{1c} is less than 7% and, if possible, to the normal range without causing episodes of hypoglycemia. Levels of less than 8.0% indicate blood sugar levels of less than 200 mg/dL; values of 11% to 12% correlate with glucose levels in excess of 300 mg/dL and indicate poor carbohydrate control. This test has superseded the *random blood sugar* determination as the best means of assessing control over time. HbA_{1c} should be checked every 6 months if diabetes is controlled (<7%) and every 3 to 6 months if it is uncontrolled (>7%) or there is a change in treatment.

For Complications

At every visit, patients with diabetes should undergo routine periodic follow-up. At every visit blood pressure should be checked, glucose logs reviewed, weight/BMI obtained, and medications and lifestyle modification measures (diet, exercise, smoking cessation) reviewed. The feet should be checked for callus, ulceration, and infection, particularly in persons with diminished sensation due to peripheral neuropathy.

Periodically, the physical examination should include a check for proliferative retinopathy, carotid bruits and others signs of central and peripheral atherosclerotic disease, and peripheral neuropathy with loss of distal sensation (best performed by using a standardized monofilament). Referral for a dilated ophthalmologic eye exam is needed annually and more frequently if retinopathy is noted.

Of particular importance is the need to test for risk factors for vascular disease, such as hypertension (see Chapter 14), hypercholesterolemia (see Chapter 15), smoking (see Chapter 54), and renal failure (see Chapter 142). Accordingly, periodic laboratory studies should include a lipid profile, urine for microalbumin, and serum creatinine.

A diabetic summary sheet placed in the patient's record makes possible quick review of the extent, severity, and progression of the disease and its complications. Teaching the patient to watch for skin, eye, neurologic, and cardiovascular changes is an important part of the monitoring effort (see later discussion).

For Adverse Effects of Drug Therapy

Patients taking *metformin* require monitoring of renal function with serum *creatinine* determination; renal insufficiency reduces metformin excretion and may lead to increased serum levels and heightened risk of *lactic acidosis*. Dose adjustment or termination of therapy needs to be considered when the serum creatinine rises to greater than 1.4 mg/dL. Persons prescribed *thiazolidinediones* require regular monitoring of *serum liver enzymes* (e.g., *ALT*; see prior discussion). Any ALT elevation in excess of three times the upper limit of normal is an indication for immediate cessation of therapy, and cessation should also be considered if any sustained increases are noted.

Persons prescribed *thiazolidinediones* have an increased risk of fluid retention and *heart failure*, necessitating monitoring of volume status and checking regularly for symptoms and signs of heart failure (see Chapter 32). Rosiglitazone use is associated with an increased risk of *myocardial infarction* (which may or may not be a class effect); patients taking this class of drugs need careful monitoring of symptoms and signs of ischemia (see Chapter 22) and further workup (see Chapter 36) if there is any suspicion clinically; a periodic check of the electrocardiogram might be helpful. Any suspicion of ischemia is an indication for terminating therapy.

PATIENT EDUCATION (60,61)

The success of a program for metabolic control depends on patient compliance. Because *weight reduction* to ideal body weight is the most important therapy that can be offered to patients with type 2 diabetes, instruction about *diet* and choosing healthful foods should take place in a setting that includes both patient and family. Sample diets can be obtained from the American Diabetic Association. The emphasis on diet therapy for the type 2 diabetic should focus more on caloric restriction than on actual percentages of carbohydrate or simple sugars.

The patient receiving insulin requires continuous education and encouragement, particularly as more-intensive insulin treatment programs are applied to patients with type 2 diabetes to limit the end-organ consequences of hyperglycemia. In many hospital-based practices and several office practices, a nurse specializing in diabetes education offers patients careful instruction in drawing up insulin into syringes (particularly if the patient is visually impaired), insulin injection techniques, and the complications of excess insulin administration and is readily available for telephone communication with patients. A syringe with *glucagon* for intramuscular injection is given to each patient in the event that the patient becomes profoundly hypoglycemic and is unable to take glucose by mouth. Oral administration of juices to an unconscious and obtunded patient may lead to pulmonary aspiration.

The importance of skin and foot care must be emphasized (see Chapter 34). Referral of elderly diabetic patients with vision loss to podiatrists for regular foot care is indicated.

INDICATIONS FOR ADMISSION AND REFERRAL

Acute hospitalization for intravenous (IV) administration of fluids is necessary for diabetic patients with protracted nausea and vomiting who are becoming dehydrated and hyperglycemic. Often, cellulitis of the foot requires IV antibiotic therapy, as does acute pyelonephritis. In general, elderly diabetic patients with pneumonia or urinary tract infections benefit from brief hospitalizations.

Regularly scheduled referral visits to the *ophthalmologist* for retinopathy screening, to the *podiatrist* for foot care, and to the *nutritionist* for dietary counseling are essential to assuring best outcomes. Referral to an endocrinologist is indicated for the diabetic patient who is subject to marked fluctuations in blood sugar with frequent episodes of hypoglycemia and hyperglycemia. *Insulin-pump* therapy may be worth considering in persons with type 1 disease difficult to control with injection therapy.

Type 1 patients who experience refractory hypoglycemia and unstable glycemic control with insulin therapy might benefit from *islet transplantation* and be considered for referral to a center with expertise in such transplantation. Such referral should be done in conjunction with a consulting endocrinologist.

When proteinuria is in the nephrotic syndrome range and the creatinine level begins to rise to greater than 2.5 to 3.0 mg/dL, referral to a *nephrologist* for management and future consideration of *dialysis* and *renal transplantation* are necessary. Indications for coronary artery bypass grafting are not different for the diabetic patient. Because of the potential severity of cholecystitis and ascending cholangitis, cholecystectomy for cholelithiasis may be a reasonable clinical choice, although more recent experience favors watchful waiting for asymptomatic cholelithiasis (see Chapter 69).

THERAPEUTIC RECOMMENDATIONS (1,8,13,15,18,19,56)

Screening and Prevention

■ Screen high-risk persons (e.g., obese, sedentary, hypertensive, hyperlipidemic) for diabetes by performing fasting and postprandial blood glucose determinations (see Chapter 93).
■ Prescribe a program of lifestyle modification for those with fasting glucose approaching 125 mg/dL and postprandial glucose approaching 200 mg/dL.
■ Implement lifestyle modification with a program of modest weight reduction (7% sustained weight loss), moderate exercise (2.5 hours/wk of walking at moderate pace), and a low-fat, low-cholesterol diet.
■ Consider adding hypoglycemic therapy if glycemic control is not sufficiently improved or lifestyle modification is not successfully implemented.

Basic Management for All Diabetic Patients

■ Attempt to normalize hyperglycemia; the goal is an HbA$_{1c}$ concentration less than 7.0% and a fasting glucose level less than 126 mg/dL.
■ Emphasize the importance of maintaining ideal body weight. For those who are obese, institute caloric restriction without compromising the regularity of meal timing.
■ Prescribe regular aerobic exercise and a low-saturated-fat, reduced-calorie, balanced diet.

- Pay assiduous attention to the diagnosis and treatment of all additional atherosclerotic risk factors, such as hypertension, hyperlipidemia, and smoking (see Chapters 26, 27, and 54).
- Teach all diabetic patients, especially those on insulin therapy, how to monitor glycemic control daily with *home blood glucose determinations*.
- Assess long-term glucose control with HbA$_{1c}$ measurements performed every 3 to 6 months.
- Carefully investigate the causes of worsening hyperglycemia (Table 102.2).
- At each visit, discuss compliance with diet, exercise, and pharmacologic programs, review results of home glucose monitoring, note any episodes of hypo- or hyperglycemia, inquire into symptoms of diabetic complications, check blood pressure, and examine feet for ulceration and infection.
- At least once a year, perform a comprehensive history and physical examination for evidence of cardiovascular and peripheral vascular diseases, neuropathy, nephropathy, and retinopathy; obtain blood urea nitrogen, creatinine, lipid profile, urinalysis, and *urine for microalbuminuria*.
- Carefully monitor *renal function* by regularly testing for *microalbuminuria* and increase in serum *creatinine*; also check *urinary sediment* for microscopic hematuria. At the first sign of nephropathy, institute tighter glycemic control and prescribe angiotensin blockade by means of an ACE inhibitor or ARB. For middle-aged patients with no sign of nephropathy or hypertension, consider instituting prophylactic ACE-inhibitor therapy, which can reduce the risk of nephropathy. When the serum creatinine level reaches 2 to 3 mg/dL, obtain a nephrology consultation.
- Exercise caution in the use of *iodinated contrast agents*, especially in the setting of renal impairment.
- Refer all diabetic patients for *diabetic retinal examination* (see Chapter 209). A dilated eye exam should be performed by an eye-care specialist to test for early detection of proliferative retinopathy every 1 to 2 years if the most recent exam is normal and more frequently as needed. Also refer promptly diabetic patients who have background retinopathy and type 1 patients who have had diabetes for 5 to 10 years and never had an eye examination to an ophthalmologist for indirect ophthalmoscopy and, if necessary, fluorescein angiography.
- Emphasize *foot care* to diabetic patients with neuropathy or vascular insufficiency. Arrange regular podiatric care for such patients.
- Perform a careful perioperative assessment of diabetic patients undergoing surgery. Pay particular attention to worsening hyperglycemia and diligently observe for infection and occult coronary artery disease, particularly in those with evidence of microvascular disease.
- Consider including a well-trained nurse, nurse practitioner, or physician assistant in the long-term management program to complement and support physician efforts at achieving glycemic control.

Patients with Type 1 Disease

- Consider early institution of *intensive insulin* therapy as soon as the "honeymoon period" ends (rising nocturnal insulin requirements) to achieve very tight control (HbA$_{1c}$ 6.0% to 7.0%), especially for highly motivated patients willing to perform multiple glucose determinations each day and self-administer insulin according to the results of each test. Consider less intensive insulin therapy or infusion pump technology for those unable to carry out an intensive insulin regimen.

For those attempting intensive insulin therapy and starting treatment as an outpatient:

- For basal control, start with a modest dose of long-acting insulin glargine (e.g., 15 U once daily administered in the evening). Alternatively, start with intermediate insulin (NPH) twice a day or longer-acting insulin detemir twice a day. If using NPH, consider giving the dose at bedtime, especially if fasting hypoglycemia is a problem. If using insulin glargine, do not mix the dose in the syringe with another insulin.
- Prescribe human recombinant insulin for newly treated diabetics to minimize risks for insulin allergy, insulin resistance, and antibody development.
- For prandial glycemic control, begin a program of rapid-acting insulin (lispro, aspart, glulisine) or one of short-acting insulin (regular), starting at 5 U administered 5 to 15 minutes before each meal for rapid-acting insulins and 15 to 45 minutes before each meal for short-acting insulin. Adjust according to the results of postprandial home glucose measurements.
- For patients achieving tight control with regular insulin but bothered by frequent hypoglycemic episodes or inconvenience of use, consider switching to a rapid-acting insulin (e.g., insulin lispro), which can be administered just 5 to 15 minutes before each meal.

For those unable to carry out an intensive insulin program or who may still be in the honeymoon period, where nocturnal insulin requirements remain small:

- Begin a twice-daily insulin regimen consisting of an intermediate-acting insulin (e.g., NPH) mixed with a short- or rapid-acting preparation administered before breakfast and before the evening meal; two thirds of the daily dose should be given in the morning and one third in the evening. The dose ratio of NPH to short- or rapid-acting insulin should be 2:1 in the morning and 1:1 in the evening. Adjust doses according to fasting, 4 p.m., and 3 a.m. glucose determinations.
- Teach the importance of regular caloric intake and regular spacing of meals to match peak insulin effects and activity schedules.
- Patients who experience refractory hypoglycemia and unstable glycemic control in response to insulin therapy should be referred for consideration of islet-cell transplantation.

Patients with Type 2 Disease

- Emphasize *weight reduction* to ideal body weight as the cornerstone of therapy for type 2 diabetes. The composition of the diet per se is less important, but the diet should have a high ratio of polyunsaturated to saturated fat and contain complex carbohydrates. Diets low in protein may be beneficial in averting diabetic nephropathy (see Chapter 142).
- Prescribe a practical program of regular exercise that fits the patient's lifestyle (see Chapter 18). Consider a program of regular moderate aerobic exercise performed three times per week for 30 to 60 minutes. Continue the exercise program irrespective of any weight loss achieved by diet alone.

If after 4 to 8 weeks of diet and exercise the treatment goals have not been achieved and the patient shows *mild to moderate glucose* intolerance (fasting glucose <240 mg/dL), then:

■ Begin oral-agent therapy with *metformin* (e.g., 500 mg twice daily, with breakfast and the evening meal), especially if the patient is overweight. Increase the dose by 500 mg every 1 to 2 weeks as needed until reaching a maximum dose of 2500 mg/d.

■ Alternatively, consider a *second-generation sulfonylurea* (e.g., 2.5 mg of *glyburide*, 5 mg of *glipizide*, or 1 mg of *glimepiride*) as initial monotherapy, particularly if there is a relative contraindication to metformin use (e.g., renal insufficiency). Increase the dose every 1 to 2 weeks as needed and consider twice-daily dosing for glyburide and glipizide to maximize control or once-daily dosing of a sustained-release glipizide. Advance until glycemic goals are achieved or maximum dose is reached (20 mg/d for glyburide and glipizide, 8 mg/d for glimepiride).

■ If after 4 to 8 weeks of monotherapy glycemic goals have not been achieved, then add a second oral agent from a different class (e.g., metformin if a sulfonylurea was given first and vice versa) or add a small dose of an intermediate-acting insulin taken before bedtime (e.g., 10 U of NPH). If the sulfonylurea was the starting drug, reduce the sulfonylurea dose to avoid the risk for prolonged hypoglycemia.

■ If after 4 to 8 weeks of two-drug oral-agent therapy control has not been achieved, then consider adding either a dose of *intermediate insulin* before bed (e.g., 10 U of NPH) or a third oral agent. Adjust the insulin dose according to the results of glucose monitoring.

■ If adding a *thiazolidinedione* (e.g., *pioglitazone, rosiglitazone*), start with a low dose (for pioglitazone, 15 mg/d; for rosiglitazone, 2 mg/d) and monitor liver function (ALT) monthly for at least the first several months, halting therapy at the first sign of persistent elevation. Consider thiazolidinediones only if other attempts have failed to achieve reasonable glycemic control and the patient is reliable, free of underlying liver or cardiovascular disease, and willing to be closely monitored.

■ If a program of insulin supplementation is considered, be aware that initially supplementing oral-agent therapy with a small bedtime dose of insulin may suffice, but usually latter stages of type 2 disease require insulin as the mainstay of the treatment program, supplemented by metformin or a thiazolidinedione (e.g., pioglitazone, rosiglitazone) to reduce insulin resistance and keep the insulin dose manageable.

■ Consider a program of intensive insulin therapy (see Table 102.1) for persons capable of complying with the requirements for frequent testing and insulin administration.

If, after 4 to 8 weeks of diet and exercise, treatment goals have not been achieved and the patient is very symptomatic or manifests *moderate to severe glucose intolerance* (fasting glucose >240 mg/dL), then:

■ Begin *insulin* therapy with an intermediate-acting insulin preparation (NPH) at a modest once-daily dose (e.g., 10 U before breakfast).

■ Specify human recombinant insulin for newly treated diabetic patients to minimize the risks for insulin allergy, insulin resistance, and antibody development.

■ Advance to use of more intensive basal and prandial insulin programs (see Table 102.2) according to the results of glucose monitoring and an estimate of patient capability.

■ If high doses of insulin, poor control, and weight gain become problems, consider adding metformin to the insulin program to improve tissue responsiveness and reduce insulin requirements and weight gain. A thiazolidinedione can also improve insulin responsiveness and control but does not halt weight gain.

Annotated Bibliography

1. American Diabetes Association. Diagnosis and classification of diabetes mellitus (position statement). Diabetes Care 2007;30(Suppl 1:S42). (*Consensus statement and authoritative compendium.*)
2. Campbell PJ, Bolli G, Cryer P, et al. Pathogenesis of the dawn phenomenon in patients with insulin-dependent diabetes mellitus. N Engl J Med 1985;312:1473. (*Physiologic studies implicating growth hormone, not catecholamines, in the preawakening rise in glucose.*)
3. Colditz GA, Willett WC, Rotnitzky A, et al. Weight gain as a risk factor for clinical diabetes mellitus in women. Ann Intern Med 1995;122:481. (*Even a modest weight gain was correlated with a significant increase in the risk for type 2 diabetes.*)
4. DeFronzo RA, Bonadonna RC, Ferrannini E. Pathogenesis of NIDDM. A balanced overview. Diabetes Care 1992;15:315. (*A comprehensive review of hyperinsulinemia and insulin resistance in the pathogenesis of type 2 diabetes.*)
5. Haffner SM, Lehto S, Ronnemaa T, et al. Mortality from coronary heart disease in subjects with type 2 diabetes and in nondiabetic subjects with and without prior myocardial infarction. N Engl J Med 1998;339:229. (*Diabetes confers a degree of risk similar to that associated with prior myocardial infarction.*)
6. Haffner SM, Miettinen H. Insulin resistance implications for type II diabetes mellitus and coronary heart disease. Am J Med 1997;103:152. (*Literature review of the relation of diabetes and insulin resistance to coronary risk and implications for therapy; 106 references.*)
7. Harris R, Donahue K, Rathore SS, et al. Screening adults for type 2 diabetes: a review of the evidence for the U.S. Preventive Services Task Force. Ann Intern Med 2003;138:215. (*Detailed review of the evidence for screening;138 references.*)
8. Reaven GM, Laws A. Insulin resistance, compensatory hyperinsulinemia and coronary heart disease. Diabetologia 1994;37:948. (*Good review of syndrome X pathophysiology.*)
9. Reiber GE, Pecoraro RE, Koepsell TD. Risk factors for amputation in patients with diabetes mellitus. A case–control study. Ann Intern Med 1992;117:97. (*Impaired circulation in the lower extremity was the most powerful predictor, along with neuropathy and low high-density-lipoprotein–cholesterol levels.*)
10. Report of the Expert Committee on the Diagnosis and Classification of Diabetes Mellitus. Diabetes Care 1997;20:1183. (*The first update of diagnostic criteria and classification in almost 20 years; does away with some categories and provides new recommendations for diagnosis.*)
11. Selvin E, Marinopoulos S, Berkenblit G, et al. Meta-analysis: glycosylated hemoglobin and cardiovascular disease in diabetes mellitus. Ann Intern Med 2004;141:421. (*Chronic hyperglycemia is associated with an increased risk for cardiovascular disease in persons with diabetes*).
12. Smieja M, Hunt DL, Edelman D, et al. Clinical examination for the detection of protective sensation in the feet of diabetic patients. J Gen Intern Med 1999;14:418. (*Evidence for the efficacy of monofilament testing.*)
13. Solomon CG, Willet WC, Carey VJ, et al. A prospective study of pregravid determinants of gestational diabetes mellitus. JAMA 1997;278:1078. (*Data from the Nurses' Health Study; advanced maternal age, family history, nonwhite ethnicity, higher body mass index, weight gain in early adulthood, and cigarette smoking were identified as risk factors.*)
14. Tesfaye S, Chaturvedi N, Eaton SEM, et al. Vascular risk factors and diabetic neuropathy. N Engl J Med 2005;352:341. (*The incidence of neuropathy was independently associated with smoking, hypertension, body mass index, and triglyceride level in addition to duration and degree of glycemic control.*)
15. The Expert Committee on the Diagnosis and Classification of Diabetes Mellitus. Follow-up report on the diagnosis of diabetes mellitus. Diabetes Care 2003;26:3160. (*An update revising some of the criteria recommended by an international expert committee in 1997.*)
16. U.S. Preventive Services Task Force. Screening for type 2 diabetes mellitus in adults: recommendations and rationale. Ann Intern Med 2003;138:212.

(Concluded that the evidence was insufficient to recommend for or against screening asymptomatic adults.)

17. Wackers FJT, Young LH, Inzucchi SE, et al. Detection of silent myocardial ischemia in asymptomatic diabetic subjects: the DIAD study. Diabetes Care 2004;27:1954. *(Silent myocardial ischemia occurs in greater than one in five asymptomatic patients with type 2 diabetes.)*

18. Ahren B. Dipeptidyl peptidase-4 inhibitors: clinical data and clinical implications. Diabetes Care 2007;30:1344. *(Good review of results with sitagliptin and vildagliptin in type 2 diabetes.)*

19. American Diabetes Association. Standards of medical care in diabetes (position statement). Diabetes Care 2007;30(Suppl 1:S4). *(A consensus position paper; 223 references.)*

20. American Diabetes Association. Nutrition recommendations and interventions for diabetes (position statement). Diabetes Care 2007;30(Suppl 1):S48). *(Evidence-based recommendations and interventions; 119 references.)*

21. Aschner P, Kipnes MS, Lunceford JK, et al. Effect of the dipeptidyl peptidase-4 inhibitor sitagliptin as monotherapy on glycemic control in patients with type 2 diabetes. Diabetes Care 2006;29:2632. *(Finds improvement in glycemic control.)*

22. Aubert RE, Herman WH, Waters J, et al. Nurse case management to improve glycemic control in diabetic patients in a health maintenance organization: a randomized, controlled trial. Ann Intern Med 1998;129:605. *(Glycemic control improved in this collaborative effort between physicians and nurse practitioners.)*

23. Aviles-Santa L, Sinding J, Raskin P. Effects of metformin in patients with poorly controlled insulin-treated type 2 diabetes mellitus: a randomized, double-blind, placebo-controlled trial. Ann Intern Med 1999;131:182. *(Strong evidence for the effectiveness of adding metformin to an insulin program.)*

24. Backonja M, Beydoun A, Edwards KR, et al. Gabapentin for the symptomatic treatment of painful neuropathy in patients with diabetes mellitus: a randomized controlled trial. JAMA 1998;280:1831. *(A placebo-controlled, randomized, controlled trial [RCT]; the treatment was found significantly to reduce pain and improve quality of life; there was no comparison with other agents.)*

25. Barnett AH, Bain SC, Bouter P, et al. Angiotensin-receptor blockade versus converting-enzyme inhibition in type 2 diabetes and nephropathy. N Engl J Med 2004;351:1952. *(Major RCT finding equivalent renal protection.)*

26. Barringer TA, Kirk JK, Santaniello AC, et al. Effect of a multivitamin supplement on infection and quality of life: a randomized, double-blind, placebo-controlled trial. Ann Intern Med 2003;138:365. *(Significant reduction was found in the rate of self-reported infection in diabetes, especially in patients with evidence of micronutrient deficiency.)*

27. Boden G, Sargrad K, Homko C, et al. Effect of low-carbohydrate diet on appetite, blood glucose levels, and insulin resistance in obese patients with type 2 diabetes. Ann Intern Med 2005;142:403. *(Two-week research unit study; weight loss and improvements in triglycerides, glycemic control, and cholesterol were noted.)*

28. Bolen S, Feldman L, Vassy J, et al. Systematic review: comparative effectiveness and safety of oral medications for type 2 diabetes mellitus. Ann Intern Med 2007;147:386. *(Meta-analysis raising question of enhanced cardiovascular risk with thiazolidinediones.)*

29. Boule NG, Haddad E, Kenny GP, et al. Effects of exercise on glycemic control and body mass in type 2 diabetes mellitus: a meta-analysis of controlled clinical trials. JAMA 2001;286:1218. *(Exercise resulted in a significant reduction in hemoglobin A [HbA_1c] independent of any effect on weight.)*

30. Brenner BM, Cooper ME, de Zeeuw D, et al. Effects of losartan on renal and cardiovascular outcomes in patients with type 2 diabetes and nephropathy. N Engl J Med 2001;345:861. *(Major RCT, demonstrating the ability of this angiotensin-receptor blocker significantly to slow progression of nephropathy in type 2 patients.)*

31. Ceglia L, Lau J, Pittas AG. Meta-analysis: efficacy and safety of inhaled insulin therapy in adults with diabetes mellitus. Ann Intern Med 2006;145:665. *(Found to be slightly less effective than subcutaneously administered short-acting insulin but more acceptable.)*

32. Chiasson JL, Josse RG, Hunt JA, et al. The efficacy of acarbose in the treatment of patients with non–insulin-dependent diabetes mellitus: a multicenter controlled clinical trial. Ann Intern Med 1994;121:928. *(The treatment provided moderate benefit when used as monotherapy or when added to an existing program.)*

33. Crowther CA, Hiller JE, Moss JR, et al. Effect of treatment of gestational diabetes mellitus on pregnancy outcomes. N Engl J Med 2005;352:2477. *(RCT; treatment reduced perinatal morbidity and improved quality of life.)*

34. DeFronzo RA, Goodman AM, and the Multicenter Metformin Study Group. Efficacy of metformin in patients with non–insulin-dependent diabetes mellitus. N Engl J Med 1995;333:541. *(Major RCT comparing metformin, glyburide, combination therapy, and placebo in obese patients.)*

35. DeFronzo RA, Ratner RE, Han J, et al. Effects of exenatide (Exendin-4) on glycemic control and weight over 30 weeks in metformin-treated patients with type 2 diabetes. Diabetes Care 2005;28:1092. *(Exenatide was well tolerated and reduced HbA_1c with no weight gain in patients failing to achieve glycemic control with metformin.)*

36. Diabetes Control and Complications Trial Research Group. The effect of intensive diabetes therapy on the development and progression of neuropathy. Ann Intern Med 1995;122:561. *(Risks for the development of neuropathy and the progression of existing neuropathy were significantly reduced.)*

37. Diabetes Control and Complications Trial/Epidemiology of Diabetes Interventions and Complications (DCCT/EDIC) Study Research Group. Long-term effect of diabetes and its treatment on cognitive function. N Engl J Med 2007;356:1842. *(An 18-year longitudinal cohort study of 1,144 patients finding no decline in cognitive function.)*

38. Diabetes Control and Complications Trial/Epidemiology of Diabetes Interventions and Complications (DCCT/EDIC) Study Research Group. Intensive diabetes treatment and cardiovascular disease in patients with type 1 diabetes. N Engl J Med 2005;353:2643. *(Intensive treatment reduced the risk of any cardiovascular disease by 42%.)*

39. Diabetes Control and Complications Trial Research Group. Effect of intensive therapy on residual β-cell function in patients with type 1 diabetes in the Diabetes Control and Complications Trial: a randomized, controlled trial. Ann Intern Med 1998;128:517. *(Early onset of intensive therapy helped to preserve beta-cell function, which facilitated control and reduced the risk for hypoglycemia.)*

40. Diabetes Control and Complications Trial Research Group. The effect of intensive treatment of diabetes on the development and progression of long-term complications in insulin-dependent diabetes mellitus. N Engl J Med 1993;329:977. *(Landmark RCT; demonstrated dramatic reductions in retinopathy, proteinuria, and clinical neuropathy.)*

41. Diabetes Prevention Program Research Group. Reduction in the incidence of type 2 diabetes with lifestyle intervention or metformin. N Engl J Med 2002;346:393. *(Multicenter RCT; both lifestyle modification and metformin prevented the onset of type 2 disease, with lifestyle modification more effective.)*

42. Drucker DJ. Dipeptidyl peptidase-4 inhibition and the treatment of type 2 diabetes: preclinical biology and mechanisms of action. Diabetes Care 2007;30:1335. *(Nice background discussion accompanying the clinical paper by Ahren, ref. 18.)*

43. Fanelli CG, Pampanelli S, Porcellati F, et al. Administration of neutral protamine Hagedorn insulin at bedtime versus with dinner in type 1 diabetes mellitus to avoid nocturnal hypoglycemia and improve control. Ann Intern Med 2002;136:504. *(Randomized, open-labeled, crossover trial; bedtime dosing was superior.)*

44. Gaede P, Vedel P, Larsen N, et al. Multifactorial intervention and cardiovascular disease in patients with type 2 diabetes. N Engl J Med 2003;348:383. *(Steno-2 study; multifactorial intervention using behavior modification and polypharmacologic therapy reduced the risk of cardiovascular and microvascular events by about 50%).*

45. Golan L, Birkenmeyer JD, Welch HG. The cost-effectiveness of treating all patients with type 2 diabetes with angiotensin-converting enzyme inhibitors. Ann Intern Med 1999;131:660. *(Finds that treating all middle-aged diabetic patients can be cost-effective.)*

46. Heine RJ, Van Gaal LF, Johns D, et al. Exenatide versus insulin glargine in patients with suboptimally controlled type 2 diabetes: a randomized trial. Ann Intern Med 2005;143:559. *(Similar improvements in glycemic control were found; there was weight loss with exenatide but also more gastrointestinal upset.)*

47. Hirsch IB. Insulin analogues. N Engl J Med 2005;353:174. *(Excellent review; 67 references.)*

48. Home PD, Pocock SJ, Beck-Nielsen H, et al. Rosiglitazone evaluated for cardiovascular outcomes—an interim analysis. N Engl J Med 2007;357:28 *(An unplanned analysis of the RECORD study; mean follow-up was only 3.75 years; the findings were inconclusive regarding the risk of hospitalization or death from cardiovascular causes; data were insufficient to establish an increased risk of myocardial infarction, but they did confirm an increased risk of heart failure.)*

49. Jovanovic-Peterson L, Peterson CM. Pregnancy in the diabetic woman. Endocrinol Metab Clin North Am 1992;21:433. *(A comprehensive review supporting the normalization of blood sugar and the management necessary to achieve tight control.)*

50. Jenkins DJA, Thomas DM, Wolever MS, et al. Glycemic index of foods: a physiological basis for carbohydrate exchange. Am J Clin Nutr 1981;34:362. *(The glycemic effects of various carbohydrates; beans cause less hyperglycemia than do potatoes or corn.)*

51. Kahn SE, Haffner SM, Heise MA, et al. Glycemic durability of rosiglitazone, metformin, or glyburide monotherapy. N Engl J Med 2006;355:2427. *(Rare head-to-head RCT; the cumulative incidence of monotherapy failure at 5 years was 15% with rosiglitazone, 21% with metformin, and 34% with glyburide.)*

52. Kerr EA, Gerzoff RB, Krein SL, et al. Diabetes care quality in the Veterans Affairs health care system and commercial managed care: the TRIAD Study. Ann Intern Med 2004;141:272. *(A cross-sectional patient survey with a retrospective review of patient records, finding that care in the reorganized Veterans Administration system was better in two of three outcome measures, but there was room for improvement in both.)*

53. Kipnes MS, Krosnick A, Rendell MS, et al. Pioglitazone hydrochloride in combination with sulfonylurea therapy improves glycemic control in patients with type 2 diabetes mellitus: a randomized, placebo-controlled study. Am J Med 2001;111:10. (*A combination of pioglitazone plus sulfonylurea significantly improved HbA$_{1c}$ fasting plasma glucose levels and had beneficial effects on serum triglyceride and high-density-lipoprotein–cholesterol levels.*)

54. Kirpichnikov D, McFarlane SI, Sowers JR. Metformin: an update. Ann Intern Med 2002;137:25. (*A review of the biguanide metformin; 102 references.*)

55. Lewis EJ, Hunsicker LG, Bain RP, et al. Effect of angiotensin-converting enzyme inhibition on diabetic nephropathy. N Engl J Med 1993;329:1456. (*There was a marked reduction in proteinuria and progression to renal failure; an important advance.*)

56. MacKenzie CR, Charlson ME. Assessment of perioperative risk in the patient with diabetes mellitus. Surg Gynecol Obstet 1988;167:293. (*End-organ consequences of diabetes, rather than hyperglycemia per se, predict infectious and renal complications of surgery.*)

57. Mayer-Davis EJ, D'Agostino R, Karter AJ, et al. Intensity and amount of physical activity in relation to insulin sensitivity: the Insulin Resistance Atherosclerosis Study. JAMA 1998;279:669. (*All forms of exercise improved insulin sensitivity.*)

58. Metchick LN, Petit WA, Inzucchi SE. Inpatient management of diabetes mellitus. Am J Med 2002;113:317. (*Discusses the need for improving glycemic control of hospitalized diabetic patients and proposes guidelines for management.*)

59. Mooradian AD, Bernbaum M, Albert SG. Narrative review: a rational approach to starting insulin therapy. Ann Intern Med 2006;145:125. (*Nice discussion of the various insulin preparations and suggestions for initiating insulin therapy.*)

60. Nathan DM, Buse JB, Davidson MB, et al. Management of hyperglycemia in type 2 diabetes: a consensus algorithm for the initiation and adjustment of therapy: a consensus statement from the American Diabetes Association and the European Association for the Study of Diabetes. Diabetes Care 2006;29:1963. (*Basic consensus guidelines; recommends early initiation of lifestyle modification and metformin.*)

61. Nissen SE, Wolski K. Effect of rosiglitazone on the risk of myocardial infarction and death from cardiovascular causes. N Engl J Med 2007;356:2457. (*Meta-analysis of 42 trials; a significant increase was found in the risk of myocardial infarction.*)

62. Purnell JQ, Hokanson JE, Marcovina SM, et al. Effect of excessive weight gain with intensive therapy of type 1 diabetes on lipid levels and blood pressure: results from the DCCT. JAMA 1998;280:140. (*Intensive therapy was found to induce weight gain, which was associated with elevations in blood pressure and lipids.*)

63. Rosenstock J, Hassman DR, Madder RD, et al. Repaglinide versus nateglinide monotherapy: a randomized, multicenter study. Diabetes Care 2004:27:1265. (*Despite similar postprandial glycemic effects, treatment with 16 weeks of monotherapy with repaglinide was significantly more effective than nateglinide monotherapy in reducing HbA1C and fasting plasma glucose.*)

64. Saudek CD, Duckworth WC, Giobbie-Hurder A, et al. Implantable insulin pump vs. multiple-dose insulin for non–insulin-dependent diabetes

65. mellitus: a randomized clinical trial. JAMA 1996;276:1996. (*A good comparison study revealing relative risks and benefits.*)

65. Shapiro AMJ, Ricordi C, Hering BJ, et al. International trial of the Edmonton Protocol for islet transplantation. N Engl J Med 2006;355:1318. (*Report of success in 36 patients.*)

66. Sigal RJ, Kenny GP, Wasserman DH, et al. Physical activity/exercise and type 2 diabetes. Diabetes Care 2004;27:2518. (*Detailed review;190 references.*)

67. Snow V, Weiss KB, Mottur-Pilson C. The evidence base for tight blood pressure control in the management of type 2 diabetes mellitus. Ann Intern Med 2003;138:587. (*Recommendations for blood pressure management in diabetes.*)

68. Stenmans S, Melander A, Groop PH, et al. What is the benefit of increasing the sulfonylurea dose? Ann Intern Med 1993;118:169. (*Little benefit is found above the equivalent of 15 mg of glyburide per day.*)

69. Tallarigo L, Giampietro O, Penno G, et al. Relation of glucose tolerance to complications of pregnancy in nondiabetic women. N Engl J Med 1986;315:989. (*Even limited degrees of glucose intolerance during pregnancy were associated with increased risks for macrosomia and its attendant complications.*)

70. Turner RC, Cull CA, Frighi V, et al. Glycemic control diet, sulfonylurea, metformin, or insulin in patients with type 2 diabetes mellitus: progressive requirement for multiple therapies (UKPDS 49). JAMA 1999;281:2005. (*The control declined markedly by 9 years after diagnosis in this report from the 20-year prospective, randomized United Kingdom Prospective Diabetes Study.*)

71. United Kingdom Prospective Diabetes Study Group. Tight blood pressure control reduced diabetes mellitus–related deaths and complications and was cost-effective in type 2 diabetes (UKPDS 38). BMJ 1998;317:703. (*Evidence for the importance of aggressive treatment of cardiovascular risk factors in diabetes.*)

72. United Kingdom Prospective Diabetes Study Group. Intensive blood glucose control with sulphonylureas or insulin compared with conventional treatment and risk of complications in patients with type 2 diabetes (UKPDS 33). Lancet 1998;352:837. (*Landmark 20-year RCT; confirmed that, as in type 1 disease, the risk for microvascular complications is reduced by tight control.*)

73. United Kingdom Prospective Diabetes Study Group. Effect of intensive blood-glucose control with metformin on complications in overweight patients with type 2 diabetes (UKPDS 34). Lancet 1998;352:54. (*The first documented reduction in macrovascular complications with intensive therapy.*)

74. United Kingdom Prospective Diabetes Study Group. A 6-year randomized, controlled trial comparing sulfonylurea, insulin, and metformin therapy in patients with newly diagnosed type 2 diabetes that could not be controlled with diet therapy (UKPDS 24). Ann Intern Med 1998;128:165. (*Therapy with an oral agent proved just as effective as insulin and caused less weight gain and fewer hypoglycemic episodes.*)

75. Vijan S, Hayward RA. Treatment of hypertension in type 2 diabetes mellitus: blood pressure goals, choice of agents, and setting priorities in diabetes care. Ann Intern Med 2003;138:593. (*Improved blood pressure control reduced the risks for cardiovascular complications; 73 references.*)

76. Yki-Jarvinen H, Ryysy S, Nikkila K, et al. Comparison of bedtime insulin regimens in patients with type 2 diabetes mellitus: a randomized, controlled trial. Ann Intern Med 1999;130:389. (*Evidence for the effectiveness of combining metformin with bedtime insulin.*)

CHAPTER 103 ■ APPROACH TO THE PATIENT WITH HYPERTHYROIDISM

DAVID M. SLOVIK

Hyperthyroidism is the clinical expression of a heterogeneous group of disorders that produce elevations of free thyroxine (T$_4$), triiodothyronine (T$_3$), or both. Well-recognized causes of hyperthyroidism include diffuse toxic goiter (Graves' disease), toxic multinodular goiter, toxic adenoma (toxic nodule),

excessive ingestion of thyroid hormone, and iodine excess (Jod-Basedow phenomenon). Transient hyperthyroidism has been noted in the settings of chronic lymphocytic (Hashimoto's) thyroiditis, subacute (granulomatous) thyroiditis, and postpartum thyroiditis. An increasingly frequent presentation is subclinical hyperthyroidism, encountered during routine screening for hypothyroidism or diagnosed during evaluation for a nonthyroid problem such as new onset of atrial fibrillation or osteoporosis.

Hyperthyroidism is relatively common and much more likely to occur in women than in men. Community-based studies have found a prevalence of 1.9% in women and 0.16% in men. Approximately 15% of recognized cases occur in persons older than the age of 60 years. The clinical presentation of hyperthyroidism in the elderly is often atypical. The primary physician should be able to recognize hyperthyroidism, identify its cause, and design a therapeutic program appropriate to the patient's underlying pathophysiology, age, clinical condition, and personal preferences. The indications and limitations of surgery, radioiodine therapy, and antithyroid agents must be understood.

PATHOPHYSIOLOGY, CLINICAL PRESENTATION, AND COURSE (1–14)

The pathophysiologic common denominator of hyperthyroidism is an excess of circulating thyroid hormone. The mechanisms responsible for this excess include stimulation of thyroid-stimulating hormone (TSH) receptors by immunoglobulins, autonomous thyroid hormone production, increased release of thyroid hormone without increased production, increased production of TSH, and intake of exogenous hormone.

Thyroid hormone stimulates calorigenesis and catabolism and enhances sensitivity to catecholamines. Excessive amounts of the hormone lead to the classic picture of *heat intolerance, nervousness, hyperactivity, tremor, increased appetite, weight loss, excessive sweating, palpitations, lid lag, stare,* and *muscle weakness.* Diarrhea or, more precisely, *frequent defecation,* may also ensue. *Muscle weakness* and *sexual dysfunction* are reported in persons with chronic disease. A reversible picture of *left-ventricular dysfunction* may emerge, and the risk of *atrial fibrillation/flutter* is increased. Elevations in *alkaline phosphatase* and *angiotensin-converting enzyme* may accompany thyrotoxicosis and persist even after treatment. The pathophysiologic significance of these elevations is unclear.

In the elderly thyrotoxic patient, the characteristic systemic manifestations of hyperthyroidism may be absent and the clinical picture, referred to as *apathetic hyperthyroidism of the elderly,* is instead dominated by *apathy, weight loss,* and otherwise *unexplained atrial fibrillation.* The condition can mimic depression and occult malignancy.

Another atypical presentation is that of subclinical hyperthyroidism, characterized by very low or undetectable levels of TSH and normal to high-normal levels of thyroid hormone. Patients may be asymptomatic or manifest subtle symptoms or signs, such as new onset of atrial fibrillation or osteoporosis (see later discussion).

Graves' Disease

Graves' disease is an autoimmune condition in which an apparent deficiency of thyroid-specific suppressor T cell lymphocytes allows a *thyroid-stimulating immunoglobulin G antibody* (*TSab*) to form. TSab (also referred to as *thyrotropin-receptor antibody*) binds to TSH receptors on the surface of thyroid cells and triggers the synthesis of excess thyroid hormone.

Other thyroid autoimmune responses are also present. Graves' disease is the most common disorder causing hyperthyroidism and accounts for 85% to 90% of cases seen in persons younger than age 40 years and for 70% in those older than age 60 years.

Ophthalmopathy

Ophthalmopathy can be a troubling accompaniment of Graves' disease, affecting about 40% of patients. It is a consequence of antibody-mediated inflammation and infiltration. TSab does not appear to be directly involved, although the onset of ophthalmopathy generally parallels that of the hyperthyroidism. Antibodies to extraocular muscle and orbital fibroblasts capable of inducing *in vitro* the pathologic changes found *in vivo* have been detected. The inflammatory infiltrate produces swelling of retroorbital tissue, which compresses orbital veins and leads to orbital edema and proptosis. Inflammatory changes of the extraocular muscles may cause diplopia. In general, the eye problems develop concurrently with the onset of hyperthyroidism and change little once established, although up to 20% of patients may experience a gradual worsening with treatment (see later discussion). Approximately 10% of patients show similar eye findings in the absence of Graves' disease. Manifestations range from lid retraction and stare, mild periorbital edema, and conjunctival inflammation to extraocular muscle dysfunction, corneal injury, and optic nerve damage. The lid lag and stare of hyperthyroidism may make the ophthalmopathy look worse than it actually is. Other associated ocular symptoms include pain, diplopia, proptosis, and blurred vision. The cosmetic changes may be among the most disturbing.

Thyroid Dermapathy (Pretibial Myxedema)

Thyroid dermapathy is a less common immune-mediated infiltrative process that affects less than 5% of patients with Graves' disease. It never occurs alone and almost always occurs in the presence of moderate or severe ophthalmopathy. The condition is characterized by the appearance of nonpitting swelling, indurated nontender plaques with brownish, reddish, dark pink, or purple color and an "orange-skin" appearance primarily limited to the skin of the pretibial area. Rarely, the lower leg can be extensively involved, giving the appearance of elephantiasis. *Thyroid acropachy,* characterized by clubbing and soft tissue swelling of the distal fingers and toes, is also rare.

Other Manifestations

The thyroid gland in Graves' disease is *diffusely enlarged,* and a *bruit* may be heard in severe cases. The classic symptoms and signs of thyrotoxicosis are common. The skin is velvety and the hair silky. *Onycholysis, vitiligo,* and *gynecomastia* are found in some cases and may suggest the diagnosis. Cardiac complications are infrequent because of the relative youth of the patient population, but a reversible *cardiomyopathy* has been identified, manifested by a fall in the ejection fraction with exercise. Heart failure is rare, but *impaired exercise tolerance* is often reported, perhaps caused by the decreased ejection fraction.

Clinical Course

The clinical course of Graves' disease usually worsens if it is untreated, although patients with mild disease may have exacerbations and remissions of unpredictable duration. After many years, mild hypothyroidism may ensue, especially in patients with small goiters and mild hyperthyroidism at the time of onset.

Toxic Multinodular Goiter (Plummer's Disease)

Toxic multinodular goiter (Plummer's disease) accounts for an increasing proportion of cases of hyperthyroidism in middle-aged and elderly persons. The condition, often associated with a long-standing simple goiter, results from diffuse hyperplasia of thyroid follicular cells whose activity becomes independent of TSH regulation. The gland is clinically and pathologically indistinguishable from the gland of patients with nontoxic multinodular goiters.

Toxic multinodular goiter tends to be more common in areas of *iodine deficiency*. Patients may have subclinical hyperthyroidism or the more typical symptoms of hyperthyroidism, but cardiovascular symptoms can dominate the clinical presentation; new onset of heart failure, atrial fibrillation, palpitations, or angina reflects the high prevalence of coexisting organic heart disease in this older population. Some may present with anorexia and constipation. Lid lag may be noted on occasion, but exophthalmos does not occur. Sometimes, apathy and weight loss are the most prominent clinical features and can be so profound as to suggest occult malignancy or severe depression.

Risk of progression to overt hyperthyroidism is about 5%/yr. Recent exposure to *iodides*—for example, iodinated contrast agents and the iodine-containing antiarrhythmic drug *amiodarone*—may precipitate overt hyperthyroidism or even thyrotoxicosis (see later discussion).

Single Toxic Nodule ("Hot" Nodule)

The autonomously functioning toxic nodule presents clinically much like the toxic multinodular goiter. The principal difference is the finding of a "hot" nodule surrounded by suppressed gland on radioiodine thyroid scan. The larger the nodule, the greater is its propensity to cause thyrotoxicosis, with the risk quite high once the nodule reaches 3 cm in diameter. Often, the onset of toxicity is first manifested by an isolated increase in serum T_3 levels; later, T_4 levels rise. Sometimes, hemorrhagic infarction terminates the overproduction of hormone and limits the progression to thyrotoxicosis.

Triiodothyronine Toxicosis

Triiodothyronine toxicosis is an important entity to consider when patients with clinically apparent hyperthyroidism have *normal T_4 levels*. The condition has been reported in association with both *diffuse* and *nodular goiters*. The clinical presentation is no different from that of hyperthyroidism caused by elevations in T_4. Isolated elevations in T_3 concentration may also occur in euthyroid patients who have no underlying thyroid disease (see later discussion).

Transient Hyperthyroidism

Transient hyperthyroidism may occur in association with *subacute (granulomatous), chronic (lymphocytic) thyroiditis* and *postpartum thyroiditis*. As noted, the mechanism appears to be uncontrolled release of hormone from an inflamed gland. Iodine uptake is reduced during the period of hyperthyroidism. The clinical manifestations of hyperthyroidism are usually mild. The course is self-limited, and hypothyroidism often follows as intrathyroidal stores of the hormone are depleted.

Iodine-Induced Hyperthyroidism (Jod-Basedow)

Iodine excess can result in unregulated thyroid hormone production especially in glands that have underlying pathology. It can develop after an iodine load—for example, contrast agents for angiography or computed tomography scanning—or with iodine-containing drugs such as *amiodarone* (see later discussion). The risk of iodine-induced thyrotoxicosis is greatest in elderly patients with large, nontoxic nodular goiters who come from areas where iodine intake is low (e.g., Europe). The problem can also occur in nonendemic cases of multinodular goiter and thyroid adenoma, in which the mechanism involves increased release of stored hormone. Characteristic laboratory findings include a low uptake of radioactive iodine and an absence of antithyroid antibodies.

Amiodarone-Induced Thyroiditis

Amiodarone, an iodinated drug with antiarrhythmic and antianginal properties, can precipitate hyperthyroidism. Type 1 amiodarone-induced thyrotoxicosis, a form of iodine-induced thyrotoxicosis, occurs in patients with underlying thyroid disease (nodular goiter, Graves' disease) and results from overproduction of thyroid hormone using iodine as a substrate. Type 2, a destructive thyroiditis, occurs in normal thyroids, and the hyperthyroidism is due to excess release, not synthesis of thyroid hormone. Distinguishing these two types can be difficult. In type 1, the gland is often enlarged because it occurs in patients with nodular goiters; in type 2, a small goiter or a small gland may be present. Color-flow Doppler studies have shown that blood flow is increased in type 1 and decreased in type 2.

Subacute Thyroiditis

Subacute thyroiditis typically follows a viral illness, producing a *tender, multinodular* gland. The occasional case associated with hyperthyroidism has an abrupt onset characterized by thyrotoxic symptoms. The erythrocyte sedimentation rate is high, and a thyroid scan characteristically shows little or no uptake of radioiodine.

Lymphocytic Thyroiditis

Lymphocytic thyroiditis resulting in hyperthyroidism is believed to be an uncommon variant of Hashimoto's disease. In some cases, it may be caused by coexisting Graves' disease. High titers of antibodies to microsomes and thyroglobulin are present. The prevalence is highest in middle-aged women and among the elderly, in whom it may go unrecognized. The gland feels rubbery and is enlarged, sometimes asymmetrically. Hypothyroidism eventually develops in a substantial number of cases.

Postpartum (Subacute Lymphocytic) Thyroiditis

Postpartum (subacute lymphocytic) thyroiditis, a previously unappreciated but surprisingly frequent problem (incidence as high as 5% in one series), can precipitate transient mild hyperthyroidism. The onset is within 3 to 6 months of delivery, and the condition often is mistaken for anxiety associated with the stress of caring for a new baby. The gland is nontender and may resemble that of Hashimoto's thyroiditis. A low uptake of radioactive iodine and the detection of antithyroid antibodies suggest an immunologic mechanism. The condition may persist for months before eventually resolving. A period of hypothyroidism may occur before the condition abates. It tends to recur with subsequent pregnancies.

Overproduction of Thyroid-Stimulating Hormone

A small number of *pituitary adenomas* produce excessive TSH. The result is a diffusely enlarged gland simulating that of Graves' disease, but ophthalmopathy does not occur. A similar clinical picture may be caused by a tumor producing human chorionic gonadotropin (hCG), such as a *hydatidiform mole* or a *choriocarcinoma*. The thyroid-stimulating activity of hCG is weak, but when it is produced in massive quantities, it can cause hyperthyroidism.

Ectopic Thyroxine Production and Intake of Exogenous Hormone

When the source of excess thyroid hormone is extrathyroidal, the thyroid gland will appear small because of the absence of TSH stimulation. A dermoid tumor of the ovary, *struma ovarii*, with elements of thyroid-like tissue, is the only neoplasm regularly capable of synthesizing excessive amounts of thyroid hormone. (Rarely, thyroid cancers can cause hyperthyroidism, but only in the context of a massive tumor burden.) The intake of thyroid hormone in excess of daily requirements (>200 μg of levothyroxine per day) may make a person hyperthyroid. Sometimes, the intake is surreptitious. The gland is small, and TSH is absent.

Subclinical Hyperthyroidism

Subclinical hyperthyroidism is characterized by low or undetectable levels of TSH in the setting of normal (usually high-

normal) levels of free T_4 and T_3. The most common cause is the excess intake of thyroid hormone, either for the treatment of hypothyroidism or for suppressing the growth of a goiter. Other causes include an autonomously functioning goiter and mild Graves' disease. Subtle symptoms or signs of thyrotoxicosis may be present. Risks associated with this state include a moderately increased frequency of atrial fibrillation in the elderly and osteoporosis in postmenopausal women. In exogenous disease, T_3 tends to be normal but thyroxine levels are either at the upper end of the normal range or frankly elevated. In endogenous disease, both the T_3 and thyroxine levels are at the upper end of normal.

DIFFERENTIAL DIAGNOSIS

The differential diagnosis of hyperthyroidism can be organized according to pathophysiology (Table 103.1). The most common cause is Graves' disease, followed by multinodular goiter, toxic adenoma, thyroiditis, and exogenous thyroid hormone. Pituitary adenoma, struma ovarii, and chorionic cancers are very rare causes.

WORKUP (7,13,15–20)

Diagnosing Hyperthyroidism

Clinical recognition of hyperthyroidism can sometimes be difficult, especially when the classic symptoms noted earlier are mild or when the condition occurs in an elderly or pregnant patient. Moreover, the correlation between symptoms and thyroid hormone levels is often poor, so that careful laboratory confirmation of the diagnosis and the severity of the condition are necessary.

Thyroid-Stimulating Hormone Determination

Determination of the serum TSH is the most sensitive way to screen for hyperthyroidism. A marked improvement in the sensitivity of the TSH assay makes it possible to diagnose hyperthyroidism solely on the basis of an absence of detectable TSH. Most patients with overt hyperthyroidism have TSH levels of less than 0.05 μU/mL. As long as the hypothalamic–pituitary axis is intact, an absence of detectible TSH represents the

TABLE 103.1

CAUSES OF HYPERTHYROIDISM

Pathophysiology	Cause
Autonomous hormone production	Toxic multinodular goiter
	Toxic adenoma
Increased hormone release	Subacute thyroiditis
	Lymphocytic (Hashimoto's) thyroiditis
	Iodide exposure
Increased glandular stimulation	Graves' disease (TSab)
	Functioning pituitary adenoma (TSH)
	Choriocarcinoma (hCG)
Exogenous hormone intake	Intake of >200 μg of levothyroxine per day
Extraglandular production	Struma ovarii
	Metastatic thyroid cancer

hCG, human chorionic gonadotropin; TSab, thyroid-stimulating antibody; TSH, thyroid-stimulating hormone.

appropriate response to too much circulating thyroid hormone. Undetectable TSH by second- or third-generation assay is diagnostic of hyperthyroidism. A normal TSH level by radioimmunoassay virtually rules out hyperthyroidism, unless a rare TSH-secreting pituitary adenoma is present.

A very low TSH level may result from severe nonthyroidal illness and from the use of drugs that suppress TSH response to thyroid hormone (e.g., glucocorticosteroids). In such circumstances, thyroid hormone levels are usually abnormal. Subclinical hyperthyroidism is suggested by a very low or undetectable TSH and thyroid hormone levels that are normal, typically at the upper end of the normal range.

Thyroid Hormone Levels

The sensitivity of second- and third-generation TSH assays has markedly reduced the need for thyroid hormone determinations in screening for hyperthyroidism. They can, however, help to confirm the diagnosis and determine the severity of disease and should be obtained when the TSH level is low or undetectable. The *free* T_4 or *free* T_4 *index* (an excellent proxy for the free T_4, calculated by multiplying the serum T_4 by the T_3 resin uptake) is the most useful and consequently the preferred determination of circulating thyroid hormone. The serum *total* T_3 concentration is elevated along with T_4 in most hyperthyroid states. In the uncommon case of T_3 toxicosis, T_3 is elevated when T_4 levels are normal.

As useful as thyroid hormone levels are for diagnosis, overreliance on them and failure to use the TSH assay can be misleading. *Euthyroid hyperthyroxemia* occurs when an increase in thyroid-binding globulin (e.g., pregnancy, estrogen use, liver disease) produces an increase in total T_4, whereas the free T_4 remains normal. More confusing are euthyroid states with increases in both free and total T_4. Patients with autoantibodies against thyroid hormones may manifest surprisingly high levels of free hormone because of interference by these immunoglobulins with the standard radioimmune assays for thyroid hormones. Acute medical, surgical, and psychiatric illnesses, in addition to intake of high doses of propranolol, amiodarone, and gallbladder dyes, can impair the peripheral conversion of T_4 to active T_3 and lead to a rise in free T_4 concentration in conjunction with a reduction in T_3 and an increase in reverse T_3. An unexpectedly normal or low T_3 level in a patient who is clinically euthyroid but has elevated T_4 and free T_4 levels should suggest the possibility of euthyroid hyperthyroxemia. The T_3 concentration helps in the differentiation.

Antithyroid Antibodies

Antithyroid antibodies (particularly those directed against *microsomal peroxidase*) are increased in both Graves' disease and lymphocytic (Hashimoto's) thyroiditis, so their diagnostic utility is limited. *Thyroid-stimulating immunoglobulin G antibody* (also referred to as *thyrotropin-receptor antibody*) can be measured to help in identifying persons with Grave's disease.

Thyroglobulin Levels

Determination serves as an elegant yet simple means of detecting a patient who is surreptitiously taking thyroid hormone—exogenous hormone use results in the suppression of thyroglobulin synthesis.

Radionuclide Thyroid Scan

The 24-hour radioiodine uptake can help to distinguish between excess endogenous thyroid synthesis (high uptake) and increased release of preformed hormone due to inflammation or glandular destruction or an extrathyroidal source (low uptake). A *"hot nodule"* is characteristic of a toxic adenoma, with little uptake by the rest of the gland. Uptake is low in patients with thyroiditis, exogenous hormone intake, extraglandular hormone production, and iodide exposure. Uptake is diffusely increased in patients with Graves' disease or a functioning pituitary adenoma. *Whole-body scanning* can identify the rare cases of extrathyroidal hormone synthesis, such as occurs in a struma ovarii or a metastasis from a thyroid malignancy.

Other Laboratory Tests

A host of nonspecific hematologic and serum chemistry abnormalities may accompany hyperthyroidism, including a mild degree of anemia, granulocytosis, lymphocytosis, hypercalcemia, hypercalciuria, and elevations in transaminases and alkaline phosphatase. These abnormalities are of little help diagnostically and do not warrant testing for them.

Identifying the Underlying Cause

Etiologic assessment should proceed once the diagnosis of hyperthyroidism has been confirmed because treatment based on such an assessment is usually the most successful.

History

Inquiry should be made into goiter, thyroid nodule, use of iodides or thyroid hormone, eye changes, recent pregnancy, or viral illness and known ovarian, pituitary, or thyroid neoplasm. A review of systems should include a search for symptoms of a pituitary tumor (see Chapters 100 and 101).

Physical Examination

Physical examination focuses on the *thyroid gland*, with a check for overall size and nodularity. A diffusely enlarged, nontender gland suggests Graves' disease; in rare instances, a TSH-secreting tumor may be responsible for such diffuse glandular stimulation. A bruit may accompany the diffusely enlarged gland of Graves' disease. An exquisitely tender, diffusely enlarged gland occurring in the context of a viral illness points to subacute thyroiditis. The gland in lymphocytic thyroiditis is nontender and diffusely, but only modestly, enlarged. A small gland indicates an extrathyroidal source of hormone. Multinodularity is consistent with a toxic multinodular goiter and also occurs in patients with Hashimoto's thyroiditis. An otherwise atrophic gland with a single nodule, especially if larger than 3 cm in diameter, strongly suggests toxic adenoma.

Extrathyroidal findings may be of diagnostic significance and should be noted. True *proptosis* (eye protrusion of greater than 20 mm from the orbital bone) is a hallmark of Graves' disease. Eye muscle dysfunction, periorbital and conjunctival edema, lid lag, and stare are also seen. *Pretibial myxedema* is also a hallmark of Graves' disease. Neck lymph nodes should be checked for enlargement; painless cervical lymphadenopathy raises the question of a thyroid malignancy. A pelvic examination and visual field testing are important to check for ovarian and pituitary sources.

Screening for Osteoporosis

Excessive amounts of thyroid hormone are associated with an increased risk for osteoporosis, especially in cortical bone, because of increased bone turnover. The risk for thyroid-induced osteoporosis and hip fracture is greatest in postmenopausal women with a history of hyperthyroidism or thyroid-suppressive therapy. Such women should have a screening *bone density examination* of the hip or wrist (sites with a predominance of cortical bone; see Chapter 144) and the spine.

PRINCIPLES OF THERAPY (11,13,21–43)

The goals of therapy are to correct the hypermetabolic state with a minimum of side effects and the smallest possible incidence of hypothyroidism. For definitive therapy, one must choose among *antithyroid drugs*, which reduce thyroid hormone synthesis, and *radioiodine* and *thyroidectomy*, which reduce the amount of thyroid tissue. Hyperthyroidism should not go untreated, particularly in the elderly, who are at risk for cardiovascular complications. *Beta-blockers* are useful for prompt, temporary control of hyperadrenergic symptoms. Moreover, not only are symptoms uncomfortable, but thyrotoxic crisis may ensue if the untreated patient unexpectedly encounters a severe stress, such as emergency surgery or acute sepsis.

Therapeutic Modalities

Beta-Blockers

These agents inhibit the adrenergic effects of excess thyroid hormone. As such, they provide excellent, prompt, symptomatic relief from many of the catecholamine-mediated manifestations of hyperthyroidism (e.g., tremor, palpitations, heat intolerance, nervousness). However, beta-blockers have no intrinsic antithyroid activity, except perhaps at very high doses (which may slow the peripheral conversion of T_4 to T_3). The control of symptoms can often be achieved within a few days, so these agents are an excellent choice for first-line therapy and preoperative treatment. Beta-blockers may suffice for the treatment of transient hyperthyroidism, but they must be used in conjunction with other treatment modalities for the definitive control of persistent disease.

Beta-blockers are particularly valuable for minimizing the major cardiac complications of hyperthyroidism (e.g., atrial fibrillation and angina; see Chapters 28 and 30). Patients with rate-related heart failure will also benefit from beta-blockade, but the condition of those with heart failure resulting from myocardial pathology may worsen with such therapy. Consequently, beta-blockade must be administered with care in elderly patients and those with preexisting heart disease (see Chapter 32).

Of the beta-blockers, propranolol is the most widely used for the control of hyperthyroidism, but other agents in this class (e.g., atenolol, metoprolol) demonstrate comparable efficacy. Those with a more sustained half-life (e.g., atenolol) are particularly useful for patients who are to undergo surgery. Adequacy of the dose is determined by monitoring the resting and exercise heart rates and the degree of symptomatic relief.

One important benefit of beta-blockade is that it becomes possible to proceed safely with thyroid surgery within 1 to 2 weeks. With antithyroid drugs (see later discussion), 6 to 8 weeks of preoperative treatment are required. The addition of *potassium iodide* to beta-blocker therapy produces more rapid and greater preoperative control in patients with Graves' disease who are to undergo thyroidectomy; it is especially useful in those whose condition is not adequately controlled on beta-blockers alone (control being defined as a resting pulse of <90 beats/min and a blunting of exercise-induced tachycardia).

Antithyroid Drugs

Methimazole and *propylthiouracil* (PTU) are the most important antithyroid agents. PTU acts by interfering with the synthesis of T_4 and blocking the peripheral conversion of T_4 to T_3, although at conventional doses, this latter effect does not appear to be clinically important. Methimazole does not have any peripheral effect but is more potent and can reverse hyperthyroidism more quickly. Both drugs suppress thyroid autoimmunity and decrease circulating thyroid-stimulating antibodies. A biochemical response to the antithyroid drugs is detectable within 1 to 2 weeks; the clinical response typically takes 4 to 8 weeks.

These antithyroid agents are widely used in *young* and *middle-aged patients*, particularly for the long-term control of *Graves' disease*. They are also used for preoperative control and in many instances for therapy before and after radioiodine ablation. The average initial dose of PTU is 300 mg/d (100 mg every 8 hours). For methimazole, the starting dose is 10 to 15 mg/d, although higher doses (e.g., 30 mg/d) may be needed for patients with large goiters or more severe hyperthyroidism. The drug can be given as a single dose because its half-life is much longer, but large doses are best given initially in divided doses to minimize gastrointestinal side effects.

Therapy is adjusted according to TSH and thyroid hormone levels, with determinations performed every 4 to 6 weeks until stabilized and then less frequently. Once control is achieved, the dose can be tapered to the lowest amount needed to maintain a euthyroid state. Usually, treatment is continued for 12 to 24 months and then halted to see if relapse occurs.

The chance for long-term remission in Graves' disease is enhanced by 1 to 2 years of antithyroid drug therapy. PTU induces a remission in approximately 50% of patients with Graves' disease who are treated for 1 to 2 years, but one third to one half of those who respond eventually relapse. Reports of a remission rate of 40% after only 3 to 5 months of antithyroid therapy initially raised hopes that a shorter course of treatment might suffice, but longer-term follow-up revealed increased rates of relapse. Combination programs in which higher doses of antithyroid medication are given in conjunction with thyroxine have not proved advantageous, and they increase the risk for adverse effects of antithyroid drugs. The risk for inducing hypothyroidism is low. For patients who relapse or fail to achieve remission, radioiodine or surgical therapy must be considered.

Adverse Effects. Common adverse effects include *skin rash*, *fever*, and *arthralgias*; these are usually not of major clinical significance. However, if fever or arthralgias develop, the drugs should be stopped because these side effects may be indicative of more severe immunologic side effects. The rare (0.2% to 0.5% of patients) but potentially fatal complication of *agranulocytosis* necessitates careful patient selection and close monitoring of therapy. The risk for agranulocytosis increases with age (beginning at about age 40 years) and is independent of the dose for PTU but is dose dependent for methimazole. Onset is usually within 2 months, rarely beyond 4 months.

Because the drop in granulocyte count is precipitous, it is not clear that close monitoring of blood counts is beneficial, but many clinicians consider it advisable during the first 4 months of therapy. Mild leukopenia is common, occurring in up to 10% of patients, and does not require cessation of treatment. If the leukocyte count falls to less than 1,500/mm³ or if patients develop fever, pharyngitis, or other symptoms of infection, therapy should be withheld.

Choice of Antithyroid Agent. The choice of antithyroid agent has been a subject of debate. With proper monitoring, either antithyroid drug is a reasonable choice. Although PTU had been more widely prescribed, *methimazole* appears *preferable* in terms of cost, hematologic side effects, more rapid reversal of hyperthyroidism and ease of administration. It also has no adverse effect on the response to radioiodine therapy when used before ablative therapy, an effect sometimes seen with PTU. At doses up to 30 mg/d, methimazole is about 30% lower in cost than a comparable dose of PTU, is less likely to induce agranulocytosis, and needs to be taken only once daily. PTU is preferable during pregnancy and breast-feeding (see later discussion).

Ablation with Radioactive Iodine (Iodine-131)

Ablation with iodine-131 was first introduced in 1942 and is widely used today, especially for older hyperthyroid patients in whom the long-term effects of radiation exposure are not a major concern. It is indicated for patients with Graves' disease when antithyroid drugs do not suffice or when the patient is elderly or noncompliant. Other uses in hyperthyroidism include the ablation of a solitary toxic nodule or toxic multinodular goiter and when surgery is contraindicated or the patient is reluctant to undergo surgery.

Advantages, Disadvantages, and Adverse Side Effects. Advantages include established efficacy, relative safety, and ease of administration. Disadvantages are delayed control of symptoms and a high incidence of hypothyroidism following therapy.

Among the *side effects* of radioactive iodine therapy, the most common complication is *hypothyroidism*. High-dose radioiodine provides predictable relief but is associated with a high incidence of early hypothyroidism (70% in the first year). The early risk for hypothyroidism is lower with low-dose regimens (15% in the first year), but they provide less control of the disease (50% of patients still hyperthyroid at 1 year). Long-term follow-up studies of patients given low-dose treatment indicate a steady increase in the cumulative incidence of hypothyroidism (75% at 11 years), suggesting that its early advantages fade with time. Regardless of the dose used, the risk for eventual hypothyroidism requires that patients be regularly reevaluated, typically at 6-month intervals.

Worsening ophthalmopathy is a concern and more common with radioiodine therapy than with other forms of antithyroid treatment for Graves' disease. Risk is exacerbated by *cigarette smoking*. As noted earlier, up to 20% of patients with Graves' disease and eye involvement predating treatment for hyperthyroidism experience an exacerbation after treatment for hyperthyroidism. Correction of hyperthyroidism does not appear to cause ophthalmopathy *de novo*, but treatment-induced hypothyroidism (which is common in patients treated with radioiodine) appears to increase the risk for worsening eye problems. The mechanism is unclear; a treatment-induced outpouring of antibody-stimulating antigen is hypothesized. The avoidance of hypothyroidism appears to be the best mode of prevention. The mode of therapy may also be germane.

Risks for cancer and *birth defects* have been long-standing concerns. The gonadal radiation dose from iodine-131 therapy is small—the equivalent of that from a barium enema or an intravenous pyelogram. To address the question of cancer risk, cohort studies have followed tens of thousands of patients for decades. Recent analyses indicate that the risk for overall cancer mortality is not increased, but the rate of thyroid cancer deaths is increased fourfold in comparison with that of patients who received other forms of therapy. Although this increase in relative risk is statistically significant, the absolute risk remains very small. Of interest, more than 1 year after treatment, a slight increase in total cancer mortality risk was noted for patients treated with antithyroid medications. More study is needed to define these comparative risks. Radioiodine therapy is also associated with increased risks for cardiovascular disease, stroke, and osteoporotic fracture. Whether this is a consequence of the therapy or the underlying thyroid status of these patients remains to be clarified.

Surgery

Surgery represents the most direct ablative approach to hyperthyroidism. The objective is to reduce the thyroid mass sufficiently to cure the hypermetabolic state without inducing a hypothyroid condition. Unfortunately, the incidence of permanent hypothyroidism is substantial, and smaller but perceptible risks for hypoparathyroidism and laryngeal paralysis exist. Moreover, hyperthyroidism may recur despite subtotal thyroidectomy in Graves' disease. Prior preparation of the patient with antithyroid drugs is required to avoid precipitating thyroid storm. Surgery is particularly useful for relieving esophageal obstruction; cosmesis and pregnancy are other indications. It is also a choice when antithyroid drugs fail or produce complications or when patients are noncompliant or refuse radioiodine. Young patients with moderate to severe disease do particularly well. However, treatment with iodine-131 has largely replaced surgery because it is less expensive and associated with less morbidity.

Iodides

Iodides are sometimes useful as supplemental agents because they can block peripheral conversion of T_4 to T_3 and inhibit hormone release. *Potassium iodide* was the earliest of the iodides to be employed. The *organic iodide radiographic contrast agents* (e.g., ipodate, iopanoate) have supplanted the inorganic iodides. However, control is sometimes problematic. Paradoxical increases in hormone release can occur. Thus, iodides are best used for preoperative control in patients who require a second drug to counter the hyperthyroidism and in those for whom beta-blockers and other antithyroid medications are contraindicated.

Treatment of Osteoporosis

Bone-preserving therapy should be considered for hyperthyroid women found to be osteoporotic, especially if they are menopausal (see Chapter 164).

Choice of Therapy

Graves' Disease

There is little consensus among thyroidologists regarding the best treatment for Graves' disease, except in the case of elderly patients, for whom *radioactive iodine* is considered the treatment of choice. Surveys of opinion regarding the treatment of middle-aged and younger patients reveal a marked diversity of opinion, which is split between antithyroid drugs and radioiodine, with surgery deemed best reserved for those who are not candidates for either. An initial trial of antithyroid drug therapy represents a reasonable starting point for treatment, supplemented by beta-blocker therapy to help establish a euthyroid state and control adrenergic symptoms. When such therapy fails to achieve control or the patient is unable to tolerate it or experiences a relapse after it has been completed, radioiodine can be considered. Despite the absence of evidence for long-term genetic risk, concern persists about giving radioiodine to patients in their reproductive years.

Contributing to the diversity of opinion is dissatisfaction with available therapies. None appears to be capable of definitively halting the underlying immunopathologic process, which remains poorly understood. Adding *thyroid replacement therapy* to antithyroid drug therapy may decrease the frequency of recurrence of Graves' disease and reduce the production of antibodies to TSH receptors, but this therapy is not commonly used.

With a host of alternative therapies available, each with its own advantages and disadvantages, it is important to individualize treatment according to the patient's needs, capabilities, and clinical status. For now, one must settle for treating the hyperthyroidism; etiologic therapy is awaited.

Treatment of Ophthalmopathy. The treatment of ophthalmopathy also remains a challenge. Etiologic therapy awaits a better understanding of the underlying disease mechanisms. Although ophthalmopathy may worsen with treatment of the hyperthyroidism, especially if hypothyroidism is induced, no evidence has been found that scaling back treatment prevents an exacerbation. However, radioiodine appears to be the modality that is most likely to worsen ophthalmopathy, perhaps because it is the most likely to induce hypothyroidism. This has led some to recommend thyroxine supplementation to prevent hypothyroidism.

Moderately high doses of glucocorticoids given at the time of antithyroid treatment can reduce the risk for ophthalmopathy, but such prophylactic therapy is not recommended for routine use because of the high incidence of adverse side effects, the inability to predict who will experience an exacerbation, and the low incidence (7%) of severe ophthalmopathy. However, patients with moderate to marked preexisting ophthalmopathy may be reasonable candidates for such prophylactic treatment. Good eye care is also a priority.

Toxic Multinodular Goiter

Radioiodine is the most common treatment, but higher doses than given for Graves' disease are needed because of the lower radioactive uptake in these glands. Elderly patients should probably be treated with *antithyroid medications* before radioactive iodine to lessen the likelihood of developing worsening symptoms after radioiodine from a radiation-induced thyroiditis. *Thyroid surgery* (near-total thyroidectomy) may be needed for patients with large goiters and compressive symptoms (difficulty in breathing and swallowing).

Toxic Nodule

Radioiodine is the treatment of choice for elderly patients with this condition. Because the rest of the gland is suppressed by the hyperfunctioning nodule, the incidence of posttreatment hypothyroidism is far less than that seen with treatment of Graves' disease. The optimal radioiodine dose remains a subject of debate. A relatively low dose of iodine-131 (5 to 15 mCi) appears to provide excellent results with minimal adverse effects (75% of patients euthyroid by 2 months and >90% within

6 months, and posttreatment hypothyroidism very rare). Surgical removal may be preferable in young patients.

Hyperthyroidism in Pregnant and Nursing Patients

The choice is between antithyroid drugs and surgery; radioiodine is contraindicated because it crosses the placenta and concentrates in the fetal thyroid. Antithyroid drug therapy is considered safer than surgery, with surgery reserved for refractory cases and patients who refuse to take their medication. Among the *antithyroid agents*, PTU is preferred; methimazole has been associated with aplasia cutis in the fetus. The risk that drug will cross the placenta and induce hypothyroidism in the fetus is small and not strictly dose related, but precipitation of hypothyroidism in the mother can compromise the fetus and should be avoided. Pregnant women with Graves' disease may transfer large amounts of TSab to the fetus and induce fetal thyrotoxicosis, even after thyroid ablation. Testing the newborn for thyrotoxicosis is essential in this setting. Evidence that treatment of pregnant thyrotoxic patients leads to impaired intellectual development in the offspring has not been found. The optimal antithyroid drug regimen for the fetal thyroid status appears to be one that maintains maternal levels of free T_4 near the upper limit of normal.

Breast-feeding mothers can transfer antithyroid medication in milk, but the amount is small, especially of PTU, and not likely to induce significant hypothyroidism. However, a discussion of potential risks and the need for careful monitoring is important.

The short-term use of *beta-blocking agents, iodides,* or both provides prompt, effective, and safe control of thyrotoxic symptoms. Symptoms improve within 2 to 7 days. Longer-term use of these agents is more problematic. Beta-blocking drugs have been linked to retarded intrauterine growth, small placenta, and postnatal bradycardia and hypoglycemia. Nevertheless, the complication rate is low, and use during pregnancy is generally safe. Extended use of iodides is riskier, with large, obstructing fetal goiters reported.

Surgery is usually reserved for the patient who has failed or is a poor candidate for medical treatment. Operative mortality, although low, still exceeds that associated with drug therapy. Before subtotal thyroidectomy, preoperative medical therapy is indicated to attain control and prevent thyroid storm.

Thyroiditis

As noted, hyperthyroidism associated with thyroiditis can be managed symptomatically with *beta-blocking agents* because spontaneous resolution is the rule. Aspirin and occasionally corticosteroids are indicated in subacute thyroiditis to control inflammatory symptoms. Type 1 amiodarone-induced thyroiditis is treated with antithyroid drugs, whereas type 2 is treated with glucocorticoids. Amiodarone need not be discontinued for treatment to be effective.

Subclinical Hyperthyroidism

The approach to management depends on the type of subclinical hyperthyroidism present.

Endogenous Subclinical Hyperthyroidism. Antithyroid treatment should not commence in persons with suspected endogenous subclinical disease until nonthyroidal disease, medications, transient causes of hyperthyroidism, and central hypothyroidism have been ruled out. If the determination is difficult and the patient is entirely asymptomatic, then holding off implementation of antithyroid treatment and repeating thyroid indices in about 2 months is a reasonable course of action. It may take 8 weeks for the TSH to normalize in persons with self-limited or nonthyroidal disease.

If subclinical hyperthyroidism is confirmed at 8 weeks yet the patient remains totally asymptomatic, then watchful waiting and retesting every 6 months is reasonable, provided the patient does not have nodular disease (which has a high likelihood of progressing to overt hyperthyroidism) or such complications as atrial fibrillation or osteoporosis. The total T_3 is important to include in the periodic testing because it may be the first of the thyroid indices to rise.

Persons with symptoms or complications of their subclinical disease should be treated at the outset, starting with small doses of antithyroid medication (e.g., methimazole 5 to 10 mg/day).

Exogenous Subclinical Hyperthyroidism. Exogenous subclinical hyperthyroidism should be treated with prompt reduction in the dose of thyroid hormone when the patient is symptomatic and serum thyroid hormone levels are at or just greater than the upper limits of normal. Repeating thyroid indices in 6 to 8 weeks can help in further adjusting dose.

Monitoring Therapy

Monitoring treatment requires attention to the clinical status and indices of thyroid function. Clinical status is assessed by taking note of any changes in weight, degree of heat intolerance, tremulousness, anxiousness, appetite, level of energy, resting heart rate, ophthalmopathy, skin texture, or skin temperature. The *TSH* level provides the best measure of the treatment endpoint (normalization of TSH) and the earliest evidence of overtreatment and development of hypothyroidism. The amount of circulating thyroid hormone can be assessed by monitoring changes in the serum concentration of *free* T_4 (or total T_3 in the case of T_3 toxicosis), but assessment is needed only when the TSH level is abnormal.

In patients with Graves' disease, monitoring the serum level of *thyroid-stimulating antibodies* also helps to predict the clinical course. Relapse is a strong possibility if antibody titers remain elevated and is less likely, although not ruled out, when titers are reduced or absent.

For patients taking antithyroid drugs, routine monitoring of the *leukocyte count* should be considered, especially for those taking PTU or more than 30 mg of methimazole per day. Risk is greatest during the first 4 months of therapy.

PATIENT EDUCATION

Patients with hyperthyroidism are often relieved to know that their "nervousness" is caused by an underlying medical illness rather than an emotional problem and that it will improve with therapy. Patients who are taking antithyroid agents need to be instructed about prompt reporting of symptoms suggestive of agranulocytosis (e.g., fever, chills, pharyngitis), especially during the first 4 months of therapy. Those with prominent exophthalmos should be warned to see the physician at the first sign of diplopia or visual impairment. Hyperthyroid mothers taking antithyroid drugs and eager to breast-feed their infants need not be prohibited from breast-feeding so long as one takes the time to explain the potential risks and the importance of careful monitoring. Patients treated with radioiodine should be told to watch for symptoms of hypothyroidism.

INDICATIONS FOR REFERRAL AND ADMISSION

Patients who are candidates for therapy with iodine-131 should undergo a thyroid scan and be seen by the endocrinologist or radiation therapist for calculation of the dose of iodine-131 to be administered. Consultation with an endocrinologist is also indicated in the management of the pregnant or lactating hyperthyroid patient and the patient with severe ophthalmopathy of Graves' disease. Visual impairment caused by severe ophthalmopathy may require hospital admission for very high dose systemic steroid therapy or surgical decompression. Referral for consideration of surgical therapy is also indicated when the patient's swallowing is obstructed and when the patient is pregnant, desires cosmetic improvement, or fails antithyroid drug therapy. Prompt hospital admission is needed if heart failure, rapid atrial fibrillation, or angina develops.

THERAPEUTIC RECOMMENDATIONS

- For prompt control of adrenergic symptoms of hyperthyroidism, regardless of underlying cause, start treatment immediately with a *beta-blocking agent* (e.g., 80 mg of propranolol per day, 50 mg of atenolol per day). Increase the dose daily until symptoms are controlled. Use with extreme caution in patients who have preexisting heart failure unrelated to thyroid disease.
- For *nonpregnant young* and *middle-aged* patients with *Graves' disease*, start *methimazole* (10 to 15 mg/d in mild cases, 15 to 30 mg/d in severe cases) in addition to the beta-blocker program. Continue both methimazole and beta-blockade for 4 to 8 weeks and then taper the beta-blocker as the antithyroid agent takes effect. Adjust the antithyroid drug dose according to the clinical status and thyroid indices (TSH, free T_4, total T_3). Use the lowest possible dose that maintains biochemical and biologic control. Monitor closely to avoid precipitating hypothyroidism. Monitor the leukocyte count if more than 30 mg of methimazole is being taken per day or if the patient is elderly.
- If a response is obtained, continue antithyroid therapy for 12 to 24 months. One can measure TSab at 12 months. If TSab is absent and the patient appears to be in remission clinically and biochemically, then try to discontinue therapy. If relapse occurs, then consider the resumption of antithyroid therapy for 12 more months or radioiodine therapy.
- For the pregnant patient with Graves' disease, consider antithyroid drug therapy, but obtain endocrinologic consultation before initiating treatment. *PTU* is preferred (starting dose is 100 mg three times daily) and can also be given to the patient who is eager to breast-feed. Risks of such therapy should be fully explained and understood by the patient. Careful monitoring of thyroid status in both mother and baby is essential. Maintain the pregnant patient's free T_4 levels near the upper limit of normal; monitor TSH closely.
- For all patients taking antithyroid medication, consider *monitoring* the *leukocyte count* every 2 to 4 weeks during the first 4 months of therapy. Stop therapy if the neutrophil count falls to less than 1,500. The risk for agranulocytosis and the need for close monitoring are greatest in elderly patients and those taking PTU or more than 30 mg of methimazole per day.
- For patients with Graves' disease who have severe symptomatic ophthalmopathy, obtain a prompt endocrinologic

consultation. Options include very high dose systemic glucocorticoids (120 to 150 mg of prednisone per day), local steroid injection, surgical decompression, and radiation therapy.

- For patients with Graves' disease who have mild to moderate ophthalmopathy, minimize the risk for worsening eye disease by avoiding posttreatment hypothyroidism. The routine use of systemic daily steroid therapy for prophylaxis of posttreatment exacerbation is not recommended but may be considered for patients who begin radioiodine treatment with moderately severe eye changes already established (20 to 40 mg of prednisone per day for the first month, followed by taper to full cessation during the next 8 weeks). For periorbital edema, advise elevating the head of the bed, and prescribe a mild diuretic (e.g., 50 mg of hydrochlorothiazide per day). Prescribe methylcellulose drops to prevent corneal drying (see also Chapter 204).
- Consider *therapy with iodine-131* for patients with a *solitary toxic nodule, a toxic multinodular goiter, elderly patients with Graves' disease*, and other patients with Graves' disease who fail or cannot be maintained on therapy with antithyroid drugs (relapse, agranulocytosis). Continue beta-blockade for the 2- to 3-month period that it takes for the radioiodine to exert its full effect on the gland. Between 3 and 6 months after the onset of treatment and at 3- to 6-month intervals thereafter, monitor TSH for evidence of hypothyroidism; correct promptly by starting thyroid replacement therapy before hypothyroidism develops.
- Refer for consideration of *surgery* any patient who has a *neck obstruction* or a *cosmetic concern* or who is *poorly compliant* in taking medication. Surgery should also be considered when antithyroid drug therapy has failed or is contraindicated. Young patients do particularly well. If surgery is contemplated, continue antithyroid or beta-blocking therapy up to the moment of surgery. Monitor for postoperative hyperthyroidism.
- Treat patients with *transient hyperthyroidism* associated with thyroiditis symptomatically with *beta-blockade* until the condition resolves on its own.
- Screen and treat hyperthyroid women for *osteoporosis* (see Chapters 144 and 164); they are at increased risk for hip fracture.

Annotated Bibliography

1. Bahn RS. Pathophysiology of Graves' ophthalmopathy: the cycle of disease. J Clin Endocrinol Med 2003;88:1939. (*A discussion of mechanical, immunologic, and cellular contributions to the development of Graves' ophthalmopathy.*)
2. Borst GC, Eil C, Burman KD. Euthyroid hyperthyroxemia. Ann Intern Med 1983;98:366. (*A detailed review of the mechanisms and syndromes of hyperthyroxemia in clinically euthyroid patients; 229 references.*)
3. Brennan MD, Powell C, Kaufman KR, et al. The impact of overt and subclinical hyperthyroidism on skeletal muscle. Thyroid 2006;16:375. (*Muscle strength is reduced in subclinical hyperthyroidism and improves with therapy.*)
4. Cappola AR, Fried LP, Arnold AM, et al. Thyroid status, cardiovascular risk, and mortality in older adults. JAMA 2006;295:1033. (*There was an association between subclinical hyperthyroidism and atrial fibrillation but not with other cardiovascular disorders or mortality.*)
5. Cantalamessa L, Baldini M, Orsatti A, et al. Thyroid nodules in Graves' disease and the risk of thyroid carcinoma. Arch Intern Med 1999;159:1705. (*The risk for thyroid cancer in nodules detected with ultrasonography was low.*)
6. Carani C, Isidori AM, Granata A, et al. Multicenter study on the prevalence of sexual symptoms in male hypo- and hyperthyroid patients. J. Clin Endocrinol Metab 2005;90:6472. (*Prevalence increased, and was reversed by normalizing thyroid hormone levels.*)
7. Chopra IJ, Hershman JM, Pardridge WM, et al. Thyroid function in nonthyroidal illnesses. Ann Intern Med 1983;98:946. (*Discusses the changes in thyroid hormone levels and their consequences in nonthyroidal illness.*)
8. Daniels GH. Amiodarone-induced thyrotoxicosis. J Clin Endocrinol Metab 2001;86:3. (*Review and discussion of this increasingly important cause of thyrotoxicosis.*)
9. Forar JC, Muir AL, Sawers SA, et al. Abnormal left ventricular function in hyperthyroidism. N Engl J Med 1982;307:1165. (*Presents evidence for a reversible cardiomyopathic state directly related to excess thyroid hormone.*)
10. Frost L, Vestergaard P, Mosekilde L. Hyperthyroidism and risk of atrial fibrillation or flutter; a population-based study. Arch Intern Med 2004;164:1675. (*The prevalence was 8.3% among 40,628 Danish registry patients; risk factors were male sex, increasing age, ischemic heart disease, congestive heart failure, and valvular disease.*)
11. Stagnaro-Green A. Postpartum thyroiditis. J Clin Endocrinol Metab 2002;57:4042. (*An excellent clinical review.*)
12. Surks MI, Sievert R. Drugs and thyroid function. N Engl J Med 1995;333:1688. (*A useful review.*)
13. Surks MI, Ortiz E, Daniels GH, et al. Subclinical thyroid disease: scientific review and guidelines for diagnosis and management. JAMA 2004;291:228. (*A detailed analysis of the evidence, noting that it is insufficient to support population-based screening but encourages individual patient assessment.*)
14. Utiger RD. Pathogenesis of Graves' ophthalmopathy. N Engl J Med 1992;326:1772. (*Reviews mechanisms, particularly in relation to the mode of antithyroid therapy.*)
15. Helfand M, Redfern CC. Screening for thyroid disease: an update. Ann Intern Med 1998;129:144. (*A thoughtful review of the evidence for screening, including a good discussion of the value of detecting subclinical hyperthyroidism.*)
16. Mariotti S, Martino E, Cupini C, et al. Low serum thyroglobulin as a clue to the diagnosis of thyrotoxicosis factitia. N Engl J Med 1982;307:410. (*An excellent way to detect surreptitious use.*)
17. Masters PA, Simons RJ. Clinical use of sensitive assays for thyroid-stimulating hormone. J Gen Intern Med 1996;11:115. (*A review that includes a discussion of the use of the assay to detect hyperthyroidism.*)
18. Ross DS, Ardisson LJ, Meskell MJ. Measurement of thyrotropin in clinical and subclinical hyperthyroidism using a new chemiluminescent assay. J Clin Endocrinol Metab 1989;69:684. (*The original report establishing the enhanced sensitivity of the assay and its use in determining and using thyroid-stimulating hormone [TSH] levels to diagnose hyperthyroidism.*)
19. Sundbeck G, Jagenburg R, Johansson PM, et al. Clinical significance of low serum thyrotropin concentration by chemiluminometric assay in 85-year-old women and men. Arch Intern Med 1991;151:549. (*Elderly persons may have a low TSH level but remain euthyroid.*)
20. Surks MI, Chopra IJ, Mariash CN, et al. American Thyroid Association guidelines for use of laboratory tests in thyroid disorders. JAMA 1990;263:1529. (*Recommends TSH measurement supplemented by free thyroxine measurement as the principal tests.*)
21. Bartalena L, Marocci C, Bogazzi F, et al. Relation between therapy for hyperthyroidism and the course of Graves' ophthalmopathy. N Engl J Med 1998;338:1998. (*Radioiodine therapy is more likely than methimazole to cause or worsen ophthalmopathy; the problem is often transient and can be prevented by treatment with prednisone.*)
22. Bartalena L, Marocci C, Tanda ML, et al. Cigarette smoking and treatment outcomes in Graves' ophthalmopathy. Ann Intern Med 1998;129:632. (*Smoking increases the risk and decreases the efficacy of corticosteroids and orbital irradiation.*)
23. Burch HB, Solomon BL, Watofsky L, et al. Discontinuing antithyroid drug therapy before ablation with radioiodine in Graves' disease. Ann Intern Med 1994;121:553. (*Suggests that antithyroid therapy before ablation has little effect on the short-term course after radioiodine therapy.*)
24. Burrow GN. The management of thyrotoxicosis in pregnancy. N Engl J Med 1984;313:562. (*A succinct but clinically useful review; 49 references.*)
25. Cooper DS. Antithyroid drugs in the management of patients with Graves' disease: an evidence-based approach to therapeutic controversies. J Clin Endocrinol Metab 2003;88:3474. (*A very thoughtful review; 66 references.*)
26. Cooper DS. Antithyroid drugs. N Engl J Med 2005;352:905. (*An excellent review; 132 references.*)
27. Cooper DS. Which antithyroid drug? Am J Med 1986;80:1165. (*Favors methimazole over propylthiouracil [PTU] for most cases.*)
28. Cooper DS, Goldminz D, Levin AA, et al. Agranulocytosis associated with antithyroid drugs. Ann Intern Med 1983;98:26. (*Increasing age and dose*

of methimazole were associated with increased risk; the risk with PTU was independent of dose.)

29. Franklyn JA, Sheppard MC, Maisonneuve P. Thyroid function and mortality in patients treated for hyperthyroidism. JAMA 2005;294:71. (*A population-based study of 2,668 individuals, noting that mortality was increased but that the association with radioactive iodine therapy disappeared if free thyroxine therapy was given for radioiodine-induced hypothyroidism.*)

30. Graham GD, Burman KD. Radioiodine treatment of Graves' disease. Ann Intern Med 1986;105:900. (*A comprehensive review of potential risks; 72 references.*)

31. Greenspan SL, Greenspan FS. The effect of thyroid hormone on skeletal integrity. Ann Intern Med 1999;130:750. (*A systematic review, finding an increased risk of osteoporosis.*)

32. Hashizume K, Ichikawa K, Sakurai A, et al. Administration of thyroxine in treated Graves' disease—effects on the level of antibodies to thyroid-stimulating hormone receptors and on the risk of recurrence of hyperthyroidism. N Engl J Med 1991;324:947. (*An intriguing approach in which adding thyroxine reduced thyroid-stimulating–antibody levels and the risk for recurrence.*)

33. Hermus AR, Duysmans DA. Treatment of benign nodular thyroid disease. N Engl J Med 1998;338:1438. (*A review that includes a discussion of the management of toxic nodular goiter.*)

34. Klein I, Becker DV, Levey GS. Treatment of hyperthyroid disease. Ann Intern Med 1994;121:281. (*A useful review.*)

35. Momotani N, Noh J, Oyanagi H, et al. Antithyroid drug therapy for Graves' disease during pregnancy. N Engl J Med 1986;315:24. (*An optimal program for the fetus appears to be one that maintains maternal free thyroxine in the mildly hyperthyroid range.*)

36. Read CH, Tansey MJ, Menda Y. A 36-year retrospective analysis of the efficacy and safety of radioactive iodine in treating young Graves' patients.

J Clin Endocrinol Metab 2004;89:4229. (*Presents long-term follow-up data suggesting that radioiodine therapy was safe in young persons.*)

37. Rittmaster RS, Abbott EC, Douglas R, et al. Effect of methimazole, with or without L-thyroxine, on remission rates in Graves' disease. J Clin Endocrinol Metab 1998;83:814. (*No benefit was found from combined therapy, and an increased risk was found for adverse drug effects from the higher doses used.*)

38. Ron E, Doody MM, Becker DV, et al. Cancer mortality following treatment of adult hyperthyroidism. JAMA 1998;280:347. (*A major cohort study, finding no increase in overall cancer mortality but a fourfold increase in thyroid cancer deaths.*)

39. Ross DS, Ridgeway EC, Daniels GH. Successful treatment of solitary toxic thyroid nodules with relatively low-dose iodine 131, with a low prevalence of hypothyroidism. Ann Intern Med 1984;101:488. (*Reports excellent efficacy and safety, and argues that high doses are unnecessary.*)

40. Singer PA, Cooper DS, Levy EG, et al. Treatment guidelines for patients with hyperthyroidism and hypothyroidism. Standards of Care Committee, American Thyroid Association. JAMA 1995;273:808. (*Consensus clinical guidelines.*)

41. Tajiri J, Noguchi S, Murakami T, et al. Antithyroid drug-induced agranulocytosis—the usefulness of routine leukocyte count monitoring. Arch Intern Med 1990;150:621. (*Presents evidence for regular monitoring.*)

42. Tallstedt L, Lundell G, Torring O, et al. Occurrence of ophthalmopathy after treatment for Graves' hyperthyroidism. N Engl J Med 1992;326:1733. (*A randomized, controlled trial, finding that iodine-131 therapy was more likely to be followed by worsening ophthalmopathy than were other therapies, especially in older patients.*)

43. Utiger RD. β-Adrenergic antagonist therapy for hyperthyroid Graves' disease. N Engl J Med 1984;310:1597. (*An editorial nicely summarizing data on the use of β-blockade.*)

CHAPTER 104 ■ APPROACH TO THE PATIENT WITH HYPOTHYROIDISM

DAVID M. SLOVIK

Hypothyroidism is a common, readily treatable disorder. Increasingly, patients present with subclinical disease detected either as part of a screening program or as a consequence of an evaluation for another medical problem, such as hypercholesterolemia. Women experience the condition much more often than men (five- to eightfold greater prevalence). The primary physician should be able to confirm the diagnosis of hypothyroidism, initiate the workup for its underlying etiology, determine when replacement therapy is indicated, and prescribe thyroid hormone with safety and precision.

PATHOPHYSIOLOGY, CLINICAL PRESENTATION, AND COURSE (1–17)

Pathophysiology

The basic mechanisms of hypothyroidism can be divided into those that impair thyroid function (*primary hypothyroidism*) and those that principally involve hypothalamic–pituitary

function (*secondary hypothyroidism*). In primary disease, the hypothalamus responds with an increased output of thyrotropin-releasing hormone (TRH), which triggers pituitary thyrotropin (TSH) secretion. This in turn stimulates thyroid gland enlargement, goiter formation, and thyroid hormone production with the preferential synthesis of triiodothyronine (T_3) over thyroxine (T_4). In secondary hypothyroidism, the TSH response is inadequate, the gland is normal or reduced in size, and both T_4 synthesis and T_3 synthesis are equally reduced.

Primary Hypothyroidism

Primary hypothyroidism may occur as a result of blockade of thyroid TSH receptors, impairment of thyroxine production, or inhibition of thyroxine release.

Hashimoto's Thyroiditis. In Hashimoto's thyroiditis, the most common form of hypothyroidism, *immune-mediated injury* may damage all three components of glandular function. The precipitants of excessive antibody production remain ill defined, but TSH receptors and microsomal enzymes (e.g., peroxidase) are among the targeted antigens. In fact, *antimicrosomal antibodies* serve as a convenient laboratory marker for the condition (see later discussion). Pathologically, a lymphocytic infiltrate and glandular enlargement are noted; frank nodularity may develop (see Chapter 95). Antibodies directed against glandular antigens can impair the response to TSH and the synthesis and release of hormone. Although most patients with Hashimoto's thyroiditis remain euthyroid, a fraction experience transient hyperthyroidism because of the premature release of thyroid hormone (see Chapter 103).

Postpartum Thyroiditis. Postpartum thyroiditis is believed to be a common variant of Hashimoto's thyroiditis (see Chapter 103), affecting up to 5% of women postpartum. Antibody production peaks 3 to 4 months after delivery and then declines. A period of transient hyperthyroidism may be followed by hypothyroidism, but most patients return to euthyroid status. The symptoms of mild hyperthyroidism may be mistakenly attributed to "tension" and are followed by fatigue and depression resulting from the onset of hypothyroidism. The symptoms resolve spontaneously within 2 to 3 months but tend to recur with subsequent pregnancies.

Radiation-Induced Hypothyroidism. Radiation-induced hypothyroidism is another leading cause of thyroid injury in the United States. It is a common and permanent consequence of iodine-131 therapy and also of external neck irradiation that exceeds 2,500 rad (used to treat lymphoma and head and neck cancers). Onset is within 3 to 6 months of treatment.

Subacute Thyroiditis. Subacute thyroiditis following a viral upper respiratory infection is a more transient form of thyroid injury. In this condition, the gland is very tender and enlarged, sometimes asymmetrically. An initial release of thyroid hormone may produce a brief period of hyperthyroidism followed by hormone depletion and glandular hypofunction, but spontaneous remission and restoration of normal thyroid function are the rule. Pathologically, a granulomatous giant-cell infiltrate and a marked reduction in iodine uptake characterize the condition. The clinical course ranges from weeks to a few months.

Subtotal Thyroidectomy and Antithyroid Drugs. Subtotal thyroidectomy produces transient hypothyroidism in most patients and permanent hypothyroidism in about half within the first year after surgery.

Drugs that have an antithyroid effect produce a rapid but reversible form of hypothyroidism, such as seen with use of the antithyroid agents *methimazole* and *propylthiouracil* in the treatment of hyperthyroidism (see Chapter 103). *Lithium*, *interferon-α*, and *interleukins* may trigger clinical hypothyroidism in a small percentage of cases, presumably by exacerbating preexisting autoimmune thyroid disease. *Amiodarone* is believed to lead to hypothyroidism by its release of iodine. *Iodide excess* impairs thyroxine synthesis and release, especially in patients with underlying thyroid disease; *iodide deficiency* inhibits hormone synthesis and, worldwide, accounts for much of the hypothyroidism and goiter seen. *Phenytoin*, *carbamazepine*, and *rifampin* increase clearance of thyroid hormone, leading to increased daily replacement requirements. The tyrosine kinase inhibitor *sunitinib* appears to be capable of triggering a destructive thyroiditis; risk appears to increase with duration of therapy.

Pregnancy. Early in pregnancy, levothyroxine requirements increase, plateauing at about 20 weeks. Mechanisms include an estradiol-related increase in synthesis of thyroxine-binding globulin and a resultant decline in the concentration of free thyroxine. The increased requirements are not a problem for euthyroid women, who respond with increased thyroxine production, but hypothyroid women may experience worsening hypothyroidism as early as 5 weeks into gestation, a time when fetal development is particularly sensitive to levels of circulating thyroid hormone.

Secondary and Tertiary Hypothyroidism (Central Hypothyroidism)

Secondary hypothyroidism is caused by *TSH deficiency* and tertiary hypothyroidism by *TRH deficiency*. Together they account for less than 1% of all hypothyroidism.

Secondary hypothyroidism occurs most commonly as a result of injury to thyrotropes by a functioning or nonfunctioning pituitary adenoma. Many other forms of sellar or suprasellar disease can produce the same net result, which is inadequate production of TSH leading to an atrophic thyroid gland and hypothyroidism. These include hypophysitis, trauma, postpartum pituitary necrosis, nonpituitary tumors, radiation, and infiltrative disease.

Tertiary hypothyroidism is caused by disorders that injure the hypothalamus or interfere with the hypothalamus–pituitary blood flow. Other hormone-producing cells of the pituitary may also be involved and cause a host of associated endocrinopathies (see Chapters 100 and 101). Primary hypothyroidism can sometimes mimic secondary disease by causing the pituitary to enlarge; however, the pituitary shrinks in response to exogenous thyroid hormone in primary disease but not in secondary disease.

Clinical Presentation

Subclinical Hypothyroidism

Along with the ability to detect early disease (see later discussion) comes the designation of subclinical hypothyroidism, defined as an asymptomatic elevation in serum TSH concentration (generally ranging from 5.5 to 10.0 mU/L, depending on the specificity desired) accompanied by thyroid hormone levels within normal limits. The general population prevalence averages 7% for women and 2.5% for men. In about 20% of patients with a TSH concentration greater than 6 mU/L, clinically symptomatic hypothyroidism develops within a period of 5 years; the incidence of clinical disease rises to almost 100% for those with a TSH level greater than 14 mU/L. Patients with high titers of antithyroid antibodies are at greatest risk for becoming overtly hypothyroid, which suggests that Hashimoto's thyroiditis plays an important role. The meaning of an isolated TSH between 6 and 10 mU/L is unclear, although some evidence has been found of an increased risk for coronary artery disease resulting from lipid abnormalities.

Clinical Hypothyroidism

The overt symptomatic manifestations of hypothyroidism reflect the decreases in metabolic rate and sensitivity to catecholamines that result from insufficient circulating thyroid hormone. Early symptoms are gradual in onset and may occur before serum free thyroxine levels fall below normal limits, although the TSH level rises as soon as circulating levels of thyroid hormone are sensed to be inappropriately low. The patient typically complains of *fatigue*, *constipation*, moderately *dry skin*, *heavy menstrual periods*, a slight *weight gain*, or *cold intolerance.* These symptoms are followed during the next few months by the development of very dry skin, coarse hair, hoarseness, continued weight gain (although appetite is minimal), and slightly *impaired mental activity* (e.g., minor diminution in psychomotor activity, visual-perceptual skills, or memory). Later, depression may become evident.

In late stages, hydrophilic mucopolysaccharide accumulates subcutaneously, producing the *myxedematous changes* that characterize the severe form of the disease. The skin becomes doughy, the face puffy, the tongue large, the expression dull, and mentation slow, even lethargic. *Muscle weakness, arthralgias, diminished hearing,* and *carpal tunnel syndrome* are also found. Daytime sleepiness in severely myxedematous patients suggests that *obstructive sleep apnea* may be occurring. *Bradycardia, pericardial effusion,* and *diastolic hypertension* may develop. *Dementia* may ensue and be only partially responsive to thyroid replacement therapy.

On examination, a *goiter* may be evident. If Hashimoto's disease is the cause, the goitrous gland may feel rubbery, non-tender, and even nodular. In the case of subacute thyroiditis, it will be very tender and enlarged, although not always symmetrically. Diffuse enlargement also occurs with hereditary defects in thyroxine synthesis or the use of iodides, *para*-aminosalicylic acid, or lithium. An atrophic gland is characteristic of secondary hypothyroidism. The heart may show signs of dilation or an effusion. Bowel sounds are diminished, and the relaxation phase of the deep tendon *reflexes* is slowed or *"hung up."*

In *secondary hypothyroidism,* signs of accompanying ovarian and adrenal insufficiency (e.g., loss of axillary and pubic hair, amenorrhea, postural hypotension) may be seen as a consequence of concurrent loss of luteinizing hormone (LH), follicle-stimulating hormone (FSH), and adrenocorticotropic hormone (ACTH) production. Myxedematous changes tend to be less marked than with primary hypothyroidism, and the gland is smaller.

Laboratory Manifestations

As noted earlier, in primary hypothyroidism, *TSH elevation* may precede clinical manifestations. The earliest development is an increase in TRH, followed by the TSH response. At this stage, thyroid hormone levels may still be reported as "within normal limits," although in reality, they are reduced from baseline. Only later does free thyroxine fall to overtly abnormal levels.

Hypercholesterolemia—an increase in low-density-lipoprotein (LDL) cholesterol and a reduction in high-density-lipoprotein (HDL) cholesterol—is often noted. Hypothyroidism is associated with a number of *anemic states.* The most common is a mild *normochromic* normocytic anemia. In addition, a microcytic anemia may ensue from iron deficiency secondary to heavy menstrual bleeding. Furthermore, a *macrocytic* picture that clears on administration of exogenous thyroid hormone is sometimes encountered. A true megaloblastic anemia resulting from vitamin B_{12} deficiency occurs in about 10% of hypothyroid patients with a macrocytic smear; the relation between hypothyroidism and pernicious anemia is unresolved, but an autoimmune mechanism is postulated.

In severe cases of myxedema, dilutional *hyponatremia* occurs as a result of inadequate renal blood flow. A warning of impending myxedema coma is a rise in arterial carbon dioxide tension, which takes place as the respiratory drive weakens.

TABLE 104.1

DIFFERENTIAL DIAGNOSIS OF HYPOTHYROIDISM

Primary Hypothyroidism
  Hashimoto's thyroiditis
  Postpartum disease (transient)
  Postirradiation disease
  Subtotal thyroidectomy
  Subacute thyroiditis (transient)
  Antithyroid drugs (lithium, PAS, PTU, methimazole, iodide excess)
  Iodide deficiency
  Infiltrative disease (hemochromatosis, amyloidosis, scleroderma)
  Biosynthetic defect, hereditary

Secondary Hypothyroidism
  Pituitary macroadenoma
  Empty sella syndrome
  Infarction
  Infiltrative disease (e.g., sarcoidosis)
  Surgery or radiation-induced injury

PAS, *para*-aminosalicylic acid; PTU, propylthiouracil.

DIFFERENTIAL DIAGNOSIS

The causes of hypothyroidism can be categorized according to whether they impair the thyroid gland (primary hypothyroidism) or the hypothalamic–pituitary axis (secondary hypothyroidism) (Table 104.1). Primary disease is far more prevalent than secondary disease. Autoimmune thyroiditis (Hashimoto's thyroiditis) accounts for most of the cases of hypothyroidism seen in the United States. Other causes of thyroid injury include idiopathic thyroid atrophy, previous radioactive iodine (iodine-131) therapy, and subtotal thyroidectomy. Women are more frequently affected than men. The prevalence of hypothyroidism increases with age. As much as 5% of the elderly population manifests evidence of hypothyroidism, most of it resulting from thyroiditis. Less common causes include neck irradiation, iodide administration, and the use of drugs, including lithium, amiodarone, and antithyroid medications. Pituitary insufficiency can result in secondary hypothyroidism. Rarely, hypothalamic disease is the source of difficulty.

WORKUP (1,2,4,6,7,12,15,16–22)

Screening for Hypothyroidism

The test of choice to screen for hypothyroidism is a serum *TSH* determination, the most sensitive and cost-effective of available tests. Modern TSH assays provide a very sensitive means of detecting hypothyroidism, often long before the patient becomes overtly symptomatic. Measurement of *thyroid hormone levels* is indicated if the TSH is elevated but not for screening because the test sensitivity is lower and the cost is no less.

Despite the ease and effectiveness of detection, considerable controversy remains regarding the value of adding a TSH determination to the periodic health examination. The frequency of hypothyroidism is low in men, and the impact of treatment on asymptomatic patients is unclear. Nonetheless, patients in subgroups with an increased prevalence of hypothyroidism might be reasonable candidates for screening, and for them a TSH determination should at least be considered. These include women older than 50 years (especially if they are hyperlipidemic) and patients with goiter, Hashimoto's thyroiditis (presence of antithyroid antibodies), recent radioiodine or external neck irradiation, or recent thyroid surgery. In addition, the prevalence of hypothyroidism is high among patients with autoimmune disorders, patients with mental dysfunction admitted to geriatric units, and women older than age 40 with such nonspecific complaints as fatigue.

Diagnosis of Hypothyroidism

Although the history (cold intolerance, skin changes, unexplained weight gain, hoarseness, fatigue, heavy periods) and physical findings (dry skin, coarse hair, goiter, "hung-up" reflexes) often suggest the diagnosis, confirmation and the detection of early disease require laboratory study.

Diagnosis of Primary Hypothyroidism

Diagnosis of primary hypothyroidism is readily achieved by demonstrating an *increased TSH level* and a *low free T$_4$ level* (or *free T$_4$ index*). The TSH is the more sensitive indicator of primary hypothyroidism and the test of choice. The designation of *subclinical hypothyroidism* is given to the asymptomatic patient with a modest elevation in TSH (6 to 10 mU/L) and a free T$_4$ index remaining within normal limits. However, the range of normal for the free T$_4$ index is wide. A single free T$_4$ determination may not detect the patient who has a modest yet physiologically important decline in hormone level because the serum concentrations may remain within normal limits. The free thyroxine level is a better measure of thyroid function than the *total T$_4$*, which is affected by changes in thyroid-binding globulin that are independent of thyroid function.

Often, measurement of total T$_3$ is routinely ordered as part of a battery of thyroid function tests. The assay is expensive to perform, and the results correlate poorly with thyroid status in the hypothyroid range and are affected by such events as a fall in peripheral conversion of T$_4$ to T$_3$, which is common in the elderly and in nonthyroidal illness. Determinations of serum cholesterol and thyroglobulin and of radioactive iodine uptake are also insensitive tests that contribute little to the diagnostic evaluation.

Diagnosis of Secondary and Tertiary Hypothyroidism

These conditions should be suspected when the TSH level is *inappropriately low* in the setting of clinically overt hypothyroidism or the TSH is low or normal in the setting of low free thyroxine levels. Concurrent amenorrhea, galactorrhea, postural hypotension, or visual field deficits also suggest pituitary–hypothalamic disease. Imaging of the sellar region is indicated. *Computed tomography* is best for detecting small lesions within the sella; *magnetic resonance imaging* is best for imaging the suprasellar region (see Chapter 100).

Diagnosis in Persons Taking Thyroid Hormone

Diagnosis in persons taking thyroid hormone but in whom hypothyroidism has not been documented can be evaluated by stopping replacement therapy. Abrupt cessation of exogenous thyroid hormone therapy is not dangerous so long as the patient has no prior history of severe hypothyroidism. Prompt and adequate (although submaximal) responses of the pituitary and thyroid gland occur when hormone intake is halted.

However, because the half-life of thyroxine is approximately 7 days, it may take about 5 weeks for full functioning of the hypothalamic–pituitary–thyroid axis to return, and testing for hypothyroidism should be delayed until then to avoid a false-positive diagnosis of hypothyroidism.

Identifying the Underlying Cause

History

History should be checked for possible etiologic factors, such as exposure to iodine-131, neck irradiation, recent viral infection, use of medications with antithyroid activity (e.g., lithium, excess iodide, amiodarone, sunitinib, interferons) or effects on thyroid hormone clearance (e.g., phenytoin, carbamazepine, rifampin), residence in an area of iodide deficiency, subtotal thyroidectomy, pituitary surgery or irradiation, recent pregnancy, and a family history of thyroid disease.

Physical Examination

Physical examination should include a careful look at the thyroid gland for size, consistency, and nodularity. An exquisitely tender gland suggests subacute thyroiditis. A nontender, diffusely enlarged gland is seen in early Hashimoto's disease, iodide deficiency, and congenital biosynthetic defects and after childbirth. A rubbery, multinodular goiter suggests more advanced Hashimoto's thyroiditis. A small gland characteristic of atrophic thyroiditis may be seen. When secondary hypothyroidism is suspected clinically, the blood pressure should be checked for postural hypotension and the visual fields for deficits.

Laboratory Investigation

Laboratory investigation is relatively limited. The *TSH* level (to differentiate primary from secondary disease) and *anti–thyroid peroxidase antibody* titer (presence of antibodies strongly suggestive of Hashimoto's thyroiditis) are the most useful. In patients with a sellar mass lesion, determination of the serum levels of *LH*, *FSH*, *ACTH*, and *prolactin* may be indicated (see Chapters 100 and 101). A *lipid profile* (see Chapter 15) should be obtained in all hypothyroid patients because it is likely to be abnormal and require attention. Those with suspected Hashimoto's disease should also have a *complete blood cell count* and a serum *vitamin B$_{12}$* determination.

PRINCIPLES OF MANAGEMENT
(1,2,4,6,12,15,22–41)

The availability of high-quality, inexpensive preparations of levothyroxine make restoration of the euthyroid state readily achievable. The issues are when to initiate therapy, how best to do so, how best to monitor the patient, and how long to continue treatment.

Subclinical Hypothyroidism

The need for replacement therapy in subclinical hypothyroidism is a matter of debate. Favoring therapy is the opportunity to correct secondary lipid abnormalities (elevated LDL cholesterol, reduced HDLs) and decrease the size of the gland if it is enlarged. In addition, some persons are actually symptomatic, although the relation of symptoms to thyroid disease is not appreciated until treatment is instituted and the patient reports feeling considerably better. This is especially true for patients with neuropsychiatric symptoms. Against treatment is the lack of evidence from prospective, controlled trials that treatment is beneficial, safe, and cost-effective. No evidence has been found that early treatment affects the natural history of the underlying cause. Lipid and symptom responses to replacement therapy in patients with only modest elevations in TSH (e.g., <10 mU/L) appear to be modest at best. Moreover, osteoporosis or atrial fibrillation can be induced with excessive treatment, which can easily occur in patients with minimally elevated TSH levels.

Given these uncertainties, a reasonable approach is to follow expectantly truly asymptomatic persons with mild elevations in TSH (<10 mU/L) and consider treating those with more substantial increases in TSH (i.e., >10 mU/L) or those with TSH levels less than 10 mU/L who are pregnant or have subtle but important manifestations of hypothyroidism (e.g., goiter, lipid abnormalities, anovulatory menses). Those who are to be managed expectantly should undergo an annual assessment that includes a TSH determination, and they should be treated if they are becoming symptomatic or the TSH increases substantially.

Clinical Hypothyroidism

For patients who are clinically hypothyroid, replacement therapy is indicated. Treatment of mild to moderate disease is best instituted gradually because hypothyroid patients are very sensitive to the effects of thyroid hormone. (An excessive rate of replacement may cause tremor, nervousness, and palpitations.) Adequate replacement should result in resolution of fatigue, loss of excess weight, and reversal of autonomic symptoms. The first signs of response are a modest loss of weight, increase in the pulse rate, and resolution of constipation. Myxedematous skin changes, pleural and pericardial effusions, and elevated creatine phosphokinase levels also normalize, but this requires more time. Most patients feel better within 2 weeks, and clinical resolution is usually complete by 3 months, although more prolonged recovery may occur. Therapy for primary hypothyroidism is continued indefinitely, except in patients with transient disease, such as those with postpartum or subacute thyroiditis.

Replacement Program

Levothyroxine remains the preparation of choice for most patients (see later discussion). A replacement dose of 100 to 125 μg/d usually suffices. The elderly tend to have a 20% lower daily requirement because of decreased T_4 clearance. Current levothyroxine replacement doses are lower than those previously cited because contemporary levothyroxine preparations are more potent.

Initiation of Therapy and Adjustment of Dose. The *starting dose* and rate of adjustment depend on age, weight, presence of chronic disease (especially coronary artery disease), severity and duration of symptoms, and pretreatment TSH level. Young, otherwise healthy patients can be started on a nearly full dose of levothyroxine (50 to 100 μg/d). In patients older than age 50 years (who are at increased risk for silent coronary disease) and those with known heart disease, more cautious replacement is indicated to avoid precipitating angina, arrhythmias (atrial fibrillation, sinus tachycardia), and even heart failure. In this setting, it is best to initiate therapy with 25 to

50 μg/d. The onset of effect is usually gradual, becoming evident in 2 to 4 weeks. One should allow 4 to 6 weeks between dose adjustments because it can take that long for a given dose to become fully effective.

The dose can be adjusted in 25- to 50-μg increments until a euthyroid state is achieved. In older patients, it is best to increase dose in 25-μg steps. If angina or other cardiac symptoms occur, the dose of thyroid hormone should be reduced. Some advocate the concurrent administration of a *β-blocking agent* (e.g., propranolol) to protect the heart from the increase in myocardial oxygen demand associated with thyroxine therapy.

Preoperative management has been a subject of concern. Coronary patients found to be mildly to moderately hypothyroid can safely undergo urgent surgery (including bypass procedures) without prior replacement. The rate of complications is no greater than that for nonhypothyroid patients, and the cardiac risks are less than when replacement therapy is initiated preoperatively. However, careful preoperative planning of anesthesia is essential because the clearance of anesthetics is reduced.

Pregnancy poses a challenge in management of hypothyroidism because thyroxine requirements increase early (as early as week 5 of gestation) and cannot be met by the affected thyroid gland. Adequate early replacement therapy is important to early fetal development. The replacement therapy dose may need to be increased by up to 50%, starting with an increase of 25 to 50 μg/d at time of diagnosis of pregnancy, and subsequently adjusted further upward according to results from monitoring of thyroid function every 4 to 6 seeks up to 20 weeks, when requirements plateau.

Replacement Preparations

The replacement preparation of choice for most patients continues to be generic levothyroxine. A host of other replacement preparations is available and aggressively promoted, including brand-name levothyroxine preparations and mixtures of levothyroxine and triiodothyronine.

Levothyroxine. Levothyroxine (l-T_4) is the preferred thyroid hormone replacement preparation, based on uniform bioavailability, cost, safety, and ease of monitoring therapy. Some of the drug is converted peripherally to T_3, so it is usually unnecessary to use the more expensive preparations containing mixtures of T_4 and T_3 (see later discussion).

In the early 1980s, variations in the biologic activity and hormonal content of some commercial preparations were reported. Quality control efforts mandated by the U.S. Food and Drug Administration have eliminated most of this variability. Although pharmacokinetic differences are found among different preparations, those that have been thoroughly tested appear to be relatively interchangeable. Nonetheless, it is probably best, if possible, to stay with a particular levothyroxine preparation as long as it appears to provide adequate replacement and a consistent performance. Using a brand-name preparation has no particular advantage.

Absorption of levothyroxine is impaired when *ferrous sulfate* or *calcium carbonate* is taken at the same time. In the acidic environment of the stomach, thyroid hormone adsorbs to iron and calcium, necessitating that levothyroxine be taken 2 hours apart from them. *Acid secretion* is required for effective absorption of levothyroxine, necessitating an increase in dose of 20% to 30% in patients with atrophic gastritis or *Helicobacter pylori* infection. Because T_3 is the pertinent feedback hormone and derives from conversion of T_4, the amount of thyroxine necessary to normalize the TSH level may produce serum free thyroxine levels in the high-normal to slightly elevated range.

Triiodothyronine. As noted, the peripheral conversion of some L-T_4 to T_3 usually obviates the need for T_3 replacement. The exclusive use of exogenous T_3 is considered inadvisable for replacement purposes, especially in older patients, because it causes rapid increases in metabolic rate and oxygen demand and can precipitate angina. Moreover, its short half-life produces wide swings in T_3 levels and makes frequent administration necessary. For these reasons, it is best to avoid T_3 as a replacement therapy and to switch any patients who are already taking T_3 exclusively to levothyroxine.

Combination Therapy. Expensive replacement preparations containing a fixed ratio of levothyroxine to triiodothyronine have been promoted by their manufacturers. As noted, such preparations are usually unnecessary because there is some peripheral conversion of L-T_4 to T_3. Although the vast majority of hypothyroid patients do just fine on levothyroxine alone, a small group of patients continue to be bothered by *neuropsychiatric symptoms* despite adequate levothyroxine replacement. Substituting T_3 for some of the L-T_4 in their replacement program has been suggested as a way to overcome neuropsychiatric refractoriness, but randomized, controlled trials and meta-analysis have failed to confirm initial reports of benefit. More to the point in such patients are consideration of major depression and need for *antidepressant therapy* (see Chapter 227). If a trial of adding T_3 is going to be attempted, it should not be done using a fixed combination preparation; rather, 12.5 μg of *triiodothyronine* should be substituted for 50 μg of the total levothyroxine dose.

Monitoring and Adjusting Replacement Therapy

Monitoring and adjusting replacement therapy is best accomplished by measuring the serum *TSH* with the sensitive TSH assay, the results of which closely correlate with physiologic measures of thyroid hormone effect. However, reliance on the TSH determination can lead to erroneous conclusions during the initial 6 to 12 months of therapy because it can take that long for the TSH level to normalize despite adequate replacement doses. *Free T_4* levels may also correlate poorly with the physiologic status during this initial period of therapy. For these reasons, objective monitoring is difficult during the start-up phase of treatment, so that reliance on symptoms and signs is necessary.

TSH Testing. TSH testing is the preferred method of monitoring, supplemented by correlation with the clinical state during periods when the TSH changes may lag behind the changes in the physiologic state (e.g., during initiation of therapy). Thus, if the patient becomes clinically euthyroid during the early phase of replacement therapy but the TSH level is still elevated, it is best to leave the dose unchanged and repeat the TSH determination in 4 to 8 weeks. If the TSH falls but remains in the hypothyroid range and the patient continues to be clinically hypothyroid, then an increase in the thyroxine dose is warranted. If the TSH level of the hypothyroid patient shows no change, then poor compliance or improper intake of L-T_4 (e.g., ingestion along with an iron or calcium supplement) may be the most likely explanation; no dose adjustment is warranted under such circumstances. If TSH is undetectable, then the replacement dose is excessive and needs adjustment.

Once the dose is properly adjusted, monitoring of replacement therapy proceeds with TSH determinations twice yearly for the first year and then yearly thereafter, unless there is clinical suspicion of need for dose adjustment.

Other Thyroid Indices. When an excessive dose is suggested by a very low or absent TSH, measurement of the *free T_4* (or *free T_4 index*, which is an excellent proxy for the free T_4) can help to determine just how excessive is the current dose.

Secondary Hypothyroidism

Treatment and monitoring must take into account the lack of TSH response and any coexisting adrenal or ovarian hypofunction. Because thyroid replacement and the resultant rise in metabolic rate can precipitate an addisonian crisis, adrenal function should be assessed with an ACTH stimulation test before replacement therapy is prescribed in any patient suspected of having secondary hypothyroidism. Patients with an inadequate ACTH response are candidates for treatment with replacement doses of glucocorticoids before levothyroxine replacement. Serum free T_4 should be measured to assess adequacy of replacement because the TSH level is low in secondary hypothyroidism.

MANAGEMENT RECOMMENDATIONS (17,18,39,41)

Screening and Diagnosis

■ Consider TSH screening for women older than 50 years (especially if they are hyperlipidemic or have complaints of fatigue); persons with Hashimoto's thyroiditis, recent radioiodine or external neck irradiation, or recent thyroid surgery; and patients with mental dysfunction admitted to geriatric units.

■ Consider screening newly pregnant women who have a strong family history of hypothyroidism or other risk factors for the condition.

■ Stop any exogenous thyroid or antithyroid medication if the reason for its use is unclear; recheck the TSH level 4 to 6 weeks after treatment is stopped.

■ Confirm the diagnosis of hypothyroidism with TSH and free T_4 or free T_4 index determinations.

■ If the patient appears clinically and biochemically hypothyroid but the TSH is not appropriately elevated, test for pituitary insufficiency.

Primary Hypothyroidism

■ If possible, stop all drugs with a potential antithyroid effect (e.g., iodides, *para*-aminosalicylic acid, lithium).

■ Begin replacement with a once-daily morning dose of levothyroxine. Initiate therapy with 50 to 100 μg/d in young, otherwise healthy patients and with 25 to 50 μg/d in older patients; the size of the dose is a function of patient age and weight, severity and duration of hypothyroidism, and the presence of underlying heart disease. Particular caution is indicated in the presence of underlying coronary disease; small starting doses are required for these patients.

■ Monitor initial therapy by TSH determination and clinical state. The goal is normalization of the TSH, but be aware that the TSH level may initially require several months to normalize despite adequate thyroid hormone replacement. If the patient is clinically euthyroid but the TSH is still elevated, continue the same dose and repeat the TSH determination in 4 to 8 weeks. A check of the free T_4 (or free T_4 index) may be of use if TSH is low or absent. Also monitor for side effects (e.g., tremor, angina, arrhythmias).

- Increase the dose in increments of 25 to 50 μg; the lower increment is appropriate for elderly patients and those with heart disease.
- Allow 4 to 6 weeks for a new dose to take full effect before considering another increase in dose.
- Patients who continue to be bothered by *neuropsychiatric symptoms* clearly referable to their hypothyroidism may benefit from a trial of *mixed therapy* in which 12.5 μg of *triiodothyronine* is substituted for 50 μg of levothyroxine. However, patients with major depression should be considered for *antidepressant* therapy (see Chapter 227) if thyroid hormone replacement is not helping.
- The average levothyroxine replacement dose for most adults is 100 to 125 μg/d; for the elderly, the average dose is 20% less.
- Avoid excessive doses of replacement therapy (TSH <0.5 mU/L) because of the risk for inducing osteoporosis.
- Once the proper dose has been achieved, monitor therapy every 6 to 12 months with a TSH determination.
- Levothyroxine is the thyroid replacement preparation of choice; select and stay with a particular manufacturer's preparation. The use of desiccated thyroid and the sole use of T_3 preparations is not recommended.
- Patients with mild to moderate hypothyroidism and underlying coronary disease need not receive replacement therapy before urgent surgery. However, careful planning of anesthesia is necessary.
- In pregnancy, increase the replacement dose of levothyroxine by 25 to 50 μg/d as soon as pregnancy is diagnosed and further adjust upward accordingly as per subsequent monitoring of thyroid function every 4 to 6 weeks up to 20 weeks of gestation.

Secondary Hypothyroidism

- Perform an ACTH stimulation test to assess adrenal reserve. If it is low, give glucocorticoids *before* prescribing thyroid replacement.
- Replace thyroid hormone as for primary hypothyroidism.
- Monitor therapy by following clinical signs and free T_4.

PATIENT EDUCATION

Euthyroid patients who are inappropriately placed on exogenous thyroid hormone for the treatment of fatigue or obesity are often reluctant to give up the medication. Documenting that their thyroid status is perfectly normal is an essential first step in taking them off the medication successfully. Often, they will agree to a request from the physician to halt thyroid hormone for 5 weeks and have their TSH and free T_4 measured. Usually, patients note little change in how they feel, and this helps to convince them that exogenous hormone is unnecessary.

Hypothyroid patients need to be warned of the danger of increasing their medication too rapidly or taking more than is prescribed. Unfortunately, some patients adjust their doses on the basis of other symptoms that they mistakenly attribute to hypothyroidism, such as symptoms of depression. All patients should be instructed to measure and record their weight regularly, and report any unexplained change of 5 lb or more. Women of childbearing age should be instructed to come for dose adjustment at the first sign of pregnancy and have their thyroid status monitored closely for at least the first half of pregnancy.

It is imperative that the patient and family be instructed about the signs of worsening hypothyroidism. Hypothyroid patients have been known to stop taking their thyroid medication. The importance of continuing therapy indefinitely must be emphasized to patients and the persons close to them.

Annotated Bibliography

1. Alexander EK, Marqusee E, Lawrence J, et al. Timing and magnitude of increases in levothyroxine requirements during pregnancy in women with hypothyroidism. N Engl J Med 2004;351:241. (*Requirements increase as early as week 5; the authors recommend an increase in replacement dose by 30% as soon as pregnancy is confirmed.*)
2. Amino N, Mori H, Iwatani Y, et al. High prevalence of transient post-partum thyrotoxicosis and hypothyroidism. N Engl J Med 1982;306:849. (*Original report; the condition was attributed to an autoimmune thyroiditis; incidence was 5%.*)
3. Basaria s, Cooper DS. Amiodarone and the thyroid. Am J Med 2005;118:706. (*Useful review.*)
4. Bauer DC, Ettinger B, Browner WS. Thyroid function and serum lipids in older women: a population-based study. Am J Med 1998;104:546. (*Women with multiple lipid abnormalities were twice as likely to have an elevated thyroid-stimulating hormone [TSH] level.*)
5. Cappola AR, Fried LP, Arnold AM et al. Thyroid status, cardiovascular risk, and mortality in older adults. JAMA 2006;295:1033. (*Major prospective cohort study; no increase in cardiovascular outcomes or mortality was found in persons with hypothyroidism, overt or subclinical.*)
6. Cappola AR, Ladenson PW. Hypothyroidism and atherosclerosis. J Clin Endocrinol Metab 2003;88:2438. (*Discusses atherosclerotic risk factors associated with hypothyroidism; 75 references.*)
7. Cooper DS. Subclinical hypothyroidism. N Engl J Med 2001;345:260. (*General review with an algorithm for the management of subclinical hypothyroidism; 44 references.*)
8. Desai J, Yassa L, Marqusee E, et al. Hypothyroidism after sunitinib treatment for patients with gastrointestinal stromal tumors. Ann Intern Med 2006;145:660. (*Hypothyroidism is a frequent complication of this type of cancer therapy.*)
9. Diez JJ, Iglesias P. Spontaneous subclinical hypothyroidism in patients older than 55 years: an analysis of natural course and risk factors for the development of overt thyroid failure. J Clin Endocrinol Metab 2004;89:4890. (*The initial TSH level was the most powerful predictor of outcomes; a mild elevation [5.0 to 9.9 mU/L] conferred a lower risk of developing overt hypothyroidism than did higher levels.*)
10. Dugbartey AT. Neurocognitive aspects of hypothyroidism. Arch Intern Med 1998;158:1413. (*Data on symptoms and their responsiveness to replacement therapy.*)
11. Gussekloo J, van Excel E, deCraen AJM, et al. Thyroid status, disability and cognitive function, and survival in old age. JAMA 2004;292:2591. (*Very elderly patients with subclinical hypothyroidism and abnormally high TSH do not experience adverse effects on daily life, depressive symptoms, or cognitive function.*)
12. Pearce EN, Farwell AP, Braverman LE. Thyroiditis. N Engl J Med 2003;348:2646. (*General review of mechanisms, clinical and biochemical changes, and types; 76 references.*)
13. Roberts LM, Pattison H, Roalfe A, et al. Is subclinical thyroid dysfunction in the elderly associated with depression or cognitive dysfunction? Ann Intern Med 2006;145:573. (*A cross-sectional study; no evidence was found for an association after controlling for comorbid conditions.*)

14. Robuschi G, Safran M, Braverman LE, et al. Hypothyroidism in the elderly. Endocrine Rev 1987;8:142. (*Comprehensive review of pathophysiology, clinical presentation, and treatment.*)

15. Rodondi N, Aujesky D, Vittinghoff E, et al. Subclinical hypothyroidism and the risk of coronary heart disease: a meta-analysis. Am J Med 2006;119:541. (*Finds evidence for increased risk [odds ratio 2.38 in pooling studies of best quality].*)

16. Surks MI, Sievert R. Drugs and thyroid function. N Engl J Med 1995;333:1688. (*Very useful review.*)

17. Surks MI, Ortiz E, Daniels GH, et al. Subclinical thyroid disease: scientific review and guidelines for diagnosis and management. JAMA 2004;291:228 (*Detailed review of the data; there was insufficient evidence to support population-based screening, but clinicians are encouraged to make individual patient assessment.*)

18. American College of Physicians. Screening for thyroid disease. Ann Intern Med 1998;129:141. (*Recommends selective screening limited to high-risk populations.*)

19. Danese MD, Powe NR, Sawin CT, et al. Screening for mild thyroid failure at the periodic health examination: a decision and cost-effectiveness analysis. JAMA 1996;276:285. (*Screening for subclinical hypothyroidism is found to be cost-effective, especially in elderly women.*)

20. Helfand M, Redfern CC. Screening for thyroid disease: an update. Ann Intern Med 1998;129:144. (*Thoughtful review of the evidence for screening; includes a detailed discussion of the value of screening for subclinical hypothyroid.*)

21. Nordyke RA, Reppun T, Madanay LD, et al. Alternative sequences of thyrotropin and free thyroxine assays for routine thyroid function testing: quality and cost. Arch Intern Med 1998;158:266. (*A literature review of cost-effectiveness; obtaining the TSH level first was found to be the most cost-effective approach to testing.*)

22. Schectman JM, Pawlson LG. The cost-effectiveness of three thyroid function testing strategies for suspicion of hypothyroidism in a primary care setting. J Gen Intern Med 1990;5:9. (*A TSH-first strategy proved best.*)

23. Bunevicius R, Kazanavicius G, Salinkevicius R, et al. Effects of thyroxine as compared with thyroxine plus triiodothyronine in patients with hypothyroidism. N Engl J Med 1999;340:424. (*A crossover study; in the group given mixed treatment, relative improvements in mood and neuropsychological functioning were noted.*)

24. Centanni M, Gargano L, Canettieri G, et al. Thyroxine in goiter, *Helicobacter pylori* infection, and chronic gastritis. N Engl J Med 2006; 354:1787. (*There was evidence that normal acid secretion is necessary for the absorption of oral thyroxine.*)

25. Chu JW, Crapo LM. The treatment of subclinical hypothyroidism is seldom necessary. J Clin Endocrinol Metab 2001;86:4591. (*The argument against treatment.*)

26. Dong BJ, Hauck WW, Gambertoglio JG, et al. Bioequivalence of generic and brand-name levothyroxine products in the treatment of hypothyroidism. JAMA 1997;277:1205. (*A pharmacokinetic study; the products were bioequivalent and interchangeable for most patients.*)

27. Danese MD, Ladenson PW, Meinert CL, et al. Effect of thyroxine therapy on serum lipoproteins in patients with mild thyroid failure: a quantitative review of the literature. J Clin Endocrinol Metab 2000;85:2993. (*The treatment lowers mean serum total and low-density-lipoprotein–cholesterol concentrations without a significant effect on serum high-density lipoprotein or triglyceride concentrations.*)

28. Escobar-Morreale HF, Botella-Carretero JI, Gomez-Bueno M, et al. Thyroid hormone replacement therapy in primary hypothyroidism: a randomized trial comparing L-thyroxine plus L-thyronine with L-thyroxine alone. Ann Intern Med 2005;142:412. (*No objective advantage was found, but patients preferred the combination therapy.*)

29. Fish LH, Schwartz HL, Cavanaugh J, et al. Replacement dose, metabolism, and bioavailability of levothyroxine in the treatment of hypothyroidism. N Engl J Med 1987;316:764. (*Detailed study of pharmacokinetics; the mean replacement dose was 112 μg/d.*)

30. Greenspan SL, Greenspan FS. The effect of thyroid hormone on skeletal integrity. Ann Intern Med 1999;130:750. (*There was an increased risk for osteoporosis, particularly in cortical bone; bone density of hip or forearm is recommended for women.*)

31. Greenspan SL, Greenspan FS, Resnick NM, et al. Skeletal integrity in premenopausal and postmenopausal women receiving long-term L-thyroxine therapy. Am J Med 1991;91:5. (*Bone loss is minimal at most when replacement therapy is carefully administered.*)

32. Grozinsky-Glasberg S, Fraser A, Nahshoni E, et al. Thyroxine-triiodothyronine combination therapy versus thyroxine monotherapy for clinical hypothyroidism: meta-analysis of randomized controlled trials. J Clin Endocrinol Metal 2006;91:2592. (*Systematic review of the best studies; no significant difference was found in outcomes.*)

33. Krugman L, Hershman J, Chopra I, et al. Patterns of recovery of the hypothalamic–pituitary–thyroid axis in patients taken off chronic thyroid therapy. J Clin Endocrinol Metab 1975;41:70. (*Full recovery of pituitary and thyroid responsiveness to thyrotropin-releasing hormone occurred in euthyroid patients by 5 weeks.*)

34. Levine HD. Compromise therapy in the patient with angina pectoris and hypothyroidism. Am J Med 1980;69:411. (*Details the difficulties of adequately controlling angina while fully correcting hypothyroidism.*)

35. Mandel SJ, Brent GA, Larsen PR. Levothyroxine therapy in patients with thyroid disease. Ann Intern Med 1993;119:492. (*Includes a detailed discussion of replacement therapy for hypothyroidism.*)

36. McDermott MT, Ridgway EC. Subclinical hypothyroidism is mild thyroid failure and should be treated. J Clin Endocrinol Metab 2001;86:4585. (*Argues for treatment.*)

37. Ross DS. Monitoring L-thyroxine therapy: lessons from the effects of L-thyroxine on bone density. Am J Med 1991;91:1. (*Outlines an approach to replacement therapy that minimizes the risk for osteoporosis by carefully titrating dose and TSH response.*)

38. Sawin CT, Geller A, Hershman JM, et al. The aging thyroid—the use of thyroid hormone in older persons. JAMA 1990;261:2653. (*Epidemiologic data showing a 10% prevalence of use in the elderly; in 10% of these patients, use was inappropriate and treatment could be discontinued.*)

39. Singer PA, Cooper DS, Levy EG, et al. Treatment guidelines for patients with hyperthyroidism and hypothyroidism. Standards of Care Committee, American Thyroid Association. JAMA 1995;273:808. (*Consensus clinical guidelines.*)

40. Singh N, Singh PN, Hershman JM. Effect of calcium carbonate on the absorption of levothyroxine. JAMA 2000;283:2822. (*Prospective cohort study; documents the reduction in absorption by adsorption to calcium, reducing bioavailability.*)

41. Toft A. Increased levothyroxine requirements in pregnancy—why, when, and how much? N Engl J Med 2004;351:292. (*An editorial recommending a 25- to 50-μg/d increase in L-thyroxine replacement dose at time of diagnosis of pregnancy, with close monitoring and further dose adjustment up to 20 weeks.*)

CHAPTER 105 ■ GLUCOCORTICOID THERAPY

DAVID M. SLOVIK

The therapeutic potency of glucocorticoids has led to their widespread use. Although benefits can be substantial, adverse effects are numerous, including serious metabolic derangements and suppression of the hypothalamic–pituitary–adrenal (HPA) axis. To maximize the therapeutic response and minimize the risks, a number of questions must be addressed before steroid therapy is initiated: (a) Is the underlying disorder of such severity that the benefits of therapy outweigh the risks? (b) Will prolonged treatment be required, or will a brief, limited course suffice? (c) Have alternative, less morbid therapies been maximally utilized? (d) Does the patient have any underlying condition that will worsen on steroid therapy or predispose to drug-induced complications? (e) Can a less suppressive regimen (e.g., alternate-day therapy or inhaled steroids) be utilized?

The primary physician must decide when and how to institute steroid therapy, whether to use daily or alternate-day treatment, and how to withdraw long-term glucocorticoid treatment safely.

ADVERSE EFFECTS (1–15)

Most adverse effects of glucocorticoids are a function of the degree of systemic absorption, dose, and duration of use. A few effects are irreversible; fortunately, most resolve within several months of termination of therapy.

Suppression of the Hypothalamic–Pituitary–Adrenal Axis

Suppression compromises the physiologic response to major stress (e.g., surgery, injury), putting the patient at risk for hypotension and hypoglycemia. Symptoms and signs include *lightheadedness*, *nausea*, *postural hypotension*, and *hypoglycemia*.

Risk of Suppression and Its Determinants

Risk correlates with the *dose* and *duration* of therapy, but it is hard to predict HPA responsiveness accurately on the basis of dose and duration alone. Other factors are believed to be operative also.

Dose and Duration of Steroid Therapy. Any patient who has received a glucocorticoid in a dose equivalent to 20 to 30 mg/d of prednisone for more than 5 days should be suspected of having some degree of HPA suppression. Prednisone at doses of 5 mg or less given once daily in the morning is generally not associated with HPA suppression. Doses greater than 5 mg/d are usually suppressive, but this also depends on the dose and the duration of therapy. Even the so-called "physiologic dose" of 7.5 mg of prednisone that supposedly corresponds

to daily endogenous glucocorticoid synthesis is suppressive in some patients. Moreover, individual patients vary widely.

Dose Scheduling. Dose scheduling has some effect on the degree of HPA suppression. *Daily* physiologic doses of glucocorticoids (e.g., 5 to 7.5 mg of prednisone) given in the morning may not cause suppression of any consequence, but if the same doses are given at night, normal diurnal cortisol secretion is inhibited. Doses just greater than the physiologic range are suppressive after about 1 month of use. *Alternate-day* therapy, in which short- or intermediate-acting preparations are taken at 8 a.m. every other day generally, does not induce clinically significant HPA suppression, nor does a *cyclic* program of 5 days of daily therapy followed by 2 to 4 weeks off therapy. However, cycles of 2 weeks on and 2 weeks off do lead to HPA suppression. A single daily pharmacologic dose of glucocorticoid produces less HPA suppression than does the same dose divided and taken at intervals during the course of the day.

Other Factors. The *renal clearance* of glucocorticoids decreases with *age*, and thus a given dose will have greater effects in older persons.

Recovery from HPA Suppression

Recovery from HPA suppression can take up to 12 months, depending on the dose and duration of treatment. Hypothalamic–pituitary function returns first, reappearing 2 to 5 months after the cessation of suppressive therapy, and is manifested by appropriate plasma adrenocorticotropic hormone (ACTH) levels, which demonstrate a normal diurnal pattern. Signs of adrenal recovery become evident at 6 to 9 months, with a return of the baseline serum cortisol level to normal. Maximal adrenal response to ACTH may not reappear until 9 to 12 months after the cessation of therapy. There is no proven method for accelerating the restoration of normal HPA function once it has been inhibited. The administration of ACTH does not seem to speed adrenal recovery.

Metabolic and Endocrinologic Side Effects

Protein and Fat

A *negative nitrogen balance* (the result of inhibition of protein synthesis and enhancement of protein catabolism) is believed to be partially responsible for reduced muscle mass, weakness, thinning of the skin, and striae formation. *Fat redistribution* accounts for the characteristic truncal obesity and cushingoid appearance. Both fat redistribution and negative nitrogen balance are minimized by using alternate-day therapy or giving no more than a physiologic dose each morning, but not by using ACTH or daily pharmacologic glucocorticoid doses. Acne is seen, more often with ACTH than with glucocorticoid use, because of stimulation of adrenal androgen production.

Glucose

Glucose intolerance is common. Mechanisms include increases in peripheral insulin resistance, gluconeogenesis, glucagon secretion, and substrate availability. Usually, the glucose intolerance is mild, does not lead to ketosis, and resolves when therapy is stopped. When carbohydrate intolerance develops, the effect appears to be dose related.

Hypertension and Fluid Retention

Hypertension and fluid retention with peripheral edema are more common when agents with mineralocorticoid effects are used, and they are not dependent on any prior elevation of blood pressure (Table 105.1). Again, the dose and duration of therapy are important factors. *Electrolyte derangements* are common, especially hypokalemia.

Enhanced Susceptibility to Infection

Enhanced susceptibility to infection results from the antiinflammatory and immunosuppressive actions of corticosteroids. Bacterial infections are common. Candidiasis and aspergillosis sometimes develop. Herpes zoster, varicella, vaccinia, and cytomegalovirus infection are the principal viral infections encountered in patients on steroids. Reactivation of tuberculosis is a well-recognized risk (see Chapter 38).

Osteoporosis

Osteoporosis develops when steroids are used for prolonged periods. The exact incidence of clinically significant bone loss is unknown, but estimates are around 50%. Bone loss is most rapid within the first 3 to 6 months of therapy. Higher doses for prolonged duration increase the risk for osteoporosis, but even as little as 5 mg of prednisone per day over time can result in bone loss. Although bone loss occurs with alternate-day and inhaled therapy, it is less than with daily oral therapy. Patients with a predisposition to osteoporosis, such as menopausal women and immobilized persons, appear to be among the most susceptible. The *axial skeleton* is affected more than the limbs, and *vertebral compression fractures* may result. *Aseptic necrosis of the femoral head* and other bones is a well-recognized and serious, but relatively rare, skeletal complication. Sometimes it may be a manifestation of the underlying illness for which corticosteroids are being given, such as rheumatoid arthritis or systemic lupus.

Gastrointestinal Effects

Gastritis, peptic ulceration, and gastrointestinal bleeding have all been attributed to steroid use. Multiple randomized, controlled trials have produced conflicting results, as have major meta-analyses examining pooled data from such trials (see Chapter 68). Hotly debated is the degree to which ulcer risk is a function of the dose and duration of exposure. The risk appears to be small until doses greater than the equivalent of 30 mg of prednisone per day are reached and continued for more than 1 month. Even then, the increase in rate of peptic ulceration is in the range of only 1% to 2%. Most peptic ulceration is caused by the concurrent use of nonsteroidal antiinflammatory agents. Antacids and food do not interfere with the absorption of oral steroid preparations.

Acute pancreatitis is noted with increased frequency in patients taking corticosteroids. *Panniculitis* is unique to iatrogenic Cushing's syndrome.

Myopathy

Myopathy may result from the prolonged intake of large doses. Proximal muscle wasting and weakness of the lower extremities are characteristic. Patients have difficulty climbing stairs and rising from a seated position. The average time of onset is 5 months into treatment. Muscle enzymes are normal. The

TABLE 105.1

COMMONLY USED GLUCOCORTICOIDS

Duration of Action	Glucocorticoid Potency[a]	Equivalent Glucocorticoid Dose (mg)	Mineralocorticoid Activity
Short Acting			
Cortisol (hydrocortisone)	1	20	Yes[b]
Cortisone	0.8	25	Yes[b]
Prednisone	4	5	No
Prednisolone	4	5	No
Methylprednisolone	5	4	No
Intermediate Acting			
Triamcinolone	5	4	No
Long Acting			
Betamethasone	25	0.60	No
Dexamethasone	30	0.75	No

[a] The values given for glucocorticoid potency are relative. Cortisol is arbitrarily assigned a value of 1.
[b] Mineralocorticoid effects are dose related. At doses close to or within the basal physiologic range for glucocorticoid activity, no such effect may be detectable.
Adapted from Axelrod L. Glucocorticoid therapy. Medicine (Baltimore) 1976;55:39, with permission.

complication is reversible, and exercise may help to minimize it. Sometimes it is difficult to distinguish between steroid myopathy and the myopathy associated with the underlying disorder it is being used to treat, for example, polymyositis.

Psychological and Behavioral Changes

Psychological and behavioral changes are particularly common in the elderly. The reported incidence ranges from 25% to 40%, mostly among patients receiving high doses. Increased appetite, mild euphoria, and insomnia are rather common at the beginning of treatment, especially with higher doses. Psychoses, which are not predictably related to dose or duration of therapy, can occur; they slowly respond to reduction or cessation of steroid use. The patient's premorbid personality may play a role. Steroid therapy can exacerbate previous psychiatric disease.

Cataracts

Cataracts of the posterior subcapsular type are reported in 10% to 35% of cases and are predominantly dose and duration dependent. A few require removal; most do not.

Adverse Effects of Inhaled Glucocorticoids

The inhaled topically active steroid preparations used for asthma are usually well tolerated and not associated with significant adverse effects, even when used daily for months at a time. However, the growing appreciation of the need for long-term therapy with inhaled steroids and the development of increasingly potent preparations (e.g., fluticasone) have raised concerns about the potential for systemic effects. Meta-analytic study finds that the risk for HPA suppression is greatest when the dose of most inhaled steroids exceeds 1.5 mg/d (>0.75 mg/d for fluticasone). Fluticasone demonstrates greater biologic activity and confers a greater risk on a milligram-per-milligram basis than beclomethasone, budesonide, and triamcinolone. Similar relationships and dose thresholds have been noted with regard to the risks for osteoporosis and posterior subcapsular cataracts. A lesser risk for ocular hypertension and glaucoma has been observed, but no evidence has been found of permanent growth retardation in children. Skin bruising parallels HPA suppression.

PRINCIPLES OF MANAGEMENT (1,2,16–24)

The challenge of glucocorticoid use is to obtain maximal therapeutic benefit with a minimum of adverse effects. In most instances, steroids do not cure disease or alter its natural history; rather, they suppress or alter the inflammatory and immunologic responses and, in doing so, reduce symptoms. Therefore, one must carefully weigh the perceived therapeutic benefit against the potential risks. The risk is negligible for a short-term course of therapy (7 to 14 days), even with high doses, which can be very effective in selected situations (e.g., acute asthma, contact dermatitis). Appetite stimulation and restlessness are the principal side effects. No long-term consequences have been noted. The decision to initiate more-prolonged steroid therapy requires additional consideration of the risks involved (see previous discussion).

Choice of Corticosteroid

Corticosteroid preparations differ principally in the duration of action and degree of mineralocorticoid activity (Table 105.1). *Short-acting agents* are less likely to cause HPA suppression, especially when prescribed for morning use in low doses as part of an alternate-day program (see later discussion). Long-acting agents are preferred for situations in which a high-dose steroid effect must be sustained (e.g., increased intracranial pressure). Mineralocorticoid activity is desirable in adrenal insufficiency but not in situations of excessive inflammation or immunoreactivity. Regardless of the agent selected, it is essential to continue maximal nonsteroidal therapy, insofar as it reduces steroid requirements.

Prednisone

Prednisone is the most widely prescribed of the glucocorticoids. Its short half-life, low cost, and negligible mineralocorticoid effect make it useful for most immunosuppressive and antiinflammatory indications. Prednisone is biologically inactive but is rapidly converted in the liver to the active form, *prednisolone*. Prednisolone is useful in the setting of severe liver failure.

Dexamethasone

Dexamethasone is the long-acting glucocorticoid of choice, being about seven times more potent on a weight basis than prednisone and having a half-life of 24 hours. This potency makes the agent useful for suppressive testing of the HPA axis.

Hydrocortisone (Cortisol)

Hydrocortisone (cortisol) is the naturally occurring glucocorticoid. It has one fourth of the glucocorticoid potency of prednisone but exerts some mineralocorticoid effect when used in pharmacologic doses. It also can be given parenterally and thus is useful in patients with adrenal suppression who need stress dose intravenous therapy (e.g., patients requiring surgery or have acute medical problems).

Florinef (9-α-Fluorohydrocortisone/Fludrocortisone)

This potent mineralocorticoid has virtually no glucocorticoid effect and is used primarily for replacement in adrenal cortical insufficiency, particularly in patients with symptomatic postural hypotension.

ACTH

Theoretically, the use of ACTH would appear to be attractive because it might avoid adrenal suppression, but it also induces undesirable mineralocorticoid and androgenic responses. Moreover, it must be given parenterally, and there is no way to know how much glucocorticoid effect is obtained from a given dose. These disadvantages limit its usefulness, although it is given by many neurologists to treat exacerbations of multiple sclerosis (see Chapter 172).

Selection of Dosing Schedule: Alternate-Day versus Daily Dosing

Most conditions that require prolonged corticosteroid treatment, such as asthma (see Chapter 48), sarcoidosis (see Chapter 51), inflammatory bowel disease (see Chapter 73), rheumatoid arthritis (see Chapter 156), and nephrotic syndrome (see Chapter 142), can be well controlled with *alternate-day therapy*, although it is often necessary to begin with a program of daily steroids when the disease is very active and symptoms are severe.

Alternate-Day Therapy

Important advantages of alternate-day treatment are avoidance of significant HPA suppression and minimization of cushingoid side effects without a substantial loss of antiinflammatory activity. It appears that the antiinflammatory effects of glucocorticoids persist longer (up to 3 days) than the undesirable metabolic effects. Other adverse effects that are reduced or eliminated by an alternate-day schedule include inhibition of delayed hypersensitivity, susceptibility to infection, negative nitrogen balance, fluid retention, hypertension, bone loss, and psychological and behavioral disturbances.

Alternate-day therapy by itself will not prevent HPA suppression if a long-acting steroid preparation is used (e.g., dexamethasone). Moreover, therapy must really be given on alternate days, with the total dose taken first thing in the morning every other day. Intermittent therapy or doses taken throughout the day every other day do not preserve HPA responsiveness.

Daily Therapy

Daily steroid therapy is indicated during acute exacerbations of disease and in the limited number of conditions that are controlled only by daily glucocorticoid administration, such as temporal arteritis (see Chapter 161) and pemphigus vulgaris. When daily therapy is necessary, HPA suppression can be minimized by having the patient take the entire daily dose first thing in the morning and by prescribing a short-acting glucocorticoid at the lowest possible dose. Daily single-dose regimens may be as effective or nearly as effective as divided-dose regimens in controlling underlying illness. However, manifestations of Cushing's syndrome are not prevented, as they are with alternate-day therapy.

Switching from Daily to Alternate-Day Schedule

Most patients who experience a remission on daily therapy are candidates for a trial of alternate-day steroids (see previous discussion for exceptions). Switching makes it possible for the patient to transfer to a program with less morbidity without a diminution in disease control. In switching, the *same total steroid dose* is continued, whereas in tapering, it is gradually reduced. Because most patients who are being switched to an alternate-day schedule have been on steroids for prolonged periods, switching should be done by gradually increasing the dose on the first day and decreasing it on the second day until a double dose is taken every other day, with no drug taken on the in-between days.

How fast the changeover can be made varies, depending on the activity of the underlying disease, duration of therapy, degree of HPA suppression, and cooperativeness of the patient. A rough guideline for switching to alternate-day therapy is to make changes in increments of 10 mg of prednisone (or its equivalent) when the daily prednisone dose is greater than 40 mg and in 5-mg increments when the daily dose is between 20 and 40 mg. For daily doses smaller than 20 mg, the changes should be made in increments of 2.5 mg. The interval between changes ranges from 1 day to several weeks and is determined empirically, based on the clinical response. It is important to keep in mind that most patients who have been on a daily steroid program for more than 2 to 4 weeks probably have some degree of HPA suppression.

Tapering and Withdrawing Steroid Therapy

Whereas rapid withdrawal of steroid therapy is possible if the underlying disease process is self-limited and there is no HPA suppression, the abrupt withdrawal of steroid therapy in the context of HPA suppression can precipitate adrenal insufficiency, a flare-up of the underlying illness, a withdrawal syndrome, or any combination of these. There is no way to speed HPA recovery, nor are specific schedules available for reducing the daily dose. One must monitor disease activity and decrease the dose empirically by small amounts, watching for flare-up of disease or signs of adrenal insufficiency, such as postural hypotension, weakness, and gastrointestinal distress.

Tapering Schedule

A commonly used empiric approach to tapering corticosteroid therapy bases the tapering program on the current daily steroid dose:

- At greater than 40 mg/d, one tapers by 10 mg/d every 1 to 2 weeks.
- At 40 mg/d, one tapers by 5 mg every 1 to 2 weeks.
- At 20 mg/d, one tapers by 2.5 mg every 1 to 2 weeks.

Tapering continues until a physiologic dose of prednisone is reached (5 to 7.5 mg/d). The patient can then be switched to 1-mg prednisone tablets or the equivalent dose of hydrocortisone, so that further reductions in dose can be made in smaller steps than is possible when 5-mg prednisone tablets are used. Weekly or biweekly reductions can then be carried out in steps of 1 mg of prednisone at a time, as permitted by disease activity.

Withdrawal Syndrome

During the tapering process, a *steroid withdrawal syndrome* develops in some patients, characterized by depression, myalgias, arthralgias, anorexia, headaches, nausea, and lethargy. Studies have failed to show a relationship between these symptoms and low cortisol levels. In most instances, symptoms are reported when levels are normal, or even elevated, but falling rapidly. HPA responsiveness has also been found to be normal in many of these patients. The mechanisms responsible for this syndrome are unknown but seem to be linked to the rapidity with which the dose is tapered.

Identification and Treatment of Steroid-Induced Adrenal Suppression

Testing for HPA Suppression

At times of anticipated stress (e.g., impending surgery), it is important to know how responsive the HPA axis is and whether supplementary steroid therapy will be needed. It is very difficult to predict the onset and duration of HPA suppression in an individual patient. The degree of suppression cannot be reliably estimated by the *basal serum cortisol* concentration, making assessment of HPA responsiveness a useful adjunct for deciding who will need supplementation.

Corticotropin (Cosyntropin) Stimulation Testing. Corticotropin (cosyntropin) stimulation testing is the most widely used approach to testing responsiveness of the HPA axis. It is a convenient, safe, and effective means of testing for suppression in the office setting. Results correlate well with cortisol levels measured during the stress of surgery. A blood sample is drawn to measure the basal serum cortisol, after which a one-ampule (250-μg) bolus of synthetic ACTH (*cosyntropin*) is injected intravenously (or may be administered intramuscularly). Subsequent cortisol determinations are drawn at 30 and 60 minutes. If the serum cortisol level at 30 or 60 minutes is greater than 18 μg/dL, then adrenal responsiveness is sufficient to sustain the patient through a stress equivalent to general anesthesia.

The test produces a few false-positive results in comparison with insulin-induced hypoglycemia (the gold standard for testing HPA function), but it is safer and more convenient to perform. False negatives may occur if central but not adrenal suppression has developed.

Corticotropin-Releasing Hormone Stimulation Test. A corticotropin-releasing hormone stimulation test can assess both ACTH and adrenal responsiveness. Sensitivity and specificity are very high, but the test is very expensive and is used predominantly in research settings.

Limitations of Testing for HPA Responsiveness. Although HPA suppression is important to detect, it is not the only factor determining the ability of corticosteroid-exposed patients to respond appropriately to stress. Some patients manifest a hypotensive response to stress despite a normally responding HPA axis, and patients with a blunted HPA response may manifest no signs of clinical adrenal insufficiency. More work is needed to elucidate the mechanisms governing stress response in steroid-treated patients.

Stress Dosing

If the patient cannot mount an adequate cortisol response, or if testing is impractical because of urgency or the unavailability of agents or assays, corticosteroid supplementation should be administered for acute stress. It is better to err on the safe side and administer stress doses of steroids if there is any uncertainty about the adequacy of the HPA axis at the time of stress. Hydrocortisone and dexamethasone are the commonly prescribed agents for stress dosing.

Hydrocortisone. Hydrocortisone is usually prescribed because it provides both glucocorticoid and mineralocorticoid effects. Depending on the severity of the stress, one administers 100 to 400 mg of hydrocortisone per day in divided doses. The lower end of the dose range is appropriate for the stress of gastroenteritis, influenza, or dental extraction. During major stress, such as trauma or surgery, the patient should be given 100 mg of hydrocortisone parenterally every 6 to 8 hours.

Dexamethasone. A prepackaged 1-mL syringe containing 4 mg of *dexamethasone* phosphate can be prescribed for the patient or family to carry for parenteral use in an emergency should medical care be unavailable and the patient become unconscious or so ill that steroids cannot be taken by mouth. The need to continue supplementation is based on the duration of the stress and the underlying state of the HPA axis.

Prophylaxis and Treatment of Osteoporosis

Patients requiring long-term daily steroid therapy are at high risk for bone loss and osteoporotic fracture, necessitating consideration of prophylaxis and treatment. Even modest doses of prednisone (e.g., 7.5 mg/d) are associated with a risk for significant bone loss when used on a daily basis for a prolonged period. Vertebral compression fractures are of particular concern because trabecular bone seems to be most affected. Bone density should be measured (see Chapter 144), especially if the patient is menopausal. Prophylactic treatment may be necessary.

Bisphosphonates (Alendronate, Risedronate)

If the patient has severe osteoporosis, is at high risk (e.g., prolonged high-dose therapy, inactivity), or has a history of vertebral compression fracture, then bisphosphonate therapy (e.g., *alendronate*, risedronate) offers the best chance for limiting bone loss. Once-weekly dosing is available, safe, and effective, provided the patient receives careful instruction on proper administration (see Chapter 164).

Estrogen

Estrogen therapy should be considered for women with menopausal symptoms and not primarily to forestall bone loss due to glucocorticoids. The risks and benefits of estrogen therapy need to be carefully weighed, especially if prolonged treatment is anticipated (see Chapters 118 and 164).

Minimizing the Risk of Inhaled Corticosteroids

The most important means of reducing the risk for systemic effects is to keep the daily dose as low as possible (i.e., <1.5 mg/d for beclomethasone, flunisolide, budesonide, and triamcinolone; <0.8 mg/d for fluticasone). The ways to accomplish this without compromising asthma control include concurrent use of a long-acting β-agonist (e.g., salmeterol) or leukotriene inhibitor (e.g., montelukast), and immunotherapy (see Chapter 48).

PATIENT EDUCATION

Steroids should be given with caution to patients whose reliability is in question because of the risk of HPA suppression and adrenocortical insufficiency. Patients on alternate-day therapy must be instructed about the importance of keeping to the alternate-day schedule and taking their medication around 8 a.m. so as to minimize the risk for suppression. Patients on a suppressive dose of steroid should be informed about the need for steroid supplementation when stress or illness occurs and should wear a medical alert bracelet or necklace and carry an emergency medical information card stating that they take a corticosteroid or have adrenal insufficiency. Patients must understand the need to contact the physician and increase the steroid dose when they are subjected to physiologic stress.

Many patients are reluctant to discontinue long-term steroid therapy because they fear recrudescence of the underlying illness or experience malaise as the drug is tapered. A detailed review of the side effects of prolonged therapy is necessary so that the rationale for reducing the dose and the desirability of eventually discontinuing corticosteroid therapy are understood and appreciated. Any change in dose and schedule should be written out. When prolonged daily high-dose therapy is required, the psychological impact of adverse effects (e.g., cushingoid features) can be lessened by informing the patient that they are likely to occur but are at least partially reversible.

THERAPEUTIC RECOMMENDATIONS (1,16–24)

- Prescribe glucocorticoids only when maximal doses of other forms of therapy have proved to be insufficient and when the risks of steroid use are outweighed by the therapeutic benefit expected.
- To minimize the steroid dose required, always try to *add steroid therapy* to the ongoing treatment program rather than replace it.
- In the setting of active autoimmune or inflammatory disease, initiate a full-strength program of daily glucocorticoid therapy with prednisone (40 to 60 mg/d, or prednisolone in cases of hepatocellular failure). When replacement therapy for adrenal cortical insufficiency is needed, use hydrocortisone (see later discussion). The long-acting *dexamethasone* is reserved for testing the HPA axis and for the rare situation in which very high dose, sustained-action therapy is required (e.g., increased intracranial pressure). All glucocorticoids can be taken with food; absorption is not impaired.
- To *minimize the risk for HPA suppression*, avoid prescribing long-acting preparations, give the entire glucocorticoid dose in the morning, or, better yet, on alternate days, and continue for the shortest possible time.
- Try initiating therapy on an *alternate-day* basis when symptoms are not severe and the condition is not one with an absolute requirement for daily treatment (i.e., temporal arteritis, pemphigus vulgaris, severe inflammatory bowel disease).
- Once control is achieved, *taper* to the lowest dose that maintains control, and terminate if possible. Tapering is carried out empirically; the patient is monitored for disease activity and evidence of adrenal insufficiency (postural hypotension, gastrointestinal upset, fatigue, muscle weakness, hypoglycemia).
- For very brief courses of corticosteroid therapy (<7 to 14 days), taper rapidly over 7 to 10 days to full cessation, provided that disease activity remains quiescent. When longer courses of therapy are required, taper more slowly, reducing the dose in 10-mg decrements when the daily dose is greater than 40 mg and in 5-mg steps when it is less than 40 mg. The *rate of tapering* is determined by disease activity and the appearance of symptoms of steroid withdrawal or adrenal insufficiency. Once the dose has been reduced to 5 mg of prednisone every other day, therapy can be stopped or switched to 5-mg hydrocortisone or 1-mg prednisone tablets and reduced in decrements of 2.5 mg of hydrocortisone or 1 mg of prednisone.
- If tapering is unsuccessful or prolonged therapy is deemed necessary, then ascertain and maintain the lowest effective dose and try *switching to an alternate-day regimen* if it is not already being used.
- When switching to alternate-day therapy, begin by modestly reducing the second day's dose and adding that amount to the first day's dose. In this manner, the same total dose is maintained. If the daily dose is greater than 40 mg, reduce the dose on the alternate day by the equivalent of 10 mg of prednisone, and if the daily dose is less than 40 mg, by 5 mg. At less than 20 mg, the increment is 2.5 mg. The interval between changes in dose is determined empirically, based on the clinical status of the patient. The endpoint of switching is attained when the previous entire 2-day dose is being given once every other day.
- If withdrawal symptoms are a problem on alternate-day therapy, a small morning dose of hydrocortisone (10 to 20 mg) given on the off day may help to alleviate symptoms without prolonging HPA suppression.
- When HPA responsiveness is in question, perform a *cosyntropin stimulation test*. Administer 250 μg parenterally, and measure serum cortisol immediately before and 30 and 60 minutes after administration.
- Because 9 to 12 months of HPA suppression may begin after as little as 2 to 4 weeks of 20 to 30 mg of prednisone daily, advise patients taking daily pharmacologic doses to supplement their steroid intake when under stress or experiencing an acute illness. In the setting of injury, surgery, or an inability to take oral medication, prescribe parenteral hydrocortisone or its equivalent. The total daily stress dose is 100 to 400 mg of hydrocortisone, given in divided doses every 6 to 8 hours. Provide a prepackaged syringe containing 4 mg of dexamethasone for intramuscular emergency use.
- To prevent or treat *steroid-induced osteoporosis,* begin by measuring the vertebral bone density. If the patient is markedly osteoporotic and postmenopausal, prescribe 70 mg of *alendronate* or 35 mg of risedronate once weekly. Instruct the patient regarding the proper intake of alendronate or risedronate to minimize the risk for esophageal irritation (see Chapter 164). Alternatively, consider estrogen replacement therapy in conjunction with calcium and vitamin D supplementation for menopausal women taking corticosteroids if the degree of osteoporosis is not severe and the risk for steroid-induced disease is not great.

Annotated Bibliography

1. Axelrod L. Glucocorticoid therapy. Medicine (Baltimore) 1976;55:39. (*A superb and comprehensive review that is slightly dated but still well worth reading; 188 references.*)
2. Boumpas DT, Chrousos GP, Wilder RL, et al. Glucocorticoid therapy for immune-mediated diseases: basic and clinical correlates. Ann Intern Med 1993;119:1198. (*An excellent National Institutes of Health conference on the topic; 98 references.*)
3. Christy NP. Pituitary–adrenal function during corticosteroid therapy: learning to live with uncertainty. N Engl J Med 1992;326:266. (*An editorial reviewing the tests for hypothalamic–pituitary–adrenal [HPA] suppression and the difficulty of predicting it.*)
4. Graeber AL, Ney RL, Nicholson WE, et al. Natural history of pituitary–adrenal recovery following long-term suppression with corticosteroids. J Clin Endocrinol Metab 1965;25:11. (*Patients took glucocorticoids for 1 to 10 years; full restoration of HPA function was noted within 1 year; hypothalamic–pituitary function returned in the first 2 to 5 months; 17-hydroxycorticosteroid levels normalized during months 6 to 9.*)
5. Krasner AS. Glucocorticoid-induced adrenal insufficiency. JAMA 1999;282:671. (*A useful case-based discussion; 34 pertinent references.*)
6. Schlagkecke R, Kornely E, Santen RT, et al. The effect of long-term glucocorticoid therapy on pituitary–adrenal responses to exogenous corticotropin-releasing hormone. N Engl J Med 1992;326:226. (*HPA responsiveness could not be reliably predicted from the dose or the duration of steroid therapy or from the basal plasma cortisol level.*)
7. Laan RF, van Riel PL, van de Putte LB, et al. Low-dose prednisone induces rapid, reversible axial bone loss in patients with rheumatoid arthritis: a randomized, controlled study. Ann Intern Med 1993;119:963. (*Evidence that even low doses can produce bone loss.*)
8. Liworth BJ. Systemic adverse effects of inhaled corticosteroid therapy: a systematic review and meta-analysis. Arch Intern Med 1999;159:941. (*Finds*

an increased risk for adrenal suppression, cataracts, and ocular hypertension, but not osteoporosis, with high-potency formulations.)

9. Messer J, Reithman D, Sacks HS, et al. Association of adrenocorticosteroid therapy and peptic ulcer disease. N Engl J Med 1983;309:21. (*A meta-analysis, finding that high-dose corticosteroids increased the risk for peptic ulcer and gastrointestinal hemorrhage, but that the relative risk was 2 and the absolute risk was 2%.*)

10. Piper JM, Ray WA, Daugherty JR, et al. Corticosteroid use and peptic ulcer disease: role of nonsteroidal antiinflammatory drugs. Ann Intern Med 1991;114:735. (*The increased risk was caused by concurrent nonsteroidal antiinflammatory drug use.*)

11. Dale DC, Fauci AS, Wolff SM. Alternate-day prednisone, leukocyte kinetics and susceptibility to infections. N Engl J Med 1974;29:1154. (*A classic article, reporting that alternate-day steroid therapy did not reduce leukocyte count, inflammatory response, or neutrophil half-life.*)

12. VanStaa TP, Leufkens HG, Abenhaim L, et al. Use of oral corticosteroids and risk of fractures. J Bone Miner Res 2000;15:993. (*A retrospective cohort study, finding that there was a dose-dependent increase in fracture risk, which declined toward baseline after the cessation of therapy.*)

13. Carella MJ, Srivastava LS, Gossain VV, et al. Hypothalamic–pituitary–adrenal function 1 week after a short burst of steroid therapy. J Clin Endocrinol Metab 1993;76:1188. (*Clinically evident adrenal insufficiency was rare after a 1-week course of steroid therapy.*)

14. Meikle AW, Tyler FH. Potency and duration of action of glucocorticoids. Effects of hydrocortisone, prednisone, and dexamethasone on human pituitary–adrenal function. Am J Med 1977;63:200. (*The intrinsic potency and the relative rate of disappearance from plasma were the two most important factors determining the relative potency of orally administered glucocorticoids.*)

15. Nielsen GL, Sorensen HT, Mellemkjoer L, et al. Risk of hospitalization resulting from upper gastrointestinal bleeding among patients taking corticosteroids: a register-based study. Am J Med 2001;111:541. (*A population-based study, noting an increased risk; the relative risk was 2.9.*)

16. Aagaard EM, Lin P, Modin GW, et al. Prevention of glucocorticoid-induced osteoporosis: provider practice at an urban county hospital. Am J Med 1999;107:456. (*Documentation of the relative lack of awareness, and suggestions for improvement.*)

17. Abdu TA, Elhadd TA, Nearly R, et al. Comparison of the low-dose short synacthen test (1 mg), the conventional-dose short synacthen test (250 mg), and the insulin tolerance test for assessment of the hypothalamo–pituitary–adrenal axis in patients with pituitary disease. J Clin Endocrinol Metab 1999;84:838. (*Presents evidence that the low-dose test may be more sensitive than the conventional test and may obviate the need for insulin tolerance testing.*)

18. Anatruda TT Jr, Hurst MM, D'Esposo ND. Certain endocrine and metabolic facets of the steroid withdrawal syndrome. J Clin Endocrinol Metab 1965;25:1207. (*A classic study, showing that the steroid withdrawal syndrome is not a consequence of inadequate serum levels of steroid.*)

19. Byyny RL. Withdrawal from glucocorticoid therapy. N Engl J Med 1976;295:30. (*Still a very practical approach.*)

20. Gleeson HK, Walker BR, Seckl JR, et al. Ten years on: safety of short synacthen tests in assessing adrenocorticotropic hormone deficiency in clinical practice. J Clin Endocrinol Metab 2003;88:2106. (*The short synacthen test remains the primary screening for adrenocorticotropic hormone deficiency.*)

21. Papanicolaou DA, Tsigos C, Oldfield EH, et al. Acute glucocorticoid deficiency is associated with plasma elevations of interleukin-6: does the latter participate in the symptomatology of the steroid withdrawal syndrome? J Clin Endocrinol Metab 1996;81:2303. (*Presents evidence suggesting that this cytokine is an important factor.*)

22. Saag KG, Schnitzer TJ, Brown JP, et al. Alendronate for the prevention and treatment of glucocorticoid-induced osteoporosis. N Engl J Med 1998;339:292. (*A randomized, controlled trial, finding that a significant improvement in bone density was achieved regardless of the baseline bone density, steroid dose, or the duration of steroid therapy.*)

23. Streeten DH, Anderson GH Jr, Bonaventrua MM. The potential for serious consequences of misinterpreting normal responses to the rapid adrenocorticotropin test. J Clin Endocrinol Metab 1996;81:285. (*An excellent discussion of pitfalls.*)

24. Streeten DH. Shortcomings of low-dose (1 mg) ACTH test for the diagnosis of ACTH deficiency states. J Clin Endocrinol Metab 1999;84:835. (*A critique of this new approach to identifying central dysfunction of the axis.*)

SECTION 8 ■ GYNECOLOGIC PROBLEMS

CHAPTER 106 ■ SCREENING FOR BREAST CANCER

Breast cancer is among the most feared illnesses that afflict women, especially in North America and northern Europe, where incidence rates are five to six times higher than in Asia and Africa. More than 170,000 women develop breast cancer each year in the United States, accounting for more than one in four cancer diagnoses among women. Of these, more than 50,000 eventually die of the disease, accounting for one in five female cancer deaths. The lifetime probability that an American woman will develop breast cancer is approximately 12%. The morbidity and mortality associated with this disease, coupled with the importance of the breasts to many women's self-image, make breast cancer a topic of intense interest.

Breast cancer is one of only a few conditions for which benefits of screening have been well documented in randomized, controlled trials, but there is controversy about which women should be screened and how often. Advances in molecular biology, including identification of breast cancer susceptibility genes, have improved our ability to estimate the risk and predict the behavior of breast cancer for some women, but the clinical introduction of these techniques poses new challenges as chemoprevention and prophylactic mastectomy become considerations. The primary care provider deals with breast cancer screening and diagnosis or associated fears on a daily basis. Knowledge of various recommendations is insufficient. Primary care providers must understand the benefits and harms of breast cancer screening and prevention and communicate these effectively to patients.

EPIDEMIOLOGY AND RISK FACTORS (1–24)

The epidemiology of breast cancer has been studied extensively. Furthermore, analysis of familial patterns and identification of breast cancer susceptibility genes have refined our understanding of risk associated with age and family history.

Age (1,5,8)

Risk of breast cancer increases with age. The median age at the time of diagnosis is about 55 years; 45% of cases occur after age 65 years. However, breast cancer is not uncommon in women younger than 40 years, in whom approximately 20% of cases occur. When breast cancer does occur earlier in life, it is more likely to be associated with a susceptibility gene. For example, before age 40 years, about 5% of non-Jewish women with breast cancer and about 25% of Jewish women with breast cancer can be expected to have BRCA1 mutations.

Family History (2–4,7,12,13,16)

Overall, a family history of breast cancer, whether among maternal or paternal relatives, increases the risk approximately two- to threefold. For women who have a family history, specific risk depends heavily on the age at onset of cancer for combinations of first-degree and second-degree relatives. For example, if one first-degree or second-degree relative had cancer diagnosed at or after age 50 years, the cumulative breast cancer risk by age 80 years is approximately 10%, not significantly different from risk for the general population. If a first-degree relative had cancer before age 50 years, cumulative risk may be as high as 20%. With a history of early onset in two first-degree relatives, the probability that the family is affected by a dominant breast cancer susceptibility gene is substantial, and cumulative cancer risk by age 80 years approaches 50%.

Susceptibility genes account for about 5% to 10% of all breast cancers. In addition to family clustering and early age at onset of disease, family history of bilateral or multifocal breast cancer and ovarian cancer suggests inherited cancer predisposition. BRCA1, which accounts for about half of all inherited breast cancer, confers a cumulative breast cancer risk of approximately 85% and an ovarian cancer risk of 50%. Women with BRCA2 mutations face approximately the same risk of breast cancer but a significantly lower (10% to 20%) risk of ovarian cancer. Many members of families affected by breast cancer susceptibility genes have indicated a preference not to be tested. In addition, the response to learning about susceptibility is varied. Some women choose to have prophylactic surgery (bilateral mastectomies and/or oophorectomies); others do not. Prophylactic surgery reduces risk by about 90%.

Because of the variability in what women want to know about their risk and what they might choose to do with that knowledge, recommendations for women with an increased-risk family history that raises concern about a specific genetic predisposition generally focus on the need for genetic counseling as the key component of evaluation for BRCA testing.

Reproductive History (5,6,11,14,15)

Generally, there is an inverse relationship between breast cancer risk and parity, but maternal age at the time of first full-term pregnancy may be the most important factor related to reproductive history. In a woman with high parity whose first birth occurs before the age of 20 years, the risk of breast cancer is one half of that of a nulliparous woman and one third of that of a woman with one or two births after the age of 30 years. It has been suggested that childbirth transiently increases the risk of breast cancer but reduces the risk in later years. Either spontaneous or induced abortion may increase risk slightly, but the association is weak and could be due to reporting bias. Lactation appears to reduce slightly the risk of premenopausal cancer.

Menstrual History

Both late menarche and early natural menopause reduce breast cancer risk. Women who experienced menarche after age 16 years have half the risk of those who experienced it earlier. Women in whom menopause occurred before age 45 years have half the risk of those in whom menopause occurred after age 55 years. Women with early surgical menopause seem to be similarly protected.

History of Benign Breast Disease (23)

The relative risk of breast cancer among women who have a history of benign breast disease compared to those who do not is roughly 1.5. However, there are complex interactions between a woman's age, family history, and the histology of the benign breast disease. Histologic appearance is strongly associated with risk. In one study, the relative risks for nonproliferative changes, proliferative changes, and atypia were 1.27, 1.66, and 4.24, respectively. For women with nonproliferative changes and no family history, there was no increased risk; this subset accounted for more than half of all women with benign disease that prompted biopsies. However, among women with a strong family history, even nonproliferative changes were associated with a relative risk of 1.62. Age is also an important factor; for example, among women younger than 45 years and older than 55 years, the relative risks conferred by a finding of atypia were 6.99 and 3.37, respectively.

Breast density is also a risk factor. Fat is radiolucent; stroma and epithelium are radiographically dense. Women who have dense tissue in 75% or more of the volume of the breast have been reported to face a risk of cancer four to six times greater than women with little or no dense tissue. One recent study that addressed the problem that breast density also reduces the sensitivity of screening mammography found a relative risk of 4.7.

History of Previous Malignancy

Approximately 10% of women who survive 10 years after the diagnosis of breast cancer will have a second primary malignancy, usually in the contralateral breast. Increased use of breast-sparing surgery for early-stage breast cancer will increase the incidence of second breast cancers; about 10% to 20% of women who choose breast-sparing surgery followed by radiation experience ipsilateral in-breast recurrences during the 10-year period after treatment of the initial tumor. Women with a history of endometrial carcinoma have slightly increased risk for breast cancer.

Diet, Drugs, and Other Factors (17–20)

Breast cancer incidence varies fivefold among different countries and is positively associated with national dietary intake of fat. Diets high in fat have produced increased rates of mammary tumors in laboratory animals. Data from case–control studies have suggested a positive association, but prospective studies, including a recent overview of studies involving more than 300,000 women and nearly 5,000 cases, have found no evidence of a positive association between dietary fat and breast cancer. The Women's Health Initiative Dietary Modification Trial among postmenopausal women failed to demonstrate a statistically significant reduction in breast cancer among women randomized to a low-fat diet, but there was a trend in that direction, with a relative risk for the intervention group of 0.91 (95% confidence interval 0.83 to 1.01). Low levels of vitamin A have also been linked to increases in risk. Obesity has been associated with minor increases in risk.

The role of drugs is controversial. Evidence for increased risk after oral contraceptive use is equivocal; risk may be slightly increased (relative risks in the range of 1.1 to 1.2) for younger women and for long-time users. Breast cancer risk from postmenopausal estrogen and combined estrogen–progestin hormone replacement therapy is also uncertain. The 16-year cohort analysis of the Nurses' Health Study found increased relative risk among women currently using hormones (1.32 for estrogen alone and 1.41 for estrogen plus progestin) as compared with postmenopausal women who had never used hormones. The Women's Health Initiative randomized trial was stopped early after a mean of 5.2 years of follow-up because of a breast cancer hazard ratio of 1.26. After the report of this finding to the public in mid-2002, there was a sharp decline in the use of hormone replacement therapy, followed by a noticeable decline in breast cancer incidence a year later.

Several studies have demonstrated an association between daily moderate alcohol consumption and modest increase in breast cancer risk. Use of antibiotics has also been associated with risk of incident and fatal breast cancer. Use of aspirin and other nonsteroidal antiinflammatory drugs (NSAIDs) has been associated with a 20% to 40% relative risk reduction in breast cancer. Prostaglandin E2 has been shown to stimulate estrogen and progesterone in laboratory experiments. A selective reduction in risk of hormone receptor–positive tumors supports the hypothesis that this is mediated by inhibition of prostaglandin synthesis. A study suggesting that women who had undergone breast augmentation had lower cancer risk received substantial media attention. However, the analysis was found to be faulty, and a subsequent analysis showed no difference in risk after breast implants.

NATURAL HISTORY OF BREAST CANCER AND EFFECTIVENESS OF CHEMOPREVENTION AND EARLY THERAPY (1–3,5,23–33)

Little can be said with certainty about the natural history of breast cancer. The few observational studies of untreated invasive breast cancer have shown widely variable tumor doubling times ranging from less than 1 week to more than 6 months.

Younger women tend to have faster-growing tumors than older women. The average time for development of an invasive tumor that can be detected by mammography for women aged 35 to 49 years is 15 months. The average time that a tumor is detectable by mammography before a clinical diagnosis is made is believed to be approximately 3 years. Again, however, progression is likely to be faster among younger women.

There is even greater uncertainty about the natural history of noninvasive breast cancer. Dramatic increases in the incidence of ductal carcinoma *in situ* (DCIS) in recent years are attributable to mammographic screening. DCIS incidence rates increased approximately 4% annually during the decade ending in 1983 and approximately 18% annually for the subsequent decade. More than 25,000 new cases of DCIS are now diagnosed among U.S. women each year. Many of these lesions appear to be slow growing, and evidence suggests that 50% or more of untreated women with DCIS would not develop invasive disease.

Therapy for early-stage breast cancer is highly effective (see Chapter 122). DCIS does not affect survival during the first 1 to 9 years after diagnosis and treatment. Women with small invasive cancers (e.g., 1 cm) and negative axillary nodes can expect a disease-free survival of 90% to 95% during the 5 to 10 years after either mastectomy or breast-conserving surgery followed by radiation. Cumulative recurrence risk rises sharply with increase in tumor size and/or metastasis to axillary lymph nodes.

Attention to breast cancer screening has dramatically increased the proportion of breast cancers that are in earlier stages of development at the time of diagnosis. Furthermore, women whose tumors are detected by screening mammography face a lower risk of recurrence independent of tumor size and other risk factors. Neither of these findings constitutes evidence for screening benefit; they may well be due to lead-time bias and time-linked bias sampling (see Chapter 3). Mammographic screening has been shown, however, to decrease breast cancer morbidity and mortality for some women. It has also been shown to result in *overdiagnosis* of breast cancer, detecting cases that never would have come to clinical attention without screening. Rates of overdiagnosis have been estimated at 5% to 50%. Extended follow-up of patients in one screening trial found a rate of 10%. Clearly, there are tradeoffs to consider. As a result, controversy remains about which women should be screened and how often.

CHEMOPREVENTION (2,3,29–33)

Chemoprevention of breast cancer with selective estrogen receptor modulators (SERMs) is an important consideration for women at high risk of breast cancer. Four trials have addressed the impact of SERMs, specifically tamoxifen and raloxifene, when taken for primary prevention of breast cancer. Two of the trials were positive and two were negative. The Breast Cancer Prevention Trial (BCPT) enrolled women with 5-year risk estimated to be higher than 1.66, equivalent to that of a 60-year-old woman with average risk. The BCPT was terminated early after finding a 49% relative risk reduction and an absolute reduction of just greater than 20 cases per 1,000 women taking tamoxifen for more than 5 years. The effect was limited to estrogen-receptor–positive (ER⁺) cancers. The BCPT also documented significant harms associated with tamoxifen, including an increased risk of endometrial cancer, stroke, deep vein thrombosis, and pulmonary embolism especially among women older than 50 years.

The Multiple Outcomes of Raloxifene Evaluation trial found a relative risk reduction in breast cancer incidence of 76% with raloxifene compared with placebo, with an absolute risk reduction of 8 cases per 1,000 women over 40 months. Again, the effect was limited to ER⁺ tumors. The two negative trials were conducted in Europe. Both the Royal Marsden Hospital Chemoprevention Trial and the Italian Tamoxifen Prevention Study compared tamoxifen with placebo and failed to find a reduction in breast cancer incidence.

Based on this evidence, the U.S. Preventive Services Task Force recommends discussing chemoprevention with selected patients at high risk for breast cancer and at low risk for the most serious adverse events. Though not supported by evidence derived from randomized trials, use of aspirin and other NSAIDS should be discussed as well. Epidemiologic studies indicate a relative risk reduction of 20% to 40%, with the effect evident for hormone receptor–positive tumors but not hormone-receptor–negative tumors.

SCREENING METHODS (1,5,8,21,34–58)

Mammography and Other Imaging Studies (1,5,8,21,34–50,52–58)

Mammography has become the cornerstone of breast cancer screening programs. Clinical trials have demonstrated that screening mammography can reduce breast cancer mortality by 25% to 30% for women aged 50 years or older. These same trials have reported no statistically significant reduction in breast cancer mortality in women aged 40 to 49 after 7 to 10 years of follow-up. The few studies that have longer follow-up for women in this age group do show a nonsignificant trend toward mortality reduction. An overview of nine randomized trials and four case–control studies estimated the relative risk for breast cancer mortality for women aged 50 to 74 years to be 0.74 (95% confidence interval, 0.66 to 0.83). For women aged 40 to 49 years, the relative risk estimate was 0.93, but the 95% confidence interval (0.76 to 1.13) included 1. A more recent systematic review of harms as well as benefits of mammography in this age group estimated that the reduction in breast cancer mortality is somewhere between 7% and 23% and that it is associated with an increased risk of mastectomy and decreased risk of adjuvant chemotherapy or hormone therapy.

The sensitivity of initial screening mammography increases with age as fat replaces more dense and radiopaque breast tissue. After age 50 years, the sensitivity approaches 95%. For women aged 30 to 39 years and 40 to 49 years, sensitivity is approximately 75% and 85%, respectively. Specificity is approximately 95% and does not vary significantly with age. However, false-positive results, including interpretations that request follow-up examination of some kind, are not at all uncommon and are a source of considerable anxiety. In one large retrospective cohort study, false-positive results, defined broadly, occurred in 6.5% of mammograms; cumulative incidence after 10 mammograms was estimated to be 50%. Cumulative incidence of false-positive mammograms leading to biopsy approached 20%. A recent systematic review suggested that these findings have little measurable long-term effect on psychological health or compliance with recommendations for subsequent screening.

It is important to note that as many as 50% of breast cancers detected after abnormal mammography in women younger than age 50 years are DCIS; in older women, DCIS accounts for only one in five cancers detected by mammography. As noted, women whose tumors are detected by screening mammography subsequently have a lower risk of distant recurrence even after adjustment for tumor size and other prognostic factors. This may be due to *lead-time bias* and *time-linked bias sampling*. Whereas this is good news for women who face life after a diagnosis of cancer made by mammography screening, it is also a reminder of the potential for *overdiagnosis* of breast cancer, as noted earlier.

Mammographic techniques have undergone many technical enhancements. It has been reported that digital mammography improves test performance, especially in the denser breasts of younger women. Computer-aided detection has also been advanced, but one study involving more than 43 facilities, 7 of which adopted this approach, reported a degradation of accuracy with an increased number of false-positive results leading to more callbacks and biopsies with no increase in cancer detection. In comparisons with state-of-the art mammography, magnetic resonance imaging shows greater sensitivity and less specificity. It is generally reserved for special situations such as defined high risk or examination of the contralateral breast of women with a recent diagnosis of breast cancer.

Physical Examination (1,5,8,45–47)

A physical examination by the patient's clinician can detect cancers that are not detected by mammography. Much of the benefit evident in the Health Insurance Plan study was derived from the physical examination rather than from mammography; only 44% of cancers in women aged 50 to 59 years and 19% of those in women aged 40 to 49 years were found on mammography alone. In the younger age group, 58% of cancers were found by physical examination alone. In the Canadian trial, in which women aged 50 to 59 years were randomized to clinical examination and mammography or clinical examination alone, clinical examination alone was as effective as the combination. However, in a recent meta-analysis of trials and case–control studies, no difference was found in mortality reduction between studies that offered both examination and mammography and those that offered mammography alone. Nevertheless, physical examination and mammography should be viewed as complementary procedures; a substantial proportion of cancers, particularly among younger women, will be missed by physicians who rely too heavily on mammography and thereby neglect careful systematic inspection and palpation of the breasts.

Breast Self-Examination (1,8,50,51)

Breast self-examination has both supporters and detractors. Surveys have disclosed that many women perform breast self-examination, but that most do not perform the procedure monthly and do not spend sufficient time to do it correctly. Age, education, marital status, having been instructed by a health professional, regular professional breast examinations, and a family history of breast cancer have all been shown to influence breast self-examination behavior. Some question the effectiveness of self-examination in the early detection of disease. A randomized trial of an intensive self-examination educational intervention among more than 250,000 factory workers in Shanghai found no difference in breast cancer mortality after 10 years of follow-up. The intervention did not appear to advance the time of diagnosis of breast cancer. However, it did increase the risk of biopsy for benign disease, thereby underscoring the potential psychological morbidity associated with self-examination. Women who are both well informed and highly motivated should not be discouraged from practicing breast self-examination.

Seven to 10 days after menses is the best time for premenopausal women who choose to practice self-examination; postmenopausal women can pick a regular calendar date, such as the first of each month.

PATIENT EDUCATION (1,5,54–58)

Many women are frightened by what they learn about breast cancer from the popular media. This is especially true for women with a family history of breast cancer, whose fears may

TABLE 106.1

ESTIMATED OUTCOMES OF FIRST-SCREENING MAMMOGRAPHY STRATIFIED BY AGE

	≤50 Years Old	≥50 Years Old
Number of women screened	1,000	1,000
Number of abnormal reports	53	71
Number of diagnostic procedures	102	132
Number of biopsies	13	25
Number of invasive cancers	1	7.5
Number of ductal carcinoma *in situ*	1	2.5

Modified from Kerlikowske K, Grady D, Barclay J, et al. Positive predictive value of screening mammography by age and family history of breast cancer. JAMA 1993;270:2444, with permission.

have been heightened by the identification of breast cancer susceptibility genes. With regard to screening and prevention, fear is more an obstacle than a motivator for many patients. The primary care provider now has greater responsibility to provide accurate information about genetic predisposition and other risk factors.

One reason that breast cancer fears may be exaggerated is frequent reference to lifetime cumulative incidence rates such as the often-cited one-in-eight or one-in-nine figures for the general population. Often, younger women do not appreciate the effect of age on breast cancer incidence and dramatically overestimate their chances of being diagnosed or dying from breast cancer in the near future. For example, a 30-year-old woman may have a 12% chance of developing breast cancer during the remainder of her lifetime, but the probability that she will develop cancer in the next 10 years is less than 5 in 1,000 and the probability that she will die of breast cancer in the same period is 1 in 1,000. For a 40-year-old woman, the comparable 10-year incidence and mortality figures are 15 in 1,000 and 2 in 1,000, respectively.

The debate about which women should receive routine mammography can best be summarized for patients by asking them to consider the likely outcomes of initial screening mammograms for women younger than 50 years and those 50 years and older, as presented in Table 106.1.

Alternatively, the discussion can focus on the mortality-reduction benefits of mammography. For example, the probability of dying in the next 15 to 20 years from breast cancer that develops in the next 10 years is reduced approximately from 0.8% to 0.7% for the 40-year-old woman, from 1.3% to 1.1% for the 50-year-old woman, from 2.0% to 1.4% for the 60-year-old woman, and from 2.5% to 1.7% for the woman who is 70 years or older. To facilitate informed choices of this kind, decision aids have been developed and evaluated. One such program designed for women age 70 years and older showed a dramatic increase in knowledge and ease in making a decision with no overall change in screening rate. Such approaches also help to address concerns about whether documented differences in racial and ethnic disparities in rates of screening reflect different preferences of different women or failure to provide equal access to and opportunity for desired health care. Practice-based systems have been developed to reach out to patients to increase access and opportunity and have been shown to increase screening rates.

CONCLUSIONS AND RECOMMENDATIONS (1–3,5,8,31,59)

- Breast cancer is common. Although risk factors allow identification of subgroups at particularly high risk, women without risk factors are nonetheless at substantial risk and should be educated about breast cancer and the benefits and harms of screening.
- Testing and counseling related to breast cancer susceptibility genes and family history must be conducted with utmost care. The implications of inherited breast cancer, including limitations of available prevention strategies, should be discussed before referral for testing.
- Breast cancer chemoprevention counseling should be provided to women who are at high risk. This should include careful description of benefits and harms and the quality of existing evidence for SERMs and aspirin and other NSAIDS.
- Breast cancer mortality is reduced 25% to 30% by mammographic screening among women aged 50 to 74 years; regular mammograms should be performed in this age group at 1- to 2-year intervals.
- Among women younger than 50 years, a modest benefit (approximately 10% mortality reduction) seems likely based on trial results, but mammography has not been proven to be beneficial. Furthermore, younger women face a higher likelihood of mammographic detection of DCIS and the subsequent difficult therapeutic decisions leading to potentially unnecessary surgery. Women in this age group should be engaged in a dialogue about their wishes regarding mammography. Ideally, this should include quantitative estimates of the benefits and harms of screening. When regular mammography is performed for women younger than 50 years, a shorter screening interval (e.g., every year) may be more appropriate.

A.G.M.

Annotated Bibliography

1. Armstrong K, Moye E, Williams S, et al. Screening mammography in women 40–49 years of age: a systematic review for the American College of Physicians. Ann Intern Med 2007;146:516. (*Few women 50 years of age or older have risks from mammography that outweigh the benefits; the evidence suggests that more women 40 to 49 years of age have such risks.*)
2. U.S. Preventive Services Task Force. Genetic risk assessment and BRCA mutation testing for breast and ovarian cancer susceptibility. Ann Intern Med 2005;143:355. (*Summarizes the U.S. Preventive Services Task Force recommendations on genetic risk assessment and BRCA mutation testing for breast and ovarian cancer susceptibility, along with the supporting scientific evidence.*)
3. Robson M, Offit K. Management of an inherited predisposition to breast cancer. N Engl J Med 2007;357:154. (*Excellent review.*)
4. FitzGerald MG, MacDonald DJ, Krainer M, et al. Germ-line BRCA1 mutations in Jewish and non-Jewish women with early-onset breast cancer. N Engl J Med 1996;334:143. (*The specific BRCA1 mutation 185delAG is strongly associated with breast cancer before age 40 years in Jewish women.*)

5. Fletcher SW, Elmore JG. Mammographic screening for breast cancer. N Engl J Med 2003;348:1672. (*Critical review.*)

6. Gammon MD, Bertin JE, Terry MB. Abortion and the risk of breast cancer. JAMA 1996;275:321. (*Discusses the potential for ascertainment bias as an explanation for occasional association.*)

7. Garber JE, Schrag D. Testing for inherited cancer susceptibility. JAMA 1996;275:1928. (*Cites the challenges associated with identifying and counseling patients with cancer-susceptibility genes.*)

8. Humphrey LL, Helfand M, Chan BK, et al. Breast cancer screening: a summary of the evidence for the U.S. Preventive Services Task Force. Ann Intern Med 2002;13:347. (*The relative risk among screened women aged 40 to 49 years is 0.85 with a 95% confidence interval of 0.73 to 0.99; see* http://www.ahrq.gov/clinic/gcpspu.htm *for updates.*)

9. Hunter DJ, Spiegelman D, Adami H, et al. Cohort studies of fat intake and the risk of breast cancer—a pooled analysis. N Engl J Med 1996;334:356. (*A meta-analysis of seven studies finding no association between total dietary fat intake and breast cancer.*)

10. Prentice RL, Chlebowski RT, Patterson R, et al. Low-fat dietary pattern and risk of invasive breast cancer. The Women's Health Initiative randomized controlled dietary modification trial. JAMA 2006;295:629. (*Among postmenopausal women, a low-fat dietary pattern did not result in a statistically significant reduction in invasive breast cancer risk over an 8.1-year average follow-up period.*)

11. Lambe M, Hsieh C, Trichopoulos D, et al. Transient increase in the risk of breast cancer after giving birth. N Engl J Med 1994;331:5. (*Evidence to support the hypothesis that pregnancy has a dual cancer risk: increasing the risk in the short term, then decreasing it.*)

12. Langston, AA, Malone KE, Thompson JD, et al. BRCA1 mutations in a population-based sample of young women with breast cancer. N Engl J Med 1996;334:137. (*BRCA1 mutations were found in 10% of women with breast cancer onset before age 35 years.*)

13. Lerman C, Narod S, Schulman K, et al. BRCA1 testing in families with hereditary breast–ovarian cancer. JAMA 1996;275:1885. (*Among family members affected by BRCA1-linked hereditary breast–ovarian cancer, 40% did not want to be tested.*)

14. Newcomb PA, Storer BE, Longnecker MP, et al. Lactation and reduced risk of premenopausal breast cancer. N Engl J Med 1994;330:81. (*A reduction in risk of approximately 20% is restricted to premenopausal women.*)

15. Newcomb PA, Storer BE, Longnecker MP, et al. Pregnancy termination in relation to risk of breast cancer. JAMA 1996;275:283. (*Reported a relative risk of 1.12.*)

16. Shattuck-Eidens D, McClure M, Simard J, et al. A collaborative survey of 80 mutations in the BRCA1 breast and ovarian cancer susceptibility gene. JAMA 1995;273:535. (*Reports on BRCA1 testing from nine laboratories.*)

17. Terry MB, Gammon MD, Zhang FF, et al. Association of frequency and duration of aspirin use and hormone receptor status with breast cancer risk. JAMA 2004;291:2433. (*Aspirin reduces the risk of hormone receptor–positive tumors but not hormone receptor–negative tumors.*)

18. Velicer C, Heckbert SR, Lampe JW, et al. Antibiotic use in relation to the risk of breast cancer. JAMA 2004;291:827. (*Use of antibiotics was associated with an increased risk of incidence and fatal breast cancer.*)

19. Writing Group for the Women's Health Initiative Investigators. Risks and benefits of estrogen plus progestin in healthy postmenopausal women. JAMA 2002;288:321. (*This trial was stopped early after a mean of 5.2 years of follow-up because of a breast cancer hazard ratio of 1.26.*)

20. Ravdin PM, Cronin KA, Howlader N, et al. The decrease in breast-cancer incidence in 2003 in the United States. N Engl J Med 2007;356:1670. (*The authors attribute the reduction to a decrease in postmenopausal estrogen use.*)

21. Boyd NF, Guo H, Martin LJ, et al. Mammographic density and the risk and detection of breast cancer. N Engl J Med 2007;356:227. (*Extensive mammographic density is strongly associated with the risk of breast cancer detected by screening or between screening tests.*)

22. Chlebowski RT, Hendrix SL, Langer RD. Influence of estrogen plus progestin on breast cancer and mammography in healthy postmenopausal women. JAMA 2003;289:3243. (*Hormone replacement therapy may stimulate breast cancer growth and hinder mammographic diagnosis.*)

23. Hartmann LC, Sellers TA, Frost MH, et al. Benign breast disease and the risk of breast cancer. N Engl J Med 2005;353:229-37. (*Detailed examination of the interaction of histology, age, and family history in determining risk.*)

24. Ernster VL, Barclay J, Kerlikowske K, et al. Incidence of and treatment for ductal carcinoma *in situ* of the breast. JAMA 1996;275:913. (*Mammography has produced an "epidemic" of ductal carcinoma in situ; treatment patterns may vary substantially in different geographic regions.*)

25. Arpino G, Laucirica R, Elledge RM. Premalignant and *in situ* breast disease: biology and clinical implications. Ann Intern Med 2005;143:446. (*Detailed review of premalignant lesions and lobular and ductal carcinoma in situ.*)

26. Hartmann LC, Schaid DJ, Woods JE, et al. Efficacy of bilateral prophylactic mastectomy in women with a family history of breast cancer. N Engl J Med 1999;340:77. (*Bilateral prophylactic mastectomy reduced the cancer risk by 90%.*)

27. Joensuu H, Lehtimaki T, Holli K, et al. Risk for distant recurrence of breast cancer detected by mammography screening or other methods. JAMA 2004;292:1064. (*Women whose tumors are detected by screening mammography face a lower risk of recurrence.*)

28. Shapiro S, Goldberg JD, Hutchinson GB. Lead time in breast cancer detection and implications for periodicity of screening. Am J Epidemiol 1974;100:357. (*The average duration of preclinical disease was previously estimated to be 20 months; the lead time was estimated to be 19 months at the initial examination and 11 to 13 months at subsequent screenings.*)

29. Cummings SR, Eckert S, Krueger KA, et al. The effect of raloxifene on risk of breast cancer in postmenopausal women: results from the MORE randomized trial. Multiple Outcomes of Raloxifene Evaluation. JAMA 1999;281:2189. (*A 76% relative risk reduction was found with raloxifene.*)

30. Fisher B, Costantino JP, Wickerham DL, et al. Tamoxifen for prevention of breast cancer: report of the National Surgical Adjuvant Breast and Bowel Project P-1 Study. J Natl Cancer Inst 1998;90:1371. (*A 49% relative risk reduction was found with tamoxifen.*)

31. Kinsinger LS, Harris R, Woolf SH, et al. Chemoprevention of breast cancer: a summary of the evidence for the U.S. Preventive Services Task Forces. Ann Intern Med 2002;137:59. (*The basis for the recommendation of the U.S. Preventive Services Task Force against the widespread use of chemoprevention for women at low or average risk; see* http://www.ahrq.gov/clinic/gcpspu.htm *for updates.*)

32. Powles T, Eeles R, Ashley S, et al. Interim analysis of the incidence of breast cancer in the Royal Marsden Hospital tamoxifen randomised chemoprevention trial. Lancet 1998;352:98. (*One of two negative trials for tamoxifen chemoprevention.*)

33. Veronesi U, Maisonneuve P, Costa A, et al. Prevention of breast cancer with tamoxifen: preliminary findings from the Italian randomised trial among hysterectomised women. Italian Tamoxifen Prevention Study. Lancet 1998;352:93. (*One of two negative trials for tamoxifen chemoprevention.*)

34. Alexander FE, Anderson TJ, Brown HK, et al. Fourteen years of follow-up from the Edinburgh randomised trial of breast-cancer screening. Lancet 1999;353:1903. (*The 13% reduction in breast cancer mortality increased to 21% after adjustment for demographics; no benefit was found for women whose cancers were diagnosed after age 50 years.*)

35. Burman ML, Taplin SH, Herta DF, et al. Interval breast cancer screening in a health maintenance organization. Ann Intern Med 1999;131:1. (*False-positive results did not decrease adherence to subsequent mammogram at the recommended interval.*)

36. Elmore JG, Barton MB, Moceri VM, et al. Ten-year risk of false-positive screening mammograms and clinical breast examinations. N Engl J Med 1998;338:1089. (*A retrospective cohort study suggesting that the cumulative risk for a false-positive result for women who undergo 10 mammograms is 50% or more; the risk for biopsy after 10 mammograms approximates 20%.*)

37. Zackrisson S, Andersson I, Janzon L, et al. Rate of over-diagnosis of breast cancer 15 years after end of Malmö mammographic screening trial: follow-up study. BMJ 2006;332:689. (*Fifteen years after the trial ended, the rate of overdiagnosis of breast cancer was 10%.*)

38. Feig SA. Strategies for improving sensitivity of screening mammography for women aged 40 to 49 years. JAMA 1996;276:73. (*Addresses the question of what to do about the 35,000 U.S. women each year in this age group who are diagnosed with breast cancer.*)

39. Kerlikowske K, Grady D, Barclay J, et al. Effect of age, breast density, and family history on the sensitivity of first screening mammography. JAMA 1996;276:33. (*Sensitivity is lower in younger women and particularly low with longer screening intervals.*)

40. Kerlikowske K, Grady D, Barclay J, et al. Likelihood ratios for modern screening mammography. JAMA 1996;276:39. (*Estimates the likelihood ratios for different mammographic interpretations.*)

41. Kerlikowske K, Grady D, Barclay J, et al. Positive predictive value of screening mammography by age and family history of breast cancer. JAMA 1993;270:2444. (*After mammography, women 15 years old and older undergo about 15 diagnostic procedures for each cancer detected; women younger than 50 years undergo 50 procedures for each cancer detected.*)

42. Kerlikowske K, Grady D, Rubin SM, et al. Efficacy of screening mammography. JAMA 1995;273:149. (*Meta-analysis combining the results of 13 studies, with the conclusion that screening mammography may be effective in reducing mortality in women of age 40 to 49 years after 10 to 12 years, but that the same benefit could likely be achieved by starting at age 50 years.*)

43. Fenton JJ, Taplin SH, Carney PA, et al. Influence of computer-aided detection on performance of screening mammography. N Engl J Med 2007;356:1399. (*Reduced accuracy of interpretation of screening mammograms.*)

44. Mandelblatt J, Saha S, Teutsch S, et al. The cost-effectiveness of screening mammography beyond age 65 years: a systematic review for the U.S. Preventive Services Task Force. Ann Intern Med 2003;139:835. (*Biennial screening after age 65 years is reasonably cost-effective.*)

45. Miller AB, Baines CJ, To T, et al. Canadian National Breast Screening Study. 1. Breast cancer detection and death rates among women aged 40 to 49 years. Can Med Assoc J 1992;147:1459. (*After 7 years of follow-up among women of age 40 to 49 years, the risk for dying from breast cancer was found to be*

higher among the women randomized to the screening intervention, which included annual physical examination and mammography.)

46. Miller AB, Baines CJ, To T, et al. Canadian National Breast Screening Study. 2. Breast cancer detection and death rates among women aged 50 to 59 years. Can Med Assoc J 1992;147:1477. *(Clinical examination alone performed as well as clinical examination and mammography.)*
47. Miller AB, To T, Baines CJ, et al. The Canadian National Breast Screening Study—1: breast cancer mortality after 11 to 16 years of follow-up. A randomized screening trial of mammography in women age 40 to 49 years. Ann Intern Med 2002;137:305. *(No risk reduction was found in this study.)*
48. Nystrom L, Andersson I, Bjurstam N, et al. Long-term effects of mammography screening: updated overview of the Swedish randomised trials. Lancet 2002;359:909. *(Follow-up of four Swedish trials for a mean of 15.8 years found a relative risk reduction of 21% for breast cancer mortality.)*
49. Moss SM, Cuckle H, Evans A, et al. Effect of mammographic screening from age 40 years on breast cancer mortality at 10 years; follow-up: a randomised controlled trial. Lancet 2006;368:2053. *(The reduction in breast-cancer mortality observed in this trial was not significant.)*
50. Olsen O, Gotzsche PC. Cochrane review on screening for breast cancer with mammography. Lancet 2001;358:1340. *(Questions the effectiveness of screening based on the quality assessment of trials; see http://www.cochrane.org for updates.)*
51. Smith-Bindman R, Chu PW, Miglioretti DL, et al. Comparison of screening mammography in the United States and the United Kingdom. JAMA 2003;209:2129. *(Recall and negative open biopsy rates are twice as high in the United States, with similar cancer detection rates.)*
52. Bains CJ, To T. Changes in breast self-examination behavior achieved by 89,835 participants in the Canadian National Breast Screening Study. Cancer 1990;66:570. *(Competence and frequency of breast self-examination increased dramatically after brief episodes of instruction.)*
53. Thomas DB, Gao DL, Ray RM, et al. Randomized trial of breast self-examination in Shanghai: final results. J Natl Cancer Inst 2002;94:1445.

(Intensive breast self-examination education failed to advance the time of diagnosis or reduce breast cancer mortality.)

54. Brewer NT, Salz T, Lillie SE. Systemic review: the long-term effects of false-positive mammograms. Ann Intern Med 2007;146:502. *(Women with false-positive results on mammography may have differences in whether they return for mammography, occurrence of breast self-examinations, and levels of anxiety compared with women with normal results.)*
55. Lehman CD, Isaacs C, Schnall MD, et al. Cancer yield of mammography, MR, and US in high-risk women: prospective multi-institution breast cancer screening study. Radiology 2007;244:381. *(Screening magnetic resonance imaging had a higher biopsy rate but helped to detect more cancers than either mammography or ultrasound.)*
56. Mathieu E, Barratt A, Davey H, et al. Informed choice in mammography screening. Arch Intern Med 2007;167:2039. *(This approach increased knowledge and assisted women in making a choice without altering the overall rate of screening.)*
57. Smith-Bindman R, Miglioretti DL, Lurie N, et al. Does utilization of screening mammography explain racial and ethnic differences in breast cancer? Ann Intern Med 2006;144:541. *(African American women are less likely to receive adequate mammographic screening that white women.)*
58. Dietrich AJ, Tobin JN, Cassells A, et al. Telephone care management to improve cancer screening among low-income women. Ann Intern Med 2006;144:563. *(Telephone support can improve cancer screening rates among women.)*
59. Chaudhry R, Scheitel SM, McMurtry EK, et al. Web-based proactive system to improve breast cancer screening. Arch Intern Med 2007;167:606. *(The breast cancer screening rate improved significantly with the practice redesign.)*
60. Qaseem A, Snow V, Sherif K, et al. Screening mammography for women 40 to 49 years of age: a clinical practice guideline from the American College of Physicians. Ann Intern Med 2007;146:511. *(Advocates an informed, personalized decision based on a weighing of the benefits and harms.)*

CHAPTER 107 ■ SCREENING FOR CERVICAL CANCER

In the United States, the annual incidence of invasive cervical cancer is roughly 13,000 cases, and the annual mortality is approximately 4,000. For an American woman, the lifetime probability of developing invasive cervical cancer is about 0.8%. Worldwide, there are approximately one-half million new cases each year and nearly 300,000 deaths. Almost all cervical cancer is caused by persistent infection with roughly 15 genotypes of human papillomavirus (HPV). The development of new vaccines shown to be efficacious in preventing infection with some of these genotypes offers great promise for the future. It will be a decade or more, however, before primary prevention has an appreciable impact, and screening for cervical cancer will be a primary care priority for the foreseeable future. The best approach to screening for cervical cancer is more uncertain now than it has been for decades. The benefits of cytologic screening with the Papanicolaou (Pap) test are undisputed, but increasing evidence suggests a role for testing for HPV DNA in cervical samples. It is important that the primary care provider stay abreast of new developments in this rapidly changing field.

EPIDEMIOLOGY AND RISK FACTORS (1–10)

Cervical cancer is caused by persistent infection with oncogenic genotypes of *HPV*. HPV types 16 and 18 have long been associated with cervical cancer; specific oncoproteins and inactivated tumor-suppressor genes have been identified. Other high-risk HPV types were recognized more recently. Nearly 100% of squamous cell cervical cancer and 75% to 95% of the precursor, cervical intraepithelial neoplasia, have detectable HPV DNA. In considering the epidemiology and risk factors for cervical cancer, it is helpful to think of infection with high-risk HPV as necessary but not sufficient. Behavior that increases the likelihood of transmission of HPV increases the risk for individuals. It is therefore not surprising that first intercourse at a *young age* (i.e., before age 18 years) and *multiple sexual partners* (four or more) have been recognized as risk factors for decades. However, only a small proportion of women who become infected with HPV progress to precancerous cervical lesions and cervical cancers. It appears that other factors influence the likelihood that infection persists rather than being cleared and leads to cancer (Fig. 107.1).

Smoking was found to be an independent risk factor for cervical cancer in a number of studies that controlled for both sexual activity and socioeconomic status. It has been hypothesized that smoking serves as a cofactor, making women more susceptible to the oncogenic effects of viruses. Similarly, oral contraceptives confer an increase in cervical cancer risk that increases with duration of use and declines after cessation. Parity and the presence of other sexually transmitted diseases are also associated with increased risk. Women infected with HIV are at

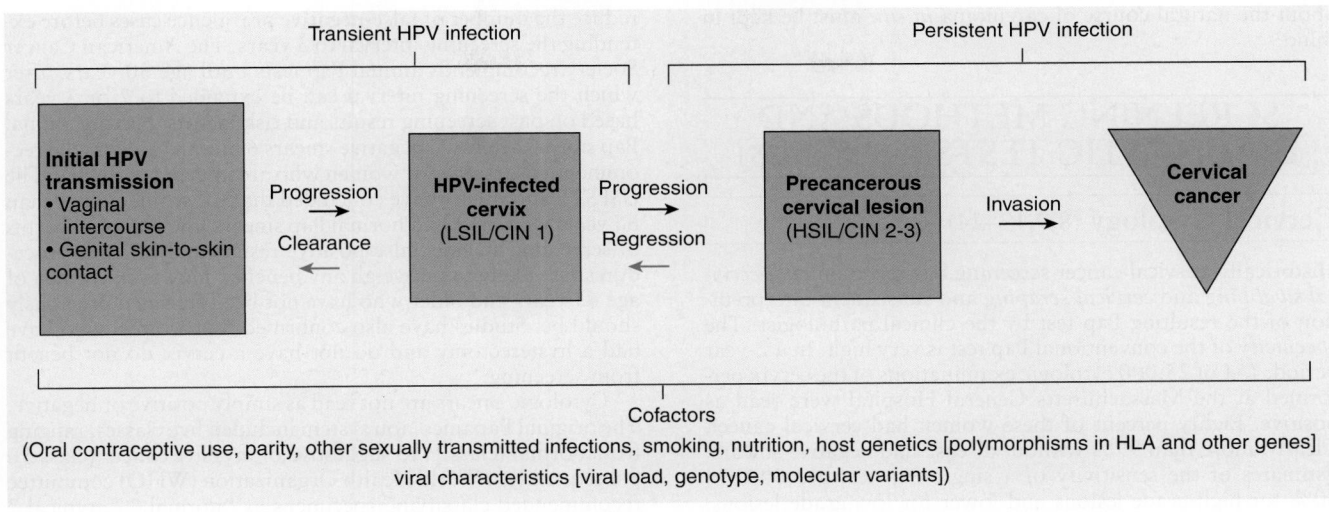

FIGURE 107.1. Full spectrum of cervical carcinogenesis, showing the preinvasive lesions that lie along the pathway from human papillomavirus (HPV) infection to cervical cancer. CIN 1, grade 1 cervical intraepithelial neoplasia; CIN 2–3, grade 2 or 3 CIN; HSIL, high-grade squamous intraepithelial lesion; LSIL, low-grade SIL. (From Lau S, Franco EL. Management of low-grade cervical lesions in young women. CMAJ 2005;173[7]:771, with permission.)

increased risk of HPV infection, and the prevalence of cervical dysplasia ranges from 10% to 60%, depending on the severity of immunosuppression.

NATURAL HISTORY OF CERVICAL CANCER, PRIMARY PREVENTION, AND EFFECTIVENESS OF THERAPY (1–4,9–16)

As noted, though most women are infected with at least one if not more HPV genotypes during their sexual life, and the majority clear the infection. Only about one third of women with HPV infections detected by DNA testing have any evident cytopathology. The peak prevalence of transient HPV infection is during the teenage years or early 20s after the initiation of sexual activity. The peak prevalence of precancerous cervical lesions occurs 10 years later and is followed by the peak prevalence of invasive cancer between 40 and 50 years of age.

Approximately 40% of high-grade squamous intraepithelial lesions eventually progress to invasive cancer if left untreated, accounting for approximately 80% of primary cervical cancers. Adenocarcinoma of the cervix accounts for the remaining 20% of invasive cervical cancer and is also associated with HPV infection.

Vaccination to prevent HPV infection is a promising primary prevention strategy for cervical cancer. Approximately 80% of cervical cancers are associated with the four "high-risk" types of HPV (types 16, 18, 31, and 45); the remaining 20% are associated with 12 other oncogenic types. HPV-16 is responsible for approximately 50% of cases and is the target of most vaccine development efforts. Vaccines were developed for both prophylactic and therapeutic purposes. Prophylactic use would focus on younger women and girls prior to the onset of sexual activity to prevent infection. It was hoped that therapeutic use would stimulate cell-mediated immune responses to recognize latent HPV infection and thereby prevent progression to high-grade intraepithelial lesions among women who have already been infected.

Gardasil (Merck) is a quadrivalent HPV-6/11/16/18 virus-like–particle vaccine that has been shown to have preventive efficacy for precancerous intraepithelial lesions related to HPV-16 and HPV-18 of 98% in the population deemed susceptible to infection. In the same trial, preventive efficacy for lesions caused by HPV-16 and HPV-18 was estimated for an-intention-to treat population at 44%. Efficacy against all high-grade cervical lesions, regardless of etiologic HPV type, in that same intention-to-treat population was estimated at 17%. Gardasil also protects against HPV-6 and HPV-11 and has been shown to be efficacious in preventing genital warts caused by those genotypes. Cervarix (GSK Biologicals) is a bivalent vaccine that has been shown to be equally efficacious prophylactically. A trial of Cervarix among women with prevalent infection, however, showed no effect on clearance of the virus.

In the absence of primary prevention, when cervical cancer does develop, the mean duration of the detectable asymptomatic period, as estimated historically from incidence and prevalence rates, is very long. For example, the mean duration of carcinoma *in situ* varies with age but averages about 10 years. The duration of asymptomatic invasive carcinoma is 5 years for all age groups. It should be emphasized that these are estimated means; the proportion of cervical cancers that become invasive early in their development is not known.

In the absence of screening, cervical cancer presents with *intermenstrual bleeding,* classically prompted by coitus. Symptoms invariably occur late in the course of the disease. There is no doubt that the earlier the clinical stage of the tumor when detected and treated, the better is the prognosis. Relative 5-year survival rates for localized and regional invasive carcinoma are about 80% and 40%, respectively. The 5-year experience of one screening program demonstrated that 86% of cases detected by cytologic screening were limited to regional invasion, whereas only 44% of those presenting symptomatically were in this early stage. Survival for carcinoma *in situ* treated with hysterectomy is essentially 100%. However, the uncertainty about the natural course of carcinoma *in situ* must be kept in mind.

SCREENING METHODS AND DIAGNOSTIC TESTS (1,8,9,17–35)

Cervical Cytology (8,9,17–24)

Historically, cervical cancer screening has relied on *endocervical swabbing* and *cervical scraping* and subsequent interpretation of the resulting Pap test by the clinical pathologist. The *specificity* of the conventional Pap test is very high. In a 2-year period, 151 of 25,000 cytologic examinations of the cervix performed at the Massachusetts General Hospital were read as positive. Eighty percent of these women had cervical cancer. Clearly, more than 99% without disease had negative smears. Estimates of the sensitivity of a single Pap test are 60% to 80% for high-grade lesions and lower for low-grade lesions. The long duration of the asymptomatic detectable period provides multiple opportunities for timely detection of abnormalities. As a result, the effective sensitivity increases substantially when two or more tests are performed at intervals of 1 year or more. Most women who present with advanced cervical cancer have never had a Pap test. False-negative results do occur, however; in one study, 17% of women developed confirmed lesions within 2 years of a negative smear. About two thirds of such false negatives are caused by *sampling error* when abnormal cells are present but not collected or properly transferred to the Pap slide. The remainder is caused by *detection error* when abnormal cells on the Pap slide are misinterpreted as normal or missed entirely.

Collection techniques have been widely studied and altered since the introduction of the Pap smear. Meta-analysis of more than 30 trials of collection techniques indicated that the once widely used Ayre's spatulas were relatively ineffective and should be replaced with extended-tip spatulas. The same study found that the combination of extended-tip spatulas and the Cytobrush produced the lowest risk of sampling error. Another approach to reducing sampling error is improved slide preparation. The U.S. Food and Drug Administration has approved a liquid-based monolayer system (ThinPrep) in which cells are placed in a fixative solution, dispersed, collected on a filter, and transferred to a microscopic slide for interpretation. Although there are not high-quality studies to demonstrate improvement in sensitivity or clinical outcomes, these procedures do reduce the frequency of unsatisfactory specimens, and such liquid-based technologies have become widely used in the United States. To minimize the risk of detection error, smears should be interpreted by an experienced cytopathologist. Other efforts to reduce detection error include developments in the automated interpretation of smears, both to enrich samples for rescreening and as a strategy to improve the efficiency of screening without a loss in sensitivity. Again, evidence for improved sensitivity and clinical outcomes is insufficient for recommending these approaches.

The *frequency* of cervical cytologic cancer screening has been controversial. Because of the usually long duration of the asymptomatic detectable period of cervical intraepithelial neoplasia, which is easily controlled and cured when detected, most authorities have moved away from recommendations for annual screening. The U.S. Preventive Services Task Force (USPSTF) recommends screening at least every 3 years beginning at age 21 years or younger if the patient is sexually active. Some advocate two screens with a short interval (e.g., 1 year) to reduce the number of false-negative prevalence cases before extending the screening interval to 3 years. The American Cancer Society recommends annual Pap tests until age 30 years, after which the screening interval can be extended to 2 or 3 years based on past screening results and risk factors. Having annual Pap smears after two negative smears 6 months apart is the recommended strategy for women who are infected with HIV. The USPSTF and others have concluded that for women older than 65 years who have had normal Pap smears, the potential harms of screening, such as false-positive results and invasive procedures, are likely to outweigh any benefits. However, women of age 65 years and older who have not been screened previously should be. Studies have also confirmed that women who have had a hysterectomy and do not have a cervix do not benefit from screening.

Cytologic smears are not read as simply positive or negative. The original Papanicolaou system included five classes, ranging from normal (class 1) to suggestive of invasive cancer (class 5). Subsequently, a World Health Organization (WHO) committee recommended classifying specimens as "normal," "atypical," "dysplasia" (mild, moderate, or severe), "carcinoma *in situ*," "invasive cervical cancer," and "adenocarcinoma." In 1988, a committee of the National Cancer Institute recommended the Bethesda System, which replaces the older class 2 "atypical" category with the designation "reactive and reparative change" to describe cellular changes in response to inflammation and other nonneoplastic processes, and "atypical squamous cells of undetermined significance". The Bethesda System also introduced the term *squamous intraepithelial lesion* (SIL), which includes two grades. Low-grade squamous intraepithelial lesions (LSILs) are consistent with HPV infection and mild dysplasia and correspond to the old class 3 mild dysplasia category. High-grade squamous intraepithelial lesions (HSILs) include the old WHO moderate and severe dysplasia and carcinoma *in situ* designations.

Women whose smears show HSIL or carcinoma *in situ* and those with smears suggestive of invasive cancer should be referred to a gynecologist experienced in the use of the colposcope. Colposcopic examination allows the gynecologist to select sites for biopsy and determine the limits of the lesion. This allows informed choice between conservative measures such as ablative and excisional measures, which are used increasingly frequently, and more extensive measures such as conization and hysterectomy. Such decisions are based not only on the size, location, and histology of the lesion, but also on the patient's age, parity, and reliability for follow-up.

TESTS FOR HPV INFECTION (1,8,9,17,25–32)

Because of the "upstream" association between HPV infection and cervical cancer, some have advocated HPV DNA testing as primary screening for cervical cancer, thereby advancing the time of diagnosis more than might be possible for cytologic screening. The argument for HPV testing can also be made on the grounds of the very limited sensitivity of cytologic screening programs. However, there are serious problems with the specificity of HPV testing. Among younger women, where reactivity is often transient, it appears to be more a marker for sexual activity than for cancer risk. For this reason, trials of HPV testing have focused on women older than age 30 years in whom a positive result is likely to indicate persistent infection. Results of early screening studies, most of which were conducted among high-risk women, were mixed. More recent studies in primary care settings allow estimates of sensitivity and specificity in populations with a low prevalence of HSIL. Sensitivity and specificity for HSIL are both approximately 80%. Estimates of sensitivity and specificity for LSIL in the primary care setting are 66% and 91%, respectively. A more recent Canadian trial of HPV DNA testing and Papanicolaou screening demonstrated sensitivity for cervical intraepithelial neoplasia grade 2 or 3 of 95% and 55%, respectively, with specificities of 94% and 97%, respectively. The addition of the HPV test to the Pap test in another study increased the proportion of women found to have grade 2 or 3 lesions by more than 50%. There was a reduction of such lesions found in subsequent screens, suggesting that HPV testing advanced the time of diagnosis. This was consistent with a randomized trial with 5-year follow-up that found that HPV screening advanced the time of diagnosis of cervical intraepithelial neoplasia grade 3 lesions.

The role of HPV testing in cervical cancer screening has not yet been defined with any certainty. A number of questions need further study. What are the true costs of any decrease in specificity associated with HPV testing in terms of increased referral rates for colposcopy and treatment? Given the earlier diagnosis made possible by HPV testing, what are the implications for the screening interval? Given the increased sensitivity of HPV testing, what are the risks of *overdiagnosis* with the detection of lesions that would have regressed or otherwise never come to clinical attention in the absence of screening? Given the potential for both earlier diagnosis and overdiagnosis, what are the implications for management of the abnormal result?

In the meantime, HPV testing may be most valuable after an abnormal cytologic finding to distinguish between women who should be followed with more intensive cytologic screening and those who can be followed otherwise. In many sites, the HPA is done as a "reflex" on the same specimen when a liquid-based cytologic sample was collected or on another suitable sample collected at the same time as the traditional Pap test. HPV testing has a clear role in determining the most effective follow-up for young women who have low-grade squamous intraepithelial lesions that may reflect recent and transient HPV infection.

It is likely that large demonstration trials in different settings using different approaches will be necessary to provide more definitive recommendations for the use of HPV DNA testing.

PATIENT EDUCATION (1,8,9,35)

There has been a sea change in our understanding of the etiology and natural history of cervical cancer over the last two decades. It is a sexually transmitted disease that can be prevented with vaccination of young women prior to the initiation of sexual activity. Exposure to the HPV infection that is causative can be ascertained and allows for earlier diagnosis than traditional cytology-based screening. There are substantial implications for patient education so as to maximize the positive impact of primary prevention and screening efforts while mitigating any negative unintended consequences,

including the anxiety and potential effect on relationships between sexual partners.

CONCLUSIONS AND RECOMMENDATIONS

- The high prevalence, long mean duration of asymptomatic detectable disease, and availability of a highly specific screening test make cervical cancer screening an important task for all primary care providers. Screening in developed countries has reduced morbidity and mortality.
- Cervical cancer is caused by transmission and persistent infection with oncogenic genotypes of HPV. Vaccination of women without evidence of prior HPV infection is highly efficacious in preventing precancerous intraepithelial lesions. Vaccination is recommended before the initiation of sexual activity.
- Because of the long duration of preinvasive detectable disease in women of reproductive age, annual screening in the absence of specific risk factors is unnecessary for most women. A 3-year screening interval has been demonstrated to be safe for women without risk factors.
- The sensitivity of cytologic screening is limited. Two initial cytologic screens with a short interval (e.g., 1 year) have been used to reduce the number of false-negative prevalence cases.
- Women who have had a hysterectomy, including removal of the cervix for indications other than cancer, do not need to have screening Pap smears.
- Having annual Pap smears after two negative smears 6 months apart is the recommended strategy for women who are infected with HIV. However, benefits for women with only 1 to 2 years of life expectancy due to late-stage HIV infection are modest.
- A cytologic smear positive for cancer or an HSIL lesion is an indication for referral to a gynecologist for further evaluation, including appropriate biopsies.
- A smear suggestive of reactive or reparative changes or mild dysplasia can be further evaluated by the nongynecologist. If a concurrent infection is evident, the smear should be repeated after specific treatment of the infection. If no infection is present, the smear may be repeated after a 3- to 6-month interval. Women with repeatedly abnormal smears should be referred for colposcopy or biopsy.
- Screening can cease after age 65 years in women with a history of regularly obtained negative smears but should be performed if not done regularly before age 65 years or if a smear has been abnormal.
- Primary screening with tests for HPV infection may prove valuable. HPV tests have been shown to be more sensitive and less specific for high-grade lesions. Evidence is insufficient to recommend primary HPV testing.

A.G.M.

Annotated Bibliography

1. Schiffman M, Castle PE, Jeronimo J, et al. Human papillomavirus and cervical cancer. Lancet 2007;370:890. (*If applied wisely, human papillomavirus (HPV)–related technology can minimize the incidence of cervical cancer and the morbidity and mortality it causes, even in low-resource settings.*)
2. Munoz N, Bosch FX, de Sanjose S, et al. Epidemiologic classification of human papillomavirus types associated with cervical cancer. N Engl J Med 2003;348:518. (*In addition to types 16 and 18, there are 13 other HPV types that confer high risk.*)
3. Schiffman MH, Brinton LA. The epidemiology of cervical carcinogenesis. Cancer 1995;76:1888. (*An excellent review of the role of HPV infection at the molecular and population levels.*)
4. Woodman CB, Collins S, Winter H, et al. Natural history of cervical human papillomavirus infection in young women: a longitudinal cohort study.

Lancet 2001;357:1831. (*The 3-year cumulative incidence of cervical HPV infection among new sexually active teenagers was 44%.*)

5. International Collaboration of Epidemiological Studies of Cervical Cancer. Cervical cancer and hormonal contraceptives: collaborative reanalysis of individual data for 16573 women with cervical cancer and 35509 women without cervical cancer from 24 epidemiological studies. Lancet 2007;370:1609. (*The relative risk of cervical cancer was increased in current users of oral contraceptives and declined after use ceased.*)

6. Kjellberg L, Hallmans G, Ahren AM, et al. Smoking, diet, pregnancy and oral contraceptive use as risk factors for cervical intra-epithelial neoplasia in relation to human papillomavirus infection. B J Cancer 2000;82:1332. (*These factors are effect modifiers that influence the association between HPV and cancer.*)

7. National Institutes of Health. Consensus Development Conference. Statement on cervical cancer. Gynecol Oncol 1997;66:351. (*An authoritative consensus statement, including the observation that half of American women with newly diagnosed invasive cervical cancer have never had a Papanicolaou smear.*)

8. U.S. Preventive Services Task Force. Guide to clinical preventive services, third edition: periodic updates (AHRQ publication No. 03-0007, March 2003). Rockville, MD: Agency for Healthcare Research and Quality. Available at: http://www.ahrq.gov/clinic/gcpspu.htm. (*Presents well-referenced, evidence-based recommendations for both cytologic screening and HPV testing; updates are regularly available at the web site.*)

9. Frazer IH. Prevention of cervical cancer through papillomavirus vaccination. Nat Rev Immunol 2004;4:46. (*Reviews vaccination trials.*)

10. Goldie SJ, Kohli M, Grima D, et al. Projected clinical benefits and cost-effectiveness of a human papillomavirus 16/18 vaccine. J Natl Cancer Inst 2004;96:604. (*Compares cost-effectiveness for different scenarios.*)

11. The FUTURE II Study Group. Quadrivalent vaccine against human papillomavirus to prevent high-grade cervical lesions. N Engl J Med 2007;356:1915. (*The vaccine [Gardasil] group had a significantly lower occurrence of high-grade cervical intraepithelial neoplasia related to HPV-16 or HPV-18 than did those in the placebo group.*)

12. Paavonen J, Jenkins D, Bosch FX, et al. Efficacy of a prophylactic adjuvanted bivalent L1 virus-like particle vaccine against infection with human papillomavirus types 16 and 18 in young women: an interim analysis of a phase III double-blind randomised controlled trial. Lancet 2007;369:2161. (*Again, vaccine [Cervarix] was found to be efficacious prophylactically.*)

13. Hildesheim A, Herrero R, Wacholder S, et al. Effect of human papillomavirus 16/18 L1 virus like particle vaccine among young women with preexisting infection. A randomized trial. JAMA 2007;298:743. (*In women positive for HPV DNA, HPV-16/18 vaccination does not accelerate the clearance of the virus and should not be used to treat prevalent infections.*)

14. Dawar N, Deeks S, Dobson S. Human papillomavirus vaccines launch a new era in cervical cancer prevention. CMAJ 2007;177:456. (*An excellent review of the characteristics of the Gardasil and Cervarix vaccines.*)

15. Goldie SJ, Weinstein MC, Kuntz KM, et al. The costs, clinical benefits, and cost-effectiveness of screening for cervical cancer in HIV-infected women. Ann Intern Med 1999;130:97. (*An analysis confirming the reasonableness of the Centers for Disease Control and Prevention recommendation for annual screening after two negative screens 6 months apart.*)

16. International Agency for Research on Cancer Working Group on Evaluation of Cervical Cancer Screening Programmes. Screening for squamous cervical cancer: duration of low risk after negative results of cervical cytology and its implications for screening policies. BMJ 1986;293:659. (*Documents diminishing returns when the screening interval is reduced to <3 years.*)

17. Nanda K, McCrory D, Myers E, et al. Accuracy of the Papanicolaou test in screening for and follow-up of cervical cytologic abnormalities: a systematic review. Ann Intern Med 2000;132:810. (*For thresholds low-grade squamous intraepithelial lesion/cervical intraepithelial neoplasia [CIN] 2 to 3, the sensitivity was 83% and the specificity was 66%; for thresholds high-grade squamous intraepithelial lesion/CIN 2 to 3, the sensitivity was 58% and the specificity was 92%.*)

18. Guglielmo R, Cuzick J, Pierotti P, et al. Accuracy of liquid based versus conventional cytology: overall results of new technologies for cervical cancer screening: randomised controlled trial. BMJ 2007;335:28. (*There was a significant increase in sensitivity for cervical intraepithelial neoplasia of grade 2 or more.*)

19. Quinn M, Babb P, Jones J, Allen E. Effect of screening on incidence of and mortality from cancer of cervix in England: evaluation based on routinely collected statistics. BMJ 1999;318:904. (*Policies that increased screening coverage to 85% of target women had a measurable effect on invasive cancer incidence.*)

20. Sawaya GF, Grady D, Kerlikowske K, et al. The positive predictive value of cervical smears in previously-screened postmenopausal women: the

Heart and Estrogen/progestin Replacement Study (HERS). Ann Intern Med 2000;133:942. (*The positive predictive value of any smear abnormality identified 1 year after a normal smear was 0% [confidence interval, 0% to 5.0%]; that of abnormalities found within 2 years was 0.9% [confidence interval, 0.0% to 3.0%].*)

21. Sawaya GF, McConnell JK, Kulasingam SL, et al. Risk of cervical cancer associated with extending the interval between cervical cancer screenings. N Engl J Med 2003;349:1501. (*Outcomes from nearly 1 million women document the safety of this approach.*)

22. Sirovich BE, Welch HG. Cervical cancer screening among women without a cervix. JAMA 2004;291:2990. (*More than 10 million women get needless screening Pap smears each year despite the U.S. Preventive Services Task Force 1996 recommendation.*)

23. Stoler MH, Schiffman M. Atypical squamous cells of undetermined significance—Low-grade Squamous Intraepithelial Lesion Triage Study (ALTS) Group. Interobserver reproducibility of cervical cytologic and histologic interpretations: realistic estimates from the ASCUS-LSIL Triage Study. JAMA 2001;285:1500. (*The interpretative variability was substantial.*)

24. Cuzick J, Sasieni P, Davies P, et al. A systematic review of the role of human papillomavirus testing within a cervical programme. Health Technology Assessment 1999;3:1. (*An excellent review, recommending pilot studies of HPV testing among women with abnormal cytology, as well as large-scale trials of primary screening.*)

25. Moss S, Gray A, Legood R, et al. Effect of testing for human papillomavirus as a triage during screening for cervical cancer: observational before and after study. BMJ 2006;332:83. (*The approach resulted in a reduction in the rate of repeat smears but an increase in rates of referral to colposcopy.*)

26. Cuzick J, Szarewski A, Terry G, et al. Human papilloma virus testing in primary cervical screening. Lancet 1995;345:1533. (*The predictive value positive was found to be 42%.*)

27. Koliopoulos G, Martin-Hirsch P, Paraskevaidis E, et al. HPV testing versus cervical cytology for screening for cancer of the uterine cervix (Cochrane review). In: The Cochrane library, Issue 1. Oxford: Update Software, 2003. (*A well-referenced, evidence-based review of the issues; see http://www.cochrane.org for updates.*)

28. Bulkmans NWJ, Berkhof J, van Kemenade FJ, et al. Human papillomavirus DNA testing for the detection of cervical intraepithelial neoplasia grade 3 and cancer: 5-year follow-up of a randomised controlled implementation trial. Lancet 2007;370:1764. (*The implementation of HPV DNA testing in cervical screening led to earlier detection of CIN3-positive lesions.*)

29. Naucler P, Ryd W, Törnberg S, et al. Human papillomavirus and Papanicolaou tests to screen for cervical cancer. N Engl J Med 2007;357:1589. (*The addition of an HPV test to the Pap test to screen women in their mid-30s for cervical cancer reduced the incidence of grade 2 or 3 cervical intraepithelial neoplasia or cancer detected by subsequent screening.*)

30. Legood R, Gray A, Wolstenholme J, et al. Lifetime effects, costs, and cost effectiveness of testing for human papillomavirus to manage low grade cytological abnormalities: results of the NHS pilot studies. BMJ 2006;332:79. (*The predicted increase in lifetime colposcopies deserves careful consideration.*)

31. Mayrand MH, Duarte-Franco E, Rodrigues I, et al. Human papillomavirus DNA versus Papanicolaou screening tests for cervical cancer. N Engl J Med 2007;357:1579. (*Compared with Pap testing, HPV testing had greater sensitivity for the detection of cervical intraepithelial neoplasia; the sensitivity of both tests used together was 100%, and the specificity was 92.5%.*)

32. Wright TC Jr, Massad LS, Dunton CJ, et al. 2006 consensus guidelines for the management of women with cervical intraepithelial neoplasia or adenocarcinoma in situ. Am J Obstet Gynecol 2007;197:340. (*Includes management recommendations for women with biopsy-confirmed adenocarcinoma in situ.*)

33. Wright TC Jr, Massad LS, Dunton CJ, et al. 2006 consensus guidelines for the management of women with abnormal cervical cancer screening tests. Am J Obstet Gynecol 2007;197:346. (Adopts *HPV testing as an adjunct to cervical cytology for screening in women 30 years of age and older.*)

34. Denny L, Kuhn L, De Souza M, et al. Screen-and-treat approaches for cervical cancer prevention in low-resource settings. A randomized controlled trial. JAMA 2005;294:2173. (*Screen-and-treat approaches are safe and result in a lower prevalence of high-grade cervical cancer precursor lesions compared with delayed evaluation at both 6 and 12 months.*)

35. Shepherd J, Weston R, Peersman G, et al. Interventions for encouraging sexual lifestyles and behaviours intended to prevent cervical cancer (Cochrane review). In: The Cochrane library, Issue 3. Oxford: Update Software, 2004. (*Emphasizes the need for gender- and culturally-sensitive interventions to reduce sexual exposure to HPV.*)

CHAPTER 108 ■ SCREENING FOR OVARIAN CANCER

Ovarian cancer is less common than breast cancer and other gynecologic malignancies; the lifetime probability is approximately 1 in 70. However, it has a high case fatality rate. Each year in the United States, more than 20,000 new cases are diagnosed and more than 15,000 women die from the disease. Ovarian cancer deaths among prominent public figures, the availability of promising diagnostic tests, and the general trend toward increased interest in disease prevention among women have focused attention on screening for ovarian cancer. The primary care provider needs to understand the epidemiology and risk factors for this disease, as well as the value and limitations of available tests, to respond appropriately to patients' questions and, when appropriate, recommend a screening intervention.

EPIDEMIOLOGY AND RISK FACTORS (1–12)

Increasing age and family history are risk factors for ovarian cancer. The annual incidence is 20 per 100,000 among women aged 30 to 50 years and increases to 40 per 100,000 among women aged 50 to 75 years. The incidence among older women is even higher when one restricts the denominator to women who have not had their ovaries surgically removed.

A family history of ovarian cancer is present in about 10% of women with the disease. Most of these women have a family history of sporadic ovarian cancer. About 5% of ovarian cancers occur among women who are members of families with inherited predisposition to cancer, including those with BRCA1 and BRCA2 mutations. For some subsets of patients with inherited predisposition, cumulative lifetime risk of ovarian cancer may be as high as 85%. For most women with *BRCA1 mutation*, however, the cumulative risk by age 70 years is closer to 25%. For women with *BRCA2 mutation,* the cumulative risk is lower—approximately 10% by age 70 years. These risks warrant consideration of prophylactic oophorectomy, as well as regular screening efforts.

A family history of the more common sporadic ovarian cancer also confers risk. The best estimate is that ovarian cancer in one first- or second-degree relative increases risk threefold. When two relatives have had the disease, risk is increased fivefold.

Use of the oral contraceptive pill and parity are associated with reduced risk of ovarian cancer in unselected women. Any use of oral contraceptives appears to reduce risk by 35% and use for 5 or more years by 50%. A case–control study indicated similar protection afforded to women with known mutations in either the BRCA1 or the BRCA2 gene. Any pregnancy reduces risk by about 50%; increasing number of pregnancies is associated with decreasing risk. Other factors, including age at first pregnancy, infertility, menstrual history, hormone replacement therapy, and dietary factors, may modify the risk of ovarian cancer, but evidence is inconclusive. Tubal ligation and possibly hysterectomy appear to be protective.

NATURAL HISTORY OF OVARIAN CANCER AND EFFECTIVENESS OF THERAPY (8,12)

Mortality rates for ovarian cancer have changed little over the last three decades. When ovarian cancer is diagnosed after clinical presentation with signs or symptoms, three of four cases have already spread beyond the ovary. Under these circumstances, the 5-year survival rate is less than 20%. In contrast, the 5-year survival rate of patients with tumor confined to the ovary was greater than 70% in older studies and is greater than 90% in recent case series.

Once diagnosed with ovarian cancer, many women report having had symptoms referable to the pelvis or to the abdomen prior to the diagnosis. Retrospective studies suggest that this is true for 95% of women, but they also document that the symptoms have very poor specificity, although some have suggested that the pattern and duration of symptoms can be indicative of early disease and that early referral for diagnostic testing deserves more attention.

Given the advanced stage at which clinical diagnosis generally occurs and the nonspecificity of symptoms, it is not surprising that there is great enthusiasm for using newer diagnostic modalities to advance the time of diagnosis and thereby reduce the burden of morbidity and mortality associated with ovarian cancer. It must be remembered, however, that we know little about the preclinical course of ovarian cancer, including variability in its biologic behavior. Any current estimates of screening benefit will be confounded by lead-time and time-linked sampling biases (see Chapter 3). No randomized trials of screening for ovarian cancer in the general population with mortality outcomes have been completed. Trials in progress include the U.K. Collaborative Trial of Ovarian Cancer Screening (UKCTOCS), the European Randomized Trial of Ovarian Cancer Screening (ERTOCS), and the NIH Prostate, Lung, Colon, Ovary (PLCO) trial in the United States. Until such trials demonstrate reduction in population mortality rates, estimates of the benefits of screening will remain tentative.

DIAGNOSTIC TESTS (8,13–26)

There has been little formal evaluation of the *pelvic examination* as a screening test for ovarian cancer among asymptomatic women. Evaluations that have been conducted comparing the physical examination with other diagnostic modalities have produced mixed results. In two studies, pelvic examination failed to detect three stage I tumors that were detected by transvaginal or abdominal ultrasound. However, in other studies, pelvic examination was able to detect early tumors. There is a general consensus that pelvic examination alone is insufficiently sensitive to be of value as a screening test.

Although early use of ultrasonography to diagnose ovarian cancer used the transabdominal approach, more recent work has focused on *transvaginal ultrasonography*, with the addition of color-flow Doppler techniques to improve specificity. The sensitivity of ultrasound has been estimated in studies of women with known ovarian cancer and in screening studies. In the former case, estimates of sensitivity ranged from 80% to 100%. Estimates were higher in the screening studies, but this may reflect failure to diagnose cancer among screened-negative study subjects. Estimates of specificity derived from screening studies range from about 75% to 97%. A recent analytic review provided summary estimates of sensitivity and specificity of 83% and 93%, respectively. Some studies have shown improvements in the specificity of transvaginal ultrasound with the addition of color-flow Doppler techniques, which can detect tumor neovascularization. Ultrasound is a safe diagnostic modality. Interpretations can be highly variable and depend on the skill of the operator. Timing the study to avoid ovulation may improve specificity. Cost, personnel, and patient inconvenience limit its use as a primary screening test. Furthermore, the limited specificity of the test results in low predictive values in the screening situation. Preliminary reports from the PLCO trial confirm the problematic aspects of transvaginal ultrasound being used as a screening rather than a diagnostic test. With nearly 40,000 women randomized to screening with transvaginal ultrasound and CA-125 (see later discussion), nearly 30,000 had at least one of the tests. Abnormal transvaginal ultrasound was found in 4.7% of women screened with this modality, but the predictive value positive was just 1%.

There is a great deal of interest in the use of *CA-125* to screen for ovarian cancer. CA-125 is an antigenic determinant on a glycoprotein that is present in the serum at elevated levels in 80% of women with epithelial ovarian cancers. CA-125 levels are also elevated in late-stage endometrial cancers and in about 60% of pancreatic cancers. Levels may also be elevated in patients with benign ovarian cysts, uterine leiomyoma, pregnancy, endometriosis, and pelvic inflammatory disease. Estimates of sensitivity derived from women with known ovarian cancer, using a reference level of 35 U/mL, range from 61% to 96%. In the screening situation, sensitivity has been estimated at 67% to 100%. However, reported sensitivities for stage I disease have ranged from 25% to 75%. The specificity of CA-125 in large screening studies, with the reference level of 35 U/mL, has been approximately 99%. Specificity is much lower in premenopausal women because CA-125 levels fluctuate with the menstrual cycle and because of a higher prevalence of the benign gynecologic conditions that are associated with elevated levels.

Given the sensitivity and specificity of CA-125 and the prevalence of ovarian cancer in the population of women older than age 50 years, the expected positive predictive value of a CA-125 level greater than 35 U/mL in that population would be 3%. If screening were restricted to women with ovarian cancer in one first-degree relative or in two or more relatives, the positive predictive values with the same reference level would be 9% and 15%, respectively. These predictive values indicate that many screened women would have false-positive results that would require invasive diagnostic evaluation, often including laparotomy.

Evidence from a pilot randomized trial combining CA-125 and ultrasound suggests that screening may be possible with a moderate number of negative biopsies. Among nearly 11,000 women screened, 468 had levels of 30 U/mL or higher. Of these, only 29 had ovarian volume estimated to be 8.8 mL or greater on ultrasonography and were referred for biopsy; 6 had cancers.

Early results of the PLCO trial, however, have not been encouraging. As noted previously, 4.7% of women screened with transvaginal ultrasound had abnormalities that needed to be pursued, but only 1% had cancers. For CA-125, the proportion with a positive result was 1.4% and the predictive value positive was 3.7%. As a result of the positive screening tests, which occurred singly or together in a total of 1,706 women, 570 women (2% of all women screened) underwent surgical procedures, including 325 laparotomies and 245 laparoscopies and/or vaginal approaches. Nineteen epithelial ovarian cancers were found, most of which were high grade and at an advanced stage.

Early work suggests that proteomic pattern recognition may play a role in improving early detection of ovarian cancer, but further evaluation is necessary to define sensitivity and specificity as well as predictive values in populations appropriate for screening. A recent technical review of the relevant evidence found nothing that would warrant use at this time and noted the worrisome promotion of these tests by manufacturers, with, in at least one case, a fall in the predictive value positive as the tested population expanded to include those with higher levels of worry than risk.

CONCLUSIONS AND RECOMMENDATIONS

- Women from families with genetic predisposition to ovarian cancer are at high risk and should be screened annually with CA-125 and ultrasound beginning at approximately age 35 years. Women known to be BRCA1-mutation carriers are at higher risk than those with BRCA2 mutations. Screening beginning at an earlier age (e.g., 25 years) on a semiannual basis may be advisable. Consideration of prophylactic oophorectomy, weighing the benefits and harms from the perspective of the particular patient, is warranted.
- Women with a family history of sporadic ovarian cancer may benefit from screening with CA-125, but because of the low predictive value and the morbidity associated with further diagnostic evaluation, *routine* screening is not recommended. However, women should be advised of the potential benefits and harms of screening. Similarly, *routine* screening is not recommended for pre- and postmenopausal women without a family history of ovarian cancer.
- Women in their childbearing years should be advised of the ovarian cancer risk reduction afforded by oral contraceptive use. This may be especially important for women with a family history or with known genetic predisposition. Women should be apprised of the potential slight increase in breast cancer risk associated with current use of oral contraceptives, but it is likely that the benefit of ovarian cancer risk reduction outweighs this potential harm.

A.G.M.

Annotated Bibliography

1. Lacey JV Jr, Greene MH, Buys SS, et al. Ovarian cancer screening in women with a family history of breast or ovarian cancer. Obstet Gynecol 2006;108:1176. (*Roughly 5% of women had positive screening tests regardless of family history; however, positive predictive value did vary: 0.7% for low-risk, 1.3% for moderate-risk, and 1.6% for high-risk women.*)

2. Burke W, Daly M, Garber J, et al. Recommendations for follow-up care of individuals with an inherited predisposition to cancer. II. BRCA1 and BRCA2. JAMA 1997;277:997. (*Recommends annual or semiannual screening starting at age 25 to 35 years.*)

3. Hankinson SE, Colditz GA, Hunter DJ, et al. A quantitative assessment of oral contraceptive use and risk of ovarian cancer. Obstet Gynecol 1992;80:708. (*The relative risk of ovarian cancer among women who had ever used oral contraceptives pills was 0.65.*)

4. Hankinson SE, Hunter DJ, Colditz GA, et al. Tubal ligation, hysterectomy, and risk of ovarian cancer: a prospective study. JAMA 1993;270:2813. (*Tubal ligation and possibly hysterectomy may reduce risk.*)

5. Hartge P, Schiffman MH, Hoover R, et al. A case–control study of epithelial ovarian cancer. Am J Obstet Gynecol 1989;161:10. (*One of many case–control studies that collectively provide highly variable estimates of relative risks.*)

6. Kasprzak L, Foules WD, Shelling AN. Fortnightly review: hereditary ovarian cancer. BMJ 1999;318:786. (*Concise review with quantitative risk estimates and advice for screening and prophylaxis.*)

7. Lacey JV Jr, Mink PJ, Lubin JH, et al. Menopausal hormone replacement therapy and risk of ovarian cancer. JAMA 2002;288:334. (*The relative risk was 1.6 for users of estrogen alone; there was no increased risk for users of progestin and estrogen combinations.*)

8. Narod SA, Risch H, Moslehi R, et al. Oral contraceptives and risk of hereditary ovarian cancer. N Engl J Med 1998;339:424. (*Risk was reduced by 50% for those with any past use and 60% for those with 6 or more years of use.*)

9. Nelson HD, Westhoff C, Piepert J, et al. Screening for ovarian cancer: brief evidence update, May 25, 2004. Available at: www.ahrq.gov/clinic/3rduspstf/ovariancan/ovcanup.htm. (*Excellent, well-referenced evidence updates.*)

10. Myers ER, Havrilesky LJ, Kulasingam SL, et al. Genomic tests for ovarian cancer detection and management. Evid Rep Technol Assess (Full Rep) 2006;145:1. (*There was no evidence for usefulness; a worrisome indication that promotion by manufacturers promotes use, with a decrease in positive predictive value.*)

11. Rodriguez C, Patel A, Calle E, et al. Estrogen replacement therapy and ovarian cancer mortality in a large prospective study of US women. JAMA 2001;285:1460. (*The relative risk was 2.2 for those who used estrogen for 10 or more years.*)

12. Kerlikowske K, Brown JS, Grady DG. Should women with familial ovarian cancer undergo prophylactic oophorectomy? Obstet Gynecol 1992;80:700. (*Weighs the risks and benefits of prophylactic surgery.*)

13. Rufford BD, Jacobs IJ, Menon U. Feasibility of screening for ovarian cancer using symptoms as selection criteria. Br J Obstet Gynaecol 2007;114:59. (*Women and their clinicians complied with referral for transvaginal ultrasound and CA-125, but no cancers were detected.*)

14. Andolf E, Jorgensen C, Astedt B. Ultrasound examination for detection of ovarian carcinoma in risk groups. Obstet Gynecol 1990;75:106. (*Pelvic examination did not detect the ovarian cancer detected by ultrasound.*)

15. van Nagell JR Jr, DePriest PD, Ueland FR, et al. Ovarian cancer screening with annual transvaginal sonography. Cancer 2007;109:1887. (*Transvaginal sonography had a sensitivity of 85.0% and a specificity of 98.7% with a positive predictive value of 14.0%.*)

16. Bell R, Pettigrew M, Sheldon T. The performance of screening tests for ovarian cancer: results of a systematic review. Br J Obstet Gynaecol 1998;105:1136. (*Estimates that between 3 and 60 women would undergo surgery for every cancer detected.*)

17. Bourne TH, Whitehead MI, Campbell S, et al. Ultrasound screening for familial ovarian cancer. Gynecol Oncol 1991;43:92. (*Women with a family history of ovarian cancer have a higher prevalence of benign ovarian abnormalities.*)

18. Buys SS, Partridge E, Greene MH, et al. Ovarian cancer screening in the Prostate, Lung, Colorectal and Ovarian (PLCO) cancer screening trial: findings from the initial screen of a randomized trial. Am J Obstet Gynecol 2005;193:1630. (*Findings that are disappointing at best; of screened women, 4.7% had positive transvaginal ultrasound with positive predictive value of 1.6%; 1.4% had positive CA-125 with positive predictive value of 4%; a total of 570 women—2% of all women screened—underwent abdominal surgery to detect 19 cancers, many of which were advanced at time of diagnosis.*)

19. Einhorn N, Sjovall K, Knapp RC, et al. Prospective evaluation of serum CA 125 levels for the early detection of ovarian cancer. Obstet Gynecol 1992;80:14. (*Prospective cohort study of 5,550 women, yielding estimates of sensitivity and specificity of 67% to 100% and 99.4%, respectively.*)

20. Jacobs IJ, Skates SJ, MacDonald N, et al. Screening for ovarian cancer: a pilot randomized trial. Lancet 1999;353:1207. (*In this randomized trial including 10,958 screened women, 468 had elevated CA-125, and 29 were referred for biopsy after ultrasound disclosed an enlarged ovary; there were 6 cancers.*)

21. Menon UA, Talaat A, Jeyarajah AR, et al. Ultrasound assessment of ovarian cancer risk in postmenopausal women with CA-125 elevation. Br J Cancer 1999;80:1644. (*Among women with elevated CA-125, ultrasound distinguished between those with baseline risk and those with relative risk >300.*)

22. Petricoin EF, Ardekani AM, Hitt BA, et al. Use of proteomic patterns in serum to identify ovarian cancer. Lancet 2002;359:572. (*A promising approach, but it needs further definition of sensitivity, specificity, and predictive values in appropriate populations.*)

23. Pittaway DE, Fayez JA. Serum CA-125 antigen levels increase during menses. Am J Obstet Gynecol 1987;156:75. (*Documents cyclic variation, which could have a profound effect on sensitivity and specificity among premenopausal women.*)

24. Schapira MM, Matchar DB, Young MJ. The effectiveness of ovarian cancer screening: a decision analysis model. Ann Intern Med 1993;118:838. (*Found a limited effect on life expectancy; not recommended for routine use.*)

25. Skates SJ, Singer DE. Quantifying the potential benefit of CA 125 screening for ovarian cancer. J Clin Epidemiol 1991;44:365. (*Presents a sophisticated mathematical model for estimating the effects of CA-125 screening.*)

26. Mironov S, Akin O, Pandit-Taskar N, Hann LE. Ovarian cancer. Radiol Clin North Am 2007;45:149. (*Reviews screening, with emphasis on transvaginal ultrasound.*)

CHAPTER 109 ■ SCREENING FOR ENDOMETRIAL CANCER

More than 95% of the cancers of the uterine corpus are adenocarcinomas arising from the endometrium. In the United States, endometrial cancer is nearly three times more common than invasive cervical cancer. There are nearly 40,000 cases and 7,500 endometrial cancer deaths among U.S. women each year. The lifetime probability of developing endometrial carcinoma is 3%. Most cases occur in women in whom risk factors are well defined. The tumors often present symptomatically at a time when cure is still possible. Diagnostic tests suitable for indiscriminate screening are not available. It is the responsibility of the primary care provider to be aware of the risk factors and limitations of diagnostic tests, to elicit the pertinent history, and to respond to worrisome symptoms.

EPIDEMIOLOGY AND RISK FACTORS (1–13)

Advancing age is an important risk factor for endometrial cancer. Most tumors occur during the sixth and seventh decades; fewer than 5% occur before age 40 years. The risk is increased among first-degree relatives of patients with endometrial cancer. Epidemiologic studies have also shown an association with cancer of the breast and cancer of the colon. The cumulative incidence of endometrial cancer by age 70 years is as high as 40% to 50% among women with hereditary nonpolyposis colorectal cancer (HNPCC), or Lynch syndrome II, compared with 3% in the general population. Women who present with endometrial cancer before age 50 years and have a family history of another HNPCC-associated cancer (colon, ovary, stomach, small bowel, renal pelvis, or ureter) may opt for genetic testing to ascertain their risks and those of family members.

Case–control studies have also demonstrated a surprisingly high prevalence of obesity and glucose intolerance among patients with endometrial cancer. Studies have estimated that the relative risks of endometrial cancer among obese women are greater than 2.0, but some estimates have been as high as 20, depending on the definition of obesity used. Among obese women, risk is associated with degree of insulin resistance ascertained by measurement of adiponectin, which is inversely associated with insulin resistance (i.e., women with low adiponectin levels are at increased risk of endometrial cancer). Up to 40% of patients with endometrial cancer in some studies have diabetes mellitus, but the strength of this association independent of obesity is unclear.

There is strong evidence that *estrogens*, either endogenous or exogenous, play a principal role in the etiology of endometrial carcinoma. The histologic precursor of endometrial cancer is atypical endometrial hyperplasia. Retrospective studies have indicated a progression from cystic hyperplasia through adenomatous hyperplasia to atypical hyperplasia, associated with unopposed estrogen effects. Prospective studies have demonstrated a cumulative incidence of carcinoma of 10% to 30% among patients with atypical endometrial hyperplasia.

A number of clinical syndromes that include ovarian estrogen excess have been associated with the increased risk of endometrial cancer. Postmenopausal women with estrogen-secreting tumors have been reported to have a 10% to 24% incidence of endometrial cancer. There is also a high incidence of cancer in patients with *polycystic ovary disease*; 19% to 25% of young women with endometrial carcinoma have underlying Stein–Leventhal syndrome. It is likely that less well-defined abnormalities of estrogen control explain the association of endometrial cancer with menstrual abnormalities and infertility. Approximately half of all women with endometrial carcinoma and 20% to 30% of married women with endometrial carcinoma are nulliparous.

The principal estrogen in postmenopausal women is estrone, which is peripherally converted from androstenedione produced in the adrenal glands. Peripheral conversion of androstenedione to estrone has been shown to be increased in patients with endometrial cancer, and estrone-to-estradiol ratios are higher. Peripheral conversion by adipose cells may be the explanatory link between obesity and endometrial cancer.

A number of retrospective case–control studies indicate that the use of *estrogens postmenopausally* substantially increases the risk of endometrial cancer. Rates of endometrial cancer among estrogen users ranged from 4 to 14 times those among control patients. Several studies demonstrated a dose–response relationship, in that the use of estrogen for longer periods of time was associated with greater risk. A program of estrogen plus progesterone for postmenopausal hormone replacement therapy is not associated with an increased risk of endometrial carcinoma.

Women who take tamoxifen as adjuvant therapy for breast cancer or for chemoprevention are also at increased risk for endometrial cancer. A meta-analysis of adjuvant therapy trials found a relative risk of 4.1 among tamoxifen users compared with women taking placebos. Case–control data suggested a 50% decrease in risk among women who have used combination birth control pills for a minimum of 12 months, with the protective effect lasting from 8 to 15 years. Women with BRCA1 and BRCA2 genes have a higher risk of endometrial cancer, but only if they have taken tamoxifen for previous breast cancer or for chemoprevention.

An inverse relationship between past or current smoking and endometrial cancer risk has been documented in a number of cohort studies, including the Nurses' Health Study.

It has been observed that endometrial cancers with poor prognostic cell types—such as clear cell or papillary serous tumors—that are not associated with endometrial hyperplasia have distinctly different risk factors. These women tend to be older, multiparous, and neither obese nor diabetic. There is little to suggest that these tumors are associated with estrogen exposure.

NATURAL HISTORY OF ENDOMETRIAL CANCER AND EFFECTIVENESS OF THERAPY (1,14)

Postmenopausal bleeding—by far the most common symptom associated with endometrial cancer—must always be pursued aggressively. Clinical studies have indicated that, depending on patient selection, cancer is the explanation for 10% to 70% of women who present with postmenopausal bleeding. In one review of more than 400 presentations of bleeding at least 2 years after menopause, 16% of patients had endometrial cancer. The likelihood of malignancy increased with the span of years since menopause.

In a series of more than 500 patients with endometrial cancer from the Mayo Clinic, nearly all presented with postmenopausal bleeding or similar symptoms; only 3% of the tumors were detected in asymptomatic women. In this series, there was little if any correlation between the duration of symptoms and the clinical stage of the tumor at the time of diagnosis. The prognosis for endometrial cancer is generally favorable. In the Mayo series, a 5-year survival rate of 75% was reported.

DIAGNOSTIC TESTS (1,15–19)

The data suggest that endometrial cancer presents with symptoms early in its natural history. There is little evidence that cytopathologic screening can appreciably advance the time of diagnosis in most patients. The diagnosis of endometrial cancer can be made on the basis of a *Papanicolaou (Pap) smear* of cells aspirated from the *vaginal pool* or scraped from the *cervical os*. However, a number of studies have indicated that the sensitivity of the Pap smear in the diagnosis of endometrial cancer is low. A retrospective review of patients with endometrial cancer who had Pap smears during the year before diagnosis found that only 18% had smears that were suggestive of cancer.

Jet wash and aspiration techniques have been used for sampling cells from the uterine cavity. These techniques proved to be less painful and effective substitutes for dilation and curettage in some diagnostic situations. However, the value of using these techniques to screen asymptomatic women for premalignant and malignant lesions has not been demonstrated.

Transvaginal ultrasound has proven to be an effective means of assessing endometrial thickness related to the probability of finding significant pathology with subsequent curettage in postmenopausal women. This approach has been advocated to monitor women at high risk of endometrial cancer, including those at iatrogenic risk due to unopposed estrogen treatment for menopause (rarely advised for women with intact uteri) or tamoxifen treatment for breast cancer. The estimation of endometrial thickness has also been advocated as a means of avoiding diagnostic curettage in postmenopausal women who experience abnormal bleeding. Its value in screening asymptomatic women has not been fully defined, although aggressive evaluation of the endometrium is generally advised for an ultrasonographic endometrial measurement of more than 8 mm. This can often be accomplished with outpatient endometrial biopsy and hysteroscopy rather than the more invasive dilation and curettage.

SUMMARY AND CONCLUSIONS

Endometrial carcinoma is a source of substantial morbidity and mortality and has well-defined risk factors. Evidence indicates that endogenous and exogenous estrogen stimulation plays an etiologic role. Although Pap smears potentially advance the diagnosis of cervical cancer, there are no tests as suitable for endometrial cancer screening. A prompt diagnostic workup, with transvaginal ultrasound preceding hysteroscopy and endometrial biopsy, must be initiated by the primary care provider in patients presenting with postmenopausal bleeding. Women affected by HNPCC, or Lynch syndrome II, are at high risk of endometrial cancer, with a cumulative incidence as high as 43% by age 70 years. Annual endometrial biopsy has been advised beginning no later than age 35 years for women known to carry HNPCC mutations, as well as those with a family member with a known mutation or a family history of colon cancer consistent with autosomal dominant predisposition. Prophylactic hysterectomy, with removal of the ovaries as well, might be preferred by women who have completed their childbearing. Transvaginal ultrasound, annually or even more frequently, is believed to be inadequate in this population.

Ultrasound followed by endometrial sampling and other diagnostic interventions should be considered for women at risk because of hormonal therapy including tamoxifen and other risk factors.

A.G.M.

Annotated Bibliography

1. Amant F, Moerman P, Neven P, et al. Endometrial cancer. Lancet 2005;366:491. (*A comprehensive review, including epidemiology, risk factors, and prevention.*)
2. Soliman PT, Oh JC, Schmeler KM, et al. Risk factors for young premenopausal women with endometrial cancer. Obstet Gynecol 2005;105575. (*Most younger patients were obese and nulliparous.*)
3. Soliman PT, Wu D, Tortolero-Luna G, et al. Association between adiponectin, insulin resistance, and endometrial cancer. Cancer 2006;106:2376. (*Insulin resistance was independently associated with endometrial cancer.*)
4. Beiner ME, Finch A, Rosen B, et al. The risk of endometrial cancer in women with BRCA1 and BRCA2 mutations. A prospective study. Gynecol Oncol 2007;104:7. (*The tamoxifen that is used for the chemoprevention or treatment of previous breast cancer confers the risk.*)
5. Viswanathan AN, Feskanich D, De Vivo I, et al. Smoking and the risk of endometrial cancer: results from the Nurses' Health Study. Int J Cancer 2005;114:996. (*The relative risk for current smokers was 0.63 and for past smokers was 0.73, with some attenuation when adjusted for body mass index.*)
6. Antunes CMF, Stolley PD, Rosenshein NB, et al. Endometrial cancer and estrogen use. N Engl J Med 1979;300:9. (*There was an overall sixfold increased risk in estrogen users; risk increased with dose and duration; stage 0 and 1 tumors were more common in estrogen users.*)
7. Centers for Disease Control Cancer and Steroid Hormone Study. Oral contraceptive use and the risk of endometrial cancer. JAMA 1983;249:1600. (*A case–control study, finding that combination pill use for >1 year had a protective effect, particularly among nulliparous women.*)
8. Horwitz RI, Feinstein AR. Alternative analytic methods for case–control studies of estrogen and endometrial cancer. N Engl J Med 1978;299:1089. (*Points out the potential of bias in case finding, but does not refute the increased risk.*)
9. Rutqvist LE, Johansson H, Signomklao T, et al. Adjuvant tamoxifen therapy for early stage breast cancer and second primary malignancies. J Natl Cancer Inst 1995;87:645. (*A meta-analysis, finding that the relative risk for endometrial cancer was 4.1.*)
10. Smith DC, Prentice R, Thompson DJ, et al. Association of exogenous estrogen and endometrial carcinoma. N Engl J Med 1975;293:1164. (*A case–control study, showing a 4.5-times-greater risk among exposed women.*)
11. The Cancer and Steroid Hormone Study of the Centers for Disease Control and the National Institute of Child Health and Human Development. Combination oral contraceptive use and risk of endometrial cancer. JAMA 1987;257:796. (*The risk reduction was 40% after 1 year of use, which lasted up to 15 years.*)
12. Watson P, Vasen HFA, Mecklin JP, et al. The risk of endometrial cancer in hereditary nonpolyposis colorectal cancer. Am J Med 1994;96:516. (*The cumulative incidence was 20% by age 70 years, compared with 3% in the general population.*)
13. Writing Group for the PEPI Trial. Effects of hormone replacement therapy on endometrial histology in postmenopausal women. JAMA 1996;275:370. (*Conjugated estrogens alone enhanced the development of endometrial hyperplasia, whereas combining them with progestins did not.*)
14. Pachecho JC, Kempers RD. Etiology of postmenopausal bleeding. Obstet Gynecol 1968;32:40. (*Sixteen percent of 401 women with postmenopausal bleeding had endometrial cancer.*)
15. Burke JR, Lehman HF, Wolf FS. Inadequacy of Papanicolaou smears in the detection of endometrial cancer. N Engl J Med 1974;291:191. (*Only 18% of Papanicolaou smears taken within 1 year of presentation with endometrial cancer were suggestive of malignancy.*)
16. Clark TJ, Voit D, Gupta JK, et al. Accuracy of hysteroscopy in the diagnosis of endometrial cancer and hyperplasia. JAMA 2002;288:1610. (*A positive likelihood ratio of 60 increased the probability of cancer from 4% to 72%; a negative likelihood ratio of 0.15 reduced the risk from 4% to 0.6%.*)
17. Koss LG, Schreiber K, Oberlander SG, et al. Detection of endometrial carcinoma and its hyperplasia in asymptomatic women. Obstet Gynecol 1984;64:1. (*Vaginal pool and endometrial sampling were used to screen 2,586 women; 17 endometrial cancers were diagnosed.*)
18. Pritchard KI. Screening for endometrial cancer: is it effective? Ann Intern Med 1989;110:177. (*Reviews the basis for the Canadian Task Force recommendation against screening.*)
19. Suh-Burgmann EJ, Goodman A. Surveillance for endometrial cancer in women receiving tamoxifen. Ann Intern Med 1999;131:127. (*A discussion that includes screening in the general population as well.*)

CHAPTER 110 ■ SCREENING FOR AND PREVENTION OF INTIMATE PARTNER VIOLENCE

Domestic violence, including intimate partner violence, is a prevalent and potentially fatal condition that frequently goes unrecognized, especially in the primary care setting. Estimates of the lifetime risk for battering for women range from 10% to 30% or even higher. Barriers to recognition include the reluctance of the patient to bring up the problem, time pressures, and physician uncertainty about how to respond effectively to the situation when it is recognized. The primary care clinician should be aware of the epidemiology and risk factors for domestic violence and intimate partner violence, the approaches to identifying patients who need help, and the resources available to intervene to reduce risk of ongoing morbidity and possible mortality.

EPIDEMIOLOGY AND RISK FACTORS (1–6)

The vast majority of victims of domestic violence are women, outnumbering men in a ratio of 9:1. The condition occurs among people of all ages and sociodemographic groups, and most often involves physical, sexual, or emotional abuse—or some combination—inflicted by an intimate partner. Prevalence rates of abuse in different clinical settings range from 4% to 44% within the last year and from 21% to 55% over a lifetime.

Pregnancy seems to be a particularly common time for intimate partner violence, with 1 in 6 women reporting physical or sexual assault during pregnancy.

A number of risk factors have been identified, including partner abuse of alcohol and/or drugs. The alcohol and smoking habits of women are also associated with abuse. In one study, women who neither smoked nor engaged in problem drinking had a 10% prevalence of abuse in the preceding year and lifetime prevalence of 39%. Those prevalences increased to 27% and 54%, respectively, for women who smoked and had drinking problems. The risks were intermediate for women who either smoked or had a drinking problem. Low income, but neither race nor education level, was associated with intimate partner violence in one study. Being single, separated, or divorced and living with a male friend or family members other than a husband were associated with higher rates of violence.

Victims of abuse, especially sexual or physical abuse, are 50% to 70% more likely to report gynecologic, central nervous system, and stress-related problems. Consequently, a wide range of office presentations is possible. Unexplained headache, pelvic pain, back pain, abdominal pain, and dyspareunia are significantly more common among abused women than among those who have never been abused. Other manifestations include worsening symptoms of a chronic condition, depression, anxiety, severe premenstrual symptoms, irritable bowel symptoms, and alcohol abuse, which may be among the presenting manifestations. Patients are at increased risk for somatization disorders, complications of pregnancy, sexually transmitted diseases, eating disorders, substance abuse, and noncompliance with medical regimens.

Repeated visits to the emergency room for "falls" or forearm injuries (sustained during attempts at self-defense) are characteristic, as are findings such as multiple ecchymoses in various stages of healing. Other characteristics of trauma include a central distribution of injuries, involvement of the head and face, and hearing loss. Being accompanied to the office or emergency room by an overly aggressive partner is also characteristic.

NATURAL HISTORY AND EFFECTIVENESS OF THERAPY (1,3–7)

Women often stay in a relationship despite progressive escalation of violence. Fear for personal safety and for the safety of other, dependent family members is often prominent. Financial constraints and social isolation are also common obstacles to taking action. Only about one third of violence victims voluntarily discuss the problem with their health care providers, and surveys have shown that in most settings providers do not routinely screen for abuse. As noted, victims of abuse are more likely to experience common symptoms. A life with chronic pain, headaches, gastrointestinal complaints, anxiety and panic disorders, and depression and suicidal ideation can be considered part of the natural history of ongoing intimate partner violence. One in every four women who attempt suicide has been a victim of domestic violence.

Interventions include advocacy and counseling support and removal from the environment where the violence occurs through the provision of "shelter stays." There is fair evidence that those who receive advocacy and counseling support after at least one night in a shelter subsequently experience lower rates of ongoing abuse. In general, however, there is very limited evidence for the effectiveness of interventions in reducing the risk of ongoing or escalating violence. Some see this as a reason not to recommend screening. Others see the lack of high-quality evidence as a reflection of the heterogeneity of victim circumstances and need, as well as the complex nature of the interventions.

SCREENING AND DIAGNOSIS (1–12)

Given the frequency and importance to health of domestic violence, there are strong arguments to be made for proactive identification of women who are experiencing intimate partner violence. Some advocate that women be screened for on a regular basis as part of the periodic health examination. Others favor a selective approach, reserving inquiries about domestic violence for patients who report chronic pain, unexplained worsening of a chronic condition, or one of the other non-specific presentations that have been associated with domestic violence. A critical requirement is that the patient be examined alone by a qualified health professional without the spouse, partner, family members, or friends being present. Although patients rarely present to the office complaining of domestic violence, they often demonstrate considerable relief and a willingness to discuss it once the subject has been broached by the primary care physician.

There is good evidence that screening instruments can identify women who are experiencing intimate partner violence. In the primary care setting, simple screening questions preceded by a general comment about the importance of checking for domestic violence usually suffice:

- Do you ever feel unsafe at home?
- Has anyone at home hit you or tried to injure you in any way?

These questions have been validated for diagnostic accuracy, demonstrating a sensitivity of 71% and a specificity of 85%. Some authorities also suggest questions that can elicit evidence of fear of a partner's intimidating or controlling behavior:

- Have you ever been afraid of your partner?
- Has anyone ever threatened you or tried to control you?

Others have proposed the mnemonic SAFE to help facilitate asking questions that address **S**afety, **A**buse, **F**riend or family awareness, and **E**mergency escape plan.

If the response to any of these questions is positive, the physician should obtain a full description of the problem and perform a pertinent physical examination for any evidence of injury. Confidentiality is essential to patient safety, and all records (including telephone numbers and billing diagnoses) should be handled carefully with patient protection as the priority.

OBTAINING HELP (6)

An essential component of the visit that uncovers domestic violence is to arrange for professional help. Information on local services can be obtained by calling the National Domestic Violence Hotline (1-800-799-SAFE). Patients appreciate knowing that the help to be offered is professional, typically free of charge, and designed to provide for safety and counseling. Having a member of the primary care team, preferably a trained social worker, help the patient access community services is often welcomed.

A.G.M./A.H.G.

Annotated Bibliography

1. McCauley J, Kern DE, Kolodner K, et al. The "battering syndrome": prevalence and clinical characteristics of domestic violence in primary care internal medicine practices. Ann Intern Med 1995;123:737. (*Of nearly 2,000 women surveyed, >5% had experienced domestic violence in the last year, >20% had as an adult, and 33% had as a child or adult.*)
2. Coker AL, Smith PH, McKeown RE, et al. Frequency and correlates of intimate partner violence by type: physical, sexual, and psychological battering. Am J Public Health 2000;90:553. (*A history of intimate partner violence of whom 77% experienced physical or sexual abuse.*)
3. Ramsay J, Richardson J, Carter YH, et al. Should health professionals screen women for domestic violence? Systematic review. *BMJ* 2002;325:314. (*Concludes that the problem is common but that there is insufficient evidence for the effectiveness and the absence of harm of screening.*)
4. Nelson HD, Nygren P, McInerney Y, et al. Screening women and elderly adults for family and intimate partner violence: a review of the evidence for the US Preventive Services Task Force. Ann Intern Med 2004;140:387. (*Concludes that the evidence is insufficient to recommend for or against screening.*)
5. Campbell J, Jones AS, Dienemann J, et al. Intimate partner violence and physical health consequences. Arch Intern Med 2002;162:1157.(*A case–control study, identifying a range of presenting bodily complaints, which include chronic pain syndromes.*)
6. Eisenstat SA, Bancroft L. Domestic violence. N Engl J Med 1999;341:886. (*An excellent and very practical review with 69 references; the source of the sample questions listed in this chapter.*)
7. Wathen CN, MacMillan HL. Interventions for violence against women: scientific review. JAMA. 2003;289:589-600. (*The identification of women experiencing violence is doable; the evidence for the effectiveness of interventions is lacking.*)
8. Feldhaus KM, Koziol-McLain J, Amsbury HL, et al. Accuracy of three brief screening questions for detecting partner violence in the emergency department. JAMA 1997;277:1357. (*Presents sensitivity and specificity data on simple screening questions.*)
9. Freund KM, Bak SM, Blackhall L. Identifying domestic violence in primary care practice. J Gen Intern Med 1996;11:44. (*An example of how very simple screening can greatly enhance detection.*)
10. Neufeld B. SAFE questions: overcoming barriers to the detection of domestic violence. Am Family Physician 1996;53:2575. (*Suggests an approach to questioning.*)
11. Feder GS, Hutson M, Ramsay J, Taket AR. Women exposed to intimate partner violence. Arch Intern Med. 2006;166:22. (*Women hoped for interactions with clinicians that would be nonjudgmental.*)
12. Rodriguez MA, Bauer HM, McLoughlin E, et al. Screening and intervention for intimate partner abuse: practices and attitudes of primary care physicians. JAMA 1999;282:468. (*A survey of 900 physicians showed that a majority of them screened, but only 6% of internists did so.*)

CHAPTER 111 ■ APPROACH TO THE WOMAN WITH ABNORMAL VAGINAL BLEEDING

SHANA L. BIRNBAUM

Abnormal vaginal bleeding is bleeding that occurs at an inappropriate time (<23 or >36 days after the last period) or in an excessive amount (persistent clots or bleeding lasting >7 days). About one half of all women presenting with this problem are over age 40 years. In these peri- and postmenopausal patients, uterine malignancy must be ruled out. Pelvic pathology is also a possibility in younger women, but disturbances of the hypothalamic–pituitary–ovarian axis resulting in anovulation are more common precipitants of abnormal bleeding. This is especially true among adolescent and immediately postadolescent women, who constitute about 20% of those presenting with abnormal bleeding. When bleeding is anovulatory and occurs in the absence of an anatomic lesion, it is sometimes referred to as "dysfunctional." The terms "anovulatory" and "dysfunctional" are often used interchangeably. The former is both more explanatory and less likely to have negative connotations for the patient.

In reproductive-age women, the differentiation of anovulatory bleeding from bleeding due to anatomic pathology in the presence of normal ovulation is the goal of the primary physician's initial evaluation and an important determinant of therapy. Pregnancy-associated bleeding is a separate diagnostic category, which must be ruled out in all women of reproductive age. Anovulatory bleeding is common for young women just beginning to ovulate and may last several years before menses become regular. It is also common as ovarian function declines in the perimenopausal woman, which may present a particular challenge because this is also a time for increased risk of endometrial cancer.

PATHOPHYSIOLOGY AND CLINICAL PRESENTATION (1–8)

Normal Menstrual Bleeding

In the absence of implantation of a fertilized ovum, the normal ovarian corpus luteum undergoes regression within 9 to 11 days of ovulation. Estrogen and progesterone production fall and menstruation ensues. The normal menstrual cycle ranges from 24 to 35 days (mean, 29 days). Cycle length shortens as menopause approaches. The menstrual period usually lasts 2 to 7 days, with most blood lost during the first few days. Presence of clots or duration of bleeding in excess of 1 week indicates excessive blood loss. Abnormal bleeding may occur in the context of normal ovulation or in its absence.

Abnormal Bleeding in the Setting of Normal Ovulatory Cycles

In normally ovulating women, abnormal vaginal bleeding may present as *menorrhagia* (bleeding that is normal in timing but excessive in amount and duration) or *intermenstrual bleeding*. Most often the cause is an *endometrial* or *cervical lesion* (Table 111.1). Occasionally, it is the presenting symptom of a *bleeding diathesis*, most often the consequence of thrombocytopenia or a qualitative platelet disorder (see Chapter 81).

Normal ovulation may be accompanied by a small amount of midcycle vaginal staining and pelvic pain (especially on the right side) referred to as *mittelschmerz*, which occurs in the context of ovarian follicle rupture and release.

Uterine Fibroids

Uterine fibroids or leiomyomas are the most common cause and account for about one third of cases. Fibroids occur in 20% to 25% of women before age 40 years and in up to one half of all women overall. However, only those fibroids that are submucosal in location and involve the uterine cavity cause bleeding, most typically menorrhagia. Because fibroids are so common, they may coexist with another cause of abnormal vaginal bleeding.

Carcinoma of the Cervix

Carcinoma of the cervix is among the more serious sources of abnormal bleeding in ovulating patients, although it accounts for only about 3% of cases. *Postcoital bleeding* and slight intermenstrual spotting are characteristic when there is surface ulceration, which may occur in early stages of the disease (see Chapter 123).

Endometrial Carcinoma

Endometrial carcinoma is more typically a disease of abnormal vaginal bleeding in postmenopausal women (see later discussion), but 20% of women have the disease while still menstruating (generally older than the age of 40 years). Heavier-than-normal periods are noted, as well as an intermenstrual watery discharge containing small amounts of blood.

Polyps, Erosions, and Infection

Cervical polyps, *cervical erosions*, and *vaginal lesions* present similarly, with slight spotting noted intermenstrually, especially after coitus. *Pelvic inflammatory disease*, usually but not

TABLE 111.1

DIFFERENTIAL DIAGNOSIS OF ABNORMAL VAGINAL BLEEDING

Ovulatory Bleeding
  Normal variant
    "Mittelschmerz"
  Anatomic lesion
    Uterine fibroids
    Cervical disease (inflammation, polyp, cancer)
    Endometrial carcinoma
    Pelvic inflammatory disease
    Intrauterine device
  Concurrent disease
    Bleeding diathesis
    Foreign body

Anovulatory Bleeding
  Hypothalamic dysfunction
    Puberty
    Perimenopausal state
    Situational stress, excessive exercise, weight loss
    Excess androgen, prolactin, cortisol; hypothyroidism
    Polycystic ovary syndrome
  Oral contraceptive use
    Inadequate estrogen dose

Postmenopausal Bleeding
  Endometrial pathology
    Fibroid
    Cancer
    Polyp
    Atrophy
  Cervical pathology
    Cancer
    Polyp
    Erosion
  Vaginal pathology
    Atrophic vaginitis

Pregnancy
  Ectopic pregnancy
  Postabortion (retained products of gestation)
  Failing pregnancy

always associated with fever, pelvic pain, and discharge, may lead to postcoital, intermenstrual, or heavy menstrual bleeding by causing cervicitis, endometritis, or salpingitis.

Foreign Bodies

Copper *intrauterine devices* (IUDs) alter the endometrial surface and can be similarly responsible for heavy menstrual bleeding or intermenstrual bleeding, whereas progesterone-releasing IUDs tend to decrease menstrual blood flow. Vaginal wall irritation from *tampon* use may lead to minor vaginal bleeding.

Anovulatory Bleeding

This type of bleeding is usually a manifestation of a disturbance within the hypothalamic–pituitary–ovarian axis. *Metrorrhagia* or *menometrorrhagia*—bleeding, sometimes heavy or prolonged, occurring at irregular intervals—is characteristic.

Hypothalamic Dysfunction

The pathophysiologic common denominator for hypothalamic dysfunction is *inadequate progesterone* production, most often due to lack of a *luteinizing hormone* (LH) *surge* at midcycle, a consequence of an alteration in the normal pattern of gonadotropin-releasing hormone (GnRH) release from the hypothalamus. This pattern is typical of patients with mild hypothalamic dysfunction, who may experience irregular menses in the context of moderate *situational stress, weight loss,* or *exercise training.* If the functional disturbance is more severe, impairing follicle-stimulating hormone (FSH) secretion and estrogen production, oligomenorrhea and amenorrhea may follow (see Chapter 112). *Hyperprolactinemia, hypothyroidism,* and excess production of *androgen* and *cortisol* can also disturb hypothalamic rhythmicity. Even *iron-deficiency anemia* has been found to inhibit ovulation.

In the ovary unruptured follicles persist, and functioning corpora lutea, the main source of progesterone, are absent. The endometrium shows hyperplasia resulting from unopposed estrogen. There is little if any secretory pattern because of the lack of progesterone. Ovulation does not occur, and anovulatory bleeding results when progesterone production returns or excessive proliferation causes sloughing of the overstimulated endometrium. There is irregularity of the menstrual interval, periods of amenorrhea, and episodes of very heavy and prolonged bleeding if there has been sufficient estrogen-induced buildup of the endometrium.

Polycystic Ovary Syndrome (PCOS)

PCOS is an incompletely understood but increasingly recognized common condition, affecting up to 8% of reproductive-age women. It represents a leading cause of chronic anovulatory bleeding. In addition to a lifelong history of irregular periods and/or amenorrhea, patients may report infertility, hirsutism, obesity, and acne. Abnormalities at multiple levels of the hypothalamic–pituitary–ovarian axis appear to contribute to androgen overproduction in the ovaries and an imbalance of gonadotropins in women with PCOS. Inadequate endogenous FSH production appears to result from disordered hypothalamic rhythmicity, with an increased frequency of hypothalamic GnRH pulses favoring pituitary production of LH over FSH. Despite their increased frequency and amplitude of LH pulses, women with PCOS rarely have adequate follicular development or estradiol levels to trigger a midcycle LH surge and ovulation. Chronic anovulation permits exposure of the endometrium to high levels of unopposed estrogen, with bleeding occurring if the endometrium is unable to sustain further growth. Unopposed endometrial estrogen stimulation may lead over time to adenomatous hyperplasia, cellular atypicality, and even endometrial carcinoma.

Hyperandrogenism, likely mediated by LH-related ovarian overproduction of *testosterone* and *androstenedione,* is another key element of PCOS, accounting for the associated hirsutism, acne, and occasional frank virilization (see Chapter 98), although the latter is uncommon. *Insulin resistance* with hyperinsulinism is common and believed to act synergistically with LH to enhance ovarian androgen overproduction. Women with PCOS are recognized to have an increased prevalence of diabetes mellitus and other risk factors for coronary disease, including dyslipidemia and hypertension. They appear to share a phenotype similar to that seen in the metabolic syndrome, with the prevalence of metabolic syndrome in women with PCOS ranging from 33% to 47%, more than twice as high as the prevalence in women without PCOS. There may be an increased risk of adverse cardiovascular events, although data are conflicting.

Puberty

The anovulatory bleeding of puberty is a consequence of immaturity of the positive-feedback mechanism responsible for the LH surge that triggers progesterone secretion. In the absence of adequate progesterone production, estrogen-withdrawal bleeding takes place. The pattern of anovulatory bleeding is irregular and may occur at any time between 22 and 45 days.

Perimenopausal Bleeding

The irregular menstrual bleeding that characterizes the perimenopausal period is also an anovulatory estrogen-withdrawal phenomenon. As the number of functioning ovarian follicles declines, insufficient estrogen is produced to cause an LH surge and ovulation. In the absence of adequate progesterone production, bleeding occurs when the endometrium can no longer sustain growth. Such perimenopausal bleeding can continue for months to years, but it eventually stops when estrogen production ceases.

Postmenopausal, Pregnancy-Related, and Breakthrough Types of Bleeding

Postmenopause

Here the major concern is cancer, although *uterine fibroids* or *endometrial atrophy* still account for most cases. Women who have had chronic unopposed estrogen stimulation are at increased risk of *endometrial carcinoma*. Early on, bleeding may be subtle and little more than minor vaginal staining (see Chapter 123). Postmenopausal women with *atrophic vaginitis*, *cervical or endometrial polyps*, or *cervicitis* from a prolapsed uterus may also experience some blood-stained vaginal discharge or minor spotting. Cervical carcinoma is uncommon after age 55 years in women who have had Papanicolaou (Pap) smears regularly but may be the cause of bleeding in the early postmenopausal period.

Pregnancy

One of the most serious causes of acute abnormal vaginal bleeding in women of reproductive age is *ectopic pregnancy*, which is characterized by delay of the regular period followed by vaginal blood spotting, often in conjunction with unilateral pelvic pain. Intraperitoneal hemorrhage can ensue if tubal rupture occurs, but this happens in fewer than 5% of cases. A *spontaneous abortion* may be heralded by onset of bleeding. *Retained products of gestation* are a very common cause of abnormal uterine bleeding after an incomplete abortion; blood loss is often heavy and may persist for more than 7 days.

Oral Contraceptives

If an oral contraceptive contains insufficient estrogen or a progestin without adequate estrogenic activity or if compliance is inadequate, then abnormal vaginal bleeding may occur. The characteristic pattern is one of *breakthrough bleeding*, or staining that occurs intermenstrually (see Chapter 119).

DIFFERENTIAL DIAGNOSIS (9)

The differential diagnosis can be divided into ovulatory, anovulatory, postmenopausal, and pregnancy-related etiologies (Table 111.1). Among postmenopausal women with bleeding, endometrial cancer accounts for 10% to 25% of cases. The majority of cases are due to benign etiologies, most commonly submucosal uterine fibroids or endometrial atrophy. In women of reproductive age, the etiology is often an anovulatory disturbance, although cancer remains a concern. As noted, girls going through puberty and perimenopausal women who complain of irregular menses are most likely to have anovulatory bleeding. In cases of ovulatory bleeding, anatomic etiologies are most common.

WORKUP (10–16)

Among women of reproductive age who complain of abnormal vaginal bleeding, the initial tasks are to rule out pregnancy and determine whether the bleeding is ovulatory or anovulatory. Postmenopausal bleeding has its own workup, which focuses on identifying the anatomic site of bleeding.

History

A careful and detailed menstrual history is essential. Most important is information on the patient's normal menstrual cycle (duration, frequency, intensity) and how the current bleeding pattern compares with it. If the patient is of childbearing age, then inquiry should be made into unprotected intercourse and symptoms of pregnancy (breast engorgement, morning sickness, cessation of normal menses). If menstrual regularity persists despite an increase in intensity or duration of flow or onset of intermenstrual staining, then an ovulatory etiology is likely. This is further supported by the presence of premenstrual symptoms, such as breast engorgement, pelvic cramping, fluid retention, and mood swings. Anovulatory bleeding is suggested by the absence of such symptoms plus complete irregularity of menstrual periods, especially if accompanied by months of amenorrhea. Although the intensity of the bleeding (e.g., by number of pads or tampons used) is difficult to quantify and varies by individual, the new onset of clots or duration of more than 7 days argues for abnormal bleeding.

Ovulatory Bleeding

History should include symptoms of a bleeding diathesis or medicines that inhibit normal clotting (see Chapter 81). Equally important is checking for dyspareunia, postcoital bleeding, vaginal discharge, pelvic pain, fever, trauma, and intrauterine device use. Risk factors for endometrial carcinoma, including use of tamoxifen, should be reviewed (see Chapter 123).

Anovulatory Bleeding

One should ask about important precipitants, such as emotional stress, weight loss, exercise, and chronic illness. If the patient is an adolescent girl, one should check for a history of irregular periods since the onset of menarche along with the common precipitants just noted. Review of medications for the use of oral contraceptives is essential, with attention to the estrogen dose and history of breakthrough bleeding. In the perimenopausal woman, menstrual irregularity and the skipping of periods suggest a functional etiology but do not rule out cancer. Androgen excess is suggested by symptoms of hirsutism and virilization (see Chapter 98) and a history of infertility. Rapid onset of hirsutism and virilization raises the possibility of an androgen-producing adrenal or ovarian tumor. A lifelong history of irregular menses, hirsutism, infertility, and obesity suggests polycystic ovary syndrome. Inquiry into galactorrhea and development of cushingoid appearance check for prolactin and cortisol excess, respectively. Any symptoms of hypothyroidism (see Chapter 104) and iron-deficiency anemia (see Chapter 79) should be noted.

Postmenopausal Bleeding

Any history of bleeding, even if just minor staining, should be taken as evidence of a possible malignancy. However, inquiry into symptomatic atrophic vaginitis and uterine prolapse may provide useful clues.

Physical Examination

All patients should be checked for *postural signs* indicative of significant intravascular volume depletion, particularly those with acute, heavy bleeding. Careful *speculum and bimanual pelvic examinations* are essential, with particular care taken to note any vaginal or cervical erosions, uterine or adnexal masses, focal tenderness, or purulent or bloody discharge. Signs of pregnancy (engorged breasts, pigmented areolae, bluish cervix, enlarged uterus) should be sought in women of reproductive age.

Suspected ovulatory bleeding necessitates concentrating on the pelvic examination, but one should also check for signs of a bleeding diathesis (petechiae, ecchymoses, splenic enlargement). The patient with *suspected anovulatory bleeding* should be carefully examined for hirsutism, virilization, cushingoid appearance, milky nipple discharge, goiter, dry skin, coarse hair, and delayed reflexes. Visual field testing is indicated if there is suspicion of a pituitary adenoma. Presence of hirsutism or virilization necessitates thorough pelvic and abdominal examinations for an ovarian or adrenal mass.

On examination of the *postmenopausal woman*, particular note should be taken of the friability of the vaginal mucosa and cervix and the presence of any uterine or adnexal masses.

Laboratory Studies

All patients of reproductive age with abnormal vaginal bleeding should be tested for pregnancy (a *serum human chorionic gonadotropin b subunit* is the most sensitive, although a urine pregnancy test maintains good sensitivity and has the advantage of immediate results; see Chapter 112). A *complete blood count* may be useful because the *hematocrit* will help to assess the severity of chronic blood loss (although not of acute hemorrhage; see Chapter 79), and a mean *red cell volume* may reveal the microcytosis of iron deficiency.

Ovulatory Bleeding

Here the goal is identification of pelvic pathology after ruling out concurrent disease that may predispose to heavy bleeding. Determinations of *blood urea nitrogen*, *creatinine*, and *platelet count* should be obtained when there is concern about a bleeding diathesis. Von Willebrand's disease should be suspected and evaluated in young women with menorrhagia since menarche, particularly if there is a family history of coagulopathy. Otherwise, one should proceed directly to transvaginal and transabdominal *pelvic ultrasound* examination or hysterosonography (infusion of sterile saline into the uterine cavity with transvaginal ultrasound). Consensus as to which should be the initial test has not been reached, although it appears that hysterosonography has substantially higher sensitivity and better specificity for detection of intracavitary abnormalities, including uterine polyps and submucosal fibroids. If ultrasound is the initial test and the lining is incompletely imaged or thickened, *hysterosonography* can provide improved visualization of the endometrial lining, revealing focal thickening, endometrial polyps, or submucosal fibroids. A *Pap smear* is indicated if the cervix appears abnormal or routine screening is due. A *cervical culture* for gonorrhea and for other pathogenic organisms is needed in the patient with pain on motion of the cervix and adnexal tenderness or with risk factors for sexually transmitted disease (see Chapter 117); an elevated *sedimentation rate* suggests pelvic inflammation.

Endometrial sampling via *office biopsy* (performed by a gynecologist) is crucial to the evaluation of ovulatory bleeding when noninvasive evaluation is unrevealing, particularly in the presence of risk factors for endometrial hyperplasia or carcinoma. In premenopausal women, as opposed to postmenopausal women, evaluation of endometrial thickness has not been shown to exclude malignancy. Office or operative *hysteroscopy*, allowing for direct visualization of the endometrium, treatment of abnormalities, and guided biopsy, is now preferred to blind diagnostic dilation and curettage. Despite its expense and invasive nature, it is considered the gold standard if bleeding persists despite a negative evaluation.

Anovulatory Bleeding

No additional studies are necessary when the etiology is evident (e.g., situational stress, puberty, chronic illness, marked weight loss). If perimenopausal bleeding is suspected, determining the *FSH* level can be confirmatory; if it is greater than 40 IU/mL, then ovarian failure is imminent. If the history or physical exam suggests thyroid disorder or hyperprolactinemia, TSH and prolactin levels are helpful. Although polycystic ovary syndrome is primarily a clinical diagnosis, a testosterone level greater than 60 ng/dL supports the diagnosis, as does an elevated free testosterone level. An LH-to-FSH ratio of greater than 2:1, although consistent with the diagnosis, is an insensitive screening test, given the variability in gonadotropin levels, and should not be used routinely. When new-onset hirsutism or virilization is noted, a serum *testosterone* is the best test. If the onset of such changes is rapid or the serum testosterone is greater than 150 ng/dL, then a functioning adrenal or ovarian neoplasm may be the source. A morning *17-hydroxyprogesterone level* can exclude the diagnosis of nonclassic congenital adrenal hyperplasia, which may clinically mimic PCOS.

Postmenopausal Bleeding

Noninvasive study for pelvic pathology is conducted as noted with *transvaginal ultrasound* and/or *hysterosonography*. If transvaginal ultrasound reveals an *endometrial stripe less than 4 mm*, the risk of cancer is quite low. Nonetheless, because concern about endometrial cancer is high in this age group, endometrial sampling is appropriate if bleeding persists or if a noninvasive study is unrevealing, particularly in the setting of hormone replacement use or tamoxifen use.

SYMPTOMATIC MANAGEMENT AND PATIENT EDUCATION (17–24)

Acute Anovulatory Bleeding

Acute anovulatory bleeding that is not severe can often be managed by the primary care physician in the office setting. To stop the abnormal bleeding, one can administer a course of oral *medroxyprogesterone* (Provera; 10 mg/d for 10 days) or a single intramuscular injection of *progesterone* (100 mg). These will convert a proliferative endometrium into a secretory one. Bleeding should stop within 24 to 48 hours of initiating progestin therapy, and menstrual flow should occur on its completion. Alternatively, combined oral contraceptives containing 30 to 35 μg of estrogen may be used at a dose of one tablet every 4 to 6 hours for 2 to 3 days, which should stabilize the endometrium and stop the bleeding. If this treatment does not stop acute bleeding, then referral for dilation and curettage and hysteroscopy is indicated.

Chronic Anovulatory Bleeding

Chronic anovulatory bleeding can be treated symptomatically by monthly administration of progesterone therapy, triggering regular endometrial shedding. This strategy protects against adenomatous changes and lowers the risk of endometrial cancer associated with long-term unopposed estrogen stimulation. A course of *medroxyprogesterone* given for 10 to 12 days of each month usually suffices. Cessation of further abnormal bleeding episodes argues strongly against a structural lesion, but resumption of such bleeding on progestin therapy necessitates further evaluation.

Ovulation may resume on this program, particularly in the young person, and periodically the treatment should be halted for 1 or 2 months to observe for the return of normal cycles. If abnormal bleeding recurs despite correction of all possible precipitating factors, then maintenance hormonal therapy may be used. In patients who do not desire pregnancy, an *estrogen-progestin* oral contraceptive preparation may be used in place of the medroxyprogesterone (see Chapter 119). Oral contraceptive therapy has the advantage of improving the hyperandrogenism that accompanies some causes of chronic anovulatory bleeding. The patient with anovulatory bleeding who desires pregnancy should be referred for consideration of medical ovulation induction. Any iron deficiency (see Chapter 82) or pelvic infection should be treated (see Chapter 117).

Nonsteroidal antiinflammatory drugs (NSAIDs) may decrease bleeding by 30% to 50%. They may also provide relief for any associated dysmenorrhea. They may be used along with oral contraceptives. *Danazol*, an androgen agonist, may be effective in reducing blood flow but has undesirable androgenic and hypoestrogenic side effects. *GnRH analogues* produce a menopausal state in women of reproductive age. They are used primarily for preoperative management of uterine fibroids and for endometrial preparation before ablation procedures. *Levonorgestrel-releasing IUDs* can be effective in reducing both ovulatory and anovulatory bleeding by decreasing endometrial proliferation.

When anovulatory bleeding is diagnosed, it is important for the patient to know that reproductive capacity is not lost, that some causes are self-limited, and that the possibility of malignancy is very low for women younger than age 30 years. Addressing any contributing factors (e.g., situational stress, dieting, excessive exercise, hypothyroidism [see Chapter 104], hyperprolactinemia [see Chapter 100], and polycystic ovary syndrome [see Chapter 112]) is essential to successful therapy.

Ovulatory Bleeding

Nonhormonal therapy is first-line treatment for menorrhagia associated with ovulatory cycles once an anatomic etiology has been excluded but may be inadequate for many women with ongoing menorrhagia affecting quality of life. *NSAIDs* have been shown to reduce blood loss in randomized trials and are also effective in treating associated dysmenorrhea. They are less effective than *danazol* or the antifibrinolytic *tranexamic acid*, which is frequently used in the United Kingdom but is not approved in the United States for menorrhagia. Hormonal options for treatment of menorrhagia include use of combined *oral contraceptives*, 21-day cycles of *oral progestin* therapy (from cycle day 5 to day 26), and the *levonorgestrel-releasing IUD (Mirena)*, which demonstrates equal long-term patient satisfaction and improvement in quality of life in studies comparing it to surgical treatment options.

Perimenopausal Bleeding

Perimenopausal bleeding may be the result of anovulatory periods, but an irregular pattern may also represent intrauterine disease. When discussed openly, the concerns that most patients already harbor can be addressed and often lessened because most cases are not likely to be cancerous. Once a structural lesion has been ruled out, symptomatic therapy with monthly *medroxyprogesterone* (10 mg/d for 10 to 12 days) can be used to correct the irregular bleeding. Therapy is continued monthly until withdrawal bleeding stops, indicating arrival of ovarian failure and menopause. A popular alternative is the use of *low-dose (20 mcg) combined oral contraceptives*, provided the patient is a nonsmoker without uncontrolled hypertension. Until menopause, some ovulatory periods may still take place and cause bleeding independent of progesterone therapy. Combined therapy will regulate such bleeding and provide the added benefit of contraception. Treatment can be stopped periodically to assess the arrival of menopause.

Breakthrough Bleeding

Patients experiencing breakthrough bleeding on low-dose estrogen oral contraceptives need to be sure they are adhering carefully to their regimen. If they are taking the medication on schedule, switching to a preparation with a higher estrogen dose or a more estrogenic progesterone is indicated.

INDICATIONS FOR ADMISSION AND REFERRAL

Immediate hospital admission is essential for any woman who is bleeding heavily and manifests signs of intravascular volume depletion. Immediate evaluation and gynecologic consultation are particularly important if ectopic pregnancy is a possibility because life-threatening hemorrhage is a real, albeit slight, risk. Gynecologic consultation should also be sought in cases of recent abortion because placental tissue may be retained. Bleeding in pregnancy is a definite indication for an emergency obstetric consultation.

Any patient with abnormal vaginal bleeding who has a mass lesion detected on pelvic examination, an abnormal-appearing cervix, an abnormal Pap test (beyond atypical squamous cells of undetermined significance), or risk factors for carcinoma of the cervix or endometrium (see Chapters 107 and 109) should be referred to the gynecologist. Consultation should be considered for any perimenopausal or postmenopausal woman who experiences the new onset of staining or abnormal bleeding while taking hormones and is essential if transvaginal ultrasound or hysterosonography suggest thickened endometrium (>4 mm) or any endometrial pathology regardless of hormone use. The risk of malignancy is increased in older women, although controversy exists as to how much; whereas one retrospective series found 23% of women with postmenopausal bleeding to have endometrial carcinoma, another series of 801 women with postmenopausal bleeding found cancer or atypical hyperplasia in only 0.76% of cases. Most experts estimate the risk of serious pathology to be 5% in women with unexplained postmenopausal bleeding. Patients younger than age 30 years with an otherwise normal examination are at very low risk and need not be referred. However, risk of cancer begins to increase at age older than 30 years, necessitating consideration of referral for invasive evaluation, especially in the ovulating patient with abnormal bleeding. For women with anovulatory bleeding who desire fertility, referral to a reproductive endocrinologist or fertility specialist is appropriate.

When medical therapy fails adequately to control chronic bleeding, there are surgical options. By this time, most women will already have been referred to a gynecologist for invasive evaluation. They may be offered endometrial ablation, hysterectomy, or placement of a levonorgestrel-releasing IUD. The primary care provider should maintain a supportive role in the decision making, ensuring that the patient is adequately informed about the harms and benefits of surgical intervention. It is especially important that women approaching menopause appreciate that their symptoms will diminish over time with watchful waiting and symptomatic therapy.

Annotated Bibliography

1. Bayer SR, DeCherney AH. Clinical manifestations and treatment of dysfunctional uterine bleeding. JAMA 1993;269:1823. (*Helpful approach to workup and symptomatic management.*)
2. Weissberg SM, Dodson MG. Recurrent vaginal and cervical ulcers associated with tampon use. JAMA 1983;250:1430. (*Case reports plus a review of the literature of what may be a frequent cause of minor abnormal vaginal bleeding.*)
3. Shangold M, Rebar RW, Wentz AC, et al. Evaluation and management of menstrual dysfunction in athletes. JAMA 1990;263:1665. (*Useful discussion with very practical recommendations; 36 references.*)
4. Berga SL, Mortola JF, Girton L, et al. Neuroendocrine aberrations in women with functional hypothalamic amenorrhea. J Clin Endocrinol Metab 1989;68:301. (*The normal pattern of gonadotropin-releasing hormone release is disturbed.*)
5. Guzick D. Polycystic ovary syndrome. Obstet Gynecol 2004;103:181. (*Excellent review of polycystic ovary syndrome [PCOS] presentation, diagnosis, pathophysiology, management, and consequences.*)
6. Ehrmann DA. Polycystic ovary syndrome. New Engl J Med 2005; 352:1223. (*Overview of the pathophysiology and evaluation of PCOS, including genetic linkages, newer treatment options, and long-term implications.*)
7. Rotterdam ESHRE/ASRM-Sponsored PCOS Consensus Workshop Group. Revised 2003 consensus on diagnostic criteria and long-term health risks related to polycystic ovary syndrome (PCOS). Hum Reprod 2004;19:41. (*These revised diagnostic criteria include two out of three of the following: oligo- and/or anovulation, clinical and/or biochemical hyperandrogenism, and polycystic ovaries, as well as exclusion of other etiologies.*)
8. Stewart EA. Uterine fibroids. Lancet 2001;357:293. (*Reviews epidemiology, evaluation, and treatment.*)
9. Brenner PF. Differential diagnosis of abnormal uterine bleeding. Am J Obstet Gynecol 1996;175:766. (*A well-organized review with emphasis on systemic disease as a contributor to abnormal uterine bleeding.*)
10. Good, A. Diagnostic options for assessment of postmenopausal bleeding. Mayo Clin Proc 1997;72:345. (*Excellent review of the advantages and disadvantages of endometrial biopsy, transvaginal ultrasound, and hysteroscopy for assessment of the endometrium in postmenopausal bleeding.*)
11. Gull B, Karlsson B, Milsom I, et al. Can ultrasound replace dilation and curettage? A longitudinal evaluation of postmenopausal bleeding and transvaginal sonographic measurement of the endometrium as predictors of endometrial cancer. Am J Obstet Gynecol 2003;188:401. (*Endometrial thickness of <4 mm excluded a diagnosis of endometrial cancer, even with 10 years of follow-up.*)
12. Archer DF, Lobo RA, Land HF, et al. A comparative study of transvaginal uterine ultrasound and endometrial biopsy for evaluating the endometrium of postmenopausal women taking hormone replacement therapy. Menopause 1999;6:201. (*Found that endometrial thickness was inconclusive among women taking hormone replacement therapy.*)
13. Isaacs JH, Ross FH. Cytologic evaluation of the endometrium in women with postmenopausal bleeding. Am J Obstet Gynecol 1978;131:410. (*A retrospective series of 143 women with postmenopausal bleeding found endometrial carcinoma in 23% of cases.*)
14. Smith-Bindman R, Kerlikowske K, Feldstein VA, et al. Endovaginal ultrasound to exclude endometrial cancer and other abnormalities. JAMA 1998;280:1510. (*A sensitivity for cancer of 96% was found using a 5-mm endometrial thickness as a threshold.*)
15. Dijkhuizen FP, De Vries LD, Mol BW, et al. Comparison of transvaginal ultrasonography and saline infusion sonography for the detection of intracavitary abnormalities in premenopausal women. Ultrasound Obstet Gynecol 2000;15:372. (*Found a sensitivity of 61% and a specificity of 96% for transvaginal ultrasound in the detection of intracavitary abnormalities vs. a sensitivity of 100% and a specificity of 85% for hysterosonography in one small series of premenopausal women, using hysterectomy specimen as the gold standard.*)
16. Clark TH, Voit D, Gupta J, et al. Accuracy of hysteroscopy in the diagnosis of endometrial cancer and hyperplasia: a systematic quantitative review. JAMA 2002;288:1610. (*Diagnostic accuracy was high for hysteroscopy in the diagnosis of endometrial cancer but only moderate for endometrial hyperplasia.*)
17. Chuong CJ, Brenner PF. Management of abnormal uterine bleeding. Am J Obstet Gynecol 1996;175:787. (*Practical review of management alternatives.*)
18. Carlson KJ, Miller BA, Fowler FJ. The Maine Women's Health Study. II. Outcomes of nonsurgical management of leiomyomas, abnormal uterine bleeding and chronic pelvic pain. Obstet Gynecol 1994;83:566. (*More than 300 women were followed with nonsurgical therapy, with most improving.*)
19. Prentice A. Fortnightly review: medical management of menorrhagia. BMJ 1999;319:1343. (*A concise review, covering differential diagnosis and diagnostic evaluation; tranexamic acid was the first choice for ovulatory bleeding from this U.K. perspective, whereas hormonal methods, including 21-day progestin and Mirena intrauterine device, are also effective.*)
20. Hurskainen R, Teperi J, Rissanen P, et al. Clinical outcomes and costs with the levonorgestrel-releasing intrauterine system or hysterectomy for treatment of menorrhagia: randomized trial 5 year follow-up. JAMA 2004;291:1456. (*Found no difference in health-related quality of life in women assigned to levonorgestrel intrauterine devices [IUDs] vs. hysterectomy for management of menorrhagia and significant cost savings in the IUD group.*)
21. Kaunitz A. Oral contraceptive use in perimenopause. Am J Obstet Gynecol 2001;185:S32. (*Reviews the advantages of oral contraceptive use in providing contraception, managing vasomotor symptoms, maintaining cycle regularity, and protecting bone health in the perimenopausal period.*)
22. Apgar BS, Kaufman AH, George-Nwogu U, et al. Treatment of menorrhagia. Am Fam Physician 2007;75:1813. (*Practical review of evaluation and treatment of menorrhagia, including both medical and surgical therapies.*)
23. Marjoribanks J, Lethaby A, Farquhar C. Surgery vs medical therapy for heavy menstrual bleeding. Cochrane Database Syst Rev 2003(2):CD003855; Update, Cochrane Database Syst Rev 2006(2):CD003855. (*A systematic review finding that surgery may be more effective at reducing bleeding at 1 year, but that the levonorgestrel-releasing IUD is equally effective at improving quality of life and may control bleeding equally well in the long term; concludes that oral therapy suits only a minority of women long term.*)
24. Lethaby A, Farquhar C, Cooke I. Antifibrinolytics for heavy menstrual bleeding (Cochrane Review). In: The Cochrane library, Issue 3. Oxford: Update Software, 2004. (*Evidence supporting the use of tranexamic acid for ovulatory bleeding, which is used in the United Kingdom but not approved for this use in the United States; see http://www.cochrane.org for updates.*)

CHAPTER 112 ■ EVALUATION OF SECONDARY AMENORRHEA

SHANA L. BIRNBAUM

Secondary amenorrhea is defined as cessation of menses for 3 or more months in a woman with previously normal cycles. The incidence of secondary amenorrhea is about 3% in unselected populations. The primary physician is frequently consulted by women who have missed one or more menstrual periods. Concerns about pregnancy and menopause are prominent. Knowing how to initiate an efficient workup for functional or structural abnormalities of the hypothalamic–pituitary–ovarian axis and knowing when to refer are important components of the primary care of women with this problem.

PATHOPHYSIOLOGY AND CLINICAL PRESENTATION (1–17)

Amenorrhea reflects an interruption in the mechanisms of normal menstruation and may result from a disturbance at the level of the hypothalamus, pituitary, ovaries, or uterus. Polycystic ovarian syndrome, one of the most common causes of amenorrhea, involves abnormalities throughout the hypothalamic-pituitary–ovarian access.

Hypothalamic Amenorrhea

Hypothalamic amenorrhea most often results from a *functional disorder of pulsatile gonadotropin-releasing hormone* (GnRH) *release* causing *loss of a luteinizing hormone* (LH) *surge* and failure to ovulate. The most profound disturbances of GnRH release may occur in the context of *marked weight loss* (<70% ideal, as in anorexia nervosa and other eating disorders; see Chapter 234), *severe emotional upset*, or *excessive exercise* (competitive athletes). Athletes in sports requiring low body weight or subjective judging (figure-skating, gymnastics) are more prone to exercise-induced hypothalamic amenorrhea. A relative caloric deficiency seems to be necessary for this type of amenorrhea because some weight-stable nonathletic women with functional hypothalamic amenorrhea exhibit evidence of subclinical eating disorders characterized by severe restriction of dietary fat. Leptin, a hormone secreted by fat cells in proportion to body fat stores, may be involved in mediating this relationship; leptin levels are lower in women with hypothalamic amenorrhea, and athletes with amenorrhea appear to lose the diurnal variation in leptin secretion. In one small study of women with hypothalamic amenorrhea, leptin administration resulted in improvement of LH pulsatility and reversal of the amenorrhea. In patients with severe functional impairment of GnRH release, estrogen levels can fall so far below normal that the patient is at risk for osteopenia; *osteoporosis* may ensue if the condition goes untreated for a prolonged period of time. This has resulted in recognition of the so-called "female athlete

triad" of amenorrhea, disordered eating, and osteopenia or osteoporosis. In the setting of significant hypoestrogenism, there is little or no endometrial proliferation, so withdrawal bleeding does not occur on uterine exposure to progesterone. Although women with severe functional hypothalamic amenorrhea can achieve a return of pulsatile GnRH release and restoration of normal periods and estrogen status with correction of the underlying problem, the bone loss may be permanent.

More commonly seen are milder functional forms of impaired GnRH release in the settings of *situational stress, excessive exercise, concurrent illness,* or *mild weight loss.* In mild functional hypothalamic disease, follicle-stimulating hormone (FSH) secretion continues at a low-normal level, allowing estrogen production, which results in endometrial proliferation. Withdrawal bleeding occurs on exposure to progesterone, whether endogenous or exogenous.

A host of endocrinopathies may cause amenorrhea by interfering with normal GnRH release. Excess production of *cortisol, androgens,* and *prolactin* has been linked to impairment of GnRH release. *Hypothyroidism* with its associated elevated thyrotropin-releasing hormone (TRH) levels may present as amenorrhea because of the ability of TRH to trigger prolactin secretion.

Drugs are sometimes responsible, including oral contraceptives and agents with dopaminergic activity (e.g., phenothiazines, risperidol, metoclopramide). Menses usually return within 2 months of stopping oral contraceptives, although "postpill amenorrhea" can last up to 6 months. More-prolonged amenorrhea suggests underlying pathology unrelated to oral contraceptive use.

Pituitary Pathology

Most *pituitary neoplasms* infrequently cause amenorrhea, but *prolactinomas* are responsible for up to one fourth of cases. Excess prolactin production *inhibits normal GnRH release* and impairs gonadotropin production. The characteristic clinical picture is one of *galactorrhea, infertility,* and *amenorrhea* (see Chapter 100). As prolactin levels rise, plasma concentrations of gonadotropins and estradiol begin to fall, resulting in amenorrhea or oligomenorrhea. Because prolactin is primarily controlled by negative inhibition from hypothalamic dopamine, an alternative mechanism for hyperprolactinemia is disruption of the pituitary stalk, as by a tumor. Most prolactinomas are small (<10 mm in diameter) and are designated as *microadenomas.* Patients with microadenomas usually have otherwise normal pituitary function, whereas those with *macroadenomas* (>10 mm) may experience reduced secretion of anterior pituitary hormones. If large enough, the tumor can displace pain-sensitive neurologic structures and cause headache; impingement on the optic chiasm may result in a visual field defect. Over time, most patients with microadenomas experience a decrease in prolactin production and a return of ovulation, even without treatment. Many patients with both micro- and macroadenomas are able to safely discontinue treatment with time. Among women who become pregnant, there is only a 1% chance that a microadenoma will undergo symptomatic enlargement, but there is a 10% to 35% risk of a macroadenoma enlarging; such women need close monitoring with visual field testing and consideration of surgical debulking before pregnancy.

Less common pituitary lesions include *sellar tumors, postpartum pituitary necrosis* (Sheehan's syndrome), *empty sella,* and *granulomatous disease* (e.g., sarcoidosis). These destructive lesions can impair functioning pituitary tissue. Growth hormone production is generally the first to suffer but does not cause symptoms. Subsequently, *reduced FSH and LH synthesis* may lead to amenorrhea, often the presenting complaint. Headache and visual field defects may follow later, along with manifestations of panhypopituitarism. In empty sella syndrome, there appears to be herniation of the arachnoid down into the sella, compressing its contents and producing a ballooning of the bony sella on x-ray. The typical patient is a woman, obese and multiparous, who complains of headache. In this syndrome, amenorrhea is caused by mild hyperprolactinemia resulting from loss of normal inhibition of prolactin secretion rather than true hypopituitarism.

Ovarian Dysfunction

Ovarian dysfunction leading to amenorrhea is characterized by marked *elevations in LH and FSH* and *low levels of estrogen and progesterone.* In all types of ovarian failure, estrogen deficiency is marked and osteoporosis may ensue.

Normal menopause results from depletion of ovarian follicles and typically occurs between 45 and 55 years of age. As estrogen production declines, gonadotropins increase, reaching extreme levels as the serum estradiol concentration drops to less than 5% of normal (about 5 pg/mL). Manifestations of the loss of normal cyclic hormone production include hot flashes, anovulatory bleeding, and missed periods, followed by total cessation of periods (see Chapter 118). *Premature ovarian failure* presents in a similar fashion, except that the patient is younger the age of 40 years. There are no associated endocrinopathies or systemic illnesses in the *idiopathic* form of premature ovarian failure, which is most common. About 4% of women presenting with premature ovarian failure will have an autoimmune oophoritis, often in combination with adrenal insufficiency and sometimes as a component of *autoimmune polyglandular syndrome.* This hereditary syndrome may present as adrenal insufficiency or ovarian, thyroid, and pancreatic endocrine dysfunction and can be accompanied by myasthenia gravis, vitiligo, or pernicious anemia. Women who experience apparent premature ovarian failure before the age of 30 years may have mosaic *Turner's syndrome* or a partial X chromosome deletion. A premutation in *the fragile X syndrome gene (FMR1)* is recognized as a relatively common finding among women with premature ovarian failure, although the mechanism is unknown; the prevalence of the premutation is as high as 14% in those women with a family history of premature ovarian failure and up to 3% in those with sporadic premature ovarian failure. Other rare genetic mutations causing early ovarian failure, such as ovarian resistance to FSH in which a somatic mutation inactivates the FSH receptor, are subjects of active investigation.

Cancer treatment may cause direct irreversible ovarian injury when *radiation therapy* is used (see Chapter 89) and potentially reversible suppression in the setting of *alkylating agent chemotherapy* (see Chapter 88). Extensive *endometriosis* may compromise ovarian function, as might mumps-related *oophoritis. Ovarian tumors* rarely destroy enough ovarian tissue to cause amenorrhea, but granulosa-cell tumors, which produce excess estrogen, and arrhenoblastomas, which synthesize excess androgen, may be responsible for amenorrhea.

Polycystic Ovary Syndrome

Polycystic ovary syndrome (PCOS), originally described as the Stein–Leventhal syndrome in 1935, is a well-recognized cause of amenorrhea, characterized clinically by *hirsutism, anovulation,* and *oligomenorrhea* or *amenorrhea.* It is present in approximately 5% to 7% of women of reproductive age and has significance beyond gynecologic repercussions. Many but not all patients are obese, sharing characteristics with metabolic syndrome, with potentially increased long-term cardiovascular risk. Similarly, many but not all patients have the bilaterally enlarged polycystic ovaries that give the syndrome its name (conversely, not all women with polycystic ovaries have the syndrome, although there is increasing evidence that women with polycystic ovarian morphology may have mild biochemical abnormalities along the PCOS spectrum). The pathophysiology of PCOS is an area of intense investigation, with abnormalities recognized at multiple levels in a complex interaction of gonadotropins, estrogens, androgens, and insulin.

Biochemical features include *androgen elevation, reduced sex hormone–binding globulins, elevated LH levels* (without a midcycle surge), *low-normal FSH levels,* and *hyperinsulinemia. Insulin resistance* is common and may play an important role in perpetuating the disease; hyperinsulinemia appears to trigger excessive ovarian production of testosterone and also inhibits hepatic synthesis of sex hormone–binding globulins. Treatment to correct hyperinsulinemia, either through insulin-sensitizing medications or with weight loss, causes many of the biochemical features of the disease to revert toward normal.

Diagnosis of PCOS had been primarily clinical, based on a 1990 National Institutes of Health consensus conference that established chronic anovulation and androgen excess (commonly manifested as hirsutism or acne) as the primary diagnostic criteria, but these were revised in a 2003 Rotterdam consensus conference to include polycystic ovaries on ultrasound. Two out of the three criteria (oligo- and/or anovulation, clinical and or biochemical signs of hyperandrogenism, and polycystic ovaries) must be present, and other causes of androgen excess, including hyperprolactinemia, late-onset congenital adrenal hyperplasia (CAH), and androgen-secreting tumor, need to be ruled out. An early-morning 17-hydroxyprogesterone drawn during the follicular phase that is less than 2 ng/mL excludes CAH.

Uterine Pathology

Endometrial scarring may occur as a consequence of radiation therapy, septic abortion, or overly vigorous curettage. Adhesions can obliterate the uterine cavity (Asherman's syndrome). Similarly, cervical trauma can result in scarring.

DIFFERENTIAL DIAGNOSIS (18)

Table 112.1 lists the causes of secondary amenorrhea, distinguishing among hypothalamic, pituitary, ovarian, and uterine

TABLE 112.1

IMPORTANT CAUSES OF AMENORRHEA

Hypothalamic Dysfunction
  Mild
    Situational stress
    Dieting, particularly dietary fat restriction
    Concurrent illness
    Increased exercise
    Drugs (phenothiazines, oral contraceptives)
    Idiopathic
  Marked
    Anorexia nervosa with severe weight loss
    Serious emotional stress or psychopathology
    Serious concurrent illness
    Competitive excessive exercise
    Excess androgen, prolactin, or cortisol
    Idiopathic

Pituitary Disease
  Prolactinoma
  Other pituitary neoplasm
  Empty sella syndrome
  Pituitary infarction (Sheehan's syndrome)
  Granulomatous disease (sarcoidosis)

Ovarian
  Menopause
  Polycystic ovary syndrome (may have hypothalamic
    etiology)
  Premature ovarian failure (idiopathic, autoimmune disease,
    radiation therapy, chemotherapy, endometriosis,
    oophoritis, FMR1 premutation)
  Follicle-stimulating hormone resistance or other genetic
    mutation

Uterine
  Obliteration of uterine cavity by intrauterine scarring and
    synechiae formation—Asherman's syndrome (overly
    vigorous curettage, septic abortion, radiation)
  Cervical scarring with resultant os closure

Endocrinopathies
  Thyroid disease
  Cushing's syndrome
  Hyperandrogenism

Pregnancy

etiologies. In one representative series of patients with secondary amenorrhea, hypothalamic dysfunction accounted for 30% of cases, polycystic ovary syndrome for 30%, pituitary disease (mostly prolactinomas) for 15%, ovarian failure for 12%, and uterine problems for about 5%.

WORKUP (19–24)

The first priority is to *rule out pregnancy*. History is reviewed for recent unprotected intercourse and symptoms of early pregnancy (e.g., morning sickness). Any possibility of pregnancy should lead directly to a *serum human chorionic gonadotropin* (hCG) *β-subunit* determination. The test is the most sensitive and specific test for pregnancy, capable of providing a definitive answer rapidly and at a much earlier stage of pregnancy than is possible with urine testing for human chorionic gonadotropin. However, the *urine human chorionic gonadotropin–precipitation slide test* is convenient because it can be performed at home on a first-morning voided urine. Given natural variation in timing of implantation, which may not occur by the time of the missed menses, and limitations of available home pregnancy test, sensitivity of a home test at the time of the missed menses (when most commercially available tests advertise 99% accuracy) may be quite low. Urine tests can achieve greater than 90% sensitivity about 6 weeks after the last menstrual period under ideal conditions, although actual sensitivity when performed by patients is closer to 75%. A negative urine test requires retesting in a week or proceeding directly to serum testing. Once the question of pregnancy is settled, evaluation for other etiologies can proceed in logical systematic fashion.

History and Physical Examination

History

History should begin with a detailed menstrual history and the circumstances of the amenorrhea. Age of menarche, character of normal cycles, timing of missed periods, and any prior pregnancies or abortions should be ascertained. A detailed psychosocial history may provide evidence for hypothalamic amenorrhea and should include inquiry into situational stresses (job, school, family, friends), emotional problems, excessive dieting, bulimia, marked weight loss, and heavy physical training. Nutritional imbalance including severe dietary fat restriction may be relevant. Oral contraceptive use and intake of other medications such as antipsychotics needs to be carefully reviewed. Family history of irregular cycles or of early menopause may suggest a familial tendency toward PCOS or premature ovarian failure.

Review of systems should include a check for hot flashes, skin changes of hypothyroidism (see Chapter 104), development or presence of hirsutism or acne, headache, visual disturbances, thyroid enlargement, breast changes or nipple discharge, increase or decrease in libido, and change in muscle mass or body habitus.

Several patterns are suggestive. Amenorrhea in the context of marked weight loss suggests anorexia nervosa (see Chapter 234). Symptoms of estrogen deficiency, including hot flashes and vaginal dryness, are more common in ovarian failure than in hypothalamic amenorrhea, despite similarly low levels of estrogen. If periods were irregular before the onset of full-fledged amenorrhea, then anovulatory bleeding was probably occurring, and one of its etiologies is likely (see Chapter 111). Amenorrhea accompanied by galactorrhea is strongly suggestive of hyperprolactinemia, which may be due to a prolactinoma, a destructive lesion of the sella, or hypothyroidism (see Chapter 100). A history of irregular periods since menarche in conjunction with hirsutism and/or obesity raises the probability of polycystic ovary syndrome. Rapid onset of amenorrhea, hirsutism, and frank virilization suggests an androgen-producing neoplasm, usually of adrenal or ovarian origin.

Physical Examination

Physical examination starts with the patient's general appearance, including low body weight, marked obesity, hirsutism, or virilization (see Chapter 98) and Cushing's syndrome. The integument is examined for signs of hypothyroidism (see Chapter 104) and adrenal disease. Vision is checked for visual field defects and the breasts for nipple discharge. On pelvic examination, note should be made of any clitoromegaly, atrophy of the vaginal mucosa, scarring of the cervical os, ovarian or adnexal masses, and uterine enlargement or masses.

Laboratory Studies

When history and physical examination are unremarkable and pregnancy has been ruled out, one needs to decide whether further evaluation is indicated. An otherwise healthy-appearing young woman undergoing situational stress can be followed

expectantly if only one or two periods have been missed and pregnancy has been ruled out. In patients with more prolonged amenorrhea (three or more cycles) or clinical evidence suggestive of more serious underlying pathology, an algorithmic approach is sometimes helpful but is best used in the context of clinical findings (Fig. 112.1). For example, a woman with amenorrhea and hot flashes should proceed directly to *FSH testing*. Some experts advocate for initial FSH testing in all women presenting with amenorrhea, given the potential for a falsely reassuring response to a progesterone challenge test

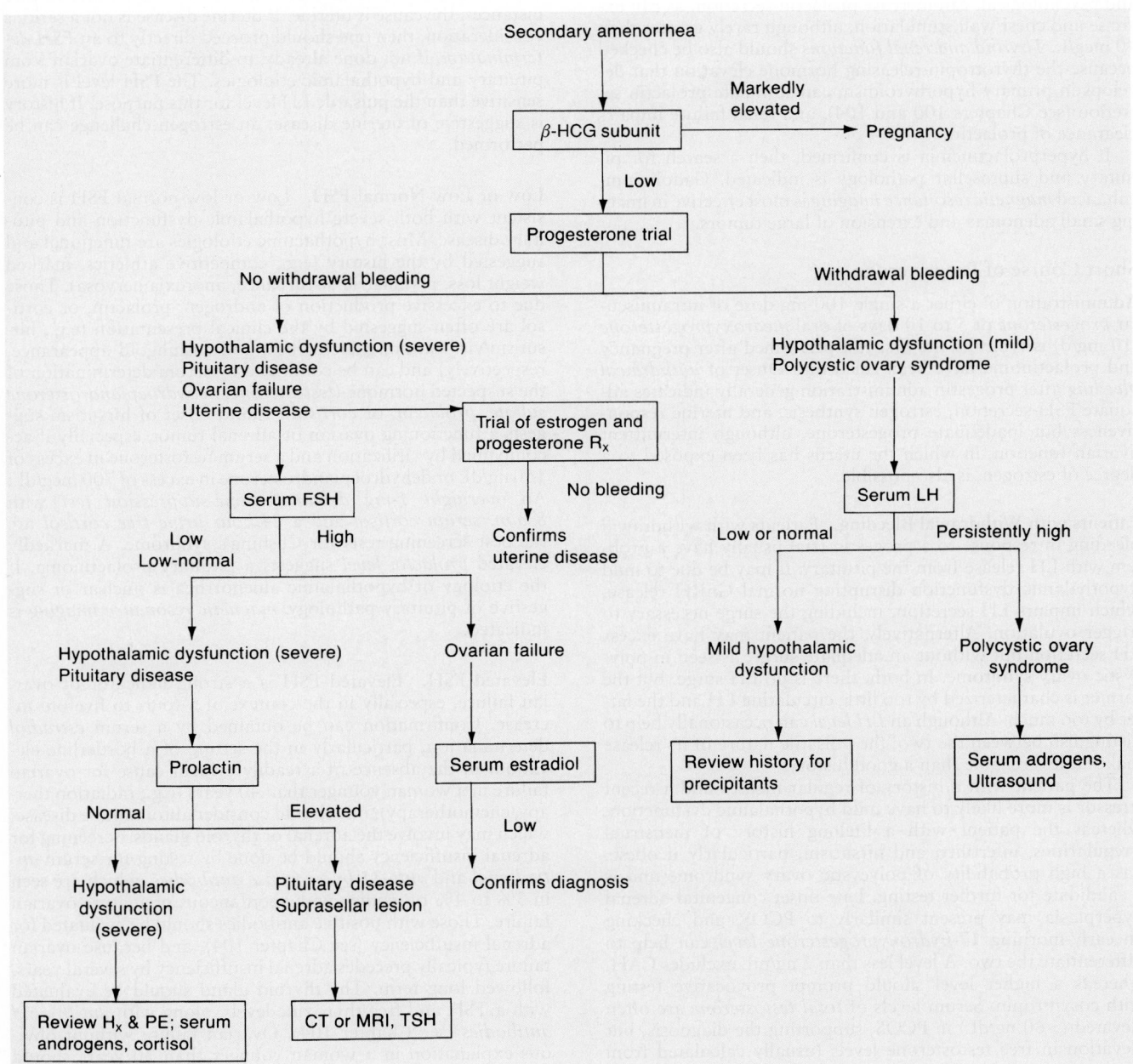

FIGURE 112.1. Initial testing of the patient with secondary amenorrhea. β-HCG, human chorionic gonadotropin, β subunit; CT, computed tomography; FSH, follicle-stimulating hormone; Hx, history; LH, luteinizing hormone; MRI, magnetic resonance imaging; PE, physical exam; r/o, rule out; Rx, prescription; TSH, thyroid-stimulating hormone.

(see later discussion) in the setting of intermittent ovarian function in women with premature ovarian failure, potentially delaying diagnosis.

There is consensus on evaluating all amenorrheic patients with a *prolactin level* because of the frequency with which hyperprolactinemia is responsible for amenorrhea, even in the absence of galactorrhea. To avoid making a false-positive diagnosis of a hyperprolactinemic condition, a borderline prolactin level (25 to 100 mcg/L) should be repeated with the patient off of all medications known to stimulate prolactin secretion, including estrogens, phenothiazines, selective serotonin reuptake inhibitors, verapamil, and reserpine. Stress, both physical and psychological, can increase prolactin secretion, as can exercise and chest wall stimulation, although rarely greater than 40 mcg/L. *Thyroid and renal functions* should also be checked because the thyrotropin-releasing hormone elevation that develops in primary hypothyroidism can stimulate prolactin secretion (see Chapters 100 and 104), and renal failure impairs clearance of prolactin.

If hyperprolactinemia is confirmed, then a search for pituitary and suprasellar pathology is indicated. Gadolinium-enhanced *magnetic resonance imaging* is most effective in imaging small adenomas and extension of large tumors.

Short Course of Progesterone

Administration of either a single 100-mg dose of intramuscular *progesterone* or 5 to 10 days of oral *medroxyprogesterone* (10 mg/d) is typically the first test performed after pregnancy and prolactinoma have been ruled out. Onset of *withdrawal bleeding* after progestin administration generally indicates adequate FSH secretion, estrogen synthesis, and uterine responsiveness but inadequate progesterone, although intermittent ovarian function, in which the uterus has been exposed to a degree of estrogen, is also possible.

Patients with Withdrawal Bleeding. Patients with withdrawal bleeding in response to a progestin trial usually have a problem with LH release from the pituitary. It may be due to mild hypothalamic dysfunction disrupting normal GnRH release, which impairs LH secretion, including the surge necessary to trigger ovulation. Alternatively, the patient may have excess LH secretion but without an adequate surge, as seen in polycystic ovary syndrome. In both, there is no LH surge, but the former is characterized by too little circulating LH and the latter by too much. Although an *LH level* can occasionally help to distinguish between the two, the pulsatile nature of its release makes it less reliable than a good history.

The patient with a history of regular menses and a recent stressor is more likely to have mild hypothalamic dysfunction, whereas the patient with a lifelong history of menstrual irregularities, infertility, and hirsutism, particularly if obese, has a high probability of polycystic ovary syndrome and is a candidate for further testing. Late-onset congenital adrenal hyperplasia may present similarly to PCOS, and checking an early-morning *17-hydroxyprogesterone level* can help to differentiate the two. A level less than 2 ng/mL excludes CAH, whereas a higher level should prompt provocative testing with cosyntropin. Serum levels of *total testosterone* are often elevated (>60 ng/dL) in PCOS, supporting the diagnosis, but elevation in free testosterone levels (usually calculated from total testosterone and sex hormone–binding globulin) are more sensitive, although not required. Similarly, an LH-to-FSH ratio greater than 2 supports the diagnosis but is insensitive as a screening test. *Ultrasonography* for detection of enlarged polycystic ovaries is now one of the Rotterdam criteria for

diagnosis of PCOS and may also be helpful in screening for endometrial hyperplasia caused by unopposed estrogen. As an aid to disease management, although not required for diagnosis, all women with PCOS should be checked for insulin resistance with a *fasting glucose* measurement or, in high-risk women such as those with obesity, metabolic syndrome, or a family history of diabetes, an oral glucose tolerance test.

Patients without Withdrawal Bleeding. Patients without withdrawal bleeding lack adequate estrogen to stimulate the endometrium and are likely to have more serious hypothalamic dysfunction, pituitary disease, or ovarian failure. In rare instances, the cause is uterine. If uterine disease is not a serious consideration, then one should proceed directly to an *FSH determination*, if not done already, to differentiate ovarian from pituitary and hypothalamic etiologies. The FSH level is more sensitive than the pulsatile LH level for this purpose. If history is suggestive of uterine disease, an estrogen challenge can be performed.

Low or Low-Normal FSH. Low or low-normal FSH is consistent with both severe hypothalamic dysfunction and pituitary disease. Most hypothalamic etiologies are functional and suggested by the history (e.g., competitive athletics, marked weight loss, psychiatric disturbance, anorexia nervosa). Those due to excessive production of androgen, prolactin, or cortisol are often suggested by the clinical presentation (e.g., hirsutism/virilization, galactorrhea, and cushingoid appearance, respectively) and can be confirmed by serum determination of the suspected hormone (*testosterone, dehydroepiandrosterone sulfate, prolactin,* or *cortisol*). Rapid onset of hirsutism suggests a functioning ovarian or adrenal tumor, especially if accompanied by virilization and a serum testosterone in excess of 150 ng/dL or dehydroepiandrosterone in excess of 700 mcg/dL. An *overnight 1-mg dexamethasone-suppression test* with *8 a.m. serum cortisol* and a *24-hour urine free cortisol* are the best screening tests for Cushing's syndrome. A markedly elevated *prolactin level* suggests a pituitary prolactinoma. If the etiology of hypothalamic amenorrhea is unclear or suggestive of pituitary pathology, *magnetic resonance imaging* is indicated.

Elevated FSH. Elevated FSH is a strong indicator of ovarian failure, especially in the context of a four- to fivefold increase. Confirmation can be obtained by a serum *estradiol* determination, particularly in the setting of a borderline elevation. In the absence of a readily evident cause for ovarian failure in a woman younger than 40 years (e.g., radiation therapy, chemotherapy), one should consider autoimmune disease, which may involve the adrenal or thyroid glands. Screening for adrenal insufficiency should be done by testing for serum *antiadrenal* and *anti–21-hydroxylase antibodies*, which are seen in 3% to 4% of women with spontaneous premature ovarian failure. Those with positive antibodies should be evaluated for adrenal insufficiency (see Chapter 104), and because ovarian failure typically precedes adrenal insufficiency by several years, followed long term. The thyroid gland should be evaluated with a TSH and free thyroxine levels, along with *antithyroid antibodies* (see Chapter 104). Ovarian failure without obvious explanation in a woman younger than 30 years should prompt *karyotype evaluation* for mosaic Turner's syndrome. As of 2006, the American College of Obstetrics and Gynecology recommends screening all women with ovarian failure before age 40 years for the presence of the fragile X syndrome premutation.

Normal FSH and Normal Estradiol. Patients with no withdrawal bleeding but normal FSH and normal estradiol are likely to have uterine pathology. History should be very suggestive (e.g., previous endometritis from abortion or delivery, vigorous curettage). Failure of a course of conjugated estrogens (1.25 mg/d for 21 days) followed by progestin (medroxyprogesterone 10 mg/d for 5 days) to induce withdrawal bleeding strongly supports the diagnosis of uterine disease and necessitates gynecologic referral for further evaluation.

SYMPTOMATIC THERAPY (25–29)

Mild Hypothalamic Dysfunction: Patients with Withdrawal Bleeding

Usually, patients with mild hypothalamic amenorrhea need only advice and reassurance (see later discussion). Their periods are likely to return quickly once the precipitant is withdrawn (whether situational stress, dieting, or exercise). There is no immediate medical need to reestablish menstrual cycles. If the condition becomes chronic, however, it is associated with prolonged unopposed estrogen stimulation of the endometrium, a risk factor for endometrial cancer. Such women should be given a periodic 5- to 10-day course of medroxyprogesterone (10 mg/d) to cause shedding of the proliferative endometrium and bring on withdrawal bleeding. Subsequently, oral contraceptives should be started if the patient desires contraception, or a withdrawal bleed should be induced every 2 to 3 months in the absence of spontaneous menses.

Severe Hypothalamic Dysfunction

When the cause is anorexia nervosa, menses will not resume until *weight* is *restored* to 90% or more of normal. Competitive athletes may have to cut down on their training program to achieve restoration of menses. They sometimes exhibit excessive weight loss and eating disorders, which contribute to the problem and require attention. Those with marked hypothalamic dysfunction due to chronic illness have to await the resolution of their underlying illness before normal menses resumes.

When severe hypothalamic amenorrhea results in inadequate secretion of both estrogen and progesterone *hormonal replacement therapy* should be considered to prevent osteoporosis, although resumption of normal menses clearly has the most beneficial effect on bone density. Inadequacy of the growth hormone access may also contribute to osteoporosis risk, particularly in anorexia nervosa. A typical replacement program includes *conjugated estrogens* (0.625 to 1.25 mg/d) on days 1 to 25 plus *medroxyprogesterone* (10 mg/d) starting on day 15 and continuing for 12 days. Alternatively, oral contraceptives may be used and are preferred by many younger women. Some authorities recommend withholding such therapy periodically (e.g., every 6 months) to see if menses have returned.

Pituitary Disease

Patients with *hyperprolactinemia* can often achieve restoration of normal GnRH release, ovulation, and menstruation with the use of the dopamine agonists *bromocriptine* and *cabergoline*, which block excessive prolactin secretion in up to 95% of cases (see Chapter 100). *Bromocriptine* should be used if fertility is desired because it has a proven safety record in pregnancy, but cabergoline is often better tolerated by patients. *Surgical resection* is reserved for patients with a pituitary tumor that imminently threatens adjacent structures (e.g., other areas of the pituitary or the optic chiasm) because even large macroadenomas often respond to medical therapy.

Patients with destructive pituitary lesions (Sheehan's syndrome, tumor, granulomatous disease) may require *replacement hormonal therapy*. The program should be tailored to the deficiencies detected. Estrogen and progesterone are usually necessary; thyroid hormone and adrenal steroids are less commonly required.

Ovarian Etiologies

Patients with premature ovarian failure should receive *estrogen/progesterone* replacement therapy until around age 50 years, when menopause would typically be expected. Transdermal or oral formulations may be used, titrated to relief of estrogen deficiency symptoms—this often requires higher doses than those used in older women (e.g., 100-mcg estrogen patch or 2 mg of oral micronized estradiol, accompanied by cyclic progesterone). If fertility is desired, the only proven successful therapy is *in vitro* fertilization with donor oocytes. Because some forms may be reversible (5% to 10% of women with premature ovarian failure may experience spontaneous ovulation and even pregnancy), a 1- to 2-month pause every year is recommended to see if there is a return of ovarian function.

Polycystic Ovary Syndrome

Not all women who suffer from infertility, hirsutism, or glucose intolerance require treatment, although evidence suggests that all women with PCOS and obesity benefit from exercise and weight loss to decrease cardiovascular risk. These lifestyle changes also have a role in restoring ovulation and fertility, although they are not always adequate. Ovulation induction with *clomiphene* and preparations of *GnRH, GnRH analogues*, and *gonadotropins* are used by fertility specialists with high rates of success. The insulin-sensitizing agent *metformin* has also been successful in stimulating ovulation in some but not all studies and may be useful in combination with clomiphene. Bilateral *wedge resection* of the ovaries, the traditional approach, is no longer in routine use. For women who do not desire fertility, *oral contraceptives*, especially those with newer progestins, including drospirinone, which has antiandrogenic properties, inhibit LH release and ovarian androgen overproduction, improve symptoms of androgen excess, regulate menses, and prevent endometrial hyperplasia. *Spironolactone* (50 to 200 mg/d) can be used in combination with oral contraceptives or as monotherapy for hirsutism, but it takes up to 6 months to show results. Glucose intolerance and hyperinsulinism are best treated by a program of weight loss and exercise, supplemented, if necessary, by oral hypoglycemics (see Chapter 102).

Uterine Disease

When the cause is granulomatous disease, treatment of the underlying disease offers the best hope for restoration of menses (see Chapters 49 and 51). Asherman's syndrome may respond to a combination of *recurettage* that severs bridging synechiae, which obliterate the uterine cavity, and *glucocorticosteroids*, which inhibit formation of new scar tissue.

PATIENT EDUCATION

Patient education occupies a central role in the management of amenorrhea. For the woman with mild hypothalamic dysfunction, addressing fears such as pregnancy, infertility, and premature menopause and reviewing how situational stresses can lead to the amenorrhea make up the principal means of treatment. Simple advice regarding degrees of exercise and dieting and how to cope with situational stresses ensures a good outcome. The competitive marathon runner with more severe hypothalamic dysfunction may care little about menses and fertility at that stage of her life but should be informed about the risk of osteoporosis and the need for hormonal replacement therapy.

Patients whose amenorrhea followed the use of oral contraceptives can be reassured that they have not been rendered infertile and that normal ovulatory periods resume in more than 99% of patients by 6 months. If conception is not desired, the need for mechanical contraception should be stressed because the incidence of spontaneous ovulation is high in this setting.

Women diagnosed with polycystic ovary syndrome need to be reassured about the options available for fertility, if that is a concern, and educated about the effect that lifestyle changes such as exercise and weight loss can have in managing their condition. Such changes may help with both the presenting complaint and long-term complications.

Women in their late 30s and early 40s who become amenorrheic fear premature menopause and its consequences. Usually, such concerns are best met by prompt assessment for ovarian failure (see prior discussion) and communication of results rather than by adopting a wait-and-see approach.

Patient education is no less important when the suspected etiology is more serious (e.g., pituitary tumor, polycystic ovary syndrome, anorexia nervosa). Sometimes, such patients may rationalize their amenorrhea, ascribing it to a benign etiology, and delay proper evaluation and treatment.

INDICATIONS FOR REFERRAL

A very significant proportion of the initial amenorrhea evaluation can be effectively carried out by the primary physician. However, referral for more intensive study and treatment is indicated when there is evidence of serious anatomic disruption (e.g., uterine synechiae), neoplasm (e.g., pituitary tumor), or marked hypothalamic dysfunction. A gynecologic or reproductive endocrine consultation can be very helpful, especially in the setting of severe functional disease, hyperprolactinemia, or premature ovarian failure. Such referral is of particular importance to the woman who desires to become pregnant, given the number of therapeutic options available. Rapid onset of hirsutism, especially if accompanied by virilization and elevations in serum androgens, suggests a functioning ovarian or adrenal tumor and necessitates prompt evaluation with endocrinologic consultation if indicated. Management of a large pituitary neoplasm that threatens adjacent structures requires the advice of a neuroendocrinologist and occasionally a neurosurgeon. Patients with idiopathic hyperprolactinemia or a microadenoma (especially those desiring to become pregnant) will appreciate a neuroendocrine consultation for confirmation of the diagnosis, counseling, and consideration of bromocriptine or cabergoline therapy.

Annotated Bibliography

1. Loucks AB, Mortola JF, Girton L, et al. Alterations in the hypothalamic–pituitary and the hypothalamic–pituitary–adrenal axes in athletic women. J Clin Endocrinol Metab 1989;68:402. (*Heavy exercise programs can disrupt these axes and lead to amenorrhea.*)
2. Fries H, Nillius SJ, Pettersson F, et al. Epidemiology of secondary amenorrhea. II. A retrospective evaluation of etiology with special regard to psychogenic factors and weight loss. Am J Obstet Gynecol 1974;118:473. (*Documents the relation of secondary amenorrhea to weight loss and stressful life events.*)
3. Perkins RB, Hall JE, Martin KA. Neuroendocrine abnormalities in hypothalamic amenorrhea: spectrum, stability, and response to neurotransmitter modulation. J Clin Endocrinol Metab 1999; 84:1995. (*Reviews the abnormal pattern of gonadotropin-releasing hormone and luteinizing hormone [LH] secretion in this disorder.*)
4. Biller BMK, Klibanski A. Amenorrhea and osteoporosis. Endocrinologist 1991;1:294. (*Estrogen production is reduced and bony changes may ensue in women with severe hypothalamic amenorrhea.*)
5. Welt CK, Chan JL, Bullen J, et al. Recombinant human leptin in women with hypothalamic amenorrhea. N Engl J Med 2004;351:987. (*Leptin administration in women with functional hypothalamic amenorrhea resulted in increased LH secretion and pulsatility, with resumption of menses in some cases.*)
6. Schlechte JA. Prolactinoma. N Engl J Med 2003;349:2035. (*Useful practical review of the management of this common problem.*)
7. Melmed S, Braunstein GD, Chang RJ, et al. Pituitary tumors secreting growth hormone and prolactin. Ann Intern Med 1986;105:238. (*Comprehensive discussion of pathophysiology, diagnosis, and treatment; 167 references.*)
8. Koppelman MC, Jaffe MJ, Rieth KG, et al. Hyperprolactinemia, amenorrhea and galactorrhea. Ann Intern Med 1984;100:115. (*Important data on the natural history of hyperprolactinemic conditions.*)
9. Falsetti L, Scalchi S, Villani MT, et al. Premature ovarian failure. Gynecol Endocrinol 1999;13:189. (*Of 40 women who were studied extensively, 18 had immunologic failure and 21 were idiopathic.*)
10. Nelson LM, Covington SN, Rebar RW. An update: spontaneous premature ovarian failure is not an early menopause. Fertil Steril 2005;83:1327.

(*Helpful review of the topic, including evaluation of potential etiologies and comorbidities, along with treatment and evidence for assisted reproductive technologies.*)
11. ACOG committee opinion. No. 338: Screening for fragile X syndrome. Obstet Gynecol 2006;107:1483. (*American College of Obstetrics and Gynecology statement on the value of screening for fragile X syndrome in all women with premature ovarian failure.*)
12. Kinigham RB, Apgar BS, Schwenk TL. Evaluation of amenorrhea. Am Family Physician 1996;53:1185. (*General review.*)
13. Guzick DS. Polycystic ovary syndrome. Obstet Gynecol 2004;103:181. (*Excellent review of complex pathophysiology.*)
14. Marx TL, Mehta AE. Polycystic ovary syndrome: pathogenesis and treatment over the long and short term. Cleve Clin J Med 2003;70:31. (*A useful review of management strategies.*)
15. Ehrmann DA. Polycystic ovary syndrome. N Engl J Med 2005;352:1223. (*A helpful overview of current knowledge of polycystic ovary syndrome [PCOS], including diagnosis, pathophysiology, etiology, and treatments; 144 references.*)
16. Revised 2003 consensus on diagnostic criteria and long-term health risks related to polycystic ovary syndrome (PCOS). Hum Reprod 2004;19:41. (*Updates the 1990 National Institutes of Health consensus on diagnostic criteria for PCOS, defining the syndrome as two of the following three cardinal features: ovarian dysfunction, hyperandrogenism, and polycystic ovary morphology.*)
17. Adams JM, Taylor AE, Crowley WF et al. Polycystic ovarian morphology with regular ovulatory cycles: insights into the pathophysiology of polycystic ovarian syndrome. J Clin Endocrinol Metab 2004;89:4343. (*Finds that women with polycystic ovarian morphology on ultrasound but regular cycles had normal gonadotropin dynamics but higher androgen and insulin levels and lower sex hormone–binding globulin levels, suggesting a mild degree of hyperandrogenism.*)
18. Reindollar RH, Novak M, Tho SPT, et al. Adult onset of amenorrhea. Am J Obstet Gynecol 1986;155:531. (*A series of 262 patients; provides a useful breakdown of etiologies.*)
19. Bastian LA, Nanda K, Hasselblad V, et al. Diagnostic efficiency of home pregnancy test kits. A meta-analysis. Arch Family Med 1998;7:465.

(The discriminating ability is greatly affected by the user; sensitivity falls from 0.91 to 0.75 when the test is performed by actual patients.)

20. Cole LA, Khanlian SA, Sutton JM, et al. Accuracy of home pregnancy tests at the time of missed menses. Am J Obstet Gynecol 2004;190:100. (*Found much lower sensitivities than claimed for 18 home pregnancy tests evaluated at different concentrations of human chorionic gonadotropin [hCG]; only 1 had adequate sensitivity to detect 95% of pregnancies at the time of missed menses.*)

21. Wilcox AJ, Baird DD, Dunson D, et al. Natural limits of pregnancy testing in relation to the expected menstrual period. JAMA 2001;286:1759. (*Based on variation in times of implantation, 10% of pregnancies are undetectable even by extremely sensitive hCG assays on the day of missed menses, and 3% may be undetectable 1 week after the missed menses.*)

22. McIver B, Romanski SA, Nippoldt TB. Evaluation and management of amenorrhea. Mayo Clin Proc 1997;72:1161. (*General review.*)

23. Laufer MR, Floor AE, Parsons KE, et al. Hormone testing in women with adult onset amenorrhea. Gynecol Obstet Invest 1995;40:200. (*In this series, 10% had abnormal follicle-stimulating hormone levels, 7.5% had abnormal prolactin levels, and 4.2% had abnormal thyrotropin-stimulating hormone levels.*)

24. Kleinberg DL, Davis JM, de Coster R, et al. Prolactin levels and adverse events in patients treated with risperidone. J Clin Psychopharmacol 1999;19:57. (*Both haloperidol and risperidone produce dose-related increases in plasma prolactin level among men and women.*)

25. Warren MP, Miller KK, Olson WH, et al. Effects of an oral contraceptive (norgestimate/ethinyl estradiol) on bone mineral density in women with hypothalamic amenorrhea and osteopenia: and open-label extension of a double-blind, placebo-controlled study. Contraception 2005;72:206. (*Extension of a randomized trial of oral contraceptives in hypothalamic amenorrhea, showing decreased markers of bone turnover on the oral contraceptives but significantly greater improvement in bone density with return of normal menses.*)

26. Grinspoon SK, Thomas L, Miller KK, et al. Effects of recombinant human IGF-1 and oral contraceptive administration on bone density in anorexia nervosa. J Clin Endocrinol Metab 2002;87:2883. (*A randomized trial in women with anorexia nervosa, showing an improvement in bone density with the combination of oral contraceptives and insulin-like growth factor-1 that was not seen with oral contraceptive use alone.*)

27. Colao A, Di Sarno A, Cappabianca P, et al. Withdrawal of long-term cabergoline therapy for tumoral and nontumoral hyperprolactinemia. N Engl J Med 2003;349:2023. (*About 30% of patients whose prolactin levels normalized with cabergoline treatment had recurrent prolactinemia within 2 to 5 years after withdrawal of therapy; recurrence was more likely if remnant tumor was present on magnetic resonance imaging, and prolactin levels were always lower than pretreatment values, suggesting that withdrawal of therapy is often safe.*)

28. Nestler JE, Jakubowicz DA. Decreases in ovarian cytochrome P450c17alpha activity and serum free testosterone after reduction of insulin secretion in polycystic ovary syndrome. N Engl J Med 1996;335:617. (*By correcting hyperinsulinemia, metformin reduced ovarian cytochrome testosterone synthesis and many of the other biochemical abnormalities of polycystic disease.*)

29. Legro RS, Barnhart HX, Schlaff WD, et al. Clomiphene, metformin, or both for infertility in the polycystic ovary syndrome. N Engl J Med 2007; 356:551. (*In this trial of 626 infertile women with PCOS, clomiphene was superior to metformin in achieving live births and equivalent to combination therapy; the conception rate among women who ovulated was lower in the metformin group than the other groups.*)

CHAPTER 113 ■ EVALUATION OF BREAST MASSES AND NIPPLE DISCHARGES

A solitary or dominant breast mass or an abnormal nipple discharge may be a harbinger of breast cancer, the most common malignancy among women. Because such a finding, whether discovered by the patient or by her physician, will raise legitimate fears, the primary physician must be able to proceed with deliberate speed in reaching a diagnosis that excludes carcinoma. Women who present with breast pain also often harbor concerns about breast cancer. In most cases assurance can be provided along with symptomatic management when necessary.

PATHOPHYSIOLOGY AND CLINICAL PRESENTATION (1–5)

Breast Mass (1–3)

Pathophysiology

A breast mass may represent proliferative changes in epithelial or mesenchymal tissue or fluid-filled cysts. The breast is a complex organ composed of epithelium, which forms acini and ducts; fibrous tissue, which provides support; and fat. It is exquisitely sensitive to its hormonal milieu. Estradiol stimulates the proliferation of epithelial cells and accompanying increases in periductal vascularity. Progesterone induces the development of acini and opposes the mesenchymal actions of estrogens.

With each menstrual cycle, the breast exhibits its own cycle of proliferation and desquamation of duct lining. However, the response of epithelium, fibrous tissue, and fat to the same hormonal stimulation is variable. Certain areas of the breast may overshoot in the monthly preparation for pregnancy, causing thickening of the breasts and lumpiness. The overgrowth may involve proliferation of fibrous tissue alone or also involve epithelial cells of the ducts and glands, leading to *fibroadenomas* or *ductal dysplasia*. Lumps can also be caused by the collection of fluids—essentially colostrum or dissolved cellular debris—which form microcysts or macrocysts. Simple cysts explain 20% to 25% of palpable masses. They are especially common in premenopausal women of age 40 to 49 years.

These physiologic events may combine to produce a breast that is *fibrocystic* in quality (hence the advice by experts to drop the term *fibrocystic disease*). Fibrocystic changes can be found clinically in approximately 50% of women during their reproductive years and histologically in 90%. Most investigators believe that benign breast disease, including neoplasms such as fibroadenomas and intraductal papillomas and fibrocystic change, represents a spectrum of responses to normal hormonal stimulation rather than distinct diseases.

Although the variable response of breast tissue to physiologic proliferative and involutional hormonal stimuli is responsible for most benign masses, there are other causes. *Infection*, usually associated with duct obstruction, can result in an inflammatory mass. Redness, warmth, and tenderness are prominent features. *Mammary duct ectasia* can result in infection and yet may simulate cancer because it can produce nipple discharge, nipple inversion, and a mass. Periareolar infection may ensue. Blunt trauma can lead to hematoma formation.

The multiple causes of benign breast lesions can be classified according to their histology and whether they confer a risk of breast cancer being diagnosed at some time in the future (Table 113.1).

The proportion of solitary or dominant breast masses that prove to be cancers varies from 5% to 20%, depending on the age of patients and at what point in the clinical process the case series is assembled. Masses noted by either patients or primary care clinicians are often not confirmed on surgical examination. The proportion of confirmed masses that prove to be cancer is higher than the proportion of all masses brought to their attention. The effect of age on the prevalence of breast cancer among women presenting with a lump is striking. Prevalence increases from 1% for women 40 years old or younger to 9% for women of age 41 to 54 years and to 37% for women of age 55 years and older.

Breast cancers derive from ductal or epithelium cells. They may invade immediately or grow *in situ*. Breast cancer in younger women tends to be *lobular* in pathologic appearance and multicentric but not calcifying or rapidly invading. *Ductal* carcinomas are prominent in older women. They are typically unicentric, readily calcified (producing the characteristic microcalcifications helpful in radiologic detection), and much more rapidly invasive than lobular lesions.

Growth is often associated with increasingly malignant behavior, characterized by the loss of estrogen and progesterone receptors, metastasis, and more aggressive local invasion. Although metastasis can occur early, it is not an invariably early event and usually does not occur in lesions less than 1 cm in diameter (unless lymphatics have been invaded). Local growth may extend to the skin or chest wall. Axillary nodes are typically the first clinical site of spread beyond the breast.

Clinical Presentation

Cancer in the breast typically presents as a painless, discrete mass. Pain is a presenting symptom in fewer than 7% of cases and is almost always accompanied by a mass. Early on, the mass may be movable; later, it can become fixed. Nipple retraction or inversion of new onset may also herald an underlying cancer. Signs of more advanced disease include skin retraction, change in breast contour, thickening or dimpling of the skin, and fixation of the mass to the chest wall. A ductal carcinoma may present as an isolated serosanguinous nipple discharge (see later discussion).

Benign lesions may be present in a manner clinically indistinguishable from that of cancers, but a few patterns are characteristic. In *fibrocystic change*, the breasts are diffusely lumpy and fibrous in quality. One breast may be more involved than the other. An isolated cyst may also be a presentation of benign disease, but those that yield blood on aspiration or recur after aspiration may be related to a malignant process.

Breast Pain (1,4)

Cyclic breast pain, occurring in the late luteal phase of the menstrual cycle, is a common problem. In one survey among American women, 58% described mild cyclic pain and 11% described moderate or severe pain. Pain was reported to interfere with normal sexual activity in nearly one half of those who experienced it and with physical activity in more than one third. Noncyclic pain, unrelated to the menstrual cycle, may be due to a cyst or mastitis. Pain arising in the chest wall can be mistaken for breast pain.

TABLE 113.1

CLASSIFICATION OF BENIGN BREAST LESIONS ON HISTOLOGIC EXAMINATION, ACCORDING TO THE RELATIVE RISK OF BREAST CANCER

Risk	Proliferation	Histologic Findings
No increase	Minimal	Fibrocystic changes (within the normal range): cysts and ductal ectasia (72%), mild hyperplasia (40%), nonsclerosing adenosis (22%), and periductal fibrosis (16%)[a]; simple fibroadenoma (15%–23%)[b]; and miscellaneous (lobular hyperplasia, juvenile hypertrophy, and stromal hyperplasia) Bengin tumors: hamartoma, lipoma, phyllodes tumor,[c] solitary papilloma, neurofibroma, giant adenoma, and adenomyoepithelioma Traumatic lesions: hematoma, fat necrosis, and lesions caused by penetration by a foreign body Infections: granuloma and mastitis Sarcoidosis Metaplasia: squamous and apocrine Diabetic mastopathy
Small increase (relative risk, 1.5–2.0)	Proliferative without atypia	Usual ductal hyperplasia, complex fibroadenoma (containing cysts >3 mm in diameter, sclerosing adenosis, epithelial calcification, or papillary apocrine changes), papilloma or papillomatosis, radial scar, and blunt duct adenosis
Moderate increase (relative risk, >2.0)	Proliferative with atypia	Atypial ductal hyperplasis and atypical lobular hyperplasia

[a]Percentage indicate the percentage of breasts examined at autopsy in which the lesion was found. Data are from Sandison AT. An autopsy study of the adult human breast; with special reference to proliferative epithelial changes of importance in the pathology of the breast. National Cancer Inst Monogr 1962;4:1.
[b]Date are from Goehring C, Morabia A. Epidemiology of benign breast disease, with special attention to histologic types. Epidemiol Rev 1997;19:310.
[c]Most phyllodes tumors are considered to be benign fibroepithelial tumors, bot some have malignant clinical and histologic features.
From Santen RJ, Mansel R. Benign breast disorders. N. Engl J Med 2005;353:275, with permission.

Nipple Discharge (1,5)

A nipple discharge that is unilateral, spontaneous, and localized to one duct should be considered pathologic. Nonlactescent unilateral breast discharges may reflect local inflammatory or neoplastic lesions, most of which are benign. Benign etiologies include chronic cystic mastopathy and intraductal papilloma. Many papillomas are not palpable. Approximately 5% of women with a breast discharge have cancer. The most worrisome nipple discharge is a bloody one, which occurs in 70% to 85% of cancers that present with a nipple discharge. However, only 25% of bloody discharges prove to be due to cancer. The discharge may predate the onset of a clinically detectable mass. The chance of a nipple discharge being associated with cancer increases with age. The onset of a lactescent nipple discharge (galactorrhea) in a woman who is not nursing may be a sign of a prolactinoma (see Chapter 100).

DIFFERENTIAL DIAGNOSIS (1–5)

The differential diagnosis of a breast mass is confusing because of lack of agreement or standardization in clinical and pathologic terminology. The category of "fibrocystic disease" has been dropped because it does not represent a pathologic state. Among lesions that come to biopsy, the most common discretely palpable solid mass is the fibroadenoma. As many as 20% of solitary or dominant breast masses are cancers.

A serous or bloody discharge may occur with intraductal papillomas, ductal ectasia, and ductal carcinoma. In one reported series, 44% of cases had papilloma or papillomatosis, 23% had ductal ectasia, 16% had fibrocystic changes, and only 11% had cancer.

WORKUP (1,2,6–17)

Breast Mass (1,2,6–11)

History

The clinical history should begin with how long ago the mass was noted and whether any change has been noted. The patient should be asked about previous diagnoses of atypical hyperplasia, lobular carcinoma *in situ*, ductal carcinoma *in situ*, or invasive cancer.

Physical Examination

The key finding is a *dominant nodule* defined as discrete and distinctly different from surrounding breast tissue or the same area on the opposite breast. Most glandular tissue is found in the upper outer quadrant of the breast and changes with the menstrual cycle. Dominant masses are characterized by their unchanging and persistent nature throughout the cycle. Breast tenderness to examination in the absence of a dominant mass is of no pathologic significance.

Much is made of the clinical characteristics of breast masses in estimating the probability of malignant disease. Easy mobility within the breast, regular borders, and a soft or cystic feel on palpation all suggest a benign process. However, these signs are not reliable; 60% of cancers are freely movable, 40% have regular borders, and 40% feel soft or cystic. A "benign" physical finding reduces the probability of cancer no further than to approximately 10%.

The young woman with multiple nodules and diffuse thickening consistent with fibrocystic change has difficult breasts to evaluate. Reexamination at different times in the menstrual cycle is often informative and reassuring when no dominant nodule emerges. A persistent solitary or dominant nodule requires biopsy.

Examination of the lymph nodes is required in all patients with a breast lump because it may provide important supporting evidence for a malignancy, especially if otherwise unexplained adenopathy is found in the ipsilateral axilla.

Mammography

In diagnostic breast centers, mammography is often performed after ultrasonography or fine-needle aspiration biopsy (FNAB). Both options have high specificity for the diagnosis of a simple cyst, thereby obviating the need for diagnostic mammography. When FNAB or ultrasound is not readily available or when they disclose a solid mass, complex cysts, or bloody cystic fluid, mammography can be a valuable diagnostic test. It must be emphasized, however, that a negative mammogram does not obviate the need for biopsy of a clinically suspicious breast mass. Studies in which the most advanced techniques were used by the most experienced clinicians repeatedly indicated that mammography has a false-negative rate of 10% to 15%.

Ultrasonography

Ultrasonography can be used to differentiate a cystic from a solid palpable mass, especially in women younger than 30 years. Ultrasonography is nearly 100% specific in the diagnosis of simple cysts when rigorous sonographic criteria are used. Therefore, when a definitive diagnosis of cyst can be made, FNAB is not necessary. Ultrasound guidance can also improve the likelihood of obtaining an adequate FNAB sample when a lump is small or far below the surface of the breast. Ultrasonography is not effective at distinguishing between benign and malignant solid lesions.

Fine-Needle Aspiration Biopsy

FNAB uses a small-gauge needle (21 to 25 gauge) to make multiple passes of solid and cystic lesions, with cytologic examination of the material obtained. It can be performed in the office or in the radiologic suite under the guidance of imaging techniques. Adequate specimens are obtained in about 60% to 85% of instances. Among adequate samples, sensitivity ranges from 65% to 98%. Sensitivity is lower in younger women, when tumors are small, and when the personnel performing the procedure are relatively untrained. Sensitivity is in the range of 92% to 98% when personnel are very experienced. Specimens characterized as malignant have a specificity exceeding 99%.

Core-Needle Biopsy

Core-needle biopsy uses a larger-diameter needle (14 to 18 gauge) to obtain tissue for histologic diagnosis. Comparison studies suggest that core-needle biopsy and FNAB have similar sensitivity and specificity. However, core-needle biopsy can more often distinguish between benign proliferative lesions with and without atypia and ductal carcinoma from invasive cancer than can FNAB.

Diagnostic Strategies

The evaluation of a dominant breast mass can most efficiently begin with either FNAB or ultrasonography. If ultrasonography shows a simple cyst, no further workup is warranted. A complex cyst of solid lump should be followed by FNAB, core-needle biopsy, or excisional biopsy. If the evaluation begins with FNAB and there is a residual lump after aspiration, repeat aspiration or excisional biopsy is indicated. If there is no residual lump after the withdrawal of clear to green fluid, there is no need for cytologic examination of the fluid. Clinical breast examination should be performed in 4 to 6 weeks. If FNAB of a solid lump is nondiagnostic, it should be followed by a repeat aspiration, a core-needle biopsy, or an excisional biopsy. FNAB read as benign combined with a negative mammogram need be followed only with a clinical breast exam in 3 to 6 months. If the mammogram is positive, additional imaging, core-needle biopsy, or excisional biopsy is indicated despite a "benign" FNAB. When atypical or suspicious cells are reported on FNAB, core-needle biopsy or excisional biopsy is indicated. FNAB read as malignant warrants referral for definitive treatment.

Nipple Discharge (1,2,12–17)

Evaluation of nipple discharge can follow a logical sequence (Fig. 113.1). The patient should undergo a careful *breast examination* that includes careful palpation, looking for a mass in the affected breast, as well as noting whether the discharge is unilateral or bilateral, spontaneous or expressible,

and localized to one or many ducts. If a mass is noted on palpation or present on an imaging study, workup should proceed as described earlier. If there is no mass and bilateral discharge is consistent with galactorrhea, thyrotropin and prolactin levels should be drawn. A unilateral discharge from multiple ducts can be followed. If the discharge is unilateral and expressed only from a single duct, one should note the quadrant of the breast from which it seems to be coming. Guaiac testing helps to detect occult blood. Cytologic examination is of limited value, with a sensitivity of less than 50%. Patients with nipple discharge that remains unexplained (especially if bloody) require referral to a surgeon experienced in evaluating breast disease, including the role of ductography and advanced imaging in the diagnosis of nipple discharge. The risk of cancer in such patients is real, and *ductal exploration* may be the only means of detecting an early ductal malignancy.

SYMPTOMATIC MANAGEMENT AND PATIENT EDUCATION (1,18)

The woman with painful breasts associated with fibrocystic change can be reassured that the discomfort is not a sign of cancer and that symptoms usually improve with the cyclical

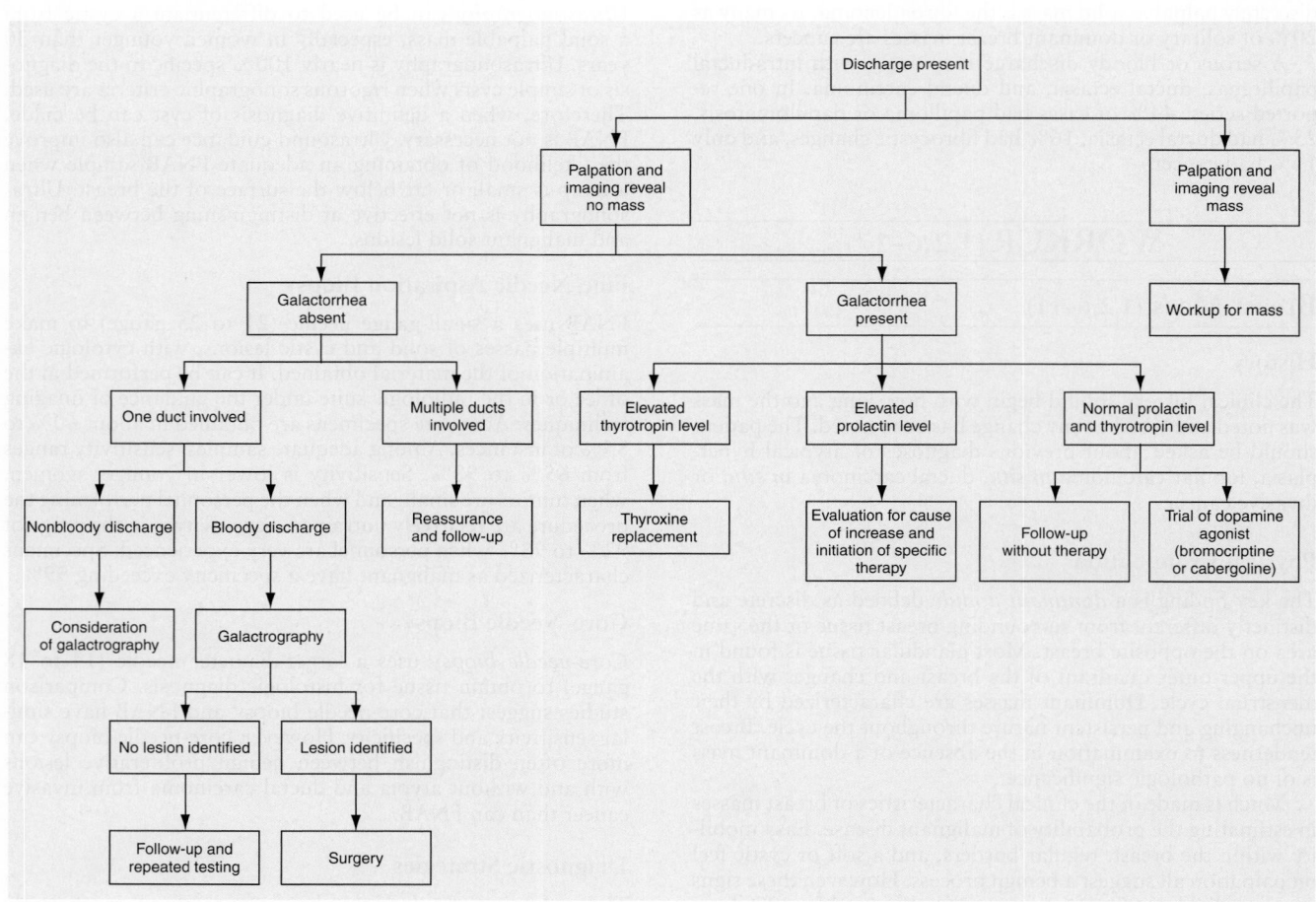

FIGURE 113.1. A logical approach to nipple discharge. In the presence of the involvement of multiple ducts, if there is a spontaneous and persistent discharge of gross blood from a single duct, galactography should be considered. (Adapted from Santen RJ, Mansel R. Benign breast disorders. N Engl J Med 2005;353:275, with permission.)

decrease in hormonal stimulation. Moreover, it is important to emphasize that the finding is not a risk factor for breast cancer. The physiologic nature of fibrocystic changes, their extremely high prevalence, and their favorable natural history can be reviewed. In one study, 85% of women with cyclic breast pain who were referred to a specialty clinic were satisfied with watchful waiting once reassurance and explanation were provided. Oral contraceptives have not been systematically studied, and it is not clear that they provide relief, but pills that contain low-dose estrogen and 19-nor progestins may be worth a trial. Commonly recommended measures include the use of a support bra or either acetaminophen, nonsteroidal antiinflammatory drugs, or aspirin. Evening primrose oil is also advised based on two randomized trials. Efficacy is variable. Gonadotropin-releasing hormone agonists have been used for severe pain.

The woman with a dominant breast mass or a bloody discharge is more concerned with the possibility of breast cancer than with symptoms. Explaining that the likelihood of a benign etiology is still greater than that of cancer can provide a modicum of reassurance and perspective while more definitive diagnostic measures are undertaken. A prompt efficient diagnostic evaluation is the best medicine.

A.G.M.

Annotated Bibliography

1. Santen RJ, Mansel R. Benign breast disorders. N Engl J Med 2005;353:275. (*A superb authoritative review of benign breast disease, including its relationship to cancer, as well as sound recommendations for diagnosis and treatment.*)
2. Britton P, Sinnatamby R. Investigation of suspected breast cancer. BMJ 2007;335:347. (*A succinct review of the role of imaging studies in the "triple assessment" of suspected breast cancer.*)
3. Ernster VL. The epidemiology of benign breast disease. Epidemiol Rev 1981;3:184. (*A thoughtful review, emphasizing the problem of case definition and reviewing the evidence for its precipitants.*)
4. Ader DN, South-Paul J, Adera T, et al. Cyclical mastalgia: prevalence and associated health and behavioral factors. J Psychosm Obstet Gynecol 2001;22:71. (*Among American women, 58% have mild cyclic pain;11% report moderate to severe pain.*)
5. Atkins H, Wolff B. Discharges from the nipple. Br J Surg 1964;51:602. (*A review of 203 cases from the Breast Clinic at Guy's Hospital, London.*)
6. Barton MB, Harris R, Fletcher SW. The rational clinical examination. Does this patient have breast cancer? The screening clinical breast examination: should it be done? How? JAMA 1999;282:1270. (*An excellent review.*)
7. Beitler AL, Hurd TC, Edge SB, et al. The evaluation of palpable breast masses: common pitfalls and management guidelines. Surg Oncol 1997;6:227. (*A surgical perspective on errors of omission and commission in the early evaluation of breast masses.*)
8. Kerlikowske K, Smith-Bindman R, Ljung B, et al. Evaluation of abnormal mammography results and palpable breast abnormalities. Ann Intern Med 2003;139:274. (*An excellent evidence-based quantitative review, including well-reasoned and clearly presented diagnostic strategies; 94 references.*)
9. Morrow M, Wong S, Venta L. The evaluation of breast masses in women younger than forty years of age. Surgery 1998;124:634. (*Masses were confirmed by surgeon examination in about 30% of women referred because of a mass detected by themselves or their physicians; carcinoma was present in 5% of each group.*)
10. Flobbe K, Bosch AM, Kessels AG, et al. The additional diagnostic value of ultrasonography in the diagnosis of breast cancer. Arc Intern Med 2003;163:1194. (*Important contributions defined.*)
11. Preece P, Baum M, Mansel R. The importance of mastalgia in operable breast cancer. Br Med J 1982;284:1299. (*Pain was the presentation in only 7% of cancers and in the absence of a mass not associated with cancer.*)
12. Cabioglu N, Hunt KK, Singletary SE, et al. Surgical decision making and factors determining a diagnosis of breast carcinoma in women presenting with nipple discharge. J Am Coll Surg 2003;196:354. (*Reviews a large series of patients with nipple discharge, including the role of ductography in diagnosis.*)
13. Gulay H, Bora S, Kilicturgay S, et al. Management of nipple discharge. J Am Coll Surg 1994;178:41. (*An extensive case series, with 448 cases of nipple discharge, of which 140 proceeded to biopsy; nearly 48% of these patients had intraductal papillomas and 14% had cancers.*)
14. Murad TM, Contesso G, Mouriesse H. Nipple discharge from the breast. Ann Surg 1982;195:259. (*Provides data on etiologies, prevalences, and presentations.*)
15. Okazaki A, Hirata K, Okazaki M, et al. Nipple discharge disorders: current diagnostic management and the role of fiber-ductoscopy. Eur Radiol 1999;9:583. (*Describes both low-tech and high-tech diagnostic approaches.*)
16. Pritt B, Pang Y, Kellogg M, et al. Diagnostic value of nipple cytology: study of 466 cases. Cancer 2004;102:233. (*The sensitivity was 85% and the specificity was 97% in this small series.*)
17. Rongione AJ, Evans BD, King KM, et al. Ductography is a useful technique in evaluation of abnormal nipple discharge. Am Surg 1996;10:785. (*Ductal abnormalities were identified in 73% of cases, most of which were explained by benign findings rather than cancer.*)
18. Mansel RE, Goyal A, Preece P, et al. European randomized multicenter trial of goserelin in the management of mastalgia. Am J Obstet Gynecol 2004;191:1942. (*The treatment was effective but was only warranted for severe pain.*)

CHAPTER 114 ■ EVALUATION OF VULVAR PRURITUS

SHANA L. BIRNBAUM

Vulvar itching can be a very annoying symptom for the patient. In the genital area, only the vulvar and perineal skin have sensory receptors that trigger the sensation of itching. However, vulvar pruritus may be secondary to a vaginal infection or due to a vulvar dermatitis or primary skin disease. In older women, it is often related to declining estrogen levels and, in rare cases, may be a manifestation of a malignancy. Estimations of the true prevalence of vulvar pruritis within the general population are difficult, and the prevalences of most of the conditions responsible for the symptom are unknown. The primary care physician should be familiar with the appearance of inflammatory, infectious, and malignant conditions of the vulva to tailor appropriate therapy and avoid delays in the detection of carcinoma.

PATHOPHYSIOLOGY AND CLINICAL PRESENTATIONS (1–7)

The most common causes of vulvar pruritus are listed in Table 114.1. Patients with vaginitis often complain of itching. In *candidal vulvovaginitis,* which the majority of women experience at some point in their life, the vulva is erythematous, often with a sharp, scalloped border demarcating the area of involvement. "Satellite" lesions are characteristic, as is the cheesy discharge of the associated vaginitis (see Chapter 117). Primary cutaneous candidiasis of the vulva can also occur without vaginitis or discharge. It is more commonly seen in women with diabetes or those who are pregnant or obese. Intense vulvar inflammation also occurs with *trichomonal infection,* and, rarely, bacterial vaginosis may present with itching. *Hidradenitis suppurativa,* which is caused by inflammation or infection of the apocrine sweat glands found in the labia majora, can cause itching or burning and progress to abscess or fistula formation.

Lesions of *herpes genitalis* are caused in most cases by herpes simplex virus type 2. The lesions, which begin as vesicles and progress to ulcers, cause burning, itching, and usually pain and tenderness of the vulva. Primary infection tends to be associated with fever, inguinal lymphadenopathy, and malaise. Vulvar lesions caused by *human papillomavirus* (HPV), also called *condyloma acuminata,* are generally multifocal and appear on the labia minora or fourchette and perineum, causing itching and occasionally vaginal discharge. The umbilicated lesions of *molluscum contagiosum* may also be pruritic,

although they are more often asymptomatic. This infection, which is generally self-limited in immunocompetent women, is also sexually transmitted. Dermatophyte lesions (tinea cruris) are a rare cause of itching in women; they are found more frequently in women using topical steroids to treat another vulvar condition.

Infestation with mites or lice can cause intense pruritis. Scabies produces papular lesions and itching, which may occur in several areas on the body, including wrists, finger webs, elbows, axillae, genitals, and buttocks. *Pediculosis pubis* (commonly known as "crabs") is confined to areas covered by hair because eggs are deposited on the hair shafts (see Chapter 195).

Vulvar irritation caused by scratching, maceration, and chemical agents is common among women and girls of all ages. Deodorants, soaps, douching agents, bubble baths, and contraceptive foams may incite allergic reactions or chemical irritations, leading to itching. An active or inactive component of a topical medication may also be the inciting agent. The vulva may appear erythematous, and edema or secondary excoriations may be present. The precipitant may be inadequate or overly aggressive genital hygiene. A warm, moist environment, which promotes infection, can occur in patients who are obese or who wear tight-fitting pants or nylon underwear. Chafing fosters maceration of the mucosa in conjunction with the itching and scratching. Elderly women who experience urinary incontinence may be forced to wear pads, which can cause irritation. Younger women who shave their pubic hair are often bothered by pruritus from a secondary folliculitis.

The term *vulvar dystrophy* has been replaced by the term *vulvar dermatoses* to describe the large group of nonneoplastic papulosquamous lesions that occur on the vulva. All of these may cause pruritus in addition to other symptoms. Any of the lesions may appear white because they are hyperkeratotic, but less than 5% are premalignant. Vulvar eczema may be either endogenous, due to atopy, or exogenous, secondary to an irritant or allergen (contact dermatitis). Chronic contact or *irritant reactions* of the vulva can cause persistent scratching and lichenification, leaving the vulva thickened and furrowed. The resultant leathery skin, termed *lichen simplex chronicus,* is the end stage of any chronic irritative or infectious disorder of the vulva that causes pruritus. *Lichen sclerosis* is an idiopathic primary disorder of the vulva characterized by depigmentation around the vaginal introitus and perianal skin in a symmetric "keyhole" pattern, with pale atrophic epidermis with fine wrinkling or scaling on a whitened dermis. It can occur in women of any age, although it is most common after menopause. If untreated, it can lead to stenosis of the vaginal introitus (although vaginal involvement itself is rare) and atrophy or fusing of vulvar structures including the labia minora. Lichen sclerosis is associated with squamous cell carcinoma of the vulva, of a type not mediated by the human papilloma virus. *Lichen planus,* another primary vulvar disorder, may present in a classic or erosive form. The classic form is characterized by "the five Ps": pruritic purple polygonal papules and plaques, which occur on both oral and genital membranes. The more common erosive form typically originates in the vaginal vestibule with erosion and erythema extending into the vaginal canal with clearly demarcated borders. It may be associated with significant distortion and destruction of vulvovaginal structures. *Psoriasis* may appear as moist red plaques with a silvery scale on the labia majora, although vulvar psoriasis may lack the typical scale. *Seborrheic dermatitis* of the vulva is uncommon but may present with scaling erythematous lesions of the vulva.

Atrophic vaginitis occurs in low-estrogen states, including postmenopause (natural and surgical) and postpartum,

---

TABLE 114.1

CAUSES OF VULVAR PRURITUS

Infections
　Candida
　Trichomonas
　Bacterial vaginosis
　Hidradenitis suppurativa
　Herpes simplex
　Human papillomavirus
　Dermatophytes
　Scabies

Dermatoses
　Lichen sclerosis
　Lichen simplex chronicus/vulvar eczema
　Lichen planus (erosive vaginitis)
　Psoriasis
　Seborrheic dermatitis

Low-Estrogen States: Atrophic Vaginitis
　Postpartum
　Postmenopausal

Premalignant/Malignant Conditions
　Vulvar intraepithelial neoplasia
　Squamous cell carcinoma
　Adenocarcinoma

Irritants
　Contact dermatitis

including lactation (see Chapter 117). The mucosa is red and thin; sometimes a mild discharge is present.

Malignancy may develop in association with dermatoses such as lichen sclerosis and possibly lichen planus; vulvar intraepithelial neoplasia may also be seen in association with HPV, especially in younger women (see later discussion). Paget's disease of the vulva, often treated as presumptive eczema when it presents with itching and burning, appears as red, scaling plaque with clear margins often involving the anal region as well. Although it is infrequent, it is associated in 5% of cases with an underlying vulvar adenocarcinoma and in up to 24% of cases with a noncontiguous adenocarcinoma.

Squamous carcinoma of the vulva is the most ominous cause of vulvar pruritus. Historically, it has been seen primarily in older women, although the age at presentation appears to be declining perhaps due to a shifting of subtype frequency away from the keratinized type found primarily in older women. This keratinized or simplex subtype is not associated with HPV infection, whereas the classic or bowenoid subtype is associated with high-risk HPV subtypes and is seen in younger women. Delay in diagnosis is common; the patient frequently gives a history of unsuccessful trials of topical agents for symptomatic relief from itching. Itching may be intense, sometimes in conjunction with a slightly bloody discharge. Squamous cell carcinoma of the vulva commonly presents with a single papule, plaque, mass, or ulcer on the labia majora or minora, although in 15% of cases multifocal or extensive lesions are found. The lesions can be red, white, or pigmented, raised or eroded, and often arise in areas already involved with premalignant change. Spread is to inguinal and deep pelvic nodes.

Vulvar intraepithelial neoplasia (VIN), which occurs in younger women (75% premenopausal), is akin to cervical intraepithelial neoplasia in its relationship to previous HPV infection, although the keratinized subtype of unifocal lesion found in postmenopausal women does not have a clear HPV association. Although half of women with VIN are asymptomatic, the most common complaint is pruritis. A certain percentage of women with VIN also have cervical intraepithelial neoplasia, necessitating a full colposcopic evaluation of both the vulva and the cervix. However, vulvar intraepithelial neoplasia progresses to malignancy at a much slower rate than cervical intraepithelial neoplasia.

DIFFERENTIAL DIAGNOSIS (8,9)

In young women, vaginitis, pediculosis, scabies, chemical irritants, and allergic reactions are the major causes of vaginal itching. The same etiologies apply to older women, but atrophic vaginitis, dermatoses, and vulvar carcinoma also become major considerations. In any woman with a persistently pruritic vulva, the possibility of a primary dermatosis should be considered.

WORKUP (9,10)

It is important to inquire about vaginal discharge, any skin rashes or conditions such as eczema or psoriasis, urinary incontinence, vulvar lesions, and other sites of itching. Possible irritants and allergies need to be identified, such as creams, soaps, bubble baths, vaginal deodorants, douches, topical medications, and contraceptive foams. The sexual history or presence of genital itching in partners or roommates may suggest infection or infestation. Information related to the duration of

the problem and responses to prior treatments can be useful. Presence of an ulceration or nodule that has persisted or grown should be ascertained. Any history of HPV or herpes simplex virus–associated lesions or abnormal Papanicolaou smears should be obtained.

The vulva and perineal skin is inspected for macules, papules, scaling, erythema, ulcerations, pigmented lesions, hypopigmentation, excoriation, rash, lice, and mites. A close look at the hair shaft may reveal lice eggs (nits), which are pathognomonic of the infestation (see Chapter 195). A speculum examination helps to identify any vaginitis or discharge (see Chapter 117). Inguinal nodes should be palpated. A wet prep or culture of the discharge for identification of an organism should be done if infection is suspected. Any suspicious lesions should be referred for biopsy and colposcopy with application of acetic acid to identify abnormalities, as should lesions that do not respond to initial treatment.

SYMPTOMATIC MANAGEMENT, PATIENT EDUCATION, AND INDICATIONS FOR REFERRAL (11–15)

The management of vulvar pruritus is most likely to be successful when a specific etiology can be identified. Self-treatments and use of potentially irritating soaps or creams should be stopped. Any infectious etiologies need to be treated. Atrophic vaginitis responds well to a topical estrogen supplementation in the form of cream, suppositories, or rings (see Chapter 117). Regular use of over-the-counter vaginal moisturizers such as Replens may be a helpful adjunct. Occasionally, a sedating antihistamine may be used at night to relieve itching and break the itch/scratch cycle. Soaking in plain warm water twice a day may be soothing and help to break this cycle. In some conditions, when the etiology is known, the short-term use of topical steroids is beneficial. Lichen simplex chronicus, eczema, and psoriasis should respond to 2 weeks of daily mid- to high-potency corticosteroid, although retreatment may be necessary. Ointments are preferred over cream preparations, which may contain ingredients more likely to trigger a contact dermatitis. Lichen sclerosis and lichen planus need treatment with a high-potency topical steroid to prevent distortion of the vulvovaginal architecture and should generally be referred to a gynecologist or dermatologist experienced in the vulvar dermatoses for management and ongoing surveillance for malignancy. Studies with topical tacrolimus and pimecrolimus have shown success in treatment of lichen sclerosis and lichen planus, but the 2005 U.S. Food and Drug Administration black box warning about risks of malignancy with use of these medications has limited their use. Persistent vulvar lesions or symptoms unresponsive to treatment should be referred to the dermatologist or gynecologist for biopsy, particularly if the etiology is unclear, given the risk for malignancy as well as the potential to treat conditions and prevent potentially severe complications.

Patients should be educated about factors that contribute to persistent vulvar irritation, including excessive hygiene or moisture (secondary to tight-fitting jeans, panty hose, nylon underwear, or exercise clothes). Such practices are common among women with vulvar complaints, and failure specifically to address these habits may prevent its resolution. Women should be encouraged to perform regular vulvar self-examination. They should be taught to use a hand mirror to inspect the vulva, looking for moles, changes in pigmentation, warts, ulcers, and sores.

Annotated Bibliography

1. Foster DC. Vulvar disease. Obstet Gynecol 2002;100:145. (*A comprehensive review of vulvar pathology and its treatment.*)
2. Jones RW, Baranya J, Stables S, et al. Trends in squamous cell carcinoma of the vulva: the influence of vulvar intraepithelial neoplasia. Obstet Gynecol 1996;60:500. (*Reviews the evolving epidemiology of vulvar squamous cell carcinoma and vulvar intraepithelial neoplasia; there is an increasing prevalence of human papillomavirus [HPV]–associated lesions in younger women.*)
3. Fischer G, Spurett B, Fischer A. The chronically symptomatic vulva: aetiology and management. Br J Obstet Gynaecol 1995;102:773. (*The most common cause was dermatitis, which occurred alone in 55% of cases and together with evidence of HPV infection in another 9%.*)
4. Bohl, TG. Overview of vulvar pruritis through the life cycle. Clin Obstet Gynecol 2005;48:786. (*A comprehensive review of different conditions causing vulvar symptoms at different life stages, covering pathophysiology, diagnosis, and management.*)
5. McKay M. Vulvitis and vulvovaginitis: cutaneous considerations. Am J Obstet Gynecol 1991;165:1176. (*A good descriptive review of vulvar dermatoses and other vulvar lesions.*)
6. Val, I, Almeida, G. An overview of lichen sclerosis. Clin Obstet Gynecol 2005; 48:808. (*A detailed review of the pathogenesis, clinical features, and management of the disorder.*)
7. Goldstein AT, Metz A. Vulvar lichen planus. Clin Obstet Gynecol 2005;48:818. (*A detailed review of etiology, clinical variants, and treatment.*)
8. Heller DS, Randolph P, Young A, et al. A five-year experience of the Columbia Presbyterian Medical Center Cutaneous-Vulvar Service. Dermatology 1997;195:26. (*The most common presenting condition was vulvar vestibulitis, at 36%, followed by lichen sclerosis and vaginitis, at 19% and 15%, respectively.*)
9. Apgar BS, Cox JT. Differentiating normal and abnormal findings of the vulva.

Am Family Physician 1996;53:1171. (*Emphasizes the tendency to overdiagnose micropapillae of the inner labia or acetowhite changes of the vulva secondary to HPV infection.*)
10. Anderson MR, Klink K, Cohrssen A. Evaluation of vaginal complaints. JAMA 2004;291:1368. (*Absence of itching makes candidiasis unlikely.*)
11. Suckling J, Lethaby A, Kennedy R. Local oestrogen for vaginal atrophy in postmenopausal women. Cochrane Database Syst Rev 2006;4: CD001500. (*Compared the efficacy and safety of various forms of topical estrogen in relieving local atrophic symptoms, finding that hormones were more effective than placebo or nonhormonal moisturizers, with most women preferring the estrogen-releasing ring.*)
12. Lotery HE, Galask RP. Erosive lichen planus of the vulva and vagina. Obstet Gynecol 2003;101:1121. (*Reports three cases of untreated lichen planus causing advanced vaginal scarring and dyspareunia, which responded to topical tacrolimus.*)
13. Berger TG, Duvic M, Van Voorhees AS, et al. The use of topical calcineurin inhibitors in dermatology: safety concerns. Report of the American Academy of Dermatology Task Force. J Am Acad Dermatol 2006;54:818. (*Review of the black box U.S. Food and Drug Administration warning and available data, finding no proof that these medications are associated with malignancy, but advocating continued investigation and use of the minimum dose possible.*)
14. Marin MG, King R, Sfameni S, et al. Adverse behavioral and sexual factors in chronic vulvar disease. Am J Obstet Gynecol 2000; 183:34. (*In a series of 530 women presenting for treatment at a specialty vulvar clinic, the majority engaged in practices that potentially exacerbated their chronic vulvar complaints.*)
15. Abramov YU, Elchalel U, Abramov D, et al. Surgical treatment of vulvar lichen sclerosis: a review. Obstet Gynecol Surv 1996;51:193. (*Review of the indications for vulvectomy, cryosurgery, and laser ablation.*)

CHAPTER 115 ■ MEDICAL EVALUATION OF FEMALE SEXUAL DYSFUNCTION

SUSAN E. BENNETT AND SHANA L. BIRNBAUM

With advances in pharmaceutical treatment of male erectile dysfunction, there has been new attention focused on understanding female sexuality with the intent to develop treatments for what has been termed *female sexual dysfunction* (FSD).

PATHOPHYSIOLOGY AND CLINICAL PRESENTATION (1–18)

Sexual difficulties are highly prevalent, with some degree of erectile dysfunction reported among 52% of all men between 40 and 70 years of age. Female sexual dysfunction, however, is harder to quantify and measure. The most widely quoted community-based survey, conducted in the United States in 1992, indicated that the prevalence of sexual problems among women is 43%. However, critics have questioned the terminology of this report, in which "difficulty" in any 2-month period was counted as a "dysfunction." In addition, the women were not asked whether the problem was severe or significant

enough to be a cause of personal distress. The most recent Kinsey Institute data indicate that physiologic measures of response during sexual activity were not predictive of a woman's satisfaction with her sexual life, whereas emotional health and relationship factors, along with overall physical health, were predictive. Although exact diagnostic criteria for the disorders of female sexual dysfunction are being debated, there is consensus that the symptoms must cause distress to the woman to be diagnostic.

Disorders of Sexual Desire

Low desire is the most common sexual problem reported by women, with prevalence rates ranging from 10% to 51% in various studies. In the Study of Women Across the Nation (SWAN), 40% of healthy midlife women reported that they rarely or never experienced spontaneous sexual desire. However, the majority of these women were satisfied with their sex lives. Aging, lengthier sexual relationship with the same partner, and loss of ovarian function correlate with lower desire. Because these are common experiences for the majority of women, low desire is not necessarily dysfunctional.

There is no evidence that hormone replacement with estrogen or progesterone improves sexual desire. A large population study in Australia failed to show a correlation between androgen levels (total and free testosterone, dehydroepiandrosterone sulfate, and androstenedione) and self-reported sexual desire and sexual satisfaction. A randomized, controlled, and double-blinded trial of testosterone administered by a transdermal delivery system showed significant improvement in the number of sexually satisfying events per month among women who had been ovariectomized before menopause. A strong placebo response, however, diminished the significance of the outcome, and the U.S. Food and Drug Administration ruled against approving the testosterone patch for women.

A recent and important interpretation of the evidence in this area holds that sexual desire is *not* the primary reason most women seek sexual activity, even if lack of desire is the most common reason women seek medical advice about their sexual health. Rosemary Basson argued that sexual desire *follows* arousal for many women, who are *willing* to accept sexual engagement with an intimate partner with the belief that desire and satisfaction will follow. The unisex linear sexual response cycle proposed by Masters and Johnson in 1966 and modified by Helen Kaplan in 1973 created the expectation that sexual desire is a prerequisite for a sexual encounter. Basson believed that this model does not reflect the sexual reality of many women.

Disorders of Sexual Arousal

Problems of arousal are less common than low sexual desire. In SWAN, 5% of women reported difficulties becoming sexual aroused. One of the problems with assessing the prevalence of arousal disorders is that many studies use vaginal lubrication as a marker of arousal. *Genital arousal* in men is penile erection, and in women, *genital arousal* is vaginal vasocongestion with associated lubrication. *Subjective arousal* is the physiologic state associated with *perceived* sexual excitement and the desire to seek continued sexual stimulation. Although there is a close relationship between penile erection and subjective arousal in men, there is a poor correlation between genital and subjective arousal in women. This is why sildenafil (marketed under the brand name Viagra) for women with the Female Sexual Arousal Disorder failed to show benefit.

Lack of subjective arousal for women is likely related to lack of clitoral stimulation and engorgement. The clitoris is widely believed to be a small structure, 1 cm in diameter and 2 cm in length. Autopsy dissections demonstrated that the clitoris is much larger, approximately 9 cm in length, with the majority of this complex structure inside the pelvis. Engorgement of the clitoris is obviously more difficult to measure than penile or vaginal engorgement, and this might explain the lack of correlation between genital and subjective arousal for women.

Disorders of Orgasm

Unlike male orgasm, there is no evidence that female orgasm is necessary for procreation. Adaptive evolutionary theory is that women have the erectile tissue and neurovascular connections for orgasm because the clitoris and penis arise from the same embryologic organ. A significant proportion of women do not experience orgasm with intercourse. A review of sexology literature found that 25% of women experienced orgasms during sexual intercourse. It is estimated that 80% of women who have never experienced orgasm can learn to become orgasmic with directed masturbation. When asked to describe what parts of their genital anatomy required the least stimulation to achieve orgasm, women in one study uniformly reported that the area above and on top of the *glans clitoris* was more sensitive by far than any other area, including the vaginal entrance and anywhere inside the vagina. A small proportion of women expel copious fluid at the time of orgasm, and this has been termed *female ejaculation.* Anatomically, there are no structures in the female genitalia large enough to contain more than a few millimeters of fluid other than the vagina and bladder. Thus, female ejaculation remains controversial.

Disorders Causing Sexual Pain

The prevalence of sexual pain disorders was reported to be 7% in the 1992 survey.

Dyspareunia is the sexual pain disorder most likely to be brought to the attention of the primary care clinician. Several mechanisms may be responsible for painful intercourse (Table 115.1), depending on whether the symptoms occur with initial insertion of the penis or deep penetration. Pain is experienced in the former case because of failure of lubrication or inadequate stimulation, vaginal or vulvar irritation, and structural impediments secondary to surgery, inflammation, or anatomic variants. Deep pain can arise from friction against inflamed tissue or by jarring of inflamed parametrial structures. The psychological contributions to dyspareunia reflect a variety of issues.

Pain on insertion can be caused by irritation of the vulva, which in turn is caused by multiple factors, including vulvovaginal infections (see Chapters 114 and 117). Ulcerative diseases like genital herpes commonly cause external pain with coitus, as do the vulvar dermatoses, including eczema, lichen planus, and lichen sclerosis. Irritation may be secondary to the use of scented soaps, shaving foam, spermicide, or a condom. A *cyst* of the *Bartholin's gland duct* occurs when mechanical irritation and the attendant inflammatory reaction obstruct the ductal lumen, causing a painful cystic swelling in the vestibule. Irritation from a previous surgery, including an episiotomy, may also be responsible for pain.

Thin vulvar and vaginal mucosal tissue, as seen in estrogen deficiency, are less resilient and more susceptible to *trauma.*

TABLE 115.1

IMPORTANT CAUSES OF DYSPAREUNIA

Pain Greatest on Insertion	Pain Greatest on Deep Penetration
Inadequate lubrication	Pelvic inflammatory disease
Vaginitis	Ovarian cyst
Incompletely ruptured hymen	Endometriosis
Bartholin's gland cyst	Pelvic adhesions
Stricture	Relaxation of pelvic support
Inadequate episiotomy	Uterine fibroids
Vulvovaginal atrophy	
Vulvar vestibulitis	
Pudendal neuralgia	
Vaginismus	

This type of vaginal atrophy is virtually universal among menopausal women, who may have insufficient lubrication even with adequate stimulation. Atrophic vaginitis is a common cause of dyspareunia. Similar symptoms and vaginal changes can be seen in any woman in a low-estrogen state, including women who are breast-feeding or postpartum, have anorexia or other causes of hypothalamic amenorrhea, or who have had pelvic irradiation. In premenopausal women, *inadequate lubrication* due to insufficient foreplay is among the most frequent causes of dyspareunia. Medications may also contribute to vaginal dryness, including low-dose oral contraceptives. Finally, scant production of vaginal secretions may reflect inadequate arousal due to anxieties about sexual intercourse or risk of infection or relationship conflicts.

Chronic vulvar vestibulitis, also known as *vulvar vestibulodynia*, is an uncommon but increasingly recognized cause of insertional dyspareunia in which pain of the vestibule is felt on vaginal entry and is associated with erythema of the vulva. A biopsy shows only chronic inflammatory changes. .

Pudendal neuralgia or *vulvodynia* is a less common cause of vulvar burning associated with unprovoked pain and little to no physical findings. *Vaginismus* is defined as involuntary spasm of the perineal muscles induced by any attempt at physical penetration. It is an important and treatable, although uncommon, cause of dyspareunia, often with a large psychogenic component in primary forms. Secondary vaginismus may be a conditioned response to vulvovaginal pain.

Deep dyspareunia may occur with endometriosis, ovarian cysts, and pelvic inflammatory disease and also from adhesions resulting from these conditions. Although a retroverted uterus is a normal variant, some women may have pain with thrusting as the uterus moves posteriorly.

DIFFERENTIAL DIAGNOSIS
(6,8–10,15–20)

Causes of problems with desire, arousal, and orgasm are listed in Table 115.2. All of the causes of dyspareunia listed in Table 115.1 should be considered according to the age of the patient and whether there is pain on insertion or on deep penetration.

WORKUP (6,8,10,15–20)

All women should be asked whether they have any concerns about their sexual functioning, including pain with intercourse,

TABLE 115.2

SECONDARY CAUSES OF SEXUAL DYSFUNCTION

Medical	Psychiatric
Cushing's disease	Bipolar disorder
Addison's disease	Anxiety disorder
Diabetes mellitus	Major depression
Hypopituitarism	Panic disorder
Hyperprolactinemia	Somatization disorder
Degenerative joint disease	Somatiform pain disorder
Hypothyroidism	
Multiple sclerosis	
Temporal lobe lesions	
Coronary heart disease	

as part of the review of systems. A positive response should elicit more detailed questioning. For all sexual problems, the clinician should take a complete history including current and previous sexual experiences and remain aware of the prevalence of sexual abuse, including incest, rape (both stranger and acquaintance), and domestic violence. It is not surprising that the patient may not be forthcoming with these experiences. Any history of sexual fears should be explored. An understanding of the patient's current sexual experience and feelings toward the partner should be sensitively obtained (see Chapter 229). Sexual problems cluster with self-reported psychological and social problems among women.

The most important question for a woman reporting any area of sexual dysfunction is whether the problem is new or longstanding. The sudden onset of loss of desire, arousal, or orgasm in a woman who was previously functioning normally suggests either major depression or an organic disorder. If dysfunction in any domain cannot be explained by depression, medication, or obvious endocrine conditions, a full medical evaluation should commence. An abrupt loss of desire should raise concern about an endocrine abnormality, such as those listed in Table 115.2. Sudden loss of arousal is unusual and would be worrisome for neurovascular disease preventing engorgement of the vagina and clitoris, such as atherosclerosis. Sudden loss of orgasm is one of the most common side effects of the selective serotonin reuptake inhibitor (SSRI) antidepressants. If a woman is not on these medications, however, loss of her ability to have an orgasm in light of no change in desire or arousal suggests neurologic disease interrupting the autonomic nerve supply to the pelvis. This would likely be associated with other neurologic deficits that would not be subtle, such as dysfunction of the urinary sphincter.

In the history of sexual pain, one needs to determine whether dyspareunia was noticed with the first experience of sexual intercourse or has developed recently, secondary to an organic disorder or a situational problem. The patient should be asked whether pain occurs before penetration, on penetration, or only after deep penetration. It is important to establish whether the patient can insert a tampon without pain; if she can, mechanical obstruction is unlikely.

The most important part of the workup for sexual pain is the pelvic examination. The physician inspects for signs of vulvovaginitis, atrophic vaginitis, narrowed introitus, cervicitis, and congenital abnormalities. Palpation may identify a uterine mass, a retroverted uterus, or tenderness, along with vaginal spasm or tenderness. The examiner should attempt to reproduce the pain with palpation using a single finger; vestibulodynia can best be assessed by application of a cotton-tipped swab to elicit point tenderness in the vestibule. The cervix should be manipulated to see whether pain is produced. A Papanicolaou smear should be obtained for cervical cytology to detect underlying malignancy if screening is not up to date. Vaginal anatomy, measured by introital caliber, length, and vulvovaginal atrophy, does not correlate with sexual function, including symptoms of dyspareunia and vaginal dryness.

A *complete blood count*, *sedimentation rate*, and *cervical culture* are indicated if there is evidence on physical examination suggesting pelvic inflammatory disease (see Chapter 116). *Wet prep* with vaginal pH can assess for *Candida* or *Trichomonas* if vulvovaginitis is suspected. *Pelvic ultrasonography* may be indicated to help define a suspected pelvic mass. Referral to a gynecologist for *laparoscopy* is indicated if endometriosis, adhesions, or an adnexal mass is under consideration.

SYMPTOMATIC MANAGEMENT, PATIENT EDUCATION, AND INDICATIONS FOR REFERRAL (2,4,5–7,10,14,18,20–22)

A healthy woman reporting low sexual desire should be reassured that this is common among women in longstanding sexual relationships and among women after menopause. She should be encouraged to enter into sexual activity with her partner, expecting desire to follow arousal. For women troubled by inadequate arousal, they should be offered advice about the benefits of effective clitoral stimulation, described in a number of books, such as *Becoming Orgasmic* by Julia Heiman and Joseph LoPiccolo. They can be reassured that many women do not achieve orgasm with intercourse, but that the majority can experience orgasm with adequate clitoral stimulation. Women who do not lubricate despite good arousal should be encouraged to use a water-soluble lubricant jelly. Contraceptive creams should not be used for lubrication because they often cause dehydration and may worsen soreness. A variety of lubricant products are available over the counter. The postmenopausal woman with an atrophic vaginal mucosa can be prescribed a topical estrogen product that is not systemically absorbed, such as the estrogen ring or slow-release estrogen suppositories (see Chapter 118). Regular sexual intercourse helps postmenopausal women to retain genital blood flow and vaginal resiliency. With aging, both men and women typically require increased erotic stimulation for adequate arousal. It is important to encourage open communication between partners, which is essential for negotiating a healthy sexual relationship over time.

Treatment of endocrine disease, such as pituitary adenomas, usually results in return of sexual desire. Controlling diabetes, hypertension, and lipids may improve arousal among women with diabetes or atherosclerosis. For women experiencing anorgasmia on SSRI antidepressants but who need to remain on their medications, addition of bupropion or buspirone might restore their abilities to achieve orgasm. Sildenafil is not effective treatment for women's sexual problems in any domain. Postmenopausal women should not be prescribed testosterone for sexual desire disorders without concomitant estrogen and progesterone replacement therapy. Furthermore, the safety and efficacy of testosterone replacement for women remains controversial.

If there is an underlying vaginal or pelvic infection, it should be treated and the patient advised to refrain temporarily from intercourse (see Chapters 116 and 117). Patients troubled by pain from herpes simplex infection can obtain relief with use of acyclovir or valacyclovir (see Chapter 193). Vulvar vestibulodynia and vulvodynia may respond to topical anesthetics (e.g., 5% xylocaine, EMLA Cream) applied before intercourse. Failure to do so should prompt referral to a gynecologist with expertise in vulvar disorders.

As noted, there is little correlation between vaginal introitus caliber or other measures of vaginal anatomy and dyspareunia. Nonetheless, the patient with an unusually narrow introitus might be referred to a gynecologist for consideration of a trial of vaginal dilators. Vaginismus may be managed by education about voluntary muscle control, relaxation, and Kegel exercises, all of which are usually best accomplished by an experienced therapist or sex therapy clinic. Referral to a gynecologist is indicated if sexual pain is due to a Bartholin's gland cyst that has not drained with warm soaks or to pain following surgery or episiotomy, or if pain is suspected to be from pelvic pathology, such as endometriosis or fibroids. Initial failure to identify or relieve dyspareunia should also prompt referral. For some women, referral to a sex therapist will be indicated when medical causes have been ruled out and basic counseling has failed (see Chapter 229). Because of the lack of evidence for pharmacologic therapy and the strong interplay with psychological and relationship issues, referral is the prudent course for the primary care clinician who has not developed special expertise in this area. It is important to be aware of well-trained resources in the community. Recognition of underlying psychopathology and psychosocial distress is also essential (see Chapter 229).

Annotated Bibliography

1. Feldman HA, Goldstein I, Hatzichristou DG, et al. Impotence and its medical and psychosocial correlates. Results of the Massachusetts Male Aging Study. J Urol 1994;151(1):54. (*One of the largest ongoing epidemiology studies of men as they age, establishing the high prevalence of erectile dysfunction.*)
2. Laumann EO, Paik A, Rosen RC. Sexual dysfunction in the United States: prevalence and predictors. JAMA 1999;281:1174. (*The condition was more prevalent in women, at 43%, than in men, at 31%.*)
3. Moynihan R. The making of a disease: female sexual dysfunction. BMJ 2003;326:45. (*Intriguing look at the evolution of female sexual dysfunction as a diagnosis, including the role of drug companies.*)
4. Bancroft J. The medicalization of female sexual dysfunction: the need for caution. Arch Sex Behav 2002;31:451. (*The director of the Kinsey Institute argues for recognition of the differences in male and female sexuality and cautions against using the male model to understand female sexuality, particularly in terms of defining what may be an adaptive response as a dysfunction.*)
5. Bancroft J, Loftus J, Long JS. Distress about sex: a national survey of women in heterosexual relationships. Arch Sex Behav 2003;32:193. (*The most recent Kinsey Institute data reveal that emotional health and relationship issues are more predictive of a woman's level of sexual satisfaction than physical measures, including orgasm.*)
6. Lightner DJ. Female sexual dysfunction. Mayo Clin Proc 2002;77:698. (*Reviews the diagnostic classification of female sexual dysfunction defined in 1998, with emphasis on the fact that symptoms must cause distress for the diagnosis to be valid.*)
7. Avis NE, Zhao X, Johannes CB, et al. Correlates of sexual function among multi-ethnic middle-aged women: results from the Study of Women's Health Across the Nation (SWAN). Menopause 2005;12:385. (*A total of 2,400 ethnically diverse midlife women in six American cities completed an initial questionnaire about various aspects of their health.*)
8. Davis SR, Davison SL, Donath S, et al. Circulating androgen levels and self-reported sexual function in women. JAMA 2005;294:91-96. (*This community-based, cross-sectional study of 1,423 women between the ages of 18 and 75 years randomly recruited in Australia reported that no single androgen level predicted sexual dysfunction.*)
9. Shifren JL, Braunstein GD, Simon JA, et al. Transdermal testosterone treatment in women with impaired sexual function after oophorectomy. N Engl J Med 2000;343:682. (*Report of a study of 75 women between the ages of 31 and 56 years who had sustained hysterectomies and oophorectomies and reported sexual distress in the domain of desire; this randomized, controlled trial of transdermal testosterone vs. placebo reported improved sexual events resulting from testosterone.*)
10. Basson R. Sexual desire and arousal disorders in women. N Engl J Med 2006;354:1497. (*A review article describing the physiology of desire and arousal among women, dysfunction in these domains, and therapeutic interventions.*)
11. Chivers ML, Rieger G, Latty E, et al. A sex difference in the specificity of sexual arousal. Psychol Sci 2004;15:736. (*Healthy young heterosexuals, homosexuals, and female transsexuals viewed erotic films and rated their degree of subjective arousal while penile plethysmography and vaginal amplitude recordings measured genital arousal.*)
12. O'Connell HE, Hutson JM, Anderson CR, et al. Anatomical relationship between urethra and clitoris. J Urol 1998;159(6):1892. (*Description by an anatomist of the clitoris based on an autopsy series of women at various ages, concluding that clinical anatomy textbooks do not accurately describe the size or location of this organ.*)

13. Lloyd EA. The case of the female orgasm: bias in the science of evolution. Cambridge, MA: Harvard University Press, 2005. (*This large review of feminist literature describes the frequency of orgasm reported by women in various studies, and critiques scientific theories about the reproductive importance of female orgasm.*)

14. Canning D, Schober JM, Meyer-Bahlberg HFL, et al. Self-assessment of genital anatomy, sexual sensitivity and function in women: implications for genitoplasty. BJU Int 2004;94:589. (*Hoping to learn why surgical correction of congenital genital abnormalities often resulted in sexual dysfunction, urologists in New York and London asked women to describe sexual sensitivity of various genital areas.*)

15. Bergeron S, Binik YM, Khalife S, et al. Vulvar vestibulitis syndrome: a critical review. Clin J Pain 1997;13:27. (*A systematic literature review of the entity that is the most common cause of dyspareunia in some series of premenopausal women.*)

16. Munday P, Buchan A. Vulval vestibulitis. BMJ 2004;328:1214. (*Reviews this common yet underdiagnosed cause of dyspareunia.*)

17. Reissing ED, Binik YM, Khalife S, et al. Vaginal spasm, pain, and behavior. An empirical investigation of the diagnosis of vaginismus. Arch Sex Behav 2004;33:5. (*Diagnostic agreement was poor in distinguishing vaginismus from dyspareunia resulting from vulvar vestibulitis based on spasm alone; the authors suggest including pain and fear of pain, pelvic floor dysfunction, and behavioral avoidance in the diagnostic criteria.*)

18. Morley JE, Kaiser FE. Female sexuality. Med Clin North Am 2003;87:1077. (*Reviews sexual response and the effect of medical problems on female sexuality, along with available therapeutics and specific counseling suggestions.*)

19. Anonymous. Drugs that cause sexual dysfunction: an update. Med Lett Drugs Ther 1992;34:73. (*The list continues to expand.*)

20. Basson R. Female sexual response: the role of drugs in the management of sexual dysfunction. Obstet Gynecol 2001;98:350. (*Emphasizes the complexity of female sexuality and the disconnect between physiologic measures and subjective experience; vasoactive drugs may affect only the former.*)

21. Kaplan SA, Reis RB, Kohn IJ, et al. Safety and efficacy of sildenafil in postmenopausal women with sexual dysfunction. Urology 1999;53:481. (*Improvements were found in lubrication and clitoral sensitivity but not in overall subjective response.*)

22. Landon M, Eriksson E, Agren H, et al. Effect of buspirone on sexual dysfunction in depressed patients treated with selective serotonin reuptake inhibitors. J Clin Psychopharmacol 1999;19:268. (*Improvement was found for 58% of patients on buspirone compared with 30% on placebo.*)

CHAPTER 116 ■ APPROACH TO THE PATIENT WITH MENSTRUAL OR PELVIC PAIN

SHANA L. BIRNBAUM

Pelvic pain is a major source of concern and morbidity for many women. Dysmenorrhea—painful periods—affects at least half of menstruating women at some time, and an estimated 10% of women are significantly impaired by the problem. Acute episodes of pelvic pain are also common and may represent potentially serious pathology. The primary care physician should be able to distinguish pain of a functional nature from that due to infection or an anatomic lesion and know when referral to a gynecologist or urgent hospital admission is indicated. The generalist should also be able to initiate treatment and educate patients about the most common causes of pelvic pain.

PATHOPHYSIOLOGY AND CLINICAL PRESENTATION (1–18)

The causes of pelvic pain can be organized into acute, chronic, and recurrent categories, with the latter group subdivided based on the relationship of the pain to the menstrual period (Table 116.1).

Acute Pain

Pelvic pain of acute onset may result from pelvic inflammatory disease, ectopic pregnancy, torsion of the fallopian tube or ovary, rupture of an ovarian cyst, or extrapelvic pathology such as acute appendicitis or ureteral stones.

Pelvic Inflammatory Disease

Pelvic inflammatory disease (PID) has long been recognized as an acute infection of the upper genital tract, including the uterus, ovaries, and fallopian tubes, which disproportionately affects young, sexually active women. It may cause little pain until the infection has spread from the cervix through the lymphatics into the parametria and fallopian tubes, which may occur weeks or even months after initial exposure to an infected partner. Subclinical PID, ranging from asymptomatic upper tract infection to mild pelvic pain, is being increasingly recognized, which has led to the current understanding of PID as a spectrum of disease with classic acute PID falling at one extreme. Thus, clinicians need to maintain a high index of suspicion, particularly in women with risk factors including young age (15 to 25 years), African American race, multiple partners, lack of barrier contraception, or prior history of sexually transmitted disease. Modern intrauterine devices (IUDs) do not appear to be associated with an increased risk of upper genital tract infections. The Centers for Disease Control and Prevention (CDC) recommend empiric treatment for young, sexually active women with pelvic pain not otherwise explained and any one of the following on exam: cervical motion tenderness, uterine tenderness, or adnexal tenderness. All three signs are typically present in the classic acute bilateral salpingitis of PID, although one side may be more involved than the other. Peritoneal signs may occur if infected discharge escapes from the fallopian tube and soils the overlying peritoneum. Tuboovarian abscess is a complication of acute PID involving formation of an inflammatory mass in the adnexa and is associated with severe unilateral pain and occasionally rupture.

TABLE 116.1

IMPORTANT CAUSES OF PELVIC PAIN

Acute Pain
  Pelvic inflammatory disease
  Ectopic pregnancy with rupture
  Torsion of the fallopian tube, ovary, or ovarian cyst
  Ruptured ovarian cyst
  Extrapelvic disease (e.g., appendicitis)

Recurrent Pain with Menstruation
  Primary dysmenorrhea
  Secondary dysmenorrhea
    Endometriosis
    Adenomyosis
    Chronic pelvic inflammatory disease
    Copper intrauterine devices

Recurrent Pain Unrelated to Menstruation
  Mittelschmerz (midcycle pain)
  Leaking ovarian cysts
  Nongynecologic pathology: adhesions, inflammatory bowel
    disease, functional bowel

Chronic Pain
  Benign neoplasms
  Malignancy
  Pelvic floor musculoskeletal pain
  Enigmatic or psychogenic pain

Chlamydia is the most common bacterial sexually transmitted disease in the United States, whereas gonorrheal infections are slowly declining; together, they account for around two thirds of PID cases. Both infections are more commonly asymptomatic than not, with only 15% of cases producing PID, and somewhat more producing an isolated cervicitis. Screening asymptomatic young women for chlamydia has decreased the incidence of PID by up to 50% in two large studies and is recommended by the CDC. Although the inciting organism in PID is sexually transmitted (usually *Chlamydia trachomatis* or *Neisseria gonorrhoeae*), polymicrobial infection is typical; other frequently seen organisms include α streptococci, *Escherichia coli* and other gram-negative rods, *Mycoplasma*, and anaerobic organisms such as *Bacteroides*. Because of the high prevalence of mixed infections in PID, treatment regimens should always include coverage for *C. trachomatis* and *N. gonorrhoeae* (see Chapter 117), along with anaerobes and the aforementioned organisms listed. Attention to local patterns of resistance is crucial; gonorrhea is now considered universally penicillin resistant, and quinolone-resistant gonorrhea is now so common that the CDC advises against fluoroquinolones for treatment of gonococcal infections.

Sequelae of PID include recurrent PID, ectopic pregnancy, infertility, and chronic pelvic or back pain. Twenty-five percent of patients with PID will have a subsequent pelvic infection. A prior episode of PID increases the risk of ectopic pregnancies 7- to 10-fold. Recurrent pelvic infections also increase the risk of infertility: One episode is associated with an 8% to 12% risk of infertility, and the risk doubles with each successive episode. Studies show a 40% to 75% infertility risk after three episodes. Asymptomatic and unrecognized pelvic infection has also been associated with tubal obstruction and infertility, as has delay in treatment for PID. Pelvic infection may also result in chronic pelvic pain in up to 20% of cases. It is increasingly evident that the sequelae of PID, including infertility, are minimized by early, effective antibiotic treatment.

Physical examination in patients with acute classic PID is notable for purulent cervical discharge, friability of the cervix, cervical motion tenderness, or adnexal tenderness. Occasionally, there may be peritoneal signs. Onset of pain during or soon after menses is typical. Abnormal vaginal bleeding occurs in one third of patients and fever in about one half. In subclinical PID, there may no signs or only minimal uterine tenderness.

Ectopic Pregnancy

Ectopic pregnancy is a much-feared cause of acute pelvic pain because catastrophic hemorrhage can result from tubal rupture. The annual incidence of ectopic pregnancies in the United States from 1970 to 1987 increased from 4.5 to 16.8 per 1,000 pregnancies and plateaued around 19 per 1,000 pregnancies in the early 1990s, the most recent data available from the CDC. The case-fatality rate, however, decreased dramatically, by almost 90% from 1979 to 1992. The drop in fatality rates is probably due to earlier diagnosis (before tubal rupture) resulting from the sensitive radioimmunoassay for human chorionic gonadotropin (hCG), high-resolution transvaginal ultrasonography, and the frequent use of laparoscopy. In most cases of ectopic pregnancy, menses is delayed by 1 to 2 weeks, followed by recurrent spotting and initially mild, generally unilateral pain. Severe hemorrhage in the setting of tubal rupture occurs in fewer than 5% of cases, causing sudden extreme pain and hypotension.

Patients with a prior history of PID (even when mild or asymptomatic), prior ectopic pregnancies, tubal surgery to enhance fertility (or for tubal sterilization), *in utero* diethylstilbestrol exposure, use of intrauterine devices, or ovulation-inducing drugs (which alter steroid hormone levels and affect tubal motility) may be predisposed to subsequent ectopic pregnancies, although the absolute risk is lower with intrauterine devices than in women without them.

Torsion

Torsion of the fallopian tube with or without ovarian involvement is seen most commonly in women of reproductive age. The adnexae may be normal except for the resulting ischemia, although ovarian cysts are seen in most cases. Severe, acute, unilateral pain and distension are found without an elevation of white blood cell count, fever, or increased sedimentation rate, unless complicated by ischemic necrosis. Most patients have an adnexal mass on ultrasound, and Doppler exam shows absent ovarian blood flow.

Ovarian Cysts

Ovarian cysts may spontaneously rupture or twist on their pedicles. Rupture can be associated with rapid blood loss, similar to a ruptured ectopic pregnancy. More commonly, only small amounts of fluid or blood are leaked, resulting in unilateral and often recurrent discomfort. Torsion of the pedicle of the cyst can cause ischemia and lead to extreme pain with acute peritoneal signs, fever, and leukocytosis.

Extrapelvic Pathology

Extrapelvic pathology that can cause acute pelvic pain includes appendicitis, kidney stones, urinary tract infections, bleeding from a Meckel's diverticulum, intestinal obstructions, and intestinal abscesses.

Chronic or Recurrent Pain

Conditions that result in recurrent or chronic pelvic pain are generally less urgent than those responsible for acute pain, but they can be problematic for patients and among the most difficult to diagnose for clinicians. Common etiologies include primary dysmenorrhea; secondary dysmenorrhea caused by endometriosis, adenomyosis, and IUDs; chronic PID; uterine fibroids; ovarian cysts; nongynecologic pathology such as adhesions, inflammatory bowel disease, or irritable bowel syndrome; and psychogenic pain. Attention to the details of the clinical presentation often yields important diagnostic clues.

Dysmenorrhea

Dysmenorrhea represents the major source of recurrent pelvic pain. It is classified as *primary* when there is no pelvic pathology and *secondary* when it occurs in the setting of an underlying gynecologic problem, such as endometriosis, PID, or IUD use. Primary dysmenorrhea affects as many as 50% of postpubertal women. It occurs in ovulatory cycles and therefore begins within a few years of menarche when the cycles become regular. The pain occurs at the onset of menstrual blood flow and generally lasts for 48 to 72 hours. It is cramping in nature and can be located in the suprapubic region, the low back, or the inner aspect of the thighs. Dysmenorrhea that begins years after the onset of regular cycles is usually secondary to gynecologic pathology.

Menstrual pain occurs because of increased prostaglandin (PG) production and release by the endometrium, which leads to abnormal uterine muscle activity. Several studies showed increased menstrual fluid prostaglandin levels (primarily PGF_{2a}) and increased circulating leukotriene and vasopressin levels in women with primary dysmenorrhea. High levels of these hormones lead to increased uterine tone and dysrhythmic contractions followed by reduction in uterine blood flow and ischemia. The pain may be from the abnormal contractions, uterine ischemia, or stimulation of sensory pain fibers by the prostaglandins and bradykinin. Nonsteroidal antiinflammatory drugs (NSAIDs), which reduce prostaglandin synthesis, are extremely effective at reducing menstrual pain.

Premenstrual Syndrome/Premenstrual Dysphoric Disorder

Many physiologic changes occur during the menstrual cycle. Women who suffer from premenstrual syndrome (PMS) appear to have an *abnormal response* to the *normal hormonal changes* associated with the menstrual cycle, particularly those in the luteal phase. The most severe form of PMS has been termed *premenstrual dysphoric disorder* (PMDD), which affects 3% to 8% of reproductive-age women and is defined by significant impairment of function. The precise mechanisms by which normal hormonal changes result in symptoms are poorly understood, but their effects on *serotonergic* and *γ-aminobutyric acid receptors* appear to be important. For example, serotonergic activity decreases in some women with PMS during the luteal phase. Personality testing done during symptomatic periods reveals abnormalities, but retesting at other stages of the menstrual cycle shows resolution of the changes, suggesting that psychological factors may be a manifestation rather than a cause of the problem. PMS is believed to be pathophysiologically distinct from dysmenorrhea, unrelated to prostaglandins, and unresponsive to nonsteroidals. It does respond rapidly to selective serotonin reuptake inhibitors (SSRIs), even when intermittently dosed during the luteal phase, supporting the importance of serotonin in the pathophysiology and a distinction from routine depression.

Symptoms, which may seriously disrupt daily activities and impair lifestyle (and must do so for PMDD to be diagnosed), include physical symptoms such as fatigue, headache, joint or muscle pain, bloating, headache, breast tenderness, or weight gain, along with psychological symptoms including irritability, food cravings, inability to concentrate, anxiety, and depression. Onset is typically 7 to 10 days before menses commence, continues through 4 days of blood flow, and is recurrent with each cycle. The diagnosis of PMS and PMDD is based on the history of symptoms and their correlation with the menstrual cycle. It is helpful to have patients keep a prospective daily chart of their symptoms and their menses for 2 or more months to assess the pattern.

Endometriosis

Endometriosis is presumed to be a common cause of secondary dysmenorrhea, although it may also be asymptomatic. Endometriosis is caused by the presence of functioning ectopic endometrial tissue, located in such places as the ovaries, uterosacral ligaments, cul de sac, and peritoneum. It occurs in 1% to 5% of reproductive women and in approximately 30% of infertile women between ages 30 and 40 years. In symptomatic women, pain can begin days or even a week before menstruation. It is usually bilateral and may radiate to the rectum or perineal region. There is frequently a history of infertility, dyspareunia, or menorrhagia. Symptoms of endometriosis depend on actively functioning endometrial tissue, with resolution at menopause. The frequency of dysmenorrhea has been found to be no different in patients with endometriosis than with normal control subjects; however, patients with extensive endometriosis (stage III or IV by laparoscopy) were more likely to have acyclic pain. Otherwise, stage of endometriosis does not affect the severity or presence of symptoms, supporting the theory that a chronic inflammatory response is responsible for the symptoms. Diagnosis of endometriosis can only be made by direct visualization of implants on laparoscopy or laparotomy, although physical findings that may suggest the disorder include tender thickening or nodularity of the uterosacral ligaments, which may cause lateral displacement of the cervix if asymmetric.

Adenomyosis

Adenomyosis is caused by the presence of functioning ectopic endometrial tissue in the myometrium. It appears to be most common in women aged 41 to 50 years. The condition can cause menorrhagia, dysmenorrhea, and an enlarged, often tender uterus, although one third of women are asymptomatic. Pain may be referred to the back and rectum. There is a slightly increased rate of endometrial carcinoma in patients with adenomyosis.

Chronic PID

Chronic PID is another source of secondary dysmenorrhea and a common cause of chronic pelvic pain in populations with a high prevalence of sexually transmitted disease. A history of previous sexually transmitted disease, dyspareunia, menstrual irregularity, backache, rectal pressure, or pelvic pain with fever is often obtained. The physical examination typically reveals tender, thickened adnexae. Bilateral involvement is characteristic, although one side may predominate.

Intrauterine Devices

Copper IUDs are an important source of secondary dysmenorrhea. Conversely, the levonorgestrel-releasing IUD is associated with a significant decrease in menorrhagia and dysmenorrhea. The rate of removal of a copper IUD because of pain and bleeding ranges from 4% to 15% within the first year. Cramping menstrual pain may occur in a woman with a newly placed IUD who has never experienced dysmenorrhea, but it usually improves within 3 to 4 months. The risk of PID does not appear to be increased with modern IUDs beyond the first several weeks after insertion.

Ovarian Cysts

Ovarian cysts are often painless unless complicated by torsion or rupture, which produces severe abdominal pain. Peripheral cysts that distend the ovarian capsule may also be painful. Chronic intermittent discomfort that is worse at the time of ovulation or in the latter half of the cycle may be seen secondary to leakage of irritant contents.

Uterine Fibroids

Uterine fibroids (leiomyomas) may produce a constant chronic ache in the pelvis or back. They may also cause urinary symptoms (increased frequency and incontinence) and bleeding, particularly when they are submucosal. Significant pain and/or obstruction of the ureters is noted usually when the uterus is larger than in 12 weeks' gestation. Severe pelvic pain and fever in a woman with a history of fibroids can suggest necrosis of the tumor.

Nongynecologic Pathology

Nongynecologic pathology may also cause chronic pelvic pain; adhesions, inflammatory bowel disease, irritable bowel syndrome, pelvic floor muscle discomfort, and interstitial cystitis are all in the differential. Of note, symptoms from irritable bowel syndrome such as pain, cramping, and change in bowel habits may also worsen in the second half of the menstrual cycle secondary to the effect of progestins on gastrointestinal motility. Interstitial cystitis, an increasingly recognized cause of chronic pelvic pain also known as painful bladder syndrome, may present with pain in the lower abdomen and dyspareunia, mimicking endometriosis. Pelvic floor muscular complaints are an increasingly recognized cause of chronic pelvic pain, present in up to 20% of women attending a chronic pelvic pain clinic.

Mittelschmerz

Mittelschmerz, or intermenstrual pain, is not a form of dysmenorrhea because it occurs in midcycle at the time of ovulation. It is more common on the right side than the left and may be accompanied by bleeding. There is some evidence that the ovary is the source of the blood loss. The pain, believed due to distention of the ovarian capsule, is harmless but annoying and a source of concern.

Enigmatic or Psychogenic Pain

The terms *enigmatic pain* and *psychogenic pain* are applied to chronic pelvic pain lasting more than 6 months without clear organic pathology. Approximately one third of laparoscopies performed for longstanding symptoms fail to reveal any pathology. Even when pathology is found, it is unclear whether it is the cause of the pain. Studies have found, for instance, that endometriosis and adhesions are as common in women without pain as in those with pain.

Numerous theories for the pain have been proposed, including pelvic vascular congestion, retrodisplacement of the uterus, and rotation of the fundus on the cervix as a universal joint (this was believed to be secondary to lacerations of the broad and cardinal ligaments from prior obstetric procedures and to cause pain because of the hypermobility of the cervix with relation to the fundus in all directions). Surgical treatments have included antefixation of a retroverted uterus, hysterectomy with or without salpingo-oophorectomy, and nerve transection procedures including presacral neurectomy and laparoscopic uterosacral nerve ablation. Although initial reports demonstrated some success with each of these techniques, most patients continued to have pain. Some studies also reported continued symptoms in patients even with total exenteration of pelvic organs, although hysterectomy does appear to be effective in relieving chronic pelvic pain in the majority of women.

Because of lack of improvement with current surgical and medical regimens and the low incidence of demonstrable pathology, attention has turned to psychogenic etiologies and treatments for patients with chronic pelvic pain. Reports have demonstrated a significant association between a childhood history of sexual abuse and chronic pelvic pain, reported in 25% of patients. Women with chronic pelvic pain have also been found to have higher rates of alcohol and drug dependency, although it is unclear whether this is in response to their chronic pain. Depression and somatization are also seen more frequently in women with chronic pelvic pain.

WORKUP

In the patient with acute pain, it is important to determine the need for immediate hospitalization. Vital signs, including temperature, and postural changes in blood pressure and pulse are essential. Physical examination should determine whether there are signs of peritoneal irritation (rigidity, percussion tenderness, rebound), presence of bowel sounds, cervical motion tenderness, or abnormal masses. Laboratory evaluation should include a *complete blood count, differential, sedimentation rate, urinalysis,* and *serum β-hCG* subunit pregnancy test. Urine hCG testing is less sensitive although highly specific; a negative *urine hCG* test within the first 6 weeks after the last menstrual period does not rule out an ectopic pregnancy.

Any patient with a high fever, orthostatic hypotension or tachycardia, or an acute abdomen should be sent immediately to the hospital, even before laboratory studies are available. However, even in an urgent situation, a few historical facts can help to establish the diagnosis. Important questions include any delay in the menstrual period, dyspareunia, IUD use, shaking chills, abnormal vaginal discharge or bleeding, recent abortion, recent sexual contacts, and the location and radiation of the pain. Development of generalized severe pain is a worrisome symptom, indicating possible peritoneal involvement, especially in conjunction with a rigid abdomen and absent bowel sounds. Unilateral pain suggests a local tubal or ovarian problem, whereas bilateral involvement is more indicative of PID or diffuse pelvic irritation. Symptoms of constipation, nausea, vomiting, diarrhea, flank pain, and dysuria need to be elicited to rule out nongynecologic etiologies such as appendicitis, acute pyelonephritis, or urethral stone.

If the pain is chronic or recurrent, a more detailed history should be obtained during the office visit, including the relationship of the pain to the menstrual cycle and a complete menstrual and obstetric history, including previous history of sexually transmitted diseases, sexual contacts, and contraception use. Onset of pain, quality and radiation of pain, and any exacerbating or ameliorating factors should be noted. Pain due to cervical, uterine, or vaginal pathology is often referred to the low back or buttock, whereas that due to tubal or ovarian problems is generally localized to one side and referred to the medial aspect of the thigh. If PMDD is suspected, patients should be asked to keep a prospective log of their symptoms for two menstrual cycles. A detailed pelvic and rectal examination should be done to look for adnexal thickening, cervical discharge, uterine masses, fixation of any structures, ovarian masses, and focal tenderness of muscles or other structures.

In addition to the tests noted earlier, *culture of the cervix* or the *rectum* for gonorrhea and chlamydia is indicated if infection is suspected. If a mass is felt, *transvaginal ultrasonography* is indicated to confirm the finding, better localize the mass, and distinguish a solid from a cystic lesion. *Laparoscopy* may be necessary to establish the diagnosis, particularly when endometriosis is suspected.

TREATMENT (5,19–34)

Acute Pelvic Pain

PID

PID may be treated on an outpatient basis if the patient is nontoxic and reliable—clinicians should have a low threshold for empiric treatment if the diagnosis is suspected. The safety and efficacy of outpatient antibiotic treatment was established in a large trial that showed no difference in short- or long-term outcomes including fertility and ectopic pregnancy. Antimicrobial regimens should include coverage for *N. gonorrhoeae* and *C. trachomatis* (see Chapter 117), as well as anaerobes and other commonly encountered organisms. Patients and their partners should be educated about safe sexual practices and the sequelae of PID to prevent subsequent infections, and partners should be empirically treated for gonorrhea and chlamydia.

Other Etiologies

Other etiologies of severe acute pelvic pain, such as *ectopic pregnancy or torsion of the fallopian tube or ovary*, are best managed by a specialist and should be referred immediately to a gynecologist. Torsion and a ruptured ectopic pregnancy require emergent surgical correction; early ectopic pregnancies are increasingly being treated medically with oral methotrexate followed by serial ultrasound and serum β-hCG measurements. Ruptured ovarian cysts may require surgery but are more typically managed expectantly with pain control.

Recurrent Pelvic Pain

Primary Dysmenorrhea

Primary dysmenorrhea can be managed symptomatically with *NSAIDs*. Lower-dose, over-the-counter formulations may be effective, although some women require higher doses or a switch to a different class of NSAID for adequate relief. Treatment is started up to 1 week before expected onset of menses and continued several days into it. Cyclooxygenase-2 inhibitors, although effective in treating dysmenorrhea, offer no benefit over traditional NSAIDs. Oral contraceptive pills (OCPs) are also effective in decreasing dysmenorrhea because they suppress ovulation, which limits the production of

arachidonic acid and thus prostaglandins in the endometrium. Women who continue to have dysmenorrhea on oral contraceptives can multicycle their pills, taking 3 to 5 months of active pills consecutively before taking the inactive pills and having menses. Initial breakthrough bleeding is more common with long cycles but usually resolves with time. OCPs and NSAIDs may be used together with good effect; women who fail to respond to this combination should be evaluated for causes of secondary dysmenorrhea. Progestins also inhibit ovulation but are less effective at reducing pain. A levonorgestrel-secreting IUD improves dysmenorrhea by up to 50% in some studies. Patient education about the mechanism of pain during menstruation may be helpful in alleviating symptoms. Locally applied heat is the best-supported nonpharmacologic intervention for dysmenorrhea and may supplement NSAIDs. There is also limited evidence to support lifestyle changes and supplements in the treatment of dysmenorrhea, with a few trials supporting a low-fat vegetarian diet, magnesium supplementation, and vitamin B supplementation, as well as exercise.

Premenstrual Syndrome/Premenopausal Dysphoric Disorder

Treatments proven effective in randomized, controlled trials and shown dramatically to reduce both the physical and psychological symptoms of PMS include the *SSRIs* and other antidepressants with serotonergic activity, along with *alprazolam (Xanax)*, which acts on γ-aminobutyric acid receptors. SSRIs are now considered first-line therapy for PMDD, with fluoxetine and sertraline the most studied. SSRIs have a more rapid onset of action than when used for depression and are effective even when therapy is limited to the luteal phase. In fact, some studies suggest that such intermittent therapy is more effective than therapy that continues through the follicular phase. There appears to be more benefit for behavioral symptoms (75% reduction) than for the physical symptoms (40% reduction). Given the hormonal basis of PMS and PMDD, it is perhaps surprising that most studies have shown no benefit to suppressing ovulation with oral contraceptives. However, two more-recent trials had modest success with use of a 24-day combined regimen containing the newer progestin drospirenone. Complete ovarian hormonal suppression by use of a *gonadotropin-releasing-hormone agonist* such as *leuprolide* ends symptoms in many PMS sufferers but is associated with long-term risks of osteoporosis. These may be mitigated by "adding back" low-dose continuous estrogen and progestin therapy. *Vitamin B_6* in doses up to 100 mg/d may reduce symptoms. Although conclusions are limited by the poor quality of most studies, a systematic review of randomized trials of vitamin B_6 suggests an odds ratio relative to placebo of overall symptom improvement of 2.32. Several randomized trials of *calcium supplementation* have demonstrated a smaller but significant effect. In one trial of more than 400 patients, symptoms were reduced by 48%, compared with 30% with placebo. Higher dietary intake of calcium and vitamin D also appear to be correlated with a lower risk of PMS. *Lifestyle changes* such as participating in regular aerobic exercise and eliminating xanthines, alcohol, and salt from the diet offer only limited improvement. PMS, unlike primary dysmenorrhea, is unresponsive to NSAID therapy.

Endometriosis

The diagnosis of this disorder is confirmed only by laparoscopy or laparotomy, and therefore it will most likely be managed by specialists. Surgical treatment with excision or ablation of visible endometriotic implants and adhesions is associated with good pain relief in the majority of women, and is considered first-line therapy for patients with severe symptoms or those who have failed to respond to medical treatment. Medical therapy of endometriosis can be highly effective, particularly for more minor symptoms. Oral contraceptive pills are an effective option for some women, particularly those with mild symptoms; they may also be used continuously or in long cycles to achieve a "pseudopregnancy" effect on the endometrial tissue. Progestin therapy inhibits endometriotic tissue growth and is effective in relieving more severe symptoms, but its oral or injectable use is associated with side effects including irregular bleeding, fluid retention, and weight gain. Such side effects may be largely avoided with use of the levonorgestrel-releasing IUD, which reduces both pelvic pain and dysmenorrhea in women with endometriosis. Danazol and GnRH agonists both inhibit gonadal function, leading to a pharmacologic menopause with excellent symptomatic relief. Danazol, an androgen derivative with progestational activity, is associated with androgenic side effects such as hirsutism, acne, and weight gain, whereas GnRH agonists typically have more hypoestrogenic side effects, such as hot flashes, osteoporosis, and vaginal dryness. "Add-back" regimens in which women are given low-dose estrogen and progesterone to prevent side effects have allowed longer-term use of these agents. In a direct, randomized trial comparing levonorgestrel IUD to GnRH agonist, both regimens resulted in equal pain relief and improvement in quality of life, with the IUD having the advantage of only a single intervention and no hypoestrogenic side effects. Combination medical and surgical therapy may be needed in some women with persistent symptoms.

Other Causes

Other causes of recurrent pelvic pain, such as IUDs, uterine fibroids, and ovarian cysts, are often managed by a gynecologist. Indications for hysterectomy for uterine fibroids are substantial bleeding, significant pelvic pain or obstruction, or anemia refractory to iron replacement.

Chronic Pelvic Pain

This problem is best managed by a combination of psychological, behavioral, and medical treatments. Primary care physicians are in a unique position to coordinate this type of therapy. Patients with chronic pain need reassurance that further diagnostic testing is unnecessary, that the physician is not abandoning them, and that there is treatment for their suffering. Psychological therapy can help to pinpoint triggers for the pain and address previous sexual trauma (if any). Behavioral therapy can help to decrease pain through relaxation techniques. Self-hypnosis may also be beneficial. Because of the frequency of concomitant depression and the known beneficial effects of the tricyclic antidepressant amitriptyline in patients with chronic pain, it may be useful to consider an antidepressant medication in some cases.

INDICATIONS FOR REFERRAL

Patients with pelvic pain and an acute abdomen should be sent immediately to the hospital with referral to a gynecologic surgeon. Women with a pelvic mass detected by physical examination should be referred, although it is helpful to obtain an ultrasound before the patient's initial visit with the gynecologist. Suspicion of chronic PID, endometriosis, adenomyosis, or other conditions best assessed by laparoscopy should prompt consultation with a gynecologist. Women with chronic pelvic pain syndrome may benefit from referral to a multimodal pain clinic, whereas those with interstitial cystitis will appreciate referral to a gynecologist or urologist experienced in managing this diagnosis.

Annotated Bibliography

1. ACOG. Technical bulletin. Chronic pelvic pain. Int J Gynaecol Obstet 1996;54:59. (*A comprehensive summary.*)
2. Beigi RH, Wiesenfeld HC. Pelvic inflammatory disease: new diagnostic criteria and treatment. Obstet Gynecol Clin North Am 2003;30:777. (*Excellent review of the importance of subclinical pelvic inflammatory disease [PID] and a discussion of etiology and treatment.*)
3. Wiesenfeld HC, Hillier SL, Krohn MA, et al. Lower genital tract infection and endometritis: insight into subclinical pelvic inflammatory disease. Obstet Gynecol 2002;100:456. (*Found a high incidence of subclinical PID in women with gonorrhea [26%] and chlamydia [27%] who reported only lower genital tract symptoms.*)
4. Scholes D, Tergachis A, Heidrich FE, et al. Prevention of pelvic inflammatory disease by screening for cervical chlamydial infection. N Engl J Med 1996;334:1362. (*The incidence of PID decreased from 18 to 8 per 10,000 woman-months when a chlamydia screening program was introduced.*)
5. Centers for Disease Control and Prevention. Sexually transmitted diseases treatment guidelines 2006. MMWR Morb Mortal Wkly Rep 2006;55 (No. RR-11). (*Treatment guidelines and diagnostic criteria for PID, emphasizing the importance of a low threshold for empiric treatment.*)
6. Grimes DA. Intrauterine device and upper-genital-tract infection. Lancet 2000;356:1013. (*Concludes that modern intrauterine devices are not associated with infection or infertility and rival tubal sterilization in efficacy.*)
7. Lipscomb GH, Stovall TG, Ling FW. Nonsurgical treatment of ectopic pregnancy. N Engl J Med 2000;343:1325. (*Reviews the safety and efficacy of methotrexate treatment of ectopic pregnancy.*)
8. Bider D, Mishiach S, Dulitzky M, et al. Clinical, surgical, and pathologic findings of adnexal torsion in pregnant and nonpregnant women. Surg Gynecol Obstet 1991;173:363. (*Case series of women with adnexal torsion at laparotomy.*)
9. French L. Dysmenorrhea. Am Family Physician 2005;71:285. (*Reviews the prevalence, pathogenesis, diagnosis, and treatment of this condition.*)
10. Dawood MY. Primary dysmenorrhea: advances in pathogenesis and management. Obstet Gynecol 2006;108:428. (*A thorough review of pathophysiology and evidence-based management, with a helpful management algorithm.*)
11. Deuster PA, Adera T, South-Paul J. Biological, social, and behavioral factors associated with premenstrual syndrome. Arch Family Med 1999;8:122. (*Prevalence in this community-based survey of women aged 18 to 44 years was 8%; associations were found with exercise, perceived stress, and alcohol consumption.*)
12. Grady-Weliky TA. Premenstrual dysphoric disorder. N Engl J Med 2003;348:433. (*Clinical review of diagnosis and treatment of this disorder.*)
13. Mortola JF. Premenstrual syndrome—pathophysiologic considerations. N Engl J Med 1998;338:256. (*An editorial summarizing current pathophysiologic understanding of premenstrual syndrome.*)
14. Schmidt PJ, Nieman LK, Danaceau MA, et al. Differential behavioral effects of gonadal steroids in women with and in those without premenstrual syndrome. N Engl J Med 1998;338:209. (*A very clever study using gonadotropin-releasing-hormone [GnRH] agonist therapy to shut down hormonal activity and then testing the effects of shutdown and replacement therapy on symptoms; showed that the suppression of activity was the only beneficial approach.*)
15. Attaran J, Falcone T, Goldberg J. Endometriosis: still tough to diagnose and treat. Cleve Clin J Med 2002;69:647. (*A useful review of treatment options.*)
16. Tu FF, As-Sanie S, Steege JF. Prevalence of pelvic musculoskeletal disorders in a female chronic pain clinic. J Reprod Med 2006;51:185. (*Found tenderness of the pelvic floor musculature in >20% of almost 1,000 women attending a chronic pelvic pain clinic.*)

17. Reiter RC. Evidence-based management of chronic pelvic pain. Clin Obstet Gynecol 1998;41:422. (*A superb review.*)
18. Walker E, Koton W, Harrop Griffiths J, et al. Relationship of chronic pelvic pain to psychiatric diagnoses and childhood sexual abuse. Am J Psychiatry 1988;145:75. (*Comparison study of women with chronic pelvic pain and women undergoing laparoscopy for infertility or tubal ligation for rates of sexual abuse, depression, alcohol, and drug use.*)
19. Ness RB, Soper DE, Helley RL, et al. Effectiveness of inpatient and out-patient treatment strategies for women with pelvic inflammatory disease: results from the Pelvic Inflammatory Disease Evaluation and Clinical Health (PEACH) randomized trial. Am J Obstet Gynecol 2002;186:929. (*No difference was found in short-term or long-term outcomes including pregnancy rates, PID recurrence, ectopic pregnancy, and chronic pelvic pain in 831 women randomized to inpatient vs. outpatient treatment of PID.*)
20. Ness RB, Trautmann G, Richter HE, et al. Effectiveness of treatment strategies of some women with pelvic inflammatory disease: a randomized trial. Obstet Gynecol 2005;106:573. (*An additional 4 years of long-term follow-up in the PEACH trial, to a mean of 84 months, found no difference in outcomes including pregnancies, live births or ectopic pregnancy, infertility, PID recurrence, or chronic pelvic pain.*)
21. Dingfelder JR. Prostaglandin inhibitors: new treatment for an old nemesis. N Engl J Med 1982;307:746. (*An editorial examining the pathophysiology and treatment of primary dysmenorrhea, with emphasis on prostaglandins.*)
22. Marjoribanks J, Proctor ML, Farquhar C. Nonsteroidal anti-inflammatory drugs for primary dysmenorrhoea. Cochrane Database Syst Rev 2003;(4):CD001751. (*A Cochrane analysis that found nonsteroidal antiinflammatory drugs [NSAIDs] to be effective in the treatment of dysmenorrhea, with insufficient evidence to determine which individual NSAID is the safest and most effective.*)
23. Baldaszti E, Wimmer-Puchinger B, Loschke K. Acceptability of the long-term contraceptive levonorgestrel-releasing intrauterine system (Mirena): a 3 year follow-up study. Contraception 2003;67:87. (*Found a 50% reduction in dysmenorrhea with the use of the Mirena intrauterine device.*)
24. Wyatt K, Dimmock P, Jones P, et al. Efficacy of progesterone and progestogens in management of premenstrual syndrome: systematic review. BMJ 2001;323:776. (*A meta-analysis indicating that progesterone and progestins do not have a clinically significant effect.*)
25. Wood SH, Mortola JF, Chan YF, et al. Treatment of premenstrual syndrome with fluoxetine: a double-blind, placebo-controlled, crossover study. Obstet Gynecol 1992;80:339. (*A well-controlled study demonstrating significant reduction [62%] in both physical and psychological symptoms with fluoxetine.*)
26. Young SA, Hurt PH, Benedek DM, et al. Treatment of premenstrual dysphoric disorder with sertraline during the luteal phase: a randomized, double-blind, placebo-controlled crossover trial. J Clin Psychiatry 1998;59:76. (*Demonstrated the effectiveness of a selective serotonin reuptake inhibitor when limited to luteal phase.*)
27. Muse KN, Cetel NS, Futterman LA, et al. The premenstrual syndrome: effects of "medical ovariectomy." N Engl J Med 1984;311:1345. (*An intriguing double-blind, placebo-controlled study showing that the use of an experimental GnRH agonist is effective in providing symptomatic relief.*)
28. Yonkers KA, Brown C, Pearlstein TB et al. Efficacy of a new low-dose oral contraceptive with drospirenone in premenstrual dysphoric disorder. Obstet Gynecol 2005;106:492. (*A randomized, multicenter, double-blind trial including 450 women, showing a decrease in daily symptom scores by at least 50% in 48% of the treatment group vs. 36% of the placebo group.*)
29. Wyatt KM, Dimmock PW, Jones PW, et al. Efficacy of vitamin B6 in the treatment of premenstrual syndrome: systematic review. BMJ 1999;318:1375. (*Overall symptoms and depressive symptoms showed improvement.*)
30. Thys-Jacobs S, Starkey P, Bernstein D, et al. Calcium carbonate and the premenstrual syndrome: effects on premenstrual and menstrual symptoms. Am J Obstet Gynecol 1998;179:444. (*Calcium in a dose of 1,200 mg/d reduced symptoms by 48%; placebo reduced symptoms by 30%.*)
31. Petta CA, Ferriani RA, Abrao MS, et al. Randomized clinical trial of a levonorgestrel-releasing intrauterine system and a depot GnRH analogue for the treatment of chronic pelvic pain in women with endometriosis. Hum Reprod 2005;20:1993. (*A multicenter, randomized trial in 82 women found significant improvement in pelvic pain with both forms of treatment, with no difference between the groups except in the frequency of bleeding, which was more in the IUD group, and hypoestrogenic effects, which was more common in the GnRH group.*)
32. Bahamondes L, Petta CA, Fernandes A, et al. Use of the levonorgestrel-releasing intrauterine system in women with endometriosis, chronic pelvic pain, and dysmenorrhea. Contraception 2007;75:S134. (*A review of the literature found improvement in pelvic pain, dysmenorrhea, and bleeding in all nine studies identified, suggesting that the levonorgestrel IUD is an effective alternative medical treatment, but emphasized the need for longer-term, controlled studies.*)
33. Carlson KJ, Nichols DH, Schiff I, et al. Indications for hysterectomy. N Engl J Med 1993;328:856. (*Discussion of the indications for hysterectomy, including uterine leiomyomas, endometriosis, and chronic pelvic pain.*)
34. Peters AAW, Van Dorst E, Jellis B, et al. A randomized clinical trial to compare two different approaches in women with chronic pelvic pain. Obstet Gynecol 1991;77:740. (*Study showing the efficacy of an integrated approach to patients with chronic pelvic pain by addressing psychological, dietary, and environmental factors in addition to somatic complaints.*)

CHAPTER 117 ■ APPROACH TO THE PATIENT WITH A VAGINAL DISCHARGE

SHANA L. BIRNBAUM

Vaginal discharge is one of the most common reasons that women consult physicians in office practice in the United States, with more than 10 million office visits per year. Most women experience at least one episode of vaginitis in her lifetime, and more than half face recurrent symptoms. Vaginal infections not only are extremely prevalent, but also result in considerable discomfort for symptomatic patients. Some vaginal infections put women at risk for upper genital tract disease and complications of a concurrent pregnancy. A history, a systematic examination of the vulva, vagina, and cervix, and a microscopic examination of the discharge enable one to identify the cause in most cases and choose the appropriate therapy. Patient education can help to allay fears, encourage compliance, and reduce recurrences.

PATHOPHYSIOLOGY AND CLINICAL PRESENTATION (1–10)

Normal vaginal discharge occurs in a quantity of 1 to 4 cm^3 per 24 hours and contains desquamated vaginal epithelial cells, secretions from cervical glands and from the uterus, and bacteria and bacterial products, including lactic acid. Under the

TABLE 117.1

COMMON CAUSES OF VAGINAL DISCHARGE

Infectious
- Bacterial vaginosis
- Vulvovaginal candidiasis
- *Trichomonas vaginitis*
- Mucopurulent cervicitis (*Chlamydia trachomatis*)
- Gonorrhea
- Condyloma acuminata
- Herpesvirus type 2
- Cytolytic vaginosis

Normal Discharge Secondary to Hormonal Changes
- Physiologic leucorrhea (midcycle cervical mucus/postintercourse)
- Atrophic vaginitis

Other
- Chemical/allergic vaginitis, foreign body
- Desquamative inflammatory vaginitis
- Erosive lichen planus
- Chronic cervicitis
- Cervical ectropion
- Cervical polyps
- Cervical and endometrial cancer
- Collagen vascular diseases

microscope, the vaginal microflora of healthy, asymptomatic women appear as moderate numbers of unclumped, rodlike organisms. These consist of a wide variety of anaerobic and aerobic bacterial genera and species dominated by *Lactobacillus*. The pH of a normal vagina in a reproductive-aged woman is between 4 and 4.5. The delicately balanced vaginal environment is easily altered by numerous internal and external influences. The amount or quality of vaginal discharge can be affected by normal changes in the body's hormonal milieu, such as midcycle mucus production with ovulation, menstruation, or the atrophic mucosal changes that occur after menopause.

The most common cause of an abnormal discharge is infection with yeast, *Trichomonas*, or the polymicrobial anaerobic overgrowth syndrome termed bacterial vaginosis (Table 117.1). Infections with organisms such as *Candida albicans* and *Trichomonas vaginalis* generally induce an inflammatory response in the vaginal wall, which is accompanied by an increased number of leukocytes in the vaginal fluid, so-called "vaginitis." The most common infection causing vaginal discharge is noninflammatory *bacterial vaginosis*, responsible for 40% to 50% of vaginal infection, followed closely by vulvovaginal candidiasis (20% to 25%) and finally trichomoniasis, which occurs less frequently (15% to 20%). The clinical presentation, including type, amount, and odor of discharge, depends in part on the underlying etiologic agent. However, the history and the physical examination do not reliably distinguish among etiologic agents, and office microscopy, potentially with a formal laboratory culture, is generally required for an accurate diagnosis and treatment.

Trichomoniasis

Trichomoniasis occurs in approximately 3 million women annually. *T. vaginalis*, a small, mobile protozoan, is not part of normal vaginal flora. It is sexually transmitted and frequently occurs in the presence of other infections. It occurs in 13% to 25% of women attending gynecologic clinics and 7% to 35% of women attending clinics for sexually transmitted diseases. It is more common in African Americans, clusters with other sexually transmitted diseases, and appears to be seen more frequently in older women. Although sexual contact is the primary mode of transmission, *T. vaginalis* can survive in hot tubs, tap water, and chlorinated swimming pools. Its sexual transmission is supported by the high prevalence (30% to 70%) in male partners of infected women and the improved cure rates of infected women whose partners are also treated. Fewer than 20% of men with *T. vaginalis* in their urine are symptomatic, and the infection may be self-limited; those that do have symptoms present with urethritis. A substantial percentage of women with trichomoniasis (10% to 50%) are also asymptomatic, but one third of asymptomatic infected women become symptomatic within 6 months.

Symptoms include a thin, malodorous discharge, pruritus, dyspareunia (caused by vulvar edema), dysuria, and increased frequency of micturition. Physical examination generally reveals vulvar erythema and edema and, occasionally, characteristic petechial hemorrhages of the external genitalia and cervix (strawberry cervix is seen by the naked eye in only 1% to 2% of patients). Vaginal discharge may be minimal or abundant, frothy, and foul smelling. Signs and symptoms alone are not sufficiently helpful to make the definitive diagnosis.

Candidiasis

Candidiasis is very common in the vagina, seen in up to half of asymptomatic women in some studies. In one private practice study, the incidence of candidiasis was 8.5%, and of these individuals, 25% were asymptomatic. In women with symptoms, complaints include vulvar pruritus and burning associated with a discharge. Symptoms are usually rather rapid in onset, classically occurring shortly before menstruation when the pH of the vagina falls. Some women are prone to vulvovaginal candidiasis after treatment with systemic antibiotics. Uncontrolled diabetes also predisposes to candidal infections, as does HIV, although usually at a more advanced stage with serious immune dysfunction. On physical examination, erythema, edema, and excoriation of the vulva are often prominent; sometimes there are pustules apparent on the skin. The discharge is typically thick, white, and adherent, often described as resembling cottage cheese.

Bacterial Vaginosis

Bacterial vaginosis, previously referred to as *Gardnerella* vaginitis or "nonspecific vaginitis," can be asymptomatic in up to 50% of women. It is the most common clinical vaginitis and occurs when the normal lactobacillus, which produces hydrogen peroxide and keeps the vaginal pH acidic, is overgrown by other components of vaginal flora, typically anaerobes such as *Gardnerella* or *Mycoplasma*. Although it is not sexually transmitted, it is more common in women with multiple or new partners and also has a high prevalence in women who have sex with women. Other risk factors are douching, intrauterine device use, and smoking. The clinical picture tends to be one of mild discomfort without significant erythema or inflammation, although in 10% to 20% of cases the vaginal burning and itching are more pronounced. Often, patients note a disagreeable "fishy" odor, particularly after unprotected intercourse. The discharge ranges from grayish to occasionally a yellow-green color. Wet mount of the discharge shows short, motile rods and characteristic *clue cells* (vaginal epithelial cells with a stippled appearance due to the adherence of bacilli on their surfaces). The diagnosis of bacterial vaginosis is made by the presence of three of the four following criteria: vaginal pH greater than 4.5; thin, gray-white, homogeneous discharge; positive amine test (fishy odor on exposure to potassium oxide [KOH]); and clue cells on saline wet prep.

Several other infectious etiologies need to be considered in the differential diagnosis of a vaginal discharge. *Mucopurulent cervicitis* caused by *Chlamydia trachomatis* or *Neisseria gonorrhoeae* (also covered in Chapter 137) is characterized by a thick, yellow-white discharge coming from the cervical os, which may be confused with a true vaginitis. Patients may complain of pruritis, purulent discharge, dysuria, or frequency, and occasionally postcoital bleeding, although pain is usually absent unless upper tract infection is present. Generally 10 or more leukocytes per microscopic field (high-power oil immersion) are seen on Gram stain examination. Erythema, friability, and ectocervical ulceration may occur. In *type 2 herpesvirus* (see Chapter 192), the infection can extend to the cervix in 75% of cases, producing ulceration, friability, and a grayish exudate in conjunction with a profuse watery discharge. In severe cases, *condyloma acuminata*, genital warts caused by papillomavirus, can cause a profuse, irritating vaginal discharge (see Chapter 194).

Atrophic Vaginitis

Atrophic vaginitis is the most common cause of vaginal discharge in older postmenopausal women and may also occur in younger woman with a hypoestrogenic state, such as postpartum or during lactation. Among postmenopausal women attending a vaginitis clinic in one study, a defined diagnosis of *T. vaginalis, C. albicans,* or bacterial vaginosis could be made in only one third of cases. Estrogen deficiency leads to thinning of the vaginal epithelium with a decrease in glycogen stores, contributing to a decline in *Lactobacillus* species and subsequent reduction in lactic acid production. The vaginal pH increases to up to 7.0, and vaginal flora changes from those listed to streptococci, coliform bacteria, and gut anaerobes; superinfection occurs more commonly in this environment. Symptoms include vaginal and vulvar burning and soreness, occasional bleeding or itching, and dyspareunia. External burning on urination is sometimes noted, resulting from localized irritation of raw and inflamed mucosa rather than from infection of the urinary tract. Examination of the vaginal mucosa reveals a thin, erythematous surface and scant watery discharge.

Other Causes

A variety of other processes cause vaginal discharge less frequently. A syndrome termed *cytolytic vaginosis* was described in the early 1990s as an overgrowth of lactobacilli causing hyperacidity with cytolysis of vaginal epithelium and a frothy white discharge. Symptoms were similar to those of a candidal infection, including dyspareunia, vulvar pruritus, white vaginal discharge, and dysuria. Other experts have not confirmed the existence of such a syndrome. *Lichen planus* is an idiopathic inflammatory mucocutaneous disease that may cause a desquamative vaginitis. Another desquamative inflammatory vaginitis, common in perimenopausal women and characterized by replacement of lactobacilli with gram-positive cocci, has been described and is responsive to clindamycin suppositories. Certain *collagen vascular diseases* can also produce a

type of vaginal inflammation and discharge. *Chronic cervicitis* can result from extensive chronic cervical inflammation and has been implicated in the pathogenesis of cervical eversion, squamous metaplasia, basal cell hyperplasia, leukoplakia, polyps, and carcinoma. The discharge is thick, tenacious, and yellowish white, and may be streaked with blood. Cervical inspection reveals edematous, grossly inflamed, and friable tissue. *Cervical ectropion* is found in 15% to 20% of healthy young women. It represents columnar epithelium that is found farther out on the exocervix, causing the cervix to appear granular and red. An increase in a nonirritating vaginal discharge consisting of mucus can be seen with a large ectropion.

DIFFERENTIAL DIAGNOSIS (1–7)

The most common cause of an abnormal vaginal discharge in women of childbearing age is infection. If an infectious etiology is not identified, other causes must be considered, including hormonal changes, allergens, and foreign bodies. The most common irritants are intrauterine devices; condoms; spermicidal foams, jellies, and creams; deodorants; sprays; soaps; and any chemical douches. Foreign bodies include forgotten tampons, condoms, diaphragms, and intrauterine devices. Some vaginal discharge is expected after conization or cauterization. Cervical polyps, uterine fibroids, and neoplasms of the vulva, vagina, uterus, ovaries, or fallopian tubes may all produce abnormal discharge (Table 117.1).

WORKUP (1–6,8–13)

History

History should include the onset of the discharge, its appearance, amount, odor (if any), and any associated symptoms. The relation of the discharge to phase of menstrual cycle, coitus, and use of medication (especially antibiotics) should be noted. Details about associated symptoms such as dysuria, pruritus, pain, dyspareunia, and skin rash provide additional information. Use of a pad or a tampon can be a precipitating factor or a sign of excessive discharge. Asking the patient for a detailed sexual history aids in understanding whether she is at particular risk for any infections; useful information includes possible exposure to sexually transmitted diseases and whether the patient's partner has a complaint of penile discharge or lesion. Known allergies need to be reviewed in conjunction with the use of spermicidal preparations and douches. Patients should be asked about the use of foreign bodies and bubble baths, soaps, or genital deodorants. A history of a previous vaginal infection, diabetes, or the recent use of antibiotics or corticosteroids needs to be considered in a search for alterations in vaginal flora or host defenses. Any self-treatment should be carefully inquired about because antifungal medication is now readily available over the counter. Women with chronic or recurrent discharge also turn to a wide range of alternative treatments, including oral and vaginal acidophilus pills, oral and vaginal yogurt, and douches with vinegar and boric acid. These self-remedies may complicate diagnosis and management.

Physical Examination

Physical examination begins with careful inspection of the vulva and vaginal canal for evidence of lesions, discharge, erythema, atrophy, or prolapse. During the speculum examination, the surface of the cervix should be examined carefully, looking for any lesions, erosion, erythema, or friability. The color, consistency, pH, and odor of the discharge can provide useful clues to the etiology. On bimanual examination, the provider should check for cervical motion tenderness and adnexal and uterine masses.

Laboratory Studies

A *wet-mount examination* of the discharge is simple and potentially diagnostic. A fresh sample is placed on a microscopic slide to which a drop or two of normal saline is added, and a cover slip is placed over the suspension. The pH should be tested and the slide examined before the sample dries and trichomonads lose motility. Although the sensitivity of the wet mount for the detection of the motile, ovoid trichomonads is low (25% to 50%), the finding is very specific and permits immediate diagnosis. The pH for *Trichomonas* is usually greater than 5.0. Although Gram and Giemsa stains show no advantage to wet mount, cultures have a sensitivity of up to 95% for the presence of trichomonads. They are often seen on conventional Papanicolaou smears, but with a sensitivity of only 60% to 70% and frequent false positives; the finding should be confirmed with culture in asymptomatic women. However, the specificity of liquid-based cervical cytology in detecting *Trichomonas* is much higher, at 99%, with a 96% positive predictive value, making treatment of asymptomatic woman with trichomonads reasonable without culture. Two point-of-care tests for trichomoniasis have been approved by the U.S. Food and Drug Administration and may be helpful in areas where microscopy is not available. The OSOM Trichomonas Rapid Test detects *Trichomonas* antigens in vaginal secretions, yielding results in 10 minutes with a sensitivity of 88% and a specificity of greater than 98%, and the Affirm VP III nucleic acid probe test evaluates vaginal secretions for *T. vaginalis*, *Gardnerella vaginalis*, and *C. albicans*, yielding results in 45 minutes, also with a higher sensitivity than microscopy and a specificity of greater than 97%.

Saline wet mounts of patients with bacterial vaginosis characteristically show few polymorphonuclear neutrophils and many (>20%) clue cells. Two additional diagnostic criteria for bacterial vaginosis are a sample pH higher than 4.5 and a positive amine test (the presence of a "fishy odor" after adding KOH to a sample).

Adding a drop of *10% KOH* to a sample of the discharge also aids in the recognition of *Candida*. The KOH dissolves most cellular material except for the filamentous hyphae and budding forms of *Candida*; the sensitivity of the test ranges from 40% to 80%. Gram stain has higher sensitivity for the detection of *Candida*. The vaginal pH with a candidal infection is closer to normal. Vaginal cultures for *Candida* are not necessary if microscopy is positive but should be done if microscopy is negative and presentation is suggestive of *Candida* and in women with recurrent or persistent symptoms. Self-diagnosis of candidal vulvovaginitis is unreliable; only approximately one third of women with self-diagnosed infections actually have evidence of candidal infection. When other causes of vaginal discharge, such as gonorrhea and chlamydia, are being considered, a Gram stain of the discharge can yield additional information (see Chapters 125 and 137), including the presence of leukocytes. Further suspicion of chlamydia or gonorrhea infection should be followed up with a nucleic acid amplification test or culture.

A few other laboratory studies may be helpful. If pelvic pain is present, a *complete blood count* evaluates for pelvic inflammatory disease. *Urinalysis* should be obtained to check for pyuria and bacteriuria, especially if there is concurrent dysuria or flank pain. Women with poorly controlled and, occasionally, new-onset diabetes mellitus can present with persistent or recurrent yeast infections, and a fasting *blood sugar* may be useful.

MANAGEMENT (14–25)

Trichomonal Vaginitis

Metronidazole or tinidazole in a single oral 2-g dose is the treatment of choice for trichomoniasis (Table 117.2), with cure rates of 90% to 95% when male partners are treated concurrently. An alternative regimen is metronidazole 500 mg orally twice daily for 7 days, which has similar cure rates but lower

---

TABLE 117.2

TREATMENT FOR COMMON VAGINAL INFECTIONS

Infection	Medication	Dosage
Candida	Butoconazole (Femstat)	Suppository, vaginal tablet, or cream for 1–7 d
	Clotrimazole (Mycelex)	Suppository, vaginal tablet, or cream for 1–7 d
	Miconazole (Monistat)	Suppository, vaginal tablet, or cream for 1–7 d
	Terconazole (Terazol)	Suppository, vaginal tablet, or cream for 1–7 d
	Tioconazole (Vagistat)	Suppository, vaginal tablet, or cream for 1–7 d
	Nystatin	Suppository or cream for 7–14 d
	Fluconazole	150 mg orally for single dose; can repeat every 72 hr for two or three doses for complicated infections
Bacterial vaginosis	Metronidazole	500 mg PO bid for 7 d
	Metronidazole 0.75% gel	5 g (one applicator full) daily for 5 days
	Clindamycin	300 mg PO bid for 7 d or 100-mg ovules intravaginally at bedtime for 3 nights
Trichomonas	Metronidazole	2-g PO single dose or 500 mg PO bid for 7 d
	Tinidazole	2-g PO single dose

Includes treatment of initial episodes only. For recurrent infections, see text. bid, twice daily; PO, orally.

compliance. Topical vaginal therapy with metronidazole gel is considerably less effective, with cure rates of less than 50%. Alternative topical regimens also have cure rates of less than 50%, and the Centers for Disease Control and Prevention (CDC) recommend metronidazole desensitization for those patients with a true allergy. Recommended therapy for treatment failure with the 2-g dose of oral metronidazole is an additional 1-week treatment with metronidazole (500 mg twice a day) or a single 2-g dose of tinidazole. For patients who fail one of those regimens, dosing regimens of either metronidazole or tinidazole 2 g every day for 5 days may be considered. Patients should be instructed to avoid alcohol for 24 hours after metronidazole therapy and 72 hours after tinidazole treatment because of their disulfiram-like effects. Other side effects include nausea and transient neutropenia. Meta-analyses have not found an association between metronidazole exposure during pregnancy and birth defects, and the drug is safe to use during pregnancy. A one-time oral dose of 2.0 g is generally recommended. Although the presence of vaginal *Trichomonas* during pregnancy has been associated with perinatal morbidity, it does not appear that treatment with metronidazole improves outcomes; some trials even suggest an increase in preterm labor. Because of these findings, some experts do not treat asymptomatic women during pregnancy.

Candidal Vaginitis

In considering treatment for candidal vaginitis, precipitants such as poorly controlled diabetes or the use of broad-spectrum antibiotics, oral contraceptives, or corticosteroids need to be addressed. Oral and intravaginal agents are equally effective for treatment of episodic, uncomplicated vulvovaginal candidiasis (cure rates 80% to 90%), and choice of treatment should be influenced by patient preference and cost. Most patients prefer the convenience of oral therapy, despite a slightly longer time to symptom relief. The U.S. Food and Drug Administration has approved fluconazole in a 150-mg tablet for single-dose treatment of yeast vaginitis; it maintains therapeutic levels in vaginal secretions for 72 hours and tends to have minimal side effects. Because fluconazole is available in a generic form, it is often less expensive than over-the-counter topical regimens of miconazole, clotrimazole, butaconazole, and tioconazole, all available in 3- and 7-day formulations, with some higher-strength, single-dose formulations also available. Symptomatic relief of vulvar irritation can be obtained by using witch hazel compresses or cool water and recovery hastened by application of nystatin or a synthetic imidazole cream directly to the vulva. Treatment of male partners is not necessary.

About 10% to 20% of women are classified as having complicated vulvovaginal candidiasis, based on severe symptoms, non-*albicans* candidiasis, host factors such as immunosuppression, poorly controlled diabetes, pregnancy, or recurrent vulvovaginal candidiasis (four or more episodes a year). For women with severe disease or an underlying debilitating medical condition, longer courses of therapy are often necessary (e.g., 7 to 14 days of topical therapy or oral fluconazole every third day for two or three doses). The lower-dose topical azole therapies applied for 7 days are recommended during pregnancy when oral medications are contraindicated. For infection with non-*albicans Candida*, particularly *C. glabrata*, treatment options include longer courses of topical agents or intravaginal boric acid, 600 mg in a gelatin capsule, administered daily for 2 weeks.

Recurrent vulvovaginal candidiasis may occur in certain genetically predisposed women, but obvious risk factors are usually absent. Each individual episode may be treated as for uncomplicated candidiasis, but some experts recommend a longer course of treatment (e.g., 7 to 14 days of topical therapy or oral fluconazole every third day for three doses), followed by antifungal maintenance regimens. Prophylactic treatment has been achieved with fluconazole 100, 150, or 200 mg weekly for 6 months. Clotrimazole vaginal suppositories, 500 mg used weekly, are an effective alternative. Unfortunately, 30% to 50% of women have recurrent candidiasis after stopping antifungal therapy. When infection is related to menstruation, 100-mg clotrimazole vaginal suppositories nightly for several days preceding menstruation may be effective.

Bacterial Vaginosis

The best results for treatment of bacterial vaginosis have occurred with *metronidazole* therapy with a usual oral dose of 500 mg twice daily for 7 days. Metronidazole intravaginal gel 0.75% for a 5-day daily (5 g) treatment is equally effective and has fewer systemic side effects. A single dose of 2 g of metronidazole is less effective and is no longer recommended by the CDC. If there are contraindications or side effects to metronidazole use, oral (300 mg twice daily for 7 days) or topical (100-mg ovules intravaginally for 3 nights) *clindamycin* is an alternative. Treatment of the sexual partner is not indicated. There has been significant controversy surrounding the treatment of asymptomatic bacterial vaginosis during pregnancy and a possible link to preterm labor. The majority of studies have shown a decreased risk of preterm labor after treatment of bacterial vaginosis in pregnant women at high risk for preterm labor, but no study supports a benefit to treatment in average-risk women. Given these data, many obstetricians choose to screen women who have had previous preterm births for bacterial vaginosis during pregnancy and treat asymptomatic infection with oral metronidazole (500 mg twice daily or 250 mg three times daily for 7 days) or clindamycin (300 mg twice daily for 7 days).

Mucopurulent Cervicitis

Mucopurulent cervicitis results from *chlamydia* or *gonorrhea*, and both should be treated unless culture or nucleic acid amplification test documents the absence of coinfection. Chlamydia responds to *doxycycline* (100 mg twice a day for 7 days) or *azithromycin* (1 g orally in a single dose, preferred when compliance is an issue). Ofloxacin and levofloxacin (300 mg twice daily and 500 mg once daily, respectively, for 7 days) are equally effective but more expensive. Gonorrhea should be treated with an intramuscular or oral cephalosporin (ceftriaxone, 125 mg intramuscularly, ×1; cefixime, 400 mg orally, ×1); quinolones are no longer recommended, given the rapid spread of quinolone-resistant gonorrhea in the United States. Treatment of the partner is crucial, and patients should be advised to abstain from intercourse for 7 days after single-dose treatment of cervicitis.

Atrophic Vaginitis

An over-the-counter vaginal moisturizer (e.g., Replens) can be used regularly for symptom relief, along with a water-soluble lubricant during intercourse, but this will not reverse the atrophic changes. *Low-dose topical estrogen* does work to restore mucosal layers of squamous epithelium in women who do not achieve adequate improvement with moisturizers. A

Cochrane review found similar efficacy to the different estrogen delivery systems, including the vaginal ring (the lowest-dose option, releasing 6 to 9 μg of estradiol daily), creams (0.5-g conjugated estrogen cream daily for 1 to 2 weeks, followed by maintenance therapy at 1 to 2 days/wk), or suppositories (a 25-μg estradiol suppository is the lowest dose available in the United States, used twice weekly). Preference trials show that the majority of women prefer the convenience of the ring, which is changed every 3 months. Systemic absorption, measured by endometrial thickness, is minimal with all of these low-dose treatment options.

PATIENT EDUCATION AND INDICATIONS FOR REFERRAL

Patient education is important whether the vaginal discharge is caused by normal physiologic changes, an infection, or a noninfectious process. All women should be educated about hormonal changes and their effect on the presence and appearance of normal physiologic vaginal discharge. Most infectious causes of vaginal discharge, except for bacterial vaginosis and candidiasis, are known to be sexually transmitted. Patients with discharge caused by *Trichomonas*, *Chlamydia*, or *N. gonorrhoeae* should be given information about the need for examination and concurrent treatment of partners and the role of barrier methods of contraception in the prevention of these infections. Women with recurrent yeast infections should be advised to avoid nylon underwear, panty hose, wet bathing suits, and tight pants.

All patients with vaginitis, especially allergic vaginitis, should be advised to avoid douches, irritant soaps, bubble baths, and genital deodorants. Patient education about personal hygiene is important. Often the patient's vulvar and vaginal discomfort is relieved after a few days of treatment, yet the patient should be encouraged to complete the treatment course and to abstain from intercourse during treatment to prevent recurrence or further irritation.

Referral for a biopsy is needed for any patient with suspicious cervical or vaginal lesions, especially if there are erosions and ulcerations that fail to clear with treatment of a known pathogen. Women with resistant or recurrent episodes of vulvovaginitis may also benefit from referral to a gynecologist with a particular competence in such disorders.

Annotated Bibliography

1. Mitchell H. Vaginal discharge—causes, diagnosis, and treatment. BMJ 2004;328:1306. (*A superb concise review.*)
2. Sobel JD. Vaginitis. N Engl J Med 1997;337:1896. (*A comprehensive and practical review.*)
3. Cleveland A. Vaginitis: finding the cause prevents treatment failure. Cleve Clin J Med 2000;67:634. (*A practical approach to office diagnosis.*)
4. Carr PL, Felsenstein D, Friedman RH. Evaluation and management of vaginitis. J Gen Intern Med 1998;13:335. (*An excellent comprehensive review with 119 references.*)
5. Kent H. Epidemiology of vaginitis. Am J Obstet Gynecol 1991;165:1168. (*Epidemiology of candidiasis, bacterial vaginosis, and trichomoniasis in the United States and Scandinavia.*)
6. Say JP, Jacyntho C. Difficult-to-manage vaginitis. Clin Obstet Gynecol 2005; 48:753. (*A thorough review of the topic, including less common diagnoses.*)
7. Hampton T. High prevalence of lesser-known STDs. JAMA 2006;295:2467. (*A brief review of a Centers for Disease Control and Prevention [CDC] report on 1,300 women attending sexually transmitted disease clinics in three cities, finding that 13% of the women became infected with Trichomonas, with incidence among black women four times higher than that among white women.*)
8. Redondo-Lopez V, Cook RL, Sobel JD. Emerging role of lactobacilli in the control and maintenance of the vaginal bacterial microflora. Rev Infect Dis 1990;12:856. (*Examines the interaction between lactobacilli and other bacterial species and the maintenance of normal vaginal flora.*)
9. Spinillo A, Bernuzzi AM, Cevini C, et al. The relationship of bacterial vaginosis, Candida and Trichomonas infection to symptomatic vaginitis in postmenopausal women attending a vaginitis clinic. Maturitas 1997;27:253. (*The three common infectious etiologies were responsible for symptoms in only one third of cases.*)
10. Faro S. Bacterial vaginitis. Clin Obstet Gynecol 1991;34:582. (*Bacterial vaginitis has a significant effect on the number of office visits per year, a woman's psychosocial well-being, and the development of subsequent obstetric/gynecologic infections.*)
11. Anderson MR, Klink K, Cohrssen A. Evaluation of vaginal complaints. JAMA 2004;291:1368. (*An absence of itching makes candidiasis unlikely; a lack of odor makes bacterial vaginosis unlikely; microscopy of the discharge is most helpful.*)
12. Landers DV, Wiesenfeld HC, Heine RP, et al. Predictive value of the clinical diagnosis of lower genital tract infection in women. Am J Obstet Gynecol 2004;190:1004. (*Discusses the limitations of signs, symptoms, and microbiologic diagnosis.*)
13. Krieger JN, Tam MR, Stevens CE, et al. Diagnosis of trichomoniasis. JAMA 1988;259:1223. (*Includes data on the sensitivity and the specificity of wet mount, cytologic study, and antibody testing.*)
14. Nyirjesy P, Weitz MV, Grody MH, et al. Over-the-counter and alternative medicines in the treatment of chronic vaginal symptoms. Obstet Gynecol 1997;90:50. (*Use is common, often when specifically treatable etiologies are present and often without the physician's knowledge.*)
15. Ferri DG, Nyirjesy P, Sobel JD, et al. Over-the-counter antifungal drug misuse associated with patient-diagnosed vulvovaginal candidiasis. Obstet Gynecol 2002;99:419. (*Only one third of women with self-diagnosed disease had evidence of candidal infection; missed diagnoses included bacterial vaginosis, mixed vaginitis, normal flora, and Trichomonas.*)
16. Caro-Paton T, Carvajal A, Martin de Diego I, et al. Is metronidazole teratogenic? A meta-analysis. Br J Clin Pharmacol 1997;44:179. (*Did not find a relationship between first-trimester exposure and birth defects.*)
17. Watson MC, Grimshaw JM, Bond CM, et al. Oral versus intravaginal imidazole and triazole anti-fungal treatment of uncomplicated vulvovaginal candidiasis (thrush). Cochrane Database Syst Rev 2001;CD 002845. (*A meta-analysis of 17 randomized, controlled trials, showing similar efficacy of oral and intravaginal antifungals; see http://www.cochrane.org for updates.*)
18. Sobel JD, Kapernick PS, Zervos M, et al. Treatment of complicated Candida vaginitis: comparison of single and sequential doses of fluconazole. Am J Obstet Gynecol 2001;185:363. (*Superior clinical and mycologic response was found with sequential dosing in a randomized trial comparing a single dose of fluconazole with two doses given 3 days apart.*)
19. Leitich H, Bodner-Adler B, Brunbauer M, et al. Bacterial vaginosis as a risk factor for preterm delivery: a meta-analysis. Am J Obstet Gynecol 2003; 189:139. (*A meta-analysis showing a twofold higher risk of preterm birth in women with bacterial vaginosis and a possible increased rate of miscarriage.*)
20. McDonald H, Brocklehurst P, Parsons J, et al. Antibiotics for treating bacterial vaginosis in pregnancy. Cochrane Database Syst Rev 2005;CD000262. (*Detection and treatment of bacterial vaginosis during pregnancy in women with a history of preterm delivery appeared to lower the rate of recurrent preterm delivery.*)
21. Livengood CH, Soper DE, Sheehan KL, et al. Comparison of once-daily and twice-daily dosing of 0. 5% metronidazole gel in the treatment of bacterial vaginosis. Sex Transm Dis 1999;26:137. (*Once-daily dosing was equally effective in this randomized trial.*)
22. Suckling J, Lethaby A, Kennedy R. Local oestrogen for vaginal atrophy in post-menopausal women. Cochrane Database Syst Rev 2003;CD001500. (*A review of 15 randomized trials found no difference among delivery methods of local estrogen, although there was patient preference for the vaginal ring.*)
23. Naessen T, Rodriguez-Macias K. Endometrial thickness and uterine diameter not affected by ultra-low doses of 17beta-estradiol in elderly women. Am J Obstet Gynecol 2002;186:944. (*Women using Estring estradiol vaginal ring for 12 months had no changes in endometrial thickness or serum estradiol levels compared to those using no treatment.*)
24. Centers for Disease Control and Prevention. Sexually transmitted diseases treatment guidelines 2006. MMWR Morb Mortal Wkly Rep 2006;55 (No. RR-11). (*Treatment guidelines for bacterial vaginosis, trichomoniasis, vulvovaginal candidiasis, chlamydia, and gonorrhea.*)
25. Centers for Disease Control and Prevention. Update to CDC's sexually transmitted diseases treatment guidelines, 2006: fluoroquinolones no longer recommended for treatment of gonococcal infections. MMWR Morb Mortal Wkly Rep 2007;56:332. (*Due to increasing prevalence of fluoroquinolone resistance in Neisseria gonorrhoeae, this class of medications is no longer recommended for treatment.*)

CHAPTER 118 ■ APPROACH TO THE MENOPAUSAL WOMAN

SHANA L. BIRNBAUM

Based on the generally accepted definition of menopause as a full year without menstrual flow in a previously menstruating woman, the incidence of menopause is 10% by age 38 years, 20% by age 43 years, 50% by age 48 years, 90% by age 54 years, and 100% by age 58 years. The mean age of menopause is 51 years. In addition, the prevalence of surgically induced menopause is estimated to be 25% to 30% of women in their mid-50s. Despite its inevitability, menopause can be difficult in a society that celebrates youthfulness. Although many of the emotional and physical changes blamed on menopause are not related to decreased estrogen levels, the cessation of menstruation has symbolic significance, and, as a result, symptoms and complaints may be unduly attributed to it. Although hormone therapy (HT) is very effective in dealing with the specific symptoms of estrogen deficiency, nonhormonal options are increasingly being used as the results of recent large-scale, randomized trials of HT continue to define risks. Previously, HT was believed to confer significant disease-prevention benefits, particularly for prophylaxis of cardiovascular disease and osteoporosis. However, the results of the Heart and Estrogen/progestin Replacement Study (HERS) and the Women's Health Initiative (WHI) contradicted earlier observational studies showing cardiovascular benefit from HT and suggested that potential harms of HT, including an increased risk of cardiovascular disease and stroke, as well as of breast cancer, may outweigh benefits for many women. This new evidence and resulting publicity has left many women uncertain about HT decisions and changed national guidelines and prescribing practices. Much remains uncertain about the effect of HT in different populations pending the results of newer trials. The primary care physician can do a great deal to help women to cope with menopause and make informed choices regarding options for symptom relief and disease prevention.

PHYSIOLOGY AND CLINICAL PRESENTATION (1–8)

The essential cause of menopause is decreased estrogen due to decreased responsiveness to follicle-stimulating hormone in aging ovaries. This results in the cessation of menses and an increase in gonadotropins. Some estrogen production continues, but its source is primarily the peripheral conversion of androstenedione. The earliest symptom of menopause is a decrease in cycle length, which may be interspersed with long anovulatory cycles. The perimenopause, with irregular cycles and menopausal symptoms, may go on for years before menses cease completely. The diagnosis of menopause is confirmed by a marked increase in the gonadotropins; maximum levels of follicle-stimulating hormone and luteinizing hormone occur within 1 to 2 years of onset and remain high for

10 to 15 years. The physiologic events are similar in surgically induced menopause, but the time course is shorter, with follicle-stimulating hormone and luteinizing hormone increasing to high levels within 20 to 30 days. Approximately 25% of women do not experience any symptoms (10% of those undergoing surgical menopause), perhaps because of nonovarian sources of estrogen production or differences in the time frame of hormone shifts.

Hot Flashes

Hot flashes, which are associated with estrogen withdrawal and resultant vasomotor instability, are among the most specific and disruptive of menopausal symptoms and generally begin during perimenopause. An intense warm sensation with sweating radiates upward from the chest to the neck and face, lasting from seconds to a few minutes before subsiding. The skin is visibly flushed and skin temperature rises due to vasodilation, with a resultant decrease in core temperature. The etiology is complex and incompletely understood, but it likely involves dysregulation of the central thermoregulatory centers in the hypothalamus, with a role for endorphins and other neurotransmitters, primarily norepinephrine and serotonin. Eating, exertion, emotional upset, and alcohol are known precipitants. As many as 20 episodes per day may occur; in most patients, the condition lasts for 2 to 3 years, but it may continue for 6 years or more. Hot flashes are usually most problematic at night, when they cause arousal and sleep disruption, which may lead to considerable morbidity, including chronic fatigue, depression and irritability, and, potentially memory, and cognition problems.

Atrophy of the Urogenital Epithelium

Atrophy of the urogenital epithelium with associated sexual dysfunction and urinary complaints is another important manifestation of estrogen decline. The vagina becomes smaller and less compliant; lubrication decreases. Women may present with complaints of itching, irritation, discharge, bleeding, or painful intercourse. Sexually active women often complain of vaginal dryness with intercourse, but they show less vaginal atrophy; regular intercourse and arousal appears to maintain vaginal blood flow and compliance. Lack of estrogen also affects urinary sphincter tone, with a resultant increase in urinary incontinence; urinary tract infections and urinary frequency are also more common. However, the hope that HT would prevent or treat urinary incontinence has not been borne out by trial results.

Sleep Disturbances

Sleep disturbances occur in many menopausal women. Most are associated with nocturnal hot flashes, but abnormalities in the sleep pattern, including a decrease in rapid-eye-movement sleep, have been documented independent of hot flashes.

Cardiovascular Disease

Cardiovascular disease is the leading cause of mortality among postmenopausal women but is seen at fairly low rates among premenopausal women. Loss of estrogen is associated with an unfavorable change in lipoprotein profile, with a decrease in high-density-lipoprotein cholesterol and an increase in low-density-lipoprotein cholesterol, providing a plausible biologic mechanism for the theory that HT would reduce cardiovascular risk. Observational studies involving tens of thousands of women suggested that as much as a 50% decrease in cardiovascular disease risk could be achieved with estrogen replacement. As a result, estrogen replacement was prescribed for millions of women with the goal of preventing heart disease. However, large-scale, randomized, controlled trials, first among women with known heart disease (the HERS trial) and subsequently among women without heart disease (the WHI trial), failed to confirm that estrogen plus progestin was effective for the secondary or primary prevention of cardiovascular disease and may in fact slightly increase the risk in primary prevention. Most recently, the estrogen-only arm of the WHI was also stopped ahead of schedule due to an increased risk of stroke, although there was no effect on cardiovascular disease. Subsequent analysis of the Nurses Health Study (NHS), a prospective, observational cohort study of more than 120,000 women, suggested that the discrepant results between observation studies and the later trials may be explained by the age of the women and the duration of the time between menopause and the initiation of HT. Women in the NHS who initiated HT near menopause had a significant reduction in coronary heart disease (CHD) risk, whereas those who began more than a decade after menopause did not. The vast majority of women in the WHI trial were older and initiated HT more than a decade after menopause. Subgroup analyses in the WHI are also consistent with the hypothesis that HT started at or near the time of menopause decreases the risk of CHD, whereas initiation later in life increases the risk, at least for the first year or so of HT.

Osteoporosis

Osteoporosis represents an important consequence of estrogen decline, with a rapid decrease in bone density occurring after menopause; decreased activity, inadequate nutrition, and the aging process may contribute. Randomized trials confirmed observational studies and demonstrated the effectiveness of HT in preventing postmenopausal osteoporosis, treating established osteoporosis, and decreasing the risk of fracture. However, newer, nonhormonal treatments, most notably the bisphosphonates, have proven to be as effective as estrogen in treating osteoporosis and are now first-line agents. Adequate calcium, vitamin D, and exercise can also decrease the risk of fracture. Risk factors for postmenopausal osteoporotic fractures include thin body build, premature surgical menopause, cigarette smoking, and heavy alcohol use. Prolonged bedrest is a potent stimulus of osteoporosis. Long-acting benzodiazepines, anticonvulsants, caffeine, and impaired visual function are other risk factors for hip fracture.

Other Symptoms

Other symptoms, such as *headache*, *nervousness*, and *depression*, which frequently occur during the climacteric, are more a reflection of the emotional stress that may be associated with this stage of life than a result of a change in hormonal milieu. Some women report feeling better emotionally on estrogen therapy, but large randomized trials have not shown a benefit in terms of quality of life. Younger, symptomatic women did report an improvement in vasomotor symptoms and sleep quality with no other quality-of-life improvements in the WHI trial, but there was a small improvement in depressive symptoms in the HERS trial. Women who experience a prolonged symptomatic perimenopausal phase may exhibit some depressive symptoms, but depression is not a consequence of the menopause itself.

Cosmetic Changes

Cosmetic changes associated with aging have been attributed by some to a decrease in estrogens, but clinical evidence is to the contrary. Breast atrophy, loss of skin turgor, and redistribution of fat to the abdomen and thighs have not been shown to be influenced by estrogen therapy and most likely are part of the more general process of aging.

PRINCIPLES OF MANAGEMENT
(1,2,4,8–50)

Short-term objectives are to alleviate any bothersome symptoms that result from estrogen deficiency and to provide support for any emotional and functional problems that may accompany this phase of life. Estrogen therapy remains the gold standard for the relief of vasomotor symptoms and urogenital atrophy and is accepted for short-term therapy at the lowest dose adequate for symptom relief. Nonhormonal approaches also exist and provide women with a choice of options for dealing with menopausal symptoms, as well as with long-term disease prevention. Given the risk–benefit ratio of HT, its long-term preventive use is no longer recommended. It is ineffective in preventing cardiovascular disease, at least for older women and those with established disease, and safer alternatives exist for osteoporosis prevention and treatment.

Hormone Therapy (1,2,4,8–45)

Many women are reluctant to use any form of hormones, given the associated negative publicity in recent years. Because symptoms such as hot flashes and vaginal dryness relate to estrogen deficiency and are most effectively treated with estrogen therapy, the clinician and patient are faced with the decision of when and if to use HT. This necessitates careful consideration of benefits and risks; for the majority of women, the risks will outweigh the benefits for long-term therapy but may support short-term therapy for symptom relief.

Benefits of Hormone Therapy

The benefits include symptom relief, reduced risk of osteoporosis and related fractures, and reduced risk of colorectal cancer.

Hot flashes severe enough to be a serious bother to the patient are an important indication for estrogen replacement.

Although in most instances the symptoms are self-limited, relief during the few years that symptoms are most severe can mean a great deal. HT is effective in relieving hot flashes in greater than 80% of women, although there is a placebo benefit of almost 30% in many trials. Sleep often improves due to a decrease in hot flashes or potentially another mechanism, although the WHI results indicate that improvement in sleep disturbance may be too small to be clinically meaningful. Atrophic vaginitis responds well to both the topical and oral administration of estrogen. Vaginal estrogen creams used at low doses (0.3 mg conjugated estrogens daily) and the estradiol-secreting vaginal ring (Estring) do not substantially increase serum estrogen levels and do not require the use of concurrent progestin in women with a uterus. Milder symptoms (e.g., mild dryness with intercourse) may respond well to use of a water-soluble vaginal lubricant such as Replens or Astroglide, obviating the need for estrogen in the woman who wants to avoid its use. Osteoporosis can be prevented by long-term prophylactic estrogen therapy. Controlled studies have shown that rates of vertebral, wrist, and hip fractures can be significantly reduced by estrogen replacement and that this protective effect is not impaired by the addition of progestin. The risk of hip fracture is reduced by 25% in women who have used estrogen in the past and to an even greater extent among current and recent users. In the WHI, estrogen plus progestin decreased the risk of hip fractures by one third and the risk of total fractures by 24%, whereas estrogen alone decreased the fracture rate by 30% to 39%. The combination of estrogen therapy in conjunction with exercise and dietary calcium supplementation is an option for the prevention of postmenopausal osteoporosis (see Chapter 164), but in light of recent trial evidence, many women and their clinicians consider the risks of long-term HT too great. Women should be strongly encouraged to engage in regular weight-bearing exercise and maintain adequate calcium intake, which can slow osteoporotic changes. Women at particular risk for osteoporosis or with known low bone density should consider additional approaches to prevention of osteoporosis such as alendronate or other biphosphonates, or raloxifene (see Chapter 164).

HT does appear to reduce the risk of colorectal cancer, as initially seen in observational studies. In the NHS, the relative risk of colorectal cancer among current hormone users was 0.65 (95% confidence interval [CI], 0.50 to 0.83). This risk reduction was confirmed in the WHI trial, in which the colorectal cancer relative risk was 0.63 (CI 0.43 to 0.92). In contrast, the estrogen-alone arm of the WHI did not show any differences in rate of colorectal cancer between estrogen and placebo.

Neither the HERS nor the WHI found a clinically significant improvement in measures of quality of life with estrogen and progestin replacement.

Risks of Hormone Therapy

Risks of HT have been increasingly well defined, and include endometrial cancer (for unopposed estrogen); breast cancer (for estrogen plus progestin); cardiovascular disease, including stroke and venous thromboembolism; urinary incontinence; and, potentially, cognitive decline and dementia.

Endometrial Cancer. Endometrial cancer is a major risk associated with the use of unopposed systemic estrogen by women with a uterus. This relationship was initially demonstrated in more than 30 epidemiologic studies evaluating the association between estrogen replacement therapy and endometrial cancer. The relative risk of endometrial cancer among estrogen users has been estimated to be as low as 2 and as high as 15; the risk

increases with the dose and duration of estrogen use. Estrogens cause hyperplasia of the endometrium, which may progress to carcinoma with prolonged continuous use. Fortunately, these tumors tend to be of low grade and in early stages when detected. Progestins, given either continuously or monthly for at least 12 days, prevent the development of endometrial hyperplasia that is otherwise associated with unopposed estrogen use. Multiple studies, including the randomized WHI and HERS trials, have examined the effect of estrogen plus progestin therapy on endometrial cancer risk, and none found a significant increase.

Breast Cancer. After considerable uncertainty, it now seems that risk of developing breast cancer increases with exposure to estrogen replacement therapy when it includes progestin as well as estrogen. Early observational studies did not always distinguish between unopposed estrogen use and combined HT, leading to inconsistent results. Stronger evidence came from a pooled analysis of 51 observational studies, which found a relative risk for breast cancer of 1.35 with 5 years of HT use; this risk increased to 1.53 when only combined regimens where analyzed. Similar trends were seen in the recent Million Women study from the United Kingdom, in which current HT use was associated with a 1.3 and 2.0 relative risk of breast cancer for estrogen alone and combined therapy, respectively. The NHS confirmed that the relative risk of developing breast cancer is a function of the duration of treatment. A duration of therapy of less than 5 years does not appear to cause a significant increase in breast cancer risk, although in the WHI an excess risk of breast cancer was evident after only 3 years of therapy (relative risk, 1.26). Postintervention follow-up of women in the WHI suggested that increased cancer risk persisted for at least 3 years after the cessation of HT. There was also a nonsignificant trend of similar magnitude toward excess breast cancer risk in the HERS trial. Of interest, the estrogen-alone arm of the WHI showed a nonsignificant trend toward *decreased* breast cancer risk (relative risk, 0.77 [CI 0.59 to 1.01]). A case–control study from Washington state also failed to demonstrate any increased risk from estrogen alone, even for long duration of use, lending support to the belief that progestin is responsible for much of the excess risk of breast cancer seen in the estrogen–progestin trials.

Cardiovascular Disease. Observational studies among tens of thousands of women indicated that coronary heart disease morbidity and mortality were markedly reduced by HT. The relative risk of cardiovascular mortality among women who were current users of HT compared to those who have never used HT ranged from 0.50 to 0.89. However, results of randomized trials failed to support a cardiovascular benefit or demonstrated increased risk. HERS, a randomized trial among women with established cardiovascular disease, showed that HT increased coronary events during the first year, after which there appeared to be a reduction in the rate of new events. That reduction was not maintained in continued follow-up; after a total of 6.8 years of follow-up, combined HT did not reduce the risk of cardiovascular events in women with a history of coronary disease.

The WHI trial of estrogen plus progestin included more than 16,000 women without heart disease and demonstrated the same early increase in coronary heart disease risk among women without prior disease. The trial was stopped early because of excess harms relative to benefits. With an average follow-up of 5.2 years, women randomized to HT were 29% more likely to have an acute coronary event. Subsequently, the estrogen-only arm of the WHI was stopped early after 7 years of follow-up due to an increased risk of stroke without any evidence of effect on cardiovascular outcomes, the primary outcome. It is important to note, however, that the vast majority of women in the WHI trial were older and initiated HT more than a decade after menopause. Subsequent analysis of the NHS, a prospective, observational cohort study of more than 120,000 women, found that women in the NHS who initiated HT near menopause had a significant reduction in CHD risk, whereas those who began more than a decade after menopause did not. Age and timing of initiation of HT may explain the discrepancy between results of the observational studies and randomized trials. The relationship between the timing of initiation of HT in relation to the stage of atherosclerosis as potential explanation for the discrepancy between results of observational studies and randomized trials is depicted in Fig. 118.1.

Consistent with observational studies, the randomized trials revealed an increased risk of thromboembolism among menopausal women on estrogen replacement, particularly with progestin. However, the absolute risk remained very low for women who were otherwise healthy and active. A history of thromboembolism is a relative contraindication to estrogen use. The relative risk of pulmonary embolus in the WHI trial was 2.13 (CI 1.39 to 3.25) but was only 1.34 (CI 0.87 to 2.06) in the estrogen-alone arm of the WHI. The incidence of DVT in the latter study did reach significance with a relative risk of 1.47 (CI 1.04 to 2.08).

Both WHI trial arms documented an increased risk of stroke in previously health women. The excess risk of stroke became apparent in the combined arm after 1 year and continued for the remainder of the study's mean follow-up of 5.2 years. The relative risk was 1.41 (CI 1.07 to 1.85). The estrogen-alone arm confirmed this elevated stroke risk, with a relative risk of 1.39 (CI 1.10 to 1.77). Although the 0.12% additional strokes per year of treatment in the estrogen-alone trial represents a very low absolute risk, it was still considered high enough to halt the trial of a preventive medicine given to healthy women.

Dementia. Initial suggestions from observational studies that women who use estrogens are at lower risk of alzheimer's disease have not been confirmed in randomized trials. The HERS trial showed no benefit with 4 years of follow-up. The WHI memory study estrogen-plus-progestin arm demonstrated slight increases in the rate of mild cognitive impairment and a definite increased risk of dementia in women receiving active hormones (hazard ratio 2.05 [CI 1.21 to 3.48]). early results from the estrogen-alone arm of the WHI also suggested a negative effect on cognitive function and dementia.

Other Adverse Effects.   Other effects of exogenous estrogen include *fluid retention, slight blood pressure elevation, gallstones* (due to a change in bile cholesterol content), *glucose intolerance, dry eyes,* and *headaches.* Often there is *recurrent uterine bleeding,* especially with cyclic progesterone use. This bleeding can complicate the clinical recognition of endometrial cancer and cause inconvenience and concern. In the NHS, estrogen replacement was associated with a twofold increase in the risk of *systemic lupus erythematosus,* but the absolute risk was very low.

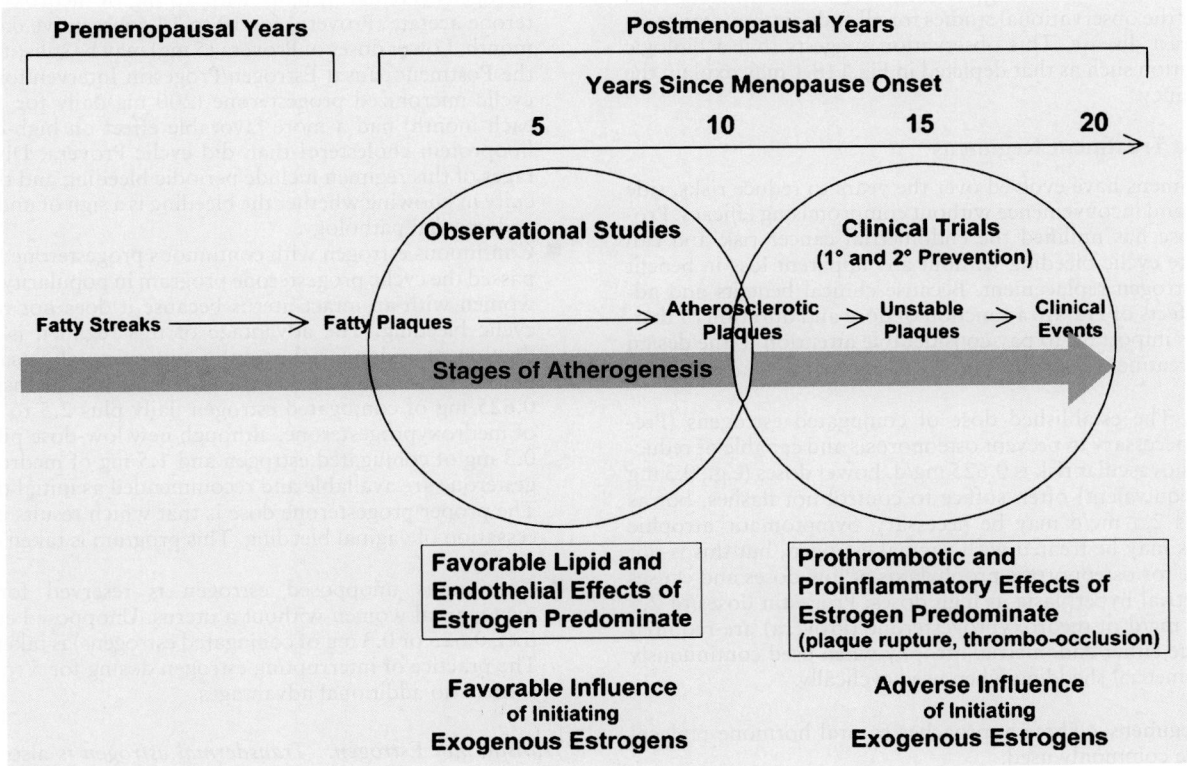

FIGURE 118.1. Timing of hormone therapy initiation and stage of atherosclerosis in observational studies and randomized, controlled trials. (From Manson JE, Bassuk S, Harman SM, et al. Postmenopausal hormone therapy: new questions and the case for new clinical trials. Menopause 2006;13:139, with permission.)

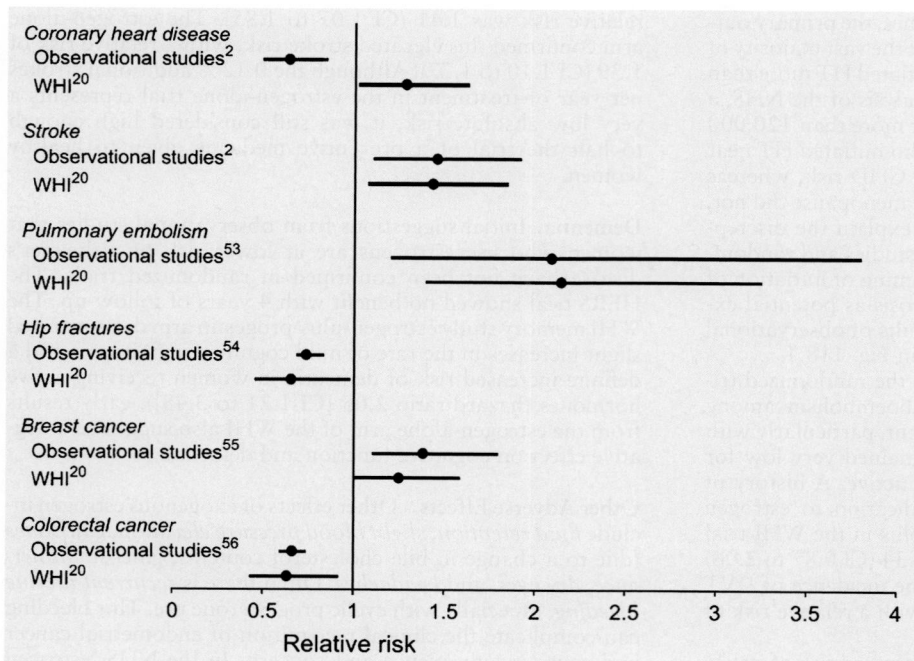

FIGURE 118.2. Comparing the effects of hormone therapy on different clinical endpoints as estimated from observational studies and the Women's Health Initiative estrogen-plus-progestin trial. (From Manson JE, Bassuk S, Harman SM, et al. Postmenopausal hormone therapy: new questions and the case for new clinical trials. Menopause 2006;13:139, with permission.)

Figure 118.2 summarizes the major benefits and harms, with relative risks drawn from the observational studies and the WHI. Of note, the findings of the WHI were consistent with those of the observational studies for all endpoints except coronary heart disease. This observation suggests that a biologic explanation such as that depicted in Fig.118.1 may explain the discrepancy.

Specific Treatment Regimens

HT regimens have evolved over the years to reduce risks, side effects, and inconvenience without compromising efficacy. Progestin use has nullified the endometrial cancer risk and can eliminate cyclic bleeding without any apparent loss in benefit from estrogen replacement. Because clinical benefits and adverse effects of HT are a function of dose and duration of therapy, it is important to pay considerable attention to the design of the treatment regimen.

Dosing. The established dose of conjugated estrogens (Premarin) necessary to prevent osteoporosis and capable of reducing cardiovascular risk is 0.625 mg/d. Lower doses (e.g., 0.3 mg or the equivalent) often suffice to control hot flashes, but as much as 2.5 mg/d may be necessary. Symptomatic atrophic vaginitis may be treated with vaginal estrogen, but this is not effective for osteoporosis prophylaxis at low doses and causes endometrial hyperplasia at high doses. Progestin doses of 2.5 to 10.0 mg/d of medroxyprogesterone (Provera) are required to induce either endometrial atrophy when used continuously or endometrial shedding when used cyclically.

Oral Regimens. Three approaches to oral hormone replacement are commonly used:

- Continuous estrogen with cyclic progesterone was the first estrogen/progesterone replacement program designed for postmenopausal women with an intact uterus. The rationale for the use of cyclic progesterone is to produce endometrial shedding so as to avoid continuous endometrial proliferative stimulation. A typical program is 0.625 mg conjugated estrogens (Premarin) daily with 10 mg of medroxyprogesterone acetate (Provera) for 10 to 14 consecutive days each month. Lower doses of Provera (5 mg) may be substituted. In the Postmenopausal Estrogen/Progestin Interventions trial, cyclic micronized progesterone (200 mg daily for 12 days each month) had a more favorable effect on high-density-lipoprotein cholesterol than did cyclic Provera. Disadvantages of this regimen include periodic bleeding and the difficulty in knowing whether the bleeding is a sign of underlying endometrial pathology.

- Continuous estrogen with continuous progesterone has surpassed the cyclic progesterone program in popularity among women with an intact uterus because it does not result in cyclic bleeding. The advantage of this regimen is the induction of endometrial atrophy and eventual cessation of uterine bleeding. A standard daily regimen has consisted of 0.625 mg of conjugated estrogen daily plus 2.5 to 5.0 mg of medroxyprogesterone, although new low-dose pills with 0.3 mg of conjugated estrogen and 1.5 mg of medroxyprogesterone are available and recommended as initial therapy. The proper progesterone dose is that which results in a full cessation of vaginal bleeding. This program is taken continuously.

- Continuous unopposed estrogen is reserved for postmenopausal women without a uterus. Unopposed estrogen (i.e., 0.625 or 0.3 mg of conjugated estrogens) is taken daily. The practice of interrupting estrogen dosing for 5 to 7 days confers no additional advantages.

Transdermal Estrogen. *Transdermal estrogen* is also an option. A patch applied twice each week produces estradiol levels similar to those resulting from oral doses of 0.625 mg of Premarin daily, and patches are available in doses ranging from 0.025 to 0.1 mg/d. Patches are also available in combination with progesterone for women who have a uterus. Another option is estrogen gel applied daily to the arm. The cost is increased with transdermal estrogen, but some women may prefer its convenience.

Topical Estrogen. *Topical estrogen* is effective for atrophic vaginitis causing dysuria or dyspareunia. Symptoms will respond to topically applied estrogen cream used as seldom as once or twice a week. Systemic absorption occurs with higher doses, raising concern about localized endometrial stimulation with prolonged daily use, but limited use on a short-term basis is probably safe. In addition, newer low-dose delivery systems, such as the low-dose estrogen-eluting vaginal ring, which is active for 3 months, and low-dose estrogen suppositories, which are used twice weekly, have minimal systemic absorption and appear to be safe for long-term use.

Duration of Therapy

Programs for symptomatic relief are usually short term, extending 1 to 2 years before attempts to withdraw HT are made. If bothersome symptoms recur, HT can be restarted with subsequent periodic attempts to withdraw therapy advised every 6 months. Tapering estrogen, by lowering either the daily dose or the number of days per week that it is administered, may make symptom recurrence less likely, although there is no definitive evidence regarding this practice.

Patient Selection

Given the serious adverse effects of HT and the fact that some of these are still poorly defined, the primary physician must exert care and judgment in selecting patients for HT. The decision to use such therapy needs to be made with full consideration of the patient's willingness to undertake the risks in exchange for specified benefits. One woman may be willing to accept the risk of breast cancer and cardiovascular disease in return for symptom relief and prevention of osteoporosis and colorectal cancer; another might not. Women should be advised of alternative prevention strategies, including exercise, calcium supplementation, vitamin D, bisphosphonates for osteoporosis (see Chapter 164), and periodic colonoscopy for the detection and removal of polyps to prevent colorectal cancer.

Monitoring

The evidence does not support definitive recommendations for monitoring women taking HT. However, because of the increased risk of breast cancer with increasing duration of HT, it is recommended that clinical breast examination and mammography be performed yearly in women taking HT, as in all women older than 50 years of age. Women taking progestins, as well as estrogens, do not need either baseline or subsequent routine endometrial evaluations.

Other Treatment Modalities (46–50)

Hot Flashes and Other Menopausal Symptoms

There are alternative treatments for hot flashes. None are nearly as effective as estrogen replacement. Selective serotonin reuptake inhibitors (SSRIs) have been effective in randomized trials. In one trial, paroxetine in a controlled-release form reduced the median number of hot flashes by 65%, compared to 39% with placebo. Similar results have been shown in trials of venlafaxine and fluoxetine. It is not clear which, if any, of these agents is preferable. The adverse effects in these SSRI trials were mod-

erate, with gastrointestinal symptoms in 10% to 20%. About 15% of women reported loss of libido, failure to reach orgasm, or both.

Clonidine is an alternative that is helpful for some women. However, trials indicate that it is only moderately more effective than placebo. Furthermore, adverse effects are quite common, with reported rates ranging from 10% to 50%. Dry mouth, drowsiness, orthostatic hypotension, and constipation dominate. Gabapentin is another neuroendocrine agent reported to reduce hot flashes, by as much as 70% in observational studies.

Soy protein from dietary sources has been promoted to help relieve hot flashes, but women must eat fairly large amounts (at least 40 g/d of products that contain about 75 mg of phytoestrogens). A meta-analysis of trials suggested a modest benefit, but the evidence is not conclusive. Pills or supplements containing isoflavones are not equivalent to dietary sources of soy and are not as effective. Black cohosh may also be effective, but in the absence of long-term data, safety concerns remain. There is no evidence to support the use of other herbs or other complementary and alternative therapies.

Prevention of Osteoporosis and Cardiovascular Disease

Advances in the prevention and treatment of osteoporosis (see Chapter 164) and cardiovascular disease provide menopausal women a host of preventive and therapeutic options for conditions related to menopause. For example, a *diet* low in fat and high in calcium, combined with regular weight-bearing aerobic *exercise*, can do much to reduce cardiovascular and osteoporotic risks. Even patients at high risk for osteoporotic disease have highly effective nonhormonal options, such as *bisphosphonates* (see Chapter 164).

Diet and exercise can slow osteoporotic changes but not as effectively as estrogen. Nevertheless, the addition of 1,200 to 1,500 mg of dietary calcium per day will compensate for the intestinal malabsorption of calcium that results from estrogen deficiency and will retard bone loss, especially when combined with regular exercise. *Vitamin D* treatment is not beneficial unless serum levels of 25-OH vitamin D_3 are low. Small doses (400 U/d) are helpful in preventing vitamin D deficiency in elderly women; large doses are unnecessary. Bisphosphonate therapy (e.g., alendronate) can reduce vertebral compression fractures by close to 50%.

Patients with worrisome lipid profiles have multiple lipid-lowering options (see Chapter 27) to supplement dietary measures. Vaginal dryness can be treated nonhormonally with a *water-soluble lubricant*, if there is a reason to avoid any estrogen exposure. Decrease in libido and/or orgasmic dysfunction that was clearly associated with the onset of menopause but persists with estrogen replacement might justify the consideration of androgen therapy (see Chapter 115).

Overly medicalizing menopause by emphasizing HT runs the risk of turning a normal phase of life into a disease state and unintentionally triggering depression. A more constructive approach is to advise the menopausal women about her options, emphasizing the range of possibilities and providing a sense that her menopause-related health status can be influenced if not fully controlled by the choices she makes.

PATIENT EDUCATION

Because the emphasis in our society is on youth and vitality, the physician has an important supportive role to play in helping the menopausal woman to adjust psychologically and maintain her sense of self-worth and well-being. Discussion of the physiologic consequences of menopause and their clinical manifestations can give the patient a rational basis for understanding her symptoms and properly attributing them. This might save many anxious phone calls and office visits. One can take advantage of this milestone to interest the patient in a program of regular exercise, attainment of ideal weight, and cessation of self-destructive habits, such as smoking. The patient needs to know that any incapacitating symptoms caused by a lack of estrogen can be controlled and that many are self-limited. During the perimenopausal period, women should be reminded to use contraception because ovulation and unwanted pregnancy may occur. Reassurance that the capacity for normal sexual activity will continue after menopause is often tremendously comforting. Lack of need for special vitamin supplements should be pointed out because the lay press heavily encourages their use, and this unnecessary expense can be considerable.

If estrogen therapy is being considered, the patient must share in the decision with full awareness of the potential risks and benefits. The need for regular follow-up and prompt reporting of any abnormal vaginal bleeding, breast masses, leg swelling, and so forth must be emphasized.

INDICATIONS FOR REFERRAL

Women with an intact uterus who are taking HT and who experience irregular vaginal bleeding that does not clear with adjustment of progesterone dose require gynecologic evaluation to rule out important endometrial pathology. The postmenopausal patient who develops major depression and does not respond to first-line antidepressant therapy and counseling should be considered for psychiatric consultation.

THERAPEUTIC RECOMMENDATIONS (1,2,4,46–50)

- *Review risks and benefits.* Decisions about treatment of postmenopausal changes require careful weighing and thorough discussion of risks and benefits. The postmenopausal woman's preferences and concerns should be elicited and addressed in the design of any program.
- *For hot flashes.* For symptomatic relief of incapacitating hot flashes, consider a trial of *oral estrogen* at the lowest dose necessary (often as little as 0.3 mg/d of conjugated estrogens). The need for continued estrogen treatment should be reevaluated regularly. Withdrawal attempts every 6 months should be made, using a tapering schedule. If the patient has an intact uterus, then add a *progestin* to the program (see later discussion). A trial of SSRI therapy may be a first best alternative for most women who cannot take estrogen or prefer to avoid hormones.
- *For atrophic vaginitis.* For atrophic vaginitis with severe dysuria or unacceptable dyspareunia, prescribe a *topical estrogen preparation* (e.g., conjugated estrogen cream) applied as seldom as once or twice a week. An estrogen-eluting vaginal ring or low-dose vaginal suppositories may be preferred as more convenient. Systemic absorption is minimal with very low doses but occurs with higher doses of estrogen cream, although its effect is uncertain. Avoid the prolonged daily use of high doses because of the risk of endometrial stimulation. In instances of painful coitus only, advise trying a *water-soluble lubricant*, especially if there is a desire to avoid estrogen exposure.
- *For depression.* Treat specifically for depression with supportive psychotherapy and/or a standard antidepressant drug regimen (see Chapter 227); HT is not a substitute.
- *For prophylaxis of osteoporosis.* Explain the need for long-term therapy and its attendant risks. Consider bisphosphonate therapy as an alternative to indefinite hormone supplementation (see Chapter 164). HT cannot replace lost bone; it is *not* a therapy for reversing established osteoporosis.
- *Oral hormone therapy regimens.* For women with an intact uterus, treat with either continuous daily estrogen combined with daily low-dose progestin (e.g., 0.3 or 0.625 mg conjugated estrogens plus 1.5 to 5.0 mg/d of medroxyprogesterone acetate or equivalent) or continuous daily estrogen plus cyclic progestin (e.g., 0.3 or 0.625 mg conjugated estrogens plus 5 to 10 mg of medroxyprogesterone acetate added on 10 to 14 consecutive days of the month). Choice should be based on desirability and acceptability of periodic vaginal bleeding, with recognition that women closer to perimenopause are more likely to have irregular bleeding on continuous therapy and may prefer cyclic therapy with predictable bleeding.
- *For women who have had a hysterectomy.* Treat with continuous daily estrogen therapy (e.g., 0.3 or 0.625 mg/d of conjugated estrogens). There is no benefit to adding a progestin.

Annotated Bibliography

1. Roberts H. Managing the menopause. BMJ 2007;334:736. (*An excellent clinical review.*)
2. North American Menopause Association. Estrogen and progestogen use in peri- and postmenopausal women: March 2007 position statement of the North American Menopause Association. Menopause 2007;14:168. (*An authoritative position statement.*)
3. Bastian LA, Smith CM, Nanda K. Is this woman perimenopausal? JAMA 2003;289:895. (*Diagnosis should be made based on menstrual history and age rather than tests.*)
4. Shanafelt TD, Barton DL, Adjei AA, et al. Pathophysiology and treatment of hot flashes. Mayo Clinic Proc 2002;77:1207. (*Useful overview.*)
5. Stearns V, Ullmer L, Lopez JF, et al. Hot flushes. Lancet 2002;360:1851. (*An excellent review; 163 references.*)
6. Utian WH, Boggs PP. The North American Menopause Society 1998 Menopause Survey. Part I. Postmenopausal women's perceptions about menopause and midlife. Menopause 1999;6:122. (*The majority of respondents were happiest and most fulfilled between the ages of 50 and 65 years.*)
7. Avis NE, Brambilla D, McKinlay S, et al. A longitudinal analysis of the association between menopause and depression: results from the Massachusetts

Women's Health Study. Ann Epidemiol 1994;4:12. (*Depression was associated with a long symptomatic perimenopause rather than with the menopause itself.*)
8. Sarrel PM. Psychosexual effects of menopause: role of androgens. Am J Obstet Gynecol 1999;180:319. (*A review of the clinical evidence, concluding that the addition of androgens to hormone therapy [HT] provided greater improvement in psychological and sexual symptoms.*)
9. Roussouw JE, Anderson GL, Prentice RL, et al. Risks and benefits of estrogen plus progestin in healthy postmenopausal women: principal results from the Women's Health Initiative randomized trial. JAMA 2002;288:321. (*The overall health risks exceeded the benefits from the use of combined estrogen plus progestin for an average 5.2-year follow-up among healthy postmenopausal U.S. women.*)
10. Manson JE, Hsia J, Johnson KC, et al. Estrogen plus progestin and the risk of coronary heart disease. N Engl J Med 2003; 349:215. (*Seemingly the last word on coronary heart disease [CHD] risk from the Women's Health Initiative [WHI] study, including subgroup analyses that showed little or no variation in the excess risk conferred by HT except for women with high baseline low-density-lipoprotein cholesterol, who face a greater excess risk.*)

11. Anderson GL, Limacher M, Assaf AR, et al. Effects of conjugated equine estrogen in postmenopausal women with hysterectomy: the Women's Health Initiative randomized controlled trial. JAMA 2004; 291:1701. (*The use of conjugated estrogens increased the risk of stroke, decreased the risk of hip fracture, and did not affect CHD incidence over an average of 6.8 years.*)

12. Stampfer MJ, Colditz GA, Willett WC, et al. Postmenopausal estrogen therapy and cardiovascular disease. Ten-year follow-up from the Nurses' Health Study. N Engl J Med 1991;325:756. (*An influential observational study, showing that the relative risk for women who have ever-used estrogen therapy was 0.6.*)

13. Grodstein F, Manson JE, Stampfer MJ. Hormone therapy and coronary heart disease: the role of time since menopause and age at hormone initiation. J Women's Health 2006;15:35. (*Women who initiated HT near menopause had a reduced risk of CHD, whereas those who did so after more than a decade did not.*)

14. Manson JE, Bassuk S, Harman SM, et al. Postmenopausal hormone therapy: new questions and the case for new clinical trials. Menopause 2006;13:139. (*Presents evidence supporting the effect of age at initiation of HT on the risk–benefit ratio.*)

15. Hsia J, Langer RD, Manson JE, et al. for the Women's Health Initiative Investigators. Conjugated equine estrogens and coronary heart disease. Arch Intern Med 2006;166:357. (*This approach provided no overall protection against myocardial infarction or coronary death, but there was a suggestion thereof in women in their 50s at initiation.*)

16. Rossouw JE, Prentice RL, Manson JE, et al. Postmenopausal hormone therapy and risk of cardiovascular disease by age and years since menopause. JAMA 2007; 297:1465. (*Women who started HT soon after menopause showed a trend toward reduced CHD risk compared to those who started later; the same was true for total mortality; the stroke risk was elevated regardless of the relation of the time of initiation of HT to menopause.*)

17. Manson JE, Allison MA, Rossouw JE, et al. Estrogen therapy and coronary-artery calcification. N Engl J Med 2007; 356:2591. (*Among women in their 50s at trial enrollment, the coronary artery calcified plaque burden was lower in those assigned to estrogen than in those assigned to placebo.*)

18. Vickers MR MacLennan AH, Lawton B, et al. Main morbidities recorded in the women's international study of long duration oestrogen after menopause (WISDOM): a randomized controlled trial of hormone replacement therapy in postmenopausal women. BMJ 2007;335:239. (*Results were consistent with the WHI.*)

19. Heiss G, Wallace R, Anderson GL, et al. Health risks and benefits 3 years after stopping randomized treatment with estrogen and progestin. JAMA 2008;299:1036. (*An increased risk of malignancy was sustained after HT, but cardiovascular risks were not.*)

20. Anderson GL, Judd HL, Kaunitz AM, et al. Effects of estrogen plus progestin on gynecologic cancers and associated diagnostic procedures. JAMA, 2003;290:1739. (*Finds a nonsignificant relative increase in ovarian cancer risk and abnormal Papanicolaou smears in the WHI study.*)

21. Barrett-Conner E. Postmenopausal estrogen therapy and selected (less-often-considered) disease outcomes. Menopause 1999;6:14. (*A 10-year literature review, addressing the evidence for positive associations with multiple conditions, including arthritis, systemic lupus erythematosus, pancreatitis, asthma, and diabetes.*)

22. Cauley JA, Robbins J, Chen Z, et al. Effects of estrogen plus progestin on risk of fracture and bone mineral density. JAMA 2003;290:1729. (*Estrogen plus progestin increased the bone mineral density and reduced the fracture risk by 24%.*)

23. Colditz GA, Hankinson SE, Hunter DJ, et al. The use of estrogen and progestins and the risk of breast cancer in postmenopausal women. N Engl J Med 1995;332:1589. (*An extended follow-up from the Nurses' Health Study, indicating a relative risk of 1.32 for women using estrogen alone and 1.41 for women using estrogen plus progesterone.*)

24. Collaborative Group on Hormonal Factors in Breast Cancer. Breast cancer and hormone replacement therapy: collaborative reanalysis of data from 51 epidemiological studies of 52 705 women with breast cancer and 108 411 women without breast cancer. Lancet 1997;350:1047. (*The risk of breast cancer in women using HT increased with increasing duration of use, reaching 1.35 after 5 years; this effect was reduced after HT cessation and s largely disappeared after about 5 years.*)

25. Espeland MA, Rapp SR, Shumaker SA, et al. Conjugated equine estrogens and global cognitive function in postmenopausal women: Women's Health Initiative Memory Study. JAMA 2004;291(24):2959. (*For women of age 65 years or older, hormone therapy had an adverse effect on cognition, which was greater among women with lower cognitive function at the initiation of treatment.*)

26. Gatspur SM, Morrow M, Sellars TA. Hormone replacement therapy and risk of breast cancer with a favorable histology: results of the Iowa Women's Health Study. JAMA 1999;281:2091. (*There was an increased risk for invasive breast cancers with a favorable prognosis.*)

27. Grady D, Brown JS, Vittinghoff E, et al. Postmenopausal hormones and incontinence: the Heart and Estrogen/Progestin Replacement Study. Obstet Gynecol 2001;97(1):116. (*Urinary incontinence was worse with HT.*)

28. Grady D, Herrington D, Bittner V, et al. Cardiovascular disease outcomes during 6.8 years of hormone therapy: Heart and Estrogen/progestin Replacement Study follow-up (HERS II). JAMA 2002;288:49. (*Lower rates of CHD events among women in the hormone group in the final years of HERS did not persist during additional years of follow-up.*)

29. Grady D, Hulley SB, Furberg C. Venous thromboembolic events associated with hormone replacement therapy. JAMA 1997;278:477. (*A randomized, controlled trial, confirming the increased risk of thromboembolic events.*)

30. Grady D, Yaffe K, Kristof M, et al. Effect of postmenopausal hormone therapy on cognitive function: the Heart and Estrogen/progestin Replacement Study. Am J Med 2002;113(7):543. (*There was no effect on cognitive function after 4 years of follow-up in the Heart and Estrogen/progestin Replacement Study.*)

31. Grodstein F, Martinez E, Platz EA, et al. Postmenopausal hormone use and risk of colorectal cancer and adenoma. Ann Intern Med 1998;128:705. (*The current use of hormones reduced the risk of colorectal cancer by 35% in the Nurses' Health Study.*)

32. Hays J, Ockene JK, Brunner RL, et al. Effects of estrogen plus progestin on health-related quality of life. N Engl J Med 2003;348. (*HT produced no significant effects on general health, vitality, mental health, depressive symptoms, or sexual satisfaction.*)

33. Hendrix SL, Cochrane BB, Nygaard IE, et al. Effects of estrogen with and without progestin on urinary incontinence. JAMA 2005;293:935. (*HT increased the incidence of all types of urinary incontinence at 1 year among women who were continent at baseline.*)

34. Hulley S, Furberg C, Barrett-Connor E, et al. Noncardiovascular disease outcomes during 6.8 years of hormone therapy: Heart and Estrogen/progestin Replacement Study follow-up (HERS II). JAMA 2002;288(1):58. (*The was an increased risk of venous thromboembolism and gallbladder surgery with HT.*)

35. Hulley S, Grady D, Bush T, et al. Randomized trial of estrogen plus progestin for secondary prevention of coronary heart disease in postmenopausal women. Heart and Estrogen/progestin Replacement Study (HERS) Research Group. JAMA 1998;280:605. (*A key study.*)

36. Kritz-Silverstein D, Barrett-Conner E. Long-term postmenopausal hormone use, obesity, and fat distribution in older women. JAMA 1996;275:46. (*HT was not associated with the weight gain and central obesity commonly seen in postmenopausal women.*)

37. MacLennan A, Lester S, Moore V. Oral oestrogen replacement therapy versus placebo for hot flushes. Cochrane Database Syst Rev 2001;(1):CD002978. (*The frequency was reduced by 77% compared to placebo, and severity also decreased; see http://www.cochrane.org for updates.*)

38. Majumdar SR, Almasi EA, Stafford RS. Promotion and prescribing of hormone therapy after report of harm by the Women's Health Initiative. JAMA 2004;292:1983. (*Tracks the effect of spending on promotion by pharmaceutical companies, as well as trial results.*)

39. Stefanick ML, Anderson GL, Margolis KL, et al. Effects of conjugated equine estrogens on breast cancer and mammography screening in postmenopausal women with hysterectomy. JAMA 2006; 295:1647. (*The protective effect was significant when noncompliers were censored; there were more mammographic callbacks, but the difference was all in those advised short-interval follow-up.*)

40. Hormone therapy.

41. Shumaker SA, Legault C, Kuller L, et al. Conjugated equine estrogens and incidence of probable dementia and mild cognitive impairment in postmenopausal women: Women's Health Initiative Memory Study. JAMA 2004;291:2947. (*Estrogen alone did not reduce dementia or cognitive impairment incidence and increased the risk for combined endpoints; pooling the data for estrogen alone and estrogen plus progestin resulted in increased risks for both endpoints.*)

42. The PEPI Writing Group. Effects of estrogen or estrogen/progestin regimens on heart disease risk factors in postmenopausal women. JAMA 1995;273:199. (*These regimens were associated with increased high-density-lipoprotein cholesterol, decreased low-density-lipoprotein cholesterol, and other favorable changes in cardiovascular risk factors.*)

43. The PEPI Writing Group. Effects of hormone replacement therapy on endometrial histology in postmenopausal women. JAMA 1996;275:370. (*Unopposed estrogen produced marked hyperplasia in 34% of cases, compared with 1% in women also taking a progestin.*)

44. Shumaker SA, Legault C, Rapp SR, et al. Estrogen plus progestin and the incidence of dementia and mild cognitive impairment in postmenopausal women: the Women's Health Initiative Memory Study: a randomized controlled trial. JAMA 2003;289(20):2651. (*Estrogen plus progestin increased the risk for probable dementia in women 65 years or older and did not prevent mild cognitive impairment in these women.*)

45. Yaffe K, Sawaya G, Lieberburg I, et al. Estrogen therapy in postmenopausal women: effects on cognitive function and dementia. JAMA 1998;279:688. (*A review of 10 observational studies and four trials, concluding that the evidence is too poor to have confidence in the modest risk reductions that have generally been reported; this skepticism seems justified, given the subsequent randomized trials.*)

46. Caiozzi G, Andrade M, Leyton V, et al. Non-hormonal therapy for hot flushes in postmenopausal women (Cochrane review). In: The Cochrane library, Issue 1. Oxford: Update Software, 2003. (*An excellent, well-referenced review; see* http://www.cochrane.org *for updates.*)

47. Kronenberg F, Fugh-Berman A. Complementary and alternative medicine for menopausal symptoms: a review of randomized, controlled trials. Ann Intern Med 2002;137:805. (*There was some evidence of effectiveness for black cohosh and foods that contain phytoestrogens, but no evidence supporting the use of other herbs or complementary and alternative medicine therapies.*)

48. Stearns V, Beebe KL, Iyengar M, et al. Paroxetine controlled release in the treatment of menopausal hot flashes. JAMA 2003;289:2827. (*There were median reductions of as much as 64% with active agent and 39% with placebo.*)

49. Tice JA, Ettinger B, Ensrud K, et al. Phytoestrogen supplements for the treatment of hot flashes: the Isoflavone Clover Extract (ICE) Study: a randomized controlled trial. JAMA 2003;290:207. (*This approach was found to be no more effective than placebo; the risks were undefined.*)

50. North American Menopause Society. Treatment of menopause-associated vasomotor symptoms: position statement of the North American Menopause Society. Menopause 2004;11:11.(*Describes the evidence for lifestyle changes, estrogens and phytoestrogens, and other nonprescription and prescription drugs, including venlafaxine, paroxetine and fluoxetine, gabapentin, clonidine, and methyldopa.*)

CHAPTER 119 ■ APPROACH TO FERTILITY CONTROL

Roughly 50% of all pregnancies in the United States are unintended. The proportion varies with the age of the woman; it is 80% among teenagers and 40% among women in their perimenopausal years. These high rates belie the general understanding that great progress has been made in contraceptive technology. The ideal contraceptive would be perfectly safe, highly effective, inexpensive, acceptable, and available. No such agent exists. The effectiveness of individual contraceptive agents is expressed in several ways. *Theoretical effectiveness* refers to the ability of the medication, device, or procedure to prevent pregnancy if applied under ideal conditions. *Use effectiveness* combines theoretical effectiveness with inherent patient-related lapses in application. *Extended-use effectiveness* adds the dimension of time, and is often expressed as the number of unintended pregnancies per 100 women per year. The primary physician should be knowledgeable about the effectiveness of contraceptive methods, including how use effectiveness is likely to vary among different patients, as well as their adverse effects, so as to help the patient or couple intelligently select the approach that suits them best.

NATURAL METHODS (1–3)

Natural methods of birth control depend on the woman being able to develop an approach to fertility awareness that she can use consistently. Faithfully practiced *rhythm*, with daily basal body temperature recording, usually results in one pregnancy every 2 years, or at least one more child than planned by the couple by their late 30s. Rhythm practiced by abstinence according to menstrual dates is less effective. Rhythm controlled by following the cervical mucus cycle is confounded by infections, dietary changes, douching habits, oral medications, the patient's understanding of her anatomy, and the availability of testing materials. One needs to understand reproductive anatomy and physiology and to have the privacy to conduct such tests. The *amenorrhea of lactation* is useful in providing an infertile period after childbirth, but the duration of ovarian inactivity in an individual is hard to predict or follow. *With-drawal* is probably the most commonly used natural contraceptive technique. Unfortunately, even when withdrawal before ejaculation is achieved, pregnancy can result from discharge of semen before ejaculation or subsequent sperm migration from the perineum. Failure rates as high as 20% have been reported.

BARRIER CONTRACEPTIVES (4–7)

Condoms

Condoms have moderate extended-use effectiveness. When properly used, this method is 85% to 95% effective. The condom is inexpensive and widely available. It requires no medical intervention or prescription. Newer, high-quality, thin condoms are affordable and mitigate concerns about the loss of sensation. Failure by means of rupture occurs rarely but is easily recognized, thereby providing the opportunity for emergency contraception as a backup (see later discussion). Most condoms are made of latex. Polyurethane condoms have been approved for people with latex sensitivity, but breakage rates are higher, and overall contraceptive effectiveness is not as well documented. The condom has protective effects against infectious agents such as HIV, *Chlamydia*, gonococci, herpes simplex virus, and possibly human papillomavirus (HPV). This effect was believed to be enhanced by nonoxynol-9, a spermicide added to the lubricant of some condoms. However, a 2002 randomized trial found that nonoxynol-9 plus condoms did not reduce rates of gonococcal or chlamydial infection compared with condoms alone. Spermicides do not appear to protect against HIV transmission.

Diaphragms

Diaphragms are synthetic latex barriers mounted on covered rims that deny access of the penis and its ejaculate to the anterior vaginal wall and cervical os. The largest diaphragm that will cover the cervix and anterior vagina from the pubis symphysis to the posterior fornix should be selected. The diaphragm should be comfortable so that the woman barely notices its presence. It should not stretch the rest of the vagina or put undue pressure on the urethra. Only significant weight changes of 25% or more of body weight require diaphragm refitting. Refitting should be performed 6 weeks or more postpartum as well. When used properly, diaphragms with a small amount of spermicidal cream or jelly are up to 95% effective. The cream facilitates insertion but need not be used in the large amounts recommended by the manufacturers because it is unpleasantly messy. Additional spermicidal cream needs to be applied intravaginally for repeated intercourse. The diaphragm is worn for 6 hours after the last coital event because this is the length of time during which sperm motility persists. It may be worn for longer periods of time, but it may then produce an unpleasant odor. It may also be worn while the patient is swimming or during menstruation.

The two most frequent complaints regarding the diaphragm are latex allergy and increased frequency of urinary tract infections. The Wide Seal diaphragm has a wider band around the rim, which puts less direct pressure on the urethra and may reduce the frequency of urinary tract infections. The woman who has experienced infections should also be advised to void after intercourse and use adequate lubrication. A physician, nurse, or trained technician must fit the diaphragm to the individual woman. The cost of the diaphragm is reasonable, but manufacturers advocate the massive use of creams, which adds to the expense. The patient must have some understanding of her anatomy and not be concerned about exploring her vagina. Some adolescents reject the diaphragm because of such concerns. For others, its use represents premeditated sexual intercourse, which they find less acceptable than spontaneous events. Women in their 20s seldom voice such a complaint. Some women cannot be fitted adequately with a diaphragm for anatomic reasons. The cervix may not protrude into the vagina adequately (absent pars vaginalis). The cervix may be displaced posteriorly by retroversion or extreme anteversion.

Cervical Caps

Cervical caps fit snugly over the cervix and are slightly more difficult to insert and remove. Their use requires significant physician or nurse instruction, and they are more costly than diaphragms. Four sizes are manufactured, and some women cannot be fit. For these reasons, they are less popular than the diaphragm. For women who have recurrent urinary tract infections, however, they are particularly useful because they do not press on the urethra. In addition, they can be worn for 48 hours, during which time intercourse may be repeated without the addition of spermicidal cream. There is evidence of a modest increase in the incidence of abnormal Papanicolaou (Pap) tests; therefore, it is recommended that a Pap test be performed 3 months after initiating the use of the cap. If the Pap smear is normal, then the woman can proceed with yearly Pap tests.

Nonprescription Barrier Methods for Women: The Lea Contraceptive, Contraceptive Sponge, and Female Condoms

Similar in some aspects to both the diaphragm and cervical cap is the *Lea contraceptive*. It is inserted before intercourse, with a spermicide, and is left in place for at least 8 and as many as 48 hours after. One size fits all, which is an advantage. Given no need for prescription, it provides enhanced access to contraception for women who prefer a barrier method. The *contraceptive sponge* is impregnated with nonoxynol-9 spermicide and is inserted deep into the vagina after moistening with water. Its manufacture was interrupted in 1995 because of concerns regarding the risk of toxic shock syndrome, but it again became available in 2005 as the *Today* sponge.

Female condoms provide another accessible option to barrier contraception approved by the U.S. Food and Drug Administration (FDA). The condom is a lubricated polyurethane pouch that lines the vagina. One outer ring lies outside the body and a smaller inner ring is pushed up toward the cervix to hold the condom in place. It gives a woman an additional choice and freedom to protect herself from sexually transmitted diseases and pregnancy. Because it is made from polyurethane, the female condom can be used by latex-allergic individuals. Female condoms appear to have failure rates similar to those of the male condom. Unfortunately, they cost about twice as much as the male condom.

Spermicidal Creams and Jellies

Spermicidal creams and jellies may have a high theoretical effectiveness, but they have lesser use effectiveness. Most contain nonoxynol-9 as the spermicidal agent. The physical nature of the creams and jellies and difficulty in their application often result in inadequately smearing the cervical os, so that sperm invasion is not prevented. Both men and women complain of the dehydrating effect of spermicidal agents and may report burning sensations. Nonoxynol-9 is toxic *in vitro* to HIV, gonococci, *Chlamydia*, and other genital pathogens, but clinical evidence does not support an *in vivo* effect; one randomized trial showed similar rates of gonococcal and chlamydial infection with condoms alone and with condoms plus nonoxynol-9. *Foams* have better physical properties, allowing more adequate smearing of the cervical os; however, foams are effective for short periods of time only, and reapplications are necessary. This increases their cost. They also contain nonoxynol-9 and may cause irritation. Failure rates up to 25% are reported. When used in conjunction with the condom, excellent pregnancy protection has been demonstrated, reaching 96% effectiveness. Like some of the barrier methods, foams have the advantage of being readily accessible in both supermarkets and drugstores, and they do not require medical instruction or prescription.

INTRAUTERINE DEVICES (8,9)

Modern intrauterine devices (IUDs) either contain copper or release a progestin. The copper devices induce an inflammatory response that prevents viable sperm from reaching the fallopian tubes. Progestin-releasing IUDs inhibit both sperm survival and nidation. The 0.1% to 0.8% first-year pregnancy rates with these IUDs are the lowest attainable with any form of reversible birth control and are comparable with those of surgical sterilization. That compliance is not an issue greatly enhances effectiveness. Another advantage is the lack of systemic effects, a major problem with oral contraceptives (see later discussion). A major limitation is expulsion, which is particularly frequent in nulliparous women. Rates as high as 19 expulsions per 100 women per year had been reported with older devices, but rates have been substantially reduced with newer devices: 3% to 10% per year for the copper device and 1% to

6% per year for those that release progestin. The copper IUD remains effective for 8 to 10 years. Progestasert IUDs, which remained effective for only 1 year, have been largely replaced with a levonorgestrel-releasing IUD (Mirena) that remains effective for 5 years. The levonorgestrel IUD reduces menstrual bleeding, causing oligomenorrhea in 70% and amenorrhea in 30% of cases. This is an advantage for women bothered by heavy bleeding and a disadvantage for those who prefer to have regular menstrual cycles. Even though not unexpected, the onset of amenorrhea warrants a pregnancy test.

Earlier IUDs increased the risk of *tubal infertility*, which greatly discouraged IUD placement, especially among nulliparous women. In 1986, the sale of all IUDs except Progestasert was discontinued. In 1988, Paragard, the current copper IUD, was approved by the FDA. The newer IUDs do not confer the same increased risk of pelvic inflammatory disease (PID) among women at low risk for sexually transmitted disease (STD). However, copper IUDs may increase the likelihood of PID and subsequent tubal infertility among women exposed to an STD and should not be inserted in women who have multiple partners or a partner with multiple partners without their being fully informed. The levonorgestrel-releasing IUD may reduce the risk of PID.

IUDs are associated with lower risk of *ectopic pregnancy* compared with no birth control but higher risk compared with hormonal methods that prevent ovulation. This is especially true for the levonorgestrel-releasing IUD; as many as 50% of pregnancies that occur with it in place are ectopic. On the rare occasions when pregnancy does occur despite IUD use, its location should be ascertained immediately.

ORAL CONTRACEPTIVES (10–41)

Combinations of synthetic estrogen and progesterone have been found to have use effectiveness rates that are significantly better than barrier methods and spermicides. Although some report failure rates as high as 5% to 10%, most report only 1 failure per 100 users per year. The combination pill prevents cyclic release of follicle-stimulating hormone (FSH) and luteinizing hormone, which are required for ovulation; alter the cervical mucus, thereby decreasing sperm motility; and alter the endometrial lining to inhibit implantation. Combination pills consist of an estrogen (ethinyl estradiol or mestranol) and a progestin (norethindrone, norgestrel, levonorgestrel, ethynodiol diacetate, desogestrel, and norgestimate). Most pill cycles are 28 days long. Pill packets contain 21 or 28 pills, depending on the brand. Twenty-eight-day packets contain placebo pills for part or all of the last week of the pill pack. Patients are instructed to start on the first Sunday of the menstrual cycle or the first day of bleeding. Extended-cycle regimens, containing 84 active pills and 7 inactive pills, became available in 2003 for women who want to reduce the frequency of menses.

Preparations

More than three dozen combination preparations are available in the United States. In general, it is most useful to renew any prescription with which a patient is satisfied, as long as the patient has no new symptoms or habits that warrant discontinuation of any oral contraceptive.

Cardiovascular risks have been a significant concern when prescribing the pill. Because of the concern that these risks might increase with estrogen dose and progestin potency, emphasis in recent years has been on the use of preparations that

have the lowest effective estrogen dose (20 to 35 μg of ethinyl estradiol) and the least progestin potency. Fortunately, the efficacy of 30 to 35 μg of estrogen for the prevention of pregnancy is about the same as that of the older, 50-μg estrogen pill.

It is best to begin with a pill containing 30 to 35 μg of ethinyl estradiol. Using the lowest possible progestin dose helps to minimize bothersome side effects such as increased appetite, steady weight gain, acne, and depression. Many newer and more expensive oral contraceptives are heavily marketed. They may offer some theoretical benefits and perhaps fewer actual ones. Currently, a line of generic birth control pills offers a range of options at a much lower cost to the patient or insurer. It is prudent to reserve the high-cost oral contraceptive pills for patients who have a medical need for a specialized contraceptive pill. A good basic pill to start with contains 1 mg of norethindrone and 35 μg of ethinyl estradiol (generic Necon 1/35, Ortho-Novum 1/35).

Patients who have a history of symptoms suggesting hyperresponsiveness to endogenous estrogens (premenstrual breast engorgement and soreness, cyclic weight gain, heavy periods) may benefit from a preparation containing a low estrogen dose and a progestin with minimal estrogenic effect (e.g., Necon 0.5/35, a generic preparation; norethindrone 0.5 mg/ethinyl estradiol 35 μg; or Ovcon with ethinyl estradiol 35 μg and norethindrone 0.4 mg). All progestins have relatively low estrogenic effect, except for ethynodiol. Similarly, a patient bothered by acne or hirsutism should be given a preparation with low androgenic progestin such as ethynodiol, desogestrel, or norgestimate (Table 119.1). Other side effects such as nausea seem to be related to estrogen content.

The disadvantages of using lower-dose agents are higher rates of spotting, breakthrough bleeding, and amenorrhea. Moreover, women who use oral contraceptives containing less than 30 μg of estrogen may experience a greater chance of pregnancy. To counteract this reduced efficacy, newer pills with 20 μg of ethinyl estradiol have lengthened the hormone cycle with as few as 2 days of hormone-free placebo in the 28-day cycle. In an attempt to improve rates of breakthrough bleeding and pregnancy associated with low-estrogen/weak-progestin formulations, manufacturers developed *biphasic* (e.g., Ortho-Novum 10/11) and *triphasic* (e.g., Ortho-Novum 7/7/7, Tri-Norinyl, Triphasil) formulations. The rationale is more closely to mimic normal ovarian patterns. Efficacy is similar to that obtained with other low-estrogen/weak-progestin preparations; no controlled evidence suggests that they are superior in terms of breakthrough bleeding. There is evidence that the monophasics are superior to triphasic pills in suppressing ovarian function and should be the pill of choice in women with a history

---

TABLE 119.1

EFFECTS OF SYNTHETIC PROGESTINS

Estrogenic	Androgenic
Ethynodiol	Norgestrel
All others have none	Levonorgestrel
	Norethindrone
	Norethindrone acetate
	Ethynodiol
	Norgestimate
	Desogestrel
	Drospirenone
In order of decreasing potency.	

of large ovarian cysts. All low-dose preparations need to be taken consistently to be maximally effective and to minimize the chances of breakthrough bleeding.

Progestin-only pills—"the minipill"—are available and prescribed for women who should not take estrogens. Lactating women, women with complex migraine headaches, women older than 35 years who smoke, and women with thromboembolic disease may be given this preparation. Other women who might fare better with the progestin-only pill include those with cardiovascular disease, hypertension, or diabetes.

It is helpful to become familiar with four or five pills and their minor differences rather than use the most recently marketed combinations. Providing the patient with full understandable information at the initiation of therapy will ward off many anxious phone calls. In particular, women should be advised that if one pill is missed, it can be made up by doubling the next dose. If two pills are missed, the patient should double the dose for the next 2 days, but barrier contraception is recommended for the remainder of the cycle. If three or more consecutive pills are missed, the pills should be stopped altogether, allowing withdrawal bleeding to occur. A new pill pack should be started 1 week after the last pill was taken. Recurrent failure to take oral contraceptives regularly is an indication for trying another form of birth control.

Because contraceptive pills are often prescribed until menopause, knowing just when to stop can be a challenge to the patient and the physician. One approach is to check FSH near the age of 50 years. The FSH should be checked on day 7 of the placebo or pill-free week. If the FSH is significantly elevated (close to 100), then it would be appropriate to stop. If the FSH is normal or midrange, then continuing the pill and rechecking the FSH in another year would be prudent.

Breakthrough bleeding is a common side effect of the pill. If it occurs late in the cycle or in the first few months of initiation of the pill, it is usually caused by too little progesterone. If it occurs early in the cycle or after years of use, it may be caused by inadequate estrogen. This problem may be temporarily resolved by having the patient take two pills a day for 3 days. The additional pills should be obtained from a separate package of pills. Women who choose the extended-cycle regimen should understand that breakthrough bleeding is likely to be more common than with the standard 28-day cycle.

If the problem recurs repeatedly after the first 3 months, then changing the pill to a stronger estrogenic or progestinal pill is appropriate. The physician should always rule out other causes of irregular bleeding, such as infection and pregnancy.

Another common complaint is that of *morning nausea*. It may be improved by having the patient take the pill with her evening meal and then consume a light breakfast daily. If the symptoms persist, switching to a lower-estrogen pill or a progesterone-only pill (e.g., Micronor) may be indicated.

Patients require follow-up care 6 to 12 weeks after the initiation of the birth control pill to check for hypertension, review proper use, and discuss side effects. Patients should then be seen yearly, checking for headaches, hypertension, breast masses, cervical abnormalities, phlebitis, and signs of cardiovascular or cerebrovascular disease.

Physicians are generally unaware of the high discontinuation rate among oral contraceptive users. Factors involved include the patient's perceptions of need and attitudes about taking medications that affect the sex organs. Oral contraceptives are expensive and require a medical prescription, which are important barriers for adolescents. Despite these factors and known side effects, birth control pills continue to be among the most used and safest birth control method for most nonsmokers.

Cardiovascular Adverse Effects

Historically, the major hazards of oral contraceptives have been related to vascular thrombosis. Relative risk estimates for myocardial infarction, thrombotic stroke, and thromboembolism for current users compared with nonusers have ranged as high as 12, 9.5, and 11, respectively. Reduction of estrogen content (e.g., to 30 or 35 μg of ethinyl estradiol or less), however, has substantially reduced these risks. At this point, there is no evidence for significant increase in cardiovascular risk for women younger than age 30 years or in nonsmoking women without other risk factors. Because of very low baseline risks in relevant populations, the additional risk of these adverse events attributable to oral contraceptive use is extremely low. For example, in the case of venous thrombosis, low-risk populations would have a baseline risk of less than 1 per 10,000 woman-years increased to 3 to 4 per 10,000 woman-years during the period of use. Studies consistently show greater increased risks *in smokers*. Mortality from myocardial infarction rises sixfold with oral contraceptive use in women older than age 40 years who are smokers. Hypertension is another factor that confers greater increased risk of adverse cardiovascular events with oral contraceptive use. This is at least partly due to further increases in blood pressure related to progestin-induced increase in aldosterone secretion and estrogen-induced increase in renin substrate.

Progestin potency is also associated with increased cardiovascular risk, possibly because of its ability to raise low-density-lipoprotein (LDL) cholesterol and lower high-density-lipoprotein (HDL) cholesterol (see Chapter 15). Initial concern that the newer progestins such as desogestrel may be related to an increase in thromboembolic disease and deep vein thrombosis has not been borne out in further studies. Any population of women provided with oral contraception will show a rise in mean blood pressure in about 3 months. Prospective studies have found that the incidence of *hypertension* increases two- to sixfold in users compared with nonusers. As noted, it is wise to check blood pressure before renewing a patient's prescription. Table 119.2 summarizes estimates of risks of cardiovascular events by age and risk factor.

Other Adverse Effects

There is a twofold increase in the risk of *gallbladder disease* in users compared with nonusers because of the increased cholesterol saturation of bile. The frequency of gallstones appears to rise after 2 years of use and to reach a plateau after 4 to 5 years of use. This risk must be balanced against the increased risk of gallbladder disease associated with multiparity. Another hepatobiliary problem is the rare development of highly vascular *hepatic adenomas*, which can rupture spontaneously, resulting in serious hemorrhage. Isolated cases have appeared in the literature; in most cases, patients had been using the pill for longer than 5 years. The actual risk is unknown. Finally, estrogen use has been associated with *cholestatic jaundice*, but oral contraceptive use does not worsen cases of mild viral hepatitis and need not be discontinued unless cholestasis or hepatocellular injury is severe.

Studies concerning the risk of breast cancer associated with the use of oral contraceptives have produced conflicting results and much controversy. Although pooled analysis of such studies suggested there may be a small but statistically significant increase in the risk of breast cancer, many of the studies examined had methodologic flaws and included the use of high-dose

TABLE 119.2

AGE-SPECIFIC ESTIMATES OF THE EXCESS RATES OF MYOCARDIAL INFARCTION, ISCHEMIC STROKE, AND VENOUS THROMBOEMBOLISM ATTRIBUTABLE TO THE USE OF LOW-ESTROGEN ORAL CONTRACEPTIVES AND PREGNANCY-RELATED MORTALITY[a]

Variable	Estimate for Given Age Range in Years		
	20–24	30–34	40–44
Number of excess cases of myocardial infarction and ischemic stroke attributable to oral contraceptive use (per 100,000 woman-yr of use)[b]			
Among nonsmokers	0.4	0.6	2
Among smokers	1	2	20
Among women with hypertension	4	7	29
Number of pregnancy-related deaths (per 100,000 live births)	10	12	45
Number of excess cases of venous thromboembolism attributable to oral contraceptive use (per 100,000 woman-yr of use)			
With norethindrone, norethindrone acetate, levonorgestrel, or ethynodiol diacetate	6	9	12
With desogestrel or gestodene	16	23	30

[a]Low estrogen was defined as <50 μg.
[b]Data are from Farley et al. (15).
From Petitti DB. Combination estrogen–progestin oral contraceptives. N Engl J Med 2003;349:1443, with permission.

preparations, which are no longer used. A more recent large-scale, observational study involving women who used low-dose preparations revealed no increase in risk, even among those with a family history of breast cancer. If there is an increased risk, it appears, at most, to be very small in most populations of women and probably only important to consider in women at high genetic risk (e.g., those who are BRCA-positive).

Systematic review suggests that the risk of cervical cancer increases with the duration of oral contraceptive use in all women and in women who are HPV-positive. Most studies have shown diminished incidences of fibroadenomas, ovarian and endometrial cancers, and benign fibrocystic disease of the breast in pill users.

Metabolic and endocrinologic effects of oral contraceptive pills are numerous. Thyroid-binding globin levels increase, which in turn raises the serum thyroxine level. Glucose tolerance falls as circulating growth hormone rises and peripheral resistance to insulin occurs. Triglyceride levels increase, sometimes dramatically, with the concurrent boost in lipoprotein production. The estrogen component tends to result in a rise in HDL cholesterol, whereas the progestin may result in a rise in LDL cholesterol. There is no evidence to suggest that the oral contraceptive pill should not be prescribed in women with hypercholesterolemia. However, it may be prudent to use a pill shown to have minimal lipid-worsening effect. Such pills are those with low doses of norethindrone (e.g., Necon 0.5/35 or Ovcon) or those with more recently developed progestins (e.g., Desogen).

A few miscellaneous effects are noteworthy. Birth control pills may increase the frequency of *migraine headache* in patients with prior migraine attacks. However, they are only contraindicated in the woman with neurologic symptoms associated with her migraine headache. Anecdotal reports of *exacerbation of lupus erythematosus* appear in the obstetric literature. Sensitivity to sunlight and chloasma (mask of pregnancy) are seen in some users and fade with discontinuation.

Certain medications such as antibiotics and seizure medications have been found to affect the efficacy of the oral contraceptive pill. Anticonvulsants such as phenytoin induce hepatic metabolism and therefore affect the circulating level of hor-

mone. Gabapentin is not metabolized and is therefore unlikely to affect contraceptive hormone levels. It is prudent to advise women who are prescribed oral antibiotics to use backup contraception for that month. However, the data to support this practice are limited.

A number of gynecologic conditions are affected by the use of these agents; the effects may be beneficial or detrimental. Patients with menstrual irregularities before oral contraceptive use will have regular pill-induced periods while taking the medication. Patients should have a full evaluation of the etiology of their irregular menses before initiation of the oral contraceptive pill. On discontinuation of the pills, some will revert to their previous irregularity. Rarely, *amenorrhea* due to ovarian suppression will persist for several months, even 1 year after pill cessation (see Chapter 112). Usually, menses return promptly, and fertility rates in the first 3 months of discontinuation are increased. Occasionally, a patient will notice nipple discharge (nonpuerperal lactation) with the use of oral contraceptives. The mechanism is not clear. No increased incidence of pituitary prolactinomas has been observed.

Many patients with *dysmenorrhea* find marked relief with oral contraceptives (see Chapter 116). If the dysmenorrhea is associated with endometriosis, the response is variable, with many patients complaining of an exacerbation of symptoms rather than relief.

With these side effects in mind, absolute and relative contraindications can be listed (Table 119.3). Patients exposed to diethylstilbestrol have used birth control pills with no evidence of either beneficial or deleterious effects.

OTHER APPROACHES TO HORMONAL CONTRACEPTION (42–48)

Subdermal Implants

Norplant was the first subdermal contraceptive widely used in the United States. It consisted of six slender Silastic tubes that

TABLE 119.3

CONTRAINDICATIONS FOR ORAL CONTRACEPTIVES

Absolute Contraindications
Thromboembolic disorders, cardiovascular disease, thrombophlebitis, or a past history of these conditions or other conditions that predispose to them
Markedly impaired liver function
Known cancers of the breast, endometrium, etc.
Undiagnosed genital bleeding
Known or suspected pregnancy
Migraine headache with focal symptoms
Smoker, >35 yr old, >15 cigarettes per day

Relative Contraindications
Age >35 yr, no focal symptoms
Migraine headache
Hypertension
Hyperlipidemia
Epilepsy
Uterine leiomyoma
History of idiopathic obstructive jaundice of pregnancy
Smoker >35 yr old, >15 cigarettes per day
Diabetes mellitus
Heart disease
Patient unreliability

continuously released the progestin levonorgestrel at a very low level for 5 years. Norplant has since been replaced by *Jadelle*, a two-rod levonorgestrel implant that is easier to insert and remove. Reported cumulative pregnancy rates are as low as 0.3 at 3 years and 1.1 at 5 years, rates comparable to IUD use and even surgical sterilization. The advantages are 5 years of continuous contraception and very low hormone levels, resulting in no clinically significant metabolic effects. The disadvantages are irregular bleeding (in 66%) lasting many months and an initial high cost. *Implanon* is a single-rod implant that provides 3 years of contraception with the slow release of the progestin etonogestrel. Effectiveness and adverse events are similar to those of Jadelle.

Intramuscular Injections

Depo-Provera has also been FDA approved for use as a contraceptive, although a warning was subsequently issued regarding a decrease in bone density during use. Medroxyprogesterone acetate 150 mg is administered intramuscularly every 3 months. Care should be taken to ensure that the woman is not pregnant initially, and it is recommended that the drug be administered during the first 5 days of the cycle. If a patient waits longer than 14 weeks between injections, a pregnancy test should be performed before her next injection. The pregnancy rate is 1% if used correctly. Disadvantages include irregular bleeding and the discomfort of patients receiving injections.

The Transdermal Patch

The transdermal contraceptive patch (e.g., Ortho Evra) delivers continuous estrogen and progestin doses while worn on the arm, abdomen, or buttock for 3 weeks (changed once per week for 3 weeks) of each 4-week cycle. In early studies, contraceptive effectiveness was similar to that of combination pills.

Compliance was better. Some adverse events—venous thromboembolism, for example—may be more frequent.

The Contraceptive Ring

Contraceptive rings (e.g., NuvaRing) were also designed to improve compliance with hormonal contraception without the need for implants or injections. They are worn intravaginally for 3 weeks of each 4-week cycle. Despite delivering lower doses of hormones, contraceptive effectiveness among compliant patients appears to equal that of oral contraceptives, although trial evidence is more limited.

EMERGENCY CONTRACEPTION (49–54)

Unplanned, unprotected intercourse is a common occurrence. It may be forced or consensual. The probability of pregnancy following unprotected intercourse during the second or third week of a woman's menstrual cycle is roughly 8%. Emergency contraceptive measures taken during the ensuing 120 hours can reduce that probability by 75% or more. Available regimens include: (a) *progestin* only (1.5 mg of single-dose levonorgestrel or two 0.75-mg doses taken 12 hours apart, the latter regimen marketed as Plan B; (b) *mifepristone* (25 to 50 mg, single dose); (c) *estrogen/progestin* (ethinyl estradiol 100 μg plus levonorgestrel 0.5 mg) repeated in 12 hours, known as the Yuzpe regimen and marketed as Preven until 2004; or (d) *high-dose estrogen* (ethinyl estradiol 0.5 mg) twice daily for 5 days. When a licensed regimen is not readily available, each dose of the Yuzpe regimen can be approximated using commonly available oral contraceptives (e.g., two Ovral tablets, four Lo Ovral tablets, four Triphasil tablets). Progestin-only contraceptive pills can be used in a similar fashion to approximate the progestin-only approach (e.g., 20 Ovrette tablets). The effectiveness of the hormonal regimens decreases over time since unprotected coitus. Nausea and vomiting may occur with estrogen-based programs and should be treated prophylactically with an antiemetic taken 1 hour before the first dose. If emesis occurs within 1 hour of taking an estrogen-containing pill, then the dose should be repeated. Advisory committees to the FDA and professional organizations have recommended that the levonorgestrel-only regimen (Plan B) be made available without prescription, as is the case in many other countries. The FDA considered the issue in May 2004 but did not give approval. Legislation in some states has made it possible for pharmacists to dispense emergency contraception directly without a physician's prescription.

Mifepristone, also known as RU-486, is an antiprogesterone. It is the only drug that interrupts pregnancy after implantation has occurred. In two randomized trials, it was 100% effective in preventing pregnancy when given within 72 hours of unprotected intercourse; delay in administration for up to 120 hours following coitus does not appear to diminish effectiveness.

Placement of a *copper IUD* within 120 hours of unprotected intercourse is also an effective option for the woman who wants continuing contraception.

ABORTION

See Chapter 121. Studies by Planned Parenthood have not found that a substantial number of American women rely on abortion as the sole method of birth control. Rather, abortion is used as a backup when other methods fail. Frequently, the necessity for an abortion initiates effective contraceptive use, particularly in those younger than age 20 years. No adverse effect of first-trimester induced abortion on future childbearing has been demonstrated. The effect of second-trimester abortions in rupturing cervical tissue is controversial. Rarely, an anomalous cervix may become incompetent, requiring *cerclage* if the patient wishes to carry future pregnancies to term. Morbidity and mortality in teenagers from induced abortion is lower than in older women.

Since 1988, mifepristone has been successfully used in Europe for medical termination of early pregnancy. It is given as an oral dose in combination with a self-administered vaginal prostaglandin analogue. It has been found to be safe, highly effective, and acceptable to women. In addition, it is being studied for other clinical uses, including the treatment of leiomyomata, endometriosis, and breast cancer, and as a potential estrogen-free contraceptive.

OVERALL RISKS

Used alone by women younger than 30 years, condoms, diaphragms, IUDs, birth control pills, and first-trimester abortion have a mortality risk of 1 to 2 per 100,000, significantly lower than the 12 per 100,000 delivery-related risk rate. After age 30 years, the risk for using birth control pills rises, especially in smokers, but it is still less than the morbidity and complications of childbearing without fertility control. The birth control pill may be prescribed to women until menopause, but it is contraindicated in a smoker past the age of 35 years. The lowest level of mortality is achieved by a combination of contraception with access to early abortion.

STERILIZATION (55-58)

In 1965, one third of the married couples in the United States used oral contraception, sterilization, or IUDs. By 1975, almost three fourths used one of these methods. Sterilization is now the most frequently used method of contraception among couples married for a decade or longer and among couples who have had all the children they want.

Vasectomy

Vasectomy is the simplest, safest, and least expensive means of sterilization. Only a few surgical instruments and local anesthesia are required. The procedure may be done in a clinic, doctor's office, ambulatory surgical day care unit, or hospital. The procedure does not lead to impotence; rather, men with problems associated with impotence may blame vasectomy. It takes about 90 days of average ejaculatory activity to completely empty the spermatic cord and accessory glands of residual sperm. Thus, the vasectomy subject should have a postoperative semen analysis before he is considered sterile. Alternative methods of birth control should be used in the interim. Circulating antibodies to sperm may be induced by foreign proteins and by sperm. The effect of elevated sperm antibodies on a man's health is not clear but has been the subject of much concern. Retrospective cohort study of more than 10,000 vasectomized men failed to support such concerns; no serious immunopathologic consequences of vasectomy were noted. Further evidence of safety emerges from case–control and cohort studies showing no relation between vasectomy and cardiovascular disease.

The only adverse effects are an increased risk of epididymitis, orchitis, and testicular changes leading to infertility (see later discussion). Some epidemiologic studies suggested an increased risk of late-onset prostate cancer, but subsequent well-designed, larger-scale, case–control studies failed to confirm the concern.

Vasectomy is not 100% effective. Recanalization when ends of the vas are tied too closely together may account for some failures. In addition, it is not 100% irreversible. Reanastomosis may be carried out with microsurgical techniques; however, only about one third of patients undergoing reanastomosis father live-born children.

Fallopian Tube Interruption (Tubal Sterilization)

Tubal sterilization is the leading form of contraception in the United States, with more than 10 million women having undergone the procedure and 1 million procedures being performed annually. Like vasectomy, the procedure is not foolproof; the pregnancy rate is 1% to 2%, depending on the type of tubal procedure performed. Of the pregnancies that do occur after tubal sterilization, a substantial proportion (0.15 to 0.65) are ectopic.

Tubal ligation is often performed as a laparoscopic procedure, often soon after a woman has given birth, when the procedure of choice is a partial salpingectomy. When not performed in the postpartum period, laparoscopic coagulation of the fallopian tubes can be accomplished as an outpatient procedure. Hysteroscopic occlusion of the tubes is a newer approach.

In general, tubal sterilization should be considered irreversible. The procedure is indicated only when it is the woman who requests it. Many requests for anastomosis of divided tubes come when the procedure is initially advocated by a physician or partner. On average, women are aged 28 to 30 years at the time of tubal sterilization; 88% are married, and only 6% have never been married. Of note, the risk of ovarian cancer appears to be reduced by tubal sterilization procedures; the mechanism is unknown.

CHOICE OF METHOD (29,59,60)

The choice of birth control is best viewed in terms of the patient's age and family expectations. *Unmarried adolescents and women in their early 20s* may use oral contraceptives with a high degree of safety and acceptability. Contraindications are infrequent in this age group, and the cost, in general, is not beyond their reach. Newer hormonal contraceptives have the advantage of lower failure rates related to problems of compliance. Diaphragms may be as effective when used correctly and consistently but often are less acceptable. Condoms are an excellent choice, given their effectiveness and protection from sexually transmitted diseases. Their use, however, depends on the motivation of the male partner as well as the woman. IUDs are effective; they are underutilized because of concerns about the risk of pelvic sepsis, which has been substantially reduced with newer devices.

For sexually active *26- to 35-year-olds*, birth control pills and newer hormonal contraceptives, as well as diaphragms and condoms, may be equally effective. Choice is simply a matter of preference. IUDs may be a very good option for women in monogamous relationships. The woman who smokes should be asked to stop tobacco use if she wants to use oral contraceptives. Many patients in this age group have completed their families and request sterilization. Nulliparous women in this age group who desire sterilization present a problem to many health care providers. If the patient is not well known to the clinic or physician, one can suggest that she practice contraception for 1 year, then undergo sterilization if she still wants to. When such advice is given, perhaps half of the patients return for the procedure. The others go elsewhere or change their minds.

For the *woman older than age 35 years*, the birth control pill may be prescribed as long as she is a nonsmoker. Diaphragms, condoms, sterilization, and, more recently, the pill and newer forms of hormonal contraception are commonly chosen by *women older than age 40 years*.

PATIENT EDUCATION (60–63)

There are few areas in primary care in which patient education is so important to decision making. Diagrammatic and written materials are available from most commercial distributors of contraceptive products, Planned Parenthood, many women's advocacy organizations, the American College of Obstetrics and Gynecology, and the American Medical Association. It is most important that information be clearly written in the patient's native language and that the patient be given an opportunity to ask questions and demonstrate her understanding. There is a clear need for women to understand their suscep-tibility to unintended pregnancy if they do not make full use of available approaches; almost one half of women surveyed after unintended pregnancy believed they could not or would not get pregnant at the time of conception.

The need to offer sympathetic and nonjudgmental counseling cannot be overemphasized. Regardless of the physician's views on abortion and birth control, the patient should be able to obtain factual information from her primary care physician or should be referred to someone who is willing to provide the information and care desired.

INDICATIONS FOR REFERRAL

Patients may need or request referral for counseling on emotional responses to sexual activity and contraceptive techniques. Referral to a social worker, sex therapist, or psychiatrist with an interest in the area may be useful, but thorough discussion between the primary physician and the patient usually suffices.

When a surgical procedure is being considered, the patient should meet with the gynecologist to discuss the issue in more detail. For patients with known medical problems, a careful history and physical examination and written referral to the specialist are helpful, so that the risks of the various procedures may be carefully discussed and therapy individualized.

A.G.M.

Annotated Bibliography

1. Jones EF, Forrest JD. Contraceptive failure rates based on the 1988 NSFG. Fam Plann Perspect 1992;24:12. (*Provides failure rates, noting that they vary more by user characteristics such as age, marital status, and poverty status than by method.*)
2. Trussell J, Grummer-Strawn L. Contraceptive failure of the ovulation method of periodic abstinence. Fam Plann Perspect 1990;22:65. (*Cites a 28% risk of pregnancy per menstrual cycle when a couple breaks any of the three most serious rules—no intercourse during mucus days and within 3 days before the day of peak fecundity and during times of stress.*)
3. Wilcox AJ, Dunson D, Baird DD. The timing of the "fertile window" in the menstrual cycle: day specific estimates from a prospective study. BMJ 2000;321:1259. (*In only about 30% of women is the fertile window entirely between days 10 and 17 of the menstrual cycle.*)
4. Cook L, Nanda K, Grimes D. Diaphragm versus diaphragm with spermicides for contraception. (Cochrane review). In: Oxford: Update Software, 2004. (*Could not distinguish between the contraceptive effectiveness of the diaphragm with and without spermicide, but does not recommend a change in spermicide use; see http://www.cochrane.org for updates.*)
5. Gallo MF, Grimes DA, Schulz KF. Non-latex versus latex male condoms for contraception (Cochrane review). In: The Cochrane library, Issue 3. Oxford: Update Software, 2004. (*Participants preferred nonlatex condoms, but breakage was more likely, with an odds ratio [OR] ranging from 2.6 to 5.0; see http://www.cochrane.org for updates.*)
6. Roddy RE, Zekeng L, Ryan KA, et al. Effect of nonoxynol-9 gel on urogenital gonorrhea and chlamydial infection: a randomized controlled trial. JAMA 2002;287:1117. (*Nonoxynol-9 plus condom use did not reduce the rates of gonococcal or chlamydial infection compared with the use of condoms alone.*)
7. Steiner MJ, Dominik R, Rountree RW, et al. Contraceptive effectiveness of a polyurethane condom and a latex condom: a randomized controlled trial. Obstet Gynecol 2003;101:539. (*The polyurethane condom was not shown to be as effective as the latex comparator condom for pregnancy prevention.*)
8. Dardano KL, Burkman RT. The intrauterine contraceptive device: an often-forgotten and maligned method of contraception. Am J Obstet Gynecol 1999;181:1. (*Despite many advantages for some women, it is used by <1% of American women who use contraception.*)
9. Hubacher D, Lara-Ricalde R, Taylor DJ, et al. Use of copper intrauterine devices and the risk of tubal infertility among nulligravid women. N Engl J Med 2001;345:561. (*The previous use of a copper intrauterine device [IUD] is not associated with an increased risk of tubal occlusion among nulligravid women, whereas infection with Chlamydia trachomatis is.*)
10. Beral V, Hermon C, Kay C, et al. Mortality associated with oral contraceptive use: 25 year follow up of cohort of 46,000 women from Royal College of General Practitioners' oral contraceptive study. BMJ 1999;318:96. (*Current and recent users had a relative risk of 0.2 for ovarian cancer and 1.9 for cerebrovascular disease.*)
11. Chan WS, Ray J, Wai EK, et al. Risk of stroke in women exposed to low-dose oral contraceptives: a critical evaluation of the evidence. Arch Intern Med 2004;164:741. (*Casts doubt on a true association between low-dose oral contraceptive pills and stroke because of the low absolute magnitude of the ORs, the severe methodological limitations, and the ORs of <1.0 in the cohort studies.*)
12. Chang CL, Donaghy M, Poulter N. Migraine and stroke in young women: case control study. BMJ 1999;318:13. (*Oral contraceptive use increases the risk of stroke associated with migraine.*)
13. Chasan-Taber L, Stampfer MJ. Epidemiology of oral contraceptives and cardiovascular disease. Ann Intern Med 1998;128:467. (*An extensive review of the literature, showing that cardiovascular risk is lower with any of the current new preparations than with prior high-estrogen-dose pills; the cardiovascular risk is significant in smokers.*)
14. Eldon MA, Underwood BA, Randinitis EJ, et al. Gabapentin does not interact with a contraceptive regimen of norethindrone acetate and ethinyl estradiol. Neurology 1998;50:1146. (*Gabapentin may be a good choice as an anticonvulsant for women on oral contraceptives.*)
15. Farley TM, Collins J, Schlesselman JJ. Hormonal contraception and risk of cardiovascular disease: an international perspective. Contraception 1998;57:211. (*Provides estimates of excess cardiovascular events attributable to low-dose contraceptive pills.*)
16. Gaspard UJ, Lefebvre PJ. Clinical aspects of the relationship between oral contraceptives, abnormalities in carbohydrate metabolism, and the development of cardiovascular disease. Am J Obstet Gynecol 1990;163:334. (*Low-dose oral contraceptives with reduced progestogen content have the least effect on glucose tolerance.*)
17. Gillum LA, Mamidipudi SK, Johnston SC. Ischemic stroke risk with oral contraceptives: a meta-analysis. JAMA 2000;284:72. (*The risk of ischemic stroke is increased in current oral contraceptive users, even with newer, low-estrogen preparations.*)
18. Hankinson SE, Colditz GA, Manson JE, et al. A prospective study on oral contraceptive use and risk of breast cancer (Nurses' Health Study, United States). Cancer Causes Control 1997;8:65. (*A cohort study of women, finding no increase in breast cancer risk in women older than 40 years of age.*)
19. Holt VL, Cushing-Haugen KL, Daling JR. Body weight and risk of oral contraceptive failure. Obstet Gynecol 2002;99:820. (*After controlling for parity,*

women in the highest body-weight quartile [≥70.5 kg] had a significantly increased risk of oral contraceptive failure [relative risk, 1.6].)

20. Kemmeren JM, Algra A, Grobbee DE. Third generation oral contraceptives and risk of venous thrombosis: meta-analysis. BMJ 2001;323:131. (*A meta-analysis, supporting the view that third-generation oral contraceptives are associated with an increased risk of venous thrombosis compared with second-generation oral contraceptives.*)

21. Kemmeren JM, Tanis BC, van den Bosch MA, et al. Risk of Arterial Thrombosis in Relation to Oral Contraceptives (RATIO) study: oral contraceptives and the risk of ischemic stroke. Stroke 2002;33:1202. (*Third-generation oral contraceptives [containing desogestrel or gestodene] confer the same risk of first ischemic stroke as second-generation oral contraceptives [containing levonorgestrel].*)

22. Mant J, Painter R, Vessey M. Risk of myocardial infarction, angina and stroke in users of oral contraceptives: an updated analysis of a cohort study. Br J Obstet Gynaecol 1998;105:890. (*A cohort study of 17,032, revealing a slight increase the risk of ischemic stroke [relative risk, 2.9] in all users and of myocardial infarction only in smokers.*)

23. Marchbanks PA, McDonald JA, Wilson HG, et al. Oral contraceptives and the risk of breast cancer. N Engl J Med 2002;346:2025. (*A large-scale, observational, case–control study, finding no increased risk of breast cancer with the use of oral contraceptives.*)

24. Miller L, Hughes JP. Continuous combination oral contraceptive pills to eliminate withdrawal bleeding: a randomized trial. Obstet Gynecol 2003;101:653. (*There were significantly fewer bleeding days.*)

25. Modan B, Hartge P, Hirsch-Yechezkel G, et al. Parity, oral contraceptives, and the risk of ovarian cancer among carriers and noncarriers of a BRCA1 or BRCA2 mutation. N Engl J Med 2001;345:235. (*The risk of ovarian cancer among carriers of a BRCA1 or BRCA2 mutation decreased with each birth but not with the increased duration of use of oral contraceptives.*)

26. Moreno V, Bosch FX, Munoz N, et al. Effect of oral contraceptives on risk of cervical cancer in women with human papillomavirus infection: the IARC multicentric case–control study. Lancet 2002;359:1085. (*The long-term use of oral contraceptives could be a cofactor that increases the risk of cervical carcinoma by up to fourfold in women who are positive for cervical human papillomavirus [HPV] DNA.*)

27. Narod SA, Risch H, Moslehi R, et al. Oral contraceptives and the risk of hereditary ovarian cancer. N Engl J Med 1998;339:424. (*A case–control study of 386 women, finding a reduced risk of ovarian cancer in women with the BRCA1 or BRCA2 gene in oral contraceptive users.*)

28. Petitti DB. Combination estrogen–progestin oral contraceptives. N Engl J Med 2003;349:15. (*An informative case discussion, with estimates of attributable risk and a summary of then-available products.*)

29. Rosenberg L, Palmer JR, Rao RS, et al. Case–control study of oral contraceptive use and risk of breast cancer. Am J Epidemiol 1996;143:25. (*A case–control study, finding an increase in relative risk in women of age 25 to 34 years.*)

30. Rosenberg L, Palmer JR, Rao RS, et al. Low-dose oral contraceptive use and the risk of myocardial infarction. Arch Intern Med 2001;161:1065. (*There was no increased risk of myocardial infarction among nonsmokers and light smokers, but users who smoke heavily may be at greatly increased risk.*)

31. Rossing MA, Standford JL, Weiss NS, et al. Oral contraceptive use and risk of breast cancer in middle-aged women. Am J Epidemiol 1996;144:161. (*A case–control study, supporting the absence of any strong association between oral contraceptive use and breast cancer risk.*)

32. Rushton L, Jones DR. Oral contraceptive use and breast cancer risk: a meta-analysis of variations with age at diagnosis, parity and total duration of oral contraceptive use. Br J Obstet Gynaecol 1992;99:239. (*A meta-analysis, revealing a relative risk of breast cancer with oral contraceptive use of 1.16 in younger women, 1.21 in nulliparous women, and 1.27 for duration of use >8 years.*)

33. Schwartz SM, Siscovick DS, Longstreth Jr WT, et al. Use of low-dose oral contraceptives and stroke in young women. Ann Intern Med 1997;127:596. (*A population-based, case–control study, finding no increase in the risk for stroke in oral contraceptive users, but raising the question of a possible increased risk in users of norgestrel-containing oral contraceptive.*)

34. Smith JS, Green J, Berrington de Gonzalez A, et al. Cervical cancer and use of hormonal contraceptives: a systematic review. Lancet 2003;361:1159. (*Compared with never-users of oral contraceptives, the relative risks of cervical cancer for durations of use of <5 years, 5 to 9 years, and ≥10 years were, respectively, 1.1, 1.6, and 2.2 for all women and 0.9, 1.3, and 2.5 for HPV-positive women.*)

35. Stampfer MJ, Willet WC, Colditz GA, et al. Past use of oral contraceptives and cardiovascular disease: a meta-analysis in the context of the Nurses' Health Study. Am J Obstet Gynecol 1990;163:285. (*A large cohort study that prospectively looked at cardiovascular events, finding no difference among past users as compared with never-users of the oral contraceptive.*)

36. Stewart FH, Harper CC, Ellertson CE, et al. Clinical breast and pelvic examination requirements for hormonal contraception: current practice vs evidence. JAMA 2001;285:2232. (*Makes the case that there is no evidence supporting the need for pelvic and breast exam before prescribing.*)

37. Tanis BC, van den Bosch AAJ, Kemmeren JM, et al. Oral contraceptives and the risk of myocardial infarction. N Engl J Med 2001;345:1787. (*Myocardial infarction risk increased among women who used second-generation oral contraceptives; inclusive evidence for users of third-generation oral contraceptives.*)

38. Van Vliet HAAM, Grimes DA, Helmerhorst FM, et al. Biphasic versus monophasic oral contraceptives for contraception (Cochrane review). In: The Cochrane library, Issue 3. Oxford: Update Software, 2004. (*Concludes that monophasic agents are preferred because of more experience and better evidence of effectiveness and safety; see http://www.cochrane.org for updates.*)

39. Vandenbroucke JP, Rosing J, Bloemenkamp KW, et al. Medical progress: oral contraceptives and the risk of venous thrombosis. N Engl J Med 2001;344:1527. (*A baseline risk of venous thrombosis of <1 per 10,000 person-years is increased to 3 to 4 per 10,000 person-years during the time when oral contraceptives are being used.*)

40. Vessey M, Painter R, Yeates D. Mortality in relation to oral contraceptive use and cigarette smoking. Lancet 2003;362:185. (*There was no harmful effect of oral contraceptive use on overall mortality.*)

41. Gallo MF, Nanda K, Grimes DA, et al. 20 mcg versus >20 mcg estrogen combined oral contraceptives for contraception. Cochrane Database Syst Rev 2005;2:CD003989. (*There was no difference in effectiveness but a somewhat higher discontinuation.*)

42. Coukell AJ, Balfour JA. Levonorgestrel subdermal implants. A review of contraceptive efficacy and acceptability. Drug 1998;55:861. (*A review of Norplant use, finding that despite a high incidence of menstrual irregularity, levonorgestrel subdermal implants are a good choice of contraceptive method in women who are looking for an alternative to an oral regimen.*)

43. Forinash AB, Evans SL. New hormonal contraceptives: a comprehensive review of the literature. Pharmacotherapy 2003;23:1573. (*Norelgestromin–ethinyl estradiol patch, etonogestrel–ethinyl estradiol vaginal ring, and medroxyprogesterone–estradiol cypionate injection all have similar efficacy and adverse-effect profiles compared with current oral hormonal contraceptives.*)

44. Gallo MF, Grimes DA, Schulz KF. Skin patch and vaginal ring versus combined oral contraceptives for contraception (Cochrane review). In: The Cochrane library, Issue 3. Oxford: Update Software, 2004. (*There was a similar effectiveness and a better compliance for the patch compared with the pill; there were no trials for the ring; see http://www.cochrane.org for updates.*)

45. Hannon PR, Duggan AK, Serwint JR, et al. The influence of medroxyprogesterone on the duration of breast-feeding in mothers in an urban community. Arch Pediatr Adolesc Med 1997;151:490. (*A prospective cohort study, finding no detrimental effect on lactation from medroxyprogesterone.*)

46. Cole JA, Norman H, Doherty M, et al. Venous thromboembolism, myocardial infarction and stroke among transdermal contraceptive users. Obstet Gynecol 2007;109:339. (*There was a twofold increase in the risk of venous thromboembolism in patch compared to pill users.*)

47. Strom BL, Berlin JA, Weber AL, et al. Absence of an effect of injectable and implantable progestin-only contraceptives on subsequent risk of breast cancer. Contraception 2004;69:353. (*No increased risk of breast cancer was associated with the use of injectable or implantable progestin-only contraceptives in women of age 35 to 64 years.*)

48. Wan LS, Stiber A, Lam LY. The levonorgestrel two-rod implant for long-acting contraception: 10 years of clinical experience. Obstet Gynecol 2003;102:24. (*This approach was effective and well tolerated.*)

49. Cheng L, Gülmezoglu AM, Van Oel CJ, et al. Interventions for emergency contraception (Cochrane review). In: The Cochrane library, Issue 3. Oxford: Update Software, 2004. (*Concludes that 1.5 mg of levonorgestrel or a low to medium dose [25 to 50 mg] of mifepristone is the best option when available; see http://www.cochrane.org for updates.*)

50. Delbanco SF, Stewart FH, Koenig JD, et al. Are we making progress with emergency contraception? Recent findings on American adults and health professionals. J Am Womens Med Assoc 1998;53:242. (*Only 11% of women knew enough about emergency contraception to use it.*)

51. Spitz IM, Bardin CW. Mifepristone (RU-486)—a modulator of progestin and glucocorticoid action. N Engl J Med 1993;329:404. (*An authoritative review of this potent abortifacient.*)

52. Task Force on Postovulatory Methods of Fertility Regulation. Comparison of three single doses of mifepristone as emergency contraception: a randomised trial. Lancet 1999;353:697. (*A dose as low as 10 mg was as effective as one of 600 mg.*)

53. Task Force on Postovulatory Methods of Fertility Regulation. Randomised controlled trial of levonorgestrel versus the Yuzpe regimen of combined oral contraceptives for emergency contraception. Lancet 1998;352:428. (*The levonorgestrel regimen was better tolerated and more effective.*)

54. von Hertzen H, Piaggio G, Ding J, et al. Low dose mifepristone and two regimens of levonorgestrel for emergency contraception: a WHO multicentre randomised trial. Lancet 2002;360:1803. (*Mifepristone and levonorgestrel do not differ in efficacy; a 1.5-mg single levonorgestrel dose can substitute for two 0.75-mg doses 12 hours apart.*)

55. Cox B, Sneyd MJ, Paul C, et al. Vasectomy and risk of prostate cancer. JAMA 2002;287:3110. (*A New Zealand national case–control study, finding no increased risk of prostate cancer.*)
56. Henkinson SE, Hunter DJ, Colditz GA, et al. Tubal ligation, hysterectomy, and risk of ovarian cancer. JAMA 1993;270:2813. (*The risk is reduced significantly by tubal ligation.*)
57. Jamieson DJ, Costello C, Trussell J, et al. The risk of pregnancy after vasectomy. Obstet Gynecol 2004;103:848. (*The cumulative probability of failure per 1,000 procedures was 9.4 at 1 year after vasectomy and 11.3 at year 2.*)
58. Peterson HB, Xia Z, Hughes JM, et al. The risk of ectopic pregnancy after tubal sterilization. N Engl J Med 1997;336:762. (*A multicenter cohort study of >10,000 women followed for 8 to 14 years after tubal sterilization; the cumulative rate of ectopic pregnancy was 7.3 per 1,000 procedures, with the bipolar technique 27 times more likely to cause ectopic pregnancy than partial salpingectomy.*)
59. Curtis KM, Chrisman CE, Peterson HB. Contraception for women in selected circumstances. Obstet Gynecol 2002;99:1100. (*There was an increased risk of cardiovascular complications with combined oral contraceptive use by women with hypertension or migraine.*)
60. Planned Parenthood. Birth control. Available at: http://www.plannedparenthood.org/bc/index.html. (*An excellent web site for patient education.*)
61. Westhoff C, Heartwell S, Edwards S, et al. Initiation of oral contraceptives using a quick start compared with a conventional start: A randomized control trial. Obstet Gynecol 2007;109:1270. (*It was better to start on the spot than to wait for menses.*)
62. Halpern V, Grimes D, Lopez L, et al. Strategies to improve adherence and acceptability of hormonal methods of contraception. Cochrane Database Syst Rev 2006;1:CD004317. (*There was little direction because of the poor quality of the research.*)
63. Nettleman MD, Chung H, Brewer J, et al. Reasons for unprotected intercourse: analysis of the PRAMS survey. Contraception 2007;75:361. (*Almost one half of the participants felt that they would not, or could not, get pregnant at the time.*)

CHAPTER 120 ■ APPROACH TO THE INFERTILE COUPLE

SHANA L. BIRNBAUM

A couple that has been engaging in regular sexual intercourse without contraception for at least 1 year without conceiving and with intent to conceive is considered infertile. After 1 year, 85% of couples attempting conception will succeed, at a rate of around 20% per cycle. From 10% to 15% of U.S. couples in their childbearing years are infertile. Although the prevalence of infertility has remained relatively stable over the last 30 years, new technologies, rising expectations, and delayed childbearing have produced significant increases in the numbers of couples seeking help. The primary physician is often the first to be consulted and is responsible for initiating a medical evaluation of the couple, along with identifying any psychological or socioeconomic barriers to conception. Although treatment is usually carried out by practitioners specializing in infertility, the primary care physician should become proficient in performing the initial assessment and knowing when referral is indicated. Principal tasks include providing accurate advice and uncovering treatable etiologies.

PATHOPHYSIOLOGY AND CLINICAL PRESENTATION

Any disorder involving the male or female reproductive system may interfere with function to a degree sufficient to cause infertility. Although the woman is frequently the first to seek consultation for infertility, a full evaluation needs to focus on both partners; invasive testing in a woman should not be done before her partner has undergone basic evaluation, given that up to 40% of infertility is attributable at least in part to male factors.

Men (1–8)

Male infertility can be classified in terms of gonadal, gonadotropic, obstructive, and functional etiologies and considered according to whether the man presents with azoospermia, oligospermia, or normal sperm counts.

Azoospermic Etiologies

Patients with primary hypogonadism affecting both spermatogenesis and testosterone synthesis have azoospermia, a low testosterone level, and elevations of luteinizing hormone (LH) and follicle-stimulating hormone (FSH). *Klinefelter's syndrome* is the archetype, usually characterized by two X chromosomes and one Y chromosome; it occurs in up to 1 in 400 phenotypic males. Even more common are Y chromosome microdeletions and translocations, which are increasingly recognized as an etiology of azoospermia and severe oligospermia; they are seen in up to 20% of infertile men.

Men with predominantly germinal compartment failure are also azoospermic but manifest relatively normal testosterone and normal LH and elevated FSH levels. *Sertoli cell–only syndrome*, and adult *mumps* orchitis and *cancer therapy*, are among the more common congenital and acquired varieties, respectively. In a study comparing childhood and adolescent cancer survivors with sibling control subjects, overall relative fertility was 85%, with radiation therapy below the diaphragm reducing it by 25% and alkylating therapy alone causing a 40% reduction.

Hypogonadotropic hypogonadism is another cause of azoospermia that may be congenital or acquired (Table 120.1). Patients present with azoospermia and low levels of FSH, LH, and serum testosterone. Congenital disease is often

TABLE 120.1

IMPORTANT CAUSES OF MALE INFERTILITY

Hypothalamic/Pituitary
Prolactinoma
Idiopathic
Drugs (e.g., alcohol, marijuana)

Testicular
Klinefelter's syndrome/Y chromosome microdeletion or
    translocation
Sertoli cell–only syndrome
Irradiation
Adult mumps
Alkylating agents

Anatomic/Functional
Obstruction of epididymis or vas
Impotence
Retrograde ejaculation
Infection
Antisperm antibodies
Idiopathic defects in sperm quantity or quality

associated with anosmia (*Kallmann's syndrome*) but may be associated with other rarer disorders. Hereditary hemochromatosis, a relatively common disorder, may cause postpubertal hypogonadotropic hypogonadism through the mechanism of excess iron deposition in the pituitary. Pituitary tumors account for much of the acquired disease; a *prolactinoma* is the most frequent etiology. Large sellar tumors (e.g., craniopharyngioma) can lead to panhypopituitarism, with features of hypothyroidism and adrenal insufficiency dominating the clinical picture. *Drugs* (including alcohol, opiates, and marijuana) can interfere with hypothalamic–pituitary function, as can any serious systemic illness, malnutrition, or obesity.

Azoospermia in association with normal levels of LH, FSH, and testosterone characterize *retrograde ejaculation* (due to diabetes or drugs) and *obstruction* of the ejaculatory system. There may be *congenital or acquired obstruction* of the epididymis and vas deferens, or the vas deferens may be congenitally absent due to mutations in chloride channels similar to those seen in cystic fibrosis. Most other types of obstruction, including that resulting from sexually transmitted infections, are more proximal, giving normal testicular size and normal semen fructose.

Oligospermic Etiologies

Patients with a large *varicocele* may present with the typical "bag of worms" appearance to the testicle, but at times the only manifestation is a faint pulsation along the spermatic vein on Valsalva maneuver or coughing. The varicocele may be unilateral (usually on the left) or bilateral. The mechanism by which varicocele results in decreased fertility is undetermined, and because 10% to 15% of fertile men have a varicocele, some authorities question the association. Repair of the varicocele by spermatic vein ligation may restore normal sperm quantity and function, but several reviews have failed to demonstrate an effect on fertility.

Another large group of oligospermic patients with normal LH and testosterone have no detectable pathology and are labeled *idiopathic*. The condition results in a quantitative or qualitative abnormality of spermatogenesis without any identifiable anatomic or endocrinologic precipitant. FSH is normal unless the sperm count falls below 20 million/mL, in which case it may begin to rise. A proportion of these men with idiopathic oligospermia are found to have Y chromosome abnormalities on genetic analysis. The acquired forms of selective tubular damage (*chemotherapy, irradiation, adult mumps*) may leave the patient oligospermic rather than azoospermic.

Men with a history of unilateral or bilateral cryptoorchidism often have spermatogenic defects, which are believed to be congenital and related to developmental defects. They may present with oligo- or azoospermia, most typically with normal LH but elevated FSH levels. Such men are at elevated relative risk for testicular cancer, although the absolute risk is still low. In milder forms of acquired *hypothalamic–pituitary dysfunction*, some spermatogenesis may be preserved. FSH and LH are low to low-normal, and testosterone is low. Prolactin may be elevated due to a *microadenoma*. In *partial androgen resistance*, testosterone and LH are elevated, whereas FSH remains normal. Depending on the degree of insensitivity, patients may present with ambiguous external genitalia, gynecomastia, and hypogonadism. *Exogenous steroid use* may also lead to oligospermia with low serum LH; testosterone levels may be normal, elevated, or low, depending on the ability of the testosterone assay to measure the exogenous androgen.

Etiologies with Normal Sperm Counts

Many patients demonstrate abnormal sperm morphology or motility and suffer from many of the same conditions as those with oligospermia (e.g., varicocele, minor Y chromosome abnormalities). In addition, *genitourinary tract infection* may cause qualitative sperm changes; leukocytes sometimes appear in the semen, although their relation to fertility is unclear. Symptomatic infection can lead to subsequent obstruction of the efferent ducts, lowering sperm counts, and should be treated. *Antisperm antibodies* are noted in some patients, and an autoimmune mechanism may be clinically important when antibodies are present in high concentrations and cause sperm agglutination. Men who have had a vasectomy reversal or testicular trauma are at particularly high risk.

Impotence or erectile dysfunction ranks as a leading, although frequently overlooked, etiology. Hormone concentrations and sperm parameters are usually normal in "functional" variants (although depression and situational stress can transiently reduce sperm counts). In organic etiologies of impotence, these parameters reflect the underlying pathology (see Chapters 132 and 229). Anatomic anomalies, such as proximal location of the urinary meatus, may lead to infertility because of deposition of sperm and semen too far from the cervical os.

Women (1–6,9–11)

Disorders of Ovulation

Disorders of ovulation are among the most frequent causes of failure to conceive, making up 20% to 40% of cases in which a female factor is responsible for the infertility. Anovulatory bleeding (irregular menses), amenorrhea, or infertility may be the presenting complaint. *Polycystic ovary syndrome* and other forms of *hypothalamic dysfunction* account for most cases (see Chapters 111 and 112). Pathophysiologically, the normal pattern of gonadotropin-releasing hormone (GnRH) release is disrupted, impairing the normal midcycle LH surge and ovulation. Occasionally, an androgen-producing tumor or late-onset congenital adrenal hyperplasia may present with anovulation and infertility. Treatment of the primary disorder can restore fertility, as can ovulation induction with medication.

Declining oocyte quality is a problem as maternal age increases. A higher incidence of chromosomal abnormalities is partially responsible, but decreased ovarian reserve with fewer, lower-quality oocytes is probably more significant. *Premature ovarian failure*, which may be autoimmune or idiopathic, occurs when ovarian reserve fails before the expected age of menopause. If it occurs before age 30 years, the possibility of mosaic Turner's syndrome or a partial X chromosome deletion should be investigated. An increasingly recognized cause of premature ovarian failure is a premutation in *the fragile X syndrome gene (FMR1)*. An important acquired source of ovarian failure is *cancer therapy* in children and adolescents (see prior discussion). In the study noted earlier comparing survivors of childhood and adolescent cancers with their siblings, overall relative fertility for women was 85%, with radiation therapy below the diaphragm reducing it by 25%. Conversely, alkylating therapy had relatively little effect.

Tubal Disorders

Tubal disorders account for about 25% of cases. *Pelvic inflammatory disease* (particularly indolent nongonococcal forms such as that due to *Chlamydia trachomatis*; see Chapters 116 and 117) is the leading cause of tubal damage. In a prospective study, 12% of those with a single episode of salpingitis had tubal occlusion, 35% of those with two infections had occlusion, and 75% of those with three or more had occlusion. Women without a known history of acute pelvic inflammatory disease who are found to have tubal occlusion have higher rates of antibodies against the agents that cause chlamydia and gonorrhea, suggesting that asymptomatic salpingitis occurs frequently. Other pelvic and abdominal infections or surgeries (such as a *ruptured appendix*) may also lead to tubal adhesions. *Postpartum infection* has an association with tubal occlusion, as does infection after induced abortion, particularly if it is inadequately treated or unrecognized. *Endometriosis*, found with much more frequency in infertile women (38% vs. 5% in one study), may cause tubal obstruction and uterine disturbances (some experts have also hypothesized an inflammatory response to account for the lower fertility rates seen in women with milder forms of endometriosis).

Uncommon causes of tubal adhesions include *pelvic trauma* from vehicular accidents, *inflammatory bowel disease*, tuberculosis, and schistosomiasis. In general, processes that cause adhesions rather than tubal epithelial damage seem to have a better prognosis.

Uterine Pathology

Uterine pathology represents about 5% of cases. *Congenital anomalies*, such as absence or duplication of the uterine fundus, often present as repeated pregnancy wastage. Complete duplication of cervix and uterus tends to diminish fertility but less so than anomalies causing distortion of a single uterine cavity. Septate and deeply arcuate uteri may be better able to maintain a pregnancy after hysteroscopic or operative repair. *Uterine fibroids* and *endometriosis* may distort or obstruct the uterine cavity, causing infertility or pregnancy loss. Resection and reresection of fibroids have been surprisingly successful. The *forgotten intrauterine device* is occasionally a cause of infertility.

Cervical Factors

Cervical factors may lead to inability to carry a pregnancy to term as well as difficulty with conception. *Cervical incompetence* may lead to repeated abortion or later-trimester pregnancy losses. The incompetence can result from inadequate innervation, disturbances in synthesis or breakdown of prostaglandin, previous cervical procedures (such as a loop excision for cervical dysplasia), or defects in muscle and collagen fibers. Incompetence of the cervix may also compromise its role in resisting the entry of infectious agents into the sterile uterine cavity.

The precise role of *cervical mucus* is not well understood, but normal viscosity and ferning are essential to conception and represent evidence of adequate estrogen stimulation and response.

Both Partners (1–5)

Interpersonal problems (see Chapter 229) are an important etiologic factor because they may lead to sexual dysfunction or inactivity. The desire for children may not be shared equally by both partners, there may be anxiety over how family responsibilities will interfere with career development, or one partner may not want to lose the economic and social freedom of being a childless couple. Transient situational problems also arise; the young professional person may be under considerable job pressure, and travel may interfere with optimal timing of intercourse for conception or lead to hypothalamic dysfunction.

DIFFERENTIAL DIAGNOSIS (1–5)

In about one third of instances, a male factor is the predominant etiology. In another one third, a female factor predominates. In the remainder, either the cause resides with both partners or the etiology is unknown; several unfavorable factors may contribute to subfertility in a particular couple. In almost one half of cases attributed to a male factor, there is either a quantitative or a qualitative sperm defect of unknown etiology. Among female factors, ovulatory disturbances account for up to 40%, tubal disorders for 10% to 30%, cervical factors for 10%, and uterine factors for about 5%. Tables 120.1 and 120.2 list some of the most important etiologies.

TABLE 120.2

IMPORTANT CAUSES OF FEMALE INFERTILITY

Hypothalamic/Pituitary
  Hypothalamic dysfunction
  Polycystic ovary syndrome
  Prolactinoma

Ovarian
  Primary failure (e.g., premature menopause)
  Irradiation

Tubal
  Pelvic inflammatory disease
  Endometriosis
  Adhesions

Uterine
  Fibroids
  Scarring (Asherman's syndrome)
  Anatomic abnormalities

Cervical
  Poor mucus quality
  Infection
  Anatomic abnormalities

WORKUP

Initial Evaluation (1–5)

The prognosis even for untreated couples is favorable (see later discussion). An extensive "infertility workup" need not be undertaken initially unless the couple is older (mid 30s and upward), has been unable to conceive despite trying seriously for more than 1 year, or has a history suggestive of a treatable etiology (e.g., oligomenorrhea, history of cancer treatment or pelvic infection). Otherwise, a reasonable approach to the first visit is to limit the assessment to a careful general history and physical examination, checking for such important causes as endocrinopathy, tumor, genitourinary tract infection, anatomic disorder, and interpersonal problems.

In the Man

History should include inquiry into drug and medication use (marijuana, alcohol, antihypertensive agents), urethral discharge, headache and other symptoms of a pituitary tumor (see Chapter 100), past history of radiation therapy or cancer chemotherapy, mumps, toxin exposure, and systemic illnesses (especially diabetes with associated retrograde ejaculation). A history of cryptoorchidism is also relevant. A sexual history that reviews the couple's relationship, sexual techniques, erectile function, and frequency of intercourse is also important.

Physical examination begins with noting general appearance and any signs of diminished androgenization (decreased body hair, gynecomastia, eunuchoid proportions). The scrotum is examined for testicular size, presence of a varicocele, hypospadias, and absent vas deferens. Soft, small testes (<4 cm in longest diameter) are consistent with primary testicular failure and pituitary–hypothalamic insufficiency. A Valsalva maneuver performed while the patient is standing may reveal a small varicocele. The urethra is observed for discharge, and the prostate and seminal vesicles are observed for tenderness and other signs of infection. If a pituitary condition is suspected, visual field testing by confrontation might reveal an important field defect, although a normal study does not rule out a mass lesion. Testing deep tendon reflexes may uncover delay in relaxation suggestive of hypothyroidism (see Chapter 104).

In the Woman

History focuses on the menstrual and reproductive history, including any abortions, miscarriages, complicated deliveries, and curettages. Asking about menstrual irregularities or episodes of amenorrhea may help to establish the presence of ovulatory dysfunction. A lifelong history of menstrual irregularities is suggestive of polycystic ovary syndrome, especially if accompanied by hirsutism, acne, or obesity. Any situational or emotional stress, marked weight loss, or excess exercise should be noted because it can lead to hypothalamic dysfunction and impairment of ovulation (see Chapters 111 and 112). Similarly, checking for symptoms of hypothyroidism (see Chapter 104), hyperprolactinemia (see Chapter 100), Cushing's syndrome (see Chapter 100), and androgen excess (see Chapter 98) may yield clues for conditions that can impair hypothalamic function. Inquiry into headaches, visual field disturbances, galactorrhea, symptoms of pituitary insufficiency (see Chapter 100), and a history of postpartum hemorrhage helps to screen for a sella turcica lesion. Checking for a history or symptoms of pelvic inflammatory disease (vaginal discharge, pelvic pain, fever, dyspareunia) is also essential. Any malignant disease history is important to note, especially if treatment included irradiation or alkylating agents. A detailed psychosocial history reviews pertinent details of the relationship, including frequency and timing of sexual activity. Loss of libido may signify psychosocial distress or hormonal dysfunction.

Physical examination focuses on checking for obesity, excessive weight loss, hirsutism, cushingoid appearance, stigmata of hypothyroidism (see Chapter 104), visual field disturbances, and goiter. Most important is a careful pelvic examination, taking special note of any ovarian, uterine, or adnexal masses, thickening, or tenderness. Examination of the cervix should include checking for erosions, discharge, polyps, masses, scarring, and pain on cervical motion. The hirsute patient is examined for clitoromegaly.

Both Partners

An empathic, supportive, nonjudgmental exploration of the marital relationship is essential; it may be best achieved by interviewing the couple together (to observe their interactions) and each partner separately.

Further Evaluation (7–16)

Couples with no evidence of serious pathology on initial evaluation can be reassured and informed that more than half of such couples go on to conceive without the aid of treatment. Those who have been trying to conceive for less than 1 year can be advised to delay further evaluation until 12 months have passed, provided they are willing to do so and have no compelling reason, including older maternal age, for proceeding directly to more extensive testing. All couples being managed expectantly, as well as those seeking preconception counseling before attempting to conceive, should be educated about the timing of ovulation and the fertile period from 5 days before ovulation to the day of ovulation (see later discussion). Couples who have failed to conceive after trying for 12 months or with a suggestive history can undergo a set of basic laboratory studies more fully to define the problem and guide further evaluation and treatment.

In the Man

The first and most important test to perform is a standardized *semen analysis,* collecting at least two specimens over a 4- to 6-week period, each after a 2- to 3-day period of abstinence. Quantitative analysis includes number of sperm per milliliter of semen (counts >20 million/mL are normal, although men with lower levels are frequently fertile) and semen volume (normal is 2 to 5 mL). Sperm motility and morphology are also evaluated, with greater than 50% motile forms and less than 30% abnormal morphology considered normal. Although these standards, established by the World Health Organization in 1999, are helpful in predicting subfertility, none is an absolute predictor of fertility, and there is substantial overlap between fertile and infertile men, as well as variability in serial samples from the same man. The percentage of sperm with normal morphology is the best predictor of fertility.

Patients with azoospermia or oligospermia are candidates for serum gonadotropin (*LH* and *FSH*) and *testosterone* determinations (measured in the morning, given its circadian pattern) because of the possibility of an underlying disorder within the hypothalamic–pituitary–testicular axis. High concentrations of gonadotropins and low or low-normal testosterone level suggest a primary gonadal problem. Low gonadotropins and testosterone characterize a pituitary–hypothalamic etiology. Normal FSH and testosterone levels and testicular size in a patient with azoospermia suggest obstruction or congenital absence of the vas deferens, particularly if sperm volume is low. Normal hormone and gonadotropin concentrations in the setting of oligospermia are characteristic of patients with varicocele or idiopathic disease. Small testes, gynecomastia, an elevated FSH, and a reduced testosterone suggest Klinefelter's syndrome. The diagnosis is confirmed by chromosomal analysis. Up to 20% of men previously diagnosed with idiopathic oligospermia are found to have microdeletions in the Y chromosome, particularly when morphology and motility are abnormal. Given this, most experts recommend further genetic testing and counseling before couples proceed to assisted reproductive technologies, given the risk of chromosomal abnormalities being passed along.

The patient with suspected pituitary disease needs a *prolactin level* and *magnetic resonance imaging* (MRI) of the sella turcica to search for a tumor. An elevated prolactin in the setting of a normal MRI may be due to a drug-induced problem or nonvisualized microadenoma; imaging should be repeated in 6 months to be sure that a microadenoma is not progressing.

The utility of more elaborate studies (e.g., antisperm antibodies, sperm–cervical mucus interaction, penetration testing) is best determined by the infertility specialist.

In the Woman

The first task is to establish that ovulation is taking place. Although regular cycles suggest ovulation, the time-tested approach to confirmation is use of a basal body *temperature chart*, which records the oral temperature each morning before rising from bed using a special thermometer graduated in tenths of degrees Fahrenheit. Ovulation is accompanied by a rise in progesterone secretion, which leads to a 0.3°F to 0.5°F rise in basal body temperature after ovulation. Given the cumbersome nature of basal body temperature charting, alternative methods are increasingly used, which appear to be equally if not more sensitive and specific when compared to a gold standard of ultrasound assessment of follicular development. A *serum progesterone* level in the midluteal phase of the cycle (days 20 to 24 after the onset of menses) greater than 6 ng/mL indicates ovulation and a functioning corpus luteum. A commercially available urinary ovulation predictor kit measures the LH surge, which precedes ovulation by 1 to 2 days. It should be used starting several days before the expected ovulation to avoid missing the surge. Endometrial biopsy has been used to assess the adequacy of the endometrium to support implantation (termed *luteal-phase defect* when the endometrium is out of phase with the cycle) but is no longer recommended because of its inability to distinguish between fertile and infertile women and a lack of proven benefit in improving pregnancy outcomes.

If the patient is anovulatory, further testing proceeds with measurement of *serum prolactin*, *FSH*, and *LH* (see Chapters 111 and 112) to evaluate for hypothalamic, pituitary, and ovarian function. The possibility of polycystic ovary syndrome is suggested by anovulation with oligomenorrhea and signs of androgen excess and should be considered along with the rarer diagnoses of androgen-secreting tumor and late-onset congenital adrenal hyperplasia. In a woman who appears to be ovulating but has failed to conceive, particularly when she is 35 years or older, ovarian reserve should be assessed. The simplest method, although lacking sensitivity, is the day 3 FSH test, in which FSH levels are measured on day 3 of the menstrual cycle; an elevated level (>10 mIU/mL) predicts poor pregnancy rates (<5% conception), regardless of age or assisted reproductive techniques. Cycle day 3 estradiol levels of less than

80 pg/mL also suggest adequate ovarian reserve and may improve the sensitivity of FSH testing. Another test is the clomiphene challenge test, in which clomiphene citrate 100 mg is given on cycle days 5 to 9, and FSH is measured on days 3 and 10. Meta-analyses comparing day 3 FSH to clomiphene challenge testing have not found a difference in their utility for predicting infertility treatment outcomes.

A *postcoital examination* has been used to assess cervical mucus function and the interaction of sperm with the cervical mucus but is now considered to lack sensitivity and predictive value in the treatment of fertility and to be intrusive without benefit. One study of 444 infertile couples found that routine use of the postcoital test did not affect the pregnancy rate at 24 months but did lead to more tests and treatment.

If, after the initial history, physical examination, and evaluation of ovulation and ovarian reserve, it appears that tubal or uterine disease may be responsible for infertility, then *hysterosalpingogram* or *laparoscopy* deserves consideration. Choice of test should be made by a gynecologist experienced in the evaluation of infertility. Hysterosalpingogram involves injection of a contrast agent into the uterus by way of a cervical catheter. Films reveal uterine and tubal anatomy and are particularly sensitive for tubal obstruction. Laparoscopy requires general anesthesia but can detect adhesions, lesser stages of endometriosis, or a nonpalpable fibroid. Tubal patency and position may also be confirmed. Another potential advantage to laparoscopy is the opportunity to treat existing pathology, such as minor endometriosis or adhesions. Negative findings on a tubal evaluation can be equally helpful in both reassuring the infertile couple and deciding on a treatment plan.

PRINCIPLES OF MANAGEMENT AND INDICATIONS FOR REFERRAL (17–26)

Studies from infertility clinics have shown that many couples go on to conceive without treatment at a rate of 1% to 2% per cycle (e.g., 44% of those with ovulation deficiency; 61% of those with endometriosis, tubal defects, or seminal deficiencies; and 96% of those with cervical factors or idiopathic infertility). A conservative approach of watchful waiting is reasonable, provided there is no evidence of tumor, infection, anatomic defect, or serious endocrinopathy. Age is also an important consideration because fecundity clearly decreases with maternal age and to a lesser degree, paternal age; whereas maternal age 35 years is often used as a cut-off, conception rates begin to slowly decline around age 30 years. Counseling is an important adjunct in helping patients make decisions (see later discussion).

When the workup suggests causative organic pathology, an appropriate referral for confirmatory testing and design of a treatment program are indicated. Couples with idiopathic infertility who are interested in assisted reproductive techniques should be referred to infertility specialists, particularly with advancing maternal age. The participation of the primary physician in the care of the couple should continue, but the subtleties of specialized care that infertility treatment require argue for referral. Successful referral depends to a large extent on proper patient selection.

Men

A neurologic or anatomic cause of *impotence*, a suspected acquired *obstructive defect*, and *varicocele* are indications for urologic consultation. Surgical ligation of a varicocele is commonly performed, but results in terms of fertility are often disappointing even though sperm counts may rise; many urologists recommend against repair unless the varicocele is symptomatic. Treatment of obstruction requires a urologist skilled in microsurgical techniques, as does vasectomy reversal. Patients with retrograde ejaculation may achieve pregnancy with alternative insemination, using semen recovered in the urine. Patients with noncorrectible obstructive defects may be candidates for sperm harvesting from the epididymis or testes with use of assisted reproductive techniques. Men with congenital absence of the vas deferens may also be candidates for sperm harvesting but should undergo genetic testing and counseling, given the possibility of mutations in the cystic fibrosis chloride channel.

Hypothalamic–pituitary disorders have a high rate of success with treatment by the reproductive endocrinologist. Patients with idiopathic hypogonadotropic disease often respond successfully to gonadotropin or GnRH administration. In the setting of a prolactinoma, bromocriptine or cabergoline often restores fertility. Larger pituitary adenomas may require neurosurgical intervention.

Idiopathic oligospermia (no evidence of a varicocele; normal LH, FSH, and testosterone levels) has no proven therapy to increase sperm counts. Clomiphene and other antiestrogens, GnRH factor, gonadotropins, and low doses of androgen have been tried but without confirmed long-term benefit. Such couples should be referred to infertility clinics for consideration of assisted reproductive techniques. Artificial insemination, *in vitro* fertilization, and, most recently, intracytoplasmic sperm injection are also available for patients with otherwise *refractory qualitative sperm defects*. Intracytoplasmic sperm injection, in which a single spermatozoon or spermatid is injected directly into an oocyte, has allowed effective treatment even for men with significant sperm abnormalities who were previously considered infertile. Prior to such techniques, men with idiopathic oligospermia or qualitative sperm defects should undergo genetic evaluation to rule out a minor chromosomal abnormality that could be passed on to their offspring.

Men who have quantitatively and qualitatively *normal sperm* and *normal LH, FSH,* and *testosterone* levels pose a challenge. When *antisperm antibodies* are found in high titers in the semen, their levels can be lowered with a course of high-dose corticosteroids. However, this therapy is no longer recommended, given the deleterious side effects of such therapy, and these couples should be referred for assisted reproductive techniques. Such techniques can also be used in cases of idiopathic infertility if the couple opts against conservative management.

Subclinical infection, especially with *Mycoplasma,* has been suggested as a cause of infertility. Culturing both partners and treating the couple if one partner is culture positive has produced inconsistent results. There is no known treatment for patients with gonadal failure or androgen insensitivity.

Women

Women with *hypothalamic dysfunction* have a good prognosis. Those with mild dysfunction are likely to resume ovulating without therapy and need only counseling at the time of initial evaluation. Those with moderate dysfunction often respond well to ovulation induction, especially when FSH, thyroid function, and prolactin remain normal. Such persons have a 50% chance of conceiving with the use of clomiphene, which is given for 3 to 5 days, followed by 1 month of waiting for either pregnancy or an ovulatory period. Patients with polycys-

tic ovary syndrome may ovulate with the combination of the insulin-sensitizing agent metformin and clomiphene or with clomiphene alone. Lifestyle changes alone, including weight loss and exercise, increase ovulation rates in such women. Patients suffering from more severe hypothalamic dysfunction who fail to respond to clomiphene may respond to synthetic GnRH therapy. GnRH is administered by parenteral pulse infusions, mimicking normal GnRH secretion. Careful dose adjustments are necessary to avoid multiple pregnancies. Only an experienced reproductive endocrinologist or infertility gynecologist should prescribe such therapy. Patients with a prolactin-secreting adenoma require neuroendocrine consultation because bromocriptine usually restores fertility (see Chapter 100).

Gynecologic referral is indicated for patients with suspected *tubal scarring, fibroids,* or *endometriosis.* Microsurgical tubal reconstruction may be required for successful repair, which leads to pregnancy in 10% to 60% of cases. If repair is not possible or not advisable given low success rates (as in bilateral proximal obstruction), assisted reproductive techniques such as *in vitro* fertilization can bypass the requirement for tubal patency.

Couples who have failed other methods or those with idiopathic infertility may be candidates for *intrauterine insemination,* in which concentrated, washed sperm are injected directly into the upper uterine cavity, often in combination with ovulation induction; *gamete intrafallopian transfer,* in which oocytes and sperm are placed into the fallopian tube; *in vitro fertilization* (IVF), in which fertilized embryos are transferred directly to the uterus; or *intracytoplasmic sperm injection* (ICSI), described previously. These are elaborate technologies that require the consultative and technical services of a specialized reproductive center. One must have adequate sperm, ovarian follicles, and a competent uterus to qualify for IVF, whereas ISCI bypasses the requirement for motile sperm. Patients may also choose to use donor eggs or donor sperm to achieve pregnancy if ovarian failure or azoospermia is the primary problem.

Couples (24–26)

Infertility resulting from a *psychosocial problem* (e.g., lack of privacy, work exhaustion, marital discord) needs to be approached with careful, empathic explanation. Some individuals may attempt to view the situation as a medical problem when there is unlikely to be a strictly medical solution. Attention needs to be directed to the home environment, work situation, and marital relationship. Infertility evaluation and treatment itself is stressful for couples, and infertile couples appear to have a lower quality of life than fertile couples, although treatment failure itself does not worsen it below baseline. Psychological distress does appear to be associated with lower success rates for assisted reproductive options, and interventions to reduce symptoms may improve pregnancy rates. When *sexual dysfunction* is detected, treatment is best directed toward it (see Chapter 229), although artificial insemination is sometimes used when there is a strong desire to have a child as soon as possible.

The infertility evaluation may lead to reconsideration and redesign of treatment regimens for *underlying medical conditions* such as cancer, diabetes, and hypertension (see Chapters 26, 88, and 89). It is also an opportunity to encourage healthy lifestyle changes in both members of the couple; smoking, marijuana use, excess alcohol intake, excess caffeine intake, and obesity clearly reduce fertility, particularly in the female partner. Women should also be encouraged to take prenatal vitamins with folic acid to prevent neural tube defects and control any preexisting medical conditions such as diabetes or hypothyroidism.

PATIENT EDUCATION (27,28)

Couples are eager for information about their chances of conceiving. At one end of the spectrum are men and women with permanent gonadal failure who have no chance of conceiving without the use of donor gametes. At the other end are those with a transient functional deficit who are likely to conceive without any treatment other than reassurance and time. The couple who remains unsuccessful after 1 year of trying can be given some reassurance as they begin to undergo evaluation. Up to one fourth of such couples achieve pregnancy within 3 months. Published findings from infertility clinics show that, overall, 25% to 35% of couples achieve conception within 1 to 2 years of registration. The percentages continue to rise over the next 4 to 5 years. The chances of conception with each cycle of IVF are 20% to 40%, depending on such factors as age of the woman and quality of the semen. Couples undergoing assistive techniques should be informed about the possible complications, including ovarian hyperstimulation and multiple gestation.

There is a slight decrease in fecundity after age 30 years and a marked decrease after age 35 years, at which point expectant management of infertility is no longer recommended. There appears to be little or no difference in prognosis between infertile couples who have conceived in the past and those who have never conceived. Patients with ovulatory problems do reasonably well; those with tubal problems have more difficulty, although improved assisted reproductive techniques are providing more options for these couples. As noted earlier, rates for live births after tubal repair range from 10% to 60%, depending on the severity and site of the scarring, quality of semen, age of the woman, and a host of other factors. Couples whose infertility involves multiple factors do less well than those in whom only one factor is identified. A proportion of these patients will conceive on their own without intervention; they also have the option of empiric assisted reproductive techniques.

The investigation of infertility provides an opportunity to educate patients about normal human reproduction and prevention of sexually transmitted disease. Education for both partners about the menstrual cycle, the best time to attempt conception (from 5 days prior to ovulation to the day of ovulation, with the most fertile days being 1 to 2 days before ovulation) and the frequency of coitus needed to achieve pregnancy (at least twice per week, and every other day before suspected ovulation) can be very helpful, sometimes even curative. The importance of using a condom to prevent spread of sexually transmitted diseases that might lead to tubal scarring cannot be overemphasized to teenagers and patients with multiple partners. Screening all young women as well as those with multiple partners for chlamydial infection and treating it when present may help to prevent tubal infertility (see Chapter 117). At times, the infertility evaluation encourages couples to make healthful lifestyle changes.

Annotated Bibliography

1. Falcone T. What the internist needs to know about infertility. Cleve Clin J Med 2001;68:65. (*Practical approach to the initial evaluation and treatment of infertility, with a focus on common etiologies.*)
2. Hanson M, Dumesic D. Initial evaluation and treatment of infertility in a primary-care setting. Mayo Clin Proc 1998;73:681. (*Reviews initial management and evaluation of infertility, including when to refer.*)
3. Whiteman-Elia GF, Baxley EG. A primary care approach to the infertile couple. J Am Board Family Pract 2001;14:33. (*A thorough clinical review of appropriate early evaluation, with emphasis on addressing male factors early in the evaluation.*)
4. Morell V. Basic infertility assessment. Primary Care 1997;24:195. (*Describes the role of the primary care provider in diagnosis, treatment, and support.*)
5. Jose-Miller AB, Boyden JW, Frey KA. Infertility. Am Family Physician 2007;75:849. (*An extensive review of the evaluation of both partners, including treatment options.*)
6. Byrne J, Mulvihill JJ, Myers MH, et al. Effects of treatment on fertility in long-term survivors of childhood or adolescent cancer. N Engl J Med 1987;317:1315. (*A retrospective cohort study; fertility rates varied by gender, site of therapy, and type.*)
7. Bhasin S. Approach to the infertile man. J Clin Endocrinol Metab 2007;92:1995. (*A helpful review of the evaluation and treatment of male infertility, with particular emphasis on the more recently recognized genetic abnormalities and their implications for counseling and treatment.*)
8. Bonde JP, Ernst E, Jensen TK, et al. Relation between semen quality and fertility: a population-based study of 430 first-pregnancy planners. Lancet 1998;352:1172. (*There was a significant overlap between sperm concentration in fertile and subfertile men, suggesting that the threshold for normal should be lower than the World Health Organization threshold of 20 million/mL.*)
9. Rosene-Montella K, Keely E, Laifer S, et al. Evaluation and management of infertility in women: the internists' role. Ann Intern Med 2000;132:973. (*An excellent review of the role of the internist in understanding, initiating evaluation for, and counseling about infertility, with particular regard to associated morbidities.*)
10. Smith S, Pfeifer SM, Collins JA. Diagnosis and management of female infertility. JAMA 2003;290:1767. (*A succinct review for the internist.*)
11. Hull MG, Cahill DJ. Female infertility. Endocrinol Metab Clin North Am 1998;27:851. (*Reviews basic investigations and summarizes cumulative pregnancy rates for alternative interventions.*)
12. Guermandi E, Vegetti W, Bianchi MM, et al. Reliability of ovulation tests in infertile women. Obstet Gynecol 2001;97:92. (*Using transvaginal ultrasonography as the gold standard, compares ovulation prediction rates in >100 women, finding that urinary luteinizing hormone and midluteal serum progesterone were superior to basal body temperature charting.*)
13. Mueller BA, Daling JR, Moore DE, et al. Appendectomy and the risk of tubal infertility. N Engl J Med 1986;315:1506. (*The risk was increased only in cases of ruptured appendix.*)
14. Oei SG, Hemerhorst FM, Bloemenkamp KW, et al. Effectiveness of the postcoital test: randomized controlled trial. BMJ 1998;317:502. (*A randomized trial of 444 infertile couples, finding no difference in pregnancy rates at 24 months but more tests and treatment.*)
15. Bukulmez O, Arici A. Assessment of ovarian reserve. Curr Opin Obstet Gynecol 2004;16:231. (*Reviews the limitations and utility of age, basal follicle-stimulating hormone level, clomiphene challenge test, and newer markers, including inhibin levels, to determine ovarian reserve.*)
16. Hendriks DJ, Mol BW, Bancsi LF, et al. The clomiphene citrate challenge test for the prediction of poor ovarian response and nonpregnancy in patients undergoing in vitro fertilization: a systematic review. Fertil Steril 2003;86:807. (*No advantage was found in the use of the clomiphene challenge test over the measurement of day 3 follicle-stimulating hormone in predicting in vitro fertilization outcomes.*)
17. Collins JA, Wrixon W, Janes LB, et al. Treatment-independent pregnancy among infertile couples. N Engl J Med 1983;309:1201. (*A retrospective review indicating that the potential for a spontaneous cure is high.*)
18. Gleicher N, Vanderlaan B, Pratt D, et al. Background pregnancy rates in an infertile population. Hum Reprod 1996;11:1011. (*The spontaneous annual pregnancy rate in this infertile population was 20%.*)
19. Schwartz D, Mayaux MJ. Female fecundity as a function of age: results of artificial insemination in 2193 nulliparous women with azoospermic husbands. N Engl J Med 1982;306:404. (*A classic study, finding a slight but significant decrease after age 30 years and a more marked decrease after age 35 years.*)
20. Moran C, Garcia-Hernandez E, et al. Prognosis for fertility analyzing different variables in men and women. Arch Androl 1996;36:197. (*Women older than 32 years had a cumulative pregnancy rate at 30 months of 31%, compared with 65% among younger women, and couples with primary infertility had a rate of 45%, compared with 88% for those with a previous pregnancy.*)

21. Evers JL, Collins JA. Assessment of efficacy of varicocele repair for male subfertility: a systematic review. Lancet 2003;361:1849. (*Found no benefit to varicocele repair using fertility as the endpoint.*)

22. Khorram O, Patrizio P, Wang C, et al. Reproductive technologies for male infertility. J Clin Endocrinol Metab 2001;86:2373. (*Reviews success rates of different assistive techniques, including in vitro fertilization, gamete intrafallopian transfer, and intracytoplasmic sperm injection.*)

23. Marcoux S, Maheux R, Berube S. Laparoscopic surgery in infertile women with minimal or mild endometriosis. Canadian Collaborative Group on Endometriosis. N Engl J Med 1997;337:217. (*A randomized, controlled trial that found an improvement in fertility after laparoscopic ablation of mild endometriosis.*)

24. El-Messidi A, Al-Fozan H, Lin Tan S, et al. Effects of repeated treatment failure on the quality of life of couples with infertility. J Obstet Gynaecol Can 2004;26:333. (*The baseline quality of life was found to be lower in infertile couples vs. fertile couples but did not decline further with treatment failure.*)

25. Van Balen F, Trimbos-Kemper TC. Factors influencing the well-being of long-term infertile couples. J Psychosom Obstet Gynaecol 1994;15:157. (*Secrecy with regard to infertility was associated with a lower sense of well-being.*)

26. de Liz TM, Strauss B. Differential efficacy of group and individual/couple psychotherapy with infertile patients. Hum Reprod 2005;20:1324. (*A literature review, finding that therapy reduced anxiety and depression and possibly increased conception rates.*)

27. Stanford JB, White GL, Hatasaka H, et al. Timing intercourse to achieve pregnancy: current evidence. Obstet Gynecol 2002;100:1333. (*Increased pregnancy rates were achieved with timed intercourse based on fertility awareness using urinary luteinizing hormone or cervical mucus changes; calendar and basal body temperature charting may miss peak fertility.*)

28. Dunson DB, Baird DD, Wilcox AJ, et al. Day-specific probabilities of clinical pregnancy based on two studies with imperfect measures of ovulation. Hum Reprod 1999;14:1835. (*Found that the highest probability of conception occurred with intercourse 1 to 2 days prior to ovulation.*)

CHAPTER 121 ■ APPROACH TO THE WOMAN WITH AN UNPLANNED PREGNANCY

SHANA L. BIRNBAUM

Approximately one half of the pregnancies that occur in the United States are unintended. Just greater than one fourth of these occur in women who are not using contraception, with the rest due to incorrect or inconsistent use or failure of a contraceptive method. More than half of the women who had a pregnancy termination in 2002 were using some form of contraception during the month they got pregnant. The majority of women had an identifiable episode for which emergency contraception could have been used to decrease the risk of pregnancy.

Similar proportions of unintended pregnancies end in abortion and in birth. The woman who suspects an unplanned or unwanted pregnancy often calls on her primary care provider to confirm the diagnosis and review her options. To provide support and assistance, the physician first must accurately diagnose the pregnancy. Because an unwanted pregnancy is a crisis in a women's life, the physician needs to be able sensitively to counsel a woman about her options without judgment or censure. If the physician feels his or her beliefs interfere with objective counseling, then referral to another provider is necessary. Awareness of the patient's social and cultural environment, including her beliefs and individual circumstances, is essential to lending appropriate support. The patient should be informed about community services available for prenatal care, medical and surgical abortion, and adoption.

CLINICAL PRESENTATIONS (1–12)

Women presenting with unplanned pregnancies have highly variable experiences. Responses to the diagnosis, coping mechanisms, and capacity to take responsibility for decision making may differ greatly from woman to woman. Most women cite multiple reasons for their decisions on what to do about an unplanned pregnancy.

A pregnancy may be untimely or unwanted because of the hardship a child would create. A limited single or dual income may be insufficient to support either a first or an additional child. Older women who believed that they had completed their childbearing years may not have the emotional, physical, or financial resources for another child. For younger women, a pregnancy may hinder opportunities for education and career advancement. Lack of a stable, long-term relationship and a feeling of being unready to parent are frequent issues. Some women who desire children may have a partner opposed to parenting or may need family or social support that is lacking. These factors may conflict with the woman's desire for motherhood (more than half of the women who undergo abortion intend to have a child in the future) or a moral opposition to abortion, creating great ambivalence. For many women, unwarranted fear that an abortion will hinder future reproductive function adds to the concern.

The woman who desires pregnancy but suffers from a chronic or life-threatening illness such as diabetes, systemic lupus erythematosus, or cancer endures unique stress when she faces an unplanned pregnancy. The pregnancy may jeopardize her health and her ability to care for her family, and she may face conflicting opinions regarding termination. In addition, the effect of pregnancy on certain disease processes is not well understood.

Many women of childbearing age are infected with HIV. The rate of transmission of HIV to the fetus in the pre-antiretroviral era was estimated to be 25% to 50%, but this has declined to less than 2% with combination antiretroviral therapy. Pregnancy does not appear to adversely affect the HIV disease process in the mother, although untreated women in the developing world have worse pregnancy outcomes. There is conflicting evidence on whether women treated with combination antiretroviral therapy, particularly during the first trimester, have a higher incidence of preterm labor than those on monotherapy or no therapy, but the overall benefits of well-controlled disease clearly outweigh the potential risks.

Substance abuse is most common among women of reproductive age, and estimates of substance use among pregnant women range from 0.4% to 27%, depending on the population surveyed. Cocaine use has been associated with lower birth weight and preterm labor along with possible congenital anomalies. Heroin use during pregnancy can lead to a withdrawal syndrome in the infant along with pregnancy complications. In addition to toxic drug effects, poor pregnancy outcomes may result from transmission of disease, hazardous behavior to support a drug habit, malnutrition, and poor prenatal care. There may be polysubstance abuse with additive effects. In addition, alcohol use remains a significant problem during pregnancy. The fetal alcohol syndrome, considered part of the fetal alcohol spectrum disorder (FASD), is manifested by intrauterine growth retardation, microcephaly, and developmental abnormalities. Subtle deficits in development and attention, without the classic phenotype, are seen with lower levels of alcohol exposure. Estimates of the prevalence of fetal alcohol syndrome range from 1 to 4.8 per 1,000, and FASD may be twice as prevalent, particularly among high-risk populations. Some substance abusers may respond to pregnancy with denial or indifference, whereas others may take the opportunity of pregnancy to engage in active substance abuse treatment. A multidisciplinary approach is most effective in caring for these patients.

Substance abuse frequently coincides with psychopathology, but any woman with a psychiatric illness presents concerns during pregnancy. Some evidence suggests that certain psychiatric disorders may worsen during pregnancy and yet remain undertreated. This is a particular concern with depression, which is common before, during, and after pregnancy—some studies estimate a prevalence of depression during pregnancy at up to 20%. There has been recent controversy surrounding the safety of pharmacologic treatment of depression with selective serotonin reuptake inhibitors (SSRIs) during pregnancy. Although multiple large observational studies have shown no increase in congenital anomalies and no long-term effects on children in terms of language, cognition, or temperament, two series demonstrated that paroxetine, especially with first trimester exposure, confers an increased risk of congenital cardiovascular anomalies, particularly ventricular septal defects. These concerns have led to a warning about the use of paroxetine in reproductive-age women. There have also been concerns raised regarding neonatal risk of transient tremor, tachypnea, and possible withdrawal symptoms with maternal third trimester SSRI use, leading to a 2004 U.S. Food and Drug Administration (FDA) warning. However, the risks of untreated maternal depression for both mother and child are significant, and include long-term cognitive and language achievement, which generally outweigh the potential effects of medication exposure. Experts generally recommend treatment of depression during pregnancy. Psychotherapy is a reasonable option for mild to moderate depression, but more severe symptoms, particularly in women with a history of good response to medication, should be treated pharmacologically, with fluoxetine and sertraline having the most safety data. Women with severe or poorly controlled psychiatric disorders, particularly psychosis or mania, may have increased birth complications resulting from poor prenatal care, concurrent substance abuse, increased incidence of homelessness, and

unrecognized physical illness. The primary care physician may be asked to provide counseling and to act as a liaison between obstetric and psychiatric providers.

Some patients undergoing amniocentesis or chorionic villus sampling to identify genetic abnormalities do so on the assumption that they will consider an induced abortion. A patient may look to her primary care provider for guidance with this difficult decision-making process, although often the assistance of a genetic counselor is indicated.

In 2002, more than 750,000 adolescents in the United States became pregnant, down almost 10% from 2000; 215,000 of those pregnancies ended in abortion. Although the teen pregnancy rate in the United States has declined substantially in the last decade and continues to decrease, it remains double or triple that of most developed countries. Consequences for the future of teenage mothers may be immense. Pregnancy may lead to dropping out of school, limited job opportunities, and dependence on the welfare system. Adolescents may intentionally or unintentionally become pregnant for various reasons. They may exhibit risk-taking behavior in response to peer pressure, to experiment, or to test parental limits. Some lonely adolescents see a child as a companion who will provide them with unconditional love. Failure to use contraception may result from lack of adequate information or availability, as well as a sense of invincibility. Risk factors for teen pregnancy include early onset of sexual activity, lower socioeconomic status, poor educational performance, coming from a single-parent family or one with a history of teen pregnancy, and other high-risk behaviors such as substance use. Teenagers may present for prenatal care at a later gestational age because of denial or lack of information about how to get help, resulting in increased morbidity and mortality from the pregnancy or termination. Children born to adolescent parents are at higher risk of cognitive and behavioral problems.

A number of presentations are particularly important because of their psychosocial circumstances. In both rural and urban areas, sexual abuse (including rape and incest) persists to a greater extent than most professional people assume. It may occur between father and daughter, but frequently involves another known adult male, such as uncle, older brother, or boyfriend. The victim may be repulsed at the thought of a baby inside her from such a traumatic experience and may not present for care until later in the pregnancy. In most states, the physician is mandated to report sexual abuse involving minors.

PRINCIPLES OF MANAGEMENT AND PATIENT EDUCATION (1,12–30)

Diagnosis

Urine pregnancy tests that measure β-human chorionic gonadotropin (βhCG) are commonly used for first diagnosis of pregnancy, either at home or in the office. Most tests are immunometric assays claiming the ability (challenged in recent studies) to detect βhCG levels from 25 to 50 mIU/mL, depending on the assay, without cross-reactivity with subunits of other hormones. Variations in time of implantation, with only 90% of pregnancies having implanted by the first day of the expected period, mean that even the most sensitive assay will fail to detect some preimplantation pregnancies, casting doubt on claims of home pregnancy tests to be 99% accurate by this time.

It may take up to 1 week or more for full sensitivity of a home pregnancy test, and accuracy is lower in actual use; positive tests or negative tests with a continued suspicion of pregnancy should be confirmed with *serum tests*. Serum radioimmunoassay tests detect lower hCG levels and appear positive earlier (7 days postconception). Serial quantitative tests can be used to assess viability of a pregnancy or possible ectopic pregnancy.

Counseling

Once a diagnosis of pregnancy is confirmed, a nonjudgmental supportive examination of the patient's feelings is needed. A thorough psychosocial history should be gathered so that her options can be fully explored and her questions about each option answered. Special attention to issues of rape and incest are necessary if this history is elicited or appears to be a possibility. Formal counseling is indicated in this instance. Community support groups may also be helpful.

Therapeutic Abortion

Abortion is one of the most common gynecologic procedures performed in the United States; about 1 in 3 U.S. women will have an abortion during her reproductive years. Data regarding the use of abortion are collected annually by the Centers for Disease Control and Prevention (CDC). After peaking around the year 1990, the number of abortions steadily declined through 2003, the last year for which data are available, although the decline has slowed in the most recent years. In 2003, the national abortion ratio (number of legal abortions per 1,000 live births) was 241, down from 344 in 1990, and the abortion rate (number of legal abortions per 1,000 women aged 15 to 44 years) was 16, down from 24 in 1990. These declines may reflect multiple factors, including more widespread contraceptive use, with long-acting contraceptives introduced in the early 1990s; lower teen pregnancy rates; a demographic shift toward older, less-fertile women in the U.S. population; and worsening access to abortion providers. In 2003, 51% of women undergoing pregnancy termination were younger than age 25 years, 82% were unmarried, and 55% were white. Abortion rates in black women are approximately three times those in white women. The majority of abortions are performed early in gestation (88% within 12 weeks, 61% within 8 weeks), with a continued increase in the percentage performed in the first 6 weeks of gestation.

Legal pregnancy termination is safe, with less than 1 death per 100,000 procedures, as opposed to more than 7 maternal deaths per 100,000 live births. Termination is safest when performed earlier in gestation. Risk increases with gestational age, maternal age, and higher parity. With legalization of abortion in the United States, morbidity has decreased dramatically. There is increased physician training and expertise; increased use of the safer suction curettage procedure rather than sharp curettage, uterine instillation, and surgical procedures; and improved access, allowing earlier procedures. However, availability in the United States has become more limited in recent years, with only 13% of U.S. counties having an abortion provider available in 2001, which means that one fourth of women seeking an abortion must travel more than 50 miles. Lack of service availability and practices regarding waiting periods, parental consent, and abortion funding may all negatively affect a woman's ability to obtain a timely and safe procedure. Additional barriers to services include cost (earlier and nonhospital procedures are cheaper than second-trimester

hospital procedures), harassment of patients at abortion facilities, and vandalism of facilities.

Preprocedure assessment includes determining any underlying medical problems that would necessitate an inpatient rather than outpatient procedure. Usual laboratory evaluation includes pregnancy testing, complete blood count, and blood type and Rh factor determination, as well as potentially screening for sexually transmitted diseases including syphilis, gonorrhea, and chlamydia. Additional studies such as HIV testing and sonography, especially if there is doubt about gestational age, can be considered. Contraception should also be addressed at this time because ovulation may occur as soon as 2 weeks postprocedure; oral contraceptives can be initiated the day after termination, and intrauterine device placement can occur with the procedure. This practice addresses the concern about frequent no-show rates for follow-up appointments. Rh immune globulin should be given after the procedure to Rh-negative unsensitized individuals. Postabortion instructions include vaginal rest (no intercourse, douching, or tampons) for 2 weeks. Because of the risk of postabortal endometritis, prophylactic antibiotics are routinely used in surgical abortions and reduce the incidence of infection by 50%.

Local anesthesia is used for first-trimester and many second-trimester procedures. Paracervical block using lidocaine, with preoperative analgesics and/or sedatives, is generally safe and inexpensive. General or spinal anesthesia is occasionally used for procedures done later in pregnancy or those requiring extensive intrauterine manipulation but carries a higher complication risk.

First-Trimester Abortions

These are performed at 12 weeks of gestation or sooner, and most in the United States are performed by suction curettage. Menstrual extraction, the least invasive procedure, is performed up to 2 weeks after a first missed period in an outpatient facility, with local anesthesia. A flexible plastic catheter is inserted with no more difficulty than performing endometrial biopsy or intrauterine device placement, and manual suction is applied. Because the procedure is done so early in pregnancy, failure to aspirate all the tissue may occur; this complication can be minimized by careful examination of extracted tissue for presence of fetal membranes at the time of the procedure. A persistent positive pregnancy test and absent postoperative bleeding should prompt further evaluation and potentially a repeat procedure. Later first-trimester terminations involve suction curettage, commonly requiring cervical dilation. Dilation may be accomplished manually with a series of cervical dilators or with osmotic dilators, which are inserted into the cervix, where they gradually absorb cervical moisture and expand; the latter are associated with a lower rate of cervical lacerations and are generally preferred. Intravaginal or oral administration of misoprostol, a prostaglandin analogue, has been shown to be effective in facilitating cervical dilation, especially in nulliparous women. A suction curette is then inserted into the uterine cavity, and suction using a cannula removes the pregnancy. The complication rate is 2 per 1,000 procedures. A small percentage (<2%) of pregnancy terminations use sharp curettage (the traditional dilation and curettage), either after suction or on its own. These are most often later first-trimester procedures (10 to 12 weeks) or earlier second-trimester procedures.

Second-Trimester Terminations

These are mostly dilation and evacuation procedures involving placement of multiple small osmotic dilators 6 to 12 hours before the procedure, which is either suction or sharp curettage, as described previously. The complication rate for dilation and curettage is 7 per 1,000 procedures. After 16 to 20 weeks of gestation, induction terminations may be performed using agents inducing labor. Intramuscular or, more commonly, intravaginal prostaglandin preparations are used to induce labor and are preferred over intrauterine instillation procedures, which have been largely abandoned because of the better safety profile of intravaginal abortifacients. Intramniotic injection of a small amount of hypertonic saline is often still used in conjunction with these vaginal prostaglandin labor induction techniques to ensure fetal demise; abortion typically occurs within 12 to 24 hours. Prostaglandins have side effects of nausea, vomiting, diarrhea, and fever, which may be treated symptomatically. Any labor induction is a hospital-based procedure, with a higher complication rate than earlier procedures, and may take several days to complete. Surgical techniques may be required if there are retained products of conception following pregnancy termination with systemic abortifacients.

Hysterotomy and *hysterectomy* are rarely performed second-trimester procedures (accounting for <0.01% of reported procedures in 2003). These have higher morbidity and mortality. Hysterectomy for pregnancy termination is generally performed only for conditions such as gynecologic cancer that require hysterectomy with a coexisting pregnancy.

In 2003, the U.S. Congress passed a law termed the Partial Birth Abortion Ban by the bill's sponsors, which bans any procedure that kills a partially delivered, living fetus. Although intended to apply to late abortions, the law does not specify a specific procedure or a gestational age. Although it makes exceptions for procedures done to save the life of the mother, it does not do so for procedures to save the health of the mother. Critics argue that the law does not adequately take into account a woman's health and privacy rights, may ignore medical standards, and erodes fundamental reproductive rights. In a 5 to 4 decision in April 2007, the U.S. Supreme Court rejected legal challenges to the ban; the consequences of this ruling are unclear.

Medical Pregnancy Termination

This is an increasingly used alternative to surgical abortion and in developing countries may be the only practical alternative— 8% of all terminations reported to the CDC in 2003 were medical abortions, an increase of almost 50% from the previous year. Extensive experience from other countries with *mifepristone*, a synthetic antiprogestin, indicates that it is safe and effective for pregnancy termination in women up to 7 weeks pregnant. The FDA recognized this fact in 2000, when it approved a pregnancy termination regimen involving mifepristone, formerly known as RU-486, followed by progestin administration. Oral misoprostol given 48 hours after oral mifeprestone is the progestin regimen approved by the FDA, but subsequent studies have shown equal or better efficacy and better tolerability with vaginal misoprostol administration.

Mifeprestone binds progesterone receptors, blocking normal activity and preventing implantation or inducing menstruation after implantation. Effectiveness of the combined regimen of mifepristone followed by misoprostol exceeds 95%. Although not FDA approved for gestations longer than 7 weeks because of lower success rates, clinical studies have also shown an efficacy of greater than 90% at 9 and even 12 weeks of gestation. Women whose pregnancies continue despite therapy should undergo a surgical abortion because pregnancies that continue after misoprostol administration are associated with congenital abnormalities in the infant; women should be counseled accordingly. An alternative approach to medical abortion

with mifepristone is the use of methotrexate, generally followed by vaginal misoprostol, or that of misoprostol alone. The former regimen is effective but lengthy (complete abortion may take up to 1 month), whereas the latter shows highly variable efficacy rates in studies.

Abortion-Related Complications

Complications are affected by time of gestation, method of procedure, and coexisting complicating illnesses. Major complications of surgical abortion, including uterine perforation, hemorrhage, and infection, occur at a rate of 1 case per 1,000 procedures. The termination needs to be repeated 2.3 times per 1,000 abortions. Presentations suggestive of these complications include bleeding, fever, abdominal pain or cramping, and uterine tenderness. Minor complications, including infection, cervical stenosis, cervical tear, and bleeding or incomplete abortion requiring resuctioning, occur in 8 per 1,000 procedures. Complication rates increase with gestational age. Complications of medical abortions include vaginal bleeding, cramping abdominal pain, and gastrointestinal side effects including nausea, vomiting, and diarrhea. Regimens using vaginal misoprostol instead of oral administration have fewer side effects, but there have been 5 reported cases of sepsis and death from *Clostridium sordelli* infection after use of vaginal misoprostol, and some experts, including Planned Parenthood, recommend avoiding its use until these have been further investigated.

A number of studies have examined women's preferences for either medical or surgical abortion. In general, women with pregnancies at earlier gestation tend to prefer medical approaches, even though the process may be more painful and associated with more days of bleeding and a longer time to completion. In one study, women who underwent medical abortion reported higher satisfaction levels; only 9% of those women would opt for a surgical abortion in the future, whereas 42% of women who underwent a surgical abortion would opt for a medical abortion.

There are no data showing that serious emotional problems result after pregnancy termination in the United States. The evidence indicates that women generally experience relief and reduced anxiety and distress after pregnancy termination. Negative emotional reactions are more common among women with prior psychiatric illnesses, second-trimester terminations, terminations of wanted pregnancies for medical or genetic reasons, or with significant ambivalence about the decision.

Women who have undergone an abortion are at no increased risk for infertility, miscarriage, ectopic pregnancy, stillbirth, or major pregnancy- or delivery-associated complication. Multiple abortions do not appear to have an effect on future childbearing, although there may be a slightly higher risk of placenta previa. Although second-trimester dilation and evacuation procedures were believed to be associated with development of an incompetent cervix, further studies have failed to demonstrate any connection.

Adoption

Placing a child for adoption is an alternative for a woman who believes it would be impossible to raise a child and who would prefer not to undergo an abortion. Women choosing this option often do so with the belief that their child will have a better upbringing than they can provide. In addition, choosing adoption may allow a woman to defer or delay parenthood, complete her education, establish economic security, or pursue goals. However, adoptions have declined significantly over the last decades; fewer than 3% of never-married women in recent years relinquished their infants. Societal acceptance of single motherhood, legalization of abortion, and establishment of programs offering financial assistance have contributed to this trend. If a woman decides to place her child for adoption, she may enlist a state-run or private agency. She should be encouraged to investigate an agency carefully to ensure that she agrees with its policies and approach. Open adoption, in which there is some future contact with the child, is becoming more common.

Keeping the Child

Keeping the child may emerge as a realistic option if a problematic social situation is amenable to change or a woman decides to adapt her current goals and plans. Identification of social supports includes extended family, as well as the woman's partner. Community agencies may facilitate this process. Adolescents need special counseling because teenage pregnancy is a serious problem resulting in poverty, child neglect, and poor maternal and child outcomes.

Birth Control

Whether a patient chooses to proceed with or terminate a pregnancy, a discussion of future contraceptive options is essential (see Chapter 119). Benefits, risks, and practicalities of each method should be discussed with each woman until she is able to choose her preferred method. Because many unwanted pregnancies and hence abortions may be traced to identifiable contraceptive failure or inconsistent use, they could be prevented by the use of emergency contraception. All women should be educated about the use of emergency contraception, which is now available over the counter to women of age 18 years and over.

Providing care to the woman faced with an unplanned and/or unwanted pregnancy is a challenge to the primary care provider. The provider must explore the patient's beliefs, fears, support network, and psychosocial history. Options must be explained thoroughly and without judgment. Only then can one formulate an appropriate care plan that incorporates the woman's circumstances and preferences.

Annotated Bibliography

1. Strauss LT, , Gamble SB, Parker WY, et al. Abortion surveillance—United States, 2003. MMWR Morb Mortal Wkly Rep 2006;55:1. (*Updated review of current trends.*)
2. Forrest JD. Epidemiology of unintended pregnancy and contraceptive use. Am J Obstet Gynecol 1994;170:1485. (*More than half of the pregnancies in the United States are unintended; of these, equal proportions end in birth and abortion.*)
3. Jones RK, Darroch JE, Henshaw SK. Contraceptive use among U.S. women having abortions in 2000–2001. Perspect Sex Reprod Health 2002;34:294. (*Greater than one half of women who had an abortion in 2000 were using contraception, but the majority of those using oral contraceptives and condoms reported inconsistent use.*)
4. Isaacs JN, Creinin MD. Miscommunication between healthcare providers and patients may result in unplanned pregnancies. Contraception 2003;68:373. (*Of the 77% of women seeking surgical abortion at a private clinic who did not know about emergency contraception, almost two thirds had an identifiable event leading to unintended pregnancy.*)
5. Finer LB. Reasons U.S. women have abortions: quantitative and qualitative perspectives. Perspect Sex Reprod Health 2005;37:110. (*The majority of women undergoing abortion in the United States cite multiple reasons.*)
6. Minkoff H. Human immunodeficiency virus infection in pregnancy. Obstet Gynecol 2003;101:797. (*A comprehensive review of this evolving topic.*)
7. Townsend CL, Cortina-Borja M, Peckham CS, et al. Antiretroviral therapy and premature delivery in diagnosed HIV-infected women in the United Kingdom and Ireland. AIDS 2007;21:1019. (*In a large surveillance study of >3,300 women with HIV, combination therapy with highly active antiretroviral therapy was associated with a higher risk of prematurity than mono or dual therapy.*)
8. Bolnick JM, Rayburn WF. Substance use disorders in women: special considerations during pregnancy. Obstet Gynecol Clin 2003;30:545. (*Helpful overview of toxicities of different substances during pregnancy, with approach to treatment.*)
9. Sokol RJ, Delaney-Black V, Nordstrom B. Fetal alcohol spectrum disorder. JAMA 2003;2990:2996. (*Overview of fetal alcohol syndrome and spectrum, with emphasis on the need for improved screening and diagnosis.*)
10. Louik C, Lin AE, Werler MM, et al. First-trimester use of selective serotonin-reuptake inhibitors and the risk of birth defects. N Engl J Med 2007;356:2675. (*Did not find a link between general selective serotonin reuptake inhibitor use and birth defects, but suggests a possible association between paroxetine and heart defects and sertraline and omphalocele, although the absolute risks remain small.*)
11. Elfenbein DS, Felice ME. Adolescent pregnancy. Pediatric Clin North Am 2003;50:781. (*Helpful review of risk factors, outcomes, and prevention.*)
12. Ventura SJ, Abma JS, Mosher WD, et al. Recent trends in teenage pregnancy in the United States, 1990–2002. Health E-stats. Hyattsville, MD: National Center for Health Statistics. Released December 13, 2006. (*Reviews the trends among the >750,000 pregnancies occurring in teenagers 15 to 19 years old.*)
13. Cole LA, Khanlian SA, Sutton JM, et al. Accuracy of home pregnancy tests at the time of missed menses. Am J Obstet Gynecol 2004;190:100. (*Only 1 of 18 brands of home pregnancy test was able to support its claim of 95% sensitivity at the time of missed menses; other tests were far less sensitive, and two gave false-positive results.*)
14. Wilcox AJ, Baird DD, Dunson D, et al. Natural limits of pregnancy testing in relation to the expected menstrual period. JAMA 2001;286:1759. (*Using an extremely sensitive human chorionic gonadotropin assay, 10% of pregnancies remained undetectable on the first day of missed menses due to delayed implantation.*)
15. Grimes DA, Creinin MD. Induced abortion: an overview for internists. Ann Intern Med 2004;140:620. (*Excellent overview of both surgical and medical abortion, intended for the internist.*)
16. Henshaw SK, Finer LB. The accessibility of abortion services in the United States, 2001. Perspect Sex Reprod Health 2003;35:16. (*In 2001, 87% of U.S. counties had no abortion provider, and one third of women aged 15 to 44 years lived in those counties.*)
17. Edwards J, Carson SA. New technologies permit safe abortion at less than six weeks gestation and provide timely detection of ectopic gestation. Am J Obstet Gynecol 1997;176:1101. (*A case series of >1,500 procedures at <6 weeks found no serious complications.*)
18. Paul M. Office management of early induced abortion. Clin Obstet Gynecol 1999;42:290. (*Good review, including procedural advances.*)
19. Council on Scientific Affairs, American Medical Association. Induced termination of pregnancy before and after Roe v Wade, trends in the mortality and morbidity of women. JAMA 1992;268:3231. (*Good review article.*)
20. Grimes DA, Schulz KF, Cates W, et al. Mid-trimester abortion by dilatation and evacuation: a safe and practical alternative. N Engl J Med 1977;296:1141. (*Compared >6,000 evacuation procedures with nearly 9,000 saline abortions and found a greater effectiveness and fewer complications for the latter.*)
21. Penney GC, Thomson M, Norman J, et al. A randomised comparison of strategies for reducing infective complications of induced abortion. Br J Obstet Gynaecol 1998;105:599. (*Routine antibiotic prophylaxis proved to be more effective and less costly than a screen-and-treat strategy in this trial.*)
22. Stewart FH, Shields WC, Hwang AC. The federal abortion ban: a clinical and moral dilemma, and international policy setback. Contraception 2004;69:433. (*Editorial objecting to the passage of the so-called "partial birth abortion law" as medically inappropriate and placing fetal rights above maternal rights.*)
23. Christin-Maitre S, Bouchard P, Spitz IM. Medical termination of pregnancy. N Engl J Med 2000;342:946. (*A review of the mechanisms of agents used for medical termination, with emphasis on their excellent safety record, high efficacy at early gestations, and acceptability.*)
24. Goldberg AB, Greenberg MB, Darney PD. Misoprostol and pregnancy. N Engl J Med 2001;344:38. (*A classic article reviewing the strong evidence for safe and effective use during pregnancy; led to an accompanying*

editorial lambasting the makers of misoprostol for not supporting its use for these indications.)

25. Chong YS, Su LL, Arulkumaran S. Misoprostol: a quarter century of use, abuse, and creative misuse. Obstet Gynecol Survey 2004;59:128. (*Comprehensive survey of the evidence for safe and effective use of misoprostol for obstetric indications, despite the lack of formal Food and Drug Administration approval until 2002.*)
26. El-Refaey H, Rajasekar D, Abdalla M, et al. Induction of abortion with mifepristone (RU 486) and oral or vaginal misoprostol. N Engl J Med 1995;332:983. (*A classic randomized study comparing oral with vaginal misoprostol, finding that vaginal misoprostol was better tolerated and more effective.*)
27. Hakin-Elahi E, Tovell HMM, Burnhill MS. Complications of first-trimester abortion: a report of 170,000 cases. Obstet Gynecol 1990;76:129.

(*A retrospective review of New York City Planned Parenthood cases; a letter in response appears in Obstet Gynecol 1990;76:1145.*)

28. Fischer M, Bhatnagar J, Guarner J, et al. Fatal toxic shock syndrome associated with *Clostridium sordelli* after medical abortion. N Engl J Med 2005;353:2352. (*Reviews the four California deaths associated with septic shock following medical abortion using intravaginal misoprostol.*)
29. Jensen JT, Harvey SM, Beckman LJ. Acceptability of suction curettage and mifepristone abortion in the United States: a prospective comparison study. Am J Obstet Gynecol 2000;182:1292. (*Greater satisfaction was seen with medical abortions, with only 9% of women saying that they would prefer surgical abortion in the future.*)
30. Adler NE, David HP, Major BN, et al. Psychological responses after abortion. Science 1990;248:41. (*Brief review of U.S. studies examining women after legal terminations.*)

CHAPTER 122 ■ MANAGEMENT OF BREAST CANCER

Breast cancer is one of the most common malignancies in the United States. About 12% of U.S. women will develop breast cancer during their lifetimes, and there are more than 170,000 cases per year. Unfortunately, despite the expanded therapeutic armamentarium for breast cancer and a trend toward increased survival, approximately 30% of women who develop the disease die from it.

Women with newly diagnosed breast cancer face a difficult and complex series of treatment decisions at a time when they may be least able to think rationally or bear the burden of decision-making responsibility. The breast cancer diagnosis evokes anger, a sense of isolation, irrational guilt, and, most of all, vulnerability. Clearly, this mix of emotions makes it difficult for the communication tasks necessary for the patient to be involved in decision making. Yet the most important determinants of the "right" decision for each patient are her attitudes toward the possible treatment outcomes and risks. New information about the relative effectiveness of alternative approaches to primary therapy and adjuvant therapy has added to the complexity of these decisions.

The primary care physician can be a critically important source of empathy, support, and information regarding treatment options. After primary treatment, with or without subsequent adjuvant therapy, the primary care provider may be principally responsible for monitoring the patient's psychosocial adjustment to breast cancer and its treatment and for evidence of disease recurrence. Finally, the primary care role is critically important in decision making about treatment for the woman with advanced breast cancer.

CLINICAL PRESENTATION AND COURSE (1–6)

Breast cancer generally occurs when women are in midlife. The median age at the time of diagnosis is about 55 years. However, breast cancer is not uncommon in women younger than 40 years of age, in whom approximately 20% of cases occur; about 10% of these younger women are pregnant at the time of diagnosis. Breast cancer rarely occurs among men; about 1,500 such cases are diagnosed annually in the United States.

The term *early-stage breast cancer* is generally applied to stage I and stage II tumors. *Stage I* disease is defined as a primary tumor of less than 2 cm in diameter with no axillary lymph node involvement (Table 122.1). Approximately 55% of patients with primary breast cancer now present with stage I disease, in part because of improved screening methods. *Stage II* disease is still considered a localized disease, but it does include involvement of axillary lymph nodes. About 25% of patients with *clinical* stage I disease turn out to have pathologic stage II disease on sampling of the axillary nodes. Of interest, a similar percentage of patients with clinical stage II disease (palpable axillary lymph nodes) turn out to have no tumor in the nodes on pathologic examination. In *stage III* disease, there is extensive tumor (>5 cm) at the primary site, and lymph nodes are larger than 2 cm with or without fixation. In *stage IV* disease, there are distant metastases.

Because of greater use of mammographic screening, cases are increasingly identified with small lesions, including those without evidence of invasion. Noninvasive cancer, or carcinoma *in situ* (CIS), is characterized as ductal or lobular based on histology and location, cytologic features, and growth patterns. These two lesions behave very differently. With ductal CIS (DCIS), mastectomy results in cure for 98% to 99% of women. Similar rates can be achieved with lumpectomy without subsequent radiation if the surgical margins are adequate. One reason for the very good prognosis after therapy is the indolent course for many cases of DCIS. Much is uncertain about the natural history, but there is evidence that many women with DCIS lesions would not progress to invasive disease if left untreated. DCIS accounts for 12% of all newly diagnosed breast cancers in the United States and 30% of cancers detected by mammography. With more than 10,000 mastectomies performed each year for DCIS, it is obvious that more information

TABLE 122.1

TABLE 122.1

CURABILITY OF BREAST CANCER BY STAGE

Stage	Tumor Extent	10-Year Disease-Free Survival (%)
I	Confined to breast	70–80
II	Involves the axillary nodes	20–40
III	Tumor >5 cm; nodes >2 cm; with or without fixation	<5
	Inflammatory	0

TABLE 122.2

PATTERNS OF RECURRENCE AND SURVIVAL IN BREAST CANCER

Pattern	Incidence (%)	Median Time (mo) Relapse	Survival
Multiple metastases	19	9	4
Pulmonary	12	36	18
Bone	26	15	29+
Effusions[a]	16	39	44
Skin and subcutaneous[b]	26	15	27+

[a]+ Minor skin nodules.
[b]+ Minor bone metastases.

and education about the clinical significance of DCIS are needed. Lobular CIS has very different treatment implications. It is not clear whether it is indeed a premalignant lesion or simply a marker for increased risk of invasive disease elsewhere in the breast(s). The incidence of invasive cancer in women with lobular CIS is about 1% per year.

Prognosis

For women with early-stage breast cancer, the prognosis is largely determined by the size of the tumor and the number of positive nodes. For women with negative nodes, 5-year cumulative recurrence rates with tumors smaller than 1 cm, 1 to 2 cm, and 2 to 5 cm in diameter are 10%, 20%, and 30%, respectively. Among women with one to three positive nodes, 40% have a recurrence within 5 years. For women with 4 to 10 nodes positive, the 5-year recurrence rate is 60% to 70%. For women with more than 10 nodes positive or with stage III disease, long-term survival is less than 5%. Inflammatory breast cancer has a worse prognosis than noninflammatory lesions.

In addition to the stage of tumor and tumor size, *estrogen receptor* and *progesterone receptor* status affect the prognosis. Patients with stage I or stage II disease whose tumors have estrogen, receptors, progesterone receptors, or both have a better prognosis than those with the same stage of disease whose tumors are receptor negative. Positive receptor status is also predictive of a positive response to hormonal therapy. Other markers also have prognostic and predictive value. Amplification of human epidermal growth factor receptor type 2 *(HER2)*, also called *HER2-neu*, and overexpression of its product in cancer cells occurs in about 15% to 20% of breast cancer cases and is associated with a poorer prognosis. As discussed later, HER2 amplification or overexpression is predictive of therapeutic response to not only the monoclonal antibody against HER2 developed for that purpose, but also to different chemotherapy regimens.

Breast cancer may metastasize to almost any site in the body, but five general categories have been distinguished, which are correlated with predictable response to therapy and prognosis (Table 122.2). It is evident that even in patients with metastatic disease, median survival may exceed 3 years, and there does not have to be significant change in quality of life when palliative radiation and chemotherapy or hormonal therapy are used throughout that period (see later discussion). More than 50% of patients with metastatic breast cancer may respond to therapy, but only a small portion (perhaps <10%) show complete regression. The median duration of response is approximately 12 to 18 months.

The clinical course of breast cancer is unique in that metastatic lesions may develop after a long period of freedom from disease, even after as long as 20 years. Thus, 5 years without evidence of metastatic spread does not indicate cure.

PRINCIPLES OF MANAGEMENT (1,2,4–44)

The therapeutic options for women diagnosed by an incisional or excisional biopsy have expanded in recent years, accompanied by greater patient participation in choice of therapy. It is no longer justified to perform a biopsy and immediate total mastectomy under the same anesthesia. Patients should be fully informed of the diagnosis, promptly staged, and advised of the therapeutic options.

Staging (4,7–9)

As in most cancers, accurate staging is essential to planning safe and effective treatment. Confirmation of early-stage disease is especially important. Traditionally, patients with no clinical evidence of metastasis underwent full *axillary lymph node dissection* to rule out regional metastasis. Although accurate and capable of reducing mortality by 5% by properly identifying the extent of disease and helping to select appropriate therapy, it is a morbid procedure that often results in axillary pain, disfigurement, tightness and limitation of movement, and troublesome chronic lymphedema of the affected limb. Sentinel node biopsy is a more limited procedure, usually involving injection of radionuclide tracer plus scintigraphic scanning to identify the draining lymph node, which is then resected and examined pathologically. In some instances, blue dye is used to help identify the sentinel node. Should the sentinel node be found positive for malignancy, the remainder of the axillary nodes are then resected for examination. The accuracy of the procedure is greater than 95%, with a false-negative rate of approximately 5% to 8%. Radionuclide bone scan is another important staging modality for breast cancer, especially in persons with positive lymph nodes. Computed tomography scanning may be used for suspected distant metastasis in such areas as liver, brain, and lung.

Primary Treatment of Early-Stage Breast Cancer (4,9,11–32)

Most women with early stage breast cancer have a choice of treatments; survival rates are comparable.

Breast-Conserving Surgery ("Lumpectomy" or "Quadrantectomy") Followed by Radiation

This approach has the obvious advantage of preserving most of the breast. Relative contraindications to breast-conserving surgery include tumors that are large relative to breast size, cancer that is near or involves the nipple, and tumors with extensive intraductal components within or adjacent to the primary tumor. In addition, women with large breasts may fare worse cosmetically with radiation therapy. Chemotherapy has been used before surgery to reduce tumor size and make breast conserving an option for more women with large tumors relative to their breast size. Termed *neoadjuvant chemotherapy*, this approach has been used increasingly in recent years. Radiation therapy after the breast-conserving option is essential. Without it, there is a 40% rate of ipsilateral breast recurrence after breast-conserving surgery. Even with radiation therapy, ipsilateral recurrences do occur, at a rate of 1% to 2% per year. These are then usually treated with mastectomy.

Mastectomy

This is preferred by some women who do not want to live with the anxiety associated with the possibility of having to deal with an ipsilateral recurrence in the breast that they chose to keep. Others prefer mastectomy simply because it does not usually involve subsequent radiation, and it thereby lets them put primary therapy behind them more quickly. However, some recent studies suggest that women who are at high risk of recurrence because of a tumor larger than 4 cm or the presence of more than four positive nodes benefit from radiation therapy after mastectomy. Innovative radiation therapy techniques, related to brachytherapy and three-dimensional conformal radiation therapy, has led to consideration of accelerated partial breast irradiation (APBI) as a potential local treatment option for women with breast cancer. APBI has been used following initial breast-conserving surgery and following a second breast-conserving procedure for an ipsilateral in-breast recurrence. Although trials have demonstrated that there is no survival difference between (a) breast-conserving surgery and radiation and (b) mastectomy, local control of the tumor is important. For every four nearer-term local recurrences following primary therapy, there is one longer-term excess breast cancer death. This recent observation in the 15-year year follow-up of the Early Breast Cancer Trialists' Collaborative indicates that local recurrence of tumor following either breast-conserving surgery or mastectomy provides additional opportunity for tumor dissemination.

After mastectomy, some women opt for breast reconstruction, whereas others feel no need for surgery for cosmetic purposes. Women considering breast reconstruction often underestimate the extent of surgery involved and often have unrealistic expectations about the cosmetic result. The primary care physician is well positioned to help the patient accurately anticipate what reconstruction and its aftermath entails.

Adjuvant Therapy of Breast Cancer

Adjuvant therapy is administered to decrease the likelihood of, or delay, cancer recurrence and death. The most commonly used chemotherapy regimens are *cyclophosphamide*, *methotrexate*, and *fluorouracil* and other regimens that include *doxorubicin* or *epirubicin*. These *anthracycline regimens* achieve improved survival with a 4% to 5% absolute benefit at 5 years in high-risk patients. A recent trial suggests that the benefit is concentrated among the 20% of women whose cancers overexpress HER2. Additional agents can provide benefit; paclitaxel has been shown to be effective following anthracycline chemotherapy in some trials. The antiestrogen *tamoxifen* administered for a period of 5 years has been the standard hormonal therapy. Substitution of the *selective aromatase inhibitor* (SAI) *exemestane* for tamoxifen for the last 2 or 3 years of the 5-year course of hormonal adjuvant therapy confers greater recurrence risk reduction than a 5-year course of tamoxifen alone. Other trials are underway to determine whether third-generation SAIs, including *anastrozole* and *letrozole*, as well as exemestane, are preferable to tamoxifen for first-line hormonal adjuvant therapy. The first and largest of many trials, the Anastrozole and Tamoxifen Alone or in Combination Trial, has reported a small but statistically significant difference (89% vs. 87%) in relapse-free survival at 3 years. In a trial of letrozole versus tamoxifen for initial adjuvant therapy, letrozole reduced the risk of an event by 30% over a mean follow-up of just more than 2 years. It will be many years, however, before we have sufficient experience with SAIs to know how long-term risks compare with those of tamoxifen. SAIs increase fracture risk and cholesterol level and may increase risk for heart disease. SAIs lead to increase in gonadotropin secretion in premenopausal women; their use is contraindicated in this situation. SAIs are also contraindicated in women with estrogen receptor–negative and progesterone receptor–negative cancer.

The effectiveness of adjuvant therapy in decreasing rates of recurrence and breast cancer death among node-positive women has been proven for some time. More recent evidence indicates that adjuvant therapy is as effective in node-negative women, with relative risk reduction by either chemotherapy or hormonal therapy—the same in node-positive and node-negative women. However, the absolute risk difference is much smaller for node-negative women because their baseline risk is lower. For example, women with two positive nodes and women with negative nodes and tumors less than 1 cm might receive the same 30% risk-reduction benefit from adjuvant chemotherapy or hormonal therapy. For the former, that means a reduction from 40% to 28%, or an increase in disease-free survival from 60% to 72%. For the node-negative woman, the same proportional benefit means a reduction from 10% to 7%, or an increase in disease-free survival from 90% to 93%. The significant morbidity associated with adjuvant therapy may or may not be justified, depending on the absolute benefit and the woman's attitudes toward the resulting tradeoffs.

Adjuvant chemotherapy has been the standard of care for premenopausal women with positive nodes, regardless of hormone receptor status, and tamoxifen has been the standard for postmenopausal women with positive nodes, particularly those with positive hormone receptor levels. Ongoing analysis by the Early Breast Cancer Trialists' Collaborative Group of individual patient experiences for tens of thousands of women who have participated in scores of randomized trials continues to refine our understanding of adjuvant therapy effects. Tamoxifen is effective regardless of age or menopausal status in women who are estrogen receptor positive or progesterone receptor positive. The effects of chemotherapy and tamoxifen are greater than either intervention alone for these women. The relatively nontoxic response has led to increasing use of tamoxifen among node-negative women who are receptor positive. Treatment of node-negative women who are receptor negative is more controversial. The source of the controversy is the question of whether the risk-reduction benefits are sufficiently great to justify the significant morbidity associated with adjuvant chemotherapy. Women who choose this option should have a clear understanding of the benefits and realistic expectations of not only transient side effects, including nausea and vomiting and alopecia, but also longer-term problems including premature menopause, osteoporosis, possible increased risk of heart disease, and cognitive dysfunction (Table 122.3).

The value of a *bisphosphonate* in the adjuvant regimen is uncertain. The antiosteolytic effect of bisphosphonates has been shown significantly to reduce the incidence of bone pain, pathologic fractures, and hypercalcemia in women with breast cancer and bone metastases (see later discussion). The adjuvant use of the bisphosphonate clodronate in women at high risk for distant metastases (with tumor cells in the bone marrow at initial staging) was shown to reduce the incidence of bony and visceral metastases by 50% in one trial. However, a subsequent trial among women at high risk for recurrence (with axillary lymph nodes positive) showed higher rates of metastases and higher mortality with clodronate.

Monitoring after Treatment of Breast Cancer (1,32)

After primary therapy, women with breast cancer should be seen at regular intervals. Psychosocial adjustments and clinical status need careful attention. A *mammogram* should be obtained annually because successfully treated women are at increased risk of a second primary tumor, which may also be curable. Follow-up *bone scan* should be undertaken only in patients who develop symptoms of bone pain. *Tumor markers* such as *CEA, CA 15-3,* and *CA 27.29* are available and sometimes ordered, but they have limited sensitivity for identification of early metastatic breast cancer, and false positives are not uncommon. There is no evidence that their use improves outcomes, and unnecessary psychological distress or false reassurance may ensue.

Treatment of Advanced Breast Cancer (34–40,42–44)

Stage III breast cancer is an inoperable local disease confined to the skin, breast, or lymph nodes. It may be treated either with systemic therapy (either hormonal or chemotherapy) to determine the effectiveness of the systemic treatment and to reduce the bulk of tumor or with local therapy, which may be either mastectomy followed by radiation therapy or radiation therapy alone. The median length of survival after effective treatment is 18 to 24 months.

The management of stage IV (metastatic) breast cancer is determined in part by sites of metastases, menopausal status and hormone receptor status, and the presence or absence of overexpression of HER2. The decision to treat and the timing of therapy depend on the presence or absence of symptoms and the growth rate of the tumor. Systemic therapy for advanced breast cancer includes hormone therapy, chemotherapy, and combination therapy, as well as the monoclonal antibody against HER2 for the roughly 20% of women whose tumors overexpress HER2. Radiation therapy is also very effective for palliation, and, as noted, bisphosphonate therapy reduces the incidence of complications associated with bony metastases.

Hormone therapy can be very effective for tumors that have high concentration of estrogen receptor protein in the cytoplasm. Tumors with progesterone receptors are also more likely to be hormonally responsive. The sites of disease most often responsive to hormones are pulmonary nodules, pleural effu-

sions, and osseous lesions. There is a much lower likelihood of response to hormonal manipulation for patients with hepatic metastases, lymphangitic pulmonary involvement, brain metastases, or skin lesions. Hormone management also depends on menopausal status. The least responsive group is that of perimenopausal women. After an initial response to hormonal therapy, a relapse usually occurs, but a subsequent secondary response to an alternative hormonal manipulation is not uncommon. For the most part, such secondary responses are short lived and are not of the quality of the initial response. It is important to recognize that the effect of hormonal therapy on tumor bulk may not be observed for 1 or 2 months, even though the agent may begin working immediately. Relief of bone pain is much more rapidly achieved.

Hormonal therapy occasionally results in exacerbation of bone pain or tumor growth. The mechanism is not known. In a small percentage of these patients, the opposite hormonal maneuver (i.e., ablation or supplementation) may induce an antitumor effect. Patients should be monitored for a period of time to determine whether tumor stimulation and serious hypercalcemia occur.

Tamoxifen, a competitive inhibitor of endogenous estrogen, binds to estrogen receptors and achieves an antitumor effect by an unknown mechanism. The drug has a low rate of toxicity and a response rate comparable with that of other forms of hormone therapy. As a result, tamoxifen has been the usual first-line hormonal therapy. More recent trials have demonstrated that both letrozole and anastrozole can achieve better rates and duration of tumor responsiveness. As a result, some oncologists now consider them to be the preferred first-line choices. Trial data for anastrozole conflict with some data indicating no difference in comparison with tamoxifen. Trials comparing exemestane and tamoxifen have shown promising early results. SAIs do not appear to increase the risk of endometrial cancer; other long-term effects of SAIs are emerging from the early trials. There are concerns about increases in cholesterol and cardiovascular risk that have yet to be fully defined.

Chemotherapy should be considered for patients with advanced disease after hormonal manipulations have failed or when they are deemed inappropriate (e.g., in receptor-negative patients). However, the likelihood of response is reduced when the tumor has proven resistant to other forms of treatment. The chemotherapeutic regimens most commonly used to manage advanced disease include the same regimens commonly used for adjuvant therapy. As with adjuvant therapy, combinations of hormonal manipulations and multidrug programs have been advocated on the basis of a possible synergistic interaction. *Trastuzumab* is increasingly used for patients with HER2-positive tumors, especially when they have become refractory to other therapies.

Breast cancer is particularly sensitive to *radiation therapy.* Metastatic bony lesions are present in more than 60% of patients with breast cancer, and lytic lesions are often associated with pain. Local radiation therapy at the relatively low doses of 2,000 to 3,500 rad may relieve pain, although persistent structural defects as a consequence of cortical bony erosion may necessitate orthopedic support and even internal fixation for weight-bearing bone structures. Another important role for radiation therapy is in palliation of patients who develop metastatic brain lesions, which occur in more than 10% of patients.

Autologous bone marrow transplantation in conjunction with high-dose chemotherapy had been used extensively in the United States among women deemed at high risk for distant metastases and death, usually because of extensive lymph

TABLE 122.3

COMMON SYMPTOMS AND PROBLEMS IN PATIENTS AFTER TREATMENT FOR BREAST CANCER

Symptom or Problem	Factors Associated with Highest Risk	Recommended Screening	Recommended Interventions[a]

Hot flashes	Chemotherapy-induced menopause
	Treatment with tamoxifen or aromatase inhibitors
		History	SSRIs[b,c]
			  Citalopram, 30 mg
			  Fluoxetine, 20 mg
			  Paroxetine (avoid if patient is receiving tamoxifen), 10–20 mg or 12.5–25 mg continuous release
			SSNRIs[b,c]
			  venlafaxine, 75 or 100 mg
			Gabapentin, 300 mg, 3 times/day[b,c]

Sexual dysfunction Loss of libido (in addition to dyspareunia)	Altered body image due to surgery, irradiation, or systemic therapy; depression	History	Sexual counseling
Dyspareunia due to vaginal dryness	Chemotherapy-induced menopause; treatment with tamoxifen or aromatase inhibitors		Nonhormonal vaginal moisturizing or lubricating preparation (polycarophil [Replens] or hydroxyethylcellulose, chlorhexidine gluconate, methylparaben, or glucono delta lactone [Astroglide]); intravaginal estradiol preparations (use with caution)[d]
Arthralgias and musculoskeletal symptoms	Treatment with tamoxifen or aromatase inhibitors (symptoms are more common with aromatase inhibitors)	History (rule out features suggestive of metastatic disease to bone, such as persistent and progressively more severe long bone or back pain, which would warrant imaging)	Conservative medical management Acetaminophen NSAIDs
Cognitive dysfunction	Diagnosis of breast cancer Of concern but not documented: chemotherapy, treatment with tamoxifen or aromatase inhibitors	History	Evaluate for Alzheimer's disease or other organic cause if progressive and severe
Depression	Diagnosis of breast cancer Of concern but not documented: chemotherapy, treatment with tamoxifen or aromatase inhibitors	History	Usual management (counseling, antidepressants)

(continued)

TABLE 122.3

COMMON SYMPTOMS AND PROBLEMS IN PATIENTS AFTER TREATMENT FOR BREAST CANCER (*Continued*)

Symptom or Problem	Factors Associated with Highest Risk	Recommended Screening	Recommended Interventions[a]
Fatigue	Diagnosis of breast cancer Chemotherapy Of concern but not documented: treatment with tamoxifen or aromatase inhibitors	History	Rule out or treat psychiatric or biologic cause (depression, anemia, hypothyroidism)
Weight gain	Chemotherapy Of concern but not documented: treatment with tamoxifen or aromatase inhibitors	History	Usual management (diet, exercise)
Osteopenia or osteoporosis	Chemotherapy-induced menopause Treatment with aromatase inhibitors Usual risk factors for osteoporosis: lean body habitus, smoking, personal or family history of osteoporotic fracture	Bone densitometry before initiation of aromatase inhibitor and every 1–2 yr thereafter	Usual management Adequate intake of calcium (1,200–1,500 mg daily) and vitamin D (400–800 IU daily)[e] Weight-bearing exercise, avoidance of smoking Bisphosphonate if indicated[f]
Cardiovascular disease	Irradiation of the left chest wall Of concern but not documented: chemotherapy-induced early menopause, treatment with aromatase inhibitors	History	Appropriate medical and lifestyle risk–reduction strategies
Congestive heart failure	Treatment with anthracyclines or trastuzumab	None Monitor left ventricular function during trastuzumab therapy	No known prophylaxis Appropriate medical management if present
Thrombosis (deep vein, cerebrovascular)	Treatment with tamoxifen	History	No proven prophylaxis Appropriate medical management if present

NSAIDs, nonsteroidal antiinflammatory drugs; SSNRIs, selective serotonin and norepinephrine reuptake inhibitors; SSRIs, selective serotonin reuptake inhibitors.

[a]Representative examples of effective interventions are shown; the list is not exhaustive.

[b]The FDA has not approved these drugs for this indication.

[c]Side effects or complications from these drugs are as follows: SSRIs — sweating, constipation, diarrhea, flatulence, anorexia, insomnia, somnolence, tremor, anxiety, blurred vision, loss of libido: bleeding hyponatremia (rare), seizure (rare), mania (rare), and suicidal thoughts or behavior (rare); SSNRIs — same, plus hypertension, hepatitis (rare); gabapentin —peripheral edema, myalgia, dizziness, hyperactivity, nystaginus, nystaginus, somnolence, tremor, mood disorder, fatigue, Stevens–Johnson syndrome (rare), and seizure (rare).

[d]Intravaginal estradiol preparations may slightly increase systemic estrogen levels (with concern about increased risk of breast cancer recurrence).

[e]Some authorities recommend 1,000 IU of vitamin D daily.

[f]Side effects or complications from bisphosphonate include esophageal irriation or ulcer; myalgias, rash; hypocalcemia, and osteonecrosis of the jaw (rare).

From Hayes DF. Follow-up of patients with early breast cancer. N Engl J Med 2007;356:2505.

node involvement. However, trials have not shown a survival benefit despite the very high morbidity associated with this approach.

CARE OF COMMON SYMPTOMS AND PROBLEMS ASSOCIATED WITH BREAST CANCER TREATMENT (1,32)

Despite real advances in treatment of breast cancer, surgery, radiation, and systemic therapy all have an effect on the quality of life. Certain symptoms are predictable and can be significantly ameliorated if the primary care provider is proactive in anticipating and eliciting them from the patient. Table 122.3 lists the most common symptoms and problems and indicates their risk factors, approaches to monitoring for them, and recommended interventions.

PATIENT EDUCATION (45–49)

Whether or not a woman has had a role in decision making about breast cancer treatment can be an important determinant of her psychosocial adjustment. Many women find reasons to blame themselves or others because of things they might have done, or might not have done, to prevent the disease. Some focus on stressful experiences and believe that they played a causative role or that they will increase the risk of recurrence and/or progression. They should be reassured that there is good evidence that this is not the case.

Young women still in their reproductive years face difficult questions about future pregnancy and childbirth. Those with early disease can be reassured that conception 6 months after completing treatment is not likely to reduce survival.

The primary care provider is well positioned to provide empathic support and vital information about the benefit and harm of alternative treatment options.

A.G.M.

Annotated Bibliography

1. Hayes DF. Follow-up of patients with early breast cancer. N Engl J Med 2007;356:2505. (*A very helpful comprehensive review including recommendations for many common symptoms and problems.*)
2. Punglia RS, Morrow M, Winer EP, et al. Local therapy and survival in breast cancer. N Engl J Med 2007;356:2399. (*A thoughtful analysis of the effect of screening on mortality and on the relationship between local control and long-term survival, concluding that historical arguments about breast cancer being a local or systemic disease underestimate its heterogeneity; failure to achieve initial local control allows some tumors to disseminate that would not have otherwise, reducing prospects for long-term survival.*)
3. Giordano SH, Buzdar AU, Hortobagyi GN. Breast cancer in men. Ann Intern Med 2002;137:678. (*A careful review of the literature.*)
4. Morrow M, Gradishar W. Breast cancer. BMJ 2002;324:410. (*Selective review of new developments, including sentinel node biopsy and the use of aromatase inhibitors.*)
5. Woo JC, Yu T, Hurd TC. Breast cancer in pregnancy. A literature review. Arch Surg 2003;138:91. (*An excellent review of prognosis and management.*)
6. Wooster R, Weber BL. Breast and ovarian cancer. N Engl J Med 2003;348:2339. (*A review emphasizing the management of patients with genetic susceptibility; 56 references.*)
7. Mirza AN, Mirza NQ, Viastos G, et al. Prognostic factors in node-negative breast cancer. Ann Surg 2002;235:10. (*Tumor size and tumor grade are the only factors that are broadly clinically useful.*)
8. Veronesi U, Paganelli G, Viale G, et al. A randomized comparison of sentinel-node biopsy with routine axillary dissection in breast cancer. N Engl J Med 2003;349:546. (*Sentinel node biopsy resulted in fewer adverse outcomes than axillary dissection in the staging of breast cancer in persons with a primary breast cancer <2 cm in diameter.*)
9. McGuire WL, Clark GM. Prognostic factors and treatment decisions in axillary-node-negative breast cancer. N Engl J Med 1992;326:1756. (*An excellent review of prognostic variables among node-negative women.*)
10. Loprinzi CL, Kugler JW, Sloan JA, et al. Lack of effect of coumarin in women with lymphedema after treatment for breast cancer. N Engl J Med 1999;340:346. (*No effect was found in this randomized trial.*)
11. Al-Ghazal SK, Fallowfield L, Blamey RW, et al. Patient evaluation of cosmetic outcome after conserving surgery for treatment of primary breast cancer. Eur J Surg Oncol 1999;24:344. (*More than 90% of women in this series were satisfied with the result.*)
12. Alderman AK, Kuhn LE, Lowery JC, et al. Does patient satisfaction with breast reconstruction change over time? Two-year results of the Michigan breast reconstruction outcomes study. J Am Coll Surg 2007;204:7. (*Differences initially found in women's general satisfaction with breast reconstruction diminish.*)
13. Early Breast Cancer Trialists' Collaborating Group. Effects of radiotherapy and surgery in early breast cancer: an overview of the randomized trials. N Engl J Med 1995;333:1444. (*Further results from the landmark meta-analysis.*)
14. Farrow DC, Hunt WC, Samet JM. Geographic variation in the treatment of localized breast cancer. N Engl J Med 1992;326:1097. (*Wide variations were found in the rates of breast-conserving surgery in different regions.*)
15. Fisher B, Anderson S, Fisher ER, et al. Significance of ipsilateral breast tumor recurrence after lumpectomy. Lancet 1991;338:327. (*Ipsilateral in-breast re-

currences occurred at a rate of 1.4% per year despite radiation after lumpectomy.*)
16. Fisher B, Redmond C, Poisson R, et al. Eight-year results of a randomized clinical trial comparing total mastectomy and lumpectomy with or without irradiation in the treatment of breast cancer. N Engl J Med 1989;320:822. (*Further evidence for the equivalence of the two primary treatment options in terms of distant recurrence and survival.*)
17. Early Breast Cancer Trialists' Collaborative Group (EBCTCG). Effects of radiotherapy and of differences in the extent of surgery for early breast cancer on local recurrence and 15-year survival: an overview of the randomised trials. Lancet 2005;366:2087. (*Differences in local treatment that substantially affect local recurrence rates would, in the hypothetical absence of any other causes of death, avoid about one breast cancer death over the next 15 years for every four local recurrences avoided and should reduce 15-year overall mortality.*)
18. Silverstein MJ, Lagios MD, Groshen S, et al. The influence of margin width on local control of ductal carcinoma *in situ* of the breast. N Engl J Med 1999;340:1455. (*Very low rates of recurrence were found in women with lumpectomy and margins of 1 cm or more with no benefit from radiation.*)
19. Hojris I, Overgaard M, Christensen JJ, et al. Morbidity and mortality of ischaemic heart disease in high-risk breast cancer patients after adjuvant postmastectomy systemic treatment with or without radiotherapy. Lancet 1999;354:1425. (*Postmastectomy radiation does not increase ischemic heart disease risk over 12 years.*)
20. Early Breast Cancer Trialists' Collaborating Group. Systemic treatment of early breast cancer by hormonal, cytotoxic, or immune therapy. Lancet 1992;339:71. (*A landmark overview and analysis of worldwide randomized trial experience with treatment of early breast cancer.*)
21. Early Breast Cancer Trialists' Collaborative Group. Multi-agent chemotherapy for early breast cancer (Cochrane review). In: The Cochrane library, Issue 3. Oxford: Update Software, 2004. (*Absolute improvement was found of 7% to 11% in 10-year survival for women younger than 50 years at presentation with early breast cancer and of about 2% to 3% for those aged 50 to 69 years.*)
22. Early Breast Cancer Trialists' Collaborative Group. Tamoxifen for early breast cancer: an overview of the randomised trials. Lancet 1998;351:1451. (*Overview of trial experience of 37,000 women who received tamoxifen for 1, 2, or approximately 5 years with or without adjuvant chemotherapy; some years of tamoxifen therapy substantially improves 10-year survival for women with estrogen receptor–positive tumors.*)
23. Early Breast Cancer Trialists' Collaborative Group. Effects of chemotherapy and hormonal therapy for early breast cancer on recurrence and 15-year survival: an overview of the randomised trials. Lancet 2005;365:1687. (*Demonstrates the persistence of the relative risk reductions previously described and quantified over 15 years.*)
24. ATAC Trialists Group. Anastrozole alone or in combination with tamoxifen versus tamoxifen alone for adjuvant treatment of postmenopausal women with early breast cancer. Lancet 2002;359:2131. (*An early trial showing a small but significant advantage for the selective aromatase inhibitor [SAI].*)
25. Coombes RC, Hall E, Gibson LJ, et al. A randomized trial of exemestane after two to three years of tamoxifen therapy in postmenopausal women with primary breast cancer. N Engl J Med 2004;350:1081. (*There was a 32%

relative risk reduction and a 4.7% absolute risk reduction when exemestane was substituted for tamoxifen for the last 2 to 3 years of a total 5-year course of adjuvant therapy.)

26. The Breast International Group (BIG 1-98 Collaborative Group). A comparison of letrozole and tamoxifen in postmenopausal women with early breast cancer. N Engl J Med 2005;353:2747. (*Adjuvant treatment with letrozole, as compared with tamoxifen, reduced the risk of recurrent disease, especially at distant sites.*)

27. Pritchard KI, Shepherd LE, O'Malley FP, et al. HER2 and responsiveness of breast cancer to adjuvant chemotherapy. N Engl J Med 2006;354:2103. (*Amplification of HER2 in breast cancer cells is associated with clinical responsiveness to anthracycline-containing chemotherapy.*)

28. Piccart-Gebhart MJ, Procter M, Leyland-Jones B, et al. Trastuzumab after adjuvant chemotherapy in HER2-positive breast cancer. N Engl J Med 2005;353:1659. (*One year of treatment with trastuzumab after adjuvant chemotherapy significantly improved disease-free survival among women with HER2-positive breast cancer.*)

29. Fisher B, Dignam J, Wolmark N, et al. Tamoxifen in treatment of intraductal breast cancer: National Surgical Adjuvant Breast and Bowel Project B-24 randomised controlled trial. Lancet 1999;353:1993. (*The addition of tamoxifen reduced cancer events over 5 years from 13.4% to 8.2%.*)

30. Gail MH, Costantino JP, Bryant J, et al. Weighing the risks and benefits of tamoxifen treatment for treating breast cancer. J Natl Cancer Inst 1999;91:1829. (*Benefits are greatest for younger women at higher risk of breast cancer.*)

31. Smith IE, Dowsett M. Aromatase inhibitors in breast cancer. N Engl J Med 2003;348:2431. (*A comprehensive clinical review; 105 references.*)

32. Rojas MP, Telaro E, Russo A, et al. Follow-up strategies for women treated for early breast cancer (Cochrane review). In: The Cochrane library, Issue 3. Oxford: Update Software, 2004. (*Regular physical examinations and yearly mammography alone are as effective as more intensive approaches in terms of timeliness of recurrence detection, overall survival, and quality of life.*)

33. Diel IJ, Solomayer EF, Costa SD, et al. Reduction in new metastases in breast cancer with adjuvant clodronate treatment. N Engl J Med 1998;339:357. (*Demonstrates a 50% reduction in both bony and visceral metastases over a median follow-up of 3 years.*)

34. Edwards AGK, Hailey S, Maxwell M. Psychological interventions for women with metastatic breast cancer (Cochrane review). In: The Cochrane library, Issue 3. Oxford: Update Software, 2004. (*Concludes that there is insufficient evidence to advocate for group psychological therapies.*)

35. Farquhar C, Basser R, Hetrick S, et al. High dose chemotherapy and autologous bone marrow or stem cell transplantation versus conventional chemotherapy for women with metastatic breast cancer (Cochrane review). In: The Cochrane library, Issue 3. Oxford: Update Software, 2004. (*Evidence that the use of high-dose chemotherapy and autograft improves progression-free survival at 1 and 2 years but has no benefit in overall survival.*)

36. Farquhar C, Basser R, Marjoribanks J, et al. High dose chemotherapy and autologous bone marrow or stem cell transplantation versus conventional chemotherapy for women with early poor prognosis breast cancer (Cochrane review). In: The Cochrane library, Issue 3. Oxford: Update Software, 2004. (*Evidence does not support use.*)

37. Hortobagyi GH, Theriault RL, Porter L, et al. Efficacy of pamidronate in reducing skeletal complications in patients with breast cancer and lytic bone metastases. N Engl J Med 1996;335:1785. (*Monthly infusions of this bisphosphonate reduced the incidence of bony complications in women with stage IV breast cancer.*)

38. Mouridsen H, Gersanovich M, Sun Y, et al. Superior efficacy of letrozole versus tamoxifen as first-line therapy for post-menopausal women with advanced breast cancer. J Clin Oncol 2001;19:2596. (*An early trial demonstrating SAI superiority.*)

39. Pavlakis N, Stockler M. Bisphosphonates for breast cancer (Cochrane review). In: The Cochrane library, Issue 3. Oxford: Update Software, 2004. (*Oral or intravenous bisphosphonates reduce the risk of skeletal event as well as increasing the time to skeletal event; see http://www.cochrane.org for updates.*)

40. Plunkett TA, Rubens RD. Biphosphonate therapy for patients with breast carcinoma. Cancer 2003;97:854. (*Details evidence for the use of biphosphonates, including uncertainty about the duration of use and their use in the adjuvant setting.*)

41. Rodenhuis S, Richel DJ, van der Wall E, et al. Randomised trial of high-dose chemotherapy and haemopoietic progenitor-cell support in operable breast cancer with extensive axillary lymph-node involvement. Lancet 1998;352:515. (*A randomized trial of 97 women with extensive axillary node metastases randomized to conventional or high-dose chemotherapy after neoadjuvant chemotherapy and primary therapy; no difference in survival was seen with a mean follow-up of 49 months.*)

42. Shenkier T, Weir L, Levine M, et al. Clinical practice guidelines for the care and treatment of breast cancer: 15. Treatment for women with stage III or locally advanced breast cancer. Can Med Assoc J 2004;170:983. (*One in a series of effective reviews.*)

43. Slamon DJ, Leyland-Jones B, Shak S, et al. Use of chemotherapy plus a monoclonal antibody against HER2 for metastatic breast cancer that overexpresses HER2. N Engl J Med 2001;344:783. (*Trastuzumab increases the clinical benefit of first-line chemotherapy in metastatic breast cancer that overexpresses HER2.*)

44. Wilcken N, Hornbuckle J, Ghersi D. Chemotherapy alone versus endocrine therapy alone for metastatic breast cancer (Cochrane review). In: The Cochrane library, Issue 3. Oxford: Update Software, 2004. (*When hormone receptors are present, treating first with endocrine therapy rather than chemotherapy is recommended except in the presence of rapidly progressive disease.*)

45. Graham J, Ramirez A, Love S, et al. Stressful life experiences and risk of relapse of breast cancer: observational cohort study. BMJ 2002;324:1420. (*Stressful life experiences are not associated with breast cancer diagnosis or recurrence.*)

46. Schover LR. The impact of breast cancer on sexuality, body image, and intimate relationships. CA Cancer J Clin 1991;41:112. (*Conflicting evidence about the comparative effects of mastectomy and breast-conserving surgery; the effect of adjuvant therapy may be underappreciated.*)

47. Pierce JP, Natarajan L, Caan BJ, et al. Influence of a diet very high in vegetables, fruit, and fiber and low in fat on prognosis following treatment for breast cancer. The Women's Healthy Eating and Living (WHEL) randomized trial. JAMA 2007;298:289. (*This approach did not reduce additional breast cancer events or mortality during a 7.3-year follow-up period.*)

48. Mutrie N, Campbell AM, Whyte F, et al. Benefits of supervised group exercise programme for women being treated for early stage breast cancer: pragmatic randomised controlled trial. BMJ 2007;334:517. (*Supervised group exercise provided functional and psychological benefit after a 12-week intervention and 6 months later.*)

49. Ives A, Saunders C, Bulsara M, et al. Pregnancy after breast cancer: population based study. BMJ 2007;334:194. (*Does not support the current medical advice given to premenopausal women with a diagnosis of breast cancer to wait 2 years before attempting to conceive.*)

CHAPTER 123 ■ MANAGEMENT OF THE WOMAN WITH GENITAL TRACT CANCER

Cancers of the genital tract account for about 20% of cancer diagnoses and 10% of cancer deaths in women. They range from the readily detectable and curable carcinoma of the cervix to the very problematic ovarian carcinoma, with its tendency to remain inconspicuous until very late. Endometrial carcinoma has come to be one of the most common genital cancers of the postmenopausal years. Cervical cancer is associated with sexual exposure to human papillomavirus (HPV) and is therefore of great concern for younger women.

Treatment of the woman with genital tract cancer is usually the province of the oncologist and gynecologist, but the primary physician remains an important part of the collaborative effort. Patient counseling, monitoring, and management of ongoing medical problems are among the important responsibilities.

CARCINOMA OF THE CERVIX (1–6)

The incidence of invasive cervical carcinoma peaks between the ages of 48 and 55 years. The peak for carcinoma *in situ* is between ages 25 and 40 years. Most women with the disease present in their 20s and 30s due to early detection from use of cytologic testing and, more recently, HPV DNA testing (see Chapter 107).

Principles of Management

Diagnosis

Postcoital bleeding should raise suspicion for the diagnosis. In most cases of early disease, the patient is asymptomatic and, as noted, detection is by screening *Papanicolaou test* and or *HPV DNA testing* (see Chapter 107). Diagnosis may be made by biopsy at the time of culposcopy following an abnormal screening test or of a grossly suspicious-looking lesion. In many cases, curative intervention occurs before invasive cancer is diagnosed. Cytologic high-grade squamous intraepithelial lesion may prompt immediate loop electrosurgical excision rather than culposcopy in older women. Immediate excision, or the "see-and-treat" approach, is not considered acceptable in adolescents.

Staging

Clinical staging of cancers is based on findings from biopsy, physical examination, and radiologic study. An estimate of extent of local disease can be made by *pelvic examination,* carefully palpating to see whether there is lateral extension to the vagina or pelvic wall. Palpating lymph nodes may detect a distant nodal metastasis, but clinical staging for involvement of pelvic nodes and the more distant paraaortic ones requires *lymphangiography* and/or *computed tomography* (CT). The latter has been especially helpful in the assessment of paraaortic nodes. Studies of *magnetic resonance imaging* suggest some usefulness in delineating local extension.

Stage of disease is designated by the TMN (tumor, metastasis, node) system (Table 123.1). Prognosis worsens with advancing stage of local disease, development of regional and distant nodal metastases (especially paraaortic nodes), and histologic grade. Risk of nodal metastasis rises with growth of tumor to greater than 4 cm, lymphovascular invasion, invasion deep into the cervical stroma, and histologic grade.

Treatment and Prognosis

Early stages of carcinoma of the cervix are curable. Patients sometimes ask the opinion of their primary physician regarding the choices of therapy for early-stage disease. Consequently, these choices are worth reviewing here.

For *stage 0 disease,* the longstanding treatment of choice has been *cold knife conization.* Alternatives excisional approaches include loop electrosurgical excision and laser conization. Ablative methods include *cryotherapy, laser ablation, electrofulguration,* and *cold coagulation. Hysterectomy* is reserved for those who have intraepithelial neoplasia at the margins of the excised specimen and for whom future childbearing is not an issue. Cure is greater than 99%.

Stage IA1 is treated with *vaginal hysterectomy* when childbearing is not an issue. When it is desired, excisional *conization* and close follow-up are the alternative if the cone margins are free of tumor. Five-year survival is greater than 90%. There is debate regarding the best approach to *stage IA2* disease. If invasion is greater than 3 mm or there is lymphovascular invasion, then these patients are usually treated like stage IB patients. If invasion is less than 3 mm and there is no lymphovascular involvement, then they are treated like IA1 patients. *Intracavitary irradiation* is another curative option.

Stages IB and IIA are treated by *radical hysterectomy* plus *pelvic lymphadenectomy* or by definitive *irradiation.* Surgery is preferred in young women because the ovarian function can be spared and the vagina is more pliable than after irradiation. In addition, radiation effects on bowel and other adjacent structures are avoided. Radiation therapy spares the need for an extensive surgical procedure and its attendant complications. With either procedure, 5-year survival is equally good, with rates averaging about 85% for patients with no pelvic node disease. If there is involvement of pelvic nodes, 5-year survival falls to about 50%.

Stages IIB and beyond are treated with *irradiation.* Five-year survival averages about 60% for patients with IIB disease and falls to about 35% for stage IIIB disease and to 20% for stage IV disease.

Concomitant chemotherapy and radiation therapy has been shown to increase overall survival and progression-free survival in women with locally advanced cervical cancer compared to

TABLE 123.1

STAGING OF CERVICAL CANCER

Primary Tumor		
0		Carcinoma *in situ*
I		Confined to uterus
	A	Preclinical invasive disease
	A1	Minimal stromal invasion
	A2	Invasion ≤5 mm
	B	Invasion ≥5 mm
II		Invasion beyond uterus but not to pelvic wall or lower third of vagina
	A	Without parametrial invasion
	B	With parametrial invasion
III		Invasion to pelvic wall, lower third of vagina, or causes hydronephrosis
	A	Only invasive to lower third of vagina
	B	Invasive to pelvic wall or hydronephrosis
IV		Invasion of bladder, rectum, or beyond true pelvis
Regional Lymph Nodes		
N0		No regional node metastasis
N1		Regional node metastasis
Distant Metastasis (includes paraaortic nodes)		
M0		No distant metastasis
M1		Distant metastasis

Adapted from Beahrs OH, Henson DE, Hutter RVP, et al., eds. Manual for staging of cancer, 3rd ed. Philadelphia: Lippincott, 1988:151, with permission.

treatment with radiation alone. It also may reduce local and distant recurrence rates. There is an increase in acute treatment toxicity; the effect on long-term side effects has not been well defined.

The high likelihood of nodal metastasis associated with advancing stages of local disease markedly lowers the chances of cure. Clinically inapparent involvement of paraaortic nodes is a particularly difficult problem, leading some to advocate surgical sampling. Prophylactic radiation to the area does not seem to improve survival.

Patient Education

Young patients need to know that carcinoma of the cervix is potentially curable and that early disease can be successfully treated without overly compromising childbearing capacity. Such knowledge ensures that the young woman with precancerous lesions will not refuse timely treatment out of fear. The clinician should, however, carefully explain the risks of preterm delivery and low birth weight that are conferred by conization and similar procedures. Older patients presenting with more-invasive disease can still obtain some comfort from knowing the prognosis remains very favorable for most stages of this disease.

CARCINOMA OF ENDOMETRIUM (7–12)

This disease continues to be the most common female genital cancer, accounting for about half of all new cases (about 33,000

per year). It predominantly strikes postmenopausal women. Peak incidence is between ages 55 and 60 years. Only 5% of cases occur in women younger than the age of 40 years. Risk factors include obesity, nulliparity, late menopause, and prolonged unopposed estrogen stimulation of the uterus (either from replacement therapy or polycystic ovary syndrome; see Chapter 111). Uninterrupted estrogen stimulation in the absence of progestin risks induction of cystic and adenomatous hyperplasia, which are considered premalignant changes. Obesity may contribute by the ability of adipose tissue to convert circulating androstenedione into estrogen. Postmenopausal bleeding (defined as uterine bleeding occurring 6 months after the onset of menopause) may be the only early clue to the development of this tumor. Occasionally, a mass is felt on routine pelvic examination.

Principles of Management

Diagnosis

Suspicion of endometrial cancer usually warrants gynecologic referral. When there is confusion about whether a pelvic mass is ovarian or uterine, ordering a *pelvic ultrasound* examination can help to make the distinction noninvasively. Abnormal uterine bleeding in the postmenopausal woman is the most common presentation. *Transvaginal ultrasound* provides estimates of endometrial thickness, which is predictive of premalignant and malignant lesions. Hospital admission for cervical dilation and fractional curettage has largely been replaced by hysteroscopic examination as an outpatient. Hysteroscopy has proved to be very well tolerated and highly accurate in the diagnosis of endometrial cancer. The sensitivity and specificity do not appear to be significantly affected by menopausal status.

Staging and Prognosis

Prognosis is a function of the extent of disease and of histologic type. The gynecologist will attempt to determine whether the problem is confined to the uterine corpus or extends into the cervix and beyond. A careful *pelvic examination*, CT, and *chest x-ray* comprise the clinical staging process. Surgical staging is based on findings at the time of hysterectomy. Histologic grade, depth of myometrial penetration, and lymph node metastases influence prognosis in patients with early-stage disease. Overall survival is about 80% for those with stage I disease (confined to the corpus), 50% for stage II disease (involves the corpus and the cervix), 27% for stage III disease (spreads beyond the uterus but within the pelvis), and 9% for stage IV disease (invades the bladder or rectum, extends beyond the pelvis).

Treatment

Patients with the *premalignant* change of adenomatous hyperplasia are usually advised to undergo *hysterectomy* because of the risk of developing cancer. However, a second option is *progestin therapy* followed by repeat curettage. Patients with *stage I* or *stage II* disease are curable when treated with *hysterectomy/bilateral salpingo-oophorectomy plus irradiation*. The addition of radiation therapy is especially useful in stage II disease. It has been shown that adjuvant radiation is used less often in obese women than nonobese women. Nonetheless, obese women have lower cancer-specific mortality. The precise type of radiation therapy depends on histologic type and degree of spread. Intracavitary and external beam treatments are considered. The treatment of *stage III* disease is individualized, determined by findings on laparotomy. Patients with more advanced disease are inoperable and treated with radiation, progestins, or chemotherapy for palliation.

Patient Education

The critical aspect of patient education regarding endometrial cancer is the need for postmenopausal women to present promptly for evaluation of uterine bleeding.

OVARIAN CARCINOMA (13–25)

Ovarian cancer ranks fourth in cancer deaths among women and leads all gynecologic cancers. Incidence increases with age, beginning shortly after menarche and continuing through the eighth decade. Risk heightens among women in their 40s, especially among those who are nulliparous. Up to 10% of cases are *familial*, with many of these demonstrating germ-line mutations of the BRCA1 gene on chromosome 17 and to lesser degree mutations in the related BRCA2 gene. Women in families with a history of ovarian cancer have a lifetime risk of the malignancy that ranges from 20% to 40%. BRCA mutations are rare in the sporadic form of the disease, and the risk is minuscule in family members with sporadic disease compared with that of women with a positive family history. Although the risk of developing the disease is greatly increased in hereditary ovarian carcinoma, the prognosis appears to be much more favorable. Among patients with advanced disease (the most common stage at presentation), those with the hereditary form that includes mutation of BRCA1 survive nearly three times as long as those with sporadic disease, making mutation at BRCA1 the most important determinant of prognosis.

Screening

Screening remains inadequate, despite the advent of transvaginal ultrasound for detection of ovarian masses and monoclonal antibody techniques for detection of the tumor-associated antigen CA-125 (see Chapter 108).

Clinical Presentation

Clinical presentation is typically late because the disease is usually silent in its early stages. More than 80% of ovarian tumors derive from the epithelial surface of the ovary, disseminating silently by surface shedding or lymph node invasion. Initial symptoms when they do occur may be extremely vague, such as nonspecific gastrointestinal complaints that seem to persist in the absence of objective evidence for bowel disease. In later stages, the disease may be manifested by an abdominal or pelvic mass or development of ascites. Almost 70% of patients have already reached advanced-stage disease at the time of initial presentation.

Diagnosis

Because the disease is so silent or nonspecific in its presentation, a high index of suspicion is required. Family history should be checked carefully for ovarian cancer. Peri- and post-

menopausal women with unexplained pelvic or abdominal complaints should have a thorough *pelvic examination* with emphasis on careful palpation of the adnexae for a mass. Ability to palpate the ovary in a postmenopausal woman is suspicious of pathologic enlargement because the ovary normally involutes to less than 2 cm in size.

A *transvaginal ultrasound* can help to confirm the presence of an ovarian mass and is superior to transabdominal study. The finding of a simple cyst less than 4 cm is unlikely to represent cancer but warrants further observation, especially in postmenopausal women who do not have functioning ovarian cysts. In women of reproductive age, ovarian enlargement is common and usually due to functioning follicular or corpus luteum cysts. These typically regress within one to three menstrual cycles. Finding a complex cyst increases the risk of malignancy to about 10% and necessitates *surgical exploration*, as does discovery of a solid mass. Spread to the opposite ovary occurs in up to 15% of cases, so the finding of bilateral disease should increase rather than decrease suspicion. CT delineates pelvic and abdominal masses, liver and pulmonary metastasis, and retroperitoneal node involvement. It can be used to assess the ovary when pelvic ultrasound study is obscured by bowel gas.

As just noted, suspicious cases require surgical exploration. Laparoscopy is not a substitute because laparoscopically guided needle aspiration or biopsy risks spilling malignant cells into the peritoneum and washings are of insufficient sensitivity.

Use of the tumor marker CA-125 to achieve earlier detection of ovarian cancer has proven disappointing, perhaps because only 50% of women with clinically detectable disease have elevated levels of the marker. In addition, many women with positive studies prove to already have advanced disease because the frequency of marker elevation increases with tumor stage and bulk. Nonetheless, a markedly elevated CA-125 in a patient with a suspicious adnexal mass only increases the importance of proceeding with surgical exploration. A negative study does not obviate the need to refer for consideration of exploration. Combining CA-125 with transvaginal ultrasound appears to have little effect on survival when used as a screening technique in the general population. Its efficacy in persons with hereditary disease may be better, but the effect on survival is unknown (see Chapter 108).

Principles of Management

Prophylaxis

Because ovarian carcinoma is hard to detect in its early stages, much attention has been directed toward prophylactic approaches to disease. The prime candidates for consideration of prophylaxis are women at very high risk (i.e., those with a family history of hereditary disease and mutation of the BRCA genes). Options include *regular screening* by CA-125 and ultrasound (see Chapter 109), *prophylactic oophorectomy*, and *oral contraceptive therapy*. Because data on efficacy and relative benefit are sparse (no randomized trials), the options need to be reviewed with each woman at high risk to help her reach a personally acceptable decision.

Prophylactic Oophorectomy. Prophylactic oophorectomy can be accomplished laparoscopically as an ambulatory surgical procedure with minimal adverse effects. It is a reasonable consideration for women with a family history of hereditary disease and BRCA mutations who have completed childbearing.

Such persons have a 20% to 40% chance of getting the disease and might be willing to undergo surgery. However, there is still a small risk (1% to 2%) of the tumor arising from a primary peritoneal site in high-risk persons with hereditary disease. Hormone replacement therapy would usually be prescribed after surgery to obviate the consequences of a surgical menopause; however, such therapy increases the relative risk of breast cancer by about 20%—a concern in this population already at increased risk for breast cancer by virtue of the BRCA1 mutation.

Oral Contraceptive Therapy. Epidemiologic observations demonstrate that the risk of ovarian cancer in unselected populations of women is reduced by approximately 50% when there is a history of long-term oral contraceptive use. A retrospective analysis of women with the BRCA mutations and a positive family history shows a similar reduction in risk with 6 or more years of oral contraceptive use. However, women with BRCA mutations are also at increased risk of breast cancer, and estrogen therapy modestly increases the relative risk of breast cancer in unselected populations. There are no data on breast cancer risk when oral contraceptive therapy is used as prophylaxis for hereditary ovarian cancer. Many women with known hereditary predisposition may well be inclined to opt for the risk-reduction benefits afforded by oral contraceptive use during their childbearing years, after which prophylactic oophorectomy may become an acceptable strategy for some women. Those opting for estrogen therapy require close monitoring and regular mammographic screening for breast cancer.

Staging and Monitoring

Staging is performed predominantly by surgical exploration. Precise staging necessitates a meticulous *laparotomy* to assess the diaphragmatic surface and the omentum and other intraabdominal sites to which spread is common. Disease limited to the ovaries is considered stage I; if confined to the pelvis, it is considered stage II. Stage III designates involvement of regional nodes or disseminated peritoneal seeding with spread to the upper abdomen. Stage IV signifies distant or visceral metastasis. Ascites and bulky peritoneal tumor are frequent manifestations of advanced-stage disease. About 75% of patients present with stage III or IV disease. In the near future, staging is likely to include genetic testing for BRCA1 status because of its important contribution to prognosis. BRCA1 status could become extremely important if it is found to predict responses to treatment modalities.

The disease most commonly recurs within the abdominal cavity. Monitoring techniques include *CA-125 levels, laparoscopic examination, ultrasonography,* and *second-look surgery.* Miliary implants on the serosal surface may go undetected by imaging studies. Elevations in CA-125 are associated with residual tumor at the time of second-look surgery.

Treatment Modalities

Although the tumor is responsive to cancer treatment measures, its bulk and spread limit the results. In advanced stages of the disease, prognosis correlates with amount of residual disease after initial surgery. Those with less than 2 cm of residual disease do better than those with greater amounts of tumor remaining. Consequently, treatment often begins with *debulking* or tumor removal. *Omentectomy* and *total abdominal hysterectomy* and *bilateral salpingo-oophorectomy* are performed, in addition to the reduction of tumor masses throughout the abdominal cavity. This is believed to lessen the host-tumor burden and increase the effectiveness of ancillary or adjunctive therapeutic modalities, such as radiation or chemotherapy.

A major advance in *chemotherapy* has been achieved with the *combination regimen of cisplatin and paclitaxel.* Complete clinical response has been achieved in more than 70% of persons with advanced stage disease (stage III or IV with residual tumor after surgery). Median survival in responding patients has increased to 38 months, a marked improvement from the 12 to 24 months achieved with older regimens. In patients appearing to respond to chemotherapy, a *second-look operation* is performed to remove residual disease, check response, and, at times, place intraperitoneal catheters for *intraperitoneal infusion* therapy with cisplatin. The regression of disease, confirmed by second-look operations, suggests that multidrug therapies should be the standard approach to ovarian cancer.

Recent trials indicate that compared with the current standard of intravenous paclitaxel plus cisplatin, intravenous paclitaxel plus intraperitoneal cisplatin and paclitaxel improves survival in women with stage III cancer who have had optimal debulking.

Radiation therapy to the pelvis or to the abdomen (for patients with disease that extends beyond the pelvis) has been advocated as a routine adjunct to surgery in patients with advanced-stage disease, although effect on survival appears to be minimal. The rationale for abdominal and pelvic irradiation is based on the fact that ovarian tumors frequently cause recurrent ascites and bowel obstruction, leading to progressive inanition.

Survival

As noted, median survival has increased dramatically. Previously more than two thirds of patients died within 1 year. Now more than two thirds of women who present with advanced disease can expect a complete clinical response to combination chemotherapy and a median survival of 38 months. Prognosis correlates with amount of residual tumor after initial surgery, stage of disease, tumor grade, age, histologic type, and BRCA1 gene status. Those with stage I or II disease, less than 2 cm of residual disease, grade I tumor, and mucinous histology have the best chance of achieving complete remission and long-term survival from postoperative therapy. Relatively young age at time of diagnosis and mutation of the BRCA1 gene are among the most powerful determinants of favorable prognosis. Median survival of those who have a mutation of BRCA1 is more than 6 years.

Patient Education

Patients with ovarian cancer have a long and difficult clinical course. Mortality rates are high, and tumor bulk leads to considerable morbidity. Women with this disease and their families need all the support, interest, and comprehensive care that one can muster (see Chapter 87). With the advent of improved chemotherapy regimens, some hope for prolongation of survival can now be offered to those with advanced disease. Careful counseling, perhaps in conjunction with genetic testing for BRCA1 status, is essential for women with a family history of ovarian carcinoma.

CARCINOMA OF THE VULVA (26)

As a disease of a readily visible area, carcinoma of the vulva lends itself to early detection and treatment. Associations between the disease and low socioeconomic class and infection with herpes simplex virus and human papillomavirus have been observed. *Vulvar intraepithelial neoplasia* (VIN) is the presumed precursor and has been associated with *lichen sclerosis*. The median age for initial presentation of VIN is 44 years; for invasive disease it is 61 years, suggesting a slowly progressive course. Presentations include a mass or growth, vulvar pruritus, and bleeding. About 20% of cases are asymptomatic. Lesions may be flat and raised or verrucal. Coloration ranges from white (leukoplakia) to brown (hyperpigmentation) to red. The term *Bowen's disease* refers to the hyperpigmented variety, and *Paget's disease* refers to the leukoplakial form. The best means of early diagnosis is a high index of suspicion. Surgical excision is the treatment of choice. More-conservative approaches are now being used to decrease short- and long-term morbidity without sacrificing chance for cure. Cure rates in excess of 90% are achievable for localized disease less than 2 cm in greatest dimension. Radiation therapy is used for nonresectable disease.

CARCINOMA OF THE VAGINA (27,28)

This is a relatively rare disease. Cancer found in the vagina is more likely to represent spread of disease from the cervix. Primary vaginal carcinomas are mostly squamous cell lesions, although those related to diethylstilbestrol exposure are of the clear cell variety. Prior irradiation may be a predisposing factor. Most lesions appear on the posterior wall and in the upper one third of the vaginal vault. The tumor spreads directly and by lymphatic channels. It may present as an ulcerated lesion or as an exophytic mass extending into the vaginal vault. Preinvasive disease is asymptomatic. Invasive disease may present as postmenopausal or postcoital bleeding. Careful inspection of the posterior and distal aspects of the vagina is important in locating the lesion. Diagnosis is made by biopsy. Carcinoma *in situ* can be treated with local excision. Laser techniques are popular. Invasive disease is treated with radiation.

A.G.M.

Annotated Bibliography

1. Schiffman M, Castle PE, Jeronimo J, et al. Human papillomavirus and cervical cancer. Lancet 2007;370:890. (*If applied wisely, human papillomavirus-related technology can minimize the incidence of cervical cancer and the morbidity and mortality it causes, even in low-resource settings.*)
2. Lee YN, Wang KL, Lin MH, et al. Radical hysterectomy with pelvic lymph node dissection for treatment of cervical cancer. Gynecol Oncol 1989;32:135. (*Excellent results for the treatment of stages IB and IIA.*)
3. Green J Kirwan TJ, Tierney J, et al. Concomitant chemotherapy and radiation therapy for cancer of the uterine cervix. Cochrane Database Syst Rev 2005 Jul 20;(3):CD002225. (*This approach improves overall and progression-free survival.*)
4. Lau SL, Franco EL. Management of low-grade surgical lesions in young women. Can Med Assoc J 2007;173:771. (*Cogent recommendations for the young woman <24 years of age depending on whether she has been sexually active for more or less than 3 years.*)
5. Kyrgiou M, Koliopoulos G, Martin-Hirsch P, et al. Obstetric outcomes after conservative treatment for intraepithelial or early invasive cervical lesions: systematic review and meta-analysis. Lancet 2006;367:489. (*Cold knife conization, large loop excision of the transformation zone, and laser conization all increased the risk of preterm delivery, low birthweight, and caesarian section to a similar degree.*)
6. Wright TC Jr, Massad LS, Dunton CJ, et al. 2006 consensus guidelines for the management of women with cervical intraepithelial neoplasia or adenocarcinoma *in situ*. Am J Obstet Gynecol 2007;197:340. (*Management recommendations for women with biopsy-confirmed adenocarcinoma in situ are included.*)
7. Clark TJ, Voit D, Gupta JK, et al. Accuracy of hysteroscopy in the diagnosis of endometrial cancer and hyperplasia. JAMA 2002;288:1610. (*A positive likelihood ratio of 60 increases the probability of cancer from 4% to 72%; a negative likelihood ratio of 0.15 reduces the risk from 4% to 0.6%.*)
8. Creutzberg CL, van Putten WL, Koper PC, et al. Surgery and postoperative radiotherapy versus surgery alone for patients with stage-1 endometrial carcinoma: multicentre randomised trial. PORTEC Study Group. Post Operative Radiation Therapy in Endometrial Carcinoma. Lancet 2000;355:1404. (*This approach seems to reduce the risk of pelvic recurrence.*)
9. Martra F, Kunos C, Gibbons H, et al. Adjuvant treatment and survival in obese women with endometrial cancer. Am J Obstet Gynecol 2008;198:89. (*No difference was found between obese and nonobese women in lymphadenectomy; obese women were less likely to have had external beam radiation therapy but had better survival.*)
10. Gusberg SB. The changing nature of endometrial cancer. N Engl J Med 1980;302:729. (*Examines the increased incidence, clinical course, and treatment.*)
11. Martin-Hirsch PL, Jarvis G, Kitchener H, et al. Progestagens for endometrial cancer (Cochrane review). In: The Cochrane library, Issue 3. Oxford: Update Software, 2004. (*Current evidence does not support the use of adjuvant progestogen therapy in the primary treatment of endometrial cancer.*)
12. Suh-Burgmann EJ, Goodman A. Surveillance for endometrial cancer in women receiving tamoxifen. Ann Intern Med 1999;131:127. (*Discussion includes the issue of screening in the general population as well.*)
13. Aslam N, Banerjee S, Carr JV, et al. Prospective evaluation of logistic regression models for the diagnosis of ovarian cancer. Obstet Gynecol 2000;96:75. (*Specificity was 91% and sensitivity was 73% for the best model using noninvasive methods.*)
14. Goff BA, Mandel LS, Melancon CH, et al. Frequency of symptoms of ovarian cancer in women presenting to primary care clinics. JAMA 2004;291:2705. (*Documents more symptoms among those who eventually had ovarian cancer diagnosed compared with those seeking care; e.g., 70% vs. 38% for bloating.*)
15. Mangioni C, Bolis G, Pecorelli S, et al. Randomized trial in advanced ovarian cancer comparing cisplatin and carboplatin. J Natl Cancer Inst 1989;81:1464. (*Establishes the role of platinum agents in the treatment of this disease.*)
16. McGuire WP, Hoskins WJ, Brady MF, et al. Cyclophosphamide and cisplatin compared with paclitaxel and cisplatin in patients with stage III and stage IV ovarian cancer. N Engl J Med 1996;334:1. (*A randomized, prospective trial establishing that the combination of paclitaxel and cisplatin is the treatment of choice, producing significant improvements in progression-free survival and overall survival.*)
17. Narod SA, Risch H, Moslehi R, et al. Oral contraceptives and the risk of hereditary ovarian cancer. N Engl J Med 1998;339:424. (*A retrospective case–control study showing a 50% to 60% reduction in risk associated with long-term oral contraceptive therapy.*)
18. Omura GA, Brady MF, Homesley HD, et al. Long-term follow-up and prognostic factor analysis in advanced ovarian carcinoma. J Clin Oncol 1991;9:1138. (*Tumor bulk, stage, and histology were among the key determinants.*)
19. Oriel KA, Hartenbach EM, Remington PL, et al. Trends in United States ovarian cancer mortality, 1979–1995. Obstet Gynecol 1999;93:30. (*Mortality rates have changed little overall but are increasing among older women and decreasing among younger women.*)
20. Rodriguez MH, Platt LD, Medearis AL, et al. The use of transvaginal sonography for evaluation of postmenopausal ovarian size and morphology. Am J Obstet Gynecol 1988;159:810. (*Documents its utility and enhanced sensitivity for disease detection.*)
21. Rubin SC, Benjamin I, Behbakht K, et al. Clinical and pathological features of ovarian cancer in women with germ-line mutations of BRCA1. N Engl J Med 1996;335:1413. (*A retrospective study, but the first evidence that mutation of the BRCA1 gene is strongly associated with a more favorable clinical course.*)
22. Rubin SC, Hoskins WJ, Hakes TB, et al. Serum CA 125 levels in surgical findings in patients undergoing secondary operations for epithelial ovarian cancer. Am J Obstet Gynecol 1989;160:677. (*The level correlates with the amount of tumor found.*)
23. Rustin GJ, Jennings JN, Nelstrob AE, et al. Use of CA 125 to predict survival of patients with ovarian cancer. J Clin Oncol 1989;7:1667. (*Those with high levels had a worse prognosis.*)
24. Armstrong DK, Bundy B, Wenzel L, et al. Intraperitoneal cisplatin and paclitaxel in ovarian cancer. N Engl J Med 2006;354:34. (*Improved survival.*)
25. Whittemore AS, Haris R, Itnyre J, et al. Characteristics relating to ovarian cancer risk: collaborative analysis of 12 US case–control studies.

Am J Epidemiol 1992;136:1184. (*A meta-analysis demonstrating a 50% reduction in the risk of ovarian cancer associated with oral contraceptive use in a general population.*)

26. Seters M Kate FJW, Beurden M, et al. In the absence of invasive carcinoma, vulvar intraepithelial neoplasia associated with lichen sclerosis is mainly undifferentiated type: new insights in histology and aetiology. J Clin Pathol 2007;60:504. (*Good discussion of etiology and pathology.*)

27. Daling JR, Madeleine MM, Schwartz SM, et al. A population-based study of squamous cell vaginal cancer: HPV and cofactors. Gynecol Oncol 2002;84:263. (*Provides estimates of incidence and risk factors.*)

28. Melnick S, Cole P, Anderson D, et al. Rates and risks of diethylstilbestrol-related clear-cell adenocarcinoma of the vagina and cervix. An update. N Engl J Med 1987;316:514. (*The risk among women exposed to diethylstilbestrol in utero is 1 in 1,000.*)

SECTION 9 ■ GENITOURINARY PROBLEMS

CHAPTER 124 ■ SCREENING FOR SYPHILIS

The prevalence of syphilis in the United States began to decline with the introduction of penicillin therapy in the 1940s, falling to about 7,000 cases in 1956. Since then, reported cases of syphilis have increased. In the 1970s, much of the increase was a consequence of infection in men who have sex with men (MSM). The AIDS epidemic produced changes in sexual behavior that have reduced the incidence of syphilis in MSM; however, syphilis has increased dramatically in African Americans, Hispanics, and inner-city residents. This trend peaked in 1990, when more than 50,000 cases of primary and secondary syphilis were reported, representing a 9% increase in just 1 year. Since then, the reported cases of syphilis declined to a low in 2000 but began steadily to increase again through 2006, once again fueled by cases among MSM and provoking concern that salutary changes in sexual behavior in response to the AIDS epidemic may be reversing.

If a patient is not identified and treated during the primary or secondary stages of the disease, the infection becomes latent and is identifiable only by means of laboratory tests until late, often irreversible, clinical manifestations appear. The prevention of destructive cardiovascular and neurologic lesions by means of appropriate screening for latent syphilis is an important task for the primary physician. Because false-positive results are common and are potentially traumatic for the patient, it is critical that the sensitivity and specificity of the various serologic tests be understood.

EPIDEMIOLOGY AND RISK FACTORS (1–5)

With the exception of infection *in utero* or, rarely, by means of blood transfusion, syphilis is transmitted exclusively by *direct sexual contact* with infectious lesions. It follows that risk increases with sexual activity. Because syphilis is readily treated with antibiotics, it is less common in populations with access to medical care. The reported incidence of syphilis in nonwhites in the United States is much higher than in whites. Rates are highest in urban areas. It must be remembered, however, when incidence rates in different populations are compared, that case reporting has been shown to be more complete in public clinics than among private practitioners.

The age-specific incidence rates parallel those of gonorrhea, with the peak incidence for both diseases occurring between ages 20 and 25 years. A diagnosis of gonorrhea, nongonorrheal urethritis, HIV infection, or another sexually transmitted disease should be considered a risk factor for syphilis. Drug abuse is an important risk factor. MSM are also at high risk. Coinfection with HIV is common in this population.

The importance of an accurate sexual history in determining the risk for syphilis is obvious. Patients with early syphilis report an average of three recent sexual contacts. The probability that syphilis will develop in a known contact following a single exposure is approximately 30%.

NATURAL HISTORY OF SYPHILIS AND EFFECTIVENESS OF THERAPY (5–9)

Treponema pallidum enters the bloodstream within a few hours after inoculation through intact mucous membranes or abraded skin. A primary lesion occurs at the site of the inoculation between 10 and 90 days after contact. The incubation period depends on the size of the inoculum but is usually less than 3 weeks. The painless chancre usually resolves within 4 to 6 weeks, ending the *primary stage*. The *secondary stage* is usually heralded by a maculopapular rash that appears approximately 6 weeks after the primary lesion has healed. When the rash subsides, after 2 to 6 weeks, untreated syphilis enters the *latent stage* (arbitrarily divided into *early latent* for the first year and *late latent* thereafter). If untreated, patients with secondary syphilis may relapse clinically during early latency.

Because anorectal or vaginal chancres are not likely to be brought to medical attention, primary syphilis is often not diagnosed among MSM or among women. Whereas more than 40% of syphilis cases are detected in the primary stage among male heterosexuals, only 23% and 11%, respectively, are detected in the primary stage among MSM and among females.

Natural history studies from Oslo, Norway, and Tuskegee, Alabama, indicate that clinically manifest tertiary disease develops in approximately one third of persons with untreated syphilis, and that evidence of cardiovascular syphilis can be found in more than one half at autopsy. In the retrospective

Oslo study, 10% of patients had clinically evident cardiovascular syphilis, 7% had neurosyphilis, and 16% had gummatous disease. The incidence of cardiovascular syphilis was higher and that of neurosyphilis was lower in the prospective Tuskegee study.

Factors that influence the progression to clinical tertiary disease are incompletely understood. Congenital syphilis or disease contracted before age 15 years does not predispose to cardiovascular tertiary disease. In general, late complications seem more likely to occur among untreated men than among untreated women.

The antibiotic regimens recommended in Chapter 141 are highly effective in eradicating early syphilis. If the response to therapy is appropriately monitored by following the quantitative Venereal Disease Research Laboratory (VDRL) test or rapid plasma reagin (RPR) titer, the risk for late complications is virtually eliminated. Antibiotic treatment of late syphilis has less predictable results. Improvement among patients with general paresis has been reported in 40% to 80% of cases. Not surprisingly, structural cardiovascular changes caused by syphilis are not reversed by antibiotic treatment.

SCREENING AND DIAGNOSTIC TESTS (5,10–12)

Two groups of serologic tests can be used to diagnose syphilis: nontreponemal tests and treponemal tests.

Nontreponemal Tests

Nontreponemal tests, first introduced by Wasserman in 1906, use *cardiolipin* antigens extracted from mammalian tissues. These tests depend on cross-reactivity with antibodies against *T. pallidum*. The *RPR test*, *VDRL test*, and *automated reagin test* are among the most widely used. Their advantages include low cost, simplicity, and automated processing for mass screening. Many of the results can be quantified to allow serologic monitoring of response to therapy.

Nontreponemal tests are well suited for *screening* because they are highly sensitive. Virtually all patients with secondary syphilis are seropositive. Most with primary disease become seropositive within 1 week of the appearance of symptoms, but in a minority, detectable antibodies fail to develop in early infection. Patients with concomitant HIV and *T. pallidum* infection usually have positive findings on serologic testing for syphilis (titers are often high). Even without treatment, 25% of patients with syphilis become seronegative in late latent disease.

A disadvantage of nontreponemal tests is that their specificity is only about 70%. *Acute false-positive reactions*, which spontaneously revert to negative within 6 months, may follow many bacterial and viral infections. *Chronic false-positive reactions* occur in patients with elevated serum globulins. Such reactions are particularly common in intravenous-drug abusers (about 25%), patients with systemic lupus (15%), and healthy elderly persons (10%). Chronic false-positive tests also occur in patients with chronic liver disease, other connective tissue diseases, myeloma, and other advanced malignancies.

Treponemal Tests

All patients with positive nontreponemal test results should be retested with specific treponemal antigens. Although these tests are more sensitive and specific than the nontreponemal tests, they are better suited for diagnostic confirmation than for screening. The *microhemagglutination–T. pallidum test* (MHATP) is now the most widely used. Others include the *fluorescent treponemal antibody-absorbed test*, the *hemagglutination treponemal test for syphilis*, and the now rarely performed *T. pallidum immobilization test*.

In general, the results of treponemal tests become positive earlier than do the results of nontreponemal tests, and they tend to remain positive throughout life. However, it has been noted that in about 13% of patients receiving prompt treatment for primary syphilis, MHATP test results become negative within 3 years of therapy.

CONCLUSIONS AND RECOMMENDATIONS

- After decades of decline, syphilis has become more common, especially among intravenous-drug abusers, the urban poor, and HIV-infected persons.
- Screening for latent disease is simple, and the late manifestations of syphilis are entirely preventable if treatment is instituted early.
- Many patients have been screened routinely at the time of marriage, during prenatal care, before giving blood, or on hospital admission. Special indications for screening include exposure to or infection with other sexually transmitted diseases, pregnancy, intravenous-drug abuse, and HIV infection.
- All patients with syphilis should be counseled about HIV infection and offered HIV testing.
- Nontreponemal tests such as the RPR or the VDRL test are appropriate for screening because of their sensitivity and simplicity. MHATP or other treponemal tests should be reserved for confirming a diagnosis suspected on the basis of clinical presentation or positive nontreponemal test results.

A.G.M.

Annotated Bibliography

1. Centers for Disease Control and Prevention. Sexually transmitted disease surveillance 2001 supplement: syphilis surveillance report. Atlanta, GA: U.S. Department of Health and Human Services, 2003. (*Incidence reached a low in 2000, followed by local increases in urban areas among homosexual men with high rates of HIV coinfection.*)
2. Centers for Disease Control and Prevention. Primary, secondary syphilis—United States, 1981–1990. JAMA 1991;265:2940. (*Presents details of the changing epidemiology of the disease.*)
3. Hutchinson CM, Hook EW. Syphilis in adults. Med Clin North Am 1990;74:1389. (*Excellent review of syphilis in adults, including serologies and treatment.*)
4. Primary and secondary syphilis among men who have sex with men—New York City, 2001. MMWR Morb Mortal Wkly Rep 2002;51:853. (*Documents the high rates of coinfection with HIV.*)
5. U.S. Preventive Services Task Force. Screening for syphilis infection: recommendation statement. Ann Family Med 2004;2:362. (*Evidence review led to*

no change in the recommendation to screen pregnant women and high-risk people.)

6. Augenbraun MH. Treatment of syphilis 2001: nonpregnant adults. Clin Infect Dis 2002;35(Suppl 2):S187. (*Evidence-based recommendations.*)
7. Clark EG, Danbold N. The Oslo study of the natural course of untreated syphilis. Med Clin North Am 1964;48:613. (*A restudy of case material of untreated syphilis collected from 1891 to 1910.*)
8. Rockwell DH, Yobs AR, Moore Jr MB. The Tuskegee study of untreated syphilis. Arch Intern Med 1964;114:792. (*A prospective 30-year study of untreated syphilis in 412 male blacks; notable for the ethical questions raised in addition to the natural history of syphilis.*)
9. Wendel GD Jr, Sheffield JS, Hollier LM, et al. Treatment of syphilis in pregnancy and prevention of congenital syphilis. Clin Infect Dis 2002;35
(Suppl 2):S200. (*Evidence-based recommendations; see* http://www.ahrq.gov/clinic/gcpspu.htm *for periodic updates and evidence summary.*)
10. Andrus JK, Fleming DW, Harger DR, et al. Partner notification: can it control syphilis? Ann Intern Med 1990;112:539. (*The answer is no because of too many anonymous sexual contacts.*)
11. Hart G. Syphilis tests in diagnostic and therapeutic decision making. Ann Intern Med 1986;104:368. (*An evaluation of available tests, with consideration of their sensitivity and specificity.*)
12. Waring GW. False-positive tests for syphilis revisited. The intersection of Bayes' theorem and Wassermann's test. JAMA 1980;243:2321. (*A reminder that as the incidence of a disease declines, so does the specificity of its screening test; the overall sensitivity of a positive result on a serologic test for syphilis was calculated to be 85%.*)

CHAPTER 125 ■ SCREENING FOR CHLAMYDIAL INFECTION

BENJAMIN DAVIS

Chlamydia trachomatis is responsible for close to 4 million cases of genitourinary tract infection each year in the United States. Transmission is by sexual contact. Because symptoms may be absent, mild, or nonspecific, treatment is often delayed or missed. Undetected or untreated infection can lead to pelvic inflammatory disease, with such consequences as tubal scarring, infertility, and ectopic pregnancy. More than 50,000 women are left sterile each year. The estimated direct and indirect costs of such adverse outcomes is in excess of $2.4 billion per year. Screening for chlamydial infection should be a consideration in the provision of routine primary care to women. Key issues are who should be screened and with what method(s).

EPIDEMIOLOGY AND RISK FACTORS (1–9)

Chlamydial infection is a sexually transmitted disease (STD) present in epidemic proportions. In 2006, 1,030,911 cases of *Chlamydia* infection were reported to the Centers for Disease Control and Prevention (CDC), a 5.6% increase over the number reported in 2005 and the largest number of cases reported to the CDC *for any condition*. The prevalence of *Chlamydia* infection varies by clinical setting. Among women seen in primary care practice, the prevalence is 3% to 5%. In family planning clinics, the prevalence increases to 9%; in STD clinics, the rate rises to 17% to 28%. Prevalence is very high among adolescents (18%), and one study of college campus women found 50% to be infected. Among female military recruits, the prevalence of chlamydial infection was 9%; the rate for the youngest recruits, 17 years of age, was 12%. Between 1987 and 1995, the reported rates of chlamydial infection increased by 281%. Although much of this rise is accounted for by increased screening, chlamydial infection is still very prevalent in the United States.

Women are at greater risk for contracting C. *trachomatis* infection than are men, and they also suffer more serious consequences. The risk in a single act of unprotected intercourse with an infected partner is 40% for women and 20% for men. The increased risk for women reflects the fact that they receive an ejaculate of infected secretions from their partner's genital tract. Men do not receive such a large inoculum unless they have an intact foreskin, which can serve as a reservoir for the woman's infected cervical secretions.

Among women with documented urogenital infection, the cervix is infected in 75% and the urethra in 50%. Endometritis can be demonstrated in about 33%; it is often clinically silent, but infection may spread to the fallopian tubes. In studies of salpingitis, *Chlamydia* is recovered from the tubes in up to 50% of subjects. Vaginal infection is rare.

Chlamydiae may also colonize the pharynx and rectum in women engaging in oral and anal sex, respectively. Among those attending an STD clinic, the rate for oral recovery of organisms was 3.2%; the rectal colonization rate was 5.2%. Rectal involvement has been noted even in the absence of rectal intercourse.

In men, the urethra is the predominant site of infection, with more than 82% having a symptomatic or visible urethral discharge. In 1% to 2% of infected men, the infection ascends to the epididymis to produce acute scrotal pain and discomfort. Men who have sex with men have higher rates of oral and anal recovery of organisms. Lymphogranuloma strains may be present.

Age is a powerful predictor of infection. Women *younger than 21 years* are at the greatest risk. Other important risk factors include having had a *new partner* in the last 2 months, *more than one partner* in the last 6 months, or a *partner known to have other partners*. Nonetheless, even among women who are monogamous or who have been sexually inactive in the last 2 months, prevalence can be as high as 7% to 10%.

Other significant predictors of chlamydial infection identified by multivariate analysis include *African American race, low level of education, unprotected intercourse, mucopurulent cervical discharge*, and *induced mucosal bleeding* on swabbing of the cervix. Among patients with *gonococcal infection*, 30% to 50% have concurrent chlamydial disease. In a large surveillance study of urban residents younger than the age of 45 years, the rate for either infection was 15% in black women, 6.4% in black men, 2.8% in white men, and 1.3% in white women. The risk of *C. trachomatis* infection was highest in the 18- to 20-year-old group (8.0%), but *Neisseria gonorrhoeae* infection was unexpectedly high in the 31- to 35-year-old group (10.2%).

SCREENING (10–17)

Screening women at risk for the disease is essential because infection is so frequently asymptomatic despite being associated with extensive inflammation of the female genital tract. The rising rate of chlamydial infection in the last decade surely reflects, in part, wider acceptance and implementation of screening programs. However, when family planning clinics (where chlamydial screening is universal) are analyzed, the rate of chlamydial infection has actually *declined* from 9% to 3% in the last decade. This very likely reflects the effect that screening programs have had on the incidence of untreated disease and quite possibly a reduction in infertility caused by chlamydial infection. In fact, a randomized, controlled trial of screening of asymptomatic women enrolled in a health maintenance organization demonstrated a 50% reduction in subsequent pelvic inflammatory disease.

DIAGNOSIS (15,16,18–22)

Clinical Recognition

In women, clinical recognition can be difficult because most patients are asymptomatic or have only minor symptoms. Although vaginal discharge, bleeding, lower abdominal discomfort, and dysuria may accompany infection, these symptoms are nonspecific and require a detailed workup in their own right (see Chapters 111, 116, 117, and 133). The only features of the history that reliably suggest the problem are the risk factors previously mentioned.

In the absence of definitive symptoms, physical findings take on additional importance. *Mucopurulent discharge*, *cervical ectopy*, *edema* in the area of ectopy, and easily *induced mucosal bleeding* have proved predictive of *C. trachomatis* infection, as has the presence of more than 10 neutrophils per high-power field. *Uterine* or *adnexal tenderness* in a patient with a mucopurulent cervical discharge is suggestive of chlamydial pelvic inflammatory disease (see Chapters 116 and 117).

In men, nongonococcal *urethritis* is the most common presentation, with dysuria, penile discharge, and the presence of more than five neutrophils per high-power field (see Chapter 136). About one third of men with chlamydial urethritis have no symptoms or signs, although pyuria may be noted. A small number experience acute testicular pain from an ascending epididymitis (see Chapter 131).

Diagnostic Tests

Culture

Culture is the gold standard for identification. However, because chlamydiae are obligate intracellular organisms, cell culture techniques similar to those used for viruses are required to isolate and identify them. Such cultures are technically difficult

and expensive, take up to 1 week, and require refrigeration of the specimen and transport to the laboratory within 24 hours.

Modifications in traditional cell culture techniques have simplified isolation of the organism. Cell monolayers set up in microtiter plates are helpful in settings in which titers are likely to be high (e.g., STD clinics). Fluorescein-conjugated monoclonal antibodies are useful for identifying chlamydial inclusions in infected monolayers. Combining both advances provides a 14% increase in diagnostic yield and sensitivity, makes second-pass testing unnecessary, and shortens test time to 3 days.

Antigen Detection

Antigen detection techniques were developed to overcome the difficulties and limitations posed by culture. *Direct immunofluorescence* staining of smears, with the use of monoclonal antibodies, and *enzyme-linked immunosorbent assay* (ELISA) of antigen eluted from swabs are commercially available. When culture is used as the gold standard, the sensitivity of the direct immunofluorescent technique in women ranges from 77% in intermediate-prevalence populations to 90% in high-prevalence ones. Specificity is greater than 95% in both. The ELISA has a sensitivity of 85% to 89% and a specificity in excess of 95%. Cost-effectiveness studies indicate that screening for *Chlamydia* infection with antigen detection techniques becomes cost-effective when the pretest probability of disease exceeds 7%. Prescreening the urine for white blood cells can facilitate identifying asymptomatic men for testing.

Nucleic Acid Amplification Techniques

Nucleic acid amplification techniques (NAATs) represent a further advance in diagnosis and have made detection possible by sampling of urine in addition to the traditional urethral or cervical swab. When a *polymerase chain reaction* or *ligase chain reaction* is used to detect minute quantities of chlamydial DNA, sensitivity rises into the 90% range and specificity to greater than 95%. The convenience of an accurate *urine test* for *Chlamydia* infection makes the polymerase chain reaction and ligase chain reaction ideal for screening high-risk, asymptomatic patients. A *Chlamydia Rapid Test* described in 2007 is a point-of-care immunoassay-based test that detects chlamydial lipopolysaccharide and has been evaluated using self-collected vaginal swab specimens, as well as clinician-collected specimens. Sensitivity and specificity have been estimated at 84% and 99%, respectively.

Screening Recommendations

For women at risk of chlamydial infection, with or without symptoms, a *C. trachomatis* NAAT such as ligase chain reaction performed on an endocervical swab offers higher sensitivity than that performed on a urine specimen. For men, an NAAT or urine test offers equivalent sensitivity to a urethral swab. Both tests have superior specificity, although positive predictive value depends on the prevalence of *Chlamydia* infection in the population screened.

EFFECTIVENESS OF TREATMENT (23,24)

Several effective treatment regimens are available for chlamydial urogenital tract infection (see Chapters 117, 135, and 141). For urethritis and cervicitis without evidence of pelvic inflammatory disease, the treatment of choice is a single 1-g oral dose of *azithromycin*. The cost is comparable to that of 1 week of *doxycycline* (100 mg twice daily) or *tetracycline* (500 mg four times daily), and ensured compliance is a major benefit. If the patient is pregnant or unable to take tetracycline or azithromycin, then 500 mg of *erythromycin* base four times daily for 7 days is recommended.

CONCLUSIONS AND RECOMMENDATIONS

- Screening for chlamydial genitourinary infection is definitely worthwhile, but universal screening is not recommended in most primary care practices because the prevalence of asymptomatic infection in this setting is likely to be below the threshold that makes universal screening cost-effective.
- In settings in which prevalence is very high (e.g., >10%), universal screening deserves consideration.
- Antigen testing becomes cost-effective among patients whose pretest risk is greater than 7%. Culturing becomes cost-effective among patients whose pretest risk is greater than 14%. DNA-based testing with polymerase chain reaction amplification lowers the prevalence threshold for cost-effective screening.
- A policy of selective screening is recommended based on a clinical estimate of the risk for chlamydial infection.
- Because the prevalence of chlamydial infection among sexually active girls and women *younger than the age of 24 years*

is high and because the risk for sterility resulting from subclinical infection is also very high, annual screening of such persons with or without symptoms has been recommended by the U.S. Preventive Services Task Force.

- The U.S. Preventive Services Task Force has recommended annual screening for women *older than the age 24* years if either of the major risk factors for chlamydial infection is present: *lack of barrier contraception* or *new or multiple partners in the preceding 3 months*.
- Those at high risk for *Chlamydia* infection should also be screened for gonorrhea (see Chapter 137) because they are at increased risk for other common STDs.
- All men presenting with a urethral discharge and all women with mucopurulent cervicitis should be screened for chlamydial infection.
- Partner notification and treatment, either by patient referral or provider referral, is a critical step in interrupting the cycle of reinfection by asymptomatic partners.
- Although antigen testing of a cervical or urethral swab is the least expensive screening method, DNA-based polymerase chain reaction technology is recommended as the testing method of choice, especially in settings of lower prevalence, because its sensitivity is superior and it allows testing of urine in addition to cervical specimens, which lowers the prevalence threshold at which screening is cost-effective.
- All young women coming for routine gynecologic care who do not desire pregnancy should be urged to insist on condom use during intercourse.

Annotated Bibliography

1. Datta SD, Sternberg M, Johnson JE, et al. Gonorrhea and chlamydia in the United States among persons 14 to 39 years of age, 1999 to 2002. Ann Intern Med 2007;147:89. (*The prevalence of Chlamydia infection was 2.2%; findings in subgroups support recommendations to screen sexually active females who are 25 years of age or younger, to retest infected females for Chlamydia infection, and to cotreat persons with gonorrhea for Chlamydia infection.*)
2. Meyers DS, Halvorson H, Luckhaupt S. Screening for chlamydial infection: an evidence update for the US Preventive Services Task Force. Ann Intern Med 2007;147:135. (*This update turned up little new evidence, confirming the basis for earlier recommendations.*)
3. US Preventive Services Task Force. Screening for chlamydial infection: US Preventive Services Task Force recommendation statement. Ann Intern Med 2007. (*Screen sexually active nonpregnant women who are 24 years of age or younger and older nonpregnant women at increased risk; the same recommendation is made for pregnant women, but with less firm evidence.*)
4. Centers for Disease Control and Prevention. *Chlamydia trachomatis* genital infections—United States, 1995. MMWR Morb Mortal Wkly Rep 1995;46:193. (*Presents epidemiologic data.*)
5. Centers for Disease Control and Prevention. Recommendations for the prevention and management of *Chlamydia trachomatis* infections, 1993. MMWR Morb Mortal Wkly Rep 1993;42(RR-12):1. (*Guidelines for screening and treating Chlamydia infection in men and women.*)
6. Chow JM, Yonekura ML, Richwald GA, et al. The association between *Chlamydia trachomatis* and ectopic pregnancy. JAMA 1990;263:3164. (*A case–control study, finding an odds ratio of 3.0 and a relative risk of 2.4; suggests that douching may increase risk.*)
7. Gaydos CA, Howell MR, Pare B, et al. *Chlamydia trachomatis* infections in female military recruits. N Engl J Med 1998;339:739. (*Presents population-based prevalence data on asymptomatic Chlamydia infection; offers a rationale for screening all women younger than age 25 years.*)
8. Howell MR, Quinn TC, Gaydos CA. Screening for *Chlamydia trachomatis* in asymptomatic women attending family planning clinics: a cost-effectiveness analysis of three strategies. Ann Intern Med 1998;128:277. (*Analysis of cohort data from two family planning clinics; finds that age-based screening provides the greatest cost savings, but that universal screening may be useful when the prevalence of infection is very high.*)
9. Turner CF, Rogers SM, Miller HG, et al. Untreated gonococcal and chlamydial infection in a probability sample of adults. JAMA 2002;287:726. (*Major surveillance study of sexually transmitted diseases in the general population;*

surprisingly high prevalences of chlamydial and gonococcal infection were found.*)
10. Aronson MD, Phillips RS. Screening young men for chlamydial infection. JAMA 1993;270:2097. (*An editorial review of the data on screening young men.*)
11. Centers for Disease Control and Prevention. Screening tests to detect *Chlamydia trachomatis* and *Neisseria gonorrhoeae* infections—2002. MMWR Morb Mortal Wkly Rep 2002;51(RR-15):1. (*Presents the Centers for Disease Control and Prevention recommendations.*)
12. Marrazzo JM, White CL, Krekeler B, et al. Community-based urine screening for *Chlamydia trachomatis* with a ligase chain reaction assay. Ann Intern Med 1997;127:796. (*Among adolescents, 9% of girls and 5% of boys were infected.*)
13. Mahilum-Tapay K, Laitila V, Wawrzyniak JJ, et al. New point of care *Chlamydia* Rapid Test—bridging the gap between diagnosis and treatment: performance evaluation study. BMJ 2007;335:1190. (*The sensitivity and the specificity were estimated to be 84% and 99%, respectively.*)
14. Phillips RS, Aronson MD, Taylor WC, et al. Should tests for *Chlamydia trachomatis* cervical infection be done during routine gynecologic visits? Ann Intern Med 1987;107:188. (*A cost-effectiveness study indicating that if prevalence is >7%, antigen testing is worth performing.*)
15. Scholes D, Stergachis A, Heidrich FE, et al. Prevention of pelvic inflammatory disease by screening for cervical *Chlamydia* infection. N Engl J Med 1996;334:1362. (*Screening asymptomatic women for Chlamydia infection results in a 50% decline in subsequent pelvic inflammatory disease.*)
16. Sellor JW, Picard L, Gafni A, et al. Effectiveness and efficiency of selective vs. universal screening for chlamydial infection in sexually active young women. Arch Intern Med 1992;152:1837. (*Two selection rules were developed by regression analysis and tested; selective testing is preferred in low-prevalence settings.*)
17. Shafer MA, Schachter J, Moncada J, et al. Evaluation of urine-based screening strategies to detect *Chlamydia trachomatis* among sexually active asymptomatic young males. JAMA 1993;270:2065. (*Prescreening the urine for white blood cells followed by antibody testing of persons with urine positive for white cells was most cost-effective.*)
18. Brunham RC, Paavonen J, Sevens CE, et al. Mucopurulent cervicitis—the ignored counterpart in women of urethritis in men. N Engl J Med 1984;311:1. (*The presence of cervical mucopus and >10 polymorphonuclear leukocytes per high-power field is predictive of Chlamydia trachomatis infection.*)

19. Johnson BA, Poses RM, Fortner CA, et al. Derivation and validation of a clinical diagnostic model for chlamydial cervical infection in university women. JAMA 1990;264:3161. (*Identifies risk factors for chlamydial infection as a means of determining who should be screened.*)

20. Phillips RS, Hanff PA, Holmes MD, et al. *Chlamydia trachomatis* cervical infection in women seeking routine gynecologic care: criteria for selective testing. Am J Med 1989;86:515. (*Multivariate study; identifies low level of education, partner with other partners, and sex with other partners as predictors of infection and indications for screening.*)

21. Stamm WE. Diagnosis of *Chlamydia trachomatis* genitourinary infections. Ann Intern Med 1988;108:710. (*Excellent review, with very useful discussion of clinical findings, culture, and antigen methods; 93 references.*)

22. Vogels WHM, van Vooster-Vader PC, Schroder FP. *Chlamydia trachomatis* infection in a high-risk population: comparison of polymerase chain reaction and cell culture for diagnosis and follow-up. J Clin Microbiol 1993;31:1103. (*Presents the test characteristics of the new DNA-based methods.*)

23. Martin DH, Mrockowski TF, Dalu ZA, et al. Controlled trial of a single dose of azithromycin for the treatment of chlamydial urethritis and cervicitis. N Engl J Med 1992;327:921. (*The treatment was found to be as effective as standard therapy.*)

24. Workanski KA, Lampe MF, Wong KG, et al. Long-term eradication of *Chlamydia trachomatis* genital infection after antimicrobial therapy. JAMA 1993;270:2071. (*Found that treatment completely eradicates the organism.*)

CHAPTER 126 ■ SCREENING FOR PROSTATE CANCER

MICHAEL J. BARRY

Prostate cancer is a common cause of morbidity and mortality among older men in the United States. The lifetime probability of a man learning that he has prostate cancer in the "prostate-specific antigen (PSA) era" is now about 18%, but the probability of death from prostate cancer is approximately 3%. This ratio of cumulative incidence to mortality indicates that most patients in whom prostate cancer is diagnosed die of something else. In fact, the lifetime risk of being diagnosed with prostate cancer depends on the intensity of screening. In the recent Prostate Cancer Prevention Trial (PCPT), after 7 years of annual digital rectal exams (DREs) and PSA tests followed by a set of biopsies, regardless of DRE and PSA results, about 25% of average-risk older men were diagnosed with prostate cancer.

Patients and clinicians face a great deal of uncertainty in making clinical decisions about the early detection and treatment of prostate cancer. These tumors are exceedingly common and have the potential to cause significant morbidity and mortality. They also have a variable, often indolent course and a higher prevalence in elderly men, whose health is often more limited by their age and other diseases. The clinician should be aware of the unpredictable natural history of the disease and the limitations of knowledge about the benefits of therapy when considering the use of screening tests for prostate cancer.

EPIDEMIOLOGY AND RISK FACTORS (1–3)

The incidence of prostate cancer increases with age. Age-specific prevalence rates derived from autopsy studies are about 15% for men in their sixth decade, 25% for those in their seventh decade, and 40% or higher for men older than 70 years. The incidence of prostate cancer rose dramatically in the United States with increasing use of the PSA test, and has now fallen to a new, higher plateau. Mortality from prostate cancer also increased with the introduction of PSA testing and is also now falling (Fig. 126.1). African Americans have a two- to three-fold higher incidence of prostate cancer. Having a brother or a father with prostate cancer increases the risk twofold. A diet high in fat (particularly red meat) may also be a risk factor, and there is some suggestion that selenium, low-dose vitamin E (at least among smokers), and tomato products (containing lycopenes) are protective. "Mega-dose" multiple vitamins (more than seven tablets a week) may increase risk. Obesity may be a risk factor, particularly for more aggressive forms of prostate cancer. Evidence linking prostate cancer with prior vasectomy has been equivocal. No strong evidence has linked prostatitis or benign prostatic hyperplasia (BPH) to the development of prostate cancer.

NATURAL HISTORY OF DISEASE AND EFFECTIVENESS OF THERAPY (4–8)

Clinical Presentation and Course

Early prostate cancers are asymptomatic; older men not infrequently have concurrent lower urinary tract symptoms caused by BPH, but there is no evidence that such symptoms increase the likelihood that a man is harboring prostate cancer. Early prostate cancers may be discovered through screening or diagnosed incidentally when men undergo prostatectomy for BPH. Advanced cancers may present with obstructive symptoms, bleeding, or bone pain due to metastases.

The prognosis of prostate cancer depends as much on the degree of histologic differentiation of the tumor as on the extent of the disease, at least before detectable metastases are evident. Histologically, prostate cancers are often heterogeneous.

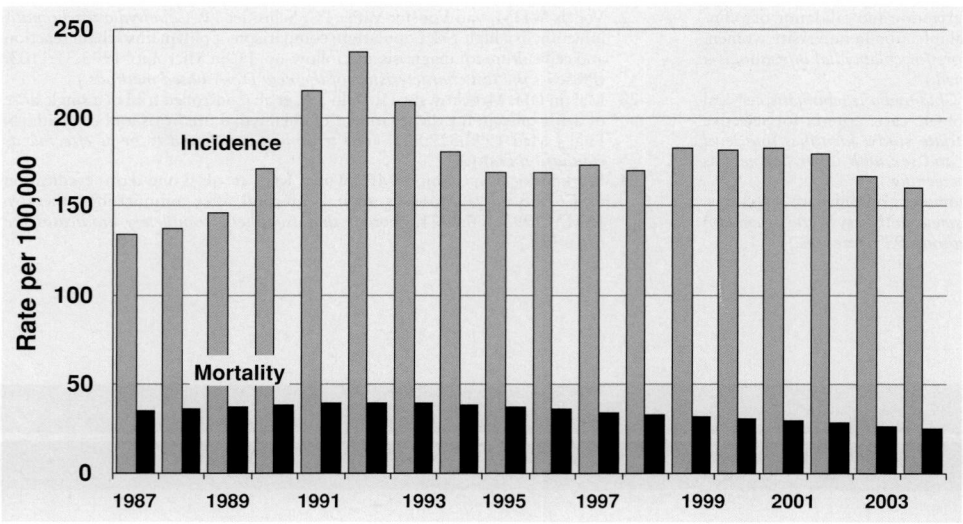

FIGURE 126.1. Incidence and mortality of prostate cancer in the United States. (National Cancer Institute. SEER Cancer Statistics Review, 1974–2004.)

Pathologists commonly assign a *Gleason score* of 1 to 5 to the most-common and next-most-common histologic patterns and add the two scores to obtain a Gleason sum ranging from 2 to 10. Cancers with Gleason sums of 2 to 4 are considered well differentiated, 5 to 7 moderately differentiated, and 8 to 10 poorly differentiated (although cancers with sums of 7 in fact behave in an intermediate fashion between moderate and poorly differentiated cancers). Most cancers discovered by screening are Gleason 6 to 7. In recent years, pathologic grading (but not the cancers themselves) has shifted so that few prostate cancers are now graded less than Gleason 6.

Clinically localized prostate cancers generally have doubling times measured in years. The prognosis of prostate cancer depends on tumor factors such as grade and patient factors such as age and comorbidity. Table 126.1 provides estimates of the 15-year probability of being alive, dying of other causes, or dying of prostate cancer for different combinations of these factors. These data were generated from men in whom cancer was diagnosed in the "pre-PSA era," with adjustment for lead time, "grade creep," and increasing life expectancy in the "PSA era."

Effectiveness of Therapy

The variability in the natural history of this disease complicates an assessment of therapeutic efficacy. Some have argued that early detection and aggressive treatment with radical

TABLE 126.1

ESTIMATES OF 15-YEAR OUTCOME PROBABILITIES FOR MEN DIAGNOSED WITH PROSTATE CANCER IN THE PROSTATE-SPECIFIC ANTIGEN ERA, BY AGE AND GLEASON SCORE

Age (yr)	15-Year Outcome	Gleason Score <7		Gleason Score 7		Gleason Score >7	
		Conservative Treatment	Curative Treatment	Conservative Treatment	Curative Treatment	Conservative Treatment	Curative Treatment
55–59	% Alive	84	84	52	64	15	41
	% Other death	16	16	17	18	13	19
	% PC death	0	0	31	18	72	40
60–64	% Alive	74	75	50	59	18	38
	% Other death	25	25	27	28	21	28
	% PC death	1	0	23	13	61	34
65–69	% Alive	61	61	45	51	23	35
	% Other death	38	38	40	41	35	42
	% PC death	1	1	15	8	42	23
70–74	% Alive	43	44	35	38	20	26
	% Other death	55	55	56	57	52	58
	% PC death	2	1	9	5	28	16

PC death, death attributed to prostate cancer.
Adapted from Parker C, Muston D, Melia J, et al. A model of the natural history of screen-detected prostate cancer, and the effect of radical treatment on overall survival. Br J Cancer 2006;94:1361, with permission.

prostatectomy or radiation therapy, either external beam radiotherapy or implantation of radioactive seeds (*interstitial radiotherapy* or *brachytherapy*), may improve survival, particularly for patients with at least a 10-year life expectancy in whom the tumor appears to be localized to the gland. However, practices have evolved in the absence of evidence for a mortality benefit from randomized clinical trials, and these treatments have side effects, including a relatively high risk of sexual dysfunction and urinary incontinence. A recent randomized trial of radical prostatectomy compared with watchful waiting was conducted among Scandinavian men younger than age 75 years with well- and moderately differentiated prostate cancer. Over 10 years, surgery resulted in a significant reduction in prostate cancer–specific mortality, from about 15% with watchful waiting to 10%, with a similar absolute decrease in overall mortality. However, it is important to recognize that men in the Scandinavian trial were generally diagnosed with a nodule or disease that was otherwise clinically evident. Another trial of radical prostatectomy among U.S. men, many of whom had their cancers detected with PSA screening, is in progress, as are trials of screening in both the United States and Europe. A trial in the United Kingdom has a treatment trial (surgery vs. radiotherapy vs. active monitoring) nested within a screening trial. In the meantime, models comparing treatment outcome using data from the pre-PSA era and taking into account factors such as lead time, "grade creep," and increasing life expectancy in the "PSA era" suggest an advantage for more aggressive treatment of Gleason 7 and particularly Gleason 8 to 10 cancers (Table 126.1).

SCREENING AND DIAGNOSTIC TESTS (9–21)

Digital Rectal Examination

Digital rectal examination for evidence of either prostate or rectal cancer is a time-honored screening maneuver, at least in the United States. Symmetric enlargement and firmness (the consistency of the tip of the nose) may be seen with BPH. Asymmetric areas of firmness or frank nodules are suggestive, and a stony, hard, asymmetric prostate is highly suggestive of malignancy. Fixation to adjacent tissue and a loss of the lateral prostate sulcus suggest local spread. Interobserver agreement regarding suspicious DRE findings is poor, even among urologists.

Test Characteristics

Test characteristics of the DRE are unknown, particularly relative to prostate biopsy as a gold standard. In the initial round of screening in the U.S. PLCO trial, 7.5% of men of age 55 to 74 years had a suspicious DRE, with an overall *positive predictive value* (see Chapter 2) for cancer of 34%. Seventeen percent of biopsies done for a DRE abnormality with a PSA less than 4 ng/mL were positive; as a result, 11% of cancers in PLCO were found by DRE alone. However, cancers diagnosed after an abnormal DRE are often found through serendipity by random biopsies distant from the palpable abnormality. About 30% of the cancers detected by DRE in modern screening studies are later found to have spread beyond the capsule of the gland. Several case–control studies have evaluated whether DRE is associated with reduced mortality from prostate cancer, with conflicting results.

Prostate-Specific Antigen

Prostate-specific antigen is a glycoprotein produced by both benign and malignant prostate epithelial tissue. Measurement of PSA can clearly find more cancers than DRE alone. Because a number of assays are commercially available, physicians should use the same assay in following serial PSAs. Elevations can be seen after cystoscopy, acute urinary retention, prostate trauma (such as a needle biopsy or prostatectomy), and with urinary tract or prostatic infection. DRE does not raise the PSA level; however, ejaculation may cause minor increases for a day or two. BPH can also produce modest PSA elevations, and separating BPH from early prostate cancer is a major clinical problem with PSA screening.

Test Characteristics

The true *sensitivity* and *specificity* of PSA have been unclear because historically only men with elevated results underwent biopsy. Gann and colleagues indirectly estimated the sensitivity of PSA to detect cancers ultimately destined to present clinically at 50% to 75%, with a specificity of about 90%; specificity deteriorates among older men or men with symptoms suggesting BPH. The predictive value of a PSA level greater than 4.0 ng/mL is about 30%, and is relatively insensitive to age because rising prevalence cancels the effect of decreasing specificity with age. The PCPT has shown that 15% of men with PSA levels less than 4.0 ng/mL have prostate cancer on biopsy, and 15% of these men have high-grade cancers. Figure 126.2 provides the probability of any histologic prostate cancer and of high-grade cancer for various PSA values less than 4.0 ng/mL. The sensitivity of PSA relative to biopsy is only about 20% for all cancers and 40% for Gleason 7 or higher cancers at this traditional cut-point. Documentation of the relatively low sensitivity of PSA has prompted some experts to recommend biopsy at lower PSA levels, whereas others have been concerned that a lower biopsy threshold will produce too many negative biopsies as well as the overdiagnosis of many clinically unimportant

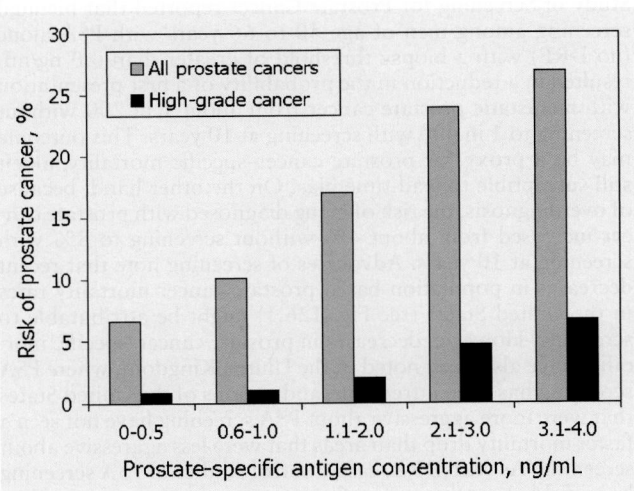

FIGURE 126.2. Probability of any histologic prostate cancer and high grade prostate cancer at biopsy for various PSA levels. (Adapted from Thompson IM, Pauler DK, Goodman PJ, et al. Prevalence of prostate cancer among men with a prostate-specific antigen level < 4.0 ng per milliliter. N Engl J Med 2004;350:2239, with permission.)

cancers. A risk calculator based on the PCPT database is available, which estimates the probability of prostate cancer at biopsy based on age, race, family history, prior biopsy results, DRE, and PSA levels (http://www.compass.fhcrc.org/edrnnci/bin/calculator/main.asp).

Prostate-Specific Antigen Derivatives

Prostate-specific antigen derivatives such as *PSA rates of change over time ("PSA velocity")* and *measures of free or complexed PSA* have been proposed to more effectively separate men with early prostate cancer from those with BPH. Increases in PSA of greater than 0.75 ng/mL yearly suggest cancer, but these calculations must be based on at least three annual values. Even smaller annual rates of change may suggest cancer among men with PSA levels less than 4.0 ng/mL at baseline. Measurements of circulating *free PSA* (not bound to macromolecules) have been suggested to avoid biopsies for false-positive results; men with higher ratios of free to total PSA are less likely to have prostate cancer. Some experts have suggested that biopsies need not be performed in men with PSA levels in the range of 4.0 to 10.0 ng/mL if free PSA comprises more than 25% of total PSA. However, only about 20% of men with these total PSA levels in this range have such a ratio, and their probability of prostate cancer still appears to be at least 10%. In addition, the levels of *complexed PSA* (PSA bound to macromolecules) can be measured directly; these measurements appear to have operating characteristics similar to those of total PSA.

Given the lack of evidence regarding the mortality benefit of screening with total PSA, no one of these PSA derivatives can be recommended over another. Similarly, recommendations for annual PSA screening, as opposed to a longer screening interval, are arbitrary.

Outcomes

No randomized trials have documented a *mortality* reduction from PSA screening. One site of the European Randomized Study of Screening for Prostate Cancer reported that biennial screening among men of age 50 to 66 years with PSA alone (no DRE) with a biopsy threshold of greater than 3.0 ng/mL resulted in a reduction in the probability of a first presentation with metastatic prostate cancer from about 1 in 200 without screening to 1 in 400 with screening at 10 years. This outcome may be a proxy for prostate cancer–specific mortality, albeit still susceptible to lead-time bias. On the other hand, because of overdiagnosis, the risk of being diagnosed with prostate cancer increased from about 4% without screening to 8% with screening at 10 years. Advocates of screening note that recent decreases in population-based prostate cancer mortality rates in the United States (see Fig. 126.1) might be attributable to screening. However, decreases in prostate cancer–specific mortality have also been noted in the United Kingdom, where PSA screening has been infrequent, and regions of the United States that were more aggressive about PSA screening have not seen a faster mortality drop than areas that were less aggressive about screening. As with DRE, case–control studies of PSA screening have yielded conflicting results.

Advocates of PSA screening point out that there is also *no convincing evidence that early detection programs do not reduce prostate cancer mortality*. As a result, groups like the American College of Physicians recommend presenting the potential benefits and known risks of PSA screening to patients and helping them to reach an informed decision about whether to undergo PSA testing. At a minimum, patients undergoing PSA screening should be informed that false-positive and false-negative PSA test and biopsy results can occur, and that no one knows whether regular PSA screening will reduce the risk of death from prostate cancer. However, even advocates of early detection and aggressive treatment generally doubt its value, at least in terms of reducing mortality, in men who have less than a 10-year life expectancy or who are about age 75 years or older with average comorbidity.

Transrectal Ultrasonography

Transrectal ultrasonography (TRUS) of the prostate is no longer widely promoted as a primary screening test because of poor sensitivity and specificity. It is, however, used to evaluate abnormalities found on DRE and PSA screening and to guide transrectal biopsy by identifying suspect hypoechoic areas. Because of the limited sensitivity of TRUS, urologists usually systematically obtain random biopsy specimens from men with an elevated PSA level when no hypoechoic areas are seen. Recently, in recognition of the relatively low sensitivity of traditional six-sample random biopsies, urologists have been taking more biopsy cores, often 10 or more. Unfortunately, even a 10- to 12-core biopsy cannot "rule out" prostate cancer, and there is considerable debate about if and when men with an initially negative set of biopsies for an elevated PSA should be rebiopsied.

CONCLUSIONS AND RECOMMENDATIONS (22,23)

- Evidence regarding DRE screening for prostate cancer is conflicting. Many U.S. clinicians, however, simply consider the DRE an extension of a thorough physical examination of older male patients.
- If a suspicious abnormality is identified on DRE in a younger patient or an older patient without significant comorbid disease who would be eligible for curative treatment, a urologic referral for biopsy should be made. A normal PSA result does not exclude cancer in the presence of a palpable abnormality.
- PSA measurement should be considered at the age of 50 years (and at age 45 years among African Americans and men with a positive family history). However, because there is no evidence that such screening reduces long-term mortality, screening is optional. Patients should understand the pros and cons of screening before undergoing the test. Early detection efforts are not indicated for men with a life expectancy of less than 10 years or after about age 75 years for men with average comorbidity.
- When to proceed to biopsy is controversial; a PSA threshold of 4.0 ng/mL is commonly used. Biopsies can be considered in men in their 50s with PSA levels greater than 2.5 ng/mL or for men with average PSA velocities greater than 0.75 ng/mL per year over at least three serial determinations.
- Screening periodicity has not been established, but repeating the PSA measurement at 1- to 2-year intervals is probably reasonable (the longer interval might be used when the initial PSA level is <2.0 ng/mL; the shorter interval if the PSA is higher or if a more accurate estimate of "PSA velocity" is desired).
- Transrectal ultrasound is not recommended as a primary screening test.

Annotated Bibliography

1. Coley CM, Barry MJ, Fleming C, et al. Early detection of prostate cancer. Part I: prior probability and effectiveness of tests. Ann Intern Med 1997;126:394. (*Synthesizes data from older autopsy studies on the histologic prevalence of prostate cancer.*)

2. Gronberg H. Prostate cancer epidemiology. Lancet 2003;361:859. (*A succinct review of genetic and dietary factors, as well as prospects for chemoprevention.*)

3. Lawson KA, Wright ME, Suar A, et al. Multivitamin use and risk of prostate cancer in the National Institute of Health–AARP diet and health study. J Natl Cancer Inst 2007;99:754. (*There was an association between excessive multivitamin use and advanced and fatal prostate cancer.*)

4. Albertsen PC, Hanley JA, Fine J. 20-year outcomes following conservative management of clinically localized prostate cancer. JAMA 2005;293:2095. (*Provides 20-year outcomes for men of different ages with tumors of different histologic types managed conservatively in the pre–prostate-specific antigen [PSA] era.*)

5. Parker C, Muston D, Melia J, et al. A model of the natural history of screen-detected prostate cancer, and the effect of radical treatment on survival. Br J Cancer 2006;94:1361. (*Uses earlier data to estimate the prognosis for men with prostate cancer diagnosed in the PSA era and treated with both conservative and aggressive management.*)

6. Bill-Axelson A, Holmberg L, Ruutu M, et al. Radical prostatectomy versus watchful waiting in early prostate cancer. N Engl J Med 2005;352:1977. (*Ther first randomized evidence for a benefit of radical prostatectomy in prostate cancer–specific and overall mortality among men with well- and moderately well differentiated prostate cancer.*)

7. Steineck G, Helgesen F, Adofsson J, et al. Quality of life after radical prostatectomy or watchful waiting. N Engl J Med 2002;347:790. (*Radical prostatectomy, compared with watchful waiting, caused more erectile dysfunction [80% vs. 45%] and urinary incontinence [49% vs. 21%].*)

8. Albertsen PC, Hanley D, Barrows, GH, et al. Prostate cancer and the Will Rogers phenomenon. J Natl Cancer Inst 2005;97:1248. (*Documents that pathologists now assign higher grades to the same prostate cancers.*)

9. Andriole GL, Levin DL, Crawford D, et al. Prostate cancer screening in the Prostate, Lung, Colorectal and Ovarian (PLCO) cancer screening trial: findings from the initial round of a randomized trial. J Natl Cancer Inst 2005;97:433. (*Provides the results of digital rectal exam [DRE] and PSA screening from the first round of the major U.S. prostate cancer screening trial.*)

10. Friedman GD, Hiatt RA, Quesenberry CP Jr, et al. Case–control study of screening for prostate cancer by digital rectal examinations. Lancet 1991;337:1526. (*A case–control study, showing that the relative risk for metastatic cancer was no lower among men who had undergone one or more rectal examinations in the preceding 10 years.*)

11. Jacobsen SJ, Bergstrahl EJ, Katusic SK, et al. Screening digital rectal examination and prostate cancer mortality: a population-based case–control study. Urology 1998;52:173. (*In contrast to the Friedman et al. study cited earlier, this study found that fatal prostate cancer was associated with a 50% lower probability of having undergone a DRE in the previous 10 years.*)

12. Richie JR, Catalona WJ, Ahmann FR, et al. Effect of patient age on early detection of prostate cancer with serum prostate-specific antigen and digital rectal examination. Urology 1993;42:365. (*A six-center screening study involving >6,000 men, providing predictive values of DRE and PSA measurement in prostate cancer for men of different ages.*)

13. Gann PH, Hennekens CH, Stampfer MJ. A prospective evaluation of plasma prostate-specific antigen for detection of prostate cancer. JAMA 1995;273:289. (*PSA measurement had a sensitivity of 73% in detecting cancers diagnosed within 4 years of the time the test serum was obtained in the Physicians' Health Study.*)

14. Thompson IM, Ankerst DP, Chi C, et al. Operating characteristics of prostate-specific antigen in men with an initial PSA level of 3.0 ng/ml or less. JAMA 2005;294:66. (*A randomized trial of finasteride to prevent prostate cancer, providing the first estimates of the sensitivity and specificity of PSA screening with biopsy as the gold standard.*)

15. Welch HG, Schwartz LM, Woloshin S. Prostate-specific antigen levels in the United States: implications of various definitions for abnormal. J Natl Cancer Inst 2005;97:1132. (*Documents the downside, in terms of the loss of specificity and increased overdiagnosis, of lowering PSA thresholds for biopsy.*)

16. Carter HB, Pearson JD, Metter JE, et al. Longitudinal evaluation of prostate-specific antigen levels in men with and without prostate disease. JAMA 1992;267:2215. (*A threshold "PSA velocity" of 0.75 ng/mL per year provided some discrimination between men with prostate cancer and men with benign prostatic hyperplasia.*)

17. Carter HB, Ferrucci L, Ketterman A, et al. Detection of life-threatening prostate cancer with prostate-specific antigen during a window of curability. J Natl Cancer Inst 2006;98:1521. (*A small study, finding that even smaller rates of change in PSA 10 to 15 years prior to diagnosis provided some prediction of eventually fatal prostate cancer among men with initially low PSA levels.*)

18. Lee R, Localio AR, Armstrong K, et al. A meta-analysis of the performance characteristics of the free prostate-specific antigen test. Urology 2006;67:762. (*Free PSA can stratify cancer risk to some degree, but it appears to add little to help in decision making regarding biopsy at this time.*)

19. Aus G, Bergdahl S, Lodding P, et al. Prostate cancer screening decreases the absolute risk of being diagnosed with advanced prostate cancer—results from a prospective, population-based randomized controlled trial. Eur Urol 2007;51:659. (*At one site of this major European trial, PSA screening resulted in a small absolute reduction in the likelihood of being first diagnosed with metastatic disease and a relatively large increase in the risk of being diagnosed with prostate cancer.*)

20. Lu-Yao GL, Albertsen PC, Stanford JL, et al. A natural experiment examining the impact of aggressive screening and treatment on prostate cancer mortality in two fixed cohorts from the Seattle area and Connecticut. BMJ 2002;325:740. (*Despite much more aggressive screening and treatment for prostate cancer in Seattle compared with Connecticut, prostate cancer mortality among Medicare-age men in these regions was the same through 11 years of follow-up.*)

21. Concato J, Wells C, Horwitz RI, et al. The effectiveness of screening for prostate cancer: a nested case–control study. Arch Int Med 2006;166:38. (*A case–control study of prostate cancer screening among veterans in New England, failing to show an association between PSA screening and lower prostate cancer mortality.*)

22. Kopec J, Goel V, Bunting PS, et al. Screening with prostate specific antigen and metastatic prostate cancer risk: a population based case–control study. J Urol 2005;1745:495. (*In this case–control study from the Toronto area, PSA screening was associated with a 35% lower risk of being diagnosed with metastatic prostate cancer.*)

23. Chan ECY, Sulmasy DP. What should men know about prostate-specific antigen screening before giving informed consent? Am J Med 1998;105:266. (*Used focus groups of physicians and patients to attempt to define what patients should be told before undergoing PSA testing.*)

CHAPTER 127 ■ SCREENING FOR ASYMPTOMATIC BACTERIURIA AND URINARY TRACT INFECTION

Efforts to detect and treat asymptomatic bacteriuria are based on the assumption that treatment reduces the likelihood of subsequent morbidity from symptomatic infection, sepsis, or chronic renal disease. The risk for such complications depends on the clinical situation, including the age and gender of the patient. For some patients, such as pregnant women, the risk is well defined and treatment is indicated; for most, however, the most significant morbidity may be related to the side effects of inappropriate treatment. It is therefore critical that the physician appreciate the implications of bacteriuria in different settings.

EPIDEMIOLOGY AND RISK FACTORS (1–7)

The prevalence of bacteriuria depends on age and gender. Among neonates, positive cultures are found in about 1% of both boys and girls. During school age, the prevalence among boys is as low as 0.03%, in comparison with 1% to 2% among girls. The prevalence among women increases by 1% of the population per decade; throughout the childbearing years, the prevalence is 2% to 4%, and by age 50 years, it has reached 5% to 10%. Elderly men are almost as likely to have bacteriuria as women because of the high incidence of prostate and other urologic disease and subsequent instrumentation in this group. Prevalence in these older age groups reaches 15%.

The greater susceptibility of younger women and girls can be explained anatomically in that a short urethra allows easier access to the bladder, so that colonization by perineal organisms is facilitated. Risk increases with local trauma associated with sexual activity and the relaxation of the pelvic supporting structures with age. Anatomic changes may also explain the higher prevalence of bacteriuria (4% to 7%) among pregnant women. Alternatively, because users of birth control pills also have an increased risk, the higher prevalence may also reflect estrogen-mediated dilation of the urethra.

The prevalence of bacteriuria is even higher in diabetic women. The relative risk for bacteriuria among women with diabetes, in comparison with nondiabetic women, is approximately 3. The risk among diabetic men is not increased.

It must be kept in mind that prevalence figures indicate the extent of bacteriuria at a single point in time. Because risk factors are shared by many, and bacteriuria frequently resolves spontaneously, as well as after therapy, the cumulative prevalence of bacteriuria is higher. By age 30 years, approximately 25% of women have experienced symptoms consistent with urinary tract infection.

Structural abnormalities (including obstruction of the urethra or ureters), significant vesicourethral reflux, neurologic lesions, and the presence of foreign bodies are important additional risk factors for bacteriuria.

NATURAL HISTORY OF ASYMPTOMATIC BACTERIURIA AND EFFECTIVENESS OF THERAPY (8–18)

Asymptomatic and symptomatic urinary tract infections have the same epidemiologic correlates. Asymptomatic infections can become symptomatic; bacteriuria can persist after symptoms have resolved. Ninety percent of women with bacteriuria have had symptoms some time in the past, and nearly 70% within the preceding year. Although both asymptomatic and symptomatic infections can resolve spontaneously, the urine is more likely to become sterile after treatment. Approximately 80% of women with bacteriuria have sterile urine after appropriate antibiotic treatment. However, follow-up studies indicate that only 55% of those treated have sterile urine at the end of 1 year. Sterile urine developed spontaneously in fully 36% of untreated bacteriuric women during the same period. Significantly, women who had recurrences of infection after treatment were more likely to have associated symptoms than those who had persistent or relapsing bacteriuria. Symptomatic infection recurs within 3 years in 40% of women. As noted, women with diabetes are more likely to have asymptomatic bacteriuria than women without diabetes, and then they are more likely to develop symptoms. In one study, 28% of women with type 2 diabetes had asymptomatic bacteriuria, and, of these, 34% developed symptoms within the ensuing 18 months.

The importance of chronic or recurrent bacteriuria as a cause of chronic renal failure has been deemphasized as diverse noninfectious etiologies for the pathologic findings of interstitial nephritis have been recognized. Patients with bacteriuria are more likely to be hypertensive. They are also more likely to have identifiable abnormalities on intravenous pyelogram, including small kidneys, delayed excretion, calyceal dilation and blunting, ureteral reflux, stones, and other obstructive lesions. However, chronic renal failure rarely occurs as a complication of urinary tract infection in the absence of structural abnormalities. Evidence indicates that such abnormalities predispose patients to both chronic renal failure and recurrent infection.

In some clinical situations, the clinician may be concerned with the possibility that chronic asymptomatic infection is a potential source of disseminated infection during instrumentation. Studies have shown that the placement of an indwelling Foley catheter is associated with a low risk of bacteremia, but the danger may be sufficient to consider treatment in the male patient with prostate disease and infection who requires more invasive instrumentation (see Chapter 140). Bacteremia has been documented in as many as 50% of male patients whose urine is infected at the time of the procedure; it is relatively rare when the urine is sterile. In elderly populations, asymptomatic bacteriuria has been associated with increased mortality. Obviously, such increased rates may be a consequence of either bacteriuria or other factors that increase the risk for both bacteriuria and death. Recent evidence suggests the latter; studies among elderly women and men found no difference between patients with and without bacteriuria when comorbidity such as cancer was controlled for.

Special risks are associated with bacteriuria during pregnancy. Asymptomatic bacteriuria, defined by repeated recovery of more than 10^5 colony-forming units per milliliter in voided urine or suprapubic aspirates positive for bacteria, occurs in approximately 5% of pregnancies. In one study, the risk for onset of bacteriuria was greatest between weeks 9 and 17 of gestation. Among women with bacteriuria identified early in pregnancy, the incidence of acute pyelonephritis without prophylactic treatment is 40%. Women with bacteriuria are nearly twice as likely to deliver low-birth-weight infants, and the relative risk for perinatal mortality in their infants has been estimated at 1.6. Randomized trials of treatment of asymptomatic bacteriuria during pregnancy have demonstrated efficacy in reducing the incidence of pyelonephritis and delivery of low-birth-weight infants.

Young women who have undergone short-term urinary catheterization experienced increased symptomatic infection over 2 weeks after catheter removal when asymptomatic bacteriuria persisted for 48 hours after catheter removal. Treatment should be considered under these circumstances.

SCREENING AND DIAGNOSTIC TESTS (19,20)

Asymptomatic bacteriuria is a laboratory diagnosis that requires careful definition. Because voided urine is easily contaminated by urethral and (in women) perineal flora during micturition, *clean-voided urine* must be cultured quantitatively. The probability of infection when a specimen contains 10^5 colony-forming units per milliliter is nearly 100% for male patients but only 80% for female patients. The finding of two such positive cultures in a female patient increases the probability of infection to 95%. False-negative findings are more likely if the patient is undergoing vigorous diuresis, if the urine is unusually acidic (pH 5.5), or if the specimen has inadvertently been contaminated with antibacterial detergents. Spurious positive cultures are more common because of unclean collection technique, contaminated collection equipment, or failure to culture the urine promptly.

The collection of a single urine specimen with 10^5 colony-forming units per milliliter during urethral catheterization has a predictive value of infection of 95%. *Catheterization* should be limited to patients requiring relief of obstruction or those who absolutely cannot cooperate with collection techniques. The risk of introducing infection during catheterization may be as high as 5%. The risk of inducing bacteremia in men with an infected urinary tract approaches 50%. When *suprapubic percutaneous bladder aspiration* is performed, either in young children or in adults with confusing problems that must be resolved, infection can be presumed if the growth of any bacteria other than skin contaminants occurs.

Nonquantitative approaches to diagnosis include microscopic examination for bacteria and clinical tests of bacterial activity, such as the reduction of nitrate to nitrite. *Dipstick nitrite testing* for bacteriuria has been shown to have a sensitivity of better than 90%, but specificity is limited and variable, ranging from 35% to 85% in different studies. This variation may be explained by differences in the prevalence of bacteria that do not reduce nitrates and variation in the time interval between the collecting and testing of urine. *Dipstick tests* for *leukocyte esterase activity* as a marker of pyuria are more sensitive but less specific. The reported sensitivity of the leukocyte esterase dipstick test for bacteriuria ranges from 72% to 97%; the reported range for specificity is 64% to 82%. Dipstick tests have been shown to be less sensitive when the prior probability of infection is low based on clinical findings. These and other nonspecific signs of urinary tract inflammation, such as the presence of microscopic pyuria or hematuria and the presence of proteinuria, may be helpful in making a presumptive diagnosis in the symptomatic patient. They may also indicate the need for urine culture when incidental abnormalities are detected in the asymptomatic patient. Confirmation of infection with *quantitative culture* technology should precede a therapeutic decision in the absence of symptoms.

CONCLUSIONS AND RECOMMENDATIONS

- Bacteriuria, both symptomatic and asymptomatic, is a common phenomenon with well-defined risk factors.
- Treatment is moderately effective in the short run, but because of high rates of spontaneous recurrence and resolution, the likelihood that bacteriuria will be noted with longer follow-up is not significantly influenced by short-term therapy.
- Symptomatic infections are generally not prevented by the treatment of asymptomatic bacteriuria in nonpregnant women.
- Although an association exists between bacteriuria and renal abnormalities, there is no evidence that this is an etiologic relationship. Furthermore, there is no evidence that the treatment of infection in the absence of urinary tract abnormalities prevents progressive renal disease.
- Screening for asymptomatic bacteriuria is recommended for pregnant women but not for other populations on a routine basis. Women who have short-term catheter placement may benefit from screening for bacteriuria 48 hours after catheter removal. Screening may be warranted in elderly men with clinical prostatism or other urologic abnormalities, before and after required instrumentation (see Chapter 140), and in patients with known renal calculi or other structural abnormalities of the urinary tract.
- Screening with reagent strips is not sufficiently sensitive to be used among patients who are at high risk and likely to benefit from detection and treatment. The screening of pregnant women should include urine culture.

A.G.M.

Annotated Bibliography

1. Colgan R, Nicolle LE, McGlone A, et al. Asymptomatic bacteriuria in adults. Am Family Physician 2006;74:985. (*A concise review of epidemiology and rationale for current recommendations.*)
2. Nicolle LE, Bradley S, Colgan R, et al. Infectious Diseases Society of America guidelines for diagnosis and treatment of asymptomatic bacteriuria in adults. Clin Infect Dis 2005;40:643. (*Authoritative recommendations for the screening and treatment of pregnant women.*)
3. Hooton TM, Scholes D, Stapleton AE, et al. A prospective study of asymptomatic bacteriuria in sexually active young women. N Engl J Med 2000;343:992. (*The same risk factors were found for asymptomatic bacteriuria and*

cystitis; 8% of those with bacteriuria developed symptomatic urinary tract infections within 1 week.)

4. Nordenstam GR, Brandberg CA, Oden AS, et al. Bacteriuria and mortality in an elderly population. N Engl J Med 1986;314:1152. (*A 9-year cohort study, finding no difference in mortality among women with and without bacteriuria, and also no difference among men when those with cancer were excluded.*)

5. Stamm WE. Prevention of urinary tract infections. Am J Med 1984;76:148. (*A thoughtful review of risk factors and preventive approaches; recommends screening only for pregnant women.*)

6. Stenquist K, Dahlen-Nilsson I, Lidin-Janson G, et al. Bacteriuria in pregnancy. Frequency and risk of acquisition. Am J Epidemiol 1989;129:372. (*A study of >3,000 pregnancies, finding that the risk for the onset of bacteriuria was greatest between weeks 9 and 17 of gestation.*)

7. Takahashi M, Loveland DB. Bacteriuria and oral contraceptives. JAMA 1974;227:762. (*Prevalence was 50% higher among oral contraceptive users.*)

8. Abrutyn E, Mossey J, Berlin JA, et al. Does asymptomatic bacteriuria predict mortality and does antimicrobial treatment reduce mortality in elderly ambulatory women? Ann Intern Med 1994;120:827. (*Treatment reduced bacteriuria; no association with mortality was found.*)

9. Asscher AW, Sussman M, Waters WE, et al. The clinical significance of asymptomatic bacteriuria in the nonpregnant woman. J Infect Dis 1969;120:17. (*A controlled trial of treatment of asymptomatic bacteriuria, concluding that screening for bacteriuria in nonpregnant women is unlikely to be of value.*)

10. Geerlings SE, Stolk RP, Camps MJ, et al. Consequences of asymptomatic bacteriuria in women with diabetes mellitus. Arch Intern Med 2001;161:1421. (*Twenty-eight percent of women with type 2 diabetes had asymptomatic bacteriuria; 34% of those women had a symptomatic infection in the next 18 months.*)

11. Harding GK, Zhanel GG, Nicolle LE, et al. Antimicrobial treatment in diabetic women with asymptomatic bacteriuria. N Engl J Med 2002;347:1576. (*Much higher relapse rates led to the cessation of a 3-day treatment regimen.*)

12. Kass EH, Zinner SH. Bacteriuria and renal disease. J Infect Dis 1969;120:27. (*An exhaustive review of the links between bacteriuria and renal disease, concluding that a causal relationship was demonstrated in cases of pyelonephri-*

tis in pregnancy and bacteremia after catheterization but not in progressive renal disease among adults.)

13. Kunin CM, Polyak F, Postel E. Periurethral bacterial flora in women. JAMA 1980;243:134. (*An intensively monitored small cohort of women with and without a history of urinary tract infection; the most notable finding was a high frequency of asymptomatic bacteriuria, with spontaneous resolution in both groups.*)

14. Nicolle LE, Mayhew WJ, Bryan L. Prospective randomized comparison of therapy and no therapy for asymptomatic bacteriuria in institutionalized elderly women. Am J Med 1987;83:27. (*No differences were noted in genitourinary morbidity or mortality; antimicrobial therapy was associated with adverse effects and a higher reinfection rate.*)

15. Romero R, Oyarzun E, Mazor M, et al. Metaanalysis of the relationship between asymptomatic bacteriuria and preterm delivery/low birth weight. Obstet Gynecol 1989;73:576. (*A meta-analysis of eight trials.*)

16. Schieve LA, Handler A, Hershow R, et al. Urinary tract infection during pregnancy: its association with maternal morbidity and perinatal outcome. Am J Public Health 1994;84:405. (*The risk for preterm delivery and low birth weight increased 1.5- to 2-fold.*)

17. Smaill F. Antibiotics for asymptomatic bacteriuria in pregnancy (Cochrane review). In: The Cochrane library, Issue 3. Oxford: Update Software, 2004. (*The treatment was effective in preventing pyelonephritis; see* http://www.cochrane.org *for updates.*)

18. Villar J, Lydon-Rochelle MT, Gülmezoglu AM, et al. Duration of treatment for asymptomatic bacteriuria during pregnancy (Cochrane review). In: The Cochrane library, Issue 3. Oxford: Update Software, 2004. (*There was insufficient evidence to recommend a duration; see* http://www.cochrane.org *for updates.*)

19. Pels RJ, Bor DH, Woolhandler S, et al. Dipstick urinalysis screening of asymptomatic adults for urinary tract disorders. II. Bacteriuria. JAMA 1989;262:1220. (*A careful review of the literature, offering estimates of sensitivity and specificity and recommendations.*)

20. Tincello DG, Richmond DH. Evaluation of reagent strips in detecting asymptomatic bacteriuria in early pregnancy: prospective case series. BMJ 1998;316:435. (*Sensitivity was too low for use in pregnant women.*)

CHAPTER 128 ■ SCREENING FOR CANCERS OF THE LOWER URINARY TRACT

Lower urinary tract cancers include tumors of the renal pelves, ureters, bladder, and urethra. These lesions can logically be considered together because of their similar cell types (>95% of these consist of transitional cells, squamous cells, or a combination of the two) and because of common epidemiologic correlates.

Cancer of the lower urinary tract is viewed by many primary physicians as a relatively benign tumor that principally affects the elderly. Nevertheless, more than 65,000 new cases occur each year in the United States, and approximately 14,000 deaths per year can be attributed to bladder cancer. The lifetime probability of incurring cancer of the bladder is approximately 3% for white men and 1% for white women. The probability of dying of bladder cancer is approximately 1% and 0.3% for white men and white women, respectively.

Risk factors, including strong associations with high relative risks for occupational exposures, have been well defined. A strong association, albeit with lower relative risk, has also been demonstrated for tobacco use. A prospective study of fluid intake and the development of bladder cancer during 10 years

suggested that a high intake of fluids decreased risk. Diagnostic tests are available, and some have been used in screening programs; new approaches focusing on urine biomarkers are in development. Although limitations in available tests and insufficient understanding of the heterogeneous natural history of bladder cancer preclude specific screening recommendations at this time, the physician should understand the epidemiology of these tumors and the potential costs and benefits of various approaches to early diagnosis in those at high risk for cancer or its recurrence.

EPIDEMIOLOGY AND RISK FACTORS (1–10)

Cancer of the lower urinary tract is a tumor of older age groups; in the United States, the mean age at the time of diagnosis is 68 years. The incidence increases at a constant rate during adult life, varying from 1 in 100,000 per year at age 20 years to

200 in 100,000 per year at age 80 years for white men. Women have approximately one third of the risk of men. In the United States, whites are twice as likely to have bladder tumors as nonwhites. Urban dwellers have consistently been shown to have a higher incidence of lower urinary tract tumors than do people who live in rural or suburban areas.

The most notable risk factor for the development of lower urinary tract cancers is *occupational exposure* to aromatic amines, which was first noted in England in 1895. Subsequently, dyestuff workers were shown to have a 10- to 50-fold increased risk for bladder carcinoma. Compounds most closely associated with bladder carcinogenesis include 2-naphthylamine and benzidine. Recent case–control studies indicate an excess risk among men who work with dyestuffs, rubber, leather, paints, and organic chemicals. It has been estimated that these occupational exposures are responsible for 18% of bladder cancer cases. As little as 2 years of exposure may be sufficient to increase the risk, but the time between exposure and subsequent cancer may be as long as 45 years.

Smoking has been implicated as a risk factor for bladder cancer in many studies, most of which indicate that smokers have a twofold increase in risk in comparison with nonsmokers. Other suggested risk factors include pelvic irradiation, which was used in the past for dysfunctional bleeding and continues to be used for cancer of the prostate, cervix, and ovaries. The abuse of phenacetin-containing analgesics is also a risk factor. Early case–control studies suggested an association with coffee consumption, but the weight of evidence does not support a significant increase in risk. Occupational exposure to hair dyes has been implicated, but there is no association with the personal use of such dyes. Exposure to diesel exhaust as a risk factor is suggested by a modest increase in incidence among truck and bus drivers.

Because direct contact of the bladder urothelium with carcinogens excreted in the urine may contribute to bladder cancer, it has been hypothesized that a high consumption of fluids could reduce risk by diluting the urine or reducing contact time. Evidence has been inconsistent, but the largest prospective study suggests that men in the highest quintile of fluid consumption face about half of the risk of those in the lowest quintile. Case–control and cohort studies also suggest that long-term use of diuretics may increase the risk for bladder cancer by as much as twofold.

NATURAL HISTORY OF LOWER URINARY TRACT CANCERS AND EFFECTIVENESS OF THERAPY (11,12)

The natural history of lower urinary tract tumors is not well defined. The prognosis at the time of diagnosis depends on both clinical stage, defined by the depth of penetration and the extent of metastases, and histologic grade of the tumor. The depth of penetration and histologic grade are often closely correlated. Urothelial tumors are grossly subdivided into papilloma, papillary carcinoma, and transitional cell carcinoma. These gross morphologic distinctions have histologic counterparts that are highly predictive of 5-year survival. Grade 1 papillary carcinoma (papilloma) has a 5-year cure or clinical control rate of approximately 95%. Grade 2 papillary carcinoma (papillary carcinoma) has a 5-year survival rate of only 25%. The outlook for grade 3 papillary and infiltrating carcinoma (transitional

cell carcinoma) is worse. The prognosis for patients with squamous carcinoma is also very poor unless the tumor is well differentiated. Clinical staging systems that distinguish among levels of tumor penetration of the bladder have also been shown to have good prognostic value. Overall, about 50% of patients with treated bladder cancer survive for 5 years. However, multiple synchronous and asynchronous tumors are the rule in lower urinary tract cancer and contribute to morbidity and eventual mortality. Hematuria is the most common presentation of lower urinary tract cancer. Other symptoms suggestive of cystitis may also occur. Although it has been claimed that 75% of tumors promptly diagnosed after a first episode of hematuria are localized, few data on this subject are available. The likelihood that screening tests, including urinalysis and urinary cytology, would significantly advance the time of diagnosis is unproven. A progression from urothelial atypia to sessile carcinoma *in situ* or papilloma to higher-grade malignancy has been postulated. Studies of the natural history of urothelial carcinoma *in situ* indicate that the majority of lesions progress to more malignant forms. Although early lesions are much less likely to be detected cytologically, 3.7% of detected tumors were *in situ* in one study. The usual synchronous and asynchronous multiplicity of such tumors makes it difficult to assess the benefits of early detection.

SCREENING TESTS (13–19)

Efforts to screen for asymptomatic bladder cancer have focused on the detection of asymptomatic hematuria with urine dipsticks and urine cytology.

Studies of *dipstick urinalysis* have been conducted in older men at increased risk for bladder cancer. Daily screening for 2 weeks or 10 serial screens conducted on a daily or weekly basis have produced at least 1 positive screen result in about 205 men. The predictive values positive for any urologic malignancy (bladder, prostate, or renal) in these two studies were 6% and 8%, respectively. One-time screening in general outpatient populations has a significantly lower yield and predictive value. In one such study, dipstick screening of more than 20,000 patients disclosed only 1 bladder cancer and 2 cancers of the prostate. In a second study, only 2% of patients with a positive screen result had any significant urologic disease. The predictive value for urologic cancer diagnosed anytime in the ensuing 3 years was 0.5%.

Urinary cytology is less sensitive but more specific than hematuria on dipstick as a screening test for lower urinary tract cancers. Reported rates of the sensitivity of cytology in detecting bladder carcinoma vary from 50% to 90%. Studies have consistently demonstrated that sensitivity increases with the grade of malignancy. Although invasive transitional cell carcinoma can regularly be detected with a sensitivity of 90% or greater, sensitivity rates for papillomas and papillary carcinomas range from 0% to 50%.

Studies of cytologic screening of high-risk populations have been conducted. In one such study, the screening of 285 exposed workers produced positive results in 31, 10 of whom had the diagnosis of cancer confirmed at cystoscopy. Within 4 years, 11 additional tumors developed among the 21 cytology-positive, cystoscopy-negative patients. Cystoscopy was also performed in the 254 workers with negative cytologic findings; only 1 case of bladder cancer was diagnosed on that examination. In general, the specificity of urinary cytology depends on the skill of the cytologist. False-positive rates as low as 1% and as high as 20% have been reported. The value of other urinary sediment abnormalities, particularly hematuria, has not been well defined. In one study of cytologic detection, hematuria was absent in 50% of true-positive cytologic diagnoses.

Because of the limited sensitivity of cytology, efforts have been made to develop *immunocytochemistry* and *proteomics* assays. The former (e.g., *Immunocyt*) use monoclonal antibodies specific to antigens expressed on transitional cell cancer cells. The latter (e.g., *NMP22 BladderChek*) is a proteomics-based assay for a nuclear matrix protein. Several comparisons of immunocytochemistry tests with cytologic examination in patients with recurrent or newly diagnosed bladder cancer have been published. In one such study, Immunocyt had a sensitivity of 60%, 75%, and 77% for grade 1, 2, and 3 transitional cell tumors, respectively, compared with sensitivities of 18%, 46%, and 64% for cytology. However, specificity for Immunocyt was 84%, compared to 95% for cytology. NMP22 BladderChek has been compared with cytology among patients at elevated risk for bladder cancer because of risk factors or symptoms of hematuria and dysuria. It had a sensitivity of 56% and a specificity of 86%, compared to 16% and 99% for cytology, respectively. Other potential urinary biomarkers are also being investigated. *Cystoscopy* and *radiographic procedures* cannot be considered screening tools. They should be reserved for patients who present with symptoms suggestive of urinary cancer or who have positive findings on cytology or with biomarker assays. Frequent follow-up cystoscopy is also part of the postoperative care of the patient with bladder cancer.

CONCLUSIONS AND RECOMMENDATIONS

- Lower urinary tract cancer is associated with significant morbidity and mortality.
- Risks of occupational exposure to dyestuffs, rubber, leather and leather products, paint, and organic chemicals have been well defined. Smoking is also associated with a significant increase in risk.
- High levels of fluid intake may reduce the risk for bladder cancer.
- Urinary cytology is an imperfect but useful screening test for high-risk groups.
- Immunocytochemistry and proteomics-based urinary assays are more sensitive than cytology, but limited specificity—false-positive rates as high as 20%—limit their applicability in routine screening.
- There is no evidence that screening significantly advances the time of diagnosis in an individual case or that early treatment influences the outcome. Nevertheless, because of the relatively high specificity and lack of morbidity associated with cytologic screening, the identification of patients at high risk because of occupational exposure, with subsequent yearly cytologic screening, may be indicated in the occupational health setting. Screening of asymptomatic smokers without a risk of occupational exposure is not recommended.

A.G.M.

Annotated Bibliography

1. Andrew AS, Schned AR, Heaney JA, et al. Bladder cancer risk and personal hair dye use. Int J Cancer 2004;109:581. (*No association was found.*)
2. Boffetta P, Silverman DT. A meta-analysis of bladder cancer and diesel exhaust exposure. Epidemiology 2001;12:125. (*A modestly increased risk was found for truck and bus drivers.*)
3. Cole P, Hoover R, Friedell GH. Occupation and cancer of the lower urinary tract. Cancer 1972;29:1250. (*A case–control study, identifying excess risk among five occupation categories: dyestuffs, rubber, leather and leather products, paint, and organic chemicals; no risk could be identified in individuals who worked with nonorganic chemicals, petroleum, or printing products.*)
4. Cole P, Monson RR, Haning H, et al. Smoking and cancer of the lower urinary tract. N Engl J Med 1971;284:129. (*Case–control data, indicating that smokers had a twofold greater risk for the development of bladder cancer.*)
5. Grossman E, Messerli FH, Goldbourt U. Does diuretic therapy increase the risk of renal cell carcinoma? Am J Cardiol 1999;83:1090. (*A systematic review of case–control and cohort studies, suggesting that the long-term use of diuretics increased the risk for bladder cancer, with an odds ratio or risk ratio of 1.5 to 2.0.*)
6. Matanoski GM, Elliott EA. Bladder cancer epidemiology. Epidemiol Rev 1981;3:203. (*An extensive review of descriptive epidemiology and risk factors, including smoking, coffee drinking, use of sugar substitutes, and occupational exposures.*)
7. Michaud DS, Spiegelman D, Clinton SK, et al. Fluid intake and the risk of bladder cancer in men. N Engl J Med 1999;340:1390. (*Men in the highest quintile for fluid intake had half of the risk of men in the lowest quintile.*)
8. Morrison AS, Buring JE. Artificial sweeteners and cancer of the lower urinary tract. N Engl J Med 1980;302:537. (*A case–control study, failing to detect a significant association between the use of artificial sweeteners and an excess risk of lower urinary tract cancer.*)
9. Piper JM, Tonascia J, Matanoski GM. Heavy phenacetin use and bladder cancer in women aged 20 to 49 years. N Engl J Med 1985;313:292. (*Analgesic abuse was the most common cause of bladder cancer in this otherwise low-risk population.*)
10. Viscoli CM, Lachs MS, Horwitz RI. Bladder cancer and coffee drinking: a summary of case–control research. Lancet 1993;341:1432. (*No significant association was found.*)
11. van der Meijden APM. Bladder cancer. BMJ 1998;317:1366. (*A review of diagnosis, prognosis, and treatment.*)
12. Heney NM, Ahmed SW, Flanagan MJ, et al. Superficial bladder cancer: progression and recurrence. J Urol 1983;30:1083. (*A useful description of the natural history of the disease.*)
13. Britton JP, Dowell AC, Whelan P, et al. A community study of bladder cancer screening by the detection of occult urinary bleeding. J Urol 1992;148:788. (*Among the 20% of men with 1 positive result in 10 screens, the predictive value for urologic malignancy was 6%.*)
14. Foot NC, Papanicolaou GN, Holmquist ND, et al. Exfoliative cytology of urinary sediments (a review of 2,829 cases). Cancer 1958;11:127. (*Sensitivity was 62% in detecting tumors of renal pelves, bladder, or ureters, 8% in renal tumors; and 15% in prostatic tumors; specificity was high.*)
15. Messing EM, Young TB, Hunt VB, et al. Comparison of bladder cancer outcome in men undergoing hematuria home screening versus those with standard clinical presentations. Urology 1995;45:387. (*Mortality during 2 years was lower among screenees.*)
16. Messing EM, Young TB, Hunt VB, et al. Home screening for hematuria: results of a multi-clinic study. J Urol 1992;148:289. (*Among 21% of patients with a positive result on one screen, the predictive value positive was 8%.*)
17. Pfister C, Chautard D, Devonec M, et al. Immunocyte test improves the diagnostic accuracy of urinary cytology: results of a French multicenter study. J Urol 2003;169:921. (*The test increased sensitivity when it was combined with cytology.*)
18. Grossman HB, Messing E, Soloway M, et al. Detection of bladder cancer using point-of-care proteomic assay. JAMA 2005;293:810. (*The procedure increased sensitivity when it was combined with cystoscopy.*)
19. Smith SD, Wheeler MA, Plescia J, et al. Urine detection of survivin and diagnosis of bladder cancer. JAMA 2001;285:324. (*One of many biomarkers under investigation.*)

CHAPTER 129 ■ EVALUATION OF THE PATIENT WITH HEMATURIA

LESLIE S.-T. FANG

Virtually every disease of the genitourinary tract can produce hematuria. The primary physician may encounter a patient with gross hematuria or may find microscopic hematuria on routine examination of the urine. Sometimes, the cause is a harmless condition, especially when asymptomatic microscopic hematuria occurs in an otherwise healthy young patient. Even with a thorough investigation, the source of the microscopic hematuria frequently is not found. At other times, particularly in patients older than the age of 50 years, hematuria may be the only symptom of genitourinary neoplasia. Its presence demands careful consideration and often a thorough investigation to ascertain the underlying cause. One needs to be able to initiate an effective workup and decide how comprehensive and invasive it should be; this includes deciding when referral for urologic evaluation or renal biopsy is necessary.

PATHOPHYSIOLOGY AND CLINICAL PRESENTATION (1–7)

Normally, fewer than 1,000 red blood cells are excreted in the urine each minute. Microscopic hematuria ensues if the rate of excretion rises to 3,000 to 4,000 red blood cells per minute; 2 to 3 red blood cells per high-power field will appear on microscopic examination of the urine. Definitions of clinically significant hematuria are somewhat arbitrary; however, the presence of more than 8 red blood cells per high-power field is considered a reasonable cutoff for separating the likelihood of a benign cause from that of potentially serious disease.

Any intrinsic lesion within the genitourinary tract involving the kidneys, ureter, bladder, prostate, or urethra can produce hematuria. Hematuria may also result from periurethral problems in the pelvis or colon, systemic diseases, bleeding diatheses, and the use of certain drugs (e.g., cyclophosphamide).

Symptoms associated with hematuria may provide important clues to etiology. The flank pain of renal colic is usually secondary to renal calculi but may occasionally be associated with the passage of clots. Frequency, dysuria, urgency, and suprapubic pain occur with inflammatory lesions of the lower urinary tract. Dull flank pain with fever and chills may accompany pyelonephritis (see Chapter 133).

Occasionally, complaints such as fever, rash, or joint pains may indicate an underlying systemic disease, ranging from postinfectious glomerulonephritis to systemic vasculitis. When a thorough workup fails to reveal an etiology, the patient is said to have "essential hematuria." Renal biopsy of such patients often shows minimal glomerular or interstitial disease. The long-term prognosis of these patients is excellent.

DIFFERENTIAL DIAGNOSIS (7–10)

Intrinsic genitourinary lesions involving the kidneys, ureters, bladder, prostate, and urethra can all produce hematuria (Tables 129.1 and 129.2).

Microscopic hematuria is most commonly associated with infection and benign prostatic hyperplasia. The prevalence of microscopic hematuria ranged from 0.18% to 16.1% in several studies. In community-based studies, the prevalence of serious underlying disease (e.g., cancer, polycystic disease) in asymptomatic microscopic hematuria is 0.1%. Even among high-risk groups (e.g., older men), the prevalence in community-based studies is only 5%. However, evaluation of 1,930 patients referred to a specialty hematuria clinic showed that 12% of the patients (mean age 58 years) had bladder cancer and 0.7% had kidney and upper tract tumors.

The differences between the prevalence of serious diseases in these studies presumably reflect referral bias in the specialty clinic population.

Causes of microscopic hematuria can be classified as either glomerular or nonglomerular in origin. Nonglomerular causes account for the bulk of microscopic hematuria. Neoplasm, nephrolithiasis, cystic disease, papillary necrosis, and disease involving the ureter, bladder, or prostate can all present with asymptomatic microscopic hematuria. Among glomerular causes, immunoglobulin A nephropathy and thin-membrane disease are the most commonly found lesions.

Rarely, periureteral inflammatory lesions in the appendix, colon, or pelvic structures produce microscopic hematuria. On occasion, a systemic illness such as lupus erythematosus, bacterial endocarditis, or rheumatic fever is the source of hematuria. Blood dyscrasias (e.g., hemophilia, sickle cell disease, polycythemia vera, and leukemia) and hemorrhagic disorders (e.g., thrombocytopenic purpura and various coagulation defects) can be responsible for the presence of red cells in the urine.

Drugs such as anticoagulants, salicylates, methenamine preparations, and sulfonamides have been known to cause hematuria. Cyclophosphamide can induce hemorrhagic cystitis or microscopic hematuria (see Chapter 88). Hematuria in a patient on anticoagulants requires evaluation because, except in instances of marked overdose of warfarin, an underlying urologic lesion is often found (see Chapter 83).

Fever, strenuous exercise, and long-distance running are among the harmless causes of microscopic hematuria in otherwise healthy patients.

Conditions occasionally mistaken for hematuria include menstrual bleeding and the intake of substances that can darken the urine, such as beets, rhubarb, and the drugs phenazopyridine (Pyridium) and rifampin. It is also possible mistakenly to believe that a patient with hemoglobinuria or myoglobinuria has hematuria.

TABLE 129.1

DIAGNOSIS IN 1,000 REFERRED CASES OF GROSS HEMATURIA

Diagnosis	Patients (%)
Kidneys	15.0
Tumor	3.5
Infection	3.0
Calculus	2.7
Trauma	2.0
Obstruction	1.5
Others	2.3
Ureters	6.5
Calculus	5.3
Tumor	0.7
Others	0.5
Bladder	39.5
Infection	22.0
Tumor	14.9
Others	2.6
Prostate	23.6
Benign hyperplasia	12.5
Infection	9.0
Tumor	2.1
Urethra	4.3
Stricture	1.7
Calculus	1.3
Others	1.3
Essential Hematuria	8.5

From Lee LW, Davis E Jr. Gross urinary hemorrhage: a symptom, not a disease. JAMA 1953;153:782, with permission.

TABLE 129.2

DIAGNOSIS IN 500 REFERRED CASES OF ASYMPTOMATIC MICROSCOPIC HEMATURIA

Diagnosis	Patients (%)
Kidneys	6.2
Calculus	3.4
Cyst	1.2
Hydronephrosis	0.6
Tumor	0.4
Others	0.6
Ureters	0.8
Calculus	0.4
Ureterocele	0.4
Bladder	8.6
Infection	6.6
Tumor	1.8
Others	0.2
Prostate	23.6
Benign hyperplasia	23.6
Urethra	23.4
Infection	21.2
Calculus	1.8
Others	0.4
Essential Hematuria	44.0

From Greene LF, O'Shaughnessy EJ Jr, Hendricks ED. Diagnosis in 500 referred cases of asymptomatic microhematuria. JAMA 1956;161:610, with permission.

If the urinary excretion rate of red cells exceeds 1 million red blood cells per minute, macroscopic or gross hematuria will result. Macroscopic hematuria is more likely to be associated with significant genitourinary tract disease. It may be the initial symptom for transitional cell carcinoma of the genitourinary tract or adenocarcinoma of the prostate. Bladder cancer is generally a disease of the elderly, with 80% of cases overall in the 50- to 79-year age group and a median age at diagnosis in women of 71 years. The incidence of bladder cancer is three to four times higher in men than in women. In the United States, bladder cancer is 1.5 times more common in whites than in African Americans. Epidemiologic evidence linking cigarette smoking and bladder cancer is strong. The relative risk of the development of bladder and urothelial cancer for smoking is 2- to 10-fold. There is evidence of an association between the development of bladder cancer and exposure to certain carcinogens. Exposure to chemical dye, commercial paint and solvents, and antioxidants used in manufacturing rubber increase the risk of bladder cancer. Chronic or recurrent urinary tract infections are also associated with the development of bladder cancer.

WORKUP (7,11–13)

The appropriate workup depends on whether the patient has macroscopic hematuria or asymptomatic microscopic hematuria, on the age and gender of the patient, and on the mode of

clinical presentation. As indicated in the previous section, the likelihood of finding a significant genitourinary tract disease is higher in patients with macroscopic hematuria, particularly in older men. Asymptomatic microscopic hematuria in young adults, on the other hand, carries a much lower risk. Evidence from five population-based studies indicates that 1% to 5% of children and adults will show evidence of microhematuria on routine urinalysis and that fewer than 2% of these patients will have a serious and treatable urinary tract disease. However, the incidence of urinary tract cancers rises dramatically with age and is more than twice as high in men as in women. An investigation of microscopic hematuria in the older male patient should therefore be pursued.

History

History is of paramount importance in narrowing the scope of the workup. A history of trauma should direct attention to possible renal, ureteral, or urethral injury. Massive hematuria is usually associated with bladder neoplasm, benign prostatic hyperplasia, or trauma. The passage of large, bulky clots implicates the bladder as the source, whereas long, shoestring-shaped clots suggest a ureteral origin. A past history of analgesic excess makes analgesic nephropathy a possibility. A prior history of nephritis requires consideration of chronic nephritis as the basis of the hematuria. A family history of renal diseases may suggest polycystic kidney disease or hereditary nephritis. Benign familial hematuria has been described and is inherited in a pattern consistent with autosomal-dominant transmission; checking for hematuria in relatives may avoid an extensive workup in otherwise healthy-appearing patients.

Harmless, self-limited forms of microscopic hematuria are suggested by a recent history of strenuous exercise, long-distance running, or a minor febrile illness.

History of smoking, occupational exposure to chemicals used in certain industries (dye, leather, or tire manufacturing), ingestion of aristolochic acid (found in some herbal weight loss preparations), or heavy phenacetin use should all be noted because these are risk factors for bladder cancer (see Chapter 128).

Physical Examination

Physical examination should include observation of any fever, hypertension, rash, purpura, petechiae, friction rub, heart murmur, or joint swelling. The presence of hypertension suggests renal parenchymal disease. The abdomen has to be examined carefully for enlargement of one or both kidneys, liver, or spleen. Thorough examination of the prostate in the male patient and the pelvis in the female patient is essential.

Laboratory Testing

The most important test in the evaluation of hematuria is the *urinalysis,* including a microscopic evaluation of the urine. A repeated urinalysis is worthwhile in patients suspected of having a self-limited or trivial cause for their hematuria, such as low-grade infection, a menstrual period, or vigorous exercise. An entirely normal result of a repeated study in a healthy young person requires no further investigation other than a follow-up urinalysis in a month or two. However, in an older patient, whose risk for malignancy is much greater, an abnormal number of red blood cells on urinalysis should be taken seriously, even if a second urine specimen is clear. A urinary tract malignancy may present in just this manner.

The *urine sediment* should be carefully examined. The presence of white cells and bacteria favors a diagnosis of cystitis; casts of white cells imply the presence of pyelonephritis or interstitial nephritis.

Red cell casts strongly suggest glomerulonephritis. The presence of dysmorphic red cells under phase-contrast microscopy is also highly suggestive of a glomerular origin of the red cells. Although helpful when present, the absence of red cell casts and dysmorphic red cells does not exclude glomerular disease.

A urine specimen should be sent for routine *culture* when pyuria is noted (see Chapter 133). Culture for urine *acid-fast bacillus* needs to be obtained if sterile pyuria and hematuria persist.

The need for further workup is determined by the probability of important underlying pathology. For example, a patient older than age 50 years is at increased risk for urinary tract cancer; it must be ruled out. In one study, evaluation of patients older than the age of 50 years presenting with asymptomatic microscopic hematuria showed that 5% had a urologic malignancy. In patients with symptomatic microscopic hematuria, the incidence of malignancy increased to 10.5%. On the other hand, an otherwise healthy young patient with an unremarkable history, normal findings on physical examination, and an otherwise benign urinary sediment need not undergo invasive testing because the likelihood of malignancy or other serious pathology is low. In a major population study, the frequency of clinically significant microscopic hematuria was 2.3%, with only 0.5% of patients having bladder or renal cell carcinoma; malignant lesions were found almost exclusively in patients older than age 50 years. A prospective analysis of 1,930 patients with microscopic hematuria demonstrated no cancer in women younger than 40 years old and no life-threatening lesions with 2.5 to 4.2 years of follow-up.

Three *first-void morning urine* specimens are sent for *cytology* in patients older than the age of 40 years with hematuria because they are at increased risk for a neoplasm. Normal findings on cytology do not rule out a malignancy (see Chapter 128); *cystoscopy* is indicated if suspicion remains. Urine cytology is less sensitive (66% and 79% in two series) than cystoscopy in the detection of bladder cancer but has high specificity (95%).

If the origin of hematuria is still unclear after the initial evaluation, imaging studies may be necessary. In patients suspected to have stone disease, *non–contrast-enhanced helical computed tomography (CT) scan* is an appropriate test. In one study, the sensitivity for detection of stone disease was 100% with helical CT and 67% with excretory urography. In patients not suspected to have stone disease, *contrast-enhanced helical CT* is the preferred imaging modality. In a prospective study, 11 patients presenting with asymptomatic microscopic hematuria underwent CT and intravenous pyelogram before cystoscopy. Sensitivity was 100% for CT and 60.5% for intravenous pyelogram, and specificity was 97.4% for CT and 90.9% for intravenous pyelogram. CT accuracy was 98.3%, compared with 80.9% for intravenous pyelogram ($p < 0.001$). In another study examining 350 consecutive patients with asymptomatic microscopic hematuria of undetermined cause, a positive diagnosis rate of 45.1% for the causes of heretofore-refractory cases of hematuria with higher sensitivity and specificity attest to the effectiveness of the *hematuric CT protocol* and support its use. CT urography should be performed first without contrast medium and then with it. This should permit reasonable evaluation of the upper tract.

Renal function is checked when renal parenchymal disease is suspected. In patients with proteinuria, a *24-hour urine collection for creatinine and protein determinations* should be performed to assess renal function and assess the degree of proteinuria quantitatively. Heavy proteinuria (>3 g/24 hr) is usually associated with glomerular lesions (see Chapter 130).

Renal angiography is reserved for evaluation of possible renal trauma, suspected renal masses, and possible arteriovenous malformations. In the presence of renal colic, the urine should be strained to detect calculi or papillae.

If clinical evidence of glomerular disease (red cell casts, dysmorphic red cells, heavy proteinuria) is present, *immunologic studies* should be performed, and a renal biopsy should be considered. The immunologic tests of diagnostic use include the following: *antinuclear antibody, anti-DNA antibody,* and complement levels [C3, C4, and CH50 (hemolytic complement)] for the diagnosis of systemic lupus erythematosus (see Chapter 130); antistreptolysin-O titer and antiDNAseB and complement levels for the diagnosis of poststreptococcal glomerulonephritis; *serum* and *urine immunoelectrophoresis* for the diagnosis of multiple myeloma; *serum immunoglobulin A* level for patients suspected of having Berger's disease (immunoglobulin A nephropathy) or Henoch–Schönlein purpura; serum *antiglomerular basement membrane antibody* levels for patients suspected of having Goodpasture's syndrome; and *anti–neutrophil cytoplasmic antibody* levels for pauciimmune glomerulonephritis and other vasculitic disease.

INDICATIONS FOR REFERRAL

The source of microscopic hematuria remains unclear in about 70% of cases after the initial studies and the imaging studies. In a patient older than age 50 years, if a distinct lesion is still not defined or a bladder lesion is suspected, it is necessary to proceed to *cystoscopy* (see Chapter 128). The procedure is particularly useful during periods of active bleeding. Careful examination of the ureteral orifices for bleeding and biopsy of suspected lesions are essential.

Patients with gross hematuria should have infection ruled out. If there is no evidence of infection, cystoscopy should be considered because gross hematuria is associated with a higher risk of urologic cancer than is microscopic hematuria. However, a proportion of patients with macroscopic hematuria would still have no diagnosis after upper tract evaluation and cystoscopy. In follow-up of these patients, most would have no further hematuria and no significant urologic abnormalities. These findings suggest that repeat cystoscopy and upper tract imaging is only warranted in patients who have recurrent bleeding after initial investigation.

Patients with evidence of glomerulonephritis should be referred to a nephrologist for consideration of *renal biopsy*, which is indicated only to establish a diagnosis that will affect the selection of therapy (see Chapter 130) and should be reserved for patients with clinical evidence of glomerular disease. The most common lesions in patients with isolated glomerular hematuria are immunoglobulin A nephropathy, Alport's disease, and thin-membrane disease.

Rarely, renal biopsy may be indicated if the preceding studies have not led to a diagnosis.

PATIENT EDUCATION

It is essential to impress on the older patient the necessity of a complete evaluation of hematuria. The high incidence of potentially curable neoplasms in patients older than 50 years (see Chapter 143) makes thorough investigation in this group mandatory.

Annotated Bibliography

1. Jones RJ, Latinovic R, Charlton J, et al. Alarm symptoms in early diagnosis of cancer in primary care: cohort study using General Practice Research Database. BMJ 2007;334:1040. (*The 3-year cumulative cancer incidence after the first episode of hematuria was 7.4% in men and 3.4% in women.*)
2. Culclasure TF, Bray VJ, Hasbargen JA. The significance of hematuria in the anticoagulated patient. Arch Intern Med 1994;154:649. (*Anticoagulation is not associated with an increased incidence or prevalence of hematuria.*)
3. Cohen RA, Brown RS. Microscopic hematuria. N Engl J Med 2003;348:2330. (*Excellent review of the clinical approach to microscopic hematuria.*)
4. Mohr DN, Offord KP, Owen RA, et al. Asymptomatic microhematuria and urologic disease: a population-based study. JAMA 1986;256:224. (*Presents community-based prevalences of underlying disease.*)
5. Nieuwhof C, Doorenbos C, Grave W, et al. A prospective study of the natural history of idiopathic non-proteinuric hematuria. Kidney Int 1996;49:222. (*A prospective study of glomerulonephritis presenting with nonproteinuria hematuria, followed up over an 8- to 14-year period; revealed no decline in renal function; such patients are at higher risk for the development of hypertension and nephrolithiasis.*)
6. Sells H, Cox R. Undiagnosed macroscopic hematuria revisited: a follow-up of 146 patients. Br J Urol 2001;88:6. (*In patients with an episode of undiagnosed macroscopic hematuria who had no abnormalities on upper tract imaging and cystoscopy, only one had a missed tumor; repeat cystoscopy and upper tract imaging is only warranted in patients who have recurrent bleeding after the initial investigation.*)
7. Sultana SR, Goodman CM, Byrne DJ, et al. Microscopic hematuria: urological investigation using a standard protocol. Br J Urol 1996;78:691. (*Urologic evaluation will reveal malignancy in 5% of asymptomatic patients older than age 50 years and in 10.5% of symptomatic patients.*)
8. Van Savage JG, Fried FA. Anticoagulant-associated hematuria: a prospective study. J Urol 1995;153:1594. (*Of 24 patients with gross hematuria, 2 had bladder cancer.*)
9. Wai CY, Miller DS. Urinary bladder cancer. Clin Obstet Gynecol 2002;45:844. (*A review of bladder cancer; 80% of bladder cancers are diagnosed in patients in the 50- to 79-year age group.*)
10. Khadra, MH, Pickard, RS, Charlton, M, et al. A prospective analysis of 1,930 patients with hematuria to evaluate current diagnostic practice. J Urol 2000; 163: 524. (*A evaluation of 1,194 male and 736 female patients with a mean age of 58 years indicated that 61% had no basis found for hematuria, 12% had bladder cancer, 13% had urinary tract infections, and 2% had stones; kidney and upper tract tumors were noted in 0.7% of patients, including some presenting with microscopic hematuria only.*)
11. Tomson C, Porter T. Asymptomatic microscopic or dipstick hematuria in adults: which investigations for which patients? A review of the evidence. Br J Urol 2002;90:185. (*A nice review touching on a number of controversial areas of evaluation.*)
12. Gray Sears CL, Ward JF, Sears ST, et al. Prospective comparison of computerized tomography and excretory urography in the initial evaluation of asymptomatic microhematuria. J Urol 2002;168:2457. (*Computed tomography resulted in a better diagnostic yield than did excretory urography.*)
13. Lang EK, Macchia RJ, Raju T, et al. Computerized tomography tailored for the assessment of microscopic hematuria. J Urol 2002;167:547. (*Use of hematuric computed tomography protocol showed a positive diagnosis rate of 45.1% for the causes of heretofore-refractory cases of hematuria, with high sensitivity and specificity.*)

CHAPTER 130 ■ EVALUATION OF THE PATIENT WITH PROTEINURIA

HASAN BAZARI

Proteinuria may be an asymptomatic finding in an apparently healthy patient or a key diagnostic finding in a patient who presents with an acute illness. The challenge for the clinician is to identify the etiology, significance, and prognosis of proteinuria and then implement the appropriate therapy when necessary. The primary care physician should have a good sense of when to refer to a nephrologist for further evaluation and treatment based on the severity of the condition and complexity of management.

PATHOPHYSIOLOGY AND CLINICAL PRESENTATION (1–8)

The normal kidney filters about 180 L of ultrafiltrate per day. The concentration of albumin in Bowman's space is 1 mg/dL. The proximal convoluted tubule reabsorbs most of the albumin and low-molecular-weight proteins that are in the ultrafiltrate. About 150 mg or less is excreted in the urine in humans daily. The excretion of higher amounts of protein warrants evaluation. The approach is guided by an understanding of underlying mechanisms. These include the following.

Overflow Proteinuria

Overflow proteinuria occurs when there is overproduction of low-molecular-weight protein that is then filtered and excreted. The classic and most prevalent example is Bence Jones proteinuria, when excessive amounts of monoclonal light chains can be found in the urine of a patient with myeloma, amyloidosis, or, rarely, monoclonal gammopathy of uncertain significance. Light chains are less well detected by the urine dipstick compared with albumin. Hence the urine dipstick may underestimate the amount of Bence Jones protein in the urine. Quantitation of the proteinuria by 24-hour urine collection or by the use of a spot urine protein:creatinine ratio allows for measurement of the degree of proteinuria.

Tubular Proteinuria

Proteinuria may occur in conditions in which there is predominantly tubular injury. In such cases the proteinuria is usually less than 1 g/d, reflecting the failure to reabsorb small, filtered proteins, as well as proteins that originate in the tubules. These are low-molecular-weight proteins when evaluated by electrophoresis.

Increased Glomerular Permeability

Most of the significant cases of proteinuria are related to loss of the permeability barrier in the glomerular basement membrane. The proteinuria can be divided into nephrotic-range proteinuria and a subnephrotic range of proteinuria. Nephrotic syndrome is a syndrome associated with greater than 3.5 g of proteinuria in 24 hours, hypertension, hyperlipidemia, and edema. Subnephrotic-range proteinuria is usually between 1 and 3.5 g per 24 hours. Although the underlying disease may be the same, the prognosis and management are significantly better for any given entity when there is subnephrotic-range proteinuria.

The earliest clinically detectable evidence of renal involvement in some diseases may be *microalbuminuria*. Microalbuminuria, which is classically associated with diabetes, is defined as the excretion of small but abnormal amounts of albumin below the level of detection by the standard screening dipstick. *Transient proteinuria* can be seen in patients in an acute illness such as fever, pneumonia, seizures, and congestive heart failure. It is presumed that there is a transient loss of the permeability barrier in these settings. It usually resolves with treatment of the underlying condition. *Orthostatic proteinuria* occurs predominantly in the upright position. The amount of protein is usually less than 1 g per 24-hour period. Understanding of the pathophysiology is incomplete; the prognosis is good.

Clinical Presentations

Proteinuria often presents as a finding on routine urinalysis. Alternatively, it may be one of several manifestations of renal disease, including significant hypertension or renal failure. In these cases, the accompanying history and clinical features often provide clues to the etiology of the renal disease.

Isolated Proteinuria

Isolated proteinuria is a condition in which there is usually less than 1 g of protein excreted in a 24-hour period. By definition, the renal function is normal and unaccompanied by hematuria, hypertension, or a systemic disease known to have renal manifestations. When biopsied, most of these patients have either normal renal histology or minor abnormalities on the renal biopsy. Occasionally, thin basement membrane disease and immunoglobulin A nephropathy may be found on the biopsy of such patients.

Patients with isolated proteinuria can be further characterized into several groups as follows.

Transient Proteinuria. This is seen as a transient increase in glomerular proteinuria that can be brought about by exercise, fever, infection, and congestive heart failure. The proteinuria resolves completely after the acute event, and patients are normal when the urine test is repeated. It is postulated that adaptive hemodynamics induces the proteinuria and that it is mediated by increased levels of angiotensin II. This usually resolves in follow-up and warrants no further evaluation.

Orthostatic Proteinuria. There is a group of patients who seem to have long-term reproducible proteinuria that occurs in the upright position. The long-term follow-up of these patients shows an excellent prognosis over a 25-year period with no evidence of the development of significant intrinsic renal disease or progression to persistent proteinuria.

Microalbuminuria. This is the earliest detectable clinical evidence of renal disease involving the changes in glomerular permeability. In a disease such as diabetes, the onset of microalbuminuria marks the onset of clinically important diabetic nephropathy and creates a clinically detectable point of intervention for the prevention of progression to overt diabetic nephropathy. Studies have shown that blood pressure control, the use of angiotensin-converting-enzyme inhibitors (ACEIs), and the use of angiotensin-receptor blocker (ARBs) slow the progression to overt diabetic nephropathy.

Persistent Isolated Proteinuria. This refers to proteinuria of less than 1 g/d and may include patients with early forms of diseases causing eventual nephrotic syndrome. The prognosis for this group is mixed, and these patients need to be evaluated and followed for the development of overt renal disease.

Proteinuria with Intrinsic Renal Disease. *Tubular proteinuria* is often less than 1 g/d, and the composition of the proteinuria is low-molecular-weight proteins. It is often accompanied by significant decrements in glomerular filtration rate.

Other Presentations

Proteinuria of greater than 1 g/d, if not from overflow proteinuria, often reflects intrinsic glomerular disease. Proteinuria of greater than 3.5 g/d, if not from overflow proteinuria, is due glomerular disease and often is associated with the nephrotic syndrome.

Nephrotic Syndrome. Nephrotic syndrome can either be associated with primary renal disease or be part of a systemic disease. Hypoalbuminemia, hypertension, hyperlipidemia, and edema often but not always accompany the syndrome. The etiology of the edema may be either low oncotic pressure from severe hypoalbuminemia or primary salt and water retention by the kidneys. The classic teaching that low oncotic pressure is the only mechanism for the development of edema in nephrotic syndrome is erroneous. Hypertension associated with renal disease can be severe but is less prominent in minimal-change disease and HIV-associated nephropathy. The hyperlipidemia of nephrotic syndrome is due the increased synthesis of low-density lipoprotein and very low density lipoprotein by the liver. Lipid-laden tubular cells form "oval fat bodies" and may be found in the urinary sediment as individual cells or as components of casts. "Maltese crosses" may be seen under polarizing light when the droplets contain large amounts of cholesterol. Other complications of the nephrotic syndrome include the hypercoagulable state as a result of loss of anticoagulants and clotting factors. The main anticoagulant that is lost in the urine is antithrombin III; the consequences of the prothrombotic state include deep venous thrombosis and renal vein thrombosis. The most common renal disease associated with renal vein thrombosis is membranous nephropathy, in which about 20% to 30% of patients may have overt or silent renal vein thrombosis. Loss of immunoglobulins can predispose to bacterial infections, and this is a particular problem in children, in whom ascites from nephrotic syndrome can predispose to spontaneous bacterial peritonitis. Loss of vitamin D attached to its binding protein can lead to deficiency of vitamin D and hypocalcemia. In patients with hypothyroidism, the onset of nephrotic syndrome can lead to changes in dosing requirement as a result of renal losses.

DIFFERENTIAL DIAGNOSIS (9–12)

The approach to proteinuria is detailed in Fig. 130.1. The evaluation should be tailored to the type, severity, and persistence of the proteinuria.

Isolated proteinuria has a limited differential diagnosis, as discussed previously. It may be transient proteinuria, orthostatic proteinuria, or persistent with early stages of diseases that could eventually cause the nephrotic syndrome.

Proteinuria with hematuria, especially if the hematuria includes the presence of dysmorphic red blood cells under phase-contrast microscopy, indicates a glomerulonephritis with a wide differential diagnosis. These findings mandate expeditious and thorough evaluation. Among the conditions that can be associated with proteinuria and hematuria are those that cause rapidly progressive glomerulonephritis, listed in Table 130.1.

Nephrotic syndrome can be caused by idiopathic intrinsic renal disease or glomerular injury associated with systemic disease. The idiopathic nephrotic syndromes are summarized in Table 130.2. Although idiopathic membranous nephropathy has been the leading cause of idiopathic nephrotic syndrome in adults, recent series show that focal and segmental glomerulosclerosis may now be more common. Minimal-change disease remains a significant cause of nephrotic syndrome in adults but is less common than in children, among whom it is by far the

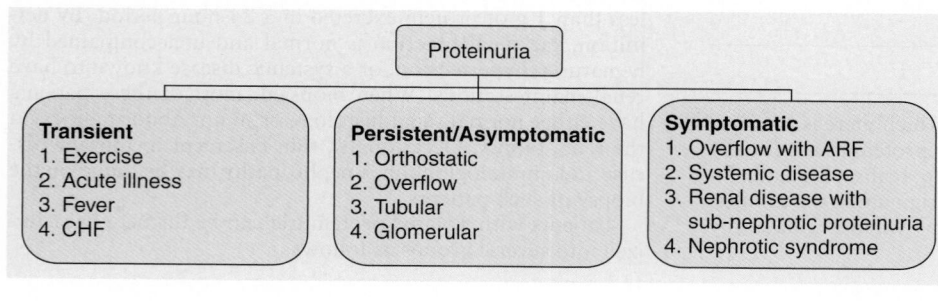

FIGURE 130.1. Approach to proteinuria. ARF, acute renal failure; CHF, congestive heart failure.

TABLE 130.1

CAUSES OF RAPIDLY PROGRESSIVE GLOMERULONEPHRITIS

Anti–glomerular basement membrane disease or
    Goodpasture's syndrome
Antineutrophil cytoplasmic antibody–positive vasculitis,
    Wegener's granulomatosis, microscopic polyangiitis,
    Churg–Strauss syndrome, pauciimmune necrotizing
    glomerulonephritis
Hypocomplementemic immune complex glomerulonephritis,
    systemic lupus, cryoglobulinemia, endocarditis,
    poststreptococcal glomerulonephritis,
    membranoproliferative glomerulonephritis
Normocomplementemic glomerulonephritis, immunoglobulin
    A nephropathy, Henoch–Schonlein purpura

leading cause. Minimal-change disease often has an abrupt and dramatic onset and is less likely to be associated with severe hypertension. Progressive renal insufficiency is rare with minimal-change disease; when it is seen it is often due to acute tubular necrosis or misclassification of focal and segmental glomerulosclerosis, which has overlapping clinical and pathologic features early in the disease.

Secondary causes of nephrotic syndrome are summarized in Table 130.3. Among these, the most common cause of significant proteinuria and nephrotic syndrome is *diabetes mellitus*, which is the leading cause of end-stage renal disease in the United States. Diabetic nephropathy is inevitably associated with the presence of diabetic retinopathy. Overt diabetic nephropathy is defined by the presence of greater than 500 mg of protein excretion in a 24-hour period, although the use of ACEIs and ARBs may mask the proteinuria. Among systemic diseases that cause nephrotic-range proteinuria, *systemic lupus* is one of the more common ones. Renal involvement in lupus can be minimally symptomatic or a cause of rapidly progressive glomerulonephritis.

Amyloidosis represents a group of diseases with a common histology and clinical spectrum but with different etiologies. All amyloid deposits share a common plasma protein called *protein P*. AL amyloidosis may be an idiopathic disease associated with the deposition of monoclonal light chains in a variety of organs. When associated with significant plasma cell infiltrates in the bone marrow, the amyloidosis is secondary to multiple myeloma. However, most often the clonal population of plasma cells in the bone marrow is not sufficient to make a diagnosis of myeloma and is referred to as primary AL amyloidosis. AA amyloidosis is a disease with the common feature of having a chronic inflammatory state such as osteomyelitis, tuberculosis, familial Mediterranean fever, and chronic draining sinuses in Crohn's disease. Transthyretin mutations are the basis of many forms of familial amyloidosis. Other forms of amyloid include the β-2 microglobulin–associated amyloidosis seen in patients with renal disease. Light-chain-deposition disease is associated with a clonal deposition of light chains in nodules mimicking diabetic nephropathy. However, the nodules usually stain for κ light chains, and there is often an underlying myeloma.

The histologic features of many of the idiopathic renal diseases can be mimicked by a variety of other conditions, including *collagen vascular disease*, *drugs*, *infections*, and *malignancies*. The response of kidneys to these various triggers highlights the limited ways in which kidneys respond to different insults and also promises further discovery of etiologies of the various causes of renal diseases currently considered idiopathic.

WORKUP (13–16)

History and Physical Examination

The history and physical examination often yield important clues to the etiology of proteinuria. The history should include a search for systemic diseases that are associated with proteinuria and renal disease, including systemic lupus, Wegener's

TABLE 130.2

IDIOPATHIC NEPHROTIC SYNDROME

Disease	Pathology	Therapy	Prognosis
Focal and segmental glomerulosclerosis	Foot process fusion by electron microscopy and segmental sclerosis by light microscopy	Steroids, cyclophosphamide, mycophenolate mofetil, cyclosporine, plasma exchange	Guarded
Membranous nephropathy	Thickening of the GBM by light microscopy, immunoglobulin G and C3 deposition along the GBM by immunofluorescence, and subepithelial electron-dense deposits on electron microscopy	Steroids, chlorambucil, cyclophosphamide, mycophenolate mofetil, cyclosporine	Good, with less proteinuria, normal creatinine
Minimal-change disease	Normal by electron microscopy and foot-process fusion by electron microscopy; normal by immunofluorescence	Steroids with cyclophosphamide, cyclosporine and mycophenolate mofetil for steroid-resistant cases	Excellent, with spontaneous and steroid-induced remission in most
Membranoproliferative glomerulonephritis	GBM thickening and immune complex deposition by immunofluorescence; subendothelial deposits by electron microscopy	Steroids, cyclophosphamide, mycophenolate mofetil	Guarded

GBM, glomerular basement membrane.

TABLE 130.3

SECONDARY CAUSES OF PROTEINURIA

Disease	Pathology	Treatment	Prognosis
Diabetes mellitus	Nodular glomerulosclerosis	ACEI, ARB, blood pressure control	Early therapy with ACEI, ARB will slow progression
AL amyloidosis	Eosinophilic, Congo red–positive deposits	Myeloma therapy	Poor
AA amyloidosis (infections such as TB, FMF, Crohn's disease, osteomyelitis)	Light chains on IF in AL	Therapy of underlying disease	Based on underlying disease
Systemic lupus	Mild mesangial to diffuse membranoproliferative; IC deposition by IF	Diffuse proliferative and membranous respond to steroids, cyclophosphamide, and mycophenolate mofetil	Responsive to therapy with steroids and cyclophosphamide or mycophenolate mofetil; prognosis related to severity of histology; mycophenolate has emerged as the favored agent over cyclophosphamide
Secondary membranous (cancers such as lung, colon; drugs such as gold, captopril; infections such as syphilis, hepatitis B, and malaria)	GBM thickening on LM, IgG and C3 deposition on IF, and subepithelial deposits on EM	Treatment of underlying disease; ACEI, ARB Withdrawal of offending agent	Prognosis based on underlying disease
Secondary minimal-change disease (drugs such as NSAIDs, Hodgkin's lymphoma)	Normal by IM and IF, podocyte foot-process fusion by EM	Withdrawal of drug or treatment of malignancy; ACEI, ARB	Prognosis related to underlying disease
Secondary FSGS (drugs such as pamidronate and heroin, infections such as HIV, obesity, reflux)	Focal and segmental sclerosis by LM; negative for immune complexes by IF and foot-process fusion by EM	Withdrawal of drug, therapy of infection, and weight loss; ACEI, ARB	Related to therapy of underlying condition or drug withdrawal
Cryoglobulinemia (myeloma, Waldenström's syndrome, hepatitis C, collagen vascular disease, and chronic infections)	MPGN by LM; immune complexes by IF and subendothelial immune complex deposits by EM	Therapy of myeloma or Waldenström's with chemotherapy; therapy of hepatitis C with interferon and ribavirin; steroids and cytotoxic therapy for severe glomerulonephritis	Myeloma and Waldenström's guarded; hepatitis C infections may respond to therapy
Bacterial endocarditis, poststrep glomerulonephritis, shunt nephritis	MPGN by LM, immune complexes by IF, and subendothelial immune complex deposits by EM	Therapy of underlying infection	Good with early treatment

ACEI, angiotensin-converting-enzyme inhibitor; ARB, angiotensin-receptor blocker; EM, electron microscopy; FMF, familial Mediterranean fever; FSGS, focal segmental glomerulosclerosis; GBM, glomerular basement membrane; IC, immune complex; IF, immunofluorescence; IgG, immunoglobulin G; LM, light microscopy; MPGN, membranoproliferative glomerulonephritis; NSAID, nonsteroidal antiinflammatory drug; TB, tuberculosis.

granulomatosis, and cryoglobulinemia. The medication history should include prescribed and over-the-counter drugs, including nonsteroidal antiinflammatory drugs. The onset of nephrotic syndrome can be dated to abrupt onset of edema and foamy urine. Illicit drug use may be the etiology of the nephrotic syndrome, as in heroin nephropathy. A history of high-risk sexual habits may lead to the suspicion of HIV-associated nephropathy. Presenting features of opportunistic infections or characteristic malignancies may also tip off the clinician to the suspicion for HIV infection. A family history of renal disease may be seen in patients with Alport's syndrome. The physical examination may also provide clues. Often the blood pressure is high in patients with renal diseases, although it may be normal in patients with amyloidosis and HIV-associated

nephropathy. The petechial rash of cryoglobulinemia or the septic emboli seen in endocarditis may be important clinical clues. There is often anasarca in patients with nephrotic syndrome. Hepatosplenomegaly, macroglossia, and carpal tunnel syndrome all may suggest amyloidosis.

Laboratory Evaluation

The evaluation of proteinuria involves a series of tests. The starting point is the *urinalysis*. The *dipstick* for protein is a very sensitive colorimetric assay; change in color is induced by the presence of proteins at a given pH. The urine dipstick is very sensitive for the presence of albumin but is much less sensitive for other proteins such as light chains. *Bence Jones protein* is better detected by *heat* and *acid tests*.

The presence of 1+ proteinuria correlates with about 30 mg/dL of albuminuria, and 3+ with greater than 500 mg/dL of proteinuria. Because the dipstick is not a quantitative measurement, small amounts of proteinuria in an oliguric patient may give the false appearance of high-grade proteinuria.

The *urine sediment* can give valuable insight into the etiology of the proteinuria. The presence of red blood cells, especially if they are dysmorphic, points to glomerular disease, and red cell casts are pathognomonic for a glomerulonephritis. The presence of white blood cells points to an acute interstitial nephritis related to an allergic reaction, an infection such as *Legionella* pneumonia, or a disease such as sarcoidosis.

A *24-hour urine collection* for the quantification of proteinuria may be valuable in the evaluation of renal disease. The collection should not include the first morning void on the first day but should include all subsequent voids, including and ending with the first morning void on the next day. Sequential collections can be used to follow the proteinuria and creatinine clearance during the course of disease in a patient or during therapy. However, the 24-hour urine collection is cumbersome and subject to inaccurate collection. Current recommendations favor the use of the *ratio of protein to creatinine* in a spot urine sample. A ratio of 3 suggests that the 24-hour protein excretion is about 3. The ratio may be inaccurate in patients with orthostatic proteinuria.

Creatinine clearance can be calculated by using a 24-hour urine for creatinine and estimating the clearance using the amount of creatinine excreted in a 24-hour period at a given serum creatinine concentration. A typical patient should produce 15 to 25 mg/kg per day, with women having relatively less muscle mass and hence less creatinine production than men. A recommended alternative is to estimate the glomerular filtration rate (GFR), using the plasma creatinine (P_{CR}, in mg/dL) and an equation derived from the Modification of Diet in Renal Disease study:

$$GFR(mL/min/1.73m^2)$$
$$= 186(P_{CR})^{-1.154}(age[years])^{-0.203}(\times 0.742 \text{ if female})$$
$$(\times 1.210 \text{ if African American})$$

Tools for the simple application of this approach are available at http://www.nkdep.nih.gov/healthprofessionals/tools/gfr—adults.htm.

The *serology studies* for the evaluation of patients with proteinuria include the following:

- *Antinuclear antibody* and, if indicated, anti–double-stranded DNA and more-specific lupus antibodies
- Complement C3 and C4 levels
- *Serum immune electrophoresis*, which identifies monoclonal gammopathy
- *Urine for Bence Jones* protein, which may be a clue to the presence of amyloidosis or multiple myeloma
- *Anti–glomerular basement antibody*, especially when there is hematuria and an active sediment; pulmonary involvement may be a clue
- *Antineutrophil cytoplasmic antibody*
- *Cryoglobulins*
- *Hepatitis B surface antigen* and *antibody* as well as hepatitis C antibody and viral titers
- *Anti-DNAse B* and *antistreptolysin O* for the diagnosis of poststreptococcal glomerulonephritis.

Renal imaging can help in selected circumstances. The presence of a single kidney may indicate the diagnosis to be sec-

ondary focal sclerosis from chronic hyperfiltration. The presence of many cysts may raise the suspicion of autosomal-dominant polycystic kidney disease. A dilated collecting system is seen in reflux with secondary focal sclerosis. Bilateral large kidneys with proteinuria may be seen in diabetes, amyloidosis, and HIV-associated nephropathy.

Older patients with nephrotic syndrome should be screened for underlying malignancies because many patients with membranous nephropathy may have an underlying malignancy. Even younger patients may have a Hodgkin's or non-Hodgkin's lymphoma. Age-appropriate cancer screening combined with a good physical examination should suffice, although additional tests may be needed such as a *chest x-ray*, and *computed tomography* scan of the lung may be done in a heavy smoker to exclude lung cancer.

Biopsies of other organs may yield a clue to the renal disease. An *abdominal fat pad biopsy* has a sensitivity of 70% to 80% for the detection of systemic amyloidosis and may make it possible to avoid a more invasive renal biopsy. Similarly, gingival and rectal biopsies may be used to make the diagnosis. *Bone marrow biopsies* are used to diagnose multiple myeloma and amyloidosis. *Renal biopsies* are used in cases of rapidly progressive glomerulonephritis, idiopathic nephrotic syndrome, glomerulonephritis of unclear etiology, chronic kidney disease of uncertain etiology, lupus nephritis for prognosis and choice of therapy, in acute renal failure of unclear etiology, and in patients with proteinuria and hematuria, in which the information may be prognostic and occasionally the information may have therapeutic implications.

INDICATIONS FOR REFERRAL

Patients with transient proteinuria that resolves do not need to be referred to a nephrologist. Patients with diabetes and microalbuminuria can be screened and treated appropriately with ACEIs or ARBs by the primary care physician without referral. The onset of overt proteinuria in a diabetic heralds the onset of overt diabetic nephropathy. A patient with concurrent retinopathy and a sediment that does not suggest glomerulonephritis can be treated with blood pressure control and the use of ACEIs and ARBs.

Patients with persistent proteinuria should be referred for evaluation, especially if there is associated renal insufficiency. Patients with nephrotic syndrome without known etiology should be referred for evaluation by a nephrologist, as should patients with an active sediment. Even orthostatic proteinuria may not be comfortably diagnosed by a primary care physician, and referral should be strongly considered.

PRINCIPLES OF MANAGEMENT (17–26)

Transient proteinuria usually resolves and needs no long-term management.

Microalbuminuria can be evaluated and managed with the addition of ACEIs or ARBs in diabetics even when the blood pressure is well within the normal range.

Persistent proteinuria of less than 1 g should be evaluated to distinguish among overflow, tubular, and glomerular etiology. Overflow proteinuria should be treated for the underlying condition producing the excess of the low-molecular-weight protein as appropriate. Tubular proteinuria should be managed to ensure that the underlying disease or toxin is eliminated.

Patients with a glomerular cause of proteinuria should be evaluated and treated for the underlying condition.

Idiopathic nephrotic syndrome is often treated with specific regimens based on the biopsy. Minimal-change disease is steroid responsive and uncommonly requires additional immunosuppression. Membranous nephropathy often responds to steroids and cytotoxic therapy. Focal and segmental glomerulosclerosis is steroid responsive about 50% of the time and may also respond to additional cytotoxic therapy. Membranoproliferative glomerulonephritis is usually unresponsive to therapy.

When the nephrotic syndrome is due to secondary causes, the treatment is often targeted to eliminating the underlying disorder. Offending drugs should be stopped. When infections are the underlying cause, the treatment should be directed to the underlying infection as in cryoglobulinemia associated with hepatitis C infection. In nephrotic syndrome associated with malignancy, the goal should be feasible resection of malignancies where appropriate. Genetic causes of nephrotic syndrome are rare and occur in young children.

When there is a nephritic component associated with proteinuria, serology followed by a biopsy is appropriate if the serologic evaluation is unrevealing. When there is rapid decline in renal function, this should be done expeditiously in the hospital. Often in the cases of rapidly progressive glomerulonephritis, empiric therapy with high doses of steroids and cyclophosphamide may be used even before a definite diagnosis is made to prevent irreversible loss of renal function.

In patients with proteinuria, there are certain common therapeutic approaches. These include the following:

- ACEI and ARB therapy. It has been demonstrated convincingly in patients with proteinuria that therapy with these agents delays the progression of chronic kidney disease. The combination of the two agents has additive effects, especially when the proteinuria is significant. These agents may be used even in the absence of hypertension.
- Blood pressure control is important in all patients with chronic kidney disease. The blood pressure goal should be less than 130/80 mm Hg.
- Aldosterone antagonists may have a role in decreasing proteinuria but may elevate potassium levels.
- Lipids are often elevated in patients with proteinuria and nephrotic syndrome and should be appropriately lowered in these patients.
- Sodium restriction to 1 to 2 g/d should be the first step in the management of edema.
- Diuretics can be important. Thiazides are often used as antihypertensives, and loop diuretics are often used for volume overload. The use of two such agents can be a powerful combination for diuresis but confers the risk of severe hypokalemia and other electrolyte abnormalities.
- Anticoagulation may be indicated for patients with deep venous thrombosis, renal vein thrombosis, or pulmonary emboli.
- Protein restriction may be indicated to prevent uremia and the progression of renal insufficiency. This should be done under the direction of a nephrologist and dietician familiar with the management of patients with chronic kidney disease (see Chapter 142).
- Vitamin D deficiency occurs both in renal disease and especially in patients with nephrotic syndrome. This should be evaluated and treated appropriately with replacement.

A.G.M.

Annotated Bibliography

1. Bernard DB. Extrarenal complications of the nephrotic syndrome. Kidney Int 1988;33:1184. (*These include edema, hyperlipidemia, hypercoagulable state, hypocalcemia, and increased susceptibility to infection.*)
2. Cirillo M, Senigalliesi L, Laurenzi M, et al. Microalbuminuria in nondiabetic patients. Relation of blood pressure, body mass index, plasma cholesterol levels, and smoking: the Gubbie Population Study. Arch Int Med 1998;158:1993. (*These cardiovascular risk factors were associated with microalbuminuria.*)
3. D'Amico G, Bazzi C. Perspectives in basic science: pathophysiology of proteinuria. Kidney Int 2003;63:809. (*An excellent, well-referenced review.*)
4. Glassock RJ. Postural (orthostatic) proteinuria: no cause for concern. N Engl J Med 1981;305:639. (*An editorial summarizing the condition and arguing that reassurance and monitoring are all that are necessary.*)
5. Robinson RR. Isolated proteinuria in asymptomatic patients. Kidney Int 1980;18:395. (*Review of pathogenesis and prognosis of isolated proteinuria.*)
6. Springberg PD, Garrett LE, Thompson AL Jr, et al. Fixed and reproducible orthostatic proteinuria: results of a 20-year follow-up study. Ann Intern Med 1982;97:516. (*Prognosis was excellent, with no renal impairment developing in the vast majority of cases.*)
7. Yamagata K, Yamagata Y, Kobayashi M, et al. A long-term follow-up study of asymptomatic hematuria and/or proteinuria in adults. Clin Nephrol 1996;45:281. (*Among patients with asymptomatic hematuria, proteinuria developed in 11% during follow-up with a mean duration of 6 years.*)
8. Ahmed Z, Lee J. Asymptomatic urinary abnormalities. Hematuria and proteinuria. Med Clin North Am 1997;81:641. (*A helpful review.*)
9. Carbone L, D'Agati VD, Cheng JT, et al. Course and prognosis of human immunodeficiency virus–associated nephropathy. Am J Med 1989;87:389. (*The condition was more common in African Americans and intravenous drug abusers; it was rapidly progressive.*)
10. Karner N, Rostaing L, Alric L. Treatment of hepatitis C-virus–related glomerulonephritis. Kidney Int 2006;69:436. (*A concise review of the current state of therapy of hepatitis C–related renal disease.*)
11. Levey AS, Lan SP, Corwin HL, et al. Progression and remission of renal disease in the Lupus Nephritis Collaborative Study. Ann Intern Med 1992;116:114. (*Prognosis is a function of the initial creatinine level and the response to initial therapy.*)
12. Abuelo JG. Proteinuria: diagnostic principles and procedures. Ann Intern Med 1983;98:186. (*A succinct review, including a detailed discussion of patients with isolated proteinuria.*)
13. Polkinghorne KR Detection and measurement of urinary protein. Curr Opin Nephrol Hypertens 2006,15:625. (*A review of the different methods for measuring proteinuria, together with a review of the data for the use of protein:creatinine ratio in assessing the degree of proteinuria.*)
14. House AA, Cattran, DC. Nephrology: 2. Evaluation of asymptomatic hematuria and proteinuria in adult primary care. Can Med Assoc J 2002;166:348. (*An excellent case-based review, with a practical diagnostic algorithm.*)
15. Levey AS, Bosch JP, Lewis JB, et al. A more accurate method to estimate glomerular filtration rate from serum creatinine: a new prediction equation Ann Intern Med 1999;130:461. (*An equation developed from the Modification of Diet in Renal Disease study provided a more accurate estimate of glomerular filtration rate.*)
16. Remuzzi G, Bengini A, Remuzzi A. Mechanisms of progression and regression of renal lesions of chronic nephropathies and diabetes. J Clin Invest 2006;116:288. (*A nice review of the mechanism of renal injury and the effect of treatment.*)
17. Bennett PH, Haffner S, Kasiske BL, et al. Screening and management of microalbuminuria in patients with diabetes mellitus: recommendations to the scientific advisory board of the National Kidney Foundation from an ad hoc committee of the Council on Diabetes Mellitus of the National Kidney Foundation. Am J Kidney Dis 1995;25:107. (*Recommends that all individuals with diabetes mellitus should be screened yearly with a spot urine albumin:creatinine ratio.*)
18. Brenner BM, Cooper ME, de Zeeuw D, et al. Effect of losartan on renal and cardiovascular outcomes in patients with type 2 diabetes and nephropathy. N Engl J Med 2001;345:861. (*Losartan reduced the incidence of a doubling of the serum creatinine concentration by 25% and end-stage renal disease by 28% but had no effect on mortality; the benefit exceeded that attributable to changes in blood pressure.*)

19. Lewis EJ, Hunsicker LG, Bain RP, et al. The effect of angiotensin-converting-enzyme inhibition on diabetic nephropathy. The Collaborative Study Group. N Engl J Med 1993;329:1456. (*Captopril slowed deterioration in renal function in insulin-dependent diabetic nephropathy and was more effective than blood pressure control alone.*)

20. Lewis EJ, Hunsicker LG, Clarke WR, et al. Renoprotective effects of the angiotensin-receptor antagonist irbesartan in patients with nephropathy due to type 2 diabetes. N Engl J Med 2001;345:851. (*Angiotensin II–receptor blocker protected type 2 diabetics against the progression of nephropathy independent of the reduction in blood pressure.*)

21. Maschio G, Alberti D, Janin G, et al. The effect of angiotensin-converting-enzyme inhibitor benazepril on the progression of chronic renal insufficiency. The Angiotensin-Converting-Enzyme Inhibition in Progressive Renal Insufficiency Study Group. N Engl J Med 1996;334:939. (*The angiotensin-converting-enzyme inhibitor benazepril protected against the progression of renal insufficiency in patients with various renal diseases but not in polycystic disease.*)

22. Mogensen CE, Keane WF, Bennett PH, et al. Prevention of diabetic renal disease with special reference to microalbuminuria. Lancet 1995;346:1080. (*A succinct review.*)

23. Nakao N, Yoshimura A, Morita Holden, et al. Combination treatment of angiotensin-II receptor blocker and angiotensin-converting enzyme inhibitor in non-diabetic renal disease (COOPERATE): a randomised control trial. Lancet 2003;361:117. (*Combination treatment safely retarded the progression of nondiabetic renal disease compared with monotherapy.*)

24. Hou FF, Zhang X, Zhang GH, et al. Efficacy and safety of benazepril for advanced chronic renal insufficiency. N Engl J Med 2006;354:131. (*A key paper, showing the efficacy of angiotensin-converting enzymes even in the setting of advanced renal insufficiency in patients without diabetes.*)

25. Bianchi S, Bigazzi R, Campese VM. Long-term effects of spironolactone on proteinuria and kidney function in patients with chronic kidney disease. Kidney Int 2006;70:2116. (*An open-label study, showing the efficacy of spironolactone when added to angiotensin-converting enzyme or angiotensin-receptor antagonists in decreasing proteinuria and slowing the rate of progression; there was a significant elevation in the potassium on spironolactone.*)

26. Tryggvason K, Patrkka J, Wartiovaara J. Hereditary proteinuria and mechanisms of proteinuria. N Engl J Med 2006;354:354. (*A review of the known mechanisms of proteinuria in genetic disorders causing this condition.*)

CHAPTER 131 ■ EVALUATION OF SCROTAL PAIN, MASSES, AND SWELLING

A mass, generalized enlargement, or acute pain involving the scrotum may be noted by the patient or discovered incidentally on physical examination. Patients with scrotal complaints are often concerned about the loss of sexual function and the possibility of cancer. The primary physician needs to be able to recognize torsion and epididymitis promptly and to differentiate benign masses from those suggestive of testicular malignancy, which require referral for urologic evaluation.

PATHOPHYSIOLOGY AND CLINICAL PRESENTATION (1–10)

Testicular Cancer

Almost all testicular neoplasms are malignant and of germ-cell origin. Fortunately, these tumors are uncommon, accounting for less than 1% of all deaths from neoplasms in men. However, testicular cancers are the most common malignancy in male patients of age 15 to 35 years, with an estimated incidence of 3 in 100,000. Incidence is increased in those with an undescended testicle and remains high even if orchiopexy is performed or the testicle is removed; the risk seems to be genetically determined. Peak incidence occurs between ages 20 and 40 years. In patients older than age 60 years, testicular lymphoma is the most common testicular malignancy.

Typically, the tumor presents as a hard, heavy, firm, nontender testicular mass that does not transilluminate, but sometimes it is smooth or even resilient in nature, and so it may be mistaken for a benign lesion, even though it blocks the trans-mission of light. Although these lesions are usually painless, about 20% cause some discomfort in the scrotum, and frank pain may be reported and tenderness noted, especially if hemorrhage into the tumor is present.

Metastasis to the retroperitoneum may cause vague pain in the back or abdomen. Spread to the chest can lead to dyspnea, cough, or hemoptysis. A palpable left supraclavicular node or epigastric mass may be noted. On occasion, extensive metastasis occurs with little evidence of the primary tumor. The metastatic lesion may be histologically different from the primary lesion. A few of these malignancies produce chorionic gonadotropin or estrogen and are associated with gynecomastia (see Chapter 99).

Nonmalignant Testicular Disease

Testicular torsion presents with acute pain and a firm, tender mass in a young patient. The annual incidence is 1 in 4,000 males younger than 25 years. The intense pain may be associated with nausea and vomiting and may be confused with an abdominal process. The condition is mostly one of adolescent boys and young men. A history of recurrent episodes of testicular pain is often present. The testicle dangles within an abnormally enlarged tunica, likened to the clapper of a bell. An attack can come on during sleep; a history of antecedent trauma is present in only 4% to 8% of cases. Torsion initially obstructs venous return, with subsequent equalization of arterial pressures leading to ischemia in as little as 4 hours.

Testicular trauma produces acute testicular pain and swelling similar to that associated with torsion or infection.

However, if the pain following trauma lasts more than 1 hour, one must consider the possibility of trauma-induced torsion. *Mumps orchitis* is usually seen 7 to 10 days after parotitis; most often, it is unilateral and accompanied by fever, swelling, pain, and tenderness. On occasion, parotitis is absent. The condition is more common in adults than in children.

Cystic and Vascular Scrotal Masses

Cystic masses containing fluid or sperm often develop spontaneously. They are slow growing and usually painless, and they may be large and fluctuant. *Hydroceles* are cystic accumulations of clear or straw-colored fluid within the tunica vaginalis or processus vaginalis. *Epididymal cysts* are common and benign. *Spermatoceles* are intrascrotal cysts containing sperm that derive from the small tubules of the epididymis. The space between the testicle and the tunica vaginalis may also fill with fluid secondary to impaired drainage or inflammation.

Varicoceles arise from incompetent venous valves. They occur on the left in 97% of cases because the left spermatic vein empties directly into the renal vein, and considerable hydrostatic pressure is transmitted into the scrotum when the valves are incompetent and the patient stands. A right-sided varicocele may occur in the context of venous obstruction or renal carcinoma. Varicoceles have a "bag of worms" appearance and are usually nontender; they decrease in size when the patient is recumbent.

Epididymitis

In men younger than age 35 years, epididymitis may occur as a consequence of gonococcal or chlamydial infection. *Ureaplasma* infection has also been implicated. Because it is a sexually transmitted disease, it may be accompanied by symptoms of urethritis (dysuria, discharge). In older men, the cause is more likely to be prostatitis, recent urinary instrumentation, or a structural lesion. Epididymitis can occur with carcinoma of the testes. Initially, tenderness and swelling are confined to the epididymis, but as the condition progresses, the inflammation may spread to the adjacent testicle, making for a large, ill-defined, tender scrotal mass.

Nontesticular Intrascrotal Malignancies

Nontesticular intrascrotal malignancies are rare and usually firm, and they do not transilluminate, which differentiates them from benign extratesticular scrotal pathology.

Inguinal Herniation

Inguinal herniation can lead to scrotal enlargement and discomfort as bowel tracks through the inguinal canal and pushes down into the scrotum.

Referred Pain

Extrascrotal sources can cause scrotal pain by stimulating one of the nerves (genitofemoral, iliofemoral, or posterior scrotal) supplying the scrotum. Scrotal examination is unremarkable.

DIFFERENTIAL DIAGNOSIS (1–8,11)

The differential diagnosis can be considered in terms of the clinical presentation. A clearly extratesticular, soft scrotal mass that transilluminates may be represent a hydrocele, spermatocele, epididymal cyst, or even generalized edema. A "bag of worms" presentation is characteristic of a varicocele. A tender, inflamed extratesticular mass is likely to be early epididymitis. Acutely painful testicular swelling may represent epididymitis, orchitis, torsion of the spermatic cord, trauma, or hemorrhage into a testicular cancer. A firm, nontender testicular nodule that does not transilluminate represents carcinoma until proven otherwise. A malignancy also has to be considered in the setting of a nontransilluminating extratesticular nodule, although benign etiologies are more common.

An extrascrotal source is suggested by pain in the absence of scrotal pathology. Causes include abdominal aortic aneurysm, ureteral colic, retrocecal appendix, retroperitoneal cancer, and prostatitis.

WORKUP (12–16)

Because testicular cancer and testicular torsion are serious but potentially curable diseases, they are prime, must-not-miss considerations in young men who present with a complaint referable to the scrotum or testicles. When torsion is suspected, the evaluation must proceed with urgency. Epididymitis is similarly curable and important to recognize because it may represent sexually transmitted disease.

History

History should include inquiry into the acuteness of symptoms, duration, clinical course, tenderness, recent trauma, urethral discharge, dysuria, fever, inguinal herniation, and concurrent infection (e.g., mumps, gonorrhea, prostatitis). A complaint of scrotal heaviness is common but nonspecific, and is found in conditions ranging from tumor to hydrocele and epididymitis. The patient's age is worth noting because testicular cancer is a disease of men younger than the age of 40 years and torsion is most common among adolescents and young men. A history of an undescended testicle raises the possibility of testicular cancer. Vague abdominal, back, or chest complaints should not be dismissed, because they may herald the onset of metastatic testicular cancer. Recurrent episodes in a young person suggest torsion (see later discussion). Concurrent flank pain, abdominal pain, prostatitis, or known extratesticular cancer suggests an extrascrotal source, especially in the absence of scrotal pathology on physical examination.

Physical Examination

When a young man presents with an acutely painful scrotum, physical examination should focus on the possibility of testicular torsion. The physical finding most sensitive for torsion is the absence of the cremasteric reflex (reflex upward movement of the testicle with stroking or pinching of the medial thigh). History and examination consistent with torsion in a patient who has had pain for less than 6 hours should lead to immediate referral for surgical exploration. The key elements of the examination in other circumstances are careful palpation of the scrotal contents and transillumination of any palpated mass. One should try to assess whether a lesion is cystic or solid, testicular or nontesticular. During inspection, the examiner should note any erythema, masses, hernias, or varices. To palpate the scrotal contents properly, one stands to the side and uses both hands, one to support the testicle and the other to feel and identify each structure, beginning with the uninvolved side. The head of the epididymis is usually situated above the testis; the body and tail run posteriorly. All are separately palpable from the testis. The normal testicle is freely movable and uniform in consistency. It is checked for abnormalities that may provide clues to disease on the involved side, such as horizontally oriented "bell clapper" mobility in a person at risk for torsion. The scrotal structures are identified and examined for tenderness, warmth, swelling, and nodularity. If a mass or a nodule is found, one attempts to determine whether it is testicular or extratesticular and whether it feels solid or cystic. The inguinal canal is examined for a hernia.

Transillumination with a penlight in a darkened room is necessary to help determine whether the lesion is cystic or solid. Cystic lesions allow the transmission of light in most instances, although a bloody exudate may not. A mass that appears to be extratesticular and cystic is most likely benign and a spermatocele, a cyst of the epididymis, or hydrocele. If it is hard, does not transilluminate, or is reported to be steadily growing, tumor must be considered, and urologic evaluation is necessary even if the mass appears to be extratesticular.

In patients suspected of having a testicular tumor, a careful check of the supraclavicular lymph nodes, chest, and abdomen is needed because more than 50% present with metastatic disease. In addition, the breasts are examined for gynecomastia. (Inguinal adenopathy does not suggest testicular cancer because the testicular lymphatics drain into the paraaortic nodes. Scrotal nontesticular lymphatics drain into the inguinal nodes.)

A tender scrotum in the absence of a mass, redness, increased warmth, or swelling should trigger a look for extrascrotal pathology. Careful examination of the abdomen for signs of appendicitis, aneurysm, and inguinal hernia is warranted, as is a check of the prostate and flanks for tenderness.

Laboratory Studies

When uncertainty persists about torsion, *testicular Doppler ultrasonography* is helpful. In testicular torsion it will show decreased blood flow; in epididymitis or orchitis, it will show increased blood flow. Radionuclide imaging is an alternative.

When a mass is noted, ultrasound is indicated to determine whether the lesion is testicular or extratesticular, solid or cystic. Measurement of human chorionic gonadotropin and α-*fetoprotein* levels is more useful for monitoring testicular cancer than for diagnosis (see Chapter 143), but a marked elevation in either is suggestive. Unfortunately, sensitivity is low; a negative study does not rule out cancer. If metastatic disease is suspected, *chest radiography* and *abdominal computed tomography* are performed as part of the staging process.

A *urinalysis* is helpful for the detection of pyuria or bacteriuria in cases suggestive of an infectious process. Semen analysis should be performed only when infertility is a concurrent complaint. A right-sided varicocele or suddenly appearing left-sided varicocele requires further evaluation because of the possibility of venous obstruction or renal carcinoma. In such cases, an *intravenous pyelogram* or *renal ultrasonography* is indicated.

When extrascrotal pathology is suspected, appropriate direction of the workup is required (see Chapters 58 and 139).

Approach to the Patient with Acute Pain and Swelling

An acutely painful, swollen testicle requires urgent assessment because if torsion of the testes is present, permanent damage may occur if treatment is not initiated within 4 hours of onset. Rates of salvage for the affected testis are 90% within 6 hours of the onset of pain, 50% within 12 hours, and 10% after 24 hours. Acute epididymitis and torsion are the two dominant considerations. Hemorrhage into a testicular cancer is a third. In an older man with concurrent prostatitis or a younger one with urethritis (see Chapter 136), epididymitis is the more likely cause of the problem. The presence of a urethral discharge, tender prostate, pyuria, or bacteriuria further supports the diagnosis of epididymitis. A firm, tender mass of acute onset in an afebrile young man with a history of prior episodes must be considered to represent torsion until proven otherwise. The diagnosis is further supported by finding a testicle with a horizontal lie on the uninvolved side. Urgent urologic consultation is necessary to determine whether the scrotum should be explored. Sometimes, it can be difficult to distinguish torsion from acute epididymitis on clinical grounds, and urgent surgical exploration is mandatory.

PATIENT EDUCATION AND INDICATIONS FOR REFERRAL

It has been suggested that teaching testicular self-examination might help shorten or eliminate the delay in presentation common in patients with testicular carcinoma. The patient with a clearly extratesticular, transilluminating scrotal lesion can be reassured that cancer is virtually ruled out and that no further evaluation for cancer is necessary other than a periodic follow-up examination. On the other hand, the person with a solid testicular mass needs prompt referral to the urologist, regardless of whether the mass is tender. Testicular cancer confined to the testicle is almost 100% curable by orchiectomy alone (see Chapter 143).

As noted, referral to a urologist should be swift in cases of suspected torsion because surgical exploration must not be delayed if a viable testicle is to be preserved. Patients in whom testicular cancer is strongly suspected are also likely to require surgical evaluation, although whenever a testicular malignancy is suspected, exploration should be conducted through an inguinal incision. Transscrotal biopsy may cause spillage of tumor into the scrotum and areas of lymphatic drainage. Any mass that cannot be confidently defined as cystic and separate from the testicle should be subjected to a urologist's examination.

A patient with varicocele should be referred if it does not deflate when he lies down, is painful, or is associated with infertility, although conception is often not achieved after correction of the varicocele (see Chapter 120). Referral to a general surgeon is needed for the patient with a poorly reducible hernia.

Most hydroceles and cystic lesions do not require surgical therapy, but the patient should be instructed to return if the enlargement becomes uncomfortable or interferes with intercourse. The patient should understand that surgery is an option that will not threaten virility or fertility. Patients may want a hydrocele removed for cosmetic reasons or for the relief of discomfort. Aspiration of a hydrocele is to be avoided.

Patients with inguinal hernias that are at risk of causing bowel strangulation should be advised to have them repaired (see Chapter 67).

A.G.M.

Annotated Bibliography

1. Ringdahl E, Teague L. Testicular torsion. Am Family Physician 2006;74:1739. (*An excellent review of diagnosis and management.*)
2. Haynes JH. Inguinal and scrotal disorders. Surg Clin North Am 2006;86:371. (*Emphasizes pediatric and adolescent conditions, but provides a very useful comprehensive review from the surgical perspective.*)
3. Cummings JM, Boullier JA, Sekhon D, et al. Adult testicular torsion. J Urol 2002;167:2109. (*The condition was found in 39% of cases in this series in men 21 years of age or older.*)
4. Davis BE, Noble MJ, Weigei IW, et al. Analysis and management of chronic testicular pain. J Urol 1990;143:936. (*A very useful discussion.*)
5. Dilworth JP, Farrow GM, Oesterling JE. Testicular tumors of nongerm cell origin. J Urol 1991;37:399. (*A comprehensive review; 126 references.*)
6. Doll DC, Weiss B. Malignant lymphoma of the testis. Am J Med 1986;81:515. (*This was the most common cause of testicular malignancy in men older than age 60 years.*)
7. Hainsworth JD, Greco FA. Testicular germ cell neoplasms. Am J Med 1983;75:817. (*A comprehensive review of evaluation and therapy; 121 references.*)
8. McGee SR. Referred scrotal pain. J Gen Intern Med 1993;8:693. (*Case reports and a review; the condition is more common than appreciated.*)
9. Williamson RCN. Death in the scrotum: testicular torsion. N Engl J Med 1977;296:338. (*A succinct discussion of the problem and its clinical diagnosis.*)
10. Witherington R, Jarrell T. Torsion of the spermatic cord in adults. J Urol 1990;143:62. (*Presentation is usually earlier in life, but adult onset does occur.*)
11. Junnila J, Lassen P. Testicular masses. Am Family Physician 1998;57:685. (*Emphasizes "must-not-miss" diagnoses: torsion, epididymitis, acute orchitis, strangulated hernia, and testicular cancer.*)
12. Haynes BE, Bessen HA, Haynes VE. The diagnosis of testicular torsion. JAMA 1983;249:2522. (*Emphasizes the importance of early diagnosis.*)
13. Krone KD, Carroll BA. Scrotal ultrasound. Radiol Clin North Am 1985;23:121. (*A comprehensive review.*)
14. Muglia V, Tucci S Jr, Elias J Jr, et al. Magnetic resonance imaging of scrotal diseases: when it makes the difference. Urology 2002;59:419. (*Ultrasound was sufficient in 97% of cases; magnetic resonance imaging was of some help in the few cases with equivocal ultrasound findings.*)
15. Richie JP, Birnholz J, Garnick MB. Ultrasound as a diagnostic adjunct for the evaluation of masses in the scrotum. Surg Gynecol Obstet 1982;154:695. (*The procedure was found to be a very useful test in indeterminate cases.*)
16. Scott RF, Bayliss AP, Calder JF, et al. Indications for ultrasound in the evaluation of the pathological scrotum. Br J Urol 1986;58:178. (*Documents the value of ultrasonography in a series of 156 men.*)

CHAPTER 132 ■ MEDICAL EVALUATION AND MANAGEMENT OF ERECTILE DYSFUNCTION

Erectile dysfunction has been defined as the inability to achieve or maintain a penile erection sufficient for satisfactory sexual intercourse. A survey among American men of age 40 to 70 years found some degree of self-reported erectile dysfunction in 52% and complete erectile dysfunction in 9.6%. Age matters. There is a 5% prevalence of complete erectile dysfunction in men 40 years old and a 25% prevalence in men 75 years old. Similar prevalences have been found in other countries. Other forms of male sexual dysfunction, including premature ejaculation, which is more common among younger men, are addressed in Chapter 229.

Recent years have seen a revolution in the evaluation and management of erectile dysfunction. Greater understanding of erectile pathophysiology led to the development and unprecedented promotion of inhibitors of phosphodiesterase type 5 (PDE-5). The availability of these drugs has affected approaches to diagnosis and treatment. The effectiveness and safety of PDE-5 inhibitors has made a therapeutic trial a reasonable approach for many men with erectile dysfunction. All of this has placed the primary care physician at the center of management decisions. With that more active role comes the responsibility fully to appreciate the level of diagnosis that is appropriate, as well as the benefits and aims of treatment.

NORMAL AND PATHOLOGIC PHYSIOLOGY AND CLINICAL PRESENTATIONS (1–12)

Normal Physiology

Penile erection is a hemodynamic process mediated by the integration of highly specialized neural and vascular mechanisms that control the rate of blood flow into and out of the highly vascular corpora cavernosa, which comprise the bulk of the penile shaft. The complex anatomy of these mechanisms is illustrated in Fig. 132.1. Blood flow is modulated by changes in the contractile state of the trabecular smooth muscle

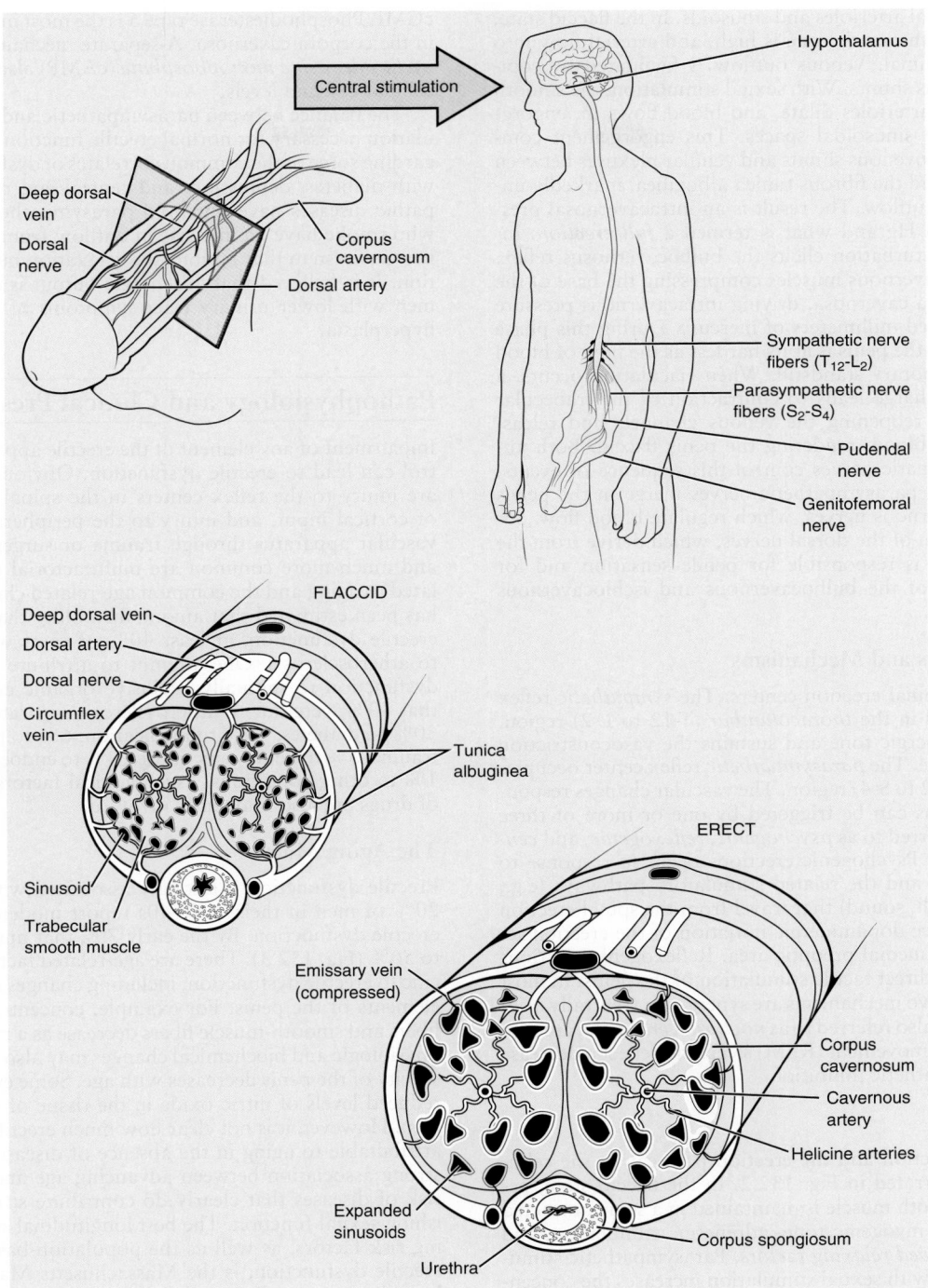

FIGURE 132.1. Anatomy of vascular and neural mechanisms of erection. Highly specialized neural and vascular mechanisms control blood flow into and out of the corpora cavernosa. Autonomic innervation is responsible for smooth-muscle relaxation, which increases blood flow into the penis when the erection pathway is triggered by direct penile stimulation or erotic stimuli. Somatic dorsal nerves are responsible for penile sensations and for functioning of the bulbocavernosus reflex. See text. (From Fazio L, Brock G. Erectile dysfunction: management update. Can Med Assoc J 2004;170:1429, with permission.)

lining the corporal arterioles and sinusoids. In the flaccid state, trabecular smooth-muscle tone is high, and arterial flow into the penis is minimal. Venous outflow is facilitated by copious arteriovenous shunts. With sexual stimulation, the smooth muscle relaxes, arterioles dilate, and blood flows in, engorging the corporal sinusoidal spaces. This engorgement compresses the arteriovenous shunts and venular plexuses between the trabeculae and the fibrous tunica albuginea, markedly impairing venous outflow. The result is an intracavernosal pressure of 100 mm Hg and what is termed a *full erection*. Intercourse or masturbation elicits the bulbocavernosus reflex, with the ischiocavernous muscles compressing the base of the engorged corpora cavernosa, driving intracavernous pressure to several hundred millimeters of mercury. During this phase of *rigid erection*, the penis is at its hardest as the flow of blood comes to a temporary standstill. When ejaculation occurs, a sympathetic discharge leads to contraction of the trabecular smooth muscle, reopening the venous channels and releasing the trapped blood, rendering the penis flaccid. Both autonomic and somatic nerves control this sequence of events. Sympathetic and parasympathetic nerves merge in the pelvis to form the cavernous nerves, which regulate blood flow. Somatic innervation of the dorsal nerves, which derive from the pudendal nerve, is responsible for penile sensation and for the functioning of the bulbocavernous and ischiocavernous muscles.

Control Centers and Mechanisms

There are two spinal erection centers. The *sympathetic* reflex center is situated in the *thoracolumbar* (T-12 to L-2) region. It controls adrenergic tone and sustains the vasoconstriction of the flaccid state. The *parasympathetic* reflex center occupies the *midsacral* (S-2 to S-4) region. The vascular changes responsible for erections can be triggered by one or more of three mechanisms, referred to as *psychogenic*, *reflexogenic*, and *centrally originated*. Psychogenic erections occur in response to erotic sensations and the related stimulatory pathways (e.g., sight, touch, smell, sound) that travel from the spinal erection centers and induce dopaminergic initiation of the erection sequence from the medial preoptic area. Reflexogenic erections are produced by direct tactile stimulation of the penis. In most instances, these two mechanisms are synergistic. Centrally originated erections, also referred to as *nocturnal erections*, are seen during rapid-eye-movement (REM) sleep and reflect a decrease in baseline sympathetic inhibition.

Mediators

Mediators of erection and the erection pathway at the cellular level are illustrated in Fig. 132.2. In the flaccid state, penile vascular smooth muscle is maintained in a semicontracted state by baseline myogenic tone, adrenergic stimulation, and *endothelium-derived relaxing factors*. Parasympathetic stimulation associated with sexual stimulation increases the concentration of *nitric oxide* in smooth muscle cells, thereby mediating the vasodilation of penile erection. High concentrations of nitric oxide are delivered to the trabecular smooth muscle by the cavernous nerves. In addition, cholinergic output stimulates endothelial nitric oxide synthase, causing an increased production of nitric oxide. The nitric oxide diffuses across the smooth muscle membrane, where it activates guanylate cyclase, stimulating the production of *cyclic guanosine monophosphate* (cGMP), which ultimately reduces cytosolic calcium concentration, causing cavernosal smooth-muscle relaxation. The pathway is regulated by phosphodiesterase enzymes that inactivate

cGMP. Phosphodiesterase type 5 is the most important isozyme in the corpora cavernosa. A separate mechanism mediated by *cyclic adenosine monophosphate* (cAMP) also decreases intracellular calcium levels.

The balance between parasympathetic and adrenergic stimulation necessary for normal erectile function offers insight regarding some of the common correlates of dysfunction. Patients with diabetes, depression, and central and peripheral neuropathic diseases have impaired parasympathetic output. Men who smoke have an increase in outflow from the sympathetic nervous system that inhibits the relaxation necessary for erection. It is believed that adrenergic output is also impaired in men with lower urinary tract symptoms of benign prostatic hyperplasia.

Pathophysiology and Clinical Presentations

Impairment of any element of the erectile apparatus or its control can lead to erectile dysfunction. Obvious organic causes are injury to the reflex centers in the spinal cord, severance of cortical input, and injury to the peripheral nerves and/or vascular apparatus through trauma or surgery. Less obvious and much more common are multifactorial explanations related to aging and the common age-related chronic diseases. It has been estimated that among men older than 50 years with erectile dysfunction, at least 40% of cases were attributable to atherosclerosis. One attempt to attribute cases of erectile dysfunction to mutually exclusive organic causes concluded that 40% were due to atherosclerosis separate from diabetes, 30% to diabetes, 15% to medication, 6% to pelvic surgery or trauma, 5% to neurogenic causes, 3% to endocrine disease, and 1% to other conditions. Psychological factors and the effects of drugs are also frequently involved.

The Aging Male

Erectile dysfunction is strongly associated with age. Roughly 20% of men in their early 40s report moderate or complete erectile dysfunction. By the early 70s, that number has grown to 50% (Fig. 132.3). There are age-related factors that are specific to erectile dysfunction, including changes in key structural elements of the penis. For example, concentrations of elastic fibers and smooth-muscle fibers decrease as a man grows older. Physiologic and biochemical changes may also contribute. Sensitivity of the penis decreases with age. Some evidence suggests reduced levels of nitric oxide in the tissue of penises of older men. However, it is not clear how much erectile dysfunction is attributable to aging in the absence of disease because of the strong association between advancing age and the increasing risk of diseases that clearly do contribute strongly to diminishing sexual function. The best longitudinal study documenting risk factors, as well as the population-based incidence of erectile dysfunction, is the Massachusetts Male Aging Study. In addition to cardiovascular disease and diabetes, submissive personality, obesity, and lower educational attainment were all associated with higher risk.

Vascular Disease

Arterial insufficiency is usually listed as a leading cause of erectile dysfunction in older men. Unexplained, progressive slowing of erection followed by decreased rigidity can be among the first symptoms of aortoiliac vascular disease when plaque obstructs the iliac arteries immediately distal to the aortic bifurcation. Erectile dysfunction develops in almost 40% of men with

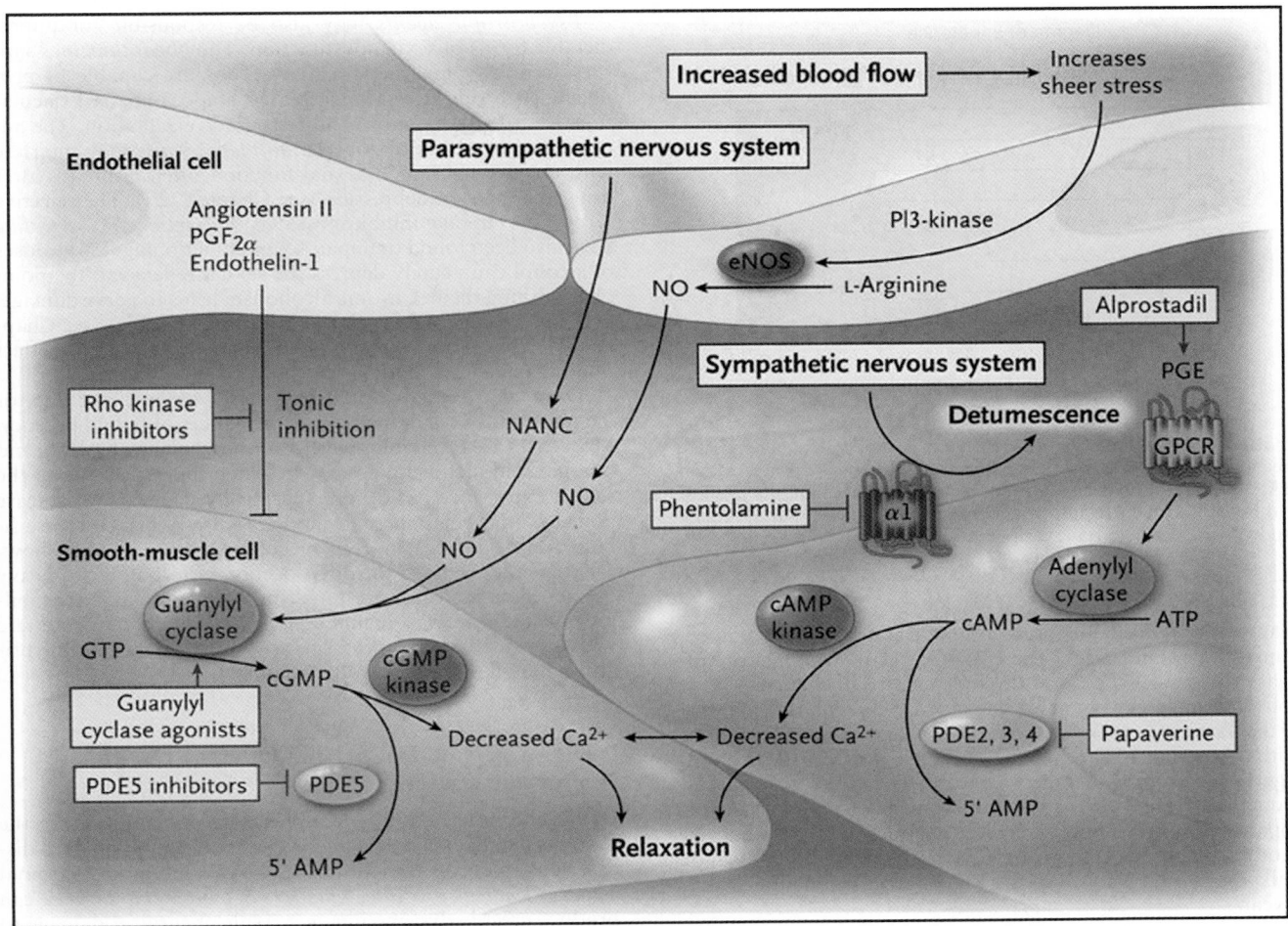

FIGURE 132.2. Mediators of erection at the cellular level. Outflow from the parasympathetic nervous system relaxes the cavernous sinusoids by increasing the concentration of nitric oxide (NO) in smooth-muscle cells. NO is the neurotransmitter in nonadrenergic, noncholinergic (NANC) fibers, and stimulation of endothelial nitric oxide synthase (eNOS) through cholinergic output causes increased production of nitric oxide. With increase in NO content, the smooth-muscle cell decreases its intracellular calcium concentration through a pathway mediated by cyclic guanosine monophosphate (cGMP), which leads to relaxation. A separate mechanism that decreases the intracellular calcium level is mediated by cyclic adenosine monophosphate (cAMP). With increased cavernosal blood flow, as well as increased levels of vascular endothelial growth factor (VEGF), the endothelial release of NO is further sustained through the phosphatidylinositol 3 (PI3) kinase pathway. Active treatments include drugs that affect the cGMP pathway (phosphodiesterase type 5 [PDE5] inhibitors and guanylyl cyclase agonists), the cAMP pathway (alprostadil), or both pathways (papaverine), along with neural-tone mediators (phentolamine and Rho kinase inhibitors). α1, α-adrenergic receptor; GPCR, G-protein–coupled receptor; GTP, guanosine triphosphate; PGE, prostaglandin E; PGF, prostaglandin F. (From McVary K. Erectile dysfunction. N Engl J Med 2007;357:2472, with permission.)

stenosis and nearly 75% of those with occlusion. Symptoms of claudication in association with erectile dysfunction, aortic or femoral bruits, and diminished peripheral pulses describe Leriche's syndrome. In some cases, the patient has the ability to initiate an erection but cannot maintain it. Patients with hypertension, diabetes, and hypercholesterolemia or who smoke are at increased risk for the compromise of penile perfusion by atheromatous disease. Radiation therapy and pelvic trauma are other risk factors for vascular injury. *Venous dysfunction* can be equally important and result from age- or lipid-induced loss of venous fibroelastic compressibility. Several authorities argue that venous dysfunction may be more important than previously suspected.

Diabetes Mellitus

Erectile dysfunction may be the presenting symptom of diabetes and is reported in up to 50% of men with the disease. Autonomic neuropathy resulting in failure of the pathways leading to vasodilation is the principal problem. In addition, endothelium-derived relaxing factor becomes deficient. Occlusive disease of larger vessels plays a much less important role

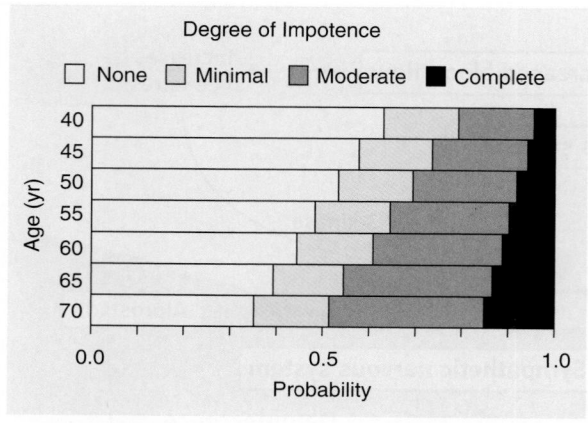

FIGURE 132.3. The probability of minimal, moderate, and complete erectile dysfunction is strongly associated with age. (From Feldman HA, Goldstein I, Hatzichristou DG, et al. Impotence and its medical and psychosocial correlates: results of the Massachusetts Male Aging Study. J Urol 1994;151:54, with permission.)

than was previously believed, although it does play an important role in some cases. The risk for erectile dysfunction appears to parallel the duration and severity of diabetes. With conventional means of achieving glucose control, the majority of diabetic men experience some degree of erectile dysfunction, with fewer than 10% achieving restoration of normal function. Aggressive control of type 1 diabetes has effected a marked reduction in the risk for the development of autonomic neuropathy. The forerunner of erectile dysfunction in the diabetic is often retrograde ejaculation. The presence of dry orgasm or milky postcoital urine augurs a loss of erectile function within 1 year.

Drugs

Although it is a common observation that drugs can interfere with sexual functioning, the precise mechanisms for the effects of particular drugs are incompletely understood. These effects are often unpredictable and may vary from patient to patient and with dose and duration. Most are reversible by reducing or discontinuing the medication.

As noted, *androgen-deprivation therapy* in the treatment of prostate cancer is now a common cause of low testosterone and resulting loss of libido. Androgen suppression with *gonadotropin-releasing-hormone* agonists (e.g., leuprolide or goserelin) is the usual approach. Antiandrogens may also be used (e.g., *flutamide, bicalutamide, nilutamide*).

Antihypertensives are frequently to blame (see Chapter 26), although less so than in the past with the decline in the use of centrally acting agents like methyldopa, clonidine, and reserpine, and diuretics leading the list. Erectile dysfunction has also been observed in patients taking antihypertensives with peripheral activity (e.g., hydralazine, thiazides, prazosin) and with beta-blockers. In patients with underlying vascular insufficiency, antihypertensives may contribute to erectile dysfunction by lowering perfusion pressure. Ganglionic blockers may inhibit parasympathetic activity from the sacral segments of the cord or sympathetic activity from the sympathetic chain. Although most antihypertensives have been implicated, the calcium-channel blockers and angiotensin-converting-enzyme inhibitors appear to interfere least with sexual function.

Psychotropic agents may also be responsible for unpredictable forms of sexual dysfunction. The *phenothiazines* suppress central sympathetic activity. They are capable of producing such side effects as decreased libido, impaired ejaculation, erectile dysfunction, and retrograde ejaculation. The anticholinergic effects of *tricyclic antidepressants* may interfere with erection, although sexual function often improves after drug treatment of depression (see Chapter 227). The selective serotonin reuptake inhibitors (SSRIs) *fluoxetine* and *sertraline* have also been found to impair sexual functioning. Large doses of alcohol can acutely depress the sexual reflexes to the point of abolishing them. Chronic alcoholism leads to nerve damage, liver failure, and high levels of circulating estrogens (see Chapter 71). *Exogenous estrogen* therapy may have a similar effect of diminishing the libido.

Drug abuse involving barbiturates, heroin, morphine, or methadone can result in major disturbances of sexual potency. Most cases are reversible. Marijuana, amyl nitrite, hashish, and lysergic acid diethylamide may heighten the perception of the sexual experience but do not specifically increase or decrease potency. Amphetamines, in moderate users, may increase libido and delay orgasm, thus prolonging the sexual act; however, erectile dysfunction often occurs with long-term, heavy use. Cocaine increases both male and female sexual excitability, but side reactions, including a flight of ideas, may interfere with sustained sexual performance. Episodes of painful priapism may develop in chronic abusers.

Pelvic Surgery or Trauma and Other Neurogenic Causes

Damage to either central or peripheral nerves can cause erectile dysfunction. Stroke, Alzheimer's disease, and Parkinson's disease cause a decrease in libido and an overinhibition of spinal centers. *Radical prostate, bladder,* or *colorectal surgery* can produce erectile dysfunction as a result of surgical damage to the pelvic autonomic nerves. The incidence of radical prostate surgery has increased dramatically in recent decades due to increased clinical detection of prostate cancer. Improved understanding of the course of these autonomic fibers has led to revised surgical techniques, such as *nerve-sparing radical prostatectomy* to lower the risk for erectile dysfunction. Some surgeons have reported good results, but the procedure cannot be performed in all cases. (See Chapter 143.) Neurogenic erectile dysfunction can also be caused by radiation therapy, which is also increasingly used for prostate cancer.

After radical *retroperitoneal lymph node dissection* for testicular tumors, ejaculatory failure may develop in young men as a result of bilateral resection of the paraaortic sympathetic ganglia, but erectile dysfunction rarely develops. *Bilateral sympathectomy* of lumbar ganglia at L-1 will inhibit ejaculatory capacity, but not orgasmic sensation, in more than half of cases. More than 75% of all men with *spinal cord injuries* demonstrate some erectile capacity, but only 25% are able to engage successfully in intercourse. The erection is reflexogenic, requiring continued penile stimulation to be maintained. Erections are totally abolished when local destruction of spinal segments S-2 to S-4 or their roots is complete. Again, the higher the location of the lesion, the better are the chances of a good erection. Ejaculation is rare when the lower thoracic and upper lumbar segments (approximately to L-3) of the cord are so extensively damaged that the nearby sympathetic components are destroyed. Sexual sensation is abolished with transection anywhere above the sacral level. Herniated intervertebral disks and metastatic cancer of the vertebral column, especially between

T-10 and L-5, which cause local swelling and destruction of spinal cord tissue, may produce a similar clinical picture.

Endocrine Diseases

The common denominator of most other endocrinopathies causing erectile dysfunction is decreased libido and a decline in serum testosterone. The most common cause for decreased androgen and resulting loss of libido is *androgen-deprivation therapy* for prostate cancer. *Hypogonadism*, whether a result of chromosomal, pituitary, or testicular disorders, involves non-development or regression of the secondary male sex characteristics, along with feeble libido and waning potency. When the cause is testicular failure, gonadotropin levels will be very high; when a pituitary or hypothalamic cause is present, gonadotropin levels will be low. *Hyperprolactinemia* is an important source of pituitary-derived erectile dysfunction. Serum testosterone levels fall as gonadotropins decline, although erectile dysfunction seems to be more closely related to the degree of prolactin elevation. A reduction in prolactin restores erectile function. Hyperprolactinemia may be idiopathic, the result of a functioning pituitary adenoma, or a consequence of *hypothyroidism* (stimulated by high levels of thyroid-stimulating hormone; see Chapter 100). It must be remembered that low levels of testosterone are involved in the pathophysiology of erectile dysfunction in a small percentage of affected men. *Addison's disease* tends to lead to loss of libido and erectile dysfunction. *Cushing's syndrome*, except when associated with adrenal carcinoma, impairs libido and potency after an initial period (weeks or months) of marked increase. *Acromegaly* leads to an early impairment of potency and a premature extinction of function. The decline in function is frequently preceded by a hyperlibidinal period.

Prostatic Disease

Benign prostatic hyperplasia (BPH) and resulting lower urinary tract symptoms are very common among men in age groups most at risk for erectile dysfunction. A number of recent studies suggested an association between BPH and erectile dysfunction, but the pathophysiologic relationship between the two is unclear. Increased sympathetic outflow and impaired nitric oxide content in the penis, prostate, and bladder have been described as possible explanations. Early evidence suggests that PDE-5 inhibitor therapy may improve urinary function, as well as erectile function.

Erectile dysfunction may be the first symptom of *prostate cancer*. Advancing centrifugal growth of neoplastic tissue in the posterior lobe of the prostate may induce local swelling and destruction of the parasympathetic fibers that run along the posterolateral aspect of the prostate. *Prostatitis* may cause painful ejaculations and even hematospermia. Premature ejaculation and postcoital fatigue occur, but erectile dysfunction is not characteristic.

Other Causes

Pelvic fracture, resulting from a crash injury in which the posterior urethra is ruptured, causes erectile dysfunction in 25% to 30% of cases. Nonperformance may result from painful intromission associated with *Peyronie's disease*, *balanitis*, acute *gonorrhea*, *herpes genitalis*, or *phimosis*. Hypospadias with a chordee of the shaft can preclude intercourse. With *priapism*, erection may be only partial and insufficient for intercourse because irreversible fibrosis of the corpora cavernosa has occurred. A large hernia or hydrocele may mechanically interfere with coitus, although potency should remain intact.

Psychogenic Conditions

Anxiety and depression are potent precipitants of erectile dysfunction. The marked sympathetic outflow that accompanies anxiety increases alpha-adrenergic tone and impedes trabecular smooth-muscle relaxation. In addition, cortical influences may inhibit sacral cord reflexes that would normally trigger erection by way of parasympathetic stimulation (see Chapter 229). Performance anxiety, relationship problems, and stress are often contributors.

DIFFERENTIAL DIAGNOSIS (1–3,6,12,13)

The differential diagnosis of erectile dysfunction is broad, as reflected in the listed description of clinical presentations. In many patients, especially the elderly, sexual dysfunction is multifactorial in origin. Both psychological and organic factors are often present, and in many instances, more than one medical condition is involved. Etiologies and contributing factors are summarized in Table 132.1.

WORKUP (1–3,6,12–15)

Advances in the pathophysiologic understanding of erectile dysfunction and the availability of safe and effective treatment in the form of *PDE-5 inhibitors* have dramatically altered the approach to workup. Before PDE-5 inhibitors, patients were often subjected to extensive laboratory investigation either before or after referral to a specialist. Now, however, a therapeutic trial of a PDE-5 inhibitor usually follows a workup that includes little more than a careful history and physical examination. It is important to distinguish erectile dysfunction from other dysfunctions such as premature ejaculation or loss of libido. The severity of erectile dysfunction can be assessed using a validated questionnaire such as the International Index of Erectile Function (IIEF). Once the presence of erectile dysfunction has been confirmed and the degree of dysfunction assessed, the evaluation can shift to differentiating psychogenic from organic disease. If psychogenic disease is deemed likely, the evaluation concentrates on underlying causes (see Chapter 229). If organic disease is more probable, then the search begins for historical and physical findings suggestive of an underlying precipitant.

History

Differentiating Organic from Psychogenic Disease

The onset of the condition, its clinical course, and its effect on morning erections help to differentiate psychogenic from organic mechanisms. A sudden onset and the preservation of erections on awakening or with masturbation are suggestive of psychogenic disease. A gradual onset and the progressive loss in duration and strength of morning erections and erections associated with masturbation and coitus are more consistent with organic disease. These distinctions are not absolute. For example, depression may be associated with a temporary loss of morning erections, mimicking organic disease. Inquiry into libido is also important. Other forms of sexual dysfunction, such as premature ejaculation, may evoke performance anxiety, which in turn may lead to erectile dysfunction.

Because an intact nervous system, blood supply, and sexual apparatus are necessary to achieve an erection, any

TABLE 132.1

CAUSES OF ERECTILE DYSFUNCTION

Aging
Structural changes
Physiological changes

Cardiovascular Disease
Peripheral vascular disease
Radiation injury
Venous dysfunction

Diabetes
Autonomic neuropathy
Vascular disease

Drugs
Gonadotropin-releasing-hormone agonists
Antiandrogens
Antihypertensives (especially beta-blockers and diuretics.)
Phenothiazines
Tricyclic antidepressants
Selective serotonin reuptake inhibitors
Protease inhibitors
H_2 antagonists
Cytotoxic agents
Exogenous estrogens
Illicit drugs

Neurogenic
Stroke
Alzheimer's disease, Parkinson's disease
Surgical injury to nerves
Spinal cord injuries
Autonomic neuropathy

Endocrine Diseases
Androgen-deprivation therapy
Hypogonadism
Hyperprolactinemia
Hypothyroidism
Addison's disease
Cushing's syndrome
Acromegaly

Psychogenic
Anxiety
Depression
Relationship issues

Other
Prostate disease
Injury to penis

occurrence of erection and ejaculation warrants careful exploration of possible psychogenic contributors. However, it is important to recognize that in the early phases of organically determined erectile dysfunction, many patients retain some erectile function and are more likely to report a decrease in number of erections, rapid detumescence after penetration, or inability to obtain a sufficiently hard erection for intercourse. Further confusing the issue, early organic disease almost always triggers performance anxiety, which exacerbates dysfunction.

Inquiry into Medical Etiologies

Of primary importance is checking for symptoms of diabetes (see Chapter 102), alcohol abuse (see Chapter 228), and atherosclerosis, particularly aortoiliac disease (see Chapter 23). Progressive difficulty in achieving erection and decreased

rigidity may be the presenting manifestation of aortoiliac insufficiency. Atherosclerotic risk factors (hypertension, smoking, diabetes, hyperlipidemia) should be noted. All medications should be reviewed, especially antihypertensives, major tranquilizers, antidepressants, other drugs with anticholinergic activity, and histamine$_2$-blockers with antiandrogenic effects (e.g., cimetidine). Careful inquiry into substance abuse is also indicated (see Chapter 235). If libido is reduced, it is worth checking for symptoms of thyroid disease (see Chapters 103 and 104), hyperprolactinemia (see Chapter 100), hypogonadism (see Chapter 120), and adrenal disease. Past medical history is reviewed for the more obvious and less common precipitants, including radical prostate or pelvic surgery, pelvic irradiation, spinal cord injury, multiple sclerosis, cancer, and pelvic fracture.

Physical Examination

The vital signs should be checked for postural fall in blood pressure (indicative of autonomic or adrenal insufficiency), the general appearance for loss of secondary sexual characteristics, and the skin for spider angiomata, palmar erythema, excessive dryness, hyperpigmentation, and other dermatologic signs of endocrinopathy. The neck is noted for goiter.

The flaccid penis is inspected for tumor, inflammation, discharge, phimosis of the foreskin, and the hard plaques of Peyronie's disease along the dorsolateral aspect of the shaft. If possible, assessment of the erect penis should be attempted, especially if disease of the shaft is suspected, so that precise information on the degree of chordee or erectile weakness can be obtained. Testicles and prostate are checked for size, masses, nodules, and tenderness. Small, soft testes suggest hypogonadism. Intrascrotal pathology such as varicocele, hydrocele, or inguinal hernia may mechanically interfere with performance and can be readily detected by a careful examination (see Chapter 131).

The aorta and femoral arteries should be palpated and auscultated for bruits and other signs of occlusive disease, especially if the patient has a history of claudication (see Chapter 23). Any femoral bruits are noted. The spine is checked for focal tenderness and evidence of cord compression (see Chapter 147). Neurologic assessment includes testing for pain sensation in the genital and perianal areas and checking the bulbocavernosus reflex to determine the integrity of second, third, and fourth sacral segments of the spinal cord. This reflex is achieved when the anal sphincter contracts around the examining finger as the glans is squeezed. A positive response indicates that S-2, S-3, and S-4 are intact. Evidence of a cortical, brainstem, spinal cord, or peripheral deficit may be an important clue to etiology.

Laboratory Studies

Ordering a routine battery of tests is rarely helpful. Moreover, no single test or set of tests rules out organic disease. The best approach is to tailor the laboratory workup to match the patient's clinical presentation.

Chemistries

A serum *glucose* determination or *hemoglobin A1c* may be ordered when diabetes is suspected (see Chapter 93). Hypothyroidism is best confirmed by an elevated level of *thyroid-stimulating hormone*. Measurement of serum total *testosterone* and *luteinizing hormone* is indicated when reduced libido accompanies erectile dysfunction but is not otherwise indicated.

Pooled samples of each (obtained 30 to 60 minutes apart) are necessary to avoid a sampling error from the large oscillations in serum concentration that can occur every few hours. A consistently low testosterone level confirms hypogonadism. Measuring luteinizing hormone and *prolactin* levels help to differentiate pituitary etiologies from primary gonadal failure (see Chapter 120). Abnormally high concentrations of total testosterone are seen with hyperthyroidism and represent an indication for testing of thyroid-stimulating hormone. If evidence of peripheral vascular disease is present, a *cholesterol* profile can help to guide therapy (see Chapter 27).

Other Studies

Other studies include attempts to confirm a loss of erectile function by monitoring for *nocturnal tumescence* in the patient who reports a total absence of erections, including those normally experienced on awakening from sleep. The physiologic basis for testing at night is the observation that 80% to 95% of young men experience erections during REM sleep. Although the percentage falls with age, nocturnal monitoring represents the most sensitive means of testing for intactness of the erectile apparatus. The absence of nocturnal tumescence indicates advanced organic disease and remains the gold standard for detecting organic erectile dysfunction. However, in early organic disease, some erectile function and morning episodes may persist. Thus, the demonstration of tumescence does not negate the need for further medical evaluation. Tumescence studies are done less frequently in the era of PDE-5 inhibitors and need not be performed before a therapeutic trial is initiated.

Most other studies are the province of the specialist in male erectile dysfunction, and they are used much less frequently. The vascular apparatus can be assessed by *Doppler ultrasonography*, both in the flaccid state and, more meaningfully, after an *intracavernosal injection* of a vascular smooth-muscle relaxant. Color flow technology provides excellent images. Papaverine alone or in combination with the alpha-blocker phentolamine can be used for the intracavernosal injection. Inability to achieve a full erection within 5 to 10 minutes of injection or an erection that is only partial or lasts less than 1 hour strongly suggests vascular disease. However, the very anxious patient with a normal vasculature may have a false-positive result because of the effect of adrenergic discharge. Patients in whom sacral neurologic injury is suspected clinically can be objectively tested by measuring the *sacral nerve reflex latency time*. One applies an electrical stimulus to the penile shaft and measures the time it takes for the bulbocavernosal muscles to contract. A time greater than 35 msec is strongly suggestive of pathology in the nerves comprising the sacral reflex arc. Referral to a specialist for this level of investigation is rarely necessary.

SYMPTOMATIC MANAGEMENT AND PATIENT EDUCATION (1–3,6,9–10,12,16–35)

Psychological Support

Erectile dysfunction can be deeply upsetting to the man and his partner. An empathic approach to educating the patient, regardless of age and marital circumstances, can be extremely helpful. Reviewing the mechanism of erection and how it is impaired provides a rational basis for diagnosis, prognosis, and treatment. Men and their partners should understand the mul-

tifactorial nature of most cases. Most patients with organic etiologies acquire performance anxieties when their ability to engage in sexual intercourse becomes impaired. Performance anxiety can also be associated with other forms of sexual dysfunction such as premature ejaculation or retrograde ejaculation. Regardless of the cause, performance anxiety can result in full loss of function in a patient who is only partially compromised physiologically. Fortunately, effective treatment is available for most men. For example, the older man with retrograde ejaculation due either to prostate surgery or diabetes can often be reassured by giving him an understanding of his condition. The man whose erectile dysfunction was preceded by premature ejaculation might benefit from treatment with SSRI (e.g., sertraline, fluoxetine) (see Chapter 229) before the initiation of treatment for the erectile dysfunction with a PDE-5 inhibitor (see later discussion).

Adjustment of Medication Program

Before prescribing medication for erectile dysfunction, it is incumbent on the physician to be sure that it is not medication induced. Patients taking an antihypertensive medication implicated in erectile dysfunction might benefit from a trial of dose reduction or from switching to an angiotensin-converting-enzyme inhibitor (e.g., captopril), a calcium-channel blocker (e.g., nifedipine), or a relatively selective beta-blocking agent (e.g., atenolol) (see Chapter 26). The patient experiencing erectile dysfunction and loss of libido with the use of cimetidine can be switched to ranitidine, which is similar in efficacy but has no antiandrogen effect. The depressed patient whose erectile dysfunction is clearly related to drug therapy can be tried on a tricyclic antidepressant with less anticholinergic activity (e.g., nortriptyline, desipramine). Switching to an SSRI (e.g., sertraline, fluoxetine) may not help because it also can impair sexual functioning. The psychotic patient with sexual dysfunction believed linked to the medication program should be referred to the psychiatrist for adjustment of the drug regimen.

Phosphodiesterase Type-5 (PDE-5) Inhibitors

Effective oral therapy for erectile dysfunction of most causes is now available. *Sildenafil* (Viagra) was the first PDE-5 inhibitor approved for use in the United States. *Vardenafil* (Levitra) and *tadalafil* (Cialis) have since also been approved. These drugs selectively inhibit PDE-5, thereby blocking metabolism of cGMP, so that concentrations are sufficient to effect the trabecular smooth-muscle relaxation necessary for engorgement of the corpus cavernosum. Nitric oxide release from the cavernous nerves is still necessary for the production of cGMP. Thus, sexual arousal and intact neural pathways are prerequisites for PDE-5-inhibitor effectiveness. For example, PDE-5 inhibitors are effective among men who have undergone radical prostatectomy for prostate cancer only if sparing of the neurovascular bundles has been possible. Effectiveness is also limited when marked vascular insufficiency limits the inflow of blood or when cavernosal fibrosis is present. However, for almost all other forms of erectile dysfunction, including those of psychogenic and mixed causes, it can be helpful. At maximum doses, a 100% improvement in erectile function is noted among responders in comparison with baseline, with successful sexual intercourse achieved in more than two thirds of attempts. Although these drugs have no effect on sexual desire, some improvement in orgasmic function does occur.

Sildenafil and vardenafil have similar pharmacokinetics, reaching peak concentrations 40 to 60 minutes after dosing and with half-lives of roughly 4 hours. Sildenafil is available in 25-, 50-, and 100-mg tablets; vardenafil is available in 10- and 20-mg tablets; and tadalafil comes in 5-, 10-, and 20-mg tablets. Tadalafil takes 2 hours to reach peak concentration and has a much longer half-life, more than 17 hours. Trials have demonstrated that effectiveness lasts 24 to 36 hours, reflecting the longer half-life. In clinical practice, there is little difference among the three in speed of onset of effect, with vardenafil taking roughly 20 minutes and sildenafil and tadalafil both taking 30 to 40 minutes. No more than one dose per day is recommended for any of the PDE-5 inhibitors. The cost of these drugs is high, averaging well above $10 per dose.

It is important to inform patients that PDE-5 inhibitors have no effect on sexual desire, despite direct-to-consumer advertising that strongly suggests otherwise, and that they work only in the context of sexual arousal. Adverse effects are transient and include *flushing, headache, visual disturbances* (alterations in hue or brightness), and *dyspepsia*. Priapism has been reported anecdotally, but there is no clear association. Similarly, nonarteritic anterior ischemic optic neuropathy has been reported, but only in high-risk individuals with long-term diabetes and hypertension, and it is not clear that there is a causative link.

PDE-5 inhibitors do cause some vasodilation, and several reported deaths have been caused by significant *hypotension*, which occurs when the drug is given concomitantly with nitrates used in the treatment of ischemic heart disease. PDE-5 inhibitors should *not* be prescribed for patients taking nitrates because of the risk for nitrate potentiation resulting in severe hypotension.

Stress-test studies suggest that men with erectile dysfunction and ischemic heart disease can use PDE-5 inhibitors without experiencing adverse cardiovascular effects, provided they are not using nitrates concurrently. Consensus recommendations have been made for men based "low," "high," and "intermediate/indeterminant" cardiovascular risk associated with sexual activity. Those considered at low risk for coital myocardial infarction or death include men with asymptomatic disease and fewer than three cardiovascular risk factors; controlled hypertension; mild, stable angina pectoris who have undergone noninvasive evaluation without evidence of ischemia; a history of revascularization with subsequent stress-testing assessment of residual ischemia; a history of myocardial infarction (>6 to 8 weeks prior) who are asymptomatic, do not exhibit treadmill-induced ischemia, or have undergone revascularization; mild valvular disease; or New York Heart Association class I left ventricular dysfunction. The recommendation for men so designated "low risk" is to initiate or resume sexual activity and treat for sexual dysfunction if necessary.

It is essential that any antianginal regimen be modified to accommodate drug therapy. PDE-5 inhibitors are contraindicated in men taking nitrates. The past use of nitrates greater than 2 weeks before the use of PDE-5 inhibitors is not considered a contraindication. It is recommended that men who develop angina during sexual activity while using a PDE-5 inhibitor should discontinue sexual activity, relax for 5 to 10 minutes, and seek emergency care if the pain persists, informing the emergency medical personnel that a PDE-5 inhibitor was taken. Patients who develop chest pain after taking sildenafil or vardenafil are advised not to take nitroglycerin for 24 hours; a 48-hour period is advised for tadalafil. Among men with heart disease or risk factors, the lowest dose (e.g., 25 mg of sildenafil) should be prescribed initially, with increase to a moderate dose (e.g., 50 mg of sildenafil) only if necessary.

Men with heart disease at other than "low risk" as defined earlier for a coital cardiac event should not initiate or resume sexual activity until their cardiac condition is stabilized (for those at "high risk") or further cardiovascular assessment has been made (for those at "intermediate/indeterminant risk").

Intracavernosal Injection Therapy

Local intracavernosal injection of smooth-muscle relaxants and alpha-adrenergic blockers has been effective in a wide variety of patients. Diabetics, patients with neurologic injury, those with psychogenic erectile dysfunction, and even some with vascular insufficiency have regained their ability to engage in successful sexual intercourse with intracavernosal injection therapy, which is a substantial advance for many patients. Follow-up of men introduced to penile injection therapy indicates that more than 70% are sufficiently satisfied to continue treatment. Of those who stop, most do so because of cost; fewer than 1 in 7 who stop do so because of ineffectiveness. However, with the advent of oral PDE-5 therapy, intracavernosal therapy has been relegated to second-line treatment.

Among the agents that have been used for intracavernosal therapy are *papaverine*, which directly relaxes trabecular smooth muscle; *phentolamine*, a short-acting, alpha-adrenergic blocker that increases arterial inflow; and *alprostadil* (an aqueous preparation of prostaglandin E1) that both relaxes smooth muscle and causes vasodilation. Within 10 to 15 minutes of injection in responding patients, an erection develops and lasts for up to 1 hour. Patients with neurologic disease and psychogenic erectile dysfunction respond most readily and require the smallest doses of medication. Underlying vascular disease is less responsive and necessitates larger doses. Alprostadil is most effective and involves the lowest risk of priapism. The most common side effect of alprostadil is pain at the injection site in 20% to 50% of cases, but this is problematic only in about 11% or cases and depends on the preparation used. Combining a modest dose of alprostadil with papaverine provides better results and less pain than papaverine plus phentolamine or larger doses of alprostadil alone. A combination of alprostadil, phentolamine, and papaverine has also been shown to be effective.

The recommended frequency of use of injection therapy is no more than three times per week and no more than once in 24 hours. Dose determination requires titration in the office and should be managed by a urologist. The optimal candidate for intracavernosal injection is the patient who has not had success with PDE-5 treatment despite an intact vascular apparatus and with the intelligence and dexterity to self-inject properly. However, even those with concurrent vascular disease may benefit, albeit with higher doses required, increasing the risk for side effects and complications. Diabetics have especially benefited because the treatment directly addresses their underlying pathophysiology.

For patients who do not have success with PDE-5 inhibitors and cannot tolerate injection therapies, *transurethral delivery* of alprostadil should be considered. This approach has been shown to be effective in about 40% of men who failed to respond to sildenafil.

Penile Implants and Other Mechanical Devices

A penile prosthesis is a consideration for the patient with refractory erectile dysfunction who expresses a serious need to regain his capacity to engage in coitus. Of the three types of prostheses available, the simpler ones (the semirigid and adjustable malleable types) have proved to be the most satisfactory. They are least likely to fail and have the fewest complications associated with their implantation and use. Although they might seem the most "natural," the inflatable prostheses have much higher breakdown and complication rates, so that surgical revision is often necessary. Reoperation rates range as high as 44%. The reservoir tends to leak, and infection is a risk on the order of 1% to 10%. Overall, patient and partner satisfaction with prostheses is in the range of 80% to 90%, with little difference reported among users of the various types. Careful counseling is required before implant surgery is elected. If the cause of erectile dysfunction is a poor interpersonal relationship, then a prosthesis is going to have little effect.

Vacuum suction devices have been used widely, especially among the elderly. A plastic cylinder is placed over the flaccid penis and connected to a hand-operated vacuum pump. The negative pressure in the cylinder facilitates passive blood flow into the penis. A band is placed at the base of the penis to retard venous outflow, and the cylinder is removed. The device works best in patients who respond to penile injection therapy and is an alternative to such therapy. Pain, ecchymoses, and difficulty ejaculating are experienced by about 10% of men. Coitus is successfully achieved in about 80% after 3 months of use. Vacuum pump use has decreased during the PDE-5 era.

Vascular Surgery

Patients with vascular insufficiency have yet to achieve consistently successful results after reconstructive surgery. Correction of aortoiliac disease often meets with disappointing results because of the high frequency of coexisting disease in distal vessels. Microsurgical techniques have been employed to correct vascular disease within the penis. Success rates range from 20% to 80%. The best results are obtained in young men with traumatic vascular injury; the worst results are in older men with diffuse atherosclerotic involvement of the cavernosal artery.

Hormone Therapy

Testosterone therapy should be reserved for patients with hypogonadism, manifested by a low serum testosterone level, and testosterone should not be used as an all-purpose sexual stimulant. It has little effect in impotent patients with normal testosterone concentrations (although it may add to frustration by increasing their libido). In such patients, particularly the elderly, the use of testosterone is associated with a high incidence of adverse effects, including sodium retention, prostatic enlargement, gynecomastia (from peripheral conversion to estrogens), and polycythemia. Patients with concurrent adenocarcinoma of the prostate may experience a serious flare of their testosterone-responsive disease.

Treatment may be intramuscular, transdermal, or oral. Meta-analysis of trials indicates that intramuscular and oral routes have equivalent effectiveness. Transdermal administration appears to be the most effective of the three routes. Patients with hyperprolactinemia-induced hypogonadism may not respond to testosterone replacement therapy because of the androgen-antagonizing effect of prolactin. Consequently, treatment of the underlying hyperprolactinemia is necessary to restore potency.

Yohimbine

Yohimbine is an alpha-blocker touted as a medical treatment for erectile dysfunction. In a double-blind, randomized study of the drug in patients with organic erectile dysfunction, it was found to be ineffective. However, it did prove helpful in a similarly designed study of patients with psychological erectile dysfunction, probably because of their high level of anxiety and sympathetic tone.

Treatment of Underlying Urologic Disease

Emerging evidence suggests that lower urinary tract symptoms due to benign prostatic hyperplasia may contribute to erectile dysfunction. There is early evidence that PDE-5 inhibitors improve urinary function symptoms but not flow rates.

At least temporary relief from the acute discomfort of prostatosis ensues from repeated prostatic massage (see Chapter 138). Selected patients with Peyronie's disease are candidates for plaque resection and replacement with a dermal skin graft. The ability to perform sexually may return after the removal of a large hydrocele or the repair of an inguinal hernia.

INDICATIONS FOR REFERRAL

Patients with urologic disease should have a urologic consultation to see whether they are candidates for surgical correction. Diabetics and other patients with otherwise refractory erectile dysfunction who have a relatively well-preserved penile vascular apparatus are reasonable candidates for referral to consider intracavernous injection therapy if they have not been sufficiently helped by PDE-5 treatment. Even those with a degree of vascular insufficiency may be candidates. The risks and benefits of prosthetic surgery can also be reviewed at the same time. Referral is best made to a urologist experienced in the treatment of erectile dysfunction. Patients found to have symptomatic aortoiliac disease require evaluation by a vascular surgeon (see Chapter 34). Endocrinologic advice is indicated for patients with elevated prolactin levels, primary hypogonadism (low levels of testosterone, high levels of luteinizing hormone), or evidence of pituitary–hypothalamic disease (low concentrations of luteinizing hormone). The rare patient suspected of harboring a cord lesion needs urgent neurologic consultation.

Psychiatric referral may be indicated when depression, anxiety disorder, or interpersonal conflict appears to be contributing significantly to erectile dysfunction. However, premature referral to a psychiatrist before an appropriate medical evaluation has been completed should be avoided because of the risk for inappropriately labeling the condition as purely psychological and alienating the patient. Referral may also be useful when the patient with organic disease fails to respond to supportive psychotherapy offered by the primary physician (see Chapter 229).

RECOMMENDATIONS

- The primary care physician can effectively evaluate and treat most men who present with erectile dysfunction. Use of a standardized questionnaire such as the IIEF should begin the evaluation. A careful history and physical examination then allows differentiation among etiologies of erectile dysfunction sufficient for decision making about the amelioration of contributing factors and the initiation of first-line therapy.

- The absence of libido may be related to depression or suggest the need for endocrine evaluation to identify men who would benefit from testosterone replacement. Careful attention to contributing psychogenic factors, including performance anxiety related to other forms of sexual function, such as premature ejaculation, should be addressed. Medications that may be contributing to erectile dysfunction should be stopped or adjusted when possible.

- First-line therapy with oral PDE-5 inhibitors should be accompanied by careful explanation about use and effectiveness. Men should understand that these agents do not directly affect libido and that sexual stimulation is necessary. Vardenafil should be taken at least 20 minutes before anticipated intercourse; sildenafil or tadalafil should be taken at least 30 to 40 minutes before sex. Sildenafil and vardenafil generally remain effective for at least 4 hours; tadalafil is effective for 24 to 36 hours after a single dose. Dosing for most men without heart disease or multiple risk factors can begin at a moderate level (e.g., 50 mg of sildenafil), decreased (e.g., to 25 mg of sildenafil) if side effects occur, or advanced (e.g., to 100 mg of sildenafil) if response is inadequate.

- Older men who have not engaged in sexual activity for some time should be questioned about exercise tolerance. If a history of recent exercise equivalent to the exertion associated with intercourse cannot be obtained, stress testing should be considered.

- Men with heart disease who can be designated at "low risk" for coital myocardial infarction or cardiac death may initiate and resume sexual activity and be treated for erectile dysfunction if necessary. PDE-5 inhibitors should not be prescribed to men taking nitrates.

- Men who do not respond to PDE-5 inhibitors should be referred to a urologist for further evaluation and consideration of second-line treatments, including intercavernosal injections.

A.G.M.

Annotated Bibliography

1. Burnett AL. Erectile dysfunction. J Urol 2006;175:S25. (*An excellent review, with emphasis on epidemiology and management, including the comparative effectiveness of phosphodiesterase type 5 inhibitors.*)
2. McVary KT. Erectile dysfunction. N Engl J Med 2007;357:2472. (*An excellent review, with emphasis on pathophysiology and treatment.*)
3. Rees J, Patel B. Erectile dysfunction. BMJ 2006;332:593. (*A concise, practical, 1-page review with clinical rather than pharmacodynamic estimates of onset and duration of effectiveness.*)
4. Bacon CG, Mittleman MA, Kawachi I, et al. Sexual function in men older than 50 years of age: results from the Health Professionals Follow-up Study. Ann Intern Med 2003;139:161. (*Lifestyle factors most strongly associated with decreased risk of erectile dysfunction [ED] were physical activity and leanness.*)
5. Esposito K, Giugliano F, Di Palo C, et al. Effect of lifestyle changes on erectile dysfunction in obese men: a randomized controlled trial. JAMA 2004;291:2978. (*Lifestyle changes are associated with improvement in sexual function in about one third of obese men with erectile dysfunction at baseline.*)
6. Fazio L, Brock G. Erectile dysfunction: management update. Can Med Assoc J 2004;170:1429. (*An excellent review of epidemiology, pathophysiology, and the comparative pharmacokinetics of phosphodiesterase type 5 inhibitors and a summary of trials.*)
7. Feldman HA, Goldstein I, Hatzichristou DG, et al. Impotence and its medical and psychosocial correlates: results of the Massachusetts Male Aging Study. J Urol 1994;151:54. (*A classic study, documenting a progressive decline in function with aging.*)
8. Fung MM, Bettencourt R, Barrett-Connor E. Heart disease risk factors predict erectile dysfunction 25 years later: the Rancho Bernardo Study. J Am Coll Cardiol 2004;43:1405. (*Mean age, body mass index, cholesterol, and triglycerides were each significantly associated with an increased risk of ED; the effect of cigarette smoking was marginal.*)
9. McVary KT, Roehrborn CG, Kaminetsky JC, et al. Tadalafil relieves lower urinary tract symptoms secondary to benign prostatic hyperplasia. J Urol 2007;177:1401. (*The effect of this treatment on symptoms was equivalent to that of alpha-blockers and finasteride; there was no effect on flow rates, which is of interest because of implications for pathophysiology.*)
10. McVary KT, Carrier S, Wessels, et al. Smoking and erectile dysfunction: evidence-based analysis. J Urol 2001;166:1624. (*An excellent critical review of the evidence, including the high degree of biologic plausibility.*)
11. Saenz de Tejada I, Goldstein I, Asadzoi K, et al. Impaired neurogenic and endothelium-mediated relaxation of penile smooth muscle from diabetic men with impotence. N Engl J Med 1989;320:1025. (*Delineates the mechanisms of diabetic erectile dysfunction, providing the basis for the use of intracavernosal smooth-muscle relaxant.*)
12. Seftel AD. Erectile dysfunction in the elderly: epidemiology, etiology and approaches to treatment. J Urol 2003;169:1999. (*A superb review of age-related changes, as well as the effect of the age-related incidence of contributing chronic diseases.*)
13. Cappeleri JC, Rosen RC, Smith MD, et al. Diagnostic evaluation of the erectile function domain of the International Index of Erectile Function. Urology 1999;54:346. (*This index appears to be useful in the clinical setting and for research.*)
14. Broderick GA, Allen GA, McClure RD. Vacuum tumescence devices: the role of papaverine in the selection of patients. J Urol 1990;145:284. (*Use of this agent led to a 94% positive predictive value.*)
15. Kessler WO. Nocturnal penile tumescence. Urol Clin North Am 1988;15:1. (*A discussion of available tests.*)
16. Arruda-Olson AM, Mahoney DW, Nehra A, et al. Cardiovascular effects of sildenafil during exercise in men with known or probable coronary artery disease. JAMA 2002;287:719. (*A randomized, placebo-controlled, crossover study in which concurrent nitrate use was prohibited, finding no adverse cardiovascular effects with the use of 25 to 50 mg of sildenafil.*)
17. Conti CR, Pepine CJ, Sweeney M. Efficacy and safety of sildenafil in the treatment of erectile dysfunction in patients with ischemic heart disease. Am J Cardiol 1999;83:29C. (*The drug was effective and safe in patients with erectile dysfunction and ischemic heart disease who were not taking nitrate therapy.*)
18. Kostis JB, Jackson G, Rosen R, et al. Sexual dysfunction and cardiac risk (the Second Princeton Consensus Conference). Am J Cardiol 2005;96:313-321. (*Presents recommendations for men at low, high, and intermediate/indeterminant risk for coital cardiac events.*)
19. Fink HA, MacDonald R, Ruths IR, et al. Sildenafil for male erectile dysfunction. A systematic review and meta-analysis. Arch Intern Med 2002;162:1342. (*A meta-analysis of 27 trials: sildenafil users had a success on 57% of intercourse attempts, compared with 21% with placebo; greater efficacy was found with higher doses.*)
20. Jain P, Rademaker AW, McVary KT. Testosterone supplementation for erectile dysfunction: results of a meta-analysis. J Urol 2000;164:371. (*A meta-analysis of 16 trials, showing a greater effect among patients with primary etiology and with transdermal administration.*)
21. Jarow JP, Burnett AL, Geringer AM. Clinical efficacy of sildenafil citrate based on etiology and response to prior treatment. J Urol 1999;162:722. (*The best predictors of satisfaction were baseline function and etiology.*)
22. Kedia S, Zippe CD, Agarwal A, et al. Treatment of erectile dysfunction with sildenafil citrate after radiation therapy for prostate cancer. Urology 1999;54:308. (*Finds a positive response for 71% of cases.*)
23. Morales A, Condra MS, Owen JA, et al. Is yohimbine effective in the treatment of organic impotence? Results of a controlled trial. J Urol 1987;137:1168. (*The answer is no for organic disease but yes for psychogenic disease.*)
24. Mulhall JP. Deciphering erectile dysfunction drug trials. J Urol 2003;170:353. (*A detailed review of methodologic issues that should be familiar to those who interpret trials of drugs used for ED.*)
25. Porst H, Padma-Nathan H, Giuliano F, et al. Efficacy of tadalafil for the treatment of erectile dysfunction at 24 and 36 hours after dosing: a randomized controlled trial. Urology 2003;62:121. (*Tadalafil 20 mg is an effective and well-tolerated treatment for ED that has a period of responsiveness of up to 36 hours.*)
26. Shabsigh R, Kaufman JM, Steidle C, et al. Randomized study of testosterone gel as adjunctive therapy to sildenafil in hypogonadal men with erectile dysfunction who do not respond to sildenafil alone. J Urol 2004;172:658. (*Testosterone gel taken with sildenafil may be beneficial in improving erectile*

function in hypogonadal men with erectile dysfunction who are unresponsive to sildenafil alone.)

27. Tomlinson J, Wright D. Impact of erectile dysfunction and its subsequent treatment with sildenafil: qualitative study. BMJ 2004;328:1037. (*Erectile dysfunction caused serious distress in these men, with marked effects on self-esteem and relationships; sildenafil increased well-being when it worked and increased distress when it did not.*)

28. O'Leary MP, Althof SE, Cappelleri JC, et al. Self-esteem, confidence, and relationship satisfaction of men with erectile dysfunction treated with sildenafil citrate. J Urol 2006;175:1058. (*Finds improvements in all measures correlating with International Index of Erectile Function scores.*)

29. Zelefsy MJ, McKee AB, Lee H, et al. Efficacy of oral sildenafil in patients with erectile dysfunction after radiotherapy for carcinoma of the prostate. Urology 1999;53:775. (*Finds significant improvement in 74% of cases.*)

30. Zippe CD, Kedia AW, Kedia K, et al. Treatment of erectile dysfunction after radical prostatectomy with sildenafil citrate. Urology 1999;52:963. (*Of those who had undergone bilateral nerve-sparing procedures, 80% responded; those who had undergone unilateral or non–nerve-sparing procedures did not respond.*)

31. Goldstein I, Lue TF, Padma-Nathan H, et al. Oral sildenafil in the treatment of erectile dysfunction. N Engl J Med 1998;338:1397. (*A placebo-controlled, dose–response study of 329 men who had erectile dysfunction with a wide variety of causes, finding a 100% improvement in function with the highest dose, with minimal side effects during 32 weeks of use.*)

32. Linet OI, Ogrinc FG, for the Alprostadil Study Group. Efficacy and safety of intracavernosal alprostadil in men with erectile dysfunction. N Engl J Med 1996;334:873. (*The men and their partners rated the sexual activity as satisfactory after 87% and 86% of the injections, respectively.*)

33. Merrick GS, Butler WM, Lief JH, et al. Efficacy of sildenafil citrate in prostate brachytherapy patients with erectile dysfunction. Urology 1999;53:1112. (*Finds a favorable response in 80% of cases.*)

34. Mulhall JP, Jahoda AE, Cairney M, et al. The causes of patient dropout from penile self-injection therapy for impotence. J Urol 1999;162:1291. (*The attrition rate was 31%; the most common reason was cost, and only 1 in 7 who quit did so because of lack of effectiveness.*)

35. Rendell MS, Rajfer J, Wicker PA, et al. Sildenafil for treatment of erectile dysfunction in men with diabetes: a randomized controlled trial. JAMA 1999;281:421. (*At 12 weeks, 56% of sildenafil patients had improved, in comparison with 10% of those on placebo.*)

CHAPTER 133 ■ APPROACH TO DYSURIA AND URINARY TRACT INFECTIONS IN WOMEN

LESLIE S.-T. FANG

Among adult women, urinary tract infection (UTI) is the most common bacterial infection. Among sexually active women, urinary tract infection has an annual incidence of 0.5% to 0.7%. More than 50% of women have a UTI in their lifetime, and 25% to 50% of women with one infection have a recurrence. Urinary tract infection accounts for an estimated 7 million office visits to physicians annually, with an estimated cost of 1.6 billion dollars. Thus, UTIs represent a significant source of morbidity among women. Evaluation by the primary physician should be directed at the detection of any anatomic abnormalities that may predispose the patient to recurrent infections. Therapy should be aimed at the eradication of infection to minimize morbidity.

PATHOPHYSIOLOGY AND CLINICAL PRESENTATION (1–11)

The evidence suggests that most episodes of UTI in adult women are secondary to *ascending infection*. Bacteria reach the bladder through the urethra and may then ascend to the kidneys through the ureters. Hematogenous spread has rarely been implicated in the pathogenesis of UTIs.

Bacteria that commonly cause UTI are found in the periurethral area in up to 20% of adult women. This *colonization* of the *vaginal introitus* has been shown to be the essential first step in the production of bacteriuria and plays an important role in recurrent UTIs. Colonization with Enterobacteriaceae occurs in postmenopausal women and is believed to account for much of the increase in susceptibility to UTI seen in this age group. Entry of bacteria into the bladder through the relatively short female urethra can occur spontaneously. In addition, *sexual intercourse* and use of a *diaphragm* are associated with increased risk of infection. The use of spermicide with a diaphragm or on a condom predisposes specifically to infection with *Staphylococcus saprophyticus*. Approximately 75% of urinary tract infections caused by *S. saprophyticus* are attributable to this exposure. Significant increases in bacteriuria follow 30% of intercourse episodes. In one study, the average 24-year-old woman who had sexual intercourse 3 days of the week had a risk of UTI that was 2.6 times greater than that of a similar female who had not had intercourse during that week. Other risk factors include history of urinary tract infections (especially before age 15 years), having a mother with a history of urinary tract infections, and exhibiting Lewis blood group antigen nonsecretor phenotypes, Le(a+b–) and Le(a–b–). The use of tampons and wiping from back to front are not risk factors for UTI.

The establishment of a bladder infection also depends on the virulence of the bacteria introduced, the number of organisms introduced, and, most important, a lapse in normal host defense mechanisms.

In patients with normal urogenital tracts, upper tract infections are caused almost exclusively by bacteria with virulence determinants. In contrast, only about 50% of cystitis strains have virulence determinants.

A number of *host defense mechanisms* normally act together to decrease the likelihood of infection. Normal voiding eliminates some organisms. Certain chemical properties of the urine are antibacterial; urine with a high concentration of urea, low pH, and high osmolarity supports bacterial growth poorly. The most important host defense mechanism is phagocytosis of bacteria that come into contact with the bladder mucosal surface. Vaginal epithelial cell characteristics also contribute. Susceptibility to UTI correlates with increases in cellular bacterial adhesiveness. Abnormalities in these host defense mechanisms result in recurrent and complicated UTIs.

In approximately 30% of cases of sustained bladder infection, the infection extends further through the ureters into the kidneys. The presence of *reflux* increases the chance that infection will ascend. Once infected urine gains access to the renal pelvis, it can enter the renal parenchyma through the ducts of Bellini at the papillary tips and then spread outward along the collecting ducts to cause parenchymal infection.

Clinical Syndromes

Urinary tract infections are associated with a number of clinical syndromes, ranging from acute urethral syndrome to pyelonephritis. Most are accompanied by dysuria, frequency, urgency, and suprapubic or flank discomfort. Other features are unique to each syndrome.

Acute Urethral Syndrome (Symptomatic Abacteriuria)

This syndrome occurs in about 10% to 15% of women who present with symptoms suggestive of UTI. Patients in this category have fewer than 10^5 organisms per milliliter on urine culture. In addition, urinalysis findings are usually unimpressive—few white blood cells (WBCs) and no bacteria. These patients can be subdivided into two groups. Approximately 70% have some degree of pyuria (more than 2 to 5 WBCs per high-power field in a centrifuged sample) and true infection, either with bacterial counts of fewer than 10^5 organisms or with *Chlamydia trachomatis*. Those with bacterial counts in the range of 10^2 to 10^4 may have early UTI with infection not yet established in the bladder. The remaining 30% have no pyuria and no infection. The cause of their dysuria is unknown. Only those without pyuria have proved to be truly abacteriuric. A subset of truly abacteriuric women with urinary frequency report chronic pelvic pain relieved by voiding, suprapubic tenderness, and dyspareunia. They have normal findings on urinalysis. Cystoscopic dilation reveals submucosal hemorrhages. The term *interstitial cystitis* has been used to designate their condition. The cause is unknown, and the course is chronic. Tricyclic antidepressants are sometimes helpful.

Asymptomatic Bacteriuria

See Chapter 126 for a discussion of this entity.

Symptomatic Bacteriuria

Symptomatic bacteriuria, in the form of cystitis or pyelonephritis, is the most common of the clinical syndromes. *Cystitis* has traditionally been believed to present primarily as frequency, urgency, dysuria, hematuria, and bacteriuria. *Pyelonephritis*, on the other hand, is generally believed to be associated with fever, flank pain, and systemic symptoms such as nausea and vomiting. Unfortunately, numerous investigations have shown that the ability to differentiate between bladder and kidney infection on clinical grounds alone is limited. Studies using bilateral ureteral catheterization directly to localize the site of infection have demonstrated that many patients with upper tract infection present with symptoms supposedly characteristic of lower tract infection. Moreover, patients whose infection

is limited to the bladder may occasionally have fever, flank pain, and systemic symptoms usually associated with pyelonephritis. Thus, the traditional clinical clues are at best imprecise for identifying the site of infection.

Recurrent Infections

Recurrent infections are characteristic of some patients. Two basic patterns of recurrence are recognized: (a) *relapse*, in which the original organism is suppressed by antimicrobial therapy and then reappears when the antibiotic is stopped, and (b) *reinfection*, in which the original organism is eradicated by antimicrobial therapy and the recurrent infection is caused by a new bacterial strain. Approximately 80% of recurrences represent reinfection. Ureteral catheterization studies have demonstrated that most reinfections occur in patients in whom infection is restricted to the bladder, whereas most relapses occur in patients with renal parenchymal infection.

Groups frequently bothered by recurrent infections include (a) sexually active women, who report a temporal relationship of urinary symptoms to intercourse; (b) patients with host defenses compromised by underlying systemic illness or residual urine in the bladder; (c) patients with upper tract infections; and (d) pregnant women.

The consequences of recurrent uncomplicated infections are, for the most part, minimal and rarely result in progressive renal impairment. However, patients with infections in the setting of vesicoureteral reflux, pregnancy, or diabetes are at greater risk. *Vesicoureteral reflux* is associated with residual urine in the bladder, ascending infection, chronic pyelonephritis, and a high risk for renal scarring, which leads to focal glomerulosclerosis, proteinuria, and progressive renal failure. Patients most likely to have vesicoureteral reflux are those who report a long history of UTIs beginning in childhood. UTI during pregnancy has been linked to increased rates of fetal complications and prematurity, especially when the infection occurs within 2 weeks of delivery. The mother has an enhanced risk for pyelonephritis. Patients with diabetes show an increased susceptibility to upper tract infection.

DIFFERENTIAL DIAGNOSIS
(1,4,5,10–13)

Dysuria

The differential diagnosis of dysuria includes *UTI*, *vaginitis*, and *urethritis*. Patients with vaginitis may occasionally be mistakenly believed to have UTI. Vaginal discharge, "external" discomfort (from urinary irritation of inflamed labial tissue), absence of frequency or urgency, and urine cultures negative for bacteria distinguish vaginitis from UTI. *Trichomonas vaginalis* and *Candida albicans* are the most commonly responsible organisms. Women with dysuria and an absence of bacterial growth on routine urine culture may have *urethritis* caused by *Neisseria gonorrhoeae* or *herpes simplex virus*, although, as previously noted, most cases are caused by *C. trachomatis* (see Chapter 125). The onset is usually gradual, dysuria is mild, and vaginal discharge may be present. Pelvic pain and vaginal or cervical discharge suggest spread of infection into the cervix and fallopian tubes, a serious development (see Chapters 116 and 117).

Pyuria typically accompanies gonococcal and trichomonal infection as well as chlamydial infection. Patients with acute urethral syndrome and no pyuria may have dysuria on the basis of *local trauma* or *irritation* rather than infection, problems that occur in postmenopausal women secondary to desiccation of vaginal and urethral tissue.

Flank Pain

Patients with *renal calculi* or *embolic infarction* may present with flank pain and hematuria, mimicking *pyelonephritis*. However, urine cultures are sterile, and no bacteria are seen on Gram's stain, as they are in UTI.

WORKUP (1,5,7,10,14–19)

The pace, extensiveness, and order of the evaluation are largely dictated by the patient's clinical presentation. Candidates for outpatient evaluation include dysuric patients with no evidence of systemic toxicity or obstruction.

Acutely Ill Patients

Patients presenting with fever, flank pain, and systemic symptoms require prompt evaluation for the possibility of urinary tract *obstruction* and superimposed infection. Such patients should be questioned about a history of diabetes, sickle cell anemia, and excessive analgesic use; patients with these problems are at higher risk for renal papillary necrosis and subsequent obstruction by sloughed papillae. Likewise, a history of renal calculi is cause for concern in this setting. The patient with any of these risk factors who appears to be toxic (high temperature, prostration) and restless on examination and who has marked tenderness in the costovertebral angle requires immediate imaging evaluation to rule out obstruction. Infection behind an obstruction constitutes a medical and urologic emergency necessitating urgent therapeutic intervention.

Dysuric Patients

History

The acutely dysuric woman should be questioned about vaginal discharge, external irritation on urination, and pain on intercourse to differentiate vaginal causes of dysuria from those referable to the urinary tract. Also helpful is a sexual history to identify risk factors for chlamydial urethritis, including new sexual partners, a partner with a penile discharge or recent urethritis, mucoid vaginal discharge, or gradual onset of symptoms. A recent history of gonorrhea or exposure to gonorrhea should be elicited.

Patients giving a history of dysuria, frequency, urgency, or back pain without vaginal discharge or vaginal irritation have a very high likelihood of urinary tract infection (96%). On the other hand, patients without dysuria and patients with vaginal symptoms are much less likely to have a urinary tract infection.

Physical Examination

One begins with a temperature determination, followed by percussion of the costovertebral angle to test for tenderness and palpation of the suprapubic region to detect discomfort and distention. The pelvic examination is indicated in patients with vaginal symptoms, any urethral discharge, or vaginal erythema, discharge, or atrophy. Cervical discharge, erosion, vesicles, or tenderness on motion must be noted.

Laboratory Studies

Urinalysis and culture are of prime importance.

Urinalysis. Urinalysis is of prime importance in the evaluation of a patient with dysuria. Proper collection of the urine specimen is essential. The clean-voided technique has withstood the test of time and minimizes contamination from vaginal and labial sources. The female patient is told to straddle or squat over the toilet and to spread the labia with the nondominant hand. This position is maintained throughout collection. With the other hand, the vulva is swabbed front to back with three sterile gauze pads soaked in sterile water or with a sponge soaked in a mild nonhexachlorophene soap. A small amount of urine is then passed. This is a urethral specimen and can be saved if bacterial or protozoan urethritis is suspected. More urine is voided and collected in a sterile cup. Alternatively, the patient can be told to slide the cup into a freely flowing stream to collect a true midstream specimen. The adequacy of collection can be confirmed by examining for epithelial cells; their presence indicates vulvar or urethral contamination.

With an elderly patient, the assistance of a family member or a nurse may be needed. When repeated contamination is suspected, *straight catheterization* of the bladder can be performed with relatively little risk.

Positive dipstick nitrite or positive leukocyte is a sensitive (75%) and specific (82%) predictor of urinary tract infection. Although microscopic examination of urine sediment or examination of Gram's stain of the unspun urine would add specificity and sensitivity, these tests are often impractical in the office setting.

Culture. The traditional criterion for infection has been a colony count of more than 10^5 organisms per milliliter; it provides high specificity but poor sensitivity. Studies using suprapubic aspirates find that half of dysuric women with "negative" urine cultures by the traditional criterion are truly infected, although the colony counts were in the range of 10^2 to 10^5. Colony counts of more than 10^2 obtained on clean-voided specimens from acutely dysuric women are diagnostic of true coliform infection. Many such women who previously were labeled as having symptomatic abacteriuria fall into this category. As noted earlier, the presence of pyuria identifies those who are infected and will respond to antibiotics.

The need to obtain a urine culture for every acutely dysuric woman with mild to moderate symptoms has been challenged. The vast majority of organisms that cause infection in this group are sensitive to the antibiotic regimens commonly prescribed (see later discussion). Even when disk-sensitivity testing designates an organism as "resistant" to an antibiotic, the resistance is only relative and the organism is usually susceptible to the much higher antibiotic concentrations found in the urine. Many authorities now recommend basing the decision to treat with antibiotics and the selection of an agent on the clinical history and the urine dipstick, with urine culture reserved for patients with a recurrence or a report of several UTIs within the past year. Empiric therapy has also been advised. In young women with uncomplicated UTIs, patients were able correctly to self-diagnose in 95% of cases. Self-treatment in these instances resulted in 92% clinical and 96% microbiologic cures with no adverse effects.

At the other extreme are patients who present acutely with severe symptoms and risk for urosepsis. They require not only urine sediment examination, Gram's stain, and culture, but also at least two sets of *blood cultures* before antibiotics are initiated.

When the urine culture is obtained, familiarity with important urinary pathogens facilitates interpretation of culture results. The most common urinary pathogen in community-acquired UTI is *Escherichia coli*, accounting for 5% to 90% of organisms grown. *Staphylococcus saprophyticus* accounts for 5% to 15% of urinary pathogens. Occasionally, the other gram-negative rods are responsible. Of the gram-positive organisms involved in UTI, enterococci, *Staphylococcus aureus*, and group B streptococci are common isolates. Diphtheroids, lactobacilli, and α-hemolytic streptococci represent contaminants.

Radiographic and Other Urinary Tract Investigations. Recurrent infection raises the specter of a structural lesion. However, as already noted, the vast majority of recurrences represent reinfection in the absence of upper tract disease or other pathology. Imaging studies including excretory computed tomography and cystoscopy in women with recurrent infection are of very low yield and are not recommended. Such radiographic and urologic evaluations should be reserved for those in whom anatomic abnormalities are suspected (e.g., onset of UTIs in childhood) or in whom obstruction is likely or renal insufficiency is developing. If there is clinical evidence of reflux, a voiding cystourethrogram should be performed to document the existence and degree of reflux. Urologic evaluation is indicated when urethral meatal stenosis is strongly suspected (see Chapter 134).

PRINCIPLES OF THERAPY (1,5,20–38)

The intensity and duration of therapy should match the patient's clinical presentation and risk for complications. In general, patients who are systemically sick require consideration for hospitalization and parenteral antibiotics, especially if they are metabolically or immunologically compromised or have an anatomic or functional defect of the urinary tract.

Acutely Ill Patients: Pyelonephritis, Urosepsis

Patients presenting with high fever, chills, flank pain, costovertebral angle tenderness, nausea, and vomiting may have upper tract or even bloodstream infection and should be hospitalized, especially if they are elderly. They require fluids, thorough evaluation for treatable precipitants (see prior discussion), and prompt initiation of parenteral antibiotics. The choice of initial antibiotic program should be consistent with the findings on urine Gram's stain, although Enterobacteriaceae account for more than 90% of cases.

Often, broad-spectrum coverage is selected in this setting because of concern for *Pseudomonas* species and other multiply resistant gram-negative rods. In addition, coverage for enterococci is usually included, although the pathogen is more common in men. *Ampicillin* plus *levofloxacin* is a reasonable and effective choice of coverage. Other alternatives for initial treatment include imipenem/cilastatin and ceftriaxone. When

culture and sensitivity results become available, the regimen can be revised to provide more focused coverage. Pyelonephritis without bloodstream invasion can be treated parenterally until fever resolves and then with oral antibiotics to complete a 14-day course. Urosepsis requires a longer course of intravenous antibiotics. However, because oral *fluoroquinolones* can achieve reasonably high serum concentration, patients can be discharged on oral fluoroquinolones once they become afebrile and can take oral intake reliably. In appropriate circumstances, imaging studies should be performed to rule out anatomic abnormalities.

Outpatient Treatment of Pyelonephritis

Otherwise healthy patients with less severe but still acutely incapacitating symptoms often have uncomplicated pyelonephritis; this can be treated entirely on an outpatient basis with 10 to 14 days of oral antibiotics, provided that the patient is reliable, can take fluids, is not seriously immunocompromised, and has no obstruction. *Trimethoprim/sulfamethoxazole* (TMS) or a fluoroquinolone (e.g., *levofloxacin, ciprofloxacin, norfloxacin*) is a reasonable choice. Up to 30% of community-acquired *E. coli* infections are now trimethoprim, ampicillin, and cephalothin resistant. With increasing ampicillin resistance among community-acquired Enterobacteriaceae, fluoroquinolone therapy is emerging as the preferred selection for outpatient treatment of pyelonephritis, with *amoxicillin/clavulanic acid* also assuming an increasingly important role. Unfortunately, rising fluoroquinolone resistance is beginning to complicate the treatment options. For infection with enterococci and *S. saprophyticus*, *amoxicillin* remains the antibiotic of choice.

Failure to respond to an antibiotic program suggests antibiotic resistance or, less commonly, an anatomic or functional abnormality. Concern over anatomic abnormality should trigger the need for radiologic evaluation and urologic consultation (see prior discussion).

Mild to Moderate Symptoms: Uncomplicated Urinary Tract Infection

Urine culture is usually not necessary in the management of patients with uncomplicated urinary tract infections. Most patients with mild to moderate symptoms have cystitis and respond well to a short course of oral antibiotics. TMS, *amoxicillin*, or *fluoroquinolone* should suffice for most cases of lower UTI, even those caused by "resistant" strains, because of the very high bladder antibiotic concentrations achieved.

Urine cultures should be considered only in a patient suspected of having a complicated urinary tract infection, if the patient did not respond to standard therapy, or if the patient has recurrent urinary tract infection.

A *3-day course* of antibiotics is usually adequate for the treatment of uncomplicated UTIs. Antibiotics that have been shown to be effective include *TMS, trimethoprim, levofloxacin,* and *ciprofloxacin*. The effectiveness of a 3-day regimen is supported by a meta-analysis that included 9,605 patients from 12 trials. The study indicated that similar symptomatic cure is achieved by antibiotic therapy for 3 days or by prolonged therapy (>5 days). Prolonged treatment, however, was more effective in obtaining bacteriologic cure. Three-day regimens with β-lactams or *nitrofurantoin* appear to be less effective than 5 or more days of therapy. *TMS* should be the first-line treatment for women presenting with acute uncomplicated UTI, in view of concern about increasing *fluoroquinolone* resistance in the community.

Suboptimal candidates for short-course therapy include patients with diabetes or a history of relapses, patients with known anatomic abnormalities, and immunocompromised patients. Such patients are best treated with a longer course of antibiotics (up to 2 weeks).

Acute Urethral Syndrome

Patients with *pyuria*, no bacteria on Gram's stain, and no clinical evidence for chlamydial, gonococcal, or other venereal forms of urethritis are considered to have acute urethral syndrome. It has been suggested that a colony count of greater than 10^2 on a midstream urine specimen be considered a positive culture in women with acute symptoms and pyuria. These patients can be treated with *a 3-day course of antibiotic therapy* in the same manner as any patient with lower tract infection. Alternatively, they can be treated with *doxycycline* (100 mg twice daily for 5 days). Doxycycline is effective against *Chlamydia* and gonococci and also most common urinary pathogens (see Chapters 125 and 137). Recurrences are common in patients with acute urethral syndrome.

Patients *without pyuria* may or may not respond to antibiotics and should also be given a trial of a *3-day course of antibiotic therapy*. Patients who fail therapy should be treated with symptomatic therapy with fluids and urinary analgesics such as phenazopyridine (Pyridium) or Uricet.

Recurrent Infection

Patients bothered by frequent symptomatic recurrences are potential candidates for preventive measures. Recurrent infection should be confirmed at least once by repeated culture. The clinical setting helps to determine the appropriate approach to therapy.

As noted earlier, recurrences in *sexually active women* are most often reinfections. Patients should be counseled about a possible association between their infections and the use of spermicides. It is also reasonable to suggest that they should attempt to have early postcoital voiding and liberal use of fluid. Cranberry juice appears to have protective efficacy. Prophylaxis at the time of intercourse with *single-tablet* therapy has proved to be effective in minimizing their frequency and severity. Drugs that have been proven to be efficacious in this manner include *TMS, nitrofurantoin, cephalexin, ciprofloxacin, norfloxacin, ofloxacin,* and *levofloxacin*.

In reliable patients with fewer than three UTIs per year, a patient-initiated *3-day course* of standard antibiotic therapy for uncomplicated UTI at the first sign of symptomatic infection has proved to be effective.

In patients with frequent recurrences, continuous antibiotic prophylaxis should be considered. Studies have shown that continuous prophylaxis would decrease recurrences by up to 95% compared with placebo. Drugs that have been shown to be efficacious in continuous prophylaxis include TMS, *trimethoprim, nitrofurantoin, cefaclor, cephalexin, norfloxacin, ciprofloxacin,* and *levofloxacin*.

A meta-analysis evaluating 10 trials involving 430 patients with recurrent infections showed that either postcoital or continuous prophylaxis appeared significantly to reduce clinical recurrences. In this study, there does not appear to be any difference between postcoital or continuous antibiotic prophylaxis.

In patients with defined anatomic abnormalities, such as significant reflux or nephrolithiasis, surgical correction to decrease the severity and frequency of recurrences should be considered.

Treatment of the Pregnant Patient

Treatment of symptomatic UTI in pregnancy is recommended because of an increased risk for upper tract infection in the mother and potential injury to the fetus (low birth weight, prematurity). Antibiotics that have been shown to be safe for use in pregnancy include *ampicillin, amoxicillin,* and oral *cephalosporins*. The combination preparation of *amoxicillin/clavulanic acid* (Augmentin) is recommended for use against organisms demonstrating resistance to multiple drugs. *Nitrofurantoin* has also been used without evidence of fetal toxicity. The fluoroquinolones should be avoided in pregnant patients.

Treatment of Asymptomatic Bacteriuria in the Elderly

Because the risk for urosepsis, renal failure, or mortality is not increased, the need for antibiotics is not urgent. The risk for symptomatic infection is increased, but the benefit of treatment is unclear. Antibiotics are indicated if obstruction is present or the patient is to undergo a genitourinary procedure.

THERAPEUTIC RECOMMENDATIONS

Table 133.1 summarizes the therapeutic recommendations for UTIs.

INDICATIONS FOR REFERRAL OR ADMISSION

Hospitalization is indicated in patients with severe symptoms such as rigors, high fever, flank pain, nausea, and vomiting. Patients with suspected obstruction and those unable to maintain oral intake also require hospitalization. Referral to a urologist is indicated if a surgically correctable anatomic abnormality is detected or suspected.

PATIENT EDUCATION
(4, 6,9,11,20, 31)

Certain general measures are important in minimizing the possibility of recurrent infection. The patient should be instructed about increasing fluid intake during symptomatic periods and maintaining urine flow around the clock. Patients with UTIs temporally related to sexual intercourse would probably benefit from voiding after intercourse. They should be advised about modifiable risk factors such as use of spermicides. Cranberry juice contains proanthrocyanidins, which can prevent the expression of P fimbrae of *E. coli* and can decrease the frequency of recurrent infections (from 36% to 16% in a 12-month follow-up in one study).

TABLE 133.1

ANTIBIOTIC REGIMENS FOR URINARY TRACT INFECTIONS IN WOMEN

Clinical Situation	Regimen
Acutely ill and toxic patient	Hospitalization; parenteral antibiotics; ampicillin plus levofloxacin if urosepsis is suspected; otherwise, a fluoroquinolone such as levofloxacin or ciprofloxacin if Gram's stain shows GNR; ampicillin if it shows GPC
Uncomplicated pyelonephritis	Oral TMS (one double-strength tablet) bid for 2 wk or levofloxacin 500 mg qd or ciprofloxacin 500 mg bid for 2 wk
Uncomplicated lower UTI	3-day course if more symptomatic with TMS (one double-strength tablet) bid, ciprofloxacin 500 mg bid, levofloxacin 500 mg qd
	7- to 10-day course if patient has diabetes, recurrent UTI, or is older than the age of 65 yr
Relapse	Same drug as for uncomplicated UTI, but continued for at least 2 wk
Acute urethral syndrome with pyuria	3-day course of TMS or fluoroquinolone as for uncomplicated UTI or doxycycline 100 mg bid for 10 d if *Chlamydia* infection is suspected
Acute urethral syndrome without pyuria	3-day course of TMS or fluoroquinolone as for uncomplicated UTI; symptomatic treatment if there is no response to antibiotics
Recurrent infection	
Sexually active	Postcoital voiding and increased fluid intake; cranberry juice; avoid spermicide use; prophylaxis with postcoital single-tablet dose of TMS or fluoroquinolone; continuous prophylaxis
Elderly patient with large postvoid residual	Prophylaxis with nightly dose of TMS (half of a single-strength tablet) or ciprofloxacin (250 mg)
Pregnancy	Ampicillin, amoxicillin, and oral cephalosporins have been shown to be safe; nitrofurantoin is safe for the fetus but potentially toxic for the mother; fluoroquinolones should be avoided

bid, twice daily; GNR, gram-negative rod; GPC, gram-positive cocci; qd, daily; TMS, trimethoprim/sulfamethoxazole; UTI, urinary tract infection.

Annotated Bibliography

1. Bent S, Nallamothu BK, Simel DL, et al. Does this woman have an uncomplicated urinary tract infection? JAMA 2000;287:2701. (*Excellent overview of the management of uncomplicated urinary tract infection.*)
2. Brown JS, Vittinghoff E, Kanaya AM, et al. Urinary tract infections in postmenopausal women: effect of hormone therapy and risk factors. Obstet Gynecol 2001;98:1045. (*Oral hormone therapy did not help prevent urinary tract infections [UTIs].*)
3. Echols RM, Tosiello RL, Haverstock DC, et al. Demographic, clinical, and treatment parameters influencing the outcome of acute cystitis. Clin Infect Dis 1999;29:113. (*A meta-analysis of six trials including more than 3,000 women with acute cystitis treated with 11 different regimens; not using a diaphragm was associated with a successful bacteriologic outcome.*)
4. Fihn SD, Boyko EJ, Chi-Ling C, et al. Use of spermicide-coated condoms and other risk factors for urinary tract infection caused by *Staphylococcus saprophyticus.* Arch Intern Med 1998;158:281. (*Nonoxynol-9 increased the risk for infection with this organism.*)
5. Fihn SD. Acute uncomplicated urinary tract infection in women. N Engl J Med 2003;349:259. (*An excellent review.*)
6. Hooten TM, Scholes D, Hughes JP, et al. A prospective study of risk factors for symptomatic urinary tract infection in young women. N Engl J Med 1996;335:468. (*An excellent prospective study showing an increased risk with recent sexual intercourse, history of recurrent infection, and use of a diaphragm with spermicide.*)
7. Hooten TM, Scholes D, Stapleton AE, et al. A prospective study of asymptomatic bacteriuria in sexually active young women. N Engl J Med 2000;343:992. (*Symptomatic urinary tract infection occurred in 8% of cases within 1 week.*)
8. Komaroff AL. Acute dysuria in women. N Engl J Med 1984;310:368. (*A review emphasizing the importance of pyuria as a sign of UTI and a predictor of response to therapy; good discussion of the acute urethral syndrome; 106 references.*)
9. Scholes D, Hooton TM, Roberts PL, et al. Risk factors for recurrent UTI in young women. J Infect Dis 2000;182:1177. (*Frequency of intercourse is the strongest risk factor; spermicide use and a new sex partner are others.*)
10. Stamm WE, Wagner KF, Cimsel R, et al. Causes of the acute urethral syndrome in women. N Engl J Med 1980;303:409. (*Patients with pyuria had infection with coliform bacteria, Staphylococcus saprophyticus, or Chlamydia trachomatis; those without pyuria had no organism isolated.*)
11. Strom BL, Collins M, West SL, et al. Sexual activity, contraceptive use, and other risk factors for symptomatic and asymptomatic bacteriuria. Ann Intern Med 1987;107:816. (*Intercourse, diaphragm use, and past history of UTI were the only independent risk factors; tampon use and wiping improperly were not.*)
12. Latham RH, Running K, Stamm WE. Urinary tract infections in young adult women caused by *Staphylococcus saprophyticus.* JAMA 1983;250:3063. (*S. saprophyticus was the second-most-common cause of UTIs, accounting for 11% of cases.*)
13. Manges AR, Johson JR, Foxman B, et al. Widespread distribution of urinary tract infections caused by a multidrug-resistant *E. coli* clonal group. N Engl J Med 2001;345:1007. (*In three geographically diverse communities, a single clonal group of trimethoprim/sulfamethoxazole [TMS]–resistant Escherichia coli accounted for half of community-acquired urinary tract infections.*)
14. Komaroff AL. Diagnostic decision: urinalysis and urine culture in women with dysuria. Ann Intern Med 1986;104:212. (*Urinalysis was the most reliable indicator of treatable infection; urine culture was of limited value except in cases of suspected upper UTI.*)
15. Krieger JN. Urinary tract infections: what's new? J Urol 2002;168:2351. (*Excellent review, including a practical approach to diagnosis and treatment.*)
16. Kunin CM, White LV, Hua TH. A reassessment of the importance of "low-count" bacteriuria in young women with acute urinary symptoms. Ann Intern Med 1993;119:454. (*It is likely to represent an early phase of UTI.*)
17. Mushlin AI, Thornbury JR. Intravenous pyelography: the case against its routine use. Ann Intern Med 1989;111:58. (*Little justification was found for its routine use in women with UTI.*)
18. Saint S, Scholes D, Fihn SD, et al. The effectiveness of a clinical practice guideline for the management of presumed uncomplicated urinary tract infection in women. Am J Med 1999;106:636. (*Use of a practice guideline decreased the use of urinalysis, urine culture, and office visits but increased the likelihood of antibiotic prescription.*)
19. Stamm WE, Counts GW, Running KR, et al. Diagnosis of coliform infection in acutely dysuric women. N Engl J Med 1982;307:463. (*A criterion of 10^5 organisms per milliliter is too insensitive for infection in this setting.*)
20. Albert X, Huertas I, Pereiró I, et al. Antibiotics for preventing recurrent urinary tract infection in non-pregnant women (Cochrane review). In: The Cochrane library, Issue 3. Oxford: Update Software, 2004. (*Extensive review documenting their effectiveness in different situations; see* http://www.cochrane.org *for updates.*)

21. Barry HC, Hickner J, Ebell MH, et al. A randomized controlled trial of telephone management of suspected urinary tract infections in women. J Family Pract 2001;50:589. (*Telephone management is equivalent to office visits in this study with a very selected low-risk patient population.*)

22. Gupta K, Scholes D, Stamm WE. Increasing prevalence of antimicrobial resistance among uropathogens causing acute uncomplicated cystitis in women. JAMA 1999;281:736. (*Documents increasing resistance to ampicillin, cephalothin, trimethoprim, and TMS.*)

23. Gupta K, Hooten TM, Roberts PL, et al. Patient-initiated treatment of uncomplicated recurrent urinary tract infections in young women. Ann Intern Med 2001;135:9. (*Eighty-eight patients self-diagnosed 172 urinary tract infections and started self-therapy; 84% had positive culture and 11% had pyuria; therapy resulted in 92% clinical and 96% microbiologic cures.*)

24. Hooton TM, Besser R, Foxman B, et al. Acute uncomplicated cystitis in an era of increasing antibiotic resistance: a proposed approach to empirical therapy. Clin Infect Dis 2004;39:75. (*Addresses concerns about the increasing resistance of common pathogens to trimethoprim.*)

25. Hooton TM, Winter C, Tiu F, et al. Randomized comparative trial and cost analysis of 3-day antimicrobial regimens for treatment of acute cystitis in women. JAMA 1995;273:41. (*TMS was the most effective treatment.*)

26. Kontiokari T, Sundqvist K, Nuutinen M, et al. Randomized trial of cranberry-lingonberry juice and *Lactobacillus* GG drink for the prevention of urinary tract infections in women. Br Med J 2001;322:1571. (*Patients randomized to receive cranberry-lingonberry juice had 16% recurrent infection in a 12-month follow-up, in comparison to 39% in the Lactobacillus GG group and 36% in the placebo group.*)

27. Kremery S, Hromec J, Tvrdikova M, et al. Newer quinolones in the long-term prophylaxis of recurrent urinary tract infections. Drugs 1999;58:99. (*Daily dosing was effective during a 12-month period in four of every five premenopausal women with a history of recurrent infection.*)

28. Lutters M, Vogt N. Antibiotic duration for treating uncomplicated, symptomatic lower urinary tract infections in elderly women (Cochrane review). In: The Cochrane library, Issue 3. Oxford: Update Software, 2004. (*No difference in effectiveness was found; see* http://www.cochrane.org *for updates.*)

29. McCarty JM, Richard G, Huck W, et al. A randomized trial of short-course ciprofloxacin, ofloxacin, or trimethoprim/sulfamethoxazole for the treatment of acute urinary tract infection in women. Ciprofloxacin Urinary Tract Infection Group. Am J Med 1999;106:292. (*These three drugs were equally effective.*)

30. Norrby SR. Short-term treatment of uncomplicated urinary tract infections in women. Rev Infect Dis 1990;12:458. (*A meta-analysis suggesting that 3-day regimens are generally more effective than 1-day programs.*)

31. Katchman, EA, Milo, G, Paul, M, et al. Three-day vs longer duration of antibiotic treatment of for cystitis in women: systematic review and meta-analysis. Am J Med 2005;118:1196. (*A meta-analysis indicating that 3-day antibiotic treatment is as effective as prolonged treatment of >5 days.*)

32. Richards D, Toop L, Chambers S, et al. Response to antibiotics of women with symptoms of urinary tract infection but negative dipstick urine test results: double blind randomized controlled trial. BMJ 2005;331:143. (*Although a negative dipstick test predicted the absence of infection, it did not predict response to trimethoprim 300 mg daily for 3 days.*)

33. Mangin D, Toop L. Urinary tract infection in primary care. BMJ 2007;334:597. (*Makes the argument for trimethoprim as first-line therapy with a switch to an alternative governed by the clinical response or lack thereof rather than on microbiologic grounds.*)

34. Schaeffer AJ, Stuppy BA. Efficacy and safety of self-start therapy in women with recurrent urinary tract infections. J Urol 1999;161:207. (*Patient initiation of norfloxacin after a dip-slide urine culture was effective in this small trial.*)

35. Stamm WE, Counts GW, Wagner KF, et al. Antimicrobial prophylaxis of recurrent urinary tract infections. Ann Intern Med 1980;92:770. (*All regimens proved to be effective and were well tolerated; there was no emergence of resistant strains.*)

36. Stamm WE, McKevitt M, Counts GW. Acute renal infection in women: treatment with trimethoprim-sulfamethoxazole or ampicillin for two or six weeks. Ann Intern Med 1987;106:341. (*Treatment for 2 weeks sufficed; TMS was better.*)

37. Stamm WE, McKevitt M, Counts GW. Is antimicrobial prophylaxis of urinary tract infections cost-effective? Ann Intern Med 1981;94:251. (*Prophylaxis became cost-effective when women had three infections per year.*)

38. Vogel T, Verreault R, Gourdeau M, et al. Optimal duration of antibiotic therapy for uncomplicated urinary tract infection in older women: a double-blind randomized controlled trial. Can Med Assoc J 2004;170:469. (*No benefit was found for the longer course in women older than age 65 years.*)

CHAPTER 134 ■ APPROACH TO INCONTINENCE AND OTHER FORMS OF LOWER URINARY TRACT DYSFUNCTION

JOHN D. GOODSON

Patients with lower urinary tract dysfunction may present with incontinence, hesitancy, dribbling, loss of stream volume or force, frequency, or urgency.

Incontinence can have a major effect on a patient and his or her family. At the least, it is an embarrassment and an inconvenience. Constant incontinence can predispose to local skin breakdown, serious infection, and social isolation. Loss of urine control requires many life adjustments and can have an effect on social interactions and levels of overall activity. In many instances, it is the culminating event that leads to nursing home placement.

Substantial progress has been made in the management of incontinence, and there are many useful strategies and interventions. The goal of therapy is to devise the most workable and effective solution possible. This takes time and interaction over multiple visits. Because even successful solutions require readjustment, an ongoing dialogue around continence is an important part of continuity of patient care for some patients.

PATHOPHYSIOLOGY AND CLINICAL PRESENTATION (1–7)

Normal Bladder Function and Continence

The *detrusor muscle* of the bladder is normally under simultaneous *sympathetic* and *parasympathetic* control. During the filling phase, sympathetic tone predominates, whereas parasympathetic tone is inhibited. The internal bladder sphincter tightens under *α-adrenergic* influence and the detrusor relaxes under *β-adrenergic* influence. During voluntary emptying, parasympathetic stimulation produces detrusor contraction; at the same time, sympathetic tone decreases, the external sphincter of the pelvic floor relaxes, and abdominal muscles tighten. Normally, the urethra is oriented to the bladder so as to facilitate continence. With the initiation of voluntary voiding, the *urethrovesicular angle* changes so as to permit full drainage. Complete bladder emptying depends on unimpeded flow.

The process of voiding usually begins with a sensation of bladder fullness mediated by proprioceptive fibers in the detrusor. A reflex arc between the detrusor and the brainstem initiates and amplifies bladder contraction by parasympathetic stimulation. This arc is under cortical inhibition. Voiding occurs with the release of inhibition and voluntary relaxation of the pelvic external sphincter.

Incontinence

The pathophysiology and clinical presentations of incontinence can be divided on clinical and mechanistic grounds into categories of detrusor instability or overactivity (urge incontinence), sphincter or pelvic incompetence (stress incontinence), reflex incontinence, detrusor hypotonia or insufficiency (overflow incontinence), and functional incontinence. Clinically, two or more processes frequently coexist to varying degrees in the same patient.

Detrusor Instability or Overactivity (Urge Incontinence)

Detrusor instability or overactivity (urge incontinence) is characterized by reduced bladder capacity resulting from excessive and inappropriate detrusor contraction. For many, the condition appears to arise as a concomitant of *aging*, although the mechanism is unclear. In some cases, it seems to be the result of *decreased cortical inhibition* of detrusor contraction. Loss of cortical input can ensue from such conditions as cerebral infarction, Alzheimer's disease, brain tumor, and Parkinson's disease. For others, the *detrusor instability* or *overactivity* is linked to *bladder irritation* from such causes as trigonitis (a common accompaniment of cystitis), chronic interstitial cystitis, postradiation fibrosis, and detrusor hypertrophy from longstanding outflow tract obstruction from urethral stricture or benign prostatic hyperplasia (BPH). Patients note a few moments of warning, frequent episodes of urgency, moderate to large volumes, and nocturnal wetting. In roughly half of patients, detrusor instability is associated with poor detrusor function. For these patients, voiding is frequent and incomplete.

Sphincter or Pelvic Incompetence (Stress Incontinence)

Sphincter or pelvic incompetence (stress incontinence) is usually a consequence of pelvic floor laxity and is the most common form of urinary incontinence in both men and women. Less frequently, it develops from *partial denervation* that reduces sphincter tone. Pelvic laxity is seen as a concomitant of normal aging or as a consequence of difficult or multiple vaginal deliveries or direct perineal injury. In some cases, a cystocele forms and further impedes control. *Estrogen deficiency* in women reduces the competency of the internal sphincter and can also cause urethral symptoms (dysuria and frequency). In men, pelvic incompetence may result from prostatic surgery, most commonly prostatectomy, although in most cases the abnormality resolves within 6 to 12 months if innervation remains largely intact. Patients complain of incontinence, which occurs predominantly at times of straining (coughing, laughing, sneezing, lifting). There is loss of small to moderate volumes of urine, very infrequent nighttime leakage, and little postvoid residual.

Reflex Incontinence

Reflex incontinence derives mostly from *spinal cord damage* above the sacral level. Interference with sensation and coordination of detrusor and sphincter activity secondary to inhibited or absent central control leads to *detrusor spasticity* and *overactivity* and *functional outlet obstruction*. The patient is unable to sense the need to void. Spinal cord injury is the most common cause. Diabetes, multiple sclerosis, tabes dorsalis, and intrinsic or extrinsic cord compression from tumor, disk herniation, or spinal stenosis are also important causes. Reflex incontinence takes place day and night with equal frequency and without warning or precipitating stress. Volumes are moderate, and voiding is frequent. Voluntary sphincter control and perineal sensation are reduced; sacral reflexes remain intact.

Detrusor Hypotonia or Insufficiency (Overflow Incontinence)

Detrusor hypotonia or insufficiency (overflow incontinence) results from longstanding *outlet obstruction, detrusor insufficiency,* or *impaired sensation*. The bladder becomes hypotonic, flaccid, and distended. Voiding consists primarily of overflow spillage. In outflow tract obstruction (most often from longstanding BPH), the detrusor is constantly overstretched and gradually becomes incapable of generating sufficient pressure to ensure bladder emptying. Often, *detrusor hypotonia or insufficiency* is a consequence of lower motor neuron damage, as occurs with injury to the sacral cord or the development of peripheral neuropathy (as in diabetes or vitamin B_{12} deficiency). Perineal sensation and sacral reflexes may be lost. Of importance, numerous medications (e.g., anticholinergics, tricyclic antidepressants) can reduce detrusor tone. Distinguishing clinical characteristics include a palpably *distended bladder* and a *large postvoid residual*. Patients void frequently, especially after fluid loads and diuretics. Incomplete emptying, slow or interrupted flow, hesitancy, and the need to strain are common complaints. There may be reports of stress incontinence. Retrograde flow of urine and increased ureteral pressures can compromise renal function if the condition is left uncorrected, and an occasional patient will present with renal failure.

Functional Incontinence

Functional incontinence refers to situations in which physical or mental disability makes it impossible to void independently, even though the urinary tract may be intact. Patients with disabling illness or simply an acute change to a bedridden state may be unable to maintain sufficient control over lower urinary function to avoid incontinence. Sedating drugs in such situations may only exacerbate the problem. Patients who are aware of their condition will describe their unsuccessful attempts to maintain continence. Patients with frontal lobe dysfunction secondary to cortical degenerative disease or normopressure hydrocephalus may be unaware of their voiding and therefore be functionally incontinent. Rarely, deliberate incontinence is part of a mental health condition.

Urinary Frequency in Conjunction with Dysuria

Frequency accompanied by dysuria is a common presentation of lower *urinary tract infection*. Inflammation of the bladder trigone and urethra are responsible for most acute symptoms. *Chronic interstitial cystitis, acute urethral syndrome,* and *chronic nonbacterial prostatis* have been implicated as causes in cases without identifiable infection, although some of these may have unapparent infection with *Chlamydia* (see Chapters 125, 133, 136, and 139). *Carcinoma* of the bladder trigone or urethra is a rare but important cause of dysuria, frequency, and symptoms of outflow tract obstruction.

Urinary Frequency in Conjunction with Difficulty Voiding

When associated with slow stream, hesitancy, and a sense of incomplete emptying, frequency is likely to be a manifestation of *outflow tract obstruction* (extrinsic or intrinsic). At first, the patient may notice only minor slowness of stream. If the obstruction persists, bladder instability may ensue and cause frequent voiding of small volumes, followed later by chronic distention and overflow incontinence (see prior discussion). Strictures, tumor (especially prostatic enlargement), and occasionally stones are responsible for most cases of obstruction. In the setting of severe constipation, the rectal vault can become sufficiently impacted that it actually blocks the urethra and prevents bladder emptying. *α-Adrenergic* agents and *β-blockers* can increase sphincter tone and impair voiding acutely, especially in patients with preexisting lower urinary tract dysfunction. *Anticholinergic drugs* may interfere with bladder contraction.

Urinary Frequency and Polydipsia

When frequency presents in association with increased thirst, it suggests a diabetic condition leading to increased urine volume and the resultant polyuria. *Diabetes mellitus* is distinguished by significant glycosuria (see Chapter 102). *Neurogenic (idiopathic central) diabetes insipidus* is manifested by sudden onset, craving for huge volumes of cold water, and prodigious urine outputs (5 to 10 L/d). Inability to concentrate the urine after overnight fluid deprivation and response to parenteral antidiuretic hormone (ADH), with formation of a concentrated urine, characterize the condition. Patients with *nephrogenic diabetes insipidus* differ from those with the neurogenic variety, in that their kidneys do not respond to intrinsic or parenteral ADH. Hypercalcemia, lithium therapy, and pregnancy are precipitants of the acquired variety. Patients with *psychogenic polydipsia* may be hard to distinguish from those with nephrogenic diabetes insipidus because they have washed out their renal concentrating system and also do not adequately respond to parenteral ADH. They do respond normally to fluid deprivation, which is a diagnostically useful finding, although some patients with neurogenic disease respond in a similar fashion (see Chapter 101).

Isolated Urinary Frequency

Isolated frequency may be a manifestation of reduced bladder capacity or a presentation of mild diabetes mellitus, mild diabetes insipidus, minor urinary tract infection, or bladder irritation. A large *extrinsic* or *intrinsic mass* impinging on the bladder can reduce its capacity and produce frequent urination, usually of small volumes, which distinguish it from other forms of polyuria. Pelvic surgery, chronic interstitial cystitis, or irradiation can have a similar effect by reducing bladder capacity. Patients who surreptitiously abuse *diuretics* rarely complain of frequency, but those who take them for therapeutic purposes are often bothered by the side effect. Nocturnal urinary frequency and occasional incontinence can represent the *mobilization of fluid* in patients with dependent edema associated with congestive heart failure or intake of certain medications, such as some of the calcium-channel blockers.

DIFFERENTIAL DIAGNOSIS (1–7)

The differential diagnosis of incontinence can be classified according to clinical presentation and mechanism (Table 134.1). The differential diagnosis of dysuria and frequency is that of urinary tract infection and its related syndromes (see Chapters 133 and 140). Most patients with difficulty voiding are men with BPH (see Chapter 138). Among other causes of difficult voiding are drugs (anticholinergics, β-blockers, sedatives), urethral stricture, congenital valves, stone, tumor, pelvic abscess, and fecal impaction. Causes of urinary frequency in the absence of other urinary tract symptoms include diabetes mellitus, diabetes insipidus, psychogenic polydipsia, diuretics, and bladder compression.

WORKUP (6–9)

The evaluation of incontinence and other lower urinary tract symptoms requires assessment of the major neuromuscular and anatomic elements involved in maintaining urinary continence and flow. Much can be gleaned from the history and physical examination, which provide important clues to the underlying pathophysiology and precipitants.

History

Assessment of incontinence begins with the collection of specific information from the patient and his or her family where appropriate. Clinical questioning should focus on the circumstances, precipitants, timing, frequency, and volume of urine loss, the presence of warning symptoms, and the intactness of perineal and bladder sensation.

When the history is sketchy, ask the patient or family to keep a *diary* of events and contributing factors. This diary should include the following: time of urination; an estimate of the volume; the symptoms associated with each void, such as leakage; and any precipitating events, such as laughing or coughing.

The history will frequently suggest the diagnosis, although there is rarely a single explanation. Incontinence triggered only by *straining, laughing,* or *coughing* indicates stress incontinence, although an occasional patient with overflow incontinence will report leakage under similar circumstances. Patients with overflow differ, in that they also experience frequent loss

TABLE 134.1

IMPORTANT CAUSES OF INCONTINENCE

Type	Mechanism	Characteristics
Detrusor Instability Bladder infection Chronic cystitis CNS disease (dementia, stroke) Detrusor hyperreflexia Detrusor hypertrophy Irradiation	Unstable detrusor	Warning; frequent episodes; nocturnal wetting; small postvoid residual, intact reflexes; normal sensation
Stress Incontinence Aging Autonomic neuropathy Estrogen deficiency Pelvic laxity Perineal injury Urologic surgery	Inadequate sphincter	On straining; small to moderate volumes; rarely at night; small postvoid volume
Reflex Incontinence Disk herniation Multiple sclerosis Spinal cord disease Tumor	Upper neurologic tract disease (autonomous bladder) Spinal cord injury Severe cortical disease	No warning or precipitants; severe neurologic disease; episodes can occur day and night; frequent; moderate volumes; loss of control and sensation; reflexes intact
Overflow Incontinence Diabetes Medications Outflow obstruction Peripheral neuropathy Sacral cord lesion Tabes dorsalis Vitamin B_{12} deficiency	Bladder outlet obstruction, lower motor neuron injury, or impaired sensation; toxic impairment of detrusor contraction	Distended bladder; history of obstructive symptoms; frequent loss of small volumes; loss of reflexes and sensation if caused by neurologic injury; large postvoid residual
Functional Incontinence Acute illness Medications Psychiatric disease	Inability to reach toilet in time	Functionally impaired patient

CNS, central nervous system.

of *small volumes* without warning or straining and are bothered by nocturnal episodes.

A history of obstructive symptoms, such as *difficulty with stream initiation* or *weakened urine flow*, suggests an etiology for the overflow physiology such BPH, urethral stricture, stone, tumor, and fecal impaction.

In contrast to those with overflow disease, patients with *frequent episodes of urgency who lose small amounts of urine yet retain perineal sensation* are likely to have detrusor instability or overactivity. Although there may be a few moments of warning, they also report nocturnal incontinence. When this is accompanied by *dysuria*, a search for urinary tract infection is indicated (see Chapters 133, 139, and 140). Frequent voiding of small volumes and urgency are also consistent with a small bladder resulting from extrinsic compression.

Reflex incontinence is suggested by a history of spinal cord injury, diabetes, multiple sclerosis, or dementia with neurologic deficits. Severe loss of cortical function is also a precipitant of detrusor instability. Furthermore, recent physical disability and confinement to bed may produce functional incontinence.

Patients with isolated *urinary frequency* should be asked about *increased thirst*, a feature consistent with diabetes mellitus and diabetes insipidus. Compulsive water drinkers with psychogenic polydipsia may deny their intake of water but gen-

erally do not report nocturia, a feature of both diabetes mellitus and diabetes insipidus. The sudden onset of intense thirst for ice-cold water is very suggestive of diabetes insipidus.

The patient and family should be carefully questioned about *medications*, especially those with anticholinergic, α-adrenergic, β-adrenergic blocking, tranquilizing, or diuretic effects (e.g., tricyclic antidepressants, major and minor tranquilizers, decongestants, and antihypertensives). Any excessive use of coffee, tea, caffeine, or alcohol should be noted.

Physical Examination

For the patient with incontinence, the examination begins by noting general appearance and any lack of attention to personal hygiene. A careful urogenital examination is essential and includes suprapubic palpation and percussion of the bladder after voiding to detect distention and masses. When appropriate, the *rectum* should be checked for impaction or *prostatic enlargement*. Absence of palpable prostatic enlargement does not rule out obstruction, especially in a patient with obstructive symptoms; median lobe encroachment on the urethra is often not palpable. Similarly, a large prostate does not predict severe obstruction.

Women with stress incontinence should be examined in the lithotomy position. *Pelvic motion* and continence should be noted during cough or Valsalva's maneuver. Testing for stress incontinence is best done with the bladder full, unless the problem is severe and requires little provocation. Check the *vaginal mucosa* for atrophic changes (red, thin mucosa with a watery discharge) indicative of inadequate estrogen. A *bimanual examination* completes the evaluation, with note taken of any uterine or adnexal masses.

Neurologic control of voiding needs to be assessed to determine the presence of any deficits above, within, or distal to the autonomic reflex arc. Checking the *bulbocavernosus reflex* tests the integrity of the arc. Normally, squeezing the clitoris or glans penis will cause anal sphincter contraction. Lack of response suggests interruption. Another means of testing the arc is to note *anal sphincter tone*. Because control of the anal sphincter is similar to that of the bladder, the examiner can indirectly estimate its competence by checking the anal tone on rectal examination and by noting the patient's ability to contract the sphincter voluntarily. Loss of sphincter tone in a patient who retains sensation suggests a motor neuron lesion within the arc.

Perineal sensation is also tested; if it is lacking, yet sacral reflexes are preserved, reflex incontinence from a lesion above the arc is suggested, such as one caused by diabetes, multiple sclerosis, or spinal cord injury. Patients with loss of both sensation and reflexes are likely to have overflow incontinence because of neurologic injury to the reflex arc. Incontinent patients who retain their reflexes and sensation have detrusor instability, stress incontinence, overflow incontinence, or a functional problem.

A mental status examination is usually not necessary to detect underlying dementia in the patient with incontinence; in most cases, the condition is apparent by the time incontinence occurs.

Laboratory Studies

Often, a careful history and examination are sufficient to arrive at a working diagnosis for the patient with lower urinary tract symptomatology. A *urinalysis* and a few simple chemistry studies (*blood urea nitrogen*, *creatinine*, and *glucose*) are appropriate for most patients. Consider a *serologic test for syphilis* in patients with overflow incontinence. All patients should have a *urinalysis* and a possible *culture* to exclude concurrent infection. *Pelvic ultrasonography* offers a noninvasive method of assessing postvoid residual and is especially useful when outflow obstruction or detrusor failure is suspected. *Straight catheterization* after voiding is a simple office technique for determining residual volume, a useful measure when overflow incontinence is in question. A volume greater than 50 mL is abnormal.

The *cystometrogram* is rarely needed but can help to sort out complicated mixed conditions. Normal persons sense bladder filling between 100 and 200 mL, have a nonurgent desire to void at 250 to 350 mL, and experience detrusor contraction at 400 to 550 mL (Fig. 134.1A). A spastic bladder will demonstrate a small capacity and recurrent uninhibited contraction (Fig. 134.1B). An atonic bladder will show a large volume and little contractile force (Fig. 134.1C).

Measurement of *urine flow* rates provides information on outflow obstruction and aids in monitoring the progression of obstruction. Normal flow rate is 10 mL/s, with more than 200 mL in the bladder. The normal curve (Fig. 134.2A) shows an early peak flow rate, whereas the curve of the obstructed bladder manifests a delayed and reduced flow rate (Fig. 134.2B).

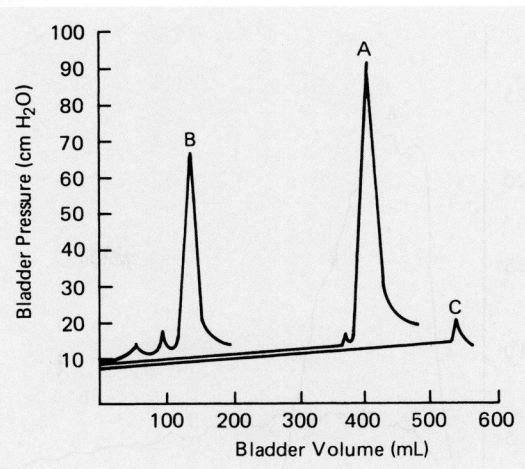

FIGURE 134.1. Cystometrogram findings. **A:** Normal pressure–volume relationship. **B:** Uninhibited neurogenic bladder. **C:** Atonic bladder.

Patients with polyuria should be checked for glycosuria, hypercalcemia, and hypokalemia. Those with normal levels should have their urine-concentrating ability tested; this is accomplished by measuring *urine osmolality* after 8 hours of *fluid restriction* (usually overnight). Normal persons and those with psychogenic polydipsia should be able to concentrate their urine to more than 700 mOsm/L after 8 hours of fluid restriction. Inability to concentrate requires further testing, including measurement of serum osmolality before and after water restriction and parenteral administration of ADH. Direct measurement of ADH may be helpful (see Chapter 101).

MANAGEMENT OF INCONTINENCE (10–28)

General Measures

Management is best guided by the mechanism(s) responsible for the incontinence, the patient's overall medical and mental status, and the capabilities of the family or caretakers (Table 134.2). However, some general measures apply to all incontinent patients:

- Restrict fluid loads, coffee, tea, and alcohol.
- Avoid all caffeinated products and related compounds, such as chocolate.
- Limit the use of diuretics, and, if necessary, give them in the morning. If twice-a-day dosing is needed, give the second dose in the early afternoon.
- Anticholinergic drugs for nonneurologic purposes should be given with care and in the lowest possible doses.
- Avoid use of indwelling catheters because of the risk for infection, exacerbation of detrusor instability, and leakage.
- Avoid use of condom catheters, except for short, well-supervised periods.
- Advise use of an adsorbent pad for patients with refractory symptoms and recommend that it be changed frequently to prevent skin breakdown.
- If long-term indwelling catheterization is unavoidable, the catheter should be inserted only by trained personnel under

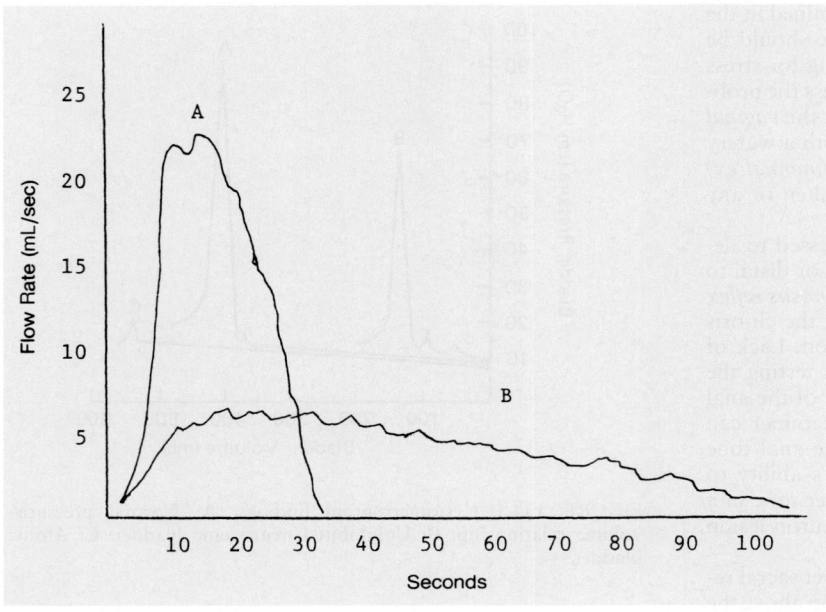

FIGURE 134.2. Urinary flow studies. **A:** Normal voiding. **B:** Obstructed voiding. The area under each curve represents the volume voided.

aseptic conditions, drained with the bag always below the patient's bladder, manipulated as little as possible, irrigated only if flow is reduced, changed if blocked, and removed if upper tract infection is suspected. Antibiotic prophylaxis is not recommended.

Detrusor Instability (Urge Incontinence)

Before symptomatic therapy is initiated, one should attend to treatable etiologic factors, such as outflow obstruction or chronic bladder irritation. In most instances, the cause cannot be identified or is not amenable to definitive treatment, so that symptomatic relief becomes the major objective. Much can be done:

- Teach the patient to void at regular, frequent intervals. From such *bladder-training* programs, patients can learn to suppress the urge to void by contracting pelvic muscles and then relaxing them slowly or by engaging in distracting activities (such as the mathematical calculations required by paying bills or the thinking required by social conversations). It is helpful to have motivated patients void initially at short, scheduled intervals, such as every 30 to 45 minutes. These intervals can be increased over time to 2 to 3 hours. Sometimes, merely keeping a voiding diary improves urinary control.
- Instruct both male and female patients in the Kegel exercises. Bladder-training programs and biofeedback programs work, but patient self-training has also been shown to be effective. Patients should be instructed to contract the pelvic muscles that control continence without contracting abdominal muscles. For example, instruct patients to contract these muscles 45 times a day, three sets of 15 contractions. Contractions should begin for 1 or 2 seconds and then advance to 10 seconds. Improvement can take several weeks.
- Provide a bedside commode or urinal for the patient.
- Initiate a trial of a tricyclic agent with anticholinergic effects, such as imipramine (10 to 25 mg, one to four times a day). Data supporting this are weak, and patients who respond

to this therapy should be periodically taken off to determine whether the treatment is still effective.
- Initiate a trial of an agent with both smooth-muscle relaxant and anticholinergic properties, such as oxybutynin (2.5 to 5 mg three times daily, lower dose for patients with stage 4 or higher chronic kidney disease [CKD] or hepatic impairment). Lower doses can be effective in the elderly, and untoward central nervous system side effects and intolerable dry mouth are thereby avoided.
- The are several selective bladder smooth-muscle relaxants that have fewer side effects than oxybutynin and may be better tolerated: tolterodine (1 to 2 mg twice daily, lower dose for patients with stage 4 or higher CKD or hepatic impairment), solifenacin (5 to 10 mg daily, lower dose for patients with stage 4 or higher CKD or hepatic impairment), trospium (20 mg once or twice daily, lower dose required for stage 4 or higher CKD), and darifenacin (7.5 to 15 mg daily, lower dose for patients with hepatic impairment). In one prospective trial, solifenacin was superior to extended-release tolterodine. All of these drugs can have an effect on cognition, even in younger patients (midlife). All these drugs should be used with caution for patients with CKD and/or hepatic impairment.

Detrusor Atony (Overflow Incontinence)

The first priority is definitive treatment of any mechanical obstruction or reversible neurologic deficit (e.g., herniated disk, vitamin B_{12} deficiency), followed by efforts to reduce the postvoid residual and prevent infection. If a fixed obstruction is present, relief may be sufficient to allow detrusor function to return.

- For both acute and chronic obstruction, place an indwelling catheter or repeatedly catheterize (every 4 to 6 hours) the patient to decompress the bladder.
- If this does not restore bladder function, then teach the patient to void while performing Credé's maneuver (suprapubic external compression) or Valsalva's maneuver.

TABLE 134.2

DRUGS USED TO TREAT INCONTINENCE

Drugs	Dose Range	Action	Side Effects	Possible Contraindications
Detrusor Instability				
Imipramine hydrochloride (Tofranil)	10–25 mg qd to qid	Decreases detrusor and increases internal sphincter tone	Dry mouth, blurred vision, constipation, postural hypotension, palpitations	Anatomic obstruction, cardiac arrhythmias, hyperthyroidism, glaucoma, hepatic or renal disease (stage 4 or higher chronic kidney disease, creatinine clearance <30 mL/min), pregnancy
Oxybutynin chloride (Ditropan)	2.5–5 mg qd to qid	Decrease detrusor tone	Same	Same
Tolterodine (Detrol)	1–2 mg bid	Selectively decreases detrusor tone	Same	Same
Solifenacin (VESIcare)	5–10 mg qd	Same	Same	Same
Trospium (Sanctura)	20 mg qd to bid	Same	Same	Same
Darifenacin (Enablex)	7.5–15 mg qd	Same	Same	Same
Detrusor Atony				
Bethanechol chloride (Urecholine)	5–25 mg bid to qid	Increases detrusor tone	Salivation, flushing, abdominal cramps, diarrhea, sweating	Anatomic obstruction, asthma, guanethidine peptic ulcer, hyperthyroidism, age
Prazosin (Minipress)	1–5 mg bid to qid	Decreases internal sphincter tone	Light-headedness	Postural hypotension
Doxazosin (Cardura)	2–8 mg qd	Same	Same	Same
Terazosin (Hytrin)	1–2 mg qd	Decreases internal sphincter tone	Same	Same
Tamsulosin (Flomax)	0.4 mg qd to bid	Selectively decreases internal sphincter tone	Same	Same
Alfuzosin (Avodart)	10 mg qd	Same	Same	Same
Sphincter Incompetency				
Imipramine hydrochloride (Tofranil)	10–25 mg qd to qid	Decreases detrusor and increases internal sphincter tone	See above	See above
Estrogen cream (in women) (Premarin)	qd initially then biw or weekly	Increases internal sphincter tone	Uterine cancer, possibly breast cancer, hypertension, cholelithiasis, glucose intolerance, thromboembolic disease	Uterine or breast malignancy, uterine fibroid tumors
Reflex Incontinence				
Prazosin (Minipress)	1–5 mg bid to qid	Decreases internal sphincter tone	See above	See above
Doxazosin (Cardura)	2–8 mg qd	Same	Same	Same
Terazosin (Hytrin)	1–10 mg qd	Same	Same	Same
Tamsulosin (Flomax)	0.4 mg qd to bid	Selectively decreases internal sphincter tone	Same	Same

bid, twice daily; biw, twice a week; qd, daily; qid, four times daily.

959

- Add an α-blocker such as prazosin (2 to 20 mg/d in divided doses), doxazosin (2 to 8 mg daily), terazosin (1 to 10 mg daily), tamsulosin (0.4 to 0.8 mg daily or in split doses), or alfuzosin (10 mg daily) to reduce sphincter resistance. Prazosin, doxazosin, and terazosin are more likely to cause clinically significant hypotension.
- Add bethanechol (25 to 50 mg/d in divided doses twice or three times a day) to augment bladder contraction. Data supporting this are weak, and patients who respond to this therapy should be periodically taken off to determine whether the treatment is still effective.
- Monitor the effects of these agents by checking postvoid residuals; patients with a residual in excess of 150 mL may require repeated sterile catheterization on an intermittent basis (three to four times per day) because the risk of recurrent infection is so high. These patients should be referred for full urologic assessment.

Sphincter Incompetence (Stress Incontinence)

The condition responds well to simple measures, beginning with exercises to strengthen the perineal muscles that terminate the urinary stream. For postmenopausal women, estrogen cream can also help. Surgical approaches are reserved for patients with persistently incapacitating difficulty.

- Instruct both male and female patients in the Kegel exercises. Bladder-training programs and biofeedback programs work, but patient self-training has also been shown to be effective. Patients should be instructed to contract the pelvic muscles that control continence without contracting abdominal muscles. For example, instruct patients to contract these muscles 45 times a day, three sets of 15 contractions. Contractions should begin for 1 or 2 seconds and then advance to 10 seconds. Improvement can take several weeks.
- For a female patient with evidence of atrophic vaginitis, prescribe a topical estrogen cream (Table 134.2). It should be applied daily for the first 3 weeks and then once or twice weekly thereafter to maintain sufficient estrogen to restore internal sphincter and urethral tone in postmenopausal women. The risk of such topical estrogen therapy is uncertain. Estrogens of any sort should be used cautiously in women with a personal history of breast cancer or thromboembolic disease (see Chapter 118). Oral estrogen therapy with or without progestin therapy worsens incontinence and should not be used for this purpose.
- Try a course of imipramine (10 to 25 mg, one to four times a day) for those with symptoms of both bladder irritability and stress incontinence. Data supporting this are weak, and patients who respond to this therapy should be periodically taken off to determine whether the treatment is still effective.
- Pessaries come in a variety of shapes and can be successfully fitted to improve continence. They must be changed and cleaned regularly. Referral should be made to a gynecologist or urologist with interest and experience.
- A penile clamp may be necessary in men who do not respond to other measures. Careful monitoring and a competent patient are necessary.

Reflex Incontinence

A major problem is a dyssynergy between bladder contraction and sphincter relaxation that results in ureteral reflux and the potential for hydronephrosis and renal function deterioration.

The bladder needs to be effectively decompressed. As a result, these patients frequently do best with a program of regular straight catheterization.

- In a patient with bladder–sphincter dyssynergy, try pharmacologically decompressing the bladder by giving an α-blocker such as prazosin (2 to 20 mg in divided doses), doxazosin (2 to 8 mg daily), terazosin (1 to 10 mg daily), tamsulosin (0.4 to 0.8 mg daily or in split doses), or alfuzosin (10 mg daily) to reduce sphincter resistance. Prazosin, doxazosin, and terazosin are more likely to cause clinically significant hypotension.
- Consider an agent used for detrusor instability if bladder capacity is small as demonstrated by straight catheterization or ultrasound, such as imipramine (10 to 25 mg, one to four times a day). Data supporting this are weak, and patients who respond to this therapy should be periodically taken off to determine whether the treatment is still effective.
- A sphincterotomy may be required to ensure bladder emptying.

Functional Incontinence

The prime effort is to ease the patient's access to a urinal, bedpan, or commode. Bedside placement is the obvious solution. For more-disabled patients, regular use of absorbent diapers, frequent straight catheterization, or, rarely, condom or indwelling catheterization can be considered.

PATIENT EDUCATION

To provide palliative relief early in the course of the evaluation, teach symptomatic measures even before the workup is completed. The use of adult diapers, pads, and scheduled voiding times, plus elimination of caffeinated beverages and alcohol and rescheduling of medication intake, can do much to lessen symptoms and the stress on patient, family, and caretakers.

With older and disabled patients, incontinence is hard for both patient and family. The primary care physician must ensure that everyone understands the problem and its cause so that no one blames the patient for being incontinent.

Many of the behavioral therapies, such as bladder training and the Kegel exercises, take time, patience, and commitment to learn. Given the annoying presence of incontinence, patients can become frustrated by the slow progress toward urine control. Reassure patients that these strategies work for many patients and reduce symptoms for most, but require time and effort.

Pharmacologic therapies are not predictably helpful. Many literature reviews have cast doubt on traditional approaches, such as the use of anticholinergics and cholinergic agonists. These interventions may help with some patients, but even in those who do seem to respond, a treatment-free interval or "drug holiday" should be considered periodically every few years.

INDICATIONS FOR REFERRAL

The incontinent patient with a suspected cord lesion or other form of neurologic injury should be promptly referred for neurologic consultation. Urologic referral is needed in cases of outflow tract obstruction, especially those severe enough to cause a hypotonic bladder and a large postvoid residual (>150 mL).

The risk for ureteral reflux and the development of hydronephrosis makes definitive therapy essential. Patients with severe sphincter dyssynergy and reflex incontinence may require a sphincterotomy if all else fails.

Patients with urge incontinence and stress incontinence are candidates for behavioral and/or biofeedback therapy if a program is available.

Women with refractory stress incontinence are candidates for reconstructive surgical efforts; referral should be made to a surgeon experienced with correcting pelvic incompetence. Minimally invasive techniques are available.

Pessaries are useful but need to be fitted by an experienced gynecologist or urologist, with an effective patient education program.

Annotated Bibliography

1. Norton P, Brubaker L. Urinary incontinence in women. Lancet 2006;367:57. (*A comprehensive review of pathophysiology, epidemiology, assessment, and treatment; 116 references.*)
2. DuBeau CE. Interpreting the effects of common medical conditions on voiding dysfunction in the elderly. Urol Clin North Am 1996;23:11. (*Reviews the mechanisms by which common medical conditions affect urinary continence.*)
3. Kozoil JA, Clark DC, Gittes RF, et al. The natural history of interstitial cystitis: a survey of 374 patients. J Urol 1993;149:465. (*Symptoms were exacerbated by acidic, alcoholic, or carbonated beverages or by tea or coffee in 50% of patients; >80% of patients had to restrict their activities.*)
4. Messing EM, Stamey TA. Interstitial cystitis. Urology 1978;12:381. (*The diagnosis should be considered in women with persistent lower urinary tract symptoms and negative findings on cultures and workup.*)
5. Ouslander JG, Schnelle JF. Incontinence in the nursing home. Ann Intern Med 1995;122:438. (*Prompted voiding and reminders by caregivers every 2 hours reduced daytime incontinence in up to one third of nursing home patients.*)
6. Resnick NM, Valla SV, Laurino E. The pathophysiology of urinary incontinence among institutionalized elderly persons. N Engl J Med 1989;320:1. (*Sixty-one percent of patients had detrusor overactivity; 50% had impaired contractility.*)
7. Resnick NM, Valla SV. Management of urinary incontinence in the elderly. N Engl J Med 1985;313:800. (*Succinct, clinically useful review; 71 references.*)
8. Glazener CMA, Lapitan MC. Urodynamic investigations for management of urinary incontinence in children and adults (Cochrane review). In: The Cochrane library, Issue 3. Oxford: Update Software, 2004. (*Evidence was insufficient to recommend for or against urodynamic studies; see http://www.cochrane.org for updates.*)
9. Brown JS, Bradley CS, Subak LL, et al. The sensitivity and specificity of a simple test to distinguish between urge and stress urinary incontinence. Ann Intern Med. 2006;144:715. (*A three-question test had acceptable sensitivities and specificities for stress and urge incontinence.*)
10. Abrams P, Freeman R, Anderstrom C, et al. Tolterodine, a new antimuscarinic agent: as effective but better tolerated than oxybutynin in patients with an overactive bladder. Br J Urol 1998;81:801. (*A prospective, randomized, controlled trial of 293 men and women with urgency or urge incontinence; oxybutynin and tolterodine were equally effective, although oxybutynin caused more side effects, mostly dry mouth.*)
11. Alhasso A, Glazener CMA, Pickard R, et al. Adrenergic drugs for urinary incontinence in adults (Cochrane review). In: The Cochrane library, Issue 3. Oxford: Update Software, 2004. (*There is weak evidence for effectiveness; see http://www.cochrane.org for updates.*)
12. Brechtelsbauer DA. Care with an indwelling catheter. Postgrad Med 1992;92:127. (*Addresses the key issues of catheter use; a succinct, well-referenced review.*)
13. Burgio KL, Goode PS, Locher JL, et al. Behavioral training with and without biofeedback in the treatment of urge incontinence in older women. JAMA 2002;288:2293. (*A randomized trial of behavioral and electronically confirmed biofeedback, behavioral and manually confirmed biofeedback, and self-administered behavioral programs; all were of nearly equal value.*)
14. Burgio KL, Locher JL, Goode PS, et al. Behavioral vs. drug treatment for urge urinary incontinence in older women. JAMA 1998;280:1995. (*Behavioral therapy produced an 80.7% reduction in incontinence episodes, in comparison with a 68.5% reduction for drug therapy and a 39.4% reduction for placebo in this randomized, controlled trial.*)
15. Fantl JA, Cardoza L, McClish DK, and the Hormone and Urogenital Therapy Committee. Obstet Gynecol 1994;83:12. (*Meta-analysis of 166 studies; all forms of estrogen subjectively improved urinary incontinence in women.*)
16. Finkbeiner AE. Is bethanechol chloride clinically effective in promoting bladder emptying? A literature review. J Urol 1985;134:443. (*Evidence for its value is weak; bethanechol may be helpful with individual patients.*)
17. Glazener CMA, Cooper K. Anterior vaginal repair for urinary incontinence in women (Cochrane review). In: The Cochrane library, Issue 3. Oxford: Update Software, 2004. (*There was insufficient evidence for comparison with physical therapy or needle suspension or laparoscopic procedures; the abdominal procedure appears to be better than vaginal repair; see http://www.cochrane.org for updates.*)
18. Grady D, Brown JS, Vittinghoff E, et al. Postmenopausal hormones and incontinence: the Heart and Estrogen/progestin Replacement Study. Obstet Gynecol 2001;97:116. (*Surprisingly, women on combination therapy had more incontinence; the role of topical estrogen or oral unopposed estrogen therapy is uncertain because it may be progestins that worsen incontinence.*)
19. Harvey MA, Baker K, Wells GA. Tolterodine versus oxybutynin in the treatment of urge urinary incontinence: a meta-analysis. Am J Obstet Gynecol 2001;185:56. (*Both are effective, but patients on tolterodine had fewer side effects.*)
20. Hay-Smith EJC, Bø K, Berghmans LCM, et al. Pelvic floor muscle training for urinary incontinence in women (Cochrane review). In: The Cochrane library, Issue 3. Oxford: Update Software, 2004. (*Evidence supports effectiveness, although studies were of marginal size and quality; see http://www.cochrane.org for updates.*)
21. Herbison P, Hay-Smith J, Ellis G, et al. Effectiveness of anticholinergic drugs compared with placebo in the treatment of overactive bladder: systematic review. BMJ 2003;326:841. (*Evidence for the value of this approach is weak; anticholinergics may be helpful with individual patients.*)
22. Holroyd-Leduc JM, Straus SE. Management of urinary incontinence in women: scientific review. JAMA 2004;291:986. (*A comprehensive review concluding that nonpharmacologic, nonsurgical approaches are effective in many cases.*)
23. Sutherland SE, Goldman HB. Treatment options for female urinary incontinence. Med Clin North Am 2004;88:345. (*Reviews the role of pelvic muscle exercises and bladder training, as well as pharmacologic approaches.*)
24. Teunissen TA, de Jonge A, van Weel C, et al. Treating urinary incontinence in the elderly—conservative therapies that work: a systematic review. J Family Pract 2004;53:25. (*Recommends starting with conservative therapies.*)
25. Womack KB, Heilman KM. Tolterodine and memory. Arch Neurol 2003;60:771. (*Documented reversible cognitive decline with tolterodine in a 46-year-old woman.*)
26. Zeitlin MP, Lebherz TB. Pessaries in the geriatric patient. J Am Geriatr Soc 1992;40:635. (*Pessaries are indicated for the control of symptomatic uterine prolapse and should be assessed frequently.*)
27. Chapple CR, Martinez-Garcia R, Selvaggi L, et al. A comparison of the efficacy and tolerability of solifenacin succinate and extended release tolterodine at treating overactive bladder syndrome: results of the STAR trial. Eur Urol 2005;48:464. (*Solifenacin was superior to extended-release tolterodine.*)
28. Kaplan SA, Roehrborn CG, Rovner ES, et al. Tolterodine and tamsulosin for treatment of men with lower urinary tract symptoms and overactive bladder. JAMA 2006; 296:2319. (*In this randomized trial of 879 men, combination therapy was superior to either alone for men with benign prostatic hyperplasia and bladder overactivity.*)

CHAPTER 135 ■ APPROACH TO THE PATIENT WITH NEPHROLITHIASIS

LESLIE S.-T. FANG

Nephrolithiasis is a significant medical problem incurring substantial morbidity and cost. One autopsy series estimated the prevalence as 1.12%. In most industrialized countries, 1% to 3% of the population may be expected to have a calculus at some time, and the likelihood that stone disease will develop in a white man by age 70 years is about 1 in 8 (lifetime incidence of up to 13%). More important, the prevalence of kidney stone disease has increased 37% in the last 20 years. Disease prevalence was 3% during the period between 1976 and 1980 and 5.2% between 1988 and 1994. Furthermore, the male-to-female ratio has changed over the last 25 years, from 3:1 male to female to less than 2:1.

The annual per capita frequency of hospitalization for nephrolithiasis is estimated at 1 in 1,000. The recurrence rate without treatment for calcium oxalate renal stones is about 10% at 1 year, 33% at 5 years, and 50% at 10 years. In the outpatient setting, the primary physician may encounter patients with a history of renal calculi, asymptomatic nephrolithiasis, or acute colic. Others may present with hematuria or urinary tract infection. One needs to identify the nature of the stone and any precipitating factors, prevent further stone formation, and know when referral for surgical intervention or lithotripsy is needed.

PATHOPHYSIOLOGY AND CLINICAL PRESENTATION (1–12)

In most industrialized countries, about 75% of stones are composed of calcium salts and usually occur as calcium oxalate and less commonly as calcium phosphate. The remaining 25% of stones are composed of uric acid, struvite or carbonic apatite, cystine, and rare stones.

Two major groups of factors are important in the pathogenesis of stones: (a) changes that increase the urinary concentration of stone constituents and (b) physicochemical changes. *Increase in concentration* can occur with reductions in urinary volume or increases in the excretion of calcium, oxalate, uric acid, cystine, or xanthine.

Calcium-Containing Stones

The majority of calcium-containing stones contain calcium oxalate; hypercalciuric and hyperoxaluric states promote stone formation. In some instances, hyperuricemia also contributes to calcium stone formation.

Hypercalciuric states can be categorized into three groups according to cause: increased gut absorption of dietary calcium, increased resorption of calcium from bone, and the presence of a renal calcium leak. Combinations of these factors can be at play in certain clinical settings. About 50% of patients with calcium stones are found to be hypercalciuric.

Hyperoxaluria is less common than hypercalciuria, but recent studies indicate that up to 30% of patients with calcium oxalate stones are hyperoxaluric. Hyperoxaluria may result from increased absorption of dietary oxalate, as occurs in patients with small-bowel disease; from increased endogenous production of oxalate, as occurs in patients with a genetic deficiency of enzymes in the glyoxalate pathway or of pyridoxine (an important cofactor in glyoxalate metabolism); or, rarely, from markedly increased ingestion of oxalate or one of its precursors.

Some patients with calcium-containing stones may be hyperuricosuric. It is believed that adsorption of glutamic acid onto a uric acid nidus allows for the growth of calcium oxalate crystals. However, a significant number of patients with calcium stones have no discernible metabolic derangement, making rational drug therapy more difficult.

Some patients with calcium-containing stones have low urinary citrate. Citrate is a potent inhibitor of stone formation, and low urinary citrate would predispose a patient to calcium stone formation.

Magnesium Ammonium Phosphate Stones (Struvite)

Struvite formation occurs in an alkaline environment and is almost invariably associated with urinary tract infection produced by a urea-splitting organism.

Uric Acid Stones

Most patients with uric acid stones have persistently acid urine, which decreases the solubility of uric acid. Some patients may be hyperuricosuric. Hyperuricosuric states are seen in patients with a high dietary intake of protein and with primary and secondary gout. In patients who have myeloproliferative disorders or are undergoing chemotherapy, significant hyperuricosuria can occur, and uric acid stones can form if adequate urine flow and alkalinization are not maintained.

Cystine Stones

Cystine stones are found exclusively in patients with cystinuria. These patients have an inherited disorder in which renal and gastrointestinal transport of cystine, ornithine, lysine, and arginine is abnormal.

Indinavir Stones

In patients on treatment for HIV with indinavir, rare instances of crystallization of indinavir with resultant stones have been reported.

Xanthine Stones

These occur in the setting of xanthinuria, an extremely rare genetic disorder of purine metabolism associated with a deficiency of xanthine oxidase. Rarely, xanthine stones may be seen in patients taking xanthine oxidase inhibitors for the treatment of uric acid disorders.

Physicochemical factors that have been identified as important in stone formation include changes in urinary pH and urinary concentrations of potential inhibitors of stone formation, such as magnesium, citrate, sulfate, organic matrix, and pyrophosphate. As noted earlier, an alkaline pH facilitates struvite formation, and an acidic pH facilitates the formation of uric acid and xanthine stones.

Magnesium, citrate, pyrophosphate, and certain anions in high urinary concentrations are potent inhibitors of stone formation. Deficiencies in one or more of the inhibitors have been identified in some patients with recurrent stones.

Three major theories have been advanced to explain stone formation and growth. The *matrix nucleation* theory suggests that some matrix substances (e.g., uric acid) form an initial nucleus for subsequent stone growth by precipitation. The *precipitation–crystallization* theory suggests that when the urinary crystalloids are present in a supersaturated state, precipitation and subsequent growth occur. The *inhibitor absence* theory postulates that the deficiency of one or more of numerous agents known to retard stone formation leads to nephrolithiasis. Evidence for and against each of these theories has been advanced; multiple factors may be involved in any patient.

Clinical Presentation

Clinical presentation is one of pain, bleeding, or silent obstruction. *Renal "colic"* is typically a constant unilateral pain, abrupt in onset, and localized to the flank when a stone sits in the upper tract and radiating into the groin when a stone lodges in the lower portion of the ureter. The presentation may be mistaken for pyelonephritis and occasionally for abdominal and pelvic processes, but the initial workup should rapidly lead to the correct diagnosis.

Any *obstruction* that occurs is usually transient and of no lasting significance; however, in some instances, it persists and may be silent and progressive. Occasionally, asymptomatic calcareous calculi are detected on abdominal x-rays film taken for other reasons. Calculi extending from one renal calix to another ("staghorn" calculi) can result in significant renal parenchymal damage, particularly in association with infection.

Natural history of stone formation is a matter of some controversy. The likelihood of *recurrence* of calcium stones with time was examined prospectively in one study of patients in whom single stones formed. An exceedingly high incidence of recurrence was found, with a mean time to recurrence of 6.78 years. With time, the incidence of cumulative recurrence approached 100%. Recurrence appeared early in half of the patients but took up to 20 years in others.

Other studies have found a more benign course. In one, a group of 101 patients was followed for an extended period (mean, 7 years); additional stone formation was observed in only one third of the patients. These differences in recurrence rates undoubtedly reflect heterogeneity among patients in the respective referral groups. In any case, the incidence of recurrence is high enough to justify evaluation and consideration of preventive treatment.

Most kidney stones pass spontaneously; however, 10% to 30% do not and may cause continuing pain, infection, or obstruction.

DIFFERENTIAL DIAGNOSIS

In the United States, about 75% of all renal calculi are composed of either calcium oxalate or calcium oxalate mixed with calcium phosphate (Table 135.1). Stones of pure uric acid account for about 10%. Struvite or magnesium ammonium phosphate stones occur almost exclusively in patients with urinary tract infections caused by urea-splitting organisms, and they constitute about 9% of all stones analyzed. Other stones occur infrequently and are composed of cystine, xanthine, and silicates.

The disease states associated with nephrolithiasis are best categorized according to the type of stones formed. In many instances, stone formation is a manifestation of systemic disease (Table 135.2).

Workup (13,14)

In the evaluation of the patient with recurrent nephrolithiasis, knowledge of the stone composition is essential to rational management. Obtaining the stone for analysis is the most important study; therefore, urine should be strained for stones when renal colic is present. Ideally, studies of the stone should include quantitative chemical analysis in addition to crystallographic examination.

History

When no stone is available for analysis, certain aspects of the clinical history can be helpful in the evaluation. The *age* of the patient at the onset of nephrolithiasis is helpful because metabolic disorders such as hyperoxaluria, cystinuria, xanthinuria, and renal tubular acidosis are often associated with stones at an early age, and idiopathic calcareous nephrolithiasis and primary hyperparathyroidism commonly develop after age 30 years. The *gender* of the patient can also be helpful; idiopathic

TABLE 135.1

TYPES OF RENAL CALCULI

Calcium oxalate	58.8%
Calcium phosphate	8.9%
Mixed calcium oxalate and phosphate	11.4%
Uric acid	10.1%
Struvite (magnesium ammonium phosphate)	9.3%
Cystine	0.7%
Miscellaneous	0.8%

TABLE 135.2

IMPORTANT CONDITIONS ASSOCIATED WITH NEPHROLITHIASIS

Calcium Stones
  Increased gastrointestinal calcium absorption
    Primary hyperparathyroidism
    Sarcoidosis
    Vitamin D excess
    Milk–alkali syndrome
    Idiopathic nephrolithiasis
  Increased bone calcium resorption
    Primary hyperparathyroidism
    Neoplastic disorders
    Immobilization
    Distal renal tubular acidosis
  Renal calcium leak
    Idiopathic hypercalciuria
  Hyperoxaluria
    Small-bowel disease
    Enzymatic deficiency
    Pyridoxine deficiency
    Increased ingestion
Magnesium Ammonium Phosphate Stones
  Alkaline environment
  Urinary tract infection caused by urea-splitting organism
Uric Acid Stones
  Increased uric acid production
    Primary gout
    Secondary gout (myeloproliferative disorder,
      chemotherapy)
Cystine Stones
  Inherited disorder for amino acid transport
Xanthine Stones
  Xanthine oxidase deficiency
  Use of xanthine oxidase inhibitor

nephrolithiasis is common in men, whereas primary hyperparathyroidism is more common in women. A *past history* of stones is invaluable if their composition has been previously determined. Any prior history of systemic illness (e.g., sarcoidosis or cancer) and any prior urinary tract infection should be noted. Having a *family history* of nephrolithiasis increases the risk for stone disease and may suggest a hereditary metabolic disorder. A careful *dietary history* should also be taken to rule out excessive protein, oxalate, or calcium intake. Consumption of apple juice and grapefruit juice has been associated with an increased risk for stone formation. Consumption of alcoholic beverages is associated with a decreased risk. It is important to check for the use of *drugs* that promote stone formation. Medications that result in an increased risk for stone formation include vitamins A, C, and D, loop diuretics, acetazolamide, indinavir (and perhaps other protease inhibitors), ammonium chloride, calcium-containing medications, alkali, and antacids. Medications may increase urinary concentrations of calcium (vitamin D, loop diuretics, calcium-containing medications, ammonium chloride), alter urinary pH (acetazolamide, ammonium chloride, and alkali), or decrease urinary concentrations of inhibitors (ammonium chloride, absorbable antacids, and alkali can decrease urinary citrate concentration).

Physical Examination

Physical examination is not particularly revealing in most cases, but the patient should be checked for evidence of a systemic disease, such as sarcoidosis (lymphadenopathy, organomegaly) and cancer (adenopathy, breast mass, and so forth).

Laboratory Evaluation

Laboratory evaluation should include *urinalysis* for determination of pH and an examination of urinary sediment for crystals. An alkaline pH suggests infection with urea-splitting organisms and struvite formation. *Urine culture* is needed. Inability to acidify the urine pH below 5.3 despite systemic acidosis suggests renal tubular acidosis. Serum should be obtained for determination of electrolytes, calcium and albumen, phosphate, uric acid, blood urea nitrogen, and creatinine levels, and a *24-hour urine* should be collected for creatinine, sodium, calcium, uric acid, citrate, and oxalate. The 24-urine collection should be done 1 to 2 months after the acute episode of stone passage. The patient should be on his or her usual diet. Collection of two or three 24-hour collections would increase the yield of detecting metabolic derangements.

Repeated determinations of *fasting serum calcium* and *phosphorus* are necessary if primary hyperparathyroidism is suspected. The serum albumin should be determined at the same time because 40% to 45% of the serum calcium is protein bound. If the serum calcium is elevated and hyperparathyroidism is suspected clinically, the diagnosis can be confirmed by obtaining a simultaneous *parathyroid hormone* determination, which should reveal an inappropriately elevated level (see Chapter 96). If the clinical presentation suggests a rare cause of nephrolithiasis, such as cystinuria or xanthinuria, special 24-hour collections of urine should be sent for study.

Roentgenographic evaluation includes a plain film of the *kidneys, ureter,* and *bladder* (KUB) and *noncontrast helical computed tomography* (CT). The flat-plate radiograph of the abdomen can provide an estimate of renal size and is important in detecting the presence of small, radiopaque stones. Staghorn calculi usually indicate magnesium ammonium phosphate or cystine stones. The latter usually have a more laminated appearance. *Noncontrast helical CT* provides better details of any renal abnormalities that may be present, in addition to the level of the obstruction caused by the renal calculus. Where available, *noncontrast helical CT with 5-mm cuts* is the diagnostic modality of choice. *Renal ultrasonography* is useful for detecting hydronephrosis but is not a substitute for noncontrast helical CT in the initial workup of urolithiasis.

The laboratory evaluation permits the identification of stones and hyperexcretory states and therefore allows rational therapy.

PRINCIPLES OF MANAGEMENT (15–25)

Because of the high incidence of stone formation and its attendant morbidity, preventive therapy is indicated in all patients with nephrolithiasis.

In general, maintenance of dilute urine by means of vigorous *fluid therapy* around the clock is beneficial in all forms of nephrolithiasis. A number of studies have indicated that the relative probability of a kidney stone forming decreases with urinary volume. Enough fluid to maintain an output of 2 to

3 L of urine needs to be taken daily. In general, 250 mL of fluid should be taken every 4 hours, and 250 mL of fluid should be taken with meals. A high fluid intake has been associated with a 40% reduction in recurrence risk. It is important also to stress nighttime fluid intake to prevent supersaturation at night. Specific therapy should be tailored to the type of stones involved.

Calcium-Containing Stones

During the last decade, dietary manipulation has become more prominent in the management of calcium-containing stones. Increasing evidence indicates that restriction of *dietary protein* is helpful in preventing the formation of calcium-containing stones. Population studies indicate a clear correlation between increased dietary protein and an increased incidence of stone formation. Protein loading in patients results in an increase in urinary excretion of both calcium and uric acid. A high dietary intake of protein also decreases urinary concentrations of inhibitors such as citrate. These metabolic abnormalities are corrected with restriction of dietary protein. *Sodium intake* should also be restricted. Restriction of dietary sodium predictably results in a decrease in urinary calcium excretion. Oxalate is a metabolic end product of glycine, and the bulk of the urinary oxalate is derived from metabolic pathways. However, in some patients, dietary excesses of oxalate can result in hyperoxaluria. These patients would benefit from a restriction of *dietary oxalate*. Evidence does not support dietary restriction of *calcium*. Calcium restriction results in an increased intestinal absorption of oxalate, which leads to hyperoxaluria in addition to mobilization of calcium from the bone because of a negative calcium balance. Cohort studies have demonstrated an inverse relationship between dietary calcium intake and stone formation. In other words, a high dietary intake of calcium decreases the risk for symptomatic stone disease. However, supplemental calcium intake has been associated with a modest increase (relative risk, 1.20) in stone formation.

Dietary manipulations have been shown to prevent further stone formation. In one series, in which patients with first-time stones were placed on a dietary program, only a 27% recurrence of stones was noted during a 5-year follow-up.

For patients with recurrent stone formation despite dietary therapy, every effort should be made to rule out underlying systemic conditions (Table 135.2) before drug therapy is initiated. Patients with underlying primary hyperparathyroidism should be treated surgically, when feasible. Drugs that can promote calcium stone formation should be stopped. Patients with sarcoidosis may benefit from steroid therapy.

Patients with calcium stones have been shown to benefit from *potassium citrate*. Potassium citrate increases citrate excretion by providing an alkali load. The induced rise in urinary citrate should inhibit the crystallization of calcium oxalate and calcium phosphate.

Thiazides decrease urinary calcium excretion, and hydrochlorothiazide (50 mg once a day) has been found to be effective in reducing recurrent stone formation. Primary hyperparathyroidism has to be ruled out before thiazides are given, to avoid hypercalcemia.

Patients with *hyperoxaluria* should have their dietary intake of oxalates limited. Tea, rhubarb, and many leafy green vegetables should be avoided. Dietary calcium, on the other hand, should not be severely restricted because severe calcium restriction has been shown to cause increases in the urinary excretion of oxalate. In the rare patient with pyridoxine deficiency, replacement would improve the hyperoxaluric state.

Patients with *hyperuricosuria* benefit from protein restriction and *allopurinol*. Reduction of the urinary uric acid concentration minimizes the likelihood of calcium oxalate crystal growth around uric acid crystals adsorbed to uric acid. Two randomized trials have shown that stone recurrence rates are lower with allopurinol treatment.

Studies in patients with no identifiable metabolic disorder should receive *potassium citrate*. Studies have demonstrated a drastic reduction in new stone formation when patients are given potassium citrate. Similar benefits have been shown with *thiazide* and *allopurinol*. In one study, six stones formed in 30 such patients, compared with a predicted 31.8 stones, during a 1- to 7-year follow-up period.

In addition to the therapeutic interventions outlined, several other, less well-evaluated modes of therapy have been advocated. Administration of *potassium magnesium citrate* increases urinary pH, urinary citrate, and magnesium and was shown in a placebo-controlled, randomized trial to be a highly efficacious in inhibiting calcium stone formation. *Slow-release neutral potassium phosphate* is a reasonably well tolerated phosphate preparation that can suppress calcitriol synthesis. Calcium absorption is reduced from the inhibition of calcitriol synthesis and from binding of calcium by phosphate in the intestinal tract, thereby correcting hypercalciuria and preventing recurrent stone formation.

Magnesium Ammonium Phosphate Stones

Magnesium ammonium phosphate stones are often very large and may have to be removed surgically. Acidification of the urine with ascorbic acid, along with a prolonged (often at least 2 months) course of appropriate *antibiotic* treatment to eradicate any *Proteus* urinary tract infection, is essential to prevent recurrences of struvite stones.

Uric Acid Stones

Efforts should be directed at reduction of uric acid excretion. Decreasing dietary protein intake and weight reduction is helpful. *Hydration* to maintain copious urine flow, *allopurinol* therapy, and *alkalinization* of the urine are the mainstays of therapy for uric acid stones. The solubility of uric acid is 100 times higher at pH 7 than at pH 4.5, and every attempt should be made to maintain alkaline urine by giving 100 to 150 mEq of *sodium bicarbonate* every 24 hours in divided doses. In patients with myeloproliferative disorders who are undergoing chemotherapy, the prophylactic use of allopurinol, saline diuresis, and alkalinization should eliminate the incidence of uric acid stone formation.

Cystine Stones

A copious urine flow and urinary pH maintained above 7.5 are important in preventing and dissolving cystine stones. D-*Penicillamine* has also been shown to be effective, but significant side effects may be encountered.

Indinavir Stones

There should be an increased index of suspicion for indinavir stones in HIV patients who present either with renal colic or acute renal failure. *Hydration*, *alkalinization*, and *cessation of indinavir* usually prevent recurrence of indinavir stones.

Xanthine Stones

Limitation of dietary purines, maintenance of urine flow, and maintenance of very high urine pH (>7.6) minimize difficulties. Prophylactic alkalinization and forced diuresis should be employed in patients with myeloproliferative disorders who are taking xanthine oxidase inhibitors.

INDICATIONS FOR ADMISSION AND REFERRAL

In a patient with renal colic, the need for hospitalization and other interventions is dictated by the clinical presentation. Patients with mild to moderate pain can be managed as outpatients with oral analgesics and instructed to maintain a high fluid intake and urine output around the clock. These patients should be told to strain the urine to retrieve calculi for stone analysis.

Patients with severe pain, nausea, and vomiting require hospitalization for intravenous hydration and pain control. In these patients, KUB and noncontrast helical CT are indicated to localize and determine the extent of the obstruction. In the majority of cases, stones will pass spontaneously. Patients with severe symptoms and persistent obstruction beyond 3 to 4 days should be referred for urologic evaluation.

Patients presenting with fever, chills, and symptoms of renal colic require hospitalization and prompt intervention. If the presence of an infection behind an obstructed ureter is indeed confirmed, antibiotic coverage (see Chapter 133) and surgical decompression are mandatory.

Surgical intervention for nephrolithiasis has changed dramatically since the introduction of *lithotripsy* and *endurologic interventions*, which have largely obviated the need for lithotomy in most patients. In lithotripsy, the stone is shattered by subjecting it to focused ultrasonic shock waves, delivered either percutaneously through a nephrostomy or extracorpo-

really. *Extracorporeal shock-wave lithotripsy* is an excellent choice for fragmentation and removal of simple stones in the kidneys and upper ureters. Its very low complication rate and high degree of efficacy are rapidly eliminating the need for surgical lithotomy in the centers where the lithotriptor is available. Because the equipment needed to perform the procedure is expensive and not always available, *percutaneous ultrasonic lithotripsy* represents an acceptable alternative and may be the preferred initial therapy for upper tract stones lodged in the ureter for more than 4 to 6 weeks. The procedure is also indicated for larger (>2.5 cm) stones. *Ureteroscopic* approaches have allowed the basketing of stones that have lodged in the ureters, obviating the need to resort to open lithotomy.

The expense and operator skill required for these technologies limit their availability to regional centers. Patients with documented stones, especially those that are located in the upper tracts and kidney or that cause continuous pain, infection, or obstruction, should be referred to such centers for intervention.

PATIENT EDUCATION

Meticulous care must be taken in giving dietary instructions. Patients should also be instructed regarding how to divide their fluid intake evenly to maintain dilute urine at all times. As noted previously, a daily fluid intake of 2 to 3 L is needed to help minimize stone formation. Consumption of apple and grapefruit juice has been associated with increased risk, and alcoholic beverages appear to decrease risk. Ingestion of cranberry juice has been shown to decrease urinary oxalate and urinary phosphate, increase urinary citrate, and decrease relative supersaturation. Because there is some evidence that soft drinks acidified solely with phosphoric acid may contribute to stone recurrence, patients might be advised to avoid them. However, most soft drinks also contain citric acid, and the combination appears to have no effect on stone recurrence. Patients who need to alkalinize their urine should be instructed in how to measure urinary pH with litmus test tapes. Long periods of immobilization should be avoided, and appropriate fluid intake should be prescribed if such situations are anticipated.

Annotated Bibliography

1. Curhan GC, Willett WC, Rimm EB, et al. A prospective study of dietary calcium and other nutrients and the risk of symptomatic kidney stones. N Engl J Med 1993;328:833. (*A high dietary intake of calcium decreases the risk for symptomatic kidney stones.*)
2. Curhan GC, Willett WC, Rimm EB, et al. Body size and risk of kidney stones. J Am Soc Nephrol 1998;9:1645. (*Body size is associated with the risk for stone formation, and the magnitude of the risk varies by gender.*)
3. Curhan GC, Willett WC, Rimm EB, et al. Family history and risk of kidney stones. J Am Soc Nephrol 1997;8:1568. (*A family history of kidney stones substantially increases the risk for stone formation.*)
4. Curhan GC, Willett WC, Rimm EB, et al. Prospective study of beverage use and the risk of kidney stones. Am J Epidemiol 1996;143:240. (*The risk decreased with the consumption of coffee and alcoholic beverages and increased with the consumption of apple juice and grapefruit juice.*)
5. Curhan GC, Willett WC, Speizer FE, et al. Beverage use and risk for kidney stones in women. Ann Intern Med 1998;128:534. (*The risk is decreased 59% by wine consumption and increased 44% by consumption of grapefruit juice.*)
6. Curhan GC, Willett WC, Speizer FE, et al. Comparison of dietary calcium with supplemental calcium and other nutrients as factors affecting the risk for kidney stones in women. Ann Intern Med 1997;126:497. (*The intake of dietary calcium was inversely associated with the risk for kidney stones, and the intake of supplemental calcium was positively associated with risk.*)
7. Frick KK, Bushinsky DA. Molecular mechanisms of primary hypercalciuria. J Am Soc Nephrol 2003;14:1082. (*Hypercalciuria is seen in up to 40% of stone formers; review of the molecular mechanism of hypercalciuria.*)
8. Goldfarb S. The role of diet in the pathogenesis and therapy of nephrolithiasis. Endocrinol Metab Clin North Am 1990;19:805. (*Excellent review of the various aspects of diet that are important to consider in the patient with nephrolithiasis, including intake of fluid, protein, calcium, oxalate, and sodium.*)
9. Goldfarb DS. Increasing prevalence of kidney stones in the United States. Kidney Int 2003;63:1951. (*There was a 37% increase in stone prevalence in the United States from the period 1976–1980 to the period 1988–1994, from 3.2% to 5.3%.*)
10. Kamel KS, Cheema-Dhadli S, Halperin ML. Studies on the pathophysiology of the low urine pH in patients with uric acid stones. Kidney Int 2002;61:988. (*A very low urinary pH is the major risk factor for uric acid stone formation; alkalinization is therefore an important modality of treatment of uric acid stones.*)
11. Madore F, Stampfer MJ, Rimm EB, et al. Nephrolithiasis and risk of hypertension. Am J Hypertens 1998;11:46. (*Prior occurrence of nephrolithiasis increases the risk for subsequent hypertension in men.*)
12. Menon M, Koul H. Clinical review: calcium oxalate nephrolithiasis. J Clin Endocrinol Metab 1993;74:703. (*An excellent review of the pathogenesis of calcium oxalate stones and management options.*)

13. Koenig CL, Lindbloom E. Accuracy of hematuria in diagnosing kidney stones. J Family Pract 1999;48:912. (*Nonhelical computed tomography is more accurate than hematuria in the diagnosis of kidney stones in patients presenting with flank pain.*)

14. Wilson DM. Clinical and laboratory evaluation of renal stone patients. Endocrinol Metab Clin North Am 1990;19:773. (*An in-depth review of the available tools for evaluation of renal stone patients.*)

15. Borghi L, Meschi T, Amato F, et al. Urinary volume, water and recurrences in idiopathic calcium nephrolithiasis: a 5 year randomized prospective study. J Urol 1996;155:839. (*A large fluid intake and a large urinary volume decrease urinary calcium concentration and prevent stone formation.*)

16. Kocara R, Plasgura P, Petrik A, et al. A prospective study of non-medical prophylaxis after a first kidney stone. Br J Urol 1999;84:393. (*Specific dietary therapy, adjusted according to a metabolic evaluation, is more effective than nonspecific general dietary recommendations in preventing the formation of a second stone.*)

17. Lee YH, Huang WC, Tsai JY, et al. The efficacy of potassium citrate based medical prophylaxis for preventing upper urinary tract calculi: a midterm followup study. J Urol 1999;161:1453. (*Potassium citrate is helpful in preventing recurrences of upper urinary calculi, decreasing the stone recurrence from 46.2% to 7.8% during a 24- to 60-month follow-up.*)

18. Lingeman JE, Woods J, Toth PD, et al. The role of lithotripsy and its side effects. J Urol 1989;141:793. (*Critical examination of the technology.*)

19. McHarg T, Rodgers A, Charlton K. Influence of cranberry juice on the urinary risk factors for calcium oxalate kidney stone formation. Br J Urol 2003;92:765. (*Cranberry juice decreases urinary oxalate and phosphate, increases urinary citrate, and decreases relative supersaturation.*)

20. Moe OW. Kidney stones pathophysiology and medical management. Lancet 2006;367:333-44. (*Update of a classic 1998 Lancet review by Pak, including a discussion of the genetics of nephrolithiasis: 139 references.*)

21. Riese RJ, Sakhaee K. Uric acid nephrolithiasis: pathogenesis and treatment. J Urol 1992;148:765. (*A review of the pathogenesis of uric acid stones and an examination of various treatment options, including allopurinol and potassium citrate therapy.*)

22. Shekarriz, B, Stroller ML. Uric acid nephrolithiasis: current concepts and controversies. J Urol 2002;168:1307. (*Excellent review of uric acid stones; discusses the importance of urinary alkalinization in the prevention of recurrent uric acid stones.*)

23. Shuster J, Jenkins A, Logan C, et al. Soft drink consumption and urinary stone recurrence: a randomized prevention trial. J Clin Epidemiol 1992;45:911. (*Reduction in the consumption of soft drinks reduced the risk for stone recurrence.*)

24. Miller NL, Lingeman JE. Management of kidney stones. BMJ 2007;334:468. (*Review of the pathogenesis of stone formation, with emphasis on the medical and lithotripsy treatment of stone disease.*)

25. Wickham JE. Minimally invasive surgery: treatment of urinary tract stones. Br Med J 1993;307:1414. (*Nice review of extracorporeal shock-wave lithotripsy and percutaneous endoscopic lithotomy.*)

CHAPTER 136 ■ APPROACH TO THE MALE PATIENT WITH URETHRITIS

JOHN D. GOODSON

A penile discharge or urethral discomfort may be the presenting manifestation of a sexually transmitted disease (STD) and, as such, requires prompt attention. Nongonococcal urethritis (NGU) has surpassed gonorrhea as the principal cause of urethral symptoms in men and has reached epidemic proportions in sexually active adolescents and college-age persons. It can occur as an isolated infection or in conjunction with gonorrhea or other STDs.

Because NGU is the most common STD among heterosexuals in the United States and is a potential source of female infertility and infant morbidity, prompt and focused efforts by the primary physician concerning the clinical manifestations combined with effective treatment have important benefits for both patients and the public health.

PATHOPHYSIOLOGY, CLINICAL PRESENTATION, AND CLINICAL COURSE (1–7)

Most penile discharges are a consequence of urethral infection or inflammation. Numerous bacterial and nonbacterial organisms can invade its mucosal lining. Organisms causing NGU are characterized by their low levels of tissue invasiveness. In older men, a discharge may result from an inflamed prostate gland or, in rare instances, a tumor.

Gonococcal Urethritis

The typical presentation of symptomatic gonococcal disease is a 2- to 4-day history of significant dysuria and a thick and purulent penile discharge. The Gram's stain reveals polymorphonuclear leukocytes and gram-negative intracellular diplococci. Systemic gonococcemia develops in approximately 3% of patients, manifested by rash, fever, and polyarthritis (see Chapter 137). *Mixed infections*, involving both gonococci and chlamydiae, occur in up to 20% of patients presenting with gonococcal urethritis. Such patients complain of persistence of symptoms after being effectively treated only for gonorrhea.

Gonococcal urethritis responds well to proper antibiotic therapy, with resolution of symptoms and no sequelae. In men, even untreated disease may resolve spontaneously within a few weeks. An asymptomatic carrier state may ensue, or a chronic low-grade discharge may remain. Stricture is a possible consequence of untreated disease.

Nongonococcal Urethritis

NGU tends to be an indolent illness of longer duration (e.g., 3 to 4 weeks). Dysuria, if present, is not as severe, and the discharge is less purulent, mucoid, sometimes scanty, or even absent. The urethral Gram's stain shows neutrophils (by definition more than 4 cells per high-power field) and, at most, a few mixed extracellular pleomorphic organisms, features that help to distinguish NGU from gonococcal infection. Only 20% of ambiguous Gram's stains (rare extracellular gram-negative diplococci) are shown by subsequent culture to represent gonococcal infection. The absence of neutrophils (<10 cells per high-power field) on analysis of the first 15 to 30 mL of urine or a urine dipstick test negative for leukocyte esterase is highly specific for urethritis (i.e., a negative test result makes infection highly unlikely).

Chlamydia trachomatis

Chlamydia trachomatis infections of the urogenital tract have reached epidemic proportions, with 20% to 50% penetration of some populations. Prevalence is greatest among sexually active adolescents and young adults, especially those younger than the age of 20 years with multiple partners. In heterosexual men, urethritis with penile discharge, dysuria, or both is the most common symptomatic clinical presentation, but 25% to 50% may manifest neither symptoms nor leukocytes on urethral swab. Proctitis can develop in homosexual men engaging in receptive anal intercourse.

In untreated cases, symptoms may wax and wane during several weeks. Spontaneous resolution can occur. Complications are rare. Prostatitis and epididymitis have been reported in untreated or poorly treated cases. Epididymitis may also be part of the initial clinical presentation. Chlamydial infection accounts for about half of the cases of epididymitis in the United States.

Female counterparts of chlamydial NGU have been identified, including mucopurulent cervicitis and urethritis (see Chapters 117, 125, and 133). The prevalence of chlamydial infection among female partners of men with chlamydial NGU is very high (almost 70%; see Chapter 125).

Ureaplasma urealyticum

Ureaplasma urealyticum is likely to be a cause of NGU, though some investigators see this organism as a nonpathogenic commensal. It may account for 10% to 40% of NGU cases and is sexually transmitted.

Mycoplasma genitalium

Mycoplasma genitalium invades epithelial cells and has emerged as a common cause of NGU, especially in male homosexual partners. The urethritis is indistinguishable from NGU of other causes.

Trichomonas vaginalis

Trichomonas vaginalis infection is a common cause of vaginitis in women and also an important source of urethritis in men. A 22% urethral prevalence was found among male partners of women with known trichomonal infection and a 6% prevalence among heterosexuals attending a clinic for STDs. About 50% of patients are symptomatic and have a discharge on examination. Others have symptoms but no visible discharge. The odds ratio for trichomonal infection in patients with nongonococcal, nonchlamydial urethritis has been found to be 3.8. The condition should be suspected in patients with symptoms but little or no discharge on physical examination.

Reactive Arthritis (Reiter's Syndrome)

The finding of genetic overlap between the histocompatibility antigen HLA-B27 (found in up to 96% of patients vs. 10% of controls) and certain *Klebsiella* and *Chlamydia trachomatis* antigens suggests that infection in susceptible persons may play a role in the pathogenesis of this form of reactive arthritis. It usually presents as urethritis in conjunction with a host of other mucocutaneous and musculoskeletal symptoms. Various combinations of conjunctivitis, iritis, fever, acute asymmetric polyarthritis (see Chapter 146), nonarticular bony pain (e.g., of the heel), circinate balanitis, keratoderma blennorrhagicum, and mucosal ulcerations may be present at any one time. The most characteristic presentation is onset of mild dysuria and a mucopurulent urethral discharge about 2 to 4 weeks after a diarrheal illness or sexual contact. Many patients present first with the urethritis, although involvement of other organ systems is frequently present in subclinical form or develops within a few weeks. Most patients with this form of reactive arthritis experience a self-limited illness of 6 to 12 months' duration, although a minority progress to chronic or recurrent symptoms in conjunction with bouts of arthritis.

Prostatitis

In older men, prostatic hyperplasia predisposes to obstruction and infection. Prostatitis may also represent infectious spread to the prostate. Minor penile discharge may be noted, exacerbated by prostatic massage. Symptoms of urinary outflow obstruction and perineal discomfort may dominate the clinical picture (see Chapters 138 and 139).

Persistence of symptomatic urethritis after appropriate antibiotic treatment of NGU has been linked to treatment-resistant strains. However, most recurrent NGU represents reinfection by an untreated sexual partner rather than infection with a resistant organism.

DIFFERENTIAL DIAGNOSIS (3,6–8)

The differential diagnosis of a penile discharge is traditionally divided into gonococcal and nongonococcal etiologies, with NGU accounting for the majority of cases. Among the causes of NGU are *Chlamydia*, *Ureaplasma*, *Mycoplasma*, and trichomonal infections of the urethra, Reiter's syndrome, prostatitis, and urethral malignancy. Chlamydial disease is responsible for about one half of cases of NGU. In up to one third of NGU cases, no pathogen is identified. Occasionally, urethral infection with herpes simplex virus or human papillomavirus may occur.

WORKUP (8)

History and Physical Examination

History

The duration and character of the discharge can be informative. Acute onset of a profuse purulent discharge usually suggests gonococcal infection. Several weeks of a more indolent, less profuse, mucoid discharge point toward a nongonococcal etiology. However, presentations overlap to some degree, and the history is not sufficient for diagnosis. A blood-tinged discharge raises the question of prostatitis or urethral tumor. Ask the patient about the number of sexual partners during the last few months and the use or nonuse of barrier contraception (important considerations in assessing risk for chlamydial infection and other STDs). Check for symptoms of prostatitis (slow stream, perineal discomfort), localized or systemic gonorrheal infection (pharyngitis, proctitis, arthritis, punctate skin lesions, sepsis), and a reactive arthritis syndrome (polyarthritis, dermatitis, conjunctivitis, bony pain). Note any history of penile warts or herpes simplex viral infection, as well as sexual contact with a partner known to have had trichomonal infection.

Physical Examination

Check the patient's temperature, and examine the integument carefully for signs of gonococcemia (fever; punctate, centrally hemorrhagic, necrotic skin lesions; tenosynovitis; polyarthritis). Similarly, check for manifestations of Reiter's syndrome, including conjunctivitis, iritis, oral or meatal mucosal ulcerations, circinate balanitis (ulceration and erythema on the penile glans), keratoderma blennorrhagicum (pustular or hyperkeratotic lesions on the soles of the feet), inflamed joints (knees, ankles, sacroiliac joints), and nonarticular bone pain (especially of the heel). Inspect the urethral meatus for herpetic lesions and warts, palpate the epididymis for tenderness and swelling, and examine the prostate for enlargement, bogginess, and tenderness. Carefully examine an acutely inflamed prostate because bacterial seeding is possible following an overly vigorous massage.

Laboratory Studies

Gram's Stain

Gram's stain of the urethral discharge should be the first study performed because it helps to distinguish gonococcal from nongonococcal disease. Even if no visible discharge is present, a swab is gently inserted into the urethral meatus and a sample obtained. A first-morning sample before urination or one several hours after urination offers the best yield. Some of the sample is plated onto Thayer–Martin medium for culture of *Neisseria gonorrhoeae* (see Chapter 137), and the remainder is placed on a glass slide and Gram's stained. The finding of polymorphonuclear leukocytes with gram-negative intracellular diplococci is highly predictive of gonococcal urethritis. The sensitivity and specificity of the Gram's stain exceed 95%. Four or more polymorphonuclear leukocytes per high-power field and mixed gram-negative and gram-positive pleomorphic extracellular organisms or leukocytes with no visible organisms are indicative of NGU. If no definite gram-negative intracellular diplococci are seen on Gram's stain, then a tentative diagnosis of NGU is appropriate. The diagnosis is confirmed by a negative gonococcal *culture*. Alternative testing for *N. gonorrhoeae* urethral infection is available with polymerase chain reaction (PCR) DNA probes or DNA amplification techniques (see Chapter 137); the latter has been approved for urine testing. Both techniques are useful for diagnosing pharyngeal or rectal infection.

Chlamydial Testing

It is not practical to culture for *Chlamydia* or *Ureaplasma* because of the expense, technical difficulty, and 2 to 3 days required to obtain results. However, antigen detection methods provide more rapid, less expensive detection of chlamydial infection. At the time an intraurethral swab is obtained for Gram's stain, a second swabbing should also be performed and the specimen saved for chlamydial testing. Such testing can be valuable, even if the patient is going to be treated presumptively for chlamydial infection, because the information thus obtained often helps to improve compliance, facilitate coun-

seling, and guide care if symptoms persist. Patients with a presumptive diagnosis of gonorrhea may also benefit from chlamydial testing because both infections can exist concurrently.

DNA amplification tests based on PCR using urine samples have proved to be reliable and predictive. These tests are 15% to 35% more sensitive than other nonculture urethral testing techniques and have greater than 99% specificity.

Direct fluorescent antibody staining of urethral smears and *enzyme immunoassay* of secretions are the most widely available antigen detection methods. The former is more sensitive and specific; the latter is cheaper and better suited for laboratories that process large numbers of specimens. They are the preferred chlamydial testing methods for men with symptomatic urethritis. Sensitivity exceeds 70% and specificity approaches 99% in symptomatic men. Sensitivity is enhanced by obtaining a specimen several hours after the last urination. Enzyme immunoassay may give a false-positive result if lower urinary tract infection is present, which makes the test less useful in older men with prostatic disease. Test results are available within 36 to 72 hours. If posttreatment testing is desired, it should not be performed until 3 weeks after completion of treatment—sufficient time for clearing of antigen. *Rapid chlamydial testing* kits are packaged for office use and provide results within 30 minutes. They also use antigen detection methods and are subject to the same false-positive results.

Other Studies

When routine cultures and Gram's stains are not diagnostic and an empiric trial of treatment for NGU is unsuccessful (see later discussion), then reevaluation and consideration of culturing for *Ureaplasma* or *trichomonads* may be appropriate. When a reactive arthritis syndrome is suspected clinically, the patient can be checked for the presence of the HLA-B27 histocompatibility antigen, although both the sensitivity and the specificity are low. Its presence is not diagnostic of Reiter's syndrome, nor does its absence rule out the condition. Bloody discharge warrants referral to a urologist for consideration of *cystoscopy*.

MANAGEMENT OF NONGONOCOCCAL URETHRITIS (9–11)

Because chlamydial infection accounts for 50% of NGU cases, ranks as the most common STD among heterosexuals in the United States, and represents a potential source of morbidity to female partners and their infants, all patients with NGU should be treated, regardless of whether definite identification of *Chlamydia* has been achieved. Female partners of NGU patients should be tested; if testing is not available, they too should be treated for presumptive chlamydial infection. Male homosexual partners should be tested. Empiric treatment of asymptomatic male homosexual partners is not recommended because of the reduced incidence of *Chlamydia* infection in this population.

Initial Treatment

The Centers for Disease Control and Prevention (CDC) recommendation for the treatment of NGU is *doxycycline* (100 mg twice daily for 7 days) or *azithromycin* (1 g orally in a single dose). Although expensive, azithromycin provides greatly enhanced ease of use and compliance. Pregnant patients and others who should not take doxycycline or azithromycin can be treated with *erythromycin base* (500 mg four times daily for 7 days; erythromycin estolate is contraindicated in pregnancy). These antibiotic regimens are usually also effective against *Ureaplasma*. *Ofloxacin* (300 mg twice daily for 7 days) is also effective for the treatment of NGU, with excellent activity against both *Chlamydia* and *Ureaplasma*. It is superior to other fluoroquinolone antibiotics for the treatment of NGU and has also proved to be effective against *N. gonorrhoeae* (see Chapter 137). *Minocycline*, a once-a-day tetracycline, appears to be as effective as doxycycline. At a dose of 100 mg daily for 7 days, vestibular toxicity is uncommon.

Management of Recurrent Nongonococcal Urethritis

Although most patients with NGU experience resolution of symptoms with onset of therapy, up to 30% relapse. Some relapses have been attributed to tetracycline-resistant strains of *Ureaplasma* and others to poor compliance with medication, reinfection, or the presence of prostatitis (see Chapter 139). It is generally better to evaluate for reinfection before resorting to empiric antibiotics. Because *erythromycin* is effective against tetracycline-resistant strains of *Ureaplasma,* it has been used for recurrent disease (500 mg four times daily for 7 days). Because *Trichomonas* are often found in patients with recurrent disease, empiric combination therapy of *erythromycin* (dose just cited) and *metronidazole* (2.0 g as a single dose or 250 mg three times daily for 1 week) is recommended by the CDC.

Treatment of Reactive Arthritis

Treatment for *Chlamydia* may shorten the duration of illness and prevent recurrences in patients who appear to have the illness on the basis of sexually transmitted chlamydial infection.

Treatment of Gonococcal Urethritis

See Chapter 137.

PATIENT EDUCATION

The most important message to patients is the importance of prevention through the use of condoms. In addition, successful treatment of the disease requires contacting and treating recent sexual partners. The asymptomatic sexual partner is an important reservoir for reinfection. Treated male patients should be told to return for follow-up evaluation if symptoms return. Female partners should undergo retesting after 3 weeks to ensure eradication of chlamydial infection. No firm data are available concerning abstinence from unprotected intercourse during the treatment period, but it seems reasonable to suggest using barrier protection with a condom for at least 7 days after treatment is completed.

RECOMMENDATIONS (9)

- Inquire into the number of sexual partners the patient had during the last few months and use or nonuse of barrier contraception.
- Check for symptoms of prostatitis, gonorrheal infection, and Reiter's syndrome and for a history of penile warts, herpes simplex viral infection, or sexual contact with a partner known to have had trichomonal infection.
- Check the patient's temperature, and examine for signs of gonococcemia and Reiter's syndrome. Also check the urethral meatus for herpetic lesions and warts and the testes and prostate for signs of epididymitis and prostatitis. Obtain a urine specimen for *Chlamydia* PCR testing.
- Obtain a urethral swab for Gram's stain and for plating onto Thayer–Martin medium for culture of *Neisseria gonorrhoeae*.
- Obtain a second swabbing for chlamydial antigen detection, either by direct fluorescent antibody staining or enzyme immunoassay.
- Alternatively, send the second swab for DNA amplification testing, which is more sensitive and specific.
- Test female partners of NGU patients; if testing is not available, treat them empirically for presumptive chlamydial infection. Male homosexual partners should also be tested but not treated empirically.
- Treat all patients with NGU for chlamydial infection, regardless of whether definite identification of *Chlamydia* has been achieved. Obtain confirmatory testing because the information often helps to improve compliance, facilitate counseling, and guide care if symptoms persist.
- Treat NGU initially with doxycycline (100 mg twice daily for 7 days) or azithromycin (1 g orally in a single dose).
- Treat documented NGU recurrences with erythromycin (500 mg four times daily for 7 days) and metronidazole (2.0 g as a single dose).
- When routine cultures and Gram's stains are not diagnostic and an empiric trial of treatment for NGU is unsuccessful, then reevaluate and consider culturing for *Ureaplasma* or trichomonads.

Annotated Bibliography

1. Krieger JN, Jenny C, Verdon M, et al. Clinical manifestations of trichomoniasis in men. Ann Intern Med 1993;118:844. (*It was found to be a cause of urethritis and to be sexually transmitted.*)
2. Marrazzo JM, White CL, Krekeler B, et al. Community-based urine screening for *Chlamydia trachomatis* with a ligase chain reaction assay. Ann Intern Med 1997;127:796. (*Risk factors for male chlamydial infection were being nonwhite, having had two or more sexual partners in previous 2 months, and not using a condom; the positive predictive value of urinary leukocyte esterase testing was 38.4%; the negative predictive value was 97.7%.*)
3. Martin DH, Pollack S, Kuo CC. *Chlamydia trachomatis* infections in men with Reiter's syndrome. Ann Intern Med 1984;100:207. (*Documents infection and an exaggerated immune response in some patients who later develop Reiter's syndrome.*)
4. McKay L, Clery H, Carrick-Anderson K, et al. Genital *Chlamydia trachomatis* infection in a subgroup of young men in the UK. Lancet 2003;361:1792. (*The condition has a 9.8% prevalence; 88% of the men were asymptomatic.*)
5. Miller WC, Ford CA, Morris M, et al. Prevalence of chlamydial and gonococcal infections among young adults in the United States. JAMA 2004;291:2229. (*Found a 3.6% prevalence of chlamydial infection; the rate was 11% in African American men.*)
6. Schwartz MA, Hooton TM. Etiology of nongonococcal nonchlamydial urethritis. Sex Transm Dis 1998;16:72. (*Most nonspecific urethritis is caused*

by organisms other than *Chlamydia*, such as *Ureaplasma urealyticum*, *Mycoplasma genitalium*, and *Trichomonas vaginalis*.)

7. Wong ES, Hooton TM, Hill CC, et al. Clinical and microbiological features of persistent or recurrent nongonococcal urethritis in men. J Infect Dis 1988;158:1098. (*Noncompliance and reinfection were the main reasons that Chlamydia and Trichomonas were often found.*)

8. Jacobs NJ, Kraus SJ. Gonococcal and nongonococcal urethritis in men. Ann Intern Med 1975;82:7. (*The sensitivity of Gram's stain was 97%, and the specificity was 98% for the diagnosis of gonococcal urethritis; 21% of specimens that were equivocal on staining were positive for gonococci on culture.*)

9. Centers for Disease Control and Prevention. Sexually transmitted diseases treatment guidelines 2002. MMWR Morb Mortal Wkly Rep 2002;51(RR-6):1. (*An excellent review of diagnostic methods and authoritative guidelines for treatment; essential reading.*)

10. Hooton TM, Wong ES, Barnes RC, et al. Erythromycin for persistent or recurrent nongonococcal urethritis. Ann Intern Med 1990;113:21. (*A 3-week course of treatment proved beneficial, especially in patients with prostatitis.*)

11. Stamm WE, Hicks CB, Martin DH, et al. Azithromycin for empiric treatment of the nongonococcal urethritis syndrome in men. JAMA 1995;274:545. (*Cure rates for Chlamydia infection were 83% for single-dose azithromycin and 90% for 7 days of doxycycline; Ureaplasma cure rates were 45% and 47%, respectively.*)

CHAPTER 137 ■ APPROACH TO THE PATIENT WITH GONORRHEA

BENJAMIN DAVIS

Like other sexually transmitted diseases, gonorrhea remains a major public health problem in the United States. Penicillinase-producing strains are now commonplace, and there is a growing problem of resistance to quinolone antibiotics. Gonorrhea ranks just behind chlamydial infection as the most common reportable sexually transmitted disease in the United States, with more than 350,000 cases reported annually and an incidence rate of 125 per 100,000. Gonorrhea is most prevalent among teenagers and young adults, with African American men and women bearing a disproportionate burden of disease, accounting for 69% of all gonorrhea cases in 2006. The incidence of gonorrhea is also increasing in men who have sex with men (MSM).

The majority of patients with sexually transmitted diseases present to an ambulatory care facility and should be diagnosed and treated in this setting. At the same time, the physician must be alert to serious systemic complications requiring hospitalization. In addition, patient education is critical to prevent inadequate treatment and recurrent infections. Finally, the responsibility of the physician must extend beyond the diagnosis and treatment of an individual patient to the identification and treatment of sexual contacts who may otherwise harbor and disseminate these infections, even if they are asymptomatic.

PATHOPHYSIOLOGY AND CLINICAL PRESENTATION (1–8)

Gonococcal infection invariably begins with the direct infection of a mucosal surface during sexual activity. Organisms may then gain access to the bloodstream to produce bacteremia and systemic spread of infection. This is most common in women, especially at the time of menstruation, but it occurs in men also. The clinical features of gonorrhea differ greatly between the sexes. Moreover, symptoms of the primary gonococcal infection may be absent or mistaken for those of another condition, making the diagnosis more difficult.

In Men

In men, clinical symptoms usually follow within 2 to 10 days of sexual exposure. The risk that a man will acquire gonorrhea after a single exposure to an infected partner is approximately 35%. Absence of symptoms does not indicate absence of infection. Indeed, up to 10% of infected men are asymptomatic carriers of the gonococcus and are fully capable of transmitting the disease. In men, gonorrhea is principally an infection of the anterior urethra, and hence the major symptom is purulent *urethral discharge*, often accompanied by urinary frequency and dysuria. Although spread of infection to the *prostate* or *epididymis* is uncommon in the antibiotic era, gonococci occasionally gain entry into the *bloodstream* to produce disseminated infection.

In Women

In women, the *cervix* is the favored site of gonococcal infection. However, up to 25% of women with gonococcal infection are asymptomatic and must be identified through epidemiologic case finding. When symptoms do occur, cervical discharge is most common. Although the vagina is usually spared, the gonococcal infection may spread downward from the cervix to produce *urethritis*, which presents as dysuria and frequency. Infection of *Bartholin's glands* presents as labial swelling and pain, and rectal infection presents as anorectal discomfort. If, on the other hand, gonococcal infection spreads upward from the cervix, more-serious processes may develop. Such upward spread is particularly likely at the time of menstruation and can produce a variety of syndromes. Gonococcal *endometritis* can cause pelvic pain and abnormal vaginal bleeding, whereas *salpingitis* characteristically leads to fever, chills, leukocytosis, and a tender adnexal mass. Both systemic and pelvic signs and symptoms are even more pronounced in frank *pelvic peritonitis*, and further intraperitoneal spread may produce gonococcal *perihepatitis* with right upper quadrant pain and tenderness.

In Both Men and Women

Primary extragenital infections are being recognized more frequently. Gonococcal infection of the pharynx is usually asymptomatic but can present as an acute *exudative pharyngitis,* with fever and cervical lymphadenopathy. Gonococcal *proctitis* may be asymptomatic but can present with anorectal discomfort, tenesmus, or rectal bleeding and discharge.

Gonococcal bacteremia is manifested by the *"dermatitis–arthritis" syndrome*. Patients have fever, chills, and other constitutional symptoms. Skin lesions are an important clue to diagnosis; these are typically pustular, hemorrhagic, or papular, are few in number, and tend to be most common on the distal extremities. *Tenosynovitis*, especially involving the extensor surfaces of the hands and feet, and *migratory polyarthritis* are typically seen. During the early stage of systemic infection, blood cultures are often positive, but joint cultures are characteristically negative. Later in the course of untreated disease, however, gonococci can produce frank *septic arthritis*. Such patients have less fever, no skin lesions, and negative blood cultures but more impressive joint swelling and pain, often with purulent synovial fluid, in which gonococci can be demonstrated by Gram's stain or culture. In rare instances, gonococci can produce *osteomyelitis* or even life-threatening bacterial *meningitis* or *endocarditis*.

DIFFERENTIAL DIAGNOSIS

The organisms besides *Neisseria gonorrhoeae* capable of producing female genital infections include *Chlamydia, Gardnerella, Trichomonas,* and *Candida* (see Chapter 117). The differential diagnosis of gonococcal salpingitis and peritonitis mainly encompasses the causes of nongonococcal pelvic inflammatory disease (see Chapter 116), but other conditions, such as appendicitis, ectopic pregnancy, hemorrhagic ovarian cysts, and endometriosis, can produce similar clinical findings and often require urgent therapy very different from that of pelvic inflammatory disease. In the male patient, the causes of nongonococcal urethritis enter the differential diagnosis (see Chapter 136). Gonococcal infection also needs to be considered among the causes of pharyngitis (see Chapter 220) and proctitis (see Chapter 66).

WORKUP (9,10)

History and Physical Examination

The diagnosis of gonorrhea requires a high index of suspicion and a careful *sexual history*. Physical examination findings in men with urethritis are usually normal except for purulent *urethral discharge*. In asymptomatic women, the physical examination findings are normal, but *cervicitis* may produce cervical inflammation, discharge, and marked cervical tenderness. *Adnexal tenderness* and fullness are signs of salpingitis and may be unilateral or bilateral in women with gonorrhea. Tubal abscesses may be suspected because of a palpable mass, and rebound tenderness is a sign of pelvic peritonitis.

Pelvic inflammatory disease caused by organisms other than the gonococcus may present similarly. Clinical features favoring the gonococcus include purulent cervical discharge, onset early in the menstrual cycle, no previous history of pelvic inflammatory disease, and exposure to a male partner with urethritis.

Laboratory Studies

A properly performed *Gram's stain* of the urethral discharge can be a highly reliable diagnostic tool. A Gram's stain is considered "positive" when biscuit-shaped, gram-negative diplococci are seen within polymorphonuclear leukocytes, "equivocal" if diplococci are only extracellular or if intracellular organisms are morphologically atypical, and "negative" if no diplococci are found. Sensitivity of the Gram's stain is more than 95% in symptomatic men but declines to 50% to 60% in those with asymptomatic urethral infection. Gram's stains are much less reliable in cervical, rectal, and pharyngeal infections.

Cultures confirming the presence of gonorrhea remain the gold standard for diagnosis. *N. gonorrhoeae* is a fragile and fastidious organism that requires special handling in the laboratory. The gonococcus is readily killed by drying, so all cultures must be plated promptly. Ideally, this should be done by the physician at the time of examination by streaking the swab across the surface of the culture medium in a Z-shaped pattern. Special culture media must be used. Although chocolate agar has been the traditional medium used, a modified *Thayer–Martin medium* is preferred for specimens obtained from genital, anal, or pharyngeal sites because the addition of antibiotics to this medium suppresses the growth of nonpathogenic *Neisseria* species and other bacteria. The culture medium should be at room temperature at the time of inoculation. Because the gonococcus requires a high carbon dioxide concentration to grow, cultures should be promptly incubated in a candle jar or carbon dioxide incubator. Nucleic acid amplification techniques are available for urine in men and for endocervical swabs in women. The sensitivity of these techniques is 97% and the sensitivity is greater than 95%. However, bacteriologic culture of the organism remains valuable diagnostically and offers the advantage of providing antimicrobial susceptibility data.

In men, cultures of the anterior urethra should be obtained. In MSM, cultures of the anal canal and pharynx are also appropriate. In women, the endocervix should be cultured by inserting a swab into the cervical os through a speculum that has been lubricated only with water.

In all women, anal cultures are indicated because rectal infection may result through direct spread from the vagina. When acute arthritis is present, *joint fluid* should be obtained by arthrocentesis and should be evaluated with cell counts, Gram's stain, and culture. *Blood* cultures are indicated in patients with fever, skin lesions, and tenosynovitis or arthritis.

PRINCIPLES OF MANAGEMENT AND THERAPEUTIC RECOMMENDATIONS (11–19)

Overcoming Antibiotic Resistance

The therapy of gonorrhea has undergone dramatic changes during the last 40 years. Penicillin had been used for decades, but during this time penicillin resistance has increased steadily. Many strains have been found to contain plasmids that produce β-lactamase. In the United States, infections with plasmid-containing strains were initially sporadic, but the number of such infections has increased dramatically and is no longer limited to a few groups of patients. More recently, high-level, chromosomally mediated penicillin resistance has emerged. A significant number of clinical isolates are also tetracycline resistant, and heavy use of spectinomycin has led to emergence of strains resistant to that agent. Since 1993, the Centers for Disease Control and Prevention (CDC) has recommended fluoroquinolones for treatment of gonorrhea. However, quinolone resistance has been on the rise in Asia, has been reported to be as high as 14% in Hawaii, and has been increasing in California. Quinolone resistance has been reported to be as high as 5% in MSM. Consequently, the CDC no longer recommends quinolones as treatment for gonorrhea in the United States.

Concurrent Infection

In addition to the problem of antibiotic resistance, the management of gonorrhea is complicated by the need to treat co-existing sexually transmitted infections. Chlamydial disease is of greatest concern, coexisting with gonococcal infection in up to 20% of men and 50% of women with sexually transmitted disease. As a result, all patients with gonorrhea should also be treated for chlamydial infection. Although much less common than chlamydial infection, incubating syphilis can be a more serious problem, and patients should be screened for syphilis (see Chapters 124 and 117). Confidential testing for HIV infection may be of benefit not only for case identification, but also for promotion of safer sexual practices (see later discussion).

THERAPEUTIC RECOMMENDATIONS (11,12)

Uncomplicated Gonorrhea (Including Urethral, Cervical, and Rectal Infection)

- Prescribe ceftriaxone (125 mg intramuscularly [IM] once) or cefixime (400 mg orally [PO] once), *plus* azithromycin (1 g PO once) or doxycycline (100 mg twice daily for 7 days). Note: Cefixime tablets are not available in the United States.
- Prescribe spectinomycin (2 g IM once) for patients who are allergic to β-lactam antibiotics (i.e., cephalosporins and penicillins).
- Prescribe erythromycin base (500 mg four times daily for 7 days) for patients who cannot take doxycycline (e.g., pregnant women and those allergic to the drug).

Disseminated Gonococcal Infection

- Hospitalize initially and begin *ceftriaxone* (1 g intravenously [IV] or IM every 24 hours for 7 days).
- Treat with higher doses of *ceftriaxone* 1 to 2 g IV every 12 hours for a more prolonged period if meningitis, endocarditis, or osteomyelitis is present.

- Treat with *spectinomycin* (2 g IM every 12 hours for 7 days) those persons who are allergic to β-lactam antibiotics.
- Discharge those who respond well to the initial 1 to 2 days of parenteral therapy, provided they return daily for IM ceftriaxone or complete 1 week of oral therapy with *ciprofloxacin* (500 mg twice daily).
- Treat also for chlamydial infection, as in uncomplicated disease.

Monitoring

Because treatment failures with ceftriaxone are rare, immediate *follow-up cultures* are not mandatory. It may be more cost-effective to delay repeated evaluation with cultures until 1 to 2 months have passed. This allows detection of reinfection and treatment failures and reinforcement of patient education. Patients treated with regimens other than ceftriaxone do require follow-up cultures 4 to 7 days after therapy has been completed.

All patients with gonorrhea should undergo *serologic testing for syphilis*. Seronegative patients treated with ceftriaxone do not require follow-up serologies because this regimen is effective for incubating syphilis. However, patients receiving other antibiotic regimens do require repeated serologic testing in 3 months. All patients with gonorrhea should be offered confidential testing for HIV infection. All gonorrhea cases should be reported to the appropriate local health department. Because many patients are asymptomatic, vigorous case finding represents the only present means of controlling this epidemic.

PATIENT EDUCATION AND PREVENTION

Health education about the prevention of sexually transmitted disease is extremely important. Properly used barrier methods of contraception are effective means of preventing gonorrhea. *Condoms* do not permit transmission of the gonococcus or *Chlamydia*. The diaphragm or contraceptive sponge may also offer some protection against gonorrhea and chlamydial infection, especially when used with a *vaginal spermicide* containing nonoxynol 9, the active ingredient in many preparations. However, diaphragms and sponges *do not reduce the risk for HIV transmission*.

Preventive measures also include attention to *partner notification*. Patients should be encouraged to notify their sexual partners of their exposure and encourage them to seek medical care. This is *patient referral*. If patients are unwilling or unable to notify their partners, then the assistance of state and local departments of public health can be enlisted. This is *provider referral*.

INDICATIONS FOR ADMISSION

Patients with disseminated disease who are febrile, who are unreliable, or who have evidence of osteomyelitis, endocarditis, or meningitis must be hospitalized. The same is true of the woman with pelvic inflammatory disease who appears toxic, pregnant, or unlikely to comply or who has pelvic pain of unclear etiology in association with peritoneal signs.

Annotated Bibliography

1. Datta SD, Sternberg M, Johnson RE, et al. Gonorrhea and chlamydia in the United States among persons 14 to 39 years of age, 1999 to 2002. Ann Intern Med 2007;147:89. (*The prevalences of gonorrhea and chlamydia were 0.24% and 2.2%, respectively.*)
2. Handsfield HH, Lipman TO, Harnisch JP, et al. Asymptomatic gonorrhea in men. N Engl J Med 1974;290:117. (*Asymptomatic men may be an important reservoir of infection; all sexual contacts should be cultured, whether male or female and whether symptomatic or not.*)
3. Hook EW, Holmes KK. Gonococcal infections. Ann Intern Med 1985;102:229. (*A highly recommended authoritative review; 157 references.*)
4. Hutt DM, Judson FN. Epidemiology and treatment of oropharyngeal gonorrhea. Ann Intern Med 1986;104:655. (*Not to be forgotten as a cause of severe pharyngitis.*)
5. Kelaghan J, Rubin GL, Ory HW, et al. Barrier-method contraceptives and pelvic inflammatory disease. JAMA 1982;248:184. (*The relative risk was 0.6 for women using barrier methods.*)
6. Klein EJ, Fisher LS, Chow AW, et al. Anorectal gonococcal infection. Ann Intern Med 1977;86:340. (*A clinical review of such infections in women and male homosexuals.*)
7. O'Brien JP, Goldenberg DL, Rice PA. Disseminated gonococcal infection: a prospective analysis of 49 patients and a review of pathophysiology and immune mechanisms. Medicine 1983;62:395. (*A comprehensive study of 49 patients and a review of the literature.*)
8. Platt R, Rice PA, McCormack WM. Risk of acquiring gonorrhea and prevalence of abnormal adnexal findings among women recently exposed to gonorrhea. JAMA 1983;250:3205. (*The risk was 50%, 86%, and 100% for one, two, and more than two exposures, respectively; spread in the upper genital tract was a common early complication.*)
9. Centers for Disease Control and Prevention. Screening tests to detect *Chlamydia trachomatis* and *Neisseria gonorrhoeae* infections. MMWR Morb Mortal Wkly Rep 2002;51(RR15):1. (*A detailed guideline report with 160 references.*)
10. Phillips RS, Safran C, Aronson M, et al. Should women be tested for gonococcal infection of the cervix during routine gynecologic visits? An economic appraisal. Am J Med 1989;86:297. (*This decision-analysis study suggests that the answer is yes in high-risk populations.*)
11. Centers for Disease Control and Prevention. Increases in fluoroquinolone-resistant *Neisseria gonorrhoeae* among men who have sex with men—United States, 2003, and revised recommendations for gonorrhea treatment, 2004. MMWR Morb Mortal Wkly Rep 2004;53:335. (*The Centers for Disease Control and Prevention recommends that fluoroquinolones no longer be used as first-line therapy in men who have sex with men.*)
12. Centers for Disease Control and Prevention. Sexually transmitted diseases treatment guidelines, 2002. MMWR Morb Mortal Wkly Rep 2002;51(RR-6). (*Expert committee consensus recommendations.*)
13. Fenton KA, Ison C, Johnson AP, et al. Ciprofloxacin resistance in *Neisseria gonorrhoeae* in England and Wales in 2002. Lancet 2003;361:1867. (*Documents the basis for growing concern.*)
14. Handsfield HH, McCormack WM, Hook EW, et al. A comparison of single-dose cefixime with ceftriaxone as treatment for uncomplicated gonorrhea. N Engl J Med 1991;325:1337. (*Oral cefixime produced results equivalent to those obtained with parenterally administered ceftriaxone.*)
15. Judson FN. Management of antibiotic-resistant *Neisseria gonorrhoeae*. Ann Intern Med 1989;110:5. (*An editorial that succinctly reviews the options.*)
16. Lyss SB, Kamb ML, Peterman TA, et al. *Chlamydia trachomatis* among patients infected with and treated for *Neisseria gonorrhoeae* in sexually transmitted disease clinics in the United States. Ann Intern Med 2003;139:178. (*Chlamydia trachomatis was found in 20% of men with confirmed gonorrhea; 4.2% of cases were resistant, compared with 2.2% and 0.7% in 2002 and 2001, respectively.*)
17. Wang SA, Harvey AB, Conner SM, et al. Antimicrobial resistance for *Neisseria gonorrhoeae* in the United States, 1988 to 2003: the spread of fluoroquinolone resistance. Ann Intern Med. 2007;147:81. (*The prevalence of penicillin resistance has declined since gonorrhea treatment with penicillin was discontinued; fluoroquinolone resistance continues to increase.*)
18. Allen S, Serufilira A, Bogaerts J, et al. Confidential HIV testing and condom promotion in Africa: impact on HIV and gonorrhea rates. JAMA 1992;268:3338. (*Condom use went up 300%, and the prevalence of gonorrhea fell by more than half.*)
19. Golden MR, Whittington WLH, Handsfield HH, et al. Effect of expedited treatment of sex partners on recurrent or persistent gonorrhea or chlamydial infection. N Engl J Med. 2005;352:676. (*The treatment reduced modestly the rates of persistent or recurrent infection.*)

CHAPTER 138 ■ APPROACH TO BENIGN PROSTATIC HYPERPLASIA

MICHAEL J. BARRY

Benign prostatic hyperplasia (BPH) is a common condition among older men, causing morbidity primarily through lower urinary tract symptoms (LUTS). The primary physician should attempt to distinguish LUTS due to BPH from the other causes of such symptoms, objectively determine symptom severity, and, when the symptoms are bothersome enough, work with the patient on a therapeutic approach to reducing symptoms while minimizing side effects. For patients who elect watchful waiting or medical therapy, regular follow-up should be instituted to monitor for symptom changes or BPH complications. The treatment of BPH has changed substantially in recent years, with increasing emphasis on nonsurgical approaches. The result is an expanded role for primary care providers in BPH management.

PATHOPHYSIOLOGY AND CLINICAL PRESENTATION (1–5)

Pathophysiology

BPH arises from *nodular hyperplasia* of prostatic stromal and glandular elements. Growth begins in the *periurethral* glandular tissue. As these nodules expand and coalesce over years, the true prostatic tissue is compressed outward and forms a "surgical capsule" around the adenomatous hyperplasia. The etiology of age-related prostatic hyperplasia is unknown, although it is reasonably well established that androgenic stimulation at the cellular level has a major influence. A better understanding of these influences on prostatic hyperplasia has led to pharmacologic interventions that can alter the natural history of the disease.

As the gland enlarges, urethral resistance to urine flow increases and *bladder muscle hypertrophy* ensues. *Detrusor instability* may develop, and emptying may become incomplete. The resulting *residual urine* predisposes to infection. *Bladder herniations* can form between the thickened, overlapping muscular bands that comprise the detrusor. These diverticula may further predispose to infection. The role of the bladder in contributing to bothersome symptoms among men with bladder outlet obstruction is becoming increasingly appreciated.

Some men with BPH develop *acute urinary retention*. The hyperplastic prostate is highly vascular and predisposed to *bleeding*; painless hematuria can occur, but alternative causes, particularly malignancy, need to be considered.

The late-stage complications of chronic retention caused by BPH include *hydroureter*, *hydronephrosis*, and *renal failure*. Fortunately, these complications are rare.

Clinical Presentation and Course

BPH manifests clinically chiefly through lower urinary tract symptoms. Although BPH is the most common cause of such symptoms among older men, other diseases can cause them also. The old term *prostatism* implies a diagnostic specificity to these symptoms that does not in fact exist; this term should be avoided. Simplistically, *voiding* symptoms (such as a weak stream, straining, hesitancy, and intermittency) have been attributed to mechanical bladder outlet obstruction, whereas *filling* symptoms (such as frequency, nocturia, and urgency) have been attributed to secondary detrusor instability. In reality, the situation is much more complex; the way in which the histologic process of BPH eventually leads to symptoms is in fact poorly understood. The severity of LUTS correlates poorly with prostate size and urodynamic measurements of the severity of bladder outlet obstruction, and some treatments (such as microwave thermotherapy) can reduce symptoms considerably without having much effect on these parameters.

It is quite common for patients to have a waxing and waning symptomatic course, with gradual deterioration through many years. Sometimes, urinary tract infection or acute retention is the first indication of bladder outlet obstruction secondary to BPH.

DIAGNOSIS (1,3,4)

The digital rectal examination of the prostate provides a rough estimate of overall gland volume but is of little help in assessing the degree of bladder outlet obstruction. Severity can be assessed by symptom frequency and a few basic laboratory studies (see later discussion). Clinicians tend to underestimate prostate size, so if the prostate feels enlarged, it usually is.

Assessing Severity of Symptoms

In older men presenting with LUTS believed likely to be caused by BPH, the clinician should first objectively document symptom severity. The seven-item *American Urological Association*

(AUA) symptom index is a quick, self-administered questionnaire that is widely used for this purpose (Fig. 138.1). Scores on individual questions can be summed to yield an *AUA symptom score* ranging from 0 to 35. Scores of 0 to 7 represent mild symptoms, 8 to 19 moderate symptoms, and 20 to 35 severe symptoms. Some clinicians use *voiding diaries* in addition to symptom scores further to assess patients' symptoms. It is especially important for clinicians to determine the extent to which the patient is bothered by his symptoms.

A *urinalysis* should be performed to check for infection or hematuria. A creatinine determination can assess renal function. Measurements of *postvoid residual urine* can be made by catheterization (>50 to 100 mL of residual urine is abnormal) or, less invasively, by transabdominal ultrasonography. However, these measurements are poorly reproducible in individual patients, and they probably help only if they are persistently and grossly increased.

Urinary flow studies are commonly performed by urologists. These tests do not require catheterization and are particularly useful in assessing patients whose presentations are atypical (e.g., younger patients or men with dominantly filling symptoms). A normal peak flow rate (>15 mL/sec) in the setting of LUTS should prompt further evaluation for alternative explanations. However, men with true bladder outlet obstruction may sometimes maintain normal flow rates by generating high bladder pressures. Similarly, men with hypotonic bladders may have low flow rates without outlet obstruction. A voided volume of less than 150 mL may produce a falsely low peak flow rate.

Imaging studies are not routinely necessary in typical cases of LUTS attributed to BPH. Radiographic assessment of the bladder and upper urinary tract is not recommended unless an elevated creatinine level, hematuria, or another specific indication is present. If necessary, transabdominal *ultrasonography* can be used to exclude hydronephrosis and assess the postvoid residual volume. Similarly, cystourethroscopy should be performed only when specifically indicated (e.g., prior genitourinary instrumentation, hematuria). More sophisticated *urodynamic studies* (cystometrics and pressure–flow studies) are best reserved for patients with conflicting results on simple tests (e.g., bothersome symptoms but a normal flow rate), neurologic disease, or prior unsuccessful prostatectomy.

Assessing Significance of Symptoms

It is essential that the physician assess the *impact of symptoms* on the patient's quality of life because the individual patient may be willing to accept a given level of symptomatology and a small risk for future BPH complications to avoid medications or surgery.

Checking for Prostate Cancer

When the digital rectal examination findings are not suggestive of prostate cancer, a test for serum *prostate-specific antigen* (PSA) is optional for men with LUTS attributable to BPH. In the recent Prostate Cancer Prevention Trial, the sensitivity of PSA for histologic prostate cancer at the traditional cut-point of 4.0 ng/mL was only about 25%, and it was about 40% for more-concerning cancers of Gleason grade 7 or higher. Specificity was 90% or higher in this study of unselected older men but is lower among men with symptoms due to BPH because benign prostatic enlargement itself can raise serum PSA. Moreover, the prior probability of subclinical prostate cancer does not seem

	not at all	less than 1 time in 5	less than half the time	about half the time	more than half the time	almost always
1. Over the past month or so, how often have you had a sensation of not emptying your bladder completely after you finished urinating?	0 ☐ 1	1 ☐ 2	2 ☐ 3	3 ☐ 4	4 ☐ 5	5 ☐ 6
2. Over the past month or so, how often have you had to urinate again less than two hours after you finished urinating?	0 ☐ 7	1 ☐ 8	2 ☐ 9	3 ☐ 10	4 ☐ 11	5 ☐ 12
3. Over the past month or so, how often have you found you stopped and started again several times when you urinated?	0 ☐ 13	1 ☐ 14	2 ☐ 15	3 ☐ 16	4 ☐ 17	5 ☐ 18
4. Over the past month or so, how often have you found it difficult to postpone urination?	0 ☐ 19	1 ☐ 20	2 ☐ 21	3 ☐ 22	4 ☐ 23	5 ☐ 24
5. Over the past month or so, how often have you had a weak urinary stream?	0 ☐ 25	1 ☐ 26	2 ☐ 27	3 ☐ 28	4 ☐ 29	5 ☐ 30
6. Over the past month or so, how often have you had to push or strain to begin urination?	0 ☐ 31	1 ☐ 32	2 ☐ 33	3 ☐ 34	4 ☐ 35	5 ☐ 36

	None	1 time	2 times	3 times	4 times	5 or more times
7. Over the last month, how many times did you most typically get up to urinate from the time you went to bed at night until the time you got up in the morning?	0 ☐ 37	1 ☐ 38	2 ☐ 39	3 ☐ 40	4 ☐ 41	5 ☐ 42

Score = sum of questions 1-7 = __ __

FIGURE 138.1. American Urological Association symptom index for benign prostatic hyperplasia. (From Barry MJ, Fowler FJ, O'Leary MP, et al. The American Urological Association Symptom Index for benign prostatic hyperplasia. J Urol 1992;148:1549, with permission.)

to be appreciably elevated in the presence of LUTS. No trials have documented that the early detection of prostate cancer improves patient outcomes (although trials have not ruled out such a benefit either). Even advocates of PSA screening do not advise the test for men with less than a 10-year life expectancy (ages 75 years and older for men with average comorbidity), given its dubious effect on mortality among these men. Nevertheless, men of any age with BPH should understand that they run a risk of harboring coincidental prostate cancer and that further tests are available if the patient and his physician wish to screen for prostate cancer (see Chapter 126).

Predicting Prognosis

PSA level, in the absence of a larger cancer, also provides a rough estimate of prostate size. The following PSA cut-points have about 70% sensitivity and specificity for a prostate size greater than 40 mL: greater than 1.6 ng/mL for age 50 to 59 years; greater than 2.0 ng/mL for age 60 to 69 years; and greater than 2.3 ng/mL for men age 70 to 79 years. Men with larger prostates and higher baseline PSA levels (particularly >3.2 ng/mL) have a higher probability of symptom progression over time, as well as higher risks of acute urinary retention and progression to prostatectomy.

PRINCIPLES OF MANAGEMENT (1,6–22)

General Measures

Most patients with LUTS attributed to BPH that are not particularly bothersome should simply be followed (*watchful waiting*). Complicating and exacerbating factors, such as infections, should be treated, and medications that impair lower urinary tract function should be eliminated if possible. In particular, *diuretics* should be stopped if possible or taken early in the day to avoid nocturnal bladder distention. Drugs that can exacerbate bladder outflow obstruction (e.g., *anticholinergics*, *tricyclic antidepressants*) should be used with care. Patients should be warned about over-the-counter *decongestants* and cough-and-cold preparations. The patient should be told to *void frequently*, take extra time to void completely, and to avoid *beverages* that are likely to produce a diuresis (coffee, tea, alcohol), particularly before bedtime. A recent trial showed that such commonsense lifestyle modifications can have a substantial effect on LUTS, similar in magnitude to the effect of medications. In a recent natural history study, even men with documented bladder outlet obstruction did remarkably well over 10 years of follow-up without active therapy.

α-Blockers

The efficacy of these agents in reducing symptoms in men with BPH has been documented in numerous clinical trials of up to 4.5 years in duration. They probably work mainly by relaxing the bladder neck and prostatic smooth-muscle tone, thereby relieving some of the "dynamic" component of obstruction. The α-blockers *doxazosin* and *terazosin* are available generically and can be given just once a day. These drugs can induce orthostatic hypotension, particularly in the frail elderly, and can cause fatigue and dizziness unrelated to blood pressure changes. Doses need to be escalated with the monitoring of supine and standing blood pressure. *Tamsulosin* and *alfuzosin* are newer α-blockers developed to reduce prostatic rather than vascular smooth-muscle tone; these agents do not appear to affect blood pressure. Whether tamsulosin and alfuzosin have fewer side effects (most of which are not blood pressure related) than doxazosin and terazosin has not been adequately tested in head-to-head clinical trials. Tamsulosin appears to cause retrograde ejaculation in about 10% of men. Because erectile dysfunction, like BPH, is common among older men, caution is required in treating both conditions medically. Because of concerns about precipitating hypotension, the phosphodiesterase type 5 inhibitor sildenafil should not be administered in doses higher than 25 mg within 4 hours of taking any α-blocker, whereas vardenafil and tadalafil should be used cautiously, starting at the lowest dose in men on a stable dose of an α-blocker, with monitoring of blood pressure.

Many physicians give α-blockers at night to reduce side effects (particularly the first dose at a particular strength), but whether the strategy accomplishes this aim is poorly documented. Doses should generally be increased (unless side effects ensue) until the patient is satisfied with the result; underdosing is one reason for treatment failure. Typical dose escalation is from 1 to 2 mg up to 4 to 8 mg daily for doxazosin or 1 to 2 mg up to 5 to 10 mg for terazosin. An extended-release formulation of doxazosin has two dose levels of 4 and 8 mg. Tamsulosin is started at 0.4 mg daily and can be increased to 0.8 mg. Extended-release alfuzosin is given in a fixed dose of 10 mg daily, after a meal. About 70% of patients report symptomatic improvement on α-blockers. In the Medical Treatment of Prostatic Symptoms (MTOPS) trial, doxazosin dramatically reduced symptomatic progression, but its effect on reducing the rates of acute retention or progression to surgery was not durable over 4 years of follow-up.

5α-Reductase Inhibitors

Finasteride and *dutasteride* block the conversion of testosterone to its metabolite dihydrotestosterone, a potent intraprostatic androgen. These drugs reduce prostate size by about 20% over 1 year of treatment. Mild improvements in symptoms and urinary flow rates relative to placebo have been demonstrated in clinical trials. The efficacy of these drugs appears to be restricted to men who have larger prostates. Long-term trials demonstrated that both drugs significantly reduced the risk for acute urinary retention or progression to prostatectomy. Because the absolute risks of these events are low, about 15 men would have to take finasteride for 4 years to prevent 1 event (acute retention or surgery). However, this *number needed to treat* drops to less than 10 among men with higher prostate volumes (>50 mL) or higher baseline levels of PSA (>3.2 ng/mL). The reductase inhibitors also seem to be effective at reducing the risk of recurrent hematuria due to BPH.

Sexual dysfunction in the form of decreased libido, impotence, or ejaculatory difficulties occurs in about 5% of men taking a 5α-reductase inhibitor. Finasteride is given at a dose of 5 mg daily and dutasteride at 0.5 mg daily; neither requires dose titration. It can take 6 to 12 months of continuous use before benefit is noted. These drugs reduce serum PSA levels by an average of 50%, which means that PSA results need to be interpreted differently among men on this drug. One common strategy is simply to double the PSA value and then interpret the results as usual.

The results of the recent Prostate Cancer Prevention Trial add further complexity to the decision regarding the use of 5α-reductase inhibitors in older men. In this trial, finasteride reduced the overall risk of a diagnosis of prostate cancer from 24% with placebo to 18% over 7 years, whereas the risk of the most dangerous high-grade cancers increased from 5.1% to 6.4%. The high incidence of prostate cancer in this trial reflected an aggressive screening strategy, including routine end-of-study biopsies. The effect of these agents on prostate cancer mortality is unknown.

Combination Therapy

In a Veterans Administration randomized trial comparing finasteride alone, terazosin alone, *finasteride and terazosin*, and placebo, the addition of finasteride to terazosin produced no additional benefit in terms of symptom relief over 1 year. However, in the MTOPS trial, adding *finasteride* to *doxazosin* reduced the cumulative risk of BPH progression (largely symptom progression or acute retention) from 10% to 5% over 4 years, translating to a number needed to treat of about 20 to prevent an additional case of progression.

Anticholinergics

Anticholinergics have traditionally been avoided in men suspected of having bladder outlet obstruction due to BPH, for fear of precipitating acute retention. However, in one trial among older men with LUTS including particularly prominent and bothersome filling symptoms, the combination of tamsulosin and tolterodine had a significantly greater effect on frequency and urgency than tamsulosin alone, with a risk of acute retention of 0.5% over 12 weeks. The role of anticholinergics, alone or in combination, in men with LUTS attributed to BPH remains to be fully defined.

Phytotherapy

Phytotherapy, or treatment with plant extracts, is widely prescribed for men with BPH by clinicians in Europe and is being used more commonly by men in the United States. The best-studied of these medications are extracts of the *saw palmetto plant (Seranoa repens)*. In recent meta-analyses of trials, these therapies were found to reduce some symptoms (especially nocturia) more than placebo. Side effects were few. Saw palmetto was roughly equivalent to finasteride at reducing symptoms; however, given the modest efficacy of finasteride, this effect is not impressive. In one recent well-conducted 1-year trial of a saw palmetto extract, no effect on symptoms was seen. Whether these extracts share the ability of finasteride to prevent future BPH complications is unknown. A problem with these treatments is that many products are available without standardization of doses.

Surgical Approaches

Prostatectomy should be strongly considered in patients who have refractory acute retention, hydronephrosis, repeated urinary tract infections due to obstruction, recurrent or refractory gross hematuria, or an elevated creatinine level that responds to a period of bladder decompression with catheter drainage. More commonly, bothersome symptoms not responding to medical therapy are an indication to consider surgery. The primary care physician must integrate the patient's report of his symptoms with an assessment of how bothered the patient is by these complaints. Surgery does provide excellent symptomatic relief in most cases, but any procedure entails risks and costs that some patients may not be willing to undertake. Furthermore, there are patients for whom surgery might not provide much benefit, particularly if concurrent detrusor abnormalities are present.

Transurethral prostatectomy (TURP) is the most common surgical procedure for BPH, with an impressive track record of effectiveness at reducing both symptoms and the risk for BPH complications. The degree of symptom reduction is, on average, much greater than that achieved with any of the medical therapies. A *retropubic* or *suprapubic ("open") prostatectomy* may be required if the gland is substantially enlarged. The mortality rate for all these operations is low (<1% for TURP). TURP has classically been said to be associated with potential complications such as incontinence and erectile dysfunction, but a Veterans Administration trial that randomized men to immediate TURP versus a strategy of watchful waiting found that the risk for these problems was no higher after TURP. On the other hand, retrograde ejaculation and resulting infertility are common complications of prostatectomy and should be discussed with the patient before operation. A transurethral incision of the prostate (TUIP) may be a good choice for younger men with small prostate glands. TUIP has been shown to be nearly as effective as TURP in providing symptom relief and carries a lower risk for retrograde ejaculation and other complications. More recently, urologists have been using laser energy or electrical vaporization to coagulate, vaporize or enucleate prostate tissue, still via a transurethral approach. These procedures seem to cause less bleeding than TURP does and can often be performed as day surgery. Recent results of holmium laser ablation and enucleation appear comparable to TURP for up to 2 years, although equipment costs are high and the procedure can be difficult to learn.

Operations for BPH leave a substantial amount of prostatic tissue in place. The postoperative risk for future malignancy is not greatly reduced. Because residual prostatic tissue may continue to grow, symptoms may recur after surgery. Patients undergo reoperation at a rate of about 1%/yr after TURP.

Device Therapies

Two newer therapies for BPH are *transurethral microwave thermotherapy* (TUMT) and *transurethral needle ablation* (TUNA). In both, a device generates heat to coagulate prostate tissue. In the former, a microwave antenna is placed in the urethra surrounded by a cooling jacket (to protect the urethra), and in the latter, radiofrequency energy is delivered directly to the prostate via intraprostatic needles. Both procedures can be performed in a single outpatient session and may be complicated by urinary retention requiring catheter drainage. In general, studies have suggested short-term symptom relief somewhat less than that obtained with TURP but greater than that

obtained with medical therapy. The mechanism of symptom relief with these treatments is unclear because the coagulated intraprostatic tissue is not removed. Long-term trials comparing the results of TUMT and TUNA with TURP or medical therapy are not available.

INDICATIONS FOR REFERRAL

A urologist should be consulted when a patient presents with strong indications for surgery, as discussed previously. In addition, consultation can be helpful when the diagnosis is unclear, particularly when evidence of an alternative cause of a patient's lower urinary tract symptoms is present. Most commonly, a consultation is called for when a patient still has bothersome symptoms despite maximal medical therapy and would like to consider a surgical intervention.

PATIENT EDUCATION

One cannot overestimate the value of patient education in the effective management of BPH. When patients are provided with information about the waxing-and-waning natural history of symptoms and the advantages and risks of the full range of treatment options, they are likely to choose differently than when exposed only to a surgical opinion. Reviewing such information enables the primary physician and the patient to make a joint management decision. A joint management strategy ensures a therapeutic approach best suited to the patient's preferences. Watchful waiting is a reasonable choice for patients without strong indications for surgery, provided the patient and the physician share a commitment to periodic review and reassessment.

TREATMENT RECOMMENDATIONS (1)

- The primary care physician should objectively assess the severity of lower urinary tract symptoms and determine their effect on the patient's quality of life.
- All patients with symptoms likely caused by BPH should have a urinalysis.
- Routine urinary tract imaging is not necessary. Upper tract imaging, preferably by ultrasonography, is indicated if hydronephrosis is a concern (a large postvoid residual urine volume or an elevated creatinine level).
- A urine flow rate measurement may be useful when symptomatology is confusing or ambiguous; it helps to identify patients who have symptoms but little evidence of obstruction (peak flow rates >15 mL/s).
- Patients should be made aware of the possible coexistence of prostate cancer and BPH and the availability of further evaluation, including PSA screening. However, the effect of early detection of prostate cancer on prostate cancer mortality is doubtful in men with a life expectancy of less than 10 years.
- Most patients can be followed expectantly unless evidence of hydronephrosis, recurrent or persistent infection, or deterioration in renal function is present. Such complications warrant prompt surgical attention. Nighttime fluids and drugs that affect lower urinary tract function should be avoided.
- Selective α_1-blocker therapy (*doxazosin, terazosin, tamsulosin,* or *alfuzosin*) can provide symptomatic improvement for many patients.

- The 5α-reductase inhibitors *finasteride* and *dutasteride* may be worth considering in patients with larger prostate glands (reflected by a palpably enlarged prostate or baseline PSA levels >3.2 ng/mL), primarily to reduce the future risk for acute retention or surgery. They are less effective than α-blocker therapy in reducing lower urinary tract symptoms in the short run.

- Urologic consultation is indicated when the diagnosis is confusing or when, despite medical therapy, the quality of life is sufficiently compromised to warrant consideration of an operation to achieve symptomatic relief.

- Less invasive treatments for BPH provide an increased array of treatment options, but *prostatectomy* remains the standard for long-term symptom relief.

Annotated Bibliography

1. AUA Practice Guideline Committee. AUA guideline on management of benign prostatic hyperplasia (2003). Chapter 1: Diagnosis and treatment recommendations. J Urol 2003;170:530. (*Definitive benign prostatic hyperplasia [BPH] management guideline from the American Urological Association, including meta-analyses of the efficacy of all BPH treatment modalities, both medical and surgical; currently in the process of being updated.*)

2. Barry MJ, Fowler FJ, O'Leary MP, et al. The American Urological Association Symptom Index for benign prostatic hyperplasia. J Urol 1992;148:1549. (*Validation of a seven-item questionnaire for assessing symptom severity in men with BPH.*)

3. Roehrborn CG, Boyle P, Gould AL, et al. Serum prostate-specific antigen as a predictor of prostate volume in men with benign prostatic hyperplasia. Urology 1999;53:581. (*Prostate-specific antigen [PSA] can be used to roughly estimate prostate size.*)

4. Roehrborn CG, McConnell JD, Lieber M, et al. Serum prostate-specific antigen concentration is a powerful predictor of acute urinary retention and need for surgery in men with clinical benign prostatic hyperplasia. Urology 1999;53:473. (*A subgroup analysis of a 4-year placebo-controlled trial, finding that men with a baseline serum PSA level >3.2 ng/mL had the greatest absolute benefit in terms of reduced risk for prostatectomy and acute retention.*)

5. Chapple CR, Roehrborn C. A shifted paradigm for the further understanding, evaluation, and treatment of lower urinary tract symptoms in men: focus on the bladder. Eur Urol 2006;49:651. (*A review emphasizing the important role of the bladder as a cause of lower urinary tract symptoms among older men.*)

6. Andriole GL, Kirby R. Safety and tolerability of the dual 5 α-reductase inhibitor dutasteride in the treatment of benign prostatic hyperplasia. Eur Urol 2003;44:82. (*Reviews clinical trial data for the newer 5α-reductase inhibitor dutasteride.*)

7. Boyle P, Gould L, Roehrborn CG. Prostate volume predicts outcome of treatment of benign prostatic hyperplasia with finasteride: metaanalysis of randomized clinical trials. Urology 1996;48:398. (*The efficacy of finasteride is best for men with larger prostates.*)

8. Bent S, Kane C, Shinohara K, et al. Saw palmetto for benign prostatic hyperplasia. N Engl J Med 2006;354:557. (*This well-conducted 1-year trial showed no effect of a saw palmetto extract on lower urinary tract symptoms.*)

9. Brown CT, Yap T, Cromwell DA, et al. Self management for men with lower urinary tract symptoms: randomised controlled trial. BMJ 2007;334:25. (*A small randomized, controlled trial, showing that instruction in lifestyle changes can have a major effect on lower urinary tract symptoms.*)

10. Gormley GJ, Stoner E, Bruskewitz RC, et al. The effect of finasteride in men with benign prostatic hyperplasia. N Engl J Med 1992;327:1185. (*Symptoms improved and flow increased, with a slight increase in the risk for sexual dysfunction.*)

11. Kaplan SA, Roehrborn CG, Rovner ES, et al. Tolteridine and tamsulosin for treatment of men with lower urinary tract symptoms and overactive bladder: a randomized controlled trial. JAMA 2007;296:2319. (*A randomized, controlled trial, suggesting that there was some marginal benefit of adding an anticholinergic to an α-blocker in a selected subset of older men with lower urinary tract symptoms, with a relatively low risk of acute retention.*)

12. Kuntz R. Current role of lasers in the treatment of benign prostatic hyperplasia (BPH). Eur Urol 2006;49:961. (*Review of the wide array of laser treatments for men with BPH.*)

13. Lepor H, Williford WO, Barry MJ, et al., for the Veterans Affairs Cooperative Studies Benign Prostatic Hyperplasia Study Group. The efficacy of terazosin, finasteride and the combination in benign prostatic hyperplasia. N Engl J Med 1996;334:533. (*Terazosin but not finasteride was effective over 1 year, and the combination was no more effective than terazosin alone.*)

14. McConnell JD, Roehrborn CG, Bautista OM, et al. The long-term effect of doxazosin, finasteride, and combination therapy on clinical progression of benign prostatic hyperplasia. N Engl J Med 2003;349:2385. (*A 4-year comparison of doxazosin, finasteride, and combination therapy, finding that combination therapy conferred the lowest risk of BPH progression.*)

15. Roehrborn CG, Van Kerrebroeck P, Nordling J. Safety and efficacy of alfuzosin 10 mg once-daily in the treatment of lower urinary tract symptoms and clinical benign prostatic hyperplasia: a pooled analysis of three double-blind, placebo-controlled studies. BJU Int 2003;92:257. (*A pooled analysis of clinical trial data regarding the latest of the alpha-blockers.*)

16. Thomas A, Cannon A, Barlett E, et al. The natural history of lower urinary tract dysfunction in men: minimum 10-year urodynamic follow-up of untreated bladder outlet obstruction. BJU Int 96:1301 2005. (*Even men with documented bladder outlet obstruction had little deterioration over 10 years of watchful waiting.*)

17. Thompson IM, Goodman PJ, Tangen CM, et al. The influence of finasteride on the development of prostate cancer. N Engl J Med 2003;349:215. (*In the Prostate Cancer Prevention Trial, finasteride reduced the risk of prostate cancer overall but increased the risk of high-grade cancers.*)

18. Wasson JH, Reda DJ, Bruskewitz RC, et al. A comparison of transurethral surgery with watchful waiting for moderate symptoms of benign prostatic hyperplasia. N Engl J Med 1995;332:75. (*A randomized trial, documenting superior symptom improvement and fewer treatment failures with surgery; however, the men managed expectantly also had relatively good outcomes.*)

19. Wheelahan J, Scott N, Cartmill R, et al. Minimally invasive non-laser thermal techniques for prostatectomy: a systematic review. BJU Int 2000;86:977. (*A review of "non-invasive" thermal therapies for men with BPH.*)

20. Wilt TJ, Ishani A, MacDonald R. Serenoa repens for benign prostatic hyperplasia. Cochrane Database Syst Rev 2002;(3):CD001423. (*Extracts of the saw palmetto plant reduced lower urinary tract symptoms more than placebo and as much as finasteride, with fewer side effects.*)

21. Wilt TJ, Mac Donald R, Rutks I. Tamsulosin for benign prostatic hyperplasia. Cochrane Database Syst Rev 2003;(1):CD002081. (*Finds small to moderate improvement in symptoms and flow compared with placebo.*)

22. Wilt TJ, Howe RW, Rutks IR, et al. Terazosin for benign prostatic hyperplasia. Cochrane Database Syst Rev 2002;(4):CD003851. (*Finds that terazosin improves symptoms and flow; effectiveness was superior to that of placebo or finasteride, similar to that of other alpha-blockers, but less than that of transurethral microwave thermotherapy.*)

CHAPTER 139 ■ MANAGEMENT OF ACUTE AND CHRONIC PROSTATITIS

JOHN D. GOODSON

Prostatitis is a common problem in primary care practice. Acute prostatitis is an infection that requires accurate recognition and prompt treatment. Chronic prostatitis is a more common condition, and its etiology is more elusive. Pain in the male perineum can arise from both infectious and noninfectious inflammation and can represent pain referred from retroperitoneal structures and low sacral nerve roots. Further complicating management is the ongoing controversy about the role of low-level commensal microorganisms that can be cultured from symptomatic patients. Experts continue to disagree about the value of extended antibiotic treatment and empiric therapy. The current scheme for classifying prostatitis syndromes has four categories (Table 139.1). Infectious agents are only found in a minority of cases. Roughly 90% of cases of chronic prostatitis are nonbacterial.

CLINICAL PRESENTATION, PATHOPHYSIOLOGY, AND COURSE (1–10)

Bacterial prostatitis presumably ensues from ascending urethral infection, reflux of infected urine, extension of rectal infection, or hematogenous spread. Gram-negative bacilli (predominantly *Escherichia coli*, *Proteus*, *Klebsiella*, and *Pseudomonas*) and *enterococci* account for most of the single isolates obtained from culture. Occasionally, *Chlamydia*, *Ureaplasma*, a virus, or *Trichomonas* may be the etiologic agent. In the immune-compromised patient, infection with fungi, such as *Aspergillus*, should be considered.

Small numbers of bacterial isolates from prostatic fluids are very difficult to interpret, especially when the organisms identified are not usually thought of as urinary tract pathogens (e.g., gram-positive organisms such as *Staphylococcus epidermidis* or *Corynebacterium* species).

When bacterial growth is associated with evidence of prostate inflammation (as defined later), then antibiotic treatment is warranted. When a specific infectious agent is not found, treatment with antibiotics may be considered; empiric therapy is a reasonable option, but the outcome may still not be satisfactory.

Acute Prostatitis

The condition is readily identified by the onset of diminished urine flow, perineal pain, dysuria, and fever. On gentle rectal examination, the gland is found to be enlarged, exquisitely tender, and boggy. Abdominal examination occasionally reveals striking bladder distention. Some patients may appear toxic at the time of presentation.

Chronic Prostatitis

In older men, the symptoms are generally those of bladder outflow obstruction, sometimes accompanied by pelvic pain. Patients complain of frequency, dribbling, loss of stream volume and force, double voiding, hesitancy, and urgency. Younger men more often complain of dysuria and dribbling, intermittent discomfort in the perineum, low back, or testicles. Some patients present initially with hematuria, hematospermia, or painful ejaculations. Rectal examination usually reveals an enlarged prostate with a variable amount of asymmetry, bogginess, and tenderness. Untreated or incompletely treated chronic prostatitis is characterized by recurrent symptomatic exacerbations, although these may be separated by long asymptomatic intervals. This has been termed *male chronic pelvic pain syndrome*.

Both acute and chronic prostatitis can cause urinary tract and systemic complications. The acutely infected gland may lead to renal parenchymal infection or bacteremia. Rarely, acute infection will progress to a well-defined abscess. Chronic infection can produce small prostatic stones, which may serve as a nidus for further inflammation and recurrent symptomatic bouts of infection.

Prostatodynia

Patients with prostatodynia complain primarily of persistent *pelvic* and *perineal* pain, but no bacterial pathogen can be identified, and no evidence of prostatic inflammation can be documented. Sometimes, the pain may be associated with urinary symptoms such as frequency, urgency, decreased stream flow, and decreased bladder capacity. As noted, some of these patients will be on extensive culturing to have small numbers of commensal gram-positive organisms in their prostate secretions, and for this reason, low-level infection with bacterial or nonbacterial agents has been believed by some to be the cause of this syndrome. However, a sizable number of patients have negative cultures, and this group remains a management challenge. Some advocate the use of α-adrenergic blockers for symptom relief. Some of these patients may have nonperitoneal causes of peritoneal pain, such as pain referred from other pelvic structures or sacral nerve root irritation.

DIFFERENTIAL DIAGNOSIS (1–5,7–9)

Acute prostatitis is readily evident by the clinical presentation and exquisitely tender prostate found on rectal examination. However, chronic prostatitis presents a more difficult

TABLE 139.1

CLASSIFICATION AND DEFINITION OF PROSTATITIS

Category I	Acute bacterial prostatitis	Acute infection
Category II	Chronic bacterial prostatitis	Persistent infection
Category III	Chronic abacterial prostatitis	No infection
IIIA	Inflammatory	WBCs in EPS or VB3 (postmassage urine)
IIIB	Noninflammatory	WBCs in EPS or VB3 (postmassage urine)
Category IV	Asymptomatic inflammatory prostatitis	WBCs in EPS or VB3 (postmassage urine) or on biopsy specimen, but no symptoms

WBC, white blood cell; EPS, expressed prostatic secretion; VB, voided bladder.
After Nickel JC. Prostatitis: myths and realities. Urology 1998;51:363, with permission.

diagnostic problem, often resembling, in clinical presentation, other common forms of urinary outflow tract obstruction, such as benign prostatic hyperplasia (see Chapter 138), prostatic carcinoma (see Chapter 143), and urethral stricture (see Chapter 134). The lower urinary tract irritative symptoms associated with chronic prostatitis may be seen with urethritis (see Chapter 136), bladder carcinoma (see Chapter 143), sphincter dyssynergy, and neurogenic bladder (see Chapter 134) (Table 134.1).

WORKUP (2–5,7,10–12)

History and Physical Examination

The pertinent history and physical examination depend on the clinical presentation. For suspected *acute prostatitis*, one needs to check for acute onset of fever, perineal pain, dysuria, and diminished urine flow. A urethral discharge is sometimes reported. On rectal examination, the prostate is found to be exquisitely tender. Examination should proceed cautiously to avoid precipitating bacteremia. The abdomen should be checked for bladder distention. For *chronic prostatitis*, one should inquire into recurrent perineal, back, or testicular discomfort, dribbling, slow stream, dysuria, and hematospermia. The prostate is enlarged, boggy, and sometimes tender on examination.

Laboratory Studies

Because the documentation of prostate inflammation and the identification of infecting organisms are essential to categorizing prostatitis, and because prostatic infection can be recurrent and elusive, it is well worth the effort to obtain *prostatic fluid* and *urine* for analysis and culture.

Expressed Prostatic Secretions

When urethritis is not suspected, then the secretions expressed by prostatic massage should be examined by Gram's stain and sent for culture. Vigorous massage should be avoided in patients with severe acute prostatitis because of the risk for inducing bacteremia. Even low levels of bacterial growth (<100,000 colony-forming units/mL) should be identified and sensitivities determined. Some laboratories require notification to do this. The presence of fewer than 10 white blood cells per high-

power field on expressed prostatic secretion (EPS) examination excludes prostatic infection with a specificity of 88%.

Pre– and Post–Prostate Massage Urines

When urethritis is not suspected clinically and no prostatic secretions can be obtained, then urine specimens can be collected before and after prostate massage (*premassage/postmassage test*). If leukocytes (>10 cells per high-power field) are present in the urine after massage when none were present before, then prostatic inflammation can be inferred. Occasionally, the *urine culture* after massage shows a single organism or mixed organisms when none were present before massage. Even low levels of bacterial growth (<100,000 colony-forming units/mL) should be identified and sensitivities determined. Some laboratories require notification to do this.

When no bacterial growth is identified on the EPS, VB3 (see later discussion), or postmassage urine despite the presence of leukocytes in any of the three, then bacterial infection has been missed, a nonbacterial infectious agent such as *Chlamydia* is present, or a noninfectious inflammation is present. Unfortunately, patients with *chronic nonbacterial* (or *abacterial*) prostatitis cannot reliably be further differentiated. At this time, the use of DNA amplification techniques such as polymerase chain reaction have not been widely studied in this situation and are not recommended. Older men who are without evidence of infection yet are bothered by lower urinary tract irritative symptoms should undergo *urine cytology* to help exclude a bladder malignancy. A bladder carcinoma located in the trigonal region can mimic chronic prostatitis.

Prostatic Fluid

The most rigorous approach is to obtain a series of specimens before and after *prostate massage*. Specimens representing urethral, bladder, and postmassage urine are collected and labeled VB1, VB2, and VB3, respectively (VB, voided bladder; see Appendix 139.1), in addition to any EPS that can be obtained as a result of massage. As noted, vigorous massage should be avoided in patients with severe acute prostatitis because of the risk for inducing bacteremia. Gram's stain of the EPS or the spun VB3 will sometimes demonstrate organisms or white blood cells (>10 cells per high-power field is abnormal).

As stated, the presence of fewer than 10 white blood cells per high-power field on EPS examination reasonably excludes prostatic infection. The EPS and VB3 show significant growth (>5,000 colony-forming units/mL), whereas the VB1 and VB2 should be sterile or have a colony count that is smaller by one order of magnitude.

Other Studies

Cystoscopy may be indicated when the diagnosis is not confirmed by urine culture data. *Blood urea nitrogen* and *creatinine* levels should be determined at the initial visit and periodically thereafter, depending on the chronicity and severity of symptoms. A *contrast spiral computed tomography* is indicated when evidence of renal deterioration or symptoms of persistent outflow obstruction are present to exclude a retroperitoneal or pelvic process. Occasionally, *lumbosacral magnetic resonance imaging* is indicated to exclude sacral nerve entrapment or impingement.

PRINCIPLES OF MANAGEMENT
(2,3,7,9,10,13–19)

Acute Prostatitis

When accompanied by severe pain, high fever, rigors, and marked leukocytosis, acute prostatitis requires *hospitalization* for *intravenous antibiotic therapy*. Such patients should be examined gently for the presence of a fluctuant prostatic mass suggestive of an abscess, which may necessitate drainage. Less toxic patients can be treated as outpatients with an oral antibiotic program. A fluoroquinolone such as *ciprofloxacin* or *levofloxacin is generally preferred*. *Trimethoprim/sulfamethoxazole* (TMS) and *doxycycline* are alternatives. Extended therapy— 4 to 6 weeks—is generally recommended to prevent acute infection from becoming established. Most other antibiotics effective against gram-negative rods (e.g., *amoxicillin*) penetrate the acutely inflamed prostate well and work satisfactorily in the acute phase of illness.

Local measures can help to reduce discomfort. Sitz baths two to three times a day for 20 minutes can relieve perineal pain. Stool softeners, antipyretics, analgesics, and bed rest are all helpful.

Bacterial and Nonbacterial Prostatitis

This condition is more difficult to eradicate. When the etiology is an infectious agent, poor penetration by oral antibiotics into the prostate limits treatment effectiveness. The identification of a target organism is the exception, and empiric therapy in this situation is unlikely to be of benefit. When a bacterial agent is identified, curative antibiotic therapy should be targeted toward the elimination of bacteria from prostatic fluid. Because the prostatic secretions are normally acidic (pH 6.5 to 7.4), the most efficacious drugs are those that readily penetrate membranes (lipid soluble) and become ionically trapped (high pH). The *fluoroquinolones*, TMS, and *erythromycin* have these characteristics and achieve good prostatic fluid levels. Because *ciprofloxacin* and TMS are more effective than *erythromycin* against gram-negative bacteria, they are preferred. TMS is not effective against enterococci. *Carbenicillin* and *doxycycline* also penetrate the prostate reasonably well. The latter is especially active against *Chlamydia* and some *Ureaplasma* organisms.

With chronic infection, the prostatic fluid becomes increasingly alkaline, which tends to reduce antibiotic penetration. As a result, prolonged treatment may be necessary. Some patients may not achieve cure even after 8 to 12 weeks of antibiotics. Cure rates with TMS range from 30% to 70%; slightly higher rates have been reported with 2 to 4 weeks of ciprofloxacin.

To demonstrate cure, the EPS or VB3 (postmassage urine) should be inspected and cultured after the treatment period. Because causative organisms are hard to identify and treatment is frequently empiric, the analysis of the prostate fluid after treatment is valuable. If evidence of infection is still present (>10 white cells per high-power field in the EPS or pus in the urine after massage), then a longer course of antibiotics may be indicated. After 12 weeks of antibiotic therapy, cure is unlikely. Some have suggested 6 to 12 months of treatment, but there are no data that clearly support this practice.

Peripheral *α-adrenergic blockers* can be used in conjunction with antibiotic therapy for both acute and chronic prostatitis to reduce symptoms. Some data suggest that these drugs also help to facilitate cure, but these studies are far from conclusive. The value of the α-adrenergic blockers declines in the more chronic cases.

The relatively low cure rate achieved with antibiotics in chronic prostatitis requires that therapeutic goals be adjusted to the patient's age. In some cases, α-adrenergic blockade can be used to control symptoms. If infection relapses and had been clearly demonstrated on culture, one TMS tablet daily appears to be an effective *suppressive regimen*. *Transurethral prostatic resection* and *total prostatectomy* provide alternatives when repeated courses of antibiotics fail. *Transurethral thermotherapy* is a less aggressive procedure, which has demonstrated symptom improvement in small trials. However, all such procedures are associated with significant morbidity, including sexual dysfunction and retrograde ejaculation with resulting infertility, and should be reserved for carefully selected patients. Recurrent infection associated with prostatic stones is an indication for removal of the gland.

Local measures can help to reduce symptoms in patients with chronic prostatitis. The patient with obstructive symptoms can try voiding while in a warm water bath with the pelvic muscles relaxed. The value of prostatic massage is a subject of debate. Many claim that *prostatic massage* relieves gland congestion in chronic cases and should be repeated every 1 to 2 weeks. (Massage of the acutely infected gland is contraindicated.) The patient should avoid alcohol, coffee, tea, or other beverages that might produce rapid bladder expansion. The physician should discontinue or reduce the dose, if possible, of anticholinergics, sedatives, and antidepressants, all of which can impair bladder function (see Chapter 134). Ejaculation is not contraindicated.

Prostatodynia or Chronic Perineal and Pelvic Pain

Patients with pain and urinary symptoms and no evidence of infection should be watched for the emergence of infection. A limited (4 to 6 weeks) course of antibiotics is unlikely to be worthwhile. Alpha-adrenergic blockade has been used with some success in these patients. Analgesics including nonsteroidal antiinflammatory drugs may be the most effective intervention.

PATIENT EDUCATION

Patients should be advised of the chronic and relapsing nature of the disease and alerted to the early signs of infection in the upper urinary tract. They can also be reassured that isolated prostatitis does not cause infertility or impotence. Local measures that can be suggested for symptomatic relief include sitz baths and voiding into a warm water bath. The importance of compliance with the prolonged antibiotic course and physician monitoring of the response to treatment needs to be stressed.

THERAPEUTIC RECOMMENDATIONS

Acute Prostatitis

- Obtain Gram's stain and culture of the EPS or VB3 (post-massage urine) and treat immediately.
- For the nontoxic patient, oral antibiotic therapy is sufficient. Prescribe ciprofloxacin (500 mg twice daily) or levofloxacin (500 mg daily) for 4 weeks. Doses of the fluoroquinolones should be adjusted for renal insufficiency. Double-strength TMS (160 mg of trimethoprim, 800 mg of sulfamethoxazole twice daily), amoxicillin (500 mg three times daily), doxycycline (100 mg twice daily), and carbenicillin indanyl sodium (1 g four times daily) are reasonable alternatives, all given for 4 weeks.

Chronic Prostatitis

- Document an infectious organism and the presence of prostatic inflammation, either with EPS examination, the premassage/postmassage test, or sequential urinary culturing.
- When a bacterial agent is identified, treat with a prolonged course of antibiotics, such as ciprofloxacin (500 mg twice daily), levofloxacin (500 mg daily), or double-strength TMS (twice daily for 8 to 12 weeks) for 4 to 6 weeks. Doses of the fluoroquinolones should be adjusted for renal insufficiency.
- After treatment, follow closely for return of infection. A second course of antibiotics with the same or an alternative drug for up to 12 weeks may be necessary in partially responsive infections.
- For patients who present with the new onset of "chronic" abacterial prostatitis, consider a 12-week course of doxycycline (100 mg twice daily), erythromycin (500 mg four times daily), or carbenicillin indanyl sodium (1 g four times daily).
- Schedule a return 1 to 2 weeks after the completion of treatment to assess the effects of therapy by checking the EPS or VB3 (postmassage urine specimen).

- Consider an α-adrenergic blocker such as prazosin (2 to 20 mg/d in divided doses), doxazosin (2 to 8 mg daily), terazosin (1 to 10 mg daily), tamsulosin (0.4 to 0.8 mg daily or in split doses), or alfuzosin (10 mg daily) to reduce sphincter resistance. Prazosin, doxazosin, and terazosin are more likely to cause clinically significant hypotension. Continue as long as the patient derives benefit, with the understanding that there is no predictable outcome.

Prostatodynia or Chronic Pelvic and Perineal Pain

- Prescribe an α-adrenergic blocker such as prazosin (2 to 20 mg/d in divided doses), doxazosin (2 to 8 mg daily), terazosin (1 to 10 mg daily), tamsulosin (0.4 to 0.8 mg daily or in split doses), or alfuzosin (10 mg daily) to reduce sphincter resistance. Prazosin, doxazosin, and terazosin are more likely to cause clinically significant hypotension. Continue as long as the patient derives benefit, with the understanding that there is no predictable outcome.
- Provide analgesia with nonsteroidal antiinflammatory drugs.

INDICATIONS FOR ADMISSION AND REFERRAL

Patients with high fever, leukocytosis, and severe perineal pain require intravenous antibiotics, antipyretics, and analgesics; hospitalization is indicated. In the presence of marked outflow obstruction, suprapubic bladder decompression may be necessary. A fluctuant prostatic mass that is suggestive of an abscess may require drainage. Until culture and sensitivity data are available, treatment of the toxic patient is directed toward gram-negative bacteria and enterococci, with parenteral administration of ampicillin and gentamicin or levofloxacin.

Patients with outflow tract obstruction or refractory chronic infection should have a urologic consultation. Patients with prostatodynia or an unexplained chronic pelvic and perineal pain syndrome should be referred to a urologist with appropriate expertise.

Annotated Bibliography

1. Brunner H, Weidner W, Schiefer HG. Studies on the role of *Ureaplasma urealyticum* and *Mycoplasma hominis* in prostatitis. J Infect Dis 1983;147:807. (*Thirteen percent of patients had documented Ureaplasma infection; >80% responded to tetracycline.*)
2. Schaeffer AJ. Chronic prostatitis and the chronic pelvic pain syndrome. N Engl J Med 2006;355:1690. (*An excellent recent review*).
3. Drach GW, Nolan PE. Chronic bacterial prostatitis: problems in diagnosis and therapy. Urology 1986;27(Suppl):26. (*When strict criteria were used, only 20% of patients referred for the evaluation of prostatitis had definitely positive results on cultures.*)
4. Krieger JN, Nyberg L Jr, Nickel JC. NIH consensus definition and classification of prostatitis. JAMA 1999;282:236. (*Presents the rationale for definitions and classification system.*)
5. Lowentritt JE, Kawahara K, Human LG, et al. Bacterial infections in prostatodynia. J Urol 1995;154:1378. (*Of 22 patients with prostatodynia, 9 had very low levels of infection documented, mostly with commensal organisms; of 7 patients treated, 5 became culture-negative and improved.*)
6. McNaughton Collins M, Stafford R, O'Leary M, et al. How common is prostatitis? A national survey of physician visits. J Urol 1998;159:1224. (*There are 2 million outpatient visits per year in the United States with a diagnosis of prostatitis.*)
7. McNaughton Collins M, MacDonald R, Wilt TJ. Diagnosis and treatment of chronic abacterial prostatitis: a systematic review. Ann Intern Med 2000;133:367. (*A systematic review of the literature, finding no evidence*

supporting the treatment of culture-negative chronic prostatitis, nor even any consensus about diagnostic criteria.*)
8. Meares EM Jr. Infected stones of the prostate gland. Urology 1974;4:560. (*These are found in 13.8% of men; most are asymptomatic, but when recurrent infection is demonstrated, the gland and stones must be removed.*)
9. Roberts RO, Lieber MM, Bostwick DG, et al. A review of clinical and pathological prostate syndromes. Urology 1997;49:809. (*The Mayo Clinic experience; the authors advocate 4 to 6 weeks of treatment for acute prostatitis and 3 to 4 months of treatment for chronic prostatitis.*)
10. Thin RN, Simmons PD. Chronic bacterial and nonbacterial prostatitis. Br J Urol 1983;55:513. (*The expressed prostatic fluid leukocyte counts for bacterial and nonbacterial prostatitis were similar; the test is highly specific but poorly sensitive.*)
11. McNaughton Collins M, Fowler FJ Jr, Elliott DB, et al. Diagnosing and treating chronic prostatitis: do urologists use the four-glass test? Urology 2000;55:403. (*For most, the answer is no; whether they do or not does not influence the use of antibiotics.*)
12. Nickel JC. Effective office management of chronic prostatitis. Urol Clin North Am 1998;25:677. (*Describes and advocates the more practical premassage/postmassage test for screening purposes; test sensitivity and specificity cannot be determined in the absence of any diagnostic gold standard.*)
13. Alexander RB, Propert KJ, Shaeffer AJ, et al. Ciprofloxacin or tamsulosin in men with chronic prostatitis/chronic pelvic pain syndrome. Ann Intern Med

2004;141:581. (*A randomized, double-blind trial, failing to show benefit from either treatment alone or the combination.*)

14. Barbalias GA, Nikiforidis G, Liatskos EN. α-Blockers for the treatment of chronic prostatitis in combinations with antibiotics. J Urol 1998;159:883. (*Concurrent use of an alpha-blocker and antibiotics was associated with a reduction in recurrence rate and improved symptom relief.*)

15. McNaughton Collins M, MacDonald R, Wilt T. Interventions for chronic abacterial prostatitis (Cochrane review). In: The Cochrane library, Issue 3. Oxford: Update Software, 2004. (*The routine use of antibiotics and alpha-blockers is not supported by the evidence; small studies examining thermal therapy are promising and merit further evaluation; an update of ref. 6; see http://www.cochrane.org for further updates.*)

16. McNaughton Collins M, Wilt T. Allopurinol for chronic prostatitis (Cochrane review). In: The Cochrane library, Issue 3. Oxford: Update Soft-

ware, 2004. (*There was only one positive trial; advises against routine use pending further study; see http://www.cochrane.org for updates.*)

17. Meares EM Jr. Long-term therapy of chronic bacterial prostatitis with trimethoprim–sulfamethoxazole. Can Med Assoc J 1975;112:225. (*A 12-week course produced an initially good response in 74% of patients, but only 31% remained cured for a 30-month follow-up period.*)

18. Nickel JC, Sorenson R. Transurethral microwave thermotherapy for non-bacterial prostatitis: a randomized double-blind sham controlled study using new prostatitis-specific assessment questionnaires. J Urol 1996;155:150. (*A >50% improvement in symptoms was noted in 7 of 10 treated patients, compared with 1 of 10 sham patients; the study was small but well conducted and offers some hope for this group of patients.*)

19. Vibhash M, Browne J, Emberton M. Role of alpha-blockers in type III prostatitis: A systematic review of the literature. J Urol 2007;177:25. (*A meta-analysis of the data, failing to demonstrate a conclusive benefit from alpha-blockers.*)

APPENDIX 139.1: URINE AND PROSTATIC FLUID COLLECTIONS IN MEN (1–3)

STANDARD CLEAN-VOIDED SPECIMEN

Specimen collection in *male patients* varies with the clinical situation. When cystitis is suspected, the patient is traditionally instructed to retract the foreskin and clean the glans penis with three moist gauze pads or soap sponges. A small amount of urine is voided into the toilet and then a midstream specimen is collected. Cleansing and retraction of the foreskin make no difference if a midstream specimen is obtained. However, omitting these steps does lead to the contamination of initial specimens. When urethritis or prostatitis is suspected, voided-bladder specimens are indicated.

EXPRESSED PROSTATIC FLUID SPECIMEN

The patient retracts the foreskin and cleans the glans penis. The physician then massages the prostate with continuous strokes. The patient should be standing, leaning forward with one arm resting on an exam table or desk and the other holding the collection container. The resulting prostatic fluid, which either comes from the meatus or is milked from the penis by the patient, is collected in a sterile container labeled EPS; this can be used for culture and Gram's stain or acid-fast stain. Vigorous prostatic massage can produce a transient bacteremia and should be avoided if acute prostatitis is suspected.

VOIDED-BLADDER SPECIMENS

The patient retracts the foreskin and cleans the glans penis. The first 10 mL are collected and labeled VB1 (Fig. 139.1). This represents a urethral specimen, which is also useful in cases of suspected urethritis (see Chapters 125 and 136). A midstream specimen is collected in the standard fashion. This is labeled VB2. The bladder must not be completely emptied. The physician then massages the prostate with continuous strokes. The patient should be standing, leaning forward with one arm resting on an exam table or desk and the other holding the collection container. The patient's toes should be pointed inward

with the heels spread. The resulting prostatic fluid, which either comes from the meatus or is milked from the penis by the patient, is collected in a sterile container labeled EPS; this can be used for culture and Gram's stain or acid-fast stain. If no fluid can be collected, the patient is told to void another 10 mL into a sterile container. This specimen, labeled VB3, represents roughly a 100:1 dilution of prostatic fluid and can be cultured or spun and stained. Vigorous prostatic massage can produce a transient bacteremia and should be avoided if acute prostatitis is suspected. If the patient has chronic prostatitis and known valvular heart disease, endocarditis prophylaxis may be necessary (see Chapter 16).

The EPS and VB3 can be inspected under the microscope for the presence of fat globules, leukocytes, and organisms. If fewer than 10 leukocytes are seen per high-power field, bacterial prostatic infection is unlikely. A Gram's stain may aid in identifying the responsible organism. With bacterial prostatitis, growth will occur in VB3 and EPS but not in VB1 and VB2. When bacterial growth is noted in both VB2 and VB3 samples, a prostatic infection may be masked by a bladder infection. In this situation, antibiotics that sterilize the bladder contents but do not penetrate the prostate (e.g., 500 mg of penicillin G four times a day orally or 100 mg of nitrofurantoin [Macrodantin] three times a day orally) may be given for 2 to 3 days before specimen collection. With bacterial prostatic infection, the EPS will still grow organisms. Urethral catheterization of male patients is rarely required for culture and should be reserved for the symptomatic relief of marked outflow obstruction.

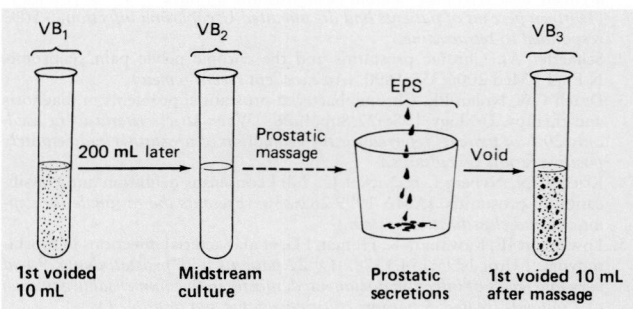

FIGURE 139.1. Segmented culture of the lower urinary tract in male patients. EPS, expressed prostatic secretion; VB, voided bladder. (Adapted from Meares EM, Stamey T. Bacteriologic localization patterns in bacterial prostatitis and urethritis. Invest Urol 1968;5:492, with permission.)

Annotated Bibliography

1. Lipsky BA, Inui TS, Plorde JJ, et al. Is the clean-catch midstream void procedure necessary for obtaining routine urine culture specimens from men? Am J Med 1984;76:257. (*Data suggest that the answer is no.*)
2. McNaughton Collins M, Fowler FJ Jr, Elliott DB, et al. Diagnosing and treating chronic prostatitis: do urologists use the four-glass test? Urology 2000;55:403. (*For most, the answer is no; whether they do or not does not influence the use of antibiotics.*)
3. Meares EM, Stamey T. Bacteriologic localization patterns in bacterial prostatitis and urethritis. Invest Urol 1968;5:492. (*A detailed description of the methodology and rationale for voided-bladder specimens.*)

CHAPTER 140 ■ MANAGEMENT OF URINARY TRACT INFECTION IN MEN

JOHN D. GOODSON

Roughly one in five urinary tract infections (UTIs) occur in men, and the lifetime cumulative incidence is about 15%. UTI is rare in young men, but the incidence begins to increase with age, particularly after the age of 50 years. By age 65 years, incidence in men equals that in women. In elderly debilitated patients confined to nursing homes, the prevalence may reach as high as 20% to 50%. The primary physician needs to know the clinical significance of UTI in men, what type of workup is indicated, and what modes of therapy are most efficient and effective.

PATHOPHYSIOLOGY, CLINICAL PRESENTATION, AND COURSE (1–15)

Young Men

UTI in young men usually represents urethritis or the introduction of bacteria through *instrumentation* (e.g., bladder catheterization for surgery). At times, a *congenital anomaly* of the urinary tract is responsible, although usually the presentation is at an earlier age. Dysuria, frequency, and urgency accompany most forms, with urethral discharge characteristic of urethritis. Most cases of urethritis are sexually transmitted in origin and respond well to treatment (see Chapter 136). The condition of patients with an anatomic defect does not improve unless the structural problem is alleviated. Patients who respond fully to a 7-day course of antibiotics are unlikely to have any serious underlying pathology.

In some young men, uncomplicated *cystitis* may develop because of exposure to uropathogenic strains of *Escherichia coli*. The exposure is seen among homosexual men engaging in anal intercourse and in heterosexual men having vaginal intercourse with a colonized partner. Lack of circumcision is a risk factor, as is HIV infection with a CD4 lymphocyte of less than 200/mm^3.

Middle-Aged Men

The increase in the rate of UTI that occurs in men of age 50 to 65 years parallels the increase in prostate size that occurs with hyperplasia of the gland. The enlargement leads to bladder outflow tract obstruction, and a postvoid residual begins to develop in the bladder. The reduced antibacterial activity of prostatic secretions among men in this age group may also contribute to infection risk. Infection of the prostate may serve as a nidus for recurrent UTI.

Elderly Men

With further prostatic enlargement, the *postvoid residual* and consequently the risk for infection continue to rise. The use of condom or urethral *catheters*, urinary incontinence, and history of a previous UTI are other risk factors for UTI in this age group. Asymptomatic bacteriuria may occur, especially among nursing home residents. Additional contributing factors include neurogenic bladder dysfunction (see Chapter 134) and *concomitant illness* (pneumonia is a common precipitant of UTI).

Despite the high prevalence of infection with pathogenic organisms, the vast majority of infected elderly men remain asymptomatic and seem to be at low risk for serious complications. However, the usual manifestations of serious, symptomatic UTI may be absent and replaced by such vague findings as "failure to thrive" or worsening mental status. Gram-negative sepsis from a urinary tract source can be life threatening. Debate continues as to whether bacteriuria per se increases mortality; studies controlling for comorbid conditions show no increase.

Bacteriology

In patients with infection caused by a single organism, *E. coli* accounts for about 25% of cases, other gram-negative rods

(*Proteus, Pseudomonas, Providencia*) for another 50%, and *enterococci* and *coagulase-negative staphylococci* for the remaining 25%. Patients with indwelling catheters and those with recurrent infections and multiple antibiotic exposures are likely to have unusual organisms with resistance to multiple antibiotics. Multiple organisms are found in as many as one third of infected nursing home patients.

WORKUP (1–3,16,17)

History and Physical Examination

In men, complaints of dysuria, frequency, and urgency have a predictive value of about 75% for UTI. The acute onset of hesitancy, nocturia, slow stream, and dribbling have a predictive value for UTI of about 33%. No symptoms differentiate upper from lower tract infection, with the possible exception of fever (which is rare in men with lower tract disease).

The temperature should be taken and a careful genitourinary tract examination performed. The urethral meatus is examined for erythema and discharge, the testes and epididymides for tenderness and swelling, and the prostate for enlargement, nodularity, and pain on palpation. In the patient with suspected acute prostatitis, palpation should be very gentle to avoid causing a bacteremia. The abdomen is checked for suprapubic distention and tenderness in the costovertebral angles.

Laboratory Studies

Urine Culture and Microscopic Examination

Unlike women, men require a urine culture because of the wider range of causative agents and their less predictable drug sensitivities. A diagnosis of UTI is justified on isolation of a pure culture of 10^3 colony-forming units (CFU) per milliliter of urine. The finding of a culture that grows fewer than 10^3 CFU/mL or the presence of three or more organisms (without one being predominant) is suggestive of contamination. A midstream urine sample or even an initial void sample without prior cleansing of the glans suffices for most clinical situations, even if the patient is uncircumcised. Sensitivity and specificity are greater than 97%. Initial and midstream urine samples correlate very well with bladder specimens ($r = .96$).

Both spun and unspun urine specimens should be examined. The spun sediment is examined for the presence of white blood cell casts (indicative of pyelonephritis) and pus, and a Gram's stain is performed to identify a predominant organism, if present. A Gram's stain of the unspun urine is also performed. The finding of a single organism or white blood cell per high-power field on a Gram's stain of the unspun urine has a sensitivity of 85% for UTI and a specificity of 60%, which are about the same as those of other rapid diagnostic methods.

Culturing the Incontinent Patient

Specimens from patients with an indwelling catheter can be obtained for culture by first cleansing the side port of the catheter with a povidone–iodine solution and then drawing up urine through a needle attached to a sterile syringe. A culture of urine drawn from an indwelling catheter is positive for organisms when 100 or more CFU/mL are present. Most patients with indwelling catheters have positive cultures.

A specimen from an incontinent patient can be obtained for culture without resorting to catheterization by cleansing the glans penis with povidone–iodine solution, applying a fresh *condom catheter* and drainage system, and collecting the first voided specimen in the drainage bag within 2 hours. The criterion for a positive study is the presence of more than 10^5 CFU/mL; lesser growth is considered to represent contamination.

Straight catheterization and direct bladder aspiration are alternative methods of obtaining urine for culture in incontinent patients. The former carries a slight risk of inducing a bacteremia (see Chapter 16); skill is required to perform the latter procedure.

Measurement of Renal Function

Some UTIs or their causes may compromise renal function. Blood urea nitrogen and creatinine are reasonable determinations. A white cell count usually contributes little to the diagnosis but may provide confirmatory evidence in the patient who appears toxic.

Imaging Studies

The dictum that all UTIs in men are complicated (i.e., caused by an anatomic or functional disruption of the urinary tract) has led many to obtain imaging studies when a UTI is detected in a male patient. Historically, this was usually an intravenous pyelogram (IVP), but recent studies suggest that the combination of plain film of the abdomen to detect urinary calculi and ultrasonography detects more abnormalities than an IVP. However, in the absence of suspected obstruction or refractory infection, there is little evidence to support imaging in male adults. (In bacteriuric infants and boys, the situation is different.) Although it is true that the prevalence of abnormalities on imaging studies is not negligible in men with UTI, the contribution of these findings to management is often minimal. Pending better data regarding who benefits most from imaging, many authorities recommend reserving the test for patients with recurrent infection, suspected upper tract obstruction, or pyelonephritis.

Determination of Residual Volume

In the elderly patient with recurrent UTI, assessment is often directed at identifying risk factors for recurrence. Residual volume is among the most prominent. *Straight catheterization* after voiding is a simple technique for determining residual volume. It entails a very low risk for infection if performed after the urine is sterilized. A volume of more than 50 mL is abnormal. Ultrasonography provides an estimate of residual volume, as does an IVP. Whether reduction in residual volume by treatment of bladder outlet obstruction reduces the risks and morbidity of UTI remains to be determined.

Testing for Prostate Involvement

In the setting of recurrent or relapsing UTI, there is usually some concern that the prostate may be harboring organisms. A *three-glass test*, which includes culture and Gram's stain of the expressed prostatic secretions (see Chapter 139), may provide objective evidence for prostatic infection. However, the test is expensive (several cultures are required), and its interpretation is uncertain (no gold standard test is available to provide a basis for comparison). Under most clinical circumstances of recurrent UTI, it is assumed that the prostate is involved to some degree, and treatment is initiated empirically without the need for such testing (see later discussion). However, when the results of testing for prostate infection would alter clinical decision making (e.g., as in planning prostate surgery), then the test may prove worthwhile.

Localization Studies

Differentiating upper from lower tract infection is helpful because of the implications for clinical course and treatment. Clinical findings are usually nonspecific. Instrumentation (ureteral catheterization, bladder washout) is the only proven method for making such a determination. The best test has been the response to an initial course of antibiotics.

Testing for Sexually Transmitted Disease in Young Patients

Sexually transmitted diseases may present with urethral symptoms and mimic UTI. Young patients with acute urethral symptoms, even if unaccompanied by discharge, need to be tested for chlamydial infection, which has reached epidemic proportions among adolescents and young adults. Urethral swabbing is carried out (see Chapters 125 and 136). Methods that can identify chlamydial infection from a urine sample are under development. In addition, any urethral discharge should be Gram's stained, examined for gonococci and leukocytes, and plated promptly on Thayer–Martin medium (see Chapter 137).

PRINCIPLES OF MANAGEMENT (7,14,18–20)

Symptomatic Infection

Initial Infection

Acute onset of a symptomatic UTI in a male patient should be treated. In the absence of evidence for serious renal parenchymal disease or marked obstruction, one can immediately start a course of oral antibiotics. The initial choice of agent is based on Gram's stain findings, pending culture results. If gram-negative rods are found, then one double-strength tablet of *trimethoprim/sulfamethoxazole* (TMS) twice daily usually suffices. If the organisms are gram-positive cocci, then *amoxicillin* (500 mg three times daily) represents a better choice. The initial program can be revised, if need be, after urine culture results and antibiotic sensitivities become available. As noted, urine culturing is important in men because of the wide range of organisms and drug sensitivities.

Unlike women, who respond well to single-dose and 3-day treatment regimens, men are customarily treated with a *7- to 10-day* course of antibiotics, based on the view that all male UTIs are at least partially "complicated." Hardly any data are available on abbreviated antibiotic regimens in men. If symptoms clear, no further evaluation or repeated culturing is necessary.

Refractory or Recurrent Infection

Failure to clear symptoms or quick relapse suggests persistence of the original infection. Prostatic involvement (about half of instances), obstruction, anatomic anomaly, or functional disease may be responsible, necessitating repeated urine culture and consideration of IVP, three-glass testing, and a prolonged course of therapy (6 to 12 weeks) with an antibiotic that both penetrates the prostate and is active against resistant organisms. Many authorities recommend the fluoroquinolone antibi-

otics in this setting (e.g., 400 mg of *norfloxacin* twice daily). Although they are one third more effective than TMS (which is also prescribed in this setting), the fluoroquinolones are several times more expensive.

About 65% to 90% of men are cured by a prolonged course of antibiotics. The variability in results depends on the frequency and severity of important underlying pathology. A patient with prostatitis and no postvoid residual has a reasonable chance for cure, but the person with a large postvoid residual is unlikely to derive lasting benefit until the underlying cause has been addressed. Looking for and correcting any treatable precipitants of infection (obstruction, bladder dysfunction, anatomic anomaly) is likely to be more productive than depending solely on repeated or prolonged courses of increasingly potent antibiotics.

Long-term antibiotic prophylaxis against symptomatic recurrences is sometimes prescribed (e.g., a double-strength tablet of TMS daily at bedtime). However, concerns about selecting for resistant strains, drug toxicity, and cost have limited this practice to a very small number of patients (those with frequent incapacitating episodes and those at high risk for a serious complication of infection). Because even the frail elderly have low rates of UTI complications, very few patients are treated with long-term antibiotics.

Asymptomatic Infection

Debate continues on the need to treat the debilitated elderly nursing home patient who has asymptomatic bacteriuria. The issue will remain moot so long as it continues to be virtually impossible to eradicate infection in many such patients, especially those who become incontinent and require indwelling or condom catheterization on a long-term basis. In those with an indwelling catheter for more than 30 days, infection becomes a near certainty. Antibiotics may temporarily clear the infection, but relapse within 4 weeks is the rule. Only those who become symptomatic derive benefit from a course of antibiotics. More important are regularly scheduled catheter changes, which reduce the risks of encrustation and obstruction. Although the incidence of bacteriuria is lower with use of a condom catheter, it still approaches 40%. A daily change of the collecting system apparatus helps to cut the rate of infection.

The role of antibiotic therapy is different for men with asymptomatic bacteriuria who are scheduled to undergo surgery and will require short-term urinary tract instrumentation.

Preoperative urine testing and treatment are essential to avoid the introduction of bacteria into the upper urinary tract and bloodstream. This is especially important for patients scheduled to undergo urologic surgery or surgery in which a foreign body is to be introduced. A fluoroquinolone antibiotic is a reasonable choice for antibiotic therapy under these conditions, but culture and sensitivity results are the best determinants of antibiotic choice.

INDICATIONS FOR REFERRAL AND ADMISSION

Any UTI patient who appears toxic or obstructed requires hospitalization. Urosepsis is a potentially life-threatening complication of UTI that necessitates high-dose parenteral antibiotics and prompt evaluation and treatment of the underlying precipitant. Symptoms of pyelonephritis and urosepsis in elderly patients may be vague (change in mental status, new onset of "failure to thrive"), so a high index of suspicion is warranted. The patient with recurrent symptomatic UTI who promptly relapses after a 6-week course of fluoroquinolone therapy

should be considered for urologic evaluation, as should the person with UTI in the context of declining renal function. An infectious disease consultant can also help in these difficult situations.

Annotated Bibliography

1. Breen DP, Wanerski GR. What is recommended workup for a man with a first UTI? Am Family Physician 2007;56:657. (*A succinct review of risk factors and yield of work-up based on their presence or absence and patient age.*)
2. Abarbanel J, Engelstein D, Lask D, et al. Urinary tract infection in men younger than 45 years of age: is there a need for urologic investigation? Urology 2003;62:27. (*The answer is no, for single episodes that respond promptly to therapy.*)
3. Andrews SJ, Brooks PT, Hanbury DC, et al. Ultrasonography and abdominal radiography versus intravenous urography in investigation of urinary tract infection in men: prospective incident cohort study. BMJ 2003;324:454. (*Plain abdominal film and ultrasonography detected more abnormalities than intravenous pyelogram.*)
4. Baldassarre JS, Kaye D. Special problems of urinary tract infection in the elderly. Med Clin North Am 1991;75:375. (*Includes the question of treating asymptomatic bacteriuria.*)
5. Barnes RC, Daifuku R, Roddy RE, et al. Urinary tract infection in sexually active homosexual men. Lancet 1986;1:171. (*Anal intercourse is a risk factor for cystitis.*)
6. Berger RE, Alexander ER, Monda GD, et al. *Chlamydia trachomatis* as a cause of acute idiopathic epididymitis. N Engl J Med 1978;298:301. (*Eight of 13 men younger than age 35 years had Chlamydia trachomatis infection; 8 of 10 men younger than 35 years had coliform infections.*)
7. Boscia JA, Abrutyn E, Kaye D. Asymptomatic bacteriuria in elderly persons: treat or do not treat? Ann Intern Med 1987;106:764. (*The evidence favors not treating.*)
8. Collins MM, Stafford RS, O'Leary MP, et al. Distinguishing chronic prostatitis and benign prostatic hyperplasia symptoms: results of a national survey of physician visits. Urology 1999;53:921. (*Pain is the distinguishing feature.*)
9. Krieger JN, Ross SO, Simonsen JM. Urinary tract infections in healthy university men. J Urol 1993;149:1046. (*The mean incidence was 5 in 10,000 men annually.*)
10. Lipsky BA. Prostatitis and urinary tract infection in men: what's new; what's true. Am J Med 1999;106:327. (*An authoritative review.*)
11. Lipsky BA. Urinary tract infections in men: epidemiology, pathophysiology, diagnosis, and treatment. Ann Intern Med 1989;110:138. (*The best review; 107 references.*)
12. Nordenstam GR, Brandberg CA, Oden AS, et al. Bacteriuria and mortality in an elderly population. N Engl J Med 1986;314:1152. (*There was no lowering of survival with bacteriuria was found when cancer is excluded.*)
13. Saint S, Lipsky BA. Preventing catheter-related bacteriuria: should we? can we? how? Arch Intern Med 1999;159:800. (*An evidence-based review, concluding that infection can be delayed but not prevented during long periods of catheterization.*)
14. Smith JW, Jones SR, Reed WP, et al. Recurrent urinary tract infections in men. Ann Intern Med 1979;91:544. (*Half of patients had underlying prostate infection and >70% grew Escherichia coli; most failed to respond to a standard 10-day course of therapy, regardless of whether they were symptomatic or not.*)
15. Spach DH, Stapleton AE, Stamm WE, et al. Lack of circumcision increases the risk of urinary tract infection in young men. JAMA 1992;267:679. (*An important risk factor for cystitis in young men.*)
16. Lipsky BA, Ireton RC, Fihn SD, et al. Diagnosis of bacteriuria in men: specimen collection and culture interpretation. J Infect Dis 1987;155:1341. (*The best study of the question, finding that initial and midstream specimens are equally valid and that meatal cleansing is unnecessary.*)
17. Ouslander JG, Greengold BA, Silverblatt FJ, et al. An accurate method to obtain urine from culture in men with external catheters. Arch Intern Med 1987;147:286. (*A useful method in incontinent persons that avoids catheterization.*)
18. Gupta K, Hooton TM, Stamm WE. Increasing antimicrobial resistance and the management of uncomplicated community-acquired urinary tract infections. Ann Intern Med 2001;135:41. (*Raises questions about the need to reassess empiric therapy practices.*)
19. Manges AR, Johnson JR, Foxman B, et al. Widespread distribution of urinary tract infections caused by a multidrug-resistant *Escherichia coli* clonal group. N Engl J Med 2001;345:1007. (*Clonal group A that was resistant to trimethoprim/sulfamethoxazole treatment accounted for a disproportionate number of resistant infections.*)
20. Stamm WE, Hooton TM. Management of urinary tract infections in adults. N Engl J Med 1993;329:1328. (*Includes an excellent discussion of urinary tract infections in the elderly; 60 references.*)

CHAPTER 141 ■ MANAGEMENT OF SYPHILIS AND OTHER SEXUALLY TRANSMITTED DISEASES

BENJAMIN DAVIS

SYPHILIS

In 1943, the dramatic efficacy of penicillin treatment for syphilis was established, and for the next 15 years the incidence of new cases of syphilis declined steadily to a low of about 6,500 in 1956. The incidence rate of syphilis peaked

in 1990 at 20.3 cases per 100,000. Between 1990 and 2000, the incidence of primary and secondary syphilis declined 90% to 2.1 cases per 100,000, which remains the lowest incidence rate since national reporting began in 1941. Between 2000 and 2002, the incidence of syphilis continued to fall for women but rose in men and, in particular, among men who have sex with men (MSM). Between 1999 and 2003, a well-described outbreak of syphilis among MSM in San Francisco was linked to Internet use for finding sexual partners, introducing a novel risk factor for sexually transmitted disease (STD) transmission, as well as an effective means for departments of public health to notify sexual contacts and prevent new cases. Syphilis continues disproportionately to affect non-Hispanic blacks at rates eightfold higher than for non-Hispanic whites, although these rates are continuing to decline.

Pathophysiology, Clinical Presentation, and Course (1–6)

Humans are the only natural reservoir of *Treponema pallidum*. Except for cases of transplacental transmission, virtually all cases are acquired by sexual contact with persons having active infectious lesions. *T. pallidum* readily penetrates abraded skin and intact mucous membranes to multiply locally and disseminate through the lymphatics and bloodstream.

The course of syphilis can be divided into primary, secondary, latent, and tertiary phases.

Primary Syphilis

The lesion of primary syphilis is the chancre, which occurs at the site of inoculation about 3 weeks after exposure. The chancre is usually located on the genitalia, but it can occur in the anal canal, on oral mucosa, on the hands, or in other locations. The lesion begins as a small papule that enlarges and undergoes superficial necrosis to produce an ulcer with a clean base and sharp margins. The chancre is typically painless, and patients are free of constitutional symptoms, although regional nodes may be enlarged. The chancre is teeming with spirochetes and is highly infectious. Even without therapy, the chancre heals completely in 2 to 6 weeks.

Secondary Syphilis

About 2 months after the primary infection, the features of secondary syphilis may appear. Secondary syphilis is a systemic disease. A flulike syndrome is common, as is generalized lymphadenopathy. The most characteristic feature of secondary syphilis is a generalized skin eruption. Lesions may be macular, papular, or papulosquamous but tend to be symmetric and uniform in size; typically, the palms and soles are involved. Patches and split papules often occur on the mucous membranes. Secondary syphilis can involve many other organs; clinical manifestations may include aseptic meningitis, hepatitis, nephritis, or uveitis. Patients with secondary syphilis are contagious. As in primary syphilis, the manifestations of secondary syphilis resolve spontaneously even without therapy, although up to 25% of patients exhibit a brief relapse of secondary lesions.

Latent and Tertiary Syphilis

Untreated patients without active lesions are considered to have latent syphilis. About two thirds of these patients remain entirely asymptomatic, but in the remaining one third, the lesions of tertiary syphilis develop, usually 10 to 40 years after primary infection. The major forms of tertiary syphilis include (a) *cardiovascular syphilis*, which is characterized by aneurysmal dilation of the ascending aorta and aortic insufficiency; (b) *neurosyphilis*, which may present as general paresis, with disorders of intellect and personality, or as tabes dorsalis, with ataxic gait, impaired pain and temperature sensation,

autonomic dysfunction, and hypoactive reflexes; and (c) *gummatous syphilis*, which is represented by slowly progressive, destructive granulomatous lesions of skin, bone, liver, or other organs.

Natural history studies from Oslo, Norway, and Tuskegee Alabama, indicate that clinically manifest tertiary syphilis develops in approximately one third of patients with untreated syphilis and that evidence of cardiovascular syphilis can be found in more than one half at autopsy. In the retrospective Oslo study, 10% of patients had clinically evident cardiovascular syphilis, 7% had neurosyphilis, and 16% had gummatous disease. The incidence of cardiovascular syphilis was higher and that of neurosyphilis was lower in the prospective (and unethical) Tuskegee study.

Infection of the Central Nervous System

Infection of the central nervous system may occur at any point in the natural history of untreated syphilis and may be more likely in HIV-positive patients. Even in the absence of neurologic symptoms, about 25% of patients with primary, secondary, or latent infection have cerebrospinal fluid (CSF) abnormalities (pleocytosis, elevated protein, positive Venereal Disease Research Laboratory [VDRL] test). Although it is not clear how many of these patients will ultimately be affected by symptomatic neurosyphilis, concern is warranted. Organisms have been detected from the central nervous system in 30% of patients with untreated primary and secondary disease.

Syphilis and HIV Disease

Patients with syphilis are at increased risk for other sexually transmitted diseases, including HIV infection. Moreover, patients with HIV infection are at increased risk for syphilis. Some studies find that HIV-infected patients have unusually high titers in their syphilis serology, whereas others find that seroconversion can be delayed or blunted by concomitant HIV infection, particularly in patients with symptomatic AIDS. In addition to being more common in HIV-infected persons, syphilis in these patients may be clinically atypical, unusually severe, or more difficult to treat successfully. Central nervous system syphilis may also be more likely in HIV-positive patients.

Congenital Syphilis

Congenital syphilis occurs as a result of transplacental transmission of spirochetes during the second or third trimester of pregnancy. Fetal loss is about 60%. Half of surviving infants have stigmata such as nonimmune hydrops, hepatosplenomegaly, rhinitis, and skin rash. Serious permanent consequences may develop in the absence of therapy. Congenital syphilis can be prevented by prompt treatment of maternal infection, and testing for syphilis is mandatory for all pregnant women, with or without symptoms.

Diagnosis (7)

Treponema pallidum cannot be cultured *in vitro*, but the diagnosis of syphilis can be made by direct visualization of treponemes from the chancre. This is a specialized technique that requires *dark-field* or *fluorescent microscopy* and very experienced observers. As a result, the diagnosis usually depends on clinical features and serologic testing.

The most widely used serologic tests for syphilis employ a nontreponemal antigen (lipoidal extract of mammalian tissues). Examples include the *VDRL*, *Hinton*, and *rapid plasma reagin* tests. These are excellent screening tests, but the false-positive rate is as high as 30%, often as the result of unrelated infections or inflammatory diseases that produce hyperglobulinemia. More-specific serologic tests use treponemal antigens and can distinguish true-positive from false-positive results. The most frequently used treponemal tests are the *microhemagglutination–T. pallidum test* and the *fluorescent treponemal antibody absorbed test*. The diagnosis of neurosyphilis may be difficult to establish conclusively. A positive CSF VDRL is very specific but insensitive for neurosyphilis. Often, the diagnosis is made by a combination of CSF abnormalities (>5 white blood cells/mm^3, elevated protein) with or without clinical symptoms (uveitis, hearing loss, posterior column spinal cord dysfunction) and a positive serum serology.

Some patients with primary syphilis manifest false-negative nontreponemal and treponemal test results. False negatives are most likely to occur in patients with infections of less than 30 days' duration. For persons with a suspect primary lesion, dark-field examination should be performed and serologic studies repeated in 10 to 14 days. For *HIV-infected* patients with suspect skin lesions and negative serology, skin biopsy may be necessary to rule out syphilis. The Warthin–Starry stain can be used to visualize organisms in biopsy specimens. Titers of the nontreponemal tests typically correlate with disease activity and should fall with effective therapy, usually to nonreactive. Some patients may harbor low-level nontreponemal antibodies for life, and such *serofast* reactions should not be interpreted as lack of cure.

Principles of Management and Therapeutic Recommendations (3, 5,7–13)

The results of treatment of early syphilis are excellent. *T. pallidum* is very sensitive to *penicillin*. Because the organism multiplies slowly, the goal is to attain long-lasting antibiotic levels. Recommendations include the following:

- For early syphilis (primary, secondary, early latent stages), treat with 2.4 million units of *benzathine penicillin* intramuscularly (IM) at a single session. Penicillin-allergic patients should receive 500 mg of oral *tetracycline* four times daily for 14 days or 100 mg of *doxycycline* twice daily for 14 days. Doxycycline and tetracycline are contraindicated in pregnancy.
- For syphilis of more than 1 year's duration (latent, tertiary, or unknown duration), treat with 2.4 million units of benzathine *penicillin* IM weekly for 3 weeks consecutively. Penicillin-allergic patients should receive 500 mg of oral *tetracycline* four times daily for 28 days or 100 mg of *doxycycline* twice daily for 28 days.
- Neurosyphilis should be treated with 18 to 24 million units of aqueous *penicillin* G intravenously, divided every 4 hours, for 14 days. Some experts recommend a single dose of 2.4 million units of benzathine penicillin IM at the end of intravenous therapy. After therapy, the cerebrospinal fluid should be reexamined every 6 months until findings are normal.
- HIV infection may increase the risk for neurosyphilis, but cerebrospinal fluid abnormalities are common in HIV-infected patients, and their presence is of uncertain significance. Lumbar puncture should be considered. There are no data to suggest that the treatment regimens prescribed for HIV-negative patients will be less effective in HIV-positive patients. HIV-infected patients should be monitored closely after therapy.

- Syphilis in pregnancy and neurosyphilis should always be treated with penicillin. Patients allergic to penicillin should be desensitized if necessary.
- A febrile reaction (the Jarisch–Herxheimer reaction), often with headache and myalgia, may occur within the first 24 hours after treatment of syphilis, especially early syphilis. Patients should be warned of this possibility, but treatment should not be delayed.

Immunity to syphilis is incomplete, and reinfection may occur, especially in patients treated with penicillin within 1 year of infection. Follow-up of patients is essential. Quantitative nontreponemal serologies at 3, 6, and 12 months after treatment help to determine the adequacy of therapy. HIV-infected patients should be followed more closely. Failure to sustain a fourfold decline in titers with therapy suggests treatment failure or reinfection, and examination of the cerebrospinal fluid should be considered. If lumbar puncture is not possible, retreatment with a regimen used for syphilis of more than 1 year's duration should be considered.

All cases of syphilis should be reported to the appropriate public health authorities so that appropriate case finding can be performed. Like all patients with sexually transmitted diseases, syphilis patients should be screened for other sexually transmitted infections, including HIV, chlamydial infection, and gonorrhea, and they should be counseled about safer-sex practices.

CHANCROID AND GRANULOMA INGUINALE (8)

Chancroid, which is endemic in some areas of the United States, is caused by the gram-negative bacillus *Haemophilus ducreyi*. It typically produces painful genital ulcers that are often accompanied by regional adenopathy. Azithromycin (1 g orally) or ceftriaxone (250 mg IM), both given as a single dose, are the treatments of choice.

Painless, slowly progressive genital ulcers are characteristic of granuloma inguinale, caused by the gram-negative bacterium *Calymmatobacterium granulomatis*. Double-strength *trimethoprim/sulfamethoxazole* twice daily or 100 mg of *doxycycline* twice daily, both for 21 days, is the treatment of choice. Both chancroid and granuloma inguinale are rare in temperate climates.

LYMPHOGRANULOMA VENEREUM (8)

Lymphogranuloma venereum is caused by *Chlamydia trachomatis,* serovars L1, L2, or L3, which are obligate intracellular organisms. In this disease, the primary genital lesion is a small, painless papule that heals spontaneously and often escapes notice. The major effect of the disease is on the regional lymphatics. Inguinal nodes enlarge and may suppurate to produce chronic draining sinuses. Scarring and lymphatic obstruction may result. Women and men who have sex with men may have proctocolitis, which can lead to rectal fibrosis, strictures, and fistulas. A 21-day course of doxycycline (100 mg twice daily) is the treatment of choice. An alternative is a 21-day course of erythromycin (500 mg four times daily).

OTHER SEXUALLY TRANSMITTED DISEASES

Gonorrhea

See Chapter 137.

Chlamydial Infection

See Chapters 125 and 136.

HIV Infection

See Chapters 7 and 13.

Genital Herpes

See Chapter 192.

Condylomata Acuminata

See Chapter 194.

Pubic Lice

See Chapter 195.

Annotated Bibliography

1. Centers for Disease Control and Prevention. Primary, secondary syphilis—U.S. 1981–1990. MMWR Morb Mortal Wkly Rep 1991;40:314. (*The changing epidemiology of syphilis.*)
2. Dylewski J, Duong M. The rash of secondary syphilis. CMAJ 2007;176:33-35. (*Effective teaching case with photographs.*)
3. Gourevitch MC, Selwyn PA, Davenny K, et al. Effects of HIV infection on the serologic manifestations and response to treatment of syphilis in intravenous drug users. Ann Intern Med 1993;118:350. (*HIV infection did not alter the clinical presentation or course of syphilis in this cohort.*)
4. Jackman JD. Cardiovascular syphilis. Am J Med 1989;87:425. (*A review of cardiovascular manifestations of tertiary disease.*)
5. Musher DM, Hamill RJ, Baughn RE. Effect of human immunodeficiency virus (HIV) infection on the course of syphilis and on the response to treatment. Ann Intern Med 1990;113:872. (*Intensive therapy and follow-up are recommended.*)
6. Musher DM. Syphilis, neurosyphilis, penicillin, and AIDS. J Infect Dis 1991;163:1201. (*Excellent review of the need for intensive therapy in HIV-infected patients.*)
7. Hart G. Syphilis tests in diagnostic and therapeutic decision making. Ann Intern Med 1986;104:368. (*A critical look at available diagnostic tests.*)
8. Centers for Disease Control and Prevention. Sexually transmitted disease treatment guidelines, 2002. MMWR Morb Mortal Wkly Rep 2002;51(RR-6):6. (*An authoritative and comprehensive reference.*)
9. Hook EW 3rd, Stephens J, Ennis DM. Azithromycin compared with penicillin G benzathine for treatment of incubating syphilis. Ann Intern Med 1999;131:434. (*Azithromycin in a single 1.0-g dose seemed to be effective.*)
10. Riedner G, Rusioka M, Todd J, et al. Single-dose azithromycin versus penicillin G benzathine for the treatment of early syphilis. N Engl J Med. 2005;353:1236. (*Single dose azithromycin is effective and may be particularly suited to developing countries; monitoring for resistance in the United States is important.*)
11. Romanowski B, Sutherland R, Fick GH, et al. Serologic response to treatment of infectious syphilis. Ann Intern Med 1991;114:1005. (*Therapeutic response must be based on illness episode and pretreatment rapid plasma reagin titer; seroconversion can occur after 36 months.*)
12. Walker GJA. Antibiotics for syphilis diagnosed during pregnancy (Cochrane review). In: The Cochrane library, Issue 3. Oxford: Update Software, 2004. (*Penicillin is the drug of choice, but uncertainty about the best regimen remains.*)
13. Woodward C, Fisher MA. Drug treatment of common STDs. Am Family Physician 1999;60:1387. (*First of a two-part series that succinctly reviews changes in the 1998 Centers for Disease Control recommendations.*)

CHAPTER 142 ■ MANAGEMENT OF THE PATIENT WITH CHRONIC KIDNEY DISEASE

HASAN BAZARI

Chronic kidney disease is an increasingly important clinical and public health problem that has received much recent attention, leading to new definitions and classification. During the next decade, the number of patients reaching end-stage renal disease in the United States is expected to double to more than 600,000 patients. Most patients with chronic kidney disease do not progress to end-stage renal disease but are at increased risk for cardiovascular disease and mortality. Over the last two decades, a wealth of evidence has accumulated regarding optimal management of patients with chronic kidney disease. The primary care physician plays a critical role in translating that knowledge into practice.

PATHOPHYSIOLOGY, CLINICAL PRESENTATION, AND COURSE (1–14)

Pathophysiology

Chronic kidney disease can result from a multitude of etiologies, including diabetes mellitus, hypertension, vascular disease, glomerulonephritis, obstruction, and cystic diseases, among others. However, among those who reach end-stage renal disease, diabetes mellitus and hypertension are the most common etiologies. Chronic kidney disease tends to be insidious and asymptomatic in the early stages. The clinical presentation can result from either the underlying disease or consequences of the kidney disease. In advanced stages of kidney disease, the symptoms are related to uremia.

Measurement of Renal Function

The serum creatinine is a poor marker of renal function. Creatinine production is related to muscle mass and is about 15 mg/kg per day in women and 25 mg/kg per day in men. The fraction of creatinine that is secreted by tubules varies from 10% to 50%, and this may play a more important role in patients with chronic kidney disease, leading to an overestimation of the glomerular filtration rate (GFR).

There are several ways to measure renal function:

- *Inulin clearance* remains the gold standard but is hard to implement and is generally not available for clinical use.
- Although the *24-hour urine collection for creatinine clearance* has been traditionally touted as the standard method for measuring renal function, there are inaccuracies that reduce its reliability, and its usefulness has been questioned.
- The *Cockcroft–Gault (CG) formula* adjusts the creatinine clearance level for age, weight, and gender, and was used widely until the Modification of Diet in Renal Disease (MDRD) equation was formulated. The CG formula is

$$\text{Creatine clearance} = \frac{(140 - \text{age [in years]} \times \text{weight [in kg]} \, (\times 0.85 \text{ for women})}{72 \times \text{serum creatine (in mg / dL)}}$$

The MDRD equation was derived from the MDRD study of the effect of protein restriction and blood pressure control on the progression of chronic kidney disease:

$$\text{GFR (mL/min/1.73 m}^2) = $$
$$186(P_{CR})^{-1.154}(\text{age})^{-0.203} \times 0.742 \text{ if female}$$
$$\times 1.210 \text{ if African American}$$

where P_{CR} is the plasma creatinine concentration (mg/dL), and age is in years. The MDRD equation is the most useful and most frequently recommended approach. Practical tools for its clinical application are available at http://nkdep.nih.gov/professionals/gfr_calculators/index.htm.
Newer methods of measuring renal function, such as the measurement of cystatin C, remain experimental and are not available for routine use.

Stages of Renal Failure

The National Kidney Foundation, through its Kidney Disease Outcomes Quality Initiative, offered new definitions of the stages of chronic kidney disease. Patients with stage 1 disease have intrinsic renal disease, such as autosomal-dominant polycystic kidney disease or diabetes with microalbuminuria, but do not have a decrement in GFR. The definition is also inclusive of compromised renal function without structural renal damage, as in patients with severe heart failure. Data from NHANES III (the National Health and Nutrition Examination Survey) indicate that 11% of the U.S. population, or 20 million people, have chronic kidney disease and 0.1% have kidney failure. The stages of chronic kidney disease are defined as follows:

Stage 1. Kidney damage with normal or increased GFR: GFR less than 90.
Stage 2. Kidney damage with mild decreased GFR: GFR 60 to 89.
Stage 3. Moderately decreased GFR: GFR 30 to 59.
Stage 4. Severely decreased GFR: GFR 15 to 29.
Stage 5. Kidney failure: GFR less than 15 (or dialysis).

Hypertension

Hypertension can be a cause or consequence of chronic kidney disease. Certain etiologies, such as renovascular disease and immunoglobulin A (IgA) nephropathy, can have severe hypertension as a presenting feature with headaches, palpitations, and dizziness. Hypertension in the context of chronic kidney disease can be difficult to control and may require multiple agents.

Proteinuria

Proteinuria is fundamental to the pathogenesis of many types of renal disease not only as a characteristic feature of these diseases, but also as a pathogenic mechanism in disease progression, as well as a target of therapy. In diabetes, microalbuminuria is the earliest clinical manifestation of diabetic nephropathy, usually occurring 6 to 7 years after onset of the diabetes in insulin-dependent diabetes mellitus. With time, the proteinuria becomes overt. Glomerular diseases are often characterized by heavy proteinuria, with patients not infrequently presenting with nephrotic syndrome including hypertension and edema. Other complications of nephrotic syndrome include deep venous thrombosis, pulmonary embolus, infections, and accelerated atherosclerosis from the accompanying hyperlipidemia. The degree of proteinuria often determines the rate of progression of the kidney disease but not in all renal diseases.

Fluid and Electrolyte Problems

Sodium and fluid retention generally occurs late in the course of kidney disease but can be a dominant feature with certain causes of chronic kidney disease. Two particular causes stand out. Bilateral renal artery stenosis classically presents with the triad of hypertension, fluid overload, and azotemia. The degree of azotemia may be mild compared with other causes of renal failure. Glomerulonephritis can also lead to salt and water retention with near-normal renal function. IgA nephropathy, lupus nephritis, cryoglobulinemia, and poststreptococcal glomerulonephritis can present with predominantly fluid retention without end-stage renal disease. In patients with underlying congestive heart failure, the kidney disease can exacerbate salt and water retention.

Conversely, there are diseases in which tubular dysfunction predominates and salt wasting and metabolic acidosis may be key features. Reflux with nephropathy can induce salt wasting, and these patients are prone to volume depletion.

Hyperkalemia often occurs in the terminal stages of kidney disease. However, it can also be a severe problem in patients in relatively early stages with certain etiologies. Of particular importance are patients with diabetic nephropathy, who often have hyperkalemia as a consequence of hyporeninemic hypoaldosteronism. The therapy of diabetic nephropathy involves the use of angiotensin-converting-enzyme (ACE) inhibitors or angiotensin-receptor blockers, both of which can worsen hyperkalemia.

Hypokalemia can also be a feature of early stages of chronic kidney disease. High renin states in renal artery stenosis can induce kaliuresis and hypokalemia. Renal tubular acidosis can also induce renal potassium wasting.

Metabolic acidosis can be seen both early and late in kidney disease. Early, the acidosis is usually of the non–anion-gap type and is related to decreased ammoniagenesis or an associated renal tubular acidosis; late in kidney disease it tends to be of the anion-gap type due to an inability to excrete organic acids.

Endocrine Problems

Important and traditionally underappreciated is the importance of calcium and phosphate metabolism. Phosphate retention and decreased 1-hydroxylation of vitamin D lead to *secondary hyperparathyroidism* very early in renal disease. The hyperparathyroidism helps to increase phosphate clearance by the kidney. *Vitamin D deficiency* leads to decreased absorption of calcium and phosphate. Hyperphosphatemia itself decreases the synthesis of 1,25-vitamin D. Fibroblast growth factor-23 (FGF-23) is a newly discovered phosphotonin that participates in phosphate excretion with parathyroid hormone in a shared role and also directly inhibits 1-hydoxylation in the kidney. This may explain the discrepancy between loss of renal mass and 1,25-vitamin D production. Vitamin D deficiency and hyperphosphatemia combine to produce progressive hypocalcemia. The bone disease that results from hyperparathyroidism is termed *osteitis fibrosa cystica*. Excessive suppression of parathyroid hormone can lead to low-turnover bone disease. Uncontrolled phosphate levels and high-calcium phosphate products can lead to premature vascular calcifications, vascular artery disease, and valvular *calcifications* causing aortic and mitral valvular disease.

Anemia

Anemia is an important consequence of kidney disease. The predominant cause of the anemia is erythropoietin deficiency. Other contributing factors may include decreases in red cell survival, mucosal bleeding, and decreased iron absorption, as well as bone marrow resistance to erythropoietin. Anemia can contribute to left ventricular hypertrophy in concert with uncontrolled hypertension. Left ventricular hypertrophy and anemia both contribute independently to poor prognosis in patients with chronic kidney disease.

Clinical Presentation and Course

Patients with kidney failure often present with a common symptom complex regardless of the etiology of their renal disease. Fatigue, decreased exercise tolerance, anorexia, and nausea tend to dominate symptomatology. *Pruritis* related to elevated phosphate and uremic toxins is also common. *Fluid overload* and *high-output congestive heart failure* from anemia may initially be mistaken for primary cardiac dysfunction. *Pericarditis* can present with pleuritic and positional chest

pain that can be worrisome for ischemic cardiac disease. Occasionally, this may progress to cardiac tamponade and present with hypotension, a globular heart, elevated neck veins, and a pulsus paradoxus. *Mucosal bleeding* can result from uremic *platelet dysfunction*. With the increased recognition of the need for optimal management of chronic kidney disease, most patients transition to dialysis or transplantation much earlier than in the past. Hence, it is less common to see *uremic encephalopathy*. When it does occur, presentation may include cognitive decline, confusion, asterixis, myoclonus, and seizures. *Seizures* may also occasionally result from severe *hypocalcemia*.

The rate of progression of chronic kidney disease can be predictable; the rate of decline in renal function, plotted as the inverse of serum creatinine, tends to be linear for chronic diseases such as diabetes and hypertension. On the other hand, inflammatory processes such as collagen vascular diseases are less predictable and are subject to both the intrinsic propensity of the disease in a particular patient and the influence of therapy. The slope of decline of renal function in chronic diseases can be mitigated by therapy such as blood pressure control and the use of ACE inhibitors.

PRINCIPLES OF MANAGEMENT (15–34)

The last two decades have seen a transition from observation and documentation of the natural history of disease to an era of active intervention leading to both a prolongation of renal function and improvement in quality of life for patients with chronic renal failure. Early recognition of chronic kidney disease and careful management of the complications are critical goals.

Blood Pressure Control

Blood pressure control is probably the most important therapeutic maneuver available to the primary care physician to slow the progression of chronic kidney disease, as evident in the MDRD study. Many other studies have confirmed the importance of blood pressure control. *ACE inhibitors* and, more recently, *angiotensin-receptor blockers* have been shown to slow progression of kidney failure more than would be expected from their effect on blood pressure control alone, especially among diabetics and patients with proteinuria. In patients with polycystic kidney disease, these agents confer no unique benefit beyond that conferred by their effect on blood pressure. The combined use of ACE inhibitors and angiotensin-receptor blockers is more beneficial than the use of either alone in patients with diabetic nephropathy. Challenges to the use of these agents include deterioration of renal function and hyperkalemia, which can be managed with sodium polystyrone sulfate. ACE inhibitors commonly induce cough; angioedema is both less common and more serious. Other agents that have been useful for blood pressure control in patients with chronic kidney disease include *thiazide* and *loop diuretics, beta-blockers, calcium-channel blockers*, and *alpha-blockers*. The most recent JNC 7 report (Joint National Committee on Prevention, Detection, Evaluation, and Treatment of High Blood Pressure) recommends a target blood pressure of less than 130/80 mm Hg for patients with chronic kidney disease.

Protein Restriction

Dietary protein intake has an effect on renal hemodynamics, as well as induction of proinflammatory cytokines. A diet rich in proteins can also lead to metabolic acidosis and the accumulation of uremic toxins. The MDRD study, undertaken to define the role of dietary protein restriction on the progression of chronic kidney disease, did not prove a clear benefit of dietary protein restriction. However, subgroup analysis of patients with early kidney disease showed some benefit. A meta-analysis also found some benefit from modest dietary protein restriction of 0.6 g/kg per day combined with tight blood pressure control. Care must be paid to the quality of protein intake and the avoidance of protein malnutrition, which can be an indication for initiation of dialysis. Controversy exists regarding the use of very low protein diets to defer dialysis, and many nephrologists are tending toward earlier and controlled transition to dialysis or transplantation preserving nutritional status.

Sodium and Potassium Management

Sodium restriction often is recommended as part of the blood pressure control measures for patients with chronic kidney disease. The usual recommendation is 2.5 g or 100 mmol of sodium intake per day in the diet. Tighter sodium restriction may be recommended for patients with severe congestive heart failure. Occasionally patients with salt-wasting nephropathy may be advised a normal or even high-sodium intake to maintain fluid balance. Concentrating defects are common, and, generally, fluid restriction is not required until the very late stages of kidney disease.

Potassium handling may vary and depend on the etiology of the kidney disease. Certain diseases such as diabetic nephropathy can have a predisposition to hyperkalemia, which makes their management particularly cumbersome. Drugs that predispose to worsening hyperkalemia such as ACE inhibitors and angiotensin-receptor blockers are also very useful in preventing progression of diabetic nephropathy, as well as other forms of renal disease associated with high-grade proteinuria. Potassium management starts with dietary restriction to 2 g/d. Tighter regulation of dietary intake may be difficult for many patients. Both thiazide and loop diuretics can help with blood pressure and volume management while helping with hyperkalemia as well. Treating metabolic acidosis with sodium bicarbonate has beneficial effects on serum potassium. Patients should be counseled on the dietary sources of potassium, as well as hidden sources such as salt substitutes. The effect of even over-the-counter medications such as nonsteroidal antiinflammatory drugs (NSAIDs), trimethoprim, beta-blockers, ACE inhibitors, angiotensin-receptor blockers, and potassium-sparing diuretics on serum potassium should be considered. When such drugs are initiated in patients with chronic kidney disease, the serum potassium should be repeated within 1 week and appropriate management implemented. Beyond dietary restriction, use of diuretics, and correction of acidosis, the best way to control potassium is with the use of the binding resin sodium polystyrene sulfate. The resin is a source of sodium, which may contribute to volume overload.

Calcium and Phosphorus Metabolism

The etiology of hypocalcemia in chronic kidney diseases is in part from elevated levels of phosphorus and vitamin D deficiency, leading to decreased calcium absorption. Decreased 1-hydroxylation of 25-hydroxy vitamin D occurs as a consequence of decreased renal mass and hyperphosphatemia as well as the role of the newly discovered phosphotonin FGF-23. The deficiency may be exacerbated in those with nephrotic syndrome with renal losses. Hypocalcemia leads to muscle weakness and, rarely, tetany. *Hyperphosphatemia* can cause pruritis. The secondary hyperphosphatemia leads to bone disease as a result of hyperparathyroidism, as well as eventual hypertrophy and autonomy of the parathyroid glands. Initial management of hyperphosphatemia is *dietary phosphate restriction* of 800 to 1,000 mg/d. *Calcium-based phosphate binders* have been used successfully to control hyperphosphatemia, and the use of *vitamin D supplementation* has been successful at controlling hyperparathyroidism. Both *calcium acetate* and *calcium carbonate* are effective as phosphate binders when taken with meals, but they are a source of calcium when taken between meals. The price of excessive suppression of the parathyroid hormone may be increased incidence of low-turnover bone disease and vascular calcifications as a result of high calcium phosphate product. Aluminum-based phosphate binders are generally avoided except for very short term use due the complications of aluminum toxicity, which include encephalopathy, microcytic anemia, and low-turnover bone disease with hypercalcemia. The recent addition of the non-aluminum–, non-calcium–based synthetic polymer *svelamar*, which binds dietary phosphate, has allowed for better parathyroid hormone control without incurring the risks of hypercalcemia and vascular calcification. Lanthanum carbonate is a new phosphate binder that has been approved for use. It binds dietary phosphate in the gastrointestinal tract and prevents absorption. In stage 3 and 4 disease, vitamin D levels of 25-hydroxy vitamin D should be measured rather than those of 1,25-hydroxy vitamin D, which tend to not reflect body vitamin D levels. When levels of 25-hydroxy vitamin D are less than 30 ng/mL and parathyroid hormone levels are elevated, the *administration of ergocalciferol (vitamin D_2)* monthly is recommended. Synthetic vitamin D analogues have been used in dialysis patients to suppress parathyroid hormone release without the significant effect on gastrointestinal absorption of calcium and phosphorus. The use of these agents has been extended to patients with chronic kidney disease. Calcimimetics have been used to suppress parathyroid hormone level in both patients in dialysis and patients with chronic kidney disease.

Metabolic Acidosis

The kidney normally excretes 1 mEq/kg per day of acid from the diet as a combination of ammonium and titratable acid. In the initial stages, acidosis is predominantly of the non–anion-gap type and is related to decreased ammonia synthesis. Acidosis leads to increased inflammation, catabolic state, and buffering of acid by bone, leading to calcium loss from bones. Guidelines recommend the maintenance of the serum bicarbonate greater than 22 mEq/L with supplementation using *sodium bicarbonate* at 0.5 to 1.0 mEq/kg per day.

Anemia

Patients with chronic kidney disease develop anemia as they progress through the stages of chronic kidney disease. Anemia contributes to left ventricular hypertrophy and is associated with increased risk of mortality that lasts for several years after the initiation of dialysis. Patients should be evaluated for anemia at stage 3 of chronic kidney disease, and other causes such as iron deficiency should be ruled out. Therapy with *recombinant human erythropoietin* should be initiated when the hemoglobin level is less than 11 g/dL or hematocrit is less than 33%. The target hematocrit is then 33% to 36%; iron supplementation is often required to avoid iron deficiency. The Correction of Hemoglobin and Outcomes in Renal Insufficiency trial demonstrated that a target hemoglobin level of 13.5 g/dL, when compared with a target hemoglobin of 11.3 g/dL, was associated with an increased risk of death, myocardial infarction, hospitalization for congestive heart failure and stroke as a composite primary endpoint. Erythropoietin at 50 μg/kg twice a week or the long-acting darbopoietin 0.45 μg/kg once a week can be used. Resistance to erythropoietin occurs with iron deficiency, hyperparathyroidism, aluminum toxicity, infection, and bone marrow processes such as malignancy. Rarely, pure red cell aplasia occurs as a result of antierythropoietin antibodies.

Cardiovascular Complications

Chronic kidney disease is an independent predictor of cardiovascular mortality; risk factors should be aggressively managed. *Hypertension management* should comply with the guideline of less than 130/80 mm Hg. *Volume management* with dietary salt restriction and the judicious use of diuretics help with blood pressure control and management of fluid status. *Lipid management* should be meticulous, aiming for low-density-lipoprotein levels of less than 100 mg/dL with drugs if lifestyle modifications are not successful. Anemia management has been previously discussed. Premature coronary and vascular calcifications are related to high calcium phosphate product. The current recommendations are the avoidance of calcium phosphate products greater than 55. Less traditional risk factors such as homocysteine, which tend to be elevated in patients with chronic kidney disease, may be important. Although it has yet to be proven whether therapy of hyperhomocysteinemia modifies the risk for cardiovascular disease, it may be advisable to screen and treat elevated homocysteine levels, given that therapy with *folic acid*, B_{12}, and *pyridoxine* is relatively benign.

Neuromuscular Complications

Patients with chronic kidney disease can develop neuropathy and muscular weakness. Muscular weakness is often exacerbated by hyperparathyroidism. More-global cognitive dysfunction, as well as lethargy and coma, supervenes in stages 4 and 5.

Medications Adjustment and Avoidance of Nephrotoxins

Drugs may have a variety of effects in patients with chronic kidney disease. Particularly vulnerable are the elderly, in whom the serum creatinine can underestimate the degree of renal dysfunction. Drugs can have hemodynamic effects that worsen renal dysfunction. Classic among these are the *ACE inhibitors* and *angiotensin-receptor blockers* in the setting of bilateral renovascular disease, as well as other precarious hemodynamic states. *NSAIDs* should be avoided both for their short-term hemodynamic effects and their potential long-term toxicity. *Contrast studies* are increasingly being done on outpatients with marginal renal reserve. Hydration with *sodium bicarbonate*, *acetylcysteine* use, and limitation of dye load are potential prophylactic measures that can be taken. Gadolinium exposure from its use in magnetic resonance imaging has been associated with nephrogenic systemic fibrosis. This has been associated with a "scleroderma-like" fibrosing condition of not only the skin, but also of organs such as the heart, lungs, and diaphragm. This has led to a U.S. Food and Drug Administration alert about such use. Physicians should avoid gadolinium exposure in patients with chronic kidney disease, especially those with stage 3 or higher, unless the risks, including increase in mortality, are outweighed by the potential value of the test and are discussed with the patient. Immediate dialysis has been recommended without evidence that dialysis decreases the risk. Other drugs that are not nephrotoxic deserve attention because their clearance or volume of distribution is affected by kidney disease. Examples include *digoxin*, *procainamide*, and *phenytoin*. Drugs excreted by the kidneys include *atenolol* and *lithium*. Careful drug level monitoring in the case of lithium and use of alternative drugs excreted by the liver such as metoprolol in the case of atenolol is recommended to avoid complications.

Planning for Dialysis and Transplantation

Access placement is a key component of the management of patients with stage 4 chronic kidney disease. The patient should first be educated regarding the choice among hemodialysis, chronic ambulatory peritoneal dialysis, and transplantation. Preemptive *transplantation* should be offered to those patients who are suitable candidates and have a living related donor. The choice of *peritoneal dialysis* or *hemodialysis* should be thoroughly discussed with the patient prior to placement of access. Although an arteriovenous fistula has to be placed at least 3 to 6 months prior to use, a peritoneal dialysis catheter can be placed several weeks prior to use. Access complications are the major cause of hospitalizations of patients on hemodialysis. Proper early planning and preparation can avoid morbidity and mortality in patients from access complications. This should be part of appropriate patient education about the options for dialysis. Patients should be instructed to save antecubital veins for potential fistula placement when they choose hemodialysis as a modality.

PATIENT EDUCATION AND SUPPORT (24,25)

Patients with chronic kidney disease benefit greatly from a collaborative relationship with the health care team, which should include nurses, dieticians, social workers, case managers, surgeon, psychiatrist, and nephrologists in addition to the primary care physician. To participate effectively, patients need extensive, supportive education about the complications of their illness and its treatments. Peritoneal dialysis options, as well as preemptive transplantation options, should be discussed and offered to appropriate patients. Nutrition is a key modality of treatment, and patients need access to an informed renal dietician to help optimize nutrition in the face of a variety of potential dietary restrictions. Patient support groups with educational sessions and disease management programs offer more-systematized ways to optimize the care of patients.

INDICATIONS FOR REFERRAL AND INITIATION OF DIALYSIS (28,32–34)

Referral to a Nephrologist

With the growing population of patients with chronic kidney disease, the optimal care of patients starts with the primary care physicians. Management of hypertension, anemia, calcium, phosphate, and lipids can and should start with the primary care physician often prior to referral to a nephrologists. The recommendation for referral is when the GFR is less than 30 mL/min, and even earlier referral will benefit some patients. Late referral is associated with higher mortality. Vascular access for those planning for hemodialysis should occur when the GFR is 30 mL/min or earlier.

Indications for Dialysis Initiation

The transition to dialysis in patients with chronic kidney disease should emphasize patient education, partnering of the patient with the health care profession, proper preparation of the patient for dialysis, anticipatory access placement, and a smooth transition to chronic dialysis. The classic indications for dialysis include hyperkalemia, acidosis, volume overload, uremic symptoms including gastrointestinal and neurologic manifestations, uremic platelet dysfunction with bleeding, and pericarditis. There has been a shift to also consider nutrition as a key indicator of uremic manifestations and initiating dialysis even when other indications are not present. The trend toward earlier initiation when the GFR is less than 15 mL/min for diabetics and 10 mL/min for nondiabetics is not yet supported by evidence.

MANAGEMENT RECOMMENDATIONS (28,32,34)

Protein and Calories

- Restriction of daily protein to 0.6 g/kg in patients with symptoms, acidosis, or blood urea nitrogen level greater than 75 mg/dL.
- Daily caloric intake of 40 to 50 cal/kg.

Fluids

- Fluid restriction may be appropriate in certain circumstances, such as in fluid overload and hyponatremia.
- In certain salt-wasting conditions in which there is a concentrating defect, increased fluid intake may be encouraged.

Hypertension

- Blood pressure control has to be less than 130/80 mm Hg in all patients with chronic kidney disease unless there is a contraindication such as cerebrovascular disease.
- ACE inhibitors and angiotensin-receptor blockers (ARBs) are the preferred agents for blood pressure control in patients with proteinuria.

- The combination of ACE inhibitors and ARBs should be used when there is heavy proteinuria refractory to one agent at maximum doses.
- Diuretics are often effective when combined with other agents.
- Other agents can be used, but dihydropyridine calcium-channel blockers may increase proteinuria.

Sodium

- Sodium restriction should be used for patients with hypertension, congestive heart failure, and nephrotic syndrome.
- Generally, administering 2 to 4 g of sodium restriction is advised, often in combination with diuretics.

Potassium

- Occasionally, patients with tubulointerstitial disease and renal tubular acidosis or patients on diuretics may need potassium supplementation.
- Hyperkalemia occurs in patients with hyporeninemic hypoaldosteronism, in advanced stages of chronic kidney disease, and often as a consequence of medications such as potassium-sparing diuretics, ACEIs, ARBs, NSAIDs, trimethoprim, and beta-blockers.
- Patients with chronic hyperkalemia should be instructed about a low-potassium diet, and if the potassium remains chronically elevated, sodium polystyrene sulfonate can be used with or without sorbitol to control the potassium.

Calcium and Phosphorous

- Secondary hyperparathyroidism occurs in the early stages of chronic kidney disease. Calcium, phosphorus, parathyroid hormone, and vitamin D levels should be measured.
- Phosphate should be controlled at the upper limits of normal with the use of calcium acetate/carbonate or the synthetic polymer svelamar.
- Parathyroid hormone levels should be kept under control but not less than 100 pg/mL by the use of 1,25-vitamin D or its analogues.
- Vitamin D deficiency should be corrected.
- The calcium phosphate product should be less than 55.

Metabolic Acidosis

- The serum bicarbonate should be maintained greater than 22 mEq/L.
- Sodium bicarbonate at 0.5 to 1 mEq/kg daily can be given to maintain normal acid–base status.

Anemia

- Erythropoietin should be initiated when the hemoglobin level is less than 11.
- Erythropoietin or darbopoietin can be used to maintain a hemoglobin level of 12 to 13.
- Iron deficiency should be prevented by iron supplementation orally or intravenously in refractory cases.

Vascular Access

- Arteriovenous fistulas are the best access for patients on hemodialysis, followed by an arteriovenous graft.
- Fistulas should be placed at least 3 to 6 months prior to anticipated initiation of dialysis.
- Peritoneal dialysis should be offered as an option for appropriate patients.

Dialysis

- Dialysis should be initiated when the GFR is less than 15 mL/min and there are symptoms.
- Dialysis adequacy should be monitored.
- Anemia management should be optimized.

- Metabolic control including calcium, phosphate, parathyroid hormone, vitamin D, and acid–base status should be continued.
- Nutrition should be optimized to increase protein intake with dialysis and increase dietary protein intake for losses in peritoneal dialysis.

Transplantation

- Early preemptive transplantation should be offered to patients who are candidates and have living donors.
- Patients who are candidates for transplantation should be listed for cadaveric transplant.
- Evaluation for transplantation should include a comprehensive evaluation for cardiovascular disease.

Annotated Bibliography

1. Stevens LA, Coresh J, Greene T, et al. Assessing kidney function—measured and estimated glomerular filtration rate. N Engl J Med 2006;354:2473. (*A concise, up-to-date summary of the current methods for estimating glomerular filtration rate and limitations of each method.*)
2. Levey AS, Boasch JP, Lewis JB, et al. A more accurate method to estimate glomerular filtration rate from serum creatinine: a new prediction equation. Modification of Diet in Renal Disease Study Group. Ann Intern Med 1999;130:461. (*An equation developed from the Modification of Diet in Renal Disease [MDRD] Study provided a more accurate estimate of glomerular filtration rate.*)
3. Cockcroft DW, Gault MH. Prediction of creatinine clearance from serum creatinine. Nephron 1976;16:31. (*The derivation included the relationship found between age and 24-hour creatinine excretion per kilogram in 249 patients aged 18 to 92 years.*)
4. Coresh J, Astor BC, Grave T, et al. Prevalence of chronic kidney disease and decreased kidney function in the adult US population: Third National Health and Nutrition Examination Survey. Am J Kidney Dis 2003;41:1. (*The prevalence of chronic kidney disease [CKD] in the U.S. adult population was 11%, or 19.2 million.*)
5. Fored CM, Ejerblad E, Lindblad P, et al. Acetaminophen, aspirin, and chronic renal failure. N Engl J Med 2001;345:1801. (*A population-based study, finding that chronic regular use of acetaminophen or aspirin was associated with a dose-dependent increase in the risk of clinically significant chronic renal failure in persons with underlying renal disease or systemic disease.*)
6. Keane WF, Eknoyan G. Proteinuria, albuminuria, risk assessment, detection, elimination (PARADE): a position paper of the National Kidney Foundation. Am J Kidney Dis 1999;33:1004. (*Reviews the evidence and offers guidelines from the National Kidney Foundation.*)
7. Coburn JW. An update on vitamin D as related to nephrology practice. Kidney Int 2003;(S87):S125. (*Reviews the role of vitamin D in pathophysiology and treatment, including evidence for elevated levels of calcium and phosphorus as factors contributing to vascular and cardiac calcification in patients with end-stage renal disease.*)
8. Gutierrez O, Isakova T, Rhee E, et al. Fibroblast growth factor-23 mitigates hyperphosphatemia but accentuates calcitriol deficiency in chronic kidney disease. J Am Soc Nephrol 2005;16:2205. (*A landmark study that identifies fibroblast growth factor-23 as a new and major modulator of calcium phosphate regulation in patients with CKD.*)
9. Levey AS, Coresh J, Balk E, et al. Clinical guidelines for chronic kidney disease: evaluation, classification, and stratification. Ann Intern Med 2003;139:137. (*Presents a definition and a five-stage classification system of CKD and summarizes the major recommendations on early detection in adults.*)
10. Shilipak MC, Sarnak MJ, Katz R, et al. Cystatin C and risk of death and cardiovascular events among elderly persons. N Engl J Med 2005;352:2049. (*A study confirming the association between CKD and cardiovascular mortality and highlighting cystatin C as a better marker of glomerular filtration rate.*)
11. Sarnak MJ, Levey AS. Cardiovascular disease and chronic kidney disease; a new paradigm. Am J Kidney Dis 2000;35:S117. (*Proposes that cardiovascular disease [CVD] and CKD are outcomes of the same underlying disorders, and argues that risk-factor-reduction strategies used to prevent CVD in the general population should also be applied to patients with CKD.*)
12. Go AS, Chertow GM, Fan D, et al. Chronic kidney disease and the risk of death, cardiovascular events, and hospitalization. N Engl J Med 2004;351:1296. (*A study establishing CKD as an independent risk factor for CVD.*)
13. Schwab SJ, Christensen RLI, Dougherty K, et al. Quantitating proteinuria by the use of protein-to-creatinine ratios in single urine samples. Arch Intern Med 1987;147:943. (*This simple single-voided test is reliable.*)
14. U.S. Renal Data Systems. Excerpts from the 2000 U.S. Renal Data Report: Atlas of End Stage Renal Disease in the United States. Am J Kidney Dis 2000;36:S1. (*Major epidemiologic data.*)
15. The ALLHAT Officers and Coordinators for the ALLHAT Collaborative Research Group. Major outcomes in high-risk hypertensive patients randomized to angiotensin-converting enzyme inhibitor or calcium channel clocker vs diuretic. The Antihypertensive and Lipid-Lowering Treatment to Prevent Heart Attack Trial (ALLHAT). JAMA 2002;288:2981. (*Thiazide-type diuretics were superior in preventing CVD.*)
16. Brenner BM, Cooper ME, de Zeeuw D, et al. Effect of losartan on renal and cardiovascular outcomes in patients with type 2 diabetes and nephropathy. N Engl J Med 2001;354:861. (*Losartan reduced the incidence of a doubling of the serum creatinine concentration by 25% and end-stage renal disease by 28% but had no effect on mortality; the benefit exceeded that attributable to changes in blood pressure.*)
17. Chobanian AV, Bakris GL, Black HR, et al. The seventh report of the Joint National Committee on Prevention, Detection, Evaluation, and Treatment of High Blood Pressure. The JNC 7 report. JAMA 2003;289:2560. (*Reviews evidence for blood pressure targets as well as indications for different antihypertensive agents, including angiotensin-converting-enzyme [ACE] inhibitors and angiotensin-receptor blockers.*)
18. Giatras I, Lau J, Levey AS, et al. Effect of angiotensin-converting enzyme inhibitors on the progression of nondiabetic renal disease: a meta-analysis of randomized trials. Ann Intern Med 1997;127:337. (*An analysis of randomized, controlled studies, finding ACE inhibitors to be more effective than other antihypertensives in reducing the risk for worsening renal failure.*)
19. Harris LE, Luft FC, Rudy DW, et al. Effects of multidisciplinary case management in patients with chronic renal insufficiency. Am J Med 1998;105:464. (*Intensive, multidisciplinary case management was of no measurable benefit for patients with modest degrees of renal failure.*)
20. Jafar TH, Stark PC, Schmid CH, et al. Progression of chronic kidney disease: the role of blood pressure control, proteinuria, and angiotensin-converting enzyme inhibition. Ann Intern Med 2003;139:244. (*A meta-analytic study with regression analysis identifying levels of blood pressure and protein excretion associated with the least risk of progression.*)
21. Levey AS, Beto JA, Coronado BE, et al. Controlling the epidemic of cardiovascular disease in chronic kidney disease: what do we know? What do we need to learn? Where do we go from here? National Kidney Foundation Task Force on Cardiovascular Disease. Am J Kidney Dis 1998;32:853. (*Reviews evidence and offers guidelines.*)
22. Lewis EJ, Hunsiacker LG, Bain RP, et al. The effect of angiotensin-converting-enzyme inhibitors on diabetic nephropathy. The Collaborative Study Group. N Engl J Med 1993;329:1456. (*Captopril slows deterioration in renal function in insulin-dependent diabetic nephropathy and is more effective than blood pressure control alone.*)
23. Lewis EJ, Hunsicker LG, Clarke WR, et al. Renoprotective effects of the angiotensin-receptor antagonist irbesartan in patients with nephropathy due to type 2 diabetes. N Engl J Med 2001;345:851. (*Angiotensin II–receptor blocker protected type 2 diabetics against progression of nephropathy independent of the reduction in blood pressure.*)

24. Martin KJ, Gonzalez EA, Gellens ME, et al. Therapy of secondary hyperparathyroidism with 19-nor-1alpha,25-dihydroxyvitamin D2. Am J Kidney Dis 1998;32(Suppl 2):S61. (*Reviews evidence for the effective control of hyperparathyroidism with paricalcitol therapy causing minimal perturbation of serum calcium and phosphorus levels.*)
25. Maschio G, Alberti D, Janin G, et al. Effect of the angiotensin-converting-enzyme inhibition on the progression of chronic renal insufficiency. The Angiotensin-Converting-Enzyme Inhibition in Progressive Renal Insufficiency Study Group. N Eng J Med 1996;329:1456. (*The ACE inhibitor benazepril protected against the progression of renal insufficiency in patients with various renal diseases but not in polycystic disease.*)
26. Mitch W, Remuzzi G. Diets for patients with chronic kidney disease, still worth prescribing. J Am Soc Nephrol 2004;15:234. (*Presents a well-argued and well-referenced case for dietary intervention despite the failure of the MDRD study to demonstrate that a low-protein diet slowed the progression of decline in glomerular filtration rate.*)
27. Ritz E, Orth SR. Primary care: nephropathy in patients with type 2 diabetes mellitus. N Engl J Med 1999;341:1127. (*An effective clinical review.*)
28. Standards of medical care for patients with diabetes mellitus. Diabetes Care 2002;25:213. (*Reviews evidence and offers guidelines.*)
29. Singh AK, Szezech L, Teng KL, et al. Correction of anemia with epoetin alfa in chronic kidney disease. N Engl J Med 2006;355:2085. (*One of two studies confirming increased risks of cardiovascular events and mortality with higher hemoglobin goals for patients with chronic kidney disease; this was also confirmed in other patients who were treated with the drug even in the absence of chronic kidney disease.*)
30. Block GA, Martin KJ, de Francisco, et al. Cinacalcet for secondary hyperparathyroidism in patients receiving hemodialysis. N Engl J Med 2004;350:1516. (*A large randomized, placebo-controlled study proving the efficacy of this calcimimetic for the control of parathyroid hormone level in patients on dialysis, improving the calcium phosphate product.*)
31. MacKinnon M, Shurraw S, Akbari A, et al. Combination therapy with an angiotensin receptor blocker and an ACE inhibitor in proteinuric renal disease: a systemic review of the efficacy and safety data. Am J Kidney Dis 2006;48:8. (*A study confirming the additive effect of angiotensin receptor blockers in patients already on ACE inhibitors.*)
32. K/DOQI clinical practice guidelines for chronic kidney disease; evaluation, classification and stratification. Kidney Disease Outcome Quality Initiative. Am J Kidney Dis 2002;39:S1. (*Practice guidelines generated by the National Kidney Foundation.*)
33. Ayanian JZ, Cleary PD, Weissman JS, et al. The effect of patients' preferences on racial differences in access to renal transplantation. N Engl J Med 1999;341:1661. (*Preferences differ, but not enough to explain the substantial racial differences in access to transplantation.*)
34. Kinchen KS, Sadler J, Fink N, et al. The timing of specialist evaluation in chronic kidney disease and mortality. Ann Intern Med 2002;162:2002. (*Late evaluation was associated with a greater burden and severity of comorbid disease, black ethnicity, lack of health insurance, and shorter duration of survival.*)

CHAPTER 143 ■ MANAGEMENT OF GENITOURINARY CANCERS IN MEN

Prostate cancer is the most common cancer in men in North America, Europe, and parts of Africa. Testicular cancer is the most common tumor in men between the ages of 15 and 35 years. The responsibilities of the primary physician in dealing with these male genitourinary cancers include prevention, screening for early disease when appropriate (see Chapter 126), counseling, support, and monitoring of patients with advanced disease. There has been a dramatic increase in the incidence of clinical prostate cancer in the United States. The effectiveness of therapeutic options that are strongly advocated by those specialists who deliver them remains unproven. Despite the uncertain benefits, these treatments do have negative effects on urinary function and sexual function. Treatment of advanced disease has been shown to contribute significantly to the frailty of older men. Different men respond differently to the uncertainty and tradeoffs. The primary care physician is well positioned to provide support and wise counsel about these issues.

CARCINOMA OF THE PROSTATE

Epidemiology and Risk Factors (1)

Carcinoma of the prostate has become the leading cancer in men in the United States, where incidence rose during the years after the introduction of prostate-specific antigen (PSA) screening. This was in part because of the detection of prevalence cases during the PSA era, but it may also have been due to increases in known and unknown risk factors. Risk for the individual man increases with advancing age; incidence and mortality rise sharply after age 50 years. By the ninth decade, more than 70% of men have at least microscopic evidence of prostate carcinoma at autopsy. Therefore, the aging of the population explains part of the increase in incidence. International age-standardized incidence rates vary dramatically from less than 10 per 100,000 men in parts of China and India to more than 100 per 100,000 in the United States, where African Americans face a 40% higher risk than whites. In addition to age and ethnic background, family history is an established risk factor; risk doubles among first-degree relatives. Candidate genes conferring prostate cancer susceptibility have been identified but account for a very small portion of genetic susceptibility. Evidence is mounting for possible pathogenetic roles for insulin growth factor, lycopene, zinc, selenium, and dietary fat. No association with benign prostatic hyperplasia or sexual activity has been found. Smoking, alcohol, vasectomy, and low levels of physical activity have been largely excluded as risk factors. Approximately 30,000 U.S. men die annually from the disease, making it the second-leading cause of cancer death among men in the United States. The lifetime risk for a 50-year-old man of developing clinical cancer is estimated to be 10%; the lifetime risk of dying from the cancer is 3%.

Pathophysiology, Clinical Presentation, and Course (2–9)

Most of the prostate cancers found at autopsy are incidental and have no clinical import. They are small in volume, well differentiated, diploid, and noninvasive, and they originate from the transition zone. Clinically important lesions are larger, less well differentiated, invasive, and nondiploid, and they usually originate from the peripheral zone. What converts microscopic pathology to clinically evident disease is a mystery. It is also unclear what percentage of all prostate cancers become clinically important. When clinically evident tumor arises in the *periphery* of the gland (posterior lobe or lamella), detection by digital examination is possible in many instances. However, fewer than 30% of new cases are now discovered by this means. Most patients now present with nonpalpable, asymptomatic lesions detected by PSA screening followed by prostate ultrasonography and biopsy (see Chapter 126). Other men present with nonspecific symptoms of urethral obstruction (see Chapter 134). Renal insufficiency resulting from prolonged urinary tract obstruction ensues in a small but important fraction. Another important minority of patients have bone pain or other manifestations of metastatic disease as the presenting complaint. Osteoblastic metastases predominate; they can be painful and are the major cause of morbidity. Metastasis to regional lymph nodes is common and usually asymptomatic.

Prognosis is a function of clinical stage at the time of diagnosis, PSA level, and histologic grade of the tumor. Because of the advanced age of this patient population, many men die from other conditions.

Clinical Staging and Tumor Grade (10–14)

Determining Extent of Local Disease

The clinical assessment begins with careful *palpation* of the prostate with a digital rectal examination (DRE). The urologist repeats the DRE and performs a transurethral ultrasound (TRUS) examination. Emphasis is on establishing tumor size and any spread into the surrounding soft tissue. Based on these findings, the tumor is classified as follows:

- T1 if it is microscopic and neither palpable nor visible on TRUS (T1a if the tumor is an incidental histologic finding in ≤5% or less of resected tissue; T1b if it is an incidental finding in >5% of resected tissue; and T1c if it is identified by needle biopsy for elevated PSA)
- T2 if it is palpable and appears to be confined to the gland
- T3 if it is protruding beyond the capsule or into the seminal vesicles
- T4 if it is fixed and extending well beyond the prostate

It must be kept in mind that the combination of DRE and TRUS understages many patients believed to have disease limited to the prostate. That is, a significant proportion of patients with clinical T1 and T2 tumors are found to have more extensive disease at surgery. Historically, as many as 50% of patients were found to have more extensive disease; in contemporary series that number is closer to 25%. Because the PSA concentration correlates with tumor volume, higher levels—for example, greater than 15 ng/mL (Hybritech assay)—suggest extension through the capsule or into the seminal vesicles.

Transrectal *ultrasonography* and *magnetic resonance imaging* (MRI) are often used to stage local disease, but the accuracy of such imaging studies has been disappointing. Newer adaptations of MRI are being developed and may prove better. Computed tomography (CT) is neither sensitive nor specific enough to be very useful. Recently, urologists have relied increasingly on tables and nomograms derived from predictive models to estimate the likelihood of organ confinement and the opportunity to effect cure with prostatectomy or, in the case of a nomo-

gram for low-volume/low-grade cancer, to select patients with a high likelihood of a good outcome with active surveillance rather than treatment. These models usually rely on clinical stage as just described, PSA level, and histologic grade in the form of a Gleason score (see later discussion).

Histologic Grading

Histologic grading is highly predictive of outcome. Biopsy specimens are scored using the *Gleason system* on a *scale of 2 to 10*. (Two separate areas are graded on a 1-to-5 scale, and those scores are added.) The more disrupted and undifferentiated the normal glandular architecture, the higher is the grade of tumor and the poorer is the prognosis.

Retrospective cohort studies indicate that men who have a Gleason score in the *range of 2 to 4* rarely die from prostate cancer in the ensuing 15 years, regardless of age at diagnosis. For men with a Gleason score in the *range of 8 to 10*, the prognosis is much worse, with 15-year case fatality rates of 80% or more except for the oldest men, who face a higher risk for death from other causes because of their age. Cancers with a Gleason score of 5 confer a prognosis similar to that for cancers with a Gleason score of 2 to 4. Gleason 7 scores are similar to Gleason 8 to 10. The prognosis for men with a Gleason 6 score is intermediate.

Metastatic Involvement. Clinical staging of local tumor involvement, PSA level, and Gleason score help in directing the approach to metastatic workup. If the PSA concentration is greater than 20 ng/mL (Hybritech assay), distant metastasis to bone is likely and a *bone scan* should be ordered. A PSA level of less than 10 ng/mL, or even less than 20 ng/mL, greatly reduces the likelihood of bony involvement and obviates the need for bone scan in a man with a tumor that appears to be confined to the gland, especially if the Gleason score is less than 7. *CT of the pelvis* and *abdomen* is often ordered to assess pelvic and retroperitoneal lymph node involvement noninvasively, but sensitivity and specificity are poor. A false-positive result under these circumstances confers a high cost if it eliminates a preferred treatment option. CTs should be reserved for men with high PSA levels or Gleason scores greater than 6. Pelvic lymphadenectomy is the only definitive means of establishing nodal disease, but its morbidity is substantial. It is typically performed when radical prostatectomy is being considered for cure.

Principles of Management (15–38)

The selection of a treatment modality depends heavily on clinical stage and on Gleason score. Because prostate tumors generally grow very slowly, patient age, comorbidity, and resulting life expectancy are important determinants, especially for moderately differentiated tumors.

Clinically Localized Disease

Patients with T1 and T2 tumors are candidates for curative therapy, with either radical prostatectomy or radiation therapy. The 10-year disease-specific survival rates for these patients are similar for both treatment modalities and approach 90%. Elderly patients with T1 tumors and low-grade histology need not be treated because survival is generally unaffected by the disease. Such patients do require regular follow-up that includes monitoring the PSA, checking the prostate, and inquiring about symptoms. This has been termed "watchful waiting," but is now more often referred to as "active surveillance." Other patients with early-stage disease may also elect this approach. The goal is surveillance sufficient to determine whether the disease is behaving in a way such that more active treatment is warranted, thereby avoiding treatment-related morbidity when treatment is not necessary. Patients with 10 or more years of life expectancy generally do have some risk for disease progression. The benefits and harms of curative therapy and active surveillance should be carefully considered.

Radiation Therapy. Most radiation oncologists consider radiation to be the standard of care for most men with clinically localized disease. Radiation may be delivered as *external beam radiation* or as interstitial *implant therapy*, termed *brachytherapy*. Compared with surgery, both forms of radiation confer relatively low morbidity. The risk of erectile dysfunction is lower with radiation than with surgery, although it increases with extended follow-up and may approximate the rates associated with surgery in the longer term. Incontinence is rare following radiation therapy compared with surgery. Bowel problems include temporary diarrhea, tenesmus, and possibly rectal bleeding. There is evidence that high-dose conformal radiation therapy lowers the rate of biochemical failure relative to conventional-dose conformal radiation.

Brachytherapy has become a mainstay of radiation therapy in many centers, but evidence is insufficient for valid long-term comparisons to be made with external beam radiation. The approach has real appeal for men who want to avoid the complications of other treatment options; nonetheless, all men considering brachytherapy should understand the limited evidence for this approach, especially young men at intermediate or high risk for long-term disease progression.

Radical Prostatectomy. It has been noted that most radiation oncologists consider radiation to be the standard of care for most men with clinically localized disease. Most urologists consider *radical prostatectomy* (RP) to be the standard for the same men. There is randomized trial evidence that RP can lower the risk of disease-specific and overall mortality in men with localized prostate cancer, but the effect was among men younger than age 65 years, and, for the most part, men in the study had clinically detected cancers. It is not clear that the same result is achievable in men with screening-detected cancers. Evidence from an observational cohort study that attempted to adjust for demographic variables, comorbidities, and tumor characteristics suggested a modest reduction in mortality over 12 years in elderly men. However, equally important in this study was the finding that only 2% of the patients followed died of prostate cancer, accounting for 6.8% and 8% of the deaths in the observation and treatment groups, respectively.

In general, morbidity is greater with RP than with radiation. Erectile dysfunction is a chief concern. In the Prostate Cancer Outcomes Study—a population-based study of 1,291 men who underwent RP for localized prostate cancer and were followed for 2 years—60% of men were unable to have an erection firm enough for intercourse 2 years after surgery. Advances in surgical technique have made the preservation of erectile function more likely, but so-called *nerve-sparing* procedures are not always possible and not always successful when they are possible. When impotence does occur after a nerve-sparing procedure, the neurovascular apparatus is more likely to be intact, allowing the capacity for erection with vasoactive agents (see Chapter 132). Although postoperative incontinence occurs in most patients, it clears by 5 weeks in more than 50%. However, it remains a long-term problem for a significant number of men: At 2 years in the Patient Cancer Outcomes Study, 1.6% of men reported no urinary control, and 7% and 42%

reported frequent or occasional leakage, respectively. *Laparoscopic prostatectomy* has been popularized in some centers and offers a significant decrease in perioperative morbidity. Evidence regarding any differences in long-term outcomes is not yet available.

Hormone Therapy. Increasingly, men with clinically localized disease at the time of diagnosis are being treated with hormonal manipulations aimed at decreasing circulating levels of testosterone. Androgen suppression with *gonadotropin-releasing hormone* (GnRH) agonists (e.g., *leuprolide* or *goserelin*) is the usual approach. Antiandrogens may also be used. Androgen deprivation has been used both as neoadjuvant and adjuvant therapy, more often among surgical patients at higher risk for "upstaging" and among patients undergoing radiation who are at high risk for disease progression. Other men are androgen deprived when the PSA level fails to fall or falls but then rises after surgery or radiation. There is some evidence for slowed disease progression, but the effect on survival and evidence sufficient confidently to define indications is lacking. There is also uncertainty about the benefits of early versus deferred androgen deprivation. Side effects and cost of therapy are substantial. Men suffer hot flashes and loss of libido and energy. Muscle wasting and osteoporosis are long-term consequences. Monthly injections of GnRH agonists or longer-lasting implants cost thousands of dollars annually. *Orchiectomy* is as effective as GnRH agonists and is substantially cheaper and easier. It does confer the same principal side effects. Its permanence can be viewed as either an advantage or a disadvantage.

Clinically Advanced Disease (31–38)

The optimal evidence-based approach to *locally advanced* (T3) disease is yet to be defined. External beam radiation may be useful for the local control of tumor but often fails to sterilize pelvic nodes, which are highly likely to be involved by tumor. Surgery fails for similar reasons. *Androgen-deprivation therapy* as described earlier is generally a central component of treatment despite its side effects. There is, however, mounting evidence that androgen deprivation contributes significantly to the progression of frailty in older men. Bone loss can be reduced and improved with once-weekly alendronate.

The mainstay of treatment for *symptomatic* metastatic disease is also androgen deprivation. Indications for androgen deprivation in the asymptomatic patient with metastatic disease are more controversial. Prostate cancers contain both hormone-dependent and hormone-sensitive cells and hormone-independent cells. Hormone-dependent cells die a programmed death in the absence of testosterone. Hormone-sensitive cells stop dividing, but hormone-independent cells continue to grow. As a result, although metastatic prostate cancer can be temporarily halted by androgen-deprivation therapy, such remissions are always temporary. Hormonal manipulation can achieve palliation in the symptomatic patient. Among asymptomatic patients, it is not clear whether hormonal manipulation should be used early in an effort to delay progression or be kept in reserve for later use.

As noted, *orchiectomy* is the time-honored standard for hormonal manipulation in prostate cancer. It can be performed easily in the outpatient setting and reduces total body androgen production by 95%. Adrenal androgen production persists.

The estrogen *diethylstilbestrol* has also been used for decades to achieve a "chemical castration." It inhibits luteinizing hormone secretion and competitively blocks circulating androgens. Doses of 3 mg daily halt testosterone production but are associated with an increased risk for thromboembolic disease. The thromboembolic risk is reduced with lower doses (e.g., 1 mg daily) and aspirin therapy, but lower doses do not suppress testosterone secretion as well. Gynecomastia is another side effect, which can be prevented by prophylactic low-dose irradiation of breast tissue. The effect is comparable to that of orchiectomy in inducing tumor regression. The combination of orchiectomy plus estrogen is no better than each used alone. Moreover, patients failing to respond to orchiectomy are unlikely to benefit from estrogen.

Because of the perception that men are negatively affected by orchiectomy, *GnRH agonists* are now used most often to achieve androgen deprivation. *Antiandrogens* block the effects of testosterone at the receptor level, which makes them useful for countering adrenal androgen secretion and the surge that accompanies early GnRH-agonist therapy. They may be steroidal (e.g., *megestrol acetate*) or nonsteroidal (e.g., *flutamide, bicalutamide, nilutamide*). These drugs cannot be used as monotherapy because they induce an increase in luteinizing hormone release that eventually stimulates sufficient testosterone secretion to overcome their blocking effect. Side effects include gynecomastia and diarrhea; chemical hepatitis sometimes develops. Although they do not induce a hypercoagulable state or gynecomastia, they do cause impotence.

Combined androgen blockade generally refers to the use of a GnRH agonist and an antiandrogen to block the effects of both testicular and adrenal androgens. The approach has been studied extensively with conflicting results. The weight of evidence suggests only a very small effect on overall survival.

Secondary hormonal therapy refers to the use of alternative agents after initial hormonal monotherapy fails. Antiandrogens such as flutamide are sometimes used. Responses occur in roughly 20% of patients and generally last an average of 6 months. Hydrocortisone, aminoglutethimide, and ketoconazole have all been used to suppress adrenal androgen production. Under investigation are the *5α-reductase inhibitors* (e.g., finasteride), which block the peripheral conversion of testosterone to its more active metabolite dihydroxytestosterone.

Much can be done to make the patient with advanced disease comfortable. In addition to the palliative measures mentioned earlier, the use of adequate analgesia (see Chapter 91) should not be overlooked.

External beam radiation is an effective means of palliation for patients with bone pain. It can prevent fracture and is used in cases of impending spinal cord compression (see Chapter 92).

Chemotherapy has been disappointing, with no agent altering survival to a significant extent. Response rates are somewhat less than 20%.

Monitoring Disease (9,15,16)

The serum *PSA* determination is used to monitor disease activity, including response to therapy. The 48-hour half-life of PSA allows it to reflect changes in tumor activity and mass quickly. The serum concentration correlates with tumor burden. Although prostatic procedures may transiently elevate the PSA level, it quickly returns to baseline, so interpretation is usually unaffected by recent examinations or procedures.

Although the *bone scan* is sensitive for the detection of bony involvement, its findings are not specific. Areas of increased uptake may reflect repair as much as damage. Thus, the test may provide confusing information when used to monitor response to therapy. It is best reserved for the initial evaluation or when bone pain of unclear significance arises.

For the asymptomatic patient not currently receiving therapy, regular inquiry into the development of *symptoms* has proved to be an economical yet effective means of monitoring. The routine repetition of blood tests and radiographic studies can become expensive and should be considered only when the result will substantively alter clinical decision making. PSA measurement after surgery or radiation therapy has become routine. Even here, however, it is worth carefully considering whether the results will affect treatment decisions or eventual outcomes. Many men express great anxiety about such routine measurement of PSA.

Patient Education and Indications for Referral and Admission (39,40)

The primary physician plays a central role in helping the patient to make informed decisions that reflect his values. For the patient with curable disease, the choice will be between radiation and radical prostatectomy. Risks of impotence, incontinence, and recurrence need to be reviewed. For the person with early metastatic disease, the issue of initiating total androgen blockade and the decision of whether to undergo orchiectomy or commit to treatment with GnRH agonists need to be faced. These difficult decisions require consultative help, but the patient will often return to the primary physician for discussion, which requires the physician to keep abreast of the options in the treatment of prostate cancer.

Referral to the urologist is indicated at the time a prostate cancer is first suspected. Careful planning of the evaluation is necessary, and a tissue sample will be needed (see Chapter 126). When curable disease is suspected, referrals to the urologist and radiation oncologist are indicated to help in choosing the optimal approach. When metastatic disease is encountered, an oncology consultation may facilitate the design of antiandrogen therapy. Urgent hospital admission is indicated if spinal cord compression is deemed imminent (see Chapter 92).

TESTICULAR CANCER

Testicular cancer is the most common malignancy in men between the ages of 15 and 35 years and is a major cause of death in this age group. Incidence has increased in recent years, with 8,000 cases per year occurring in the United States. Its seriousness and curability, both in early stages and in advanced stages, make it an important disease for the primary physician to know well. One needs to encourage self-examination, screen young men during routine checkups (see Chapter 131), and help to guide the patient with advanced disease through his illness.

Pathophysiology, Clinical Presentation, and Course (41-45)

Known predisposing factors are testicular atrophy (secondary to an undescended testicle) and Klinefelter's syndrome. Suspected risk factors include natural exposure to intrapartum estrogens, exposure to insecticides, and a prior history of a testicular tumor. Trauma is not a known precipitant.

Almost all testicular cancers are germ-cell tumors. *Seminomas* account for 40% to 50%. Most are confined to the testicle at the time of presentation. The remaining types are termed *nonseminomatous germ-cell tumors* (NSGCTs). These include *teratomas, choriocarcinomas, embryonal cell carcinomas,* and *endodermal sinus tumors*. Many are of mixed cell type. Their metastases may be less differentiated than the primary types.

Both groups commonly present as solid, painless, nontransilluminating testicular masses in young men (see Chapter 131). Some patients describe "heaviness" in the scrotum. Pain is less common. These tumors grow rapidly and spread by the lymphatics and the blood. Local extension to the epididymis occurs in 10% of cases. Occasionally, the tumor is occult at the primary site, with metastases already established. If chorionic gonadotropin is secreted (as may occur with several of the NSGCTs), gynecomastia may be an initial complaint. Disease already established in the lung may present with cough or hemoptysis.

Diagnosis and Staging (46–50)

Any solid, nontransilluminating, painless testicular mass in a young man should be presumed to represent a primary testicular cancer until proven otherwise. *Testicular ultrasonography* should be performed to obtain a more definitive determination of the location of the lesion. If it is testicular, prompt urologic consultation is required for the consideration of surgical removal of the involved testicle. Testicles with suspect lesions are subjected to *orchiectomy* through an inguinal canal approach to minimize the risk for seeding the scrotum, as might occur with a transscrotal operative procedure. If the lesion is extratesticular, urologic consultation is less urgent but still advisable. Surgical removal is less likely.

Staging Procedures and Surveillance

Staging begins with *orchiectomy* findings and proceeds to *chest radiography* and *chest CT* for metastatic disease of the chest and to *abdominal CT* for assessment of retroperitoneal lymph nodes. Circulating tumor markers also provide a means of detecting occult disease. The beta subunit of *human chorionic gonadotropin* (HCG) is always elevated in choriocarcinoma and in about half of the other NSGCTs (it is rarely elevated in pure seminoma, but a number of seminomatous cases have mixed disease and elevated HCG). *α-Fetoprotein* is produced by about 80% of patients with embryonal cell cancer. Both markers also provide an excellent means of monitoring response to therapy (see later discussion). Lactic dehydrogenase is sometimes elevated in germ-cell tumors.

False-positive rates are low for abdominal CT, but false-negative rates are as high as 30%, with the poorest results in thin persons. Previously, if no evidence of metastatic disease was found by staging studies, then an *ipsilateral complete lymphadenectomy* and a *contralateral partial lymphadenectomy* to the level of the aortic bifurcation were considered mandatory, especially for NSGCT, because of the high incidence of microscopic nodal involvement. However, lymphadenectomy is now being used less often because advances in chemotherapy have made it possible to achieve high rates of cure even if the diagnosis of metastasis is delayed. Moreover, lymph node dissection involves extensive surgery, with an attendant risk for ejaculatory failure. Finally, retroperitoneal lymph node dissection is unnecessary if the primary cancer is a seminoma and a course of radiation therapy to the nodes (which is highly curative) is being planned. *Lymphangiography* is sometimes useful in patients with seminomatous tumors whose CT results are negative. Abnormal paraaortic nodes are detected in 13% to 22% of cases.

The decision of whether to proceed with nodal dissection or opt for close surveillance with measurement of tumor markers and repeated CT is a judgment call. Factors associated with an increased risk for relapse and thus favoring node dissection include a high percentage of embryonal cell carcinoma in the primary tumor, a marked degree of local disease, and the presence of vascular or lymphatic invasion. If surveillance is elected after orchiectomy, it must be done rigorously, with monthly monitoring of tumor markers, repeat CT scanning every 2 to 3 months, and periodic physical examination. Noninvasive staging may be followed by chemotherapy, with secondary surgical exploration to evaluate the retroperitoneum after treatment.

Clinical Stages

A number of staging systems are used, with one set for seminomatous disease and another for nonseminomatous disease. Common designations are stage I or stage A for disease confined to the testis, stage II or stage B for spread to regional nodes, and stage III or stage C for spread beyond retroperitoneal nodes. Within each stage are subcategories denoting the degree of tumor burden.

Management (51–56)

Treatment decisions are based on stage, histology, and levels of tumor markers.

Seminomatous Tumors

Stage I disease is treated with inguinal *orchiectomy*, which is followed by adjuvant retroperitoneal node *irradiation* in most centers, although some now consider surveillance an option. The cure rate is close to 100%. Patients who relapse are candidates for combination chemotherapy, which is extremely effective (see later discussion). Patients with *stage IIA* disease are also treated with retroperitoneal radiation, but they no longer undergo prophylactic mediastinal irradiation because of its associated morbidity and the success of chemotherapy in treating relapses. Cure rates are still close to 100% at this stage. Patients with stage IIB and stage III disease are treated with *cisplatin-based chemotherapy*. Cure rates are greater than 90%.

Nonseminomatous Tumors

Stages I and IIA NSGCT disease are treated with *surgery only*. Surgical cure rates average 95% when lymph node dissection shows no regional disease. Even when retroperitoneal disease is detected, lymphadenectomy is likely to suffice for treatment as long as nodes are less than 3 cm in diameter. Patients with stage IIB disease have a high probability of relapse and thus are candidates for chemotherapy, as are patients with stage III disease.

Cisplatin-Based Chemotherapy

Multiple-agent chemotherapy based on cisplatin represented an important breakthrough in the treatment of testicular cancer. Even patients with distant metastatic disease now have a high probability of cure. The need for maintenance therapy has been eliminated. Even the severe nausea and vomiting associated with the use of cisplatin have become much less problematic with the advent of *ondansetron*, a serotonin receptor blocking agent capable of reducing cisplatin-induced emesis. Cisplatin-induced renal toxicity is preventable with good hydration.

Monitoring

Close monitoring of the response to therapy is essential. *HCG and α-fetoprotein* levels are used to detect subclinical relapse and failure to respond to treatment. An elevated serum marker level failing to decline with therapy suggests resistance to therapy. Its rise during follow-up indicates relapse. Patients having isolated elevations in tumor markers as the sole manifestation of relapse have nearly a 100% chance of cure when treated promptly with chemotherapy. In patients with advanced disease, a decline in HCG after initial chemotherapy is an excellent predictor of response to treatment. *Periodic physical examination* to check for the development of palpable adenopathy or an abdominal mass and chest and abdominal CT are additional components of the monitoring and surveillance processes (see prior discussion).

Patient Education

Although most of the details of care are related by the oncologist, the primary physician is often consulted by the patient and needs to be familiar with some of the basic questions regarding prognosis, treatment options, and side effects. Poor patient knowledge has been documented and contributes to delays in diagnosis, as well as overly pessimistic concerns about prognosis among many patients, who are greatly relieved to know the favorable prognosis for testicular cancer, especially those with metastatic disease. Nonetheless, treatment is not without its adverse effects. Lymph node exploration is an extensive procedure and thus not without considerable morbidity. Retrograde ejaculation and subsequent infertility are still associated risks, although they have been reduced to about 12%. The ability to achieve an erection is only rarely compromised. Radiation therapy is associated with a risk for decreased spermatogenesis in the remaining normal testicle, although shielding methods have reduced the radiation exposure and, consequently, the period of infertility associated with low sperm counts. The fear of chemotherapy can be lessened by reassurance that there are effective means of minimizing its adverse effects. If the risk of infertility is greater than 5%, sperm banking should be considered before treatment. A pretreatment sperm count may help in decision making.

A.G.M.

Annotated Bibliography

Prostate Cancer

1. Gronberg H. Prostate cancer epidemiology. Lancet 2003;361:859. (*A concise review of epidemiology and risk factors.*)
2. Albertsen PC, Hanley JA, Fine J. 20-year outcomes following conservative management of clinically localized prostate cancer. JAMA 2005;293:2095. (*Provides 20-year outcomes for men of different ages with tumors of different histologic types managed conservatively in the pre–prostate-specific antigen era.*)
3. Gittes RF. Carcinoma of the prostate. N Engl J Med 1991;34:236. (*A comprehensive review, with especially helpful discussions of staging and treatment; 150 references.*)
4. Chodak GW, Thisted RA, Gerber GS, et al. Results of conservative management of clinically localized prostate cancer. N Engl J Med 1994;330:242. (*A pooled analysis of data from >800 cases, favoring initial conservative therapy in older patients with low-grade histology.*)
5. Garnick MB, Fair WR. Prostate cancer: emerging concepts. Ann Intern Med 1996;125:118, 205. (*A comprehensive two-part review.*)
6. Johansson JE, Adami HO, Andersson SO, et al. High 10-year survival rate in patients with early, untreated prostatic cancer. JAMA 1992;267:2191. (*Watchful waiting is appropriate for those with stage A1 disease who are elderly.*)
7. Johansson JE, Holmberg L, Johansson S, et al. Fifteen-year survival in prostate cancer: a prospective, population-based study in Sweden. JAMA 1997;277:467. (*Of 642 conservatively treated men with well, moderately, and poorly differentiated disease, 6%, 17%, and 56%, respectively, died of prostate cancer during 15 years.*)
8. Johansson JE, Andren O, Andersson SO, et al. Natural history of early, localized prostate cancer. JAMA 2004;291:2713. (*Prostate cancer mortality increased from 15 per 1,000 person-years during the first 15 years to 44 per 1,000 person-years beyond 15 years of follow-up.*)
9. Stephenson AJ, Shariat SF, Zelefsky MJ, et al. Salvage radiotherapy for recurrent prostate cancer after radical prostatectomy. JAMA 2004;291:1325. (*Gleason score, preradiotherapy PSA level, surgical margins, PSA doubling time, and seminal vesicle invasion are prognostic variables for a durable response to salvage radiotherapy.*)
10. Abuzallouf S, Dayes I, Lukka H. Baseline staging of newly diagnosed prostate cancer: a summary of the literature. J Urol 2004;171:2122. (*Bone scan detected metastases in 2.3%, 5.3%, and 16.2% of patients with PSA levels of <10, 10.1 to 19.9, and 20 to 49.9 ng/mL, respectively.*)
11. Harisinghani MG, Barentsz J, Hahn PF, et al. Noninvasive detection of clinically occult lymph-node metastases in prostate cancer. N Engl J Med 2003;348:2491. (*High-resolution magnetic resonance imaging [MRI] with magnetic nanoparticles allowed the detection of otherwise undetectable lymph-node metastases in patients with prostate cancer.*)
12. Kane CJ, Amling CL, Johnstone PA, et al. Limited value of bone scintigraphy and computed tomography in assessing biochemical failure after radical prostatectomy. Urology 2003;61:607. (*Patients with biochemical recurrence after radical prostatectomy had a low probability of a positive bone scan [9.4%] or a positive computed tomography [CT] scan [14.0%] within 3 years of biochemical recurrence.*)
13. Miller DC, Hafez KS, Stewart A, et al. Prostate carcinoma presentation, diagnosis, and staging: an update from the National Cancer Data Base. Cancer 2003;98:1169. (*Compared with symptomatic patients, asymptomatic patients were more likely to have localized disease [84.6% vs. 78.2%] and well- or moderately differentiated tumors [82.2% vs. 74.6%].*)
14. Nakanishi H, Wang X, Ochiai A, et al. A nomogram for predicting low-volume/low-grade prostate cancer. Cancer 2007;110:2441. (*Presents a nomogram to predict low-volume, low-grade cancer in men with one positive core in an extended biopsy scheme for use in selecting men for active surveillance.*)
15. D'Amico AV, Whittington R, Malkowicz B, et al. Biochemical outcome after radical prostatectomy, external beam radiation therapy, or interstitial radiation therapy for localized prostate cancer. JAMA 1998;280:969. (*No difference was seen in PSA failure during 5 years for low-risk patients, but brachytherapy patients did not do as well as others if the risk was moderate or high.*)
16. D'Amico AV, Schultz D, Loffredo M, et al. Biochemical outcome following external beam radiation therapy with or without androgen suppression therapy for clinically localized prostate cancer. JAMA 2000;284:1280. (*The relative risk [RR] of PSA failure in low-risk patients treated with radiation therapy [RT] plus androgen suppression therapy [AST] was 0.5 compared with RT alone; the RRs of PSA failure in intermediate-risk and high-risk patients treated with RT plus AST compared with RT alone were 0.2 and 0.4, respectively.*)
17. Fowler FJ Jr, McNaughton Collins M, Albertsen PC, et al. Comparison of recommendations by urologists and radiation oncologists for treatment of clinically localized prostate cancer. JAMA 2000;283:3217. (*Urologists and radiation oncologists overwhelmingly recommend the therapy that they themselves deliver.*)
18. Gerber GS, Thisted RA, Scardino PT, et al. Results of radical prostatectomy in men with clinically localized prostate cancer. Multi-institutional pooled analysis. JAMA 1996;276:615. (*Ten-year disease-specific survival rates were 94%, 80%, and 77% for grades 1, 2, and 3 tumors, respectively.*)
19. Holmberg L, Bill-Axelson A, Helgesen F, et al. A randomized trial comparing radical prostatectomy with watchful waiting in early prostate cancer. N Engl J Med 2002;347:781. (*Radical prostatectomy significantly reduced disease-specific mortality, but there was no significant difference between surgery and watchful waiting in terms of overall survival.*)
20. Bill-Axelson A, Holmberg L, Ruutu M, et al. Radical prostatectomy versus watchful waiting in early prostate cancer. N Engl J Med 2005;352:1977. (*Radical prostatectomy reduced disease-specific mortality, overall mortality, and the risks of metastasis and local progression; the absolute reduction in the risk of death after 10 years was small, but the reductions in the risks of metastasis and local tumor progression were substantial.*)

21. Wong Y, Mitra N, Hudes G, et al. Survival associated with treatment vs observation of localized prostate cancer in elderly men. JAMA 2006;296:2683. (*An observational study, finding that there was a 30% relative mortality reduction over 12 years, but that only 2% of the patients died of prostate cancer.*)

22. Aeitman AL, DeSilvio ML, Slater JD, et al. Comparison of conventional-dose vs high-dose conformal radiation therapy in clinically localized adenocarcinoma of the prostate. A randomized controlled trial. JAMA 2005;294:1233. (*There was a lower risk of biochemical failure if patients received high-dose rather than conventional-dose conformal radiation; this advantage was achieved without any associated increase in Radiation Therapy Oncology Group grade 3 acute or late urinary or rectal morbidity.*)

23. Pisansky TM. External-beam radiotherapy for localized prostate cancer. N Engl J Med 2006;355:1583. (*An excellent review.*)

24. Kawakami J, Cowan JE, Elkin EP, et al. Androgen-deprivation therapy as primary treatment for localized prostate cancer. Data from cancer of the prostate strategic urologic research endeavor (CaPSURE). Cancer 2006;106:1708. (*The effect of primary androgen-deprivation therapy on quality of life needs to be compared with standard therapy, and its long-term durability should be assessed better in patients with prostate cancer.*)

25. D'Amico AV, Chen MH, Renshaw AA, et al. Androgen suppression and radiation vs radiation alone for prostate cancer: a randomized trial. JAMA 2008;299:289. (*The addition of 6 months of AST to RT resulted in increased overall survival in men with localized but unfavorable-risk prostate cancer.*)

26. Thompson IM Jr, Tangen CM, Paradelo J, et al. Adjuvant radiotherapy for pathologically advanced prostate cancer. A randomized clinical trial. JAMA 2006;296:2329. (*Adjuvant radiotherapy resulted in significantly reduced risk of PSA relapse and disease recurrence, although the improvements in metastasis-free survival and overall survival were not statistically significant.*)

27. Jhaveri FM, Zippe CD, Klein EA, et al. Biochemical failure does not predict overall survival after radical prostatectomy for localized prostate cancer: 10-year results. Urology 1999;54:884. (*At 10 years, patients with a PSA recurrence after radical prostatectomy for localized disease had an excellent overall survival that was equivalent to those without a detectable PSA.*)

28. Litwin MS, Sadetsky N, Pasta DJ, et al. Bowel function and bother after treatment for early stage prostate cancer: a longitudinal quality of life analysis from CaPSURE. J Urol 2004;172:515. (*Bowel function and bother are worse after external beam radiation but are also impaired after brachytherapy; transient impairment occurs after surgery.*)

29. Stanford JL, Feng Z, Hamilton AS, et al. Urinary and sexual function after radical prostatectomy for clinically localized prostate cancer: the Prostate Cancer Outcomes Study. JAMA 2000;283:354. (*At ≥18 months after radical prostatectomy, 8.4% of men were incontinent, and 59.9% were impotent.*)

30. Steineck G, Helgessen F, Adolfsson J, et al. Quality of life after radical prostatectomy or watchful waiting. N Engl J Med 2002;347:790. (*Erectile dysfunction [80% vs. 45%] and urinary leakage [49% vs. 21%] were more common after radical prostatectomy, whereas urinary obstruction [e.g., 28% vs. 44% for weak urinary stream] was less common.*)

31. Bolla M, Gonzalez D, Warde P, et al. Improved survival in patients with locally advanced prostate cancer treated with radiotherapy and goserelin. N Engl J Med 1997;337:295. (*Five-year overall survival was 79% with goserelin and 62% without it.*)

32. Crawford ED, Eisenberger MA, McLeod DG, et al. A controlled trial of leuprolide with and without flutamide in prostatic carcinoma. N Engl J Med 1989;321:419. (*Combination therapy was superior to monotherapy in patients with advanced disease.*)

33. Eisenberger MA, Blumenstein BA, Crawford ED, et al. Bilateral orchiectomy with or without flutamide for metastatic prostate cancer. N Engl J Med 1998;339:1036. (*The group that initially showed a benefit from long-term combination therapy, in the form of flutamide plus leuprolide, finds no additional benefit from the long-term administration of flutamide.*)

34. Loblaw DA, Mendelson DS, Talcott JA, et al. American Society of Clinical Oncology recommendations for the initial hormonal management of androgen-sensitive metastatic, recurrent, or progressive prostate cancer. J Clin Oncol 2004;22:2927. (*Reviews evidence for monotherapy and combined therapy and recommends a discussion about the pros and cons of early versus deferred androgen-deprivation therapy with the patient.*)

35. Nair B, Wilt T, MacDonald R, et al. Early versus deferred androgen suppression in the treatment of advanced prostatic cancer (Cochrane review). In: The Cochrane library, Issue 3. Oxford: Update Software, 2004. (*Limited information suggests that early androgen suppression for the treatment of advanced prostate cancer slows disease progression and reduces complications due to progression; see http://www.cochrane.org for updates.*)

36. Walsh PC, Deweese TL, Eisenberger MA. A structured debate: immediate versus deferred androgen suppression in prostate cancer—evidence for deferred treatment. J Urol 2001;166:508. (*Recommends delayed treatment in men with biochemical relapse after surgery or radiotherapy or participation in trials.*)

37. Bylow K, Mohile SG, Stadler WM, et al. Does androgen-deprivation therapy accelerate the development of frailty in older men with prostate cancer? A conceptual review. Cancer 2007;110:2604. (*The evidence indicates that androgen-deprivation therapy may accelerate the development of frailty in vulnerable older men with prostate cancer.*)

38. Greenspan SL, Nelson JB, Trump DL, et al. Effect of once-weekly oral alendronate on bone loss in men receiving androgen deprivation therapy for prostate cancer. A randomized trial. Ann Intern Med 2007;146:416. (*Bone loss that occurred with androgen-deprivation therapy was prevented and improved with once-weekly oral alendronate.*)

39. McCammon KA, Kolm P, Main B, et al. Comparative quality-of-life analysis after radical prostatectomy or external beam radiation for localized prostate cancer. Urology 1999;54:509. (*Physicians' estimates of urinary incontinence were more favorable than patients' estimates.*)

40. Litwin MS, Flanders SC, Pasta DJ, et al. Sexual function and bother after radical prostatectomy or radiation for prostate cancer: multivariate quality-of-life analysis CaPSURE. Urology 1999;54:503. (*Sexual function improved somewhat during the first year after either therapy.*)

Testicular Cancer

41. Bosl GJ, Motzer RJ. Testicular germ-cell cancer. N Engl J Med 1997;337:242. (*Excellent comprehensive review.*)

42. Huyghe E, Matsuda T, Thonneau P. Increasing incidence of testicular cancer worldwide: a review. J Urol 2003;170:5. (*There are wide international differences, but incidence has been increasing over the last 30 years in industrialized countries.*)

43. Moller H, Skakkebaek NE. Risk of testicular cancer in subfertile men: case-control study. BMJ 1999;318:559. (*In men who before the diagnosis of testicular cancer had a lower number of children than expected on the basis of their age, the relative risk was 1.98.*)

44. Nichols CR. Testicular cancer. Curr Probl Cancer 1998;22:187. (*A detailed, comprehensive review of all aspects.*)

45. Warde P, Jewett MA. Surveillance for stage I testicular seminoma. Is it a good option? Urol Clin North Am 1998;25:425. (*Presents the pros and cons of alternative approaches.*)

46. Lange PH, McIntire R, Waldmann TA, et al. Serum alpha-fetoprotein and human chorionic gonadotropin in the diagnosis and management of nonseminomatous germ-cell testicular cancer. N Engl J Med 1976;295:1237. (*The original report of the utility of these tumor markers in staging and monitoring.*)

47. Marks LB, Walker TG, Shipley WU, et al. The role of lymphangiography in staging testicular seminoma. Urology 1991;38:264. (*Yield is about 15% in patients with negative findings on CT.*)

48. Moul JW. Timely diagnosis of testicular cancer. Urol Clin North Am 2007;34:109. (*A thoughtful analytic review, documenting knowledge gaps among at-risk men.*)

49. McLeod DG, Weiss RB, Stablein DM, et al. Staging relationships and outcome in early-stage testicular cancer. J Urol 1991;146:1178. (*Excellent outcomes were achieved; 5-year survival was >90%.*)

50. Picozzi VJ, Freiha FS, Hannigan JF, et al. Prognostic significance of a decline in serum human chorionic gonadotropin levels after initial chemotherapy for advanced germ-cell carcinoma. Ann Intern Med 1984;100:183. (*A reduction in level was very predictive of an excellent long-term response to therapy.*)

51. Cubeddu LX, Hoffmann IS, Fuenmayor NT, et al. Efficacy of ondansetron (GR 38032F) and the role of serotonin in cisplatin-induced nausea and vomiting. N Engl J Med 1990;322:810. (*The use of this agent helps considerably.*)

52. Donohue JP, Foster RS, Rowland RG, et al. Nerve-sparing retroperitoneal lymphadenectomy with preservation of ejaculation. J Urol 1990;144:287. (*Advances in technique have reduced the risk for infertility.*)

53. Dunphy CH, Ayala AG, Swanson DA, et al. Clinical stage I nonseminomatous mixed germ-cell tumors of the testis: a clinicopathologic study of 93 patients on a surveillance protocol after orchiectomy alone. Lancet 1988;62:1202. (*Discusses the use of surveillance as an alternative to lymph node dissection.*)

54. Einhorn LH, Donohue J. Cis-diaminedichloroplatinum, vinblastine, and bleomycin combination chemotherapy in disseminated testicular cancer. Ann Intern Med 1977;87:293. (*The original report on this most important advance in the treatment of testicular cancer.*)

55. Williams SD, Stablein DM, Einhorn LH, et al. Immediate adjuvant chemotherapy versus observation with treatment at relapse in pathological stage II testicular cancer. N Engl J Med 1987;317:1433. (*Equivalent cure rates were achieved.*)

56. Kaufman MR, Chang SS. Short- and long-term complications of therapy for testicular cancer. Urol Clin North Am 2007;34:259. (*An extensive review of surgical and medical complications; 118 references.*)

CHAPTER 144 ■ SCREENING FOR OSTEOPOROSIS IN POSTMENOPAUSAL WOMEN

DAVID M. SLOVIK

One of the major concerns of postmenopausal women is the development of osteoporosis. Although much less appreciated, the problem is also an issue for elderly men (see Appendix 144.1). Osteoporotic fractures in aging women represent a major health problem in industrialized nations. In the United States, approximately 150,000 hip fractures occur annually in women older than the age of 65 years, with 15% to 25% of these women experiencing excess mortality or needing long-term nursing home care. Expenditures for osteoporotic fractures and their consequences are well in excess of $15 billion annually and rising with the aging of the population. The pathophysiologic mechanisms for postmenopausal osteoporosis are imperfectly understood, but the means to ensure maximal skeletal growth and strength, prevent loss of bone mass, and noninvasively evaluate bone mass are available (see Chapter 164).

The frequency and clinical significance of osteoporosis, combined with the capabilities to detect and treat it effectively so as to prevent fractures, argue strongly for screening. Many now recommend that osteoporosis screening become an essential part of the health maintenance program for women; however, data from prospective, long-term, randomized studies identifying those who are best served by screening have yet to emerge, so that clinical judgment is necessary in selecting candidates for osteoporosis screening. Effectively advising the perimenopausal woman requires a knowledge of the epidemiology of osteoporosis and of the risk factors, screening tests, and treatment modalities for this disease.

EPIDEMIOLOGY AND RISK FACTORS (1–6)

Epidemiology

As the life expectancy of women has reached the mid-80s, osteoporosis has taken on epidemic proportions, especially among white women in industrialized societies. In the United States, the prevalence of low bone density in older adults approaches 50%; a woman's risk for an osteoporotic fracture by age 80 years is approximately 40% (several times greater than the risk for breast cancer). The risk for death after a hip fracture is nearly 25%. The disability and expense attributable to the consequences of osteoporosis are enormous and growing.

Risk Factors

The National Osteoporosis Risk Assessment Study examined risk factors of low bone mineral density (BMD) and the relationship of low BMD to fracture risk in a large population-based cohort of postmenopausal women (mean age 64 years). *Age* was the greatest risk factor. Women of ages 70 to 74 years, 75 to 79 years, and older than 80 years had a 9.5-fold, 14.3-fold, and 22.6-fold risk of osteoporosis, respectively. Other risk factors for osteoporosis included *body mass index* below the 25th percentile (<23 kg/m^2), *maternal history of fracture*, and *personal history of fracture during adulthood*. Osteoporosis was associated with a fourfold increase in fracture rate (any site) at 1 year. After controlling for BMD, all of these risk factors were independently associated with fracture risk. Other epidemiologic studies have found current *cigarette smoking* and nonuse of estrogen replacement therapy to be important predictors of risk (Table 144.1).

In addition, a number of contributing risk factors have emerged. These include *lifelong inadequate intake of calcium*, *white race*, *inadequate physical activity*, *early menopause* (onset before the age of 45 years), and *excessive intake of alcohol*. All may predispose a woman to a lower bone mass and osteoporotic fractures with aging. Women in whom osteoporosis does not develop may have a larger skeletal mass, which can be increased through physical activity and calcium supplementation. Estrogen use and African American race are protective factors. Mild to moderate alcohol consumption appears to decrease the risk of osteoporosis (although it does not influence fracture risk).

Medical conditions that are *secondary causes* of osteoporosis include *Cushing's syndrome*, exogenous *glucocorticoid* administration, prolonged *heparin* therapy, *thyrotoxicosis* (including excessive replacement therapy), *hypogonadism*, *hyperprolactinemia*, *anorexia nervosa*, and *hyperparathyroidism*. However, these diseases account for only a small percentage of cases of osteoporosis.

NATURAL HISTORY AND EFFECTIVENESS OF THERAPY (5,7–13)

Natural History

The resorption and formation of bone is a continuous process throughout life. Under physiologic circumstances, the rates of these processes are equal and coupled. Skeletal mass is usually maximal by age 35 years and declines in women after age 40 years and in men after age 50 years, when the rate of new bone formation no longer equals the rate of bone resorption. The rate of decline in skeletal mass is most rapid in women within 2 years of menopause and averages 2% to 4% a year during the

TABLE 144.1

MAJOR RISK FACTORS FOR OSTEOPOROSIS IN WOMEN

Age
Family history of osteoporosis in a first-degree relative
Body mass index below the 25th percentile (<23 kg/m²)
History of fracture during adulthood
Current cigarette smoking
Nonuse of estrogen replacement therapy

first 7 years after menopause. Bone mineral content may decline by 25% to 33% during this period. Afterward, loss continues, but at a slower rate (1% to 2% a year). The areas of greatest loss include the femoral neck and lumbar vertebrae, sites rich in *trabecular bone* and subject to future fracture. *Cortical bone,* comprising 80% of skeletal bone, is lost less rapidly.

The progressive decline in skeletal mass becomes clinically manifest when fractures are sustained spontaneously or after minimal trauma. A loss of height and developing kyphosis generally indicates vertebral compression fracture. Fractures most commonly occur in the sacral and lumbar vertebrae, hip, humerus, and wrist. The clinical course and frequency of fractures in individual patients are hard to predict.

Effectiveness of Therapy

Estrogen replacement can prevent bone loss and even lead to skeletal accretion (see Chapter 164). Observational studies have consistently noted a 35% to 50% reduction in hip, wrist, and vertebral fractures in women who have used estrogen for at least 5 years after menopause. After 10 years of estrogen use, the risk for fracture decreases 75%. However, if estrogen is discontinued, bone loss rapidly ensues, and it is difficult to reverse the significant bone loss that occurs in the first few years of menopause. Beyond age 75 years, the effect of as many as 7 to 10 years of estrogen therapy started at the time of menopause is barely appreciable, which indicates that very prolonged estrogen therapy or restarting it in later years may be necessary. *Bisphosphonates* (e.g., *alendronate*) prevent bone loss and increases bone density at least as well as estrogen replacement. Fracture risk in osteoporotic patients is reduced by up to 50%. *Selective estrogen-receptor modulators* (e.g., *raloxifene*) also halt bone resorption and modestly increase bone mineral density. *Calcium supplementation* with *vitamin D* helps to preserve cortical bone mass but does not prevent bone loss to the degree that estrogen therapy does. The combination of calcium supplementation and *weight-bearing exercise* is more effective at stemming bone loss.

SCREENING TESTS (5,14–20)

Bone Densitometry

The chances for the development of significant osteoporosis and subsequent fracture cannot be adequately predicted by a review of clinical and epidemiologic risk factors. Measurement of bone mineral density is also required. Bone mineral density strongly correlates with the risk for osteoporotic fracture. The test of choice to measure bone mineral density is *dual-energy x-ray absorptiometry* (DEXA), which provides rapid, accurate screening with minimal radiation exposure. Because the bone

mineral density can vary at different sites of the body, DEXA should optimally include separate determinations at the *hip* and *spine*. The bone density at the *wrist* is also predictive of fracture, providing a reasonable approximation of body bone mineral density; the study is less expensive and of interest as an economic alternative for mass screening. Nonetheless, direct assessment of bone mineral density at the hip and spine maximizes test sensitivity and is the most accurate assessment of osteoporotic risk.

Test Interpretation

Bone mineral density measurement is expressed as the number of standard deviations from the mean for normal young adults of the same sex (*T-score*) and as the number of standard deviations from the mean for persons of the same sex and age (*Z-score*). The World Health Organization diagnostic criterion for *osteoporosis* is a *T-score of less than –2.5*. *Osteopenia* is defined as a *T-score between –1.0 and –2.5*. A *Z-score of less than –1.5* suggests a *secondary cause* of osteoporosis. The risk for osteoporotic fracture increases twofold to fourfold for every standard deviation of reduction in bone mineral density.

Cost-Effectiveness

Cost-effectiveness analysis suggests that prior to age 65 years, bone mineral density screening should be reserved for women with one or more of the major risk factors for osteoporosis. In those with no risk factors at this age, the bone mineral density measurement is discretionary. After age 65 years, bone mineral density screening appears to be cost-effective for all women. Bone mineral density screening is also appropriate at any age for patients with an underlying medical condition that might cause osteoporosis (see prior discussion).

Although many decision-analysis and cost-effectiveness studies of screening for osteoporosis have been performed, no data from long-term, prospective, randomized trials are available to confirm the value of screening. Clinical judgment and individualized decision making continue to be essential. If bone density measurement will affect clinical decision making, then screening makes sense for the individual patient. If it will not, then another compelling reason should exist.

Clinical Prediction Algorithm

A search for simpler means of determining risk of osteoporotic fracture continues. Using the extensive epidemiologic database of postmenopausal women participating in the Women's Health Initiative (WHI), investigators identified 11 independent clinical risk factors for osteoporotic hip fracture and then tested them prospectively as a predictive algorithm on a subset of WHI women who underwent DEXA bone scanning.

Test Interpretation

A point-score system based on contribution to overall risk was developed for the 11 independent risk factors identified by multivariate logistic regression analysis (age, race, current smoking, self-reported health, weight, height, history of fracture after age 54 years, parental hip fracture, current corticosteroid use, and treated diabetes). Adding the scores for each risk factor provides an overall 5-year probability estimate of hip fracture. A low score (e.g., 9) yields a probability of 0.1%; a higher score (e.g., 24) yields a probability of 5%.

Test Characteristics

The algorithm's ability to predict 5-year risk of osteoporotic hip fracture was similar to that of the DEXA scan T-score (the area under the receiver operating characteristic curve was 71% for the clinical algorithm, compared with 79% for the DEXA scan).

Cost-Effectiveness

Cost is negligible (the time to collect the data from the patient), suggesting that cost-effectiveness would be very high and the WHI algorithm very useful for initial screening at the time of menopause. Pending further validation, the algorithm could be used as a first-line approach to screening for osteoporotic hip fracture, helping to identify those at greatest risk who might benefit from early DEXA scanning and osteoporosis treatment. The algorithm requires further validation, particularly with regard to the ability to predict benefit from therapy (which the DEXA T-score provides).

RECOMMENDATIONS (21)

Although definitive benefit from screening plus prophylactic therapy remains to be demonstrated by large-scale, long-term, randomized, controlled trials, the accumulating evidence is now deemed sufficient by expert panels (e.g., the U.S. Preventive Services Task Force) to recommend screening for osteoporosis in postmenopausal women. The best guidelines for osteoporosis screening in primary care practice attempt to balance cost and outcomes and may be less aggressive than those of some advocacy organizations that seek to maximize fracture risk reduction at any cost. Based on current evidence, we recommend the following, which incorporates the guidelines of the U.S. Preventive Services Task Force:

- Screen all women older than age 65 years for osteoporosis.

- Begin screening at age 60 years for women at increased fracture risk (at least one major risk factor for osteoporosis):

1. Low body weight (<70 kg)
2. Personal history of osteoporotic fracture after age 55 years
3. Family history of osteoporotic fracture in a first-degree relative
4. Current smoking
5. Use of oral corticosteroids for more than 3 months

- Use clinical judgment to help decide when to initiate screening; consider initiating screening earlier than age 60 years in very high risk women (multiple major risk factors, such as a high score on the WHI clinical algorithm of 11 independent risk factors [age, race, current smoking, self-reported health, weight, height, history of fracture after age 54 years, parental hip fracture, current corticosteroid use, and treated diabetes]), but with the understanding that data are insufficient to prove the effect on outcomes of such earlier screening. Watch the literature for emerging data on this question.

- Order DEXA bone scanning for osteoporosis screening, provided it is available. Specify studies of the hip and the spine for the best determination of risk, but when cost is an issue, consider limiting the study to the hip, which provides a reasonable estimate of fracture risk elsewhere (a DEXA wrist study may provide an adequate lower cost alternative but needs more study). If DEXA is not available, consider a non-DEXA study of the forearm (wrist), but be aware of study limitations.

- Repeat screening biannually (or at longer intervals in persons deemed at low risk after the initial study).

- Screening is not recommended when the results will have no effect on decision making (e.g., persons already taking medication for osteoporosis prevention, refusing it, or unable to take it).

Annotated Bibliography

1. Bauer DC, Browner WS, Cauley JA, et al. Factors associated with appendicular bone mass in older women. Ann Intern Med 1993;118:657. (*Age, weight, muscle strength, and estrogen use were the major factors.*)
2. Cadarette SM, Jagal SB, Murray TM, et al. Evaluation of decision rules for referring women for bone densitometry by dual-energy x-ray absorptiometry. JAMA 2001;286:57. (*A rigorous study of the predictive value of risk factors and decision rules.*)
3. Cummings SR, Nevitt MC, Browner WS, et al. Risk factors for hip fracture in white women. N Engl J Med 1995;332:767. (*Finds a family history of osteoporosis, low body mass index, history of bone fracture as an adult, and current smoking to be the major risk factors.*)
4. Looker AC, Orwoll ES, Johnston CC Jr, et al. Prevalence of low femoral bone density in older U.S. adults from NHANES III. J Bone Miner Res 1997;12:1761. (*High prevalence was found in this major epidemiologic study.*)
5. Nelson HD, Helfand H, Woolf SH, et al. Screening for postmenopausal osteoporosis: a review of the evidence for the U.S. Preventive Services Task Force. Ann Intern Med 2002;137:529. (*A critical systematic review of evidence for the U.S. Preventive Services Task Force; 126 references.*)
6. Siris ES, Miller PD, Barrett-Connor E, et al. Identification and fracture outcomes of undiagnosed low bone mineral density in postmenopausal women: results from the National Osteoporosis Risk Assessment. JAMA 2001;286:2815. (*A major longitudinal observational study involving >200,000 women; the prevalence of low bone mineral density was nearly 50%; identifies risk factors for osteoporosis.*)
7. Black DM, Cummings SR, Karpf DB, et al. Randomised trial of effect of alendronate on risk of fracture in women with existing vertebral fractures: Fracture Intervention Trial Research Group. Lancet 1996;348:1535. (*A major study finding a 47% reduction in the rate of new fractures in comparison with a placebo group.*)
8. Cauley JA, Seeley DG, Esrud K, et al. Estrogen replacement therapy and fractures in older women: Study of Osteoporotic Fractures Research Group. Ann Intern Med 1995;122:9. (*The relative risk for nonspinal fracture was reduced by 34%.*)
9. Cummings SR, Black DM, Thompson DE, et al. Effect of alendronate on risk of fracture in women with low bone density but without vertebral fractures: results from the Fracture Intervention Trial. JAMA 1998;280:2077. (*The treatment significantly reduced the risk for hip fracture.*)
10. Eastell R. Treatment of postmenopausal osteoporosis. N Engl J Med 1998;338:736. (*A review that focuses on the evidence for the efficacy of therapy.*)
11. Eddy DM, Johnston CC Jr, Cummings SR, et al. Osteoporosis: review of the evidence for prevention, diagnosis, and treatment and cost-effectiveness analysis. Osteoporos Int 1998;8(Suppl 4):S1. (*An extensive review of the evidence; concludes that screening appears to be cost-effective, especially for women with major risk factors.*)
12. Grady D, Rubin SM, Petitti DB, et al. Hormone therapy to prevent disease and prolong life in postmenopausal women. Ann Intern Med 1992;117:1016. (*Includes a comprehensive review of the data on costs and benefits of estrogen replacement to prevent osteoporosis.*)
13. Liberman UA, Weiss SR, Broll J, et al. Effects of oral alendronate on bone mineral density and the incidence of fractures in postmenopausal osteoporosis. N Engl J Med 1995;333:1437. (*A large, randomized, controlled trial revealing a 9% increase in bone mineral density of the spine and a 6% increase at the hip; there was a 50% reduction in vertebral spine fracture.*)
14. Bates DW, Black DM, Cummings SR. Clinical use of bone densitometry: clinical applications. JAMA 2002;288:1898. (*A review of screening strategies and suggestions for improved screening.*)
15. Cummings SR, Bates DW, Black DM. Clinical use of bone densitometry: a scientific review. JAMA 2002;288:1889. (*An excellent review of the approaches to measuring bone density; 72 references.*)

16. Hui SL, Slemenda CW, Johnston CC Jr. Baseline measurement of bone mass predicts fracture in white women. Ann Intern Med 1989;111:355. (*Demonstrates the predictive value of wrist bone density measurement.*)
17. Kanis JA, Melton III LJ, Christiansen C, et al. The diagnosis of osteoporosis. J Bone Miner Res 1994;9:1137. (*World Health Organization consensus criteria for the diagnosis of osteoporosis; emphasizes the importance of bone mineral density determination.*)
18. Kellie SE. AMA Council on Scientific Affairs. Measurement of bone density with dual energy x-ray absorptiometry (DEXA). JAMA 1992;267:286. (*The test of choice for screening.*)
19. Robbins J, Aragaki AK, Kooperberg C, et al. Factors associated with 5-year risk of hip fracture in postmenopausal women. JAMA 2007;298:2389. (*Based on analysis of the Women's Health Initiative database, finds 11 independent clinical risk factors that taken together predict the 5-year risk almost as well as dual energy x-ray absorptiometry bone scan.*)
20. Shahinian VB, Kuo Y-F, Freeman JL, et al. Risk of fracture after androgen deprivation for prostate cancer. N Engl J Med 2005;352:154. (*A retrospective epidemiologic study; found a significant increase in risk.*)
21. U.S. Preventive Services Task Force. Screening for osteoporosis in postmenopausal women: recommendations and rationale. Ann Intern Med 2002;137:159. (*Evidence-based consensus recommendations.*)

APPENDIX 144.1: SCREENING FOR OSTEOPOROSIS IN MEN (1–4)

Screening for osteoporosis in men is not an established practice, mainly because there has been little study of the problem; however, this does not mean that men are not at risk. The lifetime risk of an osteoporotic fracture in men is estimated at 13%; men account for 20% to 30% of all hip fractures, and close to 50% of men who have a fracture die as a result of it. Although men do not suffer the dramatic bone loss of women, there is age-related loss, especially among those living to advanced age (>75 years). Epidemiologic study using DEXA bone scanning finds rates of osteoporosis in excess of 30% in men older than the age of 50 years.

Risk factors for osteoporosis in men are very frequent and include alcohol abuse, glucocorticosteroid therapy, and hypogonadism. The frequency and adverse effects of osteoporosis in men, coupled with the advent of DEXA scanning and demonstrated efficacy of bisphosphonate therapy (density increased and fracture risk reduced), suggest consideration of osteoporosis screening in elderly men. Although there are no studies proving the efficacy of screening and no consensus guidelines, evidence suggests that one might consider an initial DEXA screening in men at high risk, having at least one of the following risk factors:

- Advanced age (>75 years)
- Hypogonadism
- History of alcohol abuse
- Chronic glucocorticosteroid use
- History of recent fracture

Analysis of the cost-effectiveness of screening elderly men for osteoporosis suggests that screening and treatment for osteoporosis of all men older than the age of 80 years and those older than the age of 65 year with a recent history of fracture would meet standards for cost-effectiveness (cost per quality-adjusted life year <$50,000). If the cost of bisphosphonate therapy fell to less than $500/yr, screening all men older than the age of 70 years would become cost effective. Prospective study is needed for validation before widespread screening and treatment can be recommended.

A.H.G.

Annotated Bibliography

1. Hannan MT, Felson DT, Dawson-Hughes B, et al. Risk factors for longitudinal bone loss in elderly men and women: the Framingham Osteoporosis Study. J Bone Miner Res 2000;15:710. (*Community-based epidemiologic data on risk factors.*)
2. Looker AC, Orwell ES, Johnston CC, et al. Prevalence of low femoral bone density in older US adults from the NHANES III. J Bone Miner Res 1997;12:1761. (*Greater than 30% of men older than the age of 50 years have osteoporosis on dual-energy x-ray absorptiometry study.*)
3. Orwoll E, Ettinger M, Weiss S, et al. Alendronate for the treatment of osteoporosis in men. N Engl J Med 2000;343:604. (*A randomized, controlled trial; found an increased bone density and a decreased the risk of fracture.*)
4. Schousboe JT, Taylor BC, Fink HA, et al. Cost effectiveness of bone densitometry followed by treatment of osteoporosis in older men. JAMA 2007;298:629. (*A cost-effectiveness analysis; found that screening and treatment were cost-effective in men older than the age of 80 years and those older than the age of 65 years with a history of fracture.*)

CHAPTER 145 ■ EVALUATION OF ACUTE MONOARTICULAR ARTHRITIS

Acute monoarticular arthritis calls for a prompt diagnostic evaluation because of the possibility of bacterial infection, which can lead to rapid joint destruction and septic sequelae. In certain noninfectious forms of inflammation, notably crystal-induced arthropathy, quick diagnosis and treatment are also beneficial. Most patients present for care on an outpatient basis, so that the diagnosis of monoarticular arthritis is an important responsibility of the primary physician.

PATHOPHYSIOLOGY AND CLINICAL PRESENTATION (1–11)

The principal mechanisms of monoarticular arthritis can be broadly categorized as inflammatory and noninflammatory, with the inflammatory mechanisms subdivided into infectious and noninfectious.

Infectious Etiologies

Septic Arthritis

Septic arthritis may occur as a consequence of *hematogenous seeding* of the synovium in the setting of bacteremia or by *direct extension* from trauma, osteomyelitis, or placement of a contaminated joint prosthesis (which can harbor a biofilm of organisms). Early or delayed *prosthetic-joint infection* (up to 24 months after surgery) results from the placement of a contaminated appliance (intraoperative risk 1% to 2%); late infection is usually due to hematogenous seeding from dental work, skin infection, pneumonia, or urinary tract infection.

Clinically, acute septic arthritis is characterized by joint pain, effusion, erythema, warmth, and fever. Delayed prosthetic-joint infection may have a more subtle presentation, characterized by persistent joint pain and signs of implant loosening without obvious manifestations of inflammation.

Disseminated Gonorrhea

Among previously healthy, sexually active patients, disseminated gonorrhea is the most frequent cause of joint infection. Women account for two thirds of cases. Pregnancy and menstruation appear to increase the risk for dissemination, which occurs in about 1% to 3% of persons with gonorrhea (see Chapter 137). An initial bacteremic stage is characterized by fever, polyarthralgias, transient scattered tendonitis, minimal joint effusion, necrotic skin lesions, blood cultures positive for organisms, and sterile joint fluid. This phase of the illness may be followed in several days by a septic joint stage, with monoarticular or occasionally polyarticular pain, marked joint swelling, and effusion. During the septic joint stage, gonococci can be recovered from the joint in about 50% of patients.

Nongonococcal Septic Arthritis

More than 80% of cases are monoarticular, with gram-positive organisms, especially *Staphylococcus aureus*, predominating (60% of infectious cases, most of them methicillin resistant). *Streptococcus* species account for about 18%. *Gram-negative Enterobacteriaceae* also cause septic arthritis, particularly in intravenous-drug abusers, immunocompromised persons, and the chronically ill. Joint sepsis is more likely in patients with altered host defenses (diabetes, cirrhosis, immunodeficiency), previously damaged joints (rheumatoid arthritis), or prosthetic joints. Fever, chills, and joint inflammation are usually prominent, but the presentation may be devoid of systemic symptoms, especially if the patient is debilitated or immunosuppressed. A larger joint, such as a knee or a hip, is most likely to be involved. Sternoclavicular joint infection is characteristic of intravenous-drug abusers. Articular destruction can be rapid. Within 10 days of nongonococcal infection, radiographic evidence of cartilaginous and bony damage may appear. Joint injury from gonococcal arthritis is less precipitous, so that more time is available for treatment. Permanent damage is uncommon in patients who are treated.

Lyme Disease

An acute oligoarthritis can develop months after the initial infection in untreated persons, with about 60% experiencing the problem (see Chapter 160). Large joints are typically involved, especially the knees. Intermittent attacks of acute arthritis lasting weeks to months are sometimes seen, as is chronic erosive arthritis. Swelling may be more prominent than pain.

Mycobacterial Infection

HIV-infected patients are at increased risk for mycobacterial joint infection, as are persons who have had repeated glucocorticoid injections into a joint. Often, periarticular bony disease develops in addition to joint inflammation. A chronic picture remains more common than acute inflammation.

HIV Infection

An acute monoarticular or oligoarticular arthritis may be part of a syndrome accompanying the onset of HIV infection. The lower extremities are the usual site of involvement (see Chapter 13).

Noninfectious Inflammatory Etiologies

The underlying mechanism is usually crystal-induced inflammation, but occasionally one of the immunologically mediated diseases may present as monoarticular disease.

Acute Gout

Gout is a common cause of acute monoarticular arthritis. Sodium urate crystals in the synovium incite a brisk inflammatory response after they are ingested by polymorphonuclear leukocytes. The condition is found most commonly among middle-aged and older men. Onset is rapid, peaking within 12 to 24 hours. The metatarsophalangeal joint of the great toe is the classic site, but the midfoot, ankles, knees, wrists, and olecranon bursae are other important locations. Sodium urate crystals are found in the joint fluid. They are needle-like and negatively birefringent under the polarizing microscope. Although the likelihood of a gouty attack increases with serum uric acid levels, uric acid levels are not diagnostically helpful unless they are extremely high. Alcoholic binges or the new use of thiazide diuretics may precipitate gouty attacks. A mild fever may even be present. Rapid response to colchicine helps to differentiate crystal-induced arthritis from infection (see Chapter 158).

Pseudogout

Pseudogout results when crystals of calcium pyrophosphate induce joint inflammation, and it resembles gout pathophysiologically, although the clinical features differ. Knees and wrists are the most commonly affected sites. Under the polarizing microscope, weakly positively birefringent rhomboid forms of calcium pyrophosphate are revealed in the synovial fluid. Chondrocalcinosis is usually present on radiography. Pseudogout tends to occur in older patients and seems to be associated with hyperparathyroidism, hemochromatosis, and severe degenerative joint disease.

Immunologic Disease

Immunologically mediated conditions typically cause polyarthritis but may present initially as a monoarthritis. These include rheumatoid arthritis, Reiter's syndrome, ankylosing spondylitis, psoriatic arthritis, the arthritis of inflammatory bowel disease, and the arthritis of sarcoidosis (see Chapter 146).

Noninflammatory Disease

Acute traumatic causes include juxtaarticular ligament or meniscus *injury*, frank bone *fracture* extending through to the joint space, or minor trauma in patients with impaired coagulation that results in *hemarthrosis*. A variety of mechanical disorders, collectively referred to as "internal derangements" of the knee, may produce chronic recurrent pain and noninflammatory effusion. *Osteoarthritis*, characterized by the degeneration of articular cartilage with adjacent bony sclerosis and proliferation, often produces chronic, gradually increasing joint symptoms but may present as an acutely painful joint with a noninflammatory or mildly inflammatory effusion.

DIFFERENTIAL DIAGNOSIS (1,2,4,5)

The most immediately important entities in the differential diagnosis of acute monoarthritis are infection, crystal-induced arthropathy, and trauma. The gonococcus is the leading infectious agent, followed in frequency by gram-positive organisms (staphylococci, streptococci) and in compromised hosts by gram-negative coliforms. Gout and pseudogout are the important crystal-induced arthropathies.

As noted earlier, several polyarticular diseases may initially present with one acutely inflamed joint or with symptoms that are most pronounced in a single joint. These monoarticular presentations of polyarticular disease are seen in rheumatoid arthritis, Reiter's syndrome, ankylosing spondylitis, psoriatic arthritis, the arthritis of inflammatory bowel disease, and sarcoidosis.

Despite the wide range of diagnostic possibilities, it should be appreciated that recent series of monoarthritis have revealed that the most prevalent diagnoses are osteoarthritis, septic arthritis, gout, and pseudogout.

WORKUP (1–5,7–19)

The first objective is to establish whether the joint is infected. Although examination of the joint fluid is the most important diagnostic test, history and physical examination may provide useful information regarding the likelihood of infection and also its source.

History

Onset, associated symptoms, location, risk factors, and concurrent illness are essential items to check. Abrupt onset in conjunction with fever and chills points to a septic cause, as does a history of skin lesions, vaginal or urethral discharge, exposure to gonorrhea, tick bites, diabetes, concurrent rheumatoid arthritis, joint prosthesis, immunosuppression, HIV infection, intravenous-drug abuse, and previous trauma.

Acute trauma increases the probability of periarticular injury, internal derangement, and hemarthrosis. History of joint prosthesis placement raises the question of a contaminated prosthesis, even up to 24 months after surgery; a loose prosthesis may be due to the presence of indolent infection. Prior attacks are indicative of gout and pseudogout. Alcohol abuse predisposes to gout, trauma, and infection. Inflammation in the first metatarsophalangeal joint points to gout, especially in an elderly male patient; however, in patients with diabetes, extension of osteomyelitis into the joint must be ruled out. Associated back pain and stiffness raise the possibility of one of the spondyloarthropathies. Age can be a helpful clue. Pseudogout is most common in older patients. Disseminated gonococ-

cal infection, Reiter's syndrome, and ankylosing spondylitis are diseases of young people.

Physical Examination

All joints are carefully examined to ascertain the location and the nature of the problem. *Signs of inflammation* are sought (increased warmth, swelling, redness, effusion). One needs to differentiate inflammation of the joint space from a periarticular process such as tendonitis, bursitis, or cellulitis, which can be mistaken for it. Sometimes this distinction is impossible to make, but preservation of range of motion despite pain in the area reduces the likelihood of true joint involvement. The probability of a periarticular process is increased by the finding of localized tenderness that does not encompass the entire joint space. Although painful limitation of motion suggests articular disease, tendonitis and cellulitis can also cause discomfort with movement.

Once it is suspected that joint inflammation is present, the focus shifts quickly to differentiating between infectious and noninfectious causes. The patient's temperature should be taken. Almost all patients with septic arthritis are febrile (one important exception being persons with delayed prosthetic-joint infection). Low-grade fever may also be noted in gout and rheumatoid arthritis, but a high fever suggests infection. The integument is noted for necrotic lesions on the extremities (indicative of gonococcemia), the splinter hemorrhages of endocarditis, manifestations of HIV disease (see Chapter 13), needle tracks, tophi, rheumatoid nodules, pitting of the nails and other psoriatic manifestations, erythema nodosum (seen with sarcoidosis and inflammatory bowel disease), and the keratoderma blennorrhagicum and circinate balanitis of Reiter's syndrome. The eyes are examined for conjunctivitis and iritis, the fundi for signs of endocarditis, the mouth for mucosal ulceration, and the heart for murmurs. The genitalia need to be checked for signs of gonococcal urethritis and cervicitis (see Chapters 136 and 137). The spine should be examined carefully for restriction of motion and tenderness, which are indicative of spondylitis.

Laboratory Studies

No "standard" laboratory workup exists for acute monoarticular disease. Appropriate test selection should be based on the clinical presentation; only conditions suggested by the history and the physical examination are worth investigating further. Running a standard battery of "arthritis tests" is both wasteful and potentially misleading. A few guidelines for initial test selection have been suggested by the American College of Rheumatology:

- If trauma or focal bone pain is present, then the first study should be radiography of the area.
- If an effusion or other signs of inflammation are noted, then the test of first choice is joint aspiration with fluid cell count and differential to confirm the presence of inflammation.
- If no effusion or trauma is present, then testing for trigger points and tender points (see Chapter 159) is indicated to assess for tendonitis and fibromyalgia, respectively.

Examination of Joint Fluid

Aspirating and examining the joint fluid is the most important diagnostic procedure in the evaluation of acute monoarticular arthritis when evidence of inflammation is found. Taking note of the *appearance* of the joint fluid may be of help in determining the cause of arthropathy. A turbid appearance to the fluid points to inflammation; blood suggests trauma, coagulopathy, pseudogout, or neoplasm; a clear, straw-colored fluid is seen with degenerative disease and minor trauma. With sepsis, one may aspirate frank pus. The fluid should be sent promptly for *cell count* and *differential* while it is fresh, and separate samples should be put aside briefly to be sent quickly for microscopic examination for *crystals* and *organisms* and for culture if the initial fluid examination shows evidence of inflammation. A white blood cell count of greater than *2,000/mm*^{3} is suggestive of an *inflammatory process*. A predominance of *neutrophils* (>75%) confirms an inflammatory process. In gout and septic joints, the white blood cell count often exceeds 50,000/mm^3. In prosthetic-joint infection, white cell count greater than 1,700/mm^3 and neutrophils greater than 65% are associated with sensitivities for infection of 94% and 97%, respectively, and specificities of 88% and 98%, respectively, in the absence of underlying inflammatory joint disease.

Crystal examination under a polarizing lens provides the most rapid and sure method of diagnosing gout and pseudogout. However, urate crystals can often be seen under the microscope with normal light; the crystals of pseudogout are harder to identify in this manner. The *glucose* concentration is often measured; it may be suggestively low in infection and rheumatoid disease.

Bacteriologic Study

The joint fluid in a case of suspected infection should be sent for *Gram's stain* and *culturing*. Gram-positive bacteria are seen in about 80% of the cases in which they are the responsible agent. *Enterobacteriaceae* show up on Gram's stain less frequently. *Neisseria gonorrhoeae* is rarely seen. It is most important to culture the joint fluid immediately onto proper media (including Thayer–Martin plates for the detection of gonococci). Smears of the joint fluid may show organisms in the absence of a culture positive for organisms if antibiotics have already been taken. A repeated tap of the joint will improve the diagnostic yield of Gram's stain and culture if the results of the first arthrocentesis are negative. Repeatedly positive cultures provide strong evidence of infection, even if low-virulence skin organisms such as coagulase-negative staphylococci are isolated (as is common in prosthetic-joint infection).

Other Testing

When joint fluid cannot be obtained, the *complete blood cell count* and *erythrocyte sedimentation rate* are moderately helpful in distinguishing inflammatory from noninflammatory disease, but clearly the initial results of the synovial fluid examination are the most helpful in guiding further testing. If inflammatory joint fluid is sterile, a workup for connective tissue disease (see Chapter 146), Lyme disease (see Chapter 160), and sarcoidosis (see Chapter 51) must be considered. Reviewing the history and the physical examination findings for pertinent clinical clues can help to determine the extent to which testing for each of these conditions should be performed. If the fluid is frankly bloody, then determination of the prothrombin time, partial thromboplastin time, and platelet count is in order. The finding of characteristic crystals obviates the need for *serum uric acid* or *calcium* determinations; values are often normal despite an acute attack of crystal-induced disease. The serum uric acid level is useful only if it is markedly elevated. *Blood cultures* are indicated when sepsis is suspected. Culturing other possible foci of infection, such as skin lesions, urethral discharge, and the cervix, should be considered if infection is a possibility. Testing the joint fluid by polymerase chain reaction analysis for evidence of *Borrelia burgdorferi* can be diagnostic when Lyme disease is a real concern, but test availability may be limited.

Serologic Studies

A number of serologic studies are routinely offered for the assessment of arthritis. However, they are rarely diagnostic of the cause of an acute monoarticular arthritis, and false positives are common in the setting of acute inflammation. Nonetheless, they can be helpful when used carefully. Testing for *HIV antibodies* is indicated when evidence of immune compromise or high-risk sexual behavior is found (see Chapter 13). Testing for *antinuclear antibodies* and *rheumatoid factor* can help in the diagnosis of connective tissue disease, but false positives are very common, especially in the elderly and persons with other inflammatory conditions (see Chapter 146), so they should be ordered only when clinical suspicion is substantial. *Lyme antibody titers* add little to the diagnosis except in cases with strongly supporting clinical and epidemiologic evidence for *Borrelia* infection (see Chapter 160).

Radiography

Plain films are most useful when evidence of trauma or focal bone pain is present. Plain films may also reveal fracture, neoplasm, osteomyelitis, and chondrocalcinosis. A diagnosis of osteoarthritis cannot be based solely on the presence of osteoarthritic changes, but their absence makes osteoarthritis unlikely. Initial plain films in patients with an acute inflammatory arthropathy often shows little more than soft-tissue swelling, especially in early phases of the disease; in suspected septic arthritis, serial study is needed to find characteristic bony changes, such as new subperiosteal bone formation and transcortical sinus tracts.

Magnetic resonance imaging is overused, but the technology is worth considering when traumatic internal knee derangement is suspected and confirmation is required (see Chapter 152). *Bone scan* or magnetic resonance imaging is indicated if osteomyelitis is suspected.

Despite optimal efforts, many cases of acute monoarthritis elude diagnosis. In one study, one third of cases were never satisfactorily diagnosed. Fortunately, however, the majority of these patients improved, or at least did not get worse. If infection, trauma, and, less important, crystal-induced arthritis are ruled out, the evaluation can be approached less hurriedly.

SYMPTOMATIC MANAGEMENT

Until a diagnosis is established, the patient may feel better resting, immobilizing the joint, and administering ice packs. Antiinflammatory agents should be postponed for at least 12 to 24 hours so that cultures can grow and arthrocentesis can be repeated if the first result is nondiagnostic. If pain is unbearable and a diagnosis is not yet established, an analgesic without antiinflammatory effects (e.g., acetaminophen or codeine) may be used. After a second negative result of arthrocentesis, it is reasonable to institute antiinflammatory therapy even in the absence of a specific diagnosis, provided that all cultures are negative for organisms and the patient is deemed to be at very low risk for infection. More definitive therapy of acute monoarticular arthritis must be based on the underlying cause (see Chapters 137, 156, 158, and 160).

INDICATIONS FOR REFERRAL AND ADMISSION

A patient with septic arthritis requires hospital admission, treatment with intravenous antibiotics, and consultation with an infectious disease specialist. When a case of acute monoarticular arthritis remains undiagnosed but the white blood cell count is high, infection is a possibility and an infectious disease specialist should be consulted to consider an empiric course of intravenous antibiotics. The more chronic case that eludes diagnosis may benefit from a rheumatologic consultation. Closed synovial biopsy or arthroscopy may be needed.

A.H.G.

Annotated Bibliography

1. American College of Rheumatology Ad Hoc Committee on Clinical Guidelines. Guidelines for the initial evaluation of the adult patient with acute musculoskeletal symptoms. Arthritis Rheum 1996;39:1. (*Presents evidence-based consensus guidelines.*)
2. Baker DG, Schumacher HR. Acute monoarthritis. N Engl J Med 1993;329:1013. (*A clinically useful review, with an excellent section on analysis of the joint fluid; 60 references.*)
3. Edeiken J. Arthritis: the roles of the primary care physician and the radiologist. JAMA 1975;232:1364. (*Differentiates conditions with mainly clinical findings from those with specific radiographic manifestations.*)
4. Freed JF, Nies KM, Boyer RS, et al. Acute monoarticular arthritis: a diagnostic approach. JAMA 1980;243:2314. (*Discusses the prevalence of various diagnoses and which tests were useful; one third of cases were never diagnosed.*)
5. Fries JF, Mitchell DM. Joint pain or arthritis. JAMA 1976;235:199. (*Still relevant for its emphasis on clinical diagnosis and judicious use of the laboratory.*)
6. Goldenberg DL. Infectious arthritis complicating rheumatoid arthritis and other chronic rheumatic diseases. Arthritis Rheum 1989;32:496. (*There was an increased risk for infection; a comprehensive review of the issue.*)
7. Goldenberg DL, Reed JI. Bacterial arthritis. N Engl J Med 1985;312:764. (*A review of pathophysiology, risk factors, diagnosis, and therapy, emphasizing the importance of early recognition and treatment.*)
8. Holmes K, Counts G, Beaty H. Disseminated gonococcal infection. Ann Intern Med 1971;74:979. (*Arthritis occurred in almost 90% of patients with disseminated disease; a classic article describing the syndrome; 141 references.*)
9. Rowe IF, Forster SM, Seifert MH, et al. Rheumatic manifestations of human immunodeficiency virus infection. Am J Med 1988;85:59. (*The best description of joint involvement in HIV disease.*)
10. Steere AC, Schoen RT, Taylor E. The clinical evolution of Lyme arthritis. Ann Intern Med 1987;107:725. (*The multiple presentations of Lyme arthritis.*)
11. Zimmerli W, Trampuz A, Ochsner PE. Prosthetic-joint infections. N Engl J Med 2004;351:1645. (*A detailed review, with discussions of pathophysiology, as well as the approach to workup and management; 70 references.*)
12. Brown SL, Hansen SL, Linguine JJ. Role of serology in the diagnosis of Lyme disease. JAMA 1999;282:62. (*A review of the test performance of commercially available serologic kits; finds great variability among tests, low reproducibility, and disappointing sensitivity and specificity under many circumstances.*)
13. Juby AF, Davis P, McElhaney JE, et al. Prevalence of selected autoantibodies in different elderly subpopulations. Br J Rheumatol 1994;33:1121. (*Finds an increased prevalence with age; many individuals with positive test results show no signs of disease.*)
14. Pascual E, Tovar J, Ruiz MT. The ordinary light microscope: an appropriate tool for provisional detection and identification of crystals in synovial fluid. Ann Rheum Dis 1989;48:983. (*A polarizing microscope is not needed to identify urate crystals.*)
15. Shmerling RH, Delbanco T. How useful is the rheumatoid factor? Analysis of sensitivity, specificity, and predictive value. Arch Intern Med 1992;152:2417. (*The answer is that it is not too useful when ordered in low-probability situations; there are high rates of false positives and false negatives.*)
16. Shmerling RH, Delbanco T, Tosteson ANA, et al. Synovial fluid tests: what should be ordered? JAMA 1990;264:1009. (*A good discussion of the contribution of synovial fluid studies to diagnosis.*)
17. Slater CA, Davis RB, Shmerling RH. Antinuclear antibody testing. A study in clinical utility. Arch Intern Med 1996;156:1421. (*The test is often ordered in low-probability situations; positive predictive value is very low in the setting of a low clinical probability for lupus.*)
18. Trampuz, Hanssen AD, Osmon DR, et al. Synovial fluid leukocyte count and differential for the diagnosis of prosthetic knee infection. Am J Med 2004;117;556. (*Finds that these parameters were sensitive and specific for diagnosis.*)
19. Weissman BN, Hussain S. Magnetic resonance imaging of the knee. Rheum Dis Clin North Am 1991;17:637. (*A good review of the indications for its use.*)

CHAPTER 146 ■ EVALUATION OF POLYARTICULAR COMPLAINTS

Polyarticular complaints are among the most frequent in primary care practice and are often associated with considerable loss of function. Although osteoarthritis accounts for many of the more obvious cases (particularly in the elderly), the differential diagnosis can encompass a bewildering array of conditions—articular and nonarticular, inflammatory and noninflammatory (Table 146.1). Careful attention to the history and the physical examination findings helps to chart a logical course to minimize diagnostic error and maximize patient benefit. In community-practice settings, there is a high frequency of overdiagnosis of autoimmune etiologies due to excessive test ordering and misinterpretation of results.

In most instances, the workup can proceed in deliberate, sequential fashion, but its pace is best matched to that of the underlying illness. The initial evaluation should focus on answering the following basic questions:

1. Are the patient's symptoms truly articular or nonarticular?
2. Is the arthritis inflammatory or degenerative?
3. Is the problem local or systemic?
4. How sick is the patient?

DIFFERENTIAL DIAGNOSIS OF POLYARTICULAR PAIN

Inflammatory Joint Disease
  Rheumatoid arthritis
  Systemic lupus erythematosus
  Scleroderma
  Psoriatic arthritis
  Reiter's syndrome
  Ankylosing spondylitis
  Polyarticular gout
  Pseudogout
  Sarcoidosis
  Lyme disease
  Disseminated gonococcemia
  Rheumatic fever
  Hepatitis B
  Subacute bacterial endocarditis
  Vasculitis
Noninflammatory Joint Disease
  Osteoarthritis
  Hypertrophic pulmonary osteoarthropathy
  Myxedema
  Amyloidosis
  Sickle cell disease
Inflammatory Periarticular Disease
  Polymyalgia rheumatica
  Dermatomyositis, polymyositis
  Eosinophilia–myalgia syndrome
Noninflammatory Periarticular Disease
  Fibromyalgia syndrome
  Reflex sympathetic dystrophy

Adapted from Mainardi CL. Approach to the patient with pain in more than one joint. In: Kelley WN, ed. Textbook of internal medicine, 2nd ed. Philadelphia: Lippincott, 1993:1002, with permission.

PATHOPHYSIOLOGY AND CLINICAL PRESENTATION (1–17)

Pathophysiology

Polyarthritis can result from a degenerative, relatively noninflammatory process or from an inflammatory one.

Noninflammatory forms of arthritis are, in most cases, the result of breakdown in joint cartilage and secondary mechanical disruption of the joint. This can be a primary process, or it can be associated with an underlying disease, such as hemochromatosis. Signs of inflammation are minimal, although occasionally a small joint effusion may be present. Other mechanisms of noninflammatory joint injury include synovial infiltration (amyloidosis), periosteal proliferation at the ends of long bones (hypertrophic osteoarthropathy), and ischemic injury (sickle cell disease).

Inflammatory arthritis develops as a consequence of the aggregation of inflammatory cells and their products in the joint space and synovium. Infection, gout, pseudogout, and the immunologically mediated diseases—rheumatoid arthritis, lupus, the spondyloarthropathies—all produce an inflammatory type of arthritis, characterized by joint swelling, warmth, redness, effusion, and tenderness. Joint constituents may be the targets

of immunologic attack or may be caught up in a more generalized inflammatory process.

Periarticular disease involving muscles and tendons may also present as pain referable to joints, although it is not a true arthritis. Mechanisms range from autoimmune inflammatory processes to purported vasomotor instability.

Clinical Presentation: Inflammatory Polyarthritides

The hallmark of these conditions is synovitis, with manifestations of inflammation (erythema, warmth, swelling) encompassing the entire joint.

Rheumatoid Arthritis

Rheumatoid arthritis typically presents in subacute fashion with symmetric polyarthritis, although atypical forms include monoarticular and asymmetric disease. The most common sites are the wrists, proximal interphalangeal (PIP) joints, and metacarpophalangeal (MCP) joints, but elbows, neck, hips, knees, ankles, and feet may also be involved. Extraarticular manifestations include vasculitis, pulmonary nodules or interstitial fibrosis, mononeuritis multiplex, Sjögren's syndrome, and Felty's syndrome (splenomegaly, anemia, thrombocytopenia). Fatigue may dominate the early clinical presentation and precede the onset of joint symptoms. Other systemic symptoms (fever, weight loss) are prominent in severe cases. Women are more often affected than men. Morning stiffness is almost universal, with Raynaud's phenomenon a common accompaniment. Rheumatoid factor (RF) is found in approximately 75% of cases and is associated with skin nodules and more aggressive articular and extraarticular disease. Tendinous inflammation and joint destruction may ensue, producing characteristic changes (subluxation, swan neck deformities of the fingers, ulnar deviation of the wrists). Because no single clinical feature or test finding is definitive, the diagnosis requires the presence of a constellation of findings (Table 146.2). Current criteria are believed to have a sensitivity and specificity of approximately 90%.

DIAGNOSTIC CRITERIA FOR RHEUMATOID ARTHRITIS

Morning stiffness for >6 weeks
Arthritis involving three or more joint areas for >6 weeks
Arthritis of hand joints for >6 weeks
Symmetric arthritis for >6 weeks
Rheumatoid nodules
Serum rheumatoid factor in elevated titers
Radiologic changes (bony erosion in or adjacent to involved hand or wrist joints)

The presence of any four or more criteria is necessary for a diagnosis of definite rheumatoid arthritis.
Adapted from Arnett FC, Edworthy SM, Block DA, et al. The American Rheumatism Association 1987 revised criteria for the classification of rheumatoid arthritis. Arthritis Rheum 1988;31:315, with permission.

Systemic Lupus Erythematosus

Lupus usually occurs in young women, with a high prevalence in blacks. Malar rash, symmetric polyarthralgias, and nondeforming arthritis are characteristic, as is multisystem involvement, but morning stiffness and joint destruction are not as prominent as in rheumatoid arthritis (RA). Both large- and small-vessel vasculitis may occur. Oral ulcers are common. Serositis leading to pleuritis, effusion, or pericarditis develops in about one third of patients with systemic lupus erythematosus (SLE). Hematologic manifestations include leukopenia, immune thrombocytopenia, and hemolytic anemia. The most serious complications are glomerulonephritis and cerebritis.

The appearance of autoantibodies is characteristic of lupus and typically predates the development of clinical disease by years; however, their presence is not diagnostic in the absence of clinical findings and does not reliably predict the development of clinical disease. Characteristic serologic findings include positivity for *antinuclear antibody* (ANA), *antibody to native double-stranded DNA* (anti-dsDNA), and *anti-Smith* (*anti-Sm*) *antibody*. Additional serologic features may include antiphospholipid antibodies (associated with an increased risk of thrombosis and a false-positive test for syphilis), *antiribonucleoprotein* (anti-RNP, associated with manifestations of scleroderma), and *anti-Ro* and *anti-La antibodies* (also found in persons with Sjögren's syndrome).

Systemic Sclerosis (Scleroderma)

Scleroderma initially presents as hand arthralgias, mild inflammatory hand arthritis, or Raynaud's phenomenon. Florid joint inflammation is uncommon. Skin thickening, a hallmark of the condition, follows several months later. Two clinical variants are described. One is a very slowly progressive form in which visceral involvement does not become significant until after decades of activity. It is manifested by the CREST syndrome: subcutaneous calcinosis of the digits, Raynaud's phenomenon, esophageal dysmotility, sclerodactyly, and telangiectasia. In the more aggressive form, skin thickening progresses rapidly to extend to the proximal limbs and trunk (hence the term *scleroderma*), and the onset of visceral involvement is accelerated (i.e., kidneys, lung, heart, and gastrointestinal tract). The results of ANA testing are positive in most patients with diffuse organ system disease, and a *speckled pattern* is characteristic and disease specific when it corresponds to *antibody* to the nuclear enzyme *topoisomerase* (anti–Scl-70); the presence of *anti–nuclear ribonucleoprotein antibodies* is also associated with the condition.

Vasculitis

Asymmetric polyarthritis may occur as a consequence of vasculitis, either from underlying rheumatoid disease (e.g., RA, SLE), one of the antineutrophil cytoplasmic antibody (ANCA)–associated conditions (e.g., *Wegener's granulomatosis*, *microscopic polyangiitis*, *Churg–Strauss disease*, and *necrotizing pauciimmune glomerulonephritis*), or ANCA-negative disease (e.g., *polyarteritis nodosum*). The resulting vascular compromise leads to multisystem injury and a broad array of symptoms. In persons with vasculitis unassociated with rheumatoid disease, arthralgias of large joints occur in up to 50% of cases, but true synovitis develops in only a minority of patients. Skin changes (e.g., palpable purpura, livedo reticularis, ulceration) ensue due to inflammatory injury to small dermal blood vessels (see Chapter 179). The lungs and the glomeruli are commonly involved in ANCA-associated disease, but the lungs are spared in polyarteritis nodosa. Patients with ANCA-associated

disease may present with hematuria, proteinuria, hemoptysis, or pulmonary nodularity. Other features of ischemic injury include abdominal pain and peripheral neuropathy (including mononeuritis multiplex, in which there is infarction of long individual peripheral nerves such as the peroneal, ulnar, or sural). The ANCA test is positive in many cases of vasculitis, but false-positive rates are high, necessitating tissue biopsy for definitive diagnosis (see later discussion).

Mixed Connective Tissue Disease

This designation describes an indistinct clinical syndrome that contains features of systemic sclerosis, lupus, and Sjögren's syndrome. With time, the presentation usually evolves into one of these three conditions, so that some investigators have concluded that this is not a unique condition but rather an early, nonspecific clinical presentation.

Psoriatic Arthritis

Psoriatic disease has both peripheral and axial forms. The peripheral form is asymmetric, oligoarticular, and often erosive. The distal interphalangeal (DIP) joints are most often affected, and the nails are pitted. *Sausage-shaped digits* and a "*pencil-in-cup*" radiologic appearance of the affected joints caused by erosion are found in advanced disease. Psoriatic skin changes (see Chapter 187) usually predate the onset of arthritis, often by months to years, but they can be subtle. The *spondylitic form* of the disease (associated with HLA-B27 positivity) may resemble ankylosing spondylitis, but the extent of spinal involvement is less.

Reiter's Syndrome

This condition is primarily a disease of young men. Oligoarthritis, nongonococcal *urethritis*, and ocular inflammation (i.e., *conjunctivitis*, *iritis*) are the defining features. The latter two features may be fleeting and nonconcurrent. Dermatologic features include *circinate balanitis* (shallow, painless ulcers of the glans penis) and *keratoderma blennorrhagicum* (a hyperkeratosis of the feet). Onset sometimes follows a recent bacillary dysentery or chlamydial urethritis, which has led to speculation that the condition represents an immunologic cross-response in genetically predisposed hosts. *HLA-B27* positivity is common and is believed to be related to the pathogenesis (i.e., shared antigenicity with the infectious agents). Joint involvement is asymmetric and affects the lower extremities. Heel pain with plantar fasciitis and calcaneal periostitis is distinctive. Mild spondylitis is common. ANA is absent.

Ankylosing Spondylitis

The presentation begins insidiously and affects young men most severely, producing inflammation of the spinal joints and connective tissue with subsequent calcification and ossification. Characteristic radiographic findings include *sacroiliitis* and a diffuse proliferation of *syndesmophytes* leading to spinal fusion. Peripheral arthritis does occur, more often in women. In men, it tends to develop only after spinal disease has become evident. Large proximal joints such as the hips or the knees are the predominant peripheral sites. *Uveitis* and *HLA-B27* positivity are found, but their presence is not necessary for the diagnosis to be made. The arthritis of inflammatory bowel disease has many of the same features (see also Chapter 147).

Polyarticular Gout

When gout presents polyarticularly as an acute process, it almost always occurs in patients with a prior history of monoarticular or oligoarticular gouty attacks, although hyperuricemia is not always present. The acute arthritis may be migratory but usually is confined to the lower extremities. The diagnosis is made by the finding of urate crystals in synovial fluid (see Chapter 145). A chronic arthritis occurs in patients with tophaceous disease. Acute attacks may be superimposed (see Chapter 158).

Pseudogout

Like gout, pseudogout is mostly an acute monoarticular disease, but on occasion the presentation is polyarticular. Patients are usually elderly, with degenerative disease of the knees. The finding of *calcium pyrophosphate* crystals in the synovial fluid is diagnostic, although *cartilage calcification* can be seen on radiography. A subacute form, referred to as "pseudorheumatoid" arthritis, has been described, characterized by morning stiffness, synovial thickening, an elevated erythrocyte sedimentation rate (ESR), and low titers of RF.

Gonococcal Arthritis

This form of bacterial arthritis is most likely to present in polyarticular fashion. Fever is usually present, and a *papulovesicular rash* indicative of disseminated disease develops in about two thirds of cases. Initially, the patient may have diffuse polyarticular symptoms, and signs of tenosynovitis may be found in the wrists, fingers, ankles, and toes. These manifestations are followed by a purulent arthritis in a limited number of joints, usually confined to the wrists, knees, or ankles (see Chapter 137).

Acute Rheumatic Fever

Rheumatic fever causes an acute migratory polyarthritis if streptococcal infection is not treated. The abrupt onset of arthritis and fever are the predominant manifestations in adults. Both synovitis and periarticular inflammation occur, especially in the knees and ankles. Erythema of the overlying skin may be noted. Anti–DNAase B titers are elevated.

Lyme Disease

Lyme disease may begin with migratory polyarthralgias and progress about 6 months after infection in untreated patients to attacks of asymmetric oligoarthritis in large joints (especially the knees). Later, a chronic monoarticular or oligoarticular arthritis may follow. The knees are a common site of chronic involvement. *Erythema chronica migrans*, the diagnostic annular red lesion at the site of the tick bite, occurs in 50% to 80% of cases during the early phase of illness. The diagnosis of late disease can be difficult because serologic testing is imprecise (see later discussion and also Chapter 160).

Acute Viral Hepatitis B

Hepatitis B and other viral infections may present with an immune polyarthritis, often in conjunction with urticaria. The condition is symmetric, affecting the proximal joints of the hands. Onset in hepatitis B is during the preicteric phase. The condition clears spontaneously (see also Chapter 70).

Subacute Bacterial Endocarditis

Endocarditis can produce an immune-mediated polyarthritis similar to that noted with hepatitis B. Fever, petechiae, splinter hemorrhages, heart murmur, and hematuria may be seen.

Sarcoidosis

This granulomatous inflammatory disease can present with an acute arthritis of the knees, wrists, PIP joints, and ankles, accompanied by fever, simulating an infectious arthritis. Erythema nodosum, hilar adenopathy, and periarticular involvement help to differentiate the condition from other etiologies. A destructive arthritis develops in a few persons; it is asymmetric and relapsing.

Clinical Presentation: Noninflammatory Arthritides

These conditions produce joint pain with few of the manifestations of inflammation, although sometimes a small effusion or mild synovial thickening may be noted.

Osteoarthritis

The arthritis of degenerative joint disease typically presents as deep, aching joint pain that is aggravated by motion and weight bearing and by periods of inactivity. The involved joint can be enlarged as a result of osteophyte formation, but swelling is usually inconsequential because soft-tissue involvement and inflammation are minimal. In later stages, pain occurs on motion and at rest in conjunction with stiffness. Nocturnal pain after vigorous activity is common. Patients with advanced disease have pain on weight bearing and joint instability. Examination often reveals crepitus and discomfort on movement of the joint. Occasionally, slight warmth is noted in severely affected weight-bearing joints, but erythema and marked warmth are absent. Limitation of motion, malalignment, and bony protuberances from spurs are frequent findings. The joints most commonly affected include the DIP joints of the hands (with formation of Heberden's nodes), the MPC joint at the base of the thumb, hips, knees, and cervical and lumbosacral vertebral joints.

Hypertrophic Pulmonary Osteoarthropathy

This condition is associated with diffuse bony pain in the lower extremities that is worsened by dependency. New bone formation and periostosis are the source of discomfort. Articular and periarticular symptoms may be encountered. *Clubbing* is a hallmark, although it is not readily evident in about 25% of cases. Intrapulmonary disease is an important precipitant (see Chapter 45).

Hypothyroidism

Thyroid dysfunction severe enough to cause myxedema is associated with symmetric peripheral joint swelling that can mimic RA clinically, but the white blood cell count in the joint fluid is low, and no clinical signs of inflammation are present. Nonarticular neuromuscular symptoms include myalgias and hand pain related to carpal tunnel syndrome.

Amyloidosis

Synovial infiltration due to overproduction of immunoglobulin light chains can cause swelling of large joints in a symmetric distribution. Onset is gradual. An immunologic cause of arthropathy may be suspected, but the joint fluid shows no signs of inflammation or immune hyperreactivity. Concurrent involvement of skin, heart, liver, kidney, and peripheral nerves is characteristic. Carpal tunnel syndrome may be present.

Sickle Cell Disease

Sometimes, a 2- to 3-week noninflammatory arthropathy develops affecting large joints. Swelling, tenderness, and effusion predominate. The synovial fluid is noninflammatory.

Clinical Presentation: Nonarticular Disease

Polymyalgia Rheumatica

The disease polymyalgia rheumatica (PMR) develops gradually over weeks to months. Pain and stiffness of periarticular structures of the neck and shoulders are the presentation in two thirds of cases, with hip and thigh involvement accounting for the other one third. Many patients have both shoulder and thigh involvement. Morning stiffness and pain with movement are highly characteristic; muscle strength is unimpaired. Synovitis has been documented histologically; muscle biopsy specimens are usually normal or show minor inflammatory infiltrates. Sometimes, low-grade fever, weight loss, and fatigue precede the onset of musculoskeletal symptoms. The condition is usually symmetric, but if it is asymmetric, it may be mistaken for shoulder bursitis or hip arthritis. Most patients are elderly. The association with cranial arteritis makes this an important condition to recognize. Marked elevation of the ESR is characteristic. No serologic abnormalities are found (see also Chapter 161).

Myositis

Myositis of any type may present as musculoskeletal pain and be confused with polyarthritis, although weakness is typically more prominent than pain. *Polymyositis* is the prototypical inflammatory muscle disease, characterized by proximal muscle weakness, soreness, and elevated levels of muscle enzymes. It may present as *dermatomyositis* in the elderly. *Eosinophilia–myalgia* syndrome is a serious myositis observed in association with the ingestion of L-tryptophan preparations. Marked peripheral eosinophilia, muscle weakness and pain, and serum aldolase elevations comprise the initial presentation. Skin induration, pulmonary infiltrates, cardiac rhythm disturbances, and peripheral neuropathy may ensue. The risk of malignancy is significantly increased in biopsy-proven myositis, particularly for dermatomyositis (relative risk, 2.4) and a bit less so for polymyositis. In most instances the malignancy is found to be concurrent or develops within 3 years. A wide array of malignancies is found. Screening for malignancy might be undertaken with slightly increased urgency in persons with myositis but should be based on standard criteria (see Chapter 3).

Fibromyalgia Syndrome (Fibrositis, Fibromyositis)

This syndrome occurs predominantly in women. An inflammatory mechanism has been suspected (hence the "itis" designation) but never demonstrated. Characteristic manifestations include morning stiffness worsened by changes in the weather and heavy exercise, fatigue caused by disordered sleep, and tenderness at multiple symmetric *tender points* on the torso and limbs, concentrated in the upper back and the neck. The

musculoskeletal discomfort is typically diffuse and poorly localized, but exacerbations caused by extremes of joint motion may produce pain referable to the joints. All hematologic and serologic parameters are normal (see also Chapter 159).

Reflex Sympathetic Dystrophy Syndrome

This often confusing and incompletely understood condition causes diffuse musculoskeletal discomfort, swelling, weakness, and limitation of motion. A single limb is affected, usually an arm. The limb is swollen and the skin shiny, often dusky in appearance, and cool to the touch. Pain can be severe and burning. Periarticular structures are especially tender. Preceding trauma accounts for 50% of cases. A vasomotor mechanism is postulated.

DIFFERENTIAL DIAGNOSIS (1,3,5,7,11,13–16)

The causes of polyarticular complaints can be divided into articular and nonarticular categories, and these can be subdivided into inflammatory and noninflammatory conditions (see Table 146.1).

WORKUP (1–7,9,1–13,16–29)

Overall Strategy

The initial assessment of the patient who presents with multiple joint symptoms is facilitated by addressing the following questions:

1. Is the underlying disease process inflammatory or noninflammatory?
2. Is the problem systemic or focal?
3. Is it truly articular or periarticular?
4. Is vital organ function or joint integrity endangered?

In the vast majority of cases, the answers to these questions can be provided by a careful history and physical examination, supplemented by a few carefully selected blood tests and/or radiographic studies suggested by the clinical picture. It is important to keep in mind that test interpretation in the workup of polyarticular disease can be especially problematic if pretest probability (derived from history and physical examination findings) is ignored. A number of commonly ordered serologic tests useful in the diagnosis of rheumatoid disease are very sensitive but nonspecific. A positive test in itself does not constitute a diagnosis (which in most rheumatoid diseases is based primarily on clinical features; see Tables 146.2 and 146.3) nor does it necessarily predict the future development of disease (see later discussion). Routinely ordering an "arthritis panel" of blood and serologic tests without attention to pretest probability is wasteful and risks the generation of false-positive results and errors in diagnosis (see Chapter 2). The time spent obtaining a careful history and performing a focused physical examination is well worth the effort when evaluating polyarticular complaints.

A note of caution is indicated when using clinical data and official diagnostic criteria to determine pretest probability. The official diagnostic criteria for many rheumatoid diseases, although heavily weighted toward clinical findings (see Tables 146.2 and 146.3), were established to maximize diagnostic specificity, being intended primarily for use in research and epidemiologic studies. When applied to individual patients

TABLE 146.3

CONDITIONS ASSOCIATED WITH A POSITIVE ANTINUCLEAR ANTIBODY TEST

Connective Tissue Disease
  Systemic lupus erythematosus
  Drug-induced lupus
  Rheumatoid arthritis
  Sjögren's syndrome
  Systemic sclerosis
  Mixed connective tissue disease

Nonrheumatic Autoimmune Disease
  Hashimoto's thyroiditis
  Grave's disease
  Autoimmune hepatitis
  Primary biliary cirrhosis
  Primary sclerosing cholangitis

Infectious Disease
  HIV infection
  Hepatitis C

No Disease
  Advancing age

Adapted from Shmerling R. Autoantibodies in systemic lupus erythematosus—there before you know it. N Engl J Med 2003;349:1499, with permission.

(especially those with early-stage disease), these criteria may underestimate pretest probability because they emphasize the characteristic features of more-advanced stages.

History

Differentiating Articular from Nonarticular Disease

Patients complain of pain, stiffness, and loss of function and often confuse neuropathic pain, bone pain, or myalgias with arthritis. The physician should attempt to identify the anatomic basis of the symptoms by asking the patient to specify exactly where the pain is located, what aggravates it, and what functional loss has occurred. For the most part, the symptoms of joint disease are well localized to the joint and bear a logical relation to its use. Nonarticular disease rarely has a specifically articular location and does not produce loss of articular function, although range of motion may be affected to some degree. After the location of the process has been established, the underlying disease mechanism should be elucidated.

Differentiating Inflammatory from Noninflammatory Disease

One inquires into the characteristic hallmarks of inflammation: redness, warmth, soft-tissue swelling, and tenderness. If such symptoms are localized to and encompass an entire joint, one has excellent presumptive evidence for synovitis and an inflammatory process. It is important not to mistake tenderness in a segment of the joint or a small effusion as evidence of inflammation. The response to antiinflammatory agents is sometimes useful for differentiation, although most nonprescription agents, such as aspirin and other nonsteroidal antiinflammatory drugs (NSAIDs), also have analgesic activity that may provide nonspecific relief. Patients with RA reach for their

aspirin as soon as they awaken and clearly feel worse if they miss a dose. The response in patients with osteoarthritis is much less dramatic.

Elucidating a Specific Cause and Assessing Impact

The basic determinations of site and disease process help to narrow the differential diagnosis and enable a more focused consideration. Attention to other elements of the history, such as the distribution of involved joints, associated symptoms (including those suggesting systemic disease), and age and gender, facilitate identification of the cause.

By Distribution and Temporal Pattern. These are of considerable diagnostic value, so that careful inquiry about all the joints affected and the sequence of involvement is necessary. Problems that at first appear monoarticular or asymmetric may turn out to be polyarticular or symmetric on further questioning. Several patterns are quite suggestive. Symmetric noninflammatory involvement of the PIP and DIP joints, without MCP or wrist involvement and without morning stiffness, argues for osteoarthritis. Asymmetric inflammatory disease of these joints points to psoriatic arthritis. Symmetric inflammatory involvement of the MCP, PIP, carpal, or metatarsophalangeal joints supports a diagnosis of rheumatoid disease. Bilateral heel pain suggests Reiter's syndrome and the other spondyloarthropathies, as does back pain. Hip and shoulder girdle symptoms in an elderly patient with noninflammatory, nonarticular disease provide strong presumptive evidence for polymyalgia, whereas a vague distribution in conjunction with the presence of trigger points supports a diagnosis of fibromyalgia.

The temporal pattern deserves attention. A chronic, subacute, additive process is consistent with rheumatoid disease. The sudden, explosive onset of symmetric polyarthritis suggests an acute hypersensitivity reaction, such as that seen with early hepatitis B infection or penicillin allergy. A migratory pattern raises the possibilities of rheumatic fever, disseminated gonococcemia, Reiter's syndrome, and Lyme disease, among others.

By Associated Symptoms. Associated symptoms aid in the diagnosis and may provide evidence for systemic involvement. A careful review of systems is essential. *Morning stiffness* is very suggestive of rheumatoid disease, which produces maximal stiffness after inactivity. In contrast, osteoarthritis is characterized by maximal symptoms with use. If some stiffness occurs with rest in osteoarthritis, it passes quickly with activity. The acute onset of fever points to an infectious origin or a marked hypersensitivity reaction, whereas low-grade fever may herald the onset of rheumatoid disease. The development of a *rash* may be diagnostic for such conditions as SLE, gonococcemia, Lyme disease, and vasculitis (see later discussion). New onset of *Raynaud's phenomenon* raises the possibility of scleroderma, SLE, or RA. A history of chronic or bloody *diarrhea* suggests inflammatory bowel disease. Symptoms of *urethritis* and *conjunctivitis* are suggestive of Reiter's syndrome. *Sleep disorder* and *chronic fatigue* point to fibromyalgia. Chronically *dry mouth* and *dry eyes* suggest Sjögren's syndrome, a common accompaniment of RA. Systemic involvement with SLE is evidenced by reports of nasopharyngeal ulcers, pleuritic chest pain, or mental status changes.

By Age and Gender. Patients with SLE and RA are predominantly women, whereas those with Reiter's syndrome are predominantly men. The onset of rheumatic fever or ankylosing spondylitis nearly always occurs before age 40 years. The peak incidence for SLE is in the premenopausal period, although later onset is not rare. The incidence of RA is less dependent on age, with new onset occurring in elderly as well as young persons. Gout in women is mainly a postmenopausal disease; in men, it occurs at all adult ages. SLE is particularly common among black women.

By Severity. Severity and effect on daily activity help to assess the functional significance in addition to the underlying cause. Joint pain that awakens the patient at night indicates severe arthritis; alternatively, it may signify a bony or neuropathic process. Marked daily fatigue, the need for afternoon naps, weight loss, and fever all suggest active systemic illness. The assessment of the functional impact must take into account not only the severity of the condition, but also the patient's premorbid level of activity and attitudes toward work and pain.

Past Medical History and Family History. Recurrent attacks and a genetic propensity are characteristic of many conditions. Gout may present as polyarthritis, but more often one uncovers a prior history of podagra or another form of acute monoarthritis in a lower extremity. A history of travel or residence in an area endemic for Lyme disease, in addition to a history of recent tick bite, should be elicited. The spondyloarthropathies, gout, and the Heberden nodes of osteoarthritis all have a familial preponderance, which should be explored.

Social History. Any psychosocial stresses should be elicited, especially in persons presenting with vague, diffuse, poorly localized musculoskeletal symptoms free of characteristic inflammatory manifestations but accompanied by disordered sleep and marked fatigue, all of which are suggestive of fibromyalgia syndrome and are sometimes found in depression (see Chapter 227) or somatization disorder (see Chapter 230).

Physical Examination

The physical examination is basically a continuation of the same approach, with documentation of the pattern and type of joint involvement and the nature of any extraarticular disease. The myriad extraarticular manifestations of the arthritic diseases make a detailed general physical examination mandatory. Certain aspects deserve emphasis.

Skin and Integument

Important dermal clues to underlying cause include the malar rash of SLE, annular erythema chronica migrans of Lyme disease, papulovesicular lesions with a necrotic center of disseminated gonococcemia, nail pitting and scaling of psoriasis, urticarial lesions of hepatitis B infection, and palpable purpura, ulceration, or livedo reticularis of vasculitis. In a patient with suspected Reiter's syndrome, the glans penis should be checked for the ulcers of circinate balanitis and the heels for the hypertrophic changes of keratoderma blennorrhagicum. One should carefully palpate around the elbows, Achilles tendons, and pinnae and search for rheumatoid nodules and tophi, which are specific indicators of RA and gout, respectively. The nails should be examined for pitting and clubbing. Nail pitting adjacent to erosive DIP arthritis can justify a diagnosis of psoriatic arthritis in the absence of any skin psoriasis. Fingertip atrophy with healed or active ulcers suggests severe Raynaud's phenomenon and should prompt a search for the calcinosis, subungual telangiectases, and skin tightening of scleroderma. The

presence of the red, tender, subcutaneous lesions of erythema nodosum raises the possibilities of sarcoidosis and inflammatory bowel disease. Dry, doughy skin and the loss of the outer third of the eyebrows are signs of hypothyroidism.

Head, Ears, Nose, Throat, Neck, Lungs, Heart

The anterior eye should be checked for conjunctivitis and iritis, which are suggestive of Reiter's syndrome and spondylitis (see Chapter 199), and the posterior eye for retinal hemorrhages, exudates, and ischemic lesions, which are consistent with systemic lupus and vasculitis. "Cotton-wool" exudates are the most common eye lesion in SLE. The oral and nasal mucosa should be examined for ulcers, which if painful suggest SLE and if painless suggest Reiter's syndrome. Thyroid evaluation may reveal a goiter. The chest is examined for signs of effusion, pleuritis, and pericarditis. Pleural and pericardial rubs are found in RA and SLE. Heart murmurs characterize rheumatic fever and SLE, mitral valve murmurs sometimes occur in SLE, and aortic regurgitant murmurs occur in the spondyloarthropathies. The abdominal examination includes checking for splenomegaly, which is found in a variety of rheumatic diseases, including RA and SLE.

Musculoskeletal Examination

One checks for signs of serositis, noninflammatory articular disease, and periarticular disease. As emphasized earlier, inflammatory joint disease involves the entire joint; tenderness, warmth, redness, soft-tissue swelling, and often an effusion are present. In contrast, noninflammatory disease is usually associated with only focal tenderness and few, if any, signs of inflammation, although a small noninflammatory effusion may be present. The distribution of disease is noted, as are any mechanical abnormalities, such as limitation of motion, instability, subluxation, or tendon injury.

A careful look at the periarticular tissues (tendons, bursae, muscles) is also indicated. Bursitis and tendinitis commonly mimic arthritis. Subacromial bursitis and bicipital tendinitis can be confused with shoulder joint disease (see Chapter 150); lateral epicondylitis (tennis elbow) and olecranon bursitis with elbow joint disease (see Chapter 153); trochanteric bursitis with hip disease (see Chapter 151); and anserine bursitis with knee disease (see Chapter 152).

Muscle soreness and proximal muscle weakness raise the question of a myositis. Checking for characteristic *tender points* on the torso (see Chapter 159) is indicated in patients with suspected fibromyalgia syndrome.

Another important type of periarticular disease is that manifested by "frozen" joints and flexion contractures. Severe limitation of motion may occur in an intrinsically normal joint. Disuse because of neurologic disease or periarticular pain may lead to tightening of periarticular fibrous tissue and secondary contractures. The clinical presentation can be mistaken for that of arthritis, but normal radiographic findings in a joint and a lack of indicators of inflammatory arthritis, plus an awareness of a predisposing illness, lead to the correct diagnosis.

If a patient has hand stiffness or pain, a valuable screening test for finger joint and tendinous disease is *"curling."* The patient is asked to extend the MCP joints and then maximally flex the PIP and DIP joints but not to make a fist. Curling is normal if a patient can bring the fingertips into apposition with the palm. Any disease of the PIP or DIP joints interferes with curling, as does any inflammation along the dorsal extensor tendons.

For patients with a suspected spondyloarthropathy, *Schober's test* provides a useful assessment of lumbar mobility.

Two marks are made on the patient's back while the patient is standing: one at the level of the posterior iliac spine and the other exactly 10 cm above the first. When the patient bends forward maximally, the two marks should be at least 15 cm apart. An abnormal Schober's test result is nonspecific, but if an abnormal result is combined with other evidence for a spondyloarthropathy, it can advance the diagnosis.

Neurologic Examination

Evidence of peripheral neuropathy is sought by assessing motor and sensory function in the extremities, and the mental status is carefully evaluated in patients with suspected SLE and HIV infection (central nervous system involvement is a sign of serious disease).

Laboratory Studies

Approach to Testing

A large number of laboratory tests, both simple and esoteric, are routinely used in the evaluation of polyarthritic symptoms. Panels of tests are sometimes offered by laboratories as a means of "screening" for arthritic conditions. They range from a set of basic studies (e.g., ANA and RF titers, uric acid level, ESR) to elaborate panels that may include testing for anti-dsDNA, anti-Ro, anti-La, anti–Scl-70, anti-Sm, and antiribonucleoprotein. All such batteries of tests have been found to be wasteful, of little use diagnostically when ordered in the absence of clinical evidence, and a source of potentially misleading results. Perhaps it is the desire to "rule out" disease in persons with vague clinical findings that drives such testing (negative predictive value is high), but pretest probability is already very high and not improved much by further testing. The net result of such behavior is a high rate of false-positive diagnoses (especially of connective tissue disease), which can be especially harmful both psychologically and medically.

Repeated studies of workup for polyarticular complaints and rheumatoid disease demonstrate and expert panels reaffirm that the best means of diagnosing or ruling out "must-not-miss" conditions is a careful history and physical examination, complemented by thoughtfully selected tests that specifically address conditions for which at least some clinical evidence is present. Diagnostic confusion that persists at the end of the physical examination is rarely resolved by "pan-scanning" for arthritic disease. Careful patient and test selection and interpretation are especially important, particularly in the elderly because the frequency of abnormal test results in the absence of disease increases with age, especially with the most commonly ordered studies (e.g., ESR, uric acid level, ANA, and RF titers); the false-positive rate can be as high as 90%. Test selection is guided by whether the clinical assessment suggests inflammatory or noninflammatory disease.

Suspected Inflammatory Articular Disease

In this setting, a determination of the *ESR* provides useful but nonspecific confirmation of inflammatory disease activity and can be followed as a measure of disease activity. A markedly elevated reading (e.g., >60 mm/hr) suggests considerable inflammatory activity. A normal ESR in the setting of active joint symptoms reduces the probability of active inflammatory pathophysiology. However, the ESR is a relatively poor test for the detection of inflammatory disease that is in remission. *C-reactive protein* provides information similar to that of ESR and may be considered when ESR is unremarkable

yet inflammatory articular disease is still suspected. A *complete blood cell count* can be obtained at the same time to check for hematologic involvement by the underlying disease process.

If symptoms are acute and new in onset, then tests for infectious causes should be considered. *Blood cultures* are essential if endocarditis or disseminated gonococcemia is suspected. The available *Lyme antibody* assays lack specificity, so their results are difficult to interpret (see Chapter 160) and less useful than a careful clinical assessment. DNA-based assays with polymerase chain reaction technology are not widely available and are very expensive. Liver function testing (e.g., the measurement of *aminotransferases*) may help to confirm suspected viral hepatitis; hepatitis serology should follow if serum liver chemistries are abnormal.

If the duration of symptoms is more than 6 weeks, then the possibility of rheumatoid disease and other chronic forms of inflammatory joint disease need to be explored further, especially if the patient has systemic symptoms.

Rheumatoid Factor. Rheumatoid factor (RF) is a helpful test if the pretest probability of RA is intermediate and further supporting evidence is sought. In general, 70% to 80% of all patients meeting strict criteria for RA are RF-positive. The higher the RF titer, the more likely is the diagnosis of RA. RF negativity does not rule out RA; 25% of patients with RA are RF-negative. On the other hand, RF positivity does not rule in RA; it also occurs in other inflammatory conditions (e.g., SLE, subacute bacterial endocarditis, vasculitis, and even viral infection). Moreover, 5% to 15% of "normal" persons (the percentage increases with age) are RF-positive.

Antinuclear Antibody. ANA testing by indirect immunofluorescence is very sensitive (99%) for the diagnosis of SLE but lacking in specificity (50% to 85%). The test result can also be positive in other forms of connective tissue disease, nonrheumatic autoimmune conditions, infectious conditions, and even old age (see Table 146.3). The higher the ANA titer, the more likely is the diagnosis of lupus. A titer of 1:40 is usually listed as the criterion for a positive test result, but such a cutoff produces a 35% false-positive rate in a general medical setting. An ANA titer criterion of 1:160 reduces the false-positive rate to 5% while reducing sensitivity only minimally (to 95%). Titers of ANA fluctuate with time but do not necessarily parallel disease activity and typically predate the onset of symptoms by years. Patients testing positive in the absence of defining clinical manifestations should be designated as *"ANA-positive"* rather than labeled as having a connective tissue disease, which risks subjecting them to unnecessary systemic glucocorticosteroid therapy (an all-to-frequent occurrence in everyday clinical practice).

The ANA test is most useful in the setting of inflammatory polyarthritis and systemic symptoms. ANA negativity rules out SLE; however, the test is not specific enough for a positive result to rule in the condition, but it would justify further testing. As with RA, no single finding or test is diagnostic for SLE; the presence of several characteristic features is necessary to confirm the diagnosis (Table 146.4).

Because ANA positivity predates the development of clinical disease by years, it might at first glance be thought that ANA screening could improve early diagnosis. However, neither the presence of autoantibodies nor their pattern reliably predicts the development of clinical disease. Moreover, there are no known treatments for preclinical SLE or other ANA-positive diseases that will alter the clinical course in asymptomatic persons. Therefore, *ANA testing is not recommended*

TABLE 146.4

CRITERIA FOR DIAGNOSIS OF SYSTEMIC LUPUS ERYTHEMATOSUS

Malar rash
Discoid rash
Photosensitivity
Oral or nasopharyngeal ulceration
Nonerosive arthritis
Pleuritis or pericarditis
Persistent proteinuria or casts
Seizures or psychosis
Hemolytic anemia, leukopenia, or thrombocytopenia
Antinuclear antibody
Anti-DNA antibody, anti–Smith antigen antibody, or
    false-positive serologic test for syphilis.

The presence of any four or more criteria is necessary for a diagnosis of definite SLE, although many authorities accept fewer criteria in clinical practice, particularly if an antibody test result is positive.
Adapted from Tan EM, Cohen AS, Fries JF, et al. The 1982 revised criteria for the classification of systemic lupus erythematosus. Arthritis Rheum 1982;25:1271, with permission.

in the absence of supporting clinical evidence; the diagnosis of connective tissue disease still depends largely on the presence of characteristic clinical features.

Follow-up Testing If Antinuclear Antibody Test Is "Positive."
Because ANA positivity is a nonspecific finding, additional testing (Table 146.5) may be required, but only for patients with both a positive test result and supportive clinical findings. The specific nuclear constituents represented by the ANA titer function as convenient autoantigens. Testing for antibodies against these antigens can enhance diagnostic specificity but should not

TABLE 146.5

SPECTRUM OF ANTINUCLEAR ANTIBODIES IN PERSONS WITH A POSITIVE ANTINUCLEAR ANTIBODY TEST

Antibody	Significance
Anti-dsDNA	Common and specific for SLE; correlates with disease activity and with nephritis
Anti-Sm	Specific for SLE, but found in only 30% of cases; with or without correlation with disease activity
Anti-Ro	Strongly associated with Sjögren's syndrome; also appears in SLE
Anti-La	Present in Sjögren's syndrome; also in SLE (? reduced risk of nephritis)
Anti-RNP	Present in scleroderma and defines mixed connective tissue disease; present in SLE
Anti–Scl-70	Specific for systemic sclerosis, but sensitivity is low (20%)

dsDNA, double-stranded DNA; SLE, systemic lupus erythematosus; Sm, Smith antigen; RNP, ribonucleoprotein.
Adapted from Shmerling R. Autoantibodies in systemic lupus erythematosus—there before you know it. N Engl J Med 2003;349:1499, with permission.

be performed in the absence of characteristic clinical features (i.e., a reasonable pretest probability is required); otherwise, poor likelihood ratios (ratio of true positives to false positives) are likely to result. Some of these antinuclear antibodies, although considered characteristic of particular rheumatoid diseases, also appear transiently during the course of others in cascade-like fashion. This pathophysiology explains the potential for considerable overlap in antinuclear antibody findings and reemphasizes the importance of ordering and interpreting antinuclear antibody tests in the context of clinical findings.

Antibody to native dsDNA occurs in up to 70% of patients with SLE, is specific for the condition, and is also predictive of an increased risk for nephritis; it predates the onset of symptoms by nearly 2 years. Testing for anti-dsDNA is used to confirm the diagnosis of SLE in patients with suspected disease and ANA positivity. *Antibody to Smith antigen* is similarly specific but is found in only 30% of patients with SLE; correlation with disease activity is uncertain. *Anti-RNP* is a defining serologic finding of *mixed connective tissue disease*, but it is also found in scleroderma and in about 18% of lupus patients.

Antibody to Scl-70 (a nuclear topoisomerase) is highly specific for *systemic sclerosis*, but its sensitivity is low (20%). In *Sjögren's syndrome*, anti-Ro and anti-La antibodies provide 60% to 70% sensitivity and greater than 90% specificity; these antibodies are also seen in nearly half of patients with SLE and are among the first signs of autoantibody formation. *Lip biopsy* is the definitive test for Sjögren's syndrome, but it is often not necessary in the context of characteristic clinical and serologic findings.

Synovial Fluid Analysis. The analysis of joint fluid can be very useful if a joint effusion is present and the diagnosis remains undetermined. One seeks to differentiate between inflammatory and noninflammatory disease (see Chapter 145) and also to check for crystal-induced arthropathy and investigate any suspected infection (see Chapter 145). A white blood cell count greater than 2,000/mm^3 with greater than 75% polymorphonuclear leukocytes supports the presence of inflammation; a cell count less than 1,000/mm^3 indicates noninflammatory disease. A count between 1,000 and 2,000/mm^3 is ambiguous. Often, one obtains a synovial fluid white blood cell count of 5,000 to 20,000/mm^3 without crystals, bacteria, or other distinctive attributes, which allows for little more than a designation of inflammatory arthritis, type unspecified.

Serum Uric Acid. Serum urate levels are obtained unnecessarily in most arthritis patients and too often serve as the primary basis for a diagnosis of gout. The definitive diagnosis is best made by observing urate crystals in the synovial fluid. A normal serum uric acid level does not rule out the diagnosis of gout, nor does an elevated level rule it in.

Radiography. Plain films are usually of minimal diagnostic value in the early stages of inflammatory polyarthritis, showing little more than soft-tissue swelling. However, expertly reviewed *hand films* may reveal characteristic features of early joint injury from rheumatoid arthritis and facilitate diagnosis and management. In addition, early *sacroiliac films* are of value in suspected spondyloarthropathy because they may reveal sacroiliitis, a diagnostic finding. Another early radiologic change in spondyloarthropathy is squaring of the superior and inferior margins of the vertebral bodies; only later do prominent syndesmophytes appear. Films obtained during later stages may manifest more-characteristic bony changes and help to gauge disease progression.

Urinalysis and Routine Chemistries. Urinalysis is essential to screen for glomerular injury in rheumatoid disease and vasculitis. Routine serum chemistries are less rewarding, although assessing renal function by measuring *blood urea nitrogen* and *creatinine* levels is indicated in patients with proteinuria or hematuria, as is consideration of vasculitis and a check of the serum for *antineutrophil cytoplasmic antibodies.*

Antineutrophil Cytoplasmic Antibodies (ANCA). This test is useful when there is clinical suspicion of an ANCA-associated vasculitis as the cause of inflammatory polyarticular complaints. Suggestive clinical features include renal dysfunction (creatinine >2.0 mg/dL, hematuria, red cell casts), pulmonary pathology (nodularity, hemoptysis), chronic upper airway disease (sinusitis, necrosis), neurologic deficits (peripheral neuropathy, mononeuritis multiplex), and skin lesions (palpable purpura, ulceration).

Careful patient selection is essential to avoid false-positive results, especially when the indirect immunofluorescence test is used (the enzyme-linked immunosorbent assay is more specific); cross-reactions with antigens not involved in vasculitis can produce false-positive test results, most commonly in persons with rheumatoid arthritis, HIV infection, tuberculosis, endocarditis, and monoclonal gammopathy. Consensus guidelines advise ordering only in the context of at least one suggestive clinical feature to reduce the number of false-positive results and the frequency of unnecessary testing and immunosuppressive treatment.

When the test is performed on persons who have at least one of the guideline features, sensitivity is 81%, specificity 98%, positive predictive value 54%, and negative predictive value 99%. With the use of this strategy, unnecessary testing and false positives are reduced by nearly 25% without any loss in the detection of true positives. ANCA testing is negative in other vasculitides (e.g., hypersensitivity vasculitis, temporal arteritis, polyarteritis nodosa). The staining pattern of the ANCA test result (*perinuclear* [*p*] vs. *cytoplasmic* [*c*]) helps to differentiate among the causes of ANCA-associated disease.

Tissue biopsy is required for confirmation of a positive test and definitive diagnosis because ANCA's false-positive rate remains high (46%), even with use of the guidelines. *Skin* is the most accessible site when rash is present; *kidney* biopsy is of high yield when there is evidence of renal involvement. Female patients, blacks, and those with evidence of severe kidney involvement are at an increased risk of resistance to initial treatment. Patients with respiratory tract disease and *anti-PR3 antibody* positivity have a greater chance of relapse than others.

Workup should proceed expeditiously because rapid progression is possible, especially if there is evidence of severe pulmonary or renal injury. Pending results, high-dose systemic steroids can be started.

HLA-B27 Testing. Although the prevalence of HLA-B27 antigen positivity in the seronegative spondyloarthropathies is high (approximately 90%), the specificity of the test is low. About 6% to 8% of normal persons also test positive, negating the utility of HLA-B27 testing.

Suspected Noninflammatory Polyarticular Disease

In osteoarthritis, *joint radiographic findings* are abnormal by the time the patient becomes symptomatic and can confirm the diagnosis. However, degenerative changes are commonly found in asymptomatic joints also. Films of long bones can be obtained to confirm hypertrophic osteoarthropathy, but the diagnosis can usually be made clinically by the presence of clubbing.

Suspected hypothyroidism can be confirmed by a *thyrotropin* determination.

Suspected Inflammatory Nonarticular Disease

When joint complaints are vague and muscular discomfort predominates, laboratory workup should focus on polymyalgia rheumatica, polymyositis, and eosinophilic–myalgia syndrome. Small-vessel vasculitis might also be considered when suggestive multisystem findings are part of the presentation (see prior discussion). Fibromyalgia is, in part, a diagnosis of exclusion, based on ruling out these other conditions.

Polymyalgia Rheumatica. The ESR should be measured in patients with clinical evidence for polymyalgia rheumatica. A high ESR supports the diagnosis; a low one reduces the probability. If headache, jaw claudication, visual disturbance, or a tender cranial artery is noted, then evaluation for *cranial arteritis* should proceed promptly (see Chapter 161).

Polymyositis. Workup begins with measuring ESR and serum *creatine phosphokinase* and, if markedly elevated, proceeding to a consideration of *muscle biopsy.*

Eosinophilic–Myalgia Syndrome. A *complete blood cell count* and *differential* are indicated in patients with suspected eosinophilia–myalgia; if florid peripheral eosinophilia is encountered, referral for skin and muscle biopsies is indicated.

Fibromyalgia. There are no laboratory tests specific to the condition; diagnosis is based on clinical findings and the ruling out of mimicking conditions. These patients are often mistakenly diagnosed as having lupus, especially if an ANA is obtained to rule out connective tissue disease and the result is "positive" (see prior discussion and Chapter 159).

Suspected Noninflammatory Nonarticular Disease

The diagnosis of reflex sympathetic dystrophy is predominantly clinical. Plain films of the hand may show a nonspecific but suggestive patchy osteopenia. There are no tests for fibromyalgia syndrome.

INDICATIONS FOR ADMISSION AND REFERRAL

The diagnosis of polyarticular arthritis may remain uncertain. With the exception of small-vessel vasculitis and septic arthritis due to bacteremia, the underlying conditions are not immediately life threatening, and the workup can take place in the outpatient setting during several visits. Short-term risk to the patient is posed primarily by extraarticular disease, especially that due to vasculitis and infection. If any evidence of bloodstream infection, vasculitis, or involvement of the eyes, lungs, heart, kidneys, or nervous system is found, hospitalization and consultation should be promptly considered. The same recommendation pertains to persons with severe constitutional symptoms (e.g., disabling fatigue, fever, weight loss). Rheumatologic consultation is also appropriate if a patient with less serious illness remains without a diagnosis after the initial evaluation has been completed, especially if autoimmune disease is suspected but not confirmed; an empiric trial of corticosteroids is *not* indicated. A timely referral for consultation with a well-trained rheumatologist is likely to be far more productive than exhaustive serologic testing, with its high risks of false-positive results and attendant adverse consequences.

SYMPTOMATIC THERAPY

Treatment should be etiologic (see Chapters 155 through 163), but the definitive diagnosis of an inflammatory polyarthritis may take time. Pending results, and provided infection has been ruled out, the patient bothered by symptoms of joint inflammation may be given either high-dose aspirin (up to twelve 325 mg tablets daily) or a generic NSAID preparation (e.g., 400 to 800 mg of ibuprofen four times daily). Empiric therapy with systemic glucocorticosteroids is not recommended, especially if the only manifestations are vague arthralgias and ANA positivity.

A.H.G.

Annotated Bibliography

1. American College of Rheumatology Ad Hoc Committee on Clinical Guidelines. Guidelines for the initial evaluation of the adult patient with acute musculoskeletal symptoms. Arthritis Rheum 1996;39:1. (*Evidence-based consensus guidelines, with emphasis on clinical manifestations.*)
2. Arbuckle MR, McClain MT, Rubertone MV, et al. Development of autoantibodies before the clinical onset of systemic lupus erythematosus. N Engl J Med. 2003;349:1526. (*Antibodies precede the onset of clinical disease but do not predict the development of clinical disease.*)
3. Arnett FC, Edworthy SM, Bloch DA, et al. The American Rheumatism Association 1987 revised criteria for the classification of rheumatoid arthritis. Arthritis Rheum 1988;31:315. (*A collaborative study, showing a sensitivity and a specificity for the official criteria of approximately 90%.*)
4. Buchbinder R, Forbes A, Hall S, et al. Incidence of malignant disease in biopsy-proven inflammatory myopathy: a population-based cohort study. Ann Intern Med 2001;1324:1087. (*Finds a relative risk of 2.4 in persons with dermatomyositis and a slightly lower rate for polymyositis.*)
5. Goldenberg DL. Fibromyalgia syndrome a decade later: what have we learned? Arch Intern Med 1999;159:777. (*An excellent summary of diagnosis and management for the generalist, with emphasis on the importance of underlying psychosocial factors to outcomes; 156 references.*)
6. Harler NM, Franck WA, Bress NM, et al. Acute polyarticular gout. Am J Med 1974;56:715. (*A study of this uncommon presentation of a very common disease.*)
7. Hochberg MC. Updating the American College of Rheumatology revised criteria for the classification of systemic lupus erythematosus. Arthritis Rheum 1997;40:1725. (*Consensus criteria that emphasize clinical features.*)
8. Keat A. Reiter's syndrome and reactive arthritis in perspective. N Engl J Med 1983;309:1606. (*An extensive review, including a discussion of joint manifestations.*)
9. Kozin F. Reflex sympathetic dystrophy. Bull Rheum Dis 1986;36:1. (*A good summary of pathophysiologic hypotheses and clinical manifestations.*)
10. Medsger TA. Tryptophan-induced eosinophilia–myalgia syndrome. N Engl J Med 1990;322:926. (*An editorial summarizing current understanding.*)
11. Plotz PH, Dalakas M, Leff RL, et al. Current concepts in idiopathic inflammatory myopathies. Ann Intern Med 1989;111:143. (*A comprehensive review, which includes useful discussions of polymyositis and dermatomyositis.*)
12. Savige J, Gillis D, Benson E, et al. International consensus statement on testing and reporting of antineutrophil cytoplasmic antibodies (ANCA). Am J Clin Pathol 1999;111:507. (*Suggested guidelines for patient selection, with emphasis on clinical features.*)
13. Steere AC. Lyme disease. N Engl J Med 2001;345:115. (*An authoritative review, including excellent photographs of erythema migrans; 100 references.*)
14. Stone JH. Polyarteritis nodosa. JAMA 2002;288:1632. (*An excellent clinical review in a grand-rounds format; 42 references.*)
15. Wolfe F, Smythe HA, Yunus MB, et al. The American College of Rheumatology 1990 criteria for the classification of fibromyalgia: the Multicenter Criteria Committee. Arthritis Rheum 1990;33:160. (*Consensus diagnostic criteria, pending the discovery of more-definitive diagnostic findings.*)
16. Mainardi CL. Approach to the patient with pain in more than one joint. In: Kelley WN. Textbook of internal medicine, 2nd ed. Philadelphia: Lippincott, 1993:1000. (*Provides a useful categorization of the differential diagnosis, which had been adapted for use in this chapter.*)
17. Brown SL, Hansen SL, Linguine JJ. Role of serology in the diagnosis of Lyme disease. JAMA 1999;282:62. (*A review of the test performance of commercially available serologic kits; finds great variability, low reproducibility, and disappointing sensitivity and specificity.*)
18. Hogan SL, Falk RJ, Chin H, et al. Predictors of relapse and treatment resistance in antineutrophil cytoplasmic antibody–associated small-vessel vasculitis. (Ann Intern Med 2005;143:621. (*An observational study; finds that being female, being black, or having severe kidney disease is predictive of poor response to treatment; respiratory involvement and anti-PR3 positivity predict relapse.*)
19. Homburger HA. Cascade testing for autoantibodies in connective tissue diseases. Mayo Clin Proc 1995;70:183. (*Presents the argument against unselective testing.*)
20. Juby AF, Davis P, McElhaney JE, et al. Prevalence of selected autoantibodies in different elderly subpopulations. Br J Rheumatol 1994;33:1121. (*There was increased prevalence with age; many individuals with positive test results show no signs of disease.*)
21. Juby AF, Johnston C, Davis P. Specificity, sensitivity, and diagnostic predictive value of selected laboratory-generated autoantibody profiles in patients with connective tissue diseases. J Rheumatol 1991;18:354. (*Presents data on test performance characteristics.*)
22. Kahn MA, Kahn MK. Diagnostic value of HLA-B27 testing in ankylosing spondylitis and Reiter's syndrome. Ann Intern Med 1982;96:70. (*The test is usually unnecessary.*)
23. Lichtenstein MJ, Pincus T. How useful are combinations of blood tests in "rheumatic panels" in diagnosis of rheumatic diseases? J Gen Intern Med 1987;3:435. (*Finds that a positive predictive value of only 34% leads to many false-positive results.*)
24. Mandel LA, Solomon DH, Smith EL, et al. Using antineutrophil cytoplasmic antibody testing to diagnose vasculitis. Arch Intern Med 2002;162:1509. (*The use of test-ordering guidelines helped to reduce unnecessary testing and false-positive rates by about 25% without compromising the detection of vasculitis.*)
25. Narain S, Richards HB, Satoh M, et al. Diagnostic accuracy for lupus and other systemic autoimmune diseases in the community setting. Arch Intern Med 2004;164:2435. (*Finds a high frequency of overdiagnosis and unnecessary steroid use.*)
26. Slater CA, Davis RB, Shmerling RH. Antinuclear antibody testing. A study in clinical utility. Arch Intern Med 1996;156:1421. (*The test was frequently ordered in low-probability situations; positive predictive value is very low in the setting of a low clinical probability for lupus.*)
27. Shmerling RH. Autoantibodies in systemic lupus erythematosus—there before you know it. N Engl J Med 2003;349:1499. (*Presents a very useful perspective on the pathophysiologic and diagnostic significance of these antibodies.*)
28. Tan EM, Feltkamp TE, Smolen JS, et al. Range of antinuclear antibodies in "healthy" individuals. Arthritis Rheum 1997;40:1601. (*Many normal persons have an elevated antinuclear antibody titer; increasing the cutoff for a positive result to 1:160 markedly reduces the false-positive rate without significantly compromising sensitivity.*)
29. Tan EM, Chan EK, Sullivan KF, et al. Antinuclear antibodies (ANAs). Clin Immunol Immunopathol 1988;47:121. (*A comprehensive review of their diagnostic meaning and pathophysiologic significance.*)

CHAPTER 147 ■ APPROACH TO THE PATIENT WITH BACK PAIN

Back pain is the second-most-frequent complaint in primary care practice and one of the leading causes of disability. Most back pain is caused by musculoligamentous strain, degenerative disk disease, or facet arthritis and responds to symptomatic treatment. Disk disease is often responsible for recurring mild discomfort of the low back and episodes of severe back pain with sciatica. Occasionally, back pain may result from problems originating outside of the spinal axis. Serious underlying problems such as tumor, infection, or vertebral compression fracture must be kept in mind. The prevalence of back pain requires that the primary physician be skilled in assessment and conservative management and knowledgeable about the indications for referral and surgery.

PATHOPHYSIOLOGY AND CLINICAL PRESENTATION (1–9)

Musculoligamentous Strain

Muscle fibers or distal ligamentous attachments of the paraspinal muscles may tear, usually at the iliac crest or lower lumbar/upper sacral region. Resultant bleeding and spasm cause local swelling and marked tenderness at the site of injury. The patient typically presents after a specific episode of bending, twisting, or lifting. The strain is usually severe and is associated with a feeling of something giving way in the lower back. The onset of pain in the lower lumbar area is immediate. Pain radiates across the low back, often to the buttock and upper thigh posteriorly. Radiation of pain into the lower leg is rare because usually no injury to the nerve roots has occurred.

Lumbar Disk Disease

The pathophysiology of disk disease remains incompletely understood but involves degenerative changes in the disk. It is believed that degeneration and attritional changes in the lower lumbar disks are caused by the concentration of stress at the lumbosacral level. Stresses resulting from the enormous longitudinal and sheer forces that are a consequence of upright posture are aggravated by bending strain. Injury, inflammation, weakening, and tear of the disk annulus may occur and lead to localized back pain (so-called *discogenic pain*). Pain receptors in the longitudinal ligaments probably mediate the recurring attacks of local back pain, which are nonradicular and most pronounced with prolonged sitting. Eventually, the disk may become so weakened that it bulges circumferentially beyond the disk interspace. Less often, a focal or asymmetric extension beyond the interspace, termed a disk *protrusion*, develops. Extreme extension of the disk beyond the interspace has been called *extrusion*. Historically, the term *herniation* has been used

to describe all these phenomena. It has been suggested that the use of the more specific terms will sharpen our understanding of the relationship between disk disease and pain syndromes. Regardless of the vocabulary, compression and irritation of a lower lumbar or upper sacral nerve root may result, and the radicular symptoms of *sciatica* develop.

Sciatica is the symptomatic hallmark of nerve root irritation. Disk protrusion or extrusion is present in 95% of cases. It presents as sharp or burning pain radiating down the posterior or lateral aspect of the leg to the ankle or foot (depending on the specific nerve root involved). The pain may be worsened by cough, Valsalva's maneuver, or sneezing, and it is often accompanied by paresthesias and numbness. Weakness may also develop in the areas supplied by the irritated nerve root.

More than 95% of disk protrusions and extrusions occur at L-4 to L-5 or L-5 to S-1, with the L-5 and S-1 nerve roots affected, respectively. With S-1 root irritation, pain, numbness, and paresthesias involve the buttock, posterior thigh, calf, lateral aspect of the ankle and foot, and lateral toes. Calf atrophy can occur, the ankle jerk can be diminished or absent, and plantar flexion weakness may be noted. With L-5 root compression, pain radiates to the dorsum of the foot and great toe, and the only neurologic deficits may be extensor weakness of the great toe and numbness of the L-5 area on the dorsum of the foot at the base of the great toe (Fig. 147.1). In the rarer instance of high lumbar disk disease, pain radiates to the anterior thigh, and the knee jerk may be diminished or absent. Quadriceps atrophy and weakness may be found.

With lower lumbar disk disease, especially disk extrusion, lumbar paraspinal muscle spasm often occurs and limits lumbar motions. A list away from the side of the disk extrusion—so-called sciatic scoliosis—may develop, and often tenderness of the lower lumbar spine and sciatic notch is present. *Straight leg raising* (SLR) on the affected side is limited by back and leg pain that increases on ankle dorsiflexion at the extreme of the maneuver. With upper lumbar disk disease, reverse SLR often reproduces the back and anterior thigh pain (see later discussion).

The clinical course may begin with a several-year history of recurring mild mid-low back pain related to minor back strain, with symptoms clearing spontaneously within a few days. Attacks typically increase in frequency and severity at intervals of several months to several years. Finally, an episode of persistent pain accompanied by sciatica develops, often triggered by a seemingly trivial stress (e.g., bending over in the shower to pick up the soap).

Spinal Stenosis

This often-overlooked etiology is becoming better appreciated as an important cause of chronic low back and lower extremity complaints. It occurs predominantly in elderly individuals with

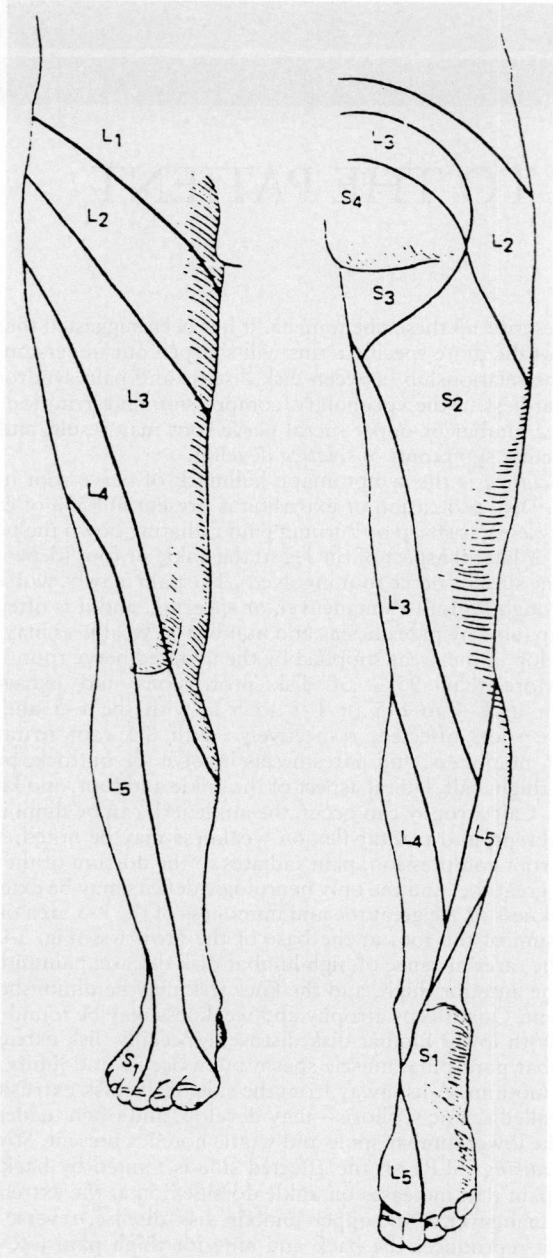

FIGURE 147.1. Dermatomes of the lower extremity. (From Finneson BE. Low back pain. Philadelphia: Lippincott, 1973, with permission.)

osteoarthritic spurring, chronic disk degeneration, and facet joint arthritis. Spinal stenosis is also found in young people who have a congenitally narrowed lumbar spinal canal. In either case, the changes narrow the canal and the neuroforamina, leading to root impingement and pain.

The characteristic symptom is pain that is worsened by standing, walking, or other activities that cause spinal extension and is relieved by rest, especially by sitting or lying down and flexing the spine and hips. Patients report pain in the low back, gluteal region, or lower extremities; often, it is bilateral. Numbness or weakness may accompany the pain in the legs.

Because symptoms are often worsened by walking and relieved by sitting down and resting, they can mimic vascular insufficiency and are sometimes referred to as *pseudoclaudication*.

On examination, the spine demonstrates good range of motion and little focal tenderness. SLR is usually normal. Minor neurologic deficits (e.g., a diminished ankle jerk) may be present, but no pattern is characteristic.

The natural history of the condition is generally favorable, with only 15% of patients reporting clinical worsening over 5 years; 70% stay the same and 10% improve. Cauda equina syndrome is very rare in spinal stenosis.

Spondylolisthesis

The term denotes forward subluxation of a vertebral body. In adults, the condition results from degenerative changes and arthritis of the facet joints, usually at L-4 to L-5 or L-5 to S-1, with forward slippage of 10% to 20% of the diameter of the vertebral body. About 70% of patients with spondylolisthesis have chronic low back pain; sciatica is infrequent. The pain is caused by strain imposed on the ligaments and intervertebral joints.

Vertebral Compression Fracture

In normal bone, this fracture requires severe flexion–compression force. It is acutely painful. Spontaneous vertebral body collapse, or pathologic fracture, is most commonly seen in elderly persons with severe osteoporosis (see Chapter 164), in patients taking long-term glucocorticoids (see Chapter 105), and in cancer patients with lytic bony metastases. Usually, the history is one of sudden back pain brought on by a minor stress. The discomfort is noted at the level of fracture, with local radiation across the back and around the trunk, but rarely into the lower extremities. The fracture is more likely to occur in the middle or lower levels of the dorsal spine, which helps to differentiate the problem from lumbar disk herniations, 95% of which occur at the level of the L-4 or L-5 disk.

Neoplasms

The most common spinal tumor is *metastatic carcinoma*. Breast, lung, prostate, gastrointestinal, and genitourinary neoplasms commonly metastasize to the spine. Purely lytic lesions, which are often caused by renal or thyroid carcinoma, are seen occasionally. *Myeloma* is the most common primary bone tumor involving the spine. About 80% of patients are older than 50 years of age.

Typically, metastasis is hematogenous to the marrow of the vertebral bodies. Involvement of the periosteum and bony destruction lead to pain, and extension to the spinal cord can produce neurologic deficits. The disk spaces are usually spared, and disk space height is maintained, helping to differentiate the condition from degenerative disease. Collapse of the vertebral body as a result of bony destruction may be difficult to differentiate from compression fracture if osteoporosis is present. Extension into the epidural space or vertebral body collapse can lead to spinal cord compression; vascular compromise by the tumor may also contribute to cord injury.

Although only 30% of persons with metastatic disease as the cause of back pain give a history of previous cancer, in those that do, the probability of spinal metastasis is high. Approximately 90% report night pain and pain unrelieved or worsened by lying down or bed rest. A history of prior malignancy, insidious increase in pain in a region atypical for disk disease (e.g., the midback), and failure to obtain relief by lying down are highly predictive of metastatic tumor.

The clinical presentation is one of insidious onset of back pain, gradually increasing in severity and aggravated by activity and lying down. Location can be anywhere in the spine, but occurrence in an area atypical for degenerative disk disease (e.g., the midback) is suggestive. A hallmark is back pain worsened by activity and worsened, or at least not relieved, by lying down. There may be focal spinal tenderness. Extension into the epidural space is heralded by increasing back pain followed by neurologic symptoms a few weeks to months later. Besides back pain, manifestations of epidural invasion include upper motor neuron signs (proximal muscle weakness, hyperreflexia, upgoing toes) sensory loss in a dermatomal distribution, and autonomic dysfunction (urinary retention, fecal incontinence). Prognosis is poor without early intervention.

Intraspinal tumors may present in the same manner as herniated disks. However, marked progression of neurologic deficits despite adequate conservative therapy is a clue to the existence of a tumor inside the spinal canal. *Extraspinal tumors* may eventually cause root impingement and simulate discogenic sciatica. Tumors of the retroperitoneum, pelvis, and large bowel may extend to the roots. This is a very late development; metastases may occur earlier.

Infection

Back pain resulting from infection is rare but important to detect. An identifiable source is found in 40% of cases; possibilities include urinary tract infection, skin abscess, indwelling catheter, and intravenous-drug abuse. *Vertebral osteomyelitis* is usually hematogenous in origin but may occasionally result from a spinal procedure, such as lumbar puncture, myelography, discography, or disk surgery. In addition to involving the vertebral bodies, it may extend into the disk space, producing a very painful *discitis*. In the absence of discitis, the presentation is typically one of dull, continuous back pain, often in conjunction with low-grade fever and spasm over the paraspinous muscles. Tenderness to percussion over the involved vertebrae is common, but fever and elevated white cell count are absent in up to half of cases. A compression fracture or an epidural abscess may ensue. *Staphylococcus aureus* accounts for about 60% of bacterial cases and enterobacteria for 30%.

Epidural abscess develops in the context of bacteremia or osteomyelitis. The infection presents as back pain, focal tenderness, and fever. Fever and spinal tenderness are present in about 85% of cases. If the condition is not promptly treated, it may extend to compromise the local blood supply to the spinal cord and rapidly progress from spinal ache to major motor and sensory deficits within hours to a few days.

Ankylosing Spondylitis and Other Spondyloarthropathies

The seronegative spondyloarthropathies (which include ankylosing spondylitis, psoriatic arthritis, reactive arthritis, and arthritis associated with inflammatory bowel disease) have both peripheral and axial skeleton manifestations. There is considerable overlap among these inflammatory joint diseases, which share involvement of the sacroiliac joints and axial skeleton, limb joints, and entheses (sites of insertion of ligaments and tendons [e.g., Achilles, patellar, plantar fascia] into bone), as well as nonarticular sites (e.g., uveal tract, skin, bowel, and aortic valve). Focal tenderness may be reported at sites of involvement. A relation to mechanical stress has been invoked to explain the distribution of findings. There is a strong association with HLA-B27 positivity, suggesting an immune pathophysiology; rheumatoid factor is negative. Male predominance is the rule.

Ankylosing spondylitis is the most common of these conditions. Its characteristic features helpful for diagnosis include low back pain of at least 3 months' duration, improvement with exercise but not with rest, limitation of lumbar spine motion and chest expansion, and bilateral sacroiliitis or severe unilateral disease. Spinal involvement is most prominent in young men; onset is gradual. Morning spinal stiffness is typical. Spinal radiographic findings are often unremarkable in the early phases, but films of the sacroiliac joints may show narrowing of the joint space and reactive sclerosis ("sacroiliitis"). Eventually, the sacroiliac joint space becomes obliterated, and fusion follows. Squaring of the vertebral bodies is the first spinal radiologic manifestation, followed by the development of syndesmophytes. Similar although less florid changes may occur in the other seronegative spondyloarthropathies.

Psychogenic Disease

Patients with *depression* may present complaining of chronic low back pain. Often, they have a history of previous back problems or onset at the time of a minor injury, with the depression amplifying the presentation and prolonging the clinical course. Mild muscle spasm may be noted on physical examination. Characteristically, the intensity of the symptoms and the degree of disability are much greater than the minor limitations found on examination would suggest. Multiple somatic symptoms are common (see Chapter 227). Other patients may have an underlying *somatization* disorder. Many of these patients appear refractory to therapy and are often unwilling to take an active role in their treatment. Some even seem to derive a sense of legitimacy and self-worth from their suffering (see Chapter 230).

Malingering implies conscious deception for the sake of obtaining gain from being ill. Inconsistencies among symptoms and physical findings typify the malingerer. These often can be brought out by distracting the patient.

Cauda Equina Syndrome

Although the spinal cord ends at the L-1 level, the collection of nerve roots that make up the cauda equina is subject to injury by any process that compromises the spinal canal below the L-1 level. Massive midline disk herniation is the most common cause of cauda compression and a serious, although very infrequent, event that requires prompt attention. In contrast to the clinical presentation of simple root impingement, the presentation in cauda equina syndrome includes urinary retention in almost 90% of cases. Another characteristic feature is *saddle anesthesia* (a reduction in sensation over the buttocks, upper posterior thighs, and perineum), which is reported by about 75% of patients. Both of these clinical findings are a consequence of sacral root compression, as is a decrease in anal sphincter tone, which is noted in about two thirds of cases. Sciatica and lower extremity motor and sensory deficits are prominent and often bilateral. Patients may report falling.

TABLE 147.1

IMPORTANT CAUSES OF LOW BACK PAIN

Mechanical (97%)	Nonmechanical Spinal Condition (1%)	Visceral Disease (2%)
Lumbar strain or sprain (70%)	Neoplasia (0.7%)	Aortic aneurysm
Degenerative disk or facet disease (10%)	Metastatic carcinoma	Renal disease
Herniated disk (4%)	Multiple myeloma	Pelvic disease
Osteoporotic compression fracture (3%)	Spinal cord tumor	Abdominal disease
Spondylolisthesis (2%)	Lymphoma, leukemia	
Trauma (<1%)	Infection (0.01%)	
Discogenic disease	Osteomyelitis	
	Epidural abscess	
	Septic discitis	
	Inflammatory disease (0.3%)	
	Ankylosing spondylitis	
	Psoriatic arthritis	
	Reiter's syndrome	
	Inflammatory bowel disease	

Adapted from Deyo RA, Weinstein JN. Low back pain. N Engl J Med 2001;344:363, with permission.

DIFFERENTIAL DIAGNOSIS (4)

The differential diagnosis of back pain can be considered in terms of underlying pathophysiology (Table 147.1). Of note, the vast majority of cases (97%) are mechanical in origin, with less than 1% due to infection, neoplasia, or inflammatory disease of the spine; about 2% represent referred pain from visceral disease due to aortic, pelvic, renal, or gastrointestinal sources.

WORKUP (2,4,5,6,8–15)

Even with the advent of sophisticated spinal imaging techniques, the history and the physical examination remain critical to the effective evaluation and management of back pain. The findings elicited are often diagnostic, and even if they are not, they can help to guide test selection and ensure timely referral. Overreliance on imaging studies often results in false-positive diagnoses.

History

In elucidating the basic features of back pain (i.e., quality, location, onset, radiation), one should also inquire specifically into symptoms that are potentially indicative of serious underlying disease (e.g., fever, progressive neurologic deficits, bilateral deficits, bladder dysfunction, saddle anesthesia, persistent pain unresponsive to bed rest or worsened by lying down). A history of recent injury and a prior history of cancer are other critical elements to be noted, as are previous therapy for back problems, recent lumbar puncture, concurrent infection, and prolonged use of high-dose corticosteroids. The presence of sciatica helps to narrow the differential diagnosis (see Table 147.1).

Aggravating and alleviating factors may have important diagnostic significance. Morning stiffness in the back that is relieved by activity suggests ankylosing spondylitis or other inflammatory conditions. Worsening or onset of symptoms with standing or walking and relief with bending or sitting is charac-teristic of spinal stenosis, whereas worsening with sitting, driving, or lifting points to lumbar disk herniation. Malignancy is suggested by pain in a location atypical for degenerative disease (e.g., the midback), as well as by pain in any location that is worsened not only with activity but also on lying supine.

Associated symptoms are critical to check for, especially fever (raising the question of epidural abscess) and neurologic deficits (suggestive of cord or root injury). Is there any difficulty in standing or climbing stairs, urinating, or maintaining fecal continence? Is there truncal or saddle anesthesia? If so, a high index of suspicion is required for cord or cauda equina injury. Typical unilateral root symptoms (pain, numbness, weakness) in a characteristic lumbosacral root distribution suggest root impingement, but bilateral radicular symptoms, especially if severe and new in onset or rapidly progressive, should raise concern about cauda equina syndrome or epidural injury.

The patient should be asked to describe the effect of the back pain on daily activities. Emotional and social stressors are sought if the severity and duration of the symptoms appear to be disproportionate to the amount of organic disease present. Under such circumstances, it is important to check for depression (see Chapter 227) and manifestations of somatization disorder (see Chapter 230).

Physical Examination

Before examining the back, one should check the abdomen, rectum, groin, pelvis, and peripheral pulses for conditions that might mimic the symptoms of spinal disease. In addition, one looks for fever, skin abscess, breast mass, pleural effusion, prostate nodule, lymphadenopathy, joint inflammation, and other signs of systemic or malignant disease that may affect the spine. Thigh and calf circumferences are measured to detect evidence of atrophy, and joint motions of the lower extremities are tested.

Back Examination

The examination of the back begins with the patient standing and the back uncovered. One checks for any abnormalities in symmetry, muscle bulk, posture, and spinal curvature.

Flexibility is assessed, with any muscle spasm or spinal segments that do not move freely noted. A description of what limits back motion is more important than an estimation of degrees of motion, which is imprecise at best. The spine is palpated for focal tenderness suggestive of tumor, infection, fracture, disk injury, and disk herniation. Sensitivity of the lower lumbar spine and sciatic notch is usually found with lower lumbar disk herniation. Sacroiliac tenderness to deep palpation is sometimes present in ankylosing spondylitis, but the finding is nonspecific. A finding of tenderness in a location atypical for degenerative disease (e.g., the midback) should raise suspicions of metastatic disease and infection.

Straight-Leg-Raising Test

This diagnostic maneuver is an important component of the assessment for disk disease. It serves as a sensitive indicator of lower lumbar disk herniation, particularly in patients with sciatica. SLR testing is based on the observation that an L-5 or an S-1 nerve root tethered by a herniated disk causes radicular pain if stretched. In the presence of a severely herniated disk, the additional root stretching causes impingement and pain, especially with an L-5 to S-1 disk injury.

Straight leg raising is performed in the supine position with passive lifting of the patient's leg at the heel while the knee is kept fully extended. The test is performed both on the side of the reported sciatica (*ipsilateral SLR testing*) and on the opposite side (*contralateral* or *crossed SLR testing*). A test result is positive if the sciatica is reproduced as the leg is elevated between 30 and 70 degrees. Reproduction of the sciatica should not be confused with hamstring muscle tightness, which can also cause discomfort on SLR, especially as elevation approaches 90 degrees. (Elevation beyond 80 degrees exerts little additional stretch on the nerve root and is not of much meaning.) If severe pain is reported on elevation and resistance occurs, yet the leg can be raised another 20 or 30 degrees when the patient is distracted, the test result is "negative" and other causes of the pain should be sought, such as hamstring muscle tightness. Dorsiflexion of the ankle at the extreme of SLR may exacerbate the pain of disk herniation on SLR testing and is particularly useful if the SLR test result is equivocal.

The earlier the onset of pain during the test, the more specific is the result and the greater is the degree of disk herniation. The test sensitivity averages 80% for ipsilateral SLR; specificity is low (about 40%). The specificity of a positive contralateral SLR test result is considerably higher (75%), but the sensitivity is only 25%. A large disk herniation with an extruded fragment is an important cause of a positive contralateral SLR result.

Much less L-4 and minimal L-2 or L-3 movement occurs during SLR testing, so that it is less useful to detect disk herniation above L-4 to L-5. Femoral nerve sensitivity is usually present with higher lumbar (L-2, L-3, or L-4) root irritation. Flexing the knee with the patient lying in a prone position may reproduce the back and anterior thigh pain of upper lumbar disk herniation.

Neurologic Examination

The examination is most efficiently performed by concentrating on the areas of compromise suggested by the history. The patient with sciatica is most likely to have deficits in the territory of the L-5 and S-1 roots and should be tested accordingly. The person with back pain radiating to the anterior thigh and associated quadriceps weakness should be tested for L-4 function. A history of suggestive of epidural injury requires a check for signs of upper motor neuron compromise (reduced proximal muscle strength, hyperreflexia, upgoing toes) and dermatomal sensory deficits at the level of suspected involvement. Concern about cauda equina syndrome should focus the physical examination on the detection of saddle anesthesia and bilateral motor and sensory deficits in the lower extremities.

Tests for *S-1 root* function (L-5 to S-1 disk) include tiptoe walking, plantar flexion against resistance, ankle deep tendon reflexes, and lateral foot sensation. A loss of plantar flexion occurs only with severe disk herniation (low sensitivity, high specificity). Tests for *L-5 root* function (L-4 to L-5 disk) include heel walking (an imprecise test), dorsiflexion of the ankle and big toe against resistance, and sensation on the anterior medial dorsal foot (Fig. 147.1). For a suspected upper lumbar disk lesion (*L-4 root*), one notes the knee deep tendon reflexes, quadriceps strength, and sensation about the medial ankle.

The sensitivity of any single neurologic test for the diagnosis of lumbar disk protrusion or extrusion is no greater than 50%, but it can be enhanced to almost 90% when clusters of findings are considered. The most accurate assessment of sensory function is attained by pinprick testing, which is most efficiently performed by limiting the examination to a few key distal dermatomal areas in the feet (see Fig. 147.1) and noting any asymmetry of response.

Responses to neurologic testing and spinal examination in patients with psychological stress may appear to be neuroanatomically inappropriate, but often they are diagnostically meaningful. Disturbances in strength or sensation that do not correspond to nerve root innervation patterns, inconsistency of responses to maneuvers, overreaction to palpation or passive movement, superficial or widespread tenderness, and pain on sham testing of spinal rotation (arms kept at sides while hips are rotated) are among the characteristic responses. The presence of three or more of these responses suggests considerable psychological overlay to the patient's back pain.

Laboratory Studies

For the majority of patients with low back pain, a careful history and a physical examination usually suffice for diagnosis at the time of the initial office visit. The utility of imaging studies is limited to a few specific situations, many of which are also indications for referral or consultation (see later discussion).

Lumbosacral Spine Films

In most instances, the routine ordering of plain lumbosacral spine films in patients presenting with back pain is low in yield and neither cost-effective nor useful for decision making. The finding of normal disk spaces does not rule out disk herniation, and the finding of a narrowed disk space does not distinguish between disk rupture and asymptomatic degeneration. The presence of osteophytes extending from the vertebral bodies indicates little more than long-existing disk degeneration and attempts at repair.

Nonetheless, early radiography of the back is indicated in some situations, as when the physician suspects (a) malignancy (patient >50 years of age, focal persistent bone pain unrelieved by bed rest, a history of malignancy); (b) compression fracture (prolonged corticosteroid therapy, postmenopausal woman, severe trauma, focal tenderness); (c) ankylosing spondylitis (young male patient, limited spinal motion, sacroiliac pain); (d) chronic osteomyelitis (low-grade fever, high sedimentation rate, focal tenderness); (e) major trauma; and (f) major neurologic deficits. Back pain localized to the high lumbar or thoracic region is also an indication for prompt spinal radiography because compression fracture and metastatic tumor are common in these areas. Although plain films might be helpful in these circumstances, they are not the imaging study of choice and should not delay proceeding to more definitive imaging with magnetic resonance imaging (MRI) or computed tomography (CT) (see later discussion).

Plain films may be needed for patients seeking compensation for back pain and for those who desire reassurance when the pretest probability of worrisome disease is very low, but test sensitivity for serious disease can be low, limiting the appropriateness of the test for reassurance purposes when pretest probability is not miniscule. For example, in early osteomyelitis, there may be no visible bony changes for at least 10 to 14 days; for spinal metastasis, the false-negative rate is 30% even in persons who present with epidural cord compression and higher in earlier stages of spinal involvement.

Computed Tomography and Magnetic Resonance Imaging

Clinical suspicion of cauda equina syndrome, epidural abscess, or cancer-related epidural spinal cord compression is an indication for urgent spinal imaging by either MRI or CT. Such imaging should be obtained as quickly as possible because of the risk of severe and irreversible neurologic damage in the absence of timely intervention.

CT and MRI are also indicated in persons being considered for surgical intervention to relieve persistent severe symptoms of disk herniation or other surgically amenable disease such as spinal stenosis. Both imaging modalities are very sensitive for the detection of lumbar disk disease and spinal stenosis and can provide anatomic detail of some surgical value. Besides being more costly, MRI often triggers a claustrophobic response, but no radiation exposure is involved.

MRI and CT should be limited to patients who are either sufficiently symptomatic that surgical intervention must be considered or are suspected of having serious systemic disease. The high sensitivity of these tests for disk disease can produce misleading results unless the patient and clinician are aware that disk bulges and protrusions are extremely common (50% and 30%, respectively) in asymptomatic people.

MRI. MRI is the test of choice in suspected cauda equina syndrome, epidural abscess, or cancer-related epidural spinal cord compression by virtue of its superiority in detecting soft-tissue pathology. In most instances, it obviates the need for myelography. MRI is the also best test for detecting early osteomyelitis and is the noninvasive test of choice for spinal cord tumors, epidural abscess, and epidural cord compression due to tumor or vertebral collapse. MRI may reveal such pathologic findings earlier than CT because it can detect marrow changes, which precede bony changes. MRI sensitivity for cancer-related back pain is estimated to be 93% and sensitivity to be 97%. MRI is superior to CT for the detection of disk pathology, including the tear of a disk annulus, manifesting a high-intensity zone on T2-weighted images in the posterior aspect of the involved disk; however, the relation between the finding and pain is not well established. There is no radiation exposure, but patients have to be able to lie in the scanner for up to 45 minutes. The presence of an implantable cardiac device is usually a contraindication to MRI scanning.

Rapid MRI is a variant of magnetic resonance technology that is quicker, less expensive, and slightly less sensitive than conventional MRI but is more sensitive than plain films. It has been suggested as an alternative to plain films and conventional MRI for the detection of cancer-related back pain. Decision-analysis study finds that it is unlikely to be cost-effective: It is associated with an incremental cost per quality-adjusted life year of additional survival of nearly $300,000, nearly six times the norm for a cost-effective modality.

CT. CT scanning is much faster, less expensive, and more readily available than MRI, but it involves radiation exposure and is less sensitive for the detection of infection, tumor, nerve injury, and disk pathology. In addition, CT does not provide the visualization of the entire spine or upper vertebrae that MRI does (desirable features if the differential diagnosis includes intraspinal tumor and disk herniation at an upper level). CT does provide excellent bony detail; contrast-enhanced study is a reasonable alternative to MRI when the latter is contraindicated, unavailable, or impractical. It can show changes in vertebral bodies caused by tumor and infection, although not as early as MRI, which can better detect early marrow changes.

Myelography

Traditional myelography has been largely replaced by MRI. It is usually performed in conjunction with CT on patients with progressive neurologic deficits, especially those with findings suggestive of injury to the spinal cord (e.g., loss of sphincter control, bilateral numbness and weakness) who have a contraindication to MRI scanning. The temptation to perform myelography in the patient with chronic refractory pain is strong, but the test should be reserved for patients with objective findings that are amenable to surgery or radiation therapy. Risks include infection, bleeding, and iatrogenic worsening of the neurologic state; the frequency of adverse effects can approach 20%.

Radionuclide Scanning

The moderately high sensitivity of the technetium bone scan for osteomyelitis and metastatic disease and its wide availability make it a reasonable consideration for the patient presenting with any combination of fever, weight loss, persistent back pain, history of malignancy, concurrent infection, and markedly elevated sedimentation rate. Gallium scanning is sometimes useful in defining soft-tissue involvement by infection or abscess formation.

Discography

This invasive diagnostic procedure is performed on patients believed to be suffering from a tear of the disk annulus. Under fluoroscopic guidance, disks are injected with contrast, which characteristically increases pain in the involved disk and helps to visualize the tear on follow-up CT scan. However, even persons without a tear might have pain on disk injection. MRI can also visualize such tears but cannot confirm the relationship between the tear and the patient's pain.

Immunoelectrophoresis

Serum and urine electrophoresis is helpful in cases of suspected multiple myeloma; crude screening with a complete blood cell count and determination of the erythrocyte sedimentation rate and serum globulin level is probably sufficient if clinical suspicion is not high. A diagnosis of myeloma must be suspected if back pain in an older person is accompanied by unexplained anemia and a very high sedimentation rate. However, such findings are quite nonspecific and may also be caused by a chronic inflammatory process.

Electromyography

Electromyography may be needed to document peripheral nerve deficits and help to select patients who require myelography.

SYMPTOMATIC MANAGEMENT AND PATIENT EDUCATION (1,2,4–6,8,16–56)

Acute Nonspecific Back Pain

Acute nonspecific back pain (no evidence of neurologic compromise or other serious pathology) is best managed conservatively because prognosis is generally very favorable. Such nonspecific acute low back resolves in about one third of patients by 1 week and in two thirds by 7 weeks.

Initial Symptomatic Relief

Initial symptomatically helpful measures include local application of *heat* or *cold* and the use of *nonnarcotic analgesics* (e.g., acetaminophen). Compared to acetaminophen, *nonsteroidal antiinflammatory agents* (NSAIDs; e.g., *ibuprofen*) provide equivalent pain relief but at the cost of increased gastrointestinal upset. NSAIDs have been shown to be effective in randomized trials and are preferred over *narcotics* for all but the first night or two of symptoms, when pain might be severe enough to warrant the temporary addition of an intermediate-strength *opioid* (e.g., oxycodone).

So-called *muscle relaxants* (e.g., *cyclobenzaprine* [Flexeril], which is chemically similar to the tricyclic antidepressants) are widely prescribed (13% of all acute back pain patients get a prescription), but controlled trials find that cyclobenzaprine adds little to the relief afforded by NSAIDs. However, meta-analysis suggests that cyclobenzaprine can be of help to patients in the very acute phase of illness, probably as a consequence of the drug's sedating effects. A less expensive alternative might be to prescribe a few days of a generic *benzodiazepine* (e.g., *diazepam* 2 to 5 mg) before bed.

Also helpful for sleep is advice regarding the most comfortable position in bed, which usually is lying supine with a pillow tucked under the knees and a small pillow folded under the nape of the neck. Alternatively, lying on one's side with the hips and knees flexed and a pillow between the knees can be helpful; lying prone usually is not.

Activity Prescription

Bed rest was formerly a mainstay of treatment, but randomized trials have demonstrated that recovery is more rapid in patients who continue their ordinary activities within the limits permitted by pain. Even for patients with continuing pain and evidence of disk protrusion or extrusion, there is little evidence to support prolonged bed rest. Deconditioning with bed rest can contribute to physical and psychological morbidity. To avoid prolonged inactivity and the deconditioning that accompanies it, patients with disk protrusion or extrusion should be encouraged to begin a reasonable activity program during the first week, consisting 20-minute walks three times a day, interspersed with several hours of bed rest. After the spine has healed sufficiently to allow sitting without pain, the patient can ease into a program of endurance exercises that may help to prevent future back problems (see later discussion), but exercises are of no benefit during the acute phase of illness.

A reasonable program of back care should be discussed after the recovery from acute symptoms allows gradual mobilization and resumption of normal activities. The patient must understand that pain is a normal protective response to injury or inflammation. Discomfort should be used as a guideline to determine the pace at which to increase activity. However, minor discomfort, stiffness, soreness, or mild aching should not interfere with progressive mobilization.

If symptoms recur or marked pain develops in relation to a specific activity or level of activity, the patient should temporarily limit activity for several days. Twisting, bending, and lifting should be avoided. If the patient undertakes a new or higher level of activity and pain increases within 24 hours, the activity should be halved each day until a tolerable level is reached and then gradually increased. The patient should be encouraged to progress as rapidly as symptoms permit.

Additional Measures: Physical Therapy, Yoga, Spinal Manipulation, Massage, and Acupuncture

Because prognosis is favorable for persons with nonspecific low back pain, additional measures beyond NSAIDs, basic back care, and the resumption of normal activity are usually not indicated for the first 3 to 4 weeks; the majority of patients recover during this time without any additional intervention. For those who experience more persistent pain, a number of additional treatment options can be considered, but most are of only modest benefit compared to patient education alone. Outcomes are strongly influenced by patient expectations of benefit from a particular modality, making patient preference an important factor to consider in the selection of treatment modality.

Physical Therapy. Randomized, controlled trials find formal physical therapy marginally better than no treatment (e.g., an educational booklet); the cost is greater, but so is patient satisfaction. Compared to spinal manipulation, functional outcomes and costs are similar. Some physical therapists also perform message therapy or spinal manipulation (see later discussion).

Yoga. Twelve weekly 75-minute sessions of yoga designed for patients with chronic back pain have been shown in a randomized trial to be more effective than exercise or the provision of a self-management book. Patients assigned to yoga had greater reductions in symptoms and disability and less need for medications when followed for 26 weeks after randomization.

Spinal Manipulation. Although very popular among patients, randomized, controlled trials find that spinal manipulation by chiropractors is only modestly better than sham therapy and other similarly worthless treatments for acute low back pain. There is no difference in outcomes when compared to effective conventional therapies; however, patient satisfaction is high and similar to that for physical therapy. Patients with herniated disks subjected to spinal manipulation are at risk for cauda equina syndrome, making this form of treatment inadvisable in persons with disk herniation. Other contraindications include the possibility of tumor, infection, compression fracture, pregnancy, previous back surgery, and neurologic deficits. Costs are high for the treatment, and no reduction in total costs has been identified. The use of a prediction rule (pain <16 days, no pain distal to the knees, one or more hypomobile lumbar segments, preserved hip internal range of motion, reduced functional capacity) has proved to be helpful in identifying persons likely to respond.

Therapeutic Massage. In randomized, controlled trials, therapeutic massage has proved to be superior to control measures, providing both short- and long-term benefit. Overall safety appears to be good, but short-term discomfort during or after a treatment is experienced by up to 15% of patients. Total costs are reduced by nearly half of patients in comparison to acupuncture and by 20% in comparison to self-care. Extrapolating from study findings to clinical practice is made somewhat difficult by the lack of standardized procedures for message.

Acupuncture. Acupuncture is rarely used in acute back pain; its efficacy has not been studied adequately in this setting.

Worthless Measures. A number of treatment modalities have been found to be devoid of benefit for acute nonspecific back pain. These include *spinal traction, facet-joint injection,* and *transcutaneous nerve stimulation.*

Disk Herniation and Discogenic Pain

The initial treatment for disk herniation is similar to that for acute nonspecific low back pain. Disk herniation tends to regress over time. Conservative therapy usually suffices, and most patients report significant improvement by 6 weeks. In those unable to tolerate symptoms, interventional measures are sometimes resorted to; however, controlled studies find little difference in pain or functional status at 1 year. Only about 10% need consideration of surgery at week 6. Spinal manipulation should be avoided due to the risk of aggravating disc herniation and causing additional neurologic impairment.

Before proceeding with any treatment, it is important carefully to check at the outset and continuously monitor for new or worsening neurologic deficits, especially for symptoms and signs of cauda equina syndrome (e.g., saddle anesthesia, severe bilateral pain, numbness, weakness, bladder and bowel dysfunction), which is a neurosurgical emergency. Their presence signifies a potential neurosurgical emergency necessitating urgent MRI spinal imaging and prompt neurosurgical consultation.

Initial Therapy

As for acute nonspecific back pain, *NSAIDs, avoidance* of back stresses, and *maintenance* of activity are the basic features of initial management (see prior discussion). In some instances, adding a short course of an *opioid analgesic* (e.g., *oxycodone* for the first few days) is needed to achieve adequate pain control; a similarly short course of *cyclobenzaprine* or a *benzodiazepine* can supplement symptomatic relief and facilitate the patient's getting a night's sleep.

Interventional Procedures—Epidural Steroid Injection

For patients with persistent, incapacitating radicular pain due to disk herniation who cannot hold out for spontaneous improvement, *epidural glucocorticoid injection* is a reasonable consideration for temporary relief. The purported mechanism of pain relief involves countering the inflammatory component of nerve injury. Several weeks to a few months of pain relief may be achieved, which can help bide time for healing and

potentially obviate the need for surgery. Controlled trials confirm a short-term benefit but reveal little effect on long-term outcomes, including the need for surgery. Contraindications include anticoagulation therapy and any evidence of local infection or discitis. In many instances, local anesthetic is added to ensure proper needle placement, which is usually done under fluoroscopy.

Two injections are typically given, spaced 3 to 4 weeks apart, with a third given if relief is only partial; however, benefit is unlikely if there is no improvement with the first injection. A *transforaminal approach* is technically more demanding but allows steroid delivery closer to the irritated nerve and the use of smaller doses; the risk of nerve root injury is greater than with the standard *interlaminar approach*. A worsening of radicular pain during the procedure is a sign of needle misplacement. Risks include postinjection headache (up to 5%), worsening radicular pain (1%), and infection. Short-term response rates are in the 50% to 75% range, but longer-term benefit is achieved in only 25% to 50% of cases. There is no evidence that repeated injections are harmful, either short term or long term. Benefit from transforaminal injection is predictive of improvement with surgical laminectomy.

Interventional Procedures—Surgery

Although most persons with lumbar disk herniation get better without surgery, those who experience (a) persistent disabling root pain despite 4 to 6 weeks of comprehensive conservative therapy or (b) progressive neurologic deficits in the lower extremities are reasonable candidates for the consideration of surgical intervention.

Diagnostic spinal imaging (CT or MRI) is indicated to help determine surgical candidacy (see prior discussion). The Spine Patient Outcomes Research Trial demonstrated that patients with herniated disks improved substantially over a 2-year period with or without surgery. The most clear-cut benefits of surgery are greater relief of sciatica and patient self-reported improvement.

An often-confusing array of surgical and invasive procedures is available. Although the selection of the best procedure is the province of the surgeon, proper referral and patient counseling by the primary physician are informed by understanding the risks and benefits of available surgical options.

Open Disk Excision (Diskectomy). *Open surgery* is the gold standard procedure for significant disk herniation. It entails removing some lamellar bone, ligamentum flavum, and medial facet to excise the herniated portion of the disk, as well as trimming any bony protrusions into the neural foramen. The operation is mandatory and urgent for patients with massive disk herniation causing a cauda equina syndrome. It is also indicated in cases of major progressive neurologic deficit due to disk herniation or extruded disk fragments that are not in continuity with the disk space.

Microsurgery (using a small incision and magnification techniques) is a variant of open diskectomy and the standard approach to this type of surgery. Results at 4 years are better than those associated with conservative treatment but are no better at 10 years. In community settings, 1-year success rates for the surgical treatment of sciatica approach 80%, with a 6% complication rate and a need for reoperation at 1 year of about 6%. Surgical mortality and infection rates are less than 0.01%; the risk of nerve injury is less than 1%. When the entire disk needs to be removed, a fusion procedure may be required, which entails lengthy incisions and muscle dissection.

In trials of persons with severe sciatica, those assigned to immediate microsurgery reported significantly better early pain relief and shorter time to recovery; however, at the 1-year mark, 95% of patients in both groups achieved full recovery with no difference in risk of adverse outcomes. These findings indicate that although disk surgery performed by an expert disk surgeon is a reasonable option for symptomatic relief, it remains optional, with no need to rush to surgery unless there is evidence of serious neurologic compromise.

Percutaneous Diskectomy. Percutaneous disk procedures, initially using chymopapain but more recently lasers, target the nucleus pulposus, removing its central portion in the hope of taking pressure off the nerve root. The herniated portion of the disk is not treated, and extruded fragments cannot be removed, which accounts for lesser efficacy compared to open disk excision. *Endoscopic diskectomy* and *electrothermal disk decompression* represent additional new approaches to percutaneous disk removal; outcomes data from controlled studies are limited, but initial results are promising.

Percutaneous Fusion and Synthetic Disk Substitutes. Attempts to reduce the morbidity of open fusion have led to laparoscopic approaches to anterior fusion and endoscopic approaches to posterior fusion. Although they are promising, these technologies are very demanding and still in their infancy; they should be approached as such, with a careful consideration of risks (e.g., longer operative time, nerve damage). Open procedures are still the approach of choice for spinal fusion. The use of bone morphogenetic proteins that enhance fusion without the need for harvested bone is becoming available, and synthetic replacement disks are under development.

Intradiskal Electrothermal Therapy. This minimally invasive form of treatment targets and attempts to repair tears in the disk annulus that are believed to be responsible for discogenic back pain. Criteria for treatment include 6 months of pain unresponsive to medical and physical therapy, pain reproduced during discography, the preservation of 50% of residual disk height, and no disk herniation. A catheter is inserted through a needle into the disk and used to position a 5-cm heating element across the identified tear. Heating the element is believed to help seal the tear and destroy annular nerve fibers. Risks include infection and disk herniation due to disk softening during the procedure. Results show significant improvement compared to placebo controls.

Management of Discogenic Pain

Discogenic pain is a less-well-established diagnostic entity, and approaches to its treatment are similarly uncertain. The initial nonsurgical approach is similar to that for disk herniation; less invasive interventional therapies offer new surgical options beyond the standard disk removal and spinal fusion for persons who fail conservative therapy.

Prevention of Relapse and Primary Prevention

Prevention of Relapse

The risk of relapse is very high, approaching 75%. A program of exercise and back hygiene can help to reduce relapse. Proper back care should become a way of life for the patient, even though acute symptoms subside with rest. The patient is advised to avoid activities that cause pain and also potentially injurious actions such as repetitive bending, twisting, heavy lifting, and shoveling snow. Increasing evidence suggests that physical therapy programs designed to improve muscle strength and flexibility are effective, helping to maintain good posture and reduce the chances of recurrent injury. Instruction sheets are often useful to supplement instruction in the office (Figs. 147.2 and 147.3). A program of mild daily exercise with more vigorous endurance exercise two to three times a week is also encouraged and appears to be more useful than traditional isometric exercises. Brisk walking for 20 minutes once or twice a day, supplemented by swimming twice weekly for up to 30 minutes, fulfills such an exercise requirement. Stationary bicycling or jogging can be substituted for swimming.

Results with braces and lumbar supports have been variable. Controlled trials have failed to confirm any benefit from the use of braces in patients with disk herniation; in fact, it is of concern that the restriction of movement may promote muscle weakness and predispose to relapse. One study found that persons with preexisting back pain who use a lumbar support at work exhibit a significant reduction in the number of days of pain, but this finding has not been confirmed.

Primary Prevention

The prevention of work-related back pain is a major occupational health objective, given that 2% of the workforce incurs a back injury annually. Predictors of back complaints include physical demands of the job, age, and job satisfaction. The data on the efficacy of lumbar supports is mixed, and no consensus has emerged on their use. Mechanical studies find little reduction in sagittal or vertical intervertebral translational forces but some reduction in intradiskal pressure and trunk motion, which helps workers to lift with less bending over. There is little effect on muscle strength. Randomized, controlled study involving cargo handlers found little benefit from an educational program or the use of lumbar support unless the worker had back pain at the time of study. Subsequent studies have also failed to find benefit from the use of back belts.

Refractory Pain

Patients with chronic refractory back pain, especially those with no clear anatomic deficit, pose one of the most difficult long-term management problems encountered in primary care practice. When due to disk herniation and accompanied by neurologic deficits, the pain is best managed by surgical intervention (see prior discussion). Surgery may also be indicated in spinal stenosis (see later discussion). In the absence of surgically correctable pathology, the approach should still be as pathophysiologic as possible, addressing likely mechanisms and protecting the patient from worthless measures.

Like all chronic pain syndromes, chronic back pain may involve multiple mechanisms that contribute to the amplification of symptoms and refractoriness to therapy (see Chapter 236). These range from social factors (e.g., *pending litigation, application for disability*) and underlying psychopathology (e.g., *depression, somatization disorder* [see Chapters 227 and 230]) to central nervous system changes that increase nerve excitability and hyperactivity (*neuroplasticity*) and perpetuate pain in the absence of ongoing nerve injury. All such factors necessitate careful exploration and targeted therapy when identified. At times, it may not be possible to eliminate the pain, but it is important to stress that the real objective is improvement in

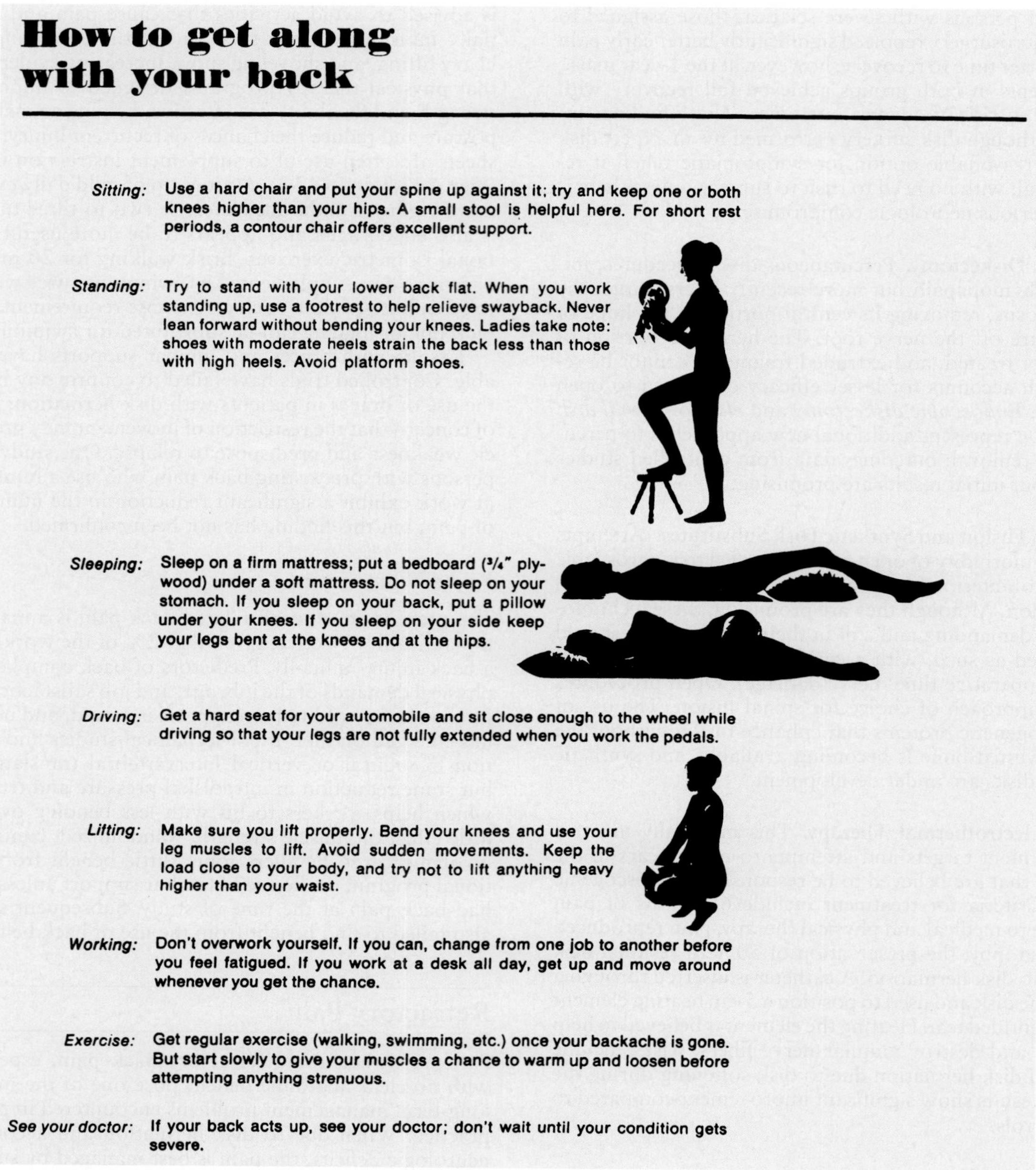

How to get along with your back

Sitting: Use a hard chair and put your spine up against it; try and keep one or both knees higher than your hips. A small stool is helpful here. For short rest periods, a contour chair offers excellent support.

Standing: Try to stand with your lower back flat. When you work standing up, use a footrest to help relieve swayback. Never lean forward without bending your knees. Ladies take note: shoes with moderate heels strain the back less than those with high heels. Avoid platform shoes.

Sleeping: Sleep on a firm mattress; put a bedboard (¾" plywood) under a soft mattress. Do not sleep on your stomach. If you sleep on your back, put a pillow under your knees. If you sleep on your side keep your legs bent at the knees and at the hips.

Driving: Get a hard seat for your automobile and sit close enough to the wheel while driving so that your legs are not fully extended when you work the pedals.

Lifting: Make sure you lift properly. Bend your knees and use your leg muscles to lift. Avoid sudden movements. Keep the load close to your body, and try not to lift anything heavy higher than your waist.

Working: Don't overwork yourself. If you can, change from one job to another before you feel fatigued. If you work at a desk all day, get up and move around whenever you get the chance.

Exercise: Get regular exercise (walking, swimming, etc.) once your backache is gone. But start slowly to give your muscles a chance to warm up and loosen before attempting anything strenuous.

See your doctor: If your back acts up, see your doctor; don't wait until your condition gets severe.

FIGURE 147.2. Sample instruction sheet describing care of the back. (Courtesy of McNeil Laboratories, Fort Washington, Pennsylvania.)

functional status. Patients are often desperate and seek treatment from a wide range of practitioners who promise relief.

There are no simple solutions to the management of these patients. Many patients do not take an active role in their treatment and frustrate the well-intentioned efforts of physicians while they continue to complain of discomfort. However, some important objectives can be achieved: the identification and treatment of underlying psychosocial factors; reduction in the severity of pain; the avoidance of inappropriate tests, addictive medications, ineffective therapies, and unnecessary surgery; and the preservation of the patient's capacity to function independently. Like most forms of chronic pain, chronic low back pain requires a comprehensive approach that includes a strong physician–patient relationship and an emphasis on

improving functional status rather than just relieving pain (see Chapter 236). The primary care physician can add considerable value by providing patient education and guidance, as well as an evidence-based approach to treatment.

Addressing Underlying Psychopathology and Social Factors

Up to one third of patients with chronic back pain suffer from depression. If depression is identified, it should be treated (see Chapter 227) regardless of whether it is the cause or the result of the patient's condition. Treatment reduces pain, and there is a trend toward improvement in activities of daily living. Both *tricyclics* and *selective serotonin reuptake inhibitors* (SSRIs) are

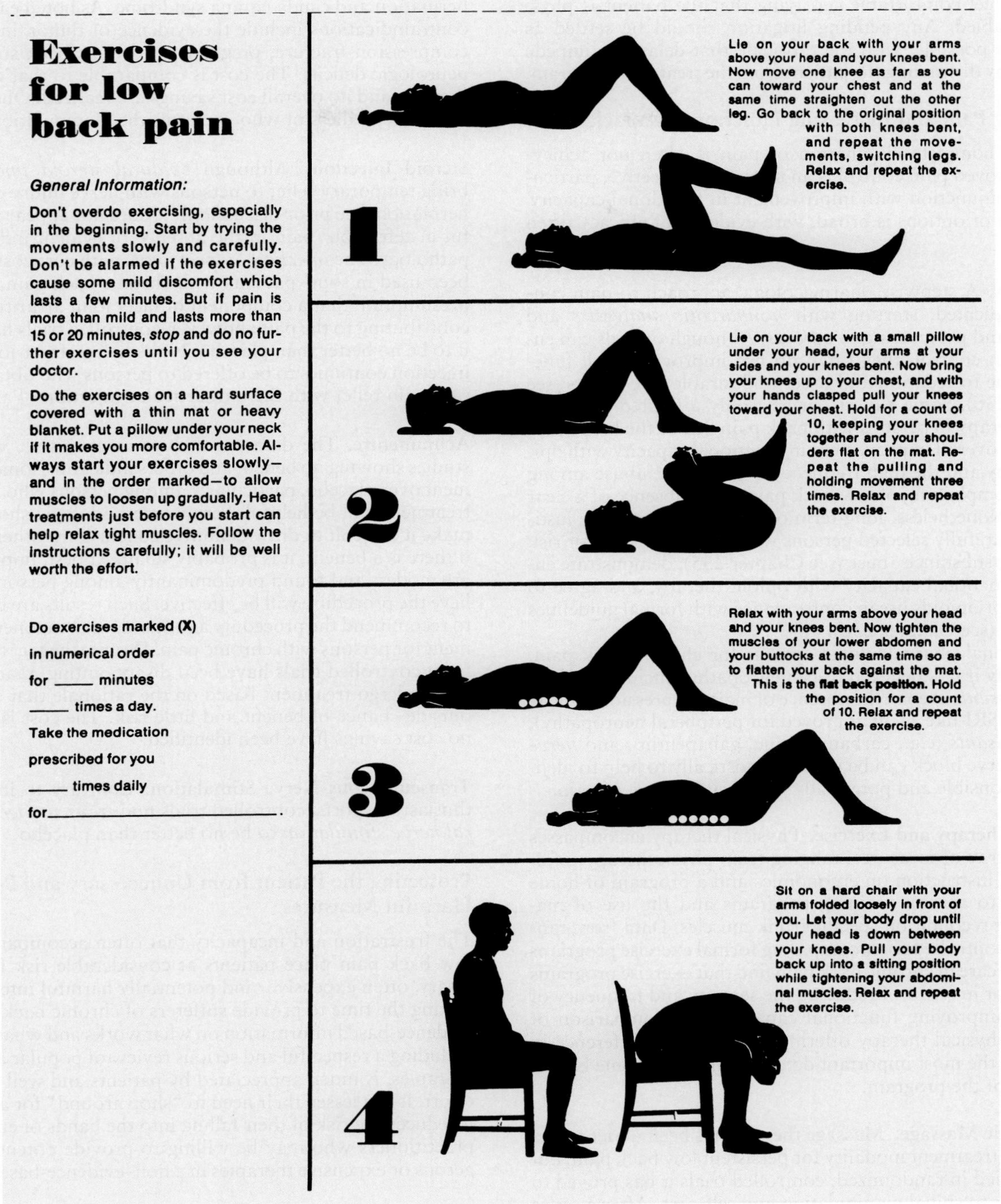

Exercises for low back pain

General Information:

Don't overdo exercising, especially in the beginning. Start by trying the movements slowly and carefully. Don't be alarmed if the exercises cause some mild discomfort which lasts a few minutes. But if pain is more than mild and lasts more than 15 or 20 minutes, *stop* and do no further exercises until you see your doctor.

Do the exercises on a hard surface covered with a thin mat or heavy blanket. Put a pillow under your neck if it makes you more comfortable. Always start your exercises slowly—and in the order marked—to allow muscles to loosen up gradually. Heat treatments just before you start can help relax tight muscles. Follow the instructions carefully; it will be well worth the effort.

Do exercises marked (X)

in numerical order

for _____ minutes

_____ times a day.

Take the medication

prescribed for you

_____ times daily

for_____.

1 Lie on your back with your arms above your head and your knees bent. Now move one knee as far as you can toward your chest and at the same time straighten out the other leg. Go back to the original position with both knees bent, and repeat the movements, switching legs. Relax and repeat the exercise.

2 Lie on your back with a small pillow under your head, your arms at your sides and your knees bent. Now bring your knees up to your chest, and with your hands clasped pull your knees toward your chest. Hold for a count of 10, keeping your knees together and your shoulders flat on the mat. Repeat the pulling and holding movement three times. Relax and repeat the exercise.

3 Relax with your arms above your head and your knees bent. Now tighten the muscles of your lower abdomen and your buttocks at the same time so as to flatten your back against the mat. This is the flat back position. Hold the position for a count of 10. Relax and repeat the exercise.

4 Sit on a hard chair with your arms folded loosely in front of you. Let your body drop until your head is down between your knees. Pull your body back up into a sitting position while tightening your abdominal muscles. Relax and repeat the exercise.

FIGURE 147.3. Sample instruction sheet describing exercises for low back pain. (Courtesy of McNeil Laboratories, Fort Washington, Pennsylvania.)

useful (see Chapters 227 and 236); tricyclics and the SSRI-like agent duloxetine may also provide pain relief to persons with chronic back pain in the absence of depression (see later discussion). For the person with a suspected somatization disorder, therapeutic efforts are best directed at helping the patient to find ways other than suffering to achieve a sense of self-worth. Attempts to "cure" such persons physically actually remove their one source (albeit maladaptive) of personal value and are bound to be sabotaged by patients unless they find something to replace their back pain. *Cognitive–behavioral therapy* has proven especially useful (see Chapters 230 and 236).

Patients with pending legal matters should be strongly encouraged to settle them as quickly as possible. If a disability determination is needed, it should be expedited. Arranging an independent evaluation may be best; this avoids jeopardizing the patient–doctor relationship, particularly if the physician does not feel comfortable certifying that the patient is physically disabled. Any pending litigation should be settled as quickly as possible, with the rationale that delay can impede recovery by distracting the patient from the treatment program.

Reducing Pain and Increasing Functional Capacity

Although complete elimination of pain is often not achievable, improved pain control is an important objective, particularly in conjunction with improvement in functional capacity. The range of options is broad, with evidence of efficacy often elusive.

Analgesics. A stepwise pharmacologic approach to pain control is indicated, starting with *nonnarcotic analgesics* and *NSAIDs* and progressing to *opioids*. Although opioids can enhance pain control, they often do not improve overall functioning due to sedation and other undesirable side effects (see Chapter 236). Some experts suggest only a limited course of opioid therapy in persons with back pain due to the lack of evidence for overall improvement in functional capacity with opioid therapy and the high frequency of substance abuse among persons complaining of low back pain in the absence of a clear etiology. Nonetheless, long-term opioid therapy may be justifiable in carefully selected persons who have no history or risk factors for substance abuse (see Chapter 235), demonstrate enhanced functional capacity with opioid therapy, and agree to contract for opioids use in conformance with formal guidelines and limits (see Chapter 236).

Additional pharmacologic options for chronic back pain, particularly if it is believed to be neuropathic, include *tricyclic antidepressants* even in the absence of major depression, *duloxetine* (an SSRI-like agent approved for peripheral neuropathy), *anticonvulsants* (e.g., carbamazepine, gabapentin), and *nerve blocks*. Nerve block can be used diagnostically to help to identify a responsible and potentially responsive source of pain.

Physical Therapy and Exercise. Physical therapy encompasses a broad array of measures, ranging from physiotherapy (individualized instruction on ergonomics and a program of home exercises) to aerobic training programs and the use of machines that recondition specific trunk muscles. Data from randomized, controlled trials comparing formal exercise programs with usual care in chronic back pain find that exercise programs are superior in terms of reducing the severity and frequency of pain and improving functional capacity. The comparison of different physical therapy offerings reveals little difference in outcomes; the most important determinant of outcome is continuation of the program.

Therapeutic Massage. Massage therapy has been underappreciated as a treatment modality for persistent low back pain, but when studied in randomized, controlled trials it has proved to be superior to spinal manipulation and self-care. After a series of treatments over 4 to 8 weeks, relief persists for up to 1 year. The initial cost is substantial, but cost savings over 1 year are achieved in comparison to spinal manipulation and self-care.

Spinal Manipulation. Spinal manipulation as practiced by chiropractors is widely applied to persons with persistent or chronic back pain, but like many other "alternative" therapies, the magnitude of improvement is modest in controlled trials and no better than that achieved with effective conventional measures. Only when compared to no treatment does spinal manipulation demonstrate significant improvement in outcomes. The procedure is contraindicated in persons with symptomatic disk herniation due to the risk of worsening disk

herniation and cauda equina syndrome. As noted earlier, other contraindications include the evidence of tumor, infection, or compression fracture, pregnancy, previous back surgery, and neurologic deficits. The cost is comparable to that of physical therapy, and no overall cost savings are realized. Outcomes are similar regardless of who performs the manipulation.

Steroid Injections. Although *epidural steroid injection* can bring temporary relief to persons with nerve injury due to disk herniation (see prior discussion), it does not appear to be helpful in refractory pain in the absence of evident inflammatory pathology. The *injection of facet joints* with corticosteroids has been used in some patients with chronic back pain, under the presumption that a component of facet joint arthritis might be contributing to the pain; however, controlled trials have shown it to be no better than placebo. Nonetheless, facet-joint steroid injection continues to be offered to persons who obtain temporary pain relief with the intraarticular injection of anesthetic.

Acupuncture. The data are at best inconclusive, with many studies showing no benefit and others indicating some improvement over placebo, particularly among persons who believe the treatment will be helpful. Serious methodologic shortcomings make it difficult to draw definitive conclusions, other than that if there is a benefit, it is probably small. At best, improvements are modest and found predominantly among persons who believe the procedure will be effective. Such results are insufficient to recommend the procedure as a standard component of treatment for persons with chronic pain. Despite the fact that results from controlled trials have been disappointing, many persons still undergo treatment based on the rationale that there is an outside chance of benefit and little risk. The cost is high, and no cost savings have been identified.

Transcutaneous Nerve Stimulation. Contrary to initially enthusiastic reports, controlled trials find *transcutaneous electrical nerve stimulation* to be no better than placebo.

Protecting the Patient from Unnecessary and Potentially Harmful Measures

The frustration and incapacity that often accompany chronic low back pain place patients at considerable risk for unnecessary, often expensive, and potentially harmful interventions. Taking the time to provide sufferers of chronic back pain with evidence-based information on what works and what does not, including a respectful and serious review of popular alternative therapies, is much appreciated by patients and well worth the effort. It can lessen their need to "shop around" for a cure, and it reduces the risk of their falling into the hands of enthusiastic practitioners who may be willing to provide potentially dangerous or expensive therapies in a non–evidence-based manner.

Preserving Capacity to Function Independently

Establishing a strong doctor–patient alliance through an understanding of and respect for the patient's perspective and psychosocial context is a prerequisite to engaging the patient in a program of self-help. The caring, concern, and responsiveness that characterize a strong relationship help to foster patient confidence and receptiveness. Even though symptoms may not disappear, it is often possible to keep the patient functioning independently through cultivation of the relationship and promulgation of a program of activity and exercise. Arranging regularly scheduled visits at intervals meaningful to the patient facilitates the sense of support and can forestall many anxious phone calls and unannounced office appearances.

Spinal Stenosis

The initial management of spinal stenosis can be conservative because the natural history of the condition includes gradual improvement over time in some patients. Nonsurgical measures commonly used include physical therapy, NSAIDs and other analgesics, and epidural corticosteroid injections. Nearly 60% of patients managed conservatively report satisfactory results at 4 years. However, for some patients the condition continues to be a frustrating source of pain and disability, leading to the consideration of surgical intervention. Although surgery is widely touted as effective and is frequently performed (spinal stenosis surgery is the most common back operation in persons older than the age of 65 years; success rates of up to 60% are reported), there are limited data from large-scale, well-designed, randomized trials comparing surgery to conservative management.

Physical Therapy

Stretching, strengthening, and aerobic exercises are typically taught with the goals of improving strength, endurance, and flexibility. Objectives include improving lumbar flexion and flattening of the lumbar lordotic curve. The formal McKenzie approach of customized exercises based on an analysis of pain response to spinal movement and postural deficiencies is among the better studied programs and is capable of producing 50% improvements in participants.

Nonnarcotic Analgesics, Antiinflammatories, and Analgesics

In the absence of studies comparing various pharmacologic approaches to pain control, nonnarcotic analgesics (e.g., acetaminophen) are a reasonable place to start. Because there is little inflammation associated with spinal stenosis, NSAIDs are used predominantly for their analgesic properties and should be used cautiously in this predominantly elderly population, which is vulnerable to their adverse effects (see Chapter 156). Opioids can have a role as part of a comprehensive treatment program, but they need to be used carefully to avoid excessive sedation and adverse consequences such as falls and automobile accidents.

Epidural Steroid Injection

Despite the fact that it is widely used, only one study has shown benefit from epidural steroid injection therapy, and there are no randomized, controlled trials. The rationale is uncertain for the use of any antiinflammatory therapy, let alone one that is delivered by invasive means, because most of the pathology is degenerative and chronic. If there is evidence of disk herniation and associated inflammation, then perhaps there might be a reason to consider steroid injection, analogous to its contribution in disk disease (see prior discussion).

Surgery

Surgery is a purely elective and reasonable consideration for persons with incapacitating disease characterized by debilitating pain and progressive neurologic impairment. There is no prophylactic indication for surgery. The procedure most commonly performed is standard *decompressive laminectomy*; if there is spondylolisthesis, *spinal fusion* is added. As noted, there have been few large-scale, long-term, randomized trials of surgery, a situation that continues to limit evidence-based decision making. However, emerging data from the best available randomized studies (which are muddied by large percentages of patients crossing over to the other treatment group) suggest modest but statistically and clinically meaningful improvements, especially in pain control. Differences in outcomes narrow over time, but they appear to persist at 2 years. Relapse rates are high, with 30% of those who undergo surgery experiencing a relapse of severe pain at 4 years and 10% requiring reoperation.

Spondyloarthropathies (7,48)

Basic therapy consists of *NSAIDs* during periods of symptomatic inflammation in conjunction with a lifelong program of *exercises* and stretching. Persistent focal inflammation due to enthesitis or synovitis can be treated with a *local injection of corticosteroid*. Enteric-coated *sulfasalazine* is helpful when NSAIDs do not suffice for the control of peripheral arthritis or when symptoms of psoriatic disease or inflammatory bowel disease flare. *Methotrexate* is used when other therapies fail, but a beneficial effect on spinal disease has not been confirmed in controlled trial. *Antibiotics* do not appear to be helpful in established cases related to chlamydial infection, but prompt treatment of chlamydial infection can help to prevent disease in susceptible populations. The most important advance in treatment has been use of parenteral *anti–tumor necrosis factor-α* (*infliximab* [Remicade] or *etanercept* [Enbrel]), which in randomized, controlled trials resulted in rapid, sustained, and significant improvements in all disease parameters. However, disease activity resumes with the cessation of these very expensive treatments.

PATIENT EDUCATION

The importance of patient education cannot be overemphasized for the person with back pain. Surveys of patients with back pain find that a lack of information is the greatest source of dissatisfaction with care. Patients suffering from a condition that suddenly disables them are extremely anxious and in need of detailed information about what has happened, what can be done, and what lies ahead. Even if the diagnosis has not been established, a review of the working differential helps one to deal with the uncertainty of the situation. The use of a model of the spine greatly simplifies explanation and helps many patients to better understand their condition. Patients with disk herniation can be reassured that the natural history of their condition is generally favorable, with most responding well to conservative therapy and very few suffering prolonged physical disability. Active patients are greatly relieved to know that jogging, stationary cycling, and swimming are not only possible but often desirable, and that the reemergence of mild to moderate discomfort with the resumption of activity is to be expected and is not a worrisome prognostic sign. At the same time, it is important to review with the patient the symptoms of serious neurologic injury that would necessitate prompt reporting and hospital admission. The rationale and anatomic basis for back hygiene measures and exercises also need to be reviewed to ensure compliance and proper implementation. A good outcome is greatly facilitated by keeping the patient well informed.

The extensive patient demand for unnecessary imaging studies and unproven therapies presents a major educational challenge to primary care physicians. A visit spent supportively eliciting the patient's perspective and objectively reviewing the relative merits of available tests and treatments (both conventional and "alternative") can be extremely helpful to the design and implementation of an effective management plan.

INDICATIONS FOR ADMISSION AND REFERRAL

Urgent Referral and Hospital Admission

Patients with rapidly progressive neurologic deficits require prompt neurologic and surgical consultations. Urgent admission and referral are indicated if symptoms suggestive of *cauda equina syndrome* or *cord compression* develop (e.g., new bilateral neurologic deficits, urinary retention, sphincter incontinence, saddle anesthesia, upper motor neuron symptoms and signs, truncal sensory loss). The same is true for patients with acute *vertebral collapse* because spinal stability may be compromised by the fracture. A suspicion of *osteomyelitis* or *epidural abscess* is an indication for immediate hospitalization and infectious disease consultation. Particularly in patients with epidural abscess, treatment must be initiated early to be effective.

Elective Referral

Back pain management often requires a multidimensional approach that benefits from the services of a number of health care professionals. An important responsibility of the primary care physician is to arrange timely and appropriate referral while continuing to maintain a close working relationship with the patient and overall control of the management program. Without compromising that relationship, referral can help to ease the burden of care, as well as provide valuable additional services.

Physical Therapy

Referral for physical therapy is an essential component of a comprehensive management program, particularly for persons with persistent symptoms. The support and patient education provided are very much appreciated, and the exercise program prescribed is one of the few evidence-based elements of an effective treatment program for persons with chronic back pain.

Surgery

If back pain due to *disk herniation* remains severe and intractable after 4 to 6 weeks of conservative therapy or if an important neurologic deficit develops or progresses (e.g., foot drop, gastrocnemius-soleus or quadriceps weakness), then further evaluation and consideration of elective surgery are indicated and referral to an orthopedist or neurosurgeon with expertise and an evidence-based approach to back problems can be helpful. Even if the patient does not have sciatica or neurologic deficits and is therefore not a candidate for surgery, the referral can serve to reassure the patient that a surgically correctable lesion is not being overlooked. Persons with disabling spinal stenosis are also reasonable candidates for surgical consultation.

Mental Health Referral

Persons with chronic pain due to or complicated by an underlying psychiatric disorder may benefit from referral to a mental health professional specifically trained in *cognitive–behavioral therapy*. Because this person is often not a psychiatrist, the referral may be easier for the patient to accept, especially if it is couched in terms of helping one to cope with pain and improve daily functioning.

Pain Center Referral

Patients with refractory chronic pain, particularly if neuropathic (see Chapter 236), may benefit from a pain center assessment and a program that might include selective nerve block and other forms of interventional treatment. Centers that can offer a comprehensive set of services in addition to injections (e.g., cognitive–behavioral therapy, physical therapy, massage) might be particularly advantageous.

Alternative Therapy Referral

A massage therapy referral can be very helpful to persons with severe acute or chronic back pain, provided a careful workup reveals no contraindications to the use of massage (see prior discussion). Some physical therapists are also trained in massage therapy and can provide the treatment as part of their overall care. Yoga has been shown to be more effective than exercise; referral to a yoga class designed for back patients should be considered if such a program is available. Referrals for chiropractic spinal manipulation and acupuncture are not recommended as standard components of care because there is little evidence these expensive modalities offer added benefit. However, a patient who has a strong belief in such therapy might achieve a good response and deserves consideration of referral.

A.H.G. A.G.M.

Annotated Bibliography

1. Baker AS, Ojemann RG, Swartz MN, et al. Spinal epidural abscess. N Engl J Med 1975;293:463. (*A classic paper describing clinical presentation.*)
2. Bates DW, Reuler JB. Back pain and epidural spinal cord compression. J Gen Intern Med 1988;3:191. (*A detailed review of this spinal presentation of metastatic disease; 52 references.*)
3. Carey TS, Garrett J, Jackman A, et al. The North Carolina Back Pain Project. The outcomes and costs of care for acute low back pain among patients seen by primary care practitioners, chiropractors, and orthopedic surgeons. N Engl J Med 1995;333:913. (*Symptoms diminished rapidly, with <20% of patients having persistent functional impairment lasting 25 days after the initial visit.*)
4. Deyo RA, Weinstein JN. Low back pain. N Engl J Med 2001;344:363. (*An excellent clinical review for the primary care physician.*)
5. Deyo RA, Loeser JD, Bigos SJ. Herniated lumbar intervertebral disk. Ann Intern Med 1990;112:598. (*A succinct, critical look at diagnostic and therapeutic modalities; 41 references.*)
6. Koes BW, van Tulder MW, Peul WC. Diagnosis and treatment of sciatica. BMJ 2007;334:131317. (*An excellent concise review.*)
7. Khan MA. Update on spondyloarthropathies. Ann Intern Med 2002;136:896. (*An excellent and extensive review; 143 references.*)
8. Kostuik JP, Harrington I, Alexander D, et al. Cauda equina syndrome and lumbar disk herniation. J Bone Joint Surg Am 1986;68:386. (*Delineates the clinical features of this important syndrome.*)
9. Waddell G, McCulloch JA, Kummel E, et al. Nonorganic physical signs in low back pain. Spine 1980;5:117. (*Describes physical findings, as noted in this chapter, suggestive of persons with psychological distress.*)
10. Deyo RA, Rainville J, Kent DL. What can the history and physical examination tell us about low back pain? JAMA 1992;268:760. (*Data on the diagnostic utility of historical and physical findings; many of its observations and conclusions are cited in this chapter.*)
11. Edelman RR, Warach S. Magnetic resonance imaging. N Engl J Med 1993;328:708. (*A major review, with a useful section on spinal imaging.*)

12. Jarvik JG, Deyo RA. Diagnostic evaluation of low back pain with emphasis on imaging. Ann Intern Med 2002;137:586. (*A systematic review, recommending imaging only for persons being considered for surgery or who have evidence of systemic disease.*)

13. Hollingworth W, Gray DT, Martin BI, et al. Rapid magnetic resonance imaging for diagnosis of cancer-related low back pain: a cost-effectiveness analysis. J Gen Intern Med 2003;18:303. (*The cost per quality-adjusted life year was nearly $300,000, making this approach hard to justify on a cost-effectiveness basis.*)

14. Jensen MC, Brant-Zawadzki MN, Obuchowski N, et al. Magnetic resonance imaging of the lumbar spine in people without back pain. N Engl J Med 1994;331:69. (*Among asymptomatic people, 52% had bulges, 27% had protrusions, and 1% had extrusions.*)

15. Liang M, Komaroff AL. Roentgenograms in primary-care patients with acute low back pain: a cost-effectiveness study. Arch Intern Med 1982;142:1108. (*The cost was high and the yield was low if films were ordered unselectively on a first visit.*)

16. Assendelft WJJ, Morton SC, Yu EI, et al. Spinal manipulative therapy for low back pain: a meta-analysis of effectiveness relative to other therapies. Ann Intern Med 2003;138:871. (*Spinal manipulation was no better than other modestly effective therapies.*)

17. Atlas SJ, Deyo RA, Keller RB, et al. The Maine Lumbar Spine Study, Part II. One-year outcome of surgical and nonsurgical management of sciatica. Spine 1996;21:1777. (*Definite improvement was seen in dominant symptoms in 71% of surgical patients and 43% of nonsurgical patients.*)

18. Atlas SJ, Keller RB, Robson D, et al. Surgical and nonsurgical management of lumbar spinal stenosis: four-year outcomes from the Maine Lumbar Spine Study. Spine 2000;25:556. (*An observational study, showing some long-term benefit, with definite improvement in dominant symptoms in 55% of surgical patients and 21% of nonsurgical patients.*)

19. Browning R, Jackson JL, O'Malley PG. Cyclobenzaprine and back pain: a meta-analysis. Arch Intern Med 2001;161:1613. (*Finds benefit over placebo, but only for the first few days.*)

20. Carette S, Leclaire R, Marcoux S, et al. Epidural corticosteroid injection for sciatica due to herniated nucleus pulposus. N Engl J Med 1997;336:1634. (*Finds no evidence for significant clinical benefit.*)

21. Carette S, Marcoux S, Truchon R, et al. A controlled trial of corticosteroid injections into facet joints for chronic low back pain. N Engl J Med 1991;325:1002. (*Find no evidence of benefit.*)

22. Cherkin DC, Deyo RA, Battie M, et al. A comparison of physical therapy, chiropractic manipulation, and provision of an educational booklet for the treatment of patients with low back pain. N Engl J Med 1998;339:1021. (*There were no clinically significant differences in outcome among the three groups; however, those seen by either a physical therapist or a chiropractor were more satisfied with their care.*)

23. Cherkin DC, Eisenberg D, Sherman KJ, et al. Randomized trial comparing traditional Chinese medial acupuncture, therapeutic massage, and self-care education for chronic low back pain. Arch Intern Med 2001;161:1081. (*Massage proved best.*)

24. Cherkin DC, Sherman KJ, Deyo RA, et al. A review of the evidence for the effectiveness, safety, and cost of acupuncture, massage therapy, and spinal manipulation. Ann Intern Med 2003;138:898. (*A systematic review, finding evidence for massage, less for manipulation, and little for acupuncture.*)

25. Childs JD, Fritz JM, Flynn TW, et al. A clinical prediction rule to identify patients with low back pain most likely to benefit from spinal manipulation: a validation study. Ann Intern Med 2004;141:920. (*Finds improved response rate in a military population.*)

26. Deen HG, Fenton DS, Lamer TJ. Minimally invasive procedures for disorders of the lumbar spine. Mayo Clin Proc 2003;78:1249. (*A helpful review for the generalist reader; 49 references.*)

27. Deyo RA, Diehl AK, Rosenthal M. How many days of bed rest for acute low back pain? N Engl J Med 1986;315:1064. (*A randomized clinical trial, showing that for patients without neuromotor deficits, 2 days of bed rest was as effective as 7 days.*)

28. Deyo RA, Walsh N, Martin D, et al. A controlled trial of transcutaneous electrical nerve stimulation (TENS) and exercise for chronic low back pain. N Engl J Med 1990;322:1627. (*Transcutaneous electrical nerve stimulation was no better than the control intervention.*)

29. Deyo RA. Conservative therapy for low back pain. JAMA 1983;250:1057. (*A review of 59 therapeutic trials; also useful for its critique of study designs.*)

30. Gorman JD, Sack KE, Davis JC. Treatment of ankylosing spondylitis by inhibition of tumor necrosis factor α. N Engl J Med 2002;346:1349. (*A randomized, controlled trial [RCT], finding that significant improvement was achieved.*)

31. Hoffman RH, Wheeler KJ, Deyo RA. Surgery for herniated disks. A literature review. J Gen Intern Med 1993;8:487. (*Finds many shortcomings in study design, but the overall impression is that properly selected patients derive some benefit from diskectomy.*)

32. Koes BW, Scholten RJ, Mens JM, et al. Efficacy of nonsteroidal anti-inflammatory drugs for low back pain: a systematic review of randomised clinical trials. Ann Rheum Dis 1997;56:214. (*Finds evidence for efficacy.*)

33. Lahad A, Malter AD, Berg AO, et al. The effectiveness of four interventions for the prevention of low back pain. JAMA 1994;272:1286. (*There was limited evidence to recommend exercise and insufficient evidence to recommend risk factor modification, mechanical supports, or education.*)

34. Malmivaara A, Hakkinen U, Aro T, et al. The treatment of acute low back pain—bed rest, exercises, or ordinary activity? N Engl J Med 1995;332:351. (*More rapid recovery was found among those who continued activity than in those treated with bed rest or exercise programs.*)

35. Mannion AF, Muntener M, Taimela S, et al. Comparison of three active therapies for chronic low back pain: results of a randomized clinical trial with one-year follow-up. Rheumatology 2001;40:772. (*The therapies were equal at 3 months, but there was some fall-off in the physiotherapy group at 12 months.*)

36. McLain RF, Kapural L, Mekhail NA. Epidural steroids for back and leg pain: mechanism of action and efficacy. Cleve Clin J Med 2004;71:961. (*A very useful clinical review for the nonspecialist; 52 references.*)

37. Mendelson G, Selwood T, Kranz H, et al. Acupuncture treatment of chronic back pain. Am J Med 1983;74:49. (*A double-blinded, placebo-controlled study, finding no difference in results.*)

38. Martell BA, O'Connor PGO, Kerns RD, et al. Systematic review: opioid treatment for chronic back pain: prevalence, efficacy, and association with addiction. Ann Intern Med 2007;146:116. (*Finds that opioids were commonly prescribed and possibly effective for short-term pain relief, but that the benefit of sustained use was unclear; there was a high prevalence of substance abuse.*)

39. Milne S, Welch MS, Brosseau L, et al. Transcutaneous electrical nerve stimulation (TENS) for chronic low back pain. Cochrane Database Syst Rev 2001:CD003008. (*No benefit was found.*)

40. Moffett JK, Torgerson D, Bell-Syer S, et al. Randomised controlled trial of exercise for low back pain: clinical outcomes, costs and preferences. BMJ 1999;319:279. (*Patients with subacute pain who participated in an eight-session exercise program did significantly better.*)

41. Pengel LHM, Refshauge KM, Maher CG, et al. Physiotherapist-directed exercise, advice, or both for subacute low back pain: a randomized trial. Ann Intern Med 2007;146:787. (*A physiotherapist-directed combined program was the best approach and was better than placebo at 6 and 12 weeks.*)

42. Peul WC, van Houwelingen HC, van den Hout WB, et al., for the Leiden–The Hague Spine Intervention Prognostic Study Group. Surgery versus prolonged conservative treatment for sciatica. N Engl J Med 2007;356:2245. (*RCT, showing improved early outcomes with surgery but no difference at 1 year.*)

43. Salerno SM, Browning R, Jackson JL. The effect of antidepressant treatment on chronic back pain: a meta-analysis. Arch Intern Med 2002;162:19. (*This approach was found to reduce pain but did little for functional status.*)

44. Shekelle PG, Adamas AH, Chassin MP, et al. Spinal manipulation for low-back pain. Ann Intern Med 1992;117:590. (*A meta-analysis, finding short-term value in patients with uncomplicated acute back pain; data were insufficient for determining utility in chronic back pain.*)

45. Sherman KJ, Cherkin DC, Erro J, et al. Comparing yoga, exercise, and a self-care book for chronic low back pain. Ann Intern Med 2005;143:849 (*Exercise was more effective in reducing symptoms, disability, and medication use than a self-care book, and yoga was more effective than exercise.*)

46. Simotas CA, Dorey JF, Hansraj KK, et al. Nonoperative treatment for lumbar spinal stenosis: clinical and outcome results and a 3-year survivorship analysis. Spine 2000;25:197. (*A cohort study, finding that most patients did reasonably well with conservative therapy.*)

47. Stevinson C, Ernst E. Risks associated with spinal manipulation therapy. Am J Med 2002;112:566. (*Quantifies the risk based on the available data.*)

48. van Tulder MW, Cherkin DC, Berman B, et al. The effectiveness of acupuncture in the management of acute and chronic low back pain: a systematic review within the framework of the Cochrane Collaboration Back Review Group. Spine 1999;24:1113. (*Finds little evidence of benefit for acute or chronic back pain.*)

49. van Tulder MW, Malmivaara A, Esmail R, et al. Exercise therapy for low back pain. Cochrane Database Syst Rev 2001;4:CD000335. (*Finds evidence for the effectiveness of exercise in chronic low back pain.*)

50. Von Korff M, Barlow W, Cherkin D, et al. Effects of practice style in managing back pain. Ann Intern Med 1994;121:187. (*Practice styles consistent with self-care for back pain yielded similar long-term pain and functional outcomes at lower cost.*)

51. Wassell JT, Gardner LI, Landsittel DP, et al. A prospective study of back belts for prevention of back pain and injury. JAMA 2000;284:2727. (*A large-scale study of thousands of employees, finding no benefit.*)

52. Weber H. Lumbar disk herniation: a controlled prospective study with 10 years of observation. Spine 1983;8:131. (*RCT comparing medical and surgical therapy, finding that earlier relief was achieved with surgery, but that no difference in outcomes was seen after 3 to 4 years.*)

53. Weinstein JN, Lurie JD, Tosteson TD, et al. Surgical versus nonsurgical treatment for lumbar degenerative spondylolisthesis. N Engl J Med 2007;356:2257. (*RCT, finding that, overall, a modest benefit was noted in surgically treated persons, with the greatest relief achieved early on.*)

54. Weinstein JN, Lurie JD, Tosteson TD, et al. Surgical vs nonoperative treatment for lumbar disk herniation. The Spine Outcomes Research Trial (SPORT) observational cohort. JAMA 2006;296:2451. (*Patients in both treatment groups improved substantially over 2 years; those who chose surgery reported greater improvement.*)

55. Weinstein JN, Tosteson TD, Lurie JD, et al, for the SPORT Investigators. Surgical versus nonsurgical therapy for lumbar spinal stenosis. N Engl J Med 2008;358:794. (*Large-scale, long-term RCT in persons without spondylolisthesis, finding evidence of benefit from surgery.*)

56. Weinstein JN, Tosteson TD, Lurie JD, et al. Surgical vs nonoperative treatment for lumbar disk herniation. The Spine Outcomes Research Trial (SPORT): a randomized trial. JAMA 2006;296:2441. (*Patients in both treatment groups improved substantially over 2 years; there were no untoward outcomes in either group.*)

CHAPTER 148 ■ EVALUATION OF NECK PAIN

The primary care physician is often faced with the patient who complains of a stiff neck; most of the time, the problem is musculoskeletal in origin. Although the majority of musculoskeletal causes are not serious, they can result in considerable discomfort. The primary care physician should be able to provide symptomatic relief to the person with a minor neck problem and to identify the patient with a serious complication of cervical spine disease, such as root compression or cord injury that requires surgical attention.

PATHOPHYSIOLOGY AND CLINICAL PRESENTATION (1–3)

Neck Strain

The most common form of neck pain is caused by *cervical paraspinal muscle spasm*, usually secondary to minor strain or prolonged, unconscious muscle contraction associated with emotional stress. The problem is usually self-limited. Neck pain caused by minor muscle ligament strain is usually self-limited if aggravating activities are avoided. A relapsing clinical course is not uncommon. Muscle spasm also occurs with cervical degenerative disease (see later discussion).

"Whiplash" Injury

Severe neck strain is seen in *cervical hyperextension* (whiplash) injury, which is typically sustained in an automobile accident. Sudden hyperextension of the neck followed by hyperflexion flexion can result in significant musculoligamentous strain. The cervical segments are forced beyond their physiologic limits, resulting in tissue failure. Shearing and compressive forces tear muscle fibers and ligaments and exert excessive pressure on the disks and zygapophyseal joints. Soft-tissue bleeding, swelling, severe muscle spasm, and joint and disk injury ensue, triggering pain. Symptoms typically increase over several hours, often becoming most severe the day after the acute event. The anterior or posterior ligaments of the cervical spine may be disrupted, but neurologic deficits are rare unless a cervical spine fracture is present that leads to root or cord compression. Refractory pain lasting more than 6 months may represent injury to a zygapophyseal joint, although other causes include the psychological stress of ongoing litigation and pending legal proceedings. The use of conventional seat belts does not prevent whiplash; force is still translated to the neck. Head restraints, if set too low, may exacerbate the hyperextension.

The clinical course is a function of the severity of injury and any preexisting mechanical or psychosocial pathology. Persons with a history of chronic pain complaints are likely to experience a prolonged course even after relatively minor injury. The same is true for those with concurrent psychosocial stress. Most other individuals experience relief within 6 months of the accident.

Degenerative Disease

Degenerative disease is a key factor, accounting for nearly 75% of cervical radiculopathy cases. Age-related reduction in disk height and degenerative changes in adjacent facet joints lead to subluxation (*cervical spondylosis*), narrowing of the neuroforamina, and encroachment on the cervical nerve roots and dorsal-root ganglia. Immobility and consolidation of the joint may ensue. Usually, the process is localized to the lower cervical levels, such as C-4 to C-5, C-5 to C-6, or C-6 to C-7. Degenerative changes and spurring at the cervical disk spaces are prominent. The condition presents as recurring neck stiffness and mild aching discomfort, with progressive limitation of neck motion over months to years. Lateral rotation and lateral flexion of the neck toward the painful side are limited; pain is precipitated or increased by such motions.

Cervical disk herniation can also lead to a narrowing of the neural foramina and the impingement of nerve roots. Herniation of the nucleus pulposus accounts for less than a one fourth of cervical radiculopathy cases. When there is concurrent compression of the dorsal root ganglia, radicular pain invariably ensues; compression of the root alone may not always trigger pain; inflammatory mediators appear to play a role in the generation of pain. Pain radiates in the distribution of the affected nerve root, and paresthesias, numbness, and weakness may be associated. The C-5, C-6, and C-7 nerve roots are most often affected. C-5 root compression results in the development of pain, paresthesias, and numbness in the anterosuperior shoulder and anterolateral aspect of the upper arm and forearm; a decreased biceps jerk and weakness of elbow flexion are found on examination. Compression of the C-6 nerve root produces symptoms in the dorsoradial aspect of the forearm and thumb, whereas C-7 impingement is indicated by altered sensation in the middle of the hand. The brachioradialis tendon reflex is affected by conditions altering C-5 and C-6, and the triceps jerk by injury to the C-7 and C-8 roots. The sensory symptoms and pain may follow different distributions, with the former being dermatomal and the latter being myotomal (see Chapter 167).

Inflammatory Disease

Rheumatoid disease can produce neck pain; it is typically worse in the morning. Concurrent symmetric polyarthropathy and subluxation at C-1 to C-2 (identifiable on plain films of the neck in flexion and extension) are characteristic. In the *spondyloarthropathies*, neck pain occurs in the context of diffuse back and sacroiliac discomfort. The earliest radiologic signs are those of sacroiliitis visible on sacroiliac joint films; advanced disease produces syndesmophytes. In *polymyalgia rheumatica*, neck pain may accompany the aching discomfort and stiffness of the shoulders and hip girdle that predominate in this condition. Polymyalgia complicated by *giant-cell arteritis* with carotid artery involvement can produce focal neck tenderness along one or both carotid arteries, sometimes referred to as *carotodynia*.

Malignancy

Tumor may infiltrate the spinal cord or the vertebral bodies and produce pain that is worse at night or while lying down. Cord involvement may be heralded by neurologic deficits in addition to the nocturnal pain.

Referred Pain

Neck pain radiating to the jaw is characteristic of *coronary ischemia*, which is usually precipitated or worsened by physical activity. Concurrent arm pain may simulate a cervical radiculopathy. *Esophageal* disease may produce pain referable to the neck; if a cancer of the esophagus extends into the prevertebral space, posterior pain may develop.

DIFFERENTIAL DIAGNOSIS (1)

The musculoskeletal causes of neck pain include muscle strain, muscle spasm, cervical spondylosis, and cervical root compression. Lymphadenopathy, thyroiditis (see Chapter 104), angina pectoris (see Chapter 20), and meningitis are important causes of cervical pain that may be mistaken for a musculoskeletal problem.

WORKUP (1,2,4)

History

Inquiry should focus on elucidating precipitating events, aggravating and alleviating factors (particularly specific neck movements), area of maximal tenderness, radiation of pain, presence of numbness or weakness in the extremities, course, past history of similar problems, history of prior or current malignancy, and previous therapeutic efforts. Warning symptoms of serious underlying pathology include concurrent fever and chills, unexplained weight loss, persistent nocturnal pain, and nuchal rigidity. Also of importance is screening for the development of myelopathy, which might be suggested by bilateral hand weakness or clumsiness, difficulty with balance, and new onset of urinary difficulties. Checking for symptoms and risk factors for myocardial ischemia rounds out the initial inquiry.

Physical Examination

Physical examination must include full visualization of the neck, thorax, and upper extremities. Neck motions are assessed, including flexion–extension, left and right lateral flexion, and left and right rotation. The neck must be carefully palpated to identify the point of local tenderness, which gives the best indication of the structure involved. Careful examination of the upper extremities is also required and should include an evaluation of tendon reflexes, strength, sensation, range of motion, and pulses. Every patient with fever and neck pain should be tested for meningeal signs. Also critical is checking for evidence of myelopathy (hyperreflexia, upgoing toes, neck flexion causing a jolt down the spine, bilateral motor and/or sensory deficits in the hands, sphincter difficulties).

Laboratory Studies

Blood tests add little to workup, except in the setting of suspected infection. Similarly, *plain films* of the neck are of limited value, except to detect fracture in persons with serious trauma or to confirm the presence of suspected degenerative disease and spondylosis, but findings may bear little relation to symptoms. In cases of nontraumatic neck strain, no imaging studies are necessary (the only finding would be loss of the normal lordotic curve).

Magnetic resonance imaging (MRI) is the test of choice when persistent neurologic compromise accompanies radicular neck pain, especially if symptoms are persistent for more than 6 to 12 weeks or steadily worsening and interventional or surgical therapy is being contemplated. Prompt MRI is indicated if there is concern about myelopathy from cervical cord compression. The test should not be ordered routinely for neck pain because test specificity is poor (up to half of asymptomatic persons have disk herniations on MRI) and cost is high. MRI has largely replaced *bone scan* for detection of spinal cord tumor. *Computed tomographic (CT) scan* is reserved for instances in which details of bony change (spurs, foraminal narrowing) or ligamentous calcification are desired.

SYMPTOMATIC MANAGEMENT (1–3,5–16)

Most causes of neck pain are self-limited and resolve with time. However, the discomfort can be considerable, so that symptomatic measures are necessary. Management of the patient presenting with chronic neck pain after an automobile accident can be problematic and challenging.

Strain

Initial Measures

Heat, *ice*, and gentle *massage* may ease muscle spasm. So-called *muscle relaxants* (e.g., *cyclobenzaprine* [Flexeril], which is chemically similar to the tricyclic antidepressants) are widely prescribed, but controlled trials found that cyclobenzaprine adds little to the relief afforded by nonsteroidal antiinflammatory drugs (NSAIDs). However, meta-analysis suggests that *cyclobenzaprine* can be of help to patients in the very acute phase of illness, probably as a consequence of the drug's sedating effects. More useful and less expensive are therapeutic doses of an NSAID (e.g., aspirin, ibuprofen), supplemented for a few days by a small nighttime dose of a generic *benzodiazepine* (e.g., 5 mg of diazepam at bedtime). Prolonged benzodiazepine use should be avoided (see Chapter 226). A soft *cervical collar* may be used to rest sore neck muscles briefly, especially at night; however, prolonged wear should be discouraged because it may lead to muscle weakening from disuse atrophy. Collar use can be supplemented by range-of-motion *exercises*, such as slow rotation clockwise and then counterclockwise multiple times each day.

Subsequent Measures

More severe strain, such as that resulting from whiplash injury, can pose a difficult management problem. Patients coming for help complaining of persistent pain may also be seeking validation and certification for liability and disability claims that can cloud the clinical picture, delay return to normal function, and strain the doctor–patient relationship. An appreciation for the degree of tissue and joint injury that can occur in severe accidents should help to minimize unnecessary skepticism, but ongoing liability claims can provide perverse incentives that compromise clinical progress. Similarly, concurrent psychosocial stress can lead to refractoriness and a prolonged clinical course. A multimodality approach is often required to get the best results.

Cervical Collar. Although patients prefer wearing a cervical collar acutely because neck movement is painful, use of the collar should be limited to the period of severe pain and eliminated as soon as the most severe pain has eased. Prolonged use of a collar beyond the initial 2 to 4 days of severe pain actually increases the duration of pain, limits the return of neck mobility, and slows the clinical course. Emphasis should be placed on return of neck function and range of motion.

Exercise. A program of range-of-motion, stretching, and strengthening exercises taught by a physical therapist can be very helpful in restoring functional capacity. In a randomized trial, patients treated with early neck mobilization and exercises experienced significantly less pain and more rapid return of function than did those randomized to 2 weeks of neck rest and a cervical collar. The exercise program in the study consisted of 10 rotational exercises performed 10 times per hour beginning no later than 96 hours after the accident. The benefits of exercise may extend well beyond the short term and can be demonstrated years later. *Exercise training* has been shown to be effective in a randomized, controlled trial of women with nonspecific chronic neck pain (absent major disk herniation). Active neck muscle training combined with aerobics and stretching performed twice weekly reduced pain and disability.

Injection, Ultrasound, Acupuncture, Spinal Manipulation. There is no evidence that *injecting anesthetic* into the tender body of a muscle in spasm speeds the resolution of the problem; injection may actually injure the muscle. *Ultrasound* and *diathermy* treatments provide subjective improvement beyond that derived from medical management but often no more so than placebo forms of these therapies. *Acupuncture* is commonly performed; evidence of efficacy is at best mixed, but most well-designed studies show no benefit, clinically insignificant benefit, or benefit limited to persons who believe in the procedure.

Spinal manipulation as performed by chiropractors gets much play in the care of chronic neck strain, but its utility, safety, and indications for use remain to be defined by properly designed prospective, randomized trials. In one of the few well-designed, randomized trials to compare medical therapy, physical therapy, and manipulation in persons with nonspecific persistent neck pain of at least 2 weeks' duration, manipulation provided the best results at 7 weeks in terms of pain relief and functional status. However, such therapy was also associated with the highest rates of adverse effects, including increased neck pain for more than 2 days (18%), headache (28%), and pain or paresthesias in the arms (13%). Moreover, there was enthusiasm for manual therapy among participants, which was a predictor of favorable outcome, raising the question of whether the benefit was due to the treatment or the belief in the treatment. Confirmation of these findings in more skeptical clinical settings is indicated before manual therapy can be considered an evidence-based component of standard therapy. Spinal manipulation is contraindicated when there is disk herniation or neurologic deficit; it may precipitate or worsen nerve root or cord compression.

Settling Disability and Liability Claims. When strain has resulted from an automobile accident or work-related event that has triggered a liability or disability claim, the patient should be encouraged to settle any lawsuit or disability claim as quickly as possible; unresolved claims can delay recovery by distracting the patient from the treatment program and creating a perverse incentive not to get better. If a disability determination is needed, it should be expedited. Arranging an independent disability evaluation may be best if the physician does not feel comfortable certifying that the patient is physically disabled; this avoids jeopardizing the patient–physician relationship.

Addressing Concurrent Psychosocial Distress. Psychosocial problems can have an important effect on chronic pain presentation and clinical course (see Chapter 236). Pain from whiplash injury is no exception, especially because the injury is usually accident related and thus accompanied by a host of major psychosocial stresses. Treating underlying depression (see Chapter 226), prescribing cognitive–behavioral therapy for persons with somatization disorder (see Chapter 230), and addressing family, job, and financial stresses can be essential to a successful outcome.

Degenerative Disease

In cases of cervical spondylosis and disk herniation associated with radiculopathy, symptomatic therapy is aimed at countering the inflammation and root compression responsible for pain.

Initial Measures

Nonsteroidal agents (e.g., generic ibuprofen or naproxen) are prescribed to treat inflammation, and a *cervical collar* may help to minimize root compression. Unlike cervical sprain, short-term immobilization (1 to 2 weeks) may be necessary in persons with mechanical neck disease; the collar should be worn continuously or at least at night until pain disappears. After pain lessens, the collar can be worn at those times when added support may be helpful, such as at night or when riding in a motor vehicle. A properly fitting collar holds the neck in gentle flexion (the neutral position); collars that produce excessive extension are to be avoided because they may aggravate root compression. Evidence supporting collar use is limited.

Home Cervical Traction

Its rationale is the relief of nerve root decompression in persons with persistent radicular pain due to cervical spondylosis or disk herniation. The evidence is of inadequate quality to make an objective determination regarding its usefulness. Nonetheless, sitting cervical traction it is a commonly applied therapy to persons with persistent or recurrent radicular pain. It is applied at home for 20 to 30 minutes, two to four times a day, with 6 to 10 pounds of weight. The cervical traction apparatus must be carefully aligned and pull slightly forward at an angle of about 20 degrees to follow the natural line in the neck (Fig. 148.1). Proper technique is essential for effective and safe use.

Epidural Injection

Either translaminar or transforaminal epidural injection of a corticosteroid (e.g., methylprednisolone) has the potential to achieve sustained pain relief in up to 60% of patients. There is an associated risk of serious complications (e.g., cord injury, brainstem infarction), which is small in expert hands but needs to be taken into consideration.

Exercises for Secondary Prevention

Active range-of-motion exercises are commonly prescribed once symptoms have eased, sometimes complemented by isometric and resistance exercises. Evidence of benefit is modest.

Surgery

Surgery is indicated for progressive or refractory disease (see Indications for Admission and Referral). Rates of long-term

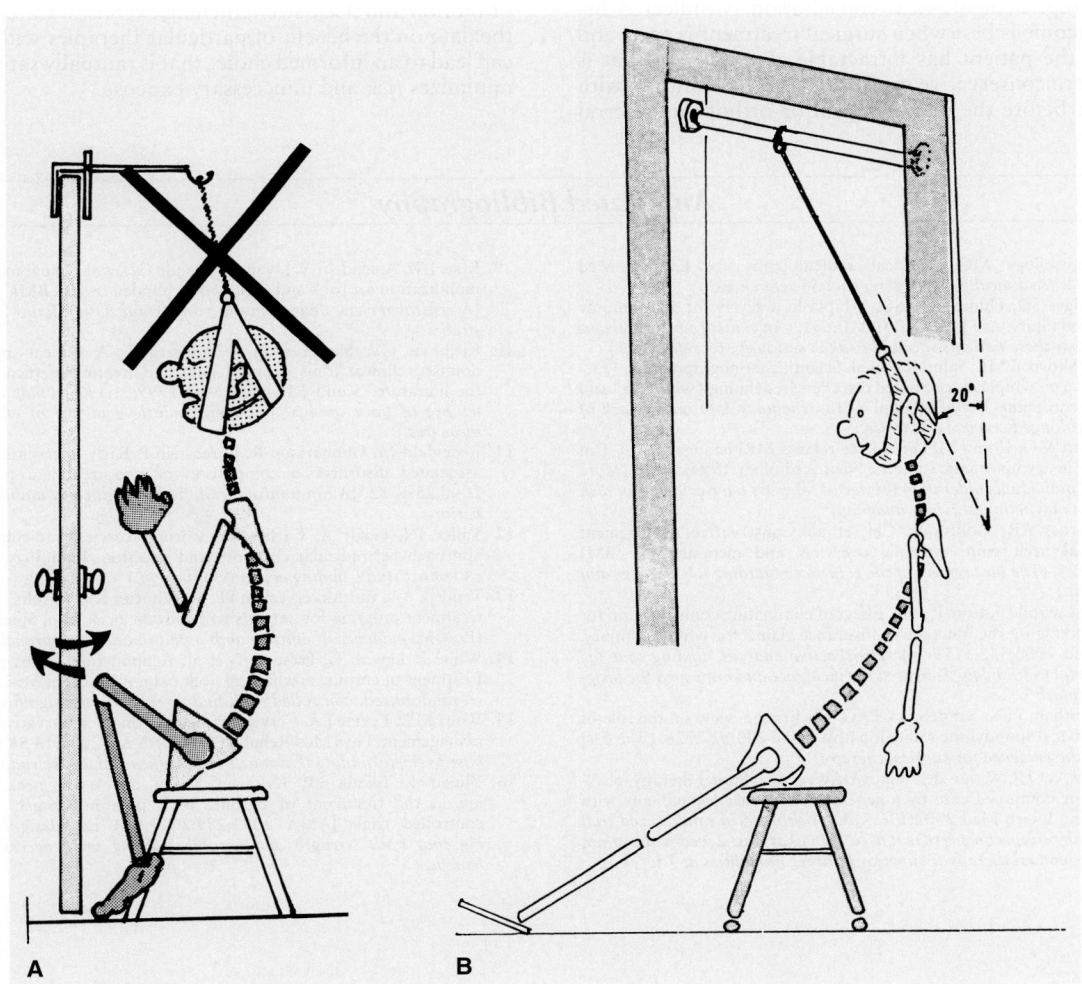

FIGURE 148.1. A: Ineffective home cervical traction with a door. The patient is too close to the door to obtain the correct angle for neck flexion. The door freely opens and closes, and so it does not permit constant traction. The patient cannot extend the legs or assume a comfortable position. This type of home traction is not recommended. **B:** Recommended home traction with a chinning bar and the sitting position. (From Cailliet R. Soft tissue pain and disability. Philadelphia: FA Davis, 1977:129, with permission.)

symptomatic relief are in the 70% range. Complications include spinal cord injury (<1%), root injury (up to 3%), and failure of screw or plate for bony repair (5%).

Measures of No Demonstrated Benefit

Ultrasound and *diathermy* treatments are harmless but of little proven benefit and probably no better than other means of delivering local heat to an area of concurrent muscle spasm. *Acupuncture* does not provide clinically significant improvement when studied in randomized, controlled trials. In those who do respond, benefit corresponds almost entirely to belief in the procedure. *Spinal manipulation* is contraindicated because of its potential to worsen root or cord compression.

INDICATIONS FOR ADMISSION AND REFERRAL (1)

Meningeal signs are an obvious indication for urgent hospitalization, as is evidence of cord compression (hyperreflexia, upturned toe, incontinence or retention, bilateral neurologic deficits); prompt neurosurgical consultation is indicated because the outcome is best when surgical treatment is early and definitive. If the patient has intractable chronic pain that is unresponsive to conservative measures, then consultation with a neurologist before the neurosurgical or orthopedic referral can sometimes be beneficial, especially to review the findings and discuss treatment options. Current indications for elective surgical intervention are MRI- or CT-confirmed root compression that corresponds to symptoms and physical findings and either persistent pain for 6 to 12 months despite conservative therapy or the progression of functionally important motor deficits.

Referral for concurrent help with psychosocial issues and/or underlying psychopathology may be necessary in persons with chronic neck pain without radiculopathy that has a strong psychosocial overlay. Cognitive–behavioral measures and multimodality care might be helpful if they are orchestrated in coordinated fashion by the primary care physician.

PATIENT EDUCATION (13)

The patient with persistent neck pain is likely to request or ask about physiotherapy and alternative therapies (e.g., diathermy, ultrasound, spinal manipulation, acupuncture). More beneficial to outcomes might be referral to a skilled physical therapist who, in a few sessions, can teach proper neck care and range-of-motion and neck-strengthening exercises. Careful review of the data on the benefit of particular therapies with the patient can lead to an informed choice that is mutually satisfactory and minimizes risk and unnecessary expense.

A.H.G.

Annotated Bibliography

1. Carette S, Fehlings MG. Cervical radiculopathy. N Engl J Med 2005;353:392. (*A clinically oriented review; 55 references.*)
2. Eck JC, Hodges SD, Humphreys SC. Whiplash: a review of a commonly misunderstood injury. Am J Med 2001;110:651. (*An evidence-based review, concluding that these patients should be taken seriously; 64 references.*)
3. Spitzer WO, Skovron ML, Salmi LR, et al. Scientific monograph of the Quebec Task Force on whiplash-associated disorders: redefining "whiplash" and its management. Spine 1990;20(Suppl 8):1S. (*Includes data on the lack of efficacy of prolonged cervical collar use.*)
4. Lehto IJ, Tertti MO, Komu ME, et al. Age-related MRI changes at 0.1 T in cervical discs in asymptomatic subjects. Neuroradiology 1994;36:49. (*More than 50% of individuals older than the age of 50 years have evidence of disk herniation on magnetic resonance imaging.*)
5. Aker PD, Gross AR, Goldsmith CH, et al. Conservative management of mechanical neck pain: systemic overview and meta-analysis. BMJ 1996;313:1291. (*The best review of the evidence regarding what works and what does not.*)
6. Cassiday JD, Carroll LJ, Cote P, et al. Effect of eliminating compensation for pain and suffering on the outcome of insurance claims for whiplash injury. N Engl J Med 2000;342:1179. (*A retrospective analysis, finding that the change in compensation law decreased the incidence and improved the prognosis for whiplash.*)
7. Fouyas IP, Statham PFX, Sandercock PAG. Cochrane review on the role of surgery in cervical spondylotic radiculopathy. Spine 2002;27:736. (*The best summary of the evidence for surgical therapy.*)
8. Hoving JL, de Vet HCW, van der Windt DAW, et al. Manual therapy, physical therapy or continued care by a general practitioner for patients with neck pain. Ann Intern Med 2002;136:713. (*A short-term randomized trial in persons with nonspecific persistent neck pain of at least 2 weeks' duration, showing that manual therapy is superior to other modalities at 7 weeks.*)
9. Koes BW, Assendelft WJ, van der Heijde GJ, et al. Spinal manipulation and mobilization for back and neck pain: a blinded review. BMJ 1991;303:1298. (*A critical review, delineating the important design flaws in manipulation studies.*)
10. Kjellman GV, Skargren EI, Lundeberg T. A critical analysis of randomised clinical trials on neck pain and treatment efficacy: a review of the literature. Scand J Rehabil Med 1999;31:139. (*Finds that most studies are of poor quality and there is little evidence of efficacy for most measures.*)
11. Rosenfeld M, Gunnarsson R, Borenstein P. Early intervention in whiplash-associated disorders: a comparison of two treatment protocols. Spine 2000;25:1782. (*A randomized trial, finding that early mobilization was superior.*)
12. Vallee JN, Feydy A, Carlier RY. Chronic cervical radiculopathy: lateral-approach periradicular corticosteroid injection. Radiology 2001;218:886. (*A cohort study, finding evidence of benefit.*)
13. Vendrig AA, van Akkerveeken PF, McWhorter KR. Results of a multimodal treatment program for patients with chronic neck pain. Spine 2000;25:238. (*Presents evidence of efficacy with a multimodality approach.*)
14. White P, Lewith G, Prescott P, et al. Acupuncture versus placebo for the treatment of chronic mechanical neck pain. Ann Intern Med 2004;141:911. (*A randomized, controlled trial, finding no clinically significant benefit.*)
15. Wolff MW, Levine LA. Cervical radiculopathies: conservative approaches to management. Phys Med Rehabil Clin North Am 2002;13:589. (*An evidence-based review, finding that much of the efficacy data are rudimentary.*)
16. Ylinen J, Takala EP, Kykanen M, et al. Active neck muscle training in the treatment of chronic neck pain in women: a randomized controlled trial. JAMA 2003;289:2509. (*A well-designed study, finding that both strength and aerobic training were necessary to achieve benefit.*)

CHAPTER 149 ■ APPROACH TO THE PATIENT WITH MUSCLE CRAMPS

Muscle cramps are prolonged, involuntary muscle contractions that can be painful and difficult to manage but rarely reflect serious underlying disease. True cramps must be differentiated from ischemic pain, contracture, tetany, dystonia, and myositis. Fluid and electrolyte disorders, medication, and endocrinologic disorders must be considered in the evaluation, although they are uncommon precipitants. Patients come in requesting symptomatic relief from these painful episodes, which can be temporarily disabling.

PATHOPHYSIOLOGY AND CLINICAL PRESENTATION (1–6)

True Cramps

True muscle cramping represents motor unit hyperactivity leading to prolonged, involuntary muscle contraction. Precipitants include unopposed contraction, electrolyte and volume shifts, and lower motor neuron disease. *Ordinary cramps* most commonly occur in the gastrocnemius muscle and the intrinsic muscles of the sole of the foot. Their nocturnal predilection appears to be related to unopposed plantar flexion of the foot in bed, which places the muscles of the calves and feet in their most shortened and therefore most vulnerable position. Without modulation by opposing muscles, the sustained contraction produces the characteristic *nocturnal leg cramp*, which is experienced as sudden, severe calf pain; often, the muscle is palpable or visibly hardened. In many instances, a voluntary contraction triggers the cramp. Passive stretching relieves it.

True cramps may be precipitated by *volume* and *electrolyte shifts*, which accounts for the fact that they frequently occur during hemodialysis and can be relieved with the administration of hypertonic dextrose. *Heat cramps* that occur during activity are a consequence of dehydration and sodium loss and respond to replenishment. *Hyponatremia* is a consistent feature of fluid-based muscle cramps. In marathon runners who suffer severe cramps, the hyponatremia can be severe, resulting from the combination of salt depletion and the drinking of large volumes of free water. Contrary to common belief, hypokalemia is not a clearly established precipitant of true muscle cramps; cramps attributable to potassium-wasting diuretics are actually uncommon and may be related to salt depletion. Ordinary cramps are often a part of symptomatic *hypoglycemia*. Muscle cramps are sometimes *drug-induced*, as may occasionally occur with *nifedipine*, *β-agonists*, and heavy *alcohol* use.

The cramp is a neural or electrical phenomenon, not primarily muscular. Electromyography shows fasciculations preceding the cramp. Cramps accompanied by clinically evident fasciculations are characteristic of *lower motor neuron diseases*, such as polio in the recovery phase, peripheral nerve injury, nerve root compression, and amyotrophic lateral sclerosis.

Other Forms of Muscle Cramping

Contractures also represent involuntary muscle contractions, but they are electrically silent and characteristically occur during exertion, not rest. They develop in persons who have inherited metabolic defects that impair the formation of adenosine triphosphate, which is needed for muscle relaxation. Most patients have McArdle's disease. Both *hyperthyroid* and *hypothyroid* disease may cause cramping. Exertional cramping has been seen in hyperthyroidism. In hypothyroidism, impaired muscle relaxation produces the "hung-up" reflexes that characterize the condition.

Tetany is a state of both motor and sensory hyperactivity associated with muscle spasm and paresthesias. The muscles of the mouth, hands, and lower extremities are typically involved, and carpopedal spasm is a characteristic manifestation, as are Chvostek's and Trousseau's signs. Hypocalcemia, hypomagnesemia, respiratory alkalosis, and hypokalemia are known precipitants. In severe cases, seizures may ensue if the condition goes uncorrected.

Occupational cramp is a form of dystonia in which muscle contractures occur in persons engaging in fine motor activities that have taken years to perfect. The typical patient is a writer or pianist whose hands curl involuntarily when he or she attempts to write or play.

Conditions Causing Cramplike Symptoms

Patients may report cramplike symptoms in the context of important medical conditions, including peripheral arterial insufficiency and statin-associated muscle injury. Autoimmune forms of myositis (dermatomyositis, polymyositis) usually present as proximal muscle weakness and possibly some soreness in the proximal muscles, but cramping is not part of the clinical picture.

Intermittent Claudication

Exercise increases the metabolic demands of skeletal muscle in the legs, necessitating a 5- to 10-fold increase in blood flow and oxygen delivery. Peripheral arterial disease causes a supply-and-demand mismatch, resulting in the characteristic exercise-induced discomfort of intermittent claudication that involves the calf muscles or thighs and quickly resolves with rest. The discomfort may range from frank pain to cramping or even numbness and may be unilateral or bilateral, depending on the state of circulation in each limb (see Chapter 23).

Statin-Associated Myopathy

Statins, which are widely used for the treatment of hypercholesterolemia (see Chapter 27), can cause muscle injury, including, in very rare instances, clinically important *myositis*

TABLE 149.1

DIFFERENTIAL DIAGNOSIS OF MUSCLE CRAMPS

True Cramps
  Ordinary (nocturnal)
  Heat induced (volume depletion, hyponatremia)
  Hemodialysis (volume and electrolyte shifts)
  Lower motor neuron disease
  Drug induced (nifedipine, β-agonists, tamoxifen, ? statins)
Dystonia
  Occupational (writer's cramp)
Tetany
  Hypocalcemia
  Hypomagnesemia
  Respiratory alkalosis
  Hypokalemia
Contracture
  McArdle's disease
  Thyroid disease
Cramplike Symptoms
  Intermittent claudication
  Statin-induced myopathy

Adapted from McGee SR. Muscle cramps. Arch Intern Med
1990;150:511, with permission.

and *rhabdomyolysis*. More commonly (1% to 5% of users),
patients may experience mild serum creatine kinase (CK) elevations, myalgias with or without elevated CK levels, minor
muscle weakness, and muscle cramps. Signs and symptoms
clear with the cessation of therapy. The mechanism of statin-
induced muscle injury is unclear, but is believed to be related
to a reduction in small regulatory proteins important for myocyte maintenance. Risk appears to be dose related and greatest
with cerivastatin. The risks of myositis and rhabdomyolysis are
exacerbated by concurrent liver or kidney disease, hypothyroidism, diabetes, and the use of drugs that increase statin
concentrations (e.g., niacin, cyclosporine, azole antifungals,
macrolide antibiotics, viral protease inhibitors, nefazodone,
verapamil, diltiazem, amiodarone). Concerns about the potentiation of statin effects with grapefruit juice intake are exaggerated; more than 1 quart/d is required.

DIFFERENTIAL DIAGNOSIS (1–6)

Table 149.1 list the causes of neurophysiologically true muscle
cramps and other forms of muscle cramping and cramplike
symptoms.

WORKUP (1–6)

History

A detailed description of the cramping is essential and should
include the setting in which the episodes occur. Those that develop at night or in the context of hemodialysis, hypoglycemia,
or heavy sweating during prolonged exertion are likely to be
true cramps, as are those coincident with the use of calcium-
channel blockers, β-agonists, and alcohol excess. Dystonic
cramping is suggested by onset with occupation-related fine

motor activity, and contracture by a lifelong onset with exercise. Associated symptoms should be reviewed for the paresthesias and carpopedal spasm of tetany, the weakness and fasciculations of lower motor neuron disease, and the cold or
heat intolerance, skin changes, and related symptoms of thyroid disease (see Chapters 103 and 104). The location of the
cramping is a less specific finding, but if calf pain is reported,
one should include intermittent claudication in the differential
diagnosis, particularly if pain is brought on by walking and
relieved promptly by rest. A review of medications is always
useful, especially for the use of statins and tamoxifen, but the
use of a potassium-wasting diuretic is not tantamount to an etiologic diagnosis because hypokalemia is rarely responsible for
true cramps (although it should be considered in the differential diagnosis of tetany). Also potentially pertinent in suspected
tetany is any distant history of thyroidectomy (with coincident
removal of the parathyroid glands).

In persons with suspected intermittent claudication, the history should also be checked for atherosclerotic risk factors and
other symptoms of arterial insufficiency (see Chapter 23). In
reviewing atherosclerotic disease and its risk factors, one also
needs to check for the use of statins and any drugs that may
increase statin serum concentration (see prior discussion).

Physical Examination

If dehydration is suspected, the physical examination begins
with a check of postural signs for a drop in blood pressure
and a rise in pulse; if dilutional hyponatremia is a concern, a
check for peripheral edema may be revealing. The skin is examined for signs of thyroid disease (see Chapters 103 and 104);
the neck for evidence of thyroidectomy; the lower extremities
for diminished or absent pulses, muscle wasting, soreness, and
fasciculations; and the nervous system for focal weakness and
absent or abnormal deep tendon reflexes. If tetany is a consideration, one can try to elicit the facial spasm of Trousseau's sign
by tapping the facial nerve or the carpal spasm of *Chvostek's
sign* by inflating the arm cuff above systolic pressure. If pulses
are diminished or absent on screening examination, a more detailed check for signs of vascular insufficiency is indicated (e.g.,
femoral bruits, dermal atrophy, skin ulceration, dependent
rubor; see Chapter 23).

Laboratory Determinations

For the majority of people who present with a clinical story of
nocturnal muscle cramps, laboratory testing is unlikely to provide additional information. Other situations do require a few
simple tests. If the patient with ordinary cramps is diabetic and
taking insulin, then testing for hypoglycemia is indicated (see
Chapter 102). If severe dehydration and hyponatremia are suspected, then determinations of serum *sodium, blood urea nitrogen*, and *creatinine* levels can guide assessment and treatment.
In the patient with possible tetany, levels of *sodium, potassium, calcium, albumin* (to interpret the calcium level), and
magnesium must be checked. Consideration of thyroid disease
is best pursued by obtaining a serum *thyrotropin* determination. For the patient with fasciculations and possible lower motor neuron disease, a *nerve conduction study* may be required.
Symptomatic persons taking a statin should have a *creatine
phosphokinase* determination obtained, but consensus guidelines do not require routine monitoring of CK levels in persons
taking statin therapy. Those with suspected peripheral arterial

insufficiency are candidates for Doppler ultrasound study (see Chapter 23).

PRINCIPLES OF MANAGEMENT AND INDICATIONS FOR ADMISSION (1,2,4–11)

Ordinary Cramps

Most ordinary cramps can be relieved or prevented by simple measures such as stretching, but more persistent and bothersome cramping may require the consideration of pharmacologic intervention. The first task is to address precipitants.

Correction of Precipitants

Patients with ordinary cramps related to dehydration and sodium depletion respond well to replacement therapy. If the patient is acutely hyponatremic from salt depletion plus excess free water intake (as in many marathon runners), simple observation may suffice as free water is excreted. Those with cramps as a consequence of hemodialysis are best treated with rapid volume expansion (infusion of hypertonic dextrose or saline solution). If hypoglycemia is responsible, then adjustment of the insulin regimen is needed (see Chapter 102). Euthyroid status should be reestablished if there is underlying thyroid disease (see Chapters 103 and 104). Altering the medication program may be necessary in cases in which β-agonists or calcium-channel blockers are believed to be responsible.

Stretching and Exercise

To relieve an established cramp, one must passively stretch the contracting muscle and gradually contract the opposing one. In some cases, this can be accomplished by simply *walking* around (which produces a relative dorsiflexion of the foot) and *stretching* the involved muscle. *Massage* of the involved muscle sometimes helps. Conscious dorsiflexion at the first sign of a leg or foot cramp may abort it; prophylactic stretching can also prevent attacks (see Chapter 18 for stretching exercise), as may positions in bed that prevent foot dorsiflexion. Swimming-induced cramps can be avoided by sacrificing the ideal kicking position of plantar flexion and maintaining a more neutral foot position.

Quinine

Quinine sulfate and its derivatives (e.g., *hydroquinine*) have been prescribed for decades for patients who have frequent incapacitating attacks of nocturnal leg cramps. Only recently have randomized, double-blind, controlled clinical trials been performed to confirm efficacy. More than two thirds of patients achieved a 50% or greater reduction in cramps, with usually mild and infrequent side effects. Regimens with low to moderate doses (200 to 300 mg daily at bedtime) provide less benefit than those with higher doses (e.g., 200 mg at supper, 300 mg at bedtime). This pattern suggests that response rates are related to the serum level attained, which can vary greatly with the age of the patient and the preparation used. Treatment effects can persist beyond the treatment period.

The risk for serious side effects is quite small but increases with dose and serum level. *Prolongation of the QT interval* on the electrocardiogram is a concern in persons who are prone to *ventricular dysrhythmias* (see Chapter 29), necessitating careful use in patients with heart disease. The QT interval should be checked before and during use; persons with prolonged QT intervals should not be prescribed quinine. *Cinchonism* (nausea, vomiting, tinnitus, hearing loss), *visual impairment*, and *ventricular arrhythmias* appear when serum levels exceed two to five times the average serum concentration. There are case reports of fatal immune *thrombocytopenia*.

The small but real risk for serious toxicity should temper one's uncritical use of quinine for this otherwise benign condition. A careful trial of quinine may be considered for those sufficiently bothered by their symptoms, first checking the QT interval on resting electrocardiogram and reviewing the risks and benefits. Starting with small doses (200 to 300 mg daily at bedtime) is best, and the platelet count should be monitored periodically. Because of the evidence for a sustained effect, it is reasonable to interrupt treatment and reassess after 2 to 4 weeks.

Other Drugs and Supplements

Some symptomatic benefit is associated with the use of *methocarbamol* and *chloroquine*, but both have considerable side effects and need to be used with care. *Vitamin E* is promoted in health food stores for the treatment of nocturnal cramps and may be sold in combination with quinine; it is no better than placebo when tested in double-blind, placebo-controlled fashion. Small-scale study suggests benefit with the calcium-channel blocker *verapamil*, although other calcium-channel blockers (e.g., nifedipine) can cause symptoms.

Occupational Cramps

These can be difficult to treat. Rest and occupational aids can be helpful; psychotherapy is not. Minor tranquilizers provide some short-term relief but little sustained benefit. Injection of botulinum toxin has been tried with some success.

Tetany

Urgent hospitalization and careful parenteral correction of the underlying electrolyte disturbances are priorities.

Statin-Related Myopathy

Using the lowest possible statin dose is important for prevention, especially when using a statin associated with increased risk (e.g., cerivastatin). Drugs that can increase serum statin levels should be used in the lowest possible doses; however, the use of such drugs is not contraindicated. Patient education is essential to the prevention of serious muscle injury, with explicit instruction given to stop statin intake at the first sign of a muscle problem (weakness, soreness, cramping) or discoloration of urine. (Most episodes of serious muscle injury were preceded by warning symptoms that were ignored.) One might consider halting statin therapy before an event associated with muscle injury, such as major orthopedic surgery or marathon running. Patients who enjoy a glass of grapefruit juice several times a week need not worry about the juice consumption being harmful, but those who drink excessive amounts daily (>1 quart) should be advised to cut back.

Asymptomatic Patients

Truly asymptomatic persons incidentally found to have an elevation in CK need not stop statin therapy as long as the increase is less than 10 times the upper limit of normal and they have cardiac risk factors strongly warranting lipid-lowering therapy. They should be reminded about the indications for halting therapy and have a thyrotropin determination performed to exclude hypothyroidism as a contributing factor. CK levels should be monitored going forward if the elevation was greater than 5 times the upper limit. If CK exceeds 10 times the upper limit of normal, consideration should be given to stopping therapy.

Symptomatic Patients

Persons with muscle complaints accompanied by CK elevation should have statin therapy stopped for several weeks (to allow any adverse biochemical events to clear) and a new statin agent tried, starting at a low dose and monitoring CK levels. If it is tolerated symptomatically and without CK elevation, then the dose can be slowly increased. If it is not tolerated or if marked CK elevation develops, then statin therapy should be abandoned.

Symptomatic persons with no elevation in CK can continue their statin therapy if symptoms are tolerable. If they are not tolerable, the drug should be stopped, and another statin can be tried after the patient has been symptom-free for about 1 month. CK levels should be followed.

Claudication-Related Cramps

See Chapter 34.

A.H.G.

Annotated Bibliography

1. McGee SR. Muscle cramps. Arch Intern Med 1990;150:511. (*A comprehensive review; 170 references.*)
2. Land SR, Wickerham L, Costantino JP, et al. Patient-reported symptoms and quality of life during treatment with tamoxifen or raloxifene for breast cancer prevention. JAMA 2006;295:2742. (*Muscle cramps were found to occur significantly more often with tamoxifen than in controls.*)
3. Naylor JR, Young JB. A general population survey of rest cramps. Age Ageing 1994;23:418. (*Documents a high incidence in the general population.*)
4. Speedy DB, Noakes TD, Schneider C. Exercise-associated hyponatremia: a review. Emerg Med 2001;13:17. (*A summary of the evidence, finding that the condition is mostly due to drinking free water.*)
5. Thompson PD, Clarkson P, Karas R. Statin-associated myopathy. JAMA 2003;289:1681. (*A comprehensive review; 100 references.*)
6. Connolly PS, Shirley EA, Wasson JH, et al. Treatment of nocturnal leg cramps. Arch Intern Med 1992;152:1877. (*Quinine but not vitamin E was found to be effective; a program of 500 mg/d relieved cramps within 3 to 5 days.*)
7. Freiman JP. Fatal quinine-induced thrombocytopenia. Ann Intern Med 1990;112:308. (*A U.S. Food and Drug Administration report of two previously well patients in whom quinine-induced thrombocytopenia was fatal.*)
8. Jansen PHP, Veenhuizen KCW, Wesseling AIM, et al. Randomized controlled trial of hydroquinone in muscle cramps. Lancet 1997;349:528. (*One of the few randomized, controlled trials in this area, finding significant benefit and relatively few side effects.*)
9. Man-Son-Hing M, Wells G. Meta-analysis of efficacy of quinine for treatment of nocturnal leg cramps in elderly people. BMJ 1995;310:13. (*Quinine significantly reduced the number of cramps and the number of nights with cramps, the former by 43% and the latter by 27%.*)
10. Man-Son-Hing M, Wells G, Lau A. Quinine for nocturnal leg cramps: a meta-analysis including unpublished data. J Gen Intern Med 1998;13:600. (*The treatment was still effective, but the relative reduction in the number of cramps fell from 43% to 21% when unpublished data were added.*)
11. Pasternak RC, Smith SC, Bairey-Merz CN, et al. ACC/AHA/NHLBI clinical advisory on the use and safety of statins. J Am Coll Cardiol 2002;40:567. (*Consensus recommendations.*)

CHAPTER 150 ■ APPROACH TO THE PATIENT WITH SHOULDER PAIN

JESSE B. JUPITER AND DAVID RING

The shoulder is a complex joint integrating three bones, four joints, and more than 15 muscles; its mobility exceeds that of all other joints. To achieve this mobility, the glenohumeral joint is less constrained and therefore less inherently stable. Shoulder pain and dysfunction are common, particularly in older patients. The majority of shoulder complaints reflect one of a few common problems that can be identified by primary care physicians. Initial treatment is usually nonoperative. The mainstay of treatment is physical therapy for strengthening of the muscles that help to stabilize the shoulder.

PATHOPHYSIOLOGY AND CLINICAL PRESENTATION (1–3)

Injury or degenerative change in the rotator cuff, bicipital tendon, or acromioclavicular joint can produce pain localized to the shoulder joint. Characteristically, focal tenderness is present and pain is aggravated during shoulder movement. Patients report difficulty in dressing, combing their hair, or reaching up. Degenerative disease of the glenohumeral joint is uncommon;

symptoms include mild stiffness, crepitus, and low-grade, aching discomfort related to vigorous or sustained use. Pain originating in or about the shoulder may be referred to the upper arm or radiate to the neck, elbow, or forearm; it does not follow a specific cervical root distribution. Although pain originating in the neck may radiate to the shoulder, it is brought on by neck motion rather than by shoulder movement and is usually not affected by shoulder position; however, poorly localized sensitivity to touch extending into the shoulder may vaguely simulate shoulder disease (see Chapter 148).

Rotator Cuff Problems (1–5)

Rotator cuff problems are the most common source of shoulder pain seen in a primary care practice; they are typically seen in patients aged 40 years or greater. Degenerative and attritional changes taking place over time in the tendons lead to structural weakening. The role of *impingement* of the rotator cuff between the greater tuberosity and the acromion is debated. As the degenerative process advances, a defect may appear in the tendons near their insertion into the proximal humerus. Use of the word *tear* in this context is commonplace, but misleading. The word *tear* implies damage that should be repaired, whereas most rotator cuff defects are unrelated to injury and asymptomatic. Furthermore, many patients with a symptomatic rotator cuff defect manage well without surgery. Rotator cuff defects are common with age even in asymptomatic shoulders. Defects are also common in the asymptomatic contralateral shoulder among patients presenting with unilateral shoulder symptoms.

Large defects of the rotator cuff affect shoulder function and can contribute to arthrosis of the glenohumeral joint. It is important to identify large defects of the rotator cuff when evaluating patients with shoulder pain. Fatty degeneration of retracted rotator cuff muscles that occurs within a few months of a large tear makes the results of repair much less predictable.

The diagnosis of *rotator cuff tendinitis* may be a misnomer because it is a degenerative rather than an inflammatory process. A better term may be rotator cuff tendinosis. This illness is best considered one of the many tendinoses and enesthopathies with onset in middle age. The diagnosis should be applied with caution to patients younger than 40 years of age. In younger patients, rotator cuff tendinitis is usually secondary to some other process, such as instability. A defect of the rotator cuff tendon in a younger person—including an isolated tear of the *subscapularis tendon*—is typically a relatively high energy injury. Such tears are rare but important to identify and repair. Careful physical examination can verify that the rotator cuff is unlikely to have a large defect (see later discussion). Any doubt merits referral to an experienced shoulder surgeon.

Most patients with pain due to rotator cuff tendon dysfunction are older than age 40 years. Pain over the deltoid, especially during overhead activities and internal rotation, and weakness of shoulder elevation and external rotation are diagnostic features. It is very common for pain from the rotator cuff to be referred to the lateral arm. Superior shoulder pain suggests acromioclavicular joint problems. Muscle atrophy over the scapula (supra and infraspinatus) suggests a large tendon defect extending posteriorly.

Biceps tendinitis of the shoulder is a diagnosis that is now rarely made in isolation. Inflammation of the tendon of the long head of the biceps is a common component of rotator cuff degeneration. Rupture of the long head of the biceps results in a "Popeye" deformity of the arm but does not affect function. This contrasts with a rupture of the distal insertion of the biceps tendon into the radius, which causes weakness of supination. Operative treatment of proximal biceps ruptures is controversial.

Glenohumeral Joint Problems (6,7)

The glenohumeral joint has little inherent stability; stability is heavily dependent on static capsuloligamentous and dynamic musculotendinous restraints. Two general categories of glenohumeral instability comprise the majority of such problems: traumatic unidirectional instability and atraumatic multidirectional instability.

Traumatic dislocation of the glenohumeral articulation almost always results in anterior dislocation of the humeral head from the glenoid articular surface of the scapula. Posterior glenohumeral dislocations are uncommon and are often related to a seizure or electric shock injury. Traumatic posterior dislocations are often fracture dislocations of the glenoid articular surface.

Traumatic anterior dislocation nearly always disrupts the anterior attachment of the glenoid labrum to the glenoid articular surface (Bankart lesion). The labrum is a ring of fibrous cartilage that helps to deepen the relatively shallow glenoid articular surface and is the site of attachment of the all-important glenohumeral ligaments. The likelihood that a patient who has had one traumatic anterior dislocation of the shoulder will have recurrent dislocations is related to the age of the patient at the time of the first dislocation. As many as 80% of patients younger than 20 years at the time of first diagnosis will have another dislocation. Older patients are less likely to have a recurrent dislocation, but tearing of the rotator cuff may occur. Recurrent anterior dislocation usually requires surgical treatment consisting of reattachment of the anterior portion of the labrum to the glenoid margin in addition to tightening of any redundant anterior capsule.

Atraumatic instability is usually related to laxity of a number of capsular restraints. In many cases, the patient may have a connective tissue disorder. Other patients, such as competitive swimmers, may develop multidirectional instability. This type of instability usually responds to a program of specific exercises intended to strengthen the dynamic muscular stabilizers of the shoulder. Athletes may also need to modify their technique; a good coach or trainer can be useful in this regard.

Patients who can actively and voluntarily dislocate their shoulder should be approached with caution. Often, a subtle underlying psychiatric condition is present. Cases in which the voluntary dislocation is habitual—often, the patient has derived some attention or reward from the ability to dislocate a shoulder—can be difficult to manage. This should be distinguished from situations in which the voluntary dislocation is positional—the patient can reproduce the instability by placing the arm in certain position but is averse to doing so.

Idiopathic adhesive capsulitis, or *frozen shoulder syndrome*, is a characteristic symptom complex of pain and tenderness located diffusely about the anterior and posterior regions of the shoulder joint capsule. It is more common among diabetic patients. The term "frozen shoulder" has, unfortunately, become imprecise. Idiopathic adhesive capsulitis should be distinguished from other forms of shoulder stiffness—posttraumatic stiffness in particular. Active and passive motions of the glenohumeral joint are limited and painful. The condition is self-limiting, although improvement of motion can take months to years. Operative treatment is controversial.

Osteoarthritis of the glenohumeral joint is relatively uncommon. It causes symptoms at rest that are exacerbated by

IMPORTANT CAUSES OF SHOULDER PAIN

Rotator Cuff
  Calcific tendonitis
  Tendinosis
  Biceps tendinosis
  Defect/tear
  Adhesive capsulitis
Glenohumeral Joint
  Instability
  Dislocation
  Arthritis
  Infection
Acromioclavicular Joint
  Arthritis
Referred
  Cervical spondylosis
  Myocardial ischemia
  Diaphragmatic irritation
  Gallbladder disease

shoulder use. The patient may note a "grinding" sound with motion. Pain, crepitation, and diminished motion may be noted on examination. Rheumatoid arthritis frequently involves the glenohumeral joint and usually gives a picture of symmetric bilateral inflammatory changes.

Acromioclavicular Arthritis

Degenerative changes of the acromioclavicular joint are common, even in asymptomatic individuals. Symptoms should be ascribed to the radiographic changes with care. The pain is typically superior rather than anterolateral as with rotator cuff tendon problems. Examination and diagnostic injection are described later.

Infection

Shoulder sepsis is typically hematogenous, but may also be postoperative or, rarely, postinjection. Laboratory analysis of the aspirate confirms the diagnosis. Operative débridement and parenteral antibiotics are required.

DIFFERENTIAL DIAGNOSIS

The causes of shoulder pain can be considered in terms of the structures that comprise the shoulder (Table 150.1). The vast majority of nontraumatic shoulder complaints are related to tendinitis.

WORKUP (1–4)

History

One should inquire about previous trauma or an inciting event, location and radiation of pain, specific limitations of movement, associated neurologic deficits, aggravating and alleviating factors, previous history of shoulder problems, and therapies used. It is important to be sure that no symptoms suggestive of angina, gallbladder disease, or diaphragmatic irritation are present. Pain resulting from myocardial ischemia usually originates in the precordial region but may present as shoulder or neck pain radiating into the arm.

Patients with symptoms suggestive of shoulder disease describe a combination of pain, loss of mobility, and weakness. Pain associated with activities above the horizontal level suggests subacromial impingement or acromioclavicular joint arthritis. Pain occurring when the patient is recumbent or trying to sleep is characteristic of rotator cuff problems. Calcific tendinitis can be a cause of severe acute shoulder pain mimicking infection or fracture. A past history of shoulder dislocations might suggest glenohumeral instability.

General Physical Examination

Before proceeding to the examination of the shoulder, it is important that the physician carefully check the neck, chest, heart, and abdomen for sources of referred pain. Cervical disease is often mistaken for a shoulder problem. Cervical root compression can sometimes be distinguished from intrinsic shoulder disease by the elicitation and reproduction of pain on lateral bending and extension of the neck toward the side of the complaint with simultaneous axial compression by the examiner (Spurling's sign). The chest is checked for effusion, pleural rub, and poor diaphragmatic movement. If the heart is examined while the patient is in pain, one can listen for transient auscultatory signs of ischemia (e.g., fourth heart sound, single second sound, mitral regurgitant murmur from papillary muscle dysfunction). The abdomen is palpated for tenderness in the right or left upper quadrant, which may signal subdiaphragmatic disease.

Shoulder Examination

The patient is comfortably seated and sufficiently disrobed to permit evaluation and comparison of both shoulders. Close *inspection* from both front and back may demonstrate asymmetry or deformity. For example, supraspinatus muscle atrophy suggests either a rotator cuff defect or suprascapular nerve disease. The patient is instructed to place the involved shoulder *actively* through a *full range of motion*, along with similar movements of the contralateral limb for comparison. This includes forward flexion, extension, abduction, and internal and external rotation. Internal rotation is best recorded as the level at which the patient can reach posteriorly, such as the buttock or thoracolumbar junction. The scapula is observed as the patient flexes the shoulder forward against resistance. Winging of the scapula can be the result of serratus anterior muscle palsy.

The patient is instructed to point out specific *sites of tenderness* (Fig. 150.1). Palpation by the examiner routinely should include the anterior aspect of the acromion, the acromioclavicular joint, the bicipital groove (which is best palpated with the humerus in about 10 degrees of internal rotation), the greater tuberosity, and the cervical spine. With the examiner's hand on the joint, the shoulder is passively put through a *range of motion* (Fig. 150.2). Limitations are noted, in addition to any palpable crepitation.

A manual *muscle test* is helpful, in particular for comparison with the uninvolved shoulder. Inability to "shrug" the shoulder suggests trapezial muscle weakness. Testing of the rotator cuff is described later. A *sensory* and *deep tendon reflex*

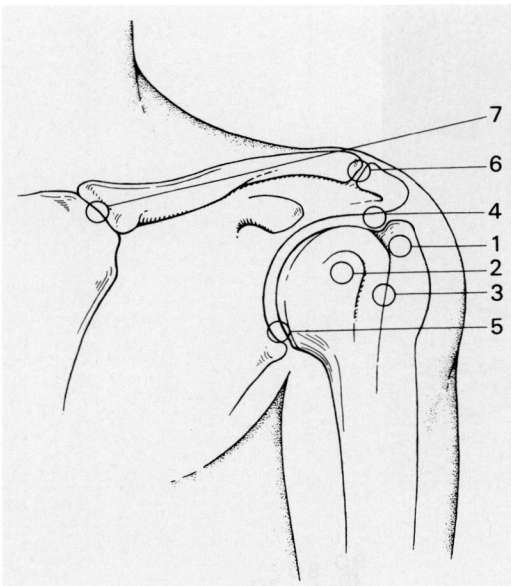

FIGURE 150.1. Discrete tender areas identified during the examination can assist with diagnosis. **1:** The greater tuberosity and site of supraspinatus tendon insertion. **2:** Lesser tuberosity, site of subscapularis muscle insertion. **3:** Bicipital groove, in which the bicipital tendon glides. **4:** Site of the subdeltoid bursa. **5:** Glenohumeral joint space. **6:** Acromioclavicular joint. **7:** Sternoclavicular joint. (Redrawn from Cailliet R. Shoulder pain. Philadelphia: FA Davis, 1973, with permission.)

examination of the upper extremity should be included in the routine shoulder evaluation.

Diagnostic Maneuvers

Several specific maneuvers are diagnostically helpful and provide a means of quick and reliable diagnosis in the office.

Impingement Signs

Neer's test is performed with the examiner standing behind the patient and bringing the involved arm to the maximum degree of forward flexion with one hand while the other functions to depress the patient's shoulder girdle. If pain is elicited in the deltoid area or beneath the acromion, inflammation of the rotator cuff tendons and *impingement* of the greater tuberosity of the humerus against the undersurface of the acromion is likely. *Hawkins' sign* tests the shoulder with internal rotation at 90 degrees of forward flexion in the plane of the scapula. Results of these tests can be confirmed if an injection of 5 mL of lidocaine (Xylocaine) into the subacromial space relieves the symptoms—the so-called *impingement test.*

Tests for Rotator Cuff Defects

Large rotator cuff defects are identified with a series of specific tests. To test the posterior portion of the rotator cuff, or infraspinatus, the arm is placed at the side with the elbow maintained against the trunk. The forearm and hand are then brought passively into maximum external rotation. The patient is asked to maintain the arm actively in this position. An external rotation lag is defined as the difference between the maximum active and passive external rotation and may

indicate a large defect in the infraspinatus tendon. The patient should also be able to place the arm up in a throwing position. Inability to hold these positions suggests a large rotator cuff defect.

The integrity of the anterior cuff (subscapularis tension) can be tested in two ways. The *lift-off test* involves maximum passive internal rotation of the arm behind the back so that the dorsum of the hand "lifts off" from the hip/back area. If the patient cannot maintain this position actively, there may be a large defect or tear in the subscapularis tendon. For the *belly press sign,* the patient is asked to place the hand flat against the abdomen with the elbow held forward in this plane. The patient is then asked to maintain the hand against the belly as the examiner pulls the hand anteriorly. A posterior swing of the elbow reflects an attempt to maintain the hand against the belly by means of extension rather than internal rotation of the shoulder, in which case a defect or tear of the subscapularis tendon may be present.

The supraspinatus is more difficult to isolate. Longstanding defects are associated with atrophy noted in the supraspinatus fossa of the scapula. Weakness of resisted abduction may be noted with the shoulder held in 90 degrees of abduction.

Tests for Acromioclavicular Joint Disease

In the *cross-arm adduction test,* symptoms are reproduced when the patient brings the involved arm across the body so that the *hand grasps the contralateral shoulder.* The result can be confirmed by having the patient repeat the maneuver after the acromioclavicular joint has been injected with 1 mL of lidocaine; a 25-gauge needle is used to enter the joint.

Tests for Glenohumeral Instability

Patients who report a feeling of imminent shoulder dislocation when the shoulder is positioned in 90 degrees of abduction and maximum external rotation—a *positive apprehension sign*—may have anterior shoulder instability. Confirmatory evidence is obtained by repeating the test with the patient supine and placing posterior pressure over the proximal humerus—the *relocation test.* The uncomfortable sensation of impending dislocation should be diminished if it is caused by anterior instability.

Multidirectional laxity is sought in an examination of other stabilizing structures. The patient is tested for laxity of the superior glenohumeral ligament by applying axial traction to the arm held at the side in external rotation. If the gap between the acromion and the humeral head is larger than that seen during testing of the opposite side—a positive sulcus sign—the superior glenohumeral ligament may be lax. Forward flexion and posterior translation of the arm may reproduce symptoms of posterior instability. Repeating the sulcus sign in internal rotation also tests the posterior capsule.

Laboratory Studies

Radiographs of the shoulder are useful in the initial evaluation. A *standard anteroposterior view* is helpful in ruling out underlying bone tumor, infection, or arthritis of either the glenohumeral or acromioclavicular joint. An anteroposterior view in the plane of the scapula rather than the body (the so-called Grache view) is the best way to evaluate the glenohumeral joint for arthritis or injury. Well-circumscribed, organized calcification reflects chronic calcification of degenerated tendons and is not particularly important. Patients who have acute, severe pain may be noted to have a more diffuse, disorganized

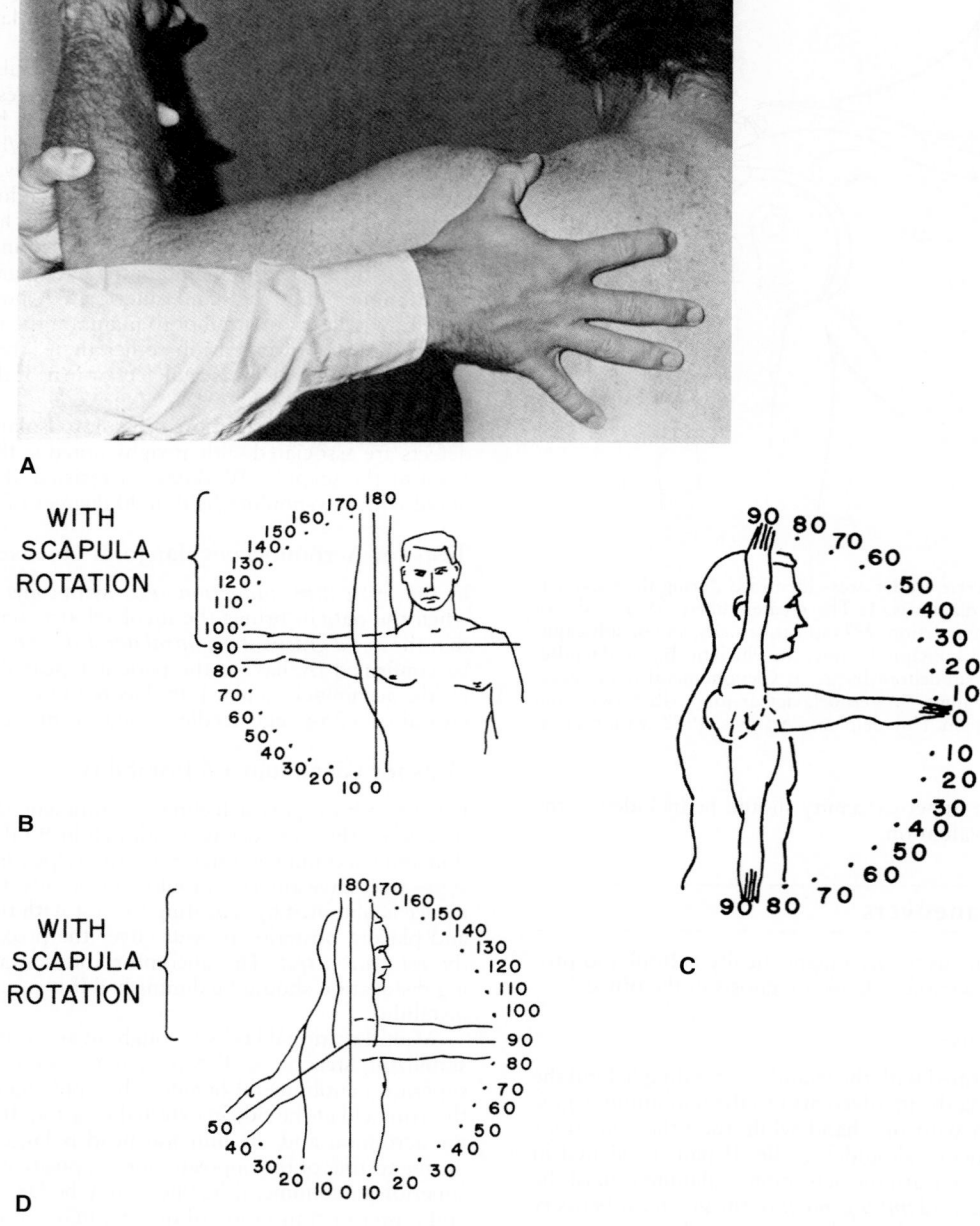

FIGURE 150.2. A: Stabilization of the scapula during testing of glenohumeral joint motion. **B:** Normal range of adduction–abduction of the shoulder with and without scapular rotation. **C:** Normal range of external–internal rotation with the upper arm at 90 degrees and the elbow held at a right angle. **D:** Normal range of flexion–extension of the shoulder with and without scapular rotation. (From Katz WA. Rheumatic diseases. Philadelphia: Lippincott, 1977, with permission.)

pattern of calcification, which suggests acute calcific tendinitis. An *axillary view* is mandatory if dislocation is suspected; it most clearly defines the relation of the humeral head to the glenoid fossa and is also helpful in the assessment of glenohumeral arthritis. In patients with chronic or recurrent dislocations, an indentation into the humeral head (or Hill–Sachs lesion) may be apparent. Cervical spine films are needed if neck motion reproduces the shoulder pain or root compression symptoms are observed (see Chapter 148).

Magnetic resonance imaging (MRI) is used to answer specific diagnostic questions that history, examination, and radiographs suggest. Because rotator cuff tendinitis and defects and acromioclavicular arthritis are common in asymptomatic individuals, the findings on MRI must be interpreted carefully in the light of the history and exam. MRI is used more often for operative planning than for diagnosis and should probably be ordered by the specialist rather than the primary care doctor. It can provide information about the size of a defect, the degree

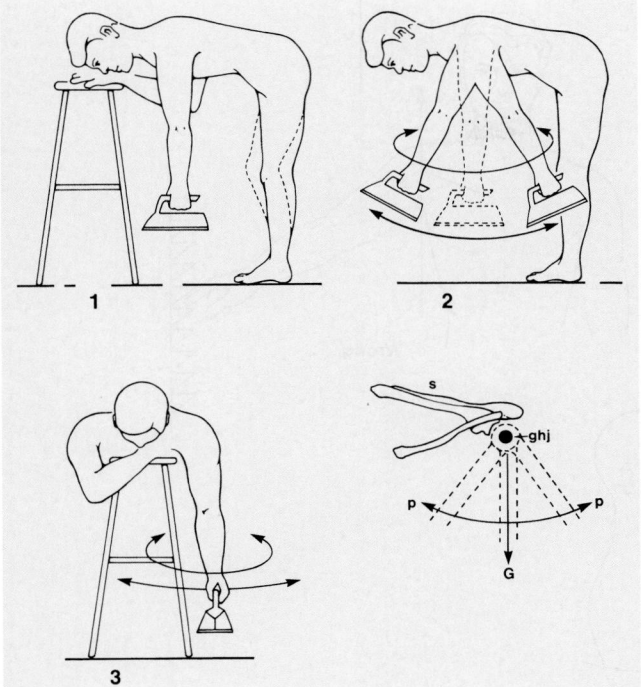

FIGURE 150.3. Active pendular glenohumeral exercise (Codman exercises). **1:** The posture to be assumed to permit the arm to "dangle" freely, with or without a weight. **2:** The arm moves in the forward and backward sagittal plane, in forward and backward flexion. A circular motion in the clockwise and counterclockwise directions is also made in increasingly larger circles. **3:** The front view of the exercise shows lateral pendular movement, actually in the coronal plane. The lower right diagram shows the effect of gravity (G) on the glenohumeral joint (ghj) with an immobile scapula (s). The p-to-p arc is the pendular movement. (Redrawn from Cailliet R. Shoulder pain. Philadelphia: FA Davis, 1973, with permission.)

of retraction, and the status of involved muscles (i.e., whether or not they have been replaced by fat). *Shoulder arthrography* was used in the past to identify a suspected rotator cuff tear but has been replaced by magnetic resonance imaging. Complex shoulder problems are increasingly evaluated using a magnetic resonance arthrogram with injected gadolinium, which is also a test best ordered by the specialist.

If infection is suspected in the joint or joint capsule, *aspiration, Gram's stain,* and *culture* are urgent so that definitive therapy can be initiated without delay (see Chapter 145). If a peripheral nerve deficit is discovered on neurologic examination, *electromyography* may help to characterize the lesion better.

SYMPTOMATIC THERAPY (1,2,5–7)

A considerable amount of symptomatic therapy can be orchestrated by the primary physician because management is largely nonoperative. Although rheumatologists and orthopedic surgeons are often asked by primary physicians to manage shoulder pain, outcomes studies adjusted for severity find no significant differences in pain relief or functional status for patients with shoulder pain managed by primary physicians, rheumatologists, and orthopedic surgeons.

Rotator Cuff Tendinitis

If a large tear of the rotator cuff is not suspected, the tendinosis can be managed with a program consisting of nonnarcotic pain medications (acetaminophen or a nonsteroidal anti-inflammatory drug; e.g., 375 mg of naproxen twice daily or 600 mg of ibuprofen three times daily) and exercises to strengthen the rotator cuff. The exercises are simple, and many patients can do them on their own with the proper equipment. Alternatively, the exercises can be supervised by a trained therapist. Commonly, a set of rubber bands providing increasing levels of resistance is used instead of small weights to exercise specific tendons and enhance their strength and performance.

If motion is restricted, the program should include specific exercises for restoring shoulder mobility. *Pendulum exercises* aid in maintaining joint mobility. With the patient bending forward at the waist, the arm is allowed to dangle and swing in forward-to-back, side-to-side, and circular patterns (Fig. 150.3). Additional exercises, such as "wall climbing" (Fig. 150.4), the use of pulleys, and recumbent active-assisted shoulder exercises using the contralateral arm are useful. The patient must be counseled to expect some mild discomfort with these exercises because they are designed specifically to stretch the joint capsule. Confidence and a sense of safety and well-being are essential components of a successful exercise program. These exercises are performed for a minimum of 15 to 30 minutes, three to four times each day.

Subacromial *injection* of a *corticosteroid* and local anesthetic is commonly used, but the results of clinical trials are mixed, and injection may not offer much more than pain relievers and exercise, although results may be a bit quicker, which appeals to patients. In patients that elect injection after honest counseling about the risks, discomforts, and debatable benefits, the subacromial joint can be entered by advancing the needle under the lateral edge of the acromion process. After the skin has been initially infiltrated with a few milliliters of lidocaine, the subacromial space is injected with 5 to 10 mL of lidocaine and 40 mg of methylprednisolone (Depo-Medrol, usually 1 mL) or an equivalent steroid (Fig. 150.5). Patients should be counseled that corticosteroid injection may acutely worsen symptoms after the anesthetic wears off. A strict limit of three total injections is recommended.

Calcific tendonitis is usually a brief but excruciating inflammation. Chronic calcification in the setting of symptoms more characteristic of tendinosis is common and likely reflects the usual tendon degeneration. Specific treatment of these chronic calcifications is controversial.

Rotator Cuff Defects ("Tears")

"Tear" is somewhat of a misnomer because the majority of these are not acute traumatic injuries but rather the results of chronic degeneration. Spontaneous healing of a torn rotator cuff is unlikely. Despite this, many patients with a "partial tear" (a debatable term that refers to degenerated tendon areas with a complete defect) or a small complete defect respond to an exercise program designed to strengthen their shoulder rotator muscles. Large, acute tears require prompt surgical treatment. In may not be possible to reconstruct very large or massive tears and defects and large defects associated with retraction and degeneration of the muscle.

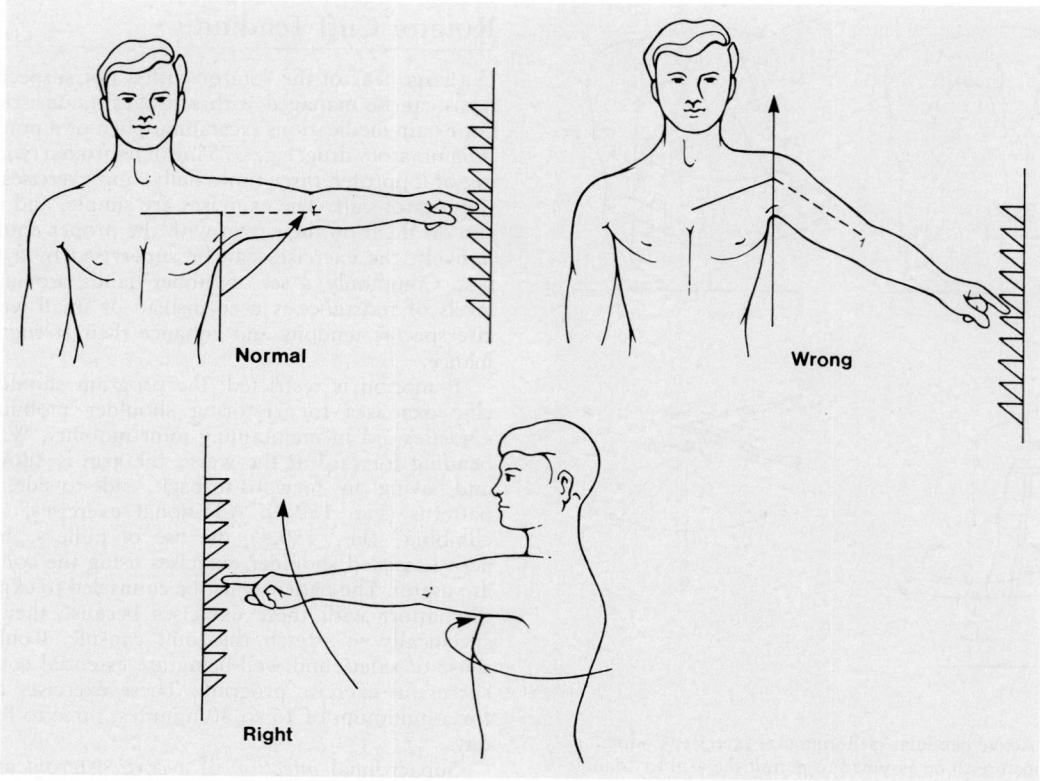

FIGURE 150.4. Correct and incorrect use of "wall-climbing" exercise. The wall-climbing exercise frequently is performed improperly. The normal arm climbs with normal scapulohumeral rhythm. If a pericapsulitis is present, the wall climb in abduction is performed with "shrugging" of the scapula, and nothing is accomplished. The wall climb should be started with the patient facing the wall and gradually turning the body until it is at a right angle to the wall. (Redrawn from Cailliet R. Shoulder pain. Philadelphia: FA Davis, 1973, with permission.)

Idiopathic Adhesive Capsulitis

Adhesive capsulitis is frustrating; the course is prolonged, and the chances for full recovery are unpredictable. The hallmark of treatment is an *active exercise program*. The patient is

instructed to precede each session with the application of local heat, either by using a heating pad or taking a warm shower, for 15 to 20 minutes. Initially, one begins by lying supine and, with the contralateral hand, bringing the involved shoulder into forward flexion. External rotation exercises are also begun; one holds a broom handle in both hands and moves from internal to

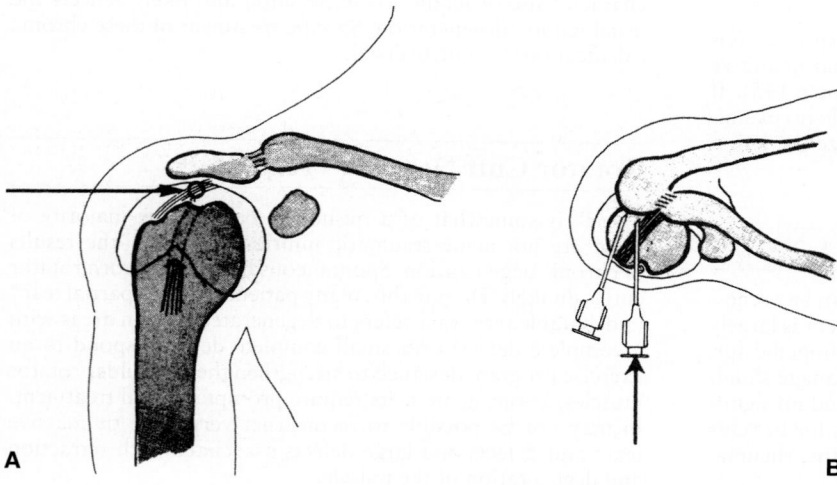

A

B

FIGURE 150.5. Site of subacromial injection. **A:** Region of supraspinatus insertion in the suprahumeral space. The region is palpable immediately below the overhanging acromion and over the greater tuberosity just lateral to the bicipital groove of the humerus. **B:** Insertion of needle viewed from above. Two directions of entrance are shown, with the arrow depicting that shown in the anterior view. (From Cailliet R. Soft tissue pain and disability. Philadelphia: FA Davis, 1977:161, with permission.)

external rotation. The patient should be encouraged to use the shoulder as much as possible in the normal activities of daily living. It is worthwhile for the patient or physical therapist to keep a weekly or monthly log regarding the shoulder motion because improvement is slow and usually occurs in small increments; objective signs of improvement help to lessen patient frustration.

Forceful manipulation of the shoulder is rarely indicated, and in fact *operative caspsulotomy* may be safer. Recently, this procedure has been performed with the arthroscope, but the indications for operative intervention are uncertain and debatable. Most people achieve a functional range of motion over time.

Glenohumeral Arthritis and Acromioclavicular Arthritis

There is no scientifically established disease-modifying treatment for glenohumeral arthritis. Treatment of this problem is palliative and largely consists in the use of pain relievers according to patient preference. Activity modification can reduce symptoms, but maintaining a high level of activity in spite of pain is not neglectful or unsafe, and patients should be given this option. The role of *cortisone injections* is debated. Improvements in total glenohumeral arthroplasty have offered a functional alternative to low-demand patients whose condition is refractory to medical management. Operative treatment of acromioclavicular arthritis consists in resection of the distal end of the clavicle, which can be accomplished either using either an open or an arthroscopic technique.

INDICATIONS FOR REFERRAL

Shoulder dislocation or instability, fractures about the shoulder, advanced acromioclavicular or glenohumeral joint arthritis, rotator cuff tears, and infection are best referred early to the orthopedic surgeon. Refractory rotator cuff tendinitis also is an indication for referral if resolution is not obtained with appropriate conservative treatment.

PATIENT EDUCATION (7)

Emphasis should be placed on the importance of active participation in the treatment program. Many patients seek only relief from pain and expect oral or injectable medication to suffice. Thorough recovery entails actively performing the exercises of the treatment program, which must be carefully taught, often with the help of a physical therapist. Repeated pain and limitation of function are bound to ensue if the exercise program is not taken seriously.

Annotated Bibliography

1. Rees JD, Wilson AM, Wolman RL. Current concepts in the management of tendon disorders. Rheumatology (Oxford) 2006;45:508. (*A review of the degenerative tendinopathies and enesthopathies of middle age.*)
2. Sachs RA, Lin D, Stone ML, et al. Can the need for future surgery for acute traumatic anterior shoulder dislocation be predicted? J Bone Joint Surg Am 2007;89(8):1665. (*A paper that addresses the risk factors and prevalence of recurrent anterior shoulder dislocation*)
3. Yamaguchi K, Ditsios K, Middleton WD, et al. The demographic and morphological features of rotator cuff disease. A comparison of asymptomatic and symptomatic shoulders. J Bone Joint Surg Am 2006; 88:1699. (*One of several studies demonstrating asymptomatic contralateral degeneration of the rotator cuff in patients with unilateral rotator cuff symptoms.*)
4. Sher JS, Uribe JW, Posada A, et al. Abnormal findings on magnetic resonance images of asymptomatic shoulders. J Bone Joint Surg Am 1995;77(1):10. (*The first of several studies demonstrating the prevalence of asymptomatic rotator cuff pathology and its increase with age.*)
5. Levine WN, Kashyap CP, Bak SF, et al. Nonoperative management of idiopathic adhesive capsulitis. J Shoulder Elbow Surg 2007;16:569. (*Emphasizes the fact that adhesive capsulitis is a self-limited condition.*)
6. Williams GR Jr, Rockwood CA Jr, Bigliani LU, et al. Rotator cuff tears: why do we repair them? J Bone Joint Surg Am 2004;86-A(12):2764. (*Reviews current concepts regarding operative and nonoperative management.*)
7. Bernstein J. In the beginning was the word. J Bone Joint Surg Am 2006;88:442. (*An editorial; discusses the importance of word choice in medicine, particularly musculoskeletal medicine.*)

CHAPTER 151 ■ EVALUATION OF HIP PAIN

Hip pain can be a major source of misery for both patient and family. The joint is essential to locomotion and weight bearing and is frequently subject to trauma and chronic mechanical stress. In the assessment of hip pain, the degree of pain and disability must be determined in addition to the underlying cause because surgery is a practical therapeutic option for disabled patients whose pain is refractory to conservative measures.

PATHOPHYSIOLOGY AND CLINICAL PRESENTATION (1–3)

The hip is supplied by the obturator, sciatic, and femoral nerves. Pain originating in or around the hip can be felt in the groin or buttock, with radiation to the distal thigh and anteromedial aspect of the knee. Occasionally, pain from the hip may be felt only in the thigh and knee. Pain occurs in the distribution of the L-2 and L-3 roots and rarely is referred to the lower leg or foot. Conversely, pain caused by a problem outside of the hip may be referred to the hip if the lesion irritates the femoral, sciatic, or obturator nerve or the nerve roots. Problems outside the hip include herniated disks in the high lumbar region, spinal stenosis, retroperitoneal or pelvic tumor, and femoral hernia; patients who have aortoiliac insufficiency may also present with hip and buttock pain (see Chapter 147).

Hip pain may be focal or diffuse, depending on the extent to which the joint and surrounding structures are involved in the pathologic process. For example, bursitis is characterized by focal pain and tenderness over the site of the bursa; synovitis is more diffuse, involving the entire joint capsule. Stiffness, limitation of motion, limp, and crepitus are frequent accompaniments of pain. Swelling is usually not evident and is difficult to detect because the joint is buried deeply in soft tissues.

The major mechanisms of hip disease include cartilaginous degeneration, synovial inflammation, tendinitis and consequent bursitis, fracture, and ischemia.

Osteoarthritis

The hip is a major site of degenerative joint disease, with the elderly being the most affected. Obesity is also a risk factor, particularly in women. The onset is often insidious, beginning with minor aching or stiffness that may be unilateral or bilateral. Symptoms are characteristically exacerbated by prolonged standing, walking, or stair climbing. Stiffness is noted when the patient gets up after sitting for long periods. The hip begins to loosen up at first with moving about, but discomfort then worsens with continued activity. As osteoarthritis gradually progresses, it results in decreasing hip motion, increasing stiffness, and increasing pain. A limp may develop as the joint architecture is disrupted, and weight bearing becomes painful. The course of the disease is usually marked by spontaneous exacerbations and remissions.

On physical examination, the patient with substantial disease characteristically holds the hip in flexion, external rotation, and adduction. An antalgic gait, Trendelenburg's sign (buttock falls when the patient stands on the opposite foot, which is indicative of abductor weakness), and limitation of hip motion with or without crepitus may be present. Pain, muscle spasm, and guarding occur when the examiner attempts to take the hip through the full range of motion. Buttock atrophy may involve the gluteus maximus posteriorly and the gluteus medius more laterally. With severe degenerative arthritis of the hip, a marked flexion deformity may develop, and pain may be felt in the hip joint even at rest (see also Chapter 157).

Rheumatoid Arthritis

The hips are rarely affected in rheumatoid disease until other joints have become involved. Pain is characteristically bilateral and associated with morning stiffness, which lessens with activity. During flares of the disease, the hip joint is tender to palpation, and capsular fullness and thickening may be felt if effusion or chronic synovitis is present. Flexion contractures occur in advanced cases (see also Chapter 156).

Ankylosing Spondylitis

Of the spondyloarthropathies, this one is unique in that the hip is sometimes affected. Concurrent sacroiliac and spinal involvement is usually present and in itself may cause pain radiating into the hip or buttock (see also Chapters 146 and 147).

Hip Fracture

At greatest risk is the frail, elderly person with a history of frequent falls and osteoporosis. Those with a history of hip fracture are at increased risk for another. The femoral neck and intertrochanteric region are common fracture sites. Loss of normal surface architecture may be associated with acute joint deformity, severe pain, guarding, and restriction of flexion and external rotation. Active straight leg raising is impaired. Competitive long-distance runners are at risk for stress fracture of the femoral neck.

Septic Arthritis

Joint infection in the hip most often follows hematogenous seeding (see Chapter 145). Because the joint is deep seated, the ordinary signs of infection may not be readily evident. Fever, hip or knee pain (caused by referral of pain), and inability to bear weight are early symptoms. The thigh is often held in flexion, and a bulging, tender joint capsule may be palpable.

Osteonecrosis/Avascular Necrosis of the Femoral Head

Also referred to as "aseptic" necrosis of the femoral head, this condition has an ischemic pathophysiology. It occurs with increased frequency in patients who take high daily doses of glucocorticoids, persons who are alcoholic, patients with hemoglobinopathies, and persons who work under conditions of increased atmospheric pressure. The mechanism of steroid-induced disease involves the proliferation of intramedullary fat, tissue hypertension, and compromised perfusion of bone. Patients report the gradual onset of focal pain and limitation of movement. Diagnostic radiographic changes include wedge-shaped areas of increased density and segmental collapse of the femoral head.

Bursitis

Inflammation of the bursa occurs as a consequence of trauma or spread of an inflammatory process. Focal pain with tenderness develops over the bursa. *Trochanteric bursitis* is felt on the lateral aspect of the hip, posterior to the trochanter. Symptoms are increased by direct pressure or hip flexion and internal rotation. Pain may worsen at night and radiate down the leg to the knee. It may occur in runners who jog on uneven surfaces and those with one leg slightly shorter than the other. *Iliopectineal bursitis* causes pain on flexion and tenderness localized to the lateral border of Scarpa's triangle. *Ischiogluteal bursitis* presents with buttock pain that is worse during prolonged sitting, occurs at night, and occasionally radiates down the leg posteriorly, simulating sciatica.

Polymyalgia Rheumatica

A disease of the elderly that is often mistaken for depression, arthritis, or bursitis, polymyalgia is characterized by bilateral aching of the hips, thighs, and shoulders in conjunction with a very high sedimentation rate. It has a strong association with cranial arteritis (see Chapter 161). Joint structures and passive range of joint motion are usually preserved.

Pigmented Villonodular Synovitis

This uncommon granulomatous disease of the synovium presents with slowly progressive pain and limitation of movement. Radiographic films show large cystic areas about the hip joint, which distinguish the condition from degenerative joint disease.

Referred Pain

Any pelvic, abdominal, or retroperitoneal process irritating the obturator muscle can cause pain that is referred to the hip. Such pain is worsened by internal rotation of the hip joint.

DIFFERENTIAL DIAGNOSIS

Hip pain is usually caused by degenerative joint disease. Other important causes include joint infection, avascular necrosis of the femoral head, bursitis, polymyalgia rheumatica, and rheumatoid arthritis. On occasion, ankylosing spondylitis or villonodular synovitis is responsible. Pain may be referred to the hip from a lumbar or pelvic problem, such as a herniated disk in the high lumbar region, retroperitoneal tumor or abscess, or obturator or femoral hernia. Aortoiliac insufficiency may present with exercise-induced hip and buttock pain.

WORKUP (1,4,5)

History

One should ascertain the onset, location, and radiation of the pain in addition to inciting and alleviating factors and the presence of numbness or weakness. It is particularly important to inquire directly about trauma, the involvement of other joints, morning stiffness, the relation of pain to activity, response to rest, steroid, or alcohol use, and current infection or fever. A few pitfalls regarding the history should be mentioned. For example, stiffness by itself is a nonspecific finding because it may occur both with degenerative disease and with rheumatoid involvement of the hip. The response to continued activity may be of more help diagnostically; stiffness usually worsens in degenerative disease and lessens in rheumatoid arthritis. Bilateral cramping hip and buttock pain that comes on with walking and is relieved by rest may actually be a sign of vascular insufficiency rather than of joint disease.

Physical Examination

The hip should be examined for deformities such as flexion or adduction contractures, which are seen with rheumatoid disease, and for fixed external rotation, which suggests a frac-ture of the femoral neck. Gait is also important to check. The hip is then put through the full range of passive motion to detect crepitus, limitation of movement, flexion contracture, muscle spasm, or guarding. The normal range of hip flexion–extension is from –20 to 90 degrees with the knee straight and from 0 to 120 degrees with the knee flexed. Normal adduction–abduction is from –20 to 90 degrees; normal internal–external rotation is from –50 to +50 degrees. One of the first movements to be limited in hip disease is internal rotation with the hip hyperextended. Palpation of the joint and individual bursae for focal tenderness and swelling is important for detecting a localized inflammatory process.

The circumference of the thigh should be measured at a fixed distance from a bony reference point, such as the tibial tubercle of the knee, the anterior superior iliac spine, or the midpatella. Atrophy is suggestive of intrinsic hip disease.

Femoral pulses should be palpated for diminution and auscultated for bruits. Pelvic and rectal examinations are helpful in searching for tumors, which may cause referred pain. The back should be examined for evidence of L-1 to L-2 or L-2 to L-3 disk herniation (see Chapter 147). Neurologic assessment of the lower extremities is needed to test for weakness, sensory loss, and reflexes.

Laboratory Studies

Hip *radiography* is essential in the assessment of hip pain. Radiography may be diagnostic of degenerative joint disease, rheumatoid arthritis, avascular necrosis, or fracture. Weight-bearing films help one judge the severity of degenerative hip disease by disclosing the extent of joint space narrowing. Sacroiliac and spine films are indicated if ankylosing spondylitis is under consideration (see Chapters 146 and 147). *Magnetic resonance imaging* is the most sensitive test for osteonecrosis of the femoral head, showing expansion of intramedullary fat before bony changes become visible. It also is more sensitive than standard radiography in the detection of stress fracture of the femoral neck.

A complete blood cell count, determination of the *sedimentation rate*, and *rheumatoid factor* analysis may be useful if a rheumatoid disease is being considered (see Chapter 146). If a septic joint is suspected, aspiration for cell count, Gram's stain, and culture is urgent (see Chapter 145).

SYMPTOMATIC THERAPY AND INDICATIONS FOR REFERRAL (1–3,5–17)

Degenerative Disease (See Also Chapter 157)

Initial Measures

Simple treatment measures for the relief of an acute exacerbation include daily periods of bed rest, analgesics (e.g., up to 1 g of *acetaminophen* four times daily), limitation of prolonged sitting or standing, and crutch or cane support. *Nonsteroidal antiinflammatory drugs* (NSAIDs) offer little benefit over pure analgesics when no signs of concurrent synovial inflammation are present. Moreover, NSAIDs increase both cost and the risk of adverse side effects (e.g., gastrointestinal toxicity, renal impairment, cardiovascular events; see Chapters 68 and 156). Sometimes a short course of *opioid* therapy is helpful for pain control during a flare.

Subsequent Management

After acute symptoms lessen, the patient can begin a program to improve functional capacity. It should include the avoidance of activities that specifically aggravate pain, daily mild *exercise* (walking short distances as tolerated) preceded by a dose of acetaminophen, cane *support* if necessary, *weight reduction* if the patient is obese, and specific daily range-of-motion and strengthening *exercises*, preferably taught by a physical therapist. Rest periods of 1 hour twice daily with local heat applied to the hip may be helpful if discomfort occurs after exercise. The benefits of weight reduction should not be overlooked. Even modest degrees of weight reduction can be remarkably helpful in alleviating pain and disability.

The dietary supplements *glucosamine* and *chondroitin sulfate* are heavily promoted for osteoarthritis. Most studies purporting benefit are poorly designed; well-designed trials fail to find significant benefit over placebo (see also Chapter 157). The cost of these supplements can be substantial, especially when taken for prolonged periods.

Consideration for Surgery

If symptoms continue to be disabling despite the maximal application of conservative measures, then *surgery* is a reasonable consideration if the patient is otherwise medically able to tolerate surgery and participate in the rehabilitation process. The use of appropriateness criteria can facilitate the selection of patients who are likely to have the best outcomes.

Results achieved from *hip reconstructive* procedures are quite good and attainable at relatively low risk. Thromboembolism is a well-recognized risk of surgery that can be effectively treated prophylactically (see Chapter 83). Risk is a function of the patient's overall medical condition but not of age per se. Medically suitable candidates older than 85 years of age can gain years of pain relief and functional improvement with hip replacement surgery without incurring unacceptable perioperative risk. However, the patient must understand and be willing and able to engage in the work of rehabilitation. Despite the relative safety of surgery, expectations for outcomes need to be realistic, and the amount of rehabilitative work necessary must be clearly understood (see also Chapter 157).

Bursitis

As an inflammatory condition, bursitis responds well to NSAID therapy (e.g., 500 mg of naproxen twice daily for 1 to 2 weeks) in conjunction with reduced activity. The jogger who has been running on uneven surfaces should change to another running surface. A *heel lift* may help the person whose legs are not the same length. If pain does not respond and if tenderness is well localized to the bursa overlying the bony prominence of the greater trochanter, a *local steroid injection* into the bursa can be attempted to provide relief. The bursa and trochanter are identified by having the patient lie in the lateral decubitus position with the involved hip exposed; the physician palpates for focal tenderness over the bony prominence of the greater trochanter. After 2 mL of 2% lidocaine has been mixed with 1 mL (40 mg/mL) of methylprednisolone (Depo-Medrol), 1 to 2 mL of the mixture is injected into the tender area overlying the bony prominence with a 25-gauge needle, inserted until it just touches the periosteal surface of the bone and then drawn back ever so slightly for the injection. Primary physicians who are unfamiliar with the technique of injecting a hip bursa should refer the patient to an orthopedist or rheumatologist.

Rheumatoid Disease

Polymyalgia rheumatica responds dramatically to low-dose steroids (see Chapter 161) and rheumatoid arthritis to high-dose aspirin or NSAIDs followed by disease-altering therapy (see Chapter 156).

Hip Fracture and Septic Arthritis

These conditions require immediate hospitalization. Early fracture repair (within 24 to 48 hours) may reduce mortality at 1 year in patients who are medically stable, but medically unstable patients need to have their medical issues attended to before undergoing surgery because prognosis can be severely affected by a postoperative medical complication. In a large-scale study from the Veterans Administration, the risk of a postoperative medical complication was 19%, with a mortality rate of 1.2% at 30 days for the 81% of patients who did not have a postoperative complication but 25% for those who did.

Hip fracture prevention in the elderly is an important responsibility of the primary care physician (see Chapter 239). Effective measures include encouraging regular modest *weight-bearing exercise* (e.g., walking), screening for and *treating osteoporosis* (see Chapters 144 and 164), carefully arranging the *home environment* for safety, and teaching *balance exercises*. The study of *hip protectors* in institutionalized frail elderly patients prone to falls has produced variable results; the best-designed studies failed to show benefit.

A.H.G.

Annotated Bibliography

1. Creamer P, Hochberg MC. Osteoarthritis. Lancet 1997;350:503. (*A comprehensive, well-written review, including a discussion of hip disease.*)
2. Hartz AJ, Fischer ME, Bril G, et al. The association of obesity with joint pain in osteoarthritis in the NAHES data. J Chron Dis 1986;39:311. (*Finds obesity to be a predictor of pain and arthritis, especially in women.*)
3. Dalinka MK, Alavi A, Forsted DH. Aseptic (ischemic) necrosis of the femoral head. JAMA 1977; 238: 1059. (*One of the original modern descriptions of the condition.*)
4. American Medical Association, Council on Scientific Affairs. Musculoskeletal applications of magnetic resonance imaging. JAMA 1989;262:2420. (*This was found to be the most sensitive imaging study for avascular septic necrosis of the femoral head and stress fracture of the femoral neck.*)
5. Paty JG. Diagnosis and treatment of musculoskeletal running injuries. Semin Arthritis Rheum 1988;18:48. (*Includes a discussion of femoral neck stress fractures and hip bursitis.*)
6. Bradley JD, Brandt KD, Katz BP, et al. Comparison of an antiinflammatory dose of ibuprofen, an analgesic dose of ibuprofen, and acetaminophen in the treatment of patients with osteoarthritis of the knee. N Engl J Med 1991;325:87. (*Pure analgesic therapy was as effective as nonsteroidal antiinflammatory drugs.*)
7. Burton KE, Wright V, Richards J. Patient's expectations in relation to outcome of total hip replacement surgery. Ann Rheum Dis 1979;38:471. (*A still useful article, making the important point that expectations are often in excess of reality; preoperative counseling is essential.*)
8. Feskanich D, Willett W, Colditz G. Walking and leisure-time activity and risk of hip fracture in postmenopausal women. JAMA 2002;288:2300. (*Data from the Nurses' Health Study—a large-scale, prospective epidemiologic study—finding that moderate levels of activity were associated with >50% reduction in the risk of hip fracture.*).

9. Griffin MR, Brandt KD, Liang MH, et al. Practical management of osteoarthritis: integration of pharmacologic and nonpharmacologic measures. Arch Family Med 1995;4:1049. (*An excellent review, with an especially good section on nonpharmacologic measures.*)
10. Grimes JP, Gregory PM, Noveck H, et al. The effects of time-to-surgery on mortality and morbidity in patients following hip fracture. Am J Med 2002;112:702. (*A retrospective cohort study, finding that delaying surgery up to 4 days to medically stabilize the patient did not adversely affect outcome.*)
11. Jones CA, Yoaklander DC, Johnston WC, et al. The effect of age on pain, function, and quality of life after total hip and knee arthroplasty. Arch Intern Med 2001;161:454. (*A community-based cohort study, finding that age was not a determinant of outcome.*)
12. Kiel DP, Magaziner J, Zimmerman S, et al. Efficacy of a hip protector to prevent hip fracture in nursing home residents: the HIP PRO randomized controlled trial. *JAMA* 2007;298:413. (*Failed to demonstrate efficacy.*)
13. Lawrence VA, Hilsenbeck SG, Noveck H, et al. Medical complications and outcomes after hip fracture repair. Arch Intern Med 2002;162:2053. (*A large series with useful outcomes and risk data, underscoring the seriousness of the problem.*)
14. Liang MH, Fortin P. Management of osteoarthritis of the hip and knee. N Engl J Med 1991;325:125. (*An overview of the approach to diagnosis and treatment.*)
15. Orosz GM, Magaziner J, Hannan EL, et al. Association of timing of surgery for hip fracture and patient outcomes. JAMA 2004; 291:1738. (*A cohort study, finding that early surgery in medically stable patients appeared to reduce the length of stay and pain but not mortality or degree of disability.*)
16. Reichenbach S, Sterchi R, Scherer M, et al. Meta-analysis: chondroitin for osteoarthritis of the knee or hip. Ann Intern Med 2007;146:580. (*A meta-analysis, finding no net benefit from chondroitin alone.*)
17. Rozendaal RM, Koes BW, van Osch GJVM, et al. Effect of glucosamine sulfate on hip osteoarthritis: a randomized trial. Ann Intern Med 2008;148:268. (*A placebo-controlled trial, showing no benefit.*)

CHAPTER 152 ■ EVALUATION OF KNEE PAIN

The knee joint is frequently the site of trauma, degenerative disease, inflammatory arthritis, and rheumatologic conditions. Disability can be considerable because of the inability to bear weight. The primary physician is frequently called on to evaluate knee pain, a complaint reported in 6% of visits. One in seven persons older than age 60 years suffer from chronic knee pain due to osteoarthritis. Such presentations can be expected to increase in frequency as the population ages. Issues that commonly arise in the course of the evaluation include the need for imaging and orthopedic referral. Using key features of the history and physical examination, the primary physician can conduct a cost-effective assessment that helps to ensure timely and appropriate but not excessive use of radiologic studies and consultations.

ical stresses. The entire joint may be painful, but often the discomfort is localized to the anterior and medial portions of the knee. Prolonged standing or walking may precipitate or worsen symptoms. Mild stiffness is common on first arising in the morning and on getting up after a long period of sitting, but unlike the situation in inflammatory arthropathies, it usually is short lived (<30 minutes) and initially improves on moving about, but it worsens with prolonged activity. Symptoms gradually progress but may take many years to become disabling. Considerable degenerative change and joint destruction can occur before serious knee pain develops. Small effusions may appear after prolonged weight bearing, but few other signs or symptoms of inflammation occur.

PATHOPHYSIOLOGY AND CLINICAL PRESENTATION (1–5)

Osteoarthritis, trauma-induced derangements of soft tissue, and inflammatory processes are the predominant mechanisms of knee pain in the adult. The pain is characteristically worsened by weight bearing and may radiate into the anterior thigh, posterior calf, or pretibial region. An inflamed joint capsule produces diffuse pain. The site of pain is characteristic of the underlying problem (Fig. 152.1). Locking of the joint suggests a loose body or torn meniscus. Hip disease occasionally presents as knee pain (see Chapter 151).

Osteoarthritis

Knee pain associated with osteoarthritis is typically chronic, although there may be acute exacerbations. Onset is typically after age 50 years and accompanied by reports of focal tenderness, "creaking" sensations, and bony deformity of the knee. Degenerative changes often originate in the medial joint compartment and patellofemoral joint, related in part to mechan-

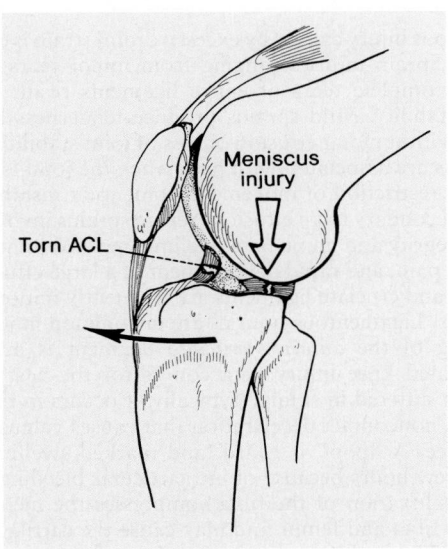

FIGURE 152.1. Cruciate ligament tear with associated meniscal damage. ACL, anterior cruciate ligament.

Rheumatoid Disease

Rheumatoid arthritis commonly affects the knees. Pain, swelling, and morning stiffness are characteristic, as is symmetric polyarticular involvement of the hands, feet, ankles, and/or wrists. Symptoms wax and wane; the course is chronic (see Chapter 156). Other rheumatoid diseases can produce a similar picture (see Chapter 146).

Acute Monoarticular Arthritis

The knee is a frequent site of septic arthritis, gout, pseudogout, early rheumatoid arthritis, rheumatic fever, palindromic rheumatism, and disseminated gonorrhea. The acute onset of unilateral swelling, pain, and generalized tenderness is the usual presentation (see Chapter 145). Motion is limited, and muscle spasm is prominent.

Degeneration or Tear of a Meniscus

An acute tear occurs as a consequence of excessive weight bearing, twisting, and/or valgus or varus stress and may be associated with the partial or complete disruption of collateral or cruciate ligaments (see later discussion). Usually, there is a history of acute trauma, typically a twisting of the leg while the foot is planted, accompanied by reports of a "pop" or a tearing sensation. If there is no accompanying ligamentous tear, it may take a few hours to days for swelling to develop, a consequence of a reactive joint effusion, but swelling can be immediate if there is concurrent tear of a ligament. A torn anterior cruciate ligament is a common precipitant of meniscal tear. If cartilaginous fragments become trapped, they cause the knee to *lock*. Chronic internal derangements caused by degeneration or tear of the meniscus produce recurrent pain and swelling and a knee that gives way, catches, or locks. Walking stairs is painful, as is squatting.

Knee Sprain/Ligamentous Injury

Ligamentous injury caused by excessive joint strain is extremely frequent. Sprain injuries ranging from minor tears of a few fibers to complete tears of entire ligaments result in a loss of joint stability. Mild sprains produce tenderness and local swelling without joint effusion or loss of joint stability. Moderate sprains are associated with pain when the joint is stressed, voluntary restriction of movement, some joint instability, and swelling secondary to an effusion. Severe sprains involve a total loss of integrity and immediate swelling, marked joint instability, severe pain, and rapid development of a large effusion. The collateral and cruciate ligaments are frequently injured in contact sports. Ligamentous injuries are uncommon in joggers.

Tearing of the *anterior cruciate* ligament is a common sports-related knee injury; it accounts for the vast majority of sprains suffered in skiing. Typically, it occurs in the setting of sudden noncontact deceleration that causes valgus twisting of the knee. A "pop" is heard, and marked swelling ensues within a few hours because of intraarticular bleeding. The resulting subluxation of the tibia compresses the meniscus between the tibia and femur and may cause the cartilage to tear (see Fig. 152.1 and later discussion). Initially after an anterior cruciate tear, the knee may function reasonably well, but instability quickly develops on the resumption of sports activity.

Tearing of the *medial collateral ligament* occurs typically in contact sports with force applied to the lateral aspect of the knee (valgus stress). The characteristic popping or tearing sensation of ligamentous or meniscal injury is reported, and swelling quickly ensues. Similarly, medially applied force can tear the *lateral collateral ligament*, and a hyperextension injury can tear the *posterior cruciate ligament*.

Chondromalacia Patellae (Patellofemoral Pain Syndrome)

Degeneration of the posterior patellar cartilage is the cause of this condition. Desiccation, thinning, fissure formation, and ultimately erosion of the cartilage occur. Mechanical factors are suspected although unproven. Chondromalacia is the most common cause of knee pain in joggers and is believed to be related to overtraining. The patient presents with retropatellar aching that is worsened by standing up, climbing stairs, or any other form of bent-knee strain; it is typically bilateral. Stiffness may develop after inactivity, but usually no locking or giving way of the knee is noted. Pain is reported in the peripatellar region and lateral aspect of the knee and can be reproduced by applying pressure against the patella with the knee actively extended. Palpable grating can be elicited at the patellofemoral joint with flexion and extension of the knee. Radiographic findings are normal until late stages, when the posterior surface of the patella becomes irregular and marginal osteophytes develop.

Baker's Cyst

Rupture of one of these popliteal fossa cysts can cause acute inflammation with pain, swelling, and limitation of knee flexion. The inflammation may extend down into the calf and simulate thrombophlebitis. Baker's cysts usually communicate with the knee joint space and most commonly occur in patients with osteoarthritis or rheumatoid disease. An unruptured cyst causes only mild aching and stiffness. Trauma may initiate a rupture.

Prepatellar Bursitis

Repeated trauma (hence the nickname "housemaid's knee") is the predominant cause. Swelling, tenderness, and occasionally erythema over the prepatellar bursae are present. The presentations of bursitis of the suprapatellar and infrapatellar bursae are similar, with findings localized to the bursal site.

Villonodular Synovitis

This granulomatous inflammatory condition involves the synovium that lines the joints, bursae, and tendon sheaths. The cause is unknown. It affects young adults, predominantly men, and presents with unilateral pain, persistent swelling, intermittent knee locking, and occasionally a palpable mass. Diagnosis requires arthroscopy or surgical exploration.

DIFFERENTIAL DIAGNOSIS

The list of conditions that can cause knee pain is extensive and includes polyarticular disease in addition to processes confined to the knee. A clinically useful classification system groups

TABLE 152.1

DIFFERENTIAL DIAGNOSIS OF KNEE PAIN (1,2,5)

Asymmetric Involvement				Symmetric Involvement			
One Knee Only		One Knee Plus Other Joints		Knees Only		Symmetric Polyarthritis	
Acute	Chronic	Acute	Chronic	Acute	Chronic	Acute	Chronic

Sprain
Strain
	Osteoarthritis
	Baker's cyst
		See Chapters 145, 146		Rheumatoid arthritis
				Juvenile rheumatoid
				  arthritis
					Osteoarthritis
					Chondromalacia
					  patellae
						See Chapter 146	

Acute gout	Chronic gout			Early phase of other rheumatoid diseases			
Meniscus tear	Chondromalacia patella				Bursitis		

Early rheumatoid
  disease
	Bursitis			Trauma	Rheumatoid
					  arthritis		

Gonococcal arthritis	Meniscal
	  injuries
					Juvenile
					  rheumatoid
					  arthritis
					Chronic gout		

Septic arthritis					Neuropathic joints		
Reiter's syndrome Bursitis Pseudogout Palindromic rheumatism Ruptured Baker's cyst Hemophilia Sickle cell disease Rheumatic fever					Hemophilia		

Adapted from Katz WA. Rheumatic diseases. Philadelphia: Lippincott, 1977, with permission.

causes of knee pain according to whether the pain is acute or chronic and whether the distribution is symmetric or asymmetric and monoarticular or polyarticular (Table 152.1). In terms of frequency of presentations in the primary care setting, osteoarthritis accounts for 34% of cases of acute knee pain, ligamentous injuries for 20%, meniscal injury for 9%, gout for 2%, and fracture for about 1.5%.

WORKUP (1–3,5–9)

History

Besides ascertaining the quality and location of pain, the alleviating and aggravating factors, and the associated symptoms such as swelling, redness, and warmth, the physician must determine whether the problem is acute or chronic, symmetric or asymmetric, and monoarticular or polyarticular. By combining a careful description of the problem with a characterization of its pattern and chronicity, one can quickly focus the evaluation onto a relatively limited set of conditions having similar clinical presentations (see Table 152.1).

Acute Unilateral Knee Pain

The first task is to ascertain whether the precipitant event was an acute injury or an acute inflammatory reaction. In some instances, a traumatic event might trigger a vigorous inflam-

matory response. If there is a clear history of trauma, then the history is explored to help identify any fracture, meniscal tear, or ligamentous injury. In the absence of trauma, other inflammatory and noninflammatory etiologies need to be considered.

In the Setting of Trauma. Although history is not particularly specific in differentiating among traumatic consequences, a few questions can be helpful: Was the knee twisted while the foot was planted (the typical cause of meniscal tear)? Was the weight-bearing knee subjected to a forceful medial, lateral, or anterior stress (the setting for a ligamentous tear)? Was there a fall or direct impact to the knee (a cause for fracture)? Associated symptoms and aggravating factors are important to explore. A report of a "popping" or "tearing" sensation at the time of injury is suggestive of both ligamentous and meniscal injury; acute onset of pain and swelling are also common to both, but delay in the onset of swelling by a few hours is more characteristic of injury confined to the meniscus, as is difficulty walking stairs and squatting. "Locking" of the knee suggests meniscal damage; "giving out" is consistent with both ligamentous and meniscal damage. Difficulty bearing weight for more than a few steps raises the question of a fracture, as does inability to flex the knee and focal tenderness at the fibular head or patella. Although history is helpful, physical examination is more specific (see later discussion).

In the Setting of Inflammation. Any report of a knee that is acutely warm, red, tender, and swollen in the absence of trauma raises the question of an inflammatory etiology. One needs to check for prior history of gout or pseudogout and symptoms of rheumatoid disease (see Chapter 146); any history of sickle cell disease or hemophilia should be noted. Also essential is inquiry into risk factors and symptoms of an infectious etiology, such as recent high-risk sexual activity, streptococcal infection, dental work, heart murmur, and tick bite, as well as concurrent rash, urethritis, purulent vaginal discharge, and conjunctivitis (see Chapter 145). On occasion, trauma may trigger an acute gouty attack.

In the Setting of Localized Swelling. When localized swelling and tenderness are noted in the absence of major trauma or diffuse joint inflammation, one needs to consider *bursitis* (when the swelling is reported at a bursal site) and a *Baker's cyst*, *popliteal vein thrombophlebitis*, and *popliteal artery aneurysm* (associated with abdominal aortic aneurysm) when the swelling is localized to the popliteal fossa.

Chronic Unilateral Knee Pain

Questioning should cover previous or recurrent trauma, as may occur occupationally; pain associated with prolonged walking, standing, or climbing stairs; knee locking; crepitus; focal swelling; and recurrent acute episodes or exacerbations. Having any three of the following has a 95% sensitivity for the diagnosis of osteoarthritis but a specificity of only 69%: age of onset older than 50 years, morning stiffness less than 30 minutes, crepitus, bone tenderness, or bone deformity. There may be acute exacerbations of pain in osteoarthritis, but usually in the context of symptoms of chronic disease.

When the pain is patellar, peripatellar, or retropatellar, especially when worsened by standing up, climbing stairs, or any other form of bent-knee strain, and the knee is stiff after inactivity but without locking or giving way, then chondromalacia patellae should be considered.

Acute Bilateral Knee Pain

When both knees are involved acutely, then the focus of inquiry should be on the symptoms of rheumatoid disease (see Chapter 146) and recent trauma.

Chronic Bilateral Knee Pain

The questioning can be similar to that for chronic unilateral disease, but rheumatoid symptoms should also be considered (see Chapter 146).

Polyarticular Presentations

When other joints are also involved, inquiry into symptoms of infectious and rheumatologic conditions is essential (see Chapter 146).

Physical Examination

Unlike the history, which can be suggestive but not very accurate, physical examination is essential to the accurate evaluation of knee complaints. The examination is tailored to the clinical presentation and suspected etiologies.

Acute Knee Injury

The task is to identify fracture, ligamentous tear, and meniscal injury. Overall sensitivity of physical examination for the tear of a meniscus or ligament is 75% to 80%; specificity is about 95%, as determined by arthroscopic and magnetic resonance imaging (MRI) study. Given the prevalence of serious knee pathology reported in primary care practice, a negative physical examination has a negative predictive value of 98.5%, making further workup unnecessary. A positive test has a positive predictive value of 50%, indicating need for further investigation (see later discussion).

Examination for Ligamentous Tear. Collateral and cruciate ligaments should be examined for stability. Collateral ligaments are tested by applying mediolateral valgus–varus strain with the knee in full extension and in 15 to 20 degrees of flexion. Tests for anterior cruciate tear include the *anterior drawer sign* and *pivot* and *Lachman tests* (Fig. 152.2). These tests range in sensitivity from 48% for the anterior drawer sign and 61% for the pivot test to 87% for the Lachman test; specificity ranges from 87% for the anterior draw sign to 93% for the Lachman test and 97% for the pivot test.

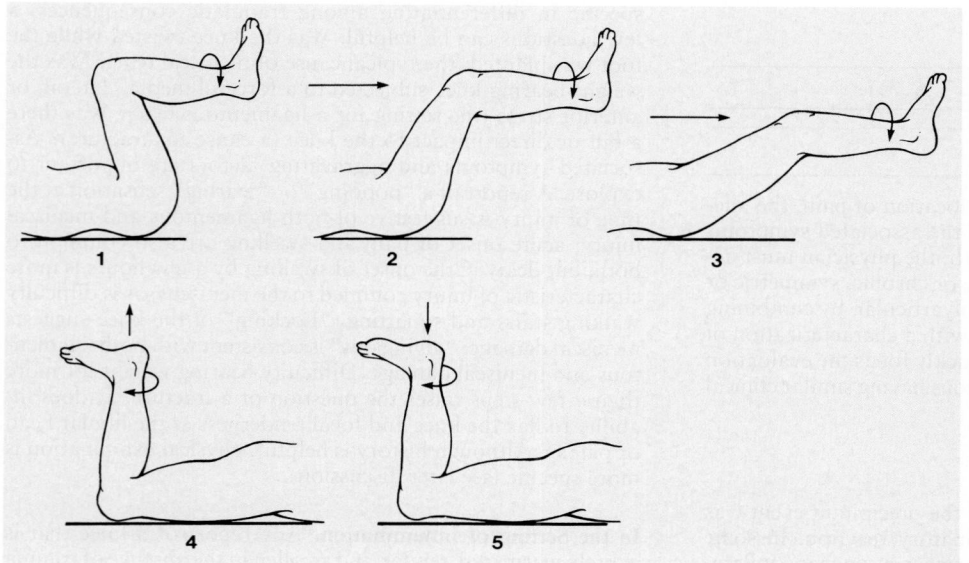

FIGURE 152.2. Meniscus signs (examination). **1–3:** McMurray test. The patient is supine with knee flexed, heel touching the buttocks at the start. The leg is internally rotated to test the lateral meniscus or externally rotated to test the medial meniscus. Then the knee is fully extended. A painful click occurs if a meniscus lesion is present. The test is more meaningful in the first phase of knee extension. Limited extension does not indicate a lesion of the anterior meniscus. **4, 5:** Apley test. The patient is prone. The leg is internally or externally rotated with simultaneous traction. Pain indicates a capsular or ligamentous lesion. Pain caused by rotation with downward pressure indicates a meniscus lesion. (Redrawn from Cailliet R. Knee pain and disability. Philadelphia: FA Davis, 1973, with permission.)

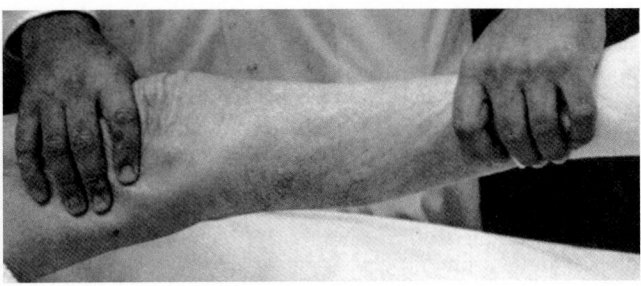

FIGURE 152.3. Testing for lateral instability of the knee by fixating the lower femur with one hand and forcibly abducting and adducting the joint while grasping the leg. (From Katz WA. Rheumatic diseases. Philadelphia: Lippincott, 1977, with permission.)

Examination for Meniscal Injury. The *joint-line tenderness test* and the *McMurray test* are performed to detect meniscal injury (Fig. 152.3). Joint-line tenderness has a sensitivity of 76% but a low specificity, 26%. The McMurray test is less sensitive (52%) but is very specific (97%).

Examination for Fracture. Patients who suffer any injury severe enough to fracture their knee are more likely to present to the emergency room than the primary physician's office, but on occasion they may present in the outpatient urgent-care setting. A key determination is need for further evaluation, especially imaging studies.

The Ottawa Decision Rule is the best-validated screening protocol for knee fracture and is used to distinguish those who need further evaluation from persons who can be followed expectantly. It is applied to persons presenting with acute knee pain associated with a fall or direct blow to the knee. Its four elements are as follows:

- Age greater than 55 years
- Isolated patellar tenderness or tenderness at the head of the fibula
- Inability to bear weight for four steps
- Inability to flex the knee more than 90 degrees

The presence of one or more of these features is associated with a very high test sensitivity for knee fracture (nearly 100%) but a very low specificity (25%). These performance characteristics make the rule particularly useful for triage but not for definitive diagnosis, which requires imaging.

Acute Joint Inflammation

Inflammation is confirmed by finding warmth, redness, swelling, and tenderness of the knee joint. The knee is examined for effusion by noting an increased knee circumference at midpatella and feeling for a distended, fluctuant capsule with a fluid wave and ballotable patella. Identifying an inflammatory knee effusion, especially one large enough to tap, provides an opportunity for potentially diagnostic joint fluid analysis (see later discussion).

When there is evidence of joint inflammation, an examination for extraarticular manifestations of inflammatory and infectious etiologies can facilitate diagnosis. Skin and integument are examined for rash, clubbing, psoriatic changes, rheumatoid nodules, pallor, alopecia, and tophi. The conjunctivae are noted for erythema and petechiae, the oral cavity for aphthous ulcers, lymph nodes for enlargement, the chest for signs of consolidation and effusion, the heart for murmurs and rubs, the abdomen for organomegaly and tenderness, the pelvis for vagi-

nal discharge and adnexal tenderness, the urethra for discharge, and the penis for balanitis. In addition, neurologic testing is indicated, particularly for meningeal signs.

When the area of inflammation and swelling localizes to the popliteal fossa, a ruptured Baker's cyst deserves consideration, as does popliteal vein thrombophlebitis, suggested by a palpable cord, tenderness along the vein, and swelling of the lower leg (see Chapter 22). Popliteal swelling in the absence of inflammation suggests a Baker's cyst but might also be a manifestation of a popliteal artery aneurysm, which requires examining for pulsatility and an audible bruit; the condition is associated with aortic aneurysm, which also needs to be checked for (see Chapter 58).

Suspected Osteoarthritis

Examination of the knee for degenerative disease should begin with inspection for distortion of normal contours and irregular bony prominences at the joint margin. It is important to note any crepitus on knee flexion, which is characteristic of degenerative disease. There should be no palpable warmth. The combination of focal bony tenderness, crepitus, bony enlargement, and no palpable warmth is associated with an 84% sensitivity and an 89% specificity; three characteristic findings raise the sensitivity to 95% but lower the specificity to about 70%. The predictive value of the combination of four physical findings is greater than 60%. When characteristic historical features (age >50 years, <30 minutes of morning stiffness) are included in consideration and two or fewer of these diagnostic findings are present, the predictive value falls to 2%.

The assessment of disease severity is facilitated by estimating the reduction in the range of motion. The knees normally extend symmetrically 180 degrees and may hyperextend an additional 5 to 10 degrees. Knee flexion is also symmetric and limited to 135 to 170 degrees by contact with posterior soft tissue or by striking of the heel against the buttock. Flexion may be limited by the presence of a cystic mass or swelling in the popliteal fossa of the osteoarthritic knee due to an unruptured Baker's cyst.

Bursitis

The bursal regions should be assessed for focal tenderness and swelling. There may be focal signs of inflammation but no joint effusion, distinguishing bursitis from other causes of knee inflammation. The finding of an angry, red, tensely swollen, very warm, very tender bursa is suggestive of a septic bursitis, especially if there is a break noted in the overlying skin.

Chondromalacia Patellae

When chondromalacia patellae is suspected, pain can be reproduced by applying pressure against the patella with the knee actively extended or by lateral displacement of the patella. Palpable grating can be elicited at the patellofemoral joint with flexion and extension of the knee.

Laboratory Studies

The key investigative questions facing the primary physician in the evaluation of knee pain are when to image and when to tap the knee. The answers to both questions depend on the clinical presentation and the associated pretest probabilities. In general, clinical evidence suggesting a cartilaginous or ligamentous problem (i.e., soft-tissue injury or internal derangement) is an indication for *MRI*, as is concern about osteonecrosis.

Plain films are indicated for suspected fracture and may add to the assessment of degenerative disease. *Computed tomography (CT)* provides additional sensitivity for the detection of subtle fractures that might be missed by plain films.

Suspected Meniscal or Ligamentous Tear

Persons with positive physical examination findings for meniscal or ligamentous tear are candidates for *MRI* of the knee. Test sensitivity ranges from 75% to 87% for ligamentous tears and from 80% to 90% for meniscal and cartilaginous tears. Specificity is in the low 90% range for all tears, except for a tear of the medial meniscus, in which case it is 80%. A positive MRI test confers at least an intermediate posttest probability. However, because of the frequency of noncontributory pathology on MRI and its lack of high specificity, some authorities recommend early orthopedic referral for confirmation of physical findings and determination of the need for additional testing (MRI or arthroscopy) rather than early MRI by the primary physician.

MRI is very expensive and should not be ordered when physical examination in persons with a negative physical examination can be followed expectantly. The test is best reserved for instances in which the clinical findings are equivocal and an invasive diagnostic procedure would otherwise be necessary. *Fiberoptic arthroscopy* is the gold standard for the diagnosis of problems in the soft tissues of the knee. Stress *plain films* are sometimes ordered to help in assessing the degree of joint stability.

Suspected Knee Fracture

Persons who meet the Ottawa criteria for knee fracture (see prior discussion) require plain films of the knee for confirmation because the decision rule's specificity for fracture is low. Reported test sensitivity of plain films ranges from 85% to 100% and specificity from 88% to 92%. Among persons who have negative knee films, options range from repeat study in 10 days if pain persists to progressing immediately to *CT scan* if clinical suspicion is high. CT can detect fractures too subtle to be seen by plain films.

Suspected Osteoarthritis

Plain films of the knee are often ordered to confirm degenerative joint disease (DJD) of the knees, but their effect on diagnosis is frequently meager. Criteria for radiologic diagnosis (sometimes referred to as the *Kellgren–Lawrence grading system*) include the presence of *osteophytes, joint-space narrowing, cystic changes* in subchondral bone, and *bony sclerosis*. Weight-bearing films are sometimes obtained to better demonstrate joint-space narrowing. These radiologic criteria have a sensitivity of 77% and a specificity of 83% for DJD of the knees. Comparing these performance characteristics with those for history and physical findings (see prior discussion) reveals that plain films correlate well with clinical findings but often add little to diagnosis in the presence of characteristic clinical features. Consequently, there is little reason to obtain them in this context. However, when only a few characteristic clinical features are present yet clinical suspicion of degenerative disease persists, the finding of osteophytes on plain films can increase the sensitivity to 91% and the specificity to 86%, making the combination of clinical features and plain films potentially useful in this setting. MRI adds little and should not be ordered if there are characteristic degenerative findings on plain films.

Plain films of the patella are of little use for early diagnosis of chondromalacia patellae because radiographic findings are normal until late stages, when the posterior surface of the patella becomes irregular and marginal osteophytes develop.

Suspected Inflammatory Disease

Arthrocentesis is indicated when there is a unilateral joint effusion, especially when it occurs in the context of other signs of inflammation. To differentiate between crystalline-induced disease and a septic process, joint fluid needs to be examined for crystals and sent for Gram's stain and cultures and determinations of white cell count, differential, and glucose concentration (see Chapter 145). Similar fluid aspiration and testing are indicated for a bursitis that appears to be septic. *Plain films* of the knee for soft-tissue calcification, a finding associated with pseudogout, are nonspecific and not sufficiently diagnostic to warrant radiologic study in this setting. With polyarticular presentations, *serologic studies* are often needed (see Chapter 146).

Inflammation concentrated in the posterior fossa suggests the differential diagnosis of a ruptured Baker's cyst versus thrombophlebitis. *Doppler ultrasound* study can usually differentiate between the two (see Chapter 22) and also helps to detect popliteal artery aneurysm, which might present as a pulsating popliteal fossa mass.

SYMPTOMATIC THERAPY AND INDICATIONS FOR REFERRAL (2,5,10–25)

Knee Sprain and Meniscal Tear

For the patient with a knee injury, acute pain responds best to a restriction of weight-bearing activities and the use of crutches. A *knee brace* is applied to provide support and prevent further injury by limiting the range of motion. Only absolutely necessary walking is allowed, and kneeling, squatting, and stair climbing are forbidden. *Aspirin* may be helpful symptomatically when used in pharmacologic doses of 2 to 4 g/d. Otherwise, any of the other nonsteroidal antiinflammatory drugs (NSAIDs) is a reasonable alternative (e.g., 375 mg of naproxen twice daily or 400 mg of ibuprofen three times daily). Once swelling subsides and the full range of motion without pain returns, rehabilitation can begin. One starts with isometric *quadriceps* and *hamstring exercises*. These help to prevent muscle atrophy, weakness, and thinning of ligamentous tissue. If the problem is one of acute severe injury and pain, especially if the knee gives way or locks and joint instability is evident, then prompt orthopedic referral is essential. Arthroscopy may be needed.

Osteoarthritis

Patients who have chronic knee pain associated with osteoarthritis have been shown to benefit from both *aerobic exercise* and *resistance exercise* in randomized trials. Quadriceps-strengthening exercises protect against new osteoarthritis in healthy knees, but a note of caution about quadriceps strengthening has emerged with regard to persons who have misaligned and lax knees. Such persons show an increased risk of progressive tibiofemoral degenerative changes when they undergo a program of quadriceps strengthening. A more customized program of exercises may be a better option, designed with the help of an experienced physical therapist. Exercise in pools—termed hydrotherapy—has been shown to be effective, as has Tai Chi.

Analgesics can be helpful in combination with an exercise program. *Acetaminophen* provides a moderate degree of pain relief equivalent to that achieved with *unselective NSAIDs* such as naproxen. *Cyclooxygenase-2 (COX-2) inhibitors* (e.g., celecoxib) are often preferred by patients because they are less upsetting to the gastrointestinal tract and, at full doses, slightly more effective than acetaminophen and lower doses of NSAIDs, but associated cardiovascular risks make their prolonged use problematic, especially in older patients (see Chapter 156).

Glucosamine, often in combination with *chondroitin sulfate*, is a popular "dietary supplement" for osteoarthritis of the knee. Well-designed, placebo-controlled trials find no overall benefit from either agent individually or the combination, with the exception of possible modest benefit in persons with moderate to severe disease (see Chapter 157). *Acupuncture* gives some relief to persons who are enthusiastic about the treatment. A meta-analysis of eight trials published through 2006 was notable for the heterogeneity of results and variable findings. Of the four largest trials, two showed significant but small effects on pain when acupuncture was compared to sham acupuncture, one showed large effects, and the fourth showed none. A subsequently published 2006 trial found that the addition of either acupuncture or sham acupuncture led to greater improvement of knee symptoms than physiotherapy and as-needed antiinflammatory drugs alone. However, a 2007 trial found no additional improvement to pain scores when acupuncture was added to advice and exercise.

Massage therapy was shown to be effective in one small randomized trial.

Arthroscopic surgery with debridement and lavage is no better than a placebo procedure. Incapacitating knee pain and end-stage joint dysfunction due to advanced degenerative disease are indications for consideration of *knee arthroplasty (replacement) surgery*. Patients who are willing and physically able to undergo joint replacement and the subsequent rehabilitation program are reasonable candidates for referral to the orthopedic surgeon. Underreferral of women has been noted, with many primary physicians not discussing the option with women who have incapacitating disease.

Chondromalacia Patellae

Symptomatic measures include acetaminophen or NSAIDs, ice, knee rest, and subsequent avoidance of knee overuse. Quadriceps-strengthening exercises are helpful. Surgery is a consideration in incapacitating cases.

Baker's Cyst

When the cyst is due to an inflammatory arthropathy, the treatment consists in injecting a long-acting corticosteroid preparation into the cyst and knee joint. When it is due to osteoarthritis or to internal knee derangement, surgical intervention to correct the underlying problem may be necessary.

Septic Arthritis or Bursitis

Septic arthritis is an indication for immediate hospitalization for intravenous antibiotic therapy. Septic bursitis should also be treated at least initially with intravenous antibiotics because an inadequately treated case can lead to serious complications.

Inflammatory Joint Disease

For initial symptomatic relief of pain and swelling due to a noninfectious etiology, NSAIDs (e.g., naproxen 500 mg twice daily) work well. However, more-etiologic, disease-modifying treatment may be required for definitive management (see Chapters 156 and 158 to 160).

Fracture

Fracture is an indication for immediate orthopedic referral.

A.H.G.

Annotated Bibliography

1. Jackson JL, O'Malley PG, Kroenke K. Evaluation of acute knee pain in primary care. Ann Intern Med 2003;139:575. (*An outstanding systematic review, providing much of the synthesized test performance data and the diagnostic approach recommended in this chapter; 217 references.*)
2. Paty JG. Diagnosis and treatment of musculoskeletal running injuries. Semin Arthritis Rheum 1988;18:48. (*A good description of overuse syndromes.*)
3. Rejeski WJ, Ettinger WH, Shumaker S, et al. The evaluation of pain in patients with knee osteoarthritis: the knee pain scale. J Rheumatol 1995;22:1124. (*Addresses the intensity of knee pain associated with six activities of daily living to obtain a summary pain intensity score.*)
4. Spector T, Harris PA, Hart DJ, et al. Risk of osteoarthritis associated with long-term weight-bearing sports. Arthritis Rheum 1996;39:988. (*Supports the hypothesis that long-term, high-intensity exercise increases risk.*)
5. Zarins B, Adams M. Knee injuries in sports. N Engl J Med 1988;318:950. (*An authoritative review, with a particularly good discussion of anterior cruciate tear and resulting meniscal injury.*)
6. Claessens AA, Schouten JS, van den Ouweland FA, et al. Do clinical findings associate with radiographic osteoarthritis of the knee? Ann Rheum Dis 1990;49:771. (*Finds good correlation between Kellgren–Lawrence grading and clinical findings.*)
7. Gelb HJ, Glasgow SG, Sapega AA, et al. Magnetic resonance imaging of knee disorders: clinical value and cost effectiveness in a sports medicine practice. Am J Sports Med 1996;24:99. (*Finds little value to the test if the clinical examination is negative for ligamentous or meniscal injury.*)
8. Koplas M, Schils J, Sundaram M. The painful knee: choosing the right imaging test. Cleve Clinic J Med 2008;75:377. (*A succinct summary for the nonspecialist.*)
9. Steill IG, Greenberg GH, Wells GA, et al. Prospective validation of a decision rule for the use of radiographs in acute knee injuries. JAMA 1996;275:611. (*Confirms the validity of the rule for imaging the knee in the setting of acute injury.*)
10. Berman, B. A 60-year-old woman considering acupuncture for knee pain. JAMA 2007;297:1697. (*A helpful review based on a case study.*)
11. Berman BM, Lao L, Langenberg P, et al. Effectiveness of acupuncture as adjunctive therapy in osteoarthritis of the knee: a randomized controlled trial. Ann Intern Med 2004;141:901. (*The procedure was modestly beneficial, but only when applied to an enthusiastic person by an enthusiastic practitioner.*)
12. Scharf HP, Mansmann U, Streitberger K, et al. Acupuncture and knee osteoarthritis. Ann Intern Med 2006;145:12. (*The addition of either acupuncture or sham acupuncture led to greater improvement than physiotherapy and as-needed antiinflammatory treatment.*)
13. Foster NE, Thomas E, Barlas P, et al. Acupuncture as an adjunct to exercise based physiotherapy for osteoarthritis of the knee: randomised controlled trial. BMJ 2007;335:436. (*Acupuncture produced no additional improvement in pain scores.*)

14. Bradley JD, Brandt KD, Katz BP, et al. Comparison of an antiinflamma-
    tory dose of ibuprofen, an analgesic dose of ibuprofen, and acetaminophen
    in the treatment of patients with osteoarthritis of the knee. N Engl J Med
    1991;325:87. (*Pure analgesic therapy was as effective as nonsteroidal anti-
    inflammatory drugs.*)
15. Clegg DO, Reda D, Harris CL, et al. Glucosamine, chondroitin sulfate, and
    the two in combination for painful knee osteoarthritis. N Engl J Med 2006;
    354:795. (*A major randomized, controlled trial [RCT], finding that, overall,
    there was no benefit of these agents alone or in combination, but there was
    a suggestion of modest benefit in persons with moderate to severe pain.*)
16. Reichenbach S, Sterchi R, Scherer M, et al. Meta-analysis: chondroitin for
    osteoarthritis of the knee or hip. Ann Intern Med 2007;l46;580. (*A meta-
    analysis, finding minimal or no effect.*)
17. Ettinger WH, Burns R, Messier SP, et al. A randomized trial comparing
    aerobic exercise and resistance exercise with a health education program in
    older adults with knee osteoarthritis. JAMA 1997;227:25. (*Aerobic exercise
    and resistance exercise were responsible for 10% and 8% improvement in
    symptoms, respectively.*)
18. Fransen M, Nairn L, Winstanley J, et al. Physical activity for osteoarthri-
    tis management: a randomized controlled trial evaluating hydrotherapy or
    Tai Chi classes. Arthritis Rheum 2007;57:407. (*RCT, finding that access to
    either hydrotherapy or Tai Chi was associated with large and sustained im-
    provement.*)
19. Perlman AI, Sabina A, Williams AL, et al. Massage therapy for osteoarthritis
    of the knee. Arch Intern Med 2006;166:2533. (*A trial of 68 patients, finding
    that this approach seemed to help.*)
20. Hawker GA, Wright JG, Coyte PC, et al. Differences between men and
    women in the rate of use of hip and knee arthroplasty. N Engl J Med
    2000;342:1016. (*An epidemiologic study, finding that women were under-
    referred.*)
21. Hochberg MC, Altman RD, Brandt KD, et al. Guidelines for the med-
    ical management of knee osteoarthritis. Arthritis Rheum 1995;38:1541.
    (*Presents comprehensive advice for the medical approach to minimizing dis-
    ability.*)
22. Kovar PA, Allegrante JP, MacKenzie CR, et al. Supervised fitness walking
    in patients with osteoarthritis of the knee. Ann Intern Med 1992;116:529.
    (*Pain and disability decreased and fitness increased.*)
23. Manheimer E, Linde K, Lao L, et al. Meta-analysis: acupuncture for os-
    teoarthritis of the knee. Ann Intern Med 2007;146:868. (*No benefit overall
    was found in placebo-controlled trials, but much placebo and expectation
    benefit was noted.*)
24. Moseley JB, O'Malley K, Petersen NJ, et al. A controlled trial of arthroscopic
    surgery for osteoarthritis of the knee. N Engl J Med 2002;347:81. (*Lavage
    and debridement were no better than placebo procedure.*)
25. Sharma L, Dunlop DD, Cahue S, et al. Quadriceps strength and osteoarthri-
    tis progression in malaligned and lax knees. Ann Intern Med 2003;138:613.
    (*Finds that quadriceps strengthening can increase disease progression in
    poorly aligned knees.*)

CHAPTER 153 ■ APPROACH TO MINOR ORTHOPEDIC PROBLEMS OF THE ELBOW, WRIST, AND HAND

JESSE B. JUPITER AND DAVID RING

As the physician of first contact, the primary care practitioner
encounters a host of elbow and distal upper extremity complaints, including pain, numbness, stiffness, a new nodule, and
swelling. The majority represent common disorders that lend
themselves to diagnosis and initial treatment by the primary
care physician. Vague, diffuse complaints of pain (often activity related) can be more difficult to diagnose and treat; the help
of the orthopedic specialist may be beneficial.

ELBOW (1–3)

Lateral Elbow Pain (Lateral Epicondylitis/"Tennis Elbow")

This term denotes pain at the origin of the extensor carpi ra-
dialis brevis (ECRB) on the lateral epicondyle of the distal
humerus. The term tennis elbow is misleading, in that there is
no evidence that playing tennis causes this disorder. The term
lateral epicondylitis is also inaccurate because pathologic specimens from operated patients have not shown any evidence of
inflammation—the histologic analyses seem to reflect a degenerative rather than an inflammatory process. It may be best to
refer to this entity as lateral elbow pain. It is one of the many
tendinoses—in this case an enesthopathy—that appear in middle age.

Lateral elbow pain has often been blamed on repetitive use
of the arm, but there is no evidence to support this contention.
Like most musculoskeletal conditions, the cause is unknown,
and the common conceptions about the illness are largely without substantiation. What is established is that the condition
is age related and seen almost exclusively in middle-aged
patients (ages 35 to 55 years). It is self-limited and usually
resolves within 6 to 12 months. Unlike other degenerative
processes such as arthritis, it is not progressive. Among the
myriad treatments that have been used for this disease, there is
meager evidence that any of them affect the natural history of
the condition, which is eventual resolution. It is not dangerous;
the worst thing that can happen as a result of this disease
process is complete detachment of the tendon origin from the
humerus, which is uncommon and does not appreciably alter
function of the elbow or wrist.

Diagnosis

The diagnosis of lateral epicondylitis or lateral elbow pain is
established by history and confirmed on examination. Patients
complain of pain over the outside of the elbow that is worse
with actions that use the wrist extensors (pouring milk, lifting

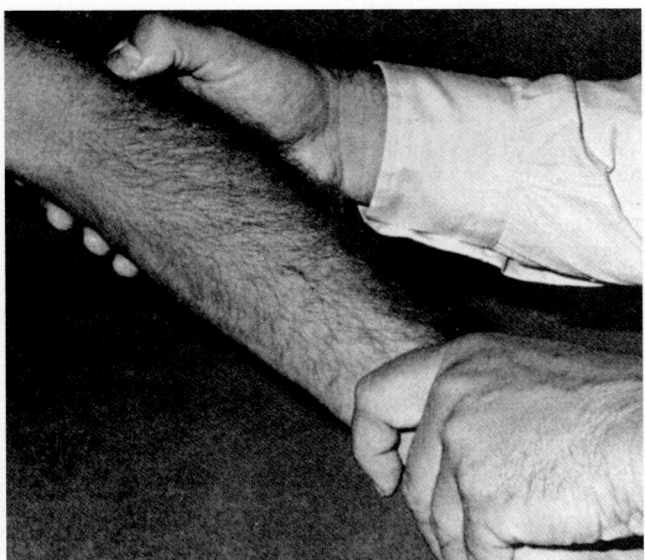

FIGURE 153.1. Technique of palpating the lateral epicondyle to elicit "point" tenderness, typical of "tennis elbow." (From Katz WA. Rheumatic diseases. Philadelphia: JB Lippincott, 1977, with permission.)

objects with the palm facing downwards, playing tennis, etc.) and that can be isolated to a point of maximal tenderness over the lateral epicondyle (Fig. 153.1). If the pain is more diffuse, not associated with specific activities, and cannot be isolated to this point, then this diagnosis should be withheld. Some surgeons have suggested the concept of a radial nerve entrapment (radial tunnel syndrome) in this circumstance, but this is controversial and we do not recommend the use of this diagnosis in a primary care setting. If the patient is between 35 and 55 years of age and has atraumatic lateral elbow pain, it is almost certainly lateral epicondylitis.

Examination discloses normal motion, maximal tenderness over the origin of the ECRB at the point of the lateral epicondyle, pain with passive wrist flexion and resisted wrist extension with the elbow extended, and a positive chair lift test (pain reproduced by lifting a chair with the palm down, but not with the palm up). There is no swelling, although patients often perceive that there is. Radiographs and other imaging are not necessary when the history and exam are characteristic and there is no history of trauma—occasionally they will show some calcification in the ECRB origin.

Management

Basic management techniques have included *antiinflammatory medications* and passive stretching and isometric strengthening of the ECRB and other radial wrist extensors. *Forearm bands* and *wrist splints* make some patients feel better and others feel worse. Doctors often recommend avoidance of any painful activity (e.g., racquet sports, handshake, forceful use of the arm in hammering or unscrewing jars, use of a screwdriver), but there is no evidence that this speeds the resolution of the disease. All of these measures are useful only to the extent that they relieve symptoms—there is no evidence that they affect the disease process. Patients should be advised that all treatments are discretionary, that active use of the arm is reasonable even with pain, and that the eventual resolution without consequence is expected regardless of the treatment and activity level.

Local *steroid injections* are commonly used, but this is probably more because patients want something done and doctors have nothing else to offer. Randomized trials suggest that steroid injection does not have an appreciable effect on lateral elbow pain. There is a risk of skin discoloration and atrophy of the subcutaneous tissues with steroid injection. Repeat injections are not advisable. The area of maximal tenderness is injected. Therapist offer corticosteroids delivered through the skin using iontophoresis among other "modalities." Many other treatments are offered (e.g., *shock wave therapy*) without established effectiveness. Randomized trials have not consistently demonstrated benefit of any treatment over the natural history of lateral elbow pain.

The abundance of these various interventions and their wide use in spite of a lack of evidence in support of their efficacy reflect the frustrating nature of this disease and the fact that patients are loathe to go without active treatment. Nonetheless, this is a relatively good diagnosis to have because it is not dangerous; it is just a nuisance that will eventually resolve.

Medial Epicondylitis ("Golfer's Elbow")

This condition is identical to lateral epicondylitis but involves the common forearm flexor origin at the humeral medial epicondyle. It is much less common. The pain is localized to the region of the medial epicondyle and is reproduced by forcefully extending the elbow against resistance with the forearm in supination and the wrist in dorsiflexion. Treatment is similar to that for lateral epicondylitis. Steroid injection in this area risks injection into the ulnar nerve—a potentially serious problem. The possibility of an ulnar nerve entrapment (cubital tunnel syndrome) should be considered.

Olecranon Bursitis

Patients who present with a swollen olecranon bursa have either chronic olecranon bursitis or septic olecranon bursitis. The latter will be obvious by virtue of the pain, redness, and warmth. In some cases of infection, there is an extensive cellulitis by the time the diagnosis is made, which may obscure the underlying bursitis. Almost all cases of septic olecranon represent spread from a contiguous soft-tissue infection or laceration. The causative organism is nearly always *Staphylococcus aureus*, and empirical antibiotic treatment is usually administered—parenteral (e.g., *cefazolin*) for severe infections and oral (e.g., *cephalexin*) for milder infections. Aspiration is reserved for severe infections, infirm or immunosuppressed patients, or infections that do not respond to empirical therapy. On rare occasions, operative débridement may be required.

If the swelling of the bursa is not associated with redness or warmth, presents with only mild discomfort, and is insidious in onset, the diagnosis is chronic olecranon bursitis. Chronic olecranon bursitis has been associated with frequent pressure on this area (e.g., chess players, draftsmen) or repetitive flexion activities, but most cases are idiopathic. On occasion the bursitis is related to an inflammatory condition such as rheumatoid arthritis or gout.

There is a longstanding tradition of avoiding aspiration or corticosteroid injection because of the possibility of introducing infection and the risk of a chronic fistula. These risks may be overstated; however, treatment with aspiration and injection is rarely curative, and chronic olecranon bursitis typically waxes and wanes chronically. The use of nonsteroidal antiinflammatory drugs (NSAIDs), ice, or compressive wrapping and the limitation of repetitive flexion and avoidance of pressure on the olecranon can help to limit swelling, but the condition is not dangerous, and none of these treatments is necessary. Surgery is considered rarely.

Nerve Entrapment Syndromes

Pain in the elbow or forearm may be secondary to compression of the ulnar nerve in the cubital tunnel. Numbness in the hand is typically the most prominent complaint—patients who complain primarily of pain are unlikely to have cubital tunnel syndrome. Entrapment neuropathies of the radial and median nerves (supinator or radial tunnel, and pronator syndromes, respectively) have been described as an occasional cause of elbow and proximal forearm pain, but these diagnoses are extremely controversial and should not be made by the primary care doctor.

With ulnar nerve compression, the typical complaint is of numbness in the small and ring fingers that wakes the patient at night and is present in the morning. During the day, bent elbow activities such as reading a book in bed are characteristic. Pain at the medial epicondyle is a minor complaint, and there may be tenderness beneath the medial epicondyle. *Tinel's sign of the elbow* (paresthesias into the small and ring fingers with tapping on the ulnar nerve at the elbow) and the *elbow flexion test* (elicitation of paresthesias with the elbow in a flexed position) are also useful. A nighttime splint that holds the elbow in relative extension (about 40 degrees of flexion) may improve sleep, but in practice the splint is often more disturbing than the numbness. If entrapment is accompanied by muscle atrophy or does not respond to simple measures, referral is required.

Septic Arthritis

Most cases of septic arthritis are the result of blood-borne infection, manifested by the rapid onset of pain, diffuse joint swelling, and erythema. Systemic symptoms are common. Septic arthritis is more common in patients with underlying conditions such as diabetes mellitus, steroid treatment, or rheumatoid arthritis. If sepsis is suspected, arthrocentesis for Gram's stain and culture of the joint fluid is required (see Chapter 145). The differential diagnosis of an acute monoarthritis includes gout and pseudogout (calcium pyrophosphate deposition), both of which can be difficult to distinguish from infection before aspiration and fluid analysis have been performed. Treatment of confirmed infection includes operative débridement and intravenous administration of organism-specific antibiotics.

Osteoarthritis

The elbow is not a common site for osteoarthritis, but arthritis may be found in association with prior fracture or dislocation. In contrast, elbow involvement is common in rheumatoid arthritis. On examination, limitation of motion, swelling, and pain are common findings. Radiographs demonstrate the extent of joint space involvement. Antiinflammatory agents provide some relief (see Chapter 156).

HAND AND WRIST (2,4–15)

Carpal Tunnel Syndrome

The primary complaint in carpal tunnel syndrome is numbness and not pain. Contrary to popular associations with computer use and repetitive activities, the cause of carpal tunnel is unknown. There is a strong genetic predisposition, and the condition is typically bilateral, although it may present in one limb decades before it presents in the other.

Diagnosis

Typically, the patient reports nocturnal symptoms, primarily numbness in the distribution of the median nerve (thumb, index finger, long finger, and radial half of the ring finger), which may be accompanied by discomfort and is relieved by shaking the hand. Thenar (base of the thumb) muscle atrophy is present in prolonged or profound median nerve compression, as is weakness of palmar abduction (pointing the thumb toward the ceiling with the palm turned up). *Tinel's sign*, elicited by tapping over the median nerve at the wrist crease, consists in "electric shocks" or paresthesias in the median nerve distribution. *Phelan's test* is performed by having the patient maintain the wrists in palmar flexion for 1 minute. *Durkan's test* is performed by pressing both thumbs over the transverse carpal ligament. The test result is considered positive and consistent with carpal tunnel syndrome if the patient's symptoms are reproduced. A negative result of Phelan's or Durkan's test or the absence of Tinel's sign does not necessarily rule out the presence of carpal tunnel syndrome.

Definitive diagnosis can be made by *nerve conduction study* and *electromyography* (EMG). Testing is indicated if the diagnosis is unclear, if nonoperative treatment does not relieve symptoms adequately, or if numbness or weakness appears. In a patient with carpal tunnel syndrome, EMG demonstrates an increase in motor or sensory latency, which is helpful in documenting the location and degree of nerve compression. Correlating the clinical findings with the neurophysiologic test results is necessary for an accurate diagnosis because as many as 50% of asymptomatic patients may have abnormal results on nerve conduction or EMG studies. Some surgeons believe that the diagnosis of carpal tunnel syndrome may be appropriate even when the EMG is normal, but this is controversial. At best this would represent very, very mild carpal tunnel syndrome that would be managed nonoperatively, and at worst a patient given the diagnosis of neurophysiologically normal carpal tunnel syndrome would receive unnecessary surgery. There is no evidence that surgery in this setting offers anything other than a placebo effect.

Management

The first line of treatment is *wrist splinting*—particularly to control night symptoms. Some suggest *steroid injections*, but these provide temporary relief at best, and injection of the median nerve must be avoided. It is most useful in patients with a significant flexor tenosynovitis (0.5 to 1 mL of dexamethasone plus 1 to 2 mL of lidocaine are used). The injection is placed just proximal to the transverse retinacular ligament in the wrist. If a paresthesia is elicited, a more superficial needle placement is made to avoid injecting into the nerve. The concept that response to steroid injection predicts response to surgery is overstated.

Surgical intervention is considered if symptoms are not controlled by splinting, if an associated thenar muscle atrophy or weakness develops, or if the motor or sensory latencies on the EMG and nerve conduction studies are extremely prolonged. A randomized, controlled trial has demonstrated that in persons with idiopathic, moderately severe disease, open surgical carpal tunnel release is superior to splinting over the long term. Predictors of a poor outcome with conservative therapy alone include age older than 50 years, presence of symptoms for longer than 10 months, constant paresthesias, triggering of flexor tendons, and positive Phalen test in less than 30 seconds. This merely reflects the inherent, progressive nature of carpal tunnel syndrome. Patients with idiopathic carpal tunnel syndrome are likely eventually to require carpal tunnel release to prevent loss of sensation and weakness of palmar abduction, although the disease typically progresses very slowly.

De Quervain's Tenosynovitis

On the dorsal aspect of the wrist, the extensor tendons to the hand and wrist course through six well-defined compartments. The first dorsal compartment contains the abductor pollicis longus and the extensor pollicis brevis and is located just proximal and radial to the anatomic "snuff box." The most common form of tendonitis at the wrist level is a nonspecific subacute or chronic inflammation of the tendons within the first dorsal compartment, or de Quervain's tenosynovitis. Pain is exacerbated by use of the thumb and is reproduced when the patient, with the wrist in ulnar deviation and palmar flexion, grasps the thumb with the adjacent digits (commonly referred to as Finkelstein's test). This test differentiates tendinitis from any underlying arthritis. The cause is unknown. It is common in new mothers within a few weeks of delivery.

As with lateral epicondylitis, the disease is self-limiting, but it tends to last for 6 to 12 months in spite of treatment. A long opponens (thumb spica) splint and oral NSAIDs will provide relief of pain. There is dispute over the effectiveness of *steroid injections*, and no controlled trials have been performed. An injection preparation such as that described for carpal tunnel syndrome is carefully placed within the first dorsal extensor compartment, which has a somewhat more radial and volar location than one might think. Surgery is not necessary but is the only known method for shortening the duration of symptoms.

Trigger Finger

Tenosynovitis also commonly involves the flexor tendons to the digits or thumb at the level of the metacarpophalangeal joints just proximal to the first annular pulley of the flexor tendon sheath. Snapping of the digit (triggering) with use and locking, or the inability to extend the proximal interphalangeal joint, are the characteristic presenting symptoms. Often, the patient perceives the triggering to be at the level of the proximal interphalangeal joint. A palpable thickening of the flexor tendon may be felt at the level of the metacarpophalangeal joint in the palm.

One or two *corticosteroid injections* will cure about 50% of trigger fingers; in the remainder of cases the patients are offered surgery. The steroid–lidocaine combination is injected just distal to the distal palmar crease, where the first annular pulley of the flexor sheath is located. The skin-related complications of steroid injections at the wrist and elbow are uncommon in the thick, glabrous skin of the hand.

Ganglion Cysts

Ganglionic cysts are the most common masses occurring in the hand or wrist and may be found in a number of sites, including the dorsum of the wrist, where the origin is the scapholunate interval. Another common location is on the radial volar surface of the wrist directly adjacent to (and not to be confused with) the radial artery. Ganglia are thought to be outpouchings of the wrist capsule and contain fluid very similar to joint fluid. Their origin (stalk) is in the wrist joint, which explains the high incidence of recurrence when treatment methods such as aspiration or the traditional home remedy of striking the cyst with a heavy object (e.g., a Bible!) are used.

Most ganglia require no treatment. *Aspiration* with a large-bore (16- or 19-gauge) needle is helpful if the diagnosis is in doubt; however, even with *steroid injection*, the recurrence rate is high. *Surgical treatment* is indicated if the cyst is painful, the appearance is unsatisfactory, or the exact nature of the mass is a concern.

Mucous Cysts

Mucous cysts, associated with degenerative arthritis of the interphalangeal joints of the digits or thumb, are outpouchings of joint fluid similar to wrist ganglia. Radiographs show joint space narrowing and, often, marginal spurs or osteophytes. Osteophytes alone are the cause of the so-called Heberden's node at the distal interphalangeal joint and Bouchard's node at the proximal interphalangeal joint. Mucous cysts are resistant to aspiration and often recur after operative resection. They occasionally become infected.

Arthritis

Degenerative joint disease commonly affects the carpometacarpal joint at the base of the thumb (see Chapter 157). Most often affecting women, the condition is associated with localized pain, decreased dexterity, and diminished grip strength. Pain and crepitus can be elicited if the examiner grasps the thumb metacarpal and compresses it onto the trapezium (grind test). Radiographic changes may vary from mild joint space narrowing to complete joint space loss and the presence of osteophytes and loose bodies.

Once recognized, mild to moderate arthritis of the trapeziometacarpal joint of the thumb can be effectively managed with *NSAIDs* and a *molded splint* worn 4 to 6 hours daily. The splint extends beyond the metacarpophalangeal joint but leaves the wrist free (a short opponens splint). It should be custom made by a trained occupational therapist.

The hand involvement in *rheumatoid arthritis* can vary from minimal pain and swelling to extensive deformity and joint destruction. Treatment includes pharmacologic and physical therapy (see Chapter 156). Tendon rupture is not uncommon; its occurrence should prompt early referral.

Hand Infections

Hand infections are potentially serious conditions, especially if they occur in a closed compartment. Presentations vary. Infection around the fingernail is termed *paronychia* and is usually caused by gram-positive organisms. Antibiotics and warm soaks suffice in mild, well-localized cases, but any spread requires referral for incision and drainage. A *felon* is a more worrisome problem because it is an infection in a closed compartment, the pulp space of the tip of the digit. The pulp is swollen, exquisitely tender, and erythematous. If not corrected, the edema can compromise arterial supply and lead to necrosis of the fingertip. Treatment includes incision, drainage, and administration of antibiotics. Early referral to a hand surgeon is essential for definitive treatment. A less troublesome infection, seen mostly in hospital personnel and children, is *herpetic infection* of the fingertip, which is characterized by the appearance of small vesicles along the pulp. It clears spontaneously, although the patient is infectious until the vesicles clear.

In *infectious flexor tenosynovitis,* the patient presents with a digit that is symmetrically swollen, painful along the entire flexor sheath, flexed, and tender on passive extension of the distal joint. Prompt recognition and, in many cases, surgical intervention are critical to preserve ultimate tendon function.

Puncture wounds, in particular human bites, may result in extremely virulent infection. Prompt and aggressive wound care, with the puncture site left open, and antibiotic treatment may abort a more serious and destructive process. Animal bites, especially from dogs and cats, can transmit *Pasteurella multocida,* which in most instances is extremely sensitive to penicillin (see Chapter 196.1).

Dupuytren's Contracture

This condition is characterized by thickening and nodularity of the palmar fascia. The overlying skin also may be invaded by proliferating fibroblasts, but other tissues and structures of the hand are spared. Flexure contraction deformities may ensue, particularly of the fourth finger. There is a genetic predisposition, and cases in men outnumber those in women by about 5:1. Smoking, alcohol abuse, and diabetes increase risk. Those with a positive family history have an earlier onset and involvement of other sites, such as the plantar fascia of the feet and Buck fascia of the penis.

Treatment is expectant; nonsurgical measures such as stretching are without benefit; local injection of collagenase appears promising for select cases. Surgery is indicated when the disease causes more than 30 degrees of contraction of the metacarpophalangeal joint or 15 degrees of fixed flexion of the proximal interphalangeal joint.

NONSPECIFIC OR IDIOPATHIC ARM PAIN

When complaints are vague and diffuse and there are no objective abnormalities, it is important not to mislabel the problem. In the absence of objective findings that imply specific pathology, it is better to admit puzzlement, reassure the patient that worrisome conditions have been ruled out (including coronary ischemia, cervical radiculopathy, polymyalgia rheumatica, shoulder tendonitis), and use a nonspecific diagnosis. Unsubstantiated use of such diagnostic labels as "repetitive strain injury," "fibromyalgia," "tendonitis," "carpal tunnel syndrome," and "thoracic outlet syndrome" may lead to unnecessary limitations of activity and inappropriate interventions. Keeping an open mind as to other sources of pain, following the patient closely for new findings, and providing psychological support (especially when a psychosocial precipitant is suspected) are very important components of care in this context. Ordering diagnostic tests in the absence of a reasonable pretest probability for a specific condition is likely further to confuse the situation because of the high risk of generating false-positive results (see Chapter 2). There is growing evidence that nonspecific arm pains are associated with heightened illness concern and ineffective copings skills and may represent a type of somatoform disorder.

Annotated Bibliography

1. Bernhang AM. The many causes of tennis elbow. N Y State J Med 1979;79:1363. (*A classic overview of the subject.*)
2. Biundo JJ Jr. Regional rheumatic pain syndromes. In: Schumacher HR Jr, ed. Primer on the rheumatic diseases, 9th ed. Atlanta, GA: Arthritis Foundation, 1988:263. (*An excellent source for clinical presentations, workup, and basic symptomatic management.*)
3. Roschmann RA, Bell CL. Septic arthritis in immunocompromised patients. Am J Med 1987;83:861. (*A good description of clinical findings; presentation is similar to that in immunocompetent patients.*)
4. Boyer MI, Hastings H 2nd. Lateral tennis elbow: "Is there any science out there?" J Shoulder Elbow Surg 1999;8:481. (*An excellent review of the current science—or lack thereof—regarding lateral elbow pain.*)
5. Anderson B, Kaye S. Treatment of flexor tenosynovitis of the hand ("trigger finger") with corticosteroids. Arch Intern Med 1991;151:153. (*A prospective study; the treatment was found to be safe and effective.*)
6. Atcheson SG, Ward JR, Lowe W. Concurrent medical disease in work-related carpal tunnel syndrome. Arch Intern Med 1998;158:1506. (*A high prevalence of underlying medical disease was found.*)
7. Atroshi I, Gummesson C, Johnsson R, et al. Prevalence of carpal tunnel syndrome in a general population. JAMA 1999;282:153. (*A large-scale epidemiologic study; the prevalence as high, and the condition was likely to be diagnosed in one in five symptomatic subjects after full evaluation.*)
8. Gerritsen AAM, de Vet HCW, Scholten JPM, et al. Splinting vs surgery in the treatment of carpal tunnel syndrome: a randomized controlled trial. JAMA 2002;288:1245. (*A well-designed study showing that surgery was superior to splinting over the long term, reflecting the effect of disease progression.*)
9. Hunt TR III. What is the appropriate treatment for Dupuytren contracture? Cleve Clin J Med 2003;70:96. (*A succinct, pathophysiologically based summary for the primary physician.*)
10. Katz JN, Lew RA, Bessette L, et al. Prevalence and predictors of long-term disability due to carpal tunnel syndrome. Am J Ind Med 1998;33:543. (*Present useful data applicable in determining who is at risk for long-term disability.*)
11. Katz JN, Simmons BP. Carpal tunnel syndrome. N Engl J Med. 2002;346:1807. (*A very useful clinical review; 49 references.*)
12. Katz JN, Larson MG, Sabra A, et al. The carpal tunnel syndrome: diagnostic utility of the history and physical examination findings. Ann Intern Med 1990;112:321. (*Analyzes the sensitivities and specificities for history and physical examination.*)
13. Katz JN, Stirrat CR, Larson MG, et al. A self-administered hand symptom diagram for the diagnosis and epidemiologic study of carpal tunnel syndrome. J Rheumatol 1990;17:1495. (*The approach has a sensitivity of 64% and a specificity of 73%.*)
14. Hakim AJ, Cherkas L, El Zayat S, et al. The genetic contribution to carpal tunnel syndrome in women: a twin study. Arthritis Rheum 2002;47:275. (*Genetics explained half of the cases of carpal tunnel syndrome where no important environmental factors were identified.*)
15. Murrell GAC. Basic science of Dupuytren's disease. Ann Hand Surg 1992;11:355. (*A good review of mechanisms of the disease.*)

CHAPTER 154 ■ APPROACH TO COMMON PROBLEMS OF THE FOOT AND ANKLE

CHRISTOPHER P. CHIODO, JESSE B. JUPITER, AND DAVID RING

Primary physicians are often consulted for advice and help regarding problems of the foot and ankle, which are extremely prevalent and can be incapacitating. Although some patients require orthopedic referral for more detailed investigation and treatment, many can be cared for by the nonspecialist physician who is knowledgeable about the diagnosis and treatment of common foot and ankle disorders and the indications for referral.

FOOT PROBLEMS (1–7)

Disorders of the foot are a major cause of frustration and disability. Although often idiopathic or the result of normal activity, foot pain can also be precipitated by structural deformity or systemic disease. Environmental factors, such as shoe type and weight-bearing surface, can also lead to the development and progression of symptoms.

The human foot has 26 bones, comprising one fourth of those in the entire skeleton, along with 100 or more ligaments, 12 extrinsic muscle insertions, and 19 intrinsic muscles. During gait, more than two times the force of body weight is borne by the foot. In normal gait, the foot assumes several roles, including that of a shock absorber, a mobile adapter to accommodate uneven surfaces, and a rigid lever to propel the limb. Limitation or excess of these primary functions places the foot at risk for acquired mechanical trauma. Classification by anatomic region (Table 154.1) helps to guide assessment. Office assessment is facilitated by familiarity with the location and manifestations of common foot problems (Fig. 154.1).

Toe and Forefoot Problems— Painful Toe Deformities

Toe Deformities—Corns

Disorders of the toes are usually related to deformities, most commonly *hammer toes*, *mallet toes*, and *claw toes*. Pain with or without development of a *corn* (clavus) is usually the primary complaint. Toe contractures develop secondary to compensatory muscle imbalances that result from years of wearing inappropriate shoes and/or from inherited foot abnormalities. The contractures can be flexible or become rigid. Wearing shoes, either prescription or commercial, that provide adequate room in the toe box is the first line of treatment. If the contractures are flexible, over-the-counter splints and pads may be helpful. In persistent or progressive disease, corrective surgery may be necessary if pain compromises daily activity.

Disorders of the First Metatarsophalangeal Joint

The most prevalent disorder of the first metatarsophalangeal (MTP) joint is a *hallux valgus* deformity, or *bunion*. Hallus rigidus can also be a problem.

Hallux Valgus—Bunions. These usually present as painful swelling on the dorsomedial aspect of the first metatarsal head, associated with lateral angulation of the great toe. Although the deformity or difficulty with shoes may be the presenting complaint, patients frequently present with secondary problems, such as hammer toes or pain underneath the other metatarsal heads (*metatarsalgia*). Narrow shoes, hindfoot malalignment (pronation), and heredity are all believed to contribute, particularly in women. The deformity is also seen in patients with rheumatoid arthritis and other inflammatory arthropathies.

On physical examination, there is tenderness over the inner side of the first metatarsal head; an inflamed bursa may also be present. The great toe is angulated laterally, and at times

TABLE 154.1

COMMON CAUSES OF FOOT PAIN

Digital Deformities
Hammer toe
Claw toe
Mallet toe

Forefoot Pain—Great Toe
Hallux valgus (bunion)
Hallux limitus/rigidus
Sesamoid disorders

Forefoot Pain—Other Structures
Tailor's bunion (bunionette)
Metatarsalgia
Morton's interdigital neuroma
Metatarsal stress fracture

Hindfoot Pain—Plantar
Plantar fasciitis
Infracalcaneal bursitis
Medial calcaneal nerve entrapment
Tarsal tunnel syndrome
Referred pain from subtalar arthritis or lumbosacral disk radiculopathy

Hindfoot Pain—Posterior
Posterior calcaneal bursitis
Exostosis ("pump bump")
Achilles tendinitis
Inflammatory arthritis

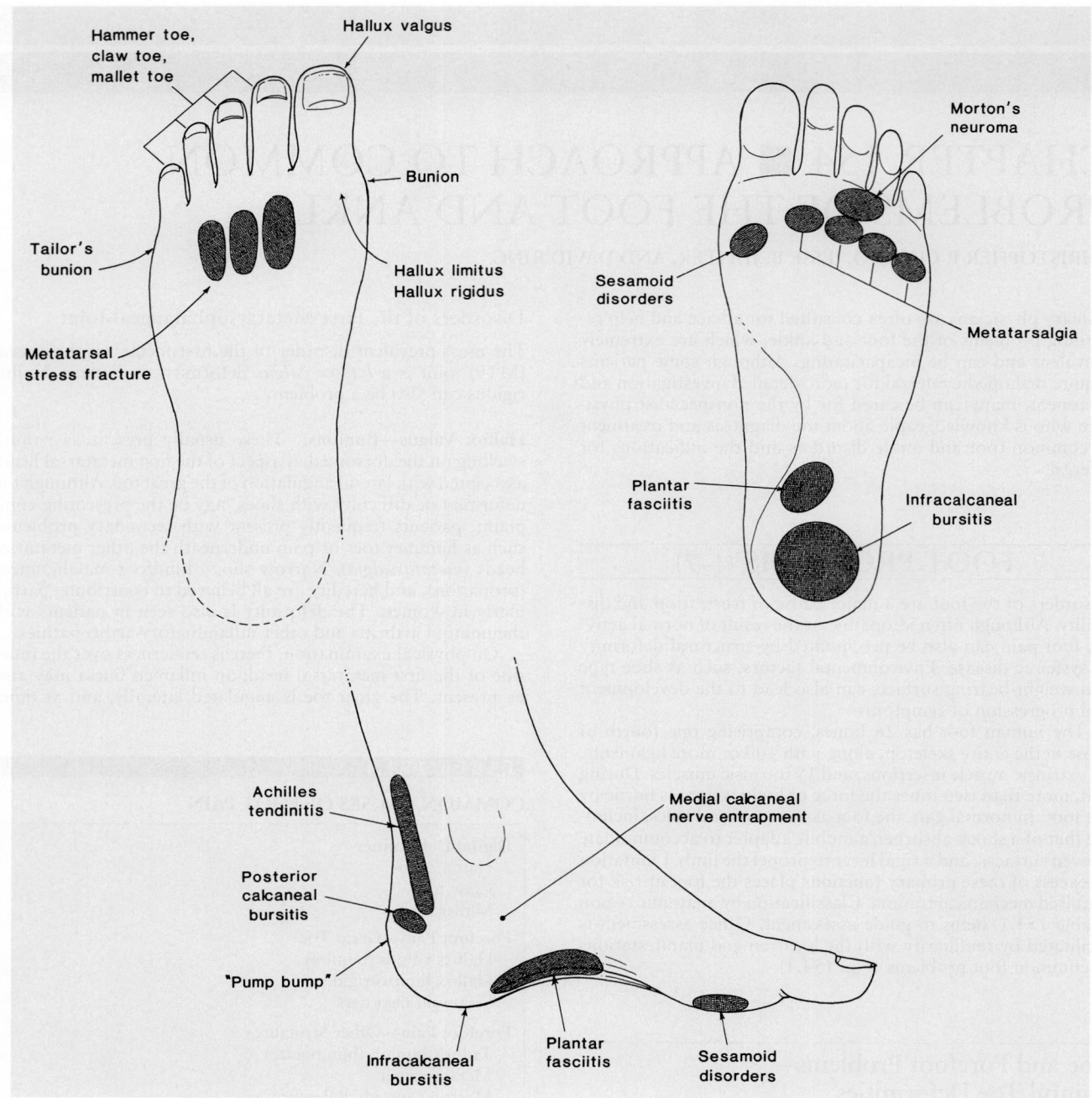

FIGURE 154.1. Sites of common foot problems.

the MTP joint cannot be passively reduced. Radiographs may show the underlying cause to be an increased angle between the first and second metatarsals (normal, <10 degrees).

Most bunions respond to nonoperative treatment. Appropriately sized shoes (with wide toe boxes), bunion splints, and orthotic devices provide symptomatic relief to many patients. In addition, stretching the shoes can be helpful. Patients should be specifically instructed to use a "ball-and-ring" shoe stretcher, a device that focally stretches just one portion of the shoe. As a last resort, surgical intervention may be necessary. The type of surgery indicated depends on the nature and degree of the underlying structural deformity. In some patients, extensive reconstruction may be required, and it is important to counsel these patients that they need more than a simple "shaving."

Hallux Rigidus. This condition is characterized by arthritis of the first metatarsophalangeal joint; it results in limited or total loss of dorsiflexion. Prominent dorsal osteophytes sometimes lead patients or providers to use the misnomer "dorsal bunion." Patients with hallux rigidus often have pain with dorsiflexion of the toe (as they push off with the foot) and complain of "jamming." If the dorsal osteophytes are large enough, finding comfortable shoes also becomes difficult.

Physical examination reveals limited mobility of the first MTP joint, especially on dorsiflexion (normal, 50 to 80 degrees). Crepitus and enlarged osteophytes may also be present. Radiographs reveal degenerative changes such as joint-space narrowing, osteophytes, and sclerosis. Chronic gouty arthritis and other inflammatory arthropathies may resemble this condition, but radiographic changes are more destructive and lytic.

Initial treatment includes limiting joint stress and use of analgesics. An orthotic device with an extension under the great toe (Morton's extension) and an extra-depth shoe should be prescribed. Limiting joint motion by stiffening the outer sole of the shoe (full-length steel shank) may also help. As with hallux valgus, using a ball-and-ring device to stretch the shoe over the prominent dorsal osteophytes may help.

Surgery involving either débridement of osteophytes ("cheilectomy") or fusion is indicated if conservative treatment is unsuccessful. In general, less advanced disease can be treated with cheilectomy, whereas more advanced disease requires joint resection. Joint replacement for hallux rigidus is controversial and under investigation.

Sesamoid Disorders. The first MTP joint contains two sesamoid bones (medial and lateral) that articulate with the plantar aspect of the metatarsal and help to serve as a fulcrum in normal joint mobility. Excessive or abnormal stress about this area can lead to pain and inflammation (*sesamoiditis*), *cartilage injury* (*osteochondritis* or *osteonecrosis*), or *sesamoid fracture*. Although a history of trauma may not be obvious, sesamoid injuries are not uncommon among runners, dancers, and other individuals who participate in high-impact activities.

On physical examination, swelling and tenderness is present on the plantar aspect of the first MTP joint; an inflamed bursa may also be appreciated in some instances. Foot radiographs should include a "sesamoid" view of the foot if a fracture is suspected. It is important to remember that bipartite (or multipartite) sesamoids are normal variants; a bone scan or magnetic resonance imaging may be needed when fracture is suspected and plain films are nondiagnostic.

Most sesamoid disorders respond to nonoperative measures, starting with rest and reduction of weight-bearing stresses. Acute fractures may require the use of a fracture boot or even a cast. Mild cases of sesamoiditis without fracture can be managed with a stiff-soled shoe and a soft insert/liner; custom orthotics providing relief under the sesamoids may also be helpful. In refractory cases, shaving or excision of the involved sesamoid may be necessary.

Disorders of the Lesser Metatarsophalangeal Joints

The second through fifth metatarsophalangeal joints ("lesser metatarsophalangeal joints") are subject to a different set of stresses than those that affect the first MTP joint. The capsule that holds the lesser metatarsophalangeal joints together (the *plantar plate*) is thickened on its plantar aspect and is especially important for stability and can be affected by both acute and chronic injury.

Acute Injury. Extreme traumatic dorsiflexion of the toe can stretch or tear the plate, resulting in tenderness to palpation on the plantar aspect and pain with passive dorsiflexion of the toe. Taping and the use of a hard-soled postoperative shoe are useful in minimizing symptoms as the injury heals.

Chronic Attenuation. Attenuation and stretching of the plantar plate over time can result in *metatarsophalangeal synovitis* and *instability*. This results in instability and maltracking of the joint, leading to inflammation and pain. Because the second metatarsal is usually longer than the other metatarsals, this condition more commonly affects the second MTP joint. Physical examination reveals tenderness of both sides of the involved joint; the toe may be passively subluxed dorsally. Initial treatment consists in using nonsteroidal antiinflammatory drugs (NSAIDs) and either taping or splinting to stabilize the joint. In a small minority of patients, surgery is necessary (tendon transfer or metatarsal osteotomy).

Bunionette. This is the fifth-metatarsal equivalent of the bunion, characterized by pain and swelling over the lateral aspect of the fifth MTP joint. An angular deformity (medial deviation) of the fifth toe may also be present. Patients typically complain of pain over the lateral aspect of the fifth metatarsal head and difficulty finding comfortable shoes. On physical examination, the lateral aspect of the fifth metatarsal head is usually tender. A local bursitis may also be present. Radiographs show an excessive angle between the fourth and fifth metatarsals, curvature of the metatarsal shaft, or an enlarged fifth metatarsal head. Shoewear modification (i.e., wider or stretched) usually helps, although surgical correction may be necessary.

Metatarsalgia. True metatarsalgia is pain with weight bearing in the vicinity of the lesser metatarsal heads. Symptoms are due to mechanical overload of the forefoot. Possible etiologies include fat pad atrophy or migration, a tight Achilles tendon, and poorly cushioned shoes. *Bunions* and *hammer toes* may also cause "secondary metatarsalgia." Often, a discrete cause of metatarsalgia cannot be identified, in which case the disorder represents a diagnosis of exclusion, reflecting an absence of other underlying conditions, such as interdigital neuroma, metatarsal stress fracture, and MTP instability.

On physical examination, the lesser metatarsal heads are tender to palpation, and one or more callosities may be present on the plantar aspect of the forefoot. The plantar fat pad may be atrophied, especially in elderly patients, along with hammertoe deformities or an Achilles tendon contracture.

Treatment entails dispersing weight away from the involved metatarsal(s); soft innersoles, molded shoes with innersoles, metatarsal bars, and orthotic devices are used. If the Achilles tendon is tight, physical therapy or the use of a night splint may be beneficial. In some situations, surgical intervention (metatarsal osteotomies, Achilles tendon lengthening, hammertoe correction, etc.) is necessary.

Metatarsal Stress Fractures. Functional overload in a lesser metatarsal (usually the second or third metatarsal) may result in a stress fracture. Stress fractures can be classified into overuse injuries, typically seen in younger active patients, or insufficiency fractures, more commonly seen in middle-aged or elderly postmenopausal women. The onset of symptoms may be insidious and in the absence of a discrete traumatic event. On exam, forefoot swelling is usually noted along with point tenderness of the involved metatarsal shaft. Early on, plain films may be negative, but bone scan or magnetic resonance imaging may show the fracture.

Healing is usually uneventful with rest and activity modification, helped by a fracture boot or hard-soled postoperative shoe for 4 to 8 weeks. In postmenopausal women or individuals with more than one stress fracture, a dual-energy x-ray absorptiometry scan should be considered to evaluate bone mineral density.

Interdigital (Morton's) Neuroma. The third intermetatarsal space is supplied by a common nerve trunk, receiving branches from both the medial and the lateral plantar nerves. Compression and irritation of this trunk by the metatarsal heads, the deep transverse intermetatarsal ligament, and the plantar weight-bearing surface are implicated. Classically, the patient is a woman who reports burning pain and cramping, most often between the third and fourth toes, aggravated by wearing closed shoes and relieved by removal of the shoe and forefoot massage. Often, there is intermittent numbness in the region between the toes.

On compressing the forefoot and pushing up in the distal third intermetatarsal space, a "click" may be felt (Mulder's sign) and the patient's symptoms reproduced. Relief is sometimes achieved through the use of wider shoes, a metatarsal bar, soft insoles, orthotic devices, NSAIDs, or local anesthetic and steroid injections. Frequently, surgical excision of the neuroma is required.

Midfoot Problems

Two common sources of midfoot pain are midfoot arthritis and the presence of an accessory navicular bone.

Midfoot Arthritis

Midfoot arthritis presents with aching or sharp pain over the top (dorsum) of the foot in conjunction with burning sensations due to prominent osteophytes irritating one or more of the sensory nerves. Midfoot tenderness and swelling may be present on examination. Plain films can confirm the diagnosis. Initial treatment consists in the use of NSAIDs and well-fitted shoes. If symptoms persist, a custom orthotic should be tried. Shaving of prominent osteophytes and/or fusion of the arthritic joints provide good results in refractory disease.

Accessory Navicular Bone

An accessory navicular is the most common accessory bone in the foot; prevalence is 10% to 15%. In most cases, the extra bone is an incidental radiographic finding, but in some patients, the accessory bone can be symptomatic. Pain is believed to originate either from irritation of the soft tissues overlying the accessory bone or from inflammation in the region of its attachment ("synchondrosis") to the main navicular bone. On exam, there is focal tenderness over the medial aspect of the midfoot. Radiographs can confirm the diagnosis. NSAIDs plus protected weight bearing with a fracture boot or custom orthotic usually suffices; sometimes surgery is required to remove the extra bone.

Hindfoot Problems

Plantar Heel Pain

Plantar (inferior) heel pain is seen in both young and old patients and can be disabling. It is often mistakenly attributed to "heel spurs," most of which are asymptomatic and unrelated to the pain.

Plantar Fasciitis. This common cause of heel pain results from inflammation of the plantar fascia at its origin on the inferior calcaneus. Typically, patients report *"first-step" pain* on getting out of bed in the morning, diminishing as the plantar fascia stretches out, only to recur after periods of inactivity. Overuse syndromes, such as jogging, can also contribute to microscopic tears. Tenderness can be elicited at the medial origin of the plantar fascia on the medial aspect of the inferior calcaneus. Although radiographs often demonstrate a plantar spur at the anterior inferior aspect of the calcaneus, this is usually not the cause of the symptoms.

Initial treatment focuses on Achilles tendon stretching exercises (see Chapter 18), activity modification, ice, NSAIDs, and use of a heel cushion to provide symptomatic relief. A night splint helps to stretch the Achilles tendon during sleep. If these measures are not effective, a 4- to 6-week trial of cast immobilization can be tried—a form of enforced complete rest. Local steroid injections can be considered but should be used sparingly due to risk of plantar fascia rupture. Both *high-energy ultrasound* and use of *magnetic insoles* have failed to demonstrate efficacy in randomized, controlled studies. Rarely, surgical release of the plantar fascia is required.

Infracalcaneal Bursitis. Infracalcaneal bursitis presents with pain or an aching sensation directly under the heel, increasing with duration of weight bearing and more pronounced as the day progresses. Examination reveals point tenderness directly under the midportion of the calcaneus; there may be some localized warmth and swelling. Treatment includes ice, massage, NSAIDs, and physical therapy. A soft heel pad, heel cup, or appropriately fabricated orthotic device to relieve direct impact on this region may also be helpful. Steroid injections should be avoided because they may result in atrophy of the fat pad that cushions the heel.

Neurologic Heel Pain. Nerve entrapment may occur when the first branch of the *lateral plantar nerve* (sometimes called *Baxter's nerve*) is compressed by the abductor hallucis muscle. The resulting symptoms and signs are very similar to those experienced with plantar fasciitis (radiating pain and tenderness on palpation of the medial side of the heel); the two conditions may coexist.

Posterior tibial nerve compression can occur due to local trauma (sprain, fracture), a space-occupying lesion (varicosity, lipoma), or foot deformity (pronation, supination) as the nerve passes behind the medial malleolus and enters a fibroosseous tunnel. The resultant *tarsal tunnel syndrome* is characterized by paresthesias, dysesthesias, numbness, and/or nocturnal pain along the plantar aspect of the foot and toes. A Tinel's sign may be elicited by percussion behind the medial malleolus, and plantar numbness is noted. Nerve conduction studies can establish the diagnosis but are not consistently abnormal. Consultation is indicated. Treatment with NSAIDs, physical therapy, orthotic devices, and local steroid injections may preclude the need for surgical release.

Lumbar radiculopathy can cause heel pain that extends in a radicular distribution (see Chapters 147 and 167).

Posterior Heel Pain

The most common cause of posterior heel pain is Achilles tendinitis; posterior heel bursitis is another etiology.

Achilles Tendinitis. Seen in both young athletic persons and the elderly, this form of tendinitis probably results from microscopic tearing of the tendon with resultant inflammation. Often, the term "tendinosis" is used interchangeably with "tendinitis." Tendinosis more specifically refers to chronic degeneration of the tendon, whereas tendinitis refers to inflammation of the tendon and surrounding tissues. In the majority of cases these two conditions coexist and are lumped together under "tendinitis."

On physical examination, the tendon is tender to palpation either directly at its insertion onto the calcaneus ("insertional" tendinitis) or a few centimeters proximal to this ("noninsertional" tendinitis) and associated with a nodule in the proximal tendon.

In acute cases, the first line of therapy is rest, even to the point of plaster immobilization. A heel lift, ultrasound, orthotics, NSAIDs, and stretching exercises are more helpful in chronic disease (usually seen in middle-aged and elderly patients). A night splint can help to provide stretching. In refractory cases, surgery is required to débride the diseased portion of the tendon. There may be some degree of pain postoperatively.

An enlarged posterior calcaneal tuberosity (*Haglund's deformity*) may contribute to the development of insertional Achilles tendinitis. Patients typically present with a tender, bony enlargement about the lateral aspect of the posterior calcaneus. Shoes with firm heel counters aggravate symptoms, and a lateral radiograph of the foot will confirm the enlarged shape of the calcaneus. The initial treatment of Achilles tendinitis associated with a Haglund's deformity is essentially the same regimen recommended for isolated Achilles tendinitis. Particular emphasis should be placed on shoewear modification, however. If surgery is necessary, the posterior bony exostosis must be removed at the same time the tendon is débrided.

Posterior Calcaneal Bursitis. Two bursae are present over the posterior heel: a superficial bursa lying between the Achilles tendon and skin, and a deep bursa located between the tendon and the calcaneus. Women who wear shoes with firm, unyielding heel counters are prone to the development of inflammation of the *superficial bursa*. Symptoms usually resolve with shoewear modification and local modalities.

Inflammation of the deeper bursa, *retrocalcaneal bursitis*, results from overuse and/or chronic degeneration of the Achilles tendon; it commonly coexists with Achilles tendinitis. Pain can be elicited by compression of the heel cord just anterior to its attachment and with passive dorsal and plantar flexion of the ankle. Treatment begins with ice followed by moist heat, NSAIDs, and rest. Formal physical therapy, heel lifts, night splints, and the use of a walking cast may be necessary with more-chronic symptoms.

Posterior Tibial Tendonitis and Insufficiency

The posterior tibial tendon courses just behind the medial malleolus of the ankle and inserts primarily onto the medial aspect of the navicular bone. This tendon is the main dynamic stabilizer of the longitudinal arch of the foot and is prone to both inflammation and chronic degeneration. With posterior tibial tendinitis, swelling and tenderness are typically present over the distal portion of the tendon (i.e., distal to the medial malleolus). Strength testing reveals pain and weakness with resisted hindfoot inversion. In more advanced cases, *posterior tibial tendon insufficiency* develops and the longitudinal arch of the foot collapses, resulting in a flatfoot deformity.

The initial treatment consists in the use of NSAIDs and the use of a custom orthotic to support the arch and decrease the stress on the tendon. In recalcitrant cases, 4 to 6 weeks in a walking cast may be beneficial. Often, surgery is necessary.

ANKLE DISORDERS (8)

Ankle Sprains

Ankle sprains are the most common orthopedic injury seen in primary care practice. Sprains range in severity from mild stretching of ligamentous fibers (*first degree*) to a tear of some portion of the ligament (*second degree*) to complete ligamentous separation (*third degree*), sometimes with avulsion of small bony fragments. Sprain usually occurs when excessive inversion or eversion stress is applied to the ankle while it is in the relatively unstable plantar-flexed position. An *inversion injury*, the most common type of sprain, causes damage to the lateral ligaments of the ankle. A sprain can occur while a person is running or even while walking on uneven surfaces. The patient may report hearing or feeling a snap or "pop." Early assessment facilitates evaluation, which may be hindered once generalized swelling sets in.

Evaluation

The history of injury is often inaccurate and may not be helpful for evaluating the extent of ligamentous damage. Instead, a careful physical examination is needed to identify the site and degree of injury, with the examiner's fingertips used to check the anterior capsule and medial and lateral ligaments (Fig. 154.2). Although significant edema commonly accompanies ligamentous injury, complete ligamentous and capsular disruption may produce remarkably little edema because of extravasation into the surrounding soft-tissue planes. Tenderness is noted over the injured ligaments, which lie anterior and inferior to the fibula; tenderness over the bone should raise the suspicion of fracture. Swelling invariably occurs, usually anterior to the lateral malleolus at the onset, and ecchymoses are common. The degree of swelling present depends on the time elapsed from the time of injury.

A useful indicator of significant injury is the *anterior draw test*. The sign may be elicited by grasping the distal tibia in one hand and the heel in the other and sliding the entire foot forward. This is done first with the ankle in neutral position and then with 30 degrees of plantar flexion. A shift of 1 or 2 mm may be normal, and the uninjured ankle should be used as a guide in this regard. With complete disruption of the anterior or lateral ligaments, one can see 4 mm or more of anterior shift as the fibers of the anterolateral ligaments lie in an anteroposterior direction.

The *talar tilt test* is also used to assess for significant injury and joint instability. In a positive test, the talus tilts as the calcaneus is adducted (Fig. 154.2). This maneuver produces a gap between the talus and the malleolus on the lateral aspect of the ankle. In the acute setting both the anterior draw and the talar tilt tests may be falsely negative because pain causes the patient to "guard" or "splint" the injured joint.

Radiography is useful in cases of moderate to severe injury to identify any associated fracture. Three standard views are obtained: anteroposterior, lateral, and mortise (an anteroposterior view with the ankle in 20 to 30 degrees of internal rotation). Stress views are usually not indicated in the acute setting. The *Ottawa rules* were developed to help determine risk of fracture and need for radiographs. Validated Ottawa rule criteria include the following:

- Pain near the malleoli, plus
- Age 55 years or older, or

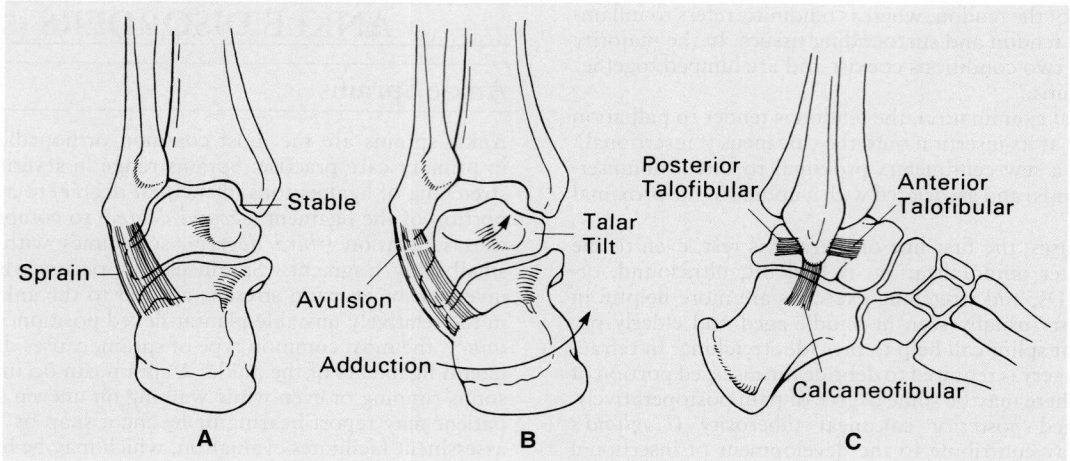

FIGURE 154.2. Lateral ligamentous sprain and avulsion. **A:** Simple sprain in which the ligaments remain intact, and the talus remains stable within the mortice. **B:** Avulsion of the lateral ligaments; the talus becomes unstable and tilts within the mortice when the calcaneus is adducted. **C:** Lateral ligaments of the ankle. The anterior talofibular and calcaneofibular ligaments are the ligaments most frequently involved in inversion injuries. (Redrawn from Cailliet R. Foot and ankle pain. Philadelphia: FA Davis, 1968, with permission.)

- Inability to bear weight both immediately after injury and currently for four steps, or
- Bone tenderness at the posterior edge or tip of either malleolus.
- Absence of these features, which are sensitive but not specific for fracture, obviates the need for radiologic study.

Management

Control of swelling is the first and immediate management priority, reducing the degree and the extent of pain. Effusion and hemorrhage may distend the joint and predispose to adhesions. An elastic bandage, ice, and elevation are helpful in controlling edema. The ankle may be placed in ice water for 15 to 20 minutes and then elevated. An ice pack can substitute for immersion. Cold application is repeated every few hours.

A soft dressing or elastic bandage is used for 1 to 2 weeks to control swelling and provide stability. When the ankle is splinted, it should be kept in neutral or slightly everted position to avoid tightening the heel cord and other posterior structures. Partial weight bearing is accomplished by the use of a crutch until pain subsides. Non–weight-bearing activities (gentle active range-of-motion exercises) can be started within 2 to 3 days. As pain subsides and swelling resolves, full weight bearing can be resumed, often with the use of a functional brace to support the ankle against inversion and eversion stresses while simultaneously allowing ankle dorsiflexion and plantar flexion.

Athletic activity, in most cases, should be postponed another 1 to 3 weeks depending on the severity of injury. With mild ligamentous laxity of the ankle and repeated minor sprains, proper taping to support the lateral structures may be necessary for competitive athletes participating in contact, running, or jumping sports. Tape strips are applied from the medial aspect to the lateral aspect of the ankle (Fig. 154.3) to hold the heel and the ankle in eversion and provide support. Exercises to strengthen the ankle evertors and the use of high-laced leather supportive shoes may also be helpful.

Ankle sprain is a potentially serious injury; if torn ligaments result in marked ankle instability (determined by examination

under anesthesia or stress radiography), cast immobilization for 4 to 8 weeks is indicated. Serious sprain requires prompt orthopedic referral to maximize chances for healing and restoration of joint stability.

Chronic Ankle Instability

In a small minority of patients who sustain ankle sprains, the injured ligaments heal in a lengthened position and are substantially weakened. This, in turn, can lead to the development of *chronic ankle instability*. Whereas some patients with chronic ankle instability complain of only a sense of weakness in their ankle, others note frequent sprains that may occur even on even

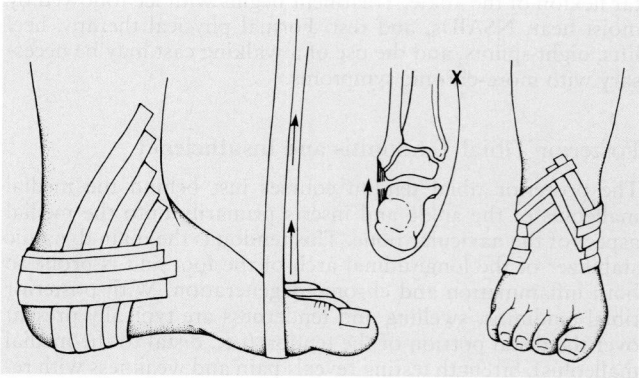

FIGURE 154.3. Taping a sprained ankle. The purpose of taping the ankle is to prevent further stretching of the injured ligaments until healing has occurred. The ankle must be inverted or everted to place the strained ligament at rest. The center figure depicts an avulsed lateral ligament. The tape here begins from inside and then runs under the foot to finish on the outer leg, holding the heel everted. The horizontal strips minimize rotation of the forefoot. (Redrawn from Cailliet R. Foot and ankle pain. Philadelphia: FA Davis, 1968, with permission.)

ground. On physical examination, tenderness is usually present over the anterolateral ankle. In addition, it may be possible gently to sublux the foot anteriorly out from underneath the leg (see prior discussion of the *anterior drawer test*). Most patients with chronic ankle instability respond to physical therapy and the use of taping or a brace. If symptoms persist, relief can be provided in the majority of cases with surgical stabilization of the ankle.

Ankle Arthritis

Ankle arthritis may result from trauma, chronic instability, infection, osteoarthritis, and systemic inflammatory disease.

Patients usually complain of deep aching pain, often on getting up in the morning or after sitting for a long period of time. The anterior joint line is tender, and both active and passive motion are substantially decreased. Radiographs reveal joint-space narrowing but may also show cyst formation, erosions, and subchondral sclerosis. Acute treatment includes NSAIDs, physical therapy, cushioned shoes, and local modalities such as radiant heat. If these measures fail, an intraarticular cortisone injection or custom brace may provide relief. If symptoms persist and significantly interfere with daily function, surgery (most often an ankle fusion) may be indicated. Ankle replacement surgery remains investigational and has not achieved the success seen in hip and knee arthroplasty.

Annotated Bibliography

1. Buchbinder B, Ptasznik R, Gordon J, et al. Ultrasound-guided extracorporeal shock wave therapy for plantar fasciitis: a randomized controlled trial. JAMA 2002;288:1364. (*No benefit was found.*)
2. Frey C, Roberts NE. Problems shoes, problem feet: what to tell women about footwear. Women's Health Primary Care 2002;5:682. (*Practical advice, with a well-illustrated patient education piece.*)
3. Gill LL. Plantar fasciitis: diagnosis and conservative management. J Am Acad Orthop Surg 1997;5:109. (*Best for emphasis on nonsurgical management.*)
4. Schepsis AA, Leach RE, Gorzyca J. Plantar fasciitis: etiology, treatment, surgical results, and review of the literature. Clin Orthop 1991;266:285. (*An excellent review of the literature and summary.*)
5. Smart GW, Taunton JE, Clement DB. Achilles tendon disorders in runners—a review. Med Sci Sports Exerc 1980;12:231. (*A good review of this common problem in runners.*)
6. Torkki M, Malmivaara A, Seitsale S, et al. Surgery vs orthosis vs watchful waiting for hallux valgus: a randomized controlled trial. JAMA 2001;285:2474. (*Surgery in carefully selected persons provided the best long-term outcome; orthoses gave short-term relief.*)
7. Winemiller MH, Billow RG, Laskowski ER, et al. Effect of magnetic vs sham-magnetic insoles on plantar heel pain: a randomized controlled trial. JAMA 2003;290:1474. (*No benefit was found.*)
8. Steill I, Wells G, Laupacis A, et al. Multicentre trial to introduce the Ottawa ankle rules for use of radiography in acute ankle injuries. BMJ 1995;311:594. (*The development of a decision rule to limit unnecessary ankle films.*)

CHAPTER 155 ■ APPROACH TO THE PATIENT WITH ASYMPTOMATIC HYPERURICEMIA

Asymptomatic hyperuricemia became commonplace when physicians began using chemistry panels that routinely included measurement of the serum uric acid. Hyperuricemia is defined as a serum uric acid concentration that exceeds the mean by at least two standard deviations. The mean (as determined by colorimetric assay, the most commonly used method) is 7.5 mg/dL for men and 6.6 mg/dL for women. By statistical definition, 2.5% of the population is hyperuricemic. The consequences of being hyperuricemic and the need for lowering the uric acid level have been subjects of debate. Some authorities have advocated prophylactic therapy in the hope of preventing acute gout, chronic tophaceous gout, stone formation, and renal failure. Others question the cost-effectiveness of such an approach and even the relationship of hyperuricemia to some of the adverse consequences attributed to it. The primary physician must decide whether and when to treat the asymptomatic patient with an elevated uric acid level.

PATHOPHYSIOLOGY AND CLINICAL PRESENTATION (1–18)

Uric acid is the end product of purine metabolism. Humans have no pathway for the further breakdown of uric acid; it must be excreted by the kidneys or the serum level will rise. The pathogenesis of hyperuricemia involves the overproduction or underexcretion of urate or both. It is estimated that one third of hyperuricemic patients are overproducers, another one third are underexcreters, and the remainder have a combined deficit.

Overproduction of uric acid is especially marked in patients undergoing treatment for myeloproliferative and lymphoproliferative malignancies and in those with severe psoriasis. Rapid cellular turnover results in the production of massive amounts of nucleic acid metabolites that are converted to uric acid. Overproduction may also develop from an increase in purine synthesis *de novo*, as occurs in patients with inborn errors of metabolism. Contrary to popular belief, excessive dietary intake of purine-rich foods is rarely responsible for hyperuricemia because dietary sources of purine make up only 10% of the uric acid pool. However, excessive intake of alcohol (>100 g of ethanol per day) results in increased urate synthesis, especially if the patient does not eat anything at the time of alcohol consumption.

Underexcretion of uric acid occurs in association with an overall decrease in the glomerular filtration or a defect in the tubular secretion of urate; uric acid is also underexcreted if another substance competes with urate for tubular secretion. A compromise in renal blood flow secondary to aging or atherosclerotic disease reduces renal urate excretion. Hyperuricemia has been noted in hypertensive patients. Although some instances may be a consequence of hypertensive renovascular injury, epidemiologic analysis suggests that most cases are caused by *thiazide* use. In addition to thiazides, low doses of *aspirin, niacin,* and *loop diuretics* reduce renal urate excretion. Excretion falls in patients with an increased proximal tubular reabsorption of sodium, which has been linked to hyperinsulinism and might account for the oft-noted, poorly understood relation between hyperuricemia and atherosclerotic cardiovascular disease. However, careful reexamination of the epidemiologic data linking hyperuricemia to an increased risk for cardiovascular disease reveals no independent causal relationship but rather an association with thiazide use for the treatment of hypertension, which is a major cardiovascular risk factor. *Fasting* that results in ketosis seems to be capable of transiently reducing urate excretion and raising the serum uric acid. *Obesity* appears to be another risk factor, especially for triggering gouty attacks associated with hyperuricemia.

More than 90% of hyperuricemic patients present asymptomatically. Most are persons who have been subjected to multiphasic screening. Half of newly discovered patients in the Framingham study were taking thiazides, and just less than 3% had elevations secondary to a concurrent illness, such as myeloproliferative disease. Risks of complications from hyperuricemia correlate with the degree of elevation in serum urate level and its duration. The well-established adverse consequences are acute gouty arthropathy, chronic gouty arthropathy, and urate kidney stone disease (see later discussion). Hyperuricemia has an association with atherosclerotic disease and renal failure, but the statistical relationship has proven not to be etiologic.

PRINCIPLES OF MANAGEMENT (3,4,7–10,12–21)

Prophylactic therapy might be indicated if lowering the uric acid level will prevent the adverse consequences of hyperuricemia. Although in some instances indefinite prophylactic treatment is indicated and effective, one needs to weigh the costs against the expected benefits,

Lowering Uric Acid

Both dietary/lifestyle and pharmacologic measures can be used (see also Chapter 158).

Dietary and Other Lifestyle Measures

Modifications in diet, alcohol consumption, and weight can be helpful, but often they are not sufficient. Dietary measures are commonly recommended for lowering uric acid and preventing gout. Purine-rich foods, such as organ meats and other meats, seafood, yeast, beer and other alcoholic beverages, legumes, oatmeal, spinach, mushrooms, asparagus, and cauliflower, have all been implicated in hyperuricemia; low-fat dairy products are believed to be protective. Epidemiologic data reveal a 40% to 50% increase in the risk of gout among persons in the highest quintile of meat and seafood intake compared to those in the lowest quintile, but there is no increase in risk among persons with a high intake of purine-rich vegetables. Those in the highest quintile of low-fat dairy-product intake have about a 40% lower risk of gout. Clinically, a purine-restricted diet is only modestly effective in lowering uric acid, due in part to the fact that only 10% of circulating purine is derived from dietary sources and to the difficulty in maintaining such a diet, which is not especially palatable. Consequently, restriction of purine intake is unlikely to be sufficient in itself as prophylactic therapy unless dietary habits or events appear to correlate strongly with gouty attacks.

If the patient is obese, weight loss should be recommended because urate levels and the risk of acute gout increase with excess weight; morbid obesity treated with bariatric surgery lowers serum urate, but starvation diets may trigger a gouty attack.

Pharmacologic Measures

The classical pharmacologic approach to treating hyperuricemia starts with a 24-hour urine collection for the measurement of urate excretion to help differentiate between overproduction (high 24-hour urinary urate) and underexcretion (low 24-hour urinary urate). In patients with gout, about 75% of cases are due to underexcretion. The findings are then used to guide the choice of agent, either one that reduces uric acid production (e.g., a xanthine oxidase inhibitor such as *allopurinol* [see Chapter 158]) or one that increases urate excretion—the uricosuric drugs *probenecid* and *sulfinpyrazone* [see Chapter 158]). However, allopurinol's convenience of use (once-daily dosing), reasonable tolerability, and efficacy for lowering serum urate irrespective of mechanism have led to the common practice of starting treatment for hyperuricemia empirically with the xanthine oxidase inhibitor and skipping 24-hour urine collection. Supporting this approach is the finding that tailoring therapy to 24-hour urate level provides no better outcomes than empiric therapy with allopurinol.

A correlate of pharmacotherapy is limiting, if possible, drugs that reduce urate excretion, including thiazides, low-dose aspirin, niacin, and loop diuretics.

Approach to Prevention of Acute Gouty Arthritis (See Also Chapter 158)

Population studies (Framingham, Normative Aging, Sudbury) confirmed that the higher the serum uric acid level, the greater is the chance of an attack of acute gout; they also confirmed that the urate concentration is the predominant determinant of risk. However, the oft-quoted 90% risk reported in the Framingham study represented a 12-year cumulative incidence figure and pertained only to 10 patients who had a uric acid level greater than 9.0 mg/dL. More relevant is the average annual incidence, which was 4.0% in the Framingham study and 4.7% in the Normative Aging study for patients with urate concentrations in the top 2%.

Implementing the dietary and lifestyle changes noted earlier that can reduce uric acid and the risk of a gouty attack is reasonable and worth doing, but to determine the utility of indefinite prophylactic pharmacotherapy that may also be required, one needs to consider the costs and benefits of preventing an attack of acute gout. The cost of lifelong prophylactic therapy can reach thousands of dollars because the mean age at the time of detection is 35 years. The prevalence of adverse drug reactions has been reported to be as high as 10% for probenecid and 25% for allopurinol. These costs appear excessive when the safety, efficacy, and minimal expense of promptly treating a single acute attack of gout with a short course of a nonsteroidal antiinflammatory drug are considered (see Chapter 158). Only if gouty attacks become disabling and frequent does the cost–benefit equation shift in favor of prophylaxis. In most instances, the intervals between recurrences of acute gout are measured in years.

Prevention of Chronic Gouty Arthritis
(See Also Chapter 158)

The issue of prophylaxis for the prevention of chronic gouty arthritis is of only minor importance because almost all patients with this condition go through a stage of acute gouty attacks before chronic joint changes develop. Thus, asymptomatic patients with no evidence of clinical gout are at little if any risk for silently falling victim to chronic gouty arthritis.

Prevention of Azotemia

Despite fears to the contrary and early studies that were confounded by high exposures to lead, chronic hyperuricemia does not appear to be a significant risk factor for the development of azotemia, nor does hyperuricemia *secondary to* renal failure pose an additional threat to the kidneys. In a prospective study from Kaiser-Permanente in which 113 patients with asymptomatic hyperuricemia and 193 controls were followed for 8 years, no difference was found in the incidence of azotemia between the two groups (1.8% vs. 2.1%). In the same study, no relation between uric acid level and risk for azotemia was found in 168 patients with clinical gout followed for 10 years. In the Normative Aging study, a creatinine level greater than 2.0 mg/dL developed in only 0.7% of the 94 patients with a uric acid level greater than 9.0 mg/dL during the 15 years of follow-up. One set of investigators calculated that a significant risk for renal injury from chronic hyperuricemia required that a uric acid level of 13.0 mg/dL in men and 10.0 mg/dL in women be sustained for 40 years. A 3-year prospective study of hyperuricemic patients with and without renal failure showed no change in renal function when allopurinol was used to normalize the serum urate concentration.

One group of hyperuricemic patients at risk for renal failure are those with myeloproliferative or lymphoproliferative malignancy who are undergoing chemotherapy. With each cytotoxic treatment comes a huge uric acid load that may trigger injurious urate crystal formation in the renal tubular cells. Acute oliguric renal failure may ensue. Such patients require pretreatment with allopurinol and vigorous hydration.

Prevention of Nephrolithiasis

The risk for nephrolithiasis in patients with asymptomatic hyperuricemia is very small. In the Kaiser-Permanente study, renal calculi occurred in 3 (2.6%) of 113 hyperuricemic patients and in 2 (1.1%) of 193 controls. In two of the hyperuricemic patients with stones, the stone was composed of calcium. The risk for the development of a stone attributable to hyperuricemia was calculated to be less than 1% annually. Among patients with gout, the control of serum uric acid was the same for those in whom stones developed and for those in whom they did not.

This minimal risk for stone development conferred by hyperuricemia alone derives from the importance of other factors in stone formation (see Chapter 135). Family history, urinary pH, and level of hydration are particularly germane. Two of the three hyperuricemic patients with stones in the Kaiser-Permanente study had a family history of nephrolithiasis. Urine acidity is a critical factor because the solubility of uric acid falls precipitously as the pH falls from 8.0 to 5.0. The amount of uric acid excreted in the urine per 24 hours has also been suggested as a factor, but careful studies have shown that the level of urinary uric acid is only a weak determinant of stone formation until extreme levels are encountered. However, dehydration is a well-established precipitant.

Urolithiasis is rarely life threatening. In a study of 1,700 patients with gout, only 1 patient experienced serious obstructive uropathy.

Prevention of Atherosclerotic Disease

Although a statistical relationship exists between hyperuricemia and atherosclerotic disease, it does not appear to be an etiologic one. Instead, the two conditions appear to share a common pathophysiologic link, namely thiazide therapy and hypertension. No evidence has been found that treating hyperuricemia lowers the risk for atherosclerotic disease.

THERAPEUTIC RECOMMENDATIONS

- Asymptomatic hyperuricemia is associated with an increased risk for acute gouty arthritis, but the cost of prophylactic pharmacotherapy in patients who have never had an attack of gout greatly exceeds the cost of treating an acute attack symptomatically, should it occur.
- Only with the development of frequent acute gouty attacks (more than three per year) is prophylactic therapy indicated, starting with lifestyle measures and empiric allopurinol therapy (see Chapter 158).
- Treatment to prevent chronic tophaceous gout need not be started until clinical evidence of gout develops.
- The evidence to justify prophylaxis to prevent renal impairment is insufficient except in patients who have a myeloproliferative or lymphoproliferative disorder and are about to be treated for it. The degree of azotemia that can be attributed to hyperuricemia is mild and clinically insignificant in most other instances.
- The risk for urolithiasis is sufficiently low to justify waiting for the development of a stone before prophylactic therapy is initiated, unless the patient has a strong family history of nephrolithiasis. However, dehydration should be avoided.
- Although hyperuricemia is associated statistically with atherosclerotic disease, the relation is not etiologic, and no cardiovascular benefit is derived from lowering the serum uric acid level.

A.H.G.

Annotated Bibliography

1. Batuman V, Maesaka JK, Haddad B, et al. The role of lead in gout nephropathy. N Engl J Med 1981;304:520. (*Detected a strong relationship between lead and nephropathy in patients with gout.*)
2. Berger LU, Yu TF. Renal function in gout: an analysis of 524 gouty subjects including long-term follow-up studies. Am J Med 1975;59:604. (*Follow-up for 12 years showed that hyperuricemia alone has no deleterious effect on renal function in ambulatory patients with gout.*)
3. Brand FN, McGee DL, Kannel WB, et al. Hyperuricemia as a risk factor of coronary heart disease: the Framingham Study. Am J Epidemiol 1985;121:11. (*Finds a statistical but not an etiologic relationship in atherosclerotic disease.*)
4. Campion EW, Glynn RJ, DeLabry LO. Asymptomatic hyperuricemia: risks and consequences in the Normative Aging Study. Am J Med 1987;82:421. (*A large epidemiologic study, with a 15-year follow-up, finding that the risk for gout with a uric acid level >9 mg/dL was 4.9% annually, and the risk for renal failure was nil.*)
5. Cappuccio FP, Strazzullo P, Farinaro E, et al. Uric acid metabolism and tubular sodium handling. JAMA 1993;270:354. (*Finds that hyperuricemia was closely linked to excessive proximal tubular reabsorption of sodium, and speculates that both are manifestations of hyperinsulinemia.*)
6. Choi HK, Mount DB, Reginato AM. Pathogenesis of gout. Ann Intern Med 2005;143:499. (*An excellent review of pathophysiology.*)
7. Choi HK, Atkinson K, Karlson EW, et al. Obesity weight change, hypertension, diuretic use, and risk of gout in men: the Health Professionals Follow-up Study. Arch Intern Med 2005;165:742. (*Obesity is a risk factor, and weight loss is protective.*).
8. Culleton BF, Larson MG, Kannel WB, et al. Serum uric acid and risk for cardiovascular disease and death: the Framingham Heart Study. Ann Intern Med 1999;131:7. (*A rigorous epidemiologic examination, finding no evidence for a causal relationship between urate level and cardiovascular risk; a previously noted link appears to be thiazide use for hypertension.*)
9. Fang J, Alderman MH. Serum uric acid and cardiovascular mortality: the NHANES I epidemiologic follow-up study, 1971–1992. JAMA 2000;283:2404. (*Epidemiologic data suggesting an independent contribution of uric acid to coronary heart disease risk.*)
10. Fessel JW. Renal outcomes of gout and hyperuricemia. Am J Med 1979;67:74. (*A prospective study, showing that the risks for renal failure and stone formation are very small and hardly justify prophylactic therapy.*)
11. Faller J, Fox I. Ethanol-induced hyperuricemia. N Engl J Med 1982;307:1598. (*Ethanol increased urate synthesis.*)
12. Hall AP, Berry PE, Dawber TR, et al. Epidemiology of gout and hyperuricemia—a long-term population study. Am J Med 1967;42:27. (*Community-based data on risk, finding that gouty attack developed during the 12 years of follow-up in 19% of those with serum urate levels between 8 and 8.9 mg/dL.*)
13. MacLaughlan MJ, Rodnan GP. Effects of food, fast, and alcohol on serum uric acid and acute attacks of gout. Am J Med 1967;42:38. (*Fasting and consumption of >100 g/d of alcohol raised urate levels; acute changes in levels precipitated gouty attacks.*)
14. Reif MC, Constantiner A, Levitt MF. Chronic gouty nephropathy: a vanishing syndrome. N Engl J Med 1981;304:535. (*An editorial summarizing the data on the lack of a relation between renal injury and most forms of hyperuricemia.*)
15. Shekarriz B, Stoller ML. Uric acid nephrolithiasis: current concepts and controversies. J Urol 2002;168:1307. (*A review of factors determining urate stone formation.*)
16. Wortmann RL. Gout and hyperuricemia. Curr Opin Rheumatol 2002;29:1942. (*A comprehensive summary of relevant studies.*)
17. Yu TF, Berger LU. Impaired renal function in gout. Am J Med 1982;75:95. (*Hyperuricemia alone did not affect renal function; renal insufficiency correlated best with coexisting hypertension, preexisting renal disease, and ischemic heart disease.*)
18. Yu TF, Gutman A. Uric acid nephrolithiasis in gout: predisposing factors. Ann Intern Med 1967;67:1133. (*A classic study of 305 patients, finding that the risk for stone formation was correlated with uric acid excretion, urine pH, serum urate level, and underlying cause.*)
19. Liang MH, Fries JF. Asymptomatic hyperuricemia: the case for conservative management. Ann Intern Med 1978;88:666. (*A well-reasoned approach to asymptomatic hyperuricemia that remains valid.*)
20. Singer JZ, Wallace SL. The allopurinol hypersensitivity syndrome: unnecessary morbidity and mortality. Arthritis Rheum 1986;29:82. (*There was a high incidence of adverse reactions; the drug is not harmless with prolonged use.*)
21. Sjostrom L, Lindroos A-K, Peltonen M, et al. Lifestyle, diabetes and cardiovascular risk factors 10 years after bariatric surgery. N Engl J Med 2004;351:2683. (*Among other outcomes, hyperuricemia was reduced.*)

CHAPTER 156 ■ MANAGEMENT OF RHEUMATOID ARTHRITIS

Rheumatoid arthritis (RA) is prevalent and accounts for considerable disability and premature death. Population surveys indicate that 3% of women and 1% of men in the United States have definite or probable RA, based on the diagnostic criteria established by the American Rheumatism Association. Prevalence increases with age, and incidence peaks in the fourth decade. The estimated annual incidence of new cases ranges from 0.5 per 1,000 to 3 per 1,000.

The management of RA has undergone a major paradigm shift with emphasis on the early use of disease-modifying agents capable of limiting immunologically mediated joint destruction. The role of the primary care physician has changed from one of managing chronic pain and disability to being responsible for early diagnosis and, in close collaboration with the rheumatologist, prompt initiation of disease-modifying therapy.

PATHOPHYSIOLOGY AND CLINICAL PRESENTATION (1–11)

Pathogenesis and Pathophysiology

Rheumatoid arthritis is an immunologically mediated chronic inflammatory disease of unknown etiology, manifested by synovitis and destructive arthritis of the diarthrodial joints. The disease model for RA posits a delayed *autoimmune reaction* triggered by a yet-to-be-identified antigenic stimulus (e.g., infectious agent, constituent of synovium or cartilage) presenting to a genetically predisposed host (e.g., genotypes *HLA-DRB1*04/04, PTPN22, STAT4, TRAF1-C5*). Research has identified *B cells, CD4 helper/inducer T cell lymphocytes, CD4* *memory T cells, plasma cells, activated macrophages,* and *neutrophils* as participants in the immunoinflammatory response. Full early T cell activation and persistence of disease activity appears to depend on a *CD80 or CD86–CD28 costimulatory signal.* Cytokines, such as *tumor necrosis factor-α, interleukin-1 and -6,* and *granulocyte-macrophage colony–stimulating factor,* are released and serve as important immune mediators, stimulating B and T cell proliferation and differentiation and activating neutrophils and monocytes. Immunoglobulin G (IgG) *rheumatoid factor* (RF) emanating from local plasma cells may form *immune complexes* with articular antigens and thereby activate *complement.*

The net result of this cellular/cytokine/complement cascade is the release of elastases and proteases by recruited neutrophils, degrading the proteoglycan coating of articular cartilage and exposing the superficial layer of collagen and chondrocytes to immune complexes. The exposed chondrocytes and cytokine-stimulated synovial fibroblasts release matrix metalloproteinases capable of degrading connective-tissue matrices and are believed to be responsible for much of the damage that occurs to articular cartilage and bone.

Pathologically, the synovium is the principal site of initial involvement. The earliest change is immunologically mediated damage to the endothelium of the microvasculature. Small-vessel lumina become obliterated by thrombi and inflammatory cells, after which new capillary formation, synovial lining cell proliferation, edema, and leukocyte infiltration take place. Neutrophils migrate into the joint space. As the inflammatory process progresses, the synovium becomes more hypertrophic, edematous, hypervascular, and further infiltrated by mononuclear cells. In severe cases, the formation of *pannus* represents an invasive synovitis with proliferation of lymphocytes, plasma cells, fibroblasts, and macrophages. Pannus is capable of eroding cartilage and bone; the process typically begins at the joint margin, then spreads over the entire cartilaginous surface. Lysosomal enzymes released from within the pannus and latent collagenases are believed to contribute to the direct erosive capacity. Often, osteopenia is seen in subchondral bone adjacent to the involved joint even before pannus has denuded the cartilage.

Clinical Presentation and Course

Initially, an effusion develops, distending the joint capsule. This is followed by damage to the articular surface and weakening of the capsule and periarticular ligaments. Secondary muscle atrophy results and leads to an imbalance of opposing muscle groups. The net effect is an unstable, weak, swollen, subluxated joint. The synovium of tendon sheaths and bursae may also be affected by the inflammatory process, so that tenosynovitis and bursitis develop.

The clinical onset of RA is usually insidious, often beginning with vague *arthralgias, morning stiffness,* and *fatigue.* In some patients, the onset is more acute. Signs of *articular inflammation* (swelling, pain, and warmth) soon follow. The small joints of the hands and feet—the proximal interphalangeals (PIPs), metacarpophalangeals (MCPs), and metatarsophalangeals (MTPs)–are typically among the first to be involved, but knees, ankles, wrists, or elbows may also be affected early on. *Tenosynovitis* is common. Initially, the arthritis may be asymmetric or may even present as a monoarticular process, but the characteristic symmetric distribution supervenes in most instances.

In an occasional patient, RA is preceded by *palindromic rheumatism,* a condition characterized by repeated episodes of transient joint pain, swelling, and redness extending beyond the joint. The condition lasts a few hours to a few days, then resolves completely without causing permanent joint injury. Fingers, wrists, shoulders, and knees are most commonly affected. Typical RA develops in about 50% of these patients.

Rheumatoid nodules appear in about 25% of patients with RA, usually as the disease progresses. These subcutaneous nodules are firm, nontender, and located principally along the extensor surface of the forearm and in the olecranon bursa. Their appearance is an unfavorable prognostic sign, as is the persistence of acute disease for more than 1 year, high serum titers of RF, and age younger than 20 years at the time of presentation.

Sustained joint inflammation lasting as little as 3 months can lead to long-term joint injury. At first, the changes are partially reversible, but as cartilage and bone erode, the injury becomes permanent.

Hands and Wrists

Characteristic hand deformities include ulnar deviation of the MCP joints, boutonnière deformities of the PIP joints, and swan-neck contractures of the fingers. In the wrists, a permanent loss of extension often occurs. A boggy, tender, dorsal wrist mass may result from tenosynovitis, and the median nerve can be compressed. The subsequent *carpal tunnel syndrome* is usually reversible, but nerve damage is permanent by the time wasting of the thenar eminence becomes obvious.

Feet

Erosion of the metatarsal heads can lead to ventral subluxation. Increased weight bearing on the inflamed heads and the formation of painful calluses result. Erosive disease may be silent in the MTP joints.

Hips and Knees

Involvement of these joints can be a source of much disability when weight bearing causes severe pain. A loss of internal rotation is the first change noted in the hip, followed by flexion contracture. One hip may predominate, even though the process is bilateral. In the knee, distention of the suprapatellar pouch by synovial effusion is common. If pressure rises rapidly, herniation of the synovium with the formation of a popliteal *Baker's cyst* can occur, and the cyst can cause severe pain if it ruptures into the calf. Loss of full knee extension is followed by flexion contractures and gait difficulties.

Other Joints

In the *elbow,* extension may be compromised, and olecranon bursitis is often present. *Shoulder* involvement presents as a subacromial or subdeltoid bursitis or as a limitation of motion. Erosion of the rotator cuff leads to painful upward subluxation of the humeral head against the acromion. In the *cervical spine,* atlantoaxial subluxation is common but usually asymptomatic. This development is potentially serious because it can lead to direct compression of the spinal cord or of the blood supply to the brainstem; fortunately, it is a rare event. When the *temporomandibular joint* is affected, pain is felt during chewing or biting, and it is difficult to open the mouth. *Avascular necrosis of the femoral head* and *vertebral osteoporosis* and collapse are usually a consequence of corticosteroid therapy.

Radiographic Manifestations

Radiographic manifestations of early disease are soft-tissue swelling around the joint and *periarticular osteopenia.* Relatively uniform narrowing of the joint space occurs as cartilage is destroyed, a finding often noted within the first 2 years of disease. *Periarticular subchondral erosion* is noted at the joint margin where pannus has developed. Finally, joint architecture is lost as the joint space is obliterated and erosion of subchondral bone progresses.

Serologic Manifestations

A variety of autoantibodies are associated with RA. The earliest serologic manifestations, which may predate the onset of clinical disease by years, are elevated levels of *IgM RF* and *antibodies to cyclic citrullinated peptide* (*anti-CCP*). About half of patients who eventually develop RA are positive for these serologic abnormalities while still appearing healthy. With the onset of symptoms, about 75% of persons with clinically definite RA will test positive for RF, but another 25% with definite RA will remain RF-negative. RF positivity is associated with skin nodules and more aggressive articular and extraarticular disease. *Antinuclear antibody* (ANA) also appears in some cases. *C-reactive protein* does not predict the risk of RA.

Extraarticular Manifestations

Extraarticular manifestations are most prominent in patients with persistent symptoms and high titers of RF (so-called seropositive disease), although up to 50% of patients with RA may show some form of extraarticular disease.

Pulmonary manifestations include *interstitial changes*, *pulmonary nodules*, and *pleuritis*. The latter is manifested by a *pleural effusion*, in which the levels of glucose (5 to 20 mg/dL) and complement are characteristically low, the leukocyte count (5,000/mm^3) is low, and the lactate dehydrogenase level is high. Accompanying *pleuritic* pain may or may not be present. An asymptomatic *pericardial effusion* also may occur.

Keratoconjunctivitis sicca (*Sjögren's syndrome*) has a strong association with RA, being found in up to 15% of patients. *Splenomegaly* is present in 5% to 10% of patients with RA, and *lymphadenopathy* is not unusual. The combination of RA, splenomegaly, and neutropenia (*Felty's syndrome*) is noted in an occasional patient. Neutropenia may be severe, but the arthritis is often quiescent. Other features include chronic leg ulceration, lymphadenopathy, and cryoglobulinemia. The risk for sepsis is high.

Vasculitis is believed to be responsible for a number of systemic manifestations, including fever, mononeuritis multiplex, Raynaud's phenomenon, chronic leg ulcers, mucosal erosions of the gastrointestinal tract, focal ischemia of the digits, and necrotizing mesarteritis. The *anemia* of chronic disease is seen in a large percentage of patients with RA.

Atherosclerotic disease is prevalent among persons with RA; cardiovascular morbidity and mortality are increased, and markers of preclinical disease, such as carotid artery atherosclerotic changes, are common. Although some treatments for RA increase cardiovascular risk (see later discussion), RA also appears to confer risk independent of other cardiovascular risk factors, perhaps related the generalized inflammation associated with the condition and its contribution to atherosclerosis (see Chapter 31).

Osteoporosis risk is doubled in RA and markedly exacerbated if steroid therapy is used.

Clinical Stages

In *stage I*, no symptoms or signs are present, just the presentation of the relevant antigen to an immunologically susceptible host. *Stage II*, in which the immune response becomes organized in the perivascular areas of the synovium, is characterized by increasing numbers of T cells, proliferation and differentiation of B cells, antibody production, synovial cell increase, and new blood vessel formation. Morning stiffness develops because fluid about the joints is increased. They are warm but not erythematous because superficial vessels are uninvolved. In *stage III*, the pathophysiologic processes of stage II continue, and extraarticular manifestations become evident. In *stage IV*, proliferating synovial membrane becomes invasive, injuring cartilage, bone, and tendons.

Clinical Course and Prognosis

The natural history of the disease is generally one of exacerbations and remissions. About 40% of patients untreated by disease-modifying therapy become disabled after 10 years, but outcomes are highly variable. Some patients experience a relatively self-limited disease, and others suffer a chronic, progressive illness. Improvements in the detection of early joint injury have provided a previously unappreciated view of how common and important early joint damage is.

It remains difficult at the outset to predict the course of an individual case, although the *HLA-DRB1*04/04 genotype*, a high serum titer of RF, extraarticular manifestations, a large number of involved joints, age less than 30 years, female gender, and systemic symptoms all correlate with an unfavorable prognosis. Insidious onset is also an unfavorable sign. Disease that remains persistently active for more than 1 year is likely to lead to joint deformities and disability. Cases in which periods of activity lasting only weeks or a few months are followed by spontaneous remission have a better prognosis. The absence of RF does not necessarily portend a good prognosis. Outcome is compromised when diagnosis and treatment are delayed. Other laboratory markers of a poor prognosis include early radiologic evidence of bony injury, persistent anemia of chronic disease, and elevated levels of the C1q component of complement.

The overall mortality for patients with RA is reported to be 2.5 times that of the general population. In those with severe articular and extraarticular disease, the mortality approaches that of patients with three-vessel coronary disease or stage IV Hodgkin's disease. Some of the excess mortality derives from infection (especially pneumonia), vasculitis, and poor nutrition, but most is attributable to complications of atherosclerotic disease. Mortality from cancer is unchanged.

Most data on rates of disability derive from specialty units caring for referred patients with severe disease. Little information is available on patients seen in primary care community settings. Estimates suggest that more than 50% of these patients remain fully employed, even after 10 to 15 years of disease, with one third having only intermittent low-grade disease and another one third experiencing spontaneous remission.

DIAGNOSIS (3,5,6,9,11–14)

The potential to prevent significant joint injury by the timely application of disease-modifying therapy places a premium on early detection. As little as 3 months of continuously active disease can lead to subclinical but important joint destruction, making it critical to identify and treat as early as possible. Impeding early recognition are the nonspecific nature of initial symptoms and signs and the absence of a single definitive laboratory test. Delay in diagnosis is common; in one study of the problem, the time to diagnosis averaged 36 months from the onset of symptoms. However, there is a constellation of clinical findings suggestive of RA and a few associated serologic changes of sufficient specificity to aid in early diagnosis.

Key Clinical Features

Although the clinical features of early rheumatoid disease can be quite nonspecific and mimicked by such illnesses as viral hepatitis (see Chapter 146), the persistence of symptoms beyond 6 weeks should quickly raise strong suspicion of RA. The presence of four or more characteristic clinical features makes for the diagnosis of "definite rheumatoid arthritis," as specified by the American Rheumatism Association; the presence of three features defines "probable" disease; and the presence of two features suggests "possible" disease. Validated diagnostic criteria include the following:

- Morning stiffness for more than 6 weeks
- Arthritis involving three or more joint areas for more than 6 weeks
- Arthritis of hand joints for more than 6 weeks
- Symmetric arthritis for more than 6 weeks
- Rheumatoid nodules
- Elevated titers of rheumatoid factor
- Characteristic radiologic changes (bony erosion in or adjacent to involved hand or wrist joints)

It is important to recognize that these criteria were developed predominantly for use in clinical research studies; some have criticized their use in patient care because they may be too specific and not sensitive enough.

Laboratory Studies

Serologic testing, although not particularly sensitive, can add some specificity to diagnosis. The presence of *IgG RF*, especially in high titers in the setting of other characteristic clinical features, helps to support the diagnosis of definite RA. Newer serologic markers, such as *anti-CCP*, are promising for their enhanced specificity and potential predictive value. *IgM RF* and IgG anti-CCP predate the onset of symptoms in about half of patients destined to develop RA, making these serologic markers potentially useful in early diagnosis.

Rheumatoid Factor

Testing for rheumatoid factor can help to support diagnosis if the pretest probability of RA is at least intermediate. In general, 70% to 80% of all patients meeting strict criteria for RA are RF-positive. The higher the RF titer, the more likely is the diagnosis of RA. However, specificity is lacking; RA positivity also occurs in other inflammatory conditions (e.g., systemic lupus, subacute bacterial endocarditis, vasculitis, and even viral infection) and in 5% to 15% of "normal" persons (the percentage increases with age). Moreover, RF negativity does not rule out RA because 20% to 30% of patients with definite RA remain RF-negative. IgM RF has been found to appear years before the onset of symptoms and may facilitate early diagnosis.

Anti–Cyclic Citrullinated Peptide (Anti-CCP)

Autoantibody testing has been sought to improve the early diagnosis of RA. The test characteristics for the presence of antibody directed against citrulline, which derives from the breakdown of arginine, appear to be promising for improving the early diagnosis of RA. Reports of specificity range from 90% to 98%, although sensitivity at the time of diagnosis can be as low as 50% to 65%, rising to 80% during advanced disease. Although it is not yet widely available and is still the subject of study, anti-CCP testing might aid in early diagnosis when ad-

ditional test specificity is desired. The test may also have some prognostic significance, being associated with erosive disease.

Genetic Testing

Although certain genotypes have been associated with poor prognosis (e.g., HLA-DRB1*04/04), and other non-HLA gene mutations have been linked to RA (e.g., *PTPN22*, *STAT4*, *TRAF1-C5*), routine genetic testing is not recommended for diagnostic purposes. Most autoimmune conditions are polygenic, involving a complex interplay of susceptibility genes. Too little is known about these genetic determinants and their interactions for such testing to be diagnostically useful at this time, but their use as prognostic indicators is promising (e.g., *HLA-DRB1*04/04* for overall prognosis and *TRAF1-C5* for the risk of anti-CCP-positive RA).

Sedimentation Rate and C-Reactive Protein

These sensitive but nonspecific measures of inflammation can be used to monitor disease activity but show little use in predicting the risk of developing clinical RA, even when measured shortly before the onset of symptoms and signs.

Radiographic Studies

Plain films of involved joints, particularly of the *hands* and *wrists*, may help in diagnosis, although many characteristic findings take months to years to appear, limiting their usefulness for early diagnosis. The earliest radiographic manifestations are soft-tissue swelling around the joint and periarticular osteopenia. Periarticular subchondral erosion of bone, a distinctive radiologic feature of RA, begins to appear within months of clinical onset at the joint margin where pannus has developed. Uniform joint-space narrowing follows later as the joint is destroyed.

Magnetic resonance imaging (MRI) has been studied as a means of improving early recognition of RA. Detection of bone edema by MRI at the time of initial presentation has been found in the research setting to be predictive of bony erosions years later. Whether the use of MRI is specific enough and the increased imaging cost offset by better outcomes remain to be determined.

PRINCIPLES OF MANAGEMENT

Goals and Strategy (15–23)

The goals are to relieve discomfort and preserve joint function, which are achievable by the use of *antiinflammatory drugs* in conjunction with *disease-modifying therapy*. The early initiation of disease-modifying therapy represents a strategic shift in the pharmacologic treatment of RA, which traditionally designated the antiinflammatory agents as first-line drugs and relegated the disease-modifying agents to a second-line role for use in refractory cases. However, the realizations that permanent joint damage starts to take place early in the course of illness and that the timely application of disease-modifying therapy can slow disease progression, preserve joint function, and limit complications triggered a fundamental reordering of priorities. Early initiation of disease-modifying therapy has become the standard of care. The best results are achieved when treatment is started within 3 months of the onset of symptoms, necessitating early diagnosis (see prior discussion). Other important elements of the disease-modifying strategy include the use of *multidrug regimens* and *biologic therapies*, particularly in persons who present with aggressive disease (e.g., systemic symptoms, a high serum titer of RF, extraarticular manifestations, a large number of involved joints, are younger than age 30 years, are women, or prove refractory to standard treatment).

The effective management of RA requires partnership with the rheumatologist to design and implement a comprehensive treatment program that is consistent with the patient's personality and fits well into the patient's lifestyle and home environment. A number of factors must be considered, including age, social and occupational responsibilities, and emotional makeup of the patient; the activity and duration of the disease; and the results of prior therapies. A balanced, multifaceted approach to therapy is most likely to provide optimal results because no single drug or treatment is effective by itself.

Despite the major advances in drug therapy, *nonpharmacologic measures* continue to be critically important in the maintenance of daily function and prevention of disability. The basic components of a program must include thorough patient education, adequate rest, and proper exercise, as well as suppression of inflammation and immune-mediated articular and vascular injury.

Pharmacologic Therapy—Antiinflammatory Agents (15,16,21,24–41)

Antiinflammatory agents continue to have an important role in the management of RA, providing both analgesic and antiinflammatory effects sufficient to achieve a reasonable degree of symptomatic relief. However, they do not prevent early joint destruction or alter the course of RA. Consequently, they are increasingly relegated to a secondary role, prescribed for short-term symptomatic relief in patients with active disease. Among agents in this category are *aspirin*, other salicylates, the nonselective *nonsteroidal antiinflammatory drugs* (NSAIDs), and the *cyclooxygenase-2* (COX-2) *inhibitors*.

Aspirin

Aspirin remains the cornerstone of antiinflammatory pharmacologic therapy for many patients and is the best-proven and least expensive agent for the treatment of RA. Its mechanism of antiinflammatory action involves the inhibition of prostaglandin synthesis. In adults younger than age 60 years, serum levels of 15 to 20 mg/dL are needed to suppress the inflammation of RA effectively. No standard dose predictably achieves this level, but usually at least 3.6 to 4.8 g/d is necessary. Because of the large dose needed and the short half-life (3 to 4 hours) of the drug, the patient must take a large number of tablets multiple times per day. The dose can be increased up to the amount at which tinnitus develops; tinnitus is a dependable and reversible sign of salicylate toxicity in adults. The most frequent adverse effect of aspirin is gastric mucosal injury, with many patients manifesting asymptomatic gastric erosions and some showing frank ulceration (see Chapter 68). Bleeding occasionally is caused by gastritis or ulceration and need not be preceded by symptoms of abdominal pain. Aspirin irreversibly inhibits platelet cyclooxygenase and impedes platelet function (see Chapter 81), causing easy bruising and a predisposition to bleeding. A single dose poisons the platelet for its entire 7-day life span. Small doses of aspirin reduce cardiovascular risk by virtue of their platelet-inhibitory effects. This beneficial effect can be blocked by the concurrent use of a nonselective NSAID (see later discussion).

Because regular aspirin use is directly injurious to the gastric mucosa, additional aspirin preparations have been marketed as less "upsetting to the stomach." *Buffered* aspirin contains bicarbonate, but the amount is insufficient to overcome ambient acid and prevent aspirin-induced mucosal injury. Slightly better tolerated are preparations such as Ascriptin, in which aspirin is combined with a more potent antacid (magnesium hydroxide and aluminum hydroxide), but the cost is markedly increased. *Enteric coating* prevents aspirin from dissolving in the stomach and minimizes the risk for direct gastric mucosal injury; however, bioavailability is delayed, so that the onset of pain relief is slower, and, again, cost is increased.

Nonacetylated Salicylates

Nonacetylated salicylates, such as *salsalate, choline magnesium salicylate,* and *sodium salicylate,* were developed to reduce the risks for gastric injury and platelet inhibition associated with aspirin yet preserve its analgesic and antiinflammatory effects. Lacking an acetyl moiety, these agents do not inhibit platelet cyclooxygenase and can be given to patients who are allergic to aspirin. However, they are still capable of causing gastric injury, and their effectiveness appears to be no better than, and in many instances less than, that of aspirin for patients with RA. The cost is much increased. *Diflunisal,* a derivative of salicylic acid, does not acetylate or break down to salicylate but does act like aspirin by virtue of its ability to inhibit prostaglandin synthesis. For patients with RA, it provides the analgesic and antiinflammatory effects of 2 to 4 g of aspirin daily, with a lower rate of gastrointestinal side effects. However, platelet inhibition does occur and can cause serious gastrointestinal bleeding. The cost of the drug is 15 times that of aspirin.

Nonsteroidal Antiinflammatory Drugs

Although aspirin and its salicylate congeners are also technically NSAIDs, the term is usually reserved for the nonsalicylate derivatives of propionic acid and related organic acids. These potent inhibitors of prostaglandin synthesis are used in RA to provide prompt symptomatic relief, which is achieved by means of their analgesic and antiinflammatory effects. The COX-2 NSAIDs, which are more selective cyclooxygenase inhibitors, have fewer adverse gastrointestinal side effects but appear to be associated with increased cardiovascular risk (see later discussion).

Mechanisms of Action. NSAIDs derive from a host of organic acids (propionic, indolacetic, phenylacetic, enolic, mefenamic) and share the ability to inhibit *cyclooxygenases* (COXs), key enzymes in prostaglandin synthesis. The COX-1 isoform is essential for renal, platelet, gastric mucosal, and vascular function; it is elaborated by the tissues it protects and is present in the serum in rather stable concentrations. The COX-2 isoform participates principally in inflammation, elaborating prostaglandins in response to cytokines and the action of macrophages; however, it may also be involved in the healing of gastric mucosa and some modulation of renal function. All the nonselective NSAIDs inhibit both isoforms of cyclooxygenase and have similar side effect profiles, including significant gastrointestinal toxicity. The promise of the COX-2–selective NSAIDs was antiinflammatory action without the adverse consequences of COX-1 inhibition (e.g., peptic ulcer and bleeding), but concerns subsequently emerged about prothrombotic effects and increased cardiovascular risk (believed to be related to blocking the formation of prostacyclin [PGI2], an arterial vasodilator).

Efficacy. On a milligram-per-milligram basis, NSAIDs are more potent than aspirin and longer acting, so that a marked reduction in the number of tablets taken and the frequency of dosing becomes possible. The degree of pain relief and anti-inflammatory effect achieved is equivalent to that of full-dose aspirin therapy. No particular NSAID (including the COX-2 agents) has consistently proved to be more effective clinically than any other when used at full doses. Nonetheless, some work better for individual patients than others. NSAIDs are sometimes compared according to their values for IC_{50} (concentration that inhibits 50%), an *in vitro* measure of drug efficiency of inhibition, but the IC_{50} has little to do with clinical efficacy. Efficacy is partially a function of dose. Persons not responding to one preparation after 2 to 4 weeks often report benefit when they try another from a different class. This may be a consequence of individual variations in the serum level attained by taking a given dose, but most differences in efficacy are usually a function of compliance with the drug regimen. Patients on agents that must be taken three or four times daily often fare better when they switch to preparations that require dosing only once or twice daily. No synergy is gained when more than one NSAID is used at a time; mechanisms of action are similar for all, and all bind to the same serum proteins. Although they provide relief from inflammatory symptoms, NSAIDs do not appear to alter the course of RA. Their principal role is to relieve symptoms of inflammation.

Adverse Effects. Most gastrointestinal (GI) side effects are related to COX-1 inhibition; adverse cardiovascular effects are believed to be related to COX-2 inhibitory effects on vascular function.

Gastric ulceration and bleeding. The integrity of the gastric mucosa depends on gastric prostaglandin activity and can be compromised by NSAIDs that inhibit COX-1. The consequences of such inhibition include dyspepsia, abdominal pain, peptic ulceration, upper gastrointestinal bleeding, and gastric perforation. The risk for clinically important ulceration is estimated to be 1% to 4% per patient-year of NSAID therapy with a nonselective agent. The risk is significantly less for COX-2–selective NSAIDs.

Risk factors for gastrointestinal complications include previous NSAID-related gastrointestinal side effects (risk of 1.4%/yr), concurrent use of prednisone (risk of 1.2/yr), advancing age (risk of 0.3%/yr for every 5 years older than the age of 50 years), and substantial disability (risk of 0.5%/yr). The total annual risk for a given patient can be estimated by summing these figures. About 15% to 25% of long-term NSAID users demonstrate gastric ulceration at endoscopy; for users of a selective COX-2 inhibitor, the figure is in the range of 5%, just slightly greater than that for placebo.

Risk generally increases with dose and duration of therapy, but up to one fourth of complications have been observed within the first month of therapy. There may be no warning symptoms preceding severe bleeding or perforation. The risk for adverse gastrointestinal effects is similar for all nonselective NSAIDs because they all inhibit gastric prostaglandin synthesis to a significant degree. The use of a prodrug preparation (e.g., nabumetone) provides no advantage because superficial erosions are much less common than with plain aspirin. The use of NSAIDs in patients with a history of peptic ulcer disease, gastrointestinal bleeding, or abdominal pain requires careful monitoring. Unlike aspirin, the nonselective NSAIDs reversibly inhibit platelet cyclooxygenase and impair platelet function only when present in the bloodstream. Nonetheless, gastrointestinal bleeding can turn into life-threatening hemorrhage with concurrent NSAID use, but NSAID-induced prolongation of the bleeding time ceases as soon as the drug is cleared from the blood.

Gastrointestinal risk can be reduced by limiting NSAID dose and duration, adding a proton-pump inhibitor (PPI) such as omeprazole or lansoprazole, using a selective COX-2 inhibitor, treating any concurrent *Helicobacter pylori* infection, and prescribing misoprostol (a gastric prostaglandin analogue) (see Chapter 68). All significantly the reduce the risk of GI adverse effects. Concurrent use of omeprazole reduces the risk to the same degree as switching to a COX-2 agent and avoids the associated cardiovascular risk. However, combination therapy is not entirely risk free, especially in high-risk persons, such as those with a history of NSAID-induced bleeding. In patients requiring long-term NSAID therapy who recently had NSAID-induced ulcer bleeding, the rate of recurrent ulcer bleeding at 6 months is about 5% for COX-2 therapy and 6.5% for NSAID plus PPI. The risk of NSAID-induced upper GI hemorrhage in patients requiring oral anticoagulation therapy is not lowered significantly by the use of a COX-2 agent, but the risk of recurrent bleeding in patients with previous NSAID-induced ulcer can be reduced by adding a PPI to COX-2 therapy. Of note, little reduction is seen in the frequency of minor gastrointestinal side effects (e.g., dyspepsia, mild nausea, diarrhea) with COX-2 drugs.

Cardiovascular effects of nonselective NSAIDs. Although there is some evidence that the antiplatelet effects of nonselective NSAIDs may reduce cardiovascular risk (at least in comparison to COX-2 drugs), there is concern that nonselective NSAIDs may interfere with the cardioprotective effects of low-dose aspirin by blocking access to the acetylation site on platelet cyclooxygenase-1. Any blockade of aspirin's platelet effects can be prevented by taking low-dose aspirin at least 2 hours before nonselective NSAID use. Whether there is an increased cardiovascular risk associated with the use of nonselective NSAIDs remains to be determined; the data are incomplete and conflicting. In addition, there are major differences among nonselective NSAIDs with respect to inhibition of COX-1 and COX-2. The literature should be watched closely.

Cardiovascular risk with COX-2 agents. A significant increase in the risk of adverse cardiovascular events and deaths (relative risk, 1.5 to 3.5) has been observed as a class effect with the use of COX-2 agents, especially if use was sustained (>18 months). These drugs block the formation of the prostaglandin vasodilator PGI2 without inhibiting platelet thromboxane (as occurs with nonselective NSAIDs), perhaps tipping the balance between prothrombotic and antithrombotic NSAID actions and increasing the risk for adverse cardiovascular events. Those agents that seem to confer the highest cardiovascular risk have been withdrawn from the market and cautions issued for the use of other COX-2 drugs that remain available (e.g., celecoxib).

Renal injury. A normal, well-perfused kidney does not depend on renal prostaglandin activity to the extent that an injured, underperfused kidney does. Under situations of hemodynamic stress, prostaglandins serve as important regulators of renal blood flow. Nonselective NSAID use may lead to fluid retention and diminished sodium excretion. Azotemia may worsen, and oliguria and renal shutdown have been reported in patients with preexisting renal disease. The control of hypertension may diminish with NSAID use. The risk for renal toxicity is greatest in the setting of inadequate renal perfusion (congestive heart failure, cirrhosis, dehydration, advanced age, use of potent diuretics). Renal injury may develop after only a few days of therapy but is reversible if NSAIDs are promptly stopped. Monitoring serum creatinine is advisable, especially in high-risk patients. Sulindac may be less nephrotoxic than other preparations because it has little effect on renal prostaglandin synthesis. NSAIDs may impair the action of antihypertensive agents. No nephrotoxicity has been reported with the prolonged use of high-dose aspirin.

No long-term data are available on the clinical effects of the COX-2 agents with regard to renal function and blood pressure control, but data suggest that the degree of risk for renal impairment in elderly persons is approximately the same as for nonselective NSAIDs. In a randomized, 6-month trial comparing celecoxib with diclofenac, the risk of an adverse renal event (hypertension, peripheral edema, renal failure) was high in both groups (24.3% vs. 30.8%) and not significantly different. The literature should be followed for longer-term data on the renal effects of COX-2 agents.

Mental impairment. The elderly are particularly susceptible. Cognitive function, mood, or personality may be altered, especially with agents that cross the blood–brain barrier (e.g., indomethacin). Confusion, poor memory, irritability, depression, lassitude, difficulty sleeping, and even paranoid behavior are among the reactions noted. Minor neurologic side effects (e.g., headache, dizziness, lightheadedness) are seen in patients of all ages.

Hepatotoxicity. A mild elevation in liver enzymes is sometimes noted, but severe hepatitis is rare. Cholestatic hepatitis has been reported. Occasional monitoring of the serum aminotransferase (transaminase) suffices; the drug is halted if levels rise to greater than the upper limits of normal.

Drug–drug interactions. NSAIDs inhibit the renal excretion of methotrexate and should not be used concurrently, especially in persons with underlying renal insufficiency.

Selection of NSAID. Because side effects are relatively similar among the traditional NSAIDs, one can use cost, frequency of dose, and response to an empiric trial (2 to 4 weeks at maximum dose) as the basis for selection. Inquiry into experience with NSAIDs can help to save time. Aspirin remains the cheapest form of antiinflammatory therapy, but frequent dosing is required, and a large number of pills must be taken each day. Generic ibuprofen is the most economical of the modern NSAIDs, but dosing three times daily is required. Generic naproxen is the least expensive of the twice-daily NSAID formulations. Generic indomethacin is also inexpensive, but its utility is limited by the frequency and severity of gastrointestinal and central nervous system side effects, especially in the elderly. Piroxicam offers once-daily dosing but at a greatly increased cost.

COX-2 agents are no longer recommended as first-line NSAID therapy because of cardiovascular safety concerns. Use should be limited to persons who cannot tolerate nonselective NSAIDs (even when complemented by PPI therapy), especially those with a history of peptic ulcer, bleeding, perforation, general debility, concurrent steroid use, or advanced age. COX-2 therapy should be avoided or at least limited to short-term, low-dose use and only in persons free of overt cardiovascular disease or multiple atherosclerotic risk factors. Prescribing a proton-pump inhibitor or misoprostol in conjunction with a nonselective NSAID may be a reasonable alternative to COX-2 use. Quickly implementing effective disease-modifying therapy

TABLE 156.1

RELATIVE COSTS OF SOME DRUGS FOR RHEUMATOID ARTHRITIS

Drug and Dosage	Relative Cost per Month
Antiinflammatory Agents	
Enteric-coated aspirin, 3.6 g/d	1.0
Ibuprofen 800 mg tid (generic)	1.2
Naproxen 500 mg bid (generic)	1.8
Celecoxib 200 mg bid	9.5
Prednisone 10 mg/d	0.4
Synthetic Disease-Modifying Agents	
Methotrexate 17.5 mg/wk	4.2
Sulfasalazine 2 g/d	2.3
Hydroxychloroquine 400 mg/d	2.4
Leflunomide 20 mg/d	15.5
Gold salts 50 mg/mo	1.0
Cyclosporine 175 mg/d	26.3
Biologic Disease-Modifying Agents	
Etanercept 25 mg SC twice weekly Others similarly expensive	63.1

bid, twice daily; SC, subcutaneously; tid, thrice daily.
Adapted from Goldring SR. JAMA 2000;283:524, with permission.

is probably a good way to limit the duration and intensity of NSAID therapy.

Corticosteroids

The oral systemic glucocorticosteroids (e.g., prednisone) occupy an intermediate position in the spectrum of pharmacologic therapies for RA, being both antiinflammatory agents capable of providing prompt symptomatic relief and immunosuppressive drugs with some disease-modifying potential. Low-dose prednisone started in the early stages of symptomatic RA may have a modest joint-sparing effect, but more confirmatory and longer-term data are needed before steroids can be considered a valuable disease-modifying treatment.

Because of the many adverse effects associated with high-dose, long-term use (see Chapter 105), corticosteroids are most often relegated to relatively short courses at low doses (e.g., 4 weeks at <10 mg/d of prednisone). Steroids are tapered to the lowest effective dose once symptoms are brought under control and discontinued as soon as other disease-modifying therapy takes hold. Such treatment helps to bridge the gap between initial presentation and the taking hold of other disease-modifying therapies. Sometimes longer courses of steroid therapy are needed to maintain symptomatic control despite the use of other disease-modifying agents. Should vasculitis or other serious systemic complications develop, high-dose therapy (e.g., prednisone 40 to 60 mg/d) is indicated.

Prolonged steroid therapy is to be avoided. Short courses of steroids that become long can produce severe *osteoporosis,* *muscle atrophy, ligamentous weakening,* and *aseptic necrosis* of the femoral head. Often, twice-daily administration is required to control symptoms adequately, which increases the risk for *hypothalamic–pituitary–adrenal suppression* (see Chapter 105). In extremely difficult situations, such as a disabling flare-up of joint disease, very low dose therapy (5.0 to 7.5 mg of prednisone per day) may be restarted to tide the patient over until additional disease-modifying therapy takes effect. The only clear indication for parenteral high-dose steroid treatment is life-threatening extraarticular disease, such as vasculitis, pericarditis, or alveolitis. Intraarticular injection of a long-acting steroid preparation may improve functional status when one large, weight-bearing joint is disproportionately inflamed. However, repeated steroid injections into the same joint may hasten its degeneration and increase the risk for infection.

Pharmacologic Therapy—Disease-Modifying Antirheumatic Drugs (DMARDs)
(15,15,21,42–59)

Major improvements in treatment outcomes have resulted from the earlier application and development of disease-modifying therapies. Disease-modifying antirheumatic drugs (DMARDs) target key elements of the immunopathologic sequence, halting or slowing disease progression and limiting permanent joint damage. No longer is disease-modifying therapy reserved for those who fail NSAID therapy; it is now implemented as soon as possible after confirmation of the diagnosis. Response rates approaching 75% are attainable. Combination therapy, using DMARDs with complementary modes of action, can improve outcomes without increasing toxic side effects (analogous to combination cancer chemotherapy). As in cancer chemotherapy, optimizing the safe and effective use of these potent drugs requires consultation and coordination with a specialist experienced in their application (in this case, a rheumatologist).

DMARD Classes and Use

DMARDS are classified as *synthetic* and *biologic* (*tumor necrosis factor [TNF] inactivators, interleukin-1 inhibitors, anti–B cell agents,* and *costimulation signal modifiers*). The first-line synthetic disease-modifying agents are *methotrexate, sulfasalazine,* and *hydroxychloroquine*; as noted, *glucocorticosteroids* also evidence some disease-modifying activity. Second-line synthetic agents in this category include *gold, penicillamine, cyclosporine,* and most recently *leflunomide*.

Disease-modifying therapy often begins with a synthetic agent, typically methotrexate, because it is effective, orally active, relatively inexpensive, and well tolerated; parenteral administration is usually required for the administration of biologic agents. Because the clinical onset of action may take weeks with synthetic DMARDs, the initial program may require concurrent short-term use of an antiinflammatory agent (e.g., low-dose prednisone; see prior discussion) promptly to bring symptoms under control. The DMARDs with the fastest onset of action are the TNF inactivators and prednisone (days), followed by methotrexate (6 weeks) and other synthetic agents (weeks to months). It is not known whether rapidly acting agents should be used initially because it is unclear whether rapid suppression of symptoms is necessary to maximize long-term outcomes. Even with early onset, the maximum effect may take longer. Biologic agents are being added in place of many older, more toxic synthetic drugs when first-line synthetic therapy proves to be insufficient.

Indefinite continuation of disease-modifying therapy appears to be necessary because disease activity returns when treatment is stopped, but the use of potent therapy at the outset may allow tapering over time. Nonetheless, even limited courses of treatment (especially with the use of biologic agents) can provide some lasting benefit (e.g., better joint preservation). More data are needed to determine the optimum duration of therapy.

Drug-related toxicity can be substantial with DMARD use (see later discussion), and the cost of treatment can be high (see Table 156.1). Nonetheless, the documented efficacy of DMARDs in this potentially disabling disease strongly argues for their early and full application.

Methotrexate

Methotrexate is an antimetabolite that inhibits purine biosynthesis, which is essential to rapidly proliferating cells (such as those of the rheumatoid pannus). Most RA patients are started on methotrexate, which has become the standard for initial disease-modifying treatment. It is effective, well tolerated, and among the fastest acting of the disease-modifying drugs, often controlling symptoms within 6 weeks. It is comparable in efficacy to the other synthetic disease-modifying agents (e.g., sulfasalazine, intramuscular gold, penicillamine).

Use. Treatment is started with low-dose therapy (e.g., 7.5 to 15.0 mg/wk) and increased as needed every 1 to 2 months in 5-mg/wk increments until signs of active joint disease resolve (effective dose range, 17.5 to 30.0 mg/wk). The liquid methotrexate preparation is the least expensive. Parenteral administration is used when high doses are needed or there are concerns with oral intake (e.g., poor response to treatment, gastrointestinal upset, stomatitis). The drug is contraindicated in pregnancy, and if it is used in women of reproductive age, then detailed patient education and birth control are essential.

Adverse Effects. Short-term, low-dose therapy is well tolerated, but *bone marrow suppression, hepatocellular injury,* and *idiosyncratic interstitial pneumonitis* can occur. The latter may lead to *pulmonary fibrosis* and is important to recognize early. Mild, nonprogressive *elevations in hepatocellular enzymes* are common and not a contraindication to continuing therapy, although the dose is often lowered, and careful monitoring is required. Longer-term therapy is often given and is well tolerated, but once the cumulative dose of methotrexate exceeds 1.5 g, the risk for *hepatic fibrosis* may begin to increase, although the probability of developing frank cirrhosis remains very low.

Alcohol use is contraindicated. Folic acid supplementation (1 to 3 mg/d) reduces the risk for drug toxicity without reducing efficacy. Aspirin and NSAIDs can slow the rate of methotrexate excretion and increase gastrointestinal toxicity. Renal dysfunction is a contraindication to use.

Monitoring of methotrexate therapy by laboratory tests includes a *complete blood cell count* (CBC), *alanine aminotransferase, albumin, blood urea nitrogen,* and *creatinine* every 4 to 8 weeks, especially at the outset of treatment. The need for *liver biopsy* after large doses have accumulated is unresolved; clinical judgment is required.

Hydroxychloroquine

Antimalarial therapy is not as effective as methotrexate but is better tolerated and therefore a reasonable selection as an initial disease-modifying therapy for patients with mild disease. At least 4 to 6 weeks of therapy is needed before results are detectable; full benefit may not be evident before 3 to 4 months.

The most serious toxic effect is *visual impairment* (even blindness) caused by drug accumulation in the retina; this complication is extremely rare when doses are limited to 200 to 400 mg/d. Regular (every 6 to 12 months) ophthalmologic screening is indicated for patients who have been taking hydroxychloroquine for years or who have renal insufficiency; the yield is very low in those who take less than 6.5 mg/kg per day. Tinnitus and vertigo are sometimes noted.

Sulfasalazine

Sulfasalazine has a long-standing record of efficacy and safety in inflammatory bowel disease and as an alternative to hydroxychloroquine for patients with mild RA. It may be superior to hydroxychloroquine. Its safety profile makes it a popular first-line disease-modifying agent to be used in combination with methotrexate or when there is a contraindication to methotrexate.

Hypersensitivity to its sulfa moiety is common, so that its use is limited in patients who are allergic to sulfa. Because of occasional *hepatocellular injury* and minor degrees of *myelosuppression*, a periodic check (every 2 to 4 weeks for 3 months, then every 3 to 4 months) of the complete blood cell count and aminotransferase levels is necessary. Gastrointestinal upset (anorexia, nausea, vomiting, diarrhea) is more common. Reversible oligospermia has been noted.

Combination Therapy with First-Line Synthetic Drugs

Combination programs are increasingly being instituted by rheumatologists if a patient's response to initial disease-modifying therapy with a single agent proves to be inadequate after several months. Combining several first-line disease-modifying agents (e.g., methotrexate, hydroxychloroquine, and sulfasalazine) achieves enhanced response rates. Not only is disease control improved, but in addition combination therapy allows smaller doses of each drug to be administered, reducing or at least minimizing the overall risk of adverse effects. Whether combination therapy should be the initial program of choice remains a subject of debate and ongoing study, but it can obviate the need for using more-toxic second-line drugs and resorting to extremely expensive biologic therapies.

Second-Line Synthetic Agents

Second-line agents in this group include older drugs that have been relegated to second-line status because of toxicity (e.g., gold, penicillamine, cyclosporine) and newer agents that have been developed as alternatives to methotrexate (e.g., leflunomide).

Leflunomide. Leflunomide is a new pyrimidine-synthesis inhibitor that interferes with the cell cycle in rapidly proliferating cells such as activated lymphocytes. Theoretically, its effects would be additive to those of methotrexate and might be useful as a complementary or alternative therapy. In placebo-controlled comparison studies with methotrexate, it demonstrated a similar degree of disease-modifying activity but not quite the same degree of tolerability, being more likely to cause diarrhea and allergic skin reactions. In combination with methotrexate, it increased response rates but also the risk of hepatic toxicity. In persons who cannot tolerate methotrexate, it may be tried as an alternative. It is contraindicated in pregnancy, necessitating the use of contraception and a negative pregnancy test before initiation of treatment. Because of a long half-life and active metabolites, the drug must be actively eliminated by using cholestyramine before a woman attempts to conceive.

Gold. Gold was the first disease-modifying agent. Because of the requirement for parenteral administration (oral therapy is of only marginal benefit), the frequency and severity of adverse effects, and the need for constant monitoring of blood and urine, gold has been relegated to a secondary role among disease-modifying agents. It is usually reserved for patients with moderate to severe disease who fail or cannot take methotrexate or combination therapy with other first-line drugs. Treatment may temporarily halt or even partially reverse articular erosion in up to 60% of cases, but fewer than 2% of patients treated have remissions that last longer than 3 years. The effects of gold are cumulative. Those who are going to respond do so by the time a total of 1,000 mg has been given. Adverse effects are often idiosyncratic and range from *rashes* and buccal cavity *mucosal ulcers* to *bone marrow suppression, glomerulonephritis, interstitial pneumonitis,* and *exfoliative dermatitis.* Most side effects are reversible if the medication is stopped immediately.

Cyclosporine. Cyclosporine was developed to provide more selective inhibition of the immune mechanisms involved in autoimmune disease while leaving other immune pathways relatively unaffected. It is a selective T cell immunosuppressor and is used as a second- or third-line agent in patients with active disease who fail combination therapy with first-line drugs. Combination with methotrexate has proved to be useful in refractory disease. Adverse effects include renal insufficiency, anemia, hypertension, and hirsutism; periodic checks of blood cell counts, renal function, and potassium levels are necessary.

Penicillamine. Penicillamine is a chelating agent that can slow aggressive disease. Adverse effects are similar to those of parenteral gold and are best mitigated by giving low doses and increasing them slowly. Fewer than 50% of patients given the drug are able to continue it for prolonged treatment. Fatal *aplastic anemia, leukopenia, agranulocytosis,* and *thrombocytopenia* can occur. Proteinuria is seen in 10% to 15% of cases and may progress to the nephrotic syndrome. Rashes and autoimmune syndromes such as myasthenia gravis have been reported. The drug is contraindicated in pregnancy. It should be reserved for those who fail to respond to all other forms of therapy and should be prescribed only under the supervision of a rheumatologist skilled in its use.

Minocycline. Minocycline is a tetracycline derivative with prominent antiinflammatory and immunosuppressive effects, including the inhibition of synovial collagenase, metalloproteinases, lymphocyte proliferation, and cell division. Randomized, placebo-controlled trials in patients requiring disease-modifying therapy have provided encouraging results, although the degree of clinical benefit appears to be modest at best. More study is required to define its efficacy and safety in comparison with other forms of disease-modifying therapy.

Cyclophosphamide and Azathioprine. The combination of these cytotoxic immunosuppressive agents had been reserved for patients with otherwise refractory disease. This therapy has been largely replaced by the use of biologic disease-modifying agents. Cyclophosphamide is used to treat systemic vasculitis. Both agents are contraindicated in pregnancy because they are *teratogenic.* The risk for malignancy is increased, especially with cyclophosphamide. Other adverse effects of cyclophosphamide include *hemorrhagic cystitis, marrow suppression,* and *sterility.* Azathioprine use is associated with gastrointestinal upset, hepatitis, and marrow depression, but the risk is low with the small doses given to patients with RA.

Biologic Agents

Advances in understanding the autoimmune and inflammatory mechanisms of RA have led to development of biologic agents for the treatment of refractory disease. Biologic therapies attempt to block key elements of the autoimmune cascade, such as the pathophysiologically important cytokines

TNF-α, interleukin-1, B cell lymphocytes, and costimulation moderator. Although they are extremely expensive and require parenteral administration, these agents can significantly improve rates of disease control, especially in patients with otherwise refractory disease. Although initial results are very encouraging and these drugs appear to be well tolerated, data from long-term study will be needed to verify efficacy, safety, and cost-effectiveness. Referral to a rheumatologist is essential when considering biologic therapy. In about half of instances of poorly controlled disease, the expense of biologic therapy can be spared by implementing a multidrug program of first-line synthetic agents (see prior discussion).

Tumor-Necrosis-Factor Inactivators. The biologic agents capable of inactivating TNF-α include *etanercept, infliximab,* and *adalimumab.* All of these agents inactivate circulating TNF-α by binding it; some also kill inflammatory cells that express TNF-α. Many patients previously unresponsive to first-line disease-modifying therapy demonstrate significant and prompt (within a few weeks) improvement in response when one of these agents is added to a standard program of disease-modifying therapy. Response rates improve two- to fivefold, with more than 70% of patients having at least a 20% reduction in symptoms.

Etanercept is a fusion protein made up of two soluble TNF receptors grafted onto the Fc portion of a human immunoglobulin molecule by recombinant methods. *Infliximab,* a monoclonal antibody that binds TNF and also kills cells that express TNF-α, was the first TNF-α inactivator. It is composed of a murine TNF-binding site grafted onto a human immunoglobulin G. *Adalimumab* is a human monoclonal antibody that binds to TNF-α; it too lyses cells that express TNF-α.

Although they are well tolerated (local irritation at the injection site is the most common adverse effect, as are headache and nausea in those receiving treatment by infusion), these agents are at least theoretically capable of impairing immunosurveillance and response. Quantitative data from long-term study on risks of opportunistic infection and cancer are not available, but case reports suggest increased risks of *tuberculosis, histoplasmosis, listeriosis,* and possibly *lymphoma.* RA also increases the risks of these conditions, so the true levels of risk are hard to ascertain. Nonetheless, all patients who are being considered for TNF-α therapy should undergo screening for tuberculosis (see Chapter 38). Persons with active infection or chronic infection should be excluded from treatment.

Because these agents are antigenic, they may generate antibody responses, but there is no evidence for these responses limiting efficacy or triggering adverse reactions. ANA positivity has been noted frequently, but cases of true drug-induced lupus are very rare. As experience with these drugs accumulates, it will facilitate determination of risk.

Interleukin-1 Inhibitors. *Anakinra* is a recombinant form of an interleukin-1 inhibitor that targets the interleukin-1 receptor. In RA, there are reduced amounts of circulating interleukin-1 inhibitor. It has proved to be effective in combination with methotrexate. Skin irritation at the injection site is the most common side effect. The absolute risk of serious bacterial infection is increased by about 1.5%, necessitating monitoring for infection. A small risk of reversible neutropenia and thrombocytopenia require monitoring of the CBC. Combination use with a TNF antagonist increases the risk of infection to an unacceptably high level.

Anti–B Cell Therapy. *Rituximab* is a chimeric anti-CD20 monoclonal antibody that attacks B cells and is primarily used in non-Hodgkin's lymphoma. Its use in RA is under study, stim-ulated by interest in the role of B cells in RA. When just two infusions are added to methotrexate therapy, the drug produces significant and lasting improvements in outcome. The risk of serious infection is low (as expected, because the treatment does not impair overall antibody production).

Selective Costimulation Modulator Therapy. *Abatacept,* a selective costimulation signal modulator, represents a new approach to RA treatment, targeting the alternative pathway to T cell activation. It produces significant clinical improvement in persons who respond inadequately to anti-TNF therapy. Experience with its use is limited, but the evidence suggests particular usefulness in persons with established disease, in which the costimulation signal is believed to play an important role in the maintenance of the inflammatory process. More data are required to determine its precise role in the management of RA.

Choice of Disease-Modifying Therapy

The choice of therapy remains largely empirical, pending the advent of genetic and other promising approaches to help predict response. The evidence of efficacy shows no clinically significant differences among synthetic disease-modifying antirheumatic drugs (DMARDs; methotrexate, sulfasalazine, and leflunomide) or the biologic DMARDs (the anti-TNF drugs adalimumab, etanercept, and infliximab). Single anti-TNF drugs produce better radiologic outcomes than those seen with methotrexate, but clinical outcomes are similar. Combinations of methotrexate and anti-TNF agents produce better response rates and outcomes than does monotherapy with either class of drug alone. In the setting of failure to respond to monotherapy, combination therapy with synthetic DMARDs improves response.

Rates and severity of short-term adverse events appear to be similar for both classes of drugs; data for rare events associated with anti-TNF drugs are limited. The risks of solid cancers and lymphomas do not appear to be increased, but rates of skin cancers are elevated. Longer-term studies are needed, as are trials in community settings.

Nonpharmacologic Measures and Other Therapies (15,21,60–68)

Despite the attention garnered by pharmacologic therapy, the importance of nonpharmacologic measures cannot be overemphasized. Controlled trials have demonstrated that nonpharmacologic programs along with detailed patient education (see later discussion) can provide as much benefit in terms of functional improvement as many pharmacologic therapies and reduce the costs of care by reducing the number of visits and time lost from work.

In addition to targeting the underlying disease process, effective management also necessitates addressing pain control, risks of complicating illnesses, and functional disability. When disease remains refractory, consideration of extreme measures is required. In a chronic disease as difficult as RA, it is not surprising that patients will try a host of remedies, often many that are neither prescribed or nor evidence based; skillful care requires being aware of such therapies and helping the patient to view them in proper perspective.

Exercise

Exercise helps to maintain range of motion and muscle strength. The goals are to strengthen supporting muscles and minimize the chances of postinflammatory contracture. Exercises that safely put involved joints through a full range of motion are taught to the patient. When pain is too severe for active exercises, isometrics can be performed, and passive exercises can be prescribed and carried out by a physical therapist. Joints with a tense effusion should not be exercised because compression of the synovium may lead to ischemic injury. Prior application of *heat* or *cold* (either may work) will facilitate the exercise program. Hot baths, paraffin soaks, or ice packs are often efficacious in loosening stiff joints. Moist heat is also useful in relieving pain and shortening the duration of morning stiffness.

Exercises involving important muscle groups are prescribed to counteract the development of atrophy, strengthen periarticular tissues, and preserve joint stability. A judicious program of walking can play a similar role. The design and execution of an exercise program can be facilitated by the participation of a physical therapist. To protect the joint from damaging stress, the patient can be instructed in the use of implements that provide a mechanical advantage. Such "joint savers" are available commercially and are most helpful for tasks requiring use of the hands.

Rest and Splinting

Rest and splinting can be helpful, but in the patient with mild to moderate disease, complete bed rest is not only unnecessary but also potentially harmful. Prolonged rest may lead to flexion contractures, osteoporosis, and muscle atrophy. Only the patient whose acute disease is severe enough to warrant hospitalization should be put to bed, in which case some benefit is derived. However, a period of rest during the day can be of considerable benefit to those patients with persistently active disease who are less ill, most of whom are usually bothered by fatigue. Selectively resting individual joints by splinting can help to relieve pain and prevent contracture of severely inflamed joints, especially those too swollen to be exercised. The principle is to maintain the joint in its physiologic position, especially during periods when the joint is stressed. Splinting of the wrist at night is the best example of this form of therapy. The pain of a patient with tenosynovitis of the wrist can be decreased and flexion deformity, with its attendant loss of grip, can be prevented. A wrist splint applied at night places the joint in 10 to 15 degrees of extension. A cervical collar worn at night can provide similar relief when the cervical spine is involved. The patient with deformed feet requires specially constructed shoes.

Dietary Measures and Supplements

Dietary measures and supplements are always appealing to patients because they offer a "natural" and presumably safe way to treat their illness. Surveys reveal that almost two thirds of patients with RA have tried dietary measures and megavitamin supplements, and about half of that group continue regular use. Although evidence of efficacy is lacking for most of these measures and supplements, an adequate *calcium* and *vitamin D* intake must be maintained because almost all patients with RA are at risk for osteoporosis, either from their disease or from its treatment. For patients taking low doses of glucocorticoids, an adequate intake of calcium and vitamin D has proved to be sufficient to prevent mineral loss. A total of 1.5 to 2.0 g of calcium daily and 400 IU of vitamin D daily is required and can be obtained by dietary measures and the use of low-cost supplements (see Chapter 164).

Claims for the efficacy of other dietary measures and supplements, usually put forward by commercial interests, continue to bombard patients; most are unproven. The results of well-designed, small-scale, prospective trials of high-dose γ-*linolenic acid* (an essential fatty acid and close precursor of

prostaglandin E1 with demonstrated antiinflammatory and immunoregulatory activity) have been promising. Essential fatty acids may also have an immunomodulatory effect independent of prostaglandin activity. The dihydro metabolite of γ-linolenic acid manifests such an effect, acting directly on T cells *in vitro* to suppress the proliferation of interleukin-dependent T lymphocytes. The value of γ-linoleic acid remains to be established by large-scale, prospective, randomized trials.

Based on studies of *fish oil supplements*, diets high in fish and plant fatty acids and low in animal fatty acids may confer a modest degree of subjective improvement. Such fatty acids are essential for the maintenance of cell membrane structure and function.

A popular diet free of additives, preservatives, fruit, red meat, herbs, and dairy products has been advocated as a treatment for RA. The only controlled, double-blinded, randomized study of this therapy failed to show any benefit in patients with long-standing, progressive, active RA.

Analgesics

In rare instances, a short course of narcotic analgesics (see Chapter 235) may be required for comfort, but with earlier and more effective treatment the need for potent analgesia should lessen.

Prevention and Treatment of Osteoporosis

The risk for the development of osteoporosis is markedly increased in RA by both inactivity and the use of glucocorticoids. Preventive measures are critical and effective. Adequate dietary calcium and vitamin D are essential components of any program for osteoporosis. All RA patients, but especially those taking corticosteroids and postmenopausal women, should undergo screening for osteoporosis by dual-energy x-ray absorptiometry bone scanning (see Chapter 144). Persons found to be osteopenic are candidates for bisphosphonate therapy (e.g., alendronate, risedronate; see Chapter 164).

Prevention and Treatment of Atherosclerotic Risk Factors

With atherosclerotic risk increased in rheumatoid arthritis, it is important to screen for and aggressively treat major cardiovascular risk factors, including hypertension, dyslipidemias, smoking, and diabetes (see Chapters 26, 27, 54, and 102). Whether reduction in the inflammation associated with rheumatoid disease has any beneficial effect on cardiovascular risk remains to be seen, but modest elevations in C-reactive protein have been identified as an independent risk factor for adverse cardiovascular events (see Chapters 15, 26, 27, 30, and 31).

Prevention and Treatment of Infection

Yearly influenza vaccination and periodic administration of the pneumonia vaccine are essential. Vaccinations should be brought up to date prior to the initiation of methotrexate, prednisone, and other potentially immunosuppressive therapies. The presence of infection is an indication to halt RA therapy and treat the infection aggressively. Persons being considered for biologic therapy need to be screened for latent tuberculosis (see prior discussion).

Surgery

Arthroplasty is an important component of therapy in patients with destroyed joints and marked disability. Hip and knee procedures are most successful; the outcome in hand, wrist, elbow, and ankle reconstructions is less certain, but rapid progress is being made. The risk for loosening of a hip prosthesis is significant (25%), even in the absence of active disease. Conventional synovectomy is generally ineffective and results in loss of joint motion; however, arthroscopic synovectomy may permit the control of particularly severe monoarticular disease involving the knee.

Total Lymphoid Irradiation and Apheresis

Total lymphoid irradiation and apheresis represent desperate attempts to inhibit the immunopathology of RA. Controlled studies of irradiation suggest some benefit in extreme situations, but the risk for infection is markedly increased. The rationale behind apheresis is to remove immune complexes and other mediators of the inflammatory process. Placebo-controlled studies have failed to show significant benefit. The selective removal of lymphocytes from peripheral blood (leukopheresis) has yielded transient mild clinical improvement in refractory cases but not of sufficient magnitude to justify the high cost. With the development of safer, more effective therapies, the demand for such extreme measures should fade.

Alternative and Complementary Measures

Patients try a wide range of alternative measures (e.g., chiropractic manipulation, special dietary supplements, biofeedback, herbal therapies, salves, magnets, acupuncture). Surveys of arthritis patients being seen by rheumatologists find that up to half tried at least one of these alternatives in the past and that nearly one fourth continue to make regular use of at least one of them. Predictors of regular use include severe pain and a college degree. Evidence of their efficacy is nonexistent for most, but some should soon be tested in randomized, placebo-controlled trials now that the National Institutes of Health is funding the formal study of these measures.

Monitoring (16)

Disease activity and response to therapy are best monitored by reproducible clinical measures, such as the duration of *morning stiffness*, the *number of tender swollen joints*, and *grip strength* (which can be measured with a blood pressure cuff). *Time required to walk 15 m* and *ring size* are also helpful. *Erythrocyte sedimentation rate* (ESR) and *C-reactive protein* (CRP) measure acute-phase reactants that are sensitive but nonspecific indicators of inflammatory activity. The *titer of RF* does not correlate with disease activity but does decrease in response to some treatments.

Outcomes research has emphasized the utility of additional measures of function, such as the answers to questions regarding psychosocial functioning and the activities of daily living included in the *Health Assessment Questionnaire* and the *Arthritis Impact Measurement Scale*. The *patient's self-assessment* and the *physician's global assessment* also demonstrate validity. Incorporating these validated parameters, the American College of Rheumatology developed the *ACR outcome measure*. The ACR 20 refers to a 20% reduction in the number of tender and swollen joints plus a similar percentage of improvements in pain, global patient and physician assessments, self-assessed physical disability, ESR, and CRP. The more demanding ACR 50 requires a 50% improvement in parameters.

Detecting early disease progression is more difficult but very important if disease-modifying therapy is to be instituted in a timely fashion. Joint-space narrowing is a specific but late radiographic sign of cartilaginous erosion that may not develop until irreversible damage has already occurred. Magnetic reso-

nance imaging has been used experimentally to detect synovial proliferation and early pannus formation, but the cost remains prohibitive for routine use. The best determinant of disease progression is the duration of symptoms.

PATIENT EDUCATION AND COUNSELING (15,21,60,61,63,65,69)

As shown in a randomized trial of the Arthritis Self-help Course (a model program of basic patient education), patient education and counseling is well worth the time invested because it helps to reduce pain, disability, and frequency of physician visits. It represents a most cost-effective intervention.

Informing the Patient of the Diagnosis

With a potentially disabling disease such as RA, the act of informing the patient of the diagnosis takes on major importance. The goal is to satisfy the patient's informational needs regarding the diagnosis, prognosis, and treatment without going into an overwhelming and excessive amount of detail. Careful questioning and empathic listening are required to understand the patient's perspective, requests, and fears. Telling patients more than they are intellectually or psychologically prepared to deal with (a common practice) risks making the experience so intense as to trigger withdrawal. On the other hand, failing to address issues of importance to the patient compromises the development of trust. The patient needs to know that the primary physician understands the situation and will be available for support, advice, and therapy as the need arises. Encouraging the patient to ask questions helps to communicate interest and caring.

Discussing Prognosis and Treatment

Patients and family do best when they know what to expect and can view the illness realistically. Uncertainty contributes heavily to the "disease" of RA. Many fear crippling consequences and dependency. The most common disease manifestations should be described. Without building false hopes, the physician can point out that spontaneous remissions are frequent and that more than two thirds of patients live independently without major disability. In addition, it should be emphasized that much can be done to minimize discomfort and preserve function. A review of available therapies and their efficacy helps to overcome feelings of depression stemming from an erroneous expectation of inevitable disability. Even in patients with severe disease, guarded optimism is now appropriate, given the host of effective and well-tolerated disease-modifying treatments that are emerging. A major fear is abandonment. Patients are relieved to know that they will be followed closely by the primary physician and health care team, working in conjunction with a consulting rheumatologist and physical/occupational therapist, all of whom are committed to maximizing the patient's comfort and independence and preserving joint function.

Dealing with Misconceptions

Several common misconceptions deserve attention. A substantial proportion of patients and their families feel that they have done something to cause the illness. Explaining that there are no known controllable precipitants helps to eliminate much unnecessary guilt and self-recrimination. Dealing in an informative, evidence-based fashion with a patient who expresses interest in alternative and complementary forms of therapy can help limit expenditures on ineffective treatments. Another misconception is that a medication has to be expensive to be helpful. Aspirin, generic NSAIDs, low-dose prednisone, and the first-line disease-modifying agents are quite inexpensive yet remarkably effective, a point that bears emphasizing. The sense that one must be treated with a COX-2 NSAID or the latest TNF inactivator can be addressed by a careful review of the overall treatment program and the proper role of such agents in the patient's plan of care. The active participation of the patient and family in the design and implementation of the therapeutic program helps to boost morale and ensure compliance, as does explaining the rationale for the therapies used.

Preserving Independence

A major goal is to preserve the patient's sense of worth and independence. However, when fatigue, morning stiffness, or specific joint disease interferes with a patient's capacity to carry out the usual responsibilities at work and at home, counseling is necessary to recommend modification of work responsibilities and perhaps retraining. With the use of occupational therapy, the treatment effort is geared to helping the patient maintain a meaningful work role within the limitations of the illness. The family plays an important part in striking the proper balance between dependence and independence. Household members should avoid overprotecting the patient (e.g., refraining from intercourse out of fear of hurting the patient) and work to sustain the patient's pride and ability to contribute to the family. Allowing the patient with RA to struggle with a task is sometimes constructive.

Supporting the Patient with Debilitating Disease

Persons with long-standing severe disease who have already sustained much irreversible joint destruction benefit from an emphasis on comfort measures, supportive counseling, and attention to minimizing further debility. Such patients need help in grieving for their disfigurement and loss of function. An accepting, unhurried, empathic manner allows the patient to express feelings. The seemingly insignificant act of touching does much to restore a sense of self-acceptance. Attending to pain with increased social support, medication, and a refocusing of attention onto function is useful. A trusting and strong patient–doctor relationship can do much to sustain a patient through times of discomfort and disability.

INDICATIONS FOR REFERRAL AND ADMISSION (15,17–19)

Referral

The importance of early diagnosis and prompt initiation of disease-modifying therapy argue for a close working relationship with a consulting *rheumatologist*. Patients who present with signs of very aggressive disease suggesting a poor prognosis and those who fail or cannot tolerate standard first-line ther-

apy should be referred for consideration of multidrug regimens and biologic therapies. Patients requiring programs associated with a high risk for serious toxicity should be periodically seen by the rheumatologist; those on programs that are better tolerated can be managed almost exclusively by the primary care physician. In all cases, a close working relationship with the rheumatologist is essential.

Referral to *physical* and *occupational therapists* is greatly appreciated by patients with active disease. The emphasis should be on teaching the patient things that can be done to improve function. Well-designed exercise and self-care programs can greatly facilitate carrying out the activities of daily living and reduce discomfort and disability.

The need for *surgical referral* is best determined by the rheumatologist, who is well trained to judge when medical therapy is insufficient. Examples of indications for surgery include carpal tunnel syndrome that persists despite corticosteroid injection, trigger-finger deformity, tendon rupture with loss of manual dexterity, and refractory dorsal wrist effusions. The patient with disabling hip or knee destruction and severe impairment of weight-bearing capacity deserves a surgical assessment regarding possible prosthetic joint replacement. Arthroscopic synovectomy may be needed for a single, very refractory joint that cannot be replaced.

Hospital Admission

When fever or other manifestations of severe extraarticular disease appear (especially signs of vasculitis or diffuse serositis), then hospital admission for workup and intravenous administration of steroids should be promptly considered.

THERAPEUTIC RECOMMENDATIONS (15,16)

- Definitively establish the diagnosis as early as possible (preferably just after 6 weeks of continuous disease activity and within the first 3 months) based on characteristic clinical findings supplemented by serologic testing (RF, anti-CCP).
- Provide a comprehensive patient and family education program that includes psychological support and strategies for maintaining the patient's activity, independence, and self-esteem (see later discussion). Use health care team members to enhance the educational and supportive efforts and work in close collaboration with the rheumatologist.
- Within 3 months of the onset of active disease, start disease-modifying therapy with a first-line synthetic agent (e.g., *methotrexate, hydroxychloroquine,* or *sulfasalazine*) or a combination of such agents, being most aggressive with persons having very active disease or indicators of a poor prognosis (e.g., genotype HLA-DRB1*04/04, high serum titer of RF, extraarticular manifestations, large number of involved joints, age younger than 30 years, female gender, systemic symptoms). Arrange rheumatologic referral for these patients.
- If there are no contraindications (pregnancy, refusal to abstain from alcohol), start with *methotrexate* (7.5 mg/wk, given orally once weekly in three divided doses, 12 hours apart, in conjunction with folic acid, 1 mg, 12 to 24 hours after methotrexate). Increase the methotrexate dose by 5 mg/wk once monthly until control is achieved or dose of 30 mg/wk reached. Increased folate proportionately to up to

3 mg/d. Closely monitor the patient for response to therapy and complications of the drug program.

- If there is a contraindication to methotrexate or the disease is mild, consider starting with hydroxychloroquine (starting at 200 mg daily) or sulfasalazine (starting at 1g twice daily). Consider adding either or both to methotrexate when the response to monotherapy is inadequate.
- Monitor first-line therapy periodically:
  - For *methotrexate*, follow the complete blood cell count, platelet count, and levels of aminotransferase, alkaline phosphatase, albumin, blood urea nitrogen, and creatinine. Inquire regularly about any pulmonary symptoms, which might be the first manifestation of interstitial pneumonitis and an indication for immediate cessation of therapy.
  - For *hydroxychloroquine*, inquire regularly about visual acuity and arrange for an ophthalmologic examination every 6 to 12 months.
  - For *sulfasalazine*, monitor the complete blood cell count, inquire about gastrointestinal symptoms, and examine the skin for rashes and pruritus.
- While waiting for disease-modifying therapy to take effect (up to 3 months may be necessary), begin antiinflammatory treatment with a generic *nonselective NSAID* for symptomatic relief (e.g., 3.6 g of enteric-coated *aspirin* daily, 800 mg of *ibuprofen* three times a day, or 500 mg of *naproxen* twice daily).
- Add proton-pump inhibition (e.g., *omeprazole*, 20 to 40 mg/d) to nonselective NSAID therapy for gastroprotection if there is a history of GI complications or GI upset. Consider substituting a *COX-2 agent* for the nonselective NSAID only if other gastroprotective measures do not suffice and the potential cardiovascular risk is deemed acceptable. Until more definitive data are available, weigh and review with the patient the potential cardiovascular risks associated with using a COX-2 agent, especially when considering a program of daily long-term COX-2 use in persons with known cardiovascular disease or multiple thrombotic cardiovascular risk factors. Be sure that the potential cardiovascular risks are deemed acceptable, especially if prolonged COX-2 therapy is anticipated.
- Use NSAIDs with care in patients with impaired renal perfusion or heart failure; monitor blood urea nitrogen and creatinine. Also prescribe cautiously to patients with a prior history of peptic ulcer disease or gastrointestinal bleeding (see Chapter 68); monitor hematocrit and test for fecal occult blood.
- For patients with very active disease inadequately controlled by initial NSAID therapy and waiting for disease-modifying therapy to take hold, consider adding a small daily dose of oral glucocorticosteroid (e.g., *prednisone*, 5 to 7.5 mg/d). Reserve daily use for patients truly limited

by symptoms, and treat with low doses (e.g., <10 mg/d) for as short a time as possible; taper to the lowest possible dose.

- If glucocorticosteroids are to be used for more than 1 month, begin a program of osteoporosis prevention that includes calcium (1.5 g/d) and vitamin D (400 to 800 IU/d) and prophylactic bisphosphonate therapy (e.g., alendronate, 35 mg/wk).
- For patients incapacitated by one disproportionately inflamed large, weight-bearing joint, consider a single *intraarticular injection* of a long-acting corticosteroid (e.g., 2.5 to 10 mg of triamcinolone acetonide, depending on joint size, mixed with 1 mL of lidocaine). Avoid repeated injections into the same joint.
- Once disease-modifying therapy begins to take hold, taper and discontinue NSAIDs and corticosteroids. Continue the disease-modifying program indefinitely.
- Prescribe a gentle exercise program to maintain range of motion and muscle strength, but avoid stressing a severely inflamed joint. Prior application of heat or cold (either may work) will facilitate the exercise program. Consult with a physical therapist to help design the program. The morning application of heat is particularly helpful before the patient engages in daily activity.
- Selectively rest severely inflamed individual joints that are too swollen to exercise. Maintain the joint in its physiologic position by splinting during periods when the joint is stressed (e.g., at night) to support weakened joints and prevent flexion contractures. Consult the rheumatologist if splinting appears to be indicated.
- Advise a daily rest period for patients bothered by generalized fatigue, but outpatients should avoid prolonged bed rest.
- Screen and treat all RA patients for osteoporosis (see Chapters 144 and 164) and for cardiovascular risk factors (see Chapters 26, 27, 54, and 102).
- Regularly immunize all RA patients for influenza and pneumococcal infection.
- Monitor disease activity and response to therapy by checking reproducible measures, such as duration of morning stiffness, sedimentation rate, number of tender swollen joints, and grip strength (have the patient squeeze a blood pressure cuff). Also monitor activities of daily living, psychosocial status, and patient's global assessment.
- Arrange for rheumatologic consultation if the patient manifests persistently active disease after treatment. It may be necessary to advance the disease-modifying regimen or alter it. Increasingly, early rheumatologic consultation and aggressive treatment may be necessary if joint destruction is to be prevented, particularly in patients with findings suggestive of a poor prognosis.

A.H.G.

Annotated Bibliography

1. Choy EHS, Panayi GS. Cytokine pathways and joint inflammation in rheumatoid arthritis. N Engl J Med 2001;344:907. (*An excellent review of disease mechanisms for the generalist clinician reader.*)
2. Davidson A, Diamond B. Autoimmune disease. N Engl J Med 2001;345:340. (*An excellent review of disease mechanisms; 163 references.*)
3. Fuchs HA, Kaye JJ, Callahan LF, et al. Evidence of significant radiologic damage in rheumatoid arthritis within the first 2 years of disease. J Rheumatol 1989;16:585. (*A disproportionate degree of joint damage was found early in the course of disease.*)
4. Guerne PA. Palindromic rheumatism: part of or apart from the spectrum of rheumatoid arthritis. Am J Med 1992;93:451. (*A modern description of the problem.*)
5. Masi AT. Articular patterns in the early course of rheumatoid arthritis. Am J Med 1983;75:16. (*Patients with multiple joint involvement at onset have a poorer prognosis than those with more limited disease.*)
6. Nielen MM, van Schaardenburg D, Reesink HW, et al. Specific autoantibodies precede the symptoms of rheumatoid arthritis: a study of serial measurements in blood donors. Arthritis Rheum 2004;50:380. (*Immunoglobulin M*

rheumatoid factor and anti–cyclic citrullinated peptide preceded active disease by years and were specific for the condition.)

7. Remmers EF, Plenge RM, Lee AT, et al. STAT4 and the risk of rheumatoid arthritis and systemic lupus erythematosus. N Engl J Med 2007;357:977. (*Loci outside the HLA complex also contributed to risk, and a shared mechanism of risk with systemic lupus erythematosus was possible.*)

8. Roman MJ, Moeller E, Davis A, et al. Preclinical carotid atherosclerosis in patients with rheumatoid arthritis. Ann Intern Med 2006;144:249. (*Rheumatoid arthritis was found to be an independent risk factor for atherosclerotic disease.*)

9. van der Heijde DM, van Riel PL, van Rijswijk MH, et al. Influence of prognostic features on the final outcome in rheumatoid arthritis: a review of the literature. Semin Arthritis Rheum 1988;17:284. (*An excellent summary of clinical and simple laboratory findings that help to predict outcome.*)

10. Van Doornum S, McColl G, Wicks IP. Accelerated atherosclerosis: an extraarticular feature of rheumatoid disease? Arthritis Rheum 2002;46:862. (*Presents evidence for heightened atherosclerotic risk.*)

11. Weyand CM, Hicok KC, Conn DL, et al. The influence of HLA-DRB1 genes on disease severity in rheumatoid arthritis. Ann Intern Med 1992;117:801. (*HLA-DRB1 genotyping helps in the early identification of patients with a poor prognosis.*)

12. Arnett FC, Edworthy SM, Bloch DA, et al. The American Rheumatism Association 1987 revised criteria for the classification of rheumatoid arthritis. Arthritis Rheum 1988;31:315. (*Widely adopted diagnostic and classification criteria based on a collaborative study of >500 patients.*)

13. McQueen FM, Benton N, Perry D, et al. Bone edema scored on magnetic resonance imaging scans of the dominant capus at presentation predicts radiographic joint damage of the hands and feet six years later in patients with rheumatoid arthritis. Arthritis Rheum 2003;48:1814. (*Evidence of utility in the early diagnosis of significant disease.*)

14. Shadick NA, Cook NR, Karlson EW, et al. C-reactive protein in the prediction of rheumatoid arthritis in women. Arch Intern Med 2006;166:2490. (*Data from the Women's Health Study, revealing no predictive value.*)

15. American College of Rheumatology Subcommittee on Rheumatoid Arthritis Guidelines. Guidelines for the management of rheumatoid arthritis: 2002 update. Arthritis Rheum 2002;46:328. (*An authoritative update of consensus guidelines, taking into account new therapies.*)

16. American College of Rheumatology. Guidelines for monitoring drug therapy in rheumatoid arthritis. Arthritis Rheum 1996;39:723. (*A set of useful guidelines for monitoring the adverse effects of nonsteroidal antiinflammatory drugs [NSAIDs] and synthetic disease-modifying agents.*)

17. Goekoop-Ruiterman YPM, deVries-Bouwstra JK, Allaart CF, et al. Comparison of treatment strategies in early rheumatoid arthritis: a randomized trial. Ann Intern Med 2007;146:406. (*Early aggressive use of disease-modifying therapy gave the best results and led to the ability subsequently to taper the program.*)

18. Lard LR, Visser H, Speyer I, et al. Early versus delayed treatment in patients with recent-onset rheumatoid arthritis: comparison of two cohorts who received different treatment strategies. Am J Med 2001;111:446. (*A prospective study, finding that early treatment was superior.*)

19. MacLean CH, Louie R, Leake B, et al. Quality of care for patients with rheumatoid arthritis. JAMA 2000;284:984. (*A cohort study, finding that a collaboration between rheumatologist and primary care physician produced the best outcomes.*)

20. Mottonen R, Hannonen P, Leirisalo-Repo M, et al. Comparison of combination therapy with single-drug therapy in early rheumatoid arthritis: a randomized trial. Lancet 1999;353:1568. (*Combination therapy was more effective and just as safe.*)

21. O'Dell JR. Therapeutic strategies for rheumatoid arthritis. N Engl J Med 2004;350:2591. (*A concise review for the generalist clinician; 121 references.*)

22. Rogers MP, Liang MH, Partridge AJ. Psychological care of adults with rheumatoid arthritis. Ann Intern Med 1982;96:344. (*An often-overlooked area; gives many practical suggestions for the effective personal care of both patient and family.*)

23. van der Heijde DM, Jacobs JWG, Bijlsma JWJ, et al. The effectiveness of early treatment with "second-line" antirheumatic drugs. Ann Intern Med 1996;124:699. (*An open-label, randomized, controlled trial [RCT], finding that disease-modifying therapy was superior to NSAIDs.*)

24. Bresalier RS, Sandler RS, Quan H, et al. Cardiovascular events associated with rofecoxib in a colorectal adenoma chemoprevention trial. N Engl J Med 2005;352:1092 (*The findings that took rofecoxib off the market; see also ref. 40.*)

25. Francis Ka Leung Chan FKL, Wong VWS, Suen BY, et al. Combination of a cyclooxygenase-2 inhibitor and a proton-pump inhibitor for prevention of recurrent ulcer bleeding in patients at very high risk: a double-blind, randomised trial. Lancet 2007;369:1621. (*Risk was reduced.*)

26. Chan FKL, Hung LCT, Suen BY, et al. Celecoxib versus diclofenac and omeprazole in reducing the risk of recurrent ulcer bleeding in patients with arthritis. N Engl J Med 2002;347:2104. (*RCT, finding similarly high rates of recurrent bleeding and renal impairment in both groups.*)

27. Chan FKL, Sung JJ, Chung SC, et al. Randomised trial of eradication of Helicobacter pylori before nonsteroidal antiinflammatory drug therapy to prevent peptic ulcers. Lancet 1997;350:975. (*This was a means of reducing NSAID gastrointestinal risk.*)

28. Clive DM, Stoff JS. Renal syndromes associated with nonsteroidal antiinflammatory drugs. N Engl J Med 1984;310:563. (*Risk was greatest in patients with impaired renal perfusion.*)

29. Cryer B, Feldman M. Cyclooxygenase-1 and cyclooxygenase-2 selectivity of widely used nonsteroidal antiinflammatory drugs. Am J Med 1998;104:413. (*An in vitro study, noting considerable variability among nonselective NSAIDs.*)

30. Federal Drug Administration. FDA issues public health advisory on Vioxx as its manufacturer voluntarily withdraws the product. Available at: http://www.fda.gov/bbs/topics/news/2004/NEW01122.html. (*Data from a large-scale, long-term, RCT, revealing a doubling of the relative risk of cardiovascular events after 18 months of continuous daily use; the drug has been voluntarily withdrawn from the market.*)

31. FitzGerald GA. Coxibs and cardiovascular disease. N Engl J Med 2004;351:1709. (*An editorial summarizing the evidence for cardiovascular risk.*)

32. Kimmel SE, Berlin JA, Reilley M, et al. Patients exposed to rofecoxib and celecoxib have different odds of nonfatal myocardial infarction. Ann Intern Med 2005;142:157. (*A case–control study, finding that the risk was significantly greater with rofecoxib use.*)

33. Kimmel SE, Berlin JA, Reilly M, et al. The effects of nonselective non-aspirin non-steroidal anti-inflammatory medications on the risk of nonfatal myocardial infarction and their interaction with aspirin. J Am Coll Cardiol 2004;43:985. (*A case–control study, providing evidence for the inhibition of aspirin's protective effect.*)

34. Kirwan JR. The effects of glucocorticoids on joint destruction in rheumatoid arthritis. N Engl J Med 1995;333:142. (*RCT, finding that early, low-dose prednisone significantly reduced the risk for radiologically detectable joint destruction.*)

35. Moreland LW, O'Dell JR. Glucocorticosteroids and rheumatoid arthritis: back to the future? Arthritis Rheum 2002;46:2553. (*A review of a new-found appreciation for the role of these agents.*)

36. Mukherjee D, Nissen SE, Topol EJ. Risk of cardiovascular events associated with selective COX-2 inhibitors. JAMA 2001;286:954. (*Retrospective data analysis, finding an increased relative risk of thrombotic cardiovascular events in persons taking cyclooxygenase-2 [COX-2] agents compared with those taking a nonselective NSAID.*)

37. Silverstein FE, Faich G, Goldstein JL, et al. Gastrointestinal toxicity with celecoxib vs nonsteroidal anti-inflammatory drugs for osteoarthritis and rheumatoid arthritis: The CLASS Study: a randomized controlled trial. JAMA 2000;284:1247. (*RCT, finding a reduced risk with the COX-2 drug.*)

38. Simon LS, Weaver AL, Graham DY, et al. Antiinflammatory and upper gastrointestinal effects of celecoxib in rheumatoid arthritis: A randomized controlled trial. JAMA 1999;282:1921. (*A large-scale, multicenter, 12-week RCT, finding that the rate of ulcers and gastrointestinal side effects was significantly reduced.*)

39. Simon LS, Mills JA. Nonsteroidal antiinflammatory drugs. N Engl J Med 1980;302:1179, 1237. (*A still useful basic review of the pharmacology and role of nonsteroidal agents in comparison with aspirin.*)

40. Solomon SD, McMurray JJV, Pfeffer MA, et al. Cardiovascular risk associated with celecoxib in a clinical trial for colorectal adenoma prevention. N Engl J Med 2005;352:1071. (*RCT, finding evidence for a class effect extending beyond rofecoxib, but not as marked a risk.*)

41. Wolf MM, Lichtenstein DR, Singh G. Gastrointestinal toxicity of nonsteroidal antiinflammatory drugs. N Engl J Med 1999;340:1888. (*An excellent review.*)

42. Bathon JM, Martin RW, Fleischmann RM, et al. A comparison of etanercept and methotrexate in patients with early rheumatoid arthritis. N Engl J Med 2000;343:1586. (*RCT, finding an improved outcome.*)

43. Bingham SJ, Buch MH, Lindsay S, et al. The impact of escalating therapy in rheumatoid arthritis patients referred for anti–tumor necrosis factor-alpha therapy. Rheumatology (Oxford). 2004;43:364. (*In half of the instances, combination therapy with first-line drugs made biologic therapy unnecessary.*)

44. Donahue KE, Gartlehner G, Jonas DE, et al. Systematic review: comparative effectiveness and harms of disease-modifying medications for rheumatoid arthritis. Ann Intern Med 2008;148:124. (*A review of the best evidence, finding little difference within classes of drugs; biologic agents were a bit more effective by radiologic criteria than synthetic agents, but not clinically; combination therapies can be more effective in patients failing to respond; adverse effects were relatively equal in severity and frequency.*)

45. Edwards JCW, Szczepanski L, Szechinski J, et al. Efficacy of B-cell–targeted therapy with rituximab in patients with rheumatoid arthritis. N Engl J Med 2004;350: (*RCT, finding that one or two infusions provided prolonged benefit, suggesting a benefit from anti–B cell therapy.*)

46. Ellenerin R, Rubin RH, Weinblatt ME. Infections and anti–tumor necrosis factor α therapy. Arthritis Rheum 2003;48:3013. (*Treatment needs to be halted in the setting of infection.*)

47. Jeurissen MEC, Boerbooms AMT, van de Putte LBA, et al. Influence of methotrexate and azathioprine on radiologic progression in rheumatoid arthritis: a randomized, double-blind study. Ann Intern Med 1991;114:999. (*Methotrexate halted disease progression and was more effective than azathioprine.*)

48. Kremer JM, Genant HK, Moreland LW, et al. Effects of abatacept in patients with methotrexate-resistant active rheumatoid arthritis: a randomized trial. Ann Intern Med 2006;144:865. (*Presents evidence of efficacy for this costimulation modulator.*)

49. Maini RN, Breedveld FC, Kalden JR, et al. Therapeutic efficacy of multiple intravenous infusions of anti–tumor necrosis factor alfa monoclonal antibody combined with low-dose weekly methotrexate in rheumatoid arthritis. Arthritis Rheum 1998;41:1552. (*Initial report, noting significant improvement in response.*)

50. Moreland LW, Baumgartner SW, Schiff MH, et al. Treatment of rheumatoid arthritis with a recombinant human tumor necrosis factor receptor (p75)–Fc fusion protein. N Engl J Med 1997;337:141. (*The original report establishing the efficacy and safety of this major new approach to treatment.*)

51. Morgan SL, Baggott JE, Vaughn WH, et al. Supplementation with folic acid during methotrexate therapy for rheumatoid arthritis. A double-blind, placebo-controlled trial. Ann Intern Med 1994;121:833. (*The risk for toxicity was significantly reduced without a compromise in efficacy.*)

52. O'Dell JR, Haire CE, Erikson N, et al. Treatment of rheumatoid arthritis with methotrexate alone, sulfasalazine and hydroxychloroquine, or a combination of all three medications. N Engl J Med 1996;333:1287. (*A carefully conducted study of the aggressive use of disease-modifying therapy.*)

53. Olsen NJ, Steiun CM. New drugs for rheumatoid arthritis. N Engl J Med 2004;350:2167. (*A clinically useful review of new biologic therapies and leflunamide;122 references.*)

54. Pinals RS, Kaplan SB, Lawson JG, et al. Sulfasalazine in rheumatoid arthritis: a double-blind, placebo-controlled trial. Arthritis Rheum 1986;29:1427. (*Establishes the utility of this agent.*)

55. Tilley BC, Alarcon GS, Meyse SP, et al. Minocycline in rheumatoid arthritis: a 48-week, double-blind, placebo-controlled trial. Ann Intern Med 1995;122:81. (*Finds that this agent was useful for patients with moderately active disease; its role in the overall treatment of rheumatoid arthritis remains to be determined.*)

56. Tugwell P, Pincus T, Yocum D, et al. Combination therapy with cyclosporine and methotrexate in severe rheumatoid arthritis. N Engl J Med 1995;333:137. (*RCT, showing improved results with combination therapy.*)

57. Ward JR, Williams J, Egger MJ, et al. Comparison of auranofin, gold sodium thiomalate, and placebo in the treatment of rheumatoid arthritis. Arthritis Rheum 1982;26:1303. (*Parenteral gold was the most effective treatment, but it was also more likely to cause renal and mucocutaneous toxicity.*)

58. Weinblatt ME, Kremer JM, Bankhurst AD, et al. A trial of etanercept, a recombinant tumor necrosis factor receptor:Fc fusion protein, in patients with rheumatoid arthritis receiving methotrexate. N Engl J Med 1999;340:253. (*Combination with methotrexate significantly increased the response without any increase in adverse effects.*)

59. Wolfe F, Michaud K. Biologic treatment of rheumatoid arthritis and the risk of malignancy: analysis from a large US observational study. Arthritis Rheum 2007;56:3381. (*There was an increased risk of skin cancers but not solid tumors or lymphoproliferative malignancies.*)

60. Bell MJ, Lineker SC, Wilkins AL, et al. A randomized controlled trial to evaluate the efficacy of community based physical therapy in the treatment of people with rheumatoid arthritis. J Rheumatol 1998;25:231. (*Presents evidence of efficacy*).

61. Bradley LA. Psychosocial factors and disease outcomes in rheumatoid arthritis. Arthritis Rheum 1989;32:1611. (*An editorial critically reviewing the role of psychological factors in outcomes.*)

62. Buckley LM, Seib ES, Cartularo KS, et al. Calcium and vitamin D3 supplementation prevents bone loss in the spine secondary to low-dose corticosteroids in patients with rheumatoid arthritis. A randomized, double-blind, placebo-controlled trial. Ann Intern Med 1996;125:961. (*Presents evidence for efficacy in patients with rheumatoid arthritis who are taking low doses of glucocorticoids.*)

63. Komatireddy GR, Leitch RW, Cella K, et al. Efficacy of low load resistive muscle training in patients with rheumatoid arthritis functional class II and II. J Rheumatol 1997;24:1531. (*Presents evidence of efficacy.*)

64. Kremer JM, Jubiz W, Michalek A, et al. Fish-oil fatty acid supplementation in active rheumatoid arthritis: a double-blinded, controlled, cross-over study. Ann Intern Med 1987;106:497. (*Finds subjective benefit, in addition to a modest reduction in leukotriene.*)

65. Kruger JMS, Helmick CG, Callahan LF, et al. Cost-effectiveness of the Arthritis Self-Help Course. Arch Intern Med 1998;158:1245. (*A well-documented example of the efficacy of a program emphasizing patient education to encourage proper self-care; demonstrated cost-effectiveness.*)

66. Leventhal LJ, Boyce EG, Zurier RB. Treatment of rheumatoid arthritis with gamma-linolenic acid. Ann Intern Med 1993;119:867. (*A small-scale study, but encouraging results were found with the use of this dietary supplement.*)

67. Mills JA, Pinals RA, Ropes MW, et al. Value of bed rest in patients with rheumatoid arthritis. N Engl J Med 1971;284:453. (*A classic study, finding that minimal benefit was obtained from enforced rest.*)

68. Rao JK, Mihaliak K, Kroenke K, et al. Use of complementary therapies for arthritis among patients of rheumatologists. Ann Intern Med 1999;131:409. (*A telephone survey study, finding a high frequency of use for complementary therapies; many patients regularly used such measures.*)

69. Lorig KR, Lubeck D, Kraines RG, et al. Outcomes of self-help education for patients with arthritis. Arthritis Rheum 1985;28:680. (*This approach was very effective, and independence was enhanced.*)

CHAPTER 157 ■ MANAGEMENT OF OSTEOARTHRITIS

Osteoarthritis (OA), the most prevalent form of arthropathy, causes symptomatic discomfort in 10% to 20% of persons older than the age of 65 years and accounts for somewhat more than 30% of visits to primary care practitioners. OA is the most common cause of disability in the elderly. Most patients have primary or idiopathic disease that is strongly associated with aging. Others present with posttraumatic and hereditary forms of the disease (e.g., chondrodystrophy, hemochromatosis, inflammatory OA, chondrocalcinosis). Although many changes are irreversible, much can be done to relieve discomfort, prevent further articular damage, and keep the patient functioning independently.

PATHOPHYSIOLOGY AND CLINICAL PRESENTATION (1–14)

Pathogenesis and Pathophysiology

Osteoarthritis is characterized by (a) the degeneration of articular cartilage and (b) the reactive formation of new bone. What causes the demise of the articular cartilage and what causes the pain are incompletely understood.

Pathogenesis and Risk Factors

The simplistic "wear-and-tear" hypothesis has been superseded by an appreciation for the role of chondrocytes in actively remodeling cartilage. Articular damage appears to be the consequence of an interplay among systemic factors affecting the health of the cartilage and local biomechanical factors. Genetic determinants account for as much as 50% of the risk of developing OA of the hands and hips and somewhat less for the knees. Defective collagen synthesis has been identified in some familial forms. Bone density and vitamin D intake also contribute. Local biomechanical determinants of risk include poor joint alignment, obesity, joint laxity, prior injury, and muscle weakness. Excessive stress from obesity can be harmful, especially in the elderly. In the Framingham Study, women who lost an average of 11 lb experienced a 50% reduction in risk of knee osteoarthritis. Running per se is neither protective nor destructive (unless the knee has been injured, in which case running hastens degenerative change). The synovial inflammation that is characteristic of rheumatoid disease appears to play only a minor role, if any, in most cases of OA.

Pathophysiology

Histologically and biochemically, the size and aggregation of *proteoglycan* monomers are reduced with age. Proteoglycan is a critical mucopolysaccharide component of the cartilage extracellular matrix and is synthesized by cartilage chondrocytes and essential for elasticity. Contributing to this reduction is increased proteolytic enzyme activity by chondrocytes. The matrix is also composed of *collagen fibrils*, which provide resiliency; these fibrils are more susceptible to damage by trauma when matrix proteoglycan declines. *Synovial collagenase* can penetrate damaged cartilage and further degrade its collagen. *Interleukin-1β* (IL-1β) participates in the degradation process. With age, bone elasticity (which provides a cushioning effect during trauma) also declines, allowing increased stress to be transmitted directly to the cartilage. Conditions that alter the mechanical relationships of joints further increase the likelihood that degenerative changes will develop.

The earliest manifestations of OA are superficial erosions of the cartilage; the response is hypertrophy and hyperplasia of chondrocytes. Early cartilaginous injury can be repaired by chondrocytes, but fissured hyaline cartilage cannot be restored. Eventually, the cartilage frays, shreds, and cracks. Underlying bone responds by remodeling, which causes trabeculae to thicken. At the joint margins, the development of hypertrophic spurs (*osteophytes*) is followed by buttressing of adjacent cortical bone (*osteosclerosis*). The joint space narrows in an irregular fashion. Cyst formation is also seen. Little *synovial reaction* occurs unless the degenerative process is rapid, a piece of cartilage dislodges, or calcium pyrophosphate crystals form and incite an acute inflammatory response (pseudogout).

Mechanism(s) of Pain

Pain is the most disabling manifestation of OA, yet its mechanism(s) remain poorly understood, reflected in the modest efficacy of current methods of pain control. There are no pain fibers in cartilage; any pain that ensues as a result of articular damage must involve adjacent pain-sensitive structures, such as the joint capsule, ligaments, synovium, periosteal bone, and bone marrow. Capsular distention is one possible source, but the injection of anesthetic into painful osteoarthritic knees usually fails to relieve pain, suggesting that the principal source(s) of pain are extraarticular.

Current research has concentrated on adjacent bone as an important source of pain. The periosteum and subchondral bone contain nociceptive nerve fibers capable of detecting injury to bone. A strong correlation has been noted between pain and marrow lesions (as identified by magnetic resonance imaging) in adjacent bone. Marrow edema has been found in bone with such lesions, suggesting an inflammatory response. If confirmed and proven causative, such a marrow response would help to explain why OA pain is often delayed until the evening and why some patients obtain better pain relief from antiinflammatory agents than from pure analgesics (see later discussion).

Clinical Presentation

Radiologic evidence of OA can be found in more than 80% of adults by age 65 years. The subset who are symptomatic complain of deep, aching joint pain that is aggravated by motion and weight bearing; sometimes it is worse at night after a day of vigorous activity. Those who come for medical attention often have a concomitant psychosocial problem. OA patients characteristically report stiffness after periods of inactivity. The involved joint can be enlarged by the formation of osteophytes, but swelling is usually inconsequential because in most instances soft-tissue involvement and effusions are minimal. In later stages, pain occurs on motion and at rest in conjunction with stiffness. Patients with advanced disease have pain on weight bearing and joint instability. Examination often reveals crepitus and discomfort on movement of the joint. Occasionally, slight warmth is noted in severely affected weight-bearing joints, but erythema and marked warmth are absent. *Limitation of motion*, *malalignment*, and *bony protuberances* from spurs are frequent findings. The joints most commonly affected include the knees, hips, distal interphalangeal (DIP) joints of the hands, carpometacarpal joint at the base of the thumb, and the joints of the cervical and lumbosacral spine.

Knees

Symptomatic knee involvement is estimated to affect as much as 10% of the population older than the age of 65 years. Obesity is a major risk factor. OA of the knee produces pain that is localized to the medial and/or lateral joint line and worsened by prolonged weight bearing and stair climbing. In later stages, crepitus is often marked and range of motion reduced. A very small effusion may be noted. The joint appears to be enlarged and feels bony. Patellofemoral joint involvement produces anterior knee pain that is exacerbated by going down stairs. On occasion, very few physical findings may be noted, although pain and radiographic changes are prominent. A skyline view of the flexed knee can reveal patellofemoral disease.

Hips

Degenerative hip disease arises in young patients with congenital dislocations or slipped femoral capital epiphyses. In the elderly, it results from wear and tear. A unilateral or asymmetric distribution is typical. The patient may describe pain that is deep in the hip and radiates into the anterior medial thigh, groin, buttock, or medial knee. The site of radiation (e.g., groin or buttock) may be the only area of reported pain. At first, pain occurs only on prolonged standing or walking, but as OA progresses, discomfort may become continuous and especially unbearable at night. The ability to engage in sexual intercourse is sometimes compromised. Loss of internal rotation during flexion is the earliest change and is as reliable as radiographic findings for diagnosis. The result of Trendelenburg's test (see Chapter 151) is positive.

Hands

Characteristic sites include the DIP joints and base of the thumb (first carpometacarpal joint); sometimes, proximal interphalangeal (PIP) joint involvement is noted. Hand disease is most common in middle-aged and elderly women, many of whom have a strongly positive family history. In some, a low-grade inflammatory response may accompany early, rapid, mucinous degenerative changes, so that the joints take on a tender, cystic inflammatory appearance. Later, osteophytes form, giving rise to characteristic bony protuberances in the DIP joints (*Heberden's nodes*) and occasionally PIP deformities (*Bouchard's nodes*) that superficially resemble those of rheumatoid disease. Eventually, all inflammatory activity resolves, and the joints are left nontender with some limitation of motion.

The base of the thumb, a site of much physical stress, is vulnerable to degenerative change. Pain develops in the region of the thenar eminence and particularly over the carpometacarpal joint. Because the thumb is so important to manual dexterity, the development of arthritis at this site may be disabling. Grip becomes impaired, and fine movements of apposition are restricted. Osteophytes are palpable and, in rare instances, may encroach on the flexor tendon sheath, causing tenosynovitis.

Cervical Spine

Degenerative changes commonly involve the posterior diarthrodial joints of the lower cervical spine (see Chapter 148). Although radiographic changes are frequent, most persons are asymptomatic. Moreover, the correlation between symptoms and radiographic findings is often poor. The patient may have pain and stiffness in the neck, but sometimes pain is reported only in the occiput, shoulder, arm, or hand. In a few instances, scapular or upper anterior chest pain is produced. Osteophytes can protrude into the foramina and impinge on nerve roots (most often C-6 and C-7), causing *radicular pain* that radiates to the shoulder, upper arms, hands, or fingers (see Chapter 167). At night, the patient may awaken with paresthesias and numbness in the arms that can be alleviated by getting up and shaking the arms. On examination, neck motion is restricted to some extent in all directions, especially lateral flexion and extension; movement reproduces or aggravates symptoms. Reactive muscle spasm and tenderness are often present, and decreased sensation, weakness, and diminished reflexes occur when root compression is marked. However, even when symptoms of root compression are reported, neurologic findings may be scant, and their absence does not rule out the complication.

Lumbosacral Spine

Degenerative changes in the lumbosacral spine involve the intervertebral disks and the apophyseal joints. With aging, the disk nucleus becomes brittle and less elastic. Herniation posteriorly or laterally through a defect in the disk annulus may occur. Intervertebral spaces narrow and marginal osteophytes form. The apophyseal joints show typical secondary degenerative changes. Disk or osteophyte encroachment on the foramina can lead to nerve root compression. The L-4, L-5, and S-1 roots are most commonly affected. The patient reports pain across the lower back with radiation into the buttock and posterior thigh, or down into the lower leg if *root compression* has occurred. Forward flexion and extension are reduced, but lateral flexion is painless. Focal areas of tenderness are common and often caused by spasm of the paraspinous muscula-

ture. Disk or osteophyte encroachment into the spinal canal can lead to *spinal stenosis*, which affects the cauda equina and exiting nerve roots. Compression of nerve roots produces *pseudoclaudication* (pain in the buttocks or thighs during prolonged standing or walking that is relieved by sitting or bending). On examination, thigh symptoms may be brought on by 30 seconds of lumbar extension, then relieved by having the patient bend forward. In addition, the patient may have a wide-based gait and neurologic deficits in the lower extremities.

Other Sites

OA may involve the great toe at the metatarsophalangeal joint to cause bony enlargement and a valgus deformity. Crepitus and pain in the temporomandibular joint are sometimes seen secondary to bruxism (grinding of the teeth because of anxiety or anger). Pain is reproduced by opening the mouth widely. Because OA is not a systemic disease, no extraarticular manifestations and no serum abnormalities occur; the sedimentation rate is normal, as is the synovial fluid in early disease. Radiographic findings are limited to the joints and include irregular narrowing of the joint space, sclerosis of subchondral bone, bony cysts, marginal osteophytes, and buttressing of adjacent bone.

Natural History of Disease

In large, weight-bearing joints, OA tends to be a progressive condition causing chronic joint pain, restricted joint motion, and resultant muscle weakness that compromises mobility. Through a period of 10 to 20 years, pain at rest develops in the majority of patients with untreated symptomatic OA of the knee, and they become unable to use public transportation; disability may ensue. An early onset of symptoms and varus deformity correlate with a poor prognosis. OA of the hip may follow a similar course. Obesity is a strong risk factor for progressive disease of the hips and knees (especially in women); heavy weight-bearing exercise is associated with an increased risk for knee disease in the elderly. Weight reduction reduces the risk. The progression of OA is typically limited to a few affected joints, and the disease does not become widespread. Clinical remissions do occur, especially in the hands, neck, and back.

DIAGNOSIS

See Chapters 145 and 146.

PRINCIPLES OF MANAGEMENT

The treatment of osteoarthritis remains largely symptomatic. Except for total joint replacement, there are no disease-modifying therapies of proven effectiveness (although some are promising; see later discussion). Nonetheless, reduction in pain and restoration of activity can be achieved with a multifaceted program. The goals are to reduce pain and muscle spasm, alleviate abnormal stresses imposed on affected joints, restore joint alignment, and enhance overall functional status. Analgesics, antiinflammatory agents, exercises, assist devices, braces, weight reduction, and surgery are among the available approaches. A host of new therapies are in various stages of development, and a large number of unproven methods are available. The primary physician has an important responsibility to help guide the patient through a daunting number of choices and ensure that the approach taken is evidence based and suits the individual well.

Pharmacologic Measures (15–28)

Analgesics and Antiinflammatory Agents

Pain relief is a top priority for most patients. Analgesics remain the predominant pharmacologic approach. Because an individual patient's response to analgesics is unpredictable, it may require a trial-and-error approach. Intermittent use of analgesics sometimes suffices, but continuous therapy is often needed in the absence of more definitive treatment. Whether to use a pure analgesic agent or a nonsteroidal antiinflammatory drug with analgesic properties is a subject of debate. Of interest, there is little long-term study data on the efficacy of analgesic therapy, even though these drugs are often taken chronically. Chronic use has raised concerns about adverse effects, both for pure analgesics and for nonsteroidals taken for OA.

Acetaminophen. Pure analgesics, such as acetaminophen, should be tried first. Results from an often-cited, well-designed study of OA patients with knee pain found acetaminophen comparable to nonsteroidal therapy (naproxen) in controlling pain and without the risk of adverse gastrointestinal effects. Other well-designed but small-scale, short-term studies failed to confirm these findings and suggested that acetaminophen is little better than placebo. Such variable findings parallel the experience of patients in everyday practice, some of whom find acetaminophen perfectly adequate, whereas others do not.

The cost of acetaminophen is low, and its long-term safety is well established. The highly publicized risk for hepatic injury is rare when doses do not exceed 4 g/d. Liver injury typically occurs only in cases of overdose or underlying alcoholic liver disease. Long-term therapy at high doses may increase the risk for renal tubular injury, but supporting data are sparse, and the risk appears to be no greater than that associated with prolonged nonsteroidal antiinflammatory drug (NSAID) use.

Nonsteroidal Antiinflammatory Drugs (NSAIDs). Current consensus guidelines relegate NSAIDs to a second-line role in OA, but a large percentage of OA patients find them preferable for pain relief. Such observations from everyday practice suggest that there might be an underappreciated inflammatory component to the pain of OA (also supported by some research into the mechanisms of OA pain; see prior discussion). More clinical and fundamental research is needed to help guide analgesic therapy, but in the meantime patients will continue to use whichever available analgesics provide them with the best pain relief over time. Those who fail acetaminophen can be started on a trial course of a generic nonselective NSAID (e.g., ibuprofen 400 mg thrice daily or naproxen 500 mg twice daily).

Because analgesic therapy is often long term in OA, the adverse effects associated with chronic NSAID use become important considerations. Peptic ulceration and gastrointestinal bleeding are the predominant risks associated with nonselective NSAID use (see Chapters 68 and 156); these can be lessened to about 5% by a number of measures, including the concurrent use of a proton-pump inhibitor (e.g., omeprazole) or the use of a cyclooxygenase-2 (COX-2) NSAID (see Chapters 68 and 156). For this reason, COX-2 drugs were very popular among patients and physicians for use in OA, but data revealed an increased risk of adverse cardiovascular events (relative risk, 1.5 to 3.5 for myocardial infarction, stroke, and death), especially with extended use (>18 months). These findings and concern

about thromboembolic potentiation prompted the withdrawal of one COX-2 agent from the market and the issuance of warnings regarding the use of the others (see Chapter 156). Both their high cost and concerns about increased cardiovascular risk have relegated the COX-2 drugs to third-line status for the treatment of chronic OA pain.

Other adverse effects of NSAIDs include renal compromise that may develop in persons with underlying renal insufficiency or heart failure (see Chapters 32 and 142). Hypertension control may also be impeded (see Chapter 26). Some elderly patients experience mental confusion while taking NSAIDs that penetrate the central nervous system (e.g., indomethacin).

Topical NSAID preparations (e.g., *diclofenac gel*) may provide modest pain relief in persons with OA of the knee or hands (the placebo benefit is high). Systemic toxicity is minimal; local skin irritation occurs in about 7%; cost is high. Animal data suggest an increased risk of UV-related skin tumors; exposure of the treated area to sunlight should be minimized.

Narcotic Analgesics. Codeine, *oxycodone*, and other narcotic analgesics should be used sparingly, if at all, and only for acute disabling pain that interferes with essential activity. *Propoxyphene* (Darvon), an opiate derivative, is taken by many patients with OA, but its analgesic potency is poor, and its potential for causing dependence is considerable—similar to that of codeine (see Chapter 236). Results from *intraarticular injection* of a narcotic analgesic have been disappointing, with fewer than 10% of persons with knee pain responding.

Antidepressants and Antispasmodics. OA patients with unrecognized and untreated depression benefit from disease-specific treatment, be it pharmacologic and/or interpersonal. Pain control improves, as does functional state and overall quality of life. Starting a generic formulation of an selective serotonin reuptake inhibitor antidepressant (e.g., fluoxetine; see Chapter 227) to supplement the analgesic program can be particularly helpful in depressed OA patients, although it may take several weeks for benefits to be fully realized.

Symptomatic Slow-Acting Drugs in Osteoarthritis

Drugs in this increasingly interesting class are believed to work by slowing the degradation of cartilage. Relief from pain and improvement in function are characteristically slow in onset but prolonged in duration, persisting even after the discontinuation of therapy.

Diacerein. Diacerein inhibits interleukin-1β, which participates in the cartilaginous degradation process. Animal studies show a moderation of cartilage loss with the intake of diacerein. Meta-analysis of mostly short-term, randomized, placebo-controlled clinical trials of use in persons with hip or knee osteoarthritis found that the drug produces statistically significant but modest (although clinically meaningful) improvements in symptoms and function. Tolerability is similar to that for NSAIDs, with diarrhea being the most common side effect (40%), but there is no increase in risk of peptic ulceration, bleeding, or cardiovascular events. There is little data on long-term use, and so the safety of chronic administration is unknown. Cost is high.

Glucosamine and Chondroitin. Classified under current federal law as "dietary supplements," glucosamine and chondroitin have become very popular with patients seeking a nonprescription approach to pain control for osteoarthritis. These substances, which occur naturally in the body and are extracted from animal products, have been used for years in veterinary medicine and are heavily promoted in the lay press by authors, manufacturers, and suppliers for use in OA; they can be sold without prescription because of their dietary-supplement designation. Annual sales are in the multimillions of dollars, and most preparations combine both substances.

Some claim that these supplements represent the first disease-modifying treatment for OA by virtue of their role in slowing cartilaginous degeneration. Glucosamine is an intermediary in mucopolysaccharide synthesis. *In vitro*, it stimulates chondrocytes to produce proteoglycans; *in vivo* basic-science evidence of beneficial effect on articular cartilage remains to be demonstrated. Chondroitin sulfate, a glycosaminoglycan touted to promote joint viscosity and cartilage repair, may partially inhibit leukocyte elastase and prevent the degradation of cartilage. Proponents view these agents as slow-acting therapies that need to be taken over a prolonged period.

Efficacy. Advocates claim that these supplements have disease-modifying potential, and some placebo-controlled radiologic studies suggest a slowing of disease progression. However, rigorous systematic reviews of pertinent published studies have found that many trials are of poor quality, overestimating the benefits of treatment and being subject to important biases, including sponsorship by the manufacturers. Moreover, accumulating data from recent randomized, placebo-controlled trials have shown little clinical benefit. In a major study of patients with osteoarthritic knee pain randomized to glucosamine alone, chondroitin sulfate alone, glucosamine plus chondroitin, celecoxib, or matched placebo (with acetaminophen as the rescue drug), supplement use failed to produce significant improvement in pain; a modest benefit was found in a small subset of patients with moderate to severe pain taking both glucosamine and chondroitin sulfate. Similar findings were noted in a subsequent randomized, placebo-controlled study of patients with hip osteoarthritis. Meta-analysis of data from the three largest, best-designed, randomized, placebo-controlled trials of chondroitin alone failed to find any significant difference in pain relief or other outcomes in persons with osteoarthritis of the hips or knees.

Safety. Both drugs appear to be well tolerated, based on available data. Although glucosamine has been linked to glucose intolerance, no evidence for an enhanced risk of glucose intolerance has been noted in the longer-term studies of up to 3 years' duration. However, given the small number of patients studied, there is insufficient data to confirm long-term safety, which is especially important for substances that are likely to be used chronically. It is also important to note that because they are dietary supplements, these preparations are not subject to any quality standards, although the U.S. Pharmacopeia (USP) has started to issue labeling of preparations that meet its standards for purity and uniformity.

Cost and Convenience. These supplements can be expensive, costing hundreds of dollars per year when taken daily. Instructions on the bottle usually recommend that three tablets be taken daily.

Physical Measures (3,6,8,29–33)

Exercise

Of the nonmedical therapies, exercise shows the most consistently beneficial results for patients with OA, especially those with disease of the knees. Restoration of favorable mechanics is essential to minimizing damage to injured joints. Strengthening the supporting muscles may help to maintain proper joint alignment.

Strengthening and *conditioning exercises* should be prescribed. *Quadriceps exercises* and a *walking program* for patients with knee involvement clearly improve exercise tolerance and decrease pain. Isometric and active exercises for the neck improve muscle tone and may sometimes help in cases of painful cervical spine disease (see Chapter 148). Exercises for the abdominal and paraspinous musculature are useful for preventing back problems (see Chapter 147). Range-of-motion exercises can also help when they are part of a comprehensive exercise program. Quadriceps exercises are among the simplest to perform and can be taught in the office. The patient is instructed to extend the knee and hold the straightened leg in a horizontal position while sitting in a chair. A program of supervised graduated isometric and isotonic quadriceps exercises can decrease pain and make it possible for the patient to walk for longer distances. A note of caution has been injected into recommendations for quadriceps exercises with the finding that some persons with knee malalignment may experience disease progression with quadriceps strengthening. Designing the exercise program with the help of a physical therapist can help to maximize safety and outcomes.

Aerobic exercise may provide some additional benefit over strengthening programs by enhancing overall conditioning. For patients with OA of weight-bearing joints, structured aerobic exercise programs with full or partial weight bearing can greatly enhance endurance, walking distance, and sense of well-being without aggravating the arthritis. A 2-month program of supervised fitness walking combined with patient education can improve functional status by close to 40% in patients with symptomatic knee disease. Gentle cycling and swimming also improve endurance, benefiting the muscle groups of the hips and knees. Participation in such conditioning programs also boosts morale considerably.

Manual physical therapy consists in active and passive range-of-motion exercises performed by physical therapists. Randomized, controlled trial of such therapy in combination with supervised exercise for OA of the knee demonstrated significant improvements in pain, stiffness, and functional capacity that persist for up to 1 year after treatment. As beneficial as exercise may be, excessive exercise may only exacerbate pain and cause further disruption of the joint. Excessive joint strain, such as results from stair climbing, should be reduced as much as possible. Supervision and patient education are essential to a successful exercise program and far superior to simply telling the patient to get more exercise.

Rest and Assist Devices

Some relief can be obtained by partially resting a very painful joint. The objective is to reduce the mechanical stress imposed on the joint. However, joint rest should be alternated with exercise to prevent muscle atrophy and worsening joint alignment. Moreover, prolonged immobility greatly disturbs cartilage metabolism.

Assist devices can help to rest or protect a diseased joint from excessive mechanical stress. The pressures on hip and knee joints generated by getting up from a toilet or low seat can be decreased by the use of handrails, grips, and a raised toilet or chair seat. An often underused approach to joint rest is the use of a *cane* in the contralateral hand, which can reduce the mechanical stress on a weight-bearing joint by as much as 50%. Embarrassment and awkwardness often make patients reluctant to use a cane, but physician encouragement and a few sessions with an occupational therapist can greatly help.

Weight Reduction

Excessive weight is one of the major risk factors for OA of the knees and hips. Epidemiologic studies show a strong correlation between obesity and the risk for symptomatic knee arthritis. Weight bearing puts mechanical stresses on the hip and knee joints that can be as much as five times the patient's weight. What is not widely appreciated is that even modest degrees of weight loss can produce substantial reductions in such mechanical stress. In community-based epidemiologic study, a 5-kg (11-lb) weight loss was associated with a 50% reduction in the risk of OA. A comprehensive program of mechanically sensible, supervised aerobic activity combined with detailed dietary counseling (see Chapter 233) should be drawn up with the help of the physical therapist and nutritionist and implemented. An assisted, supervised program is essential because obese persons with OA are otherwise likely to feel that weight loss and exercise are beyond their capacity.

Bracing, Footware, and Orthotics

Orthotic devices help to correct malalignment. Patients with hip disease resulting from or aggravated by differences in leg length may benefit from a heel lift that equalizes leg lengths. If abnormal foot pronation is causing varus stress on the knee joint, a shoe orthotic device may reduce pain and ligamentous strain on the knee. The use of such heel wedges can provide symptomatic relief in medial compartment syndrome of the knee and may obviate the need for knee replacement.

A *cervical collar* can ease neck pain by supporting the spine and resting the paraspinous musculature. It may be necessary to continue use intermittently for many weeks before significant benefit is achieved. Cervical traction may also help (see Chapter 148). A *corset* or *brace* for the back may be similarly helpful, but its use should be combined with an exercise program to avoid muscle atrophy (see Chapter 147).

Heat

Moist heat can give symptomatic relief from muscle spasm, although it has no effect on the disease itself. *Diathermy* and *ultrasound* units are expensive ways to deliver heat to deep tissues. Although many patients report improvement, controlled trials in which sham treatments were used showed no benefit. However, some patients derive considerable psychological benefit and a sense of well-being from undergoing such therapy.

Acupuncture

Most studies of acupuncture for OA are of poor quality. In the few available double-blinded studies using sham procedures as controls, acupuncture has produced inconsistent results—sometimes working, sometimes not. Results are best when both the patient and the therapist believe in the procedure. Results have not been consistently and sufficiently beneficial to justify inclusion of acupuncture in standard treatment programs, but it might be considered an option for patients who believe strongly in the procedure.

Interventional and Surgical Therapies (34–39)

Intraarticular Injections

Injections of corticosteroids and hyaluronic acid have been used for palliation, especially in cases of refractory osteoarthritis of the knee. Temporary pain relief is afforded, making injection therapy a reasonable consideration in persons with refractory pain who are awaiting joint replacement or who cannot tolerate surgery.

Glucocorticosteroids. The intraarticular injection of steroids is controversial. Use in degenerative disease of the knee (see Chapter 152) and spine (see Chapter 147) is common, but no controlled studies have documented its efficacy. The experimental finding of steroid suppression of cartilage catabolism has renewed interest in this form of therapy. However, concern remains that repeated steroid injections may accelerate joint degeneration, especially by weakening supporting structures. Little damage to articular tissue has been found with injections repeated as often as every 3 months. Nonetheless, steroid injection should be considered only when a single joint, refractory to other forms of therapy, is sufficiently inflamed and the patient sufficiently disabled that a trial of intraarticular steroids is justified. Systemic steroids have no place in the treatment of OA.

Hyaluronic Acid. A longer-acting benefit (up to 3 months) is afforded by the injection of *hyaluronic acid*, an elastoviscosity factor in normal joint fluid that declines with age. The response rate is lower than with corticosteroids, the cost is higher, and there may be some local irritation at the injection site. Patients with mild disease respond best. Hypersensitivity reactions have been reported with the use of avian-derived preparations (contraindicated in persons with allergy to eggs or feathers). The benefit for resting pain is similar to that achieved with NSAIDs; the response for pain associated with physical activity can exceed that of NSAIDs. Pseudogout has been reported as a complication of this otherwise reasonably well-tolerated treatment.

Cartilage Implantation and Grafting

New intraarticular procedures under study and being applied selectively hold promise as potential alternatives to joint replacement, especially of the knee. Patients with focal articular defects, particularly young persons who have sustained trauma, are being treated with *autogenous cartilage implantation* and *osteochondral grafting*. In the former, chondrocytes are grown from the patient's cartilage and implanted. Criteria for candidacy include normal knee alignment, absence of arthritis on the corresponding tibial surface, and preserved ligamentous joint stability. Outcomes data are promising in carefully selected patients.

Arthroscopic Surgery

Arthroscopic surgery entails debridement, smoothing of joint surfaces, and washing out of debris. Although patients often report benefit, controlled trials suggest a strong placebo effect and no long-term improvement in outcomes, unless a foreign body or internal derangement is the cause of symptoms.

Osteotomy

Osteotomy is used to correct the mechanical imbalances caused by single-compartment disease of the knee and early disease of the hip. The procedure has been popular and does seem to provide at least short-term benefit; however, few data comparing such surgical therapy with conservative management (weight loss, orthotics, exercise) are available, and the results of long-term follow-up are often disappointing. The role of such surgery may be viewed as a temporizing measure used to delay total joint replacement.

Total Joint Replacement (Arthroplasty)

Replacement of the severely osteoarthritic joint presents the most definitive form of treatment available. Advances in surgical technique, prosthetic devices, perioperative care, and thromboembolism prophylaxis have greatly improved the safety and outcomes, both short and long term. Operative and perioperative mortality risk averages less than 1% for hip and knee replacements at experienced centers. Replacement of hip and knee joints has been particularly successful. Even persons of advanced age can safely undergo arthroplasty and attain years of improved quality of life.

Indications for arthroplasty include pain at rest that interferes with sleep, inability to bear weight without severe pain, unacceptable interference with daily activity, and a requirement for narcotics to control pain. Referral for such surgery requires a comprehensive consideration of the patient's medical condition, functional status, and psychosocial state. The ability to participate physically and psychologically in a demanding program of rehabilitation is an important precondition for an optimal outcome. Ideally, the decision to refer for arthroplasty should be determined solely by patient candidacy and need, but financial barriers and racial, gender, ethnic, and regional factors should also be kept in mind and addressed if problematic.

Treatments of Possible, Unclear, or No Proven Benefit (29–33,40–45)

As in the management of any common chronic condition that is difficult to treat definitively, claims of benefit have been made for a host of unproven therapies for OA. Some are widely promoted to the public as safe, "natural" means of treatment, so that they appear particularly attractive. Evidence of efficacy is often absent when such therapies can be marketed under the rubric of "dietary supplement" without U.S. Food and Drug Administration review of their safety and effectiveness. Studies of patients with arthritis reveal that up to half are trying alternative or complementary measures, especially if they are having severe pain. Only recently are some of these widely used measures being subjected to rigorously designed clinical trials.

Diathermy, Including Ultrasound

The rationale for delivering heat by these means before exertion is that they help to relax deep tendons and muscles. Such treatment is expensive and time-consuming. As noted, in randomized, controlled trials that included sham treatment, diathermy provided no benefit over that derived from exercise alone.

Spinal Manipulation

In careful, controlled study, a short course of chiropractic manipulation of the spine appeared to provide modest relief of acute back pain caused by musculotendinous strain, similar to that afforded by conventional treatments; however, such treatment had no demonstrably beneficial effect on the chronic pain and discomfort resulting from degenerative disease of the spine; the presence of a herniated disk and root impingement were contraindications to spinal manipulation.

Wrist Bracelets

"Ionized" wrist bracelets have been promoted to help restore the balance between Yin (positive ions) and Yang (negative ions) so that bodily *chi* (energy or electrical current) will flow unimpeded. Invented in Spain in the 1970s and made of 85% cooper and 15% zinc, these bracelets are touted by the manufacturer as capable of restoring *chi* by a secret proprietary process. Cost is between $50 and $200. Double-blind study found these to be no better than placebo.

Transcutaneous Electrical Nerve Stimulation

Most of the studies that suggest benefit are poorly designed; placebo effect appears to account for most of the pain relief achieved.

Glucosamine and Chondroitin

See earlier discussion.

Acupuncture

See earlier discussion.

INDICATIONS FOR REFERRAL (46,47)

Treatment of the patient with OA requires a team approach. *Physical* and *occupational therapists* are essential to the design of a successful treatment program—teaching exercises, giving suggestions on how to perform the tasks of daily living, and providing psychological support. Referral should be made early in the course of disease for education in preventive measures and also later, when OA begins to interfere with daily activity. Early referral to the *nutritionist* is critical to the care of the obese patient. A comprehensive program of diet and exercise is needed to effect a successful weight loss effort.

Surgical consultation should be considered for the significantly disabled patient who is failing conservative management. The consultation should be explained to the patient as an opportunity to weigh treatment options rather than as an automatic capitulation to surgical intervention. The decision to refer for surgery must be made with an understanding of the risks involved and the need to undertake a vigorous postoperative exercise program. Surgery should be considered only in patients whose limitation of motion or pain has become so severe that it prevents them from living productively. They must be mentally and physically healthy enough to tolerate surgery and sufficiently motivated to carry out the exercise program needed to ensure full rehabilitation. Patients and their primary care physicians need to understand that standard arthroscopic intervention (washing and debridement), although appealing because it is less invasive, is in most instances no better than placebo. Only when internal derangement or a foreign body is documented to be the cause of disability should arthroscopic surgery become a consideration. Primary physicians need to be cognizant of and address any economic, racial, gender, and sociocultural barriers to referral and access to arthroplasty.

PATIENT EDUCATION AND PSYCHOSOCIAL SUPPORT (20,30,33)

Patients need to know that OA is not reversible, but also that much can be done to lessen pain, prevent further joint injury, and preserve, if not enhance, overall functioning. They appreciate knowing that degenerative disease is not a generalized, systemic illness. Moreover, those with cervical or lumbosacral disease can be given some hope for a spontaneous remission of their severe pain. The need to reduce weight and strengthen supporting muscles should be stressed, in addition to the importance of avoiding activity injurious to the joints and addictive analgesics. The teaching functions of the physical and occupational therapists and nutritionist are among the most critical components of the treatment program. It is important to avoid labeling the patient as "disabled" because active participation in the treatment program is essential to preservation of function. As noted, surgical options should be discussed with patients who have incapacitating pain of the hips or knees.

Because a principal determinant of presenting for care is the *psychosocial state* of the OA patient, the importance of eliciting and attending to psychosocial stresses cannot be overemphasized. A careful history that includes attention to job, family, and any financial or interpersonal problems is likely to help in the design of an effective treatment program. Identification and treatment of underlying depression (see Chapter 227) helps to improve pain control, functional status, and overall quality of life.

Prognosis is heavily influenced by how well the patient is coping psychosocially. The physician's concern and support are essential. Return visits should be regularly scheduled so that the patient can be made to feel that support and caring are being provided. A strong doctor–patient relationship helps many patients to tolerate the disease and remain active.

THERAPEUTIC RECOMMENDATIONS (47)

- Begin a comprehensive, supervised program of exercise, weight loss, and education for patients with symptomatic disease of the hips or knees.
- Provide referrals to physical and occupational therapists for the design and implementation of exercise and activity programs that strengthen quadriceps and hip muscles, increase general conditioning, avoid excessive stress on the affected joints, and ensure the proper use of assist devices.
- Obtain the services of a nutritionist to help support the obese patient in a program of weight reduction.
- Inform the patient that regular aerobic exercise is beneficial and that gentle walking, swimming, and stationary cycling are not only permissible but also desirable.
- Advise a short period (1 to 2 days) of joint rest if severe hip or knee pain flares up, but isometric and non–weight-bearing exercises should be continued and more-prolonged inactivity avoided. Limit joint stresses (e.g., stair climbing) and prescribe the use of a cane and other assist devices (e.g., railings, hand grips, elevated toilet seat).

- Consider the use of a heel lift if leg lengths are unequal and the use of a shoe orthotic device if marked foot pronation is noted. Check with an orthopedist or podiatrist if uncertain.
- Prescribe a soft cervical collar to those with cervical pain. It should be worn at all times, including the night. Four weeks or more of use may be necessary. Cervical traction is also helpful (see Chapter 148).
- For pharmacologic relief of pain, begin with acetaminophen (up to 1 g four times daily); consider a generic nonselective NSAID (e.g., naproxen, 500 mg twice daily) if acetaminophen proves insufficient. If NSAID therapy causes gastrointestinal upset or prolonged treatment is required in a person with a prior history of peptic ulcer disease or a complication of peptic ulcer disease, then add a proton-pump inhibitor (e.g., generic omeprazole, 20 to 40 mg/d) for secondary prophylaxis (see Chapter 68). Consider the use of a COX-2 agent instead of nonselective NSAID only if the potential cardiovascular risk is deemed acceptable (see Chapter 156). If analgesic/NSAID therapy proves inadequate for control of knee pain, consider a trial of a slow-acting agent (e.g., diacerein 50 mg, twice daily).
- Patients who claim that they get benefit from glucosamine/chondroitin sulfate supplements (e.g., a USP-certified preparation of glucosamine, 1,500 mg daily, and chondroitin sulfate, 1,200 mg daily) can be allowed to remain on the supplement. However, inform such patients that the evidence of efficacy and safety remains minimal and incomplete, and monitor closely for response and side effects. Do not continue indefinitely without clear evidence of benefit, although a trial period of up to 3 months may be necessary.
- Elicit and address sources of psychosocial distress; identify and treat any underlying depression (see Chapter 227).
- Avoid the use of narcotics except in the setting of an acute disabling exacerbation that is not relieved by maximal doses of nonnarcotic analgesics. Under such circumstances, consider no more than 1 to 2 days' worth of therapy with codeine sulfate or oxycodone.
- If the foregoing measures prove insufficient in patients with OA of the knees and functional impairment is severely limiting daily activity and quality of life, then consider as a temporizing measure referral for intraarticular injection of either a corticosteroid (e.g., methylprednisolone) or hyaluronic acid while more definitive therapy is pending.
- Refer for consideration of arthroplasty the patient with refractory, incapacitating disease of a major weight-bearing joint, provided that the patient is well motivated and sufficiently healthy to tolerate surgery and engage in a rehabilitation program. Age per se need not be a contraindication.

A.H.G.

Annotated Bibliography

1. Bollet AJ. Edema of the bone marrow can cause pain in osteoarthritis and other diseases of bone and joints. Ann Intern Med 2003;134:591. (*Summarizes the evidence for marrow edema as an etiologic factor.*)
2. Davis MA, Ettinger WM, Neuhaus JM, et al. Knee osteoarthritis and physical functioning: evidence from the NHANES I epidemiologic follow-up study. J Rheumatol 1991;18:591. (*There was a correlation between the severity of radiologic findings and the degree of functional impairment.*)
3. Ding C, Cicuttini F, Scott F, et al. Natural history of knee cartilage defects and factors affecting change. Arch Intern Med 2006;166:651. (*Gender, age, and body mass index were found important determinants.*)
4. Felson DT, Chaisson CE, Hill CL, et al. The association of bone marrow lesions with pain in knee osteoarthritis. Ann Intern Med 2001;134:541.

(*Presents evidence suggesting a marrow inflammatory response as an important source of pain in osteoarthritis.*)
5. Felson DT, Anderson JJ, Naimark A, et al. Obesity and knee osteoarthritis: the Framingham Study. Ann Intern Med 1988;109:18. (*Finds a strong relationship, especially in women.*)
6. Felson DT, Shang Y, Anthony JM, et al. Weight loss reduces the risk for symptomatic knee osteoarthritis in women: the Framingham Study. Ann Intern Med 1992;116:535. (*Epidemiologic data suggest that a 10-pound weight loss in obese women reduced the risk for the development of symptomatic knee pain by >50%.*)
7. Fries JF, Singh G, Morfeld D, et al. Running and the development of disability with age. Ann Intern Med 1994;121:502. (*A long-term, prospective,*

longitudinal study, finding that running markedly reduced the rate of disability but not the acceleration or postponement of osteoarthritis [OA].)

8. Gelber AC, Hochberg MC, Mead LA, et al. Body mass index in young men and the risk of subsequent knee and hip osteoarthritis. Am J Med 1999;107:542. (*Finds that there was an increased risk for OA of the knee with increased body mass index in young persons, and suggests that the cumulative weight burden may be important.*)

9. Hadler NM. Knee pain is the malady—not osteoarthritis. Ann Intern Med 1992;116:598. (*Argues that psychosocial variables are the most important determinants of who presents with knee pain.*)

10. Hamerman D. The biology of osteoarthritis. N Engl J Med 1989;320:1322. (*Slightly dated, but still one of the best basic science reviews for the generalist reader; 97 references.*)

11. Hernborg JS, Nilsson BE. The natural course of untreated osteoarthritis of the knee. Clin Orthop 1977;123:130. (*A natural history study of 94 joints in 71 patients, revealing a generally unfavorable prognosis, with pain developing at rest in the majority of patients.*)

12. Katz JN, Dalgas M, Stucki G, et al. Degenerative lumbar spinal stenosis: diagnostic value of the history and physical examination. Arthritis Rheum 1995;38:1236. (*History and physical exam were found to be very useful; reviews the key findings.*)

13. Lane NE, Bloch DA, Hubert HB, et al. Running, osteoarthritis, and bone density: initial 2-year longitudinal study. Am J Med 1990;88:452. (*No progression of OA changes was found in this group of middle-aged patients.*)

14. Salaffi F, Cavalieri F, Nolli M, et al. Analysis of disability in knee arthritis: relationship with age and psychological variables but not with radiographic score. J Rheumatol 1991;18:1581. (*Presents evidence for a strong psychosocial component.*)

15. Bradley JD, Brandt KD, Katz BP, et al. Comparison of an antiinflammatory dose of ibuprofen, an analgesic dose of ibuprofen, and acetaminophen in the treatment of patients with osteoarthritis of the knee. N Engl J Med 1991;325:87. (*An oft-cited randomized, controlled trial [RCT], showing that acetaminophen was comparable to short-term antiinflammatory therapy.*)

16. Case JP, Baliunas AJ, Block JA. Lack of efficacy of acetaminophen in treating symptomatic knee osteoarthritis. Arch Intern Med 2003;163:169. (*An example of evidence to the contrary of the Bradley study in ref. 15.*)

17. Chan FKL, Hung LCT, Suen BY, et al. Celecoxib versus diclofenac and omeprazole in reducing the risk of recurrent ulcer bleeding in patients with arthritis. N Engl J Med 2002;347:2104. (*Finds equal rates of gastrointestinal bleeding and renal insufficiency with the use of these agents.*)

18. Diclofenac gel for osteoarthritis. Med Lett Drugs Ther 2008;50:32. (*Finds a modest benefit but a high placebo effect.*)

19. Food and Drug Administration. FDA issues public health advisory on Vioxx as its manufacturer voluntarily withdraws the product. Available at: http://www.fda.gov/bbs/topics/news/2004/NEW01122.html. (*The U.S. Food and Drug Administration summary of evidence from an ongoing RCT, finding a doubling of the relative risk of cardiovascular events after 18 months of continuous daily use of Vioxx; the drug has been voluntarily withdrawn from market.*)

20. Lin EHB, Katon W, Von Korff M, et al. Effect of improving depression care on pain and functional outcomes among older adults with arthritis: a randomized controlled trial. JAMA 2003;290:2428. (*The treatment of depression improved pain control, functional status, and quality of life.*)

21. Pelletier JP, Martel-Pelletier J. The therapeutic effects of NSAIDs and corticosteroids in osteoarthritis: to be or not to be. J Rheumatol 1989;16:266. (*A discussion of their effects on the underlying disease process.*)

22. Simon LS, Lanza FL, Fipsky PE, et al. Preliminary study of the safety and efficacy of SC-58635, a novel cyclooxygenase-2 inhibitor. Arthritis Rheum 1998;41:1591. (*One of the earlier reports raising questions of cyclooxygenase-2 efficacy and safety.*)

23. Clegg DO, Reda DJ, Harris CL, et al. Glucosamine, chondroitin sulfate, and the two in combination for painful knee osteoarthritis. N Engl J Med 2006;354:795. (*A major multicenter, placebo-controlled RCT, finding no overall benefit, although modest improvement was seen in the subgroup with moderate to severe disease treated with combination therapy.*)

24. McAlindon TE, LaValley MP, Gulin JP, et al. Glucosamine and chondroitin for treatment of osteoarthritis: a systematic quality assessment and meta-analysis. JAMA 2000;283:1469. (*A critical review of the evidence, finding that study quality was questionable, publication bias likely, and benefits exaggerated, but that "some degree of efficacy [was] probable."*)

25. Petrella RJ, DiSilvestro MD, Heldebrand C. Effects of hyaluronate sodium on pain and physical functioning in osteoarthritis of the knee: a randomized, double-blind, placebo-controlled clinical trial. Arch Intern Med 2002;162:292. (*Finds a modest short-term benefit, especially for pain associated with activity.*)

26. Reichenbach S, Sterchi R, Scherer M, et al. Meta-analysis: chondroitin for osteoarthritis of the knee or hip. Ann Intern Med 2007;146:580. (*A meta-analysis, showing no net benefit from chondroitin alone.*)

27. Rintelen B, Neumann K, Leeb BF. A meta-analysis of controlled clinical studies with diacerein in the treatment of osteoarthritis. Arch Intern Med 2006;166:1899. (*Finds evidence of a significant benefit that is clinically modest.*)

28. Rozendaal RM, Koes BW, van Osch GJVM, et al. Effect of glucosamine sulfate on hip osteoarthritis: a randomized trial. Ann Intern Med 2008;148:268. (*A placebo-controlled, randomized trial, showing no benefit.*)

29. Deyle GD, Henderson NE, Matekel RL, et al. Effectiveness of manual physical therapy and exercise in osteoarthritis of the knee: a randomized controlled trial. Ann Intern Med 2000;132:173. (*Presents evidence of efficacy from a well-designed study.*)

30. Ettinger Jr WH, Burns R, Meissier SP, et al. Regular exercise reduced pain and disability from osteoarthritis of the knee. The Fitness Arthritis and Seniors Trial (FAST). JAMA 1997;227:25. (*A randomized, long-term trial, demonstrating the benefit of exercise.*)

31. Kovar PA, Allegrante JP, MacKenzie CR, et al. Supervised fitness walking in patients with osteoarthritis of the knee: a randomized, controlled trial. Ann Intern Med 1992;116:529. (*A program of patient education and supervised walking significantly improved functional status.*)

32. Minor HA, Hewett JE, Webel RR, et al. Efficacy of physical conditioning exercise in patients with rheumatoid arthritis and osteoarthritis. Arthritis Rheum 1989;32:1396. (*This approach proved to be very beneficial and can be performed without injury to the involved joints.*)

33. Pennix BWJH, Messier SP, Rejeski J, et al. Physical exercise and the prevention of disability in activities of daily living in older persons with osteoarthritis. Arch Intern Med 2001;161:2309. (*RCT, finding that aerobic and resistance exercise reduced the incidence of disability.*)

34. Arroll B, Goodyear-Smith F. Corticosteroid injections for osteoarthritis of the knee: meta-analysis. BMJ 2004;328:869. (*Finds evidence of temporary benefit.*)

35. Dieppe PA, Sathapatayavong S, Jones HE, et al. Intraarticular steroids in osteoarthritis. Rheum Rehab 1980;19:212. (*A critical look at the pluses and minuses of this controversial therapy.*)

36. LaPrade RF, Swiontkowski MF. New horizons in the treatment of osteoarthritis of the knee. JAMA 1999;281:876. (*A brief review for the general reader of autogenous cartilage implantation, osteochondral grafting, and hyaluronic acid injection.*)

37. Liang MH, Cullen KE. Primary total hip or knee replacement: evaluation of patients. Ann Intern Med 1982;97:735. (*A good review of indications, contraindications, and results.*)

38. Moseley JB, O'Malley K, Petersen NJ, et al. A controlled trial of arthroscopic surgery for osteoarthritis of the knee. N Engl J Med 2002;347:81. (*The best randomized, controlled trial to date, finding that arthroscopic surgery was no better than a placebo procedure in relieving pain and improving functional status.*)

39. Poss R. The role of osteotomy in the treatment of osteoarthritis of the hip. J Bone Joint Surg 1984;66:144. (*A review of indications, patient selection, and results.*)

40. Bratton RL, Montero DP, Adams KS, et al. Effect of "ionized" wrist bracelets on musculoskeletal pain: a randomized, double-blind, placebo-controlled trial. Mayo Clin Proc 2002;77:1164. (*Finds that this approach to be no better than placebo.*)

41. Falconer J, Hayes KW, Chang RW. Therapeutic ultrasound in the treatment of musculoskeletal conditions. Arthritis Care Res 1990;3:85. (*No benefit was found in controlled trials when this approach was compared with sham treatment.*)

42. Gaw AC, Chang LW, Shaw LC. Efficacy of acupuncture on osteoarthritic pain. N Engl J Med 1975;293:375. (*A double-blinded, controlled study, showing variable benefit.*)

43. Puett DW, Griffin MR. Published trials of nonmedicinal and noninvasive therapies for hip and knee osteoarthritis. Ann Intern Med 1994;121:133. (*The best review of the evidence and the lack thereof.*)

44. Rao JK, Mihaliak K, Kroenke K, et al. Use of complementary therapies for arthritis among patients of rheumatologists. Ann Intern Med 1999;131:409. (*These therapies had a high frequency of use; predictors of use included persistent pain and a college degree.*)

45. van Tulder MW, Cherkin DC, Berman B, et al. The effectiveness of acupuncture in the management of acute and chronic low back pain: a systematic review within the framework of the Cochrane Collaboration Back Review Group. Spine 1999;24:1113. (*Finds little evidence of benefit for acute or chronic back pain.*)

46. Skinner J, Weinstein JN, Sporer SM, et al. Racial, ethnic, and geographic disparities in rates of knee arthroplasty among Medicare patients. N Engl J Med 2003;349:1350. (*A look at factors that account for variation in rates of use.*)

47. Hochberg MC, Altman RD, Brandt KD, et al. Guidelines for the medical management of osteoarthritis. Part 1. Osteoarthritis of the hip. Part 2. Osteoarthritis of the knee. American College of Rheumatology. Arthritis Rheum 1995;38:1535. (*Evidence-based consensus guidelines.*)

CHAPTER 158 ■ MANAGEMENT OF GOUT

Gout is among the most common causes of acute monoarticular arthritis. Estimates of prevalence in the United States range from 0.3% to 2.8% of the population. Gout is predominantly a disease of adult men (sex ratio, up to 9:1). Inborn errors of purine metabolism and abnormalities of uric acid excretion account for most cases of primary gout. The expanded use of agents that decrease uric acid excretion has markedly increased the incidence of secondary gout. In the Framingham Study, almost half of new cases were associated with thiazide use. The primary physician should be able to diagnose acute gout promptly, treat it, prevent recurrences, and minimize the chances for the development of chronic gouty arthritis. Patients who present with asymptomatic hyperuricemia also require attention (see Chapter 155).

PATHOPHYSIOLOGY AND CLINICAL PRESENTATION (1–20)

The majority of patients with primary gout have a hereditary renal defect in uric acid excretion that leads to chronic hyperuricemia (see Chapter 155). Decreased renal excretion also occurs in the context of renal failure, thiazide therapy, and low doses of aspirin. Overproduction may result from myeloproliferative disease, lymphoproliferative malignancies, and severe psoriasis. Acute gout usually occurs after many years of sustained asymptomatic hyperuricemia. The higher the uric acid concentration, the greater is the risk for an acute attack, but the risk remains relatively low until very high urate levels are reached (e.g., the annual risk is 0.5% for a serum urate of 7.0 to 8.9 mg/dL and 4.9% for urate >9.0 mg/dL; see Chapter 155). The mean duration of the asymptomatic period is about 30 years. During this time, urate may be deposited in synovial lining cells and possibly also in cartilage.

Acute gout develops when uric acid crystals collect in the synovial fluid as a result of precipitation from a supersaturated state or release from the synovium. Underscoring the importance of local urate concentrations is the observation that serum uric acid is often not elevated at the time of an attack of acute gout. Trauma, a fall in temperature or pH, dehydration, starvation, excessive intake of alcohol, emotional or physical stress, and rapid changes in the serum uric acid concentration have all been implicated in the process.

As noted, a major risk factor is the use of thiazide diuretics; other risk factors include loop diuretics, obesity (especially when treated with a very low calorie diet), cyclosporine, and hypertension. In an observational study, high intakes of meat and fish compared to low intakes are associated with increased relative risks of gout (relative risks, 1.4 and 1.5, respectively), but moderate intakes of purine-rich vegetables are not. A high intake of dairy products appears to reduce risk (relative risk, 0.56).

The pathogenesis of the inflammatory response involves the phagocytosis of crystals by leukocytes in the synovial fluid, the disruption of lysosomes, the release of enzymatic products, the activation of the complement and kallikrein systems, and the release of leukocyte chemotactic factor.

Acute Gouty Arthritis

In men, the first attack is usually during the fifth decade; in women, it tends to be after age 60 years. The episode is typically monoarticular and abrupt in onset, often occurring at night. Symptoms and signs of inflammation become maximal within a few hours of onset and last for a few days to a few weeks. Untreated, symptoms of an acute attack can last for up to a few weeks, but attacks are usually self-limited, and recovery is complete.

The initial attack usually involves a joint of the lower extremity. In about half of patients, the *first metatarsophalangeal joint* is the site of inflammation (*podagra*). The tarsal joint (located at the instep), *ankle*, and *knee* are other common sites of initial attacks. Later episodes may involve a joint of the upper extremity, such as the wrist, elbow, or finger; shoulder or hip involvement is rare. More than 80% of attacks occur in a lower extremity; 85% of patients have at least one episode of podagra.

Polyarticular involvement is noted in about 5% of acute gouty attacks and may be confined to the upper extremities. Finger joint involvement is more common in women than in men and tends to present as a *Heberden's* or *Bouchard's node*. In elderly patients with gout and osteoarthritis, almost half have such nodal inflammation as the sole or initial manifestation of gout. In elderly women, the presentation of gout may be more insidious and polyarticular; multiple hand joints may be involved, with the condition resembling active rheumatoid disease.

The joint involved in an attack of acute gout appears swollen and erythematous; periarticular involvement is also common. Low-grade fever and leukocytosis may be present. A substantial fraction of patients may be *normouricemic* at the time of the acute attack. During resolution, the skin overlying the affected joint often desquamates. The clinical presentation may simulate joint infection (see Chapter 145) or even cellulitis (see Chapter 190).

Interval (Intercritical) Gout

An asymptomatic period of several years typically follows an acute attack before a second episode of acute gout takes place. The original joint or another joint may be involved in subsequent attacks. Over time, the asymptomatic intervals between acute episodes shorten. In more-advanced disease, polyarticular attacks are not uncommon, and resolution may be slower and less complete. Urate crystals may remain in the joint fluid.

Chronic Gouty Arthritis (Tophaceous Gout)

This form of gout takes years to develop. *Tophi* are typically noted an average of 10 years after the initial attack of acute gout. The risk for chronic gout is a function of the duration and severity of hyperuricemia. Tophi represent sodium urate collections surrounded by foreign-body giant-cell inflammatory reactions. They can occur in a variety of sites, including the synovium, subchondral bone, olecranon bursa, Achilles tendon, and subcutaneous tissue of the extensor surfaces of the arm. Eventually, cartilage erodes, joints become deformed, and chronic arthritis ensues. The joints of the lower extremities and hands are most commonly affected. In elderly women, the fingers may be the sole sites of involvement by gouty disease; the condition may be mistaken for rheumatoid disease, with morning stiffness and tenderness and swelling of the metacarpophalangeal and proximal interphalangeal joints. The process is insidious; the patient notes progressive aching and stiffness. Tumescences may develop over joints of the foot and make wearing shoes difficult. Fortunately, the incidence of tophaceous gout has declined markedly with the introduction of effective antihyperuricemic agents. Chronic gouty arthritis develops in fewer than 15% of patients with acute gout.

Complications

The incidence of *nephrolithiasis* among patients with clinical gout is small; the risk for new stone formation in a patient with new onset of gout is less than 1%/yr and is unrelated to the initial serum urate concentration or degree of uric acid control. Factors other than the serum urate concentration are important in stone formation and include a family history of stone formation, urine pH, hydration status, and possibly the amount of uric acid excreted by the kidneys (see Chapter 135). Stone formation is rarely dangerous; the risk for obstructive uropathy is less than 0.02%.

Concerns about the development of *chronic renal failure* as a complication of chronic hyperuricemia have been laid to rest by long-term studies (see Chapter 155). Lead intoxication is a cause in some populations; in others, it is concurrent hypertension, diabetes, cardiovascular disease, or underlying primary renal disease. *Acute renal failure* is a risk in patients undergoing chemotherapy for lymphoproliferative or myeloproliferative disease. A treatment episode may produce a uric acid load sufficient to precipitate uric acid crystals in renal tubules and elsewhere in the urinary tract, leading to acute oliguria.

Unresolved is the relation between elevations in uric acid and the risk of *cardiovascular mortality*. Epidemiologic studies suggest that elevation in uric acid is an independent risk factor for coronary heart disease (CHD), but proving a direct and independent association is made difficult by the frequent presence of important CHD risk factors (e.g., diabetes, hypertension) in patients with gout or hyperuricemia. Conversely, such cardiovascular risk factors can compromise renal function and predispose to hyperuricemia and gout.

DIAGNOSIS (4,7,10,12,15,17–19,22)

Definitive diagnosis requires *joint fluid examination* and the finding of characteristic, negatively birefringent crystals (see Chapter 145). When classic podagra appears in a patient with a prior history of gout, a clinical diagnosis can be made with reasonable confidence, but when acute monoarticular arthritis occurs in a less typical site, the full range of diagnostic possibilities must be considered (see Chapter 145). A chronic active polyarticular presentation in an older woman can be confusing because it may resemble rheumatoid disease, especially if confined to the fingers. A clue is the presence of Heberden's or Bouchard's nodes; the presence of tophi is another clue. Joint aspiration for crystal identification is needed to confirm the diagnosis. Similarly, in interval (intercritical) gout, joint aspiration and synovial fluid analysis can help to establish the diagnosis, even in the absence of an acutely inflamed joint. Aspiration can be performed on a joint that is identified by history as having been previously inflamed. *The serum uric acid* level is not helpful diagnostically because it can be normal in the presence of active inflammatory disease.

Differentiating overproduction from underexcretion can be accomplished by performing a *24-hour urine collection for uric acid*. Excretion of more than 800 to 1,000 mg/d is characteristic of overproduction. To be accurate, the test must be conducted with the patient taking a low-purine diet (false positives are possible if purine intake is not restricted) and with creatinine clearance greater than 60 mg/min (renal insufficiency reduces urate excretion and will give a falsely negative result). Other limitations include the inconvenience of the test and the inability to identify both overproduction and underexcretion.

PRINCIPLES OF THERAPY (2–6,8,9,11,14,16,17,19,21,23–32)

Acute Gouty Arthritis

Strategy

Acute symptoms can be relieved by the prompt institution of antiinflammatory therapy. Without treatment, an acute attack of gout usually resolves within 7 to 10 days, although severe episodes can last for weeks. The initiation of treatment at the very first sign of an acute attack produces a prompt and excellent therapeutic response. Delay of therapy is associated with less satisfactory results. Antiinflammatory therapy is usually continued until symptoms have resolved.

Nonsteroidal Antiinflammatory Drugs (NSAIDs)

When given in full doses, generic NSAIDs are the treatment of choice and can blunt or even terminate an attack when given within the first 24 hours after the onset of symptoms. *Indomethacin, ibuprofen,* and *naproxen* are the best studied of the NSAIDs for use in acute gout, but almost any NSAID should suffice. Persons who cannot tolerate full doses of nonselective NSAIDs due to gastrointestinal side effects (e.g., the elderly) can be treated concurrently with proton-pump inhibition (e.g., omeprazole 20 to 40 mg/d; see Chapter 68) or a cyclooxygenase-2 (COX-2) preparation, which is as effective as a nonselective NSAID (concern about adverse cardiovascular effects appears to pertain only to long-term COX-2 use; see Chapter 156). Some elderly patients may experience mental confusion with indomethacin (see Chapter 156). Delay in starting NSAID therapy compromises response because the inflammatory reaction is already well established.

Colchicine

Another alternative for patients unable to take nonselective NSAID therapy is colchicine. As with NSAIDs, colchicine treatment is most effective when given within the first 24 hours, with more than two thirds of patients responding well. Limiting colchicine's utility for an acute attack is the drug's tendency to cause *gastrointestinal upset* (nausea, vomiting, diarrhea) when taken at the necessary full doses (i.e., 0.6 mg hourly for the first 3 hours and then every 6 hours). *Bone marrow suppression* and an increased risk for *myopathy* and *neuropathy* have been reported in persons with concurrent *renal* or *hepatic insufficiency*, particularly when colchicine is administered intravenously, which is not recommended.

Glucocorticoids

Systemic glucocorticosteroids are sometimes prescribed, especially if the gastrointestinal side effects of colchicine and NSAIDs prevent their use or if patients appear to be refractory to standard first-line treatment. Parenteral therapy with a single dose of corticotropin or triamcinolone and oral therapy with a short course of high-dose prednisone or methyl prednisolone are of equal efficacy. Relief can be achieved within 24 hours. Intraarticular injection of a "depo" corticosteroid preparation is worth considering when a large, weight-bearing joint is severely affected. The use of corticosteroid therapy is associated with an increased risk of a rebound attack, often necessitating concurrent therapy with low-dose colchicine.

Interval Gout—Secondary Prevention

Although prophylactic therapy to prevent acute gouty arthritis is not necessary or cost-effective for a patient with asymptomatic hyperuricemia (see Chapter 155) or a first attack of gout, secondary prophylaxis becomes cost-effective after a patient starts having two to three attacks per year, particularly if the episodes are disabling. Intervals between future recurrences are likely to shorten without prophylactic treatment.

Strategy

Options include lowering uric acid levels by dietary and lifestyle measures, instituting chronic antiinflammatory therapy, and attending to other risk factors. Of the risk factors for recurrent gouty attacks, hyperuricemia is among the most amenable to treatment. Options include reducing purine intake (diet, lifestyle, alcohol intake), blocking urate production (allopurinol), and enhancing renal excretion (probenecid, sulfinpyrazone, and reducing drugs that limit urate excretion). The goal is to lower the uric acid concentration to less than 6.5 mg/dL, the level at which extracellular fluid becomes saturated with uric acid.

A pathophysiologic approach to secondary pharmacologic prophylaxis might base the choice of urate-lowering treatment on the 24-hour urinary excretion of uric acid. Because most persons with idiopathic disease are underexcretors, they could be identified by the 24-hour urine test. Although mechanistically logical, there is no evidence that this approach is superior to empiric treatment with allopurinol, which, unlike uricosuric therapy, poses no risk in the presence of hyperexcretion. In terms of preventing symptomatic recurrences of gout, starting pharmacologic therapy with allopurinol appears to be as effective as an approach based on the 24-hour urine test. Current standard practice is to omit the initial 24-hour collection and proceed directly to allopurinol therapy, reserving measurement of urate excretion for instances when an allopurinol program fails or is not tolerated. However, drugs that reduce urate excretion (e.g., *thiazides*, *loop diuretics*, *niacin*, low-dose *aspirin*) might be reduced or discontinued if possible; often this is not possible, and urate-lowering pharmacotherapy is required.

The allopurinol-first strategy usually suffices and is easy to implement (see later discussion); however, reducing the serum uric acid mobilizes tissue urate deposits, potentially increasing local urate concentrations and the risk of acute gout. To prevent precipitating an attack of gout during the early stages of urate-lowering therapy, treatment is started at low doses and titrated upward as evidence of urate deposits wanes. During this period, supplemental prophylaxis is provided by a program of low-dose antiinflammatory medication (e.g., colchicine).

Diet, Alcohol, and Obesity

Dietary measures can be helpful but may not suffice. Purine-rich foods, such as organ meats and other meats, seafood, yeast, beer and other alcoholic beverages, legumes, oatmeal, spinach, mushrooms, asparagus, and cauliflower, have all been implicated. In major epidemiologic study, very high intakes of meat and seafood are associated with an increased risk of gout (a relative risk of 1.5 for those in highest intake quartile compared to persons in the lowest quartile). A high intake of low-fat dairy products reduces the risk of gout (relative risk, 0.56). A high intake of vegetable sources of purines has no effect on risk.

Limiting the utility of dietary measures are that only 10% of circulating purine is derived from dietary sources, a purine-restricted diet is not especially palatable, and the degree of urate reduction by diet alone is typically modest. Consequently, the restriction of purine intake is not likely to suffice as the sole means of prophylactic therapy unless dietary habits or events appear to correlate strongly with gouty attacks.

Alcohol excess and obesity deserve attention. If a gouty attack appears to be precipitated by binge drinking, the attack can be a stimulus for discussing an alteration of drinking behavior (see Chapter 228). Similarly, gout in the context of obesity provides an opportunity to consider weight reduction efforts. Obesity is a modifiable risk factor that deserves attention, but starvation diets should be avoided because they trigger gouty attacks; a low-calorie, low-carbohydrate diet can decrease urate levels by nearly 20%. Bariatric surgery in persons with morbid obesity significantly reduces hyperuricemia.

Allopurinol

Allopurinol inhibits the production of uric acid by blocking xanthine oxidase, which converts xanthine to uric acid. Unlike uric acid, xanthine does not cause joint inflammation or stone formation. Among the advantages and reasons for the wide adoption of an allopurinol-first program are its convenience (once-daily dosing) and tolerability. In addition to usefulness in persons with idiopathic gout, the drug is also well suited for those with renal insufficiency, a history of nephrolithiasis, and hyperexcretion of uric acid. The half-life of allopurinol is about 3 hours, but its metabolites are biologically active for up to 30 hours. As a result, the drug only needs to be taken once daily. Serum urate levels fall within 1 week of initiation of therapy, but the mobilization of urate stores and the consequent risk for gouty attacks does not decline until normouricemia has been sustained for 3 to 6 months. Consequently, dose is started low and gradually titrated upward in 1- to 2-week increments; colchicine is taken concurrently.

Of the minor side effects, *rash* and *gastrointestinal upset* are among the most common. About 2% of patients experience rash. If it is mild, the rash quickly resolves with the cessation of therapy and may not recur if the drug is restarted at a low level. A recurrence of mild rash can be treated with a desensitization program (10 to 25 μg/d as an oral suspension, doubling every 3 to 14 days until full dose is achieved). However, the development of a more intense rash is associated with an increased risk of more serious hypersensitivity reactions, which occur in about 3.5% of patients. Manifestations include *fever, leukopenia, vasculitis,* and *hepatocellular injury.*

A *fulminant hypersensitivity* syndrome characterized by *desquamative rash, fever, hepatitis, eosinophilia,* and *renal failure* is the most worrisome adverse effect. Although uncommon (prevalence <0.25%), it is associated with a 15% to 25% mortality rate and occurs mostly in patients with concurrent renal insufficiency or diuretic use. Allopurinol should always be used with caution. In most instances, dose should not exceed 300 to 400 mg/d, and reduced doses are indicated in patients with renal insufficiency. The white cell count and renal function should be monitored regularly for the first several months of treatment. Drug–drug interactions are also important. The risk for drug rash is increased 10-fold by the concurrent use of *ampicillin,* and the activity of drugs metabolized by hepatic microsomal enzymes (e.g., warfarin, azathioprine) can be potentiated.

Although allopurinol is a reasonable and generally safe first-line drug for prophylaxis, it should not be prescribed casually. Careful attention to dose in renal failure and watchfulness for early signs of a serious hypersensitivity reaction help to ensure intelligent, safe use. The drug is expensive. Because the drug provides no symptomatic relief and may even precipitate an attack, it should not be started until well after an attack of gout has resolved.

Febuxostat

A nonpurine selective inhibitor of xanthine oxidase, febuxostat, has emerged as a potential alternative to allopurinol for patients with hyperuricemia and gout. The drug has been approved in Europe, and approval is awaited in the United States for use in treating hyperuricemia in patients with chronic gouty arthritis. Skin rashes and mild elevations in liver function tests are the most common side effects (occurring more frequently than with allopurinol). The finding during phase III study of an increased risk of seemingly unrelated death among persons randomized to the drug has raised concerns and prompted calls for more study before U.S. approval.

Uricosuric Agents (Probenecid, Sulfinpyrazone)

The uricosuric drugs have an excellent safety record, so they are well suited for long-term prophylactic therapy in persons who are found to be underexcretors. Probenecid and sulfinpyrazone are the principal uricosuric drugs; both act to inhibit renal tubular reabsorption of uric acid. About 80% of patients excreting less than 700 mg of uric acid daily can be effectively managed by uricosuric therapy.

Disadvantages include *frequent dosing,* a risk for precipitating *nephrolithiasis, drug–drug interactions,* and a few bothersome *side effects.* Because these agents are less convenient to use, compliance tends to be less than with allopurinol. Probenecid must be taken two to three times per day; sulfinpyrazone requires dosing three or four times daily. At the onset of therapy, uric acid excretion may reach extraordinary levels and trigger nephrolithiasis; therefore, initial doses must be modest. Generous fluid intake (2 to 3 L/d) and urinary alkalinization are also necessary. Drug–drug interactions are common. Probenecid blocks the renal excretion of penicillins and the hepatic uptake of rifampin, prolonging the half-lives of both. *Thiazides, loop diuretics,* and low doses of *salicylates* may blunt uricosuric action, but usually not enough to neutralize it. Side effects include *rash, autoimmune hemolytic anemia,* and *gastrointestinal upset.* Sulfinpyrazone is associated with a very small risk for *marrow suppression.*

Losartan

Losartan, an angiotensin II–receptor antagonist used in the treatment of hypertension and heart failure (see Chapter 26), has been found to have uricosuric activity, making it potentially useful in hypertensive patients who have a history of gout. However, cost is high and efficacy for long-term use is not well established. The drug is well tolerated and requires only once-daily dosing. It may be combined with allopurinol.

Antiinflammatory Agents (Colchicine, NSAIDs)

All urate-lowering drugs can mobilize tissue deposits of uric acid and trigger attacks of acute gout during the initial 3 to 6 months of therapy. During this period, concurrent antiinflammatory therapy is often prescribed. Both colchicine and NSAIDs are used. No definitive data are available regarding the ideal duration of concurrent antiinflammatory therapy, but most authorities recommend that it be given for 3 to 6 months or until all visible urate deposits have disappeared.

Colchicine. Once- or twice-daily low-dose colchicine for 3 to 6 months can lower the risk of a gouty attack during this period. Treatment is well tolerated, but even with low doses there is a risk for myopathy and myelosuppression. The concurrent use of drugs that inhibit drug metabolism and/or excretion (statins, macrolide antibiotics, cyclosporine) can increase colchicine levels and the risk of adverse effects. Dose is reduced in renal failure.

NSAIDs. Despite limited evidence of efficacy, some clinicians use a small daily dose of a generic NSAID rather than colchicine to enhance secondary prophylaxis in the early months of urate-lowering treatment. The potential adverse effects of chronic use (see Chapters 68 and 156) need to be carefully weighed against the expected benefits.

Chronic Gouty Arthritis

Urate-lowering therapy is also indicated in patients with tophaceous gout to prevent progressive articular damage. The prevention or relief of chronic gouty arthritis requires normalization of the serum uric acid. As the more effective and more convenient treatment, *allopurinol* is usually prescribed for patients with tophaceous gout. Often, tophi begin to resolve after several weeks of therapy. In the future, *febuxostat* may become an alternative for patients who cannot tolerate allopurinol, but concerns about its tolerability and safety remain to be resolved (see earlier discussion). A uricosuric agent is a reasonable alternative to xanthine oxidase inhibitors, provided that renal function is normal and no nephrolithiasis or excessive excretion of uric acid has been noted. Under investigation is the use of recombinant *uricase* for refractory hyperuricemia and recurrent attacks of gout. Regardless of the agent selected, concurrent antiinflammatory therapy (see prior discussion) must be given until visible urate deposits have resolved.

Renal Complications

Although the risk for a renal complication is small, attention to renal issues is required in certain instances during the management of the gouty patient (see also Chapter 155).

Nephrolithiasis

The gouty patient with an established uric acid stone should be treated with allopurinol and a high fluid intake; concurrent administration of a thiazide diuretic may be necessary (see Chapter 135). Allopurinol therapy to prevent stone formation is indicated for gouty patients with a prior history of nephrolithiasis and perhaps for those with a strong family history of kidney stones. All patients should be instructed to avoid dehydration, especially if they live in a warm, dry climate. Isolated hyperuricemia per se does not require treatment in the absence of other risk factors for nephrolithiasis (see Chapter 155).

Renal Failure

Patients undergoing chemotherapy for lymphoproliferative or myeloproliferative disease require pretreatment with allopurinol. Prolonged urate-lowering therapy has no role in the prevention of chronic renal failure in patients with gout, but avoidance of exposure to lead is important, as is the treatment of common comorbidities such as hypertension, diabetes, and cardiovascular disease.

PATIENT EDUCATION

Patients who experience an acute gouty attack are highly motivated to undertake preventive measures and are very receptive to advice. If they are obese, they should be advised to begin a concerted program of supervised weight reduction (see Chapter 233) but to avoid starvation or very low calorie diets that may only exacerbate the risk of gout. Drinkers should be warned against binges. Maintenance of good hydration needs to be stressed to those at risk for nephrolithiasis. On the other hand, patients will find it comforting to know that severe dietary restrictions are unnecessary. Fasting should be avoided because it may precipitate an attack. The importance of treating an acute attack at the first sign of illness also needs to be stressed. For the patient with interval gout, a discussion of the risks and benefits of prophylactic therapy and the importance of compliance is indicated. Those taking allopurinol should be warned of the risk of a hypersensitivity reaction and advised to cease intake immediately and call the physician at the first sign of a rash, fever, or other manifestation.

THERAPEUTIC RECOMMENDATIONS

Acute Gout

- At the first sign of an attack of acute gouty arthritis, begin a generic nonsteroidal antiinflammatory agent (e.g., 500 mg of *naproxen* three times daily). Continue full-dose treatment until symptoms resolve, then taper to cessation over 72 hours. Advise the patient that delay in starting therapy may impair the response.
- Consider application of an icepack at the outset.
- For patients unable to take NSAID therapy (e.g., those with active peptic ulcer disease), consider adding *omeprazole* 20 to 40 mg/d, using a COX-2 drug (e.g., *celecoxib* 200 mg/d), or *colchicine* (0.6 mg hourly × three doses and then four times daily). When prescribing colchicine, warn the patient that diarrhea and some upper gastrointestinal upset are likely during the course of therapy; monitor blood cell count and hepatic and renal function; avoid colchicine

use if there is renal or hepatic insufficiency. When considering a COX-2 agent, keep in mind cardiovascular risk (see Chapter 156), but the risk with short-term therapy should be minimal.
- For very severe or refractory cases of definite acute gout, consider a 7- to 10-day course of high-dose oral corticosteroids (e.g., *prednisone* 40 to 60 mg every morning); taper as clinically indicated. Intraarticular corticosteroid therapy (e.g., *methylprednisolone* 40 mg/mL) is another option if oral therapy is not feasible and just one large, weight-bearing joint is involved.
- Provide an extra supply of antiinflammatory therapy so that it will be available for prompt use in a future episode.

Interval Gout

- Recommend weight reduction (but not very low calorie diets or fasting) if the patient is obese and cessation of excess alcohol use, especially binge drinking. Consider restricting meat- and seafood-derived dietary purine intake, especially if intake is very high or if attacks are clearly precipitated by dietary events; there is no need to limit vegetable sources of purines; encourage low-fat dairy products.
- Establish that gouty attacks are sufficiently frequent (at least two to three times per year) and disabling to warrant chronic prophylactic pharmacotherapy, and, if so, that the patient is willing to take the necessary medication indefinitely.
- Begin *allopurinol* (starting at 100 mg/d) and increase by 100 mg/d every 1 to 2 weeks until a dose of 300 mg/d is reached. Adjust the dose upward if the response is inadequate. Reduce the dose in the setting of renal insufficiency and use cautiously, especially when diuretics or ampicillin are being given concurrently. Stop at the earliest sign of a hypersensitivity reaction. Consider restarting at a low dose if the drug rash was mild, but monitor complete blood cell count and hepatic and renal function closely. Consider desensitization for patients who require allopurinol but who react to it with a mild drug rash.
- If allopurinol cannot be tolerated, consider uricosuric therapy with *probenecid* or *sulfinpyrazone*, but only if the patient has normal renal function, no risk for stone disease, and a urate excretion of less than 700 mg/d (as determined by 24-hour urine collection). Therapy should be initiated in small doses (e.g., 250 mg of probenecid twice daily or 50 mg of sulfinpyrazone twice daily), and at the same time fluid intake should be kept up (2 to 3 L/d) to prevent the precipitation of uric acid in the urinary tract. Alkalinization of the urine to a pH of 6.6 is desirable during the first week of therapy but is difficult to achieve; gram doses of sodium bicarbonate are required, supplemented by acetazolamide (250 mg) before bedtime.
- Advance the uricosuric dose gradually to avoid triggering massive urate excretion. Continue high fluid intake during the early months of therapy. The maximum dose of sulfinpyrazone is 100 mg three to four times daily; for probenecid, it is 500 to 1,000 mg two to three times daily. Avoid the concurrent use of aspirin because it inhibits urate excretion.
- To reduce the risk for an attack of gout during the first 3 to 6 months of urate-lowering treatment, prescribe concurrent low-dose antiinflammatory prophylactic therapy with either *colchicine* (0.6 mg daily or twice daily) or an intermediate-acting NSAID (e.g., 250 mg of *naproxen* daily or twice daily).

- Monitor serum uric acid concentration and treat to achieve a level of less than 6.5 mg/dL, the point of supersaturation.
- Advise restriction of low-dose *aspirin, thiazides, loop diuretics,* and *niacin* to the degree possible, especially if urate-lowering therapy is not instituted. Consider losartan if thiazide therapy is necessary for the treatment of underlying hypertension.

Chronic Gouty Arthritis

- Treat as for interval gout. Continue concurrent antiinflammatory therapy until all visible manifestations of uric acid deposits have resolved, which may take 6 to 12 months.

Renal Complications

- Pretreat cancer patients with allopurinol if a large uric acid load is likely to result from an application of chemotherapy.
- Advise a marked reduction in lead exposure (e.g., home-distilled alcohol, industrial contact).
- Treat patients with urate nephrolithiasis or a strong family history of kidney stones with allopurinol (300 mg once daily) and hydration. Long-term efforts to alkalinize the urine are impractical and need not be undertaken.
- Because the risk for chronic renal failure from chronic hyperuricemia is nil, long-term urate-lowering therapy to prevent it is unnecessary.

A.H.G.

Annotated Bibliography

1. Bautman V, Maesaka JK, Haddad B, et al. The role of lead in gouty nephropathy. N Engl J Med 1981;304:520. (*An important link between gout and renal injury.*)
2. Berger L, Yu TF. Renal function in gout—an analysis of 524 gouty subjects including long-term follow-up studies. Am J Med 1975;59:604. (*A 12-year follow-up study, finding that hyperuricemia alone had no deleterious effect on renal function in ambulatory patients with gout.*)
3. Choi HK, Mount DB, Reginato AM. Pathogenesis of gout. Ann Intern Med 2005;143:499. (*An excellent review of pathophysiology.*)
4. Choi HK, Atkinson K, Karlson EW, et al. Purine-rich foods, dairy and protein intake, and the risk of gout in men. N Engl J Med 2003;350:1093. (*A large-scale, prospective, observational study, finding that the risk increased only for meat and fish but not vegetables, and was reduced with the use of low-fat dairy products.*)
5. Choi HK, Atkinson K, Karlson EW, et al. Obesity weight change, hypertension, diuretic use, and risk of gout in men: the Health Professionals Follow-up Study. Arch Intern Med 2005;165:742. (*Obesity was a risk factor and weight loss was protective.*)
6. Culleton BF, Larson MG, Kannel WB, et al. Serum uric acid and risk for cardiovascular disease and death: the Framingham Heart Study. Ann Intern Med 1999;131:7. (*A rigorous epidemiologic examination, finding no evidence for a causal relationship between urate level and cardiovascular risk; a previously noted link appeared to be thiazide use for hypertension.*)
7. Edwards NL. Gout: clinical and laboratory features. In: Klippel JD, ed. Primer on rheumatic diseases. Atlanta, GA: Arthritis Foundation, 1997:234. (*An excellent description of presentation and diagnostic features.*)
8. Fang J, Alderman MH. Serum uric acid and cardiovascular mortality: the NHANES I epidemiologic follow-up study, 1971–1992. JAMA 2000;283:2404. (*Presents epidemiologic data suggesting an independent contribution of uric acid to coronary heart disease risk.*)
9. Fessel JW. Renal outcomes of gout and hyperuricemia. Am J Med 1979;67:74. (*The risks for renal failure and stone formation were very small.*)
10. Hadler NM, Franck WA, Bress NM, et al. Acute polyarticular gout. Am J Med 1974;56:715. (*In one third of patients, the condition was confined to the upper extremities, and it sometimes occurred in the setting of a normal serum uric acid level.*)
11. Hall AP, Berry PE, Dawber TR, et al. Epidemiology of gout and hyperuricemia—a long-term population study. Am J Med 1967;42:27. (*The oft-quoted Framingham Study data, showing that the risk for acute gout rose with uric acid level.*)
12. Lally EV, Zimmerman B, Ho G, et al. Urate-mediated inflammation in nodal osteoarthritis: clinical and roentgenographic correlations. Arthritis Rheum 1989;32:86. (*A Heberden's or Bouchard's node was the initial or sole manifestation of gout in almost half of elderly patients with gout and osteoarthritis.*)
13. Lin HY, Rocher LL, McQuillan MA, et al. Cyclosporine-induced hyperuricemia and gout. N Engl J Med 1989;321:287. (*Hyperuricemia was common; gout was seen in 7% of cases.*)
14. Maclaughlan MJ, Rodnan GP. Effects of food, fast, and alcohol on serum uric acid and acute attacks of gout. Am J Med 1967;42:38. (*Fasting and consumption of >100 g of alcohol raised urate levels and often precipitated attacks.*)
15. Meyers DC, Monteagudo FSE. Gout in females: an analysis of 92 patients. Clin Exp Rheumatol 1985;3:105. (*The presentation in women may be an insidious polyarthritis rather than an acute monoarthritis.*)
16. National Task Force on the Prevention and Treatment of Obesity. Very low-calorie diets. JAMA 1993;270:967. (*The risk for triggering an acute gouty attack is low but increased in patients with prior symptomatic gout.*)
17. Terkeltaub RA. Gout. N Engl J Med 2003;349:1647. (*A succinct clinical review.*)
18. Wernick R, Winkler C, Campbell S. Tophi as the initial manifestation of gout. Arch Intern Med 1992;152:873. (*This condition was noted in the fingers of elderly women with underlying osteoarthritis, renal insufficiency, and concurrent nonsteroidal antiinflammatory drug [NSAID] use.*)
19. Wortmann RL. Gout and hyperuricemia. Curr Opin Rheumatol 2002;14:281. (*A comprehensive review by one of the field's leading authorities.*)
20. Yu TF, Berger LU. Impaired renal function in gout. Am J Med 1982;75:95. (*Hyperuricemia alone did not affect renal function; renal insufficiency correlated best with coexisting hypertension, preexisting renal disease, and ischemic heart disease.*)
21. Yu TF, Gutman A. Uric acid nephrolithiasis in gout: predisposing factors. Ann Intern Med 1967;67:1133. (*A classic study, correlating the risk for stone formation with uric acid excretion, urine pH, serum urate level, and underlying disease.*)
22. Pascual E, Batlle-Gualda E, Martinez A, et al. Synovial fluid analysis for diagnosis of intercritical gout. Ann Intern Med 1999;131:756. (*Urate crystals were found in a high percentage of patients with a history suggestive of gout but with no active joint inflammation.*)
23. Becker MA, Schumacher HR, Wortmann RL, et al. Febuxostat compared with allopurinol in patients with hyperuricemia and gout. N Engl J Med 2006;353:2450. (*A randomized, controlled trial of this new drug to lower urate production, finding that it was more effective than allopurinol in lowering uric acid but similar in the prevention of gouty attacks and not as well tolerated.*)
24. Bomalaski JS, Holtsberg FW, Ensor CM, et al. Uricase formulated with polyethylene glycol (uricase-PEG 20): biochemical rationale and preclinical studies. J Rheumatol 2002;29:1942. (*A promising new approach for refractory cases.*)
25. Fam AG, Lewtas J, Stein J, et al. Desensitization to allopurinol in patients with gout and cutaneous reactions. Am J Med 1992;93:299. (*This approach was moderately successful in persons with mild rashes.*)
26. Ferraz MB, O'Brien B. A cost-effectiveness analysis of urate-lowering drugs in nontophaceous recurrent gouty arthritis. J Rheumatol 1995;22:908. (*Treatment was found to be cost-effective after two or more attacks per year.*)
27. Groff GD, Franck WA, Raddatz DA. Systemic steroid therapy for acute gout: a clinical trial and review of the literature. Semin Arthritis Rheum 1990;19:329. (*Presents good evidence for efficacy.*)
28. Hande KR, Noone RM, Stone WJ. Severe allopurinol toxicity. Am J Med 1984;76:47. (*Describes a potentially fatal hypersensitivity syndrome.*)
29. Schlesinger N, Detry MA, Holland BK, et al. Local ice therapy during bouts of acute gouty arthritis. J Rheumatol 2002;29:331. (*Presents evidence for this commonly applied home remedy.*)
30. Siegel LB, Alloway JA, Nashel DJ. Comparison of adrenocorticotropin hormone and triamcinolone acetonide in the treatment of acute gouty arthritis. J Rheumatol 1994;21:1325. (*Both trophic and hormone therapies are effective and equally so.*)
31. Shahinfar S, Simpson RL, Carides AD, et al. Safety of losartan in hypertensive patients with thiazide-induced hyperuricemia. Kidney Int 1999;56:1879. (*Losartan reduced urate levels.*)
32. Singer JZ, Wallace SL. The allopurinol hypersensitivity syndrome. Arthritis Rheum 1986;29:82. (*There was a high mortality risk; there were many cases in patients who did not need the drug.*)

CHAPTER 159 ■ APPROACH TO THE PATIENT WITH FIBROMYALGIA

Patients with diffuse, chronic musculoskeletal pain but no evidence of arthritis account for a large number of office visits. Some of them have mild rheumatoid disease; in other cases, their symptoms are caused by bony pathology, neuropathy, and myopathy. When no source stands out, clinicians start wondering about somatization despite protests from the patient that the problem is "not in my head."

In recent years, a syndrome of diffuse and chronic musculoskeletal pain, stiffness, focal tenderness, disordered sleep, and fatigue has become increasingly recognized as an important clinical entity. The terms *fibromyalgia*, *fibrositis*, and *fibromyositis* have been used to designate it, although the "-itis" terminology has been discouraged because no inflammatory pathophysiology has been detected. Although the cause of the syndrome is unknown, it appears to be common and is estimated to have a prevalence as high as 5% among adult women, who account for 80% to 90% of cases. After osteoarthritis, fibromyalgia accounts for the most visits to rheumatologists.

PATHOPHYSIOLOGY, CLINICAL PRESENTATION, AND COURSE (1–14)

Pathogenesis

The cause of fibromyalgia is unknown. Although the symptoms suggest somatization, careful psychological studies reveal no relationship between symptoms and psychological status. Only an increased frequency of life stress has been found. Most patients are not depressed, and any onset of depression does not correlate with the level of pain. One of the most consistent findings is an alteration in central nervous system neurotransmitter metabolism and function, with abnormal levels of serotonin, norepinephrine, and substance P found. Disturbances of stage 4 (non–rapid-eye-movement) sleep are related to the symptoms. These findings suggested to some a pathophysiologic common denominator involving the neurochemistry of *sleep* and *pain perception*. *Abnormal nociception* is emerging as an important element of the explanatory model (similar to its suspected role in irritable bowel syndrome; see Chapter 74). Neuroendocrine changes have also been observed but are not sufficient to be considered etiologic.

Muscle biopsy findings and electromyographic data demonstrate no consistent or unique changes. A subset of patients with fibromyalgia have abnormal antibodies, but they appear to have concurrent connective tissue disease. Because of the overlapping of symptoms of chronic fatigue syndrome and those of fibromyalgia, a common pathophysiology has been surmised, but the pathogenesis is unknown for both conditions. Other patients have serology positive for Lyme disease, but treatment for Lyme disease usually does little to alleviate their symptoms. Some of these cases are believed to represent false-positive results that can be explained by the low specificity of Lyme serology and the high prevalence of fibromyalgia. A relation between recent infection and transient fibromyalgia syndrome has been observed in some cases of clinical Lyme disease and in some instances of acute mononucleosis, but no firm data are available to link infection with chronic symptoms.

Clinical Presentation

The typical patient is a woman in her mid-30s to mid-50s who describes chronic and *diffuse musculoskeletal pain*, *stiffness*, and *fatigue*. The pain tends to be constant, aching, and concentrated in axial regions (neck, shoulders, back, pelvis). "Stiffness" is the term often used to describe the discomfort, which is characteristically worse in the morning and exacerbated by changes in the weather, cold, humidity, sleeplessness, and stress and helped by warmth, rest, and mild exercise. Points of *focal tenderness* may be reported in the upper and lower extremities. Patients awake from sleep feeling *tired* and *unrefreshed*.

Physical examination findings are normal except for the presence of *tender points*—multiple, reproducible points of exaggerated tenderness to palpation. The tender points tend to be symmetric and located in the occiput, neck, shoulder, ribs, elbows, buttocks, and knees. Eighteen characteristic locations have been identified (Fig. 159.1).

Clinical Course

Fibromyalgia is a chronic but nonprogressive disorder. Waxing and waning with changes in the weather, degree of situational stress, and amount of rest are characteristic. The number and location of tender points tend to be stable over time. In some patients, the condition may become disabling, at least temporarily, but the clinical course overall is one of steady but nonprogressive disease. A substantial minority of patients experience spontaneous remission, and many of those who continue to have symptoms report a general improvement with time. The degree of disability can be substantial; up to one fourth of patients receive disability payments at some time during their illness. Underlying psychosocial problems are the principal determinant of disability and health care utilization in patients with fibromyalgia.

DIFFERENTIAL DIAGNOSIS (5–7,10,11)

The clinical diagnosis of fibromyalgia has been facilitated by a standardized case definition using diagnostic criteria established by the American College of Rheumatology: (a)

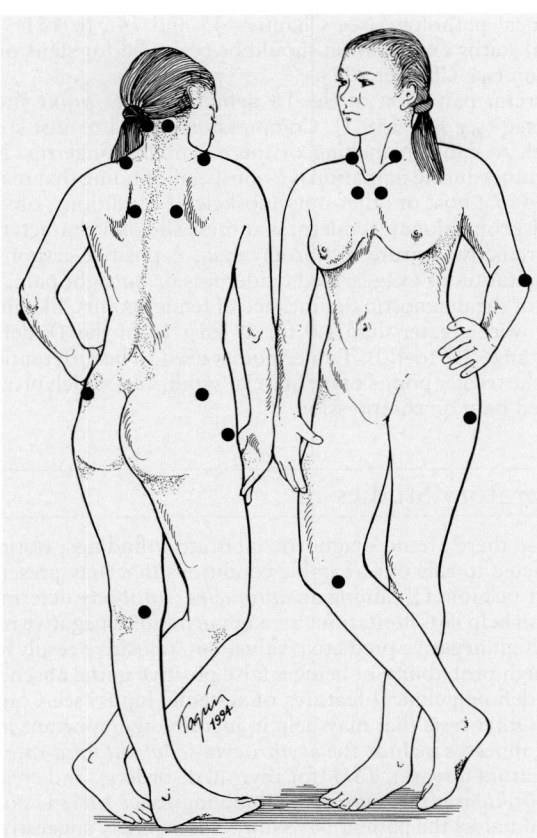

FIGURE 159.1. Tender points in fibromyalgia syndrome.

TABLE 159.1

THE AMERICAN COLLEGE OF RHEUMATOLOGY 1990 CRITERIA FOR THE CLASSIFICATION OF FIBROMYALGIA

History of Widespread Pain

Definition. Pain is considered widespread when all of the following are present: pain in the left side of the body, pain in the right side of the body, pain above the waist, and pain below the waist. In addition, axial skeletal pain (cervical spine or anterior chest or thoracic spine or low back) must be present. In this definition, shoulder and buttock pain is considered as pain for each involved side. "Low back" pain is considered lower segment pain.

Pain in 11 of 18 Tender Point Sites on Digital Palpation (Fig. 159.1)

Definition. Pain, on digital palpation, must be present in at least 11 of the following 18 tender point sites:

Occiput: bilateral, at the suboccipital muscle insertions

Low cervical: bilateral, at the anterior aspects of the intertransverse spaces at C1–C7

Trapezius: bilateral, at the midpoint of the upper border

Supraspinatus: bilateral, at origins, above the scapula spine near the medial border

Second rib: bilateral, at the second costochondral junctions, just lateral to the junctions on upper surfaces

Lateral epicondyle: bilateral, 2 cm distal to the epicondyles

Gluteal: bilateral, in upper outer quadrants of buttocks in anterior fold of muscle

Greater trochanter: bilateral, posterior to the trochanteric prominence

Knee: bilateral, at the medial fat pad proximal to the joint line

Digital palpation should be performed with an approximate force of 4 kg.

For a tender point to be considered "positive," the subject must state that the palpation was painful. "Tender" is not be considered "painful."

For classification purposes, patients are said to have fibromyalgia if both criteria are satisfied. Widespread pain must have been present for at least 3 months. The presence of a second clinical disorder does not exclude the diagnosis of fibromyalgia.

From Wolfe F, Smyth HA, Yunus MB, et al. The American College of Rheumatology 1990 criteria for the classification of fibromyalgia: the Multicenter Committee. Arthritis Rheum 1990;33:160, with permission.

---

widespread pain including axial pain for at least 3 months and (b) pain in at least 11 of 18 possible tender point sites (Table 159.1). Nonetheless, the diagnosis must not be considered established until a host of similarly presenting conditions have been ruled out, conditions that may be mistakenly labeled as fibromyalgia.

Myofascial syndromes resulting from overuse may be confused with fibromyalgia, in that tender points are characteristic of both. Unlike those of fibromyalgia, the tender points of myofascial syndrome are clustered about just one area and trigger referred pain on compression (hence the term *trigger points*). Moreover, symptoms are focal rather than diffuse. A history of onset after excessive activity or muscle strain is typical. No fatigue or sleep disorder is associated with myofascial syndrome.

Rheumatoid disease in its early or mild forms may cause diffuse musculoskeletal discomfort, morning stiffness, fatigue, and focal tenderness on physical examination. However, the tenderness appears to be less exaggerated, and results of serologic studies are abnormal. *Polymyalgia rheumatica* superficially resembles fibromyalgia, but the onset is at a much later age, symptoms are confined to the hip and shoulder girdles, few tender points are present, and the sedimentation rate is markedly elevated. *Ankylosing spondylitis* produces axial discomfort, fatigue, and focal tenderness; however, most patients with axial symptoms are men, and sacroiliitis is a defining manifestation (see Chapter 146).

Spondyloarthropathy in women can easily be mistaken for fibromyalgia because the likely symptoms are diffuse and may include chronic axial discomfort, focal spinal pain in multiple

sites, and disordered sleep. Because it is more common in men, spondyloarthropathy is not commonly considered in women, and neck pain may be more prominent than lower back pain, further confusing the picture. Clinical findings suggestive of spondyloarthropathy include a positive family history, psoriasis, inflammatory bowel disease, risk factors for Reiter's syndrome, relief of pain with exercise, sacroiliitis, and pain or tenderness at the site of insertion of a tendon or at the Achilles tendon or plantar fascia.

Chronic fatigue syndrome has been found to share many of the clinical features of fibromyalgia, including chronic, diffuse musculoskeletal pain and tender points, so that differentiation is difficult at times because both conditions are diagnosed clinically. Pain tends to be less prominent in chronic fatigue syndrome, and not all patients have tender points. Sometimes, distinguishing between chronic fatigue syndrome and fibromyalgia is impossible because of so much clinical overlap, which is not critical functionally because the approach to management is very similar for both.

Lyme disease also enters into the differential diagnosis but is readily recognized by a history of deer tick exposure, residence in an endemic area, rash, polyarthritis, and neurologic deficits (see Chapter 160). Some patients may have a transient syndrome that temporarily resembles fibromyalgia.

Hypothyroidism may be accompanied by diffuse myalgias and fatigue that simulate fibromyalgia. Differentiating features include cold intolerance, unexplained weight gain, characteristic skin changes, goiter, muscle weakness and soreness, and an elevated thyrotropin (TSH) level. Similarly, polymyositis may produce diffuse muscle achiness, but muscles are weak and diffusely sore, and the sedimentation rate and muscle enzyme levels are markedly elevated.

Depression and *somatization disorder* can cause chronic musculoskeletal pain and fatigue, but no reproducible tender points are found, and these conditions are accompanied by definite manifestations of underlying psychopathology (see Chapters 227 and 230).

The pain of *hypertrophic osteoarthropathy* may be diffuse, but tender points are minimal, and clubbing provides a unique hallmark.

WORKUP (1,5–7,10,11,14)

The diagnosis depends entirely on the history and physical examination (see Table 159.1). Laboratory studies are ordered to help rule out other conditions. Workup is also essential to gauge the effect of the illness on the patient's ability to carry out activities of daily living and to understand the patient's perspective, elements that are essential to the design of an effective management program.

History

A careful delineation of the location of the pain is essential and helps to differentiate fibromyalgia from conditions causing more-localized or regional discomfort. Inquiry into associated features such as fatigue, nonrefreshing sleep, and exacerbations associated with changes in the weather facilitate differentiation. Pertinent negatives include other somatic and affective symptoms of depression (see Chapter 227), symptoms of hypothyroidism (see Chapter 104), frank arthritis, fever, rash, muscle weakness, and a prior history of muscle injury.

Because patients with fibromyalgia often take over-the-counter supplements and herbal remedies before presenting for medical attention, it is essential to review any use at the time of the initial assessment. Similarly, it is helpful to review any nonpharmacologic treatments that might have been tried (e.g., chiropractic spinal manipulation, acupuncture, etc.). Having a complete view of what the patient has already tried can help to provide insight into the patient's perspective and help to inform treatment decisions. As noted, a review of the illness's effect on daily living is also essential.

Physical Examination

The skin, nails, mucous membranes, fundi, joints, spine, muscles, tendons, bones, and nervous system should be examined carefully for evidence of rheumatoid disease, spondyloarthropathy, myopathy, osteoarthropathy, thyroid disease,

and focal pathology (see Chapters 45 and 146 to 151). The mental status examination should be reviewed for signs of depression (see Chapter 227).

Careful palpation of the 18 defining *tender point* sites is indicated (see Fig. 159.1). Compression should be just strong enough to cause blanching of the examining fingertip. Mild discomfort during palpation is a nonspecific finding that may be elicited in a host of other musculoskeletal conditions; obvious and disproportionate tenderness at these sites is a characteristic and predictive feature of fibromyalgia. A positive response is the elicitation of exaggerated tenderness or outright pain. In a study of the diagnostic significance of tender points, likelihood ratios were greater than 1.0 for at least 13 of the 18 defined sites (range 1.2 to 4.0). Tender points need to be differentiated from the trigger points of myofascial syndrome, which produce referred pain on compression.

Laboratory Studies

Because there are no diagnostic laboratory findings, testing is conducted to rule out treatable conditions that may present in similar fashion. Obtaining an *antinuclear antibody* determination can help if its limitations are kept in mind: A negative result has a high negative predictive value, but a positive result has a very high probability of being a false positive in the absence of other defining clinical features of systemic lupus (see Chapter 146). Other tests that may help in identifying important mimicking illnesses include the *erythrocyte sedimentation rate* (for rheumatoid disease), *TSH* (for thyroid disorders), and *creatine phosphokinase* (for myositis). Obtaining *Lyme titers* is not indicated unless the patient has symptoms strongly suggestive of the disease (rash, arthritis, neurologic complaints, deer tick exposure, residence in an endemic area) because test specificity is very poor. When back pain is the predominant symptom, radiologic study of the spine or sacroiliac joints may have to be considered (see Chapter 147). When fatigue dominates the clinical picture, more extensive evaluation may be required (see Chapter 8).

PRINCIPLES OF MANAGEMENT AND PATIENT EDUCATION (1–8,15–38)

General Approach

As with any incurable and chronic pain condition of unknown cause, the principal goal is the maintenance and enhancement of functional capacity (see Chapter 236). Although it may be difficult to "cure" the pain, much can be done to help the patient remain active and productive. The large number of patients with fibromyalgia who are disabled represents a challenge to improve the medical care of persons with this condition. Key components of an effective treatment program include establishing the diagnosis; providing detailed patient education; forming a strong patient–doctor relationship; designing a medical regimen to control pain, promote sleep, and treat any concurrent depression; and initiating a program of nonmedical therapies to enhance functional capacity. In addition, it is critical to address any underlying psychosocial problems because they are a major determinant of prognosis and response to treatment. A comprehensive approach is essential; like most chronic pain syndromes, there is no "magic bullet" for treating fibromyalgia. Taking an evidence-based approach helps to minimize exposure to worthless and potentially harmful therapies. Patients with fibromyalgia often seek out and make frequent use of alternative therapies, of which the primary physician needs to be cognizant to provide the best advice.

Establishing the Diagnosis and Educating the Patient

The value of a careful workup that can confirm the diagnosis is ranked by fibromyalgia patients as one of the most valuable components of care. Knowing what the diagnosis is puts an end to the common fear that a more serious condition with a poor prognosis is responsible for symptoms. The patient feels he or she is being taken seriously. Repeated requests for further evaluation are fewer, and unnecessary or inappropriate treatments (e.g., antibiotics, steroids, nonsteroidal antiinflammatory drugs [NSAIDs]) can be avoided.

The importance of patient education cannot be overstated. Whether given individually or in a group, patient education is associated with durable improvements in scores for symptoms and overall functioning that persist long after the educational intervention has ceased. Duration of the educational effort varies in studies, but as little as an intensive 1½-day program achieves lasting differences in outcomes.

Forming an Effective Patient–Doctor Relationship

The successful care of patients with fibromyalgia requires that a trusting, understanding relationship be formed early. At the time of the initial encounter, the physician starts by eliciting the essential details of the patient's illness experience and specific concerns. Careful history taking is essential for an accurate diagnosis, and it also provides the patient with a much-needed sense of being heard. A directed physical examination pertinent to the differential diagnosis and the patient's concerns helps to reinforce the patient's confidence and feeling of being taken seriously. Taking time at the end of the visit for a focused but unhurried review of findings and their meaning is critical to consolidating the initial efforts to build a good working relationship.

Taking an Evidence-Based Approach

In the absence of a precise pathophysiologic understanding of fibromyalgia, treatment remains largely empirical; however, accumulating evidence from randomized, controlled trials makes possible an increasingly rational approach to management. Evidence-based treatment is particularly important in fibromyalgia because patients face a confusing array of treatment options and many unsubstantiated claims. Although improving in quality, studies of therapies for fibromyalgia still suffer from small sample sizes and short durations (mostly 6 to 12 weeks), limitations that will need to be overcome if study validity and generalizability are to be improved. Despite such limitations, the evidence suggests that a multimodality program combining pharmacologic measures, cognitive–behavioral therapy, and exercise is the best means of achieving symptomatic relief, enhancing physical functioning, and restoring the patient's sense of well-being.

Pharmacologic Measures

Like all chronic pain disorders, fibromyalgia appears to respond at least temporarily to drugs that affect central neurotransmission. Agents supported by evidence from reasonably well designed clinical trials include antidepressants, analgesics, and anticonvulsants (see also Chapter 236). Response rates are modest, but the degree of improvement can be substantial. A host of other agents and substances are promoted without evidence of efficacy.

Antidepressants

Even in the absence of major depression, all classes of antidepressants have produced at least a modicum of benefit in patients with fibromyalgia, lessening pain, fatigue, and sleep disturbances under controlled trial conditions. Low doses are often as effective as higher doses and are better tolerated. *Tricyclic antidepressants* are among the best studied and most consistently effective of pharmacotherapies for fibromyalgia. Well-designed, although short-duration (6- to 12-week), placebo-controlled trials show that low doses of *amitriptyline* (e.g., 25 to 50 mg) achieve significant improvements in pain, sleep, and overall functioning, although the effect on pain seems to be the least enduring. Response rates are modest (25% to 35%). *Cyclobenzaprine*, a tricyclic marketed as a "muscle relaxant," is similarly helpful. The *selective serotonin reuptake inhibitor* (SSRI) *antidepressants* (e.g., *fluoxetine*) have produced variable results, especially when low doses are used. A flexible-dose regimen (e.g., fluoxetine, 20 to 80 mg/d triturated to response) has shown considerable promise. The combination of tricyclic and SSRI therapy seems to give better results than either alone.

Promising results have also been demonstrated with *duloxetine*, a *serotonin-norepinephrine reuptake inhibitor* (SNRI). Both low-dose (60 mg/d) and higher-dose (120 mg/d) formulations produce significant reductions in symptoms and improve overall state of health; however, nearly 40% of patients drop out due to side effects or lack of perceived benefit; efficacy is similar at both doses, but side effects are greater with the larger dose. In an initial study, the SNRI venlafaxine (Effexor) failed to produce significant improvements in symptoms.

Relapse commonly occurs with the cessation of antidepressant therapy, necessitating chronic treatment. The use of generic formulations of antidepressants can help contain the cost of treatment.

Analgesics

Control of pain has been observed with use of *tramadol*, a centrally acting analgesic with low habituation potential (see Chapter 236). Combining it with *acetaminophen* has produced significant improvement. *Opioids* have not been formally studied because the risks of sustained use would probably outweigh any potential benefits; opioid use should be a last resort and limited to the short term. The injection of tender points with topical *lidocaine* has been tried, but the large number of sites that are tender, the modest responses, and the considerable amount of pain after injection make this treatment of little consequence.

Anticonvulsants and Sedatives

Pregabalin (Lyrica) and *gabapentin* (Neurontin) have been examined for use in fibromyalgia, with significant reductions in pain noted. Improvements in sleep, fatigue, and quality of life have also been achieved in randomized trials. The major adverse effect is excessive sedation, especially with larger doses. Cost is very high. Pregabalin is approved by the U.S. Food and Drug Administration for use in the condition. *Benzodiazepines* are of no proven benefit; moreover, the prolonged use that would be necessary for the treatment of fibromyalgia would be inappropriate, given the risks for benzodiazepine dependency and withdrawal (see Chapter 226).

Drugs without Efficacy

Given the absence of evidence for an inflammatory, infectious, or hormonal mechanism for fibromyalgia, it is not be surprising that results from controlled trials of *antiinflammatory agents*, *hormones*, and *antibiotics* have shown no benefit. Trials of NSAIDs and systemic corticosteroids (e.g., prednisone, 10 mg/d) have been disappointing, with the exception of a small improvement when an NSAID is added to tricyclic therapy. Despite some overlap between symptoms of fibromyalgia and those of endocrinopathies, no improvements have been noted with the administration of growth hormone, thyroid hormone, dehydroepiandrosterone, or calcitonin. Antibiotic treatment for Lyme disease has no place in the management of fibromyalgia, even in patients with positive Lyme serology. Positive serology in the absence of clinical evidence for Lyme disease is almost certainly a false-positive result. Only patients with clinical manifestations strongly suggestive of Lyme disease (rash, true arthritis, heart block, neurologic deficits) should be considered candidates for antibiotics (see Chapter 160).

Exercise and Other Physical Measures

Physical measures applied to fibromyalgia range from the well studied (e.g., aerobic exercise) to those that are frequently used by patients but without supporting evidence (e.g., chiropractic manipulation, acupuncture, and injection of tender points).

Exercise

Exercise is among the best studied of treatments for fibromyalgia. Programs of cardiovascular (aerobic) conditioning make significant contributions to reductions in pain and improvements in global functioning. Strength training and pool exercises also enhance functional state. Lesser benefit has been noted when exercise is limited to stretching and flexibility training. When exercise is part of a combination program, outcomes are further enhanced, particularly with regard to sleep and fatigue. To be effective, exercise has to be continued.

Acupuncture

A role for acupuncture is suggested by some controlled trials, but others find no benefit. Many studies are methodologically flawed. The best-designed controlled trials using patient-blinded sham treatments for the placebo group have found no differences in outcomes for pain, sleep, and well-being but do show a marked placebo effect. Like the results of acupuncture for other chronic pain conditions (e.g., for back pain; see Chapter 147), outcomes are likely influenced by the patient's belief in the procedure and the enthusiasm of the practitioner.

Chiropractic Manipulation and Massage

Data are limited for these treatment modalities despite the fact that nearly 50% of fibromyalgia patients report the use of each. The only data examining chiropractic spinal manipulation in fibromyalgia derive from a small (16-patient) uncontrolled trial, which suggested some benefit. Massage appears to reduce tender-point sensitivity and the need for analgesics.

Other Physical Measures

The injection of tender points and ultrasound treatments are widely used, but controlled data are nonexistent or too sparse to draw any conclusions. Despite claims to the contrary, there is no evidence to support the use of bracelets or magnets; a rigorously designed placebo-controlled trial of magnets revealed no benefit.

Psychological Therapies

Psychotherapeutic measures can play an important role in a comprehensive treatment program. Among the best studied is cognitive–behavioral therapy; others less well examined include relaxation techniques and hypnosis.

Cognitive–Behavioral Therapy

This form of psychotherapy redirects the patient's focus away from pain and disability and toward the restoration of function and full participation in daily life. Programs last for 1 to 6 months. Randomized, controlled trials with long-term follow-up (2+ years) find sustained significant improvements in pain and functioning. Results are best for those with symptoms of recent onset. Most cognitive–behavioral therapy is implemented as part of a multidimensional treatment program, combining cognitive restructuring, pacing of activity, and patient and family education with aerobic exercise, relaxation training, and meditation.

Other Behavioral Methods and Hypnosis

Controlled trials have shown that reductions in pain can be achieved with relaxation techniques, meditation, biofeedback, and hypnosis, which are measures that patients often employ on their own.

Spiritual Healing and Prayer

Although this is one of the most frequently practiced approaches to treatment among patients who present for comprehensive medical therapy (second only to exercise among the nonpharmacologic treatments), it is largely unstudied for efficacy.

Alternative Therapies

The list of alternative therapies is long and includes measures already discussed (e.g., chiropractic manipulation and acupuncture), as well as herbal treatments and dietary supplements (vitamins and minerals). Greater than half of fibromyalgia patients studied reported the use of supplements and "natural" remedies.

Herbal Therapies

Green tea is very popular (25% use), and *Echinacea* is taken by about one fourth of young patients. There are no data on the efficacy of these remedies, but safety is well established (see Chapters 157 and 237). A large number of other herbal remedies are used on occasion by persons suffering from fibromyalgia; many have important adverse effects on drug metabolism (e.g., *St. John's wort*), hemostasis (e.g., *Ginkgo biloba, garlic*), central nervous system activity (e.g., *kava, valerian*), and cardiovascular status (e.g., *ma huang* [ephedra]) (see Chapter 237). Inquiry into their ongoing use is essential.

Dietary Supplements

Glucosamine and *chondroitin* are taken by nearly 20% of patients. At least one vitamin or mineral is taken as a supplement by more than 80% of fibromyalgia patients. Among the most popular are vitamin C, vitamin E, magnesium, and B complex. There is no evidence of efficacy.

Refractory Disease

Patients with a chronic pain syndrome such as fibromyalgia often make repeated visits and demand help yet appear refractory to treatment efforts. They pose one of the most challenging problems encountered in office practice. Two helpful strategies for dealing with refractory fibromyalgia patients are (a) to search for and address any underlying psychosocial stresses and (b) to consider a team or multispecialty approach to management.

Identifying and Addressing Psychosocial Stresses

Patients with seemingly refractory disease should undergo a full psychosocial assessment and be carefully evaluated for psychiatric, family, occupational, and social difficulties. Although not etiologically linked to fibromyalgia, problems in these areas are the most important determinants of health care utilization and disability in fibromyalgia patients. They have little effect on the severity of symptoms, but they do determine illness behavior. Similarly, patients who perceive their symptoms to be the consequence of an injury suffered at work or in an accident also have a poor prognosis, with disability and a poor response to treatment persisting until litigation and related issues have been settled. The first step in the management of persons with refractory disease must be a thoughtful approach that directly addresses these underlying psychosocial difficulties.

Arranging Team (Multidisciplinary) Care

The multimodality approach needed for optimal management of fibromyalgia raises the question of multidisciplinary implementation. Sharing responsibility for the care of these difficult patients with members of a multidisciplinary team (e.g., psychologist, physical therapist, consulting rheumatologist) can lessen the burden of care on any one member while providing the patient with complementary inputs and perspectives. Coordination of the treatment program remains the responsibility of the primary care physician, who continues to provide the home base for care and ensures that the team plan is consistent and properly executed. The doctor–patient relationship remains intact, but the burden of care is shared and the plan is reinforced by all team members.

A.H.G.

Annotated Bibliography

1. Aaron LA, Bradley LA, Alarcon GS, et al. Perceived physical and emotional trauma as precipitating events in fibromyalgia: associations with health care seeking and disability status but not pain severity. Arthritis Rheum 1997;40:453. (*Presents evidence for the importance of psychosocial factors in prognosis.*)
2. Aaron LA, Bradley LA, Alarcon GS, et al. Psychiatric diagnoses in patients with fibromyalgia are related to health care-seeking behavior rather than to illness. Arthritis Rheum 1997;39:436. (*Discusses the importance of underlying psychiatric disease as a predictor of illness behavior.*)
3. Bennett RM. Emerging concepts in the neurobiology of chronic pain: evidence of abnormal sensory processing in fibromyalgia. Mayo Clin Proc 1999;74:385. (*A review of the conceptual basis for the chronic pain of fibromyalgia, with a focus on abnormal sensory processing.*)
4. Dailey PA, Bishop GD, Russell IJ, et al. Psychological stress and the fibrositis/fibromyalgia syndrome. J Rheumatol 1990;17:1380. (*Finds a high level of life stress.*)
5. Fitzcharles MA, Esdaile JM. The overdiagnosis of fibromyalgia syndrome. Am J Med 1997;103:44. (*Spondyloarthropathies in women was diagnosed as fibromyalgia.*)
6. Goldenberg DL. Fibromyalgia syndrome a decade later: what have we learned? Arch Intern Med 1999;159:777. (*An excellent summary of diagnosis and management for the generalist, emphasizing the importance of underlying psychosocial factors to outcomes; 156 references.*)
7. Goldenberg DL, Simms RW, Geiger A, et al. High frequency of fibromyalgia in patients with chronic fatigue seen in a primary care practice. Arthritis Rheum 1990;33:381. (*There is much overlap in the two conditions.*)
8. Kennedy M, Felson DT. A prospective long-term study of fibromyalgia syndrome. Arthritis Rheum 1996;39:682. (*The best long-term data, confirming the chronicity of disease but also a general trend toward improvement.*)
9. Simms RW, Gunderman J, Howard G, et al. The alpha-delta sleep abnormality in fibromyalgia. Arthritis Rheum 1988;31(Suppl): S100. (*The characteristic sleep disorder of fibromyalgia.*)
10. Tunks E, McCain GA, Hart LE, et al. The reliability of examination for tenderness in patients with myofascial pain, chronic fibromyalgia, and controls. J Rheumatol 1995;22:944. (*A systematic study of the test, finding that it is effective for differentiation from normal controls, but that there is some overlap with myofascial pain syndrome.*)
11. Wolfe F, Smythe HA, Yunus MB, et al. The American College of Rheumatology 1990 criteria for the classification of fibromyalgia: the Multicenter Criteria Committee. Arthritis Rheum 1990;33:160. (*Consensus diagnostic criteria, pending the discovery of more-definitive diagnostic findings.*)
12. Yunus MB, Ahles TA, Aldag JC, et al. Relationship of clinical features with psychological status in primary fibromyalgia. Arthritis Rheum 1991;34:15. (*Failure to find a relationship suggests that symptoms are independent of the patient's psychological status.*)
13. Yunus MB, Masi AT, Calabro JJ, et al. Primary fibromyalgia (fibrositis): clinical study of 50 patients with matched normal controls. Semin Arthritis Rheum 1981;11:151. (*A careful early delineation of clinical presentation and physical findings.*)
14. White KP, Harth M, Speechley, et al. A general population study of fibromyalgia tender points in noninstitutionalized adults with chronic widespread pain. J Rheumatol 2000;27:2677. (*Finds that the likelihood ratios increased for most tender points, indicating their usefulness for diagnosis.*)
15. Alfano AP, Taylor AG, Foresman PA, et al. Static magnetic fields for treatment of fibromyalgia: a randomized controlled trial. J Altern Complement Med 2001;7:53. (*A well-designed study, showing no benefit.*)
16. Almeida TF, Roizenblatt S, Benedito-Silva AA, et al. The effect of combined therapy (ultrasound and interferential current) on pain and sleep in fibromyalgia. Pain 2003;104:665. (*Presents some evidence for benefit.*)
17. Arnold LM, Hess EV, Hudson JI, et al. A randomized, placebo-controlled, double-blind, flexible-dose study of fluoxetine in the treatment of women with fibromyalgia. Am J Med 2002;112:191. (*The treatment was found to be useful for most outcome measures, but the study power was limited by sample size.*)
18. Arnold LM, Lu Y, Crofford LJ, et al. A double-blind multicenter trial comparing duloxetine to placebo in the treatment of fibromyalgia with or without major depressive disorder. Arthritis Rheum 2004;50:2974. (*The initial randomized, controlled trial showing evidence of benefit for this serotonin-norepinephrine reuptake inhibitor.*)
19. Assefi NP, Sherman KJ, Jacobsen C, et al. A randomized clinical trial of acupuncture compared with sham acupuncture in fibromyalgia. Ann Intern Med 2005;143:10. (*One of the most methodologically rigorous studies of acupuncture, finding no benefit over placebo in relieving pain, and noting a strong placebo effect.*)
20. Bennett RM, Kamin M, Karim R, et al. Tramadol and acetaminophen combination tablets in the treatment of fibromyalgia pain: a double-blind, randomized, placebo-controlled study. Am J Med 2003;114:537. (*Finds moderate benefit over 3 months.*)
21. Berman BM, Ezzo J, Hadhazy V, et al. Is acupuncture effective in the treatment of fibromyalgia? J Family Pract 1999;48:213. (*A review of seven studies, suggesting benefit.*)
22. Carette S, Bell MJ, Reynolds WJ, et al. Comparison of amitriptyline, cyclobenzaprine, and placebo in the treatment of fibromyalgia. A randomized, double-blind clinical trial. Arthritis Rheum 1994;37:32. (*A well-designed study, showing the efficacy of amitriptyline.*)
23. Crofford L, Russell IJ, Mease P, et al. Pregabalin improves pain associated with fibromyalgia syndrome in a multicenter, randomized, placebo-controlled monotherapy trial [Abstract]. Arthritis Rheum 2002;46:S613. (*A well-designed trial, showing evidence of benefit.*)
24. Fors EA, Sexton H, Gotestam KG. The effect of guided imagery and amitriptyline on daily fibromyalgia pain. J Psychiatr Res 2002;36:179. (*Finds a modest benefit.*)
25. Goldenberg DL, Burckhardt C, Crofford L. Management of fibromyalgia syndrome. JAMA 2004;292:2388. (*A very useful review of the evidence or lack thereof for treatments of fibromyalgia; 118 references.*)
26. Goldenberg DL, Mayskiy M, Mossey C, et al. A randomized, double-blind crossover trial of fluoxetine and amitriptyline in the treatment of

fibromyalgia. Arthritis Rheum 1996;39:1852. (*The selective serotonin-reuptake inhibitor was helpful for sleep disturbances and depression but not for pain.*)

27. Harris RE, Tian X, Cupps TR, et al. The treatment of fibromyalgia with acupuncture [Abstract]. Arthritis Rheum 2003;48:S692. (*A well-designed study, finding no evidence of benefit.*)

28. Leventhal LJ. Management of fibromyalgia. Ann Intern Med 1999;131:850. (*A review of the evidence for what works and what does not, with an excellent list of 119 references.*)

29. Lightfoot RW, Luft BJ, Rahn DW, et al. Empiric parenteral antibiotic treatment of patients with fibromyalgia/fatigue and a positive serologic result for Lyme disease. Ann Intern Med 1993;119:503. (*A cost-effective analysis, finding that treatment was expensive and was associated much more with antibiotic toxicity than with clinical cures.*)

30. McCain GA, Bell DA, Mai FM, et al. A controlled study of the effects of a supervised cardiovascular fitness training program on the manifestations of primary fibromyalgia. Arthritis Rheum 1988;31:1135. (*Improvement was achieved with cardiovascular training but not with simple flexibility exercises.*)

31. NIH Consensus Conference. Acupuncture. JAMA 1998;280:1518. (*Rates this approach as "may be useful as an adjunct treatment" in the management of fibromyalgia.*)

32. Rossy LA, Buckelew SP, Dorr N, et al. A meta-analysis of fibromyalgia treatment interventions. Ann Behav Med 1999;21:180. (*A systematic review, indicating benefit from cognitive–behavioral therapy.*)

33. Scudds RA, McCain GA, Rollman GB, et al. Improvements in pain responsiveness in patients with fibrositis after successful treatment with amitriptyline. J Rheumatol 1989;16:98. (*A double-blinded, crossover study, noting improvement in all parameters.*)

34. Sim J, Adams N. Systematic review of randomized controlled trials of non-pharmacological intervention for fibromyalgia. Clin J Pain 2002;18:324. (*Includes a review of herbal therapies.*)

35. Wahner-Roedler DL, Elkin PL, Vincent A, et al. Use of complementary and alternative medical therapies by patients referred to a fibromyalgia treatment program at a tertiary care center. Mayo Clin Proc 2005;80:55. (*Documents a high frequency of use in this referral population.*)

36. White KP, Nielsson WR. Cognitive behavioral treatment of fibromyalgia syndrome: a follow-up assessment. J Rheumatol 1995;22:717. (*This approach was found to be effective, with benefit lasting long after treatment was completed.*)

37. Wigers SH, Stiles TC, Vogel PA. Effects of aerobic exercise versus stress management treatment in fibromyalgia. A 4.5-year prospective study. Scand J Rheumatol 1996;25:77. (*Pain decreased; fatigue and disturbed sleep were less affected.*)

38. Worrel LM, Krahn LE, Sletten CD, et al. Treating fibromyalgia with a brief interdisciplinary program: initial outcomes and predictors of response. Mayo Clin Proc 2001;76:384. (*Evaluation of a 1½-day multimodality intervention at the Mayo clinic, finding benefit for severely impaired persons.*)

CHAPTER 160 ■ APPROACH TO THE PATIENT WITH LYME DISEASE

Lyme disease is a treatable multisystem illness caused by infection with the tick-borne spirochete *Borrelia burgdorferi*. The condition has become the most common vector-borne disease in the United States, with more than 40,000 cases reported to the Centers for Disease Control and Prevention in the last 10 years. In most instances, the acute infection can be readily diagnosed and effectively treated. The neurologic and musculoskeletal manifestations of later stages may be more subtle and resemble those of chronic fatigue syndrome, fibromyalgia, or depression. The nonspecificity of symptoms and shortcomings of available serologic tests lead to both underdiagnosis and overdiagnosis.

The primary physician needs to be skilled in the clinical recognition of early disseminated and late disease; clinically capable of differentiating it from other acute, subacute, and chronic neurologic and musculoskeletal conditions; cognizant of the limitations of diagnostic methods; and capable of prescribing an effective antibiotic program.

EPIDEMIOLOGY, PATHOPHYSIOLOGY, AND CLINICAL PRESENTATION (1–9)

Epidemiology

The spirochete causing Lyme disease is transmitted to humans by *Ixodes* ticks. *Nymph-stage* ticks feed on humans from May through July, transmitting the spirochete in the process. Endemic areas for species of the responsible tick include the northeastern coastal states, Wisconsin and Minnesota in the Midwest, and the coast of Oregon and northern California. Outbreaks in Europe and Asia have also been reported. In the U.S. eastern coastal regions and in the Midwest, the deer tick *Ixodes dammini* (*scapularis*) is the principal vector. More than one third of deer ticks carry the spirochete, which accounts for outbreaks of epidemic proportion. In the western United States, the *Ixodes pacificus* species is responsible, but the carrier rate is only 1% to 3%, and human infection is much more sporadic. The condition has also been reported in Europe and Asia.

The rising frequency of Lyme disease and its geographic spread have been linked to enlarging deer populations and concurrent suburbanization. The spirochete is transmitted horizontally to field mice, which are critical to sustaining its life cycle (deer are not, but the ticks prefer them). Human infection is a biologic dead end for the spirochete.

Human babesiosis, caused by the intracellular rickettsial parasite *Babesia microti*, is endemic to many of the same areas as Lyme disease. Transmission to humans is by the same deer tick, and the same field mice serve as the animal reservoir. The shared tick vector and animal reservoir increases the risk for concurrent infection. Approximately 10% of patients with active Lyme disease are concurrently infected with *B. microti*.

Human granulocytic ehrlichiosis is another recently appreciated rickettsial disease that is zoonotic in the same geographic sites as babesiosis and Lyme disease. No evidence of concurrent infection has been found.

Pathophysiology

The spirochete enters the bloodstream at the time of tick feeding, which usually does not occur until well after the first 24 hours of contact. After a short bloodstream phase, the organism moves out of the blood and, in seemingly trophic fashion, into the skin, synovial membranes, heart, and nervous system. After the appearance of characteristic skin lesions, there can be another period of hematogenous spread. The means by which the spirochete damages tissue is unclear; hypotheses range from direct injury to the production of antispirochetal antibodies that cross-react with tissue antigens. Patients with symptoms that persist after appropriate antibiotic therapy are suspected of having an exaggerated, sustained immune response. Such a response may account for the overlap in clinical manifestations with those of fibromyalgia and chronic fatigue syndrome, in which an immunologic pathophysiology is also suspected (see Chapters 8 and 159). The fact that patients who are positive for HLA-DR4 appear to be at increased risk for such chronic illness suggests that the severity and chronicity of disease may be related, in part, to cell-surface antigens and genetic susceptibility.

Unlike *B. burgdorferi*, the *Babesia* organism resides predominantly in the red cells and causes mostly systemic symptoms with little localization. Infection can impair host defenses and may enhance injury caused by *B. burgdorferi*.

Clinical Presentation and Course

The biting tick is usually no larger than the size of a pencil mark and often inapparent. Attachment of the tick for at least 36 hours is necessary before feeding begins and transmission of the organism takes place. A feeding nymph will appear engorged, which helps in estimating the risk of transmission when the duration of attachment is unknown. Soon after the bite, the first symptoms develop. The clinical course can be divided into three stages: (a) acute, localized disease; (b) subacute, disseminated disease; and (c) chronic disease.

Stage 1: Acute Infection

Eighty percent of infected persons manifest an expanding macular erythematous rash (*erythema migrans*) as the first clinical manifestation of *B. burgdorferi* infection (Fig. 160.1). The rash usually begins as a red macule at the site of the tick bite,

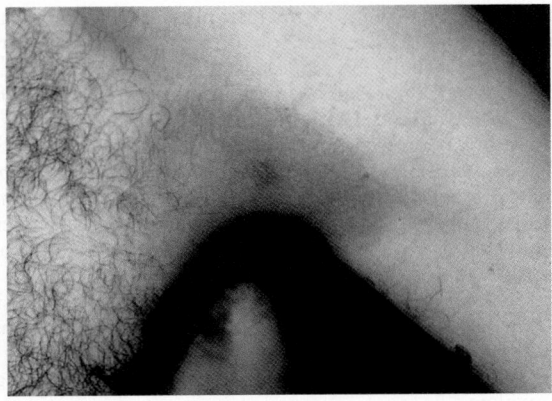

FIGURE 160.1. Erythema migrans of the axilla.

which spreads out to form a large, homogeneous lesion and later becomes annular with red secondary outer rings, an intense red outer border, and some clearing toward the center, although induration may be noted at the site of the bite. The lesion is large, averaging 15 cm. Minor constitutional *flulike symptoms* (a "summer flu") and regional *lymphadenopathy* may accompany the rash. The remaining 20% of patients have flulike symptoms without a rash or no acute-stage symptoms at all. The rash starts to fade by 3 to 4 weeks. During stage 1, the immune response is minimal.

Stage 2: Hematogenous Dissemination

Hematogenous dissemination follows the acute phase within several days to a few weeks of the tick bite and leads to a host of symptoms, mostly dermatologic, musculoskeletal, and neurologic. Constitutional symptoms may be prominent, with patients complaining of generalized *malaise* and debilitating *fatigue*. Often, bouts of severe *headache* lasting a few hours may develop, accompanied by mild neck stiffness, as may *migratory arthralgias* and musculoskeletal pain.

Dermatologic Manifestations. Dermatologic manifestations include new *annular skin lesions* smaller and less migratory than the initial one. Malar rash, diffuse erythema, and urticaria have also been noted.

Cardiac Involvement. Cardiac involvement is noted in about 5% to 10% of patients, beginning several weeks into the infection. *Transient heart block* may be a consequence, ranging from asymptomatic first-degree atrioventricular block to complete heart block with fainting. The cardiac phase lasts 3 to 6 weeks, with the most severe forms of heart block persisting for about 1 week and not requiring pacemaker placement.

Neurologic Sequestration. Neurologic sequestration ensues weeks to months after the initial infection, affecting 15% to 20% of untreated patients. It consists of a *lymphocytic meningitis* and cranial or peripheral neuropathy. The cerebrospinal fluid (CSF) shows a pleocytosis with about 100 lymphocytes/mm^3, elevated protein and normal glucose levels, and antibodies to the spirochete. A mild *encephalopathy* may ensue and produce mood changes, somnolence, and memory disturbances. A unilateral or bilateral *Bell's palsy* is the most common cranial nerve deficit. The *peripheral neuritis* presents as motor and sensory changes of the trunk or limbs in a dermatomal distribution. These neurologic manifestations can last for weeks to months.

Musculoskeletal Symptoms. Musculoskeletal symptoms evolve into frank arthritis in up to 60% of untreated patients. The onset of arthritis is variable but averages 6 months from the time of initial infection. Characteristically, self-limited attacks of acute asymmetric *monoarticular* or *oligoarticular arthritis* develop. Pain and swelling are noted in one or a few large joints. The knee is the most common site. A joint effusion may form, composed of increased numbers of neutrophils (10,000/mm^3 to 25,000/mm^3). No more than three joints are usually involved in the course of the illness. Symptoms and signs last for several days to a few weeks. After an attack, the joint returns to normal.

Stage 3: Chronic Infection

After a latent period of several months and beginning 1 year after the time of the original infection, symptoms of chronic infection begin to appear. Bouts of arthritis may become more prolonged, and chronic neurologic deficits may ensue.

Skin Changes. Most patients in the United States do not manifest skin changes in the late phases of Lyme disease, but a chronic atrophic form of *acrodermatitis* unique to Lyme disease has been observed in Europe.

Arthritis. The transient form of arthritis characteristic of disseminated disease is supplanted by a more persistent one that lasts months instead of weeks. The knee remains the most common site, and the pattern continues to be oligoarticular. Joint erosion is reported but uncommon and rarely leads to permanent loss of function. In a small percentage of patients, the arthritis persists even after a full course of antibiotic therapy. An immunologic mechanism is postulated. Over the years, the frequency of arthritic episodes declines.

Neurologic Impairment. Distal paresthesias, radicular pain, and memory loss comprise the principal neurologic manifestations of late disease, representing polyneuropathy and encephalopathy. Often, they occur concurrently. Tiredness may also be reported. In rare instances, a leukoencephalopathy with spastic paraparesis may develop. Two thirds of patients with neurologic symptoms have elevated levels of protein in the CSF, and half have Lyme antibodies in the CSF. In most patients, electrophysiologic study findings are abnormal, demonstrating evidence of axonal degeneration.

Natural History of Disease

Without treatment, 20% of patients with erythema migrans will experience spontaneous resolution and no progression of disease. Conversely, without treatment, disseminated disease develops in about 80% of patients. Attacks of oligoarthritis are common (60% to 80%) but resolve within 1 to 3 years, even without treatment. Chronic neurologic and persistent joint symptoms affect about 5% to 10% of patients. Susceptibility to late chronic disease may be genetically determined. Overall, community-based longitudinal cohort study finds that properly treated Lyme disease does not predispose to long-term disability. The view among some that Lyme disease does predispose may be a consequence of the mislabeling of incapacitated persons who do not have Lyme disease (perhaps on the basis of a false-positive serologic test).

Despite the generally favorable prognosis, a *post-Lyme syndrome/chronic Lyme disease* is described in up to one third of treated cases; it is characterized by persistence of fatigue, myalgias, and arthralgias for several more months after objective disease manifestations have resolved. A purported "molecular mimicry" leading to an autoimmune process has been postulated to account for some cases. All culture and polymerase chain reaction results are negative, and prolonged courses of antibiotics (e.g., intravenous [IV] ceftriaxone 2 g/d for 30 days followed by oral doxycycline 200 mg/d for 30 days) do not improve outcomes compared to placebo.

Concurrent Infection with *B. microti*

The symptoms of human *babesiosis* include fever, chills, sweats, arthralgias, headache, and lassitude. Patients with concurrent Lyme disease and babesiosis typically manifest what appears to be a more severe and prolonged case of Lyme disease. Marked fatigue, headache, sweats, chills, nausea, conjunctivitis, emotional lability, and splenomegaly occur more frequently than in patients with Lyme disease alone. Moreover, almost half of patients remain symptomatic for more than 3 months, whereas fewer than 5% of those with Lyme disease alone remain symptomatic for that long. Similarly, patients with concurrent babesiosis and Lyme disease appear to have a more severe case of *Babesia* infection than would be typical.

DIFFERENTIAL DIAGNOSIS
(1–3,7,10,15)

Acute and Early Disseminated Stages

Lyme disease patients with acute-phase flulike symptoms, rash, and a history of tick bite may be confused with persons having *Rocky Mountain spotted fever*, which also is tick-borne and produces an acute febrile illness with rash, musculoskeletal pain, headache, and gastrointestinal upset. However, the rash of Rocky Mountain spotted fever is different; it starts within a few days of the tick bite as an outbreak of small, blanching macules on the wrists and ankles, spreads centripetally and also to the palms and soles, and then becomes generalized and petechial. As noted previously, *human babesiosis* may mimic or exacerbate the early phases of Lyme disease and should be considered when a patient with a recent tick bite in an endemic area appears to have a particularly severe set of systemic Lyme symptoms that persist beyond 3 months. *Summertime viral illnesses* enter into the differential diagnosis in patients who present with flulike symptoms but without erythema migrans or a history of tick bite.

Patients with symptoms and signs of meningeal irritation require careful evaluation. *Viral encephalitis* is among the summer viral illnesses that may present with headache, stiff neck, and mental changes. *Bacterial meningitis* must also be considered. The erythema migrans and concurrent Bell's palsy or radiculoneuritis of Lyme disease should help to differentiate *B. burgdorferi* infection from other causes of meningeal irritation.

Late Disseminated and Chronic Stages

The presence of acute episodes of oligoarthritis raises the question of *gout, pseudogout,* and a *seronegative spondyloarthropathy* (e.g., Reiter's syndrome, psoriatic arthritis, ankylosing spondylitis). At the time of the initial presentation, *infectious arthritis* also enters into the differential diagnosis. Even early *rheumatoid arthritis* may present as a monoarticular or oligoarticular disease involving a large joint. The correct diagnosis can usually be made based on the associated clinical findings and the results of serologic testing and joint fluid analysis (see Chapters 145 and 146).

The subtle neurologic and joint manifestations of late Lyme disease can cause considerable diagnostic confusion. *Depression, fibromyalgia,* and *chronic fatigue syndrome* have manifestations that overlap with those of Lyme disease. Clinicians encountering patients with these difficult conditions may overdiagnose Lyme disease, especially if they place too much emphasis on serologic testing and too little on symptoms and signs (see later discussion and Chapters 8, 159, and 227). Adding to the confusion is the possibility that in some instances Lyme disease may be followed by a post-Lyme syndrome or may trigger fibromyalgia.

WORKUP (1–3,7,10–17)

In general, the diagnosis of Lyme disease is made clinically, by recognizing the characteristic symptoms and signs within the epidemiologic context of the illness. Serologic testing for antibody against *B. burgdorferi* can supplement the clinical evaluation, particularly in persons with an intermediate pretest probability of Lyme disease, but overdiagnosis leading to overtreatment is common (see later discussion).

Early Disease

Clinical diagnosis based on history and physical examination is necessary at this stage of the illness because characteristic serologic changes will not take place for weeks. Patients are typically those who present either with a tick bite, a rash, or a flulike illness. One inquires into any recent tick bite and other epidemiologic risk factors for Lyme disease (presence in an endemic area, walking in a wooded, brushy, or grassy area, and failure to take precautions against ticks). A history of tick bite is often absent (50% of persons with erythema migrans cannot recall tick exposure) and is not necessary for diagnosis. The nymph tick is very small (about 1 mm) and its bite is easily missed. After the nymph has fed, it will appear engorged (about twice its original size), which suggests that it has fed and transmitted the parasite. Diagnosis is strongly supported by the patient reporting a new migratory macular red rash on the trunk or limbs.

On examination, careful inspection of the skin is performed to check for the pathognomonic large erythematous homogeneous or annular lesion of *erythema migrans* (see Fig. 160.1); finding the rash is diagnostic of early Lyme disease. Most other clinical findings of early disease (e.g., fever, regional lymphadenopathy) are nonspecific. On occasion, early dissemination may occur in the presence of erythema migrans, and signs of later-stage disease (e.g., cranial nerve palsy, nuchal rigidity) may be present.

In endemic areas, patients presenting with early, nonspecific symptoms are often tested at the onset of symptoms or after a tick bite, a practice that is probably a response to patient concerns and a demand for early testing and treatment. However, it is too early to detect antibody, and the pretest probability of Lyme disease in patients with early, nonspecific symptoms is very low. Testing them at this stage maximizes the risk for false-positive and false-negative results and should be discouraged (see later discussion). Those in an endemic area with especially severe systemic symptoms should be evaluated for concurrent babesiosis (see later discussion).

Disseminated Disease

In disseminated disease, the principal clues to the diagnosis continue to be clinical. In addition to epidemiologic inquiry, a review of key historical features is necessary, including new erythematous lesions, palpitations, near-syncope, stiff neck, facial weakness (which may be bilateral), radicular pain, migratory musculoskeletal complaints, and, later, frank oligoarticular arthritis, particularly of the knee. Important physical findings include the multiple annular erythematous skin lesions of *secondary erythema migrans*, irregular pulse, nuchal rigidity, facial nerve palsy, and joint swelling with effusion. Suspicion of early disseminated Lyme disease is particularly high if the lesions of secondary erythema migrans are present. Again, when patients have particularly severe and persistent systemic symptoms, concurrent babesiosis should be suspected, and such patients should be tested accordingly.

The diagnosis can be facilitated by obtaining serum for *antibody testing*, but only in patients with sufficient clinical evidence of Lyme disease to have an intermediate (20% to 80%) pretest probability of Lyme disease (Table 160.1). For patients with meningeal signs, lumbar puncture should be considered. The CSF is sent for antibody testing in addition to cell count, differential, and chemistries. Most patients with central nervous system involvement have detectable antibody in the CSF, a pleocytosis, and an elevated protein concentration. If a joint

---

TABLE 160.1

PRETEST PROBABILITY OF LYME DISEASE BASED ON EPIDEMIOLOGY AND CLINICAL PRESENTATION

Clinical Presentation	Community Incidence 0.1%	Community Incidence 1.0%	Community Incidence 3.0%
Myalgias			
No history of rash or tick bite	0	0	0
With history of bite; no rash	0	0	0
With history of rash; no bite	0.006	0.06	0.17
With history of rash and bite	0.008	0.44	0.70
Erythema migrans only			
Typical	1.00	1.00	1.00
Atypical	0.002	0.18	0.40
Arthritis			
No history of rash or tick bite	0	0	0
History of tick bite; no rash	0	0	0
History of rash; no tick bite	0.0006	0.06	0.17

From Nichol G, Dennis DT, Steere AC, et al. Test treatment strategies for patients suspected of having Lyme disease: a cost-effectiveness analysis. Ann Intern Med 1998;128:37, with permission.

effusion is present, *arthrocentesis* is indicated. *Polymerase chain reaction* methods (see later discussion) may become useful for linking *Borrelia* infection to the arthritis.

Late Disease

The diagnosis of late disease requires careful attention to the patient's musculoskeletal and neurologic symptoms. One checks for chronic oligoarticular arthritis (particularly of the knee), memory loss, spinal radicular pain, and distal paresthesias. Patients with findings suggestive of encephalopathy should undergo a *lumbar puncture* for antibody testing of the CSF, cell count, and chemistries. Peripheral polyneuropathy can be confirmed by *electrophysiologic study*, if necessary.

Differentiating Late Lyme Disease from Other Conditions

As noted earlier, patients with *chronic fatigue syndrome* or *fibromyalgia* may be mistakenly and counterproductively labeled as having *"chronic Lyme disease." Depression* and *somatization disorder* can also mimic some of the nonspecific manifestations of these conditions and should always be considered in patients who present with fatigue and multiple nonspecific bodily complaints (see Chapters 8, 227, and 230). Tiredness and chronic neurologic and musculoskeletal symptoms are common to all of these conditions.

Distinguishing clinical features that help to differentiate late Lyme disease from the other potentially mimicking conditions include (a) oligoarticular musculoskeletal complaints that include signs of joint inflammation, (b) limited and specific neurologic deficits (memory loss, distal paresthesias, radicular pain), (c) abnormalities on CSF examination and electromyography, and (d) absence of disturbed sleep, chronic headache, depression, and tender points.

Unlike patients with late Lyme disease, these other individuals manifest (a) a persistence of symptoms independent of seropositivity, (b) an absence of positive cultures or polymerase chain reaction tests of clinical specimens, and (c) no response in controlled trials to appropriate antibiotic therapy (despite the absence of antibiotic resistance or other recognized causes of treatment failure). Complicating differentiation are (a) the ability of Lyme disease to trigger chronic fatigue syndrome and fibromyalgia and (b) the inadequate specificity of widely used serologic tests both for diagnosis and for determination of the adequacy of treatment (see following discussion).

Diagnostic Studies

Laboratory confirmation of *B. burgdorferi* infection is problematic. Antibody testing can contribute to the diagnosis but only under carefully selected conditions and at the risk of generating false-positive results. Isolation of the spirochete is not practical, and DNA detection by polymerase chain reaction technology is experimental. The diagnosis of Lyme disease is predominantly a clinical one. Laboratory testing should be used only as a supplement to the clinical findings and not as the basis for the diagnosis. Serologic and DNA tests can be helpful under certain circumstances. Urine testing for Lyme antigen is unreliable and should not be ordered.

Antibody Testing

Clinicians often turn to serologic testing for Lyme disease when the clinical picture is unclear or patient concerns are high. Serologic testing aims to detect immunoglobulin M and immunoglobulin G antibodies expressed against *B. burgdorferi* antigens in response to spirochete infection. Most so-called *first-step tests* use *enzyme-linked immunosorbent assay* (ELISA) technology for antibody detection. First-step antibody testing is sensitive; when performed more than 12 weeks after the onset of symptoms, its sensitivity ranges from 90% to 100%. However, the specificity is more modest (70% to 90%) because some *Borrelia* antigens are shared with other microorganisms, and cross-reacting antibodies are found in persons with conditions that may resemble Lyme disease (e.g., viral illnesses, other tick-borne infections, connective tissue diseases, encephalitis). Specificity can be improved by subjecting a serum sample with positive or indeterminate results by first-step assay to *Western blot testing*. This so-called *second-step test* provides enhanced specificity but is more supplementary than truly confirmatory because it detects antibodies to the same antigens as does first-step testing. Currently, 3 million serologic tests for Lyme disease are ordered annually in the United States, at a cost of nearly $100 million. In untreated persons, antibody titers become detectable several weeks into *Borrelia* infection and remain positive for years. ELISA can also detect antibody in CSF. Hyperconcentration of antibody in the CSF is strong evidence for central nervous system infection.

Pitfalls. Improper use and interpretation of Lyme serology are common, often resulting in overdiagnosis, overtreatment, and the associated adverse consequences (e.g., inappropriate health care utilization, treatment-related adverse effects, disability, and depression). The U.S. Food and Drug Administration issued a public health advisory regarding the potential for the misdiagnosis of Lyme disease when commercially available antibody assays are used. The advisory and subsequent study by the Centers for Disease Control and Prevention called attention to numerous shortcomings, such as lack of reproducibility of results, poor sensitivity when used in the early stages of illness, and unacceptably high false-positive rates when used in persons with a low pretest probability of disease. Moreover, Lyme antibodies usually persist for years after infection has cleared, so that the differentiation between active and previous infection is difficult. The proper use of antibody testing for Lyme disease needs to be understood by clinicians to avoid errors in diagnosis and resultant adverse outcomes.

Timing. Because it takes several weeks for immunoglobulin M and especially immunoglobulin G antibodies to be expressed in response to infection, antibody testing should not be ordered during the acute phase of illness. Such early testing maximizes the chances of a false-negative result, which can be greater than 50% in the first 2 weeks after the onset of symptoms. A testing strategy that uses acute-phase and later-phase sera does not appear to be cost-effective. False-negative test results can also occur when patients are treated during early stages of the disease.

Patient Selection. Antibody testing contributes best to clinical decision making when it is applied to persons with an *intermediate pretest probability* (20% to 80%) of having Lyme disease (see Table 160.1 and Chapter 2). Testing persons with a high (>80%) pretest probability contributes little to diagnosis; a negative test result does not rule out the condition, and a positive test result does not substantially increase the probability of disease. Patients with a low (<20%) pretest probability (see Table 160.1) also do not benefit because the combination of low pretest probability with high test sensitivity and insufficient specificity produces more false positives than true positives (see Chapter 2). Despite such reasons for not testing patients with a low probability of disease, many clinicians still do, often because they want to provide reassurance that the patient does not have Lyme disease. Although it is true that a negative antibody test result obtained after the acute phase of illness has passed does effectively rule out the condition, the chances of a false positive are substantial and may only aggravate the patient's concerns and disability.

Test Selection. The Centers for Disease Control and Prevention recommend a two-step testing strategy, which begins with the selection of a first-step test for initial assessment followed by Western blot testing of all "indeterminate" and "positive" sera. Theoretically, this approach has the capacity to reduce false-positive results, but its cost-effectiveness remains to be proved. With more than 40 testing kits available for Lyme antibody detection, much variability in kit performance, often poor interlaboratory and intralaboratory reproducibility, and little standardization, it is essential that one use a laboratory with skill and experience in Lyme antibody testing.

DNA Detection

Better diagnostic studies are needed to differentiate active from past infection in antibody-positive patients and to distinguish a true-positive ELISA result from a false-positive one. Short of isolating the organism (which is difficult), one can attempt to detect its DNA. Under development is the use of *polymerase chain reaction* technology to detect *Borrelia* DNA sequences in bodily fluids. Use for the detection of organisms in joint fluid has been particularly effective. Less common is detection in the cerebrospinal fluid. Preliminary studies suggest that it can be used to determine active infection in arthritic joints. Further testing is needed, but if the technique proves to be effective, it may overcome the limitations of antibody testing.

Testing for Concurrent Babesiosis

The diagnosis can be made by identifying the parasite in red cells on *Giemsa-stained thin blood smear*, but because the parasites frequently cannot be seen, test sensitivity is greatly decreased. *Indirect immunofluorescence* is the principal antibody study; a positive test result consists in a fourfold rise in titer and immunofluorescence persisting at a 1:32 dilution. *Polymerase chain reaction* assays are very sensitive and highly specific but not widely available.

PRINCIPLES OF MANAGEMENT
(1–3,5–7,9,11,12,15,18–27)

The ideal approach to management is prevention. Measures range from public health activities and personal precautions to prophylactic use of antibiotics. For established infection, antibiotics are effective against *B. burgdorferi* and the treatment of choice. Treatment is determined by the stage of disease and type of clinical manifestation. *Doxycycline* and *amoxicillin* are preferred for oral treatment programs, and *ceftriaxone* or *high-dose penicillin* is preferred when IV therapy is required. Optimal dose and duration of therapy continue to be the subject of study. Response rates are excellent, but noninfectious sequelae

may still develop in fully treated persons. Additional antibiotic therapy is without benefit in such persons. Patients with severe or prolonged systemic symptoms due to documented Lyme disease should be tested for concurrent babesiosis and treated specifically with clindamycin and quinine if the results are positive.

Many patients who lack diagnostic criteria for Lyme disease but suffer from chronic fatigue have their symptoms mistakenly attributed to Lyme disease (especially if they are antibody-positive). Such persons are commonly subjected to prolonged antibiotic treatment for presumed late Lyme disease, leading to unnecessary antibiotic exposure, no improvement in outcomes, and distraction away from potentially treatable etiologies (e.g., major depression). Such empiric use of antibiotics should be avoided.

Prophylaxis

Tick control, avoidance measures, antibiotics, and vaccination comprise the principal modalities for prevention.

Tick Control Measures

A single spraying of residential properties with an acaricide in the spring (e.g., early May) can reduce tick populations by 70% to 100%. Deltamethrin, cyfluthrin, and carbaryl are used for this purpose. Removing areas where ticks can reside, such as brush and leaf piles, and placing a wood-chip barrier between woods and one's lawn helps to cut down the spread of ticks from the forest to residential property. Deer control is not effective unless the deer population is nearly extinguished, but fencing to keep deer away may help. Bait boxes with an acaricide can be used to attract and treat rodents; treating deer with an acaricide is under study.

Avoidance Measures

Standard preventive measures begin with avoiding brushy, wooded, or grassy habitats; these include grassy dunes, but not open, sandy beaches. Tucking one's pants into one's socks is also commonly suggested. Avoidance can be enhanced by topical use of repellants and acaricides.

Diethyltoluamide (DEET) *repellants* and *acaricides* such as *permethrin* that can be applied to clothing provide added protection to persons who cannot avoid high-risk settings. DEET-containing repellants should be used with care, especially in young children, who are quite susceptible to DEET neurotoxicity. Maximum DEET concentration in the repellant should be 15% for children and 35% for adults; use on the skin of infants, on the hands and face of young children, and on cuts, abrasions, and sunburned skin should be avoided. One should apply the repellant just once daily and wash it off with soap and water after returning indoors.

Tick Removal

For the majority of patients in nonhyperendemic regions who present with a tick bite, the most practical preventive approach is simply to be sure that the tick is removed promptly and thoroughly and the patient monitored for the development of erythema migrans and other symptoms and signs of acute Lyme disease. Because it takes more than 24 to 36 hours of tick contact before spirochete transmission occurs, it is recommended that *daily checks* for ticks be performed and removal attempted if a tick is found. Proper *tick removal* is best accomplished by using a tweezers to grip the mouth parts of the tick, which is pulled straight outward with steady, gentle pressure. The fingers can be used instead of a tweezers, but gloves should be worn and the hands washed afterward. Other methods (e.g., hot match tip, alcohol, petroleum jelly, nail polish) are not effective.

Prophylactic (Postexposure) Antibiotics

Asymptomatic patients who present with a tick bite pose the question of antibiotic prophylaxis. Patients in a hyperendemic area who present within 72 hours of first recognizing and removing a tick can reduce their risk of developing Lyme disease by 87% by taking a single 200-mg dose of *doxycycline*. This is especially true if the tick was attached for more than 36 hours (the time needed for transmission of the Lyme organism). There are no study data on the efficacy of prophylactic antibiotic therapy for patients who present more than 72 hours after the tick was discovered, but some authorities recommend a prophylactic dose of doxycycline if the tick was attached for more than 72 hours.

If the tick was attached for less than 36 hours, no prophylactic antibiotic treatment is needed because transmission of *B. burgdorferi* is highly unlikely before 36 hours of attachment, especially if the tick was not engorged. Moreover, the risk of antibiotic therapy inducing a drug hypersensitivity reaction in such patients is about the same as the probability of the drug preventing Lyme disease, making prophylaxis ill advised. (A similar antibiotic regimen [200 mg of doxycycline followed by 100 mg/d for 4 days] has proven to be effective in postexposure prophylactic treatment for *tick-borne relapsing fever*, which is due to *Borrelia persica*.)

Patients who are not treated prophylactically can be reassured that the risk of developing Lyme disease is very low (especially if the tick was removed within 24 to 36 hours) and that subsequent antibiotic therapy would be fully effective should symptoms and signs develop later. Close monitoring is indicated. Patients should be aware that antibiotic prophylaxis is not a substitute for primary prevention through the wearing of proper clothing, the use of insect repellent, and the avoidance of tick-infested areas.

For the majority of patients in nonhyperendemic regions who present with a tick bite, the most practical approach is simply to be sure that the tick is removed promptly and thoroughly and the patient monitored for the development of erythema migrans and other symptoms and signs of acute Lyme disease. Occasionally, a low-risk person remains so frightened after a tick bite that a prophylactic dose of doxycycline is given for reassurance.

Vaccination

A moderately effective Lyme vaccine was developed and approved for use in high-risk settings. It has been withdrawn from the market by the manufacturer because of low use due to a requirement for multiple doses, moderate efficacy, and theoretical concerns about triggering an autoimmune response. Because the vaccine was not fully protective, avoidance measures were still needed outdoors in high-risk areas.

Stage 1: Acute Infection

The earlier antibiotic treatment is instituted, the better is the outcome and the lower are the risks for dissemination and chronic disease. Patients residing in or visiting an endemic area who develop symptoms and signs indicative of a high probability of Lyme disease (see Table 160.1) are reasonable candidates

for a prompt initiation of a full course of antibiotic therapy without serologic testing. Most others, including those with tick bites, should undergo risk assessment (see prior discussion) to determine the need for therapy. If clinical evidence suggests an intermediate pretest probability of the disease (see Table 160.1), then serologic testing should be undertaken, allowing sufficient time after the onset of symptoms for an antibody response to develop. Patients who test positive under such circumstances are also candidates for a full course of antibiotics.

Antibiotic Regimens

Doxycycline (100 mg twice daily) and *amoxicillin* (500 mg three times daily) are the agents of choice for stage 1 infection. The optimum duration of therapy for persons presenting with erythema migrans and mild to moderate systemic symptoms is 10 days. Treatment failure is very rare. For persons presenting with more-severe symptoms, treatment may be extended to 21 or even 28 days. Adding a single IV dose of *ceftriaxone* at the outset of therapy for the prevention of early central nervous system spread does not improve outcomes.

Cefuroxime (500 mg twice daily) approaches the efficacy of doxycycline. Macrolide antibiotics are less effective, and newer-generation macrolides offer no advantage over doxycycline and amoxicillin. In a carefully conducted multicenter study, a program of 7 days of *azithromycin* was associated with an unacceptably high relapse rate in comparison with 20 days of amoxicillin (16% vs. 4%).

Stage 2: Disseminated Disease

In disseminated disease, it is common for a host of organ systems to be involved, although treatment recommendations are by organ system and clinical presentation. If more than one is involved, then the most potent antibiotic program takes precedence.

Cardiac Involvement

Cardiac involvement is a potentially worrisome form of disseminated disease. Although heart block is usually self-limited, patients with a severe PR interval prolongation (>0.4 seconds) are commonly treated with IV antibiotics (*ceftriaxone* or *high-dose penicillin*) to prevent significant myocardial invasion. For those with less severe PR interval prolongation, oral doxycycline or amoxicillin prescribed for 21 to 28 days suffices.

Neurologic Involvement

Although most neurologic manifestations of disseminated disease eventually clear without treatment, antibiotic therapy is strongly recommended both to shorten the duration of symptoms and to prevent sequelae.

Facial Nerve Palsy. In the absence of evidence for meningitis, treatment can be oral with *doxycycline* or *amoxicillin* for 3 to 4 weeks.

Meningitis. Antibiotic therapy produces a prompt clinical response and shortens the clinical course substantially. Both IV *ceftriaxone* and *high-dose penicillin G* are curative. Ceftriaxone is much more expensive, but its once-daily schedule makes home administration possible and obviates a prolonged hospitalization. Lumbar puncture with CSF analysis is needed to confirm the diagnosis but not to assess the response to treatment. The duration of therapy is best determined by the clinical response. Most authorities recommend 2 to 4 weeks.

Polyneuropathy. Peripheral neuropathy and radiculopathy tend to occur in conjunction with meningitis and respond well to treatment of the meningitis. When no clinical or CSF evidence of meningitis is found, an oral program of either doxycycline or amoxicillin for 3 to 4 weeks is a reasonable alternative.

Arthritis

The migratory musculoskeletal pains and brief attacks of oligoarticular arthritis are typically self-limited, but antibiotic therapy is given to halt symptoms and prevent progression to chronic arthritis. The optimal antibiotic program has not been established. Because of the development of chronic arthritis that persists despite prolonged courses of antibiotics, antibiotic regimens have been made longer. A program of 30 days of oral *doxycycline* or *amoxicillin* (with *probenecid* to delay urinary excretion) is often recommended, with IV therapy reserved for more refractory chronic arthritis (see later discussion). Intraarticular steroids are to be avoided because they increase the risk for antibiotic failure.

Stage 3: Late Disease

Late disease tends to be more difficult to treat, with responsiveness to antibiotics often less impressive than in disseminated disease. This has led to the use of prolonged and repeated courses of antibiotics. The inability to distinguish infectious from noninfectious sequelae has hindered the design of treatment programs. With the advent of DNA detection techniques, it should be possible to make more pathophysiologically correct treatment recommendations. It is hoped that etiologic therapy will become available to persons with noninfectious sequelae.

Arthritis

Treatment is 30 days of oral *doxycycline* or *amoxicillin* (plus *probenecid*) or 2 to 3 weeks of IV *ceftriaxone* or *penicillin G*. Retreatment may be necessary but only in cases with objective evidence of persistent infection (e.g., results of polymerase chain reaction testing of synovial fluid remain positive).

Encephalopathy

Patients with Lyme disease in whom documentable memory or cognitive deficits develop in conjunction with elevations in CSF protein and antibody are candidates for antibiotic therapy. The program is identical to that for meningitis. Resolution is sometimes incomplete, and retreatment is carried out. It is unclear whether the cause in such cases is infectious. Polymerase chain reaction testing of the CSF may prove useful in making this distinction, but such testing remains to be evaluated.

Other Management Issues

Persistent Neuropsychiatric Symptoms Attributed to Lyme Disease

Patients with neuropsychiatric symptoms due to chronic fatigue syndrome, fibromyalgia, depression, or somatization disorder may request treatment for Lyme disease, especially if they seek out and test positive for Lyme antibody. Those who have no clinical evidence for Lyme disease do not respond meaningfully to prolonged intensive courses of antibiotics (e.g., IV ceftriaxone 2 g/d for 30 days followed by oral doxycycline 200 mg/d for 30 days), and such therapy should not be prescribed for them, even if they are antibody-positive. Whether the occasional patient with fibromyalgia or chronic fatigue syndrome whose illness appears to have been directly precipitated by Lyme disease will respond is unclear, but the mechanism appears unrelated to infection per se.

Pregnant Patients

Maternal–fetal transmission of infection with subsequent injury to the fetus has been reported. Antibiotic treatment should be instituted promptly in symptomatic patients. For localized early disease in which erythema migrans is the only symptom, the recommended treatment is oral *amoxicillin* for 3 weeks. For more-disseminated disease, IV *high-dose penicillin G* is required for 2 to 3 weeks. No increased risk for fetal malformation has been found in asymptomatic women who are antibody-positive. Screening asymptomatic pregnant women for Lyme antibody and treating those who test positive is not warranted.

Patients with Concurrent Babesiosis

The program of choice is a combination of *clindamycin* and *quinine*. Treatment for concurrent disease should be carried out in consultation with an infectious disease specialist familiar with the management of tick-borne disease.

PATIENT EDUCATION AND INDICATIONS FOR REFERRAL

Persons living in or visiting an area endemic for Lyme disease should be instructed to venture into tick-infested areas only after proper application of insect repellent (see prior discussion) and to cover skin surfaces with protective clothing. In addition, they should be taught to recognize the rash and other manifestations of early Lyme disease and the importance of early treatment. Parents of children should be taught the proper technique of tick removal (see prior discussion). Many fear contracting the disease with every tick bite, but they can be reassured that brief contact (<24 hours) is unlikely to result in transmission of the organism, especially if the tick is not engorged (indicative of feeding) at the time of removal.

Patients with Lyme disease benefit from being informed about the excellent response of their condition to antibiotic therapy and its very favorable prognosis. However, those with protracted symptoms that do not respond to antibiotic therapy and with no evidence of persistent infection should be informed about the possibility of a noninfectious pathogenesis that is usually self-limited but slow to resolve. It is hoped that more etiologic therapy will be available for such persons in the future.

Patients who believe that they have Lyme disease but do not require as much education about the condition as those who do. The person with depression, chronic fatigue syndrome, or fibromyalgia who insists on treatment for Lyme disease needs to know how the diagnosis is made. Those who are antibody-positive will benefit from a discussion of the minimal significance of a positive antibody test result in the absence of other defining clinical manifestations. The physician, while explaining that the probability of active Lyme disease is very low, must take care not to deny the reality and severity of the patient's symptoms. Attention should be directed to treatment of the underlying condition (see Chapters 8, 159, and 227).

Referral is indicated when the patient with strong clinical evidence of Lyme disease fails to respond to a course of appropriate antibiotic therapy. Consultation is particularly important for those with refractory neurologic deficits, debilitating arthritis, or signs of severe cardiac involvement. Referral can also be helpful to reassure the mistakenly labeled patient who does not have Lyme disease that he or she is free indeed of the condition and not in need of extended antibiotic treatment.

RECOMMENDATIONS (7,27)

Diagnosis

- Base the diagnosis of Lyme disease predominantly on clinical features (e.g., erythema migrans, relapsing oligoarthritis, heart block, facial nerve palsy) and epidemiology (e.g., community incidence).
- Use serologic testing only as a supplement to the clinical diagnosis.
- Limit serologic testing to persons with an intermediate pretest probability of Lyme disease (based on clinical presentation).
- Avoid serologic testing early in the course of the illness because of the increased risk for false-negative results.
- Consider a two-step approach to serologic testing to reduce the false-positive rate: ELISA, followed by Western blot for sera with indeterminate or positive results by ELISA.
- Use only a high-quality laboratory that has persons skilled and experienced in performing Lyme serology.
- Avoid the use of urine testing for Lyme antigen; the test is unreliable.

Treatment

- For persons with uncomplicated *stage 1 disease* (early nondisseminated disease), begin amoxicillin (500 mg three times daily) or doxycycline (100 mg twice daily) for 10 days; consider extending treatment for a total of 3 or 4 weeks in those with more-severe early disease symptoms; consider cefuroxime (500 mg twice daily) as an effective alternative; do not use the 1-week azithromycin program because of an increased risk for relapse.
- For persons with *stage 2 disease* (acute disseminated disease), treat according to the organ(s) involved:
  1. For meningitis or severe cardiac manifestations, prescribe ceftriaxone (2 g/d IV once daily for 2 to 4 weeks).
  2. For peripheral neuropathy and arthritis, treat with amoxicillin (500 mg three times daily) or doxycycline (100 mg twice daily) for 3 to 4 weeks.
- For persons with *stage 3 disease* (chronic disease), treat the arthritis initially with the same program of amoxicillin or doxycycline as for stage 2 joint disease, but consider IV ceftriaxone if the initial program fails; treat encephalitis with ceftriaxone (2 g IV once daily for 2 to 4 weeks, the same treatment as for meningitis in stage 2 disease).
- Avoid further antibiotic therapy in persons with fully treated Lyme disease manifesting persistent symptoms and those with chronic neuropsychiatric symptoms mistakenly attributed to Lyme disease.

Prevention and Prophylaxis

- Teach patients the basics of avoiding tick habitats, dressing properly, using repellants safely, and removing ticks effectively.
- Prescribe prophylactic therapy (doxycycline, single 200-mg dose) for asymptomatic patients who experience a tick bite in a hyperendemic area, especially if the tick was attached for more than 36 hours and was engorged at the time of removal and the patient presents within 72 hours of discovering the tick.
- Omit prophylactic antibiotic therapy when a tick bite occurs in a nonhyperendemic area, especially if the tick was attached for less than 36 hours and was not engorged when removed. Follow expectantly.
- Consider prophylactic antibiotic therapy for a person in a hyperendemic area who presents more than 72 hours after the discovery of a tick if the period of attachment was more than 36 hours. Also consider prophylaxis for a tick bite taking place in a hyperendemic area in a person whose follow-up is uncertain or anxiety about contracting Lyme disease cannot be allayed.

A.H.G.

Annotated Bibliography

1. Dinerman H, Steere AC. Lyme disease associated with fibromyalgia. Ann Intern Med 1992;117:281. (*Lyme disease is often confused with fibromyalgia.*)
2. Feder HM, Johnson BJB, O'Connell SO, et al. A critical appraisal of "chronic Lyme disease." N Engl J Med 2007;357:1422. (*A review of the evidence, finding no support for the designation "chronic Lyme disease."*)
3. Krause PJ, Telford III SR, Spielman A, et al. Concurrent Lyme disease and babesiosis: evidence for increased severity and duration of illness. JAMA 1996;275:1657. (*A carefully conducted community-based serologic survey and clinic-based cohort study, finding a 10% rate of concurrent infection among those with active Lyme disease; the clinical picture is one of increased severity and prolongation of systemic symptoms.*)
4. Logigian EL, Kaplan RF, Steere AC. Chronic neurologic manifestations of Lyme disease. N Engl J Med 1990;323:1438. (*Describes the presence of memory loss, radiculopathy, and leukoencephalitis.*)
5. Seltzer EG, Gerber MA, Cartter ML, et al. Long-term outcomes of persons with Lyme disease. (*A community-based, longitudinal cohort study, finding that there was no evidence of increased risk for long-term adverse effects.*)
6. Smith RP, Schoen RT, Rahn DW, et al. Clinical characteristics and treatment outcome of early Lyme disease in patients with microbiologically confirmed erythema migrans. Ann Intern Med 2002;136:421. (*An observational cohort study, showing that the finding is useful for clinical presentation and course.*)
7. Steere AC. Lyme disease. N Engl J Med 2001;345:115. (*An authoritative review, including excellent photographs of erythema migrans; 100 references.*)
8. Steere AC, Schoen RT, Taylor E. The clinical evolution of Lyme arthritis. Ann Intern Med 1987;107:725. (*The best study of the natural history of the disease, based on examination of untreated patients.*)
9. Wormser GP, KcKenna D, Carlin J, et al. Brief communication: hematogenous dissemination in early Lyme disease. Ann Intern Med 2005;142. 751. (*Patients with erythema migrans are at risk of early hematogenous spread.*)
10. Steere AC, Taylor E, McHugh GL, et al. The overdiagnosis of Lyme disease. JAMA 1993;269:1812. (*The problem results from false-positive serology.*)
11. Brown SL, Hansen SL, Linguine JJ. Role of serology in the diagnosis of Lyme disease. JAMA 1999;282:62. (*A critical review of the test performance, recommending that serologic testing be limited to those with an intermediate pretest probability of disease and that a two-step approach to testing be used.*)
12. Fix AD, Strickland T, Grant J. Tick bites and Lyme disease in an endemic setting: problematic use of serologic testing and prophylactic antibiotic therapy. JAMA 1998;279:206. (*A regional surveillance study, documenting the frequent use of unnecessary early serologic testing and empiric antibiotic therapy regardless of test results in persons with a low pretest probability of Lyme disease.*)

13. Malane MS, Grant-Kels JM, Fecer HM Jr, et al. Diagnosis of Lyme disease based on dermatologic manifestations. Ann Intern Med 1991;114:490. (*Presents excellent photographs and discussion of these findings, which are often pathognomonic.*)
14. Nocton JJ, Dressler F, Rutledge BJ, et al. Detection of *Borrelia burgdorferi* DNA by polymerase chain reaction in synovial fluid from patients with Lyme arthritis. N Engl J Med 1994;330:229. (*Presents an improved diagnostic method, and suggests that late arthritis is not caused by the persistence of organisms in the joint.*)
15. Reid MC, Schoen RT, Evans J, et al. The consequences of overdiagnosis and overtreatment of Lyme disease: an observational study. Ann Intern Med 1998;128:354. (*Documents frequent overdiagnosis and overtreatment, which lead to inappropriate health care utilization, avoidable treatment-related adverse effects, disability, and depression.*)
16. Tugwell P, Dennis DT, Weinstein A, et al. Laboratory evaluation in the diagnosis of Lyme disease. Ann Intern Med 1997;127:1109. (*An evidence-based clinical guideline recommending testing only for persons with an intermediate [20% to 80%] pretest probability of having the disease.*)
17. Wormser GP, Aguero-Rosenfeld ME, Nadelman RB. Lyme disease serology: problems and opportunities. JAMA 1999;282:79. (*An editorial review of the current state of serologic testing, suggesting strategies and discussing problems involved in testing persons who have been immunized.*)
18. Dattwyler RJ, Luft BJ, Kunkel MJ, et al. Ceftriaxone compared with doxycycline for the treatment of acute disseminated Lyme disease. N Engl J Med 1997;337:289. (*A prospective, open-label, randomized multicenter trial showing oral doxycycline to be as effective as parenteral ceftriaxone in preventing symptoms and signs of late disease.*)
19. Hayes EB, Piesman J. How can we prevent Lyme disease? N Engl J Med 2003;348:2424. (*A thoughtful review of prophylaxis; 59 references.*)
20. Klempner MS, Hu LT, Evans J, et al. Two controlled trials of antibiotic treatment in patients with persistent symptoms and a history of Lyme disease.
N Engl J Med 2001;345:85. (*A randomized, controlled trial, finding no benefit from prolonged antibiotic therapy.*)
21. Lightfoot RW, Luft BJ, Rahn DW, et al. Empiric parenteral antibiotic treatment of patients with fibromyalgia and fatigue and a positive serologic result for Lyme disease. Ann Intern Med 1993;119:503. (*In most instances, antibiotic therapy is not cost-effective.*)
22. Luft BJ, Dattwyler RJ, Johnson RC, et al. Azithromycin compared with amoxicillin in the treatment of erythema migrans: a double-blind, randomized, controlled trial. Ann Intern Med 1996;124:785. (*Amoxicillin was more likely to produce complete resolution and less likely to cause relapse.*)
23. Nadelman RB, Nowakowski J, Fish D, et al. Prophylaxis with single dose doxycycline for the prevention of Lyme disease after an *Ixodes scapularis* tick bite. N Engl J Med 2001;345:79. (*A randomized, double-blind, placebo-controlled trial, demonstrating the efficacy of single-dose prophylactic therapy after a tick bite contracted in a hyperendemic area.*)
24. Steere AC. Duration of antibiotic therapy for Lyme disease. Ann Intern Med 2003;138:761. (*An editorial summarizing the evidence.*)
25. Steere AC, Sikand VK, Meurice F, et al. Vaccination against Lyme disease with recombinant *Borrelia burgdorferi* outer-surface lipoprotein A with adjuvant. N Engl J Med 1998;339:209. (*A double-blinded, randomized, multicenter trial of >10,000 participants, finding that the rate of infection was reduced by 49% in the first year and by 76% in the second year after the third injection.*)
26. Wormser GP, Ramanathan R, Nowakowski J, et al. Duration of antibiotic therapy for early Lyme disease: a randomized double-blind, placebo-controlled trial. Ann Intern Med 2003;138:697. (*A well-designed study, finding that 10 days is sufficient.*)
27. Wormser GP, Nadelman RB, Dattwler RJ, et al. Practice guidelines for the treatment of Lyme disease. The Infectious Diseases Society of America. Clin Infect Dis 2000;31(Suppl 1):1. (*Consensus guidelines; slightly dated but still useful.*)

CHAPTER 161 ■ APPROACH TO THE PATIENT WITH POLYMYALGIA RHEUMATICA OR GIANT-CELL (TEMPORAL) ARTERITIS

Polymyalgia rheumatica (PMR) and giant-cell arteritis are believed to be manifestations of the same immunologic disease process targeting the synovium, periarticular structures, and medium- to large-sized arteries in older patients. Polymyalgia rheumatica—the milder form with minimal vasculitic injury—affects mostly white patients (especially those of Scandinavian descent); there is a 2:1 female predominance. Onset begins after age 50 years, and incidence peaks between ages 70 and 80 years. The condition is common, with an annual incidence in persons older than age 50 years of 5 per 10,000; prevalence is 50 per 10,000. The risk for developing temporal arteritis is increased.

In giant-cell arteritis (also referred to as "temporal arteritis" or "cranial arteritis"), regional vasculitic injury dominates the clinical picture, hence the designations "temporal" and "cranial." Age distribution is the same as for PMR; the condition is one fifth as prevalent. Women are more likely to be affected than men, and 40% of patients give a prior history of polymyalgia rheumatica.

The primary physician needs to be alert to these diseases, which can be subtle and nonspecific in presentation and easily dismissed as vague functional complaints or confused with other conditions. The associated risks for blindness and aortic injury make the prompt recognition and treatment of giant-cell arteritis especially critical. Because successful treatment of full-blown giant-cell arteritis necessitates prompt, long-term immunosuppressive therapy, its identification must be timely and accurate.

PATHOPHYSIOLOGY, CLINICAL PRESENTATION, AND COURSE (1–13)

The pathogenesis of these conditions is unknown but believed to be shared. A genetic susceptibility has been suggested by an association with the *HLA-DRB1*04* and *01* alleles (similar to those that predispose to rheumatoid arthritis). The antigen responsible for precipitating the immune response that targets both blood vessels and synovium has not been identified, but epidemiologic data relate the risk to several infectious agents, including parainfluenza type 1 virus, parvovirus B19, *Mycoplasma*, and *Chlamydia* species. The current pathogenetic model posits that the responsible antigen stimulates a vigorous T cell–mediated response that leads to vascular injury, synovial and periarticular inflammation, and systemic symptoms.

In this model, antigen in susceptible hosts is recognized by vascular T cells that enter large blood vessels through the vasovasorum and form clones in the vessel wall producing interferon-γ. The interferon stimulates migration and transformation of macrophages into characteristic giant-cell infiltrates. In the adventitia, macrophages produce interleukins; in the media, they produce metalloproteinases and nitric oxide. The consequences are damage to the vessel's internal elastic lamina and stimulation of intimal hyperplasia; the attempted repair is dysfunctional, in that it narrows and occludes the vessel lumen.

Whether the condition presents clinically as giant-cell arteritis or PMR appears to depend in part on the amount of interferon-γ and interleukin-2 formed. In polymyalgia rheumatica, interferon-γ levels are low; in temporal arteritis they are high, suggesting that significant levels of the interferon are necessary for full-blown arteritis to appear and/or that giant-cell arteritis is a severe form of a common underlying disease process. Of note, persons with PMR and no clinical evidence of arteritis manifest evidence of subclinical vasculitis, which supports the notion that the conditions share a common pathogenesis. Acute-phase reactants (e.g., interleukin-6, interferon-γ) produced as part of the immune/inflammatory response are the likely sources of systemic symptoms (fever, fatigue, malaise) that may predate the onset of ischemic injury and dominate the clinical picture.

Polymyalgia Rheumatica

Pathology

Biopsies reveal mild inflammation of the synovium and periarticular structures, with the infiltrate made up of macrophages and T cells (especially CD4+ helper cells), resembling the infiltrate of giant-cell arteritis. Biopsy of the temporal artery is negative, and interferon-γ levels are not elevated.

Clinical Presentation and Course

Clinically, the onset is gradual, with the condition developing over weeks or months. Bilateral pain and stiffness of periarticular structures in the *neck* and *shoulders* is the presentation in two thirds of cases, with *hip* and *thigh* involvement accounting for the other one third. Symptoms may begin unilaterally, but eventually they become bilateral. Many patients experience both shoulder-girdle and thigh discomfort. Diffuse swelling of the *hands* and *feet* occurs in some patients, with pitting edema of the dorsal surfaces being characteristic. *Morning stiffness* and pain with movement are highly characteristic. Synovitis has been documented histologically, and rotator cuff bursitis and synovitis can be demonstrated by magnetic resonance imaging. Muscle biopsy specimens are usually normal or show minor inflammatory infiltrates; muscle strength is unimpaired. Low-grade *fever*, *weight loss*, and *fatigue* may accompany the musculoskeletal symptoms and are believed to represent the systemic effects of cytokines produced as part of the inflammatory process. The erythrocyte sedimentation rate (ESR) is characteristically greater than 50 mm/hr, but an occasional patient with characteristic clinical features of PMR may have an ESR of less than 40 mm/hr and a milder form of the disease. The ESR correlates with disease activity, as do levels of other acute-phase reactants such as *interleukin-6* and *C-reactive protein*.

Polymyalgia rheumatica tends to be a self-limited illness with a duration of 1 to 2 years. Three subsets of patients have been described: One responds promptly to initial steroid therapy and has no flares after taper; the required course of steroids is relatively short. A second also responds satisfactorily but has repeated flares and requires a longer course of steroids. A third does not respond to the initial doses of steroids, so that higher initial amounts are necessary; in addition, more flares occur, and a prolonged course of steroids is required. The risk for progression to temporal arthritis appears to be low in the first group and possibly increased in the last two. The pretreatment ESR and the response of the interleukin-6 level to treatment help to identify these subsets.

As noted, PMR shares many of the immunologic features of giant-cell arteritis, which suggests that PMR may be a *forme fruste* of the later condition. The risk of developing full-blown vasculitic disease averages 10% to 15%. Why some persons progress to vasculitis whereas others experience only a mild periarticular disease is unknown.

Giant-Cell (Temporal) Arteritis

Pathology

Pathologic manifestations include histiocytic, lymphocytic, and characteristic multinucleated giant-cell infiltrations of the walls of medium-sized and large arteries originating from the aortic arch. The aortic arch and any one of these vessels can be involved, but those of the head are most often affected. The reason for this distribution is unknown. The inflammatory process tends to be segmental, producing a patchy distribution with "skip" areas. The internal elastic lamina is fragmented, and intimal proliferation develops as part of the attempted repair process, narrowing the vascular lumen and accounting for the ischemia that ensues. There is no evidence of thrombosis. The aorta does not occlude, but vasculitic involvement does subject it to aneurysmal dilation and intramural hemorrhage.

Several clinicopathologic subtypes have been identified:

1. *Cranial (temporal) arteritis* is the most common and characteristic form; granulomatous vasculitis of the temporal artery, the presence of giant cells, and high cytokine levels are classic clinical features of temporal arteritis.
2. *Large-vessel arteritis* accounts for 10% to 15% of cases; large-vessel wall injury, a risk of aortic aneurysm and rupture, stenosis of primary and secondary aortic branches, a lack of temporal artery involvement in 50% of cases, and evidence of high levels of some cytokines (e.g., interferon-γ) are found.
3. *Arteritis with systemic inflammatory symptoms* exhibits T cell infiltrates on temporal artery biopsy, high interleukin levels, fever of unknown origin, wasting syndrome, and no vascular occlusions.

Clinical Presentation and Course

The presentation may be gradual or abrupt. Early symptoms may include headache, low-grade temperature, and the aching and stiffness of PMR. *Headache* is reported in about 70% of cases and is the initial symptom in about 35%. The pain can be piercing or throbbing, often localized to the arteries of the scalp and unlike that of any previous headache. *Polymyalgia* symptoms may be the presenting manifestation in more than 50% of cases. *Constitutional symptoms* of fatigue, malaise, anorexia, and weight loss occur in the majority of patients. In about one fifth of patients, the presentation may be atypical, with *fever of unknown origin* (FUO) being a classic atypical presentation of giant-cell arteritis (accounting for about 15% of cases of FUO in patients older than the age of 65 years).

As the condition progresses, *cranial artery tenderness* and enlargement may be noted. The temporal artery is most commonly affected, but any cranial artery may become involved, as may the carotids. Ischemic symptoms such as *masseter claudication* (jaw pain with chewing) occur in one third to one half of patients. Visual manifestations are the consequence of vasculitis of the ophthalmic or posterior ciliary arteries. *Blindness*, the most dreaded manifestation, has an abrupt onset and irreversible course unless it is treated very aggressively and very early (see later discussion). Vision loss is sometimes preceded by transient visual symptoms, such as *amaurosis fugax, flashing lights, diplopia,* or *field defects.* In untreated patients, visual loss occurs in up to 50% of cases; loss in one eye increases the risk of loss in the other to 50%. Acute *hearing loss* and *vertigo* have also been reported, as has *painful dysphagia. Carotid* involvement may present as localized tenderness in the neck accompanied by *neurologic deficits.*

An *aortic arch syndrome* may occur if the arch or a major branch vessel is involved. The risk for *aortic aneurysm* and *dissection* is increased nearly 20-fold in such persons; most often, the thoracic aorta is involved, but occasionally just the abdominal portion is affected. Granulomatous inflammation of the aortic wall is found. *Subclavian occlusive disease* may cause ischemic symptoms in the arms (e.g., *Raynaud's phenomenon, claudication*); on examination, *diminished pulses* may be noted and a subclavian *bruit* heard. The temporal arteries are often spared.

The *systemic inflammatory variant* is dominated by a *wasting syndrome* of *fever, progressive weight loss, night sweats,* and *fatigue* in association with evidence of temporal artery inflammation, but often without occlusive vascular disease. Interleukin levels are high.

A *markedly increased ESR* is characteristic of all forms of the disease; a normal sedimentation rate in the absence of strongly suggestive symptoms makes the diagnosis unlikely.

A low-grade *anemia of chronic disease* and mild elevations of *serum liver enzymes* are also often present. On occasion, the anemia can be severe.

Giant-cell arteritis is a chronic illness that may last for years. Although it tends to be self-limited, the clinical course is highly variable. Complications of late disease are rare, but attempts to discontinue therapy often cause relapses.

DIAGNOSIS (9,12,14,15)

Polymyalgia Rheumatica

The diagnosis is a clinical one. Formal criteria include (a) bilateral pain, in association with morning stiffness, for at least 1 month in any two of the following: neck, shoulder girdle, and hip girdle; (b) ESR greater than 40 mm/hr by the Westergren method; (c) age older than 50 years; (d) exclusion of other diagnoses except for giant-cell arteritis; and (e) marked clinical improvement in response to 1 week of treatment with less than 15 mg of prednisone per day. Patients meeting all criteria except for an elevated ESR are, in most instances, also considered to have PMR. Seronegative rheumatoid arthritis and shoulder bursitis from mechanical overuse need to be considered in the differential diagnosis.

Giant-Cell Arteritis

The formal American College of Rheumatology criteria for the diagnosis of the temporal-arteritis variant were designed for use in research and may lack predictive value when applied to individual patients, especially those with subtypes other than cranial arteritis. Nonetheless, these criteria remain the standard for diagnosis and include (a) age at onset of symptoms older than 50 years, (b) new onset or new type of localized headache, (c) temporal artery tenderness or diminished pulse, (d) ESR greater than 50 mm/hr by the Westergren method, and (e) temporal-artery biopsy specimen showing mononuclear infiltration or granulomatous infiltration with giant cells. The presence of any three criteria constitutes evidence for the diagnosis of cranial arteritis (sensitivity, 93.5%; specificity, 91.2%). Some characteristic symptoms and signs have been omitted from the list of criteria because of their lack of sensitivity or specificity.

WORKUP (4–6,8–12,14–28)

Polymyalgia Rheumatica

The clinical evaluation entails checking the history for neck, shoulder, and hip-girdle symptoms of morning stiffness and bilateral pain with movement. The patient's age is noted, as are reports of referred pain to the upper arms and thighs and any involvement of the dorsum of the hands or feet. On examination, particular attention is paid to the shoulders, hips, and hands. Active and passive range of motion should be tested and the precise location of swelling and pain noted. Any swelling and pain of the glenohumeral joint should suggest rheumatoid arthritis rather than polymyalgia rheumatica, which is more likely to cause periarticular inflammation. Unilateral bursal pain and swelling raise the question of a rotator cuff injury, but PMR may initially present unilaterally and mimic common shoulder tendonitis (see Chapter 150). The dorsal surfaces of the hands and feet should be checked for pitting edema.

An *ESR* is the only laboratory test that contributes to the diagnosis; imaging studies are being explored, as are molecular and genetic markers. Elevation of the ESR to greater than 40 mm/hr and a marked reduction in ESR after 1 week of low-dose prednisone (e.g., 10 mg/d) support the diagnosis. *Ultrasound* and *magnetic resonance imaging* of the shoulders can identify the proximal synovitis and subacromial and subdeltoid bursitis of PMR, which are present in almost all cases, but the cost-effectiveness of such imaging remains to be determined. Imaging is sometimes used to facilitate diagnosis in atypical cases.

Patients with PMR require careful clinical evaluation for symptoms and signs of giant-cell arteritis (see later discussion).

Giant-Cell Arteritis

Diagnosis of giant-cell arteritis can be problematic because of its many subtle, confusing, and often nonspecific presentations. The best studies of diagnosis focus on the temporal-arteritis variant.

History

Of the many historical features associated with temporal arteritis, only *jaw claudication* and *diplopia* have sufficiently high likelihood ratios (LRs) (4.2 and 3.4, respectively) to be predictive of the disease. Although these features are specific, they are not sensitive; their absence does not rule out the diagnosis. Other historical features often associated with the diagnosis (e.g., fever, temporal headache, vision loss, and polymyalgia symptoms) are less predictive (LR <2), and their absence does not rule out the diagnosis. There are no symptoms associated with aortitis, but one should check for claudication symptoms and paresthesias in the upper extremities that may herald subclavian and axillary artery involvement.

Physical Examination

Abnormalities on examination of the temporal artery (e.g., beading, prominence, tenderness, reduced or absent pulsation, redness) are the most predictive of physical examination findings (positive LR 4.6, 4.3, and 2.6, respectively). They are best detected by gentle palpation along the course of the temporal artery starting just anterior to the ears and up into the temples, checking both sides simultaneously for any asymmetry suggestive of a focal lesion. The entire scalp should be examined because any cranial artery may be involved. Other signs of ischemic damage are sought, including necrotic scalp and tongue lesions and optic disk pallor. The visual fields are checked for a field cut. The absence of cranial artery abnormalities on examination significantly reduces the pretest probability (negative LR, 0.53). Examination should also include palpation of the carotid arteries for tenderness and bruits, auscultation of the subclavian arteries for bruits, and checking of the peripheral pulses of the upper extremities for diminution or loss.

Erythrocyte Sedimentation Rate

The ESR, although formally listed as a defining feature of temporal arteritis, is only modestly helpful for ruling in the condition when it is very high (LR is 1.9 for ESR >100 mm/hr); it is more helpful in reducing the probability of temporal arteritis when it is low (LR is 0.2 when ESR is <50 mm/hr). However, as many as one fourth of persons with biopsy-proven temporal arteritis may have a normal ESR.

Other Acute-Phase Reactants

Besides the ESR, several other acute-phase reactants (e.g., *interleukin-6, C-reactive protein*) are typically elevated, but their specific contributions to diagnosis are incompletely defined. When the ESR is normal, a C-reactive protein is worth obtaining; it may be elevated despite a normal ESR and help to suggest ongoing inflammation. Interleukin-6, as one of the earliest acute-phase reactants, may eventually prove to be useful for increasing test sensitivity and achieving earlier diagnosis, but because no single laboratory test can rule in or rule out giant-cell arteritis, biopsy is usually required.

Temporal Artery Biopsy

Most authorities agree that histologic confirmation should be obtained even in the setting of high pretest probability before a patient is committed to such potentially morbid therapy as long-term daily corticosteroids. In instances in which the condition can be ruled out on clinical grounds, biopsy can be omitted, but obtaining tissue is helpful to eliminating concern when some clinical suspicion remains. Patients without strong clinical evidence for the diagnosis of giant-cell arteritis and with negative biopsy results have an excellent prognosis.

Biopsy can be performed safely under local anesthesia as an ambulatory procedure; morbidity is very low. The tempo-

ral artery is usually selected, but the best results are obtained when an accessible cranial artery that feels tender or abnormal is chosen. A 2- to 4-cm specimen is optimal because the inflammatory process may be focal due to "skip" areas. A single biopsy has a sensitivity of about 90%. A negative result on frozen section does not rule out the diagnosis and is an indication for proceeding to immediate biopsy of the contralateral temporal artery. Treatment with corticosteroids before biopsy may lower the test sensitivity slightly but not by so much as to preclude immediate therapy followed by biopsy within the first 1 to 2 weeks after therapy is started.

Vascular Imaging

Noninvasive imaging studies have been applied both to help identify involved arteries for biopsy and as an alternative or complement to tissue sampling. Color duplex ultrasonography of the temporal arteries appears to be promising as an alternative or complement to temporal artery biopsy. Its sensitivity is 73% and its specificity is 100% when the finding of a dark halo about the vessel (believed to represent vessel wall edema) is used as the key diagnostic feature. Prospective study is necessary to validate the utility and cost-effectiveness of the test (which is questioned by some). Possible applications range from screening PMR patients to substituting for biopsy in persons with a very high pretest probability.

Computed tomographic angiography (CT angiography) and *magnetic resonance angiography* (MRA) are supplanting conventional angiography for the detection of extracranial vascular involvement. Key sites of concern are the aortic arch and the distal subclavian and axillary arteries, which can be imaged by these noninvasive methods. CT angiography readily detects aneurysm formation and wall irregularities but requires a significant dye load. MRA can detect aortic root dilation, stenosis or occlusion of aortic branches, and possibly wall inflammation and edema. Formal sensitivity and specificity data are limited.

Conventional arteriography is sensitive but nonspecific and unreliable diagnostically for the identification of a diseased cranial artery but has been helpful when an area must be chosen to sample after a first biopsy result has been negative. It is also used for the identification of stenosed or occluded subclavian or axillary arteries.

PRINCIPLES OF MANAGEMENT
(9,12,29–39)

Polymyalgia Rheumatica

Polymyalgia rheumatica in the absence of giant-cell arteritis characteristically responds quickly and well to modest doses of *prednisone* (e.g., 10 to 15 mg/d). Patients with severe symptoms and a very high ESR at the time of presentation may require a higher initial dose of prednisone (e.g., 20 to 30 mg/d). As the sedimentation rate falls and symptoms clear, one can begin tapering prednisone in small decrements (1 to 2.5 mg/d every 2 weeks). Therapy is titrated against symptoms and ESR. Some have suggested that following the interleukin-6 response to treatment can help to predict the dose and duration of prednisone therapy. Symptomatic flares may require restarting or increasing prednisone, after which tapering is resumed. Between months and 1 to 2 years of daily low-dose steroid therapy may be required. The most prolonged therapy and the highest doses are likely to be needed by persons who manifest a markedly elevated ESR and prominent symptoms at onset and whose serum levels of interleukin-6 fail to normalize after initial steroid treatment. To minimize the adverse effects of daily steroids, the lowest possible dose of prednisone should be prescribed, taken in the morning (see Chapter 105). Osteoporosis prophylaxis is necessary if prolonged steroid therapy is required (see Chapter 146). The steroid doses required to prevent the development of giant-cell arteritis in patients with PMR are not known nor are the determinants of risk, but it appears that the likelihood of giant-cell arteritis is low when disease activity is well suppressed. There is no evidence that alternate-day therapy is effective.

Other immunomodulator therapies have been tried. *Methotrexate* has been found to have, at best, a modest steroid-sparing effect when used in conjunction with prednisone and insufficient benefit when used alone. It might have a place in persons who cannot tolerate the necessary doses of prednisone therapy, but it should not be considered an effective substitute. Similarly, *anti–tumor necrosis factor* therapy with *infliximab* has been disappointing when low doses are added to prednisone therapy or used alone as initial treatment. More study is needed on the role of immunomodulators in polymyalgia rheumatica.

Giant-Cell Arteritis

Initiation of Steroid Therapy

The first priority is to establish control of the disease quickly to limit the risk for irreversible blindness. When the patient's pretest probability of giant-cell arteritis is high (e.g., age >70 years, new headache, palpably enlarged and tender cranial artery, jaw claudication, high ESR), it is best to begin empiric *high-dose glucocorticoid* therapy (e.g., prednisone 60 mg/d) immediately. The efficacy of lower doses for initial therapy is a subject of ongoing study. Biopsy confirmation of the diagnosis is necessary, but empiric high-dose therapy for 1 to 2 weeks before biopsy does not seriously compromise diagnosis (see prior discussion).

In most instances, the clinical response starts within 24 hours of initiation of treatment, but it can be more protracted. *Daily therapy* is needed; alternate-day schedules do not control the arteritis. To minimize adrenal suppression, prednisone should be taken once daily in the morning (see Chapter 105). Although it is not certain that permanent visual loss can be prevented in persons presenting with ischemic eye symptoms, such symptoms are treated by ophthalmologists with high-dose parenteral steroid therapy (e.g., *methylprednisolone*, 100 mg intravenously every 12 hours), started within hours of initial presentation and continued for 5 days.

Other immunosuppressive agents have been sought. *Methotrexate* was found to have no steroid-sparing effects. *Aspirin* may hold promise because it is a suppressor of interferon-γ and affords some coronary artery protection.

Tapering

The steroid dose is titrated against symptoms and sedimentation rate. To minimize the adverse effects of prolonged daily steroid therapy (see Chapter 105), the daily prednisone dose should be tapered. Tapering can be started after clinical and laboratory manifestations have normalized; it can be steady but should not be precipitous. Typically, the dose is tapered by 10% to 20% every 2 weeks. Rapid tapering of prednisone to less than 20 mg/d over the first 1 to 2 months is associated with a 30% relapse rate. More reasonable is tapering to a daily dose of 20 to 30 mg within the first 2 months and more slowly thereafter. The goal is a maintenance dose of less than 10 mg/d, but it may take more than 1 year to achieve it.

Other Immunomodulators

Anti–tumor necrosis factor therapy has been studied for its possible role in the treatment of giant cell arteritis. Initial studies using low doses of *infliximab* have shown no benefit when used for the maintenance of prednisone-induced remission.

Monitoring and Termination of Therapy

As the dose is reduced, the patient must be monitored for a recurrence of *symptoms* and elevation of the *sedimentation rate*. Some argue that the ESR is insensitive for the detection of disease reactivation and that alternative markers should be sought, such as the interleukin-6 level; more study of the question is needed.

Most patients require treatment for 2 to 3 years. Relapses occur in up to 50% of patients who attempt termination of therapy before that time. Nonetheless, the risk for blindness and other serious disease-related complications is minimal late in the course of disease, and a trial of discontinuing therapy can be attempted every 6 to 12 months after the first year. Prognosis is excellent, and life expectancy is normal. Nonetheless, the trial should be halted at the first sign of recurring symptoms or a marked rise in the ESR. Close monitoring for relapse is essential during the first 12 months that the patient is off therapy. The most common manifestation of relapse is a return of PMR symptoms, which respond to modest (2.5 to 5 mg/d) increases in prednisone dose.

Despite tapering efforts, many patients experience steroid-related side effects because of the prolonged duration of daily high-dose steroid therapy (see Chapter 105). Efforts to prevent osteoporosis should be undertaken at the outset of treatment (see Chapter 164).

Because the risk for potentially life-threatening aortic disease is increased in giant-cell arteritis, some have suggested that periodic monitoring for aortic aneurysm be part of the routine follow-up. Suggestions for monitoring range from obtaining yearly chest x-rays to screening by MR, CT, or ultrasound. Criteria for patient selection and the most cost-effective approach remain to be determined.

PATIENT EDUCATION

Patients with PMR in the absence of giant-cell arteritis can be reassured. They benefit from knowing that the risk for the development of significant arteritis is small, that the disease does not progress to disabling arthritis, and that their condition is self-limited, although it may take a few years to clear. They should be instructed to watch for symptoms of arteritis and report them promptly. The adverse effects of corticosteroid therapy need to be reviewed so that patients will use prednisone carefully and as directed and take prophylaxis for osteoporosis.

Patients with giant-cell arteritis and their families must understand the rationale for daily prednisone therapy in addition to its adverse side effects, both to ensure compliance and to provide an informed basis for long-term steroid use. Instruction in the means of minimizing steroid side effects is appreciated (see

Chapter 105). Patients can be reassured that the serious complications of giant-cell arteritis can usually be avoided by proper therapy.

INDICATIONS FOR REFERRAL AND ADMISSION

Prompt consultation with a rheumatologist is helpful when the initiation of high-dose steroid therapy for presumed giant-cell arteritis is being considered before a temporal artery biopsy can be performed, but therapy should not be delayed if consultation is not available immediately. Urgent ophthalmologic evaluation is needed if visual impairment is reported. If it is not available, one can proceed directly to hospitalization for immediate institution of high-dose parenteral corticosteroid therapy. Rheumatologic consultation is also indicated to consider the need for steroid therapy when cranial-artery biopsy results are negative but the clinical presentation strongly suggests arteritis. The occasional patient with PMR or giant-cell arteritis who does not respond adequately to steroid therapy requires a referral for reconsideration of the diagnosis and review of the treatment program.

THERAPEUTIC RECOMMENDATIONS

Polymyalgia Rheumatica

- Begin with low-dose prednisone (10 to 15 mg/d), provided that no evidence of giant-cell arteritis is present. For patients with a very high ESR and severe symptoms, consider starting prednisone at a higher dose (e.g., 20 to 30 mg/d).
- Taper in decrements of 1.0 to 2.5 mg/d every 2 weeks, titrating the dose against symptoms and ESR.
- Prescribe the lowest dose possible, to be taken in the morning.
- Continue steady tapering to full cessation of therapy if possible, monitoring symptoms and ESR for 2 years for evidence of relapse.

- Restart or increase prednisone by 5 to 10 mg/d if a flare of disease occurs; adjust the dose as needed and resume tapering as soon as remission has been achieved.
- Instruct the patient to report promptly any symptoms suggestive of giant-cell arteritis (e.g., visual disturbances, tender cranial artery, headache, fever, jaw claudication, arm claudication).

Giant-Cell Arteritis

- Begin therapy with daily high-dose glucocorticoids (e.g., 60 mg of prednisone every morning). Consider prescribing intravenous methylprednisolone (100 mg every 12 hours for 5 days) for patients who present with visual disturbances; obtain urgent ophthalmologic consultation.
- Begin reducing the initial dose by 10% to 20% every 2 weeks once symptoms have cleared and the sedimentation rate has been normalized (<40 mm/hr); aim for a daily prednisone dose of 20 to 30 mg after 1 to 2 months.
- Continue daily prednisone therapy, tapering slowly as tolerated over 12 to 18 months to the minimum dose sufficient to keep the sedimentation rate normal and the patient free of symptoms; a prednisone dose of less than 10 mg/d is often sufficient.
- Monitor symptoms and the sedimentation rate to determine the rate and extent of tapering permissible. Halt tapering if the ESR rises or symptoms return; consider increasing the prednisone dose by 2.5 to 5 mg/d if the relapse is characterized by a return of PMR symptoms; increase the dose by greater amount if vasculitic symptoms develop. After control is reestablished, resume the tapering program as before.
- Continue daily steroids for 18 to 24 months; consider a trial of phasing out therapy at that time and then every 6 to 12 months.
- After cessation of therapy, continue to monitor for recurrence of symptoms and a rise in the sedimentation rate over the next 12 months.
- Consider CT or MRI to monitor for aortic aneurysm.

A.H.G.

Annotated Bibliography

1. Ayoub WT, Franklin CM, Torretti D. Polymyalgia rheumatica: duration of therapy and long-term outcome. Am J Med 1985;79:309. (*Some patients have a 6- to 12-month course; others require therapy for up to 2 years.*)
2. Brack A, Martinez-Taboada V, Stanson A, et al. Disease pattern in cranial and large-vessel giant cell arteritis. Arthritis Rheum 1999;42:311. (*Describes subtypes, including large-vessel arteritis and aortitis.*)
3. Casselli RJ, Hunder GG, Whisnant JP. Neurologic disease in biopsy-proven giant cell (temporal) arteritis. Neurology 1988;38:352. (*Findings include acute vertigo and hearing loss in addition to visual loss.*)
4. Chmelewski WL, McKnight KM, Agudelo CA, et al. Presenting features and outcomes in patients undergoing temporal artery biopsy. Arch Intern Med 1992;152:1690. (*Presenting features did not always predict biopsy results; late disease complications were rare, but prolonged therapy was required.*)
5. Evans JM, O'Fallon WM, Hunder GG. Increased incidence of aortic aneurysm and dissection in giant cell (temporal) arteritis. Ann Intern Med 1995;122:502. (*There was a markedly increased risk for aneurysm and dissection.*)
6. Klein RG, Hunder GG, Stanson AW, et al. Large artery involvement in giant cell (temporal) arteritis. Ann Intern Med 1975;83:806. (*A classic paper, finding that the disease is not limited to the cranial arteries.*)
7. Machado EB, Michet CJ, Ballard DJ, et al. Trends in incidence and clinical presentation of temporal arteritis in Olmstead County, Minnesota, 1950–1985. Arthritis Rheum 1988;31:745. (*The best epidemiologic data, showing that clinical features are changing and that detection is occurring earlier.*)
8. Myklebust G, Gran JT. A prospective study of 284 patients with polymyalgia rheumatica and temporal arteritis: clinical and laboratory manifestations at onset of disease and at the time of diagnosis. Br J Rheumatol 1996;35:1161. (*Excellent data on clinical and laboratory manifestations.*)
9. Salvarani C, Cantini F, Boiardi, et al. Polymyalgia rheumatica and giant-cell arteritis. N Engl J Med 2002;347:261. (*An excellent general review; 77 references.*)
10. Salvarani C, Cantini F, Olivieri I, et al. Proximal bursitis in active polymyalgia rheumatica. Ann Intern Med 1997;127:27. (*Presents evidence that bursitis is the cause of the shoulder pain.*)
11. Salvarani C, Gabriel S, Hunder GC. Distal extremity swelling with pitting edema polymyalgia rheumatica. Arthritis Rheum 1996;39:73. (*This was an atypical presentation, but was important to note.*)
12. Weyand CM, Goronzy JJ. Giant-cell arteritis and polymyalgia rheumatica. Ann Intern Med 2003;139:505. (*A comprehensive review with emphasis on disease mechanisms and clinical correlations; 100 references.*)
13. Weyand CM, Goronzy JJ. Medium- and large-vessel vasculitis. N Engl J Med 2003;349:160. (*An excellent review of pathophysiology; 85 references.*)
14. Hunder GG, Bloch DA, Michel BA, et al. The American College of Rheumatology criteria for the classification of giant cell arteritis. Arthritis Rheum 1990;33:1122. (*Consensus diagnostic criteria.*)
15. Rao JK, Allen NB, Pincus T. Limitations of the 1990 American College of Rheumatology classification criteria in the diagnosis of vasculitis. Ann Intern

Med 1998;129:345. (*Finds that these criteria were less helpful for diagnosis in the individual patient.*)

16. Agard C, Ponge T, Hamidou M, et al. Role for vascular investigations in giant cell arteritis. Joint Bone Spine 2002;69:367. (*Reviews the role of computed tomography in diagnosis.*)

17. Atalay MK, Bluemke DA. Magnetic resonance imaging of large vessel vasculitis. Curr Opin Rheumatol 2001;13:41. (*A review of the contributions of noninvasive imaging methods to disease detection and monitoring.*)

18. Cantini F, Salvarani C, Olivieri I, et al. Shoulder ultrasonography in the diagnosis of polymyalgia rheumatica: a case–control study. J Rheumatol 2001;28:1049. (*Suggests a diagnostic role.*)

19. Cantini F, Salvarani C, Olivieri I, et al. Inflamed shoulder structures in polymyalgia rheumatica with normal erythrocyte sedimentation rate. Arthritis Rheum 2001;44:1155. (*Finds that imaging studies revealed inflammatory changes in the absence of erythrocyte sedimentation rate [ESR] elevation and suggests their possible use in diagnosis.*)

20. Hall S, Persellin S, Lie JT, et al. The therapeutic impact of temporal artery biopsy. Lancet 1983;2:1217. (*The procedure helped in decision making; <10% of patients with negative biopsy findings developed signs of arteritis or required steroid therapy.*)

21. Kyle V, Cawston TE, Hazleman BL. Erythrocyte sedimentation rate and C-reactive protein in the assessment of polymyalgia rheumatica/giant cell arteritis on presentation and during follow-up. Ann Rheum Dis 1989;48:667. (*ESR closely paralleled disease severity and activity in most cases, as did C-reactive protein.*)

22. Layfer LF, Banner BF, Huckman MS, et al. Temporal arteriography. Arthritis Rheum 1978;21:780. (*Arteriography was highly sensitive but not specific.*)

23. Ponge T, Barrier JH, Grolleau JY, et al. The efficacy of selective unilateral temporal artery biopsy versus bilateral biopsies for diagnosis of giant cell arteritis. J Rheumatol 1988;15:997. (*Bilateral biopsy was sometimes necessary, but careful selection could obviate the need for routinely ordering biopsies of two sites.*)

24. Robb-Nicholson C, Chang RW, Anderson S, et al. Diagnostic value of the history and physical examination in giant cell arteritis. J Rheumatol 1988;15:1793. (*Clusters of symptoms had a high sensitivity, but specificity was lacking.*)

25. Schmidt WA, Kraft HE, Vorpahl K, et al. Color duplex ultrasonography in the diagnosis of temporal arteritis. N Engl J Med 1997;337:1336. (*Sensitivity was 73% and specificity was 100%, suggesting that a positive test result might obviate the need for biopsy.*)

26. Smetana GW, Shmerling RH. Does this patient have temporal arteritis? JAMA 2002;287:92. (*A systematic review of studies of the diagnostic utility of clinical features; 72 references.*)

27. Sox HC, Liang MW. The erythrocyte sedimentation rate. Ann Intern Med 1986;104:515. (*This measure was useful for diagnosis and monitoring response to therapy.*)

28. Wong RL, Korn JH. Temporal arteritis without an elevated sedimentation rate. Am J Med 1986;80:959. (*A normal ESR does not rule out the diagnosis when other characteristic features are present.*)

29. Achkar AA, Lie JT, Hunder GG, et al. How does previous corticosteroid treatment affect the biopsy findings in giant cell (temporal) arteritis? Ann Intern Med 1994;120:987. (*Findings were not obscured by 2 weeks of prednisone.*)

30. Caporali R, Cimmino MA, Ferraccioli G, et al. Prednisone plus methotrexate for polymyalgia rheumatica: a randomized, double-blind controlled trial. Ann Intern Med 2004;141:493. (*Finds a modest potential benefit, predominantly some degree of steroid sparing.*)

31. Hoffman GS, Cid MC, Rendt-Zagar KE, et al, for the Infliximab-GCA Study Group. Infliximab for maintenance of glucocorticosteroid-induced remission of giant-cell arteritis. Ann Intern Med 2007;146:621. (*A randomized controlled trial, showing no benefit.*)

32. Hoffman GS, Cid MC, Hellmann DB, et al. A multicenter, randomized, double-blind, placebo-controlled trial of adjuvant methotrexate treatment for giant cell arteritis. Arthritis Rheum 2002;46:1309. (*Finds no adjuvant benefit.*)

33. Hunder GG, Sheps SG, Allen GL, et al. Daily and alternate-day corticosteroid regimens in the treatment of giant cell arteritis. Ann Intern Med 1975;82:613. (*Alternate-day steroids did not suffice.*)

34. Kyle V, Hazleman BL. Stopping steroids in polymyalgia rheumatica and giant cell arteritis: treatment usually lasts for 2 to 5 years. Br Med J 1990;300:344. (*The need for therapy can be prolonged.*)

35. Kyle V, Hazleman BL. Treatment of polymyalgia rheumatica and giant cell arteritis I: steroid regimens in the first 2 months. Ann Rheum Dis 1989;48:658. (*A high dose was required initially; then it could be reduced.*)

36. Rosenfeld SI, Kosmorsky GS, Klingele TG, et al. Treatment of temporal arteritis with ocular involvement. Am J Med 1986;80:143. (*High-dose intravenous steroids given acutely for 5 days offered a chance of visual recovery if started early.*)

37. Salvarani C, Macchioni P, Manzini C, et al. Infliximab plus prednisone or placebo plus prednisone for the initial treatment of polymyalgia rheumatica. Ann Intern Med 2007;146:631. (*A randomized, controlled trial, showing no benefit.*)

38. Weyand CM, Fulbright JW, Hunder GG, et al. Treatment of giant cell arteritis: interleukin-6 as a biologic marker of disease activity. Arthritis Rheum 2000;43:1041. (*Suggests a possible role for this cytokine in monitoring disease activity.*)

39. Weyand CM, Fulbright JW, Evans JM, et al. Corticosteroid requirements in polymyalgia rheumatica. Arch Intern Med 1999;159:577. (*A prospective cohort study, identifying three subgroups with different steroid requirements.*)

CHAPTER 162 ■ MANAGEMENT OF PAGET'S DISEASE

DAVID M. SLOVIK

Paget's disease of bone, or *osteitis deformans,* is a focal disorder characterized by excessive resorption and rapid, disorganized formation of new bone leading to bony deformity. Paget's disease typically involves one bone (monostotic), although more severe cases involve several bones (polyostotic). Genetic factors and viral infection are believed to play roles in pathogenesis. The incidence is 3.3% in autopsy series and 0.1% to 4.0% in radiologic studies. Approximately 2% of the U.S. population older than age 60 years has evidence of Paget's disease, most asymptomatic. Discovery is often incidental, on encountering an isolated serum alkaline phosphatase elevation or characteristic bony changes on plain films. At other times it may be noted in the workup of back or extremity pain, gait disturbance, hear-

ing loss, or high-output cardiac failure. The primary physician needs to be able to recognize the condition and know how and when to use agents that suppress osteoclastic activity.

PATHOPHYSIOLOGY AND CLINICAL PRESENTATION (1–6)

Pathophysiology

The pathophysiologic hallmarks of Paget's disease are *excessive osteoclastic destruction* and resorption of bone, followed by the *unregulated osteoblastic formation of new bone*. The initial stimulus for bone resorption is unknown, but the process culminates in an abnormal pattern of lamellar bone. Excessive local vascularity and an increase in fibrous tissue, which extends into the marrow, are characteristic. Both cortical and cancellous bone may be involved, each with several foci at different stages. The nature of the resultant bone, which is mechanically defective, distorted, and enlarged, leads to the cardinal manifestations of Paget's disease—bone pain and pathologic fractures.

Clinical Presentation

Although any bone may become involved, the common sites are *spine*, *pelvis*, *skull*, *femur*, and *tibia*. Most patients are asymptomatic, with Paget's disease presenting as an incidental finding on x-ray films or an isolated elevation in alkaline phosphatase. Those who are symptomatic present with bone pain, bony deformity, fracture, or a complication of increased marrow vascularity or bony encroachment on neural structures. About 15% of patients have very localized (so-called "monostotic") disease.

Bone pain may result from fracture or be due to lytic activity. In the latter instance, it is usually located over areas of bone where very active osteoclastic resorption is taking place. The severity of pain does not always parallel the extent of radiographic involvement. Exacerbating factors include weight bearing, muscular activity, and cold weather.

Fractures may affect the vertebrae or long bones, especially the lumbar and sacral regions of the spine and the *lesser trochanter* of the femur and the upper one third of the tibia. A history of trauma can usually be elicited, but some of these fractures may occur spontaneously. Pain may result, but vertebral fractures are often painless, although they can lead to a loss of height, kyphoscoliosis, and, in rare instances, spinal cord compression.

Bony deformity and *encroachment* are most notable in the *skull*, which may become visibly enlarged in the frontal and occipital regions. The overlying superficial blood vessels often become prominently dilated and visibly pulsatile. *Hearing loss* can ensue from the involvement of the ossicles in the middle ear, which impinge on the eighth cranial nerve in the temporal bone. *Cerebellar* and *long-tract* signs are complications of posterior fossa encroachment. Vertebral encroachment on the *spinal cord* or *nerve roots* is a rare but very serious consequence that can cause a compression syndrome leading to paraplegia. Deformity of the *long bones* is manifested as anterolateral *bowing* with resultant gait abnormalities, low back pain joint pain, and increased susceptibility to fracture.

Degenerative joint disease can ensue when hypertrophy of subchondral bone damages the overlying cartilage and causes joint dysfunction; it accounts for about 50% of the discomfort experienced by patients. Hip pain can develop from longstanding subchondral disease of the acetabulum and femoral head, leading to protrusio acetabuli. Degenerative disease of the knee joint may occur in a similar fashion if the distal femur or patella becomes pagetic.

Extensive and severe skeletal involvement increases the risk for *osteogenic sarcoma,* an uncommon but uniformly fatal cancer that affects less than 1% of pagetic patients. It is heralded by localized pain, bony enlargement, and a very high and rapidly increasing alkaline phosphatase.

Hyperuricemia leading to gouty arthritis and *hypercalciuria* resulting in renal calculi are among the biochemical consequences of disrupted bony metabolism. *Hypercalcemia* can be precipitated by immobilization. *High-output heart failure* may occur in patients with extensive Paget's disease because of the marked increase in the vascular bed.

Laboratory and Radiographic Features

Serum *alkaline phosphatase* produced by osteoblasts is usually increased and correlates with the degree of new bone formation. *Urinary hydroxyproline*—a measure of bone matrix resorption—is also increased. In most patients, these parameters are complementary markers of disease activity and parallel radionuclide uptake on *bone scan*, which is the most sensitive measure of disease activity. In patients with disease localized to a single bone, the results of standard serum and urine tests may be normal. The *bone-specific alkaline phosphatase* level provides a more sensitive determination of new bone formation, and the urinary level of *pyridinoline* and N-telopeptide (a specific component of bone matrix) are better measures of bone resorption. Although these tests are substantially more expensive than the unfractionated alkaline phosphatase, they are better indicators of disease activity, especially in persons with involvement limited to a single bone. However, the serum alkaline phosphatase correlates well with the other tests, and for routine monitoring, it alone can be measured.

Technetium bone scan demonstrates areas of increased uptake before diagnostic changes are visible on *standard radiography*. The first radiologic bony changes occur in the lytic phase and are well-demarcated areas of decalcification (seen best in the skull). With the onset of new bone formation, areas of increased density become evident, as does the expansion of bone and coarse trabeculation. In later phases, sclerosis, enlargement, and increased bone density are observed. The localized enlargement of bone that results is unique to Paget's disease and helps to distinguish it from other causes of bony sclerosis, such as prostatic cancer. Radiologic changes are most commonly evident in the pelvis, femur, and skull. A bone scan should be obtained on all patients with known or suspected Paget's disease, followed by plain radiographs of the pagetic area.

Clinical Course

Although many patients manifest slow radiologic progression, most never develop symptoms. Others are noted to have radiologic changes that remain stable; a few have rapidly progressive disease. Although clinical remission after treatment is the rule, new complications can occur in those who do not achieve full biochemical remission (see later discussion).

PRINCIPLES OF THERAPY (4,6–16)

Asymptomatic patients require no specific therapy unless the location of their disease places them at risk for a potentially serious complication (see later discussion). Localized mild bone or joint pain responds to *analgesics* (e.g., *acetaminophen* 325 mg or *ibuprofen* 400 mg, three times daily). Disease-specific therapy can halt disease progression by inhibiting bone resorption. The efficacy and safety of modern antipagetic therapy and the potentially disabling consequences of the disease have lowered the threshold for such treatment. Bisphosphonates are the primary mode of disease-specific therapy; cytotoxic agents and surgery are sometimes needed.

Indications for Disease-Specific Therapy

The management of Paget's disease has been greatly enhanced in recent years with the development of *potent bisphosphonates*, which are well tolerated, can be given by mouth or vein, and are capable of inhibiting osteoclast-mediated bone resorption without compromising bone mineralization. They produce radiographic, biochemical, and clinical improvement. Most patients with Paget's disease are considered reasonable candidates for treatment unless they are asymptomatic and the disease is confined to areas where it is unlikely to cause complications (e.g., ribs, iliac crest, sacrum, upper limbs, scapula).

Indications for Immediate Treatment

Indications include (a) severe pain in pagetic areas, (b) compression of medulla, cauda equina, or auditory nerve with neurologic deficit, (c) high-output cardiac failure, (d) hypercalcemia secondary to immobilization, (e) marked radiographic lytic lesions in long bones and skull representing a risk for fracture or brain trauma, (f) multiple fractures, (g) prevention of disfigurement when the skull is extensively involved, (h) recurrent renal calculi secondary to hypercalciuria, and (i) severe hyperuricemia and gout. Standard courses of therapy are specified, but any sign of clinical or biochemical relapse (e.g., pain, neurologic deficit, or biochemical marker greater than 20% to 30% above normal) is an indication for repeated treatment.

Indications for Prophylactic Therapy

Prophylactic therapy is indicated when orthopedic surgery is planned in an involved area and when disease is located in an area (e.g., base of the skull, spine, long bones of lower extremity, hip, or knee) where progress is likely to cause a complication.

Bisphosphonates

Bisphosphonates, which include *alendronate*, *risedronate*, *etidronate*, and *tiludronate* (oral) and *pamidronate* and *zoledronate* (intravenous), are the treatment of choice for the vast majority of patients with Paget's disease. The second-generation drugs (e.g., alendronate, risedronate) are particularly effective by mouth, as are pamidronate and zoledronate by vein. After absorption, they bind to bone and may persist there for months to years, which probably accounts for their sustained benefit long after therapy is discontinued. They markedly decrease bone turnover by inhibiting osteoclastic bone resorption. First-generation bisphosphonates (e.g., etidronate) also impair bone mineralization, a distinct disadvantage. All decrease the number of osteoclasts and induce osteoclast apoptosis. The deposition of new bone proceeds in lamellar fashion rather than in the woven pattern characteristic of Paget's disease. Patients with moderate disease respond almost completely. Bone pain decreases, and neurologic deficits lessen. The alkaline phosphatase level returns toward normal, and radionuclide uptake on bone scan decreases markedly. Hearing loss may not improve, but it ceases to worsen. Bony films may show some repair of lytic lesions. By turning off bone resorption, potent bisphosphonates may lower serum calcium, requiring calcium and vitamin D supplementation for the prevention of secondary hyperparathyroidism.

Alendronate

Alendronate is among the most effective of the available orally active bisphosphonates approved by the U.S. Food and Drug Administration (FDA). When given in full doses (40 mg/d), this second-generation bisphosphonate normalizes the alkaline phosphatase level in about half of cases and produces an overall 75% mean reduction in the alkaline phosphatase. It is superior to etidronate and calcitonin and equal to intravenous pamidronate in effectiveness. Its main drawback is gastroesophageal mucosal injury (ulcer, esophagitis), which can be minimized by taking a full 8-oz glass of water and remaining upright for at least 30 minutes. Because food nullifies absorption, alendronate must be taken on an empty stomach. A standard course of treatment is 6 months; treatment is restarted if a relapse occurs. Remissions can last from 6 months to several years. Many patients either experience a prolonged remission after a single course of therapy or respond well to repeated treatment. The remainder, who manifest more severe disease, may relapse more quickly.

Risedronate

Risedronate's efficacy is similar to that reported for alendronate (73% of patients manifest biochemical remission at 6 months, and 53% at 18 months), although no direct comparison studies have been performed. The risk of gastrointestinal mucosal injury and the need for precautions are similar to those for alendronate. The recommended dose is 30 mg/d; the duration of therapy is only 2 months. Prolonged remission can be seen. The cost of a course of treatment is about 10% less than with alendronate (i.e., the cost per tablet is much higher, but the total cost for a standard course of therapy is reduced).

Pamidronate

Pamidronate is used for moderate to severe Paget's disease, especially when Paget's disease is complicated by important neurologic deficits. It is too injurious to the gastroesophageal mucosa for oral use, but the efficacy of intravenous therapy is similar to that of oral alendronate. Its intravenous administration can be of benefit when compliance with or tolerance to long-term oral therapy is compromised. The standard dose is 30 mg/d for 3 days. The mean duration of remission is about 14 months. Inhibition of bone resorption can lower serum calcium, necessitating calcium and vitamin D supplementation. Bone mineralization is not impaired unless the cumulative dose exceeds 180 mg. Flulike symptoms may occur at high doses.

Zoledronate

Zoledronic acid is a potent intravenous bisphosphonate recently approved by the FDA for the treatment of Paget's disease of bone in a dose of 5 mg. In patients with alkaline phosphatase levels more than twice the upper limit of normal, one 15-minute intravenous infusion of 5 mg zoledronic acid resulted in 96% of patients showing a therapeutic response at 6 months, normalization of alkaline phosphatase in 89% of subjects, and prolonged remission rates. These responses were significantly better than with oral risedronate. Almost 10% of patients had a flulike syndrome after the infusion. Patients should take calcium and vitamin D to avoid the precipitation of *hypocalcemia* with infusion. There are reports of *atrial fibrillation* occurring in association with zoledronic acid use, and *osteonecrosis* of the jaw has been noted with the use of potent bisphosphonates in debilitated patients (see Chapter 164).

Etidronate

Etidronate was the first orally effective bisphosphonate; although it is still available, it is less effective than the second-generation bisphosphonates and less desirable because it can impair bone mineralization. Consequently, its use has been largely supplanted by that of the newer drugs in its class.

Tiludronate

Tiludronate is also approved for the treatment of Paget's disease in a dose of 400 mg daily for 3 months.

Calcitonin

Before the advent of the bisphosphonates, calcitonin was the only available treatment capable of inhibiting osteoclastic activity. Calcitonin is now used in settings in which second-generation bisphosphonates are not available or poorly tolerated. It can be given in conjunction with a slower-acting, first-generation bisphosphonate, such as etidronate, to control bone pain until the effects of the latter take hold. Biochemical and clinical remissions are achieved in one third of patients, improvement is noted in another one third, and the response is minimal or unsustained in the balance of cases. Urinary hydroxyproline starts to decline within a few days of onset of therapy; after a few weeks, a reduction in alkaline phosphatase and then clinical improvement are noted.

Synthetic salmon and human calcitonin preparations are commercially available. The salmon calcitonin preparation is the less expensive and it differs by just one amino acid from human calcitonin. Although up to 50% of patients manifest neutralizing antibodies to synthetic salmon calcitonin, the risk for clinically important inactivation is small. Control can be reestablished by switching to human calcitonin.

Disadvantages of calcitonin are nausea (in some patients), flushing, increased urination, and the need for parenteral administration. A nasally absorbed preparation is available but it is less effective and is not approved by the FDA for use in Paget's disease. Therapy requires considerable patient education and the ability to learn self-injection techniques. The calcitonin dose may be reduced when the disease is in remission, but a low dose needs to be continued indefinitely to prevent relapse.

Cytotoxic Agents and Surgery

Patients with serious complications of Paget's disease, such as severe *high-output heart failure* or *hypercalcemic crisis*, are potential candidates for *cytotoxic agents* capable of suppressing bone resorption (e.g., *plicamycin* [formerly mithramycin] and *dactinomycin*). These now rarely used drugs are administered intravenously to patients and require hospitalization and consultation because of risks for acute (although reversible) renal, hepatic, and hematologic toxicities; thrombocytopenia can be particularly severe.

Neurosurgical intervention is necessary in patients with spinal cord or nerve root compression syndromes. *Orthopedic procedures* such as total hip replacement and tibial or femoral osteotomy may help to restore mobility. Intraoperative bleeding is more problematic in patients with active disease, necessitating a reduction in disease activity before surgery is attempted.

Monitoring Therapy

Because initial and subsequent serum alkaline phosphatase levels are indicative of disease activity and response to therapy, regular monitoring of the serum *alkaline phosphatase* level is recommended, supplemented only if necessary by monitoring of the urinary *hydroxyproline or N-telopeptide*. Factors predictive of remission include initial values for biochemical markers, lowest posttreatment levels attained, and speed of biochemical response to the first course of therapy. Two baseline alkaline phosphatase measurements should be obtained before therapy is started, followed by monthly determinations during treatment until remission is achieved. Skeletal *radiographic films* are also helpful to have at the commencement of therapy. They are not repeated routinely except when the base of the skull or a long bone of the lower extremity is involved, where disease progression can be dangerous. The *technetium bone scan* provides an alternative baseline measure. Once remission is achieved, a follow-up measurement of the alkaline phosphatase level is indicated every 6 months. Patients with bone or joint pain or minor neurologic deficits benefit from an office check every 3 months while they remain symptomatic.

PATIENT EDUCATION AND INDICATIONS FOR REFERRAL

Patients should be instructed to *drink at least 2 L of liquid daily*, especially if they are unable to keep active, because immobilization and dehydration can precipitate hypercalcemia, hypercalciuria, and renal stone formation. Patients who are candidates for calcitonin therapy require detailed teaching by a nurse in the techniques of subcutaneous injection. Confirmation of the proper technique should be obtained before self-administration is prescribed unless another household member is going to be administering the medication.

Hospital admission and prompt neurosurgical consultation are warranted in patients who have evidence of nerve or cord compression. Admission is also indicated for severe hypercalcemia. Orthopedic surgical consultation is indicated for the person severely limited by pagetic degenerative joint disease of the hip or knee. Consultation with an endocrinologist or rheumatologist is required when initiation of specific therapy is being considered for an asymptomatic patient with radiologic or biochemical evidence of advancing disease. Referral is beneficial when standard courses of therapy fail to achieve remission and when relapse occurs.

THERAPEUTIC RECOMMENDATIONS (7)

- Follow asymptomatic patients yearly and expectantly and as long as they have no involvement of the base of the skull, spine, hip, knee, or long bones of the lower extremity; at annual visits, assess clinically and obtain an alkaline phosphatase determination.
- For those with mild to moderate pain caused by localized bony involvement or secondary degenerative joint disease, prescribe acetaminophen (e.g., 300 mg four times daily), aspirin (325 mg three times daily), or another nonsteroidal antiinflammatory drug (e.g., 400 mg of ibuprofen up to three times daily as needed or 500 mg of naproxen up to twice daily as needed) for the short-term relief of symptoms.

- For all symptomatic patients and for those with asymptomatic disease who have bony involvement in a potentially critical area (base of the skull, spine, hip, knee, or long bone of the lower extremity), obtain baseline plain x-ray films and measurement of alkaline phosphatase (consider measurement of hydroxyproline or urine N-telopeptide if alkaline phosphatase is not elevated). Then begin oral bisphosphonate therapy with a second-generation preparation (e.g., 40 mg of alendronate per day or 30 mg of risedronate per day). Specify that each dose be taken 1/2 hour before breakfast on an empty stomach with at least 8 oz of water and without lying down.
- Continue bisphosphonate therapy for the specified standard course of treatment (e.g., 6 months for alendronate, 2 months for risedronate). Monitor the alkaline phosphatase monthly until remission is achieved, then every 6 months. Consider reinstituting therapy if symptoms recur or if the alkaline phosphatase level rises to 20% to 30% above the upper limit of normal.
- Consider intravenous pamidronate (30 mg/d for 3 days) or zoledronic acid (5 mg once) for patients with moderate to severe disease, especially those ill enough to require hospitalization or who are unable to take oral alendronate or risedronate.

- Consider parenteral calcitonin (100 Medical Research Council [MRC] units given subcutaneously daily) as a means of providing short-term relief for very symptomatic patients while they are waiting for bisphosphonate therapy to take effect, especially if etidronate is being used. Once clinical and biochemical remissions have been achieved, reduce the dose to 50 MRC units and continue therapy three times a week.
- Obtain two baseline measurements of the alkaline phosphatase level and a baseline skeletal roentgenogram or bone scan before therapy is started. Follow the serum alkaline phosphatase level at monthly intervals during therapy. Also monitor the serum calcium level at the outset. Routine repetition of radiologic procedures is unnecessary, but repeating radiography periodically may help if the patient has a high-risk lesion (e.g., base of the skull, long bone of lower extremity). If fracture is suspected, another film is essential.
- Advise the patient to avoid immobilization and dehydration. Prescribe at least 2 L of liquid per day, especially if the patient is inactive. Prescribe a total daily calcium intake of 1,200 to 1,500 mg and 800 to 1,000 IU of vitamin D daily if the patient is on parenteral or second-generation bisphosphonate therapy. Monitor the serum calcium level if the adequacy of calcium intake is a concern.

Annotated Bibliography

1. Alvarez L, Guanabens N, Peris P, et al. Discriminative value of biochemical markers of bone turnover in assessing the activity of Paget's disease. J Bone Miner Res 1995;10:458. (*Finds that bone-specific alkaline phosphatase is a very sensitive marker of bone formation.*)
2. Bikle DD. Biochemical markers in the assessment of bone disease. Am J Med 1997;103:427. (*An excellent review, including data on the costs of available tests in addition to their uses and shortcomings.*)
3. Frank WA, Bries NM, Singer FR, et al. Rheumatic manifestations of Paget's disease of bone. Am J Med 1974;56:592. (*Joint disease can be an important problem for patients with Paget's disease.*)
4. Lyles KW, Siris ES, Singer FR, et al. A clinical approach to diagnosis and management of Paget's disease of bone. J Bone Miner Res 2001;16:1379. (*A general review with a good section on evaluation; 67 references.*)
5. Nagant de Deuxchaisnes C, Krane SM. Paget's disease of bone: clinical and metabolic observations. Medicine (Baltimore) 1974;43:233. (*A classic review article of clinical and biochemical manifestations.*)
6. Whyte MP. Paget's disease of bone. N Engl J Med 2006;355:593. (*A good review for the generalist reader; 50 references.*)
7. Drake WM, Kendler DL, Brown JP. 2001 Consensus statement on the modern therapy of Paget's disease of bone from a Western Alliance Symposium. Clin Ther 2001;23:620. (*Finds that alendronate and risedronate are similar in efficacy, and recommends that physician choice be based on personal experience, relative cost, and differences in dosing.*)
8. Glaser DL, Kaplan FS. Orthopedic surgery consideration in Paget's disease of bone. Clin Rev Bone Miner Metab 2002;1:159. (*When possible, medical therapy should be attempted prior to surgery to reduce the risk of intraoperative bleeding.*)
9. Hosking D, Lyles K, Brown JP, et al. Long-term control of bone turnover in Paget's Disease with zoledronic acid and risedronate. J Bone Miner Res 2007;22:142. (*After one 15-minute infusion of zoledronic acid, 5 mg, bone turnover remained within the reference range over the next 24 months*).
10. Liens D, Delmas PD, Meunier PJ. Long-term effects of intravenous pamidronate in fibrous dysplasia of bone. Lancet 1994;343:953. (*No impairment of bone mineralization is found if the total dose is <180 mg.*)
11. Meunier PJ, Vignot E. Therapeutic strategy in Paget's disease of bone. Bone 1995;17(Suppl):489S. (*Presents long-term follow-up data and a suggested approach to treatment.*)
12. Patel S, Stone MD, Coupland C, et al. Determinants of remission of Paget's disease of bone. J Bone Miner Res 1993;8:1467. (*Factors include initial values for biochemical markers, lowest posttreatment levels attained, and the speed of biochemical response to the first course of therapy.*)
13. Reid IR, Miller P, Lyles K, et al. Comparison of a single infusion of zoledronic acid with risedronate for Paget's disease. N Engl J Med 2005;353:898. (*A single 15-minute infusion produced a more rapid, more complete, and more sustained response than did daily treatment with risedronate; 88.6% of cases had a normalized alkaline phosphatase.*)
14. Reid IR, Nicholson GC, Weinstein RS, et al. Biochemical and radiologic improvement in Paget's disease of bone treated with alendronate: a randomized, placebo-controlled trial. Am J Med 1996;101:341. (*An oral dose of 40 mg/d for 6 months normalized alkaline phosphatase and improved x-ray appearance in nearly 50% of cases.*)
15. Siris ES. Goals of treatment for Paget's disease of bone. J Bone Miner Res 1999;14(S):49. (*The goals have advanced from symptomatic relief to the halting of disease progression.*)
16. Siris ES, Chines AA, Altman RD, et al. Risedronate in the treatment of Paget's disease of bone: an open label, multicenter study. J Bone Miner Res 1998;13:1032. (*Presents evidence of efficacy.*)

CHAPTER 163 ■ APPROACH TO THE PATIENT WITH RAYNAUD'S PHENOMENON

Sensitivity of the fingertips and toes to cold is a common symptom, reported in up to 10% of adults. In 3% to 5%, the response to cold or stress is characterized by bilateral blanching and discomfort in the fingers, followed by purplish discoloration and reactive erythema, the hallmarks of Raynaud's phenomenon. For some, it is an isolated problem; for others, it may represent the first manifestation of connective tissue disease, arterial occlusion, or a hematologic problem. The primary physician needs to be able to determine the probability and risk of underlying disease, perform the initial workup, and provide symptomatic relief.

PATHOPHYSIOLOGY AND CLINICAL PRESENTATION (1–7)

Alteration in dermal blood flow is a basic mechanism of thermoregulation and is also a common response to stress-induced catecholamine release. In patients with Raynaud's phenomenon, the normal vasoconstrictive responses to cold and stress are exaggerated. It may be functional (secondary to *vasospasm*), anatomic (secondary to *arterial occlusive disease*), or rheologic (secondary to *alterations in blood viscosity or red cell deformability*). *Platelet activation* appears to play a role in patients with abnormal vascular anatomy. In many instances, the pathophysiology is multifactorial. The characteristic clinical sequence begins with a rapid onset of digital blanching (vasospastic phase), which is followed by cyanosis (venospastic phase). It ends with the restoration of flow and redness (reactive hyperemia).

Clinically, Raynaud's phenomenon is classified as *primary* or *idiopathic* (Raynaud's disease) if no evidence of an associated condition can be found and *secondary* if an associated condition is present. Some have objected to this designation because secondary causes (e.g., connective tissue disease) may not become clinically evident for years.

Primary Raynaud's Phenomenon (Raynaud's Disease)

Patients with truly idiopathic disease typically experience mild symptoms that are often precipitated by emotional stress or cold. Although an episode may begin in one or two fingers, it quickly spreads symmetrically to involve all of the fingers of both hands. Attacks may occur as often as several times daily and are more frequent in winter. Peripheral adrenergic tone is believed to be especially high. Women predominate, with onset often at menarche; onset after age 40 years is much less common. Some patients manifest other vasomotor problems, such as migraine, Prinzmetal's angina, or livedo reticularis. Prog-

nosis is excellent; the risk of eventually developing connective tissue disease is less than 2%, especially if signs and serologic evidence of secondary disease (see later discussion) are absent at the time of the initial clinical presentation and do not appear over the subsequent 2 years.

A pathophysiologic relative of primary disease is drug-induced disease. *Vasoactive drugs* used to treat migraine (β-blockers, ergotamine, methysergide) have all been implicated, as has *migraine* itself. Whether drugs can cause the problem in the absence of an underlying vasomotor disorder is unclear.

Secondary Raynaud's Disease Phenomenon (Underlying Disease)

In comparison with primary disease, secondary Raynaud's phenomenon affects men as well as women and tends to appear later (often, after age 30 years). The episodes are more severe and less likely to be precipitated by emotional stress. Loss of finger pulp and skin ulcers as a consequence of ischemia may be evident. The common pathophysiologic denominator is vasoocclusion. Causes range from connective tissue disease to mechanical and atherosclerotic etiologies.

Connective Tissue Disease

Raynaud's phenomenon is associated with a wide range of connective tissue diseases, including *scleroderma*, *systemic sclerosis*, *systemic lupus erythematosus*, *mixed connective tissue disease*, and *Sjögren's syndrome*. Joint complaints and systemic symptoms may dominate the clinical picture; antinuclear antibody positivity is common (see Chapter 146).

Raynaud's phenomenon is especially prevalent in *systemic sclerosis*, occurring in more than 90% of cases. Structural narrowing of digital vessels develops as a consequence of intimal fibrosis. Abnormal vascular reactivity and platelet activation have been demonstrated. Symptoms may be especially severe, and the risk for digital ischemic injury is substantial. The compromise to digital blood flow is considerably less in patients with scleroderma.

At the time of initial presentation of Raynaud's phenomenon, the signs of sclerodermal disease and other connective tissue disorders may be subtle. *Abnormal nail-fold capillary pattern*, mild *sclerodactyly*, early *calcinosis*, or *telangiectasia* is characteristic. The presence of *antinuclear antibodies* increases the risk of eventually developing frank connective tissue disease, but its positive predictive value is only 30% in persons with Raynaud's phenomenon. More predictive is the presence of disease-specific autoantibodies (e.g., *anticentromere* and *antitopoismerase antibodies*; see later discussion). The best predictors for the development of connective tissue disorders (especially sclerodermal disease) include abnormal nail-bed capillary pattern, the presence of autoantibodies, characteristic skin lesions, abnormal pulmonary function, and esophageal dysmotility. Although predictive, none of these factors has a positive predictive value of greater than 50%. The mean onset of clinically frank disease is almost 3 years from the time of initial diagnosis of Raynaud's phenomenon, and full-blown disease may take 10 years to develop.

Other Vasoocclusive Diseases

A host of other vasoocclusive conditions can cause Raynaud's phenomenon, including *atherosclerotic disease,* occupational *vibratory injury* (jackhammer operators, welders, sheet-metal workers), and *neurovascular compression* syndromes (thoracic outlet, carpal tunnel). The neurovascular syndromes may exhibit cold sensitivity. The clinical course is a function of the underlying disease, which in some instances is reversible. *Hyperviscosity* states compromising blood flow may occur as a consequence of hematologic conditions such as *polycythemia* or *multiple myeloma.* Besides symptoms of poor peripheral blood flow (which may be severe enough to cause acrocyanosis), the clinical picture may include headache, confusion, weakness, and hematuria; relative serum viscosity is usually greater than 4. In *mixed cryoglobulinemia* due to such conditions as hepatitis C or connective tissue disease, there may be cold sensitivity, as well as purpura, arthralgias, fever, proteinuria, and reductions in serum complement levels (e.g., C3 and C4). In *cold agglutinin syndrome* (seen idiopathically and with *Mycoplasma* infection and mononucleosis), the patient complains of transient cold-induced acrocyanosis of the finger tips, ears, and tip of the nose that quickly resolves with warming. Splenomegaly and autoagglutination of blood are characteristic.

DIFFERENTIAL DIAGNOSIS (8)

The causes of Raynaud's phenomenon can be grouped according to the predominant pathophysiologic mechanism (Table 163.1), although, as noted, multiple mechanisms may be operative. About 20% of patients presenting initially with idiopathic or primary Raynaud's phenomenon prove after 2 to 3 years to have underlying connective tissue disease.

WORKUP (2,4,5,7–11)

History and Physical Examination

History and physical examination are essential in the workup of Raynaud's phenomenon because the diagnosis is determined clinically and subtle manifestations of an underlying etiology may predate the appearance of overt disease. The findings are essential to determining the need for further evaluation.

Confirming the Diagnosis

Raynaud's phenomenon can be confirmed by obtaining a history or directly observing bilateral blanching and discomfort in the fingers followed by bluish-purplish discoloration and reactive erythema in response to cold or emotional stress. At least two of the three characteristic skin changes must be present and distributed symmetrically. If the diagnosis is uncertain, one can test the patient's response to cold by immersing the hands in ice water and observing for blanching, cyanosis, and reactive hyperemia. The condition needs to be distinguished from

---

TABLE 163.1

IMPORTANT CAUSES OF RAYNAUD'S PHENOMENON

Purely Vasospastic Disease
Primary Raynaud's phenomenon (with or without migraine, Prinzmetal's angina, livedo reticularis)
Drug induced, typically in persons with primary disease (methysergide, ergotamine, ? β-blockers)

Vasospasm plus Arterial Occlusive Disease
Connective tissue disease (scleroderma, systemic sclerosis, systemic lupus, mixed connective tissue disease, Sjögren's syndrome)
Atherosclerotic disease
Occupational vascular trauma
Compression (thoracic outlet syndrome, carpal tunnel syndrome)
Toxin or substance exposure (chemotherapeutic agents, interferon, nicotine, narcotics, cyclosporine, cocaine, polyvinyl chloride)

Hemorrheologic Disease
Polycythemia vera
Paraproteinemia (multiple myeloma, Waldenström's macroglobulinemia)
Mixed cryoglobulinemia (e.g., hepatitis C, connective tissue disease)
Cold agglutinin syndrome (idiopathic, *Mycoplasma* infection, mononucleosis)

---

acrocyanosis, which is associated with persistent cyanosis exacerbated by cold.

Differentiating Primary from Secondary Disease

The initial differentiation is facilitated by attention to age at onset, gender, frequency and severity of attacks, distribution of skin changes, ischemic skin changes, manifestations of connective tissue disease, precipitating factors, associated digital swelling, and other vasomotor phenomena, such as migraine, Prinzmetal's angina, and livedo reticularis. Primary disease is suggested by onset in the teens, female gender, occurrence of multiple mild attacks every day, symmetric involvement, precipitation of attacks by stress, normal skin except for livedo reticularis, and migraine headaches. Secondary disease should be suspected in a male patient or in a female patient with onset in the mid-20s or later, moderate to severe attacks not necessarily occurring every day or in association with emotional stress, asymmetric presentation, associated finger swelling, ischemic skin ulcers, or loss of fingertip pulp.

Further Evaluation of Suspected Secondary Disease

Patients with a presentation suggestive of secondary disease should be checked carefully for additional symptoms of connective tissue disease, such as skin rash, morning stiffness, myalgias, arthralgias, joint swelling, fatigue, sicca syndrome, and fever (see Chapter 146), and of peripheral vascular disease, such as claudication, angina, and leg ulceration (see Chapter 23). Although less common, the positional symptoms of thoracic outlet and carpal tunnel syndromes (see Chapter 167) and systemic manifestations of hyperviscosity syndrome (confusion, headache, fatigue) should also be sought if the diagnosis of underlying disease is unclear. The occupational history is noted for any vibratory injury. Medications should be reviewed, and any effects on symptoms of α- or β-blockers, sympathomimetics, ergotamine, methysergide, and calcium-channel blockers noted. One should also check for exposure to chemotherapeutic agents, interferon, nicotine, narcotics, cyclosporine, cocaine, and polyvinyl chloride.

The physical examination should include a thorough check for manifestations of connective tissue disease (e.g., malar flush, sclerodactyly, petechial rash, telangiectasia, calcinosis, joint redness, swelling, and effusion). The hand and arm pulses are carefully palpated, and capillary filling is noted in the digits. Performing the Phelan test and attempting to elicit Tinel's sign can help in identifying carpal tunnel syndrome (see Chapter 153). The fingertips are felt for loss of pulp, which is indicative of ischemia, and the skin is observed for ischemic changes. Checking for enlargement of the liver or spleen is important in persons suspected of hyperviscosity syndrome.

The *nail-fold capillary pattern* should be examined carefully because an abnormal pattern is a prime predictor of connective tissue disease, especially systemic sclerosis. If available, a wide-field microscope provides excellent views of the capillary bed, but the magnification afforded by the more readily accessible handheld ophthalmoscope turned to 10 to 40 diopters may suffice. One looks at the pattern of capillary loops; asymmetry indicates dropout of capillary loops, which is characteristic and predictive of connective tissue disease, particularly systemic sclerosis.

Laboratory Testing

Patients judged to have definite primary disease on the basis of the careful history and physical examination just noted require no additional evaluation. An antinuclear antibody (ANA) test can be ordered to rule out further the risk for underlying connective tissue disease (negative predictive value of 93%), but a positive test result in the absence of other suggestive findings has a very low positive predictive value and may raise concern inappropriately. Consequently, only patients with clinical evidence suggestive of connective tissue disease should be subjected to *ANA* testing. For patients who are ANA-positive, an *anticentromere antibody* determination can help to predict the risk for development of limited systemic sclerosis (i.e., scleroderma), but the test is expensive and its contribution to overall clinical decision making needs to be considered before it is ordered. *Anti–Scl-70* is found in about one half of patients with diffuse systemic sclerosis (see Chapter 146).

Noninvasive studies of arterial flow (*digital plethysmography, arterial Doppler ultrasonography*) can confirm anatomic vascular compromise; however, similar information can often be obtained by a careful history and physical examination, and test data usually do not help differentiate among anatomic causes of the disease.

A *complete blood cell count*, *urinalysis*, and *serum globulin* determination should suffice to screen for common hematologic problems; *immunoelectrophoresis* is reserved for patients in whom myeloma or another paraproteinemia is suspected (elderly, markedly elevated globulin, anemia; see Chapter 79). A *cryoprotein* determination is indicated if other manifestations suggestive of cryoglobulinemia (arthralgias, purpura, proteinuria) are present; if obtained, C3 and C4 levels should also be checked for the consumption of complement, characteristic of the condition. A *cold-agglutinin test* is worth considering for patients with anemia and splenomegaly suggestive of cold-agglutinin syndrome.

MANAGEMENT (8,12–17)

Prevention

Regardless of the underlying cause, keeping the trunk and the extremities warm on cold days is essential. Of particular importance is *truncal warmth* because any threat to the maintenance of core body temperature is a potent stimulus to reflex peripheral vasoconstriction. *Smoking cessation* and the elimination of *passive smoking* are essential. Any drugs found to trigger episodes should be stopped or cut back.

Occupational precipitants, such as repetitive activity that leads to carpal tunnel syndrome or vibratory injury, should be reduced or eliminated. Although *pneumatic tool* operation (e.g., jackhammer) is the classic occupational association, smaller and less inertial tools that produce *high-frequency vibrations* have been found to be even more likely to cause vascular injury. Working on a vibrating or rotating tool (such as those used by welders, sheet-metal workers, carpenters, and painters) for as little as 1 to 2 hours per day can inflict vascular damage. Prevention, by limiting the number of hours such equipment is used, is the best approach but is often not feasible. Alternatively, at the first sign of symptoms, use should be markedly reduced or eliminated. Antivibration gloves and coated tool handles have not proved to be sufficient.

Symptomatic Relief

Because Raynaud's phenomenon has a strong vasoconstrictive component, it follows that vasodilators should provide symptomatic relief. Vasodilator therapy for primary disease is usually successful; secondary disease tends to be more refractory due to vessel damage.

Calcium-Channel Blockers

Calcium-channel blockers have proved to be symptomatically useful for patients with primary disease and for many with secondary disease. Their mechanism of action includes vasodilation plus some platelet inhibition. As a class, they reduce the frequency and severity of attacks by about 50% in persons with moderately severe disease. The resultant improvement in perfusion sometimes helps to speed the healing of skin ulcers. *Nifedipine* is the best studied, but any of the dihydropyridines (e.g., amlodipine, felodipine) are similarly effective. To avoid the adverse cardiovascular effects associated with short-acting dihydropyridines (see Chapters 26, 30, and 32), only a sustained-release preparation or amlodipine should be used in persons with underlying heart disease. Occasionally, headache and flushing may be troublesome, and esophageal function may worsen in patients with scleroderma. There is no evidence to suggest that vasodilator therapy alters the natural history of the underlying disease.

Sympatholytics and Angiotensin-Receptor–Blocking Agents

α-Blockers are sometimes used as an alternative to calcium-channel blockers. Only *prazosin* has been subjected to placebo-controlled trial; it has been found to be more effective than placebo but is associated with first-dose syncope and postural lightheadedness. One of the more modern α-blockers (e.g., doxazocin) may be better tolerated but has not been adequately studied. Angiotensin-receptor–blocking agents appear to be promising. In controlled trial, *losartan* provided better relief than did long-acting nifedipine in patients with scleroderma. The efficacy of angiotensin-converting-enzyme inhibitors has not been established.

Phosphodiesterase Inhibitors

Type 5 phosphodiesterase inhibitors, such as *sildenafil*, are effective vasodilators that act on vascular smooth muscle and retain vasodilatory effects even in diseased vessels. This action makes them useful in pathologic settings where vasodilation is desired (e.g., erectile dysfunction, pulmonary hypertension). Pilot study in patients with Raynaud's phenomenon found improved digital blood flow and a reduction in symptoms in nearly 70%. More testing will be required before these drugs can be recommended, but initial findings are promising. Combination therapy with a calcium-channel blocker may prove particularly effective in difficult cases by allowing the use of low doses, which might minimize side effects.

Inhibitors of Platelet Activation

Vasodilator therapy may not suffice for persons with vasospastic disease accompanied by substantial endothelial injury and platelet activation (e.g., those with systemic sclerosis). Painful episodes may persist, and ischemic skin ulcers may fail to heal. The addition of *aspirin* or *dipyridamole* to the treatment program has helped to heal some ulcers, although it has no effect on vasospastic symptoms. *Fish oil supplements* rich in omega-3 fatty acids can impair platelet activation and stimulate vasodilation through prostacyclin synthesis; paradoxically, the best responses have been noted in patients with primary disease. Intravenous *iloprost* (a prostacyclin analogue not available in the United States) both vasodilates and inhibits platelet activation; a 5-day course in persons with secondary disease can provide 3 to 5 months of relief, but oral therapy is ineffective.

Sympathectomy

Sympathectomy has been used as a measure of last resort. Patients who respond to temporary ganglionic blockade with an injected anesthetic are the best candidates for sympathectomy.

PATIENT EDUCATION AND INDICATIONS FOR REFERRAL

The major elements of patient education are preventive (see prior discussion). For patients with occupationally induced disease, a change of job or job activities must be weighed against the risk for worsening of vascular compromise. Patients with strong features of primary disease can be reassured that the risk for underlying illness is low and that their prognosis is excellent. Those with features of secondary disease associated with a risk for development of connective tissue disease need to understand their risk, but also that it may be many years before other disease manifestations appear, if they develop at all.

Referral is indicated for those with refractory symptoms, especially if symptoms are accompanied by signs of ischemia.

A.H.G.

Annotated Bibliography

1. Cherniack MG. Raynaud's phenomenon of occupational origin. Arch Intern Med 1990;150:519. (*Vibratory injury is an important and common precipitant.*)
2. Fitzgerald O, Hess EV, O'Connor GT, et al. Prospective study of the evolution of Raynaud's phenomenon. Am J Med 1988;84:718. (*A connective tissue disease developed in 19% of those who presented with no obvious evidence of underlying illness; nail-fold capillary pattern was predictive of systemic sclerosis.*)
3. O'Keeffe ST, Tsapatsaris NP, Beethan WP Jr. Increased prevalence of migraine and chest pain in patients with primary Raynaud's disease. Ann Intern Med 1992;116:985. (*Presents evidence for a common pathophysiology.*)
4. Priollet P, Vayssairet M, Housset E. How to classify Raynaud's phenomenon: long-term follow-up study of 73 patients. Am J Med 1987;83:494. (*Notes the late onset of underlying disease, and suggests a means of early identification.*)
5. Sarkozi J, Bookman AAM, Lee P, et al. Significance of anticentromere antibody in idiopathic Raynaud's syndrome. Am J Med 1987;83:893. (*The finding is predictive of scleroderma.*)
6. Spencer-Green G. Outcomes in primary Raynaud's phenomenon. Arch Intern Med 1998;158:595. (*A meta-analysis, finding that the risk for the development of connective tissue disease was approximately 12%, mostly systemic sclerosis; an abnormal nail-fold capillary pattern was the most predictive finding.*)
7. Weiner ES, Heldebrandt S, Senecal JL, et al. Prognostic significance of anticentromere antibodies and anti-topoisomerase I antibodies in Raynaud's disease: a prospective study. Arthritis Rheum 1991;34:68. (*One of the better studies of the risk for disease progression.*)
8. Wigley FM. Raynaud's phenomenon. N Engl J Med. 2002;347:1001. (*A succinct clinical review; 47 references.*)
9. Minkini W, Rabhan NB. Office nail-fold capillary microscopy using ophthalmoscope. J Am Acad Dermatol 1982;7:190. (*A look at a very simple way to make this important observation.*)
10. Spencer-Green G, Alter D, Welch G. Test performance in systemic sclerosis: anti-centromere and anti–Scl-70 antibodies. Am J Med 1997;103:242. (*Anticentromere antibody is reasonably sensitive for scleroderma; anti–Scl-70 is found in about half of patients with diffuse systemic sclerosis.*)
11. Zufferey P, Depairon M, Chamot AM, et al. Prognostic significance of nailfold capillary microscopy in patients with Raynaud's phenomenon and scleroderma-pattern abnormalities: a six-year follow-up study. Clin Rheumatol 1992;11:536. (*The disruption of the normal capillary pattern was found to be predictive.*)
12. Caglayan E, Hungeburth M, Karasch T, et al. Phosphodiesterase type 5 inhibition is a novel therapeutic option in Raynaud disease. Arch Intern Med 2006;166:231. (*An unblinded pilot study, finding improved digital blood flow and reduction of symptoms in nearly 70% of cases.*)
13. DiGiacomo RA, Kremer JM, Shah DM. Fish-oil supplementation in patients with Raynaud's phenomenon. Am J Med 1990;86:158. (*Improved tolerance was found to cold exposure in patients with primary disease.*)
14. Dziadzio M, Denton CP, Smith R, et al. Losartan therapy for Raynaud's phenomenon and scleroderma: clinical and biochemical findings in a fifteen-week, randomized, parallel-group controlled trial. Arthritis Rheum 1999;42:2646. (*This treatment was more effective than the use of sustained-release nifedipine.*)
15. Malamet R, Wise RA, Ettinger WH, et al. Nifedipine in the treatment of Raynaud's phenomenon. Am J Med 1985;78:602. (*Discusses the mechanism of action of nifedipine, and suggests some platelet inhibition.*)
16. Thompson SE, Shea B, Welch V, et al. Calcium-channel blockers for Raynaud's phenomenon in systemic sclerosis. Arthritis Rheum 2001;44:1841. (*Finds a 50% reduction in the frequency and the severity of attacks; also discusses the role for aspirin in acute ischemic crisis.*)
17. Wigley FM, Wise RA, Seibold JR, et al. Intravenous iloprost infusion in patients with Raynaud phenomenon secondary to systemic sclerosis. Ann Intern Med 1994;120:199. (*Sustained benefit was achieved with this prostacyclin analogue.*)

CHAPTER 164 ■ PREVENTION AND MANAGEMENT OF OSTEOPOROSIS

DAVID M. SLOVIK

In industrialized nations, osteoporosis is a major health problem that predisposes to incapacitating fractures and affects an estimated 10 million persons in the United States (8 million women and 2 million men); another 34 million persons have reduced bone mass. The problem is most prevalent among postmenopausal women, but it is also becoming an issue for older men as life expectancy increases (lifetime osteoporotic fracture risk in men, 15%). In the United States, more than 250,000 hip fractures occur annually, most in persons older than the age of 65 years. Osteoporotic vertebral fractures are manifested by back pain, loss of height, decreased ambulation and decreased quality of life. An estimated 750,000 vertebral fractures occur annually and are present in 5% to 10% of women by age 60 years and in 40% by age 80 years. Current annual expenditures for hip fractures alone are in excess of $15 billion. Morbidity and mortality can be substantial, with 15% to 25% of women and 30% to 40% of men needing long-term nursing home care or dying as a consequence of osteoporotic hip fracture.

The pathophysiologic mechanisms for postmenopausal osteoporosis are imperfectly understood, but the means to ensure maximal skeletal growth and strength, prevent and treat bone loss, and noninvasively evaluate bone mass are available. The primary care physician has a central role in the evaluation and management of this common and important condition.

PATHOPHYSIOLOGY AND CLINICAL PRESENTATION (1–16)

Pathophysiology

Osteoporosis is defined as a skeletal disorder characterized by impaired bone strength that predisposes to an increased risk of fracture. Bone strength is a function of *bone density* and *bone quality*. *Bone mineral density* (BMD; defined as mass of bone per unit volume) receives most of the attention because it is measurable and important. Because the strength of a bone is proportional to its density, the mechanical support of the skeleton is affected as bone mass declines. *Bone quality* is also very important to bone strength and is determined by bone architecture, turnover, microdamage, and mineralization, which are much harder to measure. For epidemiologic purposes, osteoporosis has been defined by the World Health Organization in terms of a BMD that is 2.5 or more standard deviations below the mean for a healthy young white woman (*T score of –2.5 or less*). *Osteopenia* (originally a radiologic term to indicate a reduced amount of bone mineralization) is defined in BMD terms as a *T score of –1.0 to –2.5*.

Osteoporosis can occur not only from bone loss, but also from failure earlier in life to make sufficient bone, resulting in a lower peak bone density at skeletal maturity. Osteoporosis is labeled as *primary* when it is due to the aging process and *secondary* when it is a consequence of an underlying medical condition or drug (Table 164.1). The principal mechanism of age-related disease is increased bone resorption/reduced new bone formation. Secondary osteoporosis is often a consequence of medications (e.g., glucocorticoid therapy, excessive thyroid hormone) or conditions such as malabsorption, which impair the deposition of calcium and phosphorus. The latter may also cause *osteomalacia*, a condition with inadequate mineralization, as compared to osteoporosis, which has a normal ratio of mineral to matrix, just less of it.

Increased Osteoclastic Bone Resorption and Reduced New Bone Formation

The resorption and formation of bone is a continuous process throughout life. Under steady-state physiologic circumstances, the rates of these processes are equal and coupled, with bone damage repaired and bone mass retained. Cytokines in bone and skeletal growth factors may act synergistically and serve as mediators of bone formation and resorption.

With estrogen deficiency there is an increase in bone-resorbing cytokines (e.g., interleukin-1 and tumor necrosis factor). Estrogen deficiency may also reduce bone formation directly through estrogen receptors on osteoblasts—the cells that synthesize bone matrix proteins. Estrogen deficiency also reduces the local production of growth factors such as insulin-like growth factor and transforming growth factor.

Skeletal mass is usually maximal by age 35 years and declines in women after age 40 years and in men after age 50 years, when the rate of new bone formation does not equal the rate of bone resorption. With the onset of estrogen deficiency, osteoclastic bone resorption increases. The rate of decline in skeletal mass is most rapid in women within *2 years of menopause*. The greatest and earliest loss occurs in *trabecular bone* in the *thoracic* and *lumbar vertebrae*, sites where future fracture is likely. Later in life, new bone formation is impaired.

Inadequate Deposition of Calcium and Phosphorus (Osteomalacia)

Osteomalacia is defined as the inadequate deposition of calcium and phosphorus in bone tissue matrix. It is found in 10% to 15% of patients with hip fracture and is often a result of *vitamin D deficiency*. Fractional intestinal *absorption of calcium* in elderly persons is decreased. This decline in intestinal calcium absorption appears to be caused by a *decrease in the formation of 1,25-dihydroxyvitamin D*, which is the active form of vitamin D. Vitamin D deficiency is very common especially in home-bound elderly persons, who are unlikely to eat dairy products or go out in the sun. Forty to fifty percent of patients presenting with a hip fracture have been found to be vitamin D deficient. Other causes include *impaired vitamin D metabolism*, *malabsorption*, *systemic acidosis*, and *phosphate depletion*.

TABLE 164.1

IMPORTANT CAUSES OF OSTEOPOROSIS

Primary Osteoporosis
  Aging

Secondary Osteoporosis
  Medications and substances (calcium and vitamin D
    deficiencies, excess thyroid hormone,
    glucocorticosteroids, alcohol excess, tobacco,
    anticonvulsants, excess vitamin A supplementation,
    lithium, gonadotropin-releasing hormone agonists,
    tamoxifen [in premenopausal women])
  Endocrine (hypogonadism [including androgen deprivation
    for prostate cancer], hyperparathyroidism,
    hyperthyroidism, hyperprolactinemia)
  Gastrointestinal (e.g., hepatic insufficiency, pancreatic
    insufficiency, celiac disease, other causes of fat
    malabsorption)
  Renal (renal failure, dialysis, use of phosphate-binding
    antacids)
  Systemic disease (rheumatoid arthritis, ankylosing
    spondylitis, sarcoidosis)
  Bone marrow disease (myeloma, lymphoma, leukemia,
    hemochromatosis)
  Organ transplantation

Risk Factors

The strongest measurable determinant of risk is the *BMD*, which can be measured directly (see later discussion and Chapter 144). The risk for osteoporotic fracture increases twofold to fourfold for every standard deviation of reduction in BMD. However, the BMD is not the only determinant of bone fragility and is an imperfect predictor of fracture risk in a given individual. A prior *history of fracture* is probably the strongest indicator of bone fragility and future fracture risk; self-reported humped back has a positive likelihood ratio of 3.0, also making it predictive. Meta-analytic study finds several *physical findings* predictive of osteoporosis, including weight less than 51 kg (positive likelihood [LR] ratio, 7.3), distance from the back of the head to the wall on standing upright greater than 0 cm (LR, 4.6), less than two fingerbreadths between the lowest palpable rib and the pelvic brim (LR, 3.8), and tooth count less than 20 (LR, 3.4).

Although attention to other risk factors is essential to estimating the probability of osteoporosis and risk for fracture, the predictive value of most clinical risk factors is not great because they do not account for all contributing factors. Those factors that seem to confer the greatest risk include *advanced age, low body mass index* (<22 kg/m²), *maternal history of fracture,* and *current smoking,* but the strength of these associations is only moderate. Physical *inactivity* can lead to decreased bone mass, as can intense exercise that results in *amenorrhea.* A poor *lifetime intake of calcium* is a weak risk factor.

Conversely, increased bone mass correlates strongly with *increased weight* and *strength.* In general, the loading or mechanical forces on bone are potent stimuli to osteoblastic activity and new bone formation. Height and increased age at the onset of menopause are also moderate predictors of increased bone mass. An increase in current calcium intake has only a minor effect on bone mass.

Medical conditions causing secondary disease range from endocrine disorders, gastrointestinal diseases, and chronic systemic illnesses to nutritional deficiencies and drugs (see Table

164.1) and are prominent in men and perimenopausal women. In men and perimenopausal women, secondary causes account for nearly 50% of cases. Hypogonadism (including that associated with the treatment of prostate disease), glucocorticosteroid use, and alcoholism are the most common causes in men; in perimenopausal women, they are excesses in the intake of steroids, thyroid hormone, and anticonvulsants, as well as of aromatase inhibitors used to treat breast cancer.

Drugs are an important cause; in addition to *glucocorticosteroids* and *excess thyroid hormone* replacement, recent reports suggest an increase in fragility fracture with *proton-pump inhibitors, selective serotonin reuptake inhibitors,* and *thioglitazone.* Osteoporosis can be a major problem in persons who have undergone organ transplantation due to immobilization, steroid and cyclosporine therapy, and the underlying disease for which the transplant was performed.

Clinical Presentation

The progressive decline in skeletal mass (which may approach 50%) may become clinically manifest when a *fracture* is sustained spontaneously or after minimal trauma. Fractures most commonly occur in the thoracic and lumbar vertebrae, hip, wrist, humerus, and pelvis. The clinical course and frequency of fractures in individual patients cannot be predicted; however, the development of one vertebral fracture increases the risk of another by 5-fold, and have suffered two or more vertebral fractures increases the risk by 12-fold within 1 year. *Loss of teeth* is a less-appreciated manifestation of reduced bone density, but, by correlating with reduction in quality of mandibular alveolar bone, correlates with the risk of osteoporosis. A *loss of height* and the development of *kyphosis* may indicate vertebral compression fracture, although intervertebral disk space narrowing may be part of the reason for the height loss.

Radiographically, the bones may appear *osteopenic,* indicative of a nearly 30% loss in bone mass. The characteristic x-ray appearance of the osteoporotic spine is loss of horizontal vertebral trabeculae, accentuating the end plates and producing biconcave *"codfish"* vertebrae. A *vertebral compression fracture* may be noted, manifested by a loss in vertebral height. Grade 1 fractures are defined as a 20% to 24% loss; grade 2, a 25% to 39% loss; and grade 3, a loss greater than 40%. *Pseudofractures,* generally occurring in weight-bearing long bones, are pathognomonic for osteomalacia.

The laboratory features of postmenopausal osteoporosis include normal serum levels of *calcium, phosphate, vitamin D, parathyroid hormone (PTH),* and *alkaline phosphatase,* although the alkaline phosphatase may be elevated in the context of a healing fracture. If there is osteomalacia due to inadequate vitamin D intake or absorption, there may be low or low-normal serum levels of calcium, phosphate, and *25-hydroxyvitamin D* and elevated PTH levels. Persons with an underlying pathologic state causing osteoporosis manifest laboratory evidence of the condition (e.g., low or absent thyrotropin [TSH] in hyperthyroidism, low testosterone in hypogonadism, and inappropriately elevated PTH in primary hyperparathyroidism).

WORKUP (5,8,10,12,14,17,18)

History and Physical Examination

A detailed review of historical features predictive of osteoporosis is essential, especially for identifying preexisting disease and determining the need for bone density screening. One should inquire into loss of height, loss of teeth, prior fracture, smoking, inactivity, calcium and vitamin D intake, and maternal history of osteoporosis or fracture. A review of medications is essential, including steroids, hormonal treatment for thyroid, prostate disease, and breast cancer, and anticonvulsants. Self-report of a humped back, suggestive of having sustained a silent vertebral compression fracture, is highly suggestive of having sustained a silent compression fracture.

A few key observations made during the physical examination can supplement the historical assessment. These include (a) measuring height and comparing it to the patient's recollection of height as a young adult, (b) counting teeth, (c) having the patient stand with the back against the wall and measuring the distance from the wall to the occiput, and (d) standing behind the patient, noting how many fingerbreadths occupy the space between the inferior rib margin and the superior surface of the pelvic brim. Any loss in height, a tooth count less than 20, a wall–occiput distance of greater than 0 cm, and a rib–pelvis distance of two or fewer fingerbreadths significantly increase the pretest probability of osteoporotic disease and indicate the need for bone density determination.

Measurement of Bone Mineral Density

Because bone density is the principal determinant of fracture risk, its measurement is often essential to management decisions, but the test should be ordered only if the results will affect clinical decision making. If it is already apparent from history or physical examination that the patient has had an osteoporotic fracture, then bone mineral testing may be superfluous although still helpful in monitoring patients on therapy. Although guidelines for screening are emerging (see Chapter 144), clinical judgment remains important for determining who should be tested in evaluation for suspected disease.

Dual-energy x-ray absorptiometry (DXA, DEXA) is considered by most to be the technique of choice, representing the best combination of sensitivity, technical simplicity, reproducibility, cost, and minimization of radiation exposure. The test is safe, acceptable to patients, and predictive of osteoporotic fracture risk. Its use is associated with a significant effect on outcomes, such as reduction in the incidence of hip fractures (e.g., 36% reduction over 6 years). Current guidelines recommend that all women of normal risk be tested at age 65 years and that women deemed at higher risk be tested earlier (see Chapter 144).

Measurement of *forearm BMD* or *ultrasound of the heel* provides an inexpensive approach suitable for mass screening; however, separate DXA studies of the *hip and spine* provide the best assessments of risk for a given patient because the degree of osteoporotic change may be site specific (see Chapter 144).

The DXA study expresses bone density in terms of the number of standard deviations from the mean for normal young adults of the same sex (*T score*) and as the number of standard deviations from the mean for persons of the same sex and age (*Z score*). The World Health Organization diagnostic criterion for *osteoporosis* is a *T score less than –2.5*. *Osteopenia* is defined as a *T score between –1.0 and –2.5*. The finding of a *Z score less than –1.5* suggests a *secondary cause* of osteoporosis. The risk for osteoporotic fracture increases twofold to fourfold for every standard deviation of reduction in BMD.

Workup for Osteomalacia and Other Causes of Osteopenia

Hip fracture and incidentally encountered osteopenia on radiologic study should raise concern about osteomalacia. Having a high index of suspicion for osteomalacia and other causes of osteopenia is essential because they are often treatable. *DXA study* can be obtained. As noted, the finding on DXA determination of a *Z score* of less than –1.5 suggests a secondary cause of osteopenia. *Plain films* should be reviewed with the radiologist for *pseudofractures* (pathognomic of osteomalacia). A *bone biopsy* is usually reserved for patients undergoing orthopedic procedures; it can provide definitive diagnosis of osteomalacia.

The determination of *fasting* levels of *serum calcium* and *phosphate* can help in detecting common causes of osteomalacia, as can a *25-hydroxyvitamin D* level. Hypophosphatemia may indicate a renal-phosphate wasting disorder as the cause of osteomalacia. A low serum calcium may be seen in vitamin D deficiency. Low serum levels of 25-hydroxyvitamin D are characteristic of vitamin D deficiency.

Other etiologies of osteomalacia that need to be considered include hyperthyroidism (see Chapter 103), hyperparathyroidism (see Chapter 96), anorexia nervosa (see Chapter 234), hyperprolactinemia (see Chapter 100), malignancy (e.g., myeloma, lymphoma; see Chapter 84), pernicious anemia (see Chapter 82), disease of the gastrointestinal tract (e.g., inflammatory bowel disease, chronic liver disease; see Chapters 71 and 73), rheumatoid diseases (see Chapter 156), and medications (e.g., steroids, anticonvulsants, lithium, vitamin A supplements, tamoxifen, gonadotropin-releasing hormone agonists).

Laboratory workup should be tailored to those conditions suggested by pertinent history and physical examination findings. In the absence of clinical clues, one might consider screening for secondary disease by ordering a *complete blood count* and measurements of serum *calcium* and thyrotropin (TSH).

PRINCIPLES OF THERAPY
(5,10,11,14,19–86)

The best candidates include patients with major clinical risk factors (e.g., maternal history of fracture, current smoker, small frame, lack of exercise, low calcium intake), a T score on DXA bone scanning indicative either of osteopenia (–1.0 to –2.5) or of osteoporosis (less than –2.5), clinical evidence of fracture, or radiographic evidence of osteopenia. Even persons at no increased risk can benefit from such primary preventive measures as regular exercise and ensuring adequate dietary intake of calcium and vitamin D.

A program of diet, exercise, and pharmacologic measures can reduce the risk of osteoporotic fracture in high-risk persons. Primary prevention is more effective than treating established disease, but both require attention. Outcomes are maximized by careful patient selection and the design of a treatment program customized to the patient's fracture risk, overall medical condition, lifestyle, and preferences. The pharmacologic approach to prevention and treatment has undergone a major change with the adverse findings from the Women's Health Initiative study that hormone replacement therapy is devoid of net health benefit in postmenopausal women (see Chapter 118). Current treatment options include dietary calcium and vitamin D supplementation, weight-bearing and strengthening exercise, bisphosphonates, selective estrogen receptor modulators, calcitonin, and parathyroid hormone. Estrogen, although beneficial to bone, should primarily be used to treat menopausal symptoms (see Chapter 118).

Exercise and Diet

Exercise

An important component of the preventive therapy of osteoporosis is ensuring the maximal development of skeletal mass. The amount of bone accumulated in childhood and *premenopausal women* may be critical to the appearance of osteoporosis later in life, as evidenced by the low incidence of osteoporosis in African American women (and in men), who have a greater skeletal mass than white women. Exercise and physical activity have been shown to increase skeletal mass and increase total body calcium. Physical activity, in conjunction with dietary supplementation of 1,500 mg of calcium and 400 U of vitamin D daily, offers the best hope for increasing skeletal mass during skeletal growth. However, exercise programs so intensive as to induce amenorrhea and estrogen deficiency (e.g., competitive marathon running) may lead to osteoporosis.

In *postmenopausal women*, regular weight-bearing and strengthening exercise (e.g., walking, low-impact aerobics, weight lifting, tennis) three times per week can substantially retard bone mineral loss (down to 0.5% of the baseline value per year), especially when combined with calcium and vitamin supplementation. A more ambitious program of formal exercise training (e.g., 50 minutes of walking and jogging three times per week) in combination with calcium and vitamin D supplementation may have even more pronounced effects (e.g., increase in lumbar bone mineral content). Care must be taken to ensure that the exercise program in older women is safe and does not subject the patient to an increased risk for falls or other injuries.

The efficacy of a program of exercise combined with calcium and vitamin D supplementation suggests that it should be the core of every treatment program, whether for prophylaxis or treatment of osteoporosis.

Dietary Calcium and Calcium Supplements

A daily total calcium intake of 1,200 to 1,500 mg is needed to help preserve trabecular and cortical bone mass. Although calcium therapy does not prevent bone loss to the degree that estrogen therapy does, it does represent an essential component of all treatment programs. Its effect on bone loss falls between those of estrogen and placebo. The inadequate dietary calcium intake of most women (about 600 to 800 mg/d) and the declining fractional absorption of calcium associated with aging make it important to ensure a total intake of 1,200 to 1,500 mg/d. Serious complications such as renal stones or hypercalcemia are extremely uncommon with a daily intake of elemental calcium in this range.

Dietary calcium is readily available, more nutritious, and better absorbed than calcium tablets, and it is less likely to cause kidney stones (possibly by inhibiting oxalate absorption). A cup of skim milk provides 303 mg of calcium; an 8-oz serving of low-fat yogurt provides 345 mg; a serving of canned sardines has 354 mg. However, the amount of calcium varies so much in foods and supplements that it is important to check what one is taking.

Of the *supplement preparations*, the *carbonate* salt is the least costly and has the highest amount of calcium. *Chewable preparations* are well absorbed, albeit a bit more expensive.

Splitting the daily supplement dose facilitates absorption and minimizes gastrointestinal upset. A reasonable supplemental dose of calcium is in the range of 500 to 1,500 mg/d. Larger doses, particularly in conjunction with vitamin D, may predispose the patient to hypercalcemia and hypercalciuric renal stone disease. Taking calcium carbonate supplements with meals increases absorption because of the favorable action of gastric acid.

Concern about the solubility and gut absorption of calcium carbonate has led to the marketing of other calcium preparations, most notably *calcium citrate*, which is more expensive and less dependent on gastric acid for absorption. The least expensive sources of calcium carbonate supplementation are the antacid TUMS, which comes in several strengths, ranging from 200 to 500 mg/tablet, and generic preparations, which come in strengths from 500 to 600 mg/tablet.

Vitamin D

The principal effect of vitamin D is on the gut absorption of calcium; it also directly affects osteoblasts and osteoclasts and exerts a positive effect on muscle, which reduces sway and translates into a 22% reduced risk of falls in the elderly (see later discussion). Recent evidence also suggests positive effects on immune regulation.

When vitamin D is taken together with calcium, reductions in fracture rates of 30% to 70% have been documented. The benefit appears greatest in vitamin D–deficient institutionalized and home-bound elderly persons, but it is also evident among those who are living independently in the community. When vitamin D supplementation is given in conjunction with calcium to otherwise healthy persons older than the age of 65 years with a low calcium intake, the BMD improves significantly and the risk for nonvertebral osteoporotic fracture is reduced by more than 50%.

Daily recommended dose requirements for vitamin D have been raised to a range of 800 to 1,000 IU by the National Osteoporosis Foundation, with a target serum level for *25-hydroxy vitamin D* (a measure of the vitamin D stores) greater than 32 ng/mL. At a level less than this, parathyroid hormone levels increase and the fractional absorption of calcium decreases. A generic combination preparation also containing calcium carbonate provides an inexpensive and practical approach to vitamin D supplementation. Drinking 8 oz/d of vitamin D–fortified low-fat or skim milk is a more nutritious option.

Bisphosphonates

These synthetic carbon phosphate compounds bind avidly to pyrophosphate in bone and inhibit bone resorption by osteoclasts. Bisphosphonate therapy has risen to first-line status with the advent of second-generation oral preparations (alendronate, risedronate, ibandronate) that provide enhanced efficacy, reasonable safety, and once-weekly or monthly convenience, albeit at some financial cost.

Efficacy

Long-term continuous *oral therapy* is both safe and effective. Significant increases in bone mineral density are achieved, and risks of *vertebral* and *nonvertebral fractures* are markedly decreased. Alendronate and risedronate have been shown to reduce the risks of osteoporotic fracture in the spine and *hip* by 40% to 60%. Effects on bone density appear to be cumulative. A 10-year course of full-dose therapy with alendronate increases mean bone density by about 6% in the femoral neck and nearly 15% in the lumbar spine. Similar increases are achieved with risedronate, although equivalent long-term data are not yet available. There are no prospective head-to-head comparisons of the two agents; both have also demonstrated efficacy in the prevention of bone loss and fracture associated with *corticosteroid use* and *male osteoporosis*.

Benefits are greatest when full doses are used in the setting of low bone density or prior osteoporotic fracture, but low-dose therapy in persons without established osteoporosis also provides effective primary prophylaxis against osteoporosis due to menopause and glucocorticosteroid use. A unique feature of bisphosphonate therapy is a measurable residual effect lasting for years after the cessation of treatment, which is believed to be a consequence of bisphosphonate deposition and tight bonding to bone mineral. A report comparing the fracture incidence and bone density at 10 years in patients on alendronate for either 5 or 10 years found that patients who stopped after 5 years had similar fracture rates at 10 years (except for clinical vertebral fractures) when compared to those on it for 10 years. Compared to the cessation of estrogen therapy, bisphosphonate withdrawal results in a much slower loss of bone.

The *intravenous bisphosphonate* preparations have shown improvements in BMD in postmenopausal women comparable to those of the oral medications. In a recent report, once-yearly zoledronic acid reduced spine fractures by 70% and hip fractures by 41%.

Adverse Effects and Safety

Adverse effects are an important consideration because chronic use is required. The major concerns that have emerged are upper gastrointestinal mucosal injury, osteonecrosis, a musculoskeletal pain syndrome, and atrial fibrillation.

Upper Gastrointestinal Mucosal Injury. Although no increase in the risk of upper gastrointestinal (GI) complications has been found in randomized, long-term trials comparing alendronate, risedronate, or ibandronate with placebo, postmarketing surveillance generated reports of *mucosal erosions* and *bleeding* in the esophagus, apparently related to instances in which pills failed to clear the esophagus and a chemical esophagitis resulted. These findings are seen more commonly in patients with a history of reflux. The risk of serious GI complications is low, but care is needed in patient selection and instruction (see later discussion). Concurrent use of a proton-pump inhibitor is prescribed by some clinicians to minimize GI side effects; the presence of gastroesophageal reflux disease is a contraindication to use.

Osteonecrosis. Reports of *osteonecrosis of the jaw* associated with bisphosphonate therapy have emerged and been widely reported in the lay media. A systematic review of 368 published reports of this complication found that 94% of cases occurred in cancer patients taking *intravenous bisphosphonate therapy* for bony lesions due to *multiple myeloma* or *metastatic carcinoma*; only rarely did healthy postmenopausal women taking oral bisphosphonate therapy experience the complication. The vast majority of reported cases occurred in the context of *poor dental hygiene* and *dental surgery*. Presenting manifestations include jaw numbness, pain, swelling, loose teeth, and exposed bone with failure to heal after dental surgery. The risk of jaw osteonecrosis among cancer patients taking intravenous bisphosphonate therapy is calculated at 6% to 10%; the risk associated with taking oral bisphosphonates for postmenopausal osteoporosis is unknown, but it appears to be remote in otherwise healthy women with good oral hygiene.

In sum, bisphosphonate risk appears to be greatest in debilitated persons with cancer, jaw trauma, and poor oral hygiene taking intravenous or long-duration oral therapy. One hypothesis advanced to explain the phenomenon is the oversuppression of osteoclasts, impairing removal of damaged bone and inhibiting remodeling.

In the absence of more definitive data, caution and clinical judgment are advised, particularly with the use of intravenous bisphosphonates in cancer patients and those with poor oral hygiene. A dental examination, dental prophylaxis, and any essential dental surgery are recommended before the initiation of therapy. Persons already taking oral bisphosphonate therapy should be advised to maintain good oral hygiene and get regular dental checkups and prophylaxis but not postpone necessary dental procedures. The osteonecrosis risk associated with oral surgery is probably remote in otherwise healthy postmenopausal women taking oral bisphosphonates and maintaining good oral hygiene. Nonetheless, some oral surgeons do ask about halting bisphosphonate therapy in long-term bisphosphonate users before a procedure; there is no evidence that short-term cessation of treatment it is necessary or effective in lowering osteonecrosis risk (bisphosphonates remain deposited in bone for months after the discontinuation of therapy).

Musculoskeletal Pain and Flulike Syndromes. A syndrome of incapacitating musculoskeletal pain associated with oral bisphosphonate therapy has been reported. Data on frequency, risk factors, and clinical details are sparse, but the frequency seems to be greater than that of osteonecrosis. After the infusion of intravenous bisphosphonate, a small percentage of patients have a flulike syndrome for 24 to 72 hours; myalgias may also occur.

Atrial Fibrillation. A small unexplained increase in serious atrial fibrillation was found unexpectedly in a large study of patients receiving zoledronic acid infusion. Mechanism, risk factors, and significance remain to be determined.

Use

Both oral and intravenous preparations are available.

Oral Preparations. *Alendronate, risedronate,* and *ibandronate* are approved by the U.S. Food and Drug Administration (FDA) for the prevention and treatment of osteoporosis. The second-generation bisphosphonates have become the mainstay of therapy, being well tolerated and capable of reducing risks of both vertebral and nonvertebral osteoporotic fractures. Once-weekly, twice-monthly, and monthly preparations are available, enhancing convenience and compliance. When they are used as directed, their efficacy and safety are comparable to those of daily dosing. GI complications can occur with all of the oral bisphosphonates. Oral therapy is contraindicated in persons with reflux and with motor and anatomic causes of delay in esophageal emptying.

Because oral bisphosphonate absorption is very low and inhibited by food intake and calcium, daily, weekly, and monthly preparations must be taken on an empty stomach. Antacids impair absorption and should not be used within 2 hours of intake. This requirement and the importance of ensuring complete passage through the esophagus necessitate thorough patient education on proper use (i.e., taking the pills with at least 8 oz of water on an empty stomach and remaining upright; see later discussion).

Intravenous Preparations. There are two intravenous bisphosphonates (*ibandronate* and *zoledronic* acid) approved for the treatment of postmenopausal osteoporosis. Intravenous ibandronate is given as a 15- to 30-second intravenous injection of 3 mg every 3 months; zoledronic acid is given as a 15- to 30-minute intravenous infusion of 5 mg once yearly. These agents are useful for persons who have a contraindication or intolerance to oral bisphosphonate therapy. Whether they become a primary treatment favored over oral bisphosphonates remains to be seen; more safety data are needed, particularly as relate to the risk of rapid atrial fibrillation.

Cost

In absolute terms, long-term bisphosphonate programs are expensive, but cost-effectiveness can be argued when the savings from the prevention of incapacitating fractures are taken into account. As generic versions appear in the near future, cost should come down significantly.

Selective Estrogen-Receptor Modulators

The so-called selective estrogen-receptor modulators or "*designer estrogens*" (also called *estrogen agonists/antagonists*) bind selectively to estrogen receptors and elicit a mix of agonist and antagonist responses that are tissue dependent. *Raloxifene* inhibits bone resorption through the same mechanism as estrogen but is not associated with breast cancer risk; in fact, it reduces the risk for invasive breast cancer by 50%, approximating the result of tamoxifen use. Moreover, it does not significantly affect the risk of CHD in high-risk women.

Efficacy

A modest increase (2% to 3%) in bone density occurs in the spine and hip. The reduction in the risk for *vertebral fracture* is about 50% in osteoporotic patients with or without a preexisting vertebral fracture and in osteopenic patients. A reduction in *nonvertebral fractures* has yet to be demonstrated.

Adverse Effects

Unlike hormone replacement therapy, raloxifene use is associated with a 50% *reduction* in the risk of invasive breast cancer, and there is no stimulative effect on the postmenopausal endometrium. At the doses used for osteoporosis, there is no improvement in the frequency of hot flashes, and sometimes they are exacerbated. The risk for *thrombosis* may be modestly increased, by about the same as with estrogen, but no increase in the number of strokes has been observed (although there was a higher incidence of death in those who suffered a stroke). Levels of low-density-lipoprotein cholesterol may decline.

Use

Raloxifene has been approved by the FDA for the prevention and treatment of osteoporosis. Recently the FDA approved raloxifene for the reduction in risk for invasive breast cancer in postmenopausal women with osteoporosis and in postmenopausal women at high risk for invasive breast cancer.

Estrogen/Hormone Replacement Therapy

Replacement therapy with estrogen in combination with progesterone (hormone replacement therapy [HRT]) had been the treatment of choice for the prevention of postmenopausal osteoporosis for more than a decade.

Efficacy

Estrogen stops bone loss and can produce a modest degree of skeletal mineral accretion (on the order of 2% to 4%). Observational studies have consistently noted a 35% to 50% reduction in hip, wrist, and vertebral fractures in women who used estrogen for at least 5 years after menopause. Benefit persists only as long as treatment is continued; accelerated bone loss occurs as soon as treatment stops; treatment needs to be continued indefinitely.

Adverse Effects

In addition to *pulmonary emboli*, risks of *invasive breast cancer*, *coronary disease*, and *stroke* were uncovered in large-scale, randomized trials of HRT, risks that were not recognized in earlier epidemiologic studies (see Chapter 118). The Women's Health Initiative (WHI) Randomized Trial found no net health benefit for HRT in postmenopausal women, even in those at high risk for osteoporotic fracture. Such findings have led to major revisions in recommendations for HRT use (see later discussion and Chapter 118). However, the mean age of women in the WHI was 63 years, and other analyses suggest there might be a benefit in younger women soon after menopause compared to older women.

Preparations

Conjugated estrogens derived from horse urine (thus the "marin" in Premarin) are effective when used in the established dose necessary to prevent osteoporosis (0.625 mg daily). Lower oral doses (e.g., 0.3 mg/d) and *low-dose patches* (e.g., 17β-estradiol at 14 μg/d) may suffice to control hot flashes and slow down bone loss, but efficacy in reducing fracture risk and safety of long-term use are yet to be demonstrated. Because unopposed chronic estrogen use stimulates endometrial growth and increases endometrial cancer risk (see Chapter 118), progestin doses of 2.5 to 10.0 mg/d of medroxyprogesterone (Provera) are required to induce either endometrial atrophy when used continuously or endometrial shedding when used cyclically.

Phytoestrogens (isoflavones) present in soy protein are very popular among women as a nonprescription or "natural estrogen" treatment for hot flashes; the estrogenic effect on bone afforded by even large quantities of dietary isoflavones appears to be too small to be of significance. Synthetic preparations of phytoestrogens are available. *Genistein*, the isoflavone phytoestrogen found in soy, resembles 17β-estradiol and functions as a semiselective estrogen-receptor modulator with considerably more affinity for the estrogen β-receptor in bone than the α-receptors in breast and uterus. A randomized, 24-month, placebo-controlled trial of a high-dose genistein supplement preparation revealed significantly better performance in limiting bone loss without any evident effect on endometrial thickness, but the study population was too small and the study duration too short to establish the safety of long-term use. Moreover, gastrointestinal upset caused nearly 20% of participants prematurely to terminate therapy.

Patient Selection

The risks of long-term estrogen therapy may outweigh the benefits for most women, even those at high risk of fracture. The advent of effective safe alternative therapies relegates estrogen to consideration only in persons who require estrogen for another compelling reason (e.g., incapacitating hot flashes). Only after a full consideration of risks and benefits should estrogen therapy be prescribed as a means of preventing osteoporosis. The decision to start HRT requires full discussion with the patient, not only of the potential skeletal benefit, but also of cardiovascular and cancer risks (see Chapter 118).

Calcitonin

Daily subcutaneous injections of 100 U of salmon calcitonin or 200 IU of nasally inhaled calcitonin in combination with calcium supplementation can increase the total body calcium in postmenopausal osteoporotic women by several percentage points; this increase presumably reflects an increase in skeletal mass. The risk for vertebral fracture may decline by as much as 40%, but the risk for hip fracture is not reduced, and changes in specific bones are often too small to measure. After 1 year of use, no further increase in total body calcium is noted, and total body calcium declines at the same rate as in untreated control patients. Moreover, bone loss is not prevented in early menopause.

The high cost and minimal sustained benefit of calcitonin make it a poor choice for long-term prophylaxis or treatment of osteoporosis. However, its initially positive effect on the risk for vertebral fracture and its coincident analgesic properties make it potentially useful as short-term therapy (perhaps 3 months) in elderly osteoporotic women who have sustained a painful vertebral compression fracture (see later discussion). Nasal administration is the best-tolerated route.

Parathyroid Hormone (1–34)—Teriparatide

This is the first anabolic therapy for osteoporosis that stimulates *osteoblastic activity* and the formation of new bone. Daily subcutaneous administration of this active recombinant human parathyroid hormone (1–34) fragment induces anabolic effects on bone, leading to new bone formation, particularly of trabecular bone, and improving calcium balance while producing chemically and histologically normal bone without hypercalcemia. Bone *resorption* is also increased but to a lesser degree than formation, and the overall net effect is increased bone formation. The risk of vertebral and nonvertebral fractures is significantly reduced.

Use

Because of its high cost and inconvenience, PTH therapy is reserved for severe cases (e.g., osteoporotic fracture and T score less than −2.5), especially when bisphosphonate therapy has been found to be inadequate. PTH is substituted for bisphosphonate rather than added, because of the potential inhibitory effect of bisphosphonate on PTH action. It was hoped that PTH's anabolic effects could be enhanced by combination with bisphosphonate therapy, but results have been disappointing yet variable, with inhibition rather than enhancement noted in some randomized clinical trials. The standard 20-μg daily dose is supplied in a pen containing a 28-day supply of medication, and only the 31-gauge needle has to be changed daily. It is generally well tolerated, although the initial resistance to self-injection is a barrier.

Adverse Effects

The drug is contraindicated in persons with Paget's disease of bone (who already have excess osteoblastic activity) and in cancer patients who have had external beam or implant radiation to the skeleton for bony metastases. A small increase in risk of osteosarcoma has been reported in rat studies involving doses of PTH up to 60 times the human dose for osteoporosis.

Sodium Fluoride

Sodium fluoride therapy leads to a striking increase in trabecular bone density if given in doses ranging from 40 to 60 mg/d, but cortical bone density decreases, so that skeletal fragility increases. The dense fluorotic bone is abnormal both chemically and on crystallography and has undesirable mechanical properties *in vitro*. More-promising results have been associated with long-term, low-dose fluoride therapy (20 mg/d given as monofluorophosphate) taken in conjunction with calcium. The rate of vertebral fracture is markedly reduced without the production of any noticeable adverse bony effects. More data are needed, particularly on effects on hip fracture rate. Fluoride is not approved by the U.S. Food and Drug Administration for use in osteoporosis.

Other Pharmacologic Measures (59–61)

Thiazides

Thiazide use has been associated in epidemiologic study with a one-third reduction in the risk of hip fracture. The protective effect disappears within 4 months of cessation of therapy. The responsible mechanism may involve a reduction in tubular excretion of calcium. Randomized study found that low-dose thiazide therapy (e.g., 25 mg/d of hydrochlorothiazide) helped to preserve bone mineral density in healthy older persons. Whether this directly translates into a reduced risk of fracture remains to be determined, but the magnitude of the effect on BMD approximates that of calcium and vitamin D.

Lowering of Homocysteine Levels

Several large-scale epidemiologic studies uncovered a relationship between *serum homocysteine* level and the risk of osteoporotic fracture that is independent of other known risk factors. Although vitamin B_6, vitamin B_{12}, and folic acid supplements can reduce homocysteine levels, it is premature to recommend widespread vitamin supplement use for the prevention of osteoporotic fractures in the elderly until prospective trials can confirm the significance of these findings and the efficacy of treatment.

Statins

After adjusting for other risk factors, one observational study revealed a 71% reduction in the risk of hip fracture associated with current statin use in elderly persons; other studies have yet to confirm the finding. Animal studies suggest an effect on new bone formation. The significance of these observations remains to be determined by prospective, randomized trials.

Follow-Up and Monitoring (10,13,62)

The risk for sustaining an osteoporotic fracture is related to the severity of bone mineral loss and the chance of falling. Because compliance with therapy is often poor, return visits at 6- to 12-month intervals to review and reinforce diet and exercise programs and monitor the medical regimen are warranted, especially in women with established osteoporosis. A repeat *DXA scan* in 12 to 18 months (the minimum interval for retesting) can be useful if the updated determination of bone mineral density will inform clinical decision making. Significant BMD changes (in excess of 3% in the spine and 4.5% in the hip) take 12 to 18 months to develop. A lack of improvement in BMD on the first repeated study may be a sign of poor compliance, but in patients taking bisphosphonate therapy it should not be an indication to halt or switch treatment because it may also represent a statistical deviation that is likely to be corrected on the next determination.

The clinical usefulness of measuring *biochemical markers* of bone turnover has not been established; the variability of these markers leads to 20% errors in reproducibility. Nonetheless, markers of bone formation (e.g., *bone-specific alkaline phosphatase, osteocalcin*) and bone resorption (e.g., serum *type I collagen* C and *urine N-telopeptides*) may sometimes be of benefit. Measuring urine N-telopeptides can help in determining whether a patient prescribed a bisphosphonate and not responding is taking the medication (a high urine level suggests noncompliance). Obtaining marker levels at baseline and at 3 months might eventually help in predicting response to antiresorptive treatment (especially if a 40% to 60% change is noted), but such use is not yet established.

Prevention of Falls (10,21,63,64)

Although the prevention and treatment of osteoporosis have been the focus of this chapter, the ultimate objective is to reduce the risk for fracture. Hip fracture in the elderly can be a major source of disability and a potentially life-threatening event. Community survey reveals that about one third of retirement community–dwelling persons older than the age of 75 years report at least one recent fall. Often, many factors are involved, such as sedative use, cognitive and visual impairments, gait and balance disturbances, disabled lower extremities, and foot problems.

A host of mundane but very important steps helps to reduce the risk for falling and sustaining a hip fracture; they correlate strongly with outcomes. Included among them are avoidance of long-acting tranquilizer use, treatment of impaired vision, and walking for exercise. Good *podiatric care* is essential, and physical and occupational therapy can be especially helpful in selected cases. Attention is directed toward any conditions that may impair gait or balance (see Chapters 166 and 239). Teaching balance exercise can help to reduce the risk of falls in the elderly. Patients with a neurologic or orthopedic impairment who would benefit from using a cane or a walker should be taught its proper use, both in the home and outside. Periodically, one should undertake a review of all *medications* to eliminate or reduce those that can cause postural hypotension (see Chapter 26) or sedation (see Chapters 226, 227, and 232).

Attention to the *home environment* is essential. Eliminating slippery surfaces and obstacle-laden paths, ensuring adequate illumination on stairways, installing handrails in the bathroom, and providing seating that enables easy arising all help to ensure safety. Personal items deserve attention, such as footwear that provides good stance and stability and eyeglass prescriptions that are up to date. *Hip protectors* worn by elderly osteoporotic persons at increased risk for falls can reduce the risk of hip fracture, but many falls occur at night when such protectors are not being worn, limiting the effectiveness of this intervention.

Vitamin D has a positive effect on muscle, which reduces sway and translates into a 22% reduced risk of falls in the elderly. The minimum dose required to achieve this benefit is not firmly established but appears to be 800 IU/d. A meta-analysis calculated that 15 persons would need to be treated to prevent 1 person from experiencing a fall.

Management of Fractures

The management of osteoporotic fractures involves the provision of symptomatic relief, repair (when possible), and secondary prophylaxis. Failure to recognize and treat osteoporosis in persons older than the age 50 years who present with a fracture is a common oversight and a lost opportunity to improve outcome. Wrist fractures are commonly overlooked as being related to osteoporosis. Persons older than the age of 50 years who present with a fracture should be evaluated for osteoporosis (see prior discussion) and treated aggressively. Previously untreated patients can be started on *bisphosphonate* therapy; those already taking bisphosphonate therapy who sustain a fracture should be considered for *PTH*.

Vertebral Fracture

With the exception of "burst" fractures (which require orthopedic surgical consultation; see later discussion), most vertebral fractures can be managed conservatively. *Bisphosphonates*, *raloxifene*, *calcitonin*, and *PTH* all increase spinal BMD and significantly reduce the risk for a new vertebral fracture. PTH provides the best results in terms of new bone formation and BMD compared to bisphosphonates and combination therapy, but the cost is extremely high, and cost-effectiveness is not established. Calcitonin may help to provide immediate pain relief. Determining the efficacy of therapy can be problematic in a given patient. Symptomatic improvement cannot be used to measure the response to therapy because fracture-free intervals may be long. The risk for fracture is not fully predictable by BMD because it is only one determinant of bone fragility. Despite these limitations, BMD measurement by DXA can still be helpful, particularly as an objective indicator of bony response to treatment that can help to guide therapy.

For patients who have sustained a painful osteoporotic vertebral fracture, periodic *bed rest* and adequate *analgesics* should be prescribed until the acute pain of the fracture subsides, often within several weeks. *Opioids* may be required. Thereafter, ambulation and daily exercise, such as swimming and walking, should be encouraged as tolerated. Lifting and vigorous physical activity are best avoided. *Corsets* and back *braces* (such as a Jewett-type device), if comfortable, may facilitate ambulation in formerly bedridden patients. A course of *intranasal calcitonin* is sometimes helpful in this situation because of its analgesic effect in addition to its ability to increase bone density modestly.

Vertebroplasty and *kyphoplasty* represent potentially promising orthopedic approaches to vertebral compression fracture but have yet to be subjected to carefully controlled, randomized trials and long-term follow-up. Vertebroplasty has been associated with reports of rapid pain relief, but the longer-term mechanical effects of a disproportionately strengthened vertebra are unclear. Fractures in vertebrae next to the treated vertebrae have more stress placed on them, leading to an increased incidence of subsequent fracture. Kyphoplasty is of interest for its potential to correct mechanical forces that contribute to future fracture risk.

Hip Fractures

Early repair is associated with the best outcomes. The risks of deep vein thrombosis and pulmonary embolization are high, necessitating prophylaxis (see Chapter 151).

Preventing and Treating Steroid-Induced Osteoporosis

Glucocorticoids inhibit new bone formation and calcium absorption and increase bone resorption and renal calcium excretion. Steroid-induced hypogonadism contributes to the problem in both men and women. Some degree of osteoporosis develops in more than 50% of patients on long-term steroids, and substantial bony changes can occur in as little as 3 months in persons taking high steroid doses. Even the use of topically active and inhaled preparations can produce dose-related reductions in BMD. Bone loss can be greatest during the first 3 to 12 months of steroid therapy; it then slows but persists for as long as steroid treatment continues. Some but not all bone mineral loss is reversible; the potential for recovery appears to be greatest in young persons.

Patients who will be taking systemic glucocorticoids at high doses (the equivalent of ≥20 mg/d of prednisone) or for prolonged periods (more than a few months) should be considered for prophylactic therapy. Persons requiring long-term use of inhaled steroids should be tapered to the lowest dose possible and followed with periodic bone density testing to determine the need for prophylactic treatment.

The first priorities for limiting fracture risk from systemic steroid use are to prescribe the lowest dose for the shortest time period and to use an alternate-day schedule if possible (see Chapter 105). In addition, it is essential to maintain *physical activity* and ensure adequate daily intake of *calcium* and *vitamin D. Sodium restriction* can help to improve the absorption and reduce the renal excretion of calcium. Antiresorptive therapy with *bisphosphonates* (e.g., 5 mg/d of *alendronate* or 10 mg/d in postmenopausal women; or risedronate 5 mg/d begun close to the outset of steroid use) can protect against the BMD loss during steroid therapy and reduce the chances of osteoporosis and osteoporotic fractures.

In patients already manifesting steroid-induced osteoporosis, bisphosphonate therapy (e.g., 10 mg/d of alendronate or 70 mg once weekly or risedronate 5 mg/d or 35 mg once weekly) can be used. Hypercalciuria is an indication for *thiazide* therapy (supplemented by potassium replacement or a potassium-sparing agent). Small supplements of vitamin D can be given to those who become vitamin D deficient.

PATIENT EDUCATION

Patient education is essential. The time spent educating patients about osteoporosis is extremely well spent because prevention and compliance are so important to effective management. Perimenopausal women are highly concerned about osteoporosis and are eager to discuss prevention and treatment. The full range of options and their associated risks and benefits must be reviewed and patient preferences elicited; failure to do so is likely to result in disappointing outcomes due to poor compliance. Of particular importance is addressing the change in recommendations regarding estrogen therapy (see Chapter 118). One should seek to design a program that is tailored to the patient's risk profile and lifestyle.

INDICATIONS FOR REFERRAL AND ADMISSION

Patients who develop an osteoporotic fracture while taking full doses of bisphosphonate therapy should be referred to an osteo-porosis specialist for consideration of PTH therapy and review of the overall treatment program. Those who have sustained a hip fracture need hospital admission and prompt surgical repair followed by a period of anticoagulation. The persistence of incapacitating back pain from a vertebral fracture warrants consideration of interventional therapy such as vertebroplasty. The occurrence of a "burst" fracture of the spine necessitates orthopedic consultation because the spinal cord may be at risk for injury from a bony fragment or spinal instability.

THERAPEUTIC RECOMMENDATIONS

Prevention of Osteoporosis

- Advise young women, especially if they are pregnant, to maintain a daily dietary intake of at least 1.2 to 1.5 g of *calcium* and 400 IU of *vitamin D*.
- Encourage a program of regular physical activity for all persons, including aerobic and strengthening exercises.
- Advise against important lifestyle risk factors such as smoking and alcohol excess.
- Review and advise against potential risk factors such as excess intake of vitamin A supplements, glucocorticosteroids, and thyroid hormone.
- For perimenopausal and postmenopausal women, prescribe a program of 30 minutes of *weight-bearing exercise* (e.g., walking, jogging, aerobics, dancing, tennis, weight lifting) at least three times weekly, a daily total calcium intake of 1.2 to 1.5 g, and 800 to 1,000 IU of vitamin D daily.
- If necessary, supplement the diet with *calcium carbonate* tablets (least expensive) or *calcium citrate* (more expensive, slightly better tolerated) to achieve the desired daily total; encourage supplement intake during meals to minimize gastrointestinal upset and risk for kidney stones, and encourage splitting the dose to maximize uptake and minimize gastrointestinal upset.
- Screen all women older than the age of 65 years by DXA scan of the hip and spine (see Chapter 144); perform testing earlier if major risk factors are present (e.g., maternal history of osteoporotic fracture, current smoking, history of fracture as adult, body mass index <22 kg/m^2).
- For patients with a T score greater than −1.0 (i.e., BMD within one standard deviation of the mean for young women), continue calcium, vitamin D, and exercise; repeat bone density measurement in 1 to 2 years (depending on the degree of osteoporosis risk).
- For patients with a T score between −1.0 and −2.5, begin a more aggressive prevention program and avoid delaying the initiation of therapy, because the rate of bone loss is maximal during the first few years after menopause. In addition to calcium, vitamin D, and exercise, choose one of the following based on patient preferences and total health considerations (refer also to Chapter 118):
  1. *Bisphosphonate therapy* (e.g., *alendronate*, 70 mg once weekly; *risedronate*, 35 mg once weekly; ibandronate, 150 mg once monthly) taken on an empty stomach with 8 oz of water and remaining upright 30 minutes (60 minutes for ibandronate) before breakfast; or:
  2. *Raloxifene*, 60 mg/d (also consider the risk reduction in invasive breast cancer).
- For those who refuse or cannot take such treatment but might be candidates if osteoporotic risk increased still further, monitor bone loss by DXA scan every 1 to 2 years and

reconsider treatment if the rate of loss is marked or the T score falls to less than –2.5. Continue exercise and calcium and vitamin D supplementation; avoid vitamin A supplementation, alcohol excess, and smoking.

■ Continue therapy indefinitely unless it is replaced by a therapy of nearly equal efficacy, a complication develops, or the T score falls to less than –2.5.

Established Osteoporosis

■ For asymptomatic patients who are found incidentally to have radiographic osteopenia or a bone densitometry T score of less than –2.5, begin as follows:
1. *Calcium, vitamin D,* and *weight-bearing exercise* (adjusted to minimize fracture risk) as detailed earlier, *plus*:
2. *Bisphosphonate therapy* (e.g., *alendronate,* 70 mg once weekly; *risedronate,* 35 mg once weekly; ibandronate,150 mg once monthly) taken on an empty stomach with 8 oz of water and remaining upright for 30 minutes (60 minutes with ibandronate) before breakfast; or:
3. *Raloxifene,* 60 mg/d (advantage includes risk reduction in invasive breast cancer).
■ For patients who cannot tolerate oral bisphosphonate therapy and for whom bisphosphonate therapy is contraindicated, consider *intravenous ibandronate* 3 mg every 3 months or *intravenous zoledronic* acid 5 mg once yearly. Also consider PTH (1–34), 20 μg, administered subcutaneously daily.
■ Continue therapy indefinitely unless it is replaced by a therapy of nearly equal efficacy or a complication develops.

Osteoporotic Vertebral Compression Fracture

■ Treat initially with *bed rest* and *analgesics*. When the pain subsides, begin ambulation; consider the use of a brace; follow with mild exercise such as walking or swimming. Avoid lifting and other weight-bearing stresses.
■ Consider *bisphosphonate* therapy (e.g., alendronate, 70 mg once weekly; risedronate, 35 mg once weekly; ibandronate, 150 mg once monthly) taken with the precautions noted previously.
■ Alternatively, consider intravenous ibandronate or zoledronic acid, especially in persons with a contraindication or intolerance to oral bisphosphonate therapy.
■ Consider PTH (1–34) as the initial agent, especially if the T score is less than –2.5 or as a substitute for bisphosphonate if bisphosphonate therapy proves insufficient or is not tolerated; administer PTH (1–34) subcutaneously, 20 μg daily.
■ Consider a short course of intranasal *calcitonin* (200 IU/d) for pain if marked discomfort persists.
■ Consider *raloxifene,* 60 mg/d.
■ Institute a program of *calcium* and *vitamin D* supplementation as detailed previously.

Osteoporotic Hip Fracture

■ Admit for *surgical repair* as quickly as possible; institute deep vein thrombosis prophylaxis (see Chapter 151).
■ Institute a treatment program for osteoporosis with *bisphosphonate* therapy as noted previously.
■ Also consider *PTH (1–34).*

Prevention of Glucocorticoid-Induced Osteoporosis

■ *Calcium* and *vitamin D* supplementation (as detailed previously); *plus*:
■ Consider a program of osteoporosis antiresorptive prophylaxis with a *bisphosphonate* preparation (e.g., alendronate, 35 mg once weekly, or 70 mg once weekly if postmenopausal; risedronate, 35 mg once weekly) in persons who are going to require high-dose steroids (e.g., >7.5 mg/d of prednisone) for at least a few months.
■ Give the highest priority to patients at greatest risk for osteoporosis (e.g., postmenopausal women; those with prior vertebral fracture).
■ Consider DXA determination of spinal BMD at the outset of steroid therapy to determine pretreatment risk and establish a baseline.

Annotated Bibliography

1. Bauer DC, Browner WS, Cauley JAA, et al. Factors associated with appendicular bone mass in older women. Ann Intern Med 1993;118:657. (*The best data on the risk factors for osteoporosis.*)
2. Burge R, Dawson-Hughes B, Solomon DH, et al. Incidence and economic burden of osteoporosis-related fractures in the United States, 2005–2025. J Bone Miner Res 2007;22:465 (*By 2025, the number of annual fractures and the costs are projected to grow by 50% and will surpass 3 million and $25 billion, respectively*).
3. Cummings SR, Nevitt MC, Browner WS, et al. Risk factors for hip fracture in white women. N Engl J Med 1995;332:767. (*A prospective cohort study, identifying major risk factors and the means of preventing hip fracture.*)
4. Feskanich D, Singh V, Willett WC, et al. Vitamin A intake and hip fractures among postmenopausal women. JAMA 2002;287:47. (*The long-term intake of a diet high in retinol may promote the development of osteoporotic hip fractures in women.*)
5. Fitzpatrick LA. Secondary causes of osteoporosis. Mayo Clin Proc 2002;77:453. (*An in-depth discussion of the more important secondary causes.*)
6. Gregg EW, Cauley JA, Seeley DG, et al. Physical activity and osteoporotic fracture risk in older women. Ann Intern Med 1998;129:81. (*A prospective cohort study, finding that the risk for fracture of the hip was reduced, but the risk for fracture of the spine or the wrist was not.*)
7. Holick MF. Vitamin D deficiency. N Engl J Med 2007;357:266. (*An excellent review, including treatment strategies*).
8. Hofbauer LC, Brueck CC, Singh SK, et al. Osteoporosis in patients with diabetes mellitus. J Bone Miner Res 2007;22:1317. (*Diabetes mellitus may be a risk factor for osteoporotic fractures in both type 1 and type 2 diabetes.*)
9. Israel E, Banerjee TR, Fitzmaurice GM, et al. Effects of inhaled glucocorticosteroids on bone density in premenopausal women. N Engl J Med 2001;345:941. (*A prospective cohort study, finding evidence for a dose-related loss of bone mineral density.*)
10. Khosla S, Melton LJ III. Osteopenia. N Engl J Med 2007;356:2293. (*A nice review, including recommendations for evaluation and treatment*).
11. Lukert BP, Raisz LG. Glucocorticoid-induced osteoporosis: pathogenesis and management. Ann Intern Med 1990;112:352. (*A clinically relevant discussion of disease mechanisms, followed by a review of treatment options.*)
12. McLean RR, Jacques PF, Selhub J, et al. Homocysteine as a predictive factor for hip fracture in older persons. N Engl J Med 2004;350:2042. (*Observational data from the Framingham Study, showing an independent association between homocysteine level and the risk of osteoporotic fracture in the elderly.*)
13. Michaelsson K, Lithell H, Vessby B, et al. Serum retinol and the risk of fracture. N Engl J Med 2003;348:287. (*An epidemiologic study, finding that the risk of fracture was correlated with serum retinol levels.*)

14. NIH Consensus Development Panel on Osteoporosis Prevention, Diagnosis, and Therapy. Osteoporosis prevention, diagnosis, and therapy. JAMA 2001;285:785. (*Slightly dated with regard to hormone replacement therapy, but still one of the best summaries.*)

15. Richelson LS, Wahner HW, Melton LJ, et al. Relative contributions of aging and estrogen deficiency to postmenopausal bone loss. N Engl J Med 1984;311:1273. (*A classic paper; bone loss in oophorectomized women was almost as great as that in postmenopausal women, suggesting that estrogen loss is the cause.*)

16. Shahinian VB, Kuo YF, Freeman JL, et al. Risk of fracture after androgen deprivation for prostate cancer. N Engl J Med 2005;352:154. (*A retrospective epidemiologic study, finding a significant increase in risk.*)

17. Cummings SR, Bates DW, Black DM. Clinical use of bone densitometry: a scientific review. JAMA 2002;288:1889. (*An excellent review of the approaches to measuring bone density; 72 references.*)

18. Green AD, Colon-Emeric CS, Basian L, et al. Does this woman have osteoporosis? JAMA 2004;292:2890. (*A Rational Clinical Exam study, finding that several features of the history and physical examination help in the determining risk.*)

19. Alexandersen P, Toussaint A, Christiansen C, et al. Ipriflavone in the treatment of postmenopausal osteoporosis: a randomized controlled trial. JAMA 2001;285:1482. (*A randomized, controlled trial [RCT], finding no benefit with this synthetic derivative of plant estrogen.*)

20. Aloia JF, Vaswani A, Yeh JK, et al. Calcium supplementation with and without hormone replacement therapy to prevent postmenopausal bone loss. Ann Intern Med 1994;120:97. (*Calcium produced an intermediate effect, between those of estrogen and placebo.*)

21. Barrett-Connor E, Mosca L, Collins P, et al. for the Raloxifene Use for the Heart (RUTH) trial investigators. N Engl J Med 2006;355:125. Effects of raloxifene on cardiovascular events and breast cancer in postmenopausal women. (*In 10,000 postmenopausal women with coronary heart disease [CHD] or at high risk for it, raloxifene did not significantly affect the risk of CHD, although there was an increased risk of venous thromboembolism and fatal stroke*).

22. Bischoff-Ferrari HA, Dawson-Hughes B, Willett WE, et al. Effect of vitamin D on falls: a meta-analysis. JAMA 2004;291:1999. (*Finds a 22% reduction in the rate of falls in the elderly.*)

23. Black DB, Delmas PD, Eastell R, et al. for the HORIZON Pivotal Fracture Trial. Once-yearly zoledronic acid for treatment of postmenopausal osteoporosis. N Engl J Med 2007;356:1809. (*The treatment significantly reduced the risk of vertebral, hip, and other fractures; some patients experienced atrial fibrillation.*)

24. Black DM, Cummings SR, Karpf DB, et al. Randomised trial of effect of alendronate on risk of fracture in women with existing vertebral fractures: Fracture Intervention Trial Research Group. Lancet 1996;348:1535. (*There was a 47% reduction in the rate of new fractures.*)

25. Black DM, Schwartz AV, Ensrud KE, et al. for the FLEX Research Group. Effects of continuing or stopping alendronate after 5 years of treatment. The Fracture Intervention Trial Long-term Extension (FLEX): a randomized trial. JAMA 2006;296:2927 (*There was no higher fracture risk other than that for clinical vertebral fractures compared to those who continued alendronate for 10 years.*)

26. Bone HG, Hosking D, Devogelaer JP, et al. Ten years' experience with alendronate for osteoporosis in postmenopausal women. N Engl J Med 2004;350:1189. (*Demonstrates long-term efficacy and safety.*)

27. Cauley JA, Fobbins J, Chen Z, et al. Effects of estrogen plus progestin on risk of fracture and bone mineral density: the Women's Health Initiative trial. JAMA 2003;290:1729. (*The fracture risk was reduced, but when the overall health benefit was weighed against the risks of adverse cardiovascular and cancer outcomes, no net benefit was found, even among high-risk women.*)

28. Cauley JA, Seeley DG, Esrud K, et al. Estrogen replacement therapy and fractures in older women: Study of Osteoporotic Fractures Research Group. Ann Intern Med 1995;122:9. (*The relative risk for nonspinal fracture was reduced by 34%.*)

29. Chestnut CH III, Silverman S, Andriano K, et al. A randomized trial of nasal spray salmon calcitonin in postmenopausal women with established osteoporosis: the Prevent Recurrence of Osteoporotic Fractures Study. Am J Med 2000;109:267. (*The treatment reduced the risk of vertebral fractures but not hip fractures.*)

30. Chestnut CH III, Skag A, Christiansen C, et al. for the Oral Ibandronate Osteoporosis Vertebral Fracture Trial in North America and Europe (BONE). Effects of oral ibandronate administered daily or intermittently on fracture risk in postmenopausal osteoporosis. J Bone Miner Res 2004; 19:1241. (*Both treatments reduced the risk of vertebral fractures.*)

31. Cummings SR, Black DM, Thompson DE, et al. Effect of alendronate on risk of fracture in women with low bone density but without vertebral fractures: results from the Fracture Intervention Trial. JAMA 1998;280:2077. (*The risk for hip fracture was reduced.*)

32. Cummings SR, Eckert S, Krueger KA, et al. The effect of raloxifene on risk of breast cancer in postmenopausal women. JAMA 1999;281:2189. (*The risk was reduced by nearly 50%.*)

33. Cummings SR, Palermo L, Browner W, et al. Monitoring osteoporosis therapy with bone densitometry: misleading changes and regression to the mean. JAMA 2000;283:1318. (*Suggests that a lack of response initially may be related more to test performance than to the actual response to treatment; often a very marked response is seen on follow-up determination.*)

34. Curhan GC, Willet WC, Speizer FE, et al. Comparison of dietary calcium with supplemental calcium and other nutrients as factors affecting the risk of kidney stones in women. Ann Intern Med 1997;126:497. (*The Nurses' Health Study, finding that dietary calcium reduces the risk for stones and supplemental calcium increases it.*)

35. Dawson-Hughes B, Dallal GE, Krall KA, et al. A controlled trial of the effect of calcium supplementation on bone density in postmenopausal women. N Engl J Med 1990;323:878. (*Calcium supplementation was beneficial, mostly in older women with low calcium intake.*)

36. Dawson-Hughes B, Harris SS, Krall EA, et al. Effect of calcium and vitamin D supplementation on bone density in men and women 65 years of age or older. N Engl J Med 1997;337:670. (*RCT, finding that there was modest reduction in bone loss and significant reduction in nonvertebral fractures.*)

37. Dalsky GP, Stocke KS, Ehsani AA, et al. Weight-bearing exercise training and lumbar mineral content in postmenopausal women. Ann Intern Med 1988;108:824. (*Exercise for 50 minutes three times per week plus calcium supplementation produced an increase in lumbar bone mineral content.*)

38. Delmas PD, Adami S, Strugala C, et al. Intravenous ibandronate injections in postmenopausal women with osteoporosis. One-year results from the Dosing Intravenous Administration Study. Arthritis Rheum 2006;54:1838. (*At the end of 1 year, intravenous ibandronate 3 mg every 3 months corresponded to greater bone mineral density [BMD] changes than the 2.5-mg oral daily dose*).

39. Delmas PD, Bjarnason NH, Mitlak BH, et al. Effects of raloxifene on bone mineral density, serum cholesterol concentrations, and uterine endometrium in postmenopausal women. N Engl J Med 1997;337:1641. (*The bone benefit was intermediate between that of standard hormone replacement therapy and placebo.*)

40. Ettinger B, Black DM, Bitlak BH, et al. Reduction of vertebral fracture risk in postmenopausal women with osteoporosis treatment with raloxifene: results from a 3-year randomized clinical trial. Multiple Outcomes of Raloxifene Evaluation (MORE). JAMA 1999;282:637. (*Demonstrates a 50% reduction in vertebral fracture rate.*)

41. Finklestein JS, Klibanski A, Arnold AL, et al. Prevention of estrogen deficiency–related bone loss with human parathyroid hormone: a randomized controlled trial. JAMA 1998;280:1067. (*Parathyroid hormone prevented bone loss in young women receiving pituitary suppression therapy.*)

42. Garfin SR, Yuan HA, Reiley MA. New technologies in spine: kyphoplasty and vertebroplasty for the treatment of painful osteoporotic compression fractures. Spine 2001;26:1511. (*A discussion of promising orthopedic approaches.*)

43. Greenspan SL, Emkey RD, Bone HG III, et al. Significant differential effects of alendronate, estrogen, or combination therapy on the rate of bone loss after discontinuation of treatment of postmenopausal osteoporosis. Ann Intern Med 2002;137:875. (*RCT, finding that bone loss was much slower after the cessation of bisphosphonate therapy.*)

44. Cadarette SM, Katz JN, Brookhart MA, et al. Relative effectiveness of osteoporosis drugs for preventing nonvertebral fracture. Ann Intern Med 2008;148:637. (*One of the few comparative studies available, but limited in being observational and not randomized; little difference among bisphosphonates and raloxifene noted.*)

45. Harris ST, Watts NB, Genant HK, et al. Effects of risedronate treatment on vertebral and nonvertebral fractures in women with established osteoporosis. Vertebral Efficacy with Risedronate Therapy (VERT) Study Group. JAMA 1999;282:1344. (*There was a nearly 60% reduction in risk.*)

46. Holmes MM, Rovner DR, Rothert ML, et al. Women's and physicians' utilities for health outcomes in estrogen replacement therapy. J Gen Intern Med 1987;2:178. (*The prevention of fracture was more highly valued by the women, which underscores the need for eliciting the patient's views.*)

47. Horsman A, Jones M, Francis R, et al. The effect of estrogen dose on postmenopausal bone loss. N Engl J Med 1983;309:1405. (*Notes a dose–response relationship; the required dose for conjugated estrogens was 0.625 mg.*)

48. Hosking D, Chilvers CE, Christiansen C, et al. Prevention of bone loss with alendronate in postmenopausal women under 60 years of age. Early Postmenopausal Intervention Cohort Study Group. N Engl J Med 1998;338:485. (*Presents results from the Early Postmenopausal Intervention Cohort Study, showing that the early use of alendronate was effective and well tolerated, and that a dose of 5 mg/d was better than one of 2.5 mg/d.*)

49. Jolly EE, Bjarnason NH, Neven P, et al. Prevention of osteoporosis and uterine effects in postmenopausal women taking raloxifene for 5 years. Menopause 2003;10:337. (*Women with osteopenia taking raloxifene for 5 years were significantly less likely to progress to osteoporosis than those taking placebo.*)

50. Khosla S, Burr D, Cauley J, et al. Bisphosphonate-associated osteonecrosis of the jaw: report of a task force of the American Society for Bone and Mineral Research. J Bone Miner Res 2007; 22:1479. (*The task force defined

osteonecrosis of the jaw as the presence of exposed bone in the maxillofacial region that did not heal within 8 weeks after identification by a health care worker.)

51. Khovidhunkit W, Shoback SM. Clinical effects of raloxifene hydrochloride in women. Ann Intern Med 1999;130:431. (*A useful review that the physician should read before prescribing the drug; 86 references.*)

52. LaCroix AZ, Ott SM, Ichikawa L, et al. Low-dose hydrochlorothiazide and preservation of bone mineral density in older adults: a randomized, double-blind, placebo-controlled trial. Ann Intern Med 2003;133:516. (*Low-dose therapy was found to be effective in preserving BMD in healthy older adults.*)

53. Lanza FL, Hunt RH, Thompson AB, et al. Endoscopic comparison of esophageal and gastroduodenal effects of risedronate and alendronate in postmenopausal women. Gastroenterology 2000;119:631. (*A short-term, head-to-head study, finding no difference between the treatments.*)

54. Liberman UA, Weiss SR, Broll J, et al. Effects of oral alendronate on bone mineral density and the incidence of fractures in postmenopausal osteoporosis. N Engl J Med 1995;333:1437. (*There was a 9% increase in BMD at the spine and a 6% increase at the hip, and a 50% reduction in vertebral fracture.*)

55. Lufkin EG, Wahner HW, O'Fallon WM, et al. Treatment of postmenopausal osteoporosis with transdermal estrogen. Ann Intern Med 1992;117:1. (*Finds that this treatment was effective, but that lipid changes were less beneficial than with oral therapy.*)

56. Lyles KW, Colón-Emeric CS, Magaziner JS, et al. for the HORIZON Recurrent Fracture Trial. Zoledronic acid and clinical fractures and mortality after hip fracture. N Engl J Med 2007;357:1799. (*Infusion within 90 days after the repair of a low-trauma hip fracture was associated with a reduction in the rate of new clinical fractures and improved survival.*)

57. Manson JE, Allison MA, Rossouw JE, et al. for the WHI and WHI-CACS investigators. Estrogen therapy and coronary-artery calcification. N Engl J Med 2007;356:2591. (*Women 50 to 59 years old randomly assigned to conjugated equine estrogens had a lower coronary-plaque burden and a lower prevalence of subclinical coronary artery disease after completion of the Women's Health Initiative trial of estrogen than did women receiving placebo.*)

58. McClung MR, Geusens P, Miller PD, et al. Effect of risedronate on the risk of hip fracture in elderly women. N Engl J Med 2001;344:333. (*RCT, finding that the risk was reduced in women with low BMD but not in those with risk factors other than BMD.*)

59. Neer RM, Arnaud CD, Zanchetta JR, et al. Effect of parathyroid hormone (1–34) on fractures and bone mineral density in postmenopausal women with osteoporosis. N Engl J Med 2001;344:1434. (*A landmark study, demonstrating the efficacy of the treatment.*)

60. Nguyen NG, Eisman JA, Nguyen TV. Anti-hip fracture efficacy of bisphosphonates: a Bayesian analysis of clinical trials. J Bone Miner Res 2006;21:340. (*A meta-analysis, finding that bisphosphonate treatment was associated with a reduced risk of hip fracture in postmenopausal women with osteoporosis or low BMD.*)

61. Osteoporosis Prevention Study Group. Alendronate prevents postmenopausal bone loss in women without osteoporosis: a double-blind, randomized, controlled trial. Ann Intern Med 1998;128:253. (*Low-dose therapy was well tolerated and effective.*)

62. Parker MJ, Gillespie LD, Gillespie WJ. Hip protectors for preventing hip fractures in the elderly. In: The Cochrane library, Issue 4. Oxford: Update Software, 2002. (*Finds evidence for efficacy in select groups at high risk.*)

63. Popcock NA, Eisman JA, Dunstan CR, et al. Recovery from steroid-induced osteoporosis. Ann Intern Med 1987;107:319. (*Reversal was found in these relatively young persons.*)

64. Prince RL, Smith M, Dick IM, et al. Prevention of postmenopausal osteoporosis: a comparative study of exercise, calcium supplementation, and hormone replacement. N Engl J Med 1992;325:1189. (*Bone loss was slowed or prevented by exercise plus calcium and by hormone replacement.*)

65. Recker RR, Davies M, Dowd RM, et al. The effect of low-dose continuous estrogen and progesterone therapy with calcium and vitamin D on bone in elderly women. A randomized, controlled trial. Ann Intern Med 1999;130:897. (*Low-dose therapy combined with calcium and vitamin D was as good as or better than standard-dose hormone replacement therapy in this population.*)

66. Reginster JY, Meurmans L, Zegels B, et al. The effect of sodium monofluorophosphate plus calcium on vertebral fracture rate in postmenopausal women with moderate osteoporosis: a randomized, controlled trial. Ann Intern Med 1998;129:1. (*Additional benefit was found with the use of fluoride supplement.*)

67. Riggs BL, Hodgson SF, O'Fallon WM, et al. Effect of fluoride treatment on the fracture rate in postmenopausal women with osteoporosis. N Engl J Med 1990;322:802. (*The treatment increased cancellous bone but decreased cortical bone, so that skeletal fragility was increased.*)

68. Rosen CJ, Hochberg MC, Bonnick SL, et al. Treatment with once-weekly alendronate 70 mg compared with once-weekly risedronate 35 mg in women

with postmenopausal osteoporosis: a randomized double-blind study. J Bone Miner Res 2005;20:141. (*A head-to-head, 1-year study, suggesting a greater increase in BMD with alendronate and equal tolerability, but there were no data on fracture rates.*)

69. Rosen CJ. Postmenopausal osteoporosis. N Engl J Med 2005;353:595. (*An excellent review of the nonpharmacologic and pharmacologic options.*)

70. Rubin CD, Pak SYC, Adams-Huet B, et al. Sustained-release sodium fluoride in the treatment of the elderly with established osteoporosis. Arch Intern Med 2001;161:2325. (*RCT, finding that there was a significant reduction in the risk of vertebral fracture without an increased risk of hip fracture.*)

71. Saag KG, Emkey R, Schnitzer TJ, et al. Alendronate for the prevention and treatment of glucocorticoid-induced osteoporosis. N Engl J Med 1998;339:292. (*A randomized, placebo-controlled, 48-week trial, finding an increase in BMD with alendronate.*)

72. Schairer C, Lubin J, Troisi R, et al. Menopausal estrogen and estrogen–progestin replacement therapy and breast cancer risk. JAMA 2000;283:485. (*Presents evidence that the breast cancer risk was increased and beyond that attributable to estrogen alone.*)

73. Schnitzer T, Bone HG, Crepaldi G, et al. Therapeutic equivalence of alendronate 70 mg once-weekly and alendronate 10 mg daily in the treatment of osteoporosis. Aging 2000;12:1. (*Presents evidence of equivalence.*)

74. Schoofs WMCJ, van der Klift M, Hofman A, et al. Thiazide diuretics and the risk of hip fracture. Ann Intern Med 2003;139:476. (*An epidemiologic study, demonstrating that there was an association between the use of these agents and risk, but that the effect disappeared within 3 months of cessation.*)

75. Sheikh MS, Santa Ana CA, Nicar MJ, et al. Gastrointestinal absorption of calcium from milk and calcium salts. N Engl J Med 1987;317:532. (*In these healthy young subjects, no significant differences were found.*)

76. Tang BMP, Eslick GD, Nowson C, et al. Use of calcium or calcium in combination with vitamin D supplementation to prevent fractures and bone loss in people aged 50 years and older: a meta-analysis. Lancet 2007;370:657. (*A review of 29 randomized trials, including 17 with fracture outcome, finding that fracture reduction was best with at least 1,200 mg of calcium and 800 IU of vitamin D*).

77. Tashjian AH Jr, Gagel RF. Teriparatide (human PTH(1–34)): 2.5 years of experience on the use and safety of the drug for the treatment of osteoporosis. J Bone Miner Res 2006;21:354. (*A good review of the clinical aspects of teriparatide use.*)

78. Tham DM, Gardner CD, Haskell WL, et al. Clinical review 97: Potential health benefits of dietary phytoestrogens: a review of the clinical, epidemiological, and mechanistic evidence. J Clin Endocrinol Metab 1998;83:2223. (*A thorough review of the evidence.*)

79. The Writing Group for the PEPI Trial. Effects of hormone therapy on bone mineral density. Results from the Postmenopausal Estrogen/Progestin Interventions (PEPI) Trial. JAMA 1996;276:1389. (*A randomized, double-blinded, placebo-controlled, multicenter study, finding that BMD increased at key sites with hormone replacement therapy.*)

80. Tilyard MW, Spears GFS, Thomson J, et al. Treatment of postmenopausal osteoporosis with calcitriol or calcium. N Engl J Med 1992;326:357. (*Continuous use reduced the rate of vertebral fractures.*)

81. Tinetti ME, Baker DI, McAvay G, et al. A multifactorial intervention to reduce the risk of falling among elderly people living in the community. N Engl J Med 1994;331:821. (*Because multiple factors are usually involved, treatment needs to be similarly multidimensional to be effective.*)

82. Tremaine WJ, Kholsa S. Bisphosphonates and the upper gastrointestinal tract: skeletal gain without visceral pain? Mayo Clin Proc 2002;77:1029. (*A useful editorial summarizing the evidence and arguing for careful patient selection.*)

83. Vogel VG, Costantino JP, Wickerhan DL, et al. for the National Surgical Adjuvant Breast and Bowel Project (NSABP). Effects of tamoxifen vs raloxifene on the risk of developing invasive breast cancer and other disease outcomes. The NSABP study of tamoxifen and raloxifene (STAR) P-2 trial. JAMA 2006;295:2727 (*In almost 20,000 postmenopausal women with an increased 5-year breast cancer risk, raloxifene was comparable to tamoxifen in reducing the risk for invasive breast cancer*).

84. Wang PS, Solomon DH, Mogun H, et al. HMG-CoA reductase inhibitors and the risk of hip fractures in elderly patients. JAMA 2000;283:3211. (*A case–control study, finding a 71% reduction in risk.*)

85. Woo S-B, Hellstein JW, Kalmar JR, et al. Systematic review: bisphosphonates and osteonecrosis of the jaws. Ann Intern Med 2006;144:753. (*A review of >300 reports, finding risk predominantly among cancer patients treated with intravenous bisphosphonates.*)

86. Writing Group for the Women's Health Initiative Investigators. Risks and benefits of estrogen plus progestin in healthy postmenopausal women: principal results from the Women's Health Initiative randomized controlled trial. JAMA 2002;288:321. (*Presents important risk/benefit data from a major trial.*)

CHAPTER 165 ■ APPROACH TO THE PATIENT WITH HEADACHE

AMY A. PRUITT

A complaint of headache raises numerous diagnostic possibilities. Fortunately, less than 1% of cases of headache that come to medical attention represent serious intracranial disease. Still, headache poses a diagnostic challenge for the primary physician, who must distinguish between the rare headache that represents a potentially life-threatening process and the vast majority, which are harmless. Both physicians and patients worry about headaches that are persistent, severe, sudden in onset, or different from a patient's usual headache. The primary physician's most immediate task is to identify efficiently by history and physical examination the occasional patient who requires aggressive workup. Additional priorities are to provide symptomatic relief and to diagnose the type of headache and its cause systematically while formulating a long-term plan for management.

Headache can be a difficult problem to evaluate and manage. Of patients who come for help, only one third claim they are satisfied with the care received. Fortunately for neurologists and primary physicians, recent advances in our understanding of clinical presentation and pathophysiology have greatly facilitated diagnosis and treatment.

PATHOPHYSIOLOGY AND CLINICAL PRESENTATION (1–14)

Headache may originate in either intracranial or extracranial structures, with the mechanisms and presentations of pain depending on the source.

Intracranial Sources

Intracranial sources of pain referable to the head include fibers of the fifth, ninth, and tenth cranial nerves and the upper cervical nerves, the venous sinuses, parts of the dura at the base of the skull, the dural arteries (anterior and middle meningeal), and the large arteries at the base of the brain that give rise to the circle of Willis. Brain parenchyma is not pain sensitive. Postulated *mechanisms* include (a) *traction* resulting from direct or indirect displacement of intracranial structures, (b) *distention* of intracranial arteries, (c) *inflammation* of pain-sensitive structures, and (d) *obstruction* of cerebrospinal fluid flow by a mass lesion distorting the brain contents. If the intracranial source of pain is above the tentorium, pain is usually felt in the distribution of the fifth cranial nerve. Pain from a site in the posterior fossa is usually felt in the posterior half of the head, conveyed by the glossopharyngeal and vagus nerves and also by the upper cervical spinal roots.

Mass Lesions

Mass lesions can cause headache by displacing a pain-sensitive structure. About one third of patients with a mass lesion have headache as an early symptom, often with the pain *localized to the side of the lesion*. Presentations vary widely, with none particularly diagnostic. The headache may be mild or severe, intermittent or persistent, aching, sharp, pressure-like, or even throbbing in quality. Characteristically, the headache remains in the *same location* but is *progressive*; increases in the duration and severity of pain over several months occur in conjunction with subtle changes in mental status or the development of focal neurologic deficits. As intracranial pressure increases, lying down may exacerbate the headache, as may straining at stool, coughing, or bending over, and a more generalized headache may develop. Nocturnal awakening is common but not diagnostic. Projectile vomiting is a late complication.

Brain Tumor. In brain tumor, headache may be the sole initial complaint, unaccompanied by focal neurologic deficits. However, as the condition progresses, new neurologic deficits usually ensue. *Brain abscess* may present as a mass lesion causing headache, especially in its later stages. Parenteral drug abuse, lung abscess, or parameningeal infection may serve as the source of infection. Fever and focal neurologic deficits are often absent.

Chronic Subdural Hematoma. Chronic subdural hematoma, another important mass lesion, typically presents in a subtle fashion, with head trauma followed by a symptom-free interval. The injury may be forgotten, but changes in mental status and, eventually, focal neurologic deficits begin to develop.

Pseudotumor Cerebri. This condition can mimic the clinical presentation of tumor. Characteristic features include onset of headache in an obese, young woman, papilledema on fundoscopic examination, and compressed ventricles on computed tomography.

Nonmigrainous Cerebrovascular Sources

Ischemic events may be associated with acute headache. The pain most often occurs on the side of the lesion but may be frontal or diffuse. In some instances, the headache is a consequence of the ensuing cerebral edema. *Arteriovenous malformation* and berry *aneurysm* are much-feared causes of vascular intracranial headache. Acute rupture of an aneurysm produces a headache of sudden onset that reaches maximum intensity immediately and is often accompanied by meningeal irritation. In the absence of any rupture, 10% to 15% of patients with an arteriovenous malformation may experience a chronic headache characterized by unilateral (always the same side) throbbing pain. Unlike migraine, such headaches are not associated with prodromal or other symptoms. Berry aneurysms are silent until they rupture unless they are larger than 2 cm, in which case they may present with headache similar to that caused by a mass lesion.

Migraine Headache (11)

Migraine affects about 12% of adults, and women three times more frequently than men. Despite the fact that migraine is associated with high rates of disability, most patients with migraine have never had their condition diagnosed by a doctor or treated with prescription medications. In 2007, the American Migraine Prevalence and Prevention study confirmed the stability of migraine epidemiologic profile over the last 15 years and, unfortunately, also confirmed that almost one in three patients who met criteria for migraine prophylaxis were not receiving treatment. *Family history* is present in nearly two thirds of cases, especially in patients who have a history of migraine with aura. Migraine headaches usually begin in childhood or young adult life, although in about 16% of women afflicted by migraine, the headaches first develop at the time of menopause. The condition tends to improve in many women during pregnancy, although *oral contraceptives* have been known to precipitate migraine or convert migraine without aura into migraine with aura. In roughly one in seven women with migraine, headache occurs only during the first few days of *menses*, although many women experience an exacerbation at this time. Bidirectional influences of *depression* and migraine appear to exist. The estimated relative risk for major depression associated with prior migraine is 3.2, and the adjusted relative risk for migraine associated with prior major depression is 3.1.

Mechanisms.   A number of hypotheses have been advanced to explain migraine and account for its phases. The *neurogenic–inflammatory hypothesis* enjoys considerable support. It views migraine as a primary neuronal event, with secondary neurotransmitter-mediated changes in vasculature and blood flow. Neuropeptides are believed to act as neurotransmitters at trigeminal nerve branches, precipitating an inflammatory process with vasodilation. *Serotonin receptors* are believed to be important in mediating these events, which can be triggered by a variety of stimuli (mechanical, electrical, or chemical). The clinical phenomenon of aura is now believed to be due to a slowly spreading band of "cortical depression" or decreased neuronal function.

Classification.   Migraine formerly was designated as *classic* if accompanied by prodromal symptoms (see later discussion) and as *common* if not. This taxonomy has been replaced by migraine *with aura* and *migraine without aura*. Tables 165.1 and 165.2 show the diagnostic criteria for migraine without aura and migraine with aura. Both types of migraine are accompanied by nausea and photophobia. The new classification system requires that at least two of the following be present to establish a diagnosis of migraine headache: unilateral location, pulsating quality, moderate to severe intensity, and exacerbation by physical activity. At least one of the following must accompany the headache: nausea or vomiting, photophobia, and phonophobia.

Precipitants and Complications.   Precipitants of migraine include emotional upset, menstruation, and, in some people, ingestion of tyramine- or tryptophan-rich foods (e.g., ripe cheeses, red wine, chocolate). Headache may occur shortly

---

TABLE 165.1

INTERNATIONAL HEADACHE SOCIETY DEFINITION OF MIGRAINE WITHOUT AURA (COMMON MIGRAINE)

Diagnostic Criteria
  At least five attacks
  Headache lasting 4 to 72 hr (untreated or unsuccessfully treated)
  Headache with at least two of the following characteristics:
    Unilateral location
    Pulsating quality
    Moderate or severe intensity (inhibits or prohibits daily activities)
    Aggravated by walking stairs or similar routine physical activity
  During headache, at least one of the following:
    Nausea and/or vomiting
    Photophobia and phonophobia

From Headache Classification Committee of the International Headache Society. Classification and diagnostic criteria for headache disorders, cranial neuralgias, and facial pain. Cephalalgia 1988;8(Suppl 7):1, with permission.

---

after or just before a period of psychological stress. Some patients experience a seemingly paradoxical flare-up of migraine on weekends or vacations.

The most serious complication is *ischemic stroke*. The risk is slightly increased overall and occurs predominantly in patients who have migraine with aura. In women of childbearing age with migraine, the risk of stroke increases with the use of oral contraceptives and is exacerbated by smoking and hypertension. Of some concern is the frequency of white matter lesions (especially in the posterior fossa) noted on brain magnetic resonance imaging in persons with migraine, suggesting

---

TABLE 165.2

INTERNATIONAL HEADACHE SOCIETY DEFINITION OF MIGRAINE WITH AURA (CLASSIC MIGRAINE)

Previously used terms: classic migraine; ophthalmic, hemiparesthetic, hemiplegic, or aphasic migraine

Diagnostic Criteria
  At least two attacks
  At least three of the following four characteristics:
    One or more fully reversible aura symptoms are present, indicating focal cerebral cortical or brainstem dysfunction.
    At least one aura symptom develops gradually over >4 min, or two or more symptoms occur in succession.
    No aura symptom lasts >60 min; if more than one aura symptom is present, the accepted duration is proportionally increased.
    Headache follows aura with a free interval of <60 min (it may also begin before or simultaneously with the aura).

From Headache Classification Committee of the International Headache Society. Classification and diagnostic criteria for headache disorders, cranial neuralgias, and facial pain. Cephalalgia 1988;8(Suppl 7): 1, with permission.

that migraine may be associated with increased risk of multiple subclinical strokes.

Clinical Presentation. Attacks may comprise as many as five phases: prodrome, aura, headache, termination, and postdrome. The *prodrome* is characterized by lassitude, irritability, difficulty concentrating, and nausea. Patients with *aura* often report visual phenomena (scintillating scotomata, zigzag patterns, hemianopsia, diplopia), vertigo, aphasia, or even hemiplegia preceding the onset of the *headache*, which is typically unilateral and throbbing, although it may begin as a dull sensation and take a while to reach maximum intensity. Headache *termination* usually occurs within 24 hours but sometimes not until after 48 hours. The *postdrome* phase includes feelings of fatigue, sleepiness, or irritability. Epidemiologic studies suggest that migraineurs suffer a median of about 12 attacks per year. Many have headaches both with and without aura.

Variants. A number of variants are seen. A relatively uncommon variant is *acephalgic migraine*, in which a focal neurologic deficit may evolve during an aura but is not succeeded by headache. In rare instances, the symptoms of acephalgic migraine may persist for 1 to 2 days, simulating a stroke. *Basilar migraine* produces focal symptoms referable to the posterior circulation; it is more common in children. *Vertiginous migraine* relates to patients who have an aura of dizziness preceding typical migraine attacks.

Meningitis

Infection or hemorrhage produces pain that is acute in onset, severe, generalized, and constant. Symptoms may be particularly intense at the base of the skull and aggravated by forward flexion of the neck or by leg raising in conjunction with knee extension and foot dorsiflexion. Meningitis in young people is often meningococcal or viral in origin. A major independent risk factor for meningococcal disease in such persons is living in a college dormitory. Administration of quadrivalent polysaccharide vaccine to such persons could markedly reduce risk.

Postconcussion Headache

Postconcussion headache occurs when the wrenching and displacement of pain-sensitive structures in the central nervous system during head trauma have been severe enough to cause concussion. *Postconcussion syndrome* (posttraumatic nervous instability) is a complicated, poorly characterized state manifested by chronic refractory headache, neck pain, nervousness, emotional lability, crying spells, and inability to concentrate. The symptoms are suggestive of an agitated depression following trauma; the syndrome probably represents a variant of tension-type headache. The correlation between severity of symptoms and seriousness of the injury is minimal.

Extracranial Sources

Extracranial sites of headache include the skin, fascia, muscles, and blood vessels of the scalp; the extracranial arteries; mucous membranes of the nasal and perinasal spaces; the external and middle ear; teeth; and muscles of the scalp and facial region. Problems involving the eyes, sinuses, cervical spine, temporal mandibular joints, or cranial nerves can be important sources of headache, although some common attributions are not always correct.

Tension-Type Headache

Tension headache ranks among the leading types of chronic and recurrent headache. More than 90% are bilateral and are often described as a feeling of pressure or a bandlike sensation about the head. The pain is dull and steady in most instances, characteristically worsening as the day progresses and sometimes accompanied by occipital and nuchal soreness. The headache may last days, weeks, or even months. Recording of myographic potentials from head and neck muscles reveals vigorous contractions in some but not all patients with this type of headache. Vasoconstriction can also be detected and may account for the migraine-like symptoms (nausea, throbbing pain) experienced by some patients.

Precipitants include *anxiety*, *depression*, and *situational stress*. Patients with underlying psychopathology often describe their headache pain in vivid terms (e.g., "feels like an ax" or "lightning" or "something exploding"), yet they do so without demonstrating any apparent discomfort. So psychologically engaging is the headache that many of these patients are unaware of their underlying emotional problems. Tension-type headaches may also occur secondary to muscle strain from cervical spondylosis or temporomandibular joint disease (see later discussion).

Sinusitis

True sinusitis produces a headache that characteristically is acute in onset and worse on awakening. It gets better on arising, only to worsen again as the day progresses. The patient reports a purulent nasal discharge, and pain and skin sensitivity are predominant over the involved sinus (see Chapter 219). Many patients with other forms of headache (e.g., frontal muscle-contraction headaches) mistakenly attribute their problem to "sinusitis" and self-treat with decongestants to no avail. Because the pain of sinusitis is sometimes described as throbbing in quality and can worsen when the patient bends over, it may be mistaken for migraine or the headache of a intracranial mass lesion.

Giant Cell Arteritis

Also referred to as *temporal arteritis* or *cranial arteritis*, this disease of older persons (almost all are older than age 50 years) affects medium and large arteries (especially those of the extracranial vasculature) and can cause blindness if it spreads to the ophthalmic artery. The headache may begin as a throbbing discomfort and progress to a dull, aching pain. Some patients describe burning, and others note bouts of lancinating pain. Scalp tenderness (especially when the hair is combed) localized to the involved vessel(s) is characteristic. However, the inflamed artery may not always be tender or palpable, and although the temporal artery is commonly involved, it need not be. Jaw (masticatory muscle) claudication is often part of the clinical picture, and the condition is strongly associated with *polymyalgia rheumatica* (see Chapter 161).

The most-feared complication is *blindness*, which occurs when arteritis results in occlusion of the ophthalmic artery, usually about 1 to 2 months after the onset of headache. Diplopia may precede and is predictive of visual impairment (50% risk). Once visual impairment sets in, it progresses quickly over several hours to total visual loss (see Chapter 161).

Temporomandibular Joint Dysfunction (TMJ)

TMJ has received much attention in the lay press as a common, sometimes overlooked cause of chronic refractory headache. Occasionally, the problem is caused by joint changes resulting from malocclusion. However, the problem in most cases is not malocclusion, but rather tension-induced jaw clenching and nocturnal teeth grinding (*bruxism*). Such chronic involuntary oral habits lead to masticator muscle fatigue and spasm. Chronic dull, aching, unilateral discomfort may be described about the jaw, behind the eyes and the ears, and even down the neck into the shoulders. Jaw pain, clicking sounds, and difficulty opening the mouth in the morning are characteristic. Chewing may exacerbate symptoms; locking of the jaw is common. On physical examination, masticatory muscle tenderness, mandibular hypomotility, and joint clicking and deviation on opening are noted. Molar prominences may be flat from chronic grinding of the teeth (see Chapter 225).

Cluster Headache

The pathophysiology of cluster headache is obscure, although extracerebral vasodilation appears to be a component. It occurs predominantly in middle-aged men and is the only type of headache more common in men than in women. Cluster headache is distinguished by its location, timing, and periodicity. In the most typical presentation, seen in more than 50% of cases, patients describe an intense, nonthrobbing, unilateral headache "behind the eye" that is searing, stabbing, or burning and accompanied by ipsilateral lacrimation, nasal stuffiness, and facial flushing. In 20% to 40% of cases, ipsilateral ptosis and miosis are also present. Headache typically begins a few hours after the patient goes to bed and lasts for 30 to 90 minutes. Attacks occur nightly for 2 to 3 months and then disappear, only to return several months to years later. About 10% of these patients have *chronic cluster headache*, in which attacks occur daily for 1 to 2 years; periodicity is not noted. These headaches are sometimes confused with migraine because they are unilateral and severe, but the pain is not throbbing, and most of the other defining features of migraine are lacking.

Indomethacin-Responsive Headache

Headaches in this group include chronic paroxysmal hemicrania, ice pick headache, and hemicrania continua. *Chronic paroxysmal hemicrania* is a rare cluster variant occurring predominantly among women and characterized by a similarly severe unilateral facial pain; unlike cluster, these headaches occur in short spasms of 10 to 20 minutes up to 20 or 30 times per day. Horner's syndrome and ipsilateral tearing are often noted. *Ice pick headache* occurs in patients suffering from migraine, although not exclusively. The headache is brief, sharp, and jabbing. *Hemicrania continua* differs from the other types in causing continuous unilateral aching discomfort, although it is accentuated by ipsilateral jabbing pain.

Systemic Infection and Fever

These conditions are among the most common causes of cranial vasodilation and diffuse, throbbing headache. The headache that frequently accompanies a *viral syndrome* is typical. Numerous *metabolic disturbances* and *drugs* may lead to vasodilation and headache. A pounding headache is a prominent symptom of early carbon monoxide poisoning and a common complaint of patients who take nitrates for angina or vasodilators for other conditions.

Hypertension

Moderate to severe *hypertension* (diastolic pressures >110 mm Hg) sometimes results in occipital headaches. The mechanism of the headache is unknown. The discomfort is worse in the morning and recedes as the day progresses. This headache resolves with correction of the hypertension. It should not be confused with the muscle-contraction and psychogenic headaches that account for most of the headaches occurring in hypertensive patients or with the headache caused by the increased intracranial pressure that accompanies malignant hypertension.

Ocular Sources

Headaches are often attributed to eye problems, especially when they are felt about the orbit. *Eyestrain* is often blamed for headaches, although in most instances, the attribution is incorrect, and refraction fails to improve the problem. However, in an occasional patient, astigmatism can cause difficulty when the eyes are used for close work for prolonged periods. It produces ocular muscle imbalance and sustained contraction of extraocular, frontal, and temporal muscles; aching discomfort about the orbit and the frontotemporal region results. Refraction corrects the problem. *Acute glaucoma* may produce an orbital headache of sudden onset that is accompanied by cloudy vision (see Chapters 201 and 207).

Cervical Radiculopathy

Headache is commonly the first symptom of cervical radiculopathy. The pain arises during mechanical irritation of an upper cervical root. Findings on radiography of the cervical spine are variable, ranging from normal to spondylotic. The pain is often localized to one side of the occiput or base of the skull, in conjunction with tenderness to palpation. It may start in the neck and at times even radiate to the forehead or eye. The discomfort is described as nagging or aching and is aggravated by *neck movement*. The headache tends to be worse on awakening, perhaps because of unconscious neck motion during sleep. The mechanism of pain is believed to involve entrapment of upper cervical nerve roots as they course toward the occiput through irritated nuchal ligaments and muscles. *Occipital neuralgia* is a particularly common variant. Patients describe sudden lancinating pain in the distribution of the greater occipital nerve, which may be precipitated by turning over in bed and is often relieved by sitting up.

Trigeminal Neuralgia (Tic Douloureux)

Trigeminal neuralgia (*tic douloureux*) is one of the most severe pain syndromes known. Paroxysms of lancinating facial or cranial pain occur in middle-aged or elderly patients; these may last only a few seconds but can be excruciating and recurrent. The jaw, gums, lips, or maxillary region may be involved. Characteristically, a trigger zone is located within the region of pain (see Chapter 176).

Syndrome of Chronic Daily Headache

Patients presenting with chronic daily headache (CDH) pose a clinical challenge. The International Headache Society defines the CDH syndrome as the presence of headache on more than 15 days per month for greater than 3 months. The entities comprising it are a diverse group and include *chronic migraine*, *chronic tension-type headache*, *new daily persistent headache*, *chronic cluster headache*, and *hemicrania continua*.

DIFFERENTIAL DIAGNOSIS (15)

For differential diagnosis, headache can be divided into primary and secondary headaches. The primary headache

TABLE 165.3

IMPORTANT CAUSES OF HEADACHE

Acute
  Meningitis
  Intracranial hemorrhage (stroke, rupture of aneurysm)
  Stroke
  Acute increase in intracranial pressure (mostly from
    cerebral edema or hemorrhage, including hypertensive
    encephalopathy)
  Acute glaucoma
  Acute sinusitis
  Acute metabolic disturbance (carbon monoxide poisoning,
    hypoglycemia)
  Acute viral illness
  Initial presentation of a persistent or recurrent headache
Persistent or Recurrent
  Intracranial mass lesion (neoplasm, abscess, subdural
    hematoma, large arteriovenous malformation)
  Tension-type headache
  Migraine, with and without aura
  Cluster headache
  Indomethacin-responsive headache (ice pick, paroxysmal
    hemicrania)
  Postconcussion syndrome
  Cervical spine disease
  Giant cell arteritis
  Trigeminal neuralgia
  Hypertension
  Arteriovenous malformation
  Bruxism/temporomandibular joint dysfunction
  Medications
  Substance abuse

syndromes include migraine with and without aura, cluster headache, and tension-type headache (Table 165.3).

WORKUP (1,7,8,15–17)

The first priority is to distinguish the worrisome headache from the harmless one. Headaches of concern are those that are sudden in onset, severe, or persistent. Despite the advent of elaborate imaging techniques, the history and physical examination remain indispensable.

The goal of the workup is to distinguish one of the primary headache syndromes (migraine with or without aura, cluster headache, tension-type headache) from a headache secondary to a mechanical or systemic process that would dictate a different therapy.

History

The time invested in obtaining a full description of the headache, particularly its clinical course, associated symptoms, precipitants, aggravating and alleviating factors, and patient concerns, is well worth the effort. The information obtained is often diagnostic, always critical to intelligent test selection, and essential to dealing effectively with patient worries and expectations. The medication history is also critical because a number of agents (e.g., indomethacin, nifedipine, cimetidine, captopril, nitrates, atenolol, trimethoprim/sulfamethoxazole, aspirin/dipyridamole combination [Aggrenox], oral contracep-

tives) can trigger nonspecific headaches. Drug-related intracranial hypertension can be seen with minocycline, isoretinoin, nalidixic acid, tetracycline, trimethoprim/sulfamethoxazole, cimetidine, corticosteroids, and tamoxifen.

The history pertinent to a new headache differs slightly from that for chronic or recurrent headache.

Headache of New Onset

History should include inquiry into any *associated neurologic deficits*, *fever*, or *neck stiffness*. The patient unaccustomed to having headaches who presents with the sudden onset of the "*worst headache ever experienced*" deserves prompt attention, particularly if fever, neck stiffness, ataxia, alteration in mental status, focal neurologic deficit, or visual impairment is reported. Diffuse headache in conjunction with a stiff neck and fever suggests acute meningitis. When acute headache and *stiff neck* occur in conjunction with *gait ataxia* and profuse nausea and vomiting, a midline cerebellar hemorrhage must be considered. Early recognition is important because urgent surgical treatment can be life-saving. Abrupt onset of a headache that reaches maximum intensity immediately suggests rupture of a cerebral aneurysm. Hypertensive encephalopathy may be heralded by diffuse headache, nausea, vomiting, and altered mental status. Acute fever with frontal and orbital headache is suggestive of acute sinusitis. Eye pain and blurred vision raise the possibility of acute glaucoma. New onset of headache in an elderly patient requires consideration of temporal arteritis. Acute onset of a throbbing headache should trigger inquiry into migrainous epiphenomena (prodromal and aural symptoms), febrile illness, vasodilator use, carbon monoxide exposure, drug withdrawal, and hypoglycemia. A throbbing headache accompanied neurologic deficits may be migrainous, but if deficits persist beyond 12 hours, then stroke and other causes should be considered.

Recurrent or Persistent Headache

With migraine and tension-type headaches being the most common causes of chronic or recurrent headaches and brain tumor being the most feared, the history becomes critical to the evaluation. The *clinical course* can be particularly revealing. Increases in severity, frequency, or both with time raise the question of an intracranial mass lesion, whereas a headache pattern that remains constant or waxes and wanes is more typical of tension-type or migraine headache. The nightly occurrence of headache for some time followed by symptom-free intervals is among the most characteristic features of cluster headache.

In acute headache, the severity of the pain helps to identify an increased risk for serious pathology; however, in chronic or recurrent headache, the intensity of the pain is of little value. Most patients have headaches with different degrees of pain at different times. The headache of a brain tumor may begin as a relatively minor complaint, whereas the pain of a migraine, cluster, or tension-type headache may be excruciating. Careful attention to *associated symptoms* is always essential. Inquiry into migrainous epiphenomena can be diagnostic, and eliciting a report of a new neurologic deficit strongly increases the likelihood of tumor. *Location* and *quality* are sometimes helpful, although the overlap among headaches with different causes can be considerable. Whole-head, bandlike, and occipital–nuchal distributions suggest tension-type headache, as does tightness or a pressure-like quality, but such sensations may also be reported when intracranial pressure is increased. A unilateral location and throbbing are characteristic of migraine but sometimes are reported by patients with tension-type headache.

Unilaterality and stereotypical location suggest that the headache is caused by a mass lesion.

Associated symptoms are important for the identification of other causes of chronic or recurrent headache. Temporomandibular joint pain suggests bruxism, whereas jaw claudication and scalp vessel tenderness indicate giant cell arteritis. Concurrent shoulder and hip-girdle discomfort provide supporting evidence. Neck pain raises the question of a cervical radiculopathy. Purulent nasal discharge is indicative of sinus disease. A history of head trauma, parameningeal infection, depression, situational stress, or substance abuse and a family history of headache should always be sought, and a careful medication history must be taken. Of particular concern is *rebound headache*, a pattern of headache caused by overuse of analgesic medication, particularly those preparations containing barbiturates, ergotamine compounds, or the serotonergic agonists known as triptans. Patients with rebound headache have fallen into a pattern of overuse of medication with consequent withdrawal headache.

Aggravating and *precipitating factors* deserve investigation. Headache worsened by straining, coughing, or bending over is characteristic of an intracranial mass lesion; bending over may also exacerbate the headache of sinusitis. Headache brought on by ingesting certain foods or beverages (chocolate, cheese, red wine) is typical of migraine, which is also exacerbated by noise, odors, and bright light. Alcohol may also trigger cluster headache during a period of disease activity. Migraine can be induced or exacerbated by a host of drugs, including cimetidine, ethinyl estradiol, atenolol, indomethacin, danazol, nifedipine, selegiline, and oral contraceptives.

Risk factors are important to review, especially for brain tumor (e.g., ionizing radiation, prior history of a cancer with potential for brain metastasis [breast, melanoma, lung, renal cell], AIDS, neurofibromatosis). Initial concerns about cellular telephone use being a risk factor for brain cancer were not confirmed by controlled studies, but long-term data are limited, making it impossible to rule out a long lead-time effect. Also unsubstantiated are risks from exposure to high-tension power lines, hair dyes, head trauma, and *N*-nitrosourea compounds. It should be remembered that migraine patients, particularly those with severe headache-related disability, have a high prevalence of somatic symptoms, with a synergistic relationship between major depression and high physical complaint severity (26).

Physical Examination

Acute Headache

The physical examination contributes significantly to the search for serious underlying disease. The blood pressure and temperature should be checked for elevations, the scalp for cranial artery tenderness, the sinuses for purulent discharge and tenderness, the pupils for loss of reactivity, the corneas for clouding (indicative of acute glaucoma), the disc margins for papilledema, and the neck for rigidity on anterior flexion. A neurologic examination should be performed to check for ataxia, alteration of mental status, focal deficits, and meningeal signs.

Chronic or Recurrent Headache

The physical examination begins with a check of all the areas mentioned in the evaluation of acute headache and expands into other areas based on findings from the history. For example, in a patient with a headache history that includes facial pain, the oral cavity should be examined for a trigger zone indicative of trigeminal neuralgia, the teeth for signs of bruxism, the temporomandibular joint for limitation of motion and crepitus, and the neck for signs of degenerative disease (see Chapter 148) and movements that reproduce head pain. Excessively taut muscles and focal tenderness about the shoulders, neck, and occiput are noted in many patients with tension-type headache. A careful and complete neurologic examination is essential because the finding of a fixed focal deficit is important evidence of intracranial pathology. Suspicion of a mass lesion necessitates consideration of brain abscess in addition to malignancy and subdural hematoma. Under such circumstances, the nasal cavity is examined for purulent discharge, the sinuses for tenderness, and the ears for signs of chronic otitis media (see Chapter 218). Both sinusitis and chronic otitis are potential foci for parameningeal infection that can lead to brain abscess.

Laboratory Studies

Acute Headache

Patients with acute onset of the "worst headache ever," especially if accompanied by meningeal signs or evidence of increased intracranial pressure, require prompt hospitalization. In such settings, emergency *computed tomography* is the test of choice for prompt detection of potentially life-threatening but treatable lesions (e.g., midline cerebellar hemorrhage or central nervous system mass). In patients with signs of meningeal irritation, *lumbar puncture* and examination and culture of the cerebrospinal fluid should follow computed tomography to rule out an infectious cause, provided no evidence of markedly increased intracranial pressure is found. Persons at greatest pretest risk for increased intracranial pressure are those with immunocompromise, age greater than 60 years, recent seizure, a history of central nervous system diseases, new focal neurologic deficit, or altered mental status. New onset of headache in an elderly patient, especially if accompanied by cranial artery or scalp tenderness, dictates determination of the *erythrocyte sedimentation rate* to check for giant cell arteritis. In addition, a *temporal artery biopsy* should be considered (see Chapter 161).

Chronic or Recurrent Headache

Much of the controversy and discrepancies regarding the proper evaluation of headache result from the failure to differentiate patients who present with a first headache from those who have a chronic, recurring headache. In the presence of normal physical examination findings and a headache history that does not suggest intracranial disease but classifies the patient's headache clearly into a recurring migrainous type, ancillary studies are not likely to be useful.

A disturbing trend toward uncritically ordering neuroimaging studies (*computed tomography, magnetic resonance imaging*) for all patients with recurrent or chronic headache has led to escalating costs for evaluations that provide no more information than did the initial headache history and physical examination. The probability of a patient with chronic headache and normal neurologic examination findings having a positive neuroimaging study is exceedingly small. The yield is so low that in the absence of a very worrisome history or a neurologic deficit on physical examination, an imaging study is not needed. Some feel that the reassurance value of such testing can be helpful, but most patients with benign chronic headache who fear serious underlying disease can be adequately reassured if time is taken to review the clinical findings and directly address patient concerns. Such steps are essential to providing meaningful reassurance and usually obviate the need for an otherwise medically unnecessary imaging procedure exposing the patient to radiation (for computed tomography) and to the possibility of incidental findings (for magnetic resonance imaging) that may add to overall anxiety.

Nonetheless, there are a few situations in which a neuroimaging study might still be appropriate in the absence of abnormalities on physical and neurologic examinations. These exceptions include patients with a headache of *recent onset* (<6 months) the cause of which is still not apparent after a thorough history and physical examination. In addition, those with a persistent headache that is *worsening* with time and does not fit the pattern of a tension-type headache should be considered for imaging study. When one uncovers a history of *aura symptoms* or *loss of consciousness* suggestive of a seizure (see Chapter 170), then a search for an intracranial mass lesion is warranted. If the patient or family member reports a *persistent personality change*, a tumor of the frontal or temporal regions might be suspected. Finally, if a *change in the character* of longstanding headache is noted or if the headache fails to respond to treatment directed at an initially suspected diagnosis, such as migraine, the usefulness of magnetic resonance imaging or computed tomography increases.

The efforts taken to perform a careful history and physical examination are well worth the time because these methods remain the best means for efficient test selection and accurate diagnosis of headache.

PRINCIPLES OF MANAGEMENT

Migraine (8,9,18–25)

Migraine is the one headache disorder for which relatively specific therapy exists; therefore, establishing its presence is extremely important to the patient. The neurogenic hypothesis has refocused attention from vasodilators to drugs designed to act on serotonin receptors. Several older drugs useful in the prophylaxis of migraine (e.g., methysergide, cyproheptadine) have been found to act as 5-HT$_2$ serotonin receptor antagonists. The drugs most useful in acute migraine attacks (e.g., *ergotamine*, triptans) interact with the presynaptic serotonin 5-HT$_{1D}$ and 5-HT$_{1B}$ receptors, interrupting the cycle of neurotransmitter-mediated inflammation and pain.

For most patients, the combination of a tolerable prophylactic medication with occasional use of analgesics or abortive regimens should minimize the intrusion of this highly disabling condition into their daily lives. Because most prophylactic drugs require several weeks to several months to establish efficacy, it is particularly important to maintain a strong and sympathetic relationship with each patient being treated for migraine.

Prophylaxis

Most patients with migraine can be helped by the implementation of both prophylactic and abortive measures. Once the diagnosis is established by the criteria of the most recent classification system, the physician should ascertain the frequency of disabling headache. As a general rule, if headaches are interfering with work or other activities more than once a week, it is reasonable to consider prophylactic medication. Educating the migraine-prone patient to avoid precipitants such as certain foods (cheese, chocolate, citrus fruits, nuts, red wine—although not invariably in all patients), inadequate sleep, and prolonged fasting may help to prevent some headaches. Useful information on precipitants is sometimes derived by keeping a *headache diary*.

Nonpharmacologic Measures. Prevention of attacks involves a number of *nonpharmacologic measures* in addition to drug treatment. Because migraine may be precipitated by emotional stress or psychological conflict, it is important to investigate family, work, and social circumstances to design a program of prevention. Regular *exercise* and *relaxation techniques* (see Chapter 226) may significantly decrease the frequency and severity of headaches. These activities help to reduce the impact of stress. Many patients prefer to try them before attempting other forms of therapy. Patients under significant psychological stress may benefit from informal supportive psychotherapy, which helps them to express their feelings and deal with the stress. Although extensive psychotherapy may not reduce the number of attacks, it is worth trying to pinpoint areas of stress and search with the patient for ways to resolve them. Recommending rest or a vacation may not suffice; in fact, flare-ups are common during vacations and weekends. *Biofeedback* is of unproven benefit and probably no better than relaxation exercises and other nonpharmacologic methods. The lack of adequately designed studies limits conclusions regarding biofeedback.

Pharmacologic Measures. Drug therapy should be added when nonpharmacologic measures do not suffice. Several different classes of drugs have been useful in the prophylaxis of migraine; the doses and side effects are outlined in Table 165.4. An approach of trial and error is often necessary before the appropriate medication that is most effective with the fewest side effects in any individual patient can be found. Each drug should be given at least a 2-month trial, and many patients require longer than this before full benefit is obtained.

Beta-Blockers. These are first-line prophylactic agents, capable of reducing frequency and severity of attacks by at least 50%. In most instances modest doses suffice, but sometimes such high doses are required that fatigue develops and an alternative must be sought.

Calcium-Channel Blockers. A pharmacologic alternative in persons who cannot take or tolerate high doses of beta-blockers is the calcium-channel blocker verapamil. Only the sustained-release formulation should be used, and the drug should be avoided in persons with heart failure or heart block.

Angiotensin Blockers. Both angiotensin-converting-enzyme inhibitors and angiotensin II–receptor blockers demonstrate prophylactic efficacy in migraine, suggesting a general benefit related to inhibition of angiotensin II. About one third of patients experience a greater than 50% reduction in frequency and severity of headaches; mean reduction is about 30%.

Tricyclic Antidepressants. Tricyclic antidepressants (e.g., *nortriptyline*, *amitriptyline*) are an appropriate first-line choice, especially in view of the increasingly evident relationship between migraine and major depression, but weight gain is an undesirable complication of this type of therapy.

Nonsteroidal Antiinflammatory Agents (NSAIDs). Antiinflammatory agents such as generic naproxen and ibuprofen have been useful, especially for patients with menstrual

TABLE 165.4

DRUGS FOR MIGRAINE HEADACHE PROPHYLAXIS

Drug	Recommended Dosage	Side Effects/Special Considerations
Beta-Blockers		
Propranolol	40–320 mg/d	Full beta-blockade required; 3 mo may be necessary to achieve full benefit
Nadolol	40–240 mg/d	
Atenolol	50–150 mg/d	Contraindications: congestive heart failure, asthma
Timolol	10–30 mg/d	Side effects: drowsiness, exercise intolerance, depression
Tricyclic Antidepressants		
Amitriptyline	10–150 mg/d	Efficacy in headache treatment is independent of antidepressant effect and may occur earlier and with lower doses than the antidepressant effect
Nortriptyline	10–125 mg/d	
Doxepin	10–150 mg/d	Side effects: drowsiness, urinary retention, weight gain
Calcium-Channel Blocker		
Verapamil	240–320 mg/d	May require 1 mo for perceived benefit Contraindications: congestive heart failure, heart block, atrial fibrillation, sick sinus syndrome Side effects: hypotension, atrioventricular block, headache, constipation, edema, congestive heart failure
Nonsteroidal Antiinflammatory Drug		
Naproxen	500 mg twice daily	Particularly useful for women with menstrual migraine, taken for several days perimenstruation Side effects: gastrointestinal upset, ulcers, worsening renal function in susceptible patients Contraindications: ulcer, aspirin sensitivity, renal failure
Antiepileptic Drugs		
Valproate	Titration to therapeutic level from 250 mg thrice daily	Side effects: nausea, platelet dysfunction, hair loss, hepatotoxicity; teratogenicity: neural tube defects
Topiramate	25–100 mg twice daily	Cognitive dysfunction, weight loss, renal calculi

migraine. They are prescribed for several days before, during, and after menstruation.

Antiepileptic Drugs (AEDs). Some AEDs have shown efficacy in migraine prophylaxis. *Valproate,* the only Food and Drug Administration–approved drug of this category, is useful in patients with migraine but is limited by its teratogenic potential (neural tube defects) and tendency to cause hair loss and weight gain. Of the other AEDS studied for migraine prophylaxis, *topiramate* has achieved the most promising results. Major side effects of topiramate include cognitive difficulties, weight loss, and renal calculi. However, as of 2008, this is probably the drug most frequently prescribed by neurologists for migraine prophylaxis. In doses of 200 mg/d or more, topiramate has the potential to induce metabolism of oral contraceptives, and patients should be warned to use an additional barrier method of contraception if their medication requirement is in this range.

Vitamins. Promising results in small-scale, short-term studies suggest a possible prophylactic role for high-dose *riboflavin (vitamin B$_2$)*; when given in doses of 400 mg/d, it reduces the frequency and total number of headache days, and riboflavin may be a useful adjunct to other prophylactic regimens.

Abortive Therapy

For the patient with only occasional migraine headaches and for patients with generally well-controlled but occasional se-

vere breakthrough headaches, it is important to establish an effective abortive regimen. Options range from nonpharmacologic measures, analgesics, and NSAIDs to triptans and ergot compounds. Two contrasting strategies toward abortive therapy have emerged: *stepped care* (starting with simple measures and escalating according to response within a single attack or over several attacks) and *stratified care* (treating from the start according to severity of attack). In one of the few randomized trials of treatment strategies, stratified care proved superior in terms of headache response and disability.

Selective 5-HT$_{1B/1D}$ Agonists(Triptans). The triptans have revolutionized the management of migraine headache. Several are now on the market. The participants in the "triptan wars" are outlined in Table 165.5. Both sumatriptan and the second-generation triptans are cerebral and coronary vasoconstrictors; they act by both vasoconstriction and inhibition of neurogenic inflammation. The drugs differ in their bioavailability and half-lives. A single 6-mg subcutaneous dose of sumatriptan has proved to be highly effective; it acts rapidly and is well tolerated in the treatment of severe migraine attacks. Sumatriptan is now available as a subcutaneous autoinjection formulation, tablets, and nasal spray. In general, the second-generation triptans have better oral pharmacokinetic properties than sumatriptan does, and they last longer. Therefore, the initial relief of headache is at least as good as that with oral sumatriptan, and the recurrence rate may be lower. Recurrence may be minimized with the longer-acting triptans, such as naratriptan or

TABLE 165.5

TRIPTANS

Drug (Generic/Brand)	Route	Dose (mg)	$T_{1/2}$ (hr)	Onset (hr)	Recurrence
Sumatriptan/Imitrex	SC	6[a]	2	1/6–1/4	45% (all routes)
	PO	25, 50,[a] 100	2	1–1.5	
	Nasal	5, 20[a]		1/4	
Zolmitriptan/Zomig	PO	2.5,[a] 5	3	1	22%
Naratriptan/Amerge	PO	2.5[a]	6	1	19%–28%
Rizatriptan/Maxalt	PO	5, 10[a]	1.5	1	30%
Rizatriptan/Maxalt MLT	SL	5, 10	As for PO	As for PO	As for PO
Eletriptan/Relpax	PO	40,[a] 80	4–5	1	—
Almotriptan/Axert	PO	12.5	3	1	—
Frovatriptan/Frova	PO	2.5	24	1	Very low

All: 5-HT$_{1B/1D}$ agonists, cerebral and coronary vasoconstrictors. Variable: pharmacokinetics and lipophilicity.
PO, oral; SC, subcutaneous; SL, sublingual.
[a]Preferred initial dose.

frovatriptan. A second dose of any of the triptans may be effective, but overuse of the triptans can result in a rebound phenomenon. The use of sumatriptan and other triptans should be restricted to no more than 1 to 2 days weekly.

Contraindications. Recent use of *monoamine oxidase inhibitors, uncontrolled hypertension, coronary artery disease,* and *pregnancy* are the main contraindications. Patients should not take triptans during the aura phase of the migraine, and patients with complicated auras such as hemiparesis or dysphasia should not receive triptan therapy. Those on selective serotonin-reuptake inhibitors may take triptans, but the dose of both medicines should be monitored carefully.

Side Effects. Sumatriptan injection is safe for large numbers of patients despite the fact up to 40% of patients report *chest-related symptoms* when specifically asked about them. The initial theoretical concerns about possible ischemia have been allayed by large-scale follow-up studies that found not a single clear incident of myocardial infarction within 24 hours of sumatriptan injection, no deaths, and no increased incidence of stroke.

Dihydroergotamine. The subcutaneous, intramuscular, intravenous, or nasal administration of ergot is highly effective. Parenteral administration in emergency department settings has helped to terminate severe, acute attacks of migraine. Although the vasoconstrictive effects of dihydroergotamine on peripheral arteries are minimal, it is contraindicated in patients with coronary disease, peripheral vascular disease, transient ischemic attacks, pregnancy, or sepsis. Nausea is a significant problem and may be minimized by prior intravenous administration of metoclopramide (Reglan).

Analgesics and Sedatives. Many patients find prompt use of NSAIDs quite helpful, but barbiturate-containing analgesics remain the most frequently prescribed remedy for migraine. In general, it is best to avoid the regular use of analgesics and sedatives. Popular combination analgesic and sedative formulations containing either acetaminophen or aspirin with butalbital and caffeine (e.g., *Fioricet* and *Fiorinal*) are often requested by patients because they were widely prescribed in the past. Although they may be helpful for occasional use, marked caution is warranted in prescribing such combination agents

because of their potential for habituation when used regularly in a chronic recurring condition such as migraine and because of the development of rebound headache patterns. *Narcotic analgesics* are sometimes needed, but their regular use can lead to a vicious cycle of headache, narcotic intake, drug withdrawal, more headache, and more narcotic intake (see later discussion).

Antiemetics. Nausea can be problematic but may respond to *NSAIDs,* prokinetic drugs (e.g., *metoclopramide*), or antiemetic compounds (e.g., *prochlorperazine*). The administration of antiemetics and metoclopramide 30 minutes before analgesics improves oral absorption, combats nausea, and increases the efficacy of aspirin, acetaminophen, and caffeine-containing compounds.

Minimizing Stroke Risk

Although the risk for ischemic stroke is low in patients who have migraine without aura, the odds ratio for stroke in patients who have migraine with aura is increased (to approximately 6). *Oral contraceptives,* even those with a low estrogen content of less than 50 μg, appear to cause an increase in ischemic stroke risk, with an odds ratio of about 2. Many neurologists discourage the use of oral contraceptives in patients who have migraine with aura and in older female patients who have migraine with other risk factors for stroke such as smoking or hypertension.

Cluster Headache (1)

As with migraine, both abortive and prophylactic treatments are available. One abortive treatment for an acute attack consists of inhalation of oxygen (5 to 8 L/min for 10 minutes). *Ergotamine* suppositories may be effective and can be taken at bedtime during a cluster by a patient whose symptoms occur at night. Dihydroergotamine (intramuscular or intravenous as outlined previously) is effective, as is *sumatriptan,* particularly the subcutaneous form. A corticosteroid bolus of 8 mg of dexamethasone or prednisone started at 20 mg three times a day and tapered during 2 weeks has also been helpful in aborting a cluster.

Prophylaxis for patients with chronic cluster headaches or for those with severe frequent cluster episodes includes 360 mg of verapamil daily, given in divided doses. Methysergide at a dose of 2 mg three times a day or *lithium* at doses achieving a therapeutic level identical to that for bipolar disease is useful. Sphenopalatine ganglion block performed by an anesthesiologist may provide significant temporary relief. A radiofrequency trigeminal rhizotomy is reserved for patients whose headaches are completely refractory to all of the foregoing medical therapies.

Tension-Type Headache (3,4,6,8,26,27)

For the vast majority of patients with mild or occasional tension headache, mild analgesics (aspirin, acetaminophen, non-prescription doses of NSAIDs) usually suffice. Such patients usually do not consult a physician. Patients with chronic or persistent tension-type headaches are candidates for evaluation of underlying anxiety and depression (see Chapters 226 and 227). Often, definitive treatment of such headaches requires that the underlying sources of psychological distress be addressed. *Stress reduction* measures may be of considerable help for those with an anxiety state (see Appendix 226.1), and *antidepressant therapy* may benefit depressed patients (see Chapter 227). Patients with chronic headache subsequent to trauma should be encouraged to conclude any pending legal proceedings.

Chronic Daily Headaches (6,8,26,27)

Chronic daily headache is among the most difficult types of headache encountered by primary physicians. In some patients, a migraine syndrome evolves into a daily headache more typical of tension-type headache with superimposed migrainous events. Depression, anxiety, and drug abuse may all complicate the picture at this stage. While counseling this group of patients about precipitating factors and lifestyle modification, it is important that the physician elicit a history of analgesic and ergotamine use. Ergotamine or analgesic abuse can lead to a vicious cycle of headache, medication, and headache. As the effect of a previous dose of ergotamine or analgesic wanes, headache begins to recur, which leads to further use of medication. Drug-induced sleep disturbances and psychological dependency ensue, leading to a self-sustaining rhythmic cycle of headache and medication. Thus, caution must be exerted to avoid prescribing large amounts of ergotamine or analgesics (both narcotic and nonnarcotic) for a patient with migraine or tension-type headache. Total elimination of analgesics and ergotamine compounds may improve the therapeutic results of other medications chosen for the prophylaxis of headache. Hospitalization for withdrawal of medication and institution of a comprehensive program may be beneficial.

Management of Other Conditions Causing Headache

See Chapter 225 for the treatment of temporomandibular joint dysfunction and bruxism. See Chapter 161 for the management of temporal arteritis and Chapter 219 for the treatment of sinusitis.

INDICATIONS FOR ADMISSION AND REFERRAL

Admission or Urgent Referral

Urgent hospitalization is indicated for the patient with acute onset of a severe headache accompanied by signs of meningeal irritation. Intracranial hemorrhage or meningeal infection may be responsible. Evidence of increased intracranial pressure is another indication for prompt admission. Severe, intractable migraine may require prompt hospital admission for one of the abortive treatments outlined previously. An ophthalmologist needs to be consulted at once if acute glaucoma is believed to be the cause of an acute orbital headache.

Elective Referral

Less urgent situations involving headache that deserve neurologic consultation include episodes of transient neurologic dysfunction, unilateral headache increasing in frequency and severity, change in personality, and new onset of progressive deficits suggestive of an evolving process or a mass lesion. Sometimes, patients with an intractable tension-type headache or severe migraine syndrome can benefit from the reassurance and suggestions provided by the neurologist. Dental consultation is indicated if temporomandibular joint problems appear to be refractory to conservative therapy. Surgical referral for a temporal artery biopsy may be necessary when an elderly patient is suspected of having giant cell arteritis but more definitive evidence that long-term steroid therapy is warranted is required (see Chapter 161). Ophthalmologic consultation for a vision check and assessment of the need for refraction is indicated if prolonged close work is resulting in headaches.

For patients with chronic, intractable, tension-type headache, a diagnostic consultation with a psychiatrist may serve as an important learning experience. However, many of these patients are reluctant to consider a psychological cause for their symptoms. Thus, it is important that a full medical evaluation be conducted before a psychiatric referral is suggested. This obviates any misunderstanding by patients who believe that their problem has a medical basis and view the referral as an inappropriate dismissal of their symptoms.

Annotated Bibliography

1. Bahra A. Cluster headache: a prospective clinical study with diagnostic implications. Neurology 2002;58:354. (*Emphasizes the overlap between migrainous and cluster-type headaches, with associated therapeutic implications.*)
2. Becker WJ. Use of oral contraceptives in patients with migraine. Neurology 1999;53(Suppl 1):S19. (*The odds ratio for stroke in patients who have migraine with aura and use oral contraceptives is increased.*)
3. Breslau N, Merikangas K, Bowden CL. Comorbidity of migraine and major affective disorders. Neurology 1996;44(Suppl 7):S17. (*This article reviews the first clear evidence of the existence of bidirectional influences of depression and migraine.*)
4. Bruce MG, Rosenstein NE, Capparella JM, et al. Risk factors for meningococcal disease in college students. JAMA 2001;286:694. (*Living in a dorm was an independent and powerful risk factor.*)
5. Chang CL, Monaghy M, Poulter N, et al. Migraine and stroke in young women: case–control study. BMJ 1999;318:8. (*Risk was increased and further exacerbated by oral contraceptive use, high blood pressure, and smoking.*)

6. Colas R, Munoz P, Temprano R, et al. Chronic daily headache with analgesic overuse. Neurology 2004;62:1338. (*Analgesic overuse–associated headache was most common in women in their 50s, among whom 5% met its diagnostic criteria.*)

7. DeAngelis LM. Brain tumors. N Engl J Med 2001;344:114. (*Detailed review, including clinical presentation and diagnosis; 87 references.*)

8. Gladstone J, Eross E, Dodick D. Chronic daily headache: a rational approach to a challenging problem. Semin Neurol 2003;23:265. (*Revised 2004 International Headache Society classification criteria; offers an approach to minimizing disability.*)

9. Goadsby PJ, Lipton RB, Ferrari MD. Migraine—current understanding and treatment. N Engl J Med 2002;346:257. (*This article goes beyond practical management considerations to discuss pathophysiologic mechanisms and helps to make sense of the various seemingly trial-and-error categories of medicines.*)

10. Kruit MC, van Buchem MA, Hofman PAM, et al. Migraine as a risk factor for subclinical brain lesions. JAMA 2004;291:427. (*A population-based study that found increased risk of posterior fossa subclinical brain lesions in female migraine patients with and without aura.*)

11. Lipton RB, Bigal ME, Diamond M, et al. Migraine prevalence, disease burden and the need for preventive therapy. Neurology 2007;68:343. (*Major epidemiologic data updating the American Migraine Study II from 2001.*)

12. Muscat JE, Malkin MG, Thompson S, et al. Handheld cellular telephone use and risk of brain cancer. JAMA 2000;284:3001. (*A case–control study; no evidence was found to substantiate concern, but longer-term follow-up is needed.*)

13. Silberstein SD, Merriam G. Sex hormones and headache 1999 (menstrual migraine). Neurology 1999;531(Suppl 1):S3. (*A useful review of the often-contradictory evidence about hormonal influences in migraine headache.*)

14. Stewart WF. Prevalence of migraine headache in the United States. JAMA 1992;267:64. (*This is likely to become a classic article dispelling many previously held tenets about the epidemiology of migraine.*)

15. Lipton RB, Bigal ME, Steiner TJ, et al. Classification of primary headaches. Neurology 2004;63:427. (*Overview of the revised International Headache Society criteria and presentation of a differential diagnostic approach based on these criteria.*)

16. Frishberg BM. The utility of neuroimaging in the evaluation of headache in patients with normal neurologic examinations. Neurology 1994;44:1191; Practice parameter from the American Academy of Neurology. Neurology 1994;44:1353. (*Although they admit that the yield of diagnostic investigations in patients with primary headache syndromes and normal examination findings is very low, both documents leave open the role of clinical judgment.*)

17. Katzman GL, Dagher AP, Patronas NJH. Incidental findings on brain magnetic resonance imaging from 1,000 asymptomatic volunteers. JAMA 1999;282:36. (*Although incidental lesions did occur, the vast majority of patients who had a history compatible with a primary headache syndrome and normal physical examination findings had normal results on magnetic resonance imaging.*)

18. Lipton RB, Stewart WF, Stone AM, et al. Stratified care vs step care strategies for migraine: the Disability in Strategies of Care (DISC) Study: a randomized trial. JAMA. 2000;284:2599. (*One of the only randomized, controlled trials [RCTs] comparing approaches with treatment.*)

19. Mathew NT. Antiepileptic drugs in migraine prevention. Headache 2001;41(Suppl 1):18. (*From an evidence-based perspective, antiepileptic drugs [AEDS] are superior to traditional beta-blockers and tricyclic antidepressants; when factors such as cost and safety are included, however, AEDS likely should be second-line therapy for migraine prophylaxis.*)

20. O'Quinn S, Davis RL, Herman DL, et al. Prospective large-scale study of the tolerability of subcutaneous sumatriptan injection for the acute treatment of migraine. Cephalalgia 1999;19:223. (*A multicenter open-label study of 12,339 migraine patients followed for 1 year.*)

21. Silberstein SD. Divalproex sodium in headache: literature review and clinical guidelines. Headache 1996;36:547. (*Depakote has been widely promoted for migraine headache, but its side effect profile and possible teratogenic effects limit its utility as a first-line agent in patients with migraine.*)

22. Silberstein SD, for the US Headache Consortium. Practice parameter/evidence-based guidelines for migraine headache. Neurology 2000;55:754. (*Consensus guidelines on available abortive and prophylactic therapies.*)

23. Schoenen J, Jacquy J, Lenaerts M. Effectiveness of high-dose riboflavin in migraine prophylaxis: a randomized controlled trial. Neurology 1998;50:466. (*A short-term, small-scale study finding a significant reduction in frequency and number of migraine days; the results were promising, but confirmation by longer-term, larger-scale study is needed.*)

24. Schrader H, Stovner LJ, Helde G, et al. Prophylactic treatment of migraine with angiotensin converting enzyme inhibitor (lisinopril): randomised, placebo controlled, crossover study. BMJ. 2001;322:19. (*A 20% average improvement was found in frequency and severity of headaches on average; about 20% of patients have >50% reduction.*)

25. Tronvik E, Stovner LJ, Helde G, et al. Prophylactic treatment of migraine with an angiotensin II receptor blocker: a randomized controlled trial. JAMA 2003;289:65. (*About one third of patients have >50% reduction in headache frequency and severity; the average reduction is about 30%.*)

26. Tietjen GE, Brandes JL, Digre KB, et al. High prevalence of somatic symptoms and depression in women with disabling chronic headache. Neurology 2007;68:134. (*Low education and household income, as well as depression, correlate with somatic symptoms; obesity is another interrelated risk factor for chronic migraine even after adjusting for other comorbidities.*)

27. Holroyd KA, O'Donnell FJ, Stensland M, et al. Management of chronic tension-type headache with tricyclic antidepressant medication, stress management therapy and their combination: a randomized controlled trial. JAMA. 2001;285:2208. (*RCT finding benefit from each and when used in combination.*)

CHAPTER 166 ■ EVALUATION OF DIZZINESS

AMY A. PRUITT

Dizziness can be one of the more frustrating complaints to assess; the task is often made difficult by a vague history and a large number of possible causes, ranging from psychiatric disease and cardiovascular disorders to peripheral and central defects within the nervous system. However, with a bit of patience and careful attention to the history and physical examination findings, the primary physician can conduct a remarkably sophisticated clinical evaluation, one that will help to direct further workup and treatment. With the problem of true vertigo, an additional goal of the clinical examination is at times to provide immediate bedside relief from the symptom for those patients who are found to have benign positional vertigo.

PATHOPHYSIOLOGY AND CLINICAL PRESENTATION (1–6)

The patient complaining of "dizziness" may have a malfunction of virtually any organ system, including vestibular dysfunction, cardiovascular insufficiency, psychiatric illness, metabolic derangement, multiple sensory deficits, cerebellar disease, or a combination of problems.

Vestibular Disease

Patients with vestibular disease experience *true vertigo*, which is defined as a head sensation of abnormal movement or (and the distinction does not matter) abnormal movement of the environment. Descriptive terms include not only "spinning" but also "weaving," "seasickness," "ground rising and falling," "rocking," "things moving," and "merry-go-round" sensation. Nausea, vomiting, and diaphoresis accompany severe cases. Tinnitus and hearing loss indicate associated injury to the auditory component of the eighth cranial nerve. Nystagmus is frequently found on examination (see later discussion) or can be induced.

The vestibular problem may be *central* or *peripheral*; peripheral lesions include those that are *cochlear* or *retrocochlear*. Central lesions differ from peripheral ones in that they typically present with vertigo in association with other brainstem deficits; in peripheral disease, vertigo occurs in isolation except for accompanying tinnitus or hearing loss.

Peripheral Lesions

Peripheral etiologies are characterized by absence of brainstem symptoms and signs and include benign positional vertigo, acute vestibular neuronitis, Ménière's disease, and acoustic neuroma.

Benign Positional Vertigo (BPV). In this common problem of the elderly, vertigo is experienced only in specific positions. Onset is sudden, usually within a few seconds after the triggering position has been assumed. Symptoms cease after several minutes if the patient does not move, but they resume with further change in position. In many patients, the condition resolves within 6 months; recovery is usually complete. Head trauma sometimes results in this type of temporary vertigo. The mechanism is stimulation of the labyrinth by free-floating particulate matter in the posterior semicircular canal. A less common but more persistent cause of positional vertigo is believed to be vascular compression of the vestibular nerve. Patients with this condition have constant positional vertigo and severe nausea; it has been labeled *disabling positional vertigo* to distinguish it from the more common forms of positional vertiginous disease.

Ménière's Disease. Ménière's disease ensues from idiopathic endolymphatic hydrops, with damage to the hair cells caused by swelling of the semicircular ducts. Patients report tinnitus, pressure in the ear, and hearing loss in conjunction with vertigo. Episodes are paroxysmal, last minutes to hours, and then decrease in frequency after multiple attacks, only to recur in several months or years. Hearing loss and tinnitus usually accompany the episodes of vertigo, and the hearing loss, although initially reversible, eventually becomes permanent.

Acute Labrynthitis (Vestibular Neuritis). Acute vestibular neuritis develops as a consequence of probable viral infection involving the cochlea and labyrinth. The patient reports a viral upper respiratory syndrome followed by onset of vertigo, tinnitus, and hearing loss. Symptoms resolve entirely by 3 to 6 weeks, with no residual deficits. Some patients may have no hearing loss. Many have incomplete recovery, with residual impaired balance during walking and head movement.

Ototoxins. Ototoxins can injure the peripheral vestibular apparatus, although hearing impairment usually predominates. *Streptomycin* and *gentamicin* are among the toxins that are most injurious to the vestibular portion of the eighth cranial nerve.

Acoustic Neuroma. Acoustic neuroma (benign schwannoma of the eighth cranial nerve), the most worrisome of the peripheral lesions, is retrocochlear in location. It is distinguished from the others in that it causes the retrocochlear type of hearing loss (see later discussion) and can produce serious brainstem compression if untreated. Symptoms start almost imperceptibly, with mild hearing loss, tinnitus, and vague dizziness, and may resemble those of other forms of peripheral vestibular disease. However, the clinical course is progressive and the hearing loss is asymmetric, which differentiates it from that associated with other peripheral lesions. In advanced stages of the condition, there may be cranial nerve deficits from tumor extending to the cerebellar–pontine angle and compressing exiting roots of cranial nerves.

Central Lesions

Central lesions, as already noted, are accompanied in most instances by other brainstem symptoms. In addition, the vertigo and any accompanying nystagmus can be bidirectional or vertical, which does not occur in peripheral vestibular disease.

Multiple Sclerosis. Multiple sclerosis associated with focal demyelination in the vestibular pathways of the brainstem is an important central cause of vertigo. Because of the often transient nature of attacks (days to weeks) and the subtlety of accompanying symptoms (slight facial numbness or huskiness of voice), multiple sclerosis may at first be mistaken for one of the self-limited peripheral causes of vertigo. Only with repeated episodes might the diagnosis become evident. The population afflicted with multiple sclerosis in general is younger than the patients (median age of 54 years) with canalithiasis as a cause of benign positional vertigo. In the aftermath of an acute attack, a central type of positional nystagmus may persist after the vertigo resolves. The vertigo has no characteristic features; attacks can be sudden, transient, recurrent, or persistent. Diagnosis depends on magnetic resonance imaging (MRI) evidence of discrete central nervous system lesions and a course of recurrent dysfunction and intervals of remission.

Vertebrobasilar Insufficiency. Vertebrobasilar insufficiency usually produces vertigo in conjunction with diplopia, sensory loss, dysarthria, dysphagia, hemiparesis, and other brainstem deficits. Self-limited episodes are manifestations of transient ischemic attacks (TIAs). In rare instances and almost exclusively in diabetics, transient vertigo may be the initial and sole complaint of impending infarction in the territory of the anterior inferior cerebellar artery supplying the inner ear; vertigo and/or unilateral hearing loss may be reported. Most other vertebrobasilar TIAs do not cause isolated vertigo as the sole symptom; rather, they present initially or subsequently with vertigo plus other brainstem symptoms. A subtler, progressive form of dizziness, usually without true vertigo, can be seen when multiple lacunar infarctions are present, particularly if the pons is involved. The MRI appearance of this so-called *ischemic pontine rarefaction* can be quite dramatic.

Migraine-Associated Vertigo. True vertigo is reported by up to 25% of migraine sufferers. This is an atypical form of migraine with aura. The dizziness often antedates the headache phase of the syndrome and can persist in a less vivid form after the migraine headache is over. Persons with basilar migraine may report vertigo, ataxia, dysarthria, tinnitus, and visual disturbances. At times there may be no relation to headache, making etiology more difficult to establish, but it may be suggested by a personal or family history of migraine or motion sickness.

Drugs. Drugs that suppress the reticular activating system of the brainstem (e.g., sedatives, anticonvulsants) can cause vertigo of a central nature, especially when taken in excess. Therapeutic doses of some drugs (e.g., phenytoin, carbamazepine) produce nystagmus.

Cardiovascular Disease

Cardiac and vascular insufficiency leading to inadequate cerebral perfusion can result in dizziness, which patients tend to describe as "light-headedness" or a sense of faintness (see Chapter 24). This form of dizziness is seen in patients with fixed or limited cardiac output, serious cardiac dysrhythmias, diminished vascular tone, or severe intravascular volume depletion. Symptoms typically worsen on standing and improve on lying down; postural changes in blood pressure and pulse are characteristic.

Multiple Sensory Deficits, Cerebellar Disease, and Other Causes of Disequilibrium

These neurologic problems produce sensations of *impaired balance* and *disequilibrium*. In this form of dizziness, patients report the sensation to be in the feet rather than in the head. Like light-headedness, it may come on with standing; like true vertigo, it can be aggravated by walking or turning.

Multiple Sensory Deficits

Patients with multiple sensory deficits are usually elderly and have diabetes or other conditions that impair eyesight, sense of position, and motor function. Symptoms typically worsen in the dark (because of elimination of visual positional data) and improve with the use of a cane or holding onto a railing.

Cerebellar Disease

Elderly patients with disequilibrium may also have degenerative cerebellar disease, presenting as gait ataxia and unsteadiness. Etiologies range from ischemic injury to alcohol abuse and paraneoplastic syndromes. The latter are associated with cancers of the breast, ovary, and lung and Hodgkin's disease. Onset of symptoms often postdates the clinical presentation of the cancer, and the ataxia may occur during remission due to the appearance of autoantibodies that cross-react with cerebellar antigens. The physical examination findings are notable for ataxia and other cerebellar signs. Acute disequilibrium may be caused by a midline cerebellar hemorrhage and present as severe dizziness, marked gait ataxia, headache, and stiff neck.

Psychiatric Illness

Patients with psychiatric difficulties complain of ill-defined dizziness ("I just feel dizzy"), constant "light-headedness," or a "foggy" feeling. *Depression*, *anxiety states*, and *psychosis*, in addition to the *medications* used to treat such conditions, are common precipitants. The precise mechanism of the light-

headedness is unknown, but it is thought to be related to a confusional state induced by these illnesses or by the medications used to treat them. In the case of a panic attack leading to hyperventilation (see Chapter 226), the ensuing metabolic alkalosis usually causes paresthesias and light-headedness, although sometimes vertigo is reported. Staab's article in the bibliography provides a lucid discussion of the overlap of anxiety disorders, migraines, and presyncopal states that lead to the complaint of chronic dizziness.

Metabolic Disturbances

Alterations in central nervous system metabolic homeostasis can cause dizziness resembling that associated with inadequate cerebral perfusion. The patient describes light-headedness or feeling faint. Precipitants of acute symptoms include *hypoglycemia*, *hypoxia*, *hypocarbia*, *hypercarbia*, and *drugs*.

DIFFERENTIAL DIAGNOSIS (6,7)

Conditions that cause dizziness can be grouped according to pathophysiologic mechanism (Table 166.1). Vestibular disease is divided into central and peripheral types. Central lesions are mostly caused by basilar artery disease and multiple sclerosis. Peripheral causes include acoustic neuroma, benign positional vertigo, vestibular neuronitis, Ménière's disease, and ototoxic drugs.

TABLE 166.1

DIFFERENTIAL DIAGNOSIS OF DIZZINESS

Vestibular Disease
  Benign positional vertigo
  Vestibular neuronitis and ototoxic drugs
  Ménière's disease
  Acoustic neuroma and other tumors of the cerebellopontine
    angle
  Basilar insufficiency
  Multiple sclerosis

Cardiac and Vascular Disease
  Critical aortic stenosis
  Carotid sinus hypersensitivity
  Volume depletion and severe anemia
  Autonomic insufficiency (drugs, diabetes)
  Diminished vascular reflexes of the elderly

Multiple Sensory Deficits
  Diabetes mellitus
  Cataract surgery
  Some cases of multiple sclerosis
  Cervical spondylosis
  Cerebellar disease

Psychiatric Illness
  Anxiety
  Depression
  Psychosis

Metabolic Disturbances
  Hypoxia
  Severe hypoglycemia
  Hypocapnia and hypercapnia

Cardiac and vascular diseases are a second important group. Faintness on standing may be caused by critical aortic stenosis, severe volume depletion, the use of antihypertensive drugs, autonomic insufficiency, or prolonged confinement to bed. Carotid sinus hypersensitivity results in inappropriate reduction of vascular tone.

Multiple sensory deficits are most common in diabetics and others with poor vision and peripheral neuropathies. Cervical spondylosis disturbs cervical sensory input and contributes to dizziness. Lenses used by patients following cataract surgery distort peripheral vision and can confuse their sense of position. Cerebellar dysfunction leads to a similar clinical presentation of gait unsteadiness. Less commonly, idiopathic normal-pressure hydrocephalus can present with unsteadiness of gait or disequilibrium.

Psychiatric problems are often associated with light-headedness. Patients with anxiety, depression, and psychosis report feeling light-headed. At times, tranquilizers and antidepressants are responsible. Panic attacks frequently are accompanied by feelings of light-headedness or dizziness. Metabolic disturbances affecting the central nervous system have a similar presentation; hypoxia, hypoglycemia, hypocapnia, and hypercapnia are among the most important features.

In a study of 104 consecutive cases referred for evaluation of dizziness, 38% of patients had peripheral vestibular disease, 23% had hyperventilation, 13% had multiple sensory deficits, 9% had psychiatric problems, and 5% had cardiovascular or central neurologic illness. Many cases are multifactorial.

WORKUP (5,7–12)

History

The most important initial step in the evaluation of dizziness is to obtain from the patient the best possible description of the experience and what is meant by "dizziness." A history taken without leading questions or suggested descriptions is most likely to provide meaningful clues. True vertigo suggests *vestibular disease*; faintness that is *postural* or paroxysmal implies a *cardiovascular* disorder; constant *ill-defined dizziness* or light-headedness unrelated to posture points toward a *psychogenic* cause; a feeling of *poor balance* or disequilibrium typifies *multiple sensory deficits* and *cerebellar* causes.

When the problem is light-headedness, it is worth asking whether standing or turning brings on symptoms. If standing does, the use of antihypertensive, tranquilizer, or antidepressant medications should be investigated. During the examination, postural signs, carotid upstroke, and cardiac function should be evaluated, especially for signs of hemodynamically significant aortic stenosis. If turning worsens the situation, it is important to evaluate vision, search for other sensory deficits, and check for cerebellar signs (see later discussion). If light-headedness is a constant sensation, an underlying psychiatric or metabolic disorder is likely. Anxiety and depression are frequent causes and warrant investigation (see Chapters 226 and 227).

Central versus Peripheral Disease

If the patient has *true vertigo*, then the task shifts to determining whether the lesion is *central* or *peripheral*. The most direct way of making this distinction is to inquire about brainstem symptoms (e.g., diplopia, facial numbness, weakness, hemiplegia, dysphasia). Evidence of brainstem involvement rules out a peripheral lesion. The absence of brainstem symptoms does not

rule out a central lesion but does make it improbable. Even the very confusing picture of apparently isolated vertigo resulting from vertebrobasilar insufficiency or multiple sclerosis eventually becomes clearer as accompanying brainstem symptoms become more evident. The pattern of discrete central nervous system lesions and a course of recurrent episodes followed by remissions further suggest the diagnosis of multiple sclerosis (see Chapter 172). Vertebrobasilar insufficiency should be considered in the patient with multiple atherosclerotic risk factors or a prior history of cardiovascular or cerebrovascular disease.

Distinguishing among Peripheral Causes

In the patient with a suspected peripheral lesion, the focus turns to distinguishing *cochlear* from *retrocochlear* disease, that is, relatively benign causes from acoustic neuroma. The latter has a variable presentation and can initially mimic other peripheral types of vertigo. Episodes of vertigo, tinnitus, pressure in the ear, and hearing loss may take place, simulating Ménière's disease. However, the hearing loss is slowly and steadily progressive, rather than fluctuating or episodic. The development of brainstem symptoms (facial weakness or numbness) is a late occurrence and not very helpful for early diagnosis. When doubt persists, physical examination and audiologic testing can be used to help make the differentiation between cochlear and retrocochlear disease (see later discussion).

Timing and *precipitating factors* help to elucidate most other peripheral causes of vertigo. If symptoms occur only on change of position and last but a few moments, the diagnosis is benign positional vertigo, a condition mostly affecting people older than age 60 years. It may be a recurrent problem. A single bout of severe spontaneous vertigo, sudden in onset, sometimes after a *viral illness*, is usually vestibular neuronitis. When seen in the context of inner ear infection, it is properly called *acute labyrinthitis*. Some degree of positional vertigo may remain after the acute illness resolves. Ménière's disease is suggested by acute, recurrent paroxysms of vertigo that are accompanied by *tinnitus* and temporary *hearing loss*. Tinnitus, *pressure* in the ear, and hearing loss are episodic and may precede the other symptoms. Attacks can last for hours to days; residual positional vertigo occurs in 25% of cases.

Drug History

Obtaining a thorough drug history is important. The ototoxic effects of the aminoglycoside antibiotics have been well documented; the diuretic ethacrynic acid also can cause injury to the eighth nerve, especially in patients with compromised renal function. Diuretics may be responsible for severe volume depletion. Vasodilators, phenothiazines, and antihypertensive agents can produce postural light-headedness. Antidepressants and minor tranquilizers cause some patients to feel dizzy.

Physical Examination

The *general appearance* of the patient can be quite informative (e.g., the anxious person will appear overly nervous and may hyperventilate or sigh frequently during the interview). *Blood pressure* and pulse should be measured, and changes between readings taken in the *supine* and *standing* positions should be noted. The skin is examined for pallor, the eyes for *nystagmus* (a few beats of nystagmus on extreme lateral gaze are normal), and the ears for tympanic membrane lesions and *hearing acuity* (see later discussion). The carotid arteries in the neck are checked for bruits (suggestive of cerebrovascular disease) and delay in upstroke (characteristic of severe aortic stenosis). A forceful, sustained left ventricular impulse, single second heart sound, and loud ejection quality murmur on cardiac examination also support a diagnosis of significant aortic stenosis (see Chapter 21).

A thorough and careful *neurologic examination* is essential, particularly when the possibility of central vestibular disease is being considered. Most important is examination for a brainstem lesion, which suggests central pathology or extrinsic compression by an acoustic neuroma. *Cranial nerves* V, VII, and X can be affected by a large acoustic neuroma pressing at the cerebellopontine angle of the brainstem. Testing of sensory function, peripheral vision, and gait often reveals multiple defects in elderly patients troubled by dizziness. Results of the *Romberg test* (standing with feet together, eyes closed) will also be abnormal in such patients, as well as in some with vestibular disease. The side to which the vertiginous patient sways helps to localize the lesion. Cerebellar testing helps to detect any ataxia.

Provocative Maneuvers/Vestibular Stimulation

Provocative maneuvers designed to trigger symptoms and reproduce the patient's problem can be extremely useful. Asking the anxious patient to *hyperventilate* voluntarily for 30 to 120 seconds will often reproduce "dizziness" and associated symptoms, whereas vestibular maneuvers (see later discussion) will not. *Standing up* from a supine position will cause the patient with cardiac or vascular disease to feel faint; it may trigger vertigo in the patient with vestibular disease. *Walking* and *turning* will cause a feeling of disequilibrium in the patient with multiple sensory deficits, cerebellar disease, or vestibular dysfunction. *The Fukuda step test* involves asking the patient to march in place with eyes closed. A patient with a vestibular lesion may circle toward the side of the lesion.

The Dix–Hallpike (Báránay) Maneuver. This vestibular-stimulation test serves both as a good provocative test for reproducing symptoms (useful when the description of dizziness remains unclear) and as a means of distinguishing peripheral from central vestibular disease. It is the least noxious of the standard forms of vestibular stimulation. The patient starts in a sitting position on the examination table and lies down with the head extending over the edge of the table, tilted back, and turned 45 degrees to one side. The assumption of this position need not be overly abrupt, but it should be held for at least 30 seconds. The maneuver is repeated, this time with the head turned 45 degrees to the opposite side. For a final time, the test is repeated without turning the head (Fig. 166.1).

The Dix–Hallpike maneuver provides simultaneous stimulation of all three semicircular canals. It is a useful provocative maneuver for identifying vestibular disease and potentially helpful in separating peripheral from central lesions. One asks the patient to look straight ahead and watches for onset of nystagmus (horizontal or rotatory) and reproduction of symptoms. If symptoms occur, one asks to which side things seem to be spinning; if nystagmus ensues, one notes to which side the slow phase moves. By combining these results with findings from the Romberg and Rinne tests, one can make a diagnosis of a peripheral lesion if (a) the slow phase of nystagmus moves toward the same side as the hearing loss, (b) the patient reports that the spinning is away from the side of the hearing loss, and (c) the Romberg test result is positive and the patient sways toward the side of the hearing deficit. Absence of any one of these findings suggests a central lesion.

Other findings on head position testing suggestive of central vestibular disease are immediate onset of nystagmus and vertigo (peripheral disease has a latency period of 3 to 40 seconds), failure of nystagmus and vertigo to resolve (symptoms usually disappear within 30 seconds), and failure of the patient to adapt on repeated testing.

Maneuvers Alleviating Symptoms

Maneuvers alleviating symptoms are also of diagnostic use. Getting up slowly lessens the faint feeling associated with cardiovascular causes; *rebreathing into a paper bag* reduces the light, giddy feeling that follows hyperventilation; *lying still* in one position may halt positional vertigo; touching the examiner's hand or using a *cane* to walk helps the patient with sensory deficits or cerebellar dysfunction. Withholding suspected drugs may be informative.

Testing of Hearing on Physical Exam

Simple physical examination tests of hearing can be very helpful in distinguishing central from peripheral disease and cochlear from retrocochlear peripheral disease. The *Rinne test* (see Chapter 212) identifies which eighth cranial nerve is involved and helps to differentiate between conductive and sensorineural hearing loss. Patients with a sensorineural hearing deficit may have a cochlear or a retrocochlear lesion. The distinction can be made by testing *speech discrimination*, which is easily performed in the office by whispering a series of 10 two-syllable, closely linked words (e.g., baseball, ice cream) into the patient's ear while making a sound in the other ear to limit its participation. The patient is asked to repeat each whispered word. Correctly identifying fewer than 20% of the words is very suggestive of a retrocochlear lesion (which causes a disproportionate loss of speech discrimination); a score of 70% or better indicates that the problem is cochlear. Scores in between these are indeterminate and necessitate formal audiologic testing (see Chapter 212).

Laboratory Studies

When a vestibular lesion is suspected but it is clinically difficult to differentiate a central from peripheral etiology, then additional testing is indicated.

Electronystagmography and/or Audiologic Testing

Posturographic testing by electronystagmography can help to localize the source of vestibular dysfunction if it is not apparent after history and initial physical examination and determine the need for additional study. If acoustic neuroma is suspected, then one should consider *brainstem auditory evoked response* testing, which is a cost-effective audiologic means of differentiating cochlear from retrocochlear disease. *Formal hearing testing* can help screen candidates for such testing (see Chapter 212).

Imaging Studies

MRI of the internal auditory canal and cerebellopontine angle should follow if evidence of a retrocochlear lesion emerges from the clinical examination and audiologic testing. MRI is the most sensitive test for a small intracanalicular schwannoma. However, MRI is too often obtained simply to rule out a schwannoma in any dizzy patient. The probability of a patient with vertigo and no characteristic hearing loss having a vestibular schwannoma is less than 1 in 9,000; the probability increases slightly (to 1 in 600) for patients with dizziness and asymmetric hearing loss.

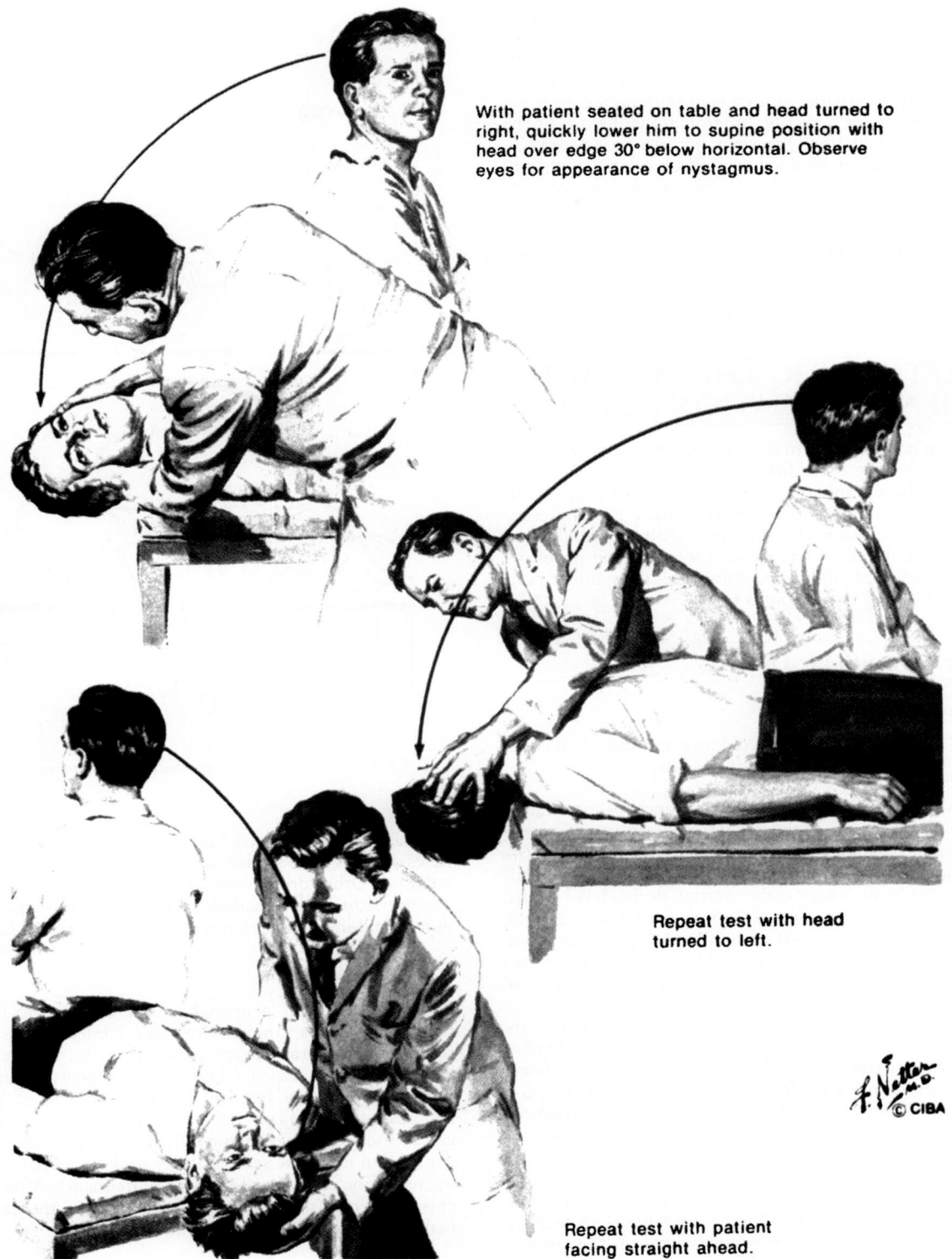

With patient seated on table and head turned to right, quickly lower him to supine position with head over edge 30° below horizontal. Observe eyes for appearance of nystagmus.

Repeat test with head turned to left.

Repeat test with patient facing straight ahead.

FIGURE 166.1. Bárány's test for vestibular disease. (©1981, Ciba Pharmaceutical Company, Division of Ciba-Geigy Corporation. Reproduced from Clinical Symposia by Frank H. Netter, M.D., with permission. All rights reserved.)

If basilar transient ischemic attacks are suggested by transient vertiginous spells accompanied by other brainstem symptoms, then *magnetic resonance angiography (MRA)* should be ordered, especially if the person has multiple atherosclerotic risk factors. MRA provides an excellent (although expensive) noninvasive means of detecting atheromatous disease of the vertebrobasilar circulation. Transient episodes of isolated vertigo are very unlikely to be due to vertebrobasilar disease, and yield from MRA is extremely low in this setting; however, persons with diabetes, who are at risk for occlusion of a branch of the anterior inferior cerebellar artery supplying the inner ear, might present in this fashion (with or without hearing loss) and be considered for MRA. Isolated lightheadedness episodes in the absence of other brainstem symptoms is rarely a sign of vertebrobasilar insufficiency and is not an indication for MRA.

SYMPTOMATIC THERAPY AND PATIENT EDUCATION (11,13–17)

Dizziness can be controlled in most instances and in some situations cured virtually at the first visit. Therapy is aimed at the underlying pathophysiology. The vast majority of people with dizziness have benign disorders. Symptomatic therapy combined with explanation and reassurance is always comforting and appreciated. In particular, patients tolerate their problems better when they know that in most instances the symptom can be controlled or will resolve on its own.

Peripheral Vestibular Disease

Benign Positional Vertigo

Treatment options range from avoidance and dislodging maneuvers to the use of vestibular suppressants.

Maneuvers. BPV responds to a bedside maneuver introduced by *Epley* and referred to as the *canalith-repositioning maneuver*. The maneuver relocates free-floating debris from the posterior semicircular canal into the vestibule of the vestibular labyrinth, where it no longer causes vertigo during head movement (Fig. 166.2). An 80% success rate after a single treatment is reported. The recurrence rate for a 30-month period is about 30%. The maneuver can be performed by primary care physicians in the office, and some patients can be taught to self-treat with this maneuver at home.

Patients with a more widespread balance problem may benefit from *balance–vestibular rehabilitation therapy* (*vestibular exercises*). When carried out under the supervision of a trained therapist, such therapy can effectively reduce positionally provoked vertigo through vestibular "retraining" (i.e., adaptation of the central nervous system to a peripheral vestibular abnormality).

Pharmacologic Therapy. The use of vestibular-suppressant drugs such as *meclizine* (25 to 50 mg every 6 hours as needed) and *promethazine* (25 mg every 6 hours as needed) is an imperfect therapy. Symptoms may be too brief to benefit from medication, and there is concern that their use may impede central adaptation. Moreover, these drugs are sedating and can cause drowsiness (which may be welcome to a patient having an acute attack but is an adverse effect in the treatment of chronic disease). Consequently, suppressant drugs are reserved for patients who have frequent incapacitating episodes and do not responded satisfactorily to avoidance efforts and the Ep-

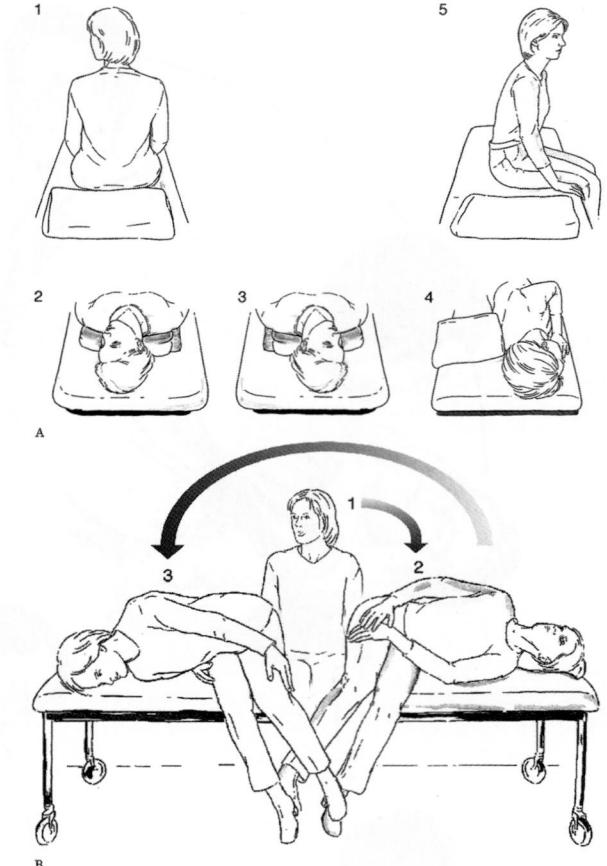

FIGURE 166.2. The canalith-repositioning maneuver.

ley maneuver. Prolonged low-dose meclizine (12.5 mg three times daily) is quite sufficient in elderly patients and causes less sedation. Other drugs used to decrease acute vertigo include *dimenhydrinate* (Dramamine; 50 mg every 6 hours), which is more rapid in onset than meclizine, and the *benzodiazepines*.

Vestibular Neuronitis

Although vestibular neuritis has been assumed to be a reactivation of herpes simplex virus type 1 infection, its does not respond to antiviral therapy with acyclovir. Under trial conditions, outcome is improved by use of glucocorticosteroids, but more study is needed before it can be recommended. Vestibular suppressants such as *meclizine* (25 mg every 6 hours as needed) can be used for symptomatic relief while the condition runs its course, but excessive sedation may be experienced, necessitating reduction in dose and tapering of frequency. After the acute episode, benign positional vertigo may ensue; the patient may benefit from a program of *vestibular exercises*.

Ménière's Disease

The condition is usually managed with *salt restriction* and mild *diuretics*. Strong empiric evidence exists for restricting salt intake to the range of 1 g of sodium per day for 6 months to 1 year. Diuretics (e.g., 250 mg of acetazolamide twice daily or 50 mg of hydrochlorothiazide twice daily) provide additional benefit. Caffeine and alcohol should be avoided.

Central Vestibular Disease

Whereas patients with peripheral causes of dizziness typically recover within months, patients with central causes of dizziness may be bothered for years. Some patients may be helped with *lorazepam* (Ativan; 1 to 2 mg twice daily). Gait training and vestibular exercises under the supervision of a trained therapist may be beneficial. In patients with chronic vertigo, the goal is to retrain the eye and body musculature to compensate for the loss of vestibular input.

Cardiovascular Faintness

Cardiovascular faintness also requires etiologic therapy supplemented by taking adequate hydration, standing up slowly, and discontinuing or reducing offending drugs (see Chapter 24). A thorough review of all medications is essential in the elderly, looking for agents that can cause postural hypotension. The patient with critical aortic stenosis should undergo evaluation for valve replacement (see Chapter 33).

Psychogenic Light-Headedness

Psychogenic light-headedness may be refractory to symptomatic therapy, although *rebreathing into a paper bag* is effective for acute hyperventilation. Treatment with an *anxiolytic* agent may help, but it can also cause symptoms (see Chapter 226). *Antidepressant* therapy is indicated when depression is the predominant cause, although a side effect of some antidepressants (e.g., tricyclics) is postural light-headedness; selective serotonin reuptake inhibitors are better tolerated (see Chapter 227).

Multiple Sensory Deficits, Geriatric Dizziness, Cerebellar Dysfunction

Patients with multiple sensory deficits benefit from attention to correctable components of the problem, such as removal of cataracts to improve vision or use of a walking stick to provide additional sensory input. Similarly, the geriatric syndrome of dizziness requires attention to all contributing factors, ranging from medications that may cause postural hypotension or central nervous system suppression to psychiatric states and sensory and vestibular dysfunctions. A multifaceted approach to treatment is needed and should not overlook simple measures that help to ensure safety and facilitate function (e.g., handrails, good lighting, use of a walker).

Most forms of gait instability due to acquired cerebellar disease do not readily lend themselves to correction. In paraneoplastic syndromes, the causative tumor may remain in remission, yet symptoms persist. Treatment of cerebellar degenerative or ischemic injury is largely supportive; avoidance of aggravating factors such as alcohol excess is important.

Annotated Bibliography

1. Alexander MP. Mild traumatic brain injury: pathophysiology, natural history, and clinical management. Neurology 1995;45:1253. (*A review of postconcussive syndrome and the frequency of complaints of dizziness.*)
2. Baloh RW. Vestibular neuritis. N Engl J Med 2003;348:1027. (*A useful case-based clinical review.*)
3. Furman JM, Cass SP. Benign paroxysmal positional vertigo. N Engl J Med 1999;341:1590. (*A good review of the pathogenesis of benign positional vertigo, with a discussion of examination and diagnostic criteria.*)
4. Hammack J, Kotanides H, Rosenblum MK, et al. Paraneoplastic cerebellar degeneration. II. Clinical and immunologic findings in 21 patients with Hodgkin's disease. Neurology 1992;42:1938. (*A good description of the condition and its underlying pathophysiology.*)
5. Savitz SI, Caplan LR. Vertebrobasilar disease. N Engl J Med 2005;352:2618. (*Makes the important point that isolated dizziness is almost never due to vascular insufficiency and that vascular studies are of little value in cases of isolated dizziness.*)
6. Tinetti ME, Williams CS, Gill TM. Dizziness among older adults: a possible geriatric syndrome. Ann Intern Med 2000;132:337. (*A population-based cross-sectional study, finding that deficits in multiple domains combine to cause the problem.*)
7. Kroenke K, Lucas CA, Rosenberg ML, et al. Causes of persistent dizziness: a prospective study of 100 patients in ambulatory care. Ann Intern Med 1992;117:898. (*Vestibular disease and psychiatric disorders were the most common causes.*)
8. Staab JP, Ruckenstein MJ. Expanding the differential diagnosis of chronic dizziness. Arch Otolaryngol Head Neck Surg 2007;133:170. (*Nearly all patients with chronic subjective dizziness can be diagnosed with a psychiatric or neurologic illness; these include anxiety disorders in nearly 60% of cases; <2% had cardiac arrhythmias.*)
9. Gizzi M, Rosenberg ML. The diagnostic approach to the dizzy patient. Neurologist 1998;4:138. (*Audiometry, vestibular testing, and neuroimaging are discussed; if the patient is dizzy but has no abnormalities on examination and if progression of asymmetric hearing loss is not documented, neuroimaging is not recommended.*)
10. Gizzi M, Riley E, Molinari S. The diagnostic value of imaging the patients with dizziness: a Bayesian approach. Arch Neurol 1996;53:1299. (*Provides a sequential strategy for workup based on pretest probabilities.*)
11. Staab JP. Chronic dizziness: the interface between psychiatry and neuro-otology. Curr Opin Neurol 2006;19:41. (*A thoughtful review and discussion.*)
12. Sullivan M, Clark MR, Katon WJ, et al. Psychiatric and otologic diagnoses in patients complaining of dizziness. Arch Intern Med 1993;153:1479. (*Psychiatric disease is common when vestibular disease is ruled out.*)
13. Epley JM. Positional vertigo related to semicircular canalithiasis. Otolaryngol Head Neck Surg 1995;112:154. (*Initial report of a postural repositioning maneuver that can cure positional vertigo.*)
14. Froehling DA, Bowen JM, Mohr D, et al. The canalith repositioning procedure for the treatment of benign positional vertigo: a randomized controlled trial. Mayo Clin Proc 2000;75:695. (*The procedure was found to be effective and able to be performed successfully by primary physicians in the office.*)
15. Radtke A, von Bevern M, Tiel-Wilck K, et al. Self-treatment of benign paroxysmal positional vertigo. Neurology 2004;63:150. (*The response rate was 95% in patients who correctly performed the procedure.*)
16. Solomon D. Benign paroxysmal positional vertigo. Curr Treat Options Neurol 2000;2:417. (*A clear outline of the diagnosis of benign positional vertigo and an excellent diagrammatic description of the canalith-repositioning procedures.*)
17. Strupp M, Zinlger V, Arbusow V, et al. Methylprednisolone, valacyclovir, or the combination for vestibular neuritis. N Engl J Med 2004;351:4. (*A randomized, controlled trial; methylprednisolone significantly improved the recovery of peripheral vestibular function, but valacyclovir did not.*)

CHAPTER 167 ■ FOCAL NEUROLOGIC COMPLAINTS: EVALUATION OF NERVE ROOT AND PERIPHERAL NERVE SYNDROMES

AMY A. PRUITT

Primary physicians are frequently asked to evaluate complaints of focal numbness, tingling, weakness, pain, or some combination of these. In general, major acute neurologic disease is not at issue during an office visit. Nevertheless, the broad range of outpatient problems encountered encompasses lesions throughout the nervous system. Disorders of the nerve roots and peripheral nerves in the upper and lower extremities are especially common. The primary physician should be able to analyze several of these syndromes. The identification and localization of such problems can facilitate a thorough neurologic evaluation and accurately segregate those cases that must be referred to a neurologist.

PATHOPHYSIOLOGY AND CLINICAL PRESENTATION (1–8)

Many peripheral nerves, because of their superficial location, are easily injured mechanically, and others are vulnerable because of specific anatomic variants or because of alterations in anatomy caused by degenerative disease.

Upper Extremity Syndromes

Cervical Radiculopathy and Myelopathy

Age-related loss of water and elasticity in cervical disks leads to increased stress on the vertebral bodies. Osteophytic spurs develop and may encroach on nerve roots. More serious but less common is encroachment on the spinal cord itself by progressive cervical spondylotic changes. Usually, a combination of radiculopathy involving the C-5, C-6, or C-7 roots (Figs. 167.1 and 167.2) and myelopathy is present. Cord compression resulting from spondylosis is indicated by radicular pain, variable weakness, diminished reflexes, and atrophy in the arms, with spastic weakness and hyperreflexia in the lower extremities.

Brachial Plexus Neuritis

Brachial plexus neuritis, a painfully disabling condition, develops in some patients after an immunization or viral infection and in others without any antecedent illness. It presents with severe pain in the shoulder and upper arm followed by weakness. Usually, the upper roots of the plexus are involved more than the lower ones. The prognosis is ultimately good, but recovery may be prolonged.

Thoracic Outlet Syndrome

A cervical rib or bony abnormality of the first rib may cause pressure on the subclavian artery or brachial plexus as it passes through the thoracic outlet (Fig. 167.1). The diagnosis is primarily clinical and is based on the presence of pain in the arm in certain positions, color changes in the hand, and a pattern of sensory loss and weakness most pronounced in the fourth and fifth fingers. Deep tendon reflexes are usually normal. A bruit may be heard over the subclavian artery. Most surgeons advocate removal of the potentially constricting structures (cervical rib, fascial band to first rib, or first rib). Shoulder exercises to improve posture are often advised first, and orthopedic advice should be sought in each case.

Long Thoracic Nerve Entrapment

This nerve arises from the brachial plexus and innervates the serratus anterior. It is vulnerable to injury in workers who lift or push heavy loads, occurs after direct trauma from heavy backpacks, and may evolve for several months after the injury. The patient notes a change in the appearance of the shoulder, and examination reveals winging of the scapula. Most cases have a good prognosis.

Carpal Tunnel Syndrome

In this disorder, the median nerve is entrapped at the carpal tunnel (Fig. 167.1) because of pressure from ligamentous thickening. Most cases are idiopathic, but the disorder may be seen with rheumatoid arthritis, pregnancy, acromegaly, hypothyroidism, fractures of the carpal bones, amyloidosis, and myeloma. Occupational causes involving repetitive traumatic actions have been implicated. A combination of pain, paresthesias, and numbness in the median nerve distribution is the earliest complaint; symptoms are often worse at night (Fig. 167.2). Later, muscle weakness (particularly of thumb abduction and apposition) occurs, and thenar atrophy may be seen. Of importance, aching pain can be felt as far up as the shoulder.

Ulnar Nerve Entrapment

The most common location of ulnar entrapment is the elbow (Fig. 167.1). Causes include fracture deformities, arthritis, faulty positioning of the arm during surgery, or repetitive occupational or recreational trauma (e.g., tennis). Sensation is usually spared in the forearm, but sensory loss occurs in the fifth finger and half of the fourth (Fig. 167.2). Wasting of the intrinsic muscles of the hand with weakness of grip occurs later. Nerve conduction studies can accurately localize the site of compression. If focal entrapment is present, repositioning of

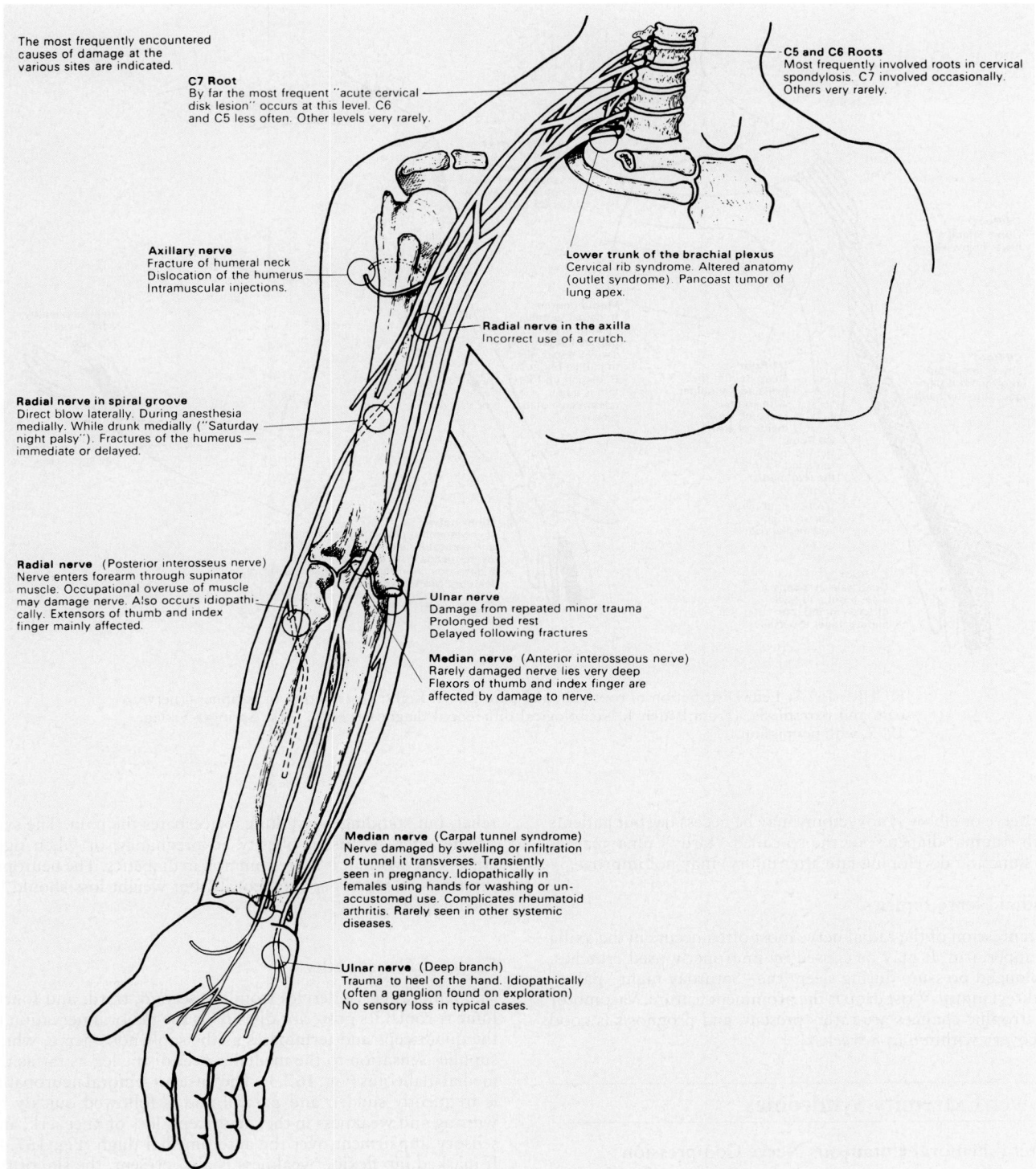

The most frequently encountered causes of damage at the various sites are indicated.

C7 Root
By far the most frequent "acute cervical disk lesion" occurs at this level. C6 and C5 less often. Other levels very rarely.

C5 and C6 Roots
Most frequently involved roots in cervical spondylosis. C7 involved occasionally. Others very rarely.

Axillary nerve
Fracture of humeral neck
Dislocation of the humerus
Intramuscular injections.

Lower trunk of the brachial plexus
Cervical rib syndrome. Altered anatomy (outlet syndrome). Pancoast tumor of lung apex.

Radial nerve in the axilla
Incorrect use of a crutch.

Radial nerve in spiral groove
Direct blow laterally. During anesthesia medially. While drunk medially ("Saturday night palsy"). Fractures of the humerus — immediate or delayed.

Radial nerve (Posterior interosseus nerve)
Nerve enters forearm through supinator muscle. Occupational overuse of muscle may damage nerve. Also occurs idiopathically. Extensors of thumb and index finger mainly affected.

Ulnar nerve
Damage from repeated minor trauma
Prolonged bed rest
Delayed following fractures

Median nerve (Anterior interosseous nerve)
Rarely damaged nerve lies very deep
Flexors of thumb and index finger are affected by damage to nerve.

Median nerve (Carpal tunnel syndrome)
Nerve damaged by swelling or infiltration of tunnel it transverses. Transiently seen in pregnancy. Idiopathically in females using hands for washing or unaccustomed use. Complicates rheumatoid arthritis. Rarely seen in other systemic diseases.

Ulnar nerve (Deep branch)
Trauma to heel of the hand. Idiopathically (often a ganglion found on exploration) No sensory loss in typical cases.

FIGURE 167.1. Peripheral nerve distribution to the upper limb. (From Patten J. Neurological differential diagnosis. New York: Springer-Verlag, 1977, with permission.)

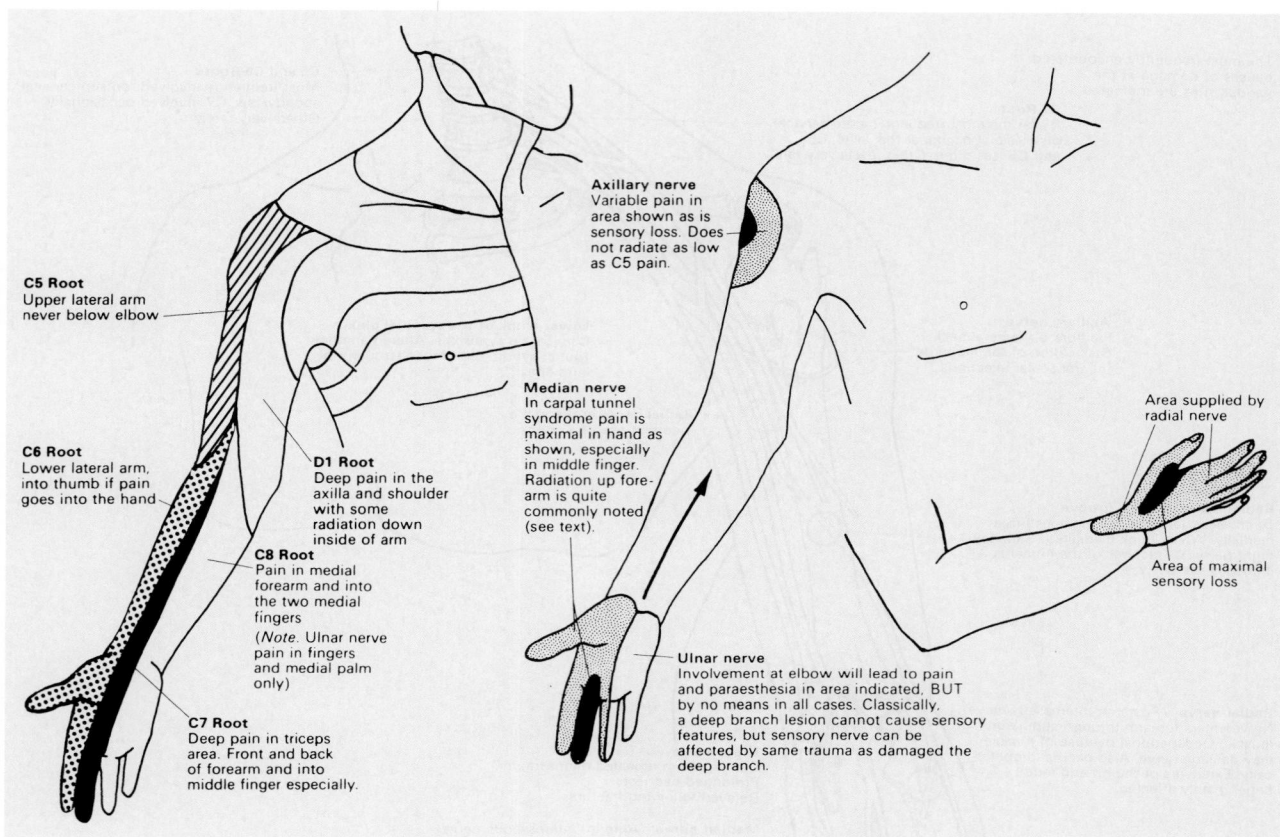

FIGURE 167.2. Left: Distribution of root pain and paresthesia. **Right:** Distribution of peripheral nerve pain and paresthesia. (From Patten J. Neurological differential diagnosis. New York: Springer-Verlag, 1977, with permission.)

the nerve or elbow synovectomy may be necessary, but patients with trauma, diabetes, or the so-called "tardy" ulnar palsies (dysfunction developing late after injury) may not improve.

Radial Nerve Injuries

Compression of the radial nerve most often occurs in the axilla or upper arm. It may be caused by improperly used crutches, prolonged pressure during sleep (the "Saturday night" palsy), or direct injury. Wrist drop is the prominent feature. Vasomotor or atrophic changes are rarely present, and prognosis is good (recovery within 6 to 8 weeks).

Lower Extremity Syndromes

Lateral Femoral Cutaneous Nerve Compression

Also known as meralgia paresthetica, this syndrome involves a nerve formed by branches arising from the second and third lumbar roots. The nerve enters the thigh in close relation to the inguinal ligament, the anterior superior iliac spine, and the sartorius muscle insertion (Fig. 167.3). It is purely sensory and supplies the anterolateral and lateral aspects of the thigh almost as far as the knee (Fig. 167.4). Compression causes an extremely unpleasant, characteristic burning pain with increased cutaneous sensitivity. Sitting or lying usually provides

relief, but standing or walking exacerbates the pain. The syndrome often occurs in obesity, in pregnancy, or when tight corsets are worn. It is more common in diabetics. The neuropathy tends to regress spontaneously, but weight loss should be encouraged.

Femoral Neuropathy

The femoral nerve derives from the second, third, and fourth lumbar roots. Its posterior division is the major innervation to the quadriceps and terminates as the saphenous nerve, which supplies sensation to the medial aspect of the leg as far as the medial malleolus (Fig. 167.3). The onset of femoral neuropathy is frequently sudden and painful and is followed quickly by wasting and weakness in the quadriceps, loss of knee jerk, and sensory impairment over the anteromedial thigh (Fig. 167.4). If marked hip flexion weakness is also present, the site of the lesion is usually in the lumbar plexus. Sensory symptoms in the saphenous distribution are uncommon in lesions of the main trunk of the femoral nerve.

Entrapment may occur in the inguinal region and from direct retroperitoneal compression by tumor or hematoma; however, the most common cause of femoral nerve injury is diabetes, presumably from diabetic nerve infarction causing thigh pain, weakness, and sensory deficit. Electromyographically, the involvement in diabetic femoral neuropathy is frequently more widespread. Although some improvement may occur, the patient is often left quite weak.

Sciatic Nerve Syndromes

The sciatic nerve arises from the lumbosacral plexus (L-4 through S-3) and terminates in the common peroneal and tibial nerves (Fig. 167.3). The tibial nerve supplies the gastrocnemius, plantaris, soleus, and popliteus muscles, and its extension into the calf, the posterior tibial nerve, supplies muscles of the calf. All of these muscles are involved in plantar flexion. The common peroneal nerve divides into the superficial and deep peroneal nerves. The latter supplies the muscles of dorsiflexion of the foot and toes. The superficial peroneal nerve innervates the muscles that evert the foot.

Sciatic nerve compression may result from tumors within the pelvis or from prolonged sitting or lying on the buttocks. Gluteal abscesses and misplaced buttock injections have caused sciatic injury. Weakness of the gluteal muscles and pain in the area of the sciatic notch imply compression within the pelvis. Lesions just beyond the sciatic notch cause weakness in the hamstrings and in all the muscles of the lower leg.

Common peroneal compression usually occurs at the level of the fibular head (Fig. 167.3) and is seen in cachectic patients following prolonged bed rest, alcoholics, diabetics, and patients placed in tight casts. Injury leads to faulty dorsiflexion and eversion of the foot, which produces a characteristic foot drop with a slapping gait. Complete or partial recovery can be expected when paralysis results from transient pressure. Treatment consists of a foot brace and careful avoidance of compressive positions.

Lumbar Disk Syndromes

Compressive neuropathies of the lower limbs must be distinguished from the very common lumbar disk syndromes. In the lumbar region, the fourth and fifth disks are most frequently affected (i.e., the disks between the L-4 and L-5 vertebral bodies and between the L-5 and S-1 vertebrae). The most common complaint is the sudden onset of severe low back pain (see Chapter 147). The inciting event is often trivial, although heavy lifting or an acute twisting motion is sometimes reported. The pain is worsened by bending forward, sneezing, or straining.

The herniated disk can compress one or more nerve roots, but a disk herniation at a particular level generally causes a distinctive picture (see Chapter 147). Herniation of the *L4-5 disc* usually affects the L-5 root, causing pain over the sciatic notch, lateral thigh, and leg; numbness of the web of the great toe and lateral leg; weakness of dorsiflexion of the great toe and foot; and no reflex changes (Fig. 167.4). Herniation of the disk between *L-5 and S-1* catches the S-1 root, producing pain down the back of the leg to the heel; numbness in the lateral heel, foot, and toe; weakness of plantar flexion; and loss of the ankle jerk (Fig. 167.4).

The clinical course is usually favorable with conservative measures (see Chapter 147).

Peripheral Polyneuropathy

When patients present with distal, symmetric sensorimotor or predominantly motor symptoms and are found to have diminished sensation or motor abnormalities in a "stocking-glove" distribution with variably hypoactive deep tendon reflexes, they are likely to have a peripheral polyneuropathy. The list of causes is extensive (Table 167.1). Although most produce some degree of motor and sensory dysfunction, usually one component predominates.

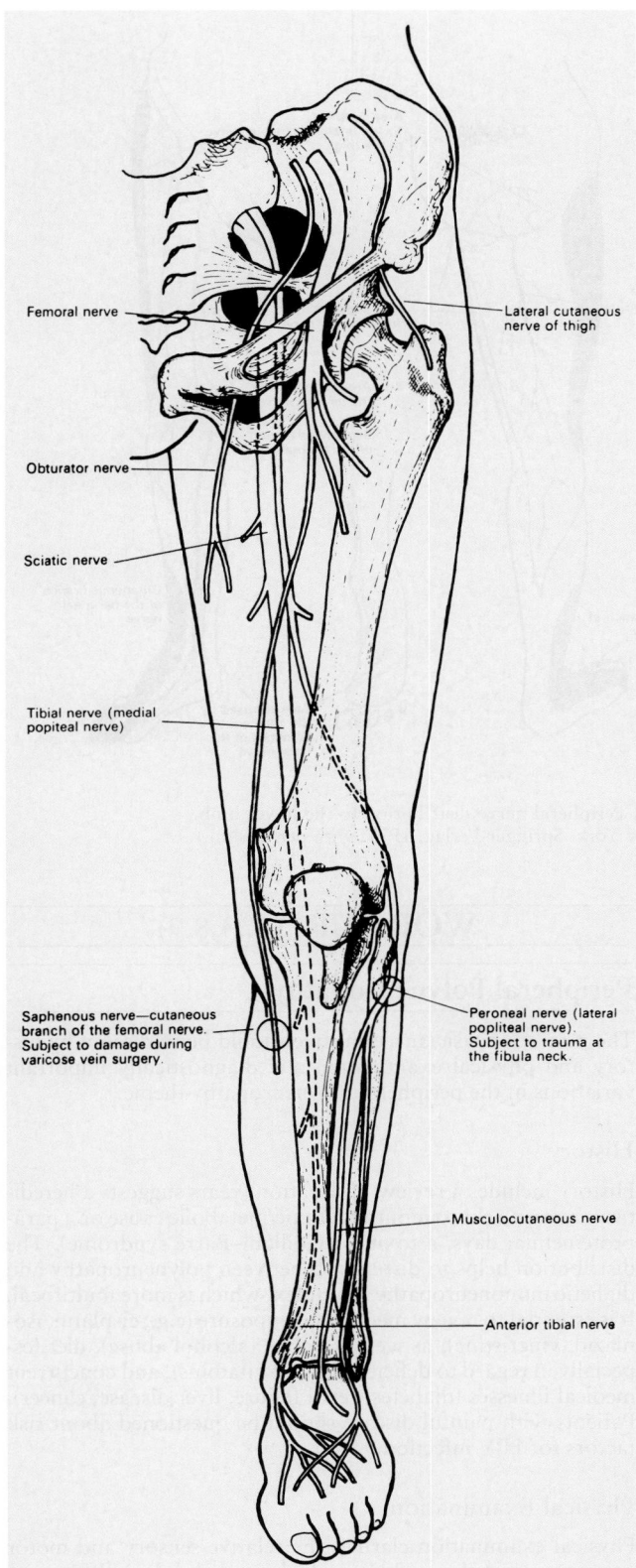

FIGURE 167.3. Peripheral nerve distribution to the lower limb. (From Patten J. Neurological differential diagnosis. New York: Springer-Verlag, 1977, with permission.)

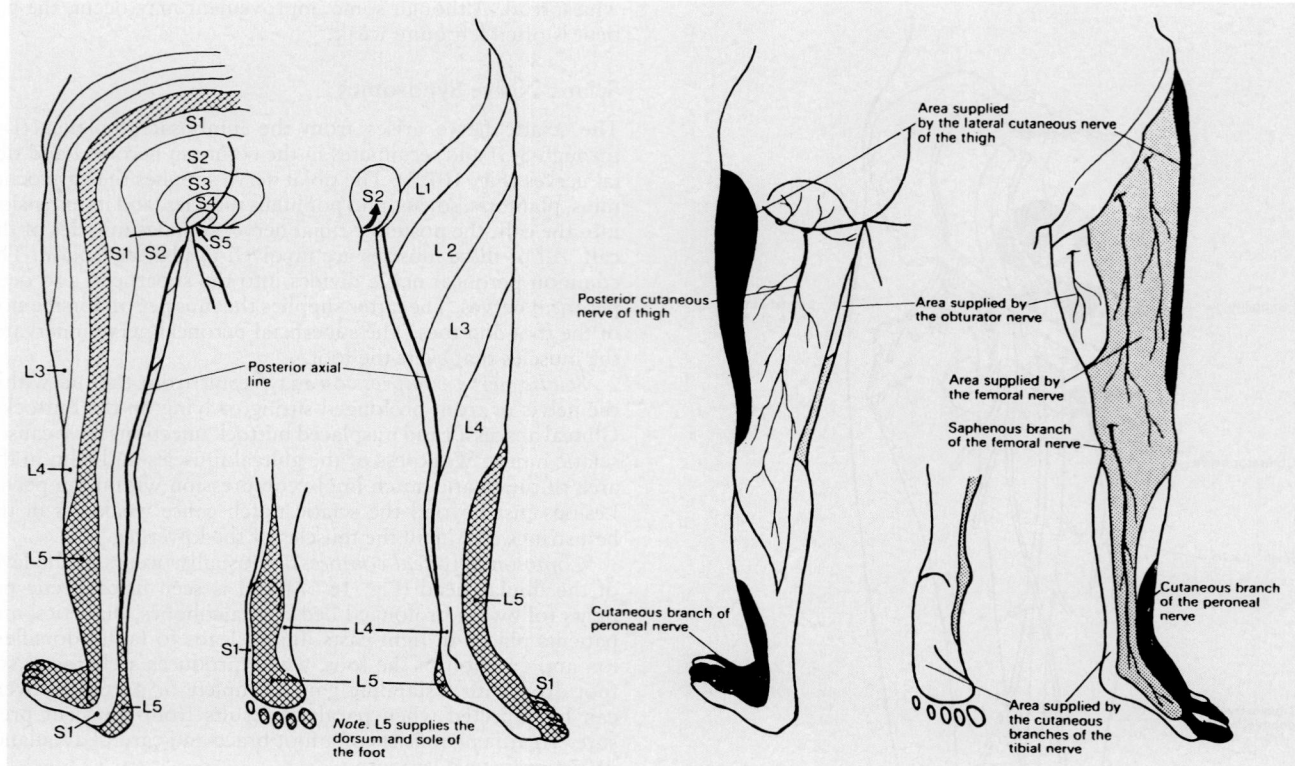

FIGURE 167.4. Left: Lumbosacral dermatomes. **Right:** Peripheral nerve distribution to the lower limb. (From Patten J. Neurological differential diagnosis. New York: Springer-Verlag, 1977, with permission.)

The most common polyneuropathies in the United States (due to diabetes and alcoholism) present principally with sensory deficits, although a more mixed picture develops later. *Diabetes* is a common source of sensorimotor polyneuropathy; symptoms respond to a tightening of glucose control (see Chapter 102). *Alcoholism, deficiencies of B vitamins, renal failure, hypothyroidism, AIDS,* and *paraneoplastic syndromes* are among the other causes.

Motor polyneuropathies include *Guillain–Barré syndrome,* an acquired autoimmune disease that is the most dramatic of the predominantly motor polyneuropathies. Its typical presentation is one of acute onset following a viral illness and rapid progression of ascending weakness over a few days in conjunction with a loss of deep tendon reflexes. Other predominantly motor polyneuropathies include those associated with *monoclonal gammopathy, toxin exposure,* and *porphyria.*

A predominantly *sensory polyneuropathy* is seen with *amyloidosis, paraneoplastic syndromes, vitamin B_6 excess,* and *Sjögren's syndrome.*

DIFFERENTIAL DIAGNOSIS (5)

The causes of peripheral polyneuropathy are extensive, varied, and best considered in terms of the rapidity of onset and whether the presentation is predominantly motor, sensory, or mixed (see Table 167.1). The differential for the more focal peripheral neuropathies is anatomic (and considered in the workups listed in the next section).

WORKUP (1,2,3,8,9)

Peripheral Polyneuropathy

The primary physician's objective should be to discern by history and physical examination any diagnostically important variations in the peripheral polyneuropathy theme.

History

History includes a review of duration (years suggests a hereditary cause; weeks to months, a toxic/metabolic cause or a paraproteinemia; days, a toxin or Guillain–Barré syndrome). The distribution helps to distinguish between polyneuropathy and diabetic mononeuropathy multiplex, which is more multifocal. It is essential to review medication exposure (e.g., cisplatin, isoniazid, vincristine), as well as habits (alcohol abuse), diet (especially in regard to deficiencies of B vitamins), and concurrent medical illnesses (diabetes, renal failure, liver disease, cancer). Patients with painful disease should be questioned about risk factors for HIV infection.

Physical Examination

Physical examination clarifies the relative sensory and motor components of the problem, which are helpful in differentiation. Signs of systemic disease may also be revealed. Diabetic peripheral neuropathic pain (DPN) is a source of major disability and is underrecognized. In a 2007 Position Statement, the American Diabetes Association recommended that all

TABLE 167.1

IMPORTANT PERIPHERAL POLYNEUROPATHIES

Predominantly Motor
  Acute (days)
    Guillain–Barré syndrome
    Diphtheria
    Porphyria
    Toxin (organophosphate exposure)
  Subacute (weeks to 1–2 yr)
    Toxin exposure (lead poisoning, glue sniffing)
    Paraproteinemia
  Chronic
    Hereditary (Charcot–Marie–Tooth disease)

Predominantly Sensory
  Acute (days)
    None
  Subacute (weeks to 1–2 yr)
    Amyloidosis
    Drug toxicity (cisplatin, vitamin B_6 excess)
    Paraneoplastic syndrome
    Sjögren's syndrome
  Chronic (years)
    Hereditary sensory neuropathy

Sensorimotor
  Acute (days)
    Toxin exposure (arsenic)
  Subacute (weeks to 1–2 yr)
    Diabetes
    Alcohol abuse
    B-vitamin deficiency
    Renal failure
    Hypothyroidism
    Connective tissue disease
    Paraneoplastic syndrome
    Drug toxicity (isoniazid, cancer chemotherapeutic agents)
    AIDS
  Chronic (years)
    Charcot–Marie–Tooth disease

Adapted from American College of Physicians. Medical Knowledge Self-Assessment Program IX. General Internal Medicine Syllabus. Philadelphia: American College of Physicians, 1991:106, with permission.

patients with diabetes be screened at least annually for DPN. The predictive value of a simple 128-Hz vibration test is excellent and should be a routine office procedure.

Laboratory Studies

Laboratory studies should include a complete blood cell count, erythrocyte sedimentation rate or C-reactive protein, and determinations of serum glucose, lipid profile, liver chemistries, blood urea nitrogen, creatinine, and thyroid-stimulating hormone. If these tests are unrevealing, vitamin B_{12}, homocysteine, methylmalonic acid, serum protein electrophoresis, antinuclear antigen, and hepatitis B and C screening can be done. HIV-antibody testing is indicated if there are risk factors for the condition. Chest radiography and immunoelectrophoresis should be performed if a paraneoplastic syndrome is suspected or possible. Patients whose neuropathy is apparent from the results of the foregoing studies (e.g., diabetic polyneuropathy) do not require additional testing. *Electromyography* (EMG) should be

seen as an extension of the clinical history and physical examination and is indicated when the diagnosis is unclear, when weakness due to primary muscle or neuromuscular junction disease is suspected, and when the differentiation between demyelinating disease and axonal polyneuropathy and between root or plexus and more-distal nerve trunk involvements can be of differential diagnostic value. The test also distinguishes upper from lower motor neuron weakness. The EMG is unlikely to answer a question that is too general, such as "explain weakness" or "total body pain—rule out neurologic process." *Nerve biopsy* is infrequently recommended; its main indication is in hereditary disorders, multifocal mononeuropathy multiplex, or asymmetric clinical syndromes, in which it can reveal such underlying conditions as vasculitis, amyloidosis, or sarcoidosis. Patients with monoclonal gammopathy may profit from tests for *antibody to myelin-associated glycoprotein* (*anti-MAG antibody*) and *anti-GM1 antibody*; these tests can identify patients who are candidates for plasmapheresis or immunosuppressive therapy.

Other Peripheral Nerve Syndromes

Identification of the nerve root or peripheral nerve syndrome and precise localization of the neurologic lesion is possible in the office setting. Assessment is facilitated by determining (a) whether the problem is peripheral (in a nerve root or peripheral nerve) or central (in the cord or above); (b) whether the problem, if peripheral, is caused by a lesion in the peripheral nerve or by nerve root injury; (c) whether evidence of cord compression (manifested by signs of myelopathy) is present, particularly in upper extremity syndromes; (d) whether evidence (in other extremities) of more widespread peripheral neuropathy is present (e.g., the diabetic patient with a femoral neuropathy who also has a diffuse peripheral neuropathy); and (e) whether weakness is caused by a muscle or nerve lesion.

The neurologic examination should be organized to address these issues and answer the following questions:

- *Is the lesion an upper motor neuron or a lower motor neuron lesion?* Fasciculations, flaccidity, and a lack of reflexes indicate a lower motor neuron lesion and suggest that the disorder originates at the anterior horn cell or peripheral nerve level. Spasticity and increased reflexes are evidence for a lesion above the anterior horn cell that supplies the involved musculature. Thus, a cervical disk at the C-6 level might decrease the biceps reflex and cause biceps weakness and atrophy while increasing reflexes and causing spasticity below that level.
- *Is the nerve dysfunction confined to one root or dermatome or to one peripheral nerve?* A positive answer to this question suggests a compression neuropathy such as a radial, ulnar, or median nerve palsy. Findings of more generalized dysfunction, such as diffusely decreased deep tendon reflexes, absent vibration sense at the ankles, and a stocking-glove pattern of sensory loss, suggest a more diffuse peripheral neuropathy. Commonly seen forms of peripheral neuropathy include those associated with diabetes mellitus, excess alcohol consumption, toxin and drug exposure, and genetic conditions such as Charcot–Marie–Tooth disease. An electromyogram can localize the individual nerve abnormality and confirm the presence of a generalized neuropathy.
- *Is the weakness caused by nerve or by muscle disease?* Weakness in conjunction with altered tendon reflexes and sensory loss suggests nerve disease. In primary muscle disease, reflexes and normal sensation are preserved. Characteristic

patterns of muscle weakness occur in the genetically determined muscular dystrophies. The toxic and metabolic myopathies produce largely proximal muscle weakness, in contrast to almost all of the primary nerve diseases, which affect distal musculature early and preferentially. Serum muscle enzyme elevations are seen in muscle disease, and some muscular disorders are associated with myotonia. The electromyogram, coupled with nerve conduction studies, can distinguish primary muscle disease from neuropathic processes.

The clinical identification of nerve root and peripheral nerve syndromes is often facilitated by the selective use of radiologic, nerve conduction, electromyographic, and serologic studies (detailed in discussions of each of the important syndromes). However, laboratory studies are usually not necessary during the initial assessment.

Cervical Radiculopathy

Radiologic assessment usually includes *cervical spinal radiography*. Unfortunately, nearly 50% of patients older than age 50 years show degenerative changes of the cervical spine on radiographic films, and these do not correlate well with the degree of abnormality found clinically in either radiculopathy or myelopathy. Nevertheless, plain films of the cervical spine with oblique views to visualize the neural foramina are often informative. *Magnetic resonance imaging* (MRI) is the best noninvasive test for assessing the degree of cervical spondylosis or disk protrusion. It should be ordered when radicular pain is severe or when a motor or sensory deficit, reflex change, or myelopathic finding is present. It may be difficult to distinguish cervical spondylotic myelopathy from other *progressive myelopathies*, which include *multiple sclerosis, subacute combined degeneration associated with vitamin B_{12} deficiency, spinal tumor,* and *syringomyelia*. Suspicion of myelopathy should prompt referral to a neurologist.

Brachial Plexus Neuritis

Clinical examination reveals variable weakness and sensory loss in the C-5 to T-1 root distributions (Fig. 167.2), with diminished deep tendon reflexes. Because many nerve roots are involved, confusion with a cervical disk problem does not usually arise. Electromyography and nerve conduction studies help to localize the abnormality. MRI of the brachial plexus with gadolinium enhancement may be valuable in excluding neoplastic disease of the plexus.

Thoracic Outlet Syndrome

The diagnosis is primarily clinical and is based on the presence of pain in the arm in certain positions, color changes in the hand, and a pattern of sensory loss and weakness most pronounced in the fourth and fifth fingers. Deep tendon reflexes are usually normal. A bruit may be heard over the subclavian artery. The differential diagnosis includes Raynaud's phenomenon, ulnar nerve entrapment at the elbow, and compression of the brachial plexus by neoplasm or fibrosis resulting from radiation.

Carpal Tunnel Syndrome

Tapping on the wrist or anywhere else along the median nerve may reproduce the pain (*Tinel's sign*). Aching pain can be felt as far up as the shoulder, but it should not distract the examiner's attention from the wrist. The differential diagnosis includes radiculopathy from cervical spine disease, but the exact loca-

tion of the pain should conform to the median nerve rather than to the distribution of just one nerve root. *Electromyography* and *nerve conduction studies* with motor and sensory conduction latencies of the median nerve provide the most useful data. Failure to respond to surgical intervention should prompt rechecking of the nerve conduction studies, careful reexamination, and consideration of the possibility of coexistent cervical spine disease or of median nerve compression higher in the forearm.

Lateral Femoral Cutaneous Nerve Syndrome

The differential diagnosis includes a lesion of the second or third lumbar roots, usually associated with low back pain radiating into the lower leg. Sensory changes in this case extend further down the leg and more medially, and iliopsoas or quadriceps weakness is present. Weakness and reflex changes do not occur in meralgia paresthetica.

Lumbar Disk Syndromes

When any combination of progressive limb weakness and numbness (especially if bilateral), uncontrollable pain, saddle anesthesia (numbness in the distribution of S-2 and S-3), and bladder and bowel dysfunction is noted, the emergent *MRI* examination (or *computed tomographic myelography* if MRI is not available) is needed to rule out *cauda equina syndrome*. Imaging of the spinal canal is required to detect any caudal compression and to rule out more unusual causes of lumbar radiculopathy, such as neurofibroma. MRI may also help in predicting the response of a patient with disk disease to conservative therapy.

SYMPTOMATIC MANAGEMENT OF PAINFUL PERIPHERAL NEUROPATHY (4–6,8,10–16)

Overall Approach

Where possible, prevention remains the best overall approach to treatment of painful peripheral neuropathies because once established, symptoms can be difficult to treat. Prompt aggressive treatment of herpes zoster (see Chapter 193) and vitamin B_{12} deficiency (see Chapter 82), tight glycemic control of diabetes (see Chapter 102), reduction of the viral load in HIV infection (see Chapter 13), and treatment of underlying malignancy are examples of preventive measures, both primary and secondary, that are effective for minimizing painful sensory neuropathy associated with these conditions.

Narcotics are often required. Despite much enthusiasm and off-label use of newer nonnarcotic analgesics (e.g., *gabapentin, pregabalin, duloxetine*), evidence-based efficacy remains limited to a few specific conditions, such as diabetes mellitus and postherpetic neuralgia. Topical therapies such as *capsaicin cream* and a *5% lidocaine patch (Lidoderm)* are sometimes used. The patch is approved by the U.S. Food and Drug Administration for postherpetic neuralgia, and the cream is applied with variable results for neuropathic pain (local burning, a delay of 2 to 3 weeks before benefit, and reversible denervation may occur). The treatment of painful polyneuropathy requires frequent adjustments of medication type and dose.

Some patients may inquire about the efficacy of *plasmapheresis*, which is extremely useful in myasthenia gravis and chronic inflammatory demyelinating polyneuropathy. It is now administered less often in acute Guillain–Barré syndrome in part because intravenous immune globulin is being increasingly used to treat this condition. Plasmapheresis is also useful in monoclonal gammopathy-associated peripheral neuropathy. Patients with other peripheral neuropathic syndromes are less likely to benefit, and the primary physician should be aware of the limited value of expensive plasmapheresis in conditions other than those mentioned.

Condition-Specific Treatments

Diabetic Peripheral Neuropathy

Beside narcotics, the *tricyclic antidepressants* (e.g., *amitriptyline, nortriptyline*) have been mainstays of therapy for diabetic neuropathic pain for years, but the advent of the newer *anticonvulsants* (e.g., *gabapentin [Neurontin], pregabalin*) and the *selective serotonin and norepinephrine reuptake inhibitor antidepressants* (e.g., *duloxetine*) provide expensive but additionally effective alternatives that may be useful in persons who cannot tolerate the side effects of the tricyclics (see Chapter 227) or high-dose narcotics. Combination use with a narcotic may be synergistic, but excessive sedation needs to be watched for.

Duloxetine Cymbalta. This selective serotonin and norepinephrine reuptake inhibitor is well absorbed, can be used twice daily, and is hepatically metabolized. Recommended dose is 60 mg/d, which under study conditions provides a 50% reduction in pain in nearly 50% of patients. Adverse effects include dizziness, nausea, somnolence, and constipation. The drug should not be used in persons with narrow-angle glaucoma; safety in pregnancy is not established. Minor transaminase elevations may be noted.

Pregabalin Lyrica. This anticonvulsant is structurally similar to gabapentin, which has been widely used off label in diabetic peripheral neuropathy. Significant reductions in pain are achieved by almost half of users. Side effects include somnolence, dizziness, and peripheral edema; weight gain has been reported as well as euphoria. Cost is high; twice-daily dosing often suffices (starting at 50 to 75 mg twice daily). Patients concurrently taking a thiazolidinedione for diabetes (e.g., pioglitazone) experience a greater weight gain and more peripheral edema. Angioedema has been reported with use. Use in pregnancy is contraindicated.

HIV Infection

The painful peripheral neuropathy associated with HIV infection has proved to be responsive to optimizing HIV virologic control on antiretroviral therapy and to removing potential neurotoxic agents (see Chapter 13). Gabapentin, pregabalin, and duloxetine have been helpful in managing symptoms. Results with the anticonvulsant *lamotrigine* (*Lamictal*) have been more variable, and a rash progressing to Stevens–Johnson syndrome has been reported. Acupuncture and tricyclic antidepressants provide no benefit.

Postherpetic Neuralgia

When prevention is unsuccessful, treatment options in addition to narcotics include the newer anticonvulsants gabapentin and pregabalin (see also Chapter 192). Combination of gabapentin with morphine has shown better results than the use of either agent alone.

INDICATIONS FOR REFERRAL AND ADMISSION (1)

Evidence of acute spinal cord or cauda equina compression is an indication for immediate neurosurgical consultation and hospitalization. The patient with symptoms and signs of a slowly progressive myelopathy requires neurologic consultation and MRI. Vitamin B_{12} deficiency, multiple sclerosis, and tumor all need to be considered in patients with a progressive myelopathy if mechanical cord compression is excluded by MRI. A root or peripheral nerve compression syndrome may require surgical repair, and the patient with such a problem will need to see a neurosurgeon or an orthopedist skilled in its treatment. Nevertheless, before referral, the primary physician should have localized the problem and instituted appropriate initial therapy.

Annotated Bibliography

1. Bella I, Chad DA. Neuromuscular disorders and acute respiratory failure. Neurol Clin 1998;16:391. (*An excellent guide to the more emergent causes of rapidly progressive weakness, with good guidelines for respiratory management and acute triage.*)
2. Darnell RB, Posner JB. Paraneoplastic syndromes involving the nervous system. N Engl J Med 2003;349:1543. (*Comprehensive review of this important and often confusing cause of peripheral neuropathy.*)
3. Dawson DM. Entrapment neuropathies of the upper extremities. N Engl J Med 1993;329:2013. (*A nice review of carpal tunnel, ulnar, and thoracic outlet syndromes.*)
4. Delamonte SM. Peripheral neuropathy in the acquired immune deficiency syndrome. Ann Neurol 1988;28:485. (*This demyelinating neuropathy is being seen with increasing frequency by primary physicians and should be recognized.*)
5. Dyck PJ. The 10 P's: a mnemonic helpful in the characterization and differential diagnosis of peripheral neuropathy. Neurology 1992;42:14. (*It is actually a difficult mnemonic, but the article is helpful in delineating the principles of classifying and reviewing peripheral neuropathy.*)
6. Galer BS. Painful polyneuropathy. Neurol Clin 1998;16:791. (*An excellent review of clinical data supporting various oral and topical medications for polyneuropathy.*)
7. Polydefkis M, Griffin JW, McArthur J. New insights into diabetic polyneuropathy. JAMA 2003;290:1371. (*A grand-rounds review.*)
8. Woolf CJ, Mannion RJ. Neuropathic pain: aetiology, symptoms, mechanisms, and management. Lancet 1999;353:1959. (*Excellent scholarly review emphasizing the mechanisms of action of available and investigational medicines.*)
9. Jarvik JG, Hollingworth W, Martin B, et al. Rapid magnetic resonance imaging vs radiographs for patients with low back pain. JAMA 2003;289:2810. (*Rapid magnetic resonance imaging [MRI] and radiographs resulted in nearly identical outcomes for primary care patients with low back pain, although physicians and patients preferred the MRI.*)
10. Sater RA, Rostami A. Treatment of Guillain–Barré syndrome with intravenous immunoglobulin. Neurology 1998;51(Suppl 5):S9. (*Excellent summary of results with apheresis, intravenous immune globulin, or both.*)
11. Shlay JC, Chaloner K, Max MB, et al. Acupuncture and amitriptyline for pain due to HIV-related peripheral neuropathy: a randomized controlled trial. JAMA 1998;280:1590. (*Randomized, controlled trial [RCT]; neither approach was found to be better than placebo.*)
12. Backonja M, Beydoun A, Edwards KR, et al. Gabapentin for the symptomatic treatment of painful neuropathy in patients with diabetes mellitus: a randomized controlled trial. JAMA 1998;280:1831. (*RCT; produced significant reductions in symptoms and accompanying depression.*)
13. Clark WF, Rock GA, Buskard N, et al. Therapeutic plasma exchange: an update from the Canadian Apheresis Group. Ann Intern Med 1999;131:453. (*The approach was found to be useful for myasthenia gravis, chronic*

inflammatory polyneuropathy, and Guillain–Barré syndrome but not useful in other polyneuropathies and most cases of multiple sclerosis.)

14. Gilron I, Bailey JM, Tu D, et al. Morphine, gabapentin, or their combination for neuropathic pain. N Engl J Med 2005;352:1324. (*RCT; all were effective, but the combination was better than either alone.*)

15. Lesser H, Sharma U, LaMoreaux L, et al. Pregabalin relieves symptoms of painful diabetic neuropathy. Neurology 2004;63:2104. (*RCT; the treatment was found to be effective in diabetic peripheral neuropathy.*)

16. Raskin J, Pritchett YL, Wang F, et al. A double-blind, randomized multicenter trial comparing duloxetine with placebo in the management of diabetic peripheral neuropathic pain. Pain Med 2005;6:346.(*RCT demonstrating efficacy in diabetic peripheral neuropathy.*)

CHAPTER 168 ■ EVALUATION OF TREMOR

AMY A. PRUITT

Tremor is defined as a regular oscillation of a body part, and it must be distinguished from other rapid, involuntary movements. Many patients assume that the development of "shakiness" is a natural concomitant of aging. The physician must determine the significance of a variety of clinically similar tremors that may have widely dissimilar diagnostic, therapeutic, and prognostic implications. Workup involves differentiating the resting tremor of early parkinsonism from essential tremor and differentiating essential tremor from an exaggerated physiologic tremor. As new specific treatments are developed, accurate clinical distinction becomes increasingly valuable. Unfortunately, it may be difficult to differentiate tremors by clinical observation alone, and evaluation requires a working knowledge of simple electrophysiologic and pharmacologic characteristics.

PATHOPHYSIOLOGY AND CLINICAL PRESENTATION (1–3)

The precise neural mechanisms of tremor are unknown despite some clinicopathologic correlations, such as the abolition of the parkinsonian and essential tremors by lesions in the ventrolateral nucleus of the thalamus. Drugs such as L-dopa, which are known to act centrally to increase catecholamines, may worsen essential tremor; this observation has led to the suggestion that β-adrenergic blockers such as propranolol may exert their therapeutic action by central antagonism of β-adrenergic receptors.

The patient most frequently reports the insidious onset of "shaking" of a limb. Very likely, the patient will have ignored the symptom initially, assuming that it was a consequence of nervousness or fatigue. However, steady progression impels the patient to see the physician. Tremors can be present during the maintenance of a posture, at rest, or during an action (intention tremor).

Postural (Physiologic) Tremors

Postural or physiologic tremors are fine tremors with a frequency of 8 to 12 Hz; they occur normally in everyone during movement and while a fixed position is held against gravity. A true physiologic tremor is defined as one that does not produce symptoms and is within the given frequency range. The movement is usually invisible to the naked eye, but it may become exaggerated by anxiety, muscular fatigue, ingestion of coffee, use of β-agonists, and hyperthyroidism. Drugs, notably lithium and tricyclic antidepressants, may also accentuate this tremor. Amplitude and frequency vary among different people and in the same person at different times.

Resting Tremors

Unlike physiologic tremors, resting tremors occur when a limb is supported against gravity and no voluntary movement is required.

Parkinson's Disease

The most common rest tremor in a relaxed, supported limb is that caused by Parkinson's disease. It characteristically begins in the fingers and may later involve the arm and the leg. Flexion and extension of the fingers, abduction and adduction of the thumbs, and pronation and supination of the wrist produce the well-known "pill-rolling" movement. Frequently, this is the symptom that brings parkinsonian patients to the physician and may occur well in advance of the bradykinesia and postural difficulties characteristic of the full-blown syndrome. The tremor is slow (3 to 8 Hz), and its electromyographic (EMG) pattern, quite unlike that of essential tremor, shows alternating discharge in antagonistic muscle groups, which is suppressed with voluntary movement. Most such patients also have some degree of postural tremor. Some parkinsonian patients may have a typical action (essential) tremor, which is worsened by L-dopa therapy. Phenothiazines and haloperidol worsen the rest tremor (see Chapter 174).

Intention (Action) Tremors

These tremors occur with and are worsened by voluntary muscle contraction.

Essential (Familial, Senile) Tremor

The major intention tremors are those labeled *essential* (also referred to as *familial* or *senile*). Half of cases are transmitted as an autosomal-dominant trait and half are sporadic. The condition is characterized by an intention tremor of the hands, head, voice, and sometimes legs or trunk. Typically, the tremor is most prominent when the hands or head are held outstretched in a position against gravity and least noticeable at rest (although the tremor of early parkinsonism may also be seen best in an outstretched hand). Tremor may be accentuated by tasks that require precision, such as writing and carrying full cups of liquid (also seen in some patients with parkinsonism). Many patients report that the ingestion of a small amount of alcohol will temporarily reduce their tremor. Essential tremor may begin at any age, although early and late adult life are the most common periods of onset (which helps to differentiate the condition from parkinsonism, which typically begins in middle age). The tremor increases with age.

Cerebellar Disease

A more dramatic action tremor is displayed by patients with cerebellar diseases and is characterized by progressively increasing amplitude of the tremor as the patient brings the limb toward a target. There is no tremor at rest. In younger patients, this is most frequently caused by multiple sclerosis, but similar clinical states may be produced by cerebellar infarction, degenerative disorders of the spinocerebellar pathways, and chronic, relapsing, steroid-sensitive polyneuropathy. This tremor is multiplanar, with large, irregular, and relatively slow (2 to 4 Hz) oscillations. The tremor often is worsened by alcohol. Propranolol has no effect, and no satisfactory therapy is available.

Other Abnormal Movements

The definition of tremor as a regular oscillation of a body part serves to distinguish it from other rapid, intermittent movements that bespeak a different neurologic state. For diagnostic, therapeutic, and prognostic purposes, several categories of abnormal involuntary movements should be distinguished from tremor. All of the following involuntary movements (and most true tremors) are greatly reduced or disappear altogether with sleep.

Tics

Tics are repetitive, coordinated, usually stereotyped movements that are seen widely in the population and increase in frequency in a given patient in response to stress. They usually involve face or hand muscles, may initially be a conscious mannerism, and usually can be suppressed by voluntary effort. *Hemifacial spasm* is a kind of oscillating movement usually beginning in a middle-aged or elderly person that is localized to the facial muscles. It is believed to be caused by degenerative lesions of the facial nucleus or peripheral nerve, but the exact mechanism is unknown, and treatment is unsatisfactory.

Asterixis

Asterixis is an irregular contraction of skeletal muscles that results in flapping of the hands; it is electromyographically coincident with brief pauses at irregular intervals. *Chorea* is an irregular, jerking movement usually involving the fingers and often accompanied by *athetosis*, in which writhing movements of limbs or trunk may be added. *Epilepsia partialis continua*

refers to a focal seizure in which continuous seizure activity may result in a somewhat rhythmic jerking of one body part. Sudden onset of the illness is the most useful distinguishing feature.

Dyskinesias

These are rhythmic, involuntary movements of the orofacial musculature resulting in tongue protrusion and chewing movements. They are important to recognize because of the frequency with which they occur as early manifestations of the tardive dyskinesia syndrome caused by the use of phenothiazines and other major tranquilizers.

DIFFERENTIAL DIAGNOSIS (3)

Tremors can be divided clinically into postural, intention, and resting types. Most postural tremors are physiologic. Among the intention tremors are the essential, senile, and cerebellar varieties. Most resting tremors are caused by Parkinson's disease. Tremors must be distinguished from other voluntary movements such as dyskinesias, tics, myoclonus, and athetosis.

WORKUP (1–3)

History

The clinical assessment of tremor is greatly aided by first ascertaining the *circumstances* under which the tremor occurs. Some tremors are present during maintenance of a posture, some during rest, and others only during an action (the intention tremors). Careful questioning will often identify the type of tremor. Common diagnostic problems include distinguishing the resting tremor of early Parkinson's disease from an essential tremor and an essential tremor from an exaggerated physiologic tremor. All of these are common, and some may in fact be present simultaneously in a given patient. *Drug history* is important because it may reveal a sympathomimetic agent, an antiepileptic drug, a selective serotonin reuptake inhibitor, or another medication that can cause or exacerbate tremor.

Physical Examination

Physical examination is directed primarily at determining whether the tremor is better or worse with activity. Patients should be asked to hold out their hands, write, perform rapid alternating movements, and touch their nose with a finger repeatedly; the objective is to detect evidence of cerebellar or extrapyramidal disease. They should be observed discretely during the history and other parts of the physical examination because calling attention to the tremor may worsen it.

Laboratory Studies

At the end of the examination, it is sometimes difficult to determine whether a tremor is primarily resting or action in quality. Moreover, many parkinsonian patients have no other extrapyramidal signs at the time they present with tremor, limiting definitive diagnosis. Under such circumstances, a tremor recording by *EMG* can help to identify the type of tremor that is present because EMG patterns are distinctive for each type. Sometimes the EMG reveals that both types of tremors are present simultaneously. *Thyroid function* should be checked in any case of tremor.

SYMPTOMATIC MANAGEMENT (3–7)

Essential Tremor

Pharmacologic Therapy

A major advance in treatment was made with the discovery of the beneficial effect of *β-blockers* (e.g., 120 mg of *propranolol* daily). Long-acting preparations are more convenient and equally effective. A decade later, the anticonvulsant drug *primidone* (Mysoline) was found to be extremely effective at reducing or eliminating essential tremor in doses far smaller than those necessary for antiepileptic activity. The mechanism of action of primidone in tremor is unknown. No consensus has been reached regarding which of these two agents is the drug of choice for tremor. Because primidone is somewhat more effective for the majority of patients, starting with a low dose of 50 mg/d and working up to as much as 250 mg/d in divided doses is a very reasonable approach to treatment. Sedation is the major side effect, but it is generally tolerated if the drug is increased slowly. Propranolol is also well tolerated in most patients, although it is relatively contraindicated in those with underlying asthma, insulin-dependent diabetes, heart block, or congestive heart failure (see Chapters 25, 32, 48, and 102).

Alprazolam (Xanax) and other benzodiazepines have been used for essential tremor and may be effective as intermittent adjunctive agents in a patient on *β*-blockers or primidone. *Topiramate* (Topamax) has been advocated for essential tremor, although its frequent impairment of cognition may make it unsuitable for many older patients; other treatment-limiting adverse effects include paresthesias and difficulty concentrating. *Alcohol intake* will reduce the tremor for about 1 hour, but recurrent use will lead to increasingly larger amounts of alcohol required to suppress the tremor.

Interventional Therapies

Continuous deep-brain stimulation through an electrode implanted in the thalamus is a promising approach to suppression, having fewer complications than ablative surgery.

Physiologic Tremor

Performance anxiety sometimes exaggerates an otherwise inconsequential physiologic tremor in performers (e.g., concert musicians, public speakers), and the problem can sometimes be alleviated by a small preperformance dose of a *β-blocker* or a short-acting *benzodiazepine* (see Chapter 226). However, too large a dose of either can have an overly sedating effect and hinder performance. Moreover, the regular use of benzodiazepines is associated with a risk for habituation (see Chapter 226), and *β*-blockers usually have little effect on baseline physiologic tremors.

Intention Tremor

Parkinson's Disease

The tremor of Parkinson's disease, although it does not respond as well as bradykinesia and rigidity to dopaminergic agents, may benefit from *anticholinergic therapy* (see Chapter 174).

Cerebellar Disease

The tremor of cerebellar disease is notoriously unresponsive, although *β*-blockers, primidone, baclofen, gabapentin, and benzodiazepines are usually tried. Wrist weights may dampen the amplitude of these tremors and make the limb more functional.

PATIENT EDUCATION AND INDICATIONS FOR REFERRAL

The cause of the tremor and the fact that it can be controlled should be discussed with the patient. Avoidance of agents that worsen symptoms must be stressed. Patients with intention tremors and cerebellar signs must be referred to a neurologist because demyelinating or hereditary degenerative diseases may be responsible. Disabling tremors refractory to simple therapy may benefit from neurologic consultation. Neurosurgical techniques to control drug-refractory essential tremor include thalamotomy and deep-brain stimulation. Patients should be referred to a center that specializes in the surgical treatment of movement disorders.

Annotated Bibliography

1. Findley LJ, Gresty MA, Halmagyi GM. Tremor, the cogwheel phenomenon and clonus in Parkinson's disease. J Neurol Neurosurg Psychiatry 1981;44:534. (*Presents classic descriptions.*)
2. Lou JS, Jankovic J. Essential tremor: clinical correlates in 350 patients. Neurology 1991;41:234. (*An excellent discussion of clinical features.*)
3. Rehman H. Diagnosis and management of tremor. Arch Intern Med 2000;160:2438. (*A useful literature review and classification of tremors; 96 references.*)
4. Gironell A, Kulisevsky J, Barbanoj M, et al. A randomized placebo-controlled comparative trial of gabapentin and propranolol in essential tremor. Arch Neurol 1999;132:129. (*The efficacies were comparable.*)
5. Koller WC. Efficacy of primidone in the treatment of essential tremor. Neurology 1986;26:121. (*Establishes the utility of the drug in a high percentage of patients.*)
6. Ondo WG, Jankovic J, Connor GS, et al. Topiramate in essential tremor: A double-blind placebo-controlled trial. Neurology 2006;66:672. (*Finds some benefit, but high doses were often needed, and impairment of cognition was seen.*)
7. Schuurman PR, Bosch DA, Possuyt PMM, et al. A comparison of continuous thalamic stimulation and thalamotomy for suppression of severe tremor. N Engl J Med 2000;342:461. (*These two therapies were equally effective for the suppression of drug-resistant tremor, but thalamic stimulation had fewer adverse effects.*)

CHAPTER 169 ■ EVALUATION OF DEMENTIA

AMY A. PRUITT

Dementia is the progressive decline of intellectual ability from a previously attained level. Speech, memory, judgment, and mood may all be altered in varying proportions. The prevalence rises rapidly with age, starting at 1% at age 60 years and doubling every 5 years to nearly 40% by the age of 85 years. An estimated 600,000 persons with advanced dementia in the United States require institutional care. With the aging of the U.S. population, the social consequences of the problem are likely to be staggering if no major changes in prevention and treatment are implemented. By 2030, when nearly 20% of the U.S. population will be older than the age of 65 years, approximately 6% will have severe dementia, and an additional 10% to 15% will have mild to moderate impairment. The current annual dementia-related expense of long-term care either at home or in a nursing facility is more than $50 billion. Dementia also accounts for more admissions and hospital inpatient days than does any other geriatric psychiatric condition. Median survival depends on age at diagnosis and can range from 3 to 20 years.

More than 55 illnesses can cause dementia. Although in one sense all are treatable, at least with psychosocial intervention, the 15% of patients with significantly reversible causes or complicating conditions are depressed or exhibit drug-induced changes in mental status. When a decline in mental functioning is noted, fear of Alzheimer's disease arises in patients and their families. Each patient requires a careful workup for dementia and proper identification of the underlying cause. Primary physicians should know how to distinguish dementia from other, more specific cortical deficits (aphasia, agnosia, isolated memory deficit) and should be able to perform a screening examination for potentially reversible disease. Prompt recognition of dementia is essential, not only for the initiation of a diagnostic workup, but also to protect the patient from avoidable harm, such as that due to a fall, drug overdose, fire, or inadequate nutrition.

PATHOPHYSIOLOGY AND CLINICAL PRESENTATION (1–10)

Definition and Description

Dementia

The term "*dementia*" refers to a syndrome characterized by *generalized* and *sustained* decline in *intellectual functioning* from a previously attained level. It is a characteristically *progressive* disorder, measurable in months or years rather than days or weeks. The decline from a previously attained level of mental ability is broad based, usually involving *memory, cognitive capacities,* and *adaptive behavior without alteration of consciousness.* Initially, the patient may be aware of some difficulties but later seems mostly not to be disturbed by them.

Mild Cognitive Impairment

It is important but not always possible to distinguish the early stages of dementia from nonprogressive cognitive changes (*benign forgetfulness*) that occur in normal aging. The term "*mild cognitive impairment*" (MCI) refers to an isolated loss of memory without problems in other cognitive domains and with intact activities of daily living. Between 6% and 25% of MCI patients progress to Alzheimer's disease or other dementia each year, and disease-modifying therapies increasingly are directed at this population.

Presentation

The onset of dementia is usually insidious, although a few conditions evolve rapidly. Patients initially may be noted to be slightly forgetful, with attention and concentration deficits and increasing repetitiousness or inconsistencies in their usual behavior. Later in the course of the process, patients may display increasingly impaired judgment, an inability to abstract or generalize, and personality changes, reacting with rigidity, perseveration, irritability, and confusion to minor changes in the environment. Affective disturbances or aggressive behavior may be prominent, and in extreme forms, patients lose all vestiges of their original personality, are unable to participate in matters of personal hygiene and nutrition, and are left helpless.

Dementia is often progressive (as in degenerative diseases), but it may be static (as in a posttraumatic brain injury state). Depending on the pathologic condition that causes dementia, indications of disease outside the areas of the brain responsible for cognitive and behavioral change may or may not be found. Concomitant disorders of extrapyramidal function are particularly common.

Some conditions that result in dementia may also cause mental retardation (e.g., Down's syndrome). Patients with dementia may or may not be psychotic, and a patient with psychosis may or may not have any evidence of cognitive decline consistent with dementia.

Epidemiologic studies of both elderly men and women find that programs of regular exercise (as modest as walking at a slow pace for 1/2 hour several times a week) are associated with significant reductions in the risk of developing dementia.

Primary Neurologic Conditions

Alzheimer's Disease

The leading cause of dementia, Alzheimer's disease accounts for well more than half of cases among the elderly and affects 15 million people worldwide. Its incidence increases with advancing age. Because many patients survive for a decade, the prevalence increases from 43% at age 65 years to 47% after age 85 years. Most cases are *sporadic*, but *familial autosomal-dominant* forms of the disease exist. Mutations in the gene for the amyloid precursor protein and the genes for *presenilin 1 and 2* cause the uncommon, dominantly inherited forms of the disease that become symptomatic before the age of 60 years, and the *e4 variant* of *apolipoprotein E* is associated with the sporadic form and some later-onset familial forms. Elevated serum levels of *homocysteine* and aspects of the *metabolic syndrome* have been found to be an independent risk factor for Alzheimer's disease, increasing the relative risk nearly twofold and offering targets for midlife intervention in the primary care setting.

No specific physical signs are characteristic, although *frontal lobe release signs* and secondary mild *extrapyramidal features* may be present. Although this disease cannot be diagnosed with certainty during life, a high probability of the diagnosis can be determined according to the criteria established by the Alzheimer's Disease and Related Disorders Work Group of 1984. Progressive *worsening of memory* with impairment of at least *one other cognitive function* is the hallmark of the disease. About two thirds of patients with moderate to severe dementia who have no other illness that can cause dementia (e.g., cerebrovascular disease, hypothyroidism) are given the diagnosis of probable Alzheimer's disease.

The diagnosis of Alzheimer's disease can be confirmed only at postmortem examination. Neuropathologic study reveals *neuronal loss*, *neurofibrillary tangles* composed of τ-protein, and *senile plaques* containing the β-amyloid peptide. Basal forebrain degeneration reduces the acetylcholine content. The loss of this transmitter correlates with memory impairment. Frequently, vascular dementia and Alzheimer's disease coexist and both pathologies are found postmortem.

Dementia with Lewy Bodies

This increasingly appreciated but probably widespread and underdiagnosed idiopathic condition has features of Alzheimer's and Parkinson's diseases, which leads to considerable diagnostic confusion and the potential for therapeutic mismanagement. Recognition is important because these patients manifest marked sensitivity to neuroleptic drugs, which may exacerbate symptoms (see Chapter 173).

The pathologic hallmarks are the widespread presence of *Lewy bodies* (intracytoplasmic inclusions) in the cortex, amygdala, hippocampus, and pars compacta of the substantia nigra and nucleus ceruleus, with a loss of neuronal density in the latter areas. Unlike patients with Alzheimer's disease, these patients have only mild brain atrophy grossly and normal density of the neocortex.

The initial presentation is often one of *visual hallucinations*, *episodic delirium*, *fluctuating cognitive difficulties*, and *parkinsonism* and *extrapyramidal motor symptoms* (dysarthria, poor coordination of voluntary movements). As in Alzheimer's disease, *short-term memory impairment* and a *progressive decline in cognition* interfere with social and occupational functioning. In early stages, the memory impairment may be mild, and periods of nearly normal functioning occur intermittently. Deficits in attention and visual–spatial and frontal–subcortical skills are nonetheless evident.

Core features include recurrent *visual hallucinations* that are well formed and detailed, fluctuating consciousness, and spontaneous motor features of *parkinsonism* and *extrapyramidal disease*. Other characteristics include falls, syncope, transient loss of consciousness, hallucinations in other domains, systematized delusions, and, as noted, sensitivity to neuroleptic medications. The rate of clinical decline is generally more rapid than that of Alzheimer's disease.

Multiinfarct Dementia

"Hardening of the arteries" with cerebral hypoperfusion has been a common, although mistaken, lay view of the cause of dementia. However, multiple strokes can leave a patient with impaired cognition and produce a true dementia, often referred to as *multiinfarct dementia*. Although the exact contribution of vascular dementia to the overall rate of dementia is a subject of debate, groups with a high prevalence of vascular risk factors (e.g., African Americans, Japanese) are at increased risk. An elderly patient with hypertension, diabetes, atrial fibrillation, or known carotid disease or who smokes should be considered at risk.

The characteristic clinical course is one of *stepwise progression* if discrete large-vessel occlusions occur and is more *gradual* if the infarctions are primarily lacunar (see Chapter 171). The infarctions may be large and heralded by clearly defined episodes of neurologic injury or develop subclinically as small lacunar strokes contributing to a slow decline in intellectual function. Magnetic resonance imaging (MRI) may reveal multiple lacunar infarctions and a loss of periventricular white matter. Most patients have evidence of upper motor neuron injury (lateralized weakness, brisk reflexes, or Babinski signs). Multiinfarct dementia is sometimes referred to as a *subcortical dementia*, characterized by apathy, slowness, and decreased memory retrieval. The development of dementia within 1 year of a first stroke is a subject of significant research.

Newly identified independent risk factors for dementia such as elevations in *low-density-lipoprotein* (LDL) *cholesterol* and *homocysteine* may exert their effect through vascular mechanisms because both are established risk factors for atherosclerotic vascular disease (see Chapter 26). Aggressive reduction in LDL cholesterol reduces the risk of stroke (see Chapter 171); whether it will reduce the risk of dementia remains to be established. Reduction in homocysteine is yet to be proven to reduce cardiovascular risk (see Chapter 31).

Mixed Disease

As patients age, the brain becomes increasingly vulnerable to insult. Moreover, the risks for vascular and degenerative diseases increase. For this reason, it is likely that a large percentage of cases of dementia in the very elderly are of a mixed type, with both vascular disease and Alzheimer's disease as underlying conditions. The significance of this notion of mixed disease is that it focuses attention on various potential causes of dementia and the importance of controlling risk factors (e.g., improving diabetic or hypertensive control).

Normal-Pressure Hydrocephalus

Normal-pressure hydrocephalus deserves special mention both because it is reversible and because it is generally overdiagnosed. The name of this entity denotes slow ventricular enlargement without cortical atrophy resulting from poor resorption of cerebrospinal fluid over the cerebral convexities. Most often, the precipitant is unknown, but the condition can occur when cerebrospinal fluid resorption is blocked as a consequence of remote meningeal inflammation or subarachnoid hemorrhage. *Dementia*, *gait disturbance*, and urinary and fecal *incontinence* comprise the classic triad. Some patients respond dramatically to ventricular–peritoneal shunting, and the diagnosis is suspected clinically and radiographically. Serial lumbar punctures with the removal of large volumes (>30 mL) of cerebrospinal fluid are undertaken to try to predict which patients will respond to this maneuver.

Space-Occupying Lesions

Space-occupying lesions such as *chronic subdural hematoma* or slowly growing *tumors* of the brain produce variable dementia, depending on their size and location. When they are located on the orbital surface of the *frontal lobe* or the medial surface of the *temporal lobe,* patients may present primarily with *cognitive defects* and no other focal signs of cerebral tumor. The development of a progressive unilateral headache (see Chapter 165), a new neurologic deficit, or a change in personality may provide a clue to the presence of a mass lesion.

Depression

Depression can produce the rapid onset of a true cognitive deficit that is reversible with appropriate treatment. Other symptoms of depression (hopelessness, low self-esteem, early-morning awakening, fatigue, anhedonia; see Chapter 227) almost always predate the onset of the dementia and help to suggest the diagnosis. Unlike patients with Alzheimer's disease, depressed patients will complain of memory loss during a mental status examination. Although depression alone can produce significant reversible cognitive impairment, severe mood disturbance may also accompany other causes of dementia, such as Alzheimer's disease or Parkinson's disease.

Other Primary Neurologic Conditions

Other primary neurologic conditions associated with dementia and specific neurologic deficits include frontotemporal dementia, *Parkinson's* disease (see Chapter 174), Wilson's disease, severe *multiple sclerosis* (see Chapter 172), Creutzfeldt–Jakob disease, neurosyphilis, and *Huntington's* disease (Table 169.1). Frontotemporal dementia is associated with predominantly frontal and temporal lobe pathologic involvement. The age of onset is usually earlier, and cognitive deficits differ from those of Alzheimer's disease, with early personality change and impairment of executive function (the ability to modify behavior in response to changing stimuli, solve problems, organize, think abstractly, and avoid perseveration). Parkinson's disease and Huntington's disease are sometimes referred to as *subcortical dementias* because they present with significant motor dysfunction and no prominent aphasia or agnosia. Proper identification is essential to initiating effective treatment and providing accurate prognostic information.

Other Causes of Dementia

Toxins, infections, metabolic disorders, and nutritional disorders may affect the brain and result in dementia (Table 169.2). Frequently, more than one pathologic cause is present.

TABLE 169.1

NEUROLOGIC DISEASES ASSOCIATED WITH INTELLECTUAL DYSFUNCTION

Disease	Physical Signs	Clinical Features
Alzheimer's disease	Frontal lobe release signs, extrapyramidal signs	Enlarged ventricles *and* cortical atrophy by CT or MRI
Normal-pressure hydrocephalus	Gait disorder,[a] incontinence	Enlarged ventricles with little or no cortical atrophy
Dementia with Lewy bodies (Lewy-body disease)	Visual hallucinations, periodic confusion, parkinsonism	Marked exacerbation of extrapyramidal symptoms with use of standard neuroleptics
Multiinfarct dementia	Focal deficits	Stepwise course; multiple areas of infarction, often subcortical, by CT or MRI
Parkinson's disease	Extrapyramidal signs[a]	Usually present only after disease has been evident for several years
Intracranial tumor	Focal signs, papilledema	Often subacute evolution, seizures possible
Neurosyphilis	Frontal lobe signs, optic atrophy, Argyll Robertson pupils	Positive serology serum and CSF
HIV infection	Variable systemic involvement	Positive HIV, cortical atrophy; dementia may be presenting symptom
Creutzfeldt–Jakob disease	Myoclonus,[a] cerebellar signs, eye movement abnormalities	Subacute course; EEG has specific abnormalities; brain biopsy diagnostic
Huntington's disease	Choreiform movements,[a] corticospinal signs	Often positive family history; caudate atrophy by CT or MRI
Multiple sclerosis	Brainstem signs, optic atrophy, corticospinal signs	Usually longstanding disease; episodic illness with remissions; often extensive white matter abnormalities by MRI
Wilson's disease	Extrapyramidal signs[a], hepatic dysfunction, Kayser–Fleischer rings[a]	Onset in adolescence or young adult life, psychiatric disorders
Progressive supranuclear palsy	Failure of vertical downgaze,[a] extrapyramidal signs[a]	Eye movement abnormalities; differentiate from Parkinson's disease; unresponsive or only transiently responsive to levodopa

CSF, cerebrospinal fluid; CT, computed tomography; EEG, electroencephalogram; MRI, magnetic resonance imaging.
[a]Invariably present; all other physical signs are neither invariably present nor pathognomonic.

TABLE 169.2

SYSTEMIC CONDITIONS ASSOCIATED WITH INTELLECTUAL IMPAIRMENT

Infectious
  Syphilis with central nervous system involvement
  HIV infection with central nervous system involvement
  Cryptococcal infection of the central nervous system

Endocrine
  Hypothyroidism and hyperthyroidism
  Panhypopituitarism
  High-dose glucocorticoid therapy

Metabolic
  Vitamin B_{12} deficiency
  Thiamine deficiency
  Niacin deficiency (pellagra)

Chemical Poisons
  Alcohol
  Metals (lead, mercury)
  Aniline dyes

Drug Intoxications
  Barbiturates
  Opiates
  Anticholinergics
  Lithium
  Bromides
  Haloperidol
  Antihypertensives

Medications/Intoxication

The patient with a progressive degenerative dementia may be taking an excess of a medication that is exacerbating the primary process, or the drug itself may be causing an apparent loss of cognitive abilities. Medications capable of producing dementia in patients without other underlying conditions include opiates and the numerous neurotropic agents available. Less obvious but frequently prescribed medications causing or aggravating dementia include the *anticholinergic preparations* used in movement disorders, *antihypertensives*, and *sedatives*. These agents are high on the list of causes of disease that can be arrested or reversed.

Infection

Any infection involving the brain can produce a picture of diffuse cognitive impairment. *Neurosyphilis*, *HIV infection* (see Chapter 13), and *cryptococcal infection* spread into the central nervous system to produce dementia, often with great regularity. Infectious agents responsible for subacute conditions like Creutzfeldt–Jakob disease and progressive multifocal leukoencephalopathy are resistant to treatment.

Endocrinologic, Nutritional, and Metabolic Disorders

This category of etiologies represents some of the more reversible causes of dementia, which tend to present with clinical manifestations of the underlying condition, as well as with altered cognitive function, although sometimes these manifestations may be subtle.

Endocrine. Thyroid dysfunction due to *hyperthyroidism* or *hypothyroidism* may lead to impaired but reversible cognitive function. In the elderly, the clinical manifestations may be ab-

sent or atypical (see Chapters 103 and 104). The administration of *high-dose corticosteroid therapy* can acutely alter cognitive function.

Nutritional. The most common nutritional disorder is *vitamin B_{12} deficiency*, which can produce dementia along with megaloblastic anemia, peripheral neuropathy, and subacute combined degeneration of the spinal cord (see Chapter 79). If it is detected and treated before the onset of permanent nerve damage, some of the deficits may resolve at least partially (see Chapter 82).

Thiamine deficiency, if untreated, may lead to Korsakoff's dementia, which is largely irreversible. Thiamine deficiency is a preventable condition seen with alcoholism, pernicious vomiting of any cause, depression, and inadequate diet. *Pellagra*, which is uncommon in developed countries, shows a dramatic response to niacin, even when mental changes have been present for a long time.

Metabolic. The metabolic derangements resulting from advanced *renal or hepatocellular failure* usually cause an encephalopathic picture that differs from true dementia in that consciousness is altered. However, milder forms of metabolic disease may exacerbate an underlying dementia, as may *dehydration*. Of the hereditary metabolic diseases associated with prominent cognitive alteration, *Wilson's disease*, *metachromatic leukodystrophy*, and the *adrenal leukodystrophies* are among the most notable.

DIFFERENTIAL DIAGNOSIS

A useful way of organizing the differential diagnosis of dementia is to divide the dementing conditions into pathologic processes that originate in the brain (see Table 169.1) and those that affect the brain secondarily, such as exogenous intoxication, infections, and metabolic derangements (see Table 169.2). Diseases that are primary in the brain may be accompanied by signs of neurologic disease other than cognitive change. Diseases that affect the brain secondarily are more likely to be accompanied by signs and symptoms of medical disease and perhaps are more reversible. Among patients presenting with dementia, Alzheimer's disease accounts for 65% of cases, vascular disease with multiple infarctions for 10% to 20%, and brain tumors for 5%; all other and unknown causes account for 10% to 15%. Among the very old (older than age 85 years), vascular dementia and Alzheimer's disease account for the vast majority of cases, but occult thyroid disease and vitamin B_{12} deficiency are also common, potentially reversible, and need to be considered in the differential.

WORKUP (1,2,4,11–18)

The goal of the workup is to distinguish dementia from other causes of mental impairment and to identify the cause as either a primary neurologic condition or a condition that secondarily affects the brain. Differentiating among neurologic conditions is essential, not only to identify and treat reversible conditions promptly, but also to optimize the care of those with incurable disease. Not all neurologic dementia is Alzheimer's disease, and not all of these conditions respond similarly to symptomatic measures (see Chapter 173). Careful workup is essential for proper management, with attention to diagnostic criteria to facilitate accurate diagnosis.

Diagnostic Criteria for Alzheimer's Disease

The diagnostic criteria established by the U.S. Department of Health and Human Services require:

■ The presence of dementia established by clinical examination and documented by the Mini-Mental State Examination or similar examination
■ Evidence of deficits in two or more areas of cognition
■ Progressive worsening of memory and other cognitive function
■ No disturbance of consciousness
■ The absence of systemic disorders or other brain disease that in and of themselves could account for the deficits

History

A careful history is the most important component of the initial evaluation. The help of a family member is critical to taking an adequate history because the patient's recall may be inadequate.

Differentiating Dementia from Other Neurologic Impairments

Differentiating dementia from other neurologic impairments requires a description by the patient or family of the specific *cognitive*, *memory*, and *behavioral problems* the patient is experiencing and the *consequences* of such deficits in the patient's daily life, such as difficulties with driving, work, or family relationships. Detailed questioning should define the *temporal course* of the illness and enable the physician to ascertain whether the process is indeed chronic and progressive, stepwise, or static.

A stepwise pattern in conjunction with focal deficits raises the question of a multiinfarct basis. An episode of severe hypotension followed by the onset of dementia points to hypoperfusion as the mechanism of what may be a static (nonprogressive) posthypoxic encephalopathy. A story of progressive, generalized intellectual impairment without alteration of consciousness is indicative of Alzheimer's disease and other neurodegenerative conditions, but multiple lacunar strokes may also be associated with this temporal pattern.

Finally, the examiner should check for important epidemiologic *risk factors* for dementia, including a prior severe episode of *head trauma*, *diabetes*, *never having been married*, and a *low level of education*.

Identifying Treatable Causes and Differentiating among Etiologies

Once dementia is strongly suspected, the history should then focus on identifying potentially treatable causes, be they primarily neurologic or secondary. The search for neurologic disease includes inquiry into risk factors and specific neurologic accompaniments. *Cardiovascular risk factors* (e.g., smoking, hypertension, hyperlipidemia, diabetes) should be ascertained for identification of the patient at risk for vascular dementia. Questioning about *gait*, *incontinence*, and a prior history of *meningitis* or *subarachnoid hemorrhage* helps to identify the patient at increased risk for normal-pressure hydrocephalus. A prior history of *head trauma*, unexplained onset of a *focal neurologic deficit*, and unilateral *headache* worsening over time are potential clues to a mass lesion. A history of *resting tremor* and *rigidity* are likely manifestations of Parkinson's disease. *Extrapyramidal symptoms* (dysarthria, poor coordination

of voluntary movements) raise the question of Lewy-body disease; if concurrent hepatocellular dysfunction is present, then Wilson's disease should be considered. Reports of vivid *visual hallucinations* suggest Lewy-body disease. *High-risk sexual behavior* raises the probabilities of HIV infection and neurosyphilis. Any symptoms or prior history of *depression* need to be reviewed (see Chapter 227). A *family history* of dementia, Down's syndrome, or psychiatric disorders is the basis for identifying patients at risk for one of the hereditary causes of dementia.

The history is also critical to identifying nonneurologic conditions that may be causing or exacerbating a loss of mental capacity. Concurrent illnesses and precipitating factors are reviewed. For example, one asks about previous *gastric surgery* (leading to vitamin B_{12} deficiency) and adequacy of *nutrition* (for thiamine, niacin, and vitamin B_{12} deficiencies). A detailed review of *medications* (particularly opiates, sedative–hypnotics, analgesics, anticholinergics, anticonvulsants, corticosteroids, centrally acting antihypertensives, and psychotropics) should be elicited. It is critical to rule out *alcohol* abuse and other forms of substance abuse (see Chapters 228 and 235). It is important to check for symptoms of *hypothyroidism* (see Chapter 104) and *pituitary insufficiency* (see Chapter 101). The *occupational history* may reveal exposure to toxic substances (e.g., aniline dyes or heavy metals).

Physical Examination

Mental Status Examination

Assessment begins with a mental status examination to confirm the presence of dementia. The complex faculties that constitute intellect are usually divided into functions, not necessarily anatomically or pathologically exclusive, that can be tested. This part of the examination should be geared both to the *detection of focal lesions* and to *signs of general brain dysfunction*.

The *Mini-Mental State Examination* has been the best studied of the cognitive tests. When results are properly adjusted for age and level of education, test sensitivity and specificity can reach as high as 90% but may be as low as 50% to 70%. The test performs best in the assessment of white persons with at least a high school education; sensitivity is reduced in highly educated persons, and specificity is compromised by having a limited educational background and being from another culture.

The mental status examination in the office should include assessment of the following elements of cortical function:

■ *Immediate memory:* recall of three objects, forward and backward recitation of digits given by the examiner, and recall of a short story.
■ *Remote memory:* response to questions about historical events of note, family milestones, or more recent happenings reported in the newspaper.
■ *Language:* naming of parts of objects, following complex commands, and generating word lists (e.g., number of animals named in 60 seconds).
■ *Visual–spatial relations:* reproducing simple drawings, drawing from memory a clock that reads 10:35, and discerning similarities among objects.
■ *Judgment and reasoning:* responding to decision-requiring situations ("finding a stamped letter" or "seeing a fire in a theater"); responding to questions like "how is an apple like a banana"?
■ *Attention and concentration:* capacity to reverse sequences, as in naming the months of the year backward.

General Physical and Neurologic Examinations

The physician should examine the patient to uncover evidence of any coexisting abnormalities that may be causing or contributing to the problem. One checks for physical evidence of neurovascular risk factors (see Chapter 171) and carefully palpates and auscultates the carotid arteries. In addition, the physician notes any signs of alcoholism (see Chapter 228), hepatocellular injury (see Chapter 71), renal insufficiency (see Chapter 142), and other systemic illnesses. Specific neurologic abnormalities, such as frontal lobe release signs (grasp, suck, snout, and root), visual field cut, limitation of extraocular movement, or abnormal papillary reaction should be elicited. Nystagmus may indicate recent drug ingestion or the presence of brainstem disease. The motor examination should pay particular attention to extrapyramidal features or involuntary movements such as tardive dyskinesias, tremors, asterixis, chorea, or myoclonus. The sensory examination may reveal evidence of peripheral neuropathy or combined system disease (vitamin B_{12} deficiency). Gait should be observed carefully; the small, rigid steps of frontal lobe gait apraxia can be distinguished from a wide-based cerebellar gait or the small steps associated with extrapyramidal disease.

Laboratory Studies

No single test can establish the presence of dementia, and a poor score on a Mini-Mental State Examination should not be the sole criterion for its diagnosis. The score should be considered clinically significant if it is corroborated by other components of the initial evaluation and history. Several clinical drug trials have confirmed what neurologic clinicians have long suspected, namely, that considerable variability in the annual Mini-Mental State Examination score is noted in patients with probable Alzheimer's disease and that variability of scores among examiners is prominent. Similarly, the existence of several different sets of criteria for vascular dementia confounds both the longitudinal assessment of patients and initial diagnostic certainty. Continuing observation over time may be necessary to establish the diagnosis for some patients and to identify complicating conditions.

Baseline Laboratory Studies

The laboratory tests recommended should be individualized, based on the patient's history and physical and mental status examination results. Because the history and physical examination limit the differential possibilities, the patient should be spared the inconvenience and costs of excessive testing. Undertesting is also hazardous because elderly patients in whom medical diseases may underlie nonspecific presentations of dementia comprise the usual patient population.

The guidelines specified by the National Institute of Aging Task Force on Mental Impairment in the Elderly have become the standard for investigating patients with dementia, and the American Academy of Neurology supplies similar guidelines for its member neurologists. Diagnostic tests should include the following:

- *Formal screening for depression* (see Chapter 227)
- *Serum vitamin B_{12}* (plus foliate if B_{12} low; see Chapter 79)
- *Thyroid-stimulating hormone*
- *Complete blood cell count* and *sedimentation rate*
- *Chemistry panel* (electrolytes, calcium, albumin, blood urea nitrogen, creatinine, transaminase, glucose) and urinalysis

- *Screening test for syphilis* (e.g., the rapid plasma reagin test; see Chapter 124), but only if the patient has a specific risk factor (e.g., history of sexually transmitted disease)
- *Screening for HIV infection* (specifically for persons with a history of high-risk sexual activity or exposure; see Chapter 7).
- *Computed tomography* (CT) or *MRI* of the head, especially when potentially treatable or preventable intracranial pathology is a consideration (see later discussion).

In addition, chest x-ray and electrocardiogram are included in some recommended lists of tests, but clinical judgment is a better determinant of their appropriateness. There is no indication for the routine use of brain single-photon emission computed tomography imaging, cerebrospinal sampling for τ protein, genetic testing for apolipoprotein E genotype, or electroencephalogram. Sampling the cerebrospinal fluid for the 14-3-3 protein may be useful when Creutzfeldt–Jakob disease is suspected and recent stroke and viral encephalitis can be excluded.

Computed Tomography and Magnetic Resonance Imaging

Neuroimaging by CT or MRI is appropriate in the presence of (a) a history suggestive of a mass lesion, (b) focal neurologic signs or symptoms, (c) dementia of abrupt onset, (d) a history of seizures, and (e) a history of stroke. Subdural hecatombs and intracranial tumors can be readily identified, especially when contrast-enhanced studies are performed, and radiologic evidence of normal-pressure hydrocephalus also may be provided. MRI with gadolinium contrast enhancement is superior to CT for the diagnosis of multiinfarct dementia and for the elucidation of problems referable to the posterior fossa. If the clinical suspicion of tumor is high, MRI is the more sensitive test.

Positron Emission Tomography (PET)

PET scanning differs from conventional neuroimaging in its ability to detect functional changes in regional brain metabolism, providing enhanced diagnostic and prognostic capabilities. Test sensitivity for the detection of neuropathologically confirmed Alzheimer's disease is 94% and specificity about 73%; for other neurodegenerative diseases, the test characteristics are similar. Clinical course can be predicted by the pattern of cerebral metabolism, with hypometabolism having a 93% sensitivity for disease progression over 2 to 3 years (the false-positive rate is 9%). The exact contributions of PET scanning to the evaluation of dementia remain to be defined, but testing in the early phases of illness holds promise for improving the accuracy of diagnosis and prognostication. A promising PET technique using special radionuclides that bind to *amyloid* and *τ protein neurofibrillary tangles* (the pathologic hallmarks of Alzheimer's disease) offers the possibility of differentiating among mild cognitive impairment, Alzheimer's disease, and normal aging.

Other Ancillary Studies

Electroencephalographic patterns may be normal even in advanced states of dementia, or nonspecific slowing of the baseline rhythm may be found. For patients who have episodes of altered consciousness and in whom seizures may therefore be suspected, this is an indicated procedure. Occasionally, the electroencephalogram may raise suspicion of a particular disease process; focal delta slowing is seen with tumor, unilateral attenuation of voltage may suggest an extracranial mass such as subdural hematoma, and excessive beta activity may be consistent with drug ingestion. Finally, Creutzfeldt–Jakob disease has a highly specific electroencephalographic pattern.

Formal neuropsychologic evaluation would be appropriate for obtaining more-specific information when the diagnosis is in doubt and is also helpful in providing additional information about the nature of impairment after focal brain injury. *Speech analysis* with speech therapy may improve patient and family communication. Formal *psychiatric assessment* may be desirable if depression is suspected in addition to dementia.

Studies of Limited or Uncertain Utility

Brain biopsy for nonneoplastic and noninfectious diseases is rarely justified. Very occasionally, progressive multifocal leukoencephalopathy or Creutzfeldt–Jakob disease is diagnosed by this technique, but MRI is emerging as a more sensitive test for the latter.

Noninvasive neurovascular studies (carotid ultrasonography, Doppler flow studies; see Chapter 171) are not of routine value in the workup of dementia unless the clinical course or physical examination findings suggest cerebrovascular disease or the MRI or CT demonstrates infarction.

Genetic Testing

Genetic testing is controversial and poses ethical issues. When the family history suggests early-onset Alzheimer's disease, tests for mutations on chromosomes 1, 14, and 21 can be considered. Clinicians can expect to be asked by patients and families about the "test for dementia"—the search for the *e4 allele* of the *gene encoding apolipoprotein E* (*APOE*e4*), which is encoded on protein 19 and has been associated with Alzheimer's disease. *APOE* genotyping is not accurate enough to serve alone as a test for Alzheimer's disease, but at least one *APOE*e4* allele can be found in 65% of pathologically confirmed cases of Alzheimer's disease. When combined with clinical evaluation, *APOE* genotyping can improve diagnostic specificity, but the test lacks sufficient sensitivity to be used to rule out Alzheimer's disease. Moreover, it is not sufficiently predictive of developing dementing illness to be of prognostic value. These features of the apolipoprotein E test should be shared with patients inquiring about the "test for Alzheimer's disease." Taking a mail order test for *APOE* genotyping should be discouraged because of the shortcomings of the test and the high probability of misinterpreting the results.

Screening for Dementia

The growing prevalence of dementia in aging populations of postindustrialized societies and the recent advent of medications that may slow the progression of common neurodegenerative diseases (see Chapter 173) raise the question of screening. The U.S. Preventive Services Task Force examined the issue and made several observations based on best evidence: (a) available screening tests have "some sensitivity but only fair specificity," (b) available drug therapy can delay disease progression by several months, but the effect on basic activities of daily living is "small at best," and (c) the generalizability of findings in research studies to patients seen in everyday clinical practice is unclear. They concluded that available evidence is insufficient to determine whether the expected benefits would be outweighed by the potential harms

(e.g., the consequences of a false-positive diagnosis) and thus recommended neither for nor against screening for dementia at this time. Use of the Mini Mental Status Examination can be helpful in identifying persons with mild cognitive impairment, who are at increased risk for developing dementia.

MANAGEMENT (1,2,4,8,9,19–26)

Prevention

The best approach to management of dementia is prevention, given the irreversibility and refractoriness to treatment of many etiologies. Recent epidemiologic and community-based observational studies suggest a number of possible approaches, as do a few randomized trials (particularly with regard to lowering cholesterol and blood pressure).

Exercise

Simple lifestyle measures, such as regular modest exercise, can significantly reduce the risk in the elderly of developing dementia. As few as 1.5 hours/wk of walking at a slow pace was associated with a 20% reduction in risk among elderly women in the Nurses' Health Study. Participation in leisure activities such as playing board games, playing musical instruments, and reading were associated with a reduced risk of dementia. These and other healthy lifestyle interventions need confirmation by prospective study better to assess their precise contributions to prevention, but there seems to be little harm in implementing them while awaiting confirmatory data.

Lowering of Cholesterol and Blood Pressure

The reduction of *LDL cholesterol* in the elderly is important to overall cardiovascular health (see Chapter 26), and mounting evidence suggests a benefit in lowering the risk of both stroke-related dementia and Alzheimer's disease. A modest reduction of blood pressure (5 to 10 mm Hg) in both hypertensive and nonhypertensive persons with previous stroke or transient ischemic attack reduces the risk of stroke-related dementia by about 20%.

Lowering of Homocysteine

More data are required before one can recommend the aggressive treatment of homocysteine elevations, but suggesting an adequate dietary intake of foods rich in folate, B_{12}, and pyridoxine is not unreasonable (see Chapters 26 and 31).

Alcohol Consumption

Moderate alcohol consumption (one to six drinks per week) is associated with a lower risk of dementia than abstention in observational study. Whether this translates into a recommendation to have a nightly drink with dinner will require substantially more confirmatory evidence. Alcohol excess is clearly harmful.

Use of Vitamin Supplements

The consumption of *"antioxidant" vitamin supplements* is very popular among the public for the purported purpose of reducing cardiovascular and dementia risks. Although there is epidemiologic evidence of an association between the intake of foods rich in antioxidant vitamins C and E and a decreased risk of Alzheimer's disease, there is no evidence that the use of antioxidant vitamin supplements confers any protection.

Alzheimer's Disease and Lewy-Body Disease

See Chapter 173.

Other Causes

Vascular Dementia

For the patient with vascular dementia, the control of such cerebrovascular risk factors as hypertension, hyperlipidemia, smoking, and diabetes mellitus is essential (see Chapters 26, 27, 54, and 102, respectively). The question of the need for endarterectomy deserves consideration when a vascular problem is strongly suspected and a significant stenosis is found (see Chapter 171). Attention to embolic risk (see Chapters 28, 33, and 83) is also critical.

Central Nervous System Infections

Patients with dementia secondary to *HIV infection* may respond to intensive antiretroviral therapy (see Chapter 13). Those with *Lyme disease* may improve with a prolonged course of parenteral antibiotics (see Chapter 160). The response of dementia to antibiotics for central nervous system involvement with syphilis is variable, but treatment should certainly be considered (see Chapter 141).

Metabolic and Toxic Etiologies

In cases of vitamin B_{12} deficiency and hypothyroidism, replacement therapy is essential (see Chapters 82 and 104). In cases of substance abuse, avoidance of the causative substance(s) is a sine qua non of treatment, complemented by the correction of any concurrent vitamin and nutritional deficiencies (see Chapters 228 and 235).

INDICATIONS FOR REFERRAL AND ADMISSION (24–26)

Referral

Some families will request a neurologic consultation when a diagnostic evaluation has been completed by the primary physician and no cause is apparent other than Alzheimer's disease. Such a consultation can provide reassurance to the family that a comprehensive workup has been performed and that the diagnosis is correct. If the primary physician has conducted a thoughtful and complete examination as outlined, the referral need not generate additional testing. If the means for conducting a full workup are not available to the primary physician, then a referral can be used to complete the evaluation. In addition, patients suspected of having a potentially treatable neurologic condition (Parkinson's disease, normal-pressure hydrocephalus, mass lesion, carotid artery disease) are candidates for neurologic or neurosurgical evaluation. Finally, when a suspected hereditary condition is under consideration, referral for confirmation and genetic counseling is indicated.

Admission

Admission to a hospital for behavioral management or for the treatment of intercurrent medical illness can be very stressful for the patient and family. Careful attention to factors associated with the development of delirium in the hospitalized patient and use of the lowest possible doses of analgesic and sedative–hypnotic medications are essential (see also Chapter 173).

Terminal care for the patient with advanced dementia involves careful assessment of and attention to quality-of-life parameters, such as bedsores and overall comfort. The role of tube feeding in patients with advanced dementia has received much attention; there is no evidence that such therapy prolongs survival or improves quality of life.

Annotated Bibliography

1. Beal MF. Clinicopathologic conference No. 7—1998. N Engl J Med 1998;338:603. (*A lucid, case-based clinical and pathologic discussion of Lewy-body disease.*)
2. Cummings JL. Alzheimer's disease. N Engl J Med 2004;351:56. (*A superb review of epidemiology, diagnosis, and management.*)
3. Grossman M. Frontotemporal dementia: a review. J Int Neuropsychol Soc 2002;8:566. (*An excellent review by the laboratory that has defined the clinical syndrome.*)
4. Kawas CH. Early Alzheimer's disease. N Engl J Med 2003;349:11. (*An excellent practical review of the clinical problem of mild cognitive impairment, risk of progression to dementia, and appropriate screening tests.*)
5. Mehta KM, Ott A, Kalmijn S, et al. Head trauma and risk of dementia and Alzheimer's disease. Neurology 1999;53:1959. (*No association was found with head trauma; no interaction was found between head trauma and the APOE*e4 allele.*)
6. Moroney JT, Tang MX, Berglund L, et al. Low-density lipoprotein cholesterol and the risk of dementia with stroke. JAMA 1999;282:254. (*A prospective, longitudinal, community-based study, finding that low-density-lipoprotein cholesterol was an independent risk factor for dementia with stroke in the elderly.*)
7. Seshadri S, Beiser A, Selhub J, et al. Plasma homocysteine as a risk factor for dementia and Alzheimer's disease. N Engl J Med 2002;346:476. (*A community cohort study, finding that plasma homocysteine was an independent risk factor for both dementia and Alzheimer's disease.*)
8. Shumaker SA, Legault C, Kuller L, et al. Conjugated equine estrogens and incidence of probable dementia and mild cognitive impairment in postmenopausal women. Women's Health Initiative Memory Study. JAMA 2004;291:2947. (*A pivotal study of estrogen therapy for dementia; negative results in fact suggested an increased risk.*)
9. Verghese J, Lipton RB, Katz MJ, et al. Leisure activities and the risk of dementia in the elderly. N Engl J Med 2003;348:2508. (*A cohort study, finding that participation in leisure activities such as playing board games, playing musical instruments, and reading were associated with a reduced risk of dementia.*)
10. Wolfson C, Wolfson DB, Asgharian M, et al. A reevaluation of the duration of survival after the onset of dementia. N Engl J Med 2001;344:1111. (*A Canadian population survey, finding a marked decrease in median survival.*)
11. Andreasen N, Minthon L, Clarber A, et al. Sensitivity, specificity, and stability of CSF-tau in AD in a community-based patient sample. Neurology 1999;53:1488. (*This agent was useful in helping to differentiate patients with Alzheimer's disease from those with dementia of other causes.*)
12. Boustani M, Peterson B, Hanson L, et al. Screening for dementia in primary care: a summary of the evidence for the U.S. Preventive Services Task Force. Ann Intern Med 2003;138:927. (*Screening tests can detect undiagnosed dementia, but test sensitivity is often low, and specificity can be wanting.*)
13. Chui HC, Mack W, Jackson JE, et al. Clinical criteria for the diagnosis of vascular dementia. Arch Neurol 2000;57:191. (*Compares four different clinical definitions of vascular dementia for reliability among raters, finding that they are not interchangeable.*)
14. Chui H, Zhang Q. Evaluation of dementia: a systematic study of the usefulness of the American Academy of Neurology's practice parameters.

Neurology 1996;49:925. (*Finds that a marked reduction in the cost of assessment was possible, and that the false-negative rate was 5%.*)

15. Holsinger T, Deveau J, Boustani M, et al. Does this patient have dementia? JAMA 2007;297:2391. (*Reviews the use of basic diagnostic tools such as the Mini-Mental State Examination to recognize mild cognitive impairment early in its course.*)

16. Mayeux R, Saunders AM, Shea S, et al. Utility of the apolipoprotein E genotype in the diagnosis of Alzheimer's disease. N Engl J Med 1998;338:506. (*At least one APOE*e4 allele was found in 65% of pathologically confirmed cases of Alzheimer's disease, but overall this was of limited use for testing.*)

17. Silverman DH, Small GW, Chang CY, et al. Positron emission tomography in evaluation of dementia: regional brain metabolism and long-term outcome. JAMA 2001;286:2120. (*A prospective cohort study, finding that abnormal regional brain metabolism was a sensitive indicator of Alzheimer's disease; a negative study was associated with good prognosis.*)

18. Small GW, Kepe V, Ercoli LM, et al. PET of brain amyloid and tau in mild cognitive impairment. N Engl J Med 2006;355:2652. (*Presents evidence on the use of positron emission tomography with a radionuclide that detects amyloid for differentiating persons with mild cognitive impairment from those with early Alzheimer's disease.*)

19. The PROGRESS Collaborative Group. Effects of blood pressure lowering with perindopril and indapamide therapy on dementia and cognitive decline in patients with cerebrovascular disease. Arch Intern Med 2003;163:1069. (*A major randomized, controlled trial, finding a reduction in risk.*)

20. U.S. Preventive Services Task Force. Screening for dementia: recommendation and rationale. Ann Intern Med 2003;138:925. (*Concludes that evidence is insufficient to recommend for or against screening at this time.*)

21. Doody RS, Stevens JC, Beck C, et al. Practice parameter: management of dementia. Report of the Quality Standards Subcommittee of the American Academy of Neurology. Neurology 2001;56:1154. (*An evidence-based review of cholinesterase inhibitors, vitamin E, selegiline, antiinflammatories, and estrogens for dementia; also covers antipsychotics and antidepressants.*)

22. Engelhart MJ, Geerlings MI, Ruitenberg A, et al. Dietary intake of antioxidants and risk of Alzheimer disease. JAMA 2002;287:3223. (*An epidemiologic study, suggesting that there is a reduction in risk with dietary intake but not evidence that supplements are indicated; see the accompanying editorial: Foley DJ, While LR. Dietary intake of antioxidants and risk of Alzheimer disease: food for thought. JAMA 2002;287:3261.*)

23. Mukamal KJ, Kuller LH, Fitzpatrick AL, et al. Prospective study of alcohol consumption and risk of dementia in older adults. JAMA 2003;289:1405. (*A case–control observational study, finding that risk was reduced by a daily drink.*)

24. Finucane TE, Christmas C, Travis K. Tube feeding in patients with advanced dementia. A review of the evidence. JAMA 1999;282:1365. (*A thoughtful review of the risks of tube feeding and the failure to prevent aspiration pneumonia, improve function, or prolong survival.*)

25. Inouye, SK, Bogardus ST, Charpentier PA, et al. A multicomponent intervention to prevent delirium in hospitalized older patients. N Engl J Med 1999;340:669. (*Finds that protocols for cognitive impairment, sleep deprivation, immobility, visual impairment, hearing impairment, and dehydration reduced the number and duration of episodes of delirium.*)

26. Mitchell SL. A 93 year-old man with advanced dementia and eating problems. JAMA 2007;298:2527.(*A thoughtful case study.*)

CHAPTER 170 ■ APPROACH TO THE PATIENT WITH A SEIZURE

AMY A. PRUITT

The occurrence of a convulsion is a dramatic and frightening event. One of every 11 Americans who lives to be 80 years old has had at least one seizure. The first experience of a seizure is likely to trigger an immediate visit to an emergency department. Retrospective clarification of a "spell" is the diagnostic challenge in the office setting. In the context of evaluating an episode of lost or altered consciousness, the primary care physician needs to consider seizure (see Chapter 24). If a seizure is likely, then one should attempt to determine its type and plan to prevent future episodes while conducting a diagnostic evaluation for the underlying cause.

PATHOPHYSIOLOGY AND CLINICAL PRESENTATION (1–5)

A *seizure* is a paroxysmal alteration in consciousness or other cerebral cortical function. It results from a synchronous activation of a population of neurons, either in one focal area or generally throughout the brain. The occurrence of a single seizure does *not* constitute *epilepsy*, which connotes recurrent, unprovoked seizures. Many people have a single seizure without recurrence—for example, as a consequence of a transient metabolic disturbance, such as severe hypoglycemia or hypoperfusion. Only about 1% of the U.S. population actually has epilepsy. Epileptic seizures can result from many different types of diseases, ranging from hereditary conditions to vascular, traumatic, and neoplastic causes. Seizures can be classified as *localization related* (previously known as *partial*) or *generalized* (Table 170.1).

Localization-Related Seizures

Localization-related seizures may begin in one area of the brain and initially produce symptoms that are referable to the region of cortex involved. *Simple* partial seizures are focal neurologic events in which consciousness remains intact, whereas in complex partial seizures, consciousness is impaired. Simple seizures may evolve into complex partial seizures, and both of these types of focal seizures may evolve into secondarily generalized seizures. The spread of symptoms may follow the cortical representation of body parts, beginning, for example, in the fingers and spreading up the arm or down the leg.

Symptoms of complex partial seizures are numerous and include coordinated, involuntary motor activity (automatisms), such as lip smacking or chewing, olfactory or gustatory hallucinations, and behavioral automatisms. Seizure activity typically begins in the temporal lobe or its connections. Premonitory symptoms include olfactory hallucinations, epigastric discomfort, and a sense of fear or *déjà vu*. At times, the symptoms may resemble those of a psychosis. Episodes last 1 to 3 minutes, followed by a period of confusion with consciousness

TABLE 170.1

INTERNATIONAL CLASSIFICATION OF EPILEPSIES AND EPILEPTIC SYNDROMES

Localization-Related (Focal, Local, Partial) Epilepsies and Epileptic Syndromes
Idiopathic with age-related onset
Benign childhood epilepsy with centrotemporal spikes
Childhood epilepsy with occipital paroxysms
Symptomatic

Generalized Epilepsies and Epileptic Syndromes
Idiopathic with age-related onset
Benign neonatal epilepsy
Childhood absence epilepsy (pyknolepsy)
Juvenile myoclonic epilepsy (impulsive petit mal)
Juvenile absence epilepsy with generalized tonic–clonic
seizures on awakening
Secondary (idiopathic or symptomatic)
West syndrome (infantile spasms)
Lennox–Gastaut syndrome

Symptomatic
Nonspecific etiology (early myoclonic encephalopathy)
Specific syndromes (epileptic seizures that may complicate
many diseases, such as Ramsay Hunt syndrome,
Unverricht's disease

usually impaired but not lost. Localization-related seizures are the most common type of epilepsy in adults, accounting for 70% of patients presenting with epilepsy after age 18 years. More than 50% of all patients with localization-related epilepsy have both partial and secondarily generalized tonic-clonic seizures.

Generalized Seizures

Generalized seizures are bilaterally symmetric and without focal onset. An episode may begin with a premonitory aura that is followed by a sudden loss of consciousness. *A tonic* phase of limb extension ensues, lasting 10 to 30 seconds, followed by a *clonic phase* of limb jerking of at least 30 seconds. The patient then becomes flaccid and comatose before regaining consciousness. *Postictal confusion* is characteristic and can last for hours, although 10 to 30 minutes is more typical. *Tongue biting* and *incontinence* are other characteristic features.

Important Precipitants of Seizures and Pertinent Misconceptions

A number of factors have been implicated as causes of seizures, including fever, stroke, alcohol and drug use, and head trauma. Although these factors are often important, a number of misconceptions about their role are prevalent and need to be addressed.

- Adults rarely have convulsions with *high fever*; a temperature higher than 102°F does not suffice to explain the occurrence of a seizure in an adult.
- Seizures are rare during the initial presentation of an *embolic stroke,* although 20% to 25% of such patients may have seizures at some time after the initial stroke.
- *Subarachnoid hemorrhage* and *lacunar strokes* rarely have seizure activity as a sequela, although *emboli* and *cortical vein thrombosis* are more likely to lead to symptomatic epilepsy.
- *Alcohol-withdrawal seizures* occur between 7 and 48 hours after cessation of drinking, with a peak at 13 to 24 hours. Usually, only one or two convulsions occur, and status epilepticus is rare. Alcohol withdrawal is more likely to produce seizures in an epileptic patient than in a nonepileptic person, and less drinking is required to precipitate a seizure in patients with epilepsy who drink alcohol. *Other drugs* are associated with seizures, either when they are taken in overdose or when they are withdrawn (Table 170.2).
- *Trauma* is frequently invoked as a cause for seizures. However, in two large studies, unless the trauma was severe, causing a loss of consciousness for more than 1/2 hour or a lobar

TABLE 170.2

DRUGS COMMONLY ASSOCIATED WITH SEIZURES

Drugs	Overdose Seizures	Withdrawal Seizures	Dose Required to Induce Seizure
Alcohol	−	+	Depends on previous drinking or underlying epilepsy
Meperidine (Demerol)	+	+	2–3 g/d,[a,b]
Propoxyphene (Darvon)	+	+	Variable
Pentazocine (Talwin)	−	−	May precipitate withdrawal from other opiates with as little as 100 mg
Barbiturates	−	+	>600 mg/d (short-acting)[b]
Meprobamate (Miltown)	−	+	>1.2 g/d[b]
Chlordiazepoxide, diazepam	−	+	Unknown—may have 7- to 8-day latency period
Phenothiazines, haloperidol	But myoclonus may occur; may cause seizures in patients with old cortical focus	−	Variable

+, occurs; −, does not occur.
[a]Overdose seizure.
[b]Withdrawal seizure.

hematoma or depressed skull fracture, the incidence of post-traumatic seizures was not greater than that in the general population. With a history of closed head trauma, epilepsy usually develops within 2 years, whereas with open head trauma, seizures may develop at a longer interval after the original injury.

DIFFERENTIAL DIAGNOSIS (1,4)

Conditions Mimicking Seizures

Several conditions can mimic seizures, either by causing focal deficits or producing episodic loss of consciousness. Among the former are transient ischemic attacks, migraine, and local pathology, such as nerve compression. Among the latter are syncopal attacks of any cause, including transient diminished cerebral perfusion resulting from cardiac conditions and transient ischemic attacks (see Chapter 171). Panic attacks and altered mental status during psychotic episodes may cause confusion with complex partial seizures.

Conditions Causing Seizures

The differential diagnosis of conditions responsible for a seizure is based largely on the age of the patient at the time of the first seizure and the type of seizure as determined by the history, especially that obtained from observers. *Primary* or *idiopathic epilepsy* is the most common cause of recurrent seizures in children, but it becomes increasingly rare in the young adult population. After age 30 years, an *underlying cause (secondary epilepsy)* becomes increasingly likely when a patient presents with a first seizure. Among patients with more than one documented seizure of any type, a cause becomes obvious after thorough investigation and a 10-year follow-up in only 23%. Only 15% of seizures generalized from the outset have a demonstrable cause, whereas underlying disorders can be found in more than 30% of seizures with a focal component. In the *young adult* population (ages 18 to 45 years), the demonstrated causes include *drugs* (usually alcohol withdrawal), *neoplasm*, and *trauma*. In the *older adult* population, underlying pathology is divided about equally among *neoplasm, trauma*, and *cerebrovascular disease*. A nonepileptic convulsion may occur in the context of a transient metabolic disturbance, such as cerebral hypoperfusion, hypoglycemia, a hyperosmolar state, or hyponatremia.

WORKUP (1,3,4)

For the patient who reports a "spell," the first step is to ascertain whether it was a seizure and, if so, to characterize its type. Identifying the type facilitates ascertaining whether the cause is likely to be primary (idiopathic) or secondary (underlying central nervous system pathology) (Table 170.1). Generalized seizures with no initial focus are usually primary. Such epilepsies are often inherited, age related, and not associated with structural lesions identified by current neuroradiographic techniques. With partial or focal seizures, the prevalence of identifiable underlying disease or abnormality in the brain is much higher.

History

An effective history requires an exact description of events from both witnesses and the patient. Reports of witnesses are especially useful because the patient's consciousness and recall of the event are likely to have been compromised. Questioning should include inquiry into the presence of an aura, focal onset, loss of consciousness, and observed injury during the convulsion. Such symptoms suggest seizure rather than syncope, although it is not possible to distinguish between them absolutely on the basis of any characteristic features.

Once it has been ascertained that a seizure has occurred, it is essential to check carefully for a history of *focal onset*, even in patients with a history of generalized seizure. The focal onset of a witnessed seizure that later became generalized may be an important clue to an underlying lesion of the central nervous system.

History is also essential for identifying *precipitants* and *underlying disease*. It should include inquiry into drugs (e.g., *alcohol, cocaine, amphetamines, antidepressants, sedatives, theophylline, insulin, diuretics), cardiac arrhythmias, valvular disease, previous malignancy, stroke*, and *head trauma*. The examiner should check for symptoms of *hyperglycemia* and *hypoglycemia* (see Chapter 102) in addition to those of meningeal irritation (*headache, stiff neck*). A *family history* of convulsions should always be sought.

Physical Examination

The physician may have the opportunity to perform the neurologic examination shortly after the seizure. A *focal residual abnormality*, such as paralysis of one arm (Todd's paralysis), may suggest a focal onset even when the witnessed event was generalized. In addition to a careful neurologic examination, the physical examination should also include a check for postural hypotension, abnormalities in heart rate and rhythm, head trauma, carotid disease, cardiac disease, systemic infection, and signs of alcohol and drug abuse (see Chapters 228 and 235).

Laboratory Studies

It is not possible by clinical means to determine definitively whether a transient or persistent neurologic event is a seizure. The American Academy of Neurology recently published a Practice Parameter on evaluation of an apparent unprovoked first seizure in an adult. Recommendations include an *electroencephalogram (EEG)*, brain imaging with *computed tomography* or *magnetic resonance imaging*, and laboratory tests such as *complete blood count, blood glucose*, and *electrolyte panel*. *Lumbar puncture* and *toxicology* screening maybe helpful as determined by the specific clinical circumstances but need not be part of the routine evaluation.

Electroencephalography

The EEG remains the most helpful laboratory diagnostic test for suspected seizure activity. An abnormal study with epileptiform features (e.g., spikes or sharp waves) supports the diagnosis of seizures and may provide information about the type of seizure disorder. However, an abnormal EEG pattern is not adequate for the diagnosis of seizures, and a normal interictal EEG pattern can be found in up to 20% of patients with purely generalized seizures.

A *sleep EEG* is obtained when partial complex seizures (temporal lobe epilepsy) are a consideration. The likelihood of detecting an abnormality is increased by obtaining the sleep study. However, because the EEG concentrates on cortical disturbances, abnormalities of deep temporal lobe or diencephalic structures may not be evident on a surface EEG.

Specialized units provide in-hospital telemetric monitoring of patients with suspected epilepsy. A Digitrace device allows for ambulatory EEG recording for periods of up to 72 hours. The patient records clinical events with a pushbutton, and the patient's experiences then can be correlated with the EEG findings.

Neuroimaging

Most neurologists would agree that *magnetic resonance imaging* of the brain without and then with *gadolinium* contrast enhancement is an important part of the workup of a patient with a first seizure. This procedure is more sensitive than *computed tomography* and may be particularly useful in demonstrating abnormalities in the medial temporal region. *Positron emission tomography* and *single-photon emission computed tomography* are new methods of examining cerebral function in patients with seizures. They may confirm the presence of an organic abnormality and provide an outline of the abnormal region for which surgical treatment of epilepsy might be considered. It is unlikely that a primary physician would refer a patient for one of these studies, but the primary physician should be aware that newer methods for differentiating generalized from localization-related seizures and selecting patients for epilepsy surgery are available in epilepsy centers.

Other Testing

Additional laboratory studies should include blood chemistries; measurement of *electrolytes*, *calcium*, and *alcohol* levels and a *toxic screen* are important. All patients with risk factors for HIV should undergo *HIV testing* (see Chapter 7). Unless evidence of infection is found or the patient presents in status epilepticus, it is no longer common practice to perform a lumbar puncture for a patient with a first seizure.

If fever is present or the history is compatible with systemic infection, lumbar puncture remains an essential part of the neurologic evaluation.

PRINCIPLES OF MANAGEMENT (1,3,6–17)

As precise a diagnosis as possible must be made before treatment is begun. This includes the phenotype of the seizure, the EEG findings, and the identification of any underlying cause or precipitating factors. The distinction between a single seizure and epilepsy is important. During the last 20 years, important advances have been made in the treatment of all seizure types. Monotherapy with one of the standard antiepileptic drugs (AEDs) (Table 170.3) provides adequate control in 70% of adult patients. In another 15% to 20%, seizures can be controlled with a combination regimen including one or two additional AEDs. Unsatisfactory control of the seizures of the remaining patients makes them candidates for surgery or experimental drug therapy. The clinician should always seek independent confirmation of seizure activity from a family member. A valuable addition to the literature is a study by Hoppe and colleagues, who convey important cautions regarding the objectivity of seizure reporting by patients. They studied patients undergoing video-EEG monitoring and found that 55% of all seizures went unreported by patients.

The Isolated Seizure

As noted earlier, an isolated convulsion does not constitute epilepsy. When a single convulsion has occurred because of a transient metabolic disturbance or drug overdose or withdrawal, it is best treated by attending to the factors that led to the disturbance. The long-term use of drugs for seizure prophylaxis in such patients is not indicated, although a short-term course may be used in the setting of alcohol or drug withdrawal (see Chapters 228 and 236). When no obvious, self-limited cause can be determined in a patient who presents with a single seizure, then prophylaxis must be considered. Social variables, such as loss of driving privileges, will influence the

TABLE 170.3

PHARMACOKINETIC SUMMARY OF ANTIEPILEPTIC DRUGS

Drug (Generic/Brand)	Indication[a]	Starting Dose[b] (mg/d)	Maintenance Dose (mg/d)	Time to Steady-State Elimination Half-Life[c] (hr)	Therapeutic State Plasma Concentration (day)	Range of Plasma Concentration (μg/mL)
Phenytoin/Dilantin	T-C, CP, SP	300	200–500	10–34	7–8	10–20
Carbamazepine/Tegretol, Tegretol-XR	T-C, CP, SP	200–400	600–1,200	14–27	3–4	4–12
Phenobarbital	T-C, CP, SP	90	90–240	46–136	14–21	10–40
Primidone/Mysoline	T-C, CP, SP	125	750–1,500	6–18	4–7	5–12[d]
Valproic acid/Depakote	A, M, T-C	750	1,000–4,000	6–15	1–2	40–100
Ethosuximide/Zarontin	A	500	500–1,500	20–60	7–10	40–120
Clonazepam/Klonopin	A, AT, M	1.5	1.5–10	20–40	—	—

[a]A, absence; AT, atonic; CP, complex partial; M, myoclonic; SP, simple partial; T-C, tonic–clonic.
[b]All doses are for adults.
[c]This is the interval at which drug levels should be checked after any adjustment in dose.
[d]Primidone is metabolized to phenobarbital, and its therapeutic concentrations are the same as those listed under phenobarbital. The value in this column refers to primidone concentration.

decision to treat. The most critical issue is to determine risk factors for recurrence. Recurrence is most common within the first 6 months after the first seizure, and more than 50% of patients who have a recurrence will have it within this period. The recurrence rate after a first unprovoked seizure varies from 36% to 77%. Risk factors for recurrence include known prior neurologic lesions, history of epilepsy in a sibling, prolonged Todd's paralysis, and EEG with generalized epileptiform discharges. The risk for recurrence after two seizures is 70%, and after a third it is nearly 80%.

Recurrent Epileptic Seizures

Principles of Pharmacologic Treatment

There are several basic tenants of pharmacologic therapy related to program design and implementation.

Choice of Agent. The treatment of choice for recurrent epileptic seizures is the administration of a *single anticonvulsant drug* appropriate for the seizure type diagnosed (Table 170.1). Most available AEDs are used to prevent the recurrence of seizures rather than to produce any specific effect on the course of established epilepsy or to prevent the development of seizures after trauma. As a group, generalized seizures respond best to treatment, and full seizure control is possible with monotherapy for as many as 80% of patients with idiopathic epilepsy.

Prior to 1990, six AEDS were available: *carbamazepine, phenobarbital, phenytoin, primidone, valproate,* and, for absence seizures, *ethosuximide.* As a class these drugs had several problems, including frequent drug–drug interactions and severe side effects in some patients (see later discussion). These disadvantages spurred development of newer drugs that are similarly effective but better tolerated (e.g., *gabapentin, lamotrigine, levetiracetam, oxcarbazepine, tiagabine, topiramate,* and *zonisamide;* see Table 170.5.)

Carbamazepine and phenytoin remain the first-line treatments for adult patients with localization-related epilepsy. When newer AEDs are compared with the older six drugs, oxcarbazepine equals carbamazepine and phenytoin in efficacy but is superior in dose-related tolerability. Gabapentin is also effective in the treatment of newly diagnosed partial epilepsy. Lamotrigine, topiramate, and oxcarbazepine are effective in a mixed population of newly diagnosed partial and generalized tonic–clonic seizures. Thus, patients with newly diagnosed epilepsy can begin standard AEDs or one of the newer drugs.

Choice of AED will depend on individual patient characteristics. The drug should be used in doses sufficient to control the seizures as completely as possible. The rates for complete control of generalized tonic–clonic seizures are similar for carbamazepine, primidone, phenobarbital, and phenytoin. Valproate is the first-choice drug of some neurologists for generalized epilepsy, but the newer AEDs lamotrigine, topiramate, and oxcarbazepine are equally good choices.

Adjusting Doses and Achieving Therapeutic Levels. When an AED is begun or the dose of the drug is altered, one must wait for five drug-elimination half-lives to elapse before the effect of the change can be assessed. To achieve immediately a steady-state concentration equal to the usual maintenance concentration, it is usually necessary to give a loading dose of drug. Therapeutic monitoring of blood levels provides a standard for each individual patient's seizure control. Levels should be checked frequently while doses are adjusted (see Table 170.3

for appropriate intervals for level checks, maintenance doses, loading doses, and therapeutic levels of AEDs).

Switching or Adding Agents. Side effects severe enough to necessitate a change in therapy occur in about 30% of patients treated with AEDs. If side effects become intolerable, the drug should be replaced with another one, also used as monotherapy (unless it becomes clear later that the patient's seizures cannot be controlled with a single drug). Side effects and interactions of drugs may become intolerable if more than one drug is required.

In switching drugs, it is best to make the transition by initially adding the new agent rather than suddenly substituting it for the original drug; this provides continued seizure protection while the serum concentration of the second drug is rising. The first drug should then be tapered and discontinued. A second drug should not be added until it has been documented that control cannot be achieved with the first drug at a high therapeutic concentration or that the dose required to achieve control produces toxic effects.

Classes of Drugs

Effective drugs are available for treating each form of epilepsy; the drug of first choice for a particular patient is the one causing the least toxicity. Three classes of antiepileptic drugs are available:

- *Type 1 drugs* (e.g., *carbamazepine* and *phenytoin*) block sustained repetitive firing—the rapid firing of action potentials that is produced by an applied depolarizing current and is dependent on the opening of increased numbers of sodium channels.
- *Type 2 drugs* (e.g., *phenobarbital, valproate,* and *benzodiazepines*), enhance γ-aminobutyric acid (GABA) inhibitory transmission and block sustained repetitive firing.
- *Type 3 drugs* (e.g., *ethosuximide*) have no effect on either postsynaptic GABAergic inhibition or sustained repetitive firing but block T-calcium currents, which appear to be important in the generation of normal rhythmic activity.

Specific Agents

Familiarity with a few of the first-line agents is helpful.

Phenytoin. For most seizure types occurring in adults, phenytoin is an appropriate drug choice. The proprietary formulation, Dilantin, is preferable to the generic formulation. Phenytoin is well absorbed orally and has a serum half-life of 22 to 30 hours. An initial loading dose must be administered. Dose-related side effects include nystagmus, ataxia, dysarthria, and blurred vision. The presence of nystagmus can be used as a crude guide to the adequacy of dose. Duration-related side effects include osteomalacia, peripheral neuropathy, folate-deficiency anemia, and cerebellar degeneration. Idiosyncratic reactions include gingival hypertrophy, hypertrichosis, spiking fevers, exfoliative dermatitis, bone marrow depression, liver abnormalities, teratogenesis during the first trimester of gestation, and neonatal coagulation defects.

Like many antiepileptic agents, phenytoin is inducer of the hepatic microsomal cytochrome P450 enzymes, altering metabolism of numerous drugs and creating important potential drug–drug interactions (Table 170.4). If hormonal contraception is chosen for birth control by a woman taking enzyme-inducing AEDs, a formulation including at least 50 μg of ethinyl estradiol or mestranol should be used (see later discussion).

TABLE 170.4

PHENYTOIN: ADVERSE EFFECTS AND DRUG INTERACTIONS

Major Adverse Effects

Dose related: nystagmus, ataxia, dysarthria, blurred vision, decrease in measured total thyroxine

Duration related: osteomalacia, peripheral neuropathy, anemia, cerebellar degeneration

Idiosyncratic: gingival hypertrophy, acne, hypertrichosis, encephalopathy

Rare, toxic: high, spiking fevers; exfoliative dermatitis; bone marrow depression; pseudolymphoma and actual lymphoma; lupus-like syndrome; teratogenesis during first trimester; neonatal coagulation defects

Interactions with Commonly Prescribed Drugs

Increased phenytoin levels with:
   Antimicrobials: chloramphenicol, isoniazid
   Anticoagulants: warfarin
   Amphetamines (but seizure threshold decreased)
   Disulfiram (Antabuse)
   Alcohol: acute ingestion raises phenytoin levels, but see below
   Antiinflammatory agent: phenylbutazone
   Anticonvulsants: ethosuximide; no consistent effect with simultaneous barbiturate administration
   Sedatives: chlordiazepoxide (Librium), diazepam (Valium), oxazepam (Serax), clonazepam (Klonopin)

Decreased phenytoin levels with:
   Alcohol: chronic ingestion

Phenytoin effects on levels of other drugs:

Insulin: may interfere with endogenous insulin release

Quinidine: decreases quinidine effect at given dose

Falsely low total thyroxine

Carbamazepine (Tegretol). This drug is another excellent first-line agent for adult-onset generalized tonic–clonic seizures and for complex partial seizures. Many patients report less fatigue and better performance while on this medication than on phenytoin, but a controlled study failed to confirm that carbamazepine is clearly superior. The major disadvantages of this medication include the necessity of multiple daily dosing and the requirement for frequent blood testing during initiation of the medication to monitor for uncommon instances of *bone marrow depression*. It, too, induces hepatic microsomal enzymes, which can speed the metabolism of other drugs.

Valproate (Depakote). For patients allergic to phenytoin or carbamazepine, valproate is a good choice of medication. Many neurologists would choose this as a first-line drug for spike-and-wave or generalized tonic–clonic epilepsy, even in the absence of EEG abnormalities. This drug also has to be given in multiple daily doses (Table 170.3). Major side effects include nausea, weight gain, hair loss, platelet dysfunction, fetal anomalies (neural tube defects), and liver dysfunction. Valproate is an inhibitor of hepatic microsomal enzymes and may potentiate other drugs.

Phenobarbital. Phenobarbital is no longer a first-line drug for generalized tonic–clonic seizures, although for patients allergic to the three first-line medications previously described, it provides good control, usually with acceptable side effects. It, too, induces hepatic microsomal enzymes.

Newer Antiepileptics. Several new AEDs have been introduced in the last decade. These are summarized in Table 170.5. The overall efficacy and safety of the new AEDs promises alternatives for many patients with refractory seizures. However, additional clinical trials and more widespread clinical use are needed to determine the exact role these drugs will play as first-line choices in epilepsy management. The older drugs remain the most cost-effective first-line drugs against localization-related and generalized epilepsy in adults.

Lamotrigine. Lamotrigine is acquiring a role as monotherapy for patients with newly diagnosed epilepsy, but the dose must

TABLE 170.5

NEW ANTIEPILEPTIC DRUGS

Name (Generic/Brand)	Indication	Initial Adult Dose (mg/d)	Maintenance Dose (mg/d, Divided Doses)	Half-Life (hr)	Special Issues
Gabapentin/Neurontin	SP, CP, T-C	300	900–4,800	5–7, if renal function normal	Few side effects, no AED interaction
Felbamate/Felbatol	CP, T-C, A, L-G	1,200	1,200–3,600	20	Hepatic failure, aplastic anemia
Lamotrigine/Lamictal	CP, T-C, A, L-G	50 no VPA 25 with VPA	300–500 no VPA 100–400 with VPA	25 monotherapy 70 with VPA	Skin rash with VPA
Topiramate/Topamax	SP, CP, T-C	50	200–600	18–30 normal renal, 60 renal failure	Kidney stones, cognitive slowing
Tiagabine/Gabitril	CP, SP, T-C	4	32–56	7–9 monotherapy 4–7 with enzyme-inducing AEDs	Dizziness, tremor
Oxcarbazepine/Trileptal	SP, CP	150	600–1,200	4–9	
Zonisamide/Zonegran	CP, SP	100	100–400	24–60	Lethargy
Levetiracetam/Keppra	CP, SP, T-C	250	500–2,000	6–8	Agitation, paranoia

A, absence; AED, antiepileptic drug; CP, complex partial; L-G, Lennox–Gastaut syndrome; SP, simple partial; T-C, tonic–clonic; VPA, valproate.

be increased very slowly to avoid potential severe rash development.

Felbamate. Felbamate carries a risk for aplastic anemia and acute hepatic failure and is reserved for selected patients in whom the benefits outweigh the risks and in whom other AEDs have failed. It should be used only under the supervision of a neurologist familiar with its adverse effect profile.

Gabapentin. Gabapentin has an excellent side effect profile, and for this reason is used as add-on therapy. As a single agent, it is not sufficiently effective in controlling most adult forms of epilepsy.

Topiramate and Oxcarbazepine. These agents are effective as add-on therapy for patients with partial and secondarily generalized tonic–clonic seizures.

Levetiracetam (Keppra). This is emerging as an extremely useful drug for the initial treatment of localization-related seizures and generalized seizures. It has few cognitive side effects, although an agitated paranoia can occur, and it does not interfere with the metabolism of other antiepileptic drugs. Since 2006, a parenteral form also has been available.

Prognosis and Duration of Pharmacologic Therapy

The prognosis is a function of the underlying condition. For *idiopathic epilepsy*, it depends on both the age at onset and type of convulsion. Patients with primary generalized seizures have the best overall prognosis. Childhood-onset seizures cease by age 20 years in more than half of cases. On average, more than half of patients are seizure-free with or without medication at 10 years after diagnosis. The probability of remaining seizure-free is highest for those patients whose seizures were generalized at the outset and were diagnosed before age 10 years. Eighty percent of recurrences develop within 5 years of discontinuation of medication. The major cause of failure to control seizures is *noncompliance,* and it has been shown that as many as one third of patients do not take their medication as prescribed.

Predictors of refractory epilepsy are failure to become seizure-free with medications, many seizures before the initiation of therapy, and inadequate response to initial treatment. For patients with correctable structural abnormalities, surgery should be considered as soon as treatment with two first-line drugs fails. In selected groups, this approach can yield an 80% seizure-free success rate (see later discussion).

Discontinuing Antiepileptic Drugs

Most neurologists require a seizure-free interval of at least 2 years before considering discontinuation of medication. The EEG is of only modest help in predicting which patients may be weaned successfully from their medications; persistent EEG abnormalities would make discontinuation of medication inadvisable, but the documentation of a normal EEG does not eliminate the risk for seizure recurrence. In a large prospective study, the risk for relapse was greatest in patients who had complex partial seizures with secondary generalization, EEG abnormalities before treatment that did not change during treatment, or a requirement for valproate. According to current American Academy of Neurology recommendations, discontinuation of AEDs can be considered for a patient who has been seizure-free for 2 to 5 years on AEDs if the patient has a single type of partial seizure, the neurologic examination findings and intelligence quotient are normal, and the EEG has normalized

with treatment. For patients not meeting this profile, the risk for recurrence may be greater than 40%.

Surgical Therapy

With the advent of sophisticated monitoring techniques for the localization of epileptic foci, surgery has begun to play an increasing role in seizure management. Many neurologists would consider referral to a center specializing in epilepsy surgery for patients who have failed several standard drugs or who require more than one drug for seizure control and experience intolerable side effects of the medical regimen. The number of surgical procedures for epilepsy rose sixfold in the United States between 1985 and 2003. It is estimated, however, that there are many more patients who might benefit from surgery who are not being referred until suboptimally late in their disease course. Although criteria for drug failure have not been definitely established, patients with *disabling partial seizures* with or without secondarily generalized seizures who have failed appropriate trials of first-line AEDs should be considered for referral to an epilepsy surgery center. Those who have anteromesial *temporal lobe seizure* foci are most likely to benefit from surgical resection, whereas the benefit of surgery for patients with localized neocortical epileptogenic regions outside the temporal is less well established.

Approach to Epilepsy in Women of Childbearing Age

Epilepsy in women of childbearing age raises special challenges. During the reproductive years, the aim of treatment is AED monotherapy, with attention given the effects of such treatment and the underlying disease on contraception, pregnancy, and breast-feeding.

Contraception

AEDs that induce hepatic microsomal enzymes decrease the effectiveness of estrogen-based hormonal contraception. If hormonal contraception is chosen for birth control by a woman taking enzyme-inducing AEDS, a formulation including at least 50 μg of ethinyl estradiol or mestranol should be used.

Pregnancy

For an epileptic woman considering pregnancy, *folic acid supplementation* should be instituted at a dose of no less than 0.4 mg daily. Concerns about the effect of pregnancy on the seizure disorder, the seizure disorder on the pregnancy, and the teratogenic potential of AEDs should be discussed. Options for considering AED discontinuation before pregnancy can be considered.

Effect of Pregnancy on Seizures. The effect of pregnancy on the severity of a seizure disorder is nil in about half of women. Of the remainder, half experience a slight worsening of seizures. Ideally, with well-controlled seizures, it would be possible to taper and discontinue the patient's medication before conception. However, one does not always have the luxury of discontinuation.

Risk of Seizures on the Fetus and Teratogenic Potential of Seizure Therapy. The risk for fetal malformations in an epileptic woman not on medication is still roughly double that of the general population, and teratogenesis has clearly been established for phenytoin (digital and craniofacial abnormalities and some cardiac defects), valproate (neural tube defects), and carbamazepine (facial anomalies and neural tube defects). Thus, the risks of continuing AEDs must be weighed against the benefits of preventing a sustained convulsion (fetal hypoxia, mechanical injury if the mother falls). Overall, women taking phenytoin still have a 94% chance of having a completely normal pregnancy outcome.

Monitoring, Testing, and Readjusting Dose during Pregnancy. During pregnancy, women with epilepsy who take carbamazepine or valproate should be offered prenatal *testing with α-fetoprotein* levels at 14 to 16 weeks' gestation. For the patient who needs to remain on AEDs during pregnancy, monthly monitoring of drug levels is important because the combination of decreased protein binding, decreased absorption, and increased metabolism and plasma volume result in lower drug levels, necessitating increase in dose. Monitoring of therapy during pregnancy should be done by ordering *non–protein-bound AED levels*.

Vitamin K Supplementation. Women taking enzyme-inducing AEDs risk becoming vitamin K deficient, necessitating an oral supplement of 10 mg/d during the last trimester of pregnancy.

Postpartum Readjustment of Therapy. The AED program needs to be readjusted for women whose dose had been increased during pregnancy. AED doses usually can be reduced to those given before pregnancy by 8 weeks after delivery.

Breast-Feeding

Should the mother taking anticonvulsant therapy elect to nurse her infant, she can be reassured that breast-feeding usually poses little problem. Some sedation in the infant is occasionally seen with phenytoin, carbamazepine, or phenobarbital. One case has been reported of an infant with thrombocytopenia and anemia, presumed to have been induced by valproate ingested through breast milk. Breast-feeding appears to be safe, without any risk for hepatic or hematologic toxicity to the infant.

INDICATIONS FOR REFERRAL AND ADMISSION

The workup of a patient with a first seizure can be accomplished by the primary care physician with a sleep-deprived EEG and magnetic resonance imaging. Antiepileptic medication usually can be initiated in the outpatient setting, and appropriate monitoring of therapeutic levels can be planned (Table 170.3).

For the patient who fails to respond to the first-choice medication or for whom side effects are intolerable, a second drug should be tried. If it appears that the patient may require two drugs for seizure control or if the organic nature of all the witnessed spells is questionable, it is appropriate to refer the patient to a neurologic specialist experienced in drug management and the techniques of EEG and telemetry. Such a referral also provides the patient with access to centers in which epilepsy surgery is performed and through which newer anticonvulsant medications can be obtained.

Differentiating between an epileptic attack and other systemic disorders or psychiatric conditions can be difficult. Nonepileptic attacks and epileptic seizures can coexist in patients with seizure disorders. Monitoring with telemetry for several days in the hospital may be necessary to clarify the diagnosis. However, hospitalization after a typical generalized

seizure is not necessary for a patient with a known seizure disorder, unless significant trauma has occurred or it is necessary to adjust the medication program under careful monitoring.

PATIENT EDUCATION

Perhaps the most important role a physician can play in caring for an epileptic patient is that of counselor, educator, and sometimes legal advocate. A longstanding relationship must be maintained with a patient whose chronic disease is surrounded by an enormous amount of superstition, prejudice, and misunderstanding. The diagnosis of epilepsy clearly imposes certain restrictions on the patient's life, so the certainty of the diagnosis in a healthy young person is imperative (see prior discussion). Patient education is especially important to the epileptic patient of childbearing age (see prior discussion).

Work

In addition to reviewing the prognosis with the patient, it is important for the physician to emphasize that even if seizures are not entirely controlled, most epileptics are able to lead productive lives. Of the nation's 4 million epileptics, 15% to 25% are unemployed, a figure higher than the national average. However, people known to have seizures are barred absolutely only from those professions that require a chauffeur's or pilot's license.

Driving

Driving laws vary from state to state, but in general, states require a *seizure-free interval of 6 months to 1 year* before reapplication for a driver's license may be made. Continued supervision by a physician is mandatory. These laws apply both to patients with generalized epilepsy and those with localization-related seizures.

Alcohol and Caffeine

The diagnosis of epilepsy does not make absolute abstention from alcohol mandatory, although the patient should be counseled that alcohol can lower the seizure threshold and that binge drinking is contraindicated. The relationship of seizures to the ingestion of large amounts of caffeine is less clear, but the patient should be counseled to use substances containing caffeine in moderation.

Surgery

Surgical procedures pose no special threat to the epileptic patient as long as medications are not discontinued. Parenteral forms of phenytoin, phenobarbital, and valproate are available. Although no parenteral form of carbamazepine is available, a rectal suppository can be prepared in many hospital pharmacies.

Hereditary Risk

Patients may worry considerably about the inheritance of seizures. Epilepsy is hereditary, although the precise genetics is not clear for all types. One fourth to one third of patients with idiopathic epilepsy have a family history of seizures. Seizures develop in 3% of the children of patients with idiopathic epilepsy. Febrile convulsions also appear to be more common in children who have afflicted relatives, as are posttraumatic seizures.

Family First-Aid Education

Families of patients with epilepsy should know the fundamentals of emergency management of seizures. They should be instructed in the positioning that protects the airway and cautioned against use of the time-honored tongue blade. It should be emphasized to the patient's family that few seizures last long enough to impair cardiopulmonary function.

THERAPEUTIC RECOMMENDATIONS (9,12,14)

- Establish an etiologic diagnosis and treat the underlying cause if possible. Symptomatic therapy can begin while evaluation is in progress.

- To prevent further convulsions, begin with a loading dose of a drug of choice appropriate to the seizure type identified. This can often be accomplished on an outpatient basis. Then begin a maintenance dose, and adjust the dose to achieve a therapeutic level, checking the level at an interval appropriate for the drug half-life.

- If seizures persist, check the serum levels of the AED and inquire into alcohol and other drug use. Add a second drug and then taper, and discontinue the first drug if the seizures cannot be controlled with the drug of first choice.

- If the seizures are controlled, have the patient continue the medication for at least 2 years. If the patient remains seizure-free for 2 to 5 years on antiepileptic drugs, a cautious attempt to taper the medication can be made if the patient also manifests a single type of seizure, normal neurologic exam, normal IQ, and electroencephalogram normalized with treatment.

- Teach the patient how to recognize the warning signals of a seizure and what to do to minimize injury. Instruct the patient about the role of alcohol in precipitating seizures.

- Educate the patient and family about prognosis, activity, and obstetric precautions.

Annotated Bibliography

1. Brown TR, Holmes GL. Epilepsy. N Engl J Med 2001;344:1145. (*A practical review for the primary physician, with especially good sections on discontinuing therapy and when to seek neurologic consultation.*)
2. Hauser WA, Rich SS, Lee JR, et al. Risk of recurrent seizures after two unprovoked seizures. N Engl J Med 1998;338:429. (*The risk approaches 90% in some subgroups.*)
3. Hoppe C, Poepel A, Elger CE. Epilepsy: accuracy of patient seizure counts. Arch Neurol 2007;64:1595. (*Data on the usefulness of such counts.*)
4. Krumholz A, Wiebe S, Gronseth G, et al. Practice parameter: evaluating an apparent unprovoked first seizure in adults, an evidence-based review. Neurology 2007;69:1996. (*Consensus recommendations of the American Academy of Neurology and the American Epilepsy Society.*)
5. Willmore LJ. Epilepsy emergencies. The first seizure and status epilepticus. Neurology 1998;51(Suppl 4):S34. (*A good summary of two important areas.*)
6. Consensus statements: medical management of epilepsy. Neurology 1998;51(Suppl 4):S39. (*Summary of American Academy of Neurology opinions on the treatment of a first seizure, the choice of medication, the management of epilepsy during pregnancy and in the elderly, and the management of status epilepticus.*)
7. Engel J, Wiege S, French J, et al. Practice parameter: temporal lobe and localized neocortical resections for epilepsy. Neurology 2003;60:538. (*Anteromesial temporal lobe resection for disabling complex partial seizures is better than continued drug treatment.*)
8. First Seizure Trial Group. Randomized clinical trial on the efficacy of antiepileptic drugs in the risk of relapse after a first unprovoked tonic–clonic seizure. Neurology 1993;43:478. (*A multicenter randomized, controlled trial; the cumulative risk for recurrence was 25% among treated patients and 51% among those not treated.*)
9. French JA, Kanner AM, Bautista J, et al. Efficacy and tolerability of the new antiepileptic drugs I: treatment of new onset epilepsy. And II treatment of refractory epilepsy. Report of the Therapeutics and Technology Assessment Subcommittee and Quality Standards Subcommittee of the American Academy of Neurology and the American Epilepsy Society. Neurology 2004;62:1252. (*An evidence-based review of seven new drugs.*)
10. Holmes LB, Harvery EA, Coull BA, et al. The teratogenicity of anticonvulsant drugs. N Engl J Med 2001;344:1132. (*A case–control study, finding an increased risk of fetal abnormalities with the use of anticonvulsants during pregnancy.*)
11. Kwan P, Brodie MJ. Early identification of refractory epilepsy. N Engl J Med 2000;342:314. (*Patients who have many seizures before therapy or who have breakthrough seizures during initial treatment are likely to have refractory epilepsy.*)
12. Mattson RH. An overview of the new antiepileptic drugs. Neurologist 1998;4(Suppl 5):S2. (*An excellent summary of felbamate, gabapentin, lamotrigine, topiramate, tiagabine, and vigabatrin; notes that extensive post-marketing data are still required to delineate optimal dosing, spectrum of efficacy, potency, and adverse effects.*)
13. American Academy of Neurology Quality Standards Subcommittee. Practice parameter: a guideline for discontinuing antiepileptic drugs in seizure-free patients—summary statement. Neurology 1996;47:600. (*Conservative criteria to be met before discontinuing drug.*)
14. Tempkin NR, Dikmen SS, Wilensky AJ, et al. A randomized double-blind study of phenytoin for the prevention of posttraumatic seizures. N Engl J Med 1990;323:497. (*Phenytoin does not prevent the development of posttraumatic seizures.*)
15. Report of the Quality Standards Subcommittee of the American Academy of Neurology. Practice parameter: management issues for women with epilepsy (summary statement). Neurology 1998;51:944. (*Important consensus recommendations.*)
16. Wiebe S, Blume WT, Girvin JP, et al. A randomized controlled trial of surgery for temporal-lobe epilepsy. N Engl J Med 2001;345:311. (*Surgery was superior to prolonged medical therapy.*)
17. Zahn CA, Morell MJ, Collins SD, et al. Management issues for women with epilepsy. Neurology 1998;51:949. (*Useful guidelines for a discussion of preconception, contraception, folate repletion, teratogenesis, and vitamin K supplementation.*)

CHAPTER 171 ■ MANAGEMENT OF TRANSIENT ISCHEMIC ATTACK AND ASYMPTOMATIC CAROTID BRUIT

AMY A. PRUITT

Stroke is the third-leading cause of death in the United States and is the leading cause of long-term disability in the older population. Although medical and surgical therapies for stroke are improving, prevention is still the most effective strategy and a major responsibility of the primary care physician. Stroke prevention through risk factor management may be a major contributor to the rapid decline during the last two decades in death rates from stroke. The cornerstone of the preventive effort is the early identification and vigorous treatment of stroke risk factors (e.g., hypertension, hypercholesterolemia, diabetes, coronary artery disease, smoking; see Chapters 26, 27, 30, 54, and 102). Atrial fibrillation, a major risk factor for embolic stroke, also requires serious attention (see Chapters 28 and 83).

Patients who present with a transient ischemic attack (TIA) or an asymptomatic carotid bruit pose the problem of stroke prevention at a more advanced stage of cerebrovascular disease. Approximately 50,000 patients with TIAs present for evaluation annually, and it is estimated that 2 million people have some degree of asymptomatic carotid stenosis. The primary physician should be able to differentiate these two conditions by history and physical examination, use appropriate noninvasive imaging and flow studies cost-effectively, and know when to initiate more-aggressive measures, such as anticoagulant therapy and surgical intervention.

PATHOPHYSIOLOGY, CLINICAL PRESENTATION, AND COURSE (1–8)

Transient Ischemic Attack

Definition

The concept of TIA has undergone refinement with the advent of new neuroimaging techniques. It currently is defined as a less-than-1-hour episode of focal dysfunction caused by brain or retinal ischemia that results in no imaging evidence of acute infarction on diffusion-weighted magnetic resonance imaging. Until recently, transient ischemic attacks were defined in timed-based fashion as episodes of temporary (<24 hours) focal cerebral dysfunction resulting from vascular disease. However, the majority of TIAs actually resolve within 1 hour, and most resolve within 30 minutes. Among patients who present with an ischemic focal deficit that lasts more than 1 hour, only 2% have resolution in 24 hours. Many patients whose deficits appear to resolve completely are found to have radiographic changes suggesting infarction. Thus, modern imaging has blurred the distinction between the old definition of TIAs, cerebral infarction with transient signs, and stroke. Regardless of definition, TIAs reside within the spectrum of ischemic events associated with a marked increase in risk of serious ischemic injury to the brain.

Pathogenesis

TIAs can develop through any of several mechanisms. In the majority of cases, emboli of platelets and fibrin or of atheromatous material that breaks off from a vessel wall (usually the carotid, but also the aortic arch) transiently occlude a cerebral or ophthalmic artery or one of its branches. Thrombus formation distal to an atherosclerotic plaque is common in tightly stenosed arteries (>75% stenosis, residual lumen <2 mm) or even in totally occluded carotid arteries, and the thrombus often serves as a source of emboli. Occasionally, the intracranial arteries are the source of emboli. This phenomenon occurs most frequently among male African Americans and should be considered in patients with no extracranial vascular or cardiac source of emboli.

The heart is the other important source of emboli. *Atrial fibrillation* greatly exacerbates stroke risk, estimated to be on the order of 3% per year (see Chapter 28). Other cardiac lesions predisposing to cerebral embolism include *mitral valve stenosis*, mitral valve *prolapse*, *calcified mitral annulus*, *ventricular aneurysm* or *dyskinesia*, atrial or ventricular *clot*, valvular *vegetation*, and interatrial *shunt*. The combination of *patent foramen ovale* and *atrial septal aneurysm* confers significantly increased risk of recurrent stroke in persons with a prior stroke of unknown origin, but a patent foramen ovale alone does not appear to pose as much of a risk, especially if it is small (<2 mm).

Transient ischemic attacks may also develop when *transient hypotension* occurs in conjunction with a hemodynamically *significant carotid stenosis* (>75% occlusion). The resulting reduction in collateral flow to the ipsilateral carotid territory can lead to transient neurologic symptoms. The reduced blood pressure rarely results in focal symptoms unless a severely stenotic lesion is already present.

Small-vessel thrombotic or *lacunar stroke* may be preceded by transient, focal neurologic deficits in as many as one third of patients who go on to have a completed stroke. The clinician must be aware that the distinction between stroke mechanisms, particularly distal emboli or large-vessel origin and small-vessel thrombotic disease, may be difficult. Because management of the two types of conditions differs considerably, it is important to be aware of syndromes that commonly are associated with small-vessel disease (pure motor hemiparesis, ataxic hemiparesis, clumsy hand dysarthria syndrome).

In certain rare instances, TIAs may be attributable to one of the following: *steal* phenomena (e.g., subclavian steal); *hyperviscosity* states (e.g., polycythemia); *vasculitis*; *coagulopathies* (e.g., antiphospholipid antibody syndrome, deficiency of factor V Leiden, protein C, protein S, or antithrombin III); and *dissection* of the carotid or vertebral artery. These underlying causes of stroke and TIA are more common in younger patients (younger than age 45 years).

Clinical Presentation

TIAs can be divided into those caused by disease in the *carotid* circulation and those that are a consequence of disease in the *vertebrobasilar* territory, but no single feature is a consistently reliable sign. For example, there is no difference between groups with normal or diseased carotid arteries in cumulative number of attacks per patient, and the presence of purely ocular or purely hemispheric symptoms also does not distinguish between the two groups. Nonetheless, certain clinical features are more likely to be associated with carotid or vertebrobasilar disease.

Carotid TIAs. Symptoms of TIA associated with carotid disease include *transient monocular blindness, clumsiness, weakness,* or *numbness of the hand,* and *disturbed speech.* Transient monocular blindness is caused by occlusion of the ophthalmic artery or branches ipsilateral to the carotid stenosis and classically is described by the patient as a "shade" or "curtain" that descends over the affected eye. In patients with symptoms suggestive of carotid disease, the detection of a carotid bruit on the same side as the symptomatic eye or cerebral hemisphere is suggestive but not diagnostic of high-grade carotid stenosis. The *nonsimultaneous occurrence of transient hemispheric episodes* and *transient monocular blindness* correlated with an 80% incidence of carotid disease.

Vertebrobasilar TIAs. Symptoms of *vertebrobasilar disease* include *binocular visual disturbance, vertigo, paresthesias, diplopia, ataxia, dysarthria, light-headedness, generalized weakness, loss of consciousness,* and *transient global amnesia.* Each of these may be an isolated symptom of disease of the posterior circulation, although isolated vertigo without other brainstem symptoms is rarely caused by vertebrobasilar occlusive disease (see Chapter 166).

Clinical Course and Risk for Stroke (5)

The *interval since the most recent TIA* appears to be the most important factor in predicting the risk for stroke. The short-term stroke risk following a TIA is substantial: In one study of prognosis following a TIA, the stroke risk was 11%, with half of the strokes occurring within 2 days of the TIA. The short-term risks of cardiovascular events, death, and recurrent TIA were 25% in the 3 months after a TIA. The risk for stroke cannot be predicted by the number of TIAs, duration of symptoms, or clinical phenomena. One validated prognostic score, the ABCD[2] score, considers diabetes status and then looks at age, blood pressure, clinical features, and duration, all risk factors for rapid progression to stroke. A low score (<4) means a 2-day stroke risk of 1% versus a high score (>5) of 8.1%. However, all patients with any type of TIA should be considered at risk for stroke, and those with TIA of recent onset (<1 month) should be evaluated urgently (see later discussion). About 50% to 75% of patients with occlusive carotid disease who have a stroke had preceding TIAs.

Asymptomatic Carotid Bruits

Incidental discovery on physical examination of an asymptomatic carotid bruit suggests the presence of an atherosclerotic lesion that has narrowed the lumen by at least 50%, to less than 3 mm. The pitch of the bruit increases with the severity of stenosis. Prolonged, very high pitched bruits suggest a residual lumen of less than 1.5 mm (>75% stenosis). Most atherosclerotic lesions causing bruits tend to be located on the posterior wall of the common carotid artery at the bifurcation, compromising flow at the origin of the internal carotid. When stenosis is tight and flow is reduced, a mural thrombus may form distally in the proximal internal carotid artery, worsening occlusion and serving as a source of emboli. Plaque ulceration may also provide a nidus for mural thrombus formation.

Stroke Risk

Epidemiologic studies indicate that asymptomatic bruits are associated with an increased risk for stroke, coronary disease, and death but not necessarily with an increased risk for stroke on the side of the bruit. In observational study, the overall risk for stroke in patients who remain asymptomatic is 1% at 1 year and 1.7% when those in whom TIAs develop are included. A major predictor of stroke is the severity of carotid stenosis, as is progression to high-grade stenosis (>75% stenosis, residual lumen <2 mm). Other risk factors include hypertension, preexisting heart disease, male gender, and a positive family history.

Cardioembolic Stroke with Transient Symptoms

In patients with cardioembolic stroke who have transient symptoms, the symptoms tend to last *several hours.* The neurologic event is maximal at onset in 80% of patients, and about 75% of emboli lodge in one of the middle cerebral arteries and cause symptoms similar to those of carotid occlusive disease. A hemispheric attack lasting longer than 60 minutes, whether single or multiple, is predictive of cardiac embolization.

DIFFERENTIAL DIAGNOSIS

The differential diagnosis of a TIA-like episode includes any condition that causes transient symptoms in a focal distribution and is not limited to those of vascular origin. Vascular mechanisms include carotid or vertebrobasilar occlusive disease, small-vessel ischemic stroke, and occlusion by emboli originating in the heart or aortic arch. *Focal seizures* (see Chapter 170) can produce symptoms similar to those of a TIA, as can the focal aura of *migraine,* which is not always followed by headache (see Chapter 165). *Hyperventilation* can produce distal tingling and numbness. *Carpal tunnel syndrome* may present with intermittent (often nocturnal) paresthesias in a median nerve distribution. Even a protruding *cervical disk* or osteophyte may produce transient focal motor or sensory symptoms (as during manipulation of the head or neck; see Chapter 167).

WORKUP (1–10)

The goals in evaluating a TIA or an asymptomatic bruit are the detection of significant vascular disease and the assessment of stroke risk. One needs to identify those patients who require aggressive intervention. In addition, if cerebrovascular disease can be ruled out as the cause, a search for other causes is required. The patient with a new onset of TIAs (<30 days) has an increased risk for stroke and should be evaluated promptly. On the other hand, a recent U.S. Preventive Services Task Force guideline recommends against screening for asymptomatic carotid artery stenosis in the general adult population.

History

For the patient with a suspected TIA, questioning should first confirm that the transient episode was indeed a TIA, based on onset and duration. Symptoms lasting longer than 24 hours exclude TIA; cessation within 10 minutes increases the probability. An episode that lasts hours might be the consequence of an embolic event. The onset of headache during resolution of the neurologic deficit is more suggestive of a migrainous episode (see Chapter 165). A careful description of symptoms may be helpful in distinguishing vertebrobasilar involvement from carotid disease (see prior discussion). In addition, the frequency of episodes, date of first onset, and presence of underlying heart disease and cardiovascular risk factors are important to ascertain because they can help to predict the clinical course. If the patient has hypertension or cardiac disease or is older (>65 years), the risk for subsequent stroke is increased. A disabling stroke is more likely to develop in patients with carotid symptoms than in those with vertebrobasilar dysfunction. The patient is at greatest risk for stroke in the first few months after the onset of TIAs.

When an apparently asymptomatic carotid bruit is found on physical examination, it is worthwhile to go back to the patient's history and check carefully for overlooked transient neurologic events. Their presence would greatly increase the significance of the physical examination finding and indicate a heightened risk for stroke.

Inquiry into a history of hypertension or heart disease and any family history of stroke further helps to determine stroke risk. Risk factors for stroke include advanced age, elevated systolic blood pressure, current smoking, and the presence of diabetes, atrial fibrillation, or coronary heart disease.

Physical Examination

Physical examination should be directed to the cardiovascular and nervous systems. One checks for *hypertension*, *atrial fibrillation*, and *heart murmurs* (see Chapters 21 and 33). Fundoscopic examination at the time visual symptoms occur may reveal an *embolus* in a *retinal artery branch*. Neurologic examination findings are likely to be normal if the examination is conducted after the TIA has passed.

Gentle palpation and auscultation of the *carotid arteries* should be performed to note upstroke, volume, and the presence of a *bruit*. As stated earlier, the presence of a bruit does not invariably herald significant stenosis (a bruit can be present with hemodynamically insignificant lesions), but in as many as 70% to 80% of cases, the bruit does indicate important ipsilateral carotid disease. The pitch of the bruit and its duration should be noted because they tend to correlate with severity of stenosis.

Laboratory Studies

Initial laboratory studies should include a *complete blood cell count* and an *erythrocyte sedimentation rate* and a determination of *glucose*, *lipid profile*, and *creatinine*. Homocysteine has been independently associated with stroke risk and should be measured, along with serum folate and vitamin B_{12} if it is elevated.

Carotid Imaging and Flow Determinations

No entirely reliable noninvasive test for carotid or vertebrobasilar disease is available. In the last two decades, great strides have been made in the noninvasive evaluation of the carotid arteries and vessels of the posterior circulation. For the assessment of suspected *carotid lesions*, the combination of *Doppler* and *B-mode ultrasonography* allows a determination of lumen size and visualization of the carotid arterial lesion. In studies comparing arteriography with duplex carotid ultrasonography, a reduction in the diameter of the carotid artery of more than 60% was associated with a residual lumen at arteriography of less than 2 mm. However, in some instances, one cannot tell whether the carotid artery is completely occluded or only tightly stenosed. The degree of thickening of the media and intima correlates well with risk of stroke and myocardial infarction and can be used as a predictor of prognosis and guide to management.

Magnetic resonance angiography increasingly is being used in lieu of standard arteriography in the preoperative assessment of symptomatic carotid disease. However, most clinical studies still require the gold standard of arteriography. The use of *transcranial Doppler* techniques helps to measure flow in the ophthalmic system, assess the hemodynamic significance of the carotid stenosis, and detect any major stenosis of the intracranial vessels.

Vertebrobasilar Imaging and Flow

For the study of the *posterior circulation, transcranial Doppler* ultrasonography provides a relatively inexpensive means of noninvasively surveying large intracranial vessels. The test measures the velocity of flow, which increases in the setting of stenosis. However, it does not provide direct anatomic information. *Magnetic resonance angiography* provides noninvasive visualization of the vertebrobasilar system.

Brain and Cerebrovascular Imaging

To detect silent or prior infarction, unsuspected hemorrhage, or nonvascular disease such as tumor, *computed tomography* or *magnetic resonance imaging* of the brain with diffusion-weighted sequences should be performed. Arteriography with the use of selective transfemoral catheterization or digital subtraction techniques should be performed only if the physician would proceed to endarterectomy in the instance of carotid disease or to anticoagulation in the case of vertebrobasilar disease. Thus, the procedure should lead to a critical management decision. The dye load involved in cerebrovascular angiography can be substantial and necessitates adequate hydration, particularly in patients with underlying renal disease or diabetes.

Cardiac Imaging and Monitoring

Transthoracic echocardiography makes it possible to identify cardiac lesions that predispose to embolization, but the yield is low in patients older than the age of 50 years without evidence of cardiac disease on physical examination (see Chapter 33). *Transesophageal echocardiography* is more sensitive and specific for detecting intracardiac and aortic sources of embolization, such as left atrial thrombus and atherosclerosis of the ascending aortic arch. It should be considered when standard echocardiography is unrevealing but clinical suspicion of embolization is strong. Ambulatory *Holter monitoring* is useful when atrial fibrillation as a precipitant of embolization is a concern and results of the *resting electrocardiogram* are normal (see Chapters 25 and 29).

Testing for Coagulopathy

Abnormalities of blood coagulation may contribute to 4% of strokes in young persons. Some authorities recommend a *coagulopathy workup* for stroke patients whose age is less than 50 years, who have prior venous disease or a family history of abnormal clotting and no other explanation for their stroke, or whose hematocrit, platelets, prothrombin time or partial thromboplastin time is abnormal. A full workup in the young stroke patient would require a test for *anticardiolipin antibodies*; measurement of *protein C* and *protein S*, *antithrombin III*, *factor V Leiden*, and *homocysteine levels*; an *antinuclear antibody test*; determination of the *erythrocyte sedimentation rate*; and *syphilis serology* (see also Chapters 22 and 81).

PRINCIPLES OF MANAGEMENT (1,11–37)

Transient Ischemic Attack

All patients with any type of TIA should be considered at risk for stroke, and because the interval since the most recent TIA appears to be the most important factor in predicting the risk for stroke, those with a recent onset (<1 month) of TIA should be evaluated and treated promptly. The physician should remember that although TIAs are predictors of stroke, myocardial infarction is still the most common cause of death in this group (annual mortality rate of 5%) and that the patient's cardiovascular status and cardiac risk factors must also be considered and addressed (see Chapters 26, 27, 30, and 31). With the caveat that optimal therapy for TIAs is an evolving area and that new information is forthcoming regularly, the following guidelines for management are recommended.

All Patients

Aggressive control of atherosclerotic risk factors combined with initiation of antiplatelet therapy constitutes the bedrock of the TIA treatment program. The importance of these measures has promoted an English group to suggest the ultimate combination pill, containing a statin, a thiazide, a beta-blocker, an angiotensin-converting-enzyme (ACE) inhibitor, folic acid, and 75 mg of aspirin.

Control of Atherosclerotic Risk Factors. Cessation of *smoking* and tight control of *blood pressure* (systolic blood pressure <140 mm Hg, diastolic blood pressure <90 mm Hg), aggressive lowering of *low-density-lipoprotein cholesterol* (<70 mg/dL), and *fasting glucose* (<126 mg/dL) significantly lower stroke risk (see Chapters 26, 27, 54, and 102). Epidemiologic studies find that programs of regular moderate aerobic *exercise* (including walking) and a diet containing weekly servings of *fish* rich in *omega-3 fatty acids* (e.g., salmon, sardines, mackerel, swordfish) are associated with markedly reduced risks of ischemic stroke. The value of lowering homocysteine is the subject of ongoing study (see later discussion).

In patients with a history of stroke or TIA, lowering blood pressure is not only safe, but it is also associated with a reduced risk of recurrent events (Heart Outcomes Prevention Evaluation [HOPE] and Perindopril Protection Against Recurrent Stroke Study [PROGRESS] trials). *ACE inhibitors* should be considered as first-line antihypertensive agents for patients with known cerebrovascular disease. Combination therapy with a low-dose *diuretic* (e.g., indapamide 2.5 mg/d or hydrochlorothiazide 12.5 mg/d) appears to offer the greatest benefit and may be instituted at the physician's discretion. Low-dose ACE inhibitor therapy should be considered for all patients with cerebrovascular disease regardless of blood pressure.

Antiplatelet Therapy. A daily *antiplatelet agent* should be prescribed. Options include aspirin, clopidogrel, ticlopidine, and a combination of aspirin and extended-release dipyridamole. *Aspirin* (50 to 325 mg/d) is recommended as initial therapy, reducing the combined risk of TIA, stroke, and death by nearly 20%. Low doses appear to be as effective as higher ones, but with fewer gastrointestinal side effects. Compared with aspirin, *clopidogrel* reduces the relative risk of a combined endpoint of ischemic stroke, myocardial infarction, and vascular death by 8.7% but at a nearly 50-fold increase in cost. *Ticlopidine* is similarly expensive and effective and has the disadvantage of being associated with a risk of neutropenia. The combination of *dipyridamole* and *aspirin* (Aggrenox) is at least as effective as clopidogrel and less costly, but it still markedly more expensive than aspirin alone.

Compared with antiplatelet therapy, *oral anticoagulation* with warfarin offers no advantage over aspirin in terms of stroke prophylaxis (Stroke Prevention In Reversible Ischemia Trial [SPIRIT]), except in persons with atrial fibrillation (see Chapter 28) and possibly in those with a major hypercoagulable state (e.g., antiphospholipid syndrome), aortic arch disease, or a patent foramen ovale (see later discussion).

Lowering Homocysteine. The benefit of identifying and treating elevated homocysteine levels remains to be demonstrated, even though such elevations are associated with an increased risk for stroke. Relative risk of vascular disease for patients in the top quintile of homocysteine levels is 2.2 compared with those in the lowest quintile; however, in a major prospective randomized trial (Vitamin Intervention for Stroke Prevention), lowering of homocysteine by high-dose vitamin therapy (B_{12}, B_6, and folate) failed to produce a reduction in rate of recurrent stroke, coronary events, or death in persons with prior stroke and a homocysteine level in the top quintile.

Symptomatic Patients with Tight (>70%) Carotid Stenosis

Patients with a tight carotid stenosis, especially those who have had recurrent TIAs or a TIA within 4 months of the current visit, require prompt attention and should be considered for *carotid endarterectomy*. If adequate radiologic support is available, these patients should undergo arteriography as soon as possible in addition to a careful cardiovascular evaluation (see Chapter 30). Because the risk for cardiovascular mortality and morbidity associated with noncardiac surgery is very high in this population, a careful cardiac assessment is an essential component of the determination of surgical candidacy. (Some physicians directly admit such patients to the hospital and immediately place them on intravenous heparin until arteriography can be performed.)

As demonstrated by the landmark North American Symptomatic Carotid Endarterectomy Trial, endarterectomy (when performed by a skilled surgical team) is superior to medical management (aspirin) for patients with recent hemispheric or retinal TIA (or nondisabling stroke) and *ipsilateral* high-grade stenosis of the *internal carotid artery*.

Less invasive approaches to carotid revascularization have been sought. Advances in *angioplasty* and *stenting* have led to trials in high-risk patients with carotid disease. Using an emboli-protection device to minimize the risk of procedure-related embolic stroke, investigators have carried out early randomized trials of angioplasty with stent placement compared with conventional endarterectomy. Although initial studies of angioplasty plus stent placement were encouraging, subsequent randomized trials found that the procedure was inferior to endarterectomy in terms of stroke and mortality. Indications for stenting are limited to persons who are poor surgical candidates and have symptomatic disease and a greater than 70% stenosis.

Symptomatic Patients with Less Severe Carotid Stenosis (<70% Stenosis)

The North American Symptomatic Carotid Endarterectomy Trial also addressed the role of surgery in patients with *less severe carotid stenosis (50% to 69%)*. For those with a recent TIA or stroke, endarterectomy lowers the risk for stroke to a greater degree than does medical management. Patients with *less than 50% stenosis* do not benefit from surgery. These patients have a cardiovascular mortality risk from noncardiac surgery equal to that of patients with critical carotid stenosis, but a lower stroke risk reports from both of these multicenter trials offer guidance on the best approach to the management of such patients.

Symptomatic Patients with Normal Carotid Vessels

Patients with transient ischemic attack and normal carotid vessels should undergo a thorough cardiac evaluation (including assessment for patent foramen ovale and aortic arch atheromatous disease) to rule out an embolic source. Oral anticoagulation with *warfarin* (International Normalized Ratio [INR] 2 to 3) is indicated for those found to be in atrial fibrillation; the incidence of stroke can be reduced by greater than 80% without a marked increase in the risk of bleeding (see Chapter 28). Aspirin can reduce the stroke risk due to atrial fibrillation by about 20% and represents an alternative for patients who have a contraindication to taking warfarin.

In the absence of atrial fibrillation, valvular heart disease, or carotid disease, the proper preventive treatment for future stroke is not clear. Possible embolic sources include atherosclerotic plaque in the aortic arch and venous clot passing through a patent foramen ovale; a hypercoagulable state may also contribute. It is common practice when a source is not evident to place patients on *aspirin* prophylactically (e.g., 325 mg/d), and some evidence is available to recommend this practice. Although aspirin may reduce the morbidity from myocardial infarction, it is unclear whether it reduces stroke from noncarotid/noncardiac sources. Observational study suggests some role for warfarin, especially in persons with aortic arch atheroma or antiphospholipid syndrome. Well-designed, randomized trials comparing aspirin with warfarin for stroke prophylaxis in such settings are underway.

Symptomatic Patients Who Cannot Tolerate Surgery, Have a Single Remote TIA, or for Whom Angiographic and Surgical Services Are Not Available

Medical therapy with aspirin and an ACE inhibitor (see prior discussion) may be elected for such persons. Risk reductions on the order of 20% are achievable.

Asymptomatic Carotid Bruit

A carotid bruit detected in an asymptomatic patient need not be considered an invariable harbinger of stroke, but it does suggest atherosclerotic carotid disease. The risk for stroke increases significantly with the severity of stenosis, onset of TIAs, and progression of the lesion. The patient should undergo a thorough, noninvasive carotid evaluation (see prior discussion) to confirm the carotid origin of the bruit, the severity of stenosis, and its hemodynamic effects. Regardless of the severity of stenosis, the recognition and *prompt reporting of any TIA symptoms* should be emphasized. Previously asymptomatic patients with high-grade stenosis (70% to 99%) who subsequently experience a TIA are at markedly enhanced risk for stroke and should be referred promptly for consideration of *surgical intervention* (see prior discussion).

Medical Therapy

Antiplatelet therapy with low-dose aspirin (60 to 325 mg/d) is recommended; higher doses are associated with an increased risk for subarachnoid hemorrhage, especially in elderly patients with hypertension. Aggressive treatment of *cardiovascular risk factors* (i.e., *hypertension, lipids, smoking, diabetes;* see Chapters 26, 27, 54, and 102) is essential, not only because the risk for coronary events is high and can be significantly reduced (see Chapter 30), but also because the risk for stroke can be lessened. For example, clinically significant reductions in the risk for stroke and stroke mortality (12% to 23%) are associated with aggressive lipid-lowering therapy with statins, reductions in risk similar to those associated with the use of antiplatelet agents. The benefit of identifying and treating elevated *homocysteine* levels remains to be ascertained, even though such elevations appear to be associated with an increased risk for stroke.

Endarterectomy

The role of carotid endarterectomy in the asymptomatic patient with a high-grade stenosis is unresolved. The cost-effectiveness of this practice needs to be questioned. In the Asymptomatic Carotid Atherosclerosis Study, a 53% reduction in *relative risk* was noted, but the *absolute risk* declined by only 1% annually in a comparison with medical therapy. Sixty-seven patients would have to undergo surgery to prevent one stroke, at an additional cost of more than $1.5 million. Moreover, because patients were a select, low-risk surgical group and the surgeons and hospitals were screened for a perioperative complication rate of only 2.3%, it is difficult to extrapolate these results to practice at large. Reported perioperative complication rates in most settings are considerably higher (e.g., 6.5% for perioperative stroke and death, including a 1.8% rate of disabling stroke). Asymptomatic patients with an occluded carotid artery and asymptomatic stenosis on the other side experience a reported perioperative complication rate after endarterectomy of 12.6%. Such levels of perioperative risk appear to outweigh any benefit obtained from elective endarterectomy.

Trials of asymptomatic persons have failed to identify a subgroup in whom prophylactic benefit clearly outweighs such operative risk. Thus, despite the temptation to conclude that these patients are at particular risk for stroke, surgery cannot yet be recommended in this asymptomatic population. Pending definitive data on medical versus surgical therapy in the truly asymptomatic patient, some authorities recommend that endarterectomy be considered for those who demonstrate a rapid progression to hemodynamically and anatomically critical stenosis (e.g., lumen <1 mm), provided that they have no active coronary disease, are not diabetic, and have an anticipated life expectancy of more than 5 years. In support of this view is the high risk for stroke; against it is the high cardiac risk associated with surgery and the absence of proven benefit. If surgery is going to be recommended, one must have access to a skilled surgical team with a proven record of low perioperative morbidity and mortality (<2%) and be sure that a careful preoperative cardiac risk assessment is carried out (see Chapters 30 and 36).

Previous Stroke

Secondary prevention of stroke in persons who are not candidates for carotid endarterectomy and have no identifiable cardiac source has long been the subject of debate. The analysis of data from well-designed randomized, controlled trials (e.g., the Warfarin–Aspirin Recurrent Stroke Study) finds that aspirin is equivalent to warfarin therapy (INR 1.4 to 2.8). Given the cost, complexity of use, inconvenience, and bleeding risks associated with warfarin, aspirin (325 mg/d) emerges as the preferred approach to secondary prophylaxis in conjunction with aggressive treatment of atherosclerotic risk factors.

INDICATIONS FOR ADMISSION (11)

The patient who calls or comes to the office complaining of new onset of a neurologic deficit that is persisting for more than 1 hour and not clearly of migrainous etiology should be sent immediately to the nearest emergency room for urgent assessment and consideration of *tissue plasminogen activator* (t-PA) therapy. Intravenous administration of t-PA can reduce the risk of progression to disabling stroke if administered within 3 hours of onset of symptoms, but careful patient selection is essential to minimize the risk of intracranial hemorrhage. Even if symptoms are resolving at the time of evaluation, administration of t-PA may be indicated, given the high risk of subsequent disabling stroke.

Annotated Bibliography

1. Albers GW, Caplan LR, Easton JD, et al. Transient ischemic attack—proposal for a new definition. N Engl J Med 2002;347:1713. (*Proposes criteria of 1 hour in duration and no deficit on imaging; notes that time is precious and that the old definition of <24 hours gives a false sense of security.*)
2. Benavente O, Eliasziw M, Streifler JY, et al. Prognosis after transient monocular blindness associated with carotid artery stenosis. N Engl J Med 1991;345:1084. (*The North American Symptomatic Carotid Endarterectomy Trial; identifies a high-risk group that has a good outcome with endarterectomy.*)
3. Bostom AG, Rosenberg IH, Silbershatz H, et al. Nonfasting plasma total homocysteine levels and stroke incidence in elderly persons: the Framingham Study. Ann Intern Med 1999;131:352. (*Elevated homocysteine levels were independently associated with stroke incidence.*)
4. Inzitari D, Eliasziw M, Gates P, et al. The causes and risk of stroke in patients with asymptomatic internal-carotid-artery stenosis. N Engl J Med 2000;342:1693. (*The risk of stroke from this lesion was found to be relatively low.*)
5. Johnston SC, Rothwell PM, Nguyen-Huynh MN, et al. Validation and refinement of scores to predict very early stroke risk after transient ischemic attack. Lancet 2007;369:283. (*The ABCD^2 [diabetes status; age, blood pressure, clinical features, and duration] score was validated.*)
6. Mas JL, Arquizan C, Lamy C, et al. Recurrent cerebrovascular events associated with patent foramen ovale, atrial septal aneurysm, or both. N Engl J Med 2001;345:1740. (*An observational cohort study; increased risk was found only in persons with both lesions.*)
7. Schuchlenz HW, Weihs W, Horner S, et al. The association between the diameter of a patent foramen ovale and the risk of embolic cerebrovascular events. Am J Med 2000;109:456. (*A cohort study suggesting that size seems to matter.*)
8. O'Leary DH, Polak JF, Kronmal RA, et al. Carotid-artery intima and media thickness as a risk factor for myocardial infarction and stroke in older adults. N Engl J Med 1999;340:14. (*The degree of wall thickness as measured by ultrasound strongly correlates with the risks of stroke and myocardial infarction.*)
9. Madden KP, Karanjia PN, Adams HPJ, et al., for the TOAST investigators. Accuracy of initial stroke subtype diagnosis in the TOAST study. Neurology 1995;45:1875. (*The absence of major computed tomography abnormalities and the presence of pure motor hemiparesis or sensorimotor presentation did not always correspond to a small-vessel [lacunar] infarction.*)
10. U.S. Preventive Services Task Force. Screening for carotid artery stenosis: U.S. Preventive Services Task Force recommendation statement. Ann Intern Med 2007;147:854. (*Makes a grade D recommendation: against screening the general population, due to the risk of false-positive results leading either to unindicated surgeries or angiography.*)
11. Alpers GW, Bates VE, Clark WM, et al. Intravenous tissue-type plasminogen activator for treatment of acute stroke: the Standard Treatment with Alteplase to Reverse Stroke (STARS) study. JAMA 2000;283:1145. (*A multicenter prospective trial performed at academic centers, demonstrating the efficacy and promise of the treatment.*)
12. Albers GW, Harat RG, Helmi LL, et al. Supplement to the guidelines for the management of transient ischemic attacks. Stroke 1999;30:2502. (*Consensus guidelines.*)
13. Albers GW. A review of published TIA treatment recommendations. Neurology 2004;62(Suppl 6):S26. (*A succinct summary of recommendations and controversies.*)
14. Albers GW, Tijssen JGP. Antiplatelet therapy: new foundations for optimal treatment decisions. Neurology 1999;53(Suppl 4):S25. (*A good summary of safety and efficacy data for ticlopidine, clopidogrel, and aspirin/dipyridamole.*)
15. Barnett HJM, Taylor WD, Eliasziw M, et al. Benefit of carotid endarterectomy in patients with symptomatic moderate or severe stenosis. N Engl J Med 1998;339:1415. (*The North American Symptomatic Carotid Endarterectomy Trial; durable benefit was found in symptomatic persons with stenosis >70%.*)
16. Bucher HC, Griffith LE, Guyatt GH. Effect of HMG CoA reductase inhibitors on stroke: a meta-analysis of randomized, controlled trials. Ann Intern Med 1998;128:89. (*The risk for stroke in hyperlipidemic patients was reduced by nearly 25%; no such result was noted with the use of resins or fibrates.*)
17. Dutch TIA Trial Study Group. Comparison of two doses of aspirin (30 mg versus 383 mg per day) in patients after a transient ischemic attack or minor ischemic stroke. N Engl J Med 1991;325:1261. (*Low-dose aspirin was as effective as higher doses in preventing stroke recurrence.*)
18. Executive Committee for the Asymptomatic Carotid Atherosclerosis Study. Endarterectomy for asymptomatic carotid artery stenosis. JAMA 1995;273:1421. (*The risk for ipsilateral stroke is reduced in selected patients if endarterectomy is performed with <3% perioperative risk.*)
19. Ferguson GG, Eliasziw M, Barr HW, et al. North American Symptomatic Carotid Endarterectomy Trial: surgical results in 1,415 patients. Stroke 1999;30:1751. (*The overall stroke and death rate was 6.5%, and the rate of disabling stroke was 1.8%; perioperative risk was not influenced by the degree of stenosis, shunting, age, or vascular risk factors.*)
20. Furlan AJ. Carotid artery stenting—case open or closed? N Engl J Med 2006;355:1726. (*An editorial summarizing the data; concludes that stenting has very limited indications and should be reserved for persons who are not surgical candidates and have symptomatic disease with at least a 70% stenosis of the internal carotid artery.*)
21. Gorelick PB, Born GV, D'Agostino RB, et al. Therapeutic benefit: aspirin revisited in light of the introduction of clopidogrel. Stroke 1999;30:1716.

(Clopidogrel provides a slight improvement in outcome compared with aspirin at 45 times the cost.)

22. Hart RG, Benavent O, McBride R, et al. Antithrombotic therapy to prevent stroke in patients with atrial fibrillation: a meta-analysis. Ann Intern Med 1999;131:492. (*Warfarin was superior to aspirin, but aspirin does offer some degree of protection.*)

23. Hobson RW, Weiss DG, Fields WS, et al. Efficacy of carotid endarterectomy for asymptomatic carotid stenosis. N Engl J Med 1993;328:221. (*A randomized, controlled trial [RCT] showing a reduction in the rate of ipsilateral neurologic events but not in the combined incidence of stroke and death.*)

24. Hu FB, Stampfer MJ, Colditz GA, et al. Physical activity and risk of stroke in women. JAMA 2000;283:2961. (*Epidemiologic data from the Nurses' Health Study; finds that exercise makes a significant independent contribution to reduction in risk.*)

25. Iso H, Hennekens CH, Stampfer MJ, et al. Prospective study of aspirin use and risk of stroke in women. Stroke 1999;30:1764. (*A 14-year follow-up in the Nurses' Health Study cohort showed benefit and safety for low-dose therapy.*)

26. Mas J-L, Chatellier G, Beyssen B, et al. for the EVA-35 Investigators. Endarterectomy versus stenting in patients with symptomatic severe carotid stenosis. N Engl J Med 2006;355;1660. (*Multicenter RCT; surgery was found to be superior to stenting in terms of stroke and death.*)

27. Meschia JF, Miller DA, Brott TG. Thrombolytic treatment of acute ischemic stroke. Mayo Clin Proc 2002;77:542. (*A succinct, evidence-based review, which includes guidance on implementation in clinical practice.*)

28. Mohr JP, Thompson JLP, Lazar RM, et al. A comparison of warfarin and aspirin for the prevention of recurrent ischemic stroke. N Engl J Med. 2001;345:1444. (*The Warfarin–Aspirin Recurrent Stroke Study [WARSS] trial, a major RCT, finds that the two are equivalent.*)

29. North American Symptomatic Carotid Endarterectomy Trial Collaborators. Beneficial effect of carotid endarterectomy in symptomatic patients with high-grade carotid stenosis. N Engl J Med 1991;325:445. (*Major RCT documenting the superiority of surgical over medical management in this group of patients.*)

30. Perry HM, Davis BR, Applegate WB, et al. Effect of treating isolated systolic hypertension on the risk of developing various types and subtypes of stroke: the Systolic Hypertension in the Elderly Program (SHEP). JAMA 2000;284:465. (*Landmark RCT showing a significant reduction in stroke risk with a lowering of systolic pressure to <160 mm Hg.*)

31. Powers WJ. Oral anticoagulation therapy for the prevention of stroke. N Engl J Med 2001;345:1493. (*An editorial succinctly summarizing the data.*)

32. PROGRESS Collaborative Group. Randomised trial of a perindopril-based blood-pressure-lowering regimen among 6,105 individuals with previous stroke or transient ischaemic attack. Lancet 2001;358:1033. (*A major European RCT, finding that angiotensin-converting-enzyme [ACE] inhibitor therapy was protective, especially when it was combined with a low dose of a mild diuretic.*)

33. The Stroke Prevention by Aggressive Reduction in Cholesterol (SPARCL) Investigators. High-dose atorvastatin after stroke or transient ischemic attack. N Engl J Med 2006;355:549. (*RCT; found a significant reduction in stroke and overall cardiovascular events but not in mortality.*)

34. Toole JF, Malinow MR, Chambless LE, et al. Lowering homocysteine in patients with ischemic stroke to prevent recurrent stroke, myocardial infarction, and death: The Vitamin Intervention for Stroke Prevention (VISP) randomized controlled trial. JAMA 2004;291:565. (*A major study; failed to demonstrate benefit, but the short follow-up period and presence of significantly more smokers in the treatment group may have contributed to failure.*)

35. Tu JV, Hannan EL, Anderson GM, et al. The fall and rise of carotid endarterectomy in the United States and Canada. N Engl J Med 1998;339:1441. (*Raises the question of whether the benefits of carotid endarterectomy in the general population are similar to those demonstrated in the clinical trials.*)

36. Wald NHJ, Law MR. A strategy to reduce cardiovascular disease by more than 80%. BMJ 2003;326:1419. (*Proposes a combination pill formulation containing a statin, a thiazide, a beta-blocker, an ACE inhibitor, folic acid, and 75 mg of aspirin.*)

37. Yadav JS, Wholey MH, Kuntz RE, et al. Protected carotid-artery stenting versus endarterectomy in high-risk patients. N Engl J Med 2004;351:1493. (*Early promising results were reported from this small-scale RCT examining a less invasive alternative to surgery.*)

CHAPTER 172 ■ MANAGEMENT OF MULTIPLE SCLEROSIS

AMY A. PRUITT

Multiple sclerosis (MS) is the most common demyelinating disease of the central nervous system (CNS), affecting approximately 2.5 million young adults worldwide. Severe disability develops in approximately 30% of patients. The manifestations of the disease are protean, and its clinical course is highly variable from patient to patient. Although most patients with MS will be under the care of the neurologist during periods of marked exacerbation, they often depend on the primary physician for initial diagnostic suspicion, help with decisions about whether, when, and with what to initiate long-term therapy, monitoring of blood tests for the treatment of adverse effects, interpretation of symptoms, treatment of intercurrent infections, discussion of the effects of pregnancy on the disease, and decisions regarding the need for referral. Consequently, the primary physician must be familiar with the range of clinical presentations for MS, its natural history, and the therapeutic options. Such knowledge facilitates the provision of proper primary care and ensures the optimal timing of referrals.

PATHOPHYSIOLOGY, CLINICAL PRESENTATION, AND COURSE (1–7)

The etiology of multiple sclerosis is unknown, but research suggests an interplay of genetic susceptibility, environmental exposure(s), and defective regulation of the immune response. Epidemiologic and virologic studies show an association between Epstein–Barr virus (EBV) infection and risk of MS, suggesting a role for EBV as a possible environmental factor in genetically predisposed persons. Antigen-specific cytotoxic T cells directed against an external antigen (e.g., an EBV protein) are believed to recognize and cross-react with myelin antigens in genetically susceptible persons, producing an autoimmune response. There is no evidence that vaccinations increase the risk of developing MS.

The consequence of immunologic cross-reactivity is a series of discrete episodes of myelin-specific *autoimmune injury* to the central nervous system, separated both in time and space. Acutely, an infiltrate of lymphocytes, macrophages, and plasma cells forms in areas of involvement. T cells are believed to initiate the process, and activated macrophages to damage the myelin. Localized edema and transient breakdown of the blood–brain barrier occur.

The chronicity of the inflammatory process results in the formation of a *plaque* or glial scar, made up of proliferated astrocytes that cluster in response to inflammatory injury of the myelin sheath. Lesions occur predominantly in the *white matter* of the brain and spinal cord; occasionally, gray matter is involved to a minor degree. *Demyelination* is characteristically focal, but axonal injury can occur early in the course of the disease. Brain atrophy also has been documented during early, clinically silent phases of the illness. Plaques are most commonly found in the optic nerves, spinal cord, brainstem, cerebellum, and periventricular areas.

After an attack, some remyelination occurs, which accounts for a partial resolution of symptoms. However, partially demyelinated axons are susceptible to dysfunction, particularly under conditions of heat stress or intercurrent infection. The finding that transected axons are common in the lesions of MS reverses a long-held pathologic axiom and suggests that early treatment is needed to prevent such irreversible damage.

Clinical Presentation

Clinical presentation is a function of the site of the inflammatory process. Attacks are by definition those that produce symptoms that last more than 24 hours.

Sensory Deficits

Transient sensory deficits are the most common initial presentation, affecting about 40% to 50% of patients. They include *paresthesias* or diminution of sensation in the upper or lower extremities. The sensory disturbance may be bilateral and symmetric, extending to involve the adjacent trunk.

Visual and Oculomotor Deficits

About 15% to 20% of patients experience *acute monocular visual loss* because of *optic neuritis*. A central scotoma, transient pain on eye movement, and decreased pupillary reaction to light (Marcus Gunn pupil) are characteristic features. *Diplopia* resulting from *internuclear ophthalmoplegia* or an oculomotor defect is another common symptom heralding MS. Bilateral internuclear ophthalmoplegia is very characteristic of MS and strongly suggests the diagnosis. A failure of adduction and coarse nystagmus in the abducting eye are noted. Other oculomotor functions remain intact.

Motor and Cerebellar Deficits

Ataxia and *intention tremor* are manifestations of cerebellar involvement. Motor deficits may occur acutely or insidiously, with the insidious variety particularly common in older patients. Legs are more likely to be involved than arms, initially

asymmetrically. However, upgoing toes (Babinski's sign) are common bilaterally, even in patients with unilateral problems.

Autonomic Deficits

Urinary difficulties (frequency, urgency, incontinence) are consequences of upper motor nerve injury in the spinal cord. The external sphincter fails to relax adequately, causing incomplete emptying. Such autonomic injury may also produce *constipation* and *impotence*.

Cerebral Deficits

Later in the course of illness, cerebral involvement may produce *memory loss*, *personality change*, and *emotional lability*. More than 60% of MS patients demonstrate abnormalities on formal neuropsychiatric testing, even if symptoms are not troubling and/or not reported.

Paroxysmal Symptoms and Fatigue

Paroxysmal symptoms may result from dysfunction of partially demyelinated axons and simulate a transient ischemic attack or focal seizure or produce an attack of tic douloureux (see Chapter 176). *Fatigue* (believed to be related to high circulating levels of immunomodulators) may be prominent and even predate exacerbations.

Clinical Course

The clinical course tends to follow one of several patterns, which are used as a basis for classification.

Relapsing–Remitting Disease

Younger patients manifest a relapsing–remitting course, characterized by attacks followed by complete or nearly complete remission. If there are any residual manifestations, they remain stable between relapses. Some patients present with a clinically isolated syndrome yet develop new, asymptomatic white matter lesions on serial brain magnetic resonance imaging without new clinical symptoms.

Secondary Progressive Disease

After years of an initial relapsing–remitting course, a secondary progressive course, with steady gradual worsening, develops in more than 50% of patients.

Primary Progressive Disease

About 10% of patients who present with MS in later life (40 to 60 years of age at onset) have a steadily progressive course; this pattern is called *primary progressive* and tends to be associated with prominent spinal cord involvement.

Relapsing Progressive Disease

A fourth possible variant of MS—actually a combination of two others—is relapsing progressive disease, which is diagnosed when patients have largely progressive disease exacerbated by acute attacks and little remission.

Prognosis

After 15 years of clinical disease, about 50% of patients are still capable of walking and 30% are able to continue working.

Frequent attacks early in the course of the disease increase the chances of disability, as does late onset, a progressive course, or early cerebellar or pyramidal involvement. In about 5% to 10% of patients, the disease seems to pursue a very "benign" course, but it is difficult to predict which patients safely can forego any disease-modifying therapy. Increasing volume of white matter lesions in persons who first present with clinically isolated disease correlates to a moderate degree with the risk of long-term disability, but number of relapses does not. Pregnancy decreases the risk of relapse, but risk increases in the postpartum period.

DIAGNOSIS (3,8–11)

The diagnosis is suggested clinically by the development of symptoms and signs suggesting *CNS white matter disease separated both anatomically and in time* (>1 month). At times, the symptoms suggest only a single lesion, but a careful physical examination reveals evidence of multiple lesions (upturned toes bilaterally, subtle internuclear ophthalmoplegia, mild afferent pupillary defect).

Diagnostic Criteria

Until recently, diagnosis was confirmed using the *Poser criteria*, which require a minimum of *two clinical episodes*, but waiting for a second episode to confirm diagnosis is increasingly undesirable, given the availability of effective disease-modifying therapy. The *McDonald criteria* take advantage of advances in technology and understanding of MS to afford earlier diagnosis. For a diagnosis of definite relapsing–remitting MS the following must be present:

1. Two clinical attacks and two objective lesions on examination; *OR*
2. One *clinical* attack and "dissemination in space and time" shown on a gadolinium-enhanced MRI demonstrating multiple lesions, some of which enhance, indicating recent disease activity; *OR*
3. One clinical attack and abnormal cerebrospinal fluid protein with oligoclonal bands.

Cerebrospinal Fluid Testing

The cerebrospinal fluid examination reveals abnormalities in 95% of MS patients. Modest increases in cell count and protein are common but nonspecific; increases in *immunoglobulin G* (IgG) and *oligoclonal IgG bands* on electrophoresis are more specific and suggest an increased risk for disseminated disease.

Neuroimaging

The most sensitive diagnostic test is *MRI*. Multiple periventricular plaques, presenting as areas of increased signal intensity on long TR–weighted and proton density–weighted images, are characteristic and found in more than 90% of patients with known MS. Patients with chronic progressive disease have more confluent periventricular and infratentorial lesions, but they are often most disabled by spinal cord lesions. However, the hyperintense white matter lesions seen on long TR–weighted images on MRI are nonspecific, and similar white matter lesions occur in normal elderly persons and patients with chronic uncontrolled hypertension, advanced

Lyme disease, and CNS vasculitis. Indeed, one of the most common reasons for referral to a neurologist is the incidental finding of lesions. A recent study from Rotterdam, albeit in a population older than age 45 years and thus not in the range for most new-onset multiple sclerosis, found asymptomatic brain lesions in greater than 10% of patients, most of whom had asymptomatic small-vessel brain infarcts (8).

Spinal MRI can be of great benefit in the diagnosis of MS. Spinal cord abnormalities are common in patients even with early-stage MS, are less likely to be confused with other diagnostic entities, and help to determine dissemination in space at the time of diagnosis.

Evoked Potentials

Visual- or *auditory-evoked potentials* are abnormal in demyelinated tracts and may serve as additional evidence of MS when MRI results require supporting data.

Tests to Rule Out Other Causes

Exclusionary blood work in all patients suspected of having MS should include *Lyme disease serology*, determination of *vitamin B_{12} levels* and *antinuclear antibody*, and possibly *HIV testing*.

PRINCIPLES OF MANAGEMENT (12–24)

The threefold goal of therapy for patients with MS is to prevent and treat relapses, treat persistent symptoms such as pain and spasticity, and retard progressive worsening of the disease. There is no cure for MS, but much can be done to reduce the symptoms of an acute exacerbation. A more difficult task is to improve the long-term course of the illness.

Efforts to treat MS have focused on suppressing the immunologically induced inflammatory response that characterizes the condition. Disease-modifying therapy is available and should be considered early in the course for patients with unfavorable prognostic markers, such as progressive disease from the onset, a short interval between the first two relapses, poor recovery from relapse, the presence of motor and cerebellar signs at onset, and multiple cranial lesions on long TR–weighted MRI. Increasingly, neurologists are treating proactively at the time of a first event that is consistent with multiple sclerosis (the clinically isolated event) even in the absence of all of the criteria for definitive diagnosis.

Evidence for efficacy in treating MS must always be interpreted with an appreciation for the highly variable and unpredictable course of MS and the difficulty of establishing measurements of disability, as well as for the adverse effects of the currently available injectable medicines.

Acute Attack

High-dose parenteral corticosteroids are the first line of treatment, capable of shortening an acute attack. As established by the Optic Neuritis Treatment Trial, 3 days of high-dose *intravenous* (IV) *methylprednisolone* (in the study it was also followed by several weeks of oral prednisone) achieves the best immediate and long-term results compared with oral prednisone alone or placebo. At 3 years, patients showed a 66% reduction in relative risk for the development of definite MS. Patients treated with oral prednisone alone did worse at 6 months than those given placebo. The worsening on oral prednisone alone is hard to explain, but oral steroids alone should not be used until more data are forthcoming. For now, a course of high-dose IV therapy is preferred, but whether it should be followed by a more prolonged course of oral prednisone is unclear because the study did not explore IV therapy without subsequent oral prednisone. Many neurologists choose not to treat a purely sensory attack, whereas they would intervene with corticosteroids for weakness or bladder dysfunction.

Relapsing–Remitting Disease

The U.S. Food and Drug Administration approved several disease-modifying/immunomodulating drugs for patients with relapsing–remitting MS. Most are recombinant versions of *interferon beta* (e.g., recombinant *interferon beta-1b* [*Betaseron*] and two different formulations of recombinant *interferon beta-1a* [*Avonex* and *Rebif*]). One, *glatiramer acetate* (*Copaxone*), is a random polypeptide containing the amino acid sequence of myelin basic protein. Removed from the market 3 months after its 2004 introduction because of three cases of progressive multifocal leukoencephalopathy, natalizumab, a recombinant monoclonal antibody against α_4-integrins that blocks migration into the CNS of activated lymphocytes, T cells, and monocytes was reintroduced in 2006 and, is another option for patients who have failed or cannot tolerated other immune-modulating drugs.

Efficacy, Administration, and Side Effects

In placebo-controlled, double-blinded multicenter trials, interferons achieved 30% to 35% reductions in relapse rates. The interferons also produced a similar rate of reduction in disease progression and reduced the number of new lesions on MRI. Primary prevention has been demonstrated with at least one preparation (Avonex) when given after a single demyelinating episode; fewer patients progressed to clinically definite MS. Efficacy can be reduced by the development of neutralizing antibodies (see later discussion).

These drugs are available only by injection. Betaseron, Rebif, and Copaxone are administered subcutaneously several times a week; Avonex is given intramuscularly once weekly.

The three interferon preparations have been associated with *flulike symptoms*, which can be severe and persistent but tend to decrease after the first year; depression can occur. *Injection-site reactions* are more common with subcutaneously administered preparations (Betaseron, Rebif, Copaxone) than those given intramuscularly (Avonex). Patients taking Copaxone have experienced uncommonly a self-limited systemic reaction of flushing, sweating, and palpitations.

Timing of Therapy

A consensus is growing that disease-modifying therapy should be initiated early in the course of MS, before irreversible disability has developed. This opinion is supported by increased clinical and MRI evidence that the inflammatory process is active in many patients during periods of clinical remission and that irreversible axonal injury accumulates with time, even during the phase of relapsing–remitting disease.

Choice of Agent

Pending large-scale, long-term, head-to-head studies comparing these therapies, choice of agent depends largely on considerations of cost, patient preference for frequency of injection, injection technique (intramuscular vs. subcutaneous), and potential side effects.

Progressive Disease

Treatment of progressive disease is more problematic.

Use of the Immunomodulating Agents

Controlled clinical trials of *interferon beta* in secondary progressive multiple sclerosis have produced variable results: One clearly found a significant delay in time to sustained progression; a second demonstrated that double-dose *interferon beta-1a* (Avonex) reduced progression according to one functional scale but not another. The role of *glatiramer* in secondary progressive multiple sclerosis is unknown. The serum of patients who continue to have clinical disease activity despite interferon therapy should be tested for *neutralizing antibodies*. These typically cause clinical difficulty only after 18 to 24 months of treatment; use of interferon beta-1b is more likely to trigger their appearance than use of the beta-1a preparation.

Despite the limited data on efficacy, most neurologists offer these disease-modifying drugs to patients with secondary progressive disease. Patients and their families need to understand that the drugs are extremely expensive and may cause several weeks of unpleasant side effects as they are started. Furthermore, patient and family must be taught how to administer them.

Patients whose disease continues to progress despite interferon or copolymer therapy may benefit from other strategies, including combination of two immune-modulating drugs and use of other immunologically active agents.

Use of Other Immunologically Active Therapies

IV *immune globulin* was used monthly for 2 years in a small study that demonstrated less worsening of disability in the active treatment group. *Immunosuppressive agents* (e.g., *methotrexate, azathioprine*) have been used, but their efficacy in progressive disability is unclear. Patients with rapidly progressive disease given a course of IV *cyclophosphamide* with or without subsequent booster injections have demonstrated stabilization over 1 year. Such nonspecific immunosuppressive treatment is fraught with significant morbidity and should be reserved for patients with rapidly progressive disease who do not respond to less toxic alternatives.

Natalizumab (see earlier discussion) reduced the frequency of relapses and the number of inflammatory lesions in an initial randomized, controlled trial of persons with secondary progressive disease and represents a promising option in this group of patients. *Plasmapheresis* has shown some benefit for patients with rapidly progressive disease, but data are limited to one small long-term study.

Mitoxantrone (*Novantrone*), a drug with potent effects on both cellular and humoral immunity, reduces the relapse rate and decreases MRI lesions in patients with relapsing–progressive or secondary progressive disease. Most side effects are self-limited or mild and include blue discoloration of sclera, urine, and stool, gastrointestinal upset, and headache. Mild leukopenia and thrombocytopenia may develop; heart failure and acute promyelocytic leukemia are risks.

All of the available drugs seem more useful for patients with recent clinical or MRI evidence of inflammatory lesions. Patients with slow progression over the years and chronic MRI changes are unlikely to respond well to these therapies. Hemmer and Hartung provide a detailed discussion of new directions in multiple sclerosis therapy.

Treatment of Complications

The primary physician is often called on to treat complications of the disease. These include paroxysms of pain and spasticity, urinary incontinence, impotence, and debilitating fatigue and depression.

Paroxysmal Symptoms or Pain and Spasticity

Lancinating pain responds to *carbamazepine* (200 mg twice daily). Low doses of *tricyclic antidepressants* (e.g., *amitriptyline* 25 to 75 mg/d) may relieve neuropathic pain and help to control *emotional lability;* higher doses are indicated for overt *depression;* selective serotonin reuptake inhibitors (SSRIs) offer another alternative (see Chapter 227). Although for insurance reasons it is difficult to obtain pregabalin for these patients, it can be helpful for pain. *Spasticity* lessens with the use of *baclofen* in low doses (started at 5 to 10 mg three times daily), but confusion, sedation, and increased muscle weakness are limiting side effects. *Diazepam* and *dantrolene* are alternatives. *Gabapentin* (Neurontin, 300 to 900 mg/d) has proven useful when there is a combination of spasticity and neuropathic pain; higher doses can cause excessive sedation.

Incontinence and Impotence

When bladder spasticity leads to urge incontinence, a drug such as *tolterodine* (Detrol) or *oxybutynin* (Ditropan; 5 to 10 mg two or three times per day) may help; both are available in long-acting preparations; anticholinergic side effects may limit dose (see also Chapter 134). Sildenafil (Viagra, 50 to 100 mg as needed) has proven useful for treatment of impotence.

Debilitating Fatigue

This may be a consequence of the illness or its treatment (e.g., with use of interferon). When due to concurrent depression, it may respond to antidepressant therapy with an SSRI (e.g., fluoxetine, 20 mg/d; see Chapter 227). When it is due to the underlying illness or its treatment, *amantadine* (Symmetrel; 100 mg two or three times per day) and *modafinil* (Provigil, 200 mg per day) have proven helpful.

PATIENT EDUCATION (2–6,8)

One of the most difficult aspects of MS is the uncertainty that accompanies the disease. If the diagnosis is in question, every effort should be made to confirm it or rule it out. Patients with MS fear becoming disabled. Providing them with as much information as possible helps them to maintain a sense of control. Even advice on handling the affairs of everyday life is greatly appreciated, such as avoiding a very hot shower that may transiently exacerbate symptoms. The value of establishing a close, supportive relationship cannot be overemphasized. Patient morale appears to be an important determinant of outcome. In randomized studies, the high frequency of remission and outright clinical improvement noted among patients randomized to placebo underscores this point.

Prognosis

Although it is hard to predict a patient's future clinical course, reasonable estimates can be made based on the clinical course to date and perhaps on some of the laboratory features noted earlier (e.g., volume of MRI lesions, serum antibody titers—although there are many caveats about their use for prognosis). Even frequent relapses in persons with relapsing–remitting disease do not portend disabling disease. Patients need to know that progression to disabling disease is not inevitable, that the prognosis is highly variable, and that in many cases the disease never becomes incapacitating. Maintaining a hopeful perspective may have a remarkably positive effect and should not be overlooked.

Advising about Pregnancy

The primary care physician may be asked about the effect of pregnancy on MS and vice versa. Many women experience a relapse-free period during pregnancy. Those being treated need alteration of therapy because the interferon preparations are Food and Drug Administration category C agents, contraindicated in pregnancy and requiring immediate cessation; glatiramer is a category B drug. Evidence indicates that pregnancy does not have a detrimental effect on the long-term course of MS. Genetic counseling should take into account that MS has a familial occurrence of about 15%, with a 10-fold difference in clinical concordance rates between monozygotic and dizygotic twins. Thus, the risk to a family member should be depicted as higher than that of the general population but still rather low. Breast-feeding is contraindicated during the use of immunomodulating therapy.

INDICATIONS FOR REFERRAL AND ADMISSION

When a diagnosis of MS is suspected on clinical grounds, a neurologic consultation can help in determining the need for further diagnostic studies (MRI, lumbar puncture with immunoelectrophoresis, evoked potentials) and in selecting a treatment modality. The beneficial outcomes beginning to be seen with early treatment make early referral appropriate and desirable. Neurologic consultation about the timing or appropriateness of interferon beta or copolymer treatments is important. In addition, patients experiencing an acute exacerbation of functional significance should be referred to a neurologist promptly for consideration of a course of high-dose IV glucocorticoid therapy. Referral to an occupational and physical therapist can greatly facilitate the maintenance of daily functioning in patients with significant motor or sensory deficits.

Annotated Bibliography

1. Ascherio A, Munger KL, Lennette ET, et al. Epstein–Barr virus antibodies and risk of multiple sclerosis: a prospective study. JAMA 2001;286:3083. (*A presentation of virologic data suggesting that there is a relationship.*)

2. Beatty WW. Cognitive and emotional disturbances in multiple sclerosis. Neurol Clin North Am 1993;11:189. (*Mild to moderate cognitive impairment is common.*)

3. Brex PA, Ciccarelli O, O'Riordan JI, et al. A longitudinal study of abnormalities on MRI and disability from multiple sclerosis. N Engl J Med 2002;346:158. (*A prospective cohort series; the volume of lesions at onset correlated moderately with the degree of long-term disability.*)

4. Confavreux C, Suissa S, Saddier P, et al. Vaccinations and the risk of relapse in multiple sclerosis. N Engl J Med 2001;344:319. (*No evidence was found of an increase in the risk of relapse.*)

5. Confavreux C, Hutchinson M, Hours MM, et al. Rate of pregnancy-related relapse in multiple sclerosis. N Engl J Med 1998;339:285. (*A large prospective study; the relapse rate decreases during and increases after pregnancy; no increased risk or special precautions are needed during pregnancy.*)

6. Confavreux C, Vukusic S, Moreau T, et al. Relapses and progression in multiple sclerosis. N Engl J Med 2000;343:1430. (*Relapses did not significantly correlate with the development of irreversible disability.*)

7. Trapp BD, Peterson J, Ransonoff RM, et al. Axonal transection in the lesions of MS. N Engl J Med 1998;338:278. (*Presents evidence of irreversible damage and the importance of treatment to prevent it.*)

8. Vernooij MW, Ikram A, Tanghe HL, et al. Incidental findings on brain MRI in the general population. N Engl J Med 2007;357:1821. (*The younger population at risk for multiple sclerosis has different etiologies but also frequent unexplained findings; the major error is to call hypertensive vascular disease multiple sclerosis.*)

9. Bot JCJ, Barkhof F, Polman CH, et al. Spinal cord abnormalities in recently diagnosed MS patients. Neurology 2004;62:226. (*Dissemination in space was found in 66.3% of patients at diagnosis if only brain magnetic resonance imaging [MRI] was used, which increased to 84.6% when spinal cord imaging was added.*)

10. McDonald WI, Compston A, Edan G, et al. Recommended diagnostic criteria for multiple sclerosis: guidelines from the International Panel on the Diagnosis of Multiple Sclerosis. Ann Neurol 2001;50:121. (*New guidelines allow laboratory support from gadolinium-enhanced MRI and from cerebrospinal fluid studies, making earlier intervention with immune-modulating drugs more likely.*)

11. Polman CH, Reingold SC, Edan G, et al. Diagnostic criteria for multiple sclerosis: 2005 revisions to the "McDonald Criteria." Ann Neurol 2005;58:840. (*Presents the current imaging criteria.*)

12. Beck RW, Cleary PA, Trobe JD, et al. The effect of corticosteroids for acute optic neuritis on the subsequent development of multiple sclerosis. N Engl J Med 1993;329:1764. (*The treatment was found to prevent the development of clinical multiple sclerosis.*)

13. Beck RW, Cleary PA, Anderson MM Jr, et al. A randomized, controlled trial of corticosteroids in the treatment of acute optic neuritis. N Engl J Med 1992;326:581. (*Presents the best available evidence for the efficacy of high-dose steroids.*)

14. European Study Group on Interferon Beta-1b. Placebo-controlled multicenter randomised trial of interferon beta-1b in the treatment of secondary progressive multiple sclerosis. Lancet 1998;352:1491. (*Evidence for efficacy includes delayed progression for 9 to 12 months; reduced relapse rate and severity; and fewer steroid treatments, hospital admissions, and new lesions on MRI.*)

15. Frohman E, Phillips T, Kokel K, et al. Disease-modifying therapy in multiple sclerosis: strategies for optimizing management. Neurologist 2002;8:227. (*Excellent guidelines for comprehensive treatment of challenges in a chronic illness requiring long-term parenteral therapy.*)

16. Hartung HP and the Mitoxantrone in Multiple Sclerosis Study Group. Mitoxantrone in progressive multiple sclerosis: a placebo-controlled, randomized, multicentre trial. Lancet 2002;360:2018. (*Data establish its efficacy in reducing disease activity and slowing disease progression; therapy was generally well tolerated.*)

17. Hemmer B, Hartung HP. Toward the development of rational therapies in multiple sclerosis: What is on the horizon? Ann Neurol 2007;62:314. (*Future treatments will need to target inflammation as well as promote neuroprotection and repair; useful to the primary care physician giving advice to a patient with worsening multiple sclerosis.*)

18. IFNB Multiple Sclerosis Study Group. Interferon beta-1b is effective in relapsing–remitting multiple sclerosis. Neurology 1993;43:665. (*The first report that the natural history of multiple sclerosis can be altered.*)

19. Jacobs LD, Beck RW, Simon JH, et al. Intramuscular interferon beta-1a therapy initiated during a first demyelinating event in multiple sclerosis. N Engl J Med 2000;343:898. (*A major randomized, controlled trial establishing the benefit of such therapy.*)

20. Kappos L, Bates D, Hartung HP, et al. Natalizumab treatment of multiple sclerosis: recommendations for patient selection and monitoring Lancet Neurol 2007;6:431. (*Includes criteria for patient selection in view of reported deaths.*)

21. Kiesier BC, Wiendl H, Hemmer B, et al. Treatment and treatment trials in multiple sclerosis. Curr Opin Neurol 2007;20:286. (*A good summary of treatment and ongoing research.*)

22. Lessell S. Corticosteroid treatment of acute optic neuritis. N Engl J Med 1992;326:634. (*An editorial recommending high-dose intravenous therapy for acute attacks.*)

23. Polman CH, O'Connor PW, Havrdova E, et al. Randomized, placebo-controlled trial of natalizumab for relapsing multiple sclerosis. N Engl J Med 2006;354:899. (*The treatment was found to reduce the risk of progression and relapse.*)

24. Rudick RA. Disease-modifying drugs for relapsing–remitting multiple sclerosis and future directions for multiple sclerosis therapeutics. Neurology 1999;56:1079. (*Succinct summary of data establishing the efficacy of interferon therapy.*)

CHAPTER 173 ■ MANAGEMENT OF ALZHEIMER'S DISEASE AND RELATED DEMENTIAS

M. CORNELIA CREMENS

According to the prevalence data from the U.S. census in 2000, approximately 4.5 million Americans suffered from Alzheimer's disease. With the aging of the U.S. population and a doubling of the prevalence of dementia for every 5 years older than the age of 65 years, the problem of caring for such patients is becoming an increasingly important medical and societal challenge. Medical care for the majority of patients with Alzheimer's disease and other dementias is usually the responsibility of the primary care physician. This role requires knowledge of the course of the illness, the best approaches to managing concomitant medical and psychiatric conditions (psychosis, anxiety, depression, behavioral disturbances), and the social services available. Skill is required in family education and counseling, the appropriate application of new therapies, and the cessation of life-prolonging therapy at the end of life.

CLINICAL PRESENTATION AND COURSE (1–8)

Dementia is a syndrome of persistent cognitive impairment in many areas of intellectual functioning, which may include memory, executive function, and language and visuospatial abilities. Changes in mood and personality are often noted early or late in the development of the illness. The various presentations of dementia depend on the area or areas of the brain that are implicated in the disease with regard to the manifestation of behavioral, neurologic, psychiatric, and cognitive symptoms. There are many types of dementia, including Alzheimer's disease, vascular dementia, Lewy body dementia, frontotemporal dementia, and numerous other subtypes or mixed dementias. With such a broad array of dementias, which are often mixed, establishing a clear diagnosis is complex, difficult, and time consuming but worth the effort (see also Chapter 169).

Mild Cognitive Impairment

The earliest stages of cognitive decline beyond those of normal aging are designated by the term *mild cognitive impairment* (MCI). MCI is viewed as a transitional stage between age-appropriate cognitive function and dementia, in which at least one domain of cognitive function declines more than expected for age but overall functional capacity remains intact. The most common presentation is that of the *"amnestic"* variety, which is characterized by subjective reports of memory loss and objective memory deficits greater than those expected for age but the relative preservation of all other cognitive functions and adequate functional capacity.

Causes include *Alzheimer's disease* and *depression*. Persons with amnestic mild cognitive impairment demonstrate nearly 10 times the risk of progressing to Alzheimer's disease as do normal individuals (about 12.5%/yr vs. 1%/yr to 2%/yr for normal persons of the same age). Other MCI subgroups include those with an isolated decline in a cognitive domain other than memory or have a combination of deficits but still function adequately. Persons with multidomain or nonamnestic impairment are at increased risk for other forms of dementia, including *vascular disease* and *Lewy body disease*.

Alzheimer's Disease

Alzheimer's disease (AD) is a slow, progressive, and eventually fatal disease, which also affects those who care for these patients. AD, the most common form of dementia in older patients, is a neurodegenerative disorder characterized not only by a decline in memory and cognition (the first symptoms to emerge), but also by a loss of the ability to care for self and the emergence of disabling and disruptive psychiatric and behavioral symptoms. The principal clinical features include memory loss, language impairment, and visuospatial deficits, followed later by gait disturbance, motor and sensory impairments, incontinence, and delusions and hallucinations. The presentation and course can be divided into early, intermediate, and advanced stages.

Early Stages

In the earliest stages of the illness (i.e., *mild cognitive impairment*; see prior discussion), most patients are mildly forgetful and complain of specific memory deficits, such as forgetting names or where they placed household items. Although the patient is concerned, there are no social or employment problems and no evidence of memory deficit during a clinical interview. Due to the preservation of social and conversational abilities, most patients are not diagnosed in the early or mild stages of AD. Clinicians in a busy primary care office may fail to see, minimize, or dismiss complaints if they are not associated with significant functional impairment. However, mild cognitive impairment is associated with a marked increase in risk for the development of AD.

With some progression, the patient enters the early stages of AD, which may be manifested by decreased performance in demanding work and social situations. Patients complain of *poor concentration*, difficulty in remembering words and names, more prominent memory loss, and confusion, and they may report that coworkers have noticed their relatively poor performance. Characteristically, there is an *inability to learn* and remember new information and difficulty in consolidating the information into memory (revealed by simple word retrieval testing or the use of a word list; see Chapter 169). Patients may present with *visual–spatial deficits* or difficulty with *speech*; they may report getting easily disoriented or lost when traveling to an unfamiliar location. *Anxiety* and/or *depression* may ensue as patients become aware of their symptoms; some begin to deny them. Changes in *personality* and *judgment* can cause problems with family and coworkers.

Intermediate Stages

As the illness progresses, patients become unable to travel alone and are unable to handle their personal finances. Memory for recent events is drastically impaired, and patients display a decreased knowledge of current events. Complex tasks are impossible, but patients remain fairly well oriented to time and person and can travel to very familiar places, such as the corner drugstore. Many patients remain aware of their deficits and are capable of understanding what is happening to them. They instinctively withdraw from previously challenging situations and may even have trouble with the activities of daily living. Difficulty with speech and language are more pronounced. Denial may become pronounced. Anxiety and depression may increase, along with suspiciousness and agitation. The most difficult behavior at this stage is wandering and pacing (balance and gait are usually preserved); the patient may get lost.

Late-Stage Disease

Patients can no longer survive without some assistance. They are unable to recall major relevant aspects of their current lives or even the names of close friends and family members. Delusions and hallucinations are common. For example, the spouse may be accused of being an impostor, or patients may talk to imaginary persons or their own reflection in the mirror. Depression, agitation, aggression, and violent behavior may occur. Frequently, patients are disoriented to time or place. However, they generally remain able to eat and use the toilet without assistance, but they may have difficulty in properly choosing and putting on clothing.

Advanced Disease

In the final stages of the disease, patients become totally incapacitated and disoriented. They eventually forget their name and may not recognize their spouse. Incontinence is common, frequently with a loss of both bladder and bowel control. Personality and emotional changes are prominent, although these changes occasionally occur even in the earliest stages of disease (see prior discussion). Eventually, all verbal abilities are lost, motor skills further deteriorate, making gait and balance nearly impossible, and patients require total care. Total dependence on the caregiver ensues, leading to caregiver stress, or "burnout" (see later discussion). Generalized cortical and focal neurologic signs and symptoms are frequently present. Death usually occurs from total debilitation or infection.

Clinical Course

The course of Alzheimer's disease from onset to death varies from 2 to 20 years. The average is about 8 to 10 years. Typically, the illness progresses at a fairly constant rate. If it has rapidly developed during the last year, it is likely to continue at that rate. A slowly progressive illness during the last 5 to 10 years suggests that the patient may survive for a number of years, especially if he or she is in otherwise good physical health. Other clinical features found to be independent predictors of more rapid progression to incapacity and death include hallucinations, paranoia, delusions, misidentification syndromes, extrapyramidal signs, and a low score on initial psychometric testing.

Dementia with Lewy Bodies (Lewy Body Disease)

Dementia with Lewy body disease (DLB) is a form of dementia often confused with other dementing illnesses, such as Alzheimer's disease and idiopathic Parkinson's disease (see Chapter 169). Accurate diagnosis is essential because of the increased sensitivity of these patients to psychotropic drugs, particularly antipsychotic agents (see later discussion).

Early on, the clinical presentation is predominated by *psychosis* (usually *visual hallucinations*) before the onset of other characteristic features. Patients may present with psychiatric, cognitive, or parkinsonian motor symptoms, which can be a source of confusion and lead to incorrect diagnosis. A progressive decline in cognition interferes with social or occupational functioning. Memory impairment may not be prominent in the earlier stages, but deficits in attention and visual–spatial and frontal–subcortical skills are often prominent.

In established disease, core clinical features include *recurrent visual hallucinations* that are well formed and detailed, *fluctuating consciousness*, and spontaneous motor features of *parkinsonism* and *extrapyramidal disease*. Other features include *falls* resulting from difficulty with movement, *syncope*, and a transient loss of consciousness resulting from suspected *autonomic dysfunction*. Hallucinations in other domains, systematized *delusions*, and *sensitivity to antipsychotic medications* are typical. The pace of clinical decline is more rapid than that of Alzheimer's disease.

PRINCIPLES OF MANAGEMENT

Once treatable causes have been ruled out (see Chapter 169), the primary care physician and practice team face the daunting challenge of caring for patients with a largely irreversible, progressively debilitating illness. Management of Alzheimer's disease involves the skillful interplay of medication to improve the patient's cognitive state and functional status, psychopharmacologic therapy, supportive care by team and family members (who often choose to maintain the patient at home), and community agencies. The approach to the patient with Lewy body disease is quite similar, with the exception of the use of antipsychotic agents.

Prevention (9,10)

Most attempts at the prevention of dementia provide, at best, modest benefit, reflecting the limits of current pathophysiologic understanding. However, even a modest delay in disease progression can result in a major reduction in care burden. Interest in prevention extends beyond lowering the risk of dementia to preserving mental function in an aging population. Lifestyle measures have shown some promise, including regular physical exercise, diets rich in fruits and vegetables, and mentally stimulating activities and exercises. In persons with mild cognitive impairment, the use of cholinesterase inhibitor therapy may transiently slow progression to Alzheimer's disease. Vitamin supplements, ginkgo, and other pharmacologic measures are popular but without evidence of efficacy.

Lifestyle Interventions

Simple lifestyle measures for elderly persons, such as regular modest *exercise* and engagement in *mentally stimulating leisure activities* (e.g., playing board games, playing musical instruments, reading), are associated with significantly reduced risks of developing dementia, including AD. As few as 1.5 hours per week of *walking* at a slow pace was associated with a 20% reduction in risk among elderly women in the Nurses' Health Study. Similar degrees of reduced risk were associated with participation in cognitively stimulating leisure activities. Cognitive training exercises reportedly negated the expected amount of normal cognitive decline in an elderly population. These and other healthy lifestyle interventions need confirmation by prospective long-term study to better assess their precise contributions to prevention, but there seems little harm in implementing them while awaiting confirmatory data.

Diet and Antioxidant Vitamin Supplements

The hypothesis that "oxidative stress" from free radical formation might damage neurons has been given much play in the lay media, spurred by commercial interests promoting the use of vitamin supplements. The hypothesis derives support from epidemiologic data and small, randomized trials revealing an association between the dietary intake of fruits and vegetables (i.e., foods rich in so-called "antioxidants") and a reduction in the risk of developing AD (risk reduction, 20% to 40%). However, randomized, controlled trials of supplement preparations containing the so-called antioxidant vitamins (e.g., C, E, β-carotene, *flavonoids*), even at high doses, have consistently failed to show any protective effect and do not support supplement use. The best nutritional advice is to adopt a well-balanced diet rich in fruits, green vegetables, grains, and nuts.

Treatment of Atherosclerotic Risk Factors

Hypertension, hypercholesterolemia, and diabetes are important risk factors for vascular dementia, and attention to the treatment of these risk factors is important. Atherosclerotic risk factors also appear to increase the risk of AD, and there is interest in applying treatments of these risk factors to the prevention of AD. Epidemiologic studies find a reduction in the risk of AD among persons taking *statin* therapy, which may exert its effect independent of lowering low-density-lipoprotein (LDL) cholesterol (LDL levels are no greater among AD patients). Randomized trials of statins for the prevention of AD are underway.

Homocysteine elevation is also associated with an increased risk of AD, but studies of the lowering of homocysteine through the use of folate, B_{12}, and B_6 supplementation in older persons with an elevation in serum homocysteine have failed to show improved cognitive performance or the prevention of progression to AD.

Cholinesterase Inhibitors and Memantine

A transient delay in progression to frank Alzheimer's disease has been observed in persons with mild cognitive impairment assigned to donepezil in a randomized, placebo-controlled trial. The significant delay in progression noted at 12 months disappeared by 36 months, but although the effects were mild and transient, they conceivably could have a meaningful effect both individually and populationwise. Such findings have encouraged the increasingly early use of cholinesterase-inhibitor therapy, starting at the time of diagnosis of mild cognitive impairment, as well as early detection (see also Chapter 169).

Avoidance of Potentially Toxic Substances

The avoidance of known toxins that can cause brain injury and dementia is important (e.g., *aniline dyes*, *heavy metals*, and perhaps very high levels of dietary *mercury*; see Chapter 169). There is no evidence that the avoidance of aluminum-containing preparations (e.g., antacids) is of any benefit , although concerns were raised when aluminum deposition was noted in the central nervous system of patients with Alzheimer's disease.

Nonsteroidal Antiinflammatory Drugs and Immunotherapy

Epidemiologic data suggest a protective effect associated with the long-term use of nonsteroidal antiinflammatory drugs (relative risk, 20%); however, data are few, and there are none from prospective study. A randomized, controlled trial is ongoing to help clarify the intriguing observational findings. Immunotherapy is being explored as an approach to preventing the buildup of β-amyloid peptide. Early vaccines had serious side effects. Work continues in this area.

Ginkgo Biloba

Despite much commercial promotion of *Ginkgo biloba* use, there is no evidence indicating a measurable preventive benefit or improvements in memory or related cognitive function in community-dwelling, non–cognitively impaired persons older than the age of 60 years or in the prevention of AD or other forms of dementia.

Hormone Replacement Therapy

Early epidemiologic data suggested some protection against the development of Alzheimer's disease in postmenopausal women using hormone replacement therapy (HRT), but more-definitive data from the Women's Health Initiative Memory Study failed to confirm the initial findings and even suggested an increase in risk of dementia (including Alzheimer's disease). Moreover, emerging safety concerns associated with long-term HRT (i.e., increased cancer and cardiovascular risks; see Chapter 118) have further dampened the initial enthusiasm for HRT use. Hormone replacement therapy is not recommended for the prevention of AD.

β-Amyloid Peptide–Reducing Drugs

Ongoing efforts are aimed at ways of reducing the accumulation of neurotoxic β-amyloid peptide, a central pathologic feature of the disease and a purported cause of brain cell death. No proven antiamyloid therapies have been identified, but much promising work is ongoing, and the literature should be followed closely for the results of studies testing experimental approaches to limiting β-amyloid peptide accumulation.

Treatment of Memory Loss and Cognitive Impairment (11–32)

Treatment entails a mix of supportive nonpharmacologic measures and drug therapy, largely with *cholinesterase inhibitors* and *N-methyl- d-aspartate* (NMDA) *antagonists*. Herbal extracts, dietary supplements, and hormone replacement therapy have received much attention but have failed to demonstrate efficacy convincingly.

Nonpharmacologic Measures—Cognitive Stimulation

At the least, cognitive stimulation can help to preserve the sleep–wake cycle and in doing so improve quality of life. Whether it improves overall cognitive function as it does in persons without dementia remains to be demonstrated. Programs are available through Alzheimer Association chapters.

Cholinesterase Inhibitors (Table 173.1)

The findings of cholinergic neuronal degeneration and depletion of acetylcholine-synthesizing enzyme (choline acetyltransferase) in Alzheimer's disease stimulated trials of *cholinesterase inhibitors* and *acetylcholine-receptor agonists* in patients with dementia, particularly those with Alzheimer's disease. Cholinesterase inhibitors increase acetylcholine levels in the cerebral cortex, which might account for the clinical improvements noted.

Efficacy. When used in patients with mild to moderate dementia, these agents produce statistically significant but clinically modest improvements in *cognition* and *global assessment*; improvements in *behavior* and *caregiver burden* are less consistently noted. There is some suggestion of delay in disease progression, but few studies are of longer than 6 months' duration, limiting the determination of this effect and the safety and efficacy of long-term use. Use for agitation or improvement in quality of life in patients with more advanced disease shows little benefit over placebo. An absence of benefit after 3 months of use makes it unlikely that there will be a beneficial response. The drugs are approved by the U.S. Food and Drug Administration (FDA) for use in mild to moderate AD.

Side Effects. The predominant side effects are gastrointestinal (e.g., nausea, emesis, diarrhea). Somnolence, headache, and occasional insomnia have been noted, and falls may occur. In

TABLE 173.1

CHOLINESTERASE INHIBITORS

Agent	Dose Range (mg)
Donepezil	2.5–10.0 (daily)
Rivastigmine	1.5–6.0 (twice daily)
Galantamine	4.0–12.0 (twice daily)
Memantine	5.0–10.0 (twice daily)
Tacrine[a]	10–40.0 (four times a day)

[a]Not often used, due to hepatotoxicity.

some patients, the abrupt discontinuation of medication results in a precipitous decline in cognition and a worsening of behavioral difficulties. Contraindications to use include poorly controlled asthma, angle-closure glaucoma, sick sinus syndrome, and left-bundle-branch block.

Preparations. The first cholinesterase inhibitor approved for the treatment of Alzheimer's disease was *tacrine* (Cognex), which demonstrated a statistically significant reduction in the rate of cognitive decline, but its high frequency of hepatotoxic effects (40% of patients), need for regular monitoring of liver function, and four-times-daily dosing schedule have limited its use, especially with the advent of safer, more convenient cholinesterase inhibitors.

Donepezil (Aricept) is the most widely used and extensively studied of the drugs in this class, showing consistent ability to improve both cognition and global functioning in persons with mild to moderate AD or vascular dementia. When used in more advanced disease, there is little meaningful improvement in quality of life. This second-generation piperidine cholinesterase inhibitor has a half-life of 70 to 80 hours and is eliminated both renally and hepatically. The starting dose is 5 mg/d, which is increased to 10 mg/d given in once-daily dosing.

Rivastigmine (Exelon) is a second-generation carbamate reversible cholinesterase inhibitor that is believed to increase acetylcholine selectively in the cortex and hippocampus. It has a half-life of 10 hours and is eliminated predominantly via the kidneys. Treatment is initiated at 1.5 mg twice daily, with the dose increased gradually to 6 mg/d and eventually up to 12 mg/d. Effects on cognition and global assessment are similar to those of the other drugs in its class; one head-to-head study with donepezil suggested a slightly better efficacy but also an increased frequency and severity of gastrointestinal side effects.

Galantamine (Reminyl) is a tertiary alkaloid cholinesterase inhibitor with a half-life of 7 hours, primarily hepatic metabolism, and minimum renal clearance. In addition to the cholinergic action, galantamine is an allosteric modulator of nicotinic receptors, which theoretically might prove advantageous for smokers. Like other drugs in its class, galantamine shows best results for cognition and global assessment and less consistent benefit for functional status and behavior. One comparison with donepezil found little difference in efficacy.

Choice of Cholinesterase Inhibitor. Tacrine should not be used, given the availability of newer cholinesterase inhibitors that are equally effective and much better tolerated. Among the latter, the dearth of head-to-head studies and the clinically minimal differences noted in available trials make the choice of agent predominantly a function of cost, side effects, and convenience.

NMDA Antagonists—Memantine (Namenda)

Glutamate overstimulation of the NMDA receptor is believed to play a role in the neurodegenerative process. Memantine, an uncompetitive antagonist of the NMDA receptor, is believed to act when there is glutamate excess and pathologic activation of this system.

Efficacy. The drug has been tested most extensively in persons with moderate to severe AD and mild to moderate vascular dementia, both as monotherapy in milder disease and in combination with cholinesterase inhibitor therapy in patients with more advanced disease. As with the cholinesterase inhibitors, findings include significant but clinically modest improvements in cognition and global assessment in persons with mild to moderate dementia. In addition, these benefits and modest improvements in quality of life and behavior have been noted in persons with more advanced disease. Effects appear to be sustained up to 6 months; there are few data on longer-term use.

Side Effects. Up to 10% of patients withdraw from therapy due to nausea, diarrhea, dizziness, or agitation.

Use. The drug is FDA approved for use in moderate to severe AD and is often prescribed in combination with a cholinesterase inhibitor; it can also be used as monotherapy for mild to moderate AD and vascular dementia. The starting dose is 5 mg once daily, advancing to 10 mg/d as tolerated.

Antioxidants (Selegiline, Vitamin E)

The reduction of free radical formation and "oxidative stress" has been the rationale for the use of antioxidants in AD. *Selegiline*, a monoamine oxidase inhibitor used in Parkinson's disease and demonstrated to slow disease progression of that illness (see Chapter 174), is believed to reduce neuronal oxidative injury and enhance cerebral catecholamine levels. α-Tocopherol (vitamin E) traps free radicals and reduces cell death *in vitro* caused by exposure to β-amyloid. In the best randomized, controlled study of such "antioxidant" therapy, very large doses of vitamin E (2,000 IU/d) modestly slowed disease progression by about 8 months and preserved function in persons with moderately severe Alzheimer's disease; similar results were obtained with selegiline, but combination therapy was no better than either agent alone, and there was no improvement in cognitive function. On the basis of such results, it is common for high-dose vitamin E (2,000 IU daily), the better tolerated of the two antioxidants, to be recommended and prescribed for moderately severe Alzheimer patients, but cost-effectiveness, safety, and long-term benefit remain to be more fully defined. Emerging concerns about the safety of long-term, high-dose vitamin E necessitate continuous reassessment. Selegiline may have a role in Lewy body disease (see later discussion).

Supplements

Many herbal preparations and dietary supplements are available and heavily promoted. Patients and family members often ask about using them (because they are "natural") in addition to prescribed medications. When tested in well-designed studies, these preparations have proved ineffective or marginally beneficial at best. On example is the popular herbal *Ginkgo biloba*, which in a single randomized study did demonstrate a slight improvement in cognitive function in a subset of AD patients and a stabilizing effect over 6 to 12 months in another, but the magnitude of benefit was of questionable clinical significance and considerably less than that observed with cholinesterase inhibitors. In addition, herbal preparations can be costly, have no dose-standardization or purity requirements, and can contain other pharmacologically active ingredients (see Chapter 237). Their use is not recommended. No evidence has been found that *lecithin* supplements have any effect.

Other Nonbeneficial Drugs

A host of drugs has been tried and found not to be helpful. *Hormone replacement therapy* was popular when initial epidemiologic studies suggested it as a possible link to reduced

TABLE 173.2

COMMONLY USED NEUROLEPTICS IN THE ELDERLY

	Sedation	Anticholinergic Effect	Extrapyramidal Effect	Hypotension
First-Generation Antipsychotics (Potency)				
Thioridazine (low) (10–50 mg)	High	High	Low	High
Perphenazine (intermediate) (0.5–5 mg)	Medium	Medium	Medium	Medium
Haloperidol (high) (0.25–2 mg)	Low	Low	High	Low
Thiothixine (high) (0.5–4 mg)	Low	Low	High	Low
Second-Generation ("Atypical") Antipsychotics				
Clozapine (Clozaril 6.25–100 mg)	High	High	Low	High
Olanzapine (Zyprexa 2.5–10 mg)	Medium	Medium	Low	Low
Quetiapine (Seroquel 12.5–300 mg)	Medium	Low	Low	High
Risperidone (Risperdal 0.25–3 mg)	Low	Low	Medium	Medium
Aripiprazole (Abilify 10–30 mg)	Low	Low	Low	Medium
Ziprasidone (Geodon 20–160 mg)	Low	Low	Low	Medium

rates of AD in postmenopausal women. Subsequent studies of estrogen alone and in combination with progesterone failed to show benefit in the treatment of AD, and data from the landmark Women's Health Initiative Memory Study suggested that hormone replacement may actually increase the risk of dementia.

Other nonbeneficial drugs include *cerebral vasodilators* (dihydroergotoxine), *ergoloid mesylates* (Hydergine), central nervous system *stimulants* (e.g., amphetamines, except for the treatment of apathy; see later discussion), *opiate antagonists* (naloxone), *neuropeptides* (vasopressin), and *glucocorticosteroids*.

Treatment of Confusion, Agitation, Disturbed Sleep, and Depression (33–39)

The neuropsychiatric consequences of Alzheimer's disease can be as disabling as the cognitive ones and may compromise care at home or in a nursing home, necessitating full implementation of nonpharmacologic measures and the consideration of pharmacologic intervention despite its risks and side effects (see Tables 173.2 to 173.4). Close monitoring and ready adjustment of drug programs are particularly important when antipsychotics, benzodiazepines, and sedative–hypnotics are prescribed. The long-term use of sedatives and psychoactive agents in the confused patient should be avoided unless persistent, extreme agitation hampers care. The regular use of sedative–hypnotic agents for sleep (see Chapter 226) is also problematic because they can cause confusion and disorientation and prolong sedation. A substantial improvement has been noted in many AD patients when the long-term use of psychotropic drugs is discontinued or reduced. If such therapy is contemplated, the lowest possible doses should be given for the shortest possible time.

Nonpharmacologic Measures

Readily implementable nonpharmacologic measures can be taught to family members for use in the home. Because these can significantly reduce agitation and depression, these measures should be fully implemented before resort is had to pharmacologic therapy (particularly the use of neuroleptics).

Assessment before Starting Pharmacotherapy

Before starting drug therapy, a check for etiologies of agitation and confusion other than dementia (e.g., medical illness, overmedication, environmental factors) should be made. Patients with Alzheimer's disease deteriorate rapidly both cognitively and behaviorally when they experience a *superimposed illness*. Coexistent medical problems, such as asthma, arthritis pain, diabetes, and congestive heart failure, should be carefully

TABLE 173.3

EFFICACY AND ADDITIONAL ADVERSE EFFECTS OF SECOND-GENERATION ANTIPSYCHOTICS

Drug	Efficacy	Hyperglycemia	Weight Gain	QT Prolongation	Neutropenia
Abilify	+/−	+/−	+/−	+/−	+/−
Clozapine	++++	++++	++++	+	+++
Olanzapine	+++	++++	++++	+	+/−
Quetiapine	++	++	+++	+/−	+/−
Risperidone	+++	++	++	+	+/−
Ziprasidone	++	+/−	+/−	++	+/−

Adapted from Second-generation antipsychotics—aripiprazole revisited. Med Lett 2005;47:81.

TABLE 173.4

ANTIDEPRESSANTS FOR DEPRESSION IN THE ELDERLY

Drug	Dose Range (mg/d)	Comments
Tricyclic Antidepressants		
Nortriptyline	10–150	Reliable blood levels
Desipramine	10–250	Mild anticholinergic
		Minimal orthostasis
Stimulants		
Dextroamphetamine	2.5–40	Agitation
Methylphenidate	2.5–60	Mild tachycardia
		Limited studies
Selective Serotonin Reuptake Inhibitors		
Fluoxetine	5–60	Akathisia
Sertraline	25–200	Anxiety/sedation
Paroxetine	10–40	Agitation
Fluvoxamine	25–300	Gastrointestinal symptoms
Citalopram	10–40	Headache
Escitalopram	5–20	Diarrhea/constipation
		Rash
Others		
Trazodone	25–250	Sedation
		Orthostasis
		Incontinence
		Hallucinations
		Priapism
Nefazodone	50–600	Pedal edema
		Rash
Mirtazapine	7.5–30	Sedation
		Weight gain
Venlafaxine	25–300 (slow-release form available)	Increase in blood pressure
		Confusion
		Lightheadedness
Bupropion	75–450 (slow-release form available)	Seizures
		Less mania/cycling
Duloxetine	30–60	Headache/nausea

See also Chapter 227.

controlled. Even a minor upper respiratory tract or urinary tract infection can worsen behavior.

Patients are susceptible to *medication-induced delirium*; a review of drug regimens is imperative. β-Blockers and anticholinergics may exacerbate confusion and should be reduced or eliminated if possible. The long-term use of sedatives and psychoactive agents in the confused patient should be avoided unless persistent, extreme agitation hampers care. As noted earlier, the regular use of sedative–hypnotic agents for sleep (see Chapter 226) is also problematic because they can cause confusion, disorientation, and prolonged sedation.

Cholinesterase Inhibitors and Memantine

These agents provide a pharmacologic option worth exploring before resort is had to psychotropic therapy, especially in persons with earlier-stage disease with mild to moderate psychiatric or behavioral difficulties. Patients with more severe symptoms (which may be the presenting complaint of family and other caregivers) show little benefit from this treatment over placebo, and some may experience worsening agitation. *Memantine* may help to ease neuropsychiatric symptoms in persons with moderately severe disease.

Neuroleptics (See Tables 173.2 and 173.3 and Appendix 173.1)

In severe or unresponsive cases, neuroleptic pharmacotherapy may be necessary. The safe and effective use of psychotropic medication in patients with Alzheimer's disease requires careful drug selection, dosing, and monitoring due to the increased risks of adverse effects and the alterations in drug uptake and metabolism that occur in the elderly (see Appendix 173.1).

Atypical ("second-generation") antipsychotics (e.g., olanzapine, clozapine, risperidone) are often tried first because of their lower side effect profile compared with first-generation neuroleptics (see Tables 173.2 and 173.3 and Appendix 173.1); however, adverse effects such as significant weight gain, marked glucose intolerance, hypotension, and parkinsonism and excessive sedation are common. One must be careful to avoid long-term use because of the risk for inducing tardive dyskinesia. Worsening of depression may occur with use in younger persons. Prolongation of the *QT interval* on electrocardiogram and an increased risk of *cardiac sudden deaths* have been reported with antipsychotic use in elderly demented patients, resulting in a "black-box" warning mandated by the FDA; although it is increased, the absolute risk remains small and less than that associated with the use of first-generation antipsychotics. A small increase in the risk of *stroke* in elderly persons has also been reported. *Neuroleptic malignant syndrome* is another rare but potentially catastrophic event associated with neuroleptic use (see Appendix 173.1).

These drugs are not FDA approved for use in elderly persons with psychotic symptoms due to advanced dementia, but often there is no other option, which accounts for their widespread use. Again, careful consideration of expected benefits and risks needs to be undertaken when considering use of antipsychotic agents; nonpharmacologic measures should be maximized before resorting to drug therapy. Controlled trials find significant benefit from the use of the popular second-generation neuroleptics, but tolerability is still low (nearly 80% of patients discontinue therapy due to intolerability or lack of efficacy), and the risk of serious adverse effects remains substantial.

Treatment of Depression (Table 173.4)

Depression is best treated with a *selective serotonin reuptake inhibitor* (SSRI; see Chapter 227). Psychotherapy is limited in what it can accomplish, but behavioral measures can be taught to the family that will limit the risk and severity of depression. Often SSRI therapy is started by the primary care physician. Patients who do not respond to one or two of these first-line agents may be considered for one of the newer antidepressants (e.g., *venlafaxine* [Effexor] or *bupropion* [Wellbutrin]) or one of the older tricyclic compounds with few anticholinergic side effects, such as *desipramine* (10 to 50 mg at bedtime) or *nortriptyline* (10 to 75 mg at bedtime). However, the use of tricyclic drugs in the elderly can be problematic, especially those agents with marked anticholinergic activity (e.g., *amitriptyline*), which may worsen memory, cause agitation, and trigger cardiac dysrhythmias (see Appendix 173.1, Table 173.4, and Chapter 227). Patients with depression who are started on antipsychotic therapy should be monitored carefully for the worsening of depression, an uncommon but important adverse effect (see Appendix 173.1).

Psychopharmacologic consultation can be helpful for the comprehensive evaluation of comorbid depression, especially if failure of two or more antidepressants has ensued.

Patients with Alzheimer's disease can have symptoms of prominent apathy and lack of motivation unrelated to comorbid depression, and these symptoms respond more robustly to stimulants (e.g., methylphenidate, dextroamphetamine, or modafinil).

Management of Severe Behavioral Disorders (40–44)

Deterioration in behavior is particularly troublesome to family members. Educating the family in how to recognize the symptoms early, approach the patient, and communicate with the physician are key steps in management. Among the disturbing behaviors cited most frequently are catastrophic reactions, severe agitation, aggression (including violent behavior), resistance to care, wakefulness, suspiciousness or paranoia, and incontinence. Wandering can also be problematic.

Catastrophic Reactions

Catastrophic reactions are massive emotional overresponses that are typically precipitated by task failure or minor stress. Hitting and violent resistance to care are extreme forms of such reactions. Most excessive emotional responses can be minimized by teaching the family to avoid or remove the precipitating task or stress, to remain quiet and calm, and to change the focus of attention gently. *Antipsychotic drugs*, *anticonvulsant drugs* (e.g., valproic acid, carbamazepine, or gabapentin), or *buspirone* sometimes help in difficult cases, but only as an adjunct to behavioral techniques (see Appendix 173.1).

Wakefulness and Night Walking

Wakefulness and night walking often deprive the caregiver of much-needed rest. Helpful environmental interventions include placing locks on each door so that the patient will not wander out of the house at night, keeping the patient physically active during the day, and not allowing a nap. An initial trial of a sedating *antidepressant* at bedtime or an *atypical antipsychotic* may benefit sleep onset and duration. Sedative–hypnotics, such as a *short-acting benzodiazepine* or *chloral hydrate*, may be helpful but might cause confusion (see Chapter 228).

Suspiciousness

Suspiciousness and accusatory behaviors are believed to result from the brain-injured person's efforts to explain misplaced possessions or misinterpreted events. If the family members understand this, their frustration, hurt, and anger may be reduced. Simple interventions, such as keeping an orderly house or making a sign pointing to where an object is kept, may help. *Atypical antipsychotics* are used more liberally when more-violent reactions occur. However, these behaviors may be dampened with the addition of a *cholinesterase inhibitor*.

Incontinence

Incontinence is typically a late manifestation of Alzheimer's disease, but when present early, it warrants a careful search for other causes, such as urinary tract infection atrophic vaginitis, constipation, mobility problems related to arthritis, and other causes of dementia, such as normal-pressure hydrocephalus (which includes incontinence as part of the diagnosis; see Chapters 134 and 169). Detrusor instability may be prominent and responsive to anticholinergic therapy, but care needs to be exercised with such pharmacologic treatment because it may cause confusion or agitation. An agent with minimal crossing of the blood–brain barrier is preferred (e.g., tolterodine [Detrol]; see Chapter 134). Conversely, drugs with anticholinergic effects may reduce bladder filling, exacerbating urge incontinence.

Inappropriate Sexual Behavior

Inappropriate sexual behavior is very uncommon in Alzheimer's disease. Family members can be reassured. In the rare instances in which it occurs, self-stimulation is the usual form. Alzheimer's patients are not sexually aggressive toward children.

Wandering

Wandering becomes an issue as the disease progresses. Without advance planning, it can become problematic. Besides making changes in supervision, home environment, and pharmacologic program, simple measures such as the use of an identification bracelet (available through the Alzheimer's Association's Safe Return Program) helps to support patient safety.

Managing the Home Environment (40–44)

As mentioned earlier, families need to be encouraged to maintain a *structured*, predictable environment for the patient. Any change can be devastating and stressful to a patient and may produce a massive emotional overresponse. A schedule in which activities such as arising, eating, taking medication, and exercise occur at the same time each day maximizes the patient's familiarity with the personal environment. At times, the use of an *orientation center* in the home, with pertinent information such as the date, time, schedule of household events, and pictures of relevant people, is very helpful.

Preventing Falls

Of particular importance to survival and quality of life is the need to reduce the risk for falls in the home. It has been clearly demonstrated that falls are one of the major predictors of reduced survival. Installing handrails, encouraging the use of a walker, and eliminating throw rugs and other obstacles can be extremely important to maximizing survival and minimizing disability. In the nursing home environment, the use of both tricyclic antidepressants and the SSRIs has been found to increase the risk for falls. The tricyclics may decrease blood pressure and cause postural hypotension. The SSRIs do not cause orthostasis, but they may cause dizziness and increase a patient's mobility. The risk for falls is dose related with any medication, which suggests that physicians should start some patients with doses less than the usual starting dose (see Appendix 173.1).

Driving

Frequently, patients will want to drive even when it is clear that they are no longer safe on the roads. The family members at times will resist stopping the patient from driving, stating that the patient is a good driver. This may be true, but the patient is at great risk of becoming lost or getting into a dangerous situation. Therefore, family education is essential. If possible, it is best to avoid direct confrontation with the patient. Simple techniques such as hiding the keys, disconnecting distributor wires, and giving the patient a nonfunctional set of keys have usually been successful in discouraging patients who are at risk from driving.

Firearms and Other Safety Considerations

All firearms should be removed from the home for obvious reasons. In addition, smoking and cooking become potentially dangerous activities. Environmental modifications, such as removing stove knobs, having a stove cut-off switch placed in an inconspicuous place, locking rooms or closets, and locking up matches, are important for safety.

Family and Caregiver Education and Support (40–46)

Some family members may react with dread and depression to the fact that their relative has Alzheimer's disease. Those members who have a preexisting psychiatric illness may de-

compensate in the setting of a family member who will need more care. Others will have suspected the diagnosis and are relieved to find an understanding physician who will be available and helpful during the course of the illness. Family members who are initially stunned and ask few questions should not have information forced on them. Careful explanation of any further tests should be provided and a follow-up appointment arranged within a week. Common questions include the following: How long will the patient live? How rapidly will the patient deteriorate? What are the chances that other family members will be affected by the disease? Is it hereditary? Is there a treatment?

Education about Hereditary Risk

Family members concerned about risk can now be more accurately informed than previously, given the availability of data from large-scale epidemiologic studies. Being a first-degree relative confers significant risk [relative risk (RR) about 2.5], as does being African American (RR, 1.6) and of female gender (RR, 1.5). Apo E genotype also is an important risk factor. Although the cumulative risk of dementia by age 85 years among first-degree relatives is high (just greater than 25% for whites and 43.7% for African Americans), the cumulative risk does not approach these levels until later in life. Graphs of cumulative risk from major epidemiologic studies can be used to help determine an individual family member's degree of risk. Establishing the degree of risk can be helpful in determining who should be followed closely, especially as advances are made in the prevention of Alzheimer's disease, so that timely intervention can be assured.

Use of the Social Worker and Collaborative Care Management

Most helpful for coping are the services of a *social worker* skilled in the management of Alzheimer's disease. Within the first few weeks after the diagnosis has been made, family members should see a social worker who is familiar with community resources, such as visiting nurse services, delivery of meals, financial aid, and nursing homes. For the patient with very early Alzheimer's disease, this may seem premature, but family members will be reassured by the knowledge that help will be available when it is needed in the future. Most families read about the illness and become acutely aware of its devastating course.

The value of a *collaborative care* approach to caring for patients and their families is becoming increasingly recognized. This approach goes beyond standard family education and care by the primary care physician to include the services of a care manager (usually an advanced practice nurse), who becomes part of the primary care team and meets with the family and patient twice monthly to assess how they are doing, especially with regard to behavioral and psychological issues. Emphasis is placed on managing the behavioral and psychologic problems rather than on enhancing cognitive function. Behavioral protocols specific to given problems are used. Such an approach has been found in randomized trial significantly to improve behavioral and psychological outcomes, for both patients and their families, without a significant increase in use of medication.

Dealing with Psychological Problems

Guilt, *unrealistic expectations*, and the assumption of *excessive responsibility* are common responses of families. In discussing these and similar issues, the physician should focus on both physical realities and the family's emotional response to the patient. One frequently encountered source of difficulty is the reversal of parent–child roles that the care of an elderly person often represents. There is no one way to handle this issue; however, in the overwhelming majority of such cases, just allowing family members to discuss these and other issues is therapeutic.

A *lack of personal time for caregivers* and *sleep disturbances* in patients are the least tolerable aspects of home care. Caregivers are at risk for depression and anxiety disorders that can hamper their ability to care for the patient. Families do best when relatives and friends visit frequently and when provisions are made for the primary caregiver to take breaks from his or her responsibilities. Visiting nurses and centers that provide day care can be invaluable. Family support is the major variable in keeping the cognitively impaired elderly patient at home.

Support Groups

Support groups can be very helpful. Even with a compassionate and empathic physician, many families feel alone with this illness and are unable to find friends who understand. Embarrassment may make them withdraw from previous social contacts. To meet the need for communication and information, families in many areas have established *volunteer organizations* that are involved in helping each other, sharing solutions to management problems, exchanging information, supporting needed legislation and research, and educating the community. These organizations welcome members who are concerned about any of the dementing illnesses, of which Alzheimer's disease is the most common. The number of such support groups is growing rapidly, and families consistently report how helpful they are. Local volunteer organizations have established a national organization, the *Alzheimer's Association*, whose goals are family support, education, advocacy, and encouragement of research. The address of the Alzheimer's Association is 919 North Michigan Avenue, Suite 1000, Chicago, IL 60611-1672; the Web address is http://www.alz.org; the telephone number is 800-272-3900. The national organization will give family members the addresses of local groups. Each family member should be encouraged to read one of the available lay books on Alzheimer's disease. *The 36-Hour Day* (see ref. 44) is required reading for anyone (including the physician) who is dealing with a person with a progressive dementing illness.

Nursing Home Placement and Care (40,41,47,48)

It is always a difficult moment when the family considers nursing home placement. Placement represents an irrevocable loss of autonomy for the patient. The decision must be approached with careful deliberation and respect for the patient. Although the family's needs are important to consider, the physician has a special obligation to the patient. If the patient created an advance directive before becoming mentally incapacitated (see Chapter 1), the choices set forth can be respected and followed. In the absence of such a directive, the physician needs to act as it appears the patient would have wanted. If a surrogate has been designated, this person can help in the decision making. The goal, first and foremost, is to help the patient.

Before any action is taken regarding nursing home placement, it is worth carefully reexamining the home situation to be sure all alternatives to placement have been explored. Have home health aides, senior day care, and similar supports been used to relieve the family's burden?

Only after all home care resources have been exhausted or found to be insufficient is it proper to proceed with placement. An appropriate site is one that can provide emotional support, reassurance, and security. One seeks a nursing home that preserves a sense of connection and closeness to others. The primary physician plays a critical role in ensuring that the placement is carried out well and serves the best interests of the patient.

As noted earlier, the use of psychoactive drugs in the nursing home environment can adversely affect alertness, mobility, and blood pressure. The risk of falls and the decline in overall functional status correlate with number and doses of drugs prescribed. Use should be kept to a minimum (see Appendix 173.1).

Often during advanced phases of the illness, when nutrition begins to decline because of difficulty in feeding, the question arises of the value of a *feeding tube*. The best available data show no benefit from tube feeding in regard to pressure sores, infections, cognitive function, pain, or risk for aspiration pneumonia. Moreover, survival does not appear to be prolonged. Most authorities discourage the practice of placing a feeding tube.

Management of Dementia due to Lewy Body Disease (49)

Although the basic principles and much of the care for this condition are nearly identical to those for Alzheimer's disease, important exceptions exist. The most important one is the need for *caution in the administration of antipsychotics*. Because patients who have dementia with Lewy bodies may present with psychotic features (e.g., vivid visual hallucinations), physicians tend to expose them early to standard first-generation antipsychotic medications (e.g., haloperidol), often before the diagnosis is recognized. The net result is a worsening or precipitation of extrapyramidal symptoms and little improvement in mental status. Because patients with Lewy body disease are very sensitive to these medications, it is best to begin with one of the *atypical antipsychotics* when treatment of hallucinosis or other psychotic features is required, taking into consideration and closely monitoring for the many adverse side effects associated with their use (see Tables 173.2 and 173.3 and Appendix 173.1). In addition, *selegiline* (5 mg twice daily) has demonstrated some ability to slow disease progression.

THERAPEUTIC RECOMMENDATIONS (50,51)

- For prevention, recommend regular exercise, mentally stimulating activities, and balanced diets rich in fruits and vegetables; discourage the use of measures lacking evidence of efficacy (e.g., "antioxidant" vitamin supplements, herbal preparations, homocysteine-lowering B vitamin supplements, hormone replacement therapy).
- Screen for mild cognitive impairment (see Chapter 169) because early treatment may at least transiently slow disease progression.
- Before initiating dementia-related treatment, recheck for reversible causes of cognitive decline (e.g., comorbid medical illness, depression, excessive medication).
- For patients with mild cognitive impairment, consider initiating cholinesterase inhibitor therapy (e.g., donepezil 5 mg/d) to temporarily slow disease progression.

■ Once a diagnosis of Alzheimer's disease or other progressive dementia has been established, decide whether to take on management responsibility or refer. Take into consideration the ability to implement a collaborative, multidisciplinary team approach (e.g., the use of a nurse practitioner to monitor behavioral and the psychological aspects of the illness and to complement physician efforts), which may facilitate achieving the best outcomes.

■ Apprise family members of the patient's diagnosis and conduct an open discussion as part of the initial management; include a family meeting with the social worker to help plan for care and provide emotional support. A referral to the Alzheimer's Association may be of benefit (http://www.alz.org or 800-272-3900), as may suggested reading (e.g., *The 36-Hour Day*; see ref. 44).

■ Advise setting up a predictable, well-structured, and safe home environment, especially one that limits the risk for falls, confusion, and overstimulation; remove dangerous objects from the home; prevent driving.

■ Recommend that the family implement a program of behavioral measures, which can be taught or offered by the local Alzheimer Association and range from cognitive stimulation to behavioral and environmental approaches that can limit depression and agitation.

■ Before considering the use of pharmacotherapy, taper and if possible discontinue all potentially contributing medications (e.g., sedatives–hypnotics, anticholinergics, antipsychotics).

■ For cognitive impairment and overall functioning in mild to moderate dementia, consider a 3-month trial of a cholinesterase inhibitor (e.g., *donepezil*, starting at 5 mg daily; *rivastigmine*, starting at 1.5 mg twice daily; or *galantamine*, starting at 4 mg twice daily). Because benefits are likely to be modest, weigh the risks and benefits before implementing and continue only if improvement outweighs side effects. Alternatively, consider a 3-month trial of monotherapy with memantine (starting at 5 mg/d).

■ For behavioral problems or mild agitation or paranoia in patients with early disease implement nonpharmacologic measures such as restructuring the living environment and counseling the family in how to respond; consider starting or increasing cholinesterase-inhibitor therapy. For those with more advanced disease, add memantine.

■ For cognitive impairment, behavioral problems, and overall functioning in moderate to severe disease consider adding memantine (starting at 5 mg/d); continue this dose for 5 to 6 weeks before increasing, because higher doses are associated with increased risk of adverse effects. Do not continue if the slowing of disease progression is not deemed an appropriate goal (e.g., in very advanced disease).

■ If a concomitant psychiatric problem (e.g., psychosis, depression, anxiety, behavioral disorder) proves to be very severe or refractory, then consider psychopharmacologic intervention, but only after full implementation of nonpharmacologic measures, including checking for and eliminating any potentially contributing factors, such as environmental precipitants, comorbid medical conditions, and medications (e.g., sedatives, β-blockers, anticholinergics, neuroleptics).

■ If, after attention to precipitants, severe agitation or psychotic or catastrophic reactions persist, then consider a trial of an *atypical/second-generation antipsychotic* agent (e.g., risperidone, starting at 0.25 mg/d; see Tables 173.2 and 173.3), but only after carefully weighing the risks and benefits and seeking psychopharmacologic consultation if necessary.

■ Monitor neuroleptic therapy closely for adverse effects (e.g., hyperglycemia, parkinsonism, excessive sedation, hypotension, and cardiac arrhythmias) and keep the treatment as brief as possible, using the smallest doses possible.

■ For major depression, begin with a low dose of an SSRI or a well-tolerated tricyclic agent (see Table 173.4 and Chapter 227). For anxiety or difficulty with sleeping, consider a low dose of an atypical antipsychotic, sedating antidepressant, or short-acting benzodiazepine (see Chapter 226), but watch for confusion and disorientation.

■ For moderately advanced Alzheimer's disease, consider the addition of *vitamin E* (2,000 IU/d) or *selegiline* to attempt to slow disease progression (if deemed appropriate), but efficacy is modest at best and the effect on outcomes is limited. Vitamin E is the better tolerated, but there are concerns about the safety of long-term use (there is a question of an increase in the risk of lung cancer).

■ For patients with Lewy body disease, consider a trial of *selegiline* (5 mg twice daily). Avoid first-generation antipsychotic agents for hallucinations because symptoms might be exacerbated; second-generation drugs may be tried (e.g., risperidone 25 mg at bedtime).

■ Actively monitor and support the principal caregiver's emotional state and physical health; encourage family members to join the local chapter of the Alzheimer's Association or a similar community support group.

■ Refer the patient to a community support group for the consideration of day care services.

■ Approach the need for nursing home placement carefully and only after home care resources have been fully utilized. Many day care programs have been established that specialize in the care of patients with Alzheimer's disease. Emphasis is on providing for the emotional and physical needs of the patient, although family preferences also deserve consideration. Many specialized care units for patients with Alzheimer's disease can provide a comfortable, stimulating, and safe environment for the patient who can no longer remain at home.

RESOURCES

Alzheimer's Association, 800-272-3900, http://www.alz.org

American Association of Retired Persons, 800-424-3410, http://www.aarp.org

Eldercare Locator, 800-677-1116, http://www.ageinfo.org/elderloc/elderb.html

Family Caregiver Alliance, http://www.caregiver.org

Health Care Financing Administration, 800-633-4227, http://www.cms.hhs.gov/medicare

National Nursing Home Data Base, http://www.medicare.gov/Nursing/Overview.asp

National Association for Incontinence, 800-252-3337 (800-BLADDER)

National Caregiving Foundation, 800-930-1357, http://www.caregivingfoundation.org

National Citizen's Coalition for Nursing Home Reform, 202-332-2275, http://www.nccnhr.org

National Hospice Foundation, 800-658-8898, http://www.hospicefoundation.org

National Institute on Aging, http://www.nih.gov/nia

National Library of Medicine, http://www.nlm.nih.gov/medlineplus

Social Security information, retirement or disability benefits, http://www.ssa.gov

Annotated Bibliography

1. Bird TD. Genetic Factors in Alzheimer's disease. N Engl J Med 2005;352:862. (*A succinct but authoritative summary.*)
2. Budson AE, Price BH. Memory dysfunction. N Engl J Med 2005;352:692. (*An excellent review of pathophysiology; 56 references.*)
3. Kawas CH. Early Alzheimer's disease. N Engl J Med 2003;349:1056. (*A clinical review for the nonspecialist, including a discussion of mild cognitive impairment; 66 references.*)
4. McKeith IG, Galasko D, Kosaka K, et al. Consensus guidelines for the clinical and pathologic diagnosis of dementia with Lewy bodies. Neurology 1996;47:1113. (*A clear outline and definition of the condition.*)
5. Naslund J, Haroutunian V, Mohs R, et al. Correlation between elevated levels of amyloid β-peptide in the brain and cognitive decline. JAMA 2000;283:1571. (*Presents evidence of its important pathologic role in Alzheimer's disease.*)
6. Petersen RC. Mild cognitive impairment as a diagnostic entity. J Intern Med 2004;256:183. (*A detailed description of the condition.*)
7. Stern Y, Min-Xing T, Albert MS, et al. Predicting time to nursing home care and death in individuals with Alzheimer disease. JAMA 1997;277:806. (*A prospective cohort study, finding that low psychometric test score, extrapyramidal signs, psychotic symptoms, short duration of illness, and age <65 years at onset are independent predictors of a poor prognosis.*)
8. Walsh JS, Welch HG, Larson EB. Survival of outpatients with Alzheimer-type dementia. Ann Intern Med 1990;113:429. (*The length of survival was more a function of the severity of disease than of its duration; wandering, falling, and behavioral problems were correlated with shortened survival.*)
9. Engelhart MJ, Geerlings MI, Ruitenberg A, et al. Dietary intake of antioxidants and risk of Alzheimer disease. JAMA 2002;287:3223. (*A prospective, large-scale, observational cohort study, finding that a 20% reduction in risk was associated with a high dietary intake of foods rich in vitamins E and C, but that no benefit was found from the use of vitamin supplements.*)
10. Veld BA, Ruitenberg A, Hofman A, et al. Nonsteroidal antiinflammatory drugs and the risk of Alzheimer's disease. N Engl J Med 2001;345:1515. (*Presents epidemiologic data suggesting a protective effect; the relative risk was 20%.*)
11. Larson EB, Wang L, Bowen JD, et al. Exercise is associated with reduced risk for incident dementia among persons 65 year of age and older. Ann Intern Med 2006;144:73. (*A prospective cohort study, finding a significant benefit of exercise.*)
12. McMahon JA, Green TJ, Skeaff CM, et al. A controlled trial of homocysteine lowering and cognitive performance. N Engl J Med 2006;354:2764. (*A randomized, controlled trial [RCT], finding no benefit in normal elderly volunteers.*)
13. Petersen RC, Thomas RG, Grundman M, et al. for the Alzheimer's Disease Cooperative Study Group. Vitamin E and donepezil for the treatment of mild cognitive impairment. N Engl J Med 2005;352:2379. (*RCT, finding that there was a short-term benefit from donepezil in slowing the progression to Alzheimer's disease, but that by 3 years there was no difference from placebo; there was no benefit whatsoever from vitamin E.*)
14. Qi D, Borenstein AR, WU, et al. Fruit and vegetable juices and Alzheimer's disease: the KAME Project. Am J Med 2006;119:751. (*There was evidence of a preventive effect, but none was observed for vitamin supplements.*)
15. Shumaker SA, Legault C, Kuller L, et al. Conjugated equine estrogens and incidence of probable dementia and mild cognitive impairment in postmenopausal women: Women's Health Initiative Memory Study. JAMA 2004;291:2947. (*No benefit was demonstrated.*)
16. Solomon PR, Adams F, Silver A, et al. Ginkgo for memory enhancement: a randomized controlled trial. JAMA 2002;288:835. (*A well-designed study, finding no benefit in normal elderly people.*)
17. Willis SL, Tennstedt SL, Marsiske M, et al. Long-term effects of cognitive training on everyday functional outcomes in older adults. JAMA 2006;296:2805. (*RCT, finding that a 10-session program produced a sustained reduction in functional decline and improved cognitive abilities*)
18. Wilson RS, de Leon CFM, Barnes LL, et al. Participation in cognitively stimulating activities and risk of incident Alzheimer disease. JAMA 2002;287:742. (*A longitudinal cohort study, finding a 33% reduction in risk.*)
19. Cummings JL, Schneider L, Tariot PN, et al. Reduction of behavioral disturbances and caregiver distress by galantamine in patients with Alzheimer's disease. Am J Psychiatry 2004;161:532. (*A well-designed study, noting reductions in behavioral problems and caregiver stress.*)
20. Cummings JL. Alzheimer's disease. N Engl J Med 2004;351:56. (*An excellent review of a variety of drugs used in the treatment of patients with Alzheimer's disease; 88 references.*)
21. DeKosky ST. Statin therapy in the treatment of Alzheimer's disease: what is the rationale? Am J Med 2005;118(12A):S485. (*Reviews the evidence for potential benefit, and argues in favor of testing.*)
22. Howard RJ, Juszczak E, Ballard CG, for the CALM-AD Trial Group. Donepezil for the treatment of agitation in Alzheimer's disease. N Engl J Med 2007;357:1382. (*RCT, finding no benefit over placebo in persons with moderately advanced disease.*)
23. Le Bars PL, Katz MM, Berman N, et al. A placebo-controlled, double blind, randomized trial of an extract of Ginkgo biloba for dementia. JAMA 1997;278:1327. (*Notes a modest benefit in patients with dementia.*)
24. Mulnard RA, Cotman CW, Kawas C, et al. Estrogen replacement therapy for treatment of mild to moderate Alzheimer disease: a randomized trial. JAMA 2000;283:1007. (*Finds no benefit, but a suggestion of adverse effect.*)
25. Oken BS, Stotzbach DM, Kaye JA. The efficacy of Ginkgo biloba on cognitive function in Alzheimer's disease. Arch Neurol 1998;55:1400. (*A meta-analysis of five clinical studies, noting a slight cognitive improvement.*)
26. Raina P, Santaguida P, Ismaila A, et al. Effectiveness of cholinesterase inhibitors and memantine for treating dementia: evidence review for a clinical practice guideline. Ann Intern Med 2008;148:379. (*An excellent review of the evidence; 84 references.*)
27. Reisberg B, Doody R, Stoffler A, et al. Memantine in moderate to severe Alzheimer's disease. N Engl J Med 2003;1333. (*One of the initial studies demonstrating the efficacy of N-methyl-d-aspartate antagonist in reducing clinical deterioration in moderate to severe disease.*)
28. Sano M, Ernesto C, Thomas RG, et al. A controlled trial of selegiline, α-tocopherol or both as treatment for Alzheimer's disease. N Engl J Med 1997;336:1216. (*A multicenter study, finding a modest but significant slowing of functional deterioration in moderately severe disease, and no additional benefit with combination therapy.*)
29. Tariot PN, Farlow MR, Grossberg GT, et al. Memantine treatment in patients with moderate to severe Alzheimer disease already receiving donepezil: a randomized controlled trial. JAMA 291:317. (*Finds improved measures of cognition, activities of daily living, behavior, and global outcome.*)
30. Teri L, Gibbons LE, McCurry SM, et al. Exercise plus behavioral management in patients with Alzheimer's disease: a randomized controlled trial. JAMA 2003;290:2015. (*A home-based program taught to caregivers improved physical health and lessened depression.*)
31. Thompson TL, Filley CM, Mitchell WD, et al. Lack of efficacy of Hydergine in patients with Alzheimer's disease. N Engl J Med 1990;323:445. (*Hydergine had been widely prescribed but never properly studied; no benefit was found in this rigorously designed, controlled study.*)
32. Trinh NH, Hoblyn HJ, Mohanty S, et al. Efficacy of cholinesterase inhibitors in the treatment of neuropsychiatric symptoms and functional impairment in Alzheimer disease. JAMA 2003;289:210. (*A meta-analytic study, demonstrating a modest benefit for this class of drugs in persons with mild to moderate disease.*)
33. Cohen-Mansfield J, Lipson S, Werner P, et al. Withdrawal of haloperidol, thioridazine, and lorazepam in the nursing home: a controlled, double-blind trial. Arch Intern Med 1999;159:1733. (*Withdrawal improved clinical status.*)
34. Howard RJ, Juszczak E, Ballard CG, et al. Donepezil for the treatment of agitation in Alzheimer's disease. N Engl J Med 2007;357:1382. (*RCT, finding that this treatment was not effective in persons with more severe agitation.*)
35. Larson EB, Kukull WA, Vuchner D, et al. Adverse drug reactions associated with global cognitive impairment in elderly persons. Ann Intern Med 1987;107:169. (*Adverse drug reactions were an important source of cognitive impairment, especially when more than four drugs were being taken.*)
36. Lipowski ZJ. Delirium in the elderly patient. N Engl J Med 1989;320:578. (*A short, very useful review; 32 references.*)
37. Schneider LS, Tariot PN, Dagerman KS, et al., for the Clinical Antipsychotic Trials of Intervention Effectiveness—Alzheimer's Disease (CATIE-AD) Study Group. Effectiveness of atypical antipsychotic drugs in patients with Alzheimer's disease. N Engl J Med 2006;355:1525. (*A multicenter, placebo-controlled, head-to-head, randomized trial, showing that adverse effects are frequent and often offset the benefits.*)
38. Schneider LS, Dagerman KS, Insel P. Risk of death with atypical antipsychotic drug treatment for dementia. Meta-analysis of randomized placebo-controlled trials. JAMA 2005;294:1934. (*Atypicals were found to be associated with a small but statistically significant increase in the risk of death compared to placebo.*)
39. Wang PS, Schneeweiss S, Avorn J, et al. Risk of death in elderly users of conventional vs atypical antipsychotic medications. N Engl J Med 2005;353:2335. (*A retrospective cohort study, finding that conventional antipsychotics were at least as likely to the increase risk of death as atypical agents.*)
40. American Academy of Neurology Ethics and Humanities Subcommittee. Practice parameter: ethical issues in the management of the demented patient. Neurology 1996;46:1180. (*Covers the patient–physician relationship, advance directives, proxy decision making, restraints, and withdrawal of life-sustaining treatment.*)
41. American College of Physicians. Cognitively impaired subjects. Ann Intern Med 1989;111:843. (*A position paper on ethical issues regarding the care of such patients.*)

42. Callahan CM, Boustani MA, Unverzagt FW, et al. Effectiveness of collaborative care for older adults with Alzheimer disease in primary care. A randomized controlled trial. JAMA 2006;295:2148. (*Finds that the use of advanced practice nurses focusing on behavioral and psychological issues was effective.*)

43. Drachman DA. Who may drive? Who may not? Who shall decide? Ann Neurol 1988;24:787. (*Analysis of the tricky regulation process and the physician's obligation to patients and others.*)

44. Mace NL, Rabins PV. The 36-hour day: a family guide to caring for persons with Alzheimer's disease, dementing illness, and memory loss in later life. Baltimore: Johns Hopkins University Press, 1999. (*Required reading for all who care for patients with dementing illnesses; excellent for family members.*)

45. Green RC, Cupples LA, Go R, et al. Risk of dementia among white and African American relatives of patients with Alzheimer disease. JAMA 2002;287:329. (*Presents epidemiologic data on risk, identifying first-degree-relative status, female gender, and African American race as important risk factors independent of apo E genotype.*)

46. Nussbaum RL, Ellis CE. Alzheimer's disease and Parkinson's disease. N Engl J Med. 2003;348:1356. (*An excellent review of the genetics.*)

47. Finucane TE, Christmas C, Travis K. Tube feeding in patients with advanced dementia. A review of the evidence. JAMA 1999;282:1365. (*There were no data to suggest that tube feeding relieves pressure sores, infections, or pain, reduces the risk for aspiration pneumonia, or increases cognitive function or survival.*)

48. Meier DE, Cassel CK. Nursing home placement and the demented patient. Ann Intern Med 1986;104:98. (*A most helpful discussion of this difficult phase of care.*)

49. Rojas-Fernandez OH, McKnight C. Dementia with Lewy bodies: review and pharmacotherapeutic implications. Pharmacotherapy 1999;19:795. (*A useful summary of psychopharmacologic management.*)

50. Doody RS, Steven JC, Beck C, et al. Management of dementia. Report of the Quality Standards Subcommittee of the American Academy of Neurology. Neurology 2001;56:1154. (*Evidence-based guidelines.*)

51. Qaseem A, Snow V, Cross JT Jr, et al. Current pharmacologic treatment of dementia: a clinical practice guideline from the American College of Physicians and the American Academy of Family Physicians. Ann Intern Med 2008;148:370. (*Consensus guidelines that find cholinesterase inhibitors and memantine of modest benefit yet worth considering for the treatment of dementia.*)

> ## APPENDIX 173.1: USE OF ANTIPSYCHOTIC DRUGS AND OTHER PSYCHOPHARMACOLOGIC AGENTS IN THE ELDERLY (1–7)

PHARMACOKINETIC AND NEUROTRANSMITTER CHANGES ASSOCIATED WITH AGING

Pharmacokinetic Changes

Significant changes in drug absorption and distribution, protein binding, hepatic metabolism, and renal excretion occur in elderly patients. Gastric pH increases, and splanchnic blood flow decreases, altering drug solubility and absorption. Total body fat rises from 10% of body weight at age 20 years to 24% at age 60 years, which increases the volume of distribution for lipid-soluble drugs, such as diazepam and its metabolites, and greatly prolongs drug half-life. In addition, total body water may decrease from 25% to 18% in the same period, so that the concentrations of water-soluble drugs, such as ethanol, are higher because of decreased reservoir size. Serum albumin levels decline by 10% to 15%; as a consequence, protein-binding sites are decreased, and more free active drug is released into the circulation, raising the risk for toxicity. Drug metabolism slows; the activity of hepatic cytochrome P450 decreases, as does demethylation. The result is higher levels of unmetabolized drug. After age 40 years, the glomerular filtration rate and renal plasma flow decline progressively. By age 70 years, the reduction is about 50%, which prolongs drug action and increases the likelihood of toxicity if the dose is not adjusted downward.

Neurotransmitter Changes

In addition to these pharmacokinetic changes, decreased levels of dopamine and acetylcholine in the central nervous system can lead to an increase in extrapyramidal and anticholinergic side effects, respectively. An increased tendency to central nervous system disinhibition in the elderly increases the likelihood of drug-associated confusion, sedation, and paradoxical reactions.

ANTIPSYCHOTICS (Tables 173.2 and 173.3)

Indications

In elderly patients with Alzheimer's disease or other forms of dementia, treatment with an antipsychotic ("*neuroleptic*") agent is indicated when paranoia, delusions, or hallucinations lead to violence and rage that pose a threat to the patient or others. However, because the use of antipsychotic drugs in the elderly is associated with an increased risk of death (see later discussion), as well as to other major adverse effects, considering their use should be undertaken only after exhausting other measures and carefully weighing risks and benefits. Antipsychotics should never be used to treat simple anxiety or uncomplicated depression, nor should they be given for long periods to patients with an *acute* psychotic episode.

Preparations

The *first-generation antipsychotics* (e.g., *thioridazine, perphenazine, haloperidol*) and the succeeding *atypical or second-generation antipsychotics* (e.g., *clozapine, quetiapine, risperidone, olanzapine, ziprasidone*) demonstrate comparable antipsychotic activity, but rates of discontinuation and net efficacy vary considerably due to differences in side effects and patients' ability to tolerate them (see Tables 173.2 and 173.3).

Adverse Effects

Antipsychotic use in the elderly is problematic because of the wide range of adverse effects, including risks of death, metabolic syndrome, and motor disturbances. The principal side effects of the first-generation agents are believed to be related to their strong antagonism of dopamine D_2 receptors and include sedation, orthostatic hypotension, motor dysfunction, and anticholinergic symptoms (see Tables 173.2 and 173.3). The atypical or second-generation antipsychotics were developed with the hope of reducing such side effects and improving tolerability and thus overall efficacy. Because they have less affinity for dopamine D_2 receptors and more for those related to serotonin and norepinephrine, these agents cause fewer motor disturbances, but they can lead to marked metabolic disruptions, including frank diabetes mellitus, hyperlipidemia, and obesity.

Increased Mortality

Short-term, risk-adjusted mortality rates in randomized, placebo-controlled trials were increased in elderly persons with dementia and neuropsychiatric symptoms (the adjusted relative risk was 1.5 with second-generation agents at 8 to 12 weeks and 2.1 with first-generation agents over 8 to 12 weeks). Retrospective cohort study found that the risk-adjusted relative risk of death was significantly greater with the use of first-generation agents than with second-generation antipsychotics (the adjusted relative risk was 1.37 at <180 days). The risk increased with dose. Mortality data on longer-term use are not available.

Because of the increased risk of death, the FDA issued a black-box warning for the use of second-generation atypical antipsychotics in elderly persons, but, as noted, the mortality risk is at least as problematic with first-generation agents. Observed causes include cardiac sudden death and pneumonia. The presumed mechanisms range from rhythm disturbances (due to QT-interval prolongation and anticholinergic activity) to aspiration (from extrapyramidal effects that compromise swallowing). Excessive sedation, postural hypotension, and motor disturbances may also threaten survival by increasing the risk of falls and subsequent life-threatening injury.

Sedation

The sedating side effects of these agents can be used therapeutically (e.g., for the patient who has trouble falling asleep or is excessively agitated during the day), but most often sedation is an unwanted side effect. Daytime sedation may cause or aggravate nighttime insomnia and also increase confusion and disorientation, making the patient more agitated.

Postural Hypotension

One of the most severe dangers entailed in the use of antipsychotics is the possibility of inducing *orthostatic hypotension*, which can lead to falls and fractures, stroke, or even heart attack. Hypotensive episodes are especially apt to occur at night when an elderly patient awakens and gets up to urinate.

Extrapyramidal Effects

Extrapyramidal symptoms (akathisia, parkinsonism, akinesia) develop in as many as 50% of all patients between the ages of 60 and 80 years taking antipsychotic therapy; those with brain damage, dementia, or Parkinson's disease are especially susceptible. The risk is greatest with potent first-generation agents, but is also possible with high doses of second-generation antipsychotics.

Akathisia is a feeling of motor restlessness associated with a subjective sensation of discomfort, often described as anxiety. Sleep is usually disturbed because the patient is unable to find a comfortable, motionless position. Sometimes, this restlessness is misinterpreted as an increase in psychotic symptoms and is treated with increased antipsychotic dose. The best initial approach to akathisia is to lower the dose or switch to another agent. Akathisia is also reported with the SSRIs.

Parkinsonism associated with antipsychotic use appears to be identical to the postencephalitic or idiopathic forms. An occasional patient will be exquisitely sensitive to this side effect,

and as little as one dose of a high-potency agent may precipitate the syndrome. Treatment involves reducing the dose and considering a switch to another agent.

Tardive Dyskinesia

Tardive dyskinesia is manifested by a wide variety of movements, including lip smacking, sucking, jaw movements, tongue writhing, chorea, athetosis, dystonia, tics, and facial grimacing. In severe cases, speech, eating, walking, and even breathing can be seriously impaired. The onset is gradual, usually developing after long-term, high-dose administration, but on rare occasions it can occur with short-term or low-dose use. Advancing age correlates not only with increased prevalence, but also with severity. Once tardive dyskinesia has developed, it is much less likely to reverse in an elderly patient than it is in a younger person.

A baseline examination before starting antipsychotic therapy and close monitoring (at least every 3 months) to detect the early signs of tardive dyskinesia (e.g., fine vermicular movements or restlessness of the tongue, mild choreiform movements of the fingers or toes, and facial tics or frequent eye blinks) are essential. No consistently effective agents are available for treatment. In view of the significant risk to the elderly patient and the ineffective treatment options, physicians should avoid the use of antipsychotic drugs in elderly patients whenever possible.

Neuroleptic Malignant Syndrome

This idiosyncratic and rare (<1%) but potentially life-threatening complication initially presents acutely with *muscle rigidity*, *high fever*, *autonomic instability*, and *confusion*. Elevated creatinine phosphokinase and *leukocytosis* are characteristic early laboratory features; *rhabdomyolysis*, *renal failure*, *aspiration*, *infection*, *seizure*, *circulatory collapse*, *respiratory failure*, and *cardiac arrest* may ensue. Treatment requires immediate halting of antipsychotic medication and emergency hospital intensive care unit admission for aggressive hydration, cooling blankets, and ventilatory and circulatory support. Incidence is greater in younger (<40 years old) men but has been reported in elderly. The use of specific drug therapies such as dopamine agonists (i.e., bromocriptine) or skeletal muscle relaxants (i.e., dantrolene) is uncertain.

Metabolic Disturbances

Some second-generation antipsychotics are associated with an increased risk of *metabolic syndrome* side effects (hyperinsulinemia, glucose intolerance, hypertension, hypercholesterolemia, low high-density-lipoprotein cholesterol, increased triglycerides). In randomized head-to-head study with first-generation agents, olanzapine caused significant increases in hemoglobin A_{1c}, total cholesterol, triglycerides, and body weight. Weight gain with *olanzapine* was as much as 2 lb/mo. Lesser degrees of metabolic disturbance were found with other second-generation drugs (see Table 173.3), and some improvement in metabolic parameters was observed with ziprasidone. *Increased prolactin* has been noted with the use of *risperidone*. When prescribed, second-generation antipsychotics require close monitoring of metabolic parameters (glucose, lipids).

Neutropenia

Neutropenia is a risk associated with *clozapine* use. Although clozapine is among the most effective drugs for the treatment of psychotic symptoms, it is usually reserved for difficult situations in which other antipsychotics fail and symptoms prove to be incapacitating. Frequent monitoring of the white blood cell count is required.

Choice of Agent

In a controlled head-to-head comparison study of first-generation and second-generation agents in nonelderly schizophrenic patients, olanzapine was found to be the best tolerated but the most likely to cause metabolic disruption (see later discussion; extrapolation from younger patients to the elderly needs to be done with caution). Consequently, these drugs should be used with caution and at the lowest possible doses in the frail elderly.

A fairly consistent relationship is found between the potency of an antipsychotic and its side-effect profile. The more potent the agent, the greater are the frequency and severity of sedation, orthostatic hypotension, anticholinergic symptoms, and extrapyramidal effects. *High-potency first-generation antipsychotics*, such as *haloperidol*, *thiothixene*, and *fluphenazine*, should be started at very low doses (e.g., 0.5 mg of haloperidol once or twice daily). These drugs are more likely than low-potency agents (e.g., chlorpromazine or thioridazine) to produce extrapyramidal symptoms in the elderly.

The second-generation agents are less likely to cause motor disturbances, and some have lower risks of sedation, anticholinergic side effects, and hypotension (Table 173.1). However, because of the potential for inducing metabolic syndrome side effects, they must be used carefully in elderly persons at increased cardiovascular risk, especially those with preexisting coronary artery disease, hypercholesterolemia, or diabetes mellitus. The risk of metabolic syndrome appears to be greatest with olanzapine and lowest with ziprasidone.

Anxiolytics

See Chapter 226.

Antidepressants

See Chapter 227.

Hypnotics

See Chapter 232.

Annotated Bibliography

1. Avorn J, Soumerai SB, Everitt DE, et al. A randomized trial of a program to reduce the use of psychoactive drugs in nursing homes. N Engl J Med 1992;327:168. (*Reduction in the unnecessary use of psychotropic drugs in this cohort with a high prevalence of dementia often led to improved functioning.*)
2. Jenike MA, Cremens MC. Geriatric psychopharmacology. Psychiatr Clin North Am (Annu Drug Ther) 1994;1:125. (*A monograph on medications and their use in the elderly.*)
3. Culpepper L. A roadmap to key pharmacologic principles in using antipsychotic. Prim Care Companion J Clin Psychiatry 2007;9:44. (*Presents clinical cases, mostly in younger patients, but illustrative of key clinical issues; useful tables.*)
3. Jenike MA. Tardive dyskinesia: special risk in the elderly. J Am Geriatr Soc 1983;31:71. (*A detailed discussion of this important complication.*)
4. Lieberman JA, Stroup TS, McEvoy JP, et al. Effectiveness of antipsychotic

drugs in patients with chronic schizophrenia. N Engl J Med 2005;353:1209. (*A major randomized, controlled trial comparing first- with second-generation antipsychotics.*)
5. Schneider LS, Kagerman KS, Insel P. Risk of death with atypical antipsychotic drug treatment for dementia: meta-analysis of randomized placebo-controlled trials. JAMA 2005;294:1934. (*Finds a significant increase in risk; the odds ratio was 1.54.*)
6. Thapa PB, Gideon P, Cost TW, et al. Antidepressants and the risk of falls among nursing home residents. N Engl J Med 1998;339:875. (*Both tricyclics and selective serotonin reuptake inhibitors increased the risk for falls in a dose-related fashion.*)
7. Wang PS, Schneeweiss S, Avorn J, et al. Risk of death in elderly users of conventional vs. atypical antipsychotic medication. N Engl J Med 2005;353:2335. (*A large retrospective cohort study, finding that the risk was significantly greater in persons taking first-generation agents.*)

CHAPTER 174 ■ APPROACH TO THE PATIENT WITH PARKINSON'S DISEASE

AMY A. PRUITT

Parkinson's disease is the second-most-common neurodegenerative disease in older Americans, affecting more than 1 million people in North America. It is characterized by tremor at rest, rigidity, and bradykinesia. The refinement of drug therapy for Parkinson's disease has brought relief to thousands of patients with this immobilizing condition. The recent development of therapy that may slow disease progression makes the early

diagnosis and treatment of Parkinson's disease particularly critical. Proper treatment requires careful timing and skillful utilization of drugs because important difficulties are associated with pharmacologic therapy. Moreover, drug efficacy declines with time, and the therapeutic response may be blunted by improper timing or inappropriate selection of antiparkinsonian agents.

Although the fine tuning of treatment for Parkinson's disease is largely in the province of the neurologist, the primary care physician is in the best position to make the diagnosis, institute therapy, and monitor the often substantial side effects associated with antiparkinsonian agents.

PATHOPHYSIOLOGY, CLINICAL PRESENTATION, AND COURSE (1–5)

Pathophysiology

Parkinson's disease is a *neurodegenerative* condition. Its most characteristic pathologic feature is a loss of *dopamine-containing* neurons; the nuclei of these neurons reside in the pars compacta of the *substantia nigra*, and the axons terminate in the *caudate nucleus* and *putamen* (the striatum). Other pigmented and nonpigmented nuclei in the brainstem and elsewhere are also affected. Associated with neuronal loss is the development of concentric hyalin inclusions in the cytoplasm of affected neurons, called *Lewy bodies*. Symptoms are believed to be related to the *imbalance* between *dopaminergic* and *cholinergic* influences on striatal tissue created by the loss of dopamine-containing neurons. Proper striatal function depends on this balance. Loss of sympathetic innervation can occur in the nigrostriatal system in the brain and in the sympathetic nervous system of the heart, leading to neurocirculatory failure.

Both genetic and environmental factors have been implicated in the development of Parkinson's disease. Their relative contributions differ for early-onset and late-onset disease.

Genetic Contributions

Gene mutations appear to be most important in hereditary forms of the disease, which typically have onset before the age of 50 years. Several gene mutations have been identified as contributory, including mutations of the *parkin gene* on chromosome 6 and the *α-synuclein gene* on chromosome 4. The products of these genes are likely to be important in pathogenesis, with α-synuclein being a major component of presynaptic terminals and Lewy bodies and the product of the parkin gene being involved in protein degradation and clearance.

In persons with the more common idiopathic form of Parkinson's disease, gene mutations probably do not play as large a role, but some evidence suggests a susceptibility function for mutations of the *tau gene*, which codes for the tau protein, a component of microtubules.

Environmental Contributions

In sporadic idiopathic Parkinson's disease with onset older than the age of 50 years, environmental factors are believed to be possibly important. The substantia nigra of patients with Parkinson's disease seems particularly vulnerable to oxidative insults. MPTP (1-methyl-4-phenyl-1,2,3,6-tetrahydropyridine, an analogue of meperidine injected by intravenous-drug abusers) and the pesticide rotenone (used in animal models of the disease) both inhibit mitochondrial complex I, impairing mitochondrial function and leading to findings nearly identical to those of idiopathic disease.

The demonstration that mitochondrial toxins can produce parkinsonism has stimulated an ongoing search for causative environmental precipitants. It is suspected that long-term, low-level exposures may be important and predate the onset of symptoms by years. Of note, being from a rural area is a risk factor for parkinsonism, as is *not* smoking. Separately, high caffeine intake is associated with a decreased risk of Parkinson's disease, suggesting a role for the adenosine receptor, which it antagonizes.

Clinical Presentation

Parkinson's disease is an affliction of middle to late adult life, although 30% of patients report recognizable symptoms before the age of 50 years. In another 40%, the disease develops between the ages of 50 and 60 years, and the remainder are older than 60 years old at the time of diagnosis. The classic syndrome of parkinsonism includes *tremor at rest, rigidity, bradykinesia, masked face, stooped posture,* and a *shuffling gait*. Although tremor is the most obvious initial finding, it is absent in 20% of patients. Parkinson's disease may begin insidiously with vague, *aching pain* in the limbs, neck, or back and with *decreased axial dexterity* before tremor is noted. *Dysarthria* may be an early feature; *dysphagia* usually occurs later. The onset of Parkinson's disease, whether primarily with tremor, rigidity, or bradykinesia, is usually asymmetric.

Subtler symptoms may also be noted, sometimes early. *Orthostatic hypotension* suggests cardiac sympathetic denervation, which can be found in many patients and may cause neurocirculatory failure. *Micrographia* (decrease in the caliber of handwriting), decrease in volume of the voice, and *anosmia* are other subtle but characteristic manifestations. *Depression* may be a feature of early disease. The estimated frequency of *dementia* (which usually develops late) varies widely, but *cognitive impairment,* including hallucinations and psychosis, develops in at least 15% to 20% of patients (some of whom are likely to have Lewy body disease; see Chapter 169). However, dementia and psychosis are not inevitable, and remediable causes of changes in mental status always need to be sought.

Clinical Course

Before the introduction of levodopa, Parkinson's disease had a fairly predictable course. At 5 years after onset, 60% of patients were severely disabled, and at 10 years, nearly 80% were. The rate of progression varied widely. Death rarely was a direct consequence of parkinsonism; rather, it was a consequence of immobility (aspiration pneumonia, urinary tract infections) or of trauma. Patients with Parkinson's disease comprise several different subgroups manifesting specific clinical patterns. It is believed that patients who present primarily with tremor have a slower course than do those for whom bradykinesia is the primary symptom. Patients who present with significant instability of posture and gait are largely an older group who are more likely to have cognitive impairment and a more rapid progression of disease.

The advent of dopaminergic agents has changed the natural history of the disease significantly. The initial benefit of levodopa therapy is one of the diagnostic criteria for the disease. Although patients with idiopathic Parkinson's disease usually respond to levodopa, the initial benefits of therapy decline for as many as one half of all treated patients after 2 or more years. Delay in onset of disability has been enhanced by the use of the monoamine oxidase B inhibitor deprenyl (see later discussion).

DIAGNOSIS (6,7)

The classic presentation of Parkinson's disease usually poses few diagnostic problems. However, several other presentations may be more problematic. These include isolated tremor at presentation, symptoms confined to half of the body (hemi-parkinsonism), and the presence of these symptoms in younger patients. Symptomatic parkinsonism can be seen in several other disorders, such as progressive supranuclear palsy and multisystem atrophy, or as a side effect of numerous medications (Table 174.1). An extrapyramidal syndrome resembling

TABLE 174.1

DIFFERENTIAL DIAGNOSIS OF PARKINSONISM

Idiopathic Parkinsonism (Parkinson's Disease)
  Infectious and postinfectious
    Postencephalitic parkinsonism (von Economo's disease)
    Other viral encephalitides
  Toxins
    Manganese
    Carbon monoxide
    Carbon disulfide
    Cyanide
    Methanol
    MPTP[a]
  Drugs
    Neuroleptics
    Reserpine
    Metoclopramide
    Lithium
    Amiodarone
    α-Methyldopa

Multisystem Degeneration
  Striatonigral degeneration
  Progressive supranuclear palsy
  Olivopontocerebellar degeneration
  Shy–Drager syndrome

Primary Dementing and Other Degenerative Disorders
  Alzheimer's disease
  Lewy body disease
  Creutzfeldt–Jakob disease

Other Central Nervous System Disorders
  Multiple cerebral infarctions (lacunar state, Binswanger's disease)
  Hydrocephalus (normal-pressure or high-pressure)
  Posttraumatic encephalopathy (pugilistic parkinsonism)

Metabolic Conditions
  Hypoparathyroidism
  Chronic hepatocerebral degeneration
  Idiopathic calcification of basal ganglia

Hereditary Disorders
  Wilson's disease
  Juvenile Huntington's disease (rigid variant)

This list is not meant to be all-inclusive. Rather, it highlights the more common disorders that may have parkinsonism as a prominent feature.
[a]1-Methyl-4-phenyl-1,2,3,6-tetrahydropyridine, a meperidine analogue used by intravenous-drug abusers.
Adapted from Koller WC. How accurately can Parkinson's disease be diagnosed? Neurology 1992;42(Suppl 1):6, with permission.

that of parkinsonism also occurs in Lewy body disease and may be mistaken for Alzheimer's disease because of the prominent dementia that ensues (see Chapters 169 and 173).

The clinical diagnosis of Parkinson's disease is based on a careful examination in which the clinician looks for physical signs other than those associated with the basal ganglia, elicits a careful drug and family history, and most likely performs at least one neuroimaging study, probably magnetic resonance imaging, to exclude significant small-vessel vascular disease, which may produce a parkinsonian-like state. Table 174.2 provides a summary of inclusion and exclusion criteria, which should help the physician in this clinical diagnosis. Among the inclusion criteria is a sustained responsiveness to levodopa therapy, with improvement lasting for 1 year or more. Many parkinsonian syndromes with other causes may show a transient response to dopaminergic agents. There are no confirmatory laboratory tests or imaging studies, but ligands that bind the dopamine transporter and are visible on single photon emission computed tomography can be helpful in the investigational setting.

The list of causes of parkinsonism includes toxins, central nervous system infections, structural lesions of the brain, and drugs. Dopamine antagonists, including neuroleptic agents and atypical neuroleptics, antiemetic drugs, valproate, and lithium all have been reported to cause parkinsonism.

PRINCIPLES OF MANAGEMENT (7–20)

Parkinson's disease cannot be cured, but advances in treatment have improved prospects for patients.

Goals and Overall Strategy

The goals of therapy are (a) to delay disease progression, (b) to relieve symptoms, and (c) to preserve functional capacity. Restoring the striatal balance between dopaminergic and cholinergic activity is at the core of efforts to achieve symptomatic relief. Inhibiting oxidative injury appears to be helpful in retarding disease progression. The patient may be able to tolerate many of the early signs of parkinsonism, which are sufficient to prompt medical consultation but, aside from provoking psychological discomfort, are not disabling. The goal of therapy is to maintain the patient at maximum function with minimal medication.

The three categories of management strategies are preventive treatment, symptomatic relief, and regenerative therapy.

Delay of Disease Progression: Preventive Treatment

If the degeneration of dopaminergic neurons in the substantia nigra and striatum is a consequence of oxidative injury, then might it be possible to interrupt the degenerative process and slow or halt disease progression with agents that inhibit oxidative activity in the central nervous system? This hypothesis has led to the study of the monoamine oxidase B inhibitors.

Selegiline (Deprenyl)

Although not universally accepted, evidence from several double-blinded, placebo-controlled studies of this monoamine oxidase B inhibitor indicates that monotherapy early in the

TABLE 174.2

CRITERIA FOR THE DIAGNOSIS OF PARKINSON'S DISEASE

Inclusion Criteria	Exclusion Criteria

Presence for 1 yr or more of two of the three cardinal motor signs:
  Resting or postural tremor
  Bradykinesia
  Rigidity
Responsiveness to levodopa therapy with moderate to marked
  improvement and duration of improvement for
  1 yr or more
	Abrupt onset of symptoms
	Remitting or stepwise progression
	Neuroleptic therapy within 1 yr
	Exposure to drugs or toxins associated with parkinsonism
	History of encephalitis
	Oculogyric crises
	Supranuclear downward or lateral gaze palsy
	Cerebellar signs
	Unexplained upper motor neuron or lower motor neuron signs
	More than one affected relative
	Dementia from the onset of disease
	Severe autonomic symptoms

Adapted from Reich SG, DeLong M. Parkinson's disease. In: Johnson R, ed. Current therapy in neurologic disease, 3rd ed. St. Louis: Mosby, 1990, with permission.

course of disease delays the onset of disability and the need to initiate levodopa therapy. It is suspected that the mechanism of benefit is protection of striatal tissue from oxidative injury, but this has yet to be proved, and the major benefit may be some direct effect of relieving symptoms.

Nonetheless, it seems reasonable to recommend this drug as initial treatment when Parkinson's disease is first diagnosed because it delays the requirement for levodopa therapy. It may also increase the time during which patients remain functional on levodopa, and, for some patients, it may decrease the levodopa requirement. This drug is given in the standard dose found to inhibit monoamine oxidase B in most patients: 5 mg given in the morning and 5 mg at noon. Side effects of tremor and dyskinesia are common when deprenyl is used in conjunction with levodopa. These are attributable to increased dopaminergic activity, which can be controlled by lowering the levodopa dose.

Other Antioxidants

In the largest and best-designed of the deprenyl studies, *tocopherol, a vitamin E analogue* with antioxidant properties, was tested. Tocopherol showed no benefit, either alone or as an enhancer of deprenyl activity. Further study of antioxidants and their prolonged effects is ongoing.

Symptomatic Relief

Whereas anticholinergic therapy was the mainstay of treatment before the advent of levodopa (see later discussion), today the most important choice of initial therapy involves a decision between *levodopa/dopa decarboxylase* preparations and a *direct dopamine agonist*. The choice may influence the chance of future motor compilations, such as drug-induced dyskinesias and "on–off" motor fluctuations. Levodopa provides superior motor benefit but is associated with a higher risk of dyskinesia.

Anticholinergic Therapy

Anticholinergic agents were the mainstay of parkinsonian therapy for more than a century, and they have remained important. Commonly used drugs are *trihexyphenidyl* (Artane)

and *benztropine* (Cogentin). These agents may be particularly beneficial for patients with tremor as a prominent symptom. Both are muscarinic blocking agents with typical anticholinergic side effects of urine retention, dry mouth, increased intraocular pressure in patients with glaucoma, and confusion (Table 174.3).

Dopamine Agonists

Treatment with one of the dopamine agonists—*bromocriptine, pergolide,* and more recently *pramipexole (Mirapex)* and *ropinirole (Requip)*—is increasingly recommended as *first-line therapy* for patients with mild to moderate parkinsonian symptoms. These medicines may suffice to control symptoms and delay for several years the need to prescribe levodopa. Their side effects are similar to those of levodopa but with less risk of dyskinesias and motor fluctuations. Recently a dopamine agonist patch with rotigotine, a nonergoline dopamine agonist, has been developed. Whether continuous rather than pulsatile dopamine delivery protects against long-term motor complications is unknown, but the U.S. Food and Drug Administration approval of the transdermal patch allows a new and well-tolerated form of drug delivery.

Since its introduction to the U.S. market, pramipexole has become the most widely prescribed drug for early parkinsonism. Recent reports of several motor vehicle accidents in patients on pramipexole or ropinirole, as a consequence of paroxysmal attacks of sleep, have led to the recommendation that patients taking these medicines refrain from driving. A possibly unique complication of pergolide is tricuspid insufficiency, resembling that associated with fenfluramine/phentermine use. In view of these findings, dopamine-agonist therapy should be initiated with a nonergot agonist.

Levodopa

Eventually, most patients experience a worsening of symptoms that requires the introduction of levodopa (in combination with a peripheral dopa decarboxylase inhibitor). Levodopa is recommended for patients who become too symptomatic to function satisfactorily despite anticholinergic therapy with deprenyl plus a dopamine agonist. By prescribing levodopa, the physician is able to offer most parkinsonian patients much benefit,

TABLE 174.3

DRUGS USED FOR THE TREATMENT OF PARKINSON'S DISEASE

Drug	Preparation	Dose	Schedule	Starting Dose	Maintenance Dose
Anticholinergic Agents (representative examples)					
Trihexyphenidyl hydrochloride (Artane)	Scored tablets Elixir	2, 5 mg 2 mg/5 mL	tid–qid	2 mg	2–10 mg
	Timed-release capsule	5 mg	qd	(Timed-release capsule may be substituted for regular Artane after maintenance dose is determined)	
Benztropine mesylate (Cogentin)	Tablets	0.5, 1, 2 mg	qd or bid	1 mg	0.5–6 mg
Dopaminergic Agents					
Carbidopa/levodopa (Sinemet)	Scored tablets 10/100 mg 25/100 mg 25/250 mg		bid–qid	50/200 mg in two divided doses	400–500 mg levodopa
Sinemet CR	50/200 mg		bid	50/200 mg bid	Variable
Bromocriptine (Parlodel)	Scored tablets	2.5 mg	bid–tid	1.25 mg qd	7.5–30 mg
	Capsules	5.0 mg			
Pergolide mesylate (Permax)	Scored tablets	0.05, 0.25, 1.0 mg	tid	0.05 mg qd	1–3 mg
Deprenyl (Eldepryl, selegiline hydrochloride)	Tablets	5.0 mg	bid	5 mg qd	10 mg
Amantadine (Symmetrel)	Capsules	100 mg	bid	100 mg qd	200 mg
Pramipexole (Mirapex)	Tablets	0.125, 0.25, 0.5, 1, 1.5 mg	tid	0.25 mg tid	Variable
Ropinirole (Requip)	Tablets	0.25, 0.5, 1, 2 mg	tid	0.25 mg tid	Variable
COMT Inhibitor					
Tolcapone (Tasmar)	Tablets	100, 200 mg	tid	100 mg tid	100 mg tid

bid, twice daily; COMT, catechol-O-methyltransferase; qd, daily; qid, four times daily; tid, thrice daily.
Adapted from Reich SG, DeLong M. Parkinson's disease. In: Johnson R, ed. Current therapy in neurologic disease, 3rd ed. St Louis: Mosby, 1990; and Lang AE, Lozano AM, Medical progress: Parkinson's disease. N Engl J Med 1998;339:1044, 1130; with permission.

---

although the drug has a number of important limitations and side effects.

Timing of Initiation. The limited duration of levodopa efficacy makes it necessary to consider carefully when to begin therapy. Weighing against early initiation of levodopa treatment is the phenomenon of a decline in its effectiveness in as many as 50% of patients after 2 years of use. This observation is the basis for the traditional view that onset of therapy should be delayed as long as possible. However, some data indicate a reduction in mortality when levodopa is started within 1 to 3 years of onset of symptoms rather than after 4 years. Clinical judgment that takes into account both of these findings is required.

Preparations and Initial Dosing. Levodopa is the naturally occurring precursor of dopamine. It crosses the blood–brain barrier and enhances dopaminergic activity. However, because much of the drug is converted peripherally by a decarboxylase into dopamine (which cannot cross the blood–brain barrier), levodopa is best given in combination with a peripheral decar-

boxylase inhibitor, such as *carbidopa*. Combination preparations containing both agents in various strengths are commonly used. In a typical starting program, the combination preparation of 25 mg of carbidopa and 100 mg of levodopa is given (e.g., Sinemet 25 to 100 mg two or three times daily; see Table 174.3). Levodopa is rapidly absorbed after oral administration, reaches its peak effect after 30 minutes to 2 hours, and has a half-life of 1 to 3 hours. The rate of absorption is decreased by the ingestion of a protein-rich meal.

Adverse Effects. Significant adverse reactions develop in many patients; *nausea, vomiting, anorexia, hypertension, dyskinesias*, and *hallucinations* can be disturbing. The nausea can be partly overcome by taking the drug with small meals. Dyskinesias include chorea, athetosis, and dystonia. They usually occur simultaneously with peak concentrations of levodopa and are best managed by having the patient take small doses of medication at frequent intervals.

Problems in Late-Stage Therapy—Wearing Off and On–Off Phenomena. With disease progression, the benefits of levodopa therapy appear to wear off more quickly, producing marked fluctuations in symptoms.

Wearing off is the recurrence of severe symptoms hours after the most recent dose of medication and is often followed by a recurrence of rigidity and bradykinesia. A *controlled-release preparation* (e.g., *Sinemet CR*) relieves this problem for some patients. The development of a sustained-release preparation of levodopa/carbidopa (e.g., Sinemet CR, 50 mg/200 mg) has been a therapeutic advance for patients afflicted with motor fluctuations. The controlled-release form can almost double the duration of effect to 5 to 6 hours. To match the effects of conventional levodopa preparations, a program of up to 25% more daily levodopa in the controlled-release form may be required. Doses administered after 6:00 p.m. can be given in the rapidly absorbed form to eliminate nocturnal side effects of the medication.

Other ways to manage wearing-off symptoms include administering drugs that reduce the metabolism of dopamine or levodopa. The *catechol-O-methyltransferase* (COMT) inhibitors (e.g., *tolcapone* [*Tasmar*] and *entacapone* [*Comtan*]) have been introduced for this purpose. Tolcapone must be used with caution because cases of fulminant hepatic failure have been reported. The physician should refer a patient requiring this therapy to a neurologist with expertise in the treatment of late-stage Parkinson's disease.

As drug efficacy declines, patients may experience the *on–off phenomenon*, with a severe fluctuation of dose–response relations and rapid onset and termination of therapeutic and adverse effects. Impairment of levodopa absorption and transport into the brain by dietary amino acids contributes to the problem. Treatment entails scheduling levodopa 1 hour before meals, *reducing protein* intake, and adding an ergot preparation (see later discussion). Use of a controlled-release formulation may also help, but the development of the "on–off" state represents an advanced form of disease and a difficult one to treat. *Drug "holidays"* have been proposed to restore sensitivity to levodopa, but results are not impressive.

Other Dopaminergic Agents in Late-Stage Disease

Bromocriptine and *pergolide* are direct *dopamine-receptor agonists*. These agents are used to enhance the therapeutic effects of levodopa and may be particularly helpful in late stages of the disease, when the conversion of levodopa to dopamine is inefficient in the degenerating substantia nigra. They are less likely than levodopa to cause dyskinesias and the on–off phenomenon. In addition, they may allow the use of lower doses of levodopa when given early on with levodopa as combined therapy.

Gabapentin (Neurontin) has shown some efficacy for patients with advanced disease and is well tolerated except for drowsiness at high doses. Small-scale, short-term study of gabapentin, which stimulates the striatal release of γ-aminobutyric acid (GABA), has produced promising results in patients with advanced disease. It is theorized that GABA stimulation may help overcome the loss of dopaminergic stimulation.

Both the direct dopamine agonists and the levodopa controlled-release preparations are likely to be prescribed by neurologists, but recognition of the necessity to move to such therapies is facilitated by the observations of the primary physician closely monitoring the patient.

Treatment of Psychiatric Symptoms

Nightmares, hallucinations, and increased sexual drive are disturbing psychiatric features of late-stage disease. Hallucina-

tions and psychosis are best treated with the atypical neuroleptic *clozapine*. Use of phenothiazines such as haloperidol should be avoided, especially if there is frank Lewy body disease (see Chapters 169 and 173). Severe depression is managed with the same medications given to patients without Parkinson's disease. However, because most of these patients are elderly, the physician must be careful of side effects of the tricyclic antidepressants (see Chapter 227). Theoretically, the combination of selegiline and a selective serotonin reuptake inhibitor is problematic, and indications for this class of drug should be carefully weighed against the possibility of inducing the *serotonin syndrome* (hypertension, tachycardia, other autonomic dysfunction, and hallucinations). *Electroconvulsive therapy* may be used in depressed patients who are not confused.

Supportive Measures

Because maintaining function is a central goal of therapy, one should not forget the value of such important adjunctive measures as *physical therapy* and *psychological support*. Physical therapy can improve functioning by helping to preserve muscle strength and flexibility. Although a central component of the supportive psychological effort involves close follow-up and detailed patient education (see later discussion), one must also be watchful for the development of depression and the need to treat it promptly and effectively (see Chapter 227).

Interventional and Investigational Therapies

Surgery and Deep-Brain Stimulation

As the pathophysiology of parkinsonism has become better understood, the role of functional neurosurgical procedures has grown. *Surgery* is reserved for disabling, medically refractory disease. When the problem is severe dyskinesia and on–off fluctuations, *unilateral pallidotomy* has been demonstrated to be effective.

Deep-brain stimulation of the globus pallidus and subthalamic nucleus is a less invasive interventional option. In randomized study, deep brain stimulation in patients younger than the age of 75 years with severe motor complications provided significantly better relief of symptoms (especially improved mobility and relief of dyskinesia) than medical therapy alone, allowing patients to achieve independent mobility after being previously in need of daily assistance; however, risk of a serious adverse event was 13% versus 4%, including one death from cerebral hemorrhage. These procedures are not as effective for bradykinesia.

Transplantation of Fetal Tissue and Stem Cells

This investigational method involves transplantation of fetal substantia nigra tissue into the striatum, which relieves the signs of parkinsonism in animals with experimental lesions of the substantia nigra. Early attempts to treat humans who had Parkinson's disease with grafts of human fetal tissue were disappointing, but work on fetal tissue and *stem cell transplantation* continues; results are promising.

Other Methods under Development

These include new drugs for inhibiting dopamine breakdown, synthesis of new dopamine-receptor agonists, and blockade of excitotoxic neurotransmitter receptors in the subthalamic nucleus. Finally, jejunal infusion of levodopa and carbidopa has been tried in an attempt to improve levodopa absorption.

PATIENT EDUCATION (19)

Patient and family education is essential to the success of therapy. The need for trial and error to obtain maximal benefit with minimal side effects must be explained. Frequent visits are needed in the initiation period and later in the course of the disease. Although therapy can be proposed optimistically, the inevitable diminution in the efficacy of therapy must be anticipated and discussed with patient and family so that they can be adequately prepared, both psychologically and practically. Patients are obviously concerned about their prognosis, and a frank discussion of what is known is usually appreciated. A number of helpful guidebooks are available for patients and their families.

THERAPEUTIC RECOMMENDATIONS (7,14)

- After other potential causes of parkinsonism have been excluded, it is appropriate to start selegiline in the early stages of disease. The daily dose is 10 mg (5 mg in the morning and 5 mg at noon). This drug may also be started in patients already taking levodopa/carbidopa in an attempt to lower the amount of levodopa needed.

- If symptoms progress to impair daily functioning despite the use of deprenyl, then start one of the dopamine agonists (e.g., pramipexole, starting at 0.125 mg three times daily); double the dose at weekly intervals until a maintenance dose of about 1 mg three times daily is reached.

- As symptoms progress, begin levodopa/carbidopa, starting at a dose of 25 mg/100 mg three times daily; adjust the dose according to the patient's response. There is no advantage to starting with a sustained-release preparation.

- Add amantadine or an anticholinergic if tremor is problematic.

- Consider a sustained-release levodopa/carbidopa preparation for dealing with on–off symptoms; prescribe the taking of medication 1 hour before meals and restrict protein intake. Obtain neurologic consultation at this stage of disease.

- Similarly, consider a COMT inhibitor (e.g., *tolcapone* or *entacapone*) for late-stage wearing-off phenomenon; again, obtain neurologic consultation. A trial of gabapentin therapy might be considered for late-stage disease but only with consultation.

- Do not overlook the important roles of physical therapy, psychological support, and recognition and treatment of depression. Refer patients to one of the excellent websites available, including http://www.apdaparkinson.org, http://www.michaeljfox.org, and http://www.parkinson.org.

- In patients with advanced, incapacitating disease, consider referral for interventional or investigational therapy, but only to a nationally recognized center with expertise in these measures.

Annotated Bibliography

1. Goldstein DS, Holmes C, Li ST, et al. Cardiac sympathetic denervation in Parkinson disease. Ann Intern Med 2000;133:338. (*Evidence that cardiac sympathetic denervation is common.*)
2. Lang AE, Lozano AM. Medical progress: Parkinson's disease (two parts). N Engl J Med 1998;339:1044, 1130. (*A superb two-part review covering pathophysiology and treatment.*)
3. Marin ER, Scott WK, Nance MA, et al. Association of single-nucleotide polymorphisms of the tau gene with late-onset Parkinson disease. JAMA 2001;286:2245. (*Evidence for a genetic contribution to idiopathic disease.*)
4. Ross GW, Abbott RD, Petrovitch H, et al. Association of coffee and caffeine intake with risk of Parkinson disease. JAMA 2000;283:2674. (*Data from the Honolulu Heart Study population showing that caffeine intake is associated with reduced risk.*)
5. Siderowf A, Stern M. Update on Parkinson disease. Ann Intern Med 2003;138:651. (*A review that includes an excellent summary of the evidence for genetic and environmental contributions to clinical disease.*)
6. Koller WC. How accurately can Parkinson's disease be diagnosed? Neurology 1992;42(Suppl 1):6. (*A particularly lucid description of the clinical diagnosis.*)
7. Nutt JG, Wooten GF. Diagnosis and initial management of Parkinson's disease. N Engl J Med 2005;353:1021. (*A comprehensive review for the generalist reader.*).
8. Deuschl G, Schade-Brittinger C, Krack P, et al. for the German Parkinson Study Group Neurostimulation Section. A randomized trial of deep-brain stimulation for Parkinson's disease. N Engl J Med 2006;355:896. (*The approach was found to be more effective than medical therapy alone.*)
9. Diamond SG, Markham CH, Hoehn MM, et al. Multi-center study of Parkinson mortality with early versus later dopa treatment. Ann Neurol 1987;22:8. (*Mortality was less in patients treated earlier than in those treated later.*)
10. Fine J, Chen R, Hutchinson W, et al. Long-term follow-up of unilateral pallidotomy in advanced Parkinson's disease. N Engl J Med 2000;342:1708. (*Sustained improvement was found in off-period contralateral signs.*)
11. Freed CRT, Greene PE, Breeze RE, et al. Transplantation of embryonic dopamine neurons for severe Parkinson's disease. N Engl J Med 2001;344:710. (*The results were largely negative, except for an improvement in motor performance in patients <60 years of age.*)
12. Krack P, Patir A, Van Biercom N, et al. Five-year follow-up of bilateral stimulation of the subthalamic nucleus in advanced Parkinson's disease. N Engl J Med 2003;349:1925. (*An uncontrolled trial; improvements were found in motor function and dyskinesia.*)
13. Jankovic J. New and emerging therapies for Parkinson's disease. Arch Neurol 1999;56:785. (*A good review of catechol-O-methyltransferase inhibitors and research on surgical therapies.*)
14. Miyasaki JM, Martin W, Sujchowersky O, et al. Practice parameter: initiation of treatment for Parkinson's disease: an evidence-based review. Neurology 2002;58:11. (*Includes evidence for a neuroprotective effect for selegiline and a recommendation for its early use.*)
15. Olson WL, Gruenthal M, Mueller ME, et al. Gabapentin for parkinsonism: a double-blind, placebo-controlled, crossover trial. Am J Med 1997;102:60. (*A small-scale, short-term study, but it shows very encouraging results in patients with advanced disease.*)
16. Parkinson Study Group. Pramipexole vs levodopa as initial treatment for Parkinson disease: a randomized controlled trial. JAMA 2000;284:1931. (*A lower incidence of any motor complication was found in patients receiving pramipexole.*)
17. Parkinson Study Group. Low-dose clozapine for the treatment of drug-induced psychosis in Parkinson's disease. N Engl J Med 1999;340:757. (*Very few side effects and excellent efficacy were found, whereas virtually all other antipsychotic agents exacerbated symptoms.*)
18. Parkinson Study Group. Effects of tocopherol and deprenyl on the progression to disability in early Parkinson's disease. N Engl J Med 1993;328:176. (*Deprenyl, but not tocopherol, was effective in delaying the onset of disability and the need for levodopa therapy.*)
19. Rascol O, Brooks DJ, Korczyn AD, et al. A five-year study of the incidence of dyskinesia in patients with early Parkinson's disease who were treated with ropinirole or levodopa. N Engl J Med 2000;342:1484. (*A 5-year trial in Europe, Canada, and Israel, showing that patients receiving ropinirole had a lower risk of dyskinesias.*)
20. Watts RL, Jankovic J, Waters C, et al. Randomized blind controlled trial of transdermal rotigotine in early Parkinson disease. Neurology 2007;68:171. (*The patients on rotigotine improved primarily in their motor scores; oral ropinirole in a prolonged-release preparation is also on the horizon.*)
21. Duvoisin RC. Parkinson's disease: a guide for patient and family, 4th ed. New York: Raven Press, 1996. (*A sensible, very useful guide for the patient and family embarking on a course of treatment for Parkinson's disease.*)

CHAPTER 175 ■ APPROACH TO THE PATIENT WITH BELL'S PALSY (IDIOPATHIC FACIAL MONONEUROPATHY)

AMY A. PRUITT

Bell's palsy denotes abrupt paralysis of the facial muscles innervated by the seventh cranial nerve. The condition encompasses 80% of all facial mononeuropathies. The primary physician should be able to distinguish Bell's palsy from other, more ominous causes of facial palsy and balance therapeutic intervention against the self-limited course and favorable prognosis of the disease.

PATHOPHYSIOLOGY, CLINICAL PRESENTATION, AND COURSE (1–7)

Pathophysiology

Satisfactory explanations for the condition are lacking, although serologic and DNA evidence implicates *herpesvirus* infection. The condition shows an increasing incidence with age, is slightly more common in the winter, and is associated with pregnancy, diabetes, and hypothyroidism. In patients younger than the age of 50 years, it is more common among women, but this gender distribution reverses in patients older than the age of 50 years. In patients with vascular risk factors, ischemia has been invoked to explain facial palsy due to subsequent edema of the facial nerve and adjacent structures.

Clinical Presentation

The onset is usually acute, with maximal deficit developing within a few hours. The motor deficit is almost always *unilateral*, and in two thirds of cases it may be accompanied by *pain* in or behind the ear. *Fever*, *tinnitus*, and mild *hearing diminution* may be present during the first few hours. Symptoms may fluctuate during the first few days after onset. Voluntary and involuntary motor responses are lost. Both *upper and lower* parts of the face are affected, a feature that distinguishes this peripheral facial nerve lesion from a central supranuclear lesion, in which only lower facial muscles are affected. Patients may report facial weakness with difficulty closing the eyelid or drooling, preauricular pain, and alterations in taste or hearing.

On examination, there is facial asymmetry. The palpebral fissure appears widened, the forehead is smooth, and the nasolabial fold is flattened on the involved side. *Bell's phenomenon* (the normal upward deviation of the eye with lid closure) is exaggerated because of weakness of the orbicularis oculi. The *corneal reflex* may be decreased on the involved side. Lacrimation is only rarely defective, and if the injury involves the nervus intermedius proximal to the geniculate ganglion, loss or *perversion of taste* on the anterior two thirds of the tongue may occur, as may *altered sensitivity to sound* (hyperacusis) due to involvement of the stapedius muscle.

Clinical Course

In 75% to 85% of cases, patients recover to a cosmetically acceptable level without treatment. Most do so within 3 weeks. Recovery is best in children; a poor prognosis has been associated with increasing age, hyperacusis, diminished taste, and severity of the initial motor deficit. The prognosis can be assessed by electromyographic (EMG) testing of the involved muscles at least 72 hours after the clinical nadir. Those with EMG evidence of extensive axonal degeneration 2 weeks after the onset of the weakness have a poorer prognosis. Those with partial or complete preservation of the compound muscle action potential amplitude have anatomic continuity of the facial nerve, partial axonal preservation, and a better prognosis. EMG is indicated only for patients with severe clinical involvement that has not improved by 7 to 10 days after onset.

Other poor outcomes in Bell's palsy result from abnormal regeneration of damaged nerve fibers. *Lacrimation* during eating or "crocodile tears" appears when fibers regrow and connect with lacrimal ducts instead of salivary glands. Abnormal movements (*facial synkinesis*) may occur if regenerating motor fibers innervate inappropriate muscles. Contracture of the involved site may be noted during voluntary movement. Seven percent of patients experience *recurrent facial paralysis*.

DIFFERENTIAL DIAGNOSIS

The distinction between Bell's palsy and other facial paralyses is usually not difficult. Approximately one third of cases of acute peripheral facial weakness are caused by trauma, varicella-zoster infection (the Ramsay Hunt syndrome), Lyme disease, sarcoidosis parotid tumors, Sjögren's syndrome, or amyloidosis or are related to diabetes mellitus, pregnancy, intranasal influenza vaccine, or Guillain–Barré syndrome. The remaining two thirds of acute facial palsies are deemed idiopathic or Bell's palsy. Tumors are not likely to present with acute facial weakness, although the seventh nerve can be involved by acoustic neuroma, pontine glioma, neurofibroma, cholesteatoma, parotid gland tumor, meningeal carcinomatosis, or lymphomatosis. Bilateral facial paralysis raises a different set of diagnostic possibilities, including Guillain–Barré syndrome (with or without HIV infection), sarcoidosis, and Lyme disease. Diseases of the neuromuscular junction such as myasthenia gravis or botulism must also be considered in the presence of bilateral facial nerve dysfunction.

WORKUP (1,3–5,8)

History and Physical Examination

The patient found to have a peripheral mononeuropathy of the seventh cranial nerve should be queried and examined for evidence of an underlying cause. The history is reviewed for facial trauma, ear infection, herpes zoster, and tick bite. Past medical history is reviewed for diabetes mellitus, sarcoidosis, and malignancy and systems for progressive hearing loss, lymphadenopathy, and facial mass or tenderness.

On examination, one checks for zosteriform lesions (see Chapter 193) on the tympanic membrane, in the external auditory canal, and behind the ear. The skin is examined for the characteristic truncal erythematous lesion of early Lyme disease (see Chapter 160) and for neurofibromas. The tympanic membrane is also checked for cholesteatoma and evidence of otitis media (see Chapter 218). The jaw is examined for tenderness and trauma to the temporal bone. The lymph nodes are palpated, as is the parotid gland. A careful neurologic examination completes the assessment, with a focus on the detection of additional neurologic deficits.

Laboratory Studies

In the patient with a characteristic history and physical findings, standard blood tests are of limited value, although they may reveal diabetes or some other medical condition associated with an increased risk for Bell's palsy. *Serologic testing for Lyme disease* (see Chapter 160) may be appropriate in highly endemic areas, as suggested by a recent study in which one fourth of summertime cases of Bell's palsy demonstrated evidence of infection with the tick-borne spirochete of Lyme disease, *Borrelia burgdorferi*. The identification of Lyme disease has important consequences for management (see later discussion and Chapter 160).

Magnetic resonance imaging (MRI) *studies* are necessary only when atypical features suggest a posterior fossa process as the cause of the seventh nerve palsy. If MRI is performed, the most common abnormality is contrast enhancement of the intracanalicular and labyrinthine segments of the facial nerve. In patients with atypical or persistent facial palsy, gadolinium-enhanced magnetic resonance imaging can help to differentiate Bell's palsy from other causes. *Lumbar puncture* is indicated only if inflammation, granuloma, or malignancy is a consideration. A mild pleocytosis of the cerebrospinal fluid has been reported in typical cases of Bell's palsy. *Electromyography* may be used to predict recovery but is not needed for diagnosis and is most informative when at least 3 weeks have elapsed after the onset of facial paralysis.

PRINCIPLES OF MANAGEMENT (1–5,9–16)

Treatment is etiologic in persons with an underlying cause. For those with idiopathic disease, most will have a self-limited course and treatment is largely supportive, the top priority being prevention of corneal injury due to lid paresis. For persons who present with severe disease and have a less favorable prognosis, steroid therapy becomes a consideration, as does treatment for herpes virus infection.

Prevention of Corneal Injury

Of greatest practical importance during the acute stage of the illness is the prevention of injury to the *cornea*, which is left exposed by weakness of the orbicularis muscle. When the lid is weak, *methylcellulose drops* should be prescribed for use twice a day and at bedtime; in addition, the lid may need to be taped shut at night. If corneal abrasion is suspected because of pain, visual impairment, or other ocular symptoms (see Chapter 201), then prompt referral for ophthalmic consultation and slit-lamp examination with fluorescein is indicated.

Corticosteroids

The prognosis for most cases of Bell's palsy is good, but some 20% to 30% of patients may have permanent facial weakness. There may be other disfiguring consequences such as synkinesia, loss of taste, and loss of tearing or hyperacusis. Therefore, early treatment is important for this significant minority of patients. The rationale for steroid therapy stems from surgical observations of facial nerve swelling during decompressive operations. In addition, more recently physicians have tended to add antiviral agents based on the observation of herpes simplex virus in the endoneurial fluid of patients with Bell's palsy. Data are limited, but evidence from placebo-controlled trials suggest a 35% improvement in chances for a full recovery (to 88%) with early use of prednisone in persons with signs suggesting an unfavorable prognosis by virtue of the severity of the facial palsy. Prednisone also appears markedly to reduce associated ear pain and frequency of chronic autonomic dysfunction when administered early in the course of illness. Diabetics respond particularly well. Nonetheless, the benefits of steroid treatment are often difficult to demonstrate because the disease has such a good prognosis. Of note, patients with Lyme disease as the underlying cause should not receive steroids, which can worsen the situation by compromising immune function.

Therapy for Herpesvirus Infection

Based on serologic and DNA evidence that herpesvirus infection is the cause of many cases of facial paralysis, some authorities now recommend institution of appropriate therapy (e.g., *famciclovir* 750 mg three times daily or 1,000 mg of *valacyclovir* twice daily for 7 to 10 days; see Chapter 192). Initial studies comparing prednisone therapy with and without antiviral therapy show only a modest benefit from the addition of antiviral therapy. More data are needed to define the role of antiviral treatment; the 2001 American Academy of Neurology guidelines concluded that corticosteroids are definitively effective and antiviral treatment is "possibly effective." More recent randomized studies found no benefit for antiviral therapy in persons with mild to moderate palsy but did find additional benefit (90% compete recovery vs. 75%) over corticosteroids alone with the use of valacyclovir in persons with severe or complete palsy (in another study acyclovir was not found to be effective).

Other Treatments

The role of *surgical decompression* is controversial. Based on the observation that nerve swelling at the narrowest point (the entrance to the meatal foramen) contributes to the deficit, randomized trials of prednisone versus decompression have been undertaken, with variable results. The risk of permanent unilateral deafness after surgery ranges from 1% to 15%. Decompression should not be performed more than 14 days after onset of paralysis.

Some patients have been followed with *electromyographic stimulation* of the muscles to hasten particularly stubborn paralyses. The possible role of electromyographic stimulation in management is unclear; it has not been subjected to controlled study.

PATIENT EDUCATION

Persons with idiopathic disease free of manifestations of poor prognosis can and should be reassured that prognosis for a full recovery is excellent. Concern about permanent disfigurement can be considerable, and such reassurance is very welcome. Even patients with signs of a less favorable prognosis can be informed that with treatment they, too, have a very good chance (>85%) of making a full or nearly full recovery. Despite the favorable prognosis, it is essential to stress the importance of keeping the cornea well hydrated and protected during the period of lid weakness.

THERAPEUTIC RECOMMENDATIONS AND INDICATIONS FOR REFERRAL

- Ascertain that the condition is indeed Bell's palsy. Check for the involvement of other cranial nerves and ear infection.

- Examine for zosteriform lesions on the tympanic membrane, in the external auditory canal, and behind the ear.

- In areas endemic for Lyme disease, examine the patient carefully for characteristic features and consider serologic testing (see Chapter 160).

- Explain the benign nature and good prognosis of the condition and caution the patient about corneal abrasion. Mention that altered taste, decreased tearing, decreased salivation, or altered sensitivity to sound may be experienced.

- Prescribe methylcellulose eye drops, to be used twice a day and at bedtime, with taping of an especially weak lid. Tarsorrhaphy may be considered when severe lid weakness exists.

- If the patient is seen within 1 week of onset of facial weakness and if no important contraindications to corticosteroid use are found (Lyme disease is a contraindication), then a short course of prednisone may be prescribed.

- Begin with prednisone 1 mg/kg of body weight every morning for 7 to 10 days. If improvement occurs or weakness does not progress during this week, the steroids may be stopped without taper. If improvement does not occur during the first week, then continue the initial dose of prednisone each morning for a total of 10 days and taper over another 10 days. If postauricular pain recurs when the dose is tapered, then reinstitute the preceding dose.

- Consider adding a course of antiviral therapy for herpesvirus infection (e.g., oral valacyclovir 500 mg twice daily for 7 days [cost about $70] or famciclovir 750 mg three times daily for 7 days; see Chapter 192) for severe or complete facial palsy.

- The same steroid course just outlined is acceptable during pregnancy, but the safety of antiviral agents in pregnancy has not been established.

- In the 10% of patients who do not achieve an acceptable recovery, autografting with a hypoglossal-to-facial anastomosis may provide reasonable cosmetic results and afford lasting protection of the eye. Patients in this category should be referred to an otolaryngologist or a neurosurgeon.

Annotated Bibliography

1. Adour KK. Diagnosis and management of facial paralysis. N Engl J Med 1982;307:348. (*A superb, succinct clinical review, not only of Bell's palsy, but also of facial paralysis resulting from herpes zoster, trauma, otitis media, neoplasms, and other causes.*)
2. Barringer JR. Herpes simplex virus and Bell palsy. Ann Intern Med 1995;124:63. (*A summary of the evidence for herpesvirus as the etiologic agent.*)
3. Gilden DH. Bell's palsy. N Engl J Med 2004;351:1323. (*Best review, covering all aspects of the clinical problem, anatomy, and treatment.*)
4. Halperin JJ. Lyme borreliosis in Bell's palsy. Neurology 1992;42:1268. (*A very high incidence of Lyme seropositivity is found in patients with Bell's palsy during the summer in endemic areas.*)
5. Katusic SK. Incidence, clinical features, and prognosis in Bell's palsy: Rochester, MN, 1968–1982. Ann Neurol 1986;20:622. (*The best available community-based data.*)
6. Keane JR. Bilateral seventh nerve palsy: analysis of 43 cases and review of the literature. Neurology 1994;44:1198. (*A different set of illnesses needs to be considered, particularly Guillain–Barré syndrome and sarcoidosis.*)
7. Kuiper H, Devriese P, deJhongh B, et al. Absence of Lyme borreliosis among patients with presumed Bell's palsy. Arch Neurol 1992;49:940. (*Almost all of the patients in this series had features atypical of idiopathic facial palsy and other systemic symptoms.*)
8. Tien R, Dillon WP, Jackler RK. Contrast-enhanced MR imaging of the facial nerve in 11 patients with Bell's palsy. Am J Neuroradiol 1990;11:735. (*Gadolinium enhancement was helpful in cases with atypical or persistent facial palsy.*)
9. Adour KK. Bell's palsy. Results of a double-blind, placebo-controlled acyclovir–prednisone and placebo–prednisone treatment study. Br Med J 1995. (*Ninety-four patients were randomized, and a better outcome was found in the group receiving the combination of prednisone and acyclovir.*)
10. Austin JR, Peskind SP, Austin SG, et al. Idiopathic facial nerve paralysis: a randomized, double-blind, controlled study of placebo versus prednisone. Laryngoscope 1993;103:1326. (*Given preferably within 24 hours of the onset of paralysis, prednisone improves cosmetic results.*)
11. DeDiego JI, Prim MP, DeSarria MJ, et al. Idiopathic facial paralysis: a randomized, prospective, and controlled study using single-dose prednisone versus acyclovir three times daily. Laryngoscope 1998;108:573. (*At 3 months, facial muscle strength was better after prednisone than after acyclovir.*)
12. Gantz BJ, Rubinstein JT, Gidley P, et al. Surgical management of Bell's palsy. Laryngoscope 1999;109:1177. (*Review of the surgical approach.*)
13. Gilden DH, Tyler, KL. Bell's palsy—is glucocorticoid treatment enough? N Engl J Med 2007;357:1653. (*An editorial examining the discrepant study results being reported.*)
14. Grogan PM, Gronseth GS. Practice parameter: steroids, acyclovir, and surgery for Bell's palsy. Neurology 2001;56:830. (*Consensus guidelines on therapies for idiopathic disease.*)
15. Hato N, Yamada H, Kohno H, et al. Valacyclovir and prednisolone treatment for Bell's palsy: a multicenter, randomized, placebo-controlled study. Otol Neurotol 2007;28:408. (*The combination was found to be more effective than either alone.*)
16. Sullivan FM, Swan IRC, Donnan PT, et al. Early treatment with prednisolone or acyclovir in Bell's palsy. N Engl J Med 2007;357:1598. (*There was no benefit of acyclovir alone or any additional benefit of acyclovir in combination with prednisolone.*)

CHAPTER 176 ■ MANAGEMENT OF TIC DOULOUREUX (TRIGEMINAL NEURALGIA)

AMY A. PRUITT

Tic douloureux is among the most excruciating of pain syndromes seen in office practice. Fifteen thousand new cases occur annually in the United States; most patients are middle-aged or elderly. Some have found the pain so intolerable that they consider suicide. The primary physician needs to know how to use available medical therapies and when to send the patient for a neurosurgical consultation.

CLINICAL PRESENTATION AND NATURAL HISTORY (1,2)

The illness is characterized by paroxysms of unilateral lancinating facial pain involving the jaw, gums, lips, or maxillary region (areas corresponding to branches of the trigeminal nerve). The maxillary and mandibular divisions are affected more frequently than the ophthalmic division. Minor, repeated contact with a trigger zone often precipitates an attack, setting off fierce pain that usually lasts up to a few minutes. Repeated paroxysms may continue day and night for several weeks. The disease is unilateral and unaccompanied by demonstrable sensory or motor deficits, features that distinguish it from trigeminal pain with other causes, such as tumor.

The condition can be chronic, although spontaneous remissions are not uncommon. Women are more often affected than men, and the incidence rises with age. The etiology of the condition is unknown. Despite much speculation, no definitive evidence links it to herpes simplex virus. The pathologic lesion found in some electron micrographs appears to be a breakdown of myelin.

Although trigeminal neuralgia may be a symptom of multiple sclerosis, which should be considered in a young adult with trigeminal neuralgia, it is infrequently the initial or sole manifestation of this disease. Similarly, trigeminal neuralgia is uncommonly the isolated symptom of a cerebellopontine angle tumor. Both diseases can be demonstrated by magnetic resonance imaging (MRI), and some authors recommend MRI for all patients with trigeminal neuralgia, although the cost–benefit ratio remains to be determined.

DIFFERENTIAL DIAGNOSIS (1,2)

Although few conditions absolutely mimic the lancinating pain of trigeminal neuralgia, pain referable to structures of the face may be similar. Conditions that should be excluded include dental disease, temporomandibular joint dysfunction, temporal arteritis, sphenoid sinusitis, and cluster headache. The preeruption pain of herpes zoster, which occurs in the distribution of the ophthalmic division of the trigeminal more frequently than in the distribution of the other two divisions,

and postherpetic neuralgia, which follows the skin eruption by a few weeks, are two other entities to be considered. Physical examination should be normal without evidence of sensory loss in the distribution of the trigeminal nerve.

Other facial pain syndromes that should be differentiated from trigeminal neuralgia include short-lasting unilateral neuralgiform headache with cranial injection and tearing (SUNCT)–related syndromes, whose common feature is significant autonomic symptomatology. These are fairly uncommon. Cluster headache is the longest-lasting and most common headache syndrome with autonomic features (15 to 180 minutes) and tends to occur at night. Paroxysmal hemicrania is a female-predominant headache syndrome and can occur up to 100 times per day with exquisite responsiveness to indomethacin. Facial pain related to sinusitis is an important exclusionary diagnosis. Usually there are other symptoms, such as nasal congestion and rhinorrhea.

PRINCIPLES OF MANAGEMENT (1–5)

Treatment is symptomatic. Because drug therapy may provide adequate control of symptoms, surgical intervention should be reserved for refractory cases. Pharmacologic agents found to be particularly useful in the condition include carbamazepine, oxcarbazepine, and baclofen.

Pharmacologic Therapy

Carbamazepine (Tegretol)

Carbamazepine is the drug of choice; it was initially tried because the paroxysmal painful attacks were believed to resemble epilepsy. Studies have shown impressive short-term effects; most patients report marked relief of pain within 24 to 72 hours. The drug is so effective that some argue that failure to respond places the diagnosis in doubt. The starting dose is 100 to 200 mg twice daily. The maintenance dose ranges from 400 to 800 mg/d and is adjusted according to serum drug levels; the therapeutic range is 5 to 12 μg/mL. An extended-release preparation of carbamazepine allows for the same total daily dose with convenient twice-daily dosing. The most common side effect is sedation.

Adverse Effects. The incidence of serious side effects (*bone marrow suppression, rash, liver injury*) is high (5% to 19%), often necessitating cessation of therapy. Marrow suppression is often reversible if the drug is stopped early. Skin rash often precedes other serious side effects; it may be erythematous and pruritic. The onset of a skin rash is an early indication to halt therapy. Annoying side effects include *nausea, diarrhea, ataxia, dizziness,* and *confusion.* Neurologic reactions are reported most commonly and affect about 15% of patients.

Initiating and Monitoring Therapy. Starting carbamazepine at a dose of 200 mg daily helps to avoid many of the annoying minor side effects. During the first 2 months of therapy, a *complete blood cell count* and *platelet count* should be obtained weekly to biweekly; later, the frequency of monitoring can be reduced to monthly. It is advisable to attempt a reduction or cessation of carbamazepine therapy at least once every 2 to 3 months. Unfortunately, by 3 years, 30% of patients no longer obtain relief by taking carbamazepine.

Oxcarbazepine (Trileptal)

Many clinicians would now consider using oxcarbazepine (Trileptal) as the initial therapy because it appears to be as effective as carbamazepine but does not require frequent liver function and blood count monitoring. However, serum sodium must be followed carefully because this is a common metabolic derangement with oxcarbazepine. The starting dose is 300 mg in the evening, and the daily dose can be titrated upward to a target daily dose of 900 to 1,800 mg in three divided doses.

Baclofen

Baclofen, an agent that enhances synaptic transmission of γ-aminobutyric acid, has been used with success in a high percentage of cases. Some even consider it the drug of choice for trigeminal neuralgia. The initial dose of 10 mg twice daily is increased slowly. The usual maintenance dose is 50 to 60 mg/d. *Sedation* and *nausea* are the most common limiting side effects. Abrupt cessation of therapy can lead to hallucinations and seizures; therefore, discontinuation must be gradual.

Combination Therapy and Use of Other Agents

Combination therapy may be necessary because trigeminal neuralgia tends to increase in severity.

Carbamazepine and Baclofen or Either with Phenytoin. These agents in combination or either in conjunction with phenytoin can provide additional relief. The usual daily dose of phenytoin that achieves therapeutic serum levels is 300 to 400 mg (see Chapter 170). Although phenytoin is not as effective as carbamazepine as monotherapy, it may be a useful add-on treatment, and parenteral phenytoin is sometimes used emergently for patients who are having a flurry of severe attacks and cannot take medicine orally.

Gabapentin (Neurontin). This drug may be prescribed if other medicines are unsuccessful, but sedation can be a limiting side effect if high doses are needed. Narcotics should be avoided because they are unlikely to be helpful for long-term control of pain and may lead to drug dependency. Off-label use of *pregabalin* and *duloxetine* is being considered in refractory cases of painful peripheral neuropathy (see Chapter 167).

Tricyclics. Amitriptyline, although useful for postherpetic neuralgia and other forms of neuropathic pain, is not helpful for trigeminal neuralgia.

Surgical Approaches

Surgical approaches can be considered when drug therapy proves inadequate and pain is incapacitating.

Percutaneous Radiofrequency Rhizotomy

This is the least invasive procedure that produces the greatest relief of symptoms and the least loss of sensation. The small pain fibers are destroyed, whereas the more heavily myelinated touch fibers that supply the relevant zone are spared. The procedure has produced lasting relief in 80% of those treated once; only 5% have experienced an undesirable loss of sensation. Late recurrences occur in up to 50% of cases at 5 years, but pain relief is achieved with a repeated procedure in these patients.

Microvascular Decompression

This procedure affords the best chance of long-term pain relief without sensory deficit but entails much more complicated surgery, reserving it for younger patients. It requires general anesthesia and a craniotomy. More than 90% of operated patients have compression of the trigeminal nerve by an artery or vein. Muscle tissue or synthetic material is used to decompress the nerve with an 85% 1-year success rate.

Formerly Used Treatment Methods

Formerly used treatment methods include *alcohol injection* or partial section of the sensory root of the fifth cranial nerve. These techniques provided pain relief, but often only for 1 to 2 years, and at the price of unacceptable permanent sensory deficits. Total *tooth extraction* is an ineffective and erroneous treatment method.

PATIENT EDUCATION

The patient needs to be told that the condition can be controlled and is often self-limited. This knowledge can prevent a distraught sufferer from attempting suicide. The physician must keep in mind the anguish that these patients may experience; they require close support. Obvious ways to prevent attacks, such as avoiding repetitive contact with the trigger zone, have usually been discovered by the patient, but they are worth mentioning. Patients treated with carbamazepine must be informed of the risk for marrow suppression and the importance of regular monitoring of the complete blood cell count.

THERAPEUTIC RECOMMENDATIONS AND INDICATIONS FOR REFERRAL

- Teach the patient to avoid repetitive contact with the trigger zone.
- Begin drug therapy for disabling and frequent episodes of pain with *carbamazepine* (100 mg twice daily, preferably in the extended-release preparation); increase the dose by 200 mg/d until control of symptoms is achieved or a dose of 800 to 1,000 mg/d is reached.
- During the first 2 months of carbamazepine therapy, monitor the complete blood cell and platelet counts weekly to biweekly; thereafter, monthly checks suffice.

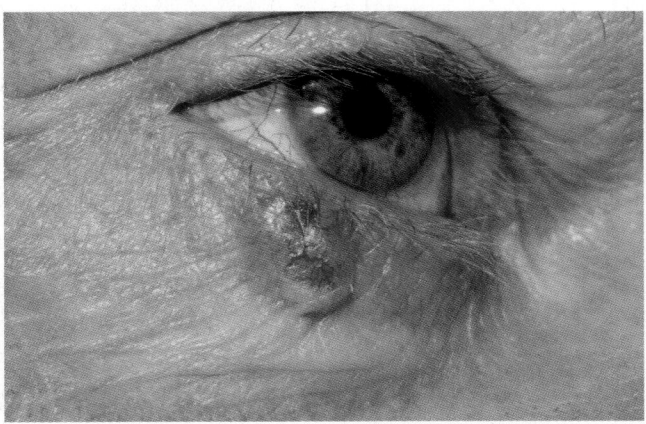

FIGURE 177.2. A typical nodular basal cell carcinoma with pearly texture and telangiectasia. (See Figure 177.2 in text.)

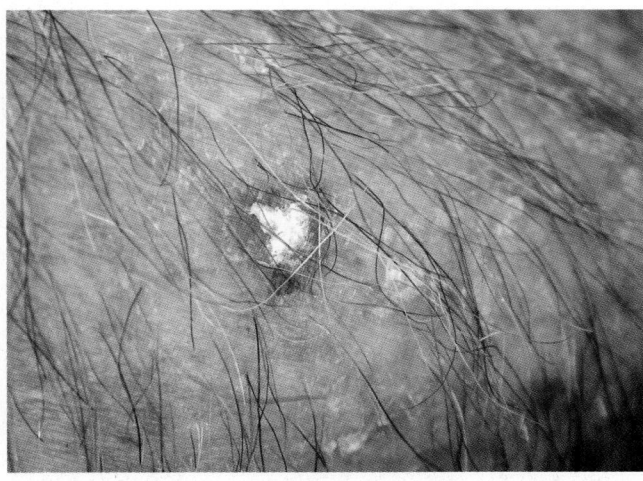

FIGURE 177.4. A keratotic papule characteristic of a hypertrophic actinic keratosis. (See Figure 177.4 in text.)

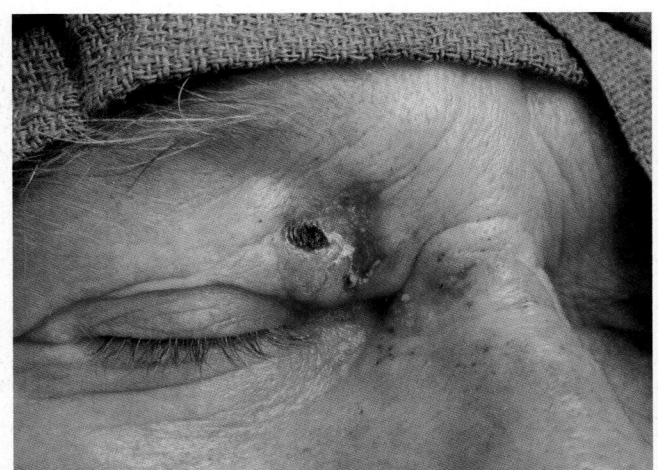

FIGURE 177.3. An ulcerated basal cell carcinoma; note the nodular and sclerotic components. (See Figure 177.3 in text.)

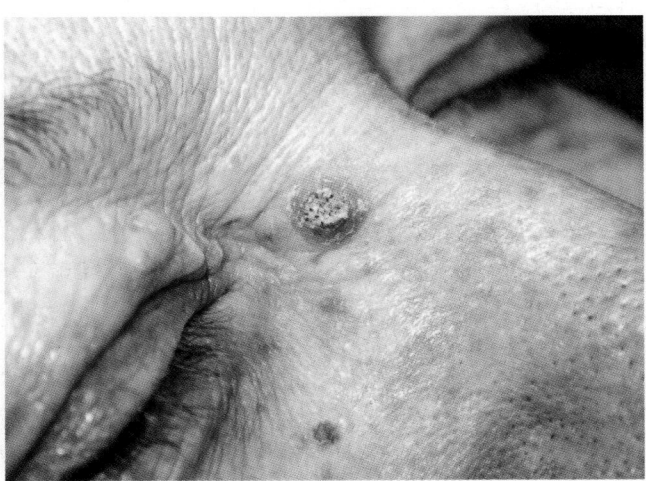

FIGURE 177.6. A keratotic papule, thicker and clinically tender, which was a squamous cell carcinoma. (See Figure 177.6 in text.)

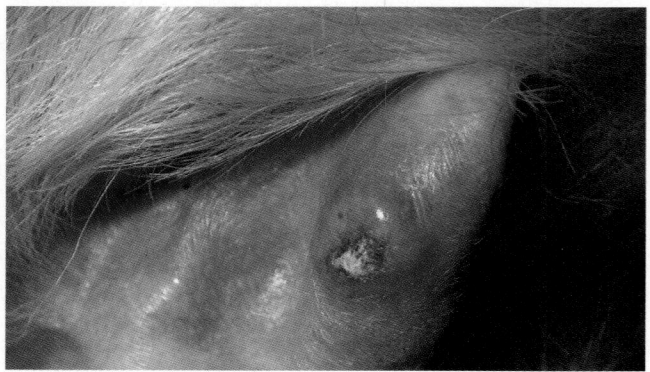

FIGURE 177.7. Keratoacanthoma with a crateriform appearance and a central keratin plug on the ear. (See Figure 177.7 in text.)

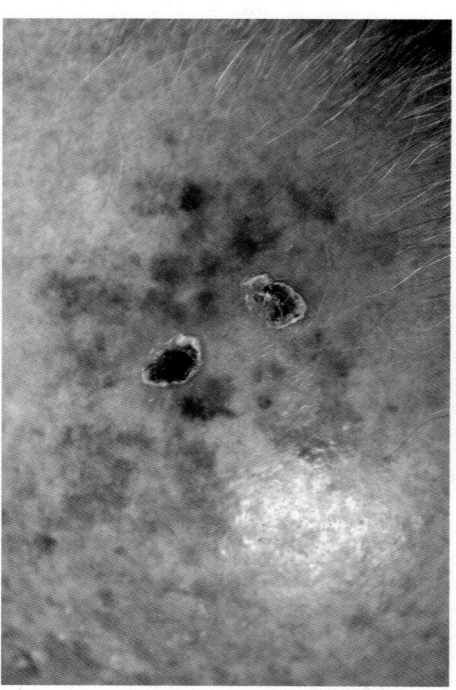

FIGURE 177.10. Lentigo maligna melanoma with indistinct borders and multiple colors. The crusts are secondary to biopsies. (See Figure 177.10 in text.)

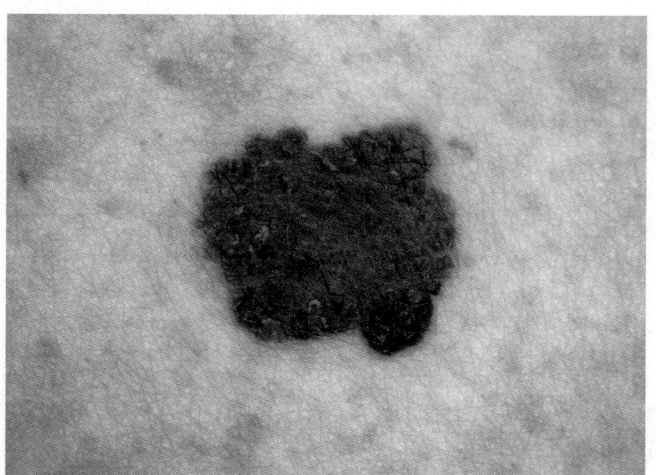

FIGURE 177.8. Superficial spreading melanoma. Note the notching, multiple colors, and regression in the center of the lesion. (See Figure 177.8 in text.)

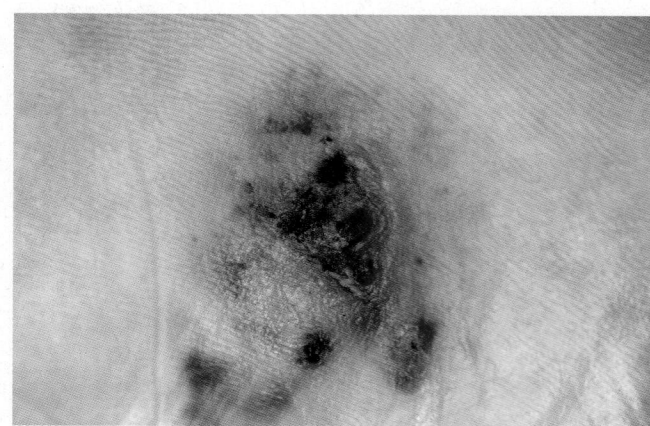

FIGURE 177.11. Acral lentiginous melanoma. There is a central vertical growth component, as well as ulceration and lateral pigment growth. This lesion was Clark level IV, 2.71 mm. (See Figure 177.11 in text.)

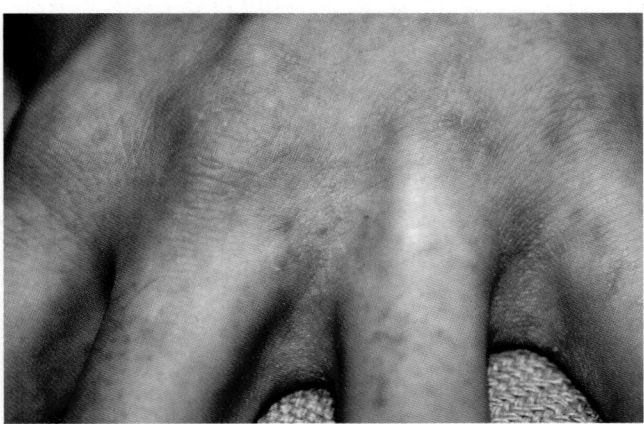

FIGURE 178.1. Papules and a single burrow (right) in the webspaces of a man with *Sarcoptes scabeii* infection. (See Figure 178.1 in text.)

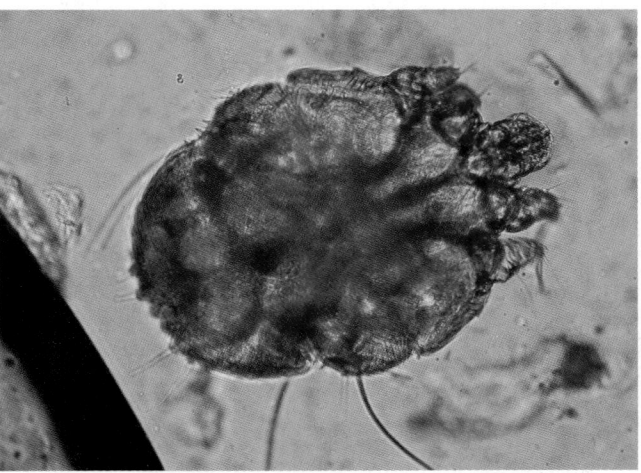

FIGURE 178.3. Scabies mite. (See Figure 178.3 in text.)

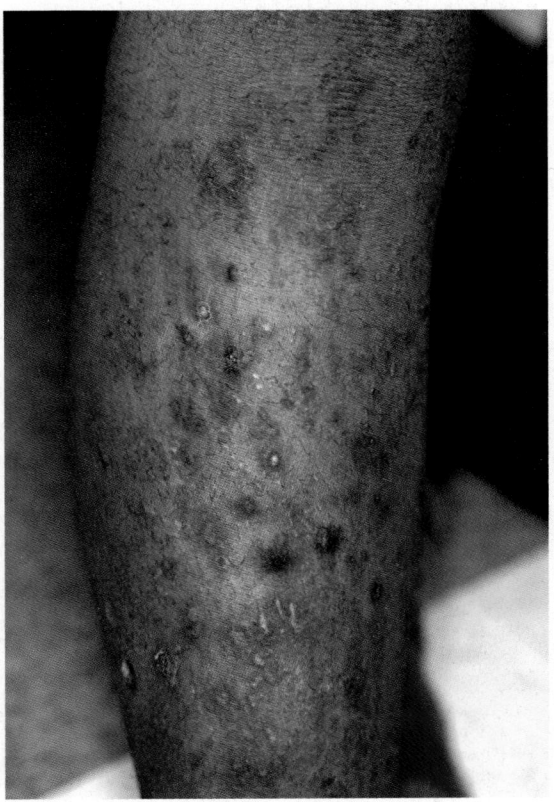

FIGURE 178.2. Multiple prurigo nodules on the leg of a man with bed bug bites. (See Figure 178.2 in text.)

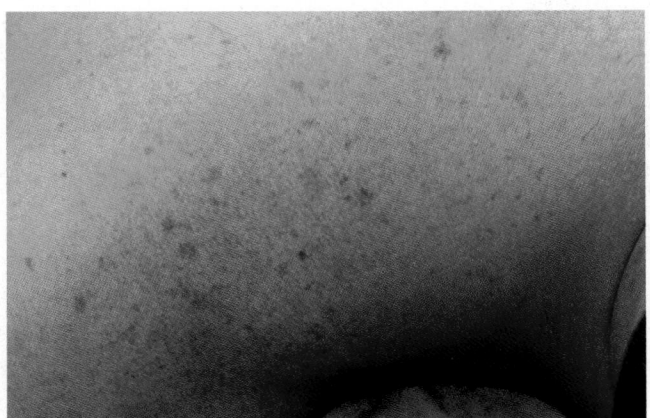

FIGURE 180.1. Solar lentigines on the shoulder after a previous blistering sunburn. (See Figure 180.1 in text.)

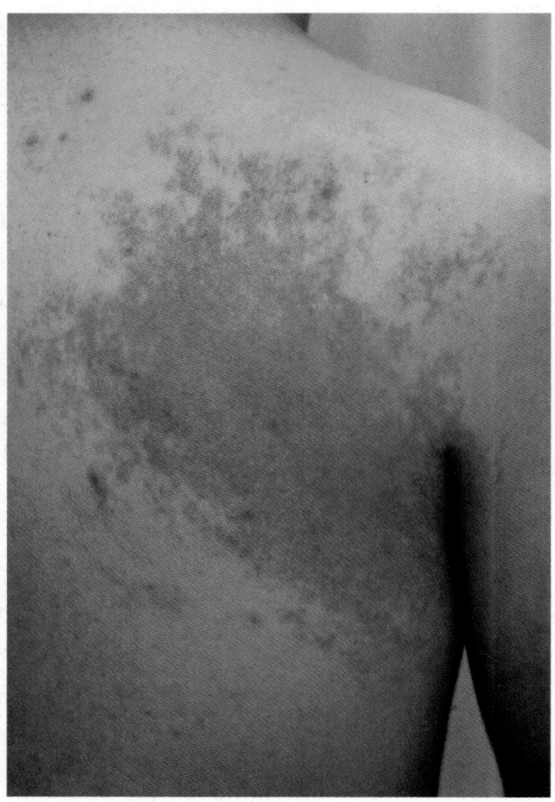

FIGURE 180.2. Becker's nevus on the shoulder of a young man. In this case, he did not have hypertrichosis. (See Figure 180.2 in text.)

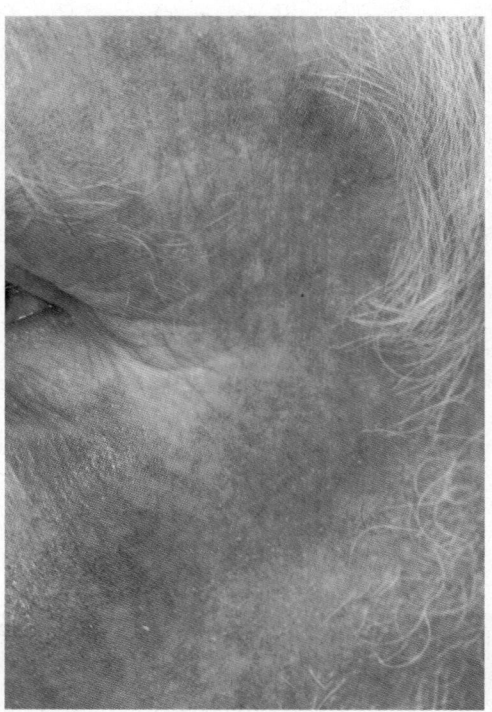

FIGURE 180.4. Brown pigmentation on a sun-exposed area from amiodarone use. (See Figure 180.4 in text.)

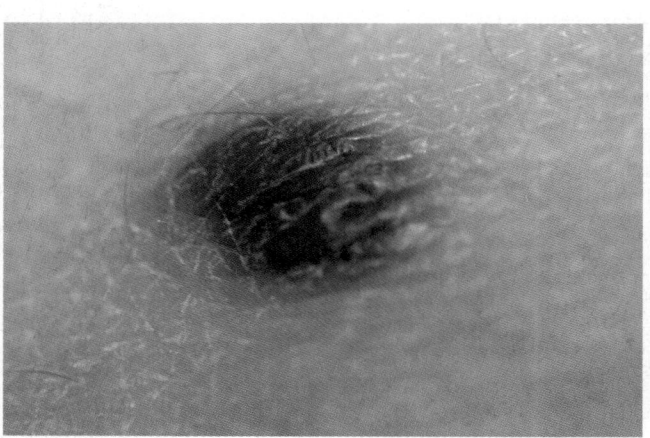

FIGURE 180.3. A dome-shaped, blue-black papule that has the characteristic features of a blue nevus. (See Figure 180.3 in text.)

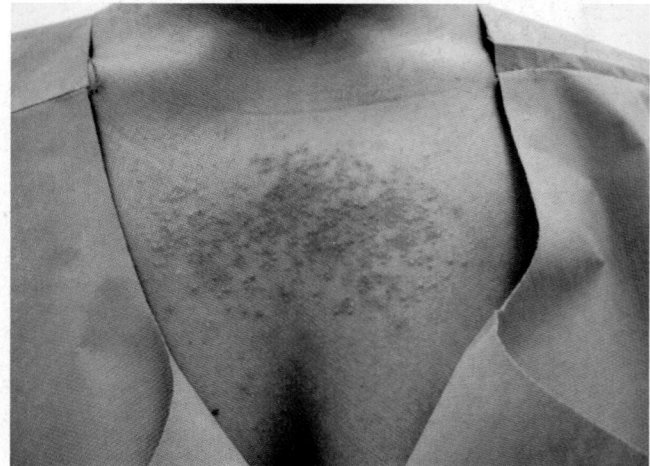

FIGURE 180.5. Postinflammatory hyperpigmentation after the resolution of papular eczema (centrally). Note the active lesions laterally. (See Figure 180.5 in text.)

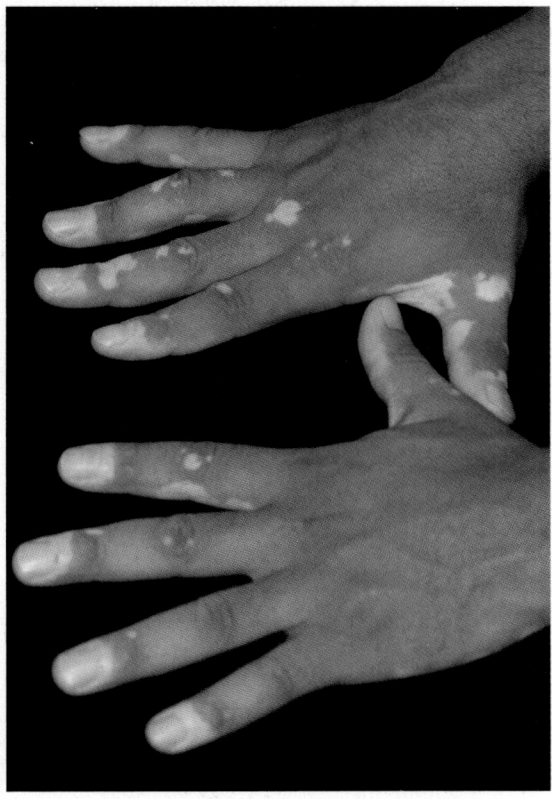

FIGURE 180.6. Vitiligo on bilateral hands. (See Figure 180.6 in text.)

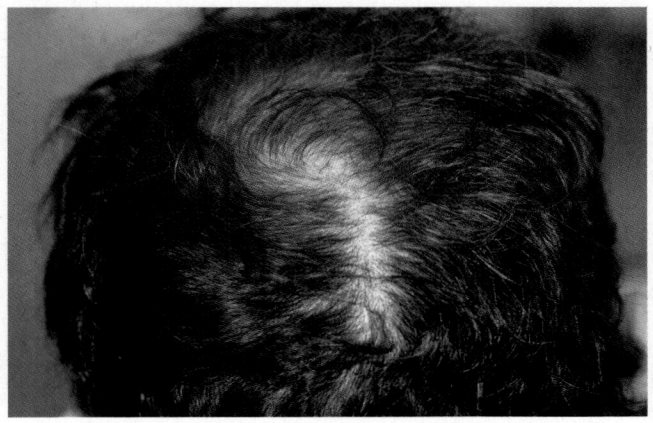

FIGURE 182.1. Male pattern alopecia in the typical "bald spot" on the occipital scalp. (See Figure 182.1 in text.)

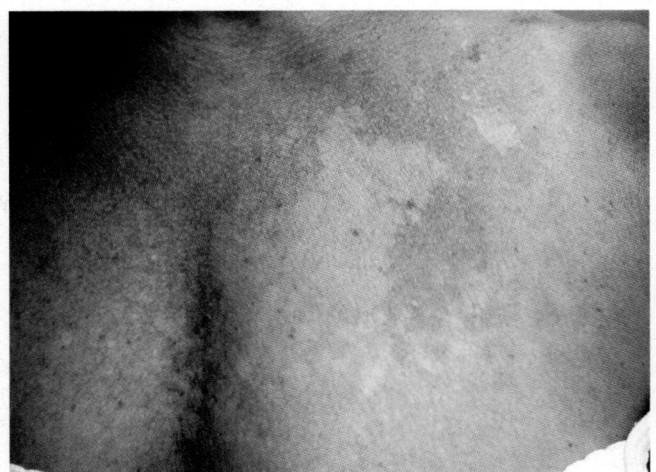

FIGURE 180.7. Hypopigmented patches after a 20-year history of tinea versicolor on the chest. (See Figure 180.7 in text.)

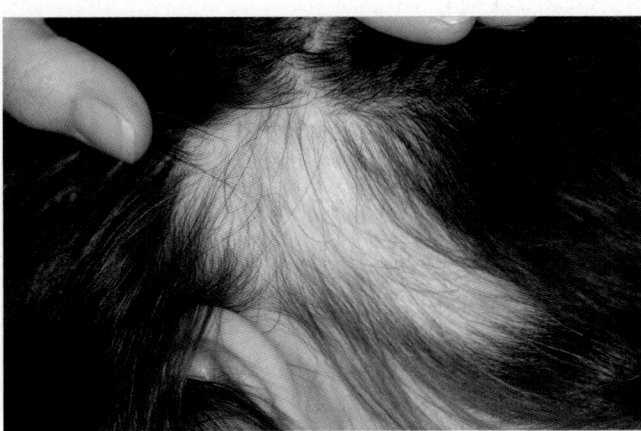

FIGURE 182.2. Alopecia areata on the temporal scalp, partially in the "ophiasis" distribution. (See Figure 182.2 in text.)

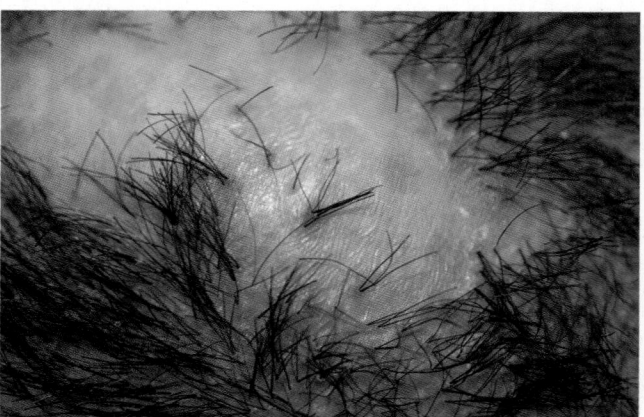

FIGURE 182.3. Scarring alopecia with "doll's hairs" (scarring encasing many hair shafts). (See Figure 182.3 in text.)

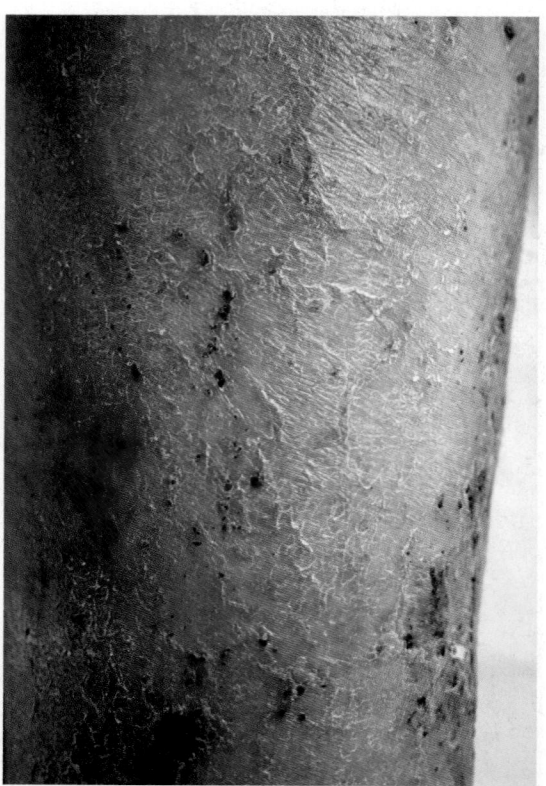

FIGURE 183.1. Erythema craquelé/severe xerosis on the shins. (See Figure 183.1 in text.)

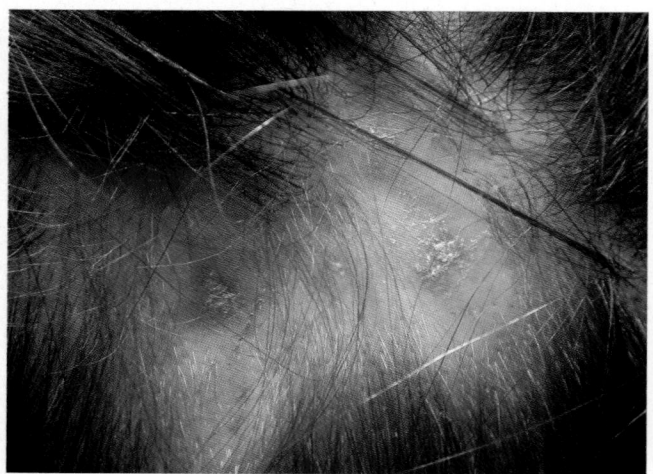

FIGURE 182.4. Chronic cutaneous lupus erythematosus causing a scarring alopecia on the scalp. (See Figure 182.4 in text.)

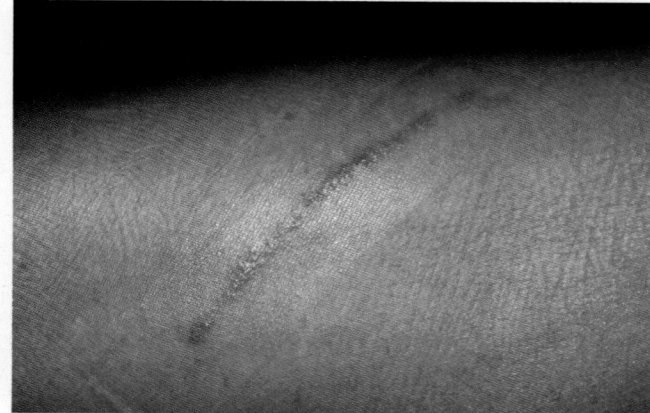

FIGURE 184.1. Linear vesicles. This pattern in characteristic of a plant allergic dermatitis—in this case, poison ivy. (See Figure 184.1 in text.)

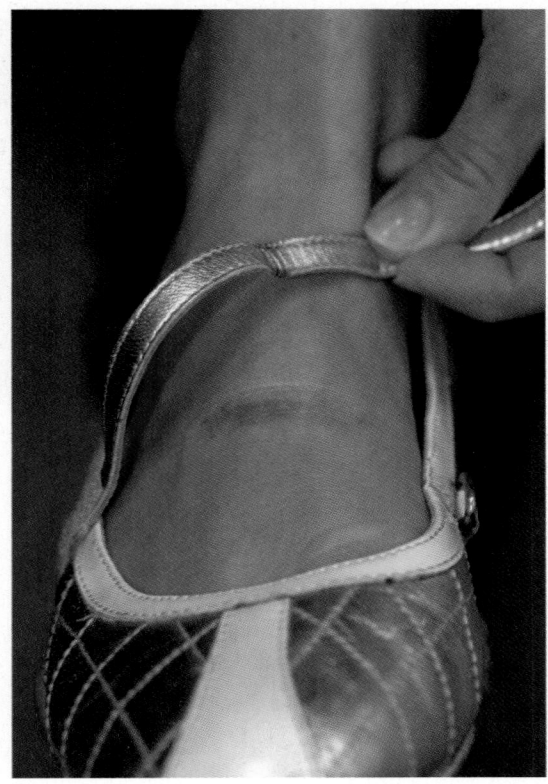

FIGURE 184.2. Allergic dermatitis from the chromates in tanned leather in a shoe; note dermatitis under the strap. (See Figure 184.2 in text.)

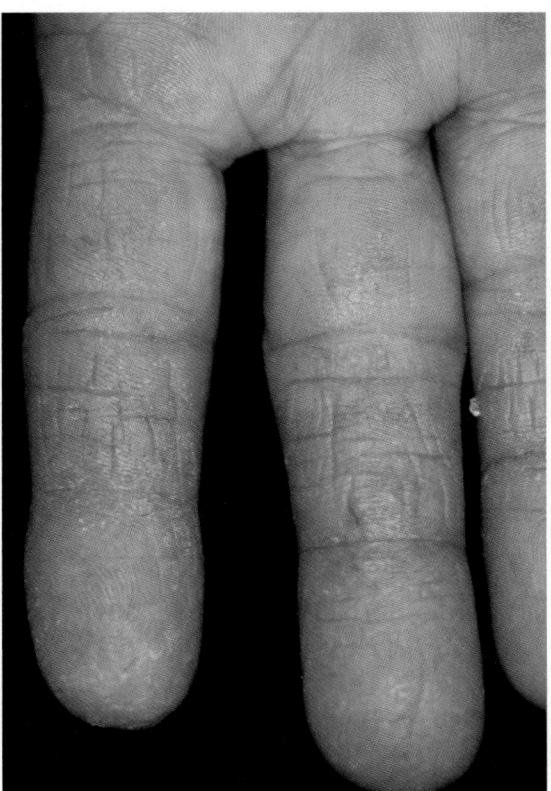

FIGURE 184.4. Chronic irritant dermatitis from frequent hand-washing. (See Figure 184.4 in text.)

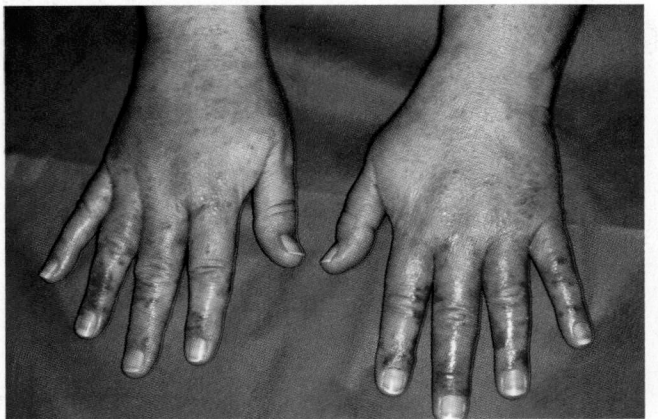

FIGURE 184.3. Rubber accelerator (carba and thiuram) allergic dermatitis from latex rubber work gloves. (See Figure 184.3 in text.)

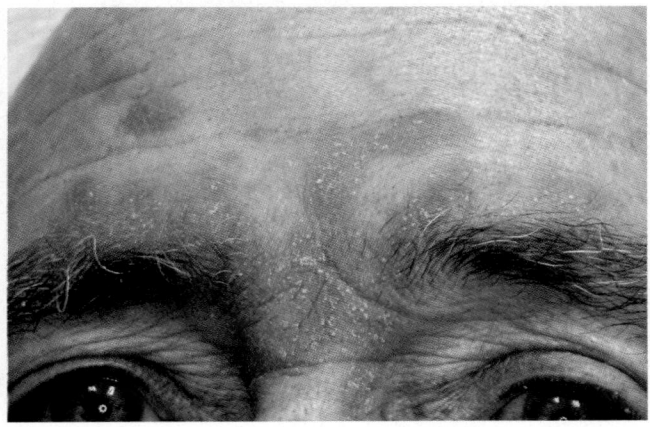

FIGURE 184.5. Seborrheic dermatitis on the glabellar region. (See Figure 184.5 in text.)

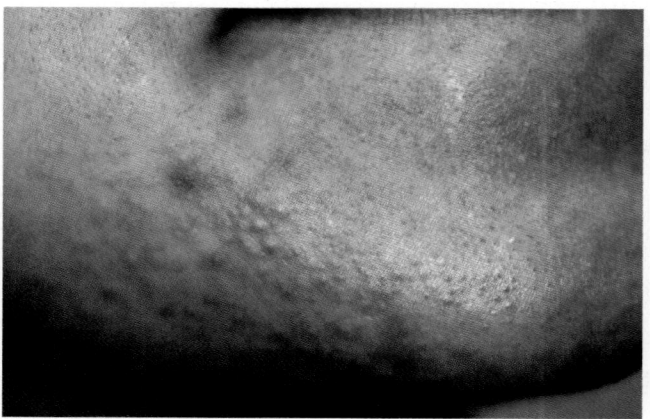

FIGURE 185.1. Comedonal acne on the chin of a young woman. (See Figure 185.1 in text.)

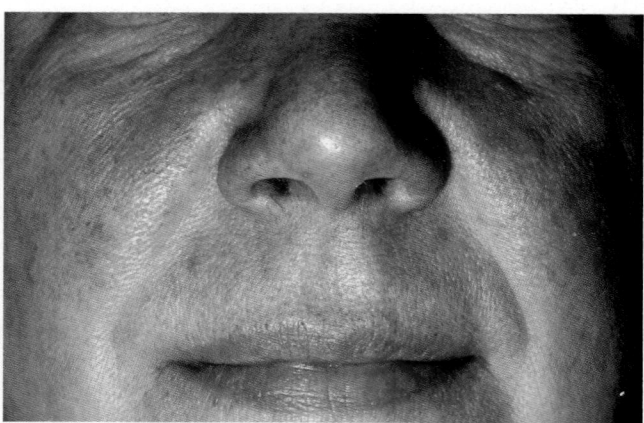

FIGURE 186.1. Papulopustular and telangiectatic rosacea. (See Figure 186.1 in text.)

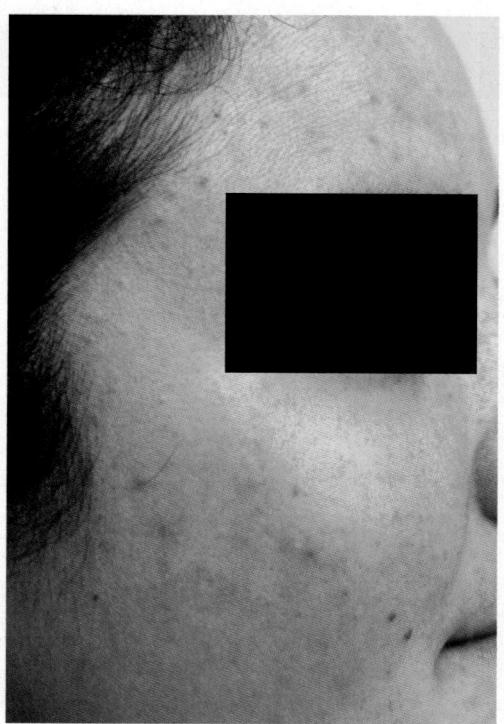

FIGURE 185.2. Mild papular and comedonal acne. (See Figure 185.2 in text.)

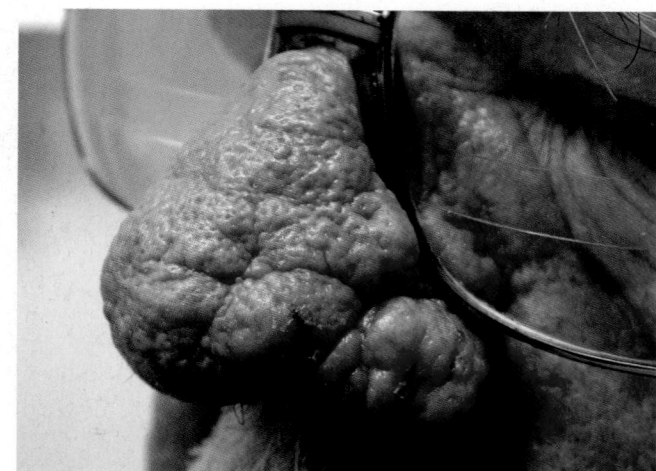

FIGURE 186.2. Severe rhinophyma in an elderly man. (See Figure 186.2 in text.)

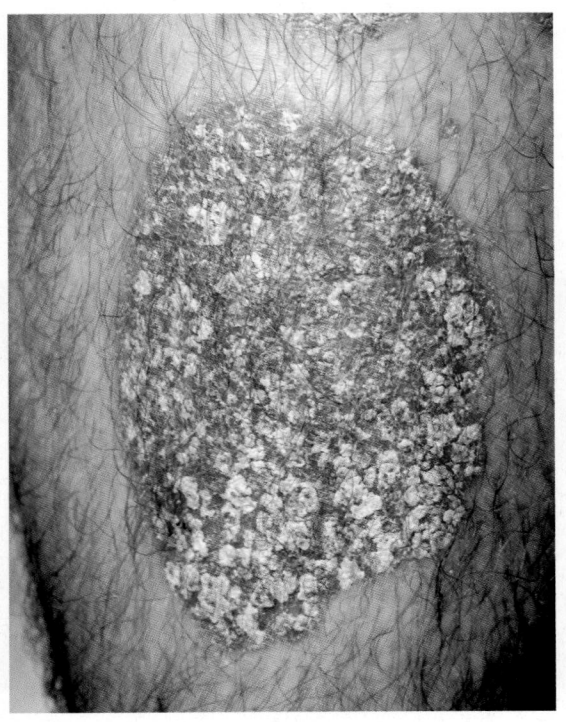

FIGURE 187.1. Typical Psoriatic Plaque on the SHIN with Micaceous Scale. (See Figure 187.1 in text.)

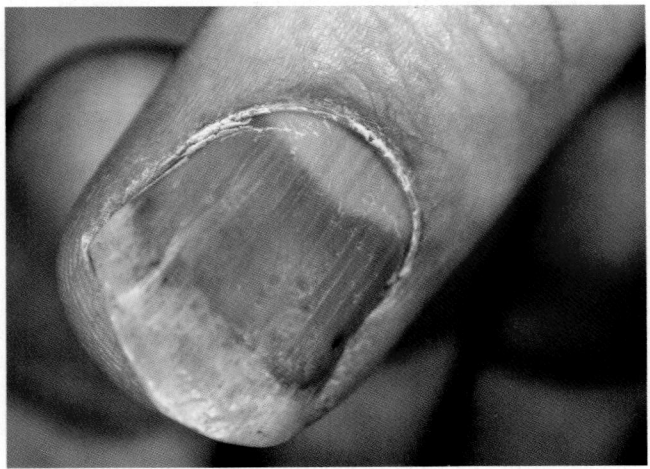

FIGURE 187.3. Typical nail finding of psoriasis with nail pitting and onycholysis. (See Figure 187.3 in text.)

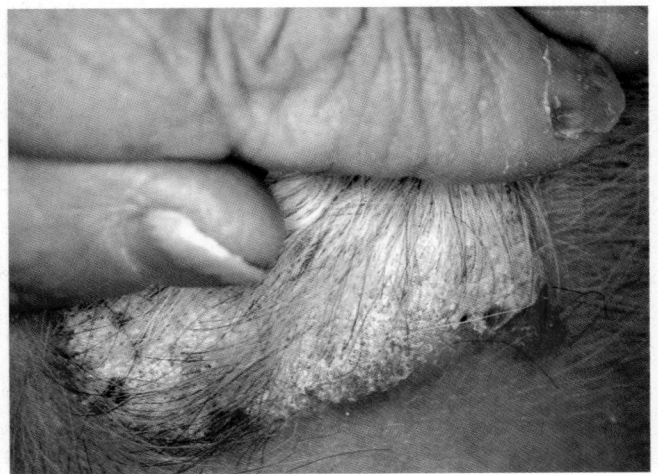

FIGURE 187.2. Scalp psoriasis with involved fingernails. (See Figure 187.2 in text.)

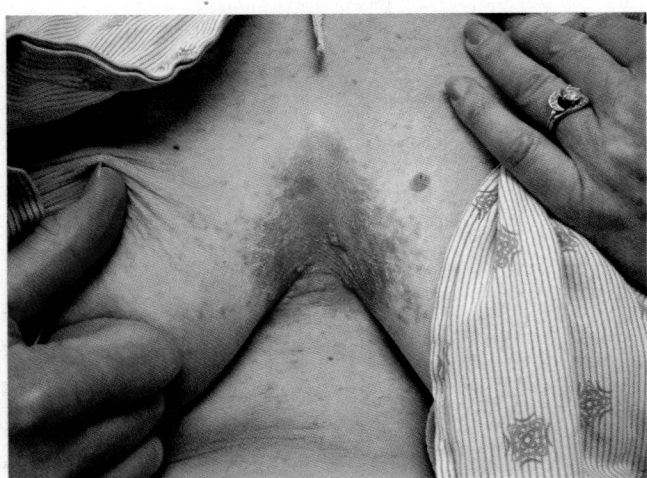

FIGURE 188.1. Inframammary candidal infection. (See Figure 188.1 in text.)

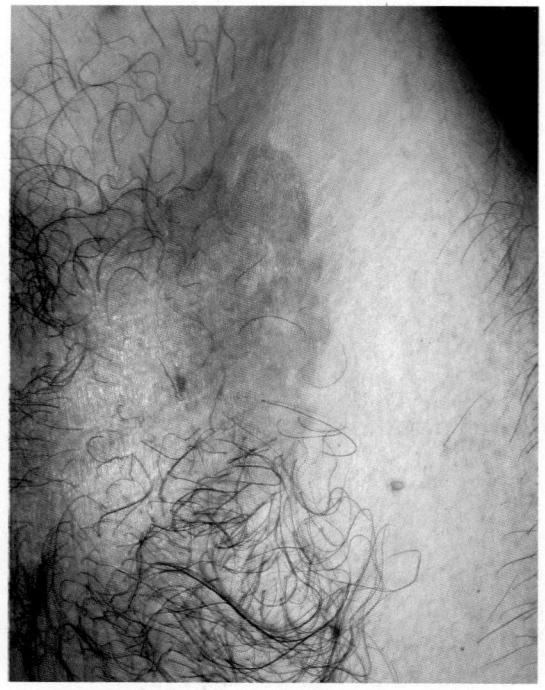

FIGURE 188.2. Clinical view of erythrasma with dull red-brown plaques in the axilla. (See Figure 188.2 in text.)

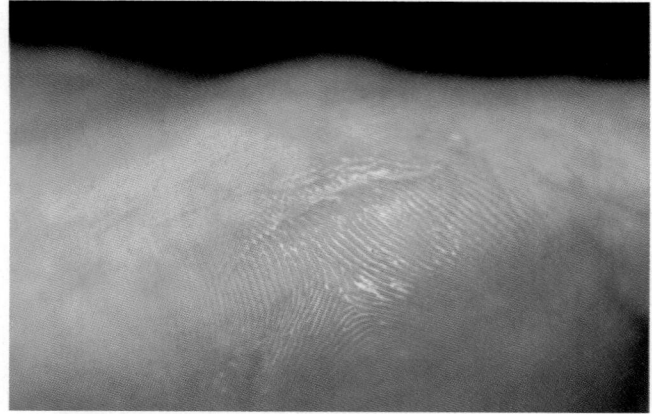

FIGURE 189.1. Callosity on the lateral border of the foot. (See Figure 189.1 in text.)

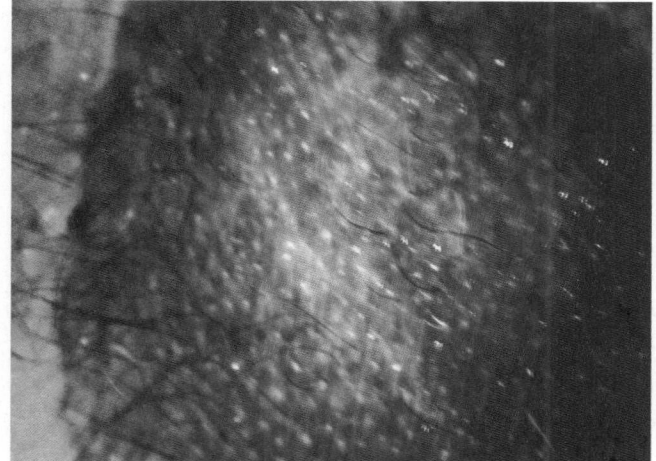

FIGURE 188.3. Coral red fluorescence from the same lesion as in Fig. 188.2, with a Wood's lamp exam. (See Figure 188.3 in text.)

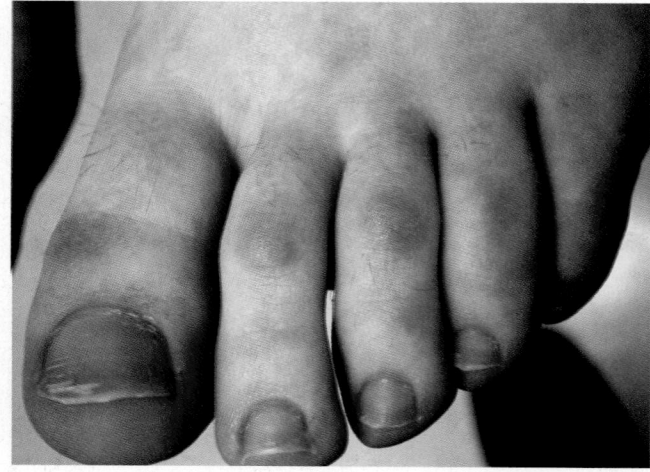

FIGURE 189.2. Callosities on the dorsal toes of an Irish step dancer. (See Figure 189.2 in text.)

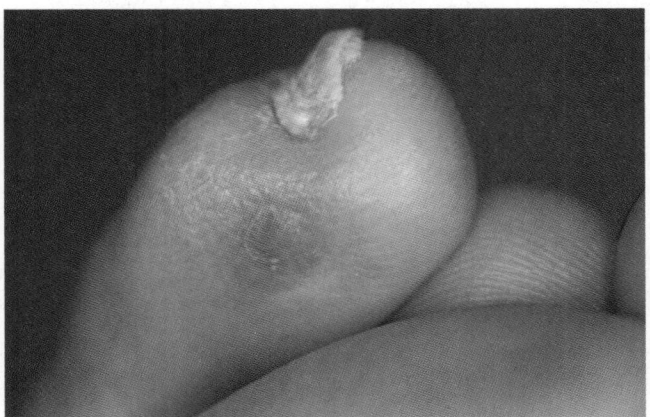

FIGURE 189.3. Heloma durum; note the lack of skin marking. (See Figure 189.3 in text.)

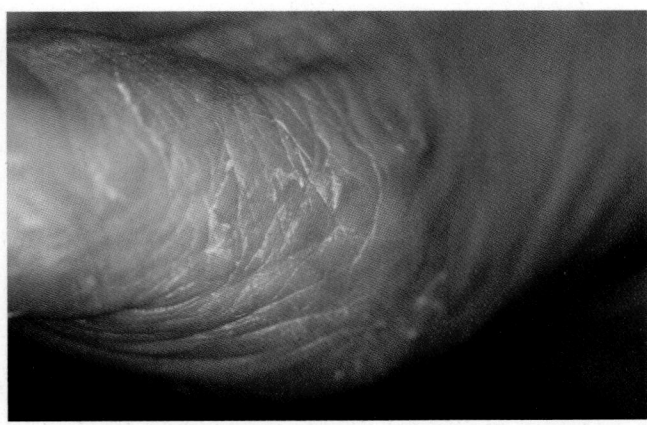

FIGURE 191.1. Tinea pedis on the side of the foot adjacent to the great toe. (See Figure 191.1 in text.)

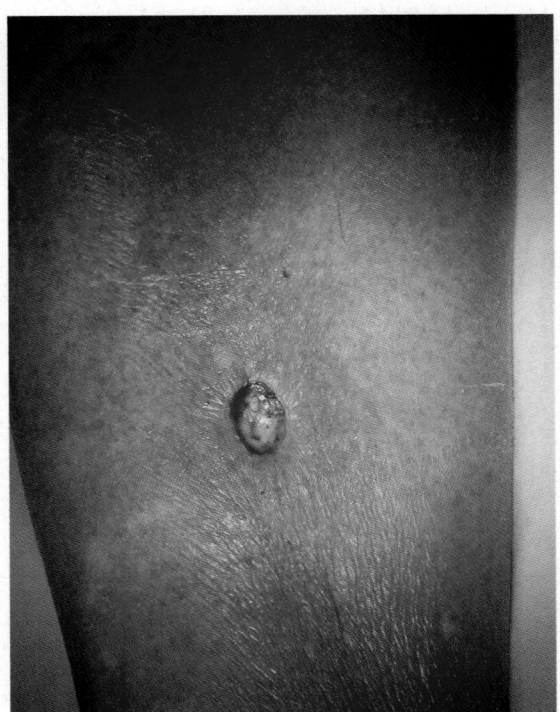

FIGURE 190.1. *Escherichia coli* infection in a shave biopsy site of an elderly immunosuppressed man. (See Figure 190.1 in text.)

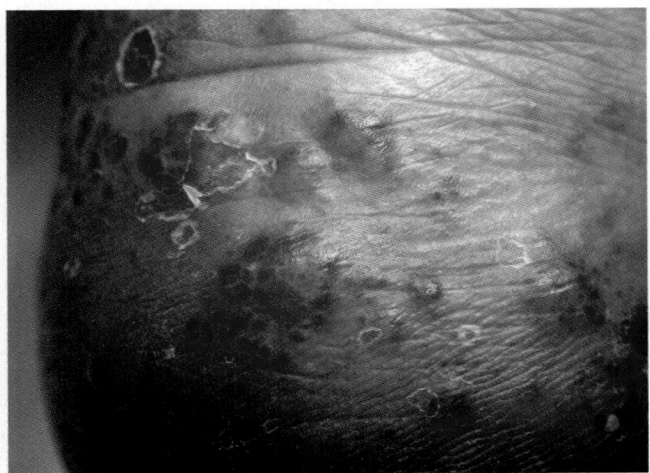

FIGURE 191.2. Multiloculated bullae, a less common presentation of tinea pedis. (See Figure 191.2 in text.)

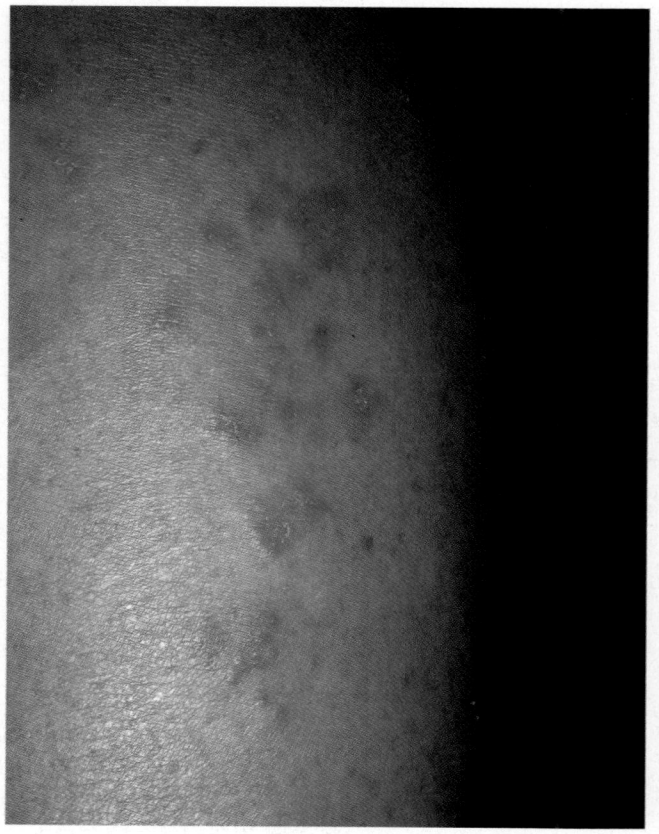

FIGURE 191.3. Majocci's granulomas on the leg. (See Figure 191.3 in text.)

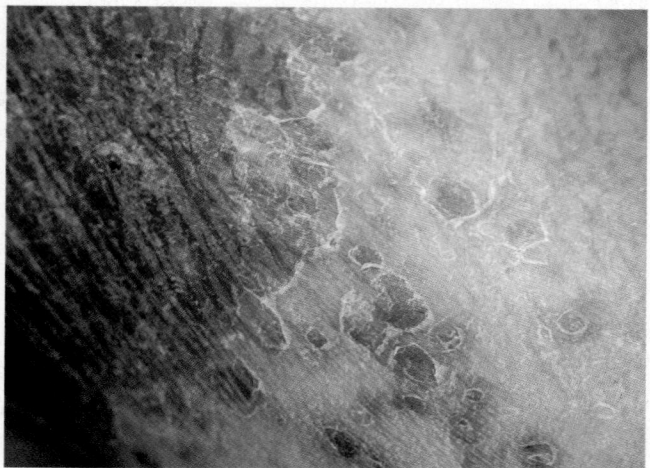

FIGURE 191.4. Cutaneous *Candida* infection with prominent satellite lesions. (See Figure 191.4 in text.)

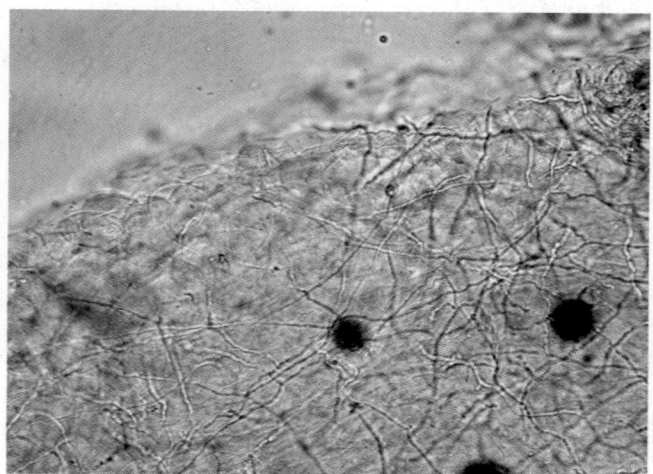

FIGURE 191.5. Positive potassium hydroxide test with prominent hyphae. (See Figure 191.5 in text.)

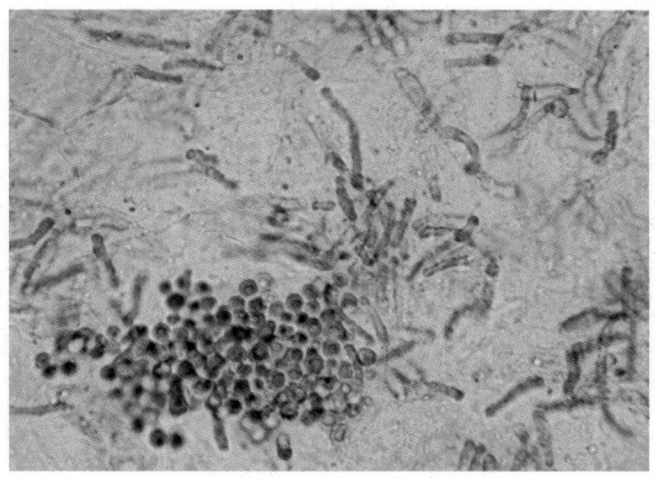

FIGURE 191.6. "Spaghetti and meatballs" appearance of *Malassezia furfur* on potassium hydroxide exam. (See Figure 191.6 in text.)

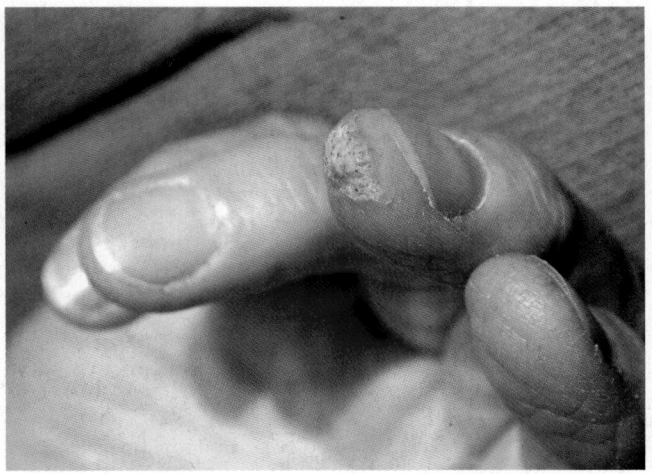

FIGURE 194.1. Common verruca vulgaris on the fingertip. (See Figure 194.1 in text.)

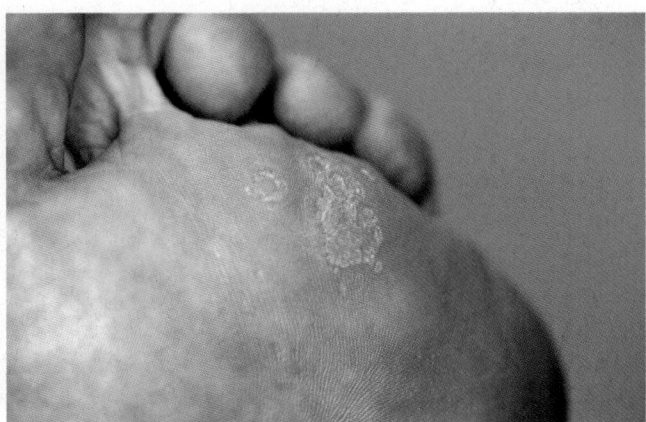

FIGURE 194.2. Plantar verruca. These lesions are often not exophytic. (See Figure 194.2 in text.)

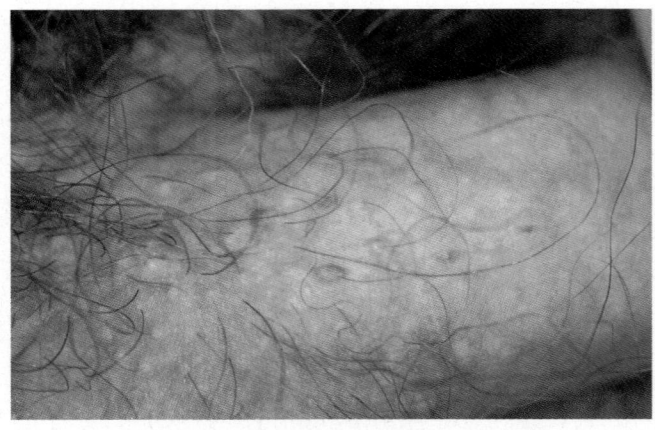

FIGURE 194.3. Condyloma on the penis. (See Figure 194.3 in text.)

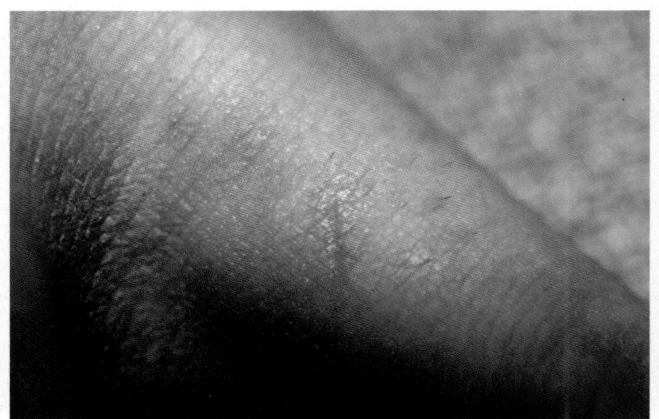

FIGURE 195.1. Scabies burrow on the finger. (See Figure 195.1 in text.)

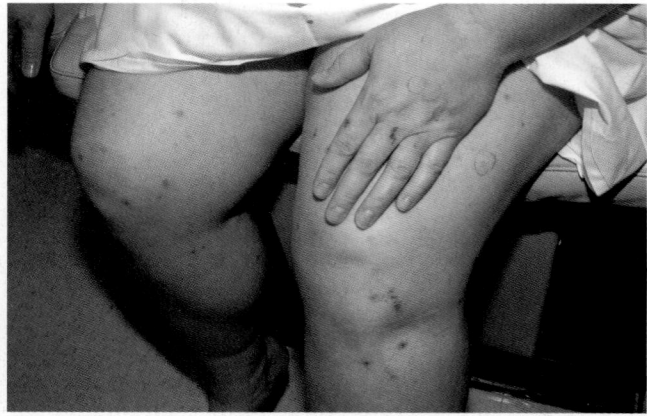

FIGURE 195.2. Crusted generalized excoriations and papules. Burrows are circled on the skin. (See Figure 195.2 in text.)

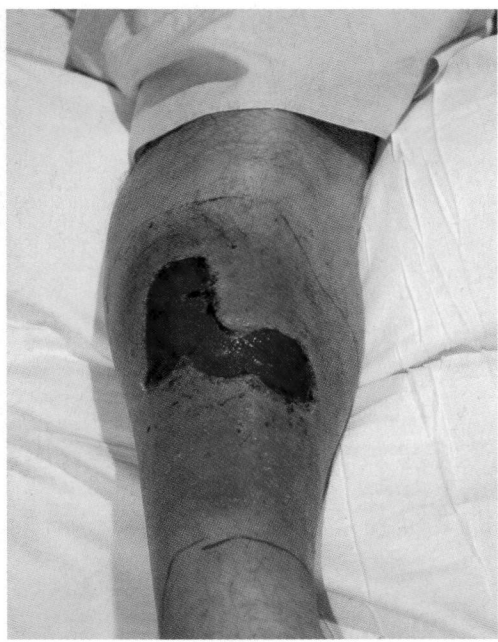

FIGURE 197.1. Large, later-stage arterial ulceration on the leg. This lesion was extremely painful. (See Figure 197.1 in text.)

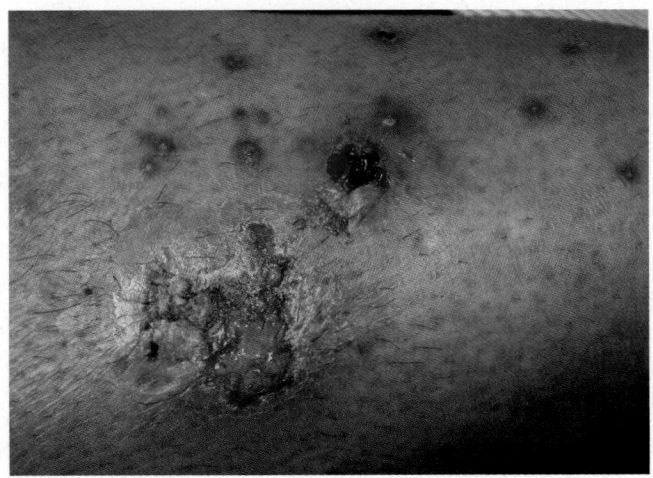

FIGURE 197.2. Pyoderma gangrenosum, early pustules and ulcerations on the shin. (See Figure 197.2 in text.)

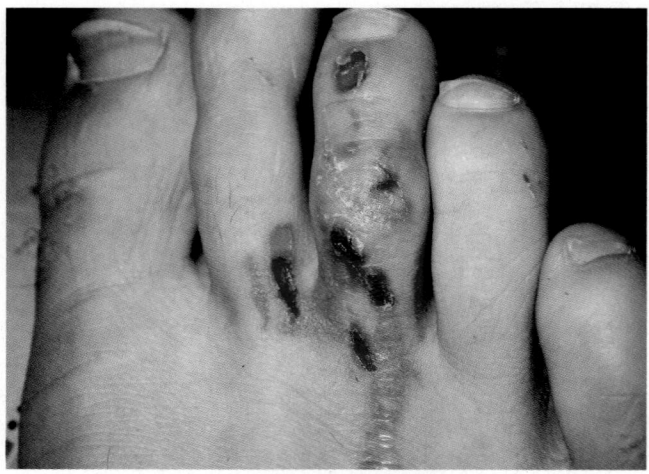

FIGURE 197.3. Ulcerations on the dorsal foot. These were caused by heating a piece of metal with a lighter and burning the foot. (See Figure 197.3 in text.)

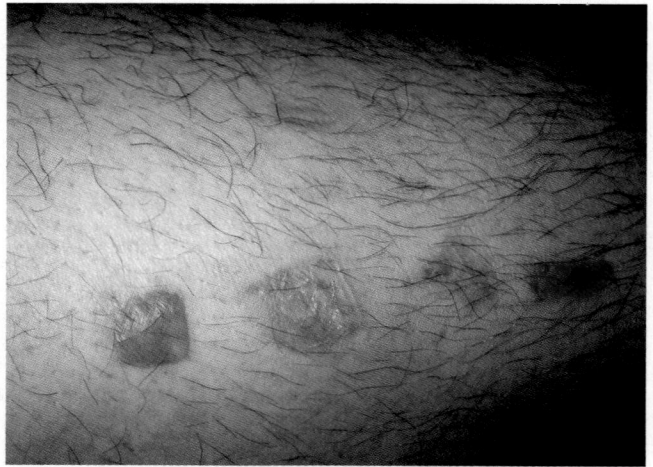

FIGURE 197.4. Quadratic bullae on the leg of the same patient as in Fig. 197.3. These were also factitial. (See Figure 197.4 in text.)

- Stop carbamazepine immediately if the white blood cell count falls to less than 3,000/mm^3 or if skin rash, easy bruising, fever, mouth sores, or petechiae develop.
- An alternative to carbamazepine is oxcarbazepine at a dose of 300 to 600 mg three times daily or *baclofen* at a dose of 10 mg twice daily. Increase the dose by 10 mg/d every 3 days until a response is achieved or a maximum of 60 mg/d is reached. Discontinue the medication gradually; do not withdraw it abruptly.
- If carbamazepine or baclofen alone is not sufficient to control symptoms, add *phenytoin* at a dose of 300 mg/d.

- If the foregoing medicines are unsuccessful, gabapentin (Neurontin) may be started at a dose of 300 mg at bedtime and then increased by 300 mg every 4 days until a total of 1,800 mg is being taken divided into three doses daily. Sedation may be a limiting side effect.
- Avoid narcotics because they are unlikely to be helpful for the long-term control of pain and may lead to drug dependency.
- Refer the patient who cannot be managed by pharmacologic measures to a neurosurgeon skilled in selective radiofrequency rhizotomy or microvascular decompression.

Annotated Bibliography

1. Dworkin RH, Backonja M, Rowbotham MC, et al. Advances in neuropathic pain: diagnosis, mechanisms, and treatment recommendations. Arch Neurol 2003;60:1524. (*A very useful review, not just about trigeminal neuralgia, but also about all types of central and peripheral neuropathic pain problems.*)
2. Solomon S, Lipton RB. Facial pain. Neurol Clin 1992;8:913. (*An excellent review of differential diagnosis and management strategies.*)
3. Fromm GH, Terrence CF, Chattha AS. Baclofen in the treatment of trigeminal neuralgia: double-blind study and long-term follow-up. Ann Neurol 1984;15:240. (*Efficacy was demonstrated.*)
4. Janetta PJ. Trigeminal neuralgia: treatment by microvascular decompression. In: Wilkins RH, Rengacharg SS, eds. Neurosurgery. New York: McGraw-Hill, 1996:3961. (*The acknowledged master of the procedure reports superb results in patients with trigeminal and glossopharyngeal neuralgia and in those with hemifacial spasm.*)
5. Kondziolka D, Lunsford LD, Flicknger JC. Stereotactic radiosurgery for the treatment of trigeminal neuralgia. Clin J Pain 2002;18:42. (*The radiosurgical target is the trigeminal nerve as it exits the brainstem, with 70% complete pain relief at 1 year.*)

SECTION 12 ■ DERMATOLOGIC PROBLEMS

CHAPTER 177 ■ SCREENING FOR SKIN CANCERS

ARTHUR J. SOBER AND PETER C. SCHALOCK

Neoplasms of the skin are among the most common cancers in humans and a source of considerable morbidity and mortality, which are largely avoidable by preventive measures and timely diagnosis and treatment. More than 1 million new skin cancers occur annually in the United States, accounting for more than 10,000 deaths. Screening for these tumors is important because they are relatively easy to diagnose in early stages, when cure is possible by simple measures; this is particularly true for melanoma. In the last decade, the incidence of melanoma in the United States has approximately doubled and overall is increasing more rapidly than that of any other cancer.

EPIDEMIOLOGY AND RISK FACTORS (1-4)

Basal Cell Carcinomas

Basal cell carcinomas are the most common malignancy in humans. They are distinctly sun related, with the majority oc-

curring on the head and neck, especially the nose and cheeks. Recently an increase in frequency has been seen on the male torso and on the legs of women. Other etiologic factors include a genetically transmitted autosomal-dominant disorder—the basal cell nevus syndrome—in which multiple basal cell carcinomas occur in relatively young persons in association with palmar pits, bone cysts, and frontal bossing. Basal cell lesions can develop in persons exposed to arsenic. Scars from radiation dermatitis and thermal burns can also provide sites favorable to the development of basal cell tumors. Previously identified disease is also a risk factor.

Once a single basal cell carcinoma has developed, the chance that a second one will ensue within 1 year is 20%. After two have developed, there is a 40% likelihood that a third or more will occur within 1 year. This observation forms the basis of annual follow-up examinations after basal cell carcinoma has been detected.

Squamous Cell Carcinomas

Most squamous cell carcinomas develop from the precursor lesion—*actinic keratosis*. Two thirds of these cancers occur on sun-exposed surfaces, with risk proportional to total accumulated *sun exposure*. Other precipitants include *arsenic*

All photos are courtesy of Peter C. Schalock.

ingestion, *radiation-induced scarring*, and *thermal burns*. Those lesions arising in sun-damaged skin usually behave in a less biologically aggressive fashion than do those that occur on unexposed surfaces and are less likely to metastasize.

Melanoma

Melanoma, although far less common than basal cell carcinoma and squamous cell carcinoma, accounts for more than 75% of skin cancer deaths. The incidence has been increasing rapidly during the last few decades and currently exceeds that for Hodgkin's disease, leukemia, pancreatic cancer, carcinoma of the thyroid, and carcinoma of the pharynx and larynx. The sex ratio for melanoma in the United States is approximately 1:1 with a modest male predominance. A second primary melanoma develops in up to 10% of nonfamilial patients; 10% have affected relatives.

Risk Factors and Precursors

Because of the rapid rise in melanoma incidence, attention has focused on melanoma risk factors and precursors. Persons with *fair skin* who tan poorly and burn easily are at greatest risk, especially those with a history of episodic, *intense sun exposure*. Blacks, Asians, and dark-skinned whites have a much lower risk.

Precursor lesions include *congenital nevi* and *dysplastic nevi* (i.e., clinically atypical moles). Although congenital nevi occur in approximately 1% of all newborns, fortunately most of these are small (≤1.5 cm in diameter). Melanoma risk has been most clearly associated with large (>20 cm) nevi. *Giant hairy nevus* (Fig. 177.1) is a form of congenital nevus associated with malignant degeneration; the overall *lifetime* risk for malignancy is about 6%. Melanomas may arise in these lesions at any time throughout life, but most often by age 10 years. Melanoma occasionally arises in smaller pigmented congenital nevi, but the exact risk is unknown.

Dysplastic nevi occur in 5% to 10% of light-skinned whites and usually are recognizable in early adolescence. Lifetime risk

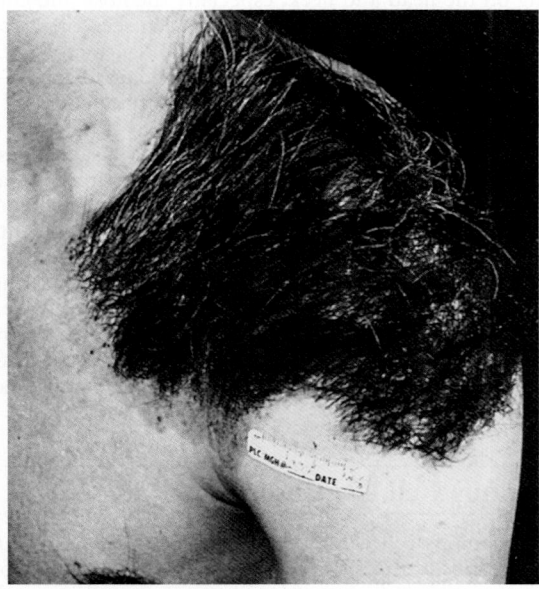

FIGURE 177.1. Giant hairy melanocytic nevus.

for melanoma is elevated severalfold in individuals with dysplastic nevi. An inherited predisposition to dysplastic nevi may contribute to the 8- to 12-fold increase in melanoma risk among first-degree relatives of patients with melanoma. In patients with dysplastic nevi and two or more first-degree relatives with cutaneous melanoma, the lifetime risk exceeds 50%. Patients with a large number (>100) of benign-appearing nevi may also be at increased risk.

NATURAL HISTORY OF SKIN CANCERS AND EFFECTIVENESS OF THERAPY (1,2,5–8)

Basal Cell Carcinomas

These cancers rarely metastasize or cause death, but they can be locally invasive and disfiguring. Metastasis usually occurs in patients who have delayed therapy for many years and who have large, locally invasive, eroded lesions. The risk for other skin cancers is increased because of their shared risk factors.

Several effective forms of therapy exist, all yielding a cure rate of approximately 95%: *surgical excision*, *radiation* therapy, *electrodessication and curettage*, and *cryotherapy* with *liquid nitrogen* applied by special spray apparatus. Treatment of the 5% that recur presents a greater challenge. The cure rate of a *recurrent basal cell carcinoma* is about 66% when the four traditional modalities just listed are applied. A special form of micrographic surgery, *Mohs' surgery*, is used for difficult, recurrent, or infiltrative basal cell carcinomas. In Mohs' surgery, the excised tissue is examined microscopically by frozen section to determine whether the tumor has been completely removed. Additional sections of skin are removed until all the borders are histopathologically clear of tumor. With Mohs' technique, cure rates of recurrent tumors exceed 90%, and those for primary tumors are better than 98%.

The use of *5-fluorouracil (5-FU)* and *imiquimod (Aldara)* topically has been advocated by some physicians for the treatment of *superficial basal cell carcinoma*. These agents may have some role in patients with multiple superficial lesions in whom other techniques cannot easily be employed.

Squamous Cell Carcinomas

Squamous cell carcinomas may begin as *actinic keratoses*, of which perhaps 1 in 1,000 annually undergoes malignant change. *Bowen's disease* represents carcinoma *in situ*, which may progress to a more advanced lesion if untreated.

Actinic Keratoses

Application of *5-FU* cream or solution twice daily for 2 to 4 weeks or *imiquimod* two times weekly for 16 weeks usually results in the destruction of these lesions. Some clinically inapparent lesions will also be destroyed by this therapy. The patient must be warned about the impressive inflammation that occurs when 5-FU or imiquimod is used. Because 5-FU is also a photosensitizing agent, treatment in late fall or winter, when solar exposure is diminished, is preferred. Imiquimod may result in local loss of pigmentation. Other effective modalities include *cryotherapy* with *liquid nitrogen* and *light desiccation*. Cryotherapy may also result in local decrease in pigmentation. If a cutaneous horn is present, *biopsy* of the lesion may be warranted to rule out the presence of a squamous cell carcinoma at the base. Actinic keratoses are extremely common and usually present no great threat to life.

Bowen's Disease

Bowen's disease (squamous cell carcinoma *in situ*) represents the next grade of neoplasia in the keratinocytic line; it is substantially less common than actinic keratoses. *Surgical removal* of the lesions of Bowen's disease is probably the most effective treatment. Alternatively, this tumor can be treated satisfactorily by *cryotherapy* with *liquid nitrogen* or *electrodessication* and *curettage*.

More-Advanced Squamous Cell Carcinomas

More-advanced squamous cell carcinomas are treated with surgical excision or radiation; the latter is usually reserved for people older than 60 years.

Melanomas

Melanomas can be divided into four histopathologic categories, each with a characteristic natural history and clinical course.

Superficial Spreading Melanoma

Superficial spreading melanoma is the most common type in the United States, representing 70% of all melanomas diagnosed. The early lesion exists for 1 to 7 years before a papule or nodule develops, which indicates that deep penetration has occurred. Before penetration, the lesion grows superficially, and its removal during this time is associated with a 5-year survival rate approaching 100%.

Nodular Melanoma

Nodular melanoma has a poorer prognosis. It may arise *de novo* or within a nevus as an invasive tumor from the onset. Even when the lesion is removed soon after it becomes clinically evident, metastasis may already have occurred in a substantial proportion of patients. This type of tumor can occur on any cutaneous surface, as can superficial spreading melanoma. Nodular melanoma represents about 15% of all melanomas. Prognosis is especially poor for those lesions found on the head and neck, particularly among older men with ulcerated lesions.

Lentigo Maligna Melanoma

Lentigo maligna melanoma, the third type, accounts for about 5% of melanomas and occurs on sun-damaged skin of older patients. It is the least aggressive of the melanomas and may be present for 5 or more years before dermal invasion develops. Prior to invasion, the lesion is termed *lentigo maligna*. Local excision with 5-mm margins is satisfactory for the treatment of lentigo maligna. In lentigo maligna melanoma, excision with wider margins is advocated. Surgical outcome in this type of tumor is almost uniformly favorable, although local recurrence is sometimes seen. It is unusual for a patient to die of disseminated lentigo maligna melanoma.

Acral Lentiginous Melanoma

Acral lentiginous melanoma occurs on palms, soles, subungual areas, and mucous membranes. This is the most common type to affect blacks and East Asians, but it may also occur in whites. The lesion begins as a flat, pigmented lesion that may be irregular in its border and pigment pattern. Early biopsy is essential to achieving cure before metastasis has occurred.

Prognosis for Melanoma

The most widely used system for estimating the prognosis of a patient with melanoma is that of Breslow, which uses the *thickness* of the primary tumor as the principal determinant. Tumor thickness is measured with an ocular micrometer on a standard microscope from the granular cell layer down to the deepest tumor cell. Lesions *with a thickness of less than 1.0 mm* have a nearly uniformly favorable prognosis (10-year survival of >90%), whereas those with a thickness of more than 4.0 mm have a fairly poor prognosis (10-year survival of <50%). In between these extremes are lesions of 1.0 to 2.0 mm (10-year survival of 80% unulcerated, 65% ulcerated) and 2.0 to 4.0 mm (10-year survival of 65% unulcerated, 55% ulcerated).

Treatment for Melanoma

Systems for determining prognosis are used to match treatment extent with the seriousness of the lesion.

Primary Melanoma. *Wide local excision* is the treatment recommended for primary melanoma. The width of excision in our institution is based on primary tumor thickness. For tumors up to 1.0 mm thick, 1.0-cm margins are recommended; 2-cm margins are recommended for tumors from 1.0 to 4.0 mm thick. *Sentinel lymph node biopsy* is useful as a staging procedure in intermediate-risk patients, enabling meaningful stratification for adjuvant therapy.

Disseminated Melanoma. Treatment remains difficult and unrewarding. Patients with advanced disease should be referred to a medical oncologist or cancer center experienced in the treatment of melanoma. Clinical trials should be considered. Because the prognosis in disseminated melanoma is poor, attempts are being made to use *adjuvant therapy* postoperatively in patients who are at high risk for recurrence. Only *interferon alfa 2b* has been shown to be beneficial in increasing disease-free survival and is approved for patients with stage III disease (nodal involvement).

The management of giant congenital nevi is controversial. Early surgical removal is necessary to reduce the risk of malignancy. Because the lifetime risk is estimated to be about 6% and the cosmetic consequences of surgery can be substantial, some advocate a wait-and-see approach with regular follow-up.

CLINICAL SCREENING AND DIAGNOSIS (1,2,9–15)

Skin cancers are unique among cancers in their accessibility and the relative ease with which a tissue diagnosis can be made.

Basal Cell Carcinomas

Basal cell carcinomas may take several forms. The typical appearance is that of a translucent *papule* with *telangiectases* over the surface (Fig. 177.2) that slowly enlarges, with subsequent development of a *central ulceration* (Fig. 177.3). This lesion has been termed the "rodent" ulcer. Basal cell carcinoma may also become pigmented in darker-skinned persons and be confused with melanoma of the nodular or superficial spreading type. Superficial forms of basal cell carcinoma exist, most commonly on

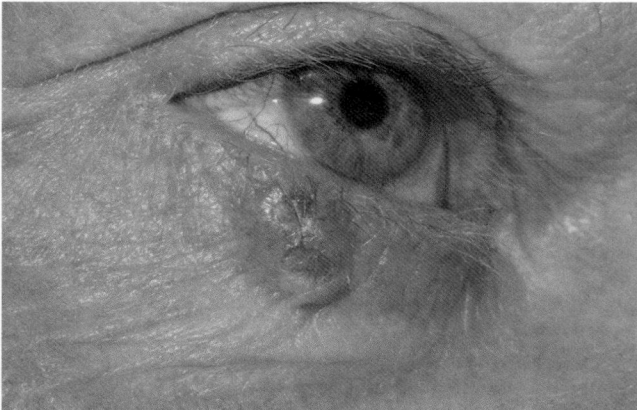

FIGURE 177.2. A typical nodular basal cell carcinoma with pearly texture and telangiectasia. (See the color insert.)

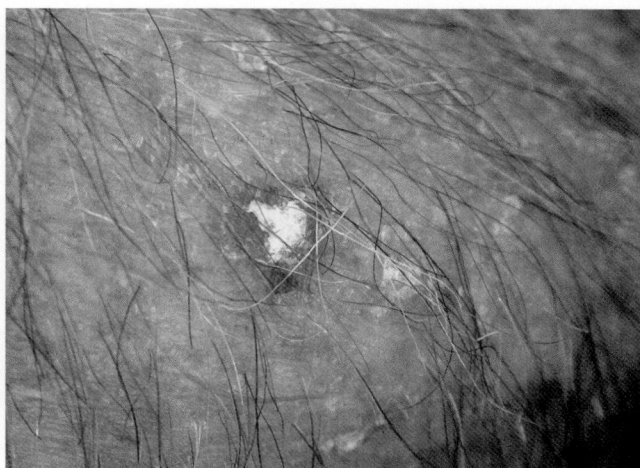

FIGURE 177.4. A keratotic papule characteristic of a hypertrophic actinic keratosis. (See the color insert.)

the back, which have the appearance of an *erythematous patch*. Superficial basal cell carcinomas are also becoming more common on the legs of women. In the sclerotic form of basal cell carcinoma, which resembles a scar (morpheaform basal cell carcinoma), nests of tumor cells are interspersed within thick fibrotic bundles. This tumor is more resistant to treatment.

The differential diagnosis of basal cell carcinoma includes dermal nevi and other appendage tumors, such as *trichoepithelioma*, which can look just like a basal cell carcinoma. On histopathologic examination of a basal cell carcinoma, proliferation of basophilic cells is seen, usually in nests surrounded by discrete lacunae located in the upper dermis. This tumor is relatively easy for the pathologist to diagnose microscopically. Because basal cell carcinomas are more common in persons who have already had one, patients should be followed on an annual basis for early detection of new lesions.

Squamous Cell Carcinoma

The precursor *actinic keratosis* appears as a scaly, erythematous patch that is flat to slightly raised; it may be single or

multiple and occurs in sun-exposed areas (Fig. 177.4). Often, this lesion is more easily felt (a sandpaper-like texture) than observed. It appears to evolve through cycles from a macular erythematous lesion to a raised scaly lesion. In the later stages, a crusted surface, and sometimes even a horn of keratin, develop. Histopathologic examination of these lesions reveals atypical keratinocytes in the basal layer of the epidermis.

Bowen's Disease

Bowen's disease, the carcinoma *in situ* stage, usually presents as a chronic, asymptomatic, nonhealing, slowly enlarging erythematous patch that generally has a sharp but irregular outline. It may resemble eczematous dermatitis but does not respond to topical steroid therapy (Fig. 177.5). Within the patch, areas of crusting are generally found. The sharp borders, chronicity, and lack of symptoms are clues that suggest the necessity of performing a biopsy. In dark-skinned patients, such as those of Mediterranean descent, these lesions may have a brownish coloration. Bowen's disease can occur on any part of the skin and on mucocutaneous sites, such as the vulva. In the vulvar area,

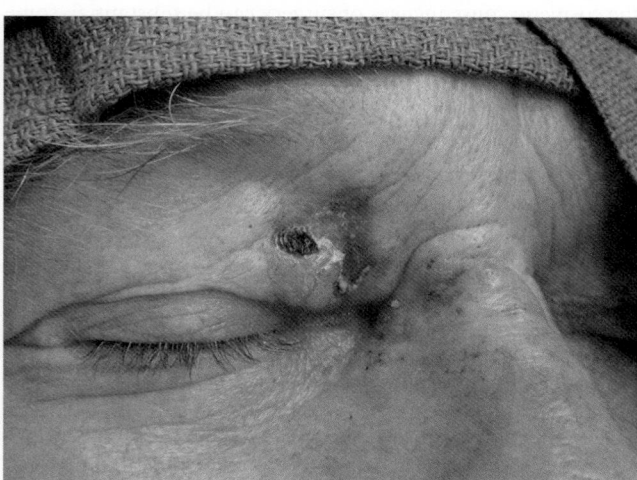

FIGURE 177.3. An ulcerated basal cell carcinoma; note the nodular and sclerotic components. (See the color insert.)

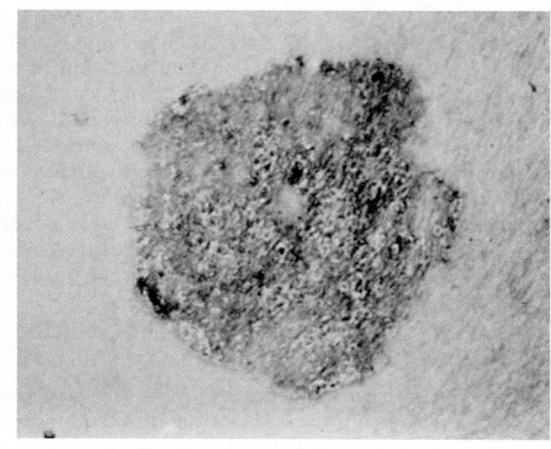

FIGURE 177.5. Bowen's disease—squamous cell carcinoma *in situ*.

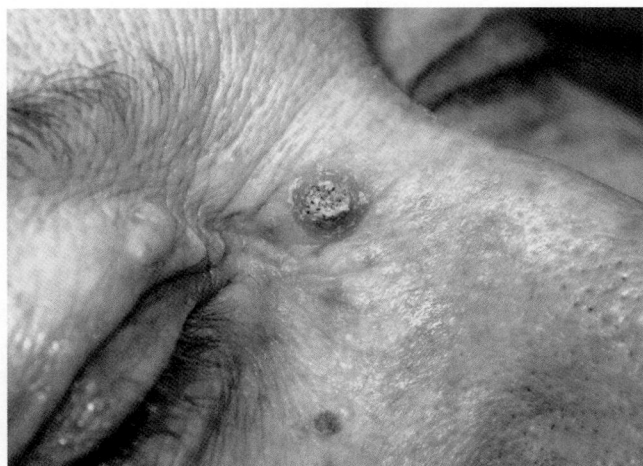

FIGURE 177.6. A keratotic papule, thicker and clinically tender, which was a squamous cell carcinoma. (See the color insert.)

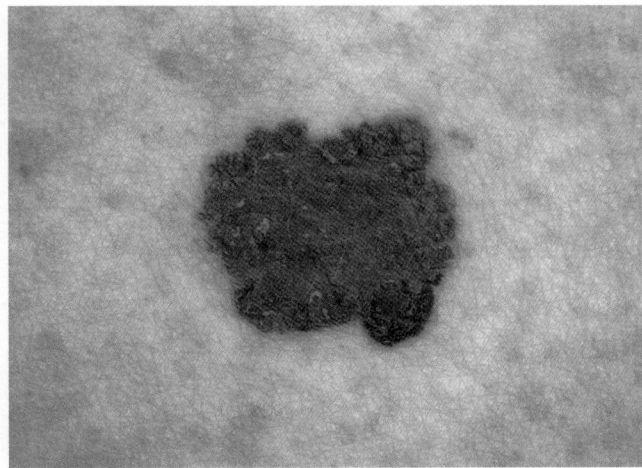

FIGURE 177.8. Superficial spreading melanoma. Note the notching, multiple colors, and regression in the center of the lesion. (See the color insert.)

the differential diagnosis includes lichen sclerosis et atrophicus, lichen simplex chronicus, squamous cell carcinoma, and, when the lesion is pigmented, melanoma. On histopathologic examination, atypical keratinocytes are noted throughout the epidermis but do not invade the dermis.

Invasive Squamous Cell Carcinoma

Invasive squamous cell carcinoma presents as a flesh-colored, asymptomatic nodule that enlarges and often undergoes ulceration and crusting (Fig. 177.6). The lesion may become keratotic and have a thickened surface. A cutaneous horn may be present. Microscopically, the squamous cell carcinoma has fingers of atypical keratinocytic cells infiltrating into the dermis. The nuclei are clearly atypical; mitoses are frequently found.

Squamous cell carcinoma may sometimes be confused with a benign keratinocytic lesion, *keratoacanthoma*, which is dome shaped and exhibits a prominent central plug (Fig. 177.7). Histopathologically, keratoacanthoma may be difficult for the pathologist to differentiate from squamous cell carcinoma. The keratoacanthoma usually exhibits more rapid growth and often regresses spontaneously.

Melanoma

The hallmarks include *asymmetry* (one half is not identical to the other) and *irregularity of the border* (sometimes a notch is present; Fig. 177.8), *variegation in the color* and *pigmentation pattern* (notably red, white, blue, and admixtures of these colors, such as grays and pinks), and *increasing size*. The recognition of suspected pigmented lesions that may represent early disease is facilitated by use of the mnemonic *ABCDE*:

A, *asymmetry* of lesion shape
B, *border* irregularity
C, *color* variegation
D, *diameter* greater than 6.0 mm (the size of a pencil eraser tip)
E, *evolution* or rapid change of the lesion

It should be emphasized that some melanomas are detected when the tumor is less than 6 mm in diameter.

Additional features seen in intermediate and advanced lesions include an *irregular raised surface* and *ulceration* or *bleeding* of the surface. Regardless of appearance, any pigmented lesion that undergoes change should be considered for biopsy. Each type of melanoma has distinguishing features clinically and histopathologically.

Superficial Spreading Melanomas

Superficial spreading melanomas have some irregularity in the border and some alteration in the regularity of pigment pattern and coloration (Fig. 177.8).

Nodular Melanoma

Nodular melanoma, which arises *de novo* or within nevi as an invasive tumor from the onset, has no radial growth component. It appears as a blue, blue-black, or gray nodule of varying size (Fig. 177.9). These lesions may be symmetric or have an irregular perimeter. Their borders are characteristically discrete and sharp. About 5% of nodular melanomas lack pigment (amelanotic melanoma). Most nodular lesions are considerably invasive at the time of diagnosis (>1 mm) and associated with a poor prognosis, especially when ulcerated and found on the head or neck in an older man.

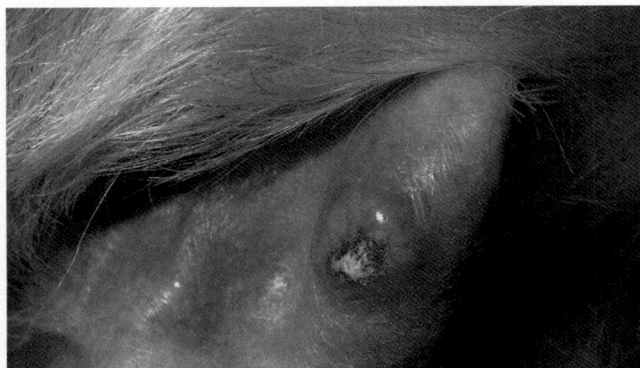

FIGURE 177.7. Keratoacanthoma with a crateriform appearance and a central keratin plug on the ear. (See the color insert.)

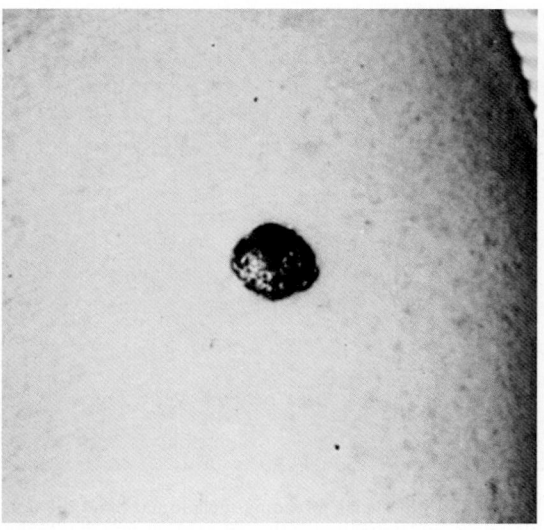

FIGURE 177.9. Melanoma, nodular type.

Lentigo Maligna

Lentigo maligna begins as a freckle-like lesion that slowly expands. It has a markedly irregular pigmentation pattern and usually an extremely irregular border (Fig. 177.10). Spontaneous regression may occur; the border may advance on one side while regressing on another, so that the lesion appears to march across the skin surface.

Acral Lentiginous

Acral lentiginous melanoma occurs on palms, soles, subungual areas, and mucous membranes, beginning as a flat, pigmented

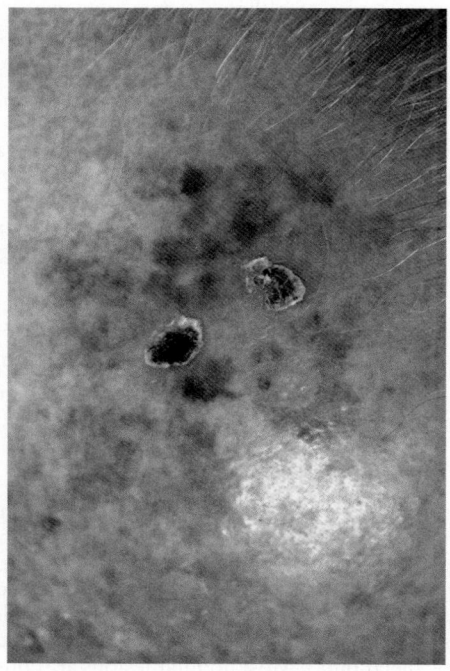

FIGURE 177.10. Lentigo maligna melanoma with indistinct borders and multiple colors. The crusts are secondary to biopsies. (See the color insert.)

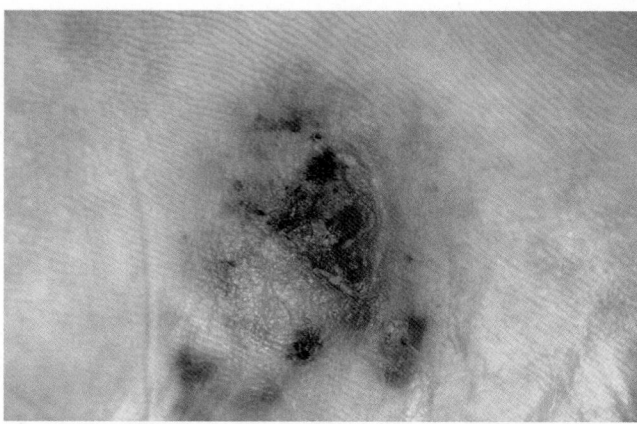

FIGURE 177.11. Acral lentiginous melanoma. There is a central vertical growth component, as well as ulceration and lateral pigment growth. This lesion was Clark level IV, 2.71 mm. (See the color insert.)

lesion that may be irregular in its border and pigment pattern (Fig. 177.11). Early biopsy is essential to achieving cure before metastasis has occurred.

The Distribution of Melanomas

The distribution of melanoma across the body surface is not uniform. In both sexes, lesions aggregate on the upper back. In female patients, the lower extremities from ankles to knees are heavily affected, but these areas are relatively spared in male patients, in whom the anterior torso is more likely to be involved. The bra and swim trunk areas are spared in females, and the swim trunk area and thighs are spared in males. Cutaneous melanomas of the head and neck are increasing in prevalence and, as noted, are associated with a worse prognosis, particularly in older men who present with nodular, ulcerated lesions.

Because a *second primary tumor* develops in up to 10% of patients with nonfamilial melanoma, it is worthwhile to examine the entire skin surface to look for a second tumor on each encounter. In familial melanoma, a second primary tumor may develop in as many as 30% of patients. Family members of patients who have had melanoma should be examined.

Differential Diagnosis of Melanoma

The preceding characteristics are sometimes found in *pigmented basal cell carcinoma* and pigmented lesions of *Bowen's disease*. In addition, odd dermal or *compound nevi*, irritated *seborrheic keratoses*, and occasionally vascular lesions can be clinically confused with melanoma. The *benign blue nevus* also shares similar clinical features. Biopsy and histopathologic evaluation are warranted if a lesion meets the criteria previously noted.

Staging of Disease.

Staging is best done by determining the depth of the lesion and noting any evidence for disease spread, especially lymphadenopathy; spread to lymph nodes occurs in 15% to 20% of persons. Sentinel-node biopsy adds prognostically useful information in persons with primary lesions of intermediate-thickness (1.2 to 3.5 mm), helping to identify individuals whose survival can be improved by immediate lymphadenectomy.

CONCLUSIONS AND RECOMMENDATIONS FOR SCREENING AND PREVENTION

Screening for skin cancer represents one of the best examples of early detection leading to an improved outcome. For example, the current 10-year survival rate for melanoma is greater than 90% if the thickness of a lesion is less than 1.0 mm and the tumor is not ulcerated. It is estimated that with education of patients and physicians about signs of disease and the importance of early diagnosis, the overall 5-year survival rate for malignant melanoma could approach 90%.

Every primary care provider should be able to recognize the common skin cancers, and patients should be taught to avoid environmental risk factors and report suspect lesions. In particular, the following precautions should be observed:

- All fair-skinned persons who sunburn easily and those with evidence of solar damage or skin cancer should be warned about the hazards of continued high-intensity solar exposure. They should be advised to avoid sun exposure between 11:00 a.m. and 2:30 p.m., the period during which 70% of exposure to harmful ultraviolet radiation occurs, and to avoid or minimize use of tanning devices, which are a source of ultraviolet radiation.

- All persons at risk for skin cancer should be advised to use a broad-spectrum sunscreen when going out into the sun. The preparation should block ultraviolet A in addition to ultraviolet B radiation and have a solar protection factor of at least 15.
- Patients with a history of exposure to arsenic or previous radiation therapy and radiation dermatitis should be watched closely for the development of cancer.
- For nonmelanoma skin cancer, patients should report to their physician any new, slowly growing, nodular or papular lesions that are flesh colored or translucent, and particularly the occurrence of any spontaneous bleeding, ulceration, or horn formation. Areas of maximum solar exposure are at greatest risk.
- For cutaneous melanoma, patients should report to their physician any pigmented lesion with an irregular border or a variation in color, especially blue, gray, or black. Any growth in a pigmented lesion or change in color should also arouse suspicion. Do not ignore head and neck regions.
- If any doubt exists about whether a skin lesion is benign, the obligation of the primary physician is either to obtain a sample of the lesion for biopsy or to refer the patient to an experienced specialist for an opinion. If patients and physicians work together, the incidence of skin cancer and the deaths associated with it can be greatly reduced

Annotated Bibliography

1. Alam M, Ratner D. Cutaneous squamous-cell carcinoma. N Engl J Med 2001;344:975. (*A comprehensive review; 71 references.*)
2. Jemal A, Siegel R, Ward E, et al. Cancer statistics, 2007. CA Cancer J Clin 2007;57:43. (*A useful source of epidemiologic data.*)
3. Karagas MR, Stannard VA, Mott LA, et al. Use of tanning devices and risk of basal cell and squamous cell skin cancers. J Nat Cancer Inst 2002;94:224. (*A case–control study of 1,500 persons; the odds ratio associated with the use of a tanning device was 1.5 for basal cell cancer and 2.5 for squamous cell cancer.*)
4. Miller AJ, Mihm MC. Melanoma. N Engl J Med 2006;355:51. (*A comprehensive review of disease mechanisms; 106 references.*)
5. Balch CM, Soong SJ, Gershenwald JE, et al. Prognostic factors analysis of 17600 melanoma patients: validation of the American Joint Committee on Cancer Melanoma Staging System. J Clin Oncol 2001;19:3622. (*Thickness and ulceration are the most important determinants of prognosis for localized melanoma.*)
6. Golger A, Young DS, Ghazarian D, et al. Incidence and prognosis of cutaneous melanoma involving the head and neck. Arch Otolaryngol Head Neck Surg 2007;133:442. (*Lesions of the head and neck had a particularly poor prognosis, especially if they were nodular and ulcerated.*)
7. Thompson SC, Jolley D, Marks R. Reduction of solar keratoses by regular sunscreen use. N Engl J Med 1993;329:1147. (*A study that supports the value of regular sunscreen use.*)
8. Tsao H, Atkins MB, Sober AJ. Management of cutaneous melanoma. N Engl J Med 2004;351:998. (*A comprehensive review*).
9. Alguire PC, Mathes BM. Skin biopsy technique for the internist. J Gen Intern Med 1998;13:46. (*A useful illustrated clinical review with a discussion of indications and technique.*)
10. Balch CM, Buzaid AC, Soong SJ, et al. Final version of the American Joint Committee on Cancer staging system for cutaneous melanoma. J Clin Oncol 2001;19:3635. (*Consensus staging system.*)
11. Elder D, Elenitsas R, Johnson BL, et al., eds. Lever's histopathology of the skin, 9th ed. Philadelphia: Lippincott Williams & Wilkins, 2004. (*An authoritative clinical and histopathologic description of cutaneous malignancies.*)
12. Rigel DS, Friedman R, Dzubow L, et al., eds. Cancer of the skin. Philadelphia: Elsevier, 2004. (*A compendium on all aspects of skin cancer.*)
13. Epstein DS, Lange JR, Gruber SB, et al. Is physician detection associated with thinner melanomas? JAMA 1999;281:640. (*A survey study, showing that physician-detected lesions were thinner and thus less advanced, evidence that screening pays off.*)
14. Morton DL, Thompson JF, Cochran AJ, et al. for the MSLT Group. N Engl J Med 2006;355:1307. (*Notes the value of this technique for staging intermediate-depth lesions and choosing therapy.*)
15. Whited JD, Grichnik JM. Does this patient have a mole or melanoma? JAMA 1998;279:696. (*Part of the Rational Clinical Examination series examining the accuracy and the yield of the skin examination.*)

CHAPTER 178 ■ EVALUATION OF PRURITUS

PETER C. SCHALOCK AND ARTHUR J. SOBER

Pruritus is an unpleasant cutaneous sensation that provokes the urge to scratch. It may be localized or generalized, or acute or chronic, and it may occur with or without skin lesions. In addition to the skin, it can occur on any epithelial surface, such as the conjunctivae, oropharynx, and anogenital region. Itching may be caused by a dermatologic condition, systemic illness, or psychological disturbance. The complaint is particularly common among the elderly, because the prevalence of itch increases with aging. It can prove especially challenging to the clinician when the etiology remains elusive and symptoms interfere with the patient's daily functioning. The primary physician should be capable of performing a reasonably detailed evaluation and providing effective symptomatic relief.

PATHOPHYSIOLOGY AND CLINICAL PRESENTATION (1–15)

Pathophysiology

The sensation of itching arises from a complex plexus of free nerve endings at the lower epidermis and dermal–epidermal junction in the skin, although an "itch receptor" remains elusive. These fibers are only found in the skin, especially concentrated in the flexor aspects of the wrist and ankles, and mucous membranes. Afferent transmission is through the myelinated A-delta and unmyelinated C fibers to the dorsal horn of the spinal cord, ascending to the contralateral spinothalamic tracts and terminating in the cerebral cortex. The scratch response is a spinal reflex and may abolish itch by central inhibition rather than attenuation of the peripheral sensory input. Many chemical mediators and modulators of itch have been suggested, including leukotriene B4, prostaglandin E2, substance P, histamine, opioid and nonopioid peptides, somatostatin, neurokinin A, leukotrienes, serotonin, kinins, acetylcholine (ACh), and prostaglandins. Histamine plays a direct link in causing itch in conditions such as urticaria and mastocytosis. Leukotriene B4 and prostaglandin E2 induce itch in human skin. ACh mediates itch in patients with atopic dermatitis.

Various external stimuli decrease the threshold for itching. These include inflammation, heat, dryness, and vasodilation. Persons vary in their response to itching. There is a psychological influence on the perception of itching, which explains why a health care worker may experience itching after attending a patient with scabies or pediculosis.

A possible classification system for itch divides this sensation into four distinct categories. *Neurogenic itch* arises from neurophysiologic dysfunction such as cholestasis or medications. *Neuropathic itch* is caused by a primary neurologic disorder. *Psychiatric itch* such as "delusions of parasitosis" is an-

other cause of pruritus. In the final category is the itch arising from skin disorders, *dermatologic itch*.

Clinical Presentation

Pruritus may be localized or generalized and can occur with or without skin lesions. Pruritus from a systemic disease can occur with or without a primary skin lesion.

Dermatologic Disease

A host of dermatologic conditions can present with itching.

Dry Skin (Xerosis). Dry skin (xerosis; see Chapter 183) is the most frequent precipitant and is particularly common in older individuals due to age-related decreased production of skin lipids. Symptoms are worse in low indoor humidity, especially in the winter or with use of air conditioning. Tangential light reveals fine scaling and cracking.

Urticaria. Urticaria (see Chapter 181) is a common skin disorder characterized by edematous, erythematous, coalescing *wheals* with pale centers. Although very itchy, urticaria generally persists for less than 24 hours, in contrast to urticarial vasculitis, which is a result of a small-vessel vasculitis, classically described clinically as burning, persisting beyond 24 hours, and associated with systemic complaints (especially gastrointestinal and musculoskeletal). Patients usually give a history of wheals and demonstrate dermographism (urticaria on stroking the skin with a blunt object).

Dermatitis Herpetiformis. Dermatitis herpetiformis can have a subtle presentation, with few skin manifestations, but vesicles are characteristic, although excoriations may obliterate them. Often, pruritus will cease once the vesicle is unroofed by scratching. An intense burning sensation often predates the appearance of skin lesions.

Scabies. Scabies can have a subtle presentation. Infestation is endemic in long-term care facilities, such as nursing homes and neuropsychiatric institutions. In persons with good hygiene, there may be fewer than 10 of the characteristic burrowing-induced skin lesions (Fig. 178.1) (see Chapter 195). At times, the only finding may be nonspecific papules caused by an immune skin response.

Atopic Dermatitis. Atopic dermatitis (also referred to by some as *eczema*) is a chronic, inflammatory, pruritic skin condition seen with increased frequency in patients with allergic rhinitis/seasonal allergies and a personal or family history of asthma (known as the "atopic triad"). A vicious itch–scratch cycle, in which scratching induces further inflammation and skin damage, often ensues. Unlike the other dermatologic disorders mentioned, atopic dermatitis lacks a primary skin lesion, and so the secondary changes produced by the inflammation are varied. A patient with chronic atopic dermatitis may exhibit scaly,

All photos are courtesy of Peter C. Schalock.

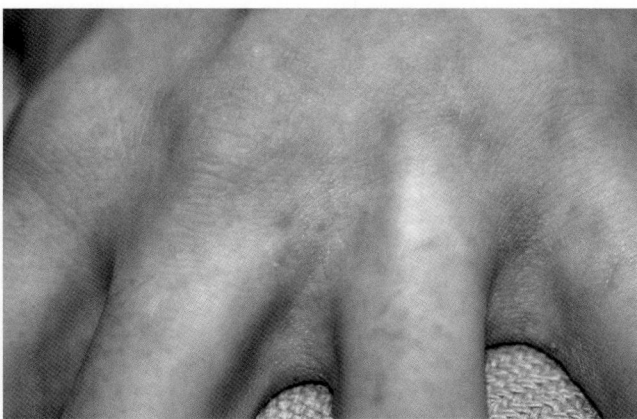

FIGURE 178.1. Papules and a single burrow (right) in the webspaces of a man with *Sarcoptes scabeii* infection. (See the color insert.)

hyper- or hypopigmented plaques with lichenification (thickened skin with accentuation of skin lines), or weeping, erythematous, and possibly superinfected papules and plaques during an acute phase.

Prurigo

Prurigo nodules are extremely pruritic, multiple, isolated hyperkeratotic nodules (Fig. 178.2) caused by a variety of

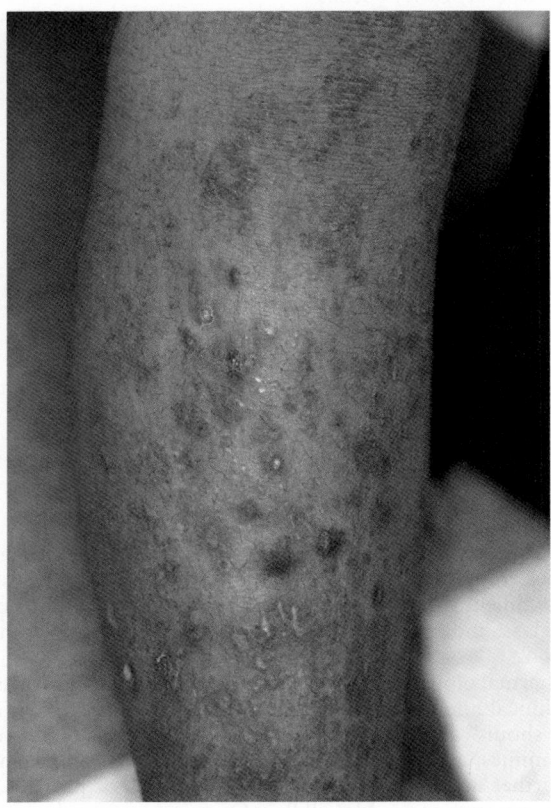

FIGURE 178.2. Multiple prurigo nodules on the leg of a man with bed bug bites. (See the color insert.)

etiologies, including atopy, pregnancy and systemic disease. Often, the cause is elusive. As in atopic dermatitis, often there is an vicious circle of itch–scratch. These nodules develop on the extremities as a result of picking rather than scratching and may be associated with an underlying anxiety disorder. Psychogenic/emotional causes are common.

Renal Disease

Pruritus may accompany severe chronic renal failure, especially in patients receiving *hemodialysis*, in which up to 80% may experience this unpleasant sensation. The pruritus of renal disease does not correlate with plasma histamine levels and is unresponsive to antihistamines. *Secondary hyperparathyroidism* causing hyperphosphatemia may contribute to pruritus in these patients. Other investigations have implicated neuropathy, anemia, general xerosis, and endopeptidases or kinins as substances that can accumulate in uremia.

Neuropathy

The main finding with neuropathy is usually paresthesia and not itching. Neuropathy often causes "pins and needles" type of sensations that evoke the desire to rub, not scratch. The most common dermatologic disease associated with pruritus is notalgia paresthetica, a condition of chronic upper back pruritus of unclear etiology, possibly from spinal nerve entrapment/trauma. Brachioradial pruritus presents as chronic intermittent pruritus of the brachioradial region of the arm and is an isolated neuropathy of the cutaneous branch of the radial nerve. Treatment for these conditions is discussed later.

Endocrine Disease

Generalized itching occurs among 4% to 11% of patients with *Graves' disease*, usually when the disease is longstanding. Increased kinin activity and augmented cutaneous blood flow resulting in elevated skin temperatures are suggested mechanisms. Hypothyroidism can also involve widespread pruritus, probably due to xerosis. The mechanisms for other endocrinopathies are poorly understood, although pruritus in diabetes may in some instances involve local irritation due to candidiasis.

Liver Disease

Among the many disorders of the liver, *obstructive cholestatic jaundice* produces the most pruritus. Itching may be especially prominent and can be the presenting manifestation in *primary biliary cirrhosis*, which occurs almost exclusively in middle-aged women. About 20% to 25% of patients with jaundice are plagued with itching, although it is rare in the absence of *cholestasis*. Nevertheless, there is little correlation between the serum bile salt concentration and itch intensity. Pruritus of cholestasis has been linked to opioid peptides and the release of proteases in the skin by the bile salts. Itching during the last trimester of *pregnancy*, called intrahepatic cholestasis of pregnancy or pruritus gravidarum, has been reported in 1% to 3% of expectant women and is believed to be cholestatic in origin, although jaundice is uncommon.

Hematologic Disease

Generalized pruritus in an elderly or middle-aged patient should prompt the clinician to consider an underlying malignancy and pursue a directed workup based on the history and physical exam. The itching affects 30% to 50% of patients with *polycythemia vera* (PCV), often on the lower extremities.

The itching is induced often by a hot shower or bath. Pruritus may precede the development of PCV by years. In *mycosis fungoides* (cutaneous T cell lymphoma), pruritus is exceedingly common and has been suggested as an adverse prognostic factor. *Hodgkin's disease* may also cause pruritus, although its role as a prognostic indicator is less than previously thought. Histamine release by an increased number of circulating basophils and cholestasis are postulated mechanisms for this type of itch. Pruritus has also been found in association with *iron-deficiency anemia*, although the mechanism is unexplained and there is no correlation between itch and disease severity. *Human immunodeficiency virus* (HIV) *infection* causes progressive itch in some patients, related possibly to hypereosinophilia, prostaglandin synthesis, and peripheral neuropathy. Pruritus has also been reported to occur in *Waldenström's macroglobulinemia*, *hypereosinophilic syndrome*, *multiple myeloma*, and *systemic mastocytosis*.

Psychiatric Disease

Patients with neurotic scratching report that they scratch even in the absence of itching. Itching is reported to occur more often at night, when other stimuli are lacking. Although the excoriations of this "neurodermatitis" may occur anywhere the patient can reach, they tend to be concentrated on the extremities. Depression and dysphoric mood are particularly common among such patients, as are serious conflict and situational stress preceding the onset of pruritus.

DIFFERENTIAL DIAGNOSIS

The conditions that cause itching may be dermatologic, systemic, or psychological in origin (Table 178.1). Skin disorders account for the vast majority. Pruritus may be localized or generalized. Localized itching is usually a sign of a primary dermatologic condition, dermatophyte infection, infestation, or psychological disorder. Generalized itching raises the possibility of a systemic condition or a psychogenic etiology, although dermatologic disease still predominates. In the older age groups, the most common cause of itching is xerosis.

WORKUP (1,3,5,7,10–12)

A search for a primary dermatologic disease or scabies infestation is the first step in the evaluation of the pruritic patient. Often a careful examination of the skin combined with a few clues from the history suggests the diagnosis. Skin diseases associated with recognizable lesions and characteristic distribution usually do not present significant diagnostic difficulty unless they are camouflaged by secondary changes like excoriations, lichenification, or infection. Systemic illnesses require a more detailed history and a physical examination that extends beyond the skin, followed by selected laboratory studies.

History

Location, associated symptoms, precipitants, clinical course, and severity (including effect on sleep and daily activity) should be carefully elicited. A detailed description of any skin changes or rashes should be included. If the patient reports little in the way of skin findings, clues to an underlying dermatologic condition should still be sought. For example, a history of atopy, asthma, or urticaria raises the probability of an allergic origin,

TABLE 178.1

CONDITIONS ASSOCIATED WITH PRURITUS

Dermatologic
  Arthropod/insect bites and stings
  Bullous pemphigoid
  Dermatitis
    Atopic dermatitis
    Contact dermatitis (allergic and irritant)
    Dermatitis herpetiformis
  Dermatophytosis
  Infestation
    Scabies
    Pediculosis
  Lichen planus
  Lichen simplex chronicus
  Pityriasis rosea
  Psoriasis
  Urticaria and dermatographism
  Varicella
  Xerosis

Psychological
  Neurotic excoriations
  Depression
  Delusions of parasitosis

Systemic
  Hyperthyroidism/hypothyroidism
  Renal failure, chronic
  Drug reaction
  Hematologic disease
    Iron-deficiency anemia
    Mycosis fungoides
    Polycythemia vera
    Paraproteinemia
    Systemic mastocytosis
  Hepatobiliary problems
    Intrahepatic cholestasis
    Extrahepatic obstruction
    Third trimester of pregnancy
  Malignancy
    Malignant carcinoid
    Lymphoma, leukemia
    Multiple myeloma
  HIV infection
  Parasitosis
    Ascariasis
    Hookworm
    Onchocerciasis
    Trichinosis

whereas concurrent pruritus in household members suggests scabies, and exacerbation in winter months points to dry skin. Environmental factors such as sunburn, "prickly heat," cats, fiberglass, and excessive drying of the skin also deserve consideration.

Pharmacologic exposure is important to review because a subclinical allergic reaction may occur with almost any drug. One should also check specifically for use of opiates, amphetamines, quinidine, aspirin, B vitamins, and nicotinamide. To further assist the clinician with evaluation of pruritus, instruments such as the McGill Pain Questionnaire or the Visual-Analog Scale may be useful.

In the setting of generalized pruritus, one should inquire about symptoms or a history of hyperthyroidism (see Chapter 103), renal failure (see Chapter 142), lymphoma (see Chapter 84), polycythemia (see Chapter 80), cholestatic liver disease (see Chapter 62), and HIV infection (see Chapter 13). Pregnancy as a cause of itch should be considered in women of childbearing age.

If the cause is not evident from the medical history, it is worth exploring psychosocial aspects of the patient's life and any relation between psychological or situational stresses and the onset of pruritus. Given the high prevalence of depression among patients with idiopathic pruritus, inquiry into symptoms of depression (see Chapter 227) may prove useful. In patients hospitalized for severe itch, consultation with a psychiatrist was of benefit for many patients.

Physical Examination

A careful and complete inspection of the skin is essential. The presence and distribution of a rash, excoriations, lichenification, and inflammatory changes should be noted, along with any evidence of xerosis (scaling and dryness). Dry skin is especially evident on the legs; tangential lighting can help reveal the subtle scaling.

If the complaint is localized pruritus, a more detailed look at the involved area is needed. The scalp is checked for psoriasis and seborrhea; the trunk for urticaria, scabies, and the well-defined lesions of contact dermatitis; the inguinal area for *Candida* or dermatophyte infection, pediculosis, tinea, and scabies; the hands for eczema, contact dermatitis, and the tell-tale interdigital lesions of scabies; the legs for neurotic excoriations, stasis dermatitis, atopic dermatitis (popliteal fossa), lichen simplex (lateral malleoli), and dermatitis herpetiformis (knees); and the feet for tinea or contact dermatitis. Atopic patients may exhibit prominent infraorbital folds (known as Dennie–Morgan lines), hyperlinear palmoplantar creases, patches of hypopigmentation on the arms and face (pityriasis alba), or horny follicular plugs on the face and extremities (keratosis pilaris).

If the pruritus is generalized and there is no evidence of primary dermatologic disease, a search for signs of a systemic condition is warranted. The skin is examined for jaundice and findings associated with HIV disease (see Chapter 13), and the sclerae are checked for icterus, the lymph nodes for enlargement, the thyroid for goiter, and the liver and spleen for organomegaly.

Laboratory Studies

Test selection should be based on findings from the history and the physical examination. Resorting initially to an extensive workup is wasteful and likely to generate false-positive results that are further frustrating to both the clinician and the patient. *Skin scrapings* are performed to confirm a clinical diagnosis of dermatophytosis or scabies (see Fig. 178.3 for an example of a scabies mite) (see Chapters 195 and 191, respectively). A *skin biopsy* examination with special stains or *direct immunofluorescence* may be required to confirm a diagnosis of one of the autoimmune bullous diseases or mastocytosis. If cutaneous T cell lymphoma is suspected, multiple skin biopsies and T cell gene rearrangement studies can be helpful. In the setting of suspected cholestasis, one should order *serum bilirubin*, *alkaline phosphatase*, and *transaminase levels* and obtain an

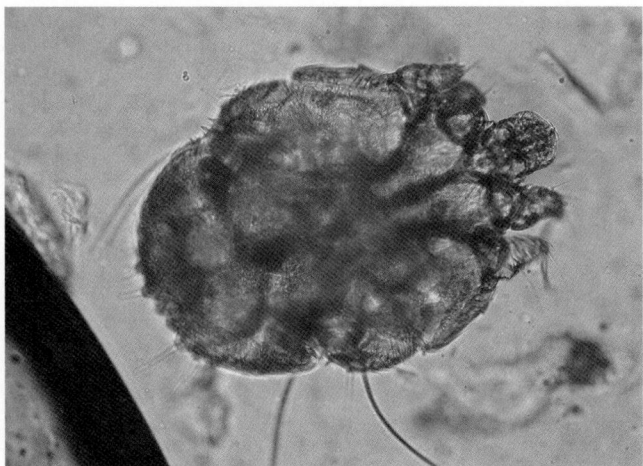

FIGURE 178.3. Scabies mite. (See the color insert.)

ultrasound of the biliary tree (see Chapter 62). If there is concern for lymphoma or carcinoid, a *chest x-ray* or *abdominal computed tomography* may be indicated (see Chapters 44 and 84). *HIV testing* is indicated if the patient has risk factors for infection (see Chapter 13).

If the diagnosis continues to be elusive, then a *complete blood count*, *blood urea nitrogen*, *thyroid-stimulating hormone*, *calcium*, *albumin*, and *globulin* are worth considering. Pruritus per se is not a predictor of malignancy and need not trigger a workup for occult malignancy in the absence of other clinical evidence for cancer.

SYMPTOMATIC THERAPY AND PATIENT EDUCATION (8–18)

To be most effective, treatment of pruritus should be based on etiology if possible. However, nonspecific symptomatic measures are often required, especially if a workup is still in progress and the itching is disturbing sleep and/or interfering with daily life. Symptomatic treatment is also indicated for refractory conditions (e.g., biliary cirrhosis). Even if little can be done for the underlying condition, relief from itching is greatly appreciated by the patient and enhances the patient–physician alliance. Avoidance of provocative factors is important, complemented by simple empiric therapy of low toxicity. Counseling the patient on how to overcome the itch–scratch–itch cycle is most beneficial.

Behavioral and Topical Measures

Behavioral Measures

Behavioral measures can be significantly helpful regardless of etiology and often reduce or eliminate itching without the need to resort to additional therapies. Patients should be told to *trim fingernails*, keep them clean to prevent infection, *rub* with their palms rather than their fingers if they have an uncontrollable urge to scratch, and cover the pruritic area with *an Unna boot*. If coffee, spices, or alcohol precipitate itching, they should be avoided. Rough clothing, particularly wool, should be avoided. *Cotton clothing* that has been doubly rinsed of detergents is preferred. *Humidification* of the indoor environment should be maintained, both when using an air conditioner and during the winter, in either case with humidifiers. Avoiding frequent, hot, prolonged showers is recommended because they eliminate the skin's lubricants and moisture, contributing to dryness. Use of *mild soaps* (Dove, Basis, Neutrogena, Purpose, Aveeno Bar) is preferred to heavily perfumed soap products or liquid soap/bodywashes, which are drying. Use of *cool to warm water* is preferred to hot water because the latter worsens itching by increasing cutaneous blood flow and transepidermal water loss. *Sponging the skin* with cool water is also effective, but it is not recommended for patients with xerosis.

Topical Measures

Physicians should be familiar with several available *lotions* and *creams*. *Emollient preparations* such as Vaseline or Aquaphor are preferred, but creams (Cetaphil, Purpose, Curel, Oil of Olay, and Aveeno) are acceptable if the patient is unwilling to use an ointment. Application immediately after showering, when the skin is partially moist, is ideal. Application of a moisturizer before bed can be helpful. Preparations containing combinations of *menthol* and *phenol* (e.g., Sarna Lotion) applied as necessary may provide symptomatic relief. *Calamine* may alleviate itching briefly but is drying; it is most useful on weeping lesions. *Pramoxine-containing products* (PrameGel, Prax, Pramosone) also may reduce itching, but topical antihistamines (diphenhydramine/doxepin) should be avoided because they can be potent sensitizers.

Topical Anesthetics. *Capsaicin*, a plant isolate that depletes substance P from C fibers, can be applied three to five times daily in cases of notalgia paresthetica, brachioradial pruritus. and pruritus from uremia. However, capsaicin may be initially poorly tolerated due to local burning. *Local anesthetics* like benzocaine, lidocaine, and tetracaine, as well as the nonionic surfactant *polidocanol*, have proven benefits, but the anesthetics, except for lidocaine, may cause a contact dermatitis. *Topical aspirin*, rather than oral administration, has demonstrated antipruritic effects, especially in patients with chronic atopic dermatitis, but this is not commercially available. *Doxepin*, a tricyclic antidepressant available as a cream, is relatively expensive and not as effective as the oral preparation and can be a potent contact sensitizer.

Topical Glucocorticosteroids. Topical glucocorticosteroids can be helpful. *Hydrocortisone* 1% or 2.5% lotion, cream, or ointment may provide symptomatic relief of itch; higher-potency corticosteroids should be restricted to specific steroid-responsive inflammatory dermatoses (such as atopic dermatitis or psoriasis) because prolonged use can cause dermal atrophy.

Systemic Measures. If environmental manipulation and topical agents are not effective, then systemic medications must be considered. The systemic medications most commonly used are oral antihistamines, especially in the more common pruritic skin conditions, atopic dermatitis, and urticaria.

Antihistamines. By occupying the histamine receptors, these agents are very effective for allergen-mediated itch; however, their sedating qualities account for much of their benefit, especially in itch not mediated by histamine. Furthermore, nonsedating second- and third-generation antihistamines are often ineffective. The sedative quality of first-generation histamine$_1$(H_1)-blocker antihistamines makes them especially useful as a bedtime medication in patients with sleep difficul-

ties. The ideal agent is found by trial and error on the basis of the placebo, sedative, and anticholinergic effects of the drug. *Hydroxyzine* (e.g., 25 mg thrice daily or 50 mg at bedtime) is among the most effective. It is mildly to moderately sedating and more effective than diphenhydramine or cyproheptadine, other commonly used antihistamines. *Diphenhydramine* is available without prescription and is very sedating. Although nonsedating, the metabolite of hydroxyzine, *cetirizine* (Zyrtec), is an excellent antipruritic agent when used in doses of 5 to 10 mg daily, after which a lower maintenance dose can be used. Nonsedating antihistamines such as loratadine (Claritin) and fexofenadine (Allegra) are useful for daytime use where histamine plays a primary role, such as in some urticarias, but are generally disappointing as antipruritics and do little to help the patient fall asleep. H_2-blockers are believed to enhance the effect of H_1-blockers, but they are generally ineffective in the treatment of idiopathic pruritus. Nonetheless, cimetidine has been reported to be useful in itching associated with polycythemia, uremia, urticaria, and Hodgkin's lymphoma.

Antiinflammatory Agents. Mild antiinflammatory agents such as *aspirin* are occasionally useful for symptomatic relief, especially if the suspected mechanism is kinin or prostaglandin mediated. *Systemic steroids* suppress itching, but they should not be used for symptomatic relief unless a severe allergic disorder is suspected and has failed to respond to conventional treatments.

Sedatives. The *benzodiazepines* can be useful in acute circumstances associated with anxiety and difficulty in falling asleep, but chronic use is to be avoided because of the risk of habituation (see Chapter 226). *Antidepressants* like paroxetine (a selective serotonin reuptake inhibitor) may help relieve itch at doses of 5 to 10 mg daily in patients with or without evidence of depression. Relief occurs in several days, too soon to be from its effect on depression. Patients should be aware that nausea and sedation are common side effects. Oral *doxepin*, a tricyclic antidepressant, at 25 to 75 mg at bedtime is particularly useful, but the physician should be aware that concurrent use of monoamine oxidase inhibitors and drugs that inhibit cytochrome P450 (such as cimetidine, imidazoles, antifungals, and macrolide antibiotics) should be discontinued. Topical doxepin is a potent sensitizer causing allergic contact dermatitis. *Pimozide,* a neuroleptic, is effective for treating delusions of parasitosis. The intravenously infused opiate antagonist *naloxone* has been shown in some studies to improve acute itch from cholestasis and the oral opioid antagonist naltrexone in cases of chronic pruritus, but further studies are warranted.

Chelating Agents. *Cholestyramine* and *colestipol* are used with benefit for cholestatic itching, including the pruritus of pregnancy. *Ultraviolet radiation* (narrow-band ultraviolet B, psoralens with ultraviolet A) can be used for renal and biliary pruritus, as well as itching associated with other systemic and primary dermatologic disorders. Recalcitrant uremic pruritus has been treated with *photochemotherapy*, intravenous *lidocaine, activated charcoal, intravenous erythropoietin, plasmapheresis*, and *parathyroidectomy*, with varying degrees of success.

Other Agents

Opioid antagonists can be helpful in uremic pruritus and in some cases of intractable generalized pruritus. The mu-opioid-receptor antagonist naltrexone may be effective in cases of cholestatic pruritus and intractable pruritus, especially itch at nighttime. The selective serotonin reuptake inhibitors, especially paroxetine, are helpful in cases of uremic pruritus. Their effect is usually rapid, probably on the serotonin type 3 receptor, thus suggesting that the α1-type receptors that cause the antidepressant effects are not involved. Mirtazapine is a presynaptic α2-adrenergic antagonist with H_1-blocking effects. It can be effective for short-term treatment of itch associated with lymphoma, uremia, and cholestasis, as well as nocturnal itch. Mirtazapine is usually effective for no more than 1 month.

INDICATIONS FOR REFERRAL

The patient with refractory or idiopathic pruritus poses a very frustrating problem, which often benefits from a dermatologic consultation and the consideration of skin biopsy. When pruritus represents a somatic response to psychological distress, it may be useful to discuss considering a mental health referral with the patient. The consultation suggests to the patient that the problem is being taken seriously and that everything is being done to address both its cause and the patient's discomfort.

Annotated Bibliography

1. Ikoma A, Steinhoff M, Ständer S, et al. The neurobiology of itch. Nat Rev Neurosci 2006;7:535. (*A well-written discussion of the pathophysiology of itch and its relation to pain; 206 references.*)
2. Paus R, Schmelz M, Biro T, et al. Frontiers in pruritus research: scratching the brain for more effective itch therapy. J Clin Invest 2006;116:1174. (*An excellent review of the neurobiology of itch.*)
3. Charlesworth EN, Beltrani VS. Pruritic dermatoses: overview of etiology and therapy. Am J Med 2002;113(Suppl 9A):25S. (*A brief but comprehensive summary and update on the recent understanding of pruritus and its treatment.*)
4. Fruensgaard K. Neurotic excoriations: a controlled psychiatric examination. Acta Psychiatr Scand 1984;69(Suppl 312):3. (*There is a high prevalence of depression; lesions are often confined to the extremities.*)
5. Fleischer AB Jr. Pruritus in the elderly. Adv Dermatol 1995;10:41. (*A review that considers evaluation and emphasizes the utility of the history for diagnosis.*)
6. Schneider G, Driesch G, Heuft G, et al. Psychosomatic cofactors and psychiatric comorbidity in patients with chronic itch. Clin Exp Dermatol 2006;31:762. (*A review of 109 inpatients with pruritus; 60% of the patients had psychiatric treatment recommended.*)
7. Greco PJ, Ende J. Pruritus: a practical approach. J Gen Intern Med 1992;7:340. (*A very useful evaluation strategy is outlined.*)
8. De Marchi S, Cecchin E, Villalta D, et al. Relief of pruritus and decreases in plasma histamine concentrations during erythropoietin therapy in patients with uremia. N Engl J Med 1992;326:969. (*Significantly decreased pruritus and lowered plasma histamine concentrations were found in 20 patients with uremia.*)
9. Kantor GR, Bernhard JD. Investigation of the pruritic patient in daily practice. Semin Dermatol 1995;14:290. (*A practical approach to evaluation and treatment, with many useful tables.*)
10. Khandelwal M, Malet PF. Pruritus associated with cholestasis: a review of pathogenesis and management. Dig Dis Sci 1994;39:1. (*A comprehensive look at this difficult problem.*)
11. Chosidow O. Scabies. N Engl J Med 2006;354:1718. (*A review of scabies infection and treatment options; 38 references.*)
12. Lober CW. Should the patient with generalized pruritus be evaluated for malignancy? J Am Acad Dermatol 1988;19:350. (*Patients with persistent pruritus do not show an increased risk for malignant disease when carefully compared with age- and sex-matched nonpruritic controls.*)
13. Paul R, Paul R, Jansen CT. Itch and malignancy prognosis in generalized pruritus: a 6-year follow-up of 125 patients. J Am Acad Dermatol 1987;16:1179. (*There was no increased risk for malignancy in persons with generalized pruritus followed for 6 years.*)
14. Wallengren J. Prurigo: diagnosis and management. Am J Clin Dermatol 2004;5:85. (*A comprehensive review of prurigo; 69 references.*)
15. Yosipovitch G, Fleischer A. Itch associated with skin disease: advances in pathophysiology and emerging therapies. Am J Clin Dermatol 2003;4:617. (*A practical review of the neurophysiologic research on pruritus with practical clinical relevance.*)
16. Breneman DL, Cardone JS, Blumsack RF, et al. Topical capsaicin for treatment of hemodialysis-related pruritus. J Am Acad Dermatol 1992;26:91. (*Topical capsaicin four times daily relieved hemodialysis-related pruritus in 10 of 14 patients.*)
17. Greaves MW. Itch in systemic disease: therapeutic options. Dermatol Ther 2005;18:323. (*A thorough review of treatment options in systemic itch.*)
18. Teofoli P, Procacci P, Maresca M, et al. Itch and pain. Int J Dermatol 1996;35:159. (*An excellent review; 98 references.*)

CHAPTER 179 ■ EVALUATION OF PURPURA

Purpura represents bleeding into the skin. In the office setting, patients present with easy bruising, spontaneous ecchymoses, or a petechial rash. Although many cases of purpura are caused by unappreciated trauma, patients who report easy bruising or spontaneous ecchymoses need to be evaluated for an underlying bleeding disorder (see Chapter 81). Those with petechial rashes may have a platelet problem, vasculitis, or a bacteremia. The primary physician should be able to make these distinctions and efficiently initiate the evaluation and any necessary referrals.

PATHOPHYSIOLOGY AND CLINICAL PRESENTATION (1–6)

The integrity of small vessels is maintained by quantitatively and qualitatively adequate platelets and by healthy connective tissue. Normally, a break in a vessel triggers prompt formation of a platelet plug followed by a fibrin clot. Purpura occurs when the integrity of the vessel wall or the mechanisms of hemostasis are disturbed.

Purpura is divided into petechial and ecchymotic categories. *Petechiae* are red macules that measure less than 3 mm in diameter; they reflect a defect in platelets or vessel walls. When caused by disturbances of platelets, petechiae appear in dependent areas, such as the ankles and lower legs (see Chapter 81). Immune-mediated inflammation of small vessels may also produce petechial macules, which sometimes progress to palpable lesions (so-called *palpable purpura*; see later discussion).

Ecchymoses are purpuric lesions larger than 3 mm in diameter. They may result from trauma or a clotting factor disorder, as well as from a vascular or platelet problem. Clotting factor dysfunction causes delayed but more prolonged blood loss, during which continuous oozing secondary to inadequate fibrin clot formation results in ecchymoses rather than petechiae (see Chapter 81).

The mechanisms of purpura can be divided into the thrombocytopenic, thrombocytopathic, coagulopathic, vascular, connective tissue, and idiopathic varieties. The first three are discussed in detail in Chapter 81. The vascular, connective tissue, and idiopathic varieties require further elaboration here.

Vascular Defects

These range from mild disruption of the endothelium to necrotizing injury. The latter are the more important.

Small-Vessel Vasculitis

Leukocytoclastic vasculitis of small vessels is capable of damaging vessel walls and causing *palpable purpura*. It may develop in the context of a *hypersensitivity reaction*, *rheumatoid disease*, *dysproteinemias*, and *systemic vasculitis* associated with positive *antineutrophil cytoplasmic antibodies (ANCAs)* (Table 179.1). Immunologically mediated, necrotizing neutrophilic infiltration of arterioles, capillaries, and venules occurs. The process can be limited to the vessels of the skin or involve small to medium-sized vessels of any organ; renal and pulmonary involvement are common and potentially life threatening in the ANCA-positive systemic vasculidities. In rheumatoid disease, the postcapillary venules are the principal site of leukocytoclastic injury; systemic involvement is the rule.

The skin lesions of leukocytoclastic vasculitis typically begin as small macules that become palpable and may turn confluent or nodular. The petechial papules do not blanch; they appear in symmetric fashion and predominate in dependent areas. Urticaria, vesicles, and necrotic ulcerations may also develop. Fever, arthralgias, myalgias, arthritis, pulmonary infiltrates, effusions, pericarditis, peripheral neuropathy, abdominal pain, bleeding, and encephalopathy can occur along with the petechial rash if systemic involvement is present. The skin commonly itches, stings, or burns. *Hematuria* and *proteinuria* indicate renal injury; pulmonary *infiltrates* suggest intrathoracic involvement.

Bacteremia

Bacteremia can lead to vascular injury and the formation of petechiae, which are sometimes palpable. Petechial lesions associated with *subacute bacterial endocarditis* are flat, do not blanch, and appear on the upper chest, neck, and extremities in addition to the mucous membranes. In *gonococcal* and *meningococcal septicemias*, petechiae develop early, become pustular, and then turn hemorrhagic and necrotic. The lower extremities are a common site for the gonococcal lesions, which resolve within 5 to 7 days. The rash of *Rocky Mountain spotted fever* begins as pink macules on the wrists, soles, ankles,

TABLE 179.1

IMPORTANT CAUSES OF LEUKOCYTOCLASTIC SMALL-VESSEL VASCULITIS

ANCA Associated
  Drug-induced ANCA associated
  Wegener's granulomatosis
  Microscopic polyangiitis
  Churg–Strauss syndrome

Immune Complex
  Rheumatoid disease (e.g., lupus, rheumatoid arthritis, Sjögren's syndrome)
  Cryoglobulinemia (mixed type)
  Drug-induced immune complex (penicillins, thiazides, aspirin, amphetamines)
  Henoch–Schönlein purpura
  Serum sickness
  Goodpasture's syndrome

Inflammatory Bowel Disease
  Ulcerative colitis
  Primary biliary cirrhosis
  Chronic active hepatitis

Paraneoplastic
  Lymphoproliferative disease
  Myeloproliferative disease
  Carcinoma

ANCA, antineutrophil cytoplasmic autoantibody.
Adapted from Jennette JC, Falk RJ, Andrassey K, et al. Nomenclature of systemic vasculitides: proposal of an international consensus conference. Arthritis Rheum 1994;37:187, with permission.

and palms. The rash spreads centripetally and by the fourth day becomes petechial and papular. Hemorrhagic, ulcerated lesions may follow.

Other Forms of Vascular Injury

In *stasis dermatitis*, petechial lesions in the legs result from capillary injury. *Scurvy* compromises the vascular endothelium, and perifollicular purpura develops because of increased capillary fragility. In *amyloidosis*, the deposition of amyloid in the skin and subcutaneous tissue causes fragile vessels, with ecchymoses forming when the skin is pinched.

Connective Tissue Defects

Defects in connective tissue can compromise vessel walls and supportive extravascular structures and lead to easy bruising. When caused by the degeneration of dermal collagen because of *age* or *corticosteroid use*, ecchymoses may develop after trivial injury and be noticed on the face, neck, dorsum of the hands, forearms, or legs. A variant is stasis or *orthostatic purpura*, which usually develops in the lower extremities of an elderly patient after a prolonged period of standing.

Idiopathic Causes

Idiopathic causes include *autoerythrocyte sensitization*, a puzzling form of purpura characterized by spontaneous, painful ecchymoses surrounded by erythema and edema. Headache, nausea, and vomiting sometimes accompany the purpura. Many patients with this condition also have pronounced psychoneurotic complaints. The mechanism is unknown, but intradermal injection of autologous red cells or DNA can reproduce the clinical picture.

Purpura simplex or *easy-bruising syndrome* is an idiopathic condition of young women in otherwise good health. All platelet and bleeding parameters are normal, and the risk for hemorrhage during surgery or childbirth is not increased.

Platelet and Clotting Factor Disorders

Platelet and clotting factor disorders are important etiologic factors and discussed in detail elsewhere (see Chapter 81).

DIFFERENTIAL DIAGNOSIS (1–5)

As noted earlier, causes of purpura can be divided into thrombocytopenic, thrombocytopathic, clotting factor, vascular, connective tissue, and idiopathic categories (see also Chapter 81). Purpura associated with trauma or drug-induced impairment of platelet function, benign purpura simplex, and senile purpura are the most common forms. Vasculitis is particularly troublesome because of the wide range of potentially important causes (Table 179.1).

WORKUP (1–5)

The workup of the patient with purpuric lesions must emphasize the history and physical examination to avoid costly, nonproductive laboratory evaluations. The clinical findings are also essential in quickly differentiating serious hematologic, vasculitic, or infectious pathologies from more-benign processes. For example, ecchymoses smaller than 6 cm and localized to such areas of trauma as the thighs are less likely to be of pathologic significance than are larger ones; palpable purpuric lesions indicate a vasculitic process; and petechial macules in dependent areas suggest a problem with platelets.

History

A careful description of the location, size, and clinical course of the purpuric lesions, along with an inquiry into associated symptoms and precipitants, constitutes the essence of the history. One should quickly screen for a bleeding diathesis by inquiring about blood loss from other sites; easy bruisability; bleeding into a joint; a history of abnormally heavy bleeding with menstruation, surgery, or dental work; and a family history of a bleeding problem. A review of medications is essential, with a focus on agents that can interfere with platelet function (e.g., aspirin, nonsteroidal antiinflammatory drugs [NSAIDs], dipyridamole, ticlopidine, sulfinpyrazone) and those associated with hypersensitivity reactions that affect platelets (e.g., antibiotics, quinidine, phenothiazines). Any history of renal or hepatocellular failure is important to note.

Patients with an early petechial rash or palpable purpura should be carefully checked for fever, pruritus, joint pain, urticaria, dry mouth/dry eyes, morning stiffness, pleuritic pain, abdominal pain, melena, hematuria, lymphadenopathy, jaundice, symptoms of inflammatory bowel disease, chronic leg edema, and paresthesias. A recent streptococcal or staphylococcal infection may be responsible for a hypersensitivity vasculitis and should be noted. Medications to be reviewed include recent use of a penicillin, a thiazide, aspirin, or amphetamines.

If fever is prominent, bacteremia must be considered, and the patient should be asked about recent purulent penile or vaginal discharge, pelvic pain, other recent infection, intravenous drug abuse, HIV infection, and history of a heart murmur or recent dental work.

Physical Examination

Physical examination begins with inspection of the skin lesions. If they appear petechial, it is useful to press a glass slide over them. Failure to blanch helps to differentiate petechiae from nonpurpuric skin lesions. However, blanching lesions must not be dismissed too hastily because telangiectases and spider angiomata are signs of conditions predisposing to purpura (see Chapter 81). Shining a light tangentially to the skin is a sensitive means of detecting elevated lesions, which may be confirmed by careful palpation. The size, number, and location of purpuric lesions should be recorded, and note should be made of whether they are palpable or macular, petechial, or ecchymotic. It is sometimes helpful to circle ecchymoses so that extension or regression can be followed objectively.

If the history suggests a bleeding problem or if the physical examination reveals petechiae in dependent areas or large ecchymoses, then the physical examination should be directed toward hematologic causes (see Chapter 81).

If palpable purpura is present, then the physical examination should include inspection for splinter hemorrhages, rheumatoid nodules, a separate malar rash, dry mucous membranes, jaundice, lymphadenopathy, pleural effusion, heart murmur, pericardial rub, hepatic abnormalities, purulent vaginal or urethral discharge, joint inflammation, and changes of stasis dermatitis.

If the history reveals only easy bruising and no evidence for hematologic or vasculitic pathology can be found, then consideration of connective tissue and idiopathic causes is in order. Does the patient appear cushingoid or have a history of long-term corticosteroid use? Is the patient elderly with multiple small ecchymotic lesions in areas of minor everyday trauma? Are the ecchymoses tender in the absence of trauma? Is the patient an otherwise healthy young woman with easy bruising and relatively small ecchymoses?

Laboratory Studies

There is no standard battery of laboratory tests for the patient with purpura. To obtain meaningful information, the selection of studies must be based on the clinical findings.

Suspected Hematologic Disease

In patients with flat petechial rashes, the presence of platelet-related disease should be checked for with a *platelet count* and possibly with a determination of the *bleeding time* (see Chapter 81). Those with large ecchymoses may have a clotting factor problem and are best screened by measuring the *prothrombin time* and *partial thromboplastin time*. Other hematologic testing may also be in order. (See Chapter 81 for more details of the hematologic evaluation.)

Suspected Vasculitis

If palpable purpura is noted, the first priorities are to rule out bacteremia and vasculitis. Two sets of *blood cultures* should be obtained at the outset, especially if fever or other manifestations of infection are noted. If there is clinical evidence of rheumatoid disease, one can screen by testing for *antinuclear antibodies* and *rheumatoid factor*, although the results may be nonspecific (see Chapter 146). Patients with concurrent pulmonary symptoms or multiorgan system complaints should have a *urinalysis* checked for proteinuria and hematuria, a serum sample sent for *ANCA determination*, and *skin biopsy* performed. In addition to histologic processing, the biopsy specimen should also be cultured and a Gram's stain performed.

If a *leukocytoclastic vasculitis* is confirmed by skin biopsy, then more-specific testing can be conducted if clinically indicated. The otherwise healthy patient with resolving skin lesions and nothing more than a recent history of using a potentially offending drug needs no further evaluation. If the lesions persist, more testing may be in order. Elderly persons are at risk for dysproteinemias; a serum *immunoelectrophoresis* should be considered. *Cryoprotein* and *serum complement* determinations may prove useful diagnostically in a young woman with leukocytoclastic histology. Testing for *ANCA* may help in the etiologic identification of cases presenting pathologically as small-vessel vasculitis. Consultation with a rheumatologist is advised in persons who are ANCA-positive or who have evidence of active rheumatoid disease.

PATIENT EDUCATION

Detailed reassurance needs to be provided to the patient with no hematologic or systemic abnormality but only *after* a thorough evaluation has been completed. In the elderly patient with senile purpura, supportive explanation that the condition is a normal concomitant of aging is often helpful. Similarly, the young woman with a syndrome of easy bruising can be reassured. Occasionally, such patients buy and take large doses of vitamins C and K in the hope of lessening easy bruising. Such self-treatment is without any proven efficacy and adds an unnecessary expense. Avoidance of aspirin and NSAIDs is better advice.

For patients who require drugs that impair platelet function or compromise connective tissue integrity, it may be necessary to advise at least a reduction in dose; otherwise, they may have to accept the cosmetic unpleasantness of ecchymoses. It may be helpful to prepare those with palpable purpura for extended testing and the possibility of a skin biopsy.

INDICATIONS FOR ADMISSION AND REFERRAL (5)

Any patient with fever and purpura requires prompt hospital admission because bloodstream infection and systemic vasculitis are possible causes. The person with evidence of bleeding from multiple sites is also best hospitalized, as is the patient with severe thrombocytopenia or marked prolongation of the prothrombin time or partial thromboplastin time.

Consultation with the rheumatologist is worthwhile to guide the evaluation and immediate treatment of the systemic-vasculitis patient, who may require high-dose corticosteroids plus additional immunosuppressive therapy.

A.H.G.

Annotated Bibliography

1. Cines DB, Blanchette VS. Immune thrombocytopenic purpura. N Engl J Med 2002;346:995. (*A comprehensive review of this perplexing autoimmune cause of purpura; 103 references.*)
2. Gibson LE, Su WPD. Cutaneous vasculitis. Rheum Dis Clin North Am 1990;16:309. (*An important cause of purpura.*)
3. Hunder GG, Arend WP, Bloch DA, et al. The College of Rheumatology 1990 criteria for the classification of vasculitis. Arthritis Rheum 1990;33:1065. (*Includes criteria for the leukocytoclastic variety.*)
4. Jennette JC, Falk RJ. Small-vessel vasculitis. N Engl J Med 1997;337:1512. (*A definitive review, with especially helpful sections on clinical presentation and diagnosis; includes discussion of antineutrophil cytoplasmic autoantibody testing; 99 references.*)
5. Jennette JC, Falk RJ, Andrassey K, et al. Nomenclature of systemic vasculitides: proposal of an international consensus conference. Arthritis Rheum 1994;37:187. (*Presents names and definitions categorized by the size of the vessels involved.*)
6. Bosch X, Guilabert A, Espinoza G, et al. Treatment of antineutrophil cytoplasmic antibody–associated vasculitis: a systematic review. JAMA 2007;298:655. (*An excellent review of treatment modalities based on clinical presentation and extent of disease.*) (See also the bibliography for Chapter 81, which includes references on clotting disorders and other hematologic causes.)

CHAPTER 180 ■ EVALUATION OF DISTURBANCES IN PIGMENTATION

PETER C. SCHALOCK AND ARTHUR J. SOBER

Disturbances in pigmentation are conspicuous and common. Patients present with concerns about general darkening, brown spots, and depigmented areas. Pigmentary alterations may be manifestations of a genetic, endocrine, metabolic, nutritional, infectious, or neoplastic disorder. Physical and chemical factors also can be important because skin color can be altered by exposure to heat, solar and ionizing radiation, trauma, medications, heavy metals, and tattoos.

PATHOPHYSIOLOGY AND CLINICAL PRESENTATION (1–9)

Hyperpigmentation

Pathophysiology

Pigmentary changes are caused by melanin being absent, increased, decreased, or abnormally placed or distributed. Hyperpigmentation may result from an increased rate of melanosome production, an increased number of melanosomes transferred to keratinocytes, or a greater size and melanization of melanosomes. Because of the Tyndall phenomenon, hyperpigmentation is perceived as blue when melanin is located deeply in the dermis.

The pathophysiologic mechanisms that produce hyperpigmentation through the melanocyte system include increased levels of adrenocorticotropic hormone (ACTH), which has a melanocyte-stimulating action; ultraviolet radiation; and certain medications. Abnormal diffuse pigmentation may manifest as a change in pigment naturally present in skin or the expression of pigment in areas for the first time, such as the mucosal membranes, palmar creases, and intertriginous areas (body folds).

Hypomelanosis, or depigmentation, may result from the genetic loss of melanocytes, destruction by inflammation, or trauma. Inflammation may be secondary to infection or burns or associated with a variety of immunologically mediated diseases. Any damage to the skin may cause hypo- or hyperpigmentation, especially in darker-skinned individuals.

Clinical Presentation

Hyperpigmentation may be circumscribed (i.e., bounded, limited, or confined to a specific areas) or diffuse.

Circumscribed Hyperpigmentation. Circumscribed hyperpigmentation includes *freckles* (ephelides), *lentigines* (simple or solar), *café-au-lait spots*, dermal *melanocytosis* (formerly known

as a "Mongolian spot"), *nevus of Ota and Ito*, *Becker's melanosis*, *melasma*, and *acanthosis nigricans*.

Freckles are small, macular lesions seen on areas exposed to the sun. Freckles may lighten in adults but darken after exposure to long-wave ultraviolet radiation. *Lentigines* are classified as solar or simple (Fig. 180.1). Both appear as macules, but lentigines are larger, darker, and differ histologically from freckles. Simple lentigines are not associated with age or sun exposure and are clinically and histologically indistinguishable from solar lentigines, which often appear after the sixth decade on sun-exposed skin. Patients call solar lentigines "liver spots" and rarely realize that "liver" refers to the color of the lesion and not to its cause.

Café-au-lait spots are congenital or acquired, light- to dark-brown macules ranging in size from 1 to 20 cm. They can be round or oval with smooth or irregular borders. The presence of multiple lesions is associated most commonly with neurofibromatosis and Albright's syndrome, among many others. *Dermal melanocytosis* refers to round or oval, ill-defined, blue-hued patches on the sacrococcygeal area of infants usually of darker skin types. They represent benign dermal pigmentation that resolves over time. *Nevus of Ito and Ota* are most often unilateral, speckled blue-gray patches located on the shoulder and scapular skin, or periorbital and facial skin, respectively. *Becker's melanosis* (or Becker's *pigmented hairy nevus*) (Fig. 180.2) is a hyperpigmented patch located on the chest, back, or shoulder with overlying hypertrichosis (hair growth) and, at times, an underlying smooth muscle hamartoma. A *blue nevus* is a dome-shaped, blue-black macule or papule usually located on the extremities (Fig. 180.3). *Melanocytic nevi* ("moles") are also circumscribed, skin colored to dark brown (depending on the individual's skin), dome-shaped papules or macules.

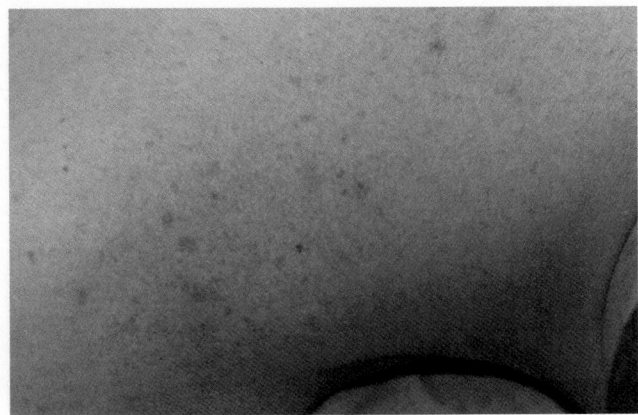

FIGURE 180.1. Solar lentigines on the shoulder after a previous blistering sunburn. (See the color insert.)

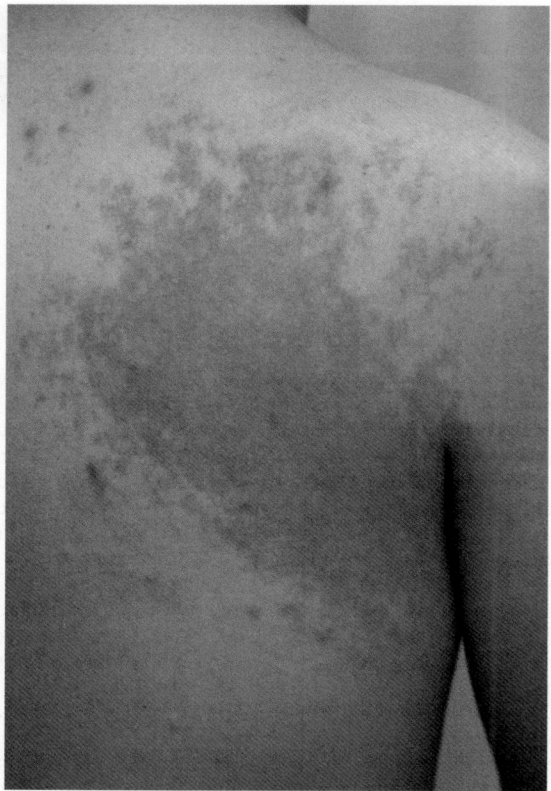

FIGURE 180.2. Becker's nevus on the shoulder of a young man. In this case, he did not have hypertrichosis. (See the color insert.)

Melasma (Greek for "black spot")/*chloasma* (pregnancy-induced melasma) is diffuse hyperpigmentation involving light brown to gray macules or patches that occur on the forehead, cheeks, and upper lip, usually in women. Sunlight exposure appears to be one of the most significant factors in developing and perpetuating the condition. In addition, hormones, especially estrogen and progesterone exposure during pregnancy, in birth control pills, or through hormone replacement therapy, substantially contribute to its development. Melasma is seen in up

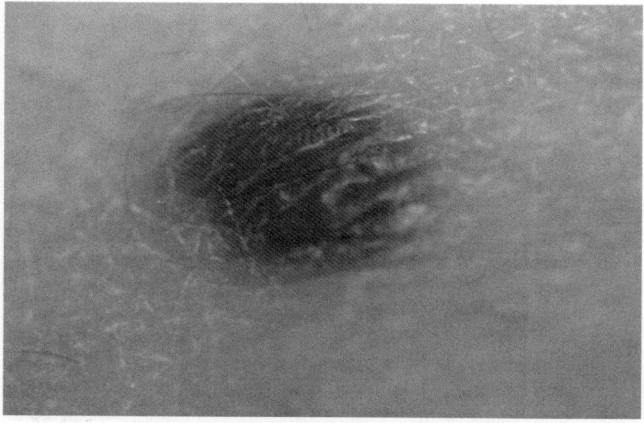

FIGURE 180.3. A dome-shaped, blue-black papule that has the characteristic features of a blue nevus. (See the color insert.)

to 70% of pregnant women and 35% of women taking oral contraceptives and in men undergoing hormone therapy for prostate cancer. On a related note, a physiologic darkening of the linea alba, pigmented nevi, nipples, and genitalia is caused by melanocyte-stimulating hormone (MSH) and increased levels of estrogen and progesterone in pregnancy.

Acanthosis nigricans presents as "velvety" textured, hyperpigmented patches located around the neck, axillae, groin, and inframammary folds. Patients are often overweight and have an underlying endocrine disorder, such as diabetes mellitus, or hyperandrogenism. The onset is usually slow and confined to skin folds and the back of the neck. In some cases, acanthosis nigricans can appear because of underlying malignancy, most often adenocarcinoma of the stomach or other gastrointestinal or genitourinary locations. Onset is rapid, often on the palms ("*tripe palms*"), and may be associated with *eruptive seborrheic keratoses* (sign of Leser–Trélat) and acrochordons. Other causes include systemic disease, medications, or genetics.

Diffuse Hyperpigmentation. Diffuse hyperpigmentation results from increased amounts of melanin in the epidermis. The color may be accentuated in sun-exposed areas, over pressure points or body folds, or in areas of trauma, such as new scars.

Addison's disease is associated with increased amounts of MSH and ACTH as a compensatory feedback response to decreased adrenal cortisol levels. Hyperpigmentation on sun-exposed sites, the genitalia, and oral mucous membranes is common and may present before the progressive lethargy and hypotension is evident.

Metabolic diseases such as *Wilson's disease, von Gierke's hemochromatosis, alkaptonuria, biliary cirrhosis, hyperthyroidism,* and *porphyria cutanea tarda* may be accompanied by diffuse melanosis. On occasion, rheumatoid arthritis, Still's disease, and scleroderma have been associated with hyperpigmentation.

Oral medications cause varying types of hyperpigmentation. Busulfan, minocycline, cyclophosphamide, clofazimine, 5-fluorouracil, psoralens, and zidovudine can produce *diffuse melanosis*, as can methotrexate, hydroxyurea, and topical nitrogen mustard. Chronic inorganic arsenic poisoning causes diffuse hyperpigmentation with normal or lighter skin areas scattered throughout, colorfully called "rain drops in the dust."

Chlorpromazine, amiodarone (Fig. 180.4), and antimalarial drugs (i.e., hydroxychloroquine) tend to produce a *bluish-gray hyperpigmentation*. Silver (argyria) and gold (chrysiasis), as well as bismuth and mercury, can accumulate in the skin and cause hyperpigmentation, depending on the dose given. *Starvation* (i.e., anorexia nervosa, bulimia, kwashiorkor, and marasmus), *hepatic insufficiency, malabsorption* syndromes, and *lymphomas* and *melanomas* may result in diffuse melanosis.

Focal Hyperpigmentation

Bleomycin can produce *linear, flagellate hyperpigmentation*. Exposure to a photosensitizer, such as oil of bergamot in perfumes and some hair preparations, can lead to *photocontact dermatitis*, which commonly appears on the neck or retroauricular skin; it is also referred to as *berloque dermatitis*. A similar compound (coumarin) in figs, parsnip, and citrus rinds causes inflammation and pigmentation in areas exposed to both the sensitizing chemical and the sun. A classic presentation is a bartender or vacationer with streaks of hyperpigmented skin on the extremities, corresponding to the circuitous path of oil and juice from citrus rind that arose on sun exposure after preparing mixed drinks.

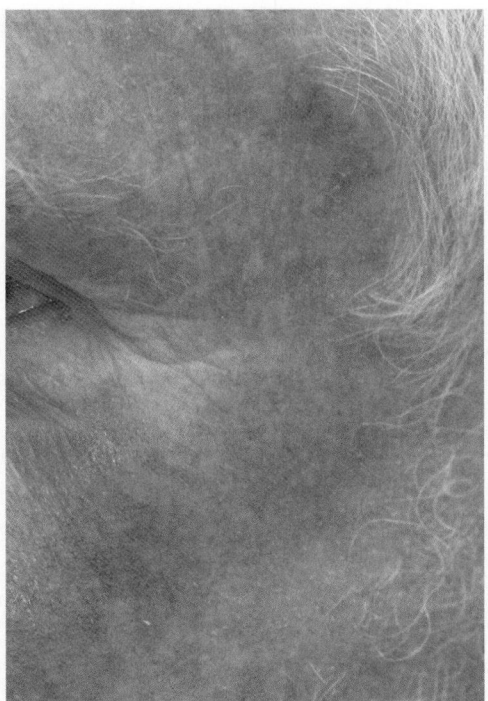

FIGURE 180.4. Brown pigmentation on a sun-exposed area from amiodarone use. (See the color insert.)

Postinflammatory hyperpigmentation is caused by a wide variety of etiologies, the common link being that the pigmentation changes follow skin inflammation (Fig. 180.5). Inflammatory disorders that affect the dermal–epidermal junction (e.g., *lichen planus*, *lupus erythematosus*) may lead to pigmentary alterations. Photosensitizing agents present in meadow grasses, citrus fruits, and edible plants may cause an exaggerated sunburn. Hyperpigmentation follows the acute inflammatory phase. Tar, pitch, and oils can induce similar changes. Physical trauma, friction, and heat may also lead to postinflammatory pigmentary changes, as may inflammatory

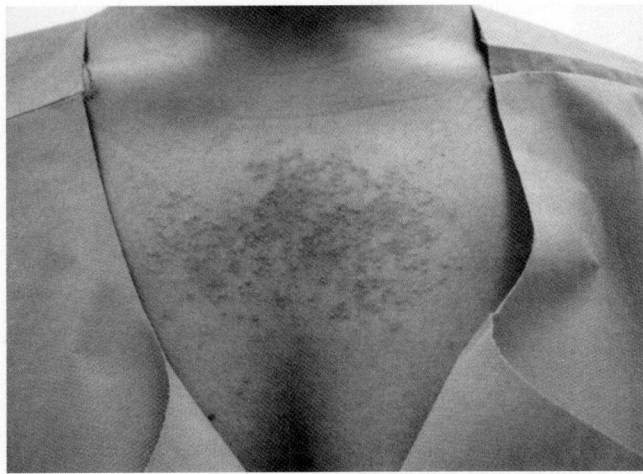

FIGURE 180.5. Postinflammatory hyperpigmentation after the resolution of papular eczema (centrally). Note the active lesions laterally. (See the color insert.)

dermatoses that stimulate melanin formation. Pigment alteration (both hyper- and hypopigmentation) is also seen after *cryogenic treatment* (i.e., liquid nitrogen), chemical peels, and laser therapy. Patients with darker skin tones in particular must be informed of the risks inherent in any of these procedures.

Other Discolorations. Yellow discoloration of the skin is seen in *carotenemia* and *jaundice;* mucous membrane involvement leads to scleral icterus with jaundice. Carotenemia, due to an inability to convert ingested β-carotene to vitamin A (as in diabetes mellitus, anorexia, and hypothyroidism) or as a result of a high intake of carrots or other carotenoid-containing vegetables, can give the skin a yellow-orange tint. The accumulation of *lycopene* from excessive ingestion of tomatoes or papaya can also tint the skin. Quinacrine, phenazopyridines, and canthaxanthin can also cause a yellowish discoloration.

Hypopigmentation

Pathophysiology and Clinical Presentation

Hypopigmentation may be hereditary or acquired.

Hereditary Conditions. Hereditary forms result in a lack or deficiency of melanin. In *albinism*, there is lack of pigment in the eyes (ocular albinism), skin, and hair (oculocutaneous albinism); melanocytes are normal in number but unable to produce melanin as a result of defective or absent tyrosinase. *Phenylketonuria* and *homocysteinuria* lead to hypopigmentation as a consequence of abnormal amino acid metabolism in the skin and hair. In *tuberous sclerosis*, "ashleaf" and small, "confetti" hypopigmented macules are observed, as are facial angiofibromas, café-au-lait macules, firm truncal plaques (collagenomas), and periungual fibromas. Hereditary absence of skin melanocytes occurs in *piebaldism* and *Waardenburg's syndrome*.

Acquired Forms. Acquired hypopigmentation is often a sequela of healed inflammatory skin conditions (e.g., infections, autoimmune disorders, and trauma).
   Vitiligo may occur in the context of other autoimmune conditions, such as pernicious anemia, Hashimoto's thyroiditis, diabetes, and Addison's disease. Onset is usually early in adult life but can occur at any age. Lesions may be symmetric and occur primarily on the face, upper trunk, fingertips and hands, genitalia, bony prominences, and periorificial skin (Fig. 180.6). In involved areas, the hair may be white (poliosis). The border of the lesion is often sharp and may be scalloped in shape. Occasionally, vitiligo assumes a segmental or zosteriform pattern. Halo nevi—centrifugal areas of depigmentation that surround a pigmented nevus—are present in 18% to 25% of cases. Premature graying of the hair may also occur. Partial repigmentation of vitiligo may occur in sun-exposed areas, but vitiliginous patches may sunburn more easily due to the lack of protective pigmentation.
   Chemical agents that interfere with tyrosinase activity (e.g., phenolic compounds, hydroquinone, sulfhydryls, and monobenzylether of hydroquinone) may cause depigmentation. Similarly, contact with rubber antioxidants, photographic processing chemicals , cosmetics (those containing benzyl alcohol), and adhesives may also cause a loss of pigment. Hypopigmentation may ensue after treatments with *liquid nitrogen* or *intralesional corticosteroids*. Other agents that may cause hypopigmentation include chloroquine, fluphenazine, azelaic acid, mercurials, and arsenic.

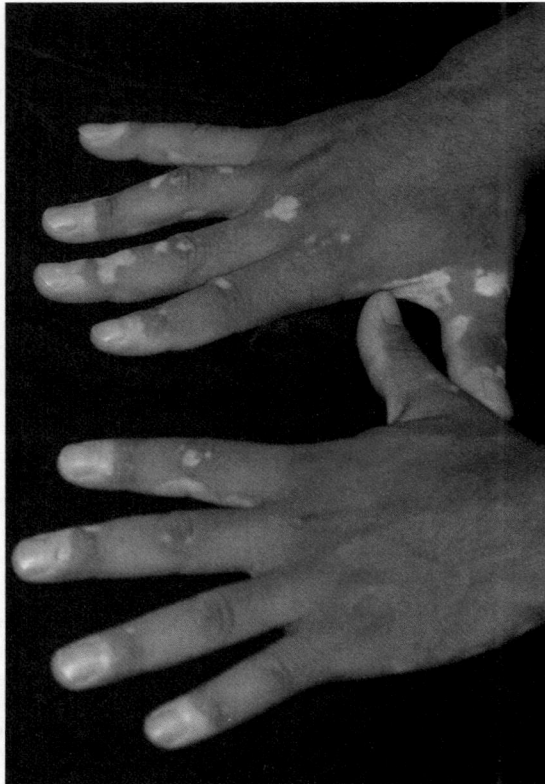

FIGURE 180.6. Vitiligo on bilateral hands. (See the color insert.)

Inflammation and infections may result in localized areas of pigment loss. Such areas may be more noticeable in dark-skinned persons. Inflammation may precede the loss of pigment (postinflammatory hypopigmentation). Multiple, hypopigmented macules 2 to 5 mm in diameter, termed *idiopathic guttate hypomelanosis*, occur in sun-exposed areas in sun-damaged individuals of any age. A host of inflammatory skin conditions (e.g., *tinea versicolor, pityriasis alba, pinta, leprosy, syphilis, erythema ab igne, sarcoidosis, scleroderma, and cutaneous T cell lymphoma* [*mycosis fungoides*]) may present as areas of hypopigmentation (Fig. 180.7).

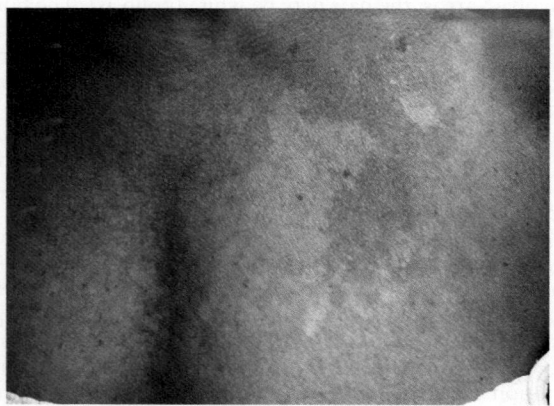

FIGURE 180.7. Hypopigmented patches after a 20-year history of tinea versicolor on the chest. (See the color insert.)

TABLE 180.1

CAUSES OF DISTURBANCES IN PIGMENTATION

Hyperpigmentation
  Circumscribed
    Freckles
    Lentigines
    Melasma/chloasma (pregnancy, estrogen, oral contraceptives)
    Postinflammatory/physical trauma
  Diffuse
    Addison's disease
    Systemic conditions (Wilson's disease, hemochromatosis, hyperthyroid, hepatic insufficiency, biliary cirrhosis, porphyria cutanea tarda, rheumatoid arthritis, scleroderma)
    Drugs (arsenic, antimalarials, chlorpromazine, busulfan, cyclophosphamide, clofazimine, gold, silver, zidovudine)
    Nutritional (pellagra, malabsorption syndromes, starvation, folic acid deficiency)
    Malignancy (lymphomas)

Hypopigmentation
  Hereditary conditions
    Partial albinism
    Tuberous sclerosis
    Piebaldism/Waardenburg's syndrome
    Phenylketonuria
    Homocysteinuria
  Vitiligo (with or without concurrent autoimmune disease, including pernicious anemia, Hashimoto's thyroiditis, male hypogonadism, diabetes mellitus)
  Dermatoses
    Tinea versicolor
    Pityriasis alba
    Eczema/postinflammatory
    Infections
  Chemical exposure
    Rubber
    Antioxidants
    Germicides
    Phenols/hydroquinones
    Other: chloroquine, fluphenazine, azelaic acid, benzyl alcohol, mercurials, arsenic

DIFFERENTIAL DIAGNOSIS (2–4,6,8,9)

Table 180.1 lists the causes of disturbances in pigmentation.

WORKUP (4,6–9)

Hyperpigmentation

The majority of localized hyperpigmented areas are postinflammatory and of cosmetic concern only, although they should be distinguished from more worrisome pigmented lesions, such as melanomas (see Chapter 177). Evaluation of the patient with localized hyperpigmentation requires an inspection of the lesions and an inquiry about previous inflammation and the use of oral contraceptives that can produce melasma.

History

Localized hyperpigmentation may arise over a period of many years (moles, solar lentigines) or relatively suddenly (postinflammatory after trauma or inflammation, melasma during pregnancy, or a Becker's nevus at adolescence), or it may be congenital or related to infancy (café-au-lait macules). Diffuse hyperpigmentation necessitates a careful history that specifies the time of onset and possible sun, chemical, or drug exposure. A complete history of all previous medication with attention to duration and dose of agents known to produce pigmentary changes should be pursued. A general review of systems should be made, and any weakness associated with Addison's disease and any itching or hepatic dysfunction associated with biliary cirrhosis should be noted. The physician should be aware of dietary behaviors that may suggest an eating disorder, lead to vitamin deficiencies and malnutrition, or involve the excessive intake of one particular food or food group.

Physical Examination

One checks for hyperpigmentation in creases and scars (characteristic of Addison's disease) and clues to obvious underlying pathology, as may occur with malignancy, hepatic insufficiency, endocrine abnormalities, or malabsorption. Magnification with a hand lens may better characterize pigmented lesions (e.g., on inspection of a mole, the more irregular the border or variably pigmented it is, the more likely it is that the mole is atypical histologically; see Chapter 177).

Laboratory Investigation

Laboratory investigation is a function of the clinical findings, with biopsy a consideration for irregular localized pigmented lesions or diffuse pigmentation.

Hypopigmentation

History

Hypopigmentation requires a careful history of approximate time of onset, family history (vitiligo, piebaldism, Waardenburg's syndrome, tuberous sclerosis, etc.), and exposure to bleaching agents, phenol-containing industrial cleaners such as those used in janitorial work, or agents used by individuals who work with adhesives/glues. Patients with vitiligo should be given a careful general review that seeks to identify associated conditions, such as pernicious anemia, thyroid disease, diabetes, or connective tissue disease.

Physical Examination

Distribution, shape, and associated signs of disease (cutaneous or systemic) assist diagnosis in many cases of infectious, autoimmune, or congenital diseases. The total depigmentation of vitiligo should be differentiated from partial postinflammatory hypopigmentation with the use of a Wood's lamp, which accentuates depigmented skin from the surrounding normal skin. Persons with vitiligo should be examined for manifestations of pernicious anemia (see Chapter 79), thyroid disease (see Chapter 104), diabetes (see Chapter 102), and collagen vascular disease (see Chapter 146).

Laboratory Studies

Hypopigmented areas should be scraped and a *potassium hydroxide wet mount* examined microscopically to diagnose tinea versicolor. Laboratory screening to test for concurrent autoimmune disease is best undertaken according to the clinical presentation but might include evaluation for serum *vitamin B$_{12}$*, *thyroid-stimulating hormone*, *antithyroid antibodies*, random *glucose*, and *antinuclear antibodies*.

SYMPTOMATIC THERAPY AND PATIENT EDUCATION (4–7,10–14)

Hyperpigmentation

In treating hyperpigmented areas, the chief symptomatic advice is strict *avoidance of sunlight*. Potent *topical corticosteroids* have a pigment-lightening effect, as do *retinoic acid* and its derivatives (*tretinoin* and *tazarotene*). Other skin-lightening agents include azelaic acid, kojic acid, mequinol (hydroquinone monomethyl ether), and monobenzylether of hydroquinone, although the last-named agent is almost exclusively reserved for permanent bleaching of patients with extensive vitiligo.

Melasma and Postinflammatory Hyperpigmentation

A commercial product, *Tri-Luma Cream*, containing a combination of 0.05% tretinoin, 0.01% fluocinolone, and 4% hydroquinone, can be effective if used daily for up to 8 weeks. It should be used with caution in darker-skinned individuals because hypopigmentation of unaffected areas can occur. Treatment continues with the combined use of a retinoid and a hydroquinone blended with a sunscreen after the 8-week Tri-Luma therapy. It is important to not continue Tri-Luma long term because topical steroid use is associated with atrophy and telangiectasias.

Other treatments for melasma include topical peels, lasers, and cryotherapy. *Chemical peeling* may be helpful in some cases. Bleaching agents may not be beneficial for deep pigment deposition, as in some cases of postinflammatory hyperpigmentation, because the melanin is often deeper. Intense pulse light, the Q-switched alexandrite, ruby, and neodymium-doped yttrium aluminum garnet *lasers, cryotherapy*, and chemical peels may benefit patients with multiple lentigines. These laser treatments have also been used to target melanin pigment in patients with melasma, but the results have been disappointing. Months of treatment can be undone in a single day (or less) of unprotected exposure to the sun.

Hypopigmentation

Hypopigmentation can usually be masked by appropriate *cosmetics* (e.g., Dermablend, Lydia O'Leary, Clinique). In some instances, repigmentation is worth consideration.

Vitiligo

To variable degrees, *repigmentation* can be achieved with topical steroids, topical tacrolimus and pimecrolimus, and psoralens plus ultraviolet A or narrowband ultraviolet B radiation. Excimer laser, surgical grafting, calcipotriene (a topical vitamin D analogue), and, if the condition is extensive, monobenzylether of hydroquinone (total depigmentation) are other available modalities. The primary care physician must assess the patient's motivation and commitment to treatment because multiple sessions over an extended period of time are required. Age, gender, and duration of vitiligo do not affect the response. Lesions on the face and abdomen tend to become repigmented more rapidly than those on the hands, feet, and bony prominences. Treatment should be supervised by a dermatologist experienced in using these agents to achieve optimal cosmetic results.

If careful workup reveals no accompanying hematologic or endocrinologic autoimmune disorders, the patient can be reassured that only the skin is affected. Others appreciate knowing that the condition is not contagious. The primary physician should advise the patient about cosmetic alternatives and help the patient to decide on an appropriate course of treatment. Because these patients may be unhappy with their body image, psychological support and counseling can be very helpful and should not be overlooked.

Annotated Bibliography

1. Dunston GM, Halder RM. Vitiligo is associated with HLA DR4 in black patients: a preliminary report. Arch Dermatol 1990;126:56. (*Certain HLA antigens may be risk factors.*)
2. Hendrix JD Jr, Greer KE. Cutaneous hyperpigmentation caused by systemic drugs. Int J Dermatol 1992;31:458. (*An excellent resource on offending agents.*)
3. Kovacs SO. Vitiligo. J Am Acad Dermatol 1998;38:647. (*An encyclopedic review of the subject; 296 references.*)
4. Ongenae K, Beelaert L, van Geel N, et al. Psychosocial effects of vitiligo. J Eur Acad Dermatol Venereol 2006;20:1. (*Most patients felt embarrassment when showing their bodies or meeting strangers.*)
5. Resnick S. Melasma induced by oral contraceptive drugs. JAMA 1967;199:601. (*A classic article; melasma developed in 29% of cases.*)
6. Ruiz-Maldonado R, Orozco-Covarrubias ML. Post-inflammatory hypopigmentation and hyperpigmentation. Semin Cutaneous Med Surg 1997;16:36. (*Presents clinical examples of both types of pigmentary change, together with management suggestions.*)
7. Schwartz RA, Janniger CK. Vitiligo. Cutis 1997;60:239. (*A succinct review; 82 references.*)
8. Stefanato CM, Bhawan J. Diffuse hyperpigmentation of the skin: a clinicopathologic approach to diagnosis. Semin Cutaneous Med Surg 1997;16:61. (*A systematic classification based on clinical and pathologic findings; 79 references.*)
9. Tal A, Gagel RF. The diagnostic dilemma of hyperpigmentation in patients with acquired immunodeficiency syndrome. Cutis 1991;48:153. (*Both zidovudine and adrenal insufficiency may be responsible; the presentation is similar for both.*)
10. Arroyo MP, Tift L. Vitiligo therapy: where are we now? J Drugs Dermatol 2003;2:404. (*A current review, extensively referenced.*)
11. Kim HY, Kang KY. Epidermal grafts for treatment of stable and progressive vitiligo. J Am Acad Dermatol 1999;40:412. (*Even progressive disease was improved after epidermal grafting with a suction blister technique.*)
12. Lepe V, Moncada B, Castanedo-Cazares JP, et al. A double-blind randomized trial of 0.1% tacrolimus vs 0.05% clobetasol for the treatment of childhood vitiligo. Arch Dermatol 2003;139:651. (*Tacrolimus, a relatively new nonsteroid ointment, was as effective as a commonly used potent topical steroid and had significantly fewer side effects.*)
13. Njoo MD, Spuls PI, Bos JD, et al. Nonsurgical repigmentation therapies in vitiligo. Meta-analysis of the literature. Arch Dermatol 1998;134:1532. (*Class III corticosteroids and ultraviolet B therapy are effective and safe treatments for localized and generalized vitiligo, respectively.*)
14. Gupta AK, Gover MD, Nouri K, Taylor S. The treatment of melasma: a review of clinical trials. J Am Acad Dermatol. 2006;55:1048. (*An excellent review comparing the more traditional and novel treatments for melasma.*)

CHAPTER 181 ■ EVALUATION OF URTICARIA AND ANGIOEDEMA

Urticaria (*hives*) is a pruritic, often immune-mediated skin eruption of well-circumscribed wheals on an erythematous base. It is estimated that up to one fifth of the population will experience an urticarial episode, with women more likely to be affected than men (especially with regard to chronic urticaria). *Angioedema* is a related condition involving the deeper layers of the skin. Approximately half of patients have urticaria with angioedema, 40% have pure urticaria, and 10% have pure angioedema. If the process occurs for less than 6 weeks, it is termed acute, but if it persists beyond 6 to 8 weeks, it is termed chronic. Most chronic urticaria resolves within 1 year, although persistence well beyond that occurs in approximately 10% of cases. The diagnostic responsibilities of the primary physician include searching for precipitants and underlying causes and distinguishing urticaria from urticarial vasculitis, a manifestation of connective tissue disease. Eliciting the cause can be diffi-

cult and is not always possible. In the absence of an identifiable and remediable precipitant, one needs to provide symptomatic relief.

PATHOPHYSIOLOGY AND CLINICAL PRESENTATION (1–8)

Urticaria

Mechanisms

Urticaria is the consequence of a mast cell release of mediators that increase vascular permeability, which leads to extravasation into the skin of protein-rich fluid from small blood vessels, usually postcapillary venules. Many mechanisms have been implicated, and much remains incompletely understood, but *mast cell activation* is usually the final common pathway. Precipitants range from physical stimuli to autoimmune mechanisms. In food-induced and some forms of drug-induced disease, ingested or infused antigens trigger mast cell activation by an *immunoglobulin E* (IgE)–mediated pathway. In other drug-induced cases (e.g., opiates, amphetamines), *direct* activation by the drug does not occur. Hyperreactivity to acetylcholine (perhaps related to inadequate production of cholinesterases) is the suspected mechanism in persons with physical urticaria. Physical urticarias may also have some degree of IgE-mediated pathophysiology. In some cases, if not a substantial proportion of them, idiopathic chronic urticaria may represent a form of *autoimmune* activation of mast cells.

Regardless of the initial trigger, *mast cell activation* remains the final common pathway, with a release of mediators from mast cells or circulating basophils increasing vascular permeability. *Histamine* serves as a principal mediator, producing a classic wheal and flare on intracutaneous injection. Transient histamine elevations even occur in the extremities of patients with physical urticarias. Other possible mast cell–derived mediators include bradykinin, eosinophilic and high-molecular-weight neutrophilic chemotactic factors, and prostaglandin D2, leukotrienes, and platelet-activating factors. Substance P may contribute to the flare that surrounds urticarial wheals. Heat, fever, emotional stress, alcohol, and the premenstrual state can exacerbate urticaria independent of the specific pathophysiology. Additional precipitants and mediators of the urticarial reaction are constantly being identified.

Clinical Presentations

The localized accumulation of fluid produces the characteristic edematous, erythematous, well-circumscribed itchy wheals, which blanch on pressure, range in size from a few millimeters to several centimeters, and manifest serpiginous borders. Individual lesions may persist for 12 to 24 hours, but most resolve spontaneously much sooner. Central clearing can lead to an annular pattern. The common final pathway for urticaria of most causes produces a rather stereotypical presentation, but each of the common types has a few distinguishing characteristics.

Food- and Drug-Induced Urticarias. The attacks tend to be brief and usually do not cause chronic urticaria, but attacks may be accompanied by angioedema. The most commonly implicated foods include *eggs, shellfish, true nuts, peanuts, fish,* and *milk,* and the most common drugs are *penicillins* and *sulfa-containing agents.* Intravenous *iodinated contrast agents, opiates,* and *amphetamines* appear to cause the direct release of mediators from the mast cells. *Aspirin* and *nonsteroidal antiinflammatory agents* (NSAIDs) produce urticaria in a dose-related nonimmunologic manner in susceptible persons, perhaps because they have an underlying abnormality in prostaglandin synthesis, which these agents block. Patients with urticarial reactions to aspirin can tolerate sodium salicylate or choline salicylate, which do not inhibit cyclooxygenase. *Latex* is an increasingly important example of a contact antigen common to medical settings that may trigger acute urticaria, angioedema, and even anaphylaxis by an IgE-mediated pathway. The latex powder that coats latex examination gloves is especially sensitizing.

Chronic urticaria is often erroneously ascribed to exposure to *food additives.* Although benzoic acid derivatives (e.g., *sodium benzoate*) and several *azo food dyes* (e.g., tartrazine and sunset yellow) have been implicated, placebo-controlled trials revealed that food additives accounted for no more than 10% of cases.

Physical Urticarias. These include dermatographism, pressure urticaria, cold urticaria, and cholinergic urticaria. In *dermatographism,* gentle stroking of the skin produces an immediate wheal and flare response. In *pressure urticaria,* the application of pressure at a right angle to the skin results in a red swelling after a latent period of up to 4 hours. In *cold urticaria,* the application of cold produces pruritic, erythematous eruptions within minutes. *Cholinergic* urticaria is characterized by tiny, 1- to 3-mm punctate lesions surrounded by erythema; they are intensely pruritic and triggered by *exercise* or a *hot shower.* Some exercise-induced disease may require prior ingestion of a food to which the patient is allergic. *Aquagenic urticaria* is characterized by tiny perifollicular hives that appear after contact with water. *Solar urticaria* develops in susceptible persons on exposure to ultraviolet light.

Autoimmune Disease. An autoimmune form of mast cell disease has been postulated and might account for many of the otherwise idiopathic cases of chronic urticaria encountered. A wheal-producing, noncytokine IgG mediator directed against the mast cell IgE receptor and causing the mast cell release of histamine has been identified in up to half of patients with chronic urticaria. Many of these patients also have autoantibodies to thyroid antigens, which perhaps accounts for the increased frequency of urticaria in persons with active *Hashimoto's thyroiditis.* Greater than 25% of persons with chronic urticaria have antithyroid antibodies or antibodies to thyroglobulin. In studies of such patients (whether euthyroid or with clinical thyroid disease), treatment with exogenous thyroid hormone to lower the level of thyroid-stimulating hormone often resulted in resolution of the urticaria. More work remains to test these hypotheses.

Infectious Diseases. The formation of antigen–antibody complexes that trigger mast cell release has been the purported mechanism of the urticaria seen in some infectious diseases. For example, in the prodromal phase of hepatitis B, symmetric arthritis of the small joints of the hands may accompany an urticarial reaction, which is believed to be complement mediated. Some patients with chronic "idiopathic" urticaria reported that their urticaria resolved with treatment for *Helicobacter pylori* infection. These observations raise the possibility that *H. pylori* antigens may be responsible for some of the "idiopathic" disease encountered.

Angioedema

The mechanisms for angioedema are basically the same as for urticaria, which accounts for the simultaneous appearance of both types of lesions in some patients. The *autoimmune mechanism* described previously for urticaria and associated with Hashimoto's thyroiditis is likely to account for a large fraction of idiopathic cases. Compared to urticaria, the extravasation of fluid in angioedema occurs in deeper layers of the skin and subcutaneous tissue, especially in the periorbital, perioral, pharyngeal, palmar, and plantar surfaces of the body. The edema is more diffuse, and the overlying skin appears normal and less itchy than in urticaria. Submucosal involvement in the upper airway and gastrointestinal tract can lead to hoarseness, life-threatening airway obstruction, nausea, vomiting, and abdominal discomfort. Sometimes, the abdominal pain is severe enough to mimic an acute abdomen. Most precipitants of urticaria can also trigger angioedema. Chronic angioedema and a few causes of acute angioedema have unique mechanisms and no associated urticaria.

Hereditary Angioedema

Hereditary angioedema is an autosomal-dominant hereditary disease characterized by reduced or defective production of the inhibitor of the first component of complement (C1 INH). In *type I,* the most common form, C1 INH levels are markedly reduced and levels of C4 are low, whereas in *type II,* the patient has normal to elevated amounts of a dysfunctional C1 INH. Half of patients have no family history of the condition. There is no urticaria.

A characteristic presentation has been described of generalized skin swelling (involving the extremities, face, genitals, and trunk) in conjunction with abdominal discomfort occurring in greater than 97% of episodes; oropharyngeal involvement is uncommon (0.3% to 0.9%). Onset early in life portends a worse prognosis with more severe episodes.

Acquired Angioedemas

In patients with certain malignancies (*adenocarcinoma, lymphoma, chronic lymphocytic leukemia*), *autoantibodies to C1 INH* may develop and lead to attacks of angioedema. C1 levels fall, as do levels of C4 and C1 INH. Such patients do not report urticaria.

The angioedema that is occasionally seen with the use of *angiotensin-converting-enzyme inhibitors* (ACEIs) appears to be mediated by bradykinins, purportedly occurring in persons who slowly metabolize kinins and experience a tissue-kinin buildup with ACEI therapy. It typically occurs shortly after the initiation of treatment with an ACEI, but it may develop at any time. Risk factors include African American race, age greater than 65 years, a history of drug rash with other agents, and seasonal allergies. The related *angiotensin II–receptor antagonists,* which do not affect bradykinins, are not associated with the same risk for angioedema.

Unlike the angioedemas related to C1 INH, the *autoimmune* form associated with antibodies against the mast cell IgE receptor often presents with chronic urticaria, as well as angioedema (see earlier discussion).

Urticarial Vasculitis

Urticarial vasculitis superficially resembles urticaria but represents a vasculitic process heralding systemic autoimmune disease (e.g., *systemic lupus, Sjögren's syndrome*). The skin lesions differ from those of urticaria, in that the wheals last for longer than 24 hours and manifest a more indolent appearance, which includes some central clearing, purpura, and residual pigmentation; the lesions hurt more than they itch. Patients also have systemic symptoms (e.g., fever, arthralgias, and abdominal pain) and may not obtain much relief from antihistamines. Laboratory studies may reveal an elevated sedimentation rate, the presence of antinuclear antibodies, and evidence of glomerulonephritis (microscopic hematuria, albuminuria). Biopsy demonstrates leukocytoclastic changes and extravasation of red cells, findings not seen with urticaria.

DIFFERENTIAL DIAGNOSIS (1–8)

The causes of acute urticaria/angioedema are usually more straightforward, whereas the causes of chronic disease tend to

TABLE 181.1

COMMON CAUSES OF URTICARIA AND ANGIOEDEMA

Acute Disease (episodes stop recurring after 6 weeks)
  Infection (viral, bacterial, fungal, parasitic)
  Foods (eggs, shellfish, nuts)
  Food additives (sodium benzoate, azo dyes such as tartrazine and yellow dye no. 5)
  Drugs, immunologic release of mediators (penicillins, sulfa-containing agents)
  Drugs, direct mediator release (intravenous iodinated contrast agents, opiates, amphetamines)
  Drugs, prostaglandin inhibition (aspirin, other nonsteroidal antiinflammatory drugs)
  Other sensitizing antigens (e.g., latex, blood transfusion)
  Insect sting
  All causes of chronic urticaria

Chronic Disease (episodes continue for 6 weeks)
  Idiopathic
  Physical urticarias
    Cold
    Pressure
    Dermatographism
    Cholinergic (exercise, hot shower, emotional stress)
    Solar
    Vibratory
  Hereditary C1 inhibitor deficiency
  Acquired angioedema (lymphoma, adenocarcinoma, chronic lymphocytic leukemia)
  Causes of acute urticaria

be more elusive because the relation to precipitants is often less clear (Table 181.1). Urticaria needs to be differentiated from urticarial vasculitis, a presentation of connective tissue disease.

WORKUP (1–9)

The history is the most useful component of the evaluation and yields clues to an underlying cause or precipitant far more often than does the physical examination or laboratory studies. Nonetheless, the latter are essential for identifying urticarial vasculitis and should not be overlooked when individual lesions persist for more than 24 hours.

History

A good description of the urticarial response is essential. Is the predominant reaction one of angioedema (suggesting possible C1 INH deficiency) or of urticaria? Do individual wheals persist for more than 24 hours (suggesting urticarial vasculitis, especially if accompanied by purpura and pigmentation), or do they clear quickly? Is there a history of onset early in life (suggesting hereditary disease)? Inquiry into illnesses, medications, foods, activities, and exposures associated with urticaria or angioedema (see Table 181.1) is essential to uncovering the proximate cause, especially in cases of acute urticarial disease. Commonly overlooked is nonprescription use of *NSAIDs* and *aspirin*; prescription use of *ACE inhibitors* should also be checked. *Latex* allergy should be considered in health care workers who present with urticaria. When a food allergy is suspected, the patient should be encouraged to keep a food diary. One should not overlook agents that may be entering through the conjunctivae, nasal mucosa, rectum, or vaginal area. Although allergy to milk and beer antigens is rare in adults, penicillin antigen may be present in dairy products and yeast in beer, factors that can precipitate urticaria in sensitized patients. It is important to determine whether exposure to pressure, cold, light, heat, or exercise precipitates lesions. A travel history can suggest a parasitic infestation. Inquiry into agents and factors that might modulate the intensity of an urticarial reaction (e.g., alcohol, NSAIDs, heat, humidity, occlusive clothing, psychological stress) can provide clinically useful information. A positive family history of angioedema is helpful, but a negative family history does not rule out C1 INH deficiency.

The review of systems should be used to check for systemic illnesses, infections, and malignancies that might present with urticaria and angioedema. Patients should be asked about night sweats, fatigue, weight loss, lymphadenopathy, recurrent peptic ulcer disease, jaundice, easy bruising, cold intolerance, dry skin, thyroid enlargement, dysuria, vaginal or sinus discharge, and pain in the teeth, joints, or sinuses.

Physical Examination

The severity of the condition and occasionally its cause are revealed by the physical examination. Dermatographism is associated with linear wheals. Small lesions with erythematous flares are typical of cholinergic urticaria. Periorbital or perioral swelling suggest angioedema. Lesions that persist for more than 24 hours and are accompanied by purpura and hyperpigmentation are characteristic of urticarial vasculitis. Careful examination of the ears, pharynx, sinuses, and teeth may help to uncover a focal infection. One should check for lymphadenopathy and hepatosplenomegaly, which suggest an underlying lymphoma or hepatocellular disease. The joints are noted for swelling, effusion, and warmth, which suggest active rheumatoid disease.

Laboratory Studies

It is usually unproductive to attempt diagnosis through the performance of an extensive panel of laboratory tests in the absence of suggestive historical and physical examination evidence. There is no standard battery of tests for the workup of urticaria and angioedema. Testing is based on clinical presentation and the associated pretest probabilities for underlying etiologies.

Clinical Evidence of Infection, Myeloproliferative Disease, or Inflammation

A *complete blood cell count, differential, erythrocyte sedimentation rate* (ESR), and *peripheral smear* are reasonable first steps in testing. If there is clinical evidence of connective tissue disease or vasculitis (e.g., fever, arthralgias, markedly elevated ESR, lesions lasting >24 hours, petechiae, purpura), then *urinalysis* and an *antinuclear antibody test* should be obtained and strong consideration given to *skin biopsy*. The biopsy sample is taken at the margin of a lesion to include normal and involved skin. Patients with chronic angioedema in the absence of urticaria are candidates for measurement of the serum *C4 complement* level; if it is low, a *C1 INH* determination should follow.

Idiopathic Disease

Idiopathic cases of chronic urticaria with angioedema might be assessed by checking for *antithyroid antibodies* and *thyroid-stimulating hormone* levels. For the patient with idiopathic urticaria and recurrent peptic ulcer disease, *serology* for *H. pylori* or a related test should be obtained (see Chapter 68).

Tests of Limited or No Value

Skin testing is of minimal value (except for suspected penicillin allergy; see later discussion), and the costly IgE *radioallergosorbent test* rarely reveals a cause in elusive cases. Mean serum levels of *IgE* are usually normal. *Radiologic* examinations are indicated only if clinical evidence suggests a focal infection or malignancy. *Stool examination* for ova and parasites is appropriate only if recent diarrheal illness or travel to endemic areas has taken place or if peripheral eosinophilia is noted. *"Cytotoxic food allergy"* testing has no scientific validity and should be firmly discouraged.

Provocative Tests

Provocative tests can help to ascertain precipitants.

For Physical Urticarias. Placing an *ice cube* on the skin may induce cold urticaria, and *stroking* can reveal dermatographism. Cholinergic urticaria may be revealed by an intradermal injection of *methacholine* (0.1 mL of a 1:500 dilution). Pressure urticaria may be elicited by *pressing* at a right angle to the skin surface and noting whether a red swelling appears at the site after a latent period of 30 minutes to 4 hours.

For Food Allergies. Placebo-controlled challenge testing for reactivity to food additives is sometimes performed by allergists, who administer capsules containing the additives in addition to placebo capsules and monitor symptoms. Such testing is not appropriate in persons with a history of asthma or airway involvement or in persons with chronic urticaria, in whom food allergy is almost never the cause.

For Drug Allergy (Penicillin). A distant history of *penicillin allergy* usually triggers avoidance of the drug and often related agents such as cephalosporins, but *skin testing* with *benzylpenicilloyl-polysine (Pre-Pen)* and *penicillin G* can help to determine the significance of the presumed allergy and the safety of future penicillin and cephalosporin use. Skin testing demonstrates the presence of IgE antibodies. Benzylpenicilloyl-polysine tests for allergy to major determinants; penicillin G in 10,000 U/mL provides testing for allergy to minor determinants. A skin prick of each with a saline control is performed, and the findings are observed 20 minutes later. A positive test is a wheal greater than 3 mm compared to a saline control. If both are negative, an intradermal test is performed next. A positive test to either is associated with a significant risk of anaphylaxis and a 50% chance of an immediate allergic reaction; a negative test to both gives a less than 3% chance of an allergic reaction to penicillin and almost no risk of anaphylaxis. A recent anaphylactic response to penicillin can result in a false-negative skin test if it is performed 1 to 2 weeks after the episode. The risk of an adverse reaction from the skin test is less than 1% and is associated with giving too high a dose or skipping the skin-pricking and going directly to intradermal injection. Contraindications include a history of Stevens–Johnson syndrome and exfoliative dermatitis.

Cephalosporin skin testing is not available, but results from penicillin skin testing can be informative. A positive reaction to penicillin is associated with a 4% risk of a reaction to cephalosporin; a negative test predicts little risk of a serious reaction to cephalosporin.

Therapeutic Trials

Therapeutic trials may be helpful in identifying a cause of acute urticaria. An elimination diet that consists of lamb, rice, string beans, fresh peas, tea, and rye crackers excludes most common food allergens. A more limited approach would be to eliminate dairy products, beer, nuts, shellfish, berries, and food additives. It is often useful to stop all drugs or change preparations or brands to eliminate tartrazine dyes or the peculiar additives of particular toothpastes or cosmetics.

Chronic urticaria poses significant diagnostic and management challenges. Trials of elimination diets have no effect on chronic urticaria or angioedema. Hospitalization for control of diet and observation is both expensive and low in diagnostic yield. A specific cause is identified in fewer than 10% of patients, and the idiopathic designation often applies even after extensive evaluation.

SYMPTOMATIC MANAGEMENT (1–13)

The best treatment is identification and avoidance of etiologic agents, but in the many instances of chronic urticaria in which this is not possible, empiric measures for symptomatic relief are indicated. Even if an etiologic diagnosis has not been made, the avoidance of substances that may aggravate symptoms (e.g., aspirin, NSAIDs, alcohol, ACE inhibitors) should be part of any program. Half of patients with urticaria alone and 25% with associated angioedema are free of lesions within 1 year; however, 10% to 20% may experience episodes for more than 20 years.

Agents

Antihistamines

Antihistamines provide excellent symptomatic control. The H_1-blockers, such as *hydroxyzine* (10 to 25 mg daily at bedtime) and *diphenhydramine* (25 to 50 mg daily at bedtime), have been the mainstay of antihistamine therapy. They are inexpensive and effective but have a sedating effect. The *nonsedating* H_1-blockers (e.g., *fexofenadine* 60 mg or *cetirizine* 10 mg every morning) are also effective and are better tolerated for daytime use. Disadvantages are their substantial cost and, with some H_1-blockers, drug–drug interactions (see Chapter 222). It is often best to use a nonsedating antihistamine during the day and a more sedating agent at night. *Chlorpheniramine* and *diphenhydramine* are useful alternatives for nighttime use because they are available over the counter and are much less expensive; chlorpheniramine can be used in pregnancy.

In refractory cases of urticaria, H_1-blockers (e.g., 400 mg of cimetidine three times daily) may improve control in combination with H_1-antihistamines. The rationale for the use of H_2-blockers is that 15% of the receptors in the cutaneous vasculature are H_2-receptors. *Doxepin*, a tricyclic antidepressant with potent H_1-blocker activity, has proved to be helpful in persons with urticaria complicated by anxiety or depression. Low doses (e.g., 25 mg twice daily or 25 mg daily at bedtime) may be useful. Doxepin should not be used concurrently with the H_1-blocker terfenadine.

Steroids and Other Drugs

For severe refractory cases, oral *glucocorticosteroids* are worth considering (see later discussion), but they must be used with care if prescribed for more than 1 to 2 weeks (see Chapter 105). Some reports suggest that the β_2-agonist *terbutaline* in fairly high doses (1.25 mg three times daily) can decrease itching and the number of episodes, but others find little benefit whether it is used alone or in combination with antihistamines. *Nifedipine*, a calcium-channel blocker, can improve the clinical appearance of lesions by interfering with mast cell activity, but overall efficacy is not impressive. *Anabolic steroids* have been used with success in hereditary angioedema (see later discussion). *Leukotriene-receptor antagonists* (e.g., *montelukast*) are better than placebo, indicating some mechanistic role for the leukotriene pathway, but there is no evidence of an additional advantage over maximal doses of H_1- and H_2-receptor antagonists.

Agents of No Proven Efficacy

Empiric trials of broad-spectrum antibiotics and antifungal agents have been advocated for the treatment of patients with idiopathic urticaria as a means of eliminating any occult infection, but there are no data to justify this hypothesis or their use. Specific treatment of infections such as sinusitis or vaginitis is appropriate only if infection is confirmed. Topical preparations of corticosteroids, antihistamines, and local anesthetics are expensive and without benefit in chronic urticaria.

Treatment Applications

Acute Attacks

Mild to moderate attacks usually respond well to a full program of oral antihistamines. Severe attacks complicated by angioedema are an indication for the prompt administration of subcutaneous aqueous *epinephrine* (0.3 mL of a 1:1,000 dilution). For severe acute urticaria uncomplicated by angioedema, a short course of systemic steroids (e.g., *prednisone* started at 40 mg/d and rapidly tapered to full cessation by 1 week) can help to provide symptomatic relief, but it should not be a substitute for a careful etiologic evaluation.

Physical Urticaria

The physical urticarias are also treated with antihistamines. *Cyproheptadine* is an H_1-blocker that is particularly useful for aquagenic, cold-induced, and dermatographic urticaria. Topical *capsaicin* has been tried in patients with cold-induced and localized heat-induced urticaria; results are variable. Antihistamines have been useful in vibratory physical urticaria. Exercise-induced urticaria can be treated by avoiding vigorous exercise, and it is important for the patient not to exercise after eating or when taking aspirin or NSAIDs.

Chronic and Refractory Urticaria

Controlling chronic urticaria requires empiricism and careful follow-up. One begins with an H_1-blocker, usually a nonsedating agent. If this fails, an H_1-blocker, such as *cimetidine*, is added. If the patient fails to respond, *doxepin* is substituted. In severe cases, a brief course of *systemic corticosteroids* (e.g., 20 to 40 mg of prednisone daily), with rapid taper after 10 to 14 days and a switch to alternate-day therapy with ultimate elimination by 3 to 4 weeks, is reasonable. Longer-term systemic steroid therapy usually fails to provide adequate control and is associated with adverse effects more serious than the condition for which it is being taken (see Chapter 105). Patients with chronic refractory disease who manifest antithyroid antibodies should be given a trial of exogenous *thyroid hormone* sufficient to lower the level of thyroid-stimulating hormone. The patient with idiopathic urticaria and positive *H. pylori* serology is a reasonable candidate for the consideration of *antibiotic therapy*, but antibiotics should not be administered unless evidence of active infection is present (see Chapter 68).

Hereditary Angioedema

An acute attack that threatens airway obstruction should be treated with subcutaneous *epinephrine* (0.3 mL of a 1:1,000 dilution). Patients with known angioedema should carry an epinephrine self-administration kit. The best treatment is the prevention of attacks. Synthetic *anabolic steroids* (e.g., danazol, stanozolol) have been used in cases of frequent or severe attacks. They appear to induce the synthesis of normally functioning C1 esterase inhibitor. Periodic monitoring of the C1 esterase inhibitor level and of liver function is required. A purified C1 INH is under development for the prophylaxis and treatment of acute attacks.

INDICATIONS FOR REFERRAL AND ADMISSION

The management of urticaria can be frustrating, and it is often useful both for physician and patient to enlist the aid of a specialist. Allergists can help evaluate patients with repeated eruptions possibly caused by food allergies that can be detected on testing, although the probability of food allergy being the cause of chronic urticaria is low. They may also perform penicillin skin testing, particularly with minor determinants. Their experience in seeing a large number of patients with urticaria helps to provides comfort and reassurance to the concerned patient. The patient with suspected urticarial vasculitis should be referred to the rheumatologist or dermatologist for skin biopsy and immunohistologic staining of the sample.

Admission for patients with acute angioedema complicated by airway symptoms or gastrointestinal symptoms may be necessary briefly for respiratory support and observation. Hospitalizations that are sometimes advocated for elimination diets are far too costly in a climate of cost containment.

PATIENT EDUCATION

It is important to educate the patient in advance of the workup that a cause is usually not found. One should emphasize the variable natural history of hives and the high probability that the lesions will disappear spontaneously, and prepare the patient for the likelihood that urticaria will recur. Patients should be instructed to avoid exacerbating factors (e.g., aspirin, NSAIDs, heat, exertion, alcoholic beverages). Specific advice, such as the avoidance of swimming in cold water for patients with cold urticaria, can be life-saving. The patient should be reassured that the medical workup will exclude serious and treatable diseases and that many options are available to shorten the process and alleviate symptoms. Eliminating unrealistic expectations can prevent the disappointment that may follow a negative workup. It is important to emphasize the overall good prognosis and the high probability that remission will occur, although it may be delayed.

Patients with a vague or distant history of penicillin allergy whose skin tests are negative can be reassured that the likelihood of a serious reaction is very small and that a penicillin or cephalosporin can be used without much risk.

A.H.G.

Annotated Bibliography

1. Bork K, Meng G, Staubach P, et al. Hereditary angioedema: new findings concerning symptoms, affected organs, and course. Am J Med 2006;119:267. (*A large retrospective series describing the characteristic clinical pattern.*)
2. Casale TB, Sampson HA, Hanifin J, et al. Guide to physical urticarias. J Allergy Clin Immunol 1989;82:758. (*Still one of the best reviews of the topic.*)
3. Charlesworth EN. Urticaria and angioedema: a clinical spectrum. Ann Allergy Asthma Immunol 1996;76:484. (*A broad overview, with an especially useful section on differential diagnosis.*)
4. Greaves MW. Chronic urticaria. N Engl J Med 1995;332:1767. (*A comprehensive, authoritative discussion, with good photographs, a practical algorithm for workup, and consideration of urticarial vasculitis; 59 references.*)
5. Kaplan AP. Chronic urticaria and angioedema. N Engl J Med 2002;346:175. (*A succinct, clinically relevant review of diagnosis and treatment, with a brief discussion of pathophysiology; 30 references.*)
6. Kostis JB, Kim HJ, Rusnak J, et al. Incidence and characteristics of angioedema associated with enalapril. Arch Intern Med 2005;165:1637. (*A large cohort study, finding that angioedema was uncommon [0.68%], and that being African American, having a history of drug rash, and being of older age were risk factors.*)
7. Soter NA. Acute and chronic urticaria and angioedema. J Am Acad Dermatol 1991;125:146. (*History was more useful than laboratory examination;*

half of the patients with urticaria alone and 25% of those with associated angioedema were free of lesions within 1 year; 20% experienced episodes for >20 years.*)
8. Wanderer AA, Bernstein IL, Goodman DL, et al. The diagnosis and management of urticaria: a practice parameter. Ann Allergy Asthma Immunol 2000;85:521. (*A practice parameter paper.*)
9. Arroliga ME, Pien L. Penicillin allergy. Cleve Clin J Med 2003;70:313. (*A practical review, with emphasis on testing for penicillin allergy.*)
10. Frieri M, Madden J. Chronic steroid-resistant urticaria. Ann Allergy 1993;70:13. (*An excellent discussion of this difficult problem for both patient and physician.*)
11. Kennard CD, Ellis CN. Pharmacologic therapy for urticaria. J Am Acad Dermatol 1991;25:176. (*Nonsedating antihistamines in combination with antidepressants or histamine$_2$-blockers may be useful.*)
12. Pollack CV Jr, Romano TJ. Outpatient management of acute urticaria: the role of prednisone. Ann Emerg Med 1995;26:5. (*A small-scale, randomized, prospective, placebo-controlled trial, finding that a 5-day course of prednisone was effective, regardless of etiology.*)
13. Rumbyrt JS, Katz JL, Schocket AL. Resolution of chronic urticaria in patients with thyroid autoimmunity. J Allergy Clin Immunol 1995;96:901. (*Patients with previously refractory urticaria responded to exogenous thyroid hormone.*)

CHAPTER 182 ■ APPROACH TO THE PATIENT WITH HAIR LOSS

PETER C. SCHALOCK AND ARTHUR J. SOBER

Alopecia may be described as the loss of hair in areas where it normally grows. The most noticeable area in which alopecia develops is the scalp, but loss of hair at other body sites may occur. Whether alopecia is a result of genetic influences, local inflammatory processes, or systemic disease, the primary care physician may be the first clinician to offer the patient a diagnosis and treatment options.

PATHOPHYSIOLOGY AND CLINICAL PRESENTATION (1–9)

Normal Hair Growth

The follicular unit is a product of proliferating and differentiating keratinocytes in the hair bulb (otherwise known as the matrix). The hair shaft (consisting of the cuticle, cortex, and medulla) is predominately hard keratin, or trichohyalin, rich in disulfide bonds. The growth of hair is cyclical, the length of the cycle varying with the location. Scalp hair grows from 2 to 6 years (anagen), enters a transition period over 2 to 3 weeks (catagen), and then involutes over 3 months (telogen). In contrast, the anagen phase for the short hairs on the extremities is between 2 and 6 months. Moreover, the longer (or shorter) the growth period, the longer (or shorter) the hair length. In healthy young persons, about 85% to 90% of all scalp hairs are in anagen, the phase of active growth. The remainder of hairs are in telogen (10% to 15%) and catagen (<1%). The number of terminal hairs on the scalp is estimated to be $250/cm^2$, with an average normal daily loss of 100 to 200 hairs, although there is considerable individual variation. Hairs that grow for long periods and rest briefly are the most susceptible to interruptions of the growth cycle, and variations in the ratio of the growth phase to the resting phase are most noticeable. Scalp hair grows at the rate of approximately 0.35 mm/d, or about 1 cm/mo, but multiple factors can affect the rate.

Hair Loss

Alopecia can be classified as *scarring* (cicatricial) or *nonscarring* (noncicatricial), depending on whether there is permanent injury to the bulge region (location of stem cells) located between the hair bulb and insertion of the erector pili muscle. The primary pathogenic mechanisms of hair loss are destruction of the hair matrix and stem cell bulge region by physical or chemical agents, infectious or immunologically mediated inflammation, metabolic diseases, and the administration of

All photos are courtesy of Peter C. Schalock.

antimetabolites or other drugs. In general, destructive agents (physical, chemical, or infectious) produce scarring alopecia, whereas systemic illnesses and drugs usually result in nonscarring alopecia.

In noncicatricial alopecia, the follicular integrity is retained, and once the inciting process subsides, there is potential for hair regrowth. In cicatricial alopecia, hair never regrows. A few conditions that begin as nonscarring alopecia may later develop into scarring alopecia with chronicity.

Nonscarring Alopecia

Alopecia is often nonscarring, with male- and female-pattern baldness accounting for most patient complaints.

Male-Pattern Hair Loss *or Baldness (Androgenetic Alopecia).* Male-pattern hair loss/baldness is symmetric, usually beginning in the frontoparietal scalp with progressive recession and vertex hair density thinning (Fig. 182.1). Its development is related to genetic predisposition and hormonal (dihydrotestosterone) activity, and it is age related. The inheritance is polygenetic or autosomal dominant, with incomplete penetrance. The process is permanent, with pigmented scalp hairs replaced by fine, unpigmented vellus hairs. Dihydrotestosterone (DHT) inhibits the growth of scalp hair, whereas it stimulates the growth of facial hair and promotes a male pattern of pubic hair growth. When DHT is taken exogenously, laboratory investigation reveals increased levels of free testosterone, sulfated dehydroepiandrosterone (DHEA-S), or both.

Female-Pattern Hair Loss. The mechanisms of female-pattern alopecia may be similar to those of male-pattern baldness, but female-pattern baldness is usually more diffuse, located centrally and in frontal scalp areas, without complete balding. Neither an androgenetic nor a genetic cause has been proven. Some cases may be due to *iron deficiency* or *thyroid disease.* Early-onset alopecia at puberty may be related to a strong family history, whereas onset of alopecia in older women (peri- or postmenopausal) may be due to genetic susceptibility combined with androgen sensitivity at the follicular level or systemic androgen excess.

Male-Pattern Hair Loss in Women. The presence of male-pattern hair loss in a female patient should provoke concern about *androgen excess,* manifested by hirsutism (growth of hair in a male distributed pattern) in mild cases and virilization (coarsening of facial features, voice deepening, and clitoral enlargement) in more serious cases. Polycystic ovary disease (Stein–Leventhal syndrome), androgen-producing ovarian and adrenal tumors (see Chapter 98), hyperprolactinemia, contraceptive pills or anabolic steroids, hepatic disease, and tumor production of ectopic androgens (usually carcinoid,

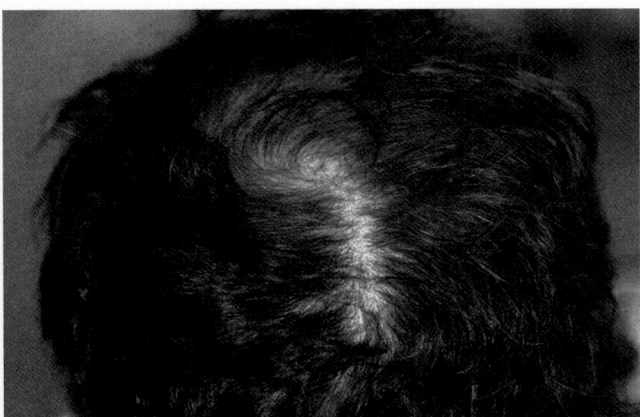

FIGURE 182.1. Male pattern alopecia in the typical "bald spot" on the occipital scalp. (See the color insert.)

choriocarcinoma, or metastatic lung cancer) are some causes of androgen excess and hirsutism.

Systemic Disease, Metabolic Abnormalities, and Medications. Nonscarring alopecia is often associated with systemic disease, a metabolic abnormality, or the use of medications. *Alopecia areata*, a condition that is believed to be an autoimmune attack on the hair follicle, results in relatively rapidly hair loss in distinct, well-defined round or oval patches (Fig. 182.2). Less common variants of alopecia areata include *ophiasis* (a bandlike pattern involving the occiput and bilateral temporal regions) and generalized patterns, where one encounters generalized thinning rather than distinct patches of hair loss. *Alopecia totalis* is the progressive loss of all scalp hair; *alopecia universalis* manifests as complete facial and body hair loss.

Presumed *autoimmune diseases* like *vitiligo*, *Hashimoto's thyroiditis*, and inflammatory bowel disease are associated with the onset of alopecia areata. The course of alopecia areata is unpredictable. Some persons have one episode, in which the development of one or several bald spots is followed by spontaneous regrowth. In others, new areas of alopecia may develop, and they become totally bald. Onset before puberty is associated with a poorer prognosis.

Diffuse hair thinning may occur in *thyroid disease* and *iron deficiency*. Less commonly, hypopituitarism and parathyroid disease produce hair loss. Alopecia is a manifestation of *connective tissue diseases*, notably systemic lupus erythematosus and dermatomyositis. Occasionally, hair loss is self-induced, a condition known as *trichotillomania*. Such patients may not be aware that they are plucking hairs, and the condition may indicate significant psychiatric disturbance.

Secondary syphilis, *HIV infection*, *superficial folliculitis*, and *tinea capitis* also produce nonscarring alopecia. Commonly used *medications* that can cause alopecia include β-blockers, tricyclic antidepressants, anticonvulsants, systemic retinoids, warfarin and heparin anticoagulants, allopurinol, antithyroid drugs, quinine, verapamil, indomethacin, sulfasalazine, haloperidol, and vitamin A in excessive doses (see Table 182.1). Antineoplastic agents such as 5-fluorouracil, paclitaxel, cyclophosphamide, and methotrexate predictably produce hair loss.

Physiologic Alterations in Follicular Cycling. Alterations in the cycling of the follicular unit may produce nonscarring hair loss, a process known as *telogen effluvium*, by altering the relation between the growing and resting phases of hair follicles. *High fever* due to illness, surgery, postpartum, medications (such as *oral contraceptives*), and even *seasonal changes* may result in rapid hair loss 2 to 4 months after the insult. However, a more chronic telogen effluvium, such as that seen in middle-aged women, may present insidiously. During pregnancy, fewer hairs are shed (due to prolonged anagen), so that fewer telogen hairs are produced. *Postpartum*, the percentage of telogen hairs increases substantially and hair is lost diffusely over several subsequent months. Postpartum alopecia resolves within 18 months, but about half of women feel they have less hair after childbirth than they did before pregnancy.

Scarring Alopecia

Cicatricial hair loss (Fig. 182.3) is a result of permanent destruction of the stem cell region. Forms of physical trauma, such as burns, radiation, physical trauma, and chronic traction, are commonly responsible. Traction alopecia usually results from braiding or the use of tight hair rollers. The pattern of hair loss depends on the styling. The process is initially reversible but progresses to fibrosis and scarring with time. The use of hot combs in combination with petrolatum to straighten hair in darkly pigmented individuals may contribute to a condition known as central centrifugal cicatricial alopecia, characterized by midline alopecia that progresses centrifugally over the scalp. This condition highlights the deleterious effects of repetitive heat, traction, and trauma to the scalp. Factitious conditions like trichotillomania may result in end-stage scarring if they are chronic. Infections, including bacterial (folliculitis decalvans and dissecting cellulitis), fungal (kerion), or viral (e.g., recurrent herpes simplex or herpes zoster), result in significant inflammation and follicular destruction. Other dermatologic conditions, such as chronic cutaneous lupus erythematosus (Fig. 182.4) (discoid lupus erythematosus), scleroderma, lichen planus (lichen planopilaris), cutaneous or metastatic neoplasms to the scalp, and infiltrative diseases like sarcoidosis, result in cicatricial alopecia.

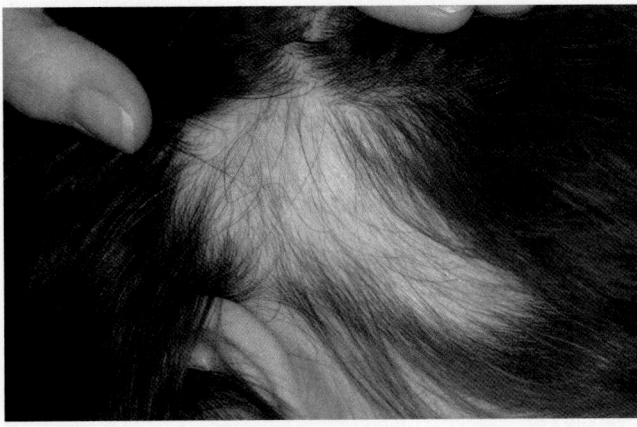

FIGURE 182.2. Alopecia areata on the temporal scalp, partially in the "ophiasis" distribution. (See the color insert.)

TABLE 182.1

DIFFERENTIAL DIAGNOSIS OF HAIR LOSS

Nonscarring Alopecia
- Androgenic
  - Male pattern
  - Female pattern
- Alopecia areata
- Post febrile infection
- Folliculitis (mild)
- Tinea capitis (ectothrix)

Human immunodeficiency virus infection
Hypothyroidism
Iron deficiency
Systemic lupus erythematosus
Syphilis
Medications
- Antineoplastics
- Antimetabolites
- Propylthiouracil

Scarring Alopecia
- Physical trauma
  - Burns
  - Radiation
  - Chronic traction
- Infection
- Bacterial folliculitis (severe)
- Fungal (endothrix)

Antidepressants
Anticonvulsants
Anticoagulants
Allopurinol, probenecid
β-Blockers
Quinine
High-dose vitamin A, isotretinoin

Oral contraceptives
Discontinuation of corticosteroids
Psychiatric
  Trichotillomania
Telogen effluvium
Crash diets
Post pregnancy

Discoid lupus erythematosus
Morphea
Lichen planopilaris
Pseudopelade
Neoplasms
Granulomatous disease
Factitial

Hair Breakage

Alopecia may arise from hair shaft abnormalities due to inherited structural defects in the hair fiber. These include monilethrix, pili torti, trichorrhexis nodosa, trichoschisis, and trichorrhexis invaginatum. There are many inherited syndromes that include hair abnormalities as a component of the syndrome, usually presenting in childhood. Referral to a pediatric dermatologist can be helpful for the diagnosis of children with hair breakage.

In general, hair loss must be differentiated from hair breakage, which results from physical or chemical stress to the shaft. The term proximal trichorrhexis is sometimes used to describe hair breakage within the first centimeter from the scalp, whereas breakage beyond this point is called distal trichorrhexis. Hair straightening can cause proximal trichorrhexis. Patients often recognize distal breakage as split ends; such breakage may be accelerated by being exposed to sunshine or swimming in chlorinated pools.

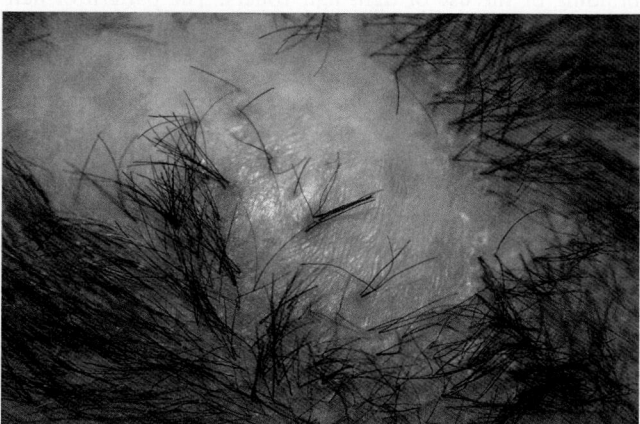

FIGURE 182.3. Scarring alopecia with "doll's hairs" (scarring encasing many hair shafts). (See the color insert.)

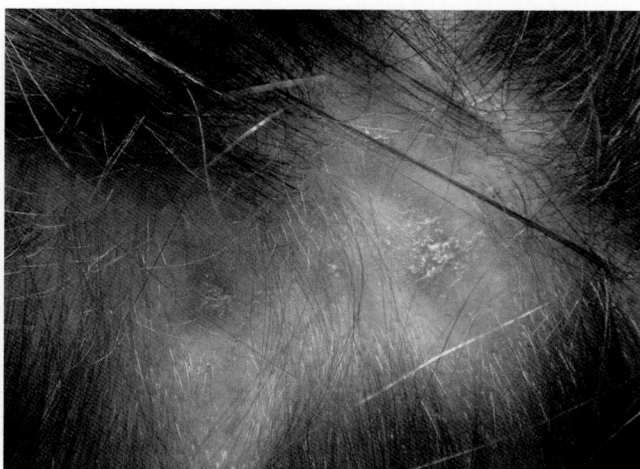

FIGURE 182.4. Chronic cutaneous lupus erythematosus causing a scarring alopecia on the scalp. (See the color insert.)

DIFFERENTIAL DIAGNOSIS
(1,4,6,7)

See Table 182.1.

WORKUP (4–8)

History

The history should begin by investigating the duration and time period over which the hair has been lost. It is especially helpful to review a family history of male- or female-pattern baldness in all patients. Has the patient been troubled only by a specific area of hair loss or by generalized hair loss? Has there been a recent or chronic stressful event or systemic illness (infectious, endocrine, autoimmune) such as hypothyroidism, systemic lupus, or iron deficiency? Is there a history of physical trauma (e.g., pulling the hair; use of curlers, bleaches, permanent wave lotions, straightening lotions, hot combs)? A review of current and previous medications is essential to the investigation, with emphasis on chemotherapeutic agents, anticonvulsants, anticoagulants, antihypertensives, colchicine, antithyroid drugs, androgens, oral contraceptives, isotretinoin, and vitamin A. Other precipitants worth noting include recent pregnancy or surgery, significant dieting, and the presence of skin conditions such as lupus, lichen planus, folliculitis, tinea, or other conspicuous inflammatory or infectious lesions.

Physical Examination

The scalp is examined carefully for areas of reduced hair growth, hair loss, and scarring. The pattern of hair loss is noted. Is it localized or diffuse? Is an androgenetic pattern present? It is essential to differentiate scarring from nonscarring alopecia, the latter presenting with preservation of follicles or small, fine, lightly pigmented hairs. The presence of short, broken hairs suggests hair pulling or trauma. One examines the surrounding areas for evidence of inflammation and induration, folliculitis, and fungal infection. If available, a Wood's light may produce a fluorescent glow in an area infected by some fungal organisms. Any area of inflammation presenting with weeping lesions, crust, or scale should be scraped for microscopic examination (see Chapter 191) and culture.

To obtain objective evidence of hair loss, it is may be useful to have the patient collect lost hairs daily within envelopes and count the total. From 50 to 200 hairs per day is within normal limits. If the circular areas characteristic of alopecia areata are seen, applying light traction to the hairs at the edge of the bald area may indicate whether disease is active at that location. If hairs come out with ease, then extension of the alopecic area is to be expected. Some dermatologists perform telogen counts by removing 100 hairs and counting how many are in the telogen phase. With this procedure, the examiner can distinguish between conditions resulting from telogen excess and those resulting from broken hairs, but it may be too time-consuming to be useful to the primary physician and is best reserved for the dermatologist experienced in its performance.

Evidence of systemic illness should be sought, including signs of hypothyroidism (see Chapter 104), lupus (see Chapter 146), iron deficiency (see Chapter 79), and sarcoidosis (see Chapter 51). One checks the woman with male-pattern hair loss for signs of hirsutism and virilization (see Chapter 98).

Examining the nails for Beau's lines (linear, longitudinal depressed bands), pitting, clubbing, or other dystrophic changes may reveal a correlation with a systemic dermatologic or medical condition.

Laboratory Studies

A *biopsy* may be helpful, particularly in cases of scarring alopecia with suspected inflammation. The decision to perform laboratory tests to detect systemic disease (e.g., *complete blood cell count, serum iron, ferritin, total iron-binding capacity, thyroid-stimulating hormone, antinuclear antibody,* androgenic hormones such as *DHEA-S* and *free testosterone*) depends on the patient history and physical findings.

PRINCIPLES OF THERAPY
(1–3,6,10–14)

The primary care physician can provide the patient with reassurance, advice, and, when appropriate, specific therapy. The treatment of alopecia essentially depends on an established diagnosis, a result of history, physical exam, and, at times, scalp biopsy. Patients who perceive excessive hair loss that is not substantiated by exam or daily hair counting of lost hair should be reassured. Sympathetic consolation and affirming a good prognosis is particularly important in women with pregnancy-related telogen effluvium. Drugs associated with hair loss should be discontinued if possible and alternatives sought. Scalp infection, either bacterial or fungal, requires directed treatment (see Chapters 190 and 191), as does any underlying dermatologic or systemic disease. Hair regrowth eventually takes place after successful therapy of nonscarring alopecia. Occasionally, purchasing a hair prosthesis (wig) or a scarf (see Chapter 88) may be helpful.

Symptomatic Measures

In the vast majority of cases of hair loss, the cause is either alopecia areata or androgenetic baldness, and treatment is symptomatic for those troubled by the cosmetic effects.

Alopecia Areata

Alopecia areata is often self-limited, but if the condition is severe, it may be worthwhile to consider specific medical therapy, which should be undertaken only by a dermatologist or physician skilled in its application. A wide range of options is available to patients, ranging from topical and systemic immunotherapy to immunomodulators and contact sensitizers. These include single or combination therapies of topical and intralesional steroids (such as using triamcinolone acetonide), oral minoxidil, topical tacrolimus, imiquimod, anthralin or squaric acid dibutyl ester, phototherapy, photodynamic therapy, systemic steroids (pulsed methylprednisolone or prednisone), or systemic cyclosporine. The efficacy of some of these agents has yet to be explored in larger series. When preparations of steroids are used intralesionally, the patient should be made aware of the potential risk for dermal atrophy, telangiectasias, and hypopigmentation. To circumvent this, small volumes of dilute steroid solutions are used (3 to 10 mg/mL of triamcinolone), and injections every month for many months may be necessary to cover a large area. Systemic corticosteroids and cyclosporine have on occasion been helpful, but their effectiveness is often lost when the drugs are discontinued, and the risks of long-term therapy (see Chapter 105) outweigh the benefits. They should be used only under exceptional circumstances and only by a dermatologist experienced in treating patients with hair problems.

Despite the substantial interest in various therapies and the literature extolling them, no approach can be judged effective enough to recommend in all occasions. Many experienced clinicians believe that treatment merely accelerates resolution in the approximately 50% of patients with alopecia areata in whom hair would spontaneously regrow in any event. Some argue that watchful waiting is the safest and most cost-effective approach.

Male-Pattern Hair Loss

Male-pattern hair loss compromises the self-image and self-confidence of many men. Available treatments include oral *finasteride* (Propecia) and topical *minoxidil*.

Finasteride. Finasteride acts on the enzyme 5α-reductase type 2, blocking the conversion of testosterone to its active metabolite, DHT, a potent androgen. In men ages 18 to 41 years, careful studies have shown that after 1 year, men treated with finasteride (1 mg daily) have higher vertex hair counts, which are maintained for up to 24 months. Fifty percent of treated men find the appearance of their hair improved. Additional studies have shown that 65% of men can regrow their hair, and therapy stops hair loss in 90% of men. A small number of adverse events are seen, but not much more than in placebo-treated patients. These include loss of libido, erectile dysfunction, or a decrease in ejaculatory volume (occurring in about 2% of cases). Serum levels of prostate-specific antigen are reduced by 40% to 50%, so that the values obtained must be doubled when being interpreted in prostate cancer screening. The ratio of bound to unbound (percentage of free) prostate-specific antigen is not affected by finasteride. Like minoxidil, continued use is necessary to sustain regrowth, and effects may not be seen until 6 months or more of use.

Minoxidil. A topical nonprescription 5% solution of the antihypertensive *minoxidil* (Rogaine) works best in younger men (<40 years) who have been bald for less than 10 years. The patient should be aware that 6 months of daily treatment might be necessary before hair growth becomes apparent, and that new hair persists only as long as the twice-daily applications are continued. New growth may be lost within 2 to 6 months of discontinuing treatment. The only common side effect is local irritation, and, although rare, patients with a low systolic pressure may experience postural hypotension with dizziness.

Many men use both finasteride and topical minoxidil. Both drugs may to some extent prevent further hair loss. In one long-term study, hair growth tended to peak at 1 year, with a slow decline in regrowth subsequently. After $4^1/_2$ to 5 years of use, nonvellus (terminal) hairs were maintained above the baseline counts.

Spironolactone and Dexamethasone. Women with male-pattern hair loss may have associated hirsutism. This combination suggests androgen excess and should be treated specific to the etiology (see Chapter 98). Symptomatically, androgen excess can be treated with spironolactone (75 to 200 mg/d for at least 6 months) or dexamethasone (0.125 to 0.250 mg at bedtime for at least 6 months). Clinically, the hirsutism may improve before the alopecia does.

Female-Pattern Alopecia

Female-pattern hair loss is an increasingly common complaint, with 40% of women experiencing cosmetically significant hair loss by the sixth decade. Women whose hair is thinning fear that they will become bald like men affected by androgenetic baldness. However, women should be informed this rarely happens. Low-strength (2%) minoxidil is approved for female pattern hair loss. Women (and men) may initially experience hair loss after initiating therapy, but decreased shedding and stimulation of new hair growth within 6 to 12 months of use can be expected. Women should not use the 5%-strength *minoxidil*, although they may use and find it more effective. It may cause hypertrichosis, and therefore precautions should be taken to avoid contact on these areas. Women of childbearing age must not take finasteride, and pregnant women should not even handle crushed or broken tablets because of the risk for development of congenital genitourinary abnormalities in male offspring. Recently, *flutamide* has been shown to be more effective than *finasteride* or *cyproterone* acetate after 1 year of use in hyperandrogenetic premenopausal women. This drug has been shown to be safe for use in postmenopausal women but has not been shown to be effective.

PATIENT EDUCATION

Education can be the most important part of the primary care provider's management of the patient with alopecia. Once the diagnosis is established and serious diseases are excluded, the patient can be reassured. Patients are often concerned that hair loss will progress, and the most useful information that can be provided is the actual likelihood of progressive or total hair loss. Even men with genetic alopecia are often reassured to know that they do not have a systemic disease. Success in the management of alopecia often depends on the physician's ability to help patients come to terms with their hair loss.

Hair Care

Advice on hair care is greatly appreciated by most patients. They should be advised to avoid alkaline pH shampoos (alkaline pH softens the hair and breaks bonds allowing for straightening) and excessive toweling or blow drying after washing. Use of a conditioner may be helpful. Combing is less injurious than brushing. If one must brush, it is useful to disentangle the hair from the brush gently and to use a brush with natural bristles or a nylon brush with rounded edges. Patients should avoid bleaching, permanent waving, straightening, using hot combs, and excessive exposure to the sun.

Hair Weaving and Transplants

Patients are often well aware of the option of a hair prosthesis but may ask the primary physician about such issues as hair weaving or hair transplants. Weaving is a relatively safe procedure performed by nonphysicians. It is a successful option, but must be repeated periodically. Hair transplants are expensive and have varying rate of success. The procedure may be painful and is usually not covered by insurance. However, it is a viable option for many patients, especially those with coarse, dark hair. Implants of artificial hair should be discouraged because they have a tendency to be unsuccessful over time or elicit a chronic foreign-body reaction.

Annotated Bibliography

1. Bolduc C, Shapiro J. Management of androgenetic alopecia. Am J Clin Dermatol 2000;1:151. (*A directed review on current pathophysiology and therapies available to the patient.*)
2. Hunt N, McHale S. The psychological impact of alopecia. BMJ 2005; 331:951. (*A concise review of psychological aspects of hair loss, especially depression and anxiety.*)
3. McKinney PA, Finkenbine RD, DeVane CL. Alopecia and mood stabilizer therapy. Ann Clin Psychiatry 1996;8:183. (*Alopecia is a common side effect in patients treated with 10% lithium, 12% valproate, and 6% carbamazepine.*)
4. Olsen E, Stenn K, Bergfeld W, et al. Update on cicatricial alopecia. J Invest Dermatol Symp Proc 2003;8:189. (*A superb technical review of scarring alopecia.*)
5. Rebora A. Telogen effluvium. Dermatology 1997;195:209. (*Distinguishing acute and chronic telogen effluvium from androgenetic alopecia.*)
6. Roberts JL. Androgenetic alopecia in men and women: an overview of cause and treatment. Dermatol Nursing 1997;9:379. (*The selective activity of finasteride against 5α-reductase reduces levels of follicular dihydrotestosterone, the hormone that leads to miniaturization of hairs.*)
7. Vafaie J, Weinberg JM, Smith B, et al. Alopecia in association with sexually transmitted disease: a review. Cutis. 2005;76:361. (*Review of sexually transmitted disease causes of alopecia, predominantly HIV and syphilis.*)
8. Shellow WVR, Edwards JE, Koo JYM. Profile of alopecia areata: a questionnaire analysis of patient and family. Int J Dermatol 1992;31:186. (*A strong family history is found in 42% of participants, and there is an association between alopecia areata and type 1 diabetes.*)
9. Whiting DA. Chronic telogen effluvium. Dermatol Clin 1996;14:723. (*This form of diffuse hair loss in women ages 30 to 60 years is characterized by an abrupt onset but a self-limited course.*)
10. Carmina E, Lobo RA. Treatment of hyperandrogenic alopecia in women. Fertil Steril 2003;79:91. (*Flutamide at 250 mg/d for 1 year was more effective than finasteride or cyproheptadine acetate in a large cohort of hyperandrogenic premenopausal women.*)
11. Hoffmann R, Happle R. Topical immunotherapy in alopecia areata. What, how and why? Dermatol Clin 1996;14:739. (*Cytokines and growth factors are involved in the pathogenesis of alopecia areata and in the therapeutic effect mediated by contact sensitizers.*)
12. Olsen EA. Topical minoxidil in the treatment of androgenetic alopecia in women. Cutis 1991;48:243. (*This study found that 2% minoxidil is effective in the treatment of female-pattern baldness; 5% minoxidil cannot be used by women.*)
13. Olsen E, Hordinsky M, McDonald-Hull S, et al. Alopecia areata investigational assessment guidelines. National Alopecia Areata Foundation. Am Acad Dermatol 1999;40:242. (*A useful resource for national guidelines and data comparison.*)
14. Price VH, Roberts JL, Hordinsky M, et al. Lack of efficacy of finasteride in postmenopausal women with androgenetic alopecia. J Am Acad Dermatol 2000;43:768. (*After 1 year of use at 1 mg/d, there was no change in hair growth or progression of loss.*)

CHAPTER 183 ■ DISTURBANCES OF SKIN HYDRATION: DRY SKIN AND EXCESSIVE SWEATING

PETER C. SCHALOCK AND ARTHUR J. SOBER

PART 1: MANAGEMENT OF DRY SKIN

Dry skin, or simple xerosis, is commonly seen during the winter months and occurs more often in the elderly. The most common clinical presentation is scaling skin with or without mild to moderate itching (see Chapter 178). A related condition is mild irritant dermatitis. This is seen particularly on the hands and the face. Fingertip fissuring is another common problem during winter months. Severe chronic dry skin can become eczematous (*asteatotic eczema*). The primary physician should recognize dry skin and use simple measures and effective patient education to relieve the symptoms.

PATHOPHYSIOLOGY AND CLINICAL PRESENTATION (1,2)

Pathophysiology

The term "dry" implies that the basic defect is a lack of water, but in reality causes of xerosis are multifactorial. As the

---

All photos are courtesy of Peter C. Schalock.

water percentage in the top layer of epidermis—the stratum corneum—drops from a normal level of 15% to 20% to below 10%, signs of xerosis such as scaling appear. Skin barrier damage causes an increase in evaporative water loss through a defective stratum corneum.

The lipids that aid in the retention of water within the stratum corneum diminish with age, low humidity, forced-air heat, or cold winter winds. Excessive use of soap, detergent, or disinfectants damages the stratum corneum and increases water loss up to 50 times the normal rate. Cigarette smoking also disrupts the skin's lipid barrier and can lead to dry skin. A familial tendency toward the development of dry skin remains incompletely defined. A variety of hygroscopic chemicals are known to retain water in the skin, including lactic acid, urea, and sodium pyrrolidine carboxylic acid. In addition, creams containing lipids similar to those in the stratum corneum can help repair the barrier function of the skin. Collectively, these substances are referred to as moisturizing agents.

Clinical Presentation

Dry skin is characterized by scaling and loss of suppleness and elasticity. The clinical appearance is one of fine scaling of the

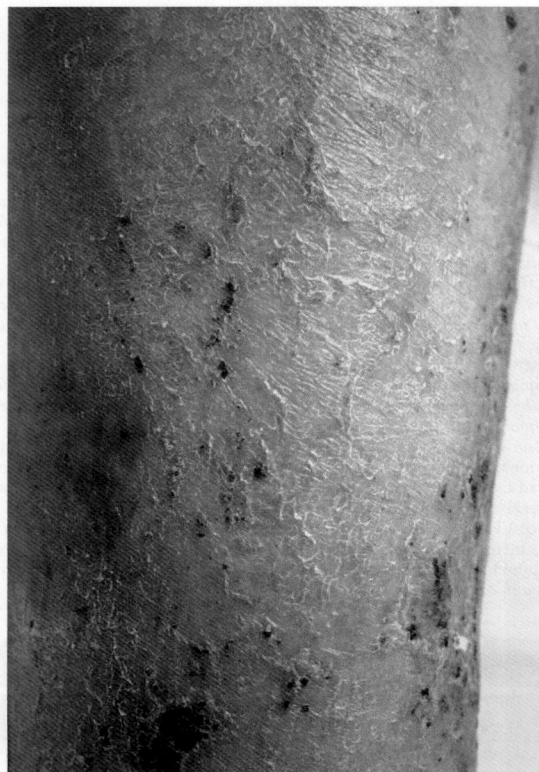

FIGURE 183.1. Erythema craquelé/severe xerosis on the shins. (See the color insert.)

lower portions of the legs. In severe xerosis, loss of elasticity leads to cracking and fissuring, producing a superficial appearance of "cracked porcelain," referred to as *eczema craquelé* (Fig. 183.1). Itching is a frequent concomitant and may lead to scratching and excoriation. Occasionally, dry skin is a consequence of hypovitaminosis A, drug reactions, hypothyroidism, or ichthyosis (vulgaris, acquired or hereditary).

PRINCIPLES OF THERAPY (1–5)

After systemic causes such as hypothyroidism have been ruled out (see Chapter 104), treatment is largely symptomatic. The goals are to prevent loss of water and restore hydration. Modalities include environmental manipulations, modifications in habits, and the judicious use of agents that hold water in the skin.

Preventive Measures

One should teach the patient to avoid very strong soaps, detergents, and excessive contact with water, which dry the skin. Many soaps are essentially detergents and are extremely dehydrating. Substituting a well-oilated soap is recommended. Daily bathing may also be too drying, although a brief, cool shower is much less drying than a bath. Teaching the patient to avoid liquid shower soaps and gels (even if the label says the are "moisturizing") can be helpful, as is adding a nonfragranced bath oil if baths are taken. Remind patients that if bath oil is used, they need to exercise caution regarding slips and falls.

It is also wise to avoid exposure to mild irritants, such as solvents, and wool clothing. It is important to humidify the indoor environment, particularly during the winter months.

Restoring Hydration

The treatment of preexisting dryness requires the addition of water and the application of hydrophobic agents. The physician should instruct patients to soak affected areas for several minutes and then apply a hydrophobic substance. Basically, most of the lotions and creams contain combinations of *petrolatum* (Vaseline), *mineral oil*, *lanolin*, *glycerin*, and *water* in proprietary blends. Ointments contain the lowest water content and are most effective. To make a cream, water and a preservative are blended in an ointment base. Lotions contain even more water and in fact can lead to further drying due to water evaporation. Plain petrolatum is inexpensive and effective, but it is not as pleasant to use as many proprietary preparations. Patients with an allergy to wool should avoid lanolin-based emollients (including Aquaphor).

A wide variety of agents are available, and patients are subjected to multimedia advertising for many of these products. *Aveeno* and *Curel lotions* are light and easily applied but are less occlusive than emollient creams. *Lac-Hydrin Five* is a 5% ammonium lactate and *Am-Lactin* is a 12% ammonium lactate that are available over the counter.

Creams containing ceramides are commercially available (*CeraVe*). Two creams have recently been approved by the U.S. Food and Drug Administration (FDA) as medical devices for treating atopic dermatitis that act to repair the barrier function. *MimyX* is a cream that is compounded with a bioactive fat—palmitoylethanolamide—which is considered lacking in atopic skin. *Atopiclair* is a moisturizer also for atopic dermatitis and contains glycyrrhetinic acid. Neither cream contains topical steroids or calcineurin inhibitors, and they are similar in their effectiveness to low-potency topical steroids.

Aquaphor and *Elta* are greasier than the aforementioned lotions and creams and are more effective in decreasing xerosis. Plain white petrolatum may be the most economical emollient.

The many expensive skin creams do little to retain moisture in the skin. Hygroscopic agents such as urea, *α-hydroxy acids*, *sorbitol*, and *glycerol* have chemical properties that retain moisture in the skin. Most moisturizers contain *propylene glycol*. If a patient experiences irritation with use of a facial moisturizer, it may be the propylene glycol that is causing the problem.

In severe cases, or to achieve more rapid results, *topical corticosteroids may be applied*. The use of Lac-Hydrin may help to relieve fissured fingertips, but sometimes a medium-potency corticosteroid ointment is required. If fissured fingertips are especially painful, the application of cyanoacrylate (Krazy Glue) can bring immediate relief, although patients can become sensitized to this compound over time.

Occasionally, oral *antipruritic agents*, such as the antihistamines, may be required for severe, generalized itching that results from xerosis (see Chapter 178). The physician should emphasize patient education to prevent recurrence.

THERAPEUTIC RECOMMENDATIONS (1–5)

■ Instruct the patient about environmental modifications to increase ambient humidity. Home humidification in winter may be useful in cold climate areas. Room temperature should be kept as low as is compatible with comfort.

- Caution the patient to avoid dehydrating soaps, solvents, or disinfectants or excessive contact with water. The skin should not be scrubbed.
- Encourage the use of bath oils and well-oiled soaps. The patient should soak in the tub for 1 to 10 minutes before the bath oil is added. Warn the patient about the potential for bath oil to cause slipping. Oils can also be applied after showering.
- Emollients should be used after showering or bathing. A variety of agents can be tried, beginning with the an inexpensive one, to find one that is acceptable.

- Lotions or creams that contain from 5% to 12% ammonium lactate help hold water in the stratum corneum.
- In the presence of eczematous change or for a patient who insists on rapid resolution, topical moderate-potency corticosteroid ointments with or without occlusion may be used.
- The most important aspect of management is patient education. The primary care provider should reinforce the adjustments that prevent the development of dryness.

Annotated Bibliography

1. Westphal SA. Unusual presentations of hypothyroidism. Am J Med Sci 1997;314:333. (*Dry skin is one of the common presentations, along with other classic signs and symptoms.*)
2. Steigleder R, Raab WP. Skin protection afforded by ointments. J Invest Dermatol 1962;38:129. (*Various ointments were compared with regard to barrier effectiveness; white petrolatum proved to be the best.*)
3. Proksch E, Lachapelle JM. The management of dry skin with topical emollients—recent perspectives. J Dtsch Dermatol Ges 2005;3:768–74. (*A detailed review of the pathophysiology and treatment of cutaneous xerosis.*)
4. Ghadially R, Halkier-Sorensen L, Elias PM. Effects of petrolatum on stratum corneum structure and function. J Am Acad Dermatol 1992;26:387. (*Petrolatum does not form or act like an impermeable membrane; rather, it permeates the interstices of the stratum corneum to allow normal barrier recovery.*)
5. Loden M. Barrier recovery and influence of irritant stimuli in skin treated with a moisturizing cream. Contact Dermatitis 1997;36:256. (*Treatment of surfactant-damaged skin with a moisturizing cream for 14 days promoted barrier recovery, as measured by water loss through the epidermis.*)

PART 2: APPROACH TO EXCESSIVE SWEATING

Excessive sweating (hyperhidrosis) is a common complaint, but it rarely signifies underlying pathology. Medical consultation may be sought because of abnormal wetness, a change in the pattern or the amount of sweating, sweaty palms, stained clothing, or offensive odor. The amount that people sweat in response to the physiologic stimuli of heat, emotion, or eating varies greatly. The interaction of the person, the environment, and the emotions influences the amount of sweating. The primary care provider must offer a scientific explanation and symptomatic management to the patient who complains of excessive sweating.

PATHOPHYSIOLOGY AND CLINICAL PRESENTATION (1)

Pathophysiology

Normal Physiology

Sweating helps to maintain temperature and fluid and electrolyte homeostasis, particularly under the environmental stresses of heat. There are two kinds of sweat glands—eccrine and apocrine. Cooling results from evaporation of eccrine sweat. Eccrine glands are concentrated on the palms and soles and are present on the face, axillae, and, to a lesser extent, the rest of the body. Heat causes sweating on the face, upper chest, and back. Sweating of the palms and soles is a characteristic response to stress. Gustatory sweating occurs on the face, particularly on the upper lip, often following ingestion of spicy foods. The eccrine glands have no anatomic relation to other cutaneous appendages.

Sebaceous and apocrine glands are closely associated with hair follicles. The apocrine glands are concentrated in the axillae, areolae, groin, and perineum. Apocrine secretions consist of minuscule viscid and milky drops that produce odor after bacteria act on them.

Eccrine sweating is controlled by neural factors or by reflex action. Thermal sweating is governed by the hypothalamus and emotional sweating by the cerebral cortex. The innervation of eccrine glands is anatomically sympathetic, but for unexplained reasons, the sweat glands are under cholinergic control and are therefore mediated by acetylcholine rather than by epinephrine.

Pathophysiology

Excess sweating may be induced by abnormalities of the autonomic nervous system. Autonomic overactivity of the sweat glands may occur without any identifiable cause. Sweating is associated with medical diseases that cause an increase in metabolic activity, so that heat must be dissipated. It is well known that sweating occurs during defervescence, particularly at night. Although the eccrine glands are under cholinergic control, epinephrine stimulates excessive sweating. Most cases of excess sweating are caused by exaggerated physiologic responses or functional variations of no pathologic consequence.

Clinical Presentation

Hyperhidrosis most commonly involves the palms, soles, or axillae. This may be a result of an increase in impulses from the central nervous system or it may reflect underlying problems with the sweat glands. A relation to emotional stress is often noted, and the problem becomes disabling if it interferes with work or social interactions. Axillary hyperhidrosis is less common than palmar or plantar hyperhidrosis. For many, it makes frequent clothing changes necessary.

DIFFERENTIAL DIAGNOSIS (1)

The most common cause of localized hyperhidrosis is the normal physiologic response to every day stress. Menopause is the leading cause of generalized sweats. Of the pathologic causes, *fever* is the most common. Night sweats raise the possibility of underlying *infectious disease* and *malignancy*. Central neurologic injury from *stroke* or tumor may produce hyperhidrosis. *Peripheral neuropathy* involving the autonomic nerves is associated with excess sweating, as are such medical conditions as *thyrotoxicosis* and, uncommonly, *pheochromocytoma*. *Parkinson's disease* may lead to increases in both sweating and sebaceous gland activity. Various *drugs*, such as antipyretics, insulin, meperidine, emetics, alcohol, and pilocarpine, may induce sweating. Gustatory sweating, although uncommon, may be caused by compensatory diabetic neuropathy, damage to the seventh cranial nerve such as during parotid surgery or trauma, the rare Frey's syndrome, or injury to the sympathetic trunk following surgery.

WORKUP (1)

History

Is the excess sweating restricted to the axillae, palms, and soles and indicative of a normal response to everyday events or is it more generalized, suggesting an underlying medical condition? If sweating occurs primarily at night, then inquiry into fever, fatigue, adenopathy, cough, sputum production, and other symptoms of infection and malignancy should be sought (see Chapter 11). Generalized sweating should also trigger questions regarding hyperthyroidism (see Chapter 103) and menopause (see Chapter 118). Paroxysms of sweating are consistent with panic disorder (see Chapter 226) and pheochromocytoma (see Chapter 19). A careful drug history is needed, with a check for use of antipyretics, insulin, meperidine, emetics, alcohol, and pilocarpine. The physician should ask whether excess sweating began relatively recently and whether it can be correlated with stress.

Physical Examination

The degree of sweating and its location are noted. If fever or generalized night sweats are reported, careful examination for underlying infection and malignancy is required (see Chapter 11). The patient should also be examined for signs of hyperthyroidism (see Chapter 103). The presence of increases in blood pressure should be noted because if the blood pressure is elevated in the setting of paroxysmal flushing and sweating, then pheochromocytoma should be considered. A careful neurologic examination is needed in patients suspected of central nervous system disease or peripheral autonomic neuropathy.

Laboratory Testing

No laboratory investigations are mandatory. Test selection is based entirely on the findings from history and physical examination. A screening "pan-scan" is of little use and is more likely to generate false-positive results than a true-positive one.

SYMPTOMATIC MANAGEMENT (1–6)

Excessive sweating can interfere with employment and social interactions. Many therapies have been used; several are effective, but some are associated with undesirable side effects.

Topical and Local Therapies

Topical Agents

The most effective topical agent for use on the hands and the axillae is a 20% alcoholic solution of *aluminum chloride hexahydrate* (Drysol). To be effective, it should be used under occlusion. A preparation of 6.25% aluminum tetrachloride (Xerac) is a less potent alternative. A clinical improvement in axillary hyperhidrosis may be seen after one to three consecutive treatments per week. Maintenance is usually possible with only one treatment per week after dryness has been achieved. Other topical therapies include 10% *formalin compresses*, which work well but can induce allergic sensitization, and formalin is a carcinogen. Buffered *glutaraldehyde* is effective but stains the skin and also induces allergic contact dermatitis.

Electrical current may be used to block sweat glands temporarily. *Topical iontophoresis* with either tap water or an anticholinergic agent and aluminum chloride can reduce sweating of the palms. Tap water units can be used at home. Response rates are greater than 80% and have been reported with an average remission of about 1 month.

Botulinum A Neurotoxin (Botox)

Botulinum A neurotoxin (*Botox*) is FDA approved for both axillary and palmar hyperhidrosis. Intradermal injection of Botox results in long-term reduction in sweating in both locations. When Botox is injected into the palm, some patients experience reversible minor weakness in their handgrip.

Surgery

In rare instances of genuinely incapacitating hyperhidrosis, surgery is sometimes considered. Axillary hyperhidrosis may be ameliorated with surgical *extirpation of the eccrine glands* in the axillae. Studies suggest that liposuction of the axillae may remove the sweat glands without altering the normal architecture. Palmar sweating may respond to *sympathectomy*, which can be performed endoscopically.

Systemic Therapy

Anticholinergic agents decrease sweating but have many undesired side effects, including dry eyes and mouth, blurry vision, constipation, and difficulty in urinating. *Phenoxybenzamine*, an adrenergic antagonist, has been reported to be successful in several cases of generalized hyperhidrosis, but it must be used carefully in persons with underlying cardiovascular disease. *Benzodiazepines* can be helpful in anxiety-related hyperhidrosis.

PATIENT EDUCATION

Patient education is crucial to the treatment of excess sweating. Providing the patient with a scientific explanation and a firm understanding of sweating is helpful in relieving anxiety. Patients with night sweats should record their temperature so that any significant febrile illness can be identified. The application of topical agents should be well explained and carefully carried out by patients. Surgical intervention for hyperhidrosis requires the patient's understanding of the risks and benefits of such a procedure and the active involvement of the primary care provider in helping the patient to reach a decision.

THERAPEUTIC RECOMMENDATIONS

- Once medical causes have been ruled out, reassure the patient that excess sweating is not the consequence of a pathologic condition.
- For axillary sweating, recommend frequent changes of clothing.
- For excess sweating of the palms or the axillae, recommend a 20% alcoholic solution of aluminum chloride hexahydrate (Drysol). An effective alternative is 6.25% aluminum tetrachloride (Xerac). It should be applied at bedtime and covered with a plastic food wrap; polyethylene or vinyl gloves can be worn if the palms are affected. In the morning, the treated areas should be washed with soap and water. Prescribe one to three consecutive treatments per week. Once dryness has been achieved, maintenance with one treatment per week should suffice.
- Electrical current may be used to block sweat glands temporarily. Use of the Drionic device daily for 1 week may relieve sweating for up to 1 month.
- Intradermal injection of botulinum toxin is should be considered as a relatively noninvasive therapy. Liposuction techniques may also be useful.
- If topical therapy and reassurance and less invasive approaches fail, sympathectomy performed via a thoracoscope may be considered for palmar or axillary disease, but only if the patient's hyperhidrosis is truly incapacitating. Referral should be made to a neurosurgeon or vascular surgeon for evaluation.

Annotated Bibliography

1. Sato K, Kang WH, Saga K, et al. Biology of sweat glands and their disorders. II. Disorders of sweat gland function. J Am Acad Dermatol 1989; 20:713. (*A definitive review with comments about therapy; 117 references.*)
2. Atkinson JLD, Fealey RD. Sympathotomy instead of sympathectomy for palmar hyperhidrosis: minimizing postoperative compensatory hyperhidrosis. Mayo Clin Proc 2003;78:167. (*Disconnection of the T2 ganglion input into the brachial plexus produces excellent results.*)
3. Benohanian A, Dansereau A, Bolduc C, et al. Localized hyperhidrosis treated with aluminum chloride in a salicylic acid gel base. Int J Dermatol 1998;37:701. (*Good and excellent results were achieved with the use of 20% to 30% aluminum chloride hexahydrate in a 4% salicylic acid gel base.*)
4. Elgart ML, Fuchs G. Tapwater iontophoresis in the treatment of hyperhidrosis. Int J Dermatol 1987;26:194. (*The device can be used at home by patients; it provides a reduction in hyperhidrosis for up to 6 weeks.*)
5. Heckmann M, Ceballos-Baumann AO, Plewig G, et al. Botulinum toxin A for axillary hyperhidrosis (excessive sweating). N Engl J Med 2001;344:488. (*A controlled trial of efficacy.*)
6. Thomas I, Brown J, Vafaie J, et al. Palmoplantar hyperhidrosis: a therapeutic challenge. Am Family Physician 2004;69:1117–20. (*A practical discussion of available therapies.*)

CHAPTER 184 ■ APPROACH TO THE PATIENT WITH DERMATITIS

PETER C. SCHALOCK AND ARTHUR J. SOBER

PART 1: ATOPIC OR CONTACT DERMATITIS

The atopic and contact dermatitides (also referred to as "*eczema*") are frequently encountered in medical practice, with a reported prevalence of atopic disease of up to 15% in Western industrialized countries. These conditions may be acute or chronic. The acute form is characterized by erythema, edema, vesiculation, oozing, crusting, and scaling. The chronic stage manifests excoriation, thickening, hyperpigmentation, and often lichenification. All are defined clinically by the observable changes in the skin, which reflect a common cutaneous reaction to a variety of pathogenetic stimuli. The clinical challenges for the primary care physician are to provide symptomatic relief and identify the underlying precipitant. These tasks can be difficult, often necessitating consultation with a dermatologist.

PATHOPHYSIOLOGY AND CLINICAL PRESENTATION (1–7)

Pathophysiology

Atopic Dermatitis

Pathogenesis remains incompletely understood, but genetic factors appear to predispose, with defects in cell-mediated

---

All photos are courtesy of Peter C. Schalock.

immunity noted, perhaps accounting for the observed increase in susceptibility to cutaneous viral infections. Many patients exhibit other forms of atopy, and two thirds have family members with asthma, hay fever, or eczema. Elevations of immunoglobulin E are seen in 40% to 80% of patients. Environmental irritants also contribute; certain fabrics, notably wool, may induce itching, and lesions are exacerbated by extremes of temperature and humidity. Psychological stress may trigger flares.

Infection may precipitate an attack. The skin of atopic persons is frequently colonized by *Staphylococcus aureus,* whereas fewer than 5% of those without atopy carry *S. aureus.* Risk of infection with *S. aureus* is markedly increased due to a deficiency in expression of the antimicrobial peptides LL-37 and HBD-2 compared to patients without atopic dermatitis. Other differences in atopic skin include the following: alteration in vascular activity, demonstrated by the formation of a white rather than a red line when the skin is stroked (white *dermatographism*); greater sweating response to acetylcholine than is seen in normal control individuals; deficiency of sebaceous gland lipids on the skin surface; lowered threshold for the release of histamine from basophils; and increased histamine levels in both skin and plasma.

Contact Dermatitis

The cause is exposure of the skin to a precipitant, which may have a purely irritant or an immunologic effect. Irritants penetrate and disrupt the stratum corneum, injuring the underlying epidermis and causing an inflammatory reaction. Irritant effects are universal and require no previous exposure. Strong acids, alkalis, detergents, and organic solvents are among the important irritants. It is extremely rare for laundry detergents to cause contact dermatitis, although the antistatic products and fragrances contained in these products can be problematic.

Immunologically mediated contact reactions occur only in patients previously sensitized to an allergen. Reactions are classified into *urticarial (type I)* and *delayed (type IV) hypersensitivity reactions.* Common sensitizing antigens for urticaria include latex rubber (most commonly in health care workers) and animal-derived proteins (from shellfish, meats, etc.); the plant oil component urushiol accounts for the delayed hypersensitivity skin reactions of poison oak and poison ivy, which typically take up to 48 hours to develop.

By patch testing, the top 10 contact allergens in the United States areas follows: nickel sulfate (16.7%), neomycin (11.6%), *Myroxilon pereirae* (balsam of Peru) (11.6%), fragrance mix (10.4%), thimerosal (10.2%), sodium gold thiosulfate (10.2%), quaternium-15 (9.3%), formaldehyde (8.4%), bacitracin (7.9%), and cobalt chloride (7.4%).

Clinical Presentation

Atopic Dermatitis

Atopic dermatitis is characterized by intense itching, which leads to scratching, eczematous change, and lichenification. In adults, the lesions characteristically involve the neck, wrists, area behind the ears, and antecubital and popliteal flexural areas. *Nummular eczema* is a variant characterized by pruritic, coin-shaped lesions on the external aspects of the extremities, the buttocks, and the posterior aspect of the trunk. The lesions may ooze, crust, and become purulent. The course varies; a few constant lesions may be present, or the num-

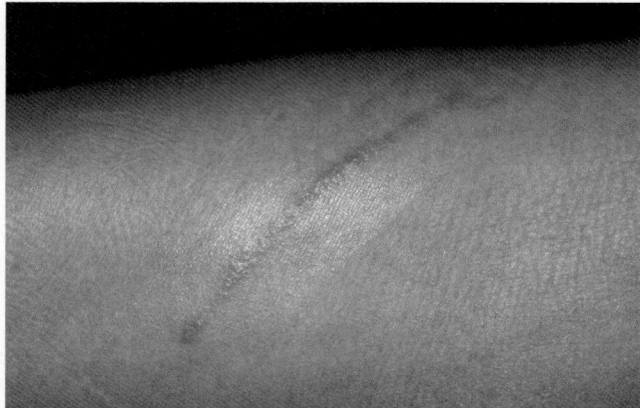

FIGURE 184.1. Linear vesicles. This pattern in characteristic of a plant allergic dermatitis—in this case, poison ivy. (See the color insert.)

ber of lesions may increase gradually. The prognosis is good, with eventual clearing for most cases, although it may take years.

Contact Dermatitis

Contact dermatitis can affect any area of the body. *Linear patterns* are pathognomonic for plant allergens (Fig. 184.1), but almost any pattern may be seen. The distribution and the location of the rash may provide clues to the irritant or allergen,

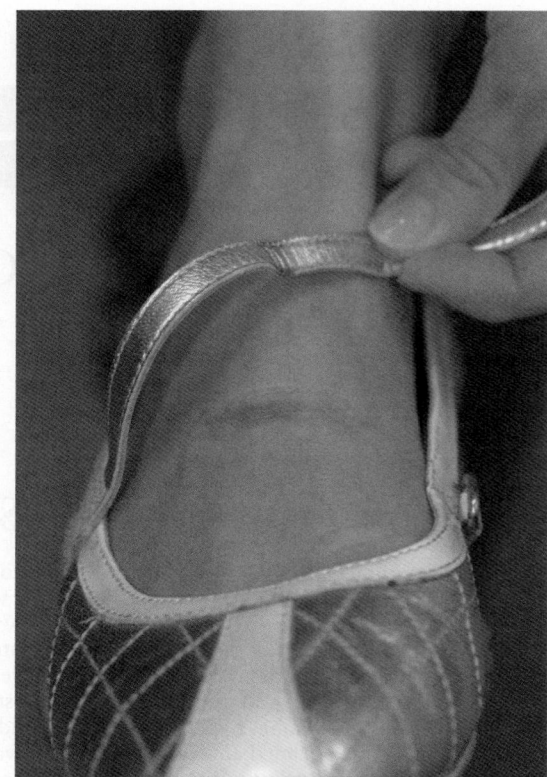

FIGURE 184.2. Allergic dermatitis from the chromates in tanned leather in a shoe; note dermatitis under the strap. (See the color insert.)

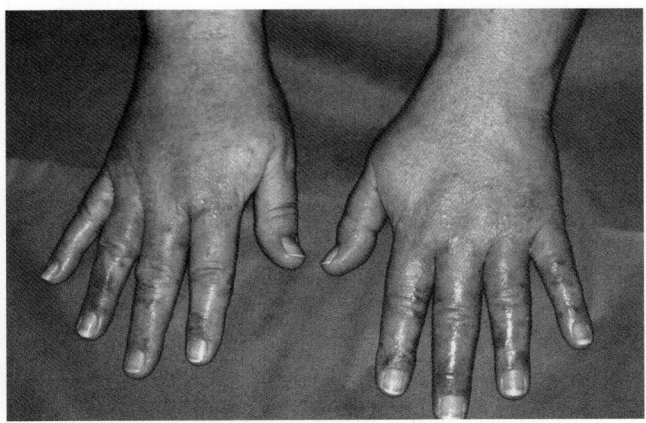

FIGURE 184.3. Rubber accelerator (carba and thiuram) allergic dermatitis from latex rubber work gloves. (See the color insert.)

such as for a shoe (Fig. 184.2) or glove (Fig. 184.3) allergy. Patch testing can help to identify the contactant.

Chronic Hand Dermatitis

Chronic hand dermatitis presents a diagnostic and therapeutic challenge that can frustrate the most experienced dermatologist. It may be irritant in nature (e.g., "housewives' hands") (Fig. 184.4), pustular (psoriasis), or vesicular (pom-

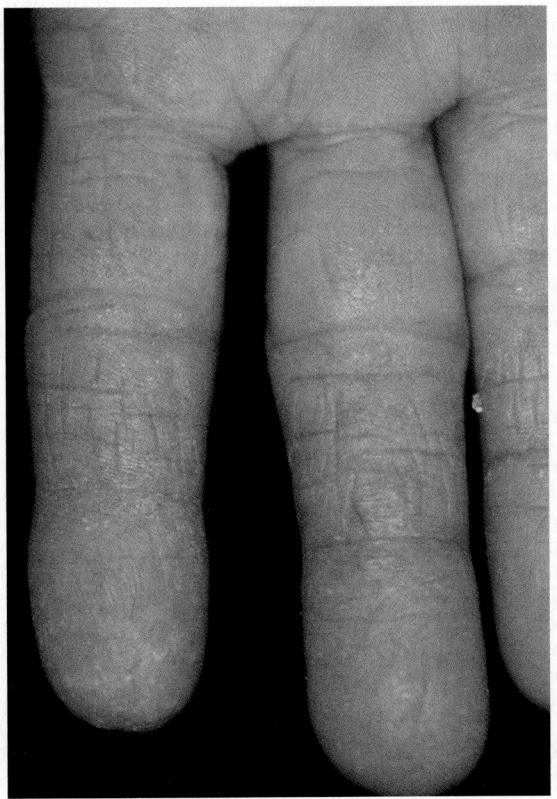

FIGURE 184.4. Chronic irritant dermatitis from frequent handwashing. (See the color insert.)

pholyx/dyshidrosis). It can occur in the context of a fungal infection with "id" reaction.

Lichen Simplex Chronicus

Regardless of the cause, chronic eczematous change may lead to *lichen simplex chronicus*. Itching can be intense, and the condition may be complicated by secondary infection. Lichen simplex chronicus can also result from localized neurodermatitis and present as a circumscribed plaque of thickened skin with increased markings, some scaling, and papulation. The occipital region is a common site. Lesions may also be seen on the wrists, thighs, or lower aspects of the legs. Women are more commonly affected. The prognosis is variable, but when rubbing is stopped, lesions regress.

PRINCIPLES OF MANAGEMENT (6–12)

The management of eczema embodies the fundamental principles of dermatologic therapy: Precipitants should be eliminated, wet lesions dried, xerotic lesions hydrated, and inflammation treated with corticosteroids or calcineurin inhibitors. Resistance to treatment should be anticipated, and if basic management fails, referral to an experienced dermatologist should be considered. A search for precipitating factors is mandatory. Topical corticosteroids are frequently an important agent in treatment.

Topical Corticosteroids

Topical steroids exert antiinflammatory, antipruritic, and antiproliferative effects. Available agents vary widely in potency, as measured by vasoconstriction assays (Table. 184.1). The strongest steroid is 500 times more effective in blanching the skin than is the weakest. Often, differences in potency are found between generic products and those with brand names.

Preparations and Their Selection

Preparations are categorized according to strength (Table 184.1). The halogenated preparations are the most potent, particularly those available in ointment formulation (see later discussion). One starts with a sufficiently potent formulation to establish control of the eczematous process and then switches to a preparation with lower potency if maintenance therapy is indicated. Because of the large number of available preparations, it is recommended that the clinician become familiar with one or two agents from each category and make the choice on the basis of cost, cosmetic acceptability, and efficacy.

Topical hydrocortisone is available over the counter in strengths that cannot exceed 1%. Mild forms of dermatitis may respond, but the patient often selects the wrong vehicle— for example, an ointment when a lotion or cream would be better.

Formulations and Application

The vehicle affects potency and cosmetic acceptability. *Ointment* formulations are more potent than *creams* and are best reserved for thick, scaling lesions or for severe xerosis. Nongreasy cream formulations are quite acceptable cosmetically and easy to use on the trunk, extremities, or face. Some atopic

TABLE 184.1

TOPICAL CORTICOSTEROID PREPARATIONS

Group 1—Highest Potency
Betamethasone dipropionate in optimized vehicle 0.05% cream, ointment, solution (Diprolene)
Clobetasol propionate 0.05% cream, ointment, solution (Temovate)
Halobetasol propionate 0.05% cream, ointment (Ultravate)
Diflorasone diacetate 0.05% cream, ointment (Psorcon)

Group 2—High Potency
Amcinonide 0.1% ointment (Cyclocort)
Betamethasone dipropionate 0.05% ointment (Diprosone)
Desoximetasone 0.25% cream and ointment (Topicort)
Fluocinonide 0.05% cream, gel, ointment, solution (Lidex)
Halcinonide 0.1% cream, ointment (Halog)

Group 3—Medium-High Potency
Amcinonide 0.1% cream (Cyclocort)
Betamethasone dipropionate 0.05% cream (Diprosone, Maxivate)
Diflorasone diacetate 0.05% cream, ointment (Psorcon)

Group 4—Medium Potency
Desoximetasone 0.05% cream (Topicort LP)
Flurandrenolide 0.05% ointment (Cordran)
Hydrocortisone butyrate 0.1% ointment (Locoid)
Hydrocortisone valerate 0.2% ointment (Westcort)
Mometasone furoate 0.1% cream, ointment (Elocon)
Triamcinolone acetonide 0.1% ointment (Aristocort, Kenalog)

Group 5—Low Potency
Alclometasone dipropionate 0.05% cream (Aclovate)
Betamethasone valerate 0.1% cream (Valisone)
Flurandrenolide 0.05% cream (Cordran)
Fluocinolone acetonide 0.025% cream (Synalar, Synemol, Fluonid)
Hydrocortisone butyrate 0.1% cream (Locoid)
Hydrocortisone valerate 0.2% cream (Westcort)
Triamcinolone acetonide 0.1% cream or lotion (Aristocort, Kenalog)

Group 6—Mild Potency
Desonide 0.05% cream (Tridesilon)
Fluocinolone acetonide 0.01% solution (Fluonid, Synalar)

Group 7—Lowest Potency
Dexamethasone 0.1% gel, ointment (Decadron)
Hydrocortisone 0.5%, 1%, and 2.5% cream, ointment, lotion (Hytone, Synacort, Nutracort)

It is recommended that the physician become familiar with and use one agent from each category, making the selection on the basis of cost, cosmetic acceptability, and efficacy.

patients itch more with ointments, and therefore creams may be better tolerated. *Gels* can be used in hairy areas and on glabrous skin, although gels are somewhat drying when used on nonhairy skin. *Lotions* are usually creamy, whereas solutions have an alcohol or propylene glycol base; in either case, lotions are more drying than creams. Specialized formulations include *aerosol sprays/foams* as well as *oils*, which are used on the scalp or to cover large areas of skin in acute dermatitis. For recalcitrant scalp dermatitis, fluocinolone acetonide oil (Derma-Smoothe FS) applied at bedtime under occlusion may

be beneficial. This preparation is in a peanut oil base, and so confirming that the patient does not have an allergy to nuts is essential before prescribing this preparation.

Occlusion of the skin enhances penetration, with up to 100 times more vasoconstriction observed if a polyethylene film is used over a given formulation than if no occlusion is used. *Steroid-impregnated tape* (*Cordran Tape*) provides occlusion as well and is useful for application to lesions that patients manipulate/scratch. Ointments are generally not occluded because folliculitis may develop.

Topical agents are normally applied two to three times daily, but retention of corticosteroid in the stratum corneum makes one or two applications per day sufficient. Because hydration of the epidermis is salutary for healing, concomitant use of a *moisturizer* is beneficial.

When a topical agent is prescribed, it is helpful to estimate the quantity of topical medication that will be required. A 2-week course of therapy applied two times daily requires at least 45 g for the face and neck, 15 g for hands, 30 g for feet, 60 g for arms or 100 g for legs, 100 to 150 g for the trunk, and 350 to 400 g for the whole body.

Adverse Effects

The potent halogenated corticosteroids are the most likely to cause *atrophy*, *telangiectasia*, *purpura*, *striae*, and *acneiform eruptions*. Restrictions are recommended for the use of certain superpotent corticosteroids—no more than 45 g of medication per week for no longer than 2 weeks. Suppression of the pituitary–adrenal axis, measured by plasma cortisol levels, may be demonstrable but is rarely clinically significant. Thin-skinned areas are especially susceptible to the development of atrophy. Less potent formulations should also be used on areas such as the face, the dorsum of the hands, intertriginous areas, and the scrotum. Only low-potency ophthalmic preparations should be used around the eye due to increased risk for glaucoma and cataract formation with longer-term use of even moderate-potency steroids in susceptible individuals. Low-potency products are also preferred in the groin and axillae because of the risk for the development of striae with more potent preparations. Purpura may be seen on the dorsal aspect of the forearms and the hands after prolonged use of potent topical agents especially in photoaged patients.

Nonsteroidal Topical Preparations

Tacrolimus and *pimecrolimus* are unique drugs that block T cell function via inhibition of calcineurin-dependent transcription of genes such as that for interleukin-2, leading to a decrease in the production of inflammatory cytokines. Tacrolimus is available in two strengths in ointment formulation, whereas pimecrolimus is available as a single-strength cream. These drugs, although expensive, have proven to be very effective in treating atopic dermatitis. They have none of the adverse side effects associated with prolonged use of topical corticosteroids and are considered cost-effective for patients who are unresponsive or poorly controlled with topical corticosteroids. The U.S. Food and Drug Administration added a black box warning for both tacrolimus and pimecrolimus in 2006 indicating that the risk for malignancy (skin cancer and lymphoma) may be increased, but no causal link has been established, and research is ongoing.

Treatment of Specific Dermatitides

Acute Eczematous Dermatitis

Acute eczematous dermatitis benefits from drying with such measures as *Burow's solution* compresses. *Systemic corticosteroids* are sometimes used on a short-term basis for generalized or incapacitating dermatitis; a 10-day program is usually required; shorter courses risk early relapse. Addition of a *topical corticosteroid* can also speed recovery. Topical corticosteroids alone may suffice in milder cases. Secondary bacterial infection may require *topical mupirocin* ointment three times per day, or systemic antibiotics may be needed if the condition is extensive.

Chronic Eczematous Dermatitis

Chronic eczematous dermatitis usually is of an irritant nature and benefits from the identification and withdrawal of possible irritants. Detergents, gasoline, polishes, and other occupational and household products should be avoided. In many cases, frequent exposure to water has a sufficient irritant effect to produce dermatitis. Frequent baths or showers, exposure to hot water, and the use of drying soaps should be reduced. Although systemic corticosteroids are contraindicated in chronic eczema, *topical steroids* are helpful and are often needed for prolonged periods. Some *coal tar* preparations are useful adjuncts in the treatment of chronic dermatitis.

Patient Education and Indications for Referral

Patients must be instructed about the proper use of topical steroids. They need to be warned specifically to avoid contact with the eyes and the eyelids (unless a low-dose ophthalmic preparation is prescribed) and to avoid using a potent topical formulation on the face. Consider recommending use of a calcineurin inhibitor (tacrolimus or pimecrolimus) for facial dermatitis instead of a steroid. If a brief course of oral prednisone therapy is necessary, the patient should be given a written schedule to ensure proper tapering and cessation within 12 to 16 days. For those with atopic disease, advice on substances to avoid is greatly appreciated. Simple measures such as clipping fingernails at bedtime and wearing cotton gloves can reduce secondary excoriation. Early identification and treatment of eczematous exacerbations helps to facilitate treatment. Patients with chronic hand dermatitis need to know that prolonged treatment may be necessary.

Chronic hand dermatitis often proves refractory to the basic measures prescribed by the primary physician. Referral to a dermatologist for more-detailed identification of precipitants and therapeutic program may be helpful.

THERAPEUTIC RECOMMENDATIONS (12)

- Identify and remove potential contacts, allergens, and irritants. Treat any skin dryness (see Chapter 183). Recommend the use of nonlatex gloves with cotton lining for wet work.
- Oozing lesions should be dried with Burow's solution compresses applied two to four times a day for 10 to 30 minutes, depending on the degree of vesiculation; colloidal oatmeal baths are indicated for more-generalized lesions.
- Suppress pruritus with a topical antipruritic (e.g., Pramosone cream/lotion or Sarna lotion) (see Chapter 178; there is minimal evidence that systemic antihistamines are effective, except for sleep).
- For acute dermatitis, begin with a corticosteroid cream. Start with the highest-potency steroid preparation necessary and reduce the potency as soon as the acute inflammation has been controlled. For extensive dermatitis, *triamcinolone* 0.1% cream, 454 g (1 lb) encourages the patient to use an adequate amount. Usually 10 to 14 days of topical therapy are necessary. If the acute process is extensive and severe, begin oral *prednisone* at a starting dose of approximately 1 mg/kg daily and taper rapidly to full cessation within 12 to 16 days.
- For chronic lichenified eruptions, treat for prolonged periods with ointment formulations of corticosteroids or, if unresponsive, steroid cream under occlusion. In refractory cases, intralesional injection of a diluted triamcinolone solution (3.0 mg/mL) by an experienced physician may be effective.
- Refer patients with refractory hand dermatitis to a dermatologist.

Annotated Bibliography

1. Breuer K, Werfel T, Kapp A. Allergic manifestations of skin diseases—atopic dermatitis. In: Crameri R, ed. Allergy and asthma in modern society: a scientific approach. Basel: Karger, 2006:76. (*Pathophysiology and new treatment options for atopic dermatitis.*)
2. Cohen DE, Brancaccio RR. What is new in clinical research in contact dermatitis? Dermatol Clin 1997;15:137. (*New and clinically relevant allergens are being discovered; patch testing is important; 53 references.*)
3. Juckett G. Plant dermatitis. Possible culprits go far beyond poison ivy. Postgrad Med 1996;100:159, 167. (*An excellent discussion of plants that cause cutaneous disease.*)
4. Ong PY, Ohtake T, Barndt C, et al. Endogenous antimicrobial peptides and skin infection in atopic dermatitis. N Engl J Med 2002;347:1151. (*Evidence for deficiency of expression of antimicrobial peptides.*)
5. Pratt MD, Belsito DV, DeLeo VA, et al. North American Contact Dermatitis Group patch-test results, 2001-2002 study period. Dermatitis. 2004;15(4):176. (*A summary of important allergens causing allergic contact dermatitis in North America.*)
6. Weidman AI, Sawicty HH. Nummular eczema. Review of the literature: survey of 516 case records and follow-up of 125 patients. Arch Dermatol 1956;73:58. (*A classic review and long-term evaluation of 125 patients.*)
7. Zasloff M. Antimicrobial peptides in health and disease. N Engl J Med 2002;347:1199. (*An editorial on the role of these skin peptides and implications for the treatment of atopic dermatitis.*)
8. Berger TG, Duvic M, Van Voorhees AS, et al. The use of topical calcineurin inhibitors in dermatology: safety concerns. Report of the American Academy of Dermatology Association Task Force. J Am Acad Dermatol 2006;54:818. (*Consensus statement.*)
9. Ellis CN, Drake LA, Prendergast MM, et al. Cost-effectiveness analysis of tacrolimus ointment versus high-potency topical corticosteroids in adults with moderate to severe atopic dermatitis. J Am Acad Dermatol 2003;48:553. (*An excellent multicenter study focusing on effectiveness and pharmacoeconomics.*)
10. Hanifin JM, Cooper KD, Ho VC, et al. Guidelines of care for atopic dermatitis, developed in accordance with the American Academy of Dermatology (AAD)/American Academy of Dermatology Association "Administrative Regulations for Evidence-Based Clinical Practice Guidelines." J Am Acad Dermatol 2004;50:391. (*Consensus guidelines.*)
11. Nghiem P, Pearson G, Langley RG. Tacrolimus and pimecrolimus: From clever prokaryocytes to inhibiting calcineurin and treating atopic dermatitis. J Am Acad Dermatol 2002;46:228. (*Why these drugs work; how they are used, as well as some off-label indications; 60 references.*)
12. Williams HC. Clinical practice. Atopic dermatitis. N Engl J Med 2005;352:2314. (*An excellent review of evidenced-based treatments for atopic dermatitis.*)

PART 2: MANAGEMENT OF SEBORRHEIC DERMATITIS

Seborrheic dermatitis affects 1% to 3% of the adult population. It is a benign but chronic inflammatory skin disease that is constitutionally determined and has no single defined cause. It can develop at any age, most commonly during infancy and after the second decade of life, with the highest prevalence in the fourth and fifth decades. Men are affected more often than women. The condition's high prevalence and incurability render it a therapeutic challenge. The primary physician should be capable of treating seborrheic dermatitis and educating the patient about chronicity and the need for continued management.

PATHOPHYSIOLOGY AND CLINICAL PRESENTATION (1,2)

Pathogenesis

The cause of seborrheic dermatitis is unclear; both endogenous factors (e.g., sebum level/hormonal influences) and exogenous precipitants (e.g., yeast species) are suspected. The anatomic localization correlates with areas of sebaceous gland concentration; quantity and composition of sebum do not appear to be key factors. Hormonal influences, fatigue, and anxiety may trigger or aggravate the condition. An etiologic relation between *Malassezia* spp. yeasts (formerly *Pityrosporum*) and seborrheic dermatitis has been postulated and is supported by the finding that topical ketoconazole and other antiyeast agents produce improvement or resolution in some patients. If treatment ceases, the number of yeast organisms increases and the problem recurs for most patients.

Clinical Presentation

Skin Manifestations

Common *dandruff* may be the mildest expression of this disease. Seborrheic dermatitis presents as *scaly patches* that are occasionally slightly papular, surrounded by minimal to moderate *erythema* (Fig. 184.5). The borders of the lesions are ill defined, and the scales may be greasy and appear yellow. The lesion is usually asymptomatic, but pruritus may occur. More extensive disease involves the forehead at the margin of the hair, eyebrows, nasal folds, and the retroauricular and presternal area. In more severe cases, intertriginous areas, the external ear canal, and the umbilicus are involved. In these areas, erythema and exudation predominate, sometimes progressing to chronic dermatitis with scaling. The scalp is most often involved, and the condition is differentiated from common dandruff by its association with erythema. At the extreme end of the spectrum, total-body erythroderma may be seen.

Associated Conditions

Seborrheic dermatitis is associated with several conditions, such as Parkinson's disease, phenylketonuria, prior cardiac fail-

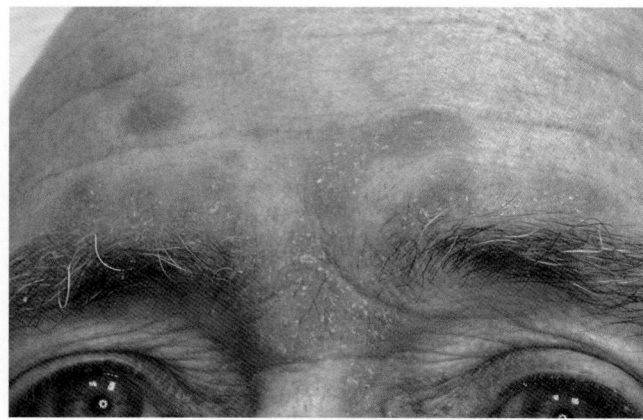

FIGURE 184.5. Seborrheic dermatitis on the glabellar region. (See the color insert.)

ure, zinc deficiency, and epilepsy. Cutaneous diseases such as rosacea and psoriasis may be associated with it. Florid manifestations of seborrhea may be an early cutaneous indicator of *HIV infection*. The dermatitis in such patients can be very extensive and resistant to therapy.

Mimicking Conditions

The differential diagnosis of seborrheic dermatitis includes psoriasis vulgaris (sebopsoriasis), atopic dermatitis, allergic contact dermatitis of the face, tinea capitis, and candidiasis.

PRINCIPLES OF MANAGEMENT (1,3–5)

As noted earlier, the condition is chronic and persistent. The approach to treatment has evolved with the growing realization of the role of *Malassezia* spp. in pathogenesis. Previously, treatment was strictly symptomatic, directed at removing scale, reducing oiliness and redness, and controlling itching. Currently, the approach is somewhat more etiologic and includes reducing the yeast count on the skin. Therapy is guided by severity, anatomic location, and relative degree of scale, erythema, oiliness, and itch.

Mild to Moderate Disease

For mild disease of the scalp, nonprescription shampoos that remove scale and provide mild antiyeast activity may suffice, but prescription shampoos and creams containing ketoconazole may be needed for more persistent disease. In refractory cases, topical steroids deserve consideration.

Nonprescription Shampoos

The scaling of scalp involvement responds well to shampoo formulations. The regular use of an over-the-counter dandruff or antiseborrheic shampoo is often sufficient. To be effective, the shampoos should generate good detergent action and be allowed to remain in contact with the scalp for at least 5 to 7 minutes. Commercially available shampoos to combat seborrhea may contain selenium sulfide, zinc pyrithione, tar, salicylic acid, and/or sulfur. Many preparations contain multiple agents but have one predominant active ingredient.

Zinc pyrithione (DHS Zinc, Head & Shoulders, Sebulon, Zincon, and ZNP Bar shampoos) and *selenium sulfide* (Selsun/Selsun Blue and prescription Exsel shampoos) have been classified as keratolytic agents. Their mode of action also appears to be cytostatic and by eliminating yeast. The combination of *sulfur* and *salicylic acid* (Sebulex, Ionil, and Vanseb shampoos) has keratolytic, mild antiyeast, and antiseptic effects. *Coal tar* is the prominent ingredient in Sebutone, Pentrax, T/Gel, and Zetar shampoos, which must be used cautiously, if at all, by people with blond, light gray, or white hair because they can change the color of the hair.

Patients should be given a list of recommended antiseborrheic agents as a guide and advised to find one suitable to their preferences for lather, odor, and efficacy. Many patients find that a shampoo works for a period and then becomes less effective, and a new product must be chosen.

Prescription Shampoos and Keratolytic Lotions

For patients with resistant seborrheic dermatitis who have tried many over-the-counter shampoos before reaching the physician, a prescription shampoo may be of benefit: A 2.5% *selenium sulfide* shampoo (Exsel or Selsun), *chloroxine* shampoo (Capitrol), ciclopirox (Loprox), or 2% *ketoconazole* shampoo (Nizoral) may be prescribed (see later discussion). Heavy crusts may be softened with keratolytic lotions (Sebizon, Sebucare) or oil-based agents (Derma-Smoothe F/S liquid, P & S liquid) before the hair is washed.

Ketoconazole (Nizoral)

Ketoconazole has proved to be very useful for topical use. Its 3- to 9-day residual effect between applications is an added advantage. Cream and shampoo formulations are available. For mild to moderate facial or chest involvement, 2% ketoconazole cream applied to the affected areas twice a day until clearing is noted often suffices. Indefinite maintenance therapy may be required once or twice weekly.

Severe Disease with Significant Erythema

Seborrhea accompanied by marked erythema may benefit from addition of a *topical corticosteroid* preparation to the treatment program. In hairy areas, a lotion, solution, spray, or gel may be applied two to four times daily. Creams should be avoided because they cause hair to become matted. Ointments are satisfactory to use at night but make the hair greasy, so that shampooing is required again in the morning. On the scalp, a fluorinated corticosteroid is acceptable. A midpotency (e.g., *betamethasone valerate*) or high-potency (e.g., clobetasol proprionate) corticosteroid in a foam base is cosmetically very acceptable but costly. Mild erythema on glabrous skin should be treated by washing with a mild soap twice a day, followed by application of 1.0% *hydrocortisone cream*. Hydrocortisone is relatively inexpensive and is considerably less likely than fluorinated topical steroids to cause telangiectasia and atrophy; a 1% concentration may be used for erythematous or papular lesions.

After initial success, a period of tachyphylaxis may ensue, requiring increased concentrations of medium-potency, non-fluorinated steroids. Telangiectasia and other signs of dermal atrophy may occur with the long-term use of these products,

and application on the face should be avoided. *Topical ketoconazole* produces no such adverse skin changes and should be part of the program in severe disease.

For moderate to severe disease not responsive to the antimycotics or topical steroids, the use of a topical calcineurin inhibitor can be beneficial. Application of *pimecrolimus* is effective in reducing both erythema and scale in moderate to severe disease within two weeks of starting the medication for many patients. This type of medication should only be used for 2 to 3 weeks at a time due to concerns associated with more prolonged use (the U.S. Food and Drug Administration added a black box warning for both tacrolimus and pimecrolimus indicating a possible increase in the risk for malignancy [skin cancer and lymphoma], but no causal link has been established, and research is ongoing).

Exudative lesions of intertriginous seborrheic dermatitis may require the application of *Burow's solution* compresses followed by a fluorinated corticosteroid lotion. Secondary bacterial infection may require the use of *oral antibiotics*.

PATIENT EDUCATION

It is reassuring for the patient to know that seborrhea is not contagious, but the chronic nature of the condition also needs to be emphasized. Its relation to stress may help to explain flares to the patient. The patient will appreciate being provided with a list of over-the-counter preparations. If topical steroid therapy is needed, the patient should be cautioned about its potential adverse effects and instructed in proper application. Patients with severe disease need to understand that reviewing for HIV risk factors and, if present, testing for HIV infection are reasonable considerations.

THERAPEUTIC RECOMMENDATIONS

- Provide the patient with a list of over-the-counter shampoos and suggest selecting one that meets personal preferences. For oily hair, advise daily shampooing daily for the first week; this can sometimes be decreased to two or three times a week for maintenance. For resistant cases, ketoconazole shampoo should be used every other day.
- For mild to moderate facial or chest involvement, 2% ketoconazole cream may be applied to the affected areas twice a day until clearing is noted. Maintenance therapy may be required once or twice weekly indefinitely.
- If erythema is present, prescribe a topical nonfluorinated corticosteroid preparation (e.g., 1% or 2.5% hydrocortisone cream) for the face; a fluorinated lotion is appropriate for the scalp (e.g., 0.1% betamethasone valerate lotion).
- Heavy crusts can be removed by softening with keratolytic lotions or oil-based agents before shampooing.
- Treat exudative intertriginous lesions with a nonfluorinated topical steroid lotion.
- Blepharitis may be treated hygienically by gentle rubbing of the eyelashes with a washcloth and No More Tears shampoo. Occasionally, a steroid-containing eye ointment, such as *Metimyd* or *Blephamide* solution, can be used, but care must be taken not to allow prolonged use.
- Consider testing for HIV in persons with severe disease and risk factors for HIV infection.

Annotated Bibliography

1. Gupta A, Madzia SE, Batra R. Etiology and management of seborrheic dermatitis. Dermatology 2004;208:89. (*An excellent overall review.*)
2. Mathes BM, Douglas NC. Seborrheic dermatitis in patients with acquired immunodeficiency syndrome. J Am Acad Dermatol 1985;13:947. (*There is a high prevalence in HIV infection; the severity is greater than usual and is associated with a poor prognosis.*)
3. Johnson BA, Nunley JR. Treatment of seborrheic dermatitis. Am Family Physician 2000;61:2703. (*An excellent primer with tabular presentation of available therapeutic options.*)
4. Shuster S, Meynadier J, Kerl H, et al. Treatment and prophylaxis of seborrheic dermatitis of the scalp with antipityrosporal 1% ciclopirox shampoo. Arch Dermatol 2005;141:47. (*When used twice weekly, the treatment is found to be effective.*)
5. Warshaw EM, Wohlhuter RJ, Liu A, et al. Results of a randomized, double-blind, vehicle-controlled efficacy trial of pimecrolimus cream 1% for the treatment of moderate to severe facial seborrheic dermatitis. J Am Acad Dermatol 2007; 57:257. (*Topical pimecrolimus was found to be effective and acceptable by elderly men.*)

CHAPTER 185 ■ MANAGEMENT OF ACNE

PETER C. SCHALOCK AND ARTHUR J. SOBER

Acne is a polygenic, multifactorial disease that in some form afflicts nearly all adolescents in the United States. It ranges in severity from a few scattered whiteheads and blackheads to disfiguring, painful, deep-seated, pus-filled, and bleeding nodulocystic lesions. About 15% of surveyed patients with acne seek medical care. The primary care physician is in a unique position to identify and treat many acne sufferers. Properly managing acne requires a thorough understanding of the development of acne in all its phases, so that therapy appropriate to the circumstances can be selected from the available modalities. Early effective treatment minimizes the physical scarring of the disease and prevents or reduces equally important psychological distress.

PATHOPHYSIOLOGY AND CLINICAL PRESENTATION (1–3)

Pathophysiology

Acne is a disease of pilosebaceous units, which are predominantly on the face and central upper back and chest. The pathogenesis of acne results from the interplay of three factors: (a) hyperkeratinization and obstruction of the follicular infundibulum caused by abnormal desquamation of the follicular epithelium, (b) androgen-stimulated increases in sebum production, and (c) colonization of the follicle by *Propionibacterium acnes,* which generates inflammation.

The initial event of acne is conversion of the loose, easily shed, horny layer of the epithelium lining the follicular duct wall to a self-adhering mass that gradually obstructs the follicular duct. This has been called "retention hyperkeratosis." A *microcomedone* is the initial lesion, a precursor to both open and closed comedones. It occurs following occlusion of the follicular ostia. An *open comedone* ("*blackhead*") is this ker-

atin plug that enlarges and does not become inflamed. The black color is due to oxidation of the tyrosine in keratin to melanin. *Closed comedones* ("*whiteheads*") form from microcomedones after 1 to 2 months, once the accumulated mass of keratin, sebum, and bacteria reaches visible size. Whiteheads may expand the duct ("pore") opening to communicate freely with the outside.

Chemotactic agents produced by bacteria within the duct attract leukocytes, leading to duct wall rupture and release of follicular contents into the surrounding dermis. This provokes a profound inflammatory response, leading to the development of *papules, pustules, nodules,* and *suppurative nodules* that are commonly but mistakenly termed "*cysts*." These inflammatory lesions may lead to permanent scarring.

Propionibacterium acnes, a normal inhabitant of the follicular canal in humans, may participate in the initiation and aggravation of inflammatory lesions by elaborating enzymes, including lipases, that act on sebum to release potentially irritating free fatty acids. Its hyaluronidase may increase permeability of the follicular duct wall, and its protease can damage the duct wall, increasing leakage of materials into the surrounding dermis. In addition, *P. acnes* produces chemotactic substances that contribute to the initiation and evolution of inflammatory lesions.

The debate about the role of *diet* and other environmental factors continues. It is hypothesized that adolescents in Westernized societies may be repeatedly acutely hyperinsulinemic due to their highly glycemic diets, which in turn may initiate an endocrine cascade (involving insulin growth factor [IGF], IGF-binding protein 3, testosterone, and retinoid signaling pathways) that affects sebaceous gland production and follicular keratinization. Whether adherence to a diet with a low glycemic load can reduce acne risk is unknown, but such diets are characteristic of non-Westernized populations that have low prevalences of acne. Milk consumption has been positively associated with the severity of acne; teenagers who consume greater amounts of cow's milk, especially skim milk, had a greater number of acne lesions and severity of acne, perhaps related to high levels of bovine hormones, including estrogens, progesterones, and precursors to androstenedione.

All photos are courtesy of Peter C. Schalock.

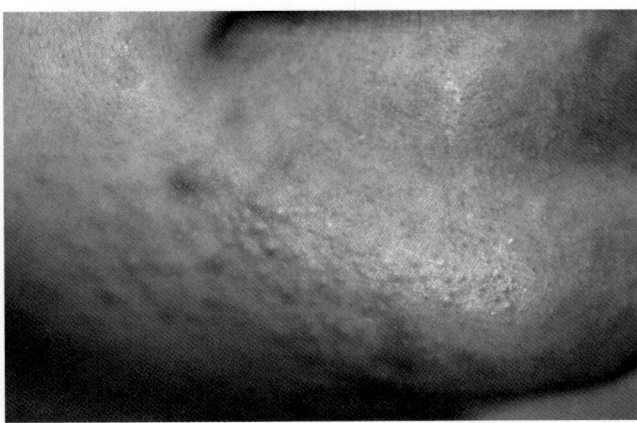

FIGURE 185.1. Comedonal acne on the chin of a young woman. (See the color insert.)

Clinical Presentations

Acne can be categorized as *obstructive* or *inflammatory;* both types of lesions may be present. Obstructive disease results from impaction of horny material, bacteria, and sebum, which dilates follicular ducts and produces *closed comedones* (*whiteheads*) and *open comedones* (*blackheads*) (Figs. 185.1 and 185.2). Leakage of intrafollicular contents from comedones into the adjacent dermis produces an inflammatory response. Depending on the degree of leakage into the dermis and the amount of material released, inflammatory lesions vary from

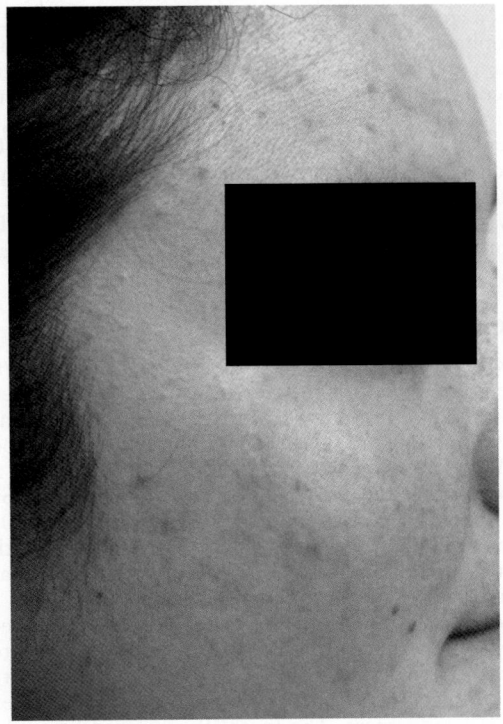

FIGURE 185.2. Mild papular and comedonal acne. (See the color insert.)

small, erythematous papules and superficial pustules to deeper pustules and larger, persistent, and occasionally suppurative nodules. Genetic immunologic factors may contribute to an exaggerated inflammatory response and more severe cystic forms of acne.

PRINCIPLES OF THERAPY (3–16)

Treatment is often initiated with topical agents, and with progression, systemic agents are added in more severely affected cases. An initial presentation of severe or scarring acne or with clear hormonal factors should hasten the use of systemic agents.

Removal of Acnegenic Factors

Eliminating precipitants is an important component of therapy. Some *cosmetics*, including makeup, hair sprays, oils, and moisturizing creams, may be capable of producing comedones, and their use should be reduced or discontinued. The physician should advise against using acnegenic *drugs* such as androgens, systemic steroids, iodides, and bromides. Other medications such as lithium and epidermal growth factor–receptor blockers (erlotinib/gefitinib) can cause acneiform reactions, but discontinuation of these medications is not typically recommended. The role of *foods* in the pathogenesis of acne is unclear, but recent epidemiologic and pathophysiologic evidence (see earlier discussion) suggests a potential benefit from the reduction of excessive *carbohydrate* and *dairy* intake (especially those forms that induce hyperinsulinism; see Chapter 102).

After precipitants have been eliminated, the goals of therapy shift to treatment of existing lesions and further prevention of new lesions. The modalities employed depend on the kind of lesions present.

Treatment of Obstructive Acne

The goals of therapy are to normalize desquamation of the follicular epithelium, promote drainage of existing comedones, and prevent development of new ones.

Retinoids

The retinoids are vitamin A derivatives that have all the desired properties for treatment of obstructive acne. *Tretinoin* (*trans*-retinoic acid; Avita, Retin-A, Retin-A Micro) is a popular first-generation retinoid used as a comedolytic agent. Skin irritation is the primary adverse effect, which can be controlled by reducing the frequency of application to minimize desquamation.

Other retinoids include adapalene and tazarotene. *Adapalene* (Differin), a synthetic lipophilic retinoid with some of the biologic activities of tretinoin, causes minimal skin irritation, making it helpful in mild cases. *Tazarotene*, a potent synthetic retinoid used in more severe cases, can be more irritating and drying than tretinoin or adapalene. Tazarotene is pregnancy category X and should be used with caution in women of childbearing potential. A negative pregnancy test is required before starting topical therapy with tazarotene.

Retinoid Precursors

Precursors of retinoic acid, *retinal* and *retinol*, are being included in over-the-counter "cosmeceutical" products. These induce much less irritation than topical tretinoin, but their efficacy has not been established.

Treatment of Mild Inflammatory Acne

Mild inflammatory acne often responds to topical agents with antibacterial or direct antiinflammatory activity.

Benzoyl Peroxide

Benzoyl peroxide is a potent bactericidal agent available in concentrations of 2.5% to 10% and in formulations that include gels, creams, lotions, and cleansers. It is often used in combination with retinoic acid. These topical agents in conjunction with oral antibiotic therapy appear to be synergistic, possibly increasing antibiotic concentration in the follicular duct.

Topical Antibiotics

Topical antibiotics are used in mild inflammatory acne to suppress *P. acnes* and provide both an active and a preventive therapy. These agents are less likely than retinoic acid or benzoyl peroxide to cause dryness or irritation, but their widespread topical use is associated with an increased prevalence of skin colonization by drug-resistant strains. Most common is resistance to erythromycin, in association with cross-resistance to clindamycin. Antibiotic preparations are available in roll-on dispensers, individually wrapped throw-away pledgets, or gels.

Intralesional Corticosteroids

Intralesional corticosteroids may hasten the involution of nodulocystic lesions, reducing the risk of permanent scarring. *Triamcinolone acetonide*, 2.0 or 2.5 mg/mL in saline injected with a 30-gauge needle directly into specific lesions, is often remarkably effective. Skin thinning in areas of injection is a danger.

Metronidazole Gel

Metronidazole gel is of well-established efficacy in acne rosacea (see Chapter 186). It has been found to be equal to systemic tetracycline therapy when applied in conjunction with 5% benzoyl peroxide cream.

α-Hydroxy Acids

Some suggest nonprescription α-hydroxy acid preparations (e.g., *glycolic acid*) for acne. These may be moderately helpful as keratolytic agents; their formulations make them cosmetically acceptable, which increases patient compliance.

Azelaic Acid

This naturally occurring dicarbonic acid has antikeratinizing, antibacterial, and antiinflammatory properties; it is somewhat less effective than benzoyl peroxide, has mild skin-lightening effects, and can induce a mild irritant contact dermatitis at the onset of therapy. It is a reasonably safe agent for use during pregnancy or lactation, if therapy is necessary.

Treatment of Severe Inflammatory Acne

This form of acne is characterized by large, deep papules and pustules and destructive, suppurating, nodular lesions and requires systemic therapy. Because *P. acnes* is believed to play an important role in the pathogenesis of inflammatory acne, systemic antibiotics have become the mainstay of therapy, with 13-*cis*-retinoic acid reserved for refractory, disabling disease.

Systemic Antibiotic Therapy

Systemic antibiotic therapy is the best means of preventing new inflammatory lesions. By suppressing *P. acnes*, the risk of enzymatic injury to the gland is markedly reduced along with the rate of new lesion formation. Four decades of experience and much evidence have established systemic antibiotic therapy as rational, effective, and remarkably safe. Response consists in a clearing of old lesions and a decrease in new lesions. After a response is observed, the dose may be gradually decreased over a period of weeks to the lowest effective maintenance dose.

Choices for systemic antibiotic therapy include *tetracycline*, a synthetic tetracycline derivative (*doxycycline* or *minocycline*), and *erythromycin*. The synthetic tetracyclines are more expensive than generic tetracycline but cause less gastrointestinal upset, require less frequent dosing, and are highly efficacious. The initial dose of doxycycline or minocycline is 100 to 200 mg daily with gradual reduction to a maintenance dose, which often can be as low as 50 mg daily day or every other day. Reports of rare but serious side effects with minocycline use (see later discussion) make doxycycline a better choice if prolonged therapy is contemplated. Erythromycin causes significant gastrointestinal upset and is less effective when compared to the tetracycline family. Azithromycin has also been reported to be as effective as minocycline in the treatment of inflammatory acne but is not a first- or second-line choice for treatment of acne.

Adverse Effects. Tetracycline and erythromycin commonly cause gastrointestinal upset. Gastrointestinal symptoms are less of a problem with tetracycline derivatives, although pill esophagitis is reported with doxycycline use. In rare instances, minocycline leads to irreversible pigmentation of the mucous membranes and sun-exposed skin and a lupus-like syndrome with positive serology, autoimmune hepatitis, and a hypersensitivity syndrome with pulmonary infiltrates. Use of tetracycline and its derivatives is associated with risk of photodermatitis, necessitating caution regarding sun exposure. There is no evidence to support the concern that systemic antibiotics used for acne impair the effectiveness of oral contraceptive therapy.

Hormonal Therapy

The *oral contraceptive* agents *Ortho Tri-Cyclen* and *Estrostep* have been approved for the treatment of acne in women, but their use can be associated with a flare of the disease on their introduction and a possible rebound flare on discontinuation. *Yasmin/Yaz* (drospirenone–ethinylestradiol) and *Alesse* (levonorgestrel–ethinyl estradiol) also can be helpful. Studies show a decrease in inflammatory lesions of 30% to 60% after 6 to 9 months of therapy. Possible interactions with oral antibiotics and all of the other issues associated with oral contraceptive use need to be taken into consideration.

Spironolactone, an antiandrogen, has been prescribed empirically for women with refractory acne. Doses of 50 to 200 mg/d are effective in two thirds of women treated, but menstrual irregularities occur in 22%, and some women experience breast tenderness. The most effective and best-tolerated dose is 100 mg/d. Due to concerns from animal studies, it should not be used in women with a family history or genetic predisposition for breast cancer. Checking a potassium level prior to therapy and occasionally during therapy is recommended.

13-*cis*-Retinoic Acid (Isotretinoin, Accutane)

13-*cis*-Retinoic acid is a powerful systemic agent for the treatment of nodulocystic inflammatory acne. A 16- to 20-week course often brings severe acne under complete control, with little or no further therapy. However, it is essential for the physician to recognize that this is a potent *teratogen*, which has caused numerous tragic birth defects. The Guidelines of Care for Acne Vulgaris published by the American Academy of Dermatology clearly state that 13-*cis*-retinoic should not be first-choice therapy and that it must be demonstrated that the patient is unresponsive to other standard therapies. In the treatment of women of childbearing potential, it should be used only in patients with severe, disfiguring, cystic acne and only with very clear instructions and monitoring.

Guidelines for Safe Use. Because of the teratogenicity of isotretinoin, use of a detailed *informed-consent* protocol is mandatory for use in women of childbearing age; a copy is given to the patient and one is kept in the patient's record. The patient is entered into the IPLEDGE website or by phone using an assigned identification number. Counseling prior to initiating therapy includes the following:

- Use of two methods of contraception simultaneously or total coital abstinence.
- Onset of contraceptive program at least 1 month before starting treatment and continuing for at least 1 month after discontinuing therapy.
- Obtaining a negative pregnancy test within 1 week before the next period.
- Initiating therapy during the second or third day of the next menstrual period.
- Monthly follow-up with monthly pregnancy testing and monthly monitoring of lipids and transaminases.
- Provision of suitable counseling should a pregnancy occur to assist in deciding on management of the pregnancy, including possible termination.

The patient is scheduled for a monthly visit, with a negative pregnancy test confirmed prior to prescribing isotretinoin. Each month, both physician and patient are required to enter the IPLEDGE website and confirm all details before the pharmacy can obtain approval to dispense the drug. The patient has 7 days from the time of the office visit to fill the prescription. If it is not filled, she must wait until 30 days have passed to again be eligible for isotretinoin. Special approval is required for physicians to participate in the IPLEDGE program.

Adverse Effects. As noted, the most serious is the risk of birth defects. The most common problem is drying of mucocutaneous tissues (lips, eyes, mouth, epidermal surfaces). Potential for elevations in transaminases and triglycerides necessitate monitoring lipids and liver function tests. Some patients experience headaches. Rare side effects include pseudotumor cerebri, idiopathic skeletal hyperostosis, pyogenic granuloma-like lesions, and arthralgias. Most of these adverse effects are reversible. Patients should be forewarned that their acne may worsen shortly after initiating therapy. Patients should avoid unnecessary procedures during and a few months after treatment because unexpected keloidal scarring has been observed when simple procedures such as dermabrasion have been performed soon after completing a course of isotretinoin.

INDICATIONS FOR REFERRAL AND PATIENT EDUCATION (8,11)

Treatment of acne often falls within the domain of the primary physician. The dermatologist should be consulted if basic topical and systemic therapies fail.

Patient education and cooperation are crucial to the success of therapy. Patients must understand the chronic nature of the process and not be discouraged when lesions continue to appear. Patients who unrealistically expect an immediate cure may become discouraged, uncooperative, and eventually angry.

A vast mythology about acne has developed. The patient should be assured that acne has no relation to masturbation, sexual activity or inactivity, constipation, dirt, or angry feelings. The patient should be helped to gain perspective and discouraged from self-examination in magnifying mirrors, which often produces a distorted self-image. Instructions for the use of topical and systemic agents must be precise and carefully followed. The patient should be reminded that therapeutic results are not achieved immediately, and treatment must be continued for an extended period of time. The most common reason for failure of therapy is lack of compliance by the patient.

THERAPEUTIC RECOMMENDATIONS (8)

- Explain the basis for treatment; patient understanding and cooperation are essential for success.
- Eliminate acnegenic drugs, such as systemic steroids or androgens, exposure to oils, and habits such as rubbing the face. Consider reducing excessive intake of concentrated carbohydrates and dairy products.

For Obstructive Acne

- Begin with a topical retinoid (*tretinoin* 0.025%, 0.05%, 0.1% or adapalene 0.1% cream or gel) applied at bedtime to dry skin; if the skin has been recently wet from cleansing, it should be allowed to dry for at least 15 minutes to minimize irritation. Consider *adapalene* or *tretinoin* in milder cases; reserve *tazarotene* for severe cases.
- Consider topical antibiotics (e.g., *clindamycin*) in the forms of lotions, solutions, or gels and/or *benzoyl peroxide* in various strengths and formulations if papules or pustules are present concurrently. Add topical benzoyl peroxide if the patient is not responsive to topical antibiotic alone.

For Severe Inflammatory Acne

- Prescribe a systemic antibiotic, (e.g., *doxycycline*, 100 mg twice daily). Start with a full dose and reduce to a maintenance dose once acne is under control, which can take up to several months.

For Severe Nodulocystic Acne Resistant to Conventional Therapy

- Consider systemic *13-cis-retinoic acid* with full awareness of its risks, especially teratogenesis, and the requirement of appropriate monitoring.

Annotated Bibliography

1. Adebamowo CA, Spiegelman D, Danby FW, et al. High school dietary dairy intake and teenage acne. J Am Acad Dermatol 2005;52:207. (*A positive association was found between acne severity and increasing consumption of milk products.*)
2. Cordain L, Lindeberg S, Hurtado M, et al. Acne vulgaris: a disease of Western civilization. Arch Dermatol 2002;138:1584. (*An interesting observational study.*)
3. Purdy S, de Berker D. Acne. BMJ 2006;333:949. (*A review discussing new discoveries in the pathogenesis of acne, as well as new and time-honored therapies.*)
4. Archer JS, Archer DF. Oral contraceptive efficacy and antibiotic interaction: a myth debunked. J Am Acad Dermatol 2002;46:917. (*Pharmacokinetic evidence demonstrates that plasma levels of oral contraceptive steroids are unchanged despite concomitant administration of antibiotic.*)
5. Bigby M, Stern RS. Adverse reactions to isotretinoin. J Am Acad Dermatol 1988;18:543. (*Review of the significant and less significant adverse reactions.*)
6. James WD. Clinical practice. Acne. N Engl J Med 2005;352:1463–72. (*An organized, succinct review of treatment options for acne; 68 references.*)
7. Cunliffe WJ, Poncet M, Loesche C, et al. A comparison of the efficacy and tolerability of adapalene 0.1% gel versus tretinoin 0.025% gel in patients with acne vulgaris: a meta-analysis of five randomized trials. Br J Dermatol 1998;139(Suppl 52):48. (*Adapalene demonstrates more rapid efficacy with greater tolerability.*)
8. Drake LA. Guidelines of care for acne vulgaris. J Am Acad Dermatol 1990;22:676. (*American Academy of Dermatology guidelines in outline form, including guidelines for the use of 13-cis-retinoic acid.*)
9. McManus P, Iheanacho I. Don't use minocycline as first line oral antibiotic in acne. BMJ. 2007;334:154. (*An evidenced-based review of the effectiveness and side effects of minocycline; recommends not using it for acne.*)
10. Humbert P, Treffel P, Chapuis JF, et al. The tetracyclines in dermatology. J Am Acad Dermatol 1991;25:691. (*A review of the use of the tetracyclines in acne, acne rosacea, and other dermatologic conditions; 99 references.*)
11. Landow K. Dispelling myths about acne. Postgrad Med 1997;102:94, 103, 110. (*An excellent three-part review.*)
12. Leyden J. The role of isotretinoin in the treatment of acne: personal observations. J Am Acad Dermatol 1998;39:S45. (*Recalcitrant acne responds well to Accutane.*)
13. Meynadier J, Alirezai. Systemic antibiotics for acne. Dermatology 1998;196:135. (*Review of the side effects and efficacy of commonly used oral antibiotics for acne.*)
14. Rodondi N, Darioli R, Ramelet AA, et al. High risk for hyperlipidemia and the metabolic syndrome after an episode of hypertriglyceridemia during 13-cis retinoic acid therapy for acne: a pharmacogenetic study. Ann Intern Med 2002;136:582. (*There are important adverse effects.*)
15. Shaw JC. Antiandrogen and hormonal treatment of acne. Dermatol Clin 1996;14:803. (*A discussion of these agents in the treatment of adult women's acne.*)
16. Sturkenboom MC, Meier CR, Juck H, et al. Minocycline and lupuslike syndrome in acne patients. Arch Intern Med 1999;159:493. (*The risk of developing a lupus-like syndrome is increased 8.5-fold in young acne patients taking minocycline.*)

CHAPTER 186 ■ MANAGEMENT OF ROSACEA AND OTHER ACNEIFORM DERMATOSES

PETER C. SCHALOCK AND ARTHUR J. SOBER

Rosacea and periorificial dermatitis produce acneiform lesions. Rosacea is particularly common, affecting between 1.5% and 10% of the population, depending on the sample. It most commonly occurs between the ages of 30 and 50 years, although it can be present in individuals both older and younger. Periorificial dermatitis typically presents in women aged 20 to 40 years. The primary care physician should be able to identify these acneiform conditions, differentiate them from other diseases, and institute proper treatment.

PATHOPHYSIOLOGY AND CLINICAL PRESENTATION (1–4)

Rosacea

Pathophysiology

Rosacea is a chronic inflammatory condition of unknown etiology. Although individuals of all ethnic backgrounds can

All photos are courtesy of Peter C. Schalock.

develop rosacea, it affects patients of Irish, Scottish, Scandinavian, and English descent more frequently. The earliest pathophysiologic change is vascular instability, with flushing attributable to a heat-regulating reflex involving the counter-current thermal exchange between the common carotid artery and the internal jugular vein; substance P and vasoactive peptides may also play a role. Ultraviolet damage with microscopic evidence of dermal elastotic degeneration is noted in most patients. *Demodex folliculorum* and *Demodex brevis* mites have been found at higher concentrations in patients with rosacea, especially those with topical steroid-induced rosacea. *Helicobacter pylori* infection may contribute to rosacea, possibly through the release of vasoactive substances such as gastrin. Studies on *H. pylori* have prompted consideration of an association between rosacea and gastritis. A statistically significant incidence of migraine headaches accompanying rosacea has been reported, perhaps indicating a background of vascular reactivity.

Clinical Presentation

Patients exhibit a spectrum of lesions involving the central face, the mildest being erythema producing a red face or ruddy

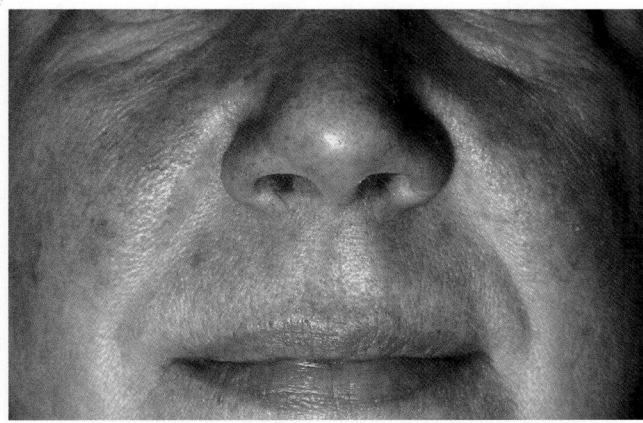

FIGURE 186.1. Papulopustular and telangiectatic rosacea. (See the color insert.)

cheeks and flushing in response to hot liquids, spicy foods, alcohol consumption, sun exposure, vasodilating drugs, or emotional factors. Additional lesions include papules and pustules, but not comedones; the latter are more specific for acne vulgaris. Telangiectasias may develop as a response to recurrent erythema and flushing, and facial edema may ensue from longstanding erythema. Fig. 186.1 shows a case of moderate rosacea. In severe rosacea, *rhinophyma,* a thick, lobulated overgrowth of connective tissue and sebaceous glands of the nose, may be a feature (Fig. 186.2). Ocular complications commonly include *blepharitis, conjunctivitis, episcleritis,* and, *infrequently, iritis* and *keratitis.*

Periorificial Dermatitis

Patients present with an erythematous, scaling, papular, or papulopustular eruption around the mouth, chin, upper lip, eyes, and nasolabial folds. The lesions are usually bilateral and symmetric. Occasionally, papulopustular lesions are widespread. Many patients report a stinging sensation associated with these lesions. The course is typically relapsing and remitting, similar to that of rosacea.

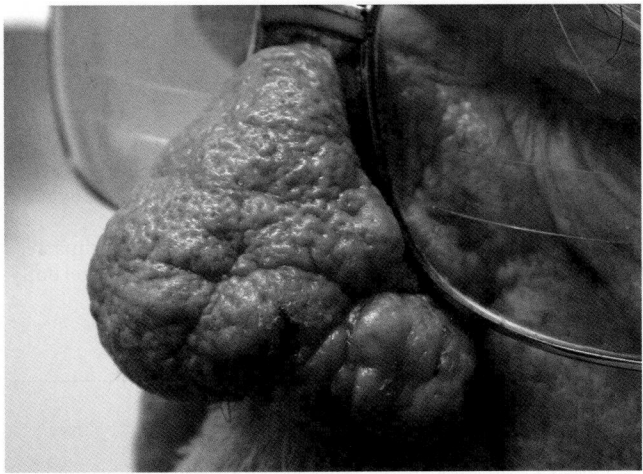

FIGURE 186.2. Severe rhinophyma in an elderly man. (See the color insert.)

The cause of periorificial dermatitis is unknown. Light sensitivity, rosacea, atopy, *Demodex* mite infestation, candidiasis, overgrowth of the yeast *Pityrosporum ovale,* and the use of fluoride toothpaste have been implicated. Some cases of perioral dermatitis have been reported as a reaction to dental resins. Controversy exists as to whether use of cosmetics and/or self-manipulation contribute to this disease. The condition can be replicated by chronic use of fluorinated corticosteroid medications.

DIAGNOSIS

Rosacea

The diagnosis is made clinically, taking care to differentiate rosacea from acne and other erythematous skin diseases such as seborrheic dermatitis, *Pityrosporum* folliculitis, contact dermatitis, eczema, and drug-induced photosensitivity. Acne presents in a younger age group and features comedones in addition to papules and pustules. Perioral dermatitis can look like rosacea, and some consider it to be a variant of rosacea. Serious systemic diseases can present similarly to rosacea, including lupus erythematosus and sarcoidosis.

PRINCIPLES OF MANAGEMENT (3,5–10)

Rosacea

Treatment involves minimizing factors that precipitate flushing or vasodilation, removing exacerbating conditions, and using topical or systemic antibiotics with antiinflammatory action.

Minimizing Precipitants

Exposure to *sunlight,* extreme heat or cold, and ingestion of hot or spicy foods or beverages, including alcohol, should be minimized. Review of medications is worthwhile for any expendable *vasodilating agents* (e.g., aminophylline, hydralazine, niacin, nitroglycerin, papaverine). Angiotensin-converting-enzyme inhibitors and simvastatin also have been reported to worsen rosacea. Sunscreens with *para-aminobenzoic acid* (PABA) are common irritants, but even *avobenzone* should be used with caution. It is most important to caution against THE use of *topical fluorinated corticosteroids,* which can result in the atrophy of skin and the development of permanent telangiectasia. Patients with rosacea should select moisturizers and sunscreens formulated for sensitive skin; physical blockers (titanium dioxide and zinc oxide) are best tolerated.

Topical Therapies

Topically applied antibiotics are the first line of symptomatic treatment.

Metronidazole and Other Topical Antibiotics. *Metronidazole* provides antiinflammatory, antimicrobial, and antioxidant activity when used topically. It is available in cream, gel, and lotion vehicles. It does not have activity against *Demodex* mites. Topical *sodium sulfacetamide,* which competes with PABA (an essential component of bacterial proliferation), can be of benefit by suppressing *Demodex* proliferation; it also possesses keratolytic properties and may help to reduce erythema.

Other Topical Therapies. Topical *azelaic acid* (Finacea) has antiinflammatory, antibacterial, comedolytic, and bleaching properties that reduce inflammatory papules and erythema; it is more effective than topical metronidazole. Topical acne therapies (e.g., *erythromycin, clindamycin, benzoyl peroxide, retinoic acid;* see Chapter 185) may prove helpful, although dryness associated with the latter two agents may limit tolerability. In patients with only mild erythema and telangiectasias, the use of topical retinoids may actually exacerbate rosacea because of their potential for cutaneous irritation and possible promotion of angiogenesis. Topical *pimecrolimus,* a nonsteroidal antiinflammatory topical agent, may be helpful in periocular rosacea.

Systemic Therapies

Patients presenting with papules, pustules, or ocular symptoms often need systemic treatment in addition to topical therapies. *Systemic antibiotics* (e.g., *tetracycline, doxycycline, minocycline,* or *erythromycin*) can be helpful in persons with moderate to severe rosacea. Systemic antibiotic therapy is often initiated in conjunction with topical measures; as patients improve, the antibiotics are tapered, leaving topical therapy for maintenance. In many cases, a 6-month course of systemic therapy is required to prevent relapse on discontinuation. For severe cases, systemic *isotretinoin* can be effective. Recent reports note some efficacy for *ketoconazole* and *clarithromycin.*

Flushing does not respond to the antiinflammatory properties of these systemic therapies and can be difficult to treat pharmacologically. Anticholinergic medications (e.g., *glycopyrrolate*), beta-blockers, clonidine, spironolactone, and psychotropic medications have been suggested. Their side effects must be weighed against potential benefits. For example, the tetracyclines can cause photosensitivity, and minocycline can cause pigmentation abnormalities, dizziness, and a lupus-like syndrome.

Laser and Surgical Management

Treatment with the *pulsed dye laser* can be useful for telangiectasias and facial erythema. Intense pulsed-light therapy may improve facial erythema. *Rhinophyma* can be treated with *carbon dioxide laser,* electrosurgery, excision, or dermabrasion. Surgical management should be performed by an experienced dermatologist or surgeon.

Periorificial Dermatitis

Patients with perioral dermatitis should avoid heavy cosmetics and topical ointments. Some practitioners also advise patients to change toothpastes or mouthwashes. Topical acne preparations that increase turnover of skin are useful, but they are often inadequate if used alone. *Hydrocortisone* 1% cream may promote rapid resolution of the dermatitis but should be discontinued as soon as possible. Fluorinated corticosteroid creams should not be used because they may exacerbate erythema and lead to telangiectasia formation. *Topical metronidazole* can sig-

nificantly reduce the number of papules but is not as effective as *systemic antibiotics. Systemic antibiotics* such as the *tetracyclines* are consistently effective in controlling perioral dermatitis, as well as rosacea. If the tetracyclines cannot be tolerated, *erythromycin* may be used instead. Systemic antibiotics can be discontinued on resolution, usually in 4 to 8 weeks.

PATIENT EDUCATION

The major element of patient education is to explain that these conditions are common and treatable but may be chronic with intermittent flares. Many patients are bothered by a single papule, whereas others can sustain the disfigurement of rosacea without complaint. Detailed review of aggravating factors is important for management and helps to make the patient a partner in the treatment of these stubborn conditions.

THERAPEUTIC RECOMMENDATIONS (3)

Rosacea

- Instruct the patient to avoid prolonged sun exposure, fluorinated steroids, fluoridated toothpaste, systemic vasodilators, and foods/beverages known to exacerbate the condition.
- Begin topical metronidazole (0.75% twice daily or 1% daily). Consider systemic antibiotics if symptoms are moderate or severe, and maintain patients on topical therapy after taper of systemic therapy.
- If topical metronidazole cannot be tolerated, use topical sulfur and sodium sulfacetamide lotions twice daily unless the patient is allergic to sulfa.
- Begin doxycycline 100 mg twice a day and continue for weeks to months followed by gradual reduction in dose to 100 mg every other day before considering cessation. Alternatively, low-dose doxycycline can be started at 40 mg once daily. Prolonged low-dose therapy may be necessary. Alternatively, minocycline 50 to 100 mg twice daily can be used.
- Suggest green-tinted makeup to provide extra coverage of red areas. Apply flesh-colored makeup over the green base.
- Refer for surgical management of persistent erythema, rhinophyma, and telangiectasia.

Periorificial Dermatitis

- Begin with doxycycline 100 mg twice daily, gradually reduced over a period of weeks after resolution has occurred. Alternatively, low-dose doxycycline at 40 mg once daily may be helpful.
- Avoid heavy cosmetics, creams, and fluoridated toothpastes.
- If a topical medication is desired, metronidazole 1% gel daily can be helpful.

Annotated Bibliography

1. Beacham BE, Kurgansky D, Gould WM. Circumoral dermatitis and cheilitis caused by tartar control dentifrices. J Am Acad Dermatol 1990;22:1029. (*Study of a series of 20 otherwise healthy women, aged 22 to 51 years; the condition probably represents an irritant contact dermatitis.*)

2. Erbagci Z, Ozgoztasi O. The significance of *Demodex folliculorum* density in rosacea. Int J Dermatol 1998;37:421. (*There was a higher mite count in rosacea patients; however, there was no correlation of counts with severity.*)

3. Powell FC. Clinical practice. Rosacea. N Engl J Med. 2005;352:793. (*Evidenced-based recommendations for the treatment of rosacea.*)
4. Rebora A, Drago F, Picciotto A. *Helicobacter pylori* in patients with rosacea. Am J Gastroenterol 1994;89:1603. (*Controversial report of an association of rosacea with Helicobacter pylori gastritis.*)
5. Liu RH, Smith MK, Basta SA, et al. Azelaic acid in the treatment of papulopustular rosacea: a systematic review of randomized controlled trials. Arch Dermatol 2006;142:1047. (*A review of five randomized, controlled trials for azelaic acid in the treatment of rosacea.*)
6. Erdogan FG, Yurtsever P, Aksoy D, et al. Efficacy of low-dose isotretinoin in patients with treatment-resistant rosacea. Arch Dermatol 1998;134:884. (*Oral isotretinoin 10 mg daily for 16 weeks was successfully used for treatment-resistant rosacea.*)
7. Pelle MT. Rosacea therapy update. Adv Dermatol 2003;19:139. (*A useful discussion of treatments and presumed mechanisms.*)
8. Elewski BE, Fleischer AB Jr, Pariser DM. A comparison of 15% azelaic acid gel and 0.75% metronidazole gel in the topical treatment of papulopustular rosacea: results of a randomized trial. Arch Dermatol 2003;139:1444. (*The use of 15% azelaic acid gel twice daily for 15 weeks demonstrated significant superiority over the use of 0.75% metronidazole gel.*)
9. Nichols K, Desai N, Lebwohl MG. Effective sunscreen ingredients and cutaneous irritation in patients with rosacea. Cutis 1998;61:344. (*The least-irritating formulation contained dimethicone and cyclomethicone.*)
10. Veien NK, Munkvad JM, Nielsen AO, et al. Topical metronidazole in the treatment of perioral dermatitis. J Am Acad Dermatol 1991;24:258. (*Tetracycline was significantly more effective.*)

CHAPTER 187 ■ MANAGEMENT OF PSORIASIS

PETER C. SCHALOCK AND ARTHUR J. SOBER

Psoriasis is a common chronic skin disease characterized by discrete and confluent erythematous papules and plaques covered with silvery white scale; its prevalence approaches 3% of the adult populations in the United States and northern Europe. Varieties include pustular and erythrodermic forms; a destructive arthritis may also develop. Patients present with cosmetic concerns and requests for relief from itching and pain. Treatment strategy depends on the type of psoriasis present, location, severity, age, and medical history. The primary physician should be able to treat mild and localized forms of the disease and be knowledgeable about approaches to more severe disease, ensuring appropriate referral and collaboration with the dermatologist.

PATHOPHYSIOLOGY AND CLINICAL PRESENTATION (1–9)

Pathophysiology

The epidermal turnover time for a cell to travel from the basal cell layer of the epidermis to the granular layer is normally 14 days. In psoriatic skin, it is reduced to 2 days. Normal cell maturation cannot take place in this short time, leading to faulty keratinization. Clinically, this process leads to *scaling*. Histologically, the epidermis is thickened, and immature nucleated cells are seen in the stratum corneum. An accompanying dilation of the subepidermal blood vessels and infiltration with mononuclear cells account for the characteristic *erythema*. Neutrophils are often seen within the stratum corneum, forming characteristic *micropustules*.

The exact causes of this abnormal cellular proliferation and inflammation are unknown, but it is conjecture that genetically predisposed persons experience T cell activation in response to antigen stimulation. Inheritance is multifactorial, with ge-

netic determinants overlapping with those of atopic dermatitis, rheumatoid arthritis, and Crohn's disease. Multiple gene loci have been identified, the most common being PSORS1 at chromosome 6p21. Affected individuals have an increased incidence of several HLA antigens, including HLA-B27 in patients with psoriatic arthritis. HLA-Cw6 is strongly associated with familial, early onset psoriasis. Psoriatic plaques are rich in activated T lymphocytes, which are capable of inducing both cellular proliferation and inflammation. Interleuking-22 (IL-22) may play a role in the thickening of the skin seen in psoriasis. IL-12 and IL-23 cytokines are overexpressed in psoriatic plaques; administration of monoclonal antibodies directed against them produces significant clinical improvement, strongly implicating these cytokines in pathogenesis. The search for responsible antigens is ongoing.

Drug-exacerbated psoriasis offers some insights into disease mechanisms: Lithium is believed to enhance the release of inflammatory mediators from neutrophils; beta-blockers decrease cyclic AMP–dependent protein kinase (an inhibitor of cell proliferation); and nonsteroidal antiinflammatory drugs can cause a buildup of the inflammatory mediator arachidonic acid. Other medications associated with exacerbations include antimalarials and interferon; a flare may follow withdrawal of systemic corticosteroids. Drug-induced exacerbations can be severe and unpredictable.

Clinical Presentation

Psoriasis usually develops in early adult life, but the disease may appear in childhood or old age; 70% of patients report onset between the ages of 16 and 22 years, usually with a positive family history and a tendency toward more severe disease. A second, less common peak is between 55 and 60 years, characterized by milder disease and little family history.

Plaque psoriasis is the most common form, presenting with well-marginated, erythematous, elevated papules or plaques, which, if not previously treated by the patient, also show thick,

---

All photos are courtesy of Peter C. Schalock.

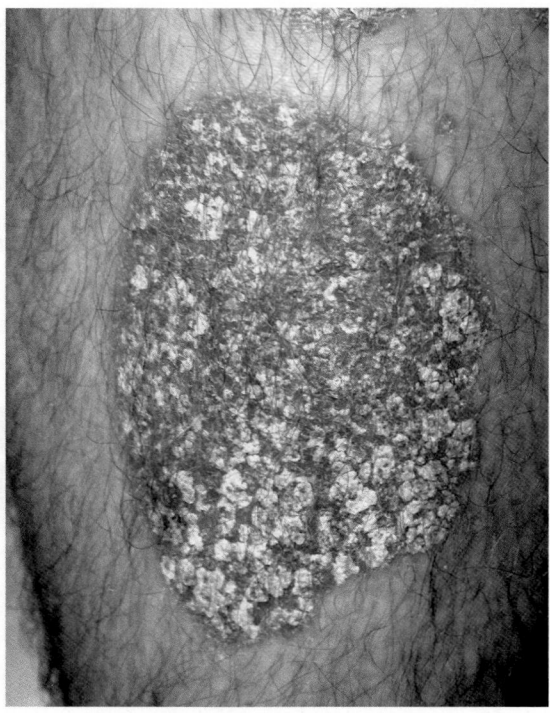

FIGURE 187.1. Typical Psoriatic Plaque on the SHIN with Micaceous Scale. (See the color insert.)

silvery scaling (Figs. 187.1 and 187.2). Removal of this scale reveals punctate bleeding points known as *Auspitz's sign*. Nails often show punctuate irregular *pitting* and a characteristic discoloration of the surface of the nail that resembles a drop of oil (Fig. 187.3). Subungual collections of keratotic material are also common, with distal separation of the nail from the nailbed. Mucous membranes are rarely involved. Commonly affected sites are extensor surfaces of the arms and legs as well as the scalp. Skin trauma increases the risk of involvement (koebnerization), and any epidermal surface may become involved, even the mucosa. Other triggering factors include

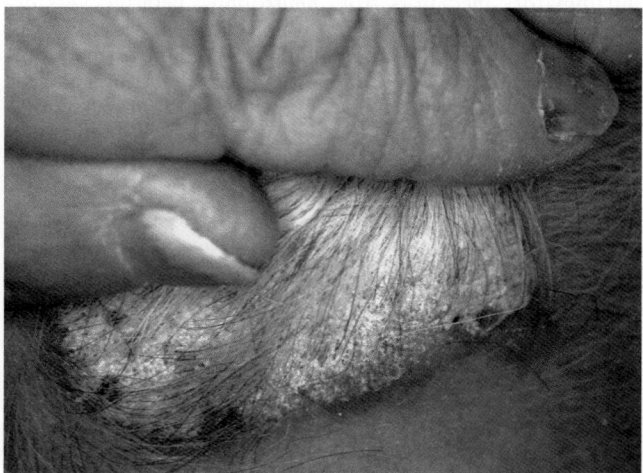

FIGURE 187.2. Scalp psoriasis with involved fingernails. (See the color insert.)

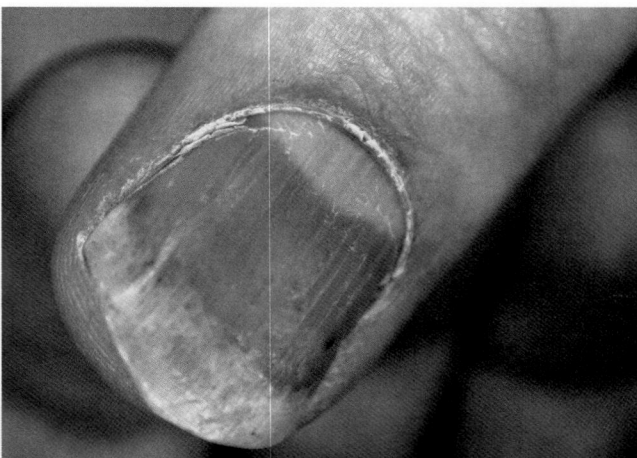

FIGURE 187.3. Typical nail finding of psoriasis with nail pitting and onycholysis. (See the color insert.)

infections (most commonly streptococcal pharyngitis), including HIV infection; hypocalcemia; psychogenic stress; drugs (see later discussion); obesity; and increased alcohol consumption and/or tobacco smoking.

Guttate psoriasis, which presents with small, discrete, erythematous papular lesions, is often preceded by a streptococcal infection. An exfoliative or *erythrodermic form* of psoriasis shows generalized erythema without any characteristic lesions of psoriasis. Localized *pustular psoriasis* with sterile pustules of the palms and soles may also be seen without other characteristic lesions. An uncommon but serious variant is *generalized pustular psoriasis*, which is often accompanied by systemic symptoms and risk of circulatory collapse. Patients with the acquired immunodeficiency syndrome may also develop extensive psoriasis that is recalcitrant to therapy.

Psoriatic arthritis can be a destructive process that is often polyarticular and asymmetric, although single joint involvement does occur. Most commonly involved are the proximal interphalangeal and distal interphalangeal joints of the hands and feet (metacarpophalangeal joints are rarely involved, in comparison to the situation with regard to rheumatoid arthritis). Classic manifestations include *sausage-shaped swelling* and deformity of the distal interphalangeal joints in association with the characteristic nail changes. Juxtaarticular inflammation produces the sausage-like swelling. Radiologic features include interphalangeal joint erosion ("*pencil-in-a-cup*" appearance) and *erosion* of the distal tufts. The skin disease usually precedes the joint disease by months to years, but arthritis may occur prior to skin findings in 10% to 15% of patients.

The clinical course of psoriasis is characterized by chronicity and seasonal fluctuations, with improvement in the summer due to sun exposure and worsening in the winter.

PRINCIPLES OF MANAGEMENT (1–27)

The basic objective is to reduce the rate of epidermal proliferation, either directly or indirectly by inhibiting dermal inflammatory and immune responses. At the same time, one needs to protect the skin from drying and other forms of injury that may precipitate a flare. Most patients have relatively localized disease (involving <20% of the body surface area); in general, topical therapy serves as their first line of treatment. However, previous failure of topical therapy, inability to apply it, rapid relapse, and presence of severe psoriatic arthritis may prompt systemic therapy.

Topical Therapy

Topical Corticosteroids

Topical corticosteroids are effective because of their antiinflammatory, antiproliferative, and immunosuppressive qualities. Preparations come in ointment, cream, lotion, gel, impregnated tape, aerosol, and foam vehicles and are classified on the basis of their relative potency (as measured by vasoconstrictive effect). Both the structure of the corticosteroid moiety and the type of vehicle delivery system used determine potency and enhance percutaneous transfer of the corticosteroid. Ointments are considered the most efficient delivery system due to the high solubility of corticosteroids in ointment bases and their relative occlusive action in comparison with other vehicles. Occlusion of localized lesions can be used to enhance the effect of a given potency of topical corticosteroid.

Topical corticosteroids commonly serve as first-line agents for mild/limited plaque disease. Their popularity derives from ease of use, convenience, rapid response, broad range of potency, varied delivery systems, patient acceptability, and wide availability. Although highly effective, topical corticosteroids applied inappropriately or over more than 20% of the body surface area can lead to adverse local and systemic effects (e.g., skin *atrophy*, *acneiform eruptions*, *adrenal suppression*; see Chapter 105). Anatomic site, extent of involvement, patient age, potency of the product, application techniques, duration, and any preexisting dermal atrophy or compromised adrenal reserve all need to be taken into account. Elderly patients have an increased risk of adverse effects.

Intermittent dosing schedules have been used to minimize the adverse topical effects of potent preparations. One regimen involves treating the psoriatic plaque with a superpotent steroid twice daily for 2 to 3 weeks, followed by application on weekends only (*weekend* or *pulse therapy*). Remissions are prolonged while avoiding the side effects of daily application. Combination programs with other classes of agents can also help spare steroid use (see later discussion).

Tars

Topical coal tar preparations are among the oldest topical therapies for psoriasis. They appear to enhance the effects of suberythemogenic ultraviolet B (UVB) light. When used alone, they are only as effective as mild to midpotency topical corticosteroids, but response improves when they are used as part of a combination program with other modalities, particularly *UVB light* (*Goeckerman program*). Patients with more than 10% of skin surface involvement are reasonable candidates for such combination therapy, and they achieve 80% to 90% remission rates without a marked increase in the risk of skin cancer. Modifications of the program allow outpatient therapy using less messy coal tar gels, followed in 2 hours by UV treatment. Four to six weeks of treatment is usually necessary to achieve maximum benefit. Topical coal tar preparations are messy, malodorous, and staining, making them inconvenient for patient use.

Tar shampoos (Zetar, Sebutone, Pentrax, T/Gel) may be of benefit to patients with scalp psoriasis. The shampoo is mas-saged in thoroughly and left on for 5 to 10 minutes; adding water and shampooing gently for several minutes helps to remove scales. Combining with overnight application of a moderate-strength topical steroid solution (e.g., Synalar solution) provides maximum effect.

Anthralin

Anthralin, one of the more effective agents for topical treatment, reduces epidermal inflammation and keratinocyte proliferation. Its efficacy matches that of class II corticosteroids, but unpleasant side effects associated with the traditional overnight application program (e.g., irritation and staining of the nonaffected perilesional skin and clothing) limit patient acceptability. Regional lymphadenopathy is a rare adverse consequence. Modifications to the traditional overnight program provide equivalent efficacy while decreasing staining and irritation. A popular *short-contact* application program uses a cream formulation (e.g., Dritho-Creme) applied for a few hours, based on the finding that anthralin penetrates faster through lesional than perilesional skin, thereby requiring less contact time than was originally believed.

Vitamin D Analogues

Vitamin D analogues act as immune modulators via the vitamin D receptor, serving as intranuclear transcription factors that bind to specific DNA sequences to modulate gene transcription activity affecting inflammation, control of epidermal growth, and keratinization. The vitamin D analogues include calcipotriene (or calcipotriol in Europe), calcitriol, and talcacitol (which is not yet approved for use in the United States).

Calcipotriene (Calcipotriol [Dovonex]). Calcipotriene, a derivative of naturally occurring vitamin D, is recommended as a first- or second-line agent for mild to moderate plaque psoriasis. It has also been shown to be safe and effective for intertriginous psoriasis. Benefits include flattening plaque and decreasing scale. The ointment formulation is more effective and more cosmetically acceptable than short-contact anthralin cream in reducing plaques and more effective than the topical steroids betamethasone 17-valerate and fluocinonide ointment, with a considerably lower rate of relapse. Response often begins within 2 weeks of treatment and continues over 6 to 8 weeks; improvement persists for up to 12 months, making it useful for both continuous and intermittent therapy.

The most common side effects are perilesional or lesional *irritation* and/or *erythema*. Patients may also develop *facial dermatitis* by inadvertent transfer to the face, necessitating advice to wash hands immediately after application. *Hypercalcemia* and *hypercalciuria* can occur if the topical dose reaches or exceeds 100 g/wk, necessitating caution when prescribing to patients with renal compromise, hypercalcemia, or a history of kidney stones. Patients with extensive psoriasis who may require a dose approaching 100 g/wk should be screened for hypercalciuria before starting treatment.

Calcitriol (1,25-Dihydroxyvitamin D_3). Calcitriol, a naturally occurring hormone with physiologic actions involved in calcium and bone metabolism (see Chapter 164), is a safe and effective topical treatment for plaque psoriasis, reducing scale production, plaque thickness, and erythema with less risk of hypercalcemia, hypercalciuria, or local cutaneous side effects than calcipotriene. It causes only minimal irritation even when applied to the face; at the low doses of calcitriol used, there is no effect on calcium homeostasis. Efficacy is somewhat less than that of calcipotriene.

Tazarotene

Tazarotene, a vitamin A derivative, selectively binds to retinoic acid receptors. Application of tazarotene 0.05% for 2 weeks decreases keratinocyte proliferation, improves abnormal keratinocyte differentiation, and decreases the expression of inflammatory markers in the skin. The gel formulation is effective in concentrations of both 0.05% and 0.1%, applied either once or twice daily; the higher-dose gel has a more rapid effect but a higher incidence of skin irritation than the lower-concentration formulation. Benefits of tazarotene over other topical agents include sustained effect (generally within 20% of final treatment levels for up to 12 weeks after treatment), rapid resolution of plaque elevation (noticed by the first week), decreased scaling (by the second week), and decreased erythema (by the end of 6 weeks). These effects are generally more rapid on lesions of the trunk and limbs than on the thicker elbow and knee lesions. Another benefit of tazarotene is its suitability for application to the face and scalp.

In comparison to other therapies, tazarotene gel (0.1% or 0.05% applied once daily for a week) is as effective as the topical corticosteroid fluocinonide 0.05% cream in reducing plaque elevation, but it is slower in effect on plaque erythema; however, after 4 weeks of treatment, the overall treatment success rates are similar. The relapse rate for tazarotene 0.1% gel is significantly lower than that for fluocinonide cream.

Tazarotene is listed as a *pregnancy category X* agent and carries a U.S. Food and Drug Administration (FDA) recommendation that women of childbearing age be checked for pregnancy before they start the medication and maintain adequate contraception for the duration of its use.

Combination Topical Therapy

Combination programs are desirable because psoriasis usually requires prolonged treatment and the long-term side effects of corticosteroids make them problematic as monotherapy.

The combination of a topical *vitamin D analogue* (e.g., *calcipotriene ointment*) and a *superpotent steroid* (e.g., *halobetasol* or *clobetasol* ointment) induces greater improvement and reduces side effects better than when either agent is used as monotherapy. Weekend steroid therapy can be combined with weekday calcipotriene ointment to increase the duration of remission. Morning treatment with calcipotriene combined with evening treatment with halobetasol ointment also enhances benefit. A combination of *calcipotriene* and *betamethasone* dipropionate in an ointment base is available for twice-daily use.

Topical corticosteroids (e.g., betamethasone dipropionate) combined with a *topical retinoid* (e.g., tretinoin 0.1%) reduce the risk of skin atrophy. *Tazarotene* in combination with a mid- or high-potency *corticosteroid* achieves greater reductions in the severity than tazarotene alone. Another potentially useful approach is the use of tazarotene and other topical agents in combination with UVB phototherapy.

Systemic Treatment of Psoriasis

Systemic treatment is indicated only for severe or incapacitating forms of the disease, such as generalized pustular psoriasis, generalized exfoliative psoriasis, psoriatic arthropathy, topical treatment failure, severe uncontrolled psoriasis (generally involving >20% of the body surface area), and socially incapacitating disease. An additional indication is acute guttate psoriasis; the use of systemic therapy may prevent this form from becoming chronic.

Phototherapy/Photochemotherapy

Phototherapy using *narrowband ultraviolet B (NBUVB) light* is quite effective for the treatment of moderate to severe psoriasis; for many, it is an effective and convenient first-line therapy. Bulbs that emit only those wavelengths (311 to 312 nm) achieve a faster response time and better clearance than broadband UVB. When compared to psoralen plus UVA (PUVA), NBUVB is equally efficacious, although patients with severe recalcitrant psoriasis often require PUVA. NBUVB is safe in pregnant women and in children because it does not require ingestion of a photosensitizer. As with other sources of UV light, carcinogenesis risk is a concern, but it is lower than that of broadband UVB or PUVA.

Photochemotherapy combines a systemic photosensitizing agent, *psoralen,* with long-wavelength (320 to 400 nm) *ultraviolet A light* (commonly referred to as *PUVA therapy*). This therapy generally produces excellent results (80% to 90% remission) in patients with otherwise recalcitrant severe disease and is reserved for them. Acute side effects include *pruritus* and *nausea* in approximately 15% of patients; *burning* may also occur. Long-term side effects include premature skin aging and carcinogenesis. The risk of *skin cancer* is increased with both UVA and PUVA therapies, the most common type being squamous cell carcinoma; melanoma is also a concern in persons undergoing long-term therapy. Regular skin checks are essential. Patients at increased risk for skin cancer (fair skin, easily sunburned, previous x-ray therapy to the skin) should not receive PUVA treatment.

Methotrexate

Methotrexate provides immunomodulation and decreases mitotic rate and DNA synthesis in the epidermis. It is effective in controlling severe disease, but the risk of serious side effects limits its use to chronic, refractory cases in male patients and women past reproductive age due to a high mutagenic potential. Doses are given once weekly. If nausea is significant, parenteral administration can be used.

Because of the drug's potential for hematopoietic, hepatic, and pulmonary toxicity (see Chapter 88), close monitoring and full patient compliance are essential. Impaired renal function increases the chances of toxicity. Hematologic status and renal and liver functions should be normal before treatment is begun, and the patient must be willing to undergo periodic blood sampling and liver biopsy if necessary during treatment to monitor for side effects. Laboratory monitoring begins with weekly, followed by monthly, blood samples. *Idiopathic pneumonitis* and *aplastic anemia* may occur, even at low doses. Although evidence of bone marrow suppression may arise, pulmonary and hepatic injury are uncommon at the doses used for treatment of psoriasis. *Hepatic fibrosis* may occur with prolonged use. The most recent consensus suggests obtaining a pretreatment liver biopsy only for patients at high risk for liver damage. The American Academy of Dermatology Consensus Panel recommends a liver biopsy for all patients after a cumulative dose of 1.5 g of methotrexate.

Systemic Retinoids (Acitretin)

Acitretin (Soriatane) is a systemic retinoid effective in erythrodermic, pustular, and chronic plaque psoriasis, but it is limited by its *teratogenicity*. Acitretin is the active metabolite of the teratogen etretinate and is reverse metabolized by endogenous esterases to etretinate, which can accumulate in fat for years. This reverse metabolization is potentiated by alcohol ingestion. If a woman has been treated with acitretin, she should avoid pregnancy for at least 3 years following acitretin therapy and not consume alcohol while taking the medication and for 2 months following cessation.

Side effects include hypertriglyceridemia, dry lips, conjunctivitis, pruritus, alopecia, color-blindness, and decreased night vision. Patients should have pretreatment measurement of liver function and triglycerides, followed by monitoring at monthly intervals. Liver biopsy is unnecessary, even with prolonged therapy.

Acitretin and Phototherapy. Acitretin monotherapy is the preferred treatment for pustular psoriasis, whereas adjunctive therapy with UV light is preferred for plaque psoriasis. Acitretin plus narrowband ultraviolet B or PUVA phototherapy has been shown to be superior to either treatment alone. The dose of acitretin or amount of total UV exposure can be reduced if they are used in combination. Increases in ultraviolet or PUVA dose, however, should be more gradual and cautious than in patients not taking systemic retinoids due to an increased risk of UV-induced erythema. After clearance of psoriasis has been achieved, the patient can be maintained on either low doses of acitretin or PUVA alone.

Cyclosporine

Cyclosporine blocks transcription of the interleukin-2 gene, decreasing production of interleukin-2 and other T cell–produced cytokines and suppressing T cell activity. More than two thirds of patients achieve significant improvement and even total clearing. However, relapse within several weeks of discontinuing treatment is common. Moreover, hypertension, renal toxicity, hirsutism, and myalgias can occur on a short-term basis, and lymphoma can occur over the longer term.

The drug is started at a low dose (2.5 mg/kg per day) and slowly increased to achieve remission. Once remission is achieved, the dose can be gradually decreased. Of two proprietary formulations of cyclosporine, Sandimmune and Neoral, the latter appears to require fewer dose increases to reach remission, aided by increased bioavailability and reduced pharmacokinetic variability. Such qualities may facilitate intermittent or pulse therapy with Neoral. Abrupt cessation of therapy may result in a relapse.

Biologics

Advances in the understanding of immune mechanisms and inflammation have resulted in promising new therapies for psoriasis. Most prominent are biologic agents whose unique mechanisms of action offer hope for more-effective, less-toxic, synergistic combination programs for persons with severe disease. Although promisingly effective, these agents are extremely expensive and have immunosuppressive action, necessitating that they be prescribed only by physicians skilled and experienced in their use.

Anti–Tumor Necrosis Factor (TNF)-α Agents. These agents, which include *infliximab (Remicade)*, *etanercept (Enbrel)*, and *adalimumab (Humira)*, bind and inactivate tumor necrosis factor-α (TNF-α), an important cytokine and mediator of inflammation. The first two are effective and FDA approved for the treatment of psoriasis and psoriatic arthritis; the last is currently approved only for the treatment of psoriatic arthritis, but it is also effective against the skin manifestations of the disease in such patients. As potent inhibitors of cytokine activity, they have several drawbacks, including very high cost, increased risk of *serious infections* (especially reactivation of latent *tuberculosis* and other fungal infections), exacerbation

of *demyelinating disease*, and a dose-dependent increased risk of *hematologic malignancy*. Some patients develop antinuclear antibodies and anti-DNA antibodies and occasionally true clinical lupus erythematosus. Heart failure is a contraindication to use of TNFα inhibitors. Purified protein derivative (PPD) testing is required before starting therapy. These agents are listed as category B agents for pregnancy.

Parenteral administration is usually required; the individual agents differ in frequency and route of administration and local reactions. Inflixamab, a chimeric (mouse–human) monoclonal antibody, requires periodic intravenous infusion by the physician. Etanercept, a fully humanized monoclonal antibody, can be administered by the patient subcutaneously twice weekly, but it causes mild to moderate injection-site reactions (erythema and/or itching, pain, or swelling) in about one third of patients. These are most prevalent in the early stages of use and then decrease, usually not resulting in discontinuation of the drug. Adalimumab is also a fully humanized monoclonal antibody.

Inhibitors of Activated T Cells. *Alefacept (Amevive)* is a human fusion protein that binds to CD2 on T cells, inhibiting T cell activation and proliferation and causing apoptosis of T cells expressing high levels of CD2. Because CD2 expression is higher on activated memory than on naive T cells, alefacept produces a selective reduction in memory T cells and the inflammatory response, providing efficacy in psoriasis without evidence of increased susceptibility to infectious disease or malignancy, including skin cancers. Weekly monitoring of CD4 T cells is recommended. Alefacept is listed as a pregnancy category B agent.

Efalizumab (Raptiva), a humanized monoclonal antibody against CD11a (which is part of a T cell surface molecule important in T cell activation, migration, and cytotoxic activity), is also effective in psoriasis. Administration is subcutaneous, once weekly. Adverse events are primarily mild to moderate *fever, headache, chills, nausea,* and *asthenia*, with incidence highest following the first infusion and decreasing with subsequent doses. Some patients have shown evidence of *exacerbation* of the disease on abrupt discontinuation of the medication, similar to that observed following the abrupt discontinuation of cyclosporine or, less commonly, methotrexate. No signs of clinical immunosuppression, hepatotoxicity, or nephrotoxicity have been noted, but there are no long-term studies. Efalizumab is pregnancy category C and should only be used in nursing mothers when the benefits to the mother clearly outweigh the risks to the baby. Mild *thrombocytopenia* (platelet counts decreasing to <50,000) has been observed in 0.3% of patients receiving efalizumab during clinical trials; platelet counts should probably be monitored.

Experimental Measures. Monoclonal Antibodies against Interleukins. Monoclonal antibodies directed against suspected pathophysiologically important interleukins, such as IL-12/23, demonstrate significant clinical efficacy with minimal serious toxicity, suggesting therapeutic promise for this experimental approach to treatment.

PATIENT EDUCATION AND INDICATIONS FOR REFERRAL (15)

For many patients, the social and psychological effects can be significant. Longstanding psoriasis can lead to loneliness and depression. Regularly scheduled visits to reinforce the details of therapy and also to render support are appreciated by the patient and family. Knowing that disease severity can be reduced through appropriate treatment is reassuring. Informed advice about what works and what does not is essential. Concerns about the condition being contagious or transmitted genetically need to be addressed. The chronic relapsing nature of the disease should be acknowledged so that patient expectations will be realistic. Preventive measures should be stressed, such as keeping the skin well hydrated and avoiding sunburn and other forms of skin trauma. Excellent support and disease information for the patient can be obtained through the National Psoriasis Foundation.

The safety and efficacy of most psoriatic regimens depend on strong patient compliance. Careful teaching that includes the rationale for a given practice is helpful, as are written instructions.

Patients with extensive, refractory, or acute pustular disease should be referred to the dermatologist for consideration of phototherapy, retinoids, antimetabolites, and immunosuppressive/biologic therapy. The development of generalized disease, especially if it is erythrodermal or pustular, requires hospitalization.

THERAPEUTIC RECOMMENDATIONS

- Treat localized, mild to moderate disease topically. Refer more extensive (>20% body surface area involvement) or refractory cases to the dermatologist.
- Emphasize the importance of keeping the skin well hydrated and avoiding sunburn and other forms of skin injury.
- Allow sun exposure if done with caution and sunburning is avoided, and do not recommend for those at increased risk for skin cancer (fair skinned, easily burned, with a history of skin irradiation).

- Review medications for potential exacerbating drugs (lithium, beta-blockers); reduce dose or substitute if possible.
- Prescribe a *topical steroid* program for the control of bothersome visible lesions. Begin with a "superpotent" preparation (e.g., Diprolene, Psorcon, Temovate, Ultravate), and change to a less potent preparation for maintenance. Only use milder steroids or calcineurin inhibitor on the face and skin folds.
- Consider *calcipotriene* or *tazarotene* as alternatives to topical steroids.
- Recommend an ointment preparation for lesions with considerable scale, although a cream may be more acceptable for daytime use and suffice for plaques with minimal scale. A twice-daily regimen of steroid application achieves the best results.
- For patients with excessive scale, recommend gentle removal by warm bathing following application of a keratolytic agent.
- For mild scalp involvement, recommend nightly use of a *tar shampoo*. It is rubbed in gently, left on for 10 minutes, and then rinsed out. For more severe scalp disease, the tar shampoo is followed by gentle application of *topical steroid lotion* (e.g., Synalar). Patients with marked scalp involvement may benefit from covering the head with a shower cap after steroid application and the use of a superpotent topical steroid lotion (e.g., Diprolene), steroid-containing scalp oil (e.g., Derma-Smoothe/FS), anthralin scalp preparation, Dovonex scalp lotion, or Tazorac gel.
- Refer patients who fail to respond and those with extensive disease to the dermatologist for consideration of *methotrexate* or other systemic therapies. Promptly admit to the hospital those who develop generalized pustular or erythrodermal disease.

Annotated Bibliography

1. Farber EM, Rein G, Lanigan SW. Stress and psoriasis: psychoneuroimmunologic mechanisms. Int J Dermatol 1991;30:8. (*Stress is associated with exacerbations; possible mechanisms are reviewed*.)
2. Granstein RD. New therapies for psoriasis. N Engl J Med 2001;345:287. (*Editorial review for the generalist reader, including a review of mechanisms*.)
3. Jullien D, Barker J. Genetics of psoriasis. J Eur Acad Dermatol Venereol 2006;20:42. (*A comprehensive, detailed review on the genetics of psoriasis*.)
4. Kupper TS. Immunologic targets in psoriasis. N Engl J Med 2003;349:1987. (*A succinct review of new developments in pathophysiology and treatment*.)
5. Krueger GG, Langley RG, Leonardi C, et al. A human interkeukin-12/23 monoclonal antibody for the treatment of psoriasis. N Engl J Med 2007;356:580. (*A significant improvement was achieved, suggesting the importance of these cytokines in the pathophysiology of the disease and a promising approach to treatment*.)
6. Naldi L, Chatenoud L, Linder D, et al. Cigarette smoking, body mass index, and stressful life events as risk factors for psoriasis: results from an Italian case–control study. J Invest Dermatol 2005;125:61. (*A study suggesting that these factors increase the risk for psoriasis*.)
7. Schon MP, Boehncke WH. Psoriasis. N Engl J Med. 2005;352:1899. (*A review of genetics, pathogenesis, and clinical features*.)
8. Zheng Y, Danilenko DM, Valdez P, et al. Interleukin-22, a T(H)17 cytokine, mediates IL-23–induced dermal inflammation and acanthosis. Nature 2007;445:648. (*A discussion of the immunology of psoriasis and the role of interleukin-22 in causing thickening of the skin*.)
9. Bleiker TO, Bourke JF, Mumford R, et al. Long-term outcome of severe chronic plaque psoriasis following treatment with high-dose topical calcipotriol. Br J Dermatol 1998;139:285. (*The treatment was shown to have long-term safety and efficacy*.)
10. Bongartz T, Sutton AJ, Sweeting MJ, et al. Anti-TNF antibody therapy in rheumatoid arthritis and the risk of serious infections and malignancies:

systematic review and meta-analysis of rare harmful effects in randomized controlled trials. JAMA 2006;295:2275. (*A meta-analysis of four randomized, controlled trials in rheumatoid arthritis patients, showing a significant increase in serious infections*.)
11. Chuang TY, Heinrich LA, Schultz MD, et al. PUVA and skin cancer: a historical cohort study of 492 patients. J Am Acad Dermatol 1992;26:173. (*High-dose therapy is associated with increased rates of squamous cell carcinoma but not of basal cell cancers*.)
12. Gilbertson EO, Spellman MC, Piacquadio DJ, et al. Superpotent topical corticosteroid use associated with adrenal suppression: clinical considerations. J Am Acad Dermatol 1998;38:3181. (*A discussion of adrenal suppression with various doses of topical corticosteroids*.)
13. Heydendael VMR, Spuls PI, Opmeer BC, et al. Methotrexate versus cyclosporine in moderate–severe chronic plaque psoriasis. N Engl J Med 2003;349:658. (*A randomized, controlled trial; no significant difference was noted*.)
14. Katz HI. Topical corticosteroids. Dermatol Clin 1995;13:805. (*A thorough review of these commonly prescribed medications*.)
15. Koo J, for the OLP 302 study group. A randomized, double-blind study comparing the efficacy, safety and optimal dose of two formulations of cyclosporine, Neoral and Sandimmune, in patients with severe psoriasis. Br J Dermatol 1998;139:86. (*Demonstrates the advantages of the Neoral formulation*.)
16. Kimball AB, Jacobson C, Weiss S, et al. The psychosocial burden of psoriasis. Am J Clin Dermatol. 2005;6:383. (*The effects can be marked*.)
17. Krueger GC, Langley RG, Leonardi C, et al. A human interleukin-12/23 monoclonal antibody for the treatment of psoriasis. N Engl J Med 2007;356:580. (*Promising results indicating a pathophysiologic role for these cytokines and a possible new avenue of treatment*.)
18. Langner A, Ashton P, Van De Kerkhof PCM, et al. A long-term multicentre assessment of the safety and tolerability of calcitriol ointment in the

treatment of chronic plaque psoriasis. Br J Dermatol 1996;135:385. (*An in-depth discussion of calcitriol.*)

19. Lebwohl M. Topical application of calcipotriene and corticosteroids: combination regimens. J Am Acad Dermatol 1997;37:S55. (*Using superpotent corticosteroids with calcipotriene results in greater improvement with fewer side effects.*)
20. Lebwohl MG, Breneman DL, Goffe BS, et al. Tazarotene 0.1% gel plus corticosteroid cream in the treatment of plaque psoriasis. J Am Acad Dermatol 1998;39:590. (*Tazarotene combined with topical corticosteroids increased efficacy and reduced adverse events*).
21. Lebwohl M, Trying SK, Hamilton TK, et al. A novel targeted T-cell modulator, efalizumab, for plaque psoriasis. N Engl J Med 2003;349:2004. (*Multicenter, double-blind, randomized, controlled trial; found the treatment to be effective*).
22. Leonardi CL, Powers JL, Matheson RT, et al. Etanercept as monotherapy in patients with psoriasis. N Engl J Med 2003;349:2014. (*A double-blind, randomized, controlled trial; the treatment was found to be effective over 24 weeks.*)

23. Lowe NJ, Prystowsky J, Bourget T, et al. Acitretin plus UVB phototherapy for psoriasis. J Am Acad Dermatol 1991;24:591. (*Greater clearing occurred with the combination than with either agent used alone.*)
24. McClure SL, Valentine J, Gordon KB. Comparative tolerability of systemic treatments for plaque-type psoriasis. Drug Saf. 2002;25:913. (*Excellent review of safety profiles of the commonly used systemic therapies for psoriasis.*)
25. Muller SA, Perry HO. The Goeckerman treatment in psoriasis: six decades of experience at the Mayo Clinic. Cutis 1984;34:265. (*The standard to which new regimens must be compared.*)
26. Roenigk HH Jr, Auerbach R, Maibach H, et al. Methotrexate in psoriasis: consensus conference. J Am Acad Dermatol 1998;38:478. (*Guidelines for treating and monitoring psoriasis patients on methotrexate.*)
27. Thomas JA, Aithal GP. Monitoring liver function during methotrexate therapy for psoriasis: are routine biopsies really necessary? Am J Clin Dermatol 2005;6:357. (*A comprehensive review of the literature regarding liver biopsy in methotrexate therapy.*)

CHAPTER 188 ■ MANAGEMENT OF INTERTRIGO AND INTERTRIGINOUS DERMATOSES

PETER C. SCHALOCK AND ARTHUR J. SOBER

Intertrigo is an inflammatory condition of body folds that presents as a moist lesion, erythema, and scaling. It is more common in obese people and is exacerbated by warm weather. The areas of involvement may include the axillary, inguinal, abdominal, and inframammary folds and the toe webs. The primary physician should be capable of distinguishing intertrigo from other eruptions of the body folds, such as erythrasma, seborrheic dermatitis, psoriasis, candidiasis, and dermatophyte infections, and of rendering appropriate treatment.

PATHOPHYSIOLOGY AND CLINICAL PRESENTATION (1–4)

Intertrigo presents as an erythematous exudative inflammation in the body folds. Patients may have soreness and itching, and with secondary infection, overt purulence may occur. The pathogenic mechanism is mechanical. Heat, moisture, and the retention of sweat produce maceration and irritation, an environment that promotes bacterial infection.

Early intertrigo is characterized by slight maceration and erythema. The moisture initially comes from eccrine sweat that cannot evaporate in the intertriginous areas because of reduced air circulation. With time, redness intensifies and the epidermis becomes eroded or denuded. Subsequent inflammation causes exudation of serous fluid. Increased moisture may lead to bacterial colonization, which accounts for the odor that is sometimes associated with intertrigo. The groin and intergluteal areas may be colonized by gram-negative organisms. Incontinence of urine or feces may exacerbate maceration and irritation in the groin and gluteal areas.

All photos are courtesy of Peter C. Schalock.

DIFFERENTIAL DIAGNOSIS (2)

Intertrigo in the Groin and Axilla

Intertrigo in the groin must be differentiated from *psoriasis*, *candidiasis*, and *tinea cruris*. Tinea cruris is a fungal infection characterized by red, scaly patches and plaques. The lesions form circinate plaques with scaly or papular borders and central clearing. After scales are scraped and 20% potassium hydroxide solution is added, the finding of hyphae in specimens under low microscopic power serves to differentiate tinea cruris from intertrigo. Candidiasis produces deep, beefy red lesions with characteristic satellite vesicopustules outside the border of the primary lesion. Involvement of the scrotum is common in candidiasis, whereas this area is often spared with tinea cruris. Psoriasis can affect all intertriginous areas. A clue to diagnosis on exam is involvement of the superior portion of the gluteal cleft (gluteal pinking).

Contact dermatitis can be caused by a variety of topical agents applied for the therapy of intertrigo or secondary to pruritus or discomfort in the affected area. Often the allergy is a secondary diagnosis in addition to other causes of intertrigo. This diagnosis should be considered in patients with recalcitrant and itchy disease.

Other diagnoses that should be considered in the groin area are erythrasma, benign familial pemphigus, Fox–Fordyce disease, and hidradenitis suppurativa. Erythrasma, caused by *Corynebacterium minutissimum*, demonstrates coral red fluorescence under the Wood's light. A condition known as *benign familial pemphigus* (Hailey–Hailey disease) should also be considered. In Hailey–Hailey disease, small blisters break

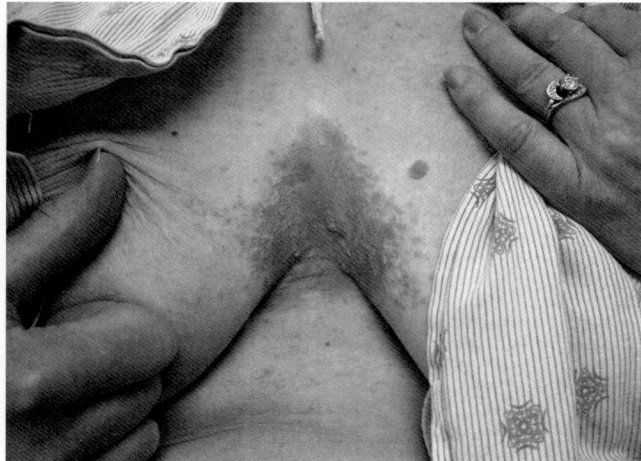

FIGURE 188.1. Inframammary candidal infection. (See the color insert.)

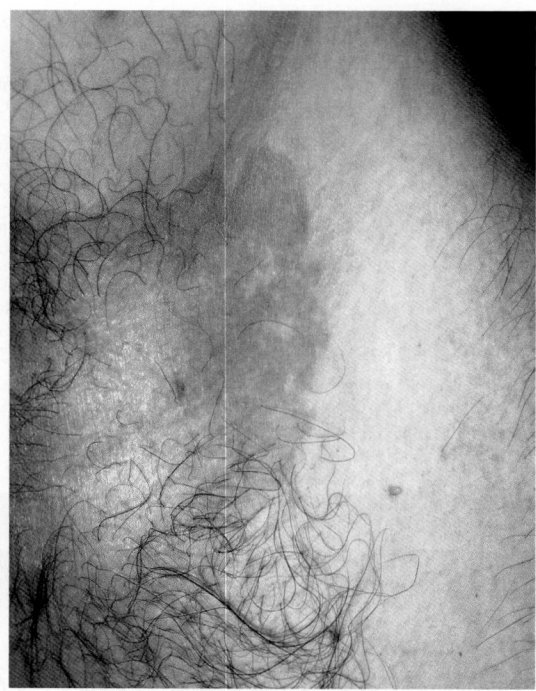

FIGURE 188.2. Clinical view of erythrasma with dull red-brown plaques in the axilla. (See the color insert.)

down to produce the eruption. If an axillary lesion is nodular or raised, Fox–Fordyce disease and *hidradenitis suppurativa* enter the differential. The groin may be affected by sexually transmitted diseases such as *condyloma*, *herpes*, *scabies*, and *pediculosis*. These produce an erythematous and pruritic eruption with characteristics that point to the underlying diagnosis (see Chapters 141, 192, 193, and 195). In severe cases of intertrigo, an underlying disease such as lichen sclerosus et atrophicus or lichen planus should be considered. Longstanding intertrigo with scratching often leads to the development of lichen simplex chronicus.

Intertrigo in the axilla needs to be differentiated from *candidiasis*, *tinea*, *erythrasma*, and *contact dermatitis*. Candidal infection presents with an erythematous eruption with satellite pustules; tinea corporis in the axilla demonstrates an active border with scale (Fig. 188.1); erythrasma has a reddish brown discoloration (Fig. 188.2) with coral fluorescence on Wood's light exam (Fig. 188.3); and contact dermatitis usually spares the axillary vault. All of these diagnoses can have presentations in both the axilla and groin.

Intertrigo of the Inframammary Region

Intertrigo in the inframammary region can occur with or without *candidal infection*.

Intertrigo of the Toe Webs

This can mimic *tinea pedis* but is usually much more macerated, malodorous, and exudative, and it is painful rather than itchy. Gram-negative organisms, often *Pseudomonas aeruginosa*, are frequently responsible for toe web intertrigo.

PRINCIPLES OF THERAPY (3,4–7)

Correcting Precipitants

The first principle of therapy is to alter the conditions that cause maceration and irritation of closely apposed skin. The goal is to *promote drying*, which can be accomplished by exposing

the intertriginous areas to air. The use of a fan can promote drying. A handheld hair dryer set to a cool setting is very effective. Addition of a nonmedicated *absorbent powder* that does not contain cornstarch is helpful. Zeasorb powder, made from corncobs, is useful (cornstarch is to be avoided because it serves as a food source and stimulates the growth of local bacteria).

The patient should be instructed to wear loose-fitting cotton clothing. Bras that provide good support are also helpful. Hot, humid environments and clothing made of wool, nylon, or synthetic fibers can precipitate or worsen intertrigo. Nylon pantyhose is a common offender. Men with groin

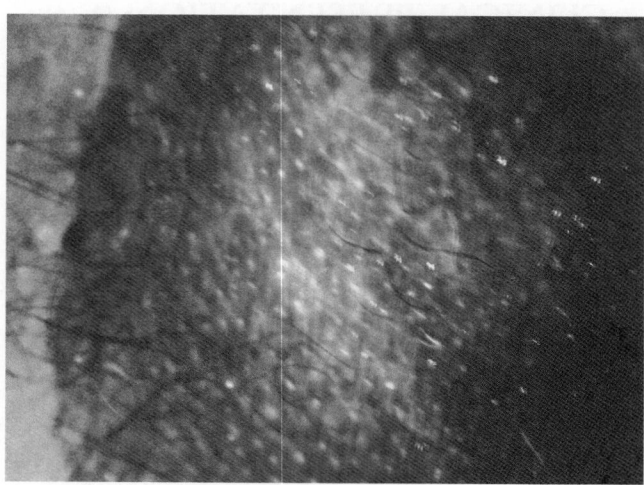

FIGURE 188.3. Coral red fluorescence from the same lesion as in Fig. 188.2, with a Wood's lamp exam. (See the color insert.)

involvement should be encouraged to wear boxer shorts rather than briefs, and women should wear cotton rather than nylon panties.

Ointments and greasy preparations of topical medications retain moisture and exacerbate the condition; they should be avoided or used sparingly. Concurrent medical conditions such as diabetes or obesity should be treated.

Exudative lesions should be treated by the application of *compresses containing Burow's solution*, prepared by adding one package or tablet to a pint of water.

Treating Secondary Infection

Any secondary infection should be treated. Pustules or scales should be examined microscopically and cultured for evidence of bacteria, yeast, and dermatophytes, after which appropriate therapy should be instituted (see Chapters 190 and 191). There is no evidence that antibacterial soaps are more effective than ordinary toilet soaps. Over-the-counter medicated powders should not be used. For intertrigo of the toe webs complicated by gram-negative infection, gentamicin cream is helpful. Toe web intertrigo can also be treated by painting gentian violet in the web spaces and having the patient use lamb's wool to separate the toes.

Treating Inflammation

As long as the area of intertriginous disease is uninfected, *topical corticosteroids* may be added to reduce inflammation. The strength of the preparation should match the severity of the condition. *Hydrocortisone cream* is an effective, safe, low-cost therapy for patients with mild to moderate inflammation. Fluorinated topical corticosteroids are useful when inflammation is more severe, but these should be applied only for short periods (1 to 2 weeks) because intertriginous striae and atrophy are common complications of more prolonged use. If a steroid sparing agent for more severe inflammation is desired, tacrolimus (*Protopic*) ointment or pimecrolimus (*Elidel*) cream may be helpful for short-term use. These medications are approved by the U.S. Food and Drug Administration for atopic dermatitis; use for intertrigo is off-label.

Combination Therapy

Some corticosteroid preparations promoted for use in intertrigo also contain an *antifungal* (e.g., *clotrimazole, clioquinol*) or *anticandidial* (e.g., *nystatin*) *agent*. These combinations are sometimes prescribed when the clinician has difficulty differentiating a fungal or candidial dermatitis from intertrigo. An additional rationale for use is treatment or prevention of secondary candidal or dermatophyte infection; however, randomized, controlled trials have failed to confirm this advantage, at least when the combination of *triamcinolone* (a medium-potency corticosteroid) and *nystatin* (Mycolog II) is compared to steroid therapy alone. Lotrisone combines medium-potency *betamethasone* with *clotrimazole*. In cases of inflammatory fungal infection, this agent is helpful. Otherwise, treatment with single agents is recommended.

Combination lotions with an alcohol base are quite drying and may sting. Some original preparations of combination formulations also contained sensitizing antibacterial agents and preservatives. Others may stain clothing yellow (e.g., Vioform-Hydrocortisone/Vytone).

PATIENT EDUCATION

The patient must understand the mechanical effects of skin occluding skin and be encouraged to dress accordingly to ensure adequate aeration and absorption of moisture. Women with large or pendulous breasts might benefit from the use of a support bra and the placement of soft cotton cloths, gauze pads, or lamb's wool between the breasts and the chest wall. The patient should be taught to inspect intertriginous zones to detect the development of erythema and maceration so that effective therapy can be instituted early. In elderly, immobile patients, the physician should educate the family or a friend to inspect intertriginous areas to prevent maceration and secondary infection.

THERAPEUTIC RECOMMENDATIONS

- Eliminate precipitating conditions. Carefully dry the area that separates folds with absorbent material, avoiding the use of paper products (paper towels); dust with drying powders; and recommend loose, absorbent clothing. In exudative lesions, a drying agent such as Burow's solution should be used as a compress.
- Advise avoidance of potential irritants/contactants in axillary eruptions.
- Treat areas with mild to moderate inflammation with topical hydrocortisone. For more severe cases, use a low- to medium-potency fluorinated topical corticosteroid for short periods only. Alternatively, tacrolimus (Protopic) ointment or pimecrolimus (Elidel) cream as a steroid sparing agent for short periods of time can also treat more severe cases of intertrigo.
- Treat any secondary bacterial or fungal infection with appropriate agents (see Chapters 190 and 191).

Annotated Bibliography

1. Bray GA. Health hazards of obesity. Endocrinol Metab Clin North Am 1996;25:907. (*Intertrigo, striae, hirsutism, acanthosis nigricans, and multiple papillomas are associated with obesity.*)
2. Janniger CK, Schwartz RA, Szepietowski JC, et al. Intertrigo and common secondary skin infections. Am Family Physician 2005;72:833. (*An excellent review of the differential diagnosis.*)
3. Holdiness MR. Management of cutaneous erythrasma. Drugs. 2002;62:1131. (*A thorough discussion of the management of erythrasma; 41 references.*)
4. Aste N, Atzori L, Zucca M, et al. Gram-negative bacterial toe web infection: a survey of 123 cases from the district of Cagliari, Italy. J Am Acad Dermatol 2001;45:537. (*The prevailing pathogen is Pseudomonas aeruginosa, but other gram-negative organisms may be involved; therapy should be directed to the control of these bacteria.*)
5. Epstein NN, Epstein WL, Epstein JH. Atrophic striae in patients with intertrigo. Arch Dermatol 1963;87:450. (*Original report of the hazard of treating intertrigo with potent topical corticosteroids.*)
6. Hedley K, Tooley P, Williams H. Problems with clinical trials in general practice—a double-blind comparison of cream containing miconazole and hydrocortisone with hydrocortisone alone in the treatment of intertrigo. Br J Clin Pract 1990;4:131. (*A well-designed study showing no difference.*)
7. Chapman MS, Brown JM, Linowski GJ. 0.1% tacrolimus ointment for the treatment of intertrigo. Arch Dermatol. 2005;141:787. (*Evidence of efficacy.*)

CHAPTER 189 ■ MANAGEMENT OF CORNS AND CALLUSES

PETER C. SCHALOCK AND ARTHUR J. SOBER

Corns and calluses are common, vexing lesions that can interfere with daily living. They may not be a presenting complaint, but the primary care physician is frequently asked about them. The tasks in the primary care setting are to provide diagnosis, simple therapy, advice on prevention, and timely referral if symptoms are refractory or disabling.

PATHOPHYSIOLOGY AND CLINICAL PRESENTATION (1,2)

Corns (helomata, clavi) and calluses (tylomata) have a common pathologic origin. *Friction* and *pressure* on the skin overlying bony prominences lead to hyperemia and proliferation of keratin. Corns often have a central, hard core that is painful if the lesion is pressed. Ill-fitting shoes are the most common cause, and the pressure of shoes on a corn may produce pain during walking (Fig. 189.1). Repeated friction may also cause callosities (Fig. 189.2).

The most common locations are on the lateral aspect of the small toe and over the metatarsal heads on the plantar aspect of the foot. *Hard corns* (heloma durum) (Fig. 189.3) have a translucent, cone-shaped avascular core with interruption of normal skin markings. *Soft corns* (interdigital heloma molle) appear as macerated white or gray lesions that are tender. The fourth and first interdigital web spaces are favored sites. Calluses, but usually not corns, may develop in persons who do not wear shoes. *Calluses* do not contain a central core and tend

to occur across the area of the metatarsal heads; normal skin markings are preserved. Women are two and a half times more likely to be bothered by corns and calluses than are men.

DIFFERENTIAL DIAGNOSIS (2)

Calluses are skin-colored or yellowish, elevated, thickened plaques that are seen in areas of friction. Calluses can be confused with plantar warts but can be distinguished from them by the preservation of normal skin markings; with verrucae, these markings are interrupted. When corns are pared down with a scalpel, one does not see the small, dark-brown-to-black dots that represent thrombosed capillaries and are characteristic of warts.

PRINCIPLES OF THERAPY (1–4)

Prevention

The primary physician's major contribution to therapy is to encourage prevention through patient education. The elimination of friction and pressure is the essence of prevention. Shoes must fit correctly, and pressure over the toes must be evenly distributed. Softer shoe materials and sandals are often helpful. Stockings must fit properly and should cushion the foot. Keeping the feet dry by using powder reduces friction. Careful

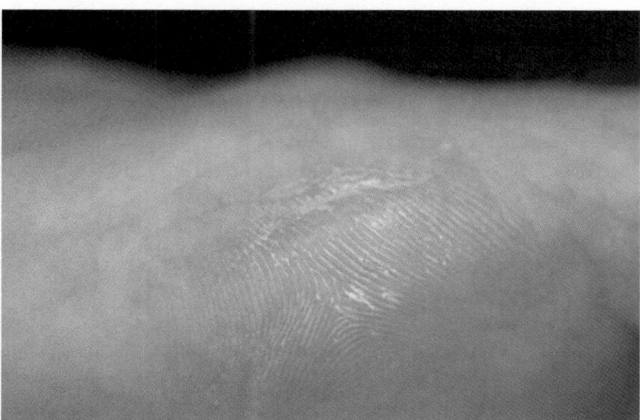

FIGURE 189.1. Callosity on the lateral border of the foot. (See the color insert.)

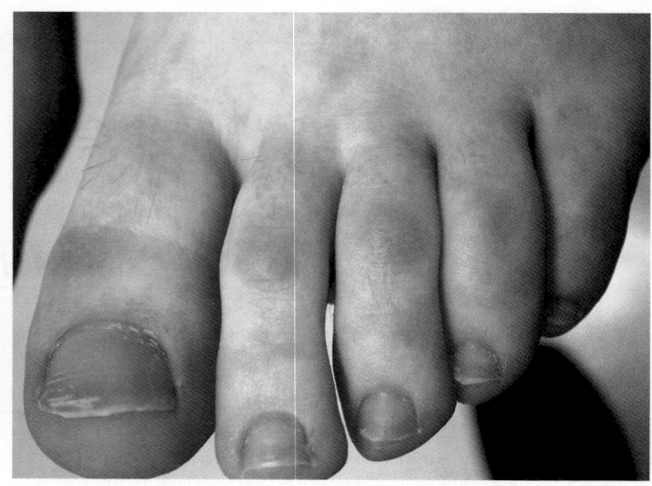

FIGURE 189.2. Callosities on the dorsal toes of an Irish step dancer. (See the color insert.)

All photos are courtesy of Peter C. Schalock.

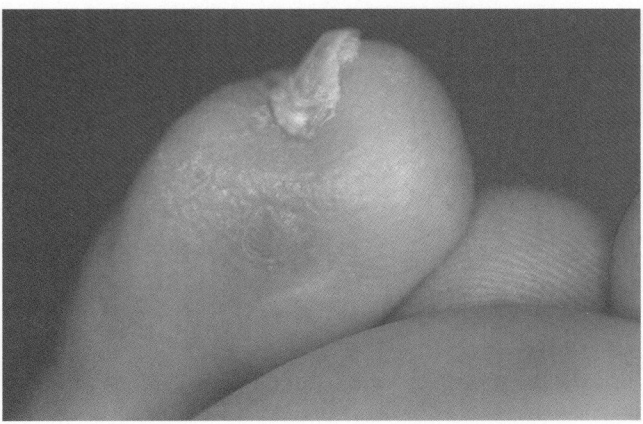

FIGURE 189.3. Heloma durum; note the lack of skin marking. (See the color insert.)

explanation of the rationale for such measures is essential to ensuring patient compliance.

Symptomatic Relief

Symptomatic relief of calluses can be achieved by *paring* hyperkeratotic lesions with a no. 10 or 15 scalpel blade. Keratin should be shaved off with the blade held parallel to the skin. Repeated strokes of the blade should be made in a direction least likely to cause penetration should the patient move suddenly. Proximal-to-distal movement is best. After a callus is removed, it is essential that previous weight-bearing trauma not be continued, or the callus will recur.

Patients can treat corns and calluses themselves by intermittent debridement with *keratolytic agents*. Salicylic and lactic acid combinations and 40% salicylic acid plasters are used to reduce the thickness of tissue. The patient should cut a piece of 40% salicylic acid plaster that is smaller than the lesion and apply it to the skin. It may be left on overnight or for as long as several days. The dressing should be removed and the foot soaked. The softened and macerated skin can be removed with a pumice stone. The plaster may be carefully reapplied as often as necessary to keep the lesions flat and asymptomatic.

The treatment of soft corns involves reducing excess perspiration. Use of absorbent *lamb's wool,* soaking the foot in potassium permanganate (1:4,000 solution), and application of silver nitrate have all been successful.

Intrinsic bone problems subject the foot to uneven pressure. Any pronation, flat foot, or medial or lateral imbalance should be treated. Padding of lesions with felt adherent padding (moleskin) or lamb's wool may prevent uneven distribution of external pressure. If the lesion is surrounded with foam rubber, pressure is distributed around the lesion rather than directly on it. If underlying bony abnormalities are suspected, x-ray films of the foot should be obtained.

INDICATIONS FOR REFERRAL

Referral to a podiatrist or orthopedic surgeon is indicated if simple measures and advice fail to reduce symptoms or recurrences. Latex, plastic, or silicone molds can be individually adapted to prevent localized pressure from producing corns or calluses. Shoes can be constructed by a podiatrist to redistribute weight and pressure. Occasionally, surgical removal of a subjacent bony prominence eliminates the source of abnormal pressure on the skin. Diabetics and other patients with impaired vascular systems should receive foot care from a podiatrist.

THERAPEUTIC RECOMMENDATIONS

- Advise the patient to avoid tight shoes with pointed toes and wear shoes that fit properly. Socks should cushion the sensitive area.
- Corns and calluses may be treated by the patient with proprietary plasters. The physician or patient can apply a keratolytic agent to the lesion in the form of a 40% salicylic acid plaster for several days. After the lesion has improved, the use of circular pads may prevent recurrence.
- Consider paring down a large lesion. Patients can perform this procedure themselves, but instruct them never to pull loose skin. Protect the tender area with moleskin after paring.
- After the lesions have been removed or pared down, ensure that the foot is not subjected to the same pressures that originally produced the problem.
- Patients with refractory lesions and lesions caused by underlying orthopedic disease should be referred to a podiatrist or orthopedist for definitive treatment of the structural problem. A molded shoe insert device may be prescribed. Diabetics and other patients with an insufficient vascular supply to the foot should be evaluated by a podiatrist.

Annotated Bibliography

1. Brainard BJ. Managing corns and plantar calluses. Physician Sports Med 1991;19:61. (*Corns and calluses arise from foot or ankle abnormalities, poorly fitting footwear, and overuse.*)
2. Singh D, Bentley G, Trevino SG. Callosities, corns and calluses. BMJ 1996;312:1403. (*An excellent review of the differences in these lesions and how to provide symptomatic relief to the patient.*)
3. Holmes GB Jr, Timmerman L. A quantitative assessment of the effect of metatarsal pads on plantar pressures. Foot Ankle 1990;11:141. (*Orthotic devices such as a metatarsal pad can be an inexpensive and effective method of reducing metatarsal pressure.*)
4. Sheard C. Simple management of plantar clavi. Cutis 1992;50:138. (*Freezing with liquid nitrogen to induce a blister followed by shaving of the crust in 3 to 4 weeks should eliminate the corn.*)

CHAPTER 190 ■ APPROACH TO BACTERIAL SKIN INFECTIONS

PETER C. SCHALOCK AND ARTHUR J. SOBER

PART 1: CELLULITIS

Cellulitis represents bacterial infection of the skin that involves the deeper subcutaneous layers. It must be differentiated from inflammatory skin changes caused by vascular insufficiency and phlebitis. Once cellulitis is identified, the primary physician needs to decide whether the patient can be managed at home on oral antibiotics or requires hospitalization. Prompt recognition and treatment of community-acquired methicillin-resistant staphylococcal skin infection is becoming a particularly important challenge.

PATHOPHYSIOLOGY AND CLINICAL PRESENTATION (1–9)

Pathogenesis

Any process that compromises the integrity of the skin allows normal skin bacteria access to the underlying subcutaneous tissue, which may initiate an inflammatory response. Trauma, stasis ulceration, ischemia, and chronic edema are common precipitants. On the lower extremity, tinea pedis may allow a site of entry. Contiguous or hematogenous spread from other sites occurs uncommonly.

Organisms and Settings

The organisms most commonly producing cellulitis are normal skin flora, with *Streptococcus pyogenes* and *Staphylococcus aureus* predominating. *Haemophilus influenzae* has been becoming less prevalent since the widespread use of the Hib vaccine.

Methicillin-resistant Staphylococcus aureus (MRSA) strains are increasingly identified in community-acquired cases of cellulitis, now accounting for most cases of skin infection seen in local emergency rooms. Although the majority of community-acquired disease still derives from health care facilities, outbreaks of community-acquired MRSA infection distinct from that associated within health care facilities have been reported among all age and socioeconomic groups, including members of contact-sports teams and attendees of child care centers. Risk factors are incompletely understood but are believed to be related in part to the high frequency of excessive antibiotic exposure (e.g., use in foods, soaps, and treatment of viral illnesses). Most cases seen involve just the skin and soft tissue, but potentially fatal invasive disease may ensue (the reported incidence is about 5%); many strains probably pro-

duce the dermonecrotic cytotoxin known as Panton–Valentine leukocidin.

Staphylococci also produce disease through their ability to multiply and produce a host of other extracellular enzymes, including α- and β-hemolysin, leukocidin, coagulase, hyaluronidase, and lipases. Streptococci produce more than 20 extracellular enzymes.

Conditions that impair the host response may predispose to skin infection by opportunistic organisms such as *gram-negative bacteria*. Skin infections with *Escherichia coli*, *Pseudomonas*, and *Klebsiella* are seen in immunosuppressed patients, diabetics, and alcoholics (Fig. 190.1). Cellulitis in the perineum may be caused by enteric aerobic and anaerobic bacteria.

Injury to mucosal surfaces predisposes to infection with *anaerobic organisms*. Anaerobic bacteria can produce hyaluronidase, proteases, neuraminidase, and extracellular enzymes, and they can also act synergistically with aerobic bacteria. Anaerobes play an important role in diabetic foot ulcers, abscesses, and traumatic wounds. Anaerobic infection also occurs in the setting of crush injuries. The degree of pain may be disproportionate to skin findings. A mixture of aerobic and anaerobic streptococci can cause fasciitis and cellulitis. Once connective tissue is involved, infection spreads along fascial planes.

In certain settings, cellulitis is caused by unusual organisms. In persons who handle fish, poultry, or meat, cellulitic infection with *Erysipelothrix rhusiopathiae* may occur. In patients with water-related injury and sometimes in those with immunosuppression, *Aeromonas hydrophila* can cause cellulitis. Animal bites or scratches are associated with cellulitis caused by *Pasteurella multocida* and *Capnocytophaga canimorsus*. *Vibrio* species have been implicated in salt-water–related injuries. Arthropod bites are portals of entry for conventional streptococcal or staphylococcal species, but one must also consider the unusual spreading cellulitis, a reaction to the toxin of a *brown recluse spider* or a *fire ant*. Another unusual cause of cellulitis simulating a septic thrombophlebitis is *Campylobacter* infection, often in the context of a concurrent enteritis.

Clinical Presentation

Cellulitis presents with local redness, heat, swelling, and tenderness that develops over a few days. Children usually present with cellulitis of the head and neck, whereas the extremities are commonly affected in adults. Fever, chills, and rigors may precede the cellulitis and herald possible bacteremia. The clinical presentation does not allow delineation of the specific microbial etiology. Red streaks extending proximally in conjunction with tender lymph nodes indicate an associated *lymphangitis*. Crepitus indicates *gas production* and suggests anaerobic

---

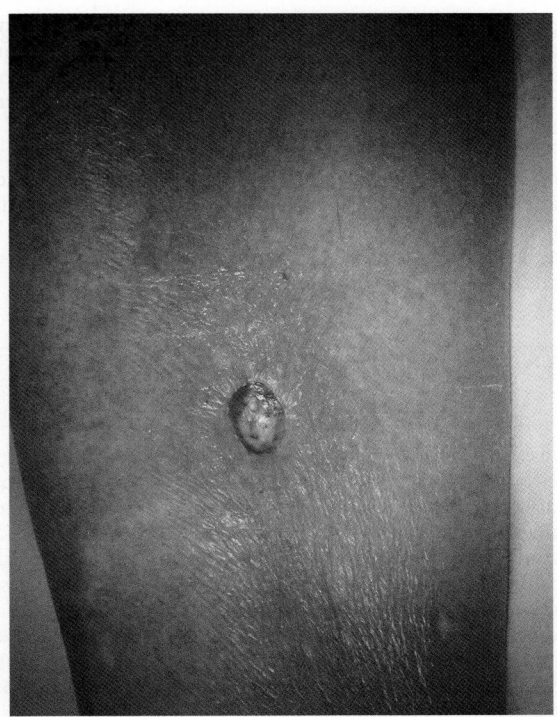

FIGURE 190.1. *Escherichia coli* infection in a shave biopsy site of an elderly immunosuppressed man. (See the color insert.)

involvement. Severe infections may be associated with bullae, pustules, or necrotic tissue.

Invasive strains of *group A streptococci* (M types 1 and 3) cause not only the usual forms of invasive streptococcal disease (scarlet fever, erysipelas, necrotizing fasciitis, myositis), but also a *toxic shock–like syndrome* associated with mucosal or cutaneous infection. Mortality is as high as 30%. Onset is abrupt, with fever, diarrhea, rigors, and pain. In many cases, pain out of proportion to the presentation can be a clue to the diagnosis. Bacteremia may be detected in 60% of cases; hematogenous spread is common.

There are no distinguishing clinical features of skin and soft-tissue infections caused by MRSA that help to differentiate them from skin infections caused by methicillin-susceptible *S. aureus*.

DIFFERENTIAL DIAGNOSIS (1,2,7–9)

Cellulitis needs to be distinguished from other causes of focal erythema, swelling, and tenderness, particularly of the lower extremities. *Superficial thrombophlebitis* may present similarly, but the inflammatory response is usually centered about the involved vein, which is tender and palpable. *Stasis dermatitis* is commonly misdiagnosed as cellulitis because both cause erythema of the lower extremity and develop in persons with severe venous insufficiency; however, cellulitis is rarely bilateral in the lower extremities, whereas stasis dermatitis is commonly bilateral. Moreover, crusting and scaling are also rare with cellulitis but common with stasis dermatitis, which has an eczematous pathophysiology. Severe *arterial insufficiency* may also cause a red lower extremity, but the erythema is typically dependent (dependent rubor), pulses are diminished or absent,

and the leg is nontender and cold. *Erythema nodosum* is indicated by lesions that are typically multiple, exquisitely tender, and often pretibial in location. It is a secondary phenomenon, and the cause needs to be ascertained. It should be remembered that cellulitis may occur concurrently with phlebitis or arterial insufficiency.

WORKUP (1–10)

The diagnosis of cellulitis is primarily clinical.

History

Once it is established that cellulitis is present, predisposing factors should be identified. A history is obtained for diabetes, congestive heart failure, recent trauma, leg edema, claudication, previous infection, tinea pedis, and loss of sensation. One should ask about intravenous drug use, occupational exposure, and any recent bites and stings. A history of fever with rigors suggests bacteremia. Community outbreaks of MRSA skin infection should be checked into, as well as exposure to members of contact-sports teams and those attending day care facilities or persons recently hospitalized or institutionalized.

Physical Examination

Note is made of the temperature, area(s) of skin involved, lymphangitic streaking, proximal lymphadenopathy, heart murmur, peripheral edema, diminished peripheral pulses, decreased sensation, and any breaks in the skin, ulceration, or atrophy. Marking the borders of the lesion with an indelible pen allows objective and rapid assessment of progression and resolution. Crepitus or foul odor is suggestive of anaerobic infection. One palpates for fluctuance and inspects the viability of surrounding tissue. Any tinea, dermatitis, venous insufficiency, or previous injury should be noted. As noted, there are no distinguishing clinical features of MRSA-related cellulitis that differentiate it from non-MRSA disease.

Laboratory Studies

A *complete blood cell count* and *differential* are helpful in gauging the severity of infection and the hematologic response. *Bacterial culture of the skin* is indicated in patients who have open or weeping wounds, abscess, or infection in unusual areas, such as the *perineum*. Material from such areas should be cultured both anaerobically and aerobically and include testing for MRSA. Because most cases of uncomplicated cellulitis in immunocompetent persons are caused by streptococci or staphylococci, culturing is not routinely performed; however, with the rise in prevalence of community-acquired MRSA infection, *culturing for MRSA* is being urged, especially in the setting of skin abscess or wound. It can be difficult to culture the offending organism from unbroken skin; there is no evidence that aspiration from the advancing margin is superior to sampling from any other area of involved skin. Any associated abscess should be incised, drained, and cultured fully before initiation of antibiotic therapy (see Part 2 of this chapter).

When rigors, fever, heart murmur, or lymphangitic or deep tissue spread is present or the patient is immunocompromised, two separate sets of *blood cultures* should be obtained before any antibiotics are administered. Blood cultures are not routinely necessary for immunocompetent patients with localized cellulitis, but if there is a local outbreak of MRSA infection or MRSA is suspected on epidemiologic grounds (member of sports team, day care attendee, recent discharge from hospital, nursing home, or prison), blood cultures should be obtained. If crepitus, fluctuance, or devitalization is present, obtain a *plain film* to look for gas production in soft tissue, which is indicative of gangrene. In cases suggestive of adjacent osteomyelitis (especially in diabetic or immunocompromised patients), a plain film may be helpful, but if infection is too early to have caused obvious bony changes, a *magnetic resonance imaging* scan may be required.

PRINCIPLES OF MANAGEMENT (1–5,7,9)

The majority of patients can be treated as outpatients with oral antibiotics and supportive measures. Concomitant foreign body should be ruled out. The edges of the erythema should be marked with ink to determine progress over the ensuing 48 hours.

Prevention

Outbreaks of MRSA and other important skin infections can be limited by handwashing, not sharing personal items, and keeping wounds clean, dry, and covered. Culturing skin wounds and infections helps in surveillance. Avoidance of unnecessary everyday antibiotic exposure (in foods, soaps, detergents, and for viral infections) may facilitate prevention and should be urged.

Antibiotics

Antibiotic coverage should target the common gram-positive organisms of the skin. There is little definitive evidence concerning antibiotic selection. In immunocompetent individuals in whom MRSA infection has been ruled out, coverage with a penicillinase-resistant penicillin, a first-generation cephalosporin, amoxicillin–clavulanate, or fluoroquinolone (adults only) is appropriate. Most prescribing guidelines still indicate using a penicillinase-resistant penicillin such as *dicloxacillin* as a first-line agent. If after 24 to 48 hours the patient is still febrile or not improving, a third-generation penicillin like amoxicillin–clavulanate, a macrolide, or fluoroquinolone should be substituted. Antibiotic therapy should continue for 10 to 14 days, depending on the rate of clinical resolution. Consider a broader-spectrum antibiotic in diabetic patients because many will have infections due to organisms other than the standard gram-positive skin flora (gram-negative aerobes).

Treatment for *MRSA infection* should be guided by culture results. Community isolates of organisms not associated with health care facilities demonstrate susceptibility to most non–β-lactam antimicrobial agents, in contrast to strains isolated from hospitalized or institutionalized patients, which are typically multidrug resistant and require vancomycin.

Supportive Measures

Supportive measures include *elevation* of the affected part and scrupulous prevention of new trauma. In patients with underlying conditions such as congestive heart failure, stasis dermatitis, and vascular insufficiency, *control of edema* and maintenance of *skin moisturization* should be instituted to restore or maintain the cutaneous barrier and help to prevent recurrent episodes. Topical antibiotics play no role in uncomplicated cellulitis if there is no ulceration.

In patients with open wounds, the risk for tetanus should be considered. If a booster of *tetanus toxoid* has not been obtained within 5 years, it should be given. Patients who have not had an initial tetanus series should receive both tetanus toxoid and tetanus immune globulin (see Chapter 6).

INDICATIONS FOR REFERRAL AND ADMISSION

Abscesses should be drained and necrotic tissues should be debrided, and so prompt surgical referral is necessary. Hospitalization and intravenous antibiotics are indicated for compromised hosts who are at risk for hematogenous spread of infection (e.g., patients with poorly controlled diabetes, alcoholics, injection-drug abusers, HIV-infected persons). Persons with community-acquired cellulitis due to MRSA should also be admitted, especially if there is evidence of spread to deeper tissues or positive blood cultures. Other indications for prompt hospital admission and intravenous antibiotics include rapidly progressive or recurrent infection, cellulitis caused by group A streptococci, the presence of subcutaneous gas or necrotizing fasciitis, and cellulitis of the orbit, face, or perineum, especially when accompanied by fever and lymphangitis. Clinical signs that suggest a need for intravenous therapy include high fever, systemic symptoms, and pain more severe than the clinical appearance would indicate.

In cases of progression despite the administration of oral antibiotics, the outpatient approach to treatment must be reconsidered. When patients appear unreliable and unable to care for themselves at home, admission is also indicated.

PATIENT EDUCATION

When a lower extremity is involved, the patient should be instructed to rest in bed and elevate the limb. Getting up to go to the bathroom is allowed, but bed rest is mandatory. Exercises and anticoagulation may be needed to reduce the possibility of thrombophlebitis in patients at increased risk (see Chapter 35). The importance of taking antibiotic therapy as instructed should be emphasized. The patient should be asked to report progress by telephone and to call if cellulitis fails to improve in 48 hours and resolve within 5 to 7 days.

THERAPEUTIC RECOMMENDATIONS

- Hospitalize patients unable to care for themselves reliably at home, and also any patient with high fever, rigors, lymphangitis, rapid progression, compromised host defenses, or involvement of the face, orbit, or perineum; also consider admission for those with MRSA infection, especially if there is evidence of spread to deeper tissues or positive blood cultures.
- Incise, drain, and culture any associated abscess (see Part 2 of this chapter) before initiating antibiotic therapy.

- Treat the patient with mild, uncomplicated non-MRSA illness on an ambulatory basis. Begin with a penicillinase-resistant penicillin (e.g., 500 mg of *dicloxacillin* four times daily, 1 hour before meals and at bedtime), and monitor closely during the next 48 hours.
- If inflammation and fever do not begin to resolve after 24 to 36 hours or if close monitoring is not possible, consider obtaining a culture and broadening coverage to a cephalosporin (e.g., cephalexin 500 mg four times daily) or a third-generation penicillin (e.g., amoxicillin clavulanate) or a fluoroquinolone. If erythema continues to progress after 48 hours, consider hospital admission.
- For patients markedly allergic to penicillin (type I hypersensitivity), start with *azithromycin* or a first-generation cephalosporin (e.g., *cephalexin*, 500 mg four times daily) if the allergy to penicillin is not well documented and was not anaphylactoid. The fluoroquinolones, such as *ciprofloxacin*, are effective against gram-negative cellulitis; however, they have only moderate antistreptococcal and antistaphylococcal activity *in vitro* and should be used cautiously in cellulitis.
- If anaerobes are suspected, then a fluoroquinolone plus *clindamycin* or *metronidazole* is indicated.
- Culture cellulitis for MRSA if it is associated with a wound, deeper tissue involvement, or epidemiologic risk factors; treat according to the results of antibiotic sensitivity testing. Pending culture results, it is reasonable to start with clindamycin, trimethoprim–sulfamethoxazole, or a long-acting tetracycline (e.g., doxycycline); linezolid is another possibility. Provide close follow-up because relapse or recurrence may occur.
- Patients with an open wound but without a recent tetanus booster within 10 years should be given tetanus toxoid.

Annotated Bibliography

1. Anaya DA, Dellinger EP. Necrotizing soft-tissue infection: diagnosis and management. Clin Infect Dis 2007;44:705. (*A useful review of diagnosis and treatment; 32 references.*)
2. Brook I, Frazier EH. Aerobic and anaerobic microbiology of infection after trauma. Am J Emerg Med 1998;16:585. (*In 32% of cases, the predominant organisms were anaerobes; in 16%, only aerobic bacteria were isolated; in 52%, mixed aerobic and anaerobic organisms were isolated.*)
3. Daum RS. Skin and soft-tissue infections caused by methicillin-resistant Staphylococcus aureus. N Engl J Med 2007;357:380. (*A very useful clinical review; 69 references.*)
4. Goldstein EJ, Citron DM, Nesbit CA. Diabetic foot infections. Bacteriology and activity of 10 oral antimicrobial agents against bacteria isolated from consecutive cases. Diabetes Care 1996;19:638. (*Staphylococcus aureus was isolated from 76% of patients; streptococci, enterococci, Enterobacteriaceae, and anaerobes were also present in about 40%; sparfloxacin and levofloxacin were the most active agents tested.*)
5. Hauser AR. Another toxic shock syndrome. Streptococcal infection is even more dangerous than the staphylococcal form. Postgrad Med 1998;104:31, 39, 43. (*Hypotension, confusion, and unexplained renal insufficiency are clues to streptococcal toxic shock syndrome; even with aggressive therapy, mortality can exceed 50%.*)
6. Klevens RM, Morrison MA, Nadle J, et al. Invasive methicillin-resistant Staphylococcus aureus infections in the United States. JAMA 2007;298:1763. (*Epidemiology, bacteriology, and genetics of this important skin infection and causative organism.*)
7. Lewis RT. Soft-tissue infections. World J Surg 1998;22:146. (*Classification of soft-tissue infections is based on the degree of localization and the presence of tissue necrosis.*)
8. Quartery-Papafio CM. Importance of distinguishing between cellulitis and varicose eczema of the leg. BMJ 1999;318:1672. (*A very useful discussion of an everyday problem.*)
9. Stulberg DL, Penrod MA, Blatny RA. Common bacterial skin infections. Am Family Physician 2002;66:119. (*A review of antibiotic choices and pathogens of skin infections.*)
10. Schmid MR, Kossmann T, Duewell S. Differentiation of necrotizing fasciitis and cellulitis using MR imaging. AJR Am J Roentgenol 1998;170:615. (*When no deep fascial involvement is seen with magnetic resonance imaging, necrotizing fasciitis can be excluded.*)

PART 2: MANAGEMENT OF PYODERMA

The common cutaneous bacterial infections include impetigo, ecthyma, folliculitis, furunculosis, and erysipelas. They must be recognized promptly by the primary physician and treated effectively with antibiotics. Awareness of increasingly resistant organisms involved in skin infections is particularly important for the primary physician.

PATHOPHYSIOLOGY AND CLINICAL PRESENTATION (1–6)

The clinical manifestations reflect a combination of factors, including the causative organism, environmental factors, area of skin involved, and host resistance. "Primary" cutaneous bacterial infections develop on normal skin and are usually initiated by a single organism, such as coagulase-positive staphylococci or β-hemolytic streptococci. *Methicillin-resistant Staphylococcus aureus* is becoming an increasingly important causative organism in community-acquired skin infection (see Part 1). "Secondary" bacterial infection refers to infection superimposed on diseased skin. Cutaneous bacterial infections may also be classified according to the depth of infection and the propensity for scarring.

Impetigo

Impetigo, a common condition caused primarily by *S. aureus* and less often by *Streptococcus pyogenes*, begins as a small, erythematous macular lesion that evolves into a *vesicle* beneath the stratum corneum. Bullous impetigo is caused almost exclusively by *S. aureus*. The thin-roofed collection of fluid ruptures easily, leaving denuded, oozing areas. A *honey-colored crust* forms as the fluid dries and collects. Intense erythema at the base of the pustule suggests a *β-hemolytic streptococcal component* to the condition. New lesions appear in the same location, and they coalesce. When the honey-colored crusts are removed, the skin appears raw and glistening. Individual lesions usually do not exceed 2 cm in size. Impetigo is seen most frequently in children, but it also occurs in adults, especially those with poor hygiene. In adults, the condition is not as contagious as it is among infants. The face is the most common site of involvement. Ordinary lesions do not produce scarring, but they may leave erythematous marks for some time. Untreated infections may last for weeks.

Ecthyma

Ecthyma is a deeper version of impetigo, usually caused by *streptococci*, but it is sometimes a sign of gram-negative sepsis or fungal infection. Erosion of the epidermis creates ulcerative, crusted lesions. The heaped-up crust conceals the underlying erosion. Healing is accompanied by some scarring because of the depth of the lesions. The legs are commonly involved, and children are more susceptible than are adults. Antecedent conditions include eczema, scabies, arthropod bites, and trauma. The *brown recluse spider bite* is characterized by necrotizing ulcer and spreading ecthyma.

Folliculitis

Folliculitis is infection of the hair follicles, usually caused by coagulase-positive *staphylococci*, and may be divided into superficial and deep types. Superficial folliculitis consists of a small pustule pierced by the hair shaft. It may be seen on the scalp or other hairy portions of the body. Occupational exposure to cutting oils and the use of coal tar products or topical corticosteroids under occlusive dressings may precipitate folliculitis. Fungal folliculitis caused by *Pityrosporum ovale* may resemble bacterial folliculitis, but it is refractory to treatment with antibiotics. The diagnosis is often made by the finding of yeastlike organisms on a potassium hydroxide wet mount, but a skin biopsy is sometimes required. Rarely, small pustules with surrounding erythema caused by *Propionibacterium acnes* may develop around the occiput in male patients. *Pseudomonas folliculitis* has been described in association with bathing in hot tubs.

Furuncles and Carbuncles

Furuncles and carbuncles may develop from a preceding folliculitis and are limited to hairy areas. A furuncle involves a single follicular unit. This erythematous lesion usually become fluctuant after 4 days. A yellowish, pointed area may be seen on the surface, and, if the lesion ruptures spontaneously, pus and necrotic tissue are extruded. The buttocks, axillae, neck, face, and waist areas are common sites of involvement. Predisposing systemic factors include diabetes, malnutrition, obesity, and hematologic disorders. Carbuncles involve multiple follicular units and are a coalescence of deep furuncles with multiple points of drainage.

Erysipelas

Erysipelas, caused by *β-hemolytic streptococci* (mainly group A, but also groups G, C, D, and B), is characterized by a peripherally spreading, infiltrated, erythematous, sharply circumscribed plaque. The lesion is warm to the touch. The face, scalp, hands, and genitals are frequently involved. Rapid evolution of the lesions is seen, and some patients have constitutional symptoms such as fever and malaise. Poor hygiene and lowered resistance promote infection. Trauma may elicit infection, and recurrent erysipelas may lead to brawny edema and lymphostasis (*elephantiasis verrucosa nostra*) in the lower extremities.

Lesions are usually diagnosed and treated on the basis of clinical appearance; however with the community emergence of resistant staphylococcal strains such as MRSA, culturing before initiation of antibiotic therapy is increasingly recommended, even for superficial infections, as well as for more destructive lesions and those that fail to improve with initial treatment. Abscesses should be incised and drained and the contents sent for culture and sensitivity before commencing antibiotics. For patients with recurrent gram-positive infections, culturing the nares and perianal areas to evaluate for colonization by MRSA and other resistant strains can be helpful.

PRINCIPLES OF THERAPY (1–11)

Physical measures are used to enhance resolution and make the skin surface less amenable to colonization by bacteria; antibiotics are given to treat responsible pathogens, prevent more invasive disease from developing, and limit recolonization.

Physical Measures

The physical measures used differ according to the pyoderma being treated. The crusts of impetigo should be debrided to expose the skin surface where bacteria are present. The use of a washcloth for this purpose is recommended. Furuncles and carbuncles are treated with hot compresses to enhance drainage. Fluctuant lesions with abscess formation usually require *incisure and drainage*. Sometimes, packing of the wound is necessary. With exudative lesions, drying compresses are required to remove detritus and desiccate the lesion. Saline solution, tap water, or Burow's solution may be applied for 10 to 20 minutes three to four times a day. Dehydration improves the appearance of the skin and destroys many organisms.

In persons with recurrent furunculosis, soaking the beard with hot water for 5 minutes before shaving and discarding blades after each use can be helpful. Separate towels, sheets, and clothing should be used and frequently laundered and changed.

Antibiotics

Topical Antibiotics and Other Local Antibacterial Measures

Topical antibiotics, such as *mupirocin* (*Bactroban*), are usually sufficient for impetigo and folliculitis, particularly when combined with cleansing and debridement. Most cases of pyoderma are caused by gram-positive organisms, and many respond to topical *clindamycin*. If antibiotic resistance is suspected, these topical agents should be avoided. Mupirocin ointment applied to the nares may help to eliminate colonization in the nares (see later discussion).

Washing with *chlorhexidine* (Hibiclens) is a valuable adjunct because of its bactericidal properties. Patients should wash the areas with the liquid two or three times daily before applying mupirocin. Antibiotic creams and ointments containing neomycin or bacitracin are rarely effective as topical therapy and commonly worsen the condition by causing an allergic contact dermatitis.

Reducing colonization is particularly important in the treatment of recurrent furunculosis. Frequent cleansing with soap, particularly *chlorhexidine*, is useful. An over-the-counter option is to use the alcohol-based hand cleansers on the affected areas twice daily (not on mucous membranes). Nails should be clipped and vigorously scrubbed. If culture from the nares or perianal skin is positive, *mupirocin* ointment should be applied twice daily. It can be used on a long-term basis to reduce bacterial carriage in the nares of patients in whom pyoderma repeatedly develops.

Systemic Antibiotics

Systemic antibiotics are indicated when constitutional symptoms are present or if the patient is not willing to treat topically; presence of MRSA infection is also an indication for systemic antibiotic therapy because of the organism's invasive potential. As noted, antibiotic selection may be based on clinical appearance, but culture-and-sensitivity testing should be performed before antibiotics are started. Pending results of such testing, *dicloxacillin* or *cephalexin* is a reasonable initial choice of systemic antibiotic; both are effective against most staphylococcal and streptococcal species that cause pyoderma; *azithromycin* is a good alternative in β–lactam-allergic patients. If MRSA is a concern, one might start with clindamycin, trimethoprim–sulfamethoxazole, or a long-acting tetracycline (e.g., doxycycline), pending results from culture testing. There is no evidence that antibiotic therapy prevents poststreptococcal glomerulonephritis.

PATIENT EDUCATION AND INDICATIONS FOR REFERRAL

A primary consideration in the therapy of all cases of pyoderma is patient education. Teaching aggressive and regular use of cleansing and debridement is central to the successful resolution of the infection. In addition, careful review of preventive measures and antibiotic use is essential.

If aggressive hygienic measures and attempts to eliminate the staphylococcal carrier state fail to prevent recurrent infection, consider treatment with rifampin, a cloxacillin or minocycline, and topical mupirocin, which is effective for eradicating nasal carriage of pathogenic staphylococci. Rifampin should not be used as a single agent because many patients will develop antibacterial resistance.

THERAPEUTIC RECOMMENDATIONS

Impetigo

- Apply compresses soaked in Burow's solution for 20 minutes two to four times daily, then debride gently with a washcloth and cleanse with a chlorhexidine-containing agent.

- Lightly apply mupirocin or fusidic acid ointment (not available in the United States, but as effective as mupirocin) to the area after drying. A nighttime application is also advised.
- Cephalexin should be used in patients with widespread disease or with systemic symptoms. Other oral penicillinase-resistant agents, such as dicloxacillin or amoxicillin–clavulanate, may be substituted.
- Advise the patient not to cover the lesions and the family to avoid using the same towel or washcloth; keep children away from the patient with impetigo.

Folliculitis

- Treat with gentle debridement and topical antibiotics, as for impetigo.

Furuncles and Carbuncles

- Treat with hot compresses until the lesions are fluctuant and spontaneous drainage occurs. Obtain some of the material drained for culture and sensitivity testing.
- Have larger lesions incised and drained if they become fluctuant; culture contents, including culturing for MRSA; check antibiotic sensitivities.
- Treat furuncles or carbuncles that are associated with cellulitis, fever, or facial location with oral antistaphylococcal antibiotics, either *cephalexin* (500 mg four times daily for 10 days) or *dicloxacillin* (250 mg four times daily for 10 days); check for the presence of MRSA and, if present, adjust the antibiotic program according to the results of sensitivity testing.
- Treat recurrent infection with a 14- to 21-day course of a systemic antibiotic and remove bacteria from potential sources, such as the skin, nares, nails, and razors and other fomites.

Erysipelas

- Treat with cool compresses and *phenoxymethyl penicillin* (500 mg four times daily) for 10 to 14 days.

Recurrent Pyoderma

- Eradicate the staphylococcal nasal carrier state. Prescribe oral *dicloxacillin* (500 mg four times daily for 10 to 14 days) in combination with topical *mupirocin* applied twice daily for at least 5 days. *Rifampin* can be used as a single agent effectively, but it should be used in combination with a cloxacillin or minocycline to prevent antibacterial resistance.

Annotated Bibliography

1. Bisno AL, Stevens DL. Streptococcal infections of skin and soft tissues. N Engl J Med 1996;334:240. (*Current concepts in the range of infections caused by this organism.*)
2. Bolognia JL, Jorizzo JL, Rapini RP, eds. Dermatology. New York: Mosby, 2003. (*A general review of bacterial skin infections.*)
3. Brown J, Shriner DL, Schwartz RA, et al. (2003). Impetigo: an update. Int J Dermatol 2003;42:251. (*A general review of impetigo.*)
4. Carroll JA. Common bacterial pyodermas. Taking aim against the most

likely pathogens. Postgrad Med 1996;100:311, 317. (*Recommended antibiotic treatment for all common cutaneous infections.*)
5. Daum RS. Skin and soft-tissue infections caused by methicillin-resistant *Staphylococcus aureus*. N Engl J Med 2007;357:380. (*A very useful clinical review; 69 references.*)
6. Odell ML. Skin and wound infections: an overview. Am Family Physician 1998;57:2424. (*A practical review of common infections.*)
7. Sadick NS. Current aspects of bacterial infections of the skin. Dermatol Clin

1997;15:341. (*A very practical review with specific recommendations; 50 references.*)

8. Bass JW, Chan DS, Creamer KM, et al. Comparison of oral cephalexin, topical mupirocin and topical bacitracin for treatment of impetigo. Pediatr Infect Dis J 1997;16:708. (*Shows the effectiveness of mupirocin as a topical agent against uncomplicated impetigo.*)

9. George A, Rubin GA. Systematic review and meta-analysis of treatments for impetigo. Br J Gen Pract 2003;53:480. (*Evidence supporting treatments for impetigo.*)

10. McLinn S. A bacteriologically controlled, randomized study comparing the efficacy of 2% mupirocin (Bactroban) with oral erythromycin in the treatment of patients with impetigo. J Am Acad Dermatol 1990;22:883. (*Two percent mupirocin was as effective as oral erythromycin.*)

11. Falagas ME, Bliziotis IA, Fragoulis KN. Oral rifampin for eradication of *Staphylococcus aureus* carriage from healthy and sick populations: a systematic review of the evidence from comparative trials. Am J Infect Control 2007;35:10614. (*Oral rifampin reduces the carrier state of Staphylococcus aureus but causes antimicrobial resistance when used as a single agent.*)

CHAPTER 191 ■ MANAGEMENT OF SUPERFICIAL FUNGAL INFECTIONS

PETER C. SCHALOCK AND ARTHUR J. SOBER

Although they are neither dangerous nor life-threatening, superficial fungal infections are prevalent, irritating, and often recurrent. They are easily diagnosed but commonly confused with nonfungal dermatoses such as impetigo (see Chapter 184) and nummular eczema. The primary physician and other health care professionals encountering such patients should be capable of providing a definitive diagnosis, cost-effective therapy, and patient education for prevention.

PATHOPHYSIOLOGY AND CLINICAL PRESENTATION (1–5)

Most of the organisms that cause superficial fungal infections are ubiquitous in nature. Fungal infection occurs when one of these ubiquitous organisms invades the superficial layers of the skin. Hereditary factors and systemic diseases like diabetes commonly contribute to susceptibility, as do local precipitants such as dampness and friction leading to skin maceration. Dermatophytes do not usually invade below the level of keratin.

Dermatophytic and candidal infections produce scaly, erythematous lesions with defined margins; multiloculated bullae may occur, especially on the feet. Characteristic presentations vary depending on the organism and area of the body involved.

Tinea Versicolor

Tinea versicolor, caused by *Malassezia globosa* and other *Malassezia* species, produces brown, pink, red, or white *scaly patches* or slightly elevated *plaques* on the chest, back, and shoulders. During the summer, it may present as areas of *hypopigmentation* often mistaken for vitiligo. Decreased pigmentation results from the inhibition of melanocytes by dicarboxylic acids produced by the yeast. Scratching a macular area raises a small amount of fine scale, suggesting the diagnosis. Examination of the skin with a *Wood's light* reveals gold or orange-brown fluorescence. The infection is confirmed by *scraping* a scaly lesion and examining it with a drop of

20% potassium hydroxide for characteristic short hyphae and spores, sometimes referred to as *"spaghetti and meatballs."*

Dermatophyte Infections

Dermatophyte infections are defined by the area of the body they affect. The most common is *tinea pedis*. This condition is characterized by blisters and/or inflammation and scale on the soles and interdigital areas of the feet (Figs. 191.1 and 191.2). *Tinea cruris* involves the groin and inner thighs and sometimes even extends onto the abdomen and buttocks. *Tinea corporis* affects other areas of the body, including the trunk and extremities; facial involvement is referred to as *tinea faciei*. *Tinea capitis*, or scalp ringworm, occurs almost exclusively in children. *Tinea barbae*, involving the bearded area, is uncommon but needs to be considered in the differential diagnosis of a facial rash. *Onychomycosis*, caused by *Trichophyton rubrum*, *Trichophyton mentagrophytes*, and *Epidermophyton floccosum*, leads to characteristic accumulation of subungual keratin, which produces a thickened, distorted, crumbling nail. *Microsporum canis*, acquired by contact with infected pet cats and dogs, is another common pathogenic fungus.

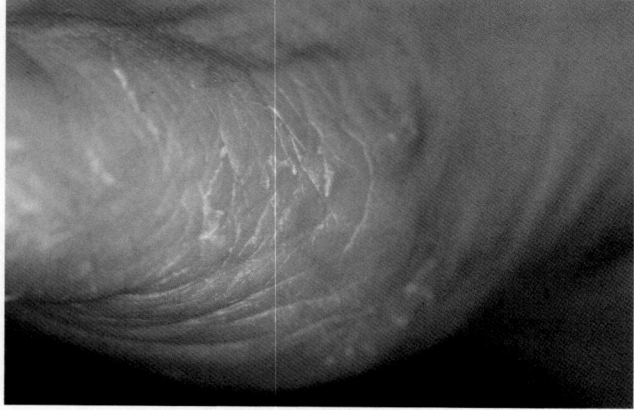

FIGURE 191.1. Tinea pedis on the side of the foot adjacent to the great toe. (See the color insert.)

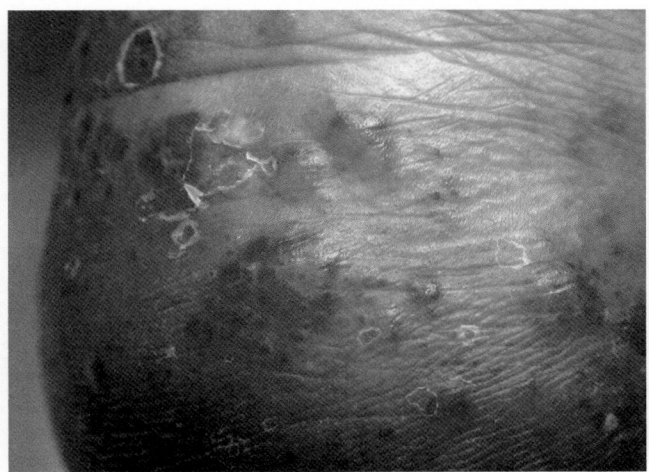

FIGURE 191.2. Multiloculated bullae, a less common presentation of tinea pedis. (See the color insert.)

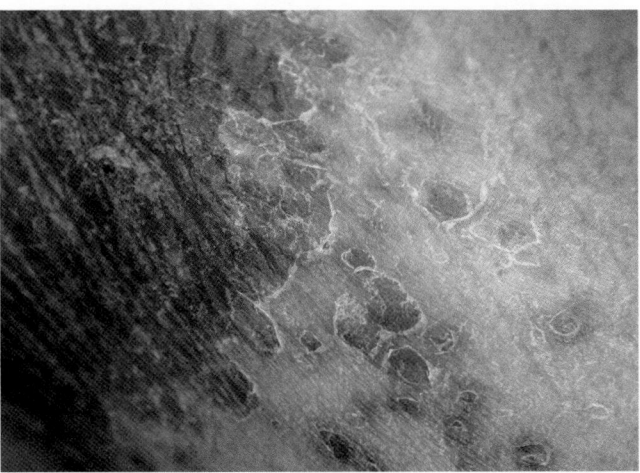

FIGURE 191.4. Cutaneous *Candida* infection with prominent satellite lesions. (See the color insert.)

Atypical presentations may be noted. The treatment of a superficial fungal infection with a topical corticosteroid can suppress inflammation without curing the infection, a state referred to as *tinea incognito*. The infection of the hair follicle by a dermatophyte is called *Majocci's granuloma* (Fig. 191.3). It is caused by *T. rubrum* infection and is most commonly seen on the legs of women. It is hypothesized to be from shaving of the legs. The fungal infection penetrates the hair shaft and causes an inflammatory/granulomatous response. *Kerion* is a vigorous inflammatory response to fungal infection of the scalp, frequently by *Trichophyton tonsurans*. A boggy, tender plaque forms on the scalp, often with lymphadenopathy. Permanent alopecia may occur in longstanding plaques.

Candida Infections

Candida infections of the skin occur principally in *intertriginous* locations, such as the axillae, groin, intergluteal folds, inframammary area, and interdigital web spaces. Crusted involvement of the labial commissures, known as *perlèche*, and involvement of the *glans penis* also occur. The presence of erythema on the glans penis and scrotum suggests a candidal rather than a dermatophyte infection. Lesions are pustular and thin walled, located on a reddish base, and often produce burning and itching. Candidiasis may be clinically suspected by the presence of characteristic smaller *satellite lesions* (papules, macules, or pustules outside the margin of the primary lesion) (Fig. 191.4).

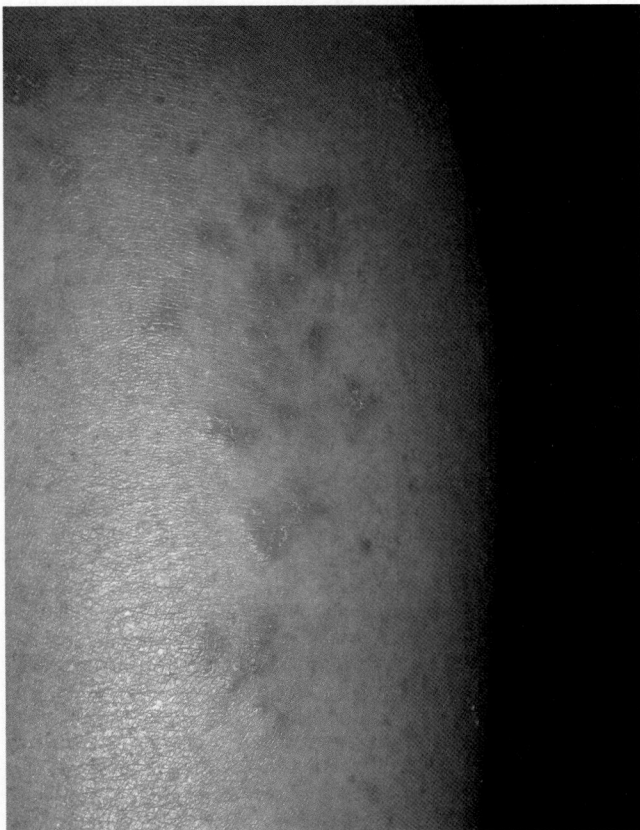

FIGURE 191.3. Majocci's granulomas on the leg. (See the color insert.)

DIAGNOSIS (1–5)

The finding of scaly, erythematous lesions with defined margins in characteristic areas of the body that promote the growth of fungi should raise suspicion of a superficial fungal infection. Satellite pustules suggest a candidal involvement. In intertriginous areas, fungal infection must be differentiated from *intertrigo* and *erythrasma*. Asymptomatic, slightly erythematous to light brown, finely scaling patches in the groin and upper thigh with little or no central clearing are characteristic of erythrasma (a corynebacterial infection). Early intertrigo is characterized by slight maceration and erythema. With time, the redness becomes more intense, and the epidermis becomes eroded or even denuded. *Psoriasis* involving the nails may lift the nail and mimic onychomycosis, but pitting is not seen with fungal infection; skin involvement with psoriasis can lead to erythematous scaling plaques and be mistaken for fungal

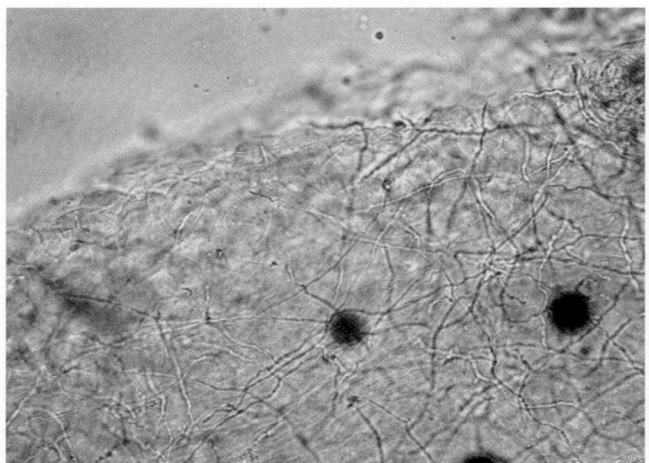

FIGURE 191.5. Positive potassium hydroxide test with prominent hyphae. (See the color insert.)

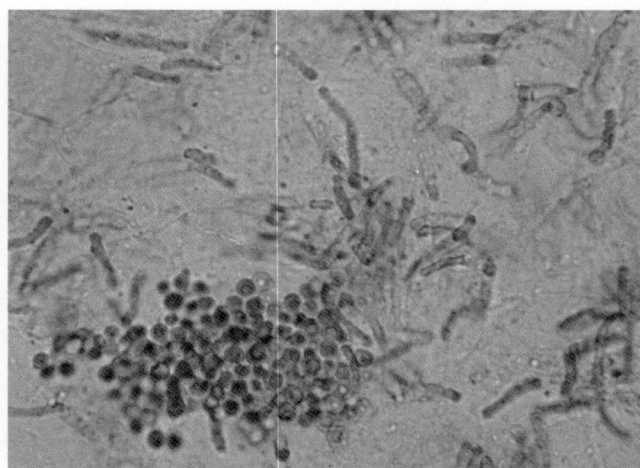

FIGURE 191.6. "Spaghetti and meatballs" appearance of *Malassezia furfur* on potassium hydroxide exam. (See the color insert.)

dermatitis, but prime areas of involvement (e.g., extensor surfaces) are quite different from those of fungal dermatitis.

Potassium Hydroxide Testing

When dermatophyte infection is suspected, microscopic examination of scrapings from an involved area of skin is helpful. To prepare a specimen for microscopic examination, the border of the lesion is scraped lightly with a no. 15 scalpel blade or the edge of a microscope slide. The scale is collected onto a clean microscope slide, and a coverslip is used to push all the scale into a small mound. Several drops of 20% potassium hydroxide solution are placed in the center of the mound of scale, and a coverslip is laid over it. The slide must be heated lightly to improve "clearing" of the epithelial cells.

Under a magnification of 40× with reduced light and a narrow aperture, threadlike hyphae can be seen crossing cell walls (Fig. 191.5). The presence of branched, septate hyphae can be confirmed by using higher power (100×) to make sure that artifacts are not being mistaken for hyphae. If budding spores and pseudohyphae are found, the diagnosis is candidal infection. Short hyphae and spores suggest pityriasis versicolor (Fig. 191.6). The wet mount should be examined within a few hours. The hyphae will dissolve after a period of time. Occasionally, a scraping must be planted on Sabouraud's dextrose agar for culturing to identify the fungal infection.

If candidal infection is identified or topical fungal infection is recurrent or extensive, one should check for conditions associated with immune compromise (e.g., HIV infection, diabetes, cirrhosis, lymphoma, steroid use, chemotherapy).

PRINCIPLES OF MANAGEMENT (1,3–16)

Effective management requires attention to predisposing factors and the proper use of antifungal agents. For example, systemically, diabetes control should be tightened and the use of immunosuppressive agents cut back. Locally, the *elimination of moisture* and the *prevention of maceration* are priorities (see later discussion and Chapter 188). Further drying of inflamma-

tory or weeping lesions can be achieved with the application of compresses containing an astringent such as aluminum acetate, available as *Burow's* tablets or packets.

Treatment should include the reduction of predisposing factors, drying of lesions, and addition of specific antifungal medication. A host of effective agents is available. One should identify and use the least expensive, most effective agent that produces the fewest side effects. Patients with fungal infections have invariably tried over-the-counter remedies before they visit the physician or other member of the primary care team. It is important to find out what they have used before prescribing the same product in its prescription version.

Antifungal Agents

Topical Agents

Four classes of topical antifungal agents are available (azoles, ethanolamines, allylamines, and polyene antibiotics). The over-the-counter preparations are the least expensive (although not necessarily inexpensive). New topical antifungal agents appear regularly and are usually the most costly (e.g., sertaconazole). Claims of unique efficacy are made for each one, but most within a given class provide similar cure rates. Most topical agents provide a cure rate of better than 85% for acute infections, but the rate is much lower for chronic infections. Topical lotions are more drying, less messy, and more useful for daytime application; a cream should be used at night.

Azoles. Azoles make up the largest class of topical antifungal agents; the older ones (*miconazole, clotrimazole*) are available without prescription. Others include *econazole* (Spectazole), *oxiconazole* (Oxistat), *sulconazole* (Exelderm), *ketoconazole* (Nizoral), and *sertaconazole* (Ertaczo). In general, these are slightly less effective than the allylamines for the treatment of tinea pedis, but the nonprescription preparations are considerably less expensive and they have better anticandidal activity than the allylamines. Econazole also has weak antibacterial effects.

Ethanolamines. This class of agents currently consists only of *ciclopirox olamine* (Loprox). As a nail lacquer (Penlac), the agent penetrates the nail plate, making it useful as an adjunct topical treatment of onychomycosis. Topical and shampoo vehicles are also available.

Allylamines. The allylamines exhibit both fungicidal and fungistatic activity, providing slightly better cure rates but at substantially higher cost. Anticandidal activity is lower. Examples include *naftifine* (Naftin) and *terbinafine* (Lamisil); *butenafine* (Mentax) has a structure similar to that of the allylamines.

Polyene Antibiotics. The topical antifungals *amphotericin* and *nystatin* represent this class, which is used for superficial candidal infection.

Combination Therapy. If marked improvement of clinical lesions and symptoms is not seen within 3 weeks, it may help to try combination therapy, with an antifungal agent from one class used during the day and another from a different class applied at night.

Oral Agents

Orally administered systemic therapy may deserve consideration if a patient's condition appears to be refractory to topical therapy and discomfort from the superficial fungal infection is sufficiently severe to outweigh the risks of treatment. Patients with onychomycosis often seek help due to refractoriness to topical therapy. The risks and benefits must be weighed carefully because adverse effects can be serious. Prime candidates include immunocompromised hosts (e.g., those with HIV infection or lymphoma undergoing chemotherapy). However, many of the systemic antifungal agents are potentially toxic to bone marrow and liver and must be used with care, especially if prolonged courses of therapy are needed or the patient has underlying liver disease. Rapid clearing of dermatophyte infection is likely to follow, but relapses are common, and recurrent courses of therapy may be necessary. An awareness of the risks associated with the commonly used oral therapies helps to inform clinical decision making.

Terbinafine (Lamisil). Terbinafine (Lamisil), a widely promoted allylamine approved for oral use in onychomycosis, causes fewer drug–drug interactions than a competing drug, itraconazole, but rare instances of serious skin reactions (e.g., Stevens-Johnson syndrome), symptomatic hepatobiliary dysfunction, severe but reversible neutropenia, and ocular lens and retinal changes have been reported. Clearance of the drug is hepatic and reduced by the concurrent use of cimetidine or terfenadine. Common side effects include gastrointestinal upset (16% of patients), headache (13%), rash (6%), liver enzyme abnormalities (3%), and taste disturbances (3%). Liver enzymes should be measured before treatment is begun and again after 6 weeks if a longer treatment course is contemplated; complete blood cell count should also be monitored.

Itraconazole (Sporanox). Itraconazole (Sporanox), an orally active azole sometimes prescribed in severe onychomycosis, commonly causes nausea and abdominal discomfort; hepatitis has been reported. Important drug–drug interactions derive from its inhibition of hepatic microsomal cytochrome systems (cytochrome P450 3A4), which can substantially increase serum concentrations of many hepatically metabolized drugs (e.g., digoxin, terfenadine, astemizole, triazolam, sulfonylureas, cisapride, felodipine, and quinidine).

Fatal cardiac arrhythmias (torsades de pointes) have occurred in patients taking terfenadine or cisapride concurrently; prolonged severe hypoglycemia may ensue in patients taking sulfonylureas. High doses can cause hypokalemia and hypertension; thrombocytopenia and leukopenia have been reported.

Griseofulvin. Use of griseofulvin, the original oral antifungal for onychomycosis, is problematic due to a long list of potential risks associated with its use. Headache, nausea, and abdominal discomfort are commonly reported. Monitoring of complete blood cell counts and liver function are required because of a tendency to cause leukopenia and hepatocellular injury; bone marrow suppression and serious hepatocellular toxicity are uncommon but serious complications. Caution is warranted in patients with lupus erythematosus because of the risk of triggering an exacerbation; the drug is contraindicated in patients with acute intermittent porphyria due to increase the frequency of attacks.

Ketoconazole (Nizoral). Immunocompromised patients with superficial fungal infection too widespread to be managed with topical therapy are candidates for systemic ketoconazole. For best results, ketoconazole should be taken with an acidic fruit juice or cola to enhance absorption. Side effects include itching, rash, and dizziness. Serum testosterone is reduced, which may lead to gynecomastia in men and menstrual irregularities in women. Mild hepatocellular injury is common; severe impairment is rare. The risk for fatal idiosyncratic hepatotoxicity is nil when ketoconazole is taken for less than 2 weeks, but the drug should be stopped immediately whenever symptomatic hepatocellular dysfunction appears.

Fluconazole (Diflucan). Fluconazole (Diflucan) is well tolerated and useful for candidal infections, but it can be teratogenic, and in rare instances is associated with hepatic necrosis, Stevens–Johnson syndrome, and anaphylaxis. Gastrointestinal upset and rash are common. A few drug–drug interactions have been noted, including potentiation of phenytoin, anti-HIV agents (zidovudine, indinavir), warfarin, and sulfonylureas.

Other Antifungal Agents. *Posaconazole.* (Noxafil) is an oral liquid approved for oropharyngeal candidiasis resistant to itraconazole and/or fluconazole and for prophylaxis and treatment of invasive *Aspergillus* and *Candida* infections in severely immunocompromised patients. *Voriconazole* (VFEND), a derivative of fluconazole and administered by intravenous or oral routes, is used for the treatment of systemic fungal infections, including resistant systemic candidiasis, aspergillosis, and other rare fungal infections such as *Fusarium*. These agents are rarely used for superficial skin infections.

Treatment of Specific Conditions

Tinea Versicolor

For effectiveness, convenience, and least expense, a 2.5% suspension of *selenium sulfide* (Selsun) or a *pyrithione zinc shampoo* (Zincon, Head & Shoulders) can be applied with a rough washcloth, allowed to remain on the affected areas for 10 to 20 minutes, and then rinsed off. Daily application for 1 week is recommended. An 87% success rate at the end of 4 weeks was found with use of this program. Topical antifungal agents are much more expensive but are useful in treating recalcitrant involvement of small areas. *Ketoconazole cream* or *shampoo* is quite effective for treating tinea versicolor.

After treatment, patients should be reexamined for continued scaling, which suggests persistent activity. Patients with no signs of persistence or relapse should be advised that depigmentation will slowly diminish.

For immunocompromised patients and patients with infection too widespread to be managed with topical therapy, *systemic ketoconazole* is worth consideration. A dose of 200 mg is prescribed daily for 7 to 10 days. For best results, ketoconazole should be taken with an acidic fruit juice or cola soft drink. An alternative method is to take 400 mg once with an acidic drink and then, after several hours, exercise to induce sweating. The patient is advised not to shower until the next day. This regimen is repeated 1 week later and can also be repeated monthly to prevent recurrence. It should be followed by topical ketoconazole shampoo lathered in the scalp and affected areas three times per week for 6 months to prevent recurrence.

Other Diffuse Forms of Tinea

In moist intertriginous areas, the patient should dry oozing lesions by applying compresses soaked in *Burow's solution* for 30 to 60 minutes one to three times daily. A nonmedicated or antifungal *powder* (such as *Zeasorb* or *Zeasorb AF*) may be used to absorb moisture. Topical treatment suffices when glabrous skin is involved, but systemic drugs should be considered if hair sheaths are involved, involvement is widespread, or folliculitis develops.

Tinea Pedis

Athlete's foot is sometimes difficult to treat. The patient must be instructed to wear nonocclusive footwear or sandals and absorbent cotton socks and to dry the feet frequently without rubbing, perhaps by using a hair dryer on low heat. *Topical antifungals* alone often suffice. The allylamines are more effective than the azoles. The allylamine *terbinafine* (*Lamisil*) cream is available over the counter. *Naftifine* cream used once daily is effective for tinea pedis and may yield better results than clotrimazole used twice daily. If a component of mild bacterial infection is suspected, econazole twice daily may be helpful. If widespread scaling with hyperkeratosis occurs ("moccasin-type" tinea pedis), *keratolytic agents* are required. The nightly application of Keralyt gel (6% salicylic acid) under occlusion, with antifungal creams used two to three times daily, may successfully treat this difficult problem. Urea 20% to 40% lotion (*Carmol 20* or *Carmol 40*) is another alternative keratolytic.

Onychomycosis and Treatment with Topical Measures

Nail involvement by fungus, especially of the toenails, is extremely refractory to topical treatment and likely to recur, although fingernail infections usually respond better than do toenail infections. Most topical agents cannot penetrate the nail plate, and cure rates are less than 10%. *Ciclopirox* (Loprox) appears to be the most effective of the topical agents; it can be applied at night under occlusion. The best-penetrating formulation of ciclopirox is as a *nail lacquer* (Penlac), which demonstrates complete cure rates of about 10% over 48 weeks of use. It is costly and recurrences are common, but it is safer than systemic therapy and worth consideration in patients where safety profile is critical. Because toenails are slow to grow, months of treatment may be necessary before improvement is noted. Keeping toenails well trimmed can also help with control. To prevent spread to uninvolved nails, nail clippers should be soaked in alcohol after use and separate ones used for involved nails and uninvolved ones.

Systemic Therapy. Often, topical therapy is insufficient, and the question of employing systemic antifungal therapy comes up. Patients with severe nail involvement that has proven refractory to topical therapy, foot pain secondary to nail deformity, diabetes, or immunodeficiency disorders that increase the risk of secondary bacterial infection are reasonable candidates for oral antifungal therapy. The value of the cosmetic benefit alone must be weighed against the cost and risks of prolonged systemic treatment. Even with successful therapy, relapse is common. Some oral preparations are heavily promoted by direct advertising to patients to generate demand. Drug–drug interactions and hepatic and renal toxicities can be significant.

Terbinafine (Lamisil) As noted, terbinafine is heavily promoted for the treatment of onychomycosis. Mycologic and clinical cure rates average about 75% at 1 year. In blinded comparison studies, results have been superior to those for itraconazole at 1 year. However, relapse rates are still in the range of 15%. This drug is taken once daily (250 mg) for 6 weeks for fingernail infections and for 12 weeks for toenail infections. Compared to itraconazole, terbinafine causes fewer drug–drug interactions, but the risk of hematologic and hepatic adverse effects are slightly greater. The risk of clinically evident hepatobiliary dysfunction is 1 in 45,000. Liver enzymes should be monitored, as should the complete blood count. Drugs affecting the clearance of terbinafine include caffeine, cimetidine, terfenadine, theophylline, and rifampin. Drug–drug interactions have been reported with beta-blockers, selective serotonin reuptake inhibitor antidepressants, tricyclic antidepressants, and monoamine oxidase inhibitors.

Itraconazole (Sporanox). Itraconazole is a broad-spectrum antifungal. Clinical cure rates of up to 90% have been reported under study conditions. More commonly achieved mycologic and clinical cure rates with a 3-month course of therapy are approximately 50% and 75%, respectively. Pulsed dosing (1 week/mo) appears to be more effective and safer than continuous therapy, which is believed due to the drug being deposited in the nail and remaining there for up to 9 months, whereas it disappears from the serum within 7 days. In pulsed dosing, a dose of 200 mg of itraconazole is given twice daily for 1 week each month, with two pulses given for fingernail infections and three or four for toenail disease. Due to the slow rate of growth of toenails, patients must be told that continued clearing is to be expected during the next several months.

The major concern with the use of the drug is its inhibition of cytochrome P450 3A4 enzyme activity, which slows the metabolism of hepatically processed drugs, increasing their potency and prolonging their duration of action. Particular caution, drug-level monitoring, and dose adjustment are required in patients taking Dilantin, digoxin, or cyclosporine. Concurrent use is not recommended in persons taking some statin preparations, hepatically metabolized benzodiazepines, terfenadine, or astemizole. Other adverse effects include liver enzyme elevations in 0.3% to 0.5% of patients and symptomatic hepatitis in 1 in 500,000 patients. The monitoring of liver function tests is recommended. Headache, gastrointestinal upset, rash, and urticaria have been noted. Cost is relatively high, especially for prolonged therapy.

Other Agents. Griseofulvin and *ketoconazole* have been replaced by less toxic, more effective oral antifungal agents for onychomycosis. Ketoconazole was formerly used to treat patients with severe disease who did not respond to griseofulvin or who could not tolerate it, but because the risk for hepatotoxicity is greatly increased during prolonged treatment, some authorities no longer recommend that it be used for this condition, especially now that less toxic alternatives are available (see earlier discussion). Baseline liver function should be documented with testing and laboratory studies repeated at least monthly. Fluconazole is an effective systemic antifungal agent; however, it is not approved for use in onychomycosis.

Design of Program. The cosmetic effects of fungal nail infection and the enhanced efficacy of available systemic agents should be weighed against the considerable expense of such therapy, its potentially serious side effects, and the need for careful monitoring and frequent blood testing. Many patients will choose to live with their fungal nail infection, especially when it is limited to the toenails. Many women find that they can substantially reduce cosmetic unsightliness by filing down the hyperkeratotic nail and covering it with nail polish. Persons with socially or physically disabling consequences of their infection or risk of serious foot infection deserve consideration of systemic therapy.

Candidal Infections

Treatment begins with attention to predisposing factors, such as the use of systemic corticosteroids, birth control pills, tetracycline, and other antibiotics and the presence of diabetes, Cushing's syndrome, and HIV infection. One proceeds to meticulous drying of the area, adequate exposure to air, and specific anticandidal therapy. Gentian violet or Castellani's paint are time-proven but quite messy remedies and have largely been abandoned. The polyene *nystatin* or the imidazole creams or lotions (e.g., *clotrimazole* cream) should be used two or three times daily, but ointments should be avoided because they maintain a moist local environment. In highly inflamed infections, initiating therapy with the combination of a topical corticosteroid cream and a light application of clotrimazole is useful. *Fluconazole* (Diflucan) is an effective oral anticandidal agent for extensive or refractory infection.

Paronychial Infection

Chronic paronychia has traditionally been associated with candidal infection, although a causal relationship has not been shown. Topical steroid therapy is more effective than antifungal therapy, and mycologic cure is not associated with clinical cure. Therefore, therapy should always consist in avoiding exposure to water and using rubber gloves with a cotton lining whenever contact with water is unavoidable. This avoidance should be accompanied by twice-daily application of a midpotency steroid such as triamcinolone 0.1% cream. An antifungal agent can be added in cases in which infection is clearly an exacerbating factor.

Angular Cheilitis (Perlèche)

Angular cheilitis (Perlèche) requires combined treatment, including correction of the primary oral abnormality to prevent leakage of saliva through the corners of the mouth and treatment of a possible secondary infection. The combination of *nystatin* and *triamcinolone acetonide* as an ointment formulation is the most effective topical agent. It should be used sparingly three times daily. Occlusive petrolatum ointment should be applied sparingly immediately before bedtime. Dental procedures should be directed at restoring the seal at the angles of the mouth. For persistent cases, the depth of the grooves of the angles may be reduced with dermal fillers. *Fluconazole* may be of value in treating persistent episodes.

INDICATIONS FOR REFERRAL

Referral to the dermatologist should be considered if a fungal infection proves refractory to conventional topical treatment and prolonged or repeated systemic therapy is being contemplated. Consultation for consideration of the risks and benefits can be quite worthwhile, as can a second look at the problem because some rare skin conditions mimic superficial fungal infections. Short courses of systemic therapy (2 weeks) entail little risk and often do not require dermatologic referral.

PATIENT EDUCATION

At the time of the first incident, patients with fungal infection should be instructed about appropriate measures to prevent recurrence.

Maintaining Dryness

Instructing the patient about how to keep the skin dry and prevent maceration is critical to both successful treatment and prophylaxis. Dryness is particularly important in tinea pedis, tinea cruris, and candidal infections. Preventive measures should be taken in areas that have shown a tendency to become infected. In addition, the patient should be told to apply powder liberally to naturally moist areas of the body and to wear cotton clothing and loose-fitting underwear. In addition, patients with tinea pedis should always wear socks and avoid sneakers and rubber-soled shoes, and the physician should encourage exposure of the feet to the air as often as possible. Finally, people who sweat profusely should change their clothing more frequently, shower, and apply nonmedicated talcum powder.

Other Advice

Fungal infections may be slow to clear. To ensure compliance, it is essential to instruct the patient carefully about the appropriate application and duration of treatment. Patients should be told to call at the first sign of recurrence and to institute appropriate drying measures and specific therapy after physician consultation.

THERAPEUTIC RECOMMENDATIONS

- Prescribe a topical preparation approved for once-a-day or twice-a-day use. This is cost-effective and is also likely to improve patient compliance. Continue treatment for 2 weeks after clinical clearance.
- Avoid prescribing creams for intertriginous areas because patients may apply the medication too heavily and thereby increase maceration. Prescribe a lotion or solution instead.
- If clearing is incomplete after 2 to 3 weeks, the short-term use of a systemic antifungal should be considered.
- For patients with onychomycosis, the expense and potential for serious adverse effects of systemic agents should be carefully weighed against the cosmetic consequences of living with the untreated condition.

Annotated Bibliography

1. Borelli D, Jacobs PH, Nall L. Tinea versicolor: epidemiologic, clinical and therapeutic aspects. J Am Acad Dermatol 1991;25:300. (*An in-depth discussion of tinea versicolor, with emphasis on treatment considerations.*)
2. Morishita N, Sei Y. Microreview of pityriasis versicolor and *Malassezia* species. Mycopathologia 2006;162:373. (*The cause of pityriasis versicolor is Malassezia globosa.*)
3. Abraham AG, Kulp-Shorten CL, Callen JP. Remember to consider dermatophyte infection when dealing with recalcitrant dermatoses. South Med J 1998;91:359. (*Cutaneous fungal infections can be mistaken for other dermatoses; an examination with potassium hydroxide can confirm the diagnosis.*)
4. Brodell RT, Elewski B. Superficial fungal infections. Errors to avoid in diagnosis and treatment. Postgrad Med 1997;101:279. (*Discusses common errors in diagnosis and treatment in the form of short vignettes.*)
5. Kovacs SO, Hruza LL. Superficial fungal infections. Getting rid of lesions that don't want to go away. Postgrad Med 1995;98:61. (*Emphasizes differential diagnosis and treatment options.*)
6. Brautigam M. Terbinafine versus itraconazole: a controlled clinical comparison in onychomycosis of the toenails. J Am Acad Dermatol 1998;38:S53. (*At 52 weeks, the mycologic cure rate was 81% with terbinafine and 63% for itraconazole.*)
7. Darkes MJ, Scott LJ, Goa KL. Terbinafine: a review of its use in onychomycosis in adults. Am J Clin Dermatol 2003;4:39. (*Terbinafine was most effective in onychomycosis in adults.*)
8. Gupta AK, Joseph WS. Ciclopirox 8% nail lacquer in the treatment of onychomycosis of the toenails in the United States. J Am Podiatr Med Assoc 2000;90:495. (*A randomized, controlled trial, finding that complete cure rates were approximately 10%.*)
9. Gupta AK, Shear NH. A risk–benefit assessment of the newer oral antifungal agents used to treat onychomycosis. Drug Safety 2000;22:1. (*A detailed presentation of the risk and benefit data and a thoughtful discussion regarding the use of these heavily promoted drugs.*)
10. Gupta AK, De Docker P, Scher RK, et al. Itraconazole for the treatment of onychomycosis. Int J Dermatol 1998;37:303. (*Both continuous and pulse regimens were safe, with few adverse effects; pulse therapy was more cost-effective.*)
11. Gupta AK, Einarson TR, Summerbell RC, et al. An overview of topical antifungal therapy in dermatomycoses. A North American perspective. Drugs 1998;55:645. (*A comprehensive review of topical therapy; 447 references.*)
12. Hart R, Bell-Syer EM, Crawford F, et al. Systematic review of topical treatments for fungal infections of the skin and nails of the feet. BMJ 1999;319:79. (*A formal, systematic review.*)
13. Hay RJ, Logan RA, Moore MK, et al. A comparative study of terbinafine versus griseofulvin in "dry-type" dermatophyte infections. J Am Acad Dermatol 1991;24:243. (*After 12 weeks of therapy, 100% of the terbinafine-treated group were clear, compared with only 45% of the group treated with griseofulvin.*)
14. Macura AB. Fungal resistance to antimycotic drugs: a growing problem. Int J Dermatol 1991;30:181. (*Some antifungal agents are only fungistatic at lower concentrations; at high concentrations, they are fungicidal.*)
15. Sanchez JL, Torres VM. Double-blind efficacy study of selenium sulfide in tinea versicolor. J Am Acad Dermatol 1984;11:235. (*Daily 10-minute application of 2.5% selenium sulfide for 1 week proved to be an effective, convenient treatment, with an 87% success rate at the end of 4 weeks.*)
16. Tosti A, Piraccini BM, Ghetti E, et al. Topical steroids versus systemic antifungals in the treatment of chronic paronychia: an open, randomized double-blind and double dummy study. J Am Acad Dermatol 2002;47:73. (*Finds that steroids were more effective than antifungals, and suggests that Candida was a cofactor but not the causative agent in paronychia.*)

CHAPTER 192 ■ MANAGEMENT OF CUTANEOUS AND GENITAL HERPES SIMPLEX

Herpes simplex virus is a ubiquitous virus that clinically affects humans. *Herpes simplex virus type 1* (HSV-1) is the prototypical infectious agent in cutaneous disease of the upper body; *herpes simplex virus type 2* (HSV-2) generally infects the genitals and the lower body, but the two types share 50% of their genetic material and may be interchangeable clinically. They differ slightly in their sensitivity to antiviral drugs and in their proclivity to cause specific disease in other organs. Serologic studies indicate a 22% prevalence for HSV-2 infection among adults in the United States. The prevalence of HSV-2 is declining, but that of genital HSV-1 is increasing.

Many patients seek confirmation of a suspected herpes infection or treatment of frequent and recurrent rashes and symptoms. The primary care physician must know how to obtain a prompt diagnosis, use the current approaches to prevention and treatment, and address the patient's concerns and negative social stigmata that often accompany genital infection.

PATHOPHYSIOLOGY AND CLINICAL PRESENTATION (1–7)

The severity and duration of symptoms are a function of the patient's state of immunity to HSV. In primary infection, pre-existing antibody protection is lacking, and symptoms tend to be more severe and longer lasting than at other stages of the illness. With time, the frequency and severity of recurrences tend to decline, especially with HSV-1 infection. Some cross-type antibody protection is also afforded, so that when a person with a prior history of HSV infection of one type contracts HSV infection of another type (i.e., first episode of nonprimary herpes), the resulting clinical presentation may be less severe than that of primary disease. In many instances, seroconversion precedes symptomatic infection by many months. Because of their inability to mount effective antibody responses, immunocompromised patients are at great risk for severe, sustained outbreaks (see Chapter 13). As noted, the prevalence of HSV-2 infection is declining as the prevalence of genital HSV-1 infection is increasing, probably due to changes in sexual behavior, such as more careful partner selection, more condom use, and/or choosing oral sex over vaginal sex.

Initial Presentation. Primary Infection

Primary infection is usually the most dramatic form of HSV disease, but the spectrum of presentations is wide, ranging from asymptomatic disease to a florid outbreak with systemic symptoms. In almost half of cases, seroconversion occurs silently, with initial symptoms not developing for many months. The characteristic lesions are *erythematous papules*, which evolve during 2 to 3 days to *vesicles* with clear fluid and then progress to *pustules*, which erode and leave superficial, tender *ulcerations*, especially in moist areas. Healing occurs within 2 to 6 weeks. *Systemic symptoms* develop in one third of men and two thirds of women; fever, malaise, nausea, headache, and myalgias are all reported. *Meningeal irritation*, manifested by headache, stiff neck, and photophobia, can occur. *Regional lymphadenopathy* is characteristic of primary infection; the nodes are enlarged, firm, and tender.

Primary HSV-1 Infection

Primary HSV-1 infection usually goes unnoticed but may present as severe *exudative pharyngitis* or *gingivostomatitis*, with high fevers and tender lymphadenopathy. The illness often is mistaken for streptococcal disease, other bacterial infections of the oropharynx, or mononucleosis. Systemic manifestations of the illness may be more prominent than local symptoms. HSV-1 infection may also present as painful *genital lesions*, a consequence of oral–genital sexual activity and an unappreciated risk factor for neonatal herpes. The old clinical dictum that HSV-1 infection does not cause genital disease is belied by the finding of equal numbers of oropharyngeal and genital presentations for persons with initial symptomatic HSV-1 infection.

Primary HSV-2 Infection

Primary HSV-2 infection also may be missed or misdiagnosed. In its most overt form, an exudative, painful, bilateral *vulvovaginitis* is seen in female patients and painful *penile ulceration* with tender inguinal nodes in male patients. The genital lesions are painful in 95% of men and 99% of women. *Cervicitis* develops in nearly three fourths of women with primary infection, manifested by vaginal discharge and intermenstrual spotting. Local symptoms increase during the first 6 to 7 days of illness and peak between days 8 and 10, gradually decreasing during the next week. Lymph nodes are enlarged, firm, and tender. Although suppurative lymphadenopathy does not occur, superimposed bacterial infections can produce this finding. Atypical presentations occur in about 15% of symptomatic persons and include urethritis, cystitis, and meningitis.

Primary genital infection usually takes place in adolescence, but it may be contracted at the time of birth. Fever and malaise occur in 67% of patients, dysuria (resulting from urethral involvement or urinary irritation of ulcers) in 63%, and tender adenopathy in 80%. In 20%, extragenital lesions appear on the hands or in the oropharynx. Complications include secondary *yeast infection* in 11%, *aseptic meningitis* in 8%, and *sacral autonomic neuropathy* leading to bladder or bowel dysfunction in 2%. *Cervical cancer* is strongly associated with HSV-2 antibodies or the presence of HSV-2, although no study or series has directly found HSV genetic material within these cancer cells. The association of HSV infection with cervical cancer may be epidemiologic rather than etiologic. Infection with HSV-2 may increase the risk of HIV infection and its transmission. Increased genital shedding and transmission of HIV-1 have been documented in persons with HSV-2 infection.

Uncommon Presentations

An unusual form of primary infection results from the implantation of virus into broken skin; this produces a *herpetic whitlow* characterized by pain, swelling, and erythema of the fingers, with pronounced adenopathy. In wrestlers, *herpes gladiatorum*, a primary herpes infection, may develop on exposed parts of the body that are inoculated during the rough activity of wrestling.

First Episode of Nonprimary Disease

In most cases, a first episode of nonprimary disease represents new infection with HSV-2 in persons with clinical and serologic evidence of HSV-1 exposure earlier in life. Patients with a past history of fever blisters or cold sores note a new onset of painful lesions of the genital skin or mucous membranes. Women are more likely to be symptomatic than man. The severity and duration of symptoms are characteristically intermediate between those of primary infection and recurrent disease—lesions are fewer in number, and healing takes place within 1 to 3 weeks. Cervicitis, urethritis, adenopathy, and systemic symptoms are minimal, if present at all.

Clinical Course and Complications

Latent Disease

After primary infection, latent disease develops in all patients, with the virus residing in the associated dorsal root ganglion and circulating along the endoneural sheath to the skin if host defenses break down. Emotional or physical stress, sunburn, and skin trauma are among the reported precipitants of recurrences. The result is a localized, self-limited form of illness with fewer lesions, which resolve more quickly than in primary infection.

Recurrent Disease

Recurrences may be symptomatic or asymptomatic.

Symptomatic. Symptomatic recurrences begin with a prodrome of tingling or discomfort in the skin, and sometimes mild systemic symptoms are present, although they are not as severe as in primary disease. Infections can recur in different distributions along the same ganglia, and heterogeneity characterizes the illness. Genital disease may recur in a nongenital area (e.g., legs or buttocks) in about 10% of cases. If both genital and nongenital lesions are present at the time of primary infection, the chance of a nongenital recurrence is close to 50%.

Although pain without rash develops in some symptomatic patients, most patients experience the characteristic *maculopapular–vesicular* eruption. The lesions become turbid as interferon is produced in the vesicles and as lymphocytes stimulated by interleukin-2, interleukin-6, and other cytokines begin controlling the infection.

Asymptomatic. Most recurrences of genital herpes are overlooked by both patient and physician because symptoms are inapparent, atypical, or truly absent. It is in this stage that viral shedding is most likely to result in transmission to sexual partners.

Viral Shedding

Viral shedding occurs during both active disease and latency. The risk for transmission is greatest in the first 96 hours after the appearance of the rash. Even without evidence of disease, silent shedding occurs in 2% to 5% of patients, particularly those with recurrent genital disease. During the initial 3 to 4 days of recurrent infection, patients can inoculate themselves in other areas (hands, eyes, periorbital areas), but secondary infections are usually brief, mild, and self-limited, and disease is not established in new regions. Eventually, reepithelialization of the skin occurs, usually without scarring. Recurrent disease sometimes takes the form of *erythema multiforme* without evidence of vesicles.

Complications

Complications of local recurrent infections are few but can be clinically important. *Secondary bacterial infections* (caused by streptococci or staphylococci) can lead to cellulitis and lymphangitis and must be anticipated. Sacral disease is associated with a risk for *hemorrhagic cystitis, dyspareunia,* and *sacral radiculopathy* (which leads to difficulty in voiding, fecal soilage, or both). It may also cause recurrent *aseptic meningitis.* Perirectal disease can cause *proctitis.* Disseminated disease is rare, even in immunocompromised patients, but lesions of autoinoculation may occur on the fingers or about the eyes. In atopic persons, HSV can produce a devastating generalized *eczema herpeticum.* Chronic pain syndromes associated with infection but without lesions are being identified more frequently. *Postherpetic neuralgia* caused by HSV-1 is described as a recurrent syndrome without clinical evidence of skin lesions. Vulvar burning alone may be an expression of HSV-2 infection. *Elsberg's syndrome* with radiculomyelopathy and acute urinary retention may also be secondary to clinically inapparent disease. HSV has been associated with an acute *retinal necrosis* syndrome presenting as eye pain and visual loss.

Neonatal Herpes

Neonatal HSV is most often the consequence of direct contact between the infant and HSV (both type 1 and type 2) during passage through the birth canal of an asymptomatic mother with active genital infection. The risk is estimated at 10% in women with recurrent or primary infection at 32 weeks and is several times higher if infection is present at term in the absence of antibody production. Congenital HSV infection frequently leads to death or severe neurodevelopmental problems. Acquisition of HSV infection early in pregnancy followed by a normal antibody response does not appear to compromise the outcome of pregnancy, but infection in the last trimester may not leave enough time for type-specific antibodies to form, so that the infant is at risk.

DIFFERENTIAL DIAGNOSIS

The differential diagnosis of genital ulceration in conjunction with inguinal lymphadenopathy includes *syphilis* and *chancroid* (see Chapter 141). Ulcerations may also be associated with noninfectious conditions, such as *Behçet's syndrome* and *inflammatory bowel disease,* or they may simply represent excoriation and secondary bacterial infection caused by vigorous sexual activity. *Syphilis* serology should always be obtained in the setting of a genital ulcer, even one that is painful. Approximately 50% of ulcerative lesions in the genital area prove to be herpetic.

WORKUP (8–11)

History

In most instances, the diagnosis is a clinical one, based on finding the characteristic lesions. However, atypical disease is common, particularly in the genital area, so that quick diagnosis is difficult. A detailed sexual history is essential (see Chapter 229) and must include inquiry about oral–genital sexual activity because HSV-1 can also be a source of genital infection. Any history of genital redness, spotting, fissures, pain, and paresthesias, even in the absence of skin lesions, should raise suspicion of genital herpes. Any prior history of fever blisters or cold sores should also be noted because it indicates prior HSV infection and helps to identify patients with a first episode of nonprimary disease.

Physical Examination

Besides helping to identify early vesicular lesions as herpetic ("dew drop on a rose petal"), the physical examination is especially important for differentiating HSV infection from other causes of genital ulcer. Unlike the very tender ulcer of HSV infection, the ulcer (chancre) of primary syphilis is indurated and painless or only minimally uncomfortable. As in genital herpes, the base is clean, and tender, firm, nonfluctuant inguinal adenopathy may be present. These findings contrast with those of chancroid, which is characterized by very tender, soft, purulent ulcerations in conjunction with sore, fluctuant lymph nodes and erythema of the overlying skin.

Laboratory Studies

Tzanck Prep and Viral Culture

Unroofing a vesicle and performing a *Tzanck test* to check for presence of multinucleate giant cells (see Chapter 193) can be very helpful in making the diagnosis clinically, but this is less specific than *viral culture,* which is also the most sensitive of the commonly available tests. The results (including typing) can be available within 2 to 3 days, which makes it of practical value. The best time to culture is within 48 hours after the onset of symptoms; the highest-yielding lesions are intact vesicles, pustules, and early moist ulcers.

Serologic Testing

Detecting *HSV antibodies* can confirm prior infection, but the information is less useful in the evaluation of an ongoing episode because titers often do not rise sufficiently, and cross-reactivity between HSV-1 and HSV-2 occurs. *Western blot* assay promises to provide sensitive and specific type-specific antibody testing, but it is not yet widely available. Most commercial laboratories are unable to provide reliable type-specific antibody testing. Serology also has the disadvantage of not producing data while the patient is clinically affected, and patients, once exposed, carry titers forever, whether or not their infection becomes reactivated. Antibody testing can be used to identify persons at increased risk for primary infection (i.e., pregnant women with no antibody titers).

DNA Probes and Monoclonal Antibody

DNA probes are under development to provide a more sensitive, specific, and rapid approach to viral detection and typing. The use of *polymerase chain reaction* assays to detect the presence of specific DNA or RNA sequences offers the most sensitive and specific means for diagnosing active disease; cost is a consideration, but once these tests become widely available commercially, their cost should decrease, and they are likely to become the test of choice. Promising monoclonal and oligoclonal detection methods are also under development. HSV-antigen detection by direct fluorescent antibody testing is of limited sensitivity, and false-negative rates are high when it is used in populations with a low prevalence of HSV infection. Typing is not achieved. Only when it is used in settings of high HSV prevalence does the predictive value of a positive test result rise sufficiently to warrant its use.

Papanicolaou Smear

Genital herpes is a major cause of type II and type III abnormalities on Papanicolaou smear and should be routinely considered if these changes are seen. It is important to differentiate this benign inflammatory abnormality from real metaplastic or anaplastic disease (see Chapter 107).

Screening for HIV Infection

Because of the increased risk of HIV infection in the setting of genital herpes simplex infection, all genital HSV patients should be screened for HIV infection (see Chapter 7).

PRINCIPLES OF THERAPY (12–22)

Goals and Strategy

Because HSV infection is incurable and characterized by self-limited symptomatic recurrences and asymptomatic recurrences in which virus is shed, the goals of therapy center on reducing the duration of symptoms, the frequency and severity of recurrences, and the risk for transmission. Because treatment is either symptomatic or prophylactic, decisions regarding the use of antiviral therapy are customized to the physical and psychosocial needs of the patient.

The treatment of *symptomatic recurrences* is most effective when it is initiated at the first sign of a relapse (during the prodromal phase); half of outbreaks can be prevented with an early start to antiviral therapy. The initiation of therapy after skin lesions have appeared is less effective, shortening the course of illness by little more than 1 day.

Suppressive therapy can be offered to persons bothered by frequent recurrences and to those who want to decrease asymptomatic viral shedding and the risk for transmission, especially to an antibody-negative partner. The risk of transmission can be reduced by 50% with a daily prophylactic dose of a nucleoside analogue.

Nucleoside Analogues

The nucleoside analogues (acyclovir, valacyclovir, and famciclovir) are the principal antiviral agents available for use against HSV. They are effective for the symptomatic treatment of primary and recurrent disease and can prevent recurrences and the shedding of virus; however, they do not cure HSV infection. The emergence of resistant strains is very rare when antiviral therapy is used in immunocompetent persons, but it has been observed in those who are immunocompromised and take these agents for prolonged periods.

Acyclovir

Acyclovir, the first of the nucleoside analogues, acts as a purine analogue substrate for viral thymidine kinase, which is uniquely activated in cells that are infected with HSV. Acyclovir is effective against both types of HSV, although HSV-1 is more sensitive. Oral acyclovir shortens viral shedding time and reduces the time to healing and crusting of lesions. The earlier the treatment is instituted, the better. The continuous use of acyclovir in patients with frequent recurrences reduces the number and severity of repeated episodes. Unfortunately, once the drug is discontinued, its effect on recurrence ceases. Long-term use is associated with slow adaptation of the virus to the drug, but clinically important resistance has not been reported. Cessation of use results in reversion to original sensitivity. One can readily treat for 12 months at a time without adverse consequences. Side effects include *nausea, headache,* and *vomiting.* Elimination is renal, and downward dose adjustment is required in the setting of azotemia. The half-life is less than 4 hours, so that frequent dosing is necessary.

The use of acyclovir for genital herpes in *pregnancy* appears to decrease dramatically the chance of fetal transmission in the last trimester, but safety remains to be established. Often, a cesarean section is advocated in these cases. Intravenous (IV) acyclovir is indicated in *immunocompromised hosts* and in persons with disseminated disease, such as meningoencephalitis. IV acyclovir produces higher, more-consistent blood levels than does oral acyclovir, which is only 15% absorbed. The oral vehicle is acceptable for mucocutaneous manifestations in immunocompetent hosts.

Topical acyclovir is of little use, although it has some limited efficacy in primary infection. Topical acyclovir is also of little use in keratoconjunctivitis, a dangerous illness; trifluorothymidine ointment plus oral or IV acyclovir should be used.

Famciclovir

Famciclovir was developed to improve the absorption and effective half-life of acyclovir so that higher serum levels could be obtained with less frequent dosing. Famciclovir is a nucleoside prodrug that is stable and well absorbed in the gastrointestinal tract and converted in the small bowel and liver to penciclovir, the active agent. The drug is effective in treating and suppressing recurrent infection and has also been used successfully for treating primary genital infection. No head-to-head studies have compared this agent with acyclovir. Adverse effects include nausea, dizziness, and headache. Drug–drug interactions are possible because the conversion of famciclovir requires hepatic oxidative metabolism. Elimination is by renal tubular excretion, so that dose reduction is necessary in the setting of renal insufficiency and the concurrent use of such drugs as probenecid. No interactions with cimetidine have been observed.

Valacyclovir

Valacyclovir, a prodrug of acyclovir, is rapidly absorbed and converted to acyclovir in its first pass through the intestines and liver. Higher serum levels of acyclovir are attained than with the oral administration of acyclovir. A regimen of 250 mg of valacyclovir four times daily provides the same serum levels as 800 mg of acyclovir five times daily. Efficacy is similar to or better than that of acyclovir and famciclovir. A potentially important finding is its ability to reduce viral shedding and transmission of HIV-1 in persons with concurrent HSV-2 and HIV-1 genital infections.

Side effects include nausea, vomiting, diarrhea, and headache. Interactions with cimetidine and probenecid are possible. The efficacy and safety of valacyclovir have not been established in immunocompromised patients and those with disseminated disease; thrombotic thrombocytopenic purpura and hemolytic/uremic syndrome have been reported in association with valacyclovir treatment in patients with advanced AIDS.

Adjuncts

Good local skin care and the use of drying agents to speed the transition from active vesicle to crusting are the essence of adjunctive therapy. Topical surfactants such as ether and chloroform seem to provide some additional relief. Some have advocated, with little evidence, the use of cimetidine because of research evidence suggesting that histamine$_2$-blockers have antiherpes activity. Vidarabine, ribavirin, bromodeoxyuridine, and ganciclovir sodium have shown some promise of antiviral activity. Care of skin lesions is especially important in the immunocompromised or eczematous host, in whom dissemination and autoinoculation can lead to serious consequences.

Some clinicians use *topical corticosteroids* to abort the progression of herpetic lesions. This empiric approach often works, although scientific evidence is lacking, and there is a theoretical concern about spread. However, no evidence has been published to document this danger.

Over-the-counter preparations such as Blistex, Campho-Phenique, and Anbesol may provide minimal symptomatic relief but do not affect the course of the eruption. Considering the long history of ineffective therapy, physicians should remain skeptical about new remedies offered.

Prevention

Condom use remains an important means of prevention. When used more than 25% of the time during sexual activity, condoms reduce the risk of transmission of infection from seropositive men to seronegative women by greater than 90%. However, no similarly protective benefit has been documented for seronegative men having sex with seropositive women, presumably because of frequent unprotected penile contact with vulvar and perianal areas (where much shedding occurs in infected women) and the likelihood of limiting condom use to times when lesions are present in the sexual partner. *Limiting sexual activity* to periods when there are no genital lesions can help to reduce risk but does not eliminate it due to the persistence of viral shedding. *Prophylactic antiviral therapy* can reduce the number and severity of outbreaks and the risk of transmission, usually without increasing the risk of a resistant strain; benefit persists only as long as medication is taken.

PATIENT EDUCATION (18)

Genital Herpes

Reassurance of the frightened patient with genital herpes (and partner) is critical. The primary care physician can help to reduce the shame and suspicion that often accompany confirmation of the diagnosis. Herpes has acquired an unjustifiably vicious reputation in the media, not only as a risk factor for neonatal tragedy, but also as a sign of sexual infidelity. Patients need to understand that genital herpes could have been acquired months to decades ago and that asymptomatic shedding of virus is the most likely mode of transmission.

Guilt can be assuaged by providing approaches to the prevention of transmission (e.g., safe sexual practices, suppressive therapy, condom use). Women of childbearing age appreciate knowing how neonatal herpes can be avoided and what they and their obstetrician can do to contribute to a safe delivery.

In educating patients about transmissibility, it is important to inform them about what constitutes a high-risk situation (e.g., unprotected sexual intercourse; oral–genital sexual activity between an infected patient and an antibody-negative partner, especially one who is pregnant). The concept of asymptomatic shedding must be appreciated by the patient. Transmission to an uninfected female partner is markedly reduced with *condom use* but is still possible. Patients with HSV-1 infection need to know that it too can be the source of genital disease, and not just HSV-2. If the presence of antibody in a sexual partner is confirmed, anxiety surrounding sexual relations can be reduced. Use of *prophylactic antiviral therapy* to limit outbreaks can also be comforting.

Pamphlets about the disease are available through the Centers for Disease Control and Prevention, the National Institutes of Health, and the American Social Health Association. These sources of information are superior to many of the lay-initiated hotlines, which tend to overplay the emotional problems. It should be emphasized that recurrent infection is far less likely to produce discomfort or pain than primary infection.

Facial Involvement

Facial lesions are always annoying and often embarrassing. Protection from sunburn and trauma should be urged, as should good local care, with the use of drying agents to speed the transition from active vesicle to crusting. Prompt antiviral therapy treatment at the first sign of an outbreak can help to limit its severity and duration. Patients are reassured by knowing that the risk for scarring is very small and that effective oral therapy is available for shortening severe episodes and reducing the risk for recurrence.

INDICATIONS FOR REFERRAL AND ADMISSION

The primary physician should consult with an obstetrician regarding the safety and advisability of antiviral treatment in the third trimester versus cesarean section at the time of delivery to prevent HSV transmission to the fetus. Patients with suspected eye involvement should be referred urgently to an ophthalmologist for eye examination and treatment with trifluorothymidine and acyclovir. The immunocompromised person in whom disease appears to be disseminating requires prompt admission for IV therapy.

THERAPEUTIC RECOMMENDATIONS

Primary Infection and Nonprimary Initial Genital Disease

- Begin a 7- to 10-day course of oral acyclovir (200 mg five times daily), valacyclovir (1,000 mg twice daily), or famciclovir (250 mg three times daily). Titrate the dose according to the response to treatment. Continue therapy until the lesions have healed. Reduce the dose for patients with renal failure. Provide a supply for use during recurrences, which are likely to develop several times in the first year after the initial infection.

Recurrent Disease

- Treat bothersome symptomatic recurrences for 5 days with acyclovir (200 mg five times daily or 400 mg three times daily), famciclovir (125 mg twice daily), or valacyclovir (500 mg twice daily). Begin treatment at the first sign of illness, preferably during the prodromal phase before skin lesions emerge.
- Consider long-term suppressive therapy for patients who have more than six to eight recurrences per year, want to minimize the risk for asymptomatic viral transmission, or are immunocompromised. Prescribe acyclovir (400 mg twice daily), famciclovir (250 mg twice daily), or valacyclovir (500 to 1,000 mg daily). Titrate the prophylactic dose to the low-

est level possible without reactivation, and continue for up to 12 months at a time.
- After 12 months, halt suppressive therapy, and reassess the need for continuation.

Prevention of Spread to Uninfected Partner

- Recommend the use of condoms, abstinence during symptomatic outbreaks, and daily chronic use of nucleoside analogue antiviral therapy (e.g., acyclovir 400 mg twice daily or valacyclovir 500 mg daily).

Additional Measures for All Patients

- Educate patients about the transmissibility of genital herpes, including the risk for genital infection associated with oral–genital sexual activity and with asymptomatic viral shedding; recommend the use of condoms when one partner is antibody-negative.
- Help the patient to keep the problem in perspective, and address common misconceptions regarding the meaning of the infection.
- Watch for secondary bacterial infection and disseminated HSV disease. In patients who are immunosuppressed, dissemination may present as gangrenous ulcers or deep-seated eschars.
- Follow genital infections closely during pregnancy; consider monitoring antibody status in the latter part of pregnancy to determine susceptibility to primary infection and the need for extra precautions or the use of suppressive therapy in an infected male partner.

A.H.G.

Annotated Bibliography

1. Benedetti JK, Zeh J, Selke S, et al. Frequency and reactivation of nongenital lesions among patients with genital herpes simplex virus. Am J Med 1995;98:237. (*About 10% of patients had nongenital lesions initially; a similar percentage had recurrences at a nongenital site.*)
2. Bierman SM. Recurrent genital herpes simplex infection. A trivial disorder. Arch Dermatol 1985;121:173. (*A good normative statement placing this illness in perspective.*)
3. Brown ZA, Selke S, Zeh J, et al. The acquisition of herpes simplex virus during pregnancy. N Engl J Med 1997;337:509. (*The neonates of antibody-negative patients who became infected in the later stages of pregnancy were at greatest risk for herpes.*)
4. Langenberg AG, Corey RL, Ashley RL et al. A prospective study of new infections with herpes simplex virus type 1 and type 2. N Engl J Med 1999;341:1432. (*A large prospective cohort study, finding that there is much overlap between types and that infection often precedes clinical presentation by many months.*)
5. Gonzales GR. Post–herpes simplex type 1 neuralgia simulating post-herpetic neuralgia. J Pain Symptom Manage 1992;7:320. (*Gives evidence that herpes simplex virus [HSV] neuralgia presents much like the postherpetic neuralgia associated with herpes zoster.*)
6. Maccato ML, Kaufman RH. Herpes genitalis. Dermatol Clin 1992;10:415. (*A review of genital HSV infection, with attention to silent shedding.*)
7. Xu F, Sternberg MR, Kottiri BJ, et al. Trends in herpes simplex virus type 1 and type 2 seroprevalence in the United States. JAMA 2006;296:964. (*A major epidemiologic study, finding that HSV-2 prevalence declining, but that there is an increase in genital HSV-1.*)
8. Dahm C, Elgas M, Kuhn JE, et al. The diagnostic significance of the polymerase chain reaction and isoelectric focusing in herpes simplex virus encephalitis. J Med Virol 1992;36:147. (*Discusses the use of polymerase chain reaction for the diagnosis of HSV infection.*)
9. Koutsky LA, Stevens CE, Holmes KK, et al. Underdiagnosis of genital herpes by current clinical and viral-isolation procedures. N Engl

J Med 1992;326:1533. (*Sensitivity is low; reviews new strategies for diagnosis.*)
10. Mckay M. Vulvodynia. Diagnostic patterns. Dermatol Clin 1992;10:423. (*Defines multiple causes, including HSV infection, of vulvar burning.*)
11. Solomon A, Rasmussen JE, Varani J. The Tzanck smear in the diagnosis of cutaneous herpes simplex. JAMA 1984;251:633. (*Viral culture was superior, but the Tzanck preparation is still a useful, cost-effective aid in early diagnosis.*)
12. Corey L, Wald A, Patel R, et al. Once-daily valacyclovir to reduce the risk of transmission of genital herpes. N Engl J Med 2004;350:11. (*A major randomized, placebo-controlled, multicenter trial in couples with one partner having a history of recurrent symptomatic disease, finding that the risk of transmission was reduced by 50%.*)
13. Diaz-Mitoma F, Sibbalk G, Shafran SD, et al. Oral famciclovir for the suppression of recurrent genital herpes: a randomized, controlled trial. JAMA 1998;280:887. (*A large-scale, multicenter European study, finding that the drug was effective and safe for suppression in persons with frequent recurrences.*)
14. Douglas JM, Critchlow C, Benedetti J, et al. A double-blind study of oral acyclovir for suppression of recurrences of genital herpes simplex virus infection. N Engl J Med 1984;310:1551. (*Oral acyclovir given for 4 months markedly reduced but did not eliminate recurrences; the natural history of recurrences was not affected.*)
15. Luby ED, Klinge V. Genital herpes: a pervasive psychosocial disorder. Arch Dermatol 1985;121:494. (*An article emphasizing the adverse effect of herpes on intimate sexual relationships.*)
16. Mertz GJ, Critchlow CW, Benedetti J, et al. Double-blind placebo-controlled trial of oral acyclovir in first-episode genital herpes simplex virus infection. JAMA 1984;252:1147. (*One of the original controlled trials of efficacy, finding that a course of acyclovir treatment shortened the duration of viral shedding, symptoms, and lesions but did not reduce subsequent recurrences.*)

17. Nagot N, Owudraogo A, Foulongne V, et al. Reduction of HIV-1 RNA levels with therapy to suppress herpes simplex virus. N Engl J Med 2007;356:790. (*A randomized, controlled trial, finding that the suppression of HSV-2 with valacyclovir led to a reduction in HIV shedding and transmission.*)

18. Spruance SL, Tyring SK, De Gregorio B, et al. A large-scale, placebo-controlled, dose-ranging trial of peroral valacyclovir for episodic treatment of recurrent herpes genitalis. Arch Intern Med 1996;156:1729. (*Treatment in the prodromal phase was most effective and prevented outbreaks in nearly half of cases.*)

19. Wald A, Zeh J, Barnum G, et al. Suppression of subclinical shedding of herpes simplex virus type 2 with acyclovir. Ann Intern Med 1996;12:8. (*A reduction of 90% in subclinical viral shedding was achieved with a standard suppressive dose of acyclovir.*)

20. Mertz GJ, Critchlow CW, Benedetti J, et al. Double-blind placebo-controlled trial of oral acyclovir in first-episode genital herpes simplex virus infection. JAMA 1984;252:1147. (*One of the original controlled trials of efficacy, finding that treatment shortened the duration of viral shedding, symptoms, and lesions but did not reduce subsequent recurrences.*)

21. Spruance SL, Tyring SK, De Gregorio B, et al. A large-scale, placebo-controlled, dose-ranging trial of peroral valacyclovir for episodic treatment of recurrent herpes genitalis. Arch Intern Med 1996;156:1729. (*Treatment in the prodromal phase was most effective and prevented outbreaks in nearly half of cases.*)

22. Wald A, Langenberg AGM, Link K, et al. Effect of condoms on reducing the transmission of herpes simplex virus type 2 from men to women. JAMA 2001;285:3100. (*This approach was found to be effective, especially in protecting seronegative women; it was much less protective in seronegative men.*)

CHAPTER 193 ■ MANAGEMENT OF HERPES ZOSTER

Herpes zoster (shingles) is a common viral cutaneous eruption that is estimated to affect 300,000 persons a year in the United States. Most cases represent reactivation of the varicella-zoster virus (VZV). The incidence increases with age and degree of host immunosuppression. A community-based study found 100 cases per 100,000 person-years between the ages of 15 to 35 years, with a rise each decade to 450 cases per 100,000 by age 75 years. The seasonal variation seen with varicella does not occur with zoster; shingles is rarely an epidemic illness. Shingles may present as a pain syndrome without vesicles and pose a diagnostic problem. The primary physician must recognize zoster, make the patient comfortable, and prevent complications.

PATHOPHYSIOLOGY AND CLINICAL PRESENTATION (1–6)

Pathophysiology and Epidemiology

Varicella, or chickenpox, usually affects people early in life; the virus then lies dormant in a nerve ganglion in a genomic state until reactivation occurs. It is suspected that every person who has had chickenpox harbors latent virus. Estimates are that 50% of all people who live to the age of 85 years will have an attack of zoster, and that approximately 10% will have at least two attacks.

The nerve root changes consist in necrosis and sometimes cyst formation. A decrease in *cellular immunity* may allow the latent virus to reactivate and spread along the nerve; clinical zoster is the result. Helper T cells and several lymphokines produced by other T cell subsets usually protect the host from reactivation. The disorder occurs with increased frequency among immunocompromised patients and the elderly, probably as a consequence of defects in cellular immunity. Humoral immunity does not appear to be an important factor; even severely infected patients show significantly elevated antibody titers to zoster, and fewer than 5% of persons born in the United States do not possess varicella antibody. Occasional outbreaks may result from trauma to a nerve in which the virus is latent.

The *risk for transmission* is low despite the fact that zoster skin lesions contain large amounts of virus. However, immunosuppressed patients and those who have never had chickenpox are at risk for transmission from persons with zoster. Although a tenuous suggestion has been made that persons with zoster are at somewhat higher than average risk for some cancers (e.g., colon cancer) due perhaps to reduced cellular immunity, the observed relative cancer risk of latent cancer is only 1.1 times that of the general population.

Clinical Presentation

The presentation is one of radicular *pain* followed by the appearance of tense, grouped *vesicles* on an erythematous base ("dew drops on a rose petal") in a *dermatomal distribution*. The pain is also dermatomal and may begin as an itch or tenderness that precedes the cutaneous lesion by 1 to 7 days. Patients describe sensations of burning, tingling, and sharp, knifelike pricking or of deep, boring discomfort. More than half of patients have a unilateral involvement of one or more thoracic dermatomes. The cranial dermatomes accounts for approximately 15% of cases, and cervical and lumbar dermatomes each accounts for approximately 10%.

The cutaneous eruption becomes pustular within a few days; crusting and healing then follow during 14 to 21 days. The crust is often dark, almost black. Scarring and atrophy can occur if the lesions are deep. Malaise, low-grade fever, and adenopathy accompany severe eruptions. The total length of the course is related to the duration of new vesicle development; vesicle formation for several days usually predicts a 2- to 4-week course, whereas vesicle formation persisting for more than 1 week predicts a longer course.

Complications

About one in eight patients experiences at least one complication; risk is higher in the elderly (approaching 50%) and in those who are immunocompromised. Major complications include *postherpetic neuralgia, keratitis, uveitis, motor deficits, infection,* and systemic involvement, such as *meningoencephalitis, pneumonia, deafness,* and *dissemination.*

Postherpetic Neuralgia. Postherpetic neuralgia is most prevalent in persons older than the age of 50 years. The pain is often excruciating and can be refractory (see later discussion). The incidence exceeds 40% in zoster patients older than the age of 60 years; the risk is also high in those with HIV infection or other immunocompromised states.

Ocular Complications. Persons with involvement of the first division of the trigeminal nerve have a nearly 50% risk of developing eye complications such as *keratitis, keratopathy, epislceritis,* and *iritis.* Vesicles on the tip of the nose were believed to indicate definite nasociliary involvement (putting the eye at risk), but recent data do not confirm this traditional view.

Disseminated Disease. The presence of more than 10 lesions outside a single dermatome of distribution is early evidence of dissemination. Patients with HIV/AIDS may have VZV infection as part of the AIDS-related complex. In most HIV cases, VZV infection presents as a typical dermatomal illness; occasionally, it is disseminated and can be complicated by hepatitis, pneumonia, meningitis, or proctitis. In immunocompromised hosts, VZV and herpes simplex infections may present in similar and atypical fashion, sometimes in unusual distributions or even without vesicles.

DIAGNOSIS (1,7–9)

The diagnosis is generally not difficult if the characteristic dermatomal rash and pain are present. The most serious diagnostic problem occurs during the prodromal phase, when patients present with a pain syndrome. Periorbital headache, unexplained back pain, or chest wall pain may represent the prodromal period of herpes zoster. Prodromal zoster pain has been mistaken for myocardial infarction, cholecystitis, and appendicitis. The characteristic eruption may not appear until 2 to 5 days later.

In patients with the characteristic rash, a *Tzanck preparation* demonstrating the presence of *multinucleated giant cells* provides strong supportive evidence of zoster. The Tzanck preparation has been found to be superior to viral isolation in the diagnosis of early lesions. In persons with atypical presentations (e.g., immunocompromised patients), confirmation may be required. Culture, although slow, allows for confirmation, but the VZV virus can be hard to recover from the swab. More sensitive, rapid, and less expensive than culturing is subjecting the sample obtained from a swab to immunofluorescence staining, which uses fluorescein-conjugated monoclonal antibodies against VZV. Finally, the diagnosis can be confirmed by the demonstration of a *rising antibody titer,* but this requires two separate determinations separated in time.

Rapid molecular diagnostic assays that detect DNA sequences of VZV by *polymerase chain reaction assay* are available for severely ill persons who present with acute but nonspecific symptoms (e.g., meningeal infection). Their high cost makes them best reserved for prompt diagnosis in inpatient settings.

PRINCIPLES OF THERAPY (1–3,10–20)

The goals of therapy are to dry the vesicles and relieve pain and prevent secondary infection and complications.

Drying Vesicles, Keeping Skin Clean, and Relieving Discomfort

Lesions can be kept clean by gently washing with plain soap and water. Covering the lesions with a sterile, nonadherent dressing can prevent irritation from contact with clothing. Drying can be facilitated by the application of a wet-to-dry compress soaked with *Burow's solution* and applied three to four times a day. If purulence or erythema suggestive of secondary infection develops, antibiotics are indicated. No data are available to support the use of prophylactic antibiotics.

Pain relief can usually be achieved with a mild analgesic such as *aspirin* or *acetaminophen,* but one should not hesitate to use *codeine* if need be. Antiviral therapy (see later discussion) often reduces pain within 72 hours and frequently alleviates the need for stronger pain relief measures. The pain of thoracic zoster can be reduced by splinting the affected area with a *tight wrap.* Trunk lesions are covered with a nonadherent dressing, and then the area is wrapped with an elastic bandage. Malaise reflects viremia and should be treated with rest. Severe local pain can be relieved with *intralesional steroid* injections (e.g., *triamcinolone,* 2 mg/mL in lidocaine). There is little evidence to suggest that pain can be relieved or the rate of healing hastened by the use of *systemic corticosteroids*; however, such treatment may reduce the incidence of postherpetic neuralgia (see later discussion).

Pruritus may be relieved by oral *antihistamines* (see Chapter 178) or by *calamine lotion,* which both reduces itching and dries the rash. *Topical capsaicin* has been tried, but with only minimal success. *Peripheral nerve block* is an invasive approach to reducing acute pain that does not respond to antiviral therapy; *sympathetic blockade* has also been tried in this setting with a modicum of success.

Shortening Clinical Course and Reducing Risk for Postherpetic Neuralgia

Antiviral therapy with *a nucleoside analogue* can markedly shorten the clinical course, reduce pain, and possibly reduce the risk of postherpetic neuralgia. The addition of systemic *glucocorticosteroid* therapy (e.g., prednisone) helps to alleviate pain and speeds the healing of lesions.

Antiviral Therapy

The antiviral agents approved for use in the United States are *acyclovir, famciclovir,* and *valacyclovir.* The "cyclovirs" are nucleoside analogues with activity against both VZV and herpes simplex virus (HSV). VZV is more resistant to these agents than is HSV, necessitating higher dose regimens for treatment. To be maximally effective, antiviral therapy must begin as early as possible and preferably no later than 72 hours after the onset of rash. Treatment started after 72 hours of onset may still of be of benefit in some patients (particularly those who show continued development of new vesicles), but the earlier the onset of nucleoside therapy, the better is the response. Those who benefit most from early initiation of antiviral therapy and are the best candidates for treatment are persons who present early with severe pain, have a large area of involvement, are older than 50 years, or have potential for ophthalmic involvement. Response, manifested by a reduction in pain and the cessation of new lesions, typically occurs within 72 hours. These agents produce a marked speeding of healing and significant reductions in the severity and duration of pain. The risk and duration of postherpetic neuralgia are also reduced.

Choice of Antiviral Agent. Acyclovir was the original agent in this class. Although it is effective, its suboptimal pharmacokinetics necessitates frequent dosing and up to 10 days of treatment at high doses (e.g., 800 mg five times daily for 7 to 10 days). The newer cyclovirs (famciclovir and valacyclovir) were developed to provide better pharmacokinetics, allowing more convenient dosing and shorter courses of treatment (e.g., famciclovir 500 to 750 mg thrice daily for 7 days; valacyclovir 1 g thrice daily for 7 days). These agents also produce fewer central nervous system side effects in the elderly (see Chapter 192) and demonstrate equal or better efficacy than acyclovir, often at lower cost. They are comparable in efficacy and preferred over acyclovir. Because the drugs are renally excreted, their doses should be reduced in persons with renal insufficiency. For immunocompetent patients, valacyclovir is the probably the more cost-effective because it is often lower in price, but in immunocompromised patients, its use is a bit more problematic due to case reports of thrombotic thrombocytopenic purpura and hemolytic/uremic syndrome. The duration of antiviral therapy needs to be extended in HIV-infected persons, with treatment continued until all lesions have cleared. These agents should not be used in pregnant women. There is no benefit from the use of topical antiviral drug preparations.

Glucocorticosteroids

Systemic steroids are prescribed in conjunction with antiviral therapy, particularly in patients older than 50 years. Data regarding efficacy are limited, but recent randomized trials suggested that a short course of high-dose therapy started early in conjunction with antiviral therapy could further speed the healing of lesions and lessen the duration and intensity of pain. The hoped-for reduction in the risk of postherpetic neuralgia remains to be proven. Steroids should not be used alone in lieu of antiviral therapy.

Steroid therapy is started at the same time as antiviral treatment. The best-studied regimen is a 3-week program of *prednisone*, in which a dose of 60 mg is given daily for the first week; the dose is then tapered to 30 mg/d during week 2 and to 15 mg/d during week 3. To minimize adverse effects, prednisone is taken in the morning with food (see Chapter 105).

Pain Medication

Around-the-clock opiates may be required, starting with short-acting agents and proceeding to sustained-release preparations if pain persists (see Chapter 236). Aside from providing comfort, the use of agents that block the central processing of pain (e.g., opioids, tricyclic antidepressants, gabapentin) has been suggested as a means of ameliorating the risk of postherpetic neuralgia. The suggestion is based on the hypothesis that postherpetic neuralgia may represent a dysfunctional central response to the initial peripheral nerve injury. Studies are underway to test this approach.

Vaccination: Zoster Vaccine

Because the incidence of shingles and the risk of postherpetic neuralgia increase with advancing age (due to a decline in cell-mediated immunity), vaccination has emerged as a key strategy for reducing the morbidity associated with the herpes zoster reactivation. The varicella-zoster vaccine stimulates T cell subsets and cytotoxic killer T cells in the elderly and significantly reduces the risk of reactivation and postherpetic neuralgia.

Efficacy and Cost-Effectiveness. In randomized, placebo-controlled trial of immunocompetent persons older than the age of 60 years, the live-attenuated zoster vaccine reduced the incidence of herpes zoster by 51% and postherpetic neuralgia by 66.5%. This vaccine is 14 times more potent than the varicella vaccine given to children to prevent chickenpox. Cost-effectiveness analysis suggests a cost per quality-adjusted life-year ranging from $14,000 to nearly $100,000, based on assumptions of efficacy, duration of effect, and vaccine cost.

Recommendations. The Centers for Disease Control and Prevention recommendation is to administer one dose of the live-attenuated zoster vaccine to immunocompetent persons older than the age of 60 years, irrespective of whether they have had a prior episode of zoster. The best candidates are those younger than the age of 70 years; advancing age blunts the immune response and vaccine efficacy.

Unresolved Issues. A number of unresolved issues remain, including cost-effectiveness, the duration of protection, use in persons aged 50 to 59 years, efficacy and safety of use in mildly immunocompromised persons (e.g., diabetes, those using low-dose steroids or tumor necrosis factor blockers), use in previously immunocompetent persons with new onset of HIV infection or about to undergo major immunosuppressive therapy, and need in persons with a previous episode of herpes zoster.

Treatment of Postherpetic Neuralgia

Postherpetic neuralgia can be one of the most severe of chronic pain syndromes. The best treatment is prevention (see prior discussion). For persons who develop the condition, *tricyclic antidepressants* remain the first line of treatment (e.g., *amitriptyline* at a starting dose of 25 mg daily at bedtime); they provide significant benefit to about 50% of patients. The *anticonvulsants gabapentin, pregabalin,* and *carbamazepine* are approved by the U.S. Food and Drug Administration for treatment of the condition; dizziness and somnolence are common side effects (see Chapters 167 and 236). *Narcotics* are not well studied for long-term use in postherpetic neuralgia, but they are often added if a first-line drug is found to be insufficient. Combination therapy has not been well studied but may prove useful if the agents used work by different pathways. Topical therapies are less effective; *capsaicin* is among the best, but its efficacy is modest, and a burning sensation may ensue with prolonged use. Similarly, a *topical lidocaine patch* can help to alleviate pain, but it may be irritating and should only be applied on healed skin.

INDICATIONS FOR REFERRAL

If any suggestion of *visual compromise* or other ocular involvement is present, prompt ophthalmologic consultation for herpetic eye care is essential to avoid scarring and permanent visual impairment. *Otic* involvement can lead to severe pain and otic nerve damage, so that referral to an ear, nose, and throat specialist is important. The patient with *herpetic skin lesions* and signs of *meningeal irritation* requires prompt hospitalization.

A.H.G.

Annotated Bibliography

1. Gilden DH, Kleinschmidt-DeMasters BK, LaGuardia JJ, et al. Neurologic complications of the reactivation of varicella-zoster virus. N Engl J Med 2000;342:635. (*The best review; 100 references.*)
2. Gnann JW Jr, Whitely RJ. Herpes zoster. N Engl J Med 2002;347:340. (*A succinct clinical review; 53 references.*)
3. Kost RG, Straus DB, Coombs FP. Post-herpetic neuralgia: pathogenesis, treatment and prevention. N Engl J Med 1996;335:32. (*One of the best reviews.*)
4. Liesegang TJ. The varicella-zoster virus: systemic and ocular features. J Am Acad Dermatol 1984;11:165. (*A superb review, with emphasis on ophthalmic disease.*)
5. Ragozzino MW, Melton LJ, Kurland LT, et al. Risk of cancer after herpes zoster. N Engl J Med 1982;307:393. (*No increased risk was found.*)
6. Yawn BP, Addier P, Wollan PC, et al. A population-based study of the incidence and complication rates of herpes zoster before zoster vaccine introduction. Mayo Clin Proc 2007;82:1341. (*A community-based study, finding that 68% of cases occurred in persons older than the age of 50 years; postherpetic neuralgia occurred in 18% of persons older than the age of 50 years and in 33% of those older than 79 years.*)
7. Dahl H, Marcoccia J, Linde A. Antigen detection: the method of choice in comparison with virus isolation and serology for laboratory diagnosis of herpes zoster in human immunodeficiency virus–infected patients. J Clin Microbiol 1997;35:345. (*A useful comparison study.*)
8. Oxman MN, Levin MJ, Johnson GR, et al., for the Shingles Prevention Study Group. A vaccine to prevent herpes zoster and postherpetic neuralgia in older adults. N Engl J Med 2005;352:2271. (*A placebo-controlled, randomized, controlled trial, finding that the vaccine was effective.*)
9. Solomon AR, Rasmussen JE, Weiss JS. A comparison of the Tzanck smear and viral isolation in varicella-herpes zoster. Arch Dermatol 1986;122:282. (*The Tzanck preparation was superior to viral isolation in diagnosing early lesions.*)
10. Watson CP, Tyler KL, Bickers DR, et al. A randomized vehicle-controlled trial of topical capsaicin in the treatment of post-herpetic neuralgia. Clin Ther 1993;15:510. (*A modest reduction in pain was achieved, but a placebo effect is hard to rule out.*)
11. Whitley RJ, Weiss H, Gnann JW Jr, et al. Acyclovir with and without prednisone for the treatment of herpes zoster: a randomized, placebo-controlled trial. Ann Intern Med 1996;125:376. (*A 3-week program of acyclovir plus high-dose prednisone not only sped healing, but also reduced pain and improved quality of life more than either drug given separately.*)
12. Wood MJ, Shukla S, Fiddian AP, et al. Treatment of acute herpes zoster: effect of early (<48 h) versus late (48–72 h) therapy with acyclovir and valacyclovir on prolonged pain. J Infect Dis 1998;178(Suppl 1):S81. (*Benefit was greatest with early treatment, but there was some still benefit even if treatment was started after 3 days.*)
13. Gershon AA, LaRussa P, Hardy I, et al. Varicella vaccine: the American experience. J Infect Dis 1992;166(Suppl 1):S63. (*Discussed the use of varicella vaccines in healthy and immunocompromised hosts.*)
14. Hornberger J, Robertus K. Cost-effectiveness of a vaccine to prevent herpes zoster and postherpetic neuralgia in older adults. Ann Intern Med 2006;145:317. (*A decision-analysis study, finds that vaccination was effective but very expensive and of uncertain cost-effectiveness [>$50,000 per quality-adjusted life-year].*)
15. Jackson JL, Gibbons R, Meyer G, et al. The effect of treating herpes zoster with oral acyclovir in preventing post-herpetic neuralgia. Arch Intern Med 1997;157:909. (*A meta-analysis, finding a 46% reduction in risk for this complication.*)
16. Kimberlin DW, Whitley RJ. Varicella-zoster vaccine for prevention of herpes zoster. N Engl J Med 2007;356:1338. (*A clinical review, recommending the use of the vaccine in healthy persons older than the age of 60 years.*)
17. Levin MJ, Barber D, Goldblatt E, et al. Use of a live attenuated varicella vaccine to boost varicella-specific immune responses in seropositive people 55 years of age and older: duration of booster effect. J Infect Dis 1998;178(Suppl 1):S109. (*Antibody response was obtained.*)
18. Rowbotham M, Harden N, Stacey B, et al. Gabapentin for the treatment of post-herpetic neuralgia. JAMA 1998;280:1837. (*A multicenter, randomized, controlled trial demonstrating a significant reduction in pain and significant improvements in sleep and quality of life.*)
19. Tyring SK, Beutner KR, Tucker BA, et al. Antiviral therapy for herpes zoster: randomized, controlled clinical trial of valacyclovir and famciclovir therapy in immunocompetent patients 50 years and older. Arch Family Med 2000;9:863. (*The two treatments were found to be equally effective.*)
20. Tyring SK, Barbarash RA, Nahlik JE, et al. Famciclovir for the treatment of acute herpes zoster: effects on acute disease and postherpetic neuralgia: a randomized, double-blind, placebo-controlled trial. Ann Intern Med 1995;123:f89. (*The treatment reduced the duration of postherpetic neuralgia by 2 months.*)

CHAPTER 194 ■ MANAGEMENT OF WARTS

PETER C. SCHALOCK AND ARTHUR J. SOBER

Warts result from skin infection with human papillomavirus (HPV). They can be cosmetically bothersome and occasionally a source of pain. Cervical involvement with some strains of the virus can lead to cervical cancer (see Chapter 107). Nongenital warts affect 7% to 10% of the general population and are among more commonly seen dermatologic problems in primary care. The primary care physician should be able to distinguish warts from other skin tumors, select effective treatment, and educate the patient in proper self-care and prevention.

All photos are courtesy of Peter C. Schalock.

PATHOPHYSIOLOGY, CLINICAL PRESENTATION, AND COURSE (1,2)

Pathophysiology

Human papillomavirus is a double-stranded DNA virus, with more than 118 types identified. It is epitheliotropic and causes tumors of the epidermis. Multiple types are oncogenic (HPV types 16, 18, 31, 33, 45, and 59), implicated in cervical carcinoma (see Chapter 107) and squamous cell carcinoma (see Chapter 177). HPV types 6 and 11 are implicated in low-risk anogenital warts. Warts can be transmitted by direct contact, autoinoculation, or, rarely, as a fomite. Young people have a high frequency of warts, which occur most commonly between the ages of 12 and 16 years. Healing can occur spontaneously, presumably through immunologic mechanisms. Approximately three fourths of warts disappear spontaneously within 2 years of their appearance, but if they are left untreated, additional warts may develop from the original ones.

Clinical Presentations

Clinical presentations vary according to site and viral strain involved. Morphologically, nongenital warts appear in three forms: the keratotic common wart, the filiform wart, and the flat wart. Most warts are asymptomatic; however, a plantar wart can be the source of considerable pain, acting as a foreign body during weight bearing. Anogenital warts may become friable, bleed, and cause discomfort. Periungual lesions may become fissured and destroy the nail matrix and nail bed.

Common Warts (Verruca Vulgaris)

The common wart (verruca vulgaris), associated with HPV-1, 2, 4, 27, or 57 infection, appears flesh colored or grayish white with a papillate, hyperkeratotic surface. The wart may be punctuated with black dots that represent thrombosed superficial capillaries, which are present in large numbers (Fig. 194.1). The common wart may appear anywhere, but frequently affects the elbows, knees, fingers, and palms. The filiform wart is more delicate and threadlike. The *flat wart* (*verruca plana*), caused by HPV-3 and 10, is smaller than the common wart. Flat warts are tan-to-flesh–colored, slightly raised papules with a relatively smooth surface. Great numbers of them may appear on the hands, in bearded areas, and on the shaved legs of women. Flat warts are easily spread and occasionally present in a linear arrangement.

Plantar Warts (Verruca Plantaris)

The plantar wart (verruca plantaris) results from infection of the plantar surface of the foot with HPV-1 or 4. It appears as a

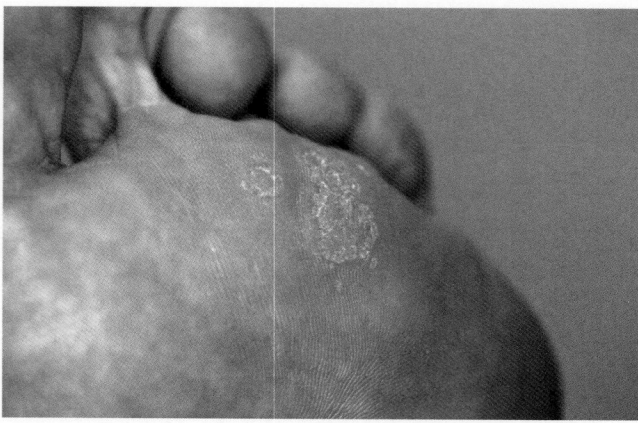

FIGURE 194.2. Plantar verruca. These lesions are often not exophytic. (See the color insert.)

small skin nodule that produces grayish or yellow interruptions in the skin lines (dermatoglyphics) of the foot (Fig. 194.2). It is less elevated than other warts because weight bearing presses it inward. These warts may be solitary, multiple, or confluent; if they are confluent, the term *mosaic wart* is used.

Genital Warts

In the genital area, four clinical morphologic types are seen: the cauliflower variety (*condyloma acuminatum*); smooth, flesh-colored papular lesions (Fig. 194.3); flat warts; and keratotic genital warts, which can mimic seborrheic keratosis. Low-risk *anogenital warts* result from the sexual transmission of HPV- 6 or 11 and grow on mucous membranes. Lesions that are high risk for dysplasia and squamous cell carcinoma are derived from infection with HPV-16, 18, 31, 33, 45, or 59. Anogenital warts range in appearance from pinpoint to cauliflower-like. Elevated, lobulated papular lesions correlate with HPV-6 and 11, whereas the flat, hyperpigmented types are high-risk lesions associated with HPV-16 and 18. Coexistent sexually transmitted diseases are common (see Chapter 141). Mucocutaneous warts may become refractory to treatment (see later discussion).

DIFFERENTIAL DIAGNOSIS

Common warts should be differentiated from *squamous cell carcinoma*, *seborrheic keratosis*, and a *cutaneous horn* arising

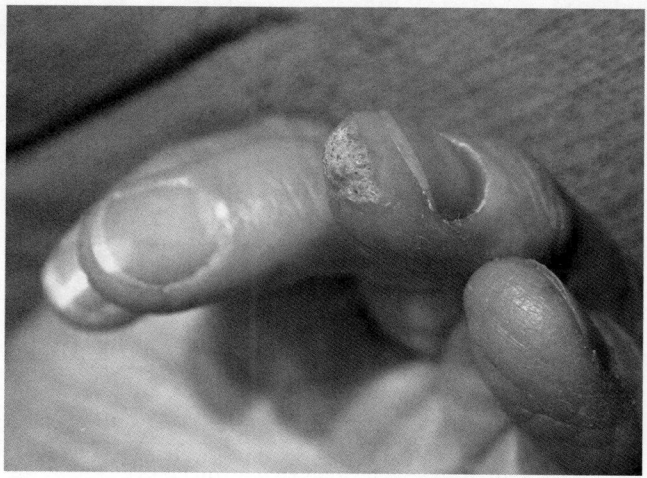

FIGURE 194.1. Common verruca vulgaris on the fingertip. (See the color insert.)

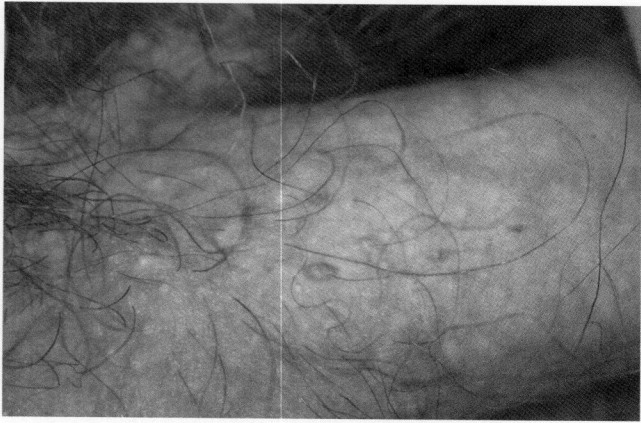

FIGURE 194.3. Condyloma on the penis. (See the color insert.)

from an actinic keratosis (see Chapter 177). The differential diagnosis also includes *Gottron's papules* (seen on the dorsal aspect of the fingers in dermatomyositis), *granuloma annulare*, *lichen planus*, *molluscum contagiosum*, *skin tags*, epidermal nevus, and *lichen nitidus*. Other lesions that patients may mistake for warts include digital *fibrous tumors* and *mucous cysts*. Multiple flat warts on the face should be differentiated from trichoepithelioma, syringoma, and the cutaneous lesions of *sarcoidosis*.

Anogenital warts must be differentiated from the *condyloma latum* of syphilis and from *squamous cell carcinoma*. The differential diagnosis also includes *pearly penile papules*, *ectopic sebaceous glands* (common after circumcision), and *nevi*. *Bowenoid papulosis* (associated with HPV-16) appears as pigmented wartlike lesions on the male and female genitalia and is a form of carcinoma *in situ*, although it has little biologic tendency to behave aggressively.

WORKUP (3–9)

The appearance is usually sufficient to indicate the diagnosis, but early genital warts can be difficult to identify. Typically, a patient comes for evaluation because warts have been found in a sexual partner. In a male patient, the penis and upper portion of the scrotum should be carefully examined. If no visible lesions are present, acetic acid can be used. Soaking the penis for 5 minutes with a gauze moistened with 5% acetic acid (white vinegar) demonstrates early lesions not previously evident. For the gynecologic examination, early warts are best demonstrated when they are made white with acetic acid. The colposcope provides magnification if necessary. However, one must remember that the use of acetic acid is very nonspecific; any disease or lesion that alters the stratum corneum will turn white with acetic acid.

PRINCIPLES OF MANAGEMENT

Not all warts need to be removed. The primary care physician should keep in mind the basic principle that warts are benign tumors that often regress spontaneously. Treatment should not be so aggressive as to produce permanent scarring. Simple and safe treatments should be employed.

Location, discomfort, cosmetic effect, and therapies available influence the decision to treat. Larger, longstanding warts and those involving the plantar, perianal, or periungual area are the most difficult to treat but among those that patients most want to have removed. The patient's occupation, skin pigmentation, and body area involved should be considered when therapy is designed. The goal is to destroy the epidermal tumor while minimizing damage to the underlying dermis. The greater the dermal injury, the greater is the risk for scar formation. Only minimal scarring should be expected or considered acceptable.

Many therapeutic measures are available; choice is based on efficacy, patient acceptability, and scarring potential of the therapy and on location, size, and type of lesion. Physicians will most likely see a self-selected group of patients for whom over-the-counter remedies have failed. It should be noted that the efficacy of few therapies beyond home use of salicylic acid or practitioner-applied liquid nitrogen are supported by well-designed, controlled clinical trials. However, there are many other potentially useful treatment modalities; the practitioner should tailor the treatment to the patient, the lesions, and the prior failed therapies.

Common Warts

Treatment options include liquid nitrogen, curettage with or without electrodessication, chemical cautery, cantharidin, imiquimod, or even duct tape application; liquid nitrogen therapy is the most effective.

Liquid Nitrogen

Freezing the lesion with liquid nitrogen applied on a cotton swab is convenient, well tolerated, often effective, and associated with a low risk for serious scarring. The freezing injury separates the epidermis containing the wart from the underlying dermis. Caution should be exercised in pigmented skin because postfreezing hypopigmentation is common with aggressive cryodestruction. Solid freezing of the lesion is usually achieved by the repeated application of liquid nitrogen with a cotton swab dipped into a Styrofoam cup containing the supercold liquid. An equally effective method that delivers the liquid nitrogen more uniformly is use of a spray canister delivery system with a nozzle. Usually two freeze–thaw cycles suffice with this method, with freeze times between 10 and 20 seconds. For larger lesions, a repeated freeze–thaw cycle may enhance efficacy. Lesions of 1 to 2 mm may be treated by supercooling the tips of serrated forceps and pinching the lesion for 10 seconds; this technique avoids excessive damage to surrounding skin.

The successfully treated wart falls off within 2 weeks. Before freezing, the thickened keratin should be pared off, but care should be taken not to cut into the profuse collection of capillaries within the wart. It is best to freeze a few millimeters of the surrounding normal tissue to facilitate separation from the underlying dermis. The patient should be warned that the area may hurt for several hours after treatment, and occasionally hemorrhagic blistering develops, especially with vigorous treatment.

If not completely cured, the wart can be retreated within 3 weeks. In difficult areas or with large lesions, multiple treatments may be necessary. Treatment with liquid nitrogen has the advantage of being quick, bloodless, and not too painful, but the liquefied gas evaporates quickly and requires storage in special containers. Commercial kits generating sticks of "dry ice" from compressed carbon dioxide gas are available, but because the sticks are not as cold as liquid nitrogen, they are not as effective and require the application of more pressure for a longer time.

Curettage with or without Electrodesiccation

Curettage with or without electrodesiccation is effective but time-consuming, and substantial scarring can result if treatment is too vigorous. Human papillomavirus is in the smoke caused by the electrodesiccation and precautions should be taken if using electrocautery on warts. *Chemical cautery* with *nitric acid* or *monochloroacetic*, *bichloracetic*, or *trichloroacetic acid* is an alternative to liquid nitrogen.

Topical Imiquimod (Aldara)

Imiquimod is an immunomodulator with antiviral and antitumor activity related to its ability to induce production of interferon-α and tumor necrosis factor-α by mononuclear cells and immature keratinocytes. In some cases, topical application of 5% imiquimod cream under occlusion has proved useful for the treatment of recalcitrant warts. For verruca vulgaris, treatment is daily and may take up to 12 weeks for complete cure. The original U.S. Food and Drug Administration approval for imiquimod was for genital warts. Treatment is three times weekly for up to 16 weeks. The major adverse effect is localized erythema. Relapse rates are low.

Other Treatments

Cantharidin, derived from the beetle *Cantharis vesicatoria*, causes blister formation by acting on epidermal mitochondria to cause cell death. The agent is applied for 2 to 4 hours and then washed off; blister formation followed by healing occurs over 1 to 2 weeks. The agent is not available in the United States but is available in Canada.

Application of *duct tape* to warts has shown promise in removing up to 85% of warts. A piece of tape slightly larger than the wart is applied and left in place for 6 days, followed by removal. Any excess keratin that remains is removed with a pumice stone or emery board and the area is left open to the air overnight after removal. One repeats the process for 2 months or until the wart resolves.

Plantar Warts

Nonsurgical methods are preferred to surgical removal because scarring in this location can cause permanent discomfort.

Salicylic Acid

The lesion should be pared and then treated with the application of 40% *salicylic acid plasters* (available over the counter), which can be held in place by strong adhesive tape for 1 to 3 days, after which the macerated skin is scraped off. This procedure is repeated for 2 to 3 weeks by the patient. Other convenient formulations include Mediplast and Dr. Scholl's Corn Remover. Medicated pad formulations containing the suspension are cut to size after the wart is pared down with an emery board. A drop of water is placed on the wart, and the pad is applied and left in place for 8 hours each day. A larger salicylic acid patch (Trans-Plantar) is indicated for treating large plantar warts. Occlusal-HP is a prescription salicylic acid–lactic acid combination that contains salicylic acid in a polyacrylic vehicle. It is quite effective for plantar warts and has also been used successfully for warts on the hands.

Liquid Nitrogen and Topical Imiquimod

Liquid nitrogen can be used on plantar warts as first-line therapy, but care should be used in weight-bearing areas because the patient may experience pain in the area for several days after therapy. There are reports of efficacy with *topical imiquimod* (Aldara; see previous discussion) applied under salicylic acid pads for recalcitrant plantar warts.

Flat Warts

The location and configuration of flat warts necessitate a slightly different approach to management. Men should switch to an electric razor if they are using a blade razor because cutting facial warts spreads them throughout the beard area. Similarly, women with flat warts on their legs must switch to an electric razor or use depilatory creams. *Tretinoin* cream or gel applied nightly has been used effectively for flat warts, especially those on the face. Adverse effects include erythema, scaling, and burning, about which the patient should be forewarned. Alternatively, 6% *salicylic acid gel* (Keralyt) is sometimes effective in treating multiple flat warts on the legs. A short course of topical *imiquimod* may be sufficient to induce regression of flat warts. *Liquid nitrogen* can be used cautiously for flat warts, depending on the location.

Genital Warts

Genital warts are upsetting to the patient and notoriously problematic to treat. Poor efficacy, inconvenience, high recurrence rates, discomfort, and high cost of standard therapies have made treatment difficult. Most therapies must be applied by the physician in the office, but new patient-applied treatments are emerging. Just as important as treatment of the warts is screening for concurrent venereal disease (see Chapters 107, 124, and 125).

Prevention of HPV Infection

HPV is found in 100% of histologic specimens from cervical cancer. A *vaccine* against the most common HPV types causing genital warts and cervical cancer is available (*Gardasil*) and should be helpful in significantly decreasing the incidence of these problems. The vaccine is effective against HPV-6, 11, 16, and 18. The U.S. Centers for Disease Control and Prevention's Advisory Committee on Immunization Practices recommends that girls 11 to 12 years of age be immunized with the quadrivalent vaccine. At the physician's discretion, girls as young as 9 years and women up to 26 years of age may be vaccinated. A second vaccine (Cervarix), which prevents infection with HPV-16 and 18, should soon be available.

Liquid Nitrogen, Heat, and Imiquimod

Liquid nitrogen is the treatment of choice for isolated small lesions of the genitals. *Hot water* has been reported useful in treating stubborn genital warts; the warts are soaked for 15 minutes twice daily in water of 43°C. The cytokine inducer *imiquimod* (see earlier discussion) has proved effective in the treatment of anogenital warts, with cure rates greater than 50% reported and very low relapse rates (10% to 13%). Local irritation occurs, but it can be applied by the patient at home and might be considered in persons in whom first-line therapies fail.

Podophyllin

Podophyllin (20% to 40%) in compound tincture of benzoin is a traditional therapy used to treat macerated genital warts. It must be applied sparingly, only to the wart, and allowed to dry thoroughly before the patient dresses. The medication is washed off by the patient 4 to 6 hours after application. Repeated treatment is the rule. Podophyllin is contraindicated in pregnancy. *Podofilox 0.2%* (Condylox) is a purified fraction of podophyllin resins available in solution and gel preparations, enabling prescription therapy to be self-applied at home. It is applied for 3 days consecutively, followed by 4 days of no treatment. Treatment is repeated if the warts persist. About two thirds of patients achieve cure after up to 8 weeks of treatment. Local reactions are usually mild to moderate and usually do not cause discontinuation of therapy.

Refractory Warts

Refractory disease poses problems for both patient and physician. Available interventions have had mixed results in placebo-controlled studies, and adverse effects can be substantial. Modalities include intra- or sublesional injection with bleomycin or interferon-α and laser therapy.

Sublesional Bleomycin

Sublesional *bleomycin*, diluted to 10 U/mL, has a distinct role in the treatment of refractory warts, both those on the hands and the plantar variety. Usually, 1 or 2 U injected beneath the wart is sufficient. Blanching occurs immediately, followed by blackening of the wart with subsequent clean sloughing. This treatment is quite painful but causes no systemic effects.

Intralesional Interferon-α

Intralesional *interferon-α* (types 2a and 2b) has been approved for the treatment of refractory genital warts. Intralesional injection of 100,000 to 500,000 units per lesion is performed three times a week for 3 weeks. Lesions clear in fewer than 50% of patients, and this treatment has the disadvantages of being painful and expensive. Treatment is occasionally associated with flulike symptoms, which are relieved with acetaminophen.

Laser

The *carbon dioxide laser* can be used for treating warts, although in many instances it is little more than an expensive method of causing tissue destruction. It is best reserved for extensive vaginal or anal warts or refractory periungual lesions. The procedure is carried out in an operating room environment. Postoperative morbidity is much less than when conventional methods are used. Another application of laser therapy is concomitant treatment of vascular-appearing warts with a *pulsed-dye laser* (585 to 595 nm), which may enhance clearance of warts by destroying the enhanced microvasculature. With the use of either laser, precautions should be taken to prevent the spread of wart virus aerosolized in the smoke plume.

PATIENT EDUCATION

Prevention entails avoiding others with warts and having warts removed so that the viral reservoir is reduced. Although warts may initially have been acquired during contact with others, biting and picking at warts may result in the formation of additional lesions. Patients with periungual warts should be cautioned that biting the warts or pulling hangnails may result in the spread of lesions to the mucosa. Patients with genital warts can be reassured that warts do not develop in everyone who is exposed, but condom use should be urged.

Treatment of warts can be both time-consuming and expensive. Recurrences are seen in at least one third of instances. The patient must be made to understand that warts are caused by a virus and that treatment usually does not completely eliminate the virus. Nonetheless, the patient can be reassured that in most instances the immune system will eventually prevent HPV from causing clinical warts despite the continued presence of the virus. The length of treatment, cost, discomfort, risk for scarring, and possible failure of therapy should be candidly discussed before treatment is initiated.

INDICATIONS FOR REFERRAL

A Papanicolaou smear showing cervical dysplasia and evidence of HPV requires referral to a gynecologist for consideration of cervical biopsy. Women with extensive involvement by vaginal warts are also candidates for gynecologic consultation and possible laser therapy. Patients with truly refractory lesions who still insist on their removal may benefit from a dermatologic or surgical consultation. If topical treatment proves ineffective, electrocoagulation or surgical excision deserves consideration. Excision of large venereal warts that do not respond to podophyllin or imiquimod is indicated to rule out malignancy.

THERAPEUTIC RECOMMENDATIONS

- Use *liquid nitrogen* for the initial treatment of common warts. This can be applied with a cotton swab or sprayed cautiously with a spray can dispenser to an area that includes a small rim of surrounding skin.
- Treat plantar warts by first paring them down carefully with a scalpel and then applying a piece of 40% *salicylic acid* plaster cut in the shape of, but slightly smaller than, the wart. Cover with occlusive adhesive tape and leave in place for 24 to 72 hours. Have the patient continue treatment at home, with gentle paring and reapplication of salicylic acid plaster as needed. Check progress regularly. Alternatively, liquid nitrogen can be used as a first-line treatment.
- Treat flat warts with topical *tretinoin* or *Keralyt*, a 6% salicylic acid gel.
- Treat moist anogenital warts with *imiquimod* for common warts or anogenital lesions. Alternatively, topical podophyllin may be used.
- If these topical treatments prove ineffective or if the patient has extensive anal or genital involvement, then refer for consultation and consideration of more aggressive therapy, such as carbon dioxide laser treatment.

Annotated Bibliography

1. Lipke MM. An armamentarium of wart treatments. Clin Med Res 2006;4:273. (*A comprehensive review covering virology, epidemiology, pathogenesis, immunology, clinical manifestations, and treatment; 301 references.*)
2. Munoz N, Bosch FX, de Sanjose S, et al. Epidemiologic classification of human papillomavirus types associated with cervical cancer. N Engl J Med. 2003;348:518. (*The association of multiple subtypes of papillomavirus with cervical neoplasia.*)
3. Beutner KR, Tyring SK, Trofatter KF Jr, et al. Imiquimod, a patient-applied immune-response modifier for treatment of external genital warts. Antimicrob Agents Chemother 1998;42:789. (*Fifty-two percent of warts were cleared, with a recurrence rate of 19%.*)
4. Bourke JF, Berth-Jones J, Hutchinson PE. Cryotherapy of common viral warts at intervals of 1, 2 and 3 weeks. Br J Dermatol 1995;132:433. (*Cure was related to the number of treatments and independent of the interval between treatments.*)
5. Edwards L, et al. Self-administered topical 5% imiquimod cream for external anogenital warts. Arch Dermatol 1998;134:25. (*A randomized, controlled trial; the cure rate was 50%.*)
6. Ordoukhanian E, Lane AT. Warts and molluscum contagiosum. Beware of treatments worse than the disease. Postgrad Med 1997;101:223. (*A discussion of etiology, natural course, and treatment options.*)
7. Street ML, Roenigk RK. Recalcitrant periungual verrucae: the role of carbon dioxide laser vaporization. J Am Acad Dermatol 1990;23:115. (*Seventy-one percent were cured after one or two treatments.*)
8. Tyring SK, Edwards L, Cherry LK, et al. Safety and efficacy of 0.5% podofilox gel in the treatment of anogenital warts. Arch Dermatol 1998;134:33. (*The overall cure rate was near 60% after 8 weeks of treatment.*)
9. Tyring SK, Arany I, Stanley MA, et al. A randomized, controlled molecular study of condylomata acuminata clearance during treatment with imiquimod. J Infect Dis 1998;178:551. (*Efficacy was demonstrated and linked to the induction of cytokine production.*)

CHAPTER 195 ■ MANAGEMENT OF SCABIES AND PEDICULOSIS

PETER C. SCHALOCK AND ARTHUR J. SOBER

Scabies and pediculosis are two arthropod parasitic skin diseases commonly seen in the primary care setting. Although accurate diagnosis, effective treatment, and preventive measures are available, infestations with scabies and lice are pandemic, affecting millions of people worldwide. The primary physician should be able to recognize the manifestations of infestation quickly and treat infestations effectively.

PATHOPHYSIOLOGY AND CLINICAL PRESENTATION (1,2)

Scabies

Infestation with the *human skin mite Sarcoptes scabiei var hominis* is an extremely common problem worldwide, with an estimated prevalence of 300 million cases. Transmission is through close personal contact, either sexual or nonsexual. Persons of all socioeconomic levels, both sexes, and all age groups can be affected. Once contracted, scabies usually persists until specific therapy is instituted.

The scabies mite is an obligate arachnid human parasite that is unable to live independent of its host for more than 24 to 36 hours; fomite transmission is rare. The mite measures 1/60 in. in length. The adult female mite attaches to and burrows into the horny layer of the skin. Copulation with a wandering male mite renders the female fertile for life. The female mite remains within her burrow for the rest of her 1-month life, laying two or three eggs a day. These eggs hatch within 3 to 4 days. Mature adults develop during the next 10 to 14 days. While in her burrow, the female mite feeds on epidermal cells. The average number of female mites on the body is 11.

Patients usually present with intense *pruritus*, which is often severe during the night. Eighty-five percent of infested persons have *burrows* on the fingers, interdigital areas, and wrists; these appear as linear marks a few millimeters in length, often with a dark dot at one end, which represents the female mite (Fig. 195.1). Other common sites for burrows are the elbows, feet, ankles, penis, scrotum, buttocks, nipples, and axillae. Vigorous scratching may lead to excoriations, eczematous plaques, crusted papules and nodules, or secondary infection (Fig. 195.2). In healthy adults, infestation is usually confined to skin below the neck. However, infant, elderly, or immunosuppressed patients may also present with head and neck lesions.

The mite is not necessarily found in all of the cutaneous lesions. The rash and accompanying pruritus reflect a sensitivity reaction to the mite, eggs, or scybala (fecal droppings). In pa-

tients who have never been infested, the pruritic rash develops after a 2- to 4-week initial asymptomatic phase of infestation. In previously sensitized patients, the eruption can occur within a few days. Antiscabietic treatment kills the mite and ova but does not remove the sensitizing dead organisms or scybala from the burrow. Thus, pruritus may continue for a few weeks after treatment, until the contents of the burrow are shed with the natural turnover of skin. Persistent postscabetic papules may occur, especially on the penis, which may require topical or intralesional injection of corticosteroids.

Crusted (Norwegian) scabies is an infrequent variant of the disease in which patients harbor a high mite load and present with hundreds of thick, keratotic papules. This form often affects patients with a decreased host defense, such as those with *HIV infection*, or without the ability to scratch, such those who have had a stroke. Crusted scabies is highly contagious because of the myriad of mites in the exfoliating scales.

Pediculosis

Human lice, which are obligate human parasites, are responsible for the diseases pediculosis capitis, pediculosis corporis, and pediculosis pubis. Transmission is through contact with infested humans, clothing, combs, or bedding. Body lice are most commonly found in people with poor personal hygiene or in indigent populations. Head lice are a public health problem among school children and affect all socioeconomic classes. Pubic lice are predominantly transmitted sexually. Human lice are the vectors for the transmission of typhus, trench fever, and louse-borne relapsing fever.

The two species of these wingless, dorsoventrally flattened, blood-sucking insects are *Pediculus humanus* (subspecies *capitis* and *humanus*), which infests the head and clothing, and *Phthirus pubis* (crab louse), which infests the pubic area. These insects measure 3 to 4 mm in length, with *Phthirus pubis* demonstrating a more rounded body in comparison with *Pediculus humanus*. Adult lice require a blood meal every 3 to 6 hours. The female insect lives 1 month and lays 7 to 10 eggs (nits) a day. These eggs hatch in about 8 to 10 days. The head louse lives on the scalp and lays eggs that are cemented onto hairs. Body lice live and lay eggs in clothing, often in the seams. The crab louse prefers axillary, eyebrow, eyelash, beard, pubic, limb, and trunk hairs and lays its eggs on these hairs. Lice may be able to survive off the human host for 3 days.

The head louse typically infests the occipital portion of the *scalp* and sometimes the postauricular region. Although few adults are present, many oval nits can be found cemented to the hair. Patients often complain of scalp *pruritus*. Cervical adenopathy may be present. Body lice cause pruritus, often

---

All photos are courtesy of Peter C. Schalock.

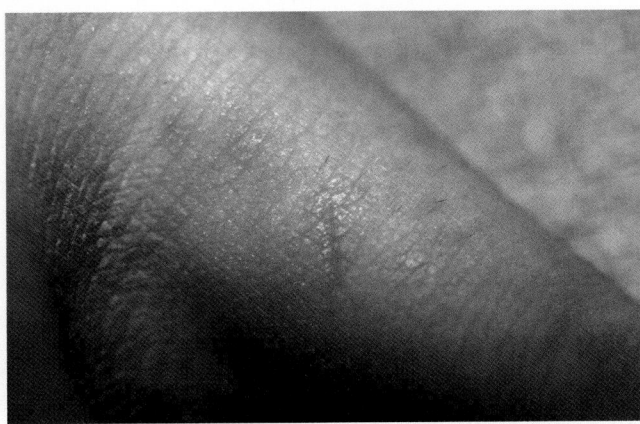

FIGURE 195.1. Scabies burrow on the finger. (See the color insert.)

representing a sensitivity reaction to lice excretions. Patients can have multiple excoriations over the trunk, and vertical excoriations are characteristic of infestation. Body lice and eggs can be seen in clothing. Pubic lice cause pruritus, often *nocturnal*. Characteristic asymptomatic, macular, blue discolorations called maculae ceruleae are sometimes seen on the trunk and thighs; the mechanism of discoloration is unknown. Lice can be seen grasping pubic hairs, and specks of brownish feces can sometimes be seen.

DIAGNOSIS (2)

Scabies

The diagnosis is suggested by finding the characteristic *burrows*. They should be sought on the hands, wrists, ankles, and genital areas, where the recovery rate is highest. A *scraping* is performed by shaving off the roof of the burrow with a scalpel, scraping the base to remove the contents, and placing the material on a microscope slide. Next, a drop of light mineral oil and a cover slip are added. Alternately, putting a drop of mineral

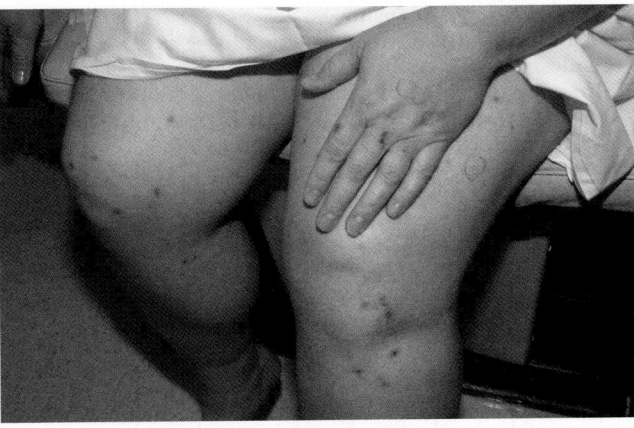

FIGURE 195.2. Crusted generalized excoriations and papules. Burrows are circled on the skin. (See the color insert.)

oil on the skin prior to scraping may aid in ensuring that all scale and mites are removed with scraping. The lowest-power objective should be used to view the specimen under a light microscope. The presence of adult mites, immature mites, ova, or tan-brown scybala confirms the diagnosis. In mineral oil, but not in potassium hydroxide, movement of the mite may be seen. In the absence of a scraping, presumptive diagnosis can be made based on the symptoms, the appearance of the rash, and the history of contacts who also have symptoms of itching.

Pediculosis

The diagnosis is made by direct examination of the involved area. Few adult lice are found at the bases of the hairs, but many nits are typically seen. Both are usually visible to the naked eye, but a hand lens and bright light may help. Nits appear as gray or white specks attached to the hair. The examination should be performed with gloves to avoid transmission. The detection of head lice is facilitated by plucking a few hairs and identifying the full or empty egg cases about 7 to 10 mm up the hair shaft. Organisms may be found at the nape and behind the ears. Pyoderma of the nape or the occiput requires that pediculosis capitis be ruled out. The underwear of a patient infected with pubic lice is often speckled with blood.

PRINCIPLES OF MANAGEMENT (2–9)

The elimination of the infestation and the relief of pruritus are the goals of treatment.

Scabies

Because infestation is from person to person, close contacts of a scabies patient should be treated even if they are free of symptoms. After the mites and ova have died, but before they are shed from the skin, pruritus may continue for a few weeks following treatment. During this time, it may be necessary to use topical corticosteroids and oral antihistamines to help control the sensitivity rash and pruritus. Occasionally, systemic steroids are required (see Chapter 105). Although theoretically the scabies mite should not be able to live without its human host, most authorities recommend that the bed linens and underwear of all household members be washed thoroughly in hot water with detergent or dry-cleaned to prevent reinfestation. The treatment of scabies is generally effective, provided that all close contacts of the patient are treated simultaneously.

Permethrin

Permethrin 5% cream, which is synthetically derived from a derivative of the chrysanthemum flower called pyrethrin, is the first-line treatment for scabies. Its toxicity in mammals is low because it is minimally absorbed and quickly reduced to inactive metabolites. Permethrin acts on the parasite nerve cell membranes and leads to paralysis. The 5% formulation is available with prescription in the United States. The patient should be treated from the ears and chin down for 8 to 12 hours; the bedding should be washed in hot water during this period. This is repeated in 1 week.

Lindane (γ-Benzene Hexachloride) Lotion

Lindane lotion was formerly the agent of choice for the treatment of scabies. Because of reports of organism resistance and neurotoxicity in infants and persons with an extensively compromised epidermal barrier, lindane has been relegated to alternative-treatment status. It should not be used in children younger than 2 years of age or in pregnant or lactating women. It has been banned in California.

Crotamiton and Malathion

Crotamiton 10% lotion is antipruritic and less successful as a scabicide than is permethrin. The cure rate after 5 consecutive days of therapy is only about 55%. *Malathion 0.5% lotion* (Ovide) is a scabicide that is now again available in the United States. It is reserved as an alternative agent.

Ivermectin

The off-label use of ivermectin, an antiparasitic medication, has been gaining popularity since it was introduced in the United States for the treatment of *Strongyloides* infestation. This macrocyclic lactone preferentially inhibits glutamate-gated chloride-ion channels in invertebrate nerve and muscle. Its affinity for human channels is low, and it does not penetrate the blood–brain barrier. Typically, a single dose of 200 to 400 μg/kg is given orally and repeated in 1 week. This has been reported to be extremely successful in treating infestation. Compliance is high because of the simplicity of treatment. A topical formulation is available and appears to be effective, but further studies are needed. There is some concern for use in elderly patients due to reports of increased mortality in older individuals in a single nursing home after treatment with ivermectin.

Pediculosis

First-Line Therapy

Permethrin 1% cream rinse shampoo is the first-line treatment for pediculosis. The 1% strength is available without a prescription in the United States. Less than 2% is absorbed, and the drug is quickly reduced to inactive metabolites. The 1% preparation is effective for the treatment of pediculosis capitis. Most other nonprescription treatments for pediculosis combine *pyrethrin*, a natural extract of chrysanthemum flowers, and a synergistic compound, *piperonyl butoxide*. The synergized pyrethrins have a wide safety margin because they are minimally absorbed through the skin. Because the nits have an undeveloped nervous system, none of these neurotoxic chemicals is completely ovicidal. Only permethrin has activity against eggs because it retains residual activity for 2 weeks and remains on the hair for 14 days after treatment. Thus, eggs that hatch after treatment can be killed. Some physicians still recommend that a second permethrin treatment be given 1 week after the first, for maximum cure rate.

Resistant Cases and Secondary Bacterial Infection

Reports of resistance to standard treatment with 1% permethrin have engendered alternative strategies, including 5% permethrin cream overnight under a shower cap, *ivermectin* as described for scabies, oral *trimethoprim/sulfamethoxazole*, and *malathion 0.5% lotion* (Ovide). Eyelash involvement may be treated with *petrolatum*, which is nonirritating and nontoxic; the lice either suffocate or slip off the greased hairs. As in scabies treatment, the use of *lindane* for the treatment of lice is no longer considered the first choice. On occasion, *secondary bacterial infection* may occur, which can be treated with the application of topical *mupirocin 2% ointment* three times daily or the administration of appropriate oral antibiotics.

Prevention

To prevent reinfestation, *asymptomatic close contacts* should be treated simultaneously. Sheets and all clothing worn in the last 3 days should be laundered in hot, soapy water or dry-cleaned. Brushes and combs should be washed in hot water for 10 to 20 minutes. Floors, furniture, and play areas should be thoroughly vacuumed to remove hairs that may have been shed with viable eggs attached.

PATIENT EDUCATION

Patient education is essential. Treatment failure is usually the result of poor patient compliance. Written instructions are helpful. A review of the foregoing preventive measures is very important.

THERAPEUTIC RECOMMENDATIONS

Scabies

- Prescribe 5% permethrin cream, to be applied from the neck down (including all body folds and creases) and left on overnight for 8 to 12 hours. The use of about 30 g is sufficient for the average adult. This is repeated in 1 week. One treatment is usually adequate. Some practitioners recommend application to the scalp also. Application beneath the nails may prevent reinfestation.
- Advise changing and cleaning underwear and bed linen during therapy.
- Treat all household members.
- A second course of treatment should be necessary only if reinfestation has occurred.
- Prescribe topical corticosteroids and oral antihistamines if rash and pruritus are bothersome; if they are severe, oral steroids can be considered.
- For crusted scabies, the use of a keratolytic agent (10% salicylic acid or 20% urea) can hasten the shedding of the affected horny layer of skin. Subungual areas should be carefully coated with permethrin cream.

Pediculosis Capitis

- Have the patient routinely shampoo without medication and thoroughly dry the hair. Excess water slows the neural activity of the insect, protecting it from the neurotoxic effects of permethrin. Sufficient permethrin 1% cream rinse should be applied to wet the hair thoroughly. It is left on for 10 minutes and then rinsed out.

■ Alternatively, recommend a synergized pyrethrins shampoo, to be applied undiluted until the infested areas are entirely wet. After 10 minutes, the areas are washed thoroughly with warm water and then dried. Because it is less effective as an ovicide, this treatment should be repeated in 7 to 10 days to kill any newly hatched lice.

■ Advise drying the hair with a clean towel after treatment with a pediculicide and removing any remaining nits with a fine-toothed comb. Nit removal is believed to reduce the chance of reinfestation.

■ Recommend that combs, clothing, and bed linens be washed.

Pediculosis Corporis and Pediculosis Pubis

■ Treatment is similar to treatment for pediculosis capitis. Permethrin 1% cream rinse or 1% cream can be applied to the body for 10 minutes before being washed off.

■ The sexual partners of patients with pediculosis pubis need to be treated.

■ Treat eyelash involvement with the application of petrolatum jelly up to five times a day for 5 to 7 days. Alternately, recommend physostigmine ophthalmic ointment 0.25%, applied to the lashes four times daily for three consecutive days.

■ Clothing and bed linens need to be washed.

Annotated Bibliography

1. Chosidow O. Clinical practices. Scabies. N Engl J Med 2006;354:1718. (*Reviews epidemiology, clinical manifestations, treatment, and prevention.*)
2. Ko CJ, Elston DM. Pediculosis. J Am Acad Dermatol 2004;50:1. (*An excellent review of pediculosis.*)
3. Burkhart CG, Burkhart CN, Burkhart KM. An assessment of topical and oral prescription and over-the-counter treatments for head lice. J Am Acad Dermatol 1998;38:979. (*Reviews the use of permethrin, pyrethrin with piperonyl butoxide, lindane, crotamiton, and ivermectin.*)
4. Cheoela EN, Abeldano AM, Pellerano G, et al. Oral ivermectin in the treatment of scabies. Arch Dermatol 1999;135:651. (*A randomized, controlled trial, finding a 95% cure rate.*)
5. Meinking T, Taplin D, Kalter DC, et al. Comparative efficacy of treatment for pediculosis capitis infestations. Arch Dermatol 1986;122:267. (*Evaluates various treatments for pediculosis and questions the widespread use of lindane.*)
6. Meinking TL, Taplin D, Hermida JL, et al. The treatment of scabies with ivermectin. N Engl J Med 1995;333:26. (*Discusses the use of a single oral 200-mg/kg dose of ivermectin to treat scabies in healthy and HIV-infected adults.*)
7. Schachner LA. Treatment-resistant head lice: alternative therapeutic approaches. Pediatr Dermatol 1997;14:409. (*Describes treatment with 5% permethrin, ivermectin, trimethoprim/sulfamethoxazole, and petrolatum.*)
8. Bigby M. A systematic review of the treatment of scabies. Arch Dermatol 2000;136:387. (*Examines the evidence for the various scabies treatments, finding a trend toward permethrin being more effective than lindane.*)
9. Barkwell R, Shields S. Deaths associated with ivermectin treatment of scabies. Lancet 1997;349:1144. (*There was an increase in deaths in elderly patients given ivermectin compared to controls.*)

CHAPTER 196 ■ MANAGEMENT OF SKIN TRAUMA: BITES AND BURNS

PART 1: ANIMAL AND HUMAN BITES

ELLIE J. C. GOLDSTEIN

Five million animal bites, leading to 800,000 medical encounters, occur in the United States each year. Patients often present to the primary physician for advice and therapy. Patients may appear shortly after injury concerned about rabies, tetanus, or the repair of a disfiguring tear. Sometimes they delay seeking care, only to present later with infection. The primary physician must provide first aid and tetanus prophylaxis, decide whether antibiotics are necessary, and estimate the risk for rabies. Human bites are less common but potentially more serious. Particularly treacherous are clenched-fist injuries, which result from striking the teeth. Bites in children and the elderly should be evaluated for abuse potential. Occlusional bites and paronychial injuries may also result in infection.

PATHOPHYSIOLOGY AND CLINICAL PRESENTATION (1–8)

Most bites result in minor trauma. Approximately 80% of patients neither need nor seek medical care. Bite wounds that produce a break in the skin allow the inoculation of bacteria that normally inhabit the skin or, more usually, the oral cavity of the biting animal. Conditions favoring infection include prior splenectomy, liver disease, immune compromise, crush injury, edema, wounds to the hand, and multiple punctures. Patients with established infection usually present more than 8 hours after having sustained an injury. Patients with preexisting edema (e.g., persons with congestive heart failure or chronic venous insufficiency, women who have undergone radical or modified mastectomy) are at risk for more-severe infection.

Animal Bites

In animal bites, the wound itself may or may not be problematic, depending on how much tearing of the skin occurs. The infecting organisms are usually the normal oral flora of the biting animal. *Pasteurella* species, including *Pasteurella multocida*, are present in 50% of animal oral cavities and in 50% of dog and 75% of cat bite wounds. Cat bites are more prone to infection than are dog bites and may lead to severe cellulitis, and approximately 20% present as abscesses. Cat-scratch disease is caused by *Bartonella henselae* and *B. quintana*, fastidious gram-negative rods; it often presents with fever and lymphadenopathy and is more frequently seen during the cold-weather months. Any patient who has undergone splenectomy or has alcoholic liver disease is prone to sepsis with *Capnocytophaga canimorsus* (formerly DF-2).

Human Bites

Human bites, especially *clenched-fist injuries*, in which damage is inflicted while the tendons and other tissues of the exterior area of the finger are stretched to full length, can be serious because they result not only in breakage of the skin, but also in exposure of the tendon and possibly the joint. As the fingers are straightened, the damaged parts relax, and infecting organisms are carried into the tissues, producing infection in wounds that may initially appear minor. If the joint capsule is penetrated, septic arthritis or osteomyelitis is a risk.

The oral flora in humans is more abundant than in that in most animals and includes *Streptococcus viridans*, *Haemophilus influenzae*, *Eikenella corrodens*, *Prevotella* species, *Porphyromonas* species, anaerobic diphtheroids, fusobacteria, and spirochetes. Wounds may also be infected by *skin flora*, such as a group A β-hemolytic streptococci (*Streptococcus pyogenes*) or staphylococci (*Staphylococcus aureus*). *Streptococcus anginosus* may be present in approximately 50% of wounds, *S. aureus* and *E. corrodens* in 30%, and anaerobes in approximately 55%, especially *Fusobacterium nucleatum* in approximately 30% and *Prevotella melaninogenica* in 20%. The presence of anaerobic bacteria is associated with more severe infection and may lead to abscess formation. Human bites are responsible for most severe bite wound infections, accounting for greater than 50% of clenched-fist injuries and 45% of occlusional bite wounds in adults requiring hospitalization. In children, bites may occur during play, but only 14% may require hospitalization. Many patients initially deny that a human bite was a cause of injury.

PRINCIPLES OF THERAPY (1–11)

Basic elements of management include characterization of the injury, vigorous cleansing, elevation, tetanus prophylaxis, and the administration of appropriate antibiotics.

Animal Bites

It is important to elicit a history of the circumstances surrounding the injury. If an animal bite occurred, the type of animal and its behavior need to be detailed, as well as whether the animal had been vaccinated and whether the attack was provoked or unprovoked. The wound should be diagrammed in the chart, with proximity to bones or joints noted. Minor animal puncture wounds should be cleansed with *soap and water* and treated expectantly without antibiotics. Copious *irrigation* of wounds with normal saline solution is an important therapeutic adjunct. Animal puncture wounds that are small and clean require no other treatment.

Rabies

Since 1967, only one or two cases of rabies in humans have been documented each year in the United States. No cases of rabies have occurred in New York City or Los Angeles for many years. Raccoon rabies is epidemic in all states along the entire eastern seaboard. In most other states, skunks and bats are the most common rabid animals. Rabies is more prevalent in cats than in dogs in the United States. Rabies is a concern if the attack is unprovoked, occurs in a rural setting, or involves a raccoon, a bat, a skunk, or an animal that is behaving in a peculiar manner. The local health department provides data regarding the local incidence of rabies and should be notified for follow-up and documentation. Patients with bat exposure, even without a known bite, should be considered for prophylaxis because a bat bite or exposure has been the most common cause for clinical rabies in humans in the United States. If rabies is considered a possibility, *human diploid cell vaccine* should be given along with *rabies immune globulin* without delay (see Chapter 6). If a person is bitten by a pet, the animal should be watched at home by the owner for 2 weeks and the bite reported to the local health department.

Tetanus

It is important to determine whether the patient has had an initial series of tetanus shots and a booster within the last 10 years. Those who have not had an initial series should be given both *tetanus toxoid* and *tetanus immune globulin* (see Chapter 6). For persons who have had the initial series but no booster in 10 years, 0.5 mL of *tetanus toxoid* should be administered intramuscularly.

Tear Wounds

Therapy for tear wounds is problematic. No controlled trials of closure versus nonclosure, with or without antibiotics, have been undertaken. The principles of therapy are to cleanse and debride the wound cautiously. After the wound has been left open for 24 hours, the edges can be approximated with adhesive strips or sutured and a 3- to 5-day course of *amoxicillin/clavulanate* prescribed (875 mg thrice daily for 3 to 5 days if the patient is >125 lb) taken with food. Secondary closures can be performed if no infection is apparent. Facial wounds may be closed and antibiotics given. It is useful to refer these patients to a plastic surgeon.

Infected Wounds

Patients who present with infection should receive debridement, drainage, cleansing, and antibiotics. *Amoxicillin/clavulanic acid* is effective against most animal bite pathogens. In penicillin-allergic patients, *doxycycline* is preferred because *P. multocida* is often resistant to erythromycin and cephalexin. *Penicillin* and *amoxicillin* are effective against *P. multocida*, streptococci, anaerobes, and *E. corrodens* but are ineffective against *S. aureus*. *In vitro* and anecdotal clinical data exist for *moxifloxacin*, which also covers most pathogens. Oral second-generation cephalosporins, such as *cefuroxime*, are active against *P. multocida* but not anaerobes.

Human Bites

Human bites are usually located on an extremity; hand wounds are the most serious. The same principles of cleansing, drainage, and debridement apply. Human bites should not be closed primarily, although edges can be approximated if the tear is severe. Antibiotics should be instituted after wound cultures are taken. *Amoxicillin/clavulanic acid (ampicillin/sulbactam*, intravenously) should be administered pending culture results to cover β-lactamase–producing oral anaerobes and gram-positive cocci, particularly *S. aureus. Ertapenem* and other intravenous carbapenems can be used but are more expensive alternatives. Infrequently, the presence of a gram-negative organism necessitates a change in antibiotic regimen. All patients previously immunized who have not had a booster in 5 years should be given 0.5 mL of *tetanus toxoid*. Follow-up is essential because of the potential for late serious infection. A risk exists for the transmission of viral pathogens such as hepatitis A, B, and C viruses and less for HIV.

Clenched-Fist Injuries

These usually require specialized care. Radiographs should be taken to rule out fractures and provide a baseline for future assessment of osteomyelitis. Extension and flexion of digits should be carefully checked and sensation tested. The third metacarpophalangeal joint is most often affected. The integrity of the joint capsule must be determined, and this may require an experienced surgeon. If the capsule is intact, the hand is cleaned, debrided, immobilized, and elevated. *Ampicillin/sulbactam, cefoxitin*, or *ertapenem* should be started and *tetanus toxoid* administered. Patients seen within 8 hours of injury with intact joint capsules can be managed as outpatients with careful follow-up. Those with torn capsules need to be admitted for surgery and treatment with intravenous antibiotics. Patients who present after 8 hours should be admitted for observation to determine whether the capsule is intact or interrupted.

THERAPEUTIC RECOMMENDATIONS AND PATIENT EDUCATION (1,3,6, 8,10–13)

- Clean all wounds vigorously with soap and water. Copiously irrigate with normal saline solution. A needle and syringe can be used to generate a high-pressure jet to cleanse puncture wounds.
- Immunize patients who have previously been immunized but have not had a booster in the last 5 years against tetanus with 0.5 mL of intramuscular tetanus toxoid.

Animal Bites

- Animal puncture wounds that are trivial and clean, without crush injury and not involving the hand, often require no other treatment.
- Treat moderate or severe fresh, *uninfected* animal tear wounds with cleansing, debridement, and *amoxicillin clavulanate* (500 to 875 mg two times daily, depending on weight, with food), followed by secondary closure in 24 to 48 hours if no signs of infection are present.
- Treat *infected* animal bite wounds with debridement, drainage, and cleansing. Culture the wound, delay wound closure until the infection subsides, and begin *Amoxicillin/clavulanic acid* (500 to 875 mg twice daily, with food). It may be used as a single agent, as may *cefuroxime* (500 mg twice daily), plus *metronidazole* if anaerobes are suspected, especially for an infected cat bite. If the patient is allergic to penicillin, use *doxycycline* (100 mg twice daily) for initial antibiotic therapy; consider *moxifloxacin* (400 mg/d) if other options are problematic.
- Advise elevation of the effected body part for resolution of edema.
- Treat for 7 to 10 days for an uncomplicated cellulitis.

Human Bites

- Treat all human bites initially with *amoxicillin/clavulanate* (875 mg, twice a day with food, orally), *ampicillin sulbactam* (intravenously), or *ertapenem* (1 g/d, intravenously); delay closure of the wound.
- Elevate the affected limb until the swelling declines, usually after 3 to 5 days.
- Immobilize clenched-fist injuries and obtain hand surgery consultation promptly.
- Instruct the patient to watch the wound for signs of infection, such as pain, redness, warmth, swelling, or purulent exudate.

Annotated Bibliography

1. Chuinard RG, D'Ambrosia RD. Human bite infections of the hand. J Bone Joint Surg 1977;59:416. (*A classic article, outlining early and aggressive surgical management, and stressing the need to determine capsule integrity.*)
2. Fallouji MA. Traumatic love bites. Br J Surg 1990;77:100. (*The underreported problem of "love" bites.*)
3. Goldstein EJC. Bite wounds and infection. Clin Infect Dis 1992;14:633. (*A review of the current literature and a guide to proper management.*)
4. Mann RJ, Hoffeld TA, Farmer CB. Human bites of the hand: 20 years of experience. J Hand Surg 1977;2:97. (*Streptococcus viridans was the most common aerobic pathogen; 44% of wounds had Staphylococcus aureus; the use of penicillinase-resistant penicillin is recommended.*)
5. Merchant RC, Fuerch J, Becker BM, et al. Comparison of the epidemiology of human bites evaluated in three US pediatric emergency departments. Pediatr Emerg Care 2005;21:833. (*A analysis, with some different findings than other pediatric studies; 14% of cases required hospitalization.*)
6. Sacks JJ, Kresnow M, Houston B. Dog bites: how big a problem? Injury Prev 1996;2:52. (*A review of the epidemiology and incidence of dog bites.*)
7. Stockheim J, Wilkinson N, Ramos-Bonan C. Human bites and blood exposures in New York City Schools. Clin Pediatr 2005;44:699. (*Reviews 734 exposures from 1999 to 2001.*)
8. Talan DA, Citron DM, Abrahamian FA, et al., and the Emergency Medicine Animal Bite Infection Study Group. The bacteriology and management of dog and cat bite wound infections presenting to emergency departments. N Engl J Med 1999;340:85. (*The bacteriology of dog and cat bite wounds and their urgent care.*)
9. Talan DA, Abrahamian FM, Moran GJ, et al., Clinical presentation and bacteriological analysis of infected human bites in patients presenting to emergency departments. Clin Infect Dis 2003;37:1481. (*An analysis of human infected bite wounds and clenched-fist injuries and their complications.*)
10. Fleisher GR. Management of bite wounds. N Engl J Med 1999;340:138. (*An editorial summarizing the current best practices.*)
11. Goldstein EJC, Citron DM, Richwald GA. Lack of *in vitro* efficacy of oral forms of certain cephalosporins, erythromycin, and oxacillin against *Pasteurella multocida*. Antimicrob Agents Chemother 1988;32:213. (*Many strains of Pasteurella multocida isolated from infected bite wounds were resistant to cephalexin, erythromycin, and oxacillin.*)
12. Moran GJ, Talan DA, Mower W, et al. Appropriateness of rabies postexposure prophylaxis treatment for animal exposures. JAMA 2000;284:1001. (*The use of prophylaxis was often inappropriate.*)
13. Taylor GA. Management of human bite injuries of the hand. Can Med Assoc J 1985;133:191. (*A well-conceived approach.*)

PART 2: MANAGEMENT OF MINOR BURNS

PETER C. SCHALOCK AND ARTHUR J. SOBER

Accidental minor burns are common. The majority of the estimated 2 million annual burn victims can be treated as outpatients. The primary physician is often asked for advice about immediate care and should render definitive treatment for localized, partial-thickness burns.

PATHOPHYSIOLOGY AND CLINICAL PRESENTATION (1–5)

Burns represent direct thermal injury to the cells of the skin and underlying structures. The clinical presentation depends on the degree of damage, which is a direct function of the intensity of heat and duration of exposure.

First-Degree Burns

These involve just the superficial layers of the epidermis. The skin is painful, red, and swollen. It blanches with pressure and shows little or no edema. Ultraviolet radiation, scalding, low-intensity steam exposure, and brief contact with a hot object are common causes. Complete recovery usually occurs within 1 week, often with peeling and sometimes with postinflammatory hyperpigmentation.

Second-Degree Burns

Involvement extends into both the epidermis and dermis; a broad distinction is made between *superficial* and *deep* burns, based on the amount of dermis involved. Deep second-degree burns involve the entire papillary dermis, with penetration to some or all of the reticular dermis. Second-degree burns present as painful red blisters or broken epidermis exposing a weeping, edematous surface. They are most often caused by scalds or brief exposure to a flame. Recovery requires 2 to 3 weeks; sometimes scarring occurs.

Third-Degree Burns

All layers of the epidermis and dermis are affected, with penetration into underlying fat and muscle. They usually result from prolonged contact with steam, hot objects, or flames and present with ulceration and tissue necrosis. They are painless because nerve tissue in the area has been destroyed. Deep tissue destruction can occur in electrical or chemical burns that may not become evident for several days.

Sunburn and Photosensitivity Reactions

Sunburn is one of the most common types of burn seen by the office-based practitioner. It represents ultraviolet injury to the skin. There are two phases: an immediate, initial, erythematous phase, which generally fades within 30 minutes after exposure, and a delayed response—what patients call sunburn—that oc-

curs 3 to 6 hours after the exposure to the sun and peaks in 12 to 24 hours. Sunburn is characterized by erythema, pruritus, and tenderness but may proceed to edema, vesiculation, and even blistering. Repeated severe sunburns at an early age increase the risk for melanoma and other skin cancers later in life (see Chapter 177). Long-term excessive exposure to ultraviolet light leads to sustained elevations in skin matrix metalloproteinases, which can degrade skin collagen and contribute to premature skin aging.

Sun-related eruptions may also occur as a result of photosensitizing medications. The primary culprits are thiazide diuretics, sulfa-containing agents, tetracyclines (particularly demeclocycline/doxycycline), griseofulvin, phenothiazines, and nalidixic acid. Topical substances, particularly furocoumarins (found in parsley, celery, carrots, and citrus fruits [especially lime], certain perfumes, and aftershave lotions) are also photosensitizing. The popular herbal compound known as St. John's wort may increase sun sensitivity.

PRINCIPLES OF THERAPY (1–8)

The first task is to assess the depth and the extent of injury. The treatment of burn wounds is based on the depth and the surface area of skin involved. The surface area of burns has traditionally been based on the "rule of nines": Each arm is considered to be 9% of the body surface area, each leg is 18%, the anterior and the posterior trunk are each 18%, the head is 9%, and the perineum and genitalia are 1%.

With the use of these classifications, the treatment of burns can proceed in an organized fashion. All second-degree burns involving more than 5% to 10% of the body surface, all third-degree burns, any burns associated with an electric current, and all burns of the ears, eyes, face, hands, feet, or perineum should be treated immediately at a major hospital familiar with burn care. A history of prolonged contact with scalding liquids, flaming clothing, or high-voltage electric current portends full-thickness damage and the need for referral, as does dry, parchment-like skin with a loss of hair follicles and sensation.

First-degree burns and second-degree burns involving less than 5% of the body surface can be treated on an outpatient basis by the primary physician with adequate wound care and follow-up, provided that the patient is reliable and the home situation amenable.

The goals of therapy are to reduce inflammation, prevent infection, relieve pain, and promote healing.

First-Degree Burns

First aid to minor burns involves the immediate application of *cold water bath or compresses* of water, milk, or oatmeal. Water temperature should be cool but not cold, around 8°C to 10°C (~50°F). Cold reduces discomfort, edema, and hyperemia and may diminish the extent of injury. The application of cold should continue for 10 to 30 minutes. Avoid ice packs or the application of ice. *No dressing* is required, just skin lubricant and instructions to return if blistering occurs. Prophylactic antibiotics appear to have little or no effect. A tetanus vaccination should be administered if the patient has not received one within the last 5 years.

Pain can usually be relieved with aspirin or acetaminophen. Aspirin or nonsteroidal antiinflammatory drugs have the advantage of suppressing inflammation and are particularly helpful in sunburn. Patients appreciate the offer of early pain relief. In cases of extensive sunburn, a topical corticosteroid lotion may provide symptomatic relief. Systemic corticosteroids do not reduce the edema associated with sunburn and are not recommended.

Second-Degree Burns

If the skin is broken, the wound requires protection so that healing can occur without infection. This involves gently *washing* the area of the burn with water and a mild antiseptic soap, such as one containing chlorhexidine. Washing is followed by gentle *irrigation* with sterile isotonic saline solution and the application of a sterile *occlusive dressing*. With chemical burns, the involved area is placed under running water for at least 15 to 30 minutes before cleansing or debridement is started. A syringe or water pick can be used to help irrigate and remove embedded debris. Devitalized tissue should be debrided (see Appendix to Section 12). Patients complaining of pain or who appear to be anxious should be given an analgesic or a sedative before the injured area is manipulated. Adherent tar can be removed after being hardened by the application of ice or softened with a topical antibiotic such as polysporin or mupirocin (Bactroban) ointment. *Tetanus prophylaxis* is indicated and includes the administration of tetanus toxoid booster to previously immunized patients (see Chapter 6).

Management of Blisters

Management is somewhat controversial. Some argue that blisters provide an excellent burn dressing and protective barrier, but others suggest that the trapped fluid can become a culture medium for bacteria. Small, thick-walled blisters probably should be left intact, whereas those that are larger, thin walled, located on hairy skin that is prone to infection, or located in areas where movement is likely to cause rupture should be removed. Removal should be complete because needle aspiration simply negates the protective barrier while retaining the potential culture medium for infection.

Prophylaxis against Infection

Topical antibiotic preparations are used. *Silver sulfadiazine cream* (1% Silvadene) is the most common choice because it is effective, easy to use, and reasonably well tolerated (it can cause a transient and self-limited fall in white cell count during the first week of use). It is contraindicated in persons allergic to sulfa and in pregnant and nursing women. Other topical agents of proven effectiveness include 11.1% *mafenide acetate cream* and 0.5% *silver nitrate solution*. The silver sulfadiazine cream is easy to apply and provides softening in addition to an antibacterial effect. The agent should be applied with a tongue depressor or glove in a layer thick enough to prevent the burn from being visible. Pain can be minimized by keeping the cream refrigerated. Silver sulfadiazine should be removed daily or every other day and reapplied. *Systemic antibiotics* are indicated only for established infection and are not appropriate for prophylaxis or outpatient use.

Dressings

Dressings have changed considerably in recent years. The newer hydrocolloid, hydrofiber, silicon, alginate, and polyurethane dressings are quite helpful for maintaining moisture in the wound bed, preventing infection. Alternatively, a dressing can be prepared by applying a nonadherent, fine mesh gauze soaked in sterile saline solution to the burn. This is then covered with a bulky dressing into which fluid can drain without passing through (see Appendix to Section 12). The patient should be examined in 2 days for pain, adenopathy, and fever, and the dressing should be checked. If no evidence of infection is seen, the dressing may remain for 5 to 7 days, after which the area is reexamined to determine the need for a dressing change.

Pain Relief

An essential part of management, pain relief starts with use of aspirin or a nonsteroidal agent such as ibuprofen. Short courses of an opioid (e.g., codeine, oxycodone) are appropriate for painful burns. Topical anesthetics may provide symptomatic relief but are not justified because of the risk for allergic sensitization. In cases of extensive sunburn, topical corticosteroid lotions may provide modest symptomatic relief.

Moisturization

Moisturizing the skin is important but often overlooked. After the burn heals, the new epithelial layer tends to dry and crack, and this problem can be reduced by the application of a moisturizer such as white petrolatum (Vaseline) or *Aveeno* lotion for 4 to 8 weeks after apparent resolution.

INDICATIONS FOR REFERRAL AND ADMISSION (1,4,6–8)

Referral for surgical consultation and hospitalization is indicated if burns exceed 10% to 15% of body area or if full-thickness burns exceed 3%. Prompt admission and surgical consultation should be considered for circumferential or full-thickness burns; involvement of the eyes, ears, other organs of sensation, hands, or perineum; evidence of inhalation injury; or serious concurrent medical conditions such as diabetes and immunosuppression. Patients who are unreliable or unable to care for themselves may also require inpatient treatment.

PATIENT EDUCATION

Patient education is critical to successful recovery from a burn. The patient and caretaker should be instructed to keep the wound clean and note erythema or inflammation, which are signs of infection. The patient should be instructed to note numbness, tingling, or a change in skin color or temperature, which may suggest that the dressing is too tight and circulation is being impaired. Explicit (often written) instructions on the removal of dressings, cleansing of the wound, reapplication of topical sulfadiazine, and treatment of dried skin are important. Patients with healed burns should be instructed to avoid exposure to direct sunlight because of increased sensitivity during the year after a burn injury. A burn provides a good opportunity to reinforce the importance of sunscreen use and to educate the patient about the warning signs of skin cancer (see Chapter 177).

The occurrence of a burn, even a minor one, is a good opportunity to reinstruct patients on the importance of burn prevention. The obvious caveats are not to smoke and to keep flammable material and matches away from children. Specific instructions on the use of pot holders, careful puncture and removal of plastic wraps from food heated in microwave ovens, and controlling the temperature of hot tap water are all helpful. Reminders about the importance of smoke detectors and maintaining an approved fire extinguisher are important. A written burn prevention checklist is a useful aid.

THERAPEUTIC RECOMMENDATIONS (1,4,6–8)

- For first-degree burns, immediately apply a cool water bath for 10 to 30 minutes.
- If the skin is broken, cleanse with a mild soap and water before applying cool water; no dressing or antibiotic is indicated for first-degree burns.
- If blistering does not occur after several days, prescribe the use of an emollient such as white petrolatum or *Aveeno* lotion.

- For severe sunburn, prescribe a gentle topical corticosteroid lotion for symptomatic relief. Aspirin or ibuprofen provides analgesia and helps to limit inflammation. Consider a brief course of systemic steroids for extensive sunburn.
- For second-degree burns, spread silver sulfadiazine (Silvadene) over the involved area in a thickness sufficient to prevent the burn from showing through. Refrigerating the sulfadiazine minimizes pain. Wrap the area with six or seven layers of gauze for protection.
- Prescribe systemic antibiotics—usually dicloxacillin—for any secondary cellulitis. Prophylactic oral antibiotics should not be used, for fear of selecting out resistant gram-negative organisms.

Annotated Bibliography

1. Deitch EA. The management of burns. N Engl J Med 1990;323:1249. (*A comprehensive discussion, including the approach to more serious burns.*)
2. Fisher GJ, Wang ZQ, Datta SC, et al. Pathophysiology of premature skin aging induced by ultraviolet light. N Engl J Med 1997;337:1419. (*The best discussion of the mechanisms of sun-induced skin damage and the implications for treatment.*)
3. Herbert K, Lawrence JC. Chemical burns. Burns 1989;15:381. (*A good review of this important category of burn injury.*)
4. Monafo WW. Initial management of burns. N Engl J Med. 1996;45:1321. (*A useful review for the nonspecialist; 50 references.*)
5. Sheridan RL, Hinson MI, Liang MH, et al. Long-term outcome of children surviving massive burns. JAMA 2000;283:69. (*Most patients were found to function well years later and enjoy a good quality of life.*)
6. Alsbjorn B, Gilbert P, Hartmann B, et al. Guidelines for the management of partial-thickness burns in a general hospital or community setting—recommendations of a European working party. Burns 2007;33:1550. (*A European consensus for outpatient management.*)
7. Rockwell WB, Ehrlich HP. Should burn blister fluid be evacuated? J Burn Care Rehabil 1990;11:93. (*Argues for the removal of even intact blisters because the fluid can be a good culture medium for bacteria.*)
8. Sheridan RL. Burn care: Results of technical and organizational progress. JAMA 2003;290:719. (*A succinct summary of advances.*)

CHAPTER 197 ■ MANAGEMENT OF SKIN ULCERATION

PETER C. SCHALOCK AND ARTHUR J. SOBER

Skin ulceration can be a troublesome, disabling, and potentially dangerous problem. Cutaneous ulcers commonly encountered in medical practice include leg and pressure ulcerations. Approximately 1% of the population is affected by venous leg ulcers. Diabetics and others with arterial insufficiency are at increased risk for ischemic ulceration and limb-threatening infection. About 20% of bed-bound or immobilized patients have pressure ulcers. The primary physician who recognizes and effectively treats early skin changes can prevent many of the debilitating consequences.

PATHOPHYSIOLOGY AND CLINICAL PRESENTATION (1–7)

Skin ulceration most commonly results from venous/arterial insufficiency or from prolonged, excessive pressure. Infectious and malignant causes are also encountered, especially in immunocompromised persons.

Venous Insufficiency

The initial manifestation of venous insufficiency is edema, usually absent on waking and severe at the end of the day. Incompetent venous valves can be associated with age, thrombophlebitis, or a hereditary tendency for the development of venous varicosities. In all three conditions, abnormally high venous pressure during ambulation causes fibrinogen to leak from the engorged capillary bed. A precapillary fibrin layer develops that is a sign of abnormal microcirculation. Some believe that this fibrin layer interferes with oxygen and nutrient exchange. Pigmentation, induration, dermatitis (*stasis dermatitis*), and finally ulceration may develop. The rupture of delicate venules releases hemoglobin, which changes to hemosiderin, producing pigmentation. Scaling and oozing develop when the skin is scratched. Vesicles may indicate a contact dermatitis caused by a topical medication. Secondary bacterial invasion occurs and may lead to cellulitis.

All photos are courtesy of Peter C. Schalock.

Stasis ulcerations develop within areas of dermatitis or indurated cellulitis. They occur most often above the medial malleolus because of its poor vascular supply and sparse subcutaneous tissue, although the entire medial lower calf has higher venous pressures. Minor trauma can precipitate ulceration. The stasis ulcers vary in size from small erosions to an ulcer that encircles the ankle. They may or may not be painful. The base of the ulcer is usually moist, with exuberant granulation tissue. Purulence indicates secondary infection.

Arterial Insufficiency

The most common cause of arterial insufficiency is *atherosclerotic disease*. The leg is cold and appears pale or cyanotic (although dependent rubor may be present), and peripheral pulses are lost or reduced. The ulcers are initially small, punctate, and superficial, but with worsening ischemia, they become larger and deeper (Fig. 197.1). Typically, they occur on the sides of the feet, the heels, the toes, and the nail beds. This type of ulceration makes up approximately 10% of leg ulcerations.

Ischemic ulcers are also associated with *hypertensive disease* and *vasculitis*. Those occurring in the context of hypertension characteristically develop over the lateral malleoli and surface of the calf. They begin as painful, blue-red plaques that soon ulcerate. A purpuric halo may surround the ulceration. Vasculitic ulcers occur in the context of connective tissue disease, hematologic and malignant conditions, and hypersensitivity reactions, beginning as palpable purpuric lesions or hemorrhagic vesicles (see Chapter 179).

Decubitus Ulcer

The pressure sore or decubitus ulcer is common in bed-ridden or semiambulatory patients. Factors contributing to the development of pressure sores include shearing forces, friction, and moisture; age per se does not. Decubitus ulcers usually occur over bony prominences. The pressure gradient occludes lymphatic vessels and overloads the microvascular system, and so waste products accumulate, and ultimately necrosis ensues. The lower part of the body and sacrococcygeal area are the predominant sites, with the hip, malleolus, and heel being other important areas.

The problem may initially present as nonblanchable erythema, soft-tissue loss, blisters, or eschar over bony prominences. Pressure ulcer severity is reflected by the stage of the lesion. Stage 1 lesions are manifested by nonblanchable erythema of intact skin. Stage 2 ulcers involve only the epidermis and the dermis. Stage 3 ulcers extend into the subcutaneous tissues and undermine the surrounding skin. Stage 4 lesions extend through deep fascia to involve muscle and may extend to the bone.

Pressure sores can lead to cellulitis, bacteremia, osteomyelitis, and even meningitis. The microbiology of decubitus ulcers is polymicrobial, and the organisms that cause the most problems, including life-threatening bacteremias, are *group A streptococci*, *Staphylococcus aureus*, *Escherichia coli*, and *Bacteroides fragilis*.

Pyoderma Gangrenosum

The condition is characterized pathologically by sterile neutrophilic infiltrates and dermal abscesses of the skin leading to tissue breakdown. Its association with minor trauma as well as with inflammatory and neoplastic conditions (e.g., inflammatory bowel and joint diseases, paraproteinemias, myeloproliferative conditions) suggests hyperactive dysfunction of neutrophils in response to an inflammatory or neoplastic stimulus. Clinical hallmarks include rapid development, pain, suppuration, violaceous discoloration, and necrotic borders (Fig. 197.2). Ulcers due to pyoderma gangrenosum are frequently confused with those due to other conditions (see Table 197.1).

DIAGNOSIS (3–7)

The differential diagnosis of skin ulceration is extensive (Table 197.1), but workup is aided by the appearance and the location

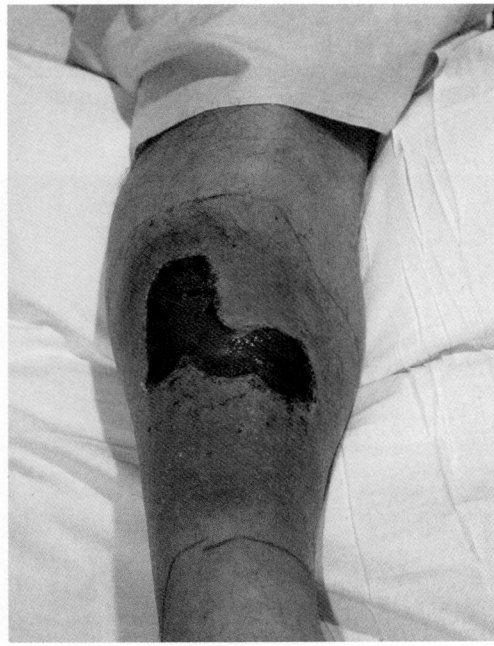

FIGURE 197.1. Large, later-stage arterial ulceration on the leg. This lesion was extremely painful. (See the color insert.)

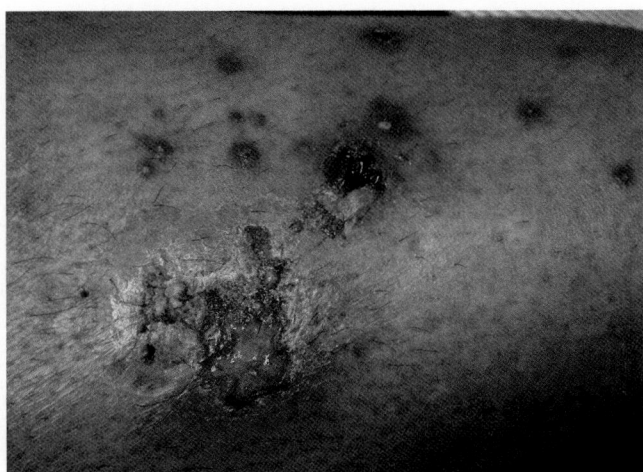

FIGURE 197.2. Pyoderma gangrenosum, early pustules and ulcerations on the shin. (See the color insert.)

TABLE 197.1

SOME IMPORTANT CAUSES OF SKIN ULCERS

Arterial occlusive disease[a]
Venous insufficiency/stasis dermatitis[a]
Pressure
Vasculitis[a]
Cutaneous involvement by internal malignancy (e.g.,
   lymphoma)[a]
Pyoderma gangrenosum
Primary skin infection (e.g., fungal—sporotrichosis)[a]
Drug-induced or exogenous tissue injury[a]
Skin malignancy (squamous and basal cell carcinoma)
Connective tissue diseases

[a]May be mistaken for pyoderma gangrenosum.
Adapted from Weenig RH, Davis MDP, Dahl PR, et al. Skin ulcers
misdiagnosed as pyoderma gangrenosum. N Engl J Med
2002;347:1412, with permission.

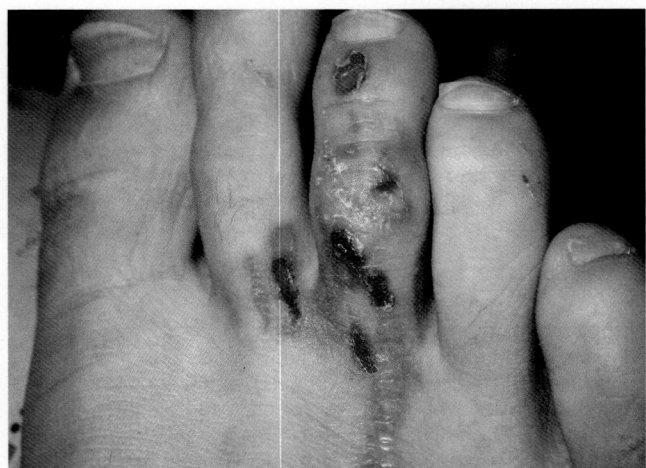

FIGURE 197.3. Ulcerations on the dorsal foot. These were caused by heating a piece of metal with a lighter and burning the foot. (See the color insert.)

of the ulcer and the clinical context in which it occurs. If it involves the lower extremity and the ulcer initially appears small, punctate, and superficial in a patient with absent pulses and a cold, pale leg (or one with dependent rubor), then peripheral atherosclerotic disease is the likely etiology. Vasculitic ulcers are suggested by associated palpable purpura and/or hemorrhagic vesicles in the setting of connective tissue disease, malignancy, or hypersensitivity reaction (see Chapter 179). Ulcers that begin as areas of nonblanchable erythema, soft-tissue loss, blisters, or eschar over bony prominences in debilitated persons are likely to be decubital in origin. Ulceration in the lower extremity occurring in the context of chronic edema, hyperpigmentation, induration, and erythema points toward venous insufficiency. Pyoderma gangrenosum is suggested by a painful, violaceous leg ulcer with irregular borders that begins as a pustule in the setting of minor trauma or concurrent inflammatory/neoplastic disease. When diagnosis is uncertain, referral for biopsy can be helpful, especially in cases of suspected vasculitis or pyoderma gangrenosum. About 10% of cases labeled as pyoderma gangrenosum are misdiagnosed. Factitial ulceration is a diagnosis of exclusion. Angulated or square borders and linear patterns may suggest this diagnosis (Figs. 197.3 and 197.4).

PRINCIPLES OF MANAGEMENT
(1–3,8–17)

Treatment of the underlying etiology is essential for sustained healing and prevention of recurrence, but many of the principles of initial ulcer management are similar, regardless of cause or location. Important objectives are to restore circulation (see Chapters 34 and 35), improve local factors, reduce pressure, remove necrotic tissue, maintain cleanliness, and prevent further injury.

Leg Ulcers

Initial General Measures

Regardless of cause, treatment of the leg ulcer begins with *washing* the leg and ankle with a mild soap. If debridement is needed, *wet-to-dry dressings* can provide cleaning and gentle debridement. Sterile gauze sponges moistened with normal

saline are applied several times daily and removed when dry. In leg ulcers with a clean base, application of an *Unna paste boot* or an *occlusive wound dressing* may encourage healing and reepithelialization as well as provide pressure. The Unna boot is a flesh-colored, gauze-roll bandage impregnated with zinc oxide, calamine, glycerin, and gelatin. *Topical enzymes* and *hydrophilic beads* are sometimes useful adjunctive agents in leg ulcers or pressure ulcers. Brief application of *topical tretinoin* solution (0.05% applied for 10 minutes followed by rinsing with normal saline) stimulated the development of granulation tissue and facilitated healing in one study.

Occlusive dressings are promoted as being capable of shortening the healing time but appear no better than wet-to-dry dressings. However, they do offer greater convenience and afford some improved pain relief compared to zinc paste and nonadherent dressings, making them worth consideration in persons with particularly painful leg ulcers. Commercially available preparations include polyurethane films (Opsite, Tegaderm, Bioclusive), polyethylene oxide hydrogels

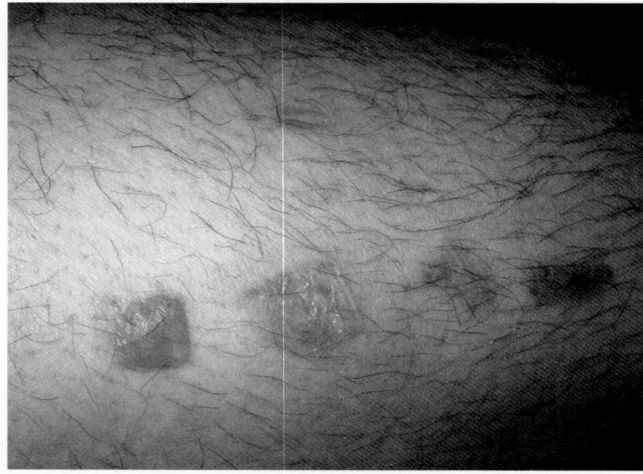

FIGURE 197.4. Quadratic bullae on the leg of the same patient as in Fig. 197.3. These were also factitial. (See the color insert.)

(Vigilon, Spenco 2nd Skin), foam dressings (Lyofoam, Allevyn), laminate dressings (Biobrane), alginate dressings (Sorbsan, Kaltostat), and hydrocolloid dressings (DuoDERM). The occlusive dressing is replaced every 3 to 7 days or sooner if it begins to leak. The patient must be warned to expect an unpleasant odor, caused by a buildup of fluid, when the dressing is removed. The optimal occlusive dressing for wound healing remains to be developed; no specific one has been proven to be better than another. DuoDerm is readily available and convenient to use. Occlusive dressings should not be used on wounds complicated by cellulitis.

The presence of cellulitis requires the use of *systemic antibiotics* (see Chapter 190). In most instances, prophylactic use of topical antibiotics (e.g., neomycin, polymyxin, bacitracin) is not recommended because of a high frequency of skin sensitization and resulting allergic dermatitis. *White petrolatum* is an excellent wound dressing in a noninfected ulceration.

Prevention of Stasis Ulcers/Treatment of Stasis Dermatitis

Stasis dermatitis of any degree should be attended to because it can lead to further ulceration. Venous insufficiency and edema should be treated (see Chapter 35). *Topical corticosteroid cream* or *ointment* is useful to reduce the inflammatory component and itching; however, they should not be applied within an ulcer because of delayed wound healing. Oozing dermatitis requires wet dressings (compresses) and bed rest with leg elevation. Acute exudative dermatitis can be soothed and dried with cool *Burow's compresses*. Scratching, use of over-the-counter medications, and placement of adhesive tape on involved areas should be avoided.

Secondarily infected dermatitis should be treated with *oral antibiotics* active against staphylococcal infection, such as *dicloxacillin, amoxicillin/clavulanate* (Augmentin), or *amoxicillin*. *Topical antibiotics* may be used in mild cases. *Topical mupirocin* is effective against a wide range of staphylococci, including methicillin-resistant organisms, and appears to be rarely sensitizing. However, its use should not be continued beyond 14 days because of the risk for the emergence of resistant species with longer use. Preparations containing *neomycin and bacitracin* should be avoided because of the tendency to induce contact sensitization and dermatitis.

External *compressive bandages* or *stockings* should be used to reduce venous pressure in the lower extremities, and compression has been shown to promote healing. Graduated compressive surgical stockings are expensive but can be helpful (see Chapter 35). The patient should apply the compression in the morning before getting out of bed. Prolonged standing should be avoided, weight loss emphasized, and periods of leg elevation encouraged. In refractory cases, *intermittent pneumatic compression* can be used as an alternative to elastic compression; it helps speed ulcer healing but requires specialized equipment and supervised use, usually in an inpatient setting.

Decubitus Ulcers

Nutritional repletion is important to reverse catabolism and to correct all factors that affect the oxygenation of tissue, such as anemia, edema, and vascular problems. *Reducing pressure on the affected area is critical.* In some cases, an alternating-pressure air mattress may be indicated. The basic principle of *debridement* is to use *wet-to-dry dressings* or an occlusive dressing. A variety of biochemical agents that dissolve debris are purported to promote healing, although double-blind evidence of their efficacy is generally lacking. Occasionally, *grafts* are required to close the ulceration.

If decubitus ulcers are complicated by infection, the *antibiotic program* should include anaerobic in addition to aerobic coverage. Even a shallow ulcer may hide a deep infective sinus or a tunnel to an osteomyelitis. A plain film may be useful to detect chronic osteomyelitis.

New measures include the use of growth factors, allografts, and platelet aggregation inhibitors. Increased appreciation for the role of growth factors in the promotion of wound healing has stimulated the testing of various topical growth factors. Nonetheless, the best treatment remains primary prevention.

PATIENT EDUCATION

With most ulcers, prevention is the key. Patients and family must be educated to look for preulcerative changes in stasis dermatitis and use compensatory measures before ulceration occurs. In patients with chronic vascular disease, advice about trimming nails, treating sores early, and seeking medical care at the first sign of a break in skin is important. For people confined to bed or a chair, the family should be educated about preventing prolonged pressure on a bony prominence.

INDICATIONS FOR REFERRAL AND ADMISSION

Failure of ulcers to heal despite good management and a compliant patient indicates the need for surgical consultation. Surgical debridement and split-thickness or full-thickness skin grafting may be necessary. If fever or other signs of bacteremia develop, then intravenous antibiotics and prompt hospitalization are needed. Mortality risk is high, especially with associated anemia and hypoalbuminemia.

THERAPEUTIC RECOMMENDATIONS

Venous Insufficiency and Stasis Dermatitis

- In all patients with changes of stasis, control edema with rest, elevation, diuretics, avoidance of dependency, and external compression with stockings or bandages.
- Treat any concurrent nutritional deficiency, hypertension, diabetes, or congestive heart failure.
- Treat pruritus with moderate-potency topical corticosteroids (e.g., triamcinolone acetonide 0.1%). Ointments are indicated if the area is dry and scaly, and creams should be used if the area is moist. Avoid application on an ulcer because corticosteroids may delay wound healing.
- Treat acute exudative dermatitis with cool Burow's compresses (1:40 dilution) two to three times daily for 30 to 60 minutes.
- Scratching and use of over-the-counter medicaments should be discouraged.

Cutaneous Ulceration

- Prescribe application of wet-to-dry dressings, followed by cleaning and gentle debridement with gauze sponges several times daily. Dilute hydrogen peroxide can be used to clean the ulcerated area.

- Occlusive dressings are worth a trial because they may ease pain, debride ulcers, and lead to healing without the need for surgical intervention.
- In the clinical setting of secondary infection, culture for aerobic and anaerobic bacteria, and treat accordingly with oral or intravenous antibiotics.
- In cases of mild skin infection, a topical antibiotic such as mupirocin can be considered for short-term use (<2 weeks), but preparations that contain neomycin or bacitracin should be avoided.

- In cases of persistent deep ulcers, underlying osteomyelitis should be considered. An x-ray may be useful.
- Refer for surgical consultation patients whose ulcers prove refractory to proper conservative management. Pinch grafting is a relatively simple approach that can be performed in the office. Culture-derived human skin–equivalent grafts (Apligraf) have been quite successful but are very expensive. Becaplermin (recombinant human platelet-derived growth factor BB) gel (Regranex) has been shown to be clinically effective in healing ulcers.
- Surgical debridement and split-thickness or full-thickness skin grafting may be necessary.

Annotated Bibliography

1. Allman RM. Pressure ulcers among the elderly. N Engl J Med 1989;320:850. (*A good discussion of risk factors.*)
2. Angle N, Bergan J. Chronic venous ulcer. Br Med J 1997;314:1019. (*A succinct review of mechanisms by which venous ulcers develop and ways to heal them.*)
3. Dharmarajan TS, Ahmed S. The growing problem of pressure ulcers: evaluation and management for an aging population. Postgrad Med 2003;113:77, 81, 88. (*Presents guidelines for both prevention and treatment.*)
4. Hofman D, Ryan TJ, Arnold F, et al. Pain in venous leg ulcers. J Wound Care 1997;6:2224. (*A prospective study of 140 patients, assessing the prevalence, severity, and diagnostic utility of pain caused by venous leg ulcers.*)
5. Phillips TJ, Dover JS. Leg ulcers. J Am Acad Dermatol 1991;25:965. (*A comprehensive review; 211 references.*)
6. Shai A, Maibach HI, eds. Wound healing and ulcers of the skin: diagnosis and therapy—the practical approach. New York: Springer-Verlag, 2005. (*A concise text discussing all aspects of skin ulceration.*)
7. Weenig RH, Davis MDP, Dahl PR, et al. Skin ulcers misdiagnosed as pyoderma gangrenosum. N Engl J Med 2002;347:1412. (*The Mayo Clinic experience with the condition and approaches to its accurate diagnosis.*)
8. Ahnlide I, Bjellerup M. Efficacy of pinch grafting in leg ulcers of different aetiologies. Acta Derm Venereol 1997;77:144. (*Of 145 therapy-resistant leg ulcers, 36% healed after pinch grafting.*)
9. De Araujo T, Valencia I, Federman DG, et al. Managing the patient with venous ulcers. Ann Intern Med 2003;138:326. (*A very useful review for primary care physicians; 103 references.*)
10. Fletcher A, Cullum N, Sheldon TA. A systematic review of compression treatment for venous leg ulcers. BMJ 1997;315:576. (*Compression systems improve the healing of venous leg ulcers and should be used routinely.*)
11. Landi F, Aloe L, Russo A, et al. Topical treatment of pressure ulcers with nerve growth factor: a randomized clinical trial. Ann Intern Med 2003;139:635. (*A randomized, controlled trial; topical nerve growth factor produced significant improvement in healing.*)
12. Limova M. New therapeutic options for chronic wounds. Dermatol Clin 2002;20:357. (*An excellent short review of newer dressings*).
13. Mol MAE, Nanninga PB, van Eendenburg JP, et al. Grafting of venous leg ulcers. J Am Acad Dermatol 1991;24:77. (*Indications and success of skin grafting of leg ulcers.*)
14. Paquettte D, Badiavas E, Falanga V. Short-contact topical tretinoin therapy to stimulate granulation tissue in chronic wounds. J Am Acad Dermatol 2001;45:382. (*This approach may be worth trying for chronic wounds; it is inexpensive and not time-consuming.*)
15. Sarkar PK, Ballantyne S. Management of leg ulcers. Postgrad Med J 2000;76:674. (*A practical review of the subject as it is handled in the United Kingdom; 100 references.*)
16. Thomas DR. Prevention and treatment of pressure ulcers: what works? what doesn't? Cleve Clin J Med 2001;68:704. (*A comprehensive review of approaches that make things better and those that make things worse; 146 references.*)
17. Lopez P, Dachs R. Effectiveness of dressings for healing venous leg ulcers. Am Family Physician 2007;75:649. (*Finds that no particular dressing is better than another.*)

APPENDIX TO SECTION 12: MINOR SURGICAL OFFICE PROCEDURES FOR SKIN PROBLEMS

PIERRE E. DE DELVA AND CHARLES J. MCCABE

SIMPLE LACERATIONS

Treatment of simple lacerations is one of the most commonly performed outpatient surgical procedures. It is estimated that lacerations account for 8 million procedures per year, most presenting to the emergency department, but a significant number arrive at the primary care physician's office. The physician must assess the wound and decide the appropriateness of repair in the office.

Evaluation and Cleansing

All lacerations should be evaluated for the *extent of injury* to surrounding structures, particularly nerves. This is most important with lacerations of the face, hand, and wrist. All injuries involving *peripheral nerves* should be referred to the emergency department; certain nerve branches can be approximated with excellent long-term benefit. All tendon injuries should receive the attention of a hand surgeon. An orthopedic surgeon should treat those lacerations complicated by bone fracture.

Several principles apply to the management of lacerations. The wound should be thoroughly *irrigated* and all *foreign material removed*. Devitalized tissue is *débrided*, and an assessment of bacterial contamination is made. The *extent of bacterial contamination* can be estimated by the mechanism of injury and the time from injury to presentation. The degree of contamination is balanced against the *anatomic location* of the injury and patient conditions that may impair wound healing. Diabetes, renal failure, obesity, and malnutrition are examples of conditions that hinder wound healing. Facial lacerations are almost always closed, given the excellent blood supply, low risk of infection, and cosmetic considerations. Wounds open for more than 12 hours generally have high bacterial counts and are at risk of infection. Wounds with high bacterial colonization should be left open and treated with dressing changes. Wounds created by animal or human bites are generally left open or are closed in a delayed manner. Bite injuries to the face can be closed, given the excellent blood supply of the face. The physician must balance the cosmetic outcome versus the risk of infection with closure.

Wound Closure

Once the decision is made to close a wound, appropriate instruments are required (Table 1). A sterile field is created, and a plan for anesthesia is made. Field blocks with lidocaine work well. Targeted nerve blocks provide anesthesia without distortion. In general, simple interrupted transcutaneous sutures with a monofilament suture should be used for wound closure (Fig. 1). The location of the wound determines the size of the suture used (Table 2). A running closure is helpful if the purpose is closure and hemostatic control. Skin edges should be everted and brought together under minimal tension. Tension at the skin can be relieved by appropriately placed subcutaneous absorbable sutures. Knots should be laid down away from the laceration line to place the tension from the knot away from the skin edge.

A *sterile dressing* is applied to the wound. In general, *antibiotics* are not necessary. The exception is wounds closed despite a high estimate of bacterial contamination. These patients should be seen in the office within 24 to 48 hours following closure to reevaluate the wound. Patients are instructed to return for suture removal at an interval determined by the location of the wound (Table 2). Wounds should be maintained dry for 48

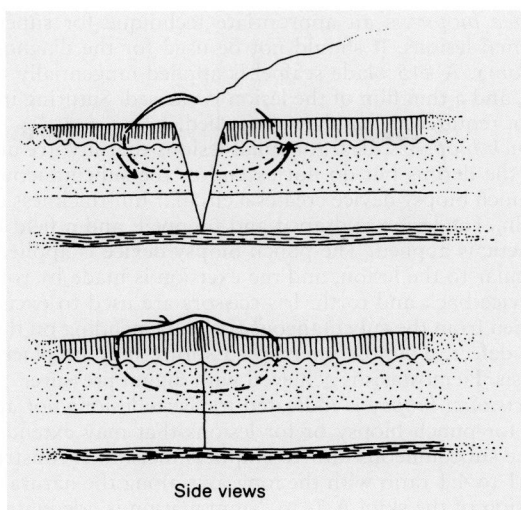

Side views

FIGURE 1. A simple interrupted stitch for skin closure. Note the path of the needle; it enters and leaves the skin at acute angles, which allows eversion of the skin edges. (From Grossman JA. Minor injuries and disorders: surgical and medical care. Philadelphia: Lippincott, 1984:52, with permission.)

hours. Soaking of the wound should be avoided for 1 week. Limiting the exposure of the wound to sunlight for several months after closure is believed to decrease the pigmentation of the scar. With careful patient and wound selection and precise technical execution, most wounds can be expected to heal with an acceptable aesthetic result.

SKIN BIOPSY

Skin cancer is the most commonly diagnosed malignancy, with squamous cell and basal cell cancer accounting for 50% of lesions. Melanoma accounts for a small percentage but is the most serious form of skin cancer. Its incidence has increased steadily (see Chapter 177). Primary care physicians are often called on not only to examine suspicious lesions, but also to provide tissue for pathologic assessment. Benign inflammatory masses and rashes may also require biopsy. Several techniques are available for the biopsy of skin lesions. The correct technique depends on the anatomic location, morphology, and expected pathologic diagnosis.

TABLE 1

LIST OF INSTRUMENTS AND SUPPLIES FOR MINOR SKIN SURGICAL PROCEDURES

Sterile drapes	Prep solution (Betadine/alcohol)
A #15 blade scalpel	Needle holder
Iris scissors	Appropriate suture
Adson forceps	18–30 gauge needles and syringe
Kelly clamp	2 × 2 and 4 × 4 gauze
Skin hooks	

TABLE 2

SUTURE SELECTION AND REMOVAL TIME BASED ON ANATOMIC LOCATION OF INJURY

Location	Sutures	Removal Time (Days)
Scalp	3-0 Nylon	10–14
Face	5-0, 6-0 Nylon	4–5
Neck	3-0, 4-0 Nylon	7–10
Trunk	3-0 Nylon	7–10
Extremities	3-0 Nylon	8–12
Hands	4-0, 5-0 Nylon	8–12
Feet	3-0, 4-0 Nylon	8–12
Oral mucosa	4-0 Vicryl	10–14
Subcutaneous space	3-0, 4-0 Vicryl	N/A

Shave biopsy is an appropriate technique for superficial epidermal lesions. It should not be used for the diagnosis of melanoma. A #15 blade scalpel is applied tangentially to the lesion, and a thin film of the lesion is excised. Suturing in usually not required. A bandage is applied.

Punch biopsy is ideal for small lesions that involve all layers of the dermis but do not extend to the subcutaneous fat. The punch biopsy device creates a circular full-thickness cut of the skin. The lesion is draped and prepped, and a field block anesthetic is applied. The punch biopsy device is applied perpendicular to the lesion, and the excision is made by rotating the device back and forth. Iris scissors are used to excise the specimen from the subcutaneous tissue. Depending on the size of the defect, a simple interrupted suture may be placed for cosmesis. Hemostasis is achieved with digital pressure.

Excisional biopsy is indicated for large lesions not appropriate for punch biopsy or for lesions that may extend deep into the subcutaneous fat. An elliptical incision is constructed in a 3:1 to 4:1 ratio with the long axis along the natural lines of tension of the skin. A 1- to 2-mm margin is adequate for a diagnostic biopsy. The incision is carried down into the subcutaneous fat. Iris scissors are used to excise the specimen from the subcutaneous fat. Interrupted nylon sutures are used to close the incision.

ABSCESS

Subcutaneous abscesses frequently present to the primary care physician. In general, patients present with a painful, indurated, and fluctuant mass. Some patients present with persistent symptoms despite antibiotic treatment. The principle of treatment of subcutaneous abscesses is drainage.

After instillation of local anesthesia, the abscess cavity is incised with a scalpel. Typically, purulence is encountered. A Kelly clamp is introduced into the wound, and all loculations and pockets are disrupted. Cultures should be obtained. The cavity is irrigated with normal saline, and hemostasis is ensured. Abscess cavities in general require at least 24 hours of drainage, which can be accomplished by a Penrose drain or gauze packing. Packing should be changed two to three times per day. Packing or the Penrose drain can be removed once the drainage is normal.

Perianal abscesses deserve special attention. A careful history and examination should precede drainage. Digital rectal exam and anoscopy can help to identify the extent of involvement. Abscesses limited to the superficial perianal area and not associated with a fistula or inflammatory bowel disease may be drained in the office. The threshold for referral to a surgeon should be low. The abscess is drained in similar fashion to the foregoing description. Care must be taken to avoid injury to the anal sphincter complex. Cultures should be sent because infection with anaerobes and/or gram-negative rods may reflect infection from the deep anal glands and higher risk of delayed fistula formation. These patients should have close follow-up. Packing can be removed when the drainage is no longer purulent. Sitz baths maintain cleanliness and promote healing.

SIMPLE PARONYCHIA

Paronychia is a soft tissue infection of the lateral nail border (Fig. 2). The patient usually complains of pain, and the area surrounding the nail base is red, swollen, and tender. The infection often forms a small abscess. Drainage relieves most symptoms.

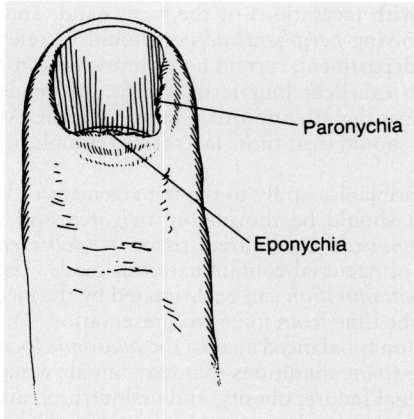

FIGURE 2. Simple paronychia. (From Grossman JA. Minor injuries and disorders: surgical and medical care. Philadelphia: Lippincott, 1984:253, with permission.)

Complete anesthesia of the finger may be accomplished with a metacarpal block (Fig. 3). After alcohol preparation of the skin over the metacarpophalangeal joint is performed, points for needle entrance are selected on the medial and lateral palmar surface of the metacarpal head. Care is taken to aspirate each time before the infiltration of 1 to 2 mL of Xylocaine without epinephrine.

The entire digit, including the metacarpal head, may be washed with a gentle soap solution, followed by application of

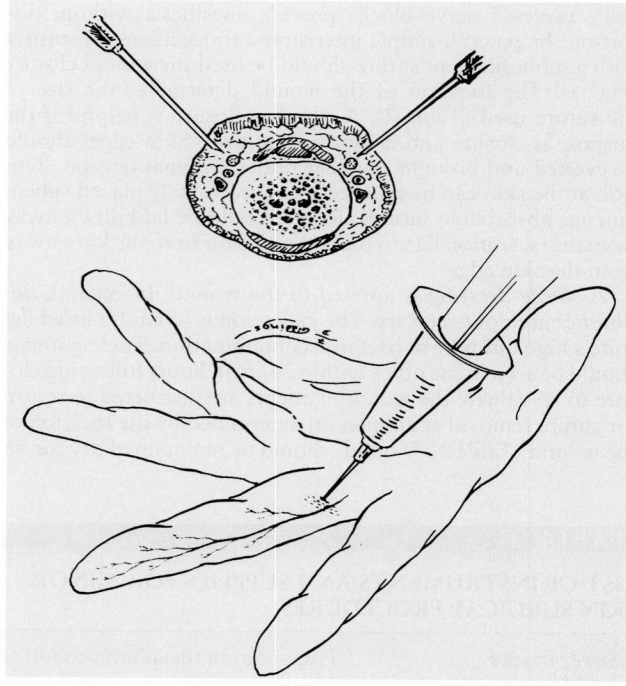

FIGURE 3. Metacarpal block. The entrance of the needle is at the palmar base of the finger, medial and lateral. The needle path is then toward the palmar metacarpal head. (From Van Way CW III, Buerk CA, eds. Surgical skills in patient care. St. Louis, MO: Mosby, 1978:55, with permission.)

a uniform layer of Betadine. Treatment of the laterally based infection involves incising the skin along the lateral edge of the nail; a small incision is made directly under the eponychium, over the swollen, fluctuant area. After drainage of purulent material, a wick may be used to prevent premature wound closure but is often not necessary. The wick is removed after 24 hours, and warm compresses are begun on a twice-daily schedule. Occasionally, a portion of the nail must be removed to establish adequate drainage, particularly if the infection has established penetration of the subungual space. Iris scissors are used to separate the nail from the underlying matrix. This dissection is carried out from the tip of the nail to the base in a vertical strip involving 1/6 to 1/4 inch of the nail surface. The nail is then incised with a #15 blade or a scissors along this vertical line. A Kelly clamp is then used to grasp the portion of nail to be removed and tease the nail from beneath the eponychium.

Xeroform or Vaseline-impregnated gauze is placed within the wound created by nail removal, taking care to place a layer between the matrix and the eponychium to ensure that nail growth can occur in the area of resection. A gauze pad covers this dressing, which is secured in place. Routine administration of antibiotics is unnecessary. However, those patients with diabetes should be placed on antistreptococcal and antistaphylococcal coverage for 7 days.

SUBUNGUAL HEMATOMA

A subungual hematoma occurs when blood accumulates between the nail and the nail matrix as a result of blunt trauma. Pressure on the nail bed causes throbbing pain. Distal phalanx fractures are often associated with large subungual hematomas and must be ruled out with a radiograph. It is important not to miss a nail bed laceration because in the long term, it may lead to nail deformity, and they are difficult to repair in a delayed fashion. Occult nail bed lacerations can be predicted by the size of the hematoma and the presence of nail avulsion or an associated distal phalanx fractures. Small subungual hematomas with minimal symptoms do not need intervention. Symptomatic subungual hematomas can be treated by trephination or removal of the nail.

Trephination involves creating a small hole to allow drainage of the hematoma (Fig. 4). A digital nerve block is not required. A small trephination is created directly over the hematoma with a needle, electrocautery, drill, or heated paper clip. Blood usually spurts from the hole, and relief is immediate. A sterile dressing is applied. Antibiotic coverage is not necessary.

Nail avulsions and hematomas greater than 50% require exploration of the nail bed because of the high incidence of nail bed lacerations. Removal of the nail is performed as described previously. Nail bed lacerations are repaired with interrupted 6-0 absorbable sutures. The nail is then returned to its normal location as a protective splint to promote comfort. A sterile dressing is then applied. Antibiotic coverage is not necessary. Fractures of the distal phalax with associated subungual hematoma should be referred to a hand surgeon.

BURNS

Burns of the skin can result from many sources: flame, steam, scald, electrical, and chemical. These agents cause variable cellular damage to the layers of epidermis, dermis, and subcutaneous fat, depending on the depth. Classification and treat-

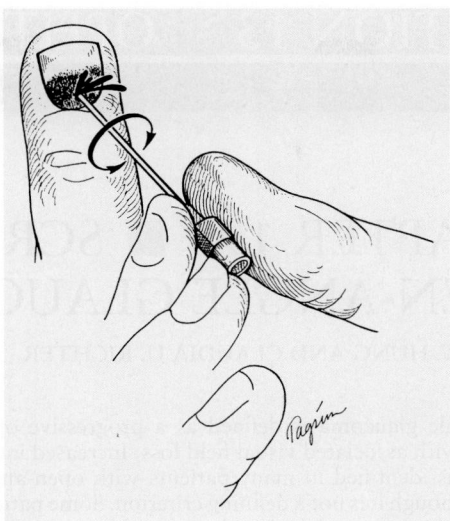

FIGURE 4. Trephination for the management of simple subungual hematoma.

ment of burn wounds is based on the depth and the surface area of skin involved. First-degree burns are those that involve the superficial layers of the epidermis. Second-degree burns involve the epidermis and dermis; a broad distinction is made between superficial and deep burns, based on the amount of dermis involved. Deep second-degree burns involve the entire papillary dermis, with penetration to some or all of the reticular dermis. Third-degree burns involve all layers of the epidermis and dermis, with penetration into underlying fat and muscle.

The surface area of burns has traditionally been based on the rule of nines. Each arm is considered 9% of the body surface area, each leg is 18%, the anterior and the posterior trunk are each 18% the head is 9%, and perineum/genitalia is 1%.

Using these classifications, the treatment of burns can proceed in an organized fashion. All second-degree burns covering more than 10% of the body, all third-degree burns, any burns associated with electrical current, and all burns of the ears, eyes, face, hands, feet, or perineum should be immediately referred to a major hospital familiar with burn care. The remaining first-degree burns and second-degree burns covering less than 10% of the body can be cared for on an outpatient basis with adequate wound care and follow-up.

Office-based management of the burn wound begins with gentle washing with soapy water. Chemical burns should undergo a generous lavage. Second-degree burns often cause blistering of the skin. Unruptured blisters should be left intact because they serve as a biologic dressing. Ruptured blisters are debrided with scissors. Most burn wounds managed in the office setting will heal with dressing changes. Silvadene cream is applied to the surface of the burn in a thin, even layer. Application with a tongue depressor works nicely. Silvadene is subsequently covered with dry gauze pads, which are secured with rolled gauze. Complete dressing change should then be done twice daily, with complete cleansing of the wound before a new dressing is applied. Healing for first-degree burns can be expected in 3 to 4 days; second-degree burns require 10 to 20 days. Scald and chemical burns can progress from second to third degree over several hours and should have close follow-up. Failure of healing should prompt referral to a burn center.

CHAPTER 198 ■ SCREENING FOR OPEN-ANGLE GLAUCOMA

JAMES W. HUNG AND CLAUDIA U. RICHTER

Open-angle glaucoma is defined as a progressive optic neuropathy with associated visual field loss. Increased intraocular pressure is identified in many patients with open-angle glaucoma, although it is not a defining criterion. Some patients with glaucoma have normal intraocular pressures, whereas some patients with elevated intraocular pressure do not have an associated optic neuropathy. Screening for glaucoma by checking eye pressures alone is insufficient. Careful fundoscopic evaluation of the optic nerve is essential, particularly for those in high-risk categories, for the identification of affected patients. The disease is typically asymptomatic until the later stages, when irreversible vision loss occurs. Therefore, it is critical that patients be identified as early as possible and appropriate treatment initiated. Once the glaucoma is diagnosed, vision loss can be prevented or minimized as the patient's intraocular pressure is controlled medically or surgically.

EPIDEMIOLOGY AND RISK FACTORS (1–6)

Open-angle glaucoma affects approximately 2.2 million persons in the United States, 50% of whom are unaware that they have a vision-threatening disease. It is a leading cause of legal blindness in the United States, and the leading cause of legal blindness among African Americans. Given the aging of the U.S. population, the number of affected persons is expected to increase to more than 3 million by 2020. It is estimated that blindness from glaucoma costs more than $1.5 billion annually in Social Security benefits, lost income tax revenues, and health care expenditures.

Important risk factors include *elevated intraocular pressure, age, African descent,* and *family history.* Glaucoma is five times more likely to occur in African Americans than in whites and leads to blindness in African Americans about four times more often than in whites. Other, less strongly correlated risk factors are myopia, diabetes, thin corneal thickness, and vasospasm (as in migraine).

Elevated intraocular pressure is one of the most important risk factors and is currently the only modifiable risk factor. Intraocular pressure in normal eyes ranges from 10 to 21 mm Hg and is skewed in distribution to the higher pressures. Patients with eye pressures of greater than 21 mm Hg without optic nerve damage are described as ocular hypertensives or glaucoma suspects. Patients with an intraocular pressure of less than 22 mm Hg but with glaucomatous nerve damage and associated visual field loss are diagnosed with normal-tension glaucoma. This entity may account for up to 15% of open-angle glaucoma cases. The pathogenesis of normal-tension glaucoma is not completely clear. Regardless of the type of glaucoma, studies have repeatedly demonstrated that lowering the intraocular pressure can stop or slow the progression of optic nerve damage.

PATHOPHYSIOLOGY, NATURAL HISTORY, AND EFFECTIVENESS OF EARLY THERAPY (7–13)

The essential pathophysiologic feature of glaucoma is loss of ganglion cell axons and the development of optic neuropathy and visual field loss. The exact mechanism of optic nerve damage has not been established and is probably due to a combination of factors. Mechanical ischemia of the optic nerve, caused by elevated intraocular pressure and increased vascular resistance or small-blood-vessel disease, can result in loss of ganglion cell axons. Increased intraocular pressure can also interfere with axoplasmic flow in the ganglion cell axons, causing cell dysfunction and death. The lamina cribrosa—the sievelike structure through which axons pass when leaving the eye—may lose support for the ganglion cell axons, resulting in interference with axonal function. Apoptosis may also play a role in the development of glaucoma. These different mechanisms of axonal damage are of variable importance in different patients, but the final result is a loss of ganglion cells and their axons, optic nerve cupping, and visual field loss.

The relationship between intraocular pressure and visual loss, as manifested by field defects, is highly variable among individuals. For instance, not every person with elevated intraocular pressure will develop glaucoma. The incidence of the development of glaucomatous field defects among patients with ocular hypertension is 5 to 10 per 1,000 per year. Therefore, the rationale that not every ocular hypertensive patient needs therapeutic intervention can be argued. However, these patients are often carefully monitored every 6 to 12 months with serial visual fields and other optic nerve evaluations in an attempt to detect progressive optic neuropathy. Glaucomatous visual field loss is irreversible, but reduction in intraocular pressure significantly reduces the risk of disease progression (optic nerve damage and visual field loss) both in early and advanced forms of disease; however, in nearly half of patients, the disease progresses despite reduction in pressure. Nonetheless, early diagnosis and treatment are important because the optic nerve becomes increasingly vulnerable to further damage once initial damage has occurred.

SCREENING METHODS (12,14–17)

No single test is sufficiently sensitive or specific for screening, but the use of a combination of measures helps to maximize disease detection. There is now a Medicare glaucoma screening benefit for patients who are at high risk of the disease. This should increase access to care and increase screening populations.

Measurement of Intraocular Pressure—Tonometry

Tonometry has been the most widely used screening test for glaucoma because it is a means of detecting its principal risk factor, increased intraocular pressure. Unfortunately, there is no level of intraocular pressure above which damage to the optic nerve and visual loss always occurs or below which glaucomatous damage never occurs.

Statistically, the mean intraocular pressure in normal adults is 15 to 16 mm Hg. Some patients with glaucoma have screening intraocular pressures less than 21 mm Hg, and many individuals with intraocular pressure repeatedly greater than 21 mm Hg do not have and may never develop glaucomatous damage. No particular value provides an optimal balance between sensitivity and specificity. A pressure value of 18 mm Hg is associated with a test sensitivity of 65% and a specificity of 65%.

The accuracy of intraocular pressure measurement is affected by corneal thickness: Thicker corneas artificially inflate eye pressure measurements, whereas thinner corneas cause underestimated measurements. The measurement of central corneal thickness assists in interpreting tonometry readings, and several nomograms have been developed to include corrective factors in eye pressure measurements and the necessary adjustments. However, intraocular pressure also needs to be interpreted in the context of risk factors and findings from the rest of the examination.

Ophthalmoscopy

Screening can be made more effective by including an assessment of optic nerve status, either by examining the appearance of the optic nerve and retinal nerve fiber layer or by testing visual functions. Changes in the contour of the optic cup in the center of the optic disc provide the first definitive evidence of glaucomatous damage. The usual cup has a round, regular contour. The cup in early glaucoma becomes notched on the superotemporal or inferotemporal rim. Later changes include an increase in the depth and width of the physiologic cup (customarily expressed as an increase in the *cup-to-disc ratio*), nasal displacement of the central retinal vessels, and progressive *pallor of the optic nerve head*. Other disc changes associated with glaucoma are asymmetric discs and disc hemorrhages. The preferred technique for optic nerve evaluation involves magnified stereoscopic visualization (as with a slit-lamp biomicroscope) through a dilated pupil.

Limits to ophthalmoscopy include wide variability among observers in assessments of optic nerve status, the need for highly trained personnel, and the possible need to dilate the pupils to allow adequate visualization. The advent of computer-assisted optic nerve imaging may improve the validity and reliability of traditional cup-to-disc ratio estimates, but expense, immobility, and complexity of use make these techniques inappropriate for mass population screenings.

Visual Field Testing

The diagnosis of glaucoma includes decreased visual function, beginning in the far peripheral vision. The utility of visual field testing is predicated on the presence of visual field defects. Typically, early defects are only identified by a formal manual or automated visual field test. However, such testing is inadequate for mass glaucoma screening because of the time and technical difficulty in performing an adequate examination, the low sensitivity of manual visual field techniques, and the low specificity of automated visual field methods.

Nerve Fiber Layer Analysis

Computer-assisted nerve fiber layer analysis may detect glaucomatous optic nerve damage before optic nerve cupping is visible or visual field defects are detectable. Various modalities include optical coherence tomography, scanning laser polarimetry, and confocal scanning laser ophthalmoscopy. These technologies have high equipment costs, a high level of operator variability, and relatively immobile machinery. In addition, nerve fiber layer analysis has a high rate of false positives and false negatives for glaucomatous damage and therefore is not practical for screening examinations.

RECOMMENDATIONS

- Glaucoma is a condition that should be screened for because it is prevalent, there is effective treatment, treatment in the asymptomatic period improves outcomes, and there are reasonable means of detection.
- Multimodality screening is required and best performed by the ophthalmologist rather than the primary care physician because it entails many of the elements of a standard ophthalmologic examination and can be done as part of it.
- The primary care physician should participate in screening for glaucoma by checking for characteristic changes in the optic cup during routine fundoscopic examination, identifying other risk factors, and directing patients to appropriate ophthalmic care.
- The frequency of screening depends on the risk factors of each patient. Asymptomatic African Americans should be screened every 3 to 5 years between ages 20 and 39 years, every 2 to 4 years between ages 40 and 64 years, and every 1 to 2 years at age 65 years and older. Other asymptomatic patients need to be screened less than every 3 to 5 years between ages 20 and 39 years, every 2 to 4 years between ages 40 and 64 years, and every 1 to 2 years at age 65 years and older.
- Automated perimetry and/or nerve fiber layer analysis may be a valuable screening adjunct in the future, but current technological costs are too high, false positives too frequent, and the equipment too immobile to recommend these at present.

Annotated Bibliography

1. Armaly MF, Krueger DE, Maunder L, et al. Biostatistical analysis of the Collaborative Glaucoma Study. I. Summary report of the risk factors for glaucomatous visual-field defects. Arch Ophthalmol 1980;98:2163. (*Identifies five risk factors related to the development of glaucomatous visual field defects: outflow facility, age, applanation pressure, cup-to-disc ratio, and pressure change after water drinking.*)

2. Sommer A, Tielsch JM, Katz J, et al. Relationship between intraocular pressure and primary open angle glaucoma among white and black Americans. The Baltimore Eye Survey. Arch Ophthalmol 1991;109:1090. (*Presents results confirming that intraocular pressure [IOP] is an important risk factor in glaucoma, but not supporting the traditional distinction between "normal" and "elevated" pressure.*)

3. Friedman D, Wolfs R, O'Colmain B, et al. Prevalence of open-angle glaucoma among adults in the United States. Arch Ophthalmol 2004;122(4):532. (*A meta-analysis of population-based studies in the United States, Europe, and Australia applied to 2000 U.S. census data, calculating the prevalence in black and white populations, as well as estimated increases in future years.*)

4. Sommer A, Tielsch JM, Katz J, et al. Racial differences in the cause-specific prevalence of blindness in East Baltimore. N Engl J Med 1991;325:1412. (*Whites are more likely to have age-related macular degeneration, and blacks are more likely to have primary open-angle glaucoma.*)

5. Tielsch JM, Katz J, Singh K, et al. A population-based evaluation of glaucoma screening: the Baltimore Eye Survey. Am J Epidemiol 1991;134:1102. (*Includes useful data on the sensitivity and specificity of screening methods, as well as prevalence data in particular populations at risk.*)

6. The Advanced Glaucoma Intervention Study (AGIS): 3. Baseline characteristics of black and white patients. Ophthalmology 1998;105:1137. (*Confirms that visual field defects in patients with open-angle glaucoma are more severe in blacks than in whites.*)

7. Wolfs RC, Klaver CC, Ramrattan RS, et al. Genetic risk of primary open-angle glaucoma. Population-based familial aggregation study. Arch Ophthalmol 1998;116:1640. (*The prevalence of glaucoma was 10.4% in siblings of patients, 1.1% in offspring of patients, 0.1% in siblings of controls, and 0% in offspring of controls.*)

8. Alward WLM. Medical management of glaucoma. N Engl J Med 1998;339:1298. (*A review of data on the efficacy of medical management that lowers pressure, showing it to be effective.*)

9. Gordon MO, Beiser JA, Brandt JD, et al. The Ocular Hypertension Treatment Study: baseline factors that predict the onset of primary open-angle glaucoma. Arch Ophthalmol 2002;120:714. (*A randomized, controlled trial, finding that pressure lowering reduced the risk of progression to early glaucoma in patients with ocular hypertension.*)

10. Leske MC, Heijl A, Hussein M, et al. Factors for glaucoma progression and the effect of treatment: the Early Manifest Glaucoma Trial. Arch Ophthalmol 2003;121:48. (*A 10% reduction in the risk of progression occurred with every 1-mm Hg drop in IOP, but 45% of treated patients had visual deterioration despite well-controlled IOP.*)

11. Janz NK, Wren PA, Lichter PR, et al. Quality of life in newly diagnosed glaucoma patients: the Collaborative Initial Glaucoma Treatment Study. Ophthalmology 2001;108:887. (*Demonstrates the efficacy of treatment to lower pressure in newly diagnosed patients.*)

12. Levi L, Schwartz B. Glaucoma screening in the health care setting. Surv Ophthalmol 1983;28:164. (*Concludes that physicians should use ophthalmoscopy in screening.*)

13. Quigley HA. Open-angle glaucoma. N Engl J Med 1993;328:1097. (*A comprehensive review; 114 references and excellent photographs.*)

14. Van Veldhuisen PC, Schwartz AL, Gaasterland DE, et al. The advanced glaucoma intervention study (AGIS): 7. The relationship between control of intraocular pressure and visual field deterioration. Am J Ophthalmol 2000;130:429. (*Documents a reduction in visual loss with reduction in pressure in persons with advanced disease.*)

15. Margolis KL, Money BE, Kopietz LA, et al. Physician recognition of ophthalmoscopic signs of open-angle glaucoma. J Gen Intern Med 1989;4:296. (*An educational program that includes good photographs of the key findings.*)

16. Mundorf TK, Zimmerman TJ, Nardin GF, et al. Automated perimetry, tonometry, and questionnaire in glaucoma screening. Am J Ophthalmol 1989;108:505. (*Tonometry alone is much less sensitive than perimetry.*)

17. Javitt J, Lee P, Lum F. The value of regular examinations to detect glaucoma and other chronic conditions among older Americans. Ophthalmology 2007;114(5):833. (*Medicare established a glaucoma screening benefit for individuals who are at high risk for the disease, and many private insurance companies followed suit.*)

CHAPTER 199 ■ EVALUATION OF THE RED EYE

NICOLETTA FYNN-THOMPSON AND CLAUDIA U. RICHTER

The red eye is the most common eye problem encountered by the primary care physician. Most cases represent benign, self-limited disorders that can be expeditiously diagnosed and treated by the primary physician; however, because redness of the eye may signal serious disease that threatens vision, the physician must be aware of the differential diagnosis and conduct a proper initial evaluation.

PATHOPHYSIOLOGY AND CLINICAL PRESENTATION (1–6)

Redness of the eye and the periocular tissues reflects *inflammation* or *hemorrhage*. Causes of inflammation include bacterial, viral, chlamydial, and fungal infections; allergic responses; immune disorders; elevated intraocular pressure; environmental and pharmacologic irritants; foreign bodies;

and trauma. Hemorrhage may be idiopathic or due to laceration, contusion, coagulopathy, concomitant infection, or strenuous activity. Much less commonly, eyelid redness may be the presenting sign of benign or malignant eyelid *neoplasms* or be due to local dermatoses or systemic immunologic disease.

The pattern of conjunctival injection provides important clues to etiology. Corneal or intraocular inflammation produces *ciliary flush*—dilation of the fine capillaries around the corneal border—which produces a red-violet halo around the cornea. Larger, deep episcleral vessels may also be engorged. Primary conjunctivitis induces diffuse vessel engorgement on the palpebral and bulbar conjunctiva without a ciliary flush. The clinical presentations of various causes of red eye are distinctive (Table 199.1).

A red eye may be due to pathology in the conjunctiva, cornea, uveal tract, eyelids, or orbit.

TABLE 199.1

SOME IMPORTANT CAUSES OF RED EYE

Conjunctival Disease
Infection (bacterial, viral, chlamydial)
Allergy
Foreign body
Subconjunctival hemorrhage
Pinguecula
Pterygium
Episcleritis
Scleritis
Abrasion

Corneal Disease
Abrasion ((with or without concomitant infection)
Herpes simplex/herpes zoster
Abrasion
Keratoconjunctivitis sicca
Exposure keratopathy
Chemical trauma
Corneal ulceration (with or without concomitant infection)

Uveal Tract Disease
Primary iritis and choroiditis
Secondary iritis (infection, trauma)
Recurrent iritis from systemic diseases

Diseases of the Eyelid and Orbit
Blepharitis
Chalazion
Hordeolum
Dacryocystitis
Cellulitis
Hemorrhage

Intraocular Disease
Acute glaucoma

Conjunctival Pathology

Conjunctivitis

Conjunctivitis is the most common cause of a red eye. Discharge with crusted eyelids stuck together in the morning, conjunctival erythema (especially of the peripheral bulbar segment), normal vision, lids, and absence of photophobia are the major manifestations. The etiology may be infectious, allergic, or chemical.

Bacterial conjunctivitis is characterized by a mucopurulent discharge and usually occurs unilaterally without preauricular adenopathy. The eyelids have a thick crust on them after a night's sleep. *Streptococcus pneumoniae*, *Staphylococcus aureus*, and *Haemophilus influenzae* are the most common etiologic pathogens. A severe, hyperacute conjunctivitis suggests *Neisseria infection*, which may scar or perforate the cornea, leading to systemic dissemination. Chronic conjunctivitis is often due to *Staphylococcus aureus* or *Moraxella lacunata*. *Chlamydial conjunctivitis*, transmitted from the genitourinary tract, occurs as bilateral *"inclusion conjunctivitis"* in sexually active young adults, differing in presentation from typical bacterial conjunctivitis by a prominent follicular conjunctival response and preauricular adenopathy. *Trachoma* is a major cause of blindness and affects approximately 400 million individuals worldwide but is rare in the United States, except among Native Americans in the Southwest. However, the

rapidly increasing rate of chlamydial cervicitis (see Chapter 115) among young women raises the risk of trachoma in a much wider population of newborns.

Viral conjunctivitis is characterized by watery, sometimes mucoid discharge, often beginning in one eye and spreading to the other eye several days later. Preauricular adenopathy is common. It may be associated with fever and pharyngitis (pharyngoconjunctival fever), particularly in children. Epidemic keratoconjunctivitis is a highly contagious adenoviral infection that may be accompanied by corneal epithelial defects in the first week and subepithelial infiltrates in the second week, sometimes causing a diminution of vision. Pseudomembranes or scarring of the conjunctiva may occur and sometimes is painful.

Allergic conjunctivitis may be associated with seasonal allergies and atopic dermatitis and is characterized by bilateral itching and tearing. Vernal keratoconjunctivitis is a chronic recurrent hypersensitivity reaction that may lead to the formation of corneal ulcers.

Bilateral sterile conjunctival inflammation can occur in patients with acne rosacea, Reiter's syndrome, and Stevens–Johnson syndrome. Patient's with *acne rosacea* may have associated lid inflammation (*blepharitis*) and develop concomitant sterile marginal corneal ulcers with chronic staphylococcal infection.

Hypersensitivity

Sensitivity to eye medications may cause erythema of the external lids, especially at the lateral canthus with an associated conjunctivitis. *Angioneurotic edema* of the lids may occur bilaterally as an allergic response to a systemic allergen—often food—or unilaterally secondary to exposure to local allergens such as topical chemicals, poison ivy, and insect bites; it develops rapidly and resolves in 1 to 2 days. Edema without erythema suggests allergy, not infection.

Pinguecula and Pterygium

Pinguecula is a yellow-white, harmless nodule of the scleral conjunctiva, usually found on the nasal side and causing mild discoloration; calcific changes may be present. The condition results from heavy exposure to ultraviolet light (actinic exposure). A more problematic consequence of ultraviolet light exposure is a *pterygium*, which is characterized by wing-shaped, fibrovascular conjunctival tissue growth and redness potentially encroaching on the cornea, with the risk of impairing vision.

Subconjunctival Hemorrhage

Subconjunctival hemorrhages are associated with minor trauma. In many instances the trauma is unapparent and seemingly without provocation. More pronounced hemorrhage usually occurs secondary to obvious trauma. Massive hemorrhage leading to proptosis and limited extraocular movements signals orbital hemorrhage, which may compromise the optic nerve and retinal circulation. Subconjunctival hemorrhages may also appear during an acute conjunctivitis. Systemic causes include impaired clotting and venous congestion (Valsalva maneuver). Clinical findings include a focal or diffuse patch of redness on the conjunctiva, without associated discharge or itching,

Foreign Body

A foreign body on the bulbar conjunctiva or under either the upper or lower lid may result in copious tearing, conjunctival injection, and a sensation that something has gotten "into" the eye. On occasion, the foreign body may be well tolerated, with the eye remaining white and quiet.

Episcleritis

This is usually a benign inflammation of superficial episcleral vessels, but in recurrent cases (associated with connective tissue disease, gout, herpes, syphilis, tuberculosis, and rosacea), the conjunctiva may manifest areas of circumscribed nodular inflammation and the patient complains of a mildly tender, red eye. Vision and lids are normal, the corneas are clear, and the conjunctivae show local raised areas of redness.

Scleritis

Scleritis—a potentially destructive, severely painful inflammation of the collagen in the sclera and deep episcleral vessels—is a rare condition associated with autoimmune connective tissue diseases, vasculitides, infectious disorders, and metabolic disorders. An experienced observer is required to make the diagnosis.

Corneal Disease

Keratitis—inflammation of the cornea—presents with a perilimbal ciliary flush, accompanied by tearing and photophobia. Dry eyes can cause intense reactions secondary to superficial keratitis, as does overuse of contact lenses (corneal hypoxia) and ultraviolet keratitis.

Corneal ulcers detected by fluorescein staining may be sterile or caused by bacteria, viruses, or fungi. A focal area of haze or opacification of the cornea is often visible. Particularly distinctive is the *"dendritic" figure* of herpes simplex keratitis, in which the epithelium stains in a fine, branching pattern. Herpes simplex and zoster may also cause broader "geographic" defects. *S. aureus* may cause a sterile infiltrate in the corneal limbus.

Corneal abrasions stain with fluorescein but have no infiltrate unless they are untreated for several days. *Hyphema* (blood layering in the anterior chamber) indicates severe trauma and requires ophthalmologic consultation. *Recurrent erosion* presents as an epithelial defect at the site of an abrasion that occurred months or years before and was often caused by organic material (e.g., a tree branch, a fingernail). It may also occur in corneal dystrophies. In both instances, it is due to a defect in epithelial adherence to the underlying stroma.

A *corneal foreign body* may cause tearing, hyperemia, and the sensation of a foreign body. This is particularly true of rust rings left by ferrous foreign bodies.

Corneal laceration with perforation is suggested by a shallow or absent anterior chamber, markedly decreased intraocular pressure, and eccentric pupil with iris prolapse into the wound.

Chemical keratoconjunctivitis is a common industrial injury due to exposure to an irritant chemical solution. The conjunctiva is uniformly red, the pupil constricted, vision decreased, the cornea hazy, and the eye painful because of spasm of the iris.

Uveal Tract Disease

Uveitis

Uveitis refers to inflammation of the uveal tract, including the iris, ciliary body, and choroid. *Iritis* (anterior uveitis) presents with eye pain, photophobia, redness, and pupillary contraction, ciliary flush, and decreased vision. It may be unilateral or bilateral; if it is unilateral, the affected pupil is smaller than that of the other eye because of iris spasm or synechiae. Flashlight examination shows a slightly cloudy anterior chamber. Slit-lamp examination discloses cells in the anterior chamber (aqueous cellular reaction) and "flare" (increased vascular permeability). Inflammatory cells, called "keratic precipitates," may collect in clusters on the posterior cornea.

Iritis and uveitis are usually idiopathic but may be associated with a large number of systemic and ocular diseases, including ankylosing spondylitis, Behçet's syndrome, sarcoidosis, and juvenile rheumatoid arthritis. Infectious and neoplastic diseases are other causes accompanied by posterior segment involvement (posterior uveitis). Ocular trauma can result in reactive iritis.

Eyelid and Orbital Disease

Blepharitis

Blepharitis results from inflammation (both infectious and noninfectious) of the structures of the lid margin and presents as lid-margin redness, scaling, and crusting. *Staphylococcal blepharitis* produces dry scales, lash loss, and sometimes conjunctivitis and corneal limbal infiltrates. *Seborrheic blepharitis* and *meibomian gland dysfunction* are associated with chronic oily secretions causing irritation and dilated vessels at the posterior lid margin in association with conjunctiva inflammation; examination of the margin may reveal inspissated sebaceous material. Meibomian gland dysfunction is frequently associated with seborrheic dermatitis and acne rosacea. Blepharitis tends to be chronic with acute flare-ups and is more common in fair-skinned people. Table 199.2 lists other causes of eyelid inflammation.

Hordeolum

Hordeolum is an acute inflammatory or infectious nodule of the meibomian glands (internal hordeolum), the glands of Zeis, or lash follicles (external hordeolum or sty). It presents as a red, tender mass near the eyelid margin. An internal hordeolum may point to either the skin or the conjunctival side of the lid, whereas an external hordeolum always points to the skin. Hordeolum may produce a diffuse superficial lid infection known as "preseptal cellulitis."

Chalazion

Chalazion is a sterile chronic granulomatous inflammation of a Zeis or meibomian gland, which may be tender and mildly inflamed or a quiet discrete mass.

Acute Dacryocystitis

This localized infection of the tear ducts and/or lacrimal sac over the lateral nose presents as focal tenderness to palpation and the expression of purulent material from the tear duct on the application of pressure.

Hemorrhage

Bleeding into the lids or forehead, either spontaneous or traumatic, may rapidly dissect along the tissue planes of the lids and cause an impressive generalized ecchymosis, which can greatly alarm the patient.

OTHER CAUSES OF EYELID INFLAMMATION

Condition	Cause
Bacterial infection	Impetigo
	Erysipelas
Viral infection	Herpes simplex
	Molluscum contagiosum
	Varicella-zoster
	Papillomavirus
Parasitic infection	*Pthirus pubis*
Immunologic skin condition	Atopic dermatitis
	Contact dermatitis
	Erythema multiforme
	Pemphigus foliaceus
	Connective tissue disorders
	Lupus erythematosus
	Dermatomyositis
Dermatoses	Psoriasis
	Ichthyosis
	Exfoliative
	Erythroderma
Benign eyelid tumors	Pseudoepitheliomatous
	hyperplasia
	Actinic keratosis
	Squamous cell papilloma
	Sebaceous gland hyperplasia
	Hemangioma
	Pyogenic granuloma
Malignant eyelid tumors	Basal cell carcinoma
	Squamous cell carcinoma
	Sebaceous cell carcinoma
	Melanoma
	Kaposi's sarcoma
Other	Neurofibromatosis
	Sarcoidosis
	Down's syndrome

Orbital Cellulitis

Orbital cellulitis is a serious infectious condition presenting as swollen, red eyelids with chemosis, exophthalmos, pain, fever, and leukocytosis. Organisms enter the orbit either directly from disruption of the normal skin barrier or through the sinuses or venous channels. If it progresses, it may lead to paresis of the third, fourth, and sixth cranial nerves or the ophthalmic division of the fifth, which are signs of the very serious complication *cavernous sinus thrombosis*.

Intraocular Disease

Acute Glaucoma

This is an ocular emergency that presents as a painful red eye with prominent ciliary flush. The pupil is mid-dilated and fixed, and the cornea is cloudy secondary to edema. Intraocular pressure exceeds 40 mm Hg and may reach 70 to 80 mm Hg. The patient reports cloudy vision, colored rings around lights (due to corneal edema), and unilateral headache, often accompanied by nausea and vomiting, which occasionally leads the physician to consider an acute abdomen. Acute glaucoma is usually due to angle closure in eyes with susceptible narrow angles, but it

may be due to inflammatory cells or red blood cells in the anterior chamber, neovascularization of the iris (rubeosis iridis), or peripheral anterior synechiae.

DIFFERENTIAL DIAGNOSIS (3,4,6)

The causes of red eye can be divided anatomically into the categories of conjunctival, corneal, uveal, eyelid–orbital, and intraocular disease (Table 199.1). Differentiation can usually be made on clinical grounds (Table 199.3).

WORKUP (3,4,6)

History

The history is directed toward ascertaining the duration of redness, the rapidity of onset, the patient's activity at the time, and the degree and quality of symptoms. Ophthalmologic history and medications should be noted. Key symptoms include visual changes, pain, itching, crusting in the morning, tearing, mucoid or purulent discharge, photophobia, and foreign-body sensation. One should note that, although it is usually helpful, the history can be misleading. For example, viral conjunctivitis may be accompanied by itching or a foreign-body sensation, or the patient may ascribe the symptoms of herpes simplex keratitis to a "chemical in the eye" because the symptoms were first noted after, for example, a home hair permanent.

Physical Examination

Accurate measurement of visual acuity, preferably at a distance, is essential. If it is abnormal, it is important to check for uncorrected optical abnormality by the use of a pinhole. Any patient with reduced vision not readily explained by a preexisting or obviously harmless condition needs to be immediately referred to an ophthalmologist. Mucus and tearing may reduce vision one or two lines at most. Corneal lesions may further reduce vision, with only partial improvement on pinhole testing; a central epithelial abrasion typically maintains vision at about 20/100 or better. Preauricular nodes should be palpated. A complete examination of the eye and fundus is important. The lid margins should be inspected for crusting, ulceration, inspissations, and masses and the conjunctiva for the distribution of redness, ciliary flush, foreign bodies (including lid eversion), and, if a slit lamp is available, follicles and papillae. Corneal clarity is noted with a flashlight, and a direct ophthalmoscope set at about +15 diopters can be used to magnify corneal details.

If *fluorescein stain* is available, it can be used in conjunction with a blue filter to visualize the cornea for abrasions, infection, and other injury. However, if there is any suspicion of corneal injury, referral is needed quickly for slit-lamp examination.

Intraocular pressure should be determined if acute angle-closure glaucoma is suspected. The depth of the anterior chamber of the other eye can be assessed by aiming a flashlight parallel to the iris (coronal plane) from the temporal side. A shallow anterior chamber is usually convex and will cast a shadow on the nasal iris.

Laboratory Studies

Most testing is done by the ophthalmologist, but the primary practitioner may attempt *conjunctival smears*, which

TABLE 199.3

THE RED EYE

	Conjunctivitis			Corneal Injury or Infection	Iritis	Acute Glaucoma
	Bacterial	Viral	Allergic			
Vision	−	−	−	↓ or ↓↓	↓	↓↓
Pain	−	−	−	+	+	+++
Photophobia	−	±	−	+	++	−
Foreign-body sensation	−	±	±	+	−	−
Itch	±	±	++	−	−	−
Tearing	+	++	+	++	+	−
Discharge	Mucopurulent	Mucoid	−	−	−	−
Preauricular adenopathy	−	+	−	*a*	−	−
Pupils	−	−	−	NL or small[b]	Small	Mid-dilated and fixed
Conjunctival hyperemia	Diffuse	Diffuse	Diffuse	Diffuse and ciliary flush	Ciliary flush	Diffuse and ciliary flush
Cornea	Clear	Sometimes faint punctate staining or infiltrates	Clear	Depends on disorder	Clear or lightly cloudy	Cloudy
Intraocular pressure	NL	NL	NL	*c*	↓,NL, or ↑	↑↑

NL, normal
[a]In herpes keratitis.
[b]Indicates secondary iritis.
[c]Very low in perforating trauma.

show polymorphonuclear leukocytes in acute bacterial conjunctivitis, lymphocytes in viral or late bacterial conjunctivitis, and eosinophils in allergic reactions. Such smears are time-consuming and generally not necessary, but they can be helpful in recurrent or recalcitrant cases. Purulent discharges should be *cultured* on blood agar and, if *Neisseria* is suspected, plated on chocolate agar and Gram's stained. Scrapings for inclusion bodies in suspected chlamydial and viral disease are usually unrewarding, and scraping and culturing an infected corneal ulcer requires an ophthalmologist.

White blood cell and *differential counts* are indicated, as are *blood cultures*, in suspected cellulitis. Clotting studies for subconjunctival hemorrhage are not indicated unless other evidence of coagulopathy is present (see Chapter 81) or the patient is being treated with anticoagulants (see Chapter 83).

PRINCIPLES OF MANAGEMENT AND INDICATIONS FOR REFERRAL (1–10)

Red eye problems associated with eye pain, visual disturbance, or corneal abnormality require immediate referral, as does acute glaucoma. In most other situations, the primary physician can provide symptomatic relief or at least first aid. A nonophthalmologist should never prescribe topical steroid or steroid–antibiotic combination drops because infection may worsen and a corneal ulcer may rapidly form and cause perforation.

Conjunctival Disease

Conjunctivitis, in the absence of photophobia, eye pain, or change in visual acuity, can be managed by the primary physician.

Viral Conjunctivitis

The infection is contagious, and live virus is shed in the tears for up to 2 weeks. The patient should be instructed to refrain from rubbing the eye and transmitting infection to the other eye or to another person. Treatment is supportive because the condition is self-limited, usually clearing within 2 to 3 weeks. Cold compresses and lubricants may decrease some of the irritation the patient experiences. Topical antibiotics (see later discussion) are commonly prescribed for 7 to10 days, based on the observation that their use shortens the duration of illness. Cases that fail to improve should be referred to the ophthalmologist.

Bacterial Conjunctivitis

Mild cases respond well to *erythromycin ophthalmic ointment* (prescribed four times a day) or *polymyxin/trimethoprim* (Polytrim) *drops* (prescribed four times a day). Improvement is usually noted in several days. Bacitracin ophthalmic ointment and sodium sulfacetamide are alternative antibiotics. Neomycin causes allergic keratitis in 5% of patients treated topically and should be avoided if possible. More potent topical antibiotics such as the aminoglycosides (e.g., gentamicin 0.3% solution) and fluoroquinolones (e.g., gatifloxacin 0.3% [Zymar] and moxifloxacin 0.5% [Vigamox]) are reserved for more severe cases, which require consideration of ophthalmic referral.

Allergic Conjunctivitis

Seasonal allergic conjunctivitis generates many requests for symptomatic relief. Treatment options range from topical therapy with decongestants, antihistamines, mast-cell stabilizers, corticosteroids, and nonsteroidal antiinflammatory drugs to sedating and nonsedating oral antihistamines. Cool compresses are also very soothing. Cost-effective management benefits from the use of over-the-counter (OTC) and generic formulations. Severe allergic conditions, as might result from a contact dermatitis, may require *topical steroid therapy*; the management of severe disease and the use of topical steroids should be the province of the ophthalmologist because of the risks of steroid-induced glaucoma and cataract.

Over-the-Counter Antihistamine/Decongestant Drops. Fast-acting combination topical preparations produce vasoconstriction, reducing hyperemia and chemosis. The recommended frequency is four times daily; however, continuous daily use can lead to reactive hyperemia. Available medications include Naphcon-A, Vasocon-A, and Visine-A. Antihistamine drops provide immediate relief of itching. Topical ketotifen (Zaditor or Alaway) are effective at twice-daily dosing.

Prescription Antihistamine/Mast-Cell Stabilizer Drops. These prescription topical combination preparations are helpful for allergic disease that is inadequately controlled by over-the-counter drops. Prescription antihistamines can provide immediate relief and include emedastine (Emadine) and levocabastine (Livostin). Mast-cell stabilizers, such as pemirolast (Alamast), Nedocromil (Alocril), Lodoxamide (Alomide), and cromolyn sodium (Opticrom), are ideal for long-term control but do not provide acute symptom relief. Combination preparations can do both; these include olopatadine (Patanol, Pataday), azelastine (Optivar), and epinastine (Elestat).

Oral Antihistamines. The OTC antihistamines are effective for many patients; the advent of nonprescription generic nonsedating preparations (e.g., *loratadine* 10 mg) has greatly lowered cost and reduced the risk of daytime sedation, obviating the need for a prescription antihistamine, which can be up to five times more costly.

Subconjunctival Hemorrhage

This usually requires only reassurance. Compresses (initially cool, then warm) and erythromycin ophthalmic ointment or a lubricating ointment may reduce discomfort in cases with marked swelling.

Conjunctival Foreign Bodies

Most foreign bodies are easily removed with a cotton swab or fine forceps; erythromycin ointment three times a day for 2 days is adequate for healing, unless an infiltrate is present, which necessitates ophthalmic consultation.

Eyelid and Orbital Disease

Topical therapies are often helpful, at times supplemented by oral antibiotics.

Blepharitis

Lid hygiene measures and topical antibiotics should suffice. One can instruct the patient to dilute Johnson's *baby shampoo* 50:50 with water and use a cotton ball to clean the lids well with the eyes closed; there are also commercially prepared eyelid cleaners (SteriLid, OCuSOFT). After rinsing with water, one applies a hot compress to the closed lids for 5 to 10 minutes and then instills *erythromycin* or *bacitracin ophthalmic ointment* in the inferior fornix. The excess is rubbed into the eyelash base. Carrying out this procedure as many as three to four times daily will improve most cases. After improvement is obtained, the lids can be maintained by nightly lid hygiene and warm compresses. An occasional stubborn case requires nightly antibiotic ointment as prophylaxis.

Chronic Blepharitis and Meibomian Gland Inflammatory Due to Acne Rosacea

In addition to topical therapy for acne rosacea, the institution of systemic treatment for the rosacea is indicated. Traditionally, this has consisted in using long-term suppressive therapy with a *low-dose cycline*-family antibiotic (e.g., tetracycline 250 mg, doxycycline 50 or 100 mg, or minocycline 50 mg once daily). Recent evidence implicating *Helicobacter pylori* in the pathogenesis of acne rosacea has led to a therapeutic regimen of a 7- to 14-day course of double- or triple-antibiotic therapy (e.g., amoxicillin, metronidazole, bismuth subsalicylate; see Chapter 68).

Hordeolum/Chalazion

Aggressive warm compresses and topical antibiotic ointment are first-line therapy. At times, incision and curettage may require an ophthalmologist.

Cellulitis

Mild cellulitis of the lid margin (preseptal cellulitis) responds to topical treatment plus oral antibiotics. *Augmentin* (875 mg two times a day) is a good first choice. Double coverage with Levaquin and Bactrim is an effective alternative for patients who are penicillin allergic. *Orbital cellulitis* and orbital cellulitis complicated by *cavernous sinus thrombosis* are medical emergencies that require immediate hospitalization for intravenous antibiotics.

Acute Dacryocystitis

Warm *compresses* and oral antibiotics are also indicated, but persistent localized abscess requires *incision* and *drainage* by an ophthalmologist.

Mild Hypersensitivity Reactions

The lids respond rapidly to discontinuation of the offending agent and application of cool compresses. Systemic antihistamines are useful in moderate reactions, and steroids are useful in severe reactions.

Traumatic Lid Ecchymoses

These can be minimized by the early application of cool compresses and ice packs. Later, warm compresses speed resolution.

Corneal Disease

Prompt referral to ophthalmologist is usually required, but a number of corneal conditions can be treated by the primary physician in the initial stages.

Corneal Ulcers

These require intensive emergency evaluation and treatment by an ophthalmologist. Patients with typical herpes simplex dendritic keratitis may be started on oral antiviral medication (acyclovir [Zovirax], famciclovir [Famvir], valacyclovir [Valtrex]) if an ophthalmologist is not immediately available.

Corneal Abrasions

Abrasions heal rapidly with *erythromycin ointment* or *topical antibiotic drops*. A tight *sterile patch* that prevents lid motion for 24 hours may be used to decrease pain; however, this is not recommended if the abrasion is due to trauma from an organic substance (e.g., a tree branch) or is related to soft contact wear. Healing is equivalent with or without a pressure patch. If the initial abrasion was sizable (roughly 25% of the cornea or more), healing should be checked in 1 to 2 days. Lesions of this size also require cycloplegic eye drops (tropicamide 1% or cyclopentolate 1%) for the relief of painful secondary iritis during healing (see iritis treatment). Pain may also need to be treated with prescription pain medications. After reepithelialization occurs, ointment applied three times daily for 4 days helps to complete the healing process.

Foreign Bodies

Vigorous *irrigation* is the best treatment. Rust rings are treated like abrasions once the foreign body has been washed away. Foreign bodies that do not wash away with irrigation can be removed with a *cotton swab*, a sterile "golf stick," or a 30-gauge needle with a syringe as a handle, but such removal should not be attempted by the nonophthalmologist unless he or she is specifically trained to do so. Rust on the surface is easily debrided, but scraping is prohibited because it can damage Bowman's membrane and cause permanent scarring. Left untreated, rust may be irritating, but it will surface and slough in 1 or 2 weeks.

Contact Lens Overwear and Ultraviolet Keratitis

Use of topical antibiotic eye drops or ointment along with a cycloplegic agent provides adequate treatment. For cases of contact lens overwear, the contact lens should be discontinued.

Suspected Corneal Laceration and Perforation

These are ophthalmic emergencies. A protective metal shield ("Fox shield") should be placed over the eye; no medication should be instilled.

Uveal Tract Disease

An ophthalmologist must evaluate and treat *primary iritis*, but treating initially with cycloplegia by tropicamide 1% or cyclopentolate 1% four times a day will prevent posterior synechia formation and relieve pain. *Iritis* secondary to corneal abrasion may be treated with these medications. The nonophthalmologist should avoid atropine because its effects persist for 1 to 2 weeks.

Intraocular Disease

Acute glaucoma should be treated by the immediate administration of *pilocarpine* 2% every 15 minutes for two to three doses to break the attack, followed by topical antiglaucomatous medications such as a *β-blocker* (timolol), an *α-agonist* (apraclonidine, brimonidine), a *topical carbonic anhydrase inhibitor* (dorzolamide, brinzolamide), and/or acetazolamide 500 mg orally or intravenously acutely to lower intraocular pressure and protect the optic nerve. Immediate attention by an ophthalmologist is necessary because the only definitive treatment is laser or surgical iridectomy.

Annotated Bibliography

---

1. Alfonso ED, Cantu-Dibildox J, Munir WM, et al. Insurgence of *Fusarium* keratitis associated with contact lens wear. Arch Ophthalmol 2006;124:941. (*The microbial spectrum of contact lens–related keratitis may be evolving, with a higher participation of Fusarium species.*)
2. Cavuoto K, Zutshi D, Karp CL, et al. Update on bacterial conjunctivitis in South Florida. Ophthalmology 2008;115(1):51. (*Reports demographics, organism occurrence, and in vitro resistance trends.*)
3. Leibowitz HM. The red eye. N Engl J Med 2000;343:345. (*An excellent review for the generalist reader; 36 references and useful photographs.*)
4. Margo CE, Mulla ZD. Malignant tumors of the eyelid: a population-bases study of non–basal cell and non–squamous cell malignant neoplasms. Arch Ophthalmol 1998;116:195. (*Addresses the less common malignancies.*)
5. Soparkar CN, Wilhelmus KR, Koch DD, et al. Acute and chronic conjunctivitis due to over-the-counter ophthalmic decongestants. Arch Ophthalmol 1997;115:34. (*The condition is a complication of prolonged use of these commonly applied agents.*)
6. Wirbelauer C. Management of the red eye for the primary care physician. Am J Med 2006;119:302. (*A review of the causes of red eye, simple diagnostic methods, and emergency management.*)
7. Frucht-Pery J, Sagi E, Hemo I, et al. Efficacy of doxycycline and tetracycline in ocular rosacea. Am J Ophthalmol 1993;116:88. (*Discusses the systemic treatment of this common and undertreated disorder.*)
8. Isenberg SJ, Apt L, Wood M. A controlled trial of povidone–iodine as prophylaxis against ophthalmia neonatorum. N Engl J Med 1995;332:562. (*Explains the basis for the change in accepted practice patterns to avoid this dreadful disease.*)
9. Ohnsman C, Ritterband D, O'Brien T, et al. Comparison of azithromycin and moxiflosacin against bacterial isolates causing conjunctivitis. Curr Med Res Opin 2007;23:2241. (*Resistance to azithromycin was more common than resistance to moxifloxacin in clinical isolates.*)
10. Parmar P, Salman A, Kalavathy CM, et al. Comparison of topical gatifloxacin 0.3% and ciprofloxacin 0.3% for the treatment of bacterial keratitis. Am J Ophthalmol 2006;141:282. (*Gatifloxacin had a significantly better action against gram-positive cocci than ciprofloxacin.*)

CHAPTER 200 ■ EVALUATION OF IMPAIRED VISION

JAMES W. HUNG AND CLAUDIA U. RICHTER

Patients with decreasing or blurred vision often refer themselves directly to an eye specialist, but at times they may first present to their primary physician. Eye disorders are common, with more than one third of the U.S. population having some ocular abnormality that may affect vision. Sudden visual loss is a medical emergency. Gradual diminution of sight can impair important activities such as driving or reading and raises the specter of eventual blindness and inability to function independently. Paradoxically, some elderly patients may not volunteer that their vision is decreasing because they consider it a natural part of aging. Consequently, the primary physician needs to screen elderly patients for treatable causes of decreased vision. In addition, the primary physician should be capable of a basic assessment that helps to ensure proper initial care and appropriate and timely referral.

PATHOPHYSIOLOGY AND CLINICAL PRESENTATION (1–5)

Anatomic orientation provides a framework for considering the pathophysiology of visual difficulties, beginning with the eyelid and cornea and working inward to internal structures including the anterior chamber, lens, vitreous, retina, and optic nerve.

Vision can become impaired when there is a change in the refractive state of the eye, opacification of the transparent ocular media, damage to the photoreceptor cells of the retina, or a lesion of the optic nerve, its radiations, or the visual cortex.

Refractive Error

Refractive error is the most common cause of decreased visual acuity. It results from the inability of the eye to focus light precisely on the retina and may be due to an abnormality in the cornea, lens, or size of the globe. Myopic patients commonly present during their teens and early 20s. Patients in their 40s may report decreased visual acuity, but in fact they simply cannot accommodate to near distances and require reading glasses. Early cataracts can increase myopia before they opacify and block the transmission of light. Uncontrolled diabetes mellitus can produce swelling of the lens and myopia, which resolves with control of the blood sugar. Sulfonamides, thiazides, and anticholinergic agents may induce myopia, causing blurred vision.

Eyelid Disease

Occasionally, sudden visual loss results from eyelids being closed by swelling due to trauma, insect bites, cellulitis, or angioneurotic edema. Acute blepharospasm secondary to ocular surface pain may be described as an inability to see.

Corneal Disease

The *cornea* is the major refracting surface of the eye, and any change in it can lead to visual disturbances. A corneal abrasion, herpes simplex virus keratitis, or ulcer causes irregularity of the corneal epithelium and opacification of the normally clear cornea. Acute glaucoma causes corneal edema. Corneal dystrophies or degenerations result in a more gradual reduction in visual acuity, often progressing over a period of years.

Anterior Chamber Disease

The anterior chamber may be opacified by inflammatory cells resulting from *iritis* or red blood cells resulting from a *hyphema*.

Lenticular Disease

Cataracts—opacifications of the lens—are a leading cause of gradual vision loss in older patients. The usual history is one of a painless slow deterioration of eyesight in the sixth, seventh, or eighth decade. However, a traumatic cataract may develop over a period of hours to days.

Vitreal Disease

Vitreous opacification occurs most often from *hemorrhage* and less commonly from *inflammation* or *infection*. Proliferative diabetic retinopathy, a retinal hole or detachment, trauma, sickle cell retinopathy, hypertension, and clotting abnormalities may cause vitreous hemorrhage. A *vitreous floater* may transiently blur vision or may be called a blind spot. Age-related *vitreal syneresis* with associated posterior vitreous detachment is a common cause of floaters. Given its association with retinal tears and detachment, patients complaining of new-onset floaters should be evaluated by an ophthalmologist.

Retinal Disease

The retinal pathology that can compromise vision ranges from degeneration, inflammation, and trauma to detachment and ischemia. Visual loss may ensue.

Age-related macular degeneration (ARMD) occurs in patients older than age 55 years and is a leading cause of legal blindness. Central vision is impaired, whereas peripheral vision remains intact. Funduscopic examination may show a loss of the foveal reflex, macular drusen, atrophy of the retinal pigment epithelium with prominent choroidal vessels, subretinal edema or hemorrhage, or a central fibrous scar. Some 15% of patients with ARMD have treatable disease, presenting with early visual symptoms and a subretinal neovascular net that can be treated. They need to be seen promptly to maximize their chances of effective treatment. Those at particular risk of developing subretinal neovascular nets have *soft drusen* or a *disciform scar* in one macula. These patients should screen their central vision daily with an Amsler grid (see Chapter 206).

Central serous retinopathy is an idiopathic spontaneous detachment of the retina in the macular area. Patients range in age from 20 to 50 years. Central vision is reduced, but recovery is usually spontaneous within a few months.

Retinal inflammation, such as that due to histoplasmosis, toxoplasmosis, cytomegalovirus, or herpes virus infections, can involve the macula or produce a vitritis, decreasing vision. *Cytomegalovirus retinitis* is of concern in HIV-infected patients and important to recognize because it is treatable. Patients with CD4 counts less than 200 are at significantly increased risk of developing cytomegalovirus retinitis. Spread to the eye is hematogenous. Ocular symptoms include new floaters and loss of vision. Funduscopic manifestations include perivascular yellow-white retinal lesions presenting as a focal white granular infiltrate with or without hemorrhage, expanding in a "brushfire" pattern.

Trauma may cause decreased visual acuity by producing macular edema or a choroidal rupture. Macular edema resolves within a few days, and visual acuity improves. A choroidal rupture causes permanent decreased visual acuity.

Retinal detachment may cause decreased visual acuity when it is extensive or may be noted as a minor field defect when it is small. Flashing lights and a shower of vitreous floaters may presage a retinal detachment. As a detachment extends, the patient may note that the visual field defect progresses like a shade being drawn. A detached retina appears ballooned forward with undulating folds.

Ischemic disease of the retina or optic nerve may lead to sudden visual loss. In *central retinal artery occlusion*, there is sudden painless profound loss of vision to hand movements or no light perception. The patient may have had previous episodes of amaurosis fugax with fleeting blindness lasting only seconds. Ophthalmoscopy reveals a pale optic disc, attenuated arterioles, "boxcar" veins, hazy edematous retina, and a cherry-red spot in the macula. Occasionally, an embolus may be seen at a bifurcation of a retinal arteriole. *Branch retinal artery occlusion* presents with a visual field defect and retinal findings of attenuated arteriole and retinal edema only in the distribution of the affected arteriole. The most common embolic sources are an atheromatous plaque in the ipsilateral carotid artery or a vegetation from a cardiac valve leaflet.

Giant-cell (temporal) arteritis is a granulomatous inflammation of the medium and large arteries in elderly people that can cause sudden visual loss (see Chapter 161). These patients (many of whom have concurrent polymyalgia rheumatica) sometimes report premonitory visual symptoms similar to amaurosis fugax. On examination, one may find a swollen optic disc, a normal optic disc, or a central retinal artery occlusion.

Central or *branch retinal vein occlusion* causes a sudden painless decrease in visual acuity. In central retinal vein occlusion, the fundus has a classic *"blood and thunder"* appearance: The veins are tortuous and dilated, and the retina is edematous and covered with flame-shaped hemorrhages. The optic disc margin is blurred. The fundus changes in branch retinal vein occlusion are similar but limited to the distribution of the involved vein. Decreased visual acuity is due to macular edema and ischemia. In central retinal vein occlusion, 20% of patients have preexisting chronic open-angle glaucoma and 50% of men have preexisting hypertension. In branch retinal vein occlusion, 75% of patients have preexisting hypertension.

Optic Nerve Disease

Inflammatory, compressive, vascular, and degenerative insults to the optic nerve may compromise vision.

Glaucoma may damage nerve fibers at the optic disc and cause visual field defects. Most visual loss due to glaucoma is gradual and progressive (see Chapter 207). Four types of visual field defects occur: paracentral scotomas occurring along the distribution of the arcuate nerve fiber bundle, arcuate scotomata, sector-shaped defects, and nasal steps. As the disease progresses, these visual field defects enlarge. Central vision remains intact until late in the disease, but even this may be lost. Acute angle-closure glaucoma produces a red eye, fixed pupil, hazy cornea, eye pain, and acute impairment of vision. Acute angle-closure glaucoma accounts for less than 5% of all glaucoma cases.

Optic neuritis—inflammation of the optic nerve—presents with a relatively acute impairment of vision in young persons (age 15 to 40 years). It is usually idiopathic, but 20% to 50% of patients eventually develop clinical multiple sclerosis. Clinically, there is progressive loss of vision over hours to days, typically unilateral with pain on eye motion, and improved visual function in the second to third week. Examination reveals an afferent pupillary defect, globe tenderness, visual field defects, and impairment of color vision. The optic nerve may appear normal.

Infiltrative or compressive lesions of the optic nerve, such as pituitary adenomas, meningiomas, gliomas, or internal carotid artery aneurysms, cause gradual visual field loss. It is unusual for lesions posterior to the optic chiasm to present with decreased visual acuity because of the decussation of fibers in the optic chiasm. Unilateral lesions, such as a tumor or a cerebrovascular accident, cause a homonymous hemianopsia or related visual field defect. Bilateral central nervous system lesions may cause profound visual loss.

Anterior ischemic optic neuropathy is produced by ischemia to the anterior portion of the optic nerve. The patient notes decreased visual acuity or a visual field defect, usually involving the superior or inferior visual field and the macula. The optic disc initially appears edematous, sometimes in just one portion, with a few flame-shaped hemorrhages. Optic atrophy follows the disc edema. The most common etiology is thrombosis of an arteriosclerotic vessel. The patients tend to be younger than those affected by giant-cell arteritis and have hypertension or diabetes mellitus.

Optic neuropathy may be due to inherited degenerative diseases, drugs, toxins, or vitamin deficiencies. Many patients complain of blurred vision at night. Rarely, these patients may be found to have true night blindness caused by retinitis pigmentosa or vitamin A deficiency. More commonly, no etiology is found; a slight decrease in visual acuity at night is common and normal.

Psychopathology

Hysteria and *malingering* account for most psychogenic cases. Patients present with subjective vision loss, but the objective eye examination and other independent measures of visual function are intact.

TABLE 200.1

CAUSES OF IMPAIRED VISION

Eyelids
  Edema
  Blepharospasm
Cornea
  Abrasion
  Infection
  Edema
  Degeneration
Anterior Chamber
  Inflammatory cells (from iritis)
  Hyphema
Lens
  Cataract
  Swelling (e.g., poorly controlled diabetes)
Vitreous
  Hemorrhage
  Floaters
Retina
  Age-related macular degeneration
  Central serous retinopathy
  Inflammation
  Trauma
  Detachment
  Diabetes
  Hypertension
Vasculature
  Central retinal artery occlusion
  Giant cell (cranial or temporal) arteritis
  Anterior ischemic optic neuropathy
  Retinal vein occlusion
Optic Nerve
  Compression (glaucoma, tumor)
Psychiatric
  Hysteria
  Malingering
Refractive Error

DIFFERENTIAL DIAGNOSIS (1–5)

The causes of visual impairment can be logically considered in terms of anatomic site affected (Table 200.1).

WORKUP (1–7)

History

It is essential to establish the onset, duration, clinical course, and pattern of visual loss. Any associated visual phenomena should be ascertained, as well as any pain. The presence of premonitory symptoms is helpful. Acute loss is suggestive of a vascular event or retinal detachment. Preceding episodes of amaurosis fugax indicate central retinal artery occlusion or giant-cell arteritis. A sudden flurry of flashes of light (photopsia) and vitreous floaters may herald a retinal detachment. Scintillating scotomata may herald a migraine headache. Progressive visual loss points to a chronic disturbance, such as cataract, macular

degeneration, or glaucoma. Previous episodes of decreased visual acuity with halos around lights and pain may indicate angle-closure glaucoma. A foreign-body sensation indicates a corneal abrasion, foreign body, or herpes simplex keratitis. The presence of other diseases, such as diabetes mellitus, hypertension, heart disease, or sickle cell anemia, may be contributory. A history of trauma is important to note, as is smoking, which is an important independent risk factor for age-related macular degeneration.

Physical Examination and Laboratory Studies

Visual acuity testing should be done formally, one eye at a time. If the patient complains of pain, a topical anesthetic such as proparacaine should be used to allow testing. If the lids are tightly swollen, it may be necessary to pry them apart forcibly. The patient should wear his or her distance glasses. A Snellen eye chart with its standardized letter sizes is most convenient. If letters cannot be read, the distance at which the patient can accurately count fingers or identify hand motions is noted. If targets cannot be seen, it is important to determine whether the eye can perceive light. Vision is rechecked with the patient looking through a pinhole to eliminate any residual refractive error.

The pupils should be examined carefully, noting size, direct and consensual reactions to light, and the presence of any afferent pupillary defect. An afferent pupillary defect may be found in optic neuritis, central retinal artery occlusion, giant-cell arteritis, and extensive retinal diseases. A fixed pupil in conjunction with a red eye is indicative of acute angle-closure glaucoma.

The conjunctiva is examined to determine whether the eye is red and inflamed or white and quiet. With the exception of trauma, acute glaucoma, and infection, the diseases that cause sudden visual loss do not cause a red eye (see Chapter 199). The cornea normally is clear with a crisp light reflex and no fluorescein stain. If a tonometer is available, the intraocular pressure should be measured.

Ophthalmoscopy is important; it should first be noted whether the fundus can be visualized or whether a dense cataract or vitreous opacity is present. If the fundus can be visualized, the optic disc is examined for papilledema or atrophy. The macula is examined, looking for a cherry-red spot, hemorrhages, and signs of ARMD. The retinal vessels are examined, with attention paid to the caliber and the presence of visible emboli. Patients older than age 50 years with sudden visual loss should have a careful check for temporal arteritis, which includes palpation of the cranial arteries for tenderness, enlargement, and loss of pulsation and determination of the erythrocyte sedimentation rate for marked elevation (see Chapter 161).

If a patient is a malingerer or hysterical, the examination of the eye will be normal, including opticokinetic responses, stereoscopic vision, and visual fields. One can quickly check opticokinetic responses by passing the front page of a newspaper before the eyes of the patient.

VISION SCREENING (8,9)

Adults with gradual onset of visual impairment often do not recognize or complain of their deficit; those with diabetes and the elderly are at particularly high risk for visual impairment. The primary physician should always take a brief ophthalmologic history complemented by Snellen chart testing of visual acuity for persons at increased risk. These two simple tasks provide high yield in the detection of important eye pathology.

Diabetics should be referred to the ophthalmologist, even if they are asymptomatic, because screening complemented by early diagnosis and treatment can prevent vision loss. Persons with diabetes are especially well served by periodic retinal examination for proliferative retinopathy, which is capable of causing loss of vision if it goes undetected and untreated (see Chapter 209). Guidelines for screening diabetic eye examinations include the following:

- For type 1 diabetes: start of screening 5 years after the initial diagnosis and yearly thereafter.
- For type 2 diabetes: screening at the time of diagnosis and yearly thereafter.

For adults with no risk factors, the frequency of a screening eye examination depends on age:

- Age 65 years or older: every 1 to 2 years
- Age 40 to 64 years: every 2 to 4 years
- Age 30 to 39 years: at least twice during the time span
- Age 20 to 29 years: at least once during the time span

SYMPTOMATIC MANAGEMENT

Patients with sudden visual loss need immediate ophthalmologic consultation. If an ophthalmologist is not immediately available, appropriate emergency measures should be taken. If giant-cell arteritis is suspected, the patient should be started at once on high-dose glucocorticosteroids (e.g., prednisone 60 mg/d) and considered for temporal artery biopsy. Some vision may be salvaged in the affected eye, and the other eye is protected (see Chapter 161).

Acute angle-closure glaucoma should be treated at once with topical pilocarpine 2% in both eyes and acetazolamide 500 mg intravenously. The pilocarpine acts therapeutically in the involved eye and prophylactically in the uninvolved eye. Other topical medications that may help lower intraocular pressure include topical β-blockers (timolol, betaxolol, levobunolol, etc.), α-agonists (brimonidine, apraclonidine), and carbonic anhydrase inhibitors (dorzolamide, brinzolamide). Pain medication and antiemetics are appropriate. If available, an osmotic agent such as intravenous mannitol should be used. All patients with acute angle-closure glaucoma need an iridectomy to prevent further attacks.

INDICATIONS FOR REFERRAL

All patients with acute loss of vision or eye trauma should be referred immediately to the ophthalmologist. Individuals suspected of having glaucoma, macular degeneration, retinal vein occlusion, or an infectious etiology and those in whom the cause of impaired vision is unclear also should have early ophthalmologic consultation. Other findings indicative of benefit from ophthalmologic referral include age older than 65 years, diabetes (see prior discussion), vision worse than 20/40 by Snellen testing, or a difference on testing of greater than two Snellen lines between the two eyes.

Annotated Bibliography

1. Whiteside MM, Wallhagen MI, Pettengill E. Sensory impairment in older adults: Part 2: Vision loss. Am J Nurs 2006;106:52. (*A good summary of simple screening measures.*)
2. Bienfang DC, Kelly LD, Nicholson DH, et al. Ophthalmology. N Engl J Med 1990;323:956. (*Overview for the general reader.*)
3. Shingleton BJ, O'Donoghue M. Blurred vision. N Engl J Med 2000;343:556. (*Discusses causes of blurred vision; 35 references.*)
4. Tielsch JM, Javitt JC, Coleman A, et al. The prevalence of blindness and visual impairment among nursing home residents in Baltimore. N Engl J Med 1995;332:1205. (*The high prevalence argues for screening in primary care practice.*)
5. Tielsch JM, Sommer A, Witt K, et al. Blindness and visual impairment in an American urban population. Arch Ophthalmol 1990;108:286. (*Presents important epidemiologic data.*)
6. Margolis KL, Money BE, Kopietz LA, et al. Physician recognition of ophthalmoscopic signs of open-angle glaucoma. J Gen Intern Med 1989;4:296. (*An educational program that includes good photographs of the key findings.*)
7. Bloom JN, Palestine AG. The diagnosis of cytomegalovirus retinitis. Ann Intern Med 1988;109:963. (*Required reading for those caring for HIV patients.*)
8. Strahlman E, Ford D, Whelton P, et al. Vision screening in a primary care practice. Arch Intern Med 1990;150:2159. (*Screening has a high yield in high-risk persons.*)
9. Singer DE, Nathan DM, Fogel HA, et al. Screening for diabetic retinopathy. Ann Intern Med 1992;116:660. (*Finds screening to be beneficial.*)

CHAPTER 201 ■ EVALUATION OF EYE PAIN

AUDREY AHUERO AND CLAUDIA U. RICHTER

Pain in the eye is most often produced by conditions that do not threaten vision, but discomfort may also result from corneal or intraocular pathology that is capable of compromising eyesight. The first responsibility of the primary physician is to determine promptly whether there is an immediate threat to vision that requires urgent therapy or quick referral to the ophthalmologist; minor problems can be treated symptomatically in the office. Pain referable to the orbit from a nonocular etiology may simulate that due to eye pathology and needs to be differentiated. Ocular pain is usually not the only presentation of eye injury or disease; redness (see Chapter 199) and impaired vision (see Chapter 200) may also ensue.

Etiologic diagnosis requires taking the entire presentation into consideration.

PATHOPHYSIOLOGY AND CLINICAL PRESENTATION (1,2)

The external ocular surfaces (lid, conjunctiva, and cornea) and the uveal tract are richly innervated to detect pain. Localization within these structures is relatively less precise because most pain localizes to the upper outer lid regardless of the location of the surface lesion. The orbit and sinuses may give rise to pain localized to the eye. Pathology confined to the vitreous, retina, or optic nerve is rarely a source of pain.

Eyelids

Inflammation of the eyelid causes tenderness and foreign-body sensation. Common causes are hordeolum (stye), trichiasis (inturned lashes), tarsal foreign bodies, cellulitis, and herpes infection. Redness and edema may accompany the pain.

Conjunctiva

Viral and bacterial conjunctivitis cause mild burning and foreign-body sensation, whereas allergic conjunctivitis primarily elicits itching (see Chapter 199). Toxic, chemical, and mechanical injuries are commonly responsible for unilateral disease with a myriad of symptoms.

Cornea

The cornea is densely innervated by pain fibers, so even a minor injury may result in considerable discomfort. Pain arises from exposure of nerve endings in the epithelium; the patient complains of a burning or foreign-body sensation and, in some cases, reflex photophobia and tearing. Blinking exacerbates the pain. Ocular surface disease from dry eye can produce discomfort (see Chapter 202).

Keratitis (inflammation of the cornea) occurs with trauma, infection, exposure, vascular disease, or decreased lacrimation. Contact lens use is an important source of microbial keratitis. Severe pain is a prominent symptom; movement of the lid typically exacerbates symptoms. If blood vessels invade the normally avascular corneal stroma, vision may become cloudy. Fluorescein stain reveals the epithelial defects quite well and allows identification with a penlight. In infectious keratitis, corneal infiltrates are sometimes visible with a penlight, appearing as white spots.

Sclera

Compared with disease of the eyelids, scleral problems are more likely to cause dull, deep pain. If the condition involves the anterior sclera, it may be readily visible as an area of redness. Tenderness on palpation of the inflamed area may be present and, rarely, pain with eye movement. The blood supply to the sclera is not extensive, and its metabolism is relatively inactive. Consequently, inflammatory conditions of the sclera tend to be rather torpid; many are associated with connective tissue disease. Posterior scleritis may present with vision loss.

Uveal Tract

Anterior uveitis or *iritis* is accompanied by a dull ache and photophobia due to the irritative spasm of the pupillary sphincter. *Posterior uveitis* without anterior involvement may be painless or cause deep-seated aching.

In *acute angle-closure glaucoma*, profound ocular and orbital pain radiating to the frontal and temporal regions accompany sudden elevation of pressure; vagal stimulation from the high pressure may result in nausea and vomiting. Often the patient gives a history of mild intermittent episodes of blurred vision preceding the onset of an attack of throbbing pain, nausea, vomiting, and decreased visual acuity; halos about lights are sometimes noted. A fixed midposition pupil, redness, and a hazy cornea may be present (see Chapter 207).

Orbit

Inflammation and rapidly expanding mass lesions may cause deep pain. Displacement of the globe and diplopia may ensue, as seen in cases of *Graves' ophthalmopathy* and *orbital tumors*. In *orbital cellulitis* there is proptosis, limitation of extraocular movement, injection, and diminished vision. *Orbital pseudotumor* often presents in a very similar fashion to orbital cellulitis. *Sinusitis* may also cause secondary orbital inflammation and tenderness on extremes of eye movement

Optic neuritis, a condition of younger patients (aged 15 to 40 years), is mostly idiopathic but 10% to 15% are associated with multiple sclerosis, and as many as 20% to 50% of patients eventually develop multiple sclerosis. Onset is sudden, and symptoms include pain on eye movement due to meningeal inflammation involving the extraocular rectus muscles at the orbital apex. Abnormal color vision and some loss of central vision also ensue. In most instances, the optic disc appears normal, but occasionally there is edema. A central scotoma may be found.

Other Sources

Mild headache referred to the orbit is associated with refractive error, ocular muscle imbalance, sinusitis, and other causes of nonocular headache, such as tension headache, cluster headache, migraine, temporal arteritis, and the prodromal phase of herpes zoster. Severe aches in the eye cannot be attributed to refractive error, nor can aches about the eye that are noted on awakening in the morning.

DIFFERENTIAL DIAGNOSIS (1,2)

The causes of eye pain can be considered anatomically (Table 201.1).

WORKUP (1,2)

The initial task is to ensure there is no threat to vision. Most intraocular conditions that cause eye pain may compromise vision. A comprehensive eye examination may be needed, and

TABLE 201.1

IMPORTANT CAUSES OF EYE PAIN

Extraocular Causes
Lid
    Hordeolum (a small abscess of the lid)
    Acute dacryocystitis
    Cellulitis
    Chalazion
Conjunctival
    Irritant exposure (prolonged sun exposure, pollution, occupational irritants, aerosol propellants, wind, dust)
    Infection (viral or bacterial)
    Lack of sleep
Corneal
    Incipient zoster
    Abrasions
    Foreign bodies
    Ulcers
    Ingrown lashes
    Contact lens abuse
    Excessive exposure to sun or other forms of ultraviolet radiation
    Infection (bacterial or viral)
Scleral
    Episcleritis
    Scleritis (connective tissue disease)

Intraocular Conditions
Anterior eye
    Acute angle-closure glaucoma
    Acute anterior uveitis (idiopathic, connective tissue disease, sarcoidosis, inflammatory bowel disease)
    Refractive error (mild pain only)
Posterior eye
    Posterior uveitis

Orbital Disease
Tumor
Inflammatory disease
Graves' ophthalmopathy
Pseudotumor oculi
Retrobulbar optic neuritis

Referred Pain from Extraocular Sources
Sinusitis
Tooth abscess
Tension, migraine or cluster headache
Temporal arteritis
Prodrome of herpes zoster
Ocular muscle imbalance

Other
Trauma

---

the primary physician can begin the assessment by focusing on a few key elements.

History

The patient should first be asked about any change in visual acuity or color vision because any report of deteriorating vision requires urgent ophthalmologic consultation. In the absence of visual compromise, the history can continue with consideration of pain quality and aggravating and alleviating factors. Deep pain suggests an intraocular problem; a foreign-body sensation points to a problem on the surface of the eye. Pain exacerbated by lid movement and relieved by cessation of lid motion points to a foreign-body or corneal lesion. Localization of a surface lesion by history is often difficult because most of the time the foreign-body sensation is felt in the outer portion of the upper lid, regardless of the lesion's location.

In considering causes of conjunctival irritation, it is important to ask about occupational exposure, trauma, sun and sun lamp exposure, and other forms of ultraviolet radiation (e.g., arc welding), as well as foreign-body contact. Photophobia is often prominent in acute anterior uveitis. History of sinusitis and headaches should be noted. A history of diplopia and displacement of the eye raises the possibility of an orbital problem. Pain worsened by eye motion may be due to retrobulbar optic neuritis, especially if it is accompanied by a loss of central vision and a normal-appearing optic disc.

Physical Examination

A handheld ophthalmoscope, penlight, fluorescein stain, and a cotton-tipped applicator for lid eversion can be very helpful for assessment of ocular conditions. First, *visual acuity*, *color vision*, and *extraocular movements* should be tested and recorded; if visual acuity is impaired, urgent referral is warranted.

The eye, lid, and conjunctiva are then inspected for masses and redness, the pupil for reactivity, the cornea for clarity, and the fundus for any abnormalities of the disc. The upper lid should be everted with a cotton-tipped applicator to check for a foreign body or chalazion. The penlight can then be used to survey the cornea for gross injury. The limbus should be examined for evidence of dilated vessels around the limbus; this *ciliary flush* is characteristic of intraocular inflammation and occurs in anterior uveitis. Often the flush cannot be seen without the aid of a slit lamp. A *cloudy cornea* in conjunction with a fixed midposition pupil is consistent with acute glaucoma; the eye may be red. A *constricted pupil* in the presence of an eye that is tearing excessively suggests anterior uveitis; in severe cases, the eye also may be reddened and the anterior chamber hazy. Finding a *central scotoma* should raise suspicion of retrobulbar neuritis; a normal-appearing disc supports the diagnosis.

In the assessment of eye pain with trauma, hyphema should be distinguished from subconjunctival hemorrhage. Hyphema presents as blood in the anterior chamber of the eye (between the cornea and the iris), suggesting internal injury; subconjunctival hemorrhage indicates blood on the surface of the eye, occurring in both traumatic and nontraumatic situations.

Fluorescein Staining

Fluorescein staining is a key component of the eye exam that can be helpful even without the use of the slit lamp. Because of the ease of bacterial (particularly pseudomonal) contamination of the fluorescein, it must be instilled by means of either a single-dose container or sterile fluorescein strips wetted with sterile saline. The strip is touched to the inferior cul de sac while the patient looks upward; the patient is then asked to blink once. The fluorescein stains into denuded areas of corneal epithelium, producing a bright green color when viewed by normal light. The intensity of staining is enhanced if the eye is illuminated with a cobalt blue light. Among the lesions that can be identified by fluorescein staining are the dendritic ulcers of herpes keratitis, abrasions, small foreign bodies, and punctate defects.

Intraocular Pressure

If pain is not clearly related to the external eye or adnexa, the intraocular pressure should be measured to rule out glaucoma, provided there is no infection and the globe is intact without external or penetrating foreign bodies.

INDICATIONS FOR REFERRAL (1,2)

Significant loss of vision always requires prompt ophthalmic evaluation. Progressive pain, redness, or discharge that fails to respond to conservative treatment must be evaluated. Care must be taken not to mistake penetrating trauma for a simple abrasion. An eccentric pupil or shallow chamber may indicate loss of aqueous humor. One should never instill antibiotic ointment if there is a possibility of a perforation. Under such circumstances, patch the eye with a metal or plastic shield, which protects the eye, and arrange referral; do not place any pressure on the globe.

SYMPTOMATIC MANAGEMENT (1–3)

Most serious causes of eye pain require prompt ophthalmologic referral, but some foreign bodies and abrasions can be managed in the office setting.

Foreign Bodies

Irrigation with normal saline from a squirt bottle, syringe without a needle, or intravenous tubing may flush out foreign material. If irrigation fails, no further attempt should be made by the nonophthalmologist to remove the foreign body if it is firmly embedded in the cornea. Use of a dry cotton-tipped applicator will only remove much normal corneal epithelium. Use of a cotton-tipped applicator or needle for foreign-body removal requires topical anesthesia, good visualization, and specific training. Patients with metal foreign bodies should have a tetanus booster if their tetanus status is not current or unknown.

Abrasions

Superficial epithelial abrasions usually heal well with prophylactic antibiotic medication (e.g., erythromycin ointment) and frequent lubricant eyedrops. Abrasions (or any ocular problem) should never be treated with topical anesthetic drops, and patching is no longer generally recommended. A very large abrasion should be referred for ophthalmologic treatment. Management may include debridement and bandaged soft contact lens placement, which allows rapid relief of pain and quicker return to normal activities but requires a more potent antibiotic regimen and a return visit to the ophthalmologist for evaluation and removal of the contact lens.

Chemical Exposure

For eye pain in the setting of suspected chemical exposure, the eyes should be copiously irrigated with saline until the pH is 7.0 and then immediate ophthalmologic referral arranged. The pH is tested using pH paper placed in the inferior fornix similarly to Schirmer's testing; the resulting color change is compared to a color pH index.

Other

Conditions such as anterior uveitis need to be referred to an ophthalmologist so that topical steroid treatment can be initiated. It is important that topical steroids not be used in the primary care setting for any ocular condition due to the risks of intraocular pressure elevation and worsening infection.

For management of conjunctivitis and glaucoma, see Chapters 199 and 207, respectively.

Annotated Bibliography

1. Bienfang DC, Kelly LD, Nicholson DH, et al. Ophthalmology. N Engl J Med 1990;323:956. (*An excellent review and overview for the general reader; 115 references.*)
2. Shingleton BJ, Hersh PS, Kenyon KR. Eye trauma. Philadelphia: Mosby, 1991. (*Still the definitive text on the subject; includes detailed sections on the management of foreign bodies and abrasions.*)
3. Peate WF. Work-related eye injuries and illnesses. Am Family Physician 2007;75:1017. (*A nice review of the evaluation and management of commonly encountered work-related ophthalmologic problems.*)

CHAPTER 202 ■ EVALUATION OF DRY EYES

CLAUDIA U. RICHTER AND AUDREY AHUERO

The normal tear film provides important protection to the eye. Defects in tear production may be a sign of systemic disease or occur as part of the aging process. As many as 14.6% of persons older than 65 years report dry eye symptoms. The primary physician's tasks include checking for underlying systemic disease, instructing patients without such disease on symptomatic measures, and referring when discomfort is persistent or changes in vision occur.

PATHOPHYSIOLOGY AND CLINICAL PRESENTATION (1–4)

Normal Tear Formation and Function

The ocular tear film performs a host of functions, including maintenance of the corneal and conjunctival epithelium, lubrication of lid motion, delivery of oxygen and uptake of carbon dioxide from the cornea, carriage of antimicrobial defenses, clearance of foreign matter and tissue debris, and smoothing of the anterior ocular surface for clear vision. The tear film is inherently unstable, depending on the interaction of its three components for stability.

The outermost layer of the tear film is lipid, excreted by the lid meibomian glands. This layer retards evaporation and counters gravitational forces on the aqueous layer. The middle layer is aqueous, secreted by the lacrimal glands, and accounts for most of the tear film. The innermost layer is mucinous, primarily secreted by conjunctival goblet cells, and attaches to the corneal epithelium. This converts the corneal surface from a hydrophobic to a hydrophilic one. Each blink redistributes and replenishes the tear film.

Pathophysiology

Dry eyes ensue from a defect in maintenance of the tear film. It is a common phenomenon of aging and may be exacerbated by medications such as diuretics and anticholinergic drugs (e.g., antihistamines, tricyclic antidepressants, bladder relaxants, and psychotropics). Risk for dry eye symptoms is particularly high when three or more drugs with known drying side effects are used concurrently. Prolonged visual efforts from reading or computer use may reduce blink rate and lead to dry eye symptoms. Environmental factors such as low humidity, dusty environments, and windy conditions can contribute.

Local eye conditions associated with dry eye include eyelid malposition, lagophthalmos, and blepharitis. Systemic pathology may result in dry eyes. *Sjögren's syndrome*, with its inflammatory cellular infiltration of the lacrimal gland, may compromise tear production; increased tear evaporation may accompany its associated rosacea and posterior and anterior blepharitis. *Cicatricial pemphigoid* and *Stevens–Johnson syndrome* produce tear deficiency from conjunctival inflammation, scarring, and goblet cell destruction.

Clinical Presentation

Patients with dry eyes complain of grittiness, itching, burning, soreness, difficulty in moving or opening the eyelids, and/or a foreign-body sensation. When ocular irritation stimulates excess reflex tearing, the patient may present paradoxically with watery eyes. Rarely, dry eyes may be so severe as to cause corneal ulceration.

DIFFERENTIAL DIAGNOSIS

The differential diagnosis of dry eyes can be organized pathophysiologically (Table 202.1). As noted, the most common cause is the generalized diminution of lacrimal secretion associated with aging (exacerbated by medications), followed by systemic conditions and environmental factors.

WORKUP (1,4–6)

History

When dryness is the chief complaint, the history should be checked for associated symptoms, such as eye irritation, tearing, burning, stinging, foreign-body sensation, photophobia, blurry vision, contact lens intolerance, redness, mucous discharge, and increased frequency of blinking. A review of environmental factors is important, including low humidity, dusty home or work environment, and exposure to wind and tobacco smoke. Medication history is reviewed (particularly in the elderly) for drugs with anticholinergic side effects. Finally, a search for symptoms suggestive of underlying systemic disease should include a check for dry mouth, joint pains, prior ocular disease or infection or surgery, and a history of rheumatoid arthritis or its symptoms.

Physical Examination

The external examination includes evaluation of the skin (e.g., rosacea), eyelids (blink rate, incomplete closure or malposition, discharge), proptosis, and cranial nerve function (e.g., cranial nerve VII palsy). Joints should be examined for signs of rheumatoid arthritis.

TABLE 202.1

PRINCIPAL CAUSES OF DRY EYES

Lacrimal Gland Dysfunction
  Age
  Systemic disease (Sjögren's syndrome, sarcoidosis,
    Hodgkin's disease)
  Anticholinergic drugs (atropine, antihistamines, tricyclics)

Compromised Eyelid Function
  Fifth or seventh nerve palsy
  Exophthalmos
  Scar formation

Mucin Deficiency
  Chemical burns
  Hypovitaminosis A
  Isotretinoin (Accutane)
  Benign ocular pemphigoid
  Trachoma

Environmental Factors
  Excessive dryness
  Excessive exposure (e.g., exophthalmos, Bell's palsy)

Lipid Abnormalities
  Chronic blepharitis
  Meibomitis

Diagnostic Tests

Routine testing is not useful for patients with mild dry eyes because it lacks sufficient sensitivity and/or specificity. For patients with severe dry eyes, the *Schirmer test* can document significant aqueous deficiency by measuring the wetting of a filter-paper strip. A folded end is hooked over the lower lid temporally, and the patient is instructed to keep the eyes lightly closed during the test. Wetting is measured after 5 minutes; less than 5 mm of wetting is considered deficient.

Evidence by history or physical examination of *Sjögren's syndrome* or *rheumatoid disease* is an indication for serologic testing, starting with an *antinuclear antibody* determination (95% sensitive in Sjögren's syndrome; specificity low) and a *rheumatoid factor* (75% sensitive; specificity low). If these screening serologic tests are positive, then follow-up testing for the more specific *anti-Ro* and *anti-La* antibodies (60% to 70% sensitivity, >90% specificity) is worth considering (see Chapter 146).

SYMPTOMATIC MANAGEMENT AND INDICATIONS FOR REFERRAL (7,8)

As long as there are no signs of ocular disease, the primary physician may instruct patients in strategies to obtain symptomatic relief. The first step is to limit or eliminate any medications that may be contributing to ocular dryness. Environmental modification may be helpful. Using a room humidifier, avoiding dusty and smoky environments, and wearing glasses and hats outdoors may all help to reduce dryness symptoms.

A trial of *lubricant eyedrops* can be helpful. Many preparations are commercially available. Topical application of one to two drops four times a day is a useful starting dose. The patient may increase or decrease the frequency as necessary to achieve and maintain comfort. Prophylactic use is especially important because drops will not provide instantaneous relief of symptoms. Topical allergic reactions to the preservatives in the drops are rare, but if it is suspected, a more expensive, preservative-free preparation can be substituted. For bedtime, a lubricant ophthalmic ointment might be useful. If environmental modifications and lubricant eyedrops and ointment do not provide adequate relief, then referral and consideration of *topical cyclosporine* (Restasis) therapy are reasonable. The latter can reduce lacrimal gland inflammation and improve tear production, relieving dry eye symptoms. Other options for treatment include inserting punctal plugs into the lacrimal puncta to minimize the outflow of tears. If punctal plugs are not tolerated, permanent occlusion of the puncta by cautery may be helpful.

The patient should be instructed to seek immediate ophthalmologic attention in the event of a red eye, visual disturbance, or eye pain. An eye specialist should be consulted when simple symptomatic treatment does not give rapid relief.

PATIENT EDUCATION

The primary care physician can help the patient to understand that dry eyes is often a chronic condition that may wax and wane, especially in older persons. Reviewing with patients the strategies for maximizing comfort is important, including instructions in the proper instillation of eyedrops (e.g., a single drop into the lower fornix without contacting the eye with the dropper; instillation of no more than one drop at a time because any more exceeds the physical capacity of the inferior fornix and is wasteful).

CONCLUSIONS AND RECOMMENDATIONS

- Check for systemic conditions.
- Minimize environmental factors and medications that can aggravate dry eye symptoms.
- Prescribe a trial of lubricant eyedrops.
- Refer to the ophthalmologist for consideration of topical cyclosporine and punctal occlusion if symptomatic measures fail.

Annotated Bibliography

1. Schein OD, Muñoz B, Tielsch JM, et al. Prevalence of dry eye among the elderly. Am J Ophthalmol 1997;124:723. (*A population-based prevalence study of 2,520 persons aged 65 years and older found that 14.6% reported dry eye symptoms.*)

2. Bergman MT, Newman BL, Johnson NC. The effect of a diuretic (hydrochlorothiazide) on tear production in humans. Am J Ophthalmol 1985;99:473. (*Hydrochlorothiazide caused a 2.1-mm decrease in wetting by Schirmer's test in 11 normal human subjects.*)

3. Nordstrom K, Norblack D, Akselsson R. Influence of indoor air quality and personal factors on the sick building syndrome (SBS) in Swedish geriatric hospitals. Occup Environ Med 1995;52:170. (*Eye irritation was reported by 23% of hospital workers and was more common in buildings with high-ventilation flow.*)
4. Schein OD, Hochberg MC, Munoz B, et al. Dry eye and dry mouth in the elderly: a population-based assessment. Arch Intern Med 1999;159:1359. (*Medications were the most common cause, accounting for the vast majority of cases; autoimmune disease was not a major factor.*)
5. Slater CA, Davis RB, Shmerling RH. Antinuclear antibody testing: a clinical study of utility. Arch Intern Med 1996;156:1421. (*A critical look at the test, finding that sensitivity was high but specificity was low.*)
6. Horwath-Winter J, Berghold A, Schmut O, et al. Evaluation of the clinical course of dry eye syndrome. Arch Ophthalmol 2003;121: 1364. (*Over an observation period of up to 8 years, appropriate treatment of the dry eye syndrome resulted in an improved or stabilized condition.*)
7. Ophthalmic cyclosporine (Restasis) for dry eye disease. Med Lett Drugs Ther 2003;45:42. (*Reviews the causes of dry eyes and the pharmacology, adverse effects, and clinical trial results for ophthalmic cyclosporine; includes cost information.*)
8. Tuberville AW, Frederick WR, Wood TO. Punctal occlusion in tear deficiency syndromes. Ophthalmology 1982;89:1170. (*Punctal occlusion provided symptomatic improvement in 97% of eyes.*)

CHAPTER 203 ■ EVALUATION OF COMMON VISUAL DISTURBANCES: FLASHING LIGHTS, FLOATERS, AND OTHER TRANSIENT PHENOMENA

CLAUDIA U. RICHTER

Flashes of light, floaters, specks, distortions, halos, and discolorations are among the transient visual phenomena reported by patients. Flashes of light (*photopsia*) and dark, moving lines and specks (*floaters*) are particularly common occurrences that are usually benign but may signal a retinal tear or detachment. Visual distortion (*metamorphopsia*) can be the presenting symptom of age-related macular degeneration. Other short-lived disturbances accompany such diverse conditions as migraine, digitalis toxicity, and acute glaucoma. The primary physician needs to know the significance of these visual phenomena and when they presage a serious ophthalmologic or systemic event that requires prompt ophthalmologic attention.

PATHOPHYSIOLOGY AND CLINICAL PRESENTATION (1–4)

Floaters

Floaters are vitreous opacities that cast a shadow on the retina. They can be single or multiple, and they characteristically move across the visual field and transiently blur vision if they cross the macula. Their presence is most notable when a person is gazing at a clear, blue sky or blank, white wall. The new onset of floaters may occur as a consequence of *vitreous detachment, a retinal tear or detachment*, or an *intraocular hemorrhage*.

Vitreoretinal traction is the principal cause of retinal tears and detachments, which can lead to sudden onset of flashes and floaters. As the vitreous gel liquefies with age, its fibrous matrix contracts and pulls away from the retina. Because the vitreous is attached to the retina at several sites, any traction can cause tearing that leads to a retinal hole. Detachment may develop by a flow of fluid from the vitreous through the hole and beneath the retina. If the tearing involves a superficial retinal vessel, hemorrhage into the vitreous may occur.

Acute or chronic intraocular inflammation and/or infection are sometimes the cause, as in the immunocompromised patient with *cytomegalovirus* (CMV) *retinitis*. The sudden appearance of one or more floaters suggests the onset of serious underlying pathology. Floaters that are multiple and longstanding are associated with *myopia* and *aging* with or without a vitreous detachment.

Flashes (Photopsia)

Flashes (photopsia) are perceptions of bright, small, flickering lights or lightning-like flashes of light. They are most vividly seen in the dark and usually occur with mechanical stimulation of the retina. They account for "seeing stars" when one suffers head trauma or coughs very hard. New onset may be a consequence of vitreous traction on the retina, leading to *retinal tear* or *detachment*. Just rubbing the eyes can cause similar symptoms. *Migraine* pathophysiology accounts for recurrent episodes, which are more complex and longer lasting (*scintillating scotoma*).

Distortion (Metamorphopsia)

Distortion (metamorphopsia) refers to the curvilinear distortion of straight lines or patterns. This visual disturbance is the consequence of an altered shape of the retinal surface, either from a collection of fluid beneath the retina or scarring on the surface. Metamorphopsia is seen with age-related *macular degeneration*, epiretinal fibrosis, and a variety of ocular diseases that cause traction on the retinal surface and/or retinal scarring.

Zigzag Lines

Migraine can produce a complex set of prodromal visual phenomena that include *zigzag lines* (sometimes referred to as *fortification phenomena*) and flashes of light with transient blind spots (*scintillating scotoma*). These may present with or without a subsequent headache. Typically, the zigzag lines occur adjacent to a gray area of shaded darkness. Both the gray area and the zigzag lines slowly expand. The visual phenomena typically end in 20 to 30 minutes with or without the onset of the headache and leave no residual visual deficit (see Chapter 165).

Halos, Discolorations, and Visual Hallucinations

The first clinical manifestations of *digitalis toxicity* may be visual (see Chapter 32) and include lightning flashes, yellow discoloration, halos, and the appearance of frost over objects. *Acute glaucoma* (see Chapter 207) also produces colored halos around lights but not lightning flashes. Visual hallucinations caused by *seizure* activity in the occipital cortex and the adjacent association area produce static light and stars. Hallucinations from the parastriate area 18 cause luminous sensations or colored flashes and rings.

DIFFERENTIAL DIAGNOSIS

The sudden onset of a visual phenomenon may be the first sign of important underlying ophthalmic or systemic pathology. Causes can be listed according to clinical presentation (Table 203.1).

TABLE 203.1

CAUSES OF FLOATERS AND FLASHING LIGHTS

Floaters
  Myopia
  Aging
  Vitreous detachment
  Retinal tear
  Retinal detachment
  Intraocular inflammation (uveitis, retinitis)
  Vitreous hemorrhage

Flashing Lights
  Vitreoretinal traction
  Retinal detachment
  Mechanical stimulation (cough, rubbing the eyes, head trauma)
  Classic migraine
  Seizure activity in the visual cortex (static light, colored flashes)

WORKUP (1–3)

History

A complete and detailed description of the visual disturbance uninfluenced by leading questions is the most important part of the history, followed by information regarding their onset, their course, and the presence of any associated symptoms (e.g., headache, decreased visual acuity). The sudden onset of flashing lights and/or floaters is highly suggestive of vitreoretinal traction, possibly in association with a vitreous detachment, retinal tear, or retinal detachment. New onset in an immunocompromised patient should suggest CMV retinitis. Flashes of light on waking and rubbing the eyes are usually harmless, as are floaters that have been present for an extended time without a marked increase in number. The patient who complains of halos needs to be checked for glaucoma (see Chapter 198). A report of lightning flashes, yellow discoloration, or frost over objects in a patient taking a digitalis preparation requires consideration of digitalis toxicity. Visual distortion should lead to a search for macular pathology.

Physical Examination

Visual acuity testing, measurement of the intraocular pressure (see Chapter 198), and careful examination of the fundus should be included. One looks for hemorrhage in the vitreous, a ballooning white area suggestive of a retinal detachment, areas of retinal inflammation, and abnormalities in the appearance of the macula suggestive of macular degenerative disease. In the immunocompromised patient, funduscopic examination should include a look for the manifestations of CMV retinitis (e.g., focal, granular, perivascular yellow-white lesions with or without hemorrhage in a "brushfire" pattern). The detection of retinal tears and small retinal detachments requires indirect ophthalmoscopy or a diagnostic contact lens examination performed by the ophthalmologist. Patients with migraine will have a normal ophthalmologic examination.

Studies

The most important study in patients with new flashes and/or floaters is *indirect ophthalmoscopy* and scleral depression done by the ophthalmologist. Patients with metamorphopsia need *fluorescein angiography*. The patient with halos needs to be checked for glaucoma by the measurement of *intraocular pressure* (see Chapter 198). The patient taking a digitalis preparation who reports visual disturbances should have a serum drug level measured (see Chapter 32).

PATIENT EDUCATION AND INDICATIONS OR REFERRAL (1–3)

Patient Education

The patient with chronic floaters in the absence of ocular disease can be reassured; prognosis is excellent, as it is for the person with visual phenomena associated with migraine. Flashes that occur with minor mechanical stimulation (cough, rubbing of the eyes) require only reassurance and explanation, as long as there is no evidence of more serious pathology.

Indications for Referral

The new onset of unexplained flashes or floaters requires urgent referral to an ophthalmologist because of the possibility of a retinal tear, retinal detachment, or an inflammatory/infectious process (e.g., CMV retinitis). Vision is best preserved when the treatment of such conditions is prompt. If the patient or examiner detects a field loss, referral is even more urgent. Metamorphopsia is also an indication for urgent referral because age-related macular degeneration has a better visual prognosis when subretinal neovascularization is treated early. A report of halos should lead to referral for evaluation of glaucoma. Visual hallucinations require workup for seizure activity and visual cortex pathology.

Patients with chronic flashes and floaters should have a complete ophthalmologic examination, including indirect ophthal-moscopy, but it is not urgent. All patients with flashes and floaters need to be warned that a sudden onset of new floaters or flashes or the appearance of a peripheral visual field defect may represent a retinal hole or detachment necessitating prompt ophthalmologic attention.

CONCLUSIONS AND RECOMMENDATIONS (1–3)

- New light flashes and floaters may represent a new retinal hole or detachment and require a prompt ophthalmologic exam.
- Metamorphopsia may represent age-related macular degeneration and requires a prompt ophthalmologic exam.
- Colored halos around lights may represent acute glaucoma and require a prompt ophthalmologic exam.

Annotated Bibliography

1. Aring CD. The scintillating scotoma. JAMA 1972;220:519. (*A detailed discussion of these migrainous visual phenomena.*)
2. Bienfang DC, Kelly LD, Nicholson DH, et al. Ophthalmology. N Engl J Med 1990;323:956. (*A succinct review of ophthalmology for the generalist reader.*)
3. Morris PH, Scheie HG, Aminlari A. Light flashes as a clue to retinal disease. Arch Ophthalmol 1974;91:179. (*A classic paper; in this series, 23% of patients had demonstrable vitreoretinal disease; of these, 16% had retinal breaks.*)
4. American Academy of Ophthalmology. Posterior vitreous detachment, retinal breaks, and lattice degeneration. Preferred Practice Pattern. San Francisco: Author, 2003. (*Practice guidelines.*)

CHAPTER 204 ■ EVALUATION OF EXOPHTHALMOS

MARK P. HATTON AND CLAUDIA U. RICHTER

Exophthalmos is defined as protrusion or proptosis of the eye. It may be a variation of normal physiognomy or a sign of systemic or orbital disease. The primary physician must be able to recognize it and evaluate the patient for a possible endocrinologic, neoplastic, or vascular cause and decide on the need for further study or referral.

PATHOPHYSIOLOGY AND CLINICAL PRESENTATION (1–5)

Pathologic forms of exophthalmos may result from inflammation, infiltration, a mass lesion, or a vascular abnormality.

Graves' Disease

The ophthalmopathy of Graves' disease occurs as a consequence of an autoimmune inflammatory process leading to infiltration of the soft tissues of the orbit. Risk factors include cigarette smoking, radioiodine therapy, persistent hyperthyroidism, and recurrence of hyperthyroidism after withdrawal of antithyroid drug therapy. Administration of prednisone at the time of radioiodine therapy can prevent treatment-induced ophthalmopathy. Pathologically, there is an inflammatory infiltrate of lymphocytes, mucopolysaccharides, and edema, followed by proliferation of fibroblasts and increase in the volume of orbital connective tissue. The proliferation of orbital fibroblasts and their fibrotic restriction of extraocular muscle movement account for the clinical picture of Graves' ophthalmopathy.

In its mildest form, there is minor lid retraction, stare, lid lag, and mild protrusion of the eye (proptosis). A particularly severe form, "malignant" exophthalmos, causes edema of the lids and conjunctiva, marked proptosis, limitation of extraocular movements, exposure keratopathy, and optic nerve compression. Although it is usually a bilateral disease, it may present unilaterally or asymmetrically.

The relatively close clinical relationship between ophthalmopathy of Graves' disease, pretibial dermopathy, and hyperthyroidism suggests a common pathophysiologic mechanism. However, the ophthalmopathy can occur in the absence of thyroid dysfunction or pretibial dermopathy. The precise pathophysiology remains to be elucidated. It may be triggered by antibodies to circulating thyroid antigen, accounting for the exacerbation seen with some treatments for thyrotoxicosis. Its precise mechanisms continue to be elucidated (see Chapter 103).

Primary Orbital Neoplasms

Primary orbital neoplasms, such as *meningiomas*, produce exophthalmos by mass effect. Some vascular lesions, such as *hemangiomas*, produce only a mass effect, whereas a *carotid-cavernous sinus fistula* may present with a diffusely congested orbit with exophthalmos, prominent episcleral vessels, and elevated intraocular pressure. Mass lesions and vascular abnormalities are unilateral processes. They may lead to diplopia, ocular irritation, and photophobia (secondary to corneal exposure). Stretching or compression of the optic nerve can impair visual acuity.

Orbital Cellulitis

Orbital cellulitis is an extremely serious, although rare, cause of proptosis. Because the orbit is bordered on three sides by paranasal sinuses, orbital infection can result from sinusitis extending directly through the lamina papyracea. Lid edema, ptosis, proptosis, chemosis, and diminished ocular movements make for a dramatic clinical presentation. Retrograde extension can lead to cavernous sinus thrombosis.

DIFFERENTIAL DIAGNOSIS

Bilateral Exophthalmos

Bilateral exophthalmos is usually caused by *Graves' disease*, but occasionally it occurs with *Cushing's syndrome*, *acromegaly*, *lithium ingestion*, *metastatic tumor*, and *orbital lymphoma*.

Unilateral Exophthalmos

Unilateral exophthalmos may be caused by *Grave's disease*, *tumor*, *inflammatory* and *infectious diseases*, *vascular abnormalities*, and *skeletal abnormalities*. Common orbital tumors include *hemangioma*, *meningioma*, and *optic nerve glioma*. Tumors extending into the orbit include those originating in the eye, lids, and paranasal sinuses. *Orbital pseudotumor* is an inflammatory lesion that can mimic a mass lesion. Inflammatory etiologies include *sarcoidosis*, *foreign body*, *orbital thrombophlebitis*, and *ruptured dermoid cyst*. Hemangioma, aneurysm, varices, carotid-cavernous fistula, and cavernous sinus thrombosis constitute important vascular etiologies. Skeletal abnormalities such as Paget's disease may also produce exophthalmos. Asymmetry of the orbits, severe unilateral myopia, facial nerve paresis, eyelid retraction, and congenital glaucoma may give the appearance of exophthalmos. Ptosis or enophthalmos of the opposite eye can mimic exophthalmos.

WORKUP

The first task is to determine whether the condition is unilateral or bilateral. Bilateral disease has a limited differential diagnosis, with Graves' disease accounting for most cases. Attention is directed toward its confirmation (see Chapter 103). The broader differential of unilateral disease necessitates a more extensive workup.

History

History should include inquiry into the time course of the exophthalmos. Old photographs are helpful in determining whether the problem is of new onset or simply a longstanding anatomic variant. Associated symptoms are also important to note. Visual acuity changes, diplopia, pain, excessive lacrimation, photophobia, and foreign-body sensation are indications of adverse effects from the exophthalmos. A prior history or current symptoms of trauma to the orbit, thyroid disease, cancer, severe sinus infection, or worsening headache should be noted.

Physical Examination

Physical examination begins with documenting the degree of exophthalmos by exophthalmoscopy. The distance to be measured is from the lateral orbital rim to the apex of the cornea with the patient looking straight ahead. The upper limit of normal is 21 to 22 mm; a difference between both eyes of 2 mm is also considered significant. Visual acuity, intraocular pressure, and extraocular muscle function should also be tested. The conjunctiva and cornea are observed for signs of drying, aided by fluorescein or rose Bengal dye if available. Color vision, pupillary reactivity, and visual fields are assessed to investigate possible optic nerve compression, which may produce a pale or swollen optic nerve head on ophthalmoscopic examination. The globe and orbit need to be auscultated for bruits and pulsation suggestive of vascular fistula. The sinuses must be checked for tenderness and discharge. In the setting of bilateral disease, the neck should be checked for goiter and bruit, the pretibial region for dermopathy, and the remainder of the examination for signs of thyroid hormone excess (see Chapter 103).

Laboratory Studies

Thyroid indices (e.g., thyroid-stimulating hormone, total triiodothyronine, free thyroxine index) should be ordered in the patient with bilateral disease, but the absence of hyperthyroidism does not rule out Graves' disease. Even in patients without evidence of thyrotoxicosis, *antibodies to thyrotropin receptors* and *peroxidase* can be detected (see Chapter 103).

Patients with unilateral exophthalmos require orbital imaging. *Magnetic resonance imaging* and/or *computed tomography* with axial and coronal views are the studies of choice in the evaluation of orbital abnormalities.

SYMPTOMATIC MANAGEMENT, PATIENT EDUCATION, AND INDICATIONS FOR REFERRAL (6,7)

Symptomatic Management and Prevention

The primary physician must be cognizant of potential ocular complications of exophthalmos and give advice for relief of minor symptoms. Periorbital and lid edema may be reduced by *elevating the head of the bed* at night. Exposure keratopathy causes a foreign-body sensation, which can be relieved by use of *artificial tear lubricants* and *taping* the *eyelids* closed at night. If such simple measures are inadequate, referral to the ophthalmologist for consideration of eyelid or orbital surgery may be necessary.

Graves' Disease (see also Chapter 103)

Preventive measures include complete cessation of smoking and effective treatment of the underlying hyperthyroidism. Treatment of the underlying Graves' disease must be done carefully in the setting of eye involvement. As noted, ophthalmopathy can worsen with some forms of therapy, perhaps due to increased release of thyroid antigen. Some authorities suggest the use of antithyroid drugs to minimize such release; others add high-dose corticosteroids to the program (e.g., prednisone, 0.5 mg/kg for 1 month, beginning a few days after radioiodine administration; see Chapter 103).

Specific treatment of Graves' ophthalmopathy is undertaken only when symptoms become severe or vision is threatened. Likelihood of progression is hard to determine, and available therapies have their own adverse effects. Nonetheless, inflammatory symptoms such as periorbital edema and ocular discomfort are treated with *corticosteroids* or *orbital radiation* in conjunction with total cessation of any smoking (smoking decreases their efficacy). Such therapy may inhibit the cytokines that perpetuate the inflammatory reaction.

Indications for Referral and Admission

Ophthalmologic consultation should be obtained early in unilateral, severe, or unexplained exophthalmos. Exophthalmos due to neoplasm requires a team approach that includes the ophthalmologist, oncologist, and radiation therapist. A suspected vascular etiology is also grounds for referral. Endocrinologic consultation is indicated for managing the ophthalmopathy of Graves' disease. Emergency admission is needed if orbital cellulitis is encountered.

PATIENT EDUCATION

Patients with Graves' disease need to know that their eye symptoms may persist or progress despite appropriate systemic therapy for the underlying disease, but also that there are approaches to limiting risk (e.g., smoking cessation, effective control of the hyperthyroidism, steroid therapy in conjunction with radioiodine). Patients with Graves' disease need to know the adverse consequences of smoking and undergo an aggressive smoking cessation program (see Chapter 54). Home measures to lessen eye discomfort and prevent eye injury, such as *elevating the head of the bed*, using *artificial tear lubricants*, and *taping the eyelids* closed at night, are important to review with the exophthalmic patient, as are symptoms warranting prompt evaluation (e.g., change in vision, ocular pain, eye injection, diplopia).

CONCLUSIONS AND RECOMMENDATIONS

- The most common cause of bilateral exophthalmos is Grave's disease.
- Unilateral exophthalmos requires orbital imaging.

Annotated Bibliography

1. Bahn RS, Heufelder AE. Pathogenesis of Graves' ophthalmopathy. N Engl J Med 1993;329:1468. (*A clinically useful review of disease mechanisms and their relation to clinical presentation and treatment.*)
2. Bartalena L, Marcocci C, Bogazzi F, et al. Relation between therapy for hyperthyroidism and the course of Graves' ophthalmopathy. N Engl J Med 1998;338:73. (*A prospective, randomized trial demonstrating an increased risk of exophthalmos with radioiodine therapy but not with methimazole; prednisone eliminated the risk.*)
3. Bartalena L, Marcocci C, Tanda ML, et al. Cigarette smoking and treatment outcomes in Graves' ophthalmopathy. Ann Intern Med 1998;129:632. (*A randomized, single-blinded study showing that cigarette smoking increased the risk of progression of exophthalmos and decreased the efficacy of treatment.*)
4. Tallstedt L, Lundell G, Torring O, et al. Occurrence of ophthalmopathy after treatment of Graves' hyperthyroidism. N Engl J Med 1992;326:1733. (*Some treatments may actually exacerbate the ophthalmopathy.*)
5. Utiger RD. Pathogenesis of Graves' ophthalmopathy. N Engl J Med 1992;326:1772. (*Mechanisms are reviewed, particularly with regard to the mode of antithyroid therapy.*)
6. Bartalena L, Marcocci C, Pinchera A. Treating severe Graves' ophthalmopathy. Bailliere's Clin Endocrinol Metab 1997;11:521. (*An excellent summary by an authority in the field.*)
7. Garrity JA, Fatourechi V, Bergstralh EJ, et al. Results of transantral orbital decompression in 428 patients with severe Graves' ophthalmopathy. Am J Ophthalmol 1993;116:533. (*A large surgical treatment series.*)

CHAPTER 205 ■ EVALUATION OF WATERY EYES

MARK P. HATTON AND CLAUDIA U. RICHTER

The presence of watery eyes reflects an increased production of tears or a decreased ability to drain them. Patients complain of watery eyes or may actually describe tears overflowing and running down their cheeks, a condition called *epiphora*. For some patients, tearing is only a mild annoyance; however, for most patients, tearing creates significant difficulty due to alteration in vision, irritation to the skin from the need to constantly wipe their eyes, or both. Consequently, a complaint of watering eyes should not be ignored. Clinicians must also recognize that tearing can be a sign of a significant underlying medical condition and may require a workup to rule out neoplastic, infectious, and inflammatory causes. A cause should be sought to improve the patient's symptoms and also identify any potential threat to the patient's health. The primary physician plays an important role in the initial evaluation.

PATHOPHYSIOLOGY AND CLINICAL PRESENTATION (1–3)

Normal Tear Production and Drainage

Tears are produced by the main lacrimal gland, which is located in the superotemporal orbit, and by accessory lacrimal glands within the eyelids. Tears leave the ocular surface via the puncta within the medial aspect of the eyelids and pass from the canaliculi to the nasolacrimal duct and into the nose. Tearing occurs when relatively more tears are produced than can be drained through the lacrimal drainage system.

Hypersecretion of Tears

Primary hypersecretion of tears has not been identified as a cause of tearing, but secondary hypersecretion, or increased tear production in response to stimulation, can occur as a result of irritation to the ocular surface (e.g., corneal abrasion), reflex tearing in the setting of severe dry eye, inflammation within the eye, aberrant regeneration after Bell's palsy, and ocular allergy. Even when the outflow pathway is patent, the relative increase in tear production will result in a watery eye.

Impaired Lacrimal Drainage

Insufficient or impeded drainage in the setting of a normal rate of tear production may also result in tearing. Abnormalities in this category may include lid malposition (e.g., ectropion), punctual stenosis, canalicular stenosis, and nasolacrimal duct obstruction. Most patients with tearing have impeded outflow as the cause rather than overproduction of tears.

Tear film movement may be obstructed by eyelid-margin lesions or conjunctival redundancy or folds. The pumping function of the lid may be impaired by *seventh nerve palsy* or conditions stiffening the lids, such as scars or *scleroderma*, or by laxity of the lids from aging. *Thyroid eye disease* may lead to tearing from corneal irritation due to proptosis and lid malposition. The puncta must be properly positioned. *Ectropion* prevents tears from gaining access to the canaliculus. *Senile ectropion* is the most common cause in the elderly and is characterized by a sagging lower lid. The punctum or the canaliculus may be occluded congenitally, by chemical or thermal injury, or by neoplasms. In addition, canalicular *infections* may cause occlusion. The most common of these are *Actinomyces israeli* (*Streptothrix*) and *Candida*. Finally, *obstruction* of the lacrimal sac and nasolacrimal duct may be idiopathic, congenital, or caused by neoplasms (particularly lymphoma), ethmoiditis, and turbinate disease. The more distal the obstruction, the more likely it is that the epiphora will be accompanied by purulent discharge or *dacryocystitis*, as the stagnant tears become infected.

DIFFERENTIAL DIAGNOSIS (3)

The differential can be organized according to the underlying pathophysiology (see Table 205.1). The most common causes are senile ectropion and increased physiologic tearing.

WORKUP (3,4)

History

A careful history often suggests the etiology. The quality, quantity, aggravating and alleviating factors, and associated symptoms should be ascertained; determining whether the tearing is unilateral or bilateral and under what conditions the tearing worsens may provide insight into the etiology. *Unilateral constant tearing* suggests insufficient lacrimal outflow, whereas intermittent *bilateral tearing* that is worse in wind and cold suggests secondary reflex tearing due to underlying dry eye. *Itching and watering eyes* together suggest ocular allergy, especially when seasonal variation is reported. Allergic rhinitis can also result in epiphora due to obstruction of the outflow pathway in the nose due to edema of the nasal mucosa. When *ocular pain* is present, consideration should be given corneal abrasions and foreign bodies, trichiasis, and intraocular inflammation. *Periocular pain* with tearing and *purulent discharge* is suggestive of dacryocystitis; *redness* or *swelling* in the region of the lacrimal sac may be noted by the patient. A history of *bloody tears* suggests malignancy along the path of the lacrimal drainage system.

The patient should be asked about systemic inflammatory disorders such as *Wegener's granulomatosis* and *sarcoidosis* and certain neoplasms, such as *lymphoma*, that can cause lacrimal outflow obstruction. The tearing patient should be

TABLE 205.1

CAUSES OF WATERY EYES

Excessive Tear Production
Keratitis
Blepharitis
Conjunctivitis
Allergy
Aberrant regeneration after Bell's palsy
Reflex tearing of dry eyes

Impaired Tear Drainage
Punctal stenosis
Canalicular stenosis
Nasolacrimal duct obstruction with or without
   dacryocystitis
Ectropion, entropion, lid laxity
Lacrimal sac or nasal mass

From Haidak DJ, Hurwitz BS, Yeung KY. Tear-duct fibrosis (dacryostenosis) due to 5-flurouracil. Ann Int Med 1978;88:657, with permission.

asked about history of malignancy and recent chemotherapy; *docetaxel* and *fluorouracil* may cause lacrimal drainage outflow obstruction; *radioactive iodine (I^{131})* may induce stenosis within the canaliculus and/or nasolacrimal duct. A history of neoplasm of the head for which the patient received *radiation therapy* should be noted because radiation can cause canalicular stenosis and severe dry eye with subsequent reflex tearing.

Physical Examination

The examination focuses on external examination of the eyelids and ocular surface, nasal examination, and slitlamp examination. The eyelids should be checked to be sure they are well-apposed to the ocular surface without ectropion on entropion. The medial canthus area should be inspected and palpated. The lacrimal sac cannot normally be felt. Fullness of the lacrimal sac, erythema of the overlying skin, or reflux of mucus or purulent material from the puncta on digital pressure suggest dacryocystitis. Tumors of the lacrimal sac and mucoceles may also result in palpable masses in the region of the medial canthus.

A basic nasal examination should be performed because obstructions within the nose can impede lacrimal drainage. Special equipment is not necessary. A light source and nasal speculum provide the ability to examine the septum, turbinates, and nasal floor. Masses, mucosal inflammation, and hypertrophic turbinates should be noted.

Tests

Any purulent discharge should be sent for Gram's stain and culture. Ophthalmologic evaluation includes *slit-lamp examination* and *fluorescein dye testing*. The slit lamp is used to identify corneal abrasions, foreign bodies, trichiasis, and intraocular inflammation. The *dye disappearance test* is a simple test in evaluating epiphora. Two percent fluorescein solution or a fluorescein strip moistened with saline solution is applied to the inferior fornix of both eyes. The volume of the tear lake is then noted with a cobalt blue–filtered light. The patient is examined 5 minutes later, at which time the relative volume of the tear lakes is determined and compared. A narrow tear strip suggests adequate lacrimal outflow, whereas elevation of the tear lake suggests obstruction of the lacrimal drainage system. The site of lacrimal drainage obstruction cannot be determined by this test.

The ophthalmologist may also evaluate the lacrimal drainage system by probing and irrigation of the canaliculi and nasolacrimal duct. This allows for localization of canalicular and nasolacrimal duct obstruction when present.

Imaging studies may also be useful in evaluating the tearing patient and should be considered when there is a history of recurrent sinus infections, bloody tears, facial trauma, or evidence of a lacrimal sac or nasal mass. *Computerized tomography* is the imaging modality of choice when bony lesions are of greatest concern; sinus images are also of good quality; *magnetic resonance imaging* gives superior soft-tissue imaging.

SYMPTOMATIC MANAGEMENT AND INDICATIONS FOR REFERRAL

Irritants must be eliminated. Dryness is treated with appropriate *lubricants* (see Chapter 202). Dacryocystitis is treated with *hot compresses* at least four times a day and *systemic antibiotics* (usually Augmentin 500 mg twice daily or erythromycin 250 mg four times a day). Patients without infection can be reassured that the condition is not harmful. Unresponsive patients should be referred to an ophthalmologist for further evaluation and treatment. In symptomatic cases, lid surgery to correct malposition or dacryocystorhinostomy to relieve nasolacrimal obstruction may be indicated.

Annotated Bibliography

1. Esmaeli B, Valero V, Ahmadi MA, et al. Canalicular stenosis secondary to docetaxel (Taxotere): a newly recognized side effect. Ophthalmology 2001;108:994. (*An example of an etiology related to cancer chemotherapy.*)
2. Schein OD, Tielsch JM, Munoz B, et al. Relation between signs and symptoms of dry eye in the elderly. A population-based perspective. Ophthalmology 1997;104:1395. (*A helpful explanation of the complex presentation of dry and wet eye complaints.*)
3. Jones LT, Linn ML. The diagnosis of the causes of epiphora. Am J Ophthalmol 1969;67:751. (*The classic paper on the subject.*)
4. Pflugfelder SC, Tseng SC, Sanabria O, et al. Evaluation of subjective assessments and objective diagnostic tests for diagnosing tear-film disorders known to cause ocular irritation. Cornea 1998;17:38. (*A comprehensive review of eye moisture disorders and approach to workup.*)

CHAPTER 206 ■ MANAGEMENT OF THE PATIENT WITH AGE-RELATED MACULAR DEGENERATION

TINA SCHEUFELE CLEARY AND CLAUDIA U. RICHTER

Age-related macular degeneration (AMD) is a major cause of vision loss in the elderly, affecting an estimated 46.2% of persons older than the age of 75 years. Advanced AMD—defined as having one eye with either geographic atrophy or neovascular AMD—affects as many as 16% of people older than the age of 80 years in the United States. With the anticipated sharp increase in the number of elderly individuals in the United States over the next 20 years, the prevalence of AMD is expected to rise dramatically from 1.75 million with advanced disease in the year 2000 to nearly 3 million by the year 2020.

Proper geriatric eye care includes early recognition of macular degeneration and prompt ophthalmologic referral so that the risk of visual impairment can be minimized. With new treatments available for neovascular AMD, 30% to 40% of patients with this type of AMD may regain some of the vision they lost if they are treated in a timely manner.

PATHOPHYSIOLOGY AND CLINICAL PRESENTATION (1–6)

Pathophysiology

The retinal pigment epithelium is critical to the maintenance of healthy retinal photoreceptors; any compromise to it can lead to a loss of vision. In macular degeneration, the retinal pigment epithelium begins to degenerate; deposits of debris called *drusen* accumulate between the epithelial cell and the underlying basement membrane (Bruch's membrane). The mechanisms are poorly understood, but inflammatory mediators probably play a role; for example, a mutation in the complement factor H gene has been identified that is associated with a two- to sevenfold increase in the risk of AMD. Other risk factors include increasing age, race (more common in whites), cardiovascular disease, atherosclerotic risk factors, sun exposure, and dietary factors (e.g., lack of antioxidants, zinc). Cigarette smoking is a potent independent risk factor, with a dose–response relationship, particularly in women.

Drusen deposits are categorized by their ophthalmoscopic appearance. *Hard* or *nodular drusen* are pinhead-sized, yellow-white lesions visible ophthalmoscopically in the macular region. *Soft* or *granular drusen* are larger and have less distinct edges. The presence of *diffuse*, or *confluent*, drusen and extensive retinal pigment epithelial changes (*hyper- or hypopigmentation*) places a patient at high risk for advanced AMD.

Detachment of the retinal pigment epithelium results from the degenerative process that both weakens and thickens Bruch's membrane. Detachment leads to visual loss as the overlying photoreceptor cells atrophy. In addition, new blood vessels may form (*neovascularization*) in response to the degenerative changes in Bruch's membrane. These fragile, abnormal new vessels leak and/or bleed underneath the retina, resulting in vision loss. If the condition is left untreated, fibrovascular scarring may ensue. Fortunately, only about 10% of people with age-related macular degeneration develop neovascularization, or wet AMD.

Clinical Presentation and Course

Because the degenerative process is concentrated in the macula, central visual acuity is most affected. Patients may complain of a loss of visual acuity that is not corrected by eyeglasses. In patients without neovascularization, the loss of visual acuity tends to be gradual. Macular examination of such persons may reveal drusen, retinal pigment epithelial changes, and/or geographic atrophy.

"Wet" versus "Dry" Macular Degeneration

The distinction is based on the presence or absence of neovascularization. Ten percent of AMD patients with neovascularization develop *"wet"* or *"exudative"* AMD. After one eye develops wet AMD, the risk to the other eye increases to 40% over the next 5 years. Close to 90% of persons with severe central vision loss have wet AMD. When neovascularization develops, vision loss may be acute. *Distorted vision* (*metamorphopsia*) may herald the onset of fluid leaking into and underneath the retina. In addition to revealing drusen, macular examination may show subretinal fluid and/or hemorrhage. Longstanding cases often develop fibrotic macular scarring.

The 90% of AMD patients without neovascularization are labeled as having *"dry"* or *nonexudative disease*, which usually has a more benign clinical course and prognosis. Nonetheless, even patients with dry AMD may lose significant vision over time due to retinal atrophy; however, the rate of vision loss is usually slow and progressive, rather than sudden.

DIAGNOSIS

Suggestive historical features include gradual or sudden loss of central visual acuity or distorted vision (*metamorphopsia*) in an elderly person. The latter suggests the development of choroidal neovascularization, or wet AMD. Metamorphopsia can be detected at home by using an *Amsler grid*, a 10 × 10-cm card with a criss-crossed grid of vertical and horizontal white lines every 5 mm and a central dot. The patient is asked to focus on the dot and note whether any of the lines appear wavy or distorted or whether any of the boxes formed by the intersecting lines are missing. Each eye is tested separately with any prescribed corrective lenses worn and the grid held at a comfortable reading distance.

Characteristic ophthalmoscopic findings are concentrated in the macular region and include drusen, irregularities in macular pigmentation, hemorrhage, subretinal fluid, and disciform scarring.

PRINCIPLES OF MANAGEMENT (1,2,5,7–11)

Prevention

Primary Prevention

Cessation of smoking is essential. Smoking is the most important known modifiable risk factor. Ongoing smoking is particularly harmful. Its identification as an independent risk factor with a dose-dependent effect makes smoking cessation a top priority (see Chapter 54).

Secondary Prevention

In addition to smoking cessation, patients with macular degeneration are encouraged to eat plenty of leafy green vegetables and at least one serving of fish a week. They may also benefit from *antioxidant vitamins* and *zinc*, based on the reduced risk of progression shown by the Age-Related Eye Disease Study (AREDS). AREDS, a major randomized trial of nutritional supplements, demonstrated a beneficial effect of high doses of antioxidant vitamins (vitamins C and E and β-carotene) and zinc supplementation in reducing progression to advanced age-related macular degeneration by 25% over 5 years. Patients who smoke should not take supplements containing β-carotene because of the reported increased risk of lung cancer with high-dose β-carotene supplementation. The AREDS II trial, a clinical trial sponsored by the National Eye Institute, will evaluate the benefit of lutein, zeaxanthin, and the omega-3 fatty acids.

Exudative (Wet) Disease (12)

The available treatments for wet AMD are evolving. Initially treatments focused on coagulation of neovascularized membrane; more-current approaches attempt to block the development of neovascularization.

Thermal laser photocoagulation, in which a thermal laser is used to coagulate the neovascular membrane, was the first treatment available. Because this treatment destroys both the abnormal neovascular membrane and the overlying normal retinal tissue, it is currently only used for neovascular membranes that do not involve the center of the vision (the fovea).

Photodynamic therapy with verteporfin was developed in the late 1990s as a treatment for neovascular lesions in the foveal zone. With this therapy, a "cold" laser is used to activate the photosensitive dye verteporfin, which is administered intravenously and selectively concentrates in areas of abnormal choroidal neovascularization.

Antiangiogenic therapy for AMD marked a dramatic advance in the treatment of wet AMD. *Anti–vascular endothe-*

lial growth factor (anti-VEGF) preparations (e.g., *pegaptanib* [*Macugen*], *bevacizumab* [*Avastin*], *ranibizumab* [*Lucentis*]) have shown ability to slow or halt disease progression, and in the case of *ranibizumab*, achieve improvement of vision. All three of these anti-VEGF drugs are injected directly into the eye.

To maximize the benefit of these therapies for wet AMD, early clinical detection of neovascularization is critical. Macular degeneration patients are instructed to watch for and promptly report any distortion of vision. Daily home use of an *Amsler grid* is an excellent and simple means of early detection. Any new defects or distortions in central vision require prompt reporting to the ophthalmologist and consideration of urgent treatment.

PATIENT EDUCATION

When AMD becomes advanced, vision may decline to 20/200 or worse, making the patient legally blind. Patients may lose the ability to do tasks that require good central vision, such as reading or driving. However, it is important to reassure them that their peripheral vision is unlikely to be affected by AMD. Patients are generally followed by their ophthalmologist every 6 months to 1 year. Smoking cessation (and avoidance of secondhand smoke) is strongly advocated (see Chapter 54). Patients are encouraged to eat a diet rich in leafy green vegetables and to have at least one serving of fish a week. AREDS-type vitamin supplements are recommended, but smokers should take a modified supplement that does not contain β-carotene. Although research is still being conducted to assess the benefit of lutein, zeaxanthin, and the omega-3 fatty acids, some ophthalmologists recommend supplemental lutein and omega-3 fatty acids.

Patients are instructed to use the Amsler grid for home self-monitoring. They should report any blurred vision, metamorphopsia, or Amsler gird changes immediately because these symptoms may signal conversion from dry to wet AMD. When vision loss is extensive, patients may benefit from low-vision aids.

INDICATIONS FOR REFERRAL

Any elderly patient suspected on the basis of history or physical examination to have macular degeneration should be referred to an ophthalmologist. Prompt referral is critical if there is a recent decline in vision or the vision is distorted because these symptoms may herald the onset of wet AMD.

CONCLUSIONS AND RECOMMENDATIONS

- Age-related macular degeneration is a major cause of vision loss in the elderly.
- Metamorphopsia or a sudden change in vision may be a symptom of wet AMD and requires urgent ophthalmologic evaluation.
- Antioxidant vitamin and zinc supplementation (AREDS formula vitamins) may reduce the progression to advanced AMD.
- Wet AMD can be treated with intravitreal anti-VEGF agents, photodynamic therapy, intravitreal steroids (usually in combination with one of these other treatments), or thermal laser.

Annotated Bibliography

1. Christen WG, Glynn RJ, Manson JE, et al. A prospective study of cigarette smoking and risk of age-related macular degeneration in men. JAMA 1996;276:1147. (*Data from the Physicians' Health Study showing a significant increase in risk with smoking.*)
2. Edwards AO, Ritter R 3rd, Abel KJ, et al. Complement factor H polymorphism and age-related macular degeneration. Science. 2005; 308:421. (*A genetic link for age-related macular degeneration.*)
3. Fine SL, Berger JW, Maguire MG, et al. Age-related macular degeneration. N Engl J Med 2000;342:483. (*An excellent review for the generalist reader; 63 references.*)
4. Friedman DS, O'Colmain BJ, Munoz B, et al. Prevalence of age-related macular degeneration in the United States. Arch Ophthalmol 2004;122:564. (*Presents important epidemiologic data.*)
5. Seddon JM, Willet WC, Speizer FE, et al. A prospective study of cigarette smoking and age-related macular degeneration in women. JAMA 1996;276:1141. (*Prospective epidemiologic data from the Nurses' Health Study, finding that cigarette smoking is a strong independent risk factor.*)
6. Klein R, Klein BE, Tomany SC, et al. Ten-year incidence and progression of age-related maculopathy: The Beaver Dam Eye Study. Ophthalmology 2002;109:1767. (*Found an increased incidence with age; soft drusen significantly increase the risk of geographic atrophy and wet macular degeneration.*)
7. AREDS. A randomized, placebo-controlled, clinical trial of high-dose supplementation with vitamins C and E and beta carotene and zinc for age-related cataract and vision loss. AREDS Report no. 8. Arch Ophthalmol 2001;119:1417. (*Both zinc and antioxidants with zinc reduced the risk of developing advanced age-related macular degeneration in patients with high-risk retinal findings.*)
8. Macular Photocoagulation Study Group. Argon laser photocoagulation for senile macular degeneration: results of a randomized clinical trial. Arch Ophthalmol 1982;100:912. (*The original report of laser therapy reducing the frequency of vision loss from 60% to 25%.*)
9. Macular Photocoagulation Study Group. Laser photocoagulation of subfoveal neovascular lesions of age-related macular degeneration: updated findings from two clinical trials. Arch Ophthalmol 1993;111:1200. (*The long-term results of a major randomized, controlled trial; laser treatment delayed the onset of severe vision loss in only a small percentage of eyes with exudative disease.*)
10. Treatment of Age-related Macular Degeneration with Photodynamic Therapy (TAP) Study Group. Photodynamic therapy of subfoveal choroidal neovascularization in age-related macular degeneration with verteporfin: one-year results of 2 randomized clinical trials—TAP report. Arch Ophthalmol 1999;117:1329. (*Verteporfin safely reduced the risk of vision loss in persons with classic choroidal neovascularization.*)
11. Gragoudas ES, Adamis AP, Cunningham ET Jr, et al. Pegaptanib for neovascular age-related macular degeneration. N Engl J Med. 2004; 351:2805. (*An original report of major benefit for the use of anti–vascular endothelial growth factor.*)

CHAPTER 207 ■ MANAGEMENT OF GLAUCOMA

LAURA C. FINE AND CLAUDIA U. RICHTER

Glaucoma is an optic neuropathy characterized by acquired atrophy of the optic nerve and loss of retinal ganglion cells and their axons. Elevated intraocular pressure and other, less well understood factors contribute to progressive optic nerve cupping and visual field loss. Glaucoma is one of the leading preventable causes of legal blindness in the United States. In managing the glaucoma patient, the ophthalmologist strives to achieve a stable range of intraocular pressures deemed likely to retard further optic nerve damage.

Management poses a challenge for the patient and the doctor because of the condition's chronic, frequently asymptomatic nature and requirement for daily use of eye medications, which may have side effects. Establishing a regimen involves attention to its effectiveness, toxicity, and impact of noncompliance on outcomes. If medications are ineffective or poorly tolerated, laser or incisional surgery needs consideration.

Although the primary physician is not responsible for the definitive diagnosis or treatment of glaucoma, it remains important to identify patients at risk (see Chapter 198), recognize early stages of optic nerve damage, and understand the systemic effects of topical and oral glaucoma medications.

PATHOPHYSIOLOGY AND CLINICAL PRESENTATION (1–3)

Pathophysiology

The intraocular pressure is maintained by the dynamic equilibrium of aqueous production and outflow. The iris divides the anterior portion of the eye into anterior and posterior chambers, which communicate through the pupil. Aqueous humor, produced by the ciliary body, fills the posterior chamber, flows through the pupil into the anterior chamber, and leaves the eye through the *trabecular meshwork*, a connective tissue filter at the angle between the iris and the cornea. The aqueous passes through the trabecular meshwork into Schlemm's canal and into the episcleral venous system.

Although *elevated intraocular pressure* is not part of the definition of glaucoma, intraocular pressure is the only modifiable risk factor. Increased intraocular pressure is caused by *obstruction to outflow*. In open-angle glaucoma, obstruction exists at a microscopic level in the trabecular meshwork. In angle-closure glaucoma, the iris obstructs the trabecular meshwork due to an anatomic variation causing pupillary block and obstruction of aqueous humor flow into the anterior chamber. Increased intraocular pressure increases vascular resistance, causing decreased vascular perfusion of the optic nerve and ischemia and direct damage to the axons in the optic nerve. The increased pressure interferes with axoplasmic flow in the ganglion cell axons, causing cell dysfunction and death, and it compresses the lamina cribrosa—the sievelike structure through which axons pass when leaving the eye. The altered supporting structure may then interfere with axonal function. These different mechanisms of axonal damage are of variable importance in different patients, but the final result is loss of ganglion cells and their axons, increased optic nerve cupping, and visual field loss.

Clinical Presentation

Open-angle glaucoma (OAG), which accounts for more than 90% of glaucoma cases, has multiple risk factors, including elevated ocular pressure, older age (>50 years), African American or Hispanic race, family history of glaucoma, and thin central cornea. There appears to be a subset of patients with low diastolic perfusion pressures (diastolic blood pressure minus intraocular pressure) who are at higher risk for OAG. The effect of concurrent cardiovascular disease, systemic hypertension, myopia, and diabetes on OAG has not been demonstrated consistently. Characteristic changes in the optic nerve and nerve fiber layer (see later discussion) suggest early glaucomatous injury and facilitate diagnosis, as does asymptomatic elevated intraocular pressure. Open-angle glaucoma is frequently called the "silent stealer of sight" because extensive optic nerve damage may occur before the patient is aware of visual field loss.

Acute angle-closure glaucoma (ACG) presents with a *painful red eye*. The physical findings include decreased visual acuity, red eye, nonreactive pupil in mid-dilation, markedly elevated intraocular pressure, redness, and corneal edema. Occasionally, the principal symptoms are nausea and vomiting, and, if the eye findings are overlooked, the patient may be mistaken to have abdominal or coronary disease. Patients with acute ACG require emergency treatment to lower intraocular pressure and immediate referral to an ophthalmologist. *Subacute* attacks of angle-closure glaucoma may present with intermittent episodes of *halos* around lights or of *painful blurred vision*. Patients susceptible to ACG can be identified by shining a light parallel to the iris plane from the temporal side of the globe: eyes with narrow angles will have a shadow fall on the nasal iris.

DIAGNOSIS (4,5)

Ophthalmoscopy

Cupping of the optic nerve is the pathognomonic finding of glaucoma. Changes in the contour of the optic cup in the center of the optic disc provide the first definitive evidence of glaucomatous damage. The usual cup has a round, regular contour. The cup in early glaucoma becomes notched on the superotemporal or inferotemporal rim. Later changes include an increase in the depth and width of the physiologic cup, nasal displacement of the central retinal vessels, peripapillary choroidal atrophy, and progressive pallor of the optic nerve head. Additional signs of glaucoma are asymmetric cupping and disc hemor-

rhages. Assessment of disc pathology is not as straightforward as measurement of intraocular pressure. It requires greater skill, but it improves sensitivity to as much as 85%, which is especially helpful in the detection of early disease. Performing pupillary dilation greatly facilitates the evaluation. Red-free illumination may aid in evaluating the retinal nerve fiber layer. Color stereophotography or computer-based image analysis of the optic nerve head and retinal nerve fiber layer are the best methods of documenting optic nerve morphology.

Measurement of Intraocular Pressure

Many randomized, controlled clinical trials demonstrate that lowering the intraocular pressure (IOP) decreases the progression of glaucomatous optic nerve damage. The IOP is measured using a contact applanation method (preferably a Goldmann tonometer). It is often helpful to record diurnal IOP fluctuations, either on the same day or on different days. The presence of elevated IOP (>21 mm Hg) in the absence of cupping indicates ocular hypertension but not necessarily glaucoma. In the presence of healthy optic nerves, the degree of IOP elevation and other risk factors (age, race, family history, central corneal thickness) guide the decision to treat.

Visual Field Testing

When cupping is noted, visual field testing is indicated to check for the characteristic peripheral field deficits. Confrontation testing by the primary physician may detect large deficits, but referral for formal visual field testing is necessary for the detection of more subtle deficits. In the ophthalmologist's office, formal testing is computerized; use of short-wavelength automated perimetry and frequency-doubling technology may detect defects earlier than standard perimetry.

Central Corneal Thickness

Ophthalmologic measurement of central corneal thickness (pachymetry) aids in the interpretation of the IOP measurement and helps to stratify patient risk. Patients with thin central corneas may have falsely low applanation pressures, whereas those with thick corneas may have falsely high applanation pressures. Ophthalmologists can correct for these measurement errors by adjusting the IOP for the degree of corneal thickness.

Gonioscopy

To differentiate open- from closed-angle glaucoma, gonioscopy is required. A mirrored contact lens is used carefully to examine the anterior-chamber angle. Other secondary causes of glaucoma can also be determined, such as angle recession due to trauma.

PRINCIPLES OF THERAPY (2–4,6–10)

Although there is no direct treatment for the optic nerve injury of glaucoma, it is possible to prevent further optic nerve damage and visual field loss by lowering the IOP. This is the only modifiable risk factor in glaucoma, and several prospective, long-term, randomized clinical trials have helped to clarify the value of lowering the IOP to inhibit the progression of glaucomatous optic neuropathy.

Chronic Open-Angle Glaucoma

Treatment to achieve and maintain the target pressure involves, in escalating order, topical medications, laser trabeculoplasty, and glaucoma surgery. Most patients are first treated topically with a β-blocker, α-agonist, topical *carbonic anhydrase inhibitor*, and/or *prostaglandin analogue* singly or in combination to reach the target pressure. Intraocular pressure, optic nerve appearance, visual field, and nerve fiber layer are monitored to watch for disease progression.

Topical β-Adrenergic Antagonists

Topical β-adrenergic antagonists decrease aqueous humor production. Ophthalmic preparations include carteolol, levobunolol, metipranolol, timolol, and betaxolol (β₁-selective). The β-blockers need to be administered once or twice daily and are well tolerated topically. However, they can have significant systemic side effects, including lethargy, depression, bronchospasm, bradycardia, hypotension, worsening of congestive heart failure, heart block, and syncope. Betaxolol, the β₁-selective blocker, is less likely to trigger bronchospasm but is also slightly less efficacious in controlling glaucoma.

α₂-Selective Adrenergic Agonists

The α₂-selective adrenergic agonists are alternatives to β-blockers and include *apraclonidine* and *brimonidine*. The α₂-selective medications decrease intraocular pressure by reducing aqueous humor production. Topical side effects of these medications include topical hyperemia and allergic conjunctivitis. Systemic side effects of α₂-selective agonists include lethargy, fatigue, drowsiness, dry mouth, and decreased blood pressure.

Carbonic Anhydrase Inhibitors

Carbonic anhydrase inhibitors decrease intraocular pressure by reducing aqueous humor production. Carbonic anhydrase inhibitors are available topically (*brinzolamide, dorzolamide*) and orally (*acetazolamide, dichlorphenamide,* and *methazolamide*). The topical carbonic anhydrase inhibitors have largely replaced the oral medications and are better tolerated. However, the oral agents are still used on a short-term basis to lower very elevated IOP before laser or surgery. The oral carbonic anhydrase inhibitors are associated with significant systemic side effects, including anorexia and weight loss, fatigue, malaise, paresthesias of fingers and toes, depression, diarrhea, metallic taste, nephrolithiasis, agranulocytosis, and aplastic anemia. The blood dyscrasias are not dose dependent and may also occur with the topical drugs. Some patients report that the drops cause a bitter taste in their mouths.

Prostaglandin Analogues

Prostaglandin analogues lower intraocular pressure by increasing uveoscleral outflow. They represent a new class of drugs for treatment of glaucoma and rival β-blockers in efficacy. *Latanoprost, travoprost,* and *bimatoprost* are administered topically once daily. These medications are well tolerated but may cause darkening of the iris and periorbital skin and conjunctival hyperemia. Systemic side effects (e.g., muscle and joint pains and allergic reactions of the skin) are uncommon.

Cholinergic Agonists

Cholinergic agonists reduce intraocular pressure by increasing aqueous outflow through the trabecular meshwork. *Pilocarpine* and *carbachol* are direct-acting agonists. The ocular effects include small pupils with dimming of vision, induced myopia with blurring of vision, cataract, and retinal detachment. Systemic side effects include headache, tremor, salivation, bronchospasm, pulmonary edema, hypertension, hypotension, bradycardia, diarrhea, and nausea and vomiting.

Adherence to Medical Therapy

Adequate treatment of glaucoma requires a high level of adherence to therapy. Frequently, this is not achieved. Patient education and informed participation in treatment decisions may improve adherence and the effectiveness of treatment.

Laser and Surgical Therapies

Laser trabeculoplasty increases aqueous outflow and effectively lowers intraocular pressure in more than 75% of initial treatments of previously unoperated eyes. Laser is generally used when glaucoma is uncontrolled by topical medication, although some ophthalmologists may perform it as initial therapy. Trabeculoplasty lowers IOP by altering the structural and/or metabolic properties of the trabecular meshwork, thereby improving aqueous outflow.

Glaucoma surgery is indicated when medical therapy and laser trabeculoplasty do not lower the intraocular pressure to a level protective of the optic nerve and visual field. The usual procedure is a *trabeculectomy*, which forms a drainage route from the anterior chamber to the subconjunctival space. If filtering surgery fails or cannot be performed, an aqueous tube shunt implant may be placed or laser cycloablation to the ciliary body performed.

Acute Angle-Closure Glaucoma

Proper management requires prompt recognition, immediate treatment to lower intraocular pressure, and urgent referral to an ophthalmologist. Topical antiglaucomatous medications such as a *β-blocker*, *α-agonist*, and/or *carbonic anhydrase inhibitor* are administered. *Topical pilocarpine* 2% is administered to facilitate breaking the pupillary block. *Acetazolamide* may be administered orally or intravenously. Laser or surgical *iridectomy* is performed to prevent recurrent attacks and is indicated prophylactically in the other eye.

Prevention

Several drugs commonly used in internal medicine may increase the risk of developing glaucoma or precipitate an angle-closure attack. *Glucocorticosteroids* lead the list of agents, especially long-term, high-dose use of nasal, topical (especially if applied to the face), inhaled, or systemic preparations; the elderly are at greatest risk. Patients requiring prolonged steroid use should be seen at least annually by the ophthalmologist.

Acute angle-closure glaucoma due to pupillary block can be precipitated by *adrenergic agents*, either locally (e.g., *phenylephrine* drops, nasal *ephedrine*) or systemically (*epinephrine*), by *anticholinergic drugs* (e.g., tricyclic antidepressants, antihistamines, bladder-active agents) and even by over-the-counter formulations. Patients with narrow angles are most at risk. If narrow angles have been diagnosed and treated with laser iridectomies, these medications can be used safely.

Sulfa-based drugs (acetazolamide, hydrochlorothiazide, and topiramate) can cause acute angle-closure glaucoma due to ciliary body edema with anterior rotation of the iris-lens diaphragm. In these cases, iridotomy is not effective. Attacks are usually reversible with discontinuation of the medicine.

Persons with systemic hypertension and coincident ocular hypertension should have their *antihypertensive* regimen increased gradually; risk of hypotensive optic neuropathy increases with precipitous lowering of systemic blood pressure. Treatment should be carried out in conjunction with the guidance of an ophthalmologist.

PATIENT EDUCATION

The first priority is to teach the patient the importance of careful follow-up examinations and compliance with the treatment regimen to preserve vision. Reviewing techniques for proper use of topical medications helps to maximize the delivery of effective doses and minimize systemic absorption. Topical drug solutions are concentrated to facilitate absorption. If excess drug runs into the lacrimal duct and down into the nose, then systemic absorption through the nasal mucosa will occur. To avoid this, the patient should be taught to occlude the lacrimal duct either by direct pressure when applying drops or by closing the eyelids for 5 minutes after applying the drops. Patients should be advised about the ocular side effects of systemic drugs and the systemic effects of their glaucoma treatments.

RECOMMENDATIONS

- Send all persons older than the age of 40 years to be examined for glaucoma. This is especially critical for patients with a family history of glaucoma or with a history of chronic corticosteroid use.
- Take note of any optic nerve cupping, asymmetry, or disc hemorrhage during routine ophthalmoscopy and refer promptly for evaluation any persons with suspicious optic nerve appearance.
- Refer urgently any person with suspected acute angle-closure glaucoma (e.g., painful red eye, decreased visual acuity, markedly elevated intraocular pressure, nonreactive pupil in mid-dilation, and corneal haziness).
- Treatment of open-angle glaucoma begins with a topical β-blocker, α-agonist, topical carbonic anhydrase inhibitor, and/or prostaglandin analogue singly or in combination to reach the target pressure. If medical therapy proves inadequate or intolerable, laser trabeculoplasty or surgery may be indicated.
- Patients taking drops require instruction in the occlusion of nasal lacrimal ducts to minimize risk of systemic absorption through the nasal mucosa.
- Have intraocular pressure, optic nerve appearance, visual field, and nerve fiber layer monitored by an ophthalmologist to watch for disease progression.
- Know the patient's ocular medications and their systemic side effects.
- Monitor intraocular pressure carefully in persons (especially the elderly) taking corticosteroids. Be aware of the medications that can precipitate angle-closure attacks (anticholinergics, sulfa-based medications, etc.); patients with glaucoma should ask their ophthalmologist if these are safe for them.

Annotated Bibliography

1. Garbe E, LeLorier J, Boivin JF, et al. Inhaled and nasal glucocorticoids and the risks of ocular hypertension or open-angle glaucoma. JAMA 1997;277:722. (*A case–control study; prolonged [>3 months] daily use at high dose increases risk.*)
2. Gordon MO, Beiser JA, Brandt JD, et al. The Ocular Hypertension Treatment Study: baseline factors that predict the onset of primary open-angle glaucoma. Arch Ophthalmol 2002;120:714. (*A randomized, controlled trial; found that lowering the intraocular pressure reduces the risk of progression to early glaucoma in patients with ocular hypertension.*)
3. Van Veldhuisen PC, Schwartz AL, Gaasterland DE, et al. The Advanced Glaucoma Intervention Study (AGIS): 7. The relationship between control of intraocular pressure and visual field deterioration. Am J Ophthalmol 2000;130:429. (*Visual fields worsened more in eyes with intraocular pressure [IOP] >17.5 mm Hg than in eyes with IOP <14 mm Hg.*)
4. Alward WLM. Medical management of glaucoma. N Engl J Med 1998;339:1298. (*A detailed review of diagnosis and medical therapy of glaucoma; 118 references.*)
5. Margolis KL, Money BE, Kopietz LA, et al. Physician recognition of ophthalmoscopic signs of open-angle glaucoma. J Gen Intern Med 1989;4:296. (*An educational program, which includes good photographs of the key findings.*)
6. Janz NK, Wren PA, Lichter PR, et al. Quality of life in newly diagnosed glaucoma patients: the Collaborative Initial Glaucoma Treatment Study. Ophthalmology 2001;108:887. (*Aggressive therapy with both methods of treatment was effective in lowering IOP; visual field loss was minimal in both groups.*)
7. Kass MA, Gordon M, Morley RE, Jr., et al. Compliance with topical timolol treatment. Am J Ophthalmol 1987;103:188-193. (*Nearly one third of patients were found to be poorly adherent to therapy.*)
8. Leske MC, Heijl A, Hussein M, et al. Factors for glaucoma progression and the effect of treatment: the early manifest glaucoma trial. Arch Ophthalmol 2003;121:48. (*There was a 10% reduction in the risk of progression with every 1–mm Hg drop in IOP; 45% of treated patients had visual deterioration despite well-controlled IOP.*)
9. Shingleton BJ, Richter CU, Bellows AR, et al. Long-term efficacy of argon laser trabeculoplasty. Ophthalmology 1987;94:1513. (*Laser therapy was effective in 50% of patients treated after 4 years.*)
10. Stewart WC, Garrison PM. Beta-blocker–induced complications and the patient with glaucoma: newer treatments to help reduced systemic adverse effects. Arch Intern Med 1998;158:221. (*A good review of adverse effects and new topical alternatives, such as prostaglandin analogues, α₂-agonists, and topical carbonic anhydrase inhibitors.*)

CHAPTER 208 ■ MANAGEMENT OF CATARACTS

CLAUDIA U. RICHTER AND LAURA C. FINE

Cataracts, or opacifications of the crystalline lens, are the leading cause of blindness worldwide. Cataracts remain an important, treatable cause of blindness and visual impairment in the United States. They are unusual in young patients, but the incidence rises sharply in later years, such that virtually all elderly patients have some degree of cataract. Because of the implications of this diagnosis, the term *cataract* is best reserved for opacities resulting in functional impairment. The primary care physician should be able to detect cataract formation, monitor its progression, advise the patient when to seek ophthalmologic consultation, help the ophthalmologist assess medical candidacy for surgery, and support the patient in the perioperative and rehabilitation phases.

PATHOPHYSIOLOGY AND CLINICAL PRESENTATION (1–4)

Most cataracts occur in the elderly and reflect *senescent change*; occasionally, they ensue from systemic disease, and they are also frequently associated with intraocular inflammation and glaucoma. *Cigarette smoking*; excess exposure to *glucocorticosteroids*, *ultraviolet B light, and lead*; and *family history* have been linked epidemiologically to cataract formation. Presenile and senile cataract formation is painless and generally progresses over months or years. Cataracts found during the early years of life are either congenital or the consequence of *diabetes*, *Wilson's disease*, *Down's syndrome*, and other metabolic diseases. *Trauma* is an important precipitant.

Senile Cataract

With age, the lens increases in thickness and weight. Continued production of lens fibers causes hardening and compression of the nucleus, known as *nuclear sclerosis*. Subsequently, the lens proteins undergo modification and aggregation, and they take on a yellow-brown discoloration, changing the transparency and refractive index of the lens. In addition, sodium and calcium concentrations increase, potassium and ascorbate levels diminish, and glutathione disappears. The underlying metabolic changes leading to senile cataract are unknown. In diabetes mellitus, excess sugar is diverted to the sorbitol pathway. An insoluble alcohol accumulates, and this osmotic load causes the protein to hydrate.

As the human lens ages, the first visual event may be a shift toward nearsightedness because of the increased refractive index and thickness of the sclerotic nucleus. As a result, the patient may temporarily experience enhanced reading vision without glasses (*second sight*), and a change in spectacles may be the only treatment needed. Eventually, the nucleus acquires a yellow-brown coloration ("brunescent cataract") and becomes progressively more opaque, affecting visual clarity. Patients may be unaware of the gradual spectral change causing a yellow cast to the visual world; they usually acknowledge it only after the cataract is removed. Visual impairment initially is more marked at distance than near, and a patient may fail a driver's license examination and still be able to read a newspaper. Loss of contrast sensitivity may cause a functional impairment out of proportion to the results of a standard high-contrast visual acuity test.

Presenile Cataract

Posterior *subcapsular cataracts* form at the back of the lens, usually centrally. This type of cataract is often responsible for the "presenile" cataract in the 40- to 50-year-old age group. It may be spontaneous but is often associated with prolonged use of topical, inhaled, or systemic *steroids* and with *diabetes mellitus*. The central location of the opacity causes the vision to worsen when the pupil becomes small, as in reading or in bright light. The refractile nature of the opacity commonly causes severe difficulty with glare, such as when driving at night. Pupillary dilation by mydriatic or cycloplegic drops or use of subdued light improves vision in such cases, as more light is allowed to enter the eye.

Traumatic Cataract

These most commonly result from intraocular foreign bodies that perforate the lens capsule, allowing the lens protein to hydrate and thereby denature and opacify. Occasionally, a lens will opacify after severe blunt nonpenetrating trauma. Electric shock and high-dose ionizing radiation may lead to lens opacification. Prolonged exposure to *ultraviolet B*, as occurs with unprotected *sun exposure*, is an important risk factor for cortical cataract formation; risk of nuclear cataract is not significantly increased.

WORKUP (5)

Initial evaluation by the primary physician includes *visual acuity* determination both near and at a distance. The lenticular opacity can be appreciated with the *direct ophthalmoscope* while attempting to visualize the fundus. If the angle is not shallow, dilation with one drop of 2.5% phenylephrine or 1% tropicamide is helpful. With the ophthalmoscope lens set at zero and standing about 12 inches from the patient, a bright red reflex is seen in the normal eye. Cataract formation is clearly seen by the *disruption of the red reflex*. Plus power (black numbers) in the ophthalmoscope of about 15 or 20 diopters will put the lens of the eye in focus as the physician approaches the eye. The fundus should be examined for retinal abnormalities, particularly macular degeneration (manifested by hemorrhage, scarring, and drusen), which can cause a loss of vision symptomatically similar to that from cataract. In all cases of visual impairment, an ophthalmic consultation is indicated.

PRINCIPLES OF MANAGEMENT
(5–11)

Conservative Measures and Indications for Surgery

In early nuclear sclerosis, an *eyeglasses prescription* may sufficiently improve vision to defer surgery. Sometimes chronic *pupillary dilation* will suffice for a patient with posterior subcapsular cataract. The only definitive treatment for cataract is surgery, and in rare instances (e.g., traumatic cataracts and very advanced senile cataracts that cause inflammation and glaucoma), emergency surgery is mandatory. However, most cataract surgery is elective and reserved for unacceptable visual impairment not improved by conservative measures. The primary indication for surgery is visual function that no longer meets the patient's needs and for which cataract surgery provides a reasonable likelihood of improved vision.

For many older persons, a major stimulus for cataract surgery is visual impairment compromising ability to drive a motor vehicle. When cataract surgery is being contemplated for the improvement of driving, a patient's total medical condition, including overall psychomotor capability, needs to be taken into account; just treating the cataract may not necessarily improve someone's ability to operate a motor vehicle safely. Nonetheless, prospective cohort study correcting for confounding factors suggests that the rate of automobile accidents in seniors with cataracts can be reduced by nearly 50% with cataract surgery.

Patient Preparation for Surgery

Cataract surgery may be performed using a variety of anesthesia techniques that include general and local (regional) or topical anesthesia. The planned mode of anesthesia is discussed with the patients so that he or she will know what to expect in terms of discomfort and consciousness level. Cataract surgery is most often performed under local anesthesia (block or topical) with mild sedation; however, because any patient movement during surgery can be disastrous, general anesthesia may be necessary in children or uncooperative patients. The primary physician can assist the ophthalmologist in assessing whether age, mental status, or medical condition makes general anesthesia appropriate. However, routine medical testing before cataract surgery has not been shown measurably to improve safety or outcomes.

There is no strong evidence favoring continuation or discontinuation of anticoagulants during cataract surgery for anticoagulated patients. The risk of discontinuing anticoagulant or antiplatelet medications depends on the condition for which they were prescribed. Generally, patients can be left on these medicines if routine cataract surgery is anticipated. Alternatives to retrobulbar injections can be considered in these patients.

Surgical Approaches

Cataract surgery is one of the most common outpatients surgeries performed annually in the United States. In 2004, a total of 1.8 million cataract procedures were performed on Medicare beneficiaries who were not enrolled in health maintenance organizations. There are several options for cataract surgery. The most common is *phacoemulsification*, which uses ultrasonic energy to break up the hard nucleus and aspirate it through a small opening (about 3 mm). The small phacoemulsification wound can be constructed as a self-sealing valve, often not requiring sutures, which allows the patient rapid return to full physical activity. Although most cataract extractions in the United States use the standard phacoemulsification technique, specific circumstances may cause the surgeon to use *extracapsular extraction*, in which the lens capsule is opened and the nucleus is removed in one piece through a large wound (about 10 mm).

Postoperatively, the surgeon prescribes topical medications (antibiotic usually in combination with both steroid and nonsteroidal drops). Final visual correction may be given as soon as 1 to 2 weeks postoperatively.

Visual Rehabilitation

Three methods of *visual rehabilitation* are available: Lens implants are the standard, but contact lenses and eyeglasses are also options.

Intraocular Lens Implantation

Lens implantation is now standard practice when not specifically contraindicated. At the time of cataract extraction (and occasionally as a secondary procedure in cases of spectacle and contact lens intolerance), the surgeon implants a delicate plastic device with optical power to replace the cataractous lens. The implant is permanent, requires no care, and restores normal optics without magnification. The implant is contraindicated in some conditions, such as chronic uveitis, which is assessed by the ophthalmologist preoperatively. Intraocular lenses continue to improve. When the optical portion is made of a flexible material such as solid silicone elastomer, acrylic, or hydrogel, the lens can be folded during insertion so that only a small wound is needed. Standard intraocular lenses (IOLs) are monofocal, and patients are often required to wear reading glasses after surgery. Newer multifocal and accommodating lenses are available; they may afford patients less dependence on bifocals and reading glasses. Adverse effects of these newer lenses include reduced contrast sensitivity, haloes around lights, and glare. Whether the improvement in near unaided acuity outweighs the potential adverse effects of multifocal/accommodating IOLs varies among patients. These newer IOLs may also involve out-of-pocket costs to patients because they are not fully covered by health insurance. They represent only a small fraction of the IOLs placed today.

Cataract Spectacles/Contact Lenses

Intraocular lens implantation is the method of choice to correct aphakia optically. When IOLs cannot be used safely, powerful spectacles or contact lenses are alternative methods of optical correction. The glasses must be powerful to compensate for the absence of the crystalline lens. In addition to thickness and weight, these spectacles magnify vision by approximately 25%, which precludes the use of a cataract lens for only one eye because a double image would result. The spectacle thickness also severely limits side vision, producing a midperipheral blind spot. Such difficulties make the adjustment to cataract glasses problematic at best, and some patients find that ambulation is nearly impossible with these spectacles. Cataract spectacles are now used only in highly unusual circumstances.

Contact lenses are optically superior to eyeglasses. Because the lens power is so much closer to that of the eye than with eyeglass lenses, magnification is only 5% to 7%, and most patients will not perceive diplopia with a contact lens, although stereoscopic acuity will be reduced. Peripheral vision will be normal. Many elderly patients have difficulty handling contact lenses, but extended-wear lenses (usually soft) may facilitate use because they may be worn for weeks to months between removals for cleaning. Use of these lenses is not without difficulty, however. Lens deposits, damage, and loss may result in frequent visits to the ophthalmologist, with high cost and time lost. Devastating infectious corneal ulcers are much more common in elderly patients with extended-wear contact lenses.

Prevention

Prevention of cataract formation is important and often overlooked. Several studies show a linkage of smoking with nuclear sclerosis. Findings from studies indicate a reduced risk of cataracts in past smokers compared with current smokers, demonstrating a benefit from *smoking cessation*. Cumulative lifetime exposure to ultraviolet-B radiation has been associated with lens opacities; therefore, *brimmed hats* and *ultraviolet-B–blocking sunglasses* are reasonable precautions to recommend to patients. Sunglasses need to be specially treated fully to prevent the penetration of ultraviolet radiation, although wearing a hat with a brim and sunglasses with plastic untreated lenses does reduce exposure. However, the darkness of a lens's tint is not necessarily a measure of protective capacity. Dark, unprotective sunglasses may actually exacerbate exposure by blocking visible light transmission, resulting in pupillary dilation and thus increasing penetration of ultraviolet radiation. Outdoor workers are at particularly high risk and should wear close-fitting protective sunglasses.

Limitation of steroid use to the lowest dose and minimum strength necessary (particularly in the elderly) is another potentially important preventive measure. The highest-quality evidence does not support a benefit from nutritional supplementation in preventing or delaying the progression of cataracts. Of interest, the Women's Health Study found that higher intakes of *fruits and vegetables* did appear to be associated with a reduced risk of cataracts. Treatment with supplements is not recommended, and there are no pharmacologic treatments known to eliminate existing cataracts or retard their progression. The association of lead exposure with cataract formation suggests that limiting such exposure might be helpful.

PATIENT EDUCATION AND INDICATIONS FOR REFERRAL

Preventive measures should be taught to all patients, with an emphasis on the use of *protective eyewear and brimmed hats* (especially for those with much sun exposure), *smoking cessation*, and *limitation* in dose and duration of *steroid use*.

For elderly patients with age-related nuclear cataracts, the primary physician should help to explain the condition and outline treatment options. Patients appreciate knowing that cataract formation is not a "growth" and that it poses no harm to the eye. Patients also need to understand that although surgical correction is highly successful in up to 99% of patients, it is not risk free. Occasionally, complications do occur. When vision is good in one eye and there are no important functional limitations, a conservative approach may be preferable to surgery. The degree of interference with daily activities (e.g., driving, reading, watching television) should be reviewed to help in decision making.

Patients with cataracts that significantly impair daily living (e.g., causing falls, prohibiting reading, or interfering with driving) should be referred for consideration of microsurgical cataract extraction with intraocular lens implantation, which has a high likelihood of dramatically improving quality of life.

Annotated Bibliography

1. Garbe E, Suissa S, LeLorier J. Association of inhaled corticosteroid use with cataract extraction in elderly patients. JAMA 1998;280:539. (*A case–control study, finding a threefold increase in the risk of cataract extraction with long-term, high-dose use.*)
2. Grisso JA, Kelsey JL, Strom BL, et al. Risk factors for falls as a cause of hip fracture in women. N Engl J Med 1991;324:1326. (*Impaired vision raises the risk of hip fracture fivefold.*)
3. Schaumberg DA, Mendes F, Balaram M, et al. Accumulated lead exposure and risk of age-related cataract in men. JAMA 2004;292:2750. (*A cohort study, finding a relationship between bone lead and the risk of cataract.*)
4. Taylor HR, West SK, Rosenthal FS, et al. Effect of ultraviolet radiation on cataract formation. N Engl J Med 1988;319:1429. (*Finds a significant relationship between ultraviolet B exposure and cortical cataract formation; argues for wearing protective eyewear in the sun.*)
5. Steinert RF, ed. Cataract: evaluation, surgery, and complications. Philadelphia: Saunders, 1995. (*A comprehensive reference text.*)
6. Centers for Medicare and Medicaid Services: Medicare leading Part B procedure codes based on allowed charges: calendar year 2002. Available at: http://www.cms.hhs.gov/datacompendium/. (*Cataract surgery was the most frequently performed operation and the largest expenditure for any Part B procedure in the Medicare program.*)
7. Owsley C, McGwin G Jr, Sloane M, et al. Impact of cataract surgery on motor vehicle crash involvement by older adults. JAMA 2002;288:841. (*A prospective cohort study with a control group, finding a nearly 50% reduction in the rate of motor vehicle accidents with cataract surgery.*)
8. Rosenthal FS, Fakalian AE, Taylor HR. The effect of prescription eyewear on ocular exposure to ultraviolet radiation. Am J Public Health 1986;76:1216. (*The use of prescription eyewear was found to cut down on ultraviolet exposure.*)
9. Christen WG, Liu S, Schaumberg DA, et al. Fruit and vegetable intake and risk of cataract in women. Am J Clin Nutr 2005;81:1417. (*Found evidence suggesting preventive benefit.*)
10. Schein OD, Katz J, Bass EB, et al. The value of routine preoperative medical testing before cataract surgery. N Engl J Med 2000;342:168. (*A randomized, prospective study; no measurable benefit was found.*)
11. U.S. Department of Health and Human Services, Agency for Health Care Policy and Research. Cataract in adults: management of functional impairment. Clinical practice guideline, number 4 (February 1993). (*A guideline for care based on a comprehensive review of the available evidence.*)

CHAPTER 209 ■ MANAGEMENT OF DIABETIC RETINOPATHY

TINA SCHEUFELE CLEARY AND CLAUDIA U. RICHTER

Diabetic retinopathy is a leading cause of blindness in the United States in people less than 65 years of age. Its incidence has increased with improved long-term survival of diabetics. The prevalence increases with the duration of the disease and is also directly related to the level of diabetic control. Therapy for diabetic retinopathy is most effective when rendered promptly. It is important for the primary physician to know when to check for retinopathy and when to refer to the ophthalmologist for more detailed evaluation and treatment if necessary. Diabetes can also cause other eye problems, including refractive changes, cataracts, glaucoma, and reversible cranial nerve palsies (see Chapters 102, 200, 207, and 208).

PATHOPHYSIOLOGY, CLINICAL PRESENTATION, AND COURSE (1–7)

Diabetic retinopathy can be subdivided into two clinical categories: nonproliferative and proliferative.

Nonproliferative Diabetic Retinopathy

Nonproliferative diabetic retinopathy is the initial manifestation of diabetic eye disease and consists of intraretinal vascular damage. Loss of capillary pericytes, thickening of basement membranes, swelling and proliferation of endothelial cells, and intravascular thrombosis occur. These changes result in both dilation of small vessels and vascular closure, leading to ischemia. In addition, there is abnormal endothelial permeability with breakdown of the normal blood–retinal barrier. Retinal capillaries become permeable to water, lipids, and large molecules, which are not adequately removed by the usual cellular pump mechanism of the adjacent retinal pigment epithelium.

Clinically, this process results in *microaneurysms, intraretinal hemorrhages, cotton-wool infarctions,* and *lipid and serous exudates* leading to *retinal edema.* Microaneurysms are abnormal outpouchings of the capillary wall that may leak fluid and lipid into the retina and sometimes thrombose. They appear as red dots in the retina, similar to the small dot-blot intraretinal hemorrhages that result from bleeding in the deep layers of the retina. Flame-shaped hemorrhages occur in the striated superficial ganglion cell layer. Cotton-wool infarcts are infarcts in the nerve fiber layer. The swollen, infarcted axons become ophthalmoscopically visible as white, feathery, soft lesions. Hard exudates are deposits of the intravascular lipid in the retina and appear as yellow, glistening, spherical aggregates of lipid, sometimes arranged in a circular pattern or circinate ring around leaking microaneurysms. Accumulation of serous fluid in the intercellular spaces of the retina results in retinal thickening or edema.

Patients with nonproliferative retinopathy are asymptomatic unless retinal edema or ischemia involves the central macula. Macular edema causes blurring or distortion followed by loss of central vision. Macular edema is the leading cause of visual loss in diabetics, especially older, type 2 patients. Hypertension and hyperlipidemia can increase the risk of and severity of macular edema.

Proliferative Diabetic Retinopathy

Proliferative diabetic retinopathy describes abnormal vascular proliferation (neovascularization) originating in the retina and extending into the vitreous cavity. This form of retinopathy generally occurs at a later stage than nonproliferative retinopathy and tends to have a worse visual prognosis without prompt treatment. There is a correlation between the duration and degree of hyperglycemia and the progression of retinopathy. Tight control (hemoglobin A1c [HbA1c] <7.0%) slows the onset and severity of retinopathy and other microvascular complications of diabetes (see Chapter 102).

The onset of proliferative disease is often preceded by severe nonproliferative changes, such as a large number of cotton-wool spots and intraretinal hemorrhages, venous beading, and small networks of weblike intraretinal vessels. As increased capillary and arteriolar closure results in widespread retinal ischemia, vasoproliferative factors trigger *neovascularization,* the hallmark of proliferative disease.

Neovascular fronds appear ophthalmoscopically as a fine network of small vessels proliferating from the optic disc, the major retinal vessels, or areas adjacent to retinal ischemia. As neovascularization progresses, dense, white, fibrotic tissue forms and adheres to the posterior vitreous. Such fibrosis can cause the vitreous to contract and pull anteriorly, rupturing the fragile network of vessels growing into the vitreous and producing a *vitreous hemorrhage* inside the eye that compromises vision. When traction is severe enough, it can elevate the retina, resulting in a *tractional retinal detachment.* If traction results in the formation of a retinal hole, a *rhegmatogenous retinal detachment* may result. Neovascularization may also occur on the iris, leading to *neovascular glaucoma* from obstruction of the trabecular meshwork.

A diabetic patient who notices small floating specks or cobwebs in the vision may have a small vitreous hemorrhage. Sudden profound loss of vision occurs most commonly in the setting of a severe vitreous hemorrhage but may also signal a retinal detachment. If the loss of vision is also accompanied by eye pain, neovascular glaucoma may have developed.

Clinical Course

The risks of developing retinopathy and its progression are a function of the duration and the severity of the disease. Smoking exacerbates the risk, and retinal pathology can progress with unanticipated speed during pregnancy. Hypertension and renal failure also increase the risk of nonproliferative and proliferative diabetic retinopathy, and hyperlipidemia increases the risk of vision loss from macular edema. The prevalence of retinopathy after 5 years of type 1 disease is 25%, rising to 60% after 10 years and 80% after 15 years. In the absence of "tight" glycemic control (HbA1c <7.0), proliferative changes are found in about 2% of type 2 patients at 5 years, increasing to 25% by 25 years; approximately 25% of type 1 patients manifest proliferative changes by 15 years. As noted, the risk of developing proliferative retinopathy can be reduced significantly by achieving tight glycemic control.

WORKUP (1)

Screening Ophthalmoscopy

Screening asymptomatic diabetic patients for retinopathy is an essential part of effective diabetic care. Screening methods for detecting diabetic retinopathy include *nondilated ophthalmoscopy*, *dilated ophthalmoscopy* performed by the ophthalmologist, and *stereoscopic fundus photography*. Fundus photography has been implemented for some populations for whom access to ophthalmologists is limited; its sensitivity for detecting retinopathy has not been definitively established. The American Academy of Ophthalmology therefore recommends that patients with access to an ophthalmologist have routine dilated examinations. Dilation allows examination of the more peripheral retina, and stereoscopic biomicroscopy allows evaluation for macular edema. Examination of the nondilated eye with a handheld ophthalmoscope is inadequate for screening because only a small area of the retina is visualized, the lack of stereopsis does not allow for detection of macular edema, and the procedure may not allow for easy detection of early neovascularization. Nonetheless, handheld ophthalmoscopic examination by the primary care physician during routine diabetes follow-up visits might serve as a potentially useful adjunct to formal ophthalmologic screening.

The natural history of diabetic retinopathy dictates the proper *screening schedule*. Screening guidelines for diabetic retinopathy jointly adopted by the American College of Physicians, the American Diabetes Association, and the American Academy of Ophthalmology include the following:

- *For type 1 diabetes*, screen annually beginning 5 years after the onset of diabetes, generally not before the onset of puberty.
- *For type 2 diabetes*, screen initially at the time of diagnosis and then annually.
- *For pregnant* diabetic women, perform dilated ophthalmoscopy each trimester, and more often depending on the severity of the retinopathy. When planning pregnancy, diabetic women should be counseled on the risk of developing or worsening retinopathy. Ideally, diabetic women should be examined prior to planning a pregnancy. No screening is needed for women with gestational diabetes.

For patients with diabetic retinopathy, a shorter follow-up interval may be necessary, depending on the severity of the retinopathy and the need for treatment. Such screening does not obviate ophthalmoscopic examination by the primary physician, who might be able to detect an important lesion in the interval between screening examinations, but nondilated ophthalmoscopy by the primary physician is no substitute for a formal eye examination by the ophthalmologist.

PRINCIPLES OF MANAGEMENT (1–15)

Prevention

Both primary and secondary prevention are achievable by tightly controlling serum glucose, as demonstrated in the two landmark multicenter, randomized, prospective controlled trials of diabetes management: the *Diabetes Control and Complications Trial* (DCCT) for type 1 disease and the *United Kingdom Prospective Diabetes Study* (UKPDS) for type 2 disease.

In the DCCT trial, type 1 patients treated with intensive insulin therapy to normalize blood glucose experienced a reduction in the risk of developing retinopathy of 76%; in those with preexisting retinopathy, the risk of progression was reduced by 54%. Transient worsening of existing retinopathy occurs during the first year of intensive treatment in about one fourth of patients and consists of soft exudates and intraretinal microvascular changes. Such changes usually disappear by 18 months with continued intensive insulin therapy, and the reduction in long-term risk of progression is the same as for patients without early progression. The DCCT study was confined to patients with type 1 diabetes with either no retinopathy or only mild retinopathy. Whether similar results can be achieved in patients with more severe retinopathy remains to be demonstrated. In *type 2 diabetes*, the UKPDS similarly revealed that tight control (HbA1c <7%) significantly reduced both the risk of developing retinopathy and its progression, as well as reducing the risk of nephropathy and neuropathy. Evolving strategies for the normalization of hyperglycemia have made tight control safer and more achievable (see Chapter 102).

The risk of accelerated progression of retinopathy may be greater in patients with proliferative or severe nonproliferative retinal disease, making close ophthalmologic follow-up essential. Patients with hypercholesterolemia are at greater risk for macular edema and more often have hard exudates in the macula that can seriously impair vision. Poorly controlled hypertension and smoking are also risk factors for the progression of retinopathy.

Treatment

Once retinopathy is detected, it requires treatment by a retinal specialist. *Laser photocoagulation* reduces the rate of vision-threatening complications from both forms of retinopathy.

Nonproliferative Retinopathy

The treatment of choice for clinically significant macular edema is *focal laser* treatment of the macular region, which reduces the rate of severe vision loss by greater than 50%. The goal is prevention of vision loss; laser treatment does not necessarily make vision better. Macular edema not responsive to focal laser is often treated with *intravitreal steroids*. Macular ischemia is not reversible. Under investigation are *anti–vascular endothelial growth factor (VEGF) agents*, which hold promise for inhibiting neovascularization.

Proliferative Retinopathy

The primary therapeutic modality for proliferative disease is *panretinal photocoagulation (PRP)*. PRP reduces the neovascular stimulus and reduces the risk of severe vision loss by 50% to 65%. Potential side effects of this type of laser include a mild reduction in vision, decreased night vision, and loss of peripheral vision. Uncommon complications include inadvertent burns to the central macula and hemorrhagic or exudative choroidal detachment, leading to angle-closure glaucoma. *Anti-VEGF agents* are being investigated for their ability to limit neovascularization. When a vitreous hemorrhage does not spontaneously clear or when dense fibrovascular proliferation or tractional retinal detachment threatens the macula, *surgery* is necessary.

Other Hyperglycemia-Related Complications

A myopic shift in the refractive error can occur due to hyperglycemia-induced osmotic swelling of the lens. Reestablishment of glycemic control can reverse this refractive shift. Diplopia due to localized demyelination of the third, fourth, or sixth cranial nerve usually recovers within 1 to 3 months. Cataracts may also form (see Chapter 208).

PATIENT EDUCATION AND INDICATIONS FOR REFERRAL

Patient Education

Patient education by the primary physician is essential to the prevention, early detection, and prompt treatment of retinopathy. Reviewing the benefits of tight glycemic control can be a potent motivating force that improves patient behavior. The importance of smoking cessation, hypertension control, regular ophthalmologic examinations, and immediate reporting of eye symptoms needs to be stressed. Prompt treatment of macular edema and proliferative diabetic retinopathy in a patient with good glycemic control should prevent severe vision loss.

Ophthalmologic Referral

Ophthalmologic referral is indicated for screening (see earlier discussion) and is urgent under the following conditions:

- Change in vision, new floaters, or eye pain.
- Discovery of retinopathy (particularly if abnormal vessels are seen suggestive of neovascularization due to proliferative retinopathy, if there are symptoms or signs of macular edema, or if there are signs of moderate-to-severe nonproliferative retinopathy).
- Loss of ability to visualize the fundus.

Treatment decisions regarding diabetic retinopathy should be made by the ophthalmologist skilled in management of retinal disease.

CONCLUSIONS AND RECOMMENDATIONS

- The prevalence of diabetic retinopathy increases with the duration of disease.
- Tight glycemic control reduces the incidence of diabetic retinopathy.
- Diabetics require routine screening for the development of retinopathy, so that treatment can be initiated to limit visual loss.

Annotated Bibliography

1. American College of Physicians, American Diabetes Association, & American Academy of Ophthalmology. Screening guidelines for diabetic retinopathy. Ann Intern Med 1992;116:683. (*Consensus recommendations for screening based on the natural history of the disease.*)
2. Chew EY, Mills JL, Metzger BE, et al. Metabolic control and progression of retinopathy. The Diabetes in Early Pregnancy Study. Diabetes Care 1995;18:631. (*Glycemic control reduces the risk of progression.*)
3. Paetkau MD, Boyd TAS, Winship B, et al. Cigarette smoking and diabetic retinopathy. Diabetes 1977;26:46. (*The risk of proliferative retinopathy rose with increasing tobacco consumption.*)
4. The Diabetes Control and Complications Trial Research Group. The effect of intensive treatment of diabetes on the development and progression of long-term complications in insulin-dependent diabetes mellitus. N Engl J Med 1993;329:977. (*Tight glycemic control reduced the risks for the development and progression of retinopathy.*)
5. The Diabetes Control and Complications Trial Research Group. The relationship of glycemic exposure (HbA1C) to the risk of development and progression of retinopathy in the Diabetes Control and Complications Trial. Diabetes 1995;44:968. (*Mean hemoglobin A1c was the dominant predictor of retinopathy progression.*)
6. The Diabetes Control and Complications Trial Research Group. The effect of intensive diabetes treatment on the progression of diabetic retinopathy in insulin-dependent diabetes mellitus. Arch Ophthalmol 1995;113:36. (*A randomized, controlled trial, showing retinopathy progression in 54.1% of cases with conventional treatment and in 11.5% of cases with intensive treatment.*)
7. UK Prospective Diabetes Study (UKPDS) Group. Intensive blood-glucose control with sulfonylureas or insulin compared with conventional treatment and risk of complications in patients with type 2 diabetes (UKPDS 33). Lancet 1998;352:837. (*A landmark 20-year randomized, controlled trial, showing that the risk of microvascular complications was reduced by tight control.*)
8. Avery RL, Pearlman J, Pieramici DJ, et al. Intravitreal bevacizumab (Avastin) in the treatment of proliferative diabetic retinopathy. Ophthalmology 2006;113:1695 e1-15. (*Examined the use of anti-vascular endothelial growth factor [VEGF] for the treatment of proliferative diabetic retinopathy.*)
9. Chun DW, Heier JS, Topping TM, et al. A pilot study of multiple intravitreal injections of ranibizumab in patients with center-involving clinically significant diabetic macular edema. Ophthalmology 2006;113:1706. (*Examined the use of anti-VEGF for the treatment of macular edema.*)
10. Cunningham ET Jr, Adamis AP, Altaweel M, et al. A phase II randomized double-masked trial of pegaptanib, an anti–vascular endothelial growth factor aptamer, for diabetic macular edema. Ophthalmology 2005;112:1747. (*Examined the use of anti-VEGF for the treatment of macular edema.*)
11. Ferris FL III, Davis MD, Aiello LM. Treatment of diabetic retinopathy. N Engl J Med 1999;341:667. (*An excellent review for the general reader, with good photographs of eye changes; includes a comprehensive list of references.*)
12. Haritoglou C, Kook D, Neubauer A, et al. Intravitreal bevacizumab (Avastin) therapy for persistent diffuse diabetic macular edema. Retina 2006;26:999. (*Examines the use of anti-VEGF for the treatment of macular edema.*)
13. The Diabetic Retinopathy Study Research Group. Photocoagulation treatment of proliferative diabetic retinopathy. Ophthalmology 1978;85:82. (*A classic paper; established the role of photocoagulation in the treatment of proliferative diabetic retinopathy.*)
14. The Diabetic Retinopathy Vitrectomy Study Research Group. Early vitrectomy for severe vitreous hemorrhage in diabetic retinopathy. Arch Ophthalmol 1985;103:1644. (*Early vitrectomy improved the outcome in type 1 diabetics.*)
15. The Early Treatment Diabetic Retinopathy Study Research Group. Photocoagulation for diabetic macular edema. Arch Ophthalmol 1985;103:1796. (*Focal photocoagulation of macular edema reduced the risk of visual loss.*)

CHAPTER 210 ■ CORRECTION OF VISION

KRISTIE J. BENNETT AND CLAUDIA U. RICHTER

Eyeglasses provide excellent and safe correction of vision, but their inconvenience and cosmetic and functional compromises cause many to seek eyeglass-free means of vision correction. With the aging of the population and the increasing prevalence of presbyopia (age-related loss of ability to view near objects), there is an increasing demand for vision correction and improved approaches to it. Primary physicians are sometimes asked about the relative merits of available means for correction of vision, especially with the advent of laser and other interventional procedures. Knowing the advantages and possible complications of the spectrum of approaches to vision correction can facilitate the patient's choice of approach and referral.

CONTACT LENSES (1–7)

Types of Contact Lenses, Advantages, and Disadvantages

Hard and Rigid Contact Lenses

Hard contact lenses were the first to be developed and were fabricated from polymethyl methacrylate. The very low oxygen permeability of such lenses limited their use to daytime wear and frequently caused corneal edema. *Rigid, gas-permeable lenses*, allowing greater oxygen permeability, have replaced the original hard design and provide improved comfort and longer wearing times. Rigid lenses require longer initial adaptation and may dislodge more frequently than soft contact lenses. However, rigid, gas-permeable lenses provide excellent vision, especially with astigmatic patients. They are relatively easy to clean and can last for several years if cared for properly. Long-term tolerance is good, and the risk of corneal ulcerations, corneal neovascularization, and infection is low. Rigid, gas-permeable lenses require skill and knowledge by the practitioner in fitting and designing the lenses, much more so than soft lenses.

Soft Lenses

Most contact lens fittings are with soft lenses. The primary clinical advantage of soft contact lenses is the good initial comfort and tolerance. They can be worn for longer periods, do not dislodge easily, and allow the patient to switch easily between contacts and glasses because there is less molding effect on the cornea. The disadvantages include less effective astigmatic correction of vision compared with rigid lenses, need for more frequent thorough cleaning and disinfection, and more frequent replacement. In addition, there is increased risk of ulcerative keratitis, neovascularization, and contact lens intolerance.

Disposable Soft Lenses

Disposables represent an attempt further to enhance convenience and long-term comfort. Disposable lenses are available as single-use, bimonthly, monthly, and quarterly types. *Daily-wear* soft contact lenses are removed for sleep and are cleaned and disinfected before insertion the following day. *Extended-wear* soft lenses were developed with the goal of allowing the patient to sleep with the lenses in for one or more nights.

Extended-Wear Lenses

First-generation extended-wear lenses were associated with an increased risk for ulcerative keratitis (see later discussion) due to hypoxia-induced corneal microcysts, stromal edema, endothelial polymegethism, and neovascularization. Improved design and materials led to a new generation of soft lenses—silicone hydrogels—approved for 7-day continuous wear in 1999, followed by 30-day continuous-wear lenses in 2001. A rigid, gas-permeable extended-wear lens was approved in 2002 for 30-day continuous wear. These lenses provide more than four times the oxygen permeability, significantly reducing risk. With the benefits of higher oxygen permeability, these lenses are also being used for daily wear.

Risk of Ulcerative Keratitis from Contact Lens Use

Ulcerative keratitis (epithelial defect over a stromal infiltrate) is an infrequent but serious complication of contact lens use that can lead to infection. *Pseudomonas aeruginosa*, a rare sight-threatening pathogen, can quickly invade the injured cornea, resulting in permanent vision loss by destroying the corneal stroma. Ulcerative keratitis can occur with soft or rigid gas-permeable lenses worn on a daily or extended-wear basis. The relative risk is 10 to 15 times greater with extended-wear lenses than with daily-wear lenses; however, severity is lower with silicone hydrogel lenses than with conventional lenses. The U.S. Food and Drug Administration (FDA) has restricted the duration of continuous wear for extended-wear lenses to between 6 and 30 days, depending on the type of lens.

Corneal response to antibiotics for keratitis therapy is usually good, but the best treatment is prevention. Practitioners and patients need to be informed about the increased relative risk of overnight lens use. Patients can reduce their risk of infection by complying with proper lens care and cleaning regime and by removing their lenses and immediately contacting their eye doctor when adverse symptoms occur.

REFRACTIVE SURGERY (8–11)

Patients with refractive errors have traditionally relied on external devices—eyeglasses and contact lenses—to obtain clear vision. Refractive surgery offers patients a method for reducing or eliminating their dependence on these prostheses. Laser *in situ* keratomileusis (LASIK) is the most advanced and predictable refractive procedure available. Intense interest in this field is stimulating rapid technological advances. Patients often ask their primary physicians for advice regarding the advisability of proceeding with such surgery, necessitating some basic knowledge about the procedures, their efficacy, and safety and criteria for patient selection.

Laser Vision Correction

Laser vision correction uses ophthalmic lasers to correct myopia (nearsightedness), hyperopia (farsightedness), and astigmatism by reshaping the cornea. The most common forms of laser vision correction are photorefractive keratectomy (PRK) and LASIK, both of which use the excimer laser. Pulses from the argon fluoride, 193-nm excimer laser precisely remove collagen from the corneal stroma, allowing controlled reshaping of the corneal and correction of refractive errors.

Photorefractive Keratectomy

In PRK, the epithelial surface is first removed. The excimer laser then is applied to the surface. Each laser pulse removes a fraction of a micrometer of tissue. In the correction of myopia, a greater amount of tissue is removed from the center of the cornea and progressively less toward the periphery, achieving a flatter corneal contour. In hyperopic correction, the pattern is reversed to create a steeper cornea. For astigmatism correction, more tissue is removed on the steeper meridian. Postoperatively, the epithelium heals across the recontoured anterior corneal stromal surface.

Laser *in Situ* Keratomileusis

In LASIK, the excimer laser energy is used in essentially the same manner as in PRK. The difference is that the surgeon first creates a flap of anterior corneal tissue, using either a microkeratome (a device with a metal blade that makes the corneal flap) or a laser keratome (IntraLase, a 1,053-nm laser that pulses to create the flap through photodisruption of the stromal tissue). After the corneal flap is lifted, reshaping excimer laser pulses are applied to the exposed stromal surface, after which the flap is replaced. As a result, the corneal surface is disrupted much less than in PRK. Return of vision is faster, the patient experiences minimal pain, and the risk of anterior corneal scarring is reduced.

Patient acceptance of LASIK has been enthusiastic. Because of the minimal wound-healing response, LASIK can treat a broader range of refractive error than PRK, but LASIK requires higher surgical skills because of the necessity to create a flap with the microkeratome or IntraLase. IntraLase offers a highly consistent flap thickness compared to the microkeratome, therefore reducing flap-related complications and the need for retreatment.

Results. In clinical trials, 66% of patients could see 20/20 or better with no glasses and 95% could see 20/40 or better, depending on preoperative refractive error and the laser used. Retreatments can be performed within several months after LASIK and 6 or more months after PRK if the refractive error is not acceptably corrected. Depending on specific patient variables, LASIK can generally treat myopia up to −14 diopters, hyperopia up to +6 diopters, and astigmatism up to 6 diopters.

Presbyopic patients need to be educated that the surgery will not eliminate their need for reading glasses.

Complications. LASIK flap complications decrease with surgeon experience and rarely lead to a decrease in visual acuity. After LASIK, patients may experience glare, halos, monocular diplopia, and dry eyes. These are generally transient and typically decrease over the first several months.

Patient Selection. Candidates are usually at least 18 years of age and have a relatively stable refractive error. Presbyopic patients will still need reading glasses. Some patients elect surgically induced monovision, leaving one eye with low myopia for near vision. *Absolute ocular contraindications* include keratoconus and irregular astigmatism. *Relative ocular contraindications* include patients with a history of herpes simplex keratitis, ocular surface disease, uncontrolled glaucoma, cataracts, and dry eyes. *Relative systemic contraindications* include uncontrolled collagen vascular diseases, immunocompromised patients, diabetes mellitus, history of keloid formation, pregnancy or nursing, and the use of systemic medications that may alter healing (e.g., corticosteroids).

Other Surgical Approaches

A number of other interventional approaches to the correction of vision are available, ranging from conductive keratoplasty (CK) and radial keratotomy to intrastromal corneal ring segments and intraocular lenses.

Conductive Keratoplasty

CK has been FDA approved for the treatment of both hyperopia and presbyopia. In this procedure the cornea is reshaped by heat from radio waves, causing contraction of collagen. Myopia is induced in the nondominant eye, correcting presbyopia. Some patients experience glare, halos, or double vision for up to 6 months or more. Persons who need very acute vision for work may still need eyeglasses. The correction is not always permanent, and eyeglasses may again be needed for reading.

Radial Keratotomy

Until 1990, radial keratotomy for myopia was the most commonly performed refractive surgery. Deep radial incisions placed in the cornea from the periphery toward the pupil cause the central curvature to flatten, optically compensating for myopia. Problems inherent in the procedure include unstable correction, fluctuation during the day, a tendency in some patients for a long-term drift toward hyperopia, vulnerability to rupture from a severe blow to the eye, irregular astigmatism, and halos from the radial scars.

Intrastromal Corneal Ring Segments

Intrastromal corneal ring segments (ICRSs), or Intacs, are small, transparent ring segments that are implanted into the nonseeing periphery of the cornea. The procedure is able to correct only myopia up to −3 diopters with no astigmatism. The two main advantages of the ICRSs are that they preserve the central corneal visual zone and are removable, allowing the cornea to return to its original state. The drawbacks of ICRSs include a limited range of correction, induced astigmatism, and slow vision recovery. However, the future of ICRSs may be for the treatment of keratoconus patients.

Intraocular Lenses

The surgical correction of myopia with an intraocular lens implanted in the phakic eye is in early investigation. Compared with corneal refractive surgery, the refractive result with phakic intraocular lenses is more predictable, the range of correction is higher, and the quality of vision is improved by decreasing optical aberrations by moving the optical correction to the intraocular plane. Serious potential complications include endothelial cell loss leading to corneal edema, iritis, cataract development, and glaucoma. Long-term follow-up of patients in controlled studies is necessary to confirm the adequacy of the elective surgical procedure. This procedure is usually reserved for higher levels of myopia and hyperopia that cannot be treated by other corrective surgeries. Surgical removal of the clear lens is occasionally considered because it uses highly refined and reliable cataract surgical technology. Risks are similar to those of cataract surgery.

Annotated Bibliography

1. Bennett ES, Weismann BA. Clinical contact lens practice. Philadelphia: Lippincott Williams & Wilkins, 2005. (*The authoritative reference.*)
2. Soft contact lenses. Med Lett Drugs Ther 1990;32:69. (*A succinct summary for the generalist.*)
3. Schein OD, Beuhler PO, Stamler VF, et al. The impact of overnight wear on the risk of contact lens-associated ulcerative keratitis. Arch Ophthalmol 1994;112:186. (*Most cases of contact lens–associated ulcerative keratitis could be prevented by eliminating overnight wear.*)
4. Schein OD, Glynn RJ, Poggio EC, et al. The relative risk of ulcerative keratitis among users of daily-wear and extended-wear soft contact lenses. N Engl J Med 1989;321:773. (*An early report of this important complication in early-generation lenses.*)
5. Schein OD, McNally JJ, Katz J, et al. The incidence of microbial keratitis among wearers of a 30-day silicone hydrogel extended-wear contact lens. Ophthalmology 2005;112:2171. (*Data on the rate of this important complication.*)
6. Efron N, Morgan PB, Hill EA, et al. Incidence and morbidity of hospital-presenting corneal infiltrative events associated with contact lens wear. Clin Exp Optom 2005;88:232. (*Data on this serious complication.*)
7. Smith RE, MacRae SM. Contact lenses—convenience and complications. N Engl J Med 1989;321:824. (*A review of the pluses and minuses.*)
8. Chaudhry IM, Conti ER, Steinert RF. Advances in refractive surgery: new options expand the scope of corrective procedures. Postgrad Med 1999;106:129. (*A good overview of the spectrum of procedures available.*)
9. U.S. Food and Drug Administration Center for Devices and Radiological Health. Summary of safety and effectiveness data. FDA-approved lasers for LASIK. Available at: http://www.fda.gov/cdrh/LASIK/lasers.htm. (*A summary of corrections treated with lasers.*)
10. Conductive keratoplasty (CK) for presbyopia. Med Lett 2004;46:49. (*A succinct critical review of the procedure.*)
11. Wilson SE. Use of lasers for vision correction of nearsightedness and farsightedness. N Engl J Med 2004;351:475. (*A useful clinical review for the generalist reader.*)

SECTION 14 ■ EAR, NOSE, AND THROAT PROBLEMS

CHAPTER 211 ■ SCREENING FOR ORAL CANCER

JOHN P. KELLY

There are more than 30,000 new cases of oral cancer each year in the United States, representing 4% of cancer cases in men and 2% in women. More than 9,000 deaths result from oral cancer yearly. Despite the ready accessibility of the oral cavity to inspection by physicians, dentists, and patients, 50% of oral cancers already have metastasized at the time of diagnosis. Perhaps that is because pain, a manifestation of advanced disease, is the symptom that most commonly leads patients to seek medical attention. When detected early, oral cancer has a very good prognosis. The primary physician has an important role in early detection. Prevention is another responsibility, given the relation of oral cancer to use of tobacco and alcohol.

EPIDEMIOLOGY AND RISK FACTORS (1–9)

The peak incidence of oral carcinoma is in the sixth decade for women and is equally frequent in each decade after the age of 50 years for men. However, the appearance of the disease in the third and fourth decades is not rare and must not be overlooked.

The use of *tobacco* in all of its forms is highly correlated with the risk of oral cancer. The frequency of oral cancer of the cheek and gum rises 50-fold among long-term users of *smokeless tobacco*. Use has reached epidemic proportions among teenage boys, causing the *Surgeon General's Report* to warn against it. Such tobacco products contain multiple carcinogens in addition to tobacco, including nitrosamines, aromatic hydrocarbons, and polonium. Pipe smokers are at increased risk for cancer of the lip. Squamous cell or epidermoid carcinoma of the lower lip also has a particularly high incidence among fair-skinned people whose occupation or residence subjects them to prolonged sun exposure.

The risk of oral cancer is high among those with heavy *alcohol* consumption. Whether this is due to a direct effect of alcohol on the oral mucosa or to associated smoking or vitamin deficiency remains to be fully elucidated.

Cancer of the tongue is highly correlated with the atrophic glossitis seen with tertiary syphilis. Cancer of the tongue is more common among nonsmokers. Mucosal atrophy from other causes is also associated with an increased incidence of oral cancers. Most notably, *chronic iron deficiency* leading to Plummer–Vinson syndrome is known to alter mucosal tissues, and this change may be related to the increased incidence of oral carcinoma. *Epstein–Barr virus* (EBV) and *papilloma virus* have been found in cells of the tongue manifesting oral hairy leukoplakia, a hyperplastic change found in patients with AIDS.

Chronic irritation of the oral mucosa by ill-fitting dentures, poorly restored teeth, or particularly spicy diets has often been mentioned as contributing to the development of oral carcinoma. However, no epidemiologic data support this view.

The precise etiology of oral cancer is unknown. The foregoing etiologic factors probably act as cocarcinogens, effecting malignant change in concert with some primary agent not yet elucidated. Increased chromosomal fragility has been found in nonsmokers who develop oral cancers.

NATURAL HISTORY (1–9)

In considering the natural history of oral cancer, it is important to address premalignant and malignant disease.

Premalignant Disease

Leukoplakia

Leukoplakia—a "white patch" on the oral mucosa—is of interest because in about 10% of instances it represents premalignant change with dysplastic features on biopsy. Clinically, it ranges from slightly raised, white, translucent areas to dense, white, opaque plaques, with or without adjacent ulceration. It is difficult to differentiate completely benign from premalignant leukoplakia except by *biopsy*. However, patients demonstrating a speckled pattern interspersed with areas of ulceration or erosion are more likely to have dysplastic disease. Lesions may occur anywhere on the oral mucosa, but those on the tongue have the greatest risk of malignant transformation. Such transformation may take anywhere from 1 to 20 years. In addition to premalignant dysplasias and squamous cell carcinoma, the differential diagnosis of oral leukoplakia includes traumatic irritation (from malposed teeth or ill-fitting dentures), chemical "burns" (typically from aspirin dissolved in the oral cavity), viral infection (so-called hairy leukoplakia seen in HIV infection), lichen planus, oral candidiasis, discoid lupus, and pemphigus vulgaris.

The risk of oral leukoplakia transforming into cancer can be predicted by an analysis of the *DNA content* of the lesion. Predictive findings include *loss of heterozygosity* and changes in ploidy (*tetraploid, aneuploid lesions*), which are associated with a 30-fold increase in risk of cancer and a 50% reduction in disease-free survival.

Erythroplasia

Erythroplasia—a red, hyperplastic area of mucosa—is highly suggestive of an early carcinoma. Although most cancer screening protocols have emphasized a search for white lesions, the predominant color in premalignant or early lesions is red, not white. In fact, whereas some white lesions may only be "premalignant," the red lesions must be considered to be true malignancies unless proven otherwise by biopsy.

Malignant Disease

The average 5-year survival rate for localized oral cancer exceeds 65% but barely reaches 30% for patients with metastatic disease. When untreated, oral carcinoma metastasizes to the regional lymph nodes of the neck, ultimately leading to respiratory embarrassment or involvement of the great vessels. Ipsilateral node involvement is most common, but metastasis to the contralateral side—especially from primary lesions of the tongue or floor of the mouth—occurs with such frequency that treatment for the control of metastatic disease is difficult. Hence, early diagnosis and control of the primary lesion are important. The lungs are the most frequently involved extranodal metastatic site.

Local recurrence is common. Many instances may actually represent new primary disease, suggesting a susceptibility of the entire oral mucosa to malignant change in affected patients. As many as one patient in five may be expected to develop a second primary oropharyngeal cancer; smokers who do not quit incur the greatest risk.

Other Oral Lesions

Other oral lesions appear black, blue, or brown. Benign conditions such as *vascular malformations, heavy metal ingestion, amalgam tattooing,* pigmented *nevi,* and the pigmentations associated with such systemic conditions as neurofibromatosis, intestinal polyposis, and Addison's disease must be differentiated from the blue-black lesion of *malignant melanoma* (see Chapter 177). Biopsy is essential if this diagnosis is suggested by the appearance of the lesion.

SCREENING AND DIAGNOSTIC PROCEDURES (1–9)

The challenge to primary care physicians is to recognize premalignant and early malignant lesions of the oral cavity. The greatest hope for improved outcome is detection before the appearance of grossly invasive disease. The ready accessibility of the oral cavity to *inspection* and the appearance of premalignant mucosal changes facilitate early detection. *Incisional biopsy* of suspicious lesions should follow. Leukoplakia and erythroplasia are the most potentially important mucosal changes.

The initial evaluation of a suspicious lesion begins with eliciting appropriate historical data to eliminate such relatively harmless lesions as the acute aspirin burn. Irritative lesions can be identified by removing or repairing jagged teeth and poorly fitting or protruding dental prostheses and following the clinical healing of the mucosal wound over a short period of time. Mucosal ulceration that fails to heal within 1 or 2 weeks after the elimination of a presumed mechanical irritation must be biopsied. In any patient with a suspicious lesion, the use of a noxious agent such as tobacco must be eliminated at the outset.

Any red or white lesion that persists for 2 weeks after initial recognition and the elimination of irritating agents requires referral for biopsy. High-risk patients—specifically those with histories of smoking and drinking—should be referred for biopsy promptly, as should any patient with a deeply ulcerative or fungating lesion.

Exfoliative cytology and *in vivo* staining with toluidine blue, although sometimes suggested as noninvasive diagnostic methods, do not provide sufficient sensitivity or specificity to take the place of incisional biopsy. A *brush biopsy technique* for screening suspicious lesions has been widely promoted in recent years, but this technique is no substitute for definitive incisional biopsy.

Any swelling beneath a normal-appearing oral mucosa must be evaluated as well. Such lesions are commonly benign and are the result of infection, bony exostosis, or mucus retention phenomena, but they may represent neoplasms of the minor salivary glands or other submucosal structures.

DNA content analysis of a biopsied leukoplastic lesion can be very helpful in determining the need for more aggressive excision versus watchful waiting. Cells that show abnormal ploidy and a loss of heterozygosity are strongly predictive of risk for malignant transformation.

Serologic markers of EBV infection (e.g., immunoglobulin A antibodies against EBV capsid antigen and neutralizing antibodies against EBV DNase) are predictive of risk for nasopharyngeal carcinoma and might be considered (if available) in high-risk populations.

RECOMMENDATIONS

- Patients should be counseled on preventive measures, especially the importance of avoiding the use of tobacco products (including smokeless tobacco) and excessive alcohol consumption.
- A thorough visual and manual examination of the lips and oral cavity should be a part of every patient's evaluation; mucosal patches that are either red or white are sought.
- A high index of suspicion must be maintained for patients with a history of smoking, drinking, and heavy exposure to sunlight.
- Atrophic or hyperplastic areas of the oral mucosa must be viewed with suspicion, particularly if they are red or white (erythroplasia or leukoplakia) and last more than 2 weeks after the cessation of smoking, drinking, and exposure to irritants.
- Referral for definitive biopsy is indicated for persistent lesions.
- If available, DNA testing should be included in the examination of the biopsy specimen.

Annotated Bibliography

1. Chien YC, Chen JY, Liu MY, et al. Serological markers of Epstein–Barr virus infection and nasopharyngeal carcinoma in Taiwanese men. N Engl J Med 2001;345:1877. (*Antibodies against Epstein–Barr virus were found to be predictive of nasopharyngeal carcinoma.*)
2. Connolly GN, Winn DL, Hecht SS, et al. The reemergence of smokeless tobacco. N Engl J Med 1986;314:1020. (*An extensive review, documenting health risks and pointing out the alarming rise in popularity of smokeless tobacco; an editorial by the Surgeon General reinforces the message.*)
3. Decker J, Goldstein JC. Risk factors in head and neck cancer. N Engl J Med 1982;306:1151. (*Reviews the epidemiology of oral malignancy, emphasizing the importance of smoking, alcohol, and poor oral hygiene.*)
4. Forastiere A, Koch W, Trotti A, et al. Head and neck cancer. N Engl J Med 2001;345:1890. (*A comprehensive review;117 references.*)
5. Greene JC, Louie R, Wycoff SJ. Preventive dentistry. II. Periodontal diseases, malocclusion, trauma, and oral cancer. JAMA 1990;262:421. (*The recommendations of the U.S. Preventive Services Task Force.*)
6. Jacobs C. The internist in the management of head and neck cancer. Ann Intern Med 1990;113:771. (*Prevention can be achieved by cessation of tobacco use and reduction in alcohol intake; early detection greatly improves prognosis and response to therapy.*)
7. Mashberg A. Erythroplasia: the earliest sign of asymptomatic oral cancer. J Am Dent Assoc 1978;96:615. (*A good illustration and description of this early malignant lesion.*)
8. Shklar G. Oral leukoplakia. N Engl J Med 1986;315:1544. (*An editorial regarding its significance.*)
9. Sudbo J, Kildal W, Risberg B, et al. DNA content as a prognostic marker in patients with oral leukoplakia. N Engl J Med 2001;344:1270. (*DNA content was a powerful predictor of risk for malignant transformation.*)

CHAPTER 212 ■ EVALUATION OF HEARING LOSS

NEIL BHATTACHARYYA

It is estimated that more than 10% of the population of the United States has a hearing problem. The problem is particularly common among the elderly, and can impair quality of life. People with seriously impaired hearing often become withdrawn or appear confused. Subtle hearing loss may go unrecognized. Patients with hearing loss often can be greatly helped, particularly if the loss is due to a conductive problem. The primary physician has the responsibility to screen and detect hearing loss, to search for an etiology, and to decide when referral to an otolaryngologist is indicated.

PATHOPHYSIOLOGY AND CLINICAL PRESENTATION (1–3)

Basic Mechanisms of Hearing and Their Impairment

Hearing impairment may result from an interference with the conduction of sound, its conversion to electrical impulses, or its transmission through the nervous system. Hearing involves an acoustic stage during which sound waves cause the tympanic membrane to vibrate. The tympanic membrane and the ossicles amplify the sound, and the oscillation of the footplate of the stapes in the oval window transmits the sound energy to the perilymph of the inner ear. The endolymph of the scala media (or cochlear duct) is wedged between the perilymph of the scala vestibuli and the scala tympani. Displacement of the basilar membrane stimulates the hair cells, converting sound waves to neural impulses, which are conveyed to the temporal lobes.

On the molecular level, during the reception of sound, potassium ions flow through the upper surface of the cochlear hair cells; the ions then recycle by flowing down to the base and supporting cells and into the endolymph. *Connexin*, the "gap protein" that allows small molecules to pass from one cell to the next, facilitates this potassium flow. It is synthesized by the cells surrounding the sensory hair cells of the cochlea and by the fibrocytes of the cochlear duct.

Interference with mechanical reception or amplification of sound, as occurs with disease of the auditory canal, tympanic membrane, or ossicles, creates *conductive hearing loss*. A conductive hearing loss is localizable to the external auditory canal or the middle ear in most cases. Degeneration or destruction of hair cells or the acoustic nerve produces *sensorineural hearing loss*, as do defects in the synthesis of connexin. Genetic studies have facilitated the uncovering of a molecular basis for hearing loss. Mutations in the gene that codes for connexin are associated with nonsyndromic hearing loss, both early in life and with aging (see later discussion). Congenital malformations of the inner ear, not necessarily hereditary, may also compromise hearing at the sensorineural level.

Conductive Hearing Loss

Conductive loss presents with diminished perception of sound, particularly for low-frequency tones and vowels. There is often a history of previous ear disease. In the Weber test, a tuning fork placed against the frontal bone or the maxillary incisors is perceived more loudly in the ear with a conductive hearing loss. The Rinne test shows that bone conduction is better than air conduction. Obstruction of the auditory canal by severely impacted cerumen, a foreign body, exostoses, external otitis, otitis media with effusion, or scarring or perforation of the drum due to chronic otitis may be responsible for the conductive loss.

Otosclerosis

Otosclerosis, a surgically remediable cause of conductive hearing loss, is a disorder of the bony labyrinth that fixes the footplate of the stapes in the oval window. Clinical otosclerosis has an estimated prevalence of about 1% among whites and 0.1% among blacks. Two thirds of the cases are seen in women. There appears to be an association between pregnancy and progression of otosclerotic hearing loss. The condition is believed to be inherited in an autosomal-dominant fashion, with varying clinical expressivity. It generally presents in the second or third decade of life.

Exostoses

Exostoses are bony excrescences of the external auditory canal. They are characteristically located in the anterior, posterior, and superior quadrants of the canal. Nearly always bilaterally symmetric, their occurrence seems to be related to repetitive exposure to cold water (e.g., as in ocean swimming). They can cause symptoms by blockage of the external auditory canal,

resulting in conductive hearing loss, or by sequestration of debris and cerumen with subsequent infection.

Glomus Tumors

Glomus tumors or paragangliomas are rare benign, highly vascular tumors derived from normally occurring glomus formations of the middle ear and the jugular bulb. Presenting symptoms include conductive hearing loss (from middle ear mass effect); spontaneous hemorrhage from the canal; and paralysis of the ninth, tenth, and eleventh cranial nerves (the jugular foramen syndrome). Pulsatile tinnitus should raise suspicion for a glomus tumor. With progression, it may involve the intracranial space or cause bony destruction of the base of the skull.

Otitis Media with Effusion

Chronic otitis media with effusion is a rare diagnosis in adults. Causes include nasopharyngeal masses, viral upper respiratory infection, allergy, and, rarely, autoimmune conditions. Ninety percent of adult middle ear effusions resolve spontaneously within 3 months. A persistent middle ear effusion in an adult requires exclusion of nasopharyngeal carcinoma, typically by nasal endoscopy.

Sensorineural Hearing Loss

Sensorineural loss arises from dysfunction of the cochlear sensorineural elements and/or of the cochlear nerve. Patients may complain that they can hear people speaking but have difficulty deciphering words because speech discrimination is poor. Shouting may only exacerbate the problem. The patient with high-frequency loss may have difficulty hearing doorbells, telephones, fire alarms, or a ticking watch and may note more difficulty in hearing the higher-pitched female or child's voice. Recruitment—an abnormally rapid increase in perceived loudness with increased sound intensity—may be present and indicates cochlear dysfunction. With Rinne testing, air conduction is perceived better than bone conduction. Tinnitus of varying degrees and intensity is often a concomitant complaint.

Presbycusis

Presbycusis is hearing loss associated with aging and is the most common cause of diminished hearing in the elderly. There are four types of presbycusis, distinguished according to the correlated pathologic changes in the cochlea. Hair cell loss and cochlear neuron degeneration are the most widely recognized changes. The hearing loss is bilaterally symmetric and gradual in onset. Most cases begin with a loss of the high frequencies with slow progression. Eventually, middle- and low-frequency sounds also become difficult to perceive (Figs. 212.1 and 212.2).

Noise-Induced Hearing Loss

Noise-induced hearing loss is of major epidemiologic and economic significance. Chronic exposure to sound levels in excess of 85 to 90 dB causes hearing loss, particularly in the frequency range around 4,000 Hz. The patient may be unaware of the problem because the speech frequencies (500 to 4,000 Hz) are initially unaffected. At first, there may be a temporary threshold shift in which there is a reversible elevation in the threshold for sound perception. The ear may feel full, or the patient may complain of a sense of pressure. If loud noise exposure ceases at this point, hearing returns to its previous level. If exposure

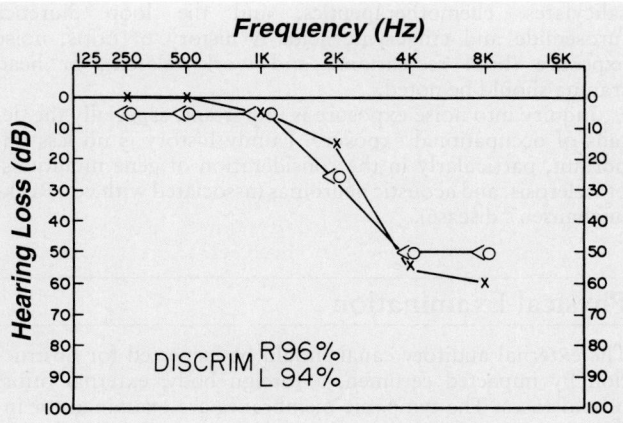

FIGURE 212.1. Presbycusis due to hair cell loss. Note the good hearing thresholds at the speech frequencies of 250 to 2,000 Hz. DISCRIM, discrimination; ×, left ear, air; ○, right ear, air; <, right ear, bone; R, right; L, left.

persists, however, a permanent threshold shift ensues. The term *acoustic trauma* more specifically relates to a particular single noise event (e.g., a shotgun blast) that induces an immediate irreversible hearing loss.

Drug-Induced Hearing Loss

The aminoglycoside antibiotics, such as gentamicin, are representative of ototoxic drugs. An early sign of gentamicin ototoxicity is disequilibrium. Monitoring antibiotic blood levels is the best, but not perfect, way to avoid such problems, adjusting dose according to peak serum levels. Restricting dosing to once daily and duration of therapy to less than 1 week also helps to reduce risk. Other potentially ototoxic drugs, including those causing symmetric sensorineural hearing loss, include furosemide, ethacrynic acid, cisplatin, quinidine, and aspirin. Aspirin doses averaging 6 to 8 g/d predictably cause tinnitus and completely reversible hearing impairment.

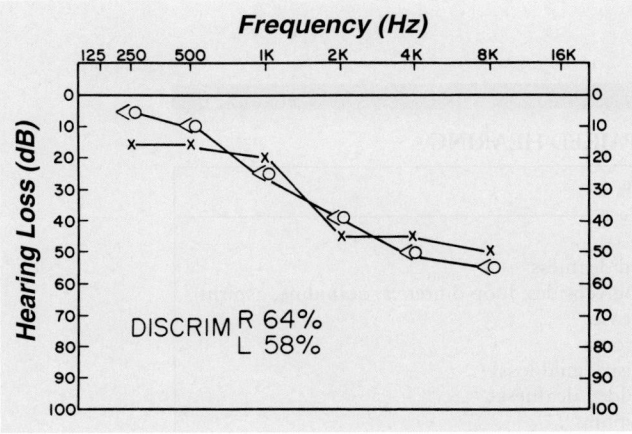

FIGURE 212.2. Late presbycusis due to loss of cochlear neurons. Note poor discrimination. DISCRIM, discrimination; ×, left ear, air; ○, right ear, air; <, left ear, bone; R, right; L, left.

Ménière's Disease

Ménière's disease manifests most commonly with a unilateral, fluctuating, low-frequency, sensorineural hearing loss, usually associated with tinnitus, a sensation of fullness in the ear, and intermittent episodes of vertigo each lasting hours to 1 to 2 days. Vertigo may be the presenting symptom of Ménière's disease, with later onset of fluctuating hearing loss. Progression of hearing loss may occur, eventually encompassing the higher frequencies as well.

Acoustic Neuromas

Acoustic neuromas—benign tumors of the eighth cranial nerve—are rare but important considerations in the evaluation of asymmetric sensorineural hearing loss, often in conjunction with disequilibrium (see Chapter 166). Speech discrimination is much worse than predicted by the pure-tone hearing loss. Symptoms progress in relentless progressive fashion.

Sudden Sensorineural Hearing Loss

Sudden sensorineural hearing loss can be due to head trauma or can appear without obvious cause or warning. In *idiopathic* sudden sensorineural hearing loss, recovery appears to be predicted by the pattern of hearing loss sustained, age (>40 years or <40 years), presence or absence of vertigo (those without vertigo fare better), and electronystagmogram pattern. The etiology of the idiopathic variant is a matter of debate, but viral infection seems to be the most likely cause. Uncommonly, an acoustic neuroma may present with sudden hearing loss. Sudden hearing loss demands expeditious referral to an otolaryngologist for further evaluation, audiometry, and possible therapy with corticosteroids and antiviral agents.

Hereditary Sensorineural Hearing Loss

Hereditary sensorineural hearing loss is generally bilaterally symmetric. Many syndromes have been identified in which hereditary hearing loss is associated with anomalies in other organ systems, but nonsyndromic hereditary hearing loss is also recognized. Among persons with isolated ("nonsyndromic") hearing loss, there is a high frequency of mutations in the gene *GJB2*, which codes for the synthesis of *connexin*. Mutations in this gene are found not only among congenitally nonsyndromic deaf children, who are usually homozygous for the mutation, but also in the carrier state among adults with late-onset isolated hearing loss. The frequency can be as high as 3% across many different populations. It is suspected that the carrier state may predispose to hearing loss later in life and account for some, if not many, cases of age-related hearing loss that are commonly encountered. More work is needed to confirm these intriguing and potentially important findings. Although screening for mutations of this gene is not difficult, the degree of hearing loss and its time of onset cannot yet be predicted. A small number of patients may exhibit a unilateral, genetically programmed sensorineural hearing loss later in life. Family history is important.

Injury

Injury to the inner ear or cochlear nerve may produce an asymmetric sensorineural hearing loss. Skull fracture, meningitis, and mumps are major etiologic factors. Trauma may also cause conductive hearing loss, for example, hemotympanum, tympanic membrane perforation, or ossicular dislocation.

Other Etiologies

Congenital Syphilis. Congenital syphilis may produce adult-onset sensorineural hearing loss. One or both ears may be affected; the course can be variable, with remissions and exacerbations. Vertigo is sometimes present as well, producing a symptom complex mimicking Ménière's disease.

Multiple Sclerosis. Multiple sclerosis should be considered when a young woman shows discrimination scores reduced out of proportion to the pure-tone thresholds (similar to the pattern seen with acoustic neuromas). The site of the lesion is retrocochlear (often in the brainstem), and there may be an associated history of optic neuritis and/or vertigo.

Perilymph Leaks or Fistulas. Perilymph leaks or fistulas may cause hearing loss, with or without vertigo, in individuals who have had inner ear surgery (e.g., stapedectomy), have sustained head trauma, or have congenital inner ear anomalies. The round and/or oval windows may be involved, and it is theorized that there is intracochlear membrane rupture as well. Surgical repair may be required. Expeditious referral to an otolaryngologist should be considered.

DIFFERENTIAL DIAGNOSIS

The causes of hearing loss can be grouped according to whether the problem is conductive or sensorineural (Table 212.1). The categorization is of practical use because the conductive defects lend themselves to correction in many instances.

WORKUP (3,5–7)

History

Evaluation of the patient with hearing loss should focus on detection of the site of lesion. This search is aided by identifying whether the impairment is conductive or sensorineural. History is of substantial importance. It is worth trying to find out the sounds or situations in which the patient has most trouble hearing. Difficulty understanding spoken words suggests sensorineural hearing loss. Inquiry into drug use is essential, focusing on aminoglycosides, quinine derivatives, salicylates, chemotherapeutics, and the loop diuretics furosemide and ethacrynic acid. A history of otitis, noise exposure (both recreational and work related), or head trauma should be noted.

Inquiry into noise exposure is important, especially the details of occupational exposure. Family history is no less important, particularly in the consideration of gene mutations, otosclerosis, and acoustic neuromas (associated with von Recklinghausen's disease).

Physical Examination

The external auditory canal should be inspected for obstruction by impacted cerumen, a foreign body, external otitis, or exostoses. The tympanic membranes are examined for inflammation, perforation, and scarring. One notes any fluid in the middle ear, although, depending on the state of the tympanic membrane, accurate detection of middle ear fluid may be challenging even for experienced clinicians. A bluish or reddish mass visible through the intact tympanic membrane may indicate a high-riding jugular bulb, an aberrant internal carotid artery, or a glomus tumor. Pneumatic otoscopy assesses tympanic membrane mobility and helps to discern the presence or absence of middle ear fluid.

Nasopharyngeal examination is indicated in patients with persisting serous otitis media, particularly if it is unilateral. If there is vertigo or suspicion of a glomus or acoustic tumor, cranial nerve examination is performed to assess central nervous system involvement (see Chapter 166).

Testing of Hearing.

The *watch tick* was an easy, although crude, method of detecting high-frequency impairment when ticking watches were common. *Whispering*, gradually increasing the intensity of the whisper, is readily performed. One asks the patient to repeat a number of words whispered into the tested ear while masking the contralateral ear (e.g., with a Barany noise box or manual occlusion of the contralateral external auditory canal). The best words are familiar bisyllabic ones in which both syllables are equally accented (e.g., pancake, hot dog). With practice, one can roughly estimate the patient's hearing thresholds.

Tuning forks can be used both to detect hearing loss and to differentiate conductive from sensorineural hearing losses

---

TABLE 212.1

COMMON AND IMPORTANT CAUSES OF IMPAIRED HEARING

Conductive	Sensorineural
Impacted cerumen	Presbycusis
Foreign body	Noise-induced deafness
Occlusive edema of auditory canal	Drugs (aminoglycosides, loop diuretics, quinidine, aspirin)
Perforation of tympanic membrane	Ménière's disease
Chronic otitis media	Acoustic neuroma
Serous otitis media	Hypothyroidism (mild loss)
External otitis	Idiopathic sudden deafness
Otosclerosis	Congenital syphilis
Exostoses	Diabetes
Developmental defects	Perilymph leak
Glomus tumors	Multiple sclerosis

(Weber and Rinne testing). A tuning fork that vibrates at a frequency of 512 Hz is acceptable; the 128-Hz tuning fork used for testing vibratory sensation is not. Testing is done to establish the threshold of perception by striking it against the heel of the hand and withdrawing it at 1 ft/s starting 1 in. from the ear until it becomes imperceptible. The distance is noted.

Differentiating Conductive from Sensorineural Hearing Loss

The *Weber* test is helpful. The normal response to a fork vibrating from a tap of the knee and placed midline on the skull is equal loudness in both ears. If there is a conductive loss, the sound will be heard more clearly in the ear with the loss. If there is a sensorineural loss in one ear, sound will be perceived as being heard in the better ear.

The *Rinne test* complements Weber testing. When the vibrating fork is placed on the mastoid process, it is heard for a period of time and then dies away. It is heard again if the same fork is promptly moved without any reactivation to the external auditory canal. Normally, sound conducted by air is heard about twice as long as a sound conducted by bone because of the greater sound transmission efficiency of the middle ear apparatus.

Alternatively, with firm application of the tuning fork against the mastoid process for a few seconds and immediate transfer to the external auditory canal, the sound should be perceived as "louder" in front of the canal when compared with the mastoid position. With a substantial (generally ≥25 dB) conductive loss, the ratio reverses. With lesser degrees of impairment, the ratio approaches 1:1. The normal ratio is preserved in sensorineural losses.

The *Schwabach test* compares the examiner's hearing by bone conduction with that of the patient's. The vibrating tuning fork is alternately placed on the mastoid process of examiner and patient. If the examiner's hearing is normal, he or she will perceive the sound for a longer time than the patient with a sensorineural deficit and for a shorter time than the patient with a conductive problem.

Laboratory Studies

An *audiogram* is an essential component of the evaluation of the patient with hearing loss. The pattern of threshold loss has considerable diagnostic and therapeutic importance, helping to establish the type of hearing loss and to localize the site of lesion. Interpretation usually requires the joint efforts of an otolaryngologist and an audiologist, but a few common patterns are useful for the primary physician to recognize (see the Appendix 212.1).

Expensive imaging technology should be used sparingly but can be helpful in carefully selected patients. *High-resolution computed tomography* of the temporal bone is used in the evaluation of certain middle ear and mastoid disorders, such as chronic infection and glomus tumors. *Magnetic resonance imaging*, particularly with gadolinium enhancement, has assumed a preeminent role in the evaluation of the patient with suspected retrocochlear disease (e.g., acoustic neuroma or multiple sclerosis). This is the test of choice when evaluating asymmetric sensorineural hearing loss.

Auditory brainstem response testing has also been found useful in the site-of-lesion testing, as has *electronystagmography* (see Chapter 166). Both tests require expert performance and interpretation and should be ordered only in consultation with consultants experienced in their use and interpretation.

Otoacoustic emissions, particularly those evoked by sound stimuli, are used to test the integrity of the outer hair cells of the cochlea, from which they are believed to emanate. Otoacoustic emissions show promise as a screening test for assessing auditory function in infants and other difficult-to-test patients.

Screening for Hearing Loss

An important aspect of geriatric care is assessment for hearing loss. In support of screening for hearing loss are the major impact hearing loss can have on quality of life, the availability of effective means of detecting and correcting hearing loss, and the ability to screen adequately in the primary care setting. The U.S. Preventive Services Task Force recommends periodic hearing assessment of all elderly persons.

The best screening methods and the optimal interval are the subjects of ongoing study. The American Academy of Otolaryngology–Head and Neck Surgery has developed a simple one-page "test" that the individual patient can self-administer to see if a hearing evaluation by an otolaryngologist is warranted.

Screening for Hearing Loss Gene Mutations

Screening for hearing loss gene mutations is technically feasible because of the frequency of mutations in *GJB2* and the ease with which these can be detected (gene size is small). However, the meaning of the findings is unclear, making proper use of the information problematic. Further study is needed, and the reader should watch the literature closely because this is a rapidly evolving aspect of hearing loss research. Adult hearing loss patients with a family history of inherited hearing loss should also be counseled on the potential need for hearing screening of their children.

SYMPTOMATIC MANAGEMENT, PATIENT EDUCATION, AND INDICATIONS FOR REFERRAL (4,7–10)

Basic Measures

The primary physician's role in the treatment of hearing loss is relatively limited, but simple advice and support are much appreciated. Elders report that cupping the hand behind the ear can be of help both in actual hearing and alerting others to speak more clearly or louder. Speech reading (interpreting what is being said by extrapolating from the words heard and the facial expressions) may also help and is facilitated by good lighting. Clear enunciation, not merely elevated volume of speech, along with directly facing the presbycusic patient while engaged in conversation and deliberately slowing the rate of speaking optimizes verbal communication. Removal of impacted cerumen or other obstruction, cessation of ototoxic drugs, and treatment of otitis media (see Chapter 218) should not be overlooked. Patients exposed to occupational or recreational noise should be advised to use *ear protection* when in a noisy environment and to avoid further exposure.

Cerumen removal may be accomplished by gentle body-temperature water irrigation using a syringe or an irrigation jet. Removal of wax, as well as some foreign bodies, may be performed using a cerumen spoon or forceps under direct visualization provided by headlight and speculum. Insects are better exterminated first by instillation of mineral oil into the canal before removal is attempted. Patients with a history of prior ear surgery (i.e., mastoidectomy) should be considered for otolaryngologic referral for cerumenectomy.

Referral

Referral to an otolaryngologist for further evaluation and treatment is indicated when a conductive etiology (such as otosclerosis or persistent serous otitis media) or a retrocochlear process (such as acoustic neuroma) is suspected or when simple symptomatic measures do not suffice. An asymmetric sensorineural hearing loss, especially when gradually progressive on serial audiometry, also warrants consideration for referral. The otolaryngologist needs to determine whether the patient is a candidate for medical or surgical therapy and whether a hearing aid is appropriate. Hearing loss resulting from traumatic rupture of the tympanic membrane also requires semiurgent referral especially when accompanied by vertigo, persistent bleeding, or profuse clear otorrhea. A true sudden hearing loss demands urgent otolaryngologic referral, typically for consideration of high-dose oral steroids and/or antiviral therapy.

Hearing Aids

A great variety of hearing aids is available on the market. Patients with sensorineural hearing losses—especially those with a flat threshold and good speech discrimination scores—benefit from amplification and deserve as much consideration as those patients with conductive hearing losses. Even those patients with steeply sloping, high-frequency sensorineural hearing loss with poor discrimination may find amplification useful. Only an adequate trial, after careful otolaryngologic evaluation and competent hearing aid fitting, can allow one to make a decision regarding the helpfulness of amplification. The advent of digital hearing aids has also lowered the threshold for prescribing hearing aids. With digital aids, substantially higher fidelity can be obtained, especially in difficult-to-amplify patterns of hearing loss, resulting in dramatic improvements in verbal communication.

APPENDIX 212.1: AUDIOMETRY

Audiometry helps to classify a hearing loss as conductive or sensorineural and subclassify it according to the pattern detected. The basic audiogram consists of pure-tone air and bone conduction testing with evaluation of speech reception threshold and speech discrimination. The minimal intensity (in decibels) at which the patient perceives each tone is charted as the threshold for that frequency. The responses are recorded as indicated in Fig. 212.3. The pure-tone air threshold curve measures both conductive and sensorineural hearing. To appreciate a conductive component to a hearing loss, bone conduction thresholds are obtained. The bone conduction audiogram bypasses the conduction system and measures cochlear/cochlear nerve capacity. In bone conduction testing, the mastoid process of each ear is directly stimulated with an oscillator or vibrator over a similar frequency spectrum and results are graphically recorded. A discrepancy between air conduction thresholds and those for bone-conducted sounds, the so-called air–bone gap, is indicative of a conductive hearing loss (Fig. 212.4).

Additional testing includes *speech reception threshold* (SRT) and *speech discrimination testing*. The SRT is defined as the lowest intensity at which the patient can correctly identify 50% of presented words. The SRT should match, within a few decibels, the average of the pure-tone thresholds. Discrimination testing evaluates speech understanding using standardized word lists. Speech discrimination that is diminished out of proportion to the measured hearing loss is suggestive of cochlear nerve pathology. Ordinarily, patients with good pure-tone thresholds should also understand speech well. Tympanomanometry is often also conducted with audiometry and measures the compliance of the tympanic membrane. A flattened tympanogram suggests middle ear fluid, and other patterns may help to identify ossicular discontinuity and other conductive hearing loss problems.

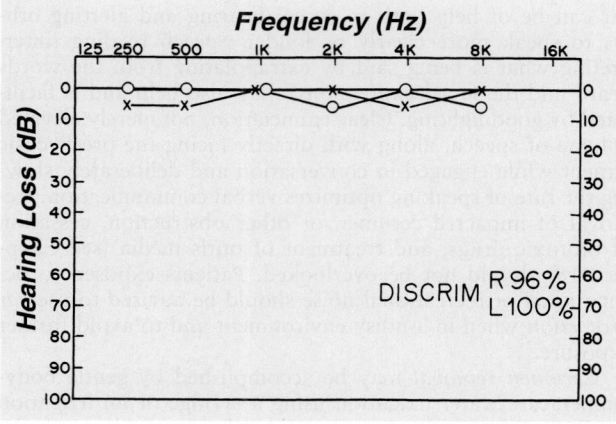

FIGURE 212.3. Normal pure-tone air audiogram. DISCRIM, discrimination; ◯, right ear, air; ×, left ear, air; R, right; L, left.

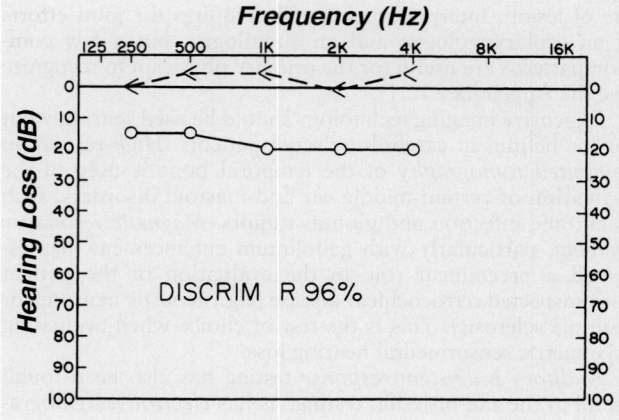

FIGURE 212.4. Air–bone gap. DISCRIM, discrimination; ◯ right ear, air; <, right ear, bone; R, right.

Annotated Bibliography

1. Morell RJ, Kim HJ, Hood LJ, et al. Mutations in the connexin 26 gene (GJB2) among Ashkenazi Jews with nonsyndromic recessive deafness. N Engl J Med 1998;339:1500. (*Mutations in the connexin gene were found in high frequency and were estimated to account for most nonsyndromic age-related hearing loss in this population.*)
2. Paterson DL, Robson JMB, Wagener MM, et al. Risk factors for toxicity in elderly patients given aminoglycosides once daily. J Gen Intern Med 1998;13:735. (*A prospective observational study in patients >70 years of age; limiting the duration of therapy to <1 week can reduce the risk of ototoxicity.*)
3. Steel KP. A new era in the genetics of deafness. N Engl J Med 1998;339:1545. (*An editorial on progress in genetic research for hearing loss; an excellent summary on connexin.*)
4. Bogardus ST Jr, Yueh B, Shekelle PG. Screening and management of adult hearing loss in primary care: clinical applications. JAMA 2003;289:1986. (*Useful case-based discussions; 42 references.*)
5. Lonsbury-Martin BL, Martin GK, McCoy MJ, et al. New approaches to the evaluation of the auditory system and a current analysis of otoacoustic emissions. Otolaryngol Head Neck Surg 1995;112:50. (*A review of otoacoustic emissions and their use in auditory evaluation.*)
6. Koike KJ, Hurst MK, Wetmore SJ. Correlation between the American Academy of Otolaryngology–Head and Neck Surgery five-minute hearing test and standard audiologic data. Otolaryngol Head Neck Surg 1994;111:625. (*Evaluates the sensitivity and specificity of this hearing screen and proposes a modification of the cutoff score.*)
7. Yueh B, Shapiro N, MacLean CH, et al. Screening and management of adult hearing loss in primary care. JAMA 2003;289:1976. (*A systematic review, finding that there was no formal confirmation of benefit, but that there are effective screening and treatment modalities; 88 references.*)
8. Consensus Conference. Noise and hearing loss. JAMA 1990;263:3185. (*Recommends several steps to limiting noise-induced hearing loss.*)
9. Gates GA, Miyamoto RT. Cochlear implants. N Engl J Med 2003;349:421. (*An update on the technology.*)
10. Larson VD, Williams DW, Henderson WG, et al. Efficacy of 3 commonly used hearing aid circuits: a crossover trial. JAMA 2000;284:1806. (*A very useful comparison trial; all proved to be beneficial, with only minor differences.*)

CHAPTER 213 ■ APPROACH TO EPISTAXIS

NEIL BHATTACHARYYA

Most spontaneous nosebleeds are self-limited. Patients present for medical care when the bleeding becomes unusually brisk or will not stop or episodes become frequent. In addition, bleeding that drains posteriorly into the oropharynx rather than anteriorly is especially daunting for patients. Severe or recurrent bleeding necessitates evaluation for nasal pathology and, less commonly, an underlying generalized disorder. The immediate therapeutic objective is control of the bleeding.

PATHOPHYSIOLOGY AND CLINICAL PRESENTATION (1–4)

Etiologies

The primary mechanisms of epistaxis involve disruption of the nasal mucosa, most commonly caused by *trauma*, *ulceration*, *bleeding disorders*, and *inflammatory* or *neoplastic conditions*.

Trauma

In patients with deviated septum or septal spurs in the anterior portion of the nose, trauma occurs easily, either from the drying effects of poorly humidified air or secondary to probing in or bumps on the nose. Nose picking, rubbing, or forceful nose blowing may also trigger bleeding when the nasal mucosa is inflamed and fragile from a viral, bacterial, or allergic cause.

Ulcerations

Ulcerations, which tend to form over septal deviations and spurs, bleed easily. Repeated mucosal exposure to cocaine leads to anoxic tissue necrosis from drug-induced intense vasospasm; perforation may result from cocaine use and cause chronic crusting and bleeding. Collagen diseases such as lupus are occasionally responsible for ulceration. The prolonged use of the widely prescribed topical nasal steroid sprays may lead to anterior septal mucosal atrophy and may be followed by frank ulcer formation or, in rare cases, septal perforation.

Bleeding Diatheses

Bleeding diatheses sometimes present as epistaxis (see Chapter 81). Nosebleeds are the most common initial presentation of *hereditary hemorrhagic telangiectasia* (Osler–Weber–Rendu syndrome) and its most frequent bleeding complication. Characteristic features include telangiectasias on the nasal mucosa, lips, and tongue; a positive family history; and onset of repeated bleeding episodes by the third or fourth decade. Adolescent boys with a nasopharyngeal angiofibroma experience repeated bouts of brisk posterior epistaxis. Sinus x-rays or computed tomographic scan imaging with contrast demonstrate a nasopharyngeal mass. Patients taking warfarin, high-dose aspirin, and other antiplatelet agents may present with complex epistaxis, sometimes with multiple sites of bleeding, unresponsive to standard conservative measures.

Inflammatory and Neoplastic Conditions

Wegener's granulomatosis, *midline granuloma*, and *nasal malignancy* share a presentation of epistaxis, unremitting sinus infection, and opacified sinuses on three-dimensional imaging. Posterior epistaxis, most commonly due to bleeding from the sphenopalatine plexus deep in the nose, is commonly attributed to hypertension, but epidemiologic studies show that few hypertensive individuals experience nosebleeds.

Site of Bleeding

Regardless of the etiology, the site of bleeding has distinguishing clinical characteristics.

Anterior Epistaxis

Active *anterior epistaxis* usually presents as unilateral, continuous, moderate bleeding from the anterior septum called Kiesselbach's plexus. Recurrent episodes of bleeding, lasting from a few minutes to 1/2 hour over the preceding few days and controlled by pinching the anterior nose, are characteristic. Most adult cases and almost all spontaneous nasal hemorrhage in children occur on the anterior aspect of the nasal septum. Most are venous, but an arterial source becomes more common with advancing age because of mucosal and vascular atrophy. Anterior epistaxis remains the most common site for patients taking antiplatelet agents. Anterior nosebleeds account for roughly 90% of all epistaxis episodes.

Posterior Epistaxis

Posterior epistaxis is associated with intermittent, very brisk arterial bleeding, with blood flowing posteriorly into the pharynx unless the patient is leaning forward. When the patient is leaning forward, the blood may run from one or both sides of the nose. Spontaneous posterior hemorrhage is more common in the older age groups and after severe facial trauma with multiple facial fractures. The vessel rupture is usually just superior or inferior to the posterior tip of the inferior turbinate on the lateral nasal wall from the sphenopalatine artery.

DIFFERENTIAL DIAGNOSIS (1–3)

The differential diagnosis of nosebleeds can be divided into local and systemic disorders (Table 213.1). The local causes are most commonly inflammatory or traumatic. More than 90% of bleeds are related to local irritation; most occur in the absence of a specific underlying anatomic lesion.

TABLE 213.1

MAJOR CAUSES OF EPISTAXIS

Local Disease	Systemic Disease
Dry indoor environment	Granulomatous disease (Wegener's, sarcoidosis)
Upper respiratory infection	Hereditary hemorrhagic telangiectasia
Chronic sinusitis	Infection (chickenpox, influenza)
Trauma (nose picking, forceful blowing)	Bleeding diathesis
Occupational exposure to irritants	Malignant hypertension
Cocaine abuse	
Angiomas	
Allergies	
Lack of humidification	
Malignancy	
Nasal steroid sprays	

WORKUP (1–3)

History

History should begin with inquiry into the amount of bleeding, duration, and frequency. After the bleeding is under control, the patient can be questioned about easy bruising, hematuria, melena, heavy menstrual periods, family history of bleeding disorders, the use of oral anticoagulants or drugs with antiplatelet effects (aspirin, etc.), occupational exposure to irritating chemicals or dust, dry home, chronic cocaine use, and repeated nose blowing or picking. Patients should be queried about any previous nasal surgery (cosmetic or otherwise) because this may affect suitability for subsequent procedures.

Physical Examination

Physical examination should be performed with the patient sitting and leaning forward so that the blood flows from the nose. This allows the physician to assess the rate and site of bleeding and to prevent the swallowing of blood, which will quickly lead to emesis. The pulse and blood pressure should be taken, and the skin, mucous membranes, and conjunctiva should be checked for rash, pallor, purpura, petechiae, and telangiectasias. Lymph nodes should be examined for enlargement, suggesting sarcoidosis, tuberculosis, or malignancy. The sinuses are percussed for evidence of sinusitis, which would raise considerations of Wegener's granulomatosis, midline granuloma, and nasal tumor.

Laboratory Studies

Laboratory studies are best ordered on the basis of findings from the history and physical examination. Patients suspected of a bleeding diathesis should have a prothrombin time test, partial thromboplastin time test, bleeding time, blood smear, and platelet count obtained (see Chapter 81). Blood work is essential for patients whose epistaxis recurs after simple cautery or nasal packing. Sinus films are appropriate for evaluating the patient with recurrent bouts of sinus pain, tenderness, and bleeding or in whom sinonasal polyposis or malignancy is suspected. Patients of Chinese descent with recurrent epistaxis must be examined for potential nasopharyngeal carcinoma.

PRINCIPLES OF MANAGEMENT (1–3)

The first objective is to stop the bleeding. The approach depends on whether the source is anterior or posterior.

Anterior Septal Bleeding

A few simple first-aid measures suffice for most cases. The patient should sit up (this reduces venous pressure) and lean forward (which prevents the swallowing of blood if the bleeding is anterior). A small piece of cotton or cotton balls soaked in a vasoconstricting nose drop such as *phenylephrine* (Neo-Synephrine) or *oxymetazoline* (Afrin) is placed in the vestibule of the nose and pressed against the bleeding site for 10 to 15 minutes with manual compression of the anterior fleshy aspect of the nose (patients often mistakenly manually compress the bony upper two thirds of the nose). The temporary packing is then removed carefully and slowly to observe for rebleeding. This will stop almost all venous types of anterior nosebleeds. *Humidification* and a *lubricant* such as petrolatum ointment promote healing.

If these remedies fail, the mucous membrane can be anesthetized by applying cotton soaked with 4% *cocaine* or 4% *lidocaine* for 5 minutes. The nose is then carefully examined, especially along the anterior septum, to determine whether exposed vasculature is the cause of bleeding. A *silver nitrate stick* can then be applied to the bleeding site and to any prominent vessels. Silver nitrate cautery should be applied carefully, and patients with a previous history of septal or nasal surgery and patients who are taking antiplatelet agents as their mucosa may become extremely friable and apt to bleed more during cautery.

Occasionally, a small artery in the septal mucous membrane will either fail to stop bleeding or rebleed a short time later. These episodes can usually be controlled by anesthetizing and recauterizing the area. This is followed by placing a small amount of *oxidized regenerated cellulose* (Surgicel) against the bleeding artery or a small *packing of petroleum gauze strip* or *Merocel sponge* soaked with *oxymetazoline* and/or *thrombin* solution, which is left in the nasal vestibule for 48 hours. Patients with nasal packing require temporary *antibiotic* coverage directed against staphylococcal species. After cautery or packing, the patient should be placed on light activity, stool softeners, and humidification. Recently, an over-the-counter product for managing anterior epistaxis has become available (Nasal-CEASE). This is a specific calcium alginate product that has been shown to cause coagulation via platelet aggregation and plasmatic coagulation and can be applied in the physician's office or even by patients at home. It has been shown to be both effective and cost-effective in the management of anterior epistaxis.

Patients with bleeding disorders require especially careful treatment to prevent abrading of the mucous membrane. Therapy involves the use of humidity, copious lubricants, and soft cotton tamponades wetted with long-acting vasoconstricting drops (*oxymetazoline 0.05%* [Afrin] nasal solution). Packing should be avoided at all costs, but if it is unavoidable, it can be accomplished with a piece of *oxidized cellulose*, which does not require removal. Further treatment is best directed at the underlying bleeding disorder.

Posterior Epistaxis

Posterior epistaxis constitutes an inherently more serious problem because of the relative rapidity of blood loss and the relatively inaccessible and poorly visualized bleeding site in the posterior nose. Initial efforts should be made to bring the bleeding under control while awaiting an otolaryngologic consult. Hematocrit, blood pressure, and pulse should be immediately obtained, and, if necessary, a sample should be sent for type and cross-match. Blood pressure should be controlled, but care must be taken not to lower the blood pressure excessively in the face of blood volume loss.

The patient should be instructed to *sit up* and *lean forward*, and if there has been a temporary interruption in the bleeding, no treatment other than *spraying* the nose with a topical anesthetic and vasoconstricting substance, such as 4% *cocaine* or *oxymetazoline 0.05%*, should be attempted. The nose should be suctioned or blown clear only when the medical personnel present are prepared to deal with brisk epistaxis.

Many cases of "posterior" epistaxis can be handled with the placement of laminated expandable *nasal tampons*. In other cases, expandable balloons with multiple ports may be placed for control of the epistaxis. After the bleeding has been stopped, short-term *nasal packing* (3 to 5 days) or *surgical control* of the bleeding may be attempted. With the advent of endoscopes, posterior epistaxis may be treated with *directed cautery*, obviating the need for extended periods of uncomfortable packing and possibly hospitalization. In rare cases, formal *anterior–posterior nasal packing* or operative *transantral ligation* of the sphenopalatine artery may be required by otolaryngologic personnel. Finally, in particularly refractory cases, endovascular arteriography with embolization may be required.

PATIENT EDUCATION

Prevention of Recurrences

Once septal bleeding is controlled in the office or emergency ward, several measures to prevent recurrences should be instituted:

- Instruct the patient on the need to avoid traumatizing the mucosa. Specifically, warn against habitual nose picking, constant rubbing with a handkerchief, and excessively forceful blowing. The fingernails of children should be trimmed short.
- Have the patient keep the septum well coated with petrolatum-based ointment such as zinc oxide, Vitamin A + Vitamin D Ointment, or an antibiotic ointment until healed, usually in 3 to 5 days.
- Teach the control of minor recurrent bleeding by the patient's use of cotton pledgets soaked in a vasoconstricting nose drop (e.g., *phenylephrine* [Neo-Synephrine] or *oxymetazoline* [Afrin]) and pressed against the bleeding site. Consider use of over-the-counter NasalCEASE.
- Explain the importance of humidifying the home environment; have the patient keep a few windows partially open, place containers of water near radiators or stoves, or install a humidifier.
- Consider patient application of a water-based lubricant applied to the rims of the nostrils to maintain mucosal moisture.

First Aid

Few patients understand the proper treatment for the care of minor nosebleeds at home; simple telephone instruction may obviate the need for an office or emergency room visit:

- Instruct the patient to *sit up* and remain calm, and *lean forward* and *pinch the side* of the nostril against the septum on the side that is bleeding to tamponade the flow.
- Then have the patient spray the nose with any of the over-the-counter nasal sprays that contain *phenylephrine* (e.g., Neo-Synephrine) or *oxymetazoline* (e.g., Afrin).
- Follow with the use of a small *pledget of cotton* lightly soaked with the spray and pressed against the bleeding portion of the septum. After 10 minutes, most nosebleeds will have stopped.
- Have the patient apply a *petrolatum-based ointment,* such as zinc oxide or Bacitracin, to the septum to prevent further drying and abrasion of the septum. It should be left in for a few days.

- Instruct the patient to limit heavy lifting, other forms of straining or bending over, intake of spicy or hot foods, hot showers, and medications that might impair hemostasis (see Chapter 81). Consider the initiation of a *stool softener*.

Reassure the patient when the nosebleed is purely a local phenomenon; many people attribute nosebleeds to hypertension and fear cerebral hemorrhage.

INDICATIONS FOR REFERRAL AND ADMISSION

Patients with *active posterior bleeding* should be admitted to the hospital immediately for emergency treatment to control the bleeding. All patients who undergo extensive posterior nasal packing need to be closely observed for signs of hypoxia and hypercarbia because posterior packing can cause airway obstruction, particularly in elderly patients, due to downward displacement of the soft palate and subsequent palatal edema and swelling or slipped packing. Unfortunately, packs must be left in place for a minimum of 5 days to be effective. Posterior packing is associated with a great deal of discomfort. Patients generally require intravenous hydration because of poor oral intake due to painful swallowing. Additional needs include antibiotics to prevent sinusitis, pain medications, and careful observation by the nursing staff for impending airway obstruction. In all cases of nasal packing, awareness of potentially devastating toxic shock syndrome must be maintained. Any form of nasal packing should not be taken lightly in the elderly or patients with known cardiopulmonary disease. Packing can often be avoided, or removed earlier, if the patient undergoes an endoscopic nasal examination and the site is visualized and electrocauterized directly, usually in the operation room. Failing this, where available, arterial embolization of the involved internal maxillary–sphenopalatine artery system can be used in life-threatening situations, most commonly when formal nasal packing and/or surgical measures have failed.

Annotated Bibliography

1. Hallberg OE. Severe nosebleed and its treatment. JAMA 1952;148:355. (*A classic article that is still very useful.*)
2. Kirchner JA. Epistaxis. N Engl J Med 1982;307:1126. (*A review of anatomy, etiology, and therapy.*)
3. Perry WH. Clinical spectrum of hereditary hemorrhagic telangiectasia (Osler–Weber–Rendu disease). Am J Med 1987;82:989. (*A detailed review of clinical presentation; nosebleeds are a major feature.*)
4. Benninger MS, Marple BF. Minor recurrent epistaxis: prevalence and a new method for management. Otolaryngol Head Neck Surg 2004;131:317. (*Introduces simple or patient product effective for typical, minor epistaxis.*)

CHAPTER 214 ■ EVALUATION OF FACIAL PAIN AND SWELLING

JOHN P. KELLY

The primary care physician often encounters patients whose presenting complaint of facial pain or swelling is related to the masticatory apparatus (teeth, gums, jaws, muscles) or salivary glands. Dental decay is the most prevalent disease in the United States and a major cause of conditions leading to facial pain and swelling. Because symptoms may be referred to nondental structures and because an odontogenic infection may involve areas of the head and neck seemingly unrelated to the teeth, the patient may first seek the advice of a physician rather than of a dentist. Prompt recognition and effective initial treatment may well prevent the development of a serious complication such as abscess formation.

PATHOPHYSIOLOGY AND CLINICAL PRESENTATION (1–4)

Odontogenic Infection

Dental decay is a multifactorial disease and encompasses dietary factors (most notably, refined carbohydrates), environmental factors (such as unavailability of fluoride ion during the production of the enamel of the teeth), and various host factors (not the least of which is the patient's oral hygiene habits). Oral bacteria use dietary carbohydrates to form plaque on the enamel of the teeth. Susceptible enamel is then decalcified, resulting in a "cavity" or carious lesion.

Tooth Decay and Inflammation of the Pulp

In its initial stages, tooth decay is asymptomatic. However, when the dentin beneath the enamel is exposed, the patient may complain of aching pain when the affected tooth comes into contact with hot, cold, or sweet substances. The frequent finding of referred pain may make localization of the offending tooth difficult and is one reason a patient may first consult the physician rather than the dentist.

Progressive decay of the tooth will result in inflammation of the pulp (*pulpitis*). The symptoms will be unchanged until the dental pulp becomes necrotic and, eventually, suppurative. The cardinal symptom becomes deep, throbbing pain on exposure to hot foods or drinks. The pain is abruptly relieved by ice or cold water. This symptom complex is distinct from the paroxysmal lancinating pain of trigeminal neuralgia, which has no relationship to extremes of temperature but may be related to eating because of the presence of trigger zones in the oral cavity (see Chapter 176).

Tooth Abscess

Simple dental decay, pulpitis, and pulpal necrosis are not associated with fever, swelling, or leukocytosis. However, when the infection of the pulp spreads beyond the confines of the tooth to involve the periodontal ligament and the adjacent alveolar bone, an acute *alveolar abscess* may ensue. In this condition, the affected tooth is tender to percussion or to masticatory forces and is mobile. The adjacent soft tissues begin to show edema, erythema, heat, and tenderness. The location of the involved tooth will determine the location of the swelling. Abscessed maxillary teeth will produce labial or infraorbital edema; an infected mandibular tooth will produce submandibular edema. Lymphadenopathy of the cervical chain can be seen in either maxillary or mandibular infection.

Complications

A facial cellulitis may result, causing fever and leukocytosis. Typically, the history reveals a preceding toothache with pain suggestive of pulpitis, followed by spontaneous regression and an asymptomatic period, corresponding to pulpal necrosis. Swelling and pain develop when the necrotic pulp becomes infected and the process spreads to adjacent anatomic structures. Further spread of infection along fascial planes or by hematogenous routes can result in life-threatening complications, such as *cavernous sinus thrombosis*, *meningitis*, *Ludwig's angina*, or *mediastinitis*. Although uncommon, such devastating complications are still seen today, even with the availability of antibiotics.

Periodontal Infection

Acute bacterial infection of the periodontal tissues is most often localized to the gingiva or mucosa adjacent to the involved tooth. The typical patient will complain of a "gum boil," and examination will reveal a discrete fluctuant swelling, which may drain easily on manual palpation.

In the late-adolescent years, infection of the soft tissue surrounding erupting third molars or wisdom teeth (pericoronitis) is common. Low-grade chronic infection may be accompanied by symptoms described as "teething"; acute infection will result in pain, swelling, and difficulty in opening the mouth (trismus) as the adjacent masticator space becomes involved.

Salivary Gland Swelling

Acute infection of the major salivary glands (parotid, submandibular, and sublingual) may be either viral or bacterial. *Viral parotitis* (mumps) occurs most frequently in school-aged children and appears either unilaterally or bilaterally. The efficacy of immunization programs has made this disease a relative rarity. Viral lymphadenopathy in the preauricular area, such as that seen in infectious mononucleosis and in cat-scratch disease, may masquerade as parotid swelling and must be considered.

Sialadenitis

Sialadenitis, bacterial infection of the salivary glands, commonly affects a single gland. The infection is generally an ascending infection in which bacteria gain access to a gland made susceptible to infection by stasis of saliva. Obstruction of the salivary duct by a stone or mucinous plug is the usual inciting event, but any low-flow state can lead to sialadenitis. The condition is frequently seen in elderly, debilitated, or postoperative patients in whom dehydration may lead to decreased salivary flow and consequent infection. The parotid gland is the usual target; involvement is more often unilateral than bilateral. Purulent drainage can be obtained from the duct orifice. Previous episodes of parotitis or congenital abnormality of the acinar structure of the parotid gland may produce sialoangiectasis, which facilitates pooling and stasis of saliva within the gland and increases the patient's susceptibility to episodes of acute infection.

Systemic Conditions

Noninfectious salivary swelling may occur with diabetes mellitus, uremia, Laennec's cirrhosis, chronic alcoholism, and malnutrition. A toxic reaction to a variety of drugs, such as iodine, mercury, and guanethidine, causes a painless bilateral parotid gland swelling. A specific triad of keratoconjunctivitis sicca, salivary gland swelling, and rheumatoid arthritis is known as *Sjögren's syndrome*. The syndrome has also been related to other chronic autoimmune connective tissue disorders, such as rheumatoid arthritis, systemic lupus erythematosus, and polyarteritis nodosa. Sjögren's syndrome may initially present without apparent systemic disease. Lymphoma may develop in a patient with longstanding Sjögren's syndrome.

Lymphoproliferative Disease

Both major and minor salivary glands may become infiltrated by a lymphoproliferative process and enlarge. Lymphoma, tuberculosis, and sarcoidosis (uveoparotid fever) have all been first diagnosed from salivary gland enlargement.

DIFFERENTIAL DIAGNOSIS

The causes of facial pain or swelling can be divided into odontogenic, nonodontogenic, and salivary gland etiologies (Table 214.1).

TABLE 214.1

IMPORTANT CAUSES OF FACIAL PAIN OR SWELLING

Odontogenic Pain
  Caries
  Pulpitis
  Periapical abscess
  Alveolar abscess

Nonodontogenic Pain
  Trigeminal neuralgia
  Temporomandibular joint dysfunction
  Myocardial ischemia (referred jaw pain)
  Giant-cell arteritis (masseter claudication)

Salivary Pain and Swelling
  Viral infection (mumps)
  Bacterial infection
  Ductal obstruction
  Sjögren's syndrome
  Lymphoproliferative disease
  Tumor
  Chemical irritant

WORKUP (1–4)

History

Evaluation of facial pain and swelling requires thorough consideration of the pain's onset, severity, quality, location, radiation, aggravating or ameliorating factors, and duration. The various stages of dental infection can be characterized by specific pain histories. For example, pain brought on by contact with hot, cold, or sweet substances is indicative of dental caries, whereas aggravation by heat and relief by cold suggest a periapical abscess. If fever and swelling ensue, an alveolar abscess must be considered. Lancinating pain precipitated by contact with a trigger zone is typical of trigeminal neuralgia; it can be distinguished by history from abscess formation because symptoms are unrelated to the temperature of the contacting substance and swelling is absent.

In the patient who complains of salivary gland enlargement, it is important to inquire about site(s) of involvement, presence of fever or tenderness, history of chronic illness, malignancy, toxin or drug exposure, and symptoms of rheumatologic disease or sicca syndrome (dry eyes, dry mouth). Unilateral painful swelling of acute onset suggests sialadenitis, especially when seen in an elderly, debilitated, or postoperative patient. A unilaterally enlarged painless parotid may be due to tumor, particularly if there is a history of progressive increase in size and extension beyond the gland. Bilateral involvement requires consideration of lymphoma and sarcoidosis and Sjögren's syndrome (which is bilateral in about half of cases).

It is important to keep in mind that episodic jaw pain may be a manifestation of coronary ischemia (see Chapter 20).

Physical Examination

A semisitting position will usually allow both patient comfort and examiner access. Although a flashlight can be used, a lighting fixture that can illuminate the oral cavity and leave the examiner with both hands free is preferable.

Inspection of the mouth for fractured, decayed, or heavily restored teeth and for heavy deposits of debris and calculus ("tartar") on the teeth and gingiva requires little experience and will direct the examiner's attention to odontogenic disease as a likely source of the pain or swelling. A dental mirror or a short-handled laryngoscopy mirror serves as a better retractor than does a wooden tongue blade. Palpation of the teeth to determine tenderness or mobility help to identify an abscessed tooth. The soft tissues should be palpated to detect the presence of indurated or fluctuant swelling adjacent to a suspicious tooth. Tenderness to percussion of a tooth, using a short, sharp tap with the dental mirror handle, is diagnostic of an abscessed tooth. The salivary glands are palpated bimanually intraorally and extraorally; the salivary duct orifices should be observed for salivary flow or purulent drainage during palpation of the individual glands. Cervical lymph nodes should be checked for enlargement and tenderness.

Laboratory Studies

Suspicion of dental caries can be confirmed by x-ray, as can abscess formation. Suspicion of malignancy necessitates consideration of *computed tomography* or *magnetic resonance imaging*. In the potentially toxic patient, a *white blood count* can be helpful, as can a *blood sugar* in the diabetic patient, and can aid in subsequent management. Suspicion of Sjögren's syndrome can be confirmed by *lip biopsy* and followed by serum *antinuclear antibody* testing to screen for underlying rheumatologic disease. Any purulent drainage should be sent for Gram's stain, culture, and sensitivity testing.

SYMPTOMATIC MANAGEMENT AND PATIENT EDUCATION (1–4)

Tooth or Periodontal Abscess

While awaiting dental evaluation, the very uncomfortable patient may require strong *analgesia* (e.g., ibuprofen 600 mg or codeine sulfate 30 mg, every 4 to 6 hours) or local anesthetic block with 2% lidocaine. Antibiotics are indicated when swelling and signs of infection are present in addition to pain. *Penicillin* remains the primary antibiotic of choice in treatment of odontogenic infection. Initiation of an oral penicillin-VK regimen of 250 to 500 mg every 6 hours is appropriate at the first recognition of swelling associated with an infected tooth or periodontal tissue.

Before certain dental work, *endocarditis prophylaxis* should be considered in patients with valvular heart disease (see Chapter 16). A single 2.0-g oral dose of *amoxicillin* 1 hour before dental procedures associated with bacteremia is the recommendation of the American Heart Association. No postprocedure antibiotic treatment is deemed necessary. *Erythromycin* is no longer recommended for patients allergic to penicillin. The preferred alternatives to penicillin are *clindamycin* (600 mg), *cephalexin* (2.0 g), and *azithromycin* (500 mg) taken orally 1 hour before the procedure.

Referral of the patient to an oral surgeon for definitive drainage of the infection at the earliest opportunity is indicated and should be made simultaneously with the prescribing of antibiotics.

Sialadenitis

Acute swelling of a salivary gland, accompanied by purulent or inspissated saliva from the involved duct, requires antibiotic treatment. Stimulation of salivary flow with sour candies and warm compresses is a helpful local measure. The submandibular gland tends to be infected with the same flora as found in odontogenic infections. Hence, *penicillin* is the drug of choice for submandibular sialadenitis. Acute bacterial parotitis, on the other hand, is associated with staphylococcal species, and one of the penicillinase-resistant antibiotics, such as *dicloxacillin*, is preferred. Antibiotic treatment for other infections that may have preceded the onset of the salivary infection can alter the oral flora and produce infection of the salivary system by unusual organisms, such as *Escherichia coli*. Thus, culturing of the purulent saliva is suggested.

Prevention

The U.S. Preventive Services Task Force has underscored the important role of the primary physician in promoting prevention of dental caries and gum disease. During the health maintenance examination, one should inquire into the time of last dental examination, examine the teeth and gums for plaque and gingival disease, urge regular brushing with a fluoride-containing dentifrice and flossing, and recommend yearly dental examination and plaque removal. Knowledge of the fluoridation status of the local public water supply is essential before the prescription of fluoride-containing vitamin preparations by primary caregivers of the pediatric population.

INDICATIONS FOR REFERRAL

Early recognition of *dental decay* and *gingival inflammation* with consequent referral to a general dentist for complete evaluation and treatment is the most effective means of preventing infection. Referral to the dentist is especially important for patients who may have their mouth *hygiene compromised* by bulimia, Sjögren's syndrome, HIV infection, or upcoming treatment for cancer (e.g., head and neck irradiation, chemotherapy). In the patient with *valvular heart disease*, full dental evaluation on a periodic basis is mandatory and is particularly indicated before consideration of a valvular prosthesis so that potential sources of dental sepsis may be eliminated. Adequate antibiotic prophylaxis for subacute bacterial endocarditis must be provided for such patients at the time dental procedures are performed (see later discussion and Chapter 16).

When physical examination indicates no other source of *facial pain*, referral for dental evaluation is indicated. Abscess formation necessitates prompt referral for definitive drainage. When the patient's clinical appearance demonstrates involvement of deep fascial spaces, as evidenced by fever, trismus, elevation of the tongue, or ophthalmoplegia, referral to an oral surgeon and admission to the hospital for parenteral antibiotics are urgent. Similarly, referral is indicated when there is concern for malignancy.

The patient with *acute salivary swelling* should be seen by an oral surgeon for radiographic examination to detect any obstructing sialoliths. Gentle dilation of the duct may help to relieve the obstruction; in some cases, surgery is necessary to remove the stone. Sialography, or examination of the salivary system with radiographic contrast injections, is contraindicated in the acute period of infection, but noninvasive imaging with computed tomography or magnetic resonance imaging has largely taken the place of sialography in nearly all cases of salivary swelling, both acute and chronic.

When salivary swelling is chronic in nature, no antibiotics are indicated. If the differential diagnosis includes Sjögren's syndrome, sarcoidosis, or lymphoma, a biopsy of one of the minor salivary glands of the lower lip will usually confirm the diagnosis without necessitating a more complex parotid biopsy.

Annotated Bibliography

1. Chow AW, Roser SM, Brady FA. Orofacial odontogenic infections. Ann Intern Med 1978;88:392. (*A comprehensive review of pertinent oral microbiology, surgical anatomy of the spread of infection, and the signs and symptoms in patients with odontogenic infection.*)
2. Wilson W, Taubert KA, Gewitz M, et al. Prevention of infective exdocarditis: guidelines from American Heart Association. Circulation 2007;116:1736. (*The most recent consensus recommendations for suba-

cute bacterial endocarditis prophylaxis; there are many important new changes.*)
3. Forastiere A, Koch W, Trotti A, et al. Head and neck cancer. N Engl J Med 2001;345:1890. (*A comprehensive review; 117 references.*)
4. Greene JC, Louie R, Wycoff SJ. Preventive dentistry: dental caries. JAMA 1989;262:3459. (*Recommendations from the U.S. Preventive Services Task Force.*)

CHAPTER 215 ■ EVALUATION OF SMELL AND TASTE DISTURBANCES

NEIL BHATTACHARYYA

The impairment of taste and smell, in addition to being intrinsically unpleasant, is annoying because it interferes with the ability to derive pleasure from food. Moreover, a diminished ability to detect noxious agents in the environment leaves the patient vulnerable to them. Patients may complain of total loss, attenuation, or perversion of these senses. Problems of smell are often reported as alterations of taste because much of the awareness of taste is olfactory. The primary physician should be capable of recognizing taste and smell disturbances that are manifestations of serious illness requiring detailed evaluation as opposed to simple forms in which symptomatic relief will suffice.

PATHOPHYSIOLOGY AND CLINICAL PRESENTATION (1–4)

Smell

The olfactory area is located high in the nasal vault above the superior turbinate. The neurons of the first cranial nerve penetrate the cribriform plate and travel to the cortex at the base of the frontal lobe on top of the cribriform plate. The most common mechanism of anosmia or hyposmia is *nasal obstruction*, which prevents air from reaching olfactory areas high in the nose. Food is tasteless while the problem persists. In most instances, such as those related to the common cold or allergic rhinitis, the process is fully reversible, but sometimes more lasting damage is done. *Chronic infection* may lead to the partial replacement of olfactory mucosa with respiratory epithelium. *Influenza* is known for its ability to cause permanent destruction of the nasal receptors especially in the elderly; the onset is often acute. Viral syndromes are also common causes of hyposmia or anosmia. Another mechanism of acute anosmia is *head trauma*, in which the nerve filaments coming through the cribriform plate are damaged due to shear injury; the prognosis for recovery after head trauma is poor. More recently, anecdotal reports have suggested that the intranasal use of zinc spray for the treatment of the common cold may be associated with acute anosmia, although overall convincing data are lacking.

More gradual onset of reduced smell is typical of an expanding *mass lesion* at the base of the frontal lobe. Meningiomas, neuroblastomas, and aneurysms of the anterior cerebral circulation are the most important sources of this problem. Upward extension of a mass lesion into the frontal lobe is manifested by a lack of initiative, personality change, and forgetfulness; posterior extension may involve the optic chiasm.

Perversion of smell (parosmia) can result from local nasal pathology, such as *empyema* of the nasal sinuses, or ozena, a chronic rhinitis of unknown etiology that causes thick, greenish discharge and crusting (see Chapter 219). In some cases, ozena is reflective of atrophic rhinitis, most commonly resulting from nasal surgeries. These patients often complain about nasal crusting and parosmia or cacosmia (a constant foul smell within the nose). *Klebsiella* and *Pseudomonas* and other polymicrobial flora are often cultured from the discharge. Olfactory hallucinations are central in origin and may present as the aura of a seizure. The responsible lesion is typically found in the area of the uncus. *Olfactory delusions* are reported by schizophrenic patients, whereas their sense of smell remains intact.

Many disorders of smell are of unknown cause. The mechanisms of reduced smell associated with *hypothyroidism*, *hypogonadism*, and *hepatitis* are not understood. Speculation has centered on the deficiencies of various trace metals, particularly copper and zinc, but replacement therapy has been disappointing.

Taste

The tongue, the seventh and ninth cranial nerves, and the hippocampal region of the cerebral cortex make up the taste apparatus. The front of the tongue detects sweet and salty tastes, the sides of the tongue sense sour tastes, and the large circumvallate papillae in the back detect bitter tastes. The pharynx also has the ability to sense taste. The taste buds are concentrated in the anterior two thirds of the tongue, which is innervated by the chorda tympani branch of the seventh cranial nerve. The posterior third of the tongue and palate are supplied by the special sensory fibers of the glossopharyngeal nerve.

The most frequent source of diminished fine taste is *impairment of smell* because the appreciation of taste is at least one-third to one-half olfactory in origin. Isolated taste impairment is 40 times less common than olfactory impairment. In addition, the taste buds may be directly injured by *alcohol use* and *smoking*. The common observation that food tastes better after these habits are terminated is due to improvement in both the olfactory receptors and the taste buds. *Aging* results in small but measurable changes in acuity for salty and bitter tastes but not for sweet or sour ones. Elderly men differ from

elderly women in that men selectively lose sensitivity to low concentrations of salt, whereas women have a more progressive loss of salt sensitivity.

Diseases and drugs that dry the mouth—for example, *Sjögren's syndrome* and *tricyclic antidepressants*—reduce the threshold for taste. Chorda tympani and seventh-nerve lesions are rarely bilateral and therefore do not produce a complete loss of taste. Cerebral mass lesions usually do not involve the hippocampal gyrus. Depression, endocrinopathies, and a host of drugs are associated with complaints of altered taste. The mechanisms are unknown, but in many instances the primary disturbance seems to be, in part, an alteration of smell. Other factors, such as poor dentition, that negatively influence oral cavity hygiene can also negatively affect the sense of taste.

DIFFERENTIAL DIAGNOSIS (1–5)

Most of the conditions that disrupt taste are annoying but not life threatening (Table 215.1). However, a disturbance in the

TABLE 215.1

SOME IMPORTANT CAUSES OF IMPAIRED TASTE

Disturbances in Smell
Injury to Taste Buds
  Age
  Smoking
  Hot liquids
  Dental disease
  Sjögren's syndrome
  Idiopathic conditions

Cranial Nerve Lesions (Seventh or Ninth, Partial Loss Only)
  Ear surgery
  Bell's palsy
  Ramsay–Hunt syndrome (herpes zoster infection of the geniculate ganglion)
  Cholesteatoma
  Cerebellopontine angle tumors (advanced disease)

Central Lesions
  Head trauma
  Tumors (rare)

Psychiatric Disorders
  Depression

Drugs
  Captopril
  Imipramine (and other tricyclic agents)
  Clofibrate
  Lithium
  L-Dopa
  Acetazolamide
  Metronidazole
  Glipizide
  Iron
  Tetracycline
  Allopurinol

Metabolic–Endocrine Conditions
  Hypogonadism
  Uremia
  Hypothyroidism
  Hepatitis
  Pregnancy

TABLE 215.2

CAUSES OF DISTURBANCES IN SMELL

Nasal
  Upper respiratory tract infection
  Polyps
  Ozena
  Chronic sinusitis
  Allergic rhinitis
  Influenza and other virus
  Chemical injury (e.g., tar, formaldehyde)
Cranial Nerve
  Trauma
  Meningioma
  Cerebral aneurysm
Cerebral Cortex
  Seizure disorder
  Meningioma
  Aneurysm
  Schizophrenia
Metabolic–Endocrine
  Hypothyroidism
  Hypogonadism
  Liver disease

sense of smell may be a sign of more serious illness (Table 215.2).

WORKUP (1–3,6,7)

Smell

History

A primary objective is to distinguish local nasal pathology from a central or cranial nerve lesion. A history of head trauma, worsening headaches, olfactory hallucinations, a change in personality, unexplained forgetfulness, visual disturbances, and a gradual onset or steady progression of symptoms suggests disease beyond the nasal cavity. A history of head congestion, nasal discharge (especially discolored discharge), allergies, sinus problems, influenza, chemical exposure, or a recent cold suggests the nose or paranasal sinuses as the source of difficulty. The physician needs to inquire about a history of previous nasal or sinus surgery. Inquiry into symptoms of hepatocellular failure (see Chapter 71) and hypothyroidism (see Chapter 104) may uncover a metabolic–endocrine etiology. A careful psychiatric history is needed when there is a description of abnormal smells in the absence of any other pathology.

Physical Examination

One can document the disorder by challenging each nostril with a representative sample of each primary odor: pungent, floral, mint, and putrid. Smell is most accurately assessed by the use of chemicals such as pyridine (garlic-like odor), nitrobenzene (bitter almond), and thiophene (burnt-rubber odor). Kits are available that contain these substances. Ammonia, which will produce a response by irritation even in the absence of olfactory powers, should be avoided. However, because noxious stimuli such as ammonia are mediated by the trigeminal nerve (rather

than the olfactory nerve), the absence of sensitivity to ammonia should alert the clinician to the possibility of malingering.

On physical examination, the head is assessed for trauma, and the nares are inspected for polyps, deviated septum, mucosal inflammation, and discharge. The sinuses are transilluminated to look for evidence of sinusitis. Fundi are checked for blurring of the disc margins, and the visual fields are tested by confrontation for evidence of optic chiasm compression. The skin, thyroid, and ankle jerks are examined for signs of hypothyroidism (see Chapter 104), and the hair, voice, muscles, and testes are examined for hypogonadism. Any jaundice, hepatomegaly, ascites, or asterixis should be noted.

Laboratory Studies

Abnormal-appearing nasal discharge may be submitted for culture or cytology, looking for bacterial infection or eosinophilic infiltrate, which may reflect significant rhinitis or associated sinusitis leading to the smell disturbance.

Sinus films should be reserved for patients with clinical evidence of sinusitis (see Chapter 219). Patients with a gradually progressive loss of smell or complete anosmia should be considered for imaging to rule out a mass lesion near the olfactory cleft. Either computed tomography or magnetic resonance imaging suffices. Incidental sinusitis leading to hyposmia may also be discovered on these imaging studies. The same principle pertains to the ordering of liver, thyroid, and gonadotropin studies (see Chapters 71, 104, and 120, respectively).

Taste

History

The initial objective of the evaluation is to localize the problem. Intracranial disease is distinctly rare, so assessment can be concentrated on disease in the mouth, in the area of chorda tympani, and the seventh nerve. Alcohol abuse, smoking, dental disease, and severe mouth dryness suggest a buccal cavity source. A history of facial palsy, herpes zoster rash about the ear, recent ear surgery, hearing problems, vertigo, and tinnitus are clues to diseases that may injure the seventh nerve. Drug use and concurrent metabolic or endocrinologic problems (see Table 215.1 and earlier discussion) deserve exploration. Isolated reduction in taste requires inquiry into smell impairment and concurrent depression. Dry eyes in conjunction with dry mouth suggests Sjögren's syndrome, especially if rheumatoid arthritis or other collagen vascular disease is present.

Physical Examination

Careful examination of the nose, ears, oral cavity, tongue, and teeth is essential. The condition of the gums and teeth is worth noting. Taste should be assessed by challenging the withdrawn tongue with sweet, salty, bitter, and sour stimuli on each side and asking the patient to indicate what he or she tastes. Lateralizing the defect on the tongue suggests a lesion of the seventh nerve, although patients rarely present with unilateral taste loss because it is difficult subjectively to appreciate. Examination of the cranial nerves needs to concentrate on the testing of olfaction, hearing, and facial motor functions.

Laboratory Studies

If history or physical examination suggests hypothyroidism, a thyroid-stimulating hormone level should be obtained; likewise, a blood urea nitrogen and creatinine should be obtained if renal disease is suspected. Sjögren's syndrome can be confirmed by lip biopsy or, less commonly, major salivary gland biopsy. Suspicion of a cerebellopontine angle tumor, typically associated with unilateral hearing loss, dizziness, or facial palsy, is an indication for computed tomography.

SYMPTOMATIC MANAGEMENT (2,4)

Smell

Local nasal pathology is often self-limited, but when chronic sinusitis or allergic rhinitis persists, definitive therapy is indicated (see Chapters 219 and 222). A short trial of high-dose oral steroids (if not contraindicated) will often help to identify reversible inflammatory nasal conditions leading to smell abnormality. The avoidance of toxic fumes (e.g., formaldehyde) and the removal of nasal polyps should also help, although the likelihood of smell recovery is inconsistent. When influenza has caused sudden, complete, and permanent loss of smell, little can be done. Ozena sometimes requires local or even systemic antibiotic therapy; saline irrigations to remove obstructing crusts are helpful (see Chapter 222). The correction of hypothyroidism improves the sense of smell. A literature has developed suggesting that zinc salts will restore normal olfaction and taste, although double-blind, controlled study finds zinc to be no better than placebo. Unfortunately, the prognosis for olfactory recovery after head trauma remains poor, with only approximately 10% of patients recovering any significant degree of smell; most patients remain hyposmic or anosmic.

Taste

Regardless of the cause of reduced taste, the patient should be encouraged to stop smoking and reduce alcohol consumption; often the development of a disability such as altered taste is sufficient motivation to get the patient to stop (see Chapter 54). If possible, medications that may impair taste should be stopped or reduced to determine what contribution, if any, they make to the taste disturbance. Any dental disease of consequence should be corrected. The same pertains to hypothyroidism (see Chapter 104). Concurrent depression may respond to a tricyclic antidepressant, but the drug may impair taste by causing a dry mouth (see Chapter 227); forewarning the patient can prevent side effects from becoming an unpleasant surprise. Disease related to the brainstem, chorda tympani, and inner ear requires referral for treatment.

INDICATIONS FOR REFERRAL

Olfactory hallucinations, change in personality, visual field defects, and the impairment of memory in conjunction with disorders of smell and multiple cranial nerve defects, vertigo, and tinnitus and altered taste are indications for neurologic consultation. Psychiatric consultation is worth considering when olfactory hallucinations are accompanied by other evidence of a thought disorder. Patients with ozena, nasal polyps, deviated nasal septum, refractory sinusitis, or a chorda tympani lesion may benefit from evaluation by the otolaryngologist. Many obstructive causes of smell disturbance can be surgically recovered. However, there seems to be an inverse correlation between the length of hyposmia and the likelihood of olfactory recovery.

Annotated Bibliography

1. Holbrook EH, Leopold DA. An updated review of clinical olfaction. Curr Opin Otolaryngol Head Neck Surg. 2006;14:23. (*A useful review, focusing on clinical analysis.*)
2. Rollin H. Drug-related gustatory disorders. Ann Otol Rhinol Laryngol 1978;87:1. (*A review of drugs that alter taste.*)
3. Schiffman SS. Taste and smell in disease. N Engl J Med 1983;308:1275. (*A two-part comprehensive review with an excellent set of references.*)
4. Weiffenbach Gordon RS. Variation in taste thresholds with human aging. JAMA 1982;247:775. (*Taste acuity declines selectively, not globally.*)
5. Pribitkin E, Rosenthal MD, Cowart BJ. Prevalence and causes of severe taste loss in a chemosensory clinic population. Ann Otol Rhinol Laryngol 2003;112:971. (*One of the few series specifically focusing on taste disturbance, with a good discussion of evaluation and management.*)
6. Seiden AM, Duncan HJ. The diagnosis of a conductive olfactory loss. Laryngoscope 2001;111:9. (*Illustrates the utility of a short course of oral steroids in distinguishing conductive/inflammatory olfactory loss from other etiologies.*)
7. Wrobel BB, Leopold DA. Clinical assessment of patients with smell and taste disorders. Otolaryngol Clin North Am. 2004; 37:1127. (*A comprehensive, well-referenced review.*)

APPENDIX 215.1: HALITOSIS

INTRODUCTION (1,2)

Halitosis is defined as a foul breath odor arising from a person's oral cavity or nasal passages. It differs from disorders of taste and smell in that the condition is typically not noticeable to the patient. The condition may be physiologic or a manifestation of oral–nasal or systemic pathology.

PATHOPHYSIOLOGY (1,2)

The most common physiologic cause is so-called morning breath. The universal condition derives from the cessation of regular salivary flow with sleep and the repopulation of the oral cavity with common oral bacterial flora. The marked reduction in salivary flow and the resulting buccal cavity stasis allow mouth flora an opportunity to feed on remaining food particles, sloughed epithelial cells, and stagnant saliva. The byproducts of bacterial metabolism cause the foul odor. Pathologic halitosis may derive from impairment of normal salivary flow (e.g., parotid disease, Sjögren's syndrome), increased presentation of bacterial substrate (periodontitis, sinusitis), or a

TABLE 215.3

SOME IMPORTANT PATHOLOGIC CAUSES OF HALITOSIS

Oral cavity: poorly fitting dental work, periodontal disease, sialadenitis, abscess
Posterior pharynx: tonsillitis, diverticulum, tumor
Sinus: sinusitis, tumor, necrotic disease
Esophagus: reflux, diverticulum, motor dysfunction
Lungs: abscess
Metabolic: renal or hepatic failure; ketoacidosis
Psychiatric: psychosis (self-perception only)

metabolic derangement (renal or hepatic failure; Table 215.3). In rare instances, the patient is the only one to note the condition, which strongly suggests a hallucination of psychiatric or epileptic origin. In younger adults, tonsillar hypertrophy leading to chronic cryptic tonsillitis may cause significant halitosis. Furthermore, chronic nasal obstruction leading to nocturnal mouth breathing may also contribute to halitosis.

WORKUP (1)

Similar to that described earlier for disorders of taste and smell, more attention should be paid to possible oral cavity pathology. It helps to begin the assessment by directly confirming the reported odor. Differentiating an oral source from a nasal one can be done by pinching the nares closed while the patient is exhaling and having the patient exhale through the nose with the mouth closed. Esophageal and gastric etiologies

may require eructation for detection. If the mouth is believed to harbor the suspected source, then the oral cavity should be examined carefully for poorly fitting dental work, periodontal disease, glossitis, tooth abscess, and tonsillar disease. The salivary glands should be checked for a free flow of clear saliva in adequate volumes. Inquiry into symptoms of nasal obstruction, nocturnal mouth breathing, and cryptic tonsillar debris can identify nasal obstruction and cryptic tonsillitis as potential etiologies. Patients with cryptic tonsillitis often expectorate small, foul-smelling, seedlike materials corresponding to tonsil debris. Pulmonary disease and metabolic dysfunction are important to consider when the oral cavity and sinus tracts appear normal. Patients who have no objective findings but are convinced of halitosis derived from an internal source have a high probability of a hypochondriacal psychosis and need psychiatric referral.

TREATMENT (1)

Treatment should be etiologic. Trying to mask the odor is far less effective than addressing its etiology. Mouthwashes are a poor substitute for good oral hygiene. Despite advertisements to the contrary, mouthwashes do little to suppress oral flora. *Oral hygiene* is particularly important in the elderly. Patients should be encouraged to floss and brush regularly, which help to remove trapped food particles and promote healthy gums. It is essential to recommend regular dental checkups, although this is often overlooked. Cryptic tonsillitis may respond to *hydrogen peroxide gargles* or Water Pik *irrigations* of the tonsillar crypts. Topical *nasal steroids* may relieve nocturnal nasal obstruction, diminishing mouth breathing. In select cases, *tonsillectomy* is curative for cryptic tonsillitis leading to halitosis.

Annotated Bibliography

1. Johnson BE. Halitosis, or the meaning of bad breath. J Gen Intern Med 1992;7:649. (*A thoughtful review of this very mundane problem; 55 references.*)
2. Krespi YP, Shrime MG, Kacker A. The relationship between oral malodor and volatile sulfur compound-producing bacteria. Otolaryngol Head Neck Surg 2006;135:671. (*Discusses the role of these bacteria and their effect on oral hygiene, with implications and directions for therapy.*)

CHAPTER 216 ■ APPROACH TO THE PATIENT WITH HOARSENESS

NEIL BHATTACHARYYA

Hoarseness is a primary symptom of laryngeal disease. Most acute episodes are self-limited and due to viral upper respiratory tract infection or voice abuse. However, the patient bothered by persistent hoarseness requires careful assessment because carcinoma of the larynx, tumor-associated damage to the recurrent laryngeal nerve, and other serious conditions may be responsible. Prompt evaluation and diagnosis maximize the chances of detecting an early lesion and achieving a cure.

PATHOPHYSIOLOGY AND CLINICAL PRESENTATION (1–3)

Pathophysiology

Vocal quality is determined by complex factors, including the gap between the vocal cords, vocal cord tension, and the rapidity of vibration. Hoarseness results from interference with normal apposition of the cords or a change in the structural integrity of the vocal fold. Inflammatory, traumatic, and neoplastic lesions cause hoarseness by altering cord structure and function. Often the quality of the voice disturbance reflects the underlying pathophysiology.

A "*breathy*" voice occurs when the vocal cords do not approximate completely, allowing air to escape during vocalization. The cords may be kept apart by tumor, polyps, or nodules. A similar presentation occurs when the cords fail to approximate due to unilateral or bilateral cord paralysis. Patients with a "breathy" voice often complain of vocal fatigue and decreased projection. Patients with hysterical aphonia purposefully hold the cords apart while speaking.

A "*raspy*" or harsh voice ensues from cord thickening due to edema or inflammation. The harshness arises from the extra effort and vocal cord strain required by the patient to generate the voice. This is the voice quality characteristic of many heavy smokers. The voice is of lowered pitch and poor clarity. Associated inspiratory or expiratory cervical stridor results from laryngeal obstruction.

A high, "*shaky*" voice or a low, soft, vibrating vocalization (vocal fry) often is a consequence of decreased respiratory force (phonasthenia). These voices characterize elderly, debilitated, or neurologically impaired (Parkinsonism) patients, who may complain of additional voice difficulties, such as change in voice pitch or poor vocal projection.

A staccato type of voice or a voice suffering from frequent changes in pitch may reflect underlying abductor or abductor spasmodic dysphonia. These are idiopathic local dystonic conditions that may or may not be associated with dystonias elsewhere in the body. This may overlap with or can be difficult to distinguish from a "tremulous" voice, which is associated with idiopathic tremor of the vocal cords; voice tremor is particularly common in the elderly.

A "*muffled*" voice occurs when the sound-generating epiglottis is muffled by supraglottic or oral pharyngeal processes. It is characteristic of epiglottitis, which may lead to airway obstruction. Although not truly "hoarseness," this cause of altered voice originates as a sore throat usually due to *Haemophilus influenzae* and may be accompanied by painful dysphagia and dyspnea. A muffled voice may also be produced by oropharyngeal or hypopharyngeal tumors, as well as by peritonsillar abscess.

Clinical Presentation

Acute Hoarseness

Acute hoarseness is associated with etiologies of acute vocal cord edema, erythema, and dysfunction.

Acute Insults

Viral infection, *voice abuse*, sudden excessive *smoking*, inhalation of *irritant gases*, *aspiration*, excessive *gastroesophageal reflux* (laryngopharyngeal reflux), and occasionally *allergic reactions* (hay fever) may result in acute hoarseness. In some instances, patients will become acutely hoarse after vocal abuse as a result of hemorrhage into the vocal fold.

Acute Laryngeal Edema. Acute laryngeal edema may present as part of a generalized edematous allergic response involving the lips, the tongue, and other hypopharyngeal tissues (angioedema). Foods are important precipitants, especially seafood and nuts; medications (especially angiotensin-converting-enzyme inhibitors) can have a similar effect. Rarely, edema can develop from hereditary deficiency of C1 esterase inhibitor, as occurs in hereditary angioneurotic edema. The voice may progress from hoarse to muffled, signaling potential airway difficulties.

Mechanical Trauma. Swelling forms in response to mechanical trauma, such as dental surgery or intubation for general anesthesia. Rarely, traumatic or difficult intubation may lead to arytenoid dislocation, creating a very weak and hoarse voice with pain on swallowing.

Croup and Epiglottitis. In the pediatric population, *subglottic* edema from viral laryngotracheal bronchitis (*croup*) can obstruct the airway. In adults, acute *epiglottitis* has been noted with increasing frequency. As noted previously, it is associated with risk of airway obstruction, especially in the setting of *H. influenzae* infection, although rapid progression to airway obstruction is rare in adults. Symptoms include fever, severe sore throat, dysphagia, dyspnea, and muffled voice.

Chronic Hoarseness

Chronic hoarseness raises questions about serious underlying pathology, although some causes are more harmless than life threatening.

Chronic Laryngitis and Contributing Factors. *Chronic laryngitis* causes a low, raspy voice, a nonproductive cough, and a "dry throat" sensation. There is usually little or no pain. The voice waxes and wanes, typically worsening as the day progresses. *Gastroesophageal reflux disease* (also known as laryngopharyngeal reflux disease) has been recognized as a common contributing factor. Another typical patient is a *heavy smoker* who continually talks, subjecting himself or herself to a combination of chemical irritation and vocal abuse. In rare instances, an infectious or chronic *inflammatory condition* (e.g., tuberculosis, mycosis, or sarcoidosis) may produce a similar picture.

Chronic Laryngeal Edema. Chronic laryngeal edema with development of dependent polyps represents another form of chronic laryngitis; it may arise in the setting of hypothyroidism, radiation therapy to the neck, or chronic sinusitis with persistent drainage and cough. Patients with this condition speak in a lowered, gravelly voice with short phonation time. Women may also present with a very low "male"-sounding voice. In severe cases, stridor may be present on deep inspiration.

Leukoplakia. Leukoplakia, another form of chronic laryngitis, is the term for the white scalelike appearance of hyperkeratotic changes involving the vocal cords. It occurs secondary to chemical irritation, especially from tobacco smoke and alcohol exposures. Symptoms include hoarseness without pain. Leukoplakia, which may be a premalignant state in 2% to 10% of cases, cannot be distinguished visually from squamous cell carcinoma *in situ* or early invasive cancer.

Contact Ulcers. Contact ulcers of the larynx occur on the posterior one third of the vocal cords, where the arytenoid cartilage is covered only by a thin layer of mucosa. Once this mucosa is abraded, an ulcer often forms. Symptoms are painful phonation and a weakened, breathy voice. Occasionally, blood-tinged sputum may be present. Chronic ulcerations may in time develop into granulations that hold the cords apart, and at times these may become large enough to cause some respiratory obstruction. The ulcerations and subsequent granulations result most commonly from acute or chronic laryngeal intubation, but classically they are the result of vocal abuse by orators who misuse their larynx by attempting to lower the pitch of their voice when speaking forcefully. Recently, gastroesophageal reflux also has been found to play a role in the development of contact ulcers.

Vocal Cord Paralysis. Vocal cord paralysis occurs with recurrent laryngeal or vagal nerve injury. Usually just one cord is paralyzed (except in patients with severe central nervous system disease), causing a weak, breathy voice. The position of the cord is affected by the amount of time that has elapsed since injury because paralyzed cords tend to move toward the midline. The degree of paralysis and the clinical presentation depend on where the neural injury is located. Injury to a vagus nerve results in the loss of all ipsilateral laryngeal muscle function and sensation, leading to aspiration and a weak, breathy voice. A more peripheral injury of the recurrent laryngeal nerve leads to little if any aspiration and a voice that is hoarse and somewhat weak but less breathy. Viral neuritis and thoracic malignancy are the most common causes; with the former, function usually returns in 6 to 9 months.

Laryngeal Carcinoma. Laryngeal carcinoma usually occurs in patients with a history of smoking and drinking. If the vocal cords are involved, progressive hoarseness is an early sign, but if the tumor arises on the epiglottis, hypopharynx, or false cords, hoarseness may be a late development. Pain secondary to ulceration is also a late symptom and is often perceived as referred otalgia, especially when swallowing. These patients may have a mildly fetid breath. Patients with a hypopharyngeal or laryngeal cancer can present with an unexplained lymph node in the neck. The voice quality is extremely variable, ranging from breathy (commonly with large exophytic lesions preventing apposition of the cords) to strained or aphonic (commonly with ulcerative or lesions eroding the vocal fold).

Vocal Cord Nodules and Polyps. Vocal cord nodules may develop when edematous cords are used excessively. With continued excess voice use, fibrous tissue begins to collect at the junction of the anterior one third and the posterior two thirds of the vocal cord. This results in a lowered, breathy voice, which can harm a singing or speaking career. Vocal cord nodules (usually bilateral) typically occur in younger patients with a history of excessive voice use. Singers, teachers, and orators are at particular risk. These patients can often describe the history of onset for the hoarseness in the way in which it affects their voice. Pain may be present as the patient increasingly strains to generate a voice. The raspy quality to the voice often becomes more prominent later in the day when additional edema sets in. Patients with vocal cord polyps (usually unilateral) may present with varied types of dysphonia, depending on the size and location of the lesion. In many cases, an odd diplophonia (two frequencies of sound generated by the larynx) can be heard. Smoking and gastroesophageal reflux disease exacerbate both of these diagnoses.

Laryngeal Dystonias and Tremors. Increasingly recognized as causes for dysphonia and hoarseness, the laryngeal dystonias are characterized by a staccato voice breaks with a strained/strangled type of speech in the case of adductor spasmodic dysphonia versus involuntary voice breaks or changes in pitch characteristic of abductor spasmodic dysphonia. These are typically diagnosed based on clinical criteria emphasizing certain characteristic voice patterns with particular speech

TABLE 216.1

IMPORTANT CAUSES OF HOARSENESS

Acute Hoarseness	Chronic Hoarseness
Acute Laryngitis	**Chronic Laryngitis**
Viral infection	Chronic or recurrent vocal abuse
Vocal abuse	Smoking
Toxic fumes	Allergy
Allergy (seasonal)	Persistent irritant exposure
Acute Laryngeal Edema	**Carcinoma of the Larynx**
Angioneurotic edema	Intrinsic to vocal cords
Infection	Extrinsic to vocal cords
Direct injury	**Vocal Cord Lesions**
Nephritis	Polyps
Acute Epiglottitis	Leukoplakia
	Contact ulcer and granuloma
	Vocal nodule (see vocal abuse)
	Benign tumors
	Vocal Cord Paralysis
	Laryngeal nerve injury (tumor, neck surgery, aortic aneurysm)
	Brainstem lesion
	Vocal Cord Trauma
	Chronic intubation
	Systemic Disorders
	Hypothyroidism
	Rheumatoid arthritis
	Virilization
	Neurologic Disorders
	Parkinson's disease
	Spasmodic dysphonia
	Laryngeal tremor
	Psychogenic

phrases. Once recognized, the spasmodic dysphonias are often effectively treated with local injections of botulinum toxin. Voice tremor is an increasingly common source of dysphonia or hoarseness in the elderly population. It may or may not be associated with hand tremor or tremor elsewhere. This is largely unresponsive to voice therapy or pharmacologic treatment.

DIFFERENTIAL DIAGNOSIS (2,3)

The causes of hoarseness are best considered in terms of acute and chronic etiologies (Table 216.1).

WORKUP (1–4)

History

The evaluation of hoarseness depends on the chronicity of the condition. One needs to determine whether the onset was sudden or gradual and the course self-limited or progressive. Difficulty in breathing or stridor suggests obstruction and is an indication for emergency hospital admission especially with acute onset. It is helpful to find out whether hoarseness is exacerbated by talking, and whether the voice completely disappeared and, if so, for how long. Any recent upper respiratory tract infection, sore throat, fever, chills, sputum, or myalgias should be noted, as well as excessive voice use. Exposure to dust, fire, smoke, or irritant fumes should be documented, as should tobacco and alcohol intake. A history of neck mass, neck surgery, intubation, or lung tumor may provide important clues to etiology. Symptoms of hypothyroidism (see Chapter 104) are worth checking for when the etiology is not readily evident. Associated symptoms of odynophagia, aspiration, otalgia, or hemoptysis should be elicited and are especially worrisome.

Physical Examination

There are two rules of thumb regarding patients with hoarseness. First, hoarseness of duration more than 2 to 3 weeks requires an examination of the larynx. Second, this examination will provide, in most cases, an immediate diagnosis.

Indirect laryngoscopy with a head light and warmed laryngeal mirror is a time-honored method and still provides the best and most rapidly obtained view of the area. A good view of the hypopharynx and larynx is somewhat difficult to obtain, but the primary physician is encouraged to try and with practice should be able to master the technique. For the gagging patient, premedication with 10 mg of diazepam orally and an analgesic throat spray (Cetacaine or Xylocaine spray) is of benefit.

Even if indirect laryngoscopy cannot be successfully carried out in the office, some clues regarding the etiology can be gleaned by a careful physical examination and observation of voice quality. One needs to examine the oropharynx and carefully palpate the thyroid and the cervical lymph nodes. The hoarse patient with an unexplained neck mass or lymph node requires a thorough check of the nose, paranasal sinuses, and nasopharynx. A breathy voice suggests poor cord apposition, which may be due to tumor, polyp, or nodule. A raspy voice is indicative of cord thickening due to edema or inflammation, as with chemical irritation, vocal abuse, and infection. The patient with a high, shaky voice or a very soft one is having trouble mounting adequate respiratory force. Dyspnea is an indication for laryngoscopy.

Laboratory Studies

Direct Laryngoscopy

For patients with uncontrollable gag reflexes, referral for examination with a *fiberoptic laryngoscope* is necessary. This instrument is introduced through the nose, requiring pretreatment of the nasal passages with 4% cocaine or combination Xylocaine–oxymetazoline solution for vasoconstriction and anesthesia. It is rare when a good laryngeal view cannot be obtained in this manner.

Other Studies

In most instances, the selection of studies depends on the findings at laryngoscopy and should be done in conjunction with the otolaryngologist. The patient with unilateral paresis of the left vocal cord may have a recurrent laryngeal nerve syndrome secondary to a tumor involving the nerve in the chest most commonly or at the skull base or neck, necessitating *chest computed tomography* scanning. If this is negative, *computed tomography of the neck and skull base* is worth considering. Pancoast tumors and carcinoma of the thyroid are unusual causes of vocal cord paralysis. The rate of unilateral vocal cord paralysis after thyroid surgery approximates 1%. If the cords appear to

be chronically edematous and there is a clinical suspicion of hypothyroidism, a check of serum *thyroid-stimulating hormone* is indicated.

Patients with a suspected carcinoma involving the larynx or with an unexplained neck node and hoarseness need a thorough evaluation of the aerodigestive tract before biopsy, facilitated by *magnetic resonance imaging scan* of the head and neck. *Small-needle biopsy* of suspicious cervical nodes can circumvent the need for some open biopsies, which should be done only under select circumstances. The patient with recurrent edematous episodes and a positive family history might have angioneurotic edema; a check of the *C1 esterase inhibitor* level is indicated. *Lateral neck soft tissue films* may be needed in the acutely dyspneic patient with suspected upper airway obstruction.

PRINCIPLES OF MANAGEMENT AND THERAPEUTIC RECOMMENDATIONS (1–4)

Regardless of causes, all patients with hoarseness should be strongly advised to *quit smoking* immediately (see Chapter 54). It is often in the setting of an associated medical problem that a smoker will finally decide to quit. Other interventions are a function of the underlying etiology.

Acute Laryngitis

The best treatment is *voice rest*. When it is necessary to speak, the patient should use a moderate voice and not whisper. Warm sialogogues, such as *hot tea with sugar and lemon*, may be helpful. Antibiotics are not indicated unless there is documented bacterial infection. *Cough suppressants*, particularly with mucolytic agents, may be helpful. *Humidity* is of benefit. Inhalation of *steam* in a hot shower or breathing through a moist, hot towel will provide immediate partial relief. When hay fever is the cause, a *topical steroid spray* such as dexamethasone or flunisolide helps to provide symptomatic relief, but steroids should not be used unless there is an allergic etiology. Acute acid reflux suppression may also hasten recovery if implicated.

Professional singers and *speakers* should be advised to rest their voice when they become hoarse (especially during upper respiratory infections) to prevent permanent injury to the vocal cords. A vasoconstricting spray and analgesics are used by professionals when use of their voice is absolutely necessary. Occasionally, professional singers may be given a short course of topical or oral steroids to get through a singing commitment, but further cord injury may ensue.

Acute Laryngeal Edema

Acute laryngeal edema represents a medical emergency; *hospitalization* is urgent. Treatment is based on the degree of swelling and subsequent airway compromise. An emergency airway is established if necessary; 0.3 mL of *adrenaline* 1:1,000 is administered subcutaneously, and steroids such as *dexamethasone* (Decadron, 12 mg) may be given intravenously. *Histamine$_1$-* and *histamine$_2$-receptor blockade* is also instituted.

Vocal Cord Nodules

Vocal cord nodules should be treated early because often (>80% of cases) they respond to voice rest and vocal therapy. Nodules that do not respond to conservative therapy can be removed; use of an *atraumatic technique* (microlaryngeal surgery, carbon dioxide laser) is mandatory. *Dependent polyps* are removed by microsurgery. Usually, *follow-up voice therapy* is helpful in preventing polyp recurrence and hastening the return to the normal voice.

Angioneurotic Edema

Angioneurotic edema does not respond well to epinephrine or glucocorticosteroids. In an acute situation, *intubation* or *tracheotomy* may be required to maintain an airway. If available, infusion of *C1 esterase inhibitor* can be given. Otherwise, treatment is prophylactic, using *anabolic steroids* with attenuated androgenic effect (e.g., *danazol* and *stanozolol*) to stimulate the synthesis of C1 esterase inhibitor. Such prophylaxis may be given for several days before planned surgery.

Temporary Unilateral Vocal Cord Paralysis

Temporary unilateral vocal cord paralysis can be treated symptomatically by the otolaryngologist through the injection of *collagen paste* into the musculature of the paralyzed cord, moving it to the midline for 3 to 6 months. This permits the functioning cord to better approximate, thereby improving vocal quality. For permanent vocal cord paralysis, *thyroplasty* and *arytenoid adduction* procedures move the paralyzed vocal cord to the midline permanently and provide excellent results. No satisfactory procedure has been developed for bilateral vocal cord paralysis, and patients are often relegated to bypass tracheotomy.

Carcinoma of the Larynx

Carcinoma of the larynx can be cured with minimal permanent morbidity, especially if detected in its early stages (T1N0). *Surgery, laser,* and *radiation* are all capable of achieving a 90% cure rate. Selection of modality depends on the type of expertise available locally and the location of the lesion. Metastases and a poor prognosis usually do not occur until the vocal cord cancer becomes larger (T3 to T4) and extends beyond the true cords. Early supraglottic carcinomas arising above the true cords can be cured in about 75% of patients with *radiation therapy, par-* *tial laryngectomy,* or a combination of the two. Larger lesions require combined *induction chemotherapy* and *radiation with surgery* for salvage, thereby sparing many larynges that otherwise might be resected. Prevention remains the best treatment; all smokers must be told to quit.

Leukoplakia is treated by *resection* of the lesion under microscopic control. With current techniques, voice outcomes remain excellent, and with resection, recurrence rates are less than 3%. Regular follow-up examinations of the larynx are necessary. Infrequently, repeated resections may be needed once or twice a year, particularly if the patient fails to limit use of irritants such as tobacco smoke.

INDICATIONS FOR REFERRAL AND ADMISSION

Referral

If the primary care physician does not feel competent to visualize the vocal cords, a decision must be made about whether to refer the patient to an otolaryngologist. Hoarseness of *duration greater than 3 weeks*, particularly when there has not been a history of an acute infectious process, requires referral. In those who have a resolving process and are at low risk for malignancy (young, nonsmoker, nondrinker), a complete otolaryngologic examination may be deferred pending full resolution.

Among patients who do undergo indirect laryngoscopy by the primary care physician, any patient with a *cord nodule, thickening,* or *paralysis* by indirect laryngoscopy requires referral, as does the patient with *persistent unexplained hoarseness* of duration more than 2 to 3 weeks and inability to tolerate indirect laryngoscopy.

Referral for *voice therapy* can help foster healthful vocal habits and is indicated for patients who experience repeated vocal trauma or who have organic disease and are in need of voice rehabilitation. A trial voice therapy may be judiciously employed for younger patients without risk factor exposure who give a clear-cut history of voice abuse. Voice therapists are also particularly adept at eliciting diagnostic features of laryngeal tremor or spasmodic dysphonia. Again, if hoarseness does not promptly resolve with voice therapy, referral for direct laryngoscopy is mandatory.

Admission

Any patient with concurrent *dyspnea/stridor* should be immediately hospitalized, especially if associated with odynophagia, dysphagia, or fever.

Annotated Bibliography

1. Frantz TD, Rasgon BM, Quesenberry CP Jr. Acute epiglottitis in adults: analysis of 129 cases. JAMA 1994;272:1358. (*The most common symptoms were sore throat and painful swallowing; muffled voice and pharyngeal erythema were the key signs; dyspnea was uncommon but important not to miss.*)
2. Garrett CG, Ossoff RH. Hoarseness. Med Clin North Am 1999;8:115. (*A comprehensive summary of the diagnosis and management for the primary care physician.*)
3. Vaughan CW. Diagnosis and treatment of organic voice disorders. N Engl J Med 1983;307:863. (*Still one of the best reviews for the general reader.*)
4. Zeitels SM, Healy GB. Laryngology and phonosurgery. N Engl J Med 2003;349:882. (*A good modern summary of new diagnostic methods and surgical treatment for common voice disorders.*)

CHAPTER 217 ■ EVALUATION OF TINNITUS

NEIL BHATTACHARYYA

Tinnitus is an important but nonspecific symptom of otologic disease. "Ringing," "buzzing," and "roaring" are terms used to describe the sensation, which can be extremely annoying and a source of concern. The occurrence of tinnitus requires assessment for potential serious and treatable otologic problems. In the absence of a specifically treatable etiology, it is still important to provide the patient with some symptomatic relief, especially at night or during quiet concentration, when tinnitus tends to be most bothersome.

PATHOPHYSIOLOGY AND CLINICAL PRESENTATION (1–5)

Tinnitus is very poorly understood. It appears to be a nonspecific manifestation of disease in the ear, cochlear nerve, or central auditory apparatus and is often (but not always) accompanied by hearing loss.

External and Middle Ear Conditions

Tinnitus may result from *impacted cerumen*, *perforation* of the tympanic membrane, or *fluid* in the middle ear, all of which "lead" to tinnitus due to the associated conductive hearing loss. The sensation is commonly described as low-pitched, intermittent, and accompanied by muffled hearing and a change in the sound of one's voice. In *otosclerosis*, tinnitus is constant but may disappear as the disease progresses. *Acute otitis media* sometimes produces a pulsating type of tinnitus that resolves as inflammation subsides. Pulsatile tinnitus is also associated with *glomus tumors* and posttraumatic *arteriovenous fistulas*.

Inner Ear and Cochlear Nerve Disease

Presbycusis, *noise-induced hearing loss*, and *acoustic trauma* can give rise to a high-pitched tinnitus that subjectively matches the frequency of greatest hearing loss. Transient tinnitus that follows acute noise exposure is a forerunner of hearing loss and a warning sign to avoid repeated exposure. *Ototoxic drugs*, such as the aminoglycoside antibiotics, may produce high-pitched tinnitus and hearing loss that often persist after the cessation of drug use. Salicylates are frequently responsible for reversible, dose-related tinnitus. *Ménière's disease* results in transient, low-pitched tinnitus that varies with the intensity of the condition's other symptoms, often worsening when vertigo and hearing loss are imminent. An *acoustic neuroma* produces a similar set of symptoms, but usually the clinical course is progressive, with unilateral or asymmetric tinnitus frequently preceding other symptoms, such as vertigo (see Chapter 166). A sudden onset of severe unilateral tinnitus may be the first presenting symptom of sudden sensorineural hearing loss, which requires immediate medical attention.

Other Sources

When ambient noise is reduced, all people will notice some head sounds. These may stem from a variety of events, ranging from the rushing of blood (most severe in aortic insufficiency) to the contraction of auditory muscles. A loss of hearing due to conductive defects may accentuate the perception of tinnitus. *Tinnitus cerebri* is described as a roaring in the head and is believed to be vascular or neurologic in origin. A *cerebral aneurysm* with an audible bruit, a jugular megabulb anomaly, *palatal myoclonus* with audible muscle contraction, and an unusually patent *eustachian tube* that transmits respiratory sounds are examples of "objective" tinnitus in which the sounds can be heard by the examiner. Tinnitus may also be associated with temporomandibular joint dysfunction (Costen's syndrome). In rare cases, intermittent tinnitus may be caused by a spasm or flutter of the tensor tympani or stapedius muscles of the middle ear.

Depressed and neurotic individuals may have less tolerance for normal head sounds and complain of them when in quiet settings. The ability to accommodate tinnitus is also subject to much individual variation. Tolerance is lessened by fatigue and emotional stress.

DIFFERENTIAL DIAGNOSIS (1,3,4)

Most tinnitus results from the same conditions that cause hearing loss, whether conductive or sensorineural, peripheral or central (see Chapter 212). Subjective complaints of ear or head noise in the absence of otologic pathology may be a concomitant of psychogenic disease. Objective tinnitus suggests cerebrovascular pathology, palatal myoclonus, or a patulous eustachian tube.

There are few data on the frequency of the various conditions responsible for tinnitus. Of interest is the fact that reports from otologic practice list as many as 50% of cases as being of unknown etiology.

WORKUP (1,3,4)

The diagnostic assessment of tinnitus follows the same pattern as that for hearing loss (see Chapter 212). Some additional points follow.

History

The pitch of the tinnitus is, unfortunately, of limited use in diagnosis, although some conditions are more likely than others to be associated with tinnitus of a certain pitch. Distinguishing pulsatile, nonpulsatile, subjective, and objective tinnitus may be more helpful. The laterality and symmetry of the tinnitus are important parts of the history. Any association of the sound with respiration, drug use, vertigo, noise trauma, or ear infection should be checked. A history of head trauma should be sought because it may be associated with an arteriovenous fistula or an aneurysm of the intrapetrous portion of the internal carotid artery. When the problem is present only at night, it suggests an increased awareness of normal head sounds. Most patients with tinnitus of otologic origin have an associated hearing defect or soon develop one, whereas those without other signs of ear disease may have vascular lesion or an accentuated awareness of normal head noises.

Physical Examination

One inspects the external ear and tympanic membrane for cerumen impaction, foreign bodies, perforation, signs of otitis media (see Chapter 218), and abnormal middle ear masses. Weber and Rinne testing should be performed to determine sensorineural or conductive hearing loss (see Chapter 212). The cranial nerves are examined for evidence of neuropathy or for signs of an acoustic neuroma or a glomus tumor. Testing for nystagmus (see Chapter 166) is worthwhile if vertigo is reported. The skull should be auscultated for a bruit if the origin of the problem remains obscure. Compression of the ipsilateral jugular vein will abolish the objective tinnitus of a jugular megabulb anomaly.

Laboratory Studies

An *audiogram* can help to identify and localize the site of the lesion underlying the hearing loss. Neuroimaging studies (e.g., *computed tomography* or *magnetic resonance imaging*) may be indicated but should not be done without first consulting an otolaryngologist to ensure proper test selection, performance, and interpretation. Gadolinium-enhanced magnetic resonance imaging may be recommended, especially in the evaluation of unilateral or asymmetric tinnitus with or without hearing loss.

Most patients with tinnitus and isolated unilateral sensorineural hearing loss on audiometry require either contrast magnetic resonance imaging of the internal auditory canals or serial audiometric follow-up.

INDICATIONS FOR REFERRAL

Referral is essential when a conductive hearing loss is discovered because many of these lesions are correctable. Suspicion of an acoustic neuroma, glomus tumor, or cerebrovascular abnormality is also an indication for consultation, especially before embarking on an expensive workup. Referral to the otolaryngologist may be necessary to satisfy the anxious patient that everything has been explored and that there is no serious or correctable underlying condition.

SYMPTOMATIC MANAGEMENT AND PATIENT EDUCATION (1,3,4,6,7)

For many patients, the priority is relief from the constant ringing, which can be very disturbing, especially at night. Drugs of all types have been tried, including nicotinic acid, vasodilators, tranquilizers, antidepressants, and seizure medications. None has proven superior to placebo. Nighttime use of a clock radio or white noise machine that shuts off after 1/2 hour of playing background music often allows the patient to fall asleep. Keeping a radio on during the day when the patient has to work in a quiet room is also helpful. Many wearable devices are promoted, such as a hearing aid (tinnitus maskers) to help mask tinnitus; they are of questionable value. *Biofeedback* may help in certain cases in which the tinnitus is related to stress. More recently, low-dose *antidepressant therapy* has been explored for tinnitus management. *Tinnitus retraining therapy* seems to hold significant promise for refractory cases. Patients may benefit from information and support provided by the American Tinnitus Association (http://www.ATA.org), which is an excellent, unbiased source of information for the patient.

Annotated Bibliography

1. Henry JA, Dennis KC, Schechter MA. General review of tinnitus: prevalence, mechanisms, effects, and management. J Speech Lang Hear Res 2005;48:1204. (*An excellent discussion, including management strategies.*)
2. Lee CA, Mistry D, Uppal S, et al. Otologic side effects of drugs. J Laryngol Otol 2005;119:267. (*An important review of side effects with respect to the ear in tinnitus.*)
3. Levine RA. Tinnitus. Curr Opin Otolaryngol Head Neck Surg 1994;2:171. (*A neurologist's perspective on the genesis of tinnitus.*)
4. Lockwood AH, Salvi RJ, Burkard RF. Tinnitus. N Engl J Med 2002;347:904. (*An excellent review for the generalist reader; 49 references.*)
5. Moller AR. Similarities between chronic pain and tinnitus. Am J Otolaryngol 1997;18:577. (*Current understanding of the mechanisms underlying chronic pain and their relevance to tinnitus.*)
6. Dobie RA. A review of randomized clinical trials in tinnitus. Laryngoscope 1999;109:1202. (*A critical analysis of data from randomized trials of treatment modalities.*)
7. Jastreboff PJ, Gray WC, Gold SL. Neurophysiologic approach to tinnitus patients. Am J Otolaryngol 1996;17:236. (*Presents the scientific basis for a treatment protocol using counseling and sound generators.*)

CHAPTER 218 ■ APPROACH TO THE PATIENT WITH OTITIS

NEIL BHATTACHARYYA

Ear discomfort from otitis media accompanying an upper respiratory tract infection is one of the more common complaints encountered in primary care practice, particularly in pediatric settings. Adults are less susceptible but no less uncomfortable when otitis sets in. Symptoms range from vague fullness to frank pain and may be accompanied by diminution in hearing. Patients may present out of concern about the safety of upcoming air travel or underwater activities, especially if over-the-counter remedies have not brought improvement. The primary care physician should be able effectively to manage most cases. Knowing the roles of antibiotics and decongestants in the treatment of otitis media is essential. Discomfort referable to the ear may also be a consequence of otitis externa. Inspection often reveals signs of otitis media or external otitis. The primary care provider should know how to recognize and treat these common conditions.

PATHOPHYSIOLOGY AND CLINICAL PRESENTATION (1–6)

Acute Otitis Media

Acute otitis media may be the consequence of abnormal *eustachian tube reflux* or *obstruction* that permits nasopharyngeal bacteria to infect the middle ear, which is normally free of organisms. Obstruction can result from mucosal edema and/or excessive mucus due to allergic or infectious etiologies. Viral nasopharyngitis is the most common cause, especially in the winter. It may produce little more than a *serous otitis*, which is generally *"sterile."* If there is bacterial invasion, a *purulent otitis media* may ensue. Of the bacterial species that can be isolated, the most common are *Streptococcus pneumoniae, Haemophilus influenzae,* and *Moraxella catarrhalis.* Viruses, *Staphylococcus aureus, Streptococcus pyogenes,* and other, less-virulent organisms are less frequently etiologic.

The principal clinical findings are ear *pain, hearing loss,* and mild to moderate *fever.* The tympanic membrane appears bulging, and an *opaque effusion* may be noted behind the drum if a purulent exudate develops in the middle ear. If pressure builds excessively, the tympanic membrane may perforate with consequent spontaneous otorrhea. A translucent *effusion* is characteristic of *serous otitis*; one may also observe apparent foreshortening of the manubrium, enhanced whiteness of the stria mallearis, and retraction of the tympanic membrane in the attic region. Most patients make a full recovery. In some patients, recurrent purulent otitis, sustained hearing loss, chronic serous otitis, or chronic otitis media may ensue.

Patients may also develop acute serous otitis media from the negative pressure changes imparted by airplane flight. In rare cases, *hemorrhage* may be evident within the drum and the middle ear space. In the absence of significant vertigo, these patients may be managed conservatively by limiting their airplane flights until resolution. Pain management may be required.

External Otitis

External otitis develops in the setting of skin breakdown in the external auditory canal, leading to inflammation of the surrounding tissues. Skin breakdown is a common denominator, whether from trauma (e.g., from a finger nail or cotton swab), excessive moisture (e.g., swimmer's ear), infection of a hair follicle, or chronic eczema. Itching, crusting, pain, redness, and/or discharge may be reported. Movement of the pinna or tragus is characteristically painful. Gram-positive bacteria, gram-negative bacteria, and fungi can be variably isolated as infectious agents.

Malignant (Necrotizing) External Otitis

Malignant external otitis is seen in immunocompromised patients and older diabetics. It develops deep in the external canal and usually represents as a *Pseudomonas* cellulitis of the canal and adjacent tissues. Characteristics include purulent discharge, granulation tissue in the external auditory canal, severe ear pain, and temporomandibular joint pain. Signs of facial nerve involvement may follow.

Chronic Otitis Media

Chronic otitis media is a consequence of untreated or recurrent acute otitis media. Bony destruction or sclerosis of mastoid air cells may result, and the tympanic membrane is often perforated, draining purulent fluid. (Marginal and attic perforations may be associated with invasive cholesteatoma.) Both aerobes and anaerobes can be cultured from the drainage, including *Staphylococcus, Streptococcus, Pseudomonas,* enteric gram-negative organisms, and *Bacteroides.* Patients report little pain or fever, except during exacerbation, but hearing loss and chronic foul otorrhea are common. Again, water exposure of a perforated tympanic membrane may spur the infectious otorrhea. Computed tomography of the temporal bone may be helpful in revealing the extent of disease of the middle ear and mastoid.

DIAGNOSIS (1–6)

Acute Otitis Media

The cornerstone of the clinical diagnosis of acute purulent otitis media is the finding of a *bulging tympanic membrane* with impaired mobility and the loss of the bony landmarks. With serous otitis media, fever and pain are absent, and although fluid is present in the middle ear, it is translucent; the tympanic membrane is retracted and the bony landmarks are present. Cultures obtained from the nasopharynx are generally not helpful in defining the infectious agent of an acute otitis media. Needle aspiration of the middle ear is occasionally used to confirm the diagnosis and to identify the causative organism; usually such *diagnostic tympanocentesis* is reserved for those cases that are unresponsive to appropriate antibiotic therapy or suspected otitic meningitis or to cases involving immunocompromised individuals.

Chronic Otitis Media and Otitis Externa

The diagnosis of chronic otitis media is suggested by the presence of a perforated drum and discharge through the perforation. Pain on movement of the pinna, erythema, and discharge in the external auditory canal are diagnostic of otitis externa. On occasion, a seemingly recurrent external otitis may reflect an unrecognized tympanic membrane perforation and chronic otitis media. Accordingly, careful otoscopic examination after resolution of the acute infection is important.

PRINCIPLES OF MANAGEMENT AND THERAPEUTIC RECOMMENDATIONS (1–7)

Acute Purulent Otitis Media

Treatment includes the use of analgesics, decongestants, and antibiotics. *Amoxicillin* is often the drug of choice. Because resistant strains of *H. influenzae* have been isolated in a substantial proportion of cases and *M. catarrhalis* may be responsible for other cases, the combination preparation *amoxicillin/clavulanate* (Augmentin) is a reasonable alternative, particularly when an initial course of amoxicillin does not suffice. For penicillin-allergic persons, *trimethoprim/sulfa* or *erythromycin* may be substituted. A *sympathomimetic decongestant* (e.g., *pseudoephedrine*) may help when the otitis occurs in the setting of an upper respiratory tract infection and eustachian tube obstruction. *Myringotomy*, although not considered therapeutic, is indicated for patients with intractable pain, progressive hearing loss, or acute mastoiditis and in those who have had a poor response to medical therapy. Antihistamines are usually contraindicated because their drying effect may lead to inspissated secretions. After the initiation of antibiotics, otalgia typically subsides in 24 to 72 hours, but the conductive hearing loss due to remaining middle ear effusion may persist for weeks or even months after the acute illness.

Acute Serous Otitis Media

Cases secondary to eustachian tube obstruction from allergy or upper respiratory infection may improve with the use of sympa-thomimetic *decongestants* (see Chapter 222). When allergy is suspected, some physicians add an *antihistamine,* but definitive evidence for its efficacy is lacking, and, as just noted, antihistamines may thicken secretions, impeding their clearance.

Chronic Otitis Media

The mainstay of therapy of chronic otitis media is careful aural toilet, with 1.5% *acetic acid irrigation* and *topical antibiotics* (ophthalmic drops tend to be less irritating). The acetic acid irrigation gently debrides accumulated debris and restores the normal acid pH of the external auditory canal. Water precautions should be instituted. Despite maximal medical therapy, *surgery* is often required. Patients should be watched for complications such as intracranial suppuration, facial paralysis, sensorineural hearing loss, and vertigo. Persistent fever and headache are ominous in the setting of otitis media (either acute or chronic) and mandate expeditious referral to an otolaryngologist. Chronic recurrent otorrhea that returns after the cessation of antibiotic eardrops raises the possibility of cholesteatoma.

Otitis Externa

Otitis externa is treated with *topical antibiotics* (e.g., eardrops containing *polymyxin, hydrocortisone,* or *neomycin*) and *analgesics.* Four drops are applied four times daily for a week, in combination with the prevention of water contamination (a cotton ball coated with petrolatum ointment usually suffices). Neomycin-containing eardrops, such as Cortisporin, can cause allergic skin reactions (especially when used over a long period). A simple patch test will identify a sensitized patient. More-severe cases of external otitis in which the canal is obstructed by edema or purulent material require referral to an otolaryngologist for *suction aspiration* of debris and the *insertion of a wick* to promote antibiotic penetration. A recent evidence-based guideline has been published by the American Academy of Otolaryngology-Head and Neck Surgery and covers this diagnosis and management in excellent detail.

Cellulitis/Malignant External Otitis

Cellulitis/malignant external otitis requires systemic antibiotic treatment that includes coverage against *Pseudomonas aeruginosa.* The infection can be life threatening in diabetics and immunocompromised hosts, necessitating prompt hospitalization, the initiation of parenteral antibiotics, and referral to an otolaryngologist for consideration of the need for debridement.

INDICATIONS FOR REFERRAL

An otolaryngologist should be consulted if acute otitis media fails to respond to medical therapy or if a complication such as tympanic membrane perforation, recurrent acute otitis, chronic serous otitis, or chronic otitis media develops. Adult patients with chronic serous otitis media require referral for examination of the nasopharynx to rule out a mass lesion obstructing the eustachian tube. The onset of persistent fever, headache, facial nerve paralysis (or other cranial neuropathy), vertigo, or sensorineural hearing loss in the setting of otologic infection mandates emergency otolaryngologic referral. As noted earlier, hospitalization for parenteral antibiotic therapy is indicated if cellulitis of the external ear develops.

PATIENT EDUCATION

General Measures

The pain of acute otitis media almost always leads the patient to seek prompt medical attention. Patients who have active external otitis or chronic otitis media with perforation of the eardrum should be instructed to avoid swimming and keep water from entering the ear. As already noted, a cotton ball coated with petrolatum ointment provides a simple yet effective barrier to water entry.

Airplane Travel

Patients with serous otitis or eustachian tube dysfunction who must travel by air without delay should use oral and intranasal *decongestants* (see Chapter 222), especially in anticipation of descent for landing, when the risk of barotrauma is greatest. *Self-inflation* of the eustachian tubes can provide symptomatic relief. The patient is instructed to pinch the nose shut, inhale deeply, close the mouth, and try to blow the nose while keeping it pinched shut.

Annotated Bibliography

1. Berman S. Current concepts: otitis media in children. N Engl J Med 1995;332:1560. (*A broad overview of the topic, with a flow chart of treatment options.*)
2. Celin SE, Bluestone CD, Stephenson J, et al. Bacteriology of acute otitis media in adults. JAMA 1991;226:2249. (*Haemophilus influenzae and Streptococcus pneumoniae were the leading causes, and antibiotics against β-lactamase–producing organisms were not necessary in most instances.*)
3. Finkelstein Y, Ophir D, Talmi YP, et al. Adult-onset otitis media with effusion. Arch Otolaryngol Head Neck Surg 1994;120:517. (*A nice review of adult otitis media, given that the literature focuses mainly on childhood otitis media.*)
4. Hendley JO. Otitis media. N Engl J Med 2002;347:1169. (*A clinically focused review for the practitioner; 35 references.*)
5. Post JC, Preston RA, Aul JJ, et al. Molecular analysis of bacterial pathogens in otitis media with effusion. JAMA 1995;273:1598. (*Polymerase chain reaction analysis of pediatric middle ear effusions detects bacterial DNA in a significant percentage of culture-negative middle ear effusions.*)
6. Rubin J, Yu VL. Malignant external otitis: insights into pathogenesis, clinical manifestations, diagnosis, and therapy. Am J Med 1988;85:39. (*Still the most comprehensive review in the general medicine literature.*)
7. Rosenfeld RM, Brown L, Cannon CR, et al. Clinical practice guideline: acute otitis externa. Otolaryngol Head Neck Surg 2006;134 (4 Suppl):S4. (*An evidence-based guideline for the diagnosis and treatment of otitis externa; worthwhile reading for clinicians encountering this diagnosis with any frequency.*)

CHAPTER 219 ■ APPROACH TO THE PATIENT WITH SINUSITIS

WILLIAM A. KORMOS

Sinusitis is an inflammation of one or more of the five paired paranasal sinuses surrounding the eyes. It is an extremely common but likely overdiagnosed condition, with more than 30 million Americans treated for acute sinusitis annually. Many patients with nasal and sinus symptoms have self-limited viral infections or allergic conditions; the physician must distinguish these patients from the patient with a bacterial infection who may require antibiotics. Although acute sinusitis is often self-limited, there is significant morbidity associated with sinusitis. The extension of infection into the central nervous system and bone may be life threatening, and patients who develop chronic sinusitis rate their quality of life similar to patients with congestive heart failure or chronic obstructive pulmonary disease.

PATHOPHYSIOLOGY AND CLINICAL PRESENTATION (1,2)

The normal sinuses are sterile structures lined with ciliated epithelium. Mucus is cleared from the sinus in a directed manner toward the ostia, or openings, which drain into the nasal cavity at the superior meatus and middle meatus. The superior meatus drains the posterior ethmoid and sphenoid sinuses, and the middle meatus drains the frontal, maxillary, and anterior ethmoid sinuses. Occlusion of these ostiomeatal complexes can lead to dysfunction of the normal sinus epithelium and bacterial infection. Although any sinus can become occluded through viral infection, anatomic abnormalities (including septal deviation, tumors, and polyps) or allergies can predispose to infection.

Acute Sinusitis

The *common cold* is actually a *rhinosinusitis* that frequently involves the paranasal sinuses. Computed tomographic study of patients with the common cold reveals that more than 85% have a self-limited paranasal sinusitis that resolves without treatment. The maxillary sinuses are the most common sites (87%), followed by ethmoidal (65%), sphenoidal (39%), and frontal (32%) involvement. Rhinorrhea and nasal stuffiness are the typical symptoms. Although symptoms may persist for well more than 10 days, those of uncomplicated viral rhinosinusitis usually start to improve by 7 to 10 days.

Failure to improve suggests bacterial superinfection. In about 0.5% to 2% of cases of the common cold, bacterial infection of the sinuses occurs, resulting in acute purulent bacterial sinusitis. It is characterized by nasal congestion, purulent nasal discharge, facial pain (which classically increases when the patient stoops forward), fever, fatigue, and other constitutional symptoms.

Bacteriology

In most cases of bacterial sinusitis, a single organism accounts for the infection; in about 25%, two organisms are present in high density. In more than three fourths of cases, the causative organism proves to be either *Streptococcus pneumoniae* or *Haemophilus influenzae*. Other potentially etiologic organisms include *Moraxella catarrhalis*, *Streptococcus pyogenes*, and anaerobes (*Fusobacterium*, *Bacteroides*, *Peptostreptococcus*). Anaerobes account for about 6% of all cases of sinusitis and usually occur in the setting of dental infections or chronic sinusitis, especially after recurrent courses of antibiotics. *Staphylococcus aureus* can be found on nasal culture, but only very infrequently is it isolated from sinus aspirates in acute sinusitis.

Viruses, especially rhinovirus and influenza virus, have been isolated alone or in combination with bacteria in 15% to 20% of patients. This may represent true causation of the sinusitis or a preceding viral infection, leading to the bacterial superinfection. *Mycoplasma pneumoniae* and *Chlamydia pneumoniae* are not believed to be important etiologies for most patients. Rarely, fungi such as *Mucor*, *Rhizopus*, and *Aspergillus* species can produce invasive sinusitis in poorly controlled diabetics, leukemics, or other immunosuppressed hosts.

Clinical Presentation

Sinus pain or pressure and purulent nasal discharge are the defining clinical features of acute sinusitis; fever is present in about half of the cases. The location of the discomfort depends on the sinuses involved. Maxillary sinusitis is the most common and produces pain and tenderness over the cheeks. The pain is referred to the teeth in some patients. Frontal sinusitis produces pain and tenderness over the lower forehead. Ethmoid sinusitis results in retroorbital pain and may have tenderness over the upper lateral aspect of the nose. Isolated sphenoid sinusitis is uncommon but can present as retroorbital, frontal, or facial pain. Purulent nasal discharge may be visualized in the middle meatus if the frontal, maxillary, or anterior ethmoid sinus is involved.

Chronic Sinusitis

Symptoms of chronic sinusitis include nasal congestion and purulent discharge, but pain and headache are usually mild or absent, and fever is uncommon. By definition, symptoms should be present for at least 2 to 3 months. The predominant organisms are *S. aureus*, Enterobacteriaceae, and anaerobic organisms, such as anaerobic streptococci and *Bacteroides* species. *H. influenzae* and pneumococcus are less important etiologies in chronic infection. The pathologic importance of anaerobes in chronic sinusitis is reflected by the predominance of anaerobes in brain abscesses of sinus origin.

Atypical organisms may be responsible for some cases in hospitalized and immunocompromised persons. *Gram-negative bacilli* may cause sinusitis in hospitalized patients who are nasotracheally intubated or immunocompromised. Fungal infection in an immunosuppressed host can lead to chronic invasive sinusitis. Fungal exposure can cause an allergic fungal sinusitis.

Complications

Complications of sinusitis are uncommon in the setting of antibiotic use but can be life threatening. The most serious are *osteomyelitis*, *orbital cellulitis*, and *cavernous sinus thrombosis*.

Osteomyelitis

Frontal sinusitis can lead to osteomyelitis of the frontal bones, especially in children. Patients present with headache, fever, and a characteristic doughy edema over the involved bone, which is termed "Pott's puffy tumor." The organisms involved are the same as those responsible for the underlying sinusitis, except that *S. aureus* may also be involved. Osteomyelitis of the maxilla is an infrequent complication of maxillary sinusitis. Orbital cellulitis is most frequently a complication of ethmoid sinusitis due to the direct extension of infection through the lamina papyracea. It usually begins with edema of the eyelids and rapidly progresses to ptosis, proptosis, chemosis, and diminished extraocular movements. Patients are usually febrile and acutely ill. Pressure on the optic nerve can lead to visual loss, which can be permanent, and retrograde spread of infection can lead to intracranial infection.

Cavernous Sinus Thrombosis

Retrograde extension of infection along venous channels from the orbit, ethmoid or frontal sinuses, or nose can produce septic cavernous sinus thrombophlebitis. These patients are highly febrile and appear "toxic." Lid edema, proptosis, and chemosis are present, but unlike uncomplicated orbital cellulitis, third, fourth, and sixth cranial nerve palsies are prominent; the pupil may be fixed and dilated; and funduscopic examination may reveal venous engorgement and papilledema. Although the process is usually unilateral at first, spread across the anterior and posterior intercavernous sinuses results in bilateral involvement. Patients may exhibit alterations of consciousness.

Intracranial Suppuration

Sinusitis can lead to intracranial suppuration either by direct spread through bone or via venous channels. A great variety of syndromes can result, including *epidural abscess*, *subdural empyema*, *meningitis*, and *brain abscess*. Clinical findings vary greatly, ranging from subtle personality changes with frontal lobe abscesses to headache, symptoms of elevated intracranial pressure, alterations of consciousness, visual symptoms, focal neurologic deficits, seizures, and, ultimately, coma and death.

DIFFERENTIAL DIAGNOSIS

The common cold and allergic or vasomotor rhinitis are by far the most common causes of "sinus" symptoms, but polyps, tumors, cysts, foreign bodies, and vasculitides such as Wegener's granulomatosis occasionally produce symptoms resembling sinusitis (see Chapter 222). Patients with migraine headaches often have bifrontal pain and nasal symptoms, leading to an erroneous diagnosis of sinus headache.

WORKUP (3–6)

Clinical findings can be very helpful in the diagnosis of sinusitis, especially when findings are considered in combination. In a prospective study comparing historical and physical findings with sinus films, no single feature had a likelihood ratio of greater than 2.5 in predicting a positive x-ray, but when five individually predictive findings (see later discussion) were considered together, the likelihood ratio rose to 6.4 if all were present and fell to 0.1 if none was found.

History

The diagnosis of sinusitis is entertained in the patient with symptoms of nasal congestion and discharge that persist beyond the expected 7 to 10 days of the common cold. The classic symptom of frontal, maxillary, retroorbital, or vertex pain that worsens on bending forward has not been found independently to predict radiographic sinusitis in several studies. A history of purulent rhinorrhea, however, has been associated with sinusitis in several studies (positive likelihood ratios of 1.5 to 3.5). In addition, a prospective study in the primary care setting comparing clinical findings and radiographs in adult males presenting with symptoms suggestive of sinusitis also revealed that maxillary toothache and poor response to decongestants were useful predictors of radiologically confirmed sinusitis (the positive likelihood ratio was 2.5 and 2.1, respectively). In a study from ear, nose, and throat practice using maxillary aspiration of purulent material for diagnosis, unilateral sinus pain also correlated with outcome. Finally, the symptom of "double sickening" (upper respiratory infection symptoms with initial improvement, followed by increasing nasal symptoms) had a positive likelihood ratio of 2.8 in one primary care study.

Risk factors such as nasal polyps, deviated nasal septum, trauma, foreign bodies, and rapid changes in altitude should be inquired about. Special attention should be paid to toxic symptoms of high fever and rigors in association with complaints suggestive of the extension of infection, such as edema of the eyelids and diplopia.

Physical Examination

One should examine the nasal cavity for purulent discharge draining from one of the turbinates and transilluminate the maxillary sinuses for impaired light transmission. Transillumination must be performed in a completely darkened room with a strong light source. The nasal cavity should also be inspected

for possible etiologies for sinus obstruction (deviated septum, nasal polyps, tumors). In a few patients, tapping the maxillary teeth may reveal a dental source of maxillary sinus infection. In the prospective study alluded to earlier, the best independent physical examination predictors of sinusitis were impaired transillumination (positive likelihood ratio, 1.6) and mucopurulent nasal discharge (likelihood ratio, 2.1). Other studies have found transillumination either more or less useful, which is partly explained by observer experience with transillumination. Palpation over the maxillary and frontal sinuses is often performed to elicit sinus tenderness. Although physicians often use this as a criterion to diagnose sinusitis, it does not appear reliably to distinguish between patients with and without sinusitis.

Laboratory Studies

As noted, the diagnosis of sinusitis remains a clinical one, albeit imprecise. The gold standard of a positive culture on sinus aspiration is too difficult and too invasive to be performed routinely for this predominantly self-limited condition. Additional testing may be appropriate in confusing cases, patients who fail to improve, patients with a suspected complication, in patients with frequent recurrences. Some studies have suggested that an elevated erythrocyte sedimentation rate or C-reactive protein is useful in diagnosing sinusitis; however, it is not common practice to obtain these tests.

Sinus Films

Confirmation of sinusitis can be achieved by finding mucosal thickening, sinus opacification, or air–fluid levels on conventional sinus x-rays. For patients with air–fluid levels or complete opacification, the positive predictive value is 80% to 100%; however, such findings are present only in 60% of cases, reducing their sensitivity. Mucosal thickening has a sensitivity of 90%, but specificity is poor. Normal sinus x-rays in a person presenting with suspected sinusitis rule out maxillary and frontal disease (negative predictive value, 90% to 100%); ethmoidal involvement is harder to exclude. For maxillary sinusitis, a single occipitomental (Waters) view is acceptable to examine the sinuses. Bone erosion can be present in chronic sinusitis.

Computed Tomography and Magnetic Resonance Imaging

The sensitivity of computed tomography (CT) is extremely high, so high that specificity is compromised (almost half of asymptomatic persons undergoing head CT for non-sinus reasons show mucosal abnormalities). CT is best reserved for complicated disease and the search for occult ethmoidal disease in patients with refractory symptoms and negative conventional x-ray studies. It has also been most useful for delineating anatomy before endoscopic surgery. Magnetic resonance imaging has proven useful for differentiating mucosal inflammation from tumor. Neither study is appropriate for patients with routine sinus infection.

Ultrasound

Ultrasound has been used in the diagnosis of sinusitis. Sensitivity is lower than for sinus x-rays, but specificity is higher. Expertise is not widely available.

Sinus and Nasal Cultures

Although used as the gold standard for research purposes, a culture of the aspirate from the maxillary sinus is negative in up to 40% of patients who undergo aspiration for suspected sinusitis. Cultures obtained from nasal swabs and even protected endoscopes are invariably contaminated with nasal flora and cannot be relied on. False-positive isolates of staphylococcal species are common.

PRINCIPLES OF MANAGEMENT AND THERAPEUTIC RECOMMENDATIONS (3,7–19)

Acute Purulent Sinusitis

The optimal treatment is controversial. The inaccuracy of the diagnosis of sinusitis and the self-limited nature of the disease have led to a discordance between microbiologic and clinical outcomes. Although sinus-aspirate studies clearly document the efficacy of antibiotics in the eradication of bacteria from infected sinuses, randomized, placebo-controlled trials find 70% rates of clearing among patients treated with nothing more than placebo. Furthermore, although many causative organisms demonstrate increasing degrees of antibiotic resistance, randomized, controlled trials show no benefit for powerful broad-spectrum antibiotics over the traditional narrow-spectrum β-lactams and sulfas. Although clear evidence is lacking, perhaps the elimination of underlying ostial obstruction through the use of decongestants is just as important as effective antibiosis. Recent guidelines advocate initial conservative treatment, with antibiotics reserved for severe symptoms or persistent moderate symptoms.

Decongestants

Decongestants are available in both topical and systemic preparations. The mixed adrenergic agonist pseudoephedrine is reasonably effective and can be administered by mouth. Popular sympathomimetic nasal sprays include phenylephrine (Neo-Synephrine) and oxymetazoline (Afrin), which is the longest acting of the topical decongestants. Patients should be instructed to spray each nostril once and then wait a minute to allow the anterior nasal mucosa to shrink. A repeat spray will then reach the upper and posterior mucosa, including the nasal turbinates and sinus ostia. This procedure can be repeated as needed every 4 hours with phenylephrine and every 12 hours with oxymetazoline for up to 3 days. Tachyphylaxis and irritation develop with prolonged topical use, but risk is minimal with short-term administration (1 to 3 days).

When there is an underlying allergic component to the nasal obstruction, one needs to consider *antihistamines* and *nasal steroids* (see Chapter 222). Antihistamines are not for routine use because in the absence of an allergic process, they may thicken secretions and worsen sinus outflow obstruction. Even in the setting of allergy-induced acute sinusitis, their use may prove problematic if they are too drying. Nasal steroids may be worth a trial if there is a history of chronic allergic rhinitis or recurrent acute sinusitis. Theoretically, steroids could impede the response to infection, but randomized trials find improved outcomes in properly selected patients; close monitoring is required. In some studies, nasal steroids have demonstrated greater symptom relief than antibiotics, highlighting the importance of inflammation in this disorder. The local application of heat may also be soothing. The inhalation of steam or water and nasal irrigation with saline can help to relieve symptoms of congestion.

Antibiotics

Patients with mild acute sinusitis may respond sufficiently well to the treatments listed and will not require antibiotics. In more severe cases of acute purulent sinusitis, antibiotics are commonly used. In randomized, controlled studies, antibiotics have demonstrated some benefit over decongestants alone, but cure rates without antibiotics remain high (approaching 70%). Many of these studies were conducted in otolaryngology clinics. The efficacy of antibiotics for sinusitis in the primary care setting has not been well established. In a randomized trial of primary care patients with at least 1 week of symptoms and at least one of the clinical predictors mentioned previously, 48% of patients in the amoxicillin group were completely improved versus 37% in the placebo group at 2 weeks. In addition, the time to improvement was approximately 3 days earlier in the antibiotic group. Another trial comparing nasal corticosteroids to amoxicillin to placebo enrolled similar patients but showed no benefit. About 70% of all patients were symptom-free at 10 days regardless of treatment.

Choice of Agent. When antibiotics are prescribed, *amoxicillin* (500 mg orally three times a day) and *trimethoprim/sulfamethoxazole* (TMS/DS, 160/800 mg twice daily) remain the best options for the initial treatment for acute sinusitis. *Doxycycline* has reasonable activity against known pathogens and may be used if the patient is allergic to penicillins and sulfa drugs.

Concern about rising prevalences of multidrug-resistant *S. pneumoniae* and β-lactamase–producing strains of *H. influenzae* (up to 40%) and *Moraxella* (100%) has stimulated the use of such broad-spectrum, penicillinase-resistant antibiotic agents as amoxicillin/clavulanate, cefuroxime, loracarbef, azithromycin, clarithromycin, and levofloxacin for the initial treatment of acute sinusitis. However, randomized, controlled trials and a recent meta-analysis failed to demonstrate any advantage for such antibiotics over amoxicillin or TMS, suggesting that β-lactamase–producing strains and multidrug resistance may not be as clinically significant as feared. Furthermore, although intermediate penicillin resistance may be present in up to 25% of pneumococci in some communities, standard full doses of amoxicillin (e.g., 500 mg three to four times a day), but not TMS or the macrolides, remain effective in achieving high rates of clinical cure. The popular second-generation macrolides such as clarithromycin and azithromycin may be less effective against the penicillin-resistant pneumococcus than previously thought, further eroding the rationale for their frequent use.

Knowledge of the prevalence of resistant strains in one's community can help to guide initial antibiotic selection and identify when an exception to the rule to start simply is appropriate. The strong presence of a very highly clinically resistant organism in the community makes it reasonable to consider starting with a broader-spectrum, penicillinase-resistant agent or a higher dose of amoxicillin (1 g three times daily).

Adverse Effects. The frequency of acute sinusitis and the common practice of unnecessary use of very expensive, very broad spectrum antibiotics have serious adverse implications not only for *cost* (10 to 20 times more costly), but also for the promotion of *antibiotic resistance* in the community and for risk of adverse effects (allergic reactions, antibiotic-induced *diarrhea*;

see Chapter 64). Such agents should be relegated to a second-line role, reserved for patients who fail to respond to amoxicillin or TMS.

Timing and Duration. Hydration and decongestant therapy can be started at the onset of symptoms to keep secretions loose and free flowing. Antibiotic therapy, with or without nasal corticosteroids, can be started if symptoms fail to start improving after 7 to 10 days, suggesting bacterial sinusitis. Although the proper duration of therapy has not been identified, it is typical to treat with antibiotics for 7 to 10 days, depending on severity and response.

Failure to Respond

Partial responses and early relapses can be treated with another week of the same program. Patients who remain unchanged after 2 full weeks of therapy or deteriorate sooner should have sinus films obtained, and a penicillinase-resistant drug should be prescribed. Further failure to respond is an indication for ear, nose, and throat referral. Surgical intervention should be avoided in acute sinusitis unless patients fail to respond to medical therapy and complications are present.

Recurrent and Chronic Sinusitis

Recurrent sinusitis is usually due to underlying allergic disease or an anatomic lesion and requires treatment of the underlying pathophysiology (see Chapter 222). Chronic sinusitis (persisting for >3 months) has a different bacteriology (see prior discussion), necessitating the consideration of broader-spectrum antibiotic coverage (e.g., *amoxicillin/clavulanate*). Treatment may need to be prolonged for several weeks. Attention also needs to be directed at underlying precipitants. Sinus irrigation or surgical drainage may be necessary.

INDICATIONS FOR ADMISSION AND REFERRAL (12)

Any patient who appears to be toxic or has clinical evidence suggestive of extension to the orbit, bone, brain, or cavernous sinus requires urgent admission for emergency assessment and high-dose intravenous antibiotics. Warning symptoms include high fever, rigors, lid edema, diplopia, pupillary abnormalities, ptosis, and palsies of extraocular movements. The patient should be seen by both an otolaryngologist and an infectious disease consultant. Antibiotic coverage is directed against both staphylococci and gram-negative rods. Surgical drainage may be urgently needed.

Referral to an otolaryngologist should be considered for patients who fail treatment with two courses of antibiotics, have anatomic abnormalities that predispose to sinusitis, or have frequent recurrences (greater than three per year). Functional endoscopic sinus surgery has provided a less invasive technique aimed at restoring normal anatomic drainage in the sinuses while preserving mucosal integrity.

PATIENT EDUCATION

Patients should understand that nasal congestion and frontal headaches are much more commonly caused by viral upper respiratory infections and allergic or vasomotor rhinitis than by true sinusitis. Nevertheless, decongestants are indicated in all these conditions to promote sinus drainage and prevent purulent sinusitis. The patient with recurrent symptoms should learn to recognize them and begin decongestant therapy, but the decision to begin antibiotics should be reserved by the physician. When antibiotics are prescribed, patients must be instructed to complete the entire course of therapy because partial treatment will encourage the development of resistant organisms.

THERAPEUTIC RECOMMENDATIONS (10–12)

Acute Sinusitis

- Ensure systemic and topical hydration (e.g., humidification, isotonic saline nasal spray) to keep secretions flowing.
- Supplement with sympathomimetic decongestants (e.g., sustained-release pseudoephedrine 120 mg twice daily); except in the setting of clear-cut allergic rhinitis, avoid the routine use of decongestants that contain antihistamines because of their drying effect, which thickens secretions and risks aggravating obstruction.
- Attend to any underlying etiologies, such as allergic rhinitis (in which the use of intranasal corticosteroids or antihistamines may be necessary; see Chapter 222).
- Observe and follow patients with mild to moderate symptoms of short duration (<1 week) for 7 to 10 days.
- For patients with marked symptoms that do not improve after 7 to 10 days, begin antibiotic treatment with *amoxicillin* (500 mg orally three times a day) or TMS/DS (160/800 mg twice daily), unless the patient is immunocompromised or there is a known highly clinically resistant organism in high prevalence in the community. If the patient is allergic to both penicillin and sulfa, consider *doxycycline* (100 mg twice daily).
- Treat with antibiotics for 7 to 14 days, supplemented by decongestants and systemic and topical hydration; continue the program for an additional 5 to 7 days if the response is not complete.
- Consider a broad-spectrum, penicillinase-resistant antibiotic agent (e.g., amoxicillin/clavulanate, 500/125 mg three times a day; cefuroxime, 250 to 500 mg twice daily; loracarbef, 200 to 400 mg twice daily; azithromycin, 500 mg on day 1 followed by 250 mg every day on days 2 through 5; clarithromycin, 500 mg twice daily; levofloxacin, 500 mg/d) *only* if there is a known highly clinically resistant organism in high prevalence in the community or if the patient fails an initial 2-week course of first-line antibiotic therapy with amoxicillin or TMS.
- Consider referral to an otolaryngologist if the patient fails two courses of antibiotics, has a suspected anatomic abnormality that predisposes to sinusitis, or has frequent recurrences (more than three per year).
- Obtain dental referral when there is suspicion of an eroding tooth abscess and add anaerobic antibiotic coverage (e.g., clindamycin or metronidazole).

Chronic Sinusitis

- Treat with a broad-spectrum, penicillinase-resistant antibiotic (e.g., amoxicillin/clavulanate, 875/125 mg twice daily).
- Refer to an ear, nose, and throat specialist for identification and definitive correction of the causative pathology.

Annotated Bibliography

1. Gwaltney JM Jr, Phillips CD, Millers RD, et al. Computed tomographic study of the common cold. N Engl J Med 1994;330:25. (*Transient occlusion of the paranasal sinuses occurs in most patients with a common cold and clears without antibiotics.*)

2. Gwaltney JM Jr, Scheld WM, Sande MA, et al. The microbial etiology and antimicrobial therapy of adults with acute community-acquired sinusitis. J Allergy Clin Immunol 1992;90:457. (*Data on the bacteriology of community-acquired disease, including amoxicillin-resistant Haemophilus influenzae.*)

3. Piccirillo JF. Acute bacterial sinusitis. N Engl J Med 2004;351:902. (*A concise review of diagnosis and treatment, advocating watchful waiting for 7 to 10 days, followed by empiric treatment with amoxicillin or trimethoprim/sulfamethoxazole [TMS] if there is no improvement.*)

4. Hueston WJ, Ebertein C, Johnson D, et al. Criteria used by clinicians to differentiate sinusitis from upper viral respiratory infection. J Family Pract 1998;46:487. (*Subjects depended on clinical features that are neither sensitive nor specific for sinusitis.*)

5. Williams JW Jr, Simel DL. Does this patient have sinusitis? Diagnosing acute sinusitis by history and physical examination. JAMA 1993;270:1242. (*A critical review of the clinical features used to make the diagnosis.*)

6. Williams JW Jr, Simel DL, Roberts L, et al. Clinical evaluation for sinusitis: making the diagnosis by history and physical examination. Ann Intern Med 1992;117:705. (*A study of adult men; there were five findings of predictive value.*)

7. Bucher HC, Tschudi P, Young J, et al. Effect of amoxicillin–clavulanate in clinically diagnosed acute rhinosinusitis. Arch Intern Med 2003;163:1793. (*A randomized, placebo-controlled trial of 252 patients diagnosed by clinical criteria.*)

8. deFerranti SD, Ioannidis P, Lau J, et al. Are amoxicillin and folate inhibitors as effective as other antibiotics for acute sinusitis? A meta-analysis. BMJ 1998;317:632. (*An analysis of 27 controlled trials with >2,700 patients, finding that no difference was apparent in the clinical cure rate between amoxicillin or TMS and newer broad-spectrum antibiotics, but that most patients were treated early rather than after a period of observation.*)

9. Dolor BJ, Witsell DL, Hellkamp AS, et al. Comparison of cefuroxime with or without intranasal fluticasone for the treatment of rhinosinusitis: the CAFFS Trial: a randomized controlled trial. JAMA 2001;286:3097. (*Intranasal steroids improved outcomes in persons with a history of chronic rhinitis or recurrent sinusitis.*)

10. Hickner JM, Bartlett JG, Besser RE, et al. Principles of appropriate antibiotic use for acute sinusitis in adults: background. Ann Intern Med 2001;134:498. (*The evidence for the position paper cited next; 52 references.*)

11. Snow V, Mottur-Pilson C, Hickner JM. Principles of appropriate antibiotic use for acute sinusitis in adults. Ann Intern Med 2001;134:495. (*Guideline from the American College of Physicians, supported by the Infectious Disease Society of America.*)

12. Rosenfeld RM, Andes D, Bhattacharyya N, et al. Clinical practice guideline: adult sinusitis. Otolaryngol Head Neck Surg 2007; 137: S1. (*A subspecialty guideline, supporting the following principles: observation is appropriate for mild cases, amoxicillin is first-line therapy, and recurrent acute sinusitis should be referred for further evaluation.*)

13. Piccirillo JF, Mager DE, Frisse ME, et al. Impact of first-line vs second-line antibiotics for the treatment of acute uncomplicated sinusitis. JAMA 2001;286:1849. (*A retrospective cohort study, finding no difference in outcomes.*)

14. Steinman MA, Gonzales R, Linder JA, et al. Changing use of antibiotics in community-based outpatient practice, 1991–1999. Ann Intern Med 2003;138:525. (*A cross-sectional study, finding that antibiotic use is decreasing, but that the use of more expensive, broad-spectrum antibiotics is increasing.*)

15. van Buchem FL, Knotterus JA, Schrijnemaekers VJJ, et al. Primary-care-based randomised placebo-controlled trial of antibiotic treatment in acute maxillary sinusitis. Lancet 1997;349:683. (*A convincing large, randomized trial of amoxicillin, showing that about 80% of patients in both placebo and treatment groups improved at 2 weeks.*)

16. Merenstein D, Whittaker C, Chadwell T, et al. Are antibiotics beneficial for patients with sinusitis complaints? J Family Pract 2005; 54:144. (*A randomized trial of 135 patients treated with amoxicillin or placebo, finding that the time to improvement was faster in the antibiotic group, with a median of 8 vs. 12 days.*)

17. Williamson IG, Rumsby K, Benge S, et al. Antibiotics and topical nasal steroid for treatment of acute maxillary sinusitis: a randomized controlled trial. JAMA 2007; 298: 2487. (*A randomized, placebo-controlled, double blind trial of amoxicillin and nasal budesonide in a factorial design, finding no benefit of either treatment.*)

18. Meltzer EO, Bachert C, Staudinger H. Treating acute rhinosinusitis: comparing efficacy and safety of mometasone furoate nasal spray, amoxicillin, and placebo. J Allergy Clin Immunol 2005; 116:1289. (*A large trial of 981 patients, finding that mometasone was superior to both amoxicillin and placebo; severe cases and patients with fever were excluded.*)

19. Williams JW Jr, Aguilar C, Cornell J, et al. Antibiotics for acute maxillary sinusitis. (Cochrane review). In: The Cochrane library, Issue 4. Oxford: Update Software, 2004. (*A systematic review of 49 trials, supporting the use of amoxicillin for first-line treatment.*)

CHAPTER 220 ■ APPROACH TO THE PATIENT WITH PHARYNGITIS

WILLIAM A. KORMOS

A wide variety of organisms may be responsible for pharyngitis, ranging from viruses and streptococci to gonococci and *Candida*. The most common concern is infection due to group A β-hemolytic strep, *Streptococcus pyogenes*, because of the associated yet completely preventable risk of rheumatic fever (see Chapter 17). Because there is no single clinical feature pathognomonic for group A β-hemolytic strep infection, diagnosis requires attention to a host of clinical parameters complemented by timely judicious testing. The objectives promptly are to identify and treat patients with *S. pyogenes* infection and to avoid delay of therapy, inconvenience, expense, and

unnecessary antibiotic exposure. The effective management of sore throat also requires an awareness of the full spectrum of etiologies and possible complications.

PATHOPHYSIOLOGY AND CLINICAL PRESENTATION (1–6)

Respiratory viruses, *Chlamydia*, *Mycoplasma*, and streptococci account for most sore throats in adults. A host of other bacteria, viruses, fungi, and spirochetes has also been identified as etiologic agents. Allergy, inhalation of irritant gases, gastroesophageal reflux, and sleep apnea are among the noninfectious causes.

Group A β-Hemolytic Strep Infection

S. pyogenes infection accounts for 5% to 38% of sore throats in adults who are subjected to throat culture. The onset of discomfort is typically acute, with difficulty swallowing often noted. Pharyngeal erythema, exudate, cervical adenopathy, and fever greater than 101°F (38.3°C) are common but by no means pathognomonic. Children with "strep throat" exhibit exudate and high fever with greater frequency than do adults with the same disease. Cough, rhinorrhea, and other symptoms of upper respiratory infection are reported in less than 25% of cases and suggest the presence of another etiology. About one fourth of adult patients give a history of recent exposure to streptococcal infection. The pharyngitis is self-limited; symptoms usually resolve within 7 to 10 days. Antibiotic therapy decreases the severity and duration of symptoms.

Complications

Suppurative complications of streptococcal pharyngitis are uncommon in the setting of antibiotic use, but they are important and require attention. In *peritonsillar cellulitis*, the tonsils become edematous and inflamed. One or both tonsils may be involved. A grayish white exudate forms in conjunction with high fever, rigors, and leukocytosis. *Peritonsillar abscess* may ensue, with a fluctuant mass palpable. Drainage is required in addition to antibiotics. Other suppurative complications include retropharyngeal and parapharyngeal space infections. *Scarlet fever* is a rare complication of strep infection in adults. It results from infection with a toxigenic strain of *S. pyogenes*.

Acute rheumatic fever is the most important nonsuppurative complication. Although its incidence has declined dramatically over the last 40 years, epidemics in the 1980s raised concern about the reemergence of this disease. The complication appears most frequently among children of age 5 to 15 years, but about 15% of hospitalized patients with rheumatic fever are older than the age of 18 years. The chances of developing rheumatic fever increase with the length of time that the organism persists in the pharynx and with the intensity of the immunologic response.

Acute glomerulonephritis is another nonsuppurative complication. Unlike rheumatic fever, it does not seem to be preventable by means of antibiotic therapy.

Other Streptococci

Group C and G streptococci can cause pharyngitis, in some populations with a frequency approaching that of group A strep. Suppurative complications are rare, and rheumatic fever and glomerulonephritis never follow. Antibiotic therapy has not been shown to be beneficial in pharyngitis due to group C and G streptococci.

Viruses

Respiratory viruses, including rhinovirus, adenovirus, parainfluenza virus, and coronavirus, are the most common causes of sore throat. Pharyngitis can be the only manifestation of illness or may be accompanied by conjunctivitis, cough, sputum production, rhinitis, and systemic symptoms. Pharyngeal erythema, exudates, tonsillar enlargement, and cervical adenopathy may be present but with less frequency than in streptococcal disease.

Epstein–Barr virus

Epstein–Barr virus (EBV) is the agent responsible for infectious mononucleosis and is the cause of sore throat in 5% to 10% of young adults. Prodromal symptoms include malaise, headache, and fatigue, followed by fever, sore throat, and cervical lymphadenopathy. Sore throat is the most common feature. The pharynx shows enlarged tonsils and erythema. About half of the patients develop tonsillar exudates, and about one third of patients have petechiae at the junction of the hard and soft palate. Both anterior and posterior cervical adenopathy may develop; generalized adenopathy often follows. Splenomegaly is noted in about half of cases, and hepatomegaly and tenderness are present in about 10%. Clinical hepatitis sometimes ensues. A faint maculopapular rash and transient supraorbital edema occasionally appear on presentation, but the rash appears in greater than 90% of patients exposed to amoxicillin. Atypical lymphocytes are often present on complete blood count, and thrombocytopenia is frequently seen.

Herpes Simplex Virus and Coxsackie A Virus

Herpes simplex virus and coxsackie A virus are other causes of pharyngitis. Herpes infection may mimic streptococcal infection with an exudative pharyngitis; shallow ulcers on the posterior palate are characteristic. Coxsackie A infection (herpangina) is characterized by vesicles and ulcers on the tonsillar pillars and soft palate.

Human Immunodeficiency Virus

Acute infection with the human immunodeficiency virus (HIV) can lead to a mononucleosis-like syndrome known as the acute retroviral syndrome. Fever, pharyngitis, lymphadenopathy, and rash are present, but the disease onset is more acute than with EBV infection. Any patient with this presentation should be assessed for HIV risk factors and tested if appropriate. Antibodies to HIV will not be present, and a viral load (quantitative HIV RNA assay) confirms the diagnosis.

Other Organisms

In patients engaging in orogenital sexual activity, gonococci can lead to sore throat, pharyngeal exudate, and lymphadenopathy but more often results in asymptomatic colonization of the pharynx. In rare instances, bacteremia may result (see Chapter 137). *Haemophilus influenzae* is a rare cause of pharyngitis in adults, but the infection can be extremely painful and complicated by epiglottitis with life-threatening airway obstruction.

Chlamydophila Pneumoniae and Mycoplasma Pneumoniae

Chlamydophila pneumoniae and *Mycoplasma pneumoniae* may account for a surprising percentage of patients presenting with pharyngitis, based on serologic evidence of infection, although the clinical significance of this finding is unclear. The diagnosis of *M. pneumoniae* is rarely made clinically in the absence of pneumonitis.

Arcanobacterium Hemolyticum

Arcanobacterium (formerly known as *Corynebacterium*) *hemolyticum* can cause pharyngitis and scarletiniform rash, particularly in teenagers and young adults. The administration of penicillin or erythromycin produces rapid improvement.

Meningococci

Meningococci are found in the pharynx in 5% to 15% of healthy people. Although sore throat may be a prodromal symptom of meningococcemia, isolated pharyngitis due to meningococcal infection is rare. Most instances of positive pharyngeal cultures for *Meningococcus* represent asymptomatic colonization.

Corynebacterium Diphtheriae

Diphtheria is rare in the United States but can occur in international travelers and cause outbreaks in unimmunized populations. The infection is characterized by the development of an adherent grayish pharyngeal exudate ("pseudomembrane") that covers the pharynx and causes bleeding if removal is attempted. Bacterial strains that produce diphtheria toxin cause myocarditis and polyneuritis.

Pneumococci and Staphylococci

Pneumococci and staphylococci commonly reside in the nasopharynx and can cause severe disease in other parts of the respiratory tract. However, they do not cause pharyngitis except under the most unusual circumstances. When these bacterial species are cultured from the pharynx in both symptomatic and asymptomatic individuals, colonization, not causation, by these organisms should be suspected. However, mixed infections with normal mouth flora do occur in debilitated patients.

Fusobacteria

Fusobacteria and spirochetes can cause gingivitis ("trench mouth") or necrotic tonsillar ulcers ("Vincent's angina"). Patients present with foul breath, pain, pharyngeal exudate, and a dirty gray membranous inflammation, which bleeds easily. A similar combination of bacteria and spirochetes can produce an extremely serious invasive gangrene of the mouth known as cancrum oris. This process occurs only in malnourished infants or patients with advanced malignancy and immunosuppression and, fortunately, is rare. *Treponema pallidum* can cause pharyngitis as part of primary or secondary syphilis. The diagnosis requires a high index of suspicion and serologic confirmation.

Yersinia Enterocolitica

Yersinia enterocolitica infection typically presents as enterocolitis, but occasionally in adults it presents as pharyngitis in the absence of enteritis. Fatalities have been reported.

Candida

Candida albicans, present in the normal mouth flora, can produce pharyngitis if antibiotics, immunosuppressive agents, or debilitating illness upsets microbial interactions or host defenses. Oropharyngeal moniliasis (thrush) can be painful and is characterized by a cheesy white exudate, which can be scraped off to demonstrate yeast forms by smear and culture. Oral moniliasis may be the first symptomatic manifestation of HIV infection (see Chapter 13).

WORKUP (2,6–11)

The first task is to attempt a clinical estimate of the risk of *S. pyogenes* infection. Often, this is done in a preliminary way over the telephone, which places a premium on risk stratification by historical features.

History

No single symptom or historical feature is diagnostic of group A β-hemolytic strep (GABHS) infection. Consequently, investigators have sought to identify symptoms that are at least independent predictors of strep infection and to see how clusters of such symptoms perform for triaging. One such triaging cluster uses the presence of *fever* and *difficulty swallowing* in support of the diagnosis of strep infection and *cough* as a *negating factor*. A score is assigned to each factor based on severity (0 through 3). The final score is derived by subtracting the score for cough from those for fever and difficulty swallowing. Based on designating a score of 2 or more as "positive" for a diagnosis of *S. pyogenes* infection, the system has a sensitivity of 85% and a specificity of 41.5%. In an adult pharyngitis population with the usual prevalence of strep (10% of sore throats due to *S. pyogenes*), a score of 6 (the highest possible score) would produce a positive predictive value of 34% for strep infection; a score of −3 (the lowest possible score) would reduce the risk to 1%. In a pharyngitis population with a high strep prevalence (prevalence, 34%), a score of 6 would indicate a 70% chance of strep infection; a score of −3 would reduce the risk to 3%. Although far from perfect, such a scheme may help in deciding who should come in for further evaluation.

History can help to determine prevalence and risk from strep infection by inquiring into exposure to family members with current documented GABHS pharyngitis and any history of prior rheumatic fever. Other factors found to be predictive of strep infection that might be elicited over the telephone include positive throat culture in the preceding year, tender anterior cervical adenopathy, temperature higher than 100.4°F, and absence of rhinorrhea and itchy eyes.

Regarding other sore throat etiologies and complications, one should ask about orogenital sexual contact, concurrent steroid or immunosuppressive therapy, and any dyspnea.

Physical Examination

Several physical findings can help to assess the probability of group A β-hemolytic streptococcal infection. *Tonsillar exudate, anterior cervical adenopathy,* or *temperature greater than 100.4°F* increase the likelihood of group A β-hemolytic streptococcal infection (see later discussion).

Examination of the pharynx is useful for identifying a less common cause of pharyngitis such as thrush, characterized by its white, cheesy exudate; gingivitis or necrotic tonsillar ulcers suggest fusobacteria and spirochetes. Associated physical findings, such as a viral exanthem, conjunctivitis, petechiae, generalized lymphadenopathy, splenomegaly, or hepatic tenderness, may provide important clues to etiology. A "sandpaper" erythematous rash with accentuation in the groin and axillae is associated with scarlet fever. Patients with severe dysphagia or dyspnea require urgent evaluation to exclude airway obstruction. If epiglottitis is suspected, the airway should not be instrumented.

Laboratory Study for Suspected Strep Pharyngitis

Prompt diagnosis and treatment of *S. pyogenes* infection has been greatly facilitated by the advent of rapid strep-antigen testing. Throat culture has been relegated to a secondary role.

Rapid Strep-Antigen Testing

Office identification of group A streptococcal pharyngitis can be achieved by taking a swab of the posterior pharynx and subjecting the specimen to rapid strep-antigen testing. For most commercially available preparations, sensitivity ranges from 85% to 90% and specificity from 95% to 99%. Small numbers of organisms are less likely to be detected. The technique for obtaining the sample is similar to that for a throat culture and includes swabbing both tonsils and posterior pharynx.

Decision-analysis study finds that rapid strep-antigen testing followed by treatment is the optimal approach to workup when the patient's pretest probability for strep infection is between 1% and 50% (which is the case for most patients). Pharyngitis patients at high risk for rheumatic fever (i.e., those with a history of rheumatic fever) and those with a very high probability of strep infection (e.g., persons in a closed population experiencing an epidemic of streptococcal pharyngitis) can forgo testing and be treated directly.

Throat Culture

Culturing a retropharyngeal swab remains the gold standard for identification of streptococcal pharyngitis and has a high sensitivity (90% to 95%) when performed correctly. A culture should be obtained when rapid antigen testing is negative yet clinical suspicion remains high. Patients with typical symptoms and signs of a viral upper respiratory infection and no historical or physical examination evidence suggestive of streptococcal infection do not need a throat culture. Some cost-effectiveness studies found that throat culture was the best approach to uniform management of all pharyngitis patients, but, as noted earlier, better results can be achieved by using pretest probability to customize one's approach to the individual patient.

Repeat culture after antibiotic treatment is not indicated because most positive cultures after treatment represent streptococcal carriers and not true infection. However, repeat culture should be performed in the patient with a history of rheumatic fever and may be considered during outbreaks of strep throat, especially when reinfection by close contacts is suspected.

In addition to the time required to obtain a result, an important shortcoming of throat culture is difficulty in differentiating infection from colonization. About 5% to 10% of adults may be carriers. Definitive identification of significant infection with the risk of rheumatic fever necessitates serologic testing for an antibody response. Such testing is of little practical use because results do not become available in time to be helpful.

Laboratory Study for Other Etiologies

Laboratory testing is indicated when the result will have an effect on management. For example, viral pharyngitis due to respiratory pathogens is essentially a clinical diagnosis and requires no laboratory investigation. On the other hand, the patient with sore throat and diffuse lymphadenopathy, splenomegaly, and pharyngeal petechiae requires evaluation for infectious mononucleosis. A heterophile antibody is a useful confirmatory test, provided there is no prior history of infectious mononucleosis. It may take as long as 3 weeks for the heterophile to become positive, necessitating a repeat test in a few weeks if it is initially negative. Alternatively, one can check serology for antibodies to Epstein–Barr virus. Immunoglobulin M (IgM) antibodies to viral capsid antigen can be demonstrated during the second week of illness, replaced later by IgG antibodies. Heterophile-negative mononucleosis may be due to cytomegalovirus infection or the acute retroviral syndrome of HIV.

The patient with a history of orogenital contact who is suspected of having possible gonococcal infection should have a throat swab plated onto Thayer–Martin media (see Chapter 137). Suspected candidal infection can be confirmed by scraping off the exudate and examining a potassium hydroxide prep for yeast forms.

PRINCIPLES OF MANAGEMENT AND THERAPEUTIC RECOMMENDATIONS (2,6,12–19)

Suspected *S. pyogenes* Infection

Rationale for Treatment

The reasons for treating strep infection are to speed symptomatic relief and prevent rheumatic fever, peritonsillar or retropharyngeal abscess, and spread of streptococcal infection. Rheumatic fever can be prevented by prompt eradication of *S. pyogenes* from the throat. The attack rate for rheumatic fever is reduced by greater than 90% if antibiotic therapy is instituted within 1 week of the onset of sore throat. However, the efficacy of prophylactic therapy is substantially reduced if there is a marked delay in initiating treatment. Starting antibiotics 2 weeks after sore throat is first noted is associated with a reduction in attack rate of only 67%, and delaying treatment until 3 weeks into the illness provides no more than a 40% reduction in attack rate.

Treatment Strategies

The approach to treatment of pharyngitis depends on the probability of strep infection, the likelihood of patient compliance, the chance of an adverse reaction to antibiotics, and the benefits of treating immediately versus waiting for culture results. The strategy begins with an assessment of the pretest probability of group A β-hemolytic streptococcal infection. A commonly used prediction rule is the modified *Centor score*, in which one point is assigned for each of the following: temperature greater than 38.0°C (100.4°F), absence of cough, swollen or tender anterior cervical nodes, and tonsillar swelling or exudate. Recognizing the lower prevalence of streptococcal infection in adults, the score subtracts one point if the patient is age 45 years or older. Table 220.1 lists approximate pretest probabilities of group A β-hemolytic streptococcal infection.

Immediate Treatment without Prior Testing. Pharyngitis patients with a history of rheumatic fever and those patients who are symptomatic with an exposure to a close contact with documented group A β-hemolytic streptococcal infection should receive immediate treatment without the need for prior testing or even an office visit. High-risk patients who have a prior history of rheumatic fever might already be on prophylactic therapy (see Chapter 17). Patients with a strongly suggestive

TABLE 220.1

PROBABILITY OF GROUP A β-HEMOLYTIC STREPTOCOCCAL INFECTION USING THE MODIFIED CENTOR SCORE

Score	Approximate Risk of Infection (%)
0	2.5
1	5
2	12
3	30
4	50

Adapted from McIsaac WJ, White D, Tannenbaum D, et al. Can Med Assoc J 1998;158:75, with permission.

clinical presentation (modified Centor score of 4) might also be candidates for empiric antibiotic therapy, but this would lead to a high percentage of these patients receiving unnecessary antibiotics. Rapid antigen testing is appropriate in these patients.

Rapid Antigen Testing Followed by Treatment of Positives. In pharyngitis patients with a moderate to high probability of strep infection (modified Centor score of 2 or more), rapid strep-antigen testing can be performed, followed by treatment of positives. In patients with a good clinical story (modified Centor score of 3 or more), a negative rapid antigen test should be followed by a throat culture, with treatment of positives as needed. Due to the low risk of rheumatic fever and suppurative complications in adults, some experts suggest forgoing cultures in adults with negative rapid strep-antigen test results. Testing for infectious mononucleosis should be considered in patients with exudative pharyngitis and adenopathy who test negative for strep.

Conservative Treatment without Testing

In patients with a low probability of infection (modified Centor score of 1 or less), diagnostic testing can be deferred. Throat cultures are more likely to identify the carrier state than active infection.

Antibiotic Program

To be effective, antibiotic therapy must completely eradicate the streptococcus from the pharynx. This can be achieved by a single intramuscular injection of 1.2 million units of *benzathine penicillin* or a 10-day course of oral *phenoxymethyl penicillin* (250 mg three or four times a day). The advantages of the intramuscular route are the certainty of full treatment and convenience. Its major disadvantage is a 5- to 10-fold increase in the incidence of serious allergic reactions to penicillin. In the patient allergic to penicillin, oral *erythromycin* (250 mg four times a day for 10 days) is an effective alternative, although there is increasing macrolide resistance in GABHS. Some antibiotics frequently prescribed for strep pharyngitis (e.g., oral *cephalosporins* and *azithromycin*) are not recommended as first-line agents because they are more expensive and/or have a less-focused spectrum of action than penicillin or erythromycin.

Recurrent Infection

The patient who returns with recurrent pharyngitis and a positive strep culture should be examined for alternative possibilities besides reinfection. The patient may have been noncompliant with oral antibiotics, and benzathine penicillin may be an appropriate option. Alternatively, the patient may be a carrier for group A streptococcus and have a concurrent noninfectious etiology for a sore throat, such as allergic rhinitis. Appropriate treatment depends on the underlying etiology. Tonsillectomy, once quite popular in children, is of uncertain benefit in adults for reducing recurrent infections or symptoms. A small randomized trial in adults suggested a reduction in symptomatic pharyngitis after tonsillectomy. Consultation with an ear, nose, and throat specialist may be considered for recalcitrant cases.

When recurrent infection is believed to be due to repeated transmission among household members ("ping-pong infection"), then another course of antibiotics aimed at eradicating the carrier state may be appropriate. Treatment regimens include a single dose of *benzathine penicillin* or *clindamycin* 300 mg twice daily for 10 days.

Other Types of Pharyngitis

The Meningococcal Carrier State

The meningococcal carrier state sometimes presents a therapeutic dilemma in terms both of selecting patients who actually need treatment and choosing antibiotics. Carriers should be treated only when there is evidence of active meningococcal disease in household or dormitory contacts. Penicillin will not eradicate the meningococcal carrier state, and because many strains are now sulfonamide resistant, rifampin should be used.

Other Bacterial Infections

The usual treatment for gonococcal pharyngitis is *ceftriaxone* 250 mg intramuscularly (see Chapter 137). *Ciprofloxacin* and *azithromycin* have also demonstrated high cure rates. In the case of diphtheria, antitoxin is necessary to prevent myocarditis and peripheral neuritis and is the mainstay of therapy. Both *erythromycin* and *penicillin* can eliminate the organism from the upper respiratory tract. In epiglottitis, hospitalization for intravenous antibiotics and observation is needed, and treatment should cover *H. influenzae*. Necrotizing pharyngitis due to fusobacterial infection responds to penicillin and good nutrition. In other bacterial etiologies of pharyngitis (*Chlamydophila*, *Mycoplasma*), antibiotics have not been shown to improve clinical outcome.

Pharyngeal Candidiasis

The patient with pharyngeal candidiasis may benefit from gargling with oral *nystatin* suspension (100,000 U/mL), 15 mL swish-and-swallow six times per day, or from using a 10-mg *clotrimazole* troche held in the mouth for 15 to 30 minutes three times each day.

Viral Sore Throat

Viral sore throats are treated symptomatically. Voice rest, humidification, and lozenges or hard candy provide some relief; saline gargling and using aspirin or acetaminophen also helps.

Patient Education (20)

Many patients call the office requesting empiric antibiotic therapy for sore throat. They assume that antibiotics are effective against most pathogens, desire prompt symptomatic relief, want to avoid the time and expense of testing, and have little fear of an adverse reaction to antibiotics. Much of the unnecessary antibiotic exposure associated with the management of pharyngitis is probably due as much to patient insistence as to the physician's desire to do something. However, studies demonstrate that patient satisfaction is not associated with receiving antibiotics but instead correlates with having the physician address patient concerns and communicating a diagnosis. Unwarranted antibiotic prescriptions also run the risk of "medicalizing" the sore throat, resulting in increased patient visits

for future episodes. When the probability of strep infection is deemed too low to warrant testing or treatment (see prior discussion), patients should be reassured that the risk is nil and that antibiotics are unlikely to provide any benefit. For the insistent person and the one with an intermediate risk by triage history, an invitation to come in for rapid antigen testing is the most reasonable advice.

The patient who proves to have *S. pyogenes* infection and elects oral antibiotic therapy should be carefully instructed on the risk of rheumatic fever and the importance of completing a full 10-day course of antibiotics. Otherwise, many patients will stop taking the medication when symptoms resolve.

Patients with recurrent strep infections and intact tonsils will ask about tonsillectomy. Reviewing the risks and benefits of tonsillectomy over medical therapy may help them to choose the treatment that best meets their needs.

Annotated Bibliography

1. Alcaide ML, Bisno AL. Pharyngitis and epiglottis. Infect Dis Clin North Am 2007;21:449. (*A review, detailing the microbiology, diagnosis, and treatment of acute pharyngitis; 83 references.*)
2. Huovinen P, Lahtonen R, Ziegler T, et al. Pharyngitis in adults: the presence and coexistence of viruses and bacterial organisms. Ann Intern Med 1989;110:612. (*A wide variety of organisms are found, including group C strep, Mycoplasma pneumoniae, and Chlamydia pneumoniae.*)
3. Ophir D, Bawnik J, Poria Y, et al. Peritonsillar abscess: a prospective evaluation of outpatient management by needle aspiration. Arch Otolaryngol Head Neck Surg 1988;114:661. (*Needle aspiration can allow the outpatient management of selected patients.*)
4. Shapiro J, Eavey RD, Baker AS. Adult supraglottis: a prospective study. JAMA 1988;259:563. (*A review of this life-threatening but uncommon Haemophilus influenzae infection.*)
5. Weisner PJ, Tronen E, Bonin P, et al. Clinical spectrum of pharyngeal gonococcal infection. N Engl J Med 1973;288:181. (*Describes the incidence, clinical features, and management of gonococcal pharyngitis.*)
6. Bisno AL, Gerber MA, Gwaltney JM, et al. Practice guidelines for the diagnosis and management of group A streptococcal pharyngitis. Clin Infect Dis 2002;35:113. (*An evidence-based guideline from the Infectious Disease Society of America, advocating the use of rapid strep testing alone in adults.*)
7. Clancy CM, Centor RM, Campbell MS, et al. Rational decision making based on history: adult sore throats. J Gen Intern Med 1988;3:213. (*Uses fever, difficulty swallowing, and cough to generate a score that predicts the probability of a positive rapid strep-antigen test.*)
8. Gerber MA, Tanz RR, Kabat W, et al. Optical immunoassay test for group A beta-hemolytic streptococcal pharyngitis. JAMA 1997;277:899. (*In >2,000 pediatric patients, a newer antigen detection test was more sensitive than standard blood agar culture and 84% sensitive compared with a gold standard broth-enhanced culture.*)
9. Hillner BE, Centor RM. What a difference a day makes: a decision analysis of adult streptococcal pharyngitis. J Gen Intern Med 1987;2:242. (*Recommends rapid strep-antigen testing for most adults with suspected strep pharyngitis.*)
10. Neuner JM, Hamel MB, Phillips RS, et al. Diagnosis and management of adults with pharyngitis: a cost-effectiveness analysis. Ann Intern Med 2003;139:113. (*A decision-analysis study, finding that throat culture for all patients was the most cost-effective and that empiric treatment was the least effective; however, when compared to observation alone, the testing or treatment strategies were not very cost-effective by current standards.*)
11. McIsaac WJ, White D, Tannenbaum D, et al. A clinical score to reduce unnecessary antibiotic use in patients with sore throat. Can Med Assoc J 1998;158:75. (*A validated predictive model for Streptococcus pyogenes infection that includes age older than 45 years as a negating factor; the sug-*

gested algorithm would result in a 48% reduction in antibiotic use in the family practice site studied.*)
12. McIsaac WJ, Kellner JD, Aufricht P, et al. Empirical validation of guidelines for the management of pharyngitis in children and adults. JAMA 2004;291:1587. (*An observational study of >750 patients, validating the modified Centor score and showing that empiric treatment of adults with high scores leads to an excess of unnecessary antibiotic prescriptions.*)
13. Humair JP, Revaz SA, Bovier P, et al. Management of acute pharyngitis in adults: reliability of rapid streptococcal tests and clinical findings. Arch Intern Med 2006; 166:64. (*A prospective study of 372 patients with a Centor score of ≥2, finding that a strategy starting with rapid strep-antigen testing was the most cost-effective and led to the most appropriate antibiotic use.*)
14. Dagnelie CF, van der Graaf Y, DeMelker RA. Do patients with sore throat benefit from penicillin? A randomized double-blind placebo controlled trial with penicillin V in general practice. Br J Gen Pract 1996;46:589. (*Treatment led to recovery 1 to 2 days earlier.*)
15. Krober MS, Bass JW, Michels GN. Streptococcal pharyngitis: clinical response to penicillin therapy. JAMA 1985;253:1271. (*Early penicillin therapy significantly ameliorated symptoms and shortened their duration.*)
16. Linder JA, Stafford RS. Antibiotic treatment of adults with sore throat by community primary care physicians: a national survey 1989–1999. JAMA 2001;286:1181. (*Data from the National Ambulatory Care Survey, showing that there was a high frequency of unnecessary antibiotic use and a use of more expensive, broader-spectrum antibiotics than those recommended.*)
17. Linder JA, Chan JC, Bates DW. Evaluation and treatment of pharyngitis in primary care practice: the difference between guidelines is largely academic. Arch Intern Med 2006;166:1374. (*Notes the failure of many primary care physicians to follow any guideline.*)
18. Paradise JL, Bluestone CD, Bachman RZ, et al. Efficacy of tonsillectomy in recurrent throat infection in severely affected children. N Engl J Med 1984;310:674. (*Rates of recurrent infection decreased in both medically and surgically treated children, with surgery producing the greater reduction.*)
19. Alho OP, Koivunen P, Penna T, et al. Tonsillectomy versus watchful waiting in recurrent streptococcal pharyngitis in adults: randomised controlled trial. BMJ 2007; 334:939. (*A randomized trial of tonsillectomy in 70 adults with more than three symptomatic infections per year, finding that tonsillectomy led to a reduction of symptomatic of group A β-hemolytic streptococcal infections at 3 months [24% vs. 3%].*)
20. Little P, Gould C, Williamson I, et al. Reattendance and complications in a randomized trial of prescribing strategies for sore throat: the medicalising effect of prescribing antibiotics. BMJ 1997;315:350. (*Patients empirically prescribed antibiotics for sore throat had a higher rate of return to the clinic for sore throat at 1 year compared with patients treated without antibiotics or with a delayed prescription.*)

CHAPTER 221 ■ APPROACH TO THE PATIENT WITH HICCUPS

Hiccup is usually a transient, innocuous symptom, but when persistent, it may become an exhausting and disabling problem. Intractable hiccup has been attributed to a host of metabolic, peridiaphragmatic, neurologic, and psychogenic conditions, but many cases are of unknown etiology. The primary physician should be able to offer the exasperated patient symptomatic relief while conducting a judicious evaluation to determine the source of difficulty.

PATHOPHYSIOLOGY AND CLINICAL PRESENTATIONS (1–3)

No useful function has been found for the hiccup, which occurs as a result of synchronous clonic spasm of intercostal muscles and diaphragm that causes sudden inspiration followed by prompt closure of the glottis and inhibition of respiratory activity. It is believed to be a reflex. There is debate about whether it is centrally mediated. The afferent pathway is from T10 to T12, and the efferent limb is along the phrenic nerve. During the hiccup, the glottis is closed. Some investigators believe that the hiccup is related more to gastrointestinal than to respiratory function. Current understanding of pathophysiology does not permit an explanation of how the presumptive etiologies operate to produce the hiccup, although the classic explanation is that it is due to stimulation of the phrenic nerve.

It is often unclear whether the reported causes of hiccup are etiologies or only associations. In a series of 220 cases seen at the Mayo Clinic, men outnumbered women by 5 to 1, and most were in their 60s. More than 90% of the women had no concurrent illness other than an emotional problem, whereas only 7% of men were labeled as having a psychogenic disorder. About 20% of men who experienced hiccup did so after undergoing intraabdominal, intrathoracic, or neurologic surgery. About 25% had a diaphragmatic hernia, another 20% had cerebrovascular disease or another central nervous system (CNS) problem, and 5% had a metabolic illness, and in 10% no associated disease or psychiatric problem was identified.

DIFFERENTIAL DIAGNOSIS (1–3)

The causes of persistent hiccup typically listed are clinical associations and cannot be considered proven etiologies (Table 221.1).

WORKUP (1–3)

Persistent hiccup that proves refractory to simple measures is an indication for further investigation. Extensive workup is usually not productive, but a check for a previously unsuspected metabolic or subdiaphragmatic process is sometimes rewarding.

History

Questioning should include inquiry into recent abdominal, thoracic, or neurologic surgery, abdominal pain (especially pain that radiates to the tip of the shoulder or is worsened by respiration), prior renal disease, excess consumption of alcohol, fever, cough, diabetes, and emotional problems. Also of help is reviewing the various methods that the patient has tried for the relief of symptoms. Any neurologic complaints should be noted.

Physical Examination

A temperature determination, a check of the tympanic membranes, percussion of the lungs for evidence of reduced diaphragmatic excursion, and auscultation for signs of an infiltrate, effusion, or pleuritis should be included. The abdomen is examined for distention, organomegaly, upper abdominal tenderness, and signs of peritonitis. A careful neurologic examination is needed if there is a history of neurologic difficulties.

Laboratory Studies

Patients with an acute bout of hiccups need no laboratory studies, but those with *refractory hiccups* that persist for days need to be evaluated for a pharyngeal, thoracic, diaphragmatic, intraabdominal, CNS, or metabolic/pharmacologic etiology. If a careful physical examination that includes a check of the tympanic membranes, pharynx, chest, heart, abdomen, and CNS is unrevealing, one should obtain a *chest x-ray* and *serum sodium, creatinine,* and *blood urea nitrogen* determinations and consider a *computed tomography of the abdomen,* concentrating on the subdiaphragmatic region. If CNS disease is suspected by the history or physical examination, a computed tomography or magnetic resonance image may help to detect the lesion of the brain. Treatment of the underlying etiology is the best means of curing refractory hiccups.

SYMPTOMATIC THERAPY AND INDICATION FOR REFERRAL (2–8)

For Self-Limited Causes

For patients with *self-limited* causes of hiccupping, several home remedies are capable of interrupting the reflex arc; others simply suppress it temporarily. *Breath holding* and breathing into a *paper bag* will decrease the frequency of hiccups, but if the underlying stimulus has not disappeared, they usually return after these maneuvers are terminated. Swallowing a

TABLE 221.1

CONDITIONS ASSOCIATED WITH PERSISTENT HICCUP

Structural Pathology
  Pericarditis
  Tumor
  Subdiaphragmatic abscess
  Pneumonia
  Pleuritis
  Myocardial infarction
  Hiatus hernia
  Peritonitis
  Gastric dilatation
  Pancreatitis
  Biliary tract disease
  Tympanic membrane Irritation
  Aortic aneurysm

Metabolic Disturbances
  Uremia
  Diabetes
  Alcoholism

Central Nervous System Disease
  Tumor
  Infection
  Surgery

Psychogenic Disease
  Hysteria
  Anorexia nervosa
  Anxiety

These are not proven etiologies.

teaspoonful of *granulated sugar* works by irritating the pharynx sufficiently to inhibit further hiccupping. A more noxious maneuver is to have the patient put his or her finger into the back of the pharynx and *stimulate the gag reflex*. Drinking from the wrong side of the glass is another gag reflex stimulant. Rubbing the nasopharynx with a cotton swab is sometimes effective. Passage of a *nasogastric tube* causing hypopharyngeal stimulation will usually work if other methods have failed. *Carotid sinus massage* can be used to provide counterirritation of the vagus nerve. Striking a blow to the chest is sometimes tried but is ill advised; case reports document sudden cardiac death (commotio cordis) with such efforts.

For Persistent or Refractory Disease

When symptoms are *persistent* and the cause remains undiagnosed or untreatable, symptomatic relief becomes an important goal. *Chlorpromazine* in doses of 25 to 50 mg intravenously will often terminate refractory hiccups and can be followed by oral maintenance therapy of 25 mg four times a day. *Metoclopramide* given intravenously, followed by oral therapy (10 mg three times a day), has also proven effective. Atropine and quinidine have been used, but with less success. *Phenytoin* (300 to 400 mg/d) and *carbamazepine* (200 mg/d) are helpful in patients with a CNS etiology.

When all other measures have failed and the hiccups remain disabling, consideration of surgical *infiltration of the phrenic nerve* is appropriate. Fluoroscopy is needed to see whether one leaf of the diaphragm is responsible and can be singled out for treatment. In addition, one needs to be sure that one leaf is not already paralyzed, a circumstance that would rule out this therapeutic option. The phrenic nerve serving the offending diaphragm is infiltrated with a long-acting anesthetic; if it works but the hiccups return, reinfiltration with alcohol or *crushing* may be necessary. If both leaves of the diaphragm are involved, one phrenic nerve is treated.

In most instances, hiccups will resolve spontaneously or respond at least partially to one of these therapeutic maneuvers.

A.H.G.

Annotated Bibliography

1. Editorial. Hiccup. Br Med J 1971;1:235. (*A succinct review of pathophysiology and the significance of the hiccup.*)
2. Samuels L. Hiccup: a ten-year review of anatomy, etiology, and treatment. Can Med Assoc J 1952;67:315. (*The classic paper on hiccups, including differential diagnosis.*)
3. Rosseau P. Hiccups. South Med J 1995;88:175. (*A useful review for the clinician.*)
4. Souadjian JV, Cain JC. Intractable hiccup: etiologic factors in 220 patients. Postgrad Med 1968;43:72. (*A classic review of 220 patients from the Mayo Clinic, presenting probable causes.*)
5. Engleman EG, Lankton J, Leakton B. Granulated sugar as treatment for hiccups in conscious patients. N Engl J Med 1971;285:1489. (*A letter reporting the successful relief of hiccups in 19 of 20 patients after they swallowed a teaspoon of ordinary dry white sugar.*)
6. Barry J, Maron BJ, Gohman TE, et al. Clinical profile and spectrum of commotio cordis. JAMA 2002;287:1142. (*A report of sudden cardiac death on the administration of a chest blow to terminate hiccups.*)
7. Salem MR, Baraka A, Rattenborg CC, et al. Treatment of hiccups by pharyngeal stimulation in anesthetized and conscious subjects. JAMA 1967;202:321. (*Therapeutic success in 84 of 86 patients by the introduction of a catheter through the nose and stimulating the pharynx at the level of C2 to C3.*)
8. Williamson BWA, MacIntyre JMC. Management of intractable hiccup. Br Med J 1977;2:501. (*A succinct review of therapeutic approaches, finding chlorpromazine and metoclopramide to be the most effective drugs; 39 references.*)

CHAPTER 222 ■ APPROACH TO THE PATIENT WITH CHRONIC NASAL CONGESTION AND DISCHARGE

NEIL BHATTACHARYYA

It is estimated that 15% to 20% of the U.S. population suffers from chronic or recurrent nasal congestion. Allergic rhinitis accounts for most such cases; vasomotor rhinitis, mechanical obstruction, drugs, and abuse of decongestants contribute to others. Much discomfort, absenteeism, and expense result. The primary physician needs to distinguish an allergic etiology from obstruction, inflammation, or vasomotor instability. Proper utilization of allergy testing and effective use of antihistamines, decongestants, and topical corticosteroids are required.

PATHOPHYSIOLOGY AND CLINICAL PRESENTATION (1–3)

Allergic Rhinitis

In atopic patients, antigen exposure stimulates the production of allergen-specific immunoglobulin E (IgE). This IgE attaches to mucosal mast cells. Subsequent exposure to the allergen leads to the formation of antigen–IgE complexes on mast cells and basophils. The formation of antigen–antibody complexes triggers an acute-phase degranulation reaction, with the release of histamine, cytokines, kinins, leukotrienes, prostaglandins, and esterases in concentrations proportional to the intensity of the antigen challenge. Hours later, a late-phase response can be demonstrated in persons with more-severe disease, manifested by a re-release of mediators (minus prostaglandins), an influx of leukocytes, eosinophils, and mononuclear cells, and an increased responsiveness to antigenic and nonantigenic stimuli. With continued allergen exposure, there is a heightened mucosal responsiveness due to an increase in the population of mast cells. The leukotriene pathway, which is active in aspirin-induced disease, can produce both early and late allergy symptoms, including sneezing, nasal itching, runny nose, and congestion.

In addition to environmental stimuli, genetic factors play a role. Antigen-specific responses are controlled by regulatory genes, and allergic rhinitis is much more common in persons with a positive family history. The relation of allergic rhinitis to reactive lower airway disease (asthma) is a subject of debate, but it appears that allergic rhinitis is neither a cause nor a consequence of it, although activation of one often accompanies activation of the other.

Nasal congestion, sneezing, and profuse watery discharge dominate the initial clinical presentation. Itching of the nose, throat, and eyes is common, as is postnasal drip, tearing, and conjunctival injection. Often the nasal mucosa appears pale and edematous. Symptoms typically vary over the course of the day. They are most severe on arising in the morning, lessen in the afternoon, and may worsen again by evening. Nighttime nasal obstruction may impede restful sleep. With continued allergen exposure, there is increased sensitivity both to allergens and to nonallergenic stimuli.

Onset of allergic rhinitis is usually during childhood but may occur at any age. Childhood cases frequently continue into adulthood. Often, the condition improves with time. The condition is seasonal when the antigen is a pollen ("hay fever") and perennial when the allergens are dusts, molds, or animal danders. Patients living in the northern half of the United States who are sensitive to tree pollen will become symptomatic in late March and early April, and those sensitive to grasses will become symptomatic in mid-May to late June. Patients affected by ragweed and other summer weeds experience difficulty in late August until the first frost. Patients with seasonal allergic rhinitis outnumber those with perennial complaints by a ratio of about 10:1. Individuals may be allergic to a number of antigens.

In some instances, the patient has all the earmarks of allergic rhinitis but no evidence of IgE mediation, and skin tests for inhaled allergens are negative. Such patients have been designated as having nonallergic rhinitis, even though their nasal secretions often contain large numbers of eosinophils and they respond to corticosteroids.

Vasomotor Rhinitis

The pathophysiology is poorly understood but is believed to involve abnormal autonomic responsiveness and vascular dilation of the submucosal vessels. IgE levels are normal, and the number of eosinophils in nasal secretions is usually, but not always, normal. Abnormal autonomic reactivity is believed to account for the nasal stuffiness or rhinorrhea sometimes occurring with emotional upset and sexual arousal. The condition may mimic perennial allergic rhinitis and is believed by some clinicians to be a diagnosis of exclusion when no allergen is identified. Others consider the condition to be a readily distinguishable entity characterized by a normal-appearing nasal mucosa and persistent nasal stuffiness without itching that is worsened by changes in ambient temperature and humidity. Although congestion is the most prominent symptom, profuse watery discharge may also be present. Sneezing is relatively absent.

Drugs

Overuse of topical nasal decongestants (e.g., *oxymetazoline, phenylpropanolamine, pseudoephedrine*) can result in a worsening of symptoms (rhinitis medicamentosa). After more than 3 days of continuous use, response to these agents becomes blunted (tachyphylaxis), leading to increased use, often on an hourly basis. Cessation results in severe rebound nasal congestion presumably due to marked reflex vasodilation. The nasal mucosa appears erythematous. The problem resolves in 2 to 3 weeks if topical decongestants are stopped. α-Adrenergic blockers can aggravate preexisting rhinitis and cause mild nasal congestion in normal patients.

Cocaine abuse is another important cause of drug-induced nasal congestion and discharge. Because cocaine is a potent sympathomimetic, the pathophysiology is analogous to that of nasal decongestant abuse. Recurrent nasal use leads to ischemic mucosal injury, atrophy, and telltale septal perforation. Aspirin-induced rhinosinusitis occurs in persons with *aspirin sensitivity,* who usually manifest the additional findings of nasal polyps and asthma. The leukotriene pathway appears to be important to mediating the allergic reaction.

Chronic Inflammatory Disease

Midline granuloma (also known as polymorphic reticulosis), an uncommon illness, causes ulcerative destruction of upper respiratory tract structures and may present as nasal stuffiness, crusting, and granulations. Steady progression leads to ulcers of the nasal septum. Most patients are older than 50 years, and many have a history of allergic rhinitis. More recently, this has been identified as a type of cutaneous T cell lymphoma. *Wegener's granulomatosis,* an immune-mediated disease of middle-aged persons, may have a similar insidious presentation with nasal obstruction, rhinorrhea, or chronic sinusitis. Necrotizing granulomatous lesions and vasculitis are found in the upper and lower airways. *Sarcoidosis* may present as bilateral nasal obstruction (see Chapter 51).

Hormonal Etiologies

Hypothyroidism and pregnancy may cause the turbinates to become pale and edematous, leading to nasal congestion. Hypothyroidism may otherwise be subclinical save for the chronic nasal obstruction. Symptoms resolve with the correction of the hypothyroidism or with delivery.

Mechanical Obstruction

Unilateral congestion, discharge, and recurrent episodes of sinusitis are characteristic of mechanical obstruction due to tumor, polyp, or deviated septum. Neoplasm is rare but is suggested by a blood-tinged discharge. *Polyps* can occur in association with allergic and vasomotor rhinitis, chronic sinusitis, aspirin-induced asthma, cystic fibrosis, and drug use. The mechanism of formation is unknown. Polyps move freely because they are pedunculated and nontender and appear as soft, pale gray, smooth structures. Patients with asthma and nasal polyps are often hypersensitive to aspirin (so-called *triad asthma*). Polyps do not regress spontaneously and may become large or multiple, causing considerable obstruction. A deviated septum is sometimes the source of obstructive

symptoms. Most are developmental and not traumatic in origin. Associated sinus occlusion is rare.

Obstruction due to crusting is seen with *atrophic rhinitis.* The condition is of unknown etiology, appears mostly in women, and is characterized by dry atrophic nasal turbinates, mucosal crusts, and a foul or fetid greenish discharge referred to as ozena. The purulent discharge is believed to be due to secondary infection. Atrophic rhinitis can also be caused by excessive nasal surgery (i.e., turbinate resection) or nasal necrosis after cocaine abuse.

DIFFERENTIAL DIAGNOSIS

The causes of nasal congestion and discharge can be organized pathophysiologically and are listed in Table 222.1.

WORKUP (4,5)

Although it is important to rule out mechanical obstruction, chronic inflammatory disease, and drug-induced illness, the most common diagnostic task is to distinguish allergic from vasomotor from structural disease.

History

The timing of symptoms can be helpful diagnostically. Nasal congestion that coincides with periods of pollination is virtually diagnostic of seasonal allergic rhinitis. Continuous waxing and waning of symptoms throughout the year, with exacerbations during the hay fever season, suggests a combination of

TABLE 222.1

IMPORTANT CAUSES OF CHRONIC OR RECURRENT NASAL CONGESTION

Allergic
  Seasonal allergic rhinitis (pollens)
  Perennial allergic rhinitis (dusts, molds)

Vasomotor
  Idiopathic (vasomotor rhinitis)
  Abuse of nose drops
  Drugs (reserpine, guanethidine, prazosin, cocaine abuse)
  Psychologic stimulation (anger, sexual arousal)

Mechanical
  Polyps
  Tumor
  Deviated septum
  Crusting (as in atrophic rhinitis)
  Hypertrophied turbinates (chronic vasomotor rhinitis)
  Foreign body (usually in children)

Chronic Inflammatory
  Sarcoidosis
  Wegener's granulomatosis
  Midline granuloma

Infectious
  Atrophic rhinitis (secondary infection)

Hormonal
  Pregnancy
  Hypothyroidism

perennial and seasonal allergic disease. When symptoms occur chronically without respect to seasons, one may be dealing with vasomotor rhinitis, perennial allergy, mechanical obstruction, or a chronic inflammatory condition. Perennial rhinitis is a possibility when the patient reports frequent "colds."

Aggravating and alleviating factors should be noted. Patients bothered by dusts are generally atopic, whereas those whose symptoms are aggravated by quick changes in temperature, emotion, or drugs fall into the vasomotor category. Use of antihypertensive agents and topical nasal decongestants needs to be explored, as does exposure to fur-bearing animals (especially cats), feathers, other possible sources of animal danders, or chemical irritants. Pollutants are often more irritating to allergic patients, but they may also cause symptoms in nonatopic people. Woodburning stoves and fireplaces are associated with chronic rhinitis and sinonasal polyposis.

Associated symptoms of potential importance include fever and a purulent nasal discharge, which suggest an infectious etiology. A cold is the most likely cause of acute discharge, but chronic discharge that is fetid, foul smelling, and accompanied by crusting indicates secondary infection as in atrophic rhinitis, Wegener's granulomatosis, and midline granuloma. Chronic sinusitis may also present with a primary symptom of nasal congestion/obstruction. Bloody discharge and unilateral obstruction suggest tumor. Mechanical obstructions are often unilateral as well. The presence of asthma or aspirin sensitivity increases the likelihood of nasal polyps and/or chronic sinusitis. Sneezing and postnasal drip are nonspecific and of little help in distinguishing among etiologies, but associated itching of the eyes, tearing, and conjunctival redness suggest an allergic mechanism.

Epidemiologic data need to be considered. Onset in childhood is typical of allergic disease, but onset of symptoms during adulthood does not rule out atopy. When chronic progressive nasal congestion develops in a middle-aged patient, particularly a woman, one must consider atrophic rhinitis or one of the necrotizing inflammatory diseases. The allergy histories of the patient's parents should be ascertained because a positive family history strongly suggests allergic disease.

Drug use and concurrent conditions are important to review, including abuse of cocaine or nasal decongestants, hypothyroidism, sarcoidosis, and pregnancy. Some intranasal medications such as intranasal migraine medications and intranasal calcitonin may also cause localized rhinitis.

Physical Examination

The nasal mucous membranes are inspected for erythema, pallor, atrophy, edema, crusting, and discharge. The presence of polyps, erosions, and septal perforations or deviations should be noted. The external appearance of the nose is often helpful: A crooked-appearing external nose often implies substantial septal deviation internally. A nasal speculum markedly improves visualization of the nasal cavity and should be used in every examination. Some findings are nonspecific. For example, a pale, boggy appearance to the mucosa is allegedly a classic sign of allergic disease, but erythema sometimes occurs in allergy, and its presence certainly does not rule it out. The posterior oropharynx may reveal purulent or mucoid discharge suggestive of infection or chronic sinusitis.

Examination of the eyes for conjunctival erythema, tearing, photophobia, and papillary edema of the lids provides supportive evidence of an allergic mechanism. Transillumination and palpation of the sinuses, pharyngeal examination for erythema and discharge, a look in the ears for evidence of otitis, cervical node examination for adenopathy, and auscultation of the chest for wheezes complete the physical examination.

Laboratory Studies

Antigen challenge is sometimes helpful when the differentiation between allergic and nonallergic disease remains difficult. *In vivo* and *in vitro* methods are used. When history provides ready identification of allergens, there is little need for skin testing, but if drastic environmental measures are being contemplated, documentation of the specific allergens is indicated.

In Vivo Testing for Allergen-Specific IgE (Skin-Prick Testing)

The procedure of choice for the detection of allergen-specific IgE continues to be *skin testing*. For environmental allergens, an epicutaneous (needle prick) test is used. (Intradermal injection should not be used because it generates a high frequency of false positives and risks severe systemic reactions.) Preparations of commonly inhaled allergens (dusts, molds, animal danders, and local pollens) are introduced by needle prick into the skin. A positive test is a wheal-and-flare reaction within 20 minutes. A positive reaction does not prove causation, only that there is sensitization to the allergen, and allergen-specific IgE present. Correlation with history and physical examination is needed to establish an etiologic role for the antigen.

Antihistamines must be omitted for 12 to 24 hours before testing to avoid a false-negative result. Dermatographism is a common cause of false-positive results, occurring in 15% to 20% of the population and necessitating the use of a saline control injection. Eczema and concurrent use of antipsychotic drugs can also interfere with interpretation. The size of the wheal and flare correlates well with the level of allergen-specific IgE. However, allergen preparations need to be standardized to avoid impairing interpretation and comparison of results.

Although many of the allergens tested by skin prick are inhaled, inhalation challenge remains predominantly a research method, used to evaluate nasal resistance after mucosal exposure.

In Vitro Testing for IgE and Other Markers of Allergy

When skin-prick testing is not available, serum tests can contribute to diagnosis. Determination of total *serum IgE* is helpful if the level is markedly elevated, but test sensitivity is low because some cases of allergic rhinitis are not associated with high serum concentrations. The same is true for the total eosinophil count. A count at the time of an exacerbation that is greater than 500 cells/mm³ suggests an allergic etiology, but the absence of peripheral eosinophilia does not rule out allergic rhinitis. *Radio allergoabsorbent testing* (RAST) is an *in vitro* means of identifying and quantifying an allergen-specific IgE. The test involves adding the patient's serum to a purified allergen absorbed to an inert particle. If the serum contains high concentrations of specific IgE antibodies to the allergen, it gives a positive test. The shortcomings of RAST are its expense and only modest sensitivity (less than that of skin testing); however, specificity is high. The test is best reserved for patients whose skin tests are equivocal and for those who cannot undergo skin testing. IgE immunoassays represent an alternative *in vitro* means of testing for specific IgE antibodies; a positive test that correlates with symptoms on natural exposure is often sufficient grounds for initiating environmental therapy.

Other Studies

Examining smears of nasal secretions for eosinophils is of limited specificity because eosinophils may be present in both vasomotor and allergic rhinitis, but an abundance is more suggestive of an allergic etiology. The smears can be informative if infection is in question because neutrophils should be present in large numbers. Plain sinus films are rarely ordered due to poor sensitivity and specificity. With purulent nasal discharge, sinus tenderness, or suspected polyposis, computed tomographic imaging of the paranasal sinuses is the test of choice, demonstrating the degree of polyposis and potentially associated sinonasal obstruction. The diagnosis of nasal obstruction/congestion is commonly facilitated by office-based nasal endoscopy. This is cost-effective, especially if first-line management with topical and/or systemic medications fail to relieve the congestion, and it offers the additional benefit of ruling out rare but potentially serious causes of nasal congestion, including benign or malignant lesions of the nasal cavity and nasopharynx.

PRINCIPLES OF MANAGEMENT AND PATIENT EDUCATION (6–18)

Allergic Rhinitis

The major components of the treatment include avoidance of responsible allergens (so-called environmental therapy) and use of antihistamines and sympathomimetics for quick symptomatic relief, topical corticosteroids or cromolyn for improved prophylaxis and control, and immunotherapy for control and prophylaxis in refractory cases.

Avoidance (Environmental) Measures

The appropriate avoidance procedures are a function of the responsible allergens and differ for seasonal and perennial disease.

Seasonal Allergic Rhinitis. Avoidance of long walks in the woods during the pollination period and staying indoors with the windows closed when symptoms are severe and the pollen count is high (e.g., hot, windy, sunny days) helps to reduce allergen exposure. Some patients find air conditioners helpful, but its filter does little to remove pollen from the air. Air conditioning simply makes it more tolerable to stay indoors with the windows closed on a hot day. The outside air intake on the air conditioner should be kept closed to avoid bringing in more pollinated air. If ragweed is a problem, daisies, dahlias, and chrysanthemums should not be kept indoors. Preventing accumulation of excess dust in the bedroom and avoiding irritants such as tobacco smoke, chemical vapors, and strong perfumes lessen symptoms.

Perennial Allergic Rhinitis. Control of perennial disease requires particular attention to allergens in the home, but recommendations should be practical. Cleaning the house and especially the bedroom with a damp mop two to three times a week will reduce dust. Humidifying the indoor environment can reduce mite and dander concentrations in the air by nearly 50%. Feather pillows should be replaced by Dacron or polyester ones, and mattresses should be covered with an elastic fabric casing. Areas where mold can collect, such as piles of old newspapers or furniture in a damp basement, should be cleaned up. A dehumidifier may prevent mold growth in very damp environments. Throwing out carpets and draperies is excessive, but new furnishings made of synthetic fabrics are preferable to cotton and wool to minimize dust collection. Humidification of air in winter also helps to reduce dusts. Patients allergic to molds should avoid having African violets and geraniums in the home. No new fur-bearing pets should be obtained. Most pets usually have to be removed from the home entirely if symptoms are disabling. Simply keeping the pet out of the bedroom does not help sufficiently because the dander circulates in the air throughout the house.

Approach to Pharmacotherapy

Patients who find allergen avoidance impractical or ineffective often request medication. The commonly used agents include *oral antihistamines*, which block mast-cell activation and the effects of histamine on end organs; inhaled cromolyn sodium and its analogues, which block degranulation of mast cells and basophils; topical corticosteroids, which inhibit cytokine production, mast-cell proliferation, and other inflammatory mediators; and sympathomimetics, which decongest by means of vasoconstriction. *Leukotriene-receptor antagonists* have recently been approved for use in allergic rhinitis, blocking a pathway that is particularly important in aspirin-induced disease.

Antihistamines

The *first-generation H_1-blockers* (e.g., *chlorpheniramine, diphenhydramine, clemastine*) provide adequate control of mild to moderate symptoms, with itching, sneezing, rhinorrhea, and conjunctival irritation responding best, but nasal congestion often persists. *Second-generation H_1-blockers* (e.g., *loratadine, fexofenadine*) are less sedating and less inhibitory of psychomotor function because their protein-bound lipophobic structure prevents their crossing the blood–brain barrier. However, they are no more effective than first-generation antihistamines. Although typically considered to be nonsedating, they have been associated with increased rates of fatigue in patients with chronic sinusitis. A *topically active antihistamine* (*azelastine*) has been developed for use as a nasal spray. About 40% of the nasal spray is absorbed systemically. Although similar in efficacy to other antihistamines, the drug's side effects (somnolence, bitter taste) and high cost make it less desirable than oral nonsedating antihistamines and inhaled steroids. However, this medication seems to be rather effective in controlling nasal hypersecretion in refractory cases.

Rapid absorption of antihistamines occurs after oral intake on an empty stomach, with onset of action within 1 to 2 hours. Intake with food may slow absorption. Duration of action ranges from 3 to 4 hours for nonsustained formulations of first-generation preparations to 12 hours for sustained-release preparations and 12 to 24 hours for second-generation H_1-blockers.

Cost

Antihistamine cost has become a major concern in an era of rapidly rising medical expenses. The prescription second-generation antihistamines are extremely expensive, costing as much as 10 times more than generic chlorpheniramine and as much as 7 times more than nasal steroids (Table 222.2). Demand for second-generation H_1-blockers has been greatly stimulated by direct advertising to patients. Approaches to cost containment in treatment of allergic rhinitis include the following:

1. Starting with a first-generation antihistamine and switching to a nonsedating preparation only if daytime sedation

TABLE 222.2

COST AND CONVENIENCE OF DRUGS FOR ALLERGIC RHINITIS

Preparation	Dose	Schedule	Relative Cost[a]
First-Generation Antihistamines			
Chlorpheniramine (generic)	4 mg	qid	1.0
Chlorpheniramine, long-acting	12 mg	bid	1.7
Brompheniramine (generic)	4 mg	qid	1.0
Diphenhydramine (generic)	25 mg	qid	1.5
Clemastine (Tavist)	1 mg	bid	8.2
Second-Generation Antihistamines			
Loratadine (generic)	10 mg	qd	3
Loratadine (Claritin OTC)	10 mg	qd	5
Cetirizine (Zyrtec)	10 mg	qd	9
Fexofenadine (Allegra)	60 mg	bid	11
Inhaled Antihistamines			
Azelastine (Astelin spray)	137 μg	bid	19
Combination Preparations			
Chlorpheniramine/pseudoephedrine	8 mg/120 mg	bid	4
Loratadine/pseudoephedrine (generic)	5 mg/60 mg	bid	7
Topical Corticosteroids			
Beclomethasone			
Beconase (also Beconase AQ)	42 μg	1-bid	8
Vancenase	42 μg	1-bid	8
Vancenase AQ	84 μg	1-qd	8
Budesonide (Rhinocort)	32 μg	2-bid	14
Flunisolide (Nasalide)	25 μg	2-bid	16
Fluticasone (Flonase)	50 μg	2-bid	16
Mometasone (Nasonex)	50 μg	2-qd	18
Triamcinolone (Nasacort AQ)	55 μg	2-qd	12
Mast-Cell Stabilizers			
Cromolyn	5.2 mg	1-tid	5
Leukotriene-Receptor Antagonists			
Montelukast (Singulair)	10 mg	qd	12

bid, twice daily; OTC, over the counter; qid, four times daily; qd, daily; tid, thrice daily.
[a]Relative average wholesale price for a 30-day supply of the lowest starting dose.

becomes a problem (tolerance to sedation commonly develops).

2. Substituting an inexpensive first-generation preparation for the nighttime dose of a twice-daily second-generation preparation.
3. Prescribing the least expensive second-generation preparation (e.g., over-the-counter loratadine [generic], providing a 50% to 75% savings).
4. Prescribing a nasal steroid preparation or intranasal cromolyn (see later discussion).

The increasing availability over the counter of previously prescription-only agents has shifted the cost of nonsedating antihistamines from the insurance plan to the patient.

Adverse Effects. Aside from anticholinergic effects and sedation, the first-generation H_1-blockers are well tolerated, as are most second-generation H_1-blockers, but an appreciation for their adverse effects, particularly in elderly patients, is important to maximizing safe use.

Anticholinergic activity can produce annoying side effects of dry mouth and constipation in some persons using first-generation agents. Preexisting urinary retention may be exacerbated. Bothersome sedation can be a problem in up to 15% of users of first-generation agents; some degrees of psychomotor and cognitive impairment can be demonstrated. When prescribing daytime use of a first-generation agent, it is important to keep in mind that psychomotor impairment may occur even without noticeable sedation, an especially important consideration in seniors (increasing the risk of falls) and in persons who operate a motor vehicle, heavy equipment, or machinery. Patients should be counseled about the potential for somnolence and psychomotor and cognitive side effects, especially if they plan to drive, operate heavy machinery, or perform complex tasks. The principal advantage of second-generation agents is the relative lack of sedative activity and cognitive/psychomotor impairment.

Reports of fatal *ventricular arrhythmias* (e.g., *torsades de pointes*) emerged with use of two second-generation agents (*terfenadine* and *astemizole*), leading to their withdrawal from the market. The episodes were related to drug-induced QT interval prolongation and occurred in situations that exacerbated prolongation of the QT interval (e.g., use of quinidine, disopyramide, or class IC antiarrhythmics; hypomagnesemia, hypokalemia) or interfered with hepatic antihistamine metabolism (e.g., concurrent use of antifungals or macrolide antibiotics). Fexofenadine, cetirizine, and loratadine do not appear to confer the same degree of risk for QT prolongation and ventricular dysrhythmias.

Sympathomimetics

Patients still bothered by marked nasal congestion despite antihistamine use may benefit from concurrent treatment with an oral sympathomimetic (e.g., pseudoephedrine). The vasoconstrictive action of adrenergic agents can help to reduce edema and secretions and counter the sedative action of antihistamines. These properties make oral sympathomimetics a useful component in over-the-counter decongestant formulations, often in combination with an antihistamine such as chlorpheniramine. All sympathomimetics are effective decongestants, but those with some β activity in addition to their vasoconstrictor α-adrenergic action (e.g., *ephedrine, pseudoephedrine*) are preferred when drowsiness is a problem. *Phenylpropanolamine* has been removed from the United States over-the-counter market because of long-term risks with cerebrovascular events, particularly in women. Longer-acting formulations of phenylephrine have substantially replaced phenylpropanolamine.

Adverse Effects. The addition of sympathomimetic therapy may provoke bothersome side effects (headache, palpitations, nervousness) or trigger harmful cardiovascular effects (e.g., elevated blood pressure, increased heart rate). Use, especially if continuous, in patients with hypertension, coronary artery disease, or heart failure is inadvisable. Persistent use of a topical sympathomimetic decongestant spray can result in tachyphylaxis; withdrawal can cause rebound nasal congestion.

Preparations. Empirical trials of various antihistamines and decongestants are often necessary to select the best agent(s) and dose(s). Combination preparations are convenient if the fixed doses match the doses needed; these preparations should not be used as initial therapy. Combination preparations containing a first-generation antihistamine and a sympathomimetic are available without prescription and are popular with many patients, who find the combination less sedating and more effective than the antihistamine alone. Second-generation antihistamines are also available in combination with a sympathomimetic. Compared with single-agent therapy, the cost of combination preparations can be high. However, sympathomimetic effects from combination therapy seem to offset some of the sedating effects of the antihistamines.

As noted, topical sympathomimetic decongestant sprays have a limited role because of tachyphylaxis with repeated use and rebound nasal congestion on withdrawal. They are best reserved for keeping the eustachian tubes patent in patients during airplane travel (see Chapter 219). A topical application of phenylephrine (Neo-Synephrine) or oxymetazoline (Afrin) spray every 3 to 4 hours while the patient is airborne should suffice, especially when preceded by an oral decongestant an hour before flight time. Rebound congestion may occur if sprays are used repeatedly for more than 3 days in a row.

Corticosteroids

For patients with persistent symptoms of seasonal or perennial allergic rhinitis, regular use of a nonabsorbable, topically active intranasal corticosteroid preparation (e.g., flunisolide, budesonide, beclomethasone, fluticasone, triamcinolone, mometasone) is becoming the treatment of choice. Nasal steroid therapy in such patients has proven to be clinically more effective and more cost-effective than chronic use of oral antihistamines. Only symptoms of allergic conjunctivitis are better controlled by antihistamines. No significant benefit is afforded by combination therapy. Once- and twice-daily nasal steroid preparations are available; cost and convenience are the principal determinants of choice (Table 222.2). Patients with dryness and crusting of the mucosa may prefer a liquid formulation rather than a powdered one. Side-effect profiles and efficacies appear to be comparable, although some claims of enhanced safety (e.g., less hypothalamic–pituitary–adrenal suppression with mometasone) remain to be confirmed. Recent literature has implicated some of the carrier agents (i.e., benzalkonium chloride) with ciliary dysfunction and even promotion of rhinitis, but this has not been borne out in subsequent studies.

Adverse Effects. Common adverse effects include mucosal irritation and friability, leading to an occasional nosebleed. Mucosal ulceration is rare. Application of the spray can cause transient burning and sneezing. Atrophic rhinitis is a risk of chronic use. Recurrent unilateral epistaxis during the use of a nasal steroid spray should raise concern for septal deviation or acquired nasal septal perforation. Colonization of the nose with *Candida* has been reported. Nasal steroid inhalers may act as carriers for bacteria, so they should be cleaned once a week with hydrogen peroxide.

At recommended doses and frequencies, significant adrenal suppression does not occur with these topical corticosteroids, even when they are used chronically. No adverse effects on adult bone metabolism have been documented, although large doses of inhaled steroids used for asthma have been associated with some increased in risk for osteoporosis, and concerns about growth retardation in children remain. Unresolved is the effect of long-term nasal-steroid use on the risk of developing cataracts and glaucoma, an association found in the elderly exposed to long-term high-dose use of inhaled and systemic glucocorticosteroids (see Chapters 105 and 208).

Intranasal Cromolyn Sodium and Nedocromil

Intranasal application of cromolyn sodium has been found to be moderately effective, making it a reasonable nonsteroidal choice in persons with less severe disease. The agent is administered either as an inhaled powder or as a dissolved liquid up to six times per day. It works by preventing degranulation of mast cells and is most effective when used prophylactically before an anticipated allergen exposure. It has benefits in both the immediate and late phases of the allergic reaction and can diminish the severity of an ongoing allergic episode. Nasal congestion is reduced. Patients with very high IgE levels are most responsive; many others are not. The agent is very safe and well tolerated, which has led to its being approved for over-the-counter use.

Nedocromil is a newer topically active mast-cell stabilizer, which is structurally different from cromolyn and possesses antiinflammatory activity. Nonetheless, its clinical efficacy in allergic rhinitis is similar to that of cromolyn, but only twice-daily administration is required.

Leukotriene-Receptor Antagonists (Montelukast)

Montelukast has been approved for use in seasonal allergic rhinitis. By blocking the leukotriene pathway, montelukast provides relief from the sneezing, nasal itching, nasal congestion, and runny nose of seasonal allergic rhinitis. Efficacy in unselected patients is about the same as that for second-generation antihistamines; the addition of montelukast does not improve outcomes in such patients but may be helpful in the subset of persons with aspirin sensitivity, in which the leukotriene pathway is believed to play an important role. The cost is very high, about three times that for over-the-counter loratadine.

Immunotherapy (Hyposensitization)

Hyposensitization is indicated as a last resort in patients who face prolonged (>6 weeks) exposure to a known allergen and who remain incapacitated despite 1 year's trial of a full program of pharmacotherapy and environmental measures. Hyposensitization reduces IgE production and stimulates the synthesis of IgG-blocking antibody. It may also induce IgE-suppressor lymphocyte activity or reduce mast-cell and basophil responsiveness. The prevention of local reaction to pollens, cat dander, and dust mites has been demonstrated in patients with allergic rhinitis. Hyposensitization involves cutaneous administration of incremental doses of allergen extract, initially at intervals of 1 to 2 weeks, progressing to intervals of 3 to 6 weeks after several months of treatment.

Immunotherapy should be considered a complement to a medical therapy because most responses are not dramatic. Skin testing for definitive identification of the causative allergen(s) is required, and frequent visits over a prolonged period mean considerable patient inconvenience and high cost. Assessment of the response to immunotherapy (improvement in symptoms, reduction in medication requirements) should be made every 6 months, and therapy should be discontinued if substantial benefit is not evident after 12 to 18 months.

Investigational Methods—Anti-IgE Antibodies

Under investigation is use of a humanized monoclonal anti–human IgE antibody (omalizumab) that binds to the mast-cell–binding site of the IgE molecule. By preventing binding, it inhibits IgE-mediated release of mast-cell mediators. In a well-designed controlled trial examining prophylactic use for seasonal allergic rhinitis, it demonstrated significant clinical benefit, reduced free IgE levels, and caused minimal side effects. The ultimate role for this novel form of prophylactic therapy remains to be more clearly defined, but the approach appears to be promising for persons who fail all other forms of treatment.

Vasomotor Rhinitis

Vasomotor rhinitis is difficult to treat. Avoidance of tobacco smoke, rapid changes in temperature or humidity, and irritant chemical vapors is helpful. *Humidification* of the home in winter is also worthwhile. Cessation of nasal spray use is essential. A change in antihypertensive medications may be needed. A mild adrenergic agent with some α activity (e.g., *pseudoephedrine*) sometimes provides partial improvement. Addition of an antihistamine for its nonspecific drying effect may give some extra relief but is ineffective by itself. A reactive depression is common in such patients; the use of an antidepressant with anticholinergic activity (e.g., *amitriptyline*) may be worth considering for both its antidepressant and drying effects.

Immunotherapy and steroids are of no proven benefit. Patients severely bothered by nasal obstruction may benefit from cryosurgical treatment of the inferior and middle turbinates; profuse rhinorrhea is occasionally treated by sectioning the parasympathetic nerve supply to the nose. Consideration of *surgical approaches* should be reserved for patients whose lives are seriously impaired by their symptoms, because chances of success are limited and the risk of complications is substantial. More recently, treatment of the obstructive symptoms of chronic rhinitis with office-based laser or radiofrequency inferior turbinate reduction has been found to be clinically valuable and cost-effective. Young patients with perennial symptoms should be considered for surgical treatment rather than year-after-year medical management.

INDICATIONS FOR REFERRAL

For the patient with allergic rhinitis whose condition is inadequately controlled on a well-designed medical regimen, referral to an allergist for skin testing and consideration of immunotherapy is a reasonable step. An allergist can also help when an allergic etiology cannot be distinguished from vasomotor rhinitis and when the antigen(s) must be identified for management purposes. Referral to an ear, nose, and throat specialist is indicated for removal of polyps or foreign bodies, management of a suspected tumor, necrotizing inflammatory condition, or atrophic rhinitis and for correction of deviated septa. Referral might also be worthwhile for patients with incapacitating vasomotor rhinitis.

THERAPEUTIC RECOMMENDATIONS

Allergic Rhinitis

- Implement avoidance and environmental measures.
- Start with a trial of a first-generation antihistamine, beginning with a twice-daily dose of a long-acting preparation (e.g., sustained-release chlorpheniramine, 8 to 12 mg). Add a small daytime dose of a shorter-acting preparation (e.g., 4 mg of chlorpheniramine) if needed and continue if well tolerated, but exercise caution in persons whose work requires unimpaired psychomotor performance (e.g., those operating machinery, heavy equipment, or a motor vehicle); avoid use in the elderly at risk for falls.
- If sedation or cognitive or psychomotor impairment is a problem and short-term treatment will suffice, then consider the short-term addition of a sympathomimetic (e.g., pseudoephedrine, 60 mg); avoid if there is hypertension or underlying heart disease.
- If sedation is a problem and longer-term therapy is needed for mild to moderate disease, then begin the least-costly twice-daily nonsedating antihistamine preparation (e.g., nonprescription loratadine or prescription fexofenadine, 60 mg every morning only); for nighttime use, recommend a nonprescription first-generation antihistamine.
- If control is inadequate, proceed to daily sustained use of a topically active, nonabsorbable, nasal corticosteroid preparation (e.g., fluticasone, one to two puffs twice daily) or cromolyn.
- Consider montelukast (10 mg once daily) in persons with aspirin sensitivity and in those who fail other measures.
- Refer for consideration of immunotherapy only those who have failed 1 year of all of the foregoing measures and in whom chronic unavoidable exposure to the offending allergen(s) is expected in the future.

Vasomotor Rhinitis

- Avoid tobacco smoke, rapid changes in temperature or humidity, and irritant chemical vapors.
- Humidify the home in winter.
- Cease any nasal spray use.
- Consider a mild adrenergic agent with some α activity (e.g., pseudoephedrine, 60 mg every 6 hours, or a 120-mg extended-release formulation twice daily).

- Add an antihistamine (e.g., loratadine).
- Consider the use of a tricyclic antidepressant with anticholinergic activity (e.g., amitriptyline, 25 to 50 mg before bed), especially if depression is concurrent.
- Omit immunotherapy and steroids.
- Refer to an ear, nose, and throat specialist for refractory symptoms, especially if there is associated nasal obstruction, and only if the patient's life is seriously impaired by symptoms.

Annotated Bibliography

1. Kay AB. Allergy and allergic disease. N Engl J Med 2001;344:30. (*An excellent review of allergic disease mechanisms; 61 references.*)
2. Naclerio RM. Understanding the pathogenesis of allergic rhinitis. J Respir Dis 1991;12(Suppl):S13. (*Describes both immediate and delayed responses to allergen change, with the late responses part of an inflammatory process.*)
3. Sousa AR, Parikh A, Scadding G, et al. Leukotriene-receptor expression on nasal mucosal inflammatory cells in aspirin-sensitive rhinosinusitis. N Engl J Med 2002;347:1493. (*Evidence for this pathway in aspirin-induced disease.*)
4. Guerin B, Watson RD. Skin tests. Clin Rev Allergy 1988;6:211. (*A good review for the practicing physician.*)
5. Ownby DR. Allergy testing: *in vivo* versus *in vitro*. Pediatr Clin North Am 1988;55:995. (*A detailed discussion of their relative merits.*)
6. Aaronson D. Comparative efficacy of H1 antihistamines. Ann Allergy 1991;67:541. (*All are equally effective for seasonal allergic rhinitis.*)
7. Agnostini JV, Le-Summers LS, Inouye SK. Cognitive and other adverse effects of diphenhydramine use in hospitalized patients. Arch Intern Med 2001;161:2091. (*Although based on a hospitalized cohort, the findings also have implications for outpatient care.*)
8. Casale TB, Condemi J, LaForce C, et al. Effect of omalizumab on symptoms of seasonal allergic rhinitis: a randomized controlled trial. JAMA 2001;286:2956. (*Found promising results for this investigational method of treatment.*)
9. Hadley JA. Overview of otolaryngic allergy management. An eclectic and cost-effective approach. Otolaryngol Clin North Am 1998;31:69. (*A nice review of cost-effective allergy management.*)
10. Juniper EF, Kline PA, Hargreave FE, et al. Comparison of beclomethasone dipropionate aqueous nasal spray, astemizole, and the combination in the prophylactic treatment of ragweed pollen–induced rhinoconjunctivitis. J Allergy Clin Immunol 1989;83:627. (*Nasal steroids were superior except for conjunctival irritation; no synergy was found from combination therapy.*)
11. Kaszuba SM, Baroody FM, deTineo M, et al. Superiority of an intranasal corticosteroid compared with an oral antihistamine in the as-needed treatment of seasonal allergic rhinitis. Arch Intern Med 2001;161:2581. (*A randomized, open-label study.*)
12. Metzger E. Comparative safety of H1-antihistamines. Ann Allergy 1991;67:625. (*A discussion of sedation and psychomotor impairment.*)
13. Pipkorn U, Pround D, Lichtenstein LM, et al. Inhibition of mediator release in allergic rhinitis by pretreatment with topical glucocorticosteroids. N Engl J Med 1987;316:1506. (*This approach blocks both immediate and late-phase responses.*)
14. Racklin RE. Clinical and immunologic aspects of allergen-specific immunotherapy in patients with seasonal allergic rhinitis and/or allergic asthma. J Allergy Clin Immunol 1983;72:323. (*A review of immunotherapy, its procedures, and its efficacy.*)
15. Ratner PH, Ehrlich PM, Fineman SM, et al. Use of intranasal cromolyn sodium for allergic rhinitis. Mayo Clin Proc 2002;77:350. (*A review of evidence in favor of efficacy; 41 references.*)
16. Weiler JM, Bloomfield JR, Woodworth GG, et al. Effects of fexofenadine, diphenhydramine, and alcohol on driving performance: a randomized, placebo-controlled trial in the Iowa driving simulator. Ann Intern Med 2000;132:354. (*Driving was poorest with diphenhydramine; drowsiness did not predict impairment.*)
17. Weiner JM, Abramson MJ, Puy RM. Intranasal corticosteroids versus oral H1-receptor antagonists in allergic rhinitis: systematic review of randomised controlled trials. BMJ 1998;317:1624. (*The best summation of the best studies; intranasal corticosteroids were superior to oral antihistamines as the first line of treatment for allergic rhinitis.*)
18. Wolthers OD, Pederson S. Knemometric assessment of systemic activity of once-daily intranasal dry-powder budesonide in children. Allergy 1994;49:96. (*Evidence of potential for growth inhibition in children, even in the absence of hypothalamic–pituitary–adrenal suppression.*)

CHAPTER 223 ■ APPROACH TO THE PATIENT WITH EXCESSIVE SNORING

NEIL BHATTACHARYYA

Snoring is essentially a lay term for the vibratory sounds produced by turbulent airflow moving the soft tissues of the upper aerodigestive tract during sleep. The complaint almost always originates from a spouse or household member whose sleep is being disturbed. Snoring may be an annoying but medically trivial problem, but when it is associated with daytime sleepiness and witnessed apneic episodes, it may be a manifestation of sleep apnea (see Chapter 46).

PATHOPHYSIOLOGY AND CLINICAL PRESENTATION (1–5)

Pharyngeal size in snorers and patients with obstructive sleep apnea is reduced compared with that in nonsnorers, with sleep apnea patients having the smallest cross-sectional pharyngeal area. The sound of snoring originates in the collapsible portion of the airway—the soft tissue between the choanae and the epiglottis. Tone in the lingual and pharyngeal muscles may be inadequate due to use of sedatives or alcohol. Structural abnormalities may contribute and include redundant or thickened lateral pharyngeal musculature, a long uvula, thickened pharyngeal folds, and flaccid tonsillar pillars. Large tonsils, cysts, or neoplasms sometimes may obstruct the airway. Mild maxillomandibular abnormalities, such as a small chin, overbite, and high hard palate, have been found to be important in women. Obstructing nasal abnormalities (e.g., severely deviated septum, polyps, sinusitis, neoplasm) may create excessive negative pressure with turbulent airflow and cause the collapse of the airway during inspiration.

Severe airway obstruction may lead to *sleep apnea*. Full obstruction interrupts ventilation and, if sufficiently prolonged and repeated, results in hypercarbia and hypoxemia. The restoration of breathing usually requires arousal from sleep. The nightly occurrence of multiple apneic episodes and disturbed sleep pattern causes daytime tiredness and hypersomnolence. Uncorrected, the condition may lead to cor pulmonale from chronic arterial desaturation. The condition is most common in obese patients but is not restricted to them (see Chapter 46).

WORKUP (5,6)

The history is most important, especially for recognition of sleep apnea. Habitual snoring, daytime sleepiness, history of motor vehicle accidents caused by falling asleep at the wheel, or witnessed apneas should trigger concern about sleep apnea. Because the condition is most common in men, with a 3:1 ratio, women with sleep apnea often go unrecognized. Delay in the diagnosis of sleep apnea is common, especially in women, because symptoms are often ignored or the presentation may be atypical (fatigue, no associated obesity or daytime sleepiness, mild maxillomandibular abnormalities). Factors associated with an increased risk for sleep apnea in snoring patients include large collar size, associated hypertension, heroic snoring (i.e., snoring that can be heard outside the bedroom), and daytime somnolence.

A careful examination of the mouth and upper airway is needed to search for obstructing anatomy. Referral for formal ear, nose, and throat evaluation may be helpful. For the patient with suspected sleep apnea, consideration of nocturnal oxygen saturation monitoring and a formal sleep study are indicated (see Chapter 46).

MANAGEMENT (5–10)

The patient with annoying but physiologically benign snoring can sometimes be helped by simple advice. The loss of excess *weight* and avoidance of *alcohol* and *sedatives* may prove beneficial. Even modest weight loss (e.g., 10 lb) can provide substantial benefit (on the order of 25% improvement). *Sleeping on one's side* rather than on the back sometimes helps to minimize upper airway collapse (an old trick is to tape a marble to the patient's back to discourage lying supine). Avoidance of the excessive neck flexion that comes from sleeping supine on several pillows can be achieved by limiting the patient to a cervical pillow placed under the nape of the neck or by elevating the entire head of the bed (as in management of reflux esophagitis). Recent randomized trials, however, have failed to show any reliable benefit from over-the-counter sprays, over-the-counter oral devices, and bedding/pillow supplements in reducing the severity of snoring.

Any nasal obstruction from chronic rhinitis should be fully treated (see Chapter 222); anatomic obstruction may benefit from a trial of an *external nasal dilator* (e.g., a Breathe Right Strip, Nose Cones). Patients whose snoring is mitigated by a trial of a topical nasal *decongestant* (e.g., oxymetazoline) may have a specific nasal cause for snoring that, when corrected, may provide substantial relief of snoring.

For patients with disturbingly refractory snoring, a more aggressive approach is to consider use of a *continuous positive airway pressure* (CPAP) device. The apparatus delivers CPAP through the nose and is usually reserved for those with sleep apnea (see Chapter 46), but it may be worth a try in households in which marital harmony and restful sleep are threatened by excessive snoring. The devices are sometimes awkward to use and not always acceptable, but newer ones are more comfortable. Consideration of dental orthosis has proven useful in preliminary studies and may be worth a referral in cases in which there is an overbite or other maxillomandibular pathology.

INDICATIONS FOR REFERRAL

Pulmonary consultation is indicated when there is concern about sleep apnea (daytime sleepiness, nocturnal apnea; see Chapter 46). An ear, nose, and throat consultation may prove useful when snoring proves intractable and appears to be associated with anatomic oropharyngeal pathology. Patients with obstructing turbinate hypertrophy, substantial nasal septal deviation, or large tonsils may be cured of their snoring with appropriate surgical therapy. In addition, relatively novel techniques for snoring reduction such as radiofrequency or laser attenuation of the soft palate (and tonsillar hypertrophy, when indicated) are minimally invasive, effective, and associated with minimal morbidity. More recently, palatal stiffening implants have demonstrated clinical effectiveness in snoring reduction in patients with primary snoring and in patients with mild to moderate obstructive sleep apnea. However, patients typically have to pay out-of-pocket for such treatments because simple nuisance snoring is not often covered by standard insurance policies.

Annotated Bibliography

1. Ayappa I, Rapoport DM. The upper airway in sleep: physiology of the pharynx. Sleep Med Rev 2003;7:9. (*An exhaustive review of upper airway physiology during sleep, useful for explaining airway physiology to patients.*)
2. Bradley TD, Brown IG, Grossman RF, et al. Pharyngeal size in snorers, nonsnorers, and patients with obstructive sleep apnea. N Engl J Med 1986;315:1327. (*Snorers have a reduced cross-sectional area; those with sleep apnea have the smallest area.*)
3. Guilleminault C, Stoohs R, Kim Y, et al. Upper airway sleep-disordered breathing in women. Ann Intern Med 1995;122:493. (*Fatigue, premenopausal status, maxillomandibular abnormalities, and mild obesity were among the prominent clinical features in this group.*)
4. Kuna ST, Sant'Ambrogio G. Pathophysiology of upper airway closures during sleep. JAMA 1991;266:1384. (*An excellent review of mechanisms of upper airway obstruction.*)
5. Schwab RJ, Gupta KB, Gefter WB, et al. Upper airway and soft tissue anatomy in normal subjects and patients with sleep-disordered breathing: significance of the lateral pharyngeal walls. Am J Respir Crit Care Med 1995;152:1673. (*A magnetic resonance imaging study of snorers, normal*

individuals, and those with sleep apnea found that thickened lateral pharyngeal muscles were more important than fat.)

6. American Sleep Disorders Association. Practice parameters for the treatment of obstructive sleep apnea in adults: the efficacy of surgical modification of the upper airway. Sleep 1996;19:152. (*An evidence-based set of guidelines for patients who failed or refused noninvasive treatment but have no obvious anatomic obstruction.*)

7. Counter P, Wilson JA. The management of simple snoring. Sleep Med Rev. 2004; 8:433 (*A good recent review of simple snoring management options.*)

8. Jennett S. Snoring and its treatment. BMJ 1984;289:335. (*A somewhat dated summary, but useful for its practical suggestions.*)

9. Peppard PE, Young T, Palta M, et al. Longitudinal study of moderate weight change and sleep-disordered breathing. JAMA 2000;284:3015. (*A 10-lb weight loss reduced breathing difficulty by about 25%; a similar weight gain produced a proportional degree of worsening.*)

10. Schmidt-Nowara WW, Meade TE, Hays MD, et al. Treatment of snoring and obstructive sleep apnea with a dental orthosis. Chest 1991;99:1378. (*A promising but preliminary report of some improvement.*)

CHAPTER 224 ■ APPROACH TO THE PATIENT WITH APHTHOUS STOMATITIS

Aphthous stomatitis (canker sores) is a common self-limited ulcerative condition of the oral mucosa. About 20% of the population is affected at one time or another. The lesions can be disturbing in appearance and very painful. The primary physician should be able to differentiate them from more serious pathology and provide symptomatic relief.

PATHOPHYSIOLOGY, CLINICAL PRESENTATION, AND COURSE (1–4)

Pathogenesis

The underlying pathophysiology is incompletely understood, but a heightened immunologic response to oral mucosal antigens appears to play an important role. There is a genetic predisposition and an increased prevalence among patients with such autoimmune diseases as Crohn's disease, chronic ulcerative colitis, Behçet's syndrome, and Reiter's syndrome. Contributing factors include deficiencies of iron, folate, and vitamin B_{12}, psychological stress, generalized physical debility, and trauma. Although vitamin and mineral deficiencies usually produce stomatitis, they have been increasingly linked to recurrent aphthous ulceration as well. In some women, flares occur premenstrually. Regardless of etiology, once mucosal breakdown has occurred, the lesions are invaded by mouth flora and become secondarily infected.

Clinical Presentation

Aphthous stomatitis develops in four clinical stages:

- *Premonitory*: tingling, burning, or hyperesthetic sensation, lasting up to 24 hours.
- *Preulcerative*: lasting from 18 hours to 3 days, characterized by moderately painful erythematous macules or papules with erythematous halos.
- *Ulcerative*: lasting 1 to 16 days, characterized by painful discrete ulcers 2 to 10 mm in diameter, occurring singly or in groups, covered by a gray-yellow membrane with a dusky erythematous halo; pain ceases during this stage.
- *Healing*: averaging 2 weeks (range from 4 to 5 weeks), usually without scarring unless lesions are very large.

Aphthous ulcers are classified according to size. Most are *minor* (i.e., <1 cm in diameter) and appear in crops of four or five. *Major lesions* are greater than 1 cm, solitary, indolent, and, as noted, may scar as they heal. Lesions are painful and may occur anywhere within the oral cavity. In two thirds of patients, recurrent lesions do not develop, but in one third, recurrences continue for up to 40 years.

DIFFERENTIAL DIAGNOSIS (3,6,7)

A host of conditions can cause oral ulcers (Table 224.1). Many are characterized by involvement beyond the oral cavity. *Pemphigus* is suggested by the presence of bullous lesions elsewhere on the body (although oral lesions may precede others by years) and a Tzanck smear from the base of the lesion showing acantholytic cells; immunofluorescence studies may be necessary if there is recurrent disease. The ulcerated mucosal lesions of *herpes simplex* infection are limited to mucosal surfaces attached to bone (e.g., the hard palate and attached gingiva), whereas aphthous ulcers may occur anywhere in the oral cavity; the Tzanck preparation shows multinucleated giant cells as it does with *herpes zoster*, which is characterized by a dermatomal skin distribution (see Chapters 192 and 193). The ulcers of *Behçet's syndrome* are identical to those of aphthous stomatitis; genital ulceration and eye involvement help to differentiate the condition from simple aphthous disease. In *hand-foot-and-mouth disease*, papulovesicular lesions with an erythematous halo appear on the hands, feet, and lips in addition to the mouth; the lesions ulcerate and then heal over 7 to 10 days. Because the condition is due to an enterovirus, the mucosal findings may be preceded by viral gastrointestinal symptoms. In *squamous cell carcinoma* of the oral cavity, there is a single ulcerated lesion

TABLE 224.1

SOME IMPORTANT CAUSES OF ORAL ULCERS

Cause	Associated Clinical Features
Aphthous ulcers	Multiple ulcers, involvement of the soft oral mucosa, e.g., tongue, floor of mouth, soft palate, and buccal and labial mucosa
Pemphigus	Bullous skin lesions, acantholytic cells on Tzanck prep
Herpes simplex	Cluster of vesicles; positive culture
Herpes zoster	Dermatomal vesicular outbreak
Behçet's syndrome	Skin findings, uveitis, urethritis, arthralgia, vascular, andneurologic involvement; not necessarily concurrent
Crohn's disease	Concurrent gastrointestinal symptoms and signs
Squamous-cell cancer	Solitary nonhealing ulcer in smoker/drinker
Hand-foot-and-mouth	Papulovesicular lesions with an erythematous halo disease appear on the hands, feet, and lips; fever, gastrointestinal upset
Lichen planus	Concurrent skin involvement
Erythema multiforme	Concurrent skin involvement

that fails to heal; a history of smoking and drinking is typically prominent (see Chapter 211).

WORKUP (2,3,5–7)

Workup concentrates on differentiating aphthous lesions from other causes of oral ulceration (see Table 224.1). *History* should focus on number of lesions, location, timeline, and associated symptoms, especially those of concurrent dermal, gastrointestinal, musculoskeletal, ocular, and urogenital systems. Checking for a history of smoking, alcohol excess, and a nonhealing single ulcer helps to identify an oral cancer (see Chapter 211). Situational stress and risk factors for iron, folate, and vitamin B_{12} deficiencies (see Chapter 79) should be noted.

The *physical examination* should identify the number, location, and appearance of the oral ulcers and any skin involvement or that of other organ systems.

Laboratory studies are of little value unless vitamin deficiencies are suspected by the history; recurrent disease should trigger testing for vitamin B_{12} deficiency. A single nonhealing ulcer requires consideration of *biopsy* to rule out squamous cell cancer of the oral mucosa. When there are concurrent skin lesions, skin biopsy may be useful. Unroofing a vesicle or bullus and performing a *Tzanck prep* can help to identify herpetic infection (multinucleated giant cells) and pemphigus (acantholytic cells).

PRINCIPLES OF MANAGEMENT (4–9)

Because etiology is usually unknown, treatment is largely empirical. Identification and correction of an existing deficiency of *folate*, *vitamin B_{12}*, or *iron* (see Chapter 82) may cure aphthous stomatitis. For lesions precipitated by emotional stress, attention to the underlying problem may help (see Chapter 226). When the chief reason for seeking medical care is concern, reassurance that the lesions will heal spontaneously and that they do not represent more serious pathology often

suffices. For patients with large lesions and those bothered badly by the discomfort, additional measures are reasonable.

In the presence of extremely painful lesions, the use of a topical anesthetic agent (e.g., *benzocaine* or *viscous lidocaine*) in the form of an oral rinse before meals may allow the patient to eat. The avoidance of abrasive foods also helps. Protective preparations (e.g., *aphthasol*, *Zilactin*, and *Ziladent* [Zilactin plus benzocaine]) adhere to the ulcer, providing a protective impermeable membrane. The topical use of *sucralfate* liquid may provide some mucosal protection. Chemical cauterization by means of *silver nitrate* sticks is used by some practitioners to treat acute lesions, but this involves the distinct possibility of destroying normal tissue and should not ordinarily be used.

Measures used to speed healing range from antibacterial rinses to corticosteroids. Rinsing with the antibacterial mouthwash *chlorhexidine* is believed to reduce ulcer duration and recurrences. *Tetracycline* rinse (250 mg in 10 cc of syrup four times a day for up to 2 weeks) may work in similar fashion. *Corticosteroids* are used to provide symptomatic relief and speed resolution (after infection and malignancy have been ruled out). *Topical* corticosteroid impregnated into a paste vehicle (e.g., Orabase), a syrup (e.g., betamethasone) or an ointment (e.g., fluocinonide) may be helpful in early superficial lesions. Systemic steroids (e.g., prednisone) may be needed for severe or progressive disease.

Colchicine, *pentoxifylline*, *topical thalidomide*, and *levamisole* have all been tried because they have immunologic and antiinflammatory actions that might be beneficial. Although results are promising, use is not established.

PATIENT EDUCATION

Besides reassurance, patient education should include recommendations for avoiding mucosal trauma and maintaining good nutrition and oral hygiene. The use of a soft-bristled toothbrush and the avoidance of foods with sharp surfaces, salt, and talking while chewing can be helpful. Patients with vitamin or mineral deficiencies can be prescribed a supplement. The possibility of recurrence in one third of patients should be explained.

A. H. G.

Annotated Bibliography

1. Graykowski EA. Aphthous stomatitis is linked to mechanical injuries, iron and vitamin deficiencies, and certain HLA types. JAMA 1982;247:774. (*A summary of evidence regarding the link to these etiologic factors.*)
2. Piskin S, Sayan C, Durukan N, et al. Serum iron, ferritin, folic acid, and vitamin B_{12} levels in recurrent aphthous stomatitis.J Eur Acad Dermatol Venereol 2002;16:66. (*Presents further evidence of an association.*)
3. Rogers RS 3rd. Recurrent aphthous stomatitis: clinical characteristics and associated systemic disorders. Semin Cutan Med Surg 1997;16:278.(*A useful summary of clinical presentations of ulcerating oral conditions.*)
4. Fairfield KM, Fletcher RH. Vitamins for chronic disease prevention in adults: scientific review. JAMA 2002;287:3116. (*A summary of evidence for vitamin deficiency and benefits from supplementation.*)
5. Fletcher RH, Fairfield KM. Vitamins for chronic disease prevention in adults: clinical applications. JAMA 2002;287:3127. (*Recommendations for supplementation.*)
6. Fischman SL. Oral ulcerations. Semin Dermatol 1994;13:74. (*Includes good review of differential diagnosis and approach to workup.*)
7. Scully C, Gorsky M, Lozada-Nur F. The diagnosis and management of recurrent aphthous stomatitis: a consensus approach. J Am Dent Assoc.2003;134:200. (*Clinical guidelines.*)
8. Barrons RW. Treatment strategies for recurrent oral aphthous ulcers. Am J Health Syst Pharm 2001;58:41.
9. MacPhail L. Topical and systemic therapy for recurrent aphthous stomatitis. Semin Cutan Med Surg 1997;16:301. (*A good review of treatments.*)

CHAPTER 225 ■ MANAGEMENT OF TEMPOROMANDIBULAR JOINT DYSFUNCTION

Temporomandibular joint (TMJ) dysfunction has received much attention in the lay press as a cause of chronic headache and facial pain (see Chapter 165). Although severe cases may require dental or oral surgical intervention, most can be managed conservatively by the primary physician.

PATHOPHYSIOLOGY AND CLINICAL PRESENTATION (1–6)

Pathophysiology

Most TMJ dysfunction is psychophysiologic in origin, the consequence of chronic *bruxism* (nocturnal jaw clenching and teeth grinding). This tension-relieving oral habit develops in response to situational and intrapsychic stresses and can lead to masticatory muscle fatigue and spasm. In most instances, the problem remains *extracapsular*, with little or no internal derangement of the TMJ. However, severe prolonged bruxism may cause *intracapsular* joint derangement, resulting in degenerative disease of the joint. *Sinovitis* from connective tissue disease, infection, or trauma is another form of intracapsular pathology. Persons with a tendency toward somatization have increased frequency of TMJ joint complaints.

Clinical Presentation

Symptoms of TMJ dysfunction include chronic, dull, aching unilateral discomfort about the jaw, behind the eyes and ears, and even down the neck into the shoulders. Jaw pain, clicking sounds, and difficulty opening the mouth widely, especially in the morning, are characteristic. Chewing may exacerbate symptoms. Locking of the jaw is common. Masticatory muscle tenderness, mandibular hypomotility, clicking, and joint deviation on opening are noted on physical examination. Molar prominences may be flat from chronic grinding. A subset of patients with symptoms referable to the TMJs also experience pain and dysfunction that extend far beyond the TMJs.

A subset of patients with TMJ complaints exhibit features characteristic of patients suffering from a *chronic pain syndrome* (see Chapter 236). They present to multiple doctors with refractory pain complaints, often extending beyond the TMJs. Not only is health care utilization high as such patients search repeatedly for a "cure," but also physician frustration is also high because nothing seems to work. Any suggestion by the physician of a "psychological" cause clashes with the patient's etiologic view and leads to a dissonant doctor–patient relationship. Such patients often seek the comfort of "TMJ" support groups.

DIAGNOSIS (1,4,5)

The hallmark of TMJ dysfunction is chronic unilateral jaw or facial pain exacerbated by jaw movement. Other causes of jaw pain worsened by jaw movement include *acute otitis media* and *parotitis*. These are distinguished by their acute onset and associated inflammatory manifestations. More subtle is the jaw claudication from *temporal arteritis* (see Chapter 161). Intracapsular TMJ disease may be differentiated clinically from extracapsular dysfunction by the presence of markedly limited jaw movement, jaw deviation on opening of the mouth, and the presence of crepitus and clicking on jaw movement. However, there is much overlap of symptoms between internal and extracapsular TMJ disease; jaw clicking may even be noted in normal persons.

Confirmation of internal derangement requires radiologic study. *Magnetic resonance imaging* (MRI) of the TMJ provides the best visualization of bony and soft tissue structures. It has become the test of choice because it is more sensitive than conventional computed tomography and free of radiation exposure. MRI test expense can be reduced substantially by imaging only the TMJ. Imaging is indicated only when internal derangement is suspected, conservative measures have failed, and more-aggressive therapy is being considered.

Patients with refractory TMJ complaints that extend well beyond the TMJs and disproportionately interfere with daily functioning should have the possibility of an underlying chronic pain syndrome explored (see Chapter 236).

PRINCIPLES OF MANAGEMENT (1–7)

Nonsurgical Measures

Because TMJ dysfunction is largely a psychophysiologic condition, treatment may begin with the primary physician inquiring into sources of stress and tension and offering counseling. Often, *cognitive–behavioral therapy* is more effective than insight-oriented approaches to psychotherapy (see Chapter 226). Most persons improve without formal psychiatric care. Less-etiologic but helpful symptomatic measures include dietary advice, local physiotherapy, analgesics, minor tranquilizers, and sometimes antidepressants.

Dietary advice includes cutting food into small pieces and using a diet that minimizes hard, repetitive chewing (e.g., no chewing gum or biting into big submarine sandwiches). *Physiotherapy* in the form of local heat and massage to the muscles of mastication helps relieve to muscle spasm and the accompanying pain. Some persons achieve relief with the application of *ultrasound* or *cold packs*. Analgesics such as aspirin and low doses of nonsteroidal antiinflammatory agents are also helpful when pain is prominent. Short-term use of a *minor tranquilizer* at bedtime (e.g., 2 mg of diazepam as needed for 35 days) can help to reduce nocturnal muscle spasm and complement

analgesic therapy. However, long-term tranquilizer use should be avoided due to the risk of dependence (see Chapter 226). The so-called muscle relaxants (e.g., Robaxin, Soma) are of no proven advantage. Patients with more-refractory pain may respond to a trial of a sedating *tricyclic antidepressant* (e.g., nortriptyline 25 mg as needed). Patients with severe grinding may benefit from the nighttime use of a custom-made *splint* or *bite guard*.

A regimen that incorporates all of these measures into a comprehensive treatment program has a success rate of greater than 75%. Patients who report refractory pain may have suffered joint damage and require consideration for regrinding or surgical intervention. When the clinical presentation is one of refractory pain accompanied by more global musculoskeletal dysfunction and disproportionately little evidence of TMJ destruction, then approaching the condition as a chronic pain syndrome may be the wisest course (see Chapter 236).

Dental and Surgical Therapies

Only the patient with severe malocclusion leading to marked joint trauma is a candidate for regrinding of the teeth. It is a therapy of limited efficacy, requiring careful patient selection. Many patients without objective malocclusion and significant joint injury are subjected needlessly to regrinding or surgical therapy. Surgical intervention is a consideration only when conservative measures have failed to provide relief *and* there is clinical evidence of internal joint derangement and secondary degenerative arthritis (see previous discussion). Under these circumstances, an MRI of the TMJs should be obtained and referral made if important degenerative changes are found.

Incapacitated patients refractory to conservative therapy yet found to have marked degenerative changes clearly linked to symptoms are potential candidates for surgery. They should be referred for consultation to an oral surgeon experienced in treating TMJ disease. There are almost no large-scale, prospective, randomized studies to guide the choice of surgery for TMJ disease. Arthroscopic approaches appear to be promising. They are reported to provide significant symptomatic relief, are minimally invasive, and have a low incidence of complications; however, long-term benefit remains to be established.

A. H. G.

Annotated Bibliography

1. American Society of Temporomandibular Joint Surgeons. Guidelines for diagnosis and management of disorders involving the temporomandibular joint and related musculoskeletal structures. 2001. Available at: www.astmjs.org/frame_guidelines.html. (*A definitive review and evidence-based guidelines.*)
2. Feinmann C, Harris M, Crawley R. Psychogenic facial pain: presentation and treatment. BMJ 1984;228:436. (*A succinct review of approaches to the psychological dimension of temporomandibular joint [TMJ] dysfunction.*)
3. Garro LC, Stephenson KA, Good BJ. Chronic illness of the temporomandibular joints as experienced by support-group members. J Gen Intern Med 1994;9:372. (*A study exploring the perspective of patients with chronic TMJ complaints, many of whom have symptoms that extend beyond the TMJs and exhibit marked health care utilization.*)
4. Guralnick W, Kaban LB, Merrill RG. Temporomandibular joint afflictions. N Engl J Med 1978;299:123. (*A classic review of mechanisms and presentation.*)
5. Kumar KL, Cooney TG. Temporomandibular disorders. J Gen Intern Med 1994;9:106. (*An excellent summary for the generalist reader, with particularly helpful suggestions for workup and conservative management; 36 references.*)
6. Wilson L, Dworkin SF, Whitney C, et al. Somatization and pain dispersion in chronic temporomandibular disorder pain. Pain 1994;57:55. (*Persons with somatization disorder are more likely to complain of chronic TMJ discomfort.*)
7. Clark GT, Delcanho RE, Goulet JP. The utility and validity of current diagnostic procedures for defining temporomandibular disorder patients. Adv Dent Res 1993;7:97. (*An excellent critical review of diagnostic measures.*)

CHAPTER 226 ■ APPROACH TO THE PATIENT WITH ANXIETY

JOHN J. WORTHINGTON III

Anxiety disorders are prevalent (the estimated lifetime prevalence is 25% in the general population) and a frequent precipitant of visits to the nonpsychiatric physician. Evaluation and management can be challenging because patients present with feelings of distress and concern about disease in the absence of objective evidence. Suffering no less from the subjective nature of their ailment, they fear something is amiss with their bodies and persistently seek an acceptable explanation and relief. The autonomic arousal accompanying anxiety may affect many organ systems and imitate physical disease. Moreover, anxiety and anxiety-like symptoms may be consequent to a variety of medical ailments and their treatments.

Anxiety is a normal human emotion. Distinguishing normal anxiety from pathologic anxiety and anxiety disorders often requires systematic evaluation and a thorough understanding of the individual patient's physical and psychological status. Underrecognized and undertreated, anxiety disorders increase the cost of medical care and render patients vulnerable to further morbidity, including demoralization, hypochondriasis, depression, and varying degrees of disability. A comprehensive and empathic assessment of the anxious patient by the primary care physician permits a reasoned and often therapeutically effective approach to the difficult problems presented.

PATHOPHYSIOLOGY AND CLINICAL PRESENTATION (1–11)

Definitions

Anxiety is the distressing experience of dread, foreboding, or panic accompanied by a variety of autonomic—primarily sympathetic—bodily symptoms. The distress, therefore, is both psychic and physical. Patients vary considerably in their tolerance to it. The new onset or exacerbation of anxiety often occurs in response to emotional or physiologic stimuli. Most individuals meet the challenge of universally anxiety-provoking situations with their personal strengths and styles of coping. When an individual's capacity for coping is overwhelmed, excessive anxiety may emerge. *Pathologic anxiety* is distinguished from the normal case by its occurrence in the absence of an objective stimulus and by its duration or intensity.

Neurotransmitter Mechanisms

Several monoamine and neuropeptide neurotransmitters are implicated in the neurobiology of anxiety. *Norepinephrine* plays a prominent role in mediating anxiety states centrally.

The locus ceruleus of the pons serves as the chief noradrenergic nucleus. Abnormal firing patterns in the locus ceruleus have been implicated in the pathophysiology of some anxiety conditions, such as panic disorder. In contrast, the inhibitory neurotransmitter γ-aminobutyric acid, which is ubiquitous in the brain, is implicated as serving an anxiolytic function within the limbic system. The resulting somatic manifestations of anxiety are principally mediated by the *sympathetic nervous system*.

Classification and Basic Components of the Clinical Presentation

The classification of anxiety disorders is largely based on clinical features (Table 226.1). In both its normal and pathologic forms, anxiety's manifestations consist of affective, cognitive, behavioral, and somatic components. The *affective component* is characterized by the experience of dread, foreboding, or panic. In its normal form, the affective component is countered by *cognitions* that make sense of or seek to neutralize the distress. In the pathologic form, other components of the clinical presentation may be exacerbated by cognitions, such as catastrophizing. A variety of *behaviors*, such as avoidance or hypervigilance, reflect the anxious state or evolve in response to it. Typical psychological presentations might include complaints of apprehension, motor tension or agitation (restlessness, edginess, jitteriness), and heightened arousal (including hypervigilance, distractibility, impaired concentration, and insomnia). The *somatic complaints* are mostly those of autonomic hyperactivity and include systemic, cardiopulmonary, gastrointestinal, urinary, and neurologic symptoms (Table 226.2).

Adjustment Disorder with Anxious Mood

Most presentations of anxiety within the medical setting are normal reactions to anxiety-provoking situations. For a limited time period, a patient may suffer symptoms similar to those of a generalized anxiety disorder (see later discussion). When a patient's capacity for coping is overwhelmed, excessive anxiety may transiently emerge until the patient is able to adjust. This state is termed *adjustment disorder with anxious mood* and typically resolves in less than 6 months. Adjustment disorders also may be heralded by other manifestations, including depressed mood and misconduct.

Generalized Anxiety Disorder

This common condition is characterized by anxiety lasting longer than 6 months and worry extending beyond a specific subject. Typically, the patient ruminates with worries over a

TABLE 226.1

ANXIETY DISORDERS AND THEIR DEFINING FEATURES

Generalized Anxiety Disorder
  Chronic anxiety lasting at least 6 months
  Concern over at least two different issues (usually many)
  Panic attacks may be present

Panic Disorder
  Episodic extreme anxiety consistent with panic attacks
  At least one of the attacks being followed by at least 1 month of one of the following:
  - Persistent concern about having additional attacks
  - Worry about the implications of the attack or its consequences (e.g., losing control, having a heart attack)
  - A significant change in behavior related to the attacks

Specific Anxiety Disorder
  Irrational fear associated with a particular stimulus

Social Anxiety Disorder
  Anxiety associated with scrutiny by others

Obsessive–Compulsive Disorder
  Obsessions (intrusive unwanted bizarre thoughts) and/or compulsions (repetitive behaviors performed in a ritualistic or stereotypical fashion)

Posttraumatic Stress Disorder
  History of severe traumatic exposure
  Subsequent anxiety symptoms lasting at least 1 month
  Reexperiencing of the trauma (e.g., flashbacks), avoidance of stimuli associated with the trauma, and increased arousal
  Syndrome may occur with delayed onset (>6 months after original trauma).

Adjustment Disorder with Anxious Mood[a]
  Anxiety develops as a maladaptive response to an identifiable stressor
  Symptoms last less than 6 months

[a]Categorized with Adjustment Disorders rather than Anxiety Disorders in the Diagnostic and Statistical Manual of Mental Disorders, 4th ed.

TABLE 226.2

SOMATIC SYMPTOMS OF ANXIETY

Type	Specific Symptoms
General	Fatigue, weakness, diaphoresis, insomnia, flushing, chills
Neurologic	Dizziness, paresthesias, derealization, near-syncope, tremulousness, restlessness
Cardiac	Palpitations, chest pain, tachycardia
Respiratory	Dyspnea, hyperventilation, choking
Gastrointestinal	Dry mouth, diarrhea, nausea, vomiting
Urinary	Frequency, urgency

(e.g., losing control, having a heart attack), or a significant change in behavior related to the attacks. Panic disorder is more common in women and in those with a positive family history of panic. Emergence of anxiety symptoms early in life, including a history of separation difficulties during childhood, also represents risk factors for panic disorder.

Many patients become disabled by anticipatory fear of subsequent panic attacks and by phobic *avoidant behavior* patterns. They avoid places with restricted escape (e.g., crowds, theaters, tunnels, elevators), fearful of being trapped during an attack. In its most extreme form, *agoraphobia* (literally, "fear of the market place"), avoidant behavior may reach a point at which a patient is afraid to leave the safety of the home or to be left alone. In rare situations, agoraphobia has also been reported to occur in the absence of panic disorder. (More commonly, the patient whose family describes him or her as "never leaving the house" has depression with loss of interest in doing activities as a prominent symptom.)

The course of panic disorder includes times of frequent panic attacks interspersed with periods of less frequent episodes, complicated by phobic avoidance and anticipatory anxiety. The paroxysmal nature of panic attacks and the prominence of autonomic symptoms may mimic cardiac or neurologic disease, causing some patients to become hypervigilant, convinced of a serious underlying medical disorder, and "doctor shoppers" in search of such a diagnosis. Such persons may become demoralized, depressed, and debilitated. Suicide risk appears to be increased in panic disorder, especially in patients with concurrent depression.

Phobias

A phobia is an irrational fear related to a specific stimulus. On exposure to that stimulus, the individual reliably manifests an anxiety response. A patient may suffer from a specific phobia of any specific stimulus. Although specific phobias commonly generate circumscribed symptoms, they may interfere with some aspect of a patient's functioning due to avoidance of the phobic stimulus or perseverance in the face of great discomfort (e.g., fear of flying leading to difficulty with travel).

Social Anxiety Disorder (Social Phobia). Patients with social anxiety disorder develop anxiety in situations in which they are the focus of attention or might be scrutinized publicly. The individual fears that he or she will act in a way (or show anxiety symptoms) that will be humiliating or embarrassing. Such patients may experience *performance anxiety* or "stage fright" but also exhibit distress in more ordinary social settings. In the *generalized type* of social anxiety disorder, the fear includes *most social situations* (participating in small groups,

variety of concerns and may have been doing this for several years with a waxing and waning course. Generalized anxiety disorder also includes an array of physical concomitants, including restlessness, fatigability, poor concentration, irritability, muscle tension, and insomnia. In addition to the persistent anxious state, the patient may describe more-discrete episodes of acute anxiety.

When sudden spells of extreme anxiety occur with prominent symptoms of sympathetic activation, they may be accompanied by feelings of impending doom, fear of dying, the sensation of panic, and the impulse to flee. Such symptoms characterize *panic attacks*, which may occasionally be experienced by patients with generalized anxiety disorder, although they are a more prominent feature in panic disorder.

Panic Disorder

Panic disorder is characterized by *recurrent unexpected panic attacks*, with at least one attack followed by no less than 1 month of persistent concern about having additional attacks, worry about the implications of the attack or its consequences dating, initiating or maintaining conversations, speaking to authority figures, attending parties, etc.). Social anxiety disorder needs to be distinguished from the more limited form of normal performance anxiety, which occurs in universally acknowledged anxiety-provoking situational settings (e.g., performing in front of a very large audience or as part of a very important event).

Obsessive–Compulsive Disorder

More common than previously recognized, obsessive–compulsive disorder (OCD) affects up to 3% of the population. It is characterized by obsessions and/or compulsions that are sufficiently severe to cause patients substantial distress or impair their ability to function.

Obsessions are unwanted intrusive thoughts of a bizarre, senseless, or extreme nature. The subject of obsessions typically includes sexual or violent themes, concerns about contamination, and preoccupations with organization or symmetry, which are very distressing to patients and may lead them to fear that they are "going crazy." The recurrent and persistent thoughts, impulses, or images themselves become a source of anxiety.

Compulsions refer to repetitive behaviors that are performed in a stereotypical or ritualized fashion, usually in response to obsessions, sometimes in an effort to neutralize them. Resisting the drive to perform compulsions causes escalating anxiety, whereas succumbing and performing them is accompanied by feelings of transient relief, followed by feelings of shame. Characteristic compulsions include hand washing (to neutralize contamination obsessions), checking behaviors (e.g., checking door locks and stove burners to counteract obsessions of uncertainty), and counting (to neutralize anxiety associated with other obsessions).

The relationship between the compulsions and obsessions may also be nonsensical or irrational. Usually patients retain insight regarding the nonsensical or extreme nature of their thoughts and behaviors, which distinguishes them from psychotic persons.

Because of the *shame* associated with the symptoms of OCD, it is not uncommon for patients to hide the disorder from friends, family, and doctors. OCD may come to the attention of primary care physicians when a patient's obsessions involve preoccupations with his or her bodily functions (e.g., urinary or bowel obsessions) or susceptibility to disease (e.g., obsessions with contamination or fear of AIDS). Rarely, the compulsions may be performed to such extreme as to pose medical risk or sequelae (e.g., dermatologic complications of hand washing).

The age of *onset* of OCD is variable, with a bimodal distribution: a male-dominated peak in the preteen years and a female-dominated peak in the third decade of life. The *clinical course* is similarly variable; symptoms may arise at any age, wax and wane, and become exacerbated in times of stress.

The etiology and underlying pathophysiology of OCD are poorly understood. It has been related genetically to Tourette's disorder and commonly occurs with *depression*. Associated disorders include *body dysmorphic disorder* (i.e., preoccupation with a defective body image) and *trichotillomania* (compulsive hair pulling).

Posttraumatic Stress Disorder

Several weeks after surviving exposure to an emotionally traumatic event or events (e.g., combat experience, natural disaster, physical assault, rape), the patient with posttraumatic stress disorder (PTSD) reports *persistent reexperiencing* of the traumatic event, via intrusive thoughts, vivid dreams, or "flashbacks." Other characteristics requisite for the diagnosis include *avoidance* of stimuli associated with the trauma, *hyperarousal* (e.g., increased startle response), and persistence of symptoms for more than 1 month. In many cases, the symptoms may continue for years. Rarely, the syndrome emerges more than 6 months after the traumatic exposure and in such cases is designated *PTSD with delayed onset*.

Patients may present for medical assistance with primary complaints of anxiety or with concerns and questions regarding the neurologic underpinnings of their symptoms. Alternatively, PTSD may develop as a consequence of medical illness or procedures (e.g., amputation or cardiac defibrillation), which by their nature represent profound trauma. Medical settings may serve to trigger reexperiencing phenomena. It is important to be aware of the entity and sensitive to the needs of its sufferers.

Substance Abuse

Anxiety is often poorly tolerated, leading some patients to seek relief through the use or abuse of anxiolytic substances. A patient's reliance on *alcohol*, *benzodiazepines* (BZDs), or any other sedating medication may reflect an unrecognized underlying anxiety disorder. Chronic use of sedating substances can lead to neural irritability and can cause or exacerbate anxiety after withdrawal. It often becomes difficult to differentiate the cause-and-effect relationship between substance abuse and anxiety. Patients with anxiety disorders are 50% more likely to be alcoholic, and, similarly, the prevalence of anxiety disorders is 50% higher in persons who suffer from alcohol abuse or dependence.

DIFFERENTIAL DIAGNOSIS (1,6,8,11)

The medical differential diagnosis of the symptoms and signs associated with anxiety includes many conditions in which there is stimulation of the sympathetic nervous system (Table 226.3). Some reports suggest that undiagnosed medical ailments are responsible for a significant number of psychiatric referrals for "anxiety." Unrecognized arrhythmias, endocrinopathies, and medication reactions may mimic anxiety disorders and vice versa.

Among the psychiatric disorders to be considered in the differential diagnosis of anxiety are the *depressive disorders*. They are among the most critical to recognize because they are common, treatable, carry a high risk of morbidity and mortality when untreated, and frequently coexist with symptoms of anxiety (see Chapter 227). Other psychiatric conditions presenting with anxiety as a prominent component include *psychosis*, *dementias*, and *drug-related disorders*.

WORKUP (1,6–8,11)

The primary care physician's evaluation of anxiety needs to include an assessment for medical causes and psychiatric diagnoses.

Assessment for Medical Causes

The list of possible medical causes is much too extensive to enable a workup that includes every possibility. A reasonable alternative is to focus on any medical conditions for which the patient is already under treatment. This includes a review of

TABLE 226.3

MEDICAL CAUSES OF ANXIETY

Type of Cause	Specific Cause
Cardiovascular	Angina pectoris, arrhythmias, congestive heart failure, hypertension, hypovolemia, myocardial infarction, syncope (of multiple causes), valvular disease, vascular collapse (shock)
Dietary	Caffeinism, monosodium glutamate ("Chinese-restaurant syndrome"), vitamin-deficiency diseases
Drug Related	Akathisia (secondary to antipsychotic drugs), anticholinergic toxicity, digitalis toxicity, hallucinogens, hypotensive agents, stimulants (amphetamines, cocaine, and related drugs), withdrawal syndromes (alcohol or sedative-hypnotics)
Hematologic	Anemias
Immunologic	Anaphylaxis, systemic lupus erythematosus
Metabolic	Hyperadrenalism (Cushing's disease), hyperkalemia, hyperthermia, hyperthyroidism, hypocalcemia, hypoglycemia, hyponatremia, hypothyroidism, menopause, porphyria (acute intermittent)
Neurologic	Encephalopathies (infectious, metabolic, and toxic), essential tremor, intracranial mass lesions, postconcussion syndrome, seizure disorders (especially of the temporal lobe), vertigo
Respiratory	Asthma, chronic obstructive pulmonary disease, pneumonia, pneumothorax, pulmonary edema, pulmonary embolism
Secreting Tumors	Carcinoid, insulinoma, pheochromocytoma

the patient's concerns, fears, and ongoing therapies. In addition, attention is directed toward the most important disorders commonly linked with anxiety, such as *dysrhythmias* (see Chapter 25), *hyperthyroidism* (see Chapter 103), and *drug reactions* or withdrawal (see Chapters 229 and 235). If the patient has a single prominent symptom or constellation of symptoms that implicate a single organ system, it is worthwhile medically to evaluate that focus in detail.

The presence of multiple physical symptoms (six or more), high patient rating of symptom severity, low patient rating of health status, physician perception of the patient encounter as difficult, and age less than 50 years are important clues for an underlying anxiety or depressive disorder. Such easily identified clinical features have been shown to be independent predictors of underlying psychopathology in patients presenting to primary physicians with bodily symptoms. Because there are effective treatments for anxiety disorders, a diagnostic trial of an anxiolytic medication might help to resolve a difficult diagnostic situation. The physician must of course bear in mind that the suppression of anxiety symptoms does not rule out a medical disorder and may even worsen it (e.g., use of BZDs for anxiety accompanying a severe asthma attack).

Assessment for Psychiatric Disorders

The physician should recall that anxiety symptoms are typically conceptualized in three dimensions: psychological, somatic, and behavioral.

Psychological

Patients suffering from an anxiety disorder may complain of somatic manifestations of anxiety but may omit history pertaining to the psychological experience. Therefore, it is important to inquire specifically about psychic manifestations such as fear, panic, the sensation of impending doom, or the impulse to flee. Reviewing the features of the various anxiety disorders sometimes helps the patient to construct a clearer clinical picture, but care must be taken not to prejudice the patient's responses or appear too eager to make a psychiatric diagnosis.

Somatic

One also needs to determine the *onset, quality, intensity,* and *duration* of symptoms, being certain to include a compassionate inquiry into recent life events and situational stressors present at the time that the symptoms emerged.

Behavioral

Identifiable *stimuli or exacerbating factors* should be noted, as well as settings that create apprehension. Development of *avoidant behaviors* should be ascertained. If a particular precipitant is identified, it is helpful to inquire into its origin (e.g., a phobia of dogs arising from a remote history of a dog bite or avoidance of elevators as a consequence of having had a panic attack in one). Often, symptoms may have arisen spontaneously, contributing to the sense that they are autonomous (as in panic disorder or OCD).

Also useful is inquiry into *strategies* used to alleviate the symptoms. This may uncover additional history about substance use, avoidance, or compulsive behaviors. *Family history* is reviewed for similar symptoms, known anxiety disorders, and related disorders such as depression or substance abuse. *History* of childhood school phobia or early patterns of timidity may be informative. Finally, a thorough physical examination is essential, checking for undisclosed sequelae of repetitive behaviors.

PRINCIPLES OF MANAGEMENT (2,6–8,11–27)

The treatment strategies for anxiety include psychotherapeutic and pharmacologic interventions; a combined approach yields the best results.

Psychotherapy

Psychotherapeutic treatments for anxiety help to alleviate symptoms through insight, education, support, and the reconditioning of behavioral patterns. Supportive, insight-oriented, and behavioral psychotherapies may be used individually or jointly. Data from the National Ambulatory Medical Care

Survey of primary care practices show a trend toward the substitution of medication for psychotherapy, a trend that raises concern about the underutilization of psychotherapy. Recognition and utilization of the contributions of psychotherapy to treatment of anxiety are important.

Supportive Psychotherapy

The hallmark of this approach is empathic listening, education, reassurance, encouragement, and guidance. The primary care practitioner frequently performs these functions, whether or not the intervention is labeled as supportive psychotherapy. In the case of anxiety, *empathic listening* helps patients to feel that another human being can appreciate their suffering and, as important, not judge them harshly because of their condition. Patients with anxiety often feel ashamed, characterizing themselves as "weak" or "silly" because of their fears and behaviors. Empathy helps to cut through the shame and loneliness. Listening and encouraging patients to relate their histories can have a cathartic effect. Many patients with anxiety disorders have hidden some or all of their suffering for years.

In addition to empathic listening, *patient education* is crucial. It begins by informing the patient of the diagnosis and explaining its origins, prognosis, and treatment plan. Increased knowledge and understanding is empowering because it promotes a sense of command and confidence while reducing feelings of uncertainty, helplessness, and isolation. Such changes themselves are anxiolytic. Fears of serious somatic illness, "going crazy," and incurable disease are alleviated. *Reassurance* serves to heal only when it addresses what is wrong and what can be done to relieve the anxiety. It must be offered in concert with true empathy and education. Reassurance in the form of "there is nothing serious," even if given in a sympathetic, nonpatronizing manner, will be demoralizing and disappointing if offered perfunctorily. Although a negative medical workup may be reassuring to some patients, the patient with an anxiety disorder is often not relieved, because he or she is still experiencing distinctive, intrusive, and distressing symptoms. Once a strategy has been developed to manage the patient's anxiety, *guidance and encouragement* are helpful to the patient in negotiating treatment trials and supervening situational stresses.

Insight-Oriented Psychotherapy

The objective with this form of therapy is to guide the patient to an understanding of the associations among circumstances, emotions, and symptoms. By exploring feelings, relationships, and actions (both past and present), the patient may develop new insights into his or her emotional makeup. This can help to reduce the symptoms of anxiety and reframe the meaning of anxiety symptoms when they do occur. Insight therapy typically requires frequent and lengthy sessions for optimal results and the skill of a good psychotherapist.

Cognitive–Behavioral Therapy (CBT)

Cognitive–behavioral therapy is especially effective for anxiety patients. It consists in reconditioning or modifying patients' behaviors or the association between a stimulus and response. Techniques include general relaxation-response training (for tolerating anxiety symptoms), *in vivo* exposure and desensitization (for phobias and avoidant behaviors), cognitive therapy (for panic and obsessions), and exposure-response prevention (for OCD). The effectiveness of each of these behavioral techniques is augmented if the patient's anxiety can be held in check. For this reason, the cognitive and behavioral therapies may be particularly well suited for combination with pharmacotherapies. As with insight-oriented psychotherapy, cognitive–behavioral therapy is best conducted by professionals specially trained in this approach.

Relaxation Techniques

Relaxation techniques are of benefit to almost anyone who suffers from anxiety. Deep muscle relaxation, autogenic exercises, and diaphragmatic breathing are taught (see Appendix 226.1). Together, these techniques help to minimize the escalating anxiety that results from autonomic dyscontrol. Their use allows patients to better tolerate moderate anxiety states, abort panic episodes, and use more-aggressive behavioral techniques.

Exposure and Desensitization

Exposure and desensitization entail gradual *reconditioning* of patients by exposing them to feared stimuli in controlled settings that minimize and allow habituation to their anxiety response. In this way, the feared stimuli become better tolerated and avoidant behaviors are eradicated as the association with the anxiety response is weakened. Similarly, the exposure-response prevention technique is used in treating OCD patients. After being exposed to a provocative stimulus, they are helped to resist the urge to perform their compulsions in response to that stimulus. Although tolerating the anxiety, they may use sanctioned relaxation techniques. Gradually, the compulsions are reduced.

Pharmacotherapy

Treatment outcomes for psychotherapy are often enhanced when pharmacotherapy is incorporated into the program. The primary goal of drug therapy is sufficient diminution of symptoms to enable performance of tasks previously impaired by anxiety, including an enhanced ability to benefit from cognitive–behavioral therapy. Patients should be informed that treatment will be of limited duration and will reduce their symptoms but not eradicate them. BZDs are still the most widely used of anxiolytics. Antidepressants, β-adrenergic blocking agents, buspirone, anticonvulsants, and neuroleptics are also used.

Benzodiazepines

For rapid specific relief of anxiety symptoms, the BZDs are regarded as the anxiolytic of choice, superior in efficacy and safety to the barbiturates and the nonbarbiturate sedatives such as meprobamate, ethchlorvynol, and glutethimide. For some patients, BZDs offer substantial or complete relief of anxiety symptoms. For others, they attenuate severe anxiety pending response to other antianxiety therapies. There is wide individual variation in clinical response, plasma levels, and dosage requirements.

Ensuring Proper Use. Overuse and drug seeking from multiple sources occur in a small percentage of patients, although rarely with the intensity and risks associated with opiates, barbiturates, and other sedatives. Nevertheless, the physician should know the patient well before prescribing BZDs and be alert for signs of concurrent alcohol or drug dependence (see Chapters 228 and 235). The efficacy of treatment should be evaluated regularly by follow-up visits, with special attention to proper use. The physician should avoid prescribing by phone, calculate exact quantities required, and remain wary of "lost prescriptions" or other signs of medication misuse. To justify continued treatment, the patient should demonstrate a decrement in anxiety, with enhanced performance or decreased avoidant behavior. Requiring the patient to be seen in person for an appointment at least every 3 months is a good guideline, as is stopping the prescription of the BZD if there is a problem with compliance (e.g., attendance at appointments). BZD overuse is uncommon in the absence of a past history of alcohol or drug abuse but can be a serious problem, at times a consequence of careless prescribing practices and inadequate patient education about proper drug use. If dose requirements escalate, especially if accompanied by addictive behaviors, referral is advised to a specialist experienced in treating this problem.

Side Effects, Tolerance, and Dependence. Side effects include sedation (especially in combination with alcohol or other sedative agents), impaired memory acquisition (including amnesia reported with single-dose triazolam use), and, rarely, disinhibition characterized by increased hostility or aggression. Alcohol and cimetidine slow hepatic BZD metabolism and increase the risk of toxicity.

Daily use of BZDs over time leads to receptor adaptation (*tolerance*) and the development of *physical dependence*. Physical dependence does not, however, imply misuse, abuse, or even loss of benefit. Rather, dependence denotes that a discontinuation syndrome will follow abrupt cessation of therapy. *Withdrawal* is usually accompanied by only mild symptoms but may include rebound anxiety, involuntary movements, insomnia, psychomotor restlessness, and perceptual changes.

Severe withdrawal symptoms are unlikely unless high doses or a high-potency preparation (especially a short-acting one) has been used daily for a prolonged time period and then halted abruptly. In such cases, a *delirium tremens*–like syndrome may develop. *Seizures* have been reported after sudden discontinuation of alprazolam after as short a time as 1 to 2 months of maintenance therapy. For less potent or long-acting BZDs, the risk of a severe abstinence syndrome is less. Chronic daily treatment is best discontinued by tapering doses over several weeks.

Selection of Agent. The available BZDs appear to be equally effective for the management of generalized anxiety symptoms when equipotent doses are used. In the future, one may see new BZDs with greater treatment specificity because heterogeneity of brain BZD receptors has been demonstrated. For now, the essential differences among BZDs are in potency and pharmacokinetics (Table 226.4). These factors determine suitability for single-dose and maintenance use and the risk of physical dependence and withdrawal.

For *single-dose use*, the desirable pharmacokinetic properties are rapid rate of onset and offset. Speed of absorption from the gastrointestinal tract is the most important factor determining onset. Capacity to traverse the blood–brain barrier is also a factor; the more lipophilic it is, the more quickly the drug enters the central nervous system. Lipophilicity also governs the rate of clinical offset by determining how rapidly the drug is redistributed into lipid stores after a single dose. Serum half-life is not relevant to the duration of action of single-dose use. *Diazepam* is rapidly absorbed and very lipid soluble, giving rapid onset and offset when used in single-dose fashion. Relatively rapid onset is usually desirable in situations in which single-dose use is prescribed.

For *maintenance use*, a drug's serum half-life is the pertinent parameter, affected by liver function and whether hepatic metabolites are active or inactive. Drugs with a short half-life are simply converted to water-soluble glucuronides and rapidly cleared by the kidneys. Their disadvantage is the potential for anxiousness and even mild withdrawal symptoms between doses. The longer–half-life agents are more likely to accumulate. However, because of the development of drug tolerance, there is little additional risk of clinically important central nervous system suppression among most users of long-acting agents. The exceptions are the elderly and those with hepatocellular disease, in whom the use of long-acting agents can lead to overwhelming drug accumulation that causes excessive sedation, drowsiness, and psychomotor impairment.

Determination of Dose. Dose must ultimately be determined empirically on a case-by-case basis. It is most prudent to begin with low doses and titrate up as necessary. Most patients suffering from anxiety of lesser intensity than panic will not benefit from doses greater than 8 mg/d of lorazepam or its equivalent. Starting doses should typically not exceed the equivalent of 4 mg/d of lorazepam in young, otherwise healthy adults who are BZD naive. In the elderly, starting and maximum doses should be approximately halved (see later discussion). Steady state takes longer to achieve using drugs with a long half-life, an important consideration when deciding how often to adjust dose. A clinically useful rule of thumb is that steady state is 90% achieved after five drug half-lives.

Antidepressants

Serotonin selective reuptake inhibitors (SSRIs) and *serotonin norepinephrine reuptake inhibitors (SNRIs)* are often used as first-line agents in the treatment of anxiety. They are among the most effective agents at eradicating the core symptoms of such anxiety conditions as panic disorder, social anxiety disorder, generalized anxiety disorder, PTSD, and OCD. As in

---

TABLE 226.4

PHARMACOKINETIC PROPERTIES OF COMMONLY USED BENZODIAZEPINES

Drug	Approximate Dose Equivalence (mg)	Relative Rapidity of Effect	Half-Life (hr)
Alprazolam (Xanax)	0.5	Fast/intermediate	12–15
Chlordiazepoxide (Librium)	10	Intermediate	5–30
Clonazepam (Klonopin)	0.25	Fast/intermediate	15–50
Clorazepate (Tranxene)	7.5	Fast	30–200
Diazepam (Valium)	5	Fastest	20–100
Lorazepam (Ativan)	1	Intermediate	10–20
Oxazepam (Serax)	15	Slower	5–15

depression, their beneficial effects are usually delayed for several weeks (see Chapter 227). Tricyclic antidepressants (TCAs) and the monoamine oxidase inhibitors (MAOIs) are generally used in the treatment of refractory patients.

Initiation of Therapy. Although the antidepressants are "first line" in terms of their efficacy, therapy is often initiated with BZDs to offer some immediate relief. Concurrently, or after anxiety symptoms are attenuated, antidepressant medication may be added. Once the antidepressant agent has become effective, some patients become entirely asymptomatic. In such instances, the BZD may be tapered down and even discontinued. In anxiety disorders, antidepressants are initiated with low doses (e.g., imipramine, 10 mg/d; fluoxetine, 10 mg/d) because brief symptom exacerbation may occur in some patients. Full antidepressant doses, if tolerated, are usually necessary. The recommended dose, for example, of paroxetine in the treatment of panic disorder is 40 mg/d.

Use in Specific Conditions. For *panic disorder*, several SSRIs (*sertraline, fluoxetine, paroxetine, paroxetine controlled release,* and *venlafaxine extended release*) have received U.S. Food and Drug Administration (FDA) indications for the treatment of *panic disorder*. There is much evidence supporting the use of the other SSRIs as well. TCAs and MAOIs have a long history of effectiveness in panic disorder. SSRIs and SNRIs may also be of utility in the treatment of generalized anxiety disorder (GAD), especially if panic attacks are present. Extended-release venlafaxine has demonstrated both short-term and long-term efficacy in persons with GAD and panic disorder.

Patients with *posttraumatic stress disorder* respond best to the initial use of antidepressants, with continuation based on treatment response and the constellation of symptoms. *OCD* patients respond especially well to SSRIs. There is some suggestion that the obsessions respond preferentially, whereas compulsions are best addressed through behavioral interventions combined with medications.

Like the other anxiety disorders, *social anxiety disorder* has been shown to be effectively treated by most of the SSRIs, with sertraline, venlafaxine extended release, paroxetine, and paroxetine controlled release gaining FDA approval. Again, MAOIs have a long history of being particularly effective for social anxiety disorder, although their safety and side-effect profile restrict their use to treatment-resistant cases.

Side Effects. See Chapter 227.

Buspirone

Buspirone is a non-BZD anxiolytic that acts as a partial serotonergic agonist and has mild anxiolytic and antidepressant effects. Because of its benign side-effect profile (nonaddicting and no withdrawal), buspirone is a reasonable alternative to BZDs in cases in which chronic anxiolysis is required, especially when substance abuse or noncompliance is a concern. Risk from overdose is low, and the drug is well tolerated. Its anxiolytic effects are modest compared with those of the BZDs, and the onset of action may take weeks, rendering the drug ineffective for single-dose use and of little help to patients with severe symptoms. Some efficacy has been reported in OCD. As a mild anxiolytic that may be taken frequently and safely, it may benefit patients with mild generalized anxiety or adjustment disorders. Treatment is initiated at doses of 5 mg three times a day and adjusted weekly in dose increments of 5 mg/d. In patients requiring more than 20 mg three times a day, referral to a specialist is recommended.

Beta-Blockers

β-Adrenergic blocking agents blunt the peripheral catecholamine-mediated manifestations of anxiety. As such, they are very useful on a short-term, as-needed basis for performance anxiety and stage fright (e.g., propranolol 10 to 20 mg as needed). In the case of a special performance, it is suggested that the patient try a test dose a few days earlier to determine both efficacy and side effects. Large doses may blunt psychomotor responses. For generally anxious patients with prominent somatic manifestations of adrenergic excess (e.g., tremor, palpitations), longer-acting β-blockers (e.g., atenolol, 50 mg/d) facilitate symptom control when used alone or in combination with BZDs. They should be used with caution, if at all, in patients with asthma, heart failure, or heart block (see Chapters 32 and 48). Moreover, they may worsen symptoms if there is an underlying depression (see Chapter 227).

Anticonvulsants

Several anticonvulsants have been shown to play an important role in the treatment of most of the anxiety disorders. Although they have yielded inconsistent results in research trials, the rationale for their use in the clinical setting is supported by neurobiologic underpinnings that make anticonvulsants a likely alternative to BZDs. *Gabapentin* and *tiagabine* have the widest use in clinic populations, usually titrated upward from their lowest dose as tolerated, and as needed for relief of anxiety.

Neuroleptics

Notwithstanding first-line interventions as described in the foregoing, approximately 40% to 70% of patients fail to reach responder status after acute treatment, with an even greater proportion remaining at least somewhat symptomatic. The rapid antianxiety and antiirritability effects of the *atypical antipsychotics* have made them relatively popular among clinicians in the treatment of refractory anxiety patients. Furthermore, in anxiety disorders, atypical antipsychotics (e.g., *aripiprazole, clozapine, olanzapine, paliperidone, quetiapine, risperidone,* and *ziprasidone*) can be effective at a fraction of the doses necessary to manage psychotic disorders. This drastically reduces such side effects as tardive dyskinesia that conventional neuroleptics pose at higher doses. Nevertheless, patients should be closely monitored for some potentially serious side effects such as prolactin elevation, weight gain, and metabolic syndromes.

Available atypical agents differ markedly in their receptor profiles; choosing among them is based mainly on their side effects, avoiding the most unpleasant side effect for that particular patient (see Chapter 173). Currently, these agents, used either as monotherapy or in combination with traditional agents, cannot be considered first-line treatment, but they do have a place for patients who remain symptomatic or fail to respond to conventional agents and/or are considered treatment refractory or intolerant. Given the notorious sensitivity to side effects of anxious patients, clinicians should favor low doses on treatment initiation and slow titration while dosing these agents.

Anxiolytic Pharmacotherapy in the Elderly

Because drug metabolism is slowed in the elderly, excessive sedation is a risk with anxiolytic therapy, especially with the use of long-acting agents.

Benzodiazepines. In most instances, nighttime use of a short-acting agent that has no active metabolites and in patients whose metabolism is relatively unaffected by aging is preferred. Lorazepam and oxazepam fulfill these requirements. Their elimination by hepatic conjugation to a water-soluble glucuronide for renal excretion changes little with age. Lorazepam is the faster in onset; oxazepam's onset is gradual. Their disadvantages include the need for frequent dosing if continuous anxiolysis is desired and rebound anxiety and insomnia if they are discontinued abruptly after prolonged use. Initial oxazepam dose is 10 mg; for lorazepam, it is 0.5 mg. Both are usually given before bed. Intake should be limited to short (5- to 10-day) courses or occasional as-needed use.

For more sustained anxiolysis, a BZD with a longer effective half-life may be required (Table 226.4). However, elimination of active drug metabolites lengthens with age, markedly prolonging drug half-life (e.g., from 20 to 90 hours for diazepam). Accumulation of active metabolites can cause diminished alertness and impair memory acquisition, mimicking dementia. Excessive sedation may cause a fall with serious injury—the risk of hip fracture rises markedly with the use of long-acting BZDs in the elderly. Initial doses should be small (e.g., the equivalent of 2 to 5 mg/d of diazepam) and increased slowly and cautiously. It may take up to 2 weeks to achieve steady-state levels after a change in dose.

Antipsychotics. In the elderly, anxiety accompanied by agitation or specific psychotic manifestations may require short-term antipsychotic therapy. The atypical antipsychotics have become first-line agents for this indication. A small dose of a high-potency typical antipsychotic such as *haloperidol* (Haldol) or *fluphenazine* (Prolixin) is another option. Lower-potency agents (e.g., chlorpromazine, thioridazine, perphenazine) necessitate the use of higher doses and increase the risk of hypotensive, cardiovascular, and anticholinergic side effects.

Antidepressants. Of the antidepressants, *SSRIs* are the best tolerated (see Chapter 227). Of the *TCAs* with anxiolytic activity, those with low anticholinergic and antiadrenergic side effects (e.g., nortriptyline) are preferred. Because antidepressant metabolism slows with age, one should start with half the usual dose and titrate up slowly.

β-Blockers. β-Blocker use requires particular caution, given the prevalence of congestive heart failure, heart block, and obstructive lung disease in the elderly and their susceptibility to such side effects as cognitive blunting, nightmares, and depression.

THERAPEUTIC RECOMMENDATIONS AND INDICATIONS FOR REFERRAL
(2,8,11,15,16,21,23–25)

General Guidelines

- Begin with supportive psychotherapy that includes explanation, empathic listening, meaningful reassurance, guidance, and encouragement.
- Teach relaxation techniques for the patient willing to use them (see Appendix 226.1).
- Consider referral for psychotherapy when there is emotional upheaval or disabling symptoms. Cognitive–behavioral

therapy is perhaps the most effective of the psychotherapies for ameliorating pathologic anxiety.
- Supplement psychotherapeutic measures with anxiolytic drug therapy to improve the patient's ability to perform daily activities previously impaired by anxiety. In most instances, use only in an adjunctive role for a limited duration. If BZD therapy is used, advise the patient of the risk of physical dependence. Inform the patient that drug treatment is likely to reduce symptoms but not eradicate them.
- Refer if there is evidence of substance abuse, either as an etiologic factor or as a mode of self-treatment.

Situational Anxiety and Adjustment Disorder

- Initiate supportive psychotherapy, including the identification of specific provocative stressors and their association with the onset of symptoms.
- If distress from anxiety impairs daily functioning, begin a short course (up to 5 days) of BZD therapy (e.g., clonazepam, 0.5 mg twice daily).
- If the distress represents one of many such episodes in a pattern of emotional upheaval, refer for insight-oriented therapy. Also refer if symptoms continue beyond the stressful period or worsen despite treatment.

Generalized Anxiety Disorder

- Initiate supportive psychotherapy and consider insight-oriented therapy to help diminish the role of psychosocial stressors.
- Consider a short course of BZD therapy for periods of exacerbation (e.g., alprazolam, 0.5 mg three times a day for up to 5 days).
- Prescribe an SSRI if there is a history of associated panic attacks or depression; e.g., begin with venlafaxine extended release (Effexor-XR), 37.5 mg twice daily, and advance the dose as tolerated to 150 mg twice daily; alternatively, paroxetine at a target dose of 40 mg daily can be used.
- Avoid chronic BZD therapy due to risk of dependence. If the patient is coming off long-term therapy, taper over several weeks according to the patient's ability to tolerate decreases. Monitor for any withdrawal symptoms (e.g., tinnitus, perceptual changes, involuntary movements).
- Consider a trial of buspirone if chronic anxiolytic therapy is desired. Begin with 5 mg three times a day and gradually advance to a maximum of 60 mg/d. Risks of physiologic dependence and withdrawal are nil, but potency is low, and it may take weeks to notice any effect.
- Refer patients with disabling chronic anxiety for psychiatric care.

Panic Disorder

- Refer patients with prominent phobic behavior and those with suicidal ideation.
- Screen for suicidality (see Chapter 227), especially if the patient is despondent; refer urgently if there is concern.
- Use pharmacologic therapy to achieve control and minimize phobic avoidance and depression. Begin therapy with a low dose of a serotonin-reuptake inhibitor (e.g., escitalopram, 10 mg daily, or paroxetine, 10 mg daily). If agitation is not

increased, proceed gradually to full antidepressant doses (e.g., escitalopram, 20 mg/d, or paroxetine, 40 mg/d).

- In situations in which the cost benefits of a generic TCA override the better tolerability of an SSRI, start with a small "test" dose (e.g., imipramine, 10 mg at bedtime, and proceed gradually as tolerated to 100 to 200 mg at bedtime). The added costs of cardiac monitoring and taking blood levels of the TCAs must be factored into the cost–benefit equation.
- Alternatively, an MAOI antidepressant may be prescribed, but dietary restriction and expertise in its use are required (see Chapter 227).
- If rapid relief is sought due to the presence of disabling phobic behavior, start with a potent BZD (e.g., alprazolam, 0.25 to 0.5 mg four times a day, or clonazepam, 0.5 mg at bedtime or twice daily), pending the onset of benefit from antidepressant therapy.
- After a period of well-being, taper BZD medication to the lowest possible maintenance dose or proceed to discontinuation.
- Weigh continued BZD use against the risk of dependence. The use of potent BZDs poses risks of dependence and severe withdrawal. Taper slowly over several weeks when discontinuing therapy that has been continuous for more than 6 weeks.
- For patients requiring longer-term maintenance therapy, it is important to continue the antidepressant medication at its full acute-phase dose.

Social Anxiety Disorder

- Refer for cognitive–behavioral therapy.
- Prescribe a BZD on an as-needed, single-dose basis to help attenuate anxiety, decrease avoidance, and facilitate daily functioning and behavioral therapy.
- Prescribe a low-dose SSRI (e.g., sertraline, 25 mg in the morning, or paroxetine controlled release, 12.5 mg in the morning), and proceed gradually to full antidepressant doses (e.g., sertraline, 150 mg in the morning, or paroxetine controlled release, 50 mg in the morning).
- For patients whose performances are compromised by ordinary "stage fright," consider a trial of a β-blocker (e.g., propranolol, 10 mg, up to 20 mg four times a day) on an as-needed basis. Give a preperformance trial dose to be sure performance is not compromised by the medication.

Specific Phobias

- Refer for cognitive–behavioral therapy.

- Consider rapidly acting single-dose BZD therapy (e.g., alprazolam, 0.25 to 0.5 mg, or diazepam, 10 mg) on an as-needed basis to provide symptomatic control in anxiety-provoking situations and to facilitate behavioral therapy.

Obsessive–Compulsive Disorder

- Refer for cognitive–behavioral therapy.
- Initiate pharmacologic therapy with an SSRI.
- Refer to an experienced psychopharmacologist for further management of the drug treatment program.

Posttraumatic Stress Disorder

- Refer to a psychiatrist specializing in the treatment of such patients. Most programs begin with an SSRI. Mood stabilizers may be helpful for prominent irritability or anger. BZDs may sometimes be helpful in the short term but must be used with caution because of the risk of substance abuse in this vulnerable population of patients.
- Refer to an experienced psychotherapist. Three psychotherapy techniques—exposure therapy, cognitive therapy, and anxiety management—are considered to be the most useful in the treatment of PTSD. Expert therapists make distinctions among the techniques, depending on which specific type of symptom presentation is most prominent. Insight-oriented psychotherapy helps to overcome emotional memories of the traumatic event; behavioral techniques may also be of benefit.

Treatment of the Elderly

- Initiate supportive psychotherapy. Consider referral to an experienced psychotherapist to assess other options, including cognitive–behavioral therapy.
- Reduce starting doses of medications by one half of the usual adult dose.
- When using BZDs for short-term anxiolysis, prescribe lorazepam or oxazepam.
- For chronic anxiolysis, use longer–half-life agents with caution and at reduced doses and dose intervals.
- If antidepressants are indicated for anxiolysis, consider an SSRI (e.g., fluoxetine) or an MAOI (see Chapter 227).
- If agitation, "sundowning," or psychotic features accompany anxiety, prescribe small doses of an atypical neuroleptic (e.g., risperidone, 0.5 mg once or twice daily).

Annotated Bibliography

1. American Psychiatric Association. Diagnostic and statistical manual of mental disorders, 4th ed. Washington, DC: Author, 1994. (*The standard for diagnosis.*)
2. APA Steering Committee on Practice Guidelines, ed. American Psychiatric Association practice guidelines for the treatment of psychiatric disorders compendium 2002. Washington, DC: American Psychiatric Publishing, 2002. (*Consensus guidelines.*)
3. Greenberg PE, Sisitsky T, Kessler RC, et al. The economic burden of anxiety disorders in the 1990s. J Clin Psychiatry 1999;60:427. (*A societal perspective on the cost of anxiety disorders.*)
4. Harman JS, Rollman BL, Hanusa, et al. Physician office visits of adults for anxiety disorders in the United States, 1985–1998. J Gen Intern Med 2002;17:165. (*Documents undertreatment and underrecognition.*)
5. Kronke K, Jackson JL, Chamberlain J. Depressive and anxiety disorders in patients presenting with physical complaints: clinical predictors and outcome. Am J Med 1997;103:339. (*Identifies a set of clinical clues that are independent predictors of underlying psychopathology in patients presenting with physical complaints.*)
6. Roy-Byrne PP, Wagner A. Primary care perspectives on generalized anxiety disorder. J Clin Psychiatry 2004;65(Suppl 13):20. (*A very useful clinical discussion.*)
7. Roy-Byrne PP, Stein MB, Russo J, et al. Panic disorder in the primary care setting: comorbidity, disability, service utilization, and treatment. J Clin Psychiatry 1990;60:492. (*Discusses improved treatment interventions for decreasing both the disability and potentially inappropriate medical service utilization.*)

8. Stein MB, McQuaid JR, Laffaye C, et al. Social phobia in the primary care medical setting. J Family Pract 1999;48:514. (*Discusses the underdiagnosis and undertreatment of a disorder that frequently presents to the primary care physician.*)

9. Weissman MM, Klerman GL, Markowitz JS, et al. Suicidal ideation and suicide attempts in panic disorder and attacks. N Engl J Med 1989;321:1209. (*Risk increased and was independent of other possible precipitants; the adjusted odds ratio was 2.6.*)

10. Yehuda R. Post-traumatic stress disorder. N Engl J Med 2002;346:108. (*An excellent review; 55 references.*)

11. Apter JT, Allen LA. Buspirone: future directions. J Clin Psychopharmacol 1999;19:86. (*A review of its clinical uses in psychiatric illness.*)

12. Brown RL, Brown RL, Saunders LA, et al. Physicians' decisions to prescribe benzodiazepines for nervousness and insomnia. J Gen Intern Med 1997;12:44. (*Reveals common misconceptions and pitfalls in the use of benzodiazepines.*)

13. Bulow K. Management of psychosis and agitation in elderly patients: a primary care perspective. J Clin Psychiatry 1999;60(Suppl 13):22. (*Presents treatment strategies for agitation in elderly patients.*)

14. Gelenberg AJ, Lydiard RB, Rudolph RL, et al. Efficacy of venlafaxine extended-release capsules in nondepressed outpatients with generalized anxiety disorder: a 6-month randomized controlled trial. JAMA 2000;283:3082. (*Evidence of efficacy in a well-designed study.*)

15. Gorman J, Shear MK, Cowley D, et al. American Psychiatric Association. Practice guideline for the treatment of patients with panic disorder. Am J Psychiatry 1998;155(Suppl):1. (*Practice guidelines developed by psychiatrists who coordinate the overall care of patients with panic disorder.*)

16. Ipser JC, Carey P, Dhansay Y, et al. Pharmacotherapy augmentation strategies in treatment-resistant anxiety disorders. Cochrane Database Syst Rev 2006;4:CD005473. (*An evidence-based review.*)

17. Mavissakalian M, Perel JM. Protective effects of imipramine maintenance treatment in panic disorder with agoraphobia. Am J Psychiatry 1992;149:1053. (*Data confirming the need for maintenance treatment to protect against relapse.*)

18. Mula M, Pini S, Cassano G. The role of anticonvulsant drugs in anxiety disorders: a critical review of the evidence. J Clin Psychopharmacol 2007;27:263. (*A review of this important emerging class of drugs.*)

19. Pollack MH. Unmet needs in the treatment of anxiety disorders. Psychopharmacol Bull 2003;37(Suppl 3):31. (*An excellent discussion*)

20. Roy-Byrne P, Stein M, Bystritsky A, et al. Pharmacotherapy of panic disorder: guidelines for the family physician. J Am Board Family Pract 1998;11:282. (*Practical clinical care by the primary care physician.*)

21. Stein DJ, Bandelow B, Hollander E, et al. World Council of Anxiety. WCA recommendations for the long-term treatment of posttraumatic stress disorder. CNS Spectr 2003;8(8 Suppl 1):31. (*Consensus guidelines.*)

22. Stein MB, Liebowitz MR, Lydiard RB, et al. Paroxetine treatment of generalized social phobia (social anxiety disorder). JAMA 1998;280:708. (*Data on the first medication approved by the U.S. Food and Drug Administration for the treatment of social phobia.*)

23. Treatment of panic disorder: the state of the art. J Clin Psychiatry 1997;58(Suppl 2). (*An entire supplement on current psychotherapeutic and psychopharmacologic treatment options.*)

24. Treatment of posttraumatic stress disorder: the expert consensus guideline series. J Clin Psychiatry 1999;60(Suppl 16):1. (*An entire journal volume devoted to treatment strategies.*)

25. Van Ameringen M, Allgulander C, Bandelow B, et al. World Council of Anxiety recommendations for the long-term treatment of social phobia. CNS Spectr 2003;8(8 Suppl 1):40. (*Consensus guidelines.*)

26. van Peski-Oosterbaan AS, Spinhoven P, Van Rood Y, et al. Cognitive–behavioral therapy for noncardiac chest pain: a randomized trial. Am J Med 1999;106:424. (*A well-designed example of the successful application of cognitive–behavioral therapy.*)

27. Williams DDR, McBride A. Benzodiazepines: time for reassessment. Br J Psychiatry 1998;173:361. (*An editorial on their proper place in the treatment armamentarium.*)

APPENDIX 226.1: STRATEGIES FOR STRESS MANAGEMENT

WILLIAM E. MINICHIELLO

Stress is not harmful when managed effectively. With the increased awareness of the impact of stress on the body has come a variety of stress-reducing techniques derived from behavior therapy. Stress management training enables the patient to condition his or her body to cope more adaptively with stress or anxiety. As part of a comprehensive treatment program, the primary care physician may choose to train the patient in one or more of the self-regulatory procedures. Relaxation training is by far the most effective of the procedures.

Before proceeding to train the patient in relaxation as a self-control procedure, the physician should advise reduction or elimination of caffeine from the patient's diet because relaxation training is aimed at lowering the patient's autonomic arousal level and caffeine augments arousal.

Progressive deep muscle relaxation, autogenic training, and diaphragmatic breathing represent the major techniques practical for use in the primary care setting.

PROGRESSIVE DEEP MUSCLE RELAXATION

Progressive deep muscle relaxation is probably the most extensively used and most effective relaxation technique for the treatment of anxiety- and stress-related problems. A brief modified version can be taught to the patient in one session. The rationale for the technique is the view that anxiety and relaxation are mutually exclusive; that is, anxiety cannot be experienced when the muscles are relaxed.

Progressive deep muscle relaxation is a simple procedure contrasting tension with relaxation. Because a person generally has very little awareness of the sensation of relaxation, the patient is asked first to tense a set of muscles as hard as he or she can until he or she can feel tension in the muscles. Then those muscles are relaxed and one tries to become aware of ("to feel internally") the difference between tension and relaxation.

This relaxation technique entails the systematic focus of attention on specific gross muscle groups throughout the body. The patient is instructed to tense each muscle group for 10 to 15 seconds, after which he or she is told to let go of the tension in the muscles, observe the difference, and relax the muscles. The sequence of tensing the muscles, letting go of the tension, and noting the difference between tension and relaxation is systematically applied to a host of muscle groups, starting at the head and ending at the toes (Table 226.5).

AUTOGENIC TRAINING

Autogenic training is a relaxation technique composed of a set of exercises that are intended to induce heaviness and warmth in the muscles through mental imagery.

Autogenic training typically involves the patient sitting comfortably in an armchair in a quiet room with the eyes closed. Verbal formulas are introduced (e.g., "my arm is heavy"), and the patient is instructed to visualize and feel the relaxation of the muscle being focused on while silently repeating and passively concentrating on that formula. The formulas, which consist of verbal somatic suggestions, are intended to facilitate concentration and "mental contact" with the parts of the body indicated by the formula.

Training consists of six psychophysiologic exercises, which are practiced several times a day. The training begins with the theme of heaviness (e.g., "my arm feels heavy and relaxed"). The second group of formulas involve warmth (e.g., "my arm feels warm and relaxed"). After warmth training, the patient

TABLE 226.5

PROGRESSIVE DEEP MUSCLE RELAXATION INSTRUCTIONS TO PATIENTS

Practice is to be done while sitting in a chair with your back straight, head on a line with your back, both feet on the floor, and hands resting on your lap. Each muscle is to be tightened, held in tightened position for 15–20 seconds, and then slowly let go while you study the difference between tension and relaxation.

Forehead. Wrinkle up your forehead by arching your eyebrows and creasing your forehead, hold the tension, and then slowly let go of the tension.

Eyes. Squeeze your eyes together tightly, hold the tension, and then slowly let go of the tension.

Nose. Wrinkle up your nose and spread your nostrils, hold the tension, and then slowly let go of the tension.

Face. Put a forced smile on your face and spread your face, hold the tension, and then slowly let go of the tension.

Tongue. Push your tongue hard against the roof of your mouth, hold the tension, and then slowly let go of the tension.

Jaws. Clench your jaws together tightly, hold the tension, and then slowly let go of the tension.

Lips. Pucker up your lips and spread them, hold the tension, and then slowly let go of the tension.

Neck. Tighten the muscles of your neck by pulling your chin in and shrugging up your shoulders, hold the tension, and then slowly let go of the tension.

Right Arm. Tense your right arm and hand by stretching them out in front of you and clenching your fist tightly, hold the tension, and then slowly let go of the tension.

Left Arm. Tense your left arm and hand by stretching them out in front of you, and then slowly let go of the tension.

Right Leg. Extend your right leg in front of you (at the height of the chair seat), tense your thigh and leg by pointing your toes inward toward your face, hold the tension, and then slowly let go of the tension.

Left Leg. Extend your left leg in front of you, tense your thigh and leg by pointing your toes inward toward your face, hold the tension, and then slowly let go of the tension.

Upper Back. Tense your back muscles by sitting slightly forward in the chair and bending your elbows and trying to get them to touch each other behind your back, hold the tension, and then slowly let go of the tension.

Chest. Tense your chest muscles by pulling your stomach in and thrusting your chest upward and outward, hold the tension, and then slowly let go of the tension.

Stomach. Tense your stomach muscles, making them hard by pushing your stomach out, hold the tension, and then slowly let go of the tension.

Buttocks and Thighs. Tense your buttocks and thighs by placing your feet squarely on the floor, pointing your toes into the floor, and forcing your heels to remain on the floor while pushing forward, hold the tension, and then slowly let go of the tension.

Practice should be engaged in twice daily for a period of 12–15 minutes. Mastery of the technique should be achieved after 2–4 weeks of twice-daily practice.

continues with passive concentration on cardiac activity (e.g., "my heartbeat feels calm and regular"). The fourth exercise focuses on breathing and respiration. In the next exercise, the patient focuses on warmth in the chest and abdomen, and in the last exercise the focus is passive concentration on cooling of the forehead.

In modern practice, the time and the six standard exercises have been condensed so that a whole round can be practiced in a very brief period of between 5 and 10 minutes. In this condensed version, the autogenic training phrases are focused primarily on the physiologic aspect used in the training, inter- spersed with general suggestions for relaxation. Each phrase is said slowly, allowing time for the patient to begin to feel some awareness of the effect of the suggestion (Table 226.6).

DIAPHRAGMATIC BREATHING

The quickest and simplest method of relaxation is to breathe slowly and deeply from the belly. Diaphragmatic breathing is an effective means of coping with and reducing stress.

TABLE 226.6

AUTOGENIC TRAINING INSTRUCTIONS TO PATIENTS

Practice is to be done while sitting in a soft, comfortable chair with your eyes closed. As attention is called to specific groups of muscles, try to *visualize* and *feel* the relaxation of those muscles. Try to let *happen* what is being suggested. Repeat each formula two or three times.

My forehead and scalp feel heavy, limp, loose, and relaxed.

My eyes and nose feel heavy, limp, loose, and relaxed.

My face and jaws feel heavy, limp, loose, and relaxed.

My neck, shoulders, and back feel heavy, limp, loose, and relaxed.

My arms and hands feel heavy, limp, loose, and relaxed.

My chest, solar plexus, and the central part of my body feel quiet, calm, comfortable, and relaxed.

My stomach feels heavy, limp, loose, and relaxed.

My buttocks, thighs, calves, ankles, and toes feel quiet, heavy, limp, loose, and relaxed.

My whole body feels quiet, heavy, limp, and relaxed.

Practice should be engaged in twice daily for a period of 6–8 minutes. Mastery of the technique should be achieved after 1–3 weeks of twice-daily practice.

TABLE 226.7

DIAPHRAGMATIC BREATHING INSTRUCTIONS TO PATIENTS

While sitting or lying down with a pillow at the small of your back:
1. Breathe in slowly and deeply by pushing your stomach out.
2. Say the word "relax" silently to yourself prior to exhaling.
3. Exhale slowly, letting your stomach come in.
4. Repeat the entire procedure 10 times consecutively, with emphasis on slow, deep breaths.

Practice should take place five times per day, with 10 consecutive diaphragmatic breaths each sitting. Mastery should be achieved after 1–2 weeks of daily practice.

For centuries, students of yoga and Zen have been aware that a mastery of breathing could slow heart rate, lower blood pressure, and calm the body. Diaphragmatic breathing involves parasympathetic nervous system stimulation. Diaphragmatic breathing prevents the possibility of hyperventilation and, after 50 to 60 seconds of such breathing, brings a feeling of quiescence to the body and reduction in bodily symptoms of stress.

Training in diaphragmatic breathing can be done either sitting or lying down. In either position, a pillow should be placed at the small of the back to force the belly out. Breathing should begin by pushing the stomach out as inhalation takes place slowly and deeply. Care should be taken to minimize the movement of the chest with each inhalation. The word "relax" should be said silently before exhaling, and the stomach should fall with exhalation. While breathing in, the stomach should be pushed out; while breathing out, the stomach should come in (Table 226.7).

CHAPTER 227 ■ APPROACH TO THE PATIENT WITH DEPRESSION

JOHN J. WORTHINGTON III AND SCOTT L. RAUCH

Most patients with depression present to primary care physicians rather than psychiatrists, often complaining of somatic symptoms such as fatigue or disturbed sleep. The frequency, treatability, and potentially serious consequences of depression make its diagnosis and management high priorities for the primary care physician. Unfortunately, the diagnosis is often not made. Sometimes it is not evident because the symptoms may masquerade as a variety of psychiatric or somatic conditions. Moreover, the stigma of psychiatric diagnosis can impede recognition of depressive illness by both patients and physicians. The primary care physician needs to be vigilant in watching for manifestations of depression and prepared to initiate further evaluation and basic treatment when symptoms or signs are encountered.

PATHOPHYSIOLOGY AND CLINICAL PRESENTATION (1–13)

Mechanisms

The purported mechanisms of depression include psychodynamic, cognitive, genetic, neuroendocrine, and neurotransmitter determinants. Depression most likely represents a complex combination of these elements. Genetic factors and/or early childhood experiences may render persons more susceptible to depression. Neurotransmitter and neurohumoral elements probably serve as important effector pathways for the development of symptoms.

Psychodynamic origins are believed to involve difficulties with formation and maintenance of self-esteem, which may occur from having hypercritical parents or being abused. In addition, growing up in an emotionally unresponsive environment may compromise learning ways effectively to cope with situational stresses. Suffering loss or failure as an adult is likely to be difficult, poorly responded to, and capable of reawakening prior painful feelings of inadequacy and worthlessness that lead to depression. Rigid dysfunctional defenses may be erected in an attempt to minimize the chances of loss or failure.

The cognitive perspective views depression as the consequence rather than as the origin of negative or distorted thinking. Subscribing to inflexible rules of conduct and unattainable goals can be a setup for failure and loss of self-esteem. Setbacks are viewed as a reflection of one's unworthiness and inadequacy.

Genetic determinants have been discovered from studies of twins, chromosomes, and pedigrees. In some pedigrees, there appears to be a dominant gene with incomplete penetrance that confers risk. A family history of affective disease is commonly elicited. Major depression is up to three times more common among first-degree relatives of people with the disorder than in the general population.

Neurotransmitter theories of depression began with the finding that reserpine could induce depression and monoamine oxidase inhibitors could reverse it. This led to the identification of altered neurotransmitter metabolism as an important biochemical concomitant of depression and to the discovery of new antidepressant drugs, each increasing the availability of a major central neurotransmitter (e.g., norepinephrine, serotonin, or acetylcholine), usually by selective inhibition of reuptake.

Neuroendocrine hypotheses derive from the observation that most neurovegetative manifestations of depression (changes in appetite, libido, diurnal rhythms) involve hypothalamic functions. In addition, links between neurotransmitter release and neurohormone activity have been identified. Corticotropin-releasing hormone is believed to play an important role, resulting in hypercortisolism. Early-morning awakening, reflecting an abnormal advance in circadian rhythm, may be one consequence.

Psychological and Somatic Manifestations

Depression's clinical presentation includes a host of psychological and bodily complaints.

Psychological Manifestations

Sadness is a very common symptom. Irritability, discouragement, loss of interest, worry, frustration, and decreased libido are the major dysphoric manifestations and may occur in the absence of overt sadness (Table 227.1). Some patients become preoccupied with physical complaints, such as pain or bowel dysfunction. Others exhibit changes in memory, concentration, or self-image. Diurnal mood variation is characteristic, with symptoms often worse in the morning and improving as the day progresses.

Depressed affect can be subtle, and at times the patient's sadness only becomes evident on talking with the physician. As depression worsens, psychomotor abnormalities may appear. Although psychomotor retardation, with slowed speech and a long latency before the patient answers questions, has been

---

TABLE 227.1

CLINICAL PRESENTATION OF DEPRESSIVE SYNDROMES

Psychological Symptoms and Signs
Mood sad, "blue," and "down"
Depressed affect
Anxiety
Irritability or anger
Anhedonia (lack of pleasure)
Loss of interest in environment
Loss of interest in activities
Loss of interest in sex (decreased libido)
Social withdrawal
Guilt (may be delusional)
Poor self-esteem
Self-deprecatory thoughts
Poor concentration or indecisiveness
Rumination or obsessive thoughts
Multiple physical complaints or hypochondriacal fears
Feelings of helplessness or hopelessness
Recurrent thoughts of death or suicide
Psychotic symptoms (e.g., delusions or hallucinations)

Neurovegetative Symptoms and Signs
Sleep disturbance (frequently early-morning awakening)
Decreased energy
Appetite disturbance (usually decreased)
Diurnal mood variation (usually worse in the morning)
Psychomotor retardation or agitation

---

thought of as the classic presentation of depression, anxiety is the much more common symptom. Nearly three fourths of patients with a depressive disorder have worry, psychic anxiety, or somatic anxiety as one of their presenting symptoms.

Somatic Manifestations

Distinctive neurovegetative symptoms include *disturbed sleep* (most commonly *early-morning awakening*), *lack of energy*, and *decreased appetite*. Neurovegetative symptoms are predictive of responsiveness to psychopharmacologic intervention. In what is termed an *atypical depression*, patients may exhibit *increased sleep* and *increased appetite* (hypersomnolence and hyperphagia).

Diagnostic Classification

Although no single classification system is universally accepted, the current standard of diagnosis in the United States is the American Psychiatric Association's *Diagnostic and Statistical Manual of Mental Disorders,* fourth edition (DSM-IV) (Table 227.2).

Major Depression (Unipolar Depression)

This is the DSM-IV term for serious depression that is accompanied by neurovegetative symptoms. The lifetime risk of developing a major depression is estimated to be 1 in 4 for women and 1 in 8 for men. Dysphoric mood typically dominates the clinical picture and is persistent. Four or more of the major neurovegetative symptoms dominate the clinical picture and are present for a minimum of 2 weeks, including appetite disturbance, sleep disturbance, psychomotor retardation or agitation, anhedonia, loss of energy, feelings of worthlessness or guilt, decreased concentration, and suicidal thoughts.

Onset is variable. Symptoms usually develop over weeks to months, but they may develop suddenly. Situational factors surrounding the onset of the illness have no bearing on the diagnosis. Historically, distinctions were made between *endogenous* and *reactive depression*, but an identifiable precipitant is no longer considered pertinent with respect to diagnosis. the frequency of episodes appears to increase with age. At least half of patients have recurrent episodes. A family history of a major affective disorder (major depression or bipolar disorder) is common. The relationship between alcoholism and depression is controversial.

Major Depression with Psychotic Features

A subclassification of major depression, this disorder has the additional features of delusions, hallucinations, bizarre behavior, or disorganized thinking.

Major Depression in the Elderly

In the elderly, depression can mimic dementia. The patient may appear withdrawn, unkempt, inattentive, or even confused. The condition may be due to depression alone or to a combination of depression and dementia. Conversely, a clinical presentation consistent with depression is much more likely to be secondary to a medical condition (infarct, brain tumor, etc.) in individuals older than 50 years.

Bipolar Disorder—Depressed Phase

Depression may be a manifestation of bipolar (*manic-depressive*) illness. The presentation of a depressive episode in a

TABLE 227.2

CLASSIFICATION OF DEPRESSIVE SYNDROMES

Major Affective Disorders

Major Depression (unipolar depression)

- Severe and episodic with prominent neurovegetative signs and symptoms
- Atypical presentations may include chronic pain, hypochondriasis, or cognitive difficulties
- May be accompanied by psychotic features
- *Treatment:* antidepressant plus psychotherapy

Bipolar Disorder (manic–depressive illness)

- Severe and episodic, with a history of a manic episode
- The depressed phase is clinically identical to major depression
- May be accompanied by psychotic features
- *Treatment:* mood-stabilizing agent (plus possibly an antidepressant in the depressed phase) plus psychotherapy

Chronic Affective Disorders

Dysthymic Disorder

- Chronic and less severe, with fewer neurovegetative symptoms
- Frequently accompanied by personality disorder
- *Treatment:* psychotherapy plus a trial of antidepressant if neurovegetative symptoms are distressing

Cyclothymic Disorder

- Less severe, chronic mood swings
- *Treatment:* mood-stabilizing agent plus psychotherapy

Organic Brain Syndrome

Organic Affective Disorder

- Depression or mania due to an organic cause
- *Treatment:* manage underlying medical problem; a trial of antidepressant if necessary

Other Conditions

Adjustment Disorder with Depressed Mood

- Time limited, in response to identifiable precipitant, without neurovegetative symptoms sufficient for major depression
- *Treatment:* psychotherapy plus a trial of antidepressant if neurovegetative symptoms are distressing

---

bipolar patient is identical to that of major depression, except that there is a history of a prior manic or hypomanic episode. *Mania* is manifested by an episode of elation or expansive mood, increased energy, decreased need for sleep, inflated self-esteem, and overinvolvement in activities, accompanied by a decreased concern for the consequences. Its diagnosis requires adequate severity substantially to impair level of functioning. *Hypomania* refers to the hallmark symptoms of mania in the absence of impaired functioning. *Bipolar I disorder* involves at least one episode of mania; *bipolar II disorder* involves at least one episode of hypomania. Prevalence is considerable, with estimates as high as 5% of the adult population (1% for bipolar I disease and 4% for bipolar II). Distinguishing between the depressions of unipolar and bipolar disorders is important

because initial treatments differ substantially (see later discussion).

Dysthymic Disorder

This category denotes a chronic low-grade depression, characterized by pervasive dysphoric mood for at least 2 years. Some patients complain of lifelong feelings of depression. Symptoms are less severe than those of major depression, and neurovegetative symptoms are fewer. Depression appears as an integral part of the patient's personality or character (hence the older term *characterologic depression*). Such patients can be frustrating to treat because of chronic dysphoria, self-pity, and development of irrational patterns of negative thinking (e.g., "Things always go wrong for me"). The physician typically develops feelings of helplessness and may unconsciously communicate a wish that the patient would go away.

Typically, onset is in adolescence or early adult life and is accompanied by other symptoms of a *personality disorder*, such as a history of difficulty with interpersonal relationships, manipulativeness, feelings of emptiness, and lack of an identity. A subpopulation of dysthymic patients seems to have an attenuated chronic form of major depression with onset later in life after a period of good functioning. Neurovegetative symptoms may be more prominent.

Dysthymia and major depression can coexist in a given patient (so-called *double depression*) when a major depressive episode evolves in the context of preexisting dysthymia. However, incomplete recovery from a major depression should be described as major depression in partial remission rather than dysthymia.

Cyclothymic Disorder

This state resembles bipolar illness, but the mood swings are less severe. These patients have a chronic mood disturbance characterized by periods of depression alternating with periods of elevated mood. Neither is of sufficient severity or duration to meet the criteria for major depressive or manic episodes. Interspersed may be periods of normal mood lasting as long as several months.

Seasonal Affective Disorder

This depressive variant is distinguished by its seasonal pattern, characteristically beginning in the fall and ending about 5 months later. It has been linked to a lack of light exposure and is more common in northern latitudes. Alterations in serotonin activity have also been noted. As in other forms of depression, sadness is the dominant affect, and fatigue and decreased libido are common. Atypical features include tendencies to overeat and oversleep. In the United States, women are more commonly affected than men (ratio, 3:1). The age of onset is typically in the 20s.

Adjustment Disorder with Depressed Mood

This occurs after a *significant life stress.* Patients usually present with depressed mood associated with feelings of hopelessness, helplessness, worthlessness, and anxiety. Their thoughts are often dominated by the problems that precipitated the episode. Sleep and appetite disturbances are common but are less severe and less persistent than in major depression. The condition is usually self-limited, lasting less than 6 months and improving when the stress is removed or the individual evolves a more adaptive coping mechanism. It is important to note that any patient with symptoms severe enough to meet the criteria for major depression (see prior discussion) should receive that diagnosis regardless of the history of a precipitant. The message that the primary care physician should gather from this chapter is that evaluating the depressive symptoms, regardless of a *suspected precipitant*, is crucial, and possibly life saving, in initiating antidepressant treatment.

Postpartum Depression

Postpartum depression affects more than 10% of new mothers, perhaps as a consequence in susceptible persons of the rapid decline in reproductive hormone levels that occur with childbirth. Those with a prior history of depression, especially postpartum depression, are at greatest risk. Other risk factors include situational stress but not mode of delivery, gender of the child, breast-feeding, or whether the pregnancy was unwanted. Clinically, symptoms of major depression appear within 4 weeks of delivery and persist for more than 2 weeks (which constitutes the formal definition of the condition); in some instances, onset may be delayed for up to 3 months postpartum. Manifestations are those of major depression, but the consequences to the newborn can be particularly serious, with disruption of normal childhood development leading to cognitive and behavioral problems.

DIFFERENTIAL DIAGNOSIS (1,14)

It is important to consider organic causes of depression, including *drug-related* etiologies, which are among the most common (Table 227.3). Chronic feelings of fatigue and dysphoria are nonspecific symptoms common to multiple medical conditions whose differential diagnosis includes *chronic fatigue syndrome*, *Lyme disease*, *fibromyalgia*, *rheumatoid disease*, and *endocrinopathies* (see Chapter 8). Patients experiencing domestic violence may present with frank major depression or multiple bodily complaints (e.g., headache, gastrointestinal symptoms, premenstrual difficulties, sexual dysfunction) mimicking depression. In addition, several psychiatric disorders can masquerade as depression, including uncomplicated bereavement, alcoholism, drug dependence, and personality disorders.

TABLE 227.3

ORGANIC ETIOLOGIES OF DEPRESSION

Drug Induced: α-methyldopa, antiarrhythmics, benzodiazepines, barbiturates and other central nervous system depressants, β-blockers, cholinergic drugs, corticosteroids, digoxin, H_2-blockers, and reserpine

Substance-Abuse Related: alcohol abuse, sedative–hypnotic abuse, cocaine and other psychostimulant withdrawal

Toxic-Metabolic Disorders: hypothyroidism or hyperthyroidism (especially in the elderly), Cushing's syndrome, hypercalcemia, hyponatremia, and diabetes mellitus

Neurologic Disorders: stroke, subdural hematoma, multiple sclerosis, brain tumor, Parkinson's disease, Huntington's disease, epilepsy, and dementias

Infectious Disorders: viral infections (especially mononucleosis and influenza), HIV with or without AIDS, and syphilis

Nutritional Disorders: vitamin B_{12} deficiency and pellagra

Other: carcinomas (especially pancreatic carcinoma) and postsurgically (especially cardiac surgery)

Uncomplicated Bereavement

Symptoms of normal grief may initially be identical to those of depression. The question of a superimposed depression should be raised if mourning continues for more than 6 months, if neurovegetative symptoms are particularly severe, if there is severe impairment in the patient's ability to function, or if psychotic symptoms emerge.

Alcoholism and Drug Dependence

Many alcoholic patients appear depressed. It is not possible to delineate which symptoms are due to alcohol and which, if any, might be due to a primary affective disorder until the patient has been fully detoxified. Other substance abuse disorders may mimic depression, especially abuse of sedative–hypnotics or withdrawal from psychostimulants.

Personality Disorders

These patients frequently complain of depressive symptoms, with periods of severe dysphoria, but their affective symptoms often fluctuate markedly with environmental changes (especially with changes in interpersonal relationships). Poor impulse control, histories of unstable relationships, and a striking quality of manipulativeness or entitlement are other clues to primarily characterologic pathology.

WORKUP (1,10–13,15–20)

The possibility of depression should always be considered in patients who present with fatigue, poor sleep, appetite disturbances, multiple bodily complaints, or expressed feelings of hopelessness or poor self-esteem. *Screening* in the primary care setting is also important and can be accomplished by asking a pair of simple questions about mood and interest during an annual checkup: "In the prior 2 weeks, have you felt down, depressed, or hopeless?" and "Have you noted a lack of interest or pleasure?"

The onset of depressive symptoms and signs in patients with chronic debilitating disorders or chronic pain can be slow and subtle and should not be overlooked. When depression is suspected, specific inquiry into its manifestations is needed. However, before proceeding with the inquiry, it is useful to complete a detailed medical history for "organic" etiologies (including elicitation of specific patient concerns) and to follow later with a detailed physical examination, especially in patients who present complaining of somatic symptomatology. Not to do so risks alienating the patient, who wants his or her medical complaints taken seriously. Also useful are a few words to explain the rationale for considering depression (e.g., "It's a serious, treatable condition and is listed as one of the important causes of the symptoms bothering you"). These few simple measures facilitate patient understanding and impart a sense of seriousness and thoroughness to the workup. In addition, they help to reduce the stigma of considering a psychiatric diagnosis.

History

The dimensions to explore include neurovegetative symptoms, multiple bodily complaints, psychosocial history, and past psychiatric history of patient and family. It is helpful and often less threatening to ask first about neurovegetative symptoms such as those relating to sleep, appetite, and energy. If the responses suggest depression, one can proceed to inquire about mood and any loss of interest in sex, family, job, and other sources of interest or pleasure. In addition, the patient should be queried about self-opinion and any self-critical feelings. With every depressed patient, it is critical to ask about suicidal thoughts and intentions (see later discussion). Also useful in the exploration of multiple bodily complaints is consideration of systemic illness that might mimic depression.

Screening for Neurovegetative Symptoms

Specific inquiry into these characteristic symptoms is facilitated by the mnemonic *SIG E CAPS* ("prescribe an energy capsule"):

S—Is your *sleep* disturbed?

I—Have you noted a loss of libido or *interest* in your usual activities?

G—Are you feeling *guilty* or having self-deprecatory thoughts?

E—Have you noticed a decrease in your *energy* level?

C—Have you been having trouble *concentrating*?

A—Have you experienced changes in your *appetite* and weight?

P—Have you been physically slowed down or sped up (i.e., experienced *psychomotor* abnormalities)?

S—Have you had thoughts of *suicide*, feelings of hopelessness, or preoccupation with issues related to death? (See later discussion for more detail.)

Checking for Multiple Bodily Complaints and Ruling Out Organicity

Patients with low energy, dysphoria, and multiple bodily complaints out of proportion to physical findings are likely to have depression, but, as noted earlier, they still require careful consideration of conditions that may present in similar fashion, such as *chronic fatigue syndrome*, *Lyme disease*, *fibromyalgia*, *rheumatoid disease*, *vasculitis*, and *endocrinopathies* (see Chapter 8 for details of workup). In addition, depression or multiple bodily complaints may be the clinical presentation of *domestic violence*. Screening for this condition can be as straightforward as asking, "At any time, has a partner ever hit you, kicked you, or otherwise physically hurt you?"

Confusion and alterations in level of consciousness strongly suggest organicity, although they are not always present. When they are, drug-induced etiologies are important to consider. Onset is usually temporally related to medication use and should be sought. Worth noting is any use of *antiarrhythmics*, *antihypertensives*, *sedative–hypnotics*, and *corticosteroids*, as well as over-the-counter agents and substances of abuse. The relation of *β-blockers* to depression remains inconclusive, but risk appears to be greatest for those that are lipophilic and readily cross the blood–brain barrier. The elderly are particularly susceptible to adverse central nervous system (CNS) effects from drugs that cross the blood–brain barrier.

Primary neuropathology should be sought when depression is accompanied by an alteration of neurologic function. *Left frontal lobe* involvement by a *mass lesion* or *stroke* may trigger a depressive syndrome. Inquiry into focal signs and symptoms helps to differentiate a structural lesion from a functional affective disorder. In some medical illnesses, depression may dominate the early clinical picture. *Pancreatic cancer* is the archetypal example. Important associated findings should be sought, including profound weight loss, vague upper abdominal discomfort, and onset of painless jaundice (see Chapter 58). *HIV infection* and emergence of *AIDS* are frequently associated with depression. In such cases, the diagnosis may be obscured by comorbid medical illness (see Chapter 13). In addition, depressive features may mistakenly be conceptualized as normal grief in response to the medical diagnosis and surrounding tragedy.

Psychosocial History

This should focus on the patient's current home environment and means of financial and emotional support. Does the patient live alone? If the patient does not, is the family environment accepting or, conversely, contributing to the patient's discomfort? The availability of responsible family members to observe and supervise the patient might mean the difference between outpatient treatment and hospitalization if the patient is very depressed or debilitated. What are the patient's daily responsibilities, and what secondary stressors arise if the patient cannot meet these obligations?

Psychiatric History of the Patient and Family

Once the issue of medical etiologies has been put to rest, one should return to eliciting a past psychiatric history. Given depression's tendency to recur, the patient should always be asked about similar episodes in the past. If there is a history of depressive or manic disease, it is important to obtain the details of treatment and treatment response; a positive family history of manic symptoms or bipolar disease should raise suspicion for bipolar disorder in the patient. A history of prior psychosis or suicidality is also important to elicit because of their risks for recurrence.

Family history can be difficult to elicit because of shame about any mental illness in the family. It helps to explain that depression is believed to run in families because of hereditary biochemical factors, not defects in character. A family history of major depression, bipolar disorder, or suicide supports a diagnosis of depression in the patient. The genetic predispositions for unipolar depression and bipolar illness are distinct.

A family history of other psychiatric diagnoses must be interpreted in the context of changing nomenclature and diagnostic criteria. In the past, mania was frequently misdiagnosed as schizophrenia. "Nervous breakdown" or "going insane" were common nonspecific terms. If family psychiatric history is present, it is worth reviewing symptoms and attempting a tentative retrospective diagnosis.

Physical Examination

The importance of a careful and detailed physical examination cannot be overemphasized, especially because most depressed patients presenting to primary physicians harbor concerns about medical illness. Specific patient concerns elicited during the history should be explicitly checked during the physical examination to facilitate the provision of meaningful reassurance. (See Chapter 8 for description of the pertinent physical examination.)

Mental Status Examination

Much of the mental status examination can be performed by taking note of the patient's appearance, affect, behavior, and responses during the history. Has the patient's condition interfered with grooming and self-care? Is there sadness, tearfulness, despondency, apathy, irritability, anxiety, or anger? Is there psychomotor retardation or agitation? Does the patient offer anything spontaneously, or is there a long period of hesitation before answering (i.e., speech latency)? Is the speech slow? Is normal inflection present?

The patient should also be asked explicitly to describe his or her *mood*. Thought is assessed for form and content. Is the patient's thought pattern clear and coherent or is it tangential, circumstantial, or nonsensical? Are there ideas of worthlessness, helplessness, hopelessness, guilt, suicidal thought, or homicidality?

Is the patient able to maintain *attention*? Distractibility may occur in depression, delirium, dementia, or severe anxiety and will interfere with the patient's overall cognitive performance. Any inattention is worth documenting by testing the ability to recall a series of random numbers (digit span). Patients should be able to repeat a series of at least five to seven numbers without error. "I don't know" answers are reflective of apathy or lack of energy associated with depression. Tests of memory, calculation, abstractions, and other higher cortical functions should be performed.

Although psychotic depression is uncommon in primary care settings, it is important not to miss this very serious condition. It should be noted whether the patient appears guarded or expresses paranoid thoughts or delusions. Inquiry into any unusual experiences, such as hearing voices or seeing things that other people do not see, provides further evidence of a thought disorder. However, unusual smells, tastes, and tactile experiences suggest an organic brain syndrome.

Evaluation for Suicidality

Depression is a potentially fatal illness. Assessment of suicide risk is an integral part of the workup of every depressed patient. About 15% of patients with major affective disorders take their lives; diagnosing and treating depression can be a life-saving medical intervention by the primary care physician. With proper intervention, most suicides can be prevented. Concurrent conditions that increase the risk of suicide include chronic alcoholism, personality disorders, and both functional and drug-induced psychoses; delusional beliefs or hallucinations may lead to self-destruction. Predicting a suicide attempt is difficult, even among patients who complain of suicidal thoughts. Assessment of risk is facilitated by specific inquiry.

Technique. Assessing risk of suicide requires attention to the patient's *thoughts* (ideas, wishes, motives), *intent* (the degree to which the patient intends to act on the thoughts), and *plans*. Inquiry necessitates a calm, empathic approach that allows expression of feelings and is free of any implied criticism. On any expression of hopelessness, helplessness, or suffering, one might begin with a rather indirect query (e.g., "Are you feeling so badly that sometimes you would prefer not to go on living?"). A positive response is followed by more direct questions about self-destructive thoughts and plans. A well-worked-out, realistic, and potentially lethal plan suggests great risk, as does the act of putting one's affairs in order.

Asking patients about suicide does not put the idea into their heads. Pitfalls include failure to ask specifically about suicidal thoughts and feelings and premature interruption of the patient who mentions suicide. Any mention of suicide must be taken seriously, and *every* depressed patient must be asked about suicide. It is an error to avoid the subject for fear of doing so. Truly suicidal patients usually are relieved to be asked about it.

Mental status, especially the patient's ability to resist suicidal thoughts, is important to consider. An extremely impulsive, psychotic, or intoxicated patient has no meaningful internal controls and requires hospitalization.

TABLE 227.4
RISK FACTORS FOR SUICIDE
History of prior attempts Depression Psychotic features present (especially command hallucinations) Substance abuse Positive family history of suicide Living alone Age: In men, the risk increases with age, peaking at 75 years; in women, the peak for completed suicide is 55–65 years Gender: Women attempt suicide three to four times more often than men, but men are successful two to three times more often than women Marital status: At great risk are those who never married; are widowed, separated, or divorced; or are married without children; those married with children are at least risk Employment: The unemployed are at greater risk than the employed; the unskilled are at greater risk than the skilled Physical illness: Of all patients who attempt suicide, 50% have a physical illness; at highest risk are those with chronic pain, diagnosed chronic disease, recent surgery, or a terminal illness

Assessment of Risk. There is no simple formula for precisely assessing suicide risk. Attention to thoughts, intent, and plans is essential, facilitated by consideration of mental status and pertinent psychosocial and demographic predictors (Table 227.4). Patients expressing suicidal thoughts, especially if accompanied by intent and plans, or who lack reliable internal controls to resist suicidal impulses require emergency psychiatric consultation. Such patients should be closely supervised and not allowed to transport themselves. Patients with severe or worsening depression who have thought about suicide but steadfastly deny intent or plans should be given a prompt confirmed appointment with a psychiatrist. Depressed patients with no suicidal thoughts, intent, or plans, a normal mental status examination, and external social supports can be treated by the primary care physician, as long as frequent visits can be arranged and the depression responds to treatment. Patients with suicide potential should never be given more than 1 g or 1 week's supply of a tricyclic antidepressant (see later discussion).

Laboratory Studies and Use of Diagnostic Instruments

There are no laboratory tests for depression. For a time there was interest in urinary catecholamine metabolites and the overnight dexamethasone-suppression test, but shortcomings in sensitivity and specificity compromised clinical utility. Depression remains a clinical diagnosis. Nonetheless, medical causes of depressed mood and neurovegetative symptoms must be ruled out (see Chapter 8). Of note, multiple sclerosis is the most common neurologic cause of depression discovered by brain magnetic resonance imaging (MRI). MRI should be considered in the workup of new-onset depression with any of the following: (a) psychotic symptoms, (b) new focal neurologic deficit, or (c) onset temporally related to head trauma.

Written Diagnostic Instruments for In-Office Evaluation

Validated diagnostic instruments are sometimes useful both for case finding and as supplements to the clinical evaluation. The

Beck Depression Inventory and the *Hamilton Depression Scale* (HAM-D) help to assess severity and can be used to follow response to therapy and clinical course. The Beck Depression Inventory is a 21-item, self-administered questionnaire. The Hamilton Depression Scale is a 21-item instrument that must be clinician administered. Both take approximately 15 minutes to complete and score. The higher the score, the more severe is the distress. Other available instruments include the Symptom-Driven Diagnostic System for Primary Care, the Medical Outcomes Study depression measure, the Quick Diagnostic Interview Schedule, and PRIME-MD. These involve 2 to 28 questions and take less than 2 to 10 minutes to administer. Test sensitivities are comparable (90% to 95%), as are test specificities (50% to 70%) for the diagnosis of major depression.

Screening for Depression

Routine screening for depression by primary care practitioners is important, given the high prevalence of depression among patients seen in office practice (up to 10%), the availability of sensitive screening tests, effective means of treatment, and the potentially serious consequences of untreated disease. The U.S. Preventive Services Task Force found the evidence for diagnosis and treatment in primary care settings sufficient to recommend screening in primary care practice. The best results are obtained when screening results are incorporated into an effective system of follow-up and treatment.

Techniques for screening include the clinical interview and use of the written case-finding instruments described earlier. Of comparable sensitivity and specificity (96% and 57%, respectively) is the two-question approach noted earlier that asks about depressed mood and anhedonia: "Over the last 2 weeks, have you felt down, depressed, or hopeless?" and "Over the last 2 weeks, have you felt little interest or pleasure in doing things?"

Because the positive predictive value of a positive screening test is relatively low (about 25% to 40% if pretest probability is 5% to 10%), positive responses to screening efforts necessitate further evaluation, as noted earlier. False-positive responses are often due to the presence of other important psychopathology, including dysthymia, other depressive syndromes, generalized anxiety disorder, panic disorder, posttraumatic stress, substance abuse, and grief reactions.

It is important to note that the effectiveness of screening depends on having a system of response in place to ensure follow-up and treatment. Persons at particularly high risk and especially good candidates for screening are those with high utilization rates of primary care services; the prevalence of mood disorders among this group can be as high as 30%.

Some also argue for including screening for bipolar disorder in primary care practice because of its high prevalence (up to 5%), treatability, and potential for misdiagnosis (confusing it with major depression; see later discussion).

PRINCIPLES OF MANAGEMENT (11,13,15,17,18,21–48)

Overall Strategy

Depression is a potentially life-threatening yet treatable condition. Most depressed patients (particularly those with major depression) can be treated as outpatients by their primary care physician. *Antidepressants* and *psychotherapy* represent the basic treatment modalities, adapted to the specific type of depressive disorder encountered. *Psychiatric referral* should be considered in severe cases and in patients with psychotic, bipolar, or characterologic qualities.

Major depression is managed with antidepressant medication in conjunction with psychotherapy, which plays a very important adjunctive role. *Bipolar disease* requires psychiatric referral; it responds well to a combination of a mood-stabilizing agent and antidepressant therapy. *Psychotic depression* is also an indication for psychiatric consultation; antipsychotics are utilized. If there is an organic cause (*secondary depression*), one treats the causative medical illness and discontinues potentially offending medications. Only if the medical condition responds slowly or is intractable are trials of an antidepressant or supportive psychotherapy indicated.

Persons with a *characterologic depression/dysthymic disorder* respond best to psychotherapy, but when neurovegetative symptoms are prominent, a trial of antidepressants is helpful because dysthymia responds to selective serotonin reuptake inhibitors (SSRIs). A patient with untreated dysthymia is five times more likely subsequently to develop an episode of major depression. *Adjustment disorder with depressed mood* can be treated by the primary care physician with supportive psychotherapy. If moderate sleep and appetite disturbances are present (as they commonly are), an antidepressant can provide symptomatic relief.

Management of major depression has two facets, psychotherapeutic and medical. The primary care physician needs to become skilled in providing supportive psychotherapy and using first-line antidepressants.

Psychotherapy (12,21–23)

Treatment begins with establishing a strong patient–physician relationship (see Chapter 1, Part 1) and providing psychological support. More intensive psychotherapy may also be beneficial. The addition of antidepressant medication improves prognosis. Psychotherapy and medication are often synergistic.

Psychological Management (Supportive Psychotherapy)

Patients with major depression benefit from supportive psychotherapy, much of which can be provided by the primary care physician. A clear, empathic, hopeful manner helps to forge a therapeutic alliance and facilitates treatment. A detailed explanation of the diagnosis combined with reassurance that depression is eminently treatable does much to calm a fearful patient and family. When patients feel hopeless or undeserving, it is useful to point out that these are the characteristic symptoms of depression and they will gradually improve.

While conveying hope and optimism, the physician must take care not to dismiss as insignificant the patient's fears, pains, and negative feelings. Many feel overwhelmed by life stresses. It is important to identify these stresses. Empathic listening and thoughtful comment can help the patient to devise strategies for coping. At the outset of treatment one should see the patient every 1 to 2 weeks for about half an hour. Appointments can then be spaced out according to the patient's needs. If a patient becomes severely depressed, agitated, or psychotic, emergency psychiatric referral should be made.

Cognitive–Behavioral Therapy

This form of psychotherapy focuses on a patient's thinking and emotional functioning, helping to motivate change by examining the consequences of one's behavior. Social problem-solving and relationship skills are emphasized. When performed by a skilled practitioner, the method is of proven efficacy in treating chronic depression; results under study conditions are comparable to pharmacotherapy, although they take a few weeks longer to achieve. When combined with pharmacotherapy, the benefits are additive, and outcomes are significantly better than with either alone. Persons with depression accompanying medical problems also benefit, manifesting improved control of their underlying medical condition through improved compliance.

Social and Environmental Interventions

A caring family willing to monitor the severely depressed patient can make the difference between outpatient management and hospitalization. Members can ensure medication compliance and follow-up appointments and minimize social isolation. Also helpful is identifying stressful elements in the patient's environment so that they might be modified. Worries about the consequences of taking time off from work and issues of confidentiality must be addressed. Helping the patient deal with these important concerns is essential and greatly appreciated.

Psychopharmacologic Therapy

The SSRIs serve as first-line antidepressants. Tricyclic antidepressants (TCAs) can be effective in patients who do not respond to initial trials of SSRIs. The monoamine oxidase inhibitors (MAOIs) and lithium are reserved for special situations.

Selective Serotonin Reuptake Inhibitors

As their name implies, the SSRIs (e.g., *fluoxetine* [Prozac, Prozac Weekly, Sarafem], *sertraline* [Zoloft], *paroxetine* [Paxil], *paroxetine* controlled-release (Paxil-CR], *fluvoxamine* [Luvox], *citalopram* [Celexa], and *escitalopram* [Lexapro]) affect CNS serotonin metabolism. All require 3 to 4 weeks of continuous use before clinical improvement becomes evident.

Efficacy. For mild to moderate depression, all of these SSRIs appear to be equal in efficacy and comparable in efficacy to the TCAs but safer and better tolerated. For severe depression, there has been controversy as to whether the SSRIs are as effective as the TCAs. Unlike the TCAs, many of which are sedating, many SSRIs have energizing or "activating" side effects, a factor favoring their selection in patients suffering anergy, apathy, and psychomotor retardation. The SSRIs have become the antidepressant of first choice, especially in circumstances in which the avoidance of tricyclic side effects is desired. Randomized, controlled trials have found the major SSRIs to be similar in efficacy, safety, and side effects. However, a period of trial and error is often necessary to determine the optimal agent and best dose for a particular patient.

Preparations and Cost. Generic equivalents of several of SSRIs are becoming increasingly available (e.g., fluoxetine), providing opportunity for major cost savings. Not coincidentally, several of the brand-name SSRIs have come to market in various slow-release formulations. Theoretically they should have fewer side effects and, because patient compliance is the biggest limiting factor in response to a trial of an antidepressant, they may be considered for patients who have demonstrated sensitivity to adverse events from prior medications. For antidepressant-naive patients, however, their first trial can begin with one of the SSRI generic equivalents.

Side Effects. These activating agents can exacerbate agitation, anxiety, and insomnia, making them problematic for depressed patients already troubled by such symptoms. The motor *restlessness* (including tremor), initial *anxiety*, and *agitation* with insomnia can be the most distressing side effects of SSRIs. Concerns about exacerbation of suicidality with SSRI use proved to be unfounded after detailed investigation. Nonetheless, it is always crucial to remain vigilant and inquire specifically about suicidal thoughts, even as patients begin to show improvement (see later discussion).

Paradoxically, up to 20% of patients experience some *sedation*. Unlike the TCAs, with their associated anticholinergic and α-blocking activity, there is little risk of orthostatic hypotension, tachycardia, heart block, blurred vision, or dry mouth. *Sexual dysfunction* has been reported, including impotence in men and decreased lubrication in women. Decreased libido and anorgasmia may occur in both men and women. These effects are reversible, but they are a common cause of discontinuation of therapy (see later discussion). Some weight gain from appetite stimulation may occur, but not to the extent associated with TCAs. *Headache, nausea,* and *diarrhea* have also been reported. All SSRIs can cause a life-threatening reaction if taken concurrently with an *MAOI*. At least 2 weeks should pass before starting an MAOI after SSRI use and 5 weeks after fluoxetine use.

Some SSRIs (fluoxetine, paroxetine, and fluvoxamine) *inhibit liver cytochrome P450 enzymes*, slowing hepatic drug metabolism and prolonging the effects of warfarin, phenytoin, and other drugs that are hepatically metabolized. Although SSRI use in *pregnancy* does not increase the risk of birth defects or retard the development of intelligence, there is a slight increase in the risk of perinatal complications when treatment is continued during the third trimester (see later discussion).

In rare instances, sudden cessation of SSRI therapy can result in a *withdrawal syndrome*, characterized by dizziness, paresthesias, tremor, anxiety, nausea, and palpitations. The risk is less than 0.1% and greatest with the use of paroxetine.

Dose. *Fluoxetine* is available in 10-, 20- and 40-mg strengths. Some patients with prominent anxiety symptoms do better to start with the lower dose. A liquid form enables even smaller starting doses. In nonelderly patients, fluoxetine can be initiated at 20 mg daily. The dose may be advanced by 10 to 20 mg/d every 4 weeks. Usually, 20 or 40 mg/d suffices. The *Physicians' Desk Reference* maximum dose is 80 mg/d, although higher doses are used to treat obsessive–compulsive disorder (see Chapter 226). Because of the drug's long serum half-life (2 to 3 days), less frequent dosing is possible for elderly persons needing less than 20 mg daily (e.g., 20 mg every 2 to 4 days).

Sertraline is started at 50 mg/d and gradually increased to therapeutic doses in the range of 100 to 250 mg/d. *Fluvoxamine* is also started at 50 mg/d and gradually increased to therapeutic doses in the range of 100 to 200 mg/d. *Citalopram* and *paroxetine* are administered in doses comparable with those of fluoxetine. All other SSRIs have shorter half-lives than fluoxetine, but dosing is still once daily. Paroxetine, fluoxetine, sertraline, citalopram, and escitalopram are also available in a liquid form.

Tricyclic Antidepressants

The TCAs are a reasonable choice for antidepressant therapy in selected persons who fail SSRI treatment. The low cost per tablet of the generic formulations weighs in their favor (although brand formulations are very expensive)

TABLE 227.5

ANTIDEPRESSANTS

Generic Name	Brand Name	Customary Initial Dose	Titrate Dose Up To
Selective Serotonin Reuptake Inhibitors (SSRIs)			
Citalopram	Celexa	20 mg/d	20–40 mg/d
Escitalopram	Lexapro	10 mg/d	10–20 mg/d
Fluoxetine	Prozac	20 mg/d	20–40 mg/d
Fluvoxamine	Luvox	50 mg/d	100–250 mg/d
Paroxetine	Paxil	20 mg/d	20–60 mg/d
Paroxetine (controlled release)	Paxil CR	25 mg/d	50–62.5 mg/d
Sertraline	Zoloft	50 mg/d	100–250 mg/d
Serotonin/Norepinephrine Reuptake Inhibitors (SNRIs)			
Duloxetine	Cymbalta	30 mg/d	60 mg/d
Venlafaxine (extended release)	Effexor-XR	37.5 mg XR bid	75–150 mg bid
Atypical Antidepressants			
Bupropion (sustained release)	Wellbutrin-SR	150 mg SR qam	150–200 mg bid
Bupropion (extended release)	Wellbutrin-XL	150 mg SR qam	300–450 mg qam
Mirtazapine	Remeron	15 mg qhs	30–45 mg qhs
Nefazodone	Serzone	50 mg bid	150–300 mg bid
Trazodone	Desyrel	50–100 mg qhs	200–600 mg/
Tricyclic Antidepressants (TCAs)			
Amitriptyline	Elavil	25 mg qhs	150–300 mg qhs
Clomipramine	Anafranil	25 mg qhs	150–200 mg qhs
Desipramine	Norpramin	25 mg qam	150–300 mg qam
Doxepin	Adapin	25 mg qhs	150–300 mg qhs
Imipramine	Tofranil	25 mg qhs	150–300 mg qhs
Nortriptyline	Pamelor	10 mg qhs	50–150 mg qhs
Protriptyline	Vivactil	10 mg qam	30–60 mg qam
Trimipramine	Surmontil	25 mg qhs	150–250 mg qhs
Monoamine Oxidase Inhibitors (MAOIs)			
Phenelzine	Nardil	15 mg bid	45–90 mg/d
Tranylcypromine	Parnate	10 mg bid	40–80 mg/d

bid, twice daily; qam, in the morning; qhs, at bedtime.

(Table 227.5). When used in properly selected patients, TCA therapy can reduce the cost of therapy by an order of magnitude, but only when used in persons who can readily tolerate the side effects. Primary care physicians should become comfortable with using at least one sedating and one nonsedating TCA compound. These agents appear to act predominantly on norepinephrine metabolism, inhibiting reuptake at CNS synapses. Some TCAs also affect serotonin and, to a lesser extent, dopamine metabolism. A large number of tricyclics is available. All are equally effective. The major differences are in the degree of *anticholinergic* and *sedative side effects*. All require 3 to 4 weeks of continuous use before clinical improvement becomes evident. Drug choice for a given patient is determined by attention to the side effects of available agents (Table 227.5). Patient comfort and compliance are facilitated by avoiding drugs with marked anticholinergic activity.

Choice of Tricyclic. In general, the TCAs tend to be sedating. Patients with severe *insomnia* might do best with a strongly sedating drug, such as *doxepin* (Adapin or Sinequan) given at bedtime. The very sedating drug *amitriptyline* (Elavil) has long been popular with physicians, but because of its strong anticholinergic side effects, it is probably not an optimal first-choice agent unless low doses suffice. The elderly and those with pro-

static hypertrophy do best with a nonsedating tricyclic that has relatively mild anticholinergic activity (e.g., *desipramine* [Norpramin] or *nortriptyline* [Aventyl or Pamelor]). Nortriptyline has the advantage among tricyclics of causing the least postural hypotension. Persons bothered by anergy and psychomotor retardation are best treated with a nonsedating, slightly activating TCA (e.g., protriptyline) or an SSRI (as per earlier discussion).

The prescribing of a *fixed-combination* preparation containing a tricyclic plus a *neuroleptic* (e.g., Triavil) or a *benzodiazepine* (e.g., Limbitrol) is irrational and should be avoided. Combinations make it difficult to achieve therapeutic levels of the tricyclic without administering too much of the other compound. Moreover, except for the depressed patient with psychotic symptoms, *typical antipsychotics* have no place in the treatment of depression. Occasionally, *atypical antipsychotics* are used for augmentation purposes in treatment-refractory patients.

Adverse Effects. Tricyclics can have *lethal* cardiovascular toxicity when taken in overdose due to severe cumulative *anticholinergic* and *α-blocking* effects. One should never write a prescription that dispenses more than 1 g of a tricyclic to a potentially suicidal patient or to a patient one does not know well. At therapeutic doses, *postural hypotension* can occur, especially in the elderly, leading to falls, fractures, and head injury. If postural hypotension is a problem, nortriptyline or an SSRI should be used. If the hypotension is always worse in the morning, it may be useful to give the nortriptyline in three divided doses. Patients should be instructed to be careful when rising from recumbency or sitting.

Before benefit is noted, patients may want to stop TCA therapy because of *dry mouth, lassitude, constipation,* or *mental clouding.* Such symptoms are common with the use of TCAs but may also result from depression. They often pass or abate with continued therapy, a reassuring fact that helps patients to continue TCA treatment. *Weight gain* is another complaint. It results from TCA-associated stimulation of appetite.

Rarely, more-severe dose-related anticholinergic symptoms occur, especially in the elderly. These include *ileus, urinary retention,* and *dysrhythmias.* In all patients older than 40 years, it is good practice to obtain a baseline electrocardiogram before starting a tricyclic. At therapeutic levels, tricyclics exert anticholinergic effects on the heart, which could cause a *rise in heart rate and conduction delay.* In patients with bundle-branch block, atrioventricular block, or sinus node disease, there is an increased risk of higher degrees of heart block. In patients without underlying conduction system disease, tricyclics rarely cause conduction problems.

Very rarely, a full *anticholinergic syndrome* develops in patients taking TCAs, characterized by agitation, delirium, and fever. The most common precipitant is simultaneous use of more than one anticholinergic drug. Most often implicated is concurrent use of thioridazine (Mellaril), anticholinergic antiparkinsonian drugs, antihistamines, antispasmodics, and over-the-counter sleep medications containing antihistamines. The number of anticholinergic compounds should be closely monitored, especially in the elderly.

Withdrawal syndrome symptoms (e.g., dizziness, paresthesias, tremor, anxiety, nausea, and palpitations) occur more frequently with abrupt cessation of TCAs than with SSRIs. Their frequency is reported to be as high as 25% to 50%, but they can be avoided by tapering before discontinuation.

Dose. Tricyclics are started at a low dose with gradual increases until the therapeutic dose range is achieved (Table 227.5). After that, trial and error is often required. Drug *serum levels* can be used to determine compliance and achievement of therapeutic serum concentrations in nonresponders. Blood levels vary widely among patients for any given oral dose due to individual differences in drug absorption and metabolism. Therapeutic serum levels have been established for imipramine, desipramine, amitriptyline, and nortriptyline (Table 227.5). For other TCAs, serum levels are useful only to ascertain compliance. Many clinical laboratories are unreliable in measuring these compounds. One should seek an experienced laboratory.

The most common cause of treatment failure is inadequate dose. In healthy nonelderly adults, a typical *starting dose* is the equivalent of 50 mg of desipramine. (Nortriptyline has twice the milligram potency of most tricyclics; thus its starting dose is 25 mg.) The daily dose is best taken at bedtime to facilitate compliance and minimize side effects. Dose can be increased by 50 mg every 3 to 4 days to a dose of 150 to 200 mg at bedtime. Doses are reduced by 50% in the elderly (see later discussion). The final dose chosen is one that provides a therapeutic response without intolerable side effects. The usual *maximum dose* is 300 mg of desipramine or the equivalent (150 mg for nortriptyline). This is easier said than done. In recent reviews, less than 10% of patients whose depression was diagnosed received a therapeutic dose of a TCA.

Atypical Antidepressants

These agents have slightly different mechanisms of action than those of the first-line SSRIs, providing them with potential benefits in selected circumstances in which SSRIs do not suffice. They are mostly the province of the psychiatrist, and unless familiar with their use, the primary physician should not prescribe one of these agents in preference to a first-line drug. However, some knowledge of their characteristics is helpful when managing patients who have been prescribed an atypical antidepressant.

Venlafaxine (Effexor). Venlafaxine is a *selective inhibitor* of both *serotonin* and *norepinephrine reuptake (SSRI/SNRI).* It is typically started at 37.5 mg twice daily (due to its short half-life) and gradually tapered up to therapeutic doses in the range of 75 to 150 mg twice daily. At its higher doses, it has more effect on norepinephrine uptake inhibition and possibly achieves a higher remission rate than other antidepressants (a question under study).

Duloxetine (Cymbalta). Duloxetine is also a selective inhibitor of both serotonin and norepinephrine reuptake. It is typically started at 30 mg at bedtime and quickly increased to its therapeutic dose of 60 mg before bed. In addition to treatment of depression, it has been approved for the treatment of painful diabetic peripheral neuropathy, making it a particularly useful agent in depressed patients suffering from this condition (see Chapter 167). The drug is well absorbed, hepatically metabolized, and requires dosing two to three times per day. Adverse effects include dizziness, nausea, somnolence, and constipation. The drug should not be used in persons with narrow-angle glaucoma; safety in pregnancy is not established. Minor transaminase elevations may be noted. Expense is high compared to that of generic formulations of SSRIs and TCAs.

Nefazodone (Serzone). Nefazodone inhibits serotonin reuptake and uniquely blocks 5-HT$_2$ receptors and mediates 5-HT-1A transmission. Results achieved with nefazodone are similar to those for SSRIs. The drug is usually started at 50 mg twice daily and gradually tapered up to therapeutic doses in the range of 150 to 300 mg twice daily.

Bupropion (Wellbutrin). Bupropion (available in sustained-release and extended-release preparations) appears to work by downregulating postsynaptic β-noradrenergic receptors. Unlike the SSRIs, there are no adverse effects on sexual function, making it helpful in depressed persons bothered by such side effects and in patients who do not respond to the SSRIs. Use of non–sustained-release preparations was associated with an increased risk of seizure activity, but availability in sustained-release preparations reduces the risk of seizure to that of other antidepressants. However, even the sustained-release (SR) form is still contraindicated in patients with a known seizure disorder or eating disorder. It is usually started at 150 mg SR in the morning and gradually tapered up to therapeutic doses in the range of 150 to 200 mg SR twice daily.

Trazodone. Trazodone (Desyrel) is a nontricyclic with efficacy similar to the that of TCAs but is generally better tolerated. The drug is sedating and particularly helpful for those who cannot sleep or tolerate anticholinergic side effects. *Postural hypotension* can be a problem in the elderly. Other common side effects include indigestion, nausea, and headaches. *Priapism,* a painful medical emergency, has been reported. Males prescribed trazodone must be warned that a sustained painful erection requires immediate medical attention. Trazodone is usually started at 50 to 100 mg at bedtime as a sleep inducer. To be used as an antidepressant, it needs to be gradually tapered up to therapeutic doses in the range of 200 to 600 mg at bedtime.

Mirtazapine. Mirtazapine (Remeron and Remeron SolTab) is associated with an increased release of both serotonin and norepinephrine. Mediation of 5-HT-1A transmission and blocking of 5-HT$_2$ and 5-HT$_3$ receptors may account for its antidepressant and *anxiolytic* effects. It is usually started at 15 mg at bedtime and gradually tapered up to therapeutic doses in the range of 30 to 45 mg at bedtime.

Monoamine Oxidase Inhibitors

MAOIs are quite useful in treating the elderly (see later discussion), being well tolerated by virtue of their lack of anticholinergic side effects. However, they do have other side effects that bear noting.

Side Effects. These drugs can be used safely, but considerable patient education on proper use and precautions is essential. The primary adverse effects are *hypotension* and *insomnia*. Hypotension is unrelated to dose and may occur up to a month after starting the drug. It rarely necessitates stopping the drug. Insomnia can be minimized by giving the last daily dose no later than 4 p.m.

Hypertensive crisis is the most serious adverse effect, caused by ingesting a large amount of *tyramine*. Dietary and drug precautions must be given. A low-tyramine diet is required, necessitating avoidance of foods such as fermented cheese, large amounts of yogurt, excessive caffeine, and chocolate, beer, and red wine. Patients can drink white wine, vodka, gin, and whiskey. A blanket warning to avoid all alcohol is not only unwarranted but may also compromise compliance. *Sympathomimetics* should be avoided, with special warning to watch for unintentional intake in many over-the-counter medications, including combination cold tablets, nasal decongestants, and appetite suppressants. *Amphetamines* are also not permitted. Treatment of a hypertensive crisis involves prompt cessation of MAOI use and the initiation of antihypertensive therapy with an α-blocker or a direct vasodilator (*phentolamine*, 5 mg given slowly intravenously, is recommended). Fever is managed by means of external cooling. Severe life-threatening reactions can also occur as a consequence of interactions between MAOIs and SSRIs or *narcotic analgesics*. A several-week period between cessation of SSRI therapy and initiation of MAOI use is required, as is psychiatric consultation before starting the MAOI.

Choice of MAOI Agent. *Tranylcypromine* (Parnate) is the preferred MAOI in the elderly because its effects last no more than 24 hours. The starting dose is 10 mg once or twice daily, and the dose is gradually increased as needed over a few weeks. Usually 20 to 30 mg daily suffices, but occasional patients require as much as 80 mg/d.

Other Agents

A host of agents have been used, ranging from anxiolytics to St. John's wort.

Anxiolytics. The benzodiazepine *alprazolam* (*Xanax*) has excellent antianxiety effects and mild antidepressant action. However, prolonged use is associated with significant risk of dependence (see Chapter 226). *Buspirone* (BuSpar) is similarly purported to have combined anxiolytic and *mild* antidepressant effects and has the advantage of a more benign side-effect profile, without risk of physiologic dependence (see Chapter 226). These agents are reasonable in cases of adjustment disorders with depressive and anxiety features, but they are not indicated for the treatment of major depression.

St. John's Wort. Fear about the use of pharmacologic agents for depression has stimulated lay interest in the use of "natural" substances for treatment (see also Chapter 238). The use of St. John's wort is reportedly widespread, but there are few large-scale, randomized, placebo-controlled trials of this herbal preparation. Those that have been completed in persons with major depression of moderate severity failed to demonstrate any benefit over placebo. Of note, the placebo effect in depression can be substantial and might account for the efficacy reported in early studies of St. John's wort that did not use placebo control. Whether the herbal preparation might be beneficial in persons with mild disease remains to be determined. Pending more data, St. John's wort should not be used in place of standard treatment for depression, which is of proven efficacy.

Selection of Antidepressant for Major Depression

Studies of efficacy find little difference among SSRIs and between SSRIs and second-generation drugs such as venlafaxine, bupropion, duloxetine, and mirtazapine. Response rates in severe depression may be higher with TCAs, but these drugs are the least well tolerated, especially in the elderly (see below).

Choice of agent should be based on the prior history of response (a good predictor), patient preference, cost, and expected side effects. Choice is best made by taking into account disease severity, patient age, degree of psychomotor retardation and sleep disturbance, and ability to tolerate anticholinergic, cardiac, and postural side effects. *Costs* are a key consideration because these drugs are likely to be used for prolonged periods of time. The generic SSRI formulations are available at a fraction of the cost of brand-name SSRIs and the brand-name TCAs (Table 227.5). Although the generic TCAs are less costly on a pill-per-pill basis, their requirements of cardiac monitoring, blood levels, and possibly more frequent office visits to manage their side effects can all contribute to a higher total cost in patients especially vulnerable to their side effects.

In the elderly and others with cardiac disease, prostatic hypertrophy, postural hypotension, or glaucoma, the SSRIs may be better tolerated. When sedation without anticholinergic activity is desired, trazodone is a reasonable choice, particularly in the elderly. For anergic, hypersomnic, or motor-retarded patients, an activating agent is best (e.g., an SSRI or bupropion-SR or desipramine). For patients with a mixture of neurovegetative symptoms, nortriptyline is reasonable, being well tolerated and free of excessive sedating, activating, anticholinergic, or antiadrenergic effects.

Monitoring and Duration of Therapy; Failure to Respond

Monitoring response to therapy can be readily accomplished by carefully reviewing symptoms and activity level. The questionnaire instruments used for the assessment of disease severity (see prior discussion) can also be used. If a patient shows little or no response to antidepressant therapy after 4 weeks at full dose (which may be 6 weeks from initiation of therapy), then the drug trial should be considered a failure. If there is doubt as to the adequacy of a dose or compliance, a serum drug level can be obtained.

Initial failure to respond is an indication for a trial of *switching* to another antidepressant. Options include trying another SSRI and switching to another class of antidepressant. In a major study of patients failing to respond to or intolerant of initial SSRI therapy with citalopram, approximately one in four achieved remission of their depression by switching to another SSRI (e.g., sertraline) or to a non-SSRI antidepressant (e.g., bupropion or extended-release venlafaxine).

Persistent failure to respond is an indication for psychopharmacologic consultation to explore whether *augmentation* therapy (i.e., adding a second agent, usually from a different class) or switching to yet another agent is the best approach. Sometimes augmentation can be the more rapid approach to achieving control, but consultation is advised.

It may also be important to reassess the patient's *use of alcohol*. It has long been known that patients who meet criteria for alcohol abuse or dependence are less likely to respond to antidepressant treatment. In a recent report, it was shown that a group of depressed outpatients who drank an average of 1 ounce of alcohol per day had a lower rate of response to an 8-week course of fluoxetine. This mild to moderate level of alcohol use was enough to decrease their chance of acutely responding to their antidepressant. Thus, patients should be encouraged to either abstain from drinking alcohol while on their antidepressant or limiting their alcohol use as much as possible.

If the response to initial therapy was promising but limited by intolerance to drug side effects, then switching to another agent in the same class with a more favorable side-effect profile might suffice (e.g., switching from amitriptyline to nortriptyline for postural hypotension).

If depression successfully remits, antidepressant medication is maintained for at least 6 to 9 months. It should be used longer among patients who have experienced moderate to severe depression and who are judged to face a high risk of recurrence, perhaps because of a history of previous episodes. Continuation-phase medication should be maintained at the same dose as was used in the acute-phase treatment. It has been shown to reduce the risk of recurrence by 70% for as long as 36 months after the acute episode. When it is time to discontinue treatment, the dose can be slowly tapered off over a period of 4 weeks while watching for the reemergence of depressive symptoms. Should symptoms recur, the dose is returned to its prior level and maintained for at least another 6 to 9 months. Major depression is a medical illness with a high rate of recurrence. After a single episode, 50% of patients subsequently have a second episode. After two episodes, the chance of having a third is approximately 80%. For patients with two or more episodes, maintenance therapy for probably 3 to 5 years is indicated. Patients with a family history of depression or bipolar disorder should also be closely evaluated for long-term maintenance therapy.

Discontinuation of Therapy Due to Drug-Associated Sexual Dysfunction

An important and commonly cited cause of discontinuation of antidepressant therapy is antidepressant-associated sexual dysfunction. Manifestations include decreased libido, erectile dysfunction, and delayed orgasm. It is estimated that 30% to 70% of patients taking SSRI antidepressants experience this side effect. The finding is prevalent even among patients who achieve remission of depression with SSRI therapy. The problem typically occurs early in treatment and tends to persist, although it may wax and wane. Among the treatment approaches studied are addition of *sildenafil* or the use of a non-SSRI such as *bupropion*, which shows the least impairment of sexual function of the antidepressants. Dose reduction and dose holiday are other options. Evidence of efficacy is strongest for the addition of sildenafil in persons who achieve remission of their depression with SSRI therapy. More than 50% of male participants in one randomized, placebo-controlled trial achieved significant improvement in most dimensions of sexual function with the use of a 50-mg dose taken 1 hour before sexual activity. Libido is the least responsive to sildenafil therapy. Because data are available only from short-term studies in men, results in women and long-term safety and efficacy remain to be established. Bupropion shows the least impairment of sexual function in controlled trials and might be considered as initial therapy where sexual dysfunction is a major concern.

Prevention of Suicide (17,37)

The best prevention is proper screening for suicidality and prompt referral at the time of initial evaluation. However, some patients are at greatest risk for suicide at the time when they are initially responding to antidepressant medication. Dysphoria may persist as energy lifts, perhaps giving the patient with suicidal thoughts adequate energy to formulate a plan and follow it through. Continuous vigilance is required, as well as care in the choice and amount of antidepressant prescribed. If there is a question of suicide risk, either a nontricyclic should be selected or no more than 1 g of a tricyclic dispensed at a time.

Treatment of Depression in the Elderly (16,38–41)

Depression is the most common psychiatric disorder of the elderly, affecting close to 1 million older Americans. Primary treatment modalities include antidepressants and, for severely affected patients, electroconvulsive therapy (ECT). Age-related changes in drug metabolism and susceptibility to drug side effects must be taken into account in the design of the treatment program (see Appendix 173.1).

Choice of Antidepressant

When anergy and psychomotor retardation predominate, the activating effects of SSRIs make them attractive. Similarly, SSRIs are an excellent first choice if there is heart block, a dysrhythmia, or postural hypotension. Of the *SSRIs*, sertraline, citalopram, and escitalopram are the least likely to interfere with hepatic drug metabolism and are preferred in patients taking drugs that are metabolized by the liver (e.g., digoxin, warfarin, phenytoin). The sedating, anticholinergic, cardiac, and postural side effects of many TCAs make their use in the elderly especially problematic. Before starting therapy, postural signs and an electrocardiogram should be performed and particular note taken of the patient's somatic symptoms and degree of psychomotor retardation. *Amitriptyline* and *imipramine* are among the most difficult to use; nortriptyline and *desipramine* are better tolerated. If sedation is desired, *trazodone* is a reasonable choice, being free of anticholinergic activity. When loss of sex drive results from SSRI therapy or is an initial concern, bupropion is a reasonable choice, having the lowest rate of sexual side effects.

Initiating and Monitoring Therapy

One starts with a *very low dose* of medication (e.g., 10 mg of fluoxetine, 25 mg of desipramine, 10 mg of nortriptyline, or 50 mg of trazodone). The dose can be raised slowly every 5 to 7 days while monitoring subjective response and heart rate and watching for anticholinergic, cardiovascular, and CNS side effects. One slows the increase in dose if tachycardia, excessive sedation, agitation, or orthostatic hypotension develops.

Often the patient is the last to recognize improvement, and family members commonly report that the patient is sleeping and eating better before the dysphoria resolves. An adequate trial may take twice as long in the elderly as in younger patients. Several studies have demonstrated patients older than 55 years not showing their response until 8 to 10 weeks.

Treating Failure to Respond

If there is little improvement after a reasonable trial at therapeutic doses, consultation is warranted to consider the use of an alternative antidepressant (e.g., MAOI) or ECT.

Use of a Monoamine Oxidase Inhibitor. MAOIs have been used sparingly in the elderly because of concern for adverse reactions. Actually, MAOIs have no anticholinergic activity and are relatively well tolerated. Many older patients who do not respond to other antidepressants improve with MAOIs. MAOI therapy should be selected and started by a psychopharmacologic consultant, but management can then shift to the primary care physician, who needs to be familiar with drug actions and side effects (see prior discussion).

Use of Electroconvulsive Therapy. Elderly patients who are psychotically depressed, severely incapacitated, refractory to or unable to take drug therapy, or in need of a rapid response should be referred for consideration of ECT. The best predictors of response are psychomotor retardation and delusions. Efficacy and safety have been well documented. Attainment of generalized seizure activity is required to achieve benefit. Customizing electrical dose to the patient's seizure threshold may help to maximize efficacy and minimize adverse effects. Electrode placement appears to be more important than electrical dose as regards amnesia, with unilateral electrode placement associated with a lower risk. Amnesia occurs for events just before and up to a few weeks after treatment. Long-term cognitive functioning is no different than that for patients treated with antidepressants. Relapses occur with high frequency, making ECT an acute treatment. Maintenance ECT is not uncommon these days. Quite often an SSRI or a TCA is prescribed for lifelong maintenance treatment in an elderly patient.

Treatment of Seasonal Affective Disorder

Light therapy is the first line of treatment. Exposure to 10,000 lux of ordinary white fluorescent light for 30 to 45 minutes at a time once or twice a day is effective. Improvement often occurs within the first week or two of therapy. Patients typically sit about 50 cm from a light box and read for the period of treatment, with the light coming in at a 45-degree angle. Improvement has been noted both with morning and nighttime treatments, although the latter may cause insomnia. Elaborate forms of lighting that more closely simulate the spectrum of sunlight are no more effective than light from a standard white fluorescent source. The intensity of light appears to be the key determinant of efficacy. SSRIs are probably as effective as light

therapy. Some clinicians use both. The efficacy of prophylactic therapy early in the winter is under study.

Treatment of Depression in Pregnancy and Postpartum (13,42,43)

Depression in pregnancy or in the postpartum period can be a serious problem, with adverse consequences for both mother and newborn. Inadequate weight gain, frank weight loss, and even malnutrition may ensue, leading to low birth weight. Suicidality is a major concern, as are failure to come for prenatal and obstetric care and difficulty caring for other children. Other consequences include the need for long-term hospitalization, marital discord, divorce, and loss of employment.

Pregnancy

The prevalence of depression in pregnancy approaches 10%. Women with depression during pregnancy are at increased risk for intrauterine growth retardation, preterm labor, placental abruption, and altered neonatal behavior. Some of these adverse effects are believed to be related to depression-induced weight loss and abnormal stimulation of the hypothalamic–pituitary–adrenal axis.

Although data are incomplete, there is no evidence that SSRI or TCA therapy during pregnancy is associated with increased risk of fetal death, growth impairment, or behavioral defects. As a class, SSRIs do not increase the overall risk of birth defects, but first trimester use of some SSRI agents has been associated with particular birth defects. Case–control epidemiologic studies suggest the following associations: between paroxetine and right ventricular outflow tract obstruction; between sertraline and omphalocele and septal defects of the heart; and between paroxetine or citalopram and anencephaly, craniosynostosis, and omphalocele. Of note, although the relative increases in risk are statistically significant, the absolute increases and overall risk remain extremely small and for most patients well below the risk of untreated depression. No associations have been found between birth defects and the use of TCIs or other SSRIs. The risk for neonatal withdrawal syndrome is increased with antidepressant use during the third trimester.

On balance, pharmacologic treatment of depression during pregnancy is preferred over withholding or discontinuing antidepressant therapy. Dose requirements change over the course of pregnancy. Increased hepatic metabolism and an increased circulating blood volume necessitate an increase in dose to about 1.6 times that prior to pregnancy. After pregnancy, dose should be reduced by 30% to 50%. Tapering several weeks before delivery can reduce the risk of a neonatal withdrawal syndrome but may compromise the control of symptoms.

Postpartum Depression

After childbirth, all women should be asked about depressed mood and anhedonia. Those who answer affirmatively should be evaluated further (see prior discussion); women with evidence of major depression should undergo specific inquiry into any intention to harm themselves or their child. Treatment options include antidepressant therapy and interpersonal psychotherapy; the former is more rapid in onset, but both are equally effective. There is no additive benefit to combining the two. SSRI pharmacotherapy is preferred over tricyclic use (much lower risk from overdose and greater response rate), but any antidepressant agent that has proven useful in the past should be among the first considerations for a new episode.

SSRI use in nursing mothers has not been associated with serious adverse effects in breast-fed children, but there are few long-term data. Little tricyclic gets into breast milk. Fluoxetine use produces the highest SSRI levels in breast-fed children. It is recommended that treatment be initiated at one half of the usual starting dose (due to increased sensitivity to medication postpartum) and continued for at least 6 to 9 months after onset of remission. The relapse rate is high (50% to 85%); longer-term therapy may be necessary.

Bipolar Disorder

Unlike major depression, bipolar disorder requires starting treatment with a *mood stabilizer* (e.g., lithium, valproate, carbamazepine), not with an antidepressant, which can trigger mania.

Lithium is the best studied of available drugs for bipolar disorder and an appropriate choice for starting treatment in the primary care setting. Effective for bipolar depression, mania, reduction in risk of suicide, and prophylaxis, the drug is inexpensive and generally safe, but with a narrow therapeutic index (the target range for serum concentration is 0.8 to 1.2 mEq/L). An extended-release preparation allows twice-daily dosing and reduced variation in serum concentration. Most adverse effects are related to serum level: rare and mild at less than 1.5 mEq/L, mild to moderate at levels from 1.5 to 2.5 mEq/L, and moderate to severe at levels greater than 2.5 mEq/L. Fine tremor, mild thirst, mild nausea, frequent urination, and generalized malaise may come with the onset of therapy and usually resolve with its continuation, but diarrhea, vomiting, drowsiness, muscular weakness, worsening polyuria, and poor coordination suggest incipient lithium toxicity. Weight gain, coordination difficulties, and mental clouding often cause patients to discontinue therapy. Hypothyroidism, renal tubular injury, and cardiac rhythm disturbances may ensue, especially at toxic doses. Regular monitoring of serum concentration and renal function (blood urea nitrogen, creatinine) is required (the drug is renally excreted). Concurrent use of thiazide therapy may increase serum level due to its enhancement of distal tubular reabsorption; nonsteroidal antiinflammatory drugs and angiotensin-converting-enzyme inhibitors increase the risk of lithium toxicity.

Antidepressant therapy is often a consideration because depression is the principal cause of disability in bipolar disease. Many bipolar patients receive an antidepressant in addition to a mood stabilizer, despite limited evidence in support of this common practice. In a major study comparing mood stabilizer therapy alone versus the addition of an antidepressant (SSRI or bupropion), no significant difference was found in the percentage of bipolar patients who achieved a durable recovery from major depressive symptoms or who experienced a flare of manic symptoms (a concern with antidepressant use).

Overall, care needs to be individualized; bipolar patients with severe depression despite lithium therapy should be referred to psychiatry for consideration of additional measures (e.g., carbamazepine, valproate, an antidepressant).

INDICATIONS FOR REFERRAL AND ADMISSION

Patients who should be referred for psychiatric consultation include those with refractory or disabling major depression, bipolar illness, psychosis, or substantial risk for suicide.

Patients who fail to respond after 1 to 2 months of appropriate antidepressant treatment should have a psychiatric consultation. Many of these patients can be referred back to their primary care physician for follow-up after one or two psychiatric appointments.

Psychiatric hospitalization is indicated for high suicide risk, lack of reliable social supports (if the depression is severe), history of previously poor response to treatment, or symptoms that are so severe that the patient requires constant observation or nursing care.

PATIENT EDUCATION (22)

Detailed patient education is a central component of supportive psychotherapy (see prior discussion). Patients who come from backgrounds that stigmatize mental illness or oppose psychotropic medication are comforted by learning of depression's "organic" pathophysiology, which helps them to comply with treatment. Compliance with antidepressant therapy is often compromised by side effects or mistaken attributions. Some patients stop their medication after only a few days if they do not notice an immediate improvement or use it only "as needed." Before initiating therapy, it is critical to review likely side effects and delayed onset of improvement. The importance of prolonged regular use must be emphasized. If the patient already has a tendency toward constipation, the prescription of a stool softener may make a tricyclic more tolerable. Patients should be instructed to report side effects rather than stopping the medication on their own and to call promptly if suicidal thoughts develop or if depression markedly worsens.

The educational process should include family and other household members. Enlisting their help in decreasing stress at home is helpful. With elderly or severely depressed patients, the family should be taught about the proper use of antidepressants and asked to monitor compliance.

THERAPEUTIC RECOMMENDATIONS (23)

- Screen for depression by asking two questions: "Over the last 2 weeks, have you felt down, depressed, or hopeless? and "Over the last 2 weeks, have you felt little interest or pleasure in doing things?"
- If the patient answers affirmatively, proceed with full evaluation that begins with screening for somatic symptoms; use the SIG E CAPS questions; screen for suicidality by asking about it directly. Also check for bipolar disease by inquiring into past manic symptoms and family history.
- If the patient appears to be at risk for suicide, has psychotic symptoms, has severe depression with no social supports, or is unable to care for himself or herself, arrange prompt psychiatric consultation with a view to possible hospitalization.
- Consider brain magnetic resonance imaging scan in the setting of new-onset depression associated with psychotic symptoms, focal neurologic deficits, or onset temporally related to head trauma.
- For patients who are deemed safe to manage on an outpatient basis, arrange for supportive psychotherapy and make any social and environmental interventions that may help; involve the family in the treatment, especially with elderly or severely depressed patients.
- For patients with major depression (or patients with other subtypes who have neurovegetative symptoms), begin

antidepressant pharmacotherapy unless there is evidence of bipolar disease, in which case a mood stabilizer should be the first line of treatment along with consideration of psychiatric consultation (see later discussion).

- Consider SSRI drugs as first-line pharmacotherapy; base the choice of agent on cost when minor differences in side-effect profiles are not clinically important; prescribe generically to limit cost (e.g., fluoxetine, 20 mg daily).
- Consider for psychopharmacologic/psychiatric referral patients who fail 4- to 6-week trials of two different SSRIs at full therapeutic doses.
- Use tricyclic antidepressants as second-line pharmacotherapy, but consider whether the patient has responded well to one in the past, the patient has rather severe depression, or SSRI therapy is not proving fully effective. Use with caution in elderly patients and those with suspected cardiac disease; obtain a baseline electrocardiogram to rule out conduction system abnormalities, and check for postural hypotension prior to initiation of treatment.
- For elderly patients, initiate pharmacotherapy at one half to one third of the standard starting doses; similarly, reduce starting doses by one half in women with postpartum depression.
- If the patient responds to the antidepressant, it should be continued for at least 6 to 9 months or longer if depression was moderate to severe and there is appreciable risk of recurrence, and then slowly tapered.
- Never prescribe more than 1 week's supply or a total of 1 g of a tricyclic if there is suicidal risk.
- Explain to patients that antidepressants must be taken regularly, that they may take 4 weeks to work, and that there may be mild side effects that do not warrant discontinuation of the drug.
- Prescribe a generic formulation whenever possible to minimize cost.
- For depression during pregnancy, strongly consider pharmacologic therapy, even during the first trimester. Review with the patient the important benefits from drug treatment and the very small increase in risk of a birth defect associated with use of some SSRIs. TCA treatment might be considered if there is concern about birth defects with some SSRIs.
- If bipolar disease is diagnosed, start treatment with a mood stabilizer (e.g., lithium carbonate, 300 mg, three times daily) rather than an antidepressant (which may exacerbate mood swings); increase the lithium dose over several days to achieve a target serum level between 0.8 and 1.2 mEq/L (obtained before the first dose of the day). If during lithium therapy severe major depression is problematic, obtain prompt psychiatric consultation before adding an antidepressant medication.

Annotated Bibliography

1. Belmaker RH. Bipolar disorder. N Engl J Med 2004;351:476. (*An excellent review with a focus on emerging knowledge of the condition; 85 references.*)
2. Brown JT, Stoudemire GA. Normal and pathological grief. JAMA 1983;250:378. (*A succinct description of normal grief and guidelines for the recognition and management of pathologic reactions.*)
3. Fawcett J, Kravitz HM. Anxiety syndromes and their relationship to depressive illness. J Clin Psychiatry 1988;44:8. (*Clarifies patterns of comorbidity.*)
4. Hays RD, Wells KB, Sherbourne CD, et al. Functioning and well-being outcomes of patients with depression compared with chronic general medical illnesses. Arch Gen Psychiatry 1995;52:11. (*Patients with depressive symptoms tended to function worse than those with other chronic medical conditions.*)
5. Kessler RC, Berglund P, Demler O, et al. The epidemiology of major depressive disorder. Results from the National Comorbidity Survey Replication (NCS-R). JAMA 2003;289:3095. (*The lifetime prevalence of depression is >16%, with a 12-month-period prevalence of nearly 7%.*)
6. Quitkin FM, Stewart JW, McGrath PJ, et al. Columbia atypical depression: a subgroup of depressives with better response to MAOI than to tricyclic antidepressants or placebo. Br J Psychiatry 1993;163(Suppl 21):30. (*Demonstrates differential responses among the antidepressants.*)
7. Roy J, Carver LA. Premenstrual syndrome, premenstrual dysphoric disorder, and beyond: a clinical primer for practitioners. Obstet Gynecol 2004;104:845. (*A practical discussion of the problem.*)
8. Schlager D, Froom J, Jaffe A. Winter depression and functional impairment among ambulatory primary care patients. Compr Psychiatry 1995;36:18. (*Winter-seasonal pain may be a common presenting symptom in seasonal affective disorder.*)
9. Scholle SH, Rost KM, Golding JM. Physical abuse among depressed women. J Gen Intern Med 1998;13:607. (*A very high incidence was found; almost all patients presented to their primary physicians rather than to mental health professionals.*)
10. Suttor B, Rummans TA, Jowsey SG, et al. Major depression in medically ill patients. Mayo Clin Proc 1998;73:329. (*A useful review of depression as a comorbid condition, including recognition and treatment.*)
11. The WPA Dysthymia Working Group. Dysthymia in clinical practice. Br J Psychiatry 1995;166:174. (*Improved knowledge of this disorder has led to a more positive approach to treatment, in which antidepressants can usefully be complemented by psychosocial measures.*)
12. Wisner KL, Parry BL, Piontek CM. Postpartum depression. N Engl J Med 2003;347:194. (*A very useful clinical review; 48 references.*)
13. American Psychiatric Association. Diagnostic and statistical manual of mental disorders, 4th ed. Washington, DC: Author, 1994. (*The standard for diagnosis.*)
14. Candilis P. The use of screening tests for detection of psychiatric disorders. In: Stern TA, Herman JB, Slavin PL, eds. MGH guide to psychiatry in primary care. New York: McGraw-Hill, 2003:643. (*A chapter describing available instruments for screening in a primary care setting.*)
15. Crawford MJ, Prince M, Menezes P, et al. The recognition and treatment of depression in older people in primary care. Int J Geriatr Psychiatry 1998;13:172. (*Diagnosis and management from the primary care perspective.*)
16. Das AK, Olfson M, Gameroff MJ, et al. Screening for bipolar disorder in a primary care practice. JAMA 2005;956. (*Presents evidence in support of screening.*)
17. Lagomasino IT, Stern TA. Approach to the suicidal patient. In: Stern TA, Herman JB, Slavin PL, eds. MGH guide to psychiatry in primary care. New York: McGraw-Hill, 1998:15. (*A chapter devoted to evaluating and treating this serious problem.*)
18. Rosenthal NE. Diagnosis and treatment of seasonal affective disorder. JAMA 1993;270:2717. (*A short but inclusive review; 44 references.*)
19. U.S. Preventive Services Task Force. Screening for depression: recommendations and rationale. Ann Intern Med 2002;136:760. (*Recommends screening in primary care practice.*)
20. Whooley MA, Avins AL, Miranda J, et al. Case-finding instruments for depression. Two questions are as good as many. J Gen Intern Med 1997;12:439. (*Identifies a simple, effective screening technique.*)
21. Alwan S, Reefhuis J, Rasmussen SA, et al. for the National Birth Defects Prevention Study. Use of selective serotonin-reuptake inhibitors in pregnancy and the risk of birth defects. N Engl J Med 2007;356:2684. (*A large epidemiologic case–control study; no overall risk was found, but did find small increases in the risk for certain birth defects associated with a few individual agents.*)
22. American Geriatrics Society, American Association for Geriatric Psychiatry. Consensus statement on improving the quality of mental health care in U.S. nursing homes: management of depression and behavioral symptoms associated with dementia. J Am Geriatr Soc 2003;51:1287. (*Consensus guidelines.*)
23. American Psychiatric Association. Guidelines for the treatment of patients with major depressive disorder (revision). Am J Psychiatry. 2000;157 (Suppl 1). (*A comprehensive statement of consensus guidelines for management.*)
24. Brody DS, Thompson II TL, Larson DB, et al. Strategies for counseling depressed patients by primary care physicians. J Gen Intern Med 1994;9:569. (*Reviews counseling techniques and adapts them for use by primary care physicians.*)
25. Chambers CD, Johnson KA, Dick LM, et al. Birth outcomes in pregnant women taking fluoxetine. N Engl J Med 1996;335:1010. (*There was no increased risk of pregnancy loss or major fetal anomalies, but there was an increased risk of perinatal complications.*)

26. Freeman MP, Freeman SA. Lithium: clinical considerations in internal medicine. Am J Med 2006;119;478. (*A succinct review of the drug, for the generalist; 70 references.*)

27. Geddes JR, Carney SM, Davies C, et al. Relapse prevention with antidepressant drug treatment in depressive disorders: a systematic review. Lancet 2003;361:653. (*The relative risk of relapse/recurrence was reduced by 70% when antidepressant therapy was continued after the acute treatment period.*)

28. Hansen RA, Gartlehner G, Lohr KN, et al. Efficacy and safety of second-generation antidepressants in the treatment of major depressive disorder. Ann Intern Med 2005;143:415. (*A systematic review; no substantial differences in efficacy was noted.*)

29. Hypericum Depression Trial Study Group. Effect of *Hypericum perforatum* (St John's Wort) in major depressive disorder: a randomized controlled trial. JAMA 2002;287:1807. (*A major multicenter randomized, controlled trial; no benefit was found in persons with moderately severe depression.*)

30. Keller MB, McCullough JP, Klein DN, et al. A comparison of sefazodone, the cognitive behavioral-analysis system of psychotherapy, and their combination for the treatment of chronic depression. N Engl J Med 2000;342:1462. (*A randomized, controlled trial, finding that the approaches were equally effective when used alone, but that the effects were additive when they were used together.*)

31. Keller MB, Kocsis JH, Thase ME, et al. Maintenance phase efficacy of sertraline for chronic depression: a randomized trial. JAMA 1998;280:1665. (*The approach was found to be well-tolerated and effective in preventing relapse and recurrence.*)

32. Kinon BJ. The routine use of atypical antipsychotic agents: maintenance treatment. J Clin Psychiatry 1998;59(Suppl 19):18. (*Guidelines for long-term management with this new generation of antipsychotics.*)

33. Kupfer DJ, Frank E, Perel JM, et al. Five-year outcome for maintenance therapies in recurrent depression. Arch Gen Psychiatry 1992;49:769. (*Long-term therapy was effective and required in those who have recurrences.*)

34. Livingston MG, Livingston HM. New antidepressants for old people? The evidence that newer drugs are much better than the old is thin. BMJ 1999;318:1640. (*An editorial that succinctly sums up the evidence.*)

35. Louik C, Lin AE, Werler MM, et al. First-trimester use of selective serotonin-reuptake inhibitors and the risk of birth defects. N Engl J Med 2007;356:2675. (*A case–control study, finding that there was no overall risk; post hoc analysis suggested a small risk of certain birth defects associated with the use of a few of the selective serotonin-reuptake inhibitors [SSRIs].*)

36. Lustman PJ, Griffith LS, Freedland KE, et al. Cognitive behavior therapy for depression in type 2 diabetes mellitus: a randomized, controlled trial. Ann Intern Med 1998;129:613. (*Evidence for efficacy in persons with depression accompanying a major medical illness.*)

37. Mulchahey JJ, Malik MS, Sabai M, et al. Serotonin-selective reuptake inhibitors in the treatment of geriatric depression and related disorders. Int J Neuropsychopharmacol 1999;2:121. (*A review of the use of SSRIs in elderly depression.*)

38. Nierenberg AA, Trivedi MH, et al. Suicide risk management for the Sequenced Treatment Alternatives to Relieve Depression Study: applied NIMH guidelines. J Psychiatric Res 2004;38:583. (*An approach to minimizing suicide risk.*)

39. Nurnberg HG, Hensley PL, Gelenberg AJ, et al. Treatment of antidepressant-associated sexual dysfunction with sildenafil. JAMA 2003;289:56. (*A 6-week randomized, controlled trial, finding a significant improvement in >50% of study participants.*)

40. Potter WZ, Rudorfer MV. Electroconvulsive therapy—a modern medical procedure. N Engl J Med 1993;328:882. (*An editorial emphasizing the important contribution of electroconvulsive therapy to the treatment of severe depression.*)

41. Roose SP, Laghrissi-Thode F, Kennedy JS, et al. Comparison of paroxetine and nortriptyline in depressed patients with ischemic heart disease. JAMA 1998;279:287. (*The SSRI was the better tolerated; the tricyclic antidepressant was associated with a significantly higher rate of adverse cardiac events.*)

42. Rush AJ, Trivedi MH, Wisniewski SR, et al. for the STAR*D Study Team. Bupropion-SR, sertraline, or venlafaxine-XR after failure of SSRIs for depression. N Engl J Med 2006;354:1231. (*A randomized, controlled trial; both switching class and trying another SSRI achieved remission in one fourth of patients who failed initial treatment with citalopram.*)

43. Scientific expert meeting: antidepressants in clinical practice. J Clin Psychiatry 1999;60(Suppl 17). (*An entire supplement devoted to the broad use of available antidepressants.*)

44. Sachs GS, Nierenberg AA, Calabrese JR, et al. Effectiveness of adjunctive antidepressant treatment for bipolar depression. N Engl J Med 2007;356:1711. (*A randomized, controlled trial; no benefit or harm was noted.*)

45. Smoller JW, Pollack MH, Lee DK. Management of antidepressant-induced side effects. In: Stern TA, Herman JB, Slavin PL, eds. MGH guide to psychiatry in primary care. New York: McGraw-Hill, 1998:483. (*A practical review of side effects and methods for managing them.*)

46. Thapa PB, Gideon P, Cost TW, et al. Antidepressants and the risk of falls among nursing home residents. N Engl J Med 1998;339:875. (*Both tricyclics and SSRIs increased the risk for falls in a dose-related fashion; although the SSRIs do not cause orthostasis, they may cause dizziness.*)

47. Wisner KL, Gleneberg AJ, Leonard AJ, et al. Pharmacologic treatment of depression during pregnancy. JAMA 1999;282:1264. (*A systematic review of the evidence.*)

48. Worthington J, Fava M, Agustin C, et al. Consumption of alcohol, nicotine, and caffeine among depressed outpatients: relationship with response to treatment. Psychosomatics 1996;37:518. (*Demonstrates a lower response in patients who drink alcohol mildly.*)

CHAPTER 228 ■ APPROACH TO THE PATIENT WITH AN ALCOHOL PROBLEM

MICHAEL F. BIERER AND ELEANOR Z. HANNA

Alcohol abuse is a national problem. Surveys reveal that 5% of U.S. adults meet criteria for alcohol abuse; up to 20% of adults attending primary care clinics have alcohol abuse or dependence. The rates of abuse and dependence in persons 18 to 29 years of age are twice those for the nation as a whole. The overall estimated societal costs of alcohol-related health problems, lost productivity, crime, accidental deaths, and fires are staggering (>$185 billion). The estimated direct cost of treatment for alcohol problems and medical consequences approaches $26 billion, with more than $18 billion for medical care alone.

Understanding every patient's drinking behavior is basic to primary care. Although the detection of plainly unhealthy levels of intake and dramatically negative health consequences of drinking are straightforward, problem drinking or specific risk may be subtler. Persons whose drinking falls into the "moderate" range may still require attention because of comorbid conditions. Risky drinking prior to the development of any resultant complications needs to be identified and modified. Timely recognition, coupled with appropriate intervention, is critical. The primary care physician is uniquely positioned to identify and address harmful patterns of alcohol use and a host of related medical and social problems.

DEFINITIONS (1–3)

Definitions

Alcoholism is an inexact but popular term, encompassing two distinct conditions: *alcohol abuse* and *alcohol dependence*. Alcohol use in excess of "*drinking in moderation*" is epidemiologically associated with excess morbidity and mortality.

Drinking in Moderation

The behavioral hallmark of moderate drinking is that it is under easy voluntary control. With the caveat that a given dose of alcohol affects different people differently, drinking in moderation may be defined quantitatively as on average two or fewer drinks per day for men and one or fewer for women and the elderly. Furthermore, for drinking to be "moderate," no single episode of drinking should exceed four drinks for men or three drinks for women, where a standard drink contains roughly 12 g, 15 mL, or 0.5 oz of alcohol (which is the approximate content of 12 oz of beer, 5 oz of wine, or 1.5 oz of liquor, respectively) (Fig. 228.1.)

Alcohol Abuse

Abuse is formally defined as a maladaptive pattern of use leading to impairment in one of several sociobehavioral domains for a 1-year period (Table 228.1).

Alcohol Dependence

Alcohol dependence is defined as a maladaptive pattern of use, resulting in substantial distress or dysfunction, characterized by at least three of seven symptoms that include tolerance, withdrawal, unsuccessful attempts at cutting down, and preoccupation with and recurrent use of alcohol despite adverse consequences in important areas of life. Patients drink more than they intend and may give up important activities because of drinking. Most problem drinkers are employed, employable, or in families, indicating that the scope of the problem extends far beyond those who meet formal diagnostic criteria.

PATHOPHYSIOLOGY, CLINICAL PRESENTATION AND COURSE (2–22)

Causes and Risk Factors

The causes of alcohol abuse and dependence are incompletely understood, but the etiology is clearly *multifactorial*. Biogenetic, sociocultural, psychological, and behavioral influences have been identified. No single factor accounts for all manifestations, but attention to each contributes to a better understanding the problem.

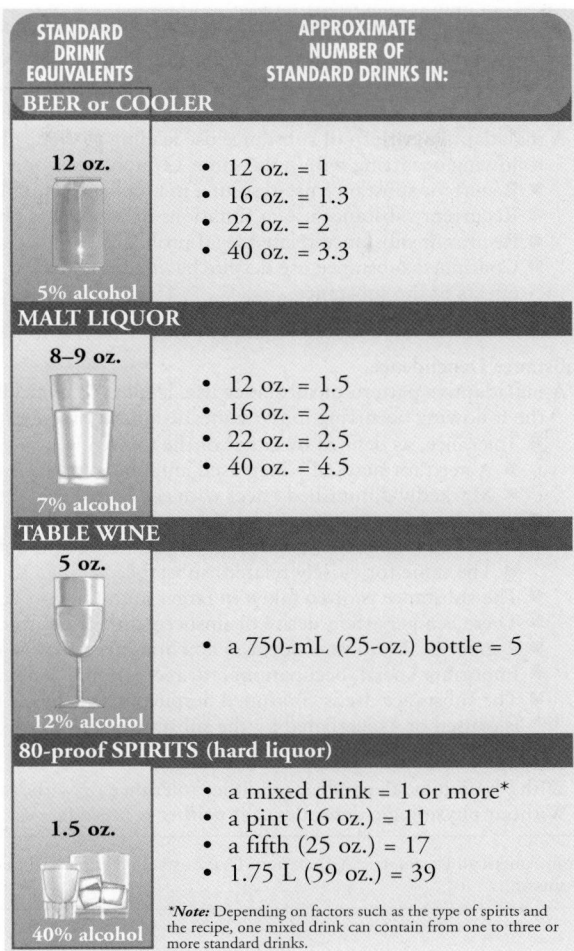

FIGURE 228.1. The standard drink. (From U.S. Department of Health and Human Services. Helping patients who drink too much: a clinician's guide. Rockville, MD: Author, 2005.)

Biogenetic Factors

Alcohol abuse clearly has genetic determinants. Genetic factors appear to influence the metabolism of alcohol and the effects of alcohol on neurotransmitters, receptors, and cell membranes. More than 100 alcohol-responsive genes and numerous genetic risk factors have been characterized, including the genes for alcohol dehydrogenase, aldehyde dehydrogenase, monoamine oxidase, and catechol-O-methyltransferase; more are likely to be identified. The *A1 allele of the D2 dopamine receptor gene* and the *G1 allele of the γ-aminobutyric acid (GABA) receptor* have been identified as independent contributors to risk. The odds ratio of developing alcohol abuse or dependence is about 10 for monozygotic twins versus about 5 for dizygotic twins. Offspring of parents with alcohol dependence frequently have an altered biologic response to alcohol, and young adult offspring with such a response are more likely to develop an alcohol diagnosis within a decade.

Sociocultural Factors

Poverty, socialization patterns, and cultural differences in the rules governing alcohol use are related to the probability of

TABLE 228.1

CRITERIA FOR SUBSTANCE ABUSE AND DEPENDENCE ACCORDING TO DSM-IV

Substance Abuse

A maladaptive pattern of substance use leading to clinically significant impairment or distress, as manifested by at least one of the following occurring within the same 12-month period:
- Recurrent substance use resulting in a failure to fulfill major role obligations at work, school, or home
- Recurrent substance use in situations in which it is physically hazardous
- Recurrent substance-related legal problems
- Continued substance use despite having persistent or recurrent social or interpersonal problems caused or exacerbated by the effects of the substance

The symptoms have never met the criteria for Substance Dependence for this class of drugs

Substance Dependence

A maladaptive pattern of substance use, leading to clinically significant impairment or distress, as manifested by at least three of the following occurring in the same 12-month time period:
- Tolerance, as defined by either of the following:
  - A need for markedly increased amounts of the substance to achieve intoxication or desired effect
  - Markedly diminished effect with continued use of the same amount of the substance
- Withdrawal as manifested by either of the following:
  - The characteristic withdrawal syndrome for the substance
  - The same (or closely related) substance is taken to relieve or avoid withdrawal symptoms
- The substance is often taken in larger amounts or over a longer period that was intended
- There is a persistent desire or unsuccessful efforts to cut down or control substance use
- A great deal of time is spent in activities necessary to obtain the substance, use the substance, or recover from its effects
- Important social, occupational, or recreational activities are given up or reduced because of substance use
- The substance use is continued despite knowledge of having a persistent or recurrent physical or psychological problem that is caused or exacerbated by the substance use

Specify If

With physiologic dependence if either tolerance or withdrawal is present
Without physiologic dependence if neither is present

From American Psychiatric Association. Diagnostic and statistical manual of mental disorders, 4th ed. [DSM-IV].Washington DC: Author, 1997; with permission.

development of disease. Parental and peer values, attitudes, and behaviors all contribute. This helps to explain the increasing use of alcohol among women and youth and use patterns of ethnic minorities, despite an overall national decline in consumption.

Psychological–Psychodynamic Factors

Underlying psychopathology (e.g., dependence conflict, depression, excessive need for power or sensation seeking, gender identification problems) contributes to predisposing a person to drink excessively, either to mask or to solve a psychological problem. Drinking in this context is viewed primarily as a symptom of the underlying psychopathology.

Behavioral Factors

Alcoholism has an element of learned behavior that is reversible, time limited, on a continuum with normal drinking behavior, and established by a series of learning and reinforcement experiences. The strength and pace of acquiring the habit vary with the intensity and rapidity of reinforcement. Social interactions, emotional stress, guilty or negative thoughts, and the need for sleep or pain relief precipitate and sustain drinking. Any of these precipitants coupled with learned expectations about the reinforcing, pleasurable effects of alcohol may initiate and maintain the drinking behavior.

The neurobiology of adaptation and tolerance affects the learning process. In the presence of reinforcing neurochemistry, environmental cues acquire greater salience, and learning is more likely to occur as the brain forges strong associations among behavior, environment, and reward, thus increasing the likelihood of repeating behavior that will lead to the reward There are many candidates for the neuroanatomic substrate of such enhanced learning, and, theoretically, many are not specific for one reinforcing drug or another.

Epidemiologic Patterns

Alcohol use varies by age, gender, and socioeconomic group.

Young People. Alcohol use and abuse among young people is high. Eighty percent of young people drink as high school seniors and 26% binge drink, a pattern that continues and increases to 40% among college students. These patterns continue into young adulthood; heavy episodic (binge) drinking is at its highest in the third decade for both men and women. Adults who began drinking or smoking regularly in their early teens suffer the most serious alcohol, drug, and psychiatric problems and often manifest the greatest proportion of familial alcohol problems.

Women. As a result of social change, women are consulting alcohol abuse clinics at double the former rates, and the gap between men and women in terms of alcohol consumption and problems continues to narrow.

The Elderly. Older patients may begin to use alcohol excessively for stress, especially in reaction to the loss of a loved one, loss of physical function or role, or other stressful transitions or because of sleep difficulties. A peak period for the onset for new alcohol-related problems is 65 to 74 years of age. The use of alcohol along with the multiple medications that are prescribed to the elderly can be especially problematic.

Ethnic Minorities. Although the total consumption of alcohol has declined somewhat in the last decade, rates of alcohol abuse have increased especially among certain ethnic groups. *Native Americans* continue to evidence high rates of alcohol diagnoses. Risk is also increasing among young *African Americans* (especially women), *Hispanics*, and *Asian* men.

Certain ethnic groups are relatively protected from alcohol dependence. Some subgroups of Asians have a form of aldehyde dehydrogenase (ALDH) that metabolizes acetaldehyde slowly, therefore yielding higher concentrations of this chemical, which is perceived as unpleasant. People with more of this isoform of ALDH enjoy drinking less than those with proportionally less and have a lower likelihood of developing dependence.

Clinical Presentation and Course

There is a wide spectrum of drinking behaviors, from drinking in moderation to frank alcohol abuse, dependence, and deterioration.

Drinking in Moderation

The use of alcohol in moderation is characterized by varying consumption and beverage according to internal cues and external circumstances. The hallmarks of moderate drinking are that it is under *voluntary control* and *does not exceed recommended maxima*. Moderate drinking may occasionally be considered either risky or problematic in a patient with signs or symptoms made worse by alcohol or with strong family histories. Such patients should be informed about the increased risk.

The At-Risk Drinker

Persons *drinking more than the recommended maxima* but *without negative consequences* and who do not meet criteria for abuse or dependence can be classified as "at-risk drinkers." Patients must drink greater more than the recommended maxima or in risky situations to fit into this category, but if there are problems stemming from drinking, then it is more useful to classify them as problem drinkers.

The Problem Drinker

Such persons experience *negative consequences of drinking*, which might be minor and of distress only to the drinker or may cause significant problems for family, friends, or colleagues. Thus, problematic drinking may range from preclinical to severe and obvious.

The Alcohol Abuser

This person meets the criteria for *heavy social drinking*, *gets drunk on occasion*, and also exhibits the negative medical, legal, social, or psychological *consequences* of excessive alcohol consumption. He or she makes or thinks of making *attempts at cutting down* or *quitting*. Functioning may vary from seemingly intact behavior to difficulty coping. The person may deny a drinking problem and blame external events or persons; denial is common even among those with multiple arrests for drunk driving. By definition, patients with alcohol abuse have not reached a severity sufficient for them to be diagnosed with dependence.

The Alcohol-Dependent Patient

The dependent patient's consumption of alcohol may be *independent of usual precipitants* or social situations, that is, the internal drive to drink is paramount and usually overwhelming. External circumstances might constrain drinking for a time, yielding a "binge-pattern" syndrome. Most continue to work, some even in high positions. Alcohol is given *high priority* in all situations (e.g., one goes to a party to drink, not to socialize). *Tolerance* to alcohol develops, and *withdrawal* symptoms (mood disturbance, tremor, nausea, sweats) may be noted during the day when the blood alcohol level drops. Drinking periodically during the day is often needed to ward off or relieve withdrawal symptoms. The patient is aware of the compulsion to drink but is difficult to reach unless family or employer notes a problem or serious medical complications develop.

The Severely Deteriorated Patient

Such individuals maintain a *near-constant state of intoxication*, having no care for their person or surroundings, and undergo periodic hospitalizations for detoxification and for medical care necessary after alcohol-related trauma or organ damage.

Natural History and Clinical Course of Alcohol Abuse

There is considerable individual variation. Onset ranges from an initial phase of social drinking to immediate heavy drinking. Early onset of drinking is associated with an increased risk of alcohol abuse, but the association is not necessarily causative. The course of alcohol dependence may be punctuated by periods of spontaneous remission. The prognosis remains relatively favorable until dependence sets in and reaches the severity that is detected clinically.

Once the addiction becomes more severe, it is difficult to break in the absence of treatment, and the clinical course is often progressive. This makes the early detection of at-risk or unhealthy alcohol use important before the patient becomes alcohol dependent. At the point of addiction, continued drinking may be punctuated by periods of abstinence or controlled drinking but usually followed by relapse and progression, especially if there is no expert intervention. Controversy continues regarding whether total abstinence is required to prevent relapse to dependent drinking.

Medical Complications

The risk of organ damage is related in part to the dose and duration of alcohol exposure, with some conditions (e.g., *alcoholic cardiomyopathy, fatty liver, alcoholic hepatitis, or anemia*) manifesting reversibility with abstinence, and others (e.g., *cirrhosis or neuropathy*) seeming to progress inexorably once organ damage has occurred. Predicting the risk of irreversible organ damage is imperfect; occasionally, resilience is afforded by abstinence and good nutrition. Risk appears to be a function of genetic predisposition, alcohol dose, and chronicity of exposure.

Cardiovascular Complications. Although moderate alcohol consumption (up to two drinks a day in white men, one in women and African American men) is associated with reductions in *coronary events* and *coronary mortality*, the consumption of more than three drinks a day is associated with an increased risk for *hypertension*. High levels of alcohol consumption place the patient at risk for paroxysms of *atrial fibrillation* (see Chapter 28) and more chronically for *alcoholic cardiomyopathy* (see Chapter 32).

Gynecologic and Reproductive Complications. Increases in the risks of *breast cancer* and *osteoporosis* are associated with drinking on average more than two standard drinks daily. (Moderate drinking is associated with a modest reduction in breast cancer mortality.) *Fetal alcohol syndrome* occurs in infants born to mothers who drink heavily during pregnancy. Features include permanently stunted growth, mental retardation, musculoskeletal abnormalities, poor coordination, and cardiac malformations. Incidence approaches 33% among pregnant women who drink more than 150 g (6.25 oz) of alcohol per day. Another one third of children born to such women l have mental retardation or severe behavior disorders. Serious maternal and infant health problems and increased infant and fetal deaths accrue among women who report drinking even as little as one drink a week during pregnancy.

In men, persistent *impotence* and *loss of libido* reflect impaired gonadotropin release and accelerated testosterone metabolism that occur as consequences of chronic alcohol excess; they predate end-stage liver disease.

Gastrointestinal Complications. *Alcoholic hepatitis, pancreatitis,* and *gastritis* may follow binge drinking. *Fatty liver* and *esophagitis* ensue from chronic use. Late-stage complications include *cirrhosis* and *oral cancers.*

Neurologic Complications. *Cerebellar degenerative disease, peripheral neuropathy, Wernicke's encephalopathy,* and *Korsakoff's dementia* are among the serious neurologic consequences of alcohol excess (see Chapters 166, 176, and 173).

DIAGNOSIS (1–3)

The fourth edition of the *Diagnostic and Statistical Manual of Mental Disorders* (DSM-IV) specifies the most widely used criteria for the formal diagnoses of alcohol abuse and alcohol dependence (see Table 228.1). Diagnosis of late-stage disease poses little difficulty. The challenge is the early detection in daily primary care practice.

WORKUP (1–3,22–27)

Overall Strategy

Formal diagnosis involves the identification of *excessive quantity* and *duration* of consumption, *physiologic manifestations* of ethanol addiction, *loss of control* over drinking, and *chronic damage* to physical health and social functioning. The tenor and words used to discuss alcohol use should be nonjudgmental and empathic. There is no great separation between the diagnostic interview and therapeutic counseling.

If problem drinking is identified, one helps the patient to understand and acknowledge the problem, its potential consequences, and the need for treatment. The objective then shifts to negotiating and carrying out an acceptable treatment plan, one that is personalized and multifaceted. These elements may be encompassed in a brief intervention and include referral for specialized care for more complex problems.

Screening

The high prevalence of alcohol abuse, its serious consequences, and good response to intervention at an early stage argue for routinely screening all adolescents and adults who come for primary care. The U.S. Preventive Services Task Force recommends universal screening and brief intervention to reduce alcohol misuse.

Drinking is addressed as would any health-related behavior, such as exercise or seat-belt use. A high index of suspicion for alcoholism is indicated for the patient who presents with a family history positive for alcoholism, anxiety, insomnia, recurrent infection, a potentially alcohol-related illness, child abuse, domestic violence, multiple psychosomatic problems, suicidality, depression, inability to articulate feelings, or interpersonal, occupational, financial, or legal problems. Recently, tobacco smoking has emerged as a marker for alcohol abuse and dependence.

The two dimensions of the screening evaluation are *quantity of* and *problems related to* the use of alcohol.

Screening for Quantity/Frequency

A simple set of questions designed to elicit quantity consumed is the first step in assessing whether a patient drinks less or greater than the recommended levels. Because beer and wine may not be recognized as "alcohol" by many patients, those who say that they do not drink should be questioned about these beverages. For patients who drink any alcohol at all, the following questions may be useful, either in a written or verbal exchange:

> "On average, how many drinks do you have per day?"
> "In the last month, what is the maximum number of drinks you've had on one occasion?"
> "In the last month, how many days per week did you typically drink any alcohol at all?"

Other, even simpler and shorter questions to screen for at-risk or hazardous drinking patterns are being validated.

Screening for Behaviors and Consequences

For the patient who consumes alcohol but in whom there is no clinical evidence or suspicion of alcohol abuse, a number of validated approaches to screening are available. These include the CAGE questions (see next paragraph) and self-administered questionnaires.

The CAGE Questions. Use of these questions is the screening test of choice (Table 228.2). In primary care settings, sensitivity for alcohol abuse or dependence with a score of 2 (the standard cutoff) ranges from 70% to 85% and specificity from 85% to 91%. In the *elderly*, in whom the prevalence of

---

TABLE 228.2

THE CAGE TEST

Have you ever felt the need to Cut down on drinking?
Have you ever felt Annoyed by criticism of drinking?
Have you ever had Guilty feelings about drinking?
Have you ever taken a morning Eye opener?

From Mayfield D, McLead G, Hall P. The CAGE questionnaire. Am J Psychiatry 1974;131:1121, with permission.

alcoholism is increased but clinical presentation may be harder to ascertain, sensitivity falls to 50%, whereas specificity remains greater than 90%. Including questions on the quantity and frequency of drinking improves detection in the elderly. The CAGE questions focus on consequences of drinking and provide a natural entry into discussions about the patient's perception of negative consequences. For example, if a patient endorses being annoyed by other's comments about his or her drinking, then exploring what aspects are annoying and what the patient thinks of them is a natural next step.

The Alcohol Dependence Scale. This 10-item, self-administered questionnaire is another popular research and screening tool in clinical settings. It can be incorporated into a previsit lifestyle screen to assess severity. Its benefits are high reliability and validity. A cutoff score of 5 identifies patients suitable for brief intervention in the physician's office.

Other Popular Tests. The Michigan Alcohol Screening Test (MAST; Table 228.3) and the Alcohol Use Disorders Identification Test (AUDIT) are widely used. The AUDIT is a 10-item questionnaire keyed to a World Health Organization hierarchy of alcohol problems. It focuses on "harmful drinking," which indicates drinking in harmful situations. A shorter questionnaire consisting of the three consumption questions of the AUDIT (the so-called AUDIT-C) performs well in detecting unhealthy drinking and DSM-IV alcohol diagnoses and may become a future standard due to its efficiency.

Clinical Assessment

A detailed drinking history is in order for all patients suspected of having an alcohol problem on the basis of any of the following:

- A positive Alcohol Dependence Scale, CAGE, Michigan Alcohol Screening Test, AUDIT, or AUDIT-C.
- A family complaint or a history of alcoholism in the family.
- A daily drinking pattern of two to three drinks accompanied by otherwise innocuous complaints that might be related to drinking (e.g., frequent nonspecific illness, accidents, gastroesophageal reflux disease, insomnia).
- A lifestyle that may promote prolonged drinking, including tobacco or drug use.
- The occurrence of intrapsychic or interpersonal problems or stressful changes in life events.
- Suggestive manifestations on physical examination, such as alcohol on the breath, spider angiomata, plethoric facies,

TABLE 228.3

THE MICHIGAN ALCOHOLISM SCREENING TEST

1. Do you feel you are a normal drinker?	(No 2)	Yes
2. Have you ever awakened in the morning after some drinking the night before and found that you could not remember part of the evening?	(Yes 2)	No
3. Does your wife (or husband or parents) ever worry or complain about your drinking?	(Yes 1)	No
4. Can you stop drinking without a struggle after one or two drinks?	(No 2)	Yes
5. Do you ever feel badly about your drinking?	(Yes 2)	No
6. Do you ever try to limit your drinking to certain times of day or to certain places?	(Yes 0)	No
7. Do your friends or relatives think that you are a normal drinker?	(No 2)	Yes
8. Are you always able to stop when you want to?	(No 2)	Yes
9. Have you ever attended a meeting of Alcoholics Anonymous?	(Yes 5)	No
10. Have you gotten into fights when drinking?	(Yes 1)	No
11. Has drinking ever created problems with you and your wife (husband)?	(Yes 2)	No
12. Has your wife (husband or other family member) ever gone to anyone for help about your drinking?	(Yes 2)	No
13. Have you ever lost friends or girlfriends/boyfriends because of drinking?	(Yes 2)	No
14. Have you ever gotten into trouble at work because of drinking?	(Yes 2)	No
15. Have you ever lost a job because of drinking?	(Yes 2)	No
16. Have you ever neglected your obligations, your family, or your work for 2 days or more in a row because of drinking?	(Yes 2)	No
17. Do you ever drink before noon?	(Yes 1)	No
18. Have you ever been told you have liver trouble?	(Yes 2)	No
19. Have you ever had DTs (delirium tremens), severe shaking, heard voices, or seen things that weren't there after heavy drinking?	(Yes 2)	No
20. Have you ever gone to anyone for help about your drinking?	(Yes 5)	No
21. Have you ever been in a hospital because of drinking?	(Yes 5)	No
22. Have you ever been a patient in a psychiatric hospital or on a psychiatric ward of a general hospital where drinking was part of the problem?	(Yes 2)	No
23. Have you ever been seen at a psychiatric or mental health clinic or gone to a doctor or clergyman for help with an emotional problem in which drinking has played a part?	(Yes 2)	No
24. Have you ever been arrested, even for a few hours, because of drunken behavior?	(Yes 2)	No
25. Have you ever been arrested for drunk driving or driving after drinking?	(Yes 2)	No

A score of 3 points or less is considered nonalcoholic; a score of 4 points is suggestive, and a score of 5 points or more indicates alcoholism

From Seizer ML. The Michigan Alcoholism Screening Test. Am J Psychiatry 1971;127:1653, with permission.

tremor, ecchymoses, peripheral neuropathy, resistant hypertension, or tachycardia.
■ Abnormal liver function tests; macrocytic anemia.

Taking a Drinking History

Patients typically do not volunteer drinking problems and request help. To the extent that a patient has protected and maintained the drinking despite significant consequences, denial is likely to be strong. Consequently, one has to use an interview technique that is kind and supportive yet firm and clear when there are serious clinical concerns or risk, such as driving under the influence or putting others at risk due to occupational impairment. Where indicated, family members, friends, and even the employer may facilitate both history taking and therapy.

The Drinking Profile. To understand the impact and dimensions of drinking, a drinking profile that goes beyond issues of quantity and frequency will prove useful and should include attention to the following:

■ Setting: time, place, and occasion for drinking.
■ Social network: the people involved with the drinking and their relationship to the patient.
■ Consumption: quantity, frequency, and rate of consumption as it relates to that of others in the drinking context and as it relates to the patient's expected consumption.
■ Pressures (internal or external) to drink.
■ Perceived benefits of drinking—what the patient "gets out of" it.
■ Perceived negative consequences.
■ Other activities related to drinking, including other drug use.

The profile is an effective tool for understanding the context and consequences of drinking. It may assist in gaining insight into the resistant patient, treating a willing patient, and educating a person with a potential problem. It also permits one to personalize treatment.

Sources of Diagnostic Error

Missing the diagnosis may be due to subtlety of presentation, use of definitions of alcoholism that do not encompass early manifestations, viewing the patient as normal so long as he or she is performing daily activities, societal acceptance of dangerous levels of alcohol intake, and general expectations of excess alcohol consumption at most social occasions. There may be unintentional collusion with the patient in denying the problem, especially if the patient is of similar or higher social status, has similar habits and lifestyle, or is attractive, verbal, and intelligent. Worry about a resistant patient's response or overidentification may lead the practitioner to avoid exploring the subject of alcohol problems fully, if at all.

MANAGEMENT (2,3,28–45)

Overall Approach

After uncovering at-risk or problematic drinking and determining whether there is alcohol abuse or dependence, the task shifts to designing a successful management program, which requires a multifaceted, personalized, long-term strategy, often conducted in collaboration with an alcohol specialty team. Therapies can be classified as pharmacologic, psychological/behavioral, and sociocultural. Selection is best done on

an individualized basis to meet the patient's specific needs, adjusted for stage of illness.

Determinants of Successful Treatment

Early detection and prompt initiation of treatment are essential to success, with success rates of 50% to 90% attained in patients abusing alcohol but without physical or social impairment. Success rates also depend on the *length of time* a person stays in treatment, *patient involvement* in goal setting and treatment planning, and continued attachment to *family* or an integrated *social network*. *Involving family members* or significant others supports the lifestyle changes that must be made, particularly when the problem drinker is a woman or young person. This ensures that the patient goes for and remains in treatment.

Other determinants of successful treatment include the use of a *personalized multifaceted* plan, an *active role* for the patient, and continuous *review*. Controversy continues regarding whether *total abstinence* is required to halt progression. Cessation certainly is necessary to halt many of the medical complications.

Role for the Primary Care Physician

The doctor—patient relationship that is so much a part of the primary care experience provides a powerful means of effecting behavioral change. When used over the course of years, the relationship permits the identification and anticipation of problems, support during difficult periods, and prevention of relapse. Long-term management solely by the primary care physician requires a willingness to be continuously available, persistently supportive, and able to shoulder a substantial care burden. Whether one intends to provide sole care for the alcohol-abusing patient or involve the specialist, the primary physician has the important initial task of assisting the patient in acknowledging the drinking problem and developing a treatment program. A relationship and an interaction based on trust and acceptance of the patient's foibles and suffering are essential. The advent of increasingly effective pharmacologic measures that help to initiate and sustain abstinence should enhance the management capabilities of the primary care physician.

Patients for whom principal management by the primary physician is realistic include those with the following:

■ Medical complications as the foremost concern
■ A strong personal tie to the primary physician
■ Good social stability
■ Only minor psychopathology
■ Intelligence and pragmatism
■ An intact and supportive social network
■ Evidence of having successfully moderated or ceased drinking in the past with a primary care physician

The transition to recovery can be long and arduous. Many false starts are to be expected. Helping a patient to deal with relapse and understanding the path that led to it are important primary care functions that minimize the likelihood of recurrence and get the patient back on the path to improvement.

Role for Specialty Care

Persons with more-serious alcohol problems will likely benefit from a coordinated, collaborative approach using the services of a specialty treatment team complementing those of the primary care physician. The incorporation of expert input often makes continued primary care management more cogent and acceptable. The team's addiction specialists, counselors, and psychiatrists can be particularly useful in helping the patient to identify and restructure destructive patterns of drinking, learn new coping skills, and deal with any underlying psychopathology. Referral and collaboration also helps to relieve the burden on the primary physician while allowing continuation of the patient–doctor relationship.

Management of the Nondependent Drinker

The Brief Intervention

For outpatients drinking more than recommended levels who do not have dependence, a program of brief, clear, and empathic discussions about changing drinking behavior has been demonstrated to reduce alcohol consumption and complications. The key components of the brief intervention are as follows:

- Making the link between the patient's drinking and potential or actual harms (psychosocial or physical).
- Giving feedback to the patient about normative drinking, such as using normative tables (Table 228.4), which is especially useful when patients have inaccurate beliefs about what is typical for their cohort.

- Reviewing the benefits of recommended change, referring predominantly to the patient's statements, beliefs, and goals, but also to objective medical findings.
- Giving clear instructions and agreement about the modification of behavior—for example, when and how to cut down to a specific level or to abstain completely.
- Instructing the patient not yet ready to change behavior to track drinking and consequences in a structured way (e.g., keeping a journal).
- Agreeing clearly about follow-up.

Follow-up is critical and cost-effective. Studies find that improved drinking persists for at least 1 year after two brief physician discussions coupled with two nurse follow-up phone calls. Telephone interventions and even mailed interventions also improve drinking outcomes.

Management of Alcohol Dependence

Patients meeting the diagnostic criteria for alcohol dependence should be advised of the likely need for expert assistance in abstaining from alcohol, but referral to a specialist or alcohol treatment program does not lessen the need for the trusting long-term relationship provided by the primary care physician. With the advent of pharmacologic therapies for dependence, care of the alcohol dependent patient is likely to begin

TABLE 228.4

CUMULATIVE PERCENTILE OF DRINKS PER WEEK

Men, age (yr)	0	1	2–3	4–5	6–8	9–12	13–19	20–29	30–39	40+
Total	32%	65%	71%	76%	80%	84%	87%	90%	93%	100%
18–20	20%	49%	59%	65%	73%	79%	85%	90%	93%	100%
21–25	19%	53%	63%	71%	78%	84%	91%	94%	97%	100%
26–29	21%	57%	68%	76%	82%	88%	93%	96%	97%	100%
30–34	25%	57%	67%	73%	80%	86%	91%	95%	97%	100%
35–39	26%	60%	68%	74%	80%	86%	91%	94%	95%	100%
40–44	27%	59%	69%	75%	81%	86%	91%	94%	96%	100%
45–49	28%	61%	70%	75%	81%	86%	92%	95%	96%	100%
50–54	32%	65%	72%	78%	84%	89%	94%	97%	98%	100%
55–59	36%	68%	74%	77%	83%	88%	93%	96%	97%	100%
60–64	45%	73%	78%	82%	87%	91%	95%	98%	99%	100%
65+	29%	61%	69%	75%	81%	86%	91%	95%	96%	100%
Women, age (yr)	0	1	2–3	4–5	6–8	9–12	13–19	20–29	30–39	40+
Total	40%	81%	86%	90%	92%	94%	96%	97%	98%	100%
18–20	27%	72%	81%	85%	90%	93%	96%	98%	99%	100%
21–25	30%	80%	88%	91%	94%	97%	98%	99%	99%	100%
26–29	32%	80%	87%	92%	94%	97%	98%	99%	99%	100%
30–34	32%	78%	86%	90%	93%	96%	98%	99%	99%	100%
35–39	35%	80%	86%	91%	94%	96%	98%	99%	100%	100%
40–44	36%	79%	86%	89%	93%	95%	97%	99%	99%	100%
45–49	42%	82%	87%	90%	94%	96%	98%	99%	99%	100%
50–54	43%	82%	88%	91%	93%	96%	98%	99%	99%	100%
55–59	50%	85%	90%	93%	95%	98%	99%	100%	100%	100%
60–64	63%	89%	92%	94%	96%	98%	99%	100%	100%	100%
65+	41%	81%	87%	91%	94%	96%	98%	99%	99%	100%

Cumulative percentile of drinks per week. The standard drink is that which contains approximately 10–15 g of ethanol (12 oz of beer, 5 oz of wine, or 2 oz of distilled spirits).
From Chan KK, Neighbors C, Gilson M, et al. Epidemiological trends for drinking by age and gender: providing normative feedback for adults. Addict Behav 2007;32:967, with permission.

emigrating to the primary care setting, but specialty referral remains an important component of the treatment program, especially for addressing major barriers to care (e.g., denial and resistance) and effecting behavioral change.

Denial

One should expect ambivalence about being diagnosed with alcohol abuse and changing one's behavior. There appears to be a relationship between the condition's severity and the likelihood of denial, which can be elicited by listening carefully to how the patient explains the findings. Suggesting a journal or a weekly log of drinking events can help to establish links between drinking and particular environmental, interpersonal, or psychologic precipitants and determine without direct confrontation exactly how much the patient drinks.

For the patient in denial, one can review the evidence on how alcohol directly affects the patient's health or stands in the way of the patient's pursuit of salient personal goals. Using screening instruments and presenting the findings in terms of a specific diagnosis or negative consequence sometimes helps to objectify the problem. If the patient continues to resist, then one can bring in family, friends, or employer to present the patient with their evidence of how destructive the drinking is. Again, these sessions should be factual, nonjudgmental discussions of the relationship of alcohol to the patient's health and behavior and its effect on those important to him or her.

Resistance to Treatment

Patients who acknowledge their drinking problem yet continue to refuse to relinquish alcohol or accept help should be handled respectfully and empathically but also firmly. Disputatious confrontation is not effective, but exploring the patient's fears and resistance can be more productive. The hostile or belligerent patient should be dealt with firmly but in a manner that enhances ability to control anger. Remember that the patient's behavior is sick and his or her anger will often be directed at the primary physician or therapist, either covertly or overtly. The ultimate goal is to help the patient gain self-control, regulation, and a sense of responsibility.

Often those who resist treatment must first *fear the loss* of something very important (e.g., spouse, job) before seeking help. It may fall on the primary physician to assist family, friends, and coworkers. One way is to develop a *contingency contract* with the patient: for example, agreeing that failure to seek and comply with treatment will result in the family's refusing the patient access to living quarters until or unless help is sought. This so-called *tough love approach*, in which *loss is seriously threatened* or carried out unless the patient goes for treatment, must be embraced by all in the patient's social circle and stained indefinitely because relapse is frequent once the danger of losing a loved one or job passes. Empty threats mean that the contingency contract is artificial and does not speak to the needs or understanding of those in the patient's life. If one is dealing with an "enabling" family or social context, it is better to present the options available, continue exploring the issue, and provide health education while treating the patient's medical problems and awaiting willingness to undergo treatment.

Should the patient agree to seek treatment, it is important to keep the waiting period brief and remind the patient a day or two ahead of the appointment.

Pharmacologic Therapy

Advances in understanding the neurobiology of alcohol dependence are spurring pharmacologic approaches to the treatment of dependent persons. Pharmacologic interventions work by decreasing the craving and physical rewards of drinking and by relieving the dysphoria and distress of abstinence. Such treatment offers a respite from alcohol consumption, enabling the patient to engage in the comprehensive, durable treatment program that is essential to long-term recovery and rehabilitation. It can also be part of a longer-term strategy to minimize the reinforcement of drinking and tip the balance toward sustained reduction of drinking and global biopsychosocial improvement. Although some object to this approach on the grounds that the cognitive and emotional work of recovery entails learning to deal with dependence's challenges, it increasingly appears that properly selected drug therapy can enhance the chances of recovery. Drug therapy can help to achieve a good early response to treatment, which is a prerequisite to later success.

Physicians need to discuss with patients the role of medication, reviewing the individual benefits and risks. Many are wary, fearing the substitution of one dependence for another. The regular use of potentially addicting agents, such as benzodiazepines, should be avoided. Medication should be prescribed with strict directions for use so that patients do not replicate escaping from a negative internal state by dint of a self-administered drug. A core goal of recovery remains the development of intra- and interpersonal, nondrug strategies. Frequent evaluation is needed.

Pharmacologic agents can be classified functionally as those that reduce the urge to drink, blunt withdrawal symptoms, or treat underlying psychiatric problems.

Topiramate. Topiramate is a GABA-receptor facilitator and inhibitor of the limbic glutaminergic pathways involved in alcohol dependence that reduces the urge to drink and facilitates abstinence. Unlike other pharmacologic treatments for alcohol problems, it can be started *without prior abstinence*, making it a candidate for initial use in persons desiring to stop or reduce drinking. When it was taken over a period of 14 weeks, study patients reduced days of heavy drinking by 50% and increased by fivefold their rate of reaching 28 or more days of continuous abstinence. Confirmation of these encouraging findings in primary care practice could make the drug a practical first-line treatment for alcohol dependence and facilitate management by the primary physician. Side effects include paresthesias, taste perversion, anorexia, and difficulty with concentration.

Naltrexone. This U.S. Food and Drug Administration–approved, pure μ-opioid antagonist appears to blunt both the craving for and the pleasurable effects of alcohol by impairing the release of dopamine in the nucleus accumbens (a neurochemical event believed to be important to reinforcement, euphoria, craving, and addiction). In theory, if a patient drinks while using the medication, the experience of *intoxication is less rewarding*. In clinical trials, the drug has demonstrated efficacy, reducing the rate of relapse to heavy drinking by 50% when paired with comprehensive services, especially coping-skills therapy. Results appear to be best in persons who describe intense cravings. It also decreases the intensity, duration, and frequency of slips or relapses. Doses of 50 mg daily are prescribed for at least 6 months in alcohol-dependent patients. An intramuscular preparation administered monthly offers the advantages of improved compliance and potentially fewer hepatic side effects, given the lack of first-pass metabolism, but comparisons with the oral formulation are not available.

Adverse effects are mostly minor, with self-limited *nausea* and *headache* being the common side effects. However, high doses may cause *hepatocellular injury*, necessitating the monitoring of liver enzymes with such use. Clinically, liver enzyme tests usually show improvement associated with decreased drinking rather than the reverse.

Contraindications include *opiate use* and *hepatocellular disease*. Patients need to understand that the drug renders the therapeutic use of opioids problematic; the drug should be held for at least 10 days prior to surgery. There is also potential opiate toxicity if naltrexone is withdrawn or stopped while opiates are administered, which is a common scenario after trauma.

Acamprosate (Calcium Acetylhomotaurinate). This synthetic analogue of calcium acetylhomotaurinate (a natural analogue of GABA) is approved for the treatment of alcohol dependence. It enhances GABA activity without being a direct agonist at the GABA receptor (the site of benzodiazepine activity). There is also some effect at other receptors (e.g., *N*-methyl-D-aspartate), but little if any effect on mood, memory, or cognition and no abuse or dependence potential.

Acamprosate increases the mean duration of sobriety by 40% and the time before full-blown resumption of heavy drinking. Benefit occurs as early as 1 month into treatment, lasts during a full year of active treatment, and persists for 1 year after treatment is discontinued. The drug is typically prescribed for 1 year in conjunction with supportive counseling services; treatment is continued irrespective of drinking episodes during that time. The addition of acamprosate to a program of naltrexone and behavioral therapy appears to offer little additional benefit.

Pharmacokinetics includes unmetabolized renal elimination and crossing of the blood–brain barrier. The drug should be used at reduced dose in moderate renal insufficiency and avoided in renal failure (creatinine clearance <30 mL/min). The dose is 666 mg three times daily for patients who weigh 60 kg or greater and 666 mg in the morning followed by two doses of 333 mg for patients whop weight less than 60 kg. Adverse effects include dose-related *diarrhea* that is relatively minor and resolves with dose reduction or cessation.

Disulfiram (Antabuse). This aversive-therapy agent was the first drug approved for the treatment of alcohol dependence. The drug sensitizes the patient to the effects of alcohol by inhibiting hepatic *aldehyde dehydrogenase*, which results in an accumulation of *acetaldehyde*. Within minutes of taking as little as 1 oz of alcohol in the presence of disulfiram, the patient experiences an increase in serum acetaldehyde concentration that leads to palpitations, flushing, diaphoresis, tachypnea, tachycardia, and shortness of breath. Nausea, vomiting, and headache develop if a greater amount of alcohol is taken. Symptoms last for about 90 minutes and usually are self-limited. Candidates require careful medical and psychiatric evaluation before initiating therapy, and a written agreement or informed consent is appropriate, given the risks entailed. The goal of using this drug is that either the patient will be motivated to avoid the worsened consequences of drinking or the experience of aversion will decrease use.

Although on balance there is a lack of good placebo-controlled trials supporting its use, there may be a role for disulfiram in specific situations. For reliable patients with a sober and helpful partner, it may be effective when the patient contracts to use the drug under scheduled supervision. The partner (significant other) in this case may witness administration by initialing a log. The drug may be used for stable patients entering a high-risk situation (e.g., a stressful period of transition such as divorce or job change) or events where drinking is common, such as weddings or reunions. The standard dose is 250 mg at bedtime.

Side effects include *drowsiness* and *lethargy*, which are countered by administering the drug before bedtime. Important drug–drug interactions occur with antihypertensive agents (e.g., potentiation of the hypotensive effect of alcohol), benzodiazepines (e.g., reduced intensity of the disulfiram reaction), tricyclic antidepressants and phenothiazines (e.g., potentiation of central nervous system effects), and drugs metabolized by hepatic microsomes (e.g., prolongation of their half-lives). Occasionally, marked *hypotension* or a *cardiac arrhythmia* may occur. Fatalities from myocardial infarction and stroke have been reported. Higher doses have resulted in death. The agent can worsen depression and schizophrenia.

Duration of therapy is individualized. Treatment should be terminated if the patient fails to keep appointments, resumes drinking, becomes pregnant or depressed, or develops abnormalities in liver function tests or cardiovascular status. Part of the informed-consent process should be a contingency plan for relapse to drinking.

Investigational Agents—Serotonergic Blockade (Ondansetron). Use of this serotonin-receptor antagonist in a randomized, controlled trial of high-risk patients with early onset alcoholism (persons who manifest increased serotonergic activity) significantly reduced alcohol intake, but confirmatory evidence is needed before a definitive contribution of serotonergic blockade to treatment is established.

Psychotherapy

Psychotherapy places emphasis on psychic restructuring and the removal of the presumed underlying psychopathology. Such treatment is important for the person whose interpersonal or psychological problems outweigh the alcohol abuse. The best candidates are patients who are socially intact, intellectually curious, and eager to be involved in the process. If concurrent treatment of the drinking is included, this can be a successful approach to patients with comorbid psychiatric disorders. Alcoholism is associated with special needs that require the therapist to take a much more active role than is typical in insight-oriented psychotherapy. One must provide structure, guidance, support, nurturance, and instruction in helping the patient to control drinking while working on the underlying conflicts and dysfunctional defense mechanisms. Behavioral–cognitive and sociocultural approaches are used.

Cognitive–Behavioral Therapies. These are based on the notion that alcoholism is a learned behavior that can be extinguished and reshaped, sometimes with controlled drinking a possible outcome. Cognitive–behavioral therapy focuses on the observables of the drinking behavior (frequency, duration, quantity, time, place, activity, age, gender, and role-appropriate drinking behaviors). It attempts to identify the precipitants to abuse and the factors that maintain and perpetuate it. Behavioral components are helpful in dealing with problems involving role changes and behaviors in specific situations.

Sociocultural Treatment

This approach emphasizes altering external factors. It includes *residential care, halfway houses,* and direct social manipulation, such as *finding jobs,* helping with *shelter and money,* and removing a person from his or her family. This is a treatment appropriate for homeless, jobless, unstable persons whose social functioning is impaired; for patients who have experienced repeated treatment failures; for young people; and for others with severe family problems. Any of these approaches and the community services that follow can be used as adjuncts to other treatments wherever necessary.

Settings for Care

Inpatient care may be necessary for detoxification and treatment of withdrawal. For achieving long-term abstinence, randomized studies show no overall advantage for residential over nonresidential treatment programs. As a result, expensive long-term inpatient care is no longer the standard for treatment of alcoholism. Only one methodologically sound randomized trial demonstrated an advantage for inpatient care, and this was part of an employee assistance program, which is itself a well-recognized determinant of success.

The net result is the current emphasis on *outpatient care*, except for the treatment of severe acute withdrawal syndrome. Inpatient care remains an option for people who have failed all other forms of treatment and who will not deal with the problems so long as they are in environments that maintain destructive drinking. It is a costly approach and should be used as a last recourse. For most patients, an outpatient program that combines psychotherapy and behavioral–cognitive approaches can be offered in primary care practices by the physician and/or staff after some training.

Community Services

Alcoholics Anonymous (AA) and other programs derived from the AA model provide the critical elements of social support, caring, and structure, which are essential to many patients. The AA program has a quasireligious orientation, making it particularly useful to the religious person. Relatively superficial involvement (e.g., two to four meetings per month) is usually not effective as the sole means of therapy but can serve as a useful adjunct to other forms of treatment. However, a person willing to dedicate to a lifetime of sobriety can achieve the goal in this carefully delineated manner. *Al-Anon and Al-Ateen* assist family members of the alcoholic. Other popular self-help groups are Women for Sobriety, which stresses individual responsibility to boost self-esteem, and Rational Recovery, which stresses using reason rather than spirituality.

Employee assistance programs can be very useful because motivation is often high. Most large companies offer such programs, and their counselors can work in tandem with physicians. They may also offer family, marital, and financial help, as may programs available through social service agencies, community guidance centers, and even state or federal agencies. *Clergy and church organizations* can be very helpful to religious persons, and they also serve as important, and often the most trusted, resources for immigrants and Hispanic and African American segments of the patient population.

Pharmacologic Therapies for Concurrent Psychiatric Conditions

Comorbid psychiatric disorders are common among patients with alcohol abuse and may require specific treatment. However, the diagnosis of comorbid psychiatric disease is complex in the setting of alcohol dependence. For example, depressive symptoms that would otherwise meet criteria for major depression are often present in the treatment-seeking patient with alcohol dependence. Diagnosis of an independent depression requires careful history taking with attention to symptoms (see Chapter 227) that were present during periods of stable, prolonged abstinence in the past, and it often cannot be made with

confidence until a period of sobriety permits observation. Similarly, anxiety and insomnia are prevalent symptoms in early recovery that frequently resolve with abstinence alone, but at times they require pharmacologic intervention. Some patients recognize their symptoms as part of the addiction syndrome and can talk themselves through rough patches; others cannot.

Cautious prescribing can be warranted, but only with full awareness of the potential risks, especially when considering the use of anxiolytics and hyponotics, with their own risk of inducing dependence. Prescribing such agents should be strictly time limited and only when both prescriber and patient understanding the ramifications. Psychoactive medications for patients in early recovery should not be prescribed on an as-needed basis. Such as-needed dosing reinforces the message that the patient should not tolerate negative symptoms without recourse to drugs. It also may direct the patient's attention to subjective states when objective recovery activities and behaviors should be taking center stage.

Anxiety

Decisions to abstain and change drinking behavior often go against decades of habitual dependence, and courage is required and trepidation is common on the part of patients. The wise admonition of Alcoholics Anonymous to take it "one day at a time" might help to ease the sense of irreversible, permanent loss conferred by giving up a trusted, if maladaptive, resource. Anxiety about maintaining abstinence is nevertheless common. Patients anxious about relapse and used to self-medicating their symptoms may feel helpless to withstand distress without pharmacologic help. Their requests for drug therapy may take on a sense of compelling urgency. Particularly anxious patients have a high probability of relapse to heavy drinking over the first year of treatment.

If anxiety is prominent, especially if it is severe or marked by panic episodes, a *selective serotonin reuptake inhibitor* (SSRI) is an appropriate first-line agent. Before a *benzodiazepine* is prescribed, consultation with an addiction psychiatrist is warranted. Caution is called for because SSRIs may precipitate mania. In this population with a particularly high prevalence of comorbid psychiatric diagnoses, including bipolar disorder, inquiring about episodes of mania when sober is critical.

Insomnia

Pharmacotherapy should be targeted to the distressing psychological symptom that most threatens recovery. If insomnia (common in the first months of recovery from alcohol) is prominent, reassurance and sleep hygiene should be the first consideration. If treatment is urgent, a sedating antidepressant such as trazodone or doxepin is a reasonable consideration. The sedating atypical antipsychotic *quetiapine* in low doses (25 or 50 mg) at bedtime usually produces improved sleep. Although the benzodiazepine-like sedatives *zolpidem (Ambien)* and *eszopiclone (Lunesta)* are touted as being nonaddicting and helpful for sleep, caution is advised with these agents in alcohol-dependent persons because of cross-tolerance between benzodiazepines and alcohol, which can subject patients to physiologic dependence.

Depression

Insomnia and anxiety might form part of a syndrome that resembles depression and would meet diagnostic criteria but for the presence of substance use. Although depression improves without antidepressant medication in many cases of alcohol dependence, pharmacologic treatment is indicated when symptoms are severe. For patients scoring high on depression symptom scales, *tricyclic antidepressants (TCAs)* have been demonstrated to confer global improvement and to enhance alcohol outcomes. Although TCAs have demonstrated efficacy, all classes of antidepressants (including *SSRIs*, but not monoamine oxidase inhibitors) may be tried. *Nefazodone* (Serzone) has demonstrated some advantage in restoring sleep architecture. In all cases, time-limited trials are preferred, with the medication tapered several months after sobriety is achieved.

Treatment of Alcohol Withdrawal

Overall Approach

The acute withdrawal syndrome (tachycardia, elevation in blood pressure, tremor, hyperreflexia, increased irritability) and its severest manifestations and complications (seizures, hallucinations, and delirium tremens) are best prevented and treated by the use of benzodiazepines. Although it is not possible to predict with certainty which patients will experience significant withdrawal syndromes, the intensity and duration of alcohol use and the abruptness of alcohol reduction are important risk factors.

Site for Care

Most patients with longstanding alcohol dependence should be offered a structured setting for withdrawal; achieving a slow, safe tapering of alcohol intake as an outpatient remains problematic in such patients but is likely to improve with the advent of improved pharmacologic measures. Consider outpatient management if the patient is reliable, has no or only mild symptoms, has no critical underlying medical illnesses that would make withdrawal particularly risky, has no prior history of severe withdrawal, and has a supportive family that can provide supervision.

The determinants for the drug treatment of withdrawal include the severity of symptoms, the past history of withdrawal, and any comorbid medical conditions. The *Clinical Institute Withdrawal Assessment–Alcohol, revised* (CIWA-Ar), is the most-validated instrument for the objective assessment of withdrawal severity and risk (Table 228.5). It use is common in inpatient settings but may also be helpful in the office. A rough clinical estimate of severity must suffice in its absence. For those with mild symptoms (e.g., CIWA-Ar score <8), no treatment is necessary other than continued monitoring unless there is a history of severe withdrawal or comorbid disease, in which case pharmacologic therapy is needed. Patients with moderate symptoms (e.g., CIWA-Ar score of 8 to 15) benefit symptomatically from treatment; those with severe symptoms (scores >15) require pharmacologic therapy because the risk of seizures is very high.

Benzodiazepines (BZDs)

Agents with prolonged activity (e.g., *diazepam, chlordiazepoxide*) appear to be more effective in preventing withdrawal seizures and in achieving a smoother withdrawal with fewer rebound symptoms than the short-acting agents; however, they are also more likely to cause sedation, particularly in the elderly and patients with liver disease. The non–hepatically metabolized BZDs (lorazepam, oxazepam) are indicated for use in persons with hepatocellular disease, but because they are shorter acting, close monitoring of the patient is needed.

Several BZD regimens have been developed and are effective when used as intended. *Fixed-dose regimens* are the standard approach to treatment. *Loading-dose programs* use a large dose of a long-acting agent (e.g., diazepam 20 mg) given at the outset and repeated until the patient is sedated. Normal drug metabolism results in tapering. *Symptom-triggered* therapy using chlordiazepoxide has been shown to decrease the mean duration of therapy and amount of drug required compared with fixed-dose treatment, but it requires close monitoring of the patient, which is usually feasible only in the inpatient setting.

Beta-Blockers

Beta-blockers such as atenolol (e.g., 50 to 100 mg/d) can help to control adrenergic symptoms and reduce BZD requirements, but they are not sufficient as monotherapy because they do not prevent seizures, hallucinations, or delirium tremens. Outpatient administration is appropriate for those with mild symptoms of withdrawal; inpatient supervision is indicated for those with more-severe symptoms or a prior history of severe withdrawal.

TABLE 228.5

TREATMENT REGIMENS FOR ALCOHOL WITHDRAWAL

Severity of Withdrawal Syndrome	Regimen
Mild (CIWA-Ar score <8)	Monitor every 4–8 hr until no worsening for 24 hr; treat as for moderate or severe disease if there is a prior history of severe withdrawal or if there is serious concurrent illness
Moderate (CIWA-Ar score 8–15)	Begin diazepam 10 mg q6h for 4 doses, then 5 mg q6h for 8 doses, or chlordiazepoxide 50 mg q6h for 4 doses, then 25 mg q6h for 8 doses; then halt and allow drug metabolism to achieve tapering
	For persons with concurrent liver disease, begin lorazepam 2 mg q6h for 4 doses, then 1 mg q6h for 8 doses
	Provide additional medication as needed when symptoms are not controlled
Severe (CIWA-Ar score >15)	Admit to inpatient facility and begin symptom-triggered regimen with hourly administration of diazepam 10–20 mg, chlordiazepoxide 50–100 mg, or lorazepam 2–4 mg and reassess hourly, repeating the dose if CIWA score >8–10

CIWA-Ar, Clinical Institute Withdrawal Assessment–Alcohol, revised; q6h, every 6 hours.
From Mayo-Smith MF. Pharmacological management of alcohol withdrawal. JAMA 1997;278:144, with permission.

Prevention

Prevention involves more than warning people of the health hazards of alcohol abuse. It requires *screening* for the early detection of alcohol abuse (see prior discussion) and providing patient-specific information. By taking a *brief drinking history* at the time of the yearly checkup, the primary physician can educate the patient and provide suitable guidelines for drinking behavior, just as one does for exercise and diet. Such very brief physician interventions or trials of advice can be easily included in an annual health maintenance visit. Randomized trials find them to be effective in reducing harmful levels of alcohol consumption.

People who do drink need to know how alcohol can affect them, how to behave responsibly when drinking (especially with regard to driving), and how to drink in a way that prevents drunkenness (Table 228.6 and Table 228.7). Individuals should know that their attitudes and behaviors will affect how their children/spouses drink. All patients should be cautioned that drinking is a dangerous way to deal with insomnia and emotional problems. Waiting-room literature and hospital and community health-education programs can complement instruction. National campaigns focus on alcohol-related accidents, crime, concomitants of abuse, and birth defects.

Approach to Alcohol Hangover

Known formally as "*veisalgia*," the alcohol hangover usually ensues after the consumption of 1.5 g/kg (five to six drinks in men and three to five drinks in women not tolerant to alcohol). The syndrome is characterized by headache, anorexia, nausea, fatigue, diarrhea, and tremulousness. Visuospatial skills, cognitive function, and job performance are impaired despite the clearing of alcohol from the bloodstream and can lead to accidents. Purported mechanisms include dehydration, an excess production of acetaldehyde from alcohol metabolism, and an accumulation of byproducts (congeners) found in dark liquors. Cytokines may play an intermediary role and account for some of the symptoms (e.g., malaise, gastrointestinal upset). Dehydration is common, leading to increases in antidiuretic hormone, cardiac output, and blood pressure; the electroencephalogram is abnormal.

The best prevention is patient education and counseling. Light to moderate drinkers need to understand that they are

TABLE 228.7

BEHAVIOR EXPECTED AT VARIOUS BLOOD ALCOHOL LEVELS

Blood Alcohol Level (mg Alcohol/ 100 mL Blood)	Behavioral Effects
0.05	Relaxation; possibility of thought, judgment, and self-control being affected
0.10	Obvious impairment of voluntary motor action; legally drunk in most states
0.20	Considerable motor impairment and loss of emotional control; definite intoxication
0.40–0.50	Unconsciousness and probable death resulting from respiratory failure

at greatest risk from acute alcohol excess; persons with heart disease should be warned that the resultant increase in cardiac work can stress their limited cardiac reserve. All patients should be warned that psychomotor and cognitive impairment can be substantial and appropriate caution is warranted.

There is a plethora of purported preventive measures and cures (e.g., *nonsteroidal antiinflammatory drugs, betablockers, carbohydrate loading, alcoholic beverages low in congeners, vitamin B$_6$, the herbal preparation Liv.52*); none is supported by evidence from randomized, controlled trials, and most have proven to be worthless. The best approach to prevention is moderation of alcohol intake and maintenance of good nutrition and hydration.

INDICATIONS FOR ADMISSION AND REFERRAL

Admission

The patient who has medically decompensated because of a complication of alcohol abuse (e.g., heart failure, pancreatitis, gastrointestinal bleeding, and hepatitis) clearly requires

TABLE 228.6

BLOOD ALCOHOL LEVEL[a]

Time Elapsed Since First Drink (hr)	Blood Alcohol Level After Given Number of Drinks (mg Alcohol/100 mL Blood)									
	1	2	3	4	5	6	7	8	9	10
1	0.01	0.03	0.05	0.08	0.10	0.13	0.15	0.17	0.20	0.22
2	0.00	0.02	0.04	0.06	0.09	0.11	0.14	0.16	0.19	0.21
3	0.00	0.005	0.02	0.05	0.07	0.10	0.12	0.14	0.17	0.19
4	0.00	0.00	0.01	0.03	0.06	0.08	0.11	0.13	0.15	0.18
5	0.00	0.00	0.00	0.02	0.04	0.07	0.09	0.11	0.14	0.18

[a]Given as a function of the number of drinks consumed in a circumscribed time period by a presumably normal 150-lb man. Women, because they are affected more quickly, require less alcohol to achieve these levels.
One standard drink is 1.5 oz of 80-proof spirits (40% alcohol), 3.0 oz of fortified wine (20% alcohol), 5.0 oz of table wine (12% alcohol), or 12.0 oz of beer (4.5% alcohol).

prompt hospital admission. Other candidates include persons with evidence of severe withdrawal (tremor, agitation, hallucinations, seizures) and those unable to tolerate a severe withdrawal syndrome (prior history of severe withdrawal, concurrent medical or psychiatric illness, chronic and severe alcohol-related illness). A free-standing detoxification center may suffice for the otherwise patient who is otherwise without complications.

Referral

Patients with major psychopathology, poor ties to the physician, or a disintegrated social network have serious drawbacks to successful treatment by even the most willing primary care physician. Such patients should be referred in a coordinated way for specialized care by the primary care physician, ensuring continuity and a personalized treatment. The primary physician can perform a major service for these patients by understanding the available specialized referral resources in the community and matching them to the patient's needs.

RECOMMENDATIONS

- Screen all patients for alcohol use and abuse; check for drinking at unhealthy levels and for problems and consequences of use.
- Establish rapport by being accepting, understanding, and respectful.
- Ally *with* the patient in pursuit of his or her goals and *against* the behavior that stands in the way, in this case drinking alcohol.
- Offer appropriate and sufficient instruction and explanation as treatment proceeds, always engaging the patient in establishing realistic goals and not pushing beyond limits.
- Provide brief, clear, patient-oriented guidance for behavior change for patients not meeting criteria for dependence.
- Maintain a proper balance of support, caring, and limit setting; remain flexible and adaptable to the patient's needs.
- Think of treatment as a series of short-term programs for developing and increasing the patient's sense of mastery; do not overlook the value of brief physician interventions.
- Have a low-threshold for referral and collaborative care with an alcohol specialty team, especially for persons who are alcohol dependent; also consider referral to community resources such as Alcoholics Anonymous.
- Set an achievable, mutually desired goal and negotiate a treatment agreement; abstinence is one possible goal, and healthier drinking is another; if serious health problems require that the patient abstain, address the issue through a supportive educational-advice session; if there is resistance to abstinence, it may still be negotiated and accomplished in the context of harm reduction; only if all else fails should there be confrontation and control in this area.
- Engage family members early; if the patient resists, seek agreement to involve them in the future if the patient cannot recover by a certain deadline.
- If a patient comes to a session drunk, kindly and calmly explain why it would be pointless to have a session, and reschedule the appointment; if this behavior continues, renegotiate the treatment agreement to include rules about it.
- Keep motivation high by having the patient define personal goals rather than rely on fears of losing health, family, friends, or job.

- Help the patient to identify, objectify, and deal with anger and other emotions to enhance emotional control.
- When the patient is ready, help to pinpoint the actual behaviors to be changed and work on them progressively; provide information, modeling, practice, feedback, and homework as the patient learns to handle feelings and develop new skills for assessing and modifying behavior.
- Encourage the self-monitoring of drinking behavior via logs, teaching the patient to detect causes, consequences, and maintaining factors and thus helping him or her to learn alternate ways of coping with the people, places, situations, and feelings associated with heavy drinking.
- Select those components of available specialized treatment programs that match the patient's needs, wants, and ability to cope.
- For patients who are rigid, repressed, and resistant to open-ended therapies, consider referral for behavioral–cognitive therapy.
- For patients with distinct psychiatric comorbidities, consider the safe use of the appropriate psychoactive drug treatment while dealing with the alcohol problem.
- For anxiety, consider an SSRI (see Chapter 226).
- For depression, consider a tricyclic or SSRI (see Chapter 227).
- Consider pharmacotherapy for patients with alcohol dependence, and obtain consultation if unfamiliar with the use of these agents. The options include the following:
  - *Topiramate* 300 mg/d for several weeks as initial drug therapy for persons still drinking but eager to stop or reduce their intake; if abstinence is achieved, consider:
  - *Naltrexone* 50 mg/d to maintain abstinence or once-monthly intramuscular administration, especially for those reporting craving for alcohol; or:
  - *Acamprosate* 666 mg thrice daily (if the patient weighs >60 kg) to maintain abstinence.
  - *Disulfiram* 250 mg/d for patients strongly motivated to attain total abstinence and specifically requesting such therapy; begin 250 mg at bedtime and renew on a monthly basis; strongly consider written informed consent.
- Use drug treatment as a complement to and a means of participating effectively in a comprehensive program of care, reevaluating the need for continued drug therapy while working on psychosocial interventions that will sustain long-term abstinence.
- Refer to a community social service agency for coordinated care and assistance for patients who are homeless, jobless, or have other serious social problems.
- For patients who have failed outpatient treatments, can afford the time, and need to be taken out of their environment to cease drinking, consider an inpatient alcohol program.
- For treatment of withdrawal:
  - Consider outpatient management if the patient is reliable, has no or only mild symptoms, has no critical underlying medical illnesses that would make withdrawal particularly risky, has no prior history of severe withdrawal, and has a supportive family that can provide supervision; otherwise, arrange inpatient care.
  - Prescribe a long-acting BZD (e.g., a fixed-schedule program of diazepam 10 mg every 6 hours for four doses, then 5 mg every 6 hours for eight doses); achieve tapering by normal drug metabolism.
  - Promptly admit unstable patients and those with other medical conditions or with symptoms suggesting

potentially severe withdrawal (e.g., tachycardia, tremor, hallucinations, increased irritability).

RESOURCE MATERIALS

The National Institute on Alcohol Abuse and Alcoholism web site http://www.niaaa.nih.gov is an excellent resource for every possible professional need; it offers ongoing publication of the latest findings and policy positions plus resource materials for medical education and health education.

The National Institute on Drug Abuse web site http://www.nida.nih.gov gives information on drugs in addition to alcohol.

The U.S. Department of Health and Human Services Substance Abuse and Mental Health Services Administration's National Drug and Treatment Referral Routing Service provides a toll-free telephone number for alcohol and drug information/treatment referral assistance. The number is 1-800-662-HELP (4357).

Self-help group directories are available online.

Annotated Bibliography

1. American Psychiatric Association. Diagnostic and statistical manual of mental disorders, 4th ed. Washington DC: Author, 1997. (*The source for diagnostic criteria for alcohol abuse and alcohol dependence.*)
2. Morse RM, Flavin DK. Joint Committee of the National Council on Alcoholism and Drug Dependence and the American Society of Addiction Medicine to Study the Definition and Criteria for the Diagnosis of Alcoholism. JAMA 1992;268:1012. (*Consensus definition and criteria.*)
3. U.S. Department of Health and Human Services. Alcohol and health, tenth special report to Congress (NIH Publication No. 00-1583). Washington, DC: Author, 2000. (*The most complete source of information on every important aspect of this subject.*)
4. Beulens JWJ, Rimm EB, Ascherio A, et al. Alcohol consumption and risk for coronary heart disease in men with hypertension. Ann Intern Med 2007;146:10. (*Presents further evidence of a specific health benefit, without mortality benefit, of alcohol consumption among men at risk for cardiovascular disease.*)
5. Breslow RA, Smothers B. Drinking patterns of older Americans: National Health Interview Surveys, 1997–2001. J Stud Alcohol 2004;65:232. (*Presents major epidemiologic data, documenting the problem in the elderly.*)
6. Chan KK, Neighbors C, Gilson M, et al. Epidemiological trends for drinking by age and gender: providing normative feedback for adults. Addict Behav 2007;32:967. (*A valuable reference, listing percentiles for consumption levels stratified by gender and age of American community-dwelling adults.*)
7. Cushman WC, Cutler JA, Hanna, EZ, et al. Prevention and Treatment of Hypertension Study (PATHS): effects of an alcohol treatment program on blood pressure. Arch Intern Med 1998;158:1197. (*A reduction in excess alcohol consumption can reduce elevations in blood pressure.*)
8. Dawson DA, Grant BF, Stinson FS, et al. Recovery from DSM-IV alcohol dependence: United States, 2001–2002. Addiction 2005;100:281. (*Presents major epidemiologic data on recovery.*)
9. Fan L, Bellinger FP, Yong-Liang GE, et al. Genetic study of alcoholism and novel gene expression in the alcoholic brain. Addict Biol 2004;9:11. (*A discussion of evidence for genetic risk factors and mechanisms.*)
10. Frezza M, di Padova C, Pozzato G, et al. High blood alcohol levels in women: the role of decreased gastric alcohol dehydrogenase activity and first-pass metabolism. N Engl J Med 1990;322:95. (*Discusses the reason women are more susceptible to the effects of alcohol.*)
11. Grant BF, Dawson DA, Stinson FS, et al. The 12-month prevalence and trends in DSM-IV alcohol abuse and dependence. United States 1991–1992 and 2001–2002. Alcohol Res Health 2006;29:79. (*The definitive statistical resource on alcohol use disorders among the adult population of the United States.*)
12. Grant BF, Stinson FS, Dawson DA, et al. Prevalence and co-occurrence of substance use disorders and independent mood and anxiety disorders. Results from the National Epidemiologic Survey on Alcohol and Related Conditions. Arch Gen Psychiatry 2004; 61:807. (*Finds high rates of concurrent substance abuse.*)
13. Gronbaek M, Becker U, Johansen D, et al. Type of alcohol consumed and mortality from all causes, coronary heart disease, and cancer. Ann Intern Med 2000;133:411. (*A Danish population study, suggesting a reduced risk with wine intake.*)
14. Hanna EZ, Faden VB, Dufour MC. The effects of substance use during gestation on birth outcome, infant and maternal health. J Substance Abuse 1997;9:111. (*Depression and substance use accounted for many adverse consequences; identifies high-risk groups.*)
15. Hanna EZ, Grant BF. Parallels to early onset alcohol use in the relationship of early onset smoking with drug use and DSM-IV drug and depressive disorders: findings from the National Longitudinal Epidemiologic Survey. Alcohol Clin Exp Res 1999;23(3):513. (*Covers the issues of youth, comorbidity, severity of illness, and familial transmission.*)
16. McKee SA, Falba T, Omalley SS, et al. Smoking status as a clinical indicator for alcohol misuse in US adults. Arch Intern Med 2007;167:716. (*Presents evidence of smoking as a risk factor for alcohol abuse.*)
17. Mendelson J, Babor T, Mello N, et al. Alcoholism and prevalence of medical and psychiatric disorders. J Stud Alcohol 1986;47:361. (*Finds a high prevalence of significant medical and psychiatric problems.*)
18. National Institute on Alcohol Abuse and Alcoholism. A call to action: changing the culture of drinking at U.S. colleges. Washington, DC: National Institutes of Health, U.S. Department of Health and Human Services, 2002. (*A useful compendium and analysis of drinking among college students, as well as a plan of action to modify the behavior.*)
19. Parker E, Noble E. Alcohol consumption and cognitive functioning in social drinkers. J Stud Alcohol 1977;38:1224. (*Drinking impairs the abstracting and adaptive abilities of social drinkers.*)
20. Pittler MH, Verster JC, Ernst E. Interventions for preventing or treating alcohol hangover: systematic review of randomized controlled trials. BMJ 2005; 331:1515. (*Finds no treatment to be effective other than moderation and avoiding dehydration.*)
21. Turner RC, Lichstein PR, Peden JG, et al. Alcohol withdrawal syndromes: a review of pathophysiology, clinical presentation, and treatment. J Gen Intern Med 1989;4:432. (*A comprehensive approach for the primary physician.*)
22. U.S. Department of Health and Human Services. The economic costs of alcohol and drug abuse in the United States 1992 (NIH Publication No. 98-4237). Washington, DC: Author, 1998. (*Documents health care costs, productivity losses, and the societal impact of alcohol- and drug-related accidents, crime, fires, and social welfare use.*)
23. Bradley KA, DeBenedetti AF, Volk RJ, et al. AUDIT-C as a brief screen for alcohol misuse in primary care. Alcohol Clin Exp Res, 2007; 31:1208. (*Finds that three questions from the Alcohol Use Disorders Identification Test provide a useful and valid screening tool.*)
24. Skinner HA, Allen BA. Alcohol dependence syndrome: measurement and validation. J Abnormal Psychol 1982;91:199. (*The original paper on this highly reliable and valid research and clinical tool that is predictive of Diagnostic and Statistical Manual of Mental Disorders diagnoses.*)
25. Soderstrom CA, Smith GS, Kufera JA, et al. The accuracy of the CAGE, the BMAST and the AUDIT in screening trauma center patients for alcoholism. J Trauma 1997;43:962. (*Presents the performance characteristics of these popularly used tests in a clinical setting.*)
26. United States Preventive Services Taskforce. Screening and behavioral counseling intervention in primary care to reduce alcohol misuse: recommendation statement. Ann Intern Med 2004;140:554. (*Strongly recommends screening and brief intervention for all adults in primary care.*)
27. U.S. Department of Health and Human Services. Helping patients who drink too much: a clinician's guide. Rockville, MD: Author, 2005. (*An extensive but handy and compact guide for screening, evaluation, and brief intervention; available on line.*)
28. Anton, RF, O'Malley SS, Ciraulo, DA, et al. Combined pharmacotherapies and behavioral interventions for alcohol dependence. The COMBINE study: a randomized controlled trial. JAMA 2006; 295:2003. (*A large, complex study, demonstrating that oral naltrexone and/or behavioral interventions improved drinking outcomes in dependent drinkers.*)
29. Brown RL, Saunders LA Bobula JA, et al. Randomized-controlled trial of a telephone and mail intervention for alcohol use disorders: three-month drinking outcomes. Alcohol Clin Exp Res 2007;31:1372. (*Finds that the approach extends the usefulness of brief interventions, both to patients with alcohol dependence and to methods other than face-to-face discussions.*)
30. Garbutt JC, Kranzler HR, Omalley SS, et al. Efficacy and tolerability of long-acting injectable naltrexone for alcohol dependence: a randomized controlled trial. JAMA 2005; 293:1617. (*Monthly intramuscular depo-naltrexone reduces drinking better than placebo; no comparison was performed between intramuscular and oral naltrexone in this study.*)
31. Garbutt JC, West SL, Carey TS, et al. Pharmacological treatment of alcohol dependence: a review of the evidence. JAMA 1999;181:1318. (*A somewhat dated but meticulous meta-analytic review, finding strong evidence for acamprosate and naltrexone and less for disulfiram.*)

32. Hanna EZ. Attitudes toward problem drinkers revisited: patient–therapist factors contributing to the differential referral of patients with alcohol problems. Alcohol Clin Exp Res 1991;15:927. (*Elucidates how stereotypes interact with patient characteristics to influence professional behavior and patient compliance.*)

33. Holder HD, Gruenewald PJ, Ponicki WR, et al. Effect of community-based interventions on high-risk drinking and alcohol-related injuries. JAMA 2000;284:2341. (*Presents evidence of efficacy.*)

34. Johnson BA, Rosenthal N, Capece JA, et al. Topiramate for treating alcohol dependence: a randomized trial. JAMA 2007;298:1641. (*A randomized, controlled trial [RCT], finding evidence for efficacy.*)

35. Johnson BA, Roache JD, DiClemente CC, et al. Ondansetron for reduction of drinking among biologically predisposed alcoholic patients: a randomized controlled trial. JAMA 2000;284:963. (*RCT, providing initial promising results in high-risk persons.*)

36. Kristol JH, Cramer JA, Krol WF, et al. Naltrexone in the treatment of alcohol dependence. N Engl J Med 2001;345:1734. (*RCT, finding that the treatment was no better than placebo in this study of older men, in which the emphasis was on abstinence.*)

37. Mark TL, Kranzler HR, Poole VJ, et al. Barriers to the use of medications to treat alcoholism. Am J Addictions 2003;12:281. (*Identifies of a host of objections and concerns about pharmacologic therapies.*)

38. Mayo-Smith MF. Pharmacological management of alcohol withdrawal. JAMA 1997;278:144. (*Protocol of the American Society of Addiction Medicine, reviewing all commonly used regimens and specifying evidence-based treatment programs.*)

39. Nunes EV, Levin FR. Treatment of depression in patients with alcohol or other drug dependence: a meta-analysis. JAMA 2004;291:1887. (*A rigorous meta-analysis, finding that outcomes depend on efficacy in treating depression.*)

40. O'Malley SS, Rounsaville, BJ Farren C, et al. Initial and maintenance naltrexone treatment for alcohol dependence using primary care vs specialty care. Arch Intern Med 2003;163:1695. (*Supports the use of naltrexone in the primary care setting, with realistic counseling support.*)

41. Pittler MH, Verster JC, Ernst E. Interventions for preventing or treating alcohol hangover: systematic review of randomized controlled trials. BMJ 2005; 331:1515. (*An objective review, pointing out the relative paucity of good information on "cures."*)

42. Saitz R, Palfai TP, Cheng DM, et al. Brief intervention for medical inpatients with unhealthy alcohol use. A randomized, controlled trial. Ann Intern Med. 2007;146:167. (*Brief interventions work.*)

43. Tournier R. Alcoholics Anonymous as treatment and ideology. J Stud Alcohol 1979;40:230. (*A still relevant critique of Alcoholics Anonymous.*)

44. Walsh DC, Hingson RW, Merrigan DM, et al. A randomized trial of treatment options for alcohol-abusing workers. N Engl J Med 1991;325:775. (*Presents the best data in support of inpatient treatment; a job-related program.*)

45. Weisner C, Ray GT, Mertens JR, et al. Short-term alcohol and drug treatment outcomes predict long-term outcome. Drug Alcohol Dependence 2003;71:281. (*Presents evidence that early success portends longer-term success.*)

CHAPTER 229 ■ APPROACH TO THE PATIENT WITH SEXUAL DYSFUNCTION

LINDA C. SHAFER

There is an important relationship between one's sexual life and emotional and physical well-being. With the advent of orally effective medication for treating erectile dysfunction and the increased interest in pharmacologic agents for treating female sexual disorders, the frequency of sexual dysfunction complaints in primary care practice has risen to nearly 15% to 20% of visits. However, the incidence of sexual problems in any medical practice is a function of the frequency with which physicians take a sexual history. Approximately 43% of women and 31% of men report some specific sexual dysfunction when questioned. Therefore, the primary care physician needs to know how to take a sexual history, perform an appropriate medical evaluation (see Chapters 115 and 132), and carry out basic types of sexual counseling and supportive therapy. More than 80% of sexual complaints can be treated successfully in the primary care setting.

DEFINITIONS (1–5)

Disorders are classified as *primary* when there has never been a period of satisfactory functioning and *secondary* when the difficulty occurs after adequate functioning had been obtained.

Male Disorders

Male Erectile Disorder

Erectile dysfunction ("impotence") is defined as the inability of a male to maintain an erection sufficient to engage in intercourse and is considered a problem if it occurs in more than 25% of attempts.

Premature Ejaculation

This condition is defined as recurrent ejaculation with minimal sexual stimulation before, on, or shortly after penetration and before the person wishes it (most often <2 minutes after penetration or on <10 thrusts).

Male Orgasmic Disorder

This disorder ("retarded ejaculation") is defined as persistent delay or absence of orgasm following normal sexual excitement. It is often restricted to failure to reach orgasm in the vagina during intercourse. Orgasm can usually occur with masturbation and/or from a partner's manual or oral stimulation. There is a persistent failure to ejaculate in the presence of a satisfactory erection. This condition must be differentiated from retrograde ejaculation.

Retrograde Ejaculation

Retrograde ejaculation is a physical impairment of internal vesicle sphincter activity. The bladder neck does not close off properly during orgasm, causing semen to spurt backward into the bladder.

Female Disorders

Frigidity is a term applied to a wide variety of conditions in the woman, from complete lack of any sexual response to various inadequacies in orgasmic response. Because it is nonspecific and has a derogatory connotation, the term has been eliminated from most recent classifications.

Female Sexual Arousal Disorder

This disorder is defined as the inability to respond to sexual stimulation with lubrication and genital vasocongestion.

Female Orgasmic Disorder

This disorder ("orgasmic dysfunction") is defined as a recurrent delay in, or absence of, orgasm following a normal sexual excitement phase, despite the ability to enjoy sexual intercourse and have normal sexual desire. Some women who can have orgasm with direct clitoral stimulation find it impossible to reach orgasm during intercourse. This is a normal variant of sensitivity requiring the pairing of direct clitoral contact with intercourse.

Vaginismus

Vaginismus is an involuntary spasm of the musculature of the outer third of the vagina, making penile penetration impossible.

Both Sexes

Dyspareunia

Dyspareunia is a condition defined as painful intercourse leading to avoidance of sexual contact.

Hypoactive Sexual Desire Disorder

This disorder ("low libido") is defined as a deficit or absence of sexual fantasies and lack of desire to engage in sexual activity.

Sexual Aversion Disorder

This disorder is defined as an active avoidance of genital sexual contact with a sexual partner.

PATHOPHYSIOLOGY AND CLINICAL PRESENTATIONS (1–11)

Pathophysiology

Organic conditions are responsible for between 50% and 85% of sexual problems in both sexes. This figure represents a dramatic shift in the understanding of the causes of sexual disorders that were once thought to be primarily of psychogenic ori-

gin. Neurogenic, hormonal, vascular, and drug-induced mechanisms are prominent (see Chapters 115 and 132). For example, diabetes mellitus is a particularly important cause of erectile dysfunction (see Chapter 102); selective serotonin reuptake inhibitor antidepressant use is associated with reduced libido.

Organically based sexual dysfunctions are usually compounded by psychological issues. There is a strong bidirectional association between *depression* and sexual dysfunction in both men and women. Although there are no rigid correlations between developmental factors and dysfunctional syndromes, sexual disorders can be related to *prior experiences*. Early sexual attitudes may be negatively shaped by parental communication that sex is bad, dirty, or sinful; by inadequate information about sex; or by myths and misconceptions such as the ever-ready penis or mutual climax. Other negative experiences range from unpleasant sexual encounters to childhood sexual abuse to rape. *Intrapsychic conflicts* extend from fear of sexual failure, to concerns about sexual identity, to profound depression.

Interpersonal issues of a sexual and nonsexual nature sometimes interfere with sexual functioning, especially in the setting of inadequate communication and lack of cooperation between partners. Sexual problems may develop from such nonsexual factors as *situational stress* and *financial pressures*. Finally, sexual difficulty may occur in the context of the *anxiety* generated by an organic illness, such as a post–heart attack fear of death.

Once a sexual problem ensues, regardless of the cause, a vicious cycle of fear of failure, anxiety, and guilt is likely to ensue and be self-perpetuating.

Clinical Presentation

Sexual dysfunction may present as the chief complaint or be an underlying or concurrent problem. Clinical presentations can be quite complex. For example, patients with sexual dysfunction may present with somatic complaints with no apparent medical cause (e.g., headache, low back pain, urinary symptoms, generalized pelvic pain, vulvar pruritus).

Male Erectile Disorder

Most normal men experience occasional erectile failure due to fatigue, too much alcohol, or any number of transient unfavorable circumstances. In the United States, it is estimated that up to 30 million men have erectile dysfunction, accounting for more than 500,000 ambulatory visits to health care professionals annually. Primary (lifelong) erectile dysfunction occurs in 1% of men younger than age 35 years. Secondary (acquired) erectile dysfunction occurs in 40% of men older than 60 years; this figure increases to 73% of men older than age 80 years. Erectile dysfunction may be the first symptom of vascular disease and should prompt further investigation. Primary impotence and longstanding secondary impotence are much more likely to be associated with medical disorders or more serious psychological issues, such as fears of intimacy, feelings of intense hostility toward women, and gender identity questions.

Premature Ejaculation

Premature ejaculation is the most common male sexual disorder, occurring in 30% to 40% of adult men. The lifetime prevalence of premature ejaculation is 15%. The psychologic causes of the disorder range from early conditioning to ambivalence and hostility toward women. Its increasing frequency has been associated with women wanting more sexual satisfaction, particularly orgasm. Once premature ejaculation occurs, it can easily be reinforced by the negative attitudes expressed by the partner. In addition, prolonged periods of no sexual activity seem to make the problem worse. If premature ejaculation occurs over a long period of time and remains untreated, secondary impotence may result. It is often easily treated in the context of a good relationship.

Male Orgasmic Disorder

Retarded ejaculation occurs most often in younger, less sexually experienced men (usually younger than age 35 years). The lifetime prevalence is 2%. Its milder form is often related to anxiety-provoking situations and has an excellent prognosis. When it is longstanding, the condition often signifies deeper-seated psychopathology, such as significant fears of rejection involved with letting go. Issues of control and commitment may be involved, as well as unconscious conflicts regarding female genitals or pregnancy. Retarded ejaculation should be considered in a couple presenting with infertility of unknown cause. The male may not have admitted his lack of ejaculation to his partner.

Female Sexual Arousal Disorder

These women present with a complete avoidance of sexual activity or an aversion to sex, which is stoically endured. The disorder has a lifetime prevalence of 60%. The condition is linked to problems of *sexual desire*, and a lack of vaginal lubrication may lead to *dyspareunia*. There is often a deep-seated conflict about sexuality, which makes the outcome less favorable. Concomitant depression and interpersonal problems and a history of medications or pelvic pathology (see Chapter 115) are other important factors.

Female Orgasmic Disorder

Orgasmic dysfunction is among the most frequent of female sexual complaints and occurs more often during the early years of sexual activity. The disorder has a lifetime prevalence of 35%. Among affected women, 30% to 40% require clitoral stimulation during intercourse to achieve orgasm; 5% to 8% present with total anorgasmia. The capacity for orgasm appears to increase with sexual experience, and that includes the aging woman. Claims that stimulation of the Grafenberg spot, or G spot, in a region in the anterior wall of the vagina will cause orgasm and female ejaculation have never been substantiated. Premature ejaculation in the male may contribute to female orgasmic dysfunction. Again, the psychologic factors involved are variable, and the prognosis for the condition is a function of which factors are responsible. These range from fears of loss of control and unrealistic expectations about sexual performance to poor partner communication. Depression must not be overlooked.

Vaginismus

Vaginismus is associated with a high incidence of pelvic pathology (see Chapter 115). The frequency of vaginismus is unknown, but the condition probably accounts for less than 10% of female sexual disorders. Lifelong vaginismus has an abrupt onset, at the first attempt at penetration, and has a chronic course. Acquired vaginismus may occur suddenly, following a sexual trauma or medical condition. A careful gynecologic examination is always warranted and, in fact, is the only definitive way to make a diagnosis. Vaginismus is one cause of *dyspareunia*. When related to psychological factors, vaginismus can be considered a conditioned response and treated behaviorally. There is often confusion about sexual anatomy and physiology, leading to fears of penetration and concerns about femininity. If the condition is longstanding, partners of these women can become seriously affected, developing secondary impotence. This disorder has been at the center of many cases of unconsummated marriages of long duration.

Dyspareunia

The overall prevalence for this condition is 20% (15% of women and 5% of men). Patients often seek medical treatment, but the physical exam is often unremarkable, with no genital abnormalities. The condition is usually chronic and results in avoidance of sex.

Hypoactive Sexual Desire Disorder

The lifetime prevalence of this condition is 40% for women and 30% for men. Low libido in one partner may reflect an excessive need for sexual expression in the other partner. Depression should be ruled out in all cases. Medical conditions causing pain, weakness, and disturbance of body image may be important triggers.

Sexual Aversion Disorder

The exact incidence is unknown, but this is a common disorder. Primary sexual aversion is higher in men, and secondary sexual aversion is higher in women. About 25% of patients meet the criteria for panic disorder. These individuals may have marital problems and may avoid sexual situations by covert strategies such as going to sleep early, traveling, neglecting personal appearance, using substances, or being overly involved at work. However, patients tend to respond naturally to sexual relations if they are able to overcome their high anxiety and initial dread.

WORKUP (1–5)

Sexual History

The sexual history should be an integral part of every medical evaluation, given the importance of sexual function to overall health, the central role that sexual dysfunction might play in somatic complaints and quality of life, and the need to review safer sexual practices. The history is most easily obtained in conjunction with performing the gynecologic and menstrual review of systems in women and the genitourinary review in men. In this way, sexual practices and concerns can be comfortably elicited in the context of routine history taking, especially if the physician displays an open, nonjudgmental, unembarrassed, and accepting attitude. One needs to take into account differences in social values, class, and age.

Helpful screening questions include "Does your present sexual functioning meet your expectations?" "Has there been a change in your sexual functioning?" "Would you like to change anything about your sexual functioning?" Additional routine questions to ask are "Have you been sexually active (or involved) with a partner in the last 6 months? (With women, men, or both?)" "Do you practice safe(r) sex?" Failure to ask HIV screening questions may result in criticism of inadequate treatment or even lead to a malpractice suit.

If a sexual problem is uncovered, the chief complaint should be explored in detail. Ask patients to describe the problem in their own words, noting its duration, circumstances, possible precipitating and alleviating factors, and severity. Avoid using "why" questions, which tend to make patients uncomfortable; use "what" questions instead. A thorough description sometimes helps to distinguish an organic from a functional etiology (see Chapters 115 and 132). For example, in the impotent male, preservation of erectile function on awakening suggests a psychological cause, as does erection with attempts at masturbation.

Also try to elicit what type of treatment the patient views as potentially helpful, be it medicine, information, or support. Clarify the patient's expectations and goals, for example, to save a marriage, or to use the problem as an excuse for an extramarital affair or divorce.

Physical Examination and Laboratory Studies

With improved understanding of the pathophysiology of sexual function and more sophisticated diagnostic testing, many sexual problems once believed to be purely psychogenic have been found to have an organic component as well. Take special note of sexual dysfunction as a common side effect of selective serotonin reuptake inhibitors, which occurs in more than 30% of patients taking the medication. Even when psychological or interpersonal problems are believed to be the principal cause of sexual dysfunction, a careful medical evaluation that includes a detailed physical examination in conjunction with a few pertinent laboratory studies is always indicated (see Chapters 115 and 132).

PRINCIPLES OF TREATMENT
(2–5,7,10–20)

The primary care physician is often the first person consulted by a patient with a sexual problem. Even the physician without formal training in sex therapy can help many patients to deal effectively with their sexual difficulties. When the problem stems from guilt and misinformation, the physician can use his or her position as an authority figure to give permission and reassurance, relabeling as "neutral" or "positive" sexual activities that the patient might fear are "bad" or "sinful," while reinforcing the normal range of sexual activities.

Educating patients and correcting misinformation is a function that should not be overlooked or underestimated. Giving permission or providing information may be all that is necessary to help many patients. An essential part of modern sexual counseling is the teaching of safer sexual practices and review of risk factors for HIV infection (see Chapters 7, 13, and 119).

Behavioral Methods

If the problem persists, a trial of behavioral methods (see later discussion) with specific suggestions to patient and partner can be helpful and is an appropriate next step. The objectives are to increase communication between partners, encourage experimentation, change the goal of sexual activity toward feeling good and away from emphasis on erection or orgasm, and relieve anxiety associated with pressure to perform at each sexual encounter. A trial of such therapy is reasonable when there is no evidence of organic illness or significant underlying psychopathology.

Pharmacologic Approaches

Medication can be prescribed for specific sexual complaints of various etiologies instead of or in conjunction with behavioral techniques. This may lead to improved sexual function without the need for referral to specialists. (See also Chapters 115 and 132.)

Male Erectile Disorder—Phosphodiesterase Inhibitors (e.g., Sildenafil, Vardenafil, Tadalafil)

Selective inhibitors of phosphodiesterase type 5 (PDE-5) facilitate erections by increasing the amount of available cyclic guanosine monophosphate (needed for vascular relaxation and erection) (see Chapter 132). Drugs in this class, which include *sildenafil* (Viagra), *vardenafil* (Levitra), and *tadalafil* (Cialis), have revolutionized the treatment of erectile dysfunction, being effective in persons with both organic and mixed psychogenic and organic impotence. Efficacy ranges from about 50% to 75% in terms of ability to obtain and sustain erection sufficient to engage in intercourse and may be improved by statins. The PDE-5 inhibitors have little effect on libido and thus may be of limited use when poor libido is the principal problem; however, in depressed men with sexual dysfunction, treatment with sildenafil is associated with a significant improvement in erectile function and sex drive, and 75% of responders have more than a 50% reduction in measures of depression. The PDE-5 inhibitors are also effective in the treatment of antidepressant-induced erectile dysfunction.

Other Drugs for Erectile Dysfunction

Yohimbine (Yocon) is approved for the treatment of male erectile disorder, but its efficacy is uncertain. Other second- and third-line orally administered agents include L-arginine (ArginMax), *phentolamine* (Vasomax), and sublingual *apomorphine* (Uprima), none of which is approved by the U.S. Food and Drug Administration (FDA) (see Chapter 132). Centrally acting melanocortin receptor agonists (in development as an intranasal preparation) appear effective, but side effects may limit utility. Topical impotence medications, including alprostadil cream (Topiglan), minoxidil solution, and nitroglycerine ointment, are under investigation. *Transdermal testosterone* helps to restore libido and erectile function in truly hypogonadal men (see Chapter 132) but is not recommended for men with normal levels of bioavailable testosterone.

Premature Ejaculation—Antidepressants

There is no FDA-approved treatment for premature ejaculation. However, both *tricyclics* and *selective serotonin reuptake inhibitors* (SSRIs) appear to be helpful in delaying ejaculation. The tricyclic *clomipramine* (*Anafranil*) is prescribed as needed 6 hours before planned intercourse. The SSRI antidepressants are prescribed for daily use to obtain the best results. *Dapoxetine*, an SSRI in phase III clinical trials, has a rapid onset and short half-life and is being studied as an on-demand treatment for premature ejaculation. *Topical anesthetics* (such as lidocaine derivatives), the most popular of which is *EMLA Cream*, can be used to slow ejaculation without the systemic side effects of antidepressants. However, these agents may cause penile numbness, resulting in erectile problems. When premature ejaculation is secondary to male erectile disorder, the PDE-5 inhibitors should be used to treat erectile dysfunction first.

Low Libido and Orgasmic Dysfunction—Transdermal Testosterone, Bupropion, Sildenafil (PDE-5 Inhibitors)

Much sexual dysfunction is a consequence of reduced libido and orgasmic dysfunction, which has triggered considerable interest in pharmacologic approaches to management.

In Women. The gradual decrease in testosterone levels that occurs with menopause has stimulated studies of hormone replacement therapy as a means of treating decreased libido in menopausal women.

Testosterone (often as a transdermal patch and usually in combination with estrogen) has been shown to improve libido, sexual arousal, and the frequency of sexual fantasies in menopausal women; however, it requires relatively high doses, which may result in acne, hirsutism, alopecia, lower high-density-lipoprotein cholesterol, and hepatic toxicity in addition to concerns about thrombosis and malignancy associated with long-term hormone replacement therapy (see Chapter 118). There are no data on the safety of long-term testosterone use in women (a testosterone patch for women failed to receive FDA approval). The patches commercially available are intended for men and release considerably greater doses of testosterone.

Estrogen itself has no demonstrable effect on libido or sexual response in the absence of vaginal or vasomotor symptoms. *Tibolone* (not FDA approved), a steroid hormone effective for osteoporosis, has been shown to increase vaginal lubrication, arousability, and sexual desire but not the frequency of sexual intercourse or orgasm.

Bupropion (*Wellbutrin*) may increase arousability and sexual response, especially in women with an underlying depression. Side effects include nervousness, insomnia, and risk of seizure. The SSRI antidepressants may actually reduce libido, causing some to consider switching to bupropion for the treatment of the underlying condition (see Chapter 227).

Sildenafil (and other PDE-5 inhibitors) fail to demonstrate effectiveness in women with orgasmic dysfunction and arousal disorder but may be of some benefit to women who exhibit greatly diminished vasocongestion. The prostaglandin *alprostadil* applied topically to the genitalia as a cream before intercourse to improve arousal has shown mixed results and may cause transient local burning. Other medications used to treat male sexual dysfunction, including yohimbine, apomorphine, melanocortin agonists, and L-arginine, are being investigated in women. *EROS-CTD*, a clitoral therapy suction device, is the only FDA-approved medical-surgical intervention for the treatment of female sexual dysfunction and can improve sexual arousal and orgasm.

In Men. Both hormone replacement and use of PDE-5 inhibitors have been the subject of study and application.

Testosterone replacement (via a transdermal patch or gel) represents an effective approach in men with poor libido and sexual dysfunction due to true *hypogonadism* (documented low levels of bioavailable serum testosterone). Routine use in aging men with sexual dysfunction in the absence of documented low bioavailable testosterone is not routinely recommended due to a host of potential medical risks, ranging from polycythemia and stroke to stimulation of a preclinical prostate cancer (see Chapter 132).

Sildenafil has been prescribed for those with low libido and/or erectile dysfunction associated with mild to moderate *depression*, resulting in significant improvement not only in sex drive and sexual function, but also in measures of depression, suggesting that some of the interplay between depression and sexual dysfunction may be amenable to the specific treatment of the sexual dysfunction. Results in other patients with diminished libido have been more variable.

TREATMENT RECOMMENDATIONS: BEHAVIORAL TECHNIQUES

Erectile Dysfunction

- First educate the patient about his ability to satisfy his partner without having penile–vaginal intercourse.
- Then begin to outline "sensate focus" exercises, which start with nongenital massage and progress to genital massage. There should be a prohibition against intercourse, even if erections occur.
- After erection is obtained by genital massage, advise the patient to progress to attempting intercourse. In the woman-superior position (woman on top of man), the woman may manually stimulate the penis, and, if erection is obtained, she may insert it into her vagina in a slow, nondemanding fashion, relieving the man of any responsibility for insertion. This may also be done with a partial erection. Gradual movement is begun. There is an emphasis on the pleasures of vaginal containment.
- Consider supplementing behavioral therapy with phosphodiesterase type 5 inhibitor therapy (e.g., *sildenafil*). Do not prescribe if nitrates are being used concurrently (risk of severe hypotension); use with caution and thorough patient education in men with underlying coronary heart disease. Avoid or use with caution in men taking α-blockers (often prescribed for benign prostatic hypertrophy).
- Consider an external vacuum constriction device.

Premature Ejaculation

- Educate the patient that his condition has little to do with the sensitivity of the penis but is usually the result of previous conditioning and anxiety.
- Suggest an increase in the frequency of sexual activity.
- Teach the *"squeeze"* technique. In this technique, the woman manually stimulates the penis. When ejaculation is approaching the point of inevitability, as indicated by the man, the woman squeezes the penis with her thumb on the frenulum, her index finger placed above, and her middle finger below the coronal ridge on the dorsal side of the penis. The pressure is applied until the man no longer feels the urgency to ejaculate (15 to 60 seconds). The squeeze technique should be repeated two or three times before ejaculation is allowed to occur.
- Once there are good results with the squeeze technique, the couple can try intercourse. In the woman-superior position, the woman remains motionless to accustom the man to vaginal containment. Gradual thrusting begins, using the squeeze technique as excitement intensifies.
- An alternative to the squeeze technique is the "stop–start" method. The woman stimulates the man to the point of ejaculation, at which time she stops the stimulation. The erection may or may not subside. She then resumes stimulating the penis. After several stop–start procedures, the man may ejaculate.
- Consider supplementing behavioral therapy with the use of *clomipramine* (Anafranil) (starting at 25 mg 6 hours before

intercourse) or an SSRI antidepressant (e.g., fluoxetine, 20 mg daily).

Retarded Ejaculation (During Intercourse)

- The woman stimulates the penis, asking for directions (verbal and physical) to enhance the feeling.
- Extravaginal ejaculation is obtained by continued stimulation. In the man's mind, the woman should become associated with ejaculatory release.
- The woman stimulates the penis manually until orgasm becomes inevitable. The penis is then inserted and the woman thrusts demandingly. Manual stimulation is repeated if there is no successful ejaculation.

Female Sexual Arousal Disorder

- Because this disorder often results from more severe psychopathology, it usually requires referral for treatment. However, on the practical side, suggestions regarding the supplemental use of lubrication such as saliva or KY jelly should be made.

Orgasmic Dysfunction

- Change the goal of sexual activity away from orgasm toward enjoyment of the experience.
- Give permission to the woman to express sexual feelings.
- Outline "sensate focus" exercises, which start with non-genital massage and progress to genital massage. Suggest the use of the back-protected position (the man in a seated position with the woman between his legs with her back against his chest) with the woman in control to alleviate self-consciousness.
- Instruct the man in stimulative techniques: He should not force responsivity but rather seek to accommodate desires; he should not approach the clitoris directly because of sensitivity.
- After success in manual genital stimulation, controlled intercourse in the woman-superior position with the man making no demands comes next. This is followed by a lateral position that allows for mutual freedom of pelvic movement.
- For women who have never experienced orgasm, suggestions regarding self-stimulation are appropriate. The use of fantasy material is most helpful.
- For women who do have orgasms with masturbation but not intercourse, the "bridge technique" may be useful. After insertion of the penis, the man can stimulate the woman (clitorally) manually or with a vibrator. This pairing can be helpful in achieving orgasm, and often after the woman experiences orgasm in this way, the need for supplementary stimulation disappears.
- Consider use of estrogen/testosterone in the postmenopausal woman who experiences orgasmic dysfunction or low libido.
- Consider EROS-CTD, a clitoral therapy suction device.

Vaginismus

- Explain to the patient and her partner that this condition is involuntary and not willfully caused. Physical demonstra-

tion of the involuntary vaginal spasm may be done by inserting a gloved finger into the vaginal entrance.

- Ask the couple to refrain from intercourse during the early treatment.
- Encourage the woman to accept larger and larger objects into the vagina in a stepwise gradual fashion. This may be accomplished with the use of graduated Hegar dilators to be used in the office and at home, or the woman may begin by using her fingers, first one and then several approximately the size of the penis. She may use her partner's fingers. Syringe containers of different sizes make good dilators.
- Suggest that the woman should gradually insert the penis while she is in the woman-superior position.

Hypoactive Sexual Desire Disorder

- Consider transdermal testosterone for men with documented hypogonadism (low bioavailable testosterone level) and for women with surgically induced menopause (in combination with estrogen). Testosterone use in men without hypogonadism and in women with physiologic menopause or other causes of low libido has not been validated.

INDICATIONS FOR REFERRAL (2–5,10)

Psychiatric Referral

After trying these medications and/or behavioral techniques, the patient's condition may still not be improved. This is often a sign that a referral to a psychiatrist or other mental professional trained in dealing with sexual problems is indicated and that the patient needs more intensive therapy. Often, direct referral to the specialist is indicated for patients with chronic psychopathology, such as those with "primary" sexual dysfunctions, gender identity questions or homosexual conflicts, marked personality disorders or significant past psychiatric history (especially of psychosis), or overt evidence of a clinical depression underlying the sexual complaint. Moreover, chronic severe problems in the relationship with one's partner signal the need for a referral.

Urologic Referral

For both organically based impotence and impotence refractory to psychological treatment, it is appropriate to refer patients to urology. Treatments include consideration of a pharmacologic erection program, such as the injection of alprostadil (Caverject) into the base of the penis, the insertion of a transurethral penile suppository of alprostadil (MUSE), external vacuum pump therapy, and surgical penile implant (see Chapter 132). The success of any such treatment requires close collaboration between the urologist and the psychiatrist. On a case by case basis, referral to specialists in gynecology, endocrinology, and/or neurology may be warranted.

PATIENT EDUCATION (2–5)

Early in one's practice, it becomes clear that patients have many sexual questions and concerns. Inadequate or inaccurate information about sexual anatomy, physiology, and practices is the basis for many sexual problems. Therefore, sex education should not be overlooked. Patients can sometimes obtain supplemental information from suggested reading material. Several popular books include *For Yourself: The Fulfillment of Female Sexuality* by Lonnie Garfield Barbach (New York, Signet, 2000); *Satisfaction: The Art of Female Orgasm* by Kim Cattrall and Mark Levinson (New York, Warner Books, 2003); *The New Male Sexuality* by Bernie Zilbergeld (New York, Bantam, 1999); *How to Overcome Premature Ejaculation* by Helen Singer Kaplan (New York, Brunner/Mazel, 1989); *The Illustrated Manual of Sex Therapy*, second edition, by Helen Singer Kaplan (New York, Brunner/Mazel, 1987); and *The Joy of Sex*, edited by Alex Comfort (New York, Crown, 2002). A

visit to answer questions that come up in the context of reading is always appreciated.

Lack of knowledge regarding safer-sex practices is a major contributor to the spread of HIV infection. Concern about HIV infection can also interfere with the enjoyment of sexual activity. Detailed review of safer-sex practices is essential (see Chapters 7, 13, and 119). Condom use is critical for those with multiple sexual partners and for monogamous partners in whom HIV status is unknown. With prudent precautions and a little creativity (e.g., making condom application an early part of foreplay), a safe and enjoyable sexual life can still be attained.

Annotated Bibliography

1. American Psychiatric Association. Diagnostic and statistical manual of mental disorders, 4th ed. Washington, DC: Author, 1994:493. (*Presents the official psychiatric criteria for sexual disorders.*)
2. Leiblum SR. Principles and practice of sex therapy, 4th ed. New York: Guilford Press, 2006. (*A comprehensive review of sex therapy.*)
3. Maurice W. Sexual medicine in primary care. New York: Mosby, 1999. (*An excellent up-to-date summary of all aspects of the diagnosis and treatment of sexual disorders.*)
4. Shafer LC. Sexual disorders and sexual dysfunction. In: Stern TA, Rosenbaum JF, Fava M, Biederman J, Rauch SL, eds. Massachusetts General Hospital Comprehensive Clinical Psychiatry. Philadelphia: Mosby/Elsevier, 2008:487.
5. Shafer L. Sexual dysfunction. In: Carlson K, Eisenstat S, eds. Primary care of women. St. Louis, MO: Mosby, 2002:415. (*An up-to-date discussion of female sexual dysfunction.*)
6. Araujo AB, Durante R, Feldman HA, et al. The relationship between depressive symptoms and male erectile dysfunction: cross-sectional results from the Massachusetts Male Aging Study. Psychosom Med 1998;60:458. (*There was a strong relationship between depression and erectile dysfunction, independent of aging.*)
7. Fava M, Rankin M. Sexual functioning and SSRIs. J Clin Psychiatry 2002;63(Suppl 5):13. (*A review article on sexual side effects from selective serotonin reuptake inhibitors, and treatment strategies.*)
8. Feldman H, Goldstein I, Hatzichristou D, et al. Impotence and its medical and psychosocial correlates: results of the Massachusetts Male Aging Study. J Urol 1994;151:54. (*Data on the prevalence of impotence in the aging population.*)
9. Laumann E, Paik A, Rosen R. Sexual dysfunction in the United States. JAMA 1999;281:537. (*A statistical analysis of the incidence of sexual disorders in the United States.*)
10. Lue TF. Erectile dysfunction. N Engl J Med 2000;342:1802. (*A comprehensive review article covering physiology and treatment options.*)
11. Thompson IM, Tangen CM, Goodman PJ, et al. Erectile dysfunction and subsequent cardiovascular disease. JAMA 2005;294:2996. (*Erectile dysfunction as a predictor of cardiovascular disease.*)
12. Andersson KE, Mulhall JP, Wyllie MG. Pharmacokinetic and pharmacodynamic features of dapoxetine, a novel drug for 'on-demand' treatment of premature ejaculation. BJU Int 2006;97:311. (*A potential new agent for the treatment of premature ejaculation.*)
13. Basson R. Sexual desire and arousal disorders in women. N Engl J Med 2006;354:1497. (*An up-to-date review.*)
14. Goldstein I, Lue T, Padma-Nathan H, et al. Oral sildenafil in the treatment of erectile dysfunction. N Engl J Med 1998;338:1397. (*The original randomized, prospective, controlled trial.*)
15. Kendirici M, Walls MM, Hellstrom WJ. Central nervous system agents in the treatment of erectile dysfunction. Urol Clin North Am 2005;32(4):487. (*A review of new agents for erectile dysfunction.*)
16. Seidman SN, Roose SP, Menza M, et al. Treatment of erectile dysfunction in men with depressive symptoms: results of a placebo-controlled trial with sildenafil citrate. Am J Psychiatry 2001;158:1623. (*Efficacy was demonstrated.*)
17. Shafer L. The patient with impotence. In Stern T, Herman J, Slavin P, eds. The MGH Guide to Primary Care Psychiatry, 2nd ed. New York: McGraw-Hill, 2004:405. (*An easy-to-read outline for the diagnosis and treatment of impotence.*)
18. Shafer L. The patient with sexual dysfunction. In Stern T, Herman J, Slavin P, eds. The MGH Guide to Primary Care Psychiatry, 2nd ed. New York: McGraw-Hill, 2004:393. (*An easy-to-read outline for the diagnosis and treatment of sexual disorders.*)
19. Shifren JL, Braunskin GD, Simon JA, et al. Transdermal testosterone in women with impaired sexual function after oophorectomy. N Engl J Med 2000;343:682. (*Trials of testosterone treatment in surgically menopausal women.*)
20. Shifren JL, Davis SR, Moreau M, et al. Testosterone patch for the treatment of hypoactive sexual desire disorder in naturally menopausal women: results from the INTIMATE NM1 Study. Menopause 2006;13:770. (*There was some evidence of efficacy but no long-term safety data.*)

CHAPTER 230 ■ APPROACH TO THE SOMATIZING PATIENT

ILANA M. BRAUN AND ARTHUR J. BARSKY III

Somatizing patients present with bodily complaints or disability out of proportion to demonstrable organic pathology. As such, they pose both diagnostic and therapeutic challenges to primary physicians and can be among the most trying and frustrating patients for which to care. Understanding causative psychopathology helps to render symptoms understandable and facilitates management.

PSYCHOLOGICAL MECHANISMS AND CLINICAL PRESENTATIONS (1–9)

Somatization has both trait- and state-like properties and occurs outside of a person's conscious awareness. Thus the somatizing patient is not lying or feigning illness. Highly somatizing patients include hypochondriacs, some depressed or anxious patients, and some patients with chronic pain.

Hypochondriasis

Hypochondriacal patients are people for whom illness, invalidism, and the pursuit of medical care have grown into *ways of life*. Somatic symptoms and medical help seeking have become a *vocabulary for communicating* with other people, a *way of responding* to stress, and a means of expressing psychological needs. Hypochondriacal patients are, on one hand, preoccupied with their bodies and their health, convinced that they have occult, serious medical disease; on the other hand, they fear disease intensely. Their concerns are remarkably persistent and are not assuaged by reassurance or thorough medical evaluation. Although they have had extensive medical care, they have found it disappointing, failing to cure or even improve their symptoms.

Clinical Presentation

Hypochondriacal *symptoms shift* and *fluctuate* over time, are often *nonspecific* and *ambiguous*, and frequently are similar to the transient benign bodily discomforts experienced by healthy individuals. When interviewed, patients with hypochondriasis talk mainly about their illnesses and their medical care and little about family, work, or hobbies. They often seem as concerned with establishing the authenticity of their complaints as with obtaining symptom relief per se. They adamantly *deny any emotional contribution* to their symptoms. This stands in sharp contrast to many patients with serious physical disease who are willing to consider the idea that anxiety and depression make their symptoms worse.

Explanatory Models

Hypochondriasis has been understood as a cognitive and perceptual process, a form of interpersonal communication, and an unconscious psychological process.

The cognitive/perceptual model suggests that hypochondriasis is a self-validating and self-perpetuating disorder of symptom amplification. Hypochondriacal patients are unusually sensitive to visceral and bodily sensation and are therefore bothered by normal physiologic sensations and minor discomforts that nonhypochondriacs ignore, dismiss, or have completely out of their awareness. Because these bodily sensations seem so intense, noxious, and disturbing, hypochondriacs readily misattribute them to serious disease.

Once the individual believes himself or herself to be sick, this belief alters subsequent somatic perceptions, and a process of *symptom amplification* begins. The belief that one is sick makes preexisting symptoms seem more intense because they are now subject to closer scrutiny. The patient's apparent worsening condition even more firmly convinces the patient that he or she is sick. These patients become *hypervigilant* for other symptoms that confirm their suspicions and ignore contradictory information indicating that they are not in fact sick. For example, an individual may notice breathlessness after climbing a flight of stairs and wonder whether this signifies the onset of heart or lung disease. With this suspicion in mind, the patient now thinks that his face looks unusually pale in the mirror when he next shaves. This too seems to provide further evidence of disease progression. Thus, a self-validating and self-perpetuating cycle of cognitive and perceptual amplification has been set in motion.

In *the interpersonal communication model*, hypochondriasis is conceptualized as a form of nonverbal communication, a way of saying something to the important people in the patient's life. The hypochondriacal patient is using a *bodily pantomime* to tell others that there is a seemingly *insurmountable life problem* that he or she is having trouble coping with or solving. The patient is asking to take "time out," saying (in a nonverbal language), "I am in a *desperate situation* and so I *need special care* and attention, unusual assistance, and support at this time." Hypochondriacal patients have unconsciously learned that illness behaviors can be used to negotiate stressful circumstances, secure support, and solicit care. It is crucial to reemphasize that hypochondriacal patients do have the symptoms they report; they are not malingering or feigning disease. Rather, they have learned over the course of their lives that assuming the sick role can help them to postpone or avoid challenge or crisis.

The unconscious psychological model posits that pain and suffering can have *unconscious meaning* and *gratification*. Bodily complaints may be amplified by a deprived and needy person who has only experienced caring and attention when sick or in pain. Suffering and illness can thus become ways of expressing and gratifying yearnings for contact, comfort, and support. Other hypochondriacal individuals may be *angry* and *hostile*, feeling rejected or wronged in some way. For them, physical symptoms offer a nonverbal means of *expressing their anger, recrimination,* and *blame* by reproaching and belaboring those around them with their suffering. Finally, symptoms and illness can unconsciously serve to *distract* some individuals from an even more painful sense of themselves as fundamentally worthless or defective as people. They can thus attribute their failures, disappointments, and rejections to a physical incapacity rather than to personal inadequacy.

Anxiety

Individuals suffering from *chronic anxiety* (see Chapter 226) focus on and become alarmed by normal bodily sensations. They report restlessness, difficulty concentrating, dry mouth, cold and clammy hands, and gastrointestinal disturbances. *Panic anxiety* has somatic manifestations that include palpitations, chest pain, tachycardia, dyspnea, choking sensations, diarrhea, sweating, tingling in hands and feet, and fainting. Such signs and symptoms may easily be misinterpreted as evidence of serious illness.

Depression

Depression's *neurovegetative symptoms* may overshadow the characteristic affective, cognitive, and behavioral changes that are part of the depressive syndrome (see Chapter 227). The chief complaint may be *headache, constipation, weakness, fatigue, abdominal pain, insomnia, anorexia,* or *weight loss.* At least one half of somatizing ambulatory medical patients are significantly depressed. These patients worry about and focus attention on their bodies. A *positive review of systems,* chronic pain, or complaints involving multiple organ systems typify the clinical presentation, and symptoms may recur with the periodicity characteristic of depressions.

Conversion Reactions

Conversion reactions are sensory or motor dysfunctions that suggest the presence of a neurologic disorder but that are actually *expressions of a psychological need* or *conflict.* The emotional distress is thought of as being "converted" into, or expressed as, physical distress. The process is entirely unconscious, so these patients are not malingering. Symptoms are either sensory or neuromuscular (e.g., weakness, paralysis, ataxia, blindness, aphasia, deafness, anesthesia, paresthesias, or seizures) and usually of short duration. Other features include a prior history of similar symptoms, major emotional stress before onset, and apparent symbolic meaning of the symptom (e.g., paralysis after losing control and striking someone or blindness after viewing a horrifying event). Other significant psychopathology is often, but not invariably, present.

Somatic Delusions

Schizophrenia, severe affective disorders, and *organic brain syndromes* are the source of somatic delusions. These are false fixed ideas that are often vivid, bizarre, or highly personalized. Unlike hypochondriacal concerns, they do not fluctuate. The individual may believe that some extraordinary change has occurred in his or her body—for example, that organs are shriveling up, body parts are deformed or missing, or foreign objects are inside an orifice or organ.

Some patients suffer from *body dysmorphic disorder,* a fixed, circumscribed delusion that they are physically deformed, although their appearance is actually unremarkable. A facial feature is often the focus. The condition is chronic, extremely disabling, causes profound social withdrawal, and can be quite difficult to treat.

Malingering and Factitious Disorder

Malingering differs from all of the aforementioned conditions in that the malingerer does not actually experience the symptoms reported and is consciously feigning disease. Malingering occurs in situations in which illness confers some obvious benefit, such as among prisoners, drug addicts, or in individuals under some legal threat. Symptoms are exaggerated, and the patient's description of them may vary with each interview. When unaware of being observed, the patient may relax the simulation and thus betray himself or herself. Such individuals are frequently sociopaths or drug addicts.

Factitious disorder is a *more severe form of malingering* in which there is no discernible advantage or gain that results from feigning illness. These patients go to extreme, self-injurious lengths to simulate abnormal physical and laboratory findings, lie about their symptoms and medical histories, and are untruthful in many other ways. Patients with factitious disorder tend to be female and are often employed in medical fields such as nursing.

DIFFERENTIAL DIAGNOSIS (2,3,7,9)

The differential diagnosis of somatization includes anxiety, depression, conversion reaction, somatization disorder, hypochondriasis, schizophrenia, malingering, and factitious disorder. Somatizing patients, of course, have the same vulnerability for medical illness as their nonsomatizing counterparts. Thus, one must take care to rule out organic causes of the patient's symptoms, just as with any other medical patient. Medical disorders that affect multiple organ systems and produce transient or recurrent nonspecific complaints (e.g., multiple sclerosis, systemic lupus, polymyalgia rheumatica, Lyme disease, myasthenia gravis, syphilis, hyperparathyroidism) pose the greatest diagnostic difficulty. Domestic violence may present with multiple, perplexing bodily complaints, especially pain complaints that may superficially resemble those of a somatization disorder (see Appendix 236.1).

WORKUP (2,3,5,7,9)

History—Step 1: Differentiating Somatization from Organic Disease

The task is not always easy, but the quality, timing, and precipitants of symptoms, as well as the patient's response to illness, attitude, and choice of words, can be of considerable help (see Chapters 8, 226, 227, and 236). The possibility of domestic violence is important to keep in mind; a few screening questions can be very helpful (see Appendix 236.1).

Quality of Symptoms

A complaint that is inconsistent with known pathophysiology is likely to be psychogenic in origin. Psychogenic sensory complaints often involve combinations of sensory modalities that are neurologically impossible (e.g., a patient reporting loss of position and vibratory sense can nonetheless walk normally; see Chapter 167). Conversion seizures, otherwise known as non-epileptic events may not involve stereotyped movements, incontinence, tongue biting, or changes in prolactin level (as epileptic events tend to). The patient with conversion blindness exhibits a withdrawal or startle reflex when a hand is flashed before the face. With conversion paralysis of the upper extremity, the patient's arm avoids striking the face when being held above it and released. In conversion paralysis of a lower extremity, a patient's attempt to lift the afflicted leg while supine will fail to invoke involuntary contractions in the contralateral leg, as is the case in neurologic disease (Hoover's sign).

Psychogenic symptoms are more likely to resemble symptoms that have afflicted someone important to the patient (a so-called *figure of identity*) or to be excessively vague or overly detailed. Inconsistent complaints and vivid, elaborate, highly personalized, or idiosyncratic descriptions are suggestive. Psychological factors may be revealed in the choice of words (e.g., "pain in the neck" or "not having a leg to stand on").

Timing and Precipitants

Psychogenic pain is typically unaffected by activity or by the passage of time, and the patient may be even more concerned with the physician accepting the authenticity of the pain than with relieving it. Although both physical and psychologic illness can be precipitated by stress, the onset of psychogenic complaints is often closely associated with *significant emotional stress*, such as the loss of a loved one or the onset of a major interpersonal conflict or sexual problem. Functional complaints are also prone to occur on the *anniversary* of a psychologically meaningful event.

Attitude Toward Symptoms

When the patient is unconcerned, inappropriately calm, or more concerned with establishing authenticity than with obtaining relief, one should suspect a strong emotional component. It must be emphasized, however, that stoical and stolid patients may also remain very unemotional when afflicted with serious organic disease. As noted, patients with psychogenic complaints who unconsciously derive considerable gain from their illness are often reluctant to consider an emotional cause for their symptoms.

History—Step 2: Defining the Underlying Psychopathology

Once a psychogenic etiology is suspected on the basis of the clinical presentation, evaluation should proceed to define the underlying psychopathology. Inquiry into precipitants, response to illness, and personality can be helpful.

Precipitants and Response to Illness

One should search the patient's history for ongoing psychologic stress, pending litigation or disability proceedings, prior medically unexplained complaints, depression, or an anxiety disorder. Details of previous medical care experiences can be revealing: A history of consulting many physicians for the same complaint or of the immediate replacement of a treated symptom with a new one helps in the diagnosis of psychogenic illness.

Personality

It is important to determine whether illness, discomfort, and disability have become a way of life and to what extent they are used to deal with emotional discomfort, interpersonal difficulties, and environmental stress. Does the patient see himself or herself as a suffering and an unfortunate person whose life is filled with disappointment, "bad luck," and defeat, as well as with illness? The angry individual may feel deprived and put upon, and therefore reproaches, accuses, and blames others for his or her state. Anger and hostility may be expressed indirectly as cynicism, sarcasm, and uncooperativeness. Finally, excessive dependence on others may be a feature of the somatizing patient's personality. One senses an overpowering hunger for care, attention, sympathy, and human contact, and the patient's attitude toward the physician may have a clinging and needy quality.

Personal Significance and Secondary Gain

What personal significance does the patient attach to his or her symptoms or to the suspected illness? Are there possible secondary gains, such as receiving sympathy, attention, and support (including financial support) from family and friends; being excused from duties, challenges, and responsibilities; and acquiring the power to influence and manipulate others by virtue of being sick?

Physical Examination and Laboratory Studies

A thorough physical examination and a careful mental status examination are essential. Not only may unexpected evidence of organic illness turn up, but also a normal examination is a prerequisite for effective reassurance and the avoidance of unnecessary laboratory testing. Checking for manifestations of conditions that can cause multiple bodily complaints (e.g., hyperparathyroidism, systemic lupus, Lyme disease, polymyalgia rheumatica, myasthenia gravis, and multiple sclerosis; see Chapters 96, 146, 160, 161, and 172) is essential.

Obtaining a few simple laboratory tests (e.g., *sedimentation rate, serum calcium*) may be in order, but only if there is some suggestive evidence from the history or physical examination. Absent clinical evidence of organic disease, there is little role for extensive testing. Elaborate testing is wasteful, and invasive studies should be avoided. Performing a test simply for the purpose of reassurance is often futile because patients who are highly anxious about their health to begin with often find some other source of concern when the result is negative. In addition, the likelihood of a false-positive result is higher than the likelihood of a true-positive result when the pretest probability of organic disease is low (see Chapter 2). For example, obtaining a sensitive but nonspecific test such as an antinuclear antibody level in the absence of clinical criteria for lupus is likely to generate a disturbing false-positive result, given that the test can be positive in up to 25% of normal persons (see Chapter 146).

PRINCIPLES OF MANAGEMENT
(3,4,7,8,10–12)

Overall Approach

Management must be directed at the underlying psychopathology and at the presenting bodily complaints. A combination of putting the complaints in perspective, emphasizing reassurance and support, and attending to the underlying personality disorder if present comprise the basic approach to management.

Putting the Complaint in Perspective

The first step is to put the complaint in perspective while still recognizing that the patient has come because of physical symptoms. When the results of the workup are presented, the reality of the symptoms should not be denied, nor should it be implied that they are imaginary or "all in your head." The patient can be told that *serious, damaging organic disease has been ruled out* and that *stress can amplify real bodily sensations and disrupt normal function*. It is important to avoid saying "there is nothing wrong" because this contradicts the patient's experience and makes him or her feel belittled and angry.

Cognitive–behavioral therapy can be very helpful in this task. Such treatment can help to target cognitive and perceptual mechanisms of illness, including overattention to bodily sensation, beliefs about symptom etiology, context in which somatization occurs, sick role behaviors, and mood. Controlled studies find that cognitive–behavioral therapy is able to achieve significant reductions in fears of illness and unnecessary medical visits.

Providing Support

Whatever their source, the symptoms are an indication of considerable distress, which the patient should be encouraged to discuss. The patient needs to know that the relationship with his or her physician will not be terminated because the medical workup is "negative" and reassured that although no serious medical disease has been found, the physician will continue to monitor symptoms for the emergence of serious disease in the future. *Follow-up visits* should be scheduled on a regular basis to provide time further to discuss personal and situational problems. By offering the patient a long-term relationship that is not contingent on the necessity of having ongoing somatic symptoms, one may remove a major stimulus for their development. Refractory cases may benefit from referral to a psychiatrist if the patient is willing.

Underlying Psychopathology and Drug-Responsive Causes

Managing the Underlying Personality Disorder

Most patients with somatization due to a personality disturbance can be managed by the primary physician. Medical intervention should be minimized when possible. Major diagnostic workups for equivocal or questionable findings should be avoided as long as it is medically responsible to do so, as should pain medication and tranquilizers. Even though medication is often requested, these patients generally do not respond to it and are especially prone to developing troublesome side effects.

To avoid struggles, the patient, especially if hostile and angry, should be involved as much as possible in therapeutic and diagnostic decisions. The physician needs to make it clear that his or her role is to *help the patient tolerate discomfort rather than to eliminate it*. The *goal* of medical management is *improved functioning* and diminished role impairment rather than outright cure. Therapeutic suggestions should be made with the caveat that although they may be helpful, they will probably not completely eliminate the problem.

The situational or psychologic need to remain distressed and symptomatic must be recognized. There is no surgical procedure that can excise, and no oral medication that can cure, the *need to be ill*. Consequently, the physician should not expect cure. The patient's self-esteem needs to be bolstered. *Acknowledging the strength to endure* suffering, tolerate discomfort, and survive misfortune is particularly gratifying to the patient. These are qualities the patient values and are a source of what little self-esteem he or she has.

Role of Drug Therapy

Unless there is an underlying drug-responsive condition such as depression or generalized anxiety disorder, nontargeted attempts to suppress somatization pharmacologically should be avoided. All too often, patients are told that their symptoms are due to their "nerves" and sent away with a prescription for a minor tranquilizer. Such an intervention frequently alienates the patient, who perceives it as a "brush off" and a paltry substitute for the physician's personal, ongoing interest and attention.

That said, it is especially important to be on the look out for depression because of its high prevalence, subtle manifestations, and good response to pharmacotherapy. Similarly, anxiety disorders, including panic disorder and generalized anxiety disorder, may often be ameliorated with antidepressants, benzodiazepines, or β-blockers, often in conjunction with cognitive and behavioral interventions (see Chapter 226).

Approach to Conversion Reactions

There are two aspects to the treatment of conversion reactions: (a) symptom remission and (b) management of the precipitating stress, internal conflict, or secondary gain in order to avoid recurrence or chronicity. The first is done through education, reassurance, and positive suggestion to reduce anxiety (these patients are often exceptionally suggestible). The patient should be assured that the disorder is known to be self-limited and that the symptoms will therefore gradually improve and finally vanish. Conversion symptoms may recur, however, unless psychotherapy is arranged to alter or neutralize the psychological forces at work.

Approach to Malingering and Factitious Disorder

Once firmly established as diagnoses, malingering or factitious disorder may be dealt with by gently confronting the patient with the physician's conclusions. Frequently, such patients will deny their psychological diagnosis and pursue medical care elsewhere. For those few patients who do remain in treatment, diagnostic and therapeutic procedures should be avoided when possible because they reinforce the patient's behavior. Any abnormal laboratory tests or physical findings must be considered suspect. In the case of factitious disorder, referrals to psychotherapy and family therapy may be of utility in helping both the patient and the members of their support system to better understand the psychological distress that precipitates illness behaviors.

INDICATIONS FOR REFERRAL

Most somatizing patients can be managed by the primary physician. Referral is indicated when a patient has accepted a psychological explanation of his or her symptoms and is willing to see a psychiatrist; when a conversion reaction, serious anxiety disorder, or psychosis is present; or when the primary physician has such a negative reaction to the patient with a personality disorder that he or she cannot serve that patient well.

Referral for *cognitive–behavioral therapy* should be considered. Getting patients to go for such therapy can be challenging, but is facilitated by a review of how they worry and how such therapy can help them to take control of their somatic symptoms and overcome their concerns about serious illness.

TREATMENT RECOMMENDATIONS

- Explain the results of the medical workup without denying or being unsympathetic to the reality of the patient's discomfort.

- Get to know the patient as a person. Inquire, for instance, how the patient spends his or her days, about psychosocial stressors, and about social supports.
- Uncouple as much as is possible medical attention from symptom flares:
- Set up appointments at regular intervals and make it apparent to the patient that physical symptoms need not be present to have access to the doctor.
- Avoid as-needed appointments when possible.
- Identify and treat any drug-responsive condition such as depression or chronic anxiety disorder (see Chapters 226 and 227).
- Avoid tranquilizer use for the nonspecific suppression of symptoms.
- In patients with somatizing personality disorders, do not attempt to remove or cure symptoms; acknowledge the suffering and offer support; avoid the use of medication and extensive workup of vague symptoms; make improved coping and improved adaptation to chronic discomfort the goal of care.
- For persons willing to explore and deal with their fears and illness concerns, consider a referral for cognitive–behavior therapy.

Annotated Bibliography

1. Abramowitz JS, Schwartz SA, Whiteside SP. A contemporary model of hypochondriasis. Mayo Clin Proc 2002;77:1323. (*A useful discussion of a conceptual model and review of cognitive–behavioral therapy.*)
2. Barsky AJ, Peekna HM, Borus JF. Somatic symptom reporting in women and men. J Gen Intern Med 2001;16:266.(*An in-depth review of gender differences in the presentation of bodily complaints; 146 references.*)
3. Barsky AJ. Clinical crossroads: a 37-year-old man with multiple somatic complaints. JAMA 1997;278:673. (*An extended discussion of a clinical case, emphasizing medical management strategies; also discusses psychiatric consultation and referral.*)
4. Barsky AJ, Wyshak G, Latham KS, et al. Hypochondriacal patients, their physicians, and their medical care. J Gen Intern Med 1991;6:413. (*Hypochondriasis causes physician frustration and impaired recognition of anxiety and depression.*)
5. Brown HN, Vaillant GE. Hypochondriasis. Arch Intern Med 1981;141:723. (*An excellent description of the psychology of hypochondriasis with many incisive clinical observations.*)
6. Campbell J, Jones AS, Dienemann J, et al. Intimate partner violence and physical health consequences. Arch Intern Med 2002;262:1157. (*Major physical consequences are noted that, together with depression and anxiety, account for the multiple bodily complaints.*)
7. Folks DG, Feldman MD, Ford CV. Somatoform disorders, factitious disorders, and malingering. In Stoudemire A, Fogel BS, Greenberg DB, eds. Psychiatric care of the medical patient, 2nd ed. New York: Oxford University Press, 2000:459. (*A thorough, comprehensive, and systematic overview; very well referenced.*)
8. Hahn SR, Kroenke K, Spitzer RL, et al. The difficult patient: prevalence, psychopathology, and functional impairment. J Gen Intern Med 1996;11:1. (*There is a high prevalence of underlying psychopathology, with multisomatoform disorder accounting for about half of difficult cases; significant functional impairment was common.*)
9. Kroenke K, Spitzer RL, Williams JBW, et al. Physical symptoms in primary care: predictors of psychiatric disorders and functional impairment. Arch Family Med 1994;3:774. (*A number of somatic and medically unexplained symptoms are powerful predictors of underlying psychiatric disease.*)
10. Allen LA, Woolfolk RL, Escobar JI, et al. Cognitive–behavioral therapy for somatization disorder—a randomized trial. Arch Intern Med 2006;166:1512. (*Finds added benefit when cognitive–behavioral therapy is made part of the treatment program.*)
11. Allen LA, Escobar JL, Lehrer PM, et al. Psychosocial treatments for multiple unexplained physical symptoms: A review of the literature. Psychosom Med 2002;64:939. (*A helpful review of management techniques for unexplained symptoms.*)
12. Kroenke K, Swindle R. Cognitive–behavioral therapy for somatization and symptom syndromes: a critical review of controlled clinical trials. Psychother Psychosom 2000;69:205. (*A thorough review of research on cognitive–behavioral therapy for somatization.*)

CHAPTER 231 ■ APPROACH TO THE ANGRY PATIENT

ILANA M. BRAUN AND ARTHUR J. BARSKY III

Patients may become angry in response to suffering caused by illness, medical error, and adverse life events, or simply as a result of the psychological threat posed by being a patient. When faced with an angry patient, the primary care physician should explore the source of the patient's anger, prevent it from interfering with therapeutic efforts, and help the patient to cope.

PSYCHOLOGICAL MECHANISMS (1–10)

Psychological Mechanisms

Anger often derives from a sense of being threatened. In the clinical setting, the threats are multifold and include dependence associated with disease, medical negligence, conflicts elsewhere in life, or the doctor–patient relationship itself. In some people, anger is a manifestation of an underlying personality disorder.

Threat from Illness

People become enraged when their wishes and aims are frustrated by disease. Illness can arouse anger when it brings with it the prospect of disfigurement, pain, lost effectiveness, lost opportunity, abandonment, or even death. Some patients are particularly sensitive to and react against the helplessness, lack of control, and enforced passivity that illness confers. Others resent that the vagaries of chance seem to have unfairly singled them out for undeserved misfortune.

Threat of Dependence and of the Doctor–Patient Relationship

Some people bristle in the role of patient. For them, participation in the doctor–patient relationship represents the threat of dependence—of allowing someone powerful to take control of and responsibility for them. Their anger functions to keep the physician at a distance. It is a defense against any closeness or attachment to the doctor that might develop.

By contrast, other patients crave such intimacy. These persons may become angry if they sense that their doctors are treating them dismissively, not taking them seriously, or not caring about their case as much as they would like.

Threats or Conflicts Elsewhere in Life

Sometimes, anger directed toward a physician is misplaced. Patients commonly besiege or reproach their clinicians in response to stresses that they are encountering elsewhere in their lives. Often in such instances, the animosity and hostility seem inappropriate to the situation and disproportionate to any provocation the doctor can identify. Usually, this misplaced anger develops when a patient is in conflict with important people in his or life, including employers and close family, to whom the patient cannot properly express his or her emotion. In a process referred to as transference, the patient can also displace onto the current doctor the anger, dissatisfaction, and disillusionment that have actually been aroused by previous physicians.

Threat of Physician Fallibility

Many patients respond to illness by investing enormous, and sometimes inordinate, faith in their physicians. Medical error, whether as a result of action or omission, can shake a patient's sense of emotional security as much as it can lead to physical suffering. Anger in this context grows not only from a belief of having been wronged, but also out of a discomforting realization that the medical system, which has been entrusted with the patient's care, is fallible.

Borderline Personality Organization

Some patients appear to live a life permeated by a quick temper, diffuse and widespread hostility, and volatile dissatisfactions and resentments. The physician is little more than an innocent bystander on whom the patient projects hostility garnered elsewhere. Some of these globally angry patients have a borderline personality disorder (although it is important to note that not all patients with this disorder are prone to such anger). In their relationships with physicians and with others, angry borderline patients are prone to extremes of emotion: idealization in one moment and storminess and turbulence in the next. Such patients relate in a dependent yet demanding fashion, exhibiting hostility toward and devaluation of the very people on whom they rely so desperately. Their frequent bouts of anger express disappointment that in the past they were denied the help that they feel they needed and deserved. Their expectation of the future is that people will be uncaring, unsympathetic, and inevitably let them down.

WORKUP (1–3,5,7,9,10)

Picking up on verbal and nonverbal clues and being aware of one's emotional response to the patient can be very helpful diagnostically.

Verbal and Nonverbal Clues

Frowns, tightened fists, clenched jaws, refusal to make eye contact, abrupt and jerky gestures, and slamming of doors may be obvious nonverbal signifiers of disgruntlement. Verbal clues include statements of demand, annoyance, resentment, cynicism, sarcasm, and negativism. Passive–aggressive acts such as stony silences and self-destructive behaviors such as failing to adhere to a medical regimen, keep appointments, or give up habits that are harmful to one's health may be more oblique expressions of anger.

Emotional Response to Patient

It is important for the interviewer to pay as close attention to his or her subjective emotional response during an interview as to objective data; reactions to the patient may provide important diagnostic clues. Feelings of anxiety, irritation, defensiveness, and guilt may develop in a physician who feels blamed and attacked. Alternatively, a sense of boredom during an examination may represent an unconscious response to anger and hostility on the part of the patient.

Recognizing the Borderline Patient

The globally angry person with borderline personality organization can be recognized by a few clinical characteristics. Interpersonal relationships are either superficial or very dependent and manipulative. Emotions are intense and labile, with extreme anger predominating. Although social and intellectual skills may be well developed, such patients frequently feel empty, and their life's trajectory is often marked by a lack of sustained fulfillment or rewarding accomplishment. Impulsive, manipulative, self-destructive behaviors predominate.

PRINCIPLES OF MANAGEMENT
(1–3,5,7,9,10)

The fundamental keys to managing the angry patient include acknowledging the patient's feelings, setting limits, exploring causes, and responding appropriately without retaliating.

Acknowledging the Patient's Feelings

Having recognized that a patient is angry, a physician can calmly and without judgment acknowledge this emotion. The doctor need not agree that the anger is justified, but simply sympathetically note in conversation its existence. This intervention introduces a quality of openness, honesty, frankness, and sensitivity into the therapeutic relationship and helps to bring about a more open give-and-take discussion. The physician should convey neither fear nor rejection of the patient's feelings, but rather should try to understand them and to be helpful. In this way, the physician demonstrates an often reassuring ability to tolerate negative emotion and conveys to the patient that anger will not destroy the therapeutic relationship.

Setting Limits

When interacting with a globally angry patient, one need not be bullied. It is possible and indeed necessary to set limits on the patient's behavior while at the same time making clear that there will be no counterattack in retribution. If the patient's hostility interferes with communication, the therapeutic regimen, or coping with illness, this should be pointed out without condemnation. The physician needs to indicate that although

he or she recognizes and acknowledges the patient's anger, it nonetheless represents a problem in its self-destructiveness.

Exploring the Causes and Responding Appropriately

It is important not only to recognize that the patient is angry, but also to learn what he or she is angry about. During the interview, the physician should note the subject matter that provokes irritation, annoyance, or hostility. If the source of the patient's anger remains obscure, the physician may explicitly comment that the patient seems angry and ask him or her to tell the physician more about it.

Having identified the frustrations and threats the patient is facing, the physician should be able to approach the patient more effectively. For the patient who is angry about being ill, a detailed exploration of exact fears and sources of despair is helpful. Even the act of ventilating his or her anxiety may help to relieve it. For the person who is angry about being thrust into the patient role, a physician might consider structuring the relationship so as to minimize those aspects that threaten the patient most. For example, if the patient most fears dependence, the physician should assume a somewhat cool, reserved, and business-like stance while still conveying support and sympathy. If the anger seems to be displaced on the physician from another situation or relationship, this may be pointed out without encouraging the patient to vent the hostility on its actual source. Finally, if the patient is angry because of perceived harm as a result of either medical care or omission of medical care, the claim should be evaluated respectfully. If true harm has been sustained or an error has been made, a direct yet sensitive explanation should be given along with a sincere apology if appropriate. There is mounting evidence to suggest that, in the face of medical errors or bad outcomes, thorough explanations, transparency, and sincere expression of regret significantly boost patient satisfaction.

Avoiding Retaliation

The physician should take care to not react defensively or with hostility and subtly retaliate against the angry and provocative patient. Maintaining a clinical distance from the situation will help the physician to see the patient's anger not as a criticism of the doctor so much as a response to the patient's worries, perceived threats, and frustrated wishes. By doing so, one is in a good position to help the angry patient, preserve the therapeutic relationship, and more effectively offer care.

INDICATIONS FOR REFERRAL
(1–3,5,9,10)

Caring for the patient with a suspected borderline personality disorder can be quite vexing. When dealing with extremes of idealization and devaluation, it is often a relief to "spread the affect" among several care providers. Psychiatric referrals can serve to confirm diagnosis, provide management suggestions, and increase the patient's overall support network. A "curbside" consult with a psychiatric colleague can help to formulate a strategy for raising the issue of consultation with the patient and successfully completing the referral. Once the referral is made, the primary physician must maintain close contact with the psychiatrist to address the tendency for such patients to see some providers as "all good" and others as "all bad."

Annotated Bibliography

1. Beckman HB. Difficult patients. In: Feldman MD, Christensen JF, eds. Behavioral medicine in primary care. Stanford, CA: Appleton & Lange, 1997:20. (*A brief but very clear and practical discussion of patient anger, together with excellent, very specific suggestions for managing it.*)
2. Crutcher JE, Bass MJ. The difficult patient and the troubled physician. J Family Pract 1980;11:933. (*Presents empirical research on the types of patients and patient problems that irritate and dismay physicians.*)
3. Gerrard TJ, Riddell JD. Difficult patients: black holes and secrets. Br Med J 1988;297:530. (*Descriptions of difficult-to-care-for patients and helpful, specific suggestions for dealing with them.*)
4. Gross R, Olfson M, Gameroff M, et al. Borderline personality disorder in primary care. Arch Intern Med 2002;162:53. (*Presents survey data from primary care practice; a borderline state was unrecognized in nearly half of instances.*)
5. Groves JE. Taking care of the hateful patient. N Engl J Med 1978;298:883. (*Includes physicians' emotional responses to patients and ways to use these responses constructively.*)
6. Hahn SR, Kroenke K, Spitzer RL, et al. The difficult patient: prevalence, psychopathology, and functional impairment. J Gen Intern Med 1996;11:1. (*Finds a high prevalence of underlying psychopathology and much functional impairment.*)
7. Kahana RJ, Bibring GL. Personality types in medical management. In: Zinberg N, ed. Psychiatry and medical practice in a general hospital. New York: International University Press, 1965. (*A classic discussion of the range of emotional meanings and responses to illness.*)
8. Lin EH, Katon W, Von Korff M, et al. Frustrating patients: physician and patient perspectives among distressed high users of medical services. J Gen Intern Med 1991;6:241. (*A very useful discussion of psychologically distressed high users of care.*)
9. Oldham JM. A 44 year-old woman with borderline personality disorder. JAMA 2002;287:1029. (*A useful case-based review of this important character disorder, which may present as anger; 53 references.*)
10. Vincent C. Understanding and responding to adverse events. N Engl J Med 2003;348:1051 (*Includes useful suggestions on how to best respond to patients who have been harmed by medical treatment.*)

CHAPTER 232 ■ APPROACH TO THE PATIENT WITH INSOMNIA

JEFFREY B. WEILBURG

Insomnia is a problem of major proportions, with up to 35% of primary care patients and up to 17% of the general population reporting at least transient difficulty with sleep; approximately 40% of the U.S. population experiences recurrent or chronic insomnia at least once in their lifetime. The condition affects persons of all ages and backgrounds but is especially prevalent in the elderly, in patients with medical or psychiatric illness, and in persons of lower socioeconomic status. It markedly reduces quality of life (to the same degree as congestive heart failure) and significantly increases the risk of motor vehicle accidents and depression. The cost of health care services provided for the treatment of insomnia exceeds $12 billion/yr in the United States, with medications accounting for more than $2 billion/yr. Given the extent and significance of the problem, it is essential that the primary care physician be skilled in the assessment and basic treatment of insomnia.

DEFINITION, PATHOPHYSIOLOGY, AND CLINICAL PRESENTATION (1–5)

Definition

The term "insomnia" is formally defined as having repeated difficulty with the initiation, duration, consolidation, or quality of sleep occurring despite an adequate opportunity for sleep and producing clinically significant impairment of social, occupational, or other daytime function.

Sleep Physiology and Pathophysiology

Sleep physiology can be examined by polysomnography, continuous all-night recording of respiration, electroencephalogram (EEG), electrocardiogram, and the monitoring of eye movements, muscle tone, and blood oxygen saturation. It helps to differentiate normal from disturbed sleep.

Normal Sleep

Normal sleep has two basic phases: *rapid eye movement (REM) sleep* and *non-REM (NREM) sleep*.

REM Sleep. REM sleep is a state of mental and physical activation. Pulse and respiration are increased but muscle tone is diminished; little body movement occurs. The brain is active, and the EEG shows a pattern similar to that seen during waking. Most dreaming occurs during REM sleep.

Non-REM Sleep. In contrast, this is a time of deep rest. Pulse, respiration, and EEG all slow, and the patient goes from light sleep, called stages 1 and 2, to deep or *delta sleep*, called *stages 3 and 4*.

REM and NREM sleep normally cycle in a reciprocal pattern, giving a typical "architecture" to the polysomnogram.

The entire cycle lasts about 90 minutes and is repeated smoothly four or five times during the night. The *ventrolateral preoptic area (VLPO)*, located in the anterior hypothalamus, appears to be a key *"sleep center."* Reciprocal inhibition between the VLPO and *"wake and alertness" centers* such as the *tuberomammillary nucleus (TMN)* in the posterior hypothalamus and other areas in the forebrain and brainstem produces alternating periods of sleep and waking.

The alternation of sleep and wake, that is, the sleep cycle, may be regulated by a "biological clock"—the suprachiasmatic nucleus (SCN)—located in the hypothalamus. The absence of light appears to be one of the signals that prompts the SCN to stimulate the pineal gland to secrete *melatonin*, which may inhibit the stimulation of wake centers by the SCN, allowing the VLPO to promote sleep.

VLPO neurons express inhibitory neurotransmitters such as *γ-aminobutyric acid (GABA)* and galanin (most available insomnia medications stimulate GABA receptors). TMN neurons secrete *histamine*, which, along with the serotonin, noradrenaline, and acetylcholine secreted by the brainstem and other centers, may stimulate the cortex and thalamus to promote alertness and wakefulness. Medications such as antihistamines, antidepressants, and stimulants may produce insomnia or sedation by affecting these neurotransmitters. Adenosine accumulates in the brain during waking. Increasing concentrations of adenosine may inhibit wake and alertness centers; *caffeine* may promote wake and may produce insomnia because it is a potent adenosine receptor antagonist.

Not all persons who sleep less than the average amount each night have insomnia. Natural *"short sleepers"* are persons who regularly have less than 7 hours of well-maintained sleep yet suffer no problems in daytime function. *Normal aging* is associated with reductions in total sleep time, sleep continuity, and slow-wave sleep but does not produce insomnia or other formal sleep disorders. Anxiety and discomfort related to these normal changes may respond to counseling but not to medication or other treatment, so it is important to distinguish normal sleep changes from the specific symptoms of insomnia.

Insomnia

Insomnia has no single or pathognomonic polysomnographic pattern. Some insomniacs have sleep times that are slightly shorter than normal, some have less stage 3 and stage 4 sleep, and some have repeated arousals, but the degree of objective polysomnographic change is often not concordant with the degree of subjective distress. Patients may report difficulty falling asleep, with *sleep latency* (time between lights out and falling asleep) consistently exceeding 60 minutes. There may be early-morning awakening. Overall, there is compromised daytime functioning.

Patients with chronic insomnia may have *high levels of physiologic arousal*, perhaps reflecting overactivity in the alertness and wake centers. Chronic insomnia may arise when patients develop *maladaptive psychological responses* to this arousal, causing some to view the condition as a secondary problem or symptom arising from a comorbid disorder. *Disorders of mood or anxiety* appear in 30% to 50% of insomnia patients; *medical disorders* (often involving *pain*) are found in approximately 10%; *substance abuse* accounts for another 10%; only about 10% appear to be *primary sleep disorders*.

Insomnia may also have a course independent of comorbid medical and psychiatric disorders, and the presence or resolution of insomnia may influence outcomes of such comorbid disorders (especially depression). As a result, insomnia, (especially chronic insomnia) is now best understood as a clinical problem in its own right (i.e., a disorder), and treatment focuses on the resolution of insomnia symptoms

Classification; Types of Insomnia

Definitions and classifications of insomnia are found in the American Psychiatric Association's *Diagnostic and Statistical Manual of Mental Disorders*, fourth edition, the American Academy of Sleep Medicine's *International Classification of Sleep Disorders*, second edition (ICSD-2), and the World Health Organization's *International Statistical Classification of Diseases and Related Health Problems*, tenth revision (Table 232.1). The ICSD-2 is particularly relevant to the primary care setting; it requires for the diagnosis that a patient complain of at least one symptom of daytime impairment related to sleep. These include the following:

- Fatigue or malaise
- Impairment in attention, concentration, or memory
- Irritability or mood disturbance
- Daytime sleepiness and reduced motivation, energy, or initiative
- A tendency toward accidents at work or while driving
- Headaches, general tension, or gastrointestinal symptoms

Some common types of insomnia include the following:

- *Insomnia related to another mental disorder*, such as mood or anxiety disorders, psychosis, personality disorders, or adjustment disorders.
- *Insomnia due to a general medical condition* (see Table 232.1)
- *Substance-induced insomnia* (Table 232.2).
- *Adjustment insomnia, or transient insomnia*, which lasts for a few days to a few weeks (<3 months) and resolves on its own; it is associated with a known life stress (e.g., financial problem, job problem, conflict, loss, travel across time zones).
- *Idiopathic insomnia, or chronic or primary insomnia*, which often begins in childhood without a known stressor and continues throughout adulthood; there is a question of its association with childhood attention-deficit/hyperactivity disorder; it may have associated psychiatric symptoms (e.g., anxiety) or personality traits, but it does not meet the formal criteria for a psychiatric disorder; polysomnography is found to be normal or only slightly abnormal.
- *Paradoxical insomnia*, a relatively common form, which is severe and persistent difficulty falling or staying asleep; there is suspected hypervigilance, excessive worry about the loss of sleep, and the view that this loss is the source of all troubles; normal polysomnography is found.
- *Psychophysiologic insomnia*, associated with excessive focus on and anxiety about falling asleep, which produces arousal and becomes associated with sleep initiation problems; sleep is good on vacation or when the patient is away from the bedroom, but there is difficulty when trying to fall asleep in the usual sleep setting.

DIFFERENTIAL DIAGNOSIS (1,2)

The causes of sleep disorders range from minor situational problems in normal persons to true insomnia, which can be primary or secondary (Tables 232.1 and 232.2). Psychiatric disorders, substance abuse, and medical conditions may present with insomnia as a major complaint.

TABLE 232.1

IMPORTANT CAUSES OF INSOMNIA

Secondary Causes
  Psychiatric Disorders
    Affective disorders: depression (major depression, dysthymia, bipolar disorder)
    Stimulating antidepressants (direct stimulant effect, production of periodic leg movements of sleep): desipramine, imipramine, bupropion, fluoxetine, sertraline
    Substance abuse
    Sedative abuse and withdrawal: alcohol, narcotics, benzodiazepines
    Stimulant abuse and withdrawal: amphetamines, cocaine, phencyclidine
    Cigarette and nicotine dependence and withdrawal
    Character disorders
    Psychosis
    Antipsychotic agent production of periodic leg movements of sleep
  Medical/Surgical Problems
    Musculoskeletal: arthritic pain, low back pain, fibromyalgia
    Cardiovascular: nocturnal angina, orthopnea, paroxysmal nocturnal dyspnea; medications: quinidine, propranolol, atenolol, pindolol, clonidine, methyldopa
    Respiratory: chronic obstructive pulmonary disease, asthma; medications: terbutaline, albuterol, salmeterol, metaproternol, phenylpropanolamine, pseudoephedrine, phenylephrine
    Endocrine: hyperthyroidism; hypothyroidism (especially if associated with sleep apnea); medications: oral contraceptive pills, cortisone and related steroids, progesterone, thyroid hormone; hot flashes and mood disturbances of menopausal syndrome; diabetes (if associated with polyuria, nocturnal hypo- or hyperglycemia, and associated autonomic changes, neuropathic pain)
    Neuropsychiatric: delirium, dementia of any type, strokes, Parkinson's disease and other neuromuscular degenerative diseases
    Urologic: nocturia, dysuria
  Primary Sleep Problems
    Sleep apnea
    Circadian rhythm disturbance
    Jet lag
    Shift work
    Delayed sleep phase syndrome
    Periodic leg movements of sleep
    Restless leg syndrome
  Miscellaneous
    Caffeine
    Over-the-counter medications
    "Diet pills"
    Environmental factors: noise, temperature

TABLE 232.2

MEDICATIONS AND SUBSTANCES THAT INDUCE INSOMNIA

Stimulants, used as medications and as substances of abuse (including caffeine found in coffee, tea, chocolate, and cola drinks)
Antihypertensives, including α- and β-blockers, calcium-channel blockers, methyldopa, and reserpine
Asthma agents and bronchodilators, including theophylline and albuterol
Corticosteroids
Decongestants, including pseudoephedrine, phenylpropanolamine, and phenylephrine
Antidepressants, including fluoxetine, bupropion, venlafaxine, phenelzine, and Parnate
Tobacco/nicotine (in cigarettes, cigars, and pipe tobacco)
Alcohol

Psychiatric Disorders

About half of all cases have a comorbid psychiatric disorder. Patients with *major depression* complain of either difficulty falling asleep or of waking in the early morning and being unable to return to sleep. Diurnal variation of mood is often noted. Severe depression with agitation may lead to markedly diminished total sleep and overall exhaustion (see Chapter 227). It is important to recognize that insomnia may be the presenting symptom of major depression, and patients with insomnia are at risk for developing depression. Insomnia may also persist after other symptoms of depression resolve.

Patients with *dysthymic disorder* (a variant of depression; see Chapter 229) often complain of feeling tired and irritable, have difficulty falling asleep, and report that they cannot get enough sleep to feel rested. Sometimes they deny feeling sad or depressed and focus only on their physical complaints. Patients in the manic phase of a *bipolar affective disorder* may report difficulty falling asleep or staying asleep, but they do not report feeling tired during waking times.

Patients with *anxiety and obsessive disorders* frequently have great difficulty falling asleep because they lie in bed and ruminate. Patients with *character disorders* such as narcissistic or *borderline character disorders* may feel angry about not being able to get the sleep they feel they are entitled to. The anger at failed efforts to sleep may produce arousal and make it increasingly difficult for them to fall asleep. *Active psychosis* of any type (e.g., schizophrenia) produces disturbed sleep and accounts for the other 10% of psychiatric insomnia. Hallucinations, delusions, and other signs and symptoms of psychotic illness present with the insomnia, facilitating recognition.

Drugs and Substance Abuse

Drugs and alcohol are present in about 10% to 15% of all patients with insomnia and may be its cause. *Alcohol* induces sedation, but the resulting sleep is often shallow, fragmented, and not restorative. Alcoholics can have prematurely "aged" sleep (i.e., shallow and short) during and for months after the cessation of drinking. *Sedatives*, especially barbiturates, when used on a regular long-term basis lead to shallow, fragmented sleep. *Rebound insomnia* and rebound anxiety prompt reuse, and tolerance leads to dose escalation, and so patients get caught in a vicious cycle. Sedatives and alcohol depress respiratory function, which can lead to sleep of very poor quality in patients with sleep apnea.

Stimulant drugs, such as amphetamines, activating antidepressants, and the phenylpropanolamine found in many over-the-counter decongestants (Table 232.3) can induce significant difficulty in falling asleep. The caffeine and other stimulant xanthines found in tea, coffee, cola drinks, and chocolate are well recognized and often used for their ability to keep one awake. In those who are sensitive, even small amounts can prevent sleep. Nicotine and other substances found in cigarette smoke disrupt sleep induction and continuity. Bronchodilators such as aminophylline and β-agonists can make sleep difficult when given before bedtime.

Medical Problems

Ten percent of cases are due principally to a medical problem. *Chronic pain* is a leading, although often overlooked, factor (e.g., that experienced by elderly persons with degenerative

---

TABLE 232.3

BEHAVIORAL APPROACHES TO INSOMNIA

Cognitive–behavioral therapy (CBT) can be used to identify and change maladaptive beliefs, behaviors, and affects around sleep

Progressive muscle relaxation can help to reduce some of the excess stimulation experience by some patients with insomnia

Stimulus-control therapy can help to break the association between bed and sleeplessness and its associated frustrations that can develop in patients with insomnia

Sleep-restriction therapy helps patients to limit the time they spend in bed to the time they actually sleep

Attention to *good sleep hygiene* helps patients to wind down, find a suitable sleep environment, get reasonable amounts of well-timed exercise, and avoid substances, such as caffeine, that may interfere with sleep

---

joint disease). *Delirium* is another important cause in the elderly, resulting from unrecognized infection or medication toxicity (as from anticholinergic agents used in over-the-counter sleep remedies). *Cardiopulmonary dysfunction* may contribute by causing orthopnea, paroxysmal nocturnal dyspnea, or nocturnal angina. *Urinary frequency* due to infection, prostatism, diabetes, or poor timing of diuretic use is another important disrupter of sleep. Often, it is the nocturia and disturbed sleep that causes the patient with prostatism finally to seek definitive therapy. Nocturia has also been noted to be a consequence of sleep apnea.

Primary Sleep Disorders

Circadian rhythm disorders may present with insomnia. In the *delayed sleep-phase syndrome*, the patient falls asleep later than the usual bedtime, sleeps well, and gets up later than is socially acceptable. This common disturbance often presents in adolescents. Other common forms are due to alternating shift work or jet travel across time zones ("*jet lag*"), in which the inability to rapidly reset one's diurnal rhythm to local time leads to insomnia. For travel westward across time zones, the typical experience is awakening in the middle of night local time (morning at home) and being unable to fall back to sleep despite feeling tired. Restful sleep is not achieved. Moreover, there is marked afternoon or early-evening sleepiness (bedtime at home). The inability to attain restful sleep culminates in exhaustion, and the patient requests help for insomnia. Endogenous disruptions of the brain's internal circadian rhythm setter can produce a similar picture.

Periodic limb movement of sleep (PLMS; formally called "*nocturnal myoclonus*") can produce poor-quality sleep in some patients and lead to the complaint of "insomnia" but more often is associated with complaints of excess daytime sleepiness or no symptoms. It is characterized by repetitive twitching of the legs or arms, which is often unrecognized by the patient but are detected during polysomnography. *Restless leg syndrome* is another motor disturbance associated with insomnia. Characteristic features include involuntary leg movements when awake and periodic leg movements when asleep (see Appendix 232.1).

Sleep apnea is a disorder characterized by repeated apneic periods due to soft-tissue upper airway obstruction followed by disruption of sleep. In severe cases, behavioral changes, pulmonary hypertension, cardiac arrhythmias, and death can occur. Patients with obstructive sleep apnea (OSA) tend to complain of marked daytime sleepiness rather than insomnia, but it is important to rule out OSA when evaluating sleep problems, given the consequences of missing the diagnosis (see Chapter 46).

WORKUP (1,2,21)

When the complaint is persistent, when sleep latency (time between lights out and falling asleep) is consistently greater than 60 minutes, and when the insomnia is associated with compromised daytime functioning, a search for an underlying etiology should be undertaken (Table 232.2).

History

A full description of the problem is essential and is facilitated by having the patient keep a *sleep log* or diary, which includes time in bed, estimate of time asleep, any awakenings, time of morning arousal, estimate of sleep quality, and comments on unusual events and any associated symptoms (e.g., orthopnea, urinary frequency, pain, palpitations). Entries are recorded by the patient directly on getting up each morning. Close attention must also be given to use of sedatives, hypnotics (including over-the-counter preparations), and stimulants (see Table 232.2). Screening for abuse of alcohol and other substances is essential (see Chapters 228 and 235). It is most important to listen carefully for and inquire directly about symptoms of depression, bipolar disease, anxiety disorder, and psychosis (see Chapters 226 and 227). Occupational and travel patterns should be noted. Whenever possible, interviewing the spouse, bed partner, or family member is of great value, particularly for symptoms suggestive of sleep apnea (e.g., excessive snoring, apneic episodes, disturbed sleep). Family members may also bring to light covert substance use or abuse that patients may minimize or deny. Past and family medical and psychiatric histories are sometimes revealing. Perimenopausal women should be asked about hot flashes.

Physical Examination

The pertinent physical examination is a function of the history. One checks for upper airway soft-tissue obstruction in the patient with suspected sleep apnea; for jugular venous distention, rales, wheezes, heaves, and gallops when there is concern about a cardiopulmonary etiology; for moist skin, tachycardia, proptosis, goiter, and tremor when hyperthyroidism is under consideration; and for prostatic enlargement in the elderly male with sleep-disturbing nocturia. Any reported sources of pain

should be evaluated and confirmed by physical examination. A careful mental status examination helps in the detection of psychiatric disease (see Chapters 226 and 227).

Laboratory Testing

Testing should be limited, selective, and based on evidence from the history and physical examination (e.g., thyroid-stimulating hormone for suspected hyperthyroidism, chest x-ray for cardiopulmonary disease, toxic screen for substance abuse). Referral to a sleep specialist is indicated if a primary sleep disorder, such as primary chronic insomnia, sleep apnea, PLMS, or circadian rhythm disorder is suspected. Polysomnography is generally not indicated in the evaluation of insomnia in primary care settings. Psychiatric evaluation is indicated when character problems interfere with diagnosis or management or if the nature of a suspected mental or emotional problem is obscure, or if insomnia persists despite resolution of mood or anxiety symptoms.

PRINCIPLES OF MANAGEMENT
(6–25)

Overall Approach (Tables 232.3 and 232.4)

For *transient insomnia*, explanation and supportive council often suffice, but time-limited courses of hypnotic medication can also be helpful and appropriate. Identification and treatment of *comorbid disorders* are important, especially in patients with

---

TABLE 232.4

BENZODIAZEPINES AND BENZODIAZEPINE-RECEPTOR AGONISTS (BZRAS) FOR SLEEP

Agent (Brand Name)	Onset	Duration	Dose (mg)	Relative Cost (Brand)	Comments
Benzodiazepine-like					
Zaleplon (Sonata)	Rapid	Short	5–10	$$$$$	May be used for awakenings at night; possible interaction with inducers of CYP 3A4
Zolpidem (Ambien)	Rapid	Short–intermediate	5–10	$$ (generic)	Potential interaction with inducers of CYP 3A4
Zolpidem (Ambien CR)	Rapid	Short–intermediate	6.125–12.5	$$$$$	
Eszopiclone (Lunesta)	Rapid	Short–intermediate	1–3		Potential interactions with ketoconazole, nefazadone, and inducers of CYP 3A4
Benzodiazepine					
Diazepam (Valium)[a]	Rapid	Long	2–5	$ ($$)	
Quazepam (Doral)[a]	Rapid	Long	15	$$ ($$$$)	
Flurazepam (Dalmane)[a]	Rapid–intermediate	Long	15–30	$$ ($$$)	
Triazolam (Halcion)[a]	Rapid–intermediate	Short	0.125–0.5	$$ ($$$)	
Estazolam (ProSom)[a]	Rapid–intermediate	Intermediate	1–2	$$ ($$$)	
Lorazepam (Ativan)[a]	Intermediate	Intermediate	1	$$ ($$$)	
Clonazepam (Klonopin)[a]	Intermediate	Long	0.5–1.0	$$ ($$)	
Oxazepam (Serax)[a]	Intermediate–slow	Short–intermediate	10–15	$$ ($$$)	
Temazepam (Restoril)[a]	Intermediate–slow	Intermediate	15	$$ ($$$)	

CYP, cytochrome P450.
[a]Generic formulation available at lower cost.

persistent insomnia; insomnia symptoms may have an independent course and should be treated when they persist. In particular, patients with insomnia persisting after resolution of primary mood or anxiety symptoms may have better immediate and long-term outcomes when the insomnia symptoms resolve. Conversely, insomnia symptoms persisting for days to weeks following usual treatments should prompt a search for a comorbid disorder,

Cognitive–behavioral therapy and other psychologically based behavioral measures (e.g., focus on *sleep hygiene, relaxation*, and *stimulus control/sleep restriction*) can be effective and should be considered as a first line of therapy, especially for patients with chronic or psychophysiologic insomnia, either alone or in combination with medication. Behaviorally based treatments are also best for patients with current or past histories of substance abuse and for many patients with anxiety and character disorders.

Pharmacologic therapy can play an important role, not only for short-term use, but also for chronic insomnia. Recent evidence suggests that hypnotics may be safe and effective in long-term (>3 months) treatment for some patients with chronic insomnia; U.S. Food and Drug Administration labeling for the newer nonbenzodiazepine hypnotics does not specify that treatment should be short term (as found for the older benzodiazepine agents), but long-term experience with these agents is limited.

Patients who engage in substance use need to achieve abstinence from alcohol and "recreational" stimulants, including caffeine and tobacco as a first step (see Chapters 54, 228, and 235). Patients with current or past histories of abuse of alcohol or other drugs or substances should generally not receive a benzodiazepine or related agent due to their increased risk of drug dependency (although most authorities now agree that patients without a personal or family history of current or past substance abuse are at low risk for addiction to hypnotics when these agents are appropriately prescribed and their use is carefully monitored).

Nonpharmacologic Methods

Behavioral treatments therapies are the backbone of nonpharmacologic treatment, providing results that rival if not exceed those of pharmacologic intervention, especially in selected populations, such as patients with underlying psychopathology.

Cognitive–Behavioral Therapy (CBT)

This approach may be as effective as hypnotics for the treatment of chronic and other kinds of insomnia and may have a more sustained positive effect than hypnotics. Although usually conducted by specially trained psychologists, CBT insomnia programs have been developed for use in primary care practices. These help patients to recognize and moderate maladaptive beliefs and habits and may be used in conjunction with other kinds of behavior manipulation, such as relaxation and sleep restriction, as well as with medication, although their concurrent use with medication may limit long-term benefit from CBT.

Relaxation

Progressive muscle relaxation, guided imagery, and related attention-focusing techniques can help to reduce excessive arousal and anxiety and may be useful for most patients with insomnia.

Stimulus Control

This approach has shown best results in patients with learned or psychophysiologic insomnia because it identifies and breaks the associations among anxiety, frustration, and related behaviors connected to sleep-onset-related problems. Stimulus control is related to education about the rules of good "sleep hygiene" (Table 232.3).

Sleep Restriction

Patients are taught how to limit time in bed to time actually asleep; this has been shown to reduce sleep latency, improve sleep continuity and quality, and reduce insomnia symptoms.

Pharmacotherapy

When behavioral methods do not suffice for chronic insomnia or short-term-only treatment is envisioned, then consideration of pharmacologic therapy is reasonable. It is essential to keep in mind the *potential adverse effects* of pharmacologic agents. Short-acting benzodiazepines and nonbenzodiazepine hypnotics have been associated with *abnormal nocturnal behaviors*, such as driving and eating, especially when used in larger-than-recommended doses or in combination with alcohol or other psychoactive agents. All sedative hypnotics can produce *cognitive* and *psychomotor impairment* (compromising the ability to drive safely), especially during time of peak serum levels. Therefore, when sedative hypnotics are considered, patients should be warned about the potential for these problems and educated to avoid concomitant alcohol or drug use, avoid driving or operating machinery after medication ingestion, and report unusual behavior or cognitive disturbance.

Falls are a serious concern with hypnotic use, especially for the elderly patient who gets up to go to the bathroom at night. Older patients, their families, and caregivers should be warned about possible gait disturbance during nocturnal ambulation. Of note, the association between sedative hypnotics and falls has recently been challenged, with some suggesting that insomnia itself may be a more important factor in the risk of falls and injury than sedative use; continued study of this issue is required.

Trends in recent years in hypnotic use include the replacement of the benzodiazepines with nonbenzodiazepine agents active at the benzodiazepine receptor.

Benzodiazepine-Receptor Agonists (BZRAs)

These nonbenzodiazepine drugs (e.g., *zolpidem* [Ambien], *zaleplon* [Sonata], and *eszopiclone* [Lunesta]) act at the benzodiazepine receptor complex, producing a clinical hypnotic effect similar to that of benzodiazepines but without many of the undesirable side effects such as disturbance of sleep architecture, daytime sedation, rebound insomnia, or marked habituation potential (although still listed by the Drug Enforcement Administration as class IV drugs due to their slight risk of inducing mild euphoria). The onset of action is rapid, reducing sleep latency (time to onset of sleep). The use of high doses can cause next-day somnolence and cognitive impairment, but less so than with benzodiazepines. Zaleplon is the shorter acting (2 to 3 hours), making it useful if the problem is limited to difficulty falling asleep or if the patient awakens in the middle of the night; it is less likely to cause residual sedation but may not prevent premature awakening. The cost for these agents is high—up to five times that of generic benzodiazepines and more for branded sustained-release formulations (which also may increase risk of daytime sedation).

Benzodiazepines

Many preparations are marketed for insomnia (see Table 232.2); none has proven to be substantially superior to any other. Most are safe and effective at low doses when used for very short periods, but all have problems associated with chronic use, including habituation, dependency, and withdrawal syndrome. Unlike the benzodiazepine-like drugs, they tend to disrupt normal sleep architecture by prolonging the first two stages of sleep and shortening deep and REM stages. Daytime drowsiness, impairment of cognitive function, and psychomotor retardation are well-described adverse effects, especially with higher doses and use of longer-acting preparations. Rebound insomnia and anxiety can occur with continuous use, necessitating the shortest possible duration of therapy and tapering to the lowest possible dose. Choice of agent can be based on cost and desired onset and duration of action (see Table 232.2).

The *short-acting* drugs are best prescribed for those whose primary problem is *falling asleep*. The *intermediate-acting* agents may be useful for those patients who complain of problems with staying asleep (sleep continuity). *Long-acting agents* are considered when daytime anxiety compounds the discomfort.

Melatonin-Receptor Agonists

Ramelteon, a specific agonist of melatonin receptors in the suprachiasmatic nucleus, is useful for patients who have problems falling asleep but does not appear to benefit those with sleep maintenance problems. Most studies indicate that 7.5 mg is the optimal dose. Ramelteon does not seem to produce rebound and may be used several times a week for more than 3 months for patients with a positive response. *Melatonin* is variably absorbed and distributed in the brain; it is not generally recommended, although it is widely used due to its availability without prescription.

Antidepressants, Buspirone, and Antipsychotics

The data supporting the use of antidepressants and buspirone for sleep disorders are very limited, but these agents are widely used in practice (e.g., *trazodone*, 25 to 50 mg ad bedtime; nortriptyline, 10 to 25 mg at bedtime, or *buspirone*, 10 to 30 mg at bedtime). They can be of particular value for patients, such as those with substance abuse, in whom typical hypnotics are contraindicated. Antipsychotic agents can relieve insomnia due to agitation in psychotic or delirious patients, but they should not be a first-line treatment for insomnia.

Antihistamines and Other Drugs

In instances in which benzodiazepines are contraindicated (e.g., a history of drug or alcohol dependence) and sedating antidepressants have not helped, some clinicians choose *antihistamines* (e.g., *diphenhydramine*, 25 to 50 mg at bedtime). Antihistamines are used in various over-the-counter sleep remedies. However, antihistamines have not been found to improve sleep and may produce delirium, urinary retention, cognitive impairment, or paradoxical excitation especially in the elderly, so this approach should be used with care, if at all. *Chloral hydrate* should rarely be used, and there is almost never a place for treating new cases of insomnia with barbiturates, meprobamate, or over-the-counter remedies. *Valerian* is a herbal preparation widely promoted for sleep; performance in clinical trials is variable and efficacy is not well established.

PATIENT EDUCATION

The overall promotion of good *sleep hygiene* is useful for many patients. Establishing a regular bed and wake time, avoiding any and all naps, having regular exercise (although not at night), using the bed only for sleeping or lovemaking (rather than reading or watching television), and getting in bed only when ready for sleep (leaving the bed if sleep is not forthcoming) are useful suggestions. Avoidance of caffeinated foods, stimulants, cigarettes, and alcohol is necessary for some sensitive patients.

Instructing patients about these basic rules of sleep hygiene and helping them to avoid trying too hard to fall asleep are often useful. Disabusing patients of the myth that everyone must have 8 hours of sleep every night makes many people feel relieved. In addition, informing patients that much of the time they spend in bed believing they are "only drowsy" is time actually spent in the lighter stages of sleep can ameliorate some patients' frustration.

THERAPEUTIC RECOMMENDATIONS

For All Patients

- Offer education regarding behavioral and relaxation measures that may help both patients with comorbid mood and anxiety disorders and those with primary insomnia; these measures may be offered first, in lieu of medication, or with medication (see Table 232.4).
- Offer education and support to an elderly patient who has normal daytime function but who is lonely or upset as his or her sleep goes through the changes associated with normal aging.

For Patients with Secondary Causes of Insomnia

- If the insomnia is related to an underlying *depressive disorder*, begin a selective serotonin reuptake inhibitor, such as *paroxetine* 20 mg or *citalopram* 20 mg, taken 1 hour before bedtime every night for 2 weeks; see the patient frequently until symptoms resolve and increase the dose as needed to fully treat the depression (see Chapter 227). If insomnia persists despite the resolution of mood symptoms, begin treatment with a hypnotic. If the insomnia is related to an anxiety disorder, use a benzodiazepine-receptor agonist (e.g., *zolpidem* [Ambien, 5 to 10 mg at bedtime] or eszopiclone [Lunesta, 1 mg at bedtime]) or the short-acting benzodiazepine *lorazepam*, 1 mg at bedtime. If the patient has a *chronic anxiety disorder* or is bothered by persistent anxiety, *clonazepam* (0.5 mg) at bedtime may be helpful (see Chapter 226).
- If *pain*, menopausal *hot flashes*, or an underlying *medical problem* is responsible, treat specifically, especially if it is interfering with quality of life, supplementing treatment if necessary with a short course of a benzodiazepine-receptor agonist or a benzodiazepine agent to help reestablish a normal sleep pattern.

■ Obtain a complete history of *alcohol* and *substance* use in every patient, checking for abuse as well as for tobacco use, caffeine intake, nonprescription drugs, and stimulants. Do not prescribe a benzodiazepine in patients with current or past alcohol or drug use problems, but do consider CBT and other behaviorally based treatments, supplemented if necessary by a nonbenzodiazepine agent such as trazodone, nortriptyline, buspirone, or ramelteon. Attend to the underlying substance abuse problem (see Chapters 228 and 235).

For Primary Insomnia

■ Begin treatment with *cognitive–behavioral therapy* (including stimulus control, relaxation, and sleep-hygiene education) and continue as necessary.

■ If symptoms remain refractory or the problem is considered a short-term issue only, consider adding a short-course of a *benzodiazepine-receptor agonist* (e.g., *zolpidem*, 5 to 10 mg at bedtime, or *eszopiclone*, 1 mg at bedtime) or a short-acting *benzodiazepine* (e.g., *lorazepam*, 1 mg at bedtime). Inform patients that the absorption of benzodiazepine-receptor agonists is slowed by a heavy, fatty meal, which may delay onset of action and falling asleep.

■ If longer-term pharmacotherapy appears necessary, consider a benzodiazepine-receptor agonist, but be aware that data are limited on safety and efficacy beyond 6 months of use, and chronic use may limit the long-term benefits of CBT. Monitor carefully for efficacy, side effects (especially in the elderly), and the development of tolerance (particularly with benzodiazepine use). In the absence of clear-cut benefit, halt drug therapy.

■ For difficulty predominantly with *sleep initiation* consider *zolpidem, zaleplon,* or the melatonin receptor agonist *ramelteon* (7.5 mg at bedtime); the latter appears to be safe for prolonged use.

■ For *sleep maintenance*, consider *eszopiclone* or the more traditional treatment with an intermediate-acting benzodiazepine such as *temazepam*. If there is awakening in the middle of the night, the shorter-acting *zaleplon* can be used.

Annotated Bibliography

1. American Psychiatric Association. Diagnostic and statistical manual of mental disorders, 4th ed. Washington, DC: Author, 1994. (*The standard for classification and diagnosis.*)
2. Diagnostic Classification Steering Committee. The international classification of sleep disorders: diagnostic and coding manual. Rochester, MN. American Sleep Disorders Association, 1990. (*Classification details.*)
3. Foley DJ, Monjan A, Simonsick EM, et al. Incidence and remission of insomnia among elderly adults: an epidemiologic study of 6800 person over three years. Sleep 1999;22(Suppl2):S366. (*A very high prevalence was noted.*)
4. National Institutes of Health. NIH state-of-the-science conference statement on manifestations and management of chronic insomnia in adults, June 13–15, 2005. Available at: http://consensus.nih.gov/2005/2005InsomniaSOS026main.htm. (*A consensus statement viewing chronic insomnia as a primary problem in its own right.*)
5. Thase ME. Correlates and consequences of chronic insomnia. Gen Hosp Psychiatry 2005;27:100. (*Finds that the treatment of depression can have a beneficial effect on the outcome of concurrent illness.*)
6. Baillargeon L, Landreville P, Verreault R, et al. Discontinuation of benzodiazepines among older insomniac adults treated with cognitive–behavioral therapy combined with gradual tapering: a randomized trial. Can Med Assoc J 2003;169:1015. (*Cognitive–behavioral therapy helped patients to taper medication and become drug-free.*)
7. Bent S, Padula A, Moore D, et al. Valerian for sleep: a systematic review and meta-analysis. Am J Med 2006;119:1005. (*Finds that study quality is wanting; there was a suggestion of modest benefit.*)
8. Brzezinski A. Melatonin in humans. N Engl J Med 1997;336:186. (*A comprehensive review; includes a basic science review of melatonin's contribution to sleep and the pharmacology of oral use.*)
9. Chesson AL Jr, Anderson WM, Littner M, et al. Practice parameters for the nonpharmacologic treatment of chronic insomnia: an American Academy of Sleep Medicine report: Standards of Practice Committee of the American Academy of Sleep Medicine. Sleep 1999;22:1128. (*Consensus guidelines for nonpharmacologic measures.*)
10. Edinger JD, Sampson WS. A primary care "friendly" cognitive behavioral insomnia therapy. Sleep 2003;26:177. (*A useful discussion of a practical program for use in primary care practice.*)
11. Holbrook AM, Crowther R, Lotter A, et al. Meta-analysis of benzodiazepine use in the treatment of insomnia. Can Med Assoc J 2000;162:225. (*An excellent review of the evidence for this approach.*)
12. Jacobs GD, Pace-Schott EF, Stickgold R, et al. Cognitive behavior therapy and pharmacotherapy for insomnia: a randomized controlled trial and direct comparison. Arch Intern Med 2004;164:1888. (*Found that cognitive–behavioral therapy was superior to zolpidem and placebo.*)
13. King AC, Oman RF, Brassington GS, et al. Moderate-intensity exercise and self-rated quality of sleep in older adults: a randomized controlled trial. JAMA 1997;227:32. (*Presents evidence that exercise improved the quality of sleep.*)
14. Krystal AD, Walsh JK, Laska E, et al. Sustained efficacy of eszopiclone over 6 months of nightly treatment: results of a randomized, double-blind, placebo-controlled study of adults with chronic insomnia. Sleep 2003;26:793. (*Presents evidence for sustained benefit of this approach for up to 6 months.*)
15. Kupfer DJ, Reynolds CF. Management of insomnia. N Engl J Med 1997;336:341. (*A comprehensive review with an excellent list of references.*)
16. Lavie P. Sleep disturbances in the wake of traumatic events. N Engl J Med 2001;345:1825. (*A comprehensive review of the sleep disturbance of post-traumatic stress disorder; 97 references.*)
17. Morin DM, Colecchi C, Steve J, et al. Behavioral and pharmacologic therapy for late life insomnia. JAMA 1999;281:991. (*A good review of the data on treating insomnia in the elderly.*)
18. Nowell PD, Mazumdar S, Buysse DJ, et al. Benzodiazepines and zolpidem for chronic insomnia: a meta-analysis of treatment efficacy. JAMA 1997;278:2170. (*Both were found to be effective, given the data on hand, but available studies are limited in scope and duration.*)
19. Ohayon MM. Severe hot flashes are associated with chronic insomnia. Arch Intern Med 2006;166:1262. (*A cohort study; the prevalence of insomnia increased markedly with the presence of hot flashes.*)
20. Mimeault V, Morin CM. Self-help treatment for insomnia: bibliotherapy with and without professional guidance. J Consult Clin Psychol 1999;67:511. (*Review of this interesting approach.*)
21. Silber MH. Chronic insomnia. N Engl J Med 2005;353:803. (*An excellent review with emphasis on management and a bent toward cognitive–behavioral therapy; 58 references.*)
22. Smith MT, Perlis ML, Park A, et al. Comparative meta-analysis of pharmacotherapy and behavior therapy for persistent insomnia. Am J Psychiatry 2002;159:5. (*There was a similar overall efficacy, with CBT better in terms of sleep latency.*)
23. Walsh JK, Pollak CP, Scharf MB, et al. Lack of residual sedation following middle-of-the-night zaleplon administration in sleep maintenance insomnia. Clin Neuropharmacol 2000;23:17. (*A randomized, controlled trial, finding evidence for a lack of residual sedation.*)
24. Walsh JK, Erman M, Erwin CW, et al. Subjective hypnotic efficacy of trazodone in DSM3-R primary insomnia. Hum Psychopharmacol 1998;13:191. (*The treatment was better than placebo but less effective than zolpidem.*)
25. Zemlan FP, Mulchahey JJ, Scharf MB, et al. The efficacy and safety of the melatonin agonist beta-methyl-6-chloromelatonin in primary insomnia: a randomized, placebo-controlled, crossover clinical trial. J Clin Psychiatry 2005;66:384. (*Finds evidence of efficacy of this melatonin derivative; best for reducing sleep latency.*)

APPENDIX 232.1: RESTLESS LEG SYNDROME

An important yet often-overlooked cause of disturbed sleep is the restless leg syndrome, a common neurologic problem with an estimated prevalence ranging from 2% to 15% of the general population. The condition is defined clinically by the following criteria: (a) irresistible urge to move the legs (akathisia) accompanied by an unpleasant leg sensation and (b) symptoms aggravated by rest, (c) alleviated by movement, especially walking, and (d) worse in the evening or night.

PATHOPHYSIOLOGY AND CLINICAL PRESENTATION (1)

The *pathogenesis* of the condition is unknown. Both hereditary and seemingly acquired forms exist, with the hereditary form manifesting onset typically before the age of 40 years, whereas those without a family history are more likely to begin experiencing symptoms after age 50 years. Purported etiologic factors include small-fiber neuropathy, dialysis, iron and folate deficiencies, and pregnancy; cigarette smoking, obesity, and sedentary lifestyle have also been implicated. Working hypotheses regarding pathophysiology center on abnormalities in the subcortical brain regarding iron, dopaminergic transmission, and circadian rhythms, with resultant loss of cortical and spinal inhibition of motor activity that occurs mostly at night.

The *clinical presentation* is likely to be dominated by a complaint of difficulty sleeping, with symptoms of restless leg being reported in the context of an inquiry into causes. The principal clinical *manifestations* of restless leg syndrome are encompassed by its definition (see prior discussion). Getting up and walking about can provide sustained relief, but with resumption of inactivity, symptoms may recur. With progression, the uncomfortable leg sensations develop earlier in the day and become increasingly severe at night. Involuntary jerking movements may be reported by the patient, and spouse or family members may note quasirhythmic limb movements during sleep (so-called periodic limb movements).

DIFFERENTIAL DIAGNOSIS AND WORKUP (1)

Restless leg needs to be distinguished from nocturnal leg cramps, which cause frank calf pain and a knot in the muscle, relieved by stretching. Paresthesias from prolonged sitting and akathisia in persons with peripheral neuropathy may worsen with sitting and mimic restless leg syndrome; however, symptoms occur only with prolonged sitting, and there are no symptoms on lying down. In persons with periodic leg movements with sleep, other etiologies need to be considered, including sleep apnea, use of neuroleptics and antidepressants, spinal cord lesions, stroke, narcolepsy, and neurodegenerative disease.

Because patients often present complaining of difficulty sleeping and not symptoms of restless leg syndrome, it is important to inquire about the condition as part of the workup for insomnia (see prior discussion). Diagnosis is clinical, based on a careful history addressing the four cardinal features that define the condition (see prior discussion). The drug history should be reviewed for medications that may affect dopaminergic transmission (e.g., antidepressants, neuroleptics, some calcium-channel blockers). There are no diagnostic physical findings. A suggestive electromyogram pattern exists, but such testing is rarely necessary. Checking serum chemistries for purported contributing factors (e.g., creatinine, ferritin, folate) is reasonable.

TREATMENT (2,3)

In many instances, symptoms are mild and sufficiently self-limited to require no treatment, but if sleep is being significantly compromised, then treatment is indicated.

Nonpharmacologic Measures

A host of nonpharmacologic measures can be helpful and include the following:

- Correcting any iron deficiency (see Chapter 82)
- Reducing or eliminating stimulants and depressants (nicotine, alcohol, caffeine)
- Curtailing as much as possible contributing medications, especially *antihistamines*, *dopamine blockers* (e.g., neuroleptics, antiemetics, metoclopramide), and *antidepressants* (both selective serotonin reuptake inhibitors and tricyclic antidepressants)
- Encouraging good sleep-hygiene measures (regular hours, avoiding perturbing activities before bed)
- Advising regular moderate exercise, including a trial of a brief walk before bed
- Messaging of limbs and hot bath or shower

Pharmacologic Measures

Pharmacologic therapy should only be considered when nondrug measures prove insufficient and symptoms are disruptive of sleep. Pharmacologic approaches are tailored to whether the patient experiences disruptive symptoms only occasionally (in which case a short-acting, rapid-onset agent is preferred) or has daily difficulties, necessitating longer-acting therapy. When symptoms are clearly related to a precipitant, treatment may be anticipatory if the precipitant cannot be avoided. Available agents include dopaminergic drugs, mild- to moderate-strength opioids, and benzodiazepines.

Dopaminergic Agents

These are among the best studied and are approved by the U.S. Food and Drug Administration for persons with nightly symptoms. Efficacy is high (approaching 90% to 100%) for both restless leg and period movement. *Levodopa* (starting at 50 mg at bedtime) is most useful for intermittent use in persons with mild to moderate symptoms because onset is fairly rapid, duration is short, and adverse side effects are minimal at such low doses (see Chapter 174). The nonergot dopaminergic agent *ropinirole* (Requip; starting at 0.25 mg, 1 to 2 hours before bed) is a longer-acting dopamine agonist (because it is nonergot, it has none of the heart-valve and fibrotic concerns of ergot-derived dopamine agonists) that is more useful in persons with daily symptoms; dose titration is necessary. *Pramipexole* (Mirapex, starting at 0.125 mg, 2 to 3 hours before bed) has similar nonergot dopamine-agonist qualities and has proven useful for continued use; however, augmentation (see later discussion) has been noted with long-term use.

Disadvantages of dopaminergic therapy include *augmentation* of symptoms (symptoms occur earlier in the day and more severely at night) associated with prolonged use and an *acute withdrawal syndrome* (severe leg restlessness for a few days) associated with sudden cessation of treatment. Use of a dopamine agonist instead of levodopa may help in preventing augmentation, as might the use of a controlled-release formulation and low doses. If augmentation develops, switching to another drug is recommended. Other adverse effects on this class include nausea, somnolence, hallucinations, and orthostatic hypotension. Impulse-control problems have been reported (gambling, hypersexual behavior, compulsive eating).

Opiates, Anticonvulsants, and Benzodiazepines

Opiates (e.g., *oxycodone*, 5 mg at bedtime) are helpful as second-line agents in persons with incapacitating disease who fail dopamine-agonist therapy, but dependence is a concern. *Anticonvulsants* (e.g., *gabapentin*, 300 mg at bedtime) represent another alternative; gabapentin was found in controlled trial to be equivalent to ropinirole in efficacy. Neither is associated with augmentation. *Benzodiazepines* and are helpful for occasional use; *clonazepam* is the best studied, but morning sedation can be problematic; shorter-acting *benzodiazepine-receptor agonist* preparations (e.g., *zolpidem*, 5 mg at bedtime) may be better tolerated. Long-term benzodiazepine use can lead to dependency (see Chapter 226) but not to augmentation.

A.H.G.

Annotated Bibliography

1. Allen RP. Controversies and challenges in defining the etiology and pathophysiology of restless leg syndrome. Am J Med 2007;120 (1A):13. (*An excellent discussion of disease mechanisms.*)
2. Earley CJ. Restless leg syndrome. N Engl J Med 2003;348:21. (*An excellent review for the clinician; 38 references.*)
3. Hening W. Current guidelines and standards of practice for restless leg syndrome. Am J Med 2007;120(1A):S22. (*A succinct, authoritative summary and review; source of many of the recommendations in this appendix; 44 references.*)

CHAPTER 233 ■ MANAGEMENT OF OBESITY

CAROLYN CRIMMINS HINTLIAN

Obesity is a major health problem in industrialized societies and has become epidemic in the United States. More than 60% of the U.S. population is *overweight* (body mass index [BMI] 25 to 29.9 kg/m^2), 30% is *obese* (BMI >30 kg/m^2), and more than 4% is *morbidly obese* (BMI >40 kg/m^2). About 20% is on some kind of weight loss program at any given time. The health risk increases when weight gain results in moderate to severe obesity. Mortality rates (all-cause, cardiovascular, and cancer related) closely parallel increases in the BMI once levels of obesity are reached.

Obesity is a chronic disease, and weight loss is not a cure, but a goal. Obesity results from a failure of normal weight and energy regulatory mechanisms. The degree of weight loss necessary to achieve many of its associated health benefits can be surprisingly modest, putting the goal within the reach of most persons. Patient requests for advice and medication are best responded to with a comprehensive assessment (see Chapter 10) and an individualized program that takes into account the patient's overall health status, as well as precipitants, preferences, and lifestyle.

The effective management of obesity starts with a careful workup of the medical and psychosocial dimensions of the problem (see Chapter 10). The assessment of associated cardiovascular risk (see Appendix 26.1) is also important. Treating etiologically and attending to concurrent obesity-related medical conditions (e.g., hypertension, hypercholesterolemia, sleep apnea, diabetes, osteoarthritis) is essential (see Chapters 26, 27, 46, 102, and 157).

The goal is to achieve the best weight possible in the context of overall health. With product and procedure claims constantly bombarding them, patients appreciate an evidence-based approach to weight loss that is tailored to their needs. Knowing the rationale, safety, and effectiveness of available treatment modalities (including popular diets, drug therapies, supplements, herbal preparations, and surgical approaches) is essential to the design of a safe and effective program. In addition, knowledge of available community resources is helpful in guiding patients to additional sources of support, education, and treatment.

PRINCIPLES OF MANAGEMENT

Goals, Strategy, and Patient Selection (1–12)

Goals

Although modest from the patient's perspective, a 5% to 10% reduction in weight is often sufficient to achieve many of the health-related benefits of weight loss (e.g., reduction in blood pressure, cholesterol, glucose intolerance, osteoarthritic complaints). This medically meaningful goal can be used as an initial target while recognizing that the request for help in losing weight may be part of a complex decision to make significant interpersonal, environmental, and lifestyle changes. Treatment goals under such circumstances might include a more profound loss of weight to correct poor self-image and the physical, social, and lifestyle consequences of obesity.

A note of caution is suggested regarding large fluctuations in body weight that might occur in the context of weight loss efforts and their aftermath. Observational data show an association between *marked shifts in weight* and an increase in all-cause mortality. The significance of the finding is debated, with some arguing that the increased mortality risk is due to the presence of multiple health risk factors in very obese persons rather than the degree of weight shift experienced.

Strategy

Because it is a chronic disease driven by a complex set of powerful and often incompletely understood etiologic factors, obesity requires a comprehensive, multidimensional program and continuous effort that includes a lifelong commitment to changes in lifestyle, behavior, and dietary practices. Major barriers to weight loss include inactivity and the ready availability of inexpensive high-carbohydrate, high-fat foods. No single measure or particular approach is effective for all persons; individual responses can be quite idiosyncratic, and there are few predictors of how well a particular measure may work.

Despite the variability in response to specific interventions, a few consensus recommendations emerge from consensus panels regarding overall strategy:

1. For overweight or obese patients not ready to lose weight, the best approach is to educate them about health risks, address other cardiovascular risk factors, and encourage the maintenance of their current weight.
2. For motivated persons who are overweight (BMI 25 to 29.9 kg/m^2) and have two or more obesity-related medical conditions or are frankly obese (BMI >30 kg/m^2), a 6-month goal of a 10% weight loss can be set (1 to 2 lb/wk) and a program of diet, exercise, and behavioral therapy prescribed. If, after 6 months, the target weight is not achieved, one can consider adding pharmacologic therapy for those at greatest risk (BMI >27 kg/m^2 plus two or more cardiovascular risk factors, or BMI >30 kg/m^2).
3. For markedly obese persons at greatest risk (BMI >35 kg/m^2 with two or more obesity-related medical conditions or BMI >40 kg/m^2), consider a surgical approach if serious and repeated attempts using the foregoing measures have been unsuccessful.

Patient Selection

In most instances, self-selection will determine who undergoes a comprehensive weight loss program because major behavioral change is required. Nonetheless, physician input can play an important motivating role in the question of who should be encouraged most to undergo an intensive program of weight reduction.

One suggested approach is to identify overweight and obese persons at greatest health risk, namely those who already manifest evidence of *hyperinsulinism* and the *metabolic syndrome*. Such persons are at particularly high risk for adverse cardiovascular events, but prognosis can be greatly improved through modest weight reduction (on the order of 5% to 10%). The identification of such persons can be performed by checking blood pressure for elevation, fasting lipid profile for a low high-density-lipoprotein (HDL) cholesterol/high triglycerides

pattern, and fasting and random blood sugars for evidence of glucose intolerance if not frank diabetes (e.g., fasting glucose approaching 126 mg/dL and random glucose approaching 200 mg/dL). Other complication-based criteria might include osteoarthritis of weight-bearing joints, marked venous insufficiency, and psychosocial dysfunction. Excess abdominal fat carries elevated health risks. Waist circumference should be used to assess abdominal fat content. A waist circumference of greater than 35 inches raises the cardiovascular risk in women.

Dietary Approaches (8,9,12–27)

"Going on a diet" is the typical first step in weight reduction, but the word "diet" implies that one is making only a temporary change in one's eating habits and patterns. Patients need to understand that the most effective diet is not a diet at all but rather a weight management program that focuses on the implementation of gradual, permanent changes in eating habits and exercise that can be followed for a lifetime. The plethora of available and often contradictory diets heavily promoted for their supposed special advantages are only as good in the long run as their degree of caloric restriction and palatability encouraging adherence. Moreover, durable weight loss and its maintenance also require a program of *regular exercise*. It is better to maintain a moderate loss over the long term than it is to achieve a greater weight loss that cannot be maintained.

Determining Daily Caloric Intake

The desired daily caloric intake needs to be determined. As a rule of thumb, reducing dietary caloric intake by 500 to 1,000 kcal/d can produce a loss of about 1 lb/wk; cutting back by as little as a 100 kcal/d can still lead to a 10-lb loss over the course of a year. More precise estimates of caloric needs and reductions are obtained by estimating the number of calories necessary to maintain an obese person's weight:

- Obese female patient: 8 to 10 calories times the present weight in pounds
- Obese male patient: 10 to 12 calories times the present weight in pounds (the lower number in the range is for the sedentary person)

From this figure, one subtracts 500 kcal/d for every pound per week that should be lost (a deficit of 3,500 calories equals a weight loss of 1 lb). All weight reduction programs should be nutritionally adequate except for calories and should include a variety of foods. Most fad diets are neither nutritionally sound nor based on proven scientific evidence (Table 233.1). Extravagant claims that a particular food or class of foods dramatically alters weight, appetite, or calorigenesis are unfounded. The cornerstones of efficacy and safety are a reduction in calories and nutritional balance. Nutrient content and the timing and number of meals and snacks are important determinants for short-term and long-term appetite control. Limiting fat calories is critical to decreasing body fat and maintaining weight loss.

When following a prescribed dietary regimen, the patient must realize that initial rapid weight loss may occur because of a negative fluid balance. After 2 to 3 weeks, the rate of weight loss slows down. Most subsequent loss reflects the catabolism of fat. Loss of fat is directly proportional to the size and duration of the energy deficit. Patients often become discouraged when they enter the slower phase. Some adjust to caloric restriction by unknowingly diminishing their expenditure of energy, one reason an exercise program is such an important adjunct (see later discussion).

TABLE 233.1

NONCOMMERCIAL, COMMERCIAL, AND CLINICAL WEIGHT LOSS PROGRAMS

Program	Approach/Method	Clients	Staff	Expected Weight Loss/Length of Program	Healthy Lifestyle Component	Comments	Availability/Cost	Headquarters
Registered dietitians in private practice	Dietitians design individual diet program according to client's lifestyle and caloric needs. Individual or group counseling may include sessions on nutrition, food preparation and recipe modification, behavior modification, and exercise.	All ages, men and women.	RD	Varies on an individual basis.	Individual and/or group counseling.	Offers individualized personalized approach to weight loss. To contact a RD in private practice, contact the American Dietetic Association (or the local state dietetic association).	Nationally. Professional organization. Usually hourly rates that vary according to the region, ranging from $85 to $150.	American Dietetic Association, Chicago, IL. http://www.eatright.org
Noncommercial								
Take Off Pounds Sensibly (TOPS)	TOPS is an international nonprofit, noncommercial weight loss support group. Members obtain an exercise and food plan and goal weight from their personal physicians. TOPS provides a supportive environment in which individuals can make slow, steady, permanent lifestyle changes necessary to reach and maintain their personal goals. The program recognizes that each person has different health conditions and weight loss goals; it helps people meet their individual needs through group support. TOPS has programs and addresses issues related to the maintenance of healthy lifestyles. Patients who have achieved their goal are an integral part of helping others in TOPS to do so. TOPS members who have reached and maintained goal weight are called KOPS (Keep Off Pounds Sensibly) and are honored accordingly.	Chapters are run on a local level by members who elect a volunteer leader. Each chapter varies in its approach according to the needs of its members, but all chapters address the complex issues involved in weight loss efforts.	Chapters frequently invite health professionals to speak at their meetings. Chapters are supported by trained field staff. Headquarters provides educational materials and a monthly magazine. A strong incentive plan with awards and recognition are woven into the program at all levels. Activities include special rallies, workshops, and recognition days, as well as low-cost, week-long retreats.	There is no set timetable to reach a goal. When a personally meaningful weight is achieved, the focus changes to maintaining that goal. Members are invited and encouraged to remain a part of TOPS as long as they need the support.	TOPS offers programs and addresses issues related to maintaining healthy lifestyles. People who have achieved their goal are an integral part of helping those in TOPS who are trying to do so.	TOPS is run by a nine-member board of directors. A medical advisor is consulted. Annual membership is $20.00 in the United States, $25.00 in Canada. This includes the monthly magazine. Local chapters charge a small weekly fee, usually no more than $5/mo. For more information about local chapters, call toll-free 1-800-932-8677.	Almost 300,000 members meet weekly in 11,700 meetings in the United States, Canada, and military bases around the world.	Milwaukee, WI. http://www.tops.org
Overeaters Anonymous	Nonprofit international organization that provides volunteer support groups worldwide patterned after a 12-step Alcoholic Anonymous program. Members are encouraged to seek professional help for individualized diet/nutrition plan and for emotional or physical problems.	Individuals who define themselves as compulsive overeaters.	Nonprofessional volunteers, who meet specific criteria, lead meetings, sit on the board, and conduct activities.	Makes no claims for weight loss.	Recommends emotional, spiritual, and physical recovery changes. No exercise or food recommendations.	Inexpensive. Provides group support. No need to follow a specific diet plan to participate. Minimal organization at the group level, so groups vary in approach. No health care providers on staff.	Nine thousand groups in 52 countries.	Rio Rancho, NM. (505) 891-2664. http://www.overeatersanonymous.org

Commercial						
Jenny Craig, Inc.	Hypocaloric diet, exercise, and lifestyle modification. Menu plans range from 1,000 to 2,300 cal, depending on the energy needs of the client. All menus are based on the Food Guide Pyramid. Jenny Craig food purchases are required at first and are gradually eliminated as the client transitions to self-planned menus.	Mostly women (90%) >18 yr of age. An adolescent program is available for ages 13–17 yr (with parental permission).	Program developed by on-staff dietitians and reviewed and approved by a Medical Advisory Board consisting of physicians, psychologists, and an exercise physiologist. All programs are delivered by trained employees who complete 56 hr of prior training. Staff also participates in weekly meetings and monthly continuing education sessions.	Anticipated weight loss is about 1% of body weight or 1–2 lb/wk. The length of the program is determined by the amount of weight that the client wants to lose.	Individual consultations are available. Information is provided on healthful eating, stress management, and building an active lifestyle. Exercise is encouraged to aid in weight loss and maintenance. Behavior modification is part of the overall goal of the program structure.	Vitamin and mineral supplements are available.
					Serves approximately 65,000 clients weekly in 660 U.S. centers (46 states), Canada, Australia, New Zealand, and Puerto Rico. Programs require a one-time enrollment fee plus approximately $72/wk for food, which decreases during the program term as fewer food purchases are made.	1135 N. Torrey Pines Road, La Jolla, CA 92037. (800) 29-JENNY. http://www.jennycraig.com Email: info@jennycraignews.com
The Solution	Family systems approach involving developmental skills for the mind, body, and spirit: nurturing (emotional therapy), limit setting (cognitive therapy), body pride (body image), good health, mastery eating, mastery living. The program encourages 30 min or more of exercise each day. Participants are educated about eating for health. No set calorie limit is recommended.	Mostly women (80%) age ≥19 yr.	The program was developed and written by a master's-level RD with input from health professionals in the fields of dietetics and nutrition, medicine, mental health, exercise, and education. The program delivery team consists of RDs and licensed mental health professionals (psychologist, family therapist, social worker, and psychiatrist). All staff must complete 20 hr of training to become certified to deliver the program. Orientation is to train those who are already certified or licensed professionals. Periodic "tune-up" training is available at annual workshops and meetings.	No more than a 1-lb weight loss per week is recommended. Each session is 12 wk for 2 hr/wk. Participants can elect to continue for more than the 12-wk session.	Counseling sessions are designed for 8–12 clients; the group forms a community, and members provide telephone support to practice methods between sessions. Positive behavior changes are emphasized in the program structure.	In the maintenance program, clients can return for 12-wk sessions any time they desire. Every 3 mo, a Saturday afternoon maintenance session for all program graduates is held.
					One hundred fifty groups meet throughout the United States. For weight loss, $275–$300 for 12 wk, including cost of materials. There is no charge for maintenance.	1623A 5th Ave San Rafael, CA 94901. (415) 457-3331. http://www.thepathway.org

(continued)

TABLE 233.1

NONCOMMERCIAL, COMMERCIAL, AND CLINICAL WEIGHT LOSS PROGRAMS (CONTINUED)

Program	Approach/Method	Clients	Staff	Expected Weight Loss/Length of Program	Healthy Lifestyle Component	Comments	Availability/Cost	Headquarters
Weight Watchers	Hypocaloric diet, exercise, and lifestyle modification. Diets range from 1,225 to 1,745 cal and are individualized for the client's energy needs for weight loss. Commercially sold Weight Watchers foods can be purchased but are optional for program participation.	Mostly women (95%) age ≥10 yr.	The program was developed by RDs and exercise physiologists. Leaders (who are Lifetime Members) deliver the program. Initial training requires 46 hr of classroom instruction.	The length of the program is determined by the individual client. Individuals must enter the maintenance program when BMI reaches 20 kg/m². Expected weight loss is up to 2 lb/wk.	Program includes group counseling sessions (individual counseling in limited areas). Information on both aerobic and resistance training exercise is provided, and exercise is encouraged to aid in weight loss and maintenance. Lifestyle modification is a component of the overall program structure.	Vitamin and mineral supplements are available.	Six hundred thousand clients are served in North America per week. There are 19,000 weekly meetings. For weight loss, there is a one-time registration fee of $16–$20 and a weekly fee of $10–$14. For maintenance, $10–$14/wk for about 6 wk until Life-time Member status is reached. There is no fee for Lifetime Members.	175 Crossways Park West, Woodbury, NY 11797-6001. (800) 651-6000. http://www.weightwatchers.com
Clinical Weight Loss Health Management Resources	Medically supervised program for high-risk or non-medically supervised for moderate-weight-loss patients combines a nutritionally complete diet with intensive lifestyle education. Options include a VLCD under medical supervision (520–800 cal/d) and Healthy Solutions, a weight loss option that includes the use of regular foods (1,000–1,600 cal/d). Both diets include the use of meal replacements. Either option is available with or without adjunctive drug therapy. Mandatory weekly 90-min group classes focus on teaching specific skills for overall health management. Health Risk Appraisal is available for every client. A long-term maintenance program and individual counseling are also available.	Contraindications: pregnancy, lactation, and acute substance abuse. VLCD requires physician's written approval for patients with comorbidities.	Program developed by MDs, RDs, RNs, and psychologists. Each location has at least one MD, RN, and health educator on staff. Participants are assigned "personal coaches" (RDs, exercise physiologists, health educators) who help dieters learn and practice weight management skills. Dieters on VLCD see MD or RN weekly.	Averages 1–5 lb/wk. The reducing phase varies according to weight loss goals but averages 12–20 wk. Maintenance program recommended for up to 18 mo. Most recent published data showed average weight loss of 65 lb (22 wk) in VLCD program. Current Health Solutions average weight loss is 20–25 lb.	Health Risk Appraisals are available for each client. Recommends clients burn a minimum of 2,000 cal/wk in physical activity. Advocates consuming a diet with no more than 30% of calories from fat per week. Decreased decision making about food choices in the weight loss phase improves compliance. All options include meal replacements.	Emphasizes exercise as a means for weight loss and control. Few decisions about what to eat. Supervised by a health professional. Requires a strong commitment to physical activity. Side effects of VLCD include intolerance to cold, constipation, dizziness, dry skin, and headaches. All options include meal replacements; diet is very high in protein, even at lower calorie levels.	More than 200 hospitals and medical settings nationwide.	Boston, MA. (617) 357-9876 or (800) 418-1367. http://www.yourbetterhealth.com

| New Directions | The New Directions system has been treating patients nationally for >10 yr. It offers two program methods: a medically supervised, low-calorie diet, comprising fortified meal replacements of 600 to 800 cal/d, and the Outlook Program, which provides 1,000–1,500 cal/d and includes fortified nutritional bars and beverages, as well as traditional foods. This is for people moderately overweight, 15–40 lb. All operations materials and patient materials are included as part of the program. The goal of the New Directions program is to give complete support (nutrition, behavioral, lifestyle, and educational) to the patient. | Contraindications: individuals <18 yr of age, pregnant and lactating women, and those with conditions such as insulin-dependent diabetes (type 1), metastatic cancer, recent myocardial infarction, liver disease requiring protein restriction, and renal insufficiency. RDs, master's-level behavioral therapists, and exercise physiologist. Outlook Programs are led by health professionals knowledgeable in dietetics, exercise, and behavior. One-on-one interaction is part of each program. Each system is headed by a physician who serves as medical director. | In the Low-Calorie Diet Program, the average weight loss is 3 lb/wk; the Outlook Program weight loss rates vary with the individual. Length of the program participation for the low-calorie program is 12–16 wk in reducing, 5–10 wk in adapting (transition to regular food), and 6–12 mo in sustaining (maintenance). Ongoing participation in each phase is strongly encouraged with each patient. Weekly classes concentrate on problem solving, lifestyle development, nutrition education, and a dieter-friendly light exercise program. | Each program emphasizes individualized care and consistent contact with health professionals. Program support includes a comprehensive treatment approach that is easy for patients to understand and to follow. Patients make few decisions about what to eat, which affords the opportunity to learn and practice effective skills to help make permanent lifestyle changes that translate into long-term success. The Outlook includes regular food with strong emphasis on lifestyle modification. These programs are medically monitored by an MD on a weekly or biweekly basis depending on patient's needs. The medical portion is usually covered by insurance. | The amount of weight necessary to lose, program choice, and medical conditions determine the cost of the program. Cost averages $110–$120/wk. Medical monitoring is about $45–$60 of the fee and is usually covered by insurance. | Robard Corporation, Medical Nutrition Division, Mt. Laurel, NJ. (800) 222-9201. http://www.robard.com |

(continued)

TABLE 233.1

NONCOMMERCIAL, COMMERCIAL, AND CLINICAL WEIGHT LOSS PROGRAMS (CONTINUED)

Program	Approach/Method	Clients	Staff	Expected Weight Loss/Length of Program	Healthy Lifestyle Component	Comments	Availability/Cost	Headquarters
Medifast	Medifast is a physician-supervised, VLCD program of fortified meal replacement containing 450–500 cal/d. Life-styles—the Medifast Program of Patient Support—prepares patients to maintain their goal weight after completing the VLCD. Medifast provides a low-calorie diet of approximately 860 cal/d for those not selected for the VLCD. Medifast also offers Take Shape, a product line that can be used as part of a weight loss or weight maintenance program.	Contraindications: those who are not ≥30% greater than ideal body weight, those who have not reached sexual and physical maturation, pregnant and lactating women, patients with recent cerebrovascular accident, bulimia, unstable angina, insulin-dependent diabetes, thrombophlebitis, active cancer, and uncompensated renal or hepatic disease.	Program supervised by a physician. At the corporate level, a medical advisory board of MDs, PhDs, and RDs is consulted on program and product development.	Physician and patient arrive at individualized goal weight. Metropolitan Life Insurance Company tables, Dietary Guidelines for Americans, and BMI charts are used as guides. Weight loss varies with individual; average weight loss is 3–5 lb/wk. Weight reduction phase lasts 16 wk and realignment lasts 4–6 wk. Maintenance is strongly encouraged for up to 1 yr.	The program includes a comprehensive education program called Life-styles that includes behavior modification, a recommended physical activity program, and nutrition education. Instruction booklets and patient guides are provided, including a quarterly newsletter to patients.	Close contact with one or more health professionals. Low-calorie level promotes rapid weight loss. Extensive product line. Must rely on company products during reducing phase. Maintenance program assists with transition to regular foods. Company products and regular foods are incorporated into the diet when VLCD is not recommended for the client.	Fifteen thousand physicians nationwide, primarily in office-based settings, and in six foreign countries. Costs for office visits, laboratory test, and Medifast products vary by individual physician. Cost is $65–$85/wk. Insurance may cover the cost of lab work and office visits.	Medifast, Inc. 11445 Cronhill Drive, Owings Mills, MD 21117. (410) 581-8042. http://www.medifastdiet.com

BMI, body mass index; RD, registered dietician; RN, registered nurse; VLCD, very low calorie diet.
From Shape Up America, American Obesity Association. Guidance for the treatment of adult obesity. Bethesda, MD: Shape Up America, 1996, with permission.

Dietary Counseling

Dietary counseling is an essential step in the educational process. It begins with the physician's endorsement (an essential component that is often overlooked). Patients need to achieve a basic understanding of the caloric and nutritional contents of foods to be able to choose intelligently. The patient also must be presented with an approach that focuses on the connections relating body, brain, and appetite. Factors that control appetite include food that is emotionally satisfying, management of stress, and exercise that suppresses hunger.

The services of a registered dietitian can be helpful in this regard because such persons are specifically trained in assessing nutritional requirements and counseling food selection and preparation. The dietitian can also review appetite-influencing factors such as exercise and the use of food for emotional satisfaction and stress management. Helping to assess and change attitudes and behaviors toward food and eating are important objectives.

The assessment integrates medical concerns with the patient's individual and family lifestyle, economic status, learning ability, and psychological needs. An individualized weight control plan is constructed to address specific needs and food preferences. Dietary changes must be gradually implemented to ensure lifelong positive eating habits. Nutrition counseling is likely to increase patient adherence to a dietary regimen and improve outcome.

Formal dietary counseling averages a reduction of –1.9 BMI units at 12 months, with a rate of change of –0.1 BMI unit per month during active counseling and a regain of 0.02 BMI units per month during subsequent maintenance. Potential predictors of weight loss include the frequency of meetings, the inclusion of exercise, diabetes, and calorie recommendations. Customizing the weight loss program to the individual needs of the patient and arranging for follow-up are important to sustaining behavioral change.

Self-Help and Commercial Weight Loss Programs

Many commercial and self-help programs are available (see Table 233.1); weight loss books are constant best sellers. Some commercial and self-help programs provide menus and a line of foods or supplements to buy; others include individual or group support. Those that just sell products are of little long-term benefit. Regarding Internet-based diet programs, interventions appear to be more effective when they include interaction with a health professional (e.g., via email) rather than being limited to web sites at which patients access information. Integrated approaches provided over the long term with frequent contacts with the practitioner that include moderate diet modification, an exercise program, and a behavioral approach are more effective, especially for mildly to moderately overweight persons. Noncommercial, community-based self-help group programs offer a low-cost alternative for those who seek the assistance of group support; however, in many instances, little professional guidance is provided. In the best-designed randomized trial of self-help versus a comprehensive commercial program, the commercial program proved superior in an intention-to-treat analysis over a 2-year period, with mean sustained weight loss of 2.9 kg compared to 0.2 kg for self-help. Compliance remains a key determinant of success, and attendance at group meetings is critical to compliance.

Fat Substitutes and Low-Fat Foods

Intensive research and development continues by food companies into substances that taste and satisfy like fat without the calories.

Olestra. This nonabsorbable mixture of sucrose esters (derived from long-chain fatty acids found in edible oils) is used as an energy-free fat substitute in the preparation of fat-free snack foods. When consumed in moderation (e.g., a 1-oz bag of potato chips), olestra is well tolerated, but excess intake is associated with diarrhea and cramping. Fat malabsorption with resultant deficiencies in lipid-soluble vitamins (A, D, E, K) is a potential risk when intake is daily and in larger quantities (potential for use in many foods as a fat substitute). The role of such fat substitutes remains to be defined, but use in a snack food as an occasional treat for the person who craves a bit of the "junk food" taste is probably harmless.

"Low-Fat, Low-Cholesterol" Processed Foods. Such foods have been popular substitutes for foods high in fat, but often they are almost as high in caloric value as the foods they replace by virtue of having a very high sugar or carbohydrate content. Even those food preparations that truly have fewer calories and less fat may provide just as much total fat and caloric intake if eaten in excess—a very common phenomenon, especially with low-fat ice cream, frozen yogurt, and baked goods. The rapid swings in glucose and insulin triggered by high intake of the refined starches and sugars in these products may actually stimulate appetite and increase consumption. Persons consuming diets rich in these foods may experience an undesirable decline in high-density-lipoprotein cholesterol if nonatherogenic essential fatty acids and monounsaturated fats are displaced from the diet by carbohydrate (see Chapter 27).

When patients substitute large quantities of "low-fat, low-cholesterol" snack foods for cholesterol-laden foods, they are likely to derive just as many calories from fat because animal fat is simply replaced in these products by *partially hydrogenated vegetable or tropical oils* (which contain *trans fatty acids* that are just as atherogenic as saturated fat and no lower in calories; see Chapter 27). This realization has led to the development of reduced-calorie snack foods that are low in *trans* fatty acids.

Reduced-Calorie Diets: Low-Carbohydrate versus Low-Fat Diets

Two basic dietary approaches to caloric restriction have emerged: one emphasizes reduction in saturated fat, the other limits carbohydrate.

Low-Fat Diet. The current mainstream dietary approach to weight reduction derives from dietary programs for hypercholesterolemia and lowering of atherosclerotic risk. These programs limit total fat, saturated fat, partially hydrogenated unsaturated fatty acids, and dietary cholesterol. They are based on the observation that saturated fat and partially hydrogenated unsaturated fatty acids are major contributors to the production of low-density-lipoprotein (LDL) cholesterol, with a lesser contribution from dietary cholesterol. Perhaps even more critical than reducing total dietary fat in this program, which is recommended for all adults, is substituting foods that provide polyunsaturated and monounsaturated fats for those rich in saturated and *trans* unsaturated fat (see Chapter 27).

When a reduction in calories ensues from the reduced intake of saturated fat, weight loss can ensue. A low-saturated-fat/reduced-calorie diet combined with an exercise program achieves sustained weight reduction and reduces cardiovascular risk. The program is of proven efficacy and safety.

Low-Carbohydrate Diet. The increased appreciation for the atherogenic and caloric pitfalls of so-called "low-fat" foods and excess carbohydrate intake combined with the difficulty many people have in restricting dietary animal fat has stimulated renewed interest in low-carbohydrate diets. Truly low-carbohydrate diets (total daily carbohydrate intake as low as 20 g/d) have been around for more than 150 years and periodically surge in popularity, triggered by claims of substantial weight loss without the need to limit dietary saturated fat. Such diets (as popularized in lay books by authors such as Dr. Robert Atkins) typically allow unlimited intake of eggs, meat, fish, fowl, and shellfish, considerable amounts of hard cheese, and modest portions of salad vegetables (lettuce, celery, spinach) and low-carbohydrate cooked vegetables (e.g., broccoli, cauliflower, squash). Some allow small additional amounts of carbohydrate (5 to 10 g) as weight loss progresses.

The purported weight loss mechanism (never confirmed) centers on a resultant ketosis from fatty acid metabolism that is believed to suppress appetite, increase energy expenditure, and/or deplete adipose tissue. Of note, only about half of persons actually achieve ketosis, yet considerably more lose weight. The popularity of these diets derives from the rapid early weight loss they induce and the liberal amounts of fat they permit. Within the first 7 to 14 days, glycogen stores quickly deplete, releasing free water. Weight loss quickly follows. After this diuretic phase, weight loss slows markedly.

Data on efficacy and safety in obese persons have been limited but are now beginning to accumulate. Although effective for achieving weight loss over the short term, low-carbohydrate diets are not easy to sustain over time. Even under study conditions, more than 25% of individuals drop out by 6 months, and beyond 6 months there is slight weight gain, suggesting difficulty maintaining very low carbohydrate intake. Changes in lipid profiles include marked reduction in serum triglycerides (as expected from low carbohydrate intake), a modest increase in HDL cholesterol, and little change in LDL cholesterol; glycemic control improves independent of weight loss.

Adverse side effects include constipation (from reduced fiber intake), headache, halitosis, muscle cramps, diarrhea, weakness, and rash. There is a self-limited increase in the blood urea nitrogen. Despite initially favorable effects on metabolic parameters in obese patients, concerns have been expressed by the American Heart Association and the American Dietetic Association about the potential for adverse long-term effects on lipids, insulin, renal function, and blood pressure from low-carbohydrate diets with their high intakes of saturated fat and protein. There are no long-term studies of important weight and metabolic outcomes in key patient populations, such as persons with diabetes, hyperlipidemia, hypertension, or coronary heart disease.

Comparison of the Two Diets. Several randomized, controlled trials are available comparing the two dietary approaches in obese persons. Although short term in duration (no longer than 12 months) and differing in patient populations and intensity of dietary programs, the studies find that low-carbohydrate diets produce significantly greater short-term reductions in weight, serum triglycerides, and glucose intolerance (independent of weight loss) and a significantly greater increase in HDL cholesterol (mean increase, 5 mg/dL). As promising as these results are, long-term studies are needed, particularly in high-risk populations, before low-carbohydrate diets can be confidently recommended for sustained use in the treatment of obesity and overweight. Of particular interest will be low-carbohydrate diets that use healthier sources of fat and protein than the slice of bacon over a fried egg that is often pictured.

Behavior Modification (9,28–32)

Behavior modification programs grew out of studies suggesting that obese persons overeat because they are stimulus bound. Behavioral treatment is directed toward the mildly to moderately obese patient. Operant conditioning techniques appear to be somewhat more effective than aversive ones. Obese patients appear to be especially prone to respond to external cues for eating. The triggering stimuli may be situational, physiologic, or emotional. The aim of the behavioral approach is to substitute an alternative eating behavior that is practical and leads to a decreased caloric intake.

Program Components

Key features of a behavior modification program include the following:

- *Describing the behavior to be controlled (self-monitoring).* Patients are instructed to keep detailed records of all eating behaviors, including specific portion sizes, time and place of eating, stimuli preceding eating that the patient is aware of, and a description of surroundings. Patients are suggested to weigh themselves weekly.
- *Modifying and controlling stimuli.* Food shopping, food preparation, and food storage habits are changed, in addition to visual cues. Meal-replacement and partial-meal-replacement programs have been studied and found to be effective as a form of stimulus control.
- *Controlling the act of eating.* The patient is taught to eat more slowly, not skip meals, take smaller bites, and place utensils on the table between bites.
- *Promptly reinforcing behaviors that delay and control eating.* Patients are advised to eat only in one room (cue elimination), have company while eating (cue supervision), develop methods of making diet food attractive (cue strengthening), arrange for deviations from the diet (problem solving), and arrange for positive feedback if they comply with exercise and diet programs.
- *Cognitive restructuring.* The patient is encouraged to transform negative, self-defeating thoughts into positive, beneficial thoughts that can help toward weight loss success.
- *Motivational approaches.* The patient is educated to focus on setting realistic goals for nutrition, weight, and physical activity.

In addition, distracting activities such as watching television or reading while eating are discouraged. Eating behavior is made to be associated with highly specific stimuli.

Both individual and group behavioral programs are available. The average length of treatment is 18 weeks. The average weight loss is 20 lb, and at 52 weeks of follow-up, almost two thirds of patients maintain that weight loss, a very positive result. Behavior modification may prove to be most helpful in helping people to maintain weight loss regardless of how it was achieved. The data suggest that it may take more behavior change to prevent weight gain after weight loss than to prevent weight gain in those who have never been obese.

Exercise (8,9,31–35)

An exercise or physical fitness component should be included in every weight loss program. Most obese persons are less active than lean people, but it is not known whether this is a cause or consequence of obesity. Energy expenditure and basal metabolic rate decrease with weight loss on calorically restricted diets. Exercise, in conjunction with a low-calorie diet, increases the metabolic rate. Increased physical activity for many obese people can promote weight loss and decrease body fat. Lean body mass is preserved when exercise and diet are combined. Obese persons use more energy and burn more body fat for the same amount of activity than persons of normal weight because the energy cost of most exercise is proportional to body weight. The amount of exercise needed to decrease body fat is related to its duration, intensity, and frequency. Exercise may also benefit the dieter by increasing feelings of self-control, reducing stress, improving appearance, and alleviating depression. Cardiovascular morbidity and mortality may be reduced.

The Exercise Prescription

Regular physical activity appears to be one of the best predictors of successful weight maintenance. A specific exercise prescription is essential. To tell a sedentary obese person to "get more exercise" is insufficient. Moreover, the dropout rate is high. Thirty percent or more of obese patients terminate physical training programs within several weeks of initiation, and as few as one third continue for up to 1 year. In some cases women have been found to not merely neglect to exercise, but to actively resist it. Exercise resistance is a conscious block against becoming physically active. To ensure compliance, the program has to be physically realistic and capable of being incorporated into the patient's daily routine. The importance of physician input and encouragement is considerable.

The intensity, duration, and frequency of exercise are proportional to the degree of weight loss achieved when combined with a dietary program, but even modest amounts of exercise achieve significant increases in weight loss in previously sedentary persons. To ensure safety, obese patients with multiple cardiac risk factors and a sedentary lifestyle may benefit from electrocardiographic stress testing before an exercise program is initiated and a detailed program of graded exercise (see Chapters 18 and 31). A good starting prescription program might entail 30 to 45 minutes of moderate-paced walking, three to five times a week. Smaller bouts of physical activity can also be beneficial—for example, parking farther away, taking the stairs, exercising while watching TV, and taking activity breaks from screens (TV, computer, and other media screens) are also important.

Pharmacologic Treatment (8,9,36–47)

Drug therapy is reserved for use in high-risk persons (BMI >27 kg/m^2 plus two or more obesity-related medical conditions or BMI >30 kg/m^2) who fail to achieve initial weight loss goals after 6 months of concerted effort with diet, exercise, and behavior modification. The weight loss benefits of available agents are modest, and side effects can be substantial, making pharmacologic therapy an adjunctive modality at best, reserved for use in high-risk patients. Such patients are likely to have multiple cardiovascular risk factors, necessitating close monitoring of drug therapy to minimize risk. Chronic administration is necessary for a sustained effect in obesity, given the chronic nature of the underlying condition.

Drug therapy is directed either at appetite suppression or impairment of nutrient absorption. Energy-expending drugs (ephedrine, thyroid hormone) are unsafe for use in the treatment of obesity.

Appetite Suppressants

The currently approved appetite suppressants increase the levels of neurotransmitters (norepinephrine, serotonin, and dopamine) believed to be active in the central nervous system control of appetite. Advances in understanding the mechanism(s) of appetite control promise a host of new, more effective agents, but at present the options are rather limited.

Norepinephrine Drugs. Although effective in suppressing appetite and achieving modest weight reduction, most adrenergic stimulants for appetite suppression have been removed from the market either because of adverse cardiovascular side effects, such as hypertensive crisis, renal failure, cardiac arrhythmias, acute psychotic episodes, stroke, and sudden death (e.g., with *ephedrine* or *phenylpropanolamine*), or because of addiction potential (e.g., *amphetamines*). With the removal of phenylpropanolamine- and ephedrine-containing preparations, there are no over-the-counter adrenergic diet pills available. Only *phentermine* (Ionamin), *diethylpropion* (Tenuate), *benzphetamine* (Didrex), and *phendimetrazine* (Bontril) remain available and only by prescription. Phentermine was a component of the infamous "fen–phen" combination but was never implicated as a cause of valvular dysfunction (see later discussion); it is the best studied and most used of the available adrenergic agents.

Careful prescribing and monitoring are essential. Tachycardia and elevation in blood pressure are common. Dry mouth, constipation, and insomnia may ensue. These agents are contraindicated in persons with hypertension, symptomatic cardiovascular disease, hyperthyroidism, or history of drug abuse. Benzphetamine and phendimetrazine are classified as Drug Enforcement Administration Schedule III agents (abuse potential). Phentermine and diethylpropion are Schedule IV drugs (less abuse potential). Because of these characteristics and adverse effects, adrenergic agents are not very popular.

Serotonin Drugs. A burst of interest in pharmacotherapy followed the publication of early studies in which the extended-release serotonergic agent *fenfluramine* was added to *phentermine* therapy. Fenfluramine increased serotonin release. Combination therapy provided synergy by acting on both adrenergic and serotonergic transmission, allowing lower doses to be used and minimizing side effects. In addition, the *dextro* form of fenfluramine, *dexfenfluramine*, proved useful as monotherapy.

Reports of *pulmonary hypertension* and *heart valve injury* on aortic and mitral valves began to appear in persons taking dexfenfluramine for more than a few months. The purported mechanism involves the adverse effects of serotonin on valvular endothelial metabolism (see Chapter 33). These reports prompted the U.S. Food and Drug Administration (FDA) to withdraw both dexfenfluramine and combination products from the market. The risk appears to be limited to those who took the drug for a minimum of 3 months, rising to as high as 20% among those treated for 18 months or more. With cessation, some improvement occurs and no progression has been found. In most instances, valve incompetence is mild, and patients remain asymptomatic. Whether asymptomatic persons will eventually become symptomatic remains to be determined, but because valve injury appears to be largely mild, the risk of developing symptomatic disease is probably low. Patients who took either of these drugs should be examined clinically for evidence of heart valve dysfunction, first by auscultation and then by cardiac ultrasonography if abnormalities are detected on physical examination.

Other serotonergic agents, such as the *selective serotonin reuptake inhibitor antidepressants*, may offer modest benefit in weight reduction if weight gain is a response to underlying depression (see Chapter 227). However, their use in nondepressed patients has produced little evidence of efficacy. Early anorectic effects appear to wear off after a few months. Tricyclic antidepressants often stimulate appetite and can be counterproductive.

Combination Activity—Sibutramine (Meridia). Structurally resembling amphetamines, sibutramine inhibits the reuptake of both norepinephrine and serotonin, increasing their central nervous system concentrations; there is also a purported effect on dopaminergic transmission. However, there is no observed increase in serotonin release (probably limiting the risk of an adverse effect on heart valves). The drug is rapidly absorbed and reaches its peak effect in 3 to 4 hours; its half-life is about 14 hours, allowing once-daily dosing. A dose-related effect on weight loss has been noted; peak doses are associated with about 12 to 15 lb of weight loss over 6 months; the effect appears to persist for up to 12 months with continued use. The starting dose is 10 mg/d.

The most common side effects are dry mouth, insomnia, headache, and constipation, as well as increase in blood pressure and heart rate. It is recommended that sibutramine not be used in conjunction with other serotonergic agents (e.g., selective serotonin reuptake inhibitors, triptans), lithium, and some analgesics (e.g., meperidine, fentanyl, dextromethorphan, pentazocine). The use of sibutramine within 2 weeks of use of a monoamine oxidase inhibitor is also to be avoided. Sibutramine is classified as a Schedule IV drug by the Drug Enforcement Agency.

Long-term studies of up to 2 years find continued efficacy, with intermittent therapy almost as effective as continuous use. One year of use in obese adolescents has been found to be safe and effective in combination with behavioral change. The cost of sibutramine therapy is high—several dollars per day.

Impairment of Food Absorption—Orlistat (Xenical, Alli). Orlistat, approved by the FDA for use in obesity, binds to and blocks the topical activity of pancreatic and gastric lipases and inhibits about 30% of gut dietary fat absorption. Randomized, double-blinded, placebo-controlled study lasting 2 years demonstrated significant weight loss (up to 10%), a reduction in weight gain, and improvements in lipid profile and insulin levels. However, about 80% of patients experienced some adverse gastrointestinal effects from the ensuing malabsorption and maldigestion that takes place (e.g., abdominal cramping, bloating, oily and greasy stools, diarrhea). Cost is high (several dollars per day). Lipid-soluble vitamin supplementation (especially vitamin D, but also vitamins A and E and β-carotene) may be necessary, taken 2 hours before or after orlistat. Longer-term data from very large samples of patients are not yet available, but 1-year study in obese adolescents found that orlistat in combination with behavioral change was reasonably well tolerated and was more effective than diet and exercise alone. More data are needed to characterize the risks associated with prolonged therapy, as well as the outcomes of cardiovascular events and other pertinent endpoints.

Herbal Therapies and Commercial Supplements. Although considerable claims are made for herbal therapies, there is neither evidence of their efficacy nor requirements for the demonstration of efficacy, safety, uniformity, purity, or labeling. No consistent listing of ingredients or standardization of preparations is available. Use of the Chinese herbal weight loss aids *chaso* and *onshido* has been associated with hepatotoxicity, which is believed to be related to the fact that they contain N-nitrosofenfluramine. Sometimes one herbal preparation is inadvertently substituted for another, resulting in serious consequences (e.g., renal toxicity). Others have been withdrawn from the market only after proving to be dangerous (see later discussion). Concerns about the safety of herbal preparations and "natural" dietary supplements have led to recommendations from scientific groups that these be avoided in the treatment of obesity.

Garcinia cambogia, an herb found in plants native to India, is claimed to lower body weight and reduce fat in humans. It is a source of hydroxycitric acid, which inhibits a citrate cleavage enzyme believed to play a role in lipogenesis. Although extracts of this herb and preparations containing hydroxycitric acid are promoted and sold commercially for weight loss, there is no evidence they are effective. In a rigorous randomized, placebo-controlled study of a concentrated extract of the herb, it failed to produce any significant weight loss or evidence of fat mobilization.

Ma huang (*ephedra*) has long been used in Chinese herbal medicine for the treatment of decongestion and asthma. It contains ephedra alkaloids, including ephedrine, which have potent sympathomimetic activity. Although ephedrine was used by physicians in the United States for asthma in the 1920s, it was abandoned with the advent of safer medications. In recent years, ephedra has made its way back into use as a component of herbal weight loss products and commercial dietary supplements, with the claim of increased energy and appetite suppression. Use became widespread, but reports of serious adverse effects (e.g., stroke and sudden death) began to emerge. Moreover, the frequency of serious adverse events was found to be orders of magnitude greater than that reported for other herbal preparations. These developments prompted the FDA to mandate the removal of all ephedra-containing products from the market.

Treatment of Morbid Obesity and Refractory Cases—Bariatric Surgery and Other Methods (9,48–58)

Very Low Calorie Diets

Very low calorie diets are sometimes considered for use in morbidly obese persons who require major weight loss. These diets, which must be administered in medical settings, severely limit calories to between 400 and 800 per day. They consist of 1.5 g of protein/kilogram of ideal body weight per day in the form of lean meat, fish, or fowl; noncaloric beverages; a multivitamin and mineral supplement containing folic acid; 1,500 mL of fluid per day; 25 mEq of potassium; and a calcium supplement. They achieve the more rapid and sustained rate of weight reduction associated with complete starvation while avoiding its inherent risks. Candidates should be at least 30% to 40% greater than their ideal weight and deemed sufficiently cardiovascularly fit to undergo such treatment, which has an arrhythmogenic potential. Goals include an optimal nitrogen balance and sparing of muscle tissue. Patients can achieve a weight loss of more than 75% fat and a concomitant decrease in waist-to-hip and waist-to-thigh ratios. The average weight loss over the 12 weeks that such a program lasts is 45 lb in fasting periods. The results achieved in combination with behavior modification appear to be promising.

The very low calorie diet is not recommended for persons who are moderately overweight or for children, adolescents, pregnant or lactating women, or the elderly. It should be avoided by patients with cardiovascular disease, essential hypertension, insulin-dependent diabetes mellitus, severe renal or hepatic impairment, active cancer, or a severe psychological disturbance. High dropout rates and poor long-term maintenance are discouraging aspects of this form of treatment.

Bariatric Surgical Treatment

Surgical intervention should be considered only after a comprehensive and sustained program of diet and exercise with or without pharmacologic measures has been unsuccessful over time and the health risks of continued obesity, particularly if morbid, outweigh the risks of surgical intervention. Surgical approaches offer an opportunity for greater and more sustained weight loss in persons with morbid obesity than any other treatment option. They range from purely restrictive gastric procedures to those that include bypass. The restrictive procedures induce a feeling of early satiety; food absorption is normal. Bypasses create some degree of nutrient malabsorption.

Candidacy. Surgical treatment had traditionally been limited to persons with *morbid obesity* (body weight >45 kg or 200% of desirable weight as defined by the Metropolitan Life Insurance Company tables; see Chapter 10), but candidacy has been extended to those with a *BMI greater than or equal to 40 kg/m²* or a *BMI greater than or equal to 35 kg/m² plus two medical complications of obesity*. With the advent of less invasive laparoscopic techniques with low perioperative risk, surgery is increasingly being offered to persons with lesser degrees of obesity (BMI 30 to 35 kg/m²).

Other criteria for patient selection include failure to achieve sustained weight reduction through extensive and repeated attempts at nonsurgical approaches, the absence of underlying endocrine disease, and psychological fitness (e.g., having an understanding of the operation and the behavioral changes needed). Contraindications range from serious concomitant medical illness (e.g., cardiopulmonary or hepatic problems precluding general anesthesia) to psychiatric disease (particularly substance or drug abuse and eating disorders such as bulimia) and plans for pregnancy. The risk increases with age. Operative mortality rates are lowest in centers with high volumes of bariatric surgery; perioperative rates are in the range of 1% to 2% for persons younger than the age of 65 years and 4% to 5% for those older than the age of 65 years. Selection should be limited to highly motivated, morbidly obese patients free of other serious medical and psychosocial problems. Adequate financial support should be available because of the frequent need for repeated hospitalizations.

Surgical Options and Choice of Procedure. Surgical options are rapidly evolving, with laparoscopic procedures being increasingly performed. Each approach has particular advantages, risks, and disadvantages (Table 233.2), necessitating a careful matching of procedure and patient. In general, laparoscopic banding procedures produce the least perioperative morbidity and mortality and offer a reasonable chance of moderate weight loss; bypass procedures achieve the greatest degree of long-term weight loss but entail much more perioperative risk. Gastric bypass appears to be more effective in promoting weight loss and long-term weight maintenance than other surgical procedures (35% reduction in weight, 70% of excess weight); 50% of excess weight is lost in the first 12 months. Long-term success rates at 5 years (BMI remaining <25 mg/kg²) have approached 90% in study settings, but under non-study conditions some regaining of weight over the subsequent 3 to 5 years takes place. A possible mechanism for the very high success rates achieved is the reduction in levels of the appetite-stimulating hormone *gherkin* seen with gastric bypass surgery but not with diet-induced weight loss.

Benefits include significant improvement if not complete resolution of glucose intolerance, hypertension, obstructive sleep apnea, and dyslipidemia. Even after 10 years of follow-up, most

---

TABLE 233.2

SURGICAL TREATMENTS FOR OBESITY

Procedure	Mechanism	Advantages	Disadvantages
Laparoscopic adjustable band	Restrictive	No anastomosis; low operative risk	Inferior weight loss Inappropriate requests for adjustment Long-term band complications
Vertical banded gastroplasty	Restrictive	No anastomosis; low operative risk	Stomal complications Frequent GERD symptoms Frequent revisions needed Inferior weight loss
RYGB	Restrictive Maldigestive	Sustained weight loss Antireflux anatomy Dumping symptoms discourage eating	Anastomosis required Dumping syndrome Obstruction, stomal problems
Duodenal switch	Restrictive/ Malabsorptive	Avoids dumping, improved wt. loss Improved reduction in comorbidities	Nutritional sequelae Technically difficult
Biliopancreatic diversion	Malabsorptive	Improved weight loss	Metabolic/nutritional sequelae Stomal ulceration Dumping syndrome, diarrhea
Very long-limb RYGB	Restrictive/ Malabsorptive	Improved weight loss in extreme cases (BMI >50 kg/m²)	Metabolic sequelae Dumping syndrome, diarrhea Stomal complications

BMI, body mass index; GERD, gastroesophageal reflux disease. RYGB; Roux-en-Y gastric bypass.
Adapted from Kendrik ML, Dakin DF. Surgical approaches to obesity. Mayo Clin Proc 2006;81(10 Suppl):S18.

improvements persist, with an average sustained weight loss of 16%.

Psychosocial benefits depend on the degree of weight loss and are independent of side effects and complications. Patients who lose significant amounts of weight become more employable and more physically active, show improvement in their sex life and self-esteem, and acquire a more gregarious outlook on life.

The risks and side effects of this procedure are substantial and require serious consideration. There is a 10% to 15% perioperative morbidity risk (e.g., deep vein thrombophlebitis, pulmonary embolization, leaks about the anastomosis, wound infection); the perioperative death rate is 0.5% to 1% at experienced centers and greater at others. After surgery, patients must be instructed to eat small amounts, eat slowly, chew carefully, avoid eating when not hungry, and take no liquids with meals. Late complications include outlet obstruction, vitamin deficiencies (thiamine, vitamin B_{12}, and foliate), partial temporary hair loss that is believed to be a result of inadequate protein intake, and an increased incidence of gallstones and gastric ulcers.

Surgical candidacy and choice of procedure are determined in conjunction with the consulting surgeon, taking into account local surgical morbidity and mortality rates, the amount of weight loss desired, the underlying medical and psychological states of the patient, and the risks for short- and long-term complications.

Suction Lumpectomy (Liposuction)

This very popular cosmetic procedure for the removal of localized fat accumulations has produced variable results. It is initiated with a subcutaneous infusion of normal saline solution mixed with 1,000 mg of lidocaine and 1 mg of epinephrine per liter to provide local anesthesia and control of bleeding. Subcutaneous fat is then removed by suction. Several liters of infuscate may be needed to remove 1 to 2 L of fat. Cosmetic success depends on the elastic properties of the overlying skin. The best candidates are persons in good physical condition who are within 30% of ideal weight but have focal areas of lipodystrophy resistant to diet and exercise. Commonly treated sites include thighs, legs, abdomen, upper arms and axillae, breasts, flanks, and back. The procedure is not effective for the treatment of peau d'orange skin changes ("cellulite"). Ultrasonic and superficial techniques have been used in attempts to improve poor skin tone.

The limited outcomes data reveal considerable psychological satisfaction, but unlike other weight loss efforts, there is no improvement in the metabolic derangements associated with obesity. Temporary loss of skin sensation, a wavy contour, and blood loss are commonly experienced. Other adverse effects include infection, extensive bruising for 2 to 3 weeks, and edema for 3 to 6 weeks. Well-documented reports of fatalities caused by lidocaine toxicity, drug–drug interactions, and venous thrombosis of the lower extremities have been published. Careful patient selection and full disclosure of the risks involved are required to help patients choose wisely.

PATIENT EDUCATION

Motivation and patient education are key factors for successful weight control. Realistic goals and expectations are critical, as is the physician's support and encouragement. The patient must be willing to alter exercise and eating patterns permanently. A number of persons will be interested in commercial or nonprofit programs and appreciate reliable information regarding their effectiveness, safety, and appropriateness (see Table 233.1). Although rapid-weight-loss programs are popular, patients need to be informed about their inadequacies for achieving long-term weight loss. Major obstacles to success need to be explored and addressed, including poor self-image, erratic eating patterns, inadequate exercise, loneliness, boredom, anger, and depression. If drug therapy is used, expectations should be realistic. Reduction to average body weight is not a realistic goal. As noted earlier, knowledge must be provided about the basic principles of nutrition, such as the caloric value of foods and practical methods for changing eating habits. Patients must take responsibility for deeply ingrained behaviors and habits, as well as for changing their environment.

Behavioral techniques are also very helpful and should include several types of action:

- Recording food intake.
- Mindful eating—becoming aware of what is going on while eating; thinking about the reason for eating these particular foods; focusing in on choice; becoming aware of how the choices made about meals and foods are nutritious or detrimental to health.
- Eating in only one place; using a smaller plate; not engaging in another activity while eating; keeping food otherwise out of sight.
- Planning meals by shopping from a list; having low-calorie foods available; taking a brown-bag lunch; having a strategy before dining out; at parties, positioning oneself away from the food table.
- Noticing if eating for emotional reasons—changing thoughts and attitudes about food, appetite, and hunger.
- Substituting an alternate activity for eating.
- Increasing physical activity.
- Implementing daily stress management techniques—meditation, relaxation techniques, yoga.

INDICATIONS FOR REFERRAL

Although the interest, involvement, and encouragement of the primary physician are critical, the implementation of a comprehensive and personalized weight loss program is often best achieved with a multidisciplinary approach. Referral to a registered dietitian is enormously helpful in providing the patient with essential nutritional information and initiating a behavioral program for the alteration of eating habits. Familiarity with community and commercial resources and their level of professional supervision is helpful when a patient requests a group approach. Before an exercise program is begun, it may be useful to refer the poorly conditioned, markedly obese patient for an electrocardiographic stress test (see Chapter 18). When emotional problems are too great for the primary physician and registered dietitian to handle, psychiatric referral should be considered. Surgical consultation should be considered only when the patient is so morbidly obese and so refractory to medical therapy that the risks associated with the surgery are less than those of remaining morbidly obese.

MANAGEMENT RECOMMENDATIONS (8,9,59,60)

- Identify and treat specifically any etiologic factors (see Chapter 10).

- Prescribe a comprehensive approach to weight management that includes a low-fat diet, dietary counseling, behavior modification, and an exercise program (see Chapter 18).
- Avoid and discourage food programs, supplements, and appetite suppressants not proven to be safe and effective. Check any patients who have been prescribed fenfluramine or dexfenfluramine in the past for evidence of valvular cardiac injury by auscultation (and cardiac ultrasonography if valvular injury is suspected by examination).
- Individualize changes in eating and exercise patterns; make them gradual to maximize the potential for long-term compliance.
- Recommend a weight loss group to those who seek the benefit of group support; suggest one that is under professional supervision. Commercial programs that include a group program and professional supervision can be beneficial, but not those that offer only food products or supplements.
- Advise a dietitian-supervised weight management program for patients who continually go from one fad diet to another.

- Warn against diets based on unsubstantiated medical claims, which may have popular appeal but are ineffective for long-term weight control.
- Restrict the use of very low calorie diets to patients more than 30% to 40% greater than their ideal weight; require medical supervision.
- Advise patients considering or seeking information on a low-carbohydrate (e.g., Atkins) diet that available data are insufficient to draw conclusions about safety and efficacy, especially with regard to sustained use. Although short-term weight loss can be impressive, long-term weight loss is hard to sustain, and potentially adverse effects on cardiovascular risk factors remain a concern.
- Consider pharmacologic intervention only for persons at very high risk for cardiovascular, metabolic, or orthopedic morbidity.
- Consider referral for surgical therapy for only those patients with life-threatening obesity who have failed all other measures.

Annotated Bibliography

1. Adams KF, Catkin A, Harris TB, et al. Overweight, obesity, and mortality in a large prospective cohort of persons 50 to 70 years old. N Engl J Med 2006;355:763. (*Presents major epidemiologic data, extending the data on the risk of excess weight to include persons who are overweight but not obese.*)
2. Blackburn G. Effect of degree of weight loss on health benefits. Obes Res 1995;3:11S. (*Finds that most health benefits are achievable with a loss of just 5% to 10% of baseline weight.*)
3. Blair SN, Shaken J, Brownell K, et al. Body-weight change, all-cause mortality, and cause-specific mortality in the multiple risk factor intervention trial. Ann Intern Med 1993;119(Part 2):702. (*A comprehensive program achieved reductions in morbidity and mortality and helped to maintain weight loss.*)
4. Headily AA, Ogden CL, Johnson C, et al. Prevalence of overweight and obesity among US children, adolescents, and adults, 1999–2002. JAMA 2004;291:2847. (*Documents the epidemic nature of the problem.*)
5. Foster GD, Warden TA, Vogt, R.A, et al. What is reasonable weight loss? Patients' expectations and evaluation of obesity treatment outcomes. J Consult Clin Psychol 1997;65:79. (*Patients' expectations are often much greater than a realistic initial goal of 10% reduction in body weight.*)
6. Katzmarzyk PT, Janssen I, Ardern CI. Physical inactivity, excess adiposity, and premature mortality. Obes Rev 2003;4:257. (*A summary of the evidence linking obesity with increased risk of death.*)
7. Kushner RF, Blatner DJ. Risk assessment of the overweight and obese patient. J Am Diet Assoc 2005;105:S53. (*Presents comprehensive assessment tools for evaluating the obese patient.*)
8. McTigue KM, Harris R, Hemphil, B., et al. Clinical guidelines. Screening and interventions for obesity in adults: summary of the evidence for the U.S. Preventive Services Task Force. Ann Intern Med 2003;139:933. (*An extensive review of the evidence; 180 references.*)
9. National Institutes of Health, National Heart, Lung, and Blood Institute. NHLBI Education Initiative. The practical guide: Identification, evaluation, and treatment of overweight and obesity in adults. 2000 (NIH Publication No.00-4084). Available at: http://www.nhlbi.nih.gov/guidelines/obesity/prctgd_c.pdf. (*Specific guidelines and useful tools for patient education.*)
10. Reaven GM. Importance of identifying the overweight person who will benefit the most by losing weight. Ann Intern Med 2003;138:420. (*Suggests that the best candidates are those with the metabolic syndrome.*)
11. U.S. Preventive Services Task Force. Clinical guidelines. Screening for obesity in adults: recommendations and rationale. Ann Intern Med 2003;139:930. (*Although the focus is on screening, the guidelines include recommendations for treatment.*)
12. Willet WC, Dietz WH, Colditz GA. Primary care: guidelines for healthy weight. N Engl J Med 1999;341:427. (*An excellent review article on body weight.*)
13. Bravata DM, Sanders L, Huang J, et al. Efficacy and safety of low-carbohydrate diets: A systematic review. JAMA 2003;289:1837. (*Finds no evidence that weight loss was related to the degree of carbohydrate restriction and insufficient data to decide for or against the use of these diets for sustained weight loss.*)
14. Dansinger ML, Gleason JA, Griffith JL, et al. Comparison of the Atkins, Ornish, Weight Watchers, and Zone diets for weight loss and heart disease

reduction. JAMA 2005;293:43. (*Benefit was related to adherence, not to the particular type of diet.*)
15. Dansinger ML, Tatsioni A, Wong JB, et al. Meta-analysis: the effect of dietary counseling for weight loss. Ann Intern Med 2007;147:41. (*Pooled data showed a moderate benefit but a falloff in results with the cessation of the counseling program.*)
16. Foster GD, Wyatt HR, Hill JO, et al. A randomized trial of a low-carbohydrate diet for obesity. N Engl J Med 2003;348:2082. (*A randomized, controlled trial [RCT], finding that individuals on the low-carbohydrate diet lost more weight at 3 and 6 months but that the difference was not significant at 1 year.*)
17. Heshka S, Anderson JW, Atkinson RL, et al. Weight loss with self-help compared with a structured commercial program: a randomized trial. JAMA 2003;289:1972. (*Presents the best available comparative data, showing that the commercial program was modestly better.*)
18. Heymsfield SB, Harp JB, Reitman JW, et al. Why do obese patients not lose more weight when treated with low-calorie diets? A mechanistic perspective. Am J Clin Nutr 2007;85:346. (*A well-designed study, failing to show evidence of efficacy.*)
19. Howard BV, Manson JE, Stefanick ML, et al. Low-fat dietary pattern and weight change over 7 years: the Women's Health Initiative Dietary Modification Trial. JAMA 2006;295:39. (*No weight gain was noted with this isocaloric diet, indicating that calories and not carbohydrate composition matters.*)
20. Freedman MR, King J, Kennedy E. Popular diets: a scientific review. Obes Res 2001;9(Suppl 1):1S. (*Presents evidence that a balanced diet was best.*)
21. Nonas C. A model for chronic care of obesity through dietary treatment. J Am Diet Assoc 1998;98(Suppl 2):S16. (*Outlines an effective dietary approach to the clinical management of the obese patient.*)
22. Samaha FF, Iqbal N, Seshadri P, et al. A low-carbohydrate as compared with a low-fat diet in severe obesity. N Engl J Med 2003;348:2074. (*RCT, finding a mean short-term loss of 5.8 kg, compared to 1.9 kg for the conventional diet, and improvements in triglycerides and insulin sensitivity but high rates of drop-out and loss to follow-up.*)
23. Schoeller DA, Buchholz AC. Energetics of obesity and weight control: does diet composition matter? J Am Diet Assoc 2005;105 (5):S24. (*A literature review, providing no support for the advantage of low-carbohydrate or high-protein diets.*)
24. St Joer ST, Howard BV, Prewitt TE. AHA science advisory. Dietary protein and weight reduction. Circulation 2001;104:1869. (*An excellent analysis of the effects of high-protein diets on health, and not recommending them.*)
25. Stern L, Iqbal N, Seshadri P, et al. The effects of low-carbohydrate versus conventional weight loss diets in severely obese adults: one-year follow-up of a randomized trial. Ann Intern Med 2004;140:778. (*At 1 year, weight loss levels were similar, but glycemic control and lipid profile were more favorable in the low-carbohydrate group.*)
26. Tsai AG, Wadden TA. Systematic review: an evaluation of major commercial weight loss programs in the United States. Ann Intern Med 2005:142:56. (*Scientific evidence documenting long-term success of commercial or self-help programs is limited.*)

27. Yancy WS, Olsen MK, Guyton JR, et al. A low-carbohydrate, ketogenic diet versus a low-fat diet to treat obesity and hyperlipidemia: a randomized, controlled trial. Ann Intern Med 2004;140:769. (*Better retention and greater weight loss were found with the low-carbohydrate diet, as well as a greater reduction in triglycerides and an increase in high-density-lipoprotein cholesterol; the diets were isocaloric.*)

28. Berkel LA, Poston WS, Reeves RS, et al. Behavioral interventions for obesity. J Am Diet Assoc 2005;105:S35. (*Presents the use of less traditional methods of behavior modification, such as Internet interventions, meal replacements, and telephone interventions.*)

29. Foreyt JP, Goodrick GK. Evidence for success of behavioral modification in weight loss and control. Ann Intern Med 1993;119(Part 2):698. (*The average weight loss was close to 20 lb, and two thirds of patients retained the loss at 1 year.*)

30. Hill JO, Thompson H, Wyatt H. Weight maintenance: What's missing? J Am Diet Assoc 2005;105:S63. (*An outline of strategies for goals in the maintenance of weight loss.*)

31. McGuire MT, Wing RR, Klem ML, et al. Behavioral strategies of individuals who have maintained long-term weight losses. Obes Res 1999;7:334. (*One ingredient was a continued exercise program.*)

32. Wing RR, Tate DF, Gorin AA, et al. A self-regulation program for maintenance of weight loss. N Engl J Med 2006;355:1563. (*RCT, finding that a program of daily weighing and face-to-face encounters proved best.*)

33. Dunn AL, Marcus BH, Kampert JB, et al. Comparison of lifestyle and structured interventions to increase physical activity and cardiorespiratory fitness: A randomized trial. JAMA 1999;281:327. (*Confirms the effectiveness of changes in daily lifestyle.*)

34. Jakicic JM, Marcus BH, Gallaher KI. Effect of exercise duration and intensity on weight loss in overweight sedentary women: a randomized trial. JAMA 2003;290:1323. (*Long-term weight loss increased with an increase in exercise, but even modest exercise achieved significant weight loss when combined with diet.*)

35. Wadden TA, Berkowitz RI, Womble LG, et al. Randomized trial of lifestyle, medication and pharmacotherapy for obesity. N Engl J Med 2005;353:2111. (*Finds that combination therapy was better than either alone.*)

36. Abenhaim L, Moride Y, Brenot F, et al. Appetite-suppressant drugs and the risk of primary pulmonary hypertension. N Engl J Med 1996;335:609. (*Risk with the use of fenfluramine.*)

37. Bent S, Tiedt TN, Odden MC, et al. The relative safety of ephedra compared with other herbal products. Ann Intern Med 2003;138:468. (*The relative risk of adverse effects was greater by more than 100-fold.*)

38. Berkowitz RI, Fujioka K, Daniels SR, et al. Effects of sibutramine treatment in obese adolescents: a randomized trial. Ann Intern Med 2006;45:81. (*One year of treatment in conjunction with behavioral change was more effective than behavioral change alone.*)

39. Chanoine J-P, Hampl S, Jensen C, et al. Effect of orlistat on weight and body composition in obese adolescents: a randomized controlled trial. JAMA 2005;293:2873 (*A 1-year trial, finding that the treatment was beneficial when used in conjunction with a program of diet and exercise.*)

40. Davidson MH, Hauptman J, DiGirolamo M, et al. Weight control and risk factor reduction in obese subjects treated for 2 years with orlistat. JAMA 1999;281:235. (*RCT, finding significant weight loss, reduction in weight gain, and improvement in lipid profile and insulin levels.*)

41. Devereux RB. Appetite suppressants and valvular heart disease. N Engl J Med 1998;339:765. (*A summary of the evidence and recommendations regarding cardiac complications and the need for the evaluation of fenfluramine users.*)

42. Dwyer JT, Allison DB, Coates PM. Dietary supplements in weight reduction. J Am Diet Assoc 2005;105:S80. (*An excellent overview of evidence on the role of dietary supplements in weight reduction.*)

43. Moyers SB. Medications as adjunct therapy for weight loss: Approved and off-label agents in use. J Am Diet Assoc 2005;105:948. (*Update on U.S. Food and Drug Administration–approved medications for weight loss and medications used off-label for weight loss.*)

44. Wirth A, Krause J. Long-term weight loss with sibutramine: a randomized controlled trial. JAMA 2001;286:1331. (*Presents evidence of continued efficacy, even when used intermittently.*)

45. Heymsfield SB, Allison DB, Vasselli JR, et al. *Garcinia cambogia* (hydroxycitric acid) as a potential antiobesity agent: a randomized controlled trial. JAMA 1998;280. (*A well-designed study, failing to show evidence of efficacy.*)

46. Saper RB, Eisenberg DM, Phillips RS. Common dietary supplements for weight loss. Am Family Physician 2004;70:1731. (*An extremely useful guide to common over-the-counter dietary supplements, giving information on supplements to recommend, caution against, or discourage use for weight loss.*)

47. Shekelle PG, Hardy ML, Morton SC, et al. Efficacy and safety of ephedra and ephedrine for weight loss and athletic performance: a meta-analysis. JAMA 2003;289:1537. (*Presents evidence of increased risk to health.*)

48. Brolin RE. Bariatric surgery and long-term control of morbid obesity. JAMA 2002;288:2793. (*A succinct but very useful review for the general reader; well illustrated.*)

49. Buchwald H, Avidor Y, Braunwald E, et al. Bariatric surgery: a systematic review and meta-analysis. JAMA 2004;292:1724. (*Finds a complete resolution of diabetes, hypertension, sleep apnea, and hyperlipidemia in a majority of patients.*)

50. Flum DR, Salem L, Elrod JA. Early mortality among Medicare beneficiaries undergoing bariatric surgical procedure. JAMA 2005;294:1903. (*Documents the risk in older patients.*)

51. Kendrick ML, Dakin GF. Surgical approaches to obesity. Mayo Clin Proc 2006;81(10 Suppl):S18. (*A good summary of the details of each particular operative approach to bariatric surgery.*)

52. Klein S, Fontana L, Young VL, et al. Absence of an effect of liposuction on insulin action and risk factors for coronary heart disease. N Engl J Med 2004;350:2549. (*Finds no benefit from this procedure.*)

53. Livington EH, Martin RF. Bariatric surgery. Surg Clin North Am 2005;85:665. (*Updated review of the comorbidities and complications after weight loss surgery.*)

54. Matarasso A, Hutchinson O. Liposuction. JAMA 2001;285:266. (*A comprehensive review; 28 references.*)

55. National Task Force on the Prevention and Treatment of Obesity. Very-low-calorie diets. JAMA 1993;270:967. (*Finds that these diets were effective and safe for short-term use under close medical supervision, and discusses means of improving outcome; 124 references.*)

56. O'Brien PE, Dixon JB, Laurie C, et al. Treatment of mild to moderate obesity with laparoscopic adjustable gastric banding or an intensive medical program. Ann Intern Med 2006;144:625. (*RCT, finding that surgery was better than medical therapy in this group with a body mass index of 30 to 35.*)

57. Rao RB, Ely SF, Hoffman RS. Deaths related to liposuction. N Engl J Med 1999;341:913. (*Based on the files of the New York State medical examiner, finding lidocaine-related adverse effects and thrombosis.*)

58. Sjostrom L, Kindroos AK, Peltonen M, et al. Lifestyle, diabetes, and cardiovascular risk factors 10 years after bariatric surgery. N Engl J Med 2004;351:2683. (*Presents long-term data from a controlled trial, showing durable improvement in most parameters.*)

59. American Dietetic Association. Adult weight management evidence-based nutrition practice guideline. ADA Evidence Analysis Library, 2007. (*A comprehensive guideline, providing the most current information on adult overweight and obesity.*)

60. National Heart Lung and Blood Institute. Guidelines on overweight and obesity: electronic textbook. Available at: http://www.nhlbi.nih.gov/guidelines/obesity/e_txtbk/index.htm. (*An electronic textbook, providing easy access to clinical guidelines.*)

CHAPTER 234 ■ APPROACH TO EATING DISORDERS

NANCY A. RIGOTTI

Anorexia nervosa, bulimia nervosa (the binge–purge syndrome), and binge-eating disorder are the principal eating disturbances of adolescents and adults. Both anorexia and bulimia are considerably more common in women and usually develop during adolescence or early adulthood. About 40% of cases of binge-eating disorder occur among boys and men. The prevalence of anorexia is approximately 1 in 200 among female adolescents and young adults in Western countries, whereas bulimia occurs in approximately 3% of women. These illnesses are psychiatric disorders that can have serious medical consequences. They extend beyond racial and socioeconomic boundaries. Because patients with these conditions often hide their problem, a high index of suspicion is required for diagnosis. Primary care physicians need to be able to recognize these disorders, evaluate and treat their medical complications, arrange and coordinate a comprehensive multidisciplinary treatment program, assist in ambulatory monitoring, and determine when a patient requires hospitalization.

PATHOPHYSIOLOGY, CLINICAL PRESENTATION, AND COURSE (1–11)

Anorexia Nervosa

Anorexia nervosa is a syndrome characterized by severe weight loss (*body weight <85% of expected* or *body mass index <17.5 kg/m²*) resulting from inadequate food intake by persons with no medical reason to lose weight. A *distorted body image* and an *intense fear of weight gain* lead to the relentless pursuit of an unreasonable and unhealthy thinness. Weight is lost in two ways. Patients with restrictive anorexia nervosa *starve* themselves. In contrast, other patients have symptoms of bulimia and lose weight by *purging* after eating, usually by vomiting or taking laxatives. Those with bulimic symptoms have a graver prognosis and more medical problems. Originally more prevalent among persons of high socioeconomic status, anorexia is now becoming more evenly distributed among socioeconomic groups.

Pathogenesis

The precise pathogenesis of anorexia is unknown but appears to be multifactorial. Neurochemical, psychological, and sociocultural factors have all been suggested as contributing factors. Neuroendocrine abnormalities are well documented (see later discussion) but these are the consequence, not the cause, of the starvation. Onset frequently coincides with a time of separation from home or the loss of a loved one. Others attribute anorexia to problems in emotional development and disturbed family interactions. Psychological studies find these patients to be bright, compulsive perfectionists who perform well at school and work. The prevalences of depression and obsessive–compulsive disorder are increased among patients with anorexia. Sociocultural pressure to be thin also contributes to the problem.

Pathophysiology

Restrictive anorexia nervosa is similar to *starvation* and can be fatal. Diets are deficient in carbohydrates and total calories, but protein and vitamin intake is relatively preserved. Consequently, vitamin deficiencies are unusual. However, inadequate nutrient intake results in a profound loss of weight, fat, and muscle mass, followed by cardiac, metabolic and endocrine, hematologic, and gastrointestinal disturbances.

Cardiac Consequences. Cardiac muscle atrophy is associated with a reduction in left ventricular wall thickness and cardiac output, but congestive failure does not occur. Sinus bradycardia is common. Electrocardiographic changes, primarily low-voltage ST-segment depression, T-wave flattening, and prolonged QT intervals, have been reported. Sudden death, which occurs in anorexia nervosa, is presumably due to ventricular arrhythmias. QT-interval prolongation, which is reversible with refeeding, may herald increased the risk of this outcome. Autopsies of some patients performed after sudden death have shown a degeneration of myocardial cells, which may predispose to arrhythmias.

Endocrine and Metabolic Consequences. Extreme weight loss produces a number of adverse endocrine and metabolic changes. Thyroid hormone metabolism is altered, with thyroxine preferentially converted to the inactive reverse 3,5,3′-triiodothyronine (T3) instead of active T3. A compensatory rise in thyrotropin (thyroid-stimulating hormone [TSH]) does not occur because the hypothalamic–pituitary response is blunted ("*sick thyroid*" syndrome). Clinical features of hypothyroidism (see Chapter 104) may ensue. Starvation also produces reversible hypothalamic–pituitary dysfunction that can lead to *hypothalamic amenorrhea* and *estrogen deficiency* (see Chapter 112). Besides weight loss, other factors yet to be identified may contribute to hypothalamic dysfunction because menstruation ceases in up to 25% of female patients with anorexia before weight loss becomes significant, and *amenorrhea* may persist after weight is regained.

Posterior pituitary function is also disrupted; a decline in vasopressin secretion leads to *central diabetes insipidus* and polyuria (see Chapter 102). In anorexia, the hypothalamus defends core temperature poorly in the face of changes in environmental temperature, so that *hypothermia* results. Many people with anorexia have *elevated plasma cortisol* levels that do not respond to an overnight dexamethasone-suppression test. However, cortisol excess is not manifested clinically, perhaps because fatty or carbohydrate substrates are lacking.

Acquired defects in lipoprotein metabolism may increase serum *cholesterol* and *carotene* levels. Blood levels of glucose, protein, amino acids, and insulin are normal or mildly reduced. Severe hypoglycemia and coma have been reported when starvation is very advanced.

Skeletal Consequences. *Osteopenia* and *osteoporosis* occur and predispose to fractures, even vertebral compression fractures in severe cases. The extent of bone loss correlates best with the degree of weight loss, although other factors, such as estrogen deficiency, cortisol excess, and poor calcium intake, may also contribute. Reversal of bone loss is most strongly associated with the restoration of body weight. Despite the potential role of estrogen deficiency, estrogen replacement is ineffective without weight gain.

Gastrointestinal Consequences. Refeeding may be followed by gastric dilation, ileus, and transient elevations of serum liver enzymes caused by fatty liver. Delayed gastric emptying explains some of the symptoms of abdominal bloating. The combination of slowed peristalsis and the meager dietary intake results in constipation.

Volume Changes. Refeeding frequently leads to fluid retention, especially in the bulimic anorectic patient, who purges and is volume depleted. Fluid retention complicates the interpretation of weight changes and frightens the patient. If fluid retention is severe, congestive heart failure may develop as the increase in intravascular volume exceeds the capacity of the weakened heart.

Hematologic Consequences. Reversible bone marrow depression is noted. Although mild anemia is common, it is rarely a consequence of iron, folate, or B_{12} deficiency. The anemia may be masked in the setting of concurrent volume depletion and may not appear until rehydration is implemented. Despite leukopenia, the patient's susceptibility to infection is not increased. Thrombocytopenia is unusual.

Clinical Presentation

Characteristically, the patient with anorexia nervosa denies she is ill, but her emaciation attracts attention. The patient typically claims to feel well and appears *unconcerned* about her emaciation. Hunger is not a complaint, but patients may report difficulty sleeping, abdominal discomfort and bloating after eating, constipation, cold intolerance, and polyuria. Amenorrhea is present in female patients. Unlike other persons who are starving, those with anorexia are not fatigued until malnutrition becomes very severe. Most are restless and physically active, and some exercise to excess. Listlessness is an ominous sign. The patient may present bundled in clothing because of cold intolerance.

On examination, the patient typically appears extremely thin, if not emaciated, but animated. Vital signs may reveal bradycardia, hypotension, and hypothermia. The skin may appear dry, pale, or yellow tinged (a consequence of carotenemia) and covered by fine, downy hair (lanugo) over the face and arms. In women, the female pattern of fat distribution disappears, but axillary and pubic hair is preserved. Acrocyanosis may be present.

Clinical Course

The disease may occur as a single episode, as repeated episodes separated by remissions, or as a chronic condition. More than half of patients relapse after an initial hospital stay for weight gain. Approximately 50% of patients have a complete recovery (i.e., regain weight and menses), 30% have partial recovery, and 10% to 20% develop a chronic illness. Bulimic symptoms, lower weight, and older age at presentation are associated with poor outcome. Even after weight is restored, the patient with anorexia may have persistent weight preoccupation, disordered eating patterns, and psychosocial problems. Up to 40% of anorexic patients develop bulimia nervosa.

The mortality rate is 0.56%/yr. Most deaths are sudden, apparently caused by cardiac arrhythmias. Fatal hypoglycemic coma has also been reported. The risk for death appears to be higher in patients whose weight loss exceeds 40% of premorbid weight (or 30% if it has occurred within 3 months). Bulimic anorectic patients with metabolic abnormalities are probably at higher risk. The risk for suicide is also increased. The mortality rate is 12 times that of age-matched unaffected persons.

Bulimia (Bulimia Nervosa)

This eating disorder is driven by *excessive concern* about *body weight* or *shape* and is characterized by *repeated episodes* of *binge eating* (at least two times per week for 3 months), during which large amounts of high-calorie foods are consumed, usually in secrecy. The binge is followed by self-deprecating thoughts and *purging, excessive exercise,* or *fasting* (at least two times per week for 3 months) to prevent weight gain. Most bulimic patients purge by inducing vomiting or using laxatives, but some use diuretics or exercise excessively. They fear losing control of their eating behavior and are ashamed when it happens. Binges may be repeated several times daily. At other times, people with bulimia may diet rigorously or take diet pills. In severe cases, the patient may have no regular eating pattern. The result of this behavior is frequent weight fluctuations but not severe weight loss.

In contrast to persons with anorexia, those with bulimia are aware that their behavior is abnormal but often conceal the illness because of embarrassment. The bulimic patient's near-normal weight permits the illness to be hidden. Detection of surreptitious vomiting or laxative abuse can be a challenge (see later discussion).

Pathogenesis

The high prevalence of alcohol and drug abuse among patients with bulimia has led some to postulate that bulimia is part of an impulse-control disorder. Depression has also been proposed as a precipitant. Changes in neurotransmitter metabolism and a response to antidepressant medication suggest a biochemical component to the condition. Cultural pressure to be thin probably contributes. People with bulimia commonly report that a diet preceded their disease. The bingeing sometimes observed when experimentally starved normal persons resume eating has led to speculation that strict dieting contributes to the onset of bulimia. Bulimia is more prevalent in individuals with type 1 diabetes, who can purge by withholding insulin after overeating. Diabetic patients with bulimia generally have worse glucose control, have poorer quality of life, and may be at greater risk of diabetic complications.

Pathophysiology

The medical consequences of bulimia depend on the specific behaviors present. Menstrual irregularities are common regardless of the purging method.

Bingeing. Bingeing has few complications, although *abdominal pain* from distention is common. Acute gastric dilation is rare but has been reported.

Chronic Induced Emesis. Repeated regurgitation of stomach contents produces *volume depletion* and a *hypochloremic metabolic alkalosis*. Dizziness, syncope, thirst, orthostatic changes in vital signs, and an elevated blood urea nitrogen occur in the volume-depleted patient. Renal compensation for the alkalosis and volume depletion causes *potassium depletion* and *hypokalemia*, which may predispose to cardiac arrhythmias, muscle cramps and weakness, paresthesias, polyuria, and constipation. T-wave flattening and U waves are seen on the electrocardiogram. Serum and urine chloride levels are low.

Reversible, painless *parotid swelling* can develop with chronic vomiting and is often accompanied by *hyperamylasemia*. Irreversible dental problems also occur. Repeated exposure of the teeth to stomach acid causes *enamel decalcification* and *erosion*. Teeth diminish in size and become discolored and sensitive to temperature changes. Many vomiters have symptoms of *reflux esophagitis*, but hematemesis is unusual. Some patients use *emetine* (ipecac) to induce vomiting. Prolonged use may cause a reversible proximal *myopathy* and a potentially fatal cardiomyopathy.

Laxative Abuse. Laxative abuse is a common and potentially dangerous form of purging. It may begin as a response to constipation and continue because of the temporary weight loss induced through *volume depletion*. Stimulant laxatives are used most often. The resultant increase in colonic motility produces *abdominal cramps*, and electrolytes are lost in a *watery diarrhea*. Volume depletion, *hyponatremia, hypokalemia*, and either *metabolic acidosis* or *alkalosis* may result. Calcium and magnesium depletion has also been reported. The irritation of intestinal mucosa or development of hemorrhoids as a result of rapid fecal transit may cause *rectal bleeding*, and rectal *prolapse* can occur. When laxative abuse stops, transient fluid retention, edema, and constipation are common.

Diuretic Abuse. Patients use diuretics more often to prevent fluid retention than to induce weight loss. Use contributes to a *hypochloremic metabolic alkalosis, hypokalemia*, and *volume depletion*. Dilutional *hyponatremia* may also occur. In contrast to vomiters and laxative abusers, patients who use diuretics do not have low urinary levels of sodium and chloride. Fluid retention transiently develops when diuretics are stopped.

Clinical Presentation and Course

Bingeing and purging may be concealed, and no physical signs are characteristic. The clinical presentation is often dominated by one of its medical complications, such as abdominal pain, diarrhea, heartburn, hypokalemia, volume depletion, hyponatremia, or parotid swelling.

Nearly half of bulimic patients remain symptomatic 6 years after the diagnosis is made, and the symptoms can persist for decades. Patients with concomitant depression, impulsivity, and personality disorders have worse prognoses for recovery.

Mortality is lower than in anorexia nervosa but higher than in an age-matched control population.

Binge-Eating Disorder

This condition, an important cause of obesity, is characterized by recurrent binge eating (at least 2 days weekly for 6 months) and marked distress associated with eating alone, too rapidly, when not hungry, or until uncomfortably full. The patient has feelings of guilt or disgust after a binge but does not purge, exercise excessively, or fast. Of the several eating disorders, this is the most common among male patients and is prevalent among the obese.

Night-Eating Syndrome

See Appendix 234.1.

DIFFERENTIAL DIAGNOSIS (1)

The differential diagnosis spans the array of conditions that may cause unexplained weight loss (see Chapter 9), secondary amenorrhea (see Chapter 112), electrolyte disturbances with volume depletion (see Chapters 59 and 64), and osteoporosis (see Chapter 164). Among them are malignancy, chronic infection, intestinal disorders (malabsorption, inflammatory bowel disease, or hepatitis), and endocrinopathies (e.g., hyperthyroidism, panhypopituitarism, adrenal insufficiency, diabetes mellitus). Tumors of the central nervous system mimic anorexia nervosa in rare cases. Psychiatric illnesses that can be confused with anorexia include depression, schizophrenia, and obsessive–compulsive neurosis (see Chapters 226, 227, and 230). Binge eating may be a manifestation of depression and, rarely, of an organic brain syndrome.

WORKUP (1,12,13)

The diagnoses of anorexia nervosa and bulimia are based exclusively on clinical findings (Table 234.1). Laboratory studies help in the detection of complications (see later discussion) and in excluding other causes of weight loss (see Chapter 9).

Anorexia Nervosa

History

The diagnosis should be suspected in patients with unexplained weight loss. The history should explore the patient's attitudes toward weight loss, desired weight, and eating habits. A *24-hour dietary recall* is more revealing than the answers to general questions about diet. Detailed weight and menstrual histories should be obtained, including the date and circumstances at the onset of weight loss, minimum and maximum weights, recent weight changes, and last normal menstrual period. One needs to ask all patients about bingeing, vomiting, and the use of laxatives, diuretics, diet pills, and emetics and to quantify daily exercise (excessive exercise is a common contributor to the weight loss).

It is also important to ask about symptoms of malnutrition (fatigue, skin or hair changes), dehydration (light-headedness,

TABLE 234.1

AMERICAN PSYCHIATRIC ASSOCIATION DIAGNOSTIC CRITERIA FOR EATING DISORDERS

Anorexia Nervosa
  Low body weight (<85% of expected weight or body mass index <17.5 kg/m²)
  Inaccurate perception of own body size, weight, or shape
  Intense fear of weight gain
  Amenorrhea (if female)

Bulimia Nervosa
  Excessive concern about body weight or shape
  Recurrent binge eating (at least twice weekly for 3 months)
  Recurrent purging, excessive exercise, or fasting (at least twice weekly for 3 months)
  Absence of anorexia nervosa

Binge-Eating Disorder
  Recurrent binge eating (at least twice weekly for 6 months)
  Marked distress with at least three of the following:
    Eating very rapidly
    Eating until uncomfortably full
    Eating when not hungry
    Eating alone
  No recurrent purging, excessive exercise, or fasting
  Absence of anorexia nervosa

Adapted from Becker AE, Grinspoon SK, Klibanski A, et al. Eating disorders. N Engl J Med 1999;340:1092, with permission; and based on the criteria specified in American Psychiatric Association. Diagnostic and statistical manual of mental disorders, 4th ed. Washington, DC: Author, 1994:539, 729.

syncope, thirst), hypokalemia (cramps, weakness, paresthesias, polyuria, palpitations), and other problems common to purgers (e.g., heartburn, abdominal pain, rectal bleeding). Because the risk for suicide is increased in patients with an eating disorder, one must *screen for suicidality* during the initial visit (see Chapter 227). Likewise, because of the increased prevalence of depression, anxiety, and personality disorders among these patients, the history should be reviewed for suggestive symptoms (see Chapters 226, 227, and 230). Exploring the psychosocial history can provide information important not only to diagnosis, but also to planning initial management.

Physical Examination

Important objectives are to assess the severity of malnutrition and dehydration and check for the development of complications. One should specifically take note of the general state of nutrition and hydration and follow with measurement of the height and weight (without street clothing). The blood pressure and pulse are checked for significant postural changes and the temperature noted for hypothermia. The skin is examined for pallor and the hair for changes of lanugo or acrocyanosis. In addition to these measures, a detailed physical examination is essential to rule out other causes of weight loss (see Chapter 9).

Laboratory Studies

Because serious volume, electrolyte, and cardiac rhythm disturbances may complicate anorexia nervosa, especially if the patient is also bulimic, one needs to obtain a full set of serum *electrolytes* plus *blood urea nitrogen*, *creatinine*, and *electrocardiogram* with rhythm strip. The finding of hyponatremia suggests excess water intake or inappropriate antidiuretic hormone secretion. Determination of the serum *calcium* (plus albumin) and magnesium is needed if a dysrhythmia is noted or laxative abuse is suspected. A *complete blood cell count* and measurement of *TSH*, *glucose*, *alkaline phosphatase*, and *gonadotropins* (see Chapter 112) may help in the initial assessment of complications of starvation, such as anemia, leukopenia, secondary hypothyroidism, hypoglycemia, fatty liver, and hypothalamic amenorrhea. If amenorrhea is persistent for 6 months or more, one should obtain a *bone mineral density* measurement to check for resultant osteopenia or osteoporosis (see Chapters 144 and 164). Unexplained weight loss may necessitate additional laboratory and imaging studies (see Chapter 9).

Bulimia

History

The diagnosis of bulimia requires a high index of suspicion because bingeing and purging may be concealed and no physical signs are characteristic. Four screening questions are helpful:

- Do you ever eat in secret?
- Does your weight affect the way you feel about yourself?
- Have any members of your family ever suffered with an eating disorder?
- Do you currently suffer with or have you ever suffered with an eating disorder?

Clues to the presence of bulimia include a preoccupation with weight and food, a history of frequent weight fluctuations, and problems common to patients who purge and become dehydrated (dizziness, thirst, syncope) or hypokalemic (muscle cramps or weakness, paresthesias, polyuria). In addition, vomiters may describe heartburn, and laxative abusers may report complain of constipation and fluid retention. When the diagnosis is suspected, the physician should ask directly about bingeing and purging and should order a determination of serum electrolytes. A direct inquiry may elicit the history from a patient seeking help but ashamed to volunteer the information.

Physical Examination

Physical examination should include a check of postural signs for evidence of volume depletion. Salivary gland enlargement or scars on the dorsum of the hand, suggestive of chronic self-induced vomiting, may be noted. The teeth should be examined for enamel erosion and discoloration.

Laboratory Studies

Most useful are the *serum and urine electrolytes*, *blood urea nitrogen*, and *creatinine* and the *electrocardiogram*. *Calcium* and *magnesium* should be measured in laxative abusers. The pattern of serum and urine electrolytes helps to determine the mode of purging. *Hypokalemic alkalosis* suggests frequent vomiting or diuretic use. A *non–anion gap acidosis* suggests laxative abuse. Some patients who vomit deny that it is voluntary. Organic causes of chronic vomiting should be excluded in these cases (see Chapter 59).

Binge-Eating Disorder

The workup focuses on the history because physical examination and laboratory findings are almost always normal, except for obese patients (see Chapter 10). It is most important to explore the patient's experiences with eating because distress characterizes the syndrome, as do feelings of disgust and guilt after a binge.

PRINCIPLES OF MANAGEMENT AND PATIENT EDUCATION (1,7,9,13–24)

Goals, Site, and Scope of Treatment

The goals of treatment are to stop the abnormal eating behaviors, restore body weight, and prevent relapse by addressing the psychological and family problems that are part of the illness. Weight restoration, the immediate goal, may require hospitalization, ideally in a psychiatric unit experienced in treating the disorder. Patients who do not meet medical criteria for hospitalization (suicidality or major electrolyte or cardiac disturbance; see later discussion), who are highly motivated for change, and who have a supportive environment can gain weight in an outpatient setting, but they require close monitoring. Several therapies produce short-term weight gain in patients with anorexia, but relapse is common, so that a comprehensive, multidimensional approach is necessary. For bulimia nervosa, outpatient treatment is usually sufficient.

Once it has been determined that hospitalization is not required, the design of the outpatient management program can proceed. The multidimensional nature of eating disorders necessitates a *multidisciplinary approach* that combines medical, nutritional, psychological, and pharmacologic measures. A *team approach* is helpful. It can be coordinated by either the primary physician or a medical specialist experienced in treating eating disorders. Close coordination and communication are essential. A set of overall treatment goals should be collectively developed, agreed on, and consistently communicated to the patient. Teamwork also helps ease the burden of treating these patients, who can be difficult when they deny the seriousness of their illness or exhibit deceptive, manipulative, angry, or distrusting behavior.

The immediate management tasks for the primary care physician are to identify and correct any potentially dangerous metabolic disturbances, set a few basic agreed-on goals, initiate a few simple behavioral measures, and arrange timely referral to persons expert in the management of eating disorders. Given the potentially life-threatening nature of some eating disorders, one should proceed with referral as quickly as possible.

Outpatient Monitoring and Treatment of Metabolic Disturbances

One monitors the *weight* and *vital signs* regularly. In bulimic patients or anorectic patients who purge, it is especially important to check *postural signs*, *cardiac rhythm*, and *serum electrolytes* at each visit. If the QT interval was prolonged on the electrocardiogram at the time of the first visit, then a *repeated electrocardiogram* is warranted, especially before any tricyclic antidepressant therapy is instituted.

The hypokalemic patient requires supplemental potassium, which must be given as *potassium chloride* to correct the metabolic alkalosis that maintains the hypokalemia. Patients should be instructed to take the supplement at a time when purging will not occur; often, this is at bedtime. Maintaining normal electrolyte levels should be a condition of continued outpatient treatment. Patients not able to maintain a normal potassium level with supplements require hospitalization.

Setting Goals and Implementing a Dietary Plan

Setting goals is an important component of care for patients with eating disorders. Several goals are optimally specified by the primary physician. The first goal is to halt the use of diuretics and laxatives as quickly as possible. Sometimes, gradual tapering of laxatives is necessary because of the onset of severe constipation. For patients with anorexia, a *weight goal* and a *minimum acceptable weight* below which hospitalization will be required should be specified. The minimum weight is usually set at 40% below the premorbid or ideal body weight. The weight goal is more difficult to determine and is often a point of disagreement between physician and patient. An estimate of desirable weight for height can be derived from standard tables (see Chapter 10). The weight goal should be at least 85% of the chart weight and, for female patients, a weight at which the patient has menstruated. Unless the patient was originally obese, it is usually close to the patient's premorbid weight. The patient and all caregivers should know of and agree to these weight guidelines. A *dietitian* can be very helpful in formulating and implementing an eating plan. Weight should be regained slowly, at a rate of 1 to 2 lb weekly, to avoid precipitating congestive heart failure. *Nutritional supplements* should be added if the patient is unable to gain weight at an acceptable rate.

Treating the Complications of Refeeding and Rehydration

During a reequilibration period of several weeks, temporary fluid retention and weight gain may occur. Patients with pedal edema can be aided by *support stockings*, *leg elevation*, mild *salt restriction*, and *reassurance* that the condition is temporary. Diuretics in the setting of volume depletion should be avoided even if edema is present because they may exacerbate the underlying metabolic and volume disturbances. To prevent constipation, patients should increase *dietary fiber* and may benefit from fiber supplements or *stool softeners*. Irritant laxative preparations are to be avoided at all costs.

Amenorrhea and *ostepenia* usually respond to an *increase in weight*. Periods return within 12 months in about 70% of those who reach 90% of their ideal weight. Estrogen replacement therapy has not shown benefit for reversing osteopenia in those who remain amenorrheic. Priority should be given to restoring normal weight and good nutrition, including an adequate intake of *calcium* (1.5 g/d) and *vitamin D* (400 IU/d). Two small studies using *bisphosphonates* plus calcium and vitamin D found an improvement in bone mass, even in the absence of weight gain. Further data on safety and efficacy of bisphosphonates are needed before their use becomes standard practice.

Psychotherapy

Because of the complex nature of eating disorders and the increased probability of serious underlying psychopathology (not to mention suicide risk), psychiatric referral for specialized multimodality care is best. Individual or group *psychotherapy*, *cognitive–behavioral therapy (CBT)*, and *family therapy* are all used. Patients with early-onset anorexia appear to respond well to family therapy. Those with bulimia respond well to CBT provided in a group or individual setting (and perhaps supplemented by psychopharmacologic treatment; see later discussion); so do patients with pure binge-eating disorder. For bulimia, CBT reduces symptoms (e.g., frequency of purging) and appears to be more effective than insight-oriented psychotherapy.

Psychopharmacologic Therapy

Unlike mild to moderate depression, in which treatment with antidepressants by primary physicians is relatively straightforward, the eating disorders are best treated with psychopharmacologic therapy only by physicians skilled and experienced in their management. One reason is the increased risk for concurrent drug and alcohol abuse, particularly among patients with bulimia.

Bulimia

Psychopharmacologic intervention is helpful in patients with bulimia. *Antidepressants* reduce the frequency of bingeing episodes, even in the patients without coexistent depression, but they are most effective when used in conjunction with psychotherapy. A combination of antidepressants and CBT may be more effective than either treatment alone, whereas antidepressants alone are less effective than CBT alone. A broad range of antidepressant agents are effective; these include *selective serotonin reuptake inhibitors* (SSRIs; e.g., fluoxetine, up to 60 mg/d), tricyclics (e.g., amitriptyline, desipramine, and imipramine, up to 300 mg/d), monoamine oxidase inhibitors (e.g., phenelzine and isocarboxazid), and others (e.g., bupropion and trazodone). A 2003 meta-analysis of 19 trials did not find evidence that any antidepressant was superior to others.

Anorexia Nervosa

In contrast, antidepressant medications have not been demonstrated to reduce symptoms or produce weight gain in anorexia nervosa. Even after weight was regained, *fluoxetine* (at 60 mg/d) did not sustain recovery better than placebo in a randomized, controlled trial.

Binge-Eating Disorder

In binge-eating disorder, antidepressants have shown promise.

PATIENT EDUCATION

The physician needs to inform the patient of the seriousness of his or her illness and its complications. The connection between the eating disorder, symptoms, and laboratory abnormalities should be explained in detail. For anorectic patients, the consequences of starvation and the necessity of weight gain must be emphasized. Patients who purge need to understand the potential consequences of their behavior (e.g., irreversible erosion of tooth enamel, cardiac arrhythmias) and the ineffectiveness of laxative or diuretic use for achieving real weight loss. Patients who have been starving themselves or abusing laxatives or diuretics should be instructed in the likelihood of transient discomfort (e.g., edema, constipation, bloating) as they stop purging and begin to eat.

INDICATIONS FOR ADMISSION AND REFERRAL

As noted earlier, anorexia is a potentially life-threatening condition. Medical criteria for hospitalization include the following: (a) loss of more than 40% of premorbid or ideal weight (or 30% if within 3 months), (b) rapid progression of weight loss, (c) presence of cardiac arrhythmias, (d) persistent hypokalemia unresponsive to outpatient treatment, and (e) symptoms of inadequate cerebral perfusion or mentation (syncope, severe dizziness, listlessness). The patient should understand that anorexia is a life-threatening illness and that the first priority is to protect life. Psychiatric hospitalization may be required for behavior beyond the patient's control or for incapacitating depression.

When outpatient management is deemed appropriate for a patient, referrals for psychiatric care and nutritional counseling are essential. It is best to select persons with expertise in the care of patients with eating disorders because treatment can be difficult. For patients with tooth enamel erosion caused by chronic emesis, a dental consultation should be obtained.

TREATMENT RECOMMENDATIONS (1,16)

Effective treatment is a multidisciplinary effort, likely to require a coordinated team approach that includes care by mental health and nutritional professionals. The guidelines that follow pertain to the role of the primary physician:

- At the time of the first visit, assess the degree of malnutrition, dehydration, and electrolyte disturbance and decide whether care should proceed on an inpatient or outpatient basis.
- Be sure that other causes of weight loss and its complications have been ruled out (see Chapters 9, 25, 59, 103, and 112).
- Obtain expert psychiatric and nutritional consultations; organize and coordinate a multidisciplinary team approach to management.
- Educate the patient about the medical complications of the illness.
- Set medical guidelines for outpatient management:
  1. Minimum acceptable weight
  2. Weight goal
  3. Weight gain of 1 to 2 lb per week for underweight patients
  4. Maintenance of normal electrolytes
  5. Compliance with concomitant psychiatric or psychological treatment
- Monitor weight, postural signs, cardiac rhythm, and electrolytes.
- Treat any hypokalemia with *potassium chloride*.
- Consider antidepressants to control symptoms in bulimic patients.
- Address and treat any endocrinologic complications (see Chapters 104 and 112).

- Anticipate and treat complications of refeeding and rehydration (edema, constipation).
- Hospitalize the patient in the following circumstances:
  1. Weight loss is in excess of 40% (or 30% if within 3 months)
  2. Weight loss is rapidly progressive

3. Cardiac arrhythmias develop (urgent)
4. Persistent hypokalemia is present and unresponsive to outpatient treatment
5. Syncope, severe dizziness, or listlessness develops (urgent)
6. Severe depression develops (urgent if patient becomes suicidal)

Annotated Bibliography

1. Becker AE, Grinspoon SK, Klibanski A, et al. Eating disorders. N Engl J Med 1999;340:1092. (*An excellent and authoritative review; 69 references.*)
2. Bo-Linn GW, Santa Ana CA, Morawski SG, et al. Purging and calorie absorption in bulimic patients and normal women. Ann Intern Med 1983;99:14. (*There was no reduction in calories absorbed; the mechanism of weight loss is fluid loss from the colon.*)
3. Bruce B, Wilfley D. Binge eating among the overweight population: a serious and prevalent problem. J Am Diet Assoc 1996;96:58. (*Documents the important contribution of binge eating to obesity and reviews approaches to treatment.*)
4. Ho PC, Dweik R, Cohen MC. Rapidly reversible cardiomyopathy associated with chronic ipecac ingestion. Clin Cardiol 1998;21:780. (*A diffuse, gradually reversible myopathy was found, characterized by proximal muscle weakness and electrocardiographic abnormalities.*)
5. Keel PK, Mitchell JE. Outcome in bulimia nervosa. Am J Psychiatry 1997;154:313. (*Useful outcomes data; about half of patients do very well.*)
6. Mannucci E, Rotella F, Ricca V, et al. Eating disorders in patients with type 1 diabetes: a meta-analysis. J Endocrinol Invest 2005;28:417. (*Bulimia, but not restrictive anorexia nervosa, is more common in type 1 diabetics.*)
7. Mehler PS. Bulimia nervosa. N Engl J Med 2003;349:875. (*A practical summary of the presentation and treatment of bulimia for clinicians.*)
8. Miller KK, Lee EE, Lawson EA, et al. Determinants of skeletal loss and recovery in anorexia nervosa. J Clin Endocrinol Metab 2006;91:2931. (*Improvement in spinal bone density was associated with a return of menses, whereas improvement in hip bone density was linked to weight gain.*)
9. Mitchell JE, Crow S. Medical complications of anorexia nervosa and bulimia nervosa. Curr Opin Psychiatry 2006;19:438. (*A summary of recent publications on medical issues.*)
10. Roche F, Barthelemy JC, Mayaud N, et al. Refeeding normalizes the QT rate dependence of female anorexic patients. Am J Cardiol 2005;95:277. (*Prolonged QT intervals on the electrocardiogram, which may increase the risk of sudden death, are reversible with refeeding.*)
11. Zipfel S, Lowe B, Reas DL, et al. Long-term prognosis in anorexia nervosa: lessons from a 21-year follow-up study. Lancet. 2000;355:721. (*Of 84 patients followed, 51% recovered fully, 10% had chronic anorexia, and 16% died of anorexia-related causes.*)
12. Cotton MA, Ball C, Robinson P. Four simple questions can help screen for eating disorders. J Gen Intern Med 2003;18:53. (*Questions useful for the primary care setting.*)
13. Mehler P. Diagnosis and care of patients with anorexia nervosa in primary care settings. Ann Intern Med 2001;134:1048. (*A good summary of clinical care of anorectic patients;* see www.psych.org/clin_res/guide.bk42301.cfm *for a revised guideline.*)
14. Agras WS, Walsh T, Fairburn CGT, et al. A multicenter comparison of cognitive–behavioral therapy and interpersonal psychotherapy for bulimia nervosa. Arch Gen Psychiatry 2000;57:459. (*Cognitive–behavioral therapy was superior to interpersonal psychotherapy.*)
15. Agras WS, Rossiter EM, Arnow B, et al. One-year follow-up of psychosocial and pharmacologic treatment for bulimia nervosa. J Clin Psychiatry 1994;55:179. (*Combination therapy was found to give the best results.*)
16. American Psychiatric Association. Practice guideline for the treatment of patients with eating disorders. Am J Psychiatry 2002;159:1246. (*Consensus guidelines.*)
17. Bacaltchuk J, Hay P. Antidepressants versus placebo for people with bulimia nervosa. Cochrane Database Syst Rev 2003;4:CD003391. (*A meta-analysis of 19 trials found that a number of antidepressants were better than placebo at reducing bingeing episodes in patients with bulimia; no one antidepressant was clearly superior to others.*)
18. Claudino AM, Hay P, Lima MS, et al. Antidepressants for anorexia nervosa. Cochrane Database Syst Rev 2006;1:CD004365. (*A systematic review found few high-quality studies and no evidence that antidepressants improved weight gain or reduced eating disorder symptoms in anorexia nervosa.*)
19. Golden NH, Iglesias EA, Jacobson MS, et al. Alendronate for the treatment of osteopenia in anorexia nervosa: a randomized, double-blind, placebo-controlled trial. J Clin Endocrinol Metab 2005;90:3179. (*In 32 adolescents with osteopenia and anorexia nervosa, alendronate improved bone density better than placebo.*)
20. Klibanski A, Biller BMK, Schoenfeld DA, et al. The effects of estrogen administration on trabecular bone loss in young women with anorexia nervosa. J Clin Endocrinol Metab 1995;80:898. (*The disappointing results suggest that other factors besides estrogen deficiency are involved in the osteoporosis associated with this condition.*)
21. Miller KK, Grieco KA, Mulder J, et al. Effects of risedronate on bone density in anorexia nervosa. J Clin Endocrinol Metab 2004;89:3903. (*In a nonrandomized trial, risedronate increased bone gain in 10 women with anorexia nervosa.*)
22. Romano SJ, Halmi KA, Sarkar NP, et al. A placebo-controlled study of fluoxetine in continued treatment of bulimia nervosa after successful acute fluoxetine treatment. Am J Psychiatry 2002;159:96. (*Presents the rationale for longer term-pharmacotherapy.*)
23. Walsh BT, Kaplan AS, Ettia E, et al. Fluoxetine after weight restoration in anorexia nervosa: a randomized controlled trial. JAMA 2006;295:2605. (*Fluoxetine was no better than placebo in maintaining weight gain after initial treatment for anorexia nervosa.*)
24. Walsh BT, Wilson GT, Loeb KL, et al. Medication and psychotherapy in the treatment of bulimia nervosa. Am J Psychiatry 1997;154:523. (*Combination therapy was found to be complementary.*)

APPENDIX 234.1: NIGHT EATING SYNDROME

Night-eating syndrome is a little studied but potentially important form of disturbed eating and sleeping. As originally described, it is characterized by morning anorexia, evening hyperphagia, and insomnia. Prevalence estimates range from 1.5% of the general population to as much as 25% among very obese persons, although the condition can also occur in nonobese individuals. The condition can be a source of both disturbed sleep and obesity.

PATHOPHYSIOLOGY AND CLINICAL PRESENTATION

The cause of the syndrome remains unknown, but a distinctive circadian pattern was noted, which included nighttime awakening with consumption of food and concordant reductions in the usual nighttime surges of melatonin and leptin and loss of normal daily cycling of plasma cortisol levels. The interplay of these hormones and cortisol releasing hormone provides potential clues to the underlying pathophysiology and the relationship of the condition to situational stress. Dietary composition is high in carbohydrate, which increases serum serotonin and the bioavailability of tryptophan for transport into the brain (helping to restore sleep).

The condition differs from bulimia and binge eating not only in its predominantly nocturnal timing but also in the amount of calories consumed, which are substantially fewer than for bulimics and binge eaters. It differs from the eating behaviors associated with sleep walking and related conditions. Clinical course is unknown.

DIAGNOSIS

At present, diagnosis remains clinical, possibly supported by observing the characteristic pattern of reductions in nocturnal melatonin and leptin and increase in cortisol (recognizing these may be nonspecific). Differentiation from other eating disorders (see above) and sleep disorders (see Chapter 232) can be difficult, and these disorders may be concurrent. The condition needs to be differentiated from night-walking and associated night eating, where alertness is impaired and there is amnesia of the event.

MANAGEMENT

Since psychosocial stress appears to be a precipitant, attention to it appears to be a reasonable first line of treatment. Similarly, identification and treatment of any concurrent sleep or eating disorders (e.g., restless leg syndrome, sleep apnea) are likely to be helpful. The observed dietary and hormonal abnormalities have led to suggestions about use of SSRI agents to increase serotonin or possible benefit from exogenous melatonin or measures that might nocturnally raise leptin and reduce cortisol (e.g., a CRH receptor antagonist). Much more work is needed before such measures can be recommended for use in primary care practice. Referral is indicated when the problem appears to be compromising quality of life.

A.H.G.

Annotated Bibliography

1. Birketvedt GS, Florholmen J, Sundsfjord J, et al. Behavioral and neuroendocrine characteristics of the night-eating syndrome. JAMA 1999;282:657. (*Study elucidating key features of the syndrome.*)

2. Yager J. Nocturnal eating syndromes: to sleep, perchance to eat. JAMA 1999;282:689. (*Editorial summarizing current knowledge.*)

CHAPTER 235 ■ APPROACH TO DRUG ABUSE AND DEPENDENCE

E. NALAN WARD

The person suffering from drug abuse or dependence poses diagnostic and management challenges to the primary care clinician and represents one of the foremost public health problems in the United States. According to National Survey on Drug Use and Health 2006 data, an estimated 20.4 million persons in the United States of age 12 years or older are current (past month) illicit drug users. Marijuana is the most commonly used illicit drug, followed by prescription pain medications in nonmedical users. Regional differences include high methamphetamine use in the West and the Midwest and opioid abuse in the Northeast. Prescription analgesics seem to be the entry point into opioid abuse and dependence.

Illicit drug abuse and dependence lead to high-risk dysfunctional behavior that disrupts interpersonal relationships and destroys lives, playing major roles in accidents, crime, domestic violence, and lost productivity. Intravenous drug use strongly contributes to the spread of AIDS and other infectious diseases such as hepatitis C. The comorbidity of substance abuse and psychiatric illness is particularly devastating. About half of individuals with a dependence on an illicit drug have another psychiatric illness (Fig. 235.1).

Despite the pervasive penetration of illicit drug use problems into all aspects of the culture, the ability of health care providers to assess and intervene has lagged far behind the current state of knowledge. Of an estimated 22.6 million persons of age 12 years or older classified with substance dependence or abuse in the last year, only 4.0 million received some kind of treatment. Unfortunately, physicians frequently treat the sequelae without directly addressing the underlying problem.

DEFINITIONS (1)

Changes in the Vocabulary of Substance Abuse

The vocabulary of substance abuse disorders has undergone change as the emphasis has shifted from physical or physiologic dependence (manifested by tolerance and a withdrawal syndrome on abstinence) to behavioral abnormalities. In addition, because the terms "*addiction*" and "*addict*" have gained many imprecise and pejorative meanings, they are

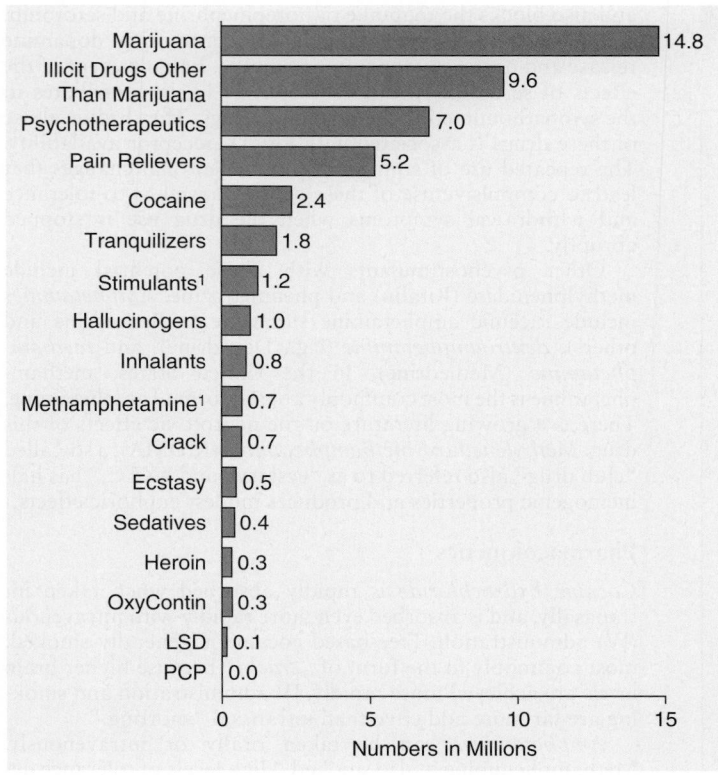

Drug	Numbers in Millions
Marijuana	14.8
Illicit Drugs Other Than Marijuana	9.6
Psychotherapeutics	7.0
Pain Relievers	5.2
Cocaine	2.4
Tranquilizers	1.8
Stimulants[1]	1.2
Hallucinogens	1.0
Inhalants	0.8
Methamphetamine[1]	0.7
Crack	0.7
Ecstasy	0.5
Sedatives	0.4
Heroin	0.3
OxyContin	0.3
LSD	0.1
PCP	0.0

FIGURE 235.1. Past-month use of specific illicit drugs among persons aged 12 years or older: 2006. LSD, lysergic acid diethylamide; PCP, phencyclidine. 1, . . . (From Office of Applied Studies. Results from the 2006 National Survey on Drug Use and Health (NSDUH): national findings (DHHS Publication No. SMA 07-4293). Rockville, MD: Substance Abuse and Mental Health Services Administration, 2007.)

not used by the World Health Association or the American Psychiatric Association, which instead divides *substance use disorders* into *substance dependence* and *substance abuse* (Table 235.1). Nonetheless, many experts prefer use of the term "addiction" because it is less likely to be confused with "physical dependence," which may not be associated with compulsive, out-of-control behaviors.

Definitions of Specific Terms

Addiction: compulsive, persistent drug-seeking and drug-taking behavior despite serious psychosocial and/or physical consequences.

Substance abuse: illegal, maladaptive, or dangerous use of a substance, but not implying dependence.

Substance dependence: the same meaning as "addiction" and used interchangeably with it.

Physical dependence: development of physical tolerance and a physical withdrawal syndrome, not necessarily pathologic drug-seeking behavior.

PATHOPHYSIOLOGY AND CLINICAL PRESENTATION (1–10)

General Pathophysiology of Drug-Use Disorders

Drug-use disorders are complex disorders caused by biopsychosocial factors. With prolonged drug exposure in vulnerable persons, neurons in key circuits undergo molecular adapta-

tions. Neurons in the *locus coeruleus* appear to adapt to prolonged opiate exposure and fire at abnormally high rates when opiates are abruptly withdrawn, thereby triggering much of the physical withdrawal syndrome. The *mesolimbic dopamine system* provides powerful *reinforcement behaviors* with important survival value (e.g., sexual activity) by producing a sense of euphoria on stimulation. The most addictive of drugs (e.g., cocaine, amphetamines, opiates, alcohol, and nicotine) are believed to tap into this "brain reward" system by mimicking or enhancing the action of endogenous neurotransmitters such as dopamine or endorphins.

It has been hypothesized that the drugs that produce these adaptive responses in the mesolimbic dopamine system cause the core symptoms of substance use disorders. A subset of these responses also produces adaptive changes in other neurons that lead to physical dependence. When the drug is stopped, the person feels that the world is intolerable without it. In this model, the pathologic behaviors (e.g., denial, manipulations) of the person with a substance use disorder become more understandable. The key motivational system in the person's brain has been usurped by drugs. Without the drug, the person experiences strong negative emotions, an inability to feel pleasure, and an intense craving for the drug.

Why some people become addicted during the course of drug use and others do not and why some people recover and some do not are not fully understood. Individual vulnerability appears in part *genetic*, such as the linkage of the dopamine receptor gene to multiple substance dependences. Developmental *experiences*, chronic *pain*, current levels of *distress*, and complex social factors, including *family* and *peer relationships* and the availability of valued behavioral alternatives, are all contributors to individual vulnerability. *Psychiatric disorders* are a significant risk factor in substance use disorders and complicate diagnosis and treatment. The debate over the origins of

TABLE 235.1

CRITERIA FOR SUBSTANCE ABUSE AND DEPENDENCE

Substance Abuse

A maladaptive pattern of substance use leading to clinically significant impairment or distress, as manifested in one (or more) of the following, occurring within a 12-month period:

- Failure to fulfill major role obligations at work, school, or home
- Recurrent use in situations in which it is physically hazardous (e.g., driving an automobile)
- Recurrent use related to legal problems
- Continued use despite persistent or recurrent social or interpersonal problems caused by substance use

The symptoms have never met the criteria for Substance Dependence of this class of substance

Substance Dependence

A maladaptive pattern of substance use leading to clinically significant impairment or distress, as manifested by three (or more) of the following occurring at any time in the same 12-month period:

Tolerance, as defined by either of the following:

- Need for markedly increased amounts of the substance to achieve intoxication or effect
- Markedly diminished effect from the same amount of substance

Withdrawal, as manifested by either of the following:

- Withdrawal syndrome for the substance
- The same substance taken to relieve withdrawal symptoms

Substance taken in larger amounts or for a longer period of time than was intended

Persistent desire or unsuccessful efforts to cut down or control substance use

A great deal of time spent in activities necessary to obtain the substance

Important social, occupational, or recreational activities given up because of substance use

The substance use continued despite knowledge of having a persistent physical or psychological problem that is likely to have been caused or exacerbated by the substance

Adapted from the diagnostic criteria specified in American Psychiatric Association. Diagnostic and statistical manual of mental disorders, 4th ed. Washington, DC: Author, 1994, with permission.

substance use disorders is not simply one of semantics; the inability of people to stop using alcohol, tobacco, or other drugs baffles or angers many physicians.

Cocaine, Amphetamines, and Other Central Nervous System Stimulants

These agents act by increasing synaptic dopamine in the mesocoricolimbic dopamine system (dopamine neurons in the ventral tegmental area and its projections in the nucleus accumbens and prefrontal cortex). *Cocaine* binds to dopamine transporter and inhibits the reuptake of dopamine in the synapse and also blocks the reuptake of norepinephrine and serotonin. *Amphetamine* acts predominantly by promoting dopamine release and decreases dopamine reuptake. Enhancement of the effects of serotonin and norepinephrine likely contributes to the sympathomimetic effects of these drugs. The chronic abuse of these drugs is associated with low D_2-receptor availability. The repeated use of stimulants causes neuronal changes that lead to compulsive use of these drugs, as well as to tolerance and withdrawal symptoms when the drug use is stopped abruptly.

Other psychostimulants with abuse potential include methylphenidate (Ritalin) and phenmetrazine. *Amphetamines* include racemic amphetamine sulfate (e.g., Benzedrine and others), *dextroamphetamine* (e.g., Dexedrine), and *methamphetamine* (Methedrine). In the United States, methamphetamine is the most commonly abused form of amphetamine. There is a growing literature on the neurotoxic effects of this drug. *Methylenedioxymethamphetamine* (MDMA), a so-called "club drug" also referred to as "ecstasy" and "XTC," has hallucinogenic properties and produces modest euphoric effects.

Pharmacokinetics

Cocaine hydrochloride is rapidly absorbed when taken intranasally, and is absorbed even more rapidly with intravenous (IV) administration. Free-based cocaine is generally smoked, most commonly in the form of *"crack."* Because higher brain levels are achieved more rapidly, IV administration and smoking are far more addictive than intranasal "snorting."

Amphetamines can be taken orally or intravenously. Methamphetamine is also smoked. High levels of tolerance develop in persons who use amphetamine on a regular basis, so that increasing doses of the drug become necessary. These people are at high risk for the development of a paranoid psychosis. MDMA is absorbed orally; immediate effects last 3 to 6 hours; residual effects (anxiety, cognitive impairment, paranoia) may persist for weeks. Perhaps the most important difference between cocaine and amphetamine derivatives is in half-life; the effects of amphetamine last longer than those of cocaine. These differences in half-life lead to different use patterns.

Clinical Effects and Patterns of Abuse

Cocaine and amphetamine produce many of the same clinical effects, the most important of which is *euphoria*—which is a sense of increased energy and confidence—as well as sympathomimetic actions. With increased dose and duration, they may also produce *restlessness, anxiety, hostility, hypersexuality,* and *paranoia.* Other effects include tachycardia, hypertension, fever, and tremor. With dependence, patients may exhibit jitteriness, weight loss, depression, and a lack of energy. *Cocaine* is often taken in *binges* to maintain drug-induced euphoria because the effects are short lived. At the termination of a *binge*, a predominantly psychophysiologic withdrawal syndrome called *crash* is often evident, characterized by severe dysphoria, anhedonia, fatigue, and a craving for cocaine.

Amphetamine may also be used in binges, but many people take the drug orally on a daily basis. They may start taking amphetamine to control weight or decrease fatigue. At low doses, it increases wakefulness and physical activity and causes euphoria and hypersexuality. At higher doses, it can cause anxiety, irritability, insomnia, and paranoia.

In the club setting, persons use *MDMA* for its disinhibitory effects, which may induce feelings of euphoria and hallucinations. The substance has a reputation as an aphrodisiac.

Use during all-night dance parties ("raves," "trances") has led to deaths caused by the combination of the drug plus many hours of intense exertion, lack of hydration, hyperthermia, and rhabdomyolysis. MDMA also produces muscle twitching and bruxism.

Overdosing with cocaine or amphetamine produces tachyarrhythmias, perspiration or chills, nausea or vomiting, hypertension, high fever, seizures, delirium, paranoia, psychosis, coma, and cardiovascular collapse. Stroke and myocardial infarction have been reported with crack use.

Despite their similarities, cocaine and amphetamine do not parallel each other in popularity. Cocaine use among the middle class has declined markedly; however, use among "hardcore" cocaine-dependent persons has persisted particularly in the form of crack cocaine. Amphetamine was popular before the start of the most recent cocaine epidemic and is now resurgent in the form of methamphetamine produced in "garage laboratories."

Opiates

Opiates produce their effects by binding to endogenous opiate receptors; therapeutically, this produces analgesia; less potent opiates are also used as antitussives and antidiarrheal agents. The most highly abused opiates (*heroin*; less commonly *morphine* or *meperidine*) interact predominantly with μ-type opiate receptors and are generally injected intravenously; other abused opiates (*oxycodone* and *hydromorphone*) are most often taken orally. Heroin may also be smoked. *Controlled-release oxycodone HCl* has the a similar effect at the opiate receptor, but when crushed and used in an abusive fashion it becomes a rapid-release drug with the same abuse potential as other opiate-receptor agonists.

Clinical Effects and Patterns of Abuse

Opiates produce an initial sense of euphoria (a "rush"), especially after IV injection, smoking, or crushing, which is followed by a sense of tranquility and then sleepiness and mental clouding. Respiratory depression, sedation, and loss of motor control occur when large amounts are abused. When tolerance and dependence develop with repeated consumption, increasing doses are required to achieve the desired euphoria. Tolerance to the respiratory depressant effects of opiates develops approximately in parallel. Tolerance to opiate-induced pupillary constriction does not develop.

Unlike alcohol, opiates do not directly produce serious organ pathology. *Constipation* is the major side effect and may represent a significant problem (e.g., in patients being treated for cancer pain). Other effects of opioids are sensation of *urinary urgency, miosis, hypotension,* and *infertility.*

As opiates produce high levels of *physiologic dependence,* repeated use of the drug is needed to prevent withdrawal symptoms. IV injection of the drug is a widely used method of administration and commonly involves sharing needles. This results in hepatitis C, HIV infection, endocarditis, infection of the local injection site, and other complications of unsterile self-injection.

Overdoses

Overdoses of opiates may be lethal because of *respiratory depression.* Overdosing is most frequent when the heroin dose is purer than what the addicted person is accustomed to,

when tolerance levels are miscalculated after detoxification, and when the user is inexperienced.

Withdrawal

In general, clinically significant withdrawal symptoms do not occur with less than 2 weeks of opioid use, unless the person has a previous opioid dependence. Withdrawal from opiates is quite uncomfortable, both physically and psychologically, but not lethal. Various factors influence the severity of withdrawal symptoms, such as specific drug used (long acting vs. short acting), total daily amount used, duration and regularity of use, and psychological and individual factors.

Withdrawal from heroin may begin 6 to 12 hours after the last dose in dependent persons and is manifested by tearing, rhinorrhea, yawning, sweating followed by sleep disturbance, dilated pupils, drug craving, loss of appetite, piloerection ("goose flesh" or "cold turkey"), irritability, tachycardia, hypertension, tremor, nausea, vomiting diarrhea, chills, fever, agitation and severe muscle cramps.

The hyperactivity of noradrenergic neurons in the locus coeruleus is responsible for an increase in blood pressure, heart rate, respiration, sweating, and diarrhea, whereas increases in cyclic adenosine monophosphate in opioid receptors and changes in the dopamine neurons of the ventral tegmental area seem to be responsible for dysphoria, craving, and relapse.

Sedative–Hypnotics

The sedative–hypnotics include the *benzodiazepines, barbiturates,* and *barbiturate-like drugs* (e.g., glutethimide, ethchlorvynol). These agents enhance the inhibitory effects of γ-aminobutyric acid (GABA$_A$) receptors in the brain. Because *ethyl alcohol* similarly affects these receptors, marked sedation is associated with concurrent use.

Benzodiazepines are most commonly prescribed for the short-term treatment of insomnia and for anxiety disorders (see Chapters 226 and 232). They can cause dependence with long-term use, and so they must be slowly tapered after a course of treatment. The likelihood of dependence is greater with high-potency, short-acting compounds (e.g., alprazolam, triazolam) than with low-potency, long-acting compounds (e.g., diazepam, chlordiazepoxide).

Flunitrazepam is fast-acting benzodiazepine that is abused in club settings and associated with *date rape.* Commonly referred to as "*Rophies,*" the "*date-rape pill,*" or the "*forget-me pill,*" when combined with alcohol it induces sedation and antegrade amnesia. Victims may have the tasteless, colorless agent added to their drink, rendering them susceptible to sexual exploitation. Although abuse and addiction may occur, it is relatively uncommon for the benzodiazepines to produce addictive behaviors (compulsive nonmedical use) except in patients with a prior history of drug abuse. Prolonged benzodiazepine use, carefully monitored, may be necessary for patients with disabling anxiety disorders (see Chapter 226).

The *barbiturates,* in comparison to the benzodiazepines and similarly acting compounds, have a greater potential for abuse, overdose, and drug–drug interactions (by inducing hepatic microsomal enzymes). The barbiturates are usually used as anticonvulsants and for headaches; phenobarbital has value in treating benzodiazepine withdrawal.

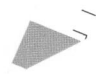

Clinical Effects and Patterns of Abuse and Withdrawal

When abused, the sedative–hypnotics produce disinhibition, which appears very similar to alcohol intoxication; disinhibition is often followed by slurry speech, incoordination, unsteady gait, nystagmus, and impairment in attention or memory. This can be followed by heavy sedation, stupor, and coma when used in high quantities. *Overdosing* with barbiturates produces respiratory depression and coma and may cause death. Benzodiazepines are not likely to be lethal when taken alone in overdose, but when combined with alcohol, they can cause death from respiratory depression.

Withdrawal from sedative–hypnotic drugs produces tachycardia, hypertension, fever, tremulousness, hyperreflexia, anxiety, restlessness, insomnia, and anorexia. Seizures and delirium may occur and may be severe. Unlike opiate withdrawal, sedative–hypnotic withdrawal may be fatal.

Marijuana

Marijuana is produced from the dried leaves and flowers of the hemp plant, *Cannabis sativa*. The active ingredient, *D-9-tetrahydrocannabinol (THC)*, acts by binding to an endogenous THC receptor in the brain, the normal function of which is unknown. During the last decade, the clonal selection of hemp plants for high THC content has markedly increased the potency of marijuana sold on the street.

Marijuana is generally smoked, although it is occasionally taken orally, and produces a feeling of relaxation, mild euphoria, and increased sociability. Physical symptoms and signs include mild tachycardia, dry mouth, and conjunctival injection. The most common short-term adverse consequence is an acute panic reaction, which may occur in inexperienced users, especially after they have smoked high-potency marijuana. Rarely, large doses of high-potency marijuana can produce *hallucinations*, *paranoia*, and *delirium*. Marijuana is far less addictive than cocaine, amphetamine, opiates, alcohol, nicotine, or barbiturates, but some habitual users appear to be dependent. Long-term heavy users manifest cognitive impairment (memory difficulties and inattention). Prolonged use may also impair testosterone secretion and lead to *gynecomastia*. Early use of marijuana (before age 17 years), peer pressure, and the social context of obtaining and using marijuana are important risk factors for the abuse of other drugs and for the development of drug-related problems.

Hallucinogens

The hallucinogens, or psychedelic compounds, are a group of structurally diverse compounds that appear to act by mimicking the actions of serotonin at certain of its receptor subtypes. The most widely used hallucinogens are the indolalkylamine compounds, including D-*lysergic acid diethylamide* (LSD), *dimethyltryptamine*, and *psilocybin* (which is the active ingredient in *"magic" mushrooms*), and the phenylethylamine compounds, such as the "designer" club drug *MDMA* (see prior discussion), and *mescaline* (derived from the peyote cactus). The hallucinogen *ketamine* is a veterinary anesthetic with effects similar to those of *phencyclidine* (see later discussion).

Clinical Effects and Patterns of Abuse

LSD produces both *sympathomimetic* and *perceptual* effects. The sympathomimetic effects, such as increased pulse rate, blood pressure, and mydriasis, generally precede the perceptual changes, which include visual illusions, hallucinations, confusion among sensory modalities (synesthesias), depersonalization, and altered time perception. Most LSD "trips" last 8 to 12 hours. The predominant effects of psilocybin and mescaline are similar to those of LSD.

The most common immediate adverse effect of hallucinogen use is a *panic reaction* or "bad trip." Extreme agitation or *delirium* occurs rarely, although it occurs often as a result of exposure to additional drugs or adulterants, particularly *phencyclidine*. In such circumstances, a toxic screen should be obtained.

Patients in whom *psychotic episodes* develop after hallucinogen use are difficult to sort out. Generally, the history of psychiatric disturbance precedes the use of the hallucinogen. *Flashbacks*, which consist of brief, recurrent visual illusions or hallucinations, may occur for months or, rarely, for several years after hallucinogen use.

Hallucinogens do not appear to be physically addictive. Their major dangers relate to the state of intoxication they produce, in which judgment is markedly impaired and panic reactions possible. These predispose to accidents, violence, and suicide (which may be inadvertent). In addition, animal data demonstrate that MDMA is highly toxic to serotonin neurons in the brain. Whether MDMA produces lesions of the serotonin system in humans is not known but is a concern.

Phencyclidine and Ketamine

Phencyclidine, like marijuana and other hallucinogens, does not produce a physiologic withdrawal pattern in humans, but a psychological abstinence syndrome is observed that includes depression, craving, and fatigue. Most important is the variable presentation of intoxication and overdose with diverse behavioral and psychological manifestations (delirium, psychosis, catatonia, mania, depression, extreme agitation, and violence) or with physiologic manifestations (nystagmus, hypertension, tachycardia, hyperreflexia that may lead to rhabdomyolysis, renal failure). The behavioral and physiologic effects can occur together or in stages that complicate the diagnosis and treatment, and they can progress to life-threatening stupor and coma in which the patient is unresponsive to pain. A careful history is mandatory, as is constant awareness in the acute setting of the possibility of phencyclidine intoxication.

Ketamine ("vitamin K," "special K") is a popular club drug that has sedative, hallucinogenic, and euphoric properties—hence its attractiveness for recreational use. It resembles phencyclidine, but its duration of action is shorter. At high doses, it produces tachycardia, hypertension, amnesia, delirium, and motor difficulties; abusers may present with chest pain and rhabdomyolysis. Flashbacks may occur, and memory may be impaired for several days.

1,4-Butanediol/γ-Hydroxybutyrate

Butanediol is an anesthetic agent converted on ingestion to γ-hydroxybutyrate (GHB), which is an active metabolite of the inhibitory neurotransmitter GABA. It has anesthetic qualities and induces a sense of euphoria and sexual disinhibition, making it a popular club drug referred to as "GHB," "Grievous Bodily Harm," "G," "Liquid Ecstasy," and "Georgia Home Boy." Outside the United States, the drug is used as an anesthetic. Sources from inside the United States include γ-butyrolactone (GBL), which has been sold as a supplement in health food stores and over the Internet; it is converted to GHB on ingestion. GHB can also be produced by mixing of GBL with sodium hydroxide. Toxic effects include vomiting, respiratory depression, seizures, short-duration coma, and death. Addiction and withdrawal have also been reported.

Alcohol and Tobacco

See Chapters 54 and 228.

DIAGNOSIS (1,11–15)

The diagnosis of substance abuse and substance dependence requires the presence of a cluster of behavioral, cognitive, and physiologic findings (see Table 235.1).

WORKUP (1,11–15)

Screening for Substance Abuse

Given its prevalence, harmful health consequences, and potential treatability, substance abuse should be screened for as part of the routine prevention and health maintenance examination for adults. Particular attention needs to be paid to persons who present with suggestive history or physical findings (Table 235.2). The effectiveness of screening has been has been extensively demonstrated and proven to be superior to routine medical advice or nonspecific alcohol or drug counseling. When combined with referral and treatment, it can decrease the frequency and severity of drug and alcohol use, reduce the risk of trauma, and increase the percentage of patients who enter specialized substance abuse treatment.

Screening instruments can be useful for substance-abuse identification. The *Drug Abuse Screening Test (DAST-20)* and the *Alcohol, Smoking and Substance Involvement Screening Test* (ASSIST; see http://www.sbirt.samhsa.gov) are the most commonly used tools with proven research validity and clinical utility. They are as useful complement to an office workup.

History

Broaching the Subject

The best means of screening is by history. Because drug use may be an emotionally charged issue, it should be addressed after some rapport with the patient has been established and discussed nonjudgmentally. It is important that the physician feel comfortable in obtaining the history, neither apologizing for asking nor suggesting blame. Apologizing ("I have to ask these questions" or "I'm sure this doesn't apply to you, but") may actually make it more difficult for the substance-abusing patient to respond honestly. Again, the importance of a nonjudgmental approach to getting an accurate history and forming a therapeutic relationship cannot be overemphasized (see http://www.niaaa.nih.gov).

Clues to its Presence

Clues leading to the presence of substance use problems include significant *psychosocial change* or *stresses* such as recent marriage or relationship difficulties, *loss of employment*, decline in *school performance*, or *legal difficulties*.

Basic Inquiry

When a problem is suspected, inquiry is directed toward obtaining basic information, including age of first use, frequency, symptoms of tolerance, withdrawal, difficulty cutting down, time spent obtaining and taking the drugs, effects on social, medical, mental functioning, and continued use despite recognized adverse consequences. Past treatment history, periods of

---

TABLE 235.2

HISTORICAL AND PHYSICAL FINDINGS SUGGESTIVE OF SUBSTANCE ABUSE

Substance	History	Physical Findings
Opiates	Fever HIV infection Hepatitis B Pneumonia, tuberculosis	Needle tracks, petechiae, murmur Lymphadenopathy, rash Jaundice, hepatomegaly/tenderness Pulmonary consolidation
Sedatives	Depression Seizures Lethargy, amnesia	Psychomotor retardation, sadness Observed convulsion Cognitive impairment
Stimulants	Agitation Nasal congestion Stroke, focal deficits Chest pain, infarction Syncope, palpitations	Delirium Perforated septum; mucosal edema New neurologic deficits New S_4 gallop, single S_2 Arrhythmia, enlarged heart, S_3
Hallucinogens	Psychosis, hallucinations Enlarged breasts in male patient	Disordered thinking Gynecomastia
Alcohol	See Chapter 228	
Any substance	Withdrawal syndrome	Tremor, tachycardia, agitation, fever

Adapted from Shine RD. The diagnosis of drug dependence by primary care providers. J Gen Intern Med 1991;6(Suppl):S32, with permission.

TABLE 235.3

URINE DRUG TESTING

Substance	Time Window for Testing
Alcohol	12 hr
Cocaine	24–72 hr
Benzodiazepines	24–72 hr
Heroin	24 hr
Methadone	72 hr
Buprenorphine	72 hr
Amphetamines	48 hr
Marijuana	3–30 days
Phencyclidine	3–10 days

abstinence, longest abstinence in the past, and relapses provide information on the progression and severity of the drug use problem.

Physical Examination

Physical examination should include a check for manifestations of intravenous drug abuse (e.g., fever, tachycardia, icterus, needle puncture marks and "tracks," hand edema, heart murmur, thrombophlebitis, abscesses). Other signs to check for include hypertension, papillary constriction, ulceration and perforation of the nasal septum, mucosal congestion, gynecomastia, lymphadenopathy, liver enlargement, tremor, and cognitive impairment. Less specific but more common clues include poor hygiene or unkempt appearance, poor nutrition, and a change in alertness or pattern of speech.

Laboratory

When substance abuse is suspected, a *toxicology screen* with urine and blood testing may be helpful. For patients suspected of abusing alcohol, it is best to check the blood or use a breathalyzer. For suspected opioid-abusing patients, in addition to checking for opioids, it is important to check for methadone and buprenorphine separately because these do not produce opioid-positive results in routine urine tests (Table 235.3) Also part of the workup are complete blood count and differential, blood chemistry profile, hepatitis panel, syphilis serology, pregnancy test for females, tuberculin skin test, chest x-ray, and electrocardiogram in patients older than 40 years of age. HIV testing (see Chapter 13) should be done with the patient's consent.

PRINCIPLES OF MANAGEMENT
(1,12,14,16–23)

Overall Approach

Substance abuse treatment may be divided into two phases: the *initiation* of abstinence in the short term and the *maintenance* of abstinence in the long term. The disorders are best approached as chronic, relapsing, progressive diseases.

Even after successful treatment, patients remain at high risk for relapse. Relapses should be seen not as failures of treatment, but as recurrent disease and as occasions to reinstate abstinence and subsequently to redouble efforts to maintain abstinence.

Establishing mutual trust is a critical task for effective management. Mutual mistrust has been well documented in studies of the interactions of physicians providing primary medical care to opiate-addicted patients. Proactive but nonconfrontational approaches that are well matched to a patient's stage of motivation can help to build mutual trust.

Getting the Patient into Care—Matching Approach with Motivation

The best chance of successful intervention, even with severe dependence and high levels of denial, is to match the patient's motivational state with treatment approach. This can be done by using the standard stage-of-change construct for achieving behavioral change.

In the *precontemplative stage*, the patient does not recognize a problem and a labeling, coercive approach will fail. The best strategy is to be empathic in demonstrating to the patient the problems (such as liver disease or loss of employment) that can result from substance abuse. Even in the face of patient resistance, an empathic, nonjudgmental approach will often lead to more-open discussion.

In the *contemplation stage,* the patient recognizes a problem but is ambivalent about stopping, and the treatment strategy is to use the ambivalence to demonstrate the downside of the substance use. Similarly, with the *planning stage,* the treatment should be designed to help the patient and family to plan concrete steps to implement to change. Then, in the *action stage* with support (Alcoholic Anonymous is a good example) the patient carries out behavioral changes that result in abstinence.

In the *maintenance stage*, the focus is relapse prevention: high-risk behavior is examined and changed before a return to precontemplation. It is important to honor confidentiality, but it useful to include the family in matching the treatment with the stage of change. Forceful confrontation will almost always result in increased resistance and withdrawal from treatment. Keeping information about referral resources close at hand helps to take advantage of the patient's motivation. Although an intoxicated patient has impaired judgment and insight, he or she often remembers an empathic, nonjudgmental clinician and seeks help later.

Comprehensive Substance Abuse Treatment

Comprehensive substance abuse treatment is best left to specialists and specialized organizations, although advances in pharmacotherapy hold promise for some treatment in the primary care setting (see later discussion). Treatment programs vary according to the patient and the substance, but successful programs have several characteristics in common:

- *Evaluation* for comorbid psychiatric or medical disorders (the presence of a comorbid psychiatric disorder worsens prognosis).
- *Education* about the effects of the drug and the nature of addiction.

- Use of *mutual support groups* such as Alcoholics Anonymous or the similarly organized Narcotics Anonymous.
- *Individual psychotherapy.*
- *Family involvement* and the promotion of a sense of belonging, and the use of other supportive measures such as exercise, meditation, and discussion of spirituality, which may include organized religion.
- Emphasis on *abstinence* and *rehabilitation.*

Importance of Abstinence

Most treatment programs stress a combination of abstinence and rehabilitation. Although there have been reports of alcoholic patients returning safely to controlled drinking, it is impossible to identify such persons ahead of time. It appears that for most people who have been drug dependent, a single use reawakens the strong positive feelings and individual vulnerabilities that produced the dependence to begin with and also loosens restraint. Thus, complete abstinence is clearly the best way to avoid relapse.

Pharmacologic Therapy

Advances noted earlier in understanding the pathophysiology of substance abuse have led to new avenues of pharmacologic intervention. They provide the opportunity to expand treatment to more patients and improve adherence by making possible treatment in the primary care setting. Combination with counseling appears to be the best approach to pharmacologic therapy.

For Opiate Dependence. *Opioid agonist substitution* is the primary approach to preventing withdrawals and cravings and blocking the euphoric effects of heroin and other illicit opioid drugs.

Methadone is an orally active opiate agonist that does not induce euphoria when used in proper doses and has been the mainstay of this approach, which is restricted to outpatient treatment programs only and regulated under federal and state laws. Methadone maintenance therapy is of proven efficacy in retaining persons in treatment and reducing illicit drug use. It permits opioid-dependent patients to stabilize their lives and avoid the dangers of IV drug abuse. Administration is restricted to specially licensed treatment centers where patients must come to have their dose administered and taken under direct observation. At these programs, in addition to methadone treatment, patients are provided with weekly individual and group therapies. Patient treatment with other involved health care professionals is coordinated to ensure optimal care. Patients are required to provide random samples for urine toxicology. Compliant patients can earn "take home" privileges up to 6 to 13 doses at a time. The need to expand treatment beyond methadone clinics has been a stimulus to the development of alternative approaches to pharmacotherapy.

Buprenorphine is a partial opioid agonist with an intrinsic activity of 40% at the μ receptor (which makes it a weak opioid) and is the first U.S. Food and Drug Administration (FDA)–approved self-administered medication for the office-based treatment of opioid addiction. A waiver to prescribe buprenorphine for opioid addiction is required. The drug's high affinity at the μ receptor, weak opioid effects, and slow dissociation rate make it well suited for maintenance therapy. It is classified as a Schedule III drug by the FDA, and is available for outpatient use as a sublingual tablet in combination with the opioid antagonist *naloxone* (Suboxone) in 2 : 0.5 ratio. Naloxone is not absorbed sublingually, but its presence limits IV abuse potential of the sublingual tablet because it is active if the sublingual pill is crushed and injected. In randomized, controlled trials, more than 50% of patients treated in the outpatient setting with this medication showed no evidence of opioid use in urine testing at 4 weeks and adverse effects no greater than those of placebo. Research is under way to identify the best strategies for use in the primary care setting, with weekly counseling by nurses in combination with drug distribution appearing to be effective and showing much promise for expanding the number of opioid-dependent persons coming under care and adhering to therapy.

For Cocaine Dependence. Specific pharmacologic treatment to diminish craving is not available for cocaine (despite limited success with *desipramine* and *dopamine agonists*). *Acupuncture* is no better than placebo.

Treatment of Acute Overdoses and Toxic Reactions

An overdose or toxic reaction should be treated in the emergency department setting. The details of such treatment are beyond the scope of this book, but some highlights are included here to aid in decision making and triage:

- *Cocaine*: no specific cocaine antagonist; treatment is aimed at relieving symptoms and providing cardiovascular support.
- *Opiates*: cardiovascular and airway supportive care; *naloxone* (Narcan), an opiate antagonist, is administered intravenously; the usual dose is 0.01 mg/kg; an average dose is approximately two ampules (0.8 mg); its half-life is shorter than the half-life of heroin, so continuous observation and possibly repeated dosing are necessary.
- *Sedative–hypnotics*: airway and cardiovascular support; the benzodiazepine antagonist *flumazenil* is available, but clinical experience is limited.
- *Marijuana*: for panic reaction, offering reassurance that the feeling will pass, and ensuring that the patient is in a safe environment.
- *Hallucinogens*: for a "bad trip," reassurance and maintenance of a safe environment; rarely, 1 to 2 mg of *lorazepam* orally (or its equivalent) for agitation; for extreme agitation or delirium, 2 mg of lorazepam every 2 hours (or the equivalent) as needed. Physical restraint is often more provoking than beneficial and is particularly dangerous with the extreme agitation and muscle injury that accompany phencyclidine use. It is essential to obtain a toxic screen to search for adulterants and additional drugs. For flashbacks, reassurance is best.

INDICATIONS FOR ADMISSION AND REFERRAL

Patients who are physically dependent on sedative–hypnotics, alcohol-dependent patients with a history of severe withdrawal symptoms, persons with serious complicating medical or psychiatric conditions, and those who have previously failed to improve with outpatient treatment should be referred for inpatient treatment. Detoxification can be safely performed on an outpatient basis in appropriate cases, but a comprehensive specialized program is required. Opiate inpatient detoxification protocols are based on the following:

■ Substitution of the long-acting oral opiate methadone for short-acting injected opiates, such as heroin, with a taper during 4 days to 2 weeks, depending on the setting; or

■ Use of the opiate agonist/antagonist buprenorphine, which can be given intramuscularly or sublingually during a course of 4 to 5 days.

All detoxification programs must be accompanied by strong psychological and social support, education, and planning for long-term treatment that should include, whenever possible, the continued support and involvement of the primary care physician.

Annotated Bibliography

1. American Psychiatric Association. Diagnostic and statistical manual of mental disorders, 4th ed., text revision. Washington DC: Author, 2000. (*The standard reference.*)
2. Substance Abuse and Mental Health Services Administration. Results from the 2006 National Survey on Drug Use and Health: national findings (DHHS Publication No. SMA 07-4293). Rockville, MD: Author, 2007. (*Presents the best epidemiologic data documenting major use.*)
3. Cami J, Farre M. Drug addiction. N Engl J Med 2003;349:975. (*A comprehensive review of neurobiology and pathophysiology; 105 references.*)
4. Cherubin CE, Sapira JD. The medical complications of drug addiction and the medical assessment of the intravenous drug user: 25 years later. Ann Intern Med 1993;119:1017. (*An important review for the primary care physician.*)
5. Levine SR, Brust JCM, Frutell N, et al. Cerebrovascular complications of the use of the "crack" form of alkaloidal cocaine. N Engl J Med 1990;323:699. (*Finds that the major adverse effect was not fully appreciated.*)
6. Lynskey MT, Heath AD, Bucholz KK, et al. Escalation of drug use in early-onset cannabis users vs co-twin controls. JAMA 2003;289:427. (*A cross-sectional twin study, showing that the effect of peers and the social context of use were powerful determinants.*)
7. McClellan AT, Lewis DC, O'Brien P, et al. Drug dependence, a chronic medical illness: implications for treatment, insurance, and outcomes evaluation. JAMA 2000;284:1689. (*A thoughtful piece on dependence as a medical condition.*)
8. Solowij N, Stephens RS, Roffman RA, et al. Cognitive functioning of long-term heavy cannabis users seeking treatment. JAMA 2002;287:1123. (*A retrospective, cross-sectional study, finding impairments in memory and attention.*)
9. Tinsley JA, Watkins DD. Over-the-counter stimulants: abuse and addiction. Mayo Clin Proc 1998;73:977. (*A good review of this often-overlooked area of addiction, emphasizing the abuse of ephedrine and phenylpropanolamine.*)
10. Zvosec DL, Smith SW, McCutcheon JR, et al. Adverse events, including death, associated with the use of 1,4-butanediol. N Engl J Med 2002;344:87. (*Documents the serious side effects from this popular "club drug."*)
11. Allen PA, Litten RZ. Screening instruments and biochemical screening tests. In: Principles of addiction medicine, 2nd ed. Chevy Chase, MD: American Society of Addiction Medicine, 1998:263. (*A comprehensive guide, with a good section on screening methods.*)
12. Galanter M, Kleber HD, eds. Textbook of substance abuse treatment, 3rd ed. Washington DC: American Psychiatric Publishing, 2004. (*An authoritative resource.*)
13. Center for Substance Abuse Treatment. Medication-assisted treatment for opioid addiction in opioid treatment programs (DHHS Publication No. SMA 05-4048). Rockville, MD: Substance Abuse and Mental Health Services Administration, 2005. (*Presents screening and treatment strategies and evidence of efficacy.*)
14. Conigliaro J, Delos Reyes C, Parran TV, et al. Principles of screening and early intervention. In: Graham AW, Schultz TK, Mayo-Smith MF, et al., eds. Principles of addiction medicine, 3rd ed. Chevy Chase, MD: American Society of Addiction Medicine, 2003. (*Authoritative discussion.*)
15. Shine D. The diagnosis of drug dependence by primary care providers. J Gen Intern Med 1991;6(Suppl):S32. (*A useful discussion of basic approaches to recognition in the office.*)
16. Center for Substance Abuse Treatment. Clinical guidelines for the use of buprenorphine in the treatment of opioid addiction. (DHHS Publication No. SMA 04-3939). Rockville, MD: Substance Abuse and Mental Health Services Administration, 2004. (*Consensus guidelines for the pharmacologic treatment of opioid addiction.*)
17. DiClemente C, Prochaska J, Fairhurst S, et al. The process of smoking cessation: an analysis of precontemplation, contemplation, and preparation stages of change. J Consult Clin Psychol 1991;59:295. (*A classic study of the stages-of-change model.*)
18. Fiellin DA, Pantalon MV, Chawarski MC, et al. Counseling plus buprenorphine–naloxone maintenance therapy for opioid dependences. N Engl J Med 2006;355:365. (*Compares two programs for use in the primary care setting, finding that both were effective for increasing compliance and use.*)
19. Fudala PJ, Bridge TP, Herbert S, et al. Office-based treatment of opiate addiction with a sublingual-tablet formulation of buprenorphine and naloxone. N Engl J Med 2003;349:949. (*A randomized, controlled trial [RCT], demonstrating the efficacy and safety of opioid treatment in an office-based setting.*)
20. Johnson RE, Chutuape MA, Strain EC, et al. A comparison of levomethadyl acetate, buprenorphine, and methadone for opioid dependence. N Engl J Med 2000;343:1290. (*RCT, showing equal efficacy.*)
21. Merrill JO, Rhodes LA, Deyo RA, et al. Mutual mistrust in the medical care of drug users: the key to the "narc" cabinet. J Gen Intern Med 2002;17:327. (*Qualitative analysis study revealing a significant degree of mistrust and suggesting means for overcoming it.*)
22. National Institute on Drug Abuse. Available at: http://www.clubdrugs.org. (*A helpful web site for information on substance abuse in the club setting.*)
23. Sees KL, Delucchi KL, Masson C, et al. Methadone maintenance vs. 180-day psychosocially enriched detoxification for treatment of opioid dependence: a randomized controlled trial. JAMA 2000;283:1303. (*Methadone maintenance was the more effective treatment in terms of reducing heroin use and high-risk behaviors.*)

APPENDIX 235.1: ADULT ATTENTION-DEFICIT/HYPERACTIVITY DISORDER

Attention deficit/hyperactivity disorder (ADHD), characterized by difficulties with inattention, hyperactivity, and impulsivity, was once believed to only affect children, but recent longitudinal, controlled studies confirm the lay impression that the condition persists and can affect adults. About 4% of adults in the United States are estimated to suffer from the condition (there is some question of overdiagnosis in the United States because the prevalence is reported to be about 1% in Europe). The condition may occur in the context of and complicate other mental health problems, such as substance abuse, depression, and anxiety. The frequency, potential disruptiveness, and co-existence of the problem with other mental health conditions make its recognition by the primary care physician important to timely and effective management.

PATHOPHYSIOLOGY AND CLINICAL PRESENTATION (1–6)

The adult form of ADHD is hereditary and associated with structural and functional abnormalities detectable on anatomic and functional neuroimaging studies. The frontocortical area of the brain seems to be the most involved. There is evidence of neurotransmitter dysfunction, especially with catecholamine regulation of dopamine and norepinephrine release. In addition, there appears to be an increased density of dopamine transporter in the striatum of the brain—the site of

TABLE 235.4

DIAGNOSTIC CRITERIA FOR ATTENTION-DEFICIT/HYPERACTIVITY DISORDER

A. Either (1) or (2):
  (1) inattention: six (or more) of the following symptoms of inattention have persisted for at least 6 months to a degree that is maladaptive and inconsistent with developmental level:
     (a) often fails to give close attention to details or makes careless mistakes in school work, work, or other activities
     (b) often has difficulty sustaining attention in tasks or play activities
     (c) often does not seem to listen when spoken to directly
     (d) often does not follow through on instructions and fails to finish school work, chores, or duties in the workplace (not due to oppositional behavior or failure to understand instructions)
     (e) often has difficulty organizing tasks and activities
     (f) often avoids, dislikes, or is reluctant to engage in tasks that require sustained mental effort (such as schoolwork or homework)
     (g) often loses things necessary for tasks or activities (e.g., toys, school assignments, pencils, books, or tools)
     (h) is often easily distracted by extraneous stimuli
     (i) is often forgetful in daily activities
  (2) hyperactivity–impulsivity: six (or more) of the following symptoms of hyperactivity–impulsivity have persisted for at least 6 months to a degree that is maladaptive and inconsistent with developmental level:
     Hyperactivity
     (a) often fidgets with hands or feet or squirms in seat
     (b) often leaves seat in classroom or in other situations in which remaining seated is expected
     (c) often runs about or climbs excessively in situations in which it is inappropriate (in adolescents or adults, may be limited to subjective feelings of restlessness)
     (d) often has difficulty playing or engaging in leisure activities quietly
     (e) is often "on the go" or often acts as if "driven by a motor"
     (f) often talks excessively
     Impulsivity
     (g) often blurts out answers before questions have been completed
     (h) often has difficulty awaiting turn
     (i) often interrupts or intrudes on others (e.g., butts into conversations or games)
B. Some hyperactive–impulsive or inattentive symptoms that caused impairment were present before age 7 years.
C. Some impairment from the symptoms is present in two or more settings (e.g., at school [or work] and at home).
D. There must be clear evidence of clinically significant impairment in social, academic, or occupational functioning.
E. The symptoms do not occur exclusively during the course of a pervasive developmental disorder, schizophrenia, or other psychotic disorder and are not better accounted for by another mental disorder (e.g., mood disorder, anxiety disorder, dissociative disorders, or a personality disorder).

From American Psychiatric Association. Diagnostic and statistical manual of mental disorders, 4th ed., text revision. Washington, DC: American Psychiatric Association, 2004, with permission.

action of many pharmacologic agents used to treat the condition. Geneticstudies suggest a role for genes coding for proteins that affect neurotransmitters at brain synapses, especially dopamine,norepinephrine, and serotonin.

Characteristic clinical features include symptoms of *inattention, hyperactivity,* and *impulsivity* (Table 235.4) that begin in *childhood* and continue into adulthood. Although most patients continue to manifest most of the same symptoms they had as children, the inattention tends to be the most problematic and most notable in adult life, whereas hyperactivity and impulsivity tend to lessen with age. Concurrent psychopathology is common. Persons with ADHD have an increased risk of

substance abuse, smoking, anxiety, and *depression.* Moreover, up to 20% of persons with substance abuse have ADHD, and similar ADHD frequencies are seen in persons with anxiety, depression, and bipolar disease.

DIAGNOSIS (1,2,7–9)

The diagnosis is made clinically, based on history of defining criteria established by the American Psychiatric Association and described in the *Diagnostic and Statistical Manual of Mental Disorders,* fourth edition (see Table 235.4). Patient recall and reports of partners have proven to be reliable and correlate well with findings from formal evaluations. The confirmation of patient reports by clinical interview is recommended, as is the use of validated questionnaire instruments (e.g., the Conners Rating Scales). Assessments for concurrent anxiety, depression, and substance abuse (see Chapters 226, 227, and 235) are indicated because of the high frequency with which they occur with ADHD.

MANAGEMENT (2,8–11)

Management is best carried out by those experienced and skilled in dealing with the condition, especially if there is also concurrent psychopathology evident. Data on treatment efficacy for adult ADHD are much more limited than they are for children, with few modalities subjected to large-scale, prospective, randomized trials. There are no published treatment guidelines.

Modalities supported at least by a modicum of evidence include *cognitive–behavioral therapy* and pharmacotherapy using *stimulants* (methylphenidate, amphetamine, pemoline), *antidepressants* (tricyclics, bupropion), and *nonstimulant noradrenergic agents* (e.g., atomoxetine,). These drugs are believed to work in ADHD by altering the levels of dopamine and norepinephrine at the synapse. Those with FDA approval include *atomoxetine (Strattera)*, a *mixed amphetamine salts* preparation (*Adderall*), and *dexmethylphenidate (Focalin)*.

Concerns have arisen about long-term ADHD drug use in adults, especially with regard to stimulants and their potential for adverse cardiovascular effects, such as *tachycardia* and *hypertension*. Blood pressure should be monitored with use. *Nervousness* is also a common side effect, and *sleep difficulties* might develop. Physicians prescribing these agents in persons with underlying heart disease or cardiovascular risk factors should take these potential adverse cardiovascular effects into account. There is no evidence that taking stimulants for ADHD begets *substance abuse*, and some that it may prevent it.

PATIENT EDUCATION AND INDICATIONS FOR REFERRAL (9)

Patients who are not doing well in life and have clear evidence of adult ADHD are grateful to learn that they have a medical condition that can be helped. Persons who have no evidence for the condition but blame their fate on it need to be corrected so that they can focus more clearly and effectively on the root causes of their true problems.

Mental health referral is indicated for confirmation of the condition and management. The unsettled approach to treatment necessitates care in the referral to ensure care by a psychiatric specialist skilled in both offering cognitive–behavioral approaches and managing the psychopharmacology of adult AD/HD. The high frequency of concurrent psychopathology underscores the importance of referral.

Annotated Bibliography

1. American Psychiatric Association. Diagnostic and statistical manual of mental disorders, 4th ed., text revision. Washington, DC: American Psychiatric Association, 2004. (*The diagnostic bible of psychiatry.*)
2. Biederman J, Faraone SV. Attention-deficit hyperactivity disorder. Lancet 2005;366:237. (*Includes a good review of disease mechanisms.*)
3. Hervey AS, Epstein JN, Curry JF. Neuropsychology of adults with attention-deficit hyperactivity disorder: a meta-analytic review. Neuropsychology 2004;18:485. (*An excellent review of neuropathophysiology.*)
4. Kessler RC, Adler L, Barkley R, et al. The prevalence and correlates of adult ADHD in the United States: results from the National Comorbidity Survey Replication. Am J Psychiatry 2006;163:716. (*The best data on U.S. prevalence.*)
5. Levin FR, Evans S, Kleber HD. Prevalence of adult attention-deficit/hyperactivity disorder among cocaine abusers seeking treatment. Drug Alcohol Depend 1998;52:15. (*Evidence of concurrent attention-deficit/hyperactivity disorder in substance abusers.*)
6. Weiss G, Hechtman L, Milroy T, et al. Psychiatric status of hyperactives as adults: a controlled prospective 15-year follow-up of 63 hyperactive children.

J Am Acad Child Psychiatry 1985;24:211. (*Early data establishing that the condition continues into adulthood.*)
7. McCann BS, Roy-Byrne P. Screening and diagnostic utility of self-report attention deficit hyperactivity disorder scales in adults. Compr Psychiatry 2004;45:175. (*Documents much misdiagnosis by self-reports and by screening instruments.*)
8. Okie S. ADHD in adults. N Engl J Med 2006;354:2637. (*An informal, thoughtful discussion of the topic, with consideration of many of the controversies surrounding the problem.*)
9. Wilens TE, Faraone SV, Biederman J. Attention-deficit/hyperactivity disorder in adults. JAMA 2004;292:619. (*A review for the generalist clinician and a critical look at the evidence; 43 references.*)
10. Wilens T, Faraone S, Biederman J, et al. Does stimulant therapy of attention-deficit/hyperactivity disorder beget later substance abuse: a meta-analytic review of the literature. Pediatrics 2003;111:179. (*The summation of the evidence says that the answer is no.*)
11. Wilens T. Drug therapy for adults with attention-deficit hyperactivity disorder. Drugs 2003;63:2395. (*A review of trials.*)

CHAPTER 236 ■ APPROACH TO THE PATIENT WITH CHRONIC NONMALIGNANT PAIN

Chronic pain is a highly prevalent problem, affecting up to 17% of persons in the United States and costing an estimated $70 billion each year. Many clinicians find patients with chronic pain an emotional and intellectual challenge, in part because of the many myths surrounding the issue (Table 236.1).

Unlike acute pain, chronic pain tends to be more multifactorial, less amenable to "cure," and more influenced by psychological and social factors. It typically requires continuous long-term management. These characteristics necessitate an appropriate adjustment of expectations and approach by both clinician and patient to achieve a satisfactory outcome. The principal goal is improvement in quality of life and function rather than complete elimination of the pain.

PATHOPHYSIOLOGY AND CLINICAL PRESENTATIONS (1–4)

Definition and the Biopsychosocial Model of Pain

Pain is defined by the International Association for the Study of Pain as "an unpleasant sensory and emotional experience arising from actual or potential tissue damage." Pain is an inherently subjective phenomenon, originating from a biologic source and modified by psychological and social factors. Perceptions and reports of pain and its severity rely heavily on a person's psychosocial context. For this reason, the biopsychosocial model is useful in the conceptualization of pain.

Biologic Components

Pain derives from afferent signals of nociceptive fibers in the periphery, triggered by tissue damage or the threat of damage (nociceptive pain) or by direct neuronal activation (neuropathic pain). These afferent nociceptive fibers course back to the central nervous system via the spinothalamic tracts to both somatosensory and frontal cortices. Modulation networks from the frontal cortex and hypothalamus create a final conscious perception. These networks are the medium by which psychological factors and the psychosocial context alter the sensation of pain.

The biologic component of chronic pain is less well understood than that of acute pain. It appears that many patients suffering from chronic pain do so with a minor biologic stimulus or occasionally even without one once the process has begun. Psychological and social factors clearly play a larger role in modulating the perception and perpetuating it. Perpetuation likely occurs via neuronal sensitization and the aforementioned modulation networks.

In neuronal sensitization, the threshold for activating nociceptors is lowered by repetitive stimuli. The continuous triggering of nociceptive fibers generates pain even when the stimulus is minimal. Modulatory factors include expectation, whereby the sensation of pain is heightened by the anticipation of its arrival. This is related to the effects of norepinephrine on sympathetic input to nociceptive fibers; it lowers their threshold for activation and even activates them directly. A well-known corollary to the modulation of pain through expectation is the placebo effect, which is still poorly understood but clearly decreases an individual's perception of pain via neuronal modulation.

Psychological Components

Besides modulating pain, psychological components may actually be considered as a cause (i.e., primary) or an effect (i.e., secondary) of chronic pain. Primary psychological considerations include whether the patient has a major depression (see Chapter 227), anxiety disorder (see Chapter 226), somatoform disorder or personality disorder (see Chapters 227 and 230), or substance abuse problem (see Chapter 235) or whether the patient is malingering (Table 236.2).

Most of these disorders cause a heightened awareness of somatic sensations, a charged emotional state, and a sense of expectation. Heightened awareness results in an inability to suppress stimuli that the individual might otherwise be capable of suppressing. A charged emotional state sensitizes nociceptive fibers to stimuli, which also creates an enhanced conscious perception of pain.

Secondary psychological processes such as depression and anxiety are common among patients with chronic pain, as is secondary substance abuse if the patient self-medicates with alcohol or narcotics. These secondary processes may also contribute to modulating and perpetuating a sensation of pain.

TABLE 236.1

MYTHS SURROUNDING CHRONIC PAIN

Patients' complaints stem from secondary gains; they do not really suffer "pain"

Patients with chronic pain are inherently noncompliant and manipulative

Patients given opiates will refer manipulative friends

Opiates in therapeutic doses will cause respiratory depression

Patients given opiates will become "addicted"

Giving patients opiates for chronic nonmalignant pain will result in investigations by state and federal review boards

Chronic pain can be fixed

TABLE 236.2

PSYCHOLOGICAL AND SOCIAL FACTORS CONTRIBUTING TO CHRONIC PAIN

Psychological Factors	Social Factors
Major depression (primary or secondary)	Domestic violence
Anxiety disorders (primary or secondary)	Daily activities causing pain
Somatoform disorders	Activities hindered by pain
Personality disorders	Work hindered by pain
Substance abuse (primary or secondary)	Work contributing to pain
Malingering	Secondary gain

Social Contributors

These encompass elements in the home, in the work environment, and at leisure (see Table 236.2). Although the home environment may serve as a potential source of relief and support for the patient with chronic pain, more often it contributes to the presentation, as with domestic violence. Pain may even serve as a cause for escape from a troubled home situation to the doctor. Likewise, a person's leisure and work environments may contribute to or be hindered by pain. Social factors can drive the sensation of pain into a chronic state if secondary gain is a possibility (e.g., ongoing litigation, worker's compensation).

Categorizations of Pain

Pain can be categorized by either clinical presentation (acute vs. chronic; diffuse vs. localized) or underlying mechanism (neuropathic vs. nociceptive; biologic vs. psychosocial).

Acute versus Chronic Pain

In general, acute pain emanates from an identifiable biologic stimulus, is self-limited, does not have much of a psychological component, and is more amenable to pure pharmacologic intervention. Chronic pain is that which lasts longer than a typically expected time for healing, or 3 to 6 months. It can be further subclassified as chronic nonmalignant pain or chronic malignant pain (see Chapter 90). Chronic nonmalignant pain, on the other hand, may or may not have an identifiable biologic stimulus, is by definition not self-limited, has greater psychosocial underpinnings, and is less amenable to pure pharmacologic intervention.

Diffuse versus Localized Pain

Some patients present with total body pain or pain that migrates from one site to another. These cases tend to have dominant psychosocial components. Most patients present with pain localized to a certain anatomic region, which remains consistent over time. The most common presentations include pain localized to one of five regions: head and face, nonaxial musculoskeletal structures, low back, abdomen and pelvis, and peripheral nerves.

Nociceptive versus Neuropathic Pain

Nociceptive pain develops from actual or potential tissue or organ damage. Somatic nociceptive pain is typically attributable to specific anatomic areas or structures. Patients present with pain that is well localized and stabbing, throbbing, or achy. Visceral nociceptive pain, being organ based, is less well localized and typically more dull and cramping.

Neuropathic pain, on the other hand, derives from direct nerve stimulation. This may occur with or without a nociceptive component. The pain is typically characterized as burning, tingling, and lancinating, often occurring in a dermatomal distribution. A sensory deficit may accompany the pain. Sensitization can lead to the nerves firing in the absence of any peripheral stimulus. Examples of neuropathic pain include postherpetic neuralgia, diabetic neuropathy, sciatica, trigeminal neuralgia, reflex sympathetic dystrophy, and phantom limb pain.

Predominantly Biologic versus Predominantly Psychosocial

The balance of biologic and psychosocial components may vary tremendously. Some cases have a primarily biologic cause with no evidence of psychiatric pathology (e.g., a functional, well-adjusted octogenarian with severe osteoarthritis). Others present with the subjective report of pain but no objective findings and go on to meet formal criteria for a primary psychiatric disorder (e.g., a young professional suffering from hypochondriasis).

The majority of patients presenting with chronic pain are somewhere in between these two extremes, with a combination of both biologic and psychosocial components. Quantification of overlap has not been performed extensively in patients presenting with chronic pain, although some data exist. For example, comorbid major depression is found in 8% to 50% of patients presenting with chronic pain, with dysthymia seen in more than 75%. Anxiety disorders (both panic attack and generalized anxiety disorder) are seen in more than 50%.

DIFFERENTIAL DIAGNOSIS

Any differential diagnosis for chronic pain must include both biologic and psychosocial factors. The biologic causes are best considered in terms of pain location (Table 236.3). The psychosocial determinants are essential considerations in assessing factors that may trigger, sustain, or aggravate pain (see Table 236.2).

WORKUP

The heterogeneity of chronic pain complaints and the variety of mechanisms and presentations necessitate an exploration of both biologic and psychosocial dimensions of the problem. The workup should define the patient's psychosocial context, classify the pain process precisely, and determine the likelihood of serious underlying biologic pathology.

Defining the Psychosocial Context

All patients presenting with chronic pain must be screened carefully for depression, anxiety, evidence of a somatoform disorder or personality disorder, substance use/abuse, and possible secondary gain. Clues suggesting a primary psychological or social cause include depressed or anxious affect, history of substance abuse, multiple unrelated sites of pain, onset in adolescence, history of difficult social interactions, and absence

TABLE 236.3

DIFFERENTIAL DIAGNOSES OF CHRONIC PAIN BASED ON LOCATION

Location	Differential of Reversible Etiologies		
Headache/Facial Pain (see Chapters 165 and 214)	Tension	Sinusitis	Glaucoma
	Migraine	Chronic otitis	Medication
	Cluster	Chronic meningitis	Trigeminal neuralgia
	Temporal arteritis	Abscess	Postconcussive
	Large AVM	Subdural	Glaucoma
	Hypertension	Tumor	Bruxism
	Dentalgia	TMJ	Sialadenitis
Musculoskeletal Pain (see Chapters 147–154)	Fibromyalgia	Rheumatoid arthritis	Paget's disease
	PMR	Osteoarthritis	Tumor
	Polymyositis	Gout/pseudogout	Cramps
	Dermatomyositis	SLE	Bursitis/tendinitis
	Drug myositis	Osteomyelitis	Reflex sympathetic dystrophy
	Hypothyroidism	Trichinosis	Sickle cell disease
	Trauma	Lyme disease	Secondary syphilis
Low Back Pain (see Chapter 147)	Chronic disk disease	Osteoporotic fracture	Tumor (bone/retroperitoneum)
	Sciatica	Spinal stenosis	Seronegative spondylosis
	Vertebral osteoarthropathy	Epidural abscess	
Abdominal/Pelvic Pain (see Chapters 58 and 116)	Irritable bowel	IBD	Kidney stones
	Biliary colic	Diverticulitis	Chronic pyelonephritis
	Esophagitis	Gastritis/PUD	Polycystic kidney
	Pancreatitis	Hepatitis	Endometriosis
	Parasitosis	Tumor (GI/GU/GYN)	Ovarian cysts
	Aortic aneurysm	Abdominal angina	PID/TOA
	Sickle cell disease	Poisoning (e.g., lead)	FMF
	Medicines	Internal hernias	Porphyria
		PMS	
Peripheral Nerve Pain (see Chapter 167)	DM neuropathy	B_{12} deficiency	Charcot–Marie–Tooth disease
	HIV neuropathy	CTDz	Hypothyroidism
	Paraneoplastic	Renal failure	Poisoning (EtOH, Pt, INH)

AVM, arteriovenous malformation; CTDz, connective tissue disease; DM, diabetes mellitus; EtOH, ethanol; FMF, familial Mediterranean fever; GI, gastrointestinal; GU, genitourinary; GYN, gynecologic; IBD, inflammatory bowel disease; INH, isoniazid; PID, pelvic inflammatory disease; PMR, polymyalgia rheumatica; PMS, premenstrual syndrome; PUD, peptic ulcer disease; Pt, platinum; SLE, systemic lupus erythematosus; TMJ, temporomandibular joint; TOA, tuboovarian abscess.

of a clear pathophysiologic mechanism (Table 236.4). Home, work, and leisure activities should be reviewed in depth for possible precipitating and aggravating social factors (see Chapter 110 for a more detailed discussion of screening for domestic violence).

Classifying the Process

The classic cardinal features of pain should always be documented: onset/duration, quality/severity, location/spread, alleviating/aggravating factors, and associated symptoms. Circumstances surrounding the onset of the pain, in addition to the location of pain and associated symptoms, are all particularly helpful in determining whether a patient's presentation might relate to a biologically plausible process or is predominantly psychological or psychosocial in origin. These features also help to determine whether the pain is acute or chronic, localized or diffuse, somatic or visceral, and nociceptive or neuropathic. Correct classification helps to guide further workup and management.

Patients of different cultural backgrounds describe pain quality in distinctively different terms, so that some basic cultural understanding is necessary to interpret the complaint of pain properly. For example, patients of Caribbean descent often describe abdominal pain as *grippée*, whereas Southeast Asians may use temperature to describe abdominal pain, and Latinos refer to many sensations as *nervios*. Pain severity can be assessed by standard severity scales, most of which are cross-culturally reproducible. Examples include the visual analogue pain scale or 1-to-10 rating scales. These scales may also be useful when applied to stepwise pharmacologic management, so it is worth documenting severity during the workup.

SIGNS THAT PSYCHOSOCIAL FACTORS ARE PREDOMINANT IN A PATIENT'S CHRONIC PAIN

The patient admits *depression* or *anxiety* that predates the pain

The pain began in adolescence or at time of trauma (suggests *pain disorder or posttraumatic stress disorder*)

The patient has a history of *substance abuse*

There are multiple, unrelated sites of pain over time (suggests *somatization disorder*)

There is no demonstrable pathophysiologic mechanism to explain the physical symptoms

There is a history of difficult social interactions to suggest a *personality disorder*

There is evidence of physical, sexual, or emotional *abuse*

There is potential for or history of the patient pursuing secondary gains, such as litigation reward or worker's compensation (suggests malingering)

Determining the Likelihood of Serious Underlying Biologic Pathology

If the pain complaint is relatively new, has little in the way of associated psychiatric symptoms, and is accompanied by constitutional or other objective findings, then the likelihood of a primary biologic process increases markedly and the workup can focus on the appropriate physical examination and laboratory testing.

PRINCIPLES OF MANAGEMENT (3,5–22)

Initial Measures

A systematic, multidimensional approach is crucial to achieving a successful outcome for the patient with chronic pain (Fig. 236.1). Simultaneously addressing the biologic and psychosocial components helps to assure the patient that the

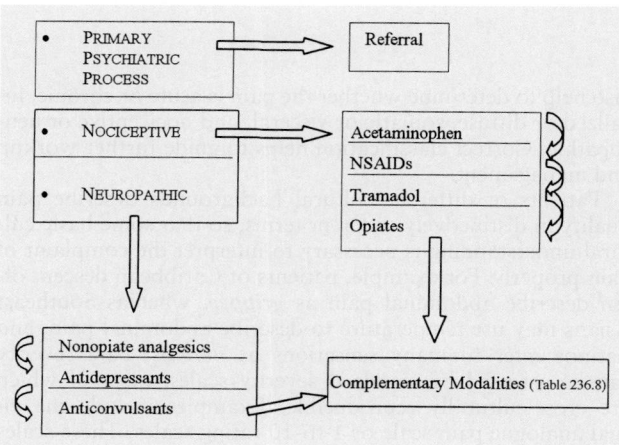

FIGURE 236.1. Sample approach to the management of patients with chronic pain. NSAIDs, nonsteroidal antiinflammatory drugs.

validity of the complaint is not in question; as a result, compliance with psychiatric referral is improved, should it be needed.

Symptomatic Relief

Early symptom relief is a priority, especially in persons with a suspected primary biologic mechanism. The intervention is usually pharmacologic, tailored to whether the pain is primarily nociceptive or neuropathic in origin. A stepwise approach is recommended, beginning with pain medications that have the greatest benefit-to-risk ratio (Table 236.5). The goal is to provide enough analgesia that daily activity can be sustained. Complementary approaches to pain control may be needed when medications do not suffice.

Early Psychiatric Referral

Early referral is essential if the initial evaluation reveals evidence for a primary psychiatric or psychosocial problem (e.g., anxiety, depression, somatization disorder, domestic violence). Effective management may require formal psychiatric input, including psychopharmacologic intervention, psychotherapy, and social interventions. Patients with what appears to be a psychiatric process secondary to the chronic pain are better managed by first addressing the biologic cause of the pain rather than by early psychiatric referral because attention to biologic factors is likely to improve both processes at once. However, even after biologic issues are attended to, it may help to focus on the dysfunctional behaviors and thinking associated with chronic pain. For this purpose, cognitive–behavioral therapy appears well suited.

Cognitive–Behavioral Therapy. Cognitive–behavioral therapy attempts to transform patterns of negative attitudes and behaviors into more productive thoughts, emotions, and actions. This is accomplished by training the patient to recognize current responses and to develop healthier responses and the skills to execute them. Evidence of efficacy is accumulating in a wide variety of chronic pain settings, ranging from low back pain to tension headache. Cognitive–behavioral therapy appears to be one of the most promising of psychotherapeutic approaches to the management of chronic pain. Results are best when the therapy is carried out by specifically trained individuals.

Nociceptive (Nonneuropathic) Pain (5–11)

Treatment begins with nonnarcotic analgesics and advances to narcotic agents as required. Nonnarcotic analgesics are first-line treatment for nociceptive pain, with acetaminophen being the first step for most situations.

Acetaminophen

Its mechanism of action is unknown, but it continues to be the drug of choice of the American College of Rheumatology and the National Kidney Foundation for the treatment of chronic pain. Acetaminophen at 1,000 mg four times daily is as effective as nonsteroidal antiinflammatory drugs (NSAIDs). This dose of acetaminophen is safe in those patients who drink fewer than five alcoholic beverages per day and have no known hepatic dysfunction. The most common side effect is mild gastrointestinal upset.

Nonsteroidal Antiinflammatory Drugs

NSAIDs are an excellent choice for nociceptive pain due to inflammatory disease. Aspirin is the prototypic NSAID, being

TABLE 236.5

OVERVIEW OF MEDICATIONS USED TO TREAT PAIN

Generic Name	Brand Name	Initial Oral Dose (mg)	Maximum Oral Dose (mg)	Comments
Nonnarcotic Analgesics				
Acetaminophen	Tylenol	500–1,000 q4–6h	1,000 qd	Reduce dose with alcohol use or known liver disease
Tramadol	Ultram	50–100 q6h	400/d	Nausea, vomiting, diarrhea; seizures with antidepressants
Nonsteroidal Antiinflammatory Drugs				
Aspirin	Ecotrin, Bayer	325–650 q4–6h	650 q4h	Dyspepsia/peptic ulcer disease
Ibuprofen	Advil, Motrin, Nuprin	200–800 q6h	800 q6h	GI/renal
Naproxen	Naprosyn, Aleve	250–500 q12h	500 q12h	GI/renal
Etodolac	Lodine	200 q8h	400 q8h	GI/renal
Indomethacin	Indocin	25–50 q8h	50 q8h	GI/renal
Ketorolac	Toradol	10 q6h	10 q4h	GI/renal (use <5 days)
Salsalate	Disalcid	500 bid	1,000 tid	GI/renal
Celecoxib	Celebrex	100 bid	200 bid	Less GI toxicity
Opioid Analgesics				
Codeine	In Tylenol Nos. 2–4	15 q4h	60 q4h	Nausea, vomiting, constipation Sedation, respiratory depression
Oxycodone	In Percocet	5 q6h	10 q4h	Same as codeine
Oxycodone SR	OxyContin	10 q12	30 q8h	Same as codeine
Morphine	Roxanol elixir	10 q6h	30 q4h	Same as codeine, pruritus
Morphine SR	MS Contin	60 q12	180 q8h	Same as codeine
Hydromor-phone	Dilaudid	2 q6h	2 q4h	Same as codeine
Methadone	Dolophine	20 q8	20 q4h	Same as codeine
Meperidine	Demerol	50 q4h	150 q3h	Same as codeine, seizure from metabolites
Fentanyl patch	Duragesic	25 g/hr q72h	200 g/hr q72h	Same as codeine
Anticonvulsants				
Gabapentin	Neurontin	100 qhs	1,200 tid	Sedation
Baclofen	Lioresal	5q8	20 q6h	Sedation
Phenytoin	Dilantin	150 qd	300 qd (level)	Multiple—refer to PDR; follow levels
Carbamazepine	Tegretol	200 q8	400 q8h (level)	Sedation; follow levels
Clonazepam	Klonopin	0.5 q6	1–5 q6h	Sedation
Antidepressants				
Doxepin	Sinequan	25 bid	100 q8h	High sedation/low arrhythmia; anticholinergic++
Amitriptyline	Elavil	25 qhs	75 bid	High sedation/high arrhythmia; anticholinergic++
Imipramine	Tofranil	75 qhs	75 bid	Moderate sedation/high arrhythmia; anticholinergic++
Nortriptyline	Pamelor	25 qhs	25 q6h	Moderate sedation/high arrhythmia; anticholinergic+
Desipramine	Norpramin	25 qhs	150 bid	Low sedation/high arrhythmia
Paroxetine	Paxil	20 qd	50 qd	GI upset, insomnia, nervousness, sedation, sexual dysfunction
Fluoxetine	Prozac	20 qd	80 qd	GI upset, insomnia, nervousness, sedation, sexual dysfunction

q3h, q4h, q4–6h, q8h, q12h, q72h: every 3, 4, 4–6, 8, 12, 72 hr, respectively; qd, daily; bid, twice daily; tid, thrice daily; qhs, at bedtime; GI, gastrointestinal; PDR, *Physicians' Desk Reference*.

directly analgesic in addition to being antiinflammatory; it is the milligram-for-milligram equivalent of acetaminophen. However, its long-term use for chronic pain is complicated by the risk of gastrointestinal ulceration and bleeding. *Nonselective NSAIDs* (e.g., ibuprofen, naproxen) provide analgesia comparable to aspirin and acetaminophen and synergism with opioids (see later discussion), but gastrointestinal toxicity can be substantial. Concurrent use of a proton-pump inhibitor (e.g., omeprazole, lansoprazole) or misoprostol reduces the risks of peptic ulceration and bleeding (see Chapter 68). Use is also problematic in the settings of hypertension, heart failure, and renal insufficiency (see Chapters 26, 32, and 142). The more *selective cyclooxygenase-2 inhibitor NSAIDs* cause less gastrointestinal toxicity, but cardiovascular risk increases two- to threefold when high doses are used for prolonged periods of time; careful patient selection and consideration of risks and benefits are essential to safe use (see Chapters 155 and 156).

Tramadol

This centrally acting analgesic has dual effects; it acts primarily as a monoamine (norepinephrine and serotonin) reuptake inhibitor that blocks pain transmission in the spinal cord and secondarily as a blocker of central nervous system μ-opioid receptors. It has a very low potential for abuse. Comparative studies in patients with osteoarthritis have shown it to be equivalent in analgesic effect to naproxen and propoxyphene. It is rapidly absorbed, with a peak effect at 2 hours and a half-life of 6 hours. It is metabolized by the liver, then excreted by the kidneys. Its benefits include a relative lack of potential for abuse and respiratory depression in comparison with opiates, but it still causes many side effects, including nausea, drowsiness, sweating, and constipation. Slowly titrating the dose upward can minimize the transient nausea. Tramadol might be considered as an opiate alternative once acetaminophen has failed in disease states without much objective inflammation, such as osteoarthritis.

Antidepressants

Although more effective for neuropathic pain (see later discussion), the tricyclics and the serotonin-norepinephrine reuptake inhibitors (e.g., duloxetine—agents that act on norepinephrine) exhibit some efficacy in persons with nociceptive pain, particularly patients suffering from fibromyalgia (see Chapter 159).

Opiates

Opiates are the most potent class of analgesics for the treatment of chronic nociceptive pain. They are effective for a host of other pain syndromes, including neuropathic pain, which traditionally had been deemed unresponsive (see later discussion). Many clinicians agonize over whether to prescribe opiates for chronic nonmalignant pain, a difficulty usually stemming from misconceptions (Table 236.1). Perhaps the most pervasive misconception is the idea that patients placed on long-term therapy with opiates will become "addicts." Although tolerance is common with prolonged use, pathologic drug-seeking behavior is unlikely when patients are carefully selected and opiate therapy is properly prescribed and supervised. Important issues associated with chronic opiate use for pain control include the efficacy of long-term use and the effect of increasing dose on safety and efficacy.

Addiction, Substance Abuse, and Tolerance. Distinctions must be made among the terms substance abuse, addiction, and tolerance because many clinicians erroneously equate them. *Substance abuse* implies the problem of dangerous use of an agent, with or without physical dependence. The term *addiction* implies compulsive substance use and an inability to control intake despite negative consequences. *Tolerance* to narcotics has nothing to do with abuse or addiction; it merely implies a physical dependence in which a higher dose of an agent is required over time to achieve the same effect. It is a well-recognized phenomenon associated with long-term narcotic use.

Two types of tolerance have been described, associative (learned) and nonassociative (adaptive); they involve different neurotransmitter systems. The learned form is responsive to environmental cues; the adaptive one entails cellular downregulation or desensitization of opioid receptors (particularly in spinal cord dorsal horn cells), which can lead to enhanced pain sensitivity, especially with the prolonged use of high opiate doses. The patient reports increased tenderness to touch and noxious stimuli, similar to that seen in neuropathic pain. In addition to tolerance-induced desensitization of opiate receptors, chronic opioid administration can lead to enhanced nociception. Both mechanisms can decrease the efficacy of pain control. There is no known relation between any particular dose regimen or opiate formulation and the risk of tolerance.

Contracting. Patients receiving narcotics and enrolled in a chronic pain program with contracting for routine follow-up have a less than 3% chance of becoming addicts or abusers if they have not been addicts or abusers previously. A current or prior history of abuse or addiction is a relative but not an absolute contraindication to long-term narcotic use because many such patients will adhere to the terms of a contract (Fig. 236.2). Such a contract allows for the tapering and discontinuation of a narcotic whenever a clinician fears that an abusive or addictive situation is developing. Narcotics can be prescribed for any patient who meets a few criteria for their use (Tables 236.6 and 236.7). Opioid analgesics all affect the μ-receptor but differ in their potency, onset, duration of action, and route of administration.

Dose-Related Side Effects and Proper Acute and Chronic Dosing. Dose-related side effects in the short term tend to be similar for all opiates and include nausea, vomiting, constipation, urinary retention, pruritus, sedation, and respiratory depression (when given in toxic doses). To minimize them, one starts with low doses and titrates upward. Underdosing is a common mistake at the outset of therapy. In the absence of sedation, one should not hesitate to increase the dose to achieve adequate pain relief.

Tolerance develops to all acute side effects except constipation. Chronic constipation can be debilitating, necessitating prophylactic treatment. Standard approaches include the use of bulk and osmotic agents in conjunction with the opioid program. Contrary to common belief, the chronic use of a stimulant laxative (e.g., senna) is safe and effective and should be considered when osmotic and bulk agents do not suffice (see also Chapter 65).

Because chronic opioid use at high doses is associated with increased nociception and the development of tolerance (which can lead to neuropathic pain), its dosing should be regulated carefully. The concept of a dose ceiling for opioid use in chronic pain is emerging among pain experts. Subsequent to establishing the minimally effective dose, the maintenance dose (usually a moderate one) should be continued with only minimal escalation. A need for escalation in dose should trigger a search for progression of the underlying disease, a repeat of the dose-adjustment phase, and, if unsuccessful, consideration of opioid rotation (starting at a lower dose) or weaning followed by

I, _____,
realize that my provider has decided to try to relieve my suffering partly with the use of opiate analgesics (pain medicines). I recognize that these medicines have both risks and benefits, which have been explained to me by my provider, and that these medicines are only one component of my pain treatment regimen.

I understand that to receive continuing care by my provider for my chronic pain, I must adhere to the following mutual expectations:

1. Pain medicines will be used *only as directed* for my pain. I will **NOT:**
   - suddenly stop taking these medicines;
   - use them other than for treating my pain;
   - increase the dose without discussion with my provider;
   - share them with others.

2. I will receive narcotics *only from my provider* and from no one else, including ER staff.

3. I will have my prescriptions filled *at only one pharmacy* of my choice, which I have clearly specified with my provider.

4. I will ask my provider for *refills on a predetermined schedule,* asking only when I still have at least 4 days' worth of medication remaining.

5. Refills will be given *only at my provider's office.* They will not be mailed.

6. I will adhere to requests for *random drug testing* should my provider ask me.

7. It is *my responsibility* to protect my prescriptions from loss, theft, or damage. A police report will be required for any theft before my provider will consider replacing them. If a second loss, or theft or damage occurs, I realize my provider may choose to not replace them.

8. These pain medicines are only one component of my treatment strategy. I agree to *adhere to other aspects of my care* as discussed with my provider.

_____
Patient signature   Date

_____
Provider signature   Date

FIGURE 236.2. Patient–provider contract for the long-term use of opioids. ER, emergency room.

abstinence and restarting. The latter methods take advantage of differences in effects on the μ-receptors among different opioids (incomplete cross-tolerance) and changes in receptor sensitivity with cessation of treatment.

Choice of Agent. *Oxycodone* is useful for chronic nonmalignant pain, being formulated for oral administration and without the side effects of long-acting morphine due to active metabolites that cause histamine release. However, the sustained-release *OxyContin* formulation is widely abused, especially when the tablet is crushed and injected. *Methadone is* a useful consideration when drug rotation is indicated; it can be started at half the dose-equivalent of the previous agent, but its long-half life increases the risk of dose accumulation.

Several narcotic preparations are best avoided, including butorphanol because it is a combination agonist–antagonist.

TABLE 236.6

CRITERIA FOR GIVING A PATIENT OPIATES FOR CHRONIC NONMALIGNANT PAIN

Patient reports subjective chronic pain on more than one occasion consistently

This pain inhibits functioning and decreases quality of life

Reversible causes have been addressed

Conservative measures (including over-the-counter medications) have been tried with inadequate response

Patient does not meet formal criteria for substance abuse or other *primary psychiatric disorder (depressive/anxiety/somatoform/personality disorders)* or malingering

There are no other contraindications to opiates (e.g., liver disease, operator of heavy machinery, drug tested at work)

Patient is capable of adhering to a simple contract about appropriate follow-up and opiate use

Meperidine likewise should be avoided because its metabolites tend to cause seizures. Narcotics in a fixed combination with acetaminophen (e.g., Percocet) should probably be avoided because of their high street value and the danger of acetaminophen overdose with dose escalations. Patients, however, should be encouraged to take maximal doses of acetaminophen simultaneously for synergy.

Neuropathic Pain (3,5,12–14)

Neuropathic pain is characteristically more resistant to pharmacologic interventions than is nociceptive pain, but new drugs and combination approaches are enhancing pain control, especially for painful peripheral neuropathy. Antidepressants (tricyclics, selective serotonin reuptake inhibitors, serotonin/norepinephrine reuptake inhibitors), anticonvulsants (gabapentin, pregabalin, baclofen, carbamazepine, phenytoin), opioids, and topical capsaicin cream constitute the main pharmacologic modalities. The combination of an anticonvulsant (e.g., gabapentin) with morphine has proven to be particularly effective.

TABLE 236.7

GENERAL PRINCIPLES TO FOLLOW WHEN PRESCRIBING NARCOTICS FOR CHRONIC PAIN

1. Have the patient sign a simple *contract* (see Fig. 236.2) with a "two strikes and you're tapered to zero" approach; stick to all the terms of the contract tightly; it may be used to encourage adherence to medical advice in other important realms.
2. Treat pain *proactively* before chronic patterns and secondary psychiatric comorbidities become ingrained
3. Use *long-acting agents* as around-the-clock treatments, avoiding short-acting medications for long-term use; use the same medication in short-acting formulation during the initial titration phase and for occasional breakthroughs
4. Monitor *functional endpoints* more than analgesia, although both are important
5. Maintain close *follow-up*

Antidepressants

All three major classes of antidepressants (tricyclics, selective serotonin reuptake inhibitors, and serotonin/norepinephrine reuptake inhibitors) provide proven pain relief, either alone or in combination with other classes of agents.

Tricyclics (TCIs). These drugs are often a first-line of treatment in neuropathic pain, having a rapid onset of action, no addiction potential, and good affordability (most are available as generic formulations); their anticholinergic side effects usually limit tolerability (see Table 236.5 and Chapter 227). Patients with a wide range of neuropathic pain syndromes (e.g., postherpetic neuralgia, diabetic peripheral neuropathy, tension and migraine headache, rheumatoid arthritis, low back pain) demonstrate benefit. When added to opioid therapy, TCAs enhance pain control. Doses required for analgesia can be much lower than those needed to treat affective disorders.

Selective Serotonin Reuptake Inhibitors. This class of antidepressants is not nearly as effective as the TCAs for neuropathic pain. In the setting of tension headache, paroxetine and fluoxetine have both been shown to provide some benefit, although citalopram did not. For migraine headaches and fibromyalgia, fluoxetine has shown conflicting results. For diabetic neuropathy, paroxetine and citalopram both showed some benefit but not of the same order as the TCA imipramine.

Serotonin-Norepinephrine Reuptake Inhibitors (SNRIs). Although they are not the first antidepressants for use in pain to act via both serotonin and norepinephrine pathways (several of the TCAs also do), the SNRIs show considerable promise. Unlike the tricyclics, they do not have strong anticholinergic side effects and tend to be better tolerated and nearly as efficacious. However, most preparations are not available generically, making them very expensive for prolonged use.

Duloxetine (*Cymbalta*) has demonstrated efficacy in painful diabetic peripheral neuropathy, carrying U.S. Food and Drug Administration (FDA) approval for use in this condition. The drug is well absorbed, can be used twice daily, and is hepatically metabolized. The recommended dose is 60 mg/d, which under study conditions provides a 50% reduction in pain in nearly 50% of patients. Adverse effects include confusion, dizziness, nausea, somnolence, hypertension, and constipation. The drug should not be used in persons with narrow-angle glaucoma; safety in pregnancy is not established. Minor transaminase elevations may be noted, and a withdrawal syndrome has been noted in some patients.

Venlafaxine (*Wellbutrin*; see Chapter 227) provides pain control equivalent to that of the TCA imipramine in patients with painful peripheral neuropathy.

Anticonvulsants

The anticonvulsants are believed to work by blocking the conduction of nociceptive fibers. *Phenytoin* and *carbamazepine* were the first drugs of this class to be used for neuropathic pain, providing relief in trigeminal neuralgia. Hematologic side effects can be problematic (e.g., bone marrow suppression, anemia, drug–drug interactions; see Chapter 176). *Gabapentin* has emerged as a heavily promoted and popular anticonvulsant for neuropathic pain, being comparable in efficacy to the older drugs but having less risk of adverse effects. It is generally well tolerated, but sedation (particularly in the elderly) necessitates starting with a low dose and gradually titrating upward. Considerable off-label use in peripheral neuropathy is common.

Pregabalin (*Lyrica*) is structurally similar to gabapentin and is FDA approved for use in diabetic peripheral neuropathy

and postherpetic neuralgia. Fifty-percent reductions in pain are achieved by almost half of users. Side effects include somnolence, dizziness, and peripheral edema; weight gain has been reported as well as euphoria. Cost is high; twice-daily dosing often suffices (starting at 50 to 75 mg twice daily). Patients concurrently taking a thiazolidinedione for diabetes (e.g., pioglitazone) experience a greater weight gain and more peripheral edema. Angioedema has been reported with use. Use in pregnancy is contraindicated.

Baclofen is a gabapentin agonist and is also generally well tolerated. It is used primarily for painful spasticity (e.g., in patients with spinal cord injury).

Capsaicin Cream

Capsaicin cream impedes afferent pain impulses by depleting substance P from sensory nerve fibers. It has been used in postherpetic neuralgia with some success, but it must be applied several times a day to provide sufficient pain relief. It often causes severe burning at the site of application for the first 1 to 2 weeks of treatment, so that concurrent use of topical lidocaine is necessary during this period.

Opiates

Well-designed studies have found moderate doses of opiates to be capable of controlling neuropathic pain for up to 32 weeks. The efficacy of longer-term therapy is unknown, and the effect on overall functioning is variable. Because *methadone* is long acting and does not result in the downregulation of opiate receptors that leads to tolerance and increased neuropathic sensitivity, it has been suggested as a potentially useful opioid for chronic neuropathic pain. However, its very long and unpredictable half-life may lead to the accumulation of respiratorily suppressive drug levels. Consequently, it should be used in small doses and is best reserved for patients with opiate tolerance and dose-escalation problems. In such settings, half-strength doses of methadone may serve well in a drug-rotation program.

Calcium N-Channel Blockers

See later discussion.

Complementary Modalities (15–20)

When therapeutic goals are not achieved with initial pharmacologic and psychosocial interventions, complementary modalities can be explored. Some of the many complementary modalities have more data behind them than others (Table 236.8).

Acupuncture

Acupuncture has been increasing in popularity among patients and physicians during the last three decades. More than 1 million patients make more than 5 million visits for treatment with acupuncture in the United States annually. Acupuncture has been applied to many conditions besides pain (e.g., asthma, depression), but its principal contribution is in pain management, the focus of a National Institutes of Health Consensus Statement.

Mode of Action. Acupuncture stems from traditional Chinese medicine, which holds that body energy (*Qi*, pronounced "chee") becomes imbalanced, causing disease. This imbalance is believed to be corrected by manipulating specific channels, called meridians, through which energy flows. This view predates the Western approach of mind–body dualism, which

TABLE 236.8

OVERVIEW OF COMPLEMENTARY APPROACHES TO THE TREATMENT OF CHRONIC PAIN

	Headache	Musculoskeletal	Low Back	Abdominal/Pelvic	Peripheral Nerve
Acupuncture	++	+++	++	+[a]	
Behavioral	+++[b]	++[c]	++[c]	+[d]	+[e]
Chiropractic			−		
Invasive		+	+	+	+[f]

[a] Menstrual cramps.
[b] See text for details.
[c] Relaxation, cognitive–behavioral therapy.
[d] Relaxation, hypnosis.
[e] Relaxation.
[f] Radiculopathy.

emphasizes disease as a purely biologic phenomenon. The biologic mechanism of acupuncture is becoming better understood. The procedure appears to trigger serotonin release in the central nervous system and to increase circulating levels of endogenous opioids. Naloxone can block the therapeutic effects of acupuncture.

Evidence of Efficacy. The few randomized, controlled trials that have been performed often suffer from methodologic shortcomings, such as inadequate sample sizes and problems with controls. Even "sham" acupuncture, in which needles are placed randomly, has been shown to provide pain relief. Comparisons among studies are difficult because there are many different ways of applying the needles with regard to location and manipulation. Manipulation is performed either manually, electrically, or through moxibustion (the combustion of a specific herb at the needle insertion site). Belief in the efficacy of the treatment is a major predictor of the outcomes observed.

The strongest evidence for efficacy has been demonstrated in cases of postoperative pain and nausea related to chemotherapy or pregnancy. Efficacy has also been demonstrated in myofascial pain, but results have been disappointing for pain relief in spinal disorders. Some studies support the efficacy of acupuncture in treating headaches, osteoarthritis, fibromyalgia, carpal tunnel syndrome, and menstrual cramps.

Adverse Effects. The incidence of adverse effects appears to be exceedingly low, certainly lower than that of commonly accepted pharmacologic interventions for chronic pain. Of the nearly 200 reported complications of acupuncture, viral hepatitis was by far the most common, stemming from a time when needles were not sterilized properly. All needles currently used by regulated providers conform to FDA safety regulations. Other, very rare complications include pneumothorax (with emphysema), ecchymoses (with anticoagulation), preterm induction of labor (in pregnant women), and conduction problems (with pacemakers when electrical stimulation of needles is used).

Indications for Use. Although it is popular and relatively safe, acupuncture's contribution to the management of chronic pain appears to be modest, being best for short-term problems such as postoperative pain. Effects overall appear to be short lived. Patients with chronic pain that appears to be refractory are often willing to "try anything," placing considerable pressure on the primary physician to make or at least acquiesce to a referral; most patients will go for treatment regardless. The best approach is to share efficacy data with patients to help them make an informed decision. Better data will help to define the role of acupuncture in treatment algorithms and drive improved standardization of training, licensing, supervision, and reimbursement. If referral of a patient to a physician acupuncturist is being considered, information can be obtained through the American Academy of Medical Acupuncture (http://www.medicalacupuncture.org).

Behavioral Therapies

Busy primary care providers classically overlook behavioral interventions. A recent review of complementary medicine in the United States showed that millions of Americans are already using these techniques, although most of their primary care providers remain unaware of this and are unfamiliar with the techniques. The importance of behavioral approaches in the treatment of chronic pain, however, cannot be overemphasized, because the risk is negligible and benefit has been demonstrated. In addition to cognitive–behavioral therapy (see prior discussion), the array of complementary behavioral therapies ranges from relaxation to hypnosis and biofeedback.

Data on these behavioral techniques are insufficient to suggest that one complementary technique be used over another for a particular condition. However, several meta-analyses have suggested positive effects of multimodal behavioral approaches, particularly for headache, joint pain, and back pain. Referral might be considered in properly selected patients as part of a comprehensive pain control program.

Relaxation. The goal is to train patients to control their focus of conscious attention. The two components are (a) repetitive focus on a word, phrase, sound, prayer, body sensation, or muscular activity and (b) adoption of a passive attitude toward intruding thoughts. Techniques include paced respiration, progressive muscle relaxation, concentration meditation, and movement meditation. Once patients master these techniques, they are capable of decreasing their perception of pain and level of arousal. There is sufficient evidence for efficacy in reducing chronic pain to recommend considering use in a variety of medical conditions.

Hypnosis. Hypnosis aims at selective focus of attention but adds a suggestive phase to reinforce new responses to pain. The presuggestion phase involves pure focus of attention (e.g., with relaxation techniques). The suggestive phase is geared toward specific goals, such as analgesia. The postsuggestive phase involves imprinting for continued use of a new behavior. Evidence of efficacy is accumulating with regard to tension headache, temporomandibular joint pain, and irritable bowel syndrome.

Biofeedback. Biofeedback involves education about physiologic responses to painful stimuli and ways to exercise voluntary control over these responses. Measurements are made with electromyography, electroencephalography, thermometers, and cardiac monitors. These tools allow patients to see their physiologic response to pain, and they are coached on techniques for affecting these responses. This leaves patients feeling more in control of their pain. Moderate evidence for the efficacy of biofeedback has been noted in the treatment of tension and migraine headaches.

Spinal Manipulation

Spinal manipulation is widely used by chiropractors, particularly for acute and chronic low back pain. More than half of patients being treated with manipulation by chiropractors have chronic low back pain. Although spinal manipulation has shown some benefit in controlled trials, the approach is only modestly better than no treatment and no better than other conventional therapies. Numerous consensus statements discourage the use of and referral for spinal manipulation (see Chapter 147).

Invasive Techniques (21,22)

Invasive techniques gained popularity in the 1980s after extensive studies showed them to be effective in patients with terminal cancer. Their use has now been extended to patients with nonmalignant chronic pain, based on the results of limited studies. These interventions are never used as monotherapy. They are added only when more-conservative measures have been ineffective and clinical evidence is available to suggest a possible benefit, especially in the setting of neuropathic pain. Invasive techniques are performed primarily by anesthesiologists in pain centers.

Local Anesthetics

Local anesthetics (e.g., *topical lidocaine*, intrathecal *bupivacaine*) may be given in the form of epidural or plexus blocks; sympathetic blocks are performed with opioids. These techniques are primarily used for acute pain states, but occasionally they are used for acute flares of chronic states (e.g., reflex sympathetic dystrophy). Neurolytic blocks with alcohol have primarily been used in patients with chronic abdominal cancer pain, but one retrospective study showed efficacy for lumbar sympathetic neurolytics in reducing the pain of patients with inoperable claudication.

Intrathecal Opioids

When given as an intrathecal or epidural injection, morphine has been quite effective in end-stage cancer patients who are unable to take oral opiates to therapeutic levels because of side effects. These techniques have been extended to some patients with chronic nonmalignant pain; a significant reduction of pain was achieved in 60 of 80 patients under study conditions. The patients included had chronic low back pain that surgery failed to alleviate, postherpetic neuralgia, and peripheral nerve injury. More than half of the patients had mild systemic side

effects (constipation, urinary hesitancy, nausea, impotence, nightmares, pruritus); approximately 20% also had system malfunctions, and a few experienced epidural hematoma, infection (epidural abscess, pocket infection, meningitis), or cerebrospinal fluid leaks. The current recommendations are that this should remain a method of last resort, to be used only after a patient has passed a psychological evaluation and responded favorably to a 3-day test of intrathecal opiates before the pump is implanted.

Intrathecal N-Type Calcium-Channel Blockers—Ziconotide (Prialt)

Ziconotide is a synthetic version of the venom from a sea snail and is the first of a new class of nonnarcotic analgesics for pain control that block N-type calcium channels in spinal cord neurons responsible for pain transmission. The drug requires a pump to patients with intractable pain who have failed to achieve adequate relief with narcotics; most candidates for use are those with terminal disease in whom the side effects of confusion, difficulty walking, and hallucinations would not be barriers to being given the drug.

Pain Centers

"Pain centers" have become increasingly numerous during the last decade as pain management has become recognized as a discipline in its own right. Centers range from small clinics offering only one type of intervention to large entities offering a multidisciplinary approach. They are directed by physicians (anesthesiologists, internists, psychiatrists) and may be staffed by nurses, physical therapists, psychologists, and social workers.

Pain specialists can be located through the American Pain Society (847-375-4715) or the American Academy of Pain Medicine (http://www.painmed.org). Information on more than 200 multidisciplinary centers can be found via the Rehabilitation Accreditation Commission (520-325-1044).

PATIENT EDUCATION AND INDICATIONS FOR REFERRAL

The principal objective is to redirect the patient's expectations toward a gradual improvement in functioning and quality of life rather than complete elimination of pain. Patients benefit from understanding that chronic pain has biologic and psychosocial components, which necessitates a multidisciplinary approach to therapy.

General internists should be able to manage their patients' pain medications and treat secondary psychiatric comorbidities. They must also determine the need for and coordinate appropriate referrals as follows:

- To mental health professionals for suspected underlying psychiatric illness and/or consideration of cognitive–behavioral therapy.
- To a substance abuse counseling program if an abuse problem is uncovered.
- To a social service program if overwhelming social factors are a factor (e.g., domestic violence).
- To a pain center, primarily if complex neuropathic pain is a factor or if invasive techniques are a consideration.

THERAPEUTIC RECOMMENDATIONS (5)

- View chronic pain as a chronic disease. Treatment goals must focus on improvement in functioning and quality of life rather than on the elimination of pain.
- Consider the psychosocial aspects of pain as much as the biologic aspects. Identify and address primary psychiatric processes and treat secondary processes along with the pain.
- Classify the biologic aspect of a patient's pain as primarily nociceptive or neuropathic, localize it, and consider reversible causes of pain for the various sites.
- Treat nociceptive pain stepwise, starting with nonopiate analgesics or NSAIDs and advancing to opiates as necessary. Tylenol remains the initial nonopiate of choice unless there is an inflammatory etiology, in which case aspirin or an NSAID is indicated. Long-term NSAID use predisposes to gastrointestinal toxicity, which can be obviated by concomitant omeprazole or misoprostol use or switching to a cyclooxygenase-2 preparation (which should be used only after consideration of the doubled to tripled risk in cardiovascular mortality).
- Do not hesitate to prescribe opiates on a long-term basis in properly selected patients who meet the following criteria:
  - Cause of pain established
  - Nonnarcotic therapy proven inadequate
  - Benefits of narcotic therapy outweigh risks
  - Treatment goals established

- Prescribe opioid therapy in a disciplined and controlled manner, using the following elements of a comprehensive approach:
  - Start therapy at low standard doses and adjust the dose upward as tolerated over 4 to 8 weeks to achieve desired pain control and establish a maintenance dose
  - Halt if pain control is not achieved or side effects are intolerable
  - Maintain stable moderate dose
  - Require monthly refills in person; reassess every 3 months
  - Base efficacy not only on pain control, but also on overall functioning
  - If control is insufficient, necessitating an escalation of dose, check for progression of underlying disease and repeat the dose-adjustment phase to reach a new stable dose
  - If this fails, consider opioid rotation, starting at a lower dose, or taper the current opioid to abstinence and then restart if necessary
- Treat neuropathic pain variably with antidepressants, anticonvulsants, and topical capsaicin cream as appropriate. Opiates at moderately high doses are an option when other drugs fail.
- Use a multidisciplinary approach. Consider directed referrals to psychiatry (primary psychiatric disorders, behavioral training) and pain centers (invasive techniques, acupuncture) when appropriate.

A.H.G.

Annotated Bibliography

1. Asbury A, Fields HL. Pain due to peripheral nerve damage: an hypothesis. Neurology 1984;34:1587. (*Proposes a mechanism.*)
2. Bovie J. Central pain. In: Wall PD, Melzack R, eds. Textbook of pain. Edinburgh: Churchill Livingston, 1994:871. (*An excellent section on mechanisms and presentation.*)
3. Bair MJ, Robinson RL, Waton W, et al. Depression and pain comorbidity. Arch Intern Med 2003;163:2433. (*A review of the literature on this important association; 173 references.*)
4. Gureje O, Von Korff M, Simon GE, et al. Persistent pain and well being. A World Health Organization study in primary care. JAMA 1998;280:147. (*Presents the epidemiology of the problem and its effect in primary care practice.*)
5. Ballantine JC, Mao J. Opioid therapy for chronic pain. N Engl J Med 2003;349:1943. (*A comprehensive review, with excellent sections on the adverse consequences of long-term therapy at high doses and an overall strategy for use, which is adopted in this chapter; 101 references.*)
6. Burchman SL, Pagel PS. Implementation of a formal treatment agreement for outpatient management of chronic nonmalignant pain with opioid analgesics. J Pain Symptom Manage 1995;10:556. (*A prospective Veterans Administration study, showing the success of patients on contract.*)
7. Katz WA. Pharmacology and clinical experience with tramadol in OA. Drugs 1996;52S:39. (*An overview of 20 years of experience with the drug.*)
8. Portenoy RK. Opioid therapy for chronic nonmalignant pain: a review of the critical issues. J Pain Symptom Manage 1996;11:203. (*An extensive, very readable overview, synthesizing the available numbers for predicting the risk of opiates to patients and proposing guidelines, which should be prospectively studied.*)
9. Tannenbaum H, Davis P, Russell AS, et al. An evidence-based approach to prescribing NSAIDs in musculoskeletal disease: a Canadian consensus. Can Med Assoc J 1996;155:77. (*A clear overview of nonselective nonsteroidal antiinflammatory drugs.*)
10. Turk DC, Brody MC, Okifuji EA. Physicians' attitudes and practices regarding the long-term prescribing of opioids for non-cancer pain. Pain 1994;59:201. (*A primary survey of 7,000 physicians, with a 27% response rate, suggesting that physicians acted more on their biases and inexperience than on germane data.*)
11. Wald A. Is chronic use of stimulant laxatives harmful to the colon? J Clin Gastroenterol 2003;36:386. (*A thoughtful review of the evidence, concluding that the answer is no.*)
12. Backonja M, Beydoun A, Edwards KR, et al. Gabapentin for the symptomatic treatment of painful neuropathy in patients with diabetes mellitus. JAMA 1998;280:1831. (*A randomized, controlled trial, finding that there was a 40% reduction in pain at 8 weeks, and that 23% of patients in the treatment group experienced somnolence and 24% experienced dizziness.*)
13. Jung AC, Staiger T, Sullivan M, et al. The efficacy of SSRIs for the management of chronic pain. J Gen Intern Med 1997;12:384. (*A straightforward review of 19 randomized, clinical trials.*)
14. Raja SN, Hawthornthwaite JA, Pappagallo, et al. Opioids versus antidepressants in postherpetic neuralgia: a randomized, placebo-controlled trial. Neurology 2002;59:1015. (*Presents an example of opioid efficacy in chronic neuropathic pain.*)
15. Cherkin DC, Deyo RA, Battie M, et al. A comparison of physical therapy, chiropractic manipulation, and provision of an educational booklet for the treatment of patients with low back pain. N Engl J Med 1998;339:1021. (*Treatments were only marginally better than education alone.*)
16. Milne S, Welch V, Brosseau L, et al. Transcutaneous electrical nerve stimulation (TENS) for chronic low back pain. Cochrane Database Syst Rev 2001;(2):CD003008. (*Finds no benefit.*)
17. NIH Consensus Conference. Acupuncture. JAMA 1998;280:1518. (*National Institutes of Health [NIH] data-driven consensus recommendations on complementary therapies; the statement is available at the web site http://consensus.nih.gov.*)
18. NIH Panel. Integration of behavioral and relaxation approaches into the treatment of chronic pain and insomnia. JAMA 1996;276:313. (*NIH data-driven recommendations on behavioral techniques.*)
19. Shekelle PG, Adams AH, Chassin MR, et al. Congruence between decisions to initiate chiropractic spinal manipulation for low back pain and appropriateness criteria in North America. Ann Intern Med 1998;129:9. (*Fifty-four percent of patients treated by chiropractors were not considered "appropriate," and the vast majority of these were patients with chronic low back pain.*)
20. Truk DC, Meichenbaum D. A cognitive–behavioral approach to pain management. In: Wall PD, Melzack R, eds. Textbook of pain. Edinburgh: Churchill Livingston, 1994:1337. (*A good review of an increasingly important modality.*)
21. Zenz M, et al. Role of invasive methods in the treatment of chronic pain. Acta Anaesthesiol Scand Suppl 1997;111:181. (*A brief overview of invasive techniques, with a plea for more conservative use.*)
22. Winkelmuller M, Winkelmuller W. Long-term effects of continuous intrathecal opioid treatment in chronic pain of non-malignant etiology. J Neurosurg 1996;85:458. (*A reduction of pain was achieved in >50% of cases, but there was a complication rate of 16%.*)

CHAPTER 237 ■ HERBAL SUPPLEMENTS COMMONLY USED AS COMPLEMENTARY OR ALTERNATIVE THERAPY

ERNIE-PAUL BARRETTE

In 1993, the U.S. Food and Drug Administration (FDA) proposed removing herbal therapies from the over-the-counter market, but a vigorous letter-writing campaign resulted instead in passage of the Dietary Supplement Health and Education Act (DSHEA) in 1994. DSHEA allowed the marketing of all supplements (defined broadly to include herbs, vitamins, minerals, and amino acids) to be expanded with information regarding uses based on "structure and function." Unfortunately, DSHEA does not require any evidence of efficacy or safety, nor does it define any standards of quality. The use of alternative medicines, including herbal preparations, has dramatically increased since the passage of DSHEA. It is critical that the primary care physician be conversant with the various preparations, claims for their effectiveness and supporting evidence, and known risks, including drug interactions. This therefore presents detailed reviews of evidence regarding the preparations most commonly encountered in primary care.

UNDERSTANDING THE EVIDENCE (1,2)

The number of published clinical trials of herbal medicines is substantial. Many of the trials, however, are in journals that are inaccessible or not published in English. Most lack adequate controls, have poorly defined inclusion criteria, and measure outcomes that are not validated or not clinically relevant. Many are simply too short in duration or enroll too few participants to provide substantive clinical information. This chapter reviews the best evidence supporting the use of several herbal therapies for specific indications. In addition, pertinent safety concerns are discussed.

In Germany, a commission was formed to evaluate the many herbs claimed to have therapeutic value. Members of the "Commission E" included physicians, pharmacists, naturopathic physicians, and scientists. They published several hundred monographs in the German Federal Register. These monographs have been recently translated and now constitute a repository of information and evidence regarding herbal preparations. This resource represents extensive experience in Europe regarding botanical medicines. Monographs with both positive and negative recommendations are included, along with discussions of adverse effects, drug interactions, use during pregnancy and nursing, specific indications, and doses. Unfortunately, no references are provided. In addition, only a positive or a negative recommendation is provided. Thus, neither the strength of the evidence nor the vigor of the recommendation can be determined.

COMMONLY USED HERBAL PREPARATIONS

Echinacea for Upper Respiratory Infections (1–4)

Extracts of three species, *Echinacea purpurea, E. angustifolia*, and *E. pallida,* are promoted for both the treatment and prevention of upper respiratory infections. *Echinacea* was used by Native Americans as an antiseptic and analgesic and was listed in the National Formulary until the introduction of synthetic antibiotics. The Commission E recommended *Echinacea* for "supportive therapy for colds and chronic infections of the respiratory tract." Unfortunately, no standardized extract exists. Multiple species, various methods of extraction, and different parts of the plant are used, and additional herbal and homeopathic agents are frequently included with preparations of *Echinacea*. All of these factors make a comparison of the literature and products very difficult.

Evidence for Efficacy

A systematic review from the Cochrane collaboration collected all the trials of monopreparations of *Echinacea* in the prevention or treatment of the common cold. Sixteen trials, including 22 comparisons of an *Echinacea* preparation versus a control group, were included in the analysis. Most comparisons were to placebo, and two were to no-treatment groups. Side effects were similar to those with placebo.

For Treatment. Fourteen trials addressed the *treatment* of an acute upper respiratory infection. Most trials were felt to be of reasonable to good quality. The reviewers felt that 9 trials showed a significant benefit over placebo, 1 trial showed a trend toward benefit over placebo, and 4 trials showed no benefit over placebo. Due to the multiple *Echinacea* preparations used, firm conclusions could not be drawn.

For Prevention. None of the three comparisons to placebo showed an effect over a placebo on the duration and severity of upper respiratory infections. The authors concluded that the benefit of *Echinacea* for the prevention of upper respiratory infections may exist but has not been demonstrated in rigorous randomized trials.

One recent study was less supportive. The trial compared three preparations of *E. angustifolia* to placebo. Participants were exposed to rhinovirus. Both prophylactic treatment starting 7 days prior to viral exposure and treatment starting with viral exposure were studied. There was no statistically significant benefit of any of the three preparations for prevention or severity of symptoms.

Safety

Anaphylaxis, acute asthma, urticaria, erythema nodosum, and maculopapular rash have been reported. Because of its immune-stimulating properties, *Echinacea* is not recommended for persons with autoimmune disorders.

Ginkgo biloba for Dementia and Memory Enhancement in Normal Older Persons (1,2,5–14)

Ginkgo biloba extracts have been used in Chinese herbal medicine for centuries. Use has increased in Europe during the last 30 years, and it is now the most prescribed herbal medicine in Germany. It is among the top three herbal products consumed in the United States. Most products are based on a standardized extract, EGb 761, which contains 22% to 27% flavone glycosides (quercetin, kaempferol, isorhamnetin) and 5% to 7% terpene lactones (2.8% to 3.4% ginkgolides A, B, and C; 2.6% to 3.2% bilobalide). EGb 761 is now off patent and may be used by any manufacturer. Unfortunately, another standardized extract process is also used, LI 1370. Although LI 1370 specifies 25% flavone glycosides and 6% terpenoids, the different process may result in different concentrations of individual ingredients. It is not known whether the active ingredient is a specific component or a combination. The Commission E approved *Ginkgo biloba* for use in dementia syndromes, specifically primary degenerative dementia, vascular dementia, and mixed forms. They also approved it for intermittent claudication, vertigo, and tinnitus.

Evidence for Efficacy

The body of research regarding potential mechanisms of action is extensive; these include scavenging free radicals, blocking platelet-activating factor, increasing blood flow, stabilizing membranes, and decreasing capillary fragility, among others.

For Use in Alzheimer's Disease. A rigorous meta-analysis has been conducted of published studies regarding the use of *Ginkgo biloba* in Alzheimer's disease. Inclusion criteria eliminated all but 4 of 57 articles addressing *Ginkgo biloba* and dementia; these trials included a total of 424 participants. Studies ranged in length from 12 to 26 weeks. All four trials used EGb 761. The analysis reported a significant mean effect size of 0.40 ($p <.0001$). The result was described as a modest benefit on cognitive function in Alzheimer's disease and was felt to be similar to the benefit of donepezil. The 4 studies reported inconsistent results with regard to noncognitive outcomes, including functional status measures. Since this meta-analysis, several European studies have shown mixed results. The separate issue of whether *Ginkgo biloba* prevents dementia is unresolved, although it is often taken for this specific purpose. Two large randomized trials with approximately 3,000 patients accrued

are ongoing: the Ginkgo Evaluation of Memory study in the United States and the GuidAge study in France).

For Use in Normal Older Persons. Extrapolating from the modest benefit in Alzheimer's patients, promoters of *Ginkgo biloba* claim that the substance improves memory and cognitive performance in normal older persons. Many seniors take *Ginkgo*-containing products in the hope of improving their mental functioning, making *Ginkgo* one of the top-selling herbal remedies in the United States. However, trials have not shown consistent benefit for nondemented older persons. In the best randomized trial, 230 patients of age 60 years or older and without significant neurologic or psychiatric illness were randomized to either *Ginkgo*, 40 mg three times daily, or matching placebo. Participants completed 14 standardized tests of memory, language, and concentration before the trial and at the end of 6 weeks. All 14 tests of cognitive function, as well as ratings by participants' family members, showed no difference between the groups. However, a similar 6-week trial of 180 mg daily versus placebo in 262 adults of age 60 years or older did show improvement in some of the objective outcomes.

Safety

Because one of the known effects of *Gingko biloba* is antagonism of platelet-activating factor, it is not surprising that several cases of severe *bleeding* during its use have been reported. These include spontaneous bilateral subdural hematomas, subarachnoid hemorrhage, subdural hematoma, intracerebral hemorrhage, and spontaneous hyphema. Because of these antiplatelet effects and the reports of associated bleeding complications, *Ginkgo* should be avoided in patients with bleeding disorders and in those taking warfarin or drugs with antiplatelet effects.

Kava-Kava for Anxiety (1,2,15–22)

The botanical name of kava-kava is *Piper methysticum* ("intoxicating pepper"). Kava-kava has been used in Pacific Island communities for centuries for its relaxing and tranquilizing effects. It continues to be used in Micronesia, Melanesia, and Polynesia. Captain James Cook first reported its use to the West. The Commission E has given kava a positive rating for the "condition of nervous anxiety, stress, and restlessness."

Evidence for Efficacy

Kava was first studied by German scientists in the 19th century, and in the 1950s, animal studies showed a sedative, analgesic, anticonvulsant, and muscle-relaxant effect. The active agents are believed to be the kavalactones (pyrones), primarily kawain, dihydrokawain, methysticin, and dihydromethysticin. Although the results of early studies with D,L-kawain suggested a benefit in treating anxiety, all recent trials have used an extract standardized to the content of kavalactones. A systematic review and meta-analysis of kava for the treatment of anxiety included seven trials. The authors concluded that kava was superior to placebo for the short-term treatment of anxiety. Methodologic limitations of several of these trials, however, limit enthusiasm for kava. The best evidence supporting the use of kava is a double-blinded, randomized, controlled multicenter trial comparing kava (100 mg three times daily, 70% kavalactones) with placebo. Enrollment consisted of 101 patients with generalized anxiety disorder, adjustment disorder with anxiety, agoraphobia, and specific phobia as defined in the revised third edition of the *Diagnostic and Statistical Manual of Mental Disorders*. The trial lasted 24 weeks and used

Hamilton Rating Scale for Anxiety (HAMA) scores with an intent-to-treat analysis as the primary outcome. The HAMA score improved in both arms, but the improvement was significantly greater with kava (30.7 to 17.1) than with placebo (31.4 to 20.3; $p = .02$) by 8 weeks. Both arms showed continued improvement for 16 weeks and then plateaued. The benefit of kava persisted from 8 weeks to the end of the trial. At 24 weeks, the HAMA scores remained improved with kava (kava, 30.7 to 9.7; placebo 31.4 to 15.2; $p < .001$). Adverse effects were minimal.

Safety

In large, observational trials, adverse effects have been rare. In several small trials, a worsening of cognitive function and coordination were seen, as expected with benzodiazepines but not with kava. Heavy, prolonged use of kava results in a well-described skin disorder characterized by dry, yellow scaling. There are case reports of dystonic reactions in five patients, including torticollis, generalized choreoathetosis, and oral–lingual dyskinesia. A single controversial report described a semicomatose state in a man who combined kava with alprazolam. Of greatest concern are the reports of hepatotoxicity, including fulminant liver failure requiring transplantation.

Milk Thistle for Hepatitis and Cirrhosis (1,23–28)

Milk thistle (*Silybum marianum*) has a 2,000-year history of use by herbalists. Although it was reported to relieve many conditions, it is currently promoted primarily for liver and biliary disorders. The active ingredient is called *silymarin*, which is composed of three isomeric compounds (silibinin, silydianin, and silychristin). From 20% to 40% of silymarin is concentrated in the bile. Milk thistle has been used in Europe for 30 years. The Commission E recommends its use as supportive treatment for chronic inflammatory liver conditions.

Evidence for Efficacy

For Treatment of Acute Viral Hepatitis. For acute *viral hepatitis,* the evidence is inconsistent. In trial of 57 patients with acute hepatitis A or B, treatment with 140 mg of silymarin three times daily for 3 to 4 weeks normalized bilirubin and aspartate aminotransferase (AST) levels more frequently than did placebo ($p < .05$). However, silymarin had no effect on the clearance of hepatitis B surface antigen, a more important clinical marker. In another study, of 52 nonalcoholic male patients with acute hepatitis B randomly assigned to silymarin (70 mg three times daily) or no treatment, no effect was seen on alanine aminotransferase (ALT), AST, and bilirubin levels or on the clearance of hepatitis B surface antigen. Although milk thistle is recommended by naturopathic physicians for acute hepatitis, little evidence is available to support its use.

For Treatment of Alcoholic Hepatitis. Many studies have been published on the use of milk thistle for alcoholic hepatitis. Unfortunately, most trials include very few participants, are short in duration, or are poorly controlled. In a large trial for alcoholic hepatitis, 106 men received either milk thistle (420 mg/d) or placebo. Participants were enrolled after admission to a military hospital because of elevations in AST or ALT for longer than 1 month. Although alcoholism was the presumed underlying condition, 20% of the men denied alcohol use. After 4 weeks, treatment with silymarin resulted in a significant decrease in ALT and AST levels; no improvement was noted with placebo. Liver biopsy also showed an improvement with treatment in comparison with placebo. However, although 90 biopsies were performed at the start of the trial, only 29 were performed at 4 weeks, which may have influenced the result.

Another trial of 116 participants, all with histologically confirmed alcoholic hepatitis, compared silymarin (420 mg/d) with placebo. After 3 months, significant improvements, noted in both arms in laboratory test results and histologic findings, suggested no benefit from the addition of milk thistle to adequate supportive care. Not surprisingly, in the information prepared by supplement manufacturers, these negative trial findings are rarely discussed.

For Treatment of Cirrhosis. Two trials addressed the use of milk thistle in cirrhosis. In an oft-quoted European multicenter study, 170 participants were entered in a trial comparing silymarin (140 mg three times daily) with placebo for 2 to 6 years (mean follow-up of 41 months). Cirrhosis was confirmed by biopsy in 70% of cases. Fifty-four percent of the participants in each arm were alcoholic. Exclusion criteria included end-stage liver disease, primary biliary cirrhosis, malignancies, and immunosuppressive therapy. Noncompliant participants were withdrawn from the analysis. At 2 years, overall survival was trending better with silymarin ($n = 105$, 77% vs. 67%; $p = .07$), and at 4 years, cumulative survival was improved with silymarin ($n = 29$, 58% vs. 38%; $p = .036$). Survival benefit was limited to alcoholics ($p = .01$) and to those rated Child's class A on entry. Unfortunately, more of the alcoholic patients receiving placebo continued to drink (73% vs. 55%), and more of the subjects rated Child's class C on entry were assigned to placebo (11% vs. 3%). Both of these factors, which favor milk thistle, may have influenced the analysis. This study represents the best evidence supporting milk thistle.

A similar European randomized, double-blinded, controlled multicenter trial compared milk thistle (150 mg three times daily) with placebo. Two hundred participants with biopsy-confirmed alcoholic cirrhosis were enrolled. Exclusion criteria included other causes of cirrhosis and the use of colchicine, penicillamine, or corticosteroids. One hundred twenty-five participants completed the 2-year follow-up. Survival was not improved at 2 years or at 5 years (odds ratio, 1.01; 95% confidence interval [CI], 0.46 to 2.22). The retrospective testing of stored sera, which was available for 75 of the 200 participants, showed 29 to be positive for hepatitis C. Among these 29, treatment may have been protective (silymarin deaths, 0 in 13; placebo deaths, 4 in 16; $p = .059$).

Safety

No serious adverse effects have been reported.

St. John's Wort for Depression (1,2,29–35)

The history of St. John's wort (*Hypericum perforatum*) as a herbal agent dates back 2,000 years. The use of *Hypericum* for mood problems continued into the 19th century but was forgotten early in the 20th century. During the last 30 years, Europe has produced an extensive literature. In 1984, the Commission E gave St. John's wort a positive rating for use in psychovegetative disturbances, depressive moods, and anxiety or nervous unrest. St. John's wort is the most commonly prescribed antidepressant in Germany. After press and television coverage of a meta-analysis with positive findings in 1996, the sales of St. John's wort in the United States rose from $20 million to $200 million during the next 2 years. It remains one of the top 10 herbal remedies consumed in the United States.

Evidence for Efficacy

Evidence suggests that the active ingredients are naphthodianthrones, primarily hypericin, pseudohypericin, and protohypericin. Although monoamine oxidase inhibitor activity is seen *in vitro,* this does not appear to be clinically important. The exact mechanism of St. John's wort is not known, but the best evidence supports effects on γ-aminobutyric acid (GABA), serotonin, and norepinephrine receptors. The hypericin content of St. John's wort varies from 0.06% to 0.75%, depending on the time of harvest and the quality of the plants. A standardized extract, LI 160, based on the content of hypericin has been used in most studies. However, recent studies suggested that another component of St. John's wort, hyperforin, may be the active agent. The content of hyperforin ranges from 2% in the flowers to 4.5% in the fruit. If hyperforin is the active agent and the most commonly used standardized extract, LI 160, is titrated to hypericin, then the clinical efficacy may vary from batch to batch. Despite the extensive knowledge of the components of St. John's wort and their actions in model systems, lingering uncertainties regarding which component or components are the most clinically relevant will continue to confound efforts to standardize preparations and treatment trials.

Five systematic reviews and meta-analyses reviewed the greater than 25 trials of St. John's wort for depression. All reported a benefit over placebo in mild to moderate depression. In one analysis of St. John's wort the relative benefit was 1.9 (CI, 1.2 to 2.8). In addition, eight trials showed St. John's wort to be equivalent to low doses of tricyclic antidepressants. Many valid criticisms of these early trials (prior to 1999) have been raised, relating to their short duration, small sample size, inadequate blinding, poorly defined entry criteria, low depression severity, and use of low doses of tricyclic antidepressants.

More-recent trials have been published with improved methodology. In the first three-arm study, 263 participants with moderate depression were randomized to St. John's wort, imipramine, or placebo for 8 weeks. St. John's wort improved the mean Hamilton Rating Scale for Depression (HAM-D) score significantly more than placebo and to a degree similar to imipramine. The trial had a high placebo response and only a trend to the improvement of imipramine compared to placebo. The dose of St. John's wort was higher than usual (350 mg three times daily), whereas the dose of imipramine was lower than recommended (100 mg/d). A recent French trial randomized to St. John's wort or placebo for 6 weeks 375 participants with a diagnosis of mild to moderate Major Depression according to the fourth edition of the *Diagnostic Statistical Manual of Mental Disorders.* St. John's wort improved HAM-D scores more than placebo ($p = 0.037$) and had a higher response rate (52.5% vs. 42.3% with placebo). In contrast to the two positive reports from Europe, two recent U.S. trials were negative. The first trial compared St. John's wort to placebo for 8 weeks in 200 participants. Significant improvement occurred in both arms, with St. John's wort no better than placebo. One criticism of this trial was that the participants enrolled had chronic depression (duration of current depression, 2.3 to 2.7 years). However, those with a history of failing to respond to an antidepressant in the current episode or failing more than one trial of antidepressants in the past were excluded. Another trial compared St. John's wort (300 mg three times daily titrated up to 1,500 mg/d), sertraline (50 to 100 mg/d), and placebo. The 340 participants with Major Depression were followed for

8 weeks. In the primary analysis, neither St. John's wort nor sertraline improved depression scores more than placebo. Why these U.S. trials of St. John's wort were negative when so many European trials showed benefit remains controversial. Another trial compared St. John's wort to fluoxetine and placebo. This smaller trial enrolled 135 participants with major depression and followed them for 12 weeks. Depression scores improved in all arms, but the greatest improvement was in the St. John's wort arm. The difference was significant when compared with fluoxetine and trended to superiority compared with placebo.

Safety

Adverse effects, which are generally mild, include gastrointestinal upset, dizziness, sedation, restlessness, and fatigue. St. John's wort may cause photosensitivity in fair-skinned patients, which can be severe at high doses. The induction of mania has been reported. It should not be used during pregnancy and should not be combined with other antidepressants. Significant interactions with drugs have been seen. The serotonin syndrome occurred when St. John's wort was added to patients on stable doses of sertraline, paroxetine, trazodone, and nefazodone. St. John's wort causes the selective induction of hepatic cytochrome P450 3A4 activity. There have been many reported cases of drug interactions with St. John's wort (e.g., cyclosporine, warfarin, theophylline, HIV protease inhibitors, oral contraceptives, etc.), resulting in more rapid clearance of the drug. Significant clinical events have resulted, such as transplant rejection.

Saw Palmetto for Benign Prostatic Hyperplasia (1,2,36–39)

Saw palmetto (*Serenoa repens*) is a plant native to the southeastern United States. Native Americans used the extract of the dried fruit from this dwarf palm for urinary difficulties, among other conditions. It was adopted by naturopathic physicians in the 19th century and is primarily promoted as a treatment for benign prostatic hyperplasia (BPH). In Germany, 90% of prescriptions for BPH are herbal medicines. Almost all of these prescriptions are for saw palmetto alone or with additional herbal agents. Saw palmetto received a positive rating for BPH by the Commission E.

Evidence for Efficacy

One systematic review of the literature from 1966 to 1997 was able to identify 18 trials, 16 of which were double blinded. Randomized, controlled trials of symptomatic BPH were included that lasted for at least 30 days. Ten trials compared saw palmetto with placebo, 2 trials compared saw palmetto with finasteride, and the remaining trials used products containing saw palmetto and other phytotherapeutic agents. The mean study duration was 9 weeks (range, 4 to 48 weeks), and 9.6% of participants were lost to follow-up (range, 4% to 15%).

The results of this meta-analysis showed a modest benefit. An improvement in self-rated symptoms (risk ratio, 1.72; 95% CI, 1.21 to 2.44, favoring saw palmetto) was seen in 6 studies. Nocturia improved in 10 trials (weighted mean difference, –0.76 episodes per night; 95% CI, –1.22 to –0.32). Saw palmetto increased peak urine flow rates in 8 trials (weighted mean difference, 1.93 mL/s; 95% CI, 0.72 to 3.14 mL/s). Because the natural history of BPH involves slow changes and some improvement in a subset of patients, the results of trials of less than 6 months' duration represent weak evidence. In addition, in the large trials of pharmaceutical agents for BPH, a robust placebo response was seen. In some of the trials with saw palmetto, little change occurred with placebo. The authors of the review felt that blinding was adequate in only 9 of the 18 studies.

Two specific trials addressed these concerns and provided stronger evidence. A European double-blinded, randomized, controlled multicenter trial compared β-sitosterol with placebo in men who had symptomatic BPH. This trial enrolled 200 men, who received 20 mg of β-sitosterol three times daily or placebo for 6 months. The self-reported symptoms measured with the International Prostate Symptom Score (IPSS) improved (IPSS mean change, -7.4 with treatment vs. -2.1 with placebo; $p <.01$). Peak urine flow rates were significantly better with β-sitosterol (baseline 9.9 mL/s to 15.2 mL/s at 6 months) than with placebo (baseline 10.2 mL/s to 11.4 mL/s at 6 months; $p <.01$).

Another European multicenter trial compared saw palmetto with finasteride without a placebo arm. In this 6-month, double-blinded study, 1,098 men with symptomatic BPH were randomized either to 160 mg of saw palmetto twice daily and finasteride placebo or to 5 mg of finasteride and saw palmetto placebo. Quality-of-life scores and the IPSS improved equally with the two treatments (-37% for saw palmetto vs. -39% for finasteride), whereas the peak urine flow rates improved slightly more with finasteride (from 10.6 ± 2.8 to 13.3 ± 6.7 mL/s with saw palmetto, and from 10.8 ± 3.1 to 14.0 ± 7.4 mL/s with finasteride; $p = .035$). Values for prostate-specific antigen (PSA) decreased 41% with finasteride but did not change with saw palmetto. Sexual dysfunction was seen somewhat more often with finasteride.

However, a rigorous trial done in the United States showed no benefit. This study enrolled 225 men with moderate to severe symptoms of BPH and followed then for 1 year. There were no significant differences in the primary outcomes (symptom index scores or maximal urinary flow rate) or secondary outcomes (e.g., quality of life) between saw palmetto and placebo. The strength of this study was the careful attention to blinding. With this result from a careful trial, the modest benefit seen in the earlier trials needs to be questioned.

Safety

Minimal adverse effects have been reported.

Valerian for Insomnia (1,40–42)

Valerian (*Valeriana officinalis*) has been used for more than 100 years as a hypnotic and mild tranquilizer. With the advent of barbiturates, it was dropped from the U.S. National Formulary and U.S. Pharmacopoeia. It remains popular as a hypnotic in Europe, where it is usually combined with hops, passionflower, lemon balm, and lavender. The Commission E gave valerian a positive rating for "nervous sleep disturbances." The active components are not known, and its mechanism is poorly understood. Proposed mechanisms involve binding to GABA or serotonin receptors and inhibition of the breakdown of GABA. The FDA lists valerian as GRAS (generally recognized as safe), and it is approved as a flavoring agent.

Evidence for Efficacy

Several studies suggest a benefit with valerian. However, most of the trials have serious deficiencies, such as small enrollment ($n = 8, 10, 14, 12$), enrollment of normal participants rather than participants with sleep disturbances, and use of nonvali-

dated symptom scores. In the largest trial, 166 volunteers received nine samples (three each of placebo, 400 mg of aqueous valerian extract, and a commercial herbal sedative containing 120 mg of valerian with 60 mg of hops) to be taken on nonconsecutive nights. One hundred twenty-eight participants completed the trial (23% dropout rate). Sleep latency and sleep quality were better on the nights when valerian was taken than on placebo nights. Subset analysis showed the benefit to be limited to self-described poor sleepers. Of interest, the commercial preparation of valerian with hops was no different from placebo.

In the most rigorous study, 121 patients with insomnia were enrolled in a double-blinded, randomized, controlled multicenter trial comparing valerian (600 mg, 70% alcohol extract standardized to 0.4% to 0.6% valerenic acid) with placebo for 28 days. Patients who had major depression and were taking medications were excluded. A marked placebo response suggested adequate blinding. At 14 days, a significant improvement was noted on the Clinical Global Impression Scale with treatment. By 28 days, valerian significantly improved sleep in comparison with placebo on three standardized scales. This study suggests that the benefit of valerian occurs slowly, during 4 weeks. If this is true, the results of earlier studies lasting 1 to 7 days are difficult to accept. Valerian is usually standardized to the content of valerenic acid (usually 0.8%). However, in the absence of a standardized extract procedure and because of uncertainty regarding the active component, different commercial products may vary in efficacy. Relative proportions of the components vary with season of harvest and species harvested. This adds further uncertainty to any comparison.

Safety

Adverse effects are rare and generally mild. A possible withdrawal reaction was reported after general anesthesia in a patient who had taken valerian (530 mg to 2 g) five times a day for "many years." Tachycardia, high-output cardiac failure, delirium, and oliguria were noted and responded to benzodiazepine. In general, valerian should not be used with other sedating medications.

Ephedra for Weight Loss and Performance Enhancement (1,43–45)

Extract of the Asian ephedra species *Ephedra sinica* is a traditional Chinese herbal preparation (*Ma huang*) rich in sympathomimetics and used for millennia for difficulty in breathing. It was also once popular in the United States before the advent of safer sympathomimetic decongestants and bronchodilators. Until recently *Ma huang* was included in almost all herbal weight loss supplements and many herbal energy "booster" supplements or performance enhancers (popular with body builders and athletes). With the passage of the DSHEA, herbal extracts taken as dietary supplements may be marketed directly to the public with an educational component, that is, labeling with a "structure function" claim. Thus ephedra may be labeled to assist with weight loss but cannot be labeled to treat obesity because only drugs legally treat diseases. However, the predominant component of ephedra is ephedrine. Synthetic ephedrine is a licensed drug with the accompanying regulatory oversight. It is a quirk of the regulations that allowed the plant extract of ephedra to be sold as an herbal supplement, which it clearly is, although it contains the chemical ephedrine, which, when sold alone, is treated as a drug.

Efficacy

Ephedra's actions relate to its strong sympathomimetic content, particularly from ephedrine, but also from pseudoephedrine, phenylpropanolamine, and norpseudoephedrine. A meta-analysis of ephedra for weight loss showed modest short-term weight loss (approximately 0.9 kg/mo) over placebo. No trial was longer than 6 months. The same meta-analysis concluded there was no evidence to support the use of ephedra for improving athletic performance.

Safety

Because it is a potent sympathomimetic extract, ephedra has long been recognized as a potentially hazardous substance, but its classification as an herbal preparation/dietary supplement and consequent exemption from FDA approval enabled makers of nonprescription weight-loss and performance-enhancing products to incorporate it into many of their offerings. Tragically, but not surprisingly, a flurry of reports appeared of serious and often fatal cardiac and neurologic events associated with its use, the most notable being the death of a major league baseball pitcher who was using an ephedra-containing weight-loss product during spring training. In the most comprehensive analysis of reports of ephedra-related adverse events, investigators found ephedra use to be nearly 100 to 700 times more dangerous than that of other popular herbal preparations, such as kava and *Ginkgo*. Based on much evidence, the FDA banned the sale of ephedra in dietary supplements in 2004.

Annotated Bibliography

1. Blumenthal M, senior ed. The complete German Commission E monographs. Boston: Integrative Medicine Communications, 1998. (*The collected monographs of Commission E, which constitute the best repository of evidence.*)
2. Ernst E. The risk–benefit profile of commonly used herbal therapies: ginkgo, St. John's wort, ginseng, *Echinacea*, saw palmetto, and kava. Ann Intern Med 2002;136:42. (*A concise review of all systematic reviews and meta-analyses of the listed herbal supplements.*)
3. Linde K, Barrett B, Wölkart K, et al. *Echinacea* for preventing and treating the common cold. *Cochrane Database Syst Rev* 2006(1):CD000530. (*Nine of 16 trials showed a significant treatment benefit; none of three trials showed preventive efficacy; see http://www.cochrane.org for updates.*)
4. Turner RB, Bauer R, Woelkart K, et al. An evaluation of *Echinacea angustifolia* in experimental rhinovirus infections. N Eng J Med 2005;353:341. (*No benefit.*)
5. Oken BS, Storzbach DM, Kaye JA. The efficacy of *Ginkgo biloba* on cognitive function in Alzheimer disease. Arch Neurol 1998;55:1409. (*Describes the result as a modest benefit on cognitive function in Alzheimer's disease similar to that of donepezil.*)
6. Kleijnen J, Knipschild P. *Ginkgo biloba*. Lancet 1992;340:1136. (*Only 8 of 40 trials met inclusion criteria.*)
7. Le Bars PL, Katz MM, Berman N, et al. A placebo-controlled, double-blind, randomized trial of an extract of *Ginkgo biloba* for dementia. JAMA 1997;278:1327. (*The only U.S. trial in the meta-analysis, noting improvement on functional scales.*)
8. Solomon PR, Adams F, Silver A, et al. *Ginkgo* for memory enhancement. A randomized controlled trial. JAMA 2002;288:835. (*No difference was found between groups in all 14 tests of cognitive function, as well as in ratings by participants' family members.*)
9. Mix JA, Crews WD. A double-blind, placebo-controlled, randomized trial of *Ginkgo biloba* extract EGb 761 in a sample of cognitively intact older adults: neuropsychological findings. Hum Psychopharmacol 2002;17:267. (*A 6-week trial in 262 adults age 60 years or older, showing improvement in some of the objective outcomes.*)
10. Rowin J, Lewis SL. Spontaneous bilateral subdural hematomas associated with chronic *Ginkgo biloba* ingestion. Neurology 1996;46:1775. (*A case report.*)
11. Vale S. Subarachnoid haemorrhage associated with *Ginkgo biloba*. Lancet 1998;352:36. (*A case report.*)
12. Gilbert GJ. *Ginkgo biloba*. Neurology 1997;48:1137. (*A case report.*)
13. Matthews MK. Association of *Ginkgo biloba* with intracerebral hemorrhage. Neurology 1998;50:1933. (*A case report.*)
14. Rosenblatt M, Mindel J. Spontaneous hyphema associated with ingestion of *Ginkgo biloba* extract. N Engl J Med 1997;336:1108. (*A case report.*)
15. Singh YN, Blumenthal M. Kava: an overview. Herbalgram 1997;39:34. (*A review, including colorful history of centuries-old use.*)
16. Pittler MH, Ernst E. Efficacy of kava extract for treating anxiety: systematic review and meta-analysis. J Clin Psychopharmacol 2000;20:84. (*Kava was superior to placebo for the short-term treatment of anxiety.*)
17. Volz HP, Kieser M. Kava-kava extract WS 1490 versus placebo in anxiety disorders—a randomized placebo-controlled 25-week outpatient trial. Pharmacopsychiatry 1997;30:1. (*The Hamilton Rating Scale for Anxiety score improved in both arms, but the improvement was significantly greater with kava [30.7 to 17.1] than with placebo [31.4 to 20.3]; p = .02] by 8 weeks.*)
18. Norton SA, Ruze P. Kava dermopathy. J Am Acad Dermatol 1994;31:89. (*Prolonged use of kava results in a well-described skin disorder characterized by dry, yellow scaling.*)
19. Spillane PK, Fisher DA, Currie BJ. Neurological manifestations of kava intoxication. Med J Aust 1997;167:172. (*Case reports of dystonic reactions.*)
20. Schelosky L, Raffauf C, Jendroska K, et al. Kava and dopamine antagonism. J Neurol Neurosurg Psychiatry 1995;58:639. (*Case reports of dystonic reactions.*)
21. Almeida JC, Grimsley EW. Coma from the health food store: interaction between kava and alprazolam. Ann Intern Med 1996;125:940. (*A single controversial report describing a semicomatose state in a man who had combined kava with alprazolam.*)
22. Center for Food Safety and Applied Nutrition, U.S. Food and Drug Administration. Consumer advisory. Kava-containing dietary supplements may be associated with severe liver injury, March 25, 2002. Available at: http://www.cfsan.fda.gov/~dms/addskava.html. (*Kava-containing products have been associated with liver-related injuries, including hepatitis, cirrhosis, and liver failure, in >25 reports of adverse events in other countries.*)
23. Magliulo E, Gagliardi B, Fiori GP. Zur Wirkung von Silymarin bei der Behandlung der akuten Virushepatitis. Med Klin 1978;73:1060. (*A small study of acute hepatitis A and B, showing improved alanine aminotransferase [ALT] with silymarin but no change in hepatitis B surface antigen.*)
24. Flisiak R, Prokopowicz D. Effect of misoprostol on the course of viral hepatitis B. Hepatogastroenterology 1997;44:1419. (*Fifty-two nonalcoholic male patients with acute hepatitis B were randomly assigned to silymarin or no treatment, with no effect on alanine ALT, aspartate aminotransferase [AST], and bilirubin levels or on the clearance of hepatitis B surface antigen.*)
25. Salmi HA, Sarna S. Effect of silymarin on chemical, functional, and morphological alterations of the liver. Scand J Gastroenterol 1982;17:517. (*Among 106 men with alcoholic hepatitis, treatment with silymarin for 4 weeks resulted in a significant decrease in ALT and AST levels; no improvement was noted with placebo.*)
26. Trinchet JC, Coste T, Levy VG, et al. Traitement de l'hépatite alcoolique par la silymarine. Une étude comparative en double insu chez 116 malades. Gastroenterol Clin Biol 1989;13:120. (*No benefit was found from the addition of milk thistle to adequate supportive care.*)
27. Ferenci P, Dragosics B, Dittrich H, et al. Randomized controlled trial of silymarin treatment in patients with cirrhosis of the liver. J Hepatol 1989;9:105. (*This flawed study represents the best evidence supporting milk thistle.*)
28. Parés A, Planas R, Torres M, et al. Effects of silymarin in alcoholic patients with cirrhosis of the liver: results of a controlled, double-blind, randomized and multi-center trial. J Hepatol 1998;28:615. (*Survival was not improved at 2 years or at 5 years.*)
29. Linde K, Ramirez G, Mulrow CD, et al. St. John's wort for depression—an overview and metaanalysis of randomised clinical trials. BMJ 1996;313:253. (*A meta-analysis with positive findings; sales in the United States rose from $20 million to $200 million during the next 2 years.*)
30. Williams JW, Mulrow CD, Chiquette E, et al. A systematic review of newer pharmacotherapies for depression in adults: evidence report summary. Ann Intern Med 2000;132:743. (*The relative benefit over placebo was 1.9.*)
31. Philipp M, Kohnen R, Hiller KO. *Hypericum* extract versus imipramine or placebo in patients with moderate depression: randomized multicentre study of treatment for eight weeks. BMJ 1999;319:1534. (*Two hundred sixty-three subjects with moderate depression were randomized to St. John's wort, imipramine, or placebo for 8 weeks; the effect of St. John's wort on the mean Hamilton Rating Scale for Depression [HAM-D] score was significantly greater than that of placebo and similar to that of imipramine.*)
32. Lecrubier Y, Clerc G, Didi R, et al. Efficacy of St. John's wort extract WS 5570 in major depression: a double-blind, placebo-controlled trial. Am J Psychiatry 2002;159:1361. (*St. John's wort improved HAM-D scores more than placebo and had a higher response rate.*)

33. Shelton RC, Keller MB, Gelenberg A, et al. Effectiveness of St. John's wort in major depression. JAMA 2001;285:1978. (*A U.S. trial in which significant improvement occurred in both arms, with St. John's wort not better than placebo.*)

34. Hypericum Depression Trial Study Group. Effect of *Hypericum perforatum* (St John's Wort) in major depressive disorder: a randomized controlled trial. JAMA 2002;287:1807. (*A trial comparing St. John's wort, sertraline, and placebo, finding that neither St. John's wort nor sertraline improved depression scores more than placebo.*)

35. Fava M, Alpert J, Nierenberg AA, et al. A double-blind, randomized trial of St. John's wort, fluoxetine, and placebo in major depressive disorder. J Clin Psychopharmacol 2005;25:441. (*A trial showing that St. John's wort was significantly better than fluoxetine and that, when it was compared to placebo, a trend to significance was noted.*)

36. Wilt TJ, Ishani A, Stark G, et al. Saw palmetto extracts for treatment of benign prostatic hyperplasia. JAMA 1998;280:1604. (*A meta-analysis, showing a modest benefit.*)

37. Berges RR, Windeler J, Trampisch HJ, et al. Randomised, placebo-controlled, double-blind clinical trial of b-sitosterol in patients with benign prostatic hyperplasia. Lancet 1995;345:1529. (*Two hundred men were randomized to β-sitosterol or placebo for 6 months, with the former having a significantly greater mean change in International Prostate Symptom Score [IPSS], –7.4 with treatment vs. –2.1 with placebo.*)

38. Carraro JC, Raynaud JP, Koch G, et al. Comparison of phytotherapy (Permixon) with finasteride in the treatment of benign prostate hyperplasia: a randomized international study of 1,098 patients. Prostate 1996;29:231. (*Quality-of-life scores and the IPSS improved equally with the two treatments, whereas peak urine flow rates improved slightly more with finasteride.*)

39. Bent S, Kane C, Shinohara K, et al. Saw palmetto for benign prostatic hyperplasia. N Engl J Med 2006;354:557. (*A U.S. trial comparing saw palmetto with placebo in 225 men for 1 year, finding no benefit with saw palmetto in any outcome; overall, this is the most methodologically sound trial.*)

40. Leathwood PD, Chauffard F, Heck E, et al. Aqueous extract of valerian root (*Valeriana officinalis* L.) improves sleep quality in man. Pharmacol Biochem Behav 1982;17:65. (*Sleep latency and sleep quality were better on the nights when valerian was taken than on placebo nights.*)

41. Vorbach EU, Görtelmeyer R, Brünig J. Therapie von Insomnien. Wirksamkeit und Verträglichkeit eine Baldrianpräparats. Psychopharmakotherapie 1996;13:109. (*A study suggesting that the benefit of valerian occurs slowly, during 4 weeks.*)

42. Garges HP, Varia I, Doraiswamy PM. Cardiac complications and delirium associated with valerian root withdrawal. JAMA 1998;280:1566. (*A possible withdrawal reaction was reported after general anesthesia in a patient who had taken valerian five times a day for "many years."*)

43. Shekelle PG, Hardy ML, Morton SC, et al. Efficacy and safety of ephedra and ephedrine for weight loss and athletic performance. JAMA 2003;289:1537. (*A meta-analysis showing modest short-term weight loss.*)

44. Bent S, Tiedt TN, Odden MC, et al. The relative safety of ephedra compared with other herbal products. Ann Intern Med 2003;138:468. (*Ephedra use was 100 to 700 times more dangerous than that of other popular herbal preparations, such as kava and ginkgo.*)

45. U.S. Food and Drug Administration White Paper on Ephedra. Evidence on the safety and effectiveness of ephedra: implications for regulation. Available at: http://www.fda.gov/bbs/topics/NEWS/ephedra/whitepaper.html. (*The Food and Drug Administration proposed a black box warning.*)

CHAPTER 238 ■ CARING FOR THE ADOLESCENT PATIENT

LAURENCE J. RONAN

Primary care physicians whose practices involve mostly older adults need to know the basics of adolescent preventive care because many adolescents will present to their offices for care. Most experts on adolescence recommend annual visits to a physician between the ages of 11 and 21 years, with a complete physical examination at least once each in early adolescence (ages 11 to 14 years), middle adolescence (ages 15 to 17 years), and late adolescence (ages 18 to 21 years).

The emphasis during the annual visit is on prevention and health promotion. The majority of adolescent deaths are due to preventable causes, predominantly accidents, homicides, and suicides. Motor vehicle accidents are the leading cause of death of adolescents and young adults. The major causes of adolescent morbidity include pregnancy, sexually transmitted diseases, substance abuse, smoking, physical violence, and depression. Young adults (ages 20 to 24 years) have five times the mortality of younger adolescents (ages 10 to 14 years). Because the leading causes of mortality and morbidity are unintended injury or are largely preventable, the focus of care for adolescents is on primary as well as secondary prevention (Table 238.1). Both biomedical and psychosocial issues should be addressed. Adolescent care emphasizes the cultivation of healthy lifelong habits to prevent heart disease and cancer in particular.

CONSENT (1–3)

In general, parents are responsible for giving consent for their children's care until the child reaches the age of 18 years. Adolescents, however, have a greater right than do younger children to participate in their health care decisions. Practitioners should review their state laws regarding the specific services that minors may obtain without the consent of their parents. These services usually are related to pregnancy, birth control, abortion, the evaluation and treatment of sexually transmitted diseases (including HIV infection), substance abuse, and sexual assault. Some states also include outpatient mental health services. "Emancipated" minors have the legal right to give consent for their care. These adolescents are married, have children, serve in the military, live apart from their parents, or are homeless. "Mature minors"—adolescents who understand the risks and benefits of treatment and its alternatives—also have the legal right to give consent.

HISTORY TAKING (1–3)

Adolescence is a dynamic time in the life cycle and is associated with rapid and dramatic changes in physical, social, and

TABLE 238.1

RECOMMENDED PREVENTIVE HEALTH SERVICES BY AGE AND PROCEDURE

History/Exam	All Years
Health guidance	Review development, diet, and physical activity, healthy lifestyles,[a] and injury prevention each year from ages 11 to 21 yr
Screening history	Review eating disorders, sexual activity,[b] alcohol and other drug use, tobacco use, abuse, school performance, depression, and risk for suicide each year from ages 11 to 21 yr
Physical assessment	Determine blood pressure and body mass index annually from ages 11 to 21 yr; perform a comprehensive examination once each during early (11–14 yr), middle (15–17 yr), and late (18–21 yr) adolescence
Test	**Ages 11–21 Years**
Cholesterol	Perform screening test once if family history is positive for early cardiovascular disease or hyperlipidemia
Tuberculosis	Screen if positive for exposure to active tuberculosis or patient lives/works in a high-risk situation, e.g., homeless shelter, health care facility
Gonorrhea, chlamydia, syphilis, human papilloma virus	Screen at least annually if sexually active
HIV	Screen annually
Pap smear	Screen annually if sexually active or if ≥18 yr
Hematocrit or hemoglobin	Determine for girls with heavy menses, weight loss, eating disorders, or who are extremely athletic
Human papillomavirus DNA	Screen annually if sexually active or if ≥ 18 yr

[a]Includes counseling regarding sexual behavior and avoidance of tobacco, alcohol, and other drug use.
[b]Includes history of unintended pregnancy and sexually transmitted diseases.
Adapted from AMA Guidelines for Adolescent Preventive Services (GAPS). American Medical Association, Adolescent Health On-Line. Available at: http://www.ama-assn.org/ama/upload/mm/39/gapsmono.pdf. With permission.

emotional development. The adolescent health history focuses on five contextual and developmental domains:

1. Social and emotional development
2. Physical development and health habits
3. Sexual development
4. Family functioning
5. School performance

The unique aspects of the five developmental domains should be explored in each stage of adolescence—early, middle, and late. A convenient acronym for remembering important psychosocial questions in the adolescent interview is HEADS: home environment, education/employment, activities/exercise, drugs, sexuality, and suicide/depression.

Early Adolescence: Ages 11 to 14 Years

Early adolescence heralds the start of dramatic physical changes. Girls undergo rapid spurts of growth, the development of pubic hair and breasts, and changes in the distribution of body fat. Generally, puberty begins in girls 2 to 3 years earlier than in boys. Boys acquire deeper voices, larger testicles, and pubic hair, and acne frequently develops. Early adolescents are preoccupied with looks and anxious about physical changes. In addition, early teenagers move from elementary to middle school, where academic demands are higher, autonomy is greater, and socialization is increased. Their thinking, although increasingly abstract, is for the most part still concrete and oriented to the present. Early teens are focused on self, family, and peers. Sexual exploration and recreational drug experimentation begin. The profound biologic, emotional, and psychological changes experienced by early teens stress the family as they challenge limits and rules and also explore new and sometimes risky behaviors.

Middle Adolescence: Ages 15 to 17 Years

By middle adolescence, the physical development of girls is complete, and most boys are well on their way to the completion of puberty. Although the thinking of middle adolescents remains concrete, many of them are progressing from concrete to abstract, formal, operational thinking. Friends become hugely important. Middle teens also become aware of the larger world and social issues. The growing need for autonomy places teens in conflict with family rules. Middle teens are very aware of academic pressures and are anxious about school and sports performance. They can obtain work permits and driver licenses.

Late Adolescence: Ages 18 to 21 Years

Pubertal development is complete. The late adolescent focuses on vocational and personal development. Older teens are legally responsible for themselves, often living separately from parents and struggling with decisions about further schooling, jobs, or the military. High-risk behaviors peak at this stage, including promiscuity, substance abuse, and eating disorders.

PHYSICAL EXAMINATION (1–4)

Measure and plot on a standard sex-specific growth chart the adolescent's height and weight. Determine the patient's body mass index. Document a blood pressure measurement at every annual visit. Evaluate for scoliosis. Look for evidence of physical abuse. Examine the adolescent's teeth for cavities, malocclusion, gingivitis, and congenital dental anomalies. Determine the Tanner stage or Sexual Maturity Rating, and keep a copy of one of these two charts in the office for reference. For girls, provide instruction in breast self-examination and inspect the external genitalia. Perform a pelvic examination with Papanicolaou smear annually for all girls who are sexually active or 18 years of age or older. Examine boys for gynecomastia and hernias. Check the testicles for abnormal masses or congenital anomalies (boys with a history of undescended testes or a single testicle are at high risk for testicular cancer are). Check the skin for acne.

LABORATORY EVALUATION (1–3,5–9)

Perform a random *cholesterol* determination on teenagers who have a positive family history for early cardiovascular disease or hyperlipidemia. Adolescents who are unsure of their family history should also be screened. Girls with heavy menses, weight loss, or eating disorders or who are extremely athletic should have a screening hematocrit or hemoglobin determination.

Only adolescents at increased risk for exposure to tuberculosis require *tuberculin (purified protein derivative) skin testing*. These risks include exposure to tuberculosis, homelessness, a history of incarceration, immigrant status, HIV infection or living with an HIV-infected person, and illicit drug use. It is reasonable to test once between the ages of 11 and 16 years if the teenager has no risk factors (see also Chapter 38).

Sexually active teenagers should be screened for sexually transmitted diseases. The frequency of screening is controversial. Usually, girls are screened during each annual pelvic examination, which should include a cervical culture for gonorrhea, immunologic testing of cervical fluid for *Chlamydia* infection, *serologic testing* for *syphilis*, and visual inspection of the genitalia. Adolescent females should be screened for cervical cancer with a *Papanicolaou smear* and human papillomavirus (HPV) DNA at age 18 years or at the onset of sexual intercourse. For boys, screening consists of *urine DNA* or *leukocyte esterase* analysis for *gonorrhea* and *Chlamydia* infection, serologic testing for syphilis, and visual inspection of the genitalia for HPV (see also Chapters 107, 117, 124, 125, and 136).

The clinician should offer *HIV testing* to all adolescents. The Centers for Disease Control and Prevention (CDC) recommend that HIV testing be a routine part of annual medical care, regardless of risk status. High risk includes the use of intravenous drugs, previous infection with a sexually transmitted disease, blood transfusion before 1985, exchange of sex for money or drugs, homelessness, a history of more than one sexual partner in the last 6 months, male homosexuality, or a sexual partner with any of the foregoing risk factors for HIV infection (see also Chapter 7).

IMMUNIZATIONS (7,8)

See also Chapter 6. Ensure that the teenager's immunizations are up to date at every clinical encounter. (See Fig. 238.1 for a recommended immunization schedule for persons 7 to 18 years old.) *Tetanus–diphtheria toxoid, measles, mumps,* and *rubella* (MMR) vaccine, and *hepatitis B vaccine* should be given to the adolescent if the previously recommended doses were missed, not documented, or given before the recommended minimum age (the recommended minimum age for completion of the second dose of MMR vaccination is 4 to 6 years; for varicella vaccination, 12 to 18 months; and for the third dose of hepatitis vaccine, 6 to 18 months). By 11 to 12 years of age, the teenager is due for the tetanus booster if more than 5 years have elapsed since his or her last dose. The adolescent should have three doses of hepatitis B vaccine, two doses of MMR vaccine, and a varicella vaccine if he or she has not had chickenpox. For incompletely immunized or unimmunized adolescents (especially newly arrived immigrants), follow the recommendations of the *Red Book* (the most recent edition of the report of the Committee on Infectious Diseases, American Academy of Pediatrics) or the MMWR QuickGuide (published by the CDC) regarding catch-up immunization schedules for adolescents (see Fig. 238.2 for a catch-up schedule for persons 7 to 18 years old). Adolescents with chronic illness or immunosuppression require *pneumococcal vaccine* and annual *influenza vaccine;* this includes all adolescents with asthma. College freshman, especially those who live in group settings and dormitories, require *meningococcal vaccine.* Schools routinely request documentation; make certain that the medical records regarding the patient's immunization status are kept up to date.

Human Papillomavirus Vaccines

The American College of Immunization Practices and American College of Gynecology recommend that all girls and women between 9 and 26 years of age receive immunization with the HPV vaccine. This vaccine has demonstrated efficacy against HPV infection, which leads to cervical cancer, the second-most-common malignancy in women.

The quadrivalent HPV 6/11/16/18 L1 VLP vaccine (Gardasil) is administered in three doses at 0, 2, and 6 months. The safety profile is considered excellent. The duration of immunity is unknown. Vaccination does not replace cervical screening, nor does it treat cytologically evident disease or infection.

ANTICIPATORY GUIDANCE (1–3,10–13)

Prevention of Injury and Violence

The use of seat belts reduces motor vehicle fatalities by 45% and the rate of serious injury by 50%. In 80% of road fatalities, the victim was not wearing a seat belt. Counsel adolescents to use seat belts. In addition, advise the use of other safety devices, such as bicycle and motorcycle helmets, protective gear

Vaccine ▼ / Age ▶	7–10 years	11–12 YEARS	13–14 years	15 years	16–18 years
Tetanus, Diphtheria, Pertussis[1]	See footnote 1	Tdap		Tdap	
Human Papillomavirus[2]	See footnote 2	HPV (3 doses)		Series	
Meningococcal[3]	MPSV4	MCV4		MCV4[3] / MCV4	
Pneumococcal[4]		PPV			
Influenza[5]		Influenza (Yearly)			
Hepatitis A[6]		HepA Series			
Hepatitis B[7]		HepB Series			
Inactivated Poliovirus[8]		IPV Series			
Measles, Mumps, Rubella[9]		MMR Series			
Varicella[10]		Varicella Series			

Range of recommended ages

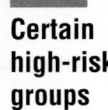
Catch-up immunization

Certain high-risk groups

This schedule indicates the recommended ages for routine administration of currently licensed childhood vaccines, as of December 1, 2006, for children aged 7–18 years. Additional information is available at http://www.cdc.gov/nip/recs/child-schedule.htm. Any dose not administered at the recommended age should be administered at any subsequent visit, when indicated and feasible. Additional vaccines may be licensed and recommended during the year. Licensed combination vaccines may be used whenever any components of the combination are indicated and other components of the vaccine are not contraindicated and if approved by the Food and Drug Administration for that dose of the series. Providers should consult the respective Advisory Committee on Immunization Practices statement for detailed recommendations. Clinically significant adverse events that follow immunization should be reported to the Vaccine Adverse Event Reporting System (VAERS). Guidance about how to obtain and complete a VAERS form is available at http://www.vaers.hhs.gov or by telephone, 800-822-7967.

1. **Tetanus and diphtheria toxoids and acellular pertussis vaccine (Tdap).** *(Minimum age: 10 years for BOOSTRIX® and 11 years for ADACEL™)*
   - Administer at age 11–12 years for those who have completed the recommended childhood DTP/DTaP vaccination series and have not received a tetanus and diphtheria toxoids vaccine (Id) booster dose.
   - Adolescents aged 13–18 years who missed the 11–12 year Td/Tdap booster dose should also receive a single dose of Tdap if they have completed the recommended childhood DTP/DTaP vaccination series.
2. **Human papillomavirus vaccine (HPV).** *(Minimum age: 9 years)*
   - Administer the first dose of the HPV vaccine series to females at age 11–12 years.
   - Administer the second dose 2 months after the first dose and the third dose 6 months after the first dose.
   - Administer the HPV vaccine series to females at age 13–18 years if not previously vaccinated.
3. **Meningococcal vaccine.** *(Minimum age: 11 years for meningococcal conjugate vaccine [MCV4]; 2 years for meningococcal polysaccharide vaccine [MPSV4])*
   - Administer MCV4 at age 11–12 years and to previously unvaccinated adolescents at high school entry (at approximately age 15 years).
   - Administer MCV4 to previously unvaccinated college freshmen living in dormitories; MPSV4 is an acceptable alternative.
   - Vaccination against invasive meningococcal disease is recommended for children and adolescents aged ≥2 years with terminal complement deficiencies or anatomic or functional asplenia and certain other high-risk groups. See *MMWR* 2005;54(No. RR-7):1–21. Use MPSV4 for children aged 2–10 years and MCV4 or MPSV4 for older children.
4. **Pneumococcal polysaccharide vaccine (PPV).** *(Minimum age: 2 years)*
   - Administer for certain high-risk groups. See *MMWR* 1997;46(No. RR-8):1–24, and *MMWR* 2000;49(No. RR-9):1–35.
5. **Influenza vaccine.** *(Minimum age: 6 months for trivalent inactivated influenza vaccine [TIV]; 5 years for live, attenuated influenza vaccine [LAIV])*
   - Influenza vaccine is recommended annually for persons with certain risk factors, health-care workers, and other persons (including household members) in close contact with persons in groups at high risk. See *MMWR* 2006;55 (No. RR-10):1–41.
   - For healthy persons aged 5–49 years, LAIV may be used as an alternative to TIV.
   - Children aged <9 years who are receiving influenza vaccine for the first time should receive 2 doses (separated by ≥4 weeks for TIV and ≥6 weeks for LAIV).
6. **Hepatitis A vaccine (HepA).** *(Minimum age: 12 months)*
   - The 2 doses in the series should be administered at least 6 months apart.
   - HepA is recommended for certain other groups of children, including in areas where vaccination programs target older children. See *MMWR* 2006;55 (No. RR-7):1–23.
7. **Hepatitis B vaccine (HepB).** *(Minimum age: birth)*
   - Administer the 3-dose series to those who were not previously vaccinated.
   - A 2-dose series of Recombivax HB® is licensed for children aged 11–15 years.
8. **Inactivated poliovirus vaccine (IPV).** *(Minimum age: 6 weeks)*
   - For children who received an all-IPV or all-oral poliovirus (OPV) series, a fourth dose is not necessary if the third dose was administered at age ≥4 years.
   - If both OPV and IPV were administered as part of a series, a total of 4 doses should be administered, regardless of the child's current age.
9. **Measles, mumps, and rubella vaccine (MMR).** *(Minimum age: 12 months)*
   - If not previously vaccinated, administer 2 doses of MMR during any visit, with ≥4 weeks between the doses.
10. **Varicella vaccine.** *(Minimum age: 12 months)*
    - Administer 2 doses of varicella vaccine to persons without evidence of immunity.
    - Administer 2 doses of varicella vaccine to persons aged ≤13 years at least 3 months apart. Do not repeat the second dose, if administered ≥28 days after the first dose.
    - Administer 2 doses of varicella vaccine to persons aged ≥13 years at least 4 weeks apart.

FIGURE 238.1. Recommended immunization schedule for persons aged 7 to 18 years. (From MMWR QuickGuide. Recommended Immunization Schedules for Persons 0–18 Years—United States, 2007. MMWR Morb Mortal Wkly Rep 2007;55(51/52):Q1.)

The table provides catch-up schedules and minimum intervals between doses for children whose vaccinations have been delayed. A vaccine series does not need to be restarted, regardless of the time that has elapsed between doses. Use the section appropriate for the child's age.

		CATCH-UP SCHEDULE FOR PERSONS AGED 4 MONTHS–6 YEARS			
Vaccine	Minimum age for Dose 1	Minimum interval between doses			
		Dose 1 to Dose 2	Dose 2 to Dose 3	Dose 3 to Dose 4	Dose 4 to Dose 5
Hepatitis B[1]	Birth	4 weeks	8 weeks (and 16 weeks after first dose)		
Rotavirus[2]	6 weeks	4 weeks	4 weeks		
Diphtheria, Tetanus, Pertussis[3]	6 weeks	4 weeks	4 weeks	6 months	6 months[3]
Haemophilus **influenzae type b[4]**	6 weeks	4 weeks if first dose administered at age <12 months **8 weeks (as final dose)** if first dose administered at age 12–14 months **No further doses needed** if first dose administered at age ≥15 months	4 weeks[4] if current age <12 months **8 weeks (as final dose)[4]** if current age ≥12 months and second dose administered at age <15 months **No further doses needed** if previous dose administered at age ≥15 months	**8 weeks (as final dose)** This dose only necessary for children aged 12 months– 5 years who received 3 doses before age 12 months	
Pneumococcal[5]	6 weeks	4 weeks if first dose administered at age <12 months and current age <24 months **8 weeks (as final dose)** if first dose administered at age ≥12 months or current age 24–59 months **No further doses needed** for healthy children if first dose administered at age ≥24 months	4 weeks if current age <12 months **8 weeks (as final dose)** if current age ≥12 months **No further doses needed** for healthy children if previous dose administered at age ≥24 months	**8 weeks (as final dose)** This dose only necessary for children aged 12 months– 5 years who received 3 doses before age 12 months	
Inactivated Poliovirus[6]	6 weeks	4 weeks	4 weeks	4 weeks[6]	
Measles, Mumps, Rubella[7]	12 months	4 weeks			
Varicella[8]	12 months	3 months			
Hepatitis A[9]	12 months	6 months			
		CATCH-UP SCHEDULE FOR PERSONS AGED 7–18 YEARS			
Tetanus, Diphtheria/ Tetanus, Diphtheria, Pertussis[10]	7 years[10]	4 weeks	8 weeks if first dose administered at age <12 months 6 months if first dose administered at age ≥12 months	6 months if first dose administered at age <12 months	
Human Papillomavirus[11]	9 years	4 weeks	12 weeks		
Hepatitis A[9]	12 months	6 months			
Hepatitis B[1]	Birth	4 weeks	8 weeks (and 16 weeks after first dose)		
Inactivated Poliovirus[6]	6 weeks	4 weeks	4 weeks	4 weeks[6]	
Measles, Mumps, Rubella[7]	12 months	4 weeks			
Varicella[8]	12 months	4 weeks if first dose administered at age ≥13 years 3 months if first dose administered at age <13 years			

1. **Hepatitis B vaccine (HepB).** (*Minimum age: birth*)
   - Administer the 3-dose series to those who were not previously vaccinated.
   - A 2-dose series of Recombivax HB® is licensed for children aged 11–15 years.
2. **Rotavirus vaccine (Rota).** (*Minimum age: 6 weeks*)
   - Do not start the series later than age 12 weeks.
   - Administer the final dose in the series by age 32 weeks. Do not administer a dose later than age 32 weeks.
   - Data on safety and efficacy outside of these age ranges are insufficient.
3. **Diphtheria and tetanus toxoids and acellular pertussis vaccine (DTaP).** (*Minimum age: 6 weeks*)
   - The fifth dose is not necessary if the fourth dose was administered at age ≥4 years.
   - DTaP is not indicated for persons aged ≥7 years.
4. *Haemophilus influenzae* **type b conjugate vaccine (Hib).** (*Minimum age: 6 weeks*)
   - Vaccine is not generally recommended for children aged ≥5 years.
   - If current age <12 months and the first 2 doses were PRP-OMP (PedvaxHIB® or ComVax® [Merck]), the third (and final) dose should be administered at age 12–15 months and at least 8 weeks after the second dose.
   - If first dose was administered at age 7–11 months, administer 2 doses separated by 4 weeks plus a booster at age 12–15 months.
5. **Pneumococcal conjugate vaccine (PCV).** (*Minimum age: 6 weeks*)
   - Vaccine is not generally recommended for children aged ≥5 years;
6. **Inactivated poliovirus vaccine (IPV).** (*Minimum age: 6 weeks*)
   - For children who received an all-IPV or all-oral poliovirus (OPV) series, a fourth dose is not necessary if third dose was administered at age ≥4 years.
   - If both OPV and IPV were administered as part of a series, a total of 4 doses should be administered, regardless of the child's current age.

7. **Measles, mumps, and rubella vaccine (MMR).** (*Minimum age: 12 months*)
   - The second dose of MMR is recommended routinely at age 4–6 years but may be administered earlier if desired.
   - If not previously vaccinated, administer 2 doses of MMR during any visit with ≥4 weeks between the doses.
8. **Varicella vaccine.** (*Minimum age: 12 months*)
   - The second dose of varicella vaccine is recommended routinely at age 4–6 years but may be administered earlier if desired.
   - Do not repeat the second dose in persons aged <13 years if administered ≥28 days after the first dose.
9. **Hepatitis A vaccine (HepA).** (*Minimum age: 12 months*)
   - HepA is recommended for certain groups of children, including in areas where vaccination programs target older children. See *MMWR* 2006;55(No. RR-7):1–23.
10. **Tetanus and diphtheria toxoids vaccine (Td) and tetanus and diphtheria toxoids and acellular pertussis vaccine (Tdap).** (*Minimum ages: 7 years for Td, 10 years for BOOSTRIX®, and 11 years for ADACEL™*)
   - Tdap should be substituted for a single dose of Td in the primary catch-up series or as a booster if age appropriate; use Td for other doses.
   - A 5-year interval from the last Td dose is encouraged when Tdap is used as a booster dose. A booster (fourth) dose is needed if any of the previous doses were administered at age <12 months. Refer to ACIP recommendations for further information. See *MMWR* 2006;55(No. RR-3).
11. **Human papillomavirus vaccine (HPV).** (*Minimum age: 9 years*)
   - Administer the HPV vaccine series to females at age 13–18 years if not previously vaccinated.

FIGURE 238.2. Catch-up immunization schedule for persons aged 4 months to 18 years who start late or who are 1 or more months behind. (From MMWR QuickGuide. Recommended Immunization Schedules for Persons 0–18 Years—United States, 2007. MMWR Morb Mortal Wkly Rep 2007;55(51/52):Q4.)

for rollerblading and skate boarding, and appropriate athletic protective devices. Ask the teenager about access to weapons.

Mental Health

Screen for depression and suicidal ideation. Risk factors include poor school performance, family dysfunction, substance abuse, physical or sexual abuse, and previous suicide attempts or plans. Note that the vegetative signs associated with adult depression (e.g., sleep disturbance, lack of interest, decreased concentration) can be part of normal adolescent development. Moreover, adolescent depression may masquerade as vague somatic complaints, such as abdominal pain or headaches. Suicidal ideation requires immediate referral. Recurrent or serious depression necessitates consultation with a mental health professional.

The journal *Pediatrics* has published new guidelines to aid primary care physicians in identifying, assessing, and treating depression in adolescents.

Use every clinical encounter—routine, urgent care, emergency care, and sports preparticipation examinations—to identify adolescents at high risk for depression. Use a standardized depression tool (i.e., Columbia Depression Scale). Risk factors include previous episodes, family history, family conflict, substance abuse, trauma, and psychosocial adversity. Once a high-risk patient is identified, monitor over time for the development of a depressive disorder.

If a depressed adolescent is identified, interview parents and family/caregivers and include some assessment of functional impairment in school and home. This will need to be done within the context of the limits of confidentiality. The adolescent needs to know, however, that the clinician will involve the parents and legal authorities when the risk of harm to the adolescent or others is present.

Develop a written treatment plan with specific goals. Also connect with community and school-based mental health resources. Establish an emergency communication mechanism (who will contact whom and when) for handling increased suicidality or acute crisis. Develop a safety plan, should the adolescent become suicidal or a danger to others, including restricting access to weapons.

For mild depression, a period of structured observation is appropriate; for moderate to severe depression, involve a mental health specialist. Monitor patients for the adverse effects of selective serotonin reuptake inhibitors.

Nutrition and Exercise

Counsel adolescents about a healthy diet, safe weight management, and regular exercise. Refer adolescents who are above the 95th percentile of the sex-specific body mass index for age growth charts to professional nutritionists. Screen for faddist diets, anorexia and bulimia, and the use of anabolic steroids by athletes. Recommend dietary supplements of calcium (1,000 mg/d) and folic acid (400 mg/d) for female adolescents. Explore with the patient plans for exercise, whether organized or informal sports and activities outside of the home.

Sexuality

Discuss sex frankly. Explore early adolescents' understanding of sexuality. Discuss responsible sexual behavior, including abstinence. Educate about birth control, stressing the use of latex condoms to prevent sexually transmitted diseases and especially HIV infection. Provide birth control and instructions on appropriate use.

Abuse of Tobacco, Alcohol, and Other Substances

Ask about smoking and the use of alcohol and other drugs during the last 6 months. Educate about the harmful effects of substance abuse. Explore family history, frequency and amount of use, and circumstances surrounding use. Encourage participation in community peer self-help groups. Determine social and psychological factors that prompt the use of drugs and refer to social services and mental health professionals as necessary.

Abuse

Screen all adolescents annually for a history of physical, emotional, and sexual abuse. Pursue aggressively any suspicion, asking about circumstances and people involved. Be aware of local reporting requirements to state offices. Involve mental health and social services professionals early in all suspected cases of abuse.

SPECIAL ISSUES AND NEED FOR REFERRAL (1,2,8–12)

Sports Participation: Screening Student Athletes for Cardiovascular Abnormalities

There are 10,000,000 American high school and college adolescents who participate in some form of organized sports activity. The primary care internist is sometimes called on to perform preparticipation screening for cardiovascular abnormalities.

This screening is an attempt to identify unsuspected cardiovascular diseases that result in sudden death in athletes. In the United States, most of these deaths are due to hypertrophic cardiomyopathy (36%), with congenital coronary artery anomalies (17%), myocarditis (6%), arrhythmogenic right ventricular cardiomyopathy (4%), mitral valve prolapse (4%), and a variety of other cardiovascular causes (coronary artery disease, aortic stenosis, congenital heart disease) accounting for the rest.

The American Heart Association released updated guidelines in 2007 for screening student athletes. The recommendations are unchanged from the 1996 guidelines and include the following:

1. Undertake the 12-element cardiovascular-targeted personal and family history and physical examination (see Table 238.2).
2. Repeat examinations every 2 years for high school students and every year for college athletes.
3. Routine use of the 12-lead electrocardiogram is not recommended for mass screening, so use it only in cases in which there is an abnormal history or physical examination finding on the 12-element screening.

The restriction in the last recommendation is controversial, especially in light of an Italian study in 2006 that reported a 90% decrease in sudden death in athletes since the implementation of a national screening program that includes the routine use of the electrocardiogram.

TABLE 238.2

THE 12-ELEMENT AMERICAN HEART ASSOCIATION RECOMMENDATIONS FOR PREPARTICIPATION CARDIOVASCULAR SCREENING OF COMPETITIVE ATHLETES

Medical history[a]
  Personal history
    1. Exertional chest pain/discomfort
    2. Unexplained syncope/near-syncope[b]
    3. Excessive exertional and unexplained dyspnea/fatigue associated with exercise
    4. Prior recognition of a heart murmur
    5. Elevated systemic blood pressure
  Family history
    6. Premature death (sudden and unexpected, or otherwise) before age 50 years due to heart disease in one or more relatives
    7. Disability from heart disease in a close relative <50 yr of age
    8. Specific knowledge of certain cardiac conditions in family members; hypertrophic or dilated cardiomyopathy, long-QT syndrome or other ion channelopathies, Marfan's syndrome, or clinically important arrhythmias
  Physical examination
    9. Heart murmur[c]
    10. Femoral pulses to exclude aortic coarctation
    11. Physical stigmata of Marfann's syndrome
    12. Brachial artery blood pressure (sitting position)[d]

[a]Parental verification is recommended for high school and middle school athletes.
[b]Judged not to be a neurocardiogenic (vasovagal); of particular concern when related to exertion.
[c]Auscultation should be performed in both supine and standing positions (or with Valsalva maneuver) specifically to identify murmurs of dynamic left ventricular outflow tract obstruction.
[d]Preferably taken in both arms.
Maron BJ, Thompson PD, Ackerman MJ, et al. Recommendations and considerations related ot preparticipation screening for cardiovascular abnormalities in competitive athletes: 2007 update. Circulation 2007;115:1643.

Scoliosis

Scoliosis is a lateral curvature of the spine associated with rotation of the involved vertebrae. Although scoliosis may be associated with chronic illness (neurofibromatosis, cerebral palsy, Marfan's syndrome, poliomyelitis), the most common type is idiopathic, generally beginning at age 8 to 10 years and progressing during growth through adolescence. It is classically asymptomatic. The clinician screens for scoliosis with the forward bend test and visual inspection for rib cage deformation and waistline asymmetry. A positive result on screening warrants imaging with a scoliosis plain film series—radiography of the entire spine in both the posterior and lateral planes with the patient in the standing position. All curves greater than 15 degrees require referral to an orthopedic specialist if spinal growth is not completed (adolescent girls usually complete spinal growth 18 to 24 months after menarche).

Eating Disorders

Between 5% and 10% of adolescent girls and young women have an eating disorder. The diagnosis of anorexia nervosa and bulimia nervosa is made through the history. Ask about recurrent dieting, body image, interruption of menses, and physical activity. Assess for the use of laxatives and diuretics, self-induced vomiting, and starvation. Except in extreme cases, the physical examination findings and results of the laboratory evaluation are normal. In anorexia, weight loss greater than 10% of previous weight or a body mass index less than the 5th percentile suggests the diagnosis. Be alert to patients who diet when not overweight, have distorted body image, or whose body mass index is less than the 5th percentile. Use laboratory findings to exclude other causes of weight loss, such as hyperthyroidism, inflammatory bowel disease, diabetes, and connective tissue disorders (see Chapters 73, 102, 103, and 104). Once the diagnosis has been made, treatment should be carried out by a multidisciplinary team that includes the primary clinician, a psychologist or psychiatrist, and a nutritionist skilled in the management of eating disorder problems (see Chapter 234).

School Failure

Not uncommonly, an adolescent, or more likely the adolescent's parent, turns to the clinician for an explanation of poor academic performance. The differential diagnosis for academic failure in adolescence is broad, and more than one factor is often involved. A thorough history, physical examination, and appropriate laboratory studies should serve to identify psychological (depression, anxiety) and physical (hearing, visual) problems, chronic disease (asthma, neurologic dysfunction), learning disorders (attention deficit disorders), drug abuse, limited intellectual ability (developmental delay), and social difficulties (dysfunctional family life, poor peer relations, abuse). Coordinate with the patient's parent, teacher, and school counselor. Many school districts are mandated to provide neuropsychological testing to aid in both diagnosis and treatment strategies.

Hypertension

About 2% to 5% of adolescents are hypertensive. Definitions of normal, borderline, and high blood pressure in adolescence involve calculating the teen's percentile for age and height. Normal is less the 90th percentile, high normal is between the 90th and 95th percentiles, and high (hypertension) is a systolic or diastolic pressure equal to or greater than the 95th percentile on three separate occasions.

Consider secondary causes of hypertension, including renal disease, oral contraception, and the use of drugs such as cocaine or steroids. The medical history focuses on growth and development, past illnesses (especially during the neonatal period and infancy), and family history. On physical examination, look for evidence of end-organ damage. Tailor the laboratory evaluation as the clinical situation warrants, and obtain a urinalysis, values for blood urea nitrogen, creatinine, and electrolytes and a complete blood cell count. Consider renal ultrasonography and echocardiography (see Chapters 14 and 19).

Obesity

The journal *Pediatrics* recently released an updated set of recommendations regarding child and adolescent obesity. The recommendations are based on more than 300 studies published since 1995 and include guidelines and evaluation tools.

Teenagers with a body mass index between the 85th and 90th percentiles are at high risk for obesity and require diet assessment and counseling. Adolescents with a body mass index greater than the 95th percentile for age and sex require aggressive nutrition counseling and benefit from a multidisciplinary approach that involves diet, exercise, and counseling (see Chapters 10 and 233). Special attention should be given when the adolescents have a strong family history of premature heart disease, obesity, or diabetes or if the patient has hypertension, hyperlipidemia, or rapid weight gain.

Gynecomastia

In the majority of male adolescents (60% to 70%), transient enlargement of one or both breasts develops during transition through Tanner stages II to III as a normal part of puberty. Type I idiopathic gynecomastia is usually unilateral (20% of cases are bilateral) and tender; it consists of a firm mass below the areola. Type II is the more generalized breast enlargement found in obese adolescents. Although more than 95% of cases of gynecomastia are idiopathic and resolve spontaneously, be alert to pathologic causes: drugs; Klinefelter's syndrome; adrenal, pituitary, and testicular tumors; hypothyroidism; and hepatic dysfunction. Most cases of gynecomastia resolve within a period of months to 2 years and require only reassurance and support to the anxious teen. On occasion, because of severe psychological damage or a persistent problem, either pharmacologic treatment (e.g., danazol) or surgical intervention is required (see also Chapter 99).

WEB SITES

American Academy of Pediatrics: http://www.aap.org

American Medical Association, Adolescent Health On-Line: http://www.ama-assn.org/ama/pub/category/1947.html

Bright Futures: http://www.brightfutures.org

Centers for Disease Control and Prevention, Division of Adolescent and School Health (DASH): http://www.cdc.gov/HealthyYouth

National Adolescent Health Information Center: http://nahic.ucsf.edu

North American Society for Pediatric and Adolescent Gynecology (NASPAG): http://www.naspag.org

Red Book Online: http://aapredbook.aappublications.org

Society for Adolescent Medicine: http://www.adolescenthealth.org

Annotated Bibliography

1. Aten CB, Gotlieb EM, eds. American Academy of Pediatrics Section on Adolescent Health. Caring for adolescent patients, 2nd ed. Elk Grove Village, IL: American Academy of Pediatrics, 2005. (*An excellent resource.*)
2. Hagan JF. Bright Futures. Guidelines for health supervision of infants, children, and adolescents, 3rd ed. Elk Grove Village, IL: American Academy of Pediatrics. 2007. (*A compendium of guidelines, including those for adolescents.*)
3. Schmidt R, White L. Internists and adolescent medicine. Arch Intern Med 2002;162:1150. (*A good review of the essentials for internists.*)
4. National High Blood Pressure Education Working Group on High Blood Pressure in Children and Adolescents. The fourth report on the diagnosis, evaluation, and treatment of high blood pressure in children and adolescents. Pediatrics 2004;114:555. (*Concensus reccommendations.*)
5. National Cholesterol Education Expert Panel on Blood Cholesterol Levels in Children and Adolescents. Highlights of the report of the Expert Panel on Blood Cholesterol Levels in Children and Adolescents. Pediatrics 1992;89:495. (*Evidence-based consensus guidelines.*)
6. Committee on Nutrition, American Academy of Pediatrics. Cholesterol in childhood. Pediatrics 1998;101:141. (*An updated statement, reviewing evidence, screening, and treatment strategies).*
7. American Academy of Pediatrics. The red book 2006. Report of the Committee on Infectious Diseases, 27th ed. Elk Grove Village, IL: Author, 2006 (*Concensus reccommendations.*)
8. Recommended Immunization Schedules for Persons 0–18 Years—United States, 2007. MMWR Morb Mortal Wkly Rep 2007;55(51/52):Q1. (*Current recommendations; an erratum was published: MMWR Morb Mortal Wkly Rep 2007;56(2):32.*)
9. Maron BJ, Thompson PD, Ackerman MJ, et al. Recommendations and considerations related to pre-participation screening for cardiovascular abnormalities in competitive athletes: 2007 update. Circulation 2007;115;1643. (*An important update.*)
10. Cheung P, Zuckerbrot R, Jensen PS, et al. Guidelines for adolescent depression in primary care (GLAD-PC): II. Treatment and ongoing management. Pediatrics 2007;120:1313. (*An excellent resource for this complex problem.*)
11. Zametikin AJ, Alter MR, Yemini T. Suicide in teenagers: assessment, management and prevention. JAMA 2001;286: 3120. (*An excellent, well-referenced, grand rounds presentation.*)
12. Becker A, Grinspoon S. Current concepts: eating disorders. N Engl J Med 1999;340:1092. (*An excellent review for the primary care physician.*)
13. Krebs NF, Himes JH, Jacobson D, et al. Assessment of child and adolescent overweight and obesity. Pediatrics 2007;120;S193. (*Key task.*)

CHAPTER 239 ■ APPROACH TO FRAILTY IN OLDER ADULTS

CLAUS HAMANN AND KENNETH L. MINAKER

Care of older adults embraces a four-phase continuum: successful aging with no overt diseases; independent function despite established diseases; frailty, with dependent, more vulnerable function due to accumulated deficits; and preterminal condition, or end of life. At each stage, balanced individualized strategies for health promotion, disease and disability prevention, and restoration and palliation offer opportunities for improving quality of life. Frailty is a clinical syndrome with predominant musculoskeletal, nutritional, and neuropsychiatric manifestations and, in its preclinical manifestations, a potential phenotype. Most frail older adults have chronic illnesses affecting multiple organ systems, diminishing physiologic reserve and making them vulnerable to destabilization. They require the support of other persons to function optimally. Frail older adults are at greater risk of dying than the nonfrail, often due to infection complicating coexistent illnesses. Frailty usually has a long prodrome that offers many opportunities for remediation; if left unattended, it leads to an accelerated pace of decline—"*failure to thrive.*" Identifying risks for frailty, preventing frailty and its consequences, and treating frailty are the central challenges of the primary physician caring for older adults.

PATHOPHYSIOLOGY AND CLINICAL PRESENTATION (1–14)

Frailty is a clinical syndrome with predominant musculoskeletal, nutritional, and neuropsychiatric manifestations. It comprises *diminished muscle strength, decreased physical activity, easy fatigability, slow, unsteady gait, increased risk and fear of falling, poor appetite and unintentional weight loss,* and, often, *impaired cognition and depression.*

Endocrine and immune antecedents for the frailty cycle have been identified. Serum levels of *growth hormone* and *insulin-like growth factor-1* decline progressively during aging, and an association with frailty has been proposed. Age-dependent changes in *testosterone, erythropoietin,* and other hormones also appear to herald frailty in the elderly, particularly via their effects on muscle mass, strength, and bone density. These changes may contribute to the activation of *catabolic cytokines (e.g., interleukin-6), C-reactive protein,* and markers of coagulopathy, such as *fibrinogen* and D-*dimer.* In addition, periodontal disease, pulmonary disease, bladder infections, renal insufficiency, and diverticula may stimulate *chronic, low-level inflammation.* Women appear to be twice as likely to develop frailty as men, perhaps due to lower protective levels of baseline lean body mass, testosterone, and growth hormone and greater dysregulation of *cortisol.*

Nutritional factors may contribute to frailty. These include *early satiation,* or the "anorexia of aging," arising from signals in the stomach and from changes in the central feeding drive, in particular from a decrease in the opioid-rewarding properties for fatty foods. Diminished nutritional drive may also be caused by higher leptin levels associated with lower testosterone in aging men and by increased cytokines from common inflammatory conditions.

Physical frailty is associated with a reduction in the fasting rate of *muscle protein synthesis,* which contributes to muscle protein wasting in advancing age. Sarcopenia is also partly due to the apoptosis of myocytes. *Bone loss* ensues from inactivity, hormonal changes, deficient calcium and vitamin D, and decreases in calcium absorption (see Chapter 164). Many of these molecular events can be at least partially reversed through physical exercise.

ASSESSMENT (15–17)

Many patients and their caregivers volunteer advancing age as the primary reason for frailty. Although age is a risk factor for frailty and illness in general, it should not be invoked reflexively because it can lead to the erroneous conclusion that "since I can do nothing about your advancing age, I can do nothing about your frailty." Instead, a two-pronged approach is recommended: first, a traditional search for medical causes, and second, a specific geriatric assessment that identifies frailty factors, refines disability assessment, and tests for physical performance and mental status. Review of medications and assessment for adverse drug effects are especially important components of the evaluation (see Chapters 166, 169, 173, and 219).

Standard Medical Evaluation

The assessment should be directed at preexisting conditions, such as congestive heart failure (see Chapter 32), renal insufficiency (see Chapter 142), and chronic lung disease (see Chapter 47), that are commonly unstable and may contribute to clinical deterioration. Infection, anemia, hypo- or hyperthyroidism, malignancy, and depression may be subclinical and require consideration. Hypogonadism, hypoadrenalism, and hypopituitarism sometimes enter the differential diagnosis. Medications should be reviewed in detail; having all medications brought in for the visit can reveal nonadherence and potential drug–drug and drug–disease interactions.

Geriatric Assessment

In addition to the standard medical evaluation, the history and physical examination can identify specific manifestations of frailty, including the following:

- *Exhaustion*: "Everything was an effort," or " I could not get going" for at least half of the previous week.
- *Unintentional weight loss*: loss of 10% or more of body weight during the last year, or (lower threshold) 10 lb (4 kg) over 5 years; body weight less than numerical age is pathognomonic.
- *Inactivity*: less than 20 minutes of brisk walking per week
- *Immobility*: taking 7 or more seconds to walk 15 feet.
- *Weakness*: diminished grip strength, measured using a handheld dynamometer

Having an increasing number of these *frailty factors* predicts worsening mobility and limitation in activities of daily living, as well as increased risk for hospitalization and death. The clinician further inquires into difficulty with six *activities of daily living (ADL)*:

- Shopping for personal items like toiletries or medicines
- Managing money (keeping track of expenses or paying bills)
- Doing light housework (washing dishes, straightening up, or light cleaning)
- Walking across the room
- Transferring from bed or chair and back
- Bathing or showering

Refined from traditionally longer lists of ADL items, these six items identify 93% of community-living older adults vulnerable to frailty, having difficulty functioning independently, and in need of help. A history of other geriatric syndromes contributing to or resulting from frailty—delirium, falls, urinary incontinence, and constipation—should be sought. Social isolation, financial hardships, and caregiver strain also need to be noted.

As part of the physical examination, one asks the patient to stand up without using the arms, stand with eyes closed, and then with eyes open walk across the room; this helps to assess the need for strength and gait training. Nutritional insufficiency can be detected in less than 4 minutes using the well-validated Mini-Nutritional Assessment–Screening Form, which quantifies loss of appetite and weight, recent acute psychological or physical disease, dementia and/or depression, impaired mobility, and low body mass index. Checking for poor dentition—a risk factor for poor nutrition—is also essential. During the visit, the patient's recall, use of language, visual/spatial abilities, thinking, and mood are noted to check for depression and cognitive impairment, which are major determinants of frailty.

PRINCIPLES OF MANAGEMENT (18–25)

The goals are to reverse or minimize remediable causes of frailty and to prevent worsening function. Acute exacerbations and treatable elements of chronic diseases are addressed, but the clinical approach must go beyond standard organ system–based treatments to include the prescription of exercise and improved nutrition. Such an approach is part of a comprehensive prevention and treatment strategy that includes the use of community resources and social supports.

Because frail patients often need the support of many caregivers and the expertise of multiple health professionals, programs in specialized comprehensive geriatric assessment, chronic disease management, caregiver support, and health promotion have been developed and shown to be effective. Geriatric assessment and treatment guidelines for such demanding problems as altered mentation (see Chapter 169), gait disorders, falls, and fractures (see Chapters 164 and 166), and urinary incontinence (see Chapter 134) can improve care but require a team approach for best results. An interdisciplinary effort extends the capabilities of the primary physician but also requires a careful restructuring of practice to ensure optimal coordination. Frail elders challenge the current professional and physical environments of ambulatory primary care practices. New practice and reimbursement paradigms are being developed to facilitate the delivery of high-quality care. Electronic health records may assist by streamlining documentation, facilitating communication, and providing test results and decision support, especially for prescribing medications.

Exercise Program

Exercising for 30 to 60 minutes three times per week reduces markers of frailty after 3 to 6 months. An exercise program of progressively increasing intensity is prescribed, encompassing the four principal modalities of exercise and scaled to an elderly patient's specific capabilities. The assistance of a therapist or trainer at a fitness or senior center can be very helpful. If standing from the chair is difficult or requires the use of arms, then *resistance exercises* are the first priority. Resistance exercise acutely and dramatically increases the rate of muscle protein synthesis and contributes to muscle hypertrophy and improved muscle strength in frail older men and women. If standing balance is impaired, then *balance exercises* are next. When strength and balance progress, the patient starts *aerobic exercise* and then adds *flexibility training*.

Supplementing the exercise program with the administration of *growth hormone* is not indicated. Although body composition may change, the impact on functional status is nil, and long-term safety in the elderly has not been established. Moreover, there is no incremental benefit over strength training alone.

The exercise prescription to prevent or treat frailty actually applies to the entire lifespan, but for older adults and especially for those who are more frail, it is a necessity for maintaining and improving quality of life. In a program modeled on the staged approach to health behavior change (precontemplation, contemplation, preparation, action, and maintenance), the clinician engages the patient to take first and next steps beyond current, generally low levels of activity. By strengthening bone and preventing falls, the exercise program is essential to the prevention of osteoporotic fractures. When combined with a nutritional program of calcium and vitamin D supplementation and augmented by antiresorptive therapy as indicated, it can markedly reduce the risk of osteoporotic fracture and the devastating consequences that often follow (see Chapter 164).

Nutritional Support

Oral supplementation of calcium and vitamin D is essential for the prevention of fractures in persons whose intake is insufficient (see Chapter 164). Such insufficiency is common, especially among nursing home residents. Increasing the quantity of protein and calories by the use of fortified shakes or commercial preparations is of proven benefit in older adults at risk from malnutrition, such as patients recently discharged from hospital, and is a prerequisite for successful physical activity. Referring the caregiver to publicly available nutrition information and the patient to a nutritionist is often very helpful. There is no evidence to support use of "antioxidant" vitamin supplements (see Chapter 31), megadoses of vitamins, or "natural" supplements such as *Ginkgo biloba* (see Chapter 173).

THERAPEUTIC RECOMMENDATIONS

Exercise Program

A suggested schedule combines resistance, balance, and flexibility training starting at 2 days/wk, adding aerobic training starting at 1 day/wk, and increasing eventually to an alternate-day schedule: aerobic training on Mondays, Wednesdays, and Fridays; resistance, balance, and flexibility training on Tuesdays and Thursdays; and makeup or extra sessions on the weekend, as desired. Consider the following:

- Resistance: two to three sessions per week, one to three sets of 8 to 12 repetitions, starting at 70% to 80% of the one-repetition maximum weight and increasing the weight progressively as tolerated, for 8 to 10 major muscle groups.
- Balance: from 1 to 7 days/wk, one to two sets of 4 to 10 dynamic postures (climbing up and down stairs, standing on one leg, Tai Chi postures).
- Aerobic: three to seven sessions per week, 20 to 60 minutes of weight-bearing, low-impact exercise, starting at 40% of predicted maximum heart rate (220 beats/min minus age) and increasing workload as tolerated to 60%.

- Flexibility: from 1 to 7 days/wk, one slow, sustained 20-second stretch of each major muscle group.

Dietary Program

- Prescribe a daily total calcium intake of 1.0 to 1.5 g, which can be taken as a mix of low-fat dairy product servings and calcium carbonate supplements.
- Ensure 400 to 800 IU of vitamin D daily, either as part of the dairy product intake or as a vitamin supplement.
- Recommend a diet that is high in fruits and vegetables and low in saturated fat and concentrated carbohydrates; be sure it provides several grams of fiber and sufficient high-quality protein for the patient's weight (limit protein intake in renal failure).
- Consider a generic daily vitamin supplement preparation that provides 100% of the recommended daily allowance of major vitamins and minerals; discourage the use of megadose supplements, "antioxidant" preparations (see Chapter 31), and preparations with "natural" substances of no proven benefit (e.g., *Ginkgo biloba*; see Chapters 173 and 237)
- Consider family and patient resources for additional educational support and instructions (e.g., Nutrition and the Aging Adult, available at: http://www.intelihealth.com/IH/ihtIH/WSIHW000/22030/22035/34061.html?d=dmtContent.)

Annotated Bibliography

1. Inouye SK, Studenski S, Tinetti ME, et al. Geriatric syndromes: clinical, research and policy implications of a core geriatric concept. J Am Geriatr Soc 2007;55:794. (*Conceptualizes advancing age and functional, mobility, and cognitive impairments as risk factors, with pathophysiology shared between frailty and geriatric syndromes.*)
2. Ahmed N, Mandel R, Fain MJ. Frailty: an emerging geriatric syndrome. Am J Med 2007;120:748. (*A thorough clinical review, highlighting a two-step approach: treating illnesses causing frailty, then treating sarcopenia with exercise and nutrition.*)
3. Cohen HJ. In search of the underlying mechanisms of frailty. J Gerontol Med Sci 2000;55A:M706. (*An editorial linking chronic inflammation to the decreased physiologic reserve characterizing frailty.*)
4. Ershler WB. Biological interactions of aging and anemia: a focus on cytokines. J Am Geriatr Soc 2003;51:S18. (*Presents the data linking the age-associated rise in interleukin-6 to age-associated diseases and to frailty.*)
5. Fried LP, Tangen CM, Walston J, et al. Frailty in older adults: evidence for a phenotype. J Gerontol Med Sci 2001;56:M146. (*The first study to distinguish among frailty, disability, and comorbidity in a population-based study and to propose measures of frailty that are useful in practice, although the study was limited by the exclusion of neurocognitive aspects of frailty.*)
6. Bergman H, Ferrucci L, Guralnik J, et al. Frailty: an emerging research and clinical paradigm–issues and controversies. J Gerontol 2007;62:731. (*Presents a spectrum of definitions, from "accelerated aging" to "phenotype," important for the clinical characterization of frailty.*)
7. Lamberts SW. The endocrinology of gonadal involution: menopause and andropause. Ann Endocrinol 2003;64:77. (*Reviews the state of the science on the menopause, andropause, adrenopause, and somatopause and concludes that hormone replacement is not recommended.*)
8. Sarkisian CA, Lachs MS. "Failure to thrive" in older adults. Ann Intern Med, 1996;124:1072. (*Deconstructs this diagnostic term into the broad differential categories of dementia, depression, malnutrition and physical disability, so that "failure to thrive" does not become "failure to diagnose."*)
9. Walker RF. Is aging a disease? Aging Male 2002;5:147. (*Workshop proceedings, reviewing the biology of aging and frailty and cautioning against growth hormone and testosterone replacement.*)
10. Walston J. Frailty—the search for underlying causes. Sci Aging Knowledge Environ 2004;28:pe4. (*Emphasizes the need to link molecular mechanisms such as oxidative damage and telomere shortening to the multiple physiologic system dysfunctions in frailty.*)
11. Morley JE. Anorexia, sarcopenia, and aging. Nutrition 2001;17:660. (*Reviews the hormones contributing to anorexia and the decreased nutrition seen in frail elders.*)
12. Nass R, Park J, Thorner MO. Growth hormone supplementation in the elderly. Endocrinol Metab Clin North Am 2007;36:233. (*Summarizes the evidence, finding that the answer is still no.*)
13. Yarasheski KE. Exercise, aging, and muscle protein metabolism. J Gerontol A Biol Sci Med Sci 2003;58:M918. (*Summarizes evidence that decreased muscle protein synthesis contributes to frailty and that resistance exercise reverses this decrement.*)
14. Marzetti E, Leeuwenburgh C. Skeletal muscle apoptosis, sarcopenia and frailty at old age. Exp Gerontol 2006;41:1234. (*Reviews the evidence for myocyte apoptosis and inflammatory medications as causes of sarcopenia and its partial reversal through physical exercise.*)
15. Vellas B, Villars H, Abellan G, et al. Overview of the MNA—its history and challenges. J Nutr Health Aging 2006;10:456. (*Reviews the nutritional assessment instrument most commonly used worldwide, the Mini Nutritional Assessment, which is available at http://www.mna-elderly.com/practice/forms/MNA_english.pdf.*)
16. Saliba D, Orlando M, Wenger NS, et al. Identifying a short functional disability screen for older persons. J Gerontol Med Sci 2000;55A:M750. *Identifies a shorter list of activities of daily living for more efficient screening in clinical practice.*
17. Stuck AE, Siu AL, Wieland GD, et al. Comprehensive geriatric assessment: a meta-analysis of controlled trials. Lancet 1993;342:1032. (*A landmark review, showing that programs with control over medical recommendations and extended ambulatory follow-up were more likely to be effective.*)
18. Fiatarone Singh MA. Exercise comes of age: rationale and recommendation for a geriatric exercise prescription. J Gerontol Med Sci 2002;57A:M262. (*A major review of the benefits of exercise in preventing and treating age-associated diseases, deconditioning, and frailty.*)
19. Prochaska JO, Velicer WF. The transtheoretical model of health behavior change. Am J Health Promotion 1997;12:38. (*A Classic explanation of the dominant model for health behavior change.*)
20. Milne AC, Potter J, Avenell A. Meta-analysis: protein and energy supplementation in older people. Ann Int Med 2006;144:37. (*An updated review of Milne AC, Potter J, Avenell A. Protein and energy supplementation in elderly people at risk from malnutrition. Cochrane Database Syst Rev 2005(2):CD003288; concluding from 55 mostly low-quality trials that*

supplementation leads to a modest weight gain but no lower mortality or hospital length of stay.)

21. Aetna InteliHealth. Nutrition and the aging adult. Available at: http://www.intelihealth.com/IH/ihtIH/WSIHW000/22030/22035/ 34061. html?d=dmtContent. (*Practical dietary advice for seniors from the Aetna Insurance Co. health web site, the content for which is reviewed by the faculty of the Harvard Medical School.*)

22. Rothman AA, Wagner EH. Chronic illness management: what is the role of primary care. Ann Intern Med 2003;138: 256. (*Proposes a new chronic care model.*)

23. Senior Services. Project Enhance. Available at: http://www.seniorservices.org/ wellness/wellness.htm#HealthEnhancement. (*A successful program of elder health promotion run by a nonprofit social services agency in the state of Washington.*)

24. Reuben DB, Roth C, Kamberg C, et al. Restructuring primary care practices to manage geriatric syndromes: the ACOVE-2 intervention. J Am Geriatr Soc 2003;51:1787. (*Describes the efficient collection of patient data and prompts for care processes, patient education, and clinician decision support in the incorporation of geriatric protocols in office settings.*)

25. Tinetti ME. Preventing falls in elderly persons. N Engl J Med. 2003;348:42. (*A case-based review that describes the interventions available for each factor in the assessment of fall risk performed for every older patient, especially the frail.*)

Page numbers followed by f indicate figures; page numbers followed by t indicate tabular material.